Normal Respiration and Blood Pressure Readings for Children

Average Respiratory Rates at Rest (Breaths/Minute)

Age	Rate (breaths/minute)
Newborn	35
1-11 months	30
2 years	25
4 years	23
6 years	21
8 years	20
10 years	19
12 years	19
14 years	18
16 years	17
18 years	16-18

Systolic Blood Pressure During the First Year

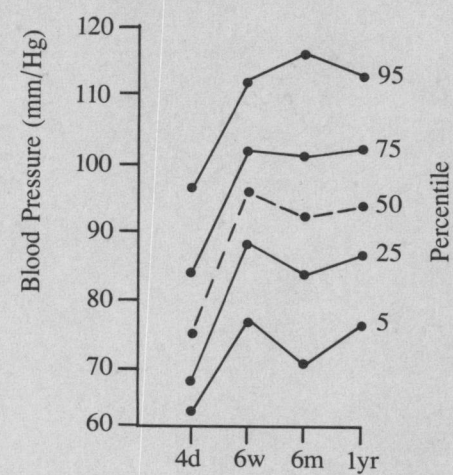

Redrawn from de Swiet, M., Fayers, P., and Shinebourne, E.: Systolic blood pressure in a population of infants in the first year of life: the Brompton study, Pediatrics **65**(5): 1028-1035, 1980. Copyright American Academy of Pediatrics, 1980.

Blood Pressure Percentiles (Right Arm, Seated)

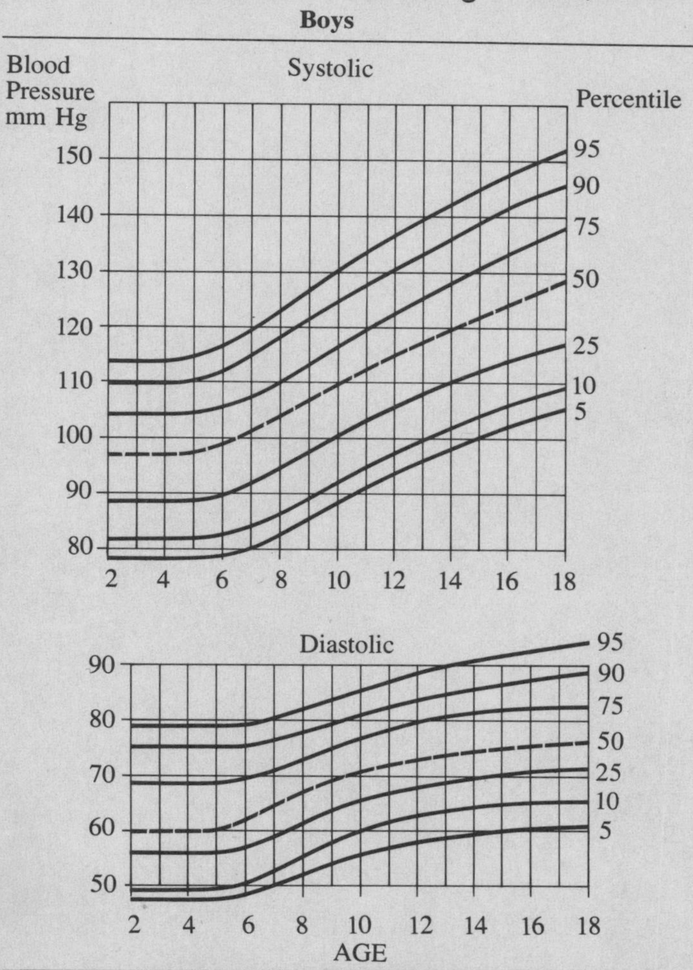

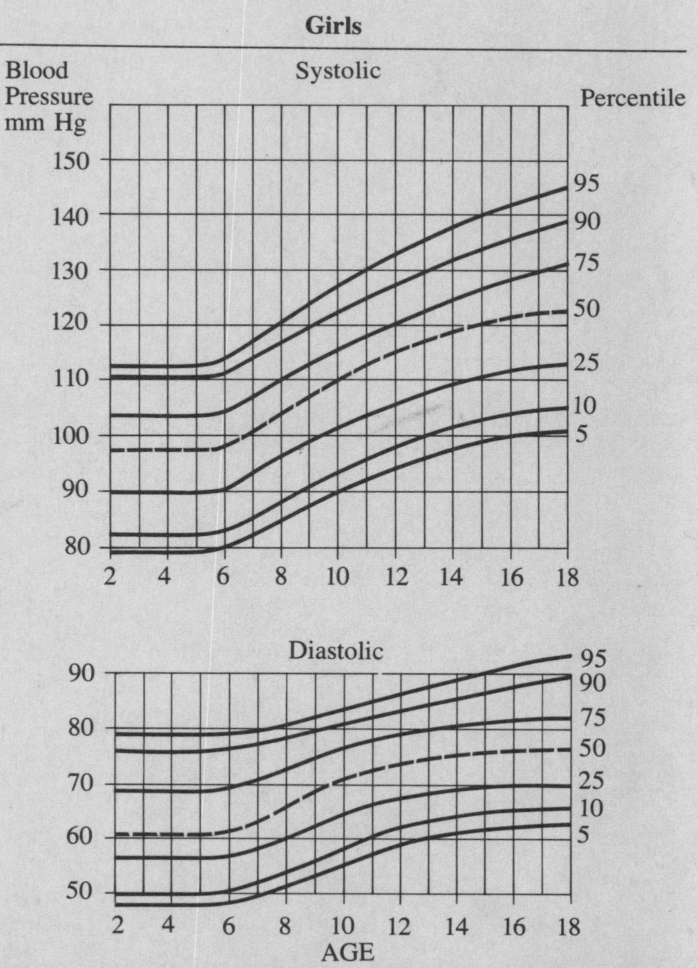

Boys

Blood Pressure mm Hg — Systolic — Percentile

Girls

Blood Pressure mm Hg — Systolic — Percentile

Diastolic

AGE

Nursing Care

of Infants and Children

Yvonne Spencer

C. C. N. Y.

Nursing

rsing Care
ofnts and Children

cille F. Whaley, R.N., Ed.D.

Consultant, Parent-Child Nursing;
Professor Emeritus, San Jose
State University, San Jose, California

ma L. Wong, R.N., M.N., P.N.P.

Nurse Counselor in Private Practice;
Consultant, Department of Education,
Saint Francis Hospital, Tulsa, Oklahoma

Third Edition
with 570 illustrations

The C. V. Mosby Company

St. Louis • Washington, D.C. • Toronto   1987

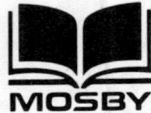

MOSBY

A TRADITION OF PUBLISHING EXCELLENCE

Editor: Alison Miller
Developmental editor: Linda L. Duncan
Project editor: Carlotta Seely
Production editors: Kathleen L. Teal, Judith Bamert
Manuscript editors: Linda Kocher, Peggy Fagen,
    Helen Hudlin, Jan L. Gardner, Elisabeth Heitzeberg

Cover design: John Rokusek

Unit and chapter opener photography:
Units 5, 12, 14 and Chapters 1, 3, 6, 7, 9, 10, 14-16, 20, 22, 25-27,
    30-32, 34, 37, 39, 40 © 1986 G. Robert Bishop

Cover art:
Mary Cassatt, THE BATH, *c. 1891. Canvas, 99.1 × 66 cm.*
Courtesy of The Art Institute of Chicago, Illinois
Robert A. Waller Fund

Third Edition

The C.V. Mosby Company
11830 Westline Industrial Drive, St. Louis, Missouri 63146

Library of Congress Cataloging-in-Publication Data

Whaley, Lucille, F.
    Nursing care of infants and children.

    Includes bibliographies and index.
    1. Pediatric nursing.   I. Wong, Donna L.
II. Title.   [DNLM: 1. Pediatric Nursing.   WY 159 W552n]
RJ245.W47   1986   618.92′00024613   86-23850
ISBN 0-8016-5407-6

C/D/D   9 8 7 6 5 4 3 2 1   02/D/215

To Bert, Kathy, and Reen
for their support and encouragement
Their presence in my life makes it all worthwhile
Lucille F. Whaley

To my family
Ting, Nina, and Rudy
for the love, sunshine, and
support that make it all possible
Donna L. Wong

Preface

The third edition of this book represents our ongoing efforts to provide a comprehensive guide for those involved in the ever-expanding field of pediatric nursing. The basic philosophy and purpose remain unchanged, and we have retained the features of the first and second editions that were so generously received by the health professionals who share our goals. The content is extensive, including normal growth and development, infant and child assessment, and both common and unusual health problems; consequently, the book remains large. It incorporates both the traditional and the expanded roles of the nurse and is based on a firm theoretic foundation from biologic, physical, and behavioral sciences.

GENERAL OVERVIEW AND MAJOR REVISIONS

The same general approach to presentation of content has been preserved from the first edition, although much content has been added, deleted, and condensed and rearranged within this framework for better organization and use of space and minimum duplication. The first part of the book again considers infancy and childhood in a developmental context, stressing the importance of the nurse's role in health promotion and maintenance, as well as in the care of common health problems. The remainder of the book presents the more serious health problems for infants and children that are not peculiar to any age-group and that frequently require hospitalization.

Unit One provides a longitudinal view of the child as an individual on a continuum of developmental changes from birth through adolescence and as a member of a family unit maturing within a culture and a community. Chapter One includes a discussion of morbidity and mortality in infancy and childhood and child health care from an historical perspective. Because of the importance of injuries as the leading cause of death in children, an overview of this topic has been added. The nursing process, with emphasis on nursing diagnosis, and the role of the nurse in caring for infants and children are discussed.

The child in the context of family, culture, and community has been elaborated and broadened to emphasize this important influence on development. The addition of Chapter 2 provides the opportunity to expand the discussion of social, cultural, and religious influences on child development and health promotion, including socioeconomic factors, customs and folkways, and health beliefs and practices. The addition of a chapter devoted to the family further emphasizes the importance of this social group on the health and welfare of children. Family theories establish the tone of the chapter, which has been expanded to include a variety of parenting situations that reflect contemporary society.

The basic overview of child development maintains the same general organization, but has been modified to reflect a more theoretic approach to personality development and learning. Biologic systems development is deemphasized in this chapter and discussed more fully in relation to major systems dysfunction later in the book. Themes established in this chapter are expanded in subsequent chapters devoted to age-specific developmental phenomena, including major theories of child development, nutrition, factors that influence growth and development, and play, which figures prominently in the life of both well and ill children. The basic needs of all infants and children are summarized. New to this chapter are introductions to spiritual development in children, the effect of temperament on childrearing, development of self-concept, and childhood stresses and fears.

Unit Two is concerned with the principles and skills of nursing assessment, including communication and interviewing, observation, physical and behavioral assessment, and health guidance. Chapter 6 contains guidelines for communicating with both children and their families and a detailed description of a health assessment, including a new and extensive discussion of family assessment and additional information on nutritional assessment. Chapter 7 continues to provide a comprehensive approach to physical examination and developmental assessment, with new material added on skinfold measurement, vision testing, and specific developmental instruments.

Unit Three stresses the importance of the neonatal period, a time of greatest risk to survival, and includes the addition of several health problems encountered in the vulnerable first month of life. Some of the additions to this unit include increased emphasis on the family during the birth process and in those instances when a newborn is critically ill or dies, and home care for phototherapy. Congenital hypothyroidism is now discussed in Chapter 9, rather than in Chapter 38, because of the emphasis on preventing the disorder through newborn screening. Assessment of gestational age is presented in Chapter 8, instead of in Chapter 10, because of its use as a routine procedure, rather than its restriction to high-risk neonates.

Chapter 10 strongly stresses the nurse's role in care of the high-risk newborn and the importance of astute observations to the survival of this vulnerable group of infants. New entries include meconium aspiration syndrome, persistent pulmonary hypertension of the newborn, polycythemia/hyperviscosity syndrome, and the effect of maternal smoking on the fetus and newborn. Rapid advances in the field of neonatal care also necessitated a major revision of previous content. The basic content of congenital defects in Chapter 11 remains essentially similar to that in previous editions with updated management and expanded discussions of cranial deformities and psychologic effects of genitourinary defects.

Units Four through Seven present the major developmental stages outlined in Unit One, which are expanded to provide a broader concept of these stages and the health problems most often associated with them. Special emphasis is placed on the preventive aspects of care. The chapters on health promotion have been reorganized to follow a standard approach that is used consistently for each age-group. New areas and those receiving expanded coverage are moral and spiritual development, development of body image, social development (including play), temperament, fears, stress, nutrition, common breast-feeding problems, sleep and activity, and dental health. Theoretic concepts are emphasized and have been expanded in some areas. New content has been included on the gifted child, daycare during the early years, discipline techniques, sleep problems, sports participation and injuries, eating disorders, smoking, and additional skin problems such as sunburn, cold injury, trauma and foreign bodies, cat scratch fever, neurofibromatosis, and lyme disease.

The chapters on health problems have also been reorganized primarily to reflect more typical and age-related concerns. Consequently, some topics previously discussed in these chapters, such as otitis media, pharyngitis, urinary tract infection, and hypertension, have been moved to the appropriate discussions of biologic systems dysfunction. Parasitic infections are discussed in much greater detail and are now presented in Chapter 16, rather than Chapter 18, because of the increased prevalence and concern with diseases such as giardiasis in the younger age-groups.

Unit Eight deals with children who have the same developmental needs as growing children but who, because of congenital or acquired physical, cognitive, or sensory impairment, require alternative interventions to facilitate development. A major revision in this unit is the addition of Chapter 23, Impact of Life-Threatening Illness on the Child and Family, and the deletion of the unit on The Child with a Potentially Terminal Illness. This change reflects the current advances in treating children with cancer. Children with cancer can no longer be labeled as terminally ill; rather they are now children with a chronic illness that has an uncertain outcome. Consequently, the special needs of the child and family are addressed in both Chapters 22 and 23. Extensive information has been added to Chapter 22 on the family's adjustment to a child with special needs and nursing interventions to optimally meet those needs. Because of increased survival in many serious childhood illnesses, attention is given to the problems faced by the maturing adolescent. The focus in Chapter 23 is primarily on the impact of life-threatening illness and death on the child and family. New additions include sections on bereavement, hospice and home care, tissue donation, the child's right to die, and the impact of the death on siblings.

Unit Nine is concerned with the impact of hospitalization on the child and the family and continues to present a comprehensive overview of the stressors imposed by hospitalization and nursing interventions to prevent or eliminate them. Chapter 26 has been reorganized to reduce redundancy of information and greatly expanded discussions of play and pain assessment and management have been added. A new section on discharge planning and home care has been included and provides the basic concepts for implementing home care for children with complex health needs. Chapter 27 continues to present information on the safe implementation of procedures with children but now includes a comprehensive discussion of preparation for procedures and compliance. Information has been added on legal issues pertaining to children, such as children as research subjects, and the focus of surgical care has been expanded to include perioperative care—an aspect of pediatrics that has received little attention.

Units Ten through Fourteen consider serious health problems of infants and children primarily from biologic systems orientation, which has the practical organizational value of permitting health problems and nursing considerations to relate to specific pathophysiologic disturbances. Some important changes are evident in these chapters, including those that reflect such advancements in pediatric care as improved survival in childhood cancer and earlier and more successful correction of congenital heart defects. The chapter on cancer is now included in this section rather than with life-threatening disorders. We have maintained a conceptual approach to the discussions of health problems and have provided generous cross-referencing to minimize repetition of content. All of the chapters in these units have been updated, and several discussions have been greatly expanded, such as common respiratory problems, asthma, urinary tract infections, diabetes, cancer treatment, and nursing care related to such topics. Some important content added includes a discussion of hypoplastic left heart syndrome, cardiomyopathy, acquired immune deficiency disease, and tissue transplantations, in particular bone marrow and heart.

NEW FEATURES

The third edition incorporates several new features to both expand the coverage of nursing care of infants and children and to facilitate the use of the text. Although there has always been a strong emphasis on the family as the unit of care, more information has been included concerning cultural influences on the family and health care practices, family theory, current changes within the family structure, and family assessment. To emphasize care components directed toward family members, the subheading, Support the Family, has been added under Nursing Considerations.

Developments within nursing theory have been incorporated throughout this text with the integration of the most current nursing diagnoses from the Seventh Conference of the North American Nursing Diagnoses Association Classification of Nursing Diagnosis both in the nursing care summaries and in other aspects of practice as appropriate, for example, in the nursing admission history. There is increased emphasis on research and ethics. Not only is research, especially nursing research, integrated throughout the chapter text, but a new feature, Questions and Controversies, has been added to help stimulate awareness of areas in which research can guide nursing practice and areas in which scientific investigation is still needed. Ethical issues are also explored with the hope of creating thoughtful insight into difficult problems that often confront nurses in practice.

With the present emphasis on the optimum development of children and on cost containment within the health care industry, the concept of home care has been greatly expanded, both from a broad conceptual view and in terms of specific areas of specialized care such as home apnea monitoring, dialysis, and the ventilator-assisted child. Since community services are so essential to the extension of care beyond the hospital setting, a new appendix, Resources for Families and Health Care Professionals, has been added. This compilation of organizations providing assistance in almost every aspect of physical, financial, and emotional care is offered in addition to the list of specific organizations and other resources that are included throughout the chapters. Every effort has been made to check the accuracy and availability of cited resources, and we invite comments regarding other helpful resources that can be included in the next edition.

To help the student consolidate the large amount of material presented in the text, many tables and boxes have been added. Content on emergency treatment of several common and/or life-threatening conditions has been outlined in a special Emergency Treatment box, which is clearly designated by a red tab on the page and a listing of the boxes on the inside front cover. Each chapter begins with an outline to provide an overview of the material to be discussed and concludes with Concept Summaries to emphasize information that is most essential to the understanding of pediatric nursing.

In addition to updating content and including new material throughout the text, several topics have been added to augment the discussions of growth and development for each age-group. These include body image, moral development, spiritual development, temperament, and stress. Theoretic foundations are presented as appropriate, and numerous practical suggestions for the implementation of the concept are included, such as identifying and dealing with childhood stress and childrearing practices that complement the child's temperament pattern. Also, most chapters in Units Ten through Fourteen present an overview of assessment of the particular biologic system, including expected findings from the history, physical examination, laboratory tests, and special diagnostic procedures that assist the nurse in identifying health deviations. Finally, we take pride in our extensive and current bibliography, in which the majority of entries are less than five years old, reflecting the most recent social, behavioral, medical, and nursing applications to pediatric health care.

Just as children and their families bring with them a vast and unique background that affects their role within the health care system, so it is that each nurse brings to each child and family an individual set of characteristics and values that will affect their relationship. Although we have attempted to present a total picture of the child in each age-group both in wellness and in illness, no one child, family, or nurse will be found in this book. We hope that each page, chapter, and unit builds a foundation on which the nurse can begin to construct the ideal of comprehensive individualized nursing care for infants and children.

Lucille F. Whaley
Donna L. Wong

Acknowledgments

With each edition of *Nursing Care of Infants and Children* more and more of our colleagues have become involved in the revision of the book. We are grateful to the many nursing faculty, practitioners, and students who have offered their comments, commendations, and suggestions. We again extend thanks to those institutions that have welcomed us to the units providing care to infants and children: Saint Francis Hospital, City of Faith, and Children's Medical Center, Tulsa, Oklahoma; Children's Hospital, St. Louis, Missouri; Santa Clara Valley Medical Center, San Jose, California; Stanford University Medical Center, Palo Alto, California; and El Camino Hospital, Mountain View, California. We appreciate the efforts of the library staffs of these institutions and of Hillcrest Medical Center, Tulsa, Oklahoma, especially Peggy Cook, for assisting in the extensive research needed to update the book, and Barbara Brown, Milton J. Chatton Medical Library, for her generosity with library facilities.

We are especially indebted to the many families who allowed us to take photographs and those individuals who share with us photographs of family members and patients. Special thanks are extended to Patti Muller, R.N., Ed.D., Director of Educational Resources, John Roy, Medical Photographer, and Dorothy Manning, Graphics Coordinator for the generous use of their facilities at Saint Francis Hospital. We also thank the following individuals who made special efforts to arrange or take photographs for us: Connie Morain Baker, Child Life Specialist, University of California Davis Medical Center, Sacramento, California; G. Robert Bishop and Pat Watson, photographers, St. Louis; Anne Kunke and Vicki Meyer, Newborn Nursery, Santa Clara Valley Medical Center, San Jose, California; Betty Stuart, Ogden, Utah; Roy Garibaldi and the yearbook staff at San Lorenzo High School; Betty Baggett, San Jose, California; Kathy Callaham, Public Relations Director, Children's Medical Center, Tulsa, Oklahoma; Mark Capehart, Pediatric Orthopedist, Tulsa, Oklahoma; Maggie Cavness, Head Nurse, Arkansas Children's Hospital, Little Rock, Arkansas; Earl Fillmore, Salt Lake City, Utah; Barbara Eppler, Rozelle Hardaway, Marilyn Knoy, and Jody Shelton, Saint Francis Hospital, Tulsa, Oklahoma; and Katherine Patterson, Head Nurse, University of Kansas Medical Center, Kansas City, Kansas. We are especially grateful to our own "resident" photographers, Ting Kin Wong and Bert Whaley, for the many long hours they have spent in their darkrooms. We again wish to thank George Wassilchenko, Oral Roberts University, for the additional illustrations he has contributed to this book and to Vicky Raine, Illustrator, Saint Francis Hospital, and Kathleen Whaley for the new drawings they have prepared.

No book is ever a reality without the dedication and perseverance of the editorial staff, and although it is impossible to list every individual at The C.V. Mosby Company who made exceptional efforts to produce this text, we are especially grateful to Dave Carroll, Linda Duncan, Carlotta Seely, and Kathleen Teal for their patience and committment to excellence. In addition, we wish to thank our typists, Maureen Whaley and Ann French, for the superb job they did and their efforts in meeting very stringent deadlines.

As always, we wish to thank the members of our family, Bert, Maureen, and Kathy Whaley, Ting and Nina Wong, and Rudy Mitchko, whose devotion, patience, and forbearance are a constant source of support and encouragement. Truly, without their willingness to assume many of the tasks necessary to produce a text of this size and their sacrifices, which allowed us the time needed to revise it, this book would never have been completed. And lastly, we thank each other for a friendship and respect that grows deeper with each edition. Throughout the long and stressful process of writing and rewriting we have shared our skills and knowledge that we feel are essential to the publication of this text.

Lucille F. Whaley
Donna L. Wong

Reviewers

A number of colleagues provided reviews of specific content areas. Their constructive criticisms and suggestions have been invaluable in ensuring accurate and up-to-date material that reflects current clinical practice. To the following individuals we express our sincere gratitude:

Connie Morain Baker, M.S.

Child Life Specialist
University of California
Davis Medical Center
Sacramento, CA

Jo Barr, R.N., M.S.

Specialist, Neurosurgical Nursing
Santa Clara Valley Medical Center
San Jose, CA

Nadine Beavers, R.N.

Clinical Nursing Coordinator
Pediatrics/PICU
Stanford University Hospital
Stanford, CA

Betty Johnson Benton, R.N.

Nursing Supervisor
Medical Oncology
Saint John Medical Center
Tulsa, OK

Judith A. Brown, R.N., M.S.N.

Bacone College of Nursing
Muskogee, OK

Mark Capehart, M.D.

Pediatric Orthopedist
Eastern Oklahoma Orthopedic Center
Tulsa, OK

Lynn Clutter, R.N., M.S.N.

Clinical Nurse Specialist, Educator
Department of Pediatrics
City of Faith
Tulsa, OK

Janice C. Childs, R.N., M.S.N.

Professor of Nursing
University of Virginia
Charlottesville, Virginia

Karen Dunne, R.N., B.A.

Clinical Nursing Supervisor
Children's Hospital at Stanford
Palo Alto, CA

Alma Fandal

John F. Kennedy Child Development Center
Denver, CO

Vivian Filer, R.N., M.S.N.

Professor of Nursing
Santa Fe Community College
Santa Fe, New Mexico

Beverly A. Foerder, R.N., M.S.N., Ed.D.

Professor of Nursing
University of Washington
Seattle, Washington

Patricia Frost-Hartzer, R.N., M.S.N.

Nursing Education Coordinator
Children's Hospital at Stanford
Palo Alto, CA

Mary Fran Hazinski, R.N., M.S.N.

Clinical Nurse Specialist
Pediatric ICU Children's Hospital
Vanderbilt University Medical Center
Nashville, TN

Eleanor A. Hedenkamp, R.N., M.S.

Pediatric Cardiovascular Nurse Specialist
Department of Nursing Service
Stanford University Medical Center
Stanford, CA

Caryn Hess, R.N., M.S.

Formerly Assistant Professor
University of Oklahoma
College of Nursing
Tulsa, OK

Mary Ellen Honeyfield, R.N., M.S.

The Children's Hospital
Denver, CO

Patricia A. Jamerson, R.N., M.S.N.

Chief Nurse
Pediatrics/Family Practice
City of Faith
Tulsa, OK

Samuel T. Jones, M.D.

Trinity Lutheran Hospital
Kansas City, MO

Teri Joyer, R.N., M.S.N.

Nurse Manager, Perinatal Services
Children's Hospital and St. Luke's Hospital
Denver, CO

Christina Algiere Kasprisin, R.N., M.S.

Quality Assurance Coordinator, Nursing
Department of Education
Saint Francis Hospital
Tulsa, OK

Sylvia M. Kerr, R.N., M.S.

Associate Professor
College of Nursing and Applied Health Sciences
University of Tulsa
Tulsa, OK

Patricia M. Klopovich, R.N.,C., M.N.

Clinical Nurse Specialist
Pediatric Hematology/Oncology
University of Kansas Medical Center
Kansas City, KS

Marilyn Knoy, R.N.

Patient Care Supervisor of Newborn Nursery
Saint Francis Hospital
Tulsa, OK

Regina D. Maroncelli, B.A., M.C.H.

Managing Director
Georgia Poison Control Center
Adjunct Professor of Clinical Pharmacy
Mercer University School of Pharmacy
Atlanta, GA

Mayo Marsh, R.N., B.S.

Clinical Coordinator
Arthritis Treatment Center
Children's Hospital at Stanford
Palo Alto, CA

Liza McCrory, R.N., B.S.N.

Case Coordinator
Medi-Kid, Inc.
Children's Medical Day Care
Jacksonville, FL

Vicki Meyer, R.N.

Head Nurse
Newborn Nursery
Santa Clara Valley Medical Center
San Jose, CA

Kristie Nix, R.N., M.S.

Assistant Professor
College of Nursing and Applied Health Sciences
University of Tulsa
President of BELT (Buckle Every Little Tot)
Tulsa, OK

Beverlee E. Redding, B.S.N.

Nurse Specialist
Pediatric Oncology Clinic
Hospice Consultant
Saint John Medical Center
Tulsa, OK

Linsay K. Manuel, M.Ed.

Exercise Test Technologist (A.C.S.M.)
Physical Performance Center
Tulsa, OK

Kiyo Sato-Viacrucis, M.N., P.H.N.

Consultant, Private Practice
Sacramento, CA

Donald Segal

Executive Director
Association for Brain Tumor Research
Chicago, IL

Jody Shelton, R.N.

Formerly Patient Care Supervisor of Pediatrics
Saint Francis Hospital
Tulsa, OK

Cynthia Spencer, R.Ph.

Manager, Regulatory Affairs
CooperBiomedica, Inc.
Mt. View, CA

Nancy Stevens, R.N., M.S., C.P.N.P.

Assistant Professor
Division of Nursing
Northeastern State University
Tahlequah, OK

Martha Thompson, R.N., M.S., M.A.

Professor of Nursing
San Jose State University
San Jose, CA

Janet K. Williams, R.N., M.A.

Genetic Associates in Pediatrics
Division of Medical Genetics
The University of Iowa
Iowa City, IA

David Wilson, R.N., M.S.

Nutrition Support Coordinator
Saint Francis Hospital
Tulsa, OK

Deborah M. Wright, R.N.

Charge Nurse
Psychosomatic Unit
Children's Hospital at Stanford
Palo Alto, CA

Tamra Yong, R.N., M.S.N.

Professor of Nursing
Dekalb Community College
Clarkston, Georgia

Contents

Inside Front Cover
Pediatric emergencies; normal pulse, temperature, respiration, and blood pressure readings for infants and children

Inside Back Cover
Conversion tables

Unit One

Children, Their Families, and the Nurse

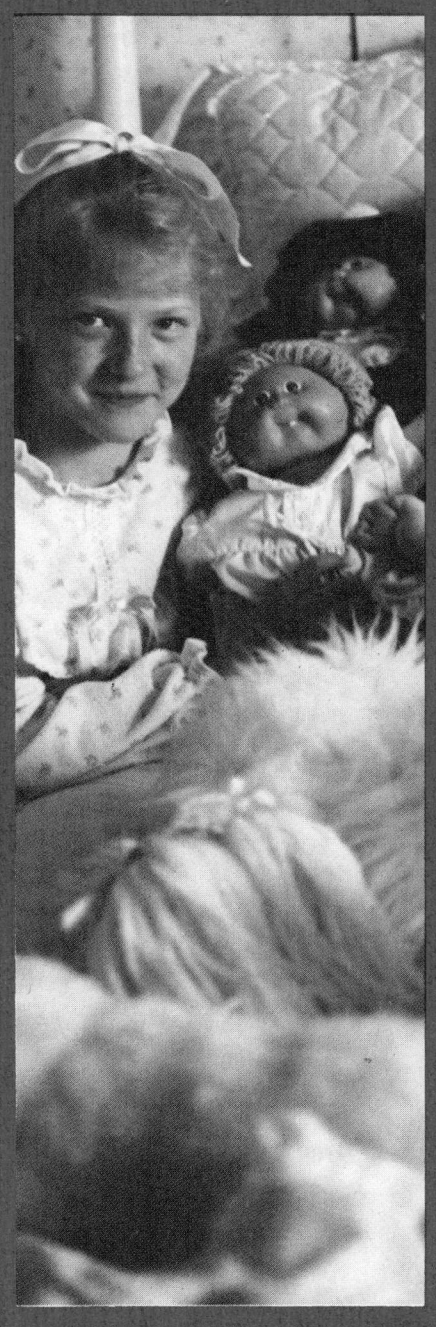

Chapter 1, *Perspectives of Pediatric Nursing*, emphasizes a child-centered rather than a disease-centered approach to nursing of infants and children. Childhood health is viewed from the perspective of mortality and morbidity trends at various ages, with special attention to injuries, the leading cause of death. A historical overview of child health care in the United States serves as a basis for understanding changes that have occurred in pediatrics. Nursing is viewed as a process and the nurse as a person who can work effectively with infants and children and help create conditions in which others, particularly parents, can function more effectively in child care.

Chapter 2, *Social, Cultural, and Religious Influences on Child Health Promotion*, considers the way in which the societal and cultural background of the family affects children, their health, and their relationships. The emphasis is on differences in health practices, environmental influences, and perspectives on health and health care providers.

Chapter 3, *Family Influences on Child Health Promotion*, is concerned with children in their family setting. It includes selected family theories, family constellations, and the way in which the family influences development. The child's place within the family is examined with emphasis on the role of family members in shaping the child's attitudes and behavior.

Chapter 4, *Growth and Development of Children*, provides a vertical or longitudinal view of the alterations that take place during growth and development and serves as a preface to the horizontal age-specific discussions in the chapter on health promotion. Children are presented as unique individuals on a life-long developmental continuum; they differ physiologically, morphologically, and emotionally from adults, from other children, and from the children they were and will become.

Chapter 5, *Hereditary and Prenatal Influences on Health Promotion of the Child and Family*, discusses genetic and prenatal factors that affect the growth and health of children. It includes cytogenetic disorders, major inheritance patterns, and effects of heredity on common diseases and conditions. Factors that influence the developing organism are discussed briefly. The major emphasis is on the nurse's role in dealing with families coping with genetic disease or disability.

Chapter 1

Perspectives of Pediatric Nursing

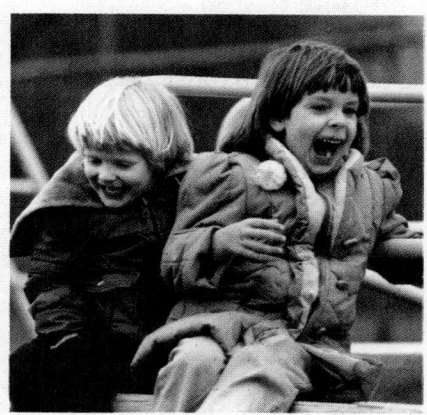

Health care of children has changed dramatically in the past century. It has paralleled society's changing view of children from "miniature adults," whose value to the community was measured in productivity, to a recognition and appreciation of children as unique individuals with special needs and qualities. There has been a shifting focus in child care from treatment of disease to prevention of illness and promotion of health. Nurses are no longer solely involved in the episodic care of children during an acute illness. They are increasingly responsible for providing comprehensive, distributive care that attempts to meet the needs of children and their families.

This chapter presents an overview of child health through discussion of past and present trends in childhood mortality and morbidity, with special attention to injuries, the leading cause of death in children. It offers a brief history of the evolution of child health care in the United States. The role of the pediatric nurse in both traditional and extended-role situations is also discussed. The process of nursing children and families is briefly reviewed because it is the basis of all nursing action.

Health During Childhood

Health is a complex phenomenon. As defined by the World Health Organization (WHO), it is "a state of complete physical, mental, and social well-being and not merely the absence of disease." Despite this broad definition, health is traditionally assessed by observing *mortality* (death) and *morbidity* (illness) rates over a period of time. Therefore the *presence* of disease becomes a prime indicator of health.

Based on these parameters, the health of children in the United States is better than ever before. As is discussed in the following sections, mortality rates for all ages of children have dropped dramatically since the beginning of the 1900s. However, there remains cause for concern (U.S. House, 1984):

1. The infant and child death rate is still high in the United States when compared to rates in some other well-developed countries.
2. Depending on race, nonwhite children have up to a 50% higher mortality rate than white children.
3. The United States rate for teenage childbearing is higher than those of 28 other developed countries; pregnancies of mothers less than 19 years of age result in almost twice as many low-birth-weight neonates as pregnancies of mothers 20 and older.
4. The poverty rate for children has increased in recent years; 21% of all children live in poverty (defined as annual income of $9862 for a family of four), and for nonwhite children this figure is doubled.
5. Other areas of concern are immunization levels among preschool children, malnutrition, increasing incidence of tuberculosis in Asian and Hispanic populations, dental problems, accidents, substance abuse, and suicide.

Information concerning mortality and morbidity is important to nurses. Such data yield significant information about (1) the causes of death and illness, (2) high-risk age-groups for certain disorders or hazards, (3) advances in treatment and prevention, and (4) specific areas of health counseling. Nurses who are aware of such information can better guide their planning and delivery of care.

MORTALITY

Figures describing rates of occurrence for events such as death in children are often referred to as *vital statistics*. Mortality statistics describe the incidence or number of individuals who have died over a specific period of time. They are usually presented as rates per 100,000 population because of their lower frequency of occurrence. Such rates are calculated from a sample of death certificates.

In the United States the National Center for Health Statistics (NCHS), under the Department of Health and Human Services (DHHS) (formerly the Department of Health, Education and Welfare), Public Health Service, has the responsibility for collection, analysis, and dissemination of data on the health of the American people. Because of the complexity of compiling such data, statistics may vary in different reports. For example, figures may be *estimated* (from previously collected data), *provisional* (from temporary current data), or *final* (from complete provisional data). It is not unusual for final statistics to be published 2 or more years after original collection of the data.

Causes of death are categorized according to the International Classification of Diseases (ICD). The ICD is revised approximately every 10 years. As of 1975 the Ninth Revision has been used. This has produced many changes in the classification system, making comparisons between causes of death before and after 1976 difficult. This should be kept in mind when reviewing mortality statistics from different sources and for various time intervals. For example, the causes of infant death are markedly different in the Eighth and Ninth Revisions. In the Ninth Revision there is the addition of respiratory distress syndrome and sudden infant death syndrome in the list of 10 leading causes of death.

Infant Mortality

Infant mortality rate is defined as the number of deaths per 1000 live births during the first year of life. It may be further divided into *neonatal* (first 28 days of life) and *postneonatal* (29 days to 1 year) mortality. In the United States there has been a dramatic decrease in the infant mortality rate. At the beginning of the twentieth century the mortality

Table 1-1 Infant mortality for 20 countries with population over 2 million, 1983 (rate per 1000 live births)

COUNTRY	RATE
Finland	6.2*
Japan	6.2
Sweden	7.0
Switzerland	7.6
Denmark	7.7*
Norway	7.9*
Netherlands	8.4*
Canada	8.5
France	9.0
Singapore	9.4
Australia	9.6
Spain	9.6*
Ireland	9.8
Hong Kong	9.9
United Kingdom	10.2*
Federal Republic of Germany	10.3
German Democratic Republic	10.7*
United States of America	11.2
Belgium	11.3*
Austria	11.9*

From Wegman, M.E.: Annual summary of vital statistics—1984, Pediatrics **76**(6):861–871, 1985.
*Provisional data.

rate was about 200 per 1000 live births; in 1984 the provisional infant mortality rate dropped to 10.6 per 1000, the lowest rate ever recorded in the United States. This decrease has primarily been a result of infectious disease control and nutritional advances during the early 1900s and the advent of antibiotic and antibacterial agents in the late 1930s.

However, when viewed from a worldwide perspective, the United States lags significantly behind other well-developed countries. In 1983 it ranked eighteenth among the 25 countries with the lowest infant mortality rates, with Finland and Japan having the lowest rate (Wegman, 1985) (Table 1-1). This is far behind neighboring countries such as Canada, which ranked eighth.

Birth weight is considered the major determinant of neonatal death in the developed countries of the world. There is an inverse relationship with birth weight and mortality; that is, the lower the birth weight, the higher the mortality. The relatively high incidence of very-low-birth-weight infants in the United States is considered a key factor in its higher neonatal mortality rates when compared to other countries.

While there has been a steady and significant decline in infant mortality, the number of deaths occurring in the first year of life is still proportionately high when compared with mortality rates at other ages. This is true of other countries, such as Canada (Table 1-2). As Table 1-3 shows, the infant death rate in the United States is greater than the cumulative rates for ages 1 through 54 years. It is not until age 55 and over that the death rate begins to exceed the infant death rate. The major causes of infant death are presented in Table 1-4.

During the first half of this century neonatal mortality rates had not shown the remarkable reduction observed in infant mortality. In the early 1960s attention focused on perinatal health care in an effort to decrease the number of deaths. As a result, the neonatal mortality rate declined from 20 per 1000 live births in 1950 to an estimated rate of

6.8 per 1000 in 1984. This drop has largely been the result of better treatment of perinatal illnesses, particularly asphyxia, immaturity, respiratory disorders, and gastrointestinal problems. As Table 1-4 demonstrates, the majority of the 10 leading causes of death during infancy continue to occur during the perinatal period; almost 75% of all infant deaths occur within the first 20 days of life.

Although a number of perinatal problems have benefited from improved treatment, congenital anomalies continue to be the leading cause of infant mortality, accounting for about 22% of those deaths. The incidence of most birth de-

Table 1-3 Death rates by age, United States, 1984 (estimated rates per 100,000 in specified group)

AGE (YEARS)	RATE
Under 1	1077.8
1-4	50.1
5-14	25.1
15-24	98.5
25-34	123.1
35-44	205.5
45-54	531.7
55-64	1289.6
65-74	2864.4
75-84	6416.5
85 and over	14,890.1

From National Center for Health Statistics: Annual summary of births, marriages, divorces, and deaths; United States, 1984. Monthly vital statistics report 33(13):6, DHHS Pub. No. (PHS) 85–1120, Sept. 26, 1985.

Table 1-4 Leading causes of death in infants under 1 year of age, United States, 1984 (estimated rates per 100,000 live births)

RANK	CAUSES OF DEATH	RATE
1	Other conditions originating in the perinatal period	272.7
2	Congenital anomalies	228.1
3	All other causes	170.2
4	Sudden infant death syndrome	131.7
5	Respiratory distress syndrome	103.9
6	Disorders relating to short gestation and unspecified low birth weight	93.3
7	Intrauterine hypoxia and birth asphyxia	26.2
8	Pneumonia and influenza	17.0
9	Birth trauma	8.9
10	Certain gastrointestinal diseases	7.6

From National Center for Health Statistics: Annual summary of births, marriages, divorces, and deaths: United States, 1984. Monthly vital statistics report 33(13):8, DHHS Pub. No. (PHS) 85-1120, Sept. 26, 1985.

Table 1-2 Death rates for children, Canada, 1981 (rates per 1000 population)

AGE (YEARS)	RATE		
	TOTAL	MALE	FEMALE
Under 1	9.6	10.8	8.4
1-4	0.5	0.6	0.5
5-9	0.3	0.3	0.3
10-14	0.3	0.4	0.2
15-19	0.9	1.4	0.5
20-24	1.0	1.6	0.5

From Vital statistics, vol. I: Births and deaths: 1981, Statistics Canada, Minister of Supply and Services, 1983.

Table 1-5 Reported incidence of selected congenital malformations, United States (including Puerto Rico), 1982

RANK	MALFORMATION	RATE*
1	Hypospadias	52.5
2	Patent ductus arteriosus	26.9
3	Clubfoot without central nervous system defects	24.5
4	Ventricular septal defect	14.7
5	Cleft lip with or without cleft palate	8.8
6	Down syndrome	7.9
7	Hydrocephalus without spina bifida	5.5
8	Spina bifida without anencephaly	4.8
9	Cleft palate without cleft lip	4.7
10	Anencephaly	3.3
10	Reduction deformity	3.3
11	Rectal atresia and stenosis	3.0
12	Tracheoesophageal fistula	1.8
13	Renal agenesis	1.7

Modified from Centers for Disease Control, Morbidity and mortality weekly report, Annual summary—1982, **32**(54):85-86 Dec. 1984.
*Per 10,000 total births.

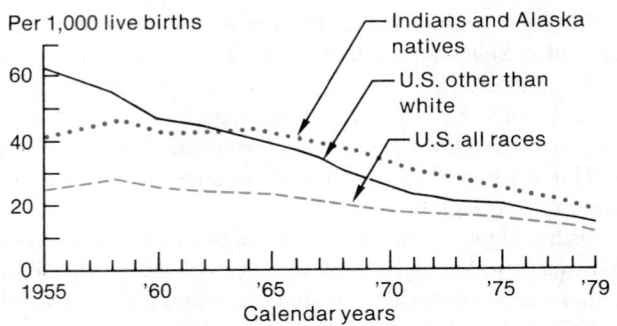

Fig. 1-1. Comparison of infant mortality rates among races other than white in the United States.
From Indian Health Service Chart Book Series, June 1984, U.S. Department of Health and Human Services, Public Health Service, Health Resources and Services Administrations, p. 20.

Table 1-6 Leading causes of death in children at selected age intervals, United States, 1983 (rates per 100,000)

AGES 1-4	RATE	AGES 5-14	RATE	AGES 15-24	RATE
All causes	55.9	All causes	26.9	All causes	96.0
Accidents	21.8	Accidents	12.7	Accidents	48.5
Congenital anomalies	6.5	Cancer	3.9	Homicide	12.4
Cancer	4.7	Congenital anomalies	1.4	Suicide	11.9
Heart disease	2.5	Homicide	1.0	Cancer	5.6
Homicide	2.3	Heart disease	0.9	Heart disease	2.6

From National Center for Health Statistics: Advance report of final mortality statistics, 1983. Monthly vital statistics report **34**(6):18-20, Suppl. (2), DHHS Pub. No. (PHS) 85-1120, Sept. 26, 1985.

Table 1-7 Number of children dying at selected age intervals according to sex and race, United States, 1983 (of 100,000 born alive)

AGE INTERVAL (YEARS)	WHITE		ALL OTHER	
	MALE	FEMALE	MALE	FEMALE
Under 1	1079	860	1832	1518
1-5	224	172	336	254
5-10	145	102	186	144
10-15	158	94	191	117
15-20	573	226	535	228

From National Center for Health Statistics: Annual report of final mortality statistics, 1982. Monthly vital statistics report **34**(6):13-15, Suppl. (2), DHHS Pub. No. (PHS) 85-1120, Sept. 26, 1985.

fects has neither substantially decreased nor increased (Table 1-5). Some notable exceptions are a slight decline in spina bifida and anencephaly and an increase in heart defects. The increased incidence of patent ductus arteriosus is probably due to improved survival of low-birth-weight infants and better diagnosis, but the increase in ventricular septal defect is likely to reflect a true increase. The relative stability of the incidence of congenital anomalies suggests the need for discovering and implementing improved prevention strategies (Kalter and Warkany, 1983).

When infant mortality rates are categorized according to race, a disturbing difference is seen. The infant mortality rates for whites are considerably lower than for all other races in the United States, with blacks having almost twice the rate for whites. Although the birth rate of both groups has declined, the gap has remained fairly constant. One encouraging note is that the gap in mortality rates between nonwhite races has been narrowing. Since the Indian Health Service assumed responsibility for the health of American Indians and Alaska Natives in 1955, infant mortality has declined by 75% (Fig. 1-1).

Childhood Mortality

After 1 year of age there is a dramatic change in the causes of death, with injuries (accidents) the leading cause until people reach their early forties. Injuries account for about 45% of all childhood deaths from ages 1 to 14 years (Table 1-6). In young adults aged 15 to 24, injuries, homicide, and suicide are responsible for about 75% of all deaths. Because of their critical importance in child health, injuries are discussed separately on p. 9 and suicide on p. 905.

The total number of deaths is also significant when each age-group is compared (Table 1-7). The school-age years have the lowest incidence of deaths. However, a sharp rise occurs during later adolescence, primarily from injuries, homicide, and suicide, all potentially preventable conditions.

Violent deaths have been steadily increasing among children. Homicide accounts for more than 10% of all deaths among adolescents and young adults—about 7% in whites and 30% in blacks. Approximately 25% of all victims are in this age-group, placing these young people at greater risk than the rest of the population. Males are three to four times more likely to be murdered and about five times more likely to be murderers than are females (Surgeon General's Report, 1979). Over 40% of murderers are under 21 years old; therefore child homicide appears to be a problem of the young killing the young (Jason, Gilliland, and Tyler, 1983).

The causes of increased violence against children are not fully understood. In young children the increase may represent more accurate identification of child abuse. In adolescents it may reflect an unhealthy preoccupation with violence and unresolved social tensions. Prevention lies in a better understanding of the social and psychologic factors that lead to the high rates of homicide and suicide. Nurses need to be especially aware of young people who are depressed, repeatedly in trouble with the criminal justice system, or associated with groups known to be violent. Prevention requires identification of these youngsters as well as therapeutic intervention by qualified professionals.

The general trend in racial differences that occurs in infant mortality is also apparent in childhood deaths. As Table 1-7 demonstrates, for all ages and for both sexes (with the exception of males 15 to 20 years) whites have fewer deaths. For all ages and for both racial groups male deaths outnumber female deaths. The lowest death rate occurs during the school-age years.

The absence of infectious diseases as a leading cause of death is testimony to the role antibacterial agents and immunizations have played in the declining mortality rates and the specific causes of death. More effective treatment of severe infections has resulted in other disorders becoming more prominent in the list of leading killers. Most notable among these are the neoplasms. (The incidence of cancer in children is discussed in Chapter 36.)

MORBIDITY

Morbidity statistics describe the prevalence of a specific illness in the population at a particular time. These are generally presented as rates per 1000 population because of their greater frequency of occurrence. Unlike mortality statistics, morbidity is very difficult to define. Morbidity may denote acute illness, chronic disease, or disability. The source of data also greatly influences the resulting statistics. Common sources include reasons for visits to physicians, diagnosis for hospital admission, or household interviews. The following discussion is intended to present an overview of illness in children from a variety of perspectives.

Childhood Morbidity

Acute illness may be defined as symptoms severe enough to limit activity or require medical attention. According to the National Health Survey, children under 5 years of age have about 3.5 acute illnesses per year with 8.8 days of restricted activity. Children 5 to 14 years of age have 2.9 episodes and 9.4 days of disability. As a general rule acute illness is less common in children under 6 months of age, increases thereafter until 3 or 4 years of age, and then gradually decreases throughout middle and older childhood. There is a slight peak again during the first year or two of school, probably as a result of increased exposure to new contagions (Green and Haggerty, 1984).

Infections account for nearly 80% of all childhood illnesses, and respiratory infections lead the list, occurring two to three times as often as all other illnesses combined. The chief illness of childhood is the common cold; the average child has one or two colds per year. Diseases of the respiratory system account for 25% of the hospitalizations for children under 1 year, 33% of the admissions for children 1 to 9, and 20% of admissions for the 10- to 14-year age-group (National Center, 1985). One third of all children annually have at least one episode of some other infection, such as gastrointestinal infection (Pless, 1978).

Injury-related morbidity is also significant, especially since less than one in 1000 injuries is fatal. About 37% of children suffer an injury each year that results in at least 1 restricted activity day (Guyer and Gallagher, 1985). Children 6 to 16 years miss 14 million days of school per year because of injuries (Collins, 1985). Between 40,000 and 50,000 children are permanently injured each year (Greensher, 1984).

From the perspective of seeking medical care, more children from white families have acute illnesses than those from black families. However, the illnesses reported by black mothers are more likely to be severe, probably in part a result of different attitudes toward health care.

Probably the most important aspect of morbidity is the degree of disability. Disability can be measured in days off from school or days confined to bed and can be the result of acute or chronic disorders. (The incidence of chronic disorders is discussed in Chapter 22.) On the average a child loses 5.6 days of school per year. Boys miss somewhat more school than girls, chiefly because of injuries. Of all

Table 1-8 Mortality from leading types of injuries, United States, 1980 (rates per 100,000 population in each age-group)

	AGE (YEARS)			
TYPE OF ACCIDENT	UNDER 1	1-4	5-14	15-24
Males				
All causes	1284.6	63.9	33.9	150.1
Accidents (all types)	32.1	26.6	17.4	80.7
Motor vehicle	6.0 (2)*	8.7 (1)	8.4 (1)	56.3 (1)
Drowning†	3.1 (5)	6.4 (2)	3.3 (2)	7.5 (2)
Fires and burns	4.2 (4)	5.4 (3)	1.5 (3)	1.5 (5)
Firearms	—	—	1.1 (4)	2.3 (3)
Ingestion of food/object	7.2 (1)	1.0 (4)	—	—
Mechanical suffocation	5.2 (3)	—	—	—
Falls	—	0.6 (5)	0.4 (5)	—
Poisoning	—	—	—	1.9 (4)
Accidents as percent of all deaths	2.5%	42%	51%	56%
Females				
All causes	1023.3	52.1	22.2	51.6
Accidents (all types)	23.6	18.5	8.7	21.7
Motor vehicle	5.5 (1)	7.2 (1)	5.0 (1)	17.3 (1)
Drowning	2.0 (5)	3.2 (3)	0.9 (3)	0.8 (2)
Fires and burns	3.5 (4)	4.0 (2)	1.3 (2)	0.7 (3)
Firearms	—	—	0.3 (4)	0.3 (5)
Ingestion of food/object	4.9 (2)	0.7 (4)	—	—
Mechanical suffocation	3.9 (3)	—	—	—
Falls	—	0.6 (5)	0.2 (5)	—
Poisoning	—	—	—	0.6 (4)
Accidents as percent of all deaths	2.3%	36%	39%	42%

Modified from National Center for Health Statistics, Public Health Service, U.S. Department of Health and Human Services, as cited in Accident Facts, Chicago, 1985, National Safety Council.
*Indicates rank among the leading types of accidents.
†Exclusive of deaths in water transportation.

children under 17 years of age more than 95% are not disabled in any way, about 2% have mild disability, another 2% have moderate disability, and 0.2% are severely disabled (Pless, 1978).

Although childhood is a time of relative health, it is the rare child who never becomes ill. Most children experience one or more episodes of acute illness annually and may be disabled for a short time. The rapidity with which children become ill often causes great anxiety for parents, who fear that the illness is serious. Part of nurses' intervention is education of parents regarding the usual types of childhood illness and recognition of those symptoms that require treatment, such as signs of respiratory distress or dehydration. Nurses should also be aware of signs of potentially fatal illnesses. However, the future progress in decreasing childhood morbidity, as in childhood mortality, rests more on parent education than on scientific discoveries such as the antibiotic. Nurses play a vital role in advancing child care through health promotion.

The New Morbidity

In addition to disease and injury, children face other problems that can significantly alter their health. These include behavioral, social (family), and educational problems that are sometimes referred to as the "new morbidity" or "pediatric social illness." Examples of such conditions include child abuse and neglect, nonorganic failure to thrive, injuries, childhood adjustment disorders, learning disorders, and attention deficit disorder. Estimates on the incidence of these problems vary, but they probably represent at least 5% and as much as 25% to 30% in specific age-groups, social classes, and medical facilities (Starfield, 1980).

One of the dilemmas of the new morbidity is its identification in children. For example, the proportion of children with these problems is *greater* than the number of visits children make to health care facilities with a "new morbidity" diagnosis. Consequently many children seen at a health center have another primary disorder, usually somatic, and are only then diagnosed with a psychosocial and psychosomatic problem. There is greater emphasis from health professionals on organic deviations than on mental or social ones, and since insurance companies generally do not reimburse for counseling required in the care of psychosocial problems, there is a distinct disincentive to diagnose them. However, children do have such problems, and those working with children, especially nurses in primary care facilities, need to be aware of their potential existence and to deliberately investigate them.

Although no conclusive characteristics have been identified for children with new morbidity problems, some findings are significant in terms of defining a high-risk group. These include children (1) from the lowest socioeconomic strata, (2) ages 7 to 14 years, (3) of male gender, (4) from one-parent families, (5) with a presenting complaint of a chronic physical disorder, (6) with reading skills below grade level, and (4) with higher rates of school absenteeism (Goldberg and others, 1984; Nader and others, 1981).

INJURIES—THE LEADING KILLER

Injuries, the leading cause of death in children over age 1 year, have not shown the dramatic declines seen in other areas of childhood mortality (Table 1-8). Some of the reasons include (Committee on Trauma Research, 1985):

1. Injury has traditionally been regarded as an unavoidable accident or a behavioral problem, rather than a health problem. The term *accident* suggests a chaotic, random event that is "luck" or "chance"; the term *injury* is preferred because it connotes a sense of responsibility and control.
2. Injury control, including research, has not received high priority or sufficient financial support. No central agency coordinates or is responsible for reducing the incidence of injuries.
3. Research on injuries has not been based on a theoretical framework, as has been done with diseases. There is a need to view injuries in terms of *host,* the affected person, *environment,* the time and place, and *agent,* the object that is the direct cause.

Host and Agent

The type of injury and the circumstances surrounding it are closely related to normal growth and developmental behavior (see box). As children develop, their innate curiosity impels them to investigate activities and to mimic the behavior of others. This is essential in order to acquire competency as an adult, but it predisposes them to numerous hazards during childhood.

The developmental stage of the child partially determines the types of injuries that are most likely to occur at a specific age and thus helps provide clues to preventive measures. For example, small infants are helpless in any environment, and when they begin to roll over or otherwise propel themselves, they can fall from unprotected surfaces. The crawling infant with a natural tendency to place objects in the mouth is at risk of aspiration or poisoning. The mo-

---

CHILDHOOD INJURIES: RISK FACTORS

Sex—preponderance of males; difference mainly due to behavioral characteristics

Temperament—children with difficult temperament profile (see p. 110), especially children with attention deficit disorder

Stress—predisposition to increased risk-taking and self-destructive behavior; general lack of self-protection

Alcohol and drug use—associated with higher incidence of motor vehicle injuries, drownings, homicide, and suicide

Developmental characteristics—mismatch between child's developmental level and skill required for activity, for example, minibike injuries
  Natural curiosity to explore environment
  Desire to assert self and challenge rules
  Older child—desire for peer approval and acceptance

Cognitive characteristics (age specific)
  Infancy—sensorimotor: explores environment through taste and touch
  Young child—object permanence: actively searches for attractive object
    Cause and effect: unaware of consequential dangers
    Transductive reasoning: may fail to learn from experiences, for example, falling from step is not perceived as same type of danger as climbing a tree
    Magical and egocentric thinking: cannot comprehend danger to self or others; cannot take place of others to realize danger; if thinking something is safe, believes it to be so
  School-age child—transitional cognitive processes: unable to fully comprehend causal relationships; attempts dangerous acts without detailed planning regarding consequences
  Adolescent—formal operations: preoccupied with abstract thinking and loses sight of reality; may lead to feeling of invulnerability

---

bile toddler with the instinct to explore and investigate and the ability to run and climb is subject to a variety of injuries, including falls, burns, and collision with objects. As children grow older, their absorption with play often makes them oblivious to environmental hazards such as street traffic or water, and the need to conform and gain acceptance compels older children and adolescents to accept challenges and dares. Although the highest incidence of injury is in children less than 9 years of age, most fatal injuries occur in later childhood and adolescence.

Children's personalities can be a factor in their susceptibility to injuries. The bright, alert, and adventuresome child is apt to have more injuries than the dull, passive, or less curious child. Boys at all ages have more injuries than girls, and this tendency increases as the child gets older.

The pattern of deaths caused by injuries, especially from motor vehicles, drowning, and burns, is remarkably consistent in most Western societies, such as Canada. Table 1-8 compares the leading causes of deaths from injuries for each age-group according to sex. The overwhelming cause of death in children over 1 year is motor vehicle fatalities, including passenger, pedestrian, bicycle, and motorcycle deaths (Fig. 1-2). Even though the *percentage* of infants dying from motor vehicle injuries is small compared to the total number of deaths in that age-group, infants less than 6 months of age are at highest risk for motor vehicle passenger deaths. Factors that may be responsible are the greater frequency of their being held on an adult's lap or being

placed on the front seat (Pless and Stulginskas, 1982).

From 1978 to 1982 nearly 3400 child passengers under 5 years of age were killed in traffic injuries and an additional 250,000 were injured. One encouraging note is that the incidence of vehicular injuries, especially among young children, has been declining, probably as a result of child passenger restraint laws (see Questions and controversies, p. 12). Currently, all states in the United States have enacted legislation requiring young children to be properly restrained in motor vehicles.

When accidental deaths are compared according to sex and age, the causes of death differ. Drowning and burns are the second and third leading causes of death in boys aged 1 to 14, but the order is reversed in girls (Fig. 1-3). In addition, firearms are a major cause of death in males but not in females (Fig. 1-4). During infancy, more males succumb to death from aspiration than do females (Fig. 1-5). More than half of all poisonings occur in children under 2 years of age (Fig. 1-6). By age 4 to 5 years, nonintentional poisonings are uncommon. However, another increase occurs in the 15- to 24-year age-group, usually represents suicide (especially females) or drug abuse, and is the fourth leading cause of death from injury.

Analyzing deaths from specific types of injuries by age and sex is useful in identifying high-risk groups. When comparing accidental deaths to other causes of childhood mortality, it is clear that preventing injuries offers the greatest promise for improving survival. Nurses certainly play a major role in providing anticipatory guidance to parents and older children regarding hazards during each age period.

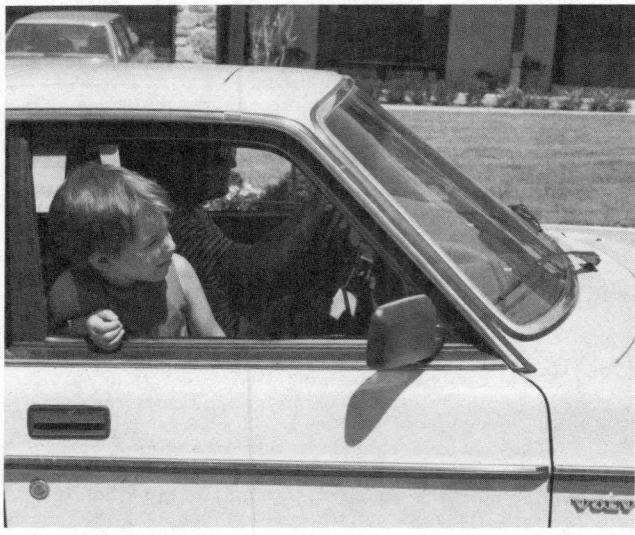

Fig. 1-2. Motor vehicle injuries are the leading cause of death in children over 1 year of age.

A

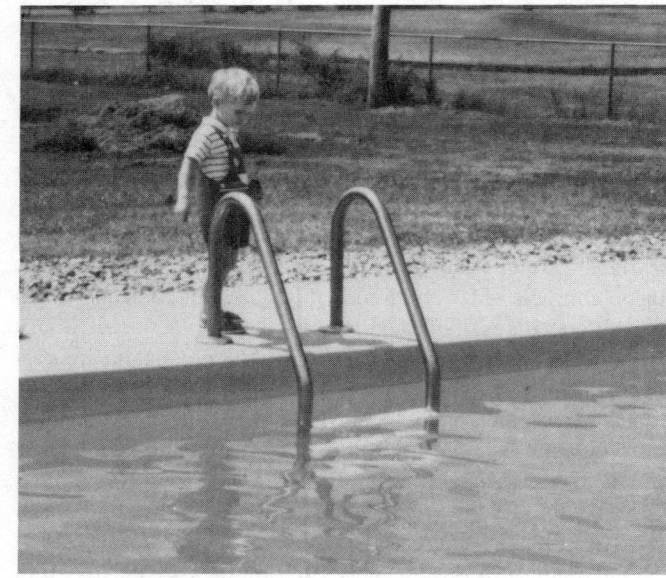

B

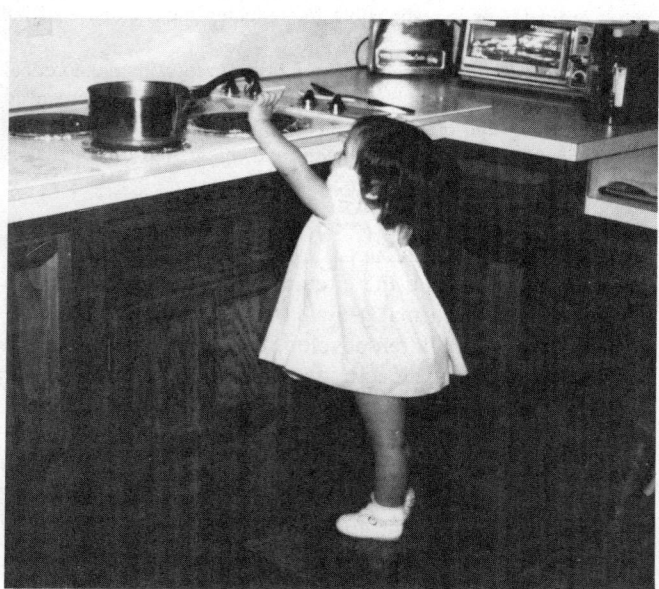

Fig. 1-3. **A,** Drowning is the second leading cause of death in boys and the third in girls ages 1 to 14 years. **B,** Burns are the second leading cause of death from injury in girls and the third in boys ages 1 to 14 years.

Environment

A number of unrelated and seemingly ordinary things appear to contribute to injuries. Often an injury occurs when there is a minor family illness and especially when the mother is ill, pregnant, tired, or just about to begin a menstrual period. Injuries frequently occur when the parent is rushed, tells the child, "Don't do that!" but is too busy to see that the direction is carried out. Illness, death of a family member, relocation, and continuous tense relationships between parents are prominent factors contributing to injuries. More injuries occur in single-parent families than two-parent families.

A higher incidence of injuries takes place from Thursday through Saturday. On Saturday, when both parents are usually at home, the routine is disrupted and each parent thinks the other is watching the child. Injuries are lowest on Sunday, when adults have more leisure time and are able to supervise children more carefully. Injuries are more apt to occur when the child is in the care of an unfamiliar person or a sibling who is too young for such responsibility, when the child changes surroundings, or when he is hungry or

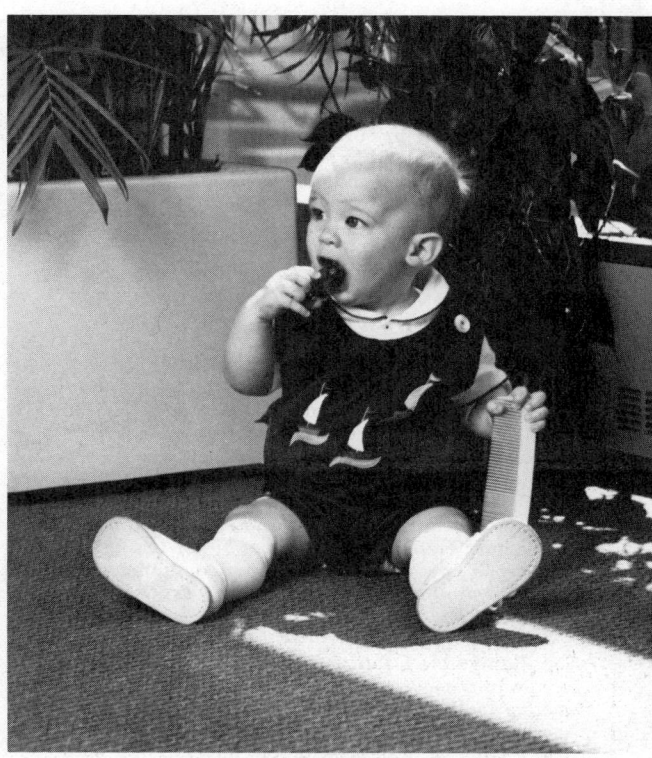

Fig. 1-5. Aspiration is the leading cause of death from injury in infants, especially in males.

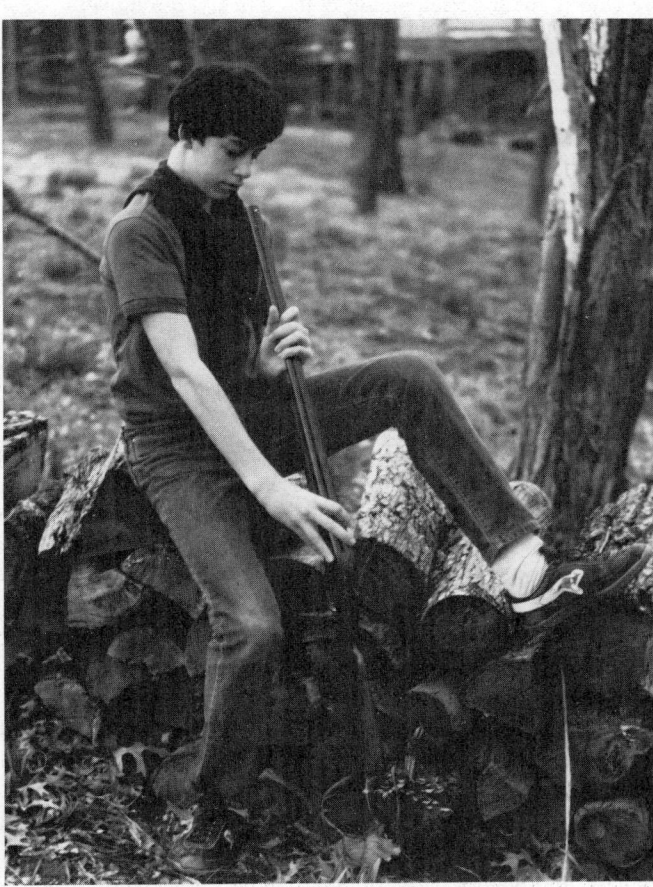

Fig. 1-4. Firearms are the fourth leading cause of death in boys and girls ages 5 to 14 years and the third leading cause in boys ages 15 to 24.

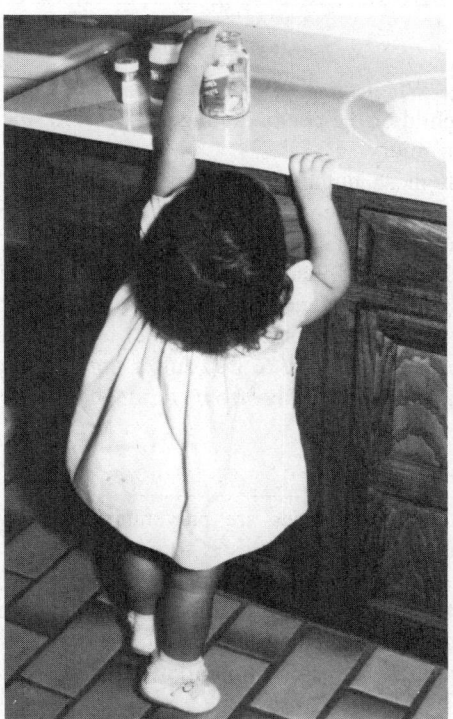

Fig. 1-6. Poisoning causes a considerable number of injuries in children under 4 years of age, but it is the fourth leading cause of death from injury in both sexes ages 15 to 24.

Questions and Controversies

How effective are injury prevention programs and what role have nurses played in education and research aimed at reducing the incidence of injuries in children?

The most effective interventions for injury prevention have been passive strategies and legislation. Rivara (1985b) predicts that the use of 12 currently available preventive strategies could reduce childhood deaths from injuries by 26% in the United States. These include:

1. Child passenger protection laws, which have reduced motor vehicle deaths in young children and could further reduce fatalities by 90% and disabling injuries by 67% (National Transportation Safety Board, 1983).

2. The Federal Hazardous Substance Labeling Act and the Poison Prevention Packaging Act, which have significantly reduced the number of poisonings by limiting the number of tablets in a container, using child-resistant closures, and limiting exposure to the toxin (Walton, 1982).

3. The Flammable Fabrics Act and the use of smoke detectors in homes, which have been effective in reducing deaths from burns (Miller and others, 1982).

4. Use of window guards, which reduced falls from windows in one city by 50% (Spiegel and Lindaman, 1977).

Unfortunately, nurses have been involved in little research related to injury prevention. One study found that nurses were the least cited source of information concerning auto safety for newborns (Righi and Krozy, 1983). Among published research on motor vehicle safety, Arneson and others (1985) have identified problems parents encountered in using child car restraints and actions taken to alleviate them. Adams (1982) found that education concerning car seats was not effective in increasing seat belt usage among school-age children. Two important factors positively affecting usage were the child's liking to wear the belt and parental use of restraints. Such research can provide health professionals with effective interventions in eliminating perceived barriers. Nurses have also been involved in developing and coordinating loaner car restraint programs.

Nurses are in an excellent position to initiate research and promote safety. Further studies could focus on the effectiveness of safety education during prenatal care versus in the nursery, the inclusion of both parents versus one parent in safety education, and comparison of different educational methods to identify those that are most effective. Injury prevention, including safety checks regarding parents' knowledge of car and home safety, could be completed in the nursery, during well child visits or hospitalizations, and at daycare centers and schools.

---

traveling. When there is increased stress on the part of either the child or the person taking care of him, there is more risk of an injury.

The highest number of injuries occurs in the home, especially in children younger than 6 years. Older children have almost as many injuries outside the home, especially at school and recreational sites. Recent attention has focused on the incidence of injuries on farms, where many children reside and work. Nearly 300 children and adolescents die each year and 23,000 suffer nonfatal trauma from farm injuries, especially from farm machinery (Rivara, 1985a).

Injury Prevention

Theoretically all injuries are preventable, and one of the chief nursing responsibilities is to anticipate and recognize where safety measures are applicable (see also Questions and controversies, above). Injury prevention necessitates protection, education, and legislation. The two major strategies for injury prevention in children are:

1. **Passive strategies,** which provide automatic protection by product and environmental design, for example, the use of automatic seat belts or airbags. Such devices require no active participation by the individual and have the greatest success rate.

2. **Active strategies,** which *persuade* individuals to change their behavior for increased self-protection, such as using seat belts voluntarily, or *require* compliance with safety regulations, such as laws that mandate use of safety restraints in young children. Persuasion through education has been much less effective than legislated change.

The preventive aspects of child care are an ongoing part of health promotion throughout childhood. To protect the child from injury, persons who are responsible for children need to be aware of the normal behavior characteristics that render children vulnerable to injuries and to be alert to factors in the environment that create a hazard to their safety. Parents and others are often surprisingly unaware of their child's developmental progress and capabilities. Anticipatory guidance regarding developmental expectations serves to alert the parents to the type of injuries that are most likely to occur at any given age and to environmental circumstances that might precipitate an injury. For example, infants must not be left where they can fall or roll over and toddlers must not be given objects or toys with small removable parts or sharp edges or given unsupervised access to places where they can fall, drown, or be burned.

Very early in the parent-child relationship the parents need to learn how to provide a safe environment for their child, what kinds of behaviors they can expect of the child at various stages in their development, and their responsibility for the safety of their children. This is particularly important for first-time parents. Safety responsibility in such areas as purchase of nursery furniture, including a car seat, should begin *before* the child is born.

It cannot be assumed that parents of one or more children are familiar with all areas of child safety. Moreover, the addition of a new child brings up the issue of sibling rivalry and the unwelcome but realistic possibility that the new child may be at risk from a jealous older sibling. For example, the parents should be cautioned against leaving the infant alone with the older child who feels threatened by the newcomer.

Providing a safe environment for the child involves the combined efforts of family, nurses, and community. At each age level there are environmental attractions that are hazardous to the safety of the child. The specific hazards vary according to season (drowning, injuries related to winter heating devices), geographic area (water injuries in areas with swimming pools, rivers, lakes; heater burns in cold climates), and socioeconomic level (lead poisoning and street injuries in slum areas, bicycle injuries in middle-class areas).

Safety should be an intrinsic element of nursing practice. Nurses who themselves practice safety, who are alert to safety needs in the environment, and who recognize the need for safety education contribute to injury reduction. The special problems and preventive measures are discussed as appropriate throughout the book and are related to the various age levels and conditions that predispose to specific hazards.

EVOLUTION OF CHILD HEALTH CARE IN THE UNITED STATES

Children in colonial America were born into a world with many hazards to their health and survival. Epidemics were common and no control or treatment was known. Physicians were few and only a small number had any formal training. Midwives also were untrained, basing their practice on past experiences. Books providing information on child care and feeding were scarce and, when available, were useful only to a minority of literate parents.

Medical care by physicians was limited to wealthy European families who lived in or could travel to more developed cities. Children who lived on farms were mainly cared for by another family member or by a competent neighbor. Traveling medicine men, with their various forms of quackery, were common. Black children who were bought as slaves or born to slaves had only as much care as their owner was able or willing to provide (Scott and Winston, 1976). American Indian children were treated for disease according to the tradition of each tribe, which was often a mixture of medicine, magic, and religion (Sayre and Sayre, 1976). With the colonization of America the Indians were

exposed to many new diseases, which were fatal to large numbers of them.

Statistics on childhood mortality during the colonial period are largely unavailable. Epidemic diseases were prevalent, however, and included smallpox, measles, mumps, chicken pox, influenza, diphtheria, yellow fever, cholera, and whooping cough, but the disease that surpassed all others as a cause of childhood death was dysentery. Sometimes entire families succumbed to this illness. Other diseases that were major contributors to childhood illness were the "slow epidemic" of tuberculosis, nutritional diseases, and accidents (Schmidt, 1976).

Although scientific knowledge was accumulating, especially from work done in Europe, there were no organized efforts in the United States to apply that knowledge to the care of the sick. It was not until the Industrial Revolution was well underway in the nineteenth century that the consequences of childhood illness and injury and the effect of child labor, poverty, and neglect became more widely recognized. The end of the nineteenth century is often regarded as the dark ages of pediatrics, and the first half of the twentieth century as the dawn of improved health care for children (Cone, 1976).

The study of pediatrics began in the last half of the 1800s, particularly under the influence of a Prussian-born physician, Abraham Jacobi (1830-1919), who is referred to as the Father of Pediatrics (Leopold, 1957). He was awarded the first professorship in pediatrics in America in 1870, started pediatric departments in several New York hospitals, and was one of the founders of the American Pediatric Society in 1888. With several other physicians he pioneered in the scientific and clinical investigation of childhood diseases. One outstanding achievement was the establishment of "milk stations," where mothers could bring sick children for treatment and learn the importance of pure milk and its proper preparation.

The crusade for pure milk helped bring the dairy industry under legal control and led to the establishment of infant welfare stations. The remarkable decline in infant mortality since 1900 has been achieved through prevention and health-promoting measures such as improved sanitation and pasteurization of milk. Before these regulations existed, the unsanitary milk supply was a chief source of infantile diarrhea and bovine tuberculosis. Cows were often kept in filthy stables and fed garbage and distillery wastes. Milk from cows fed distillery wastes was reported to make infants "tipsy." Some of the cows were so diseased with tuberculosis that they had to be raised on cranes to be milked (Cone, 1976).

At about the same time increasing concern developed for the social welfare of children, especially those who were homeless or employed as factory laborers. The work of one such reformer, Lillian Wald, had far-reaching effects on child health and nursing. She founded the Henry Street Settlement in New York City, which eventually provided nursing service, social work, and an organized program of so-

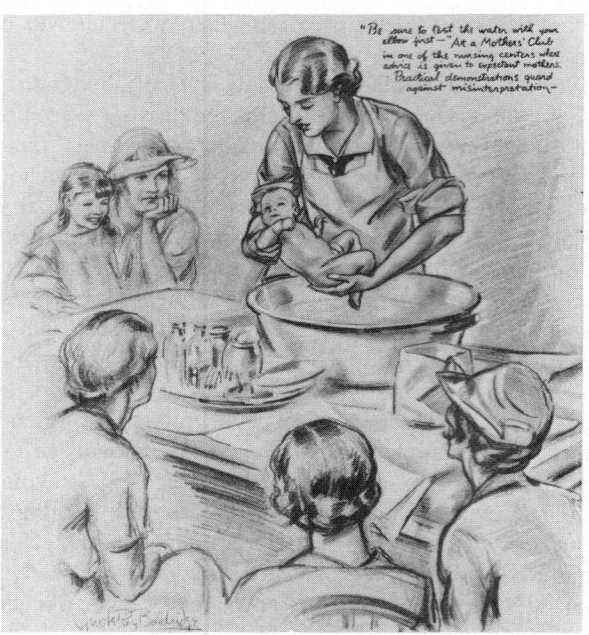

"Be sure to test the water with your elbow first — At a Mothers' Club in one of the nursing centers where advice is given to expectant mothers. Practical demonstrations guard against misinterpretation—"

Fig. 1-7. Cyrus Leroy Baldridge, *Be Sure to Test the Water with Your Elbow First*. Drawing from the 1938 pamphlet the ''Henry Street Visiting Nurse Service.'' Mugar Memorial Library, Boston University, Massachusetts.

By permission from the Henry Street Settlement Urban Life Center. In Donahue, M.P.: Nursing: the finest art—an illustrated history, St. Louis, 1985, The C.V. Mosby Co., p. 343.

cial, cultural, and educational activities (Fig. 1-7). Wald is regarded as the founder of public health or community nursing. She was instrumental in establishing the role of the first full-time school nurse, Lina Rogers. Soon other nurses were employed to teach parents and children about the prevention or need for treatment of minor skin conditions, malnutrition, and other impairments or illnesses identified in the school. An outgrowth of nursing involvement in school health was the development of pediatric courses and specialized clinical experience in schools of nursing (Williams, 1971).

As more causes of disease were identified, there was an emphasis on isolation and asepsis. In the early 1900s children with contagious diseases were isolated from adult patients. Parents were prohibited from visiting because they might transmit disease to and from the home. Even toys and personal articles of clothing were kept from the child. It was not until the 1940s and the famous work of Spitz and Robertson on institutionalized children that the effects of isolation and maternal deprivation were recognized. This brought forth a surge of interest in the psychologic health of children and resulted in changes for hospitalized children, such as rooming-in, sibling visitations, child life (play) programs, prehospitalization preparation, parent education, and hospital schooling.

Influenced by social reformers such as Lillian Wald, national leaders began to take action to improve children's living conditions. In 1909 President Theodore Roosevelt called the first White House Conference on Children. It focused on care of dependent children and attempted to address the deplorable working conditions of youngsters. As a result of this conference, the U.S. Children's Bureau was established under the jurisdiction of the Department of Labor, since at that time laws to regulate child labor were seen as the greatest need. Later, the Bureau was placed under the Department of Health, Education and Welfare (now the Department of Health and Human Services). White House conferences have been held approximately every 10 years to address the welfare, health, education, social, economic, and psychologic needs of children.

The establishment of the Children's Bureau in 1912 marked the beginning of a period of studies of economic and social factors related to infant mortality, maternal deaths, and maternal and infant care in rural areas, all of which created the basis for stimulating better standards of care for mothers and children. This helped lead to the first Maternity and Infancy Act (Sheppard-Towner Act) in 1921, which provided grants to states to develop a Division of Maternal and Child Health as a unit of the health department. However, this bill eventually lapsed because of opposition from those who viewed it as a socialist movement.

In 1935 Congress passed a much broader Maternal and Child Health program under Title V of the Social Security Act. The program consisted of three proposals: (1) aid to dependent children, (2) maternal and child health services, including Crippled Children's Services (CCS) (now the Special Child Health Services), and (3) child welfare services. The first programs provided by Title V were prenatal and postnatal clinics, child health clinics, and training of professional personnel.

Since 1935 numerous other federal programs have been developed. The Select Committee on Children, Youth and Families report, ''Federal Programs Affecting Children'' (U.S. House, 1984), lists 71 federal programs. Some of those that have had a major impact on maternal and child health include:

1. **Medicaid.** In 1965 Medicaid was created under Title XIX of the Social Security Act to reduce financial barriers to health care for the poor. It is the largest maternal-child health program. A major project under Medicaid is the Child Health Assessment Program (CHAP), which provides services for a large number of pregnant women and children.

2. **AFDC.** Aid to Families with Dependent Children was established by the Social Security Act of 1935 as a cash grant program to enable states to aid needy children without fathers.

3. **MCH Services Block Grant.** The Maternal and Child Health Services Block Grant provides health services to mothers and children, particularly those with low income or limited access to health services. Its primary purposes are to reduce infant mortality, reduce the incidence of preventable disease and handicapping conditions among children, and increase the availability of prenatal, delivery, and postpartum care to eligible mothers.

4. **Alcohol, Drug Abuse, and Mental Health Block Grant.** Established by the Omnibus Budget Reconciliation Act of 1981, the block grant provides funds to states for (1) projects to support prevention, treatment, and rehabilitation related to substance abuse and (2) grants to community mental health centers for the identification, assessment, and treatment of severely mentally disturbed children and adolescents.

5. **Social Services Block Grant.** Established under Title XX of the Social Security Act, this block grant provides states with funds for child daycare, protective and emergency services, counseling, family planning, home-based services, information and referral, and adoption and foster care services.

6. **WIC.** In 1966 the Special Supplemental Food Program for Women, Infants, and Children (WIC) was passed. It provides nutritious food and nutrition education to low-income, pregnant, postpartum, and lactating women and to infants and children up to age 5. Other nutrition programs include Food Stamps, National School Lunch Program, School Breakfast program, and Child Care Food Program, which provides financial assistance for nutritious meals to children in daycare centers, family and group daycare homes, and Head Start centers.

7. **Education for All Handicapped Children Act (P.L. 94-142).** In 1975 P.L. 94-142 was passed to provide a free appropriate public education to all handicapped children from ages 3 to 21 and to provide for those supportive services (speech, counseling, and so on) that ensure the benefit of special education.

One of the most drastic changes in health care delivery has been the establishment of a prospective payment system based on diagnosis related groups (DRGs). The DRG categories allow pretreatment (prospective) billing for almost all United States hospitals reimbursed by Medicare. With hospitals now financially responsible when Medicare patients exceed the allotted admission stay, more patients are being discharged early. This has created an immense need for home care and other sources of community-based services. The exact impact DRGs will have on pediatric care is uncertain, but with containment of health care cost a national priority, it is inevitable that some form of prospective payment will affect children. Nurses need to be aware of the changing economics and prepared to meet the challenges.

Pediatric Nursing

Nursing of infants and children is consistent with the definition of nursing as "the diagnosis and treatment of human responses to actual or potential health problems" (Nursing, 1980). Its purpose is to promote the highest possible state of health in each child. It consists of preventing disease or injury; assisting children, including those with a permanent handicap or health problem, to achieve and maintain an optimum level of health and development; and treating or rehabilitating children who have health deviations.

ROLE OF THE PEDIATRIC NURSE

Pediatric nurses are involved in every aspect of a child's growth and development. Nursing functions vary according to regional job structures, individual education and experience, and personal career goals. Just as clients (children and their families) present a vast and unique background, so it is that each nurse will bring to the clients an individual set of variables that will affect their relationship. No matter where pediatric nurses practice, their primary concern is the welfare of the child and family.

Family Advocacy

Although the nurse is responsible to self, the profession, and the institution of employment, primary responsibility is to the recipient of nursing services, the child and family. The nurse must work with members of the family, identifying their goals and needs, and plan interventions that best meet the defined problems. As a consumer advocate the nurse has the goal of ensuring that families are aware of all available health services, informed adequately of treatments and procedures, involved in the child's care when possible, and encouraged to change or support existing health care practices. The pediatric nurse is aware of the United Nations Declaration of the Rights of the Child (see box, p. 16) and practices within these guidelines to ensure that every child receives optimum care.

Of special significance is the nurse's role as child advocate. The following Pediatric Bill of Rights, composed by a 10-year-old child, clearly states the child's views regarding true "rights."

1. Any person regardless of age has the right to refuse pedeatric care.
2. Any person regardless of age has the right to pick there own pedeatrision, if there a girl they can pick a girl, if there a boy they can pick a boy.
3. Any person regardless of age has the right to not take there medicen if they dont want to.
4. Any person regardless of age has the right not to wear those paperthings at the doctors office.
5. Any person regardless of age has the right not to get weighed at the doctors office.*

Unfortunately, most of these "rights" are not in the child's best interest when health care is needed. However, they emphasize the need for nurses to consider the child's feelings and to individualize care to allow for personal preferences, fears, and dislikes. Throughout the text there are innumerable examples relating to special needs of children in various age-groups. As child advocate the nurse uses this knowledge to adapt care for the child's optimum physical and emotional well-being. Examples of this may be fostering the parent-child relationship during hospitalization, preparing the child before any unfamiliar treatment or procedure, allowing the child privacy, providing play activities

*Andreasen, S.: Pediatrics **55**(3):370, 1975. Copyright American Academy of Pediatrics 1975.

UNITED NATIONS DECLARATION OF THE RIGHTS OF THE CHILD

Preamble

Whereas the peoples of the United Nations have, in the Charter, reaffirmed their faith in fundamental human rights, and in the dignity and worth of the human person, and have determined to promote social progress and better standards of life in larger freedom,

Whereas the United Nations has, in the Universal Declaration of Human Rights, proclaimed that everyone is entitled to all the rights and freedoms set forth therein, without distinction of any kind, such as race, color, sex, language, religion, political or other opinion, national or social origin, property, birth or other status,

Whereas the child, by reason of his physical and mental immaturity, needs special safeguards and care, including appropriate legal protection, before as well as after birth,

Whereas the need for such special safeguards has been stated in the Geneva Declaration of the Rights of the Child of 1924, and recognized in the Universal Declaration of Human Rights and in the statutes of specialized agencies and international organizations concerned with welfare of children,

Whereas mankind owes to the child the best it has to give

Now therefore the general assembly proclaims

This Declaration of the Rights of the Child to the end that he may have a happy childhood and enjoy for his own good and for the good of society the rights and freedoms herein set forth, and calls upon parents, upon men and women as individuals and upon voluntary organizations, local authorities and national governments to recognize these rights and strive for their observance by legislative and other measures progressively taken in accordance with the following principles:

Principle 1

The child shall enjoy all the rights set forth in this Declaration. All children, without any exception whatsoever, shall be entitled to these rights, without distinction or discrimination on account of race, color, sex, language, religion, political or other opinion, national or social origin, property, birth or other status, whether of himself or of his family.

Principle 2

The child shall enjoy special protection, and shall be given opportunities and facilities, by law and by other means, to enable him to develop physically, mentally, morally, spiritually and socially in a healthy and normal manner and in conditions of freedom and dignity. In the enactment of laws for this purpose the best interests of the child shall be the paramount consideration.

Principle 3

The child shall be entitled from his birth to a name and a nationality.

Principle 4

The child shall enjoy the benefits of social security. He shall be entitled to grow and develop in health; to this end special care and protection shall be provided both to him and to his mother, including adequate pre-natal and post-natal care. The child shall have the right to adequate nutrition, housing, recreation and medical services.

Principle 5

The child who is physically, mentally or socially handicapped shall be given the special treatment, education and care required by his particular condition.

Principle 6

The child, for the full and harmonious development of his personality, needs love and understanding. He shall, wherever possible, grow up in the care and under the responsibility of his parents, and in any case in an atmosphere of affection and of moral and maternal security; a child of tender years shall not, save in exceptional circumstances, be separated from his mother. Society and the public authorities shall have the duty to extend particular care to children without a family and to those without adequate means of support. Payment of state and other assistance toward the maintenance of children of large families is desirable.

Principle 7

The child is entitled to receive education, which shall be free and compulsory, at least in the elementary stages. He shall be given an education which will promote his general culture, and enable him on a basis of equal opportunity to develop his abilities, his individual judgment, and his sense of moral and social responsibility, and to become a useful member of society.

The best interests of the child shall be the building principle of those responsible for his education and guidance; that responsibility lies in the first place with his parents.

The child shall have full opportunity for play and recreation, which shall be directed to the same purposes as education; society and the public authorities shall endeavor to promote the enjoyment of this right.

Principle 8

The child shall in all circumstances be among the first to receive protection and relief.

Principle 9

The child shall be protected against all forms of neglect, cruelty and exploitation. He shall not be the subject of traffic, in any form.

The child shall not be admitted to employment before an appropriate minimum age; he shall in no case be caused or permitted to engage in any occupation or employment which would prejudice his health or education, or interfere with his physical, mental or moral development.

Principle 10

The child shall be protected from practices which may foster racial, religious and any other form of discrimination. He shall be brought up in a spirit of understanding, tolerance, friendship among peoples, peace and universal brotherhood and in full consciousness that his energy and talents should be devoted to the service of his fellow men.

CODE FOR NURSES

1. The nurse provides services with respect for human dignity and the uniqueness of the client unrestricted by considerations of social or economic status, personal attributes, or the nature of health problems.
2. The nurse safeguards the client's right to privacy by judiciously protecting information of a confidential nature.
3. The nurse acts to safeguard the client and the public when health care and safety are affected by the incompetent, unethical, or illegal practice of any person.
4. The nurse assumes responsibility and accountability for individual nursing judgments and actions.
5. The nurse maintains competence in nursing.
6. The nurse exercises informed judgment and uses individual competence and qualifications as criteria in seeking consultation, accepting responsibilities, and delegating nursing activities to others.
7. The nurse participates in activities that contribute to the ongoing development of the profession's body of knowledge.
8. The nurse participates in the profession's efforts to implement and improve standards of nursing.
9. The nurse participates in the profession's efforts to establish and maintain conditions of employment conducive to high-quality nursing care.
10. The nurse participates in the profession's effort to protect the public from misinformation and misrepresentation and to maintain the integrity of nursing.
11. The nurse collaborates with members of the health professions and other citizens in promoting community and national efforts to meet the health needs of the public.

American Nurses' Association, 1976, 1985. Reproduced with permission of the American Nurses' Association.

for expression of fear, aggression, or loss of control, and respecting cultural differences relating to child-rearing practices.

The nurse is aware of the needs of children and works with all caregivers to ensure that these fundamental requirements are met. This often necessitates that the nurse expand the boundaries of practice to less traditional settings. The nurse may be involved in education, political/legislative change, rehabilitation, screening, administration, and even engineering and architecture. Regardless of how removed from direct patient care individual nurses become, they continue to foster health care practices that promote the well-being of children by incorporating knowledge of child growth and development into particular roles of practice. For example, as educator the nurse has the primary responsibility of helping others learn about and care for children. The audience for this information may be other nurses, parents, school teachers, other members of the health team, or the general public. In some states nurses are involved in mass media programs for immunization of all children.

Not infrequently, the role of family advocate conflicts with other roles of the nurse, such as those imposed by the institution. Inflexible rules, regulations designed for purposes of administration rather than optimum child welfare, and relationships with other professionals who are not knowledgeable of children's needs can create tremendous conflicts and challenges for the nurse who is dedicated to caring for the family in light of individual needs. Although there are rarely easy solutions to such dilemmas, the nurse can use the professional Code of Ethics for guidance (see box). A code of ethics provides one means for professional self-regulation. In the past the Code for Nurses, adopted by the American Nurses' Association in 1950, was more prescriptive, identifying codes of both personal and professional behavior, describing appropriate relationships with physicians and other health team members, and identifying certain responsibilities of the nurse as a citizen and employee. The present code focuses on the nurse's accountability and responsibility to the client and emphasizes the nursing role as an independent professional role that upholds its own legal liability.

Nurses may also face ethical issues regarding patient care, such as the use of life-saving measures for severely handicapped newborns or the terminally ill child's right to die. Throughout the text such dilemmas are addressed under a section titled "Questions and Controversies." The conflicting ethical arguments are presented to help nurses clarify their value judgments when confronted with similar sensitive issues.

Illness Prevention/Health Promotion

The emerging trend toward health care has been prevention of illness and maintenance of health, rather than treatment of disease or disability. Nursing has kept pace with this change, especially in the area of child care. In 1965 specialized programs for *pediatric nurse associates/practitioners* began to develop that have led to several specialized ambulatory or primary care roles for nurses. The thrust of these programs has been to educate nurses beyond the basic preparational stage in areas of child health maintenance so that all children can receive high-quality care. The practitioner programs have expanded to prepare school nurse practitioners, hospital nurse practitioners, and other specialists, such as the developmental pediatric nurse practitioner. Although the curriculum varies from program to program, the course content generally includes history taking, physical diagnosis, growth and development, health education, counseling, common childhood problems, and planning care for individuals and groups.

The *clinical nurse specialist* role has been developed in an attempt to provide expert nursing care. The term *nurse clinician* is based on a primary philosophy of clinical competence in direct patient care. The clinical specialist is competent in providing nursing care during all stages of illness or wellness and functions in any of the settings where patients may be found—the hospital, home, community, clinic, or long-term facility. The clinical specialist role has developed within each of the traditional specialty areas as well as in other areas. The educational preparation includes a graduate degree in nursing that may incorporate the practitioner skills.

The pediatric clinical nurse specialist plays an important role in the care of children, performing all the functions of the pediatric nurse. In addition, however, the clinical specialist should serve as a role model to the staff for clinical practice, a researcher to validate nursing observations and interventions, a change agent within the health care system, and a consultant/teacher to the health care team.

Obviously, the thrust of these nurse practitioner programs is prevention. However, it is not limited to them. Every nurse involved with child care must practice within the overall dimension of preventive health. Regardless of the identified problem, the role of the nurse is to plan care that fosters every aspect of growth and development. Based on a thorough assessment process, problems related to nutrition, immunizations, safety, dental care, development, socialization, discipline, or schooling frequently become obvious. Once the problem is identified, the nurse acts to intervene directly or to refer the family to other health persons or agencies.

The best approach to prevention is education and anticipatory guidance. In this book each chapter on health promotion includes sections on anticipatory guidance. An appreciation of the hazards or conflicts of each developmental period enables the nurse to guide parents regarding childrearing practices aimed at preventing potential problems. One of the most significant examples is safety. Since each age-group is at risk for special types of injuries, preventive teaching can help prevent most injuries, thus significantly lowering permanent disability and mortality from injuries in children.

Prevention also involves less obvious aspects of child care. Besides preventing physical disease or injury, the nurse's role is also to promote mental health. For example, it is not sufficient to administer immunizations without regard for the psychologic trauma associated with the procedure. Optimum health involves the practice of good medicine with a humane approach to health care; the nurse is often the one professional capable of ensuring "humanity." Because of current educational emphasis on holistic care, the extended and less formal interaction with the family, and the nursing role within the health team, the nurse's role is often one of *facilitator* of care rather than direct intervenor.

Health Teaching

Health teaching is inseparable from family advocacy and prevention. Health teaching may be a direct goal of the nurse, such as during parenting classes, or may be indirect, such as informing parents and children of a diagnosis or medical treatment, encouraging children to ask questions about their bodies, referring families to health-related professional or lay groups, and supplying patients with appropriate literature. Anticipatory guidance is one of the most important types of health teaching.

Health teaching is often one area in which nurses feel competent because it involves translating information rather than receiving messages, translating them, and planning intervention. In other words, it is a concrete, structured type of communication as opposed to other emotionally laden, nondirected types of interaction. However, the nurse focuses on giving appropriate health teaching with generous feedback and evaluation to promote learning.

Support/Counseling

Attention to emotional needs requires support and sometimes counseling. Frequently, the role of child advocate or health teacher is supportive by the very nature of the individualized approach. Support can be offered in many ways, the most common of which include listening, touching, and physical presence. The last two are most helpful with children because they facilitate nonverbal communication.

Counseling involves a mutual exchange of ideas and opinions that provides the basis for mutual problem solving. Although it is similar to health teaching, its focus is broader and more intense because it frequently implies some crisis or upsetting event that needs intervention. It involves support as well as teaching, techniques to foster expression of feelings or thoughts, and approaches to help the family cope with stress. Optimally counseling not only results in a resolved problem but also helps the family attain a higher level of functioning, greater self-esteem, and closer relationships (Satir and others, 1975). Although counseling is often the role of nurses in more specialized areas, counseling techniques are discussed in various sections of the text to help students and nurses cope with immediate crises and refer families for additional professional assistance.

Therapeutic Role

The most basic of all nursing roles is the restoration of health through caregiving activities. Nurses are intimately involved with meeting the physical and emotional needs of children, including feeding, bathing, toileting, dressing, security, and socialization. Although they are responsible for instituting physicians' prescriptions, they are also held singularly accountable for their own actions and judgments regardless of written orders.

A significant aspect of restoration of health is continual assessment and evaluation of physical status. Indeed, the concentrated focus throughout the text on physical assessment, pathophysiology, and scientific rationale for therapy is to assist the nurse in decision making regarding health status. Only when aware of normal findings can the nurse intelligently identify and document deviations. In addition, the pediatric nurse never loses sight of the emotional and developmental needs of the individual child, which can significantly influence the course of the disease process.

The therapeutic role frequently includes rehabilitation. Through expanding roles nurses are increasingly responsible for health care of handicapped children. For example, school nurses or pediatric nurse practitioners are involved in programs for severely developmentally disabled children in order to facilitate their attendance in regular classes (Del Campo and Josephson, 1978).

Coordination/Collaboration

The nurse, as a member of the health team, collaborates and coordinates nursing services with the activities of other professionals. Working in isolation does not serve the child's best interest. First, the concept of "holistic care" can only be realized through a unified interdisciplinary approach. Second, aware of individual contributions and limitations to the child's care, the nurse must collaborate with other specialists to provide for high-quality health services. Failure to recognize limitations can be nontherapeutic at best and destructive at worst. For example, the nurse who feels competent in counseling when really inadequate in this area may not only prevent the child from dealing with a crisis but may also retard his future success with a qualified professional.

Even nurses who practice in isolated geographic areas widely separated from other health professionals cannot be considered independent. Every nurse works interdependently with the child and family, collaborating on needs and interventions so that the final care plan is one that truly meets the child's needs. Unfortunately, this is one aspect of collaboration and coordination that is lacking in health care planning. Often numerous disciplines work together to formulate a comprehensive approach without consulting with clients regarding their ideas or preferences. The nurse is in a vital position to include consumers in their care, either directly or indirectly, by communicating their thoughts to the health team.

Research

Practicing nurses rarely consider themselves researchers, yet they are the individuals most likely to observe human responses to health and illness. Unfortunately few nurses systematically record or analyze such observations. For example, pediatric nurses devise innovative methods to encourage children to comply with treatments. Only if these interventions are shared with other nurses, especially through publications, can a body of knowledge on nursing practice develop.

Research also implies a questioning of *why* something is effective and *if* there is a better approach. Evaluation is essential to the nursing process and research is one of the best evaluators. Therefore nurses need to be more involved in research and in applying research findings to their practice. Throughout the text research relevant to nursing of children and families is incorporated as appropriate and is also highlighted in the Questions and Controversies section. Research findings are presented to encourage nurses to base their practice on theoretical foundations, not intuition, and additional questions may be proposed in the hope of stimulating research in a particular area.

Health Care Planning

Up to this point the nurse's role has been viewed through the nucleus of a family. However, the nursing role is far more extensive and includes the community or society as a whole. Traditionally nurses have been involved in public health care, on either a distributive or an episodic basis. Rarely, however, have nurses been involved in health care planning, especially on a political or legislative level. Their role must also involve the decision-making body of government. Nursing, as the largest health profession, needs to have a voice, especially as family/consumer advocate. This does not mean that the nurse must hold public office. Rather it suggests knowledge and awareness of community needs, interest in government formulation of bills, support of politicians to ensure passage (or rejection) of significant legislation, and active involvement in groups dedicated to the welfare of children, such as professional nursing societies, Parent-Teacher Organizations, parent support groups, religious organizations, and voluntary organizations.

Health care planning involves not only providing new services but also promoting the highest quality of existing ones. Nursing needs to ensure the excellence of its own profession through each individual member, who practices according to the Code of Ethics and Standards of Practice. Pediatric nurses are obligated to follow the Standards of Maternal and Child Health Nursing (see box, p. 20). They should also be involved in making certain their colleagues implement the standards, through education, role modeling, and supervision.

Throughout the text the highest standards of nursing practice are continually reflected in the emphasis on thorough assessment, focus on scientific rationale as the basis for care, summary of nursing care goals and responsibilities, and comprehensive discussion of growth and development. Family-centered principles are continually evident in the consideration of dynamics affecting the child, parents, siblings, and extended members. The nurse is viewed as a vital component of the health care delivery system. Although nursing functions are clearly outlined, nursing responsibilities must be equally emphasized. It is hoped that the roles briefly described here will be studied, practiced, and implemented to the ultimate benefit of all children.

Future Trends

The present shift in focus from treatment of disease to promotion of health is likely to further expand nurses' roles in ambulatory care, with prevention and health teaching receiving a major emphasis. As prospective payment becomes a certainty in pediatric care, the need for home care and community health services will necessitate that nurses become more independent and highly skilled beyond the traditional care settings. Both of these trends are illustrated throughout the book with increased emphasis on prevention through anticipatory guidance, child health and family assessment, and discharge planning and home care.

Technologic advances will also influence pediatric nurses' roles. Increasing technical skills related to patient care, as well as the demand for computer knowledge in the work setting, are inevitable future trends. As more positions are created in the health care system that do not require a nursing background, such as "patient care educator," nurses will be required to continually update their knowl-

AMERICAN NURSES' ASSOCIATION STANDARDS OF MATERNAL-CHILD HEALTH NURSING PRACTICE

Standard I
Maternal and child health nursing practice is characterized by the continual questioning of the assumptions upon which practice is based, retaining those which are valid and searching for and using new knowledge.

Standard II
Maternal and child health nursing practice is based upon knowledge of the biophysical and psychosocial development of individuals from conception through the child-rearing phase of development and upon knowledge of the basic needs for optimum development.

Standard III
The collection of data about the health status of the client/patient is systematic and continuous. The data are accessible, communicated and recorded.

Standard IV
Nursing diagnoses are derived from data about the health status of the patient.

Standard V
Maternal and child health nursing practice recognizes deviations from expected patterns of physiologic activity and anatomic and psychosocial development.

Standard VI
The plan of nursing care includes goals derived from the nursing diagnoses.

Standard VII
The plan of nursing care includes priorities and the prescribed nursing approaches or measures to achieve the goals derived from the nursing diagnoses.

Standard VIII
Nursing actions provide for client/patient participation in health promotion, maintenance and restoration.

Standard IX
Maternal and child health nursing practice provides for the use and coordination of all services that assist individuals to prepare for responsible sex roles.

Standard X
Nursing actions assist the client/patient to maximize his health capabilities.

Standard XI
The client's/patient's progress or lack of progress toward goal achievement is determined by the client/patient and the nurse.

Standard XII
The client's/patient's progress or lack of progress toward goal achievement directs reassessment, reordering of priorities, new goal setting and revision of the plan of nursing care.

Standard XIII
Maternal and child health nursing practice evidences active participation with others in evaluating the availability, accessibility and acceptability of services for parents and children and cooperating and/or taking leadership in extending and developing needed services in the community.

From American Nurses' Association, *Standards of Maternal-Child Health Nursing Practice,* American Nurses' Association, Kansas City, 1973.

edge and prove their unique contribution. While such demands may appear overwhelming, they also provide challenge and creativity.

PROCESS OF NURSING CHILDREN AND FAMILIES

Planning and implementing nursing care to meet the needs of infants and children require a systematic approach to decision making. The problem-solving process consists of five operational phases: assessment, nursing diagnosis, plan formulation, implementation, and evaluation. It involves both cognitive and operational skills. How successfully the process is carried out depends on such factors as the nurse's level of competence, the formation of the nurse-child-family relationship, and the goals and capabilities of the family members.

Assessment

Assessment is a continuous process that is operative at all phases of problem solving and is the foundation for decision making. Derived through multiple nursing skills, it consists of the purposeful collection, classification, and analysis of

data from a variety of sources. To ensure an accurate and comprehensive assessment, the nurse must consider information about the patient's biophysical, psychologic, sociocultural, and spiritual background.

Nursing Diagnosis

Analysis and synthesis of the collected data result in problem identification. In order to solve a problem it is essential to acknowledge that it exists and to describe its nature. The problem may involve an unmet need, an unrealized expectation, an interrupted process, or a community crisis. In some instances no actual problem is identified but present health practices or coping mechanisms may need to be maintained. Potential problems may be recognized because of the identified risk, such as an infection or a skin problem. *Nursing diagnoses* are used to describe these problems or concerns.

One currently accepted definition states that a nursing diagnosis is ''a clinical judgment about an individual, family, or community derived through the deliberate, systematic process of data collection and analysis which provides for the prescription of definitive therapy for which the nurse is

NURSING DIAGNOSES ACCORDING TO FUNCTIONAL HEALTH PATTERNS*

Health perception–health management pattern (HP-HMP)
Growth and development, altered (specify)
Health maintenance, alteration in
Infection, potential for
Injury: potential for
    A. Poisoning, potential for
    B. Suffocation, potential for
    C. Trauma, potential for
Noncompliance (specify)

Nutritional-metabolic attern (N-MP)
Body temperature, alteration in: potential
Fluid volume, alteration in: excess
Fluid volume deficit, actual
    1. Failure of regulatory mechanism
    2. Active loss
Fluid volume deficit, potential
Growth and development, altered (specify)
Hyperthermia
Hypothermia
Thermoregulation, ineffective
Nutrition, alteration in: less than body requirements
Nutrition, alteration in: more than body requirements
Nutrition, alteration in: potential for more than body
    requirements
Oral mucous membranes, alteration in
Swallowing, impaired
Skin integrity, impairment of: actual
Skin integrity, impairment of: potential
Tissue integrity, impaired

Elimination pattern (EP)
Bowel elimination, alteration in: constipation
Bowel elimination, alteration in: diarrhea
Bowel elimination, alteration in: incontinence
Growth and development, altered (specify)
Incontinence, functional
Incontinence, reflex
Incontinence, stress
Incontinence, total
Incontinence, urge
Urinary elimination, alteration in patterns
Urinary retention

Activity-exercise pattern (A-EP)
Activity intolerance
Activity intolerance, potential
Airway clearance, ineffective
Breathing pattern, ineffective
Cardiac output, alteration in: decreased
Diversional activity, deficit
Gas exchange, impaired
Growth and development, altered (specify)
Home maintenance management, impaired
Mobility, impaired physical (level 0 to 4)†
Self-care deficit: feeding, bathing/hygiene,
    dressing/grooming, toileting
    A. Self-feeding deficit (level 0 to 4)†
    B. Self-bathing deficit (level 0 to 4)†
    C. Self-dressing/grooming deficit (level 0 to 4)†
    D. Self-toileting deficit (level 0 to 4)†

Tissue perfusion, alteration in: cerebral,
    cardiopulmonary, renal, gastrointestinal, peripheral

Sleep-rest pattern (SRP)
Growth and development, altered (specify)
Sleep pattern disturbance

Cognitive-perceptual pattern (CPP)
Comfort, alteration in: chronic pain
Comfort, alteration in: pain
Growth and development, altered (specify)
Knowledge deficit (specify)
Neglect, unilateral
Sensory-perceptual alteration: visual, auditory,
    kinesthetic, gustatory, tactile, olfactory
Thought processes, alteration in

Self-perception–self-concept pattern (SP-SCP)
Anxiety
Fear
Growth and development, altered (specify)
Hopelessness
Powerlessness
Self-concept, disturbance in: body image, self-esteem,
    role performance, personal identity

Role-relationship pattern (RRP)
Communication, impaired: verbal
Family process, alteration in
Grieving, anticipatory
Grieving, dysfunctional
Growth and development, altered (specify)
Parenting, alteration in: actual or potential
Social interaction, impaired
Social isolation
Violence, potential for: self-directed or directed at
    others

Sexuality-reproductive pattern (SxRP)
Growth and development, altered (specify)
Rape trauma syndrome
Sexual dysfunction
Sexuality patterns, altered

Coping-stress tolerance pattern (CSTP)
Adjustment, impaired
Coping, family: potential for growth
Coping, ineffective family: compromised
Coping, ineffective family: disabling
Coping, ineffective individual
Growth and development, altered (specify)
Post trauma response

Value-belief pattern (VBP)
Growth and development, altered (specify)
Spiritual distress (distress of the human spirit)

*Nursing diagnoses include those approved by the North American Diagnosis Association in April 1986. Functional Health Patterns from
Gordon (1982). Abbreviations shown here are used to designate Functional Health Patterns in Nursing Care Summaries.
†Suggested code for functional level classification:
    0 Completely independent
    1 Requires use of equipment or device
    2 Requires help from another person for assistance, super-
      vision, or teaching
    3 Requires help from another person and equipment or
      device
    4 Is dependent, does not participate in activity

accountable'' (Shoemaker, 1984). Currently accepted nursing diagnoses are listed in the boxed material according to 11 functional health patterns (Gordon, 1985). The functional health patterns serve as a framework for organizing a nursing assessment and standardizing data collection. Additional research is needed to broaden the list, especially for specialty areas such as pediatrics. However, these nursing diagnoses are the beginning of a scientific basis for nursing practice.

Throughout the text the nursing care summaries incorporate nursing diagnoses that relate to the specific condition or disorder. They are identified by the symbol shown in the box title on p. 21 and listed in order of the functional health patterns, which are identified by an appropriate abbreviation. Since nursing diagnoses should only prescribe interventions that the nurse can independently perform, a separate section for nursing interventions related to medical management is included.

Plan Formulation

Plan formulation is the decision-making phase of the process. With a specific nursing diagnosis identified, the nurse designs a plan of action to meet a goal (objective or expected outcome). A design for action involves the selection of a plan based on scientific principles derived from a variety of disciplines. Interventions are chosen that are most likely to achieve the desired consequence with a minimum of risk to the persons involved.

Implementation

The phase of implementation begins when the nurse puts the selected intervention into action and accumulates feedback regarding its effects. The feedback returns in the form of observation and communication and provides a data base on which to evaluate the outcome of the nursing intervention. Throughout the implementation stage, the patient's physical safety as well as psychologic comfort are the main concerns.

Evaluation

Evaluation is the last step in the decision-making process. The nurse gathers, sorts, and analyzes data to determine if (1) the goal has been met, (2) the plan requires modification, or (3) another alternative should be considered. This evaluation either completes the nursing process or serves as the basis for selection of other alternatives for intervention in solving the specific problem.

Primary Nursing

Inherent in the decision-making process is accountability. Nurses are responsible for their actions, in both the legal and the ethical senses. Part of the trend in nursing practice is a deeper commitment to accountability. One of the outgrowths of this has been the movement toward *primary nursing*. Primary nursing involves 24-hour responsibility and accountability by one nurse for the care of a small group of patients. The primary nurse becomes the bedside

nurse, with few if any duties delegated to other staff. If responsibilities are shared, it is usually with an associate primary nurse who maintains continuity of care when the primary nurse is not on duty.

One of the traditional problems with primary nursing is providing consistency in scheduling the same nurse and associate. An approach that minimizes this difficulty is to designate one primary nurse and as many associates as are needed to ensure that the same group of nurses care for the child. This *primary core team* necessitates that at least one nurse be assigned to the patient for each shift and that additional nurses be assigned for these individuals' days off. By identifying the core team in advance for a specific period, all the nurses working with the child can plan care jointly, with the primary nurse maintaining overall responsibility.

The philosophy of primary care is supported throughout the discussion of nursing of children and families. In some instances the one-to-one relationship between child and nurse is emphasized because of its therapeutic benefit, such as in nonorganic failure to thrive. However, primary nursing is universally a supportive intervention in pediatric nursing because it provides a consistent caregiver for the child and focuses on the family unit as an integral component in the planning and implementation of care.

CONCEPT SUMMARIES

- Health, as defined by WHO, is "a state of complete physical, mental, and social well-being and not merely the absence of disease."

- Although the infant mortality rate in the United States is at an all-time low, the United States lags significantly behind other well-developed countries, such as Finland, Japan, and Canada.

- Birth weight is the leading determinant of neonatal death in developed countries.

- Injuries are the leading cause of death in children over age 1 year.

- Childhood morbidity, although difficult to define, encompasses acute illness, chronic disease, and disability.

- Eighty percent of childhood illnesses are attributable to infections, with respiratory infections occurring two to three times as often as all other illnesses combined.

- The "new morbidity," or "pediatric social illness," refers to behavioral, social, and educational problems that can significantly alter a child's health.

- Children's developmental stage and their environment are important determinants in the prevalence of injuries at a given age and thus help to direct preventive measures.

- Two strategies for injury prevention in children are (1) *passive*, which provides automatic protection by product and environmental design; and (2) *active*, which persuades people to change their behaviors for increased self-protection.

- The pediatric nurse's roles include family advocacy, illness prevention/health promotion, health teaching, support/counseling, therapeutic role, coordination/collaboration, research, and health care planning.

- With the shift in focus from treatment of disease to promotion of health, nurses' roles may expand in ambulatory care, with emphasis on prevention and health teaching.

- The process of nursing children and families includes accurate and comprehensive *assessment*, analysis and synthesis of assessment data to arrive at a *nursing diagnosis*, *plan formulation*, *implementation* of the plan, and *evaluation* of interventions.

- Primary nursing involves care and accountability by one nurse for a small patient population.

REFERENCES

Adams, D.: Children's response to a belt restraint program, Pediatr. Nurs. **8**(1):28-30, 1982.

Arneson, S., and others: Factors affecting parental use of child automobile safety restraints, Child. Health Care **13**(4):181-186, 1985.

Collins, J.: Persons injured and disability days due to injuries, United States, 1980-1981, Vital and Health Statistics, Series 10, No. 149, DHHS Pub. No. (PHS) 85-1577, National Center for Health Statistics, Public Health Service, Washington, DC, March 1985.

Committee on Trauma Research, Commission on Life Sciences, National Research Council and the Institute of Medicine: Injury in America: a continuing public health problem, Washington, DC, 1985, National Academy Press.

Cone, T.E., Jr.: Highlights of two centuries of American pediatrics, 1776-1976, Am. J. Dis. Child. **130**:762-775, July 1976.

Del Campo, E., and Josephson, D.: Accommodating the severely retarded child in our schools, Am. J. Maternal Child Nurs. **3**:34-37, 1978.

Goldberg, I.R., and others: Mental health problems among children seen in pediatric practice: prevalence and management, Pediatrics **73**(3):278-292, 1984.

Gordon, M.: Manual of nursing diagnosis, New York, 1985, McGraw-Hill Book Co.

Green, M., and Haggerty, R.: Episodic problems. In Green, M., and Haggerty, R., editors: Ambulatory pediatrics III, Philadelphia, 1984, W.B. Saunders Co.

Greensher, J.: Prevention of childhood injuries, Pediatrics (suppl.) **74**(5):970-975, 1984.

Guyer, B., and Gallagher, S.S.: An approach to the epidemiology of childhood injuries, Pediatr. Clin. North Am. **32**(1):5-15, 1985.

Guyer, B., Talbot, A.M., and Pless, I.B.: Pedestrian injuries to children and youth, Pediatr. Clin. North Am. **32**(1):163-174, 1985.

Jason, J., Gilliland, J.C., and Tyler, C.W., Jr.: Homicide as a cause of pediatric mortality in the United States, Pediatrics **72**(2):191-197, 1983.

Kalter, H., and Warkany, J.: Congenital malformations: etiologic factors and their role in prevention, part I, N. Engl. J. Med. **308**:424-431, Feb. 1983; part II, **308**:491-497, March 1983.

Leopold, J.: Abraham Jacobi. In Veeder, B.S., editor: Pediatric profiles, St. Louis, 1957, The C.V. Mosby Co.

McCarthy, E., and Kozak, L.J.: Hospital use by children: United States, 1983, DHHS Pub. No. (PHS) 85-1250, 1985.

Miller, R., and others: Pediatric counseling and subsequent use of smoke detectors, Am. J. Public Health **72**:392-393, 1982.

Nader, P., and others: The new morbidity: use of school and community health care resources for behavioral, educational and social-family problems, Pediatrics **67**(1):53-60, 1981.

National Center for Health Statistics, P.M. Golden: Charting the nation's health: trends since 1960, DHHS Pub. No. (PHS) 85-1251, 1984.

National Transportation Safety Board: Safety study: child passenger protection against death, disability, and disfigurement in motor vehicle accidents, Washington, DC, 1983, U.S. Government Printing Office.

Nursing: a social policy statement, Kansas City, MO, 1980, American Nurses' Association.

Pless, I.: Current morbidity and mortality among the young. In Hoekelman, R.A., and others: Principles of pediatrics: health care of the young, New York, 1978, McGraw-Hill Book Co.

Pless, I., and Stulginskas, J.: Accidents and violence as a cause of morbidity and mortality in childhood, Adv. Pediatr. **29**:471-495, 1982.

Righi, F., and Krozy, R.: The child in the car: what every nurse should know about safety, Am. J. Nurs. **83**(10):1421-1424, 1983.

Rivara, F.: Fatal and nonfatal farm injuries to children and adolescents in the United States, Pediatrics **76**(4):567-573, 1985a.

Rivara, F.: Traumatic deaths of children in the United States: currently available prevention strategies, Pediatrics **75**(3):456-462, 1985b.

Satir, V., and others: Helping families to change, New York, 1975, Jason Aronson, Inc.

Sayre, J.W., and Sayre, R.F.: American children and the "children of nature," Am. J. Dis. Child **130**:716-723, July 1976.

Schmidt, W.M.: Health and welfare of colonial American children, Am. J. Dis. Child. **130**:694-701, July 1976.

Scott, R., and Winston, M.: The health and welfare of the black family in the United States, Am. J. Dis. Child **130**:704-707, July 1976.

Shoemaker, J.: Essential features of nursing diagnoses. In Kim, M.J., McFarland, G., and McLane, A.: Classification of nursing diagnoses: proceedings of the Fifth National Conference, St. Louis, 1984, The C.V. Mosby Co.

Spiegel, C., and Lindaman, F.: Children can't fly: a program to prevent childhood morbidity and mortality from window falls, Am. J. Public Health **67**(12):1143-1147, 1977.

Starfield, B.: Psychosocial and psychosomatic diagnoses in primary care of children, Pediatrics **66**(2):159-163, 1980.

Surgeon General's Report on Health Promotion and Disease Prevention: Healthy people, DHEW Pub. No. (PHS) 79-55071, 1979.

U.S. House of Representatives, Select Committee on Children, Youth, and Families: Children, youth, and families: 1983, a year-end report, Washington, DC, 1984, U.S. Government Printing Office.

U.S. House of Representatives, Select Committee on Children, Youth, and Families: Federal programs affecting children, Washington, DC, 1984, U.S. Government Printing Office.

Walton, W.: An evaluation of The Poison Prevention Packaging Act, Pediatrics **69**(3):363-370, 1982.

Wegman, M.E.: Annual summary of vital statistics—1984, Pediatrics **76**(6):861-871, 1985.

Williams, J.K.: The pediatric nurse in the past hundred years, Clin. Proc. Child. Hosp., Jan. 1971, pp. 18-23.

BIBLIOGRAPHY

Mortality and Morbidity

Better health for our children: a national strategy, The Report of the Select Panel for the Promotion of Child Health, vol. I, Major findings and recommendations, DHHS Pub. No. (PHS) 79-55071, 1981.

Bloom, B.: Changing infant mortality: the need to spend more while getting less, Pediatrics **73**(6):862-866, 1984.

Graham, G.: Poverty, hunger, malnutrition, prematurity, and infant mortality in the United States, Pediatrics **75**(1):117-125, 1985.

McArney, E.: Adolescent pregnancy and childbearing: new data, new challenges, Pediatrics **75**(5):973-975, 1985.

McCune, Y.D., Richardson, M.M., and Powell, J.A.: Psychosocial health issues in pediatric practices, parents' knowledge and concerns, Pediatrics **74**(2):183-190, 1984.

Miller, C.: The health of children, a crisis of ethics, Pediatrics **73**(4):550-558, 1984.

National Center for Health Statistics: Health, United States, 1984, DHHS Pub. No. (PHS) 85-1232, 1984.

Newberger, E.H., and others: Pediatric social illness: toward an etiologic classification, Pediatrics **60:**178, Aug. 1977.

Shapiro, S., and others: Changes in infant morbidity associated with decreases in neonatal mortality, Pediatrics **72**(3):408-415, 1983.

Withrow, C., and Fleming, J.W.: Pediatric social illness: a challenge to nurses, Issues Compr. Pediatr. Nurs. **6:**261-275, 1983.

Injuries

American Academy of Pediatrics, Committee on Research, Committee on Accident and Poison Prevention: Reducing the toll of injuries in childhood requires support for a focused research effort, Pediatrics **72**(5):736-737, 1983.

Bass, J.L., Gallagher, S.S., and Mehta, K.A.: Injuries to adolescents and young adults, Pediatr. Clin. North Am. **32**(1):31-39, 1985.

Bergman, A.: Use of education in preventing injuries, Pediatr. Clin. North Am. **29**(2):331-338, 1982.

Boyce, W., and others: Epidemiology of injuries in a large, urban school district, Pediatrics **74**(3):342-349, 1984.

Cogbill, T., Busch, H., and Stiers, G.: Farm accidents in children, Pediatrics **76**(4):562-566, 1985.

Friedman, I.M.: Alcohol and unnatural deaths in San Francisco youths, Pediatrics **76**(2):191-193, 1985.

Garrettson, L.K., and Gallagher, S.S.: Falls in children and youth, Pediatr. Clin. North Am. **32**(1):153-162, 1985.

Gorman, R., and others: A successful city-wide smoke detector giveaway program, Pediatrics **75**(1):14-18, 1985.

Hingson, R., Merrigan, D., and Heeren, T.: Effects of Massachusetts raising its legal drinking age from 18 to 20 on deaths from teenage homicide, suicide, and nontraffic accidents, Pediatr. Clin. North Am. **32**(1):221-233, 1985.

Holroyd, H.J.: Why accidents happen, Pediatr. Ann. **12**(10):722-724, 1983.

Krassner, L.: TIPP usage, Pediatrics (suppl.) **74**(5):976-980, 1984.

McLoughlin, E., and Crawford, J.D.: Burns, Pediatr. Clin. North Am. **32**(1):61-75, 1985.

Rivara, F.: Epidemiology of childhood injuries, Am. J. Dis. Child. **136:**399-405, May 1982.

Rivara, F., and Barber, M.: Demographic analysis of childhood pedestrian injuries, Pediatrics **76**(3):375-381, 1985.

Robertson, L.S.: Motor vehicles, Pediatr. Clin. North Am. **32**(1):87-94, 1985.

Spyker, D.A.: Submersion injury: epidemiology, prevention, and management, Pediatr. Clin. North Am. **32**(1):113-125, 1985.

Steele, P., and Sypker, D.: Poisonings, Pediatr. Clin. North Am. **32**(1):77-86, 1985.

Temple, A.R.: Poison prevention education, Pediatrics (suppl.) **74**(5):964-969, 1984.

Widome, M.D.: Occasional but serious accidents, Pediatr. Ann. **12**(10):761-768, 1983.

Zuckerman, B.S., and Duby, J.C.: Development approach to injury prevention, Pediatr. Clin. North Am. **32**(1):17-29, 1985.

Evolution of Child Health Care

Bloch, H.: Jewish children in colonial times, Am. J. Dis. Child. **130:**711-713, July 1976.

Brodie, B.: Children: a glance at the past, Am. J. Maternal Child Nurs. **7**(4):219-225, 1982.

Coleman, J.R., and Smith, D.S.: DRGs: opportunity or crisis? Pediatr. Nurs. **10**(5):321-323, 1984.

Cone, T.E., Jr.: History of American pediatrics, Boston, 1980, Little, Brown & Co.

Donahue, M.P.: Nursing: the finest art, an illustrated history, St. Louis, 1985, The C.V. Mosby Co.

DRGs and pediatrics, ACCH News **7**(5):1, 1985.

Fleming, J.: Maternal-child nursing in the decade ahead, Am. J. Maternal Child Nurs. **10**(6):369-376, 1985.

Holaday, B.: Changing views of infant care 1914-1980, Pediatr. Nurs. **7**(1):21-25, 1981.

Mitchell, K., and Hargin, R.: Our children: an economic priority, Pediatr. Nurs. **11**(2):82, 1985.

Noyes, E.J.: Children: a priority? Nurs. Econ. **3:**136-139, May/June 1985.

Pokras, R.: Diagnosis-related groups using data from the National Hospital Discharge Survey: United States, DHHS 1981, Pub. No. (PHS) 84-1250, 1984.

Radbill, S.X.: Reared in adversity: institutional care of children in the 18th century, Am. J. Dis. Child. **130:**751-761, July 1976.

Rogers, D., and others: Some observations on pediatrics: its past, present, and future, Pediatrics (suppl.) **67**(5):776-784, 1981.

Schmidt, B.J.: Current outlook for children around the world, Pediatrics **74**(2):294-295, 1984.

Shaffer, F.A.: DRGs: history and overview, Nurs. & Health Care **4**(7):388-396, 1983.

Smith, C.E.: DRGs: making them work for you, Nursing 85 **15**(1):34-41, 1985.

Sonstegard, L.: Health care costs: every nurse's problem, Am. J. Maternal Child Nurs. **10**(2):87-90, 1985.

Pediatric Nursing

American Academy of Pediatrics, Committee on School Health: School nurse practitioner, Pediatrics **65**(3):665-666, 1980.

Andreoli, K.G., and Guillory, M.M.: Arenas for practicing health promotion, Family & Community Health **5**(4):28-40, 1983.

Arbeiter, J.S.: The big shift to home health nursing, RN **47**(11):38-45, 1984.

Boehm, S.: Research as a basis for changing nursing practice, Topics Clin. Nurs. **7**(2):39-44, 1985.

Brown, B., and Chard, M.: Nurse practitioners: a review of the literature, 1965-1979, American Nursing Association Pub. **I-VIII:**1-24, 1980.

Chaisson, G.M.: Patient education: whose responsibility is it and who should be doing it? Nurs. Admin. Q. **4:**1-11, 1980.

Craft, M., and Pflederer, D.: Practice setting and the successful pediatric clinical specialist, Pediatr. Nurs. **8**(3):187-189, 1982.

Dailey, C.P.: Teaching parents and children preventive health behaviors, Fam. Commun. Health **7**(4):34-43, 1985.

Fond, K.: Child advocacy: ideas for action, Pediatr. Nurs. **5:**18-19, 1979.

Greensher, J.: How anticipatory guidance can improve control of childhood "accidents," Pediatr. Consult **3**(2):1-8, 1984.

Huckabay, L.M.: A strategy for patient teaching, Nurs. Admin. Q. **4:**47-54, 1980.

Hymovitch, D.: How children, mothers, and nurses view primary and team nursing, Am. J. Nurs. **80**(11):2041-2045, 1980.

Kohnke, M.F.: The nurse as advocate, Am. J. Nurs. **80**(11):2038-2040, 1980.

Laffrey, S.: Health promotion: relevance for nursing, Topics Clin. Nurs. **7**(2):29-38, 1985.

Lancaster, W., McIlwain, T., and Lancaster, J.: Health marketing: implications for health promotion, Fam. Comm. Health **5**(4):41-51, 1983.

MacQueen, J.C.: The challenge of the PNP/A movement, Pediatr. Nurs. **5**(4):31-35, 1979.

Marram, G., Barrett, M., and Bevis, E.: Primary nursing: a model for individualized care, ed. 2, St. Louis, 1979, The C.V. Mosby Co.

Meister, S.: Building bridges between practice and health policy, Am. J. Maternal Child Nurs. **10**(3):155-157, 1985.

Mullen, P.D.: Promoting child health: channels of socialization, Fam. Comm. Health **5**(4):52-68, 1983.

Murphy, M.A., Gitterman, B.A., and Silver, H.K.: Hospital nurse practitioners: a trial approach, Pediatr. Nurs. **11**(4): 269-273, 1985.

Oberst, M.: Integrating research and clinical practice roles, Topics Clin. Nurs. **7**(2):45-53, 1985.

Rogers, F.B.: A model for parent education, Image **13:**86-88, Oct. 1981.

Storch, J.L.: Consumer rights and health care, Nurs. Admin. Q. **4:**107-115, 1980.

Tartaglia, M.: Nursing diagnosis: keystone of your care plan, Nursing 85 **15**(3):34-37, 1985.

William, M.K.: An historical perspective: the pediatric nurse associate, Pediatr. Nurs. **5**(2):32-33, 1979.

Chapter 2

Social, Cultural, and Religious Influences on Child Health Promotion

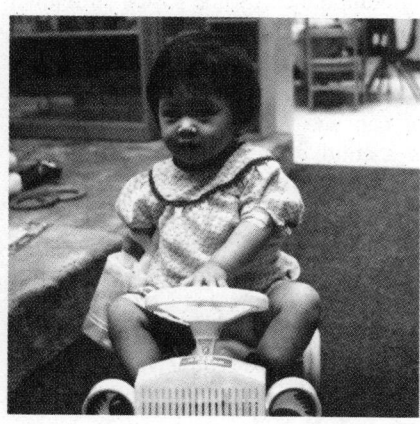

Culture
  Social roles
    Primary group influence
    Secondary group influence
    Guilt and shame orientation
  Subcultural influences
    Ethnicity
    Social class
    Poverty
    Affluence
    Occupation
    Religion
    Schools
    Peer cultures
    Biculture
  The child and family in America
    Minority-group membership
  Cultural shock

Cultural Influences on Health Care
  Susceptibility to health problems
    Hereditary factors
    Socioeconomic factors
  Customs and folkways
    *Relationships with health care
      providers*
    Food customs
  Health beliefs and practices
    Health beliefs
    Health practices
    *Folklore related to prenatal
      influences*
  Religious beliefs
  Attitude of the nurse

The future of any society depends on its children. If it is to survive, the society must make provision for their care, nurture, and socialization. Cultural survival depends on whether the customs and values of the culture are transmitted from one generation to the next through the medium of the family. The culture into which children are born outlines the roles of their parents, structures their relationships with other people, and determines much of the behavior they acquire. A holistic view of any child requires that nurses develop some understanding of the ways that culture contributes to the development of social and emotional relationships and influences childrearing practices and attitudes toward health. This includes an awareness of the nurse's own cultural frame of reference and a concerted effort to recognize and appreciate the views and beliefs of the health care recipients.

Culture

Culture is the "acquired knowledge people use to interpret experience and generate behavior" (Spradley, 1981) and differs from both race and ethnicity. *Race* is defined as "a division of mankind possessing traits that are transmissible by descent and sufficient to characterize it as a distinct human type" (Webster's, 1973) and refers to the three recognized types: caucasoid, negroid, and mongoloid. *Ethnicity* is the affiliation of a set of persons who share a unique cultural, social, and linguistic heritage (Werner, 1979). *Socialization* is the process by which children acquire the beliefs, values, and behaviors considered desirable or appropriate by the culture.

A culture is composed of individuals who share a set of values, beliefs, practices, and information that is learned, integrative, social, and satisfying. Culture is not a surface veneer that covers a basic outlook shared by all human beings but an ingrained orientation to life that serves as a frame of reference for individual perception and judgment. People from one culture differ from those in other cultures in the ways they think, solve problems, perceive, and structure the world. Culture is, essentially, the way of life of a group of people that incorporates experiences of the past, influences thought and action in the present, and transmits these traditions to future group members. However, to survive in an ever-changing world, cultures undergo constant change, consciously and unconsciously, by assuming new elements and abandoning old ones, making modifications to meet the needs of the group, and finding new ways to solve life's problems.

The observable components of a culture, such as material objects (dress, art, utensils, and other artifacts) and actions, are sometimes termed the *material, overt,* or *manifest culture; nonmaterial covert culture* refers to those aspects that cannot be observed directly, such as the ideas, beliefs, customs, and feelings of the culture. Related to the large culture are many *subcultures,* each with an identity of its own (Leininger, 1978).

The culture in which children are reared determines the type of food they will eat, the language they will speak, the ideals of behavior they will follow, and the way they will conduct themselves in social roles. To be acceptable members of the culture, children must learn how the culture expects them to behave toward others in the group. In turn, they learn how they can expect others to behave toward them.

Cultures and subcultures contribute to the uniqueness of child members in such a subtle way and at such an early age that the child grows up to feel that his beliefs, attitudes, values, and practices are the "correct" or "normal" ones; those of other cultures may be viewed as "deviant" or "wrong." A set of values learned in childhood is apt to characterize children's attitudes and behavior for life, guiding their long-range strivings and monitoring their short-range, impulsive inclinations. Thus every ongoing society socializes each succeeding generation to its cultural heritage.

The manner and sequence of the growth and development phenomenon are universal and fundamental features of all children; however, the variations in behavioral responses that children display to similar events are believed to be determined by cultures. Inborn temperament and modes of behavior that prompt children to behave in their own preferred and highly individual manner may be in harmony or in conflict with the culture. Such forces as heredity and maturation impose limits on the influence that parents and other social groups may bring to bear.

The culture fosters and reinforces those behaviors deemed desirable and appropriate; it attempts to depress or extinguish those at conflict with cultural norms. Some cultures encourage aggressive behaviors in their children; others favor amiability and compliance. Some foster individual resourcefulness and competition; others emphasize cooperation and submission to group interest. The child from a culture that values cooperation will not respond to a challenge such as, "I'll bet you can eat your breakfast faster than Johnny can," whereas a child from a culture that emphasizes individual achievement will be stimulated by the challenge.

Cultures may also differ in whether status in the group is based on age or on skill. Even children's play and their types of games are culturally determined. In some cultures children play in groups composed of members of the same sex; in others they play in mixed-sex groups. In some cultures team games predominate; in others most play is limited to individual games.

Standards and norms vary from culture to culture and location to location; a practice that is accepted in one area may meet with disapproval or create tension in another. The extent to which cultures tolerate divergence from the established norm varies among cultures and subcultural groups. Although conformity provides a degree of security, it is a decided deterrent to change.

SOCIAL ROLES

Much of children's self-concept is derived from their ideas about their social roles. Roles are cultural creations; therefore, the culture prescribes patterns of behavior for persons in a variety of social positions. All persons who hold similar social positions have the obligation to behave in a particular manner. A role prohibits some behaviors and allows for others. Because it delineates and clarifies roles, the culture is a significant influence on the development of children's self-concept, that is, the attitudes and beliefs they have about themselves.

A social group consists of a system of roles carried out in both primary and secondary groups. A *primary group* is characterized by intimate, continued face-to-face contact, mutual support of the members, and the ability to order or constrain a considerable proportion of individual members' behavior. Two such groups are the family and the peer group, both of which exert a great deal of influence on the child. *Secondary groups* are groups that have limited, intermittent contact and in which there is generally less concern for members' behavior. These groups offer little in terms of support or pressure toward conformity except in rigidly limited areas. Examples of secondary groups are professional associations and church organizations (also considered in relation to subgroups).

A concept of social role also depends largely on whether a child is reared in a primary- or secondary-group community. Children are subjected to perceptively different forms of parental training in these two types of environments.

Primary Group Influence

In a primary-group community (for example, some contemporary rural, religious, or ethnic communities), all members know each other, most belong to the same subgroups, and all are concerned about each member's behavior. There is a high degree of material and psychologic support among the community members, and since there is one traditional set of values that the entire group agrees on and supports, there is little conflict of values. In a stable community where the members remain within comparatively defined limits and relatives are likely to live close together, young members have ample opportunity to observe and absorb the practices and customs of the culture. Any member of the community feels justified in evaluating and censuring the conduct of another member.

Children reared in a primary-group community learn that there is only one acceptable way to respond to any given situation. The entire group agrees, and any tendency to deviate is met with collective disapproval. It is the parents' duty to see that the children learn and adhere to social roles and modes of behavior defined and strengthened by the views of the community.

Secondary Group Influence

The childrearing orientation in a secondary-group environment, such as urban communities, differs considerably from that of a primary-group community. An urban community is dynamic and rapidly changing. Many of the traditional behaviors and values do not meet the needs of changing society. Consequently parents are often uncertain about what to teach their children. They may wish to rear their children with values consistent with their own, but the differences in experience between the generations are too great. As a result, they often grant their children autonomy in some areas of decision making early in the developmental process, and other secondary groups assume a greater influence. The children are exposed to an assortment of social groups with diverse sets of values and expectations. None of the groups is highly dominant in its influence; therefore the children are exposed to an eclectic set of values, some in agreement and some at conflict with the others. From these they must ultimately select those that they determine to be best for them and adopt them to form a consistent set of roles and behaviors to be incorporated into the self-concept.

Guilt and Shame Orientation

Conditioning children to feel either guilt or shame for misdeeds is used by a culture to control social behavior—to internalize the norms and expectations of others. Some cultural groups value a well-developed conscience (superego) and condition their children to feel guilt following wrongdoing. The offender wants to purge himself and gets an uncomfortable physical feeling. Since guilt is based within the individual, successful conditioning produces self-regulated persons who punish themselves without their being caught in the act of wrongdoing.

In many cultural groups guilt is lacking and social controls are based on the use of shame. The offender does not want anyone to see him when he has been guilty of a wrongful deed. Sometimes children in these groups learn that anything is acceptable as long as one is not caught; the shame results when the forbidden act is found out by others.

Although both techniques are used by members of both primary- and secondary-group communities, shame is apt to be more successful in a primary-group community because most behaviors are quite public. In secondary-group communities it is less effective; persons are not as apt to be caught and, if caught, can join a group that is unaware of the misdeed. Guilt probably has a greater influence on behavior in urban communities and, although it is characteristic of most American cultures, many authorities believe that the trend in urban America is shifting away from a guilt orientation. Rapid changes in the American culture leave parents unsure of their own values; therefore much of their function is abandoned to the school and peers. Peers are notorious for the use of shame as a disciplinary technique.

SUBCULTURAL INFLUENCES

Except in rare situations, children grow and develop in a blend of cultures and subcultures, those smaller groups within a culture that possess many characteristics of the larger culture while contributing their own particular values. In a large, complex society such as the United States, different groups have their own set of standards, values, and expectations within the collective ways of the large culture. Most were formed when groups of people clustered together by preference, by external pressures from the majority culture, or by geographic isolation. Although many cultural differences are related to geographic boundaries, subcultures are not always restricted by location.

There are even subcultures related to the age stages of development that have traditions, games, loyalties, and rules. Age-related subcultures are easily identified in the behavior of school-age children and adolescents. The culture is handed down by word of mouth from one "generation" to the next, and its rituals and behavior standards are highly resistant to outside influence.

Children's membership in a cultural subgroup is, for the most part, involuntary. They are born into a family with a specific ethnic and/or racial heritage, socioeconomic level, and religious beliefs. Although in the complex American society there are countless subcultures and considerable variation in the way of life, those subcultures that seem to exert the greatest influence on childrearing are ethnicity, social class, and occupational role.

Ethnicity

Ethnicity is the classification of or affiliation with any of the basic groups or divisions of mankind or any heterogeneous population differentiated by customs, characteristics, language, or similar distinguishing factors. Ethnic differences extend to many areas and include such manifestations as family structure, language, food preferences, moral codes, and expression of emotion. Some standards of behavior result from the cultural heritage of the specific ethnic group as, for example, the traditional role of the father. Others reflect the interaction between subcultures, most notably between members of the majority culture and a minority subculture.

To establish their place in the group, children learn how to adhere to a mode of behavior that is in accordance with standards distinctive to the group and learn how they can expect others to behave toward them. They take their cues from observing and imitating those to whom they are exposed. For example, children of a racial minority form a perception of their role as a group member by observing the manner in which role models within the subgroup respond to treatment by people outside the subgroup. When they see group members display an attitude of inferiority, they assume this to be the appropriate behavior. These perceptions are then incorporated into their own self-concept.

In the United States the cross-cultural lines are becoming blurred as subcultures are assimilated and blended into the larger culture (Fig. 2-1). Although ethnic differences in childrearing are probably diminishing, they remain important. It is particularly difficult for persons to attempt to maintain an identity with a subculture while living and conforming to the requirements of the larger culture. Universal customs and language of the dominant culture used in commercial and educational systems are different from those of the minority culture. Often the values are in conflict. Consequently children reared in this environment are confused about roles and values, and they usually adopt those of the more influential or higher-status culture. Youth, in particular, are influenced by the locally dominant group.

Ethnocentrism. Ethnocentrism is the emotional attitude that one's own ethnic group is superior to others, that one's values, beliefs, and perceptions are the correct ones, and that the group's ways of living and behaving are the best way. This implies that all other groups are inferior and that their ways are not in the best interests of the group. This attitude strongly influences the ability of one person to evaluate the beliefs and behaviors of others objectively. This inherent viewpoint of individuals tends to bias their interpretation and understanding of the behavior of others.

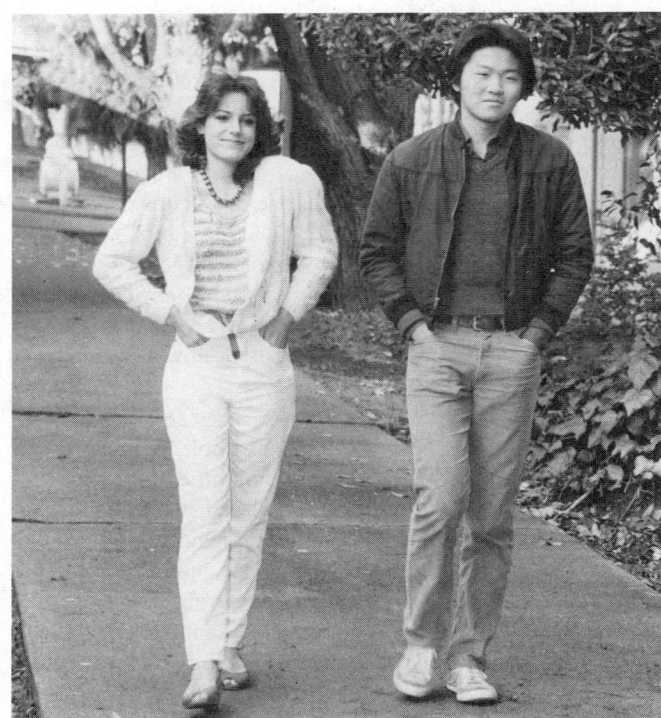

Fig. 2-1. Youngsters from different cultural backgrounds interact within the larger culture.
Photography by Garibaldi, San Lorenzo, CA.

Social Class

Those who have made extensive studies conclude that although these are exceptions, probably the greatest influence on childrearing practices and their consequences is the social class of the family into which a child is born. Differences in childrearing goals and practices as well as attitudes toward health have been found to be greater between social classes than between races or ethnic groups. In America social class and socioeconomic level are essentially synonymous, inasmuch as the factor by which a social class is defined are education, occupation, area of residence, and family income. Since children are reared differently by parents who vary in respect to these factors, social class can be expected to produce substantial variation in their upbringing.

Upper- and middle-class children live in an enriched environment that provides material comforts and broader opportunities. The parents are usually educated, and other authority figures such as teachers with whom the children are routinely in contact are usually from a middle-class background and have activities and expectations for the children that are similar to those of the parents. Parents have occupations that require judgment, creativity, and resourcefulness, and these attributes are fostered in their children.

Because members of the upper classes, or the power elite, do not participate in studies, information on childrearing practices in these groups is limited. Attitudes toward children appear to be generally permissive; however, much of the actual child care is delegated to surrogates, such as housekeepers, governesses, or private schools. The mother serves as an arbitrator between the children and the servants.

Although differences in parental behavior in different social classes are less marked than they have been in the past, one of the distinctions that is observed in middle classes but not in lower classes is the willingness to delay gratification. The uncertainty of their life leads members of the lower classes to take advantage of gratifications when they are available. This characteristic has caused lower classes to be labeled as present oriented, whereas middle classes seem to be future oriented. With better job security through unionization, unemployment compensation, and other welfare features, some segments of the lower classes are finding life more predictable. They are less apt to seize gratifications lest the opportunity vanish and are beginning to develop long-range goals, including an increased interest in education for their children. Middle-class parents have higher educational and occupational aspirations for their children and use long-range planning to meet these goals (Shaffer, 1985).

Intellectual skills. There appear to be differences in intellectual skills and scholastic achievement between children in the upper and middle classes and those in the lower classes. The more apparent differences lie in the areas of abstract thinking and manipulation. Although the relative merits of testing techniques and standards are a matter of question, there is a higher incidence of academic failure in children from the lower class with its attendant dropout rate. It has been found that lower-class parents value the concrete and tangible rather than the abstract and are therefore less inclined to encourage these qualities in their children. Their own educational level discourages these parents from reading to their children and providing other means for learning in the home. There are no role models in the family to support the value of education, and numerous provisions for intellectual growth are restricted by cost. To compound this, lower-class neighborhoods have the poorest schools, and the children are often hampered in their learning by poor health and inadequate nutrition. In addition children from the lower classes are often penalized within the school because they do not possess the symbols, attitudes, and behaviors characteristically valued by the dominant class group. There is a social class bias in educative influence. Most teachers come from the middle classes and school board members are from middle and upper classes.

Communication skills. Any concept that occurs to a person can be expressed in his language. However, ease of communication and use of language codes vary among the social classes. Language is much more restricted in the lower classes, and the classes are more easily differentiated by grammar than by pronunciation. Persons in the middle classes use different grammar from those from the lower classes and are able to express more complicated ideas; persons in the lower classes use very simple grammar and are

unable to express abstractions. Middle classes are able to communicate readily in both primary groups and secondary groups whereas lower class communication is more primary group oriented. Nonverbal communication can be culturally determined also. Many expressions may have different meanings in different cultures.

These communication differences are highly significant in relation to school achievement. School is constructed around the elaborate language codes of the middle class; therefore children from the lower classes must learn these language skills, which places them at a decided disadvantage. This is particularly true for bilingual children and children from ethnic groups who have developed a dialect unique to their own group. For example, black English, essentially another language and treated as such, is not spoken by other groups, including middle-class blacks. Many regional dialects and variations in language usage must be taken into consideration when communicating with persons from these groups.

Aspirations. Middle-class parents are positively oriented toward change, whereas working-class parents remain tradition oriented. Consequently the working class emphasizes conformity to parental values and external regulations, whereas middle-class parents are more concerned with producing self-directed children. This may reflect the occupation orientation of the different classes. Middle-class occupations tend to involve more self-direction and getting ahead; lower-class occupations tend to be standardized with direct supervision. Middle-class parents encourage their children in activities that foster achievement and that they believe will make them well-rounded adults. They involve their children in such activities as dancing lessons, athletics, and scouting. Working-class parents tend to be more concerned that their children grow up to be moral, upright, and religious. Lower-class parents are less interested in the direction of the children's activities than with their conduct; they are more concerned that the children stay out of trouble.

With few exceptions, parents in all classes love their children and in a broad sense have similar goals regarding childrearing. Differences lie in the parental behavior toward the children in attempting to help them to reach these goals. Lower-class parents are more restrictive and rely on coercive techniques in child training. They stress obedience and conformity, and the most frequently used form of discipline for undesirable behavior is physical punishment. Middle-class parents are more apt to make use of manipulative techniques such as reasoning and drawing on the child's sense of guilt. They tend to scold and use isolation rather than physical punishment. There is more concern regarding the *intent* of the act than the *consequence* of the act. It is believed that upper-class parents are more permissive and foster desirable behavior through positive reinforcement. Overall these differences tend to be small, and the general trend is in the direction of less coerciveness at all levels.

The very poor in the society who consistently exist on or

below the poverty level live in a perpetual state of despair. Their limited skills give them no bargaining power in the job market, and the education needed to improve their status is beyond them. The poor desire better things for their children but are trapped in a circular pattern that perpetuates their life condition. Their powerlessness to control their fate or condition is a source of fatalism and resignation that is characteristic of the group in general. Optimism, when it is manifest, is more likely to be expressed in terms of luck or chance. This fatalistic attitude is a significant impediment to occupational and educational aspirations and to seeking health care.

Poverty

Closely related to but distinguished from social class is the condition known as poverty. It is a relative concept and is usually associated with the general standards of a population. An *absolute standard* of poverty attempts to delimit some basic set of resources needed for adequate existence; a *relative standard* reflects the median standard of living in a society (Bauwens and Anderson, 1984) (see also p. 37). That is, what appears to be deprivation in one area may be a standard or norm in another.

The term *poverty* implies both visible and invisible impoverishment. *Visible poverty* refers to lack of money or material resources, which includes insufficient clothing, poor sanitation, and deteriorating housing. *Invisible poverty* refers to social and cultural deprivation such as limited employment opportunities, inferior educational opportunities, lack of or inferior medical services and health-care facilities, and an absence of public services (Spector, 1979). Poverty has also been defined in terms of values: "a condition of being in want of something that is needed, desired, or generally recognized as having a value" (Valentine, 1968) and psychologically in terms of deprivation and helplessness:—deprivation of the minimum adequate provisions for physical life and also of adequate sensory, social, and emotional stimuli for normal development (Bauwens and Anderson, 1984). It is a condition in which the predominant feature is inequality—inequality of both means and privileges.

As a result of his observations Lewis (1961) coined the expression "culture of poverty" to describe those caught in a way of life that is self-perpetuating and reinforced in succeeding generations just as any other culture. This concept is challenged by others (Valentine, 1968; Leacock, 1971) who maintain that this view is not consistent with the accepted notion of culture in anthropology and probably represents a bias on the part of the observers. In addition they fear that supporters of the concept will use it as rationale for withdrawing public aid and support to these groups.

Factors related to poverty. Throughout the United States there are groups of people, geographically segregated, who constitute what is known as "pockets of poverty." These are seen in the dense urban areas, such as the ghettos, and many rural areas, especially those that are geographically isolated from needed facilities and services. The nonurbanized regions identified as poverty areas in the United States are Appalachia, the deep South, the lower Southwest, and northern New England (Spector, 1979).

Certain ethnic or racial groups are overrepresented in the impoverished population. The most obvious of these are the blacks, Latinos, and Native Americans. Even more critical is the plight of the migrant farm workers. The migrant Latinos, who constitute a majority of migrant workers in the Southwest, are victims of dual minority group membership (occupational and ethnic) and are further isolated by language.

Migrant families. One of the most disadvantaged groups are migrant farm workers and their children. The low position of these families on the economic scale and their rootless, mobile existence subjects them to inadequate sanitation, substandard housing, social isolation, and lack of educational and medical facilities. This is espcially deleterious to the children. Schooling and health care are inadequate. Children are apt to live in a number of localities and attend a variety of schools in the course of a year with no continuity in either education or health care. Because both parents work in the fields, children receive little adult supervision; therefore, accident rates are high and meals are erratic. Except where prohibited by law, children are even recruited to work in the fields along with the adults.

Some migrants have a home base to which they return at the end of a growing season; others travel continuously, migrating north in summer and south in winter. With most there is little if any integration into the dominant culture; therefore migrant groups suffer social isolation. Groups who travel together, especially those with the same ethnic background, develop a cohesiveness and form their own set of values and customs. Sometimes a migrant family will leave the migration stream and become a part of a permanent community. However, this involves adaptation to a new environment and life-style that can be stress provoking to these families.

Affluence

On the opposite end of the socioeconomic spectrum are the children of affluent members of society. Although they can live within the warmth of a positive family relationship, many of them appear to be just as deprived as the poverty stricken (Grinker, 1978). Wealth does not provide protection against many of life's problems and disappointments, especially in the area of parent-child relationships. Like their counterparts in the poverty groups, children of the affluent suffer from discrimination, inadequate parenting, or unsatisfactory role models.

Children of the wealthy suffer most from lack of parental contact. There may be long separations from loving, caring parents because of social or business interests. Some have a cold, sometimes hostile parent, who is rarely available to the children. Even their places of residence contribute to their isolation and loneliness. Purchased parent surrogates such as servants, sports professionals (such as tennis or swimming instructors), and private school personnel provide their adult companionship and authority. The children of the wealthy are especially subject to psychologic problems, and emotional abuse is not uncommon.

Many children from wealthy families, just like those from poor families, seem to thrive and flourish, making positive contributions to their families and society. However, a large number grow up to display a lack of motivation or self-discipline and boredom. They are suspicious of others, finding it difficult to believe they are liked for themselves and not for their money or position, and they do not trust others enough to enter into true friendships.

Occupation

Many authorities believe that the occupational environment of the family head correlates more closely than does social class with the direction of childrearing and the values parents attempt to convey to their children. There appear to be differences in the way of life between "individuated-entrepreneurial" and "welfare-bureaucratic" occupations (Leslie, 1982). Entrepreneurial occupations include the smaller and more traditional enterprises, such as small businesses, sales, and professionals such as medicine, that require self-reliance and independence. Income depends on hard work, individual initiative, and risk taking.

The concept of welfare-bureaucracy is based on large organizational structures. Bureaucracy implies specialization and supervision governed by a set of rules; welfare refers to the job security offered by the organization. In organizational occupations the risk taking is minimum and there is more adjustment to and dependence on others.

Entrepreneurs believe the world to be more harsh than do organizational workers and they rear their children in a more authoritarian manner. They emphasize self-control, self-denial, and responsible independence with a vigorous and control-oriented approach to life. They lean toward more rigid delineation of sex roles and a more traditional orientation to family life. Organizational parents tend toward more permissive childrearing style that fosters passivity, dependency, and some degree of impulse expression. A concern for group approval (outer-directedness) takes precedence over development of the individual (inner-directedness). They are more socially minded and usually allow their children more freedom. The general trend toward passivity and outer-directedness among young Americans may be rooted in this philosophy.

The social values of the family are also related to social class differences in occupation. Parents in middle-class occupations that require initiative, independent judgment, and the ability to deal with others promote self-direction in their children. Working-class occupations are generally those that require conformity and obedience, values that are emphasized by working-class parents. It appears that children are encouraged more in higher social classes and are more likely to develop positive identification with the parent, which leads to higher occupational aspirations and achievements in the children.

Religion

Probably the most influential factor in shaping the culture of the United States is the Judeo-Christian faith. Many immigrants came to the country for religious freedom and established a religious and moral atmosphere that affected everyone. However, there are individual differences that are part of the general culture.

The religious orientation of the family dictates a code of morality and a meaning for life's mysteries as well as behavior standards (Fig. 2-2). The religious affiliation influences the family's attitudes toward education, male and female role identity, and attitudes regarding their ultimate destiny. It may determine the school that the children attend, the companions with whom they associate, and often their mate selection. In many cultures the religious beliefs are such an integral part of the culture that it is difficult to distinguish one from the other. In a few instances, such as the Oneida and Amish communities, religion is the basis of a common way of life that determines where the children are reared and a totally individualistic life-style. (See also Religious beliefs, p. 45)

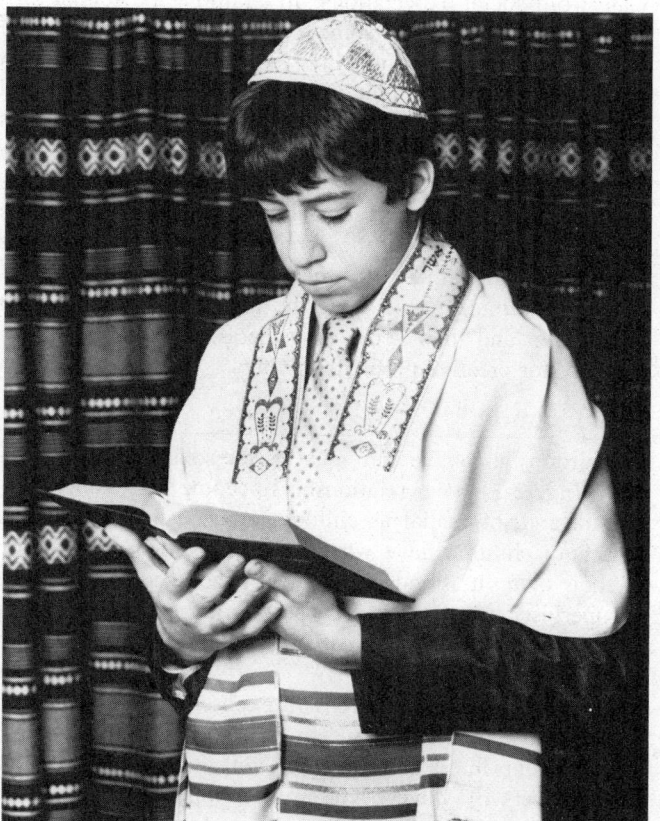

Fig. 2-2. A boy during his bar mitzvah ceremony.
Photography by G. Robert Bishop.

Schools

When children enter school, their radius of relationships extends to include a wider variety of peers and a new focus of authority. Although parents continue to exert the major influence on the children, in the school environment teachers have the most significant psychologic impact on their development and socialization. The function of teachers is primarily limited to teaching, but, like parents, they are concerned about the emotional welfare of the children. Both parents and teachers must constrain behavior, and both are in a position to enforce standards of conduct.

Socialization. Next to the family the schools exert the major force in providing continuity between generations by conveying a vast amount of culture from the older members to the young. In this way children are prepared to carry out the traditional social roles they are expected to assume as adults in society. School is the center of "cultural diffusion" wherein the cultural standards of the larger group are mediated to the local community. It governs what is taught and, to a large extent, how it is taught. School rules and regulations regarding attendance, authority relationships, and the system of sanctions and rewards based on achievement transmit to the child the behavioral expectations of the adult world of employment and relationships. School is often the only institution in which children systematically learn about the negative consequences of behaviors that deviate from social expectations. In addition, the school provides an opportunity for some children to participate in the larger society in rewarding ways (Schwartz, 1975) and often provides avenues for social mobility for both students and teachers. Through education individuals in the lower classes are offered the opportunity for further education and the capacity to move up in the social strata.

Teachers have the responsibility for transmitting the knowledge and values of the dominant culture, that is, those values on which there is broad consensus. They are expected to stimulate and guide the intellectual development of children and their sense of esthetics and to foster their capacity for creative problem solving.

Peer Cultures

Peer groups also have an impact on the socialization of children (Fig. 2-3). Peer relationships become increasingly important and influential as children proceed through school. In school children have what can be regarded as a culture of their own. It is most apparent in the school and in the unsupervised play group. The play group presents this culture in a much purer form than does the school, which is partly produced by adults.

During their lives children are exposed to value systems such as those of the family, ethnic group, and social class. In peer-group interaction they are confronted with a variety of these sets of values. The values imposed by the peer group are especially compelling because children must accept and conform to them in order to be accepted as members of the group. When the peer values are not too different

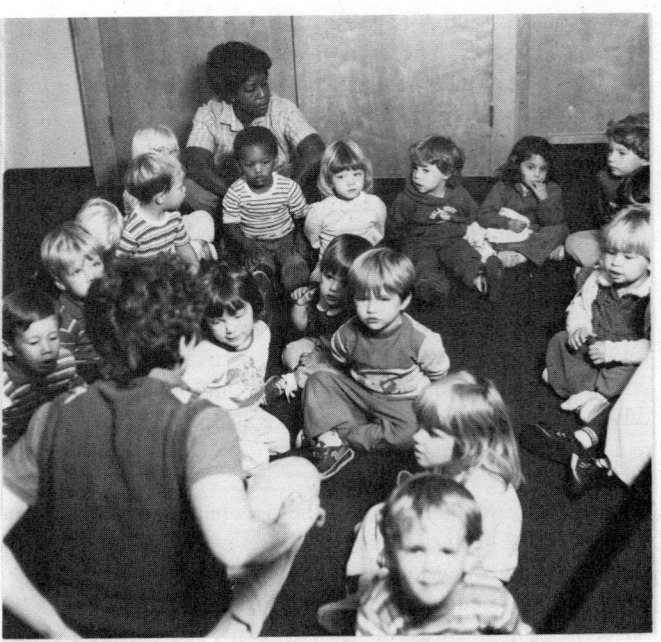

Fig. 2-3. Children from a variety of cultural and ethnic backgrounds begin to socialize in the daycare setting. Photography by John Roy, Saint Francis Hospital, Tulsa, OK.

from those of family and teachers, the mild conflict created by these small differences serves to separate children from the adults in their lives and to strengthen the feeling of belonging to the peer group.

The kind of socialization provided by the peer group depends on the special subculture that develops from the background, interests, and capabilities of its members. Some groups support school achievement, others focus on athletic prowess, and still others are decidedly antithetic to educative goals. Scholastic achievement is strongly related to the value system of the peer groups. Many conflicts between teachers and students and between parents and students can be attributed to fear of rejection by peers. There is always a conflict between what is expected from parents regarding academic achievement and what is expected from the peer culture. This is especially pronounced in high school and will be discussed further in Chapter 19.

Although it has neither the traditional authority of the parents nor the legal authority of the schools for teaching information, the peer group manages to convey a substantial amount of material to its members. Children's need for the friendship of their peers brings them into an increasingly complex social system. The world of the peer group is different from the adult world and, through peer relationships, children learn ways in which to deal with dominance and hostility and to relate with persons in positions of leadership and authority. Another function of the peer subculture is to relieve boredom and to provide recognition that individual members do not receive from teachers and other authority figures.

Children have a culture all their own, with secrets, mores, and codes of ethics with which they promote feelings of group solidarity and detachment from adults. They have traditions and folkways that are transferred from "generation to generation" of school children and that have a great influence over the behavior of all members of the group. There are age-related games and other activities and, as children move from one level to the next, folkways of the younger group are discarded as those of the new are adopted. For, example, a school-age child rides a bicycle to school; the high-school student does not. As they advance children are forward oriented only—they look forward with anticipation but look backward with contempt.

Biculture

Some children are exposed to the values, role relationships, and life-styles of two cultures—a virtual "straddling" of two cultures. This is sometimes observed in the play group but usually is not a significant factor until children enter school. Children of one culture must unlearn some of the established practices of one culture in order to become socialized in the other, especially in role relationships. For example, Latino children are taught to look away when scolded; in United States' schools the teacher expects direct eye contact—"Look at me when I speak to you." Children learn new roles and social behavior more rapidly than their adult counterparts.

This biculture is particularly marked in language differences. The bilingual child is said to be at a disadvantage in school situations of the dominant culture, and a great deal of controversy has arisen regarding the benefits and detriments of bilingual education. On the one hand those supporting bilingual education adhere to the principle that children will understand more readily and perform more realistically (especially in testing situations) if learning is directed in their own language; others contend that children living in a dominant culture should adopt the ways of that culture, including language.

Another aspect of biculture occurs when children meld the elements of the dominant culture and the minority culture with the characteristics of a subculture that is uniquely their own. This has been observed among blacks in the United States (Cole, 1970; Valentine, 1971).

THE CHILD AND FAMILY IN AMERICA

America is an aggregate of numerous Old and New World cultures that are blended with the unique heritage of pioneering frontiersmen. Models of childrearing appear to reflect the history of the country. The early philosophic standards of the Protestant ethic, which resulted in that pleasureless, . hard-driven, independent individual represented to some extent by the entrepreneurial philosophy discussed earlier, is gradually being replaced in contemporary American society by the social ethic, which emphasizes a group-oriented and other-directed philosophy.

The frontier background of the American culture has also contributed to the overall orientation to life and childrearing. There has always been a basic optimistic view of the world, a belief that things can be better and that the children can and will be better off than the parents. This hopeful outlook and a general future orientation together with the possibility of upward social mobility have created a pervasive overall attitude of optimism. Increasing development of self-confidence and autonomy in children is fostered and encouraged. Children are generally permitted a greater degree of freedom than in more tradition-oriented cultures, where a child born in one social class will remain in that class for his lifetime.

Family life in America is characterized by increasing geographic and economic mobility. Here there is less reliance on tradition, families are fragmented, and there is limited opportunity to transmit and acquire the traditional and accepted customs of a culture. Consequently young adults rely to a greater extent on the professed experts, peers, and the mass media for acquisition of acceptable patterns of behavior, including childrearing practices. Each generation, as it adapts to the new, discards the inadequacies of previous generations. This often constitutes a source of confusion and frustration as parents attempt to adjust to rapid changes; tradition and precedent no longer meet needs and challenges of rapid change that require new approaches and innovation for problem solving. Competent parents attempt to determine the comparatively stable, essential components of the culture and transmit these to their children. Awareness of an attention to changing cultural norms during childrearing helps the parent to adapt to the new demands of the culture that are different from those they learned as children.

Children in America grow up with a number of adults who differ from one another but who all provide input to them as role models, teachers, and standards for behavior. Most of the children live in some form of nuclear family located in sharply differentiated neighborhoods determined by income and ethnic status within a highly technical, largely urban society. Class differences in childrearing still persist, but they are becoming less divergent as a result of the increased homogeneity of the culture. Working classes still tend to be more tradition oriented, whereas the middle classes are more positively oriented toward social change. There are still differences in time orientation and attitudes toward education and in maternal behavior, but these differences are changing perceptibly.

Minority-Group Membership

In addition to the problems and risks encountered by all children in the course of development, a small percentage of children are particularly vulnerable to hostility, derogation, and discrimination from children and adults of the majority group. America abounds with racial, ethnic, and religious minority groups. Although the effects of a minority status can apply to any of them, the greatest impact is on blacks, the largest minority.

Studies in the past indicate that early in life children become aware of their racial or ethnic status and of the discriminatory attitudes of the majority culture toward their group. The direct effects of discrimination are anger and low self-esteem, which become manifest in a variety of behaviors. Inner conflicts and suppressed hostility that focus children's attention inward may be factors in the failure of many children to achieve in other areas.

Because of many other factors, for most blacks membership in the black minority also implies membership in the lower levels of social structure. This lower-class, lower-caste status is often characterized by broken homes, dominance of maternal authority, impoverished and deteriorating neighborhoods, environmental encouragement of delinquency, and frequently parent-child friction and antagonism.

Evidence indicates that changes in attitudes are slowly taking place in some groups and in some places. With growing awareness, interest, and understanding by increasing numbers of the majority group, which has accompanied the recent emergence of racial and ethnic pride, minority-group children are becoming more secure and confident in their racial or ethnic identity. Individuals vary in their reactions to membership in a minority group, and much of this variation can be attributed to familial factors. As with all children, the most important influences on development of the positive self-image are warm, understanding parents who take an active interest in fostering their children's growth. Parents who accept their children and react positively and constructively rather than in a negative and self-defeating manner will help their children develop feelings of self-worth, self-esteem, and self-acceptance. The more adequate children feel, the more positive will be their attitudes toward both majority and minority children, the greater will be their ability to withstand prejudice and intolerance, and the less will be their need for counteraggressive behavior.

CULTURAL SHOCK

The term *cultural shock* describes the "feelings of helplessness and discomfort and a state of disorientation experienced by an outsider attempting to comprehend or effectively adapt to a different cultural group because of differences in cultural practices, values, and beliefs" (Leininger, 1978). This occurs with both clients and health care providers who move from one culture to another culture or setting. This can be persons who immigrate to a new country (such as the Asian refugees) or persons from a subcultural group who must adjust to the ways of an unfamiliar subgroup (such as children entering the school subculture or clients who enter the hospital subculture). Cultural shock is characterized by the inability to respond to or function in a new or strange situation.

Numerous factors influence the reactions to a new environment. Language barriers, including dialects and jargon (such as medical language) specific to a subcultural group,

inhibit effective communication. Habits and customs (such as different role behaviors or etiquette) and differences in attitudes and beliefs are puzzling to the stranger in the new environment. The outsider experiences an intense sense of isolation and feelings of loneliness and nonrelatedness. Nurses entering an unfamiliar cultural situation can reduce the cultural shock by becoming familiar with the cultural groups with which they work and by learning tolerance of the values, beliefs, and customs of these groups.

Immigrants and refugees from cultures in which children are taught to respect and obey their elders and in which females are considered inferior to males, such as most Asian cultures, may find difficulty dealing with the consequences of Western egalitarianism. When children enter the school system, they learn to question authority and are confronted with the movement for equality of the sexes in all aspects of life. This often creates conflict within the family, especially in families such as the Vietnamese, who consider education highly valuable for their children.

Cultural Influences on Health Care

Cultural beliefs and practices are an important part of data gathering in the nursing assessment. Nurses continually encounter beliefs and practices that may facilitate or impede nursing interventions, including attitudes toward family planning, food habits, and folkways that are firmly entrenched in the culture. The language of the client may be different from that of the larger culture, or there may be regional or ethnic peculiarities in the use of basic English. Subcultural influences, such as some religious beliefs and practices, may be in conflict with standard health practices and therapeutic interventions.

SUSCEPTIBILITY TO HEALTH PROBLEMS

Some groups of people are more susceptible and others more resistant to certain illnesses than are persons from other groups. An innate susceptibility is acquired through generations of evolutionary changes that take place within constrained or segregated populations. The proximity to disease, environmental factors, and the general physical status are significant factors associated with health problems.

Hereditary Factors

The genetic constitution of individuals as groups influences the degree to which they are susceptible to a specific disorder. It may be the result of an inherent lack of resistance to a disease organism, a trait that is an advantage in one environment but which places the possessor at a disadvantage in another, or it may be the consequence of intermarriage within a relatively narrow range of geographic, ethnic, or religious restrictions.

A geographic constraint is illustrated by the classic example of the common communicable disease rubeola. The rubeola virus, or the populations that were continually exposed to it, became altered in such a way that the disease was considered to be a universal disease of childhood from which the majority of children suffered without ill effects. When other populations (for example, the inhabitants of the Hawaiian Islands) were exposed to the virus by explorers and missionaries, they experienced a violent response that resulted in high mortality.

Another communicable disease, tuberculosis, appears to be more prevalent in certain ethnic groups such as the Native Americans of the Southwest, Vietnamese immigrants, and Mexican-Americans (Brownlee, 1978; Orque, 1983). In many populations it is difficult to determine how much the increased incidence can be attributed to ethnic factors and how much is related to the life-styles in the lower social strata.

A number of diseases show ethnic or racial differences. For example, Tay-Sachs disease, characterized by early neurologic deterioration and mental retardation, affects primarily Ashkenasi Jewish families, particularly those of Northeastern European origin, while Sephardic Jewish families appear to be no more at risk for the disease than other populations. The incidence of cystic fibrosis is highest in whites, it is almost nonexistent in Orientals, and the rare affected blacks are usually in areas where there is apt to be mixed ancestry. Some selected genetic disorders that are more prevalent in certain populations are listed in Table 2-1. Racial and ethnic differences are further considered in relation to diseases and defects as they are discussed throughout the book.

Other groups appear to have a predisposition for certain diseases. Cardiovascular disease, pneumonia, and diabetes are especially high among blacks, Mexican-Americans are more likely to suffer from pneumonia than their Anglo counterparts, and Native Americans have particularly high rates of dysentery, pneumonia, and suicide (Bullough and Bullough, 1972).

Common food items and drugs may cause health problems in certain racial groups. For example, persons with glucose-6-phosphate dehydrogenase (G-6-PD) deficiency develop acute hemolytic anemia after they ingest fava (horse or broad) beans or certain drugs such as aspirin preparations, sulfonamides, or primaquine. The deficiency is the most common enzyme abnormality and is found in a large percentage of people around the world, especially those of Mediterranean, African, Near Eastern, and Asian origin (Cohen, 1984).

The sensitivity to foods containing lactose is a common hereditary characteristic of several cultural groups; 70% to 90% of blacks, Asians, and Native Americans and approximately 10% of whites have an intolerance to lactose (Overfield, 1977). This usually does not become a problem until the child reaches 3 to 5 years of age. However, lactose-intolerant children become uncomfortable with distention, flatus, and diarrhea after ingesting milk or milk products. Unknowing but well-meaning health workers may be responsible for these symptoms in their clients when they prescribe these items as a source of protein and calcium.

An example of resistance to disease, or selective advantage, of a population is found in persons who possess the sickle cell trait. Persons with sickle cell trait are highly resistant to a form of malaria and, in the parts of the world where the organisms are prevalent, there is a high frequency of the trait. However, in an environment where malaria is not a threat, possession of the trait has no advantage and only the negative aspects of the condition remain (risk of sickle cell anemia in offspring).

Physical characteristics. Among racial groups there are observable differences in physical appearance. The most obvious are skin and hair coloring and texture. Skin color is determined by the amount of melanin pigment present in the skin. Persons from countries located near the equator have darkly pigmented skin, which serves to protect the skin from the year-round exposure to the sun's rays; persons from the northern countries have very light skin, which provides for maximum exposure to the sun's rays (necessary for vitamin D metabolism) during the short daylight hours. There can be wide variations in skin color between these two extremes in terms of geographic origin or from intermixing of dark and light skin color.

As a consequence of the dark pigmentation, the detection of skin color changes can be difficult and requires modification of assessment techniques. For example, vasomotor alterations, cyanosis, and jaundice observable in the skin are not easily recognized in very dark or black skin. Variations in the skin color can alter the appearance of the skin in a given circumstance. For example, pallor in a light-skinned person appears white or chalky, brown-skinned persons will appear yellow-brown, and a black-skinned person will appear ashen gray (Bloch and Hunter, 1981).

Skin thickness is deceiving in some black children. Measurement of skinfold thickness, a common tool for nutritional assessment, consistently measures thinner in black children regardless of nutritional state (Malina, 1971). Also, black persons are subject to keloid formation in scar tissue more often than persons of other racial backgrounds.

Variations in the newborn are often related to racial or ethnic origin. For example, newborn infants of Asian and black parents are smaller than infants of white parentage, and bluish pigmented areas (mongolian spots) on the sacral region are a common observation on Oriental, black, Native American, and Mexican-American infants.

Evaluation of stature and body build reveals some racial tendencies. Oriental children are usually smaller at all ages and black children are taller and heavier between ages 5 and 14 than white children of the same age (see growth measurements, Appendix C). This difference in stature can lead to misinterpretation of health status and capabilities. A black child who appears normal for his age may, in fact, be underdeveloped when compared to other black children (Bloch, 1983). In communication and education a child who is smaller than the average may appear precocious and one

Table 2-1 Distribution of selected genetic traits and disorders by population or ethnic group

ETHNIC OR POPULATION GROUP	GENETIC OR MULTIFACTORIAL DISORDER PRESENT IN RELATIVELY HIGH FREQUENCY	ETHNIC OR POPULATION GROUP	GENETIC OR MULTIFACTORIAL DISORDER PRESENT IN RELATIVELY HIGH FREQUENCY
Åland Islanders	Ocular albinism (Forsius-Erikkson type)	Jews	
Amish	Limb-girdle muscular dystrophy (IN—Adams, Allen counties) Ellis-van Creveld (PA—Lancaster county) Pyruvate kinase deficiency (OH—Mifflin county) Hemophilia B (PA—Holmes county)	*Ashkenazi*	Tay-Sachs disease (infantile) Niemann-Pick disease (infantile) Gaucher disease (adult type) Familial dysautonomia (Riley-Day syndrome) Bloom syndrome Torsion dystonia Factor XI (PTA) deficiency
Armenians	Familial Mediterranean fever Familial paroxysmal polyserositis	*Sephardi*	Familial Mediterranean fever Ataxia-telangiectasia (Morocco) Cystinuria (Libya) Glycogen storage disease III (Morocco)
Blacks (African)	Sickle cell disease Hemoglobin C disease Hereditary persistence of hemoglobin F G6PD deficiency, African type Lactase deficiency, adult β-Thalassemia	Oriental	Dubin-Johnson syndrome (Iran) Ichthyosis vulgaris (Iraq, India) Werdnig-Hoffman disease (Karaite Jews) G6PD deficiency, Mediterranean type Phenylketonuria (Yemen) Metachromatic leukodystrophy (Habbanite Jews, Saudi Arabia)
Burmese	Hemoglobin E disease		
Chinese	Alpha thalassemia G6PD deficiency, Chinese type Lactase deficiency, adult		
Costa Rican	Malignant osteopetrosis	Lapps	Congenital dislocation of hip
Druze	Alkaptonuria	Lebanese	Dyggve-Melchoir-Clausen syndrome
English	Cystic fibrosis Hereditary amyloidosis, type III	Mediterranean people (Italians, Greeks)	G6PD deficiency, Mediterranean type β-Thalassemia Familial Mediterranean fever
Eskimos	Congenital adrenal hyperplasia Pseudocholinesterase deficiency Methemoglobinemia	Navaho Indians	Ear anomalies
French Canadians (Quebec)	Tyrosinemia Morquio syndrome	Polynesians	Clubfoot
Finns	Congenital nephrosis Generalized amyloidosis syndrome, V Polycystic liver disease Retinoschisis Aspartylglycoasaminuria Diastrophic dwarfism	Polish	Phenylketonuria
		Portugese	Joseph disease
		Nova Scotia Acadians	Niemann-Pick disease, type D
Gypsies (Czech)	Congenital glaucoma	Scandinavians (Norwegians, Swedes, Danes)	Cholestasis-lymphedema (Norwegians) Sjögren-Larsson syndrome (Swedes) Krabbe disease Phenylketonuria
Hopi Indians	Tyrosinase positive albinism		
Iceland	Phenylketonuria		
Irish	Phenylketonuria Neural tube defects	Scots	Phenylketonuria Cystic fibrosis Hereditary amyloidosis, type III
Japanese	Acatalasemia Cleft lip/palate Oguchi disease	Thai	Lactase deficiency, adult Hemoglobin E disease
		Zuni Indians	Tyrosinase positive albinism

From Cohen, F.L.: Clinical genetics in nursing practice, Philadelphia, 1984, J.B. Lippincott Co., pp. 23-24. Data from Damon, A.: Race, ethnic group and disease, Soc. Biol. **16**:69, 1969; Der Kaloustian, V.M., Maffah, J., Loiselet, J.: Genetic diseases in Lebanon, Am. J. Med. Genet. **7**:187, 1980; Goodman, R.M.: Genetic disorders among the Jewish people, Baltimore, 1979, Johns Hopkins University Press; McKusick, V: Mendelian inheritance in man, ed. 5, Baltimore, 1978, Johns Hopkins University Press; Ramot, B.: Genetic polymorphisms and diseases in man, New York, 1974, Academic Press; Stanbury, J.B.: The metabolic basis of inherited disease, New York, 1983, McGraw-Hill; Ferak, V., Genčík, A., and Genčíkova, A.: Population genetical aspects of primary congenital glaucoma, Hum. Genet. **61**:193, 1982.

who is larger might appear to be slow. Expectations determined on this basis can be detrimental to the child.

Visual problems vary among different racial groups. There is a high percentage of Chinese persons with myopia while few white and even fewer blacks and American Indians have this problem. Color blindness is more common in Europeans and East Indians than other groups (Brues, cited in Overfield, 1977).

Socioeconomic Factors

The most overwhelming adverse influence on health is socioeconomic status. A higher percentage of lower-class individuals are suffering from some health problem at any one time than are those in any other group. The sum of all aspects of their situation contributes to and compounds health problems; this includes crowded living conditions and poor sanitation, which facilitate transfer of disease. There is a higher incidence of lead poisoning in children from lower-class families, where there is more ready access to lead paint and other lead-containing compounds or utensils, such as pottery with lead-containing glazes.

In the lower classes, children are less likely to be immunized against preventable diseases than are children in the upper and middle classes. Lack of funds or inaccessibility to health services inhibits treatment for any but severe illness or injury. Sometimes health care is inadequate because of ignorance. In some areas a disorder is so commonplace that it is looked on as unavoidable; it is not recognized as something that requires (or is amenable to) treatment. The parents may not have information regarding causes, treatment, outcome of the illness, or preventive measures.

Upper- and middle-class parents are more likely to seek treatment for many more types of symptoms than are lower-class parents, and they are more concerned with detecting and preventing illness in their children. The disinclination of lower-class families to use preventive health services is probably another symptom of the fatalistic approach to problems and a time orientation that is concentrated on the present rather than the future. Preventive dental care, immunization, and prenatal care are examples of such health services. The incidence of prematurity is highest in the lower classes. Significantly, lower-class parents have a low participation rate in local health programs and are more likely to practice home treatment.

Poverty. A high correlation between poverty and the prevalence of illness has long been observed. Impoverished families suffer from poor nutrition; they have little if any preventive health care, inadequate health maintenance, and very limited access to health services. Health care often ranks low on their list of priorities. Day to day needs of food, clothing, and lodging take precedence as long as the ailing person feels able to perform activities of daily living.

Poor families are denied access to many health institutions for emergency or other hospital care. Frequently they must travel long distances to service centers that are willing to assume their care. In an emergency they must find money

for taxi fare, borrow an automobile, or seek other means of transportation. They must find care for dependents, such as other infants and small children, or have them accompany them when taking the ill child for care. Families tend to delay preventive care indefinitely unless health services are relatively accessible. They are more likely to consult folk practitioners or other persons within their community. Even in areas where medical facilities are available, underutilization has not been significantly altered in spite of elimination of financial obstacles (Spector, 1979).

Poor nutrition accounts for many health problems in the lower classes. Lack of funds results in a diet that may be seriously lacking in essential food substances, especially protein, vitamins, and iron. This often leads to nutritional deficiency disorders and growth retardation in children. In many the total intake is insufficient to support normal growth. Unstructured eating patterns and irregularly scheduled mealtimes can also contribute to erratic food intake and a proportionately larger consumption of nonnourishing snacks.

Because of deficient preventive care, dental problems are more prevalent. Lack of standard immunizations together with reduced resistance from poor nutrition render the exposed children in poor segments of the population vulnerable to communicable diseases. Poor sanitation and crowded living conditions also contribute to the higher incidence and perpetuation of illness. In general poor people become ill more frequently and remain ill for longer periods of time than persons in the general population.

Migrant families. Migrants generally suffer more illness, both acute and chronic, than does the general population. They are subject to the unhealthy environments, poverty, and insufficient medical care; their health-seeking behavior in general is an illness- or injury-oriented recourse to medical care. Affected persons will postpone seeking care for themselves or their children until physical pain or suffering are almost unbearable (O'Brien, 1982).

When medical care is provided to a family, follow-up care is usually impossible because of their transient lifestyle. Compliance to medical therapies is primarily related to accessiblity and availability. For example, medications provided by health workers are more likely to be taken than those that must be obtained at a pharmacy. In addition, medications are often discontinued following self-perceived recovery. Treatment regimens that do not interfere with work or family responsibilities are most likely to be adhered to. Their entire approach to health care is described by O'Brien (1982) as ''pragmatic survivalism,'' a concept ''symbolizing a pattern of health-illness attitudes and behaviors that focus on the achievement and maintenance of low-level wellness in the most practical manner possible for the continuance of productive life.''

The health problems of migrant children appear to be dental caries, upper respiratory infections, skin lesions, otitis media, and growth and development delay (Steffen and Francis, 1978). Poor nutritional status is evident, especially iron, riboflavin, and vitamin A deficiencies.

CUSTOMS AND FOLKWAYS

Nurses are becoming increasingly aware of the need to consider cultural differences in clients when providing health care. An understanding of the various beliefs regarding the causation of illness and disease as well as traditional health practices is essential to successful intervention. The more nurses know about the values, beliefs, and customs of other ethnic groups, the better able they are to meet the needs of these families and to gain their cooperation and compliance.

Relationships with Health Care Providers

The manner of relating with health care providers differs considerably among cultural groups. One area of conflict to some nurses is the attitude toward time and waiting that is part of some cultures. The time orientation of Hispanic and black ethnic groups is in the present. For example, blacks are very flexible in their time orientation; a black family may be late for or miss appointments because other issues take precedence over the appointment and they may not communicate this to the health agency (Bloch, 1983). Hispanics, too, have a very relaxed view of time. Whereas the dominant culture in the United States says that "time flies," the Hispanic says, "time walks." The Japanese, on the other hand, consider time to be valuable and to be used wisely. They tend to be punctual for medical appointments and assiduous in following prescribed regimens (Hashizume and Takano, 1983). A Vietnamese family will subordinate time to values considered to be more significant, such as propriety. They may be late for an appointment because of an overextended visit by a friend in their home. The Vietnamese do not hurry personal visits in order to maintain social harmony (Orque, 1983).

In many cultural groups the mother assumes the responsibility for health care; in others both parents are involved equally in relationships with health workers. A somewhat different approach is apparent in some of the Oriental cultures. For example, the father in Vietnamese families, as unquestioned head of the family, is traditionally the family member who interacts with persons outside the family unit. Therefore, he is the one who represents the family in health matters. In the Hispanic family the father, as head of the house, makes decisions regarding illness and treatment of family members, but the grandmother in the extended family is consulted regarding child care. Usually the family confers with other members before reaching a decision regarding treatment or hospitalization of a child. The Arab family also relies on others to give advice and guidance in a time of crisis (Meleis, 1981). A Japanese father may appear to be passive and uninvolved but actually is involved according to his own cultural standards (Tseng and others, 1982).

Nurses should make themselves aware of any specific attitudes regarding the manner of approach to a child in a given culture. Navajo Indians do not like a stranger near their infants. It is feared that the stranger may "witch" the child and cause him harm. On the other hand, if a stranger, particularly a woman, lavishes attention on a Latino infant

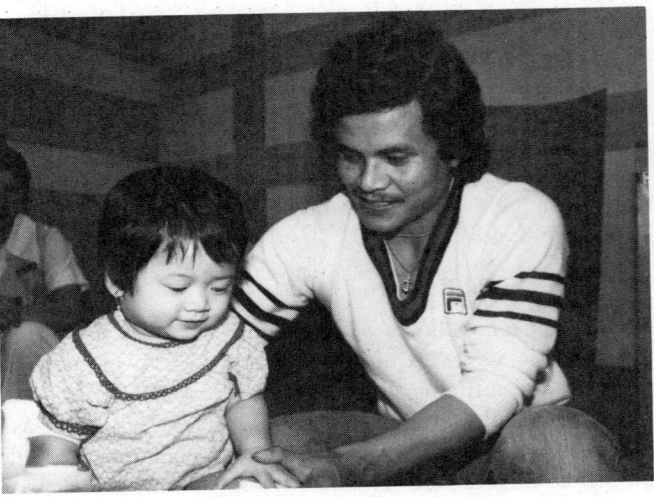

Fig. 2-4. A father with his hospitalized child.
Photography by Connie Baker, Sacramento, CA.

but fails to touch him, he will develop symptoms of the "evil eye" (see p. 42). A Vietnamese family may become upset if a newborn is admired at length for fear the evil spirits will overhear and desire the infant (Hollingsworth, Brown, and Brooten, 1980).

Some ethnic groups consider a child's admission to the hospital a family affair, with all members gathering to support and console the child and his parents. In others, such as the Samoan family, the family is willing to relinquish the care of the child to the hospital authority without interference. Their visits with the child are short, although intense, but this behavior may be misinterpreted by the hospital staff as disinterest or abandonment.

All ethnic groups are proud people who are entitled to be treated with dignity and respect. Family members are addressed by their last names; many groups consider it an affront to be called by their first names. Stereotyping is to be condemned. Persons are individuals who are evaluated in relation to their cultural standards, needs, and preferences (Fig. 2-4).

Nurses who are members of a majority culture may encounter tension and distrust in a child from a minority culture as a result of the child's learned conception or relationships with other persons in the majority group. Based on these perceptions, minority children often suspect that nurses may have hostile feelings toward them and fear ill treatment. When such children are hospitalized, this feeling compounds the feelings of loneliness, helplessness, and retribution that accompany fearful happenings and separation from families. The reverse situation may be encountered by a nurse from a minority culture attempting to meet the needs of a child who has been conditioned to view the nurse's cultural or ethnic group as inferior.

Communication. Communication is basic to all human relationships, but it may be a source of distress and misunderstanding between persons from different ethnic groups, especially if the languages are different. Ideally, conversations with families who are unable to speak the dominant language are best conducted by a health care worker who speaks the language of the family. This is not always possible, however, and it may be necessary to engage the services of an interpreter. However, use of an interpreter can be a source of misunderstanding if the interpreter is unfamiliar with the medical terminology or if there are no corresponding words in the second language to express the ideas and concepts under discussion (see Communicating with families through an interpreter, p. 191).

Some persons with poor or limited language comprehension may simply smile and nod in agreement if they do not understand the questions or directives. It is vital that the family fully understand all implications of a child's care and management before they sign permits for special procedures or assume responsibility for his care. It is not uncommon for a Vietnamese or a Japanese family to indicate ''yes'' when in fact they mean ''no'' in order to avoid social disharmony. They tend to use indirectness rather than confrontation and may become evasive when direct questioning makes them feel uncomfortable (Chen-Louie, 1983; Orque, 1983).

Nonverbal communication is a practiced art in many American Indian tribes, and the members are highly sensitive to body language. They emphasize periods of silence to formulate thoughts in preparation for speech and often remain silent after listening to statements by others in order to properly assimilate what has been said. Interruption, interjection, or haste to arrive at abrupt conclusions is perceived as immature behavior.

Eye contact is viewed differently in cultures. It is not uncommon for persons in some ethnic groups to avoid eye contact and become uncomfortable when conversing with health workers. A Vietnamese patient may not look directly into the nurse's eyes, as a sign of respect (Orque, 1983). Some Native Americans will make eye contact during the initial greeting but continued, unwavering eye contact is considered insulting and disrespectful (Wilson, 1983).

There may be reluctance on the part of families to question or otherwise initiate contact with health professionals. In the Asian cultures, for example, it is considered a sign of disrespect to question those who are viewed as persons of authority (Orque, 1983). A Japanese family may wait silently rather than ask or question. They believe that the health professionals know best and will meet their needs without being asked (Hashizume and Takano, 1983). It is also important to avoid criticism. Criticism can cause the Japanese American to ''lose face,'' to make him feel ashamed, which is highly undesirable.

It is necessary to speak slowly and carefully when conversing with families who have poor language comprehension. Many persons are able to read and write English better than they can speak or understand it. Also, the dominant language usually takes over in anxiety-provoking situations, even in persons who are able to communicate satisfactorily under ordinary circumstances.

Terms of address and use of first and last names varies among cultures and can create confusion in institutions. For example, in Asian cultures, the family name is given first in respect for the family and the given names follow. Therefore all siblings in a family have the same first name (in some families it may be the middle names that are the same). Ethiopians use no last names but have a very complex system whereby women retain their last names after marriage and the paternal grandfather's name becomes a child's last name.

Although all people share the basic emotions, there are decided ethnic variations in the way emotions are expressed. In some cultures (for example, persons of Latin or Jewish backgrounds) emotions are expressed openly and members are accustomed to share their sorrows and joys with family and friends. Conversely, Nordic and Asian groups are more restrained in expressing emotion.

Nurses caring for persons of another culture will be better able to communicate if they understand the common names used to describe symptoms and diseases: for example, *miseries* (pain) and *locked bowels* (constipation) in black people and *caida de la mollera* (fallen fontanel from dehydration), *susto* (fright), and *la diarrhea* (diarrhea) in Latinos.

Food Customs

Food customs and symbolism of various cultural, ethnic, and religious groups have become an integral part of their lives. Although in a large country such as the United States most persons have adopted the eclectic food habits that have evolved over countless generations, many ethnic and geographic food traditions and preferences are retained. Special holidays, ceremonies, and life experiences such as births, birthdays, weddings, and death are often marked by special food items or feasts. In many cultures specific food practices are followed during pregnancy in the belief that certain foods damage the developing fetus.

The distinctive food customs of ethnic groups are a product of their native environment, determined by availability. Fish is a staple food of persons living near the ocean, such as people from Japan, Polynesia, and Scandinavia. Fruit and vegetable preferences are also directly related to the climate in which these grow naturally or can be cultivated. The types of grain that are ethnically associated are also those that grow best in their native lands. For example, rice is the staple grain of the Orient and Pacific islands, wheat of the temperate climates of Europe, rye in Scandinavia, and corn of the North American Indians. The diet of the Eskimo is predominantly fish and meat, depending on which is the most easily procured in the area. Even in the continental United States there are regional favorites, like rice, hominy grits, and okra in the southern states. In some cultures food is highly spiced, in others foods tend to be bland. Table 2-2 lists the food items common to all cultures and Table 2-3 outlines some of the foods associated with some specific ethnic groups.

There are a number of restrictions related to food items. Some have a physiologic origin, such as lack of dairy foods in the diets of some persons of African or Asian ancestry in whom a hereditary lactase deficiency prevents digestion of

Table 2-2 Foods common to most ethnic food patterns

MEAT AND ALTERNATES	MILK AND MILK PRODUCTS	GRAIN PRODUCTS	VEGETABLES	FRUITS	OTHERS
Pork* Beef Chicken Eggs	Milk, fluid Ice cream	Rice White bread Noodles, macaroni, spaghetti Dry cereal	Carrots Cabbage Green beans Greens (especially spinach) Sweet potatoes or yams Tomatoes	Apples Bananas Oranges Peaches Pears Tangerines	Fruit juices

From Endres, J.B., and Rockwell, R.E.: Food, nutrition, and the young child, St. Louis, 1980, The C.V. Mosby Co., p. 18.
*May be restricted due to religious custom.

Table 2-3 Characteristic food choices for six groups

VEGETABLES	FRUITS	MEATS AND ALTERNATIVES	GRAIN PRODUCTS	OTHERS
Black Broccoli, corn, greens (mustard, collard, kale, turnips, beet, etc.), lima beans, okra, peas, pumpkin	Grapefruit, grapes, nectarine, plums, watermelon	Sausage, pigs feet, ears, etc., bacon, luncheon meat, organ meats, turkey, catfish, perch, red snapper, tuna, salmon, sardines, shrimp, kidney beans, red beans, black-eyed peas, peanuts, and peanut butter	Corn bread, hominy grits, biscuits, muffins, cooked cereal, crackers	Chitterlings, salt pork, gravies, buttermilk
Hispanic-American Avocado, chilies, corn, lettuce, onion, peas, potato, prickly pear (cactus leaf called *nopales*), zucchini	Guava, lemon, mango, melons, prickly pear (cactus fruit called *tuna*), zapote (or sapote)	Lamb, tripe, sausage (*chorizo*), bologna, bacon, pinto beans, pink beans, garbanzo beans, lentils, peanuts, and peanut butter	Tortillas, corn flour, oatmeal, sweet bread (*pan dulce*)	Salsa (tomato-pepper, onion relish), chili sauce, guacamole, lard (*manteca*), pork cracklings
Japanese Bamboo shoots, broccoli, burdock root, cauliflower, celery, cucumbers, eggplant, gourd (*Kampyo*), mushrooms, napa cabbage, peas, peppers, radishes (daikon or pickles called *takuwan*), snow peas, squash, sweet potato, turnips, water chestnuts, yamaimo	Apricot, cherries, grapefruit, grapes, lemon, lime, melons, persimmon, pineapple, pomegranate, plums (dried pickled *umeboshi*), strawberries	Turkey, raw tuna or sea bass (*sashimi*), mackerel, sardines (*mezashi*), shrimp, abalone, squid, octopus, soybean curd (*tofu*), soybean paste (*miso*), soybeans, red beans (*azuki*), lima beans, peanuts, almonds, cashews	Rice crackers, noodles (whole-wheat noodle called *soba* or *udon*), oatmeal	Soy sauce, Nori paste (used to season rice), bean thread (*konyaku*), ginger (*shoga*; dried form called *denishoga*)

From Endres, J.B., and Rockwell, R.E.: Food, nutrition, and the young child, St. Louis, 1980, The C.V. Mosby Co., pp. 182-183. Modified from Nutrition during pregnancy and lactation, California Department of Public Health, revised 1975.
NOTE: Foods common to all ethnic groups have been omitted.

Table 2-3 Characteristic food choices for six groups—cont'd

VEGETABLES	FRUITS	MEATS AND ALTERNATIVES	GRAIN PRODUCTS	OTHERS
Chinese Bamboo shoots, bean sprouts, bok choy, broccoli, celery, Chinese cabbage, corn, cucumbers, eggplant, greens (collard, Chinese, broccoli, mustard, kale), leeks, lettuce, mushrooms, peppers, scallions, snow peas, taro, water chestnuts, white turnips, white radishes, winter melon	Figs, grapes, kumquats, loquats, mango, melons, persimmon, pineapple, plums, pomegranate	Organ meats, duck, white fish, shrimp, lobster, oyster, sardines, soybeans, soybean curd *(tofu)*, black beans, chestnuts *(kuri)*	Barley, millet	Soy sauce, sweet and sour sauce, mustard sauce, ginger root, plum sauce, red bean paste
*Vietnamese** Bamboo shoots, bean sprouts, cabbage, carrots, cucumbers, greens, lettuce, mushrooms, onions, peas, spinach, yams	Apple, banana, egg-fruit *(o-ma)*, grapefruit, jackfruit, lychee, mandarin, mango, orange, papaya, pineapple, tangerine, watermelon	Beef, blood, brain, chicken, duck, eggs, fish, goat, kidney, lamb, liver, pork, shellfish, soybeans	French bread, rice, rice noodles, wheat noodles	Fish sauce, fresh herbs, garlic, ginger, lard, MSG, peanut oil, sesame seeds, sesame seed oil, vegetable oil
Indian (East) Cauliflower, carrots, cucumber, corn-gourds, leeks, eggplant, beets, radishes, hot pepper, bell pepper, peas, French beans, okra, pumpkin, red and white cabbage, mung sprouts, bean sprouts, potatoes, tapioca root, sweet potatoes	Oranges, limes, grapes, watermelon, mango, guava, honeydew, chiku, cantaloupe, pineapple, green, yellow, and red bananas, berries, custard apples	Lamb, beef, duck, chicken, shrimp, catfish, buffalo, sunfish, sardines, fresh crab, lobster, peanuts, cashews, almonds, chickpeas, split peas, black-eyed peas, dry mung beans	Rice pancakes wheat chapati, puri, mixed grain flour bread	Fresh coconut juice, curries, tomato sauce, tamarind sauce, dried grain curries *(pulses)*, yogurt-curry garnished with coriander (fresh leaves)

*Information supplied by Hanh-Trang Tran-Viet, Carbondale, Ill.

foods containing lactose. This is seldom a problem in infants and young children, but some sensitive older children can develop uncomfortable symptoms from ingestion of milk or milk products. Others have religious restrictions, such as kosher foods and food preparation of the Orthodox Jewish faith and the vegetarian diet of Seventh Day Adventists (see Vegetarian diets, p. 531).

Children in a strange environment, such as the hospital, feel much more comfortable when they are served foods to which they are accustomed. The hospital food often tastes strange and bland, especially to the child who enjoys the highly seasoned foods of his culture. The family may be concerned that he is receiving the appropriate ''hot'' or ''cold'' food to maintain or achieve a balance of foods as determined by his culture (see discussion on p. 42). Where possible, it is advisable to provide children's ethnic foods

or allow families to bring favorite foods that are not available on the hospital menu. Concern for differences in food habits and patterns projects an attitude of respect of the family's ethnic or religious heritage.

HEALTH BELIEFS AND PRACTICES

The nurse encounters people of many different racial and ethnic origins in the process of meeting the health needs of children and families. Some of these families have become so enculturated to the majority culture that their health beliefs and practices are consistent with those of the health care system. There are still numerous families, however, whose traditional practices and beliefs are an integral part of their daily lives. It is important for health care workers to be aware that ''other people may live by different rules and priorities from those of the health care provider, and these rules and priorities decisively influence health-related behavior'' (Bauwens and Anderson, 1984).

Health Beliefs

The beliefs related to the cause of illness and the maintenance of health are an integral part of the cultural heritage of families. Often inseparable from religious beliefs, they influence the way that families cope with health problems and the way that they respond to health care providers. Predominant among most cultures are beliefs related to natural forces, supernatural forces, and imbalance between forces.

Natural forces. The most common natural forces held responsible for ill health if the body is not adequately protected include cold air entering the body, impurities in the air, or other natural sources. For example, the Latino or Chinese mother will overdress the infant in an effort to keep cold wind from entering the child's body. The Chinese believe that cold weather, rain, or wind are responsible for ''cold'' conditions (Chen-Louie, 1983). They also believe that an innate energy called *chi* enters and leaves the body through mouth, nose, and ears and flows through the body in definite pathways, or meridians, at specific times and locations. Lack of *chi* and blood is believed to be a cause of fatigue, low energy, and a variety of ailments.

In the black culture natural phenomena such as phases of the moon, seasons of the year, and planet positions are believed to affect the body and its processes; therefore health maintenance is strongly associated with the ability to read ''the signs'' (Bloch, 1983). Some cultures consider such behavior as overeating, overwork, anxiety, and inadequate food and sleep as natural causes of illness (Orque, 1983). Most Native Americans consider health to be a state of harmony with nature and the universe (Wilson, 1983).

Supernatural forces. High on the list of causes of illness are forces beyond comprehension and logical explanation. Evil influences such as voodoo, witchcraft, or evil spirits are viewed in some cultures as causes of adverse health, especially those illnesses that cannot be explained by other means.

A health belief that is common among people from Latin America, Mediterranean, Near East, some Asian, and some African societies is the concept of the ''evil eye'' (*mal ojo* is the Hispanic term). It is part of the concept of health as a state of balance; illness is a state of imbalance (see below). Strength and power are associated with the evil eye; therefore, as long as an individual's strength and weakness remain in balance, he is unlikely to become a victim of the evil eye. Weaknesses are not necessarily physical. For example, an excess of some emotion, such as envy, can create a weakness. Infants and small children, because of immature development of their internal strength-weakness states, are especially vulnerable to the gaze of the evil eye (Pasquale, 1984). Consequently, evil eye serves to rationalize an inexplicable onset of illness in children who display such

symptoms as restlessness, crying, diarrhea, vomiting, and fever.

Although seldom expressed to health care providers, the belief that a witch can cast a spell over another person at the request of someone who wishes him ill is found in Hispanic and African cultures. The victim is often tortured in effigy by pins driven into a doll at the location where the intended victim is to be hurt (Hollan, 1978).

Imbalance of forces. The concept of balance or equilibrium is widespread throughout the world. One of the most common imbalances supported by the Hispanic, Filipino, Chinese, and Arab cultures is that which exists between ''hot'' and ''cold.'' This belief is reputedly derived from Hippocratic theory of humoral pathology, which states that illness is caused by an imbalance of the four humors: phlegm, blood, black bile, and yellow bile (Abril, 1977). Hot and cold describe certain properties and conditions completely unrelated to temperature. Diseases, areas of the body, foods, and illnesses are classified as either ''hot'' or ''cold.'' In Chinese health belief the forces are termed *yin* (cold) and *yang* (hot) (Chen-Louie, 1983). In order to maintain health and prevent illness these hot and cold forces must be kept in balance.

Illness is treated by restoring normal balance through the application of appropriate ''hot'' or ''cold'' remedies. A ''cold'' condition such as a respiratory disease is believed to be caused by exposure to cold weather, rain, or cold wind entering the body; it is treated by administration of ''hot'' foods, herbs, or drugs. Menstruation is considered to be a ''hot'' condition; therefore, women are cautioned against ingesting ''hot'' foods that might increase menstrual flow or produce cramping. Ingesting too much of either ''hot'' or ''cold'' foods can also be interpreted as a cause of illness.

Health care workers who are aware of this belief are better able to understand why some persons refuse to eat certain foods. It is often useful to discuss the diet with family to determine their feelings and beliefs regarding food choices. It is possible to help families devise a diet that contains the necessary balance of basic food groups prescribed by the medical subculture while conforming to the beliefs of the ethnic subculture.

The hot-cold food classification may have adverse effects. For example, newborn infants are often started on evaporated milk formulas. Evaporated milk is considered to be a hot food while whole milk is viewed as a cool food. Infants tend to develop rashes, which are believed to be caused by ''hot'' foods; in such cases parents may decide to switch to whole milk. However, parents fear that it is dangerous to change too rapidly, so they often feed the child some type of neutralizing substance, which may create additional health problems (Murillo-Rohde, 1980). Such a problem might be averted if the family's preference is determined before discharge from the hospital and a formula prescribed that is agreeable to both the family and the physician.

Health Practices

There are numerous similarities among cultures regarding prevention and treatment of illness. All cultures have some types of home remedies that they apply before seeking help from other persons. Within the ethnic community folk healers who are endowed with the ability to "cure" maladies are sought for special situations and when home remedies are unsuccessful. There is the *curandero* (male) or *curandera* (female) of the Mexican-American community whose healing powers are believed to be a gift from God. The Asian consults a herbalist, knowledgable in medicines, and/or an ethnic physician practiced in Asian therapies, including acupuncture, acupressure, and moxibustion (application of heat). Native Americans consult a variety of healers with specific skills and knowledge. Specialized medicine persons diagnose illness, provide nonsacred treatments (usually by way of massage and herbs), and care for souls. Other specialists perform services or affect cures through spiritual means.

The folk healers are very powerful persons in their community and have the ability to acquire information about an illness without resorting to probing questions. They "speak the language" of the family who seeks help and often combine their rituals and potions with prayer and entreaties to God. They also are able to create an atmosphere conducive to successful management. Furthermore, they exhibit a sincere interest in the family and their problem (Baca, 1978).

Often it will be found that the folk remedies are compatible with the medical regimen and can be used as a means to reinforce the treatment plan. For example, most of the foods contraindicated for a person with peptic ulcer are "hot" foods and would be avoided by his belief system. Also, aspirin (a "hot" medication) is an appropriate therapy for "cold" diseases such as the common cold and arthritis (Murillo-Rohde, 1980). It is not uncommon to discover that a folk prescription has a scientific basis.

To overcome the effect of the evil eye usually requires specialized rituals conducted by the appropriate practitioner. For example, the Chicano curandera ascertains that the condition is truly the result of the evil eye by performing an assessment ritual and, upon a confirmed diagnosis, performs a curative ritual. There are prescribed rituals for other maladies such as the *moller caida*. Sometimes the faith in the folk practitioner delays obtaining needed medical treatment, although the practitioner will usually suggest medical care if his or her ministrations are unsuccessful.

Health practices of different cultures may also present problems of assessment and interpretation. For example, the Vietnamese practice of "coining" may produce weltlike lesions on the child's back when a coin, held on edge, is repeatedly rubbed lengthwise on the oiled skin to rid the body of the disease (Feldman, 1984). Another such custom is the Old World practice of cupping (also practiced by the Vietnamese). A container, such as a tumbler, bottle, or jar, containing steam is placed against the skin surface to "draw out the poison" or other evil. When the heated air within the container cools, a vacuum is created that produces a bruise-like blemish on the skin directly beneath the mouth of the container (Asnes and Wisotsky, 1981; Holland and Sweeney, 1985). Both of these remedies can be misdiagnosed as evidence of "child abuse."

Other cultural health remedies that are detrimental to health include eating clay or excessive amounts of salt. A mercury compound, *azogue* (the Spanish name for quicksilver), is commonly used in Mexico and sometimes sold illegally to low-income Latino families in the United States as a "remedy" for diarrhea. Alert health care workers know that the drug can cause permanent central nervous system damage. A careful history can reveal these practices, but it may require the collaboration of a folk healer to convince a user to stop the practice.

Faith healing and religious rituals are closely allied with many folk-healing practices. Wearing of amulets, medals, and other religious relics believed by the culture to protect the individual and facilitate healing is a common practice. It is important for health workers to recognize the value of this practice and keep the items where the family has placed them or nearby. It offers comfort and support and rarely impedes medical and nursing care. If an item must be removed during a procedure it should be replaced, if possible, when the procedure is completed. The reason for its temporary removal is explained to the family and they are reassured that their wishes will be respected.

Although most subcultures in the large developed countries have become acculturated to the Western medical system, many still maintain faith in traditional healing practices and practitioners. When the folk practices do not interfere with the welfare of the patient, they need not be discouraged. Often a compromise can be reached that accomplishes the goal of the nurse while it maintains the dignity and self-esteem of the client.

Folklore Related to Prenatal Influences

Since ancient times the striking appearance of abnormal human development has been of concern, as evidenced by descriptions in primitive drawings and on clay tablets, and has served as the origin of numerous legendary and mythologic creatures. Consequently the processes of pregnancy and birth have been surrounded with strongly held beliefs and superstitions that involve taboos and prescriptions for behavior directed toward assuring the well-being of the unborn child. Even in the face of scientific advances, these superstitions and folkways have survived for generations and may still persist in various forms as part of a cultural heritage. The degree to which these beliefs are expressed depends on the strength of the cultural influence, the attitudes of the individual families, and the confidence and credibility engendered by the health care providers.

One of the most universal explanations of defective development has been maternal impressions. It has been a widespread belief that the appearance of the unborn child will be improved if the pregnant woman looks at beautiful people or things. The same concept in reverse has been used to explain birth defects. For example, if a pregnant woman was frightened by a rabbit, it was believed that her child would be born with a cleft lip; a microcephalic infant was attributed to the mother's seeing a monkey during pregnancy; and the mother's viewing a person with missing limbs would cause the unborn child to be similarly affected. Activities such as a mother reaching her arms above her head, walking in circles, or tying knots were believed to cause the umbilical cord to be knotted or twisted around the neck of the fetus. Even the shape of birthmarks and other skin defects is sometimes believed to reflect maternal impressions. For example, eating strawberries by the mother is associated with nevi. Articles of apparel or adornment, food cravings, emotions such as fright and anger, undesirable thoughts, and the time and manner of announcing the pregnancy are all believed to influence the well-being of the unborn child.

Expectant mothers who are able to rationalize the illogical nature of the beliefs will, through a normal fear of having an abnormal infant, conform to the superstitions. In most instances these customs are relatively harmless and are not in conflict with sound health practices. However, there are situations when conformity to cultural or subcultural beliefs may compromise the health and well-being of either mother or fetus, for example, the practice of eating clay. Understanding and judicious management on the part of nurses and other health care workers are required to explore with the mother all the ramifications of the practice without creating undue stress and guilt in the mother.

Not all of these beliefs are unfounded. There is evidence that maternal emotions may indeed affect the fetus. Prolonged stimulation of the autonomic nervous system caused by extreme stress or long-term anxiety produces physiologic changes in the maternal system, such as increased heart rate, vasoconstriction, and decreased gastric motility. In addition to the indirect effect produced by constriction of uter-

Table 2-4 Religious beliefs that affect nursing care

RELIGION	BELIEFS ABOUT BIRTH AND DEATH		BELIEFS ABOUT DIET AND FOOD PRACTICES
Adventist (Seventh Day Adventist; Church of God)	**Birth:**	Opposed to infant baptism Baptism in adulthood	Meat prohibited in some groups No alcohol, coffee, or tea
Baptist (27 groups)	**Birth:**	Opposed to infant baptism Believers baptize by immersion as adults	Some groups condemn coffee, tea, and alcohol
	Death:	Counsel and prayer with clergy, family, patient	
Black Muslim	**Birth:**	No baptism	Prohibit alcohol, pork and meat of dead animals, or foods traditional among American blacks, e.g., corn bread, collard greens
	Death:	Carefully prescribed procedure for washing and shrouding dead	
Buddhist Churches of America	**Birth:**	No infant baptism Infant presentation	No requirements or restrictions Some sects are strictly vegetarian Discourage use of alcohol and drugs
	Death:	Last rite chanting often practiced at bedside soon after death Priest should be contacted	
Church of Christ Scientist (Christian Science)	**Birth:** **Death:**	No baptism No last rites	No requirements or restrictions

Data from Recognizing your patients' spiritual needs, Nursing 77 **7**(12):64-68, 1977; Beliefs that can affect therapy, Pediatr. Nurs. **5**(3):40-43, 1979; Carpenito, L.J.: Nursing diagnosis: application to clinical practice, Philadelphia, 1985, J.B. Lippincott Co.; Kozier, B., and Erb, G.: Fundamentals of nursing, ed. 2, Menlo Park, CA, 1983, Addison-Wesley Publishing Co.; Spector, R.E.: Cultural diversity in health and illness, New York, 1979, Appleton-Century-Crofts; personal communications.

ine blood flow, the stress hormones cross the placental membrane to affect the fetus directly. Assisting the expectant mother to deal with her stresses or securing counseling services for her is part of the nursing considerations.

RELIGIOUS BELIEFS

Religion influences the life-styles of most cultures. Among many groups illness, injury, or death is believed to be sent by God as a punishment for sin. Some may believe that health workers will be unable to help a person whom God is punishing and may express a fatalistic attitude toward treatment, stating that it is "the will of God." Others view it as a test of strength, as the testing of Job in the Bible, and strive to remain faithful and overcome the conflicts.

Religious affiliation has implications for many health-related functions and procedures. It is comforting to the family of an ill child to have this need recognized and re-spected. Nurses need to determine if there are any special considerations related to spiritual practices that are important to the family. Dietary restrictions are clarified, especially in denominations in which there may be a number of variations. Where specific religious practices do not interfere with the health of the child or his therapy (such as fasting), the wishes of the family are respected. Family members are asked whether they want a clergy member present and whether they prefer hospital staff to call or to do this on their own.

It is important to determine the wishes of the family regarding baptism, rites or practices related to death, and other religious rituals (such as circumcision, communion, or use of amulets or icons). An important role of the nurse is to be aware of spiritual needs of families and convey an attitude of concern for this important element of the child's care. Religion, which offers families understanding and spiritual support, is a valuable asset to health care. Characteristics of selected religions are outlined in Table 2-4.

Text continued on p. 54.

BELIEFS REGARDING MEDICAL CARE	COMMENTS
Some believe in divine healing and practice annointing with oil and use of prayer May desire communion or baptism when ill Believe in man's choice and God's sovereignty Some oppose hypnosis as therapy	Sabbath: Saturday for many Accept Bible literally
"Laying on of hands" (some) May encounter some resistance to some therapies Believe God functions through physician Some believe in predestination; may respond passively to care	Some practice glossolalia (speaking in tongues)
Faith healing unacceptable Always maintain personal habits of cleanliness	General adherence to Moslem tenets overlaid, in many instances, by antagonism to whites especially Christians and Jews Do not indulge in activities (such as sleeping) more than is necessary to health
Illness believed to be a trial to aid development of soul; illness due to Karmic causes May be reluctant to have surgery or certain treatments on holy days Cleanliness believed to be of great importance Family may request Buddhist priest for counseling	In harmony with modern science Optimistic outlook; teach ways to overcome fears, anxieties, apprehension
Deny the existence of health crisis; see sickness and sin as errors of mind that can be altered by prayer Oppose human intervention with drugs or other therapies; however, accept legally required immunizations Many adhere to belief that disease is a human mental concept that can be dispelled by "spiritual truth" to extent that they refuse all medical treatment	Many desire services of Practitioner or Reader; will sometimes refuse even emergency treatment until they have consulted a Reader Unlikely to donate organs for transplant

Continued.

Table 2-4 Religious beliefs that affect nursing care—cont'd

RELIGION	BELIEFS ABOUT BIRTH AND DEATH		BELIEFS ABOUT DIET AND FOOD PRACTICES
Church of Jesus Christ of Latter Day Saints (Mormon)	**Birth:**	No baptism at birth Infant is "blessed" by church official at first opportunity after birth (in church) Baptism by immersion at 8 years	Prohibit tea, coffee, alcohol Encourage sparing use of meats Fasting for 24 hours on first Sunday each month (from after evening meal Saturday until evening meal Sunday)
	Death:	No special rites	
Eastern Orthodox (Turkey, Egypt, Syria, Rumania, Bulgaria, Cyprus, Albania, etc.)	**Birth:**	Most believe in infant baptism by immersion 8 to 40 days after birth	Restrictions depend on specific sect
	Death:	Last rites obligatory for impending death	
Episcopal (Anglican)	**Birth:**	Infant baptism mandatory; urgent if poor prognosis*	Abstain from meat on fast days May fast on Wednesday, Friday, during Lent, and before Christmas Some fast for 6 hours before receiving Holy Communion
	Death:	Last rites available but not mandatory	
Friends (Quakers)	**Birth:**	No baptism Infant's name recorded in official book	No requirements or restrictions Most practice moderation Avoid alcohol and illicit drugs
Greek Orthodox	**Birth:**	Baptism considered important Performed 40 days after birth If not possible to baptize by sprinkling or immersion, Church allows child baptism "in the air" by moving the child in the form of a cross* as appropriate words are said	Church prescribed fast periods—usually occur on Wednesday, Friday, and during Lent; consist of avoiding meat and (in some cases) dairy products If health compromised, priest may be contacted to convince family to forego fasting
	Death:	Last rites, administration of Sacrament of Holy Communion Should be performed while dying person is still conscious	
Hindu	**Birth:**	No ritual	Many dietary restrictions Beef and veal not eaten Some strict vegetarians
	Death:	Special prescribed rites Priest pours water into the mouth of dead child, ties a thread around neck or wrist to signify blessing (should not be removed) Family washes body and is particular about who touches body	
Islam (Muslim/Moslem)	**Birth:**	No baptism	Prohibit all pork products Daylight fasting practiced during ninth month of Muhammadan year (Ramadan)
	Death:	Patient must confess sins and beg forgiveness before death; family should be present Family washes and prepares body, then turns it to face Mecca Only relatives and friends may touch body	
Jehovah's Witness	**Birth:**	No baptism	Eat nothing to which blood has been added; can eat animal flesh that has been drained
	Death:	No last rites	

BELIEFS REGARDING MEDICAL CARE

COMMENTS

Devout adherents believe in divine healing through annointment with oil and "laying on of hands" by church officials (elders)
Medical therapy not prohibited

Married adults wear special undergarments
May request Sacrament on Sunday while in hospital
Financial support for sick available through well-funded welfare system
Discourage cremation

Annointment of the sick
No conflict with medical science

Discourage cremation

Some believe in spiritual healing
Rite for annointing sick available but not mandatory

Religious icons very important
Communion four times yearly: Christmas, Easter, June 30, and August 15; may be mandatory for some

---

No special rites or restrictions

Believe in plain speech and dress
Pacifists

Each health crisis handled by ordained priest; deacon may also serve in some cases
Holy Communion administered in hospital
Some may desire Sacrament of the Holy Unction performed by priest

Oppose euthanasia
Believe every reasonable effort should be made to preserve life until termination by God
Discourage autopsies that may cause dismemberment
Prefer burial to cremation

Illness or injury believed to represent sins committed in previous life
Accept most modern medical practices

Cremation preferred

Faith healing not acceptable unless psychologic condition of patient is deteriorating; performed for morale
Ritual washing after prayer; prayer takes place five times daily (upon rising, midday, afternoon, early evening, and before bed); during prayer, face Mecca and kneel on prayer rug

Older Muslims often have a fatalistic view that may interfere with compliance to therapy
May oppose autopsy

Adherents are generally absolutely opposed to blood transfusions; individuals can sometimes be persuaded in emergencies
May be opposed to modern science, including medicine

Often possible to obtain a court order appointing a hospital official as temporary guardian to consent to a child's transfusion when parents refuse consent
Autopsy approved only as required by law

Continued.

Table 2-4 Religious beliefs that affect nursing care—cont'd

RELIGION	BELIEFS ABOUT BIRTH AND DEATH		BELIEFS ABOUT DIET AND FOOD PRACTICES
Judaism (Orthodox and Conservative)	Birth:	No baptism Ritual circumcision of male infants on eighth day; performed by Mohel (ritual circumciser familiar with Jewish law and aseptic technique) Reform Jews favor ritual circumcision, but not as a religious imperative	Strict kosher dietary laws with complex proscriptions and prescriptions for preparation Allowed only meat from animals that are vegetable eaters, are cloven hoofed, and chew their cud; fish that have scales and fins Prohibit any combination of meat and milk. Milk products served first can be followed by meat in a few minutes; not the reverse, however (Reform Jews usually do not observe kosher dietary restrictions) Fasting for 24 hours on Day of Atonement (Yom Kippur) and Tisha Bab Matzo replaces leavened bread during Passover week
	Death:	Remains are ritually washed by members of the Ritual Burial Society Burial should take place as soon as possible	
Lutheran	Birth:	Baptize only living infants 6 to 8 weeks after birth	No requirements or restrictions
	Death:	Last rites optional	
Mennonite	Birth:	No baptism in infancy Baptism during early or middle teens	No requirements or restrictions
Methodist	Birth:	No baptism at birth; performed on children or adults	No requirements or restrictions
	Death:	No ritual	
Nazarene	Birth:	Baptism optional	No requirements or restrictions Alcohol prohibited
	Death:	No last rites	
Pentecostal (Assembly of God, Four-square)	Birth:	No baptism at birth Baptism by complete immersion after age of accountability	Abstain from alcohol, eating blood, strangled animals, or anything to which blood has been added Some individuals may resist pork
	Death:	No last rites	
Orthodox Presbyterian	Birth:	Infant baptism by sprinkling*	No requirements or restrictions
	Death:	Last rites not a sacramental procedure; scripture reading and prayer	
Roman Catholic	Birth:	Infant baptism mandatory; especially urgent in poor prognosis, when it may be performed by anyone*	Fasting or abstaining from meat mandatory on Ash Wednesday and Good Friday; fasting optional during Lent; no meat on Fridays during Lent as general rule Most hospital patients exempt from fasting Some older Catholics may adhere to older rule of eating fish on Friday
	Death:	Rite for Annointing of the sick is mandatory Family or patient may request annointing if prognosis is grave	
Russian Orthodox	Birth:	Baptism by priest only	No meat or dairy products on Wednesday, Friday, and during Lent
	Death:	Traditionally after death arms are crossed, fingers set in a cross	
Unitarian Universalist	Birth:	Some practice infant baptism; most consider it unnecessary	No requirements or restrictions
	Death:	No ritual	

*See Baptism, p. 393.

BELIEFS REGARDING MEDICAL CARE	COMMENTS
May resist surgical procedures during Sabbath, which extends from sundown Friday until sundown Saturday Demand medical care for illness Seriously ill are exempt from fasting	Oppose all forms of mutilation, including autopsy; body parts not donated or removed, amputated limbs, organs, or surgically removed tissues should be made available to family for burial Donation or transplantation of organs requires rabbinical consent Generally oppose prolongation of life after irreversible brain damage
If grave prognosis, family may request annointing and blessing of sick or visit by church official	Accept scientific developments
No illness rituals Deep concern for dignity and self-determination of individual that would conflict with shock treatment or medical treatment affecting personality or will	
Communion may be requested before surgery or similar crisis	Encourage donation of body or body parts to medical science
Church official administers communion and laying on of hands Adherents believe in divine healing but not exclusive of medical treatment	Cremation permitted
No restrictions regarding medical care Deliverance from sickness is provided for in atonement; may pray for divine intervention in health matters and seek God in prayer for themselves and others when ill	Some insist illness is divine punishment; most consider it an intrusion of Satan
Communion administered when appropriate and convenient Blood transfusion accepted when advisable Pastor or elder should be called for ill person Believe science should be used for relief of suffering	Full forgiveness granted for any illness connected with a sin
Encourage anointing of sick, although this may be interpreted by older members of church as equivalent to the old terminology "extreme unction" or "last rites"; they may require careful explanation if reluctance associated with fear of imminent death	Family may request that major amputated limb be buried in consecrated ground Transplant accepted as long as loss of organ does not deprive donor of life or functional integrity of body Autopsy acceptable Religious articles important
Cross necklace is important and should be removed only when necessary and replaced as soon as possible Adherents believe in divine healing, but not exclusive of medical treatment	Opposed to autopsy, embalming, or cremation
Believe God helps those who help themselves Some may prefer not to have clergy visit them in hospital	Cremation preferred to burial

Table 2-5 Cultural characteristics related to health care of children

CULTURAL GROUP	HEALTH BELIEFS	HEALTH AND DIET PRACTICES
Asian Americans Chinese	A healthy body viewed as gift from parents and ancestors and must be cared for Health is one of the results of balance between the forces of *yin* (cold) and *yang* (hot), energy forces that rule the world Illness caused by imbalance Believe blood is source of life and is not regenerated *Chi* is innate energy Lack of *chi* and blood results in deficiency that produces fatigue, poor constitution, and long illness	Goal of therapy is to restore balance of *yin* and *yang* Acupuncturist applies needles to appropriate meridians identified in terms of *yin* and *yang* Acupressure and *tai chi* replacing acupuncture in some areas Moxibustion is application of heat to skin over specific meridians Wide use of medicinal herbs procured and applied in prescribed ways Folk healers are herbalist, spiritual healer, temple healer, fortune healer Meals may or may not be planned to balance hot and cold Use of condiment, e.g., monosodium glutamate, may create difficulty with some diet regimens

Japanese	Three major belief systems:
	  Shinto religious influence
	    Humans inherently good
	    Evil caused by outside spirits
	    Illness caused by contact with polluting agents, e.g., blood, corpses, skin diseases
	  Chinese and Korean influence
	    Health achieved through harmony and balance between self and society
	    Disease caused by disharmony with society and not caring for body
	  Portuguese influence
	    Upholds germ theory of disease
		Believe evil removed by purification
		Energy restored by means of acupuncture, acupressure, massage, and moxibustion along affected meridians
		Kampō medicine—use of natural herbs
		Believe in removal of diseased parts
		Trend is to use both Western and Oriental healing methods
		Care for disabled viewed as family's responsibility
		Take pride in child's good health
		Seek preventive care, medical care for illness
		Older persons avoid some food combinations (e.g., milk and cherries, watermelon and crab) and believe pickled plums to have special properties

Vietnamese	Good health considered to be balance between *yin* (cold) and *yang* (hot) Believe person's life has been predisposed toward certain phenomena by cosmic forces Health believed to be result of harmony with existing universal order, harmony attained by pleasing good spirits and avoiding evil ones Belief in *am duc*, the amount of good deeds accumulated by ancestors Many use rituals to prevent illness Practice some restrictions to prevent incurring wrath of evil spirits	Family uses all means possible before using outside agencies for health care Fortune-tellers determine event that caused disturbance May visit temple to procure divine instruction Use astrologer to calculate cyclical changes and forces Regard health as family responsibility; outside aid sought when resources run out Certain illnesses considered only temporary (such as pustules, open wounds) and ignored Seek generalist health healers May use special diets to prevent illness and promote health Lactose intolerance prevalent
Filipino	Believe God's will and supernatural forces govern universe Illness, accidents, and other misfortunes are God's punishment for violations of His will Widely accept "hot" and "cold" balance and imbalance as cause of health and illness	Some use amulets as a shield from witchcraft or as good luck pieces Catholics substitute religious medals and other items

Sources: Bloch, 1983; Chen-Louie, 1983; Chow, 1976; Char, 1981; Ehling, 1981; Greathouse and Miller, 1981; Hashizume and Takano, 1983; Holland and Sweeney, 1985; Hoolingsworth, Brown, and Brooten, 1980; Jacques, 1976; Lacay, 1981; Monrroy, 1983; Orque, 1983; Sodetaini-Shebata, 1981.

FAMILY RELATIONSHIPS	COMMUNICATION	COMMENTS
Extended family pattern common Strong concept of loyalty of young to old Respect for elders taught at early age—acceptance without questioning or talking back Children's behavior a reflection on family Family and individual honor and "face" important Self-reliance and self-restraint highly valued; self-expression repressed Males valued more highly than females; women submissive to men in family	Open expression of emotions unacceptable Often smile when do not comprehend	Do not react well to often painful diagnostic workup; are especially upset by drawing of blood Deep respect for their bodies and belief it best to die with bodies intact; therefore may refuse surgery Believe in reincarnation Older members fear hospitals; often believe hospital is a place to go to die Children sometimes breast-fed for up to 4 or 5 years Milk intolerance relatively common
Close intergenerational relationships Family provides anchor Family tends to keep problems to self Value self-control and self-sufficiency Concept of *haji* (shame) imposes strong control; unacceptable behavior of children reflects on family Many adopt practices of contemporary middle class Concern for child's missing school may result in sending to school before fully recovered from illness	*Issei*—born in Japan; usually speak Japanese only *Nisei, Sansei,* and *Yonsei* have few language difficulties New immigrants able to read and write English better than to speak or understand it Make significant use of nonverbal communication with subtle gestures and facial expression Tend to suppress emotions Will often wait silently	Generational categories: *Issei*—1st generation to live in U.S. *Nisei*—2nd generation *Sansei*—3rd generation *Yonsei*—4th generation *Issei* and *Nisei*—tolerant and permissive childrearing until 5 or 6, then emphasis on emotional reserve and control Cleanliness highly valued Time considered valuable and used wisely Tendency to practice emotional control may make assessment of pain more difficult
Family is revered institution Multigenerational families Family is chief social network Children highly valued Individual needs and interests are subordinate to those of family group Father is main decision maker Women taught submission to men Parents expect respect and obedience from children	Many immigrants are not proficient in speaking and understanding English May hesitate to ask questions Questioning authority is sign of disrespect; asking questions considered impolite Use indirectness rather than forthrightness in expressing disagreement May avoid eye contact with health professionals as a sign of respect	Consider status more important than money Children taught emotional control Time concept more relaxed—consider punctuality less significant than other values, i.e., propriety Place high value on social harmony
Family is highly valued with strong family ties Multigenerational family structure common, often with collateral members as well Personal interests are subordinated to family interests and needs Members avoid any behavior that would bring shame on the family	Immigrants and older persons may not be able to speak or understand English	Tend to have a fatalistic outlook on life Believe time and providence will solve all

Continued.

Table 2-5 Cultural characteristics related to health care of children—cont'd

CULTURAL GROUP	HEALTH BELIEFS	HEALTH AND DIET PRACTICES

American black	Illness classified as:
	   Natural—affected by forces of nature without adequate protection, e.g., cold air, pollution, food and water
	   Unnatural—evil influences, e.g., witchcraft, voodoo, hoodoo, hex, fix, rootwork; symptoms often associated with eating
	Believe illness sent by God as punishment, e.g., parents punished by illness or death of child
	Believe serious illness can be avoided
	May resist health care because illness is "will of God"
		Self-care and folk medicine very prevalent
		Folk therapies usually religious in origin
		Attempt home remedies first; poorer people do not seek help until illness serious
		Usually seek help from:
		   "Old lady"—woman in community with a common knowledge of herbs; consults regarding pediatric care
		   Spiritualist—has received gift from God for healing incurable diseases or solving personal problems; strongly based in Christianity
		   Priest (voodoo priest/priestess)—most powerful healer
		   Root doctor—meet need for herbs, oils, candles, and ointments
		Prayer is common means for prevention and treatment

Hispanic American Mexican-American (Latino, Chicano, Raza-Latino)	Health beliefs have strong religious association Believe in body imbalance as a cause of illness, especially imbalance between *caliente* (hot) and *frio* (cold) or "wet" and "dry" Some maintain good health is a result of "good luck"—a reward for good behavior Illness prevented by performing properly, eating proper foods, and working proper amount of time; accomplished through prayer, wearing religious medals or amulets, and sleeping with relics at home Illness is a punishment from God for wrongdoing, forces of nature, and the supernatural	Seek help from *curandero* or *curandera*, especially in rural areas Curandero(a) receives his/her position by birth, apprenticeship, or a "calling" via dream or vision Treatments involve use of herbs, rituals, and religious artifacts Practice for severe illness—make promises, visit shrines, offer medals and candles, offer prayers Adhere to "hot" and "cold" food prescriptions and prohibitions for prevention and treatment of illness
Puerto Rican	Subscribe to the "hot-cold" theory of causation of illness Believe some illness caused by evil spirits and forces	Infrequent use of health care systems Seek folk healers—use of herbs, rituals Consult spiritualist medium for mental disorders *Santeria* is system and practitioners are called *santeros* Treatments classified as "hot" or "cold"

Native American (numerous tribes)	Believe health is state of harmony with nature and universe
	Respect of bodies through proper management
	All disorders believed to have aspects of supernatural
	Violation of a restriction or prohibition thought to cause illness
	Fear of witchcraft
	May carry objects believed to guard against witchcraft
	Theology and medicine strongly interwoven
		Medicine persons:
		   Altruistic persons who must use powers in purely positive ways
		   Persons capable of both good and evil—perform negative acts against enemies
		   Diviner-diagnosticians—diagnose but do not have powers or skill to implement medical treatment
		   Specialists—use herbs and curative but nonsacred medical procedures
		   Medicine persons—use herbs and ritual
		   Singers—cure by the power of their song obtained from supernatural beings, effect cures by laying on of hands

FAMILY RELATIONSHIPS	COMMUNICATION	COMMENTS
Strong kinship bonds in extended family; members come to aid of others in crisis Less likely to view illness as a burden Augmented families common (unrelated persons living in same household) Place strong emphasis on work and ambition	Alert to any evidence of discrimination Place importance on nonverbal behavior May use nonstandard English or "black English" Use "testing" behaviors to assess personnel in health care situations before seeking active care May use more paranoid responses than other groups Best to use simple, direct, but caring approach	High level of caution and distrust of majority group Social anxiety related to tradition of humiliation, oppression, and loss of dignity Will elect to retain dignity rather than seek care if values are compromised Strong sense of peoplehood High incidence of poverty Black minister a strong influence in black community Visits by family minister are sought, expected, and valued in helping to cope with illness and suffering
Traditionally men considered breadwinners, women homemakers Males are considered big and strong (*macho*) Strong kinship; extended families include *compadres* (godparents) established by ritual kinship Children valued highly and desired, taken everywhere with family Many homes contain shrines with statues and pictures of saints	May use nonstandard English Most bilingual; many only speak Spanish May have a strong preference for native language and revert to it in times of stress	High degree of modesty—often a deterrent to seeking medical care Youngsters often reluctant to share communal showers in schools Relaxed concept of time—may be late for appointments Magicoreligious practices common May view hospital as place to go to die
Family usually large and home-centered—the core of existence Father has complete authority in family—family provider and decision-maker Wife and children subordinate to father Children valued—seen as a gift from God Children taught to obey and respect parents; corporal punishment to ensure obedience	May use nonstandard English Spanish speaking or bilingual Strong sense of family privacy—may view questions regarding family as impudent	Relaxed sense of time Pay little attention to *exact* time of day Suspicious and fearful of hospitals
Extended family structure—usually includes relatives from both sides of family Elder members assume leadership roles	Most continue to speak their Indian language as well as English Nonverbal communication	Time orientation—present Respect for age Going to hospital associated with illness or disease; therefore may not seek prenatal care since pregnancy viewed as natural process

ATTITUDE OF THE NURSE

To begin to understand and to deal effectively with families in a multicultural community or in a unicultural community that is different from one's own, it is most important that nurses be aware of their own attitudes and values regarding a way of life, including health practices. Nurses, too, are a product of their own cultural background and education. Frequently, nurses and other health care workers are not aware of their own cultural values and how those values influence their thoughts and actions. Those who are aware of their own culturally founded behavior are more sensitive to cultural behavior in others. To recognize that a behavior may be characteristic of a culture rather than an "abnormal" behavior places nurses at an advantage in their relationships with families. When nurses respect cultural differences of a family, they are able to postpone judgment until it is determined whether the behavior is distinctive to the individual or a characteristic of the culture. What appears to be puzzling behavior may simply be the customary response in the culture (e.g., expression of emotion).

Cultural standards and values, the family structure and function, and past experiences with health care influence a family's feelings and attitudes toward health, their children, and health care delivery systems. It is often difficult for nurses to be nonjudgmental and objective in working with families whose behaviors and attitudes differ from or conflict with their own. To be aware of one's own feelings and attitudes as well as to respect those of the family are essential to a helping relationship and achievement of nursing goals. To rely on one's own values and experiences for guidance can result only in frustration and disappointment. It is one thing to know what is needed to deal with a health problem; it is often quite another to implement a fruitful course of action unless nurses work within the cultural and socioeconomic framework of the family.

It is beneficial to make an effort to adapt ethnic practices to the health needs of the family rather than attempt to change long-standing beliefs. To aid their efforts to understand and respect the cultural beliefs of families, nurses should have a readily available resource file containing pertinent information about the cultural and subcultural characteristics of the community in which they practice (e.g., traditional practices related to infant feeding practices and the time and manner of weaning and toilet training). Bridging cultural gaps in delivery of health care to children requires the establishment of a close relationship with families and other influential persons in the community (such as the local folk healer) and periodic assessment of one's own attitudes and behaviors and those of other health workers toward people of other racial or ethnic origins.

Some characteristics of selected cultures are outlined in Table 2-5.

CONCEPT SUMMARIES

- Nurses have a responsibility to understand how culture affects the development of social and emotional relationships, childrearing practices, and attitudes toward health.

- Culture is defined as "acquired knowledge people use to interpret experience and generate behavior."

- Race is "a division of mankind possessing traits that are transmissible by descent and sufficient to characterize it as a distinct human type."

- Ethnicity is the affiliation of a set of persons who share a unique cultural, social, and linguistic background.

- Socialization is the process by which children acquire the beliefs, values, and behaviors considered desirable or appropriate by the culture.

- A culture is composed of individuals with a set of values, beliefs, practices, and information that is learned, integrative, social, and satisfying.

- A child's self-concept evolves from ideas about his social roles.

- Primary groups are characterized by intimate contact, mutual support, and behavior constraint among members.

- Secondary groups have limited intermittent contact, little mutual support, and no pressure for conformity.

- Guilt and shame are two behaviors commonly conditioned in children to control social behavior.

- Important subcultural influences on children include ethnicity, social class, poverty, affluence, occupation, religion, schools, peers, and biculture.

- A trend that has significantly influenced the American family is increasing geographic and economic mobility.

- Membership in a minority group presents special challenges for children, although changes in societal attitudes are slowly taking place.

- Cultural shock refers to a person's feeling of helplessness and disorientation while trying to adapt to a different cultural group and its practices, values, and beliefs.

- Hereditary and socioeconomic forces play an important role in a child's susceptibility to health problems.

- Drug response, food sensitivity, disease resistance, physical characteristics, and disease states may demonstrate ethnic or cultural variations.

- Because verbal and nonverbal communication is an important cultural consideration, nurses need to acknowledge and respect their patients' practices in order for productive interaction to occur.

- Cultural beliefs related to cause of illness and maintenance of health may focus on natural forces, supernatural forces, or imbalance of forces.

- In planning and implementing patient care, nurses need to strive to adapt ethnic practices to the family's health needs rather than attempt to change long-standing beliefs.

REFERENCES

Abril, I.F.: Mexican-American folk beliefs: how they affect health care, Am. J. Maternal Child Nurs. **2:**168-173, 1977.

Asnes, R.S., and Wisotsky, D.H.: Cupping lesions simulating child abuse, J. Pediatr. **99:**267-268, 1981.

Baca, J.E.: Some health beliefs of the Spanish speaking. In Martinez, R.A., editor: Hispanic culture and health care, St. Louis, 1978, The C.V. Mosby Co.

Bauwens, E., and Anderson, S.: Social and cultural influences on health care. In Stanhope, M., and Lancaster, J.: Community health nursing, St. Louis, 1984, The C.V. Mosby Co.

Beliefs that can affect therapy, Pediatr. Nurs. **5**(3):40-43, 1979.

Bloch, B.: Nursing care of black patients. In Orque, M.S., Bloch, B., and Monrroy, L.S.A.: Ethnic nursing care, St. Louis, 1983, The C.V. Mosby Co.

Bloch, B., and Hunter, M.L.: Teaching physiological assessment of black persons, Nurse Educator **6**(1):24-27, 1981.

Brownlee A.T.: Community, culture, and care, St. Louis, 1978, The C.V. Mosby Co.

Bullough, B., and Bullough, V.: Poverty, ethnic identity, and health care, New York, 1972, Appleton-Century-Crofts.

Carpenito, L.J.: Nursing diagnosis: application to clinical practice, Philadelphia, 1983, J.B. Lippincott Co.

Char, E.L.: The Chinese American. In Clark, A.L., editor: Culture and childrearing, Philadelphia, 1981, F.A. Davis Co.

Chen-Louie, T.: Nursing care of Chinese American patients. In Orque, M.S., Bloch, B., and Monrroy, L.S.A.: Ethnic nursing care, St. Louis, 1983, The C.V. Mosby Co.

Chow, E.: Cultural health traditions: Asian perspectives. In Branch, M.F., and Paxon, P.P., editors: Providing safe nursing care for ethnic people of color, New York, 1976, Appleton-Century-Crofts.

Clark, A.L., editor: Culture and childrearing, Philadelphia, 1981, F.A. Davis Co.

Cohen, F.L.: Clinical genetics in nursing practice, Philadelphia, 1984, J.B. Lippincott Co.

Cole, J.B.: Culture: negro, black, and nigger, Black Scholar **1:**40-44, 1970.

Ehling, M.B.: The Mexican American (El Chicano). In Clark, A.L., editor: Culture and childrearing, Philadelphia, 1981, F.A. Davis Co.

Feldman, K.W.: Pseudoabusive burns in Asian refugees, Am. J. Dis. Child **138:**768-769, 1984.

Flynn, B.C., and Miller, M.H.: Current perspectives in nursing: social issues and trends, St. Louis, 1980, The C.V. Mosby Co.

Greathouse, B., and Miller, V.G.: The black American. In Clark, A.L., editor: Culture and childrearing, Philadelphia, 1981, F.A. Davis Co.

Grinker, R.R.: The poor rich: the children of the super-rich, Am. J. Psychiatry **135:**913-916, 1978.

Hashizume, S., and Takano, J.: Nursing care of Japanese patients. In Orque, M.S., Bloch, B., and Monrroy, L.S.A.: Ethnic nursing care, St. Louis, 1983, The C.V. Mosby Co.

Henderson, G., and Premeaux, M., editors: Transcultural health care, Menlo Park, CA, 1981, Addison-Wesley Publishing Co.

Holland, S., and Sweeney, E.: Vietnamese children and families: the impact of culture, Washington, DC, 1985, Association for Care of Children's Health.

Holland, W.R.: Mexican American medical beliefs: science or magic? In Martinez, R.A., editor: Hispanic culture and health care, St. Louis, 1978, The C.V. Mosby Co.

Hollingsworth, A.O., Brown, L.P., and Brooten, D.A.: The refugees and childbearing: what to expect, RN **43**(11):45-48, 1980.

Jacques, G.: Cultural traditions: a black perspective In Branch, M.F., and Paxton, P.P.: Providing safe nursing care for ethnic people of color, New York, 1976, Appleton-Century-Crofts.

Lacay, G.: The Puerto Rican in mainland America. In Clark, A.L., editor: Culture and childrearing, Philadelphia, 1981, F.A. Davis Co.

Leacock, E.: The culture of poverty: a critique, New York, 1971, Simon & Schuster.

Leininger, M.: Transcultural nursing, New York, 1978, John Wiley & Sons.

Leslie, G.R.: The family in social context, ed. 5, New York, 1982, Oxford University Press.

Lewis, O.: The children of Sanchez, New York, 1961, Random House, Inc.

Malina, R.M.: Skinfolds in American negro and white children, Am. J. Diet. Assoc. **59:**34-40, 1971.

Meleis, A.I.: The Arab American in the health care system, Am. J. Nurs. **81:**1180-1183, 1981.

Murillo-Rohde, I.: Health care for the Hispanic patient, Crit. Care Update **7**(5):29-36, 1980.

O'Brien, M.E.: Pragmatic survivalism: behavior patterns affecting low-level wellness among minority group members, Adv. Nurs. Sci. **4**(3):13-26, 1982.

Orque, M.S.: Nursing care of Filipino American patients. In Orque, M.S., Bloch, B., and Monrroy, L.S.A.: Ethnic nursing care, St. Louis, 1983, The C.V. Mosby Co.

Orque, M.S.: Nursing care of South Vietnamese patients. In Orque, M.S., Bloch, B., and Monrroy, L.S.A.: Ethnic nursing care, St. Louis, 1983, The C.V. Mosby Co.

Overfield, T.: Biologic variation: concepts from physical anthropology, Nurs. Clin. North Am. **12:**19-26, 1977.

Pasquale, E.A.: The evil eye phenomenon, Home Health Care Nurse **2**(3):32-35, 1984.

Salzer, J.L., and Nelson, N.A.: Health care of Ethiopian refugees, Pediatr. Nurs. **9:**449-452, 1983.

Schwartz, A.J.: The schools and socialization, New York, 1975, Harper & Row, Publishers, Inc.

Shaffer, D.C.: Developmental psychology: theory, research and application, Monterey, CA, 1985, Brooks/Cole Publishing Co.

Sodetani-Shibata, A.E.: The Japanese American. In Clark, A.L., editor: Culture and childrearing, Philadelphia, 1981, F.A. Davis Co.

Spradley, B.W.: Community health nursing, Boston, 1981, Little, Brown & Co.

Spector, R.E.: Cultural diversity in health and illness, New York, 1979, Appleton-Century-Crofts.

Steffen, M.L., and Francis, J.: Transcultural nursing experiences and care with migrant children. In Leininger, M.: Transcultural nursing: concepts, theories, and practice, New York, 1978, John Wiley & Sons.

Stringfellow, L., Liem, N.D., and Liem, L.D.: The Vietnamese in America. In Clark, A.L., editor: Culture and childrearing, Philadelphia, 1981, F.A. Davis Co.

Tseng, W., and others: Cross-cultural differences in parent-child assessment: U.S.A and Japan, Int. J. Soc. Psychiatry **28:**305-317, 1982.

Valentine, C.A.: Culture and poverty, Chicago, 1968, University of Chicago Press.

Valentine, C.A.: Deficit, difference, and bicultural models of Afro-American behavior, Harvard Educ. Rev. **41:**141-144, 1971.

Webster's New Collegiate Dictionary, 1973.

Werner, E.E.: Cross-cultural child development: a view from the planet earth, Monterey, CA, 1979, Brooks/Cole Publishing Co.

Wilson, U.M.: Nursing care of American Indian patients. In Orque, M.S., Bloch, B., and Monrroy, L.S.A.: Ethnic nursing care, St. Louis, 1983, The C.V. Mosby Co.

BIBLIOGRAPHY
General

Anderson, A.B., and Frideres, J.S.: Ethnicity in Canada: Theoretical perspectives, Toronto, 1981, Butterworths.

Bauwens, E.E.: The anthropology of health, St. Louis, 1978, The C.V. Mosby Co.

Bauwens, E.E., and Anderson, S.: Social and cultural influences on health care. In Stanhope, M., and Lancaster, J.: Community health nursing, St. Louis, 1984, The C.V. Mosby Co.

Beliefs that can affect therapy, Pediatr. Nurs. **5**(3):40-43, 1979.

Bonaparte, B.: Ego defensiveness, open-closed mindedness, and nurses' attitude toward culturally different patients, Nurs. Res. **28**:166-172, 1979.

Brink, P.J.: Value orientations as an assessment tool in cultural diversity, Nurs. Res. **33**:198-203, 1984.

Bullough, V.L., and Bullough, B.: Health care for the other Americans, New York, 1982, Appleton-Century-Crofts.

Carpio, B.: The adolescent immigrant, Can. Nurse **7**(3):27-29, 1981.

Chen-Louie, T.T.: Bicultural experiences, social interactions, and health care implications. In Reinhardt, A.M., and Quinn, M.D., editors: Family-centered community nursing, vol. 2, St. Louis, 1980, The C.V. Mosby Co.

DeFriese, G.H., and Hetherington, J.S.: Child health and the problem of access to care, Fam. Commun. Health **4**(3):71-83, 1982.

DeGracia, R.T.: Cultural influences on Filipino patients, Am. J. Nurs. **79**:1412-1414, 1979.

Dobson, S.: Bringing culture into care, Nurs. Times **78**:2106-2109, 1982.

Flynn, B.C., and Miller, M.H.: Current perspectives in nursing: societal issues and trends, St. Louis, 1980, The C.V. Mosby Co.

Fong, C.M: Ethnicity and nursing practice, Topics Clin. Nurs. **7**(3):1-10, 1985.

Frenkel, S.I. and others: Does patient contact change racial perceptions? Am. J. Nurs. **80**:1340-1342, 1980.

Germain, C.P.: Cultural concepts in critical care, Crit. Care. Q.**5**(3):61-78, 1982.

Harwood, A., editor: Ethnicity and medical care, Cambridge, MA, 1981, Harvard University Press.

Hautman, M.A., and Harrison, J.K.: Health beliefs and practices in a middle-income Anglo-American neighborhood, Adv. Nurs. Sci. **4**(3):49-63, 1982.

Idler, E.L.: Definitions of health and illness, Soc. Sci. Med. **13A**:723-731, 1979.

Johnston, M.: Cultural variations in professional and parenting practices, J. Obstet. Gynecol. Nurs. **9**:9-13, 1980.

Johnston, M.: Folk beliefs and ethnocultural behavior in pediatrics, medicine or magic, Nurs. Clin. North Am. **12**:77-84, 1977.

Kleinman, A.: Patients and healers in the context of culture, Berkeley, 1980, University of California Press.

Kleinman, A., and others: Culture, illness and care: clinical lessons from anthropologic and cross-cultural research, Ann. Intern. Med. **88**:251-258, 1978.

Kozier, B., and Erb, G.: Fundamentals of nursing, ed. 2, Menlo Park, CA, 1983, Addison-Wesley Publishing Co.

Kubricht, D.W., and Clark, J.A.: Foreign patients: a system for providing care, Nurs. Outlook **30**:55-57, 1982.

LaFargue, J.P.: Mediating between two views of illness, Topics Clin. Nurs. **7**(3):70-77, 1985.

Lash, M.E.: Community health nursing in a minority setting, Nurs. Clin. North Am. **15**(2):339-348, 1980.

Leininger, M.: Cultural diversities of health and nursing care, Nurs. Clin. North Am. **12**:5-18, 1977.

Linley, J.F.: Mothers' attitudes regarding health care for their children, J. Maternal Child Health **9**:37-39, 1984.

Lipson, J.G., and Meleis, A.I.: Culturally appropriate care: the case of immigrants, Topics Clin. Nurs. **7**(3):48-56, 1985.

Louie, K.B.: Transcending cultural bias: the literature speaks, Topics Clin. Nurs. **7**(3):78-84, 1985.

Low, S.M.: The cultural basis of health, illness and disease, Soc. Work Health Care **9**(3):13-23, 1984.

Mandelbaum, J.K.: The food square: helping people of different cultures understand balanced diets, Pediatr. Nurs. **9**:20-21, 1985.

Marchant, R.: Caring for hospitalized inner-city children, Pediatr. Nurs. **11**:129-131, 1985.

Noble, G.P.: Social considerations in northern health care, Can. Nurs. **74**:16, 18, 1978.

O'Brien, M.E.: Transcultural nursing research—alien in an alien land, Image **13**:37-39, 1981.

Orque, M.S., Bloch, B., and Monrroy, L.S.A.: Ethnic nursing care, St. Louis, 1983, The C.V. Mosby Co.

Ruiz, M.C.J.: Open-mindedness, intolerance of ambiguity and nursing faculty attitudes toward culturally different patients, Nurs. Res. **30**:177-181, 1981.

Shubin, S.: Nursing patients from difference cultures, Nursing 80 **10**(6):78-81, 1980.

Stern, P.N.: Solving problems of cross-cultural health teaching, Image **13**:47-50, 1981.

Sue, D.W., and Sue, D.: Barriers to effective cross-cultural counseling, J. Counsel. Psychol. **24**:420-424, 1977.

Tripp-Reimer, T.: Research in cultural diversity, West. J. Nurs. Res. **6**:353-355, 1984.

Tripp-Reimer, T., Brink, P.J., and Saunders, J.M.: Cultural assessment: content and process, Nurs. Outlook **32**:78-82, 1984.

White, E.H.: Giving health care to minority patients, Nurs. Clin. North Am. **12**:27-40, 1977.

Socioeconomics

Henry, B.M., and DiGiacomo-Geffers, E.: The hospitalized rich and famous, Am. J. Nurs. **80**:1426-1429, 1980.

Mason, D.J.: Perspectives on poverty, Image **13**:82-85, 1981.

O'Brien, M.E.: Reaching the migrant worker, Am. J. Nurs. **83**:895-897, 1983.

Wingert, W.A., and Halfman, L.P.: Migrant health question, Pediatr. Nurs. **5**(6):19-20, 1979.

Religion

D'Antonio, W.V.: The American Catholic family: signs of cohesion and polarization, J. Marriage Family **47**:395-402, 1985.

Ellis, D.: What happened to the spiritual dimension? Can. Nurs. **76**(9):42-43, 1980.

Gershan, J.A.: Judaic ethical beliefs and customs regarding death and dying, Crit. Care Nurse **5**(1):32-34, 1985.

Kim, M.J., McFarland, G.K., and McLane, A.M., editors: Classification of nursing diagnosis: proceedings of the Fifth National Conference, St. Louis, 1984, The C.V. Mosby Co.

Shelly, J.A.: Spiritual care: Planting seeds of hope, Crit. Care Update **9**(2):7-15, 1982.

Stoll, R.T.: Guidelines for spiritual assessment, Am. J. Nurs. **79**:1574-1577, 1979.

Thornton, A.: Reciprocal influences of family and religion in a changing world, J. Marriage Family **47**:381-394, 1985.

Ethnic Groups: Asian American

Aquino, C.J.: The Filipino in America. In Clark, A.L., editor: Culture and childrearing, Philadelphia, 1981, F.A. Davis Co.

Aslam, M., and others: Asian medicine: in the best tradition? The unani system of classifying food and disease as hot or cold, Nurs. Mirror **153**:34-36, July 22, 1981.

Brown, B.S.: Growing up healthy: the Chinese experience, Pediatr. Nurs. **9**:255-257, 1983.

DeGracia, R.T.: Cultural influences on Filipino patients, Am. J. Nurs. **79**:1412-1414, 1979.

DeGracia, R.T.: Health care of the American Asian patient, Crit. Care Update **6**(12):19-28, 1979.

Dung, T.N.: Understanding Asian families: a Vietnamese perspective, Child. Today **13**(2):1012, 1984.

Egan, M.G.: A family assessment challenge: refugee youth and foster family adaptation, Topics Clin. Nurs. **7**(3):64-69, 1985.

Floriani, C.M.: Southeast Asian refugees: life in a camp. Am. J. Nurs. **80**:2028-2030, 1980.

Gordon, V.C., Matousek, I.M., and Lang, T.A.: Southeast Asian refugees: life in America, Am. J. Nurs. **80**:2031-2036, 1980.

Grosso, C., and others: The Vietnamese American family . . . and grandma makes three, Am. J. Maternal Child Nurs. **6**:177-180, 1981.

Joe, V.: A new lifestyle in a new land, the Can. Nurse **7**(3):6-10, 1981.

Kwok, A.W.H.: Culture conflict: a study of the problems of Chinese immigrant adolescents in Canada, Can. Nurs. **78**(3):32-34, 1982.

Leyn, R.B.: The challenge of caring for child refugees from Southeast Asia, Am. J. Maternal Child Nurs. **3**:178-182, 1978.

Muecke, M.A.: Caring for Southeast Asian refugee patients in the USA, Am. J. Public Health **73**:431-438, 1983.

Pickwell, S.M.: Primary health care for Indochinese refugee children, Pediatr. Nurs. **8**:104-107, 1982.

Rocereto, L.V.: Selected health beliefs of Vietnamese refugees, J. School Health **51**:63-64, 1981

Rorabaugh, M.L.: The pediatric nurse practitioner in Southeast Asia: a personal account, Pediatr. Nurs. **9**:263-266, 1983.

Schultz, S.L.: How Southeast-Asian refugees in California adapt to unfamiliar health care practices, Health Soc. Work **7**:148-156, 1982.

Stern, P.N.: Solving problems of cross-cultural health teaching: the Filipino childbearing family, Image **13**:47-50, 1981.

Yeatman, W., and Dang, V.: Coa Gia (coin rubbing), JAMA **244**:2748-2749, 1980.

Ethnic Groups: Black American

Capers, C.F.: Nursing and the Afro-American client, Topics Clin. Nurs. **7**(3):11-17, 1985.

Levy, D.R.: White doctors and black patients: influence of race on the doctor-patient relationship, Pediatrics **75**(4):639-643, 1985.

Powers, B.A.: The use of orthodox and black American folk medicine, Adv. Nurs. Sci. **4**(3):35-47, 1982.

Roberson, M.H.B.: The influence of religious beliefs on health choices of Afro-Americans, Topics Clin. Nurs. **7**(3):57-63, 1985.

Stokes, L.G.: Delivering health services in a black community. In Reinhardt, AM., and Quinn, M.D., editors: Current practice in family-centered community nursing, St. Louis, 1977, The C.V. Mosby Co.

Ethnic Groups: Hispanic American

Brown, M.S.: How to cure the "evil eye," Nursing 75 **5**(7):66H, 1975.

Chesney, A.P., and others: Mexican American folk medicine: implications for the family physician, J. Fam. Pract. **11**:567-574, 1980.

daSilva, G.C.: Awareness of Hispanic cultural issues in the health care setting, Assoc. Care Child. Health **13**(1):4-10, 1984.

Foreman, J.T.: *Susto* and the health needs of the Cuban refugee population, Topics Clin. Nurs. **7**(3):40-47, 1985.

Gonzales-Swafford, M.J.: Ethno-medical beliefs and practices of Mexican-Americano, Nurs. Pract. **8**(10):29-30, 32, 34, 1983.

Guendelman, S.: At risk: health needs of Hispanic children, Health Soc. Work **10**:183-190, 1985.

Guendelman, S.: Developing responsiveness to the health needs of Hispanic children and families, Soc. Work Health Care **8**(4):1-15, 1983.

Herrera, T., and Wagner, N.N.: Behavioral approaches to delivering health services in a Chicano community. In Reinhardt, A.M., and Quinn, M.D., editors: Current practice in family-centered community nursing, St. Louis, 1977, The C.V. Mosby Co.

Mardiros, M.: A view toward hospitalization: the Mexican American experience, J. Adv. Nurs. **9**:469-478, 1984.

Martinez, R., editor: Hispanic culture and health care—fact, fiction, folklore, St. Louis, 1978, The C.V. Mosby Co.

Richardson, L.: Breakthrough to nursing, Part 2: Folk medicine in a Hispanic population, Imprint **29**:72-77, 1982.

Tamez, E.G.: Familism, machismo, and child rearing practices among Mexican Americans, J. Psychosoc. Nurs. **19**(9):21-25, 1981.

Zepeda, M.: Selected maternal-infant care practices of Spanish-speaking women, J. Obstet. Gynecol. Nurs. **11**:371-374, 1982.

Ethnic Groups: Native American

Backup, R.W.: Health care of the American Indian patient, Crit. Care Update **7**(2):16-22, 1980.

Kniep-Hardy, M., and Burkhardt, M.A.: Nursing the Navajo, Am. J. Nurs. **77**:95-96, 1977.

Primeaux, M.: Caring for the American Indian patient, Am. J. Nurs. **77**:91-94, 1977.

Primeaux, M.H.: American Indian health care practices; a cross-cultural perspective, Nurs. Clin. North Am. **12**:55-65, 1977.

Rosenblum, E.H.: Conversation with a Navajo nurse, Am. J. Nurs. **80**:1459-1461, 1980.

Satz, K.J.: Integrating Navajo tradition into maternal-child nursing, Image **14**:89-91, 1982.

Ethnic Groups: Other Cultures

Drakulic, L., and Tanaka, W.: The east indian family in Canada. Can. Nurse **7**(3):24-26, 1981.

Gershan, J.A.: Judaic ethical beliefs and customs regarding death and dying, Crit. Care Nurs. **5**:32-34, 1985.

Macdonald, A.C.: Folk health practices among north costal Peruvians: implications for nursing, Image **13**:51-55, 1981.

Meleis, A.I., and Sorrell, L.: Arab American women and their birth experiences, Am. J. Maternal Child Nurs. **6**:171-176, 1981.

Tripp-Reimer, T.: Barriers to health care: variations in interpretation of Appalachian client behavior by Appalachian and non-Appalachian health professionals, West. J. Nurs. Res. **4**:179-191, 1982.

Tripp-Reimer, T.: Retention of a folk-healing practice (matiasma) among four generations of urban Greek immigrants, Nurs. Res. **32**:97-101, 1983.

Tripp-Reimer, T., and Friedl, M.C.: Appalachians: a neglected minority, Nurs. Clin. North Am. **12**(1):41-54, 1977.

Wiggins, L.R.: Health and illness beliefs and practices among the Old Order Amish, Health Values **7**(6):24-29, 1983.

Chapter 3

Family Influences on Child Health Promotion

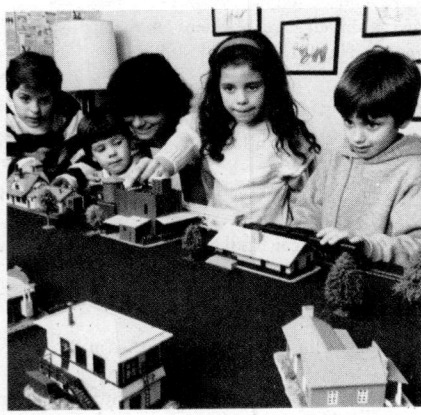

Family Theories
Developmental theory
Structural-functional theory
Interactional theory
Exchange theory
Systems theory
Conflict theory
Family Structure and Function
Functions of the family
Family structure
Nuclear family
Single-parent family
Binuclear family
Reconstituted family
Extended family
Polygamous family
Communal family
Gay family
Family structure and social class
Family Roles and Relationships
Parental roles
Role learning
Types of roles
Continuity and discontinuity
Role-structuring in children

Family size and configuration
Family size
Spacing of children
Sibling interaction
Ordinal position
Multiple births: twins
Parenting
Parenthood
Motivation for parenthood
Preparation for parenthood
Goals of parenting
Parental development
Transition to parenthood
Parental factors affecting transition to parenthood
Support systems
Essentials of parenting
Parenting behaviors
Dimensions of childrearing
Parental styles of control
Shaping behavior
Patterns of parental discipline
Disciplinary strategies
Age of the child
Communicating with children
Influence of the "experts"
Special Parenting Situations
Parenting the adopted child
Motivation
Sources of adoptive children
Preparation for adoption
Parenting adopted children
Special adoptive situations
Parenting and divorce
Impact of divorce on children
Developmental tasks
Custody and parenting partnerships
Single-parenting
Single fathers
Parenting in reconstituted families
Parenting in dual-career families
Working mothers

Societies, to maintain and perpetuate themselves, have established institutions designed for the express purpose of rearing and educating their children. The primary institution that accepts this responsibility is the family, and, as the basic interpersonal group, it is a universal characteristic of all human societies. The family provides each newborn member of society with legitimacy, that is, a family connection (usually symbolized by a family name) and an ascribed position in the societal strata. It serves as the link between individual members and the larger society (Johnson, 1984). Socialization patterns and the organization of roles and relationships within the community are largely determined in the context of the family (WHO, 1978).

Although the structure and subordinate goals of the family vary among and within cultures and change at different times and in different places, the overall purpose of the family is to provide for the future of a society and the stability of its culture. During the long time required for human infants to reach a level of independence, individual families assume the responsibility for their rearing, although such families differ considerably in form, complexity, and goals of socialization.

The term *family* has many meanings, has provided a fertile field for study, and has been defined in a number of ways and for a number of purposes according to the individual's own frame of reference, value judgment, or the discipline (Johnson, 1984). For example, biology describes the family as fulfilling the biologic function of perpetuation of the species. Psychology emphasizes the interpersonal aspects of the family and its responsibility for personality development. Economics views the family as a productive unit providing for material needs, while sociology depicts it as the social unit that reacts with the larger society. Others define family in relation to the persons that comprise the family unit: *consanguinal* (blood relationships), *affinal* (marriage relationships), and *fictive* (invented relationships, such as godparents or groups who call themselves a family). Still others attempt to describe the family as a combination of these elements or in terms of what a family ought to be.

There is no consensus regarding the definition of family. Helvie (1981) defines family as a "primary group of people living in a household in consistent proximity and intimate relationships." A similar definition describes family as "a small social system made up of individuals related to each other by reason of strong reciprocal affections and loyalties, and comprising a permanent household (or cluster of households) that persists over years and decades" (Terkelson, 1980). Probably one of the most all-encompassing definitions advanced describes family as "the coexistence of more than one human being involving continuous, presumably permanent, sharing of living facilities, a perception of reciprocal obligations, a sense of commonness, and sharing of certain obligations toward each other and towards others" (Mauksch, 1974).

Traditionally a family has been conceptualized as a group with the belief that both a mother and father are needed to rear a child. Nearly all societies grant a very high rank to the married status and, although this concept has undergone considerable modification, considerable emotion has been generated about some of the newer concepts of family—such as communal families, single-parent families, and homosexual families. To maintain the viability of the family, each culture has devised standards of familial behavior, systems that reward those who support or conform to these standards, and systems that punish those who do not.

Recently the concept of family has been broadened to include a variety of family styles and other combinations of persons sharing a common dwelling. Consequently, the term *household* has become the more descriptive term and one that is being used more frequently. According to this concept a household includes such nontraditional groups as (1) persons who have never married and who have no family or other form of union but who are members of a household, (2) the one-parent family consisting of a single parent and child(ren), (3) two homosexuals living together in a stable union, and (4) stable consensual unions, with or without

children (WHO, 1978). A household can also consist of a single, never-married person or married persons who choose not to have children. Although the concept of household is recognized and appreciated, the term *family* will be used consistently throughout this book to indicate the relationships between dependent children and one or more protective adults. It also implies relationships with other dependent selves, that is, siblings. Family members share a sense of belonging to their own family that deeply affects their lives.

Basically, families can be described as belonging to the following categories:

1. *The family of orientation.* The basic reproductive unit composed of a man and a woman with a fertile sexual relationship and their offspring—the family into which one is born.
2. *The family of procreation.* The family that an individual helps to form, usually by marriage, and in which he or she may become a parent.

Nevertheless, regardless of the way one chooses to define it, the composition of its membership, or the relationships among its members, a "family" is what the client considers it to be.

Family Theories

A theory can be described as a formulation concerning apparent relationships among certain observed phenomena that has been verified to some degree and, therefore, has predictive value. Numerous theories have been applied to families to describe and predict events and interactions; however, three have been identified that remain viable and readily distinguishable from one another: developmental theory, structural-functional theory, and interactional theory. Others include exchange theory, systems theory, and conflict theory.

DEVELOPMENTAL THEORY

Developmental theory is an outgrowth of several theories of development. Foremost among the developers are Duvall (1977), who described eight developmental tasks of the family throughout its life span, derived from Erikson's eight stages of man (see p. 113), and Rogers (1962), who incorporated role theory into the developmental concept. The family is described as a small group, semiclosed system of personalities that interacts with the larger cultural social system. As an interrelated system, changes do not occur in one part without a series of changes in other parts.

Developmental theory employs a family life-cycle approach to compare the changing structure, function, and roles of the family at various stages of development, focusing on time as the central dimension (Bower and Jacobson, 1978). The theory delineates developmental tasks for the family much like the individual developmental tasks dis-

Table 3-1 Duvall's development stages of the family

STAGES	TASKS
Stage I: Marriage and an independent home: the joining of families	Reestablish couple identity Realign relationships with extended family Make decisions regarding parenthood
Stage II: Families with infants	Integrate infants into the family unit Accommodate to new parenting and grandparenting roles Maintain the marital bond
Stage III: Families with preschoolers	Socialize children Parents and children adjust to separation
Stage IV: Families with school children	Children develop peer relations Parents adjust to their children's peer and school influence
Stage V: Families with teenagers	Adolescents develop increasing autonomy Parents refocus on midlife marital and career issues Parents begin a shift toward concern for the older generation
Stage VI: Families as launching centers	Parents and young adult establish independent identities Renegotiate marital relationship
Stage VII: Middle-aged families	Reinvest in couple identity with concurrent development of independent interests Realign relationships to include in-laws and grandchildren Deal with disabilities and death of older generation
Stage VIII: Aging families	Shift from work role to leisure and semiretirement or full retirement Maintain couple and individual functioning while adapting to the aging process Prepare for own death and dealing with the loss of spouse, and/or siblings, and other peers

Modified from Wright, L.M., and Leahey, M.: Nurses and Families: a guide to family assessment and intervention, Philadelphia, 1984, F.A. Davis Co.

cussed in relation to personality development. Central to the theory is an emphasis on individuals as persons as opposed to the roles they assume in and outside the family (see also Parental roles, p. 65).

Family developmental tasks are defined as those growth responsibilities that arise at a specific stage in the life of the family, which if successfully achieved, lead to satisfaction and success with later tasks, while failure leads to family unhappiness (Duvall, 1962). As in any other developmental task, the family meets and copes with each family task that arises at progressive stages in its life cycle. These stages are delineated on the basis of transitions and adjustments required by its members at each stage (Table 3-1). Although the family system as a whole is important, it depends on the behavior of its members, and achievement of family developmental tasks at each family life-cycle stage is interrelated with the simultaneous accomplishment of the individual developmental task of each member (Bower and Jacobson, 1978). Individual and family developmental tasks must be completed before other goal-directed tasks being attempted can be mastered.

STRUCTURAL-FUNCTIONAL THEORY

Structural-functional theory, one of the dominant orientations in modern sociology, has been most systematically applied by Parsons (Rodman, 1965). In analyzing families, this theory focuses less on family change and more on the interrelatedness, interdependence, and integration between family members and all aspects of society and its subcultures, particularly the occupational subsystem. *Structure* refers to the arrangement of roles that comprise a social system; *function* is the contribution made by an activity or role to the whole and the consequences of the activity for the system. The family is described as a social system with members that have specific roles and functions. The family process is directed toward maintaining an equilibrium between the complementary roles within the family—for example, husband-wife, father-daughter, mother-son, or wife–mother-in-law.

Internal relationships involve the division of labor between family members and the functions of these divisions for family maintenance. "Expressive" roles are seen in integrative or solidifying activities that bring emotional satisfaction to the family members. "Instrumental" roles are activities that occur external to the family but that also include satisfactory goal attainment of the family. Traditionally, expressive roles have been assigned to the wife-mother while the husband-father has assumed the instrumental roles. However, the classic breadwinner husband, homemaker wife, and two children now comprise only a small proportion of families in developed countries.

From a structural-functional viewpoint, the major goal of the family is socialization of its members in society—those broader and multiple social groups outside the family. The actions of each family member, as part of a family unit, affect how others will behave and how the family unit relates to other groups within the society. Family members must learn role behavior appropriate for living and interacting harmoniously with their neighbors, finding success in their occupations, and influencing the way their community is governed or changed (Bower and Jacobson, 1978).

Structural-functional theory focuses primarily on integration of the family within the occupational system. In the United States the status of the family is closely associated with the occupation of the breadwinner(s) since income, prestige, and life-style are derived from the occupation. In most instances the occupational roles are segregated from the familial roles; although, in some families, the work is conducted within the household. Not uncommonly, family obligations must be subordinated to occupational ones, including the need for geographic and social mobility. Occupational opportunities often conflict with family ties: young people leave the family when entering the occupational field or a spouse ceases to support the occupational advances of the wage-earner.

INTERACTIONAL THEORY

Interactional theory, which views the family as a unit of interacting personalities, was first advanced by Burgess (1926). The focus is on family interactions only, not on broader social systems. The family is described as a unit of interacting personalities that exists as long as the interaction takes place. Individuals have a position, or a status, in the family structure because they possesses attitudes and behaviors that are consistent with the norms and expectations of culturally and socially defined roles. They play these roles in interactions within the group, and the responses of others in the family serve to reinforce or to challenge the individual's role behaviors. A role cannot exist without some other role toward which it is oriented. Basic to the interactional approach is communication, since actions of the family result from the communication process.

Family members communicate by the use of symbols. Not only do individuals within the family structure react to the actions of the others, they interpret and define those actions (Rank and LeCroy, 1983). For example, a child not only reacts to a parent's actions but also to the meaning that both attach to the actions. Thus the individual lives in a symbolic as well as a physical environment. Interaction is a dynamic process in which one's concept of the role of another is continually being tested (Bower and Jacobson, 1978). The product of this testing process is the stabilization or the modification of one's own role (Turner, 1962). (See also Family roles and relationships, p. 65).

EXCHANGE THEORY

Exchange theory, one of the most current theories, provides a rationale to explain human interactions and to advance propositions for predicting behaviors. It is based on the assumption that individuals interact through the give-and-take of a broad range of commodities, resources, or skills and that all individuals have needs, the fulfillment of which constitutes a reward. Also individuals attempt to maximize rewards and minimize costs in their exchanges in order to obtain the most profitable outcomes. Behavior is positively reinforced when it is associated with reward and negatively reinforced when it is associated with punishment (Singelmann, 1972). Therefore knowledge of a person's needs, anticipations, and expectations is important if the appropriate reinforcement is to be employed.

A disadvantage of the theory is that proponents are unable to define exactly what constitutes a reward. Social interaction, nevertheless, is viewed as a complex exchange of mutually rewarding activities in which the reception of needed benefits is contingent on the delivery of a returned favor. The rule of "distributive justice" (Homans, 1958) or "fair exchange" (Blau, 1964), furthermore, claims that rewards are proportional to the cost of their attainment. There are limits beyond which individuals do not pursue self-gain. In order to deliver a benefit in exchange for other benefits, a supply of specific benefits are needed that have required previously invested resources. For example, once individuals have acquired needed skills, they can use these skills with little cost to themselves, but the investment of time and energy in acquiring the skills has been very costly.

Exchange theory helps explain how individuals find meaning in material and nonmaterial goods. Rewards have symbolic significance for those involved and are rewards only insofar as the interactants assign that meaning to them (Singelmann, 1972). In the family, however, interactions, because of their repetitiveness and emotional ties, cannot be viewed as merely responses to a reward (Bower, 1978). The feelings and interactions are much more complex. Exchange theory accords little attention to the social, ecologic, or situational aspects of family interactions.

SYSTEMS THEORY

According to systems theory the family is defined as a group of individuals of at least two generations with ties of affection and responsibility who live in proximity and who share mutual goals (Sargent, 1983). A system is "a set of objects together with relationships between the objects and between their attributes" (Hall and Fagan, 1956). It has organization, purpose, and a feedback mechanism. Living systems are open systems that exchange energy and information with their environment, and the family, viewed as an open system, follows the principles derived from general systems theory. These include (Carter and McGoldrick, 1980):

Circular causality—a change in one family member creates a change in other members which, in turn, results in a new change in the original changed member.

Nonsummativity—the family as a whole is different from the sum of the individual attributes of its members—"the whole is greater than the sum of its parts."

Equifinality—the outcome of any family problem or task depends to a large extent on the current family organization.

Communication—interpersonal messages, transmitted verbally or behaviorally, by a family member precipitate a response from other members.

Regulation—recurrent patterns of interaction become rules that determine role behaviors by which family members are governed.

Constancy and change—the family maintains homeostasis of the family life cycle, fluctuating between periods of stability and change while maintaining its integrity through direct responses to deviation.

CONFLICT THEORY

Grounded in the Marxist philosophy of class conflict, conflict theory is based on the assumption that conflict is natural and inevitable in all human interaction and should not be viewed as bad or disruptive (Eshleman, 1981). When family members are in conflict, the goal is how to manage and resolve the conflict, not how to avoid it. Family situations involve perpetual give-and-take, and harmony can be satisfactorily maintained only through negotiation (Sprey, 1979).

Conflict arises from a variety of sources but the most frequent is a perceived unequal exchange between marriage partners. The outcome can be continued conflict, dissolution of the relationship, or resolution of the conflict. Resolution of the conflict requires three ingredients (Beckman, 1978): (1) open communication, (2) accurate perceptions regarding the degree and nature of conflict, and (3) constructive efforts to resolve conflict. Efforts include a willingness on the part of each member to consider the point of view of the other, alternative solutions, and to be willing to compromise if necessary.

Family Structure and Function

Structure is a manner of organization or the arrangement of a number of parts that are interrelated in specified, recurring ways. Function refers to a special duty or performance required in the course of work or activity. The structure of a family may vary according to the composition of its component parts and according to its life cycle. Both structure and function are altered and modified as the needs of the family change.

FUNCTIONS OF THE FAMILY

Authorities agree families serve society in many ways. They play a vital role in the economy since they produce and consume goods and services. They also are the basic unit for replacing dying members of the society. Furthermore, society, to maintain its continuity, must transmit its knowledge, customs, values, and beliefs to the young. However, where children are not an economic necessity, their primary function is to receive and to give love. Not only do they appear to be loved more, but they are loved as children for a longer period. Children bring very little predetermined behavior into the world with them; therefore they depend on their families to meet the primary requirements for growth and development and to establish for them an atmosphere of security. Although goals for socialization and childrearing practices differ from one culture to another, in most societies the family appears to have three major objectives in relation to children: caregiving, nurturing, and training.

FAMILY STRUCTURE

The family structure, or family composition, consists of individuals, each with a socially recognized status and position, who interact with one another on a regular, recurring basis in socially sanctioned ways. When members are gained or lost through events (e.g., marriage, divorce, birth, death, abandonment, incarceration), the family composition is altered and roles must be redefined or redistributed.

Traditionally the family structure refers to either *nuclear* or *extended families*. However, family composition has assumed new configurations in recent years, with the single-parent family becoming a prominent form. In any case, the predominant structural pattern in any society depends to a large extent on the mobility of families as they pursue economic goals and as relationships change. It is not uncommon for children to belong to several different family groups during their lifetime. In general, extended families are associated with agricultural societies, whereas small conjugal units are characteristic of more advanced, industrialized societies.

Nuclear Family

The nuclear, or conjugal, family consists of a man, his wife, and their children (natural or adopted) who live in a common household. This is the reproductive unit in which the marital tie (legally or otherwise sanctioned) is the chief binding force. A strongly functional nuclear family is the prototype of human relationships and the basic unit from which more complex familial forms are composed. In some instances one or more additional persons (e.g., a relative, friend, foster child, or others) may reside in the same household. Nuclear families can be combined into larger units in one of two ways: through plural marriage (polygamous families) or through extension of the parent-child relationship (extended family). Some authorities classify childless couples as a nuclear family because it is a conjugal alliance with the theoretic potential for reproduction.

The nuclear family, the predominant structure in America, is more characteristic of an urban, mobile society. It is highly adaptable, with the ability to adjust and reshape its structure when needed. It is free to move where there is opportunity for higher income with concomitant improvement in other areas such as social class and prestige. It is not economically bound to a geographic area nor dependent on the cooperative efforts of other members. The family members are employed on an individual basis, and economic resources are in the form of money. The present-day family must purchase the services of specialized individuals and groups, whereas previously these needs and services were met on a cooperative basis by the extended family members.

Although extended families residing in the same household are rapidly disappearing in American society, the isolated nuclear family without relatives within easy visiting distance is uncommon. This is most often seen where there has been extreme mobility of separate generations, such as wide geographic separations or marriages into different social strata, religious backgrounds, or roles. Most consanguineous family members maintain contact through visits, telephone calls, letters, and gift exchanges. Having no relatives readily available for advice and assistance with child care, as is common in extended families, parents in some nuclear families are more likely to turn to "experts" for childrearing guidance.

The majority of nuclear families in America are associated with an extended kinship network of nuclear families living in separate households but in close geographic proximity. This concept, sometimes referred to as a modified extended family, describes a meaningful aspect of daily existence that is reflected in frequent visiting and the exchange of services and financial aid. This family association meets the members' psychologic needs to a greater extent than do experts, friends, or organizations. It is not uncommon for families to reject the opportunity for social or economic advancement rather than leave such kinship associations.

Affiliative relationships. Although the nuclear family is predominantly a legally sanctioned institution, there are a number of families in which the attachment is only affiliative, that is, nonmarital cohabitation. These families consist primarily of two adults, the "couple households" (Macklin, 1980), but may include children. The mother and father live together, often with children from previous matings, and share family responsibilities. However, the family unit is less stable and relationships are subject to change. Instability of the social environment in the home has been associated with juvenile delinquency, which appears to be related

to the number of family constellations (changes in the adult members of the household) experienced during childhood. This is probably a reflection of repeated adjustment to a variety of authority figures (Mednick and Baker, 1980).

Single-Parent Family

The single-parent family, a result of recent social phenomena, is now recognized as a family and has emerged partially as a consequence of women's rights movements wherein more women (and men) have established separate households because of divorce, death, desertion, or illegitimacy. In addition, a more liberal attitude in the courts has made it possible for single persons, both male and female, to adopt children, whereas, previously, rigid prerequisites specified that both a father and a mother must be present in the home. A significant number of single families also result from a single mother who wishes to have a child but does not choose to have a husband.

Although single-parent families are usually headed by the mother, it is becoming increasingly common for fathers to be awarded custody of dependent children in divorce settlements, and both single males as well as single females are finding it easier to adopt children. Unmarried mothers, choosing to keep and raise their children rather than place them for adoption or marry, are absorbed into the extended family. For instance, in the lower-lower class of the United States (especially lower-class blacks) where the incidence of illegitimacy is highest, the maternal grandmother is usually available to care for the children (Whitehead, 1978). Therefore, with the increased psychologic independence of women as a whole and the increased acceptability of illegitimacy in society, more unmarried women are deliberately choosing mother-child families. The problems of these single-parent families are discussed on p. 89.

Binuclear Family

Binuclear family is a term used to describe the situation that allows parents to continue the parenting role while terminating the spousal unit (Ahrons, 1979). The degree of cooperation between households and the time the child spends with each can vary. In *joint custody* the court assigns divorcing parents equal rights and responsibilities to the minor child or children. These alternate family forms are efforts on the part of those concerned to view divorce as a process of reorganization and redefinition of a family rather than as a family dissolution. Joint custody and co-parenting are discussed further in relation to special parenting situations, p. 88.

Reconstituted Family

Reconstituted families, also referred to as stepfamilies, are those in which one or both of the married adults have children from a previous marriage residing in the household. The term *blended families* or *combined families* more often refers to families composed of parents and the children each of them brings from a previous marriage. It is estimated that

10% to 15% of all households in the United States are reconstituted families (Espinoza and Newman, 1979) and that 10% of children under age 18 are living with a natural parent and a stepparent (Glick, 1979). The most common stepfamily consists of a mother, her children, and a stepfather (Perkins and Kahan, 1979). The problems of the reconstituted family are further discussed on p. 90.

Extended Family

The extended, or consanguineous, family is one mode of combining nuclear families into larger units through the parent-child relationship. It consists of the nuclear family plus lineal or collateral relatives. More often it is composed of two or more residential units of three or more generations affiliated through extension of the parent-child relationship, that is, grandparents, parents, and grandchildren. An extended family can be compounded of either monogamous or polygamous relationships. Broader views recognize the affiliation of collateral relatives as an extended family—not necessarily organized into nuclear families.

Extended family structure is more functional in areas where land is the basis of wealth and sustenance. Today the best examples of extended family units can be found among successful farmers, Native Americans, and certain recent immigrants. Here the family serves as the basic social, educational, and productive unit providing services and sharing resources. Extended families may form under conditions of either extreme poverty in order to pool resources or extreme wealth in order to consolidate resources (Winch, 1977). Extended families direct cooperative efforts for common goals; the needs of the individual are sublimated to the welfare of the family enterprise and survival. The children learn early in life to respect their elders, and this value is

reinforced through observation of their parents' behavior toward older family members (Fig. 3-1).

In the extended family, childrearing is often a shared responsibility. Relatives are always present and available to help young mothers with household chores and childcare activities. Daily lives of the children are organized around the needs and requirements of the family with assigned tasks and obligations. Family ties between the nuclear unit and the main extended family are strong, although there is a high degree of competition between individual nuclear units for acquisition of power and resources.

Polygamous Family

Although it is not legally sanctioned in the United States, sometimes the conjugal unit can be extended by the addition of spouses in polygamous matings. Polygamy generally refers to either wives (*polygyny*) or, very rarely, husbands (*polyandry*). Many societies practice polygyny that is further designated as *sororal*, in which the wives are sisters, or *nonsororal*, in which the wives can be unrelated. Sororal polygyny is widespread throughout the world and, although plural marriages produce problems of adjustment for the members, co-wives who are sisters are more likely to get along with each other and display less jealousy than co-wives who are not. Most often mothers and their children share a husband and father, usually with each mother and her children maintaining a separate household, particularly when the wives are unrelated.

A special form of sororal polygyny is the *sororate* in which a cultural rule specifies that the preferred mate for a widower is the sister of his deceased wife. In a sororate, the marriages are successive rather than concurrent.

Where it exists, polygamy is usually accorded a higher status than monogamy. It may be limited to ruling families or to high-status persons and tends to be practiced by a small segment of the population. This is probably a result of economic factors and because of the unequal sex ratio in some areas at the time of biologic maturity.

Communal Family

The communal family emerged, as have all previous experimental communities, from a disenchantment with most contemporary life choices. Although communal families may have divergent beliefs, practices, and organization, the basic impetus for formation has been dissatisfaction with social systems and life goals of the larger communities and with the nuclear family structure, in particular, as it exists either from an ideologic or a practical perspective. Relatively uncommon today, communal groups share common ownership of property and goods; in cooperatives there is private ownership of property, but certain goods and services are shared and exchanged cooperatively without monetary consideration. There is strong reliance on group members and material interdependence. Both provide collective security for nonproductive members, share homemaking and

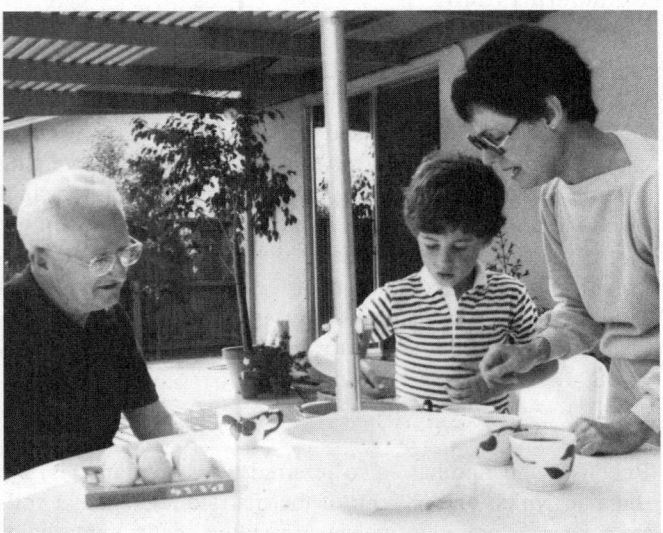

Fig. 3-1. Children benefit from interaction with grandparents even when they do not share the same household.

childrearing functions, and help overcome the problem of interpersonal isolation or loneliness.

Unlike the traditional extended family, nuclear units in a commune may come and go at will. There is no consanguineous tie between the units. The mother-child tie is strong during infancy and early childhood, but many parents are happy to relinquish older children to the care of others. Although the parents maintain primary responsibility for the health and well-being of the children, the children are free to form close relationships with a number of adults in the commune and are encouraged to do so.

Gay Family

A same-sex, or homosexual, family is one in which there is a marital or common-law tie between two persons of the same sex who have adopted children or in which one or both partners have natural children from a heterosexual mating. Unfortunately little research is available on the spousal unit in same-sex relationships or on the effects of growing up as a child in these households.

Family Structure and Social Class

In family structure, as with other aspects of childrearing, there are greater differences related to social class than any other variable. In the upper-upper class, or the old aristocracy, the nuclear family is firmly imbedded in an extended kinship structure. It is primarily patrifocal in that the older husband-father is the unilateral authority. The family's source of wealth is supervised by male family members, controlled by the eldest, and handed down from one generation to the next. In the lower-upper and upper-middle classes family ties are the most loosely attached. This is the most highly mobile element of the population—both socially, economically, and geographically—all of which encourage separation from extended family relationships.

The tendency in the lower-lower class is toward matrifocal family units. Since the family unit is often torn apart by continual economic stress, the mother-child relationship is the strongest and most intimate tie. There is a higher rate of divorce, illegitimacy, and desertion in this segment of society. Husband and wife are often emotionally separated by unfulfilled expectations. The father, who has few personal or economic assets (and who is more often than not an economic burden), has difficulty establishing a dominant role in the family. In this class the mother is often more easily employed than the father, and she is eligible for welfare benefits when there are minor dependent children; therefore, the mother-child dyad is predominant. Frequently there are three generations—grandmother, mother, and children—living in an extended structure, sharing the economic burden and child care.

Kin ties are stronger among lower- and working-class families than middle-class families. This is particularly true in relation to the kin network among lower-class American blacks where interaction, co-residence, and exchange of mutual aid are stronger than in white families (Allen, 1978) and family composition displays more variability. Such a strong network probably serves as a means for helping families and individuals cope with poverty and contribute resources needed for upward mobility. Nor does the upward mobility of members alter these close relationships (McAdoo, 1978).

Family Roles and Relationships

Each individual has a position, or status, in the family structure, and each occupant of a position plays culturally and socially defined roles in interactions within the group. Within prescribed guidelines for behavior set by the culture, subcultures (including the family group) establish variations in role definition and may specify different requirements for playing the same role. Each family has its own traditions and values and sets its own standards for interaction within and outside the family group. Each determines the experiences the children should have, those they are to be shielded from, and how each of these experiences meets the needs of family members. Conformity to group norms is directly related to the strength and nature of group ties. Where family ties are strong, social control is highly effective, and most members play their roles willingly and with commitment.

PARENTAL ROLES

In all family groups the socially recognized status of father and mother exist with socially sanctioned roles that prescribe appropriate sexual behavior and childrearing responsibilities. The guides for behavior in these roles serve to control sexual conflict in society and provide for prolonged care of children. The degree to which parents are committed and the way they play their respective roles are influenced by a number of variables. Each individual is affected by a unique socialization experience.

Role definitions are changing as a result of the changing economy and the women's liberation movement. Women are achieving equality with men in education, more of them are entering the labor force, and the number of women who choose to have fewer children or none at all is increasing. During childhood, particularly in the upper and middle classes, the trend is toward deemphasizing the basic male-female characteristics of aggression, dependence, and achievement. As the role of the woman changes, there must necessarily be a change in the complementary role of the male. Fathers are taking a more active role in childrearing and household activities, which is most evident in middle-class families. Marital roles, on the other hand, are most segregated in the lower classes. Redefinition of sex roles in the American family is taking place, but a cultural lag of the persisting traditional role definitions creates role conflicts in many of these families.

ROLE LEARNING

Roles are learned through the socialization process. During all stages of development children learn and practice, through interaction with others and in their play, a set of social roles and something of the characteristics of other roles. They behave in patterned and more or less predictable ways because they learn roles that define mutual expectations in typical and recurring social relationships. Role conceptions are transmitted by socializing agents (parents, peers, authority figures) who use positive and negative sanctions to ensure conformity to their norms. Role behaviors positively reinforced by rewards such as love, affection, friendship, and honors are strengthened. Negative reinforcement takes the form of ridicule, withdrawal of love, expressions of disapproval, or banishment.

Types of Roles

The types of roles that are learned can be broadly classified as follows:

Ascribed roles are those that are strictly defined by the culture, and very little deviation is allowed in modifying them. Ascribed roles apply to general traits such as sex, age, kinship, social class, and ethnic origin. There are culturally determined behaviors that must be adhered to regarding these roles, and they are expected to be learned in the home. For example, a child who attempts to change an ascribed role (such as sex) will be confronted with serious problems.

Achieved roles are those acquired through effort, and children must do something to attain them. Achieved roles include educational, occupational, religious, and recreational roles. These are based on performance and are acquired through satisfaction of specified requirements. The direction of these role achievements is strongly influenced by values conveyed to the children by their parents. For example, some parents believe that a college education is essential; others encourage children to seek occupational gratification. Achievement of athletic prowess is highly valued by some parents; musical accomplishment is esteemed by others.

Adopted roles are those that are sometimes transient, such as the role of patient or traveler. More often adopted behavior patterns become fixed into what are known as character roles and apply to the unique behaviors that the child displays in a given situation. Such roles as the leader, the follower, the prankster, the deceiver, the show-off, or the honest one are examples of adopted roles. They are frequently adopted when playing the role meets a need or is the response to a complementary role in another.

Assumed roles are those related to fantasy and are especially important in childhood. This is one of the dominant means for children's adjustment and socialization. Children continually assume roles of persons they observe in their environment. The environment is a primary resource for learning the conduct that befits their position or status. Assumed roles only become a problem if they persist into the world of reality. For example, a child who persistently plays an infantile role is severely hampered in relationships with peers; a girl who consistently fantasizes that she is a boy may be unable to assume a mothering role at the appropriate time.

Continuity and Discontinuity

Anthropologists who make a study of societies throughout the world have determined that there are decided differences from culture to culture in the continuity with which young children are prepared for adult roles. In some cultures children begin to learn adult roles and behaviors at a very early age and continue to do so throughout childhood. For example, cultures that value courage and aggressiveness continuously encourage these behaviors in their children. In other cultures children are taught roles and behaviors that are in direct opposition to those they are expected to assume as adults. For example, in the United States, children are expected to be submissive in childhood but dominant as adults. Continuity in the rearing of females in Western cultures has generally been more consistent in terms of role identification than is that experienced by males. With expanding female roles, however, this continuity is becoming less apparent. Another example of role discontinuity is related to attitudes toward sexuality. Many cultures are highly restrictive regarding sexual activity throughout childhood, but the same cultures become permissive or even demanding in adulthood; others are thoroughly permissive at all ages.

Role-Structuring in Children

One responsibility of the family is to develop in the children culturally appropriate role behavior. Children learn to perform in expected ways consistent with their position in the family and culture at a very early age. The observed behavior of each child is a single manifestation—a combination of social influences as well as individual psychologic processes. In this way the uniting of the child's intrapersonal system (the self) with the interpersonal system (the family) is comprehended simultaneously as the conduct of the child.

Role-structuring initially takes place within the family unit, where the children fulfill a set of roles and respond to the complementary roles of their parents and other family members. The roles of the children are shaped primarily by the parents, who apply direct or indirect pressures in an attempt to induce or force children into the desired patterns of behavior or direct their efforts toward modification of the role responses of the child on a mutually acceptable basis. Each set of parents has their own techniques, and each will determine the course that the process of socialization is to follow (see Shaping behavior, p. 77).

Children respond to life situations according to behaviors learned in reciprocal transactions. As they acquire important role-taking skills, their relationships with others change. They become proficient at understanding others as they acquire the ability to discriminate their own perspectives from those of others. The children who get along well with others and attain status in the peer group have well-developed role-taking skills (see Selman's stages of role taking, p. 116).

FAMILY SIZE AND CONFIGURATION

The size and composition of the family directly influences child development. No two children grow in exactly the same environment, although identical twins more nearly approximate this. For example, in a nuclear family with two children—even of the same sex—one will live in a family with an older sibling, whereas the other will be reared in a family with a younger sibling. In a family where there is a 10-year age span among the children, one may be born to a 20-year-old mother, the other to a 30-year-old mother. For the child in each situation the environment is different.

Family Size

Parenting practices differ between small and large families. In small families more emphasis is placed on the individual development of the children. Parenting is intensive rather than extensive, and there is constant pressure to measure up to family expectations. Children's development and achievement are measured against that of other children in the neighborhood and social class. In small families there is more democratic participation by the children than in larger families. Adolescents in small families identify more strongly with their parents and rely more on parents for advice. They have well-developed, autonomous inner controls as contrasted with adolescents from larger families who rely more on adult authority. In small families there is more opportunity for democratic participation by all the children.

Children in a large family are able to adjust to a variety of changes and crises. There is more emphasis on the group and less on the individual (Fig. 3-2). Cooperation is essential, often because of economic necessity. The large number of persons sharing a limited amount of space requires a greater degree of organization, administration, and authoritarian control. The control is wielded by a dominant family

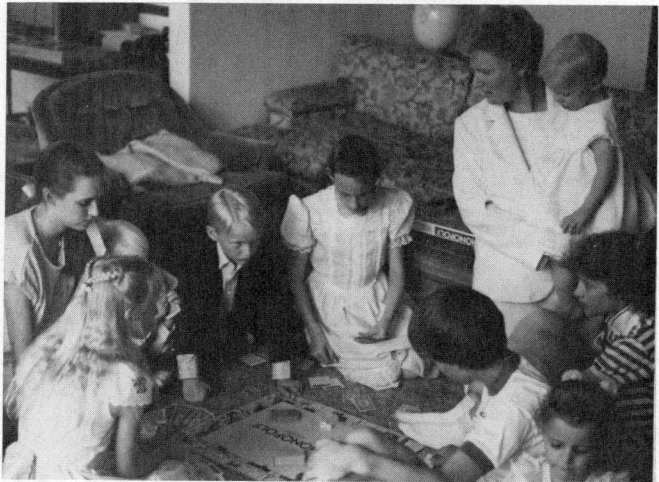

Fig. 3-2. Innumerable relationships and activities are possible in a large family.
Photography by Earl Fillmore, Salt Lake City, UT.

member—a parent or an older child. The number of children reduces the intimate, one-to-one contact between the parent and any individual child. Consequently children turn to each other for what they cannot get from their parents. The reduced parent-child contact encourages individual children to adopt specialized roles in an attempt to gain recognition in the family.

Discipline is often administered by older siblings in large families. Siblings are usually better attuned to what constitutes misbehavior, and sibling disapproval or ostracism is frequently a more meaningful disciplinary measure than parental spankings. In situations such as death or illness of a parent, an older sibling assumes responsibility for the family at considerable personal sacrifice. Large families seem to generate a sense of security in the children fostered by sibling support and cooperation. However adolescents from a large family are more peer oriented than family-oriented.

Spacing of Children

Age differences between siblings affects the childhood environment but to a lesser extent than does the sex of the siblings. The arrival of a sibling has the greatest impact on the older child, and a 2- to 4-year difference in age appears to be most threatening. When the older child is very young, his self-image is too immature to be threatened. At an older age he is better able to understand the situation and therefore less likely to see the newcomer as a threat, although he does feel the loss of his only-child status.

In general, the narrower the spacing between siblings, the more the children influence one another, especially in emotional characteristics; the wider the spacing, the greater the influence of the parents. Also, younger children tend to identify with older siblings. Consequently they assume some of the personality characteristics of the older child. Girls with brothers frequently have more "traditionally" masculine characteristics than girls raised with sisters. They are, on the whole, more aggressive, ambitious, and perform better on tests of intellectual ability, probably related to the more stimulating environment created by competitive, aggressive boys. Boys with older sisters, especially if the age difference is slight, are generally less aggressive and daring than boys raised with older boys, probably a reflection of the identification process and the greater power exerted by the older sibling (Maccoby, 1980).

Sibling Interaction

Relationships between siblings in the family group duplicate, to some extent, many of the social interaction experiences of later years. Through relationships with siblings, children learn patterns of loyalty, competition, dominance, and other interactional skills. Such factors as whether a child is the firstborn, a middle child, or the youngest child or whether there is 1 or 6 years separation from the closest sibling affects the child's view of the world and his relationship with others inside and outside the family. None of

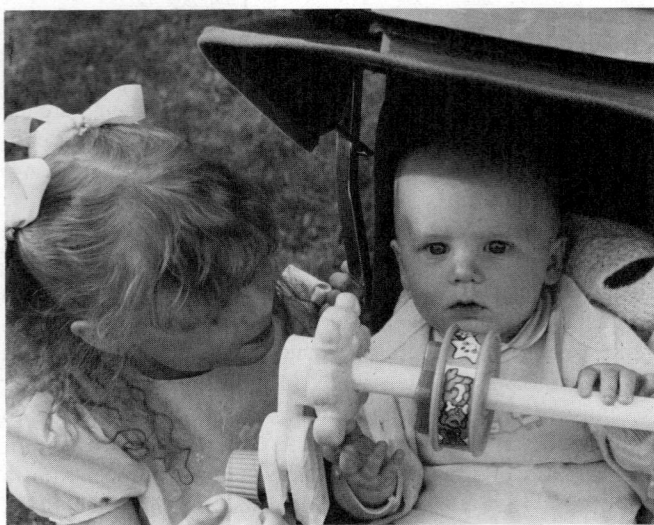

Fig. 3-3. Older children may have some doubts about a younger sibling.
Photography by Earl Fillmore, Salt Lake City, UT.

these characteristics are absolute, however, nor do they apply to all children and all parents. The potential effects depend on all other intrafamilial factors operating, such as parenting practices, the number of children in a family, and age, sex, and birth order difference between older and younger siblings (Fig. 3-3).

Sibling rivalry begins at an early age (see p. 606). It has been observed that the character of interactions between children and their parents are much more positive than between siblings (Baskett and Johnson, 1982). Children often talk to, laugh with, and display affection toward their parents, but direct behaviors such as hitting, yelling, and various annoying physical antics toward their siblings. Brothers and sisters are more coercive than parents and tend to respond less positively to a sibling's social overtures. Quarrels are most often initiated by the older sibling and become more frequent and intense as the younger child becomes more mature and is better able to retaliate. Same-sex siblings engage in more positive interaction than cross-sex siblings. Much of this behavior can be attributed to maternal behaviors. Mothers have been observed to direct more attention to the younger sibling who differs in gender from the older one (Dunn and Kendrick, 1981).

Although competition is commonplace among siblings, especially those who are nearly the same age, there are positive aspects of sibling interactions. Positive social responses outnumber negative ones in total interactions between siblings and acts of kindness are typically more common than hateful or rivalrous conduct. In many societies older children are the principal caregivers of infants and toddlers, and school-age children often assume some care of younger children in other cultures. Even older preschool children become sources of emotional support to younger ones in situations when parents are not around.

Older siblings become role models for younger ones who imitate their behavior and often take over toys abandoned by them. Older children also serve as teachers, which is of benefit to both the younger and the older children (Fig. 3-4).

Ordinal Position

It has been observed for some time that the birth position of children affects their personalities. Parents treat children differently, and sibling interactions are different depending on the children's position within the family. Also, power is unequally distributed among siblings. Older siblings attempt to dominate younger ones; therefore, younger siblings develop interpersonal skills, the ability to negotiate, and an ability to accept unfavorable outcomes to a greater extent than older siblings. Later-born children are obliged to interact with other siblings from birth and seem to be more outgoing and make friends more easily than firstborns (Steelman and Powell, 1985). However children vary tremendously and these generalizations represent averages and do not apply in all situations.

Firstborn children. Firstborn children are more achievement-oriented than children born later and exhibit strong drive and ambition. They usually receive more physical punishment than younger children and are allowed to show more aggression toward their younger siblings. They have stronger consciences and are usually more self-disciplined, inner-directed, and prone to feelings of guilt, which may account for a higher intellectual achievement. Firstborn children are better represented in college populations than are younger siblings. Although they are more likely to have tasks imposed on them, oldest children seem to experience fewer frustrations in the family setting than do younger siblings. They are better planners and tend to identify with parents and to measure themselves by adult standards.

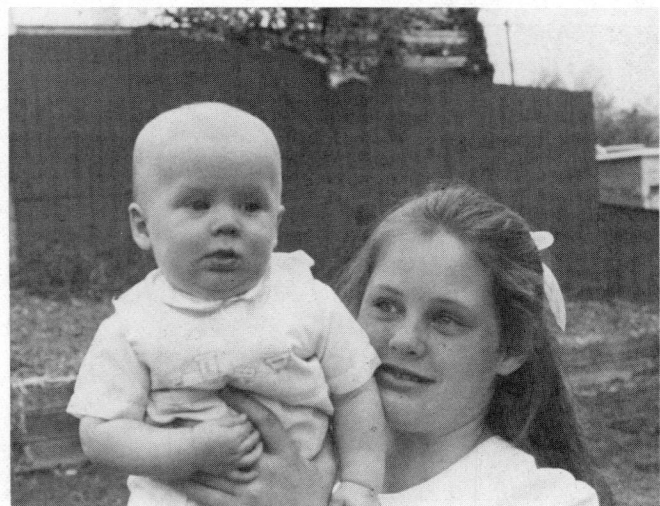

Fig. 3-4. Older school-age children can take responsibility for the care of younger children.
Photography by Earl Fillmore, Salt Lake City, UT.

First children are more likely to be the most wanted children. Born to relatively inexperienced parents, they are the recipients of all the parental uncertainties, unskilled experimentation, and a great deal of the adult attention and pressure. Parents expect more from them than from later children, tend to be more tense, and worry more about them. Parents, having had the experience of one child, are more relaxed when the second arrives, and they tend to be less strict and less preoccupied with the parental role. The close, intense attention that the eldest receive contributes to their adult orientation.

Firstborn children also appear to be more likely to suffer birth trauma, neonatal problems, and congenital anomalies (Prasad and Prasad, 1978). In addition, there is a larger percentage of premature births and stillbirths among firstborn children.

Middle children. Later-born children reflect the decrease in the amount of parental attention and anxieties. They are more difficult to characterize because they represent a variety of status—for example, the second daughter of three, the second son of four, or the third of five but the first of their sex. The middle position is the least stable of ordinal positions, and one in which the children never benefit from all the parental attention as do the oldest and the youngest. There are more demands on them for help with household tasks, they are praised less often for good behavior, and they receive less of the mother's time for pleasurable activities. While parental attention is focused on the oldest and the youngest, middle children learn adaptability and the art of compromise but are less stimulated toward achievement. They are more popular with their classmates than are firstborn children but less popular than youngest children.

Youngest children. On the whole, mothers are warmer toward the youngest child than the oldest and middle child, and the youngest child receives little physical punishment. The youngest child is less dependent than a firstborn and more apt to be left to manage things for himself. Younger children are usually more backward than the firstborn in language development and articulation. They appear to be less tense, more affectionate, and more good-natured than the firstborn, and they tend to identify more with the peer group than with parents. The older and middle children are usually assigned more tasks in the family than are younger ones, and the middle children more so than the older ones.

The only child. Being the only child in a family has traditionally been considered to be a disadvantage. Only children have been described as selfish, spoiled, dependent, and lonely. However, research indicates that there are no essential differences between a child reared alone and one who is reared with one or more siblings. They display no more evidence of maladjustment or self-centeredness than any other children and tend to strongly resemble firstborn children in such respects as higher educational goals. Only

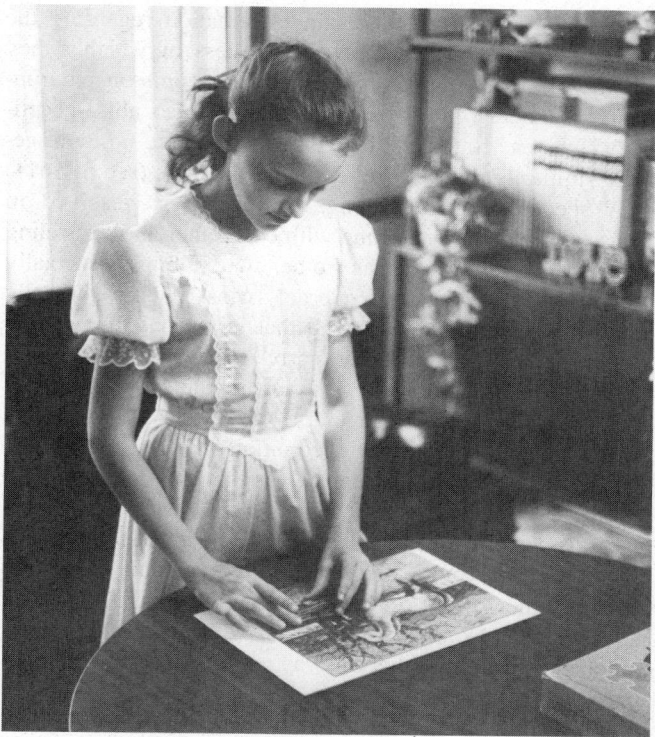

Fig. 3-5. Children without siblings learn to entertain themselves. Photography by Earl Fillmore, Salt Lake City, UT.

children perform better on cognitive tests, are more mature and cultivated, are more socially sensitive, and demonstrate superiority in language facility (Fig. 3-5).

Only children also enjoy the advantage of having parents who, without the distraction of other children, are able to devote more time to them, talk to them, and stimulate them in intellectual activities. However, parents also exert greater pressure for mature behavior at an early age and for achievement. Relative isolation from peers contributes to intellectual pursuits and encourages a rich fantasy life, independence, and originality.

The effects of onliness on personality are questionable. Only children do not have the stereotyped concept of sex-appropriate behavior and often exhibit some characteristics associated with both sexes, but the significant influence is the quality of the parent-child relationship. Because of the wide differences among parents, a typical personality cannot be assigned to the only child. An unusually large number of only children live with a single parent, primarily as a result of divorce, and parents of only children tend to be somewhat older (Pines, 1981).

Multiple Births: Twins

Twins have always been a source of interest and have provided an appealing theme for dramatists and novelists. The distinctive characteristics of the two types of twins have also been of special interest to both geneticists and environmentalists in their efforts to obtain information regarding the "nature-nurture" controversy. Regardless of whether they are identical or fraternal, twins share a common environment. Identical (monozygotic) twins are also alike genetically, whereas fraternal (dizygotic) twins share no more genetic similarity than any other pair of siblings (see p. 161).

A special kind of sibling relationship is observed in twins, although getting along with each other and quarreling is not too different from any other two siblings, especially if they are different-sex fraternal twins. Twins generally tend to work out a relationship that is reasonably satisfactory to both and demonstrate early independence from parental attention. They develop a remarkable capacity for cooperative play and considerable loyalty and generosity toward each other. It is not uncommon for them to evolve a private language between themselves that may interfere with development of the family language.

In a twinship, one member of the pair, to a greater or lesser extent, is more dominant, outgoing, and aggressive than the other, often to the consternation of their parents. However, the seemingly more passive twin is able to accomplish as much and get his way as frequently as the more aggressive twin.

It has also been observed that there is a difference in behavior between identical and fraternal twins. Whereas there is near unison in the actions of identical twins (although they alternate in assuming the leadership), fraternal twins, even of the same sex, do not display this quality. Sibling rivalry can be quite pronounced in fraternal twins, especially in mixed-sex twins. A demanding, rapidly developing girl can be particularly troublesome to her twin brother.

Identical twins also differ in their response to the tendency of some parents to treat twins exactly alike. The present philosophy is to determine the degree to which the children demonstrate an inclination toward togetherness. Some twins thrive best when they are constantly in each other's company; others prefer more individuality and separateness. The conservative approach is to allow the children to follow their natural inclinations. Early years of togetherness are often the basis of the children's security. To separate them too early may produce unnecessary stresses. The tendency is to foster individual differences as they are evidenced in order to ease the process of separation when it becomes advisable.

Any multiple birth attracts the interest of others and parents should be prepared for the added attention the twins will attract, including the interest of researchers who will ask the parents' permission to include their children in studies of twins. Friends and relatives will lavish attention on them and people on the street stop to admire the children.

Parental adjustment. The entrance of any new member into a household creates a number of stresses, but with multiple births two or more new members must be incorporated into the family at the same time. The problems are obvious. Two infants must be provided with physical care including feeding, diapering, and all the purchasing and

preparation that accompany the care of any infant. Scheduling becomes crucial and each advancement in development brings new problems and adjustments—for example, space and sleeping arrangements, selecting a stroller and other equipment. Care must be observed in selecting toys. As play becomes a serious business some toys that would be safe and appropriate for a single child become weapons when two infants share a playpen. It is a good idea to select different toys for the children as they grow older and encourage sharing.

It is especially important for parents to maintain relationships with each other and other family members. It is doubly important for parents to arrange time together as often as possible. The **National Organization of Mothers of Twins Clubs, Inc.*** has local chapters throughout the United States to offer information and support to parents of twins and is highly recommended as a resource for all new parents of twins. The **Twins Foundation†**—an organization founded by a group of twins and designed to aid twins and other multiples—is recommended for older children.

Another problem faced by parents of twins occurs at the time of birth. Not only are the parents faced with double the work and care of the newborns, but the process of attachment may also be impeded. The mother first forms an attachment to the twins as a unit before she is able to form an attachment to each child individually (see p. 332). While in the hospital the mother should be allowed to interact with both infants together as well as with each infant individually (Abbink and others, 1982). As they develop, the children, who are facing the task of differentiating themselves from their environment, must learn to differentiate themselves not only from the mother but from one another as well.

Forming separate attachments is especially difficult if one of the twins must remain in the hospital. Therefore it is recommended that, if possible, both infants should stay in the hospital until they can be discharged together (Jimenez and Jungman, 1980). However, this would be impractical when one is a seriously ill infant who requires lengthy care.

It has been found that there is an increased risk for child abuse and neglect among families with twins (Groothuis, and others, 1982). The increased stress related to the care of two young children is probably a factor, but it has been demonstrated that large families and inadequately spacing of children predispose to child abuse. Families with a multiple birth incorporate both of these factors.

Promoting individuation. All children proceed through a separation-individuation process as they grow and develop. For twins the process is complicated in a number of ways. Unlike singletons, twins lack a perception of separateness and the close physical and emotional attachment between them inhibits development of individuality. In ad-

---

*5402 Amberwood Lane, Rockville, MD 20953.
†P.O. Box 9487, Providence, RI 02940-9487.

PROMOTING INDIVIDUATION OF TWINS

Select different-sounding names.

Take separate photographs of the children (beginning at birth) so each child will have a picture of "me." Be certain to label each picture.

Avoid dressing children alike.

Use their given names. Avoid referring to them as "the twins."

Take each child on separate short outings occasionally while the other is at home with another family member or a sitter.

Build a one-to-one relationship with each child.

Hold and cuddle each child. Provide frequent body contact with each one.

Play and participate in learning with each child and to the same extent as with a singly born child.

Provide toys according to individual preferences, needs, and interests.

Entertain each as much as feasible. Avoid leaving them to entertain each other for long periods of time.

Provide separate rooms, if possible.

Praise each child individually and, preferably, at different times.

Discipline twins individually.

Provide seperate feeding and care schedules according to the needs of the individual child.

Arrange for frequent opportunities for individual contact with other adults.

Encourage play with other children the same age.

Modified from Sater, J.: Appraising and promoting a sense of self in twins, Am. J. Matern. Child Nurs. 4:218-226, 1979.

dition, twin children are frequently thought of and treated as a unit and efforts they make in the direction of individuality are often impeded by others (Sater, 1979). There are a number of ways in which parents and others can aid twins in achieving individuation. The accompanying box outlines suggestions for behaviors that promote individuation.

Parenting

The biologic route to parenthood is the same regardless of cultural background, age, or the motivation of the couple. Although the impulse for sexual union is spontaneous and not seasonally limited, the union for purposes of procreation can be timed according to needs and desires of the family and based on rational attachment to and the care and welfare of another individual, a great deal of which involves total dependency. It is a developmental stage in the life cycle, one which may be viewed by the parents as an endurance contest, a dismal failure, or the most rewarding and pleasurable experience of their lives.

There are ties that bind the parents to their children throughout a lifetime. Parenthood never truly ends until the death of the parent. As in all developmental processes, parenthood is influenced by past experiences, and current events affect the future of the parents. Many events and feelings regarding the past are brought out as parents care for their own children. In addition, the child is a reflection of the parent. If parents like what they see in the child, their own self-esteem is increased. A successful relationship with a child builds the parents' self-image and contributes to a better acceptance of themselves.

PARENTHOOD

A characteristic in all societies is that adults are expected to become parents and to be gratified by the experience. Pressures of tradition, sentiment regarding the state of motherhood, and religious exhortations to fulfill divine commands of fertility profoundly influence decision making, since conformity to social-role expectations is a strong influence in family planning.

Motivation for Parenthood

Conscious and unconscious motivation may enter into the decision to initiate a pregnancy. For a number of parents the motivation is based on the simple assumption that all normal people get married and have children. For many it provides proof of their biologic adequacy or demonstrates their adulthood. Some may wish to fulfill a parent's wish for grandchildren or to perpetuate the family name and fortune. To have a child in an attempt to cement a tenuous marriage is a hazardous motive. A corollary to this is the woman who desires a child to compensate for the lack of a meaningful relationship with her husband and to combat a feeling of inner loneliness and boredom. A child may be the only means for some persons to fulfill the urge to create something of value. Some persons have children in order to experience the full potential of their sexuality. In a few societies childless persons are not considered to have reached full maturity until they have children. Other motivating factors include the need to seek stimulation and novelty, to have power, to influence a life, or to compete with others. However, in most instances the couple sincerely wishes to become parents.

The decisions for second and subsequent children may be as varied as the initial motivation for parenthood. Parents may reason that a single child will benefit from interaction with a sibling to provide companionship, sharing, and experience with conflict in human relationships. Occasionally disappointment with a first child may prompt parents to try again in the hope for a more gratifying experience. Many find parenthood a satisfying experience and enjoy the presence of children. In other families the advent of a child is an unplanned event that is met with mixed emotions or, in many lower-class families, with a passive fatalism.

The number of children that a couple choose to have is an individual matter. Whether this choice is fulfilled may depend on how effectively the couple practices contraception as well as on their changing values and attitudes toward more or fewer children. Family-size preferences do not remain the same throughout marriage. Factors that are likely to influence family size are social class, religion, race, type of conjugal-role relationships, and the social-psychologic aspects of sexual relations. If a time comes when all parenthood becomes a matter of choice without religious, societal, or family pressures, it might be interesting to speculate on what types of people will choose to become parents.

Preparation for Parenthood

There is little or no evidence to support the existence of a "parental instinct" or a "maternal instinct." There appear to be no internal mechanisms to guide parental behavior; therefore parental behaviors must be learned through the socialization process. Adults in America as a whole are ill-prepared for the monumental task of parenthood. Education in American schools is notably deficient in courses that are relevant to most aspects of family life, such as sex, child care, home management, and interpersonal relationships. There are programs designed to prepare for childbirth during pregnancy, but few that prepare young adults for the life process. Some new parents have had limited experience caring for younger siblings or for the children of siblings, while the experience of others has been confined to occasional baby-sitting for neighbors during adolescence.

New parents approach parenthood with meager experience and scant knowledge, although no other task can compare, in overall consequences, with that of rearing a human being. Parents learn by trial and error, committing the same mistakes that have been committed by countless other parents, but they somehow manage to accomplish the task, becoming more skilled with each additional child. Tradition rather than rational planning furnishes the chief norms for childrearing.

The empiric preparation for parenthood is begun in the parent's own childhood. It has been established that the amount and quality of parenting that individuals have experienced in their own childhood significantly influence their later relationships with others and their ability to assume the role of parents in adulthood. By observation and imitation of their own parents and other role models—such as acquaintances, married siblings, and persons in the mass media—individuals learn culturally defined, sex-appropriate roles. Their own parents are probably the only persons that parents observe intimately in the parental role; this results in a *generational continuity*—parents rear their own children in much the same way as they themselves were reared—which is evident in the way that individuals fulfill their parental role.

Goals of Parenting

The family, in order to fulfill one of its primary functions, provides for the caregiving, nurturing, and training of children. In the process of childrearing, parents have three basic goals for their children (LeVine, 1974):

1. A *survival goal*—to promote the physical survival and health of their children, thereby ensuring that the children live long enough to produce children of their own.
2. An *economic goal*—to foster the skills and behavioral capacities that the children will need for economic self-maintenance as adults.
3. A *self-actualization goal*—to foster behavioral capabilities for maximizing cultural values and beliefs.

Parental Development

Parents proceed through parental developmental stages as a function of individual adult developmental tasks. In the process of parent-child development, the behavior of each influences the behavior of the other. The ways in which the child and the parents influence one another are discussed in subsequent chapters at greater length in relation to each major stage of child development. Briefly, development of a parental sense can be divided into four phases (Friedman, 1957):

1. **Anticipation.** Looking forward to parenthood, a young couple thinks about and discusses becoming parents and the way in which they will rear their children. They wonder what changes will develop in their relationship and what kind of parents they will be.
2. **Honeymoon.** This is the early interpersonal adjustment to the infant in which an attachment is formed between the parents and the child and new role-learning takes place. The transition in self-image from a nonparent to a parent is made.
3. **Plateau.** The long middle period of parental development parallels child development:
   The child as infant—parents learn to interpret the child's needs
   The child as toddler—parents learn to accept growth and development
   The child as preschooler—parents and child learn to separate
   The child as grade-schooler—parents learn to accept rejection and still be supportive
   The child as teenager—parents begin to rebuild their lives
4. **Disengagement.** This phase ends the active parental role, usually at the time of the child's marriage.

TRANSITION TO PARENTHOOD

The transition to parenthood is abrupt. Although a couple has anticipated the child's arrival, birth means the sudden imposition of totally dependent care 24 hours a day for the new member of the family. Some have described the birth of an infant as a crisis and it may very well be a crisis if the event is perceived as disturbing old habits and relationships ad eliciting new responses. It requires role changes, destroys or significantly modifies former relationships, and means adjusting to new role realignments. Whereas previously the roles of a couple were husband and wife, they now become, in addition, father and mother. It is difficult to adjust to being parents, but it is a normal human experience and a tool for personal growth.

The advent of a new family member requires that the family cope with greater financial responsibilities, a possible loss of income, changes in sleeping habits, and less time for husband and wife to spend with each other (especially if it is a firstborn) and/or with other children. If the events are perceived as aversive, it could well disrupt the husband-wife bond (Miller and Sollie, 1980). Some investigators find that the birth of a first child results in a reduction of spousal intimacy and affection while others report that the adjustment to parenthood is only mildly stressful. It appears that the impact of a new baby on the marital relationship is less severe or disruptive when the parents are older, conceive after the marriage ceremony, and have been married longer before conceiving (Belsky, 1981). In other words, mature, well-adjusted couples who have chosen to be parents are more likely to experience fewer difficulties as they make the transition to parenthood. However, numerous other factors can affect this adjustment.

Parental Factors Affecting Transition to Parenthood

The birth of an infant is a highly significant event that alters the behavior of both mothers and fathers. No amount of preparation can truly and fully prepare prospective parents for the constant and immediate needs of an infant. The importance of early parent-infant interactions are addressed in the discussion of the neonate, especially early mother-infant bonding and the attachment process (see p. 330). Some of the predominant factors affecting parenting are the age of the parents, the quality of the parental relationship, the amount of previous experience with childrearing, parental support systems, and the effects of stress on parental behavior.

Parental age. The most satisfactory age for childbearing has been established as the years between 18 and 35. During this time parents are considered to be in optimum health and with a predicted lifespan that allows sufficient time and vigor to raise a family. Increased lifespan and the trend toward dual careers and the desire for financial security before childbearing, however, has altered childbearing behaviors.

Statistics indicate that the age at which parents begin their families has increased recently. There has been a substantial increase in the birth rate for women aged 35 to 39 years of age. At the same time there has been a significant reduction in the birth rate of women in the 15 to 19 age group and, to a lesser degree, for women aged 20 to 24. Clearly, the tendency to delay childbearing that began in the 1970s is well established in the United States (Monthly Vital Statistics Report, September, 1985). One of the obvious outgrowths of the increased rate of first births for older parents is a subsequent decrease in the numbers of subsequent children born to a family.

Research has determined that age of parents has an effect on mother-child interactions. Older mothers are quite responsive to their children and appear to derive more pleasure from interactions with their children (Ragozin and others, 1982). Younger mothers express less favorable attitudes about childrearing and are likely to be less responsive to their infants. The problem of teenage parents is discussed as it applies to the adolescent in Chapter 20 (see p. 866).

Previous experience. Parents appear to be more relaxed and experience less conflict in disciplinary relationships with later born than with firstborn children. They have had experience with and are more cognizant of normal growth and development expectations. However much is contingent on the spacing of subsequent children. Frustrations can increase when parents are faced with two or more children who do not vary significantly in age. However, children are able to entertain one another and older children assume some responsibility for the care of younger children, thereby allowing parents more freedom for some activities. (See also discussion of Family size, p. 67.)

Marital relationship. The birth of an infant is highly significant and usually alters the behavior of both mothers and fathers and may even affect the quality of their relationship. For example, sex-typing of new parents is affected. New mothers feel more "feminine" and exhibit more feminine behaviors and engage in fewer masculine activities, thus behaving in the more traditionally sex-typed manner. On the other hand, new fathers become less traditionally sex-typed. Although they maintain the frequency of masculine role behaviors, fathers display an increase in feminine activities and their self-concept becomes less "masculine" (Feldman and Aschenbrenner, 1983).

Marital relationships can affect infants indirectly when the behavior of one parent influences the behavior of the other. For example, marital tension or strife can alter a mother's caregiving routines and interfere with her enjoyment of her infant (Belsky, 1981), or both parents may be unresponsive to their infant. As indicated in the discussion of family theories, every family member influences the behavior of every other member—even very early in the transition to parenthood.

More positive indirect effects occur in situations where parents serve as sources of mutual support and encouragement (Crnic and others, 1983). For example, fathers are more involved with their infants in families where the parents frequently discuss their infants. Even infants who may be at risk for later emotional problems, as determined by the Brazelton Neonatal Assessment Scale, will establish satisfying relationships with their parents unless the parents are unhappily married (Belsky, 1981).

Father involvement. Until recently the bulk of research and concern has been related to mother-infant interactions partly because mothers attend more to their infants than fathers do and partly because of the stereotypic view of motherhood. However, current practices that encourage early father-infant interaction have indicated that fathers ap-

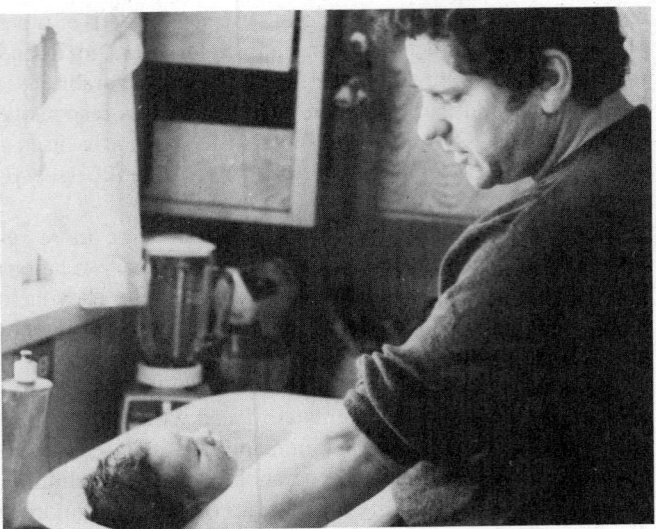

Fig. 3-6. Fathers assume care of their children soon after birth.
Photography by Anne Kunke, San Jose, CA.

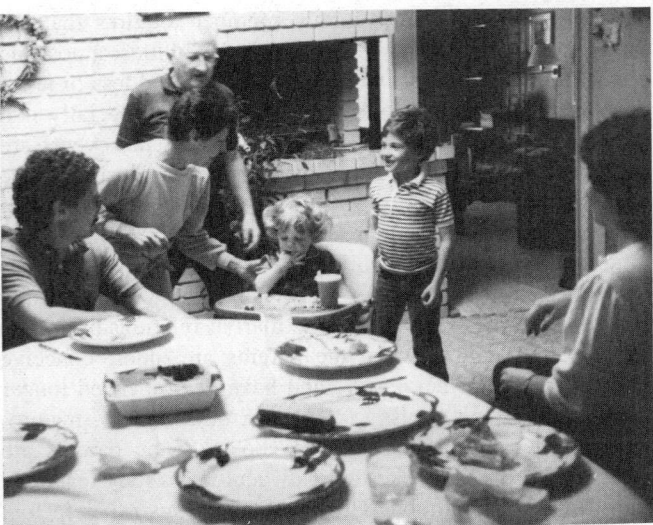

Fig. 3-7. Maintaining relationships with the extended family is important.

pear to be just as intrigued with their newborns as mothers are (see Paternal engrossment, p. 333). Even fathers who have little initial contact with their neonates will become involved with them over the next few months (Easterbrooks and Goldberg, 1984), although the type of interaction will be different from that of the mother (Fig. 3-6). For example, whereas mothers are likely to hold, soothe, care for, or play quietly with their infants, fathers are more boisterous, engaging in more physically stimulating activities that infants seem to enjoy. However fathers are more than simply playmates. They are often successful at soothing a distressed infant. Furthermore, a secure attachment to the father can help offset the consequences of an insecure attachment to the mother (Main and Weston, 1981).

Effects of stress. The effect of stress on parental behavior cannot be denied. Parents who are tired, worried, ill, or feeling unable to control the events that affect their lives may not exhibit the patience, understanding or take the time to reason with or otherwise cope with their children's behavior that they would at other times. They often find it difficult to set aside their own immediate needs in order to respond to their children. Under stressful conditions parents are less responsive to their children, are less likely to play with them, talk with them, and help them.

One of the areas in which parents, especially the mother, are subject to stress is balancing parenthood and a career. The change from more or less equal roles to that of more stereotyped roles is a source of stress to some families. The problems of dual-career families are discussed further on p. 91.

Infant characteristics. The behavior of the infant and child can also influence initial adjustment and subsequent childrearing. Parents of temperamentally difficult infants find more disruption of activities than parents with more quiet infants. Parents of children who require special care

often encounter problems not only with their children but with the quality of their relationships with each other as well. Both of these issues are discussed in association with each stage of child development and in relation to the chronically ill or disabled child in Chapter 22.

Support Systems

Successful adaptation to the stress of transition to parenthood involves at least two types of family resources (McCubbin and Paterson, 1982). First are the internal resources of the family, such as *adaptability* and *integration*. Changing from an orderly, predictable life to a relatively disordered, unpredictable one is a universal adaptation families must make. Rigid schedules are impossible to maintain and former activities must be curtailed or abandoned. Adaptation is reflected in learning to be patient, becoming better organized, and becoming more flexible.

Integration involves an attempt of the couple to continue some activities in which they were engaged before the advent of parenthood. In this way couples are able to maintain a sense of continuity and appreciate the importance of the husband-wife relationship. In some families the birth of an infant brings the couple closer together, increases their interdependence, and expands their feelings of unity and cohesion. The adjustment to parenthood can be facilitated when parents discuss their own role expectations and the role expectations of the spouse. This is especially important for first-time fathers.

The second kind of resource for coping with stress is the use of coping strategies that strengthen the organization and functioning of the family. These include the use of community resources, use of social support, and the adoption of a future orientation. Interpersonal supports that provide information, advice, and caretaking are derived from friends, relatives, and neighbors. Relationships with family, friends, and community are essential (Fig. 3-7). Arranging for time away from the infant (child or children) is beneficial. Fathers can assume care of the family to allow the mother some time to herself at home or away from the home, even for an afternoon or evening. Adoption of a future orientation provides reassurance to parents that things will get better, that they will cope, and that it is realistic to plan for the time when they are able to engage in self-fulfilling activities.

It is also reassuring to know that others experience ambivalent feelings toward parenthood and share the same difficulties and frustrations. Exchanging ideas and experiences with other parents provides an opportunity to voice concerns and to learn new ways of coping with the multiple problems of childrearing. Whether it is family, friends, or community resources, parents need persons to whom they can turn for advice, comfort, and assistance—persons with whom they can share the joys and difficulties of childrearing (Wilson, 1978).

ESSENTIALS OF PARENTING

There are some essential types of knowledge and skills parents need in order for them to feel more comfortable in the parenting role. Experience in having been nurtured as a child is an essential component of successful parenting. Parenting does indeed begin in the parents' own childhood. Parents tend to rear their children in much the same manner as they themselves were reared.

Parents need external supports including such concrete resources as are needed by all persons, that is, living space, heat, food, clothing, medical care, financial means for acquiring these, and ways to manage other expenses. Intangible sources of support needed for successful parenting have been discussed in relation to transition to parenthood in the previous section. Each family's situation and needs are unique to that family and require different types of support than another family. Also the family's needs change with alterations in circumstance (Wilson, 1978).

Skills that parents must learn include a basic understanding of childhood growth and development and the way in which it affects behavior. The behavior of infants and children is less bewildering and mysterious when parents are able to anticipate and prepare for it. Parents also need to know some of the basic skills needed to feel comfortable, for example, physical care skills, such as bathing, feeding, and the use of play to facilitate child development and interpersonal interactions.

Probably the most important skills used by parents are interpersonal skills. Infants communicate their needs to others by crying and parents must learn to interpret and respond to this basic communication. As children grow and develop, their interpersonal skills change and become more complex. Both parents and children expand their ability to communicate their needs, to respond to the needs of others, and to become sensitive to the feelings of others. The complex issues of interpersonal interactions, language development,

and communication are an integral part of this book and are addressed in all aspects of family and child care management.

PARENTING BEHAVIORS

It is impossible to discuss parent personalities and all the parental attitudes and behaviors that influence the personality development of children; volumes have been written on the significance of interactions between parents and their children. Parents' overall acceptance of a child and their disciplinary orientation have a profound impact on the way in which children view themselves and relate with others; adults' attitudes as parents are influenced by their conception of their roles in relation to children. Childrearing may be viewed as restricting and controlling child behavior, as taming the child's innate rebellious and uncivilized nature, or as guidance to provide a suitable role model for the child to emulate. Much depends on the parents' own background, their mental health, their attitudes toward childrearing in general, and their attitudes toward any individual child. A parent sees each child differently, and feedback provided by certain types of children may inadvertently create undesired attitudes in a parent.

Dimensions of Childrearing

There are infinite variations in the way parents rear their children. Some are related to cultural influences; others by social class and economic resources. Differences are found even within these narrower confines. The results of numerous studies suggest that parents that do differ from one another do so in two major dimensions.

Permissiveness-restrictiveness. Permissiveness and restrictiveness refers to the degree of autonomy that parents allow their children. Some parents exercise close, restrictive control over much of children's behavior. They limit their children's freedom of expression by imposing many demands and actively surveying their children's behavior to ensure that they comply with rules and regulations. Permissive parents make few demands and allow their children considerable freedom in exploring their environment, expressing their opinions and emotions, and making decisions about their activities. Many find a balance between the two extremes. It is not uncommon to find that many parents become less restrictive as both they and their children mature.

Warmth-hostility. Although almost all parents feel affection for their children, how openly or frequently this affection is expressed and the degree to which affection is mixed with feelings of rejection or hostility vary considerably from parent to parent. Warmth implies a human closeness, pliancy, pleasure, attention, attachment, tenderness, and deep common involvement. Parents described as warm and nurturant are those who often smile at, praise, and encourage their children while limiting their criticisms, punishments, and signs of disapproval.

Within the wide range of families the amount of affection that parents show their children may vary considerably and be influenced by cultural factors and individual differences in the personality and temperament of both the parents and children. Children who come from homes in which they are loved and accepted display socially acceptable behavior and are generally good-natured, cheerful, friendly, cooperative, and emotionally stable. Because they are loved and accepted themselves, they are able to form satisfactory relationships with others.

The terms *cool* or *cold* convey the impression of distance, rigidity, displeasure, and lack of attention and personal involvement. Cool, hostile, or rejecting parents are quick to criticize, belittle, punish, or ignore their children while limiting their expressions of affection or approval. It is important to be aware that these measures of parental warmth or coldness reflect parental behavior in a large number of situations. For example, a parent may be cool and rejecting when a child misbehaves but warm and affectionate in other contexts. Such a parent would be considered high in parental warmth. On the other hand a parent who demonstrates warmth when the child praises him or her but who is critical, punitive, or indifferent in most other situations would be classified as aloof and rejecting.

Rejection. A small minority of parents display a rejecting attitude toward their children that appears in a number of forms and occurs for a number of reasons. Rejection may be subtle or blatant and manifestations may be extensive, ranging from neglect and belittling to emotional and physical abuse. Rejecting parents overtly or covertly express feelings of dislike for the child, indicate that the child is unwanted, or state that caring for the child is burdensome. Children who are rejected develop feelings of insecurity and inferiority; they believe that if they are unworthy of parental love, they must be of no value. Many develop an avoidant relationship with the rejecting parent(s). Others attempt to win parental affection through attention-getting behaviors that frequently serve only to compound the rejecting behavior of the parents. When these tactics fail, the child may become either hostile and aggressive or withdrawn and submissive.

Sometimes rejected children find social acceptance and adjustment through identification with peers, but more often they develop feelings of isolation, inadequacy, and generally lowered self-esteem. A persistent pattern of rejection can have pervasive and long-range effects on a child's personality. The problems of disturbed parent-child relationships that are severely damaging to children are discussed in relation to failure-to-thrive syndrome, the abused child, and some of the emotional problems of childhood.

Parental Styles of Control

The extent to which parents restrict children's behavior or allow them autonomy and freedom significantly affects the psychologic atmosphere in the home. Although there are variations and degrees in parenting styles, they can generally be described as either authoritarian, permissive, or authoritative.

Authoritarian. Authoritarian, or dictatorial, parents try to control their children's behavior and attitudes through unquestioned mandates. They establish rules and regulations or a standard of conduct that they expect to be followed rigidly and unquestioningly. They value and reward absolute obedience, mute acceptance of their word, and unfailing respect for the family's principles and beliefs. They forcefully punish any behavior that is contrary to parental standards. Parental authority is exercised with little explanation and little involvement of the child in decision making. The message is: "Do it because I say so."

Punishment need not be corporal but may be stern withdrawal of their love and approval. The familiar saying—"Children are to be seen, not heard"—typifies this type of childrearing. Careful training often results in rigidly conforming behavior in the children, who tend to be sensitive, shy, self-conscious, retiring, and submissive. They are more apt to be courteous, loyal, honest, and dependable but docile. These behaviors are more typically observed when parental arbitrary power assertion is accompanied by close supervision and a reasonable level of affection. If not, arbitrary power assertion is more likely to be associated with both defiant and antisocial behavior (Maccoby, 1980).

Permissive. At the other extreme are permissive, or laissez-faire, parents who exert little or no control over their children's actions. These well-meaning parents sometimes confuse permissiveness with license. They avoid imposing their own standards of conduct and allow their children to regulate their own activity as much as possible. These parents consider themselves to be resources for the children, not role models. If rules do exist, the parents explain the underlying reason, encourage the children's opinions, and consult them in decision-making processes. They employ lax, inconsistent discipline, do not set sensible limits, and do not prevent the children from upsetting the home routine. The parents rarely punish the children, since most behavior is considered acceptable. Consequently, the children, in effect, control the parents. Children of submissive parents are often disobedient, disrespectful, irresponsible, aggressive, and generally defiant of authority.

Authoritative. Authoritative, or democratic, parents combine some childrearing practices from both the foregoing extremes. They direct their children's behavior and attitudes by emphasizing the reason for rules but negatively reinforce deviations. They respect the individuality of each of their children and allow them to voice their objections to family standards or regulations. Parental control is firm and consistent but tempered with encouragement, understanding, and security. Control is focused on the issue, not on withdrawal of love or the fear of punishment. They foster "inner-directedness," a conscience that regulates behavior based on feelings of guilt or shame for wrongdoing, not on fear of being caught or punished. Parents' realistic standards and reasonable expectations produce children with high self-esteem who are self-reliant, self-assertive, inquisitive, content, and highly interactive with other children.

The most successful type of childrearing seems to be the authoritative method. Parents do not set rigid, arbitrary limits but maintain firm control, particularly in areas of parent-child disagreement. Permissiveness, necessary for children to develop their full potential, is tempered with reasonable and consistent setting of limits. Parental power is shared and both parents provide leadership but listen to what the children have to contribute. There is more flexibility in decision-making and demands on the children, and discipline is more apt to be based on reasoning with encouragement of verbal give-and-take. However, it is very clear that parents are the final authority in areas of dispute. This approach to childrearing is more likely to facilitate the development of competence in children, which is evidenced by independent and responsible behavior on the part of the children.

SHAPING BEHAVIOR

Because children live in an organized society, they must be prepared to accept restrictions on their behavior. Discipline is not punishment. Rather it is the teaching of desirable behavior. Children need to learn the rules governing behavior in the home, the neighborhood, the school, and the community at large. To learn acceptable behavior that permits them to live enjoyably with themselves and others, children need the steady, firm guidance of loving parents and others in authority roles. Good discipline provides children with protection from dangers (from within and without) and relieves them of the burden of decisions that they are not prepared to make, yet allows them to develop independence of thought and action within a secure framework.

Children who learn to live within reasonable rules are happier and more secure children. Without the stabilizing influence of controls, children feel uncertain and insecure. Too often, inexperienced and insecure parents fear the loss of a child's love, suffer feelings of guilt over disciplinary action, or may even relinquish their authority to the child. To discipline is to teach reality. Sensible, mature parents establish fair rules and regulations in the home and then see that they are carried out. Parents should never exploit children's love for them as a means to control their children. Children's anxiety lest they lose that love is already great. Discipline based on love of the child and carried out with conviction, confidence, and consistency will produce a self-reliant, buoyant, and self-controlled child.

Patterns of Parental Discipline

Each set of parents has their own techniques and each will determine the course that the process of socialization is to follow. They may apply direct or indirect pressures in an attempt to induce or force children into the desired patterns of behavior, or they may direct their efforts toward modification of the behavioral responses of the child on a mutually acceptable basis.

Power-assertion. When parents force the child into submission to their wishes, they use power-assertive techniques. Control is exercised by taking advantage of greater physical strength and/or control over the family's resources. Power assertion relies on the child's fear of punishment for its effect and does not appeal to the child's inner resources. The most common of the power-assertive approaches, *coercion*, represents a hostile, aggressive threat of punishment (physical or verbal) if the child does not acquiesce to the parents' demands. A child responds to this type of technique either with defiance or with submission as an expression of futility.

Withdrawal of love. Withdrawal of love is a direct but nonphysical expression of anger, disappointment, or disapproval when the child misbehaves. Parents may express ridicule or dislike by explicitly stating negative feelings or refusing to listen or speak to the child. They may withdraw affection through behaviors such as ignoring, isolating, turning away from the child, or threatening to leave the child. Withdrawal of love has a decided punitive quality.

Induction. In contrast to the foregoing disciplinary tactics, induction is a relatively nonpunitive form of discipline in which the parents attempt to reason with their children. They appeal to the child's affection or respect for others. The goal of inductive discipline is to help children understand (1) why it is necessary to follow various rules and regulations, (2) why their transgressions are wrong, and (3) how they might alter their behavior to prevent future transgressions or undo whatever harm they have done (Shaffer, 1985).

Disciplinary Strategies

Within the frameworks described in the foregoing sections, parents employ various strategies for controlling and shaping behavior. Each of the strategies may have different effect on the children. It is impossible to discuss all forms of parental control. Some types of control are briefly discussed in the following section. Others are included in chapters related to children of various age-groups.

It is generally acknowledged that to be effective discipline must be appropriate to the age of the child and to the magnitude of the transgression. Disciplinary measures are more effective when they administered "early," as the child prepares to commit the prohibited act, rather than "late," when the harm has been done. It also appears that the effectiveness of punishment increases as its intensity increases, as long as the punitive consequences are not so intense that they interfere with effective learning or are perceived by the child as "cruel and unusual." Also disciplinary action should be consistent and tempered with affection. Punishment delivered by a person who has established a warm and affectionate relationship with a child is much more likely to inhibit unacceptable behavior than the same punishment administered by a cold or impersonal agent (Park, R.D., as cited in Shaffer, 1985.)

Behavioral control techniques. Control can mean *restriction*—the setting of rather narrow limits on the child's range of activities (parents impose many don'ts on children). Parents can *demand* that children do something that they do not wish to do, often expecting a high level of responsibility for the age of the children. *Strict* parents enforce rules and do not yield to a child's attempts at coercion. Parents can be *intrusive* when they interfere in a child's plans and relationships.

With *coaxing* parents attempt to elicit desired behavior by enticing the child with the promise of rewards in exchange for compliance. This may tend to create a false sense of power in the child; he may respond with defiance or he may comply in order to receive the gratification.

By *postponing,* parents attempt to alter behavior when they delay dealing with the conflict in the hope that it will resolve without further action. It may provide time to further assess the situation, but intervening factors may reduce or intensify the difficulty.

Parents use *evaluation* when they approve, disapprove, praise, blame, compare, or otherwise place a value judgment on the child's behavior. The child is uncomfortable because if he is "good" he will be expected to remain good; if he is "bad" he will be expected to change.

Parents may attempt to manipulate a situation by *masking,* that is, withholding information or substituting incorrect information to resolve a conflict. This technique tends to create an atmosphere of distrust and insecurity in the relationship.

Parents sometimes try *role reversal* in the attempt to control the child's behavior. The parent may say, "I think I see what you mean, but. . . ."

Role-modification techniques. The goal of role-modification techniques is to achieve a measure of understanding between family members and, unlike the techniques discussed in the foregoing section, they are based on a reciprocal role relationship. *Humor* enables one to appreciate and adapt to the other's point of view with a minimum of discomfort. When parents can expose the inconsistencies in a situation or appeal to a child's sense of the absurd, this is usually effective in relieving tension.

Sometimes it becomes necessary to enlist the aid of a third party to explore the problem with them. *Arbitration,* or mediation, is best performed by a person who has skills not available to the parents or the children but who has information regarding the dynamics of the situation.

Exploration of the various aspects of the problem provides both parents and children with the opportunity to look at alternatives and to propose and reject possible solutions in their attempt to arrive at an agreement. Use of this technique demonstrates a respect for the wishes and goals of the other and a willingness to search for a mutually satisfactory solution to the problem.

Compromise usually follows arbitration or exploration and refers to a problem solution that involves concessions on the part of both parties but to the detriment of neither. It requires the appraisal of each person's position and goals

and the ability to reach a reasonable agreement without submission by one in order to "keep the peace."

Role clarification is probably the most successful approach to establish complementary role relationships in the family. In situations requiring role adjustment or modification, parents are the persons who determine appropriate role responses in relation to cultural and family expectations. If they can appropriately evaluate the child's role position and their reciprocal role responses, they can assist the child in managing the specific role situation with a minimum of disequilibrium.

Consolidation is the integrated effect of redistributing goals and rewards as a consequence of various role-modification techniques. Successful consolidation, as a result of learning to work through and synthesize new roles, brings a closer unity and a higher level of complementariness to the relationships of family members.

Age of the Child

Change in parental behavior reflects the changes in needs and competencies of the children as well as changes in parental expectations. The routine caretaking of the infancy stage progresses to more noncaretaking activities such as play and visual-vocal exchanges. During the toddler years behavior-shaping and discipline are accomplished primarily through the medium of physical manipulation. The children are physically removed from hazardous situations or mischievous activity to those of the parents' choosing. Fragile and dangerous objects are placed out of reach. Older children are approached with reasoning, moral exhortation, and the giving or withholding of privileges.

However, parents function in terms of their perceptions of children's abilities. For example, stubbornness that may be amusing in a 2-year-old becomes annoying in a child of 3½ or 4 years and is often interpreted as intentional behavior, manipulation, or a deliberate attempt to anger the parents. Indeed children increasingly are able to assess the motives and perspectives of adults and older children and manipulate others for their own purposes. On the other hand, less perceptive parents may either "baby" their children or attribute to them more advanced maturity than they actually possess.

COMMUNICATING WITH CHILDREN

When children are infants communication takes place along well-defined lines. Parents become attuned to the infant's basic needs and respond in a fairly ordered way (Fig. 3-8). Gradually, however, children's personalities emerge while, at the same time, they become increasingly able to move about without assistance. With the advent of language at about 2 years of age an entirely new dimension enters the parenting process.

Empathy, the ability to step outside oneself and share the feelings of another, is the basic concept underlying satisfactory communication. However, empathy must be translated into empathetic language to be communicated effectively.

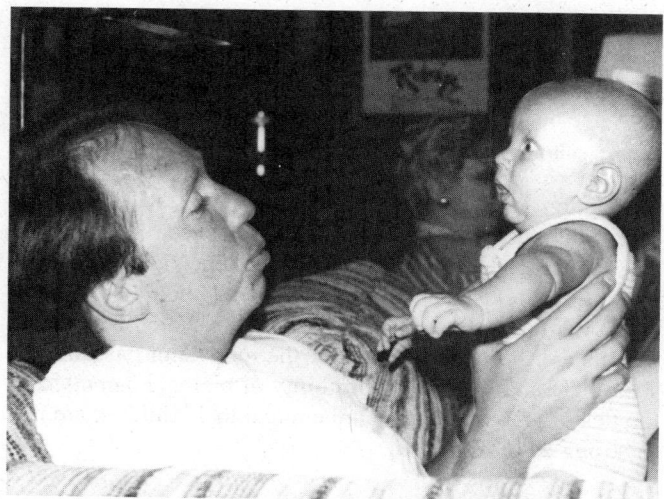

Fig. 3-8. Parents communicate with their children in a variety of ways.

Photography by Vicki Meyer, San Jose, CA.

Children's feelings must be aknowledged without concession to their demands. For example, a child who is reluctant to go to bed can be approached with a statement such as, "I know you want to stay up and be with us and you're upset about it. But it is your bedtime." It is a great relief to children to feel that they are understood. It tends to help them accept things that are difficult for them and to decrease their defenses.

Lengthy explanations of the parents' justification or instant solutions do not help children understand and cope with a situation. If an adult can get to the root of what is bothering children and help them clarify the feelings behind what they are saying, they can usually find their own way of coping with the problem. Listening to what children are really saying provides clues to the children's feelings. Parents all too often talk *at* their children rather than *with* their children.

Parents should not be reluctant to express what they are feeling. Children need to know how parents feel about their behavior and need parents to state their expectations clearly. Genuine expression of feelings without attacking the child's character or arousing hostility is a hallmark of effective communication. Use of "I" messages rather than "you" messages express personal feelings without accusation and help children develop a sense of self. For example a parent who says, "I don't like having my clothes pulled" will achieve more cooperation than with a judgmental statement such as "You are being a pest." When parents attack the behavior and not the children, they preserve their children's dignity and sense of self-worth.

To develop successful relationships and avoid conflicts, children need to know what is expected of them. It is best to establish only those rules that the parents care about enough to enforce consistently. Setting clear limits appropriate to the age, needs, and personalities of the children help children learn to control their own behavior. They can

be allowed some independence and freedom to negotiate within that framework. Whenever possible, parents can offer a choice within the prescribed limits. A parent who is having difficulty getting a child to take a bath would do well to offer the choice of method ("Do you want to take a bath or a shower?") not a choice of whether to take a bath or not. Allowing children some choice, where possible, provides them with some control in their lives and fosters independent thinking.

Directives stated positively are more likely to gain cooperation from children. For example, "Eat breakfast first, then play," rather than "You can't go out until you eat your breakfast." Endless explanations are wasted. The shorter the communication, the more effective it is.

The goal of communication with children is to help them behave more appropriately and to avoid conflict. Parents who learn to communicate with their children feel more in control of themselves. As children learn to imitate effective communication skills they, too, become better able to apply them not only at home but also to situations outside the home. What children observe has a greater impact than messages parents preach.

For additional suggestions see Communicating with children, p. 192.

INFLUENCE OF THE "EXPERTS"

Evidence indicates that there have been decided shifts in the overall philosophy of childrearing during the twentieth century. Directions on childrearing, with parental roles and practices defined by the experts, have been transmitted as advice to parents through a steady flow of pamphlets, books, and articles. Recent changes in the opinions of these experts are the result of alterations in the concept of child development and behavior and of research into the effects of parent-child interaction.

The earlier view of childcare that advocated rigid scheduling, early weaning and toilet training, and prohibition of devices that provided the child with passive pleasures (such as pacifiers) has been replaced by an easier, warmer, and more relaxed approach toward coping with child behavior that emphasizes "tender loving care" as the basis for satisfactory physical and emotional well-being. Some believe, however, that this approach generates too much permissiveness and produces some undesirable long-term consequences. The current trend in parenting manuals is to reassure parents that they will not be "perfect" parents, that mistakes are allowed, and that they should keep trying to do a good job of rearing their children while, at the same time, they should be encouraged to be relaxed, spontaneous, and to enjoy their children. These manuals attempt to convey the idea that parents are more capable than they think they are.

Parents turn to guidebooks because of an optimistic belief in progress, a faith in the future, and a typical desire to do better—better than they have been doing, better than their own parents, and better than their relatives and neighbors. Through these popular how-to parent books, parents can gain some of the accumulated knowledge of significant researchers in child development that they would be unable to acquire by attempting to read and synthesize the original texts. These guidebooks do not attempt to provide all the answers and are less authoritarian than those of the past. Most are written on the assumption that parents want to raise successful children and need support to view themselves as competent adults whose decisions are valid. Parents must deal with parenting problems on the spot at the same time that they are assimilating helpful advice and new information. They must be made to feel confident in their values and judgment during this process.

Since popular parenting manuals vary in their approaches, it is probably best to suggest that parents review some of those that are available and select at least two for use rather than to rely on the advice of a single resource. In addition to the three most widely sold authors of childrearing books—Haim G. Ginott (*Between Parent and Child* and *Between Parent and Teenager*), Fitzhugh Dodson (*How to Parent*), and Benjamin Spock (*Baby and Child Care*)—there are at least 300 others, including those of Lee Salk, Thomas Gordon, and Bruno Bettelheim.

One of the primary deficiencies in how-to books is a disregard for alternate life-styles, cultural variations, or class differences in the population. With few exceptions, the standard manuals concentrate on early childhood growth and development, on the family as an isolated entity, and still portray the mother as the primary caregiver. The working mother is ignored, or discouraged, and daycare is seldom mentioned. The implication is that mothers and fathers have distinct roles to play in raising children, and that these roles more closely resemble those of yesterday's life-styles than those encountered in this more complex society. In addition, few depict the family as a dynamic system in which each member interacts with and influences other members.

Fortunately some books have appeared that offer guidelines for single parents, adoptive parents, parents with a child who is disabled, stepparents, and families in the process of divorce. These are primarily authored by individuals who offer help based on their own experiences or by authorities who have made a study of a special problem. Parents can receive some assistance from these supplemental publications to help them cope with the additional stresses imposed by their special circumstances.

Special Parenting Situations

Parenting is a demanding task under the most ideal circumstances, but when parents and children are faced with situations that deviate from what is considered to be the norm the potential for family disruption is increased. Some of the issues that are encountered frequently are divorce with accompanying problems of single parenthood and/or reconstituted families. Adoption and dual-career families, too, have special difficulties. The problems associated with children of alcoholic parents, parents with physical disabilities, or incarcerated mothers are ones that are not addressed in the following discussions but may be topics that the reader may wish to investigate.

PARENTING THE ADOPTED CHILD

"Adoption is the method provided by law to establish the legal relationship of parent and child between persons who are not so related by birth, with the same rights and obligations that exist between children and their natural parents" (Child Welfare League of America, 1968). Adoptive parents are those who, whatever the motivation, assume the sociologic and ethical responsibility of biologic parents, and the ties of affection between them and their children are just as strong as biologic ties.

Motivation

Persons are motivated to adopt a child for different reasons. Most instances involve an adopting couple who find it impossible to have children of their own, and agencies in the past regarded this as the major criterion for placement of adoptable children. However today many people consider adoption for other reasons. There are some who feel a responsibility to provide a home for a child who needs one; others who are able to have more children of their own but are seriously concerned about overpopulation and elect to increase their family through adoption; many with families who are finding "room for one more" with whom to share their love.

Single, divorced, and widowed persons who believe that they have love and security to offer a child are seeking to adopt. Unfortunately for persons wishing to adopt a child, the demand for white infants with no physical or mental problems far exceeds the supply. However there has been an increase in the number of children with special needs, formerly considered to be unadoptable, who are finding homes through the adoptive process. These include children with disabilites, older children, children who are of minority or mixed racial ancestry, and children from foreign countries. However, the attitude that adoptive parents want only a "perfect" child has been so ingrained that healthcare workers are often unaware that there are families who have enough love and nurturing capacity to accept a child with an "imperfection."

The decision to adopt should be mutual, and various attitudes and feelings must be examined before the couple can assume the responsibility for an adopted child. Most adults assume that they will be able to have children of their own. To discover that they are unable to do so is often accompanied by feelings of inferiority, doubts about masculinity or femininity, and feelings of guilt or blame in relation to the spouse. These feelings and frustrations, superimposed on the anxious waiting for pregnancies, feelings of loss, and the endless medical procedures to establish infertility, provide an adoptive couple with their own unique preparation for parenthood.

Whatever motivates a couple to seek adoption as an alternative means to acquire a family, the decision should be based on emotionally healthy needs. The welfare of the child should be the primary consideration in placement, and such motives as the need to strengthen an unstable marriage, to treat emotional problems (including grief over death of a child), or to treat psychogenic sterility should be carefully explored. Also, when adoption satisfies the needs of only one of the two parents, the outcome is questionable.

Sources of Adoptive Children

In the past the major source of adoptable infants were socially unsanctioned pregnancies, primarily of unwed mothers since society accords a very high rating to the married status. Although adoption as a means of creating a family is openly acceptable, having children outside the marriage state is generally met with societal disapproval. However, with the widespread use of contraception, more liberalized abortion laws, and more liberal attitudes toward single parents, the number of these children available for adoption has decreased significantly.

Almost half the adoptable children in the United States are adopted by relatives, either extended family members or stepparents. Nonrelative adoptions are primarily arranged through licensed social agencies. A small proportion are arranged independently by individuals such as physicians, nurses, clergymen, and lawyers. It is well-recognized that the safest and most satisfactory adoptions are those conducted through a licensed social agency, either public or

voluntary. Some of the advantages and disadvantages of independent and agency adoptions are summarized in Table 3-2.

Risks related to adoption are usually less than those encountered in family life. Careful screening of infants can detect all but the more obscure defects, and subsequent development of defects or illnesses is no less predictable than in natural families. However, inherent emotional difficulties may be intensified in the case of adoption. Common reactions to adoption include: anxiety associated with the waiting period until adoption is legally final, uncertainty regarding whether adoption is the right choice, parents' concerns about their ability to love and parent the child, and coping with the reactions and questions of relatives, other children (if any) in the family, and friends. However bonding can be as strong and immediate for adoptive parents and children as it is for natural parents—sometimes even stronger (see p. 330).

Preparation for Adoption

Unlike natural parents who prepare for their child's birth with prenatal classes and support of friends and relatives, adoptive parents have few sources of support and preparation for the new addition to their family. Nurses who offer services to adoptive parents can provide the information, support, and reassurance needed to reduce parental anxiety regarding the adoptive process and refer them to state parental support groups that provide guidance for adoptive par-

Table 3-2 Advantages and disadvantages of agency and independent adoptions

DEFINITION	ADVANTAGES	DISADVANTAGES
Agency adoption—placement by a certified or authorized public agency	Legal safeguards for both relinquishing and adoptive parents Natural parents and adoptive parents are unknown to each other Relinquishing parent receives counseling services Careful social study of adoptive family Agency services to adoptive parents extend through the adjustment period Agency, which maintains custody of medical and other information, remains an available resource to parents and medical personnel Cost minimal	Delay in placement Placement policies of individual agencies may limit opportunities for placement of some children Not available in all areas Legal and health services vary in quality from place to place and depend on availability of legal and medical staff supervision
Independent adoption—placement by persons other than an authorized agency, such as physicians, lawyers, nurses, clergymen	Faster than agency adoptions No investigation of adopting family An alternative when unable to secure agency adoption	No guarantee of child's anonymity Limited number or lack of safeguards (legal, medical, social) Limited opportunity for selective placement Cost may be high; this may even be a profit-making venture of the intermediaries Frequently the child is not legally free for adoption at the time of placement

ents. Such sources can be contacted through a state or county welfare office or the **North American Council on Adoptable Children (NACAC)***. Prospective parents seeking information on international adoptions can contact **Families Adopting Children Anywhere†**.

Preadoption counseling should include measures to help parents overcome feelings of inadequacy and to make preparations for receiving the child, such as instruction in infant care. Adoptive parents need to prepare for the possibility that the confidentiality or the identity of the biologic parents may not be guaranteed. Some agencies even advise the adoptive parents to maintain an ongoing information store about the natural parents so that they can answer the child's questions and thereby reduce the excessive fantasizing that children may engage in later during identity formation.

Parenting Adopted Children

Most problems faced by adoptive parents are no different from those encountered by natural parents. All parents want to be good parents, but this desire is often intensified in adoptive parents. The mother, in particular, believes that she must be a better parent than the biologic mother would have been and, if she harbors any feelings about unmarried parents who relinquish children, this may affect her feelings toward the child.

The sooner infants enter their adoptive home the better for purposes of parent-infant attachment, while the more caregivers the infant has had before adoption, the more problems are likely to be encountered in attachment. The infant must break the bond with the previous caregiver and form a new bond with the adoptive parents. The difficulties in forming an attachment will depend on the amount of time the infant has spent with earlier caregivers such as the birthmother, nurse, or adoption agency personnel (Clore and Newberry, 1981).

Siblings, adopted or natural who are old enough to understand, are part of the family and should be included in decisions regarding the commitment to adopt. All the children should be treated the same and receive equal amounts of time. Neither adopted nor natural children should be made to feel that they are different or inferior, nor should they be given special consideration (Fig. 3-9).

Acceptance by extended family members and friends may create additional stresses for the family. Parents are encouraged to discuss the issue of adoption with other members of the family, especially the grandparents, whose feelings and attitudes about adoption may not be compatible. This may be a particularly difficult problem when the adopted children are members of different ethnic groups. It should be made clear to everyone that the child is the parents' child, not their "adopted" child.

Issues of origin. The task of telling children that they are adopted is a cause of deep concern and anxiety. Unfortunately there are no clear-cut guidelines for parents to fol-

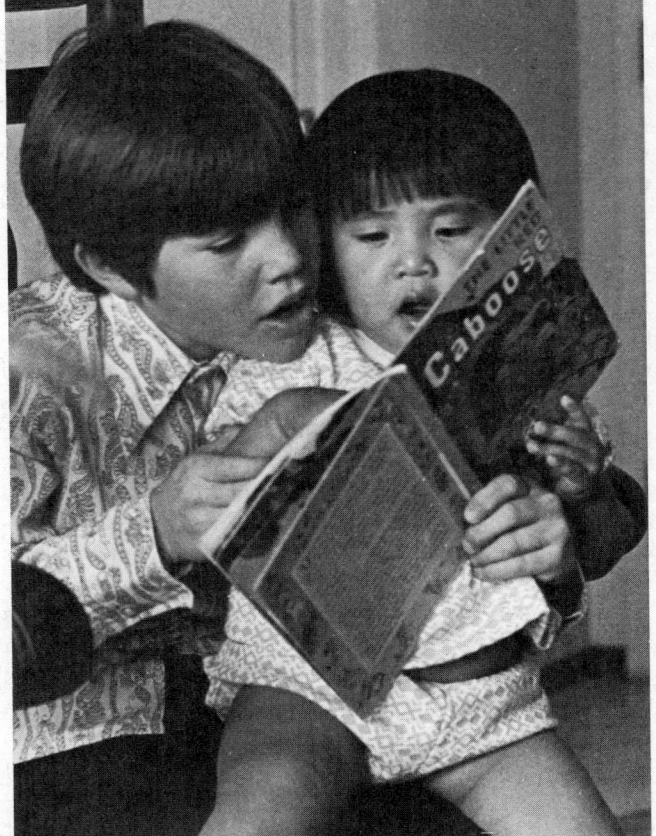

Fig. 3-9. A big brother reads a story to his adopted sister.

low in determining precisely when and at what age children are ready for the information, and parents are naturally reluctant to present the children with such unsettling news. However, it is an important aspect of their parental responsibilities, and, although they may be tempted to withhold the fact from the child, it is an essential component of the child's identity.

The timing seems to arise naturally as parents become aware of the child's readiness. Most authorities believe that children should be informed at an age young enough so that, as they grow older, they do not remember a time when they did not know that they were adopted. The time must be right for both the parents and the child and is highly individual; it may be when children ask where babies come from, at which time children can also be told the facts of their adoption. If they are told in such a way as to convey the idea that they were active participants in the selection process, they will be less apt to feel that they were abandoned victims in a helpless situation. For example, parents can tell a child that his behavior when they were looking for a child led them to believe that he wanted to go with them. It is wise for parents who have not previously discussed adoption to tell children that they are adopted before the children enter school to avoid third parties inadvertently telling the children before the parents have the opportunity. Complete honesty between parents and children usually

---

*2001 S St. NW, Washington, DC 20009.
† Box 28058, Northwood Station, Baltimore, MD 21239.

strengthens the relationship, and children should be encouraged to ask questions (Clore and Newberry, 1981).

Parents can anticipate many of the questions, although children may hesitate to ask questions about the birthparents, hoping that the adoptive parents will initiate the discussion. This is probably one of the most difficult tasks facing adoptive parents. However it is not so much what is said to the children but the attitudes and feelings that are communicated. Children should be told about their illegitimacy, if this is an actuality, and the most complete picture as possible of the birthparents should be provided (Clore and Newberry, 1981).

Parents can anticipate some behavior changes following the disclosure—especially in children who are older. Children may use the fact of their adoption as a weapon to manipulate and threaten parents. There is the inevitable "My real mother would not treat me like this," or "You don't love me as much because I'm adopted." Statements such as these hurt parents and increase their feelings of insecurity so that as parents they may become overpermissive. Adopted children need the same undemanding love as any other child combined with firm discipline and limit setting.

Adolescence. The time of adolescence may be an especially trying time for parents of adopted children. The normal confrontations of adolescents and parents may assume more painful aspects in adoptive families. Adolescents may use their adoption as a tool in defying parental authority or as a justification for aberrant behavior. As they attempt to master the task of identity formation, the feeling of abandonment by their natural parents may come to awareness or may be intensified. Sex differences in reacting to adoption may surface. It has been shown that girls have more difficulty accepting their sexuality since they may not be able to identify with a nonfertile female parent.

The children fantasize about their parents, and they may feel the need to discover the identity of their natural parents in order to define themselves and their identity—one of the major tasks of adolescent development. It is important for parents to keep lines of communication open and to reassure the youngsters that they understand the feelings of needing to search for their identities. In some states birth certificates are made legally available to adopted children when they come of age. It is important for parents to be honest with questioning adolescents and to tell them of this possibility (the parents themselves are unable to provide this for them; it is the children's responsibility if they wish).

A candid approach that may or may not be suitable for the adoptive situation is the "open adoption" program described in the book *Dear Birthmother*.* The mother who gives her child for adoption is invited to write an explanatory letter to the child and the adoptive parents, who usually respond with a letter and pictures. It is a voluntary exchange, handled through the agency that keeps all names and addresses confidential. When these exchanges are eventually read by the adopted children it helps them realize the circumstances of their adoption.

Special Adoptive Situations

The difficulty in finding infants to adopt has created an increased opportunity for adoptive parents to provide homes for children with special needs. The additional burdens of care for children with physical or emotional disabilites are no different from those of naturally born children with similar problems, with the possible exception that adoptive parents are aware of the nature of the disabilites before they receive the children. However adoption of older children and/or those of a different racial or ethnic origin pose some special problems for both parents and children.

Older children. Adopting older children constitutes an emotional experience for everyone concerned—children, parents, siblings (if any), and, often, extended family members. It involves a commitment on the part of both the adopting family and the adopted child. Adoptive families should learn as much as possible about the child before they make a final commitment.

Children awaiting adoption are usually from foster homes, group homes, or institutions. Visits between the potential adoptive family and the child can take place in the child's present home or on some type of outing during which the individuals involved are able to interact, such as on a picnic or a trip to the zoo or a playground. Visits by the child to the home of the adoptive family begin with short excursions such as an afternoon, then a day, followed by a weekend, or a week. The number and frequency of visits depend on the needs of the child and the family. During the visits the child and the family determine whether or not they will be able to make a commitment (Brockhaus and Brockhaus, 1982).

One of the difficulties of rearing adopted older children is helping them to deal with having had another set of parents. The children may have lost, in addition to their biologic parents, siblings, grandparents, friends, and personal possessions. Often they have lived in several foster homes in which they formed attachments. They need time and assistance in working through the grief process that is an integral part of any loss. At the same time they must adjust to a new household and relationships. A child who has experienced many losses and disappointments finds adjustment more difficult and takes a longer period of time to overcome fear of rejection and to develop affectionate ties to the new family. They grieve for those they left behind and may be afraid to love in case they must again move on.

Children who are adopted after age 2 maintain an image of the previous parenting persons that may cause the adopting parents some insecurity. The parents may not feel as close to these children as they would to those who are adopted in infancy. It is necessary that the children who can remember them maintain an image of the natural parents. As they grow, children are able to clearly distinguish between the parents who loved and cared for them and those who were merely responsible for their birth. Some of the

---

*Authors: K. Silber and P. Speedlin. Available through a Lutheran agency, 1037 S. Alamo, San Antonio, TX 78210.

early difficulties of adaptation are related to the change in surroundings, a change that is difficult for all children.

Early in the process of forming lasting relationships the families alter routines and activities to accommodate the children and avoid conflicts. The children are excited but somewhat frightened that they will be unable to behave in such a way that will assure acceptance and prevent their being sent away. Eventually the parents and the children are unable to maintain the host-houseguest roles and behaviors and begin a stormy period of adjustment. Children continually test families who must repeatedly reassure the children that they are wanted. Children may withdraw or act angry for months. Many conflicts can arise, particularly in the area of parental expectations and discipline. Children's past experiences, good and bad, are brought to the fore, especially during holidays. Although the children are relieved and happy to be in a new home, they often miss the familiar times and relationships. During this time the families may require considerable support and encouragement from sources outside the immediate family unit.

Eventually expectations become more realistic and family members learn to cope more effectively. The children are increasingly able to integrate past with present. They develop trust and confidence in the parents and all the members develop into a family unit with autonomy, stability, and identification (Brockhaus and Brockhaus, 1984).

Cross-racial adoption. Adoption of children of racial backgrounds different from that of the family are relatively commonplace. In addition to the problems faced by adopted children of any age, children of a cross-racial adoption must deal with their differentness. It is advised that parents who adopt such children do everything to preserve the adopted children's racial heritage.

Adoptive parents are urged to investigate the culture of their children's country, maintain their children's family name as a middle name (in some cultures this is a link to the village of their ancestors), and teach children the history and heros of their native country. Persons from the children's country can provide information about eating and sleeping patterns that will help the family make the adopted children's adaptation easier. Even music, a few words of the native language, and foods from their native country will appeal to the children's senses.

Although the children are full-fledged members of an adopting family and citizens of the adopted country, those with a foreign appearance or other decided racial characteristics may create problems outside the family. Bigotry exists that may appear among relatives and friends. Strangers may make thoughtless comments and talk about the children as though they were not members of the family. It is vital that the family make it clear to others that this is their child and a cherished member of the family.

PARENTING AND DIVORCE

In recent years there has been a marked change in the stability of families that is reflected in increased rates of divorce, single-parenthood, and remarriage. It is now estimated that 40% to 50% of current marriages in the United States will end in divorce. In 1984 1,155,000 couples divorced—a divorce rate of 4.9 per 1000 population compared with a marriage rate of 10.5 per 1000 population (Annual Summary, 1985). As a result, over 1 million children experience divorce each year.

Authorities agree that marital factors within the home significantly influence the development of children. Children from a happy, relaxed atmosphere in the home are less likely to have a negative outlook than are those from stressed homes. The effect of the parents' inability to adapt influences the adjustment and personality growth of young children. The interpersonal tension created by parental insecurity and anxiety is communicated to children, who often do not have the ego resources to cope with these feelings of tension and the vague threat of a change in their world. Even in the best divorces there will be fear, pain, uncertainty, and other emotional effects (see box below).

Since a function of parenthood is to provide for the security and emotional welfare of the child, disruption of the family structure often engenders strong feelings of guilt in the parents. Some may feel resentment toward the child—who is making the situation more difficult—and may attempt to compensate with overprotective behavior and excessive concern for the child's welfare. Some even blame the children for their problems. Children become scapegoats and find themselves dragged into their parent's problems. Some children take advantage of this opportunity to play one parent against the other.

During a divorce, parental capacity is diminished. The parents are much too preoccupied with their own feelings,

---

STAGES OF THE DIVORCE PROCESS

Acute phase
The decisive separation of the married couple with legal steps of filing for dissolution of the marriage and, usually, the departure of the father from the home. The duration of this phase lasts from several months to over a year and is accompanied by familial stress and chaotic ambience.

Transitional phase
Adults and children assume unfamiliar roles and relationships within a new family structure. The phase is often accompanied by a change of residence, a reduced standard of living and altered lifestyle, a larger share of the economic responsibility shouldered by the mother, and radically altered parent-child relationships.

Stabilizing phase
Postdivorce family reestablishes a stable, functioning family unit. Remarriage frequently occurs with concomitant changes in all areas of family life.

Modified from Wallerstein, J.S.: Children of divorce: stress and developmental tasks. In Garmezy, N., and Rutter, M., editors: Stress, coping, and development in children, New York, 1983, McGraw-Hill Book Co.

needs, and life changes to be available and supportive to their children. Newly employed parents, usually mothers, are likely to leave children with new sitters, in strange settings, or alone after school. Searching for and establishing new relationships impinge on time that can be spent at home, including weekends that may have formerly been spent with the children. Moreover, divorcing parents need to know what to do, and there are few acceptable models on which they can rely.

When adults find themselves alone for the first time in years, they may become frightened and begin to depend on their children. Such children may be forced to grow up too quickly and assume the responsibility of an absent parent or become a substitute for the absent parent. Assumption of adultlike roles places an enormous burden on children. Role reversal frequently takes place wherein the child supports the adult and is burdened not only with his own problems but with many of the parents' problems as well.

Disorder is characteristic in the custodial household following separation and divorce, coercive types of control, inflammable tempers in both parents and children, reduced parental competence, and greater sense of parental helplessness is common. There is greater disorder, poorly enforced discipline, and diminished regularity in enforcing household routines. Noncustodial parents also are seldom prepared for the role of visitor and may not have a residence suitable for children's visits. They may be concerned about maintaining the arrangement over the years to follow (Wallerstein, 1983).

Impact of Divorce on Children

The conventional belief has been that unhappily married couples should stay together for the good of the children; however research indicates that the eventual escape from parental conflict may be the most positive outcome of divorce for many children (Hetherington, 1981). Children who are under the continual stress of intact but unhappy homes often feel more secure and happy after the marital relationship is dissolved, if one of the parents is able to form a family of more quality. In fact, a couple might well *divorce* for the good of the children (Wallerstein and Kelly, 1980). However, in a number of situations the children continue to experience open parental discord for a considerable time following marriage dissolution (Wallerstein, 1983). In many ways divorce is similar to a surgical procedure—a cure for a problem when "medical" methods fail—with trauma, convalescence, and the aftermath of permanent scars.

The impact of divorce on children depends on a variety of factors, including the age and sex of the children, the outcome of the divorce, and the quality of parental care during the years following the divorce—how much love and understanding will continue after parental separation and how much genuine concern and affection exist for the child. Most children go through two phases when adjusting to a divorce: a *crisis phase,* which often lasts for a year or longer and is accompanied by an emotional upheaval that affects the relationship with the custodial parent, and an *adjustment phase,* in which children settle down and begin to adapt to life in a single-parent home (Hetherington, 1981).

Complications sometimes associated with divorce include efforts on the part of one parent to subvert the child's loyalties to the other, abandonment to other caregivers, and adjustment to a stepparent. In 90% of divorce cases the mother receives custody of the child; this has an effect on the male child's identification with a father figure in addition to all the other ramifications of living in a family without a father or in a single-parent family. Many divorced mothers with small children move in with parents, other relatives, or friends in some kind of dependent or sharing arrangement.

Children may feel a sense of shame and embarrassment concerning the family situation. Such feelings cause children to see themselves as different, inferior, or unworthy of love, especially if they feel any responsibility for the family dissolution. Although the social stigma attached to divorce no longer produces the emotions it has in the past, it may still exist in some small towns where attitudes can serve to reinforce children's negative self-image. The lasting effects of divorce depend on the children's and the parents' adjustment to the transition from an intact family to a single-parent family and, often, to a reconstituted family.

Telling the children. Many parents do not tell their children about the divorce either because they do not know what to tell the children or because they believe that the children will not understand. Although news of a pending divorce is an unhappy shock, most children are remarkably resilient and are more capable of accepting painful realities and stresses than parents expect. What is difficult for children to handle is the anxiety, uncertainty, and confusion of not knowing what is happening to their families. Children need to be told early in the process and to be told truthfully what is taking place. Frank disclosure, even when painful, helps to build trust and provides children with the security of knowing what is going on.

If possible, the initial disclosure should include both parents and all siblings, followed by later discussions with children individually. Plenty of time should be set aside for the discussions and they should take place during a period of calm, not after an argument. Parents who physically hold or touch their children provide them with a feeling of warmth that is reassuring. The discussions should include the reason for the divorce—minimizing blame—and reassurance that the divorce is not the fault of the children. Children can have guilt feelings as though they have somehow failed or are being punished for misbehavior. They wonder what role they played in the divorce or failure to keep the family together. Children assume that they have a tremendous power over parents (some actually do).

Parents need not fear open expression of their emotions. Tears express love and if parents cry, it offers permission for children to cry also. Children need to ventilate their feelings. They normally feel anger and resentment and should be allowed communicate these feelings without punishment. Parents need to listen to what the children are saying in order to gain an understanding of what they are experiencing.

The primary concern of children involved in family dissolution is to understand what will happen to them. They have feelings of terror and abandonment, see themselves apart from the family, feel alone and isolated, and long for consistency and order in their lives. They fear the uncertain future and need to know where they will live, who will take care of them, if they will be with their siblings, and if there will be enough money to live on. They worry that they might be left alone—if parents can divorce one another, can they not divorce the children? They need help in deciding what to tell their friends and teachers. They wonder if the parents will marry someone else. They need to be taught that relationships change, how to deal with new relationships, and that they will still retain the love and affection of the parents.

Age-related responses to divorce. A divorce is an unsettling experience and one that few children feel positive about for several years afterward. Previously it was believed that divorce had a greater impact on younger children, but more recent observations indicate that there is little age-related difference in the impact of divorce on children. The feelings and behaviors of children may differ according to age (see box below) but all suffer stresses second only to the stress produced by the death of a parent.

Egocentric preschoolers, who see and understand things only in relation to themselves, assume themselves to be the cause of parental distress and interpret the separation as punishment. They feel sadness and strong feelings of responsibility for the loss of the absent parent. Moreover, they consciously fear that they may be abandoned by the remaining parent. Consequently it is essential to establish some kind of stability for these children; otherwise they will convert their energies to restabilization efforts rather than to growth and development. They need frequent, repeated, and concrete explanations of what is going to happen to them, how they will be cared for, and assurance that something new will take the place of the old and that they will not be deserted. In order that they do not imagine things, explanations, such as where they will live, who will prepare their meals when the parent is at work, and when they will see the absent parent again, should be specific. They need to focus on reality.

School-age children are able to deal with parental separation better than younger children even though they feel

---

FEELINGS AND BEHAVIORS OF CHILDREN RELATED TO DIVORCE

Infancy
Effects of reduced mothering or lack of mothering
Increased irritability
Disturbance in eating, sleeping, and elimination
Interference with attachment process

Early preschool children (ages 2-3 years)
Frightened and confused
Blame themselves for the divorce
Fear of abandonment
Increased irritability, whining, tantrums
Regressive behaviors, (e.g., thumbsucking, loss of elimination control)
Separation anxiety

Later preschool (ages 3-5 years)
Fear of abandonment
Blame themselves for divorce with decreased self-esteem
Bewilderment regarding all human relationships
Become more aggressive in relationships with others, (e.g., siblings, peers)
Engage in fantasy to seek understanding of the divorce

Early school-age (ages 5-6 years)
Depression and immature behavior
Loss of appetite and sleep disorders
May be able to verbalize some feelings and understand some divorce-related changes
Increased anxiety and aggression
Feel abandoned by departing parent

Middle school-age (ages 6-8 years)
Panic reactions
Feelings of deprivation—loss of parent, attention, money, and secure future
Profound sadness, depression, fear, and insecurity
Feelings of abandonment and rejection
Fear regarding the future

Middle school-age (ages 6-8 yrs)—cont'd
Difficulty expressing anger at parents
Intense desire for reconciliation of parents
Impaired capacity to play and enjoy outside activities
Decline in school performance
Altered peer relationships—become bossy, irritable, demanding, and manipulative
Frequent crying, loss of appetite, sleep disorders
Disturbed routine, forgetfulness

Later school-age (ages 9-12 years)
More realistic understanding of divorce
Intense anger directed at one or both parents
Divided loyalties
Able to express feelings of anger
Ashamed of parental behavior
Feel the need for revenge; may wish to punish parent they hold responsible
Feel lonely, rejected, and abandoned
Altered peer relationships
Decline in school performance
May develop somatic complaints
May engage in aberrant behavior such as lying, stealing

Adolescence (ages 12-18 years)
Able to disengage themselves from parental conflict
Feel a profound sense of loss—of family, childhood
Feelings of anxiety
Worry about themselves, parents, siblings
Express feelings of anger, sadness, shame, embarrassment
May withdraw from family and friends
Disturbed concept of sexuality
May engage in acting-out behaviors

Questions and Controversies

Is it better for children to remain in a home in which there is conflict and dissention between the parents or in a divorced family where the conflict is reduced or eliminated?

Divorce has been shown to have adverse effects on the social and/or cognitive development of children. Children of divorced parents show increased behavioral problems, developmental regression, and disturbed social relationships compared to children from intact homes (Raschke and Raschke, 1979). Research also indicates that predivorce conflict in the home is associated with poor adjustment of children (Hetherington, 1981). However, children living in homes where there is parental conflict have more behavior problems than do children from divorced homes where the parents no longer show a high level of conflict (Kurdek and Siesky, 1980). In view of the findings in the literature, perhaps the question should be: What level of conflict in an intact marriage must be reached before the negative effects of that conflict on the children exceed the potential negative effects of divorce?

intense pain, loneliness, and deprivation. Younger children are preoccupied with the departure of one parent, usually the father, and grieve openly and long for his return, fearing replacement. Older children are more likely to perceive one parent as responsible, become angry with both parents, and express this anger with behavior distressing to one parent. School performance may be affected because they are unable to focus on learning; therefore teachers and school counselors should be informed so that they have a better understanding of alterations in the children's behavior and performance. Somatic complaints may be observed such as gastrointestinal complaints, headaches, asthma, a low energy level, fatigability, clumsiness, and susceptibility to injury. Often children must move to an unfamiliar environment and new neighborhood and form new relationships in addition to coping with the alteration in their family structure. They almost invariably wish for the parents to reunite.

Adolescents may be highly resentful since their lives are already sufficiently difficult and stressful. Although they are able to comprehend the divorce and are less likely to feel responsibility, adolescents find the divorce of their parents extraordinarily painful. An adolescent's sexual identity is affected by disturbed parental relationships, a precipitous deidealization of both parents, and concern about their own future as a marital partner. They are anxious about the availability of money for future needs. However, the separation of the parents may provide some space in which the the older adolescent can develop an emotional detachment from the family and individualization—normal developmental tasks of adolescence.

Sex differences. Some observers have noted sex differences in the way children respond to the stress of divorce and living in a single-parent family. The primary effect of absence of either parent from the home is that children ex-

perience difficulty adjusting to and developing of a sexual identity. This is more marked when the parental absence occurs early in the child's life and when it is the same-sex parent. Girls from homes where fathers are absent depend more on their mothers and show some anxiety about relationships with males during adolescence. Boys from homes without fathers tend to be less aggressive, more apt to have emotional and social problems, and demonstrate cognitive patterning more similar to that of girls. Overprotectiveness, extreme indulgence, and often prolonged physical contact with the mother over many years may contribute to serious sex-identity problems in male children.

Children from homes in which one or both parents are frequently absent are highly susceptible to peer group influence; this appears to be related to lack of attention and concern at home rather than to a positive attraction of the peer group. In addition, the peer group frequently serves a role identification function for young males from homes where the father is absent or ineffectual.

Other investigators have found that the effects of marital disharmony and divorce are more powerful and enduring in boys than in girls (Hetherington, 1981; Wallerstein and Kelly, 1980). Perhaps boys who show a poor adjustment to divorce are those who were very close to their fathers (Shaffer, 1985). Boys who are raised in homes where the father has custody seem to be better adjusted than those living with their mothers; girls living with their fathers are less well adjusted than those living with their mothers (Santrock and Warshak, 1979). Regular visits by the father appear to help children, especially boys, to make a positive adjustment to life in a single-parent family (Hess and Camara, 1979). One factor that seems to predict children's postdivorce relations with their parents is the quality of their relationship with each parent in the year *preceding* the divorce (Fine, Moreland, and Schwebel, 1983).

Developmental Tasks

Wallerstein (1983) describes six developmental tasks in an attempt to conceptualize the responses of children to divorce over a period of time. The first two must be dealt with immediately, others within the first few months. Successful mastery of the early tasks is linked with maintenance of developmental pace and resumption of school following an expected diminished learning effectiveness and academic performance. Later tasks are associated with a more leisurely pace and extend over the remainder of the growth period.

Task I: Acknowledge the marital disruption. The first and simplest task for children is to acknowledge the marital rift and grasp the immediate aftermath. This involves sorting out reality from the many fantasies that loom large in their attempts to understand and visualize the consequences of the situation. An additional obstacle is posed by their intense feelings that impart an ever-present sense of threat. Mastery of this first developmental task depends on the child's accuracy of perception, the emotional and intellectual capacity to understand the course of events, and the ability to master terrifying and disturbing fantasies. All of these are influenced by the developmental maturity of the child and the ability of the parents to provide satisfactory explanations concerning the disturbing aspects of the situation.

Task II: Regain a sense of direction and freedom to pursue customary activities. An early task for children is to resume their normal activities with appropriate pleasure, energy, and sustained interest, in spite of worry and preoccupation with the crisis at home. This involves some mastery over the anxieties about the collapsing family structure. Patient and loyal friends, concerned teachers, and/or other outsiders interested in the children's welfare should be available to provide the support needed to facilitate the process.

Task III: Deal with the loss and feelings of rejection. Probably the most difficult tasks facing the children are assimilating the grief, and mourning the loss of one parent from the home, and coping with the partial or total loss of that parent. The children must also overcome a profound sense of rejection and humiliation engendered by the parent's departure while, at the same time, maintaining the love and attention of that parent to ensure continuation of the relationship. Diminished self-esteem as well as a feeling of vulnerability to rejection and loss of another loving relationship can persist in children for a period of years.

Task IV: Forgive the parents. Working through the anger that children feel toward one or both parents is a major task. Their expressions of anger tend to distance them from the parent and are often manifested in behaviors designed to harass and punish the parent. One of the difficulties associated with the anger that children feel is the fact that they still love and depend on the parent and have a mutual need for forgiveness and partnership in a postdivorce family. Some of the anger is resolved as they develop a newly close relationship with one parent—a relationship that grows from a mutual need and interdependence.

Task V: Accept the permanence of the divorce and relinquish longings for the restoration of the predivorced family. Acceptance of the permanence of the divorce is closely related to successful mastery of the feelings elicited by departure of one parent. Children tend to cling to fantasies of affecting a reconciliation—fantasies that often extend beyond the remarriage of one or both parents. The divorce can only become accepted as permanent when it no longer stirs acute anxieties but is associated with relief of conflict and gratification with the current situation. Acceptance is also conditioned by the developmental maturity of the children as they achieve psychologic separation from the one parent and perceive the needs, experiences, and motivations of the parents as different from their own.

Task VI: Resolve issues of relationship. The final developmental task for children is not restricted to children of divorce but is common to all children who reach adolescence and is probably the major task. This is "to achieve realistic hope regarding future relationships and the enduring ability to love and be loved." To accomplish this task, children must revise and reformulate judgments regarding the events and work to understand the parents' marital failure. Successful completion of the task may require the support and encouragement of persons outside the immediate family who serve as models or as mentors. In the end children should be able to build substitute value systems or find persons to love and who love them in return.

Custody and Parenting Partnerships

Traditionally when parents separated the mother was given custody of the children. Now both parents and courts are seeking alternatives. The present belief is that neither fathers nor mothers should be awarded custody automatically. Rather, custody should be awarded to the parent who is best able to provide for the children's welfare.

In 90% of divorce cases the mother still receives custody of the child with visitation agreements for the father. However, more courts are now awarding custody to fathers. Men usually make more money and can offer more material benefits than many women are able to provide. The incidence of delinquent support payments to custodial mothers is a matter of universal knowledge and concern. The single-parent family is commonplace, but many divorced mothers with small children move in with parents, other relatives, or friends in some kind of dependent or sharing arrangement. No matter what type of custody arrangement is awarded, the primary consideration is the welfare of the children.

Characteristics of the various types of post-separation parenting arrangements are outlined in the box on p. 89. This typology derived from studies by Durst, Wedemeyer, and Zurcher (1985) includes joint custody (discussed later) but does not address the issue of divided custody in which the custody of the children is divided between the parents. The problems of custodianship when the mother or the father is awarded custody of the children are discussed in relation to single-parenthood (see next section).

Joint custody. When both parents believe that they are equally capable of raising the children and both want custody, joint custody is a viable alternative that is becoming more common. Co-parenting offers substantial benefits for the family: children can be close to both parents, and life with each parent can be more normal as opposed to a disciplinarian mother and a fun-and-games father.

Parents consider themselves as full partners in parenting and do not base this definition on amount of time spent with the children. The advantage of this arrangement is that neither parent feels more powerful or dominant than the other, and each is more likely to get dependable, mature adult help with problems of childrearing. The relationship between the parents is one of cooperation but limited to matters related to parental functioning.

The joint custody plan can be almost anything that both parents agree on, but both parents must be truly dedicated to making it work. It usually assumes one of two forms (Charnas, 1983). First, the children reside with one parent

PARENTING PARTNERSHIPS

Type I: Mother and nonparent father
Father never enters fathering role
Mother assumes sole responsibility for child from birth
Father's contact with children infrequent and unpredictable
Father does not engage in guidance or caretaking of children
Father functions as entertainer only
Spousal boundaries highly variable—communication usually written

Type II: Mother and father as friends
Father had participated in childcare before divorce
Mother has responsibility for children
Father maintains predictable schedule of visits for some time, often 2 to 3 days per month; overnight stays frequent
Father-child interaction is primarily "father as friend"
Close relationship between parents based on common interests, past history, and mutual affection

Type III: Mother and restricted father
Court-ordered inflexible visiting schedule for father
Father feels restricted; mother satisfied with visiting arrangement
Father's parenting role ambiguous
Father participates little in children's development
Considerable hostility between spouses
Low level of communication between spouses
Parents often need intermediary for communication

Type IV: Timesharing parents
Equal sharing of children in terms of time
Lack of shared decision-making
Low level of communication between parents
Each parent functions as "sole custodian"—each functions independently, not cooperatively
Burden of smooth-running arrangement primarily children's responsibility

Type V: Co-parents
Parents are full partners in parenting
Joint decision-making
Clear, flexible boundaries between spousal and parental subsystems
Timesharing variable

From Durst, P.L., Wedemeyer, N.V., and Zurcher, L.A.: Parenting partnerships after divorce: implications for practice, Soc. Work **30:** 423-428, 1985.

rangement is more effective when each parent maintains some personal regard and civility toward the other.

Variations of joint custody are endless. However, to be successful, the parents must place a high value on the commitment to provide as normal parenting as possible and be able to separate their marital conflicts from the parenting roles. The parents can expect some differing views on child-rearing just as parents in intact families. Another requisite is that the children should have access to both parents unless the physical or psychologic welfare of the children is in jeopardy. In some cases of joint custody, the children live with neither parent. For example, the child lives at a school and alternates vacations and holidays between the father and the mother.

Divided custody. Another parenting option is divided, or split, custody. For example, sons might live with the father and the daughters with the mother. The arrangements vary according to the needs and desires of the families. Children visit with the other parent and children. Most such families maintain an open-house policy whereby children are free to visit with little or no interference with their outside activities. The cooperation between parents is as variable as in other forms of custody. This arrangement usually requires flexibility and the ability of both families to work together to make it a success.

SINGLE-PARENTING

Single-parent status is acquired by means of divorce, separation, death, or through birth or adoption of a child by a single person. Over the past two decades the proportion of children living with two parents has decreased dramatically, while the proportion of children living with only the mother has almost doubled (U.S. Bureau of the Census, 1982). In addition, there has been an increase in the proportion of children who are born out-of-wedlock and most of whom will probably never live with two natural parents (Hofferth, 1985). It is has been determined that 40% to 50% of children in the United States spend some time in a single-parent home (Clark-Stewart, 1982; Hetherington, 1981).

Although more never-married women than ever before voluntarily elect single parenthood, the bulk of this discussion is directed toward the single-parent family created as a consequence of marital dissolution. Many of the problems are the same. However, the never-married parent is not burdened with the emotional adjustments related to a family history that accompany a divorced single parent.

Single parenthood is accompanied by an altered self-image as well as by the need for another realignment of role. The physical separation from a spouse is not always accompanied by psychologic separation. There are many unresolved feelings associated with the separation. Feelings of anger, remorse, guilt, retaliation, mixed feelings of hatred and love, and sorrow for oneself can maintain an emotional relationship for some time following the physical separation. For each parent this separation is accompanied by

with liberal visitation but, unlike sole custody of one parent, both parents are still the children's legal guardians who participate together in childrearing. This type is especially advantageous for participants whose job or geographic location prevents easy access to the children or for those who have difficulty cooperating.

Second, the parents alternate the physical care and control of the children on a reasonably equitable basis while maintaining shared parenting responsibilities legally. This type of custody arrangement works well for families who live in closer proximity and whose occupations allow an active role in the care and rearing of the children. The ar-

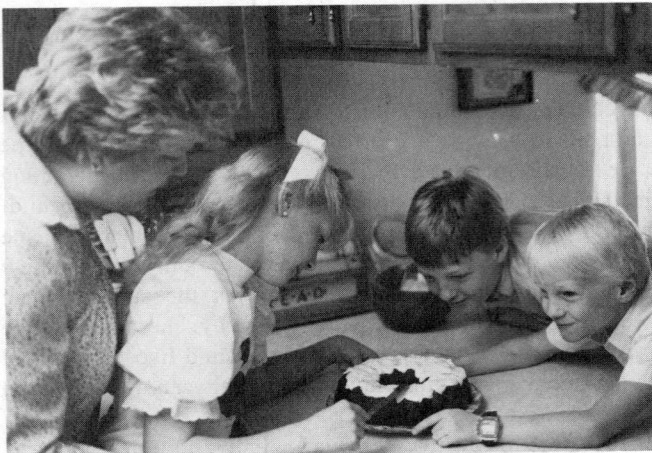

Fig. 3-10. Single parents take every opportunity to engage in activities with their children.
Photography by Earl Fillmore, Salt Lake City, UT.

mourning and resolving and facing true feelings about one-self. It takes time but can be facilitated by working through these feelings with understanding friends, relatives, or professionals such as psychologists, social workers, or nurses.

Being the sole provider in all areas of childcare places a stress on the parent both economically and emotionally. New role responsibilities for women means evaluating their wage-earning capacity. Many mothers have never worked outside the home. Following divorce, families headed by mothers must often manage on a fraction of the income to which they were accustomed when the father was present. This frequently necessitates moving to more modest housing in a poorer neighborhood, often away from the friends and neighbors who have been sources of emotional support. When the mother begins to work she has less time to spend with the children, is frequently fatigued, and can become more erratic and inconsistent in parenting (see Working mothers, p. 92).

The more financial and emotional support the mother receives from the noncustodial parent, the better she is able to cope with parenting tasks. Custodial mothers who have cordial relationships with their ex-husbands are more sensitive to the needs of the children and the regular involvement of the father is associated with better adjustment of the children.

In the process of resolution, the single parent must cope with loneliness and fewer family interactions. The feeling of being isolated from all but the children may create parent-child relationships in which the parent and child are either overly attached to eah other or in constant conflict. The reaction of the parent is to devote extra attention to the child because of feelings of guilt, lowered self-esteem, and as a protection against intimacy with other adults. Children feel that the burden of the parent's happiness or unhappiness is on their shoulders (Fig. 3-10).

There is a need on the part of the parent for social contacts and a life separate from the children for the emotional growth of both parent and child. The single parent can find support and encouragement from **Parents Without Partners**, an organization designed to meet the needs of this increasingly important group.*

Single Fathers

Fathers who have custody of their children have many of the same problems as divorced mothers. They feel overburdened by the responsibility, are depressed, and are concerned about their ability to cope with the emotional needs of the children, especially the needs of the girls (Hetherington, 1981). The lack of homemaking skills is characteristic of most fathers. They find it difficult at first to coordinate household tasks, school visits, and other activities associated with managing a household alone. Fathers often demand more assistance with household tasks and more independence from their children than custodial mothers do, and they are likely to make use of alternative caregiving and support systems.

PARENTING IN RECONSTITUTED FAMILIES

Approximately half of all children from broken homes will experience yet another major change in their lives within 3 years of a divorce—a return to a nuclear family and the sudden acquisition of a stepparent when the custodial parent remarries. Most reconstituted families involve a mother, her children, and a stepfather; less often it is a father with children and a stepmother. Sometimes two single-parent families join to form a single household (see box, p. 91).

Entrance of a stepparent into a ready-made family requires adjustments for all the family members. Some obstacles to the role adjustments and the family problem-solving include disruption of previous life-styles and interaction patterns, complexity in the formation of new ones, and lack of social supports (Nelson and Nelson, 1982). There is no formula that can guarantee success in forming a new family, but most authorities agree that flexibility and family communication are essential. There should be complete honesty and roles must be clearly defined, including the role of the noncustodial parent. Use of finances are determined from the beginning—who is responsible for expenses related to the children including food, clothing, education, and use of support moneys (if any).

Stepparenting. The role of stepparent is unclear and often confusing. He or she is in the awkward position of having to share a role with the parent who is missing from the original family in such functions as financial support, education, and coordinating visits when the parent is living and in carrying out moral, religious, and other responsibilities if the parent is dead. The reality of the natural parent's

*International Headquarters, 7910 Woodmont Ave., Washington, DC 20014.

presence, whether he or she is dead or alive, is important to the stepchildren's development of their own identity, but this complicates the role of stepparent. There is almost always the elements of mistrust, fear of failure, and a sense of vulnerability in a reconstituted family.

A stepparent plays three roles, and it is difficult to determine which role to assume in the process of rearing a stepchild. One is the role of *parent* in matters of discipline, planning family experiences, and setting limits on behavior; another is *stepparent* when plans and activities must be shared with the absent natural parent; and a third is that of a *nonparent* when the stepparent steps aside to allow the spouse to manage those things of which the stepparent is not or does not wish to be a part.

The stereotype of wicked stepmother and cruel stepfather has done little to foster healthy relationships with stepchildren, and stepparents usually go to great lengths in an attempt to avoid this image. They studiously avoid taking sides with stepchildren or minimize involvement with them as much as possible. Sometimes the natural parent at home feels guilty about separating the children from their other parent and restrains the stepparent from an authority position, thus rendering the stepparent powerless in a parental role. Sometimes the parent may wish that the stepparent would totally assume the parental role.

Many factors that affect childrearing can interfere with the relationship between parent and stepparent. The child may serve to constantly remind the parent of the previous relationship; an unresolved relationship between the natural parents may interfere with full development of the new relationship; and the feelings and attitude of the stepchild toward the stepparent may inhibit relationships. A stepchild may feel guilty about liking a stepparent better than the absent parent, especially when the outside parent "uses" the child as a go-between in an attempt to destroy the new family relationship. In this situation the best approach is to tell the child that the natural parent failed as a marriage partner, not as a parent, although children eventually realize this.

The stepparent who has replaced a dead parent is in a more difficult position. In this situation guilt and idealization, part of the normal grief process, may become intensified in the children. Overidealization and an attempt to hold onto the dead parent causes some children to make unfair and discriminating comparisons. Probably the best approach on the part of the stepparent is to be frank about the good points of the deceased parent but not to agree with the comparison and avoid defensiveness.

Sources of guidance and support for stepfamilies can be found in numerous publications and from groups, such as local chapters of **The Stepfamily Association of America,*** an organization that offers education and supportive services for stepfamilies. In many situations the relationship produces satisfaction for both the children and the stepparent. The children have warm feelings toward the stepparent and

---

*28 Allegheny Avenue, Suite 1307, Baltimore, MD 21204.

> ## TIPS FOR 'LIVING IN STEP'
>
> 1. Let relationships develop slowly and naturally. Don't expect too much too soon, from the children, from your spouse, or from yourself.
> 2. Don't criticize or belittle lost (or new) parents, or try to erase or replace them. Stepparents are additional parents.
> 3. Expect confused feelings, anxieties, competition for attention, bids for loyalty. Decide on standards of discipline and behavior and stick to them.
> 4. Communicate. Don't pretend everything is fine if it isn't. Look at problems squarely and deal with them openly.
> 5. If you need help, admit it and get it. Read a book, get counseling, join a support group, call a family meeting.
>
> From Stein, B.: Yours, mine, and ours: a look at stepfamilies, Growing parent, 12(9):1-5, 1984.

gain undersanding and maturity that they would not have achieved without a stepparent.

Effects on children. Most children from divorced families want to live in a two-parent home. Studies have found that remarriage of parents does not appear to cause problem behavior or negative attitudes toward self and others in stepchildren. In stepfather families, boys display more warmth, higher levels of self-esteem, less anxiety, and less anger than boys in intact families. Girls in stepfather families are more anxious than those in intact families and displayed more anger toward their mothers than boys do. Boys are also warmer than girls toward their stepfathers (Santrock and others, 1982). Girls also demonstrate less positive verbal and more negative problem-solving behavior toward their stepparent than do boys (Clingempeel, Brand, and Ievoli, 1984). It is believed that behavior of girls is probably related to the behaviors of the mothers than the behavior of the stepfather.

PARENTING IN DUAL-CAREER FAMILIES

No change in family lifestyle has had more impact than the large numbers of women entering the workplace. As women moved away from the traditional homemaker pattern, the numbers of dual-earner families increased dramatically until they now comprise 52% of married couples in the United States (U.S. News and World Report, 1983). This trend is unlikely to diminish. As a result, the family is subjected to considerable stress as members attempt to meet the challenge of the often competing demands of occupational needs and those regarded as necessary for a rich family life.

Role definitions are frequently altered to arrange an equitable division of time and labor, as well as to resolve conflicts between earlier and later norms, especially those re-

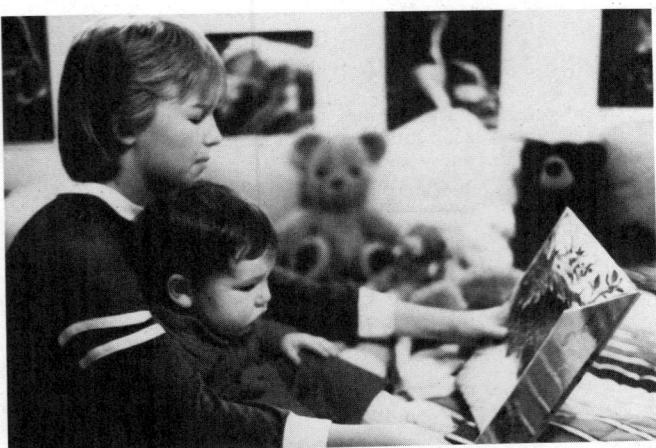

Fig. 3-11. Working mothers make a special effort to spend time with their children.
Photography by Wayne Kunke, San Jose, CA.

lated to the traditional norms of the culture. Overload is a common source of stress in a dual-career family, and social activities are significantly curtailed. Time demands and scheduling are major problems and, when there are children, the demands can be even more intense. In fact dual-career couples may increase the strain on themselves in order to avoid creating stress for their children, although there is no evidence to indicate that the dual-career lifestyle, as such, is stressful to children. However, the stress experienced by the parents may affect the children indirectly.

Working Mothers

Much has been written and a variety of conclusions drawn regarding the effects of mothers working outside the home. Mothers work for several reasons. Most work for purely economic reasons, either because they are the sole support of the family, or to supplement a husband's inadequate income, or to provide the family with a higher standard of living. Others work as a response to the boredom of housework or simply to meet their own ego needs.

Regardless of the mother's motivation, the consensus is that any deleterious effects on the children are related to the *quality* of the mother-child interaction rather than the *quantity* of time spent with the children. Quality time means not only a warm and loving relationship but time that is stimulating and enriching for both parent and child. Planning time to be alone with the children, engaging in activities that are enjoyable for both and being honest when fatigue inhibits active play, and simply being with the children (even inviting them to assist with tasks) as often as possible constitutes quality time (Fig. 3-11).

The mother's relationship to the rest of the family depends to a large extent on her own feelings and reactions to working and to her job. Although most mothers feel some guilt about leaving their children in the care of others, those who feel secure and happy in their work usually reflect this attitude in the home and in relationships with other members of the family. Sometimes, however, the mother feels guilty about leaving the children so that she can pursue a career or a job, particularly if she enjoys the outside activity. If she compensates for guilt feelings by overindulgence toward the children, they may feel more insecure and take advantage of her vulnerability with demanding behavior. On the whole, children of working mothers are self-reliant, do well in school, and show relatively few ill effects of the separation.

Many factors are related to the effect that a mother's absence has on the children: the age of the child (very young children feel the impact of the mother's absence more than older children), the attitude of the father toward the wife's employment, the regularity with which she is away from the family, and the availability and quality of substitute child care. Substitute child care, either inside or outside the home, should be selected carefully and evaluated regularly (see p. 517).

CONCEPT SUMMARIES

- Although there is no agreement about the definition of *family*, families may be grouped into the following broad categories: family of orientation and family of procreation.

- Theories that have been used to describe families include developmental theory, structural-functioning theory, interactional theory, exchange theory, systems theory, and conflict theory.

- Family composition refers to individuals with socially recognized statuses and positions who interact on a recurring basis in socially sanctioned ways.

- Although the traditional family structure has been nuclear or extended, in recent years other forms, such as the single-parent family, have emerged.

- Roles within the family may be ascribed, achieved, adopted, or assumed.

- Family size and positioning within the family structure have a strong impact on a child's development.

- Interpersonal skills and a basic understanding of childhood growth and development are two essential areas of focus for parents.

- Parents tend to demonstrate one of three dimensions of childrearing: permissiveness-restrictiveness, warmth-hostility, and rejection.

- Parents shape a child's behavior through discipline, which may take the form of power-assertion, withdrawal of love, or induction.

- Marital factors within the home significantly influence a child's development. The impact of divorce on a child depends on age and sex, outcome, and quality of parental care following the divorce.

REFERENCES

Abbink, C., and others: Bonding as perceived by mothers of twins, Pediatr. Nurs. **8:**411-413, 1982.

Ahrons, C.R.: The binuclear family: two households, one family, Altern. Lifestyles **2:**499-515, 1979.

Allen, W.R.: Black family research in the United States: a review, assessment, and extension, J. Compar. Fam. Stud. **9:**301-313, 1978.

Annual Summary, Washington, DC, 1985, U.S. Government Printing Office.

Baskett, L.M., and Johnson, S.M.: The young child's interaction with parents versus siblings: a behavioral analysis, Child Dev. **53:**643-650, 1982.

Beckman, L.J.: Couples' decision-making processes regarding fertility. In Tauber, K.E., Burgess, L.L., and Sweet, J.A., editors: Social demography, New York, 1978, Academic Press, Inc.

Belsky, J.: Early human experience: a family perspective, Dev. Psychol. **17:**3-23, 1981.

Blau, P.: Justice in social exchange, Soc. Inquiry **24:**193-206, 1964.

Bower, F.L.: Exchange theory and family study, unpublished manuscript, 1978.

Bower, F., and Jacobson, M.: Family theories: frameworks for nursing practice. In Archer, S., and Fleshman, R., editors: Community health nursing: patterns and practice, North Scituate, MA, 1978, Duxbury Press.

Brockhaus, J.P.D., and Brockhaus, R.H.: Adopting an older child—the emotional process, Am. J. Nurs. **82:**288-291, 1982.

Burgess, E.W.: The family as a unit of interacting personalities, The Family **7:**3-9, 1926.

Carter, E., and McGoldrick, M., editors: The family life cycle, New York, 1980, Gardner Press.

Charnas, J.F.: Joint child-custody counseling—divorce 1980s style, Soc. Casework **64:**546-554, 1983.

Child Welfare League of America: Standard for adoption services, New York, 1968, The League.

Clarke-Stewart, K.A.: Daycare, Cambridge, MA, 1982, Harvard University Press.

Clingempeel, W.G., Brand, E., and Ievoli, R.: Stepparent-stepchild relationships in stepmother and stepfather families: a multimethod study, Fam. Rel. **33:**465-472, 1984.

Clore, E.R., and Newberry, Y.S.G.: Nurse practitioner guidance for the adoptive family from birth to adolescence, Pediatr. Nurs. **7**(6):16-25, 1981.

Crnic, K.A., and others: Effects of stress and social support on mothers and premature and full-term infants, Child Dev. **54:**209-217, 1983.

Dunn, J., and Kendrick, C.: Social behavior of young siblings in the family context: differences between same-sex and different-sex dyads, Child Dev. **52:**1265-1273, 1981.

Durst, P.L., Wedemeyer, N.V., and Zurcher, L.A.: Parenting partnerships after divorce: implications for practice, Soc. Work **10:**423-428, 1985.

Duvall, E.R.: Family development, ed. 5, Philadelphia, 1977, J.B. Lippincott Co.

Easterbrooks, M.A., and Goldberg, W.A.: Toddler development in the family: impact of father involvement and parenting characteristics, Child Dev. **55:**740-752, 1984.

Espinoza, R., and Newman, Y.: Step-parenting, DHEW Publication No. (ADM)78-579, Washington, DC, 1979, U.S. Government Printing Office.

Eshleman, J.R.: The family: an introduction, ed. 3, Boston, 1981, Allyn & Bacon, Inc.

Feldman, S.S., and Aschenbrenner, B.: Impact of parenthood on various aspects of masculinity and femininity: a short-term longitudinal study, Dev. Psychol. **19:**278-289, 1983.

Fine, M.A., Moreland, J.R., and Schwebel, A.I.: Long-term effects of divorce on parent-child relationships, Dev. Psychol. **19:**703-713, 1983.

Freidman, D.: Parent development, Calif. Med. **86:**25-28, 1957.

Glick, P.C.: Children of divorced parents in demographic perspective, J. Soc. Issues **35:**170-182, 1979.

Groothuis, J.R., and others: Increased child abuse in families with twins, Pediatrics **70**(5):769-773, 1982.

Hall, A., and Fagan, D.: Definition of a system, General Systems Yearbook, 1956.

Helvie, C.: Community health nursing: theory and process, New York, 1981, Harper & Row, Publishers, Inc.

Hess, R.D., and Camara, K.A.: Post divorce family relationships as mediating factors in the consequences of divorce for children, J. Soc. Issues **35:**79-96, 1979.

Hetherington, E.M.: Children and divorce. In Henderson, R.W., editor: Parent-child interaction: theory, research, and prospects, New York, 1981, Academic Press, Inc.

Hetherington, E.M., Cox, M., and Cox, R.: The aftermath of divorce. In Contemporary readings in child psychology, ed. 2, New York, 1981, McGraw-Hill Book Co.

Hofferth, S.L.: Updating children's life course, J. Marr. Fam. **47:**93-115, 1985.

Homans, G.C.: Social behavior as exchange, Am. J. Soc. **63:**597-606, 1958.

Jimenez, S.L., and Jungman, R.G.: Supplemental information for the family with a multiple pregnancy, Am. J. Matern. Child Nurs. **5:**320-325, 1980.

Johnson, R.: Promoting the health of families in the community. In Stanhope, M., and Lancaster, J.: Community health nursing, St. Louis, 1984, The C.V. Mosby Co.

Kurdek, L.A., and Siesky, A.E., Jr.: Effects of divorce on children—the relationship between parent and child perspectives, J. Divorce **4:**85-99, 1980.

LeVine, R.A.: Parental goals: a cross-cultural view, Teach. Coll. Rec. **76:**226-239, 1974.

Maccoby, E.E.: Social development: psychological growth and the parent-child relationship, New York, 1980, Harcourt Brace Jovanovich, Inc.

Macklin, E.D.: Nontraditional family forms: a decade of research, J. Marr. Fam. **42:**175-192, 1980.

Main, M., and Weston, D.R.: The quality of the toddler's relationship to mother and to father: related to conflict and the readiness to establish new relationships, Child Dev. **52:**932-940, 1981.

Marriage: It's back in style, U.S. News and World Report, June 20, 1983.

Mauksch, H.: A social science basis for conceptualizing family health, Soc. Sci. Med. **8:**521-527, 1974.

McAdoo, H.P.: Factors related to stability in upwardly mobile black families, J. Marr. Fam. **40:**761-766, 1978.

McCubbin, H.I., and Patterson, J.M.: Family adaptation to crisis. In McCubbin, H.I., Cauble, E., and Patterson, J.M., editors: Family stress, coping, and social support, Springfield, IL, 1982, Charles C Thomas, Publisher.

Mednick, B., and Baker, R.: Consequences of family structure and maternal state for child and mother's development, Final report, NICHD (contract N 01-HD-82807), 1980.

Miller, B.C., and Sollie, D.L.: Normal stresses during the transition to parenthood, Fam. Rel. **29:**459-465, 1980.

National Center for Health Statistics: Annual summary of births, marriages, divorces, and deaths, Monthly Vital Statist. Rep. **33:**1-3, 1985.

Nelson, M., and Nelson, G.K.: Problems of equity in the reconstituted family: a social exchange analysis, Fam. Rel. **31:**223-231, 1982.

Perkins, T.F., and Kahan, J.P.: An empirical comparison of natural-father and stepfather family systems, Fam. Process **18:**175-183, 1979.

Pines, M.: Only isn't lonely (or spoiled or selfish), Psychol. Today **15**(3):15-19, 1981.

Prasad, R., and Prasad, A.: Survival sequence of infants: a factorial analysis, J. Biosoc. Sci. **10:**17-22, 1978.

Ragozin, A.S., and others: Effects of maternal age on parenting role, Dev. Psychol. **18:**627-634, 1982.

Rank, M.R., and LeCroy, C.W.: Toward a multiple perspective in family theory and practice: the case of social exchange theory, symbolic inter-actionalism, and conflict theory, Fam. Rel. 32:442-448, 1983.

Rodman, H.: Talcott Parsons' view of the changing American family. In Rodman, H., editor: Marriage, family, and society, New York, 1965, Random House, Inc.

Raschke, H.J., and Raschke, V.J.: Family conflict and children's self-concepts: a comparison of intact and single parent families, J. Marr. Fam. 41:367-374, 1979.

Rogers, R.H.: Improvement in the construction and analysis of family life cycle categories, Kalamazoo, MI, 1962, Western Michigan University.

Santrock, J.W., and Warshak, R.A.: Father custody and social development in boys and girls, J. Soc. Issues 35:112-125, 1979.

Sargent, A.J.: The family: a pediatric assessment, J. Pediatr. 102:973-976, 1983.

Sater, J.: Appraising and promoting a sense of self in twins, Am. J. Matern. Child Nurs. 4:218-226, 1979.

Shaffer, D.R.: Developmental psychology: theory, research, and applications, Monterey, CA, 1985, Brooks/Cole Publishing Co.

Singelmann, R.B.: Exchange as symbolic interaction: convergences between two theoretical perspectives, Am. Soc. Rev. 37:414-424, 1972.

Sprey, J.: Conflict theory and the study of marriage and the family. In Burr, W.R., and others, editors: Contemporary theories about the family, vol. 2, New York, 1979, The Free Press.

Steelman, L.C., and Powell, B.: The social and academic consequences of birth order: real, artifactual, or both? J. Marr. Fam. 47:117-124, 1985.

Terkelson, K.: Toward a theory of the family cycle. In Carter, E., and McGoldrick, M., editors: the family life cycle: a framework for family therapy, New York, 1980, Gardner Press, Inc.

Turner, R.H.: Role-taking: process versus conformity. In Arnold, M.R., editor: Human behavior and social processes, Boston, Houghton Mifflin Co., 1962.

U.S. Bureau of the Census: Marital status and living arrangements: March 1981, Curr. Pop. Rep. Series P-20, No. 372, Washington, DC, 1982, U.S. Government Printing Office.

Wallerstein, J.S.: Children of divorce: stress and developmental tasks. In Garmezy, N., and Rutter, M., editors: Stress, coping, and development in children, New York, 1983, McGraw-Hill Book Co.

Wallerstein, J.S., and Kelly, J.B.: California's children of divorce, Psychol. Today, Jan. 1980, pp. 67-76.

Whitehead, T.L.: Residence, kinship and mating as survival strategies: a West Indian example, J. Marr. Fam. 40:817-828, 1978.

WHO: Health and the family: studies in the demography of family life cycles and their health implication, Geneva, Switzerland, 1978, The Organization.

Wilson, A.L.: Parenting in perspective, Fam. Comm. Health 3:65-77, 1978.

Winch, R.F.: Familial organization: A quest for determinants, New York, 1977, The Free Press.

BIBLIOGRAPHY
General

Aldous, J., Osmond, M.W., and Hicks, M.W.: Men's work and men's families. In Burr, W.R., and others: Contemporary theories about the family, vol. I, New York, 1979, The Free Press.

Baranowski, E.: Childbirth education classes for expectant deaf parents, Am. J. Matern. Child Nurs. 8:143-146, 1983.

Barranti, C.C.R.: The grandparent/grandchild relationship: family resource in an era of voluntary bonds, Fam. Rel. 34:343-352, 1985.

Brandt, M.A.: Consider the patient part of the family, Nurs. Forum 11:19-23, 1984.

Brandt, P.A.: Social support and life change during early family development. In Chinn, P.L., and Leonard, K.B.: Current practice in pediatric nursing, vol. 3, St. Louis, 1980, The C.V. Mosby Co.

Brody, C.J., and Steelman, L.C.: Sibling structure and parental sex-typing of children's household tasks, J. Marr. Fam. 47:265-273, 1985.

Callan, V.J.: Comparisons of mothers of one child by choice with mothers wanting a second birth, J. Marr. Fam. 47:155-164, 1985.

Clements, I.W., and Roberts, F.B., editors: Family health: a theoretical approach to nursing care, New York, 1983, John Wiley & Sons, Inc.

Fsife, B.L.: A model for predicting the adaptation of families to a medical crisis: an analysis of role integration, Image 17:108-112, 1985.

Gerald, R.L.: The family in social context, ed. 5, New York, 1982, Oxford University Press.

Hymovich, D., and Barnard, M.U.: Family health care, New York, 1979, McGraw-Hill Book Co.

Jensen, M.D., and Bobak, I.M.: Maternity and gynecologic care: the nurse and the family, St. Louis, 1985, The C.V. Mosby Co.

Kaufman, D.H.: An interview guide for helping children make health-care decisions, Pediatr. Nurs. 11:365-367, 1985.

Klaus, M.H., and Kennell, J.H.: Parent-infant bonding, ed. 2, St. Louis, 1982, The C.V. Mosby Co.

Lamb. M.E.: Mothers, fathers, and children in a changing world. In Tyson, R.L., Call, J., and Galenson, E., editors: Infancy in a changing world, New York, 1985, Basic Books, Inc., Publishers.

Leslie, G.R.: The family in social context, ed. 5, New York, 1982, Oxford University Press Inc.

McCubbin, H.I., and Figley, C.R., editors: Stress and the family: coping with normative transitions, New York, 1983, Brunner/Mazel, Inc.

Newman, B.M., and Newman, P.R.: Development through life: a psychosocial appoach, ed 3, Homewood, IL, 1984, The Dorsey Press.

Reinhardt, A.M., and Quinn, M.D.: Family-centered community nursing: a sociocultural framework, St. Louis, 1980, The C.V. Mosby Co.

Sciarillo, W.G.: Using Hymovich's framework in the family-oriented approach to nursing care, Am. J. Matern. Child Nurs. 5:242-248, 1980.

Stone, L.J., and Church, J.: Childhood and adolescence: a psychology of the growing person, ed. 5, New York, 1984, Random House, Inc.

Streff, M.B.: Examining family growth and development: a theoretical model, Adv. Nurs. Sci. 3(4):61-69, 1981.

Wright, L.M., and Leahey, M.: Nurses and families: a guide to family assessment, Philadelphia, 1984, F.A. Davis Co.

Family Theories

Hurley, P.M.: Family assessment: systems theory and the genogram, Child. Health Care, 10:76-82, 1982.

Nye, F.I.: Is choice and exchange theory the key? J. Marr. Fam. 42:21-233, 1980.

Family Structure

Blanton, J.: Communal child rearing: the Synanon experience, Altern. Lifestyles 3:87-116, 1980.

Jacques, J.M., and Chason, K.J.: Cohabitation: its impact on marital success, Fam. Coord. 28:35-39, 1979.

Jordheim, A.E.: Alternate lifestyles and the family. In Reinhardt, A.M., and Quinn, M.D., editors: Family-centered community nursing, vol. II, St. Louis, 1980, The C.V. Mosby Co.

Family Configuration

Abramovitch, R., Corter, C., and Pepler, D.J.: Observations of mixed-sex sibling dyads, Child Dev. 51:1268-1271, 1980.

Cornold, C., and Faltori, L.C.: Age spacing firstborns and symbiotic dependence, J. Pers. Soc. Psychol. 33:431-434, 1977.

Falbo, T.: Only children and interpersonal behavior: an experimental and survey study, J. Appl. Soc. Psychol. 8:244-253, 1978.

Falbo, T., and Polit-O'Hara, D.F.: Only children: what do we know about them? Pediatr. Nurs. 11:356-360, 1985.

Foley, K.L.: Caring for the parents of newborn twins, Am. J. Matern. Child Nurs. 4:221-226, 1979.

Goshen-Gottstein, E.R.: The mothering of twins, triplets, and quadruplets, Psychiatry 70:769-773, 1982.

Gromada, K.: Maternal-infant attachment: the first step toward individualizing twins, Am. J. Matern. Child Nurs. **6:**129-134, 1981.

Kidwell, J.S.: Number of siblings, sibling spacing, sex and birth order: their effects on perceived parent-adolescent relationships, J. Marr. Fam. **43:**50-64, 1981.

Mercy, J.A., and Steelman, L.C.: Familial influence on the intellectual attainment of children, Am. Soc. Rev. **47:**532-542, 1982.

Minnett, A.M., Vandell, D.L., and Santrock, J.W.: The effects of sibling status on sibling interaction: the influence of birth order, age spacing, sex of child, and sex of sibling, Child Dev. **54:**1064-1072, 1983.

Paulhus, D., and Shaffer, D.R.: Sex differences in the impact of number of older and number of younger siblings on scholastic aptitude, Soc. Psychol. Q. **44:**363-368, 1981.

Samuels, H.R.: The effect of older sibling on infant locomotor exploration of a new environment, Child Dev. **51:**607-609, 1980.

Stainton, M.C.: The effect of ordinal position or birth order on child development, Nurs. Forum **19**(2):165-179, 1981.

Zajonc, R.B., Markus, H., and Markus, G.: The birth order puzzle, J. Pers. Soc. Psychol. **37:**1325-1341, 1979.

Parenthood and Parenting

Benzon, L., and Lastowka, T.: Developing a parent education program in an ambulatory care setting, J. Assoc. Care Child. Hosp. **8:**21-25, 1979.

Bishop, B.: A guide to assessing parenting capabilities, Am. J. Nurs. **76:**1784-1787, 1976.

Boger, R., and Kurnetz, R.: Perinatal positive parenting: hospital-based parenting support for first-time parents, Pediatr. Basics No. 24, pp. 4-7, 10, 1985.

Brandt, P.A.: Stress-buffering effects of social support on maternal discipline. Nurs. Res. **33:**229-234, 1984.

Brandt, P.A.: Social support and life change during early family development. In Chinn, P.L., and Leonard, K.B.: Current practice in pediatric nursing, vol. 3, St. Louis, 1980, The C.V. Mosby Co.

Briggs, E.: Transition to parenthood, Matern. Child Nurs. J. **8**(2):69-83, 1979.

Bromberg, D., and Shumway, J.: Psychosocial factors in parenting, Pediatr. Ann. **9:**256-262, 1980.

Brown, J.B.: Infant temperament: a clue to childbearing for parents and nurses, Am. J. Maternal Child Nurs. **2:**228-232, 1977.

Callan, V.J.: Comparisons of mothers of one child by choice with mothers wanting a second birth, J. Marr. Fam. **47:**155-164.

Cameron, J.: Year-long classes for couples becoming parents, Am. J. Maternal Child Nurs. **4:**358-362, 1979.

Damrosch, S.P., Lenz, E.R., and Perry, L.A.: Use of parental advisors in the development of a parental coping scale, Am. J. Matern. Child. Nurs. **14:**103-109, 1985.

Goldberg, W.A., and Easterbrooks, M.A.: Role of marital quality in toddler development, Dev. Psychol. **20:**504-514, 1984.

Gordon, S., Lerner, L., and Keefe, F.: Responsive parenting: an approach to training parents of problem children, Am. J. Comm. Psychol. **7**(1):45-56, 1979.

Grusec, J.E., and Kuczynski, L.: Direction of effect in socialization: a comparison of the parent's versus the child's behavior as determinants of disciplinary techniques, Dev. Psychol. **16:**1-6, 1980.

Holden, G.W.: Avoiding conflict: mothers as tacticians in the supermarket, Child Dev. **54:**233-240, 1983.

Hollen, P.: Parents' perceptions of parenting support systems, Pediatr. Nurs. **8:**309-313, 1982.

Johnston, M.: Cultural variations in professional and parenting patterns, JOGN Nurs. **9**(7):9-13, 1980.

Jones, F.A., Green, V., and Krauss, D.R.: Maternal responsiveness of primiparous mothers during the post-partum period: age differences, Pediatrics **65:**579-583, 1980.

Kiernan, B., and Scoloveno, M.A.: Fathering, Nurs. Clin. North Am. **12:**481-490, 1977.

Lovell, M.C., and Fiorino, D.L.: Combating myth: a conceptual framework for analyzing the stress of motherhood, Adv. Nurs. Sci. **1**(4):75-84, 1979.

Mulhern, R.K., and Passman, R.H.: Parental discipline as affected by sex of parent, sex of child, and the child's apparent responsiveness to discipline, Dev. Psychol. **17:**604-613, 1981.

Riley, D., and Cochran, M.M.: Naturally occurring childrearing advice for fathers: utilization of the personal social network, J. Marr. Fam. **47:**275-286, 1985.

Slevin, K.F.: Motherhood, culture, and change, Pediatr. Nurs. **8:**405-408, 1982.

Smoyak, S.A.: Introduction: symposium on parenting, Nurs. Clin. North Am. **12:**447-455, 1977.

Steffensmeier, R.H.: A role model of the transition to parenthood, J. Marr. Fam. **44:**319-323, 1982.

Stewart, R.B.: Sibling attachment relationships: child-infant interactions in the strange situation, Dev. Psychol. **19:**192-199, 1983.

Ventura, J.N.: Parent coping behaviors, parent functioning, and infant temperament characteristics, Nurs. Res. **31:**269-273, 1982.

Webster-Stratton, C., and Kogan, K.: Helping parents parent, Am. J. Nurs. **80:**240-241, 1980.

Wheeler, K.G.: The crisis of the first child. In Chinn, P.L., and Leonard, K.B.: Current practice in pediatric nursing, vol. 3, St. Louis, 1980, The C.V. Mosby Co.

Adoption

Braff, A.M.: Telling children about their adoption: new alternatives for parents, Am. J. Maternal Child Nurs. **2:**254-259, 1977.

Brockhaus, J.P.D., and Brockhaus, R.H.: Adopting an older child—the legal process. Am. J. Nurs. **82:**292-294, 1982.

Hill, M., and Peltzer, J.: A report of thirteen groups for white parents of Black children, Fam. Rel. **31:**557-565, 1982.

Leonard, K.B.: The challenge of adoption. In Chinn, P.L., and Leonard, K.B., editors: Current practice in pediatric nursing, vol. III, St. Louis, 1980, The C.V. Mosby Co.

Sherwen, L.N., Smith, D.W., and Cueman, M.A.: Common concerns of adoptive mothers, Pediatr. Nurs. **10:**127-130, 1984.

Smith, D.W., and Sherwen, L.N.: Mothers and their adopted children: the bonding process, New York, 1983, Tiresias Press.

Smith, D.W., and Sherwen, L.N.: The bonding process of mothers and adopted children, Top. Clin. Nurs. **6**(3):38-48, 1984.

Sokoloff, B.: Should the adopted adolescent have access to his birth records and his birth-parents? Clin. Pediatr. **16:**975, 1977.

Sokoloff, B.: Adoptive families: needs for counseling, Clin. Pediatr. **18:**184-190, 1979.

Walker, L.O.: Identifying parents in need: an approach to adoptive parenting, Am. J. Maternal Child Nurs. **6:**118-123, 1981.

Zimmerman, B.M.: The exceptional stresses of adoptive parenthood, Am. J. Maternal Child Nurs. **2:**191-197, 1977.

Divorce

Abarbanel, A.R.: Shared parenting after separation and divorce: a study of joint custody, Am. J. Orthopsychiatry **49:**320-329. 1979.

Ahrons, C.R.: Divorce: a crisis of family transition and change, Fam. Rel. **29:**533-540, 1980.

Booth, A., and Edwards, J.N.: Age at marriage and marital instability, J. Marr. Fam. **47:**67-75, 1985.

Coucouvanis, J.A., and Solomons, H.C.: Handling complicated visitation problems of hospitalized children, Am. J. Matern. Child Nurs. **8:**131-134, 1983.

Derdeyn, A.P.: Children in divorce: intervention in the phase of separation, Pediatrics **60:**20-27, 1977.

Dudding, G.S.: Counseling children through their parents' divorce, Issues Compr. Pediatr. Nurs. **2**(3):40-51, 1977.

Ellison, E.S.: Issues concerning parental and children's psychosocial adjustment, Am. J. Orthopsychiatry **53:**73-81, 1983.

Engebretson, J.C.: Stepmothers as first-time parents: their needs and problems, Pediatr. Nurs. **8:**387-390, 1982.

Fergusson, D.M., Horwood, L.J., and Dimond, M.E.: A survival analysis of childhood family history, J. Marr. Fam. **47**(2):287-295, 1985.

Futterman, E.H.: After the civilized divorce, Child Pyschiatry **19:**525-530,1980.

Greif-Brown, J.: Fathers, children, and joint custody, Am. J. Orthopsychiatry **49:**311-319, 1979.

Hetherington, E.M.: Divorce: a child's perspective, Am. Psychol. **34:**851-858, 1979.

Jackson, P.L.: Caring for children from divorced families, Am. J. Maternal Child Nurs. **8:**126-130, 1983.

Jellinek, M.S., and Slovik, L.S.: Divorce: impact on children, N. Engl. J. Med. **305:**557-560, 1981.

Jenkins, J.A.: For the kids' sake, TWA Ambassador **16**(3):16-22, 1983.

Kappelman, M.M., and Black, J.: Children of divorce: the pediatrician's responsibility, Pediatr. Ann. **9**(9):48-64, 1980.

Kulka, R.A., and Weingarten, H.: The long-term effects of parental divorce in childhood on adult adjustment. J. Soc. Issues **35**(4):50-78, 1979.

Lebowitz, M.L.: Divorce and the American teenager, Pediatrics **76:**695-698, 1985.

Lowery, C.R.: Child custody in divorce: parents' decisions and perceptions, Fam. Rel. **34:**241-249, 1985.

Lowery, C.R., and Settles, S.A.: Effects of divorce on children: differential impact of custody and visitation patterns, Fam. Rel. **34:**455-463, 1985.

Mitchell, A.K.: Adolescents' experiences of parental separation and divorce, J. Adoles. **6:**175-187, 1983.

Parish, G.D.: Perceptions of personal and familial adjustment by children from intact, single-parent, and reconstituted families, Psychol. Schools **21:**166-174, 1983.

Price-Bonham, S., and Balswick, J.O.: The noninstitutions: divorce, desertion, and remarriage, J. Marr. Fam. **42:**225-238, 1980.

Rankin, R.P., and Maneker, J.S.: The duration of marriage in a divorcing population: the impact on children, J. Marr. Fam. **47:**43-52, 1985.

Raschke, H.J., and Raschke, V.J.: Family conflict and children's self-concepts: a comparison of intact and single-parent families, J. Marr. Fam. **41:**367-374, 1979.

Schilling, L.S.: The effects of divorce on children: a perspective for the pediatric health care provider, J. Assoc. Care Child. Health **11:**92-96, 1983.

Tableman, M.: Overview of programs to prevent mental health problems of children, Public Health Rep. **96:**38-44, 1981.

Terr, L.C.: Child snatching: A new epidemic of an ancient malady, J. Pediatr. **103:**152-156, 1983.

Wallerstein, J.S., and Kelly, J.B.: Children and divorce: a review, Soc. Work **24:**468-475, 1979.

Wallerstein, J.S., and Kelly, J.B.: Effects of divorce on the visiting father-child relationship, Psychiatry **137:**1534-1539, 1980.

Single Parenting

Bowman, M.E., and Ahrons, C.R.: Impact of legal custody status on fathers' parenting postdivorce, J. Marr. Fam. **47:**481-488, 1985.

Burns, C.E.: The hospitalization experience and single-parent families: a time of special vulnerability, Nurs. Clin. North Am. **19:**285-293, 1984.

Grief, G.L.: Children and housework in the single father family, Fam. Rel. **34:**353-357, 1985.

Grief, G.L.: Single fathers rearing children, J. Marr. Fam. **47:**185-191, 1985.

Hanson, S.: Single custodial fathers and the parent-child relationship, Nurs. Res. **30:**202-204, 1981.

Hoeffer B.M.: Single mothers and their children. In Chinn, P.L., and Leonard, K.B.: Current practice in pediatric nursing, vol. III, St. Louis, 1980, The C.V. Mosby Co.

Hughes, C.B., and Scoloveno, M.: The single father, Top. Clin. Nurs. **6**(3):1-9, 1984.

Jack, M.S.: The single-parent family: an issue in nursing, Issues Compr. Pediatr. Nurs. **2**(3):30-39, 1977.

Kelly, J., and Wallerstein, J.: Brief interventions with children in divorcing families, Am. J. Orthopsychiatry **47:**23-29, 1977.

McRae, M.: An approach to the single parent dilemma, Am. J. Maternal Child Nurs. **2:**164-167, 1977.

Meagher, M.A.K.: Separation, divorce, and subsequent coping problems of single-parent families. In Reinhardt, A.M., and Quinn, M.D., editors: Family-centered community nursing, vol. 2, St. Louis, 1980, The C.V. Mosby Co.

Tankson, E.A.: The single parent. In Johnson, S.H.: High-risk parenting, Philadelphia, 1979, J.B. Lippincott Co.

Weinberg, T.S.: Single fatherhood: How is it different? Pediatr. Nurs. **11:**173-175, 1985.

Stepfamilies

Cherlin, A., and McCarthy, J.: Remarried couple households: Data from the June 1980 current population survey, J. Marr. Fam. **47**(4):23-30, 1985.

Clingempeel, W., Ievoli, G., and Brand, E.: Structural complexity and the quality of stepfather-stepchild relationships, Fam. Proc. **23:**547-560, 1984.

Ganong, L.H., and Coleman, M.: The effects of remarriage on children: a review of the empirical literature, Fam. Rel. **33:**389-406, 1984.

Jacobson, D.S.: Stepfamilies, Child. Today **9**(1):2-6, 1980.

Kleinman, J., Rosenberg, E., and Whiteside, M.: Common developmental tasks in forming reconstituted families, J. Mar. Fam. Ther. **5:**79-86, 1979.

Pink, J.E.T., and Wampler, K.S.: Problem areas in stepfamilies: cohesion, adaptability, and the stepfather-adolescent relationship, Fam. Rel. **34:**327-335, 1985.

Poppen, W.A., and White, P.N.: Transition to the blended family, Elem. Sch. Guid. Coun. **19:**50-61, 1984.

Ransom, J.W.: A stepfamily in formation, Am. J. Orthopsychiatry **49:**36-43, 1979.

Santrock, J.W., and others: Children's and parents' observed social behavior in stepfather families, Child Dev. **53:**472-480, 1982.

Stern, P.M.: Conflicting family culture: an impediment to integration in stepfamilies, J. Psychosoc. Nurs. Ment. Health Serv. **20**(10):27-33, 1982.

Visher, E.B., and Visher, J.S.: Common problems of stepparents and their spouses, Am. J. Orthopsychiatry **48:**252-262, 1978.

Dual-Career Family

Clore, E.R.: The working mother with young children, Child Care Newsletter **4**(1):4-6, 1985.

Committee on Psychosocial Aspects of Child and Family Health, American Academy of Pediatrics: the mother working outside the home, Pediatrics **73:**874-875, 1984.

Floge, L.: The dynamics of child-care use and some implications for women's employment, J. Marr. Fam. **47:**143-154, 1985.

Heins, M., and others: Attitudes of pediatricians toward maternal employment, Pediatrics **72:**283-290, 1983.

Kutzner, S.K., and Toussie-Weingarten, C.: Working parents: the dilemma of child rearing and career, Top. Clin. Nurs. **6**(3):30-37, 1984.

Sinal, S.H., and Herndon, A.: Attitude of pediatricians toward maternal employment and substitute child care, South. Med. J. **77:**726-729, 1984.

Zambana, R., Hurst, M., and Hite, R.: The working mother in contemporary perspective: a review of the literature, Pediatrics **64:**862-868, 1979.

Chapter 4

Growth and
Development
of Children

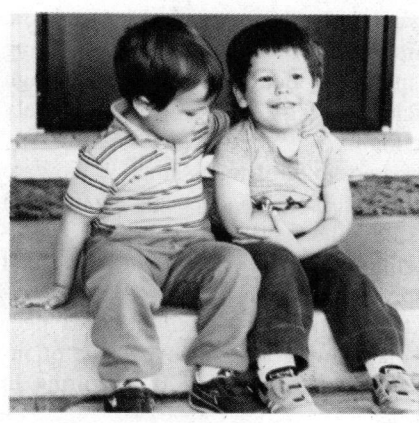

Children grow and develop in response to a predetermined plan that governs the physical and, to some extent, the behavioral changes continually taking place in their bodies and minds. Growth and development are complex processes involving numerous components that are subject to a wide variety of influences. All facets of the child's body, mind, and personality develop simultaneously, although not independently, and emerge at varying rates and sequences.

Physical growth begins at the time of conception; behavior and personality do not develop until after birth. Each aspect of development, such as the organ systems and personality components, has a timetable for growth, maturation, or elaboration. Because of the dynamic, ever-changing nature of the developmental process, a condition or behavior that is normal at one age is considered to be abnormal if it persists into subsequent stages of development.

This chapter is devoted to some of the ongoing maturational changes in children from a longitudinal perspective. The reader is introduced to the general progression and flow of developmental changes that take place throughout childhood. Also included are preliminary discussions of some of the major concepts and needs that accompany, are precipitated by, or in some way influence normal development. In subsequent chapters the topics introduced here are elaborated in discussions of major developmental stages to provide a holistic view of a child at a specific stage in development.

Growth and Development

Human beings begin their existence with a physical, biochemical, and mental potential that is contained in the genes they receive from each of their parents and that determines their ultimate developmental capacity. Equally influential in shaping the individual throughout a lifetime is the environment, which is neither constant nor dependable. At the present time hereditary factors cannot be altered, but the environment is subject to varying degrees of manipulation.

FOUNDATIONS OF GROWTH AND DEVELOPMENT

Growth and development, usually referred to as a unit, expresses the sum of the numerous changes that take place during the lifetime of an individual. The entire course is a dynamic process that encompasses several interrelated dimensions.

Growth implies a change in quantity and results when cells divide and synthesize new proteins. This increase in number and size of cells is reflected in increased size and weight of the whole or any of its parts.

Maturation, which literally means to ripen, is described as aging or as an increase in competence and adaptability. It is usually used to describe a qualitative change, that is, a change in the complexity of a structure that makes it possible for that structure to begin functioning or to function at a higher level. Sometimes maturation designates the unfolding of traits inherent in the organism.

Differentiation is primarily a biologic description of the processes by which early cells and structures are systematically modified and altered to achieve specific and characteristic physical and chemical properties, although it is sometimes used to describe one of the trends in development—mass to specific.

Development is a gradual growth and expansion. It too involves a change, in this instance from a lower to a more advanced stage of complexity. Development is the emerging and expanding of the individual's capacities through growth, maturation, and learning to provide progressively greater facility in functioning.

All of these processes are interrelated. Although they are simultaneous, ongoing processes, none occurs apart from the others. The child's body becomes larger and more complex; the personality simultaneously expands in scope and complexity. Very simply, growth can be viewed as a *quantitative* change, and development as a *qualitative* change. Children "grow" by maintaining a positive balance of increase over loss in size; they "grow up" by maturing in structure and function.

Stages of Growth and Development

Most authorities in the field of child development conveniently categorize child growth and behavior into approximate age stages or in terms that describe the features of an age-group. The age ranges of these stages are admittedly arbitrary, and since they do not take into account individual differences, they cannot be applied to all children with any degree of precision. However, this categorization affords a convenient means to describe the characteristics associated with the majority of children at periods when distinctive developmental changes appear and specific developmental tasks* must be accomplished. It is also significant for nurses to know that there are characteristic health problems peculiar to each major phase of development. The sequence of descriptive age periods and subperiods that are used here and elaborated in subsequent chapters include:

Prenatal period: conception to birth
EMBRYONIC: conception to 8 weeks
FETAL: 8 to 40 weeks (birth)
A rapid growth rate and total dependency make this one of the most crucial periods in the developmental process. The relationship between maternal health and certain manifestations in the newborn emphasizes the importance of adequate prenatal care to the health and well-being of the infant.

---

*A developmental task is a set of skills and competencies peculiar to each developmental stage that children must accomplish or master in order to deal effectively with their environment.

Infancy period: birth to 12 or 18 months

NEONATAL: birth to 28 days

INFANCY: 1 to approximately 12 months

The infancy period is one of rapid motor, cognitive, and social development. Through mutuality with the caregiver (mother), the infant establishes a basic trust in the world and the foundation for future interpersonal relationships. The critical first month of life, although part of the infancy period, is often differentiated from the remainder because of the major physical adjustments to extrauterine existence and the psychologic adjustment of the mother.

Early childhood: 1 to 6 years

TODDLER: 1 to 3 years

PRESCHOOL: 3 to 6 years

This period, which extends from the time children attain upright locomotion until they enter school, is characterized by intense activity and discovery. It is a time of marked physical and personality development. Motor development advances steadily. Children at this age acquire language and wider social relationships, learn role standards, gain self-control and mastery, develop increasing awareness of dependence and independence, and begin to develop a self-concept.

Middle childhood: 6 to 11 or 12 years

Frequently referred to as the "school age," this period of development is one in which the child is directed away from the family group and is centered around the wider world of peer relationships. There is steady advancement in physical, mental, and social development with emphasis on developing skill competencies. Social cooperation and early moral development take on more importance with relevance for later life stages. This is a critical period in the development of a self-concept.

Later childhood: 11 to 19 years

PREPUBERTAL: 10 to 13 years

ADOLESCENCE: 13 to approximately 18 years

The tumultuous period of rapid maturation and change known as adolescence is considered to be a transitional period that begins at the onset of puberty and extends to the point of entry into the adult world—usually high school graduation. Biologic and personality maturation are accompanied by physical and emotional turmoil, and there is redefining of the self-concept. In the late adolescent period the child begins to internalize all previously learned values and to focus on an individual, rather than a group, identity.

Methods of Studying Growth and Development

The early growth period in the human being extends over a longer time than that of any other mammalian species. The long period of childhood allows for more elaborate brain development, body growth, and the development of those characteristics of personality that distinguish man from lower animals. During these early years children prepare for adulthood in several dimensions: they increase in size and acquire increasingly intricate motor capacities, their personality emerges, and they assimilate their culture.

To determine whether or not growth and development have taken place, the child can be compared to a representative group of children at the same point in time (cross-sectional method), or the same child can be measured and compared at different points in time (longitudinal method). Standards or norms for the study of developmental

progress have been established by these two contrasting methods.

The *cross-sectional* method, which tests or measures the characteristics of a number of children representing the various ages or stages of development, is the more common. The observations of children are made at the same point in time. For example, a group of schoolchildren, ages 6 to 12 years, are measured for specific characteristics such as height, weight, mental ability, motor ability, or vocabulary. The data collected and averaged on a group of 6-year-old children, for instance, provide information on the expected achievement of a child in that age-group. If large groups are used, the results are expressed as averages, but the meaning of these results is directly related to the similarities within the groups, such as race, sex, and socioeconomic level. Most norms or averages are determined in this way and are helpful when comparing groups. For instance, the average height of 8-year-old children in Chicago can be compared with the average height of 8-year-old Mexican children. This method is especially useful to establish norms for a given age-group with or without other factors.

The *longitudinal* method is often used to determine growth trends and rates. Each child in a group of children is observed and measured periodically over a number of years and through successive stages of growth and development. This approach is also useful in assessing the long-term or delayed effects of an early experience, such as a prolonged illness, malnutrition, or maternal rejection. Although the longitudinal method is more difficult to carry out, the growth and development of a child can be compared at any moment with a representative group of children and can be followed through successive stages to determine the speed and direction of that child's distinctive growth.

Patterns of Growth and Development

There are definite and predictable patterns in growth and development that are continuous, orderly, and progressive. These patterns, sometimes referred to as trends or principles, are universal and basic to all human beings. Although they are more apparent with respect to physical growth, most of these patterns apply to psychologic and social growth as well. Growth and development follow predetermined trends in direction, sequence, and pace, but each human being accomplishes these in a manner and time unique to that individual.

Directional trends. Growth and development proceed in regular, related directions or gradients and reflect the physical development and maturation of neuromuscular functions (Fig. 4-1). The first pattern is the *cephalocaudal,* or head-to-tail, direction. The head end of the organism develops first and is very large and complex, whereas the lower end is small and simple and takes shape at a later period. The physical evidence of this trend is most apparent during the period before birth, but it also applies to postnatal behavioral development. Infants achieve structural control of the head before the trunk and extremities, hold their back erect before they stand, use their eyes before their

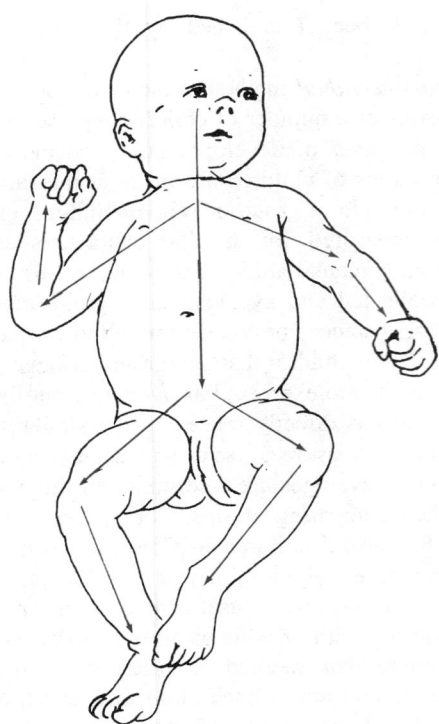

Fig. 4-1. Directional trends in growth.

hands, and gain control of their hands before they have control of their feet.

Second, the *proximodistal*, or near-to-far, trend applies to the midline-to-peripheral concept. A conspicuous illustration is the early embryonic development of limb buds, followed by rudimentary fingers and toes. In the infant, shoulder control precedes mastery of hands, the whole hand is used as a unit before the fingers can be manipulated, and the central nervous system develops more rapidly than the peripheral nervous system.

These trends or patterns are bilateral and appear to be symmetric; each side develops in the same direction and at the same rate as the other. For some of the neurologic functions, this symmetry is only external because of unilateral differentiation of function at an early stage of postnatal development. For example, by the age of approximately 5 years the child has demonstrated a decided preference for the use of one hand over the other, although previously he had used either one.

The third trend in directional growth, *mass to specific* (sometimes referred to as differentiation), describes development from simple operations to more complex activities and functions. From very broad, global patterns of behavior, more specific, refined patterns emerge. All areas of development (physical, mental, social, emotional) proceed in this direction. Through the processes of development and differentiation, early embryonal cells with vague, undifferentiated functions progress to an immensely complex organism composed of highly specialized and diversified cells, tissues, and organs. Generalized development will precede

specific or specialized development; gross, random muscle movements take place before fine muscle control. The child will at first run and jump for the sake of motion, but eventually these activities take the more complex form of a race or hopscotch. Infants will respond to people in general before they recognize and prefer their mothers.

Sequential trends. In all dimensions of growth and development there is a definite, predictable sequence. It is orderly and continuous, with each child normally passing through every stage. Each stage is affected by those preceding it and affects those that follow. Sequential patterns have been described for motor skills such as locomotion and use of hands, and types of behavior such as language and social skills. Children crawl before they creep, creep before they stand, and stand before they walk. Children first play alone, then with others in increasing numbers and increasingly complex activities.

New biologic parts and behaviors arise out of and build on those already established. This continuity with the past, or *epigenesis,* serves as a foundation for the future and requires interaction with a suitable environment at the proper time. In very early physical development, fingers arise from webbed appendages on limb buds, the nervous system develops from a neural plate derived from an area of embryonic ectoderm, and sexual organs differentiate from a morphologically neutral primitive gonad. Later, facets of the personality are built on the early foundation of trust. The child babbles, then forms words and, finally, sentences; writing emerges from scribbling.

Sensitive periods. There are limited times during the process of growth when children interact with a particular environment in a specific manner. The terms *critical periods, sensitive periods,* and *optimal periods* have been applied to those times in an organism's lifetime when it is more vulnerable to positive or negative influences. Colombo (1982) describes a ''critical'' period as one when the developing organism is more sensitive to beneficial stimulation or more susceptible to detrimental influence. Fox (1970) recommends the use of *critical* to indicate those times when specific aspects of development require a trigger and the term *sensitive* to indicate those times when the organism is especially vulnerable to adverse influences. Moltz (1973) describes the term *optimal* as more appropriate when the situation implies possible recovery and suggests that the term *critical* should be limited to those periods from which no recovery is possible.

The quality of interactions during these sensitive periods determines whether the effects on the children will be beneficial or harmful. The character and extent of the interaction's consequences depend on the nature of the environmental influences and the stage of development. For example, physiologic maturation of the central nervous system is influenced by adequacy and timing of contributions from the environment, such as stimulation and nutrition. The first 3 months of prenatal life is a sensitive period for physical growth. During this period of accelerated growth and differentiation, specific organs and systems are most vulnerable to environmental influences; the earlier the impact, the more far-reaching are the effects.

The terms *critical, sensitive,* and *optimal periods* apply to all aspects of growth and development. During fetal development there are times during the period of tissue differentiation when interference by a detrimental influence can alter the normal course of events. Such alterations can produce a physical or mental defect that can have either minor or far-reaching effects (see Teratogenesis, p. 167).

Psychologic development also appears to have sensitive periods when an environmental event has maximum influence on the developing personality. Observers have identified periods in development when behavior patterns are most readily acquired. For example, primary socialization occurs during the first year, when infants make their initial social attachments and establish a basic trust in the world. At this time a warm relationship with the caregiver is fundamental to a healthy parent-child relationship (Mitchell and Mills, 1983) (see Attachment, p. 330).

The sensitive period concept might also be applied to readiness for learning skills such as toilet training or reading. In these instances there appears to be an opportune time when the skill is best learned. However, if the skill is not learned at this time, acquisition at a later time is still possible. The optimum time for school entry has been based on the readiness to acquire the specific types of skills learned in the school setting.

Developmental pace. Although there is a fixed, precise order to development, it does not progress at the same rate or pace in all children. There are periods of accelerated growth and periods of decelerated growth in both total body growth and growth of subsystems. The very rapid growth rate before and after birth gradually levels off throughout early childhood. Relatively slow during middle childhood, the rate increases markedly at the beginning of adolescence and levels off in early adulthood.

The focus of development and growth shifts at successive stages in development. For instance, the head grows most rapidly before birth, while other body parts grow more slowly; after birth other structures grow faster than the head. This growth pattern accounts for shifts in body proportion, facial characteristics, and voice. Similarly, one type of development seems to take precedence over another during various periods of growth. At times of rapid physical growth, other development may reach a plateau. For example, when children begin to walk, the thrills of upright locomotion take precedence over other activity such as speech, and they may not learn any new words for 3 to 4 months. Schoolwork may suffer during the early adolescent growth spurt.

Cycles of behavior. Observation of child behavior over the course of development indicates that behavioral trends follow a more or less regular cyclic pattern of equilibrium and disequilibrium as children mature (Ilg and Ames, 1955). Periods in which children appear to be relatively tranquil and untroubled are followed by periods of disequilibrium (Table 4-1). At about ages 2, 5, and 10 years they have little difficulty with feelings within themselves or with the world around them.

Each of these relatively smooth stages is followed by a brief period of disturbed, troubled, and generally "broken up" behavior at 2½, 5½ to 6, and 11 years of age when children are at odds with the environment and with themselves. These stages are followed again by periods of relative calm at 3, 6½, and 12 years of age, when the children seem to be in good balance and happy with themselves and their environment.

During the next phase, in which there is a pronounced focus of their attention inward, children become introspective and thoughtful. They incorporate outer impressions and experiences to mull over, think about, and digest. At these ages, about 3½, 7, and 13 years, the inner process may be expressed differently at the various age stages. Children 3½ years old may exhibit general emotional instability, such as a variety of fears, hand tremor, stumbling, poor spatial orientation, whining, and a high, tremulous voice. Older children, better able to withstand the stresses of this inwardizing, are more apt to express this stage in marked sensitivity and touchiness, excessive withdrawal and moroseness, and a pessimistic attitude toward life in general.

Extreme expansiveness is characteristic of the ages 4, 8, and 14 years. Children at these ages are noticeably outgoing, so much so that they may be in danger of expanding too much. For example, the 4-year-old child may wander from home, the 8-year-old child may attempt hazardous activities (such as bicycle riding in the street) and get hurt, and the 14-year-old adolescent may become tangled in multiple and conflicting social plans. Less is known about ages 4½, 9, and 15 years, although each is characterized by behavior that is less outgoing than in the previous stage. During these periods children are less well balanced and have been frequently described as "neurotic." Again, relative stability and equilibrium follow at 5, 10, and 16 years.

Individual Differences

Each child grows in his or her own unique and personal way. Great individual variation exists in the age at which

---

Table 4-1 Summary of behavior cycles

AGES (YEARS)	BEHAVIORS
2, 5, 10	Smooth, consolidated
2½, 5½-6, 11	Breaking up
3, 6½, 12	Rounded, balanced
3½, 7, 13	Inwardized
4, 8, 14	Vigorous, expansive
4½, 9, 15	Inwardized-outwardized, troubled, "neurotic"
5, 10, 16	Smooth, consolidated

developmental milestones are reached. The sequence is predictable; the exact timing is not. Rates of growth vary from one individual to another, and measurements are defined in terms of ranges to allow for individual differences among children. Some children are fast growers, others are moderate, and some are slower to reach maturity. For example, periods of fast growth, such as the pubescent growth spurt, may begin earlier or later in some children than in others. Children may grow fast or slow during the spurt and may finish sooner or later than other children. The sex of the child is an influential factor because girls seem to be more advanced in physiologic growth at all ages.

Terminal points and optimum tendency. The terminal points in growth vary immensely from one child to another. For example, some individuals will grow until reaching a height of over 180 cm (6 feet), another will cease growing at 150 cm (5 feet); the majority will achieve varying heights between the two. Females as a group reach both height and weight terminal before males, with average terminal height in males exceeding that for females.

There appears to be a tendency for organisms to strive for optimum developmental potential in both structure and function. When environmental factors interfere with normal development for a time (e.g., during periods of inadequate food supply or illness), children's bodies will usually make up for the interrupted period and return to their characteristic pattern of growth. For instance, children born prematurely will demonstrate delayed development during the early months but will usually "catch up" to others of the same age by the time they enter school. However, if the deprivation is severe or occurs throughout a critical period, development may be permanently impaired.

Interrelatedness. Children develop as whole beings, not in pieces and parts. They are a product of the past environment in which they have grown and their current stresses and satisfactions. Factors affecting one part will influence others. For example, children deprived of love and affection will be delayed in physical and mental development. Although there are exceptions, children who deviate from the average with respect to one aspect of growth will probably deviate in others.

Secular Trend in Growth and Development

Measurements and observations recorded over the past century indicate a significant worldwide trend in the rate and age of maturation. Children from widely different populations are maturing earlier and becoming larger at each age. There appears to be a slight but not so marked increase in average adult height because, although children are growing faster, they also stop growing sooner. On the average young men reach their full height at approximately age 20, whereas in 1900 they did not reach their final height until about 25. The average size increase since 1900 is near 1 cm (⅜ inch) per decade in height, 1 kg (2½ pounds) in weight in preschool children, and 2.5 cm (1 inch) and 2.5 kg (5½ pounds) per decade during puberty. In girls the age of menarche has advanced progressively.

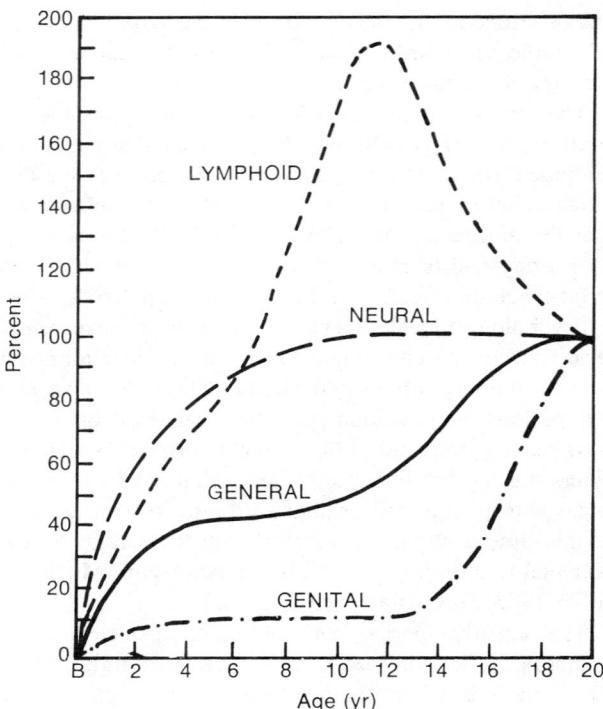

Fig. 4-2. Growth rates for body as a whole and three types of tissues. *Lymphoid type:* thymus, lymph nodes, and intestinal lymph masses; *neural type:* brain, dura, spinal cord, optic apparatus, and head dimensions; *general type:* body as a whole, external dimensions, and respiratory, digestive, renal, circulatory, and musculo-skeletal systems.

Modified from Harris, J.A., and others: The measurement of man, Minneapolis, 1930, University of Minnesota Press.

Many theories have been advanced to explain this phenomenon. Improved environmental factors, such as nutrition and socioeconomic conditions, are important factors, as well as the sharp decrease in infant mortality during this century. Since body size is an inherited trait, the tendency toward the selection of mates from wider geographic areas is an important factor. The trend appears to reach a plateau in populations with optimum environments, which suggests there is a maximum end point.

BIOLOGIC GROWTH AND DEVELOPMENT

As children grow, their external dimensions change. These changes are accompanied by corresponding alterations in structure and function of internal organs and tissues, reflecting the gradual acquisition of physiologic competence. These alterations, although progressive and interdependent, are not a uniform process but are characterized by cycles of accelerated and slow development that vary from organ to organ and system to system. Each part has its own rate of growth, and many growth rates are directly related to alterations in the size of the child (e.g., heart rate). Skeletal muscle growth approximates whole body growth; brain, lymphoid, adrenal, and reproductive tissues follow distinct and individual patterns (Fig. 4-2).

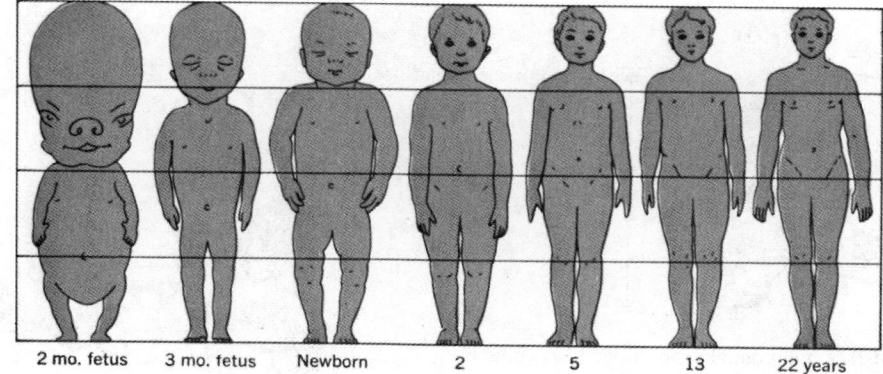

Fig. 4-3. Changes in body proportions from before birth to adulthood.
From Crouch, J.E., and McClintic, J.R.: Human anatomy and physiology, ed. 2, New York, 1976, John Wiley & Sons, Inc.

External Proportions

Variations in the growth rate of different tissues and organ systems produce significant changes in body proportions during childhood. The cephalocaudal trend of development is most evident in total body growth as indicated by these changes (Fig. 4-3). During fetal development the head is the fastest growing part, and at 2 months of gestation the head comprises 50% of total body length. During infancy growth of the trunk predominates; the legs are the most rapidly growing part during childhood; then, in adolescence, the trunk once again elongates. In the newborn the lower limbs are one third of the total body length but only 15% of the total body weight; in the adult the lower limbs comprise one half of the total body height and 30% of total body weight. As growth proceeds, the midpoint in head-to-toe measurements gradually descends from a level even with the umbilicus at birth to the level of the symphysis pubis at maturity.

The first year is a period of rapid growth dominated by lengthening of the trunk and accumulation of subcutaneous fat. When infants begin to walk, their large head, heavy trunk, and protruberant abdomen atop short, bowed legs force them to walk with a wide stance, outward rotation of the hips, and everted feet. The high center of gravity created by this disproportionate bulk causes infants to walk unsteadily and contributes to frequent falls.

After the first year and extending to puberty, the legs grow more rapidly than any other part. The bowlegged appearance disappears with locomotion, the abdomen is held in, and the body becomes slender and elongated. Until puberty this slender, long-legged build is characteristic of both sexes; in similar clothes and hairstyle the two sexes are indistinguishable. With the onset of puberty there is a marked alteration in body proportion when all structures show the effects of the pubertal growth spurt. The feet and hands are first to increase in rate of growth; therefore during this transient period they appear large and ungainly in relation to the rest of the body, often a source of embarrassment to the adolescent. The trunk again grows faster than the legs so

that a large portion of the increase in height at adolescence is a result of trunk growth.

Since the legs continue to grow until puberty, early-maturing children have shorter than average legs, and the legs of later-maturing children are longer. Inasmuch as the onset of puberty is approximately 2½ years earlier in girls, for a while girls are larger than boys, and girls' legs are shorter than boys' legs. Laterality of growth follows rapid linear growth; both boys and girls proceed to "fill out" during the later stages of adolescent growth.

One of the more outstanding features of changing body proportion is shoulder and hip breadth as a result of hormone secretion from the maturing gonads. Shoulder and hip growth increases in both sexes, but the shoulder width in boys is considerably greater than in girls. The anteroposterior hip diameter increases in girls, and the female pelvis becomes wider, shallower, and roomier than the male pelvis. The differences in deposition of fat produce the distinctive feminine contours in girls, whereas boys lose subcutaneous fat.

Physique. Physique refers to the body form, build, or shape of an individual. A number of classfication systems have been advanced that attempt to describe specific body types. The most important was developed by Sheldon (1940), who described three general body types: *endomorphic,* "soft and round" persons with short, fat builds; *mesomorphic,* well-muscled, thick chested, and broadshouldered persons; and *ectomorphic,* tall and thin persons. Children seldom exhibit these three body builds in pure form, but every body contains all three components in varying degrees. Consequently, current classification systems expand on these forms with rating scales that incorporate all components. Body build is primarily of interest in determining exercise and sports participation.

Facial proportions. Facial proportions show characteristic changes during childhood. In infancy and early childhood the face is small in relation to the skull (Fig. 4-4). The size of the cranial vault reflects the advanced development of the brain. The brain has achieved 25% of its adult

A

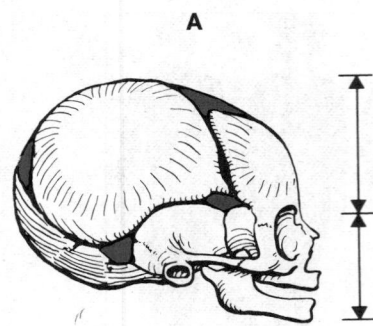

B

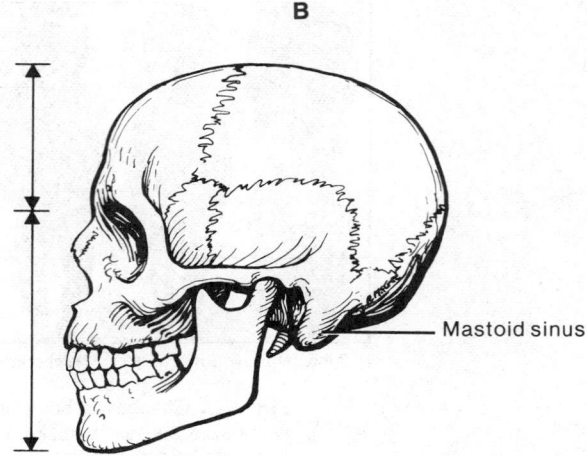

— Mastoid sinus

Fig. 4-4. Comparison of face and cranial proportions in **A,** infant, and **B,** adult, skulls. Note differences in relative size of face and angle of mandible, absence of mastoid sinus in infant, and absence of fontanels (red) in adult.

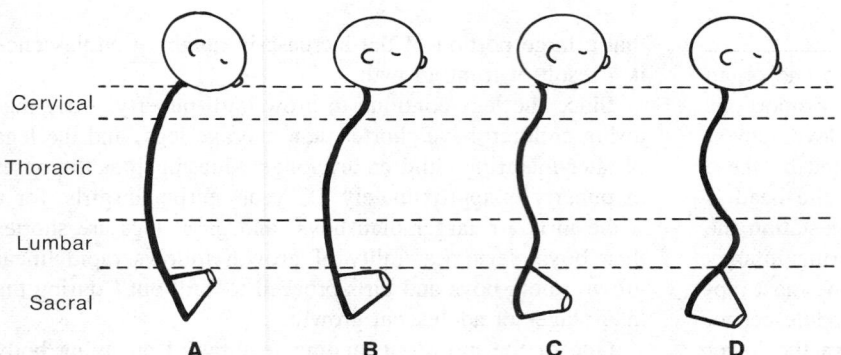

Cervical

Thoracic

Lumbar

Sacral

A   B   C   D

Fig. 4-5. Development of spinal curvatures. **A,** Newborn infant. **B,** Cervical secondary curvature. **C,** Lumbar secondary curvature. **D,** Lordosis.

size at birth and 66% at the end of 1 year. Over 90% of the growth of the brain cavity has been reached by the end of the fifth year, and 98% has been achieved at age 15 years.

After the first year the facial skeleton grows more rapidly than the brain case. The principal growth occurs in the jaws as they enlarge to accommodate the teeth and in the muscles of mastication as they develop. The face grows first in width and then in length so the child's face appears to emerge from underneath his skull, particularly during adolescence.

The size of the face relative to the skull has implications for health in the infant and young child. The large, heavy cranium is the primary site of injury in falls. The changing dimensions of the face alter the diameter and angle of ear structures, particularly the external auditory meatus and the eustachian tube. The latter contributes significantly to the incidence of middle ear infection.

Posture. Posture is also altered by growth and maturation of various structures. Within the narrow confines of the uterus the prenatal posture is one of total flexion. The spine curves with the head and extremities bent upon the child. The bones in the vertebral column of the newborn form two primary curvatures, one in the thoracic region and one in the sacral region (Fig. 4-5, *A*). Both are forward, concave curvatures that rely largely on the shape of their component bones. The thoracic curve is relatively stable, and movement is limited in scope and amount by thin, intervertebral

discs and oblique spinous processes. The sacral curve eventually becomes fused and permanently fixed.

As the infant gains control of his head, at approximately 3 months of age, a secondary curvature appears in the cervical region (Fig. 4-5, *B*). This curve, unlike the primary curvatures, is convex forward, and its mobility is maintained by thick intervertebral discs and the tension of muscles stretched across its convexity.

To maintain a sitting posture, another secondary curvature develops in the lumbar region (Fig. 4-5, *C*). Like the cervical curve, the lumbar curve is convex, mobile, depends largely on intervertebral discs, and is controlled by the large postural muscles of the spine. When children assume an upright posture in their initial efforts to walk, they compensate for a high center of gravity and the weight of a large liver by an exaggerated lumbar curvature, or *lordosis* (Fig. 4-5, *D*). With advancing skill in locomotion there is a gradual progression toward normal upright posture. When situations cause a delay in holding up the head or sitting, the secondary curvatures may fail to develop at the expected time.

Biologic Determinants of Growth and Development

The most prominent feature of childhood and adolescence is physical growth. Throughout the developmental process various tissues in the body undergo changes in growth, composition, and structure. In some tissues the changes are continuous (e.g., bone growth and dentition); in others significant alterations occur at specific stages (e.g., appearance of secondary sex characteristics). Satisfactory growth achievement is most commonly judged in terms of increase in body weight, height, and skeletal growth, and when compared with standardized norms, a child's developmental progress can be determined with a high degree of confidence. Table 4-2 and Fig. 4-6 indicate the general trends in height and weight gain during childhood.

Height. Linear growth, or height, occurs almost entirely as a result of skeletal growth and is considered to be a stable measure of general growth. It is not uniform throughout life, but when maturation of the skeleton is complete, linear growth ceases. The maximum growth in length occurs before birth, but the newborn continues to grow at a rapid, though slower, rate. As the months pass, the growth rate rapidly decelerates. By 2 years of age children normally have achieved 50% of their adult height. By age 4 birth length has usually doubled.

At approximately 3 years of age the child begins a relatively stable and steady growth rate of 5 to 6 cm (2 to 2½

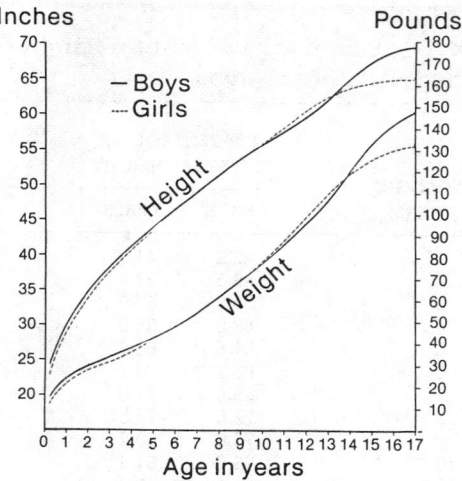

Fig. 4-6. Average height and weight curves for boys and girls. The earlier increase for girls at adolescence is clearly shown. Most girls are larger than boys between ages 11 and 13, probably a result of earlier influence of sex hormones on physical growth.

From Lowrey, G.H.: Growth and development of children, ed. 8, Chicago, 1986, Year Book Medical Publishers, Inc.

Table 4-2 General trends in height and weight gain during childhood

AGE	WEIGHT*	HEIGHT*
Infants		
Birth-6 months	Weekly gain: 140-200 g (5-7 oz) Birth weight doubles by end of first 6 months†	Monthly gain: 2.5 cm (1 inch)
6-12 months	Weight gain: 85-140 g (3-5 oz) Birth weight triples by end of first year	Monthly gain: 1.25 cm (½ inch) Birth length increases by approximately 50% by end of first year
Toddlers	Birth weight quadruples by age 2½ Yearly gain: 2-3 kg (4½-6½ lb)	Height at age 2 is approximately 50% of eventual adult height Gain during second year: about 12 cm (4¾ inches) Gain during third year: about 6-8 cm (2⅜-3¼ inches)
Preschoolers	Yearly gain: 2-3 kg (4½-6½ lb)	Birth length doubles by age 4 Yearly gain: 5-7.5 cm (2-3 inches)
School-age children	Yearly gain: 2-3 kg (4½-6½ lb)	Yearly gain after age 7: 5 cm (2 inches) Birth length triples by about age 13
Pubertal growth spurt Females—10-14 years	Weight gain: 7-25 kg (15-55 lb) Mean: 17.5 kg (38⅛ lb)	Height gain: 5-25 cm (2-10 inches); approximately 95% of mature height achieved by onset of menarche or skeletal age of 13 Mean: 20.5 cm (8¼ inches)
Males—11-16 years	Weight gain: 7-30 kg (15-65 lb) Mean: 23.7 kg (52⅛ lb)	Height gain: 10-30 cm (4-12 inches); approximately 95% of mature height achieved by skeletal age of 15 years Mean: 27.5 cm (11 inches)

*Yearly height and weight gains for each age-group represent averaged estimates from a variety of sources.
†A study has shown the mean time for doubling of birth weight to be 3¾ months (Neumann and Alpaugh, 1976).

Table 4-3 Percentage of mature height attained at different ages

CHRONOLOGIC AGE (YEARS)	PERCENTAGE OF EVENTUAL HEIGHT	
	BOYS	GIRLS
1	42.2	44.7
2	49.5	52.8
3	53.8	57.0
4	58.0	61.8
5	61.8	66.2
6	65.2	70.3
7	69.0	74.0
8	72.0	77.5
9	75.0	80.7
10	78.0	84.4
11	81.1	88.4
12	84.2	92.9
13	87.3	96.5
14	91.5	98.3
15	96.1	99.1
16	98.3	99.6
17	99.3	100.0
18	99.8	100.0

From Bayley, N.: Growth curves of height and weight for boys and girls, scaled according to physical maturity, J. Pediatr. **48:**187-194, 1956.

inches) per year that continues for the next 9 years. (Occasionally a child will exhibit a transitory midgrowth height increase at age 6 or 7.) This long midgrowth period is ended by a sudden and marked acceleration, the adolescent growth spurt. Although there is wide variation, this increase, which begins about ages 10½ to 11 in girls and 12½ to 13 in boys, lasts approximately 2 to 2½ years. During this time a boy may add 20 cm (8 inches) to his height and a girl 16 cm (6½ inches). Usually, 98% of the terminal height is reached by age 16½ in girls but not until age 17¾ in boys (Table 4-3).

From analysis of data derived from longitudinal studies, it is possible to state the percentage of terminal height that has been achieved at any given age and to predict the future height of an individual from measurements taken in childhood. Predictions are of little value until the second year of life. By this time the child has usually compensated for any deviations related to prematurity or other prenatally influenced deviations. Variability in the onset of puberty may also alter the predictive value in this age-group.

Such predictions are valuable tools to help parents and their slow-maturing children accept the child's unique pattern of growth and to help these puzzled children understand why they are different from their taller age-mates. Predictions are sometimes useful in preventing possible disappointment in the preparation for occupations or careers that have height restrictions and require early beginning preparation (e.g., ballet dancing). More importantly, if parents are satisfied that a child's apparently small size merely reflects the normal expectations based on their own adult size, they will be less likely to force-feed the child, which can result in obesity or food refusal and poor appetite. For the young girl whose predicted adult height is excessively tall, this early indication provides time to initiate therapy, if advisable, and to help the child develop the capacity to deal with the potential problems associated with this trait.

Weight. At birth, weight is more variable than height and to a greater extent is a reflection of the intrauterine environment. The rate of weight gain increases rapidly for a short time after birth but soon decreases markedly. After the second year the "normal" rate of weight gain, just as the growth rate in height, assumes a steady annual increase—approximately 2 to 2.75 kg (4½ to 6 pounds) per year—until the adolescent growth spurt. The weight gain usually lags behind the gain in height by about 3 months.

Lifetime weight gain is subject to numerous intrinsic and extrinsic factors that are discussed as they apply to specific situations or conditions. Growth responses become apparent by changes in weight before they appear in other aspects of growth. Weight gain is usually considered to be an indication of satisfactory growth progress in a child and is probably the best index of nutrition and growth. However, it may be difficult to determine if this increase in weight is caused by healthy tissue development or by an unhealthy deposition of fat or accumulation of fluid.

Bone age and dentition. Both bone age determinations and state of dentition are used as indicators of development. Since both are discussed elsewhere (for bone age, see p. 107; see pp. 108, 519, and 726 for dentition), neither is elaborated here.

Skeletal Growth and Maturation

Growth of the skeleton follows a genetically programmed developmental plan that not only furnishes the best indicator of general growth progress but also provides the best estimate of biologic age. Some degree of assessment can be achieved by observation of facial bone development (i.e., nasal bridge height, prominence of malar eminences, and mandibular size), but the most accurate measure of general development is the determination of osseous maturation by radiography. Skeletal age appears to correlate more closely with other measures of physiologic maturity (e.g., onset of menarche) than with chronologic age or height. This "bone age" is determined by comparing the mineralization of ossification centers and advancing bony form to age-related standards. Skeletal maturation begins with the appearance of centers of ossification in the embryo and ends when the last epiphysis is firmly fused to the shaft of its bone.

In the healthy child skeletal growth and development consist of two concurrent processes: (1) the creation of new cells and tissues (growth), and (2) the consolidation of these tissues into a permanent form (maturation). Early in fetal life closely packed connective tissue forms cartilage, which enlarges within the forming structures and builds successive layers on the surface of the mass. Bone formation begins

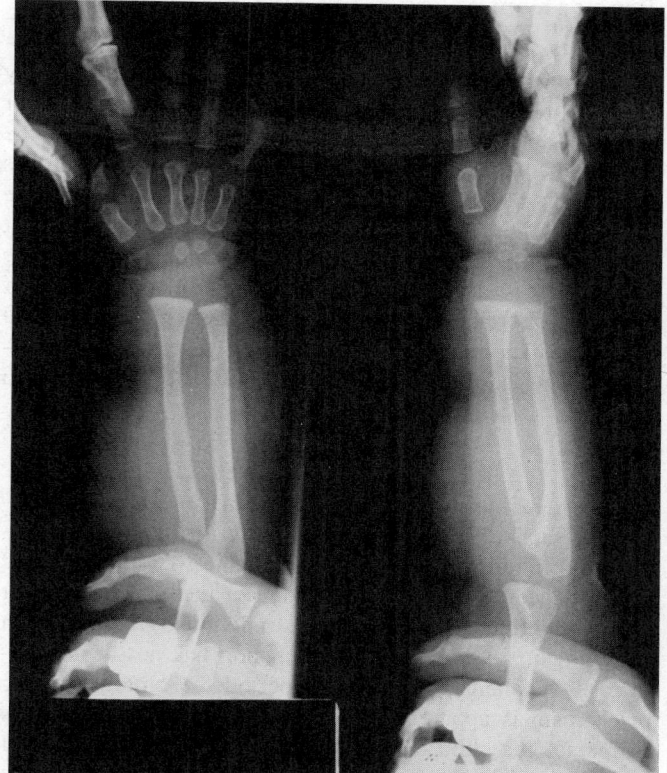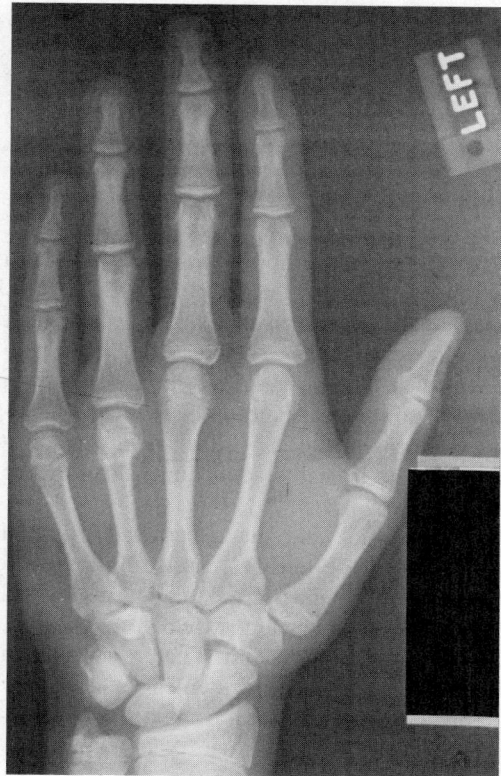

Fig. 4-7. Radiographs illustrating bone age in children, **A,** 8-month-old (note complete ossification in adult fingers). **B,** 14-year-old; epiphyses visible.

A, Courtesy Dr. Mark Capehart, Tulsa, OK.

during the second month of fetal life, when calcium salts are deposited in the intercellular substance (matrix) to form calcified cartilage first and then true bone. There are some differences in this bone formation. In small bones the bone continues to form in the center and cartilage continues to be laid down on the surfaces. Bones of the face and cranium are laid out in a tough membrane and directly ossified into bone during fetal life.

In long bones ossification takes place in two centers. It begins in the diaphysis (the long central portion of the bone) from a "primary" center and continues in the epiphysis (the end portions of the bone) at "secondary" centers of ossification. Situated between the diaphysis and the epiphysis, an epiphyseal cartilage plate unites with the diaphysis by columns of spongy tissue, the metaphysis. At this site the active growth in length takes place, and interference with this growth site by trauma or infection can result in deformity. Under the influence of hormones, principally pituitary growth hormone and thyroid hormone, bones increase in circumference by the formation of new bone tissue beneath the membrane surrounding the bone (periosteum) and in length by proliferation of cartilage.

Over the growth period of approximately 19 to 20 years, this development can be divided into three distinct but overlapping phases: (1) ossification of the diaphysis, (2) ossifi-

cation of the epiphysis, and (3) invasion and subsequent replacement of growth cartilage plates with bony fusion of epiphysis and diaphysis. These changes do not take place in all bones simultaneously but appear in a specific order and at a specific time. Although the speed of bone growth and amount of maturity at specific ages vary from one child to another, the order of ossification is constant.

The first centers of ossification appear in the 2-month-old embryo, and at birth the number is approximately 400, about half the number at maturity. New centers appear at regular intervals during the growth period and provide the basis for assessment of "bone age." Postnatally, at 5 to 6 months of age, the earliest centers to appear are those of the capitate and hamate bones in the wrist. Therefore radiographs of the hand and wrist provide the most useful areas for screening to determine skeletal age, especially before age 6 years (Fig. 4-7). A common rule of thumb is:

Age in years + 1 =
        Number of ossification centers in the wrist.

These centers appear earlier in girls than in boys.

Skeletal development advances until maturity through growth of ossification centers and lengthening of long bones at the metaphysis and cartilage plates. Linear growth can continue as long as the epiphysis is separated from the diaphysis by the cartilage plate; when the cartilage disappears, the epiphysis unites wih the diaphysis and growth ceases. Epiphyseal fusion also follows an orderly sequence; thus the timing of epiphyseal closure furnishes another medium for measuring skeletal age.

Lymphoid Tissues

Lymphoid tissues contained in the lymph nodes, thymus, spleen, tonsils, adenoids, and blood lymphocytes follow a distinctive growth pattern unlike that of other body tissues. These tissues are small in relation to total body size, but they are well developed at birth. They increase rapidly to reach adult dimensions by 6 years of age and continue to grow. About age 10 to 12 years the tissues reach a maximum development approximately twice their adult size, followed by a rapid decline to stable adult dimensions by the end of adolescence.

Lymph nodes are large, and the superficially located nodes are often palpable. The tonsils, massive during early childhood, become inconspicuous in the adult. The thymus gland beneath the sternum, a prominent feature in infancy, may be impossible to detect in an adult. The growth pattern of lymphatic tissues parallels the development of immunity and probably reflects the repeated exposure to new infectious agents.

Dentition

The course of dentition is sometimes divided into four major stages: (1) growth, (2) calcification, (3) eruption, and (4) attrition. The primary teeth arise as outgrowths of the oral epithelium during the sixth week of embryonic life and begin to calcify during the fourth to sixth months. Tooth buds form at 10 different points in each arch and eventually become the enamel organs for the 20 primary (deciduous) teeth. All the buds are present at birth, but the amount of enamel laid down varies with each set of teeth.

Teeth are divided into quadrants of the mandible and maxilla and are named for their location in each quadrant of the dental arch, such as central incisor, lateral incisor, and first and second molars. Teeth are also named after their specific function in the mastication of food. The knifelike or scissorslike, central and lateral incisors cut the food. The single pointed cuspids, also called *canines,* tear the food. The two premolars, called *bicuspids* because of their two-pointed crown, crush the food. The permanent molars, which have four or five cusps, grind the food.

The teeth and their care are discussed further in relation to time of eruption (see pp. 519 and 726). Because of its relative regularity, the eruption of teeth is sometimes used as a criterion for developmental assessment, especially the 6-year molar, which seems to be the most universally consistent in timing. However, dental maturation does not correlate well with bone age and is less reliable as an index of biologic age. Retarded eruption is more common than accelerated eruption and may be caused by heredity or may indicate health problems such as endocrine disturbance, nutritional factors, or malposition of teeth.

Development of Organ Systems

All tissues and organ systems undergo changes during development. Some are striking; others are more subtle. Many have implications for assessment and care. Since the major importance of these changes relates to their dysfunction, the developmental characteristics of various systems and organs are discussed throughout the book as they relate to these areas. Physical characteristics and physiologic changes that vary with age are included in age-group descriptions. For example, the relationship of surface area to body mass is of primary importance during very early development; physical characteristics related to hormonal changes are most significant during adolescence and are discussed as they apply to problems associated with this phase.

Catch-Up Growth

When there has been a secondary cause of growth deficiency, such as severe illness or acute malnutrition, recovery from the illness or the establishment of an adequate diet will produce a dramatic acceleration of the growth rate that usually continues until the child's individual growth pattern is resumed. Although the phenomenon has not been satisfactorily explained, during this period the biologic timing mechanism is apparently unaffected. When the problem is corrected, the child tends to catch up to the developmental stage at which he would be normally. For example, the newborn exhibits a transitory weight loss shortly after birth and then rapidly regains the weight. In addition, during the early months of life the developmental achievements of the prematurely born infant lag behind those of full-term infants of the same chronologic age. The deficit in the attainment of developmental landmarks closely corresponds to the degree of prematurity; however, the differences become less conspicuous as the infant matures. The child usually catches up to age-mates during the preschool years.

Catch-up growth involves growth in both length and weight, but the extent of inadequacy depends on the timing, severity, duration, and character of the source of the secondary deficiency. In general, any serious interruption in progress will have an impact, although small, on the ultimate size of the individual. Growth retardation that is prolonged or that occurs during a sensitive period may not be compensated. Catch-up growth applies to those tissues that can increase in size and to those that still retain the capacity to increase cell numbers. Growth deficiency in tissues such as the brain results in a permanent deficit when the problem occurs during a sensitive period in its development.

PHYSIOLOGIC CHANGES

Physiologic changes that take place in all organs and systems are discussed as they relate to dysfunction. Others, such as pulse and respiratory rates and blood pressure, are an integral part of physical assessment (see p. 229). In addition, there are changes in basic functions including metabolism, temperature, and patterns of sleep and rest.

Metabolism

Metabolism—all chemical and energy transformations in the body—is affected by an assortment of intrinsic and extrinsic factors (e.g., body size, age, sex, emotions, exercise, climate, hormones, environmental temperature). Therefore metabolic needs vary among individuals and within each individual. The rate of metabolism when the body is at rest (basal metabolic rate, or BMR) demonstrates a distinctive change throughout childhood. Highest in the newborn infant, BMR closely relates to the proportion of surface area to body mass, which changes as the body increases in size. Most authorities consider surface area to be the best estimate of the amount of functioning protoplasm present in the organism (see p. 1131 for computation of surface area). In both sexes the proportion decreases progressively to maturity. The BMR is slightly higher in boys at all ages and further increases during pubescence over that in girls.

The rate of metabolism determines the caloric requirements of the child. The basal requirement of infants is about 110 to 120 kcal/kg (50 to 55 kcal/lb) of body weight and decreases to 40 to 50 kcal/kg (18 to 23 kcal/lb) at maturity (Table 4-4). The daily water requirements show a similar modification (see Table 28-3, p. 1159). Children's energy needs vary considerably at different ages and with changing circumstances. The greatest proportion of calories in infancy is used for basal metabolic needs and growth.

The energy requirement to build tissue steadily decreases with age, following the general growth curve; however, exercise needs vary with the individual child and may be considerably more. For short periods (e.g., during strenuous exercise) and more prolonged periods (e.g., illness), the needs can be very high. For example, each degree of fever increases the basal metabolism 10% with a corresponding fluid requirement. The *specific dynamic action* (SDA) refers to the energy required to ingest and assimilate food. A very small portion of ingested calories is lost in stools during normal metabolism, but much more may be lost in this way when the child suffers from conditions that impair digestion or absorption.

Temperature

Body temperature, reflecting metabolism, displays the same decrement from infancy to maturity (see inside front cover). Following the unstable regulatory ability in the neonatal period, heat production steadily declines as the infant grows into childhood. Individual differences of 0.5 to 1° F are normal, and occasionally a child normally displays an unusually high or low temperature. Beginning at approximately 12 years of age, girls display a temperature that remains relatively stable, while the temperature in boys continues to fall for a few years longer. Females maintain a temperature slightly above that of males throughout life.

Even with improved temperature regulation, infants and young children are highly susceptible to temperature fluctuations. Body temperature responds to changes in environmental temperature and is increased with active exercise, crying, and emotional upset. Infections can cause a higher and more rapid temperature increase in infants and young children than in older children. In relation to body weight, an infant produces more heat per unit than children near maturity. Consequently, during active play or when heavily clothed, an infant or small child is likely to become overheated.

Motor Development

Closely allied to biologic development and maturation is the development of basic motor responses. Children's ability to perform motor functions depends on the state of maturation of bones, muscles, and nervous system and follows the patterns of development described earlier in the chapter. As in all maturation processes motor behavior follows a developmental sequence (Zaichkowsky, Zaichkowsky, and Martinek, 1980):

Reflexive or **rudimentary movements** are those rudimentary behaviors that are acquired during infancy and form the foundation of all other movements, including sitting, crawling, creeping, reaching, standing, and walking.

General fundamental skills are common to all children and develop during early childhood. The order in which both rudimentary and fundamental skills normally develop is the same for all children but there is wide variation in children's abilities to perform skills. Fundamental skills include such activities as running, jumping, balancing, catching, and throwing.

Specific skills develop during later childhood as general fundamental skills become more refined, fluid, and automatic. There is greater emphasis on form, accuracy, and adapatability and children begin to apply these skills to sports and other activities that require body movement.

Specialized skills evolve slowly from late childhood through adolescence and depend on the amount of repetition and concentrated application.

Table 4-4 Average daily requirements for calories and protein through adolescence

AGE (YEARS)	ENERGY (CAL/KG OF BODY WEIGHT)	PROTEIN (G/KG OF BODY WEIGHT)
Infants		
0-½	115	2.2
½-1	105	2.0
Children		
1-3	100	1.8
4-6	85	1.5
7-10	85	1.2
Males		
11-14	60	1.0
15-18	42	0.8
Females		
11-14	48	1.0
15-18	38	0.8

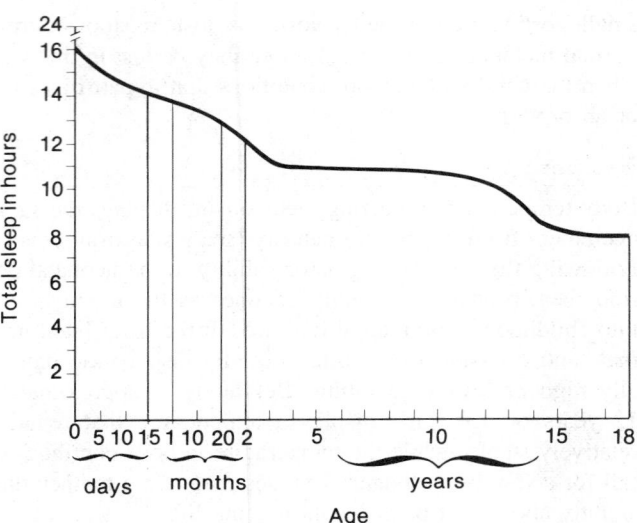

Fig. 4-8. Changes in number of hours of sleep with increasing age.

Sleep and Rest

Sleep, a protective function in all organisms, allows for repair and recovery of tissues following activity. As in most aspects of development, a wide variation exists among individual children and ages of children in the amount and distribution of sleep. As the child matures, not only does a change occur in the quantity of time he spends in sleep but also in the quality of that sleep.

The length of time spent in sleep decreases throughout childhood. Newborns sleep nearly all the time not occupied with feeding and other aspects of their care. Larger newborns sleep for longer periods than smaller ones because of their larger stomach capacity. The total time spent in sleep gradually decreases, and infants remain awake for longer periods and sleep longer at night. During the second year most children sleep through the night and take one or two naps during the day. By the time they are 3 years old, most children have eliminated the second nap; this pattern continues until age 4 or 5. After age 5 the child has usually given up daytime naps, except in those cultures in which an afternoon nap or siesta is customary. From ages 5 to 10 sleep time remains relatively constant and then declines sharply during adolescence.

Alterations take place in the percentage of sleep time spent in each of the two different identified sleep cycles: (1) active sleep characterized by irregular pulse and expirations, many body movements, and short, rapid eye movements (paradoxic, or REM, sleep); and (2) quiet sleep in which breathing and heartbeat are regular and body and eye movements are absent (slow-wave, or non-REM, sleep).

The sleep of the newborn infant consists of approximately 50% REM sleep, in contrast to approximately 20% in the older child. The large amount of active REM sleep in early infancy is believed to serve as an endogenous source of stimulation to the higher brain centers and is important

for normal development at a time when exogenous sources are minimal because of the short periods of arousal. The decrease in REM sleep as development progresses may indicate that with longer periods of wakefulness, the more mature brain has less need for this endogenous stimulation. The deep, restful non-REM sleep increases proportionately with age; children who have recently given up napping take a longer time to get into REM sleep during the initial sleep cycle than do either older or younger children, which suggests they are more fatigued. Spontaneous awakening during sleep is relatively uncommon in childhood and adolescence. The changes in sleep in relation to age are illustrated in Fig. 4-8.

TEMPERAMENT

Temperament is defined as "the manner of thinking, behaving, or reacting characteristic of an individual" (Chess and Thomas, 1985) and refers to the way a person deals with life. From the time of birth, children exhibit marked individual differences in the way they respond to their environment. These differences significantly influence the way others, particularly parents, respond to them and their needs. Temperament is a categoric term with no implications of good or bad, and without etiologic connections, and as with other characteristics, it is influenced by the environment as development progresses.

A genetic basis has been suggested for some differences in temperament. It has been found from studies of young children that identical twins are more alike than fraternal twins in temperamental attributes (Goldsmith and Gottesman, 1981; Matheny, 1980). Differences have also been noted relative to ethnic origin. For example, Caucasian infants have been found to be more irritable and difficult to comfort than Chinese-American infants (Freedman, 1979).

Temperamental Characteristics

The characteristics of behavioral individuality, derived from parental interviews, were identified, categorized, and rated in the New York Longitudinal Study (NYLS) of child behavior. The following temperamental attributes were established from analysis of the information (Chess and Thomas, 1983):

1. **Motor activity level** describes the activity level of the child's motility.
2. **Rhythmicity (regularity)** refers to the predictability and/or unpredictability of the child in the time of various functions.
3. **Approach-withdrawal** reflects the initial response to a new stimulus. *Approach* responses are positive, displayed by activity or expression; *withdrawal* responses are negative expressions or behaviors.
4. **Adaptability** reflects the ease with which the child adapts or adjusts to new or altered situations.
5. **Threshold of responsiveness** refers to the amount of stimulus required to evoke a response in a given situation.

6. **Intensity of reaction** reflects the degree to which the child expresses himself or reacts, regardless of quality or direction.
7. **Quality of mood** reflects the amount of happy, joyful behavior compared to unhappy, crying, whining behavior.
8. **Distractibility** refers to the ease with which a child's attention or direction of behavior can be diverted.
9. **Attention span and persistence** refers to the length of time a child pursues a given activity (*attention*) and the continuation of an activity in spite of obstacles (*persistence*).

Temperamental Categories

Further analysis of the NYLS data revealed that most of the behavior characteristics cluster in constellations or combinations. For example, highly active children are frequently irritable and irregular in behaviors such as sleeping, feeding, and elimination, whereas passive children are more likely to be good natured and regular in their habits. These temperamental patterns appear to persist over time and can affect children's adjustment to a variety of settings and situations throughout childhood.

From these observations, most children can be placed in one of three common categories based on their overall pattern of temperamental attributes. However, there are wide ranges in degree of manifestations, and varying combinations can be observed within normal limits. Approximately 30% of children do not appear in any of the following three groups (Chess and Thomas, 1983):

1. **The easy child.** Easy-going children are even-tempered, regular, and predictable in their habits, and have a positive approach to new stimuli. They are open and adaptable to change, and display a mild to moderately intense mood that is typically positive. Approximately 40% of NYLS children fall into this category.
2. **The difficult child.** Difficult children are highly active, irritable, and irregular in their habits. Negative withdrawal responses are typical and they require a more structured environment. These children adapt slowly to new routines, people, or situations. Mood expressions are usually intense and primarily negative. They exhibit frequent periods of crying, and frustration often produces violent tantrums. This group comprises about 10% of the NYLS children.
3. **The slow-to-warm-up child.** Slow-to-warm-up children typically react negatively and with mild intensity to new stimuli and, unless pressured, adapt slowly with repeated contact. They respond with only mild but passive resistance to novelty or changes in routine. They are quite inactive and moody but show only moderate irregularity in functions. Fifteen percent of children in the NYLS studies demonstrate this temperament pattern.

Significance of Temperament

Observations indicate that children who display the difficult or slow-to-warm-up patterns of behavior are more vulnerable to the development of behavior problems in early and middle childhood. Any child can develop behavior problems if there is dissonance between the child's temperament and his environment. Demands for change and adaptation that are in conflict with children's capacities can become excessively stressful. However, authorities emphasize that it is not children's temperament patterns that place them at risk but the degree of *fit* between children and their environment, specifically their parents, that determines the degree of vulnerability. The greater the dissonance between the child's temperament and the ability of the parents to accept and deal with the behavior, the greater the likelihood of subsequent behavior problems (Chess and Thomas, 1983). (See Failure to thrive, p. 567.)

Early identification of temperament provides a useful tool for caregivers in anticipating probable areas of difficulty or risk associated with development. For example, "difficult" children may be prone to colic in infancy, active children require more vigilance to prevent injury, and school entry will require different approaches for children with different temperaments.

Several parental questionnaires have been devised to facilitate assessment of temperament. The most widely used are those developed by Carey and McDevitt (1978). Nurses who employ these assessment tools are better able to help parents interpret their children's behavior and to provide anticipatory guidance regarding numerous aspects of childrearing. The concept of temperament is also discussed in relation to child development at various ages and coping with the experiences of hospitalization.

Development of Mental Function and Personality

Personality and cognitive skills develop in the same manner as biologic growth, and many aspects depend on physical growth and maturation. This is not a comprehensive account of the multiple facets of personality and behavior development. Many aspects are integrated with the child's emotional and social development in later discussion of various age-groups.

THEORETIC FOUNDATIONS OF PERSONALITY DEVELOPMENT (FREUD)

According to Freud, all human behavior is energized by psychodynamic forces, and this psychic energy is divided among three components of personality; the id, the ego, and the superego. The *id* is the inborn component that is driven by instincts. The id obeys the pleasure principle of immediate gratification of needs regardless of whether the object or action can actually do so. The *ego* serves the reality principle. It functions as the conscious or controlling self that is able to find realistic means for gratifying the instincts while blocking the irrational thinking of the id. The *superego* functions as the moral arbitrator and represents the ideal. It is the mechanism that prevents individuals from expressing undesirable instincts that might threaten the social order.

Psychosexual Development

Freud also considered the sexual instincts to be significant in the development of the personality. However, he used the term *psychosexual* to describe any *sensual pleasure*. Many simple body functions, considered asexual in the usual sense, were viewed as "erotic" activities by Freud and these activities were thought to be motivated by the general life force he called the *sex instinct*. Personality development was viewed as the growth or unfolding of these instincts.

According to Freud's theory, during childhood certain regions of the body assume a prominent psychologic significance as the source of new pleasures, and new conflicts gradually shift from one part of the body to another at particular stages of development. Each stage builds on the previous one, and the maturation of the sex instinct leaves distinct imprints on the developing psyche. Freud believed that children who encounter severe conflicts at any stage may be reluctant to move to the next phase, causing further development to be arrested or impaired. In addition, they may retreat to earlier stages of development if they experience too much anxiety or too many conflicts at a subsequent stage of development (see also Table 4-5).

The oral stage (birth to 1 year). During infancy the major source of pleasure-seeking centers on oral activities such as sucking, biting, chewing, and vocalizing. Children

may prefer one of these practices over the others, and the preferred method of oral gratification can provide some indication of the personality they develop. Examples of oral personality traits are pessimism or optimism, determination or submission, gullibility or suspiciousness, admiration or envy, and cockiness or self-belittlement (DiCaprio, 1983).

The anal stage (1 to 3 years). Interest during the second year of life centers on the anal region as sphincter muscles develop and children are able to withhold or expel fecal material at will. At this stage the climate surrounding toilet training can have lasting effects on children's personalities. Examples of anal personality traits are stinginess or overgenerosity, constrictedness or expansiveness, rigid punctuality or tardiness, stubbornness or acquiescence, and orderliness or messiness.

The phallic stage (3 to 6 years). During the phallic stage the genitals become an interesting and sensitive area of the body. Children recognize differences between the sexes and become curious about the dissimilarities. This is the period associated with the controversial issues of the Oedipus and Electra complexes, penis envy, and castration anxiety. Examples of phallic personality traits are brashness or bashfulness, stylishness or plainness, gaiety or sadness, blind courage or timidity, and gregariousness or isolationism.

Table 4-5 Summary of personality, cognitive, and moral development

STAGE	PSYCHOSEXUAL STAGES (FREUD)	PSYCHOSOCIAL STAGES (ERIKSON)	COGNITIVE STAGES (PIAGET)	MORAL JUDGMENT STAGES (KOHLBERG)
I Infancy (Birth to 1 yr)	Oral sensory	Trust vs mistrust	Sensorimotor (birth to 18 mo)	
II Toddlerhood (1-3 yr)	Anal-urethral	Autonomy vs shame and doubt	Preoperational thought, preconceptual phase (transductive reasoning) (2-4 yr)	Preconventional level
III Early childhood (3-6 yr)	Phallic-locomotion	Initiative vs guilt	Preoperational thought, intuitive phase (transductive reasoning) (4-7 yr)	
IV Middle childhood (6-12 yr)	Latency	Industry vs inferiority	Concrete operations (inductive reasoning and beginning logic)	Conventional level
V Adolescence (13-18 yr)	Genital	Identity and repudiation vs identity confusion	Formal operations (deductive and abstract reasoning)	Postconventional or principled level
VI Early adulthood		Intimacy and solidarity vs isolation		
VII Young and middle adulthood		Generativity vs self-absorption		
VIII Later adulthood		Ego integrity vs despair		

The latency period (6 to 12 years). During the latency period children elaborate on previously acquired traits and skills. Physical and psychic energy are channeled into acquisition of knowledge and vigorous play.

The genital stage (age 12 and over). The last significant stage begins at puberty with maturation of the reproductive system and production of sex hormones. The genital organs become the major source of sexual tensions and pleasures, but energies are also invested in forming friendships and preparation for marriage.

THEORETIC FOUNDATIONS OF PERSONALITY DEVELOPMENT (ERIKSON)

The theory of personality development advanced by Erikson (1963) is the most widely accepted and used. Although built on Freudian theory, it emphasizes a healthy personality as opposed to a pathologic approach. It involves predictable age-related stages during which specific changes are assumed to take place. Erikson also uses the biologic concepts of critical periods and epigenesis, describing key conflicts or core problems the individual strives to master during critical periods in personality development. Successful completion or mastery of each of these core conflicts is built on the satisfactory completion or mastery of the previous core conflict.

Psychosocial Development

At each stage of psychosocial development, children are confronted with a unique problem requiring the integration of personal needs and skills with social demands and cultural expectations. Erikson refers to the individual's efforts to adjust as a *crisis*. Crisis in this context implies the normal stresses as opposed to an extraordinary set of events. The tension produced by societal demands must be reduced in order that the favorable outcome can be achieved.

Each psychosocial stage has two components, the favorable and unfavorable aspects of the core conflict, and progress to the next stage depends on resolution of this conflict. No core conflict is ever mastered completely but remains a recurrent problem throughout life. No life situation is ever secure. Each new situation presents the conflict in a new form. For example, when children who have satisfactorily achieved a sense of trust encounter a new experience (e.g., hospitalization), they must again develop a sense of trust in those responsible for their care in order to master the situation.

Erikson's eight stages or "psychosocial crises" are outlined in the following segments. The lasting outcome, or ego quality (Erikson, 1978), of each stage, achieved through a central process (Newman and Newman, 1984), provides the resources for coping. Specific persons in the environment become the key socializing agents in the process (Shaffer, 1984). All eight stages are included since the later age stages are important to family functions and have an impact on the development of children. Table 4-5 summarizes the developmental theories.

Trust vs mistrust (birth to 1 year). The first and most important attribute of a healthy personality to develop is a basic trust. Establishment of basic trust dominates the first year of life and describes all the child's satisfying experiences at this age. Corresponding to Freud's oral stage, it is a time of "getting" and "taking in" through all the senses. It exists only in relation to something or someone; therefore consistent, loving care by a mothering person is essential to development of trust. *Mistrust* develops when trust-promoting experiences are deficient or lacking or when basic needs are inconsistently or inadequately met. Shreds of mistrust are sprinkled throughout the personality, but through the process of mutuality with the primary caregiver the individual develops the ego quality *hope*, an enduring belief that one can attain one's deep and essential wishes. The result is faith and optimism.

Autonomy vs shame and doubt (1 to 3 years). Corresponding to Freud's anal stage, the problem of autonomy can be symbolized by the holding on and letting go of the sphincter muscles. The development of autonomy during the toddler period is centered around children's increasing ability to control their bodies, themselves, and their environment. They want to use their powers to do things for themselves, using their newly acquired motor skills of walking, climbing, and manipulating and mental powers of selection and decision making. Negative feelings of *doubt* and *shame* arise when children are made to feel small and self-conscious, when their choices are disastrous, when others shame them, or when they are forced to be dependent in areas in which they are capable of assuming control. The central process for achieving autonomy is imitation and the key socializing agents are the parents. The favorable outcomes are *self-control* and *willpower*.

Initiative vs guilt (3 to 6 years). This stage corresponds to Freud's phallic stage and is characterized by vigorous, intrusive behavior, enterprise, and a strong imagination. Children explore the physical world with all their senses and powers. They develop a conscience. No longer guided only by outsiders, children respond to an inner voice that warns and threatens. Children sometimes undertake goals or activities that are in conflict with those of parents or others, and being made to feel that their activities or imaginings are bad produces a sense of *guilt*. Children must learn to retain a sense of initiative without impinging on the rights and privileges of others. The central process is identification and the key socializing agent is the family. The lasting outcomes are *direction* and *purpose;* the courage to imagine and pursue is a valued goal.

Industry vs inferiority (6 to 12 years). This stage correlates with the latency period of Freud. Having achieved the more crucial stages in personality development, children are now ready to be workers and producers. They want to engage in tasks and activities they can carry through to completion; they need and want real achievement. Children learn to compete with others and to cooperate, and they learn the rules. It is a decisive period in their social relationships with others. Feelings of inadequacy and *inferiority* may develop if too much is expected of them or if they believe that they cannot measure up to the standards set for them by others. The key socializing agents are teachers and peers and the central process is education. The ego quality developed from a sense of industry is *competence*, the free exercise of skill and intelligence in the completion of tasks.

Identity vs role confusion (12 to 18 years). Corresponding to Freud's genital stage, this period is characterized by rapid and marked physical changes. Previous trust in their bodies shaken, children become overly preoccupied with the way they appear in the eyes of others as compared with their own self-concept. Adolescents struggle to fit the roles they have played and those they hope to play with the current roles and fashions adopted by their peers, to integrate their concepts and values with those of society, and to come to a decision regarding an occupation. Inability to solve the core conflict results in *role confusion*. The central processes are peer pressure and role experimentation; the key socializing agent is the society of peers. The outcome of successful mastery is devotion and *fidelity*, the ability to sustain loyalties freely committed in early adolescence to others and loyalties freely pledged in later adolescence to values and ideologies.

Intimacy vs isolation (early adulthood). A sense of intimacy is established on a sense of identity. *Intimacy* is the capacity to develop an intimate love relationship with another and intimate interpersonal relationships with friends, partners, and other significant persons. Without intimacy the individual feels *isolated* and alone. The central process is mutuality among peers and the key socializing agents are lovers, spouses, and close friends. The favorable outcome is affiliation and *love*, the capacity for mutuality that transcends childhood dependency.

Generativity vs stagnation (young and middle adulthood). Central to this stage of development is the creation and care of the next generation. The essential element is to nourish and nurture. It may be directed toward one's own children, children of others, or other products of creativity. The individual who fails in this component of personality development becomes self-absorbed and *stagnant*. The key socializing agents are the spouse, children, and cultural norms and the central process is person-environment fit and creativity. The favorable outcome is production and *care*, the commitment to be concerned for what has been generated.

Ego integrity vs despair (old age). A sense of integrity results from satisfaction with life and acceptance of what has been; *despair* arises from remorse for what might have been. The central process is introspection and the favorable outcome is renunciation and *wisdom*, the detached yet active concern with life in the face of death.

THEORETIC FOUNDATIONS OF COGNITIVE DEVELOPMENT (PIAGET)

The term *cognition* refers to the process by which developing individuals become acquainted with the world and the objects it contains. Children are born with inherited potentialities for intellectual growth, but they must develop into that potential through interaction with the environment. By assimilating information through the senses, processing it, and acting on it, they come to understand relationships between objects and between themselves and their world. With cognitive development, children acquire the ability to reason abstractly, to think in a logical manner, and to organize intellectual functions or performances into higher-order structures.

The best-known theory regarding children's thinking, and a more comprehensive one than those already described, has been developed by the Swiss psychologist Jean Piaget (1969). He believes intelligence enables individuals to make adaptations to the environment that increase the probability of survival and that through their behavior individuals establish and maintain equilibrium with the environment.

According to Piaget, children progress through a series of stages of mental activity in an orderly and sequential manner. The mechanisms that enable them to adapt to new situations and to move from one stage to the next are assimilation and accommodation. By *assimilation* children incorporate new knowledge, skills, ideas, and insights into cognitive schemes (Piaget uses the term *schema**) already familiar to them. To new situations that do not fit into an established schema, children *accommodate*. They change and organize existing schema to solve more difficult tasks and form new schema. Children's understanding of a new experience is based on all relevant previous experiences. They achieve equilibrium over and over again by applying schemas already available to them. Thus children achieve an accurate understanding of reality and come to deal with increasingly complex problems in an increasingly effective manner.

Development of Logical Thinking

Piaget believes there are four major stages in the development of logical thinking. Each is derived from and builds on the accomplishments of the previous stage in a continuous, orderly process. The course of intellectual development is both maturational and invariant and is divided into the following periods, subperiods, and stages (ages are approximate).

Sensorimotor (birth to 2 years). The sensorimotor stage of intellectual development consists of six substages (see p. 503) that are governed by sensations through which simple learning takes place. Children progress from reflex activity through simple repetitive behaviors to imitative behavior. They develop a sense of "cause and effect" as they direct behavior toward objects and solve problems primarily through trial and error. They display a high level of curiosity, experimentation, and enjoyment of novelty. As a result of interactions with their environment, children begin to develop a sense of self as they are able to differentiate themselves from their environment.

---

*A schema is a pattern of action and/or thought.

Children become aware that an object has *permanence*, that it exists even though it is no longer visible. The awareness of object permanence is extremely important because it is prerequisite for all other mental activity. All concepts begin with or involve objects in one way or another (Elkind, 1979). Toward the end of the sensorimotor period children begin to use language, and representational thought appears as they imitate the behavior of others, even in the absence of these other persons.

Preoperational (2 to 7 years). The predominant characteristic of this period of intellectual development is *egocentricity*. Egocentricity in this sense does not mean selfishness or self-centeredness, but rather the inability to put oneself in the place of another. Children interpret objects and events not in terms of general properties, but in terms of their relationships or their use to them. They are unable to see things from any perspective other than their own; they cannot see another's point of view, nor can they see any reason to do so.

Preoperational thinking is concrete and tangible. Children cannot reason beyond the observable, and they lack the ability to make deductions or generalizations. Thought is dominated by what they see, hear, or otherwise experience. However, they are increasingly able to use language and symbols to represent objects in their environment. Through imaginative play, questioning, and interacting, they begin to elaborate concepts and make simple associations between ideas. One of the most salient features of preoperational thought is lack of conservation or reversibility; children at this stage cannot understand that for every action or operation there is an action or operation that cancels it. For example, children in this age-group are unable to grasp the idea that a ball of clay can be changed and brought back to the original shape. In the latter stage of this period their reasoning is *intuitive* (e.g., the stars have to go to bed just as they do), and they are only beginning to deal with problems of weight, length, size, and time.

Concrete operational (7 to 11 years). During this period thought becomes increasingly logical and coherent. Children are able to classify, sort, order, and otherwise organize facts about the world to use in problem solving. They develop a new concept of permanence—conservation (see p. 708). They realize that volume, weight, and number remain the same even though outward appearances are changed. They are able to deal with a number of different aspects of a situation simultaneously. They do not have the capacity to deal in abstraction; they solve problems in a concrete, systematic fashion based on what they can perceive. Reasoning is inductive. Through progressive changes in thought processes and relationships with others, thought becomes decentered. Children can consider points of view other than their own. Thinking has become socialized.

Formal operational (12 to 15 years). Formal operational thought is characterized by adaptability and flexibility. Adolescents can think in abstract terms, use abstract symbols, and draw logical conclusions from a set of observations. They can make hypotheses and test them; they can consider abstract, theoretic, and philosophic matters. Although they may confuse the ideal with the practical, they can deal with and resolve most contradictions in the world.

THEORETIC FOUNDATIONS OF SOCIAL LEARNING

Learning occurs when behavior changes as a result of experience, and learning theories attempt to explain the ways in which controlled changes in the environment produce predictable changes in behavior. Basically children acquire new behaviors and produce alterations in existing behaviors through (1) forming associations through conditioning and (2) observing models.

Conditioning (Skinner)

Conditioning is learning by association, that is, establishing a connection between a stimulus and a response. In *classical,* or Pavlovian, conditioning two events that occur simultaneously or close together in time come to have similar meanings to the child and thus evoke the same response. For example, infants learn very early to associate the sight of the mother's face and the sound of her voice with feeding and other pleasant sensations. Consequently the infant will cease crying or somehow indicate pleasure when she speaks or enters the infant's visual field. This type of learning appears to be the predominant form that takes place during infancy, particularly in the first 6 months, before the development of motor control.

Operant, and *instrumental,* conditioning involve the use of rewards or reinforcements to encourage the performance of specific behaviors. Reinforcing desired responses whenever they occur increases the likelihood that they will be repeated. These reinforcements can be inner satisfactions or externally applied reward systems. Behavior that is not in some way reinforced or rewarded will be extinguished. The principles of instrumental conditioning are especially applicable to learning that takes place naturally in toddlers and preschool children. These children can appreciate the significance of rewards and punishments even though they may not be able to conceptualize the context or framework in which they are operating. A substantial proportion of early childhood learning, such as acquisition of motor skills, consists of simple operant conditioning.

Avoidance conditioning discourages undesired behaviors through the use of punishment and fear of punishment. The effectiveness of rewards and punishments depends on the child's subjective assessment of the reward or punishment. Some rewards are not reinforcing, and punishments do not generate fear if they are inappropriate to the development level, emotional stage, or value system of the individual child. Punishment is effective in controlling behavior, but it must be correctly timed, brief, appropriate to the child and the undesired behavior, and tempered with love.

Operant conditioning is the basis of behavior-modification procedures that have achieved varying degrees of success in speech therapy and in modifying behavior in overly

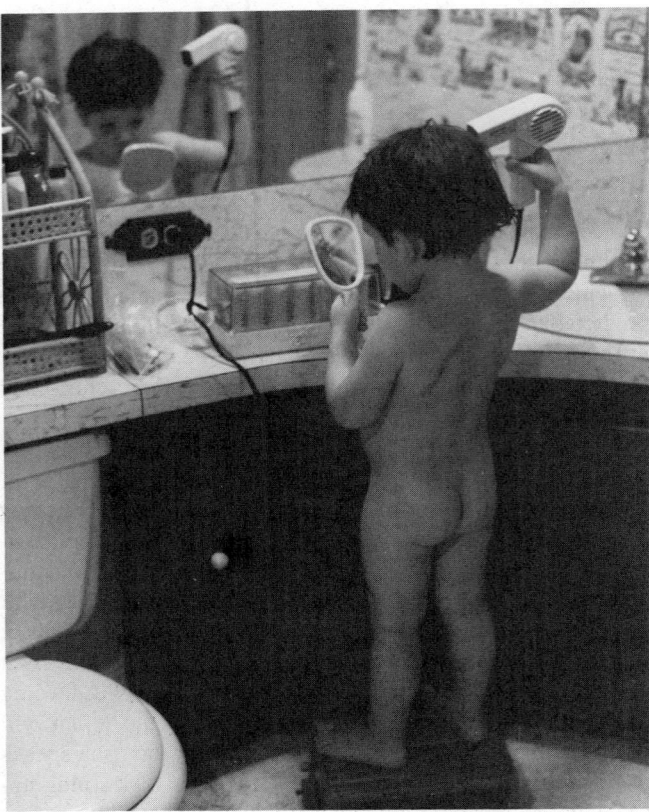

Fig. 4-9. Children learn by imitating the behavior of others. (Proper safety precautions should be observed when children use electrical appliances.)
Photography by Anne Kunke, San Jose, CA.

aggressive and mentally retarded children. Behavior is shaped by reinforcing closer and closer approximations to the behavior being taught.

Modeling or Observational Learning (Bandura)

Much of childhood learning takes place because of children's innate tendency to observe and imitate the behavior of those who are significant in their lives. Children learn many new behaviors from observing parents, siblings, and peers. Learning is immediate, and children can often correctly imitate a behavior on the first attempt. They are more apt to imitate those whom they believe to be prestigious and those whom they see being rewarded for their behavior.

As children gain more complex cognitive skills and the use of language, learning assumes broader dimensions, involving creativity, problem solving, and abstract conceptualization. Modeling requires no reinforcement, although in most situations a child imitates a behavior because he is in some way reinforced for doing so. A child may proudly proclaim he is doing something ''just like mommy and daddy.'' Apparently modeling is its own reward (Fig. 4-9).

Role Learning in Children

A *role* is a set of duties, rights, obligations, and expected behaviors that accompanies a given position in a social

structure. Children are expected to play a variety of roles such as son or daughter, sister or brother, student, classmate, and playmate. They learn and practice these roles and learn something of the characteristics of other roles through interaction with others and in their play. Children will behave in patterned and more or less predictable ways because they learn roles that define mutual expectations in typical and recurring social relationships (see also p. 66).

Individuals bring their own unique temperaments, skills, and values to the interpretation and enactment of the roles they play. Because most roles exist independently of the individuals who play them, the functions and norms associated with any given role influence the way persons play the roles and the responses of the people associated with those persons (Biddle, 1979). For example, expectations about the role of teacher affect the behavior of persons playing that role and those expectations serve as a guide to others in the evaluation of persons in that role.

As their relationships expand, children also become increasingly proficient in understanding other people. They develop the ability to distinguish their own perspectives from those of their companions through role-taking (Selman, 1980). This ability is acquired in a progressive developmental sequence that parallels the invariant cognitive stages of Piaget (see p. 114). Selman's stages of social role-taking are:

0. **Egocentric or undifferentiated perspective** (approximately 3 to 6 years). Children are unaware of any perspective other than their own—whatever is right for them is agreeable to others.
1. **Social-informational role-taking** (approximately 6 to 8 years). Children recognize that people can have perspectives that differ from their own but only because these persons have received different information. Children are unable to think about the thinking of others and imagine how others will react to an event.
2. **Self-reflective role-taking** (approximately 8 to 10 years). Children know that their own and others' viewpoints may conflict even when they receive the same information. They are able to consider another's point of view and recognize that others can place themselves in their shoes. Consequently, children are able to anticipate another's reactions to their behavior but are unable to consider their own and another's perspective at the same time.
3. **Mutual role-taking** (approximately 10 to 12 years). Children can consider their own and another's point of view simultaneously and realize that others are able to do the same. They can also assume the perspective of a disinterested child and anticipate the way the active participants (self and other) will react to the viewpoint of either participant.
4. **Social and conventional system role-taking** (approximately 12 to 15 years). Young persons now attempt to understand the perspective of another by comparing it with that of the social system in which they operate. They expect others to consider and assume perspectives on events congruent with most persons in their social group.

The ability to interact successfully with other people is closely related to role-taking skills. Relationships change as children recognize that others have different motives and intentions. For example, in Selman's stage 1 a friend is someone who not only lives nearby but also does nice things (Fig. 4-10); at stage 2 the term *friend* implies a reciprocal relationship with mutual respect, kindness, and affection (Furman and Bierman, 1983). In adolescence friendship becomes a relationship of common interests and values with a reasonably well-coordinated outlook on life, and a "friend" becomes someone with whom intimate information can be shared (Berndt, 1982). It has also been found that children who are adept in role-taking abilities are better able to establish intimate friendships (McGuire and Weisz, 1982) and are more popular with classmates (Kurdek and Krile, 1982).

SEX-ROLE IDENTIFICATION

From the moment of birth children are treated differently by their families based on their biologic sex. Almost immediately infants are placed in male or female categories with given names that clearly indicate a sex, dressed in pink if girls or blue if boys, and referred to as either "he" or "she." Thus information regarding a sexual identity is conveyed to children and to the world, and along with these overt messages a set of sex-related attitudes toward them emerges. The outcome of the identification process depends on the characteristics of the parents and other role models, the innate capacities and preferences of the child, and the cultural and familiar value placed on his or her sex.

Families recognize the importance of sex differences and even in infancy treat boys differently from girls. Parental attitudes and expectations regarding sex-appropriate behaviors, acquired from their own upbringing, influence how they react to their children from infancy. These attitudes and expectations are transmitted to infants first in subtle, then in

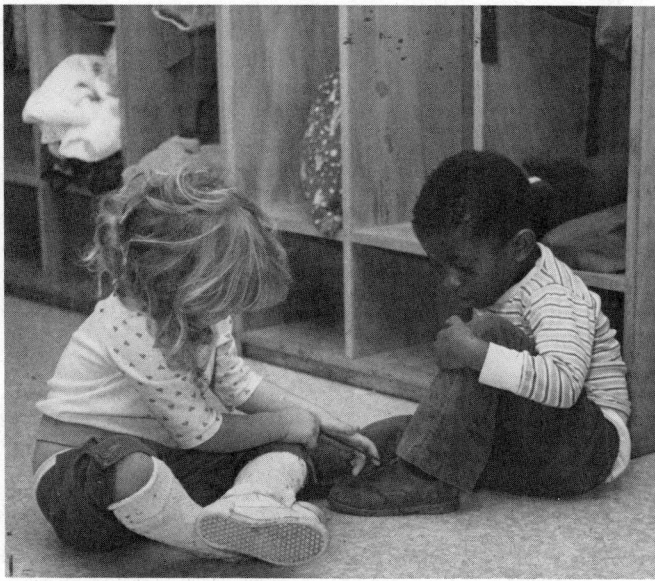

Fig. 4-10. A friend is someone who does nice things.
Photography by John Roy, Saint Francis Hospital, Tulsa, OK.

more obvious, ways. For example, family members relate to infants differently: little girls are handled more tenderly; little boys are stimulated with boisterous activity and vigorous motor play. Families provide sex-appropriate toys and encourage play consistent with the sex-role expectations of the children.

Development of Sex-Role Identification

Four dimensions appear to be involved in the development of sex-role identification. Children (1) learn to apply appropriate gender labels to themselves, (2) acquire sex-appropriate standards of behavior, (3) develop a preference for being the sex that they are, and (4) identify with their parent of the same sex.

Gender label. The gender label is achieved early and subtly through imitation of the parents' expressions as they refer to children's gender, for example, "That's a good girl" or "That's a good boy". Since it is such an important and basic component of children's total identity, the appropriate gender must be assigned as soon as possible in rare cases where the sex of the infant is in doubt (see p. 479). The gender orientation has more effect on development than does chromosomal determination of sex.

Sex-role standards. Beginning when children are toddlers, sex role standards are differentiated and continuously developed throughout childhood. By the time children are 3 years old, they know whether they are boys or girls, and they have acquired considerable knowledge of and a preference for sex-appropriate behaviors. They can differentiate one sex from the other even before they learn anatomic differences; 2-year-old children can identify others as girls or boys based on external appearances.

Preschool children have definite impressions of masculinity and femininity, and they are reflected in overt play. Most children in this age-group engage in stereotyped sex-appropriate play activities. Little girls are more likely to play at housekeeping, taking care of dolls, dressing up, and cooking; boys choose trucks, blocks, and more physically active play. Boys are generally more aggressive in their play, and in disagreements with peers they are more apt to react with shouting or fighting. Girls tend to be more dependent and introverted in their play (Maccoby, 1980). With the strong women's movement, more liberal views regarding sex-role typing, and the unisex trend in all areas of interaction, these sex-associated characteristics are less apparent than they have been in the past. However, the United States, like most cultures, still has a strong masculine orientation with males generally accorded more privileges than females.

Families expect children to learn appropriate sex-role behavior early and to deviate little from it. Each family has its own concept of what constitutes male or female attributes and the types of sex-linked behavior they wish to cultivate in their children. These beliefs are conveyed to the children by a variety of means, and parents exert special efforts to gain compliance with their expectations. Experiences the children are exposed to, toys selected for them, and activities they are encouraged to participate in all reflect some aspect of the family's sex-role conformity to standards of achievement, competition, self-assertiveness, and independence with control of feelings and repression of emotions. With girls the family usually places more emphasis on passive activities and development of interpersonal sensitivity, docility, interrelatedness with others, and nurturance.

In the case of boys the prohibition against effeminate behavior is very strong. Boys are rewarded less often for displaying behavior considered appropriate for their sex, but they are discouraged from exhibiting undesirable behavior by negative reinforcement. Parents emphasize the things that boys should *not* do or be, that is, those things that might label them as "sissies." Avoidance of the opposite sex-role behavior is a major means of sex-role learning in the American culture, especially for boys. This emphasis seems to be stronger in lower-class families, where sex roles are more clearly defined and segregated. In middle-class homes sex-role differentiation is less clear-cut. Mothers often work outside the home, and male role models are more apt to help with behaviors traditionally assigned to the female, such as housework and baby-sitting.

The family situation may be more influential for sex-role development of girls than of boys, since boys are more apt to learn much of their masculine behaviors from role models outside the home. For example, in lower-class black families in which the father is frequently absent, a male child often associates with gangs to learn a masculine role, whereas a Hispanic youth who has a male model in the home may join such gangs to escape the paternal dominance and be free to express his masculine role.

Girls, on the other hand, are dealt with more leniently in America. Their role is less rigidly defined than that of boys. Girls are permitted to engage in masculine games and activities, to wear pants, and to be a tomboy without strong cultural disapproval. This greater variance may create some confusion in establishing a sex-role identity. A girl's acceptance of a parental role model depends a great deal on whether the role model of her mother is congruent with the girl's concept of a sex role.

Gender preference. Gender preference for the sex children are born is acquired over a long time and depends on several things. Children will prefer to be a member of their own sex when their behaviors and competence closely approximate the sex-role standards, when they like their parent of the same sex, and when they believe their sex is valued. The sexes are not always valued equally in all cultures nor in all families. In cultures where males are more highly valued and are given higher status, boys are likely to develop a firm preference for their sex. However, girls in these cultures may be less certain regarding their gender assignment, even to the point of rejecting their sex group. A deterrent to sex-role preference by children can exist in families where the parents, at a specific birth, had hoped strongly for a child of the opposite sex. The environmental cues within the family will convey to these children that the opposite sex is a preferred one.

Gender identity. The process by which children style themselves after their parent of the same sex and internalize that parent's values and outlook is *identification*. Most children wish to be like their parent of the same sex, and although the motivation for identification is still unsettled, children are more willing to share these parental attributes when they are able to see a degree of similarity between themselves and their parents. Children become aware of the similarity when they perceive actual physical and psychologic similarities, adopt parental behaviors, and are told of similarities by others. Once this identification is formed, it can be strengthened by the continued positive conception of the role model or weakened if the child does not perceive the model as desirable. Identification is not a total, all-or-nothing happening. To some extent children identify with both parents, and as their sphere of social contacts widens, they identify with peers and other adults outside the family.

THEORETIC FOUNDATIONS OF MORAL DEVELOPMENT (KOHLBERG)

Children develop moral reasoning in an invariant developmental sequence. To understand the stages in the development of moral judgment, it is important to be aware of the stages of logical thought and the relationship to cognitive development as well as to moral behavior. According to Piaget there are three stages of reasoning: intuitive, concrete operational, and formal operational. When they enter the stage of concrete logical thought at about age 7 years, children are then able to make logical inferences, classify, and deal with quantitative relationships about concrete things. Not until adolescence are they able to reason abstractly with any degree of competence.

Stages of Moral Development

Moral development is based on cognitive developmental theory and consists of the following three major levels, each with two stages (Kohlberg, 1975).

Preconventional morality. The preconventional level parallels the preconceptual level of cognitive development and intuitive thought. At this level morality is external since children conform to rules imposed by authority figures. Culturally oriented to the labels of good/bad and right/wrong, children integrate these labels in terms of the physical or pleasurable consequences of their actions. The two stages of this level are:

Stage 1: The punishment-and-obedience orientation. The child determines the goodness or badness of an action in terms of its consequences. He avoids punishment and obeys unquestioningly those who have the power to determine and enforce the rules and labels. He has no concept of the underlying moral order that supports these consequences.

Stage 2: The instrumental-relativist orientation. The right behavior consists of that which satisfies the child's own needs (and sometimes the needs of others). Although elements of fairness, reciprocity, and equal sharing are evident, they are interpreted in a very practical, concrete manner without the elements of loyalty, gratitude, or justice.

Conventional level. At this stage children are concerned with conformity and loyalty, actively maintaining, supporting, and justifying the social order as well as personal expectations of those significant in their lives. They value the maintenance of family, group, or national expectations regardless of consequences. This level correlates with the concrete operational stage in cognitive development and consists of two stages:

Stage 3: *The interpersonal concordance* or *"good boy–nice girl" orientation.* Behavior that meets with approval and pleases or helps others is viewed as good. Conformity to the norm is the "natural" behavior, and one earns approval by being "nice."

Stage 4: *The "law and order" orientation.* Obeying the rules, doing one's duty, showing respect for authority, and maintaining the social order is the correct behavior. The rules and authority can be social or religious, depending on which is most valued.

Postconventional, autonomous, or principled level. At this level children have reached the cognitive formal operational stage and endeavor to define moral values and principles that are valid and applicable beyond the authority of the groups and persons holding these principles. This level is not associated with the individual's identification with these groups. Level 3 also has two stages:

Stage 5: *The social-contract, legalistic orientation.* Correct behavior tends to be defined in terms of general individual rights and standards that have been examined and agreed on by the entire society. Although procedural rules for reaching consensus become important with emphasis on the legal point of view, there is also emphasis on the possibility of changing law in terms of societal needs and rational considerations. Agreement and contract outside the legal realm are binding elements of obligation.

Stage 6: *The universal-ethical–principle orientation.* Self-chosen ethical principles guide decisions of conscience. These are abstract but universal principles of justice and human rights with respect for the dignity of the persons as individuals. It is believed that few persons reach this stage of moral reasoning.

SPIRITUAL DEVELOPMENT

Spiritual beliefs are closely related to the moral and ethical portion of children's self-concepts and as such must be considered as part of children's basic needs assessment. Children need to have meaning, purpose, and hope in their lives and the need for confession and forgiveness is present even in very young children. The research in spiritual development is both limited and subject to criticism, particularly in relation to age-stage theories. However, the stage theories provide a useful means for the reader to assess the approximate level of development for any given child.

Stages of Spiritual Development

Fowler (1974) has identified four stages in the development of faith that parallel and are closely associated with cognitive and psychosocial development.

Stage 0: Undifferentiated. This stage of development encompasses the period of infancy when children have no concept of right or wrong, no beliefs, and no convictions to guide their behavior. However, the beginnings of a faith are established with the development of basic trust through their relationships with the primary caregiver.

Stage 1: Intuitive-projective. Toddlerhood is primarily a time of imitating the behavior of others. Children imitate the religious gestures and behaviors of others without comprehending any meaning or significance to the activities. During the preschool years children assimilate some of the values and beliefs of their parents. Parental attitudes toward moral codes and religous beliefs convey to children what they consider good and bad. Children follow parental beliefs as part of their daily lives rather than through an understanding of their basic concepts.

Stage 2: Mythical-literal. Through the school-age years spiritual development parallels cognitive development and is closely related to children's experiences and social interaction. Most children have a strong interest in religion during the school-age years. The existence of a deity is accepted, and petitions to an omnipotent being are important and expected to be answered; good behavior is rewarded and bad behavior is punished. Children's developing conscience bothers them when they disobey. They have a reverence for many thoughts and matters and are able to articulate their faith. They may even begin to question its validity.

Stage 3: Synthetic-convention. As children approach adolescence they become increasingly aware of spiritual disappointments. They recognize that prayers are not always answered (at least on their own terms). They begin to reason, to question some of the established parental religious standards, and to drop or modify some religious practices.

Stage 4: Individuating-reflexive. Adolescents become more skeptical and begin to compare the religious standards of their parents with others. They attempt to determine which to adopt and incorporate into their own set of values. They also begin to compare religious standards with the scientific viewpoint. It is a time of searching rather than reaching. Adolescents are uncertain about many religious ideas but will not achieve profound insights until late adolescence or early adulthood.

LANGUAGE DEVELOPMENT

Children are born with the mechanism and capacity to develop speech and language skills. However, they will not speak spontaneously. The environment must provide a means for them to acquire these skills. Speech requires intact physiologic function of (1) the respiratory system, (2) speech control centers in the cerebral cortex, and (3) articulation and resonance structures of the mouth and nasal cavities. In addition, acquisition of language requires (1) an intact and discriminating auditory apparatus, (2) intelligence, (3) a need to communicate, and (4) stimulation.

The rate of speech development varies from child to child and is directly related to neurologic competence and intellectual development. All children go through the same sequence of stages in prelingual speech. These stages are summarized in Table 25-8, p. 1043. Preceding speech, gesture allows a small child to communicate satisfactorily. As speech develops, gesture recedes but never disappears entirely. Evidence has shown that early speech stimulation is important to the development of normal speech; therefore those responsible for the child's care should provide auditory stimulation and verbal feedback. Continual relationships with others enhance the desire to acquire greater vocabulary and communication skills.

At all stages of language development, children's comprehension vocabulary is greater than their expressed vocabulary. The acquisition of vocabulary and language keeps pace with cognitive advancement, and children begin to use words as substitutes for action. The growth of children's vocabulary reflects a continuing process of modification that involves both the acquisition of new words and the expanding and refining of word meanings previously learned. By the time they begin to walk, children are able to attach a name to objects and persons.

The first parts of speech used are nouns, sometimes verbs (e.g., go), and combination words (e.g., bye-bye). Following the use of the first meaningful words, children begin to relate words to one another to form simple and then more complex sentences. Responses are usually structurally incomplete during the toddler period, although the meaning is clear. Next they begin to use adjectives and adverbs to qualify nouns, followed by adverbs to qualify nouns and verbs. Later, pronouns and gender words are added (e.g., he and she). By the time children enter school they are able to use simple, structurally complete sentences that average five to seven words.

A common rule of thumb that is helpful in evaluation of early speech acquisition is *the number of words in an average response should correspond to the chronologic age of the child* (Goda, 1970). For example, a 2-year-old child might say, "Me do"; a 3-year-old might add a word, "Me do it"; and a 4-year-old child might say, "Let me do it."

Girls are more advanced in language development than boys. Firstborn children develop language earlier than do later-born children, and children of multiple births (twins, triplets) develop language later than children of single births. Delayed, lack of, or impaired speech can result from a variety of sources, including congenital structural defects of the mouth and nasopharynx, a hearing deficit, neurologic dysfunction (including mental retardation), maternal deprivation, and emotional factors. Some of these factors are discussed in relation to health problems in which impaired speech is a symptom or a consequence. It is also important to note that some of the organ systems and organs on which speech depends, such as the respiratory system for gas exchange and the tongue for eating, are responsible for higher priority functions that take precedence over the lesser important function of communication. During illness or trauma children may direct their limited energy to the more vital functions of these systems, breathing and eating.

DEVELOPMENT OF SELF-CONCEPT

Self-concept is all the notions, beliefs, and convictions that constitute an individual's knowledge of self and that influence one's relationships with others. It is not present at birth but develops gradually as a result of the individual's unique experiences within the self, with significant others, and with the realities of the world (Stuart and Sundeen, 1983). However, the self-concept is subjective and therefore may or may not reflect reality.

The content of the self-concept differs at various stages of development and results from the cognitive capacities and the dominant motives of individuals coming in contact with stage-related cultural expectations. In infancy self-concept is primarily an awareness of one's independent existence learned in part as a result of social contacts and experiences with other people. The process becomes more active during toddlerhood as children explore the limits of their capacities and the nature of their impact on others (Newman and Newman, 1984).

School-age children are more aware of differences in perspectives among people, social norms, and moral imperatives. They are sensitive to social pressures and become preoccupied with issues of self-criticism and self-evaluation. Because school-age children depend on adults for material and emotional resources, the self-concept is likely to be most vulnerable during this time. Little change in self-concept occurs during early adolescence when children anxiously focus on their physical and emotional changes and peer acceptance. Self-concept crystallizes during later adolescence as young people review and evaluate their childhood experiences and organize their self-concept around a set of values, goals, and competencies (Newman and Newman, 1984).

Body Image

Body image is the subjective concepts and attitudes that individuals have toward their own bodies as objects in space. Central to the concept of self, body image is the picture of the body formed in the mind, including feelings about size, function, appearance, and potential. The picture appears to be a learned phenomenon that may be conscious or unconscious and may be cognitive and/or emotional. It includes present and past perceptions and is continually modified by new perceptions and experiences.

Development of body changes during growth. Infants receive input about their bodies through self-exploration and sensory stimulation from others. As they begin to manipulate their environment they become aware of their bodies as separate from others. Toddlers learn to identify the various parts of their bodies and are able to use symbols to represent objects. Preschoolers become aware of the wholeness of their bodies and discover the genitals. Exploration of the genitals and the discovery of differences between sexes become important. There is only a vague concept of internal organs and functions (Stuart and Sundeen, 1983; Selekman, 1983).

School-age children begin to learn about internal body structure and function and become aware of differences in the body size and configurations of others. They are highly influenced by the cultural norms of society and the fads of the times. Children whose bodies deviate from the norm are often subject to criticism and ridicule.

Adolescence is the age when children become most concerned about the physical self. The familiar body changes and the new physical self must be integrated into the self-concept. Adolescents face conflicts over what they see and what they visualize as the ideal body structure. Body image formation during adolescence is a crucial element in the shaping of an identity, the psychosocial crisis of adolescence.

Self-Esteem

Self-esteem is described as the affective component of the self and the self-concept is the cognitive component; however, the two are almost indistinguishable and the terms are often used interchangeably (Stanwyck, 1983). *Self-esteem* is a personal, subjective judgment of one's worthiness derived from and influenced by the social groups in the immediate environment and the individual's perceptions of how he or she is valued by others. Self-esteem is primarily a function of being loved and of gaining the respect of others.

Self-esteem is a product of both competence and social acceptance that changes with development. Throughout childhood children experience an increased ability to differentiate components of competence, an increased concern with a variety of significant others who may give or withhold approval, and an increased capacity to experience guilt when internal norms for either competence or social acceptance are violated (Newman and Newman, 1984). *High self-esteem* is described as a feeling based on unconditional acceptance of oneself as a worthy and important being (Stuart and Sundeen, 1983).

Highly egocentric toddlers are unaware of any difference between competence and social approval. They are the center of their world, and to them all positive experiences are evidence of their importance and value. Preschool and early school-age children, on the other hand, are increasingly aware of the discrepancy between their competencies and the abilities of more advanced children. They are expected to evaluate a situation and anticipate the consequences of their behavior before they act. The acceptance of adults and peers outside the family group becomes more important to them. Since these valued persons may not be as proud of their achievements or as understanding of their limitations as their families are, their recently acquired capacity for guilt may lead to anxiety over failure, and they will be more vulnerable to feelings of worthlessness and depression. As their competencies increase and they develop meaningful relationships, their self-esteem rises. Their self-esteem is again at risk during early adolescence when they are defining an identity and sense of self in the context of their peer group.

Unless children are continually made to feel incompetent and of little worth, a decrease in self-esteem during vulnerable periods is only temporary. Transitory periods of lowered self-esteem at the stages of development are expected when they must set new goals or when there are very obvious discrepancies in competence. A constant source of anxiety arises from the endless number of separations that occur in the process of acquiring autonomy, independence, and individuality. As an expression of their own urgencies, parents often set overambitious goals for their children and expect them to perform beyond the limits of their capacity. Also, children's attempts at autonomy and achievement are often thwarted by parental overprotection, because either the parents fear the children will be hurt or the parents find it more convenient to do things for them.

Factors that Influence Development

Children are engaged in a continuous, dynamic, and reciprocal relationship with their environment in order to achieve and maintain an equilibrium. This equilibrium, or balance, is continually upset and regained through numerous and varied complex interactions. It is impossible to include a discussion of all the complex and interrelated factors that influence the development of children as unique individuals. However, some of the major areas of importance are presented.

PHYSIOLOGIC FACTORS

Children are affected by physical factors such as the climate, physiologic influences such as their innate characteristics and susceptibilities, the value system of their families and culture, and psychologic influences such as the quality of parenting and the number, sex, and personalities of the significant persons in their lives. Some factors that may be facilitated, modified, or otherwise influenced by nursing interventions are mentioned in this section, although specific activities and elaboration are discussed elsewhere when appropriate.

Heredity

Inherited characteristics have a profound influence on development. The sex of the child, determined by random selection at the time of conception, directs both his pattern of growth and the behavior of others toward him. In all cultures attitudes and expectations are different with respect to the sex of the child. Sex plus other hereditary determinants strongly affect growth rate and the end result of that growth. A high correlation exists between parent and child with regard to traits such as height, weight, and rate of growth.

Most physical characteristics, including shape and form of features, body build, and physical peculiarities, are inherited and can influence the way children grow and interact with their environment. The child's heritage may cause a deviation from established physical standards for growth and development. For example, Japanese children are smaller than average at all ages. Some children are taller and heavier than the average from early childhood and usually achieve their linear growth sooner. Black children weigh slightly less than their white peers during the years 6 to 12 and have somewhat shorter sitting height and longer legs at all ages. Black girls begin the pubertal growth spurt at a slightly earlier age than white girls and for a brief period are slightly taller (Lowrey, 1986).

The relative importance of heredity and environment in molding development has been deliberated by scientists, educators, and health professionals. It is now commonly accepted that the end product is not a result of the *action* of one or the other of these processes but the *interaction* of one with the others. For example, children who receive genes for above-average height can only achieve full potential with an optimum environment, including good diet, love, and freedom from disease. On the other hand, children who inherit genes for less-than-average height will never attain a height greater than their programmed stature even in a superior environment. Children with limited intellectual capability can never excel in a field that requires highly intellectual skills, no matter to what extent they are pushed. But children with superior mentality will be wasted without an environment that stimulates and encourages their innate capacity.

The area that has provoked the greatest controversy is the contribution of heredity and environment to behavior characteristics and intelligence. Intellectual diversity of individuals is undisputed, but the extent to which large human groups differ in intelligence on a genetic basis is continually challenged. Infant and early childhood stimulation programs and innovative educational techniques at all levels of intellectual endowment have substantiated the positive influence of environmental stimulation on achievement. On the other hand, early childhood deprivation and the alarming effects of inadequate nutrition during critical periods of development are areas of concern to health professionals.

The influences on behavior traits are more difficult to assess. The culture dictates that some hereditary characteristics (e.g., sex) imply conformity to specific behavioral expectations. Many dimensions of personality that appear to be hereditary (e.g., the degree of responsiveness or unresponsiveness, activity level, extroversion or introversion, the degree of deliberateness or impulsiveness) and various constitutional traits (e.g., beauty, ugliness, physical defor-

mity, sensory handicaps, learning impairment) affect the way others react to children and the interpersonal behavior children display in response. When a child displays undesirable behavior, careful evaluation is required to determine the degree to which the behavior can be attributed to his interpersonal environment or to hereditary influences. This determination can be a significant factor in assessing whether or not the child would profit from therapy or if the child should be removed from that environment.

Differences in health and vigor of children may be attributed to hereditary traits. An inherited physical or mental defect or disorder will alter or modify a child's physical and/or emotional growth and interactions. The extent to which handicapping conditions interfere with the child's growth and well-being are considered in relation to numerous disabilities throughout the remainder of the book.

Neuroendocrine

It has been suggested there may be a growth center in the hypothalamic region responsible for maintaining genetically determined growth patterns. It is believed that some functional relationship between the hypothalamus and the endocrine system exists that influences growth. There is also evidence, based on observations of denervated skeletal muscles, that the peripheral nervous system may influence growth, because muscles deprived of nerve supply degenerate. Many of these effects are not sufficiently explained by disuse or diminished blood supply. For example, nail growth on an extremity with a severed nerve will lag behind the nail growth on the corresponding extremity, but the growth returns to normal with regeneration of the nerve. There is no satisfactory explanation for this revived growth rate; the process may involve a chemical substance secreted by nerve cells that modifies the growth and repair processes.

Hormones. Probably all hormones affect growth in some fashion. Three hormones—growth hormone, thyroid hormone, and androgens—when given to persons deficient these hormones, stimulate protein anabolism and thereby produce retention of elements essential for building protoplasm and bony tissue. It appears that each of the hormones that has a significant influence on growth manifests its major effect at a different period of growth:

Growth hormone, or **somatotropin,** is produced by the hypothalamus and exerts its main effect on linear growth through proliferation of cartilage cells of the epiphyseal plates until the time of epiphyseal closure at puberty. It also maintains the normal rate of synthesis of body protein and appears to inhibit synthesis of fat and the oxidation of carbohydrate.

Thyroxine and **triiodothyronine,** secreted by the thyroid gland, stimulate metabolism and are important for growth and maturation of bones, teeth, and brain. The amount secreted is believed to decline somewhat during childhood until the growth spurt of puberty, when the decline is interrupted.

Calcitonin, also secreted by the thyroid, influences ossification and development of bone.

Androgens, secreted by the adrenal cortex, influence development of bone and muscle.

Testosterone and **estrogen** stimulate production of germ cells (spermatozoa and ova) and development of secondary sex characteristics. Estrogen has an inhibitory effect on epiphyseal growth; therefore linear growth ceases when estrogen activity is accelerated.

Upright Posture

Evidence indicates that the amount of time infants spend in the vertical position influences the age they reach important motor milestones. For example, infants who are placed in the upright posture develop accelerated muscular growth and strength in legs, neck, and trunk that promotes development of motor skills (Thelen and Fisher, 1982). This is partially supported by observations that infants from Third World countries who are carried vertically in slings walk at an earlier age than children in Western countries who spend more time in the horizontal position. Also, very young infants (2 to 8 weeks old) who are held upright and allowed to practice the ''stepping'' reflex walk at an earlier age than infants who do not receive this early experience (Zelazo, Zelazo, and Kolb, 1972). Thus experience may be as important as maturation in determining motor development.

Sex

The sex of the child has some influence on growth and development, although it is not always apparent which differences are related to cultural expectations as opposed to innate characteristics. Extensive research (Maccoby and Jacklin, 1974) indicates there are few actual differences but many myths regarding differences between girls and boys. There is no substantial evidence to indicate that girls are more social and suggestible, lack motivation to achieve, have a lower self-esteem, or are better at learning by rote than boys. Nor is there validity to the myth that boys are more analytic and better at high-level tasks than girls. In most studies boys and girls are equally dependent on caregivers, equally susceptible to persuasive communications, and equally motivated to achieve.

There are sex differences that influence behavior in childhood. In general, boys are more aggressive than girls, both physically and verbally. Boys also more frequently engage in rough and tumble play and aggressive fantasies as well as direct forms of aggression. This behavior persists through the college years, although aggression diminishes with age in both sexes. Competitive behavior has been observed more often in boys than in girls in some studies, but there is some question as to the validity of this; other studies find the sexes to be similar in this aspect. Both sexes are alike in their willingness to explore a novel environment.

Studies differ in regard to differences between the activity levels of boys and girls, which may reflect the situations in which the measurements were conducted. The play of both boys and girl is equally organized and planned. Some studies find that boys seem to have more difficulty sitting still, engage in more exploratory behavior, and are stimulated to bursts of high activity in the presence of other boys. Boys exhibit greater impulsiveness and have difficulty resisting distractions, as reflected by the greater incidence of injuries in boys at all ages. However, boys tend to be outside more than girls, and many activities are influenced by motivational factors such as fear, anger, and curiosity.

Both sexes are highly responsive to social situations, although there are some sex differences in social relationships. Boys and girls show interest in confronting social stimuli (e.g., human faces and voices), in imitating models, and in understanding the emotional reactions and needs of others. However, boys have a more extensive sphere of relationships, are highly oriented toward a peer group, and congregate in large groups, whereas girls are more likely to associate in pairs or small groups and become involved in a more intense relationship with a few close friends. Girls appear to be more concerned with the welfare of the group and therefore are more apt to compromise in situations involving conflict.

The sexes are similar in overall self-confidence and self-satisfaction but differ in the areas in which they seem to feel the greatest self-confidence. Boys are apt to view themselves as more powerful and with more control over events. They respond to a challenge, especially when it appeals to their ego or competitive feelings, in order to attain a higher level of achievement. Little difference exists between the sexes regarding motivation to achieve, although some studies find girls to be superior in this respect.

During childhood girls are more likely to comply with adult commands and directions. However, this ready compliance does not extend to relationships with peers. Boys, on the other hand, appear to be more concerned about maintaining status in the peer group, which may render them more vulnerable to pressures and challenges from the group.

There are differences in verbal, visual-spatial, and mathematic abilities. Girls exceed boys in verbal abilities (understanding and producing language, comprehension of difficult material, creative writing) in early life, probably the result of earlier maturation, although many studies find no such difference during the school-age years. The difference becomes more apparent beginning with preadolescence and extends through adolescence. Although there appear to be no differences during childhood, boys exhibit superiority in visual-spatial tasks and mathematical skills, which becomes apparent in adolescence. There are no differences observed between girls and boys in the performance of analytic and nonanalytic tasks.

Girls have always been considered to demonstrate more nurturant or helping behavior than boys, but this is not established to the satisfaction of child psychologists. Girls between the ages of 6 and 10 are more often seen behaving in nurturing ways than boys, but many studies of nursery school children have not observed this difference. Much of this type of behavior is the result of imitation and modeling; as with other popular beliefs about differences between girls and boys, there is little basis in fact. It may be a result of selective attention of casual observers whose ideas are confirmed or strengthened by behaviors that are consistent with their prior beliefs. Behavior inconsistent with expectations is more likely to go unnoticed, and consequently entrenched ideas are perpetuated.

Disease

Altered growth and development is one of the clinical manifestations in a number of hereditary disorders. Growth impairment is particularly marked in skeletal disorders, such as the various forms of dwarfism and at least one of the chromosomal anomalies (Turner syndrome). Many of the disorders of metabolism, such as vitamin D–resistant rickets, mucopolysaccharidoses, and the numerous endocrine disorders, interfere with the normal growth pattern. In other disorders the tendency is toward the upper percentile of height, for example, Klinefelter syndrome and Marfan syndrome.

Many chronic illnesses associated with varying degrees of growth failure are related to congenital cardiac anomalies and respiratory disorders such as cystic fibrosis. Any disorder characterized by the inability to digest and absorb body nutrients will have an adverse effect on growth and development. These include the malabsorption syndromes and defects in digestive enzyme systems. Almost any disease state that persists over an extended period, particularly during a critical period of development, may have a permanent effect on growth. For example, children on long-term corticosteroid therapy exhibit growth retardation.

Children in a prolonged state of disequilibrium caused by illness, such as chronic infections, are under a constant inner stress that inhibits their response to adult demands and contributes to their difficulty in managing stimulting environmental experiences. Behaviors that these children display as they cope with outside stimuli as well as inner irritations can be misinterpreted as distractibility and lack of persistence toward a goal. A prolonged illness that occurs in the second year during the phase of rapid acquisition of motor control and autonomy may cause a child to lose the natural impetus peculiar to this stage of development. Such a child may remain passive and require special stimulation to develop the independence that would have developed spontaneously under normal circumstances.

PHYSICAL ENVIRONMENT

Some physical conditions have been shown to have some effect on growth, although their influence is less evident than factors such as heredity, nutrition, or hormonal excesses or deficiencies.

Season, Climate, and Oxygen Concentration

There is some evidence that season and climate may have an influence on growth. Growth in height appears to be faster in the spring and summer months, whereas growth in weight proceeds more rapidly during the autumn and winter. These observations have not been satisfactorily explained. This phenomenon may have a hormonal basis, or it may be related to seasonal differences in activity levels.

It was formerly believed that persons living in a warm climate were smaller than those from a cold climate. However, it is much too difficult to separate the effects of climate from other factors such as race, nutrition, or disease. There does seem to be more evidence regarding the effects of hypoxia on growth. Children with disorders that produce a chronic hypoxia are characteristically small when compared with children of the same chronologic age. In addition, children native to high altitudes are smaller than those living at sea level. These observations have been supported by animal studies, although there are no substantiating studies with human subjects.

Environmental Hazards

Hazards in the environment are a source of concern to health care providers and others interested in health and safety. No aspect of the potential dangers of daily living has escaped investigation by some group or individual, and more types and sources of environmental pollution are detected as populations and technology expand. Physical injuries are the most prevalent consequences of environmental dangers and these are discussed extensively throughout the book as they apply in relation to age, specific hazards, and selected physical disabilities. The harmful agents most often associated with health risks are chemicals and radiation.

The sources and routes of exposure to chemical hazards are surprisingly extensive. Water, air, and food contamination from a variety of origins are well documented and discussed. Newer, recognized sources of exposure are substances carried home (usually from the workplace) on clothes or other objects, chemicals secreted in breast milk (especially prescribed drugs and nicotine), and contamination within well-insulated homes (especially from disinfectants and burning of substances that produce toxic fumes) (Rogan, 1980).

The harmful effects of large doses of radiation are unquestioned although the long-term consequences are still under investigation. The effects of low-dose or short-term radiation are still debatable as are the safe vs harmful dosage levels.

Socioeconomic Level

Evidence indicates that the socioeconomic level of children's families has a significant impact on children's body size. At all ages children from upper- and middle-class families are taller than comparative children of families in the lower socioeconomic strata. Girls from upper- and middle-class families also reach menarche up to 3 months earlier than girls from the lower socioeconomic levels.

The cause of these differences is less definite although the general health and nutrition of lower socioeconomic levels are probably significant factors. Nutritious food sources (especially proteins) are scarce, and other factors (e.g., larger family size and regularity in eating, sleeping, and exercise) may play a role.

NUTRITION

Probably the single most important influence on growth is nutrition. Dietary factors regulate growth at *all* stages of development, and their effects are exerted in numerous and complex ways. Adequate nutrition provides the essential nutrients in the amount and balance necessary to sustain physiologic needs. These needs vary widely according to age, level of activity, and environmental conditions. Inadequacies in any or all of these essential nutrients will be reflected in altered growth.

The nutritional requirements of childhood are directly related to the rate and direction of growth. During the rapid prenatal growth period, faulty nutrition may negatively influence development from the time of implantation of the ovum until birth. The nutritional needs are met entirely through the maternal system; as a result, maternal deficiencies or abnormalities in the supplementary intrauterine structures will be manifest in fetal development.

During infancy and childhood the demand for calories is relatively great, as evidenced by the rapid increase in both height and weight. Protein and caloric requirements are higher at this time than at almost any period of postnatal development. As the growth rate slows with its concomitant decrease in metabolism, a corresponding reduction in caloric and protein requirement occurs (see Table 4-4). Growth is uneven during the periods of childhood between infancy and adolescence, when there are plateaus and small growth spurts. The child's appetite fluctuates in response to these variations until the turbulent growth spurt of adolescence, when adequate nutrition is extremely important but may be subject to numerous emotional influences. The child's caloric intake must equal his energy output plus that needed for growth. It is estimated that the average child (e.g., the 6- to 10-year-old child) expends 55% of his energy for metabolic maintenance, 25% for physical activity, 8% in fecal loss, and 12% for growth.

Adequate nutrition is closely related to good health throughout life, and an overall improvement in nourishment is evidenced by the gradual increase in size and early maturation of children in this century. In the growing child, inadequate nutrition is dangerous, particularly during those periods critical for growth. Inadequate nutrition has the greatest impact during the critical periods of rapid cell division. For example, normal development of the central nervous system depends on adequate nutrition during fetal life and throughout the first 2 years of postnatal life.

Malnutrition

The term *malnutrition* in its strictest sense is usually used to describe undernutrition, primarily that resulting from insufficient caloric intake. However, malnutrition may result from the following: (1) a dietary intake that is quantitatively or qualitatively inadequate, or both, including overnutrition; (2) disease that interferes with appetite, digestion, or absorption while increasing nutritional requirements; (3) excessive physical activity or inadequate rest; or (4) disturbed interpersonal relationships and other environmental or psychologic factors. Severe malnutrition during the critical periods of development, particularly the first 6 months of life, is positively correlated with diminished height, weight, and intelligence scores. The importance of nutrition as a vital aspect of health promotion during all phases of the illness-wellness continuum is included as it relates to developmental phases and specific health problems.

INTERPERSONAL RELATIONSHIPS

Relationships with significant others play an important role in development, particularly in emotional, intellectual, and personality development. Not only do the quality and quantity of contacts with other persons exert an influence on growing children, but the widening range of contacts is essential to learning and the development of a healthy personality (Fig. 4-11). During the formative years, culturally determined, age-appropriate behaviors are reinforced and consequently repeated. Thus patterns of reward, punishment, and modeling continually modify children's individuality of character and temperament. Children behave in a manner that elicits rewards from the persons most significant in their lives.

Significant Others

Mothers or mothering persons are unquestionably the most influential persons during early infancy. They meet the infants' basic needs of food, warmth, comfort, and love, provide stimulation for their senses, and facilitate their expanding capacities. Through these individuals children learn to trust the world and feel secure to venture in increasingly

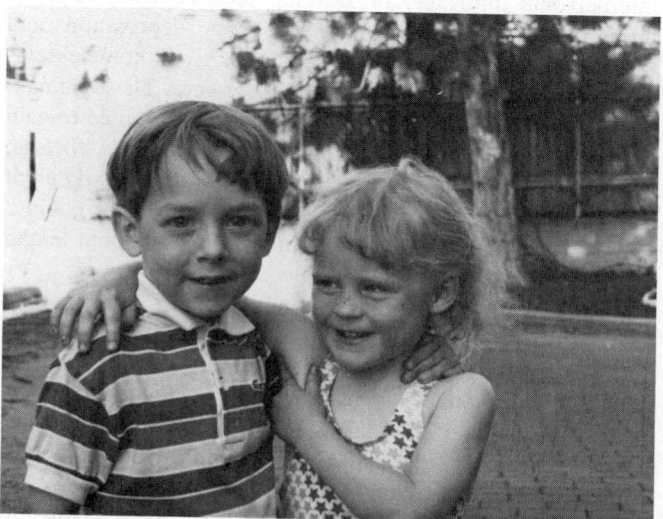

Fig. 4-11. Preschool children develop friendships outside the family group.

Photography by Earl Fillmore, Salt Lake City, UT.

wide relationships. Through constant reinforcement children learn the behaviors that bring satisfaction to the nurturing persons and incorporate them. Eventually these behaviors become self-motivating. For example, children learn that evacuating the bowel in a proper receptacle produces a positive response from the parents, resulting in a lifetime behavioral pattern.

As they get older, children seek approval from a widening sphere of persons including other members of their family, their peers, and to a lesser degree other authority figures (e.g., teachers). The increasing importance of the peer group in determining the behavior of school-age children and adolescents is well documented. However, it is the quality of the parent-child relationship that determines to a large extent the impact of peer influence on a child.

Generally the parents are most influential in assisting children to assume sex-role identification. Parents define and reinforce acceptable sex-role behavior and provide sex-appropriate role models for the children. In the absence of a suitable sex-role model in the family setting, children may adopt some characteristics of the opposite-sex parent or sibling. Frequently children identify with a teacher or other significant person of the same sex.

Siblings are children's first peers, and the way they learn to relate to each other affects later interactions with peers outside the family group. For example, firstborn children who are accustomed to a position of leadership with siblings tend to assume the same position with peers; younger children are more often followers. Ease in relationships with peers of the same or opposite sex is frequently associated with similar associations in the home.

Emotional Deprivation

The most prominent feature of emotional deprivation, particularly during the first year, is developmental retardation. Much of the information regarding the adverse effects of interpersonal influences on development has been acquired through retrospective studies of gross deprivation and trauma. The most notable instances invoved homeless infants who were placed in institutions for care. These infants, who did not receive consistent mothering care, failed to gain weight even with an adequate diet; they were pale, listless, and immobile, and unresponsive to stimuli that usually elicit a response in the normal infant, such as a smile or cooing. If the emotional deprivation continues for a sufficient length of time, the child does not survive infancy.

Harlow's classic experiments with infant monkeys illustrate the far-reaching effects of emotional and social deprivation in infancy (Harlow and Harlow, 1962). In these experiments the monkeys were raised by substitute, inanimate "mothers" made of cloth-covered wire from whom they derived nourishment and a measure of comfort but no mothering. These monkeys developed abnormal play and sex behavior. The few who bore offspring were unable to "mother" them. However, those who were allowed peer associations developed normal play and social-sex behavior. By correlating these findings with retrospective studies of

human infants in comparable age-groups, attempts have been made to explain some of the behaviors observed in these children in later interpersonal relationships.

Although the most remarkable examples of emotional deprivation were first recognized among infants in institutions, the term *masked deprivation* has been used to describe children who are reared in homes where there is a distorted mother-child relationship or otherwise disordered home environment. Infants do not thrive if the mothering person is hostile, fearful of handling them, or indifferent to them and their needs. Such children exhibit poor growth even though they are apparently free of physical disease. Children past the age of infancy who evidence physical underdevelopment are also retarded in bone age. These same infants and children display "catch-up" growth in a changed environment (Gardner, 1972).

STRESS IN CHILDHOOD

Stress has been defined and described by numerous authorities from both a physiologic and an emotional point of view. Most discussions are centered on adult responses, but children are frequently among the most affected victims of a wide range of threatening events. Most research related to children has been restricted to specific stressors and stress-provoking experiences such as hospitalization, separation and loss, and pain. A description of all the stressors to which children are exposed is beyond the scope of this segment; however, the more common manifestations and stressful events are discussed briefly. Since stress is a normal aspect of life, stressors and some coping strategies are discussed in relation to specific situations throughout the book.

Although children are not strangers to stress, some children appear to be more vulnerable than others. Children's age, temperament, life situation, and state of health affect their vulnerability and reactions to stressful events. The stressful affect and the coping reactions that are generated depend in a special way on the developmental level of the specific child. Young children are likely to become fearful of stressors, whereas older children are more likely to become angry. Also, the reaction to a probable stressful event is partly a result of the degree to which children believe they understand the incentive. For example, if children are subject to teasing or jeering by age-mates for a physical characteristic (e.g., ethnic membership), less anger is generated if they believe the hostility is a reflection of the aggressors' irrational prejudice and not their own properties. Physical avoidance of the source of the stress (in this case, the tormentors) or an alternative activity reduces the time spent in thinking about the stress (Kagan, 1983).

Parents and other caregivers can evaluate children for their vulnerability (see box, p. 127) and to recognize signs of stress (see box, p. 128) in order to help them deal with stresses before they become overwhelming. If a number of stresses are imposed on children at the same time, the children are more vulnerable. When a succession of stresses

VULNERABILITY TO STRESS

A capable child is:
  spontaneous
  active, energetic
  happy
  capable of getting excited about good things
  resourceful
  confident
  opinionated but open to new ideas
  reflective
  thoughtful, sensitive to others
  physically affectionate
  able to confront people when concerned or upset about
      something
  willing to take risks
  fond of self
  relaxed
  responsible
  helpful
  cooperative
  able to express feelings easily
  able to feel things intensely

A capable child also:
  has a sense of direction
  has goals and ambitions
  has a sense of humor
  has good eye contact
  can postpone gratification
  seeks help when he needs it
  owns up to his mistakes

A vulnerable child is:
  overly sensitive, shy
  moody, irritable
  withdrawn, preoccupied
  hesitant
  frequently sick without organic cause
  constantly in need of reassurance

  defenseless
  given to overuse of the phrase "I don't know"
  lonely and not able to make friends
  dependent, clinging
  frequently frightened
  isolated
  secretive, noncommunicative
  defensive
  resistant to being touched or hugged
  clumsy, accident prone
  belligerent, uncooperative
  easily angered
  constantly complaining
  stubborn
  subject to frequent unexplained aches and pains
  unable to concentrate
  impatient
  unable to regulate eating, taking in either too
      much or too little
  generally negative in attitude
  impulsive
  often tired
  a poor performer in school and capable
      of doing better
  overactive, frenetic

A vulnerable child also:
  has problems going to sleep
  has poor eye contact
  has a nervous laugh
  has nervous tics
  stutters
  grinds his teeth
  has frequent severe nightmares
  bites his nails
  wets his bed
  lies or distorts
  takes things that don't belong to him

From Saunders, A., and Remsberg, B.: The stress-proof child: a loving parent's guide, New York, 1984, Holt, Rinehart & Winston, pp. 10-12.

produces an excessive stress load, children may experience a serious change in health and/or behavior. An adaptation of the Holmes and Rahe stress scale for adults appears in the box on p. 128, which provides a tool to alert parents or caregivers to situations children experience that are not always viewed by adults as stressful.

It is most important that parents and persons working with children understand the nature of childhood stress and ways it can be recognized or anticipated. Caregivers must *listen* to children so they are aware of children's fears and concerns and must let them know that they are important and what they say matters. Physical contact is comforting and reassuring to children. Simply holding, touching, and hugging children is both relaxing and comforting and facilitates communication.

Coping

Coping refers to a special class of individual reactions to stressors—specifically, a reaction to a stressor that resolves, reduces, or replaces the affect state classified as stressful.

Any strategy that provides relaxation is effective in reducing stress, and most children have their own natural methods, for example, withdrawal, physical activity, reading, listening to music, working on a project, or taking a nap. The list is endless. Some turn to parents to solve their problems, or they develop socially unacceptable strategies such as cheating, stealing, or lying (Kuczen, 1982).

Children can be taught stress-reduction techniques to use in coping. First, they must be helped to recognize signs of tension in themselves and then taught any of a variety of appropriate strategies—special exercises, relaxation and breathing, imaging, and numerous other simple activities. Most of the stress-reducing strategies discussed on p. 1071 in relation to managing pain are effective for any stress situation.

Probably the most useful tool that children can learn is how to solve problems. When children can view any new situation as a problem to be solved and an opportunity to learn, they are not vulnerable to the control of others. It provides them with a sense of mastery over their own lives

WARNING SIGNS: CHILDHOOD STRESS

Bed-wetting
Boasts of superiority
Complaints of feeling afraid or upset without being able to identify the source
Complaints of neck or back pains
Complaints of pounding heart
Complaints of stomach upset, queasiness, or vomiting
Compulsive cleanliness
Compulsive ear tugging, hair pulling, or eyebrow plucking
Cruel behavior toward people or pets
Decline in school achievement
Defiance
Demand for constant perfection
Depression
Dirtying pants
Dislike of school
Downgrading of self
Easily startled by unexpected sounds
Explosive crying
Extreme nervousness
Extreme worry
Frequent daydreaming and retreats from reality
Frequent urination or diarrhea
Headaches
Hyperactivity, or excessive tension or alertness
Increased number of minor spills, falls, and other accidents
Irritability
Listlessness or lack of enthusiasm
Loss of interest in activities usually approached with vigor
Lying
Nightmares or night terror
Nervous laughter
Nervous tics, twitches, or muscle spasms
Obvious attention-seeking
Overeating
Poor concentration
Poor eating
Poor sleep
Psychosomatic illnesses
Stealing
Stuttering
Teeth grinding (sometimes during sleep)
Thumb-sucking
Uncontrollable urge to run and hide
Unusual difficulty in getting along with friends
Unusual jealousy of close friends and siblings
Unusual sexual behavior, such as spying or exhibitionism
Unusual shyness
Use of alcohol, drugs, or cigarettes
Withdrawal from usual social activities

From Kuczen, B.: Childhood stress: don't let your child be a victim, New York, 1982, Delacorte Press.

STRESS SCALE FOR CHILDREN

Life event	Value
1. Death of a parent	100
2. Divorce of parents	73
3. Separation of parents	65
4. Parent's jail term	63
5. Death of a close family member (e.g., grandparent)	63
6. Personal injury or illness	53
7. Parent's remarriage	50
8. Suspension or expulsion from school	47
9. Parent's reconciliation	45
10. Long vacation (summer, etc.)	45
11. Parent or sibling illness	44
12. Mother's pregnancy	40
13. Anxiety over sex	39
14. Birth or adoption of a new baby	39
15. New school or classroom or new teacher	39
16. Money problems at home	38
17. Death or moving away of close friend	37
18. Change in studies	36
19. More quarrels with parents (or parents quarreling more)	35
20. Change in school responsibilities	29
21. Sibling going away to school	29
22. Family arguments with grandparents	29
23. Winning school or community awards	28
24. Mother or father going to work or stopping work	26
25. School beginning or ending	26
26. Family's living standard changing	25

Life event	Value
27. Change in personal habits (e.g., bedtime, homework, etc.)	24
28. Trouble with parents (e.g., lack of communication, hostility, etc.)	23
29. Change in school hours, schedule of courses	23
30. Family's moving	20
31. New sports, hobbies, family recreation activities	20
32. Change in church activities (more involvement or less)	19
33. Change in social activities (e.g., new friends, loss of old ones, peer pressures)	8
34. Change in sleeping habits, giving up naps, etc.	16
35. Change in number of family gettogethers	15
36. Change in eating habits (e.g., going on or off diet, new way of family cooking)	13
37. Vacation	13
38. Christmas	12
39. Breaking home, school, or community rules	11

Add up the points for items that have touched the child's life in the last twelve months.
Score below 150, the child is carrying an average stress load.
Score between 150 and 300, the child has a better-than-average chance of showing some symptoms of stress.
Score over 300, the child's stress load is heavy and there is a strong likelihood for experiencing a serious change in health and/or behavior.

From Saunders, A., and Remsberg, B.: The stress-proof child: a loving parent's guide, New York, 1984, Holt, Rinehart & Winston, pp. 72-73.

and reinforces the fact that they have within themselves the ability and information to handle whatever comes their way. Problem-solving skill gives them the confidence to know where and how to seek help when they need it.

Childhood Fears

Fear is a normal function, a self-preservation signal that mobilizes the physiologic resources of the organism. *Fear* and *anxiety* are often used interchangeably, and the physical reactions to both are almost identical. *Fear* is an emotional reaction to a specific real or unreal threat or danger; *anxiety* refers to a general uneasiness, apprehension, or feeling of impending doom. Fear is a momentary reaction to danger based on a low estimate of one's own power. Fearful children perceive a threat (person, animal, or situation) as being stronger than themselves and thus capable of harming them. When the balance of power is altered, the fear disappears. For example, children's fears can be alleviated by the presence of an adult whom they perceive as a source of protection; or fear can be overcome by familiarity with the source of the threat, such as a dog or a dark room. Anxiety is general, lasting, internally generated, and reflects overall feelings of weakness, ineptitude, and helplessness (Wolman, 1978).

In childhood the distinction between fear and anxiety is important because childhood fears are specific, and except for the specific fear (or fears), children are happy and active. Childhood fears are limited problems and most are alleviated with growth and children's increased self-confidence and faith in themselves. Unrealistic fears are abandoned with maturation and learning to be replaced by realistic fears. As with other stresses, there are individual differences in the susceptibility to fear, and certain fears are age-related (see the discussions of specific age-groups for age-related fears). Fears that are likely to persist into adulthood are fear of physical danger, death, sickness, body injury, physical assault, car accidents, airplane crashes, and war.

Children often come to fear things they did not fear at a younger age because of their lack of awareness (e.g., a busy street), or they may become fearful of familiar things. With the development of imaginative ability, imaginary creatures and situations may become a source of fear. Also, children with superior intelligence are likely to be more aware of real dangers, are less likely to succumb to imaginary fears, and have fewer fears than other children. These observations are probably related to cognitive capacities (Wolman, 1978).

Coping with fears is the same as coping with other stresses. To help children overcome their fears, parents and others should not shame or show disapproval for their fears, encourage their unreasonable fears, overprotect them, or force them into a situation they fear. For example, throwing a fearful child into deep water will probably increase a fear of water to the point of a lasting phobia. Parents can serve as models by demonstrating strength, decisiveness, and self-confidence. For instance, the parents can take their children by the hand and gently guide them into shallow water or

around a dark room. Desensitization by gradually facing the fearsome object or situation (see p. 721) is effective with children. Parents can allow their children to express their fears and encourage them to cope with certain dangers. Most of all, parents need to make them feel that they will always be loved and will be protected whenever necessary.

INFLUENCE OF THE MASS MEDIA

There is no doubt that the communications media provide children with a means for extending their knowledge about the world in which they live and have contributed to narrowing the differences between classes.

Reading Materials

The oldest form of mass media—books, newspapers, and magazines—contributes to children's competence in almost every direction, as well as providing enjoyment. Recognition of the impact of reading matter used in the schools on the value system and socialization processes prompted reevaluation of textbook content in terms of the biased presentation of male and female role models, the sugar-coated view of life situations, and the unrealistic, biased history of minority groups.

Fairy tales, for generations the mainstay of young children's literature, for a time suffered condemnation as sexist, overly violent in content, and riddled with unfavorable stereotypes, such as the wicked stepmother, dwarfs, and physical unattractiveness associated with evil. They are now believed to provide an excellent medium for explaining puzzling and important topics such as death, stepparents, and inner feelings and turmoils.

Comic books and other pulp reading material have been popular in every generation, usually at the expense of literature provided by schools, libraries, and parents. Many children have nothing else to read. The easy reading, quick action, and adventure in brief episodes seem to fulfill a need for children who are striving to understand both aggression in others and their own impulses. Reading ability, intelligence, and school adjustment apparently have no relationship to the number and type of comic books read. Most comic books appear to be relatively harmless to the majority of children and are in some ways even beneficial. Comic books seem to have only a minor influence on acquisition of beliefs, values, and behaviors. The popularity of this medium has prompted some educators to encourage translations of literature into comic book form in order to stimulate the interest of students in the classics.

Movies

Movies, not closely bound to reality and often portraying an assortment of socially approved behaviors, perhaps make a contribution to children's value systems, but they do provide opportunities for desirable social learning. On the other hand, children, especially adolescents, flock to the "macho" movies and those whose heroes resort to violent resolution of problems, such as the use of karate techniques and wild automobile chases. The carry-over of these influences into daily life and relationships may account in part for the increase in violent behavior of young persons.

Television

The medium that has the most impact on children in America today is television, which has become one of the most significant socializing agents in the life of young children. The content of programs and commercials provides multiple sources for acquiring information, modeling behaviors, and observing value orientations. Besides producing a leveling effect on class differences in general information and vocabulary, TV exposes children to a wider variety of topics and events than they encounter in day-to-day life. Television always has time to talk to children and is a form of access to the adult world.

Ninety-eight percent of households in the United States have a TV set, usually situated prominently in the most used room. Children between the ages of 3 and 11 watch an average of 3 to 4 hours of TV a day and by the time they reach age 18, will have spent more time watching television than in any other single activity except sleeping (Liebert, Sprafkin, and Davidson, 1982). Similar findings have been reported on TV usage in Australia, Canada, and some European countries (Murray, 1980).

Much of the adverse influence of TV depends on the susceptibility of the individual child. Television is a solitary activity and as such increases passivity and decreases physical activity and social interaction. Insecure children with strong feelings of rejection may become addicted to the medium in order to meet a need they are unable to satisfy in other ways. It encourages low energy and apathy and may contribute to development of obesity in susceptible children (Dietz and Gortmaker, 1985). Too often TV can become a substitute for play and other activities. Research indicates that children who do not have TV available read comic books, go to movies, listen to the radio, or engage in roughly equivalent forms of entertainment (Huston and Wright, 1982). Also, popular children who engage in sports and extracurricular activities tend to read often as well as watch a lot of TV.

Most programming stresses the triumph of good over evil, but with an unrealistically rapid resolution of problems, including moral dilemmas, often accompanied by pain or violence. Programs fail to portray the complex internal dynamics that are generally part of children's moral dilemmas. Physical solutions to problems are common with violence as the first alternative for problem solving. Several factors encourage the learning or performing of TV-influenced behaviors:

Age: Younger children focus on behaviors rather than on motives or consequences. They view alternatives in a concrete manner and they are unable to differ between central and peripheral plot information. Small children remember various assorted items in the program, for example, they remember the *act*, not the motive or consequences.

Identification with characters or situations: Children will more often imitate behaviors of persons and situations similar to those in their own lives.

Reward and punishment syndrome: Children will imitate behaviors they see rewarded or *not* punished when it is expected. They are less likely to repeat an act they see punished; their attention is immediately attracted when they see an act committed that they know should be punished but is not.

Opportunity to reproduce behaviors: Children will imitate behaviors when given the right environment or when violence seems an accepted solution. When children see a situation on television, they will use this information when they encounter a similar situation that requires a solution.

Motivation to reproduce behaviors: Children will imitate behavior when given the appropriate incentives: expectation of reward or lack of punishment. Some children have self-control; others do not.

Violence and aggression. Controversy continues regarding the favorable vs deleterious effects of television viewing. There is ample documentation to implicate television as a source for learned antisocial behavior. For example, it has been shown that viewing violence on television adds aggressive strategies to the children's repertoire of responses. Consequently, in a real-life situation children may imitate the aggressive behavior of television models, and their aggressive expressions are more hostile and destructive than they would be otherwise (Lefkowitz and Huesmann, 1980). These children may prefer violent programs and even believe that violent depictions are an accurate portrayal of everyday life (Eron and others, 1983). They become sensitized to violence and therefore are likely to tolerate aggressive behaviors they witness in real-life altercations. Incidences have also been reported in which parents' inappropriate behavior toward their children was attributed to television models (Wharton and Mandell, 1985).

There is a decided *relationship* between observed violence and the acceptance of violence, although no controlled studies have proven a cause-and-effect relationship. Parents can help children evaluate TV violence by pointing out the subtleties children miss, such as the aggressor's motives and intentions, and the unpleasant consequences the perpetrators suffer as a result of their aggressive acts. Often the consequence is separated from the act by a commercial and children cannot make the correlation. Parents can stress the purpose of the programs—primarily entertainment—and explain why they like or dislike something on TV, for example, "This show is trying to tell you that crime does not pay and, if one does wrong, one will go to jail." Explanations and discussions can take place between shows (with the volume turned down), and young children can learn from older children as well as from adults. These discussions can be very effective when begun early and carried out consistently.

Prosocial modeling. On the positive side, television has been shown to be a positive influence on children's abilities to deal with a variety of social issues, such as divorce, the arrival of a new baby, discrimination, honesty, and helpfulness. Children who view educational programming (e.g., ''Mister Rogers' Neighborhood'' and ''Sesame Street'') for a long period of time become more affectionate, considerate, cooperative, and helpful toward their playmates. This is especially true when adults watch with them and encourage them to discuss the shows and to role-play the prosocial lessons they observe (Coates, Pusser, and Goodman, 1976).

The social stereotypes including sex-roles, ethnicity, and family are influenced by television. Males on TV outnumber females nearly two to one and are typically portrayed as high-status individuals who are more powerful, dominant, rational, and intelligent than women (Gerbner and others, 1980). A large percentage of nonwhite characters are depicted as very poor people who work at service occupations, are prone to violence, and are involved in illegal activities (Liebert, Spratkin, and Davidson, 1982). The ways that racial and ethnic characters are portrayed on television can have an impact on the way the majority culture views minority persons and on the self-image of minority children.

Academic achievement. There is evidence to indicate that some educational television programs, such as ''Sesame Street,'' have a positive influence on cognitive development of children, especially disadvantaged preschool children (Minton, 1975). However, TV is a one-way medium in which the viewer is a passive recipient as opposed to an active processor of information. There is a significant negative correlation between the number of hours children spend watching TV and their reading grades (Ridley-Johnson, Cooper, and Chance, 1983) and reading comprehension scores (Morgan and Gross, 1980).

Commercial messages. The average child in the United States is exposed to nearly 20,000 TV commercials each year. Many of these extol the virtues of various toys, fast-food items, high-sugar treats, and other articles that the parents may not wish to purchase (Barcus and Wolkin, 1977). Although young children do not actually purchase products, they continually ask for products they have seen advertised. When parents deny requests, conflicts often ensue (Atkin, 1978). In addition to the resentment and anger toward adults, peer relationships may be affected when children evaluate peers on the basis of whether or not they possess a valued object popularized in commercials (Gorn, Goldberg, and Kanungo, 1976).

The effect of TV advertising on health and safety behaviors is also a concern. Children see vitamins and medications in commercial messages and are convinced of their value, even asking for specific products when they do not feel well (Rossiter and Robertson, 1980). Although few television characters smoke on prime time television, many consume alcohol; and seat belts are used in only 23% of commercials involving driving (Gerbner and others, 1982).

Interventions. It is clear that parents need to supervise the amount and type of TV programs their children watch and to teach their children how to watch TV. It is especially important to identify at-risk children and control their view-ing. House rules that specify the type and amount of television help children understand limits, and video-recorded selections of appropriate programs can be substituted for less desirable offerings. Parents need to carefully monitor cable and other pay TV programming, since these popular options present more uncensored programming. Locked boxes are available for cable receivers that allow families to prevent children from viewing ''R'' rated or other programs when unsupervised. The effects of Music Television Video (MTV) on young viewers has yet to be evaluated.

It is permissible to use the TV as a ''baby-sitter'' under certain circumstances; for example, it can keep the children quiet while the parent gets organized after a difficult day and thus can prevent an explosive situation.

Nurses and parents can be powerful forces in influencing the media. They can watch closely for an increase in violence and other undesirable programming and complain if they believe it is not appropriate.

Role of Play in Development

Through the universal medium of play children learn what no one can teach them. They learn about their world and how to deal with this environment of objects, time, space, structure, and people. They learn about themselves operating within that environment—what they can do, how to relate to things and situations, and how to adapt themselves to the demands society makes on them. It has been said that play is the *work* of the child. In play children continually practice the complicated, stressful processes of living, communicating, and achieving satisfactory relationships with other people. In addition, while promoting and advancing development and relationships, play is an intrinsically satisfying activity—something children do for the fun of it (Rubin, Fein, and Vandenberg, 1983).

CLASSIFICATION OF PLAY

From a developmental point of view, patterns of children's play can be categorized according to *content* and *social character*. In both there is an additive effect; each builds on past accomplishments, and some element of each is maintained throughout life. At each stage in development the new predominates.

Content of Play

The content of play involves primarily the physical aspects of play, although social relationships cannot be ignored. The content of play follows the directional trend of the simple to the complex.

Social-affective play. Play begins with social-affective play, wherein the infant takes pleasure in relationships with people. As adults talk, fondle, nuzzle, and in various ways elicit a response from the infant, the infant soon learns to provoke parental emotions and responses with such behaviors as smiling, cooing, or initiating games and activi-

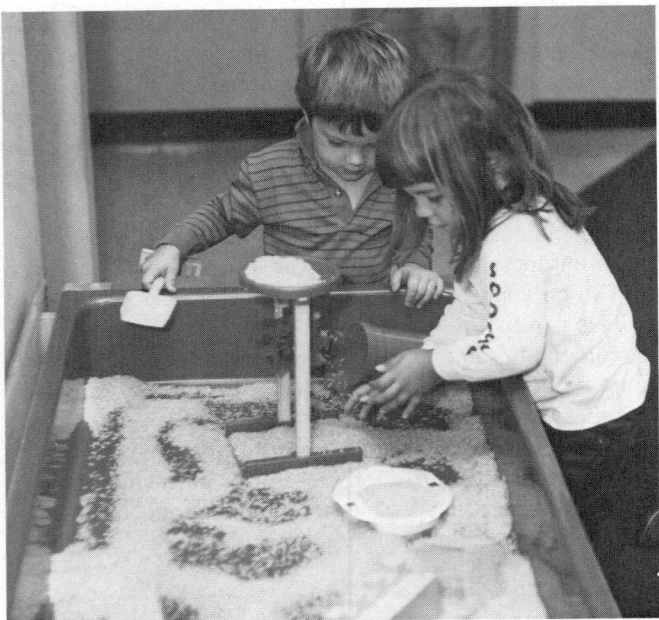

Fig. 4-12. Children derive pleasure from handling raw materials. Photography by John Roy, Saint Francis Hospital, Tulsa, OK.

ties. The type and intensity of the adult behavior with children vary among cultures.

Sense-pleasure play. Sense-pleasure play is a nonsocial stimulating experience that originates from without. Objects in the environment—light and color, tastes and odors, textures and consistencies—attract a child's attention, stimulate his senses, and give pleasure. Pleasurable experiences are derived from handling raw materials (water, sand, food), from body motion (swinging, bouncing, rocking), and from other uses of senses and abilities (smelling, humming) (Fig. 4-12).

Skill play. Once infants have developed the ability to grasp and manipulate, they persistently demonstrate and exercise their newly acquired abilities through skill play, repeating an action over and over again. The element of sense-pleasure play is often evident in the practicing of a new ability, but all too frequently the determination to conquer the elusive skill produces pain and frustration (e.g., learning to ride a bicycle).

Unoccupied behavior. In unoccupied behavior the child is not playful but focuses his attention momentarily on anything that strikes his interest. The child daydreams, fiddles with clothes or other objects, or walks aimlessly. This role differs from the onlooker, who actively observes the activity of other.

Dramatic play. One of the vital elements in the child's process of identification is dramatic play, also known as *symbolic* or *pretend play*. It begins in late infancy (11 to 13 months) as children engage in simple pretending with familiar activities, such as eating, sleeping, or drinking from a cup. In toddlerhood the activities are still primarily those that are familiar. As children enter the preschool stage their play becomes farther removed from everyday activities and much more complex. Dramatic play is the predominant form of play in the preschool child.

Once children begin to invest situations and people with meanings and to attribute affective significance to the world, they can pretend and fantasize almost anything. By acting out events of daily life, children learn and practice the roles and identities modeled by the members of their family and society. Their toys, replicas of the tools of society, provide a medium for learning about adult roles and activities that may be puzzling and frustrating to them. Interacting with the world is one way children get to know it. The simple, imitative, dramatic play of the toddler, such as using the telephone, driving a car, or rocking a doll, evolves into more complex, sustained dramas of the preschooler, which extend beyond common domestic matters to the wider aspects of the world and the society, such as playing policeman, storekeeper, teacher, or nurse (Fig. 4-13). Older children work out elaborate themes, act out stories, and compose plays.

Games. Children in all cultures engage in games alone and with others. Solitary activity involving games begins as very small children participate in repetitive activities and progress to more complicated games that challenge their independent skills, such as solving puzzles, solitaire, and

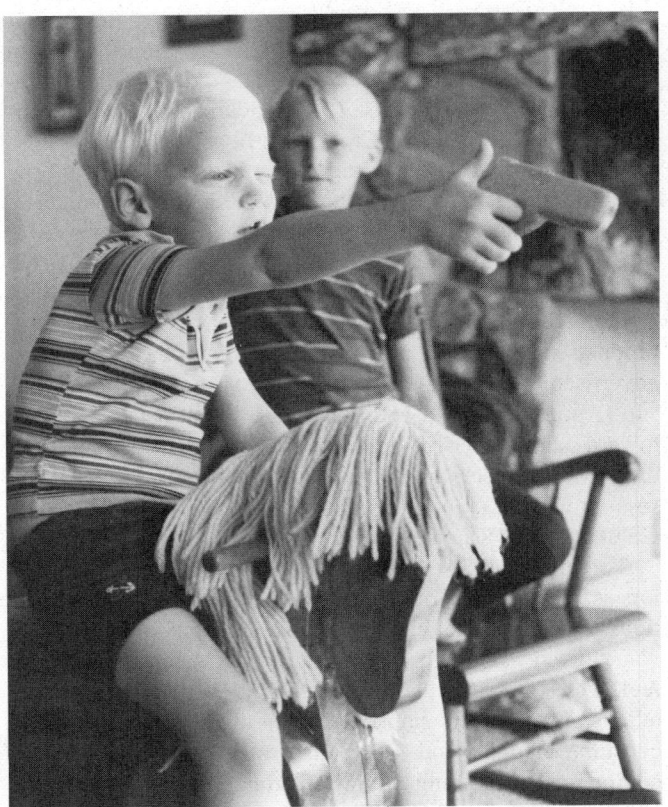

Fig. 4-13. Preschoolers spend considerable time in pretend play. Photography by Earl Fillmore, Salt Lake City, UT.

computer or video games. When children interact with others, games assume the same developmental trends. Very young children participate in simple, *imitative games* such as pat-a-cake and peekaboo.

Preschool children learn and enjoy *formal games* that begin with ritualistic, self-sustaining games, such as ring-around-a-rosy and London Bridge. With the exception of some simple board games, preschool children do not engage in *competitive games*. They do play competitively but find it difficult not to take competition seriously. Preschoolers hate to lose and will try to cheat, want to change rules, or demand exceptions and opportunities to change their moves. Competitive games are the province of school-age children and adolescents who enjoy a variety of games including cards, checkers, chess, and physically active games such as baseball.

Social Character of Play

The play interactions of infancy are between the child and an adult. Children continue to enjoy the company of an adult but are increasingly able to play alone. As age advances, interaction with age-mates increases in importance and becomes an essential part of the socialization process. Through interaction, the highly egocentric infant, unable to tolerate delay or interference, ultimately acquires concern for others and the ability to delay gratification or even to reject gratification at the expense of another. A pair of toddlers engage in a good deal of combat because their personal needs cannot stand delay or compromise. By the time they reach age 5 or 6 years, children are able to arrive at a compromise or make use of arbitration, usually after each child has attempted but failed to gain his own way. Through continued interaction with peers and the growth of conceptual abilities and social skills, children are able to increase participation with others.

Onlooker play. During onlooker play the child watches what other children are doing but makes no attempt to enter into the play activity. There is an active interest in observ-

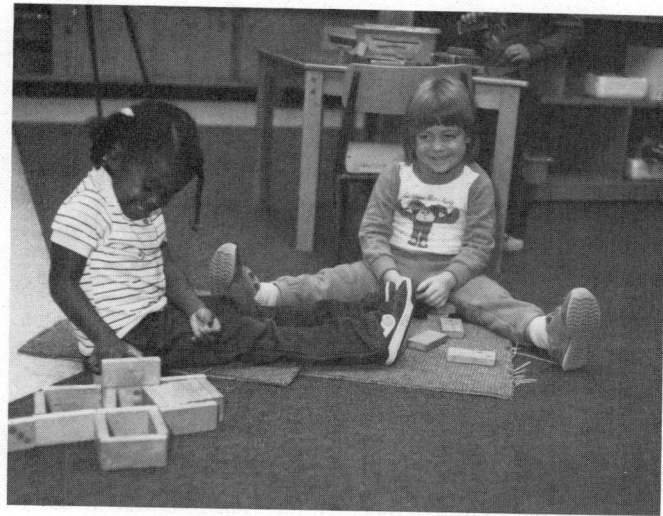

Fig. 4-15. Associative play.
Photography by John Roy, Saint Francis Hospital, Tulsa, OK.

ing the interaction of others but no movement toward participating. Watching television is a common example of the onlooker role.

Solitary play. Children who independently play alone with toys different from those used by other children in the same area are engaging in *solitary play*. They enjoy the presence of other children but make no effort to get close or speak to them. Their interest is centered on their own activity, which they pursue with no reference to the activities of the others.

Parallel play. During parallel activities children play independently but among other children. They play with toys like those the children around them are using, but as each child sees fit, neither influencing nor being influenced by the other children. Each plays beside, but not with, other children (Fig. 4-14). There is no group association. Parallel play is the characteristic play of the toddler, but it may also occur in other groups of any age. Individuals who are involved in a creative craft with each person separately working on his own project are engaged in parallel play.

Associative play. When children play together and are engaged in a similar or even identical activity, but there is no organization, division of labor, leadership assignment, or mutual goal, the play is *associative*. Children borrow and lend play materials, follow each other with wagons and tricycles, and sometimes attempt to control who may or may not play in the group. Each child acts according to his own wishes; there is no group goal (Fig. 4-15). For example, two children play with dolls, borrowing articles of clothing from each other and engaging in similar conversation, but neither directs the other's actions nor establishes rules regarding the limits of the play session. There is a great deal of behavioral contagion: when one child initiates an activity, the entire group follows the example.

Cooperative play. Cooperative play is organized, and

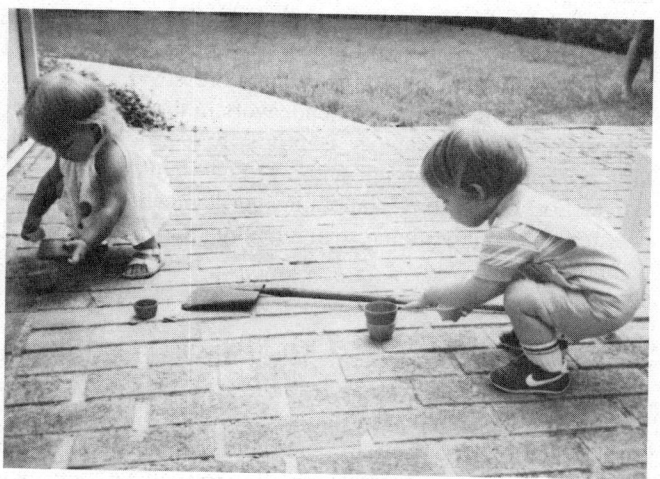

Fig. 4-14. Parallel play.

the child plays in a group *with* other children. The children discuss and plan activities for the purposes of accomplishing an end—to make something, to attain a competitive goal, to dramatize situations of adult or group life, or to play formal games. The group is loosely formed, but there is a marked sense of belonging or not belonging. The goal and its attainment require organization of activities, division of labor, and playing roles. The leader-follower relationship is definitely established, and the activity is controlled by one or two members who assign roles and direct the activity of the others. The activity is organized to allow one child to supplement another's function in order to complete the goal.

FUNCTIONS OF PLAY

The specific values of play or the functions that it serves throughout childhood include sensorimotor development, intellectual development, socialization, creativity, self-awareness, and therapeutic and moral value.

Sensorimotor Development

Sensorimotor activity is a major component of play at all ages and is the predominant form of play in infancy. Active play is essential for muscle development and serves a useful purpose as a release for surplus energy. Through sensorimotor play, children explore the nature of the physical world. Infants gain impressions of themselves and their world through tactile, auditory, visual, and kinesthetic stimulation. Toddlers and preschoolers revel in body movement and exploration of things in space. Children continue to engage in sensorimotor play, although with increasing maturity, the play becomes more differentiated and involved. Whereas very young children run for the sheer joy of body movement, older children incorporate or modify the motions into increasingly complex and coordinated activities such as races, games, roller skating, and bicycle riding.

Intellectual Development

Through exploration and manipulation, children learn colors, shapes, sizes, textures, and the significance of objects. They learn the significance of numbers and how to use them, they learn to associate words with objects, and they develop an understanding of abstract concepts and spatial relationships, such as up, down, under, and over. Activities like puzzles and games help them develop problem-solving skills. Books, stories, films, and collections expand knowledge and provide enjoyment as well. Play provides a means to practice and expand language skills. Through play children continually rehearse past experiences to assimilate them into new perceptions and relationships. Play helps children comprehend the world in which they live and distinguish between fantasy and reality.

Socialization

From very early infancy children show interest and pleasure in the company of others (Fig. 4-16). Their initial social

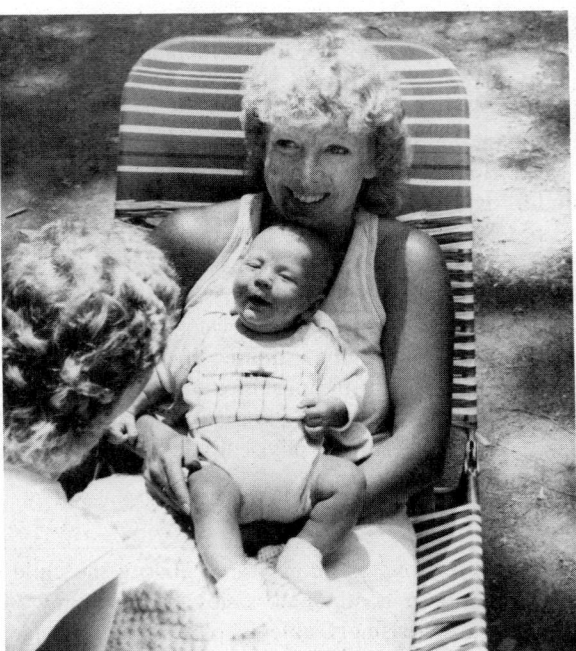

Fig. 4-16. The socialization process begins in early infancy.
Photography by Bill Meyer, San Jose, CA.

contact is with the mothering person, but through play with other children, they learn to establish social relationships and solve the problems associated with these relationships. They learn to give and take, which is more readily learned from critical peers than from more tolerant adults. They learn the sex role that society expects them to fulfill as well as approved patterns of behavior and deportment. Closely associated with socialization is development of moral values and ethics. Children learn right from wrong, the standards of the society, and to assume responsibility for their actions.

Creativity

In no other situation is there more opportunity to be creative than in play. Children can experiment and try out their ideas in play through every medium at their disposal, including raw materials, fantasy, and exploration. Creativity is stifled by pressure toward conformity; therefore striving for peer approval may inhibit creative endeavors in the school-age or adolescent child. Creativity is primarily a product of solitary, as opposed to group, activity. Once children feel the satisfaction of creating something new and different, they transfer this creative interest to situations outside the world of play.

Self-Awareness

Beginning with active explorations of their bodies and awareness of themselves as separate from the mother, the process of self-identity is facilitated through play activities. Children learn who they are and what their place is in the world. They become increasingly able to regulate their own behavior, to learn what their abilities are, and to compare their abilities with those of others. Through play children are able to test their abilities, assume and try out various roles, and learn the effect their behavior has on others.

Therapeutic Value

There is no doubt that play is therapeutic at any age. It provides a means for release from the tension and stress encountered through the environment. In play children can express emotions and release unacceptable impulses in a socially acceptable fashion. Children are able to experiment and test fearful situations and can assume and vicariously master the roles and positions they are unable to perform in the world of reality. Children reveal much about themselves in play. Children are able to communicate to the alert observer through play the needs, fears, and desires they are unable to express with their limited language skills. Throughout their play children need the presence and acceptance of adults to help them control aggression and channel their destructive tendencies.

Moral Value

Although children learn at home and at school those behaviors considered right and wrong in the culture, the interaction with peers during play contributes significantly to their moral training. Nowhere is the enforcement of moral standards so rigid as in the play situation. If they are to be acceptable members of the group, children must adhere to the culturally accepted codes of behavior—fairness, honesty, self-control, and consideration for others. Children soon learn that their peers are less tolerant of violations than are adults, and to maintain a place in the play group they must conform to the standards of the group.

CHARACTERISTICS OF PLAY

There are several aspects of play that display developmental changes and that differentiate children's play from adult play.

Tradition

In general the play of small children varies little from generation to generation within a culture. Each generation of children imitates the play of the preceding generation; in this way the more satisfying forms of play are perpetuated. Many types of play are characteristic of all cultures, for example, playing with balls, some form of doll, or some type of walking toy to help a child just beginning to walk to maintain balance.

Seasonal changes are accompanied by traditional forms of toys and play activities. Sledding and ice skating are popular in winter; jump rope, bicycling, and roller skating are played in spring and summer.

Time and Age

The amount of time that children spend in play decreases with age. Older children have less time available for play because of an increase in schoolwork and other responsibilities. With advancing age and development, the number and variety of play activities diminish and become less physically active, but the time spent in specific activities increases as interests narrow and the attention span lengthens. The number of playmates decreases with age as children progress from play with anyone available to play with a few selected and special age-mates.

Children's play can be divided into the following four categories: (1) imitative, (2) exploratory, (3) testing, and (4) model building. At all ages each of these types is evident in children's play, but one type will predominate over the others at specific ages. For example, imitative play can be seen in the infant who mimics the actions of another (pat-a-cake), but it reaches its peak in the dramatic play of preschoolers who play "house," "astronaut," or "school." It can also be observed in circular group singing and rhythmic games such as ring-around-a-rosy.

As children grow older, play activities become less spontaneous, more formal and structured, and increasingly sex appropriate. Whereas infants and small children of both sexes play in much the same way, by the time they enter school, children engage in activities deemed appropriate for their sex. Little boys in particular are clearly aware they do not play with certain toys, and they avoid their girl playmates.

Patterns of Development

Throughout childhood certain play activities are popular at one age and not at another. These activities are so consistent and predictable that childhood is sometimes divided into age stages according to the types of play characteristic of each particular phase of development.

Exploratory stage: This stage lasts from approximately 3 months of age to near the end of the first year. It consists mostly of grasping, holding, and examining articles, and exploration via creeping or crawling.

Toy stage: The toy stage begins in the first year and reaches a maximum at 7 to 8 years of age.

Play stage: During this period, school-age children's play repertory increases. Interest in toys diminishes, whereas interest in games, sports, and hobbies increases.

Daydreaming stage: This stage is characteristic of older children and pubescents playing the martyr misunderstood and mistreated by everyone or the hero or beauty admired by everyone (Fig. 4-17).

As they grow older, children also use materials in more meaningful ways. For example, an infant or small child first uses a block as something to handle or throw, then as something to represent another object, such as an airplane or car. To older children a block is a building material with which they can construct increasingly complex structures. Instead of representative objects, they require replicas of cars and airplanes. Eventually these materials are discarded altogether.

TOYS

Toys are the inanimate objects with which children interact, and cognitive development appears to be related to the va-

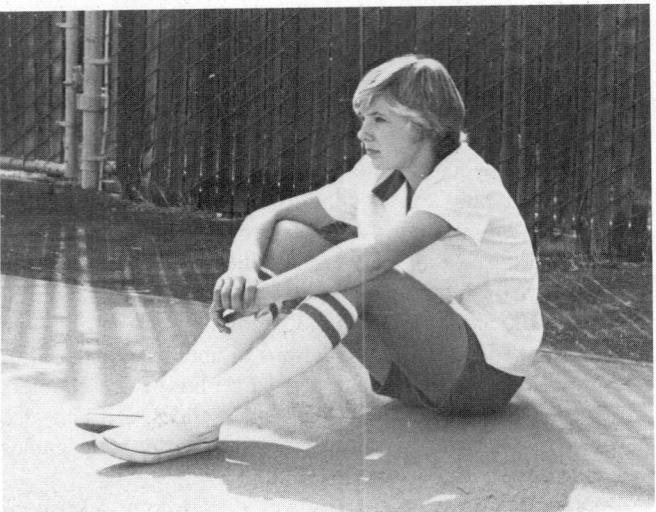

Fig. 4-17. Daydreaming is characteristic of pubescent children.

riety and accessibility of objects for children to explore, experiment with, and come to know. Access to playthings, particularly during the earlier years, correlates with the accessibility of caregivers who make objects available, react to children's response to the objects, encourage further exploration, and talk about what is happening. Consequently, although they can be significant in themselves, playthings assume an especially important aspect as a medium of social interchange.

Selecting Toys

Toys are tools that facilitate learning and the developmental progress (described earlier in Functions of play). Because they can be employed in a variety of ways, raw materials or multidimensional toys are best for enhancing skills and stimulating the imagination. Through manipulation, playthings such as boxes, clay, and blocks can assume a multitude of symbolic objects and inspire creative impulses. "Educational" toys are less flexible.

Physical properties are learned from toys such as balls, blocks, and clay. Motor skills, manipulative skills, and social skills are acquired through the use of toys. Games with rules and a prescribed format help children to understand the rules and values of society. Toys enhance the learning of sex roles and occupational roles.

Play materials need not be expensive or elaborate. Infants and small children derive enjoyment from simple kitchen utensils such as wooden spoons and small plastic plates to bang, pot lids to clang together, and a nest of measuring spoons to rattle. Empty cartons, especially oversized ones used to pack furniture for shipping, can assume the function of clubrooms, hideaways, and other private places. A large mound of dirt (3 to 4 feet high) can become a place for small children to roll toy cars and balls and dig holes during summer and a place for sliding in winter. Paper is a fascinating and versatile raw material for children of any age,

and most books on toy materials include recipes for play dough and finger paint.

Toy Safety

Selection of toys and play equipment is a joint effort between parents and children, but evaluation of their safety is the responsibility of the adult. Government agencies do not inspect and police all toys on the market. Therefore adults who purchase, supervise purchases, or allow children to use play equipment need to evaluate such equipment for its safety, including toys that are gifts or those are purchased by the children themselves. Children need toys and activities that increase their sense of competence but that do not create a threat to their health and safety (see box, p. 137).

Needs of Infants and Children

All children are basically alike. They follow the same pattern of development and maturation, while at the same time, their hereditary, cultural, and experiential backgrounds make each child a distinct and unique individual. They differ in their rate of growth, their ultimate size and capabilities, and the way in which they respond to their environment. However, regardless of the stage of development, the state of health, or the situation, *the child is first of all a child.*

THE HEALTHY CHILD

Children need ample physical room to grow as well as support from the adults in their environment. Because they do not have the resources for coping with the world, children need to be surrounded by caring people who are willing to share their pleasures and help them through troubling times. Although the emphasis and classification may vary according to the interpreter, the essential needs of children during all stages of development are physical, biologic, and emotional needs, including love, emotional security, discipline, independence, and self-esteem.

Physical and Biologic Needs

First of all, children's basic physical and biologic needs for food, water, air, warmth, elimination, and shelter must be met. Infants, except for limited reflex responses, are totally dependent on adults for satisfaction of even the most basic needs. As development proceeds, children begin to communicate their needs verbally and nonverbally and to assume increasing responsibility for their basic need gratification.

Those who care for children come to understand the physical changes that take place during the process of development and the special needs generated by these changes, for example, the nature and quantity of the food intake, the method and frequency of feeding, and the amount of sleep and activity that change during childhood.

GUIDELINES FOR TOY SAFETY

When selecting a toy:

Select toys that suit the skills, abilities, and interests of the child.

Select toys that are safe for the specific child; look for a label that indicates the intended age-group. Toys that are safe at one age may not be safe for another.

Make certain all parts are present and directions for use are clear and appropriate to the child.

Check for safety labels such as "flame retardant" or "flame resistant."

Select toys durable enough to survive rough play.

Select toys light enough that they will not cause harm if one falls on a child.

Look for toys with smooth, rounded edges. Avoid toys with sharp edges that can cut or sharp points. Points on the inside of the toy can puncture if the toy is broken.

Avoid toys with any small parts that can be swallowed or aspirated, especially for children under 3 years of age.

Avoid toys with any shooting or throwing objects that can injure eyes. This includes toys into which other missiles, such as sticks or pebbles, might be used as substitutes for the intended projectiles. Arrows and darts used by children should have blunt tips and be manufactured from resilient materials; make certain tips are securely attached.

Make certain that materials in toys are nontoxic.

Avoid toys that make loud noises that might be damaging to a child's hearing. Even some squeaking toys are too loud when held close to the ear.

Remove and discard plastic wrapping from toys that could suffocate a child.

Make certain an older child understands that a toy inappropriate for smaller children should be kept out of the hands of younger brothers and sisters.

Teach the child the proper way to unplug an electric toy—pull on the plug, not the cord.

Teach the child the safe use of utensils that under certain circumstances can cause injury—scissors, knives, needles, heating elements, or loops, long string, or cord (a potential for strangulation in very young children).

Teach children to beware of electrical appliances and even electrically operated playthings. Children are unfamiliar with the hazards of electricity in association with water.

Provide a safe place for the child to store toys.

Select a toy chest or toy box that is ventilated, is free of self-locking devices that could trap a child inside, and has a lid designed not to pinch a child's fingers or fall on a child's head.

Teach the child to store toys safely in order to prevent accidental injury from stepping or falling on a toy.

Check all toys periodically for breakage, loose parts, and other potential hazards.

Check movable parts to make certain they are attached securely to the toy. Sometimes pieces that are safe when attached to the toy become a danger when detached.

Repair or discard broken toys.

Make certain that toys are constructed with nontoxic materials, and use only paint labeled "nontoxic" to repaint toys, toy boxes, or children's furniture.

Sand sharp wooden toys or splintered surfaces smooth.

Examine all outdoor toys regularly for rust and weak or sharp parts that could become a danger to a child.

Maintain toys in good repair, without signs of possible hazards such as sharp edges, splinters, weak seams, rust; keep electrical cords and plugs in good condition.

Health and safety hazards associated with every phase of development require provisions for the child's physical safety, including prevention of injuries and disease and education of children, families, and communities regarding these potential threats to health and well-being.

Love and Affection

The single most important emotional need of children is to be loved and to feel secure in that love. Children strive above all else to gain the love and acceptance of those who are significant in their lives. When they feel secure in this love, they are able to withstand the normal crises associated with growing up and those unexpected crises (e.g., illness or loss) that are superimposed on the anticipated course of development.

Children cannot receive too much love. However, this love must be communicated to them through words and actions that tell them they are loved, not for their actions or achievement, but for what they are or simply *because they are*. Although love is closely associated with discipline, independence, and other factors that influence the child's self-concept, it should be an undemanding, accepting love that is indispensable to the development of a healthy personality. Unconditional love, freely bestowed, helps establish a sense of security and a positive sense of self within children that will persist throughout their lifetime (Fig. 4-18). Children must know they are loved and that whatever happens they can depend on this love. For many children spiritual love is a very significant source of complete, undemanding love. Without the security of loving relationships, children may become tense and insecure and develop undesirable behavior patterns as they attempt to obtain that love or try to compensate for its loss.

The primary source of love, particularly during infancy, is the parent, usually the mother or mothering person. The establishment of this early love attachment (or bonding) profoundly influences subsequent interpersonal relationships. With ever-widening relationships, children need the love and acceptance of others. They need to feel they are wanted, accepted, and belong in whatever relationships are important to them at each stage of development.

Parents may truly love their children but be unable to communicate this love to them. Parents who are insecure in their parenting skills frequently seek advice and reassurance

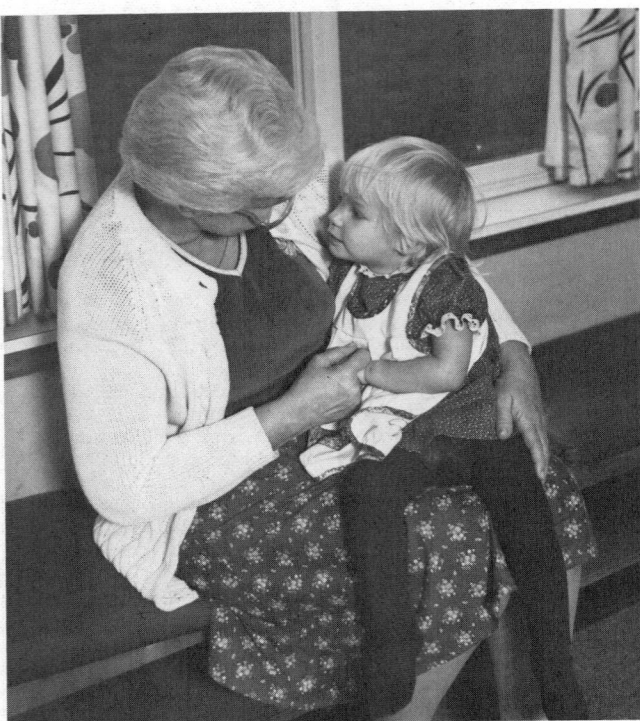

Fig. 4-18. A grandmother is a primary source of unconditional love and comfort.
Photography by John Roy, Saint Francis Hospital, Tulsa, OK.

from health professionals. Nurses aware of indications of parental insecurity will be able to provide assistance and reassurance that can preserve and enhance the parent-child relationship and build a sense of confidence in the parent.

Security

Closely allied to the need for love is the need for a sense of security. As they grow and develop in a complex world, children encounter many threats to their sense of security. Indeed, most childhood behavior problems are associated with an element of insecurity. Every change in themselves or their environment creates a feeling of uncertainty. Faced with confusing, conflicting adjustments, young children need the security provided by relatively stable situations and dependable human relationships. The degree to which they can cope with these stresses depends on the patience and support they receive from those most closely involved in their care.

A multitude of factors exists that can generate a feeling of insecurity in children. Ordinarily the parents, who are sources of comfort, guidance, and encouragement, provide a measure of security in an insecure world. To achieve this security, children need the warm acceptance of loving parents, a stable family unit, and judicious handling of stress-provoking situations such as sibling rivalry, relocation to a new neighborhood, and illness in themselves or other members of the family. A disturbed home environment caused by such factors as marital discord, illness of a parent or family member, or death of a family member can shatter their equilibrium.

Infants are disturbed by physical threats, such as hunger, cold, or discomfort. Small children are physiologically disturbed by emotions such as anger, fear, and grief, which they can release only in overt behavior. They can obtain a measure of relief from these feelings by the reassurance that their physical needs will be met, restraints will be placed on their behavior, and expectations that keep pace with their inner controls will be held. Rejection by significant persons, social ineptitude, and physical handicaps often produce insecurity in a child. The number and variety of stressful factors originating within or outside the child are often difficult to determine; therefore those responsible for the child's care must be alert for cues that reveal threats to this sense of security.

Discipline and Authority

Because children live in an organized society, they must be prepared to accept restrictions on their behavior. Discipline is not punishment. Rather it is the teaching of desirable behavior. Children need to learn the rules governing behavior in the home, the neighborhood, the school, and the community at large. To learn acceptable behavior that permits them to live enjoyably with themselves and others, children need the steady, firm guidance of loving parents and others in authority roles. Good discipline provides children with protection from dangers within and without and relieves them of the burden of decisions they are not prepared to make, yet allows them to develop independence of thought and action within a secure framework.

Children who learn to live within reasonable rules are happier and more secure children. Without the stabilizing influence of controls, children feel uncertain and insecure. Too often, inexperienced and insecure parents fear the loss of a child's love, suffer feelings of guilt over disciplinary action, or even relinquish their authority to the child. To discipline is to teach reality. Sensible, mature parents establish fair rules and regulations in the home and then see that they are carried out. Parents should never exploit children's love for them as a means to control their children. Children's anxiety lest they lose that love is already great. Discipline based on love of the child and carried out with conviction, confidence, and consistency will produce a self-reliant, buoyant, and self-controlled child.

Dependence and Independence

As children grow and mature, they are increasingly able to direct their own activities and to make more independent decisions. However, there are great fluctuations in their ability to function independently. Even with a compelling inner drive to master and achieve, they are not always able to cope with difficult and frustrating problems or conflicts. All children feel the urge to grow up and move toward maturity, but they have at their disposal only those energies not being used to maintain mastery over old conflicts. Independence should be permitted to grow at its own rate.

Periods of regression and dependence are not only normal but are often necessary and helpful. If children feel sufficiently comfortable and content in a situation or relationship and reasonably certain that they can return to this safety and security, they will venture into the untried and untested on their own. If they feel doubtful concerning their abilities to cope, regression to a more comfortable level of competence allows them to replenish their inner resources and prepare to move ahead once again. Independence grows out of dependence; one cannot be considered as distinct from the other.

Children will learn independence of thought and decision making provided the opportunity is not withheld from them. If they are pushed into acting independently before they feel themselves ready, they may withdraw from independence. When they choose not to relinquish the joys of independence and autonomy or move ahead to new worlds of independence, they will dawdle. Parents, teachers, nurses, and others responsible for the child's care must be able to adjust their expectations and support to meet the child's needs of the moment. It is important to recognize when to help and when not to help children experiment with their immature and imperfect self-control, when to make demands requiring children's utmost ability, and when to allow them to function temporarily on a more immature level. They need these freedoms and controls in the process of becoming mature, self-reliant adults.

Self-Esteem

In order to develop and preserve self-esteem, children need to feel that they are worthwhile individuals who are in some way different from, superior to, and more lovable than any other individual in the world. They need recognition for their achievements and the approval of parents and peers. Parents and other authority figures can foster a positive self-concept by providing appropriate encouragement and recognition for achievement and by discouraging inappropriate behaviors. However, when authority figures express disapproval, they must convey to a child that the *behavior* is unacceptable, not the child. Constructive communication, such as the use of ''I'' messages, conveys feeling and needs without destroying the child's self-esteem.

Children who experience warm, affectionate relationships with their family and who are aware of their parents' acceptance and positive attitudes toward them are more accepting of themselves. Children who have a strong sense of their own worth are confident, able to initiate activities, explore their environment, and take risks in their behavior when confronted with new or novel situations. They approach tasks and relationhips with the expectation that they will be well-received and successful. Such is the focus of nursing—to allow children and their families to grow and to prosper from their experiences in times of both health and illness.

CONCEPT SUMMARIES

- Heredity and environmental factors are influential in shaping an individual.

- Growth describes a change in quantity and occurs when cells divide and synthesize new proteins.

- Maturation, a qualitative change, describes the aging process or an increase in competence and adaptability.

- Differentiation refers to a biologic description of the processes by which early cells and structures are modified and altered to achieve specific and characteristic physical and chemical properties.

- Development involves change from a lower to a more advanced stage of complexity.

- Growth, maturation, differentiation, and development are interrelated processes.

- There are five major developmental phases: prenatal period, infancy period, early childhood, middle childhood, and later childhood.

- Cross-sectional studies of growth and development measure the characteristics of a number of children representing the various ages or stages of development.

- Longitudinal studies focus on each child in a group of children, with the child measured periodically over a number of years and through successive stages of growth and development.

- There are three trends in growth and development: directional, sequential, and secular.

- Temperament is the way of thinking, behaving, and reacting and includes motor activity, rhythmicity, approach-withdrawal, adaptability, threshold of responsiveness, intensity of reaction, quality of mood, distractibility, attention span, and persistence. Three common categories of temperament include the easy child, the difficult child, and the slow-to-warm-up child.

- Freud contributed to personality development with his theories on id, ego, superego, and psychosexual development.

- Erikson's theory of psychosocial development focuses on the individual's efforts to adjust, or crisis. His eight stages of psychosocial crises are trust vs mistrust, autonomy vs shame and doubt, initiative vs guilt, industry vs inferiority, identity vs role confusion, intimacy vs isolation, generativity vs stagnation, and ego integrity vs despair.

- Piaget's theory of cognitive development purports that children progress through stages of mental activity in an orderly, sequential manner that enables them to make adaptations to the environment that increase the probability of survival. His four stages of intellectual development are sensorimotor, preoperational, concrete, and formal.

- Social learning, as presented by Skinner, is achieved through both operant and avoidance conditioning.

- Bandura believes that children learn by the innate tendency to observe and imitate behavior of significant persons in their lives.

- Children learn sex roles through identification with parents.

- Moral development, as described by Kolberg, assumes three stages: preconventional morality, conventional morality, and autonomous morality.

- Spiritual development proceeds through the following stages: undifferentiated, intuitive-projective, mythical-literal, synthetic-convention, and individuating-reflexive.

- Development of self-concept occurs through a child's interactions and observations of his own experiences with others and with the environment.

- Environmental conditions that may affect growth include season, climate, oxygen concentration, hazards, and socioeconomic level.

- Nutrition is perhaps the single most important influence on growth.

- Play is the work of the child; through play children learn about themselves, others, and their environment.

- Play serves important functions in sensorimotor development, intellectual development, socialization, creativity, and self-awareness, and it has therapeutic and moral value.

- Aside from meeting physical and biologic needs, it is the responsibility of parents and caregivers to provide love and affection and promote security, discipline and authority, dependence and independence, and self-esteem.

REFERENCES

Atkin, C.: Observation of parent-child interaction in supermarket decision-making, J. Marketing **42**:41-45, 1978.

Barcus, F.E., and Wolkin, R.: Children's television: an analysis of programming and advertising, New York, 1977, Praeger Publishers.

Berndt, T.J.: The features and effects of friendship in early adolescence, Child Dev. **53**:1447-1460, 1982.

Biddle, B.J.: Role theory: expectations, identities, and behaviors, New York, 1979, Academic Press, Inc.

Carey, W.B., and McDevitt, S.C.: Revision of the infant temperament questionnaire, Pediatrics **61**:735-739, 1978.

Chess, S., and Thomas, A.: Temperamental differences: a critical concept in child health care, Pediatr. Nurs. **11**:167-171, 1985.

Chess, S., and Thomas, A.: Individuality: dynamics of individual behavioral development. In Levine, M.D., and others, editors: Developmental-behavioral pediatrics, Philadelphia, 1983, W.B. Saunders Co.

Coates, B., Pusser, H.E., and Goodman, I.: The influence of "Sesame Street" and "Mister Rogers' Neighborhood" on children's social behavior in the preschool, Child Dev. **47**:138-144, 1976.

Colombo, J.: The critical period concept: research, methodology and theoretical issues, Psychol. Bull. **81**:260-275, 1982.

DiCaprio, N.S.: Personality theories: a guide to human nature, ed. 2, New York, 1983, Holt, Rinehart & Winston General Book.

Dietz, W.H., and Gortmaker, S.L.: Do we fatten our children at the television set? Obesity and television viewing in children and adolescents, Pediatrics **75**:807-812, 1985.

Elkind, D.: The child and society, New York, 1979, Oxford University Press, Inc.

Erikson, E.H.: Childhood and society, ed. 2, New York, 1963, W.W. Norton & Co., Inc.

Erikson, E.H.: Reflections on Dr. Borg's life cycle. In Erikson, E.H., editor: Adulthood, New York, 1978, W.W. Norton & Co., Inc.

Eron, L.D., and others: Age trends in the development of aggression, sex-typing, and related television habits, Dev. Psychol. **19**:71-77, 1983.

Fowler, J.W.: Toward a developmental perspective on faith, Religious Educ. **69**:207-219, 1974.

Fox, M.W.: Overview and critique of stages and periods in canine development, Dev. Psychobiol. **2**:37-54, 1970.

Freedman, D.G.: Ethnic differences in babies, Hum. Nature **2**:36-43, 1979.

Furman, W., and Bierman, K.L.: Developmental changes in young children's conception of friendship, Child Dev. **54**:549-556, 1983.

Gardner, L.J.: Deprivation dwarfism, Sci. Am. **227**:76-82, 1972.

Gerbner, G., and others: The "mainstreaming" of America: violence profile no. 11, J. Communication **30**:10-29, 1980.

Gerbner, G., and others: Health and medicine on television, N. Engl. J. Med. **305**:901-904, 1982.

Goda, S.: Speech development in children, Am. J. Nurs. **70**:276-278, 1970.

Goldsmith, H.H., and Gottesman, I.I.: Origins of variation in behavioral style: a longitudinal study of temperament in young twins, Child Dev. **52**:91-103, 1981.

Gorn, G.J., Goldberg, M.E., and Kanungo, R.N.: The role of educational television in changing the intergroup attitudes of children, Child Dev. **47**:277-280, 1976.

Harlow, H.F., and Harlow, M.K.: Social deprivation in monkeys, Sci. Am. **203**:136-146, Nov. 1962.

Huston, A., and Wright, J.C.: Effects of communications media on children. In Kopp, C.B., and Krakow, J.B., editors: The child: development in a social context, Reading, MA, 1982, Addison-Wesley Publishing Co., Inc.

Ilg, F.L., and Ames, L.B.: Child behavior, New York, 1955, Harper & Brothers.

Kagan, J.: Stress and coping in early development. In Garmezy, N., and Rutter, M., editors: Stress, coping, and development in children, New York, 1983, McGraw-Hill Book Co.

Kohlberg, L.: The cognitive-developmental approach to moral education, Phi Delta Kappan **56**:670-677, 1975.

Kuczen, B.: Childhood stress, New York, 1982, Delacorte Press.

Kurdek, L.A., and Krile, D.: A developmental analysis of the relation between peer acceptance and both interpersonal understanding and perceived social self-competence, Child Dev. **53**:1485-1491, 1982.

Lefkowitz, M.M., and Huesmann, L.R.: Concomitants of television violence viewing in children. In Palmer, E.L., and Dorr, A., editors: Children and the faces of television, New York, 1980, Academic Press, Inc.

Liebert, R.M., Sprafkin, J.N., and Davidson, E.S.: The early window: effects of television on children and youth, New York, 1982, Pergamon Press, Inc.

Lowrey, G.H.: Growth and development of children, ed. 8, Chicago, 1986, Year Book Medical Publishers, Inc.

Maccoby, E.E., and Jacklin, C.N.: The psychology of sex differences, Stanford, CA, 1974, Stanford University Press.

McGuire, K.D., and Weisz, J.R.: Social cognition and behavioral correlates of preadolescent chumship, Child Dev. **53**:1478-1484, 1982.

Matheny, A.P.: Bayley's Infant Behavior Record: behavioral components and twin analysis, Child Dev. **51**:1157-1167, 1980.

Minton, J.: The impact of Sesame Street on readiness, Soc. Educ. **48**:141-151, 1975.

Mitchell, K., and Mills, N.M.: Is the sensitive period in parent-infant bonding overrated? Pediatr. Nurs. **9**(2):91-94, 1983.

Moltz, H.: Some implications of the critical period hypothesis, Ann. N.Y. Acad. Sci. **223**:144-146, 1973.

Murray, J.P.: Television and youth: 25 years of research and controversy, Boys Town, NE, 1980, Boys Town Center for the Study of Youth Development.

Neumann, C.G., and Alpaugh, M.: Birth-weight doubling time: a fresh look, Pediatrics **57**:469-473, 1976.

Newman, B.M., and Newman, P.R.: Development through life: a psychosocial approach, ed. 3, Homewood, IL, 1984, The Dorsey Press.

Piaget, J.: The theory of stages in cognitive development, New York, 1969, McGraw-Hill Book Co.

Ridley-Johnson, R., Cooper, H., and Chance, J.: The relation of children's television viewing to school achievement and IQ, J. Educ. Res. **20:**294-297, 1983.

Rogan, W.J.: The sources and routes of childhood chemical exposures, J. Pediatr. **97**(5):861-865, 1980.

Rossiter, J.R., and Robertson, T.S.: Children's dispositions toward proprietary drugs and the role of television drug advertising, Public Opinion Q. **44:**316-329, 1980.

Rubin, K.H., Fein, G., and Vandenberg, B.: Play. In Hetherington, E.M., editor: Carmichaels manual of child psychology: social development, New York, 1983, John Wiley & Sons, Inc.

Selekman, J.: The development of body image in the child: a learned response, Top. Clin. Nurs. **5**(1):13-21, 1983.

Selman, R.L.: The growth of interpersonal understanding, New York, 1980, Academic Press, Inc.

Shaffer, D.R.: Developmental psychology: theory, research, and applications, Monterey, CA, 1984, Brooks/Cole Publishing Co.

Sheldon, W.H.: The varieties of human physique, New York, 1940, Harper & Row, Publishers, Inc.

Stanwyck, D.J.: Self-esteem through the life span, Top. Clin. Nurs. **6**(2):11-28, 1983.

Stuart, G.W., and Sundeen, S.J.: Principles and practice of psychiatric nursing, ed. 2, St. Louis, 1983, The C.V. Mosby Co.

Thelen, E., and Fisher, D.M.: Newborn stepping: an explanation for a disappearing reflex, Dev. Psychol. **18:**760-775, 1982.

Wharton, R., and Mandell, F.: Violence on television and imitative behavior: impact on parenting practices, Pediatrics **75:**1120-1123, 1985.

Wolman, B.B.: Children's fears, New York, 1978, Grosset & Dunlap.

Zaichkowsky, L.D., Zaichkowsky, L.B., and Martinek, T.J.: Growth and development: the child and physical activity, St. Louis, 1980, The C.V. Mosby Co.

Zelazo, P.R., Zelazo, N.A., and Kolb, S.: "Walking" in the newborn, Science **176:**314-315, 1972.

BIBLIOGRAPHY
General

Committee on Genetics and Environmental Hazards: Special susceptibility of children to radiation effects, Pediatrics **72:**890, 1983.

Conway, B.L.: Pediatric neurologic nursing, St. Louis, 1977, The C.V. Mosby Co.

Dashiff, C.J.: Coaching developmental differentiation, Top. Clin. Nurs. **1**(3):11-20, 1979.

Dembo, M.H.: Teaching for learning, ed. 2, Santa Monica, CA, 1981, Goodyear Publishing Co., Inc.

Gifford, S., and Lieberman, B.I.: Evaluation of growth charts, Issues Comp. Pediatr. Nurs. **4**(2):1-25, 1980.

Harlow, H.F., and Harlow, M.K.: Learning to love, Am. Sci. **54:**244-272, 1966.

Havighurst, R.J.: Developmental tasks and education, ed. 3, New York, 1972, David McKay Co., Inc.

Kaluger, G., and Kaluger, M.F.: Human development: the span of life, ed. 3, St. Louis, 1984, The C.V. Mosby Co.

Lewis, C.E., Siegel, J.M., and Lewis, M.A.: Feeling bad: exploring sources of distress among pre-adolescent children, Am. J. Public Health **74:**117-122, 1984.

Little, D.L.: Written explanation of temperament scores, Pediatrics **75:**275-277, 1985.

McCall, R.B.: Nature-nurture and the two realms of development: a proposed integration with respect to mental development, Child Dev. **52:**1-12, 1981.

Miller, R.W.: Chemical and radiation hazards to children: highlights of a meeting, J. Pediatr. **101:**495-497, 1982.

Mullen, P.D.: Promoting child health: channels of socialization, Fam. Comm. Health **6**(1):52-68, 1983.

Mussen, P.H., Conger, J.J., and Kagan, J.: Child development and personality, ed. 5, New York, 1979, Harper & Row, Publishers, Inc.

Petrillo, M., and Sangay, S.: Emotional care of the hospitalized child, ed. 2, Philadelphia, 1980, J.B. Lippincott Co.

Phillips, J.L.: The origins of intellect: Piaget's theory, San Francisco, 1969, W.H. Freeman & Co. Publishers.

Post, E.M., and Richman, R.A.: A condensed table for predicting adult stature, J. Pediatr. **98:**440-442, 1981.

Shaffer, D.R.: Developmental psychology: theory, research, and applications, Monterey, CA, 1985, Brooks/Cole Publishing Co.

Snow, M.E., Jacklin, C.N., and Maccoby, E.E.: Sex-of-child differences in father-child interaction at one year of age, Child Dev. **54:**227-232, 1983.

Stone, L.J., and Church, J.: Childhood and adolescence, ed. 5, New York, 1984, Random House, Inc.

Withrow, C., and Fleming, J.W.: Pediatric social illness: a challenge to nurses, Issues Comp. Pediatr. Nurs. **6:**261-275, 1983.

Zachman, M., and others: Bayley-Pinneau, Roche-Wainer-Thissen, and Tanner height predictions in normal children and in patients with various pathologic conditions, J. Pediatr. **93:**749-755, 1978.

Physical Growth and Development

Sherwen, L.N.: Separation: the forgotten phenomenon of child development, Top. Clin. Nurs. **5:**1-11, 1983.

Tanner, J.M., and Davies, P.S.W.: Clinical longitudinal standards for height and height velocity of North American children, J. Pediatr. **107:**317-329, 1985.

Temperament

Blosser, C.: Avoiding potential behavior problems in children, Pediatr. Nurs. **5**(3):11-15, 1979.

Persson-Blennow, I., and McNeil, T.F.: Temperament characteristics of children in relation to gender, birth order, and social class, Am. J. Orthopsychiatry **51**(4):710-713, 1981.

Plomin, R., and Rowe, D.C.: A twin study of temperament in young children, J. Psychol. **97:**107-113, 1977.

Rothbart, M.K.: Measurement of temperament in infancy, Child Dev. **52:**569-578, 1981.

Ventura, J.N.: Parent coping behaviors, parent functioning, and infant temperament characteristics, Nurs. Res. **31:**269-273, 1982.

Moral and Spiritual Development

Betz, C.L.: Faith development in children, Pediatr. Nurs. **7**(2):22-25, 1981.

Dettmore, D.: Spiritual care: remembering your patients' forgotten needs, Nursing **14**(10):46, 1984.

Elkind, D.: Origins of religion in the child. In Elkind, D.: The child and society, New York, 1979, Oxford University Press, Inc.

Fish, S., and Shelly, J.A.: Spiritual care: the nurse's role, Downers Grove, IL, 1978, Inter-Varsity Press.

Mahon, K.A., and Fowler, M.D.: Moral development and clinical decision-making, Nurs. Clin. North Am. **14**(1):3-12, 1979.

McCown, D.E.: Moral development in children, Pediatr. Nurs. **10:**42-44, 1984.

Ryan, J.: The neglected crisis, Am. J. Nurs. **84:**1257-1258, 1984.

Shelly, J.A.: Spiritual care: planting seeds of hope, Crit. Care Update **9**(12):7-15, 1982.

Stoll, R.I.: Guidelines for spiritual assessment, Am. J. Nurs. **79:**1575-1577, 1979.

Nutrition

Committee on Nutrition: Toward a prudent diet of children, Pediatrics **71:**78-80, 1983.

Dwyer, J.T.: Family nutrition and the health care team, Issues Comp. Pediatr. Nurs. **1**(5):1-21, 1977.

Endres, J.B., and Rockwell, R.E.: Food, nutrition, and the young child, ed. 2, St. Louis, 1985, The C.V. Mosby Co.

Forbes, G.B.: Nutrition and growth, J. Pediatr. **1:**40-43, 1977.

Georgieff, M.K., and others: Effect of neonatal caloric deprivation on head growth and 1-year developmental status in preterm infants, J. Pediatr. **107:**581-582, 1985.

Jackson, R.L.: Long-term consequences of suboptimal nutritional practices in early life, Pediatr. Clin. North Am. **24:**63-70, 1977.

Pipes, P.L.: Nutrition in infancy and childhood, ed. 3, St. Louis, 1985, The C.V. Mosby Co.

Walker, W.A., and Hendricks, K.M.: Manual of pediatric nutrition, Philadelphia, 1985, W.B. Saunders Co.

Williams, S.R.: Nutrition and diet therapy, ed. 5, St. Louis, 1985, The C.V. Mosby Co.

Stress and Fear

Garmezy, N.: Stressors of childhood. In Garmezy, N., and Rutter, M. editors: Stress, coping, and development in children, New York, 1983, McGraw-Hill Book Co.

Miller, S.R.: Children's fears: a review of the literature with implications for nursing research and practice, Nurs. Res. **28:**217-223, 1979.

Rutter, M.: Stress, coping, and development: some issues and some questions. In Garmezy, N., and Rutter, M., editors: Stress, coping, and development in children, New York, 1983, McGraw-Hill Book Co.

Television

Comstock, G.A.: Influences of mass media on child health behavior, Health Educ. Q. **8**(1):32-38, 1981.

Dail, P.W., and Way, W.L.: What do parents observe about parenting from prime time television, Fam. Rel. **34:**491-499, 1985.

Devney, R., and Bensenten, R.W.: Television and children, Minn. Med. **62:**833-837, 1979.

Galst, J.P., and White, M.A.: The unhealthy persuader: the reinforcing value of television and children's purchase-influencing attempt at the supermarket, Child Dev. **47:**1089-1096, 1976.

McCown, D.: TV: its problems for children, Pediatr. Nurs. **5**(2):17-19, 1979.

Morgan, M., and Gross, L.: Television viewing, IQ, and academic achievement, J. Broadcasting **24:**117-133, 1980.

Pearl, D., Bouthilet, L., and Lazar, J.: Television and behavior: ten years of scientific progress and implications for the eighties, vols. 1 and 2, Washington, D.C., 1982, U.S. Department of Health and Human Services.

Rothenberg, M.B.: In my opinion . . . role of television in shaping the attitudes of children, Child. Health Care **13:**148-150, 1985.

Sheiman, D.J.: Effects of televised drug commercials on children, Pediatrics **65:**678, 1980.

Tower, R.B., and others: Differential effects of television programming on preschoolers' cognition, imagination, and social play, Am. J. Orthopsychiatry **49:**265-281, 1979.

Weiss, J.C.: Television violence and children, Del. Med. J. **51:**217-219, 1979.

Zuckerman, D.M., and Zuckerman, B.S.: Television's impact on children, Pediatrics **75:**233-240, 1985.

Play

Axelsson, A., and Jerson, T.: Noisy toys: a possible source of sensorineural hearing loss, Pediatrics **76:**574-578, 1985.

Bellack, J.P., and Fleming, J.W.: Theoretical practical aspects of play: a universal need. In Fore, C., and Poster, E.C., editors: Meeting psychosocial needs of children and families in health care, Washington, D.C., 1985, Assoc. Care Child. Health.

Betz, C.L., and Poster, E.C.: Incorporating play into the care of the hospitalized child, Issues Comp. Pediatr. Nurs. **7:**343-355, 1984.

Brown, C.C., and Gottried, A.W., editors: Play interactions: the role of toys and parental involvement in children's development, 1985, Johnson & Johnson Baby Products Company.

Singer, W.Q.D., and Lutner, L.: Trauma from toy boxes, J. Pediatr. **100:**242, 1982.

Tizard, B., and Harvey, D., editors: Biology of play, Philadelphia, 1977, J.B. Lippincott Co.

Chapter 5

Hereditary and Prenatal Influences on Health Promotion of the Child and Family

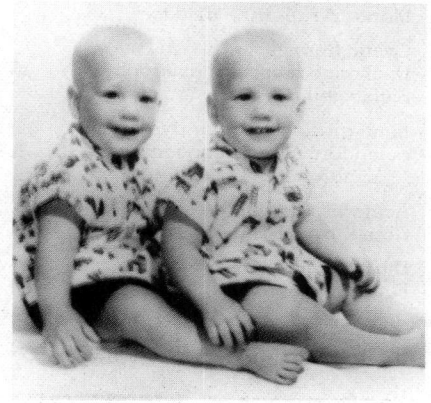

Child development begins before birth and is directed by the action of many genetic mechanisms controlled by a strict chronology. But no less significant are the influences of environment, particularly during the time of critical differentiation. The physical, biochemical, and mental characteristics of the child include not only those traits that create the individuality of each child but also those characteristics that produce unpleasant symptoms or undesirable physical abnormalities that are interpreted as disease.

Numerous defects and diseases seen frequently in the population show an increased incidence in some families or under certain environmental conditions. Parents and health workers alike are concerned with the probability that a specific disease or disorder will recur in a family. To better counsel families and to anticipate probable problems, the nurse needs (1) a fundamental understanding of the principles of genetics and the importance of heredity as an etiologic factor in diseases and disorders of childhood and (2) a knowledge, even rudimentary, of the sequence and organ relationships of early development in order to appreciate the significance of disturbances during this crucial time that produce congenital malformations—the source of major pediatric nursing problems. This chapter is concerned with some genetic factors that play a role in growth and development, some prenatal and postnatal environmental influences that can alter the normal course of events, and counseling the family regarding problems related to hereditary disorders.

Genetic Influences on Health

Hereditary influences on health and disease are assuming increasing importance to persons in the health professions. Medical science has made rapid advances in the control of infectious diseases and nutritional disorders that formerly accounted for the major share of deaths in infancy. At the same time, contributions from the fields of biochemistry and cytology have established a genetic basis and the means for identification of an increasing number of diseases and defects. Consequently there has been a corresponding increase in the proportion of conditions in which genetic factors are prominent, especially in the pediatric population.

HEREDITY IN HEALTH PROBLEMS

There is probably a genetic component in all disease processes. In some disorders the genetic defect is known; in others the precise nature of the genetic component is more obscure. In some the disorder is apparent at birth; in others the manifestations do not appear for weeks, months, or years (Table 5-1). Some diseases and disorders are determined by the genetic constitution of the individual, such as muscular dystrophy, Marfan syndrome, and Down syndrome. Other diseases, although genetically determined, do not become clinically apparent until environmental factors precipitate the onset of symptoms. For instance, an infant with phenylketonuria, a disorder caused by lack of an enzyme essential for the metabolism of the protein phenylalanine, does not display any symptoms until a sufficient amount of milk containing the protein is ingested. Also the serious effects of sickle cell anemia develop under conditions of lowered oxygen tension.

Other diseases result primarily from environmental factors. These include most infectious diseases and trauma. Development of the disease depends on environmental contact with the etiologic agent, but there is strong evidence to indicate a decided genetic element in the susceptibility to most diseases (for example, tuberculosis, poliomyelitis, and measles in some populations). However, the bulk of common diseases and disorders have varying degrees of genetic influence. This category contains most of the birth defects, the allergic disorders, many neurologic defects, and some metabolic diseases.

Definitions

To facilitate a discussion of genetic influence on the health of children, it is necessary to clarify some of the terms used to describe hereditary conditions.

Table 5-1 Characteristic age of onset for some genetic diseases

AGE OF ONSET	CONDITION
Lethal during prenatal life	Some chromosome aberrations Some gross malformations
Present at birth	Congenital malformations Chromosomal aberrations, e.g., Down syndrome Some forms of adrenogenital syndrome Some forms of deafness
Soon after birth	Phenylketonuria Galactosemia Sometimes cystic fibrosis
Infancy	Tay-Sachs disease Werdnig-Hoffman disease Maple syrup urine disease
Early childhood	Cystic fibrosis Duchenne muscular dystrophy Sickle cell anemia
Near puberty	Limb-girdle muscular dystrophy Some forms of adrenogenital syndrome
Young adulthood	Acute intermittent porphyria Hereditary juvenile glaucoma
Variable onset age	Diabetes mellitus (0 to 80 years) Facioscapulohumeral muscular dystrophy (2 to 45 years) Huntington chorea (15 to 65 years) Myotonic dystrophy (birth to old age)

congenital The condition is present at birth. The disorder may be brought about by genetic causes, nongenetic causes, or a combination of these.

familial A disorder that "runs in families" or is present in more members of a family than would be expected by chance.

genetic The disorder is caused by a single harmful gene, by several genes, or by a deviation in chromosome number or structure. It may or may not be apparent at birth.

inherited (heritable, hereditary) Synonymous with genetic, although in the past often used to describe a disorder that appeared in parent and offspring over several generations.

genotype The genetic constitution that determines the physical and chemical characteristics of an individual.

phenotype The physical or chemical characteristics of an individual, produced by the interaction of the environment on the genotype.

homozygous Having the same genes at a given position (locus) on a pair of chromosomes.

heterozygous Having dissimilar genes at a given position (locus) on a pair of chromosomes.

Classification of Genetic Diseases

Genetic diseases can usually be classified into one of the following three broad categories according to the hereditary factors that produce the observed effect:

1. Chromosomal aberrations in which there is addition, loss, or structural alteration of a chromosome; for example, Down syndrome, Klinefelter syndrome, and Turner syndrome
2. Disorders that are caused by mutation of a gene or genes and that are distributed in families according to the basic mendelian inheritance patterns; for example, cystic fibrosis, hemophilia, muscular dystrophy, and phenylketonuria
3. The common diseases and disorders that are multifactorial, that is, result from a complex interaction of both genetic and environmental factors; for example, diseases such as diabetes mellitus and peptic ulcer and congenital defects such as cleft lip or palate, congenital heart disease, and congenital hip dysplasia

CYTOGENETIC DISORDERS

An aberration is defined as a deviation from that which is normal or typical. Chromosome aberrations, or cytogenetic disorders, are deviations in either structure or number of a chromosome, and the consequences in either situation can be readily observed in the affected individual. Although the types of cytogenic disorders are not as varied as those caused by a single gene, the incidence for many of the specific abnormalities is significantly higher than any of the single-gene (monogenic) disorders.

A structural aberration involves loss, addition, rearrangement, or exchange of some of the genes of a chromosome. If there is sufficient remaining genetic material to render the organism viable, structural alterations can produce an endless variety of clinical manifestations. Also fragile, or weak, sites have been identified on both autosomes and on the X chromosome and have been associated with physical and mental abnormalities, such as the "fragile X" syndrome.

Deviations in chromosomal number involve the gain or loss of a chromosome and are designated with the suffix -*somy*. A cell that contains one less than the total number of chromosomes is called a *monosomy* because of the loss of one member of a chromosome pair; a cell that contains one more than the total number of chromosomes resulting from the addition of an extra member to a normal pair is called a *trisomy*. A number of deviations that are compatible with life occur in humans, especially those involving the sex chromosomes, but the more serious outcomes are related to abnormalities of the autosomes. Trisomies are the chromosomal aberrations encountered most commonly by health workers.

The clinical consequences that attend variations in chromosome number frequently consist of discrete, identifiable syndromes, particularly in regard to the trisomies (see Tables 5-1 and 5-2). The chromosomal structural anomalies form a more diverse group of reported physical deviations with few recognized syndromes. Some of the chromosomal disorders, such as Down syndrome, can be identified on the basis of physical characteristics; others require chromosomal analysis to establish a chromosomal abnormality as a causative factor. Many of these unidentified cases have been massed together and labeled with the dubious title "funny-looking kid" or, more recently, "unique-looking child." Although these terms are used in many areas, they serve no useful purpose and are, therefore, not employed in nursing assessments. Nurses are expected to use terminology that correctly describes and communicates specific features.

A standard nomenclature has been established by an in-

Table 5-2 Common autosomal aberrations

SYNDROME	CHROMOSOMAL ABNORMALITY AND NOMENCLATURE	AVERAGE INCIDENCE (LIVE BIRTHS)	MAJOR CLINICAL MANIFESTATIONS
Cri du chat	Deletion of short arm of B (No. 5) chromosome—46,XY,5p–		Distinctive weak, high-pitched, mewlike cry resembling the cry of a cat; small head; hypertelorism; failure to thrive; severe mental retardation—profound with age
Trisomy 13 (Patau)	Trisomy of group D (No. 13) chromosome—47,XY,13+	1:4,000-10,000	Multiple anomalies, including cleft lip and palate (frequently bilateral); ear malformations; microphthalmia; polydactyly; eye defects; mental retardation; early death
Trisomy 18 (Edwards)	Trisomy of group E (No. 18) chromosome—47,XY,18+	1:3,500-7,500	Deformed and low-set ears; micrognathia; rocker-bottom feet; overlapping (index over third) fingers; prominent occiput; hypertelorism; failure to thrive and early death; mental retardation
Trisomy 21 (Down)	Trisomy of group G (No. 21) chromosome—47,XY,21+ (trisomy); 46,XY,D–,G–(DqGq)+ (translocation); 46,XY/47,XY,21+ (mosaic)	1:650-1,100	Brachycephaly with flat occiput; inner epicanthal folds; small ears, nose, and mouth with protruding tongue; muscular hypotonia; broad, short hands with stubby fingers and transverse palmar crease; broad, stubby feet with wide space between big and second toes; mental retardation; variable life expectancy

ternational group of geneticists for designating chromosome anomalies (Paris Conference, 1971; 1975). The interested reader will find this information in any genetics or cytogentics textbook.

Causes of Chromosome Defects

There is considerable speculation regarding the precise cause of chromosome errors. Ionizing radiation has been found to be a cause of chromosome breaks, rearrangements, and nondisjunction—especially the large doses from radiographic tests and studies (mother) and from occupational exposure (father). The duration of unstable, or fragile, abnormalities may disappear in 3 to 5 years; stable, or permanent, alterations probably persist for more than 20 years. It is difficult to determine the effect on germ cells, however.

Autoimmune diseases appear to have a role in the pathogenesis of nondisjunction during cell division. Viruses have also been implicated, especially in relation to chromosome breakage.

Most of the information regarding factors that cause chromosome errors is related to parental age. The incidence of trisomic births corresponds strongly with increasing maternal age, regardless of the number of pregnancies. For example, the risk for trisomy 21, or Down syndrome, increases dramatically for mothers more than 40 years of age (see p. 1001 for further discussion). There is no positive explanation for this observation. However, throughout a lifetime the germ cells are vulnerable to a variety of exogenous influences and to the normal effects of the aging process. Recent evidence indicates that increasing paternal age is also a factor, although the coincidence of increasing maternal age and increasing paternal age hampers such investigation. Currently the risk appears to be significant only in men older than 55 years of age.

Maldistribution of Chromosomes

The complex nature of cell division makes it highly susceptible to mechanical error, which can occur during the critical processes of germ cell (gamete) formation and in the early divisions of the zygote following fertilization (nondisjunction). In a few cases the unequal distribution of genetic material results from fusion of two nonhomologous chromosomes to form one large chromosome (translocation). Both mechanisms are described in this segment.

Nondisjunction. The mechanism that is considered to be responsible for maldistribution of chromosomes in the majority of cases is nondisjunction during meiosis. *Disjunction* refers to the separation and migration of chromosomes during cell division; failure of this process is termed *nondisjunction*. The consequence of this prolonged attachment during division is an unequal distribution of chromosomes between the two resulting cells. Nondisjunction can take place during ova formation or sperm formation and can involve autosomes or sex chromosomes. The ratio of trisomic gametes that are produced depends on whether nondisjunction occurs during the first or second meiotic division. The types of germ cells that can be formed and the results when they unite with normal gametes are illustrated in Fig. 5-1.

Nondisjunction that occurs during early cell division following fertilization will result in an individual with mixed cell lines. The types of cells and their ratio depend on

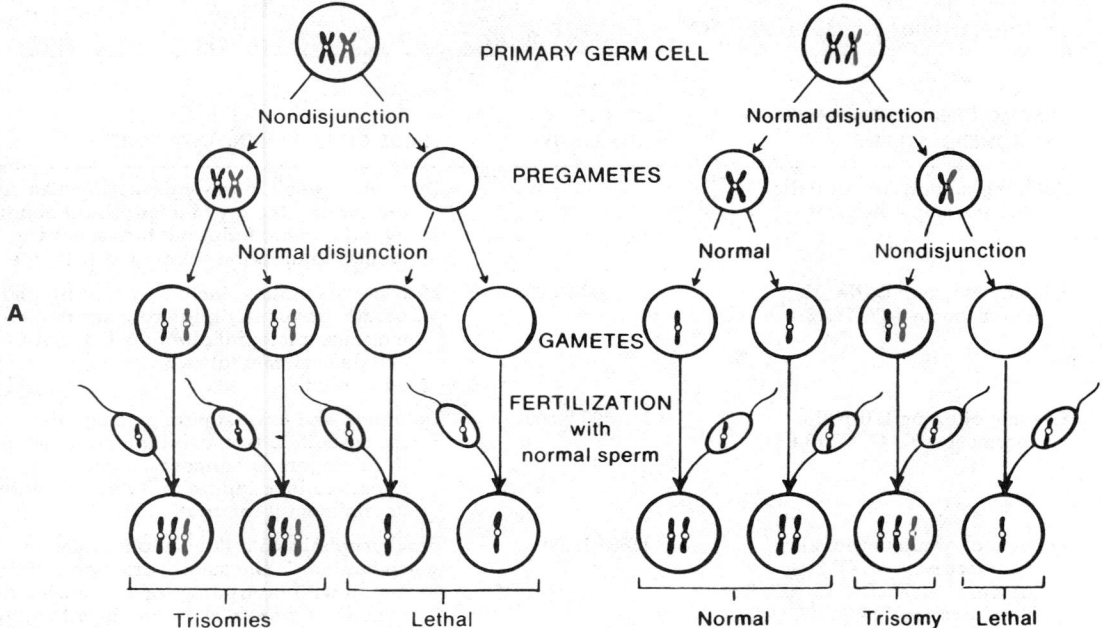

Fig. 5-1. Mechanisms of maldistribution of chromosomes during meiosis in ovum and fertilization with normal sperm. **A,** During first meiotic division. **B,** During second meiotic division. Only one mature ovum is formed, but all are illustrated to better visualize four possible gametes and consequences of fertilization.

whether nondisjunction occurs at the first or later divisions. Nondisjunction during the first division produces two cell types: half will contain 45 chromosomes, and half will contain 47 chromosomes (Fig. 5-2, *A*). Nondisjunction that occurs in one of the normal cells during the second division will produce cells with both normal and abnormal chromosome constitutions (Fig. 5-2, *B*). An individual whose cells display mixed chromosome counts is called a *mosaic*. Because monosomic cells are nonviable (with the exception of the X monosomy, which is discussed later), most mosaic individuals have an intermixture of normal and trisomic cells. The extent of clinical manifestations is determined by the type of tissues that contain cells with abnormal chromosomal numbers and may vary from near normal to a fully manifested syndrome. If a germ cell contains a trisomy, it will be transferred to half the gametes, with a 50% risk that it will be transmitted to the offspring.

Translocation. *Translocation* is a defect in chromo-somal structure that occurs when one chromosome becomes attached to another to create one large chromosome. Translocations can occur between any two chromosomes, although those encountered most commonly are those between wishbone-shaped chromosomes, the best known being the fusion of a D group chromosome (13, 14, 15) and a G group chromosome (21, 22) or between two G group chromosomes. Because the cells of a person with a translocated chromosome have the normal amount of genetic material, no physical abnormalities are associated with its possession even though the total chromosomal count is only 45. The attached chromosomes give the appearance of one large chromosome and, because they behave as a single chromosome during cell division, can be transmitted from parent to offspring. During the first meiotic division of gamete formation in such cases, there may be a balanced or an unbalanced distribution of genetic material. Fig. 5-3 shows the possible distribution of genetic material during germ cell

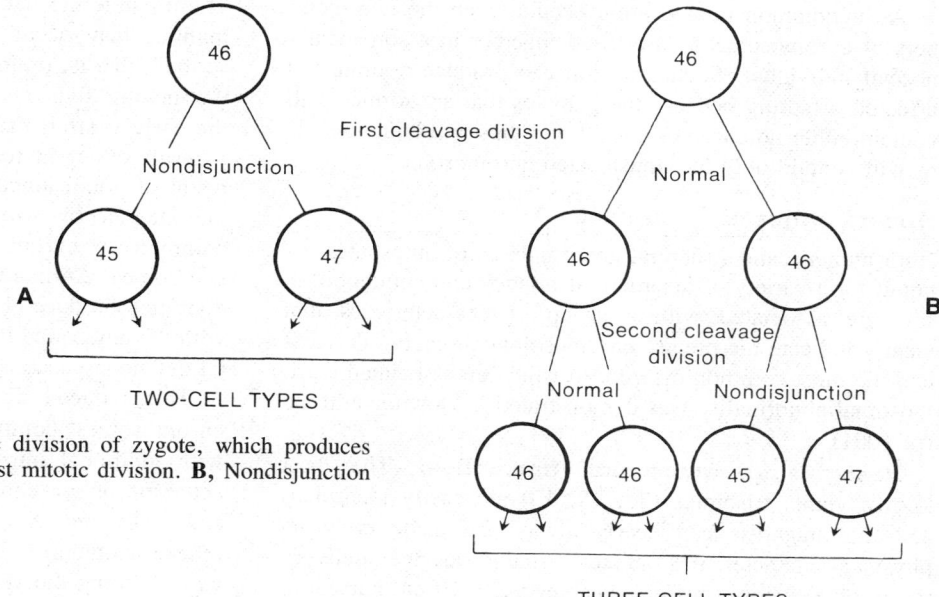

Fig. 5-2. Nondisjunction in early mitotic division of zygote, which produces mosaic genotype. **A,** Nondisjunction at first mitotic division. **B,** Nondisjunction during second mitotic division.

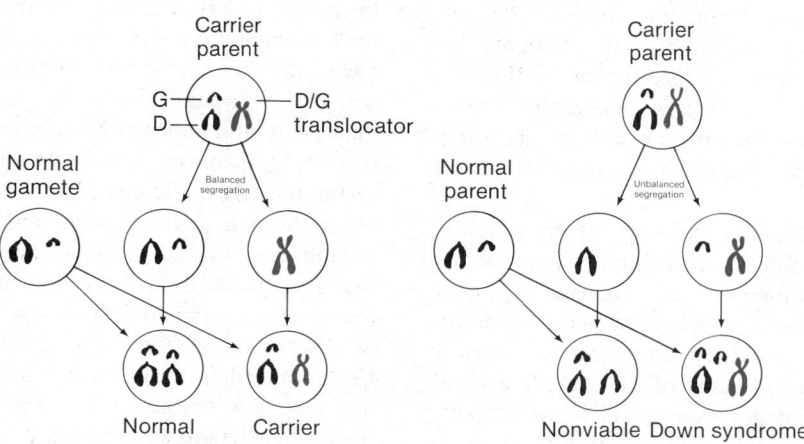

Fig. 5-3. Possible offspring from mating of somatically normal carrier of D/G translocation with genetically and somatically normal individual. D/G = translocated chromosomes D and G.

formation and the results of the combination of these various cells with gametes of normal chromosomal constitution. Persons who are clinically affected because of a translocation have extra chromosome material, although their chromosome count is 46.

Unlike nondisjunction, translocation is not related to increasing parental age. A child affected as a result of a translocated chromosome often has parents in the younger age groups. There is frequently a history of spontaneous abortion in previous pregnancies, or there may be a family history of abortions. Usually one parent is found to be a carrier of the translocated chromosome, displaying normal characteristics but a chromosomal complement of 45 chromosomes.

In a situation where a parent has a translocation involving a group D or G chromosome, the chances for an affected offspring are estimated to be 1:5 when the mother is the carrier and less than 1:20 when the father carries the translocation.

An uncommon translocation occurs when the two members of chromosome 21 are fused together in a somatically normal individual. Such a person can produce nothing but affected offspring because the gametes that are formed will contain either no chromosome 21 and thus will be nonviable or will contain only the translocated chromosome.

Abnormalities of Autosomes

Both numeric and structural abnormalities of autosomes account for a variety of disorders of infancy and childhood. A few are associated with a group of characteristics that clearly indicate the precise chromosomal anomaly. The first and the most common disorder in which an associated chromosomal abnormality was demonstrated is Down syndrome (p. 1001).

Recognizing autosomal anomalies. The best known viable trisomies (21, 18, 13) are easily identified, and the diagnosis can nearly always be made early on physical characteristics alone—usually in the delivery room or newborn nursery (Table 5-2). Often nurses in the newborn nursery see an infant who has a facial appearance that sets him apart from other infants. The infant may have no obvious congenital malformations, but on closer inspection he may evidence other variations, the sum of which disclose the specific features of known syndromes. These peculiar features or defects are often the result of chromosomal abnormalities and first attract the observer's attention.

It need not be appearance only that suggests more careful scrutiny of such infants. They may exhibit hypotonia and other neurologic manifestations such as an unusual cry, poor feeding behavior, or abnormal reflex responses. These observations in appearance have been shown to be clinically significant in the diagnosis of most of the identified chromosomal abnormalities and are also useful in recognizing many syndromes associated with other disorders having a genetic basis. Less is known about the features of the deletion syndromes.

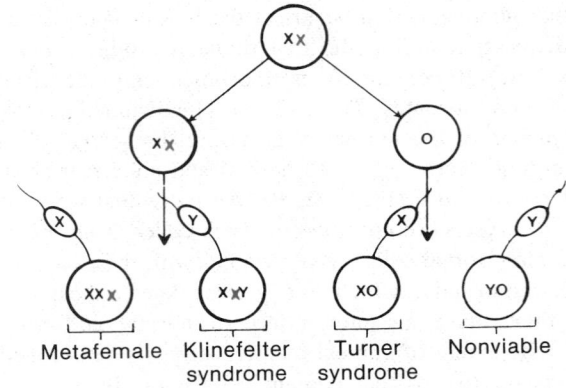

Fig. 5-4. Nondisjunction of X chromosomes in ovum fertilized by normal sperm to produce more common sex chromosomal aberrations.

Abnormalities of Sex Chromosomes

The possible mechanisms by which sex chromosome abnormalities may occur are the same as those previously described, that is, prefertilization nondisjunction during one of the meiotic divisions of gametogenesis in either parent or in the early postfertilization divisions of the zygote. Most are a result of an increase in sex chromosomal number as a result of nondisjunction during meiosis. Fig. 5-4 illustrates the manner by which nondisjunction produces the more common sex chromosomal defects—Klinefelter and Turner syndromes. An increase in the number of sex chromosomes does not produce the profound effects that are associated with the autosomal trisomies, although some degree of mental deficiency accompanies a number of them.

This reduced disability in children with multiple sex chromosomes, compared with the severe effects in children with additional autosomes, is attributed to an unusual characteristic of sex chromosomes—*X inactivation.* In all body cells only one X chromosome is biologically active; the other (or others) is in some way "switched off," or *inactivated,* during the very early divisions of the zygote and remains so throughout life. This inactivated chromosome can be easily observed through a microscope as a condensed dark-staining mass lying on the periphery of the cell nucleus—the *sex chromatin,* or *Barr body.* It is established that the maximum number of chromatin bodies is one less than the total number of X chromosomes in that cell nucleus (Fig. 5-5); therefore female somatic cells are normally chromatin positive (containing one active and one inactive X chromosome), and male cells are chromatin negative (containing only one X chromosome). Inasmuch as sex chromatin is visible in 20% to 50% of cells, the sex chromatin test provides a convenient means to determine the presence or absence of inactivated X chromosomes in somatic cells. Cells scraped from the buccal mucosa are usually used for this test. Sex chromatin can also be detected in polymorphonuclear leukocytes, where it appears as a drumsticklike mass attached to one of the nuclear lobes of the cell. Although seldom recommended because of its questionable re-

Table 5-3 Common sex chromosome abnormalities

SYNDROME	CHROMOSOMAL NOMENCLATURE	PHENOTYPE	INCIDENCE (LIVE BIRTHS)	CLINICAL MANIFESTATIONS
Turner	45,X	Female	1:2500-8000 female births	Short stature; webbed neck; low posterior hairline; shield-shaped chest with widely spaced nipples; sterile
Triple X, or super-female	47,XXX (can also be 48,XXXX or 49,XXXXX)	Female	1:850-1250 female births	Normal female characteristics; usually mentally retarded, mental deficiency in others; fertile
XYY male	47,XYY (can also be 48,XYYY or mosaic)	Male	1:840-1000 male births	Usually normal sex development; tendency to be tall with long head; poor coordination; may demonstrate aberrant behavior
Klinefelter	47,XXY (48,XXYY, 48,XXXY, 49,XXXXY, and so on, mosaics)	Male	1:500-1000 male births	Tall with long legs; hypogenitalism; sterile; male secondary sex characteristics may be deficient; may demonstrate aberrant behavior
Fragile X	46,XY 46,XX	Predominantly male	Not established	Normocephaly or macrocephaly; prominent mandible; large ears; macroorchidism; mental retardation

liability (Opitz, Shapiro, and Uehling, 1979), the test may be performed when a sex chromosomal abnormality is suspected in an infant.

A number of sex chromosomal abnormalities have been described, and some are listed in Table 5-3. The more common of these, Klinefelter and Turner syndromes, will be discussed further in relation to developmental problems of later childhood (pp. 856 and 857). Some general characteristics of chromosomal abnormalities of sex chromosome numbers are:

1. There is a direct relationship between the male or female phenotype and the presence or absence of a Y chromosome. It appears that the Y chromosome is essential for development of male characteristics.
2. The severity of defects is not related to the number of extra X chromosomes, except for mental retardation, which increases proportionately with each X chromosome.
3. The presence of more than one Y chromosome appears to have variable but as yet not well-defined effects on the phenotype.

Recently a disorder, the ''fragile X'' syndrome, has been recognized that is attributed to a fragile (unstable) site, or specific point, on the X chromosome. It appears at the same point in a given family and demonstrates an X-linked inheritance pattern. This disorder is discussed further in relation to mental retardation, one of its predominant features (see p. 1006).

MONOGENIC (SINGLE GENE) DISORDERS

Disorders for which a simple, definite inheritance pattern can be identified are rare individually, but collectively they

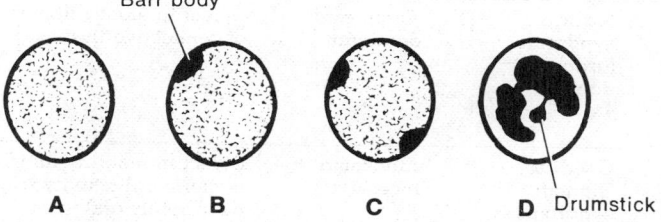

A   **B**   **C**   **D** Drumstick

Fig. 5-5. Sex chromatin, or Barr body. **A,** No sex chromatin is found in normal male somatic cells. **B,** One Barr body is normal in female somatic cells. **C,** Two Barr bodies are found in cells with three X chromosomes (XXX or XXXY). **D,** The drumstick is found in many polymorphonuclear leukocytes of normal female.

constitute a significant portion of health problems seen in infants and children. They can involve any system in the body. They can be of such minor importance that they have little effect on the child, or so severe as to cause serious disability or to be incompatible with life.

Conditions that can be directly attributed to a single gene are distributed in families in characteristic patterns according to the basic mendelian principles. Genes are either dominant or recessive in their effect, and most disorders caused by a single gene can be recognized readily by the simple family patterns that they display.

Some generalizations can be made regarding diseases and malformations caused by a single gene on either the autosomes or sex chromosomes. Disorders resulting from structural defects seem to be primarily the result of dominant genes; most metabolic defects appear to be caused by recessive genes. Dominant traits are seen more frequently and are usually less severe than are recessive traits. This is probably because of the "double-dose" effect. Whereas recessive traits are only manifest when both genes are present, a dominant disorder usually involves a single gene from a heterozygous parent. The presence of a normal gene appears to overcome the effect of a recessive gene and to reduce the severity of a dominant gene.

Codominance occurs when both genes of a heterozygous pair are expressed equally; neither is recessive to the other.

This is characteristic of the major blood groups, such as the ABO blood groups in which both the A and the B antigens are dominant. The O trait, without antigens, behaves as a recessive gene. This is clearly illustrated by type AB blood.

Some examples of single gene disorders are outlined in Table 5-4, including the inheritance pattern, basic defect, and manifestations.

Table 5-4 Partial list of single-gene disorders

DISEASE	INHERITANCE	BASIC DEFECT	MANIFESTATIONS	THERAPY
Achondro-plasia	Autosomal dominant	Defect in ossification at epiphyseal plate (growth portion of bones)	Very short limbs; large head; lordosis	Supportive
Adrenogenital syndrome	Autosomal recessive	21-Hydroxylase deficiency; failure of hydrocortisone synthesis in adrenal cortex	Virilization	Hydrocortisone
Albinism (ocular)	Autosomal recessive	Deficiency of tyrosinase; failure to convert tyrosine to dopa, and, hence, lack of melanin synthesis	Lack of pigment in skin, hair, and eyes; eye defects	Symptomatic; avoid exposure to sunlight; ophthalmologic care
Marfan syndrome (arachno-dactyly)	Autosomal dominant	Defect in elastic fibers of connective tissues	Tall and thin, with long tapering fingers; poorly developed musculature; associated defects include aortic aneurysm, dislocation of optic lens, winged scapula	Supportive; surgical correction of deformities
Chediak-Higashi syndrome	Autosomal recessive	Defect in mobility and bactericidal activity in neutrophils and macrophages	Recurrent infections; oculocutaneous albinism, photophobia; nystagmus	Ascorbic acid
Crigler-Najjar syndrome	Autosomal recessive	Glucuronyl transferase deficiency; inability to convert indirect bilirubin to direct bilirubin	Jaundice; spasticity; opisthotonos; early death	Supportive
Cystic fibrosis	Autosomal recessive	Unknown; defect in mucus-secreting glands; sweat glands secrete abnormal amounts of sodium chloride	Meconium ileus in newborn; celiac syndrome; pulmonary disease; failure to thrive	Chest physiotherapy; inhalation therapy; antibiotics; pancreatic enzymes
Cystinosis (Fanconi syndrome)	Autosomal recessive	Renal transport mechanism	Skeletal abnormalities; cystine crystals in tissues; chronic acidosis; polyuria; photophobia; early death	Vitamin D; supplementary actinium and phosphorus; penicillamine (?)
Familial hypothy-roidism	Autosomal recessive	Deficiency of iodotyrosine deiodinase	Lethargy; stunted growth; mental retardation	Early administration of thyroid hormone
Galactosemia	Autosomal recessive	Deficiency of galactose-1-phosphate uridyl transferase; inability to convert galactose to glucose	Failure to thrive; mental and motor retardation; cataracts; jaundice; hepatomegaly; cirrhosis of the liver	Eliminate galactose from diet
Gaucher disease	Autosomal recessive	Glucocerebrosidase deficiency	Hepatosplenomegaly; slow development; strabismus; difficulty feeding; laryngospasm; opisthotonos	Supportive

Table 5-4 Partial list of single-gene disorders—cont'd

DISEASE	INHERITANCE	BASIC DEFECT	MANIFESTATIONS	THERAPY
Glucose-6-phosphate dehydrogenase deficiency (G-6-PD deficiency)	X-linked recessive	Deficiency of G-6-PD	Asymptomatic under normal circumstances; certain drugs (primaquine, acetanilid, sulfanilamide, napthalene) and ingestion of fava beans produce hemolytic anemia and jaundice	Avoid agents that precipitate clinical symptoms
Hemophilia A	X-linked recessive	Deficiency of blood factor VIII prevents coagulation of blood	Uncontrollable bleeding after trauma, may be spontaneous; hematomas in any tissue; bleeding in joints, especially elbow, knee, and ankle, eventually causing stiffness and deformity	Blood transfusion; prophylactic administration of cryoprecipitates, lyophilized concentrates; plasma (fresh); prevention of trauma
Hemophilia B	X-linked recessive	Deficiency of blood factor IX prevents coagulation of blood	Same but less severe than hemophilia A	Plasma (fresh); lyophilized concentrates
Holt-Oram syndrome	Autosomal dominant	Unknown	Skeletal defects of upper limb, usually hand; cardiac defects	Surgical correction of cardiac defect
Hunter syndrome	X-linked recessive	Defect in metabolism of mucopolysaccharides	Coarse features; dwarfism; less severe than Hurler syndrome; progressive mental deterioration	Supportive
Hurler syndrome	Autosomal recessive	Defect in metabolism of mucopolysaccharides	Coarse features; dwarfism; clouding of cornea; more severe than Hunter syndrome; mental retardation; early death	Supportive
Hypophosphatasia	Autosomal recessive	Deficiency of alkaline phosphatase	Skeletal abnormalities	Supportive
Maple syrup urine disease	Autosomal recessive	Defective metabolism of branched-chain amino acids	Onset in early infancy; neurologic disorders; odor of urine similar to that of maple syrup	Diet low in branched-chain amino acids
McArdle syndrome	Autosomal recessive	Deficiency of muscle phosphorylase	Muscle weakness	Glucagon injections
Muscular dystrophy	Autosomal dominant; autosomal recessive; X-linked recessive	Unknown; appears to be caused by metabolic disturbance unrelated to nervous symptom	Progressive weakness and wasting of skeletal muscles, with increasing disability and deformity; most severe form, X-linked Duchenne type, is fatal in second or early third decade	Symptomatic and supportive; prevention of deformities
Nephrogenic diabetes insipidus	Autosomal dominant (?), X-linked recessive (?)	Failure of renal tubules to respond to antidiuretic hormone	Polyuria with low specific gravity; polydipsia	Prevent dehydration; thiazide diuretics
Neurofibromatosis (von Recklinghausen disease)	Autosomal dominant	Defective nerve growth factor and reduced receptors for cell surface lymphocyte epidermal growth factor	Highly variable; café au lait spots; auxillary freckling; multiple neurofibromas; developmental delay; seizures; scoliosis; CNS tumors; short stature; speech defects; learning disabilities	Symptomatic; supportive

Table 5-4 Partial list of single-gene disorders—cont'd

DISEASE	INHERITANCE	BASIC DEFECT	MANIFESTATIONS	THERAPY
Niemann-Pick disease	Autosomal recessive	Disturbed lipid metabolism that leads to excessive sphingomyelin in reticuloendothelial cells in CNS	Progressive neurologic deterioration; blindness; hepatomegaly; death in early childhood	Supportive
Osteogenesis imperfecta	Autosomal dominant, autosomal recessive	Defect in maturation of collagen	Skeletal defects: multiple fractures; blue sclera; loose joints and skin; progressive deafness	Orthopedic repair of fractures; supportive
Phenylke-tonuria	Autosomal recessive	Deficiency of phenylalanine hydroxylase	Blond hair; blue eyes, fair skin; eczema; mental retardation; seizures; bizarre behavior	Diet low in phenylalanine; supportive
Retino-blastoma	Autosomal dominant	Malignant tumor of retina	Onset before age 2 years; cat's eye reflex; strabismus; red, painful eye, often with glaucoma; blindness	Radiation therapy; enucleation
Severe combined immune deficiency	Autosomal recessive, X-linked recessive	Deficiency in T, B cells, cell-mediated immunity, antibody	Marked susceptibility to infection; failure to thrive	Bone marrow transplantation; supportive
Sickle cell anemia	Autosomal dominant	Abnormal hemoglobin structure (Hb S instead of Hb A); deoxygenation produces changes in red blood cell shape that cause these cells to obstruct blood flow in small vessels; destruction of sickled cells	Presence of characteristic sickle-shaped red blood cells; chronic hemolytic anemia; episodes of pain from tissue ischemia caused by occlusion of small blood vessels; symptoms directly related to tissues and organs involved	Supportive; no definitive treatment; palliative therapy during acute attacks
Tay-Sachs disease (amaurotic familial idiocy)	Autosomal recessive	Deficiency of hexosaminidase; defect in synthesis of gangliosides	Predominantly in Ashkenazi Jews; progressive neurologic deterioration; blindness, cherry-red spot in macula; early death	Supportive
Thalassemias	Autosomal recessive	Impaired protein synthesis of hemoglobin that results in shortened red blood cell survival time	Severe, fatal anemia in major forms; most do not survive childhood	Palliative; blood transfusion and sometimes splenectomy; supportive
Tyrosinosis	Autosomal recessive	Deficiency of p-hydroxyphenylpyruvic acid oxidase	Hepatosplenomegaly	Supportive
Vitamin D–resistant rickets (hypophos-phatemic)	Autosomal recessive, autosomal dominant, X-linked dominant (?)	Defect in phosphate reabsorption in renal tubules	Rachitic symptoms; retarded linear growth	Calciferol; administration of phosphorus; megadoses of vitamin D, with care to avoid toxic effects
von Gierke disease	Autosomal recessive (?)	Deficiency of G-6-PD; inability to reconvert glycogen to glucose	Hepatomegaly; vomiting; hypoglycemia; convulsions; coma; usually early death	High-protein diet; supportive; no definitive therapy
von Wille-brand disease	Autosomal dominant	Deficiency of portion of blood factor VIII molecule	Prolonged bleeding time; bleeding from mucous membranes; increased bruising	Administration of cryoprecipitates

Table 5-4 Partial list of single-gene disorders—cont'd

DISEASE	INHERITANCE	BASIC DEFECT	MANIFESTATIONS	THERAPY
Werdnig-Hoffmann disease	Autosomal recessive	Unknown; atrophy of anterior horn cells in spinal cord and motor nuclei in brainstem	Onset before age 2 years and usually apparent at birth; "floppy" infant; lies in frog position; fatal in childhood—the earlier the onset, the earlier death occurs	Symptomatic; supportive
Wilson disease	Autosomal recessive	Deficiency of plasma protein ceruloplasmin; disturbed copper metabolism	Progressive lenticular degeneration with neurologic deterioration; cirrhosis of liver; renal calculi	Administration of copper chelating agent penicillamine
Wiscott-Aldrich syndrome	X-linked recessive	Deficiency of T, some B cells; decreased cell-mediated immunity, antibody	Bleeding in infancy; recurrent infection; eczema	Platelet transfusion, immune globulin, antibiotics; supportive

Variation in Gene Action

Several factors influence the way in which genes behave or are manifest. The most notable of these is *mutation*. The genetic material, although remarkably stable, is subject to structural or chemical alteration, but when the genetic material changes, the mutant gene remains unchanged and is transmitted to future generations.

Mutations usually occur naturally *(spontaneous)*, or can be *induced* by a variety of external agents, or *mutagens*, including temperature, certain chemicals, and radiation. Other factors may influence gene mutation. For example, the incidence of mutation increases with parental age, especially that of the father. This phenomenon is most apparent in the autosomal dominant disorders.

A number of other variables are observed in many disorders that modify the basic inheritance patterns. The degree to which a gene exerts its effect or the differences in effects that a given gene may produce sometimes appear to contradict the established concepts of inheritance and, again, are more apparent in dominant disorders. These include:

penetrance The regularity with which an inherited trait is manifest in the person who carries the gene. When a gene produces its effect on the phenotype each time it is present in the genotype, it is said to be *fully penetrant* or to exhibit *complete penetrance*. For example, achondroplasia (a form of dwarfism) is always evident whenever the gene is present. If a trait is not recognized in a person who carries the responsible gene, it is said to be *nonpenetrant* in that individual. This phenomenon accounts for what appears to be skipped generations. For instance, retinoblastoma, a tumor of the retina, is 80% penetrant because 20% of the children who carry the gene do not develop the tumor (Cohen, 1984). (See p. 1608 for further discussion of the various genetic causes of retinoblastoma.)

variable expressivity The degree of severity of, or the variability in, the manifestations seen in persons of a particular genotype. For instance, polydactyly can be expressed as any number of extra digits, or the extra digits may be fingers in one generation and toes in another. The severity of a disorder may be so mild as to be almost undetected or so severe that the affected individual is totally incapacitated.

pleiotropy The multiple, different, and seemingly unrelated effects associated with a particular disorder; the varied clinical features that constitute a syndrome. For example, Marfan syndrome, a disorder of the elastic fibers of connective tissue, may be manifest in an individual by any or all of the symptoms associated with it—aortic aneurysm, dislocation of the optic lens, or any of a number of skeletal deformities.

linkage Some genes are located too closely together on a chromosome, so that they segregate and migrate together during cell division, and therefore, the characteristics they produce always appear together in the phenotype.

heterogeneity The same or similar manifestations that result from (1) different mutant genes at the same location on a chromosome or (2) from mutant genes at different locations on a chromosome (such as the hemophilias that produce defects in coagulation and the muscular dystrophies that produce muscular weakness but which exhibit different inheritance patterns).

Autosomal Inheritance Patterns

The major inheritance patterns are described with stylized models indicating the mendelian ratios that can be predicted in each type. Because there are 44 autosomes and only two sex chromosomes, the majority of hereditary disorders are a result of defective genes on an autosome.

Autosomal dominant inheritance. Characteristics of a condition caused by a dominant gene on an autosome include the following (Fig. 5-6):

1. Males and females are affected with equal frequency.
2. Affected individuals will have an affected parent (unless the condition is caused by a fresh mutation).
3. Half the children of a heterozygous affected parent will possess the defective gene, although it may be nonpenetrant.
4. Unaffected children of affected parents will have unaffected children (unless the gene is nonpenetrant).

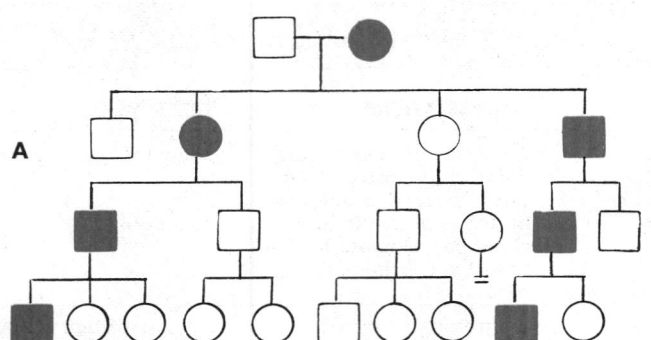

Fig. 5-6. Autosomal dominant inheritance pattern occurring in four generations. **A,** Pedigree chart. **B,** Possible offspring of mating between normal parent and one with autosomal dominant trait.

5. Traits can be traced vertically through previous generations—a positive family history.

Usually the first case in a family appears suddenly as the result of a fresh mutation and, depending on the degree of disability the condition imposes on the individual, will either die out or continue to be passed on through several generations. Incomplete penetrance is common, and there is wide variability in expression. The basic defect, probably a structural protein, is unknown in most autosomal dominant disorders; therefore, screening of undetected persons, including prenatal diagnosis, is usually not possible. Later onset is common. Examples of an autosomal-dominant disorder include achondroplasia, polydactyly, and Marfan syndrome.

Autosomal recessive inheritance. Characteristics of a condition caused by a recessive gene on an autosome include the following (Fig. 5-7):

1. Males and females are affected with equal frequency.
2. Affected individuals will have unaffected parents who are heterozygous for the trait.
3. There is a one in four chance that any child of two unaffected heterozygous parents will be affected.
4. Two affected parents will have affected children exclusively.
5. Affected individuals married to unaffected individuals will have normal children, all of whom will be carriers.
6. There is usually no evidence of the trait in previous generations—a negative family history.

Children who display an autosomal recessive disorder will always be homozygous for that trait. The heterozygous person, with only one gene for a rare recessive disorder, remains undetected in the population. It is estimated that each person carries from three to eight genes for such a severe genetic disease. However the probability of mating between two persons who carry the same gene is highly unlikely. If they are blood relatives the likelihood is increased. The chances are also increased if the mating occurs between persons who select a mate because of geographic, ethnic, or religious restrictions. For example, there is a higher risk that Ashkenazi Jews will be carriers of the gene for Tay-Sachs disease. The age of onset for autosomal recessive disorders is early, and, because they are usually biochemical defects, heterzygote detection and prenatal diagnosis are often possible. Examples of an autosomal recessive disorder include cystic fibrosis, phenylketonuria, and galactosemia.

X-Linked Inheritance Patterns

Genes on the X chromosome differ from those on the Y chromosome; therefore, the transmission of traits caused by these genes will vary according to the sex of the individual who carries the gene. The two X chromosomes in the female are alike in gene constitution, with two genes for each trait. Genes on the X chromosome have no counterpart on the Y chromosome; therefore a characteristic determined by a gene on the X chromosome is *always* expressed in the male. One of the most significant aspects of X-linked inheritance is the absence of father-to-son transmission. Although it is essential for development of the male phenotype, the Y chromosome carries no known medically significant characteristics.

X-linked dominant inheritance. Characteristics of a condition caused by a dominant gene on an X chromosome include the following (Fig. 5-8):

1. Affected individuals will have an affected parent.
2. All the daughters but none of the sons of an affected male will be affected.
3. Half the sons and half the daughters of an affected female will be affected.
4. Normal children of an affected parent will have normal offspring.
5. There are no carriers.
6. The inheritance pattern shows a positive family history.

Superficially this pattern resembles an autosomal dominant inheritance pattern. This type of inheritance is relatively uncommon, and because the effects in the male are severe and usually fatal, transmission of the gene takes place primarily in the female. An example of an X-linked dominant disorder is hypophosphatemic vitamin D–resistant rickets.

X-linked recessive inheritance. Characteristics of a disorder caused by a recessive gene on the X chromosome include the following (Fig. 5-9):

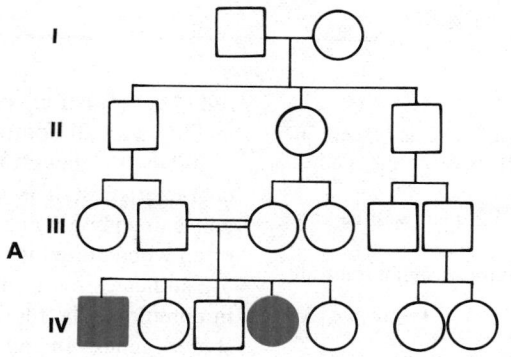

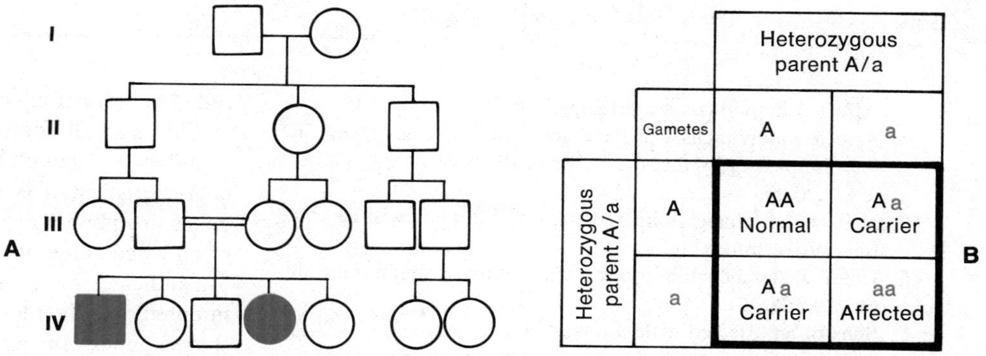

Fig. 5-7. Autosomal recessive inheritance pattern. **A,** Pedigree chart. **B,** Possible offspring of mating between two parents with recessive gene on an autosome.

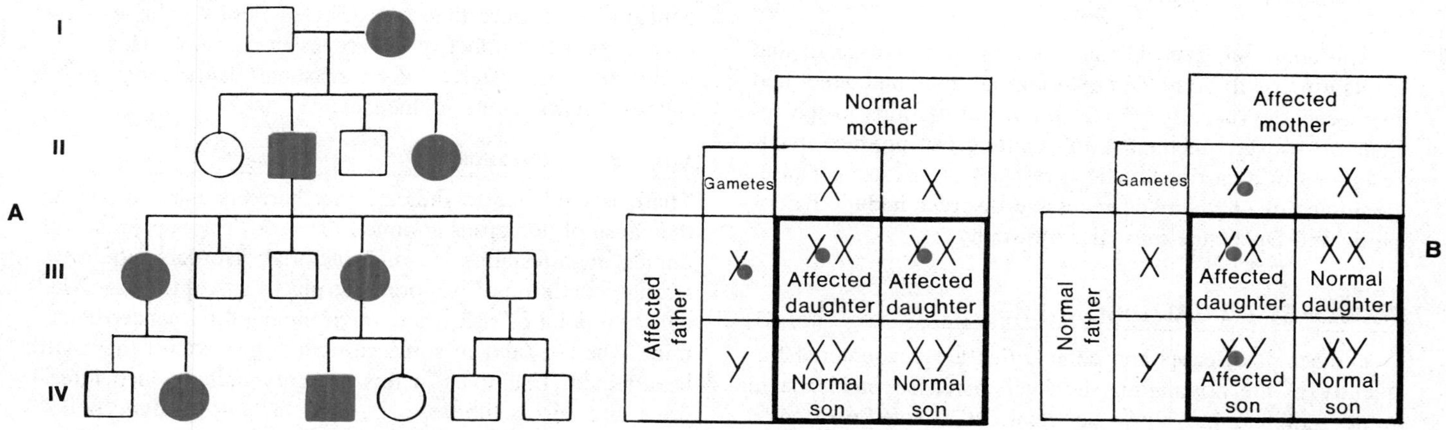

	Heterozygous parent A/a	
Gametes	A	a
A	AA Normal	Aa Carrier
a	Aa Carrier	aa Affected

(left side label: Heterozygous parent A/a)

B

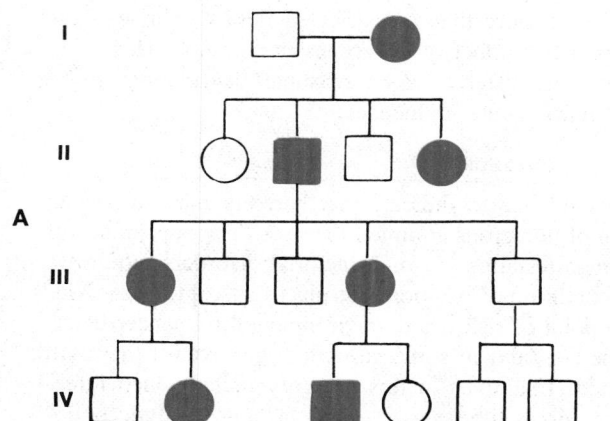

A

	Normal mother	
Gametes	X	X
X (●)	XX ● Affected daughter	XX ● Affected daughter
Y	XY Normal son	XY Normal son

(left label: Affected father)

	Affected mother	
Gametes	X ●	X
X	XX ● Affected daughter	XX Normal daughter
Y	XY ● Affected son	XY Normal son

(left label: Normal father)

B

Fig. 5-8. X-linked dominant inheritance pattern. **A,** Pedigree chart. **B,** Sex differences in offspring ratios in X-linked dominant inheritance. ● = Dominant allele on X chromosome.

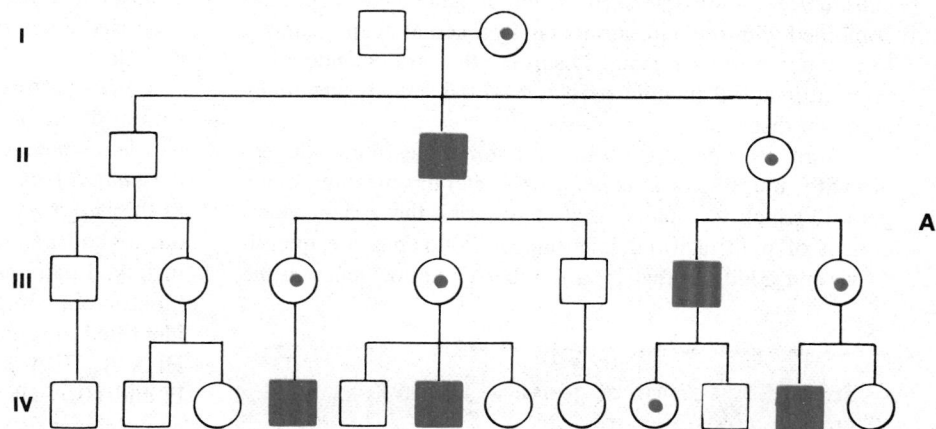

A

Fig. 5-9. X-linked recessive inheritance pattern. **A,** Pedigree chart. **B,** Sex differences in offspring ratios in X-linked recessive inheritance. ○ = Recessive allele on X chromosome.

	Normal mother	
Gametes	X	X
X ○	XX ○ Carrier daughter	XX ○ Carrier daughter
Y	XY Normal son	XY Normal son

(left label: Affected father)

	Carrier mother	
Gametes	X	X ○
X	XX Normal daughter	XX ○ Carrier daughter
Y	XY Normal son	XY ○ Affected son

(left label: Normal father)

B

1. Affected individuals are principally males.
2. Affected individuals will have unaffected parents (except in the rare possibility that the father is affected and the mother is a carrier).
3. Half of the female siblings of an affected male will be carriers of the trait.
4. Unaffected male siblings of an affected male cannot transmit the disorder.
5. Sons of an affected male are unaffected.
6. Daughters of an affected male are carriers.
7. The unaffected male children of a carrier female do not transmit the disorder.

The abnormal gene behaves as any recessive gene; that is, its effect will be hidden by a normal dominant gene, and two genes are usually present for manifestations in the female. However, unequal X inactivation can produce manifestations in a carrier female. Fresh mutations are not rare. Examples of an X-linked recessive disorder include hemophilia and Duchenne muscular dystrophy.

MULTIFACTORIAL DISORDERS

A number of diseases and defects that are encountered frequently in the population show an increased incidence in some families, but show no clear-cut affected-unaffected classification. Although the incidence is higher than would be expected by chance, no specific mode of inheritance can be identified. In some, environmental factors appear to play an important role. These are the conditions classified as *multifactorial*—disorders in which a genetic susceptibilty combined with the appropriate environmental agents interact to produce a disease state. Disorders that are considered to be multifactorial include most congenital defects and many common diseases.

A term used in relation to, and sometimes interchangeably with, multifactorial is *polygenic* (literally meaning many genes), which is usually used to describe the genetic component of multifactorial inheritance. Polygenes are quantitative and additive; that is, a number of minor genes in the

right combination produce a given characteristic—each making a small contribution to the total effect.

When the laws of inheritance are applied to polygenic characteristics, it is expected that relatives will have more genes in common and that these genes will be expressed more often when united with a similar combination of genes. Table 5-5 indicates the proportion of genes that relatives can have in common. The more distant the relationship, the fewer the shared genes. In families where there is an increased incidence of a disorder, the frequency in first-degree relatives may be 3 to 15 times that in the population as a whole. The appearance of more than one affected family member indicates a greater number of polygenes in common. However, socioeconomic differences or seasonal distribution might suggest environmental influences.

Common Diseases

There is evidence to indicate that heredity plays a role in the cause of numerous common diseases. The appearance of clinical manifestations in multifactorial disorders requires a strong genetic predisposition that places susceptible individuals at a point of risk where environmental influences determine whether (and in some cases to what extent) they will be affected. Examples in this category include such infectious diseases as tuberculosis, rubeola, and paralytic poliomyelitis. In some diseases a genetic trait can be identified. For example, the development of peptic ulcer occurs more frequently in persons with type O blood; however, environmental stresses are also important etiologic factors. Other diseases with multifactorial causes include diabetes mellitus, psoriasis, many of the juvenile osteochondroses, and schizophrenia.

HLA system. The inherited histocompatibility antigens, similar to the blood group antigens, have been implicated in the development of many diseases. These antigens, termed the *human leukocyte antigen* (HLA) system and also known as the *major histocompatibility complex* (MHC), are present on the cell membrane of almost all body cells. They occur in linked pairs and are inherited in the same manner as the blood group antigens. A number of these antigens have been identified and have been classified as follows: class 1—the HLA-A, HLA-B, and HLA-C antigens; class 2—the HLA-D and HLA-DR (D-related) antigens; and class 3—certain complement factors with genes in the HLA region.

A relationship between the HLA system has been shown for several disorders, for example, insulin-dependent diabetes mellitus, hemochromatosis, psoriasis vulgaris, celiac disease, myasthenia gravis, and several forms of arthritis. Most notable is the striking association between HLA-B27 and idiopathic ankylosing spondylitis in 90% to 95% of affected persons. Although significant associations have been identified in only a few disorders, risk estimates can be determined regarding the frequency with which one of these diseases develops in an individual carrying a specific HLA antigen compared with the frequency of the disease in persons who do not carry the HLA antigen.

Table 5-5   Portion of genes in common in various relationships

RELATIONSHIP	PROPORTION OF GENES IN COMMON
First-degree relatives	
Parent, child, sibling	½
Second-degree relatives	
Grandparent, grandchild, uncle, aunt, nephew, niece, half-sibling	¼
Third-degree relatives	
First cousins	⅛
Second cousins	1/32

Drug sensitivity. Drug sensitivity of varying degrees is very common; some people are sensitive to the effects of a given drug, whereas others are resistant. Pharmacogenetics is that branch of genetics concerned with drug responses and their genetic modification. In many drug-sensitive persons a mode of inheritance can be identified, but the disease is not manifest unless the individual is exposed to the drug in question. Examples of disorders precipitated by contact with a drug are malignant hyperthermia, which occurs in some anesthetized patients; the porphyrias, in which symptoms are produced by exposure to alcohol or certain drugs; and glucose-6-phosphate dehydrogenase (G-6-PD) deficiency, in which affected persons develop a hemolytic crisis when they take certain drugs, are exposed to naphthalene mothballs, or ingest fava beans.

A number of persons show a resistance or sensitivity to certain drugs. For example, there is a genetically related ability of some persons to resist the anticoagulant coumadin and for some individuals to metabolize the antituberculin drug isoniazid more slowly than others. Many other disorders display altered responses to therapeutic agents, such as occurs with phenylketonuria and catecholamines, Down syndrome and atropine, and familial dysautonomia and norepinephrine.

Congenital Anomalies

Congenital anomalies, or birth defects, are errors of morphogenic development present at birth. They can arise at any stage of development and present wide variability in determining factors as well as in type, extent, and frequency of defects. The development of an organism, especially during embryogenesis, is an intricate process in which all parts must be properly integrated to ensure a coordinated whole. The rate must be such that one part is ready when needed by another part; otherwise, either part may cease to grow or may deviate from its normal path. Some defects result when a state, present in one phase of development as a normal condition, persists into another phase as abnormal. For example, a cleft lip is normal in a young embryo and a patent ductus arteriosus is essential during fetal life. Any agent that interferes with these complex processes will produce a defect in development ranging in severity from an insignificant local anomaly to complete degeneration.

A few congenital defects are clearly caused by a single gene, some are associated with chromosomal abnormalities, and others are produced by known intrauterine environmental factors. However many of the more common and severe defects (e.g., cleft lip and palate, pyloric stenosis, central nervous system malformations, cataracts, and congenital heart disease) appear to be consistent with polygenic inheritance.

Nongenetic factors can produce a congenital anomaly that imitates, or is indistinguishable from, one genetically determined. Such a condition is termed a *phenocopy*. For example, deafness, hypothyroidism, and cataracts can all be caused by mutant genes, but they may also be caused by exogenous agents. Deafness can be a result of a number of different agents, rubella virus can cause congenital cataracts, and lack of iodine in a child can produce hypothyroidism.

In addition, many single-gene and chromosome abnormalities have a physical or mental defect as a clinical manifestation. Some of these include cleft lip and palate, clubfoot, congenital dislocated hip, congenital heart defects, and mental retardation. Assigning a cause of mental retardation presents a particularly difficult problem. Mental retardation is a manifestation of a variety of syndromes, both single-gene and chromosomal, and numerous environmental agents are known to be damaging to brain tissue, for example, lack of oxygen as a result of anesthesia or drugs during labor and delivery. For these reasons it is extremely important that such exogenous factors be ruled out before any given congenital defect is labeled hereditary.

Because of the steady decline in infant mortality from other causes, congenital anomalies are responsible for an ever-increasing proportion of all deaths in infancy and constitute an increasing proportion of infants requiring intensive newborn care. Many defects, such as cleft lip, deformed limbs, or meningomyelocele, are readily apparent in the newborn infant; others, such as congenital heart disease or absent kidney, may not become evident until days, weeks, or even years after birth. Some defects are of such minor significance that they have little or no effect on survival or the quality of life; others are so severe as to be incompatible with life or are a serious threat to survival. There is also a high correlation between the incidence of congenital anomalies and the infant who is small for gestational age. The more severe the growth retardation, the more likely the chance for abnormal development.

Classification. Congenital anomalies constitute such a large and heterogeneous group of defects that are so variable in type and causation that there has been no satisfactory method for classifying them. It is now recommended that congenital defects be classified from a pathogenic orientation that reflects the probable processes leading to abnormal development. The classification recognizes both heredity and environmentally induced errors of morphogenesis and provides more acurate and descriptive terminology. Following are terms used to describe the various alterations of form or structure (Spranger and others, 1982):

malformation A morphogenic defect of an organ, part of an organ, or larger region of the body resulting from an intrinsically abnormal developmental process. Examples of malformations are clawhand and polydactyly.

disruption A morphologic defect of an organ, part of an organ, or a larger region of the body resulting from the extrinsic breakdown of or interference with an originally normal developmental process. Classic examples of disruptions are the limb deficiencies caused by thalidomide and the defects caused by maternal rubella infection.

deformation An abnormal form, shape, or position of a part of the body caused by mechanical forces. An example of a deformation is the equinovarus foot, which may be the result of intrauterine crowding or lower limb paralysis caused by a meningomyelocele.

dysplasia An abnormal organization of cells into tissue(s) and its morphologic result(s), that is, the process and the consequences of dyshistogenesis. For example, the defects of osteogenesis imperfecta will affect all the bones in the body.

General terminology applied to defects of morphogenesis helps to further describe the anomalies:

agenesis Absence of a body part caused by absence of the primordial tissue, or anlage.

aplasia Absence of a body part caused by failure of the normal primordia to develop.

atrophy Decreased development of a mass of tissue or an organ as a result of a decrease in cell size or number.

hyperplasia, hypoplasia The overdevelopment or underdevelopment of an organ or tissue that results from an increase or decrease in the number of cells.

hypotrophy, hypertrophy A decrease of or increase in the size of organs, tissues, or cells.

pathogenesis The mechanisms leading to an abnormal structure, form, or function.

Multiple anomalies are not uncommon and tend to appear together in patterns or relationships. The following terms describe the type of relationship and the probable cause or genesis of the patterns of morphogenic defects (Spranger and others, 1982):

polytropic field defect A pattern of anomalies derived from the disturbance of a single developmental field. A developmental field is a region or part of an embryo that responds as a coordinated unit to embryonic interaction, that is, the influence of one developmental tissue on another. Examples of fields are the midline and the limbs.

sequence A pattern of multiple anomalies derived from a single known or presumed prior anomaly or mechanical factor. For example, the meningomyelocele sequence of lower limb paralysis, muscle wasting, clubfoot, incontinence, urinary tract infection, and renal damage.

syndrome A pattern of multiple anomalies thought to be pathogenetically related and not known to represent a single sequence or a polytropic field defect, for example, Down syndrome or Marfan syndrome.

association A nonrandom occurrence in two or more individuals of multiple anomalies not known to be a polytropic field defect, sequence, or syndrome. An example is the simultaneous occurrence of kidney defects and low-set ears.

THERAPEUTIC MANAGEMENT OF GENETIC DISEASE

There is no cure for genetic disease at present, although preventive and corrective therapy is helping to reduce the harmful effects in an increasing number of conditions. Genetic research is making progress in the art of altering the genetic material directly. Meanwhile the major goal of therapy is modification of the internal or external environment to correct or minimize the effects of the genetic defect.

Therapeutic Modalities

The therapeutic modalities available for genetic disorders are few when compared with the infinite variety of conditions afflicting the population, but with increased understanding of the basic defects and the technical advances being made, an increasing number are becoming amenable to treatment.

Surgical repair. Surgical repair of structural defects has made it possible to prolong life in a number of multifactorial disorders, such as congenital heart disease and pyloric stenosis. Numerous facial and limb deformities can be altered by plastic and reconstructive techniques. In cases of familial polyposis coli, surgical removal of the colon eliminates the countless polyps that invariably become cancerous. Splenectomy prevents the trapping of abnormal blood cells in that organ in several hereditary disorders of red blood cells. Early diagnosis and enucleation in retinoblastoma have reduced the mortality from this dreaded eye tumor.

In the last few years there has been some interest in fetal surgery for some life-threatening anomalies, particularly urinary tract abnormalities. Although some procedures are possible, such as decompression of the hydronephrotic kidney or hydrocephalic ventricles, the Council on Scientific Affairs of the American Medical Association has issued a resolution that emphasizes the need for further animal experimentation before the practice can be considered safe and beneficial.

Diet modification. In disorders in which an enzyme deficiency causes a toxic accumulation of a substance or its by-products, restricting the intake of foods containing the offending substance often prevents irreversible damage from the improper metabolism of these compounds. Examples include the low-phenylalanine diet prescribed for children with phenylketonuria, elimination of dairy products containing lactose for infants and children with hereditary lactase deficiency, avoidance of foods containing or producing galactose for children with galactosemia, and a diet low in branched-chain amino acids for infants and children with maple syrup urine disease.

Product replacement. In some deficiency diseases, supplying the missing product that cannot be synthesized prevents undesirable effects. For example, thyroid extract is prescribed to prevent the damaging effects of hypothyroidism, and providing the missing blood factors prevents life-threatening and debilitating hemorrhages in the hemophilias. Other examples are insulin for diabetes mellitus, growth hormone for pituitary dwarfism, and corticosteroids for adrenogenital syndrome.

Avoidance of drugs or other substances. In drug-induced disease, such as glucose-6-phosphate dehydrogenase (G-6-PD) deficiency and the porphyrias, avoidance of the drugs that precipitate a reaction provide a simple preventive measure.

Removal of toxic substances. Removal of toxic substances that accumulate in vital tissues as a result of a hereditary disease can prevent disabling complications. Some of the deleterious effects of hemochromatosis, a hereditary disorder characterized by an excess accumulation of iron in the liver, heart, and pancreas, can be reduced with the removal of iron by periodic venisection. Excess copper that accumulates in the liver and brain in Wilson disease can be removed by administration of chelating agents.

Immunologic prevention. The administration of immunoglobulin to Rh-negative mothers following birth of an Rh-positive infant is effective in preventing Rh-antibody formation that causes hemolytic disease of the newborn in subsequent births.

Transplantation. Replacement of nonfunctioning organs with normal organs is increasing the survival of children with defective organs because the problems of tissue incompatibility are better controlled. Examples of organ transplants include kidneys in hereditary polycystic kidneys, heart in severe cardiac myopathy, liver in hepatic atresia, pancreas in diabetes mellitus, and bone marrow in hereditary diseases affecting the blood-forming organs, such as thalassemia.

Cofactor administration. Diet supplements can be given when the body is unable to synthesize or effectively use some substances needed as cofactors in metabolism, such as vitamin B_{12} in pernicious anemia, in which absorption of this vitamin is impaired.

Recombinant DNA. The transfer of modified genetic material from one organism (a virus) to another causes the viral DNA to become integrated into the cellular DNA of the recipient cell. This recombinant DNA multiplies, producing the missing substance (such as insulin) in the cells of the recipient.

Gene transfer. Fragments of DNA from a normal gene can be introduced directly into a recipient cell lacking such a gene. This approach has been attempted in humans with the transfer of normal gene copies of beta hemoglobin into bone marrow cells in an effort to treat a form of beta thalassemia. It may also hold promise in sickle cell anemia.

Other therapies. Other methods such as enzyme repression and competitive inhibition are providing effective treatment in some metabolic disorders. Future therapies include the possibility of replacement or stabilization by injection or oral administration of a substance that the patient lacks.

Environmental Manipulation

Inherited diseases or defects for which there is no therapeutic modality can be modified to enhance the quality of life for the affected individual. Some examples of environmental manipulation include hearing aids for deaf children, glasses or vision enhancers such as enlarged print and books in braille for the visually impaired, mobilizing devices such as braces and wheelchairs for persons with muscle and bone impairment, prosthetic devices for limb deficiencies, and infant stimulation programs to maximize the potential of mentally retarded children.

GENETICS AND SOCIETY

There is no doubt that diseases constitute a significant portion of world health problems, and the advantages of improving the human race are seldom questioned. Controversy exists, however, between those who advocate improvement in the species by selective breeding and those who recommend providing a better environment. Improvement of the race through altering the genetic makeup of the individual is termed *eugenics;* improvement of the human race by modifying the environment is called *euthenics.*

Eugenics

Eugenics is essentially planned breeding designed to alter future generations. Such practice has been successfully used for many years by animal and plant breeders in developing superior food products. For many persons any discussion of controlling heredity creates visions of Hitler's interpretation and misuse of directed evolution, some racial groups view it as the code word for genocide, and religious groups protest that it is tampering with God's creation. Eugenics can be further segregated into *positive eugenics* and *negative eugenics.*

Positive eugenics. Positive eugenics is the attempt to encourage reproduction among individuals who are considered to possess superior or beneficial characteristics. Suggested means for accomplishing this purpose include selected mating of individuals who are considered to possess superior traits. Other methods are the establishment of sperm banks, with sperm from a small, select number of donors to be frozen and used to impregnate a large number of suitable women, and the production, asexually, of replicas of desirable persons by cloning (replacing the cell nucleus of a fertilized ovum with the nucleus of a cell from the desired individual; asexual reproduction). Some of the qualifications considered superior might be physical characteristics, socially desirable behavior, and superior intellect, as well as absence of genetically determined defects or disease.

Questions and Controversies

Should society allow a couple to have children when one or both have a severely disabling condition known to be hereditary that inhibits or impairs their ability to function?

In order to solve such a dilemma a number of issues need to be addressed. How is the competence or incompetence of the involved family to be determined (Kilpack, 1985)? Do all persons have the same right to procreate as persons without a physical or mental disability? If society is to have a voice in such decisions, society will need to determine what constitutes a "disabling condition." Who will determine whether a condition is disabling (physicians, lawyers, politicians)? How will such a decision be enforced (Kilpack, 1985)?

Questions and Controversies

Should parents be permitted prenatal diagnosis for sex determination unrelated to X-linked disease?

Prenatal ultrasonography and chromosome analysis from amniotic fluid allow determination of sex before birth. It has long been employed for detecting sex in carrier mothers at risk of passing a sex-linked disorder to a male offspring. Parents are also informed of the sex of the fetus when amniocentesis is performed to rule out a chromosome anomaly or some other undesirable disorder. The technique could easily be employed for sex determination alone. To date, the long-term effects on society if parents are allowed to selectively terminate a pregnancy with a fetus of the "wrong sex" are unknown. However, it is well-known that a male is the preferred firstborn (Fletcher, 1979).

Negative eugenics. Negative eugenics is the discouragement or prohibition of reproduction among individuals who are considered to be physically or mentally handicapped. Voluntary or legal prohibition of reproduction by persons with these characteristics might be accomplished with marriage laws, sterilization, and abortion. The arguments for and against the relative merits and objections of eugenics will continue for years to come.

Euthenics

An opposite point of view is taken by those who support euthenics, which advocates the modification of the environment to allow the genetically abnormal individual to live a relatively normal life. Examples of euthenic measures are prescription glasses for nearsighted persons and special schools for the deaf. Medical treatments such as special diets for children with inborn errors of metabolism, hormone replacement such as insulin for diabetic persons and thyroid for persons with cretinism, and special orthopedic appliances and prosthetic devices can be considered environmental manipulation. Providing better nutrition and home environment for children during the growing stages and educational and social stimulation are prime examples of euthenics.

Prenatal Influences on Health

The period from conception to birth is the most mysterious and least known phase of the life cycle. It is the period when the fewest outside demands are placed on the organism, but at the same time it is fraught with dangers that may have lifelong consequences. Recognition of the tremendous importance of this period of rapid growth and change has focused interest on fetal development, the relationship between prenatal events and infant health, and the factors that influence the well-being of the individual during this and subsequent stages of life.

PRENATAL DEVELOPMENT

When they begin their existence, human beings bear no resemblance to the complex organisms into which they will develop. In fact, during the very early stages they are indistinguishable from any other animal species. The early zygote contains no structures that remotely correspond to any of the organs and tissues that will make up the fully developed individual. Development consists of two distinct but interrelated processes: growth and differentiation.

Fetal Growth

Growth results when cells divide and synthesize new proteins and is reflected in increased size and weight. It is accomplished by two mechanisms: (1) *hyperplasia*, an increase in cell numbers, and (2) *hypertrophy*, an increase in cell size. Hyperplasia is the predominant form of growth during the embryonic period; although the rate decreases during later stages of gestation, cell division continues in

---

Table 5-6 Milestones in human development before birth

4 WEEKS	8 WEEKS	12 WEEKS	16 WEEKS
External appearance			
Body flexed, C-shaped	Body fairly well formed	Nails appearing	Head still dominant but erect
Arm and leg buds present	Nose flat, eyes far apart	Resembles human	Face looks human
Head at right angles to body	Digits well formed	Head erect but disproportionately large	Eyes, ears, and nose approach typical appearance on gross examination
	Head elevating	Skin pink, delicate	Arm/leg ratio proportionate
	Tail almost disappeared		Scalp hair appears
	Eyes, ears, nose, and mouth recognizable		Rapid growth
			Skin red and transparent
			Motor activity present
Crown-to-rump measurement (cm)			
0.4-0.5	2.5-3	6-8	11.5-13.5

variable degrees throughout childhood. Hypertrophy is more prominent during later periods of growth.

There is a growth pattern that is typical for each organ and tissue, but all organs progress from a stage characterized by increase in cell number to one of growth by increase in cell size. If there is interference with the growth pattern of an organ, the overall result is a reduction in the size and weight of that organ. However the consequences of the inhibiting factor depend on whether the insult is inflicted during a period of hyperplasia or a period of hypertrophy. Interruption of growth during cell enlargement is usually only temporary and can be overcome with proper intervention. Interference with growth during a period of cell proliferation is likely to cause irreversible growth retardation of that organ with permanent deficit in overall cell numbers.

The overall prenatal growth pattern shows that the most rapid gain in length precedes the gain in weight. The most rapid linear growth takes place during mid–fetal life; the most rapid gain in weight occurs in late fetal life.

Differentiation

Differentiation is the process by which early cells are systematically modified and specialized to form all the tissues that are necessary to assure an organized, coordinated individual. It is accomplished by various mechanisms (controlled mitotic division, shifts in intracellular activity, tissue movement [migration], increase in size, increase in number, controlled cellular death, aggregation of like cells, and inductive interaction between different tissues) in a specified, sequential order. Each step in the differentiation process depends on successful completion of a previous step. Anything that interferes with one of these steps, such as a mutant gene or environmental agent, will cause an arrest in the development of that particular tissue or organ. Divergence from the normal course of development will result in maldevelopment of a part or, if it occurs at an early age, a sequence of distortions causing more severe or multiple malformations.

There appears to be a relationship between the incidence of one congenital anomaly and the presence of additional anomalies in an affected child. For example, there is a striking association between malformed ears and kidney abnormalities that reflects a common developmental stage. The knowledge of the stage of development for a variety of organs and systems provides a valuable clue for the examiner. When one defect is observed, closer scrutiny may reveal defects in another organ or system related to the same stage of development.

Organogenesis

The first 8 to 12 weeks of fetal life are particularly critical to the survival of the organism. During this time of extremely rapid development and change, the beginnings of all major organ systems are formed, and the embryo begins to acquire the specific functions needed to integrate these organs and organ systems into an organized, coordinated whole. This is also the period during which the organism is most vulnerable to environmental hazards.

The overview of the major changes in the development of organs and systems outlined in Table 5-6 provides some indication of the anatomic and physiologic characteristics present in an infant born at various stages of gestation. Although growth and development are proportionately greater in the early weeks, the rate is somewhat uneven and variable.

MULTIPLE BIRTHS

A deviation in early development that occurs with variable frequency is multiple births. Twins are not uncommon in the population, but triplets are rare and quadruplets or quintuplets are extremely unusual. In any of these situations the offspring can be of the like or unlike sex, that is, derived from a single ovum, from multiple ova, or a combination of the two, which can involve one or more cell divisions. The cause of twinning is unknown, but the increase in the num-

20 WEEKS	24 WEEKS	28 WEEKS	32 WEEKS	36 WEEKS	40 WEEKS
Vernix caseosa appears Lanugo hair appears Legs lengthen considerably Sebaceous glands appear	Body lean but fairly proportioned Skin red and wrinkled Vernix caseosa present Sweat glands forming	Lean body, less wrinkled and red Nails appear	Subcutaneous fat beginning to collect More rounded appearance Skin pink and smooth Has assumed delivery position	Skin pink, body rounded General lanugo disappearing Body usually plump	Skin smooth and pink; copious vernix caseosa Moderate to profuse hair Lanugo on shoulders and upper body only Nasal and alar cartilage apparent
16-18.5	23	27	31	35	40

Continued.

Table 5-6 Milestones in human development before birth—cont'd

	4 WEEKS	8 WEEKS	12 WEEKS	16 WEEKS
Approximate weight (g)	0.4	2	19	100
Musculoskeletal system All somites present		First indication of ossification—occiput, mandible, and humerus Fetus capable of some movement; definitive muscles of trunk, limbs, and head well represented	Some bones well outlined; ossification spreading Upper cervical to lower sacral arches and bodies ossify Smooth muscle layers indicated in hollow viscera	Most bones distinctly indicated throughout body—outline of fetal skeleton visible on radiographs Legs well developed Joint cavities appear Muscular movements can be detected
Circulatory system Heart develops; double chambers visible; begins to beat Aortic arches and major veins completed Primitive plasma begins to circulate		Main blood vessels assume final plan Enucleated red cells predominate in blood	Blood forming in marrow and begins in spleen	Heart muscle well developed Blood formation alive in spleen
Gastrointestinal system Stomach at midline and fusiform Conspicuous liver Esophagus short Intestine a short tube		Intestinal villi developing Small intestines coil within umbilical cord Palatal folds present Liver very large—begins to synthesize and store chemicals and new blood cells Digestive juices forming	Bile secreted Palatal fusion complete Intestines have withdrawn from cord and assume characteristic positions Swallowing movements detectable	Meconium in bowel Some enzyme secretion Anus open Functional gastrointestinal tract Liver synthesizes fatty acids and begins to store carbohydrate Swallowing and sucking present
Respiratory system Primary lung buds appear		Pleural and pericardial cavities forming Branching bronchioles Nostrils closed by epithelial plugs	Lungs acquire definite shape Vocal cords appear Respiratory movements detectable	Elastic fibers appear in lungs Terminal and respiratory bronchioles appear Frequent respiratory movements
Renal system Rudimentary ureteric buds appear		Earliest secretory tubules differentiating Bladder-urethra separates from rectum	Kidney able to secrete urine Bladder expands as sac	Kidney in position Attains typical shape and plan
Nervous system Well-marked midbrain flexure No hindbrain or cervical flexures Neural groove closed		Cerebral cortex begins to acquire typical cells Differentiation of cerebral cortex, meninges, verticular foramina, cerebrospinal fluid circulation Ventricles large relative to cortex Spinal cord extends entire length of spine	Brain structural configuration roughly complete Cord shows cervical and lumbar enlargements Fourth ventricle foramina developed	Cerebral lobes delineated Cerebellum assumes some prominence

20 WEEKS	24 WEEKS	28 WEEKS	32 WEEKS	36 WEEKS	40 WEEKS
300	600	1100	1800-2100	2200-2900	3200+
Sternum ossifies Fetal movements strong enough for mother to feel		Astragalus ossifies	Middle fourth phalanges ossify Permanent teeth primordia indicated	Distal femoral ossification centers present Firm grasp	
	Blood formation increases in bone marrow and decreases in liver				
Enamel and dentin depositing Ascending colon recognizable					
Nostrils reopen Increased vascularity of lungs	Alveolar ducts and sacs present Primitive respiratory-like movements begin Lecithin begins to appear in amniotic fluid Eyelids free to open	Surfactant forming on alveolar surfaces	Lecithin/sphingomyelin ratio 1.2:1 Weak cry	Lecithin/sphingomyelin ratio $\geq 2:1$ Deep respiratory movements	Pulmonary branching only two-thirds complete
				Formation of new nephrons ceases	
Brain grossly formed Cord myelination begins Spinal cord ends at level of S1	Cerebral cortex layered typically Neuronal proliferation in cerebral cortex ends	Appearance of cerebral fissures; convolutions rapidly appearing Hiccups occur		Spinal cord ends at level of L3	Myelination of brain begins

Continued.

Table 5-6 Milestones in human development before birth—cont'd

	4 WEEKS	8 WEEKS	12 WEEKS	16 WEEKS
Sense organs	Eye and ear appearing as optic vessel and otocyst	Primordial choroid plexuses develop Eyes converging rapidly Internal ear developing	Earliest taste buds indicated Characteristic organization of eye attained	General sense organs differentiated
Genital system	Genital ridge appears (fifth week)	Testes and ovaries distinguishable External genitalia sexless but beginning to differentiate	Sex recognizable Internal and external sex organs specific	Testes in position for descent into scrotum Vagina open

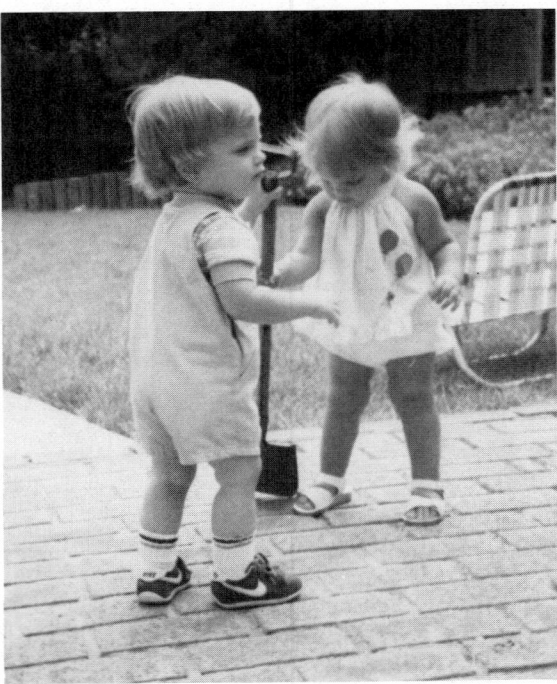

Fig. 5-10. Different sex dizygotic, or fraternal, twins.

ber of larger multiples (quintuplets, sextuplets) during recent years has been associated with the administration of fertility drugs to the mother.

Twins

It is well known that twins are of two distinct types: *identical,* or *monozygotic* (MZ); and *fraternal,* or *dizygotic* (DZ). These two types are separate and apparently unrelated phenomena. Dizygotic twins are derived from the fertilization of two ova that are released nearly simultaneously from the

ovary. They may be of like sex or opposite sexes, and they differ both physically and in genetic constitution (Fig. 5-10). They are merely siblings who happen to be born at the same time. Monozygotic twins are the result of one fertilized ovum that becomes separated at a very early stage, of development, with each part developing into a complete individual. Monozygotic twins are always alike in both gene complement and physical characteristics, including sex (Fig. 5-11). The term ''identical,'' used to describe monozygotic twins, is not entirely accurate, because no two individuals are ever exactly alike in every detail.

The frequency of twin births varies according to ethnic origin, maternal age, and heredity, and these differences are related almost exclusively to the incidence of dizygotic twins. Monozygotic twins occur with relatively uniform frequency in all populations (approximately 1:200 to 285 births) and appear to be random events. Dizygotic twinning, on the other hand, shows variable frequency among racial populations, the highest being in the black races and the lowest in the Asian races, with the white races somewhere in the intermediate range. In the United States the overall twinning rate is approximately 1:80 pregnancies and consists of one third monozygotic and two thirds dizygotic twins.

Dizygotic twinning becomes increasingly common with advancing maternal age, rising to a maximum between ages 35 and 39 years and then decreasing rapidly. Maternal age has little if any effect on the monozygotic twinning rate. Monozygotic twinning is unaffected by heredity, but dizygous twins show a marked familial tendency. The tendency toward dizygous twinning is a hereditary trait expressed only in the females. There is an increase in twins among relatives of mothers of twins (for example, female siblings and offspring of dizygotic twins) but not among relatives of the fathers (for example, brothers of dizygotic twins and

20 WEEKS	24 WEEKS	28 WEEKS	32 WEEKS	36 WEEKS	40 WEEKS
Nose and ear ossify		Eyelids reopen Retinal layers completed; light receptive Pupils capable of reacting to light	Sense of taste present Aware of sounds outside mother's body Moro reflex present Pupillary light reflex present		
	Testes at inguinal ring in descent to scrotum		Testes descending to scrotum		Testes in scrotum Labia majora well developed

offspring of a dizygotic twin). Fathers, however, do appear to transmit the disposition toward double ovulation to their daughters.

Determination of zygosity. It is important to distinguish between monozygotic and dizygotic twins for two reasons. First, monozygotic twin studies serve as a useful tool in the scientific study of the influence of heredity and environment on developmental phenomena and disease processes. Second, because there is an ever-increasing need for transplant donors and because truly successful organ or tissue transplantation is possible only between genetically identical individuals, identification of monozygotic twins is a very practical consideration. The earlier this distinction is made, the more useful the information will be. Methods used to determine zygosity are examination of fetal membranes or comparing and contrasting of physical similarities

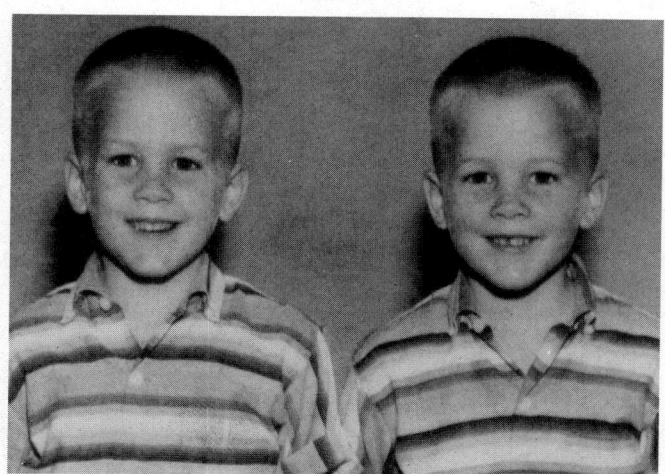

Fig. 5-11. Monozygotic, or identical, twins.
Photography courtesy Betty Baggett.

and differences between members of a pair of twins. It can be established that a pair of twins is not monozygotic, but not with absolute certainty.

Twins of different sexes or with obvious differences in physical characteristics such as hair or eye color or ear shape are dizygotic. Blood group comparisons are the most reliable physical means to distinguish types of twins. Monozygotic twins always possess identical blood groups; dizygotic twins may be alike or may differ in any or all blood group systems. If a single difference is found, it can be concluded that the pair is dizygotic.

Examination of fetal membranes provides an early means of differentiating between monozygotic and dizygotic twins of like sex. Dizygotic twins have two separate and distinct placentas and membranes, both amnion and chorion (Fig. 5-12). In some instances, if the implantations are close together on the uterine wall, the placentas may grow together, giving the impression of one placenta.

Monozygotic twins may have single or separate placentas and membranes, depending on the time during early development when division has taken place. If during the blastomere stage the cells do not separate and two inner cell masses form, the two embryos will develop within a single chorion but with individual amnions. Rarely the embryos will develop within a single amnion. If the early cells separate, the two zygotes formed from this separation will implant separately and form their own amnion and chorion in much the same manner as dizygotic twins (Fig. 5-13). Late division produces "mirror" twins; when it is later and incomplete, the result is conjoined, or "Siamese," twins. Twins that are enclosed in a single chorion (monochorionic) can be regarded as monozygotic twins; however, in other cases the distinction is not certain, inasmuch as both types of twins can have two amnions, chorions, and placentas or a single placenta.

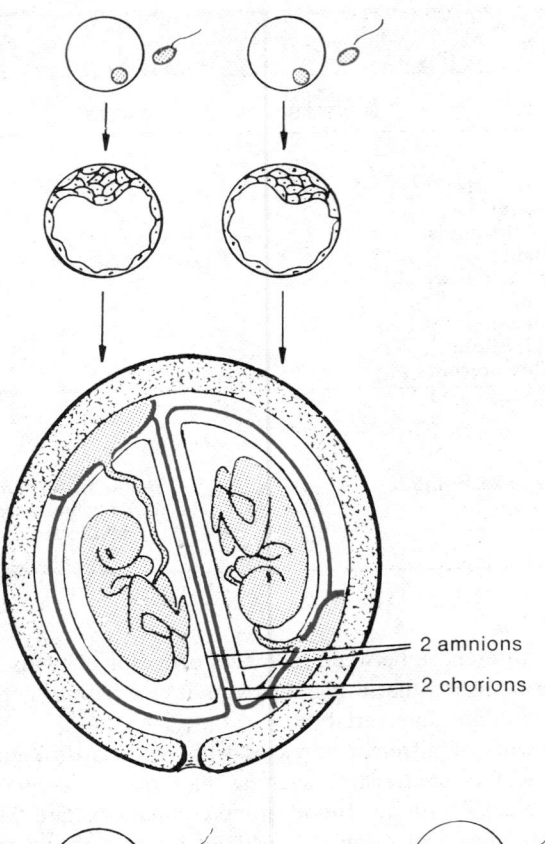

Twin studies. The study of twins is a method that has been proven of value in providing information about the roles of heredity and environment in the development of specific traits. Because monozygotic twins have the same genotype, a disease or trait appearing with higher frequency in them than in dizygotic twins suggests a genetic origin. Because both types normally grow up under the same or similar conditions, any differences that appear in dizygotic but not in monozygotic pairs can be attributed to differences in genotypes. Differences that appear in both monozygotic and dizygotic twins must be the result of environmental influences, although these are usually difficult to determine. If both members of a pair of twins display the trait under observation, they are said to be *concordant* for that trait; if only one of a pair of twins displays the trait, the twins are said to be *discordant* for that trait.

Fig. 5-12. Formation of dizygotic twins. There is fertilization of the two ova, two implantations, two placentas, two chorions, and two amnions.

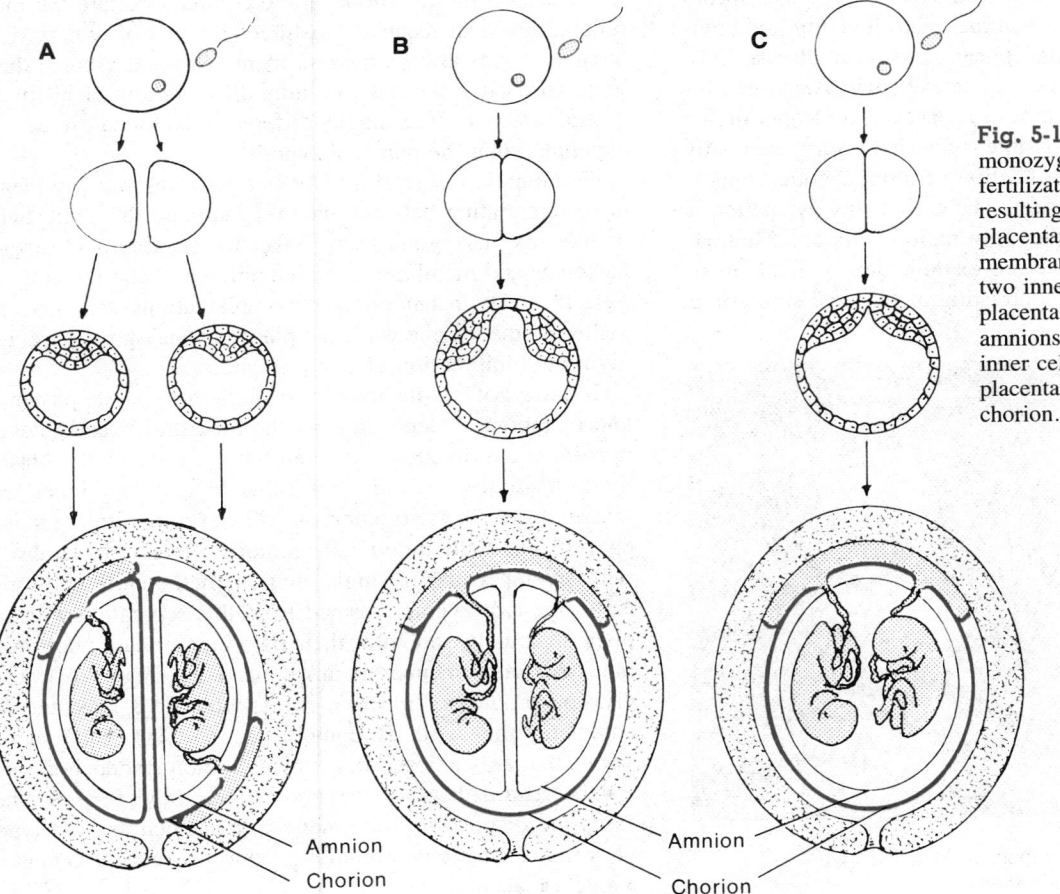

Fig. 5-13. Formation of monozygotic twins. **A,** One fertilization; blastomeres separate resulting in two implantations, two placentas, and two sets of membranes. **B,** One blastomere with two inner cell masses, one fused placenta, one chorion, separate amnions. **C,** Later separation of inner cell masses, with fused placenta and single amnion and chorion.

ENVIRONMENTAL INFLUENCES ON PRENATAL DEVELOPMENT

During intrauterine life the developing organism is protected to a great extent by the environment provided by the mother; however, this protection is not complete. Numerous internal and external factors can produce injury to the embryo, especially during periods of rapid growth or differentiation. The impact of these factors depends on the nature of the environmental change and the developmental stage of the embryo at the time of exposure.

Sensitive Periods in Prenatal Development

Every organ, system, and body part goes through a period during which it experiences the most rapid cell division and differentiation. During this time the organism displays a marked susceptibility to injurious influences. These specific stages of crucial developmental advancement are termed *sensitive,* or *critical periods,* and the major impact of environmental factors on development always coincides with these periods.

The developing organism is most highly susceptible, especially to structural disturbance, during the period of organogenesis. The sensitive periods for all organs or parts do not occur simultaneously. A part that is susceptible to adverse influences at one particular time may be resistant to the same influence at other periods of development. At the same time another part may be highly sensitive at the moment.

Susceptibility to environmental influences decreases as organ formation advances—the younger the organism and the fewer the number of cells, the greater the extent of involvement when an adverse influence is applied. During the preimplantation period, the embryo is generally considered to be relatively resistant to environmental influences. The impact at this phase either damages all or a majority of the dividing cells, with subsequent abortion, or it damages only a few. During the period of intensive differentiation most teratogenic agents are highly effective and may produce a variety of deformities. The type of defect that is produced depends on which organ is most susceptible at the time of application. The susceptibility to teratogenic influences decreases rapidly in the later periods of development, which are characterized by growth and elaboration of established organs. Fig. 5-14 indicates the approximate times of critical differentiation for some of the major organs and systems.

Teratogenesis

Teratogenesis (from the Greek *teratos,* monster, and *genesis,* production) refers to the origin or method by which prenatal growth processes are disturbed to produce a structural

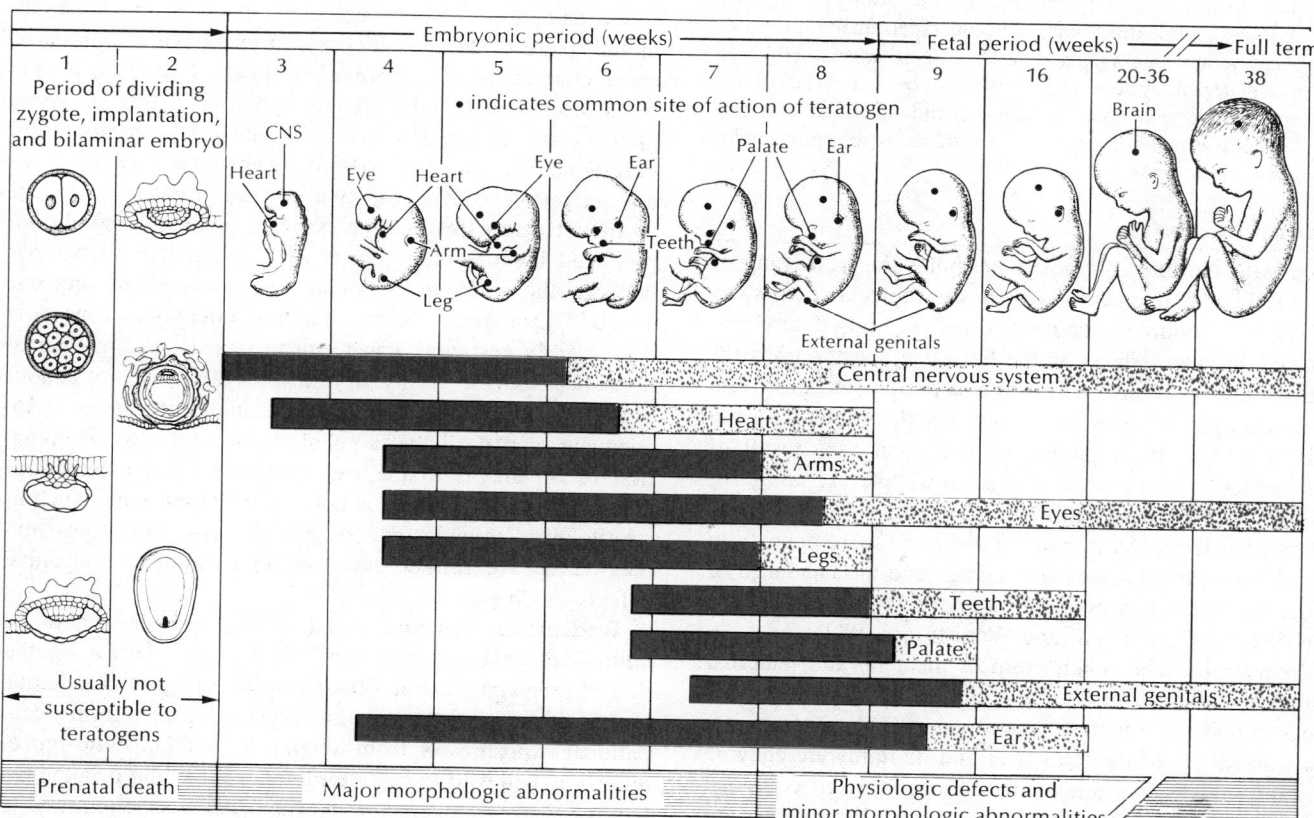

Fig. 5-14. Sensitive, or critical, periods in human development. Solid color denotes highly sensitive periods; stippled color indicates stages when embryo is less sensitive to teratogens.

From Moore, K.L.: The developing human: clinically oriented embryology, ed. 2, Philadelphia, 1977, W.B. Saunders Co.

or functional defect. An agent capable of producing such an adverse effect is called a *teratogen*. In recent years the study of defective development *(teratology)* has been broadened to include any birth defect—morphologic, biochemical, or behavioral—induced at any stage of gestation that is detected at birth *(fetotoxic)* or later in life *(developmentally toxic)*.

Principles of teratology. As a result of data gathered from retrospective studies and animal experiments, a few basic principles have emerged that present some insight into the probability of children being affected by specific teratogens:

1. The susceptibility of the organism to teratogenic factors is determined by the stage of development.
2. The effect of a teratogen depends on genetic predisposition. There are indications that a teratogenic agent accentuates the incidence of those defects that occur sporadically, implying underlying genetic instabilities.
3. A single teratogen may produce a variety of anomalies. For example, it has been established that rubella infection of the mother can produce a variety of defects, including cataracts, deafness, heart anomalies, and mental retardation.
4. A variety of teratogenic agents may produce similar anomalies; for example, viruses, chemicals, and radiation can all produce a mental deficit.
5. Teratogenic anomalies may be indistinguishable from hereditary malformations (phenocopies), for example, inherited deafness and deafness caused by maternal rubella.
6. Many teratogenic agents have little or no adverse effect on the maternal system and may even be beneficial to the mother. For example, the drug thalidomide, an effective hypnotic drug, nontoxic to the mother, is severely teratogenic to the fetus.

Prenatal Influences

Before birth the maternal host determines the well-being of the fetus by the manner in which she protects, favors, or deprives it. An unfavorable maternally imposed environment may produce effects on the fetus that are of a transient nature with few, if any, deleterious consequences or effects serious enough to cause long-range health problems in the infant or child. Health problems that occur as a result of some of these factors are discussed in Chapter 11 and elsewhere in the book as appropriate.

Parental age. As in genetic disorders there appears to be a relationship between maternal age and the incidence of postnatal deficiencies, especially motor and perceptual deficits (Gillberg, Rasmussen, and Wahlström, 1982).

Chemicals. The relationship of the fetal and maternal circulations allows for the interchange of chemical substances across the placental membrane. The limited metabolic capabilities of the fetal liver and its immature enzyme and transport systems render the unborn child ill equipped for maintaining homeostasis when chemical disturbances are imposed by the mother. This includes both substances produced by the mother in response to a disease state (such as diabetes) and exogenous substances ingested or inhaled by the mother.

The teratogenic effect of drugs is not believed to have an effect on developing tissue until day 15 of gestation, when tissue differentiation begins to take place. Before that time drugs usually have little effect on the embryo, because drugs are not believed to have a significant affinity for undifferentiated tissue. Also, until implantation takes place, at approximately 7 days after conception, the embryo is not exposed to maternal blood that contains the drug. However some drugs may affect the uterine lining, making it unsuitable for implantation. Drugs administered between days 15 and 90 may produce an effect if the tissue for which it has an affinity is in the process of differentiation at that time (see Fig. 5-14). After 90 days, when differentiation is complete, the embryo is believed to be relatively resistant to teratogenic effects of drugs (Luery, 1985).

It has been estimated that women take an average of four or five drugs—either prescription or over-the-counter preparations—during their pregnancy. In addition, hormones, frequently administered as drugs, are often classified as such. To help ensure that fewer women will inadvertently take some chemical that might be harmful to the fetus, labels on medications are now required to include information regarding the possible teratogenic effects of the drug. The Food and Drug Administration has established categories that indicate known or suspected potential of a drug to produce birth defects.

To date, alcohol does not contain a warning label, although there is strong evidence that excessive use produces some characteristic malformations in the fetus (see p. 485 for a discussion of fetal alcohol syndrome). Infants whose mothers are addicted to narcotic analgesics are small for gestational age and are at risk for having withdrawal following delivery (see Drug-addicted infants, p. 418).

Infectious agents. The range of pathologic conditions produced by infectious agents is large, and the difference between the maternal and fetal effects caused by any one agent is also great. Some maternal infections, especially during early gestation, can result in fetal loss or malformations because the ability of the fetus to handle infections organisms is limited. The fetal immunologic system is inadequate, and the fetus is unable to prevent the dissemination of organisms to the various tissues. Some infectious agents known to produce abnormalities in the fetus, such as rubella virus, toxoplasma, cytomegalovirus, and herpes simplex virus, are further discussed in relation to congenital defects in Chapter 11.

Radiation. Ionizing radiation has been shown to be both mutagenic and teratogenic in humans. Pelvic irradiation of pregnant women—from natural background radiation that is present everywhere in varying degrees, from occupational exposure, or from diagnostic or therapeutic procedures—is believed to be hazardous to the embryo, although the extent of teratogenicity and the exact dosage required to induce somatic change are still under consideration. Radiation may damage the conceptus at any time during its prenatal existence, and it is known that rapidly dividing and differentiating cells, such as those of the embryo, have increased radiosensitivity. As with other teratogens, the type of effect produced is closely correlated with the stage of development at which the radiation exposure occurs.

Although data are incomplete, there are indications that a larger number of chromosome abnormalities occur in children born to parents who have been exposed to increased preconception radiation. The increased likelihood they have been exposed to more radiation is consistent with the observation that chromosome abnormalities are highest in infants of older mothers, and there is an increased frequency of occupational exposure to radiation in chromosomally abnormal fetuses. To help prevent the possibility of radiation damage it is advisable (1) to avoid unnecessary radiation exposure, such as elective radiographs, in women of childbearing age except during the 2 weeks immediately following menstruation, (2) to ask if pregnancy is a possibility, and (3) to advise both men and women who have lower abdomen or pelvic radiographs to avoid conception for several months (Cohen, 1984). Also the harmful effects of maternal radioactive iodine (RAI) therapy on the fetal thyroid gland has led to the conclusion that pregnancies that occur during RAI therapy should be terminated.

Mechanical factors. The intrauterine environment minimizes the possibility of trauma to the fetus; however, during the later months of gestation, maintaining an attitude of complete flexion in the cramped quarters of the uterus predisposes the fetus to a number of deformities, for example, metatarsus varus, torticollis, and dislocation of the hip.

Defects sometimes occur as the result of amniotic bands or adhesions between the amnion and the fetus, such as the constriction of fetal limbs by bands of amniotic tissue that inhibit the growth of distal segments. Decrease in the production of amniotic fluid may create deformities of varying degrees as a result of the restriction of intrauterine space, for example, malformations of the jaw and ribs, asymmetry of the head, and compression marks on the body.

Temperature. There is increasing evidence to indicate that fetuses may be adversely affected by the high temperatures to which they are subjected when expectant mothers indulge in the environment of a hot tub or sauna. With the increasing popularity of these innovations, nurses should advise pregnant women to seek the advice of their physicians before extensive use of such items.

Nutritional factors. The human conceptus has no store of nutrients to sustain vital functions during the prenatal period; therefore it must rely on the mother as its single source of nutrition. A number of related factors, acting alone or in combination, influence fetal access to nutrients. These include reduction of maternal intake of specific nutrients and the general nutritional state of the mother. The chronically malnourished mother has few nutritional reserves available for fetal use, and the accumulated effects of lifetime nutritional deficiency may produce physiologic and anatomic structural defects that impair the mother's ability to support pregnancy and contribute to difficulties during labor. The

teenage mother who has special nutritional requirements for meeting her own growth needs may compete with the fetus for available nutrients. Diet fads, such as the Zen macrobiotic diet and some of the new vegetarian diets, seriously compromise the health of both the mother and the fetus (see p. 553).

Current information indicates that the restriction of calories and protein during prenatal development profoundly affects the size, viability, postnatal growth, and behavior of children. The timing and duration of nutritional deprivation appear to be crucial. Of greatest concern are the consequences of dietary restriction at the time the brain is undergoing the most rapid growth and development. Insufficient nutrients to the fetus during the time of rapid brain cell division result in permanent deficiency in brain cell numbers. The long-term consequences of nutritional deficiency may be manifest as cognitive, behavioral, and language retardation. There is a highly complicated relationship between maternal intake, postnatal environmental conditions, and the intellectual functions of offspring that is worthy of further exploration.

Maternal health. Because the physiologic well-being of the fetus depends on the maternal environment in which it grows, any disorder that affects the maternal system will have some effect on the fetal system. Some of the specific disorders and related problems (such as diabetes mellitus and substance abuse) are discussed in Chapter 10 and elsewhere in the text.

Maternal smoking. It is well established that mothers who smoke during pregnancy have a higher incidence of spontaneous abortion, complications of pregnancy, and premature delivery. The infants of these women have lower Apgar scores, lower birth weight, lower chance of survival, and decreased size throughout childhood. Offspring of these mothers demonstrate lower mental functioning, increased chance of malformations, hyperkinetic behavior, and lower scholastic ability in childhood, probably related to oxygen deprivation and exposure to the products of cigarette smoke. Nicotine and carbon monoxide decrease the oxygen supply and blood flow to the uterus and cause vasoconstriction in fetal organs, including the brain. It has also been shown that there is an increase in prenatal mortality in a household where the father smokes.

Other factors. Other factors capable of affecting the fetus adversely include:

1. Physical factors such as high altitude
2. Maternal disease such as toxemia of pregnancy, metabolic disorders such as diabetes and thyroid disease, and vascular diseases such as heart disease, lupus erythematosus, hypertension, and the hemoglobinopathies
3. Isoimmunization from maternal-fetal blood incompatibility
4. Prenatal diagnostic and therapeutic procedures

Care of Mother and Fetus

The importance of early and adequate prenatal care for the expectant mother cannot be overemphasized. Ideally preparation for childbirth begins in the mother's own childhood with a healthy physical environment and warm, affectionate parent-child relationships. It is well known that chronic exposure to substandard living conditions, poor nutrition, and inadequate health supervision are interrelated circumstances that contribute to fetal and infant morbidity and mortality, the most widely used indicator of the status of maternal and infant health care.

Nurses have always been important providers of health services to mothers and children. Now, with their expanding role as independent nurse practitioners, nurses' opportunities and responsibilities for maternal and infant health are assuming even broader dimensions. Careful assessment and monitoring of maternal health, anticipation of possible problems, and appropriate intervention will increase the likelihood of a successful outcome of pregnancy for both mother and infant. For more extensive discussion of the problems related to prenatal and intrapartum care of the mother and fetus, the reader should consult an authoritative textbook of maternity nursing.*

Impact of Hereditary Disorders on the Family

The presence of a genetically or prenatally derived disorder presents multiple problems and concerns to the family and to health workers. The disorder may have been present in a family for generations, or it may appear suddenly in a family. In either situation the family is faced with decisions regarding their reproductive future.

GENETIC SCREENING

Tests to detect the presence of a defective gene are rapidly assuming greater importance in management of genetic disorders as more defects are identified and techniques are developed for easy application. With the success of several well-organized or legislated programs and their significance in the prevention of disease or of the damaging effects of disease, an increasing number of programs are gaining acceptance and support. It is probable that with improved technology, mass screening for numerous defects may eventually be a routine procedure. However, to be truly effective, screening programs depend on education of both health professionals and the public regarding these programs. The religious, moral, and ethical issues revolving around screening and prenatal diagnosis are extensive and beyond the scope of this discussion; therefore only a few are mentioned, and the reader is encouraged to investigate these issues further in other resources.

*Highly recommended textbooks are Jensen, M.D., and Bobak, I.M.: Maternity and gynecologic care: the nurse and the family, ed. 3, St. Louis, 1985, The C.V. Mosby Co.; and Bobak, I.M., and Jensen, M.D.: Essentials of maternity nursing, St. Louis, 1984, The C.V. Mosby Co.

Purposes of Screening

Genetic screening is presumptive identification of an unrecognized genotype in individuals or populations. There are several purposes for this screening: (1) to detect the presence of disease, incipient or overt, (2) to provide reproductive information, and (3) to gain information concerning the incidence of a disorder in the population.

Screening for disease. The rationale for screening for disease is to discover persons who (1) have the disease, either manifest or incipient, or (2) may, in time or under special circumstances, develop the disease. The purpose of this knowledge is to anticipate serious consequences and provide the individual with treatment and management that will prevent, reverse, or diminish the adverse effects of the disorder. An example is the generalized, systematic screening of all newborn infants for phenylketonuria (PKU), hypothyroidism, and galactosemia. The mass screening programs have indicated that many of these disorders are more prevalent than formerly believed. Others that are included in some screening programs are hemocystinuria, maple syrup urine disease, sickle cell disease and other hemoglobinopathies, tyrosinemia, histidinemia, Hartnep disease, adenosine deaminase deficiency, and various other aminoacidurias and urea cycle disorders.

Screening for reproductive information. Screening for heterozygotes (carriers) can detect unaffected persons

Questions and Controversies

Should parents have the right to refuse permission for routine screening of their newborn to detect the presence of a disease for which therapy is now available? Should screening be required to detect the presence of a disease for which no therapy is presently available?

Screening for some biochemical defects (phenylketonuria, hypothyroidism, galactosemia) is mandatory or common practice (American Academy of Pediatrics, 1982). Initiation of treatment before irreversible damage occurs has improved the quality of life for persons with these disorders, and the cost of the screening has been less that the cost to society for institutional care of untreated victims. It has also eliminated much of the financial and other less tangible burdens to the family; that is, the cost and burden of special diets or medication is less burdensome than the care and management of a disabled child.

However, some parents strenuously object to screening procedures on the basis of religious and personal biases. Should they be given the option of refusal, inasmuch as these diseases are not a threat to other infants or children? On the other hand, if the screening is mandatory, are the parents in fact asking health professionals to break the law in submitting to their wishes?

Technology is available for detection of many more diseases for which there is no available remedy. Should the child and family be subjected to the procedures when no help can be offered? On the other hand, persons with a disorder for which there is at present no remedy can be contacted if one should be come available. However, screening for these diseases is expensive.

Questions and Controversies

Should routine genetic screening be performed for a disease with no known adverse clinical consequences? Also, should incidental but unexpected findings of genetic screening be disclosed? To whom?

Some argue that screening for a disease with no known clinical repercussions is desirable because it allows follow-up that may reveal subtle consequences unrecognized before (Cohen, 1984). However, there is no reason to subject children and families to the stress of screening procedures if there is no visible evidence of disease and no untoward symptoms.

Sometimes screening information alters family relationships. Disruption of parent-child bonding can occur in the newborn period. The common consequences of detecting a genetic disease in a child are blaming, overprotectiveness of the child with impaired psychologic development, and guilt feelings in the family. Knowledge that they have a disease can seriously alter identity formation in adolescents. It makes them "different" from their peers, and persons who are carriers of a genetic disease often exhibit an altered self-concept.

Unexpected information that might seriously alter family relationships include nonpaternity and discovery of a disorder other than the one for which the individual was screened (Korsch, 1984).

Questions and Controversies

Should parents of an unborn child known to have a disorder involving a serious mental defect be allowed to continue the pregnancy when they will be unable or unwilling to care for the child after birth? Can society deny services to the child after birth because of the family's decision, or, if the society must assume responsibility for care of the child, should society have a voice in the decision?

The physical, emotional, and monetary burdens of lifetime care for a child with a physical or mental defect can drain the resources of many families and institutions. Some families are incapable of providing adequate care for a child with physical or mental defects. Institutions are continually faced with diminished funding for the care of these children.

1. Malformations that are best corrected after delivery at term, e.g., gastrointestinal atresia, omphalocele, intact spina bifida, skeletal deformities
2. Disorders that may require preterm delivery for early correction, e.g., obstructive hydronephrosis, hydrops fetalis, obstructive hydrocephalus, gastroschisis or ruptured omphalocele, intestinal ischemia or necrosis secondary to volvulus
3. Anomalies that may require cesarean delivery, e.g., conjoined twins, giant omphalocele, large hydrocephalus, large or ruptured meningomyelocele, large sacrococcygeal teratoma
4. Conditions that may require medical treatment before birth, e.g., erythroblastosis fetalis, pulmonary immaturity (surfactant deficiency), cardiac arrhythmia
5. Defects that interfere with development and may require intrauterine surgical relief, e.g., diaphragmatic hernia, urethral obstruction, aqueductal stenosis
6. Conditions that provide information on which to base a decision to terminate a pregnancy, usually a fatal or debilitating disorder such as anencephaly, severe anomalies associated with chromosome abnormalities, renal agenesis or bilateral polycystic kidneys, and some inherited chromosomal, metabolic, and hematologic abnormalites

Prenatal diagnosis by amniocentesis has become relatively commonplace. Although it carries a certain amount of risk, this technique has been employed to detect a variety of inborn errors of metabolism, chromosomal abnormalities, some central nervous system abnormalities, and sex of the fetus in sex-related disorders. Other techniques available in selected medical facilities include ultrasonography, fetoscopy, chorionic villi sampling, and fetal blood sampling. Amniography, fetography, and radiography are used less often. Fetal cell isolation from maternal serum is possible and may be an alternative to diagnosis of neural tube defects if mass screening by amniocentesis is not feasible.

with certain genes who, when they mate with an individual who carries a similar gene, are at high risk of producing an affected offspring. These individuals are thus provided with the knowledge they need for use in decisions about family planning. Carriers of a number of diseases can be detected by laboratory tests, but because of the rarity of these diseases, mass screening is not feasible except in persons known to be at risk. Persons at risk include close relatives of persons with an inborn error of metabolism or other detectable disorder, or certain ethnic populations known to have a high incidence of a specific disease such as sickle cell anemia in blacks, Tay-Sachs disease in Ashkenazi Jews, and thalassemia in persons of Mediterranean ancestry.

Screening for epidemiologic information. Public health officials may use screening as a method of monitoring the incidence of diseases or malformations in a population in order to detect environmental or other causes that might significantly influence incidence of the disorder. For example, the observation that the incidence of a syndrome was significantly increased in a population 8 to 10 months after a rubella epidemic led to the discovery that this disease has a significant damaging impact on the unborn child during the first trimester of pregnancy.

Prenatal Diagnosis

A variety of techniques are available for diagnosing a number of diseases and defects in the fetus. As more and more diseases can be diagnosed prenatally and parents at risk are recognized early, these procedures provided the means to detect the following (Adzick, Flake, and Harrison, 1985):

Significance of Screening to Families

Mass screening programs have not been enthusiastically endorsed and carried out by all members of the health professions or wholeheartedly accepted by the public—especially compulsory screening. The reasons for this resistance are justified in many instances. Many physicians are unfamiliar with the techniques required for genetic screening, and some of the tests are not completely accurate. The cost of screening for a variety of genetic defects is beyond the means of most childbearing families, and the stigma attached to the carriers of a disease is a prohibiting factor. However, with the success of several well-organized or legislated programs and their significance in the prevention of disease or of the damaging effects of disease, an increasing number of programs are gaining acceptance and support.

In the majority of situations families support screening for genetic disease. They express a sense of relief to know their status: it is comforting to be assured that they do not carry the defective gene, or to have the information on which to make decisions when they are found to be carriers. Screening of infants for disease in the newborn period is supported by the vast majority of families, and many prefer to have the procedure performed as a nursery routine without their consent. Families have a strong desire to know what is being done to their infants, and knowledge of the procedure can lessen anxiety and help them prepare for possible consequences, such as repeat tests.

Much of family concern regarding screening centers around the issues of informed consent and the use to be made of the information from the screening. Some states require written consent, some specify the tests to be performed, and some describe the risks, benefits, and the right to be informed of uncertain results, including the process in the event of an abnormal finding. Institutions may provide classes for families to explain the screening program, provide verbal explanation, or distribute written materials. In some areas exemptions from mandated screening is allowed in certain situations, such as objections on religious grounds if there is a conflict with religious practices and beliefs of an established church. Others impose penalties for noncompliance (Cohen, 1984).

The nature and purposes of the procedure should be clearly explained to clients in language that they can understand. The issue of divulging unexpected findings is subject to debate. It is not unusual to detect one disorder while screening for another. Also, if a genetic trait is detected in a child but not in a parent (such as the sickle cell trait), the question of paternity can become an issue. It is also important to help families understand the meaning of false positive and false negative results of testing.

Release of information to persons other than the family is subject to debate. At present the reporting of genetic findings is not mandatory, as it is for certain contagious diseases, and it is questionable whether this would be desirable. A family may not wish for other family members or even the family physician to receive the results of screening. Third parties who might make use of such information are insurance companies and employers. All of these possibilities should be made clear to families in order to provide them with some selective control.

The social stigma attached to the carrier of a defective gene may be a side effect of screening. In some families such knowledge is a source of embarrassment and damaging to the self-esteem of its members. Teenagers are especially vulnerable to the effects of knowing they carry a specific defective gene at a time when identity formation and peer approval are extremely important. Cultural views regarding this knowledge can have profound effects on the members of some ethnic groups. In some cases, social status within the cultural group can be impaired.

Probably the most important area for nursing practice is teaching. Families need an understanding of why the screening is proposed, what the results mean, and how the family can interpret false positive and false negative results. Parents are concerned, and their anxiety is greater when they have not received sufficient information about the screening or testing process and its significance for the health of their infant (Sorenson, and Mangione, 1984). The need for retesting, no matter what the reason, can be extremely stressful to families, and they also have a right to know who assumes the cost of the screening—the family or the state. The nurse is a valuable resource person in making families aware of alternatives and in helping them select the one that best suits their particular situation.

Prenatal screening. The primary dilemma faced by families when a disorder is diagnosed prenatally is the option for terminating the pregnancy. When the disorder is one of major disability, the problem involves the care and management of the affected infant. Parents may choose to terminate a pregnancy in which the child will require special care that the parents are unable or unwilling to provide. A more difficult decision involves a relatively minor defect, such as cleft lip, for which there is definitive therapy but such therapy is beyond the family's physical, emotional, or financial resources.

Prenatal diagnosis of fetal sex is becoming more popular with expectant parents. When the pregnancy is at risk for an X-linked recessive disorder, such as Duchenne muscular dystrophy, there is a 50% chance that a male offspring will be affected, and many families choose to terminate a pregnancy involving a male fetus. However, there is also a 50% chance that the infant will be unaffected. More controversial is the issue of determining sex to satisfy parental curiosity or as a means of sex selection.

GENETIC COUNSELING

In recent years the significance of heredity as an etiologic agent in disease and disability has assumed a more prominent place in the nursing care of infants and children. With the expanded recognition of genetic diseases and defects, an increasingly well-informed public, assuming more responsibility for the quality of future populations, is creating a justified demand for accurate information regarding risks to present and future generations. The actual number of persons who need advice is relatively small compared with those who have many other health problems, but their need is great. When expert counseling is not accessible, these persons may become victims of well-meaning but uninformed quasi-professionals or misguided relatives and acquaintances.

It is estimated that only a small proportion of persons who need counseling are seen by professional counselors. Many families who might benefit from counseling do not recognize the need, or this special need is not apparent to those who supervise their care. Unfortunately, families who need counseling are rarely referred to counselors unless they themselves request the service. Nurses in the field of infant and child care continually encounter genetic diseases and families in which there is a risk that a disorder may be transmitted to an offspring. It is a responsibility of nurses to be alert to situations in which families could benefit from genetic counseling, to become familiar with facilities in their areas where genetic counseling is available, and to learn the basic principles of heredity. In this way they will be able to direct individuals and families to take advantage of needed counseling services and to be active participants in the counseling process. They should be knowledgeable regarding special services that are available to help in management and support of affected children.

A comprehensive definition of genetic counseling prepared by a group of eminent medical geneticists states that genetic counseling is a communication process which deals with the human problems associated with the occurrence, or risk of occurrence, of a genetic disorder in a family. This process involves an attempt by one or more appropriately trained persons to help the individual or family (Fraser, 1974):

1. Comprehend the medical facts, including the diagnosis, the probable course of the disorder, and the available management
2. Appreciate the way heredity contributes to the disorder, and the risk of recurrence in specified relatives
3. Understand the options for dealing with the risk of recurrence
4. Choose the course of action which seems appropriate to them in view of their risk and their family goals and act in accordance with that decision
5. Make the best possible adjustment to the disorder in an affected family member and/or to the risk of recurrence of that disorder

Clients

The clients, or persons who seek advice, must first be aware that there is a genetic problem or potential problem. They may be referred by a family physician, a specialist, a nurse, a friend, or a relative, or they may seek counseling as a result of information in the media. Some simply view genetic counseling as a new service of which they should take advantage.

Clients may or may not be affected themselves, but may request genetic counseling about the heritability of a trait that may be deleterious, beneficial, or merely troublesome. Clients may be a young couple contemplating marriage or childbearing who are concerned about a disorder in one of their families, no matter how remote the relationship. They may seek advice because they are related. A couple who are both members of a population at risk for certain diseases may wish to determine whether they carry the harmful gene (e.g., blacks and sickle cell anemia, Ashkenazi Jews and Tay-Sachs disease, or persons of Mediterranean ancestry and thalassemia). A couple planning adoption may seek counseling regarding a prospective child. More often persons who inquire about the possibility of recurrence of a disease or disorder are parents of a child with a specific disease or defect that significantly impairs fitness who are concerned that they might produce another similarly affected child. This advice may be sought before the couple initiates another pregnancy, after the mother is already pregnant, or after the birth of another child. There may be concern regarding the risk to unaffected siblings of the affected child or to the affected child's future children.

Some families may need counseling regarding the advisability of sterilization, artificial insemination, prenatal diagnosis, or termination of a pregnancy. Infertility or recurrent abortion in a family may indicate a need for counseling. Occasionally a counselor becomes involved in cases of disputed paternity, questioned maternity (when it is suspected that infants have been substituted for one another at birth), rape, and incestuous matings. Delayed or abnormal sexual development may also be a reason to seek genetic advice.

Objectives of Genetic Counseling

The major objectives of genetic counseling are (1) to advise families and answer questions regarding the risks of recurrence when a member of the family has a disorder that might be genetically determined, (2) to alert the medical profession to the possibility that a particular child may be born with a genetic abnormality, and (3) to prevent an increase in the number of children with serious handicaps and ultimately to reduce the proportion of these children who are born.

Advising families. More than ever before, parents plan and feel responsible for their children. They need to know the risk in *their particular situation* and how it relates to the random risk for *any* prospective parents. It has been found that when families understand the risks involved they normally make sensible decisions regarding family planning.

Special risk situations. When health personnel are alerted to the possibility of an inherited disease in a family, this knowledge makes possible the early detection and subsequent treatment of the disease. This is increasingly important as treatments are becoming available for more genetically determined diseases and is especially true in situations where treatment is effective only when initiated early. History of a condition in an older sibling, such as phenylketonuria or galactosemia, provides a clue for specific and thorough testing for the condition in a newborn. In this way early therapy can be initiated when indicated, thus minimizing or eliminating the effects of the disease or defect.

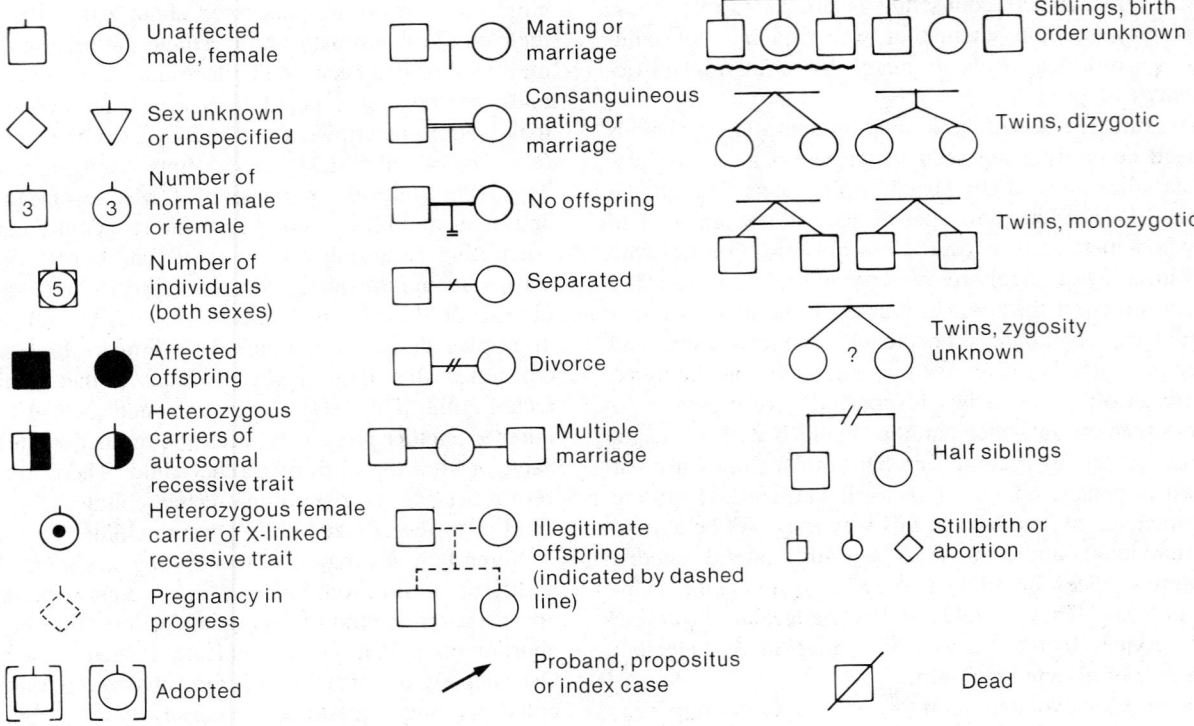

Fig. 5-15. Common pedigree symbols.

Reducing numbers of affected children. Inasmuch as it is now possible to detect the carrier state in an increasing variety of single-gene defects, this aspect of genetic counseling is assuming greater importance and offers hope in preventing disabling disease. Persons with a family history of one of these hereditary disorders, or those in an ethnic group at risk for a particular disease, are able to ascertain before initiating a pregnancy whether they are carriers of the gene for a severe defect. In these instances the genetic counselor is able to advise the couple on the risks for a specific defect occurring in any pregnancy with a high degree of accuracy. New techniques for prenatal diagnosis of chromosomal aberrations and an increasing number of metabolic defects have created the means for detecting an affected fetus early in pregnancy. Such information provides the expectant couple with the prospect of a severely affected child the option to terminate the pregnancy or the opportunity to prepare for the problems associated with care of the child.

Information Essential for Genetic Counseling

Unlike a medical prognosis that predicts the outcome of a disease, a genetic prognosis directly involves other persons: the affected child, members of the immediate family, relatives, and future offspring. Effective genetic counseling requires a thorough evaluation of each situation. Information from which the counselor derives risks of recurrence is acquired from several sources: an accurate diagnosis, a thorough family history, and an extensive knowledge of genetics.

Accurate diagnosis. The first and most important component in the counseling process is an accurate diagnosis. The disease may be diagnosed by the attending physician who refers the family for counseling, or the physician may call on the services of a counseling unit for a definitive diagnosis by special biochemical or cytogenetic tests, particularly in cases of very rare and unusual syndromes. There are about 2000 known inherited disorders, many of which have similar clinical manifestations but totally different modes of inheritance. For example, symptoms in the early stages of severe X-linked muscular dystrophy appear much like those of the more mild autosomal recessive and autosomal dominant varieties, autosomal recessive neurogenic muscular atrophies, and nongenetic poliomyelitis. The significance of the risks related to each type of disorder is readily apparent. It is especially difficult to assign a cause to deafness and mental retardation.

Family history. A careful, detailed family history is necessary to the counseling process. Not only does it provide a picture of the *proband* (the affected person, or *index case*) in relation to other family members, but it may also serve to identify other persons who are similarly affected or who may be at risk to produce affected children. Analyzing the pattern of affected members of the family may assist in confirming a tentative diagnosis or in determining the level of risk in multifactorial inheritance.

The person taking a family history must allow a liberal amount of time. When possible, it is best to include both parents in the interview in order to elicit information about relatives on both sides of the family. Medical records, birth

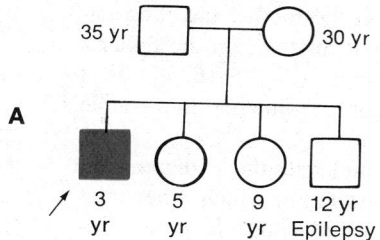

Fig. 5-16. Construction of a pedigree. **A,** Proband, siblings, and parents; **B,** maternal relatives; **C,** paternal relatives added.

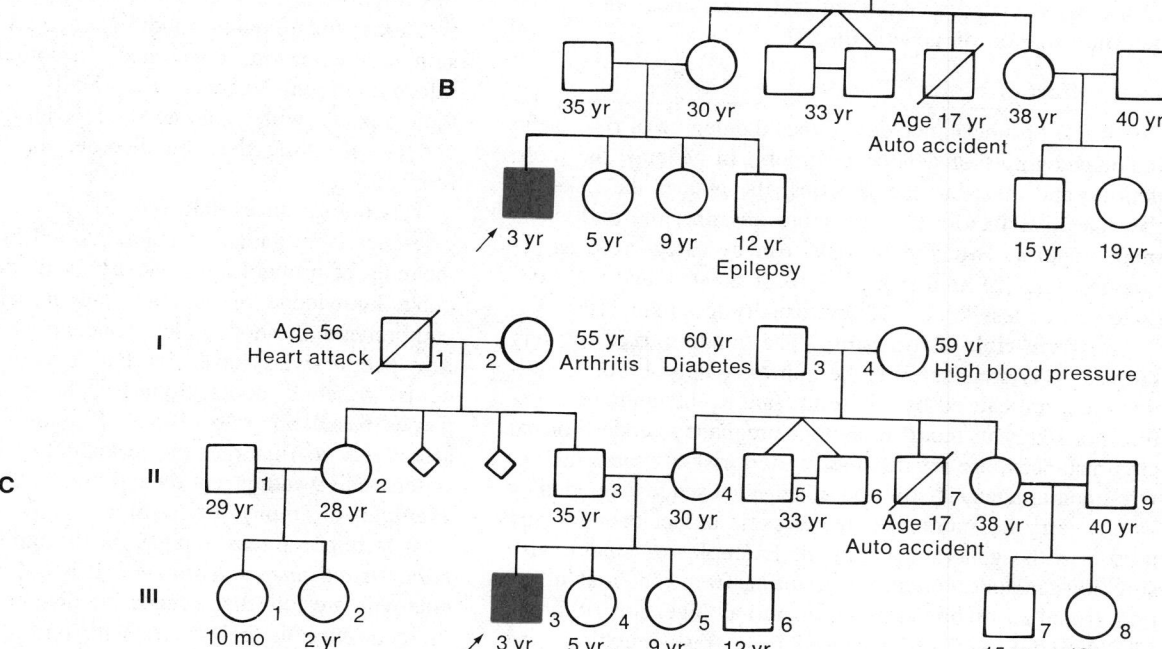

and death records, family bibles, and photograph albums are helpful resources, and persons being interviewed should be instructed to bring such items if they are available. It may be necessary to consult other members of the family. The level of education and the degree of understanding vary widely among informants and influence the reliability of the information. There may be reticence on the part of informants, particularly if they view the disorder as something to be ashamed of or in some way threatening. Sometimes true relationships may be concealed, such as illegitimacy.

The family history is recorded in the form of a pedigree chart or family tree (in some disciplines the pedigree chart is termed a *genogram*) using standard symbols to indicate persons, relationships, and significant details related to them (Fig. 5-15). It is important to include information about births—live births, stillbirths, and abortions; matings—legally sanctioned, consanguineous, multiple, unwed, and other complex relationships; and health of family members, including any diseases or disorders, and death and causes of death. Sometimes the place of birth and ethnic background are significant. For example, the incidence of Tay-Sachs

disease is higher in Ashkenazi Jews from eastern Europe than in Jews from other geographic origins. Also, when a pedigree chart is being evaluated, the fact that a sister died in infancy as a "blue baby" might be genetically significant, whereas a healthy sibling who drowned at age 1 year would not. Information concerning first-degree relatives is most important and should be complete.

Construction of a pedigree begins with the affected child (proband), who is designated with an arrow, and the outcome of *all* the mother's pregnancies (Fig. 5-16, *A*). Significant information about a pregnancy should be noted, such as bleeding, anemia, roentgenograms, or infectious diseases. Matings are represented by a bar, with males usually indicated on the left. Siblings, including stillbirths and abortions, are designated by arabic numerals in order of birth. Generations are represented by roman numerals, the earliest at the top. Next the medical history of the maternal relatives is explored, beginning with the mother's siblings and the outcome of her mother's pregnancies (Fig. 5-16, *B*). Details concerning the general health or death of maternal grandparents, nieces, nephews, uncles, aunts, and first cousins are included in a family history if the mother has information about them. Information about relatives on the father's side is gathered in the same manner (Fig. 5-16, C). It is important at this point to determine whether the couple might be related in any way.

When a family history is completed, the pedigree will reflect either a *positive family history,* in which other relatives are affected with the same disorder, or a *negative family history,* in which the proband is an isolated case.

Knowledge of genetics. In order to counsel families regarding their particular problem, a counselor must have a thorough understanding of genetic principles, a knowledge of the risks related to multifactorial inheritance, and up-to-date information on genetic diseases.

Estimation of Risks

The mode of inheritance determines the degree of risk in the major categories of genetic disorders. In general, the more definite and clear-cut the genetics, the greater the risks; as the causative factors become more obscure, the outlook is more hopeful. Broadly the risks can be categorized as (1) random risk, (2) high risk of 1:10 or greater, and (3) moderate risk of less than 1:10 and usually less than 1:20.

Random-risk situations. The random risk for any pregnancy is considered to be approximately 1:30. Conditions that are caused by environmental agents and are therefore not likely to recur in another pregnancy, under normal circumstances, are regarded as random risks. Unless the environmental agent is still operative, a subsequent pregnancy would carry no more risk of the same defect than for any person in the general population. Examples of random-risk situations include conditions resulting from maternal infection (rubella, toxoplasmosis), maternal ingestion of drugs (thalidomide), a disorder caused by a fresh mutation, and most chromosomal abnormalities. Continued exposure to harmful environmental agents, such as maternal alcoholism, radiation exposure, or teratogenic pollutants, may alter the risk factor.

High-risk situations. When the condition is caused by a factor that segregates during cell division (genes and chromosomes), the probability of an affected offspring can be predicted with a high degree of accuracy. Examples of high-risk situations include all disorders caused by a single mutant gene and chromosome abnormalities caused by a translocation.

Moderate-risk situations. The largest group of conditions is considered to be moderate risks. These include the multifactorial disorders that appear to "run in families" and are greater than the risks for the population as a whole. Risk recurrence in these disorders is *empiric.* That is, it is not based on genetic theory but on prior experience and observation of the disorder in other families that have been recorded in the literature. To arrive at an empiric risk estimate, the counselor applies knowledge of the frequencies that have been observed in other families with a similar condition to the incidence of the disorder in the family under consideration. When more than one member of a family is affected, the risks of recurrence are substantially increased, especially if these persons are near relatives. Examples of moderate risk situations include common disorders such as cleft lip and palate, pyloric stenosis, spina bifida, and congenital heart defects and common diseases such as diabetes mellitus, schizophrenia, and hypertension.

Interpretation of Risks

When explaining risk estimates, the counselor does not attempt to make recommendations or decisions for consultants. The counselor provides appropriate and accurate information about the nature of the disorder, the extent of the risk involved, the probable consequences, and alternative solutions, but remains nondirective, leaving the final decision to the persons concerned. In some instances genetic information will increase the family's distress; in others their anxiety will be reduced, depending on their makeup and the meaning that the disorder has for that particular family.

It is helpful to explain risks in different ways and to use examples from games of chance to aid in understanding the meaning of probabilities. Most persons do not have an adequate knowledge of genetics and human biology to fully comprehend these complex concepts. However, there are few people who have not had experience with flipping coins, baseball pools, lotteries, horse racing, and other games based on probabilities. Flipping coins can be used effectively to illustrate the probabilities in single-gene disorders, and weather reports and horse racing are well-known examples of empiric risk estimates.

It is important to impress on the family that *each pregnancy is an independent event.* It is not uncommon for parents who are told that a recessive disorder carries a 1:4 risk of recurrence to feel secure with one affected child. They incorrectly reason that because they already have one affected child the next three will be unaffected. Chance has no memory; the risk is 1:4 for each and every pregnancy.

Nurses and Genetic Counseling

Nurses skilled in counseling techniques are in a unique position to help meet the counseling needs of families in which there is a genetic disease or disorder. Public health nurses work with a family in a close, sustained relationship and earn the family's confidence and trust; genetics nurse specialists, with advanced preparation in genetic theory, are assuming a prominent position on counseling teams; and practitioners in the specialty areas of maternity and pediatric nursing are constantly involved with families in which there is a genetic defect. Nurses are frequently the persons who recognize clues that indicate a genetics-related problem, who assist the family in obtaining the needed services for diagnosis and treatment, and who provide follow-up care.

Counseling services. The most efficient counseling service consists of a group of specialists that may include physicians, geneticists, psychologists, biochemists, cytologists, nurses, social workers, and other auxiliary personnel. The services are most often under the leadership of a physician trained in medical genetics, who assumes responsibility for the medical aspects of the problem. The counseling service may serve only as a referral group, or it may conduct a regular clinic service. Most often it is associated with a large medical center, many of which have extensive outreach programs. There are numerous specialty clinics that deal with specific genetic disorders (such as cystic fibrosis, muscular dystrophy, hemophilia, diabetes) and provide their own genetic counseling services. Unfortunately, these units are concentrated in and around large metropolitan areas. As a result, counseling is not always accessible to the large number of persons who would benefit from the service.

It is a nurse who is frequently the family's initial contact with a counseling service. An intake interview is conducted before the primary counseling session or diagnostic workup to assess the needs of the family and attempt to reduce their anxiety; therefore, ample time should be allotted. Ideally, both spouses should attend, but small children should be excluded. If possible, childcare facilities should be made available as part of the counseling service. If this is impossible, some distraction in the form of toys and play equipment can be provided. In the interview the nurse takes a family history for pertinent information and explains the clinic procedures carefully. Many families are concerned about such things as whether they will be required to undress, if blood is to be drawn, if they can accompany the child during the visit, or if they will be told what to do about reproduction. Families who have a relaxed and nonstressful initial discussion are able to gain more from a counseling session.

Follow-up care. The success of counseling is measured by the way in which the family uses the information presented to them. Maintaining contact with the family or referral to an agency that can provide a sustained relationship—usually the public health agency in their locality— is one of the most important aspects of the counseling process. Some families do not choose to have follow-up visits, but in most instances these visits make the family feel that they have not been abandoned and facilitate the process of adjustment to the problem.

Follow-up visits to the counseling service or in the home provide the family with the opportunity to ask questions that they did not ask on previous visits. Often the family members have not really "heard" the information presented to them or have misinterpreted what they have heard, so that it may be necessary to repeat and reinforce counseling. In some disorders a diagnosis in one family member places relatives at risk and is an indication for further screening.

One very important aspect of follow-up care is support and assistance in management of the affected child. For example, a disorder such as phenylketonuria requires conscientious diet management; therefore, it is important to make certain that the family understands and follows instructions. Children born subsequently must be carefully observed for early detection of symptoms. Genetic and specialty clinics devote a great deal of their time and efforts in helping families cope with the consequences of genetic disease.

Nurses should be prepared to help families arrive at tentative decisions regarding the future, including family planning, education or institutionalization of a handicapped child, plans for adoption, and many other problems related to their specific problems. Initial and ongoing assessments of the family's coping abilities, resources, and support systems are vital in order to determine their need for additional assistance and support. Also nurses should be alert for evidence of risk factors that indicate poor adjustment, (e.g., child abuse, divorce, or other maladaptive behaviors). Locating agencies and clinics specializing in a specific disorder or its consequences that can provide services (e.g., equipment, medication, and rehabilitation), educational programs, and parent groups are all part of the nurses' resources.

Emotional Needs of Families

It requires time and understanding to deal with the emotional tension and anxiety generated in families who are faced with the prospect of a genetic disorder. Knowledge of and the ability to deal with the range of psychologic responses and all their ramifications (e.g., the grief reaction, guilt, anger, and coping mechanisms) are essential components of the nursing role in genetic counseling. Many of these factors determine the degree to which a counselor's message is understood and influence the family's attitudes and the use they make of counseling information. Awareness and understanding of these feelings make the difference between a genetic informant and a genetic counselor.

Timing of the counseling requires careful evaluation. Some families may not be ready to listen immediately after a diagnosis is made; many do not listen effectively the first time information is presented to them. Families who seek genetic counseling, spontaneously or by referral, are apprehensive and know that decisions made on the basis of the information that they receive may alter their lives significantly and may even alter their view of themselves. There may be numerous blocks to getting information across to families. Often they are so angry or frightened that they do not hear what is being said to them; they may feel guilty, embarrassed, or somehow inferior or inadequate. It is sometimes necessary to wait a week or more to allow the family sufficient time to absorb the initial impact of the situation before they are ready to assimilate any new information.

It is important early in counseling to get a clear understanding of the family's initial concerns, their state of knowledge about the disease, their attitudes and beliefs concerning the condition, and to determine the kind and amount of information they need or want. Some are not sure they should be at a counseling service. Whether the persons needing help are parents who have given birth to an affected child, relatives of an affected individual, or persons who have been identified as carriers of a deleterious gene, their feelings, attitudes, and fears must be dealt with.

It is almost certain that the counselor will be misunderstood. Most clients do not understand what they hear, and because misunderstandings are so prevalent, the follow-up interviews are especially important. Some clients say they want to know all about the disease and its implications, but this may not be true. Information often seems to go "in one ear and out the other." Others really do want to know and will ask questions until they understand. Careful interviewing and assessment will determine the extent and type of information needed and desired by the clients.

Guilt and self-blame are very natural and universal reactions. Nurses must deal with parents' feelings of guilt about carrying "bad genes" or having "made my child sick." For example, the young father of a child with Down syndrome refused to submit to chromosome analysis for fear he might be identified as a carrier of a translocated chromosome and thought he could not endure the guilt this knowledge would generate. Often the counseling person is in a position to absolve the parents of guilt by explaining the random nature of segregation during both gamete formation and fertilization. Sometimes there is comfort in knowing that everyone carries defective genes and that it is mere chance that a particular couple happens to carry the same abnormal gene. Reactions may be different in situations where one member can pinpoint the "blame" (dominant or X-linked disorders), whereas there is some reassurance in recessive disorders for the couple to know that it is not just one of them who carries the defective gene. Anxieties generated by old wives' tales, superstitions, and misconceptions can be dispelled.

It is important to stress that there is nothing shameful about an inherited or congenital defect and to emphasize any appropriate remedy. Families have a tendency to be more ashamed of a hereditary disorder than of one caused by self-indulgence, such as alcoholism. The threat of a hereditary "taint" often creates intrafamilial strife, hostility, and marital disharmony, sometimes to the point of family disintegration. Relatives frequently cease reproduction after the diagnosis of a hereditary defect, or the decision to marry may be deferred on the basis of a disorder, even a remote one, in a partner's family. While people may understand the situation intellectually, this does not help them emotionally. A large and vital part of the nurse's role in genetic counseling is that of sympathetic and supportive listener.

Burden of genetic defect. The way in which members of a family respond to the probability of a genetic disorder will depend a great deal on the nature of the condition and the burden, actual or perceived, that it may place on them. A burden is considered to be the total amount of distress, economical and emotional, that is placed on persons, their families, and society by the birth of an affected child—the anticipated burden as well as the threat of disability. Various factors that are associated with disorders produce a burden in different ways to determine the total impact on a family. These include severity, chronicity, age of onset, mortality, morbidity, presence or absence of chronic pain, mental retardation, and cosmetic disfiguration.

There is a great deal of variability in the ability of individuals and families to withstand stress, and persons respond differently to probabilities. A degree of risk that is reassuring to one may be threatening or intolerable to another. Also two individuals will respond differently to a hazard that both perceive as threatening. Some parents will choose to have children even in the face of high risk; others believe that even a moderate risk is too much to take. Some may risk having a child with a disorder that produces a minor defect or even one that causes early death but elect not to risk having a child with a life-long disability. The longer the duration of the disability, the greater the financial and emotional burden.

In some disorders, such as Down syndrome, the burden of the disease rests primarily on the family rather than on the affected child. In diseases with severe crippling effects, such as muscular dystrophy, the impact of the disease affects both the child and the family.

All of these matters confront a family when they must make a decision about whether to risk a pregnancy that might result in a child with a disability, and nurses should be prepared to explore these probabilities with them. Decisions are often irrevocable; therefore the choice must be mutually achieved. Parents who elect to have children in spite of a fairly high risk of recurrence can be helped by education. By learning about the disorder, they will be alert to signs of the disease so that early treatment can be initiated to minimize the ill effects of the disorder.

Barriers to effective counseling. Obstacles to the use of genetic counseling involve the attitudes of both the family and the counselor. Frequent obstacles to an objective use of information are religious attitudes toward conception and opposition to sterilization and to abortion in situations where there is a high risk of recurrence or where prenatal diagnosis has indicated a defective fetus. Many persons fatalistically accept "the will of God." Another obstacle is the right of the individual—the right of the fetus to come to full term and the right of parents to conceive. A person with a high risk of producing a disabling condition in an offspring may believe that he or she is entitled to the same rights as anyone else, including the right of procreation.

Differences in the ability to comprehend what is said probably interfere most with effective use of counseling information. Clients vary in experiences, education, and intellectual level, and even with careful explanation many are still unable to understand the basic fundamentals of inheritance. They may be able to repeat information but fail to grasp its significance.

Sometimes nurses themselves create barriers with their own biases. There are some diseases that have a special impact on individual nurses, and in such cases it is difficult to be nonjudgmental. Families may become defensive if they believe that the nurse is bringing undue pressure to bear on their decision. Others may pressure the nurse to make the decision for them. "What would you do if you were in this situation?" is a common question. In some instances nurses (intentionally or unintentionally) do influence families. They are often tempted to direct the decisions of the clients, especially less intelligent persons who may be judged to be less responsible for their actions. In genetic counseling families should be given all the facts and possible consequences, then assisted, without coercion, in their problem solving. However, the decision concerning a course of action should be left to them.

CONCEPT SUMMARIES

- Diseases or disorders may be traced to genetic factors, environmental factors, or a combination of both.

- Genetic diseases are classified as those produced by chromosomal aberrations, those produced by gene mutation or distribution, and those resulting from a complex interaction of both genetic and environmental factors.

- The causes of chromosome defects are complex and may involve exposure to radiation, autoimmune disease, and/or parental age.

- Nondisjunction refers to the failure of chromosomes to separate and migrate during cell division, resulting in an unequal distribution of chromosomes between the two resulting cells.

- Translocation occurs when one chromosome attaches to another to create one large chromosome.

- Klinefelter and Turner syndromes, two common sex chromosomal abnormalities, result from an increase in sex chromosomal number.

- Monogenic, or single gene, disorders are attributed to gene distribution in families in characteristic patterns.

- Modification in basic inheritance patterns that is seen in many disorders may be caused by specific gene behavior such as mutation, penetrance, variable expressivity, pleiotropy, linkage, and heterogeneity.

- The majority of hereditary disorders are caused by defective genes on an autosome.

- Monozygotic, or identical, twins are alike in both gene complement and physical characteristics; dizygotic, or fraternal, twins differ both physically and genetically.

- Congenital anomalies may occur at any stage of development and demonstrate wide variability in causative factors.

- A pathogenic classification of congenital anomalies describes alterations of form or structure, such as malformation, disruption, deformation, and dysplasia.

- Management of genetic disease may include such measures as surgical repair, modification of diet, product replacement, transplantation, and immunologic prevention.

- Eugenics refers to measures aimed at controlling heredity in order to alter future generations.

- Euthenics involves attempts to modify the environment to allow a genetically abnormal person to live a relatively normal life.

- Prenatal development comprises fetal growth, differentiation, and organogenesis and is strongly influenced by parental age, chemicals, infectious agents, radiation, mechanical factors, temperature, nutrition, maternal health, and maternal smoking.

- Genetic screening is aimed at detecting the presence of disease, providing reproductive information, and gaining information about the incidence of a disorder in the population.

- Genetic counseling for families alerts them to their special risk situations and helps to reduce the number of children with hereditary disorders.

REFERENCES

Adzick, N.S., Flake, A.W., and Harrison, M.R.: Recent advances in prenatal diagnosis and treatment, Pediatr. Clin. North Am. **32**:1103-1116, 1985.

American Academy of Pediatrics, Committee on Genetics: New issues in newborn screening for phenylketonuria and congenital hypothyroidism, Pediatrics **69**:104-106, 1982.

Cohen, F.L.: Clinical genetics in nursing practice, Philadelphia, 1984, J.B. Lippincott Co.

Fletcher, J.C.: Ethics and amniocentesis for fetal sex identification, N. Engl. J. Med. **301**:550-552, 1979.

Fraser, F.C.: Genetic counseling, Am. J. Hum. Genet. **26**:636-659, 1974.

Gillberg, C., Rasmussen, P., and Wahlström, J.: Long-term follow-up of children born after amniocentesis, Clin. Genet. **21**:69-73, 1982.

Kilpack, V.: Ethical issues in procedural dilemmas in measuring patient competence. In Chinn, P.L., editor: Ethical issues in nursing, Rockville, MD, 1986, Aspen Systems.

Korsch, B.M.: What do patients and parents what to know? What do they need to know? Pediatrics (Suppl.), 1984, pp. 917-919.

Luery, N.M.: Drugs in pregnancy, Am. Druggist, **192**:102-104, 1985.

Opitz, J.M., Shapiro, S.S., and Uehling, D.T.: Genetic causes and workup of male and female infertility, Postgrad. Med. **65**:247-252, 1979.

Paris Conference (1975), Supplement (1975): Standardization in human cytogenetics. Birth Defects: Original Article Series, vol. II, no. 9, New York, 1975, The National Foundation.

Sorenson, J.R., and Mangione, T.W.: Parental response to repeat testing of infants with ''false-positive'' results in a newborn screening program, Pediatrics **73**(2):183-187, 1984.

Spranger, J., and others: Errors of morphogenesis: concepts and terms, J. Pediatr. **100**:160-165, 1982.

BIBLIOGRAPHY
General

Anderson, C.E., Rotter, J.I., and Zonana, J.: Hereditary considerations in common disorders, Pediatr. Clin. North Am. **25**:539-556, 1978.

Bergsma, D., editor: Birth defects. Atlas and compendium, ed. 2, New York, 1979, The National Foundation.

Cohen, F.L.: Clinical genetics in nursing practice, Philadelphia, 1984, J.B. Lippincott Co.

Giller, E.L., and others: Psychosocial care in a medical genetics clinic, Gen. Hosp. Psychiatry **3**:171-178, 1981.

Hall, J.G., and others: The frequency and financial burden of genetic disease in a pediatric hospital, Am. J. Med. Genet. **1**:417-436, 1978.

Hilton, B., and others, editors: Ethical issues in human genetics, New York, 1973, Plenum Press.

Jackson, L.G., and Schimke, R.N.: Clinical genetics, New York, 1979, John Wiley & Sons, Inc.

Lessick, M.L., Van Putte, A.W., and Rowley, P.T.: Assessment of evaluation of hospitalized pediatric patients with genetic disorders, Clin. Pediatr. **20**:178-183, 1981.

McKusick, V.A.: Mendelian inheritance in man, ed. 6, Baltimore, 1983, Williams & Wilkins.

Milunsky, A., editor: Genetics and the Law II, 1980, New York, Plenum Press.

Moore, K.L.: The developing human: clinically oriented embryology, ed. 2, Philadelphia, 1977, W.B. Saunders Co.

Naeye, R.L., and Peters, E.C.: Working during pregnancy: effects on the fetus, Pediatrics **69**:724-727, 1982.

Powledge, T.M., and Fletcher, J.: Guidelines for the ethical, social, and legal issues in prenatal diagnosis, N. Engl. J. Med. **300**:168-172, 1979.

Scriver, C.R., and others: Genetics and medicine: an evolving relationship, Science **200**:952-958, 1978.

Sepe, S.J., and others: Genetic services in the United States, JAMA **248**:1733-1735, 1982.

Shaw, M.W.: Genetic services: necessity or luxury? Am. J. Med. Genet. **15**:373-378, 1983.

Smith, D.W.: Recognizable patterns of human malformation, ed. 3, Philadelphia, 1982, W.B. Saunders Co.

Stainton, M.C.: The fetus: a growing member of the family, Family Rel. 34:321-326, 1985.

Thompson, J.S., and Thompson, M.W.: Genetics in medicine, ed. 3, Philadelphia, 1980, W.B. Saunders Co.

Turner, J.H., Hayashi, T.T., and Pogoloff, D.D.: Legal and social issues in medical genetics, Am. J. Obstet. Gynecol. 134:83-99, 1979.

Weiss, J.O.: Psychosocial stress in genetic disorders: a guide for social workers, Soc. Work Health Care, 6(4):17, 1981.

Williams, J.K.: Pediatric nurse practitioners' knowledge of genetic disease, Pediatr. Nurs. 9:119-121, 1983.

Cytogenetic Disorders

Bender, B., and others: Speech and language development in 41 children with sex chromosome anomalies, Pediatrics 71:262-267, 1983.

Bocian, M., and Mohondas, T.: Recent cytogenetic advances and implications for pediatric practice, Pediatr. Clin. North Am. 25:517-538, 1978.

Miller, R.W.: Birth defects and cancer due to small chromosomal deletions, J. Pediatr. 96:1031, 1980.

Nyhan, W.L.: Cytogenetic diseases. Clin. Symp. 35(1) entire issue, 1983.

Puck, M.H., and others: Parents' adaptation to early diagnosis of sex chromosome anomalies, 16:71-79, 1983.

Rovet, J., and Netly, C.: The triple X chromosome syndrome in childhood recent empirical findings, Child. Dev. 54:831-845, 1983.

Schwartz, S., and Palmer, C.G.: Chromosomal findings in 164 couples with repeated spontaneous abortions: with special consideration to prior reproductive history, Hum. Genet. 63:28-34, 1983.

Stene, J., and others: Paternal age and Down's syndrome: data from prenatal diagnosis, Hum. Genet. 59:119, 1981.

Uchida, I.A.: Radiation-induced nondisjunction, Environ. Health Perspect. 31:13,1979.

Wilkins, L.E., and others: Clinical heterogeneity in 80 home-reared children with cri du chat syndrome, J. Pediatr. 102:528-529, 1983.

Monogenic (Single Gene) Disorders

Sinclair, L.: Metabolic disease in childhood, Oxford, Blackwell Scientific Publications, 1982.

Multifactorial Disorders

Benirschke, K., and others: Developmental terms—some proposals: first report of an international working group, Am. J. Med. Genet. 3:297-302, 1979.

Cohen, M.M., Jr.: The child with multiple birth defects, New York, 1982, Raven Press.

Golub, H.L.: Infant cry: a clue to diagnosis, Pediatrics 69:197-201, 1982.

McDevitt, H.O.: The HLA system and its relation to disease, Hosp. Pract. July 15, 1985, pp. 57-72.

Peter, D.: HLA antigens and disease, Diagn. Med. 4:54-81, 1981.

Schaller, J.G., and Hansen, J.A.: HLA relationships to disease, Hosp. Pract. May 1981, pp. 41-49.

Wilson, G.N.: Recurrence risks of malformations, J. Reprod. Med. 27:607-612, 1982.

Therapeutic Management

Cederbaum, S.D.: Introduction to recombinant DNA, Pediatrics 74:408-410, 1984.

Dunn, P.: Surgery for the unborn, Nurs. Life 4(5):19-21, 1984.

Gaffney, S.E.: Intrauterine fetal surgery: the ramifications for nurses, Am. J. Maternal Child Nurs. 10:250-254, 1985.

Merz, B.: Gene therapy: correcting the errors in life's blueprint, Med. World News 25(19):46-50, 1984.

Prenatal Influences: Developmental Defects

Bank, K.M., and others: Reproductive hazards in the work place, Fam. Comm. Health 6(1):44-56, 1983.

Benirschke, K., and others: Developmental terms—some proposals: first report of an international working group, Am. J. Med. Genet. 3:297-302, 1979.

Chernoff, G.F., and Jones, K.L.: Fetal preventive medicine: teratogens and the unborn baby, Pediatr. Ann. 10:210-217, 1981.

Kalter, H., and Warkany, J.: Congenital malformations: etiologic factors and their role in prevention, Part I, N. Engl. J. Med. 308:424-431, 1983.

Kalter, H., and Warkany, J.: Congenital malformations, Part II, N. Engl. J. Med. 308:491-497, 1983.

McNall, L.K., and Collea, J.V.: Environmental influences on embryonic and fetal development. In McNall, L.K., and Galeener, J.T., editors: Current practice in obstetric and gynecologic nursing, vol. 2, St. Louis, 1978, The C.V. Mosby Co.

Opitz, J.M.: The developmental field concept in clinical genetics, J. Pediatr. 101:805-809, 1982.

Schenzel, A.A.G.L., and others: Monozygotic twinning and structural defects, J. Pediatr. 95:921-930, 1979.

Stevenson, R.E.: The fetus and newly born infant: influences of the prenatal environment, ed. 3, St. Louis, 1981, The C.V. Mosby Co.

Prenatal Influences: Chemicals

Bibbo, M., and others: Follow-up study of male and female offspring of DES-exposed mothers, Obstet. Gynecol. 49:1-8, 1977.

Council on Scientific Affairs: Fetal effects of maternal alcohol use, JAMA 249:2517, 1983.

Done, A.K.: Drug toxins and dysmorphic syndromes, Emerg. Med. 15(7)39:42-43, 1983.

Gullekson, D.J.K., and Temple, A.R.: Maternal drug use during the prenatal period, Fam. Comm. Health 1(3):31-41, 1978.

Jaffe, J.M.: Influence of drug exposure of the father on perinatal outcome, Clin. Perinatol. 6:21-36, 1979.

Luke, B.: Maternal alcoholism and fetal alcohol syndrome, Am. J. Nurs. 77:1924-1926, 1977.

Luke, B.: Megavitamins and pregnancy: a dangerous combination, Am. J. Maternal Child Nurs. 10:18-23, 1985.

Pregnancy categories for prescription drugs, FDA Drug Bull. 12(3):24, 1982.

Reid, J.D.: Effects of selected OTC medications on the unborn and newborn, Nurse Pract. 8(8):43, 46-47, 49-50, 1983.

Shepard, T.H.: Catalog of teratogenic agents, ed. 3, Baltimore, 1980, Johns Hopkins University Press.

Shepard, T.H.: Counseling pregnant women exposed to potentially harmful agents during pregnancy, Clin. Obstet. Gynecol. 26:478-483, 1983.

Shepard, T.H.: Detection of human teratogenic agents, J. Pediatr. 101:810-815, 1982.

Shepard, T.H.: Teratogenicity of therapeutic agents, Curr. Prob. Pediatr. 10(2):3-54, Dec. 1979.

Sokya, L.F., and Joffe, J.M.: Male-mediated drug effects on offspring, Prog. Clin. Biol. Res. 36:49-66, 1980.

Weeks, H.F.: Perinatal pharmacology, Am. J. Maternal Child Nurs. 5:143, 1980.

Wicklund, S.: Special report: drugs for two in pregnancy, Am. J. Nurs. 82:980-981, 1982.

Zacharias, J.: A rational approach to drug use in pregnancy, J. Obstet. Gynecol. Nurs. 12:183-187, 1983.

Prenatal Influences: Infectious Agents

Alford, C.A., Pass, R.F., and Stagno, S.: Chronic congenital infections: common environmental causes for severe and subtle birth defects, Birth Defects 19(5):187-192, 1983.

Claypool, J.M.: Rubella protection for maternal child health care providers, Am. J. Maternal Child Nurs. 6:53-56, 1981.

Committee on Fetus and Newborn: Perinatal herpes simplex virus infections, Pediatrics **66:**147-148, 1980.

Hayden, G.F., and others: Subclinical congenital rubella infection associated with maternal rubella vaccination in early pregnancy, J. Pediatr. **96:**869-872, 1980.

Michaelis, J., and others: Prospective study of suspected associations between certain drugs administered during early pregnancy and congenital malformations, Teratology **27:**57, 1983.

Sever, J.L.: Infections in pregnancy: highlights from the collaborative perinatal project, Teratology **25:**227, 1980.

Sever, J.L.: Infectious causes of human reproductive loss. In Porter, I., and Hook, B., editors: Human embryonic and fetal death, New York, 1980, Academic Press.

Stagno, S.: Toxoplasmosis, Am. J. Nurs. **80:**720-722, 1980.

Prenatal Influences: Radiation and Temperature

Brent, R.L.: Radiation teratogenesis, Teratology **21:**281-298, 1980.

Brent, R.L.: The effects of embryonic and fetal exposure to x-ray, microwave and ultrasound, Clin. Obstet. Gynecol. **26:**484-510, 1983.

Brent, R.L.: The effects of ionizing radiation, microwaves, and ultrasound on the developing embryo: clinical interpretations and applications of the data, Curr. Probl. Pediatr. **14**(9):1-87, 1984.

Pleet, H., Graham, J.M., and Smith, D.W.: Central nervous system and facial defects associated with maternal hyperthermia at 4 to 14 weeks' gestation, Pediatrics **67:**785-789, 1981.

Prenatal Influences: Nutritional Factors

Beer, S.: What?! No meat?! Pediatr. Nurs. **3**(3):16-19, 1977.

Dwyer, J.T.: Family nutrition and the health care team, Iss. Compr. Pediatr. Nurs. **1**(5):1-21, 1977.

Evans, D., and others: Intellectual development and nutrition, J. Pediatr. **97:**358-363, 1980.

Forbes, G.B.: Nutrition and growth, J. Pediatr. **91:**40-43, 1977.

Prenatal Influences: Maternal Smoking

Berman, S.M., Hogue, C.J.R., and Marks, J.S.: Maternal cigarette smoking: effect on infant birth weight (Letter), JAMA **253:**1391-1392, 1985.

Deibel, P.: Effects of cigarette smoking on maternal nutrition and the fetus, J. Obstet. Gynecol Nurs. **9:**333-336, 1980.

Etzel, R.A., and others: Clinical and laboratory observations: urine cotinine excretion in neonates exposed to tobacco smoke products in utero, J. Pediatr., **107**(1):146-148, 1985.

Garn, S.M., and others: Effect of maternal cigarette smoking on Apgar scores, Am. J. Dis. Child **135:**503-506, 1981.

Huch, A., Danko, J., and Huch, R.: Smoking and pregnancy, J. Perinat. Med. **10:**55-57, 1982.

Kariniemi, V., and others: Effects of smoking on fetal heart rate variability during gestational weeks 27 to 32, Am. J. Obstet. Gynecol. **149:**575-576, 1984.

Longo, L.D.: Some health consequences of maternal smoking: issues without answers, Birth Defects **18**(3A):13-31, 1982.

Luck, W., and Nau, H.: Exposure of the fetus, neonate, and nursed infant to nicotine and cotinine from maternal smoking (Letter), N. Engl. J. Med. **311:**672, 1984.

McKay, S.R.: Smoking during the childbearing year, Am. J. Maternal Child Nurs. **5:**46-50, 1980.

Merritt, T.A.: Smoking mothers affect little lives, Am. J. Dis. Child **135:**501-502, 1981.

Mochinzuki, M., and others: Effects of smoking on fetoplacental-maternal system during pregnancy, Am. J. Obstet. Gynecol. **149:**413-420, 1984.

Naeye, R.L., and Peters, E.C.: Mental development of children whose mothers smoked during pregnancy, Obstet. Gynecol. **64:**601-607, 1984.

Nieburg, P., and others: The fetal tobacco syndrome, JAMA **253:**2998-2999, 1985.

Smoking and fetal growth retardation, Briefs **44:**151, 1980.

Witter, R., and King, T.M.: Cigarettes and pregnancy, Prog. Clin. Biol. Res. **36:**83, 1980.

Genetic Screening

Beaudet, A.L.: Genetic diagnostic studies for mental retardation, Curr. Probl. Pediatr. **8**(5):3-47, 1978.

Benzie, R.J.: Antenatal genetic diagnosis: current status, Can. Med. Assoc. J. **120:**685-692, 1979.

Berry, H.K.: Neonatal screening: the spectrum of metabolic disorders, Part 3, Diagn. Med. **7**(3):39-41, 44, 46, 1984.

Brusilo, S.W., and others: Screening for lethal genetic disease, Pediatrics **70:**647, 1982.

Committee on Genetics: New issues in newborn screening for phenylketonuria and congenital hypothyroidism, Pediatrics **69:**104, 1982.

Davies, B.L., and Doran, T.A: Factors in a woman's decision to undergo genetic amniocentesis for advanced maternal age, Nurs. Res. **31:**56-59, 1982.

Faden, R.R., and others: Parental rights, child welfare, and public health: the case of PKU screening, Am. J. Publ. Health **72:**396-400, 1982.

Faden, R.R., and others: A survey to evaluate parental consent as public policy for neonatal screening, Am. J. Publ. Health **72:**1347, 1982.

Fisher, D.A.: Second International Conference on Neonatal Thyroid Screening: progress report, J. Pediatr. **103:**653-654, 1983.

Fleischer, A.C., Kirchner, S.G., and Thieme, G.A.: Prenatal detection of fetal anomalies with sonography, Pediatr. Clin. North Am. **32:**1523-1536, 1985.

Fraser, F.C., and Forse, R.A.: On genetic screening of donors for artificial insemination, Am. J. Med. Genet. **10:**399, 1981.

Furlong, R.M., and Berkowitz, R.L.: Intrauterine treatment: meeting the psychosocial needs of the family, Health Soc. Work **10:**55-62a, 1985.

Hammer, R.M., and Tufts, M.A.: Chorionic villi sampling for detecting fetal disorders, Am. J. Maternal Child Nurs. **11:**29-31, 1986.

Harvey, E.B., and others: Prenatal x-ray exposure and childhood cancer in twins, N. Engl. J. Med. **312:**541-545, 1985.

Holtzman, N.A.: Ethical issues in the prenatal diagnosis of phenylketonuria, Pediatrics **74:**424-427, 1984.

Holtzman, N.A., and others: Effect of informed parental consent on mothers' knowledge of newborn screening, Pediatrics **72:**807-812, 1983.

Holtzman, N.A.: Pitfalls of newborn screening (with special attention to hypothyroidism): when will we ever learn? Birth Defects **19**(5):111, 1983.

Holtzman, N.A., Leonard, C.O., and Farfel, M.R.: Issues in antenatal and neonatal screening and surveillance for hereditary and congenital disorders, Ann. Rev. Publ. Health **2:**219, 1981.

Mamunes, P.: Neonatal screening tests, Pediatr. Clin. North Am. **27:**733, 1980.

Nussbaum, R.L., and others: Newborn screening for sickling hemoglobinopathies, Am. J. Dis. Child. **138:**44-48, 1984.

Paul, T.D., Naylor, E.W., and Guthrie, R.: Urine screening for metabolic disease in newborn infants, J. Pediatr. **96:**653-656, 1980.

President's Commission for the Study of Ethical Problems in Medicine and Biomedical and Behavioral Research: Screening and counseling for genetic conditions, 1983, Washington, D.C., Government Printing Office.

Rozovky, L.E., and others: Genetic screening: public health and the law, Can. J. Public Health **72:**15-16, 1981.

Scriver, C.R.: Genetic screening: implications for preventive medicine, Am. J. Publ. Health **73:**243, 1983.

Sorensen, J.R., and others: Parental response to repeat testing of infants with "false-positive" results in a newborn screening program, Pediatrics **73:**183-187, 1984.

Stephenson, S.R., and Weaver, D.D.: Prenatal diagnosis—a compilation of diagnosed conditions, Am. J. Obstet. Gynecol. **141**:319-343, 1981.

Summer, G.K., and Shoaf, C.R.: Developments in genetic and metabolic screening, Fam. Comm. Health **4**(4):13-30, 1982.

Worthington, S: Genetic screening, J. Obstet. Gynecol. Nurs. (Suppl.) **13**(2):32s-37s, 1984.

Genetic Counseling

Abramovsky, I., and others: Analysis of a follow-up study of genetic counseling, Clin. Genet. **17**:1, 1980.

Alder, R.: It doesn't end with death: grieving and genetic counseling, Clin. Pediatr. **18**:767-768, 1979.

Bocian, M.E., and Kaback, M.M.: Crisis counseling: the newborn infant with a chromosomal anomaly, Pediatr. Clin. North Am. **25**:643-650, 1978.

Council on Scientific Affairs: Genetic counseling and prevention of birth defects, JAMA **248**:224-229, 1982.

Feingold, M.: Genetic counseling and congenital anomalies, Pediatr. Rev. **2**(5):155-158, 1980.

Fibison, W.J.: The nursing role in the delivery of genetic services, Health Care Women **4**:1-15, 1983.

Fitzimmons, E.: Genetic counseling: learning to keep counsel, Nurs. Mirror **153**(11):48-50, 1981.

Harper, P.S.: Practical genetic counseling, Baltimore, 1981, University Park Press.

Kelly, P.T.: Dealing with dilemma: a manual for genetic counselors, New York, 1977, Springer-Verlag.

Kenen, R.H.: Genetic counseling: the development of a new interdisciplinary occupational field, Soc. Sci. Med. **18**:541-549, 1984.

Kessler, S., editor: Genetic counseling: psychologic dimensions, New York, 1979, Academic Press, Inc.

Korsch, B.M.: What do patients and parents want to know? What do they need to know? Symposium of Pediatric Patient Educations: Challenge for the 80s, 1983.

LaRochelle, D.: Prenatal genetic counseling: ethical and legal interfaces with the nurse's role, Health Care Women **4**:77-92.

Lebel, R.R.: Ethical issues arising in the genetic counseling relationship, White Plains, NY, 1978, National Foundation March of Dimes.

Lippman-Hand, A., and Fraser, F.C.: Genetic counseling: provision and reception of information, Am. J. Med. Genet. **3**:113, 1979.

Lippman-Hand, A., and Fraser, F.C.: Genetic counseling—the post counseling period: I. Parents' perceptions of uncertainty, Am. J. Med. Genet. **4**:51, 1979.

Lippman-Hand, A., and Fraser, F.C.: Genetic counseling—the post counseling period: II. Making reproductive choices, Am. J. Med. Genet. **4**:73-89, 1979.

Seller, M.J.: Ethical aspects of genetic counselling, J. Med. Ethics **8**:185, 1982.

Sheffield, L.: Genetic counseling, Aust. Nurs. J. **11**:1-4, Mar. 1982.

Smith, R.W., and Antley, R.M.: Anger: a significant obstacle to informed decision making in genetic counseling, Birth Defects **15**(5C):257, 1979.

Thurman, T.F.: Genetic counseling: practical concepts about risks and risk management, Consultant **25**(6):50-52, 56, 1985.

Tishler, C.L.: The psychological aspects of genetic counseling, Am. J. Nurs. **81**:733-734, 1981.

Valentine, G.H.: The reproductive counseling process, Clin. Pediatr. **16**:233-238, 1977.

VanRegemorter, N., and others: Congenital malformations in 10,000 consecutive births in a university hospital: need for genetic counseling and prenatal diagnosis, J. Pediatr. **104**:386-390, 1984.

Weiss, J.O.: Psychosocial stress in genetic disorders: a guide for social workers, Soc. Work Health Care **6**(6):17-21, 1981.

Wilson, G.N.: Counseling parents of children with genetic disorders, Feelings & Their Med. Signif. **25**:(4)13-16, 1983.

Unit Two

Assessment of the Child and Family

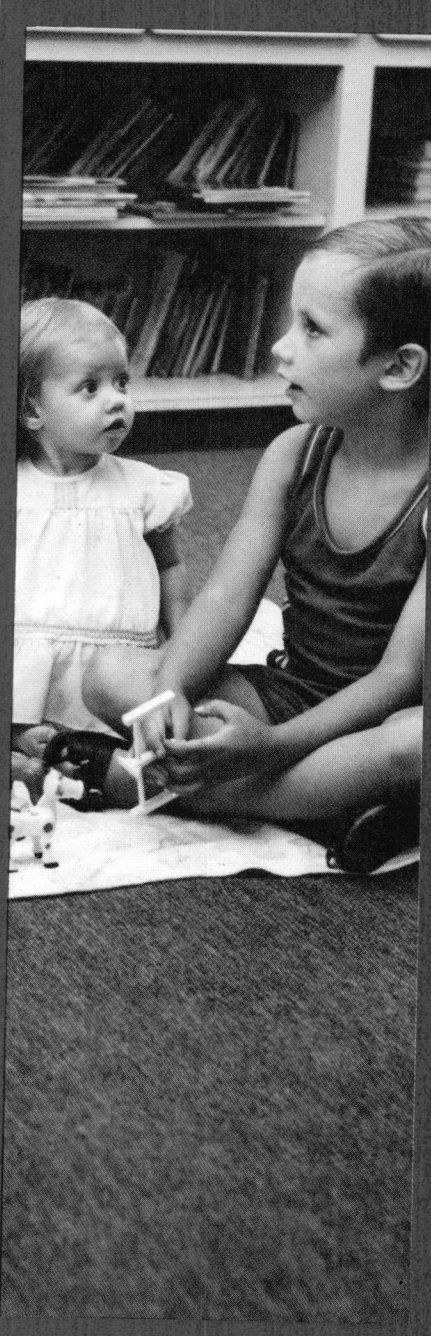

Assessment is fundamental to the nursing process. Establishing a data base on which to formulate a nursing diagnosis, plan interventions, and evaluate outcomes of care is essential whether the nurse is caring for a child who is well or ill. Assessment facilitates identification of present problems and prevention of future ones. Although the assessment process primarily focuses on the child, it permits an exploration into family dynamics and often is the first clue to cultural, environmental, socioeconomic, or religious traditions that influence the child's total well-being.

Assessment primarily involves some form of communication. Chapter 6, *Communication and Health Assessment of the Child and Family,* is concerned with general aspects of communication as they relate to the nurse, parent, and child. It also discusses the interview process specifically in terms of history-taking, with special emphasis on assessment of the family and nutrition.

Chapter 7, *Physical and Developmental Assessment of the Child,* deals with the procedures and skills required to perform a complete pediatric physical assessment, including sensory and developmental testing. Findings primarily related to normal structure and function are emphasized, with notation of those deviations that require referral and further evaluation.

Chapter 6

Communication and Health Assessment of the Child and Family

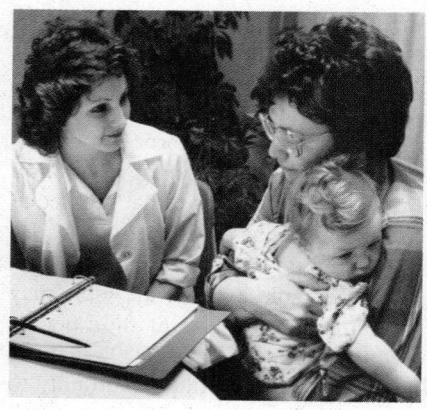

Communication is essential to the nursing of children. It is the most important skill used in assessment of children and their families and the most important feature in forming trusting relationships with them. Communication consists of all those behaviors by which one person, consciously or unconsciously, affects another. All behavior transmits a message: even the attempt not to communicate creates a particular impression. Inherent in communication are the power of observation, the use of all the senses, and the intangible reaction of intuition.

This chapter is concerned with the communication process as it relates to health assessment. In the first section, strategies for communication and interviewing are reviewed and specific suggestions for communicating with parents and children are presented. The second section deals with a particular type of interview—the health history. It is presented in some detail to give nurses the opportunity to learn to take a history, as well as to facilitate understanding those histories recorded by other members of the health team. Because of the importance of the family and nutrition in ensuring optimal emotional and physical health, special sections on family and nutritional assessment are included.

Communication

Communication may be verbal, nonverbal, or abstract. *Verbal* communication may involve language and its expression, such as vocalizations in the form of laughs, moans, and squalls, or the implications of what is not said in light of what has been said. *Nonverbal* communication is often called body language and includes gestures, movements, facial expressions, postures, and reactions. *Abstract* communication takes such forms as play, artistic expression, symbols, photographs, and choice of clothing. Because it is possible to exert greater conscious control over verbal communication, it is a less reliable indicator of true feelings, especially in relationships with children.

Many factors influence the communication process. To be successful (gratifying), communication must be appropriate to the situation, properly timed, and clearly delivered. This implies that nurses understand and use techniques of effective communication. Verbal and nonverbal messages must be congruous; that is, two or more messages sent via different levels must not be contradictory.

Nurses need to recognize their own feelings and attempt to recognize those of the persons with whom the communicative interchange takes place. Biases and judgments interfere with all aspects of the process. The tendency to approve or disapprove of another's statements inhibits positive reactions. In addition, the transmission and reception of messages may be altered by influences of intimacy or distance, trust and mistrust, security and insecurity, or caring and not caring on the part of the participants. The value of effective communication is increased understanding between the nurse, child, and family. Since nursing of infants and children always involves the inclusion of a caregiver, nurses must be able to communicate not only with children of all ages but with the adults in their lives as well.

VERBAL COMMUNICATION—THE POWER OF WORDS

Words shape reality, and thus they hold tremendous power. One can change another's perception of reality by the choice of words each uses (Cassell, 1980a). For example, if the diagnosis of cancer is always referred to as a tumor, cyst, malignancy, or carcinoma, the person may never really know that he has cancer. Consequently he may assume less responsibility for his care than if he were aware of his condition's seriousness. By learning to recognize how patients and health professionals use language to manipulate reality, one can also learn how to change one's perceptions and communicate more effectively.

Avoidance Language

Probably the most common way people try to alter reality is by avoiding words that truly describe it. For example, euphemisms such as "passed on" are used instead of the word "death." Avoidance language usually indicates that a person wants to hide something, especially feelings. As a rule, accepting a person's use of euphemisms only serves to perpetuate his fears and never helps him deal with them. In contrast, use of straightforward, precise, descriptive language lends perspective to the situation and allows the person to discuss his fears. Most often, imagined fears are far greater than the actual reality. (For a discussion of explaining death to children, see p. 962.)

Distancing Language

Sometimes people use impersonal words to shield themselves from the painful reality of a situation. For example, parents may state that they know *someone* with a child who is slow and actually be talking about personal fears regarding *their* child. By realizing that parents need to talk about this difficult subject, the nurse can provide sensitive statements that ease them into discussing their situation.

One of the dangers in supporting distancing language is that the parent may effectively deny that a problem exists. To return to the previous example, if the issue of retardation is never approached directly but is allowed to be "someone else's problem," the parents may not be able to make decisions for special schools or individualized training.

Sometimes distancing is desirable because the topic may be too painful to discuss directly. The use of third-person technique (p. 195) or symbolic language (p. 959) may be very therapeutic in allowing an individual the opportunity to indirectly approach a subject and receive feedback but still remain in control.

NONVERBAL COMMUNICATION— PARALANGUAGE

In addition to the spoken word, messages are relayed through nonverbal means, or paralanguage, which involves pitch, pause, intonation, rate, volume, and stress in speech (Cassell, 1980b). Young children become very adept at understanding paralanguage; long before they know the meaning of words, they sense anxiety or fear by the rise in pitch or the accelerated rate of the mother's voice. By careful attention to the spoken word, nurses can better understand the meaning of another's verbal message and more accurately control their own paralanguage.

Because most people do not exert conscious control over paralanguage, it is a valuable clue to such things as feelings and concerns. For example, *pausing* may signify a need to formulate thoughts, recall information, or sometimes fabricate a story. Frequent pauses, however, often make the speaker sound unsure of himself. Long pauses may mean that the individual needs more information.

Rate is another characteristic that gives unspoken messages. Talking too fast usually makes the speaker sound glib and insensitive. Talking slowly with a firm tone and appropriate pauses conveys authority. Therefore, a person is much more likely to "hear" instructions if the latter approach is used. Children, in particular, respond attentively to a slow, even, steady voice.

Confirming and Disconfirming Behaviors

People respond to each other through *confirming behaviors*, such as nodding the head, using direct eye contact, repeating or requesting clarification, and making appropriate comments, or *disconfirming behaviors*, such as tapping fingers or a foot, turning away from the speaker, avoiding eye contact, and interrupting (Heineken and Roberts, 1983). Since there is a reciprocal relationship between such behaviors, nurses need to use confirming behaviors to receive confirmation in return. This "mirroring" effect is particularly evident in children because of their sensitivity to nonverbal cues.

Guidelines for Communication and Interviewing

The most widely used method of communicating with parents on a professional basis is the interview process. Interviewing, unlike social conversation, is a specific form of goal-directed communication. As nurses converse with parents, they endeavor to focus on the parents to determine the kind of persons they are, their usual mode of handling problems, whether help is needed, and the way in which they react to counseling. It requires time and patience to develop interviewing skills, but there are some guiding principles and some obstacles to be avoided that facilitate this process.

ESTABLISHING A SETTING FOR COMMUNICATION

Part of the success in interviewing depends on the type of physical and psychologic setting the interviewer constructs. Appropriate introduction, role clarification, explanation of the reason for the interview, preliminary acquaintance with the family, and assurance of privacy and confidentiality are prerequisites for establishing a setting conducive to communication.

Appropriate Introduction

Nurses should introduce themselves to, and ask the name of, each family member who is present. During the interview, each person is addressed by name. If there is any question about using the person's first or last name, common courtesy should be the guiding rule. Asking individuals which name they wish to be called conveys respect, and it also communicates a personal interest in each family member.

At the beginning of the visit, the nurse can include the child in the interaction by asking him his name, age, and other information. Nurses often direct all questions to the adult, even when the child is old enough to speak for himself. This serves to terminate one extremely valuable source of information, the patient himself. If the child is included, the general rules for communicating with children are followed (p. 192).

Role Clarification and Explanation of the Interview

During the introduction it is also necessary to clarify the nurse's particular role in the health setting. For example, nurses performing interviews may be pediatric nurse practitioners, inpatient staff nurses, clinic nurses, office nurses, visiting nurses, or school nurses. Since the format resembles a medical history, the nurse needs to clarify the reason for eliciting this information. A parent is much more likely to reveal personal information about the child and family if the relevance and importance of the interview are stressed. If this is not done, parents may refuse to elaborate on certain areas because they feel it has no bearing on the "problem." In addition, since more than one member of the health team may take a history during the course of a hospital admission, it is important to clarify the reason for each interview.

Another reason for role clarification is education of the health consumer. With expanded roles in nursing, it is not unusual for families to think that the examiner is a physician, not a nurse. Role clarification is especially important because some parents may feel deceived if they later are made aware of the nurse's identity. Since the general consumer acceptance of pediatric nurse practitioners has been very favorable, it is also important to acknowledge the expertise of the nurse by emphasizing the nurse's role.

Preliminary Acquaintance

Because of the personal and private nature of an in-depth interview, the person being interviewed must trust the interviewer in order to reveal such extensive information. Therefore, it is best to begin with some general conversation. Comments such as, "How have things been since your last visit?" "Tell me about Johnny," or (to the child) "What do you think is going to happen today?" allow the parent or child to express his main concern in a casual, relaxed atmosphere.

The preliminary acquaintance conversation also reveals how responsive the informant may be to questions. For example, using open-ended statements may lead the parent into a lengthy detailed discussion. In this case it is more beneficial to direct questions toward specific answers in order to avoid tangential remarks. At other times a parent may respond to open-ended questions with only minimal information, in which case the continued use of open-ended questions probably will reveal more data than "yes" or "no" type questions.

Assurance of Privacy and Confidentiality

The place where the interview is conducted is almost as important as the interview itself. The physical environment should allow for as much privacy as possible with distractions, such as interruptions, ambient noise, or other visible activity, kept to a minimum. At times it may be necessary to turn off a television or radio. The environment should also have some play provision for young children to keep them occupied during the parent-nurse interview (Fig. 6-1).

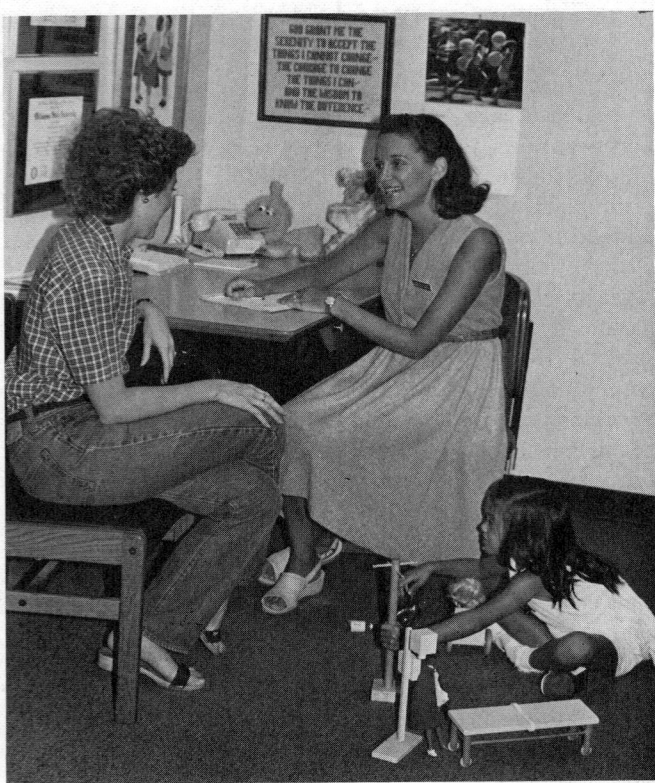

Fig. 6-1. Child plays while nurse interviews parent.

Parents who are constantly interrupted by their children are unable to concentrate fully and tend to give short, brief answers to terminate the interview as quickly as possible.

Confidentiality is also an essential component of the initial phase of the interview. Since the interview is usually shared with other members of the health team or the teacher (as in the case of students), it is the interviewer's responsibility and obligation to inform the parents of the confidential limits of the conversation. If there is any concern regarding confidentiality, such as talking to a parent suspected of child abuse or a teenager contemplating suicide, the nurse must deal with this directly and inform the person that in such instances confidentiality cannot be ensured.

Communicating with Families

Communicating with the family is a triangular process involving the nurse, parents, and child. Although the following discussion focuses primarily on this triad, in many circumstances significant others, for example, siblings, relatives, or other caregivers, may be part of the communication process.

COMMUNICATING WITH PARENTS

Although the parent and child are separate and distinct entities, relationships with the child are frequently mediated via the parent, particularly in the case of younger children. For the most part, information about the child is acquired by direct observation or is communicated to the nurse by the parents. Usually it can be assumed that because of the close contact with the child, the information imparted by the parent is reliable. Making an assessment of the child requires input from the child (verbal and nonverbal), information from the parent, and the nurse's own observations, including assessment of the child and interpretation of the relationship between the child and the parent. Counseling and guidance must be directed to the caregiver of infants and small children; when children are old enough to be active participants in their own health maintenance, the parent becomes a collaborator in health care.

Encouraging the Parent to Talk

Interviewing parents not only offers the nurse an opportunity to determine the health and developmental status of the child but also offers information about all factors that influence the child's life. Whatever the parent sees as a problem should be a concern of the nurse. These problems are not always easy to identify. Nurses need to be alert for clues and signals by which a mother communicates worries and anxieties. Careful phrasing with broad open-ended questions such as "What is Jimmy eating now?" provides more information than several single-answer questions such as "Is Jimmy eating what the rest of the family eats?" that can be answered with "yes" or "no."

Sometimes the parent will take the lead without stimulation. Other times it may be necessary for the nurse to direct another question based on an observation such as "Connie seems unhappy today," or "Does it bother you when David cries?" If the parent appears to be tired or distraught, the nurse might ask, "What do you do to relax?" or "Do you get any help with the children?" A comment such as "You handle the baby very well. Have you had a lot of experience with babies?" to a new mother who appears comfortable with her first child gives her positive reinforcement and provides an opening for any questions she might have regarding the care of her infant. Often all that is required to keep the parent talking is a nod and saying "yes," or "un-huh."

When attempting to elicit feelings and covert problem areas, it is best to avoid beginning a question with "Does . . .," "Did . . .," or "Is . . .," which usually require only a single response. In addition, asking questions such as, "Do you have any problem with your son at school?" subtly implies a lack of parental skills and evokes defensiveness. Instead, it is helpful to say "What . . .," "How . . .," "Tell me about . . .," and encourage elaboration with "You were saying . . .," "You say that . . .," or reflecting back key words or phrases, such as "He was depressed?" Open-ended questions are nonthreatening and encourage description.

Directing the Focus

Ability to direct the focus of the interview, while allowing for maximum freedom of expression, is one of the most difficult goals in effective communication. One approach is the use of open-ended or broad questions, followed by guiding statements. For example, if the parent proceeds to list the other children by name, the nurse can also say, "Tell me their ages, too." If the parent continues to describe each child in depth, which is not the purpose of the interview, the nurse can redirect the focus by stating, "Let's talk about the other children later. You were beginning to tell me about Paul's activities at school." This approach conveys interest in the other children but focuses the data collection on the patient.

In the event that the parent has suggested that a problem exists with one of the other children, the nurse should reintroduce this subject at the end of the interview to assess the need for further family follow-up. Saying to the parent, "Before you were mentioning that your older son is having trouble in school. Tell me what you see as the problem," reintroduces this subject but only in terms of the possible problem.

Listening

Listening is the most important ingredient for effective communication. When listening is truly aimed at understanding the client, it is an active process that requires concentration and attention to all aspects of the conversation—verbal, nonverbal, and abstract. One of the greatest blocks to listening is environmental distraction and premature judgment.

The attitudes and feelings of the nurse are easily injected into an interview. Often nurses' perceptions of a parent's behavior are influenced by their own perceptions, prejudices, and assumptions, which may include racial, religious, and cultural stereotypes. What may be interpreted as passive hostility or disinterest in a parent may be shyness or an expression of anxiety. For example, direct eye contact is frequently regarded as a sign of paying attention. However, in many American Indian tribes, looking into another's eyes is considered disrespectful. Therefore, judgments about "listening" need to be made with an appreciation of cultural differences (Primeaux, 1977).

Although it is necessary to make some preliminary judgments, the nurse must attempt to listen with as much objectivity as possible by clarifying meanings and attempting to see the situation from the parent's point of view. Effective interviewers use conscious control over their reactions, responses, and the techniques they employ.

Use of minimal verbal activity with active listening facilitates parent involvement. It is tempting to spend time explaining, describing, and interpreting health information when the opportunity presents itself. However, it is possible to provide effective health education by properly timing the information and presenting only as much as is necessary at the moment.

Careful listening facilitates the use of clues, verbal leads, or signals from the interviewer to move the interview along. Frequent references to an area of concern, repetition of certain key words, or a special emphasis on something or someone serve as cues to the interviewer for the direction of inquiry. Concerns and anxieties are usually mentioned in a casual, offhand manner. Even though they are casual, they are important and deserve more careful scrutiny to identify problem areas. For example, a parent who is concerned about a child's habit of bed-wetting may casually mention that the child's bed was "wet this morning."

Because the interview is almost always triangular—nurse, child, and parent—the parent may wish to convey information in such a way as to prevent the child from hearing it. This requires active listening on the part of the nurse to hear the unspoken message. The following example illustrates this point:

During a routine health visit the nurse performed a complete history and physical examination on a 4-year-old girl. The child was accompanied by her mother, who appeared to be a reliable, well-informed, and talkative informant. During the child's birth history, the mother gave all the information asked. However, during the family history, the mother stated to the nurse, "I had a hysterectomy 6 years ago." Because the nurse gave no indication of acknowledging the significance of this statement, the mother repeated it, only this time she stressed the "6 years." The nurse, who had not been listening as attentively as she should have, realized that the mother was telling her something very important. The mother raised her eyebrows and gently shook her head "no," warning the nurse not to explore this area too openly. The nurse correctly read the cues and stated, "Let's return to your health history later."

At the completion of the physical examination, the nurse brought the child to the Health Center's playroom and took the opportunity to investigate this contradictory information of a "4-year-old child born to a woman with a hysterectomy 6 years ago." The mother revealed that this child was adopted. The mother was greatly concerned about the fact that the child was unaware of this and requested the nurse's advice.

Fortunately the nurse had "listened" carefully enough to realize the significance of this woman's concern and allowed her the opportunity to discuss it in private.

Listening is also helpful in assessing reliability. For example, the answers elicited at the beginning of the interview may differ from those at the end, when the parent feels more confident in revealing problems. It is important to identify any discrepancies and reintroduce those topics for further investigation.

Using Silence

Silence as a response is often one of the most difficult interviewing techniques to learn. It requires a sense of confidence and comfort on the part of the interviewer to allow the interviewee space in which to think uninterrupted. Silence permits the interviewee to sort out thoughts and feelings, to search for responses to questions, and allows for sharing of feelings in which two or more people absorb the emotion to its depth.

Sometimes it is necessary to break silence and reopen communication. This should be done in such a way that the person is given a choice to continue talking about what is important to him. Breaking a silence by introducing a new topic or by prolonged talking essentially terminates the interviewee's opportunity to use the silence. Suggestions for breaking the silence include statements such as, "Is there anything else you wish to say?" "I see you find it difficult to continue; how may I help?" or "I don't know what this silence means. Perhaps there is something you would like to put into words but find difficult to say."

Being Empathic

Empathy means feeling and participating in the inner feelings of another while remaining objective. The empathic interviewer attempts to see the world from the interviewee's perspective and to understand him as much as possible. Empathy differs from sympathy, which is subjectively thinking or feeling like the other person. While important and necessary at times, sympathy is not always therapeutic in the helping relationship.

Some individuals are naturally empathic and easily "feel" with another person. However empathy can be learned by attending to the verbal and nonverbal language of the interviewee. Neurolinguistic programming (NLP), which is concerned with the manner of accessing and un-

Questions and Controversies

What are parents' concerns and what kinds of support are beneficial?

Two studies demonstrate that a minority of parents' concerns (about 30%) are related to medical problems. Over half are child/family concerns, such as eating, sleeping, crying, parenting skills, language development, socializing the child, discipline, safety, and adjustment to divorce; about 15% are nutritional concerns, such as breast-feeding, weaning, and eating habits (Ryberg and Merrifield, 1984; Hickson and others, 1983). Ryberg and Merrifield have developed the Parents' Needs Assessment Questionnaire to assist health care professionals in identifying parents' concerns.

Many parental concerns warrant supportive intervention. However, little research has been done on the effectiveness of different kinds of support and the impact of this effort. Wasserman and others (1984) report on the effectiveness of three supportive behaviors: (1) encouragement, the expression of positive reinforcement or good feelings in regard to a parent's actions; (2) reassurance, assuagement of a parent's concern or worry; and (3) empathy, the expression of intellectual appreciation of a parent's situation. Reassurance was used most frequently, followed by encouragement and empathy. Nurse practitioners provided significantly more reassurance and more total support than physicians.

To evaluate the impact of providing different kinds of support, the researchers compared visit outcomes as measured by various methods with mothers who received high or low levels of support. Mothers exposed to high levels of encouragement had significant improvement in their opinions of clinicians and higher satisfaction. Mothers exposed to higher levels of empathy had higher satisfaction and greater reduction in concerns. No significant differences in outcome were found for high levels of reassurance. From this study it appears that empathy, the least used form of support, is the most beneficial, encouragement is somewhat less helpful, and reassurance, the most used type of support, is least beneficial.

derstanding information, is an excellent method of increasing empathic communication and will be discussed later (p. 195).

Providing Reassurance

Most parents want to be "good" parents and have at least some anxiety about their ability to function in this role. Questionable behavior on the part of children tends to cast doubt on their success as parents. When feelings of parental adequacy are threatened, anxiety rises. Parents want and need reassurance that they are handling the task of parenthood; thus it is important that nurses do not communicate in a manner that is threatening to the parents' self-esteem. For example, the statement, "Johnny is sleeping in his own room, of course," injects the interviewer's values into the situation. The mother is most likely to respond affirmatively because she feels that the nurse wants to hear this or else that she is not behaving correctly as a mother.

Parents need to have the nurse show an interest in them as individuals as well as in the children. Questions such as, "How do you manage?" or "What do you do when things get difficult?" provide an opportunity for parents to express concerns that are not directly related to the children. Being able to vent feelings to an accepting and impartial listener assists parents to recoup resources for problem solving and coping.

Parents are reassured to know that they have feelings and problems that are shared by other parents. All want to be assured that their children are developing normally, and most have some concerns about feeding, sleep, behavior, and discipline. Occasionally parents do have negative feelings toward their children and need to know that such ambivalence is normal. If the nurse has determined that there is no physical or emotional problem underlying the reaction, parents can gain a measure of reassurance in knowing that this is a common feeling. The parent and nurse can work together to find possible avenues for coping with these feelings.

Defining the Problem

In order to arrive at a solution to a problem or concern, the nurse and the parent must agree that one exists. If neither believes that there is a problem, there is certainly no need to create one. Sometimes the parent may believe that there is a problem that the nurse is unable to see. For example, a mother was overly concerned about every small sniffle, sneeze, or cough in her infant who had been carefully examined and found to be healthy with no evidence of a respiratory problem. On careful questioning, the nurse discovered that a previous child had died of pneumonia in infancy. Consequently the nurse was able to better understand the mother's concern. Once the nurse acknowledges the mother's fear, she can help the mother deal with her special anxieties about her infant and teach her how to recognize when there is need for concern.

Occasionally the nurse identifies a problem that the parent denies exists. In this case the nurse should pursue the situation and either find a way to deal with the situation or enlist the aid of other health team members. For example, the parents of a child with Down syndrome may refuse to believe that their child is different from any other child of the same age. They may say, "He is just a little slow" and "All the child needs to do is to try harder." A child with an obvious behavior problem may be described by the parents as "just stubborn" or "just behaving that way to spite us." Such statements may be clues that the parents have not progressed past the stage of denial in adjusting to the disability.

Solving the Problem

Once the problem is identified and agreed on by parent and nurse, they can begin to arrive at a solution. A parent who is included in the problem-solving process is more apt to follow through with a course of action. Such questions as "What have you tried so far?" or "What have you thought about doing?" provide leads for exploration and give the parents the feeling that their ideas and solutions are worthwhile. These can be followed by "What prevents you from trying that?" "That sounds like a good plan," and "You seem to be stumped. Have you considered trying this?" Such approaches reinforce rather than belittle parents' efforts to solve problems and encourage participation.

Sometimes a parent arrives at a solution that the nurse does not consider to be the best alternative. If it can be ascertained that it will do no harm and the parents are convinced of its merits, it is usually best to allow them to continue with the plan. A course of action is more likely to be carried out when parents can reach their own conclusions. However, when parental decisions may be hazardous, nurses are obligated to discuss the risks with the family and try to reach a more beneficial solution. Whenever possible, decisions should be theirs with the nurse serving as a *facilitator* in problem solving.

Providing Anticipatory Guidance

The ideal way to handle a problem is to prevent it—to deal with it *before* it becomes a problem. The best preventive measure is anticipatory guidance. One of the most significant areas in pediatrics is injury prevention through appropriate anticipatory guidance. Beginning prenatally, parents need specific instructions on home safety. Because of the child's maturing developmental skills, home safety changes must be implemented early to minimize risks to the child.

Many normal developmental changes can disturb unprepared parents, such as a toddler's diminished appetite, negativism, altered sleeping patterns, and anxiety toward strangers. Such topics are discussed in the chapters on health promotion to provide the nurse with knowledge to counsel parents.

Avoiding Blocks to Communication

There are a number of blocks to communication that can severely affect the quality of the helping relationship. Some of the more common blocks include:

Socializing
Giving unrestricted and sometimes unasked-for advice
Offering premature or inappropriate reassurance
Giving overready encouragement
Defending a situation or opinion
Using stereotyped comments or cliches
Limiting expression of emotion by asking directed, close-ended questions
Interrupting and finishing the person's sentence
Talking more than the interviewee
Forming prejudged conclusions
Deliberately changing the focus

Communication blocks can be corrected by careful analysis of the interview process. One of the best methods for improving interviewing skills is audio- and/or videotape feedback. With supervision and guidance, the interviewer can recognize the blocks and consciously avoid them.

Communicating with Families Through an Interpreter

Sometimes communication is impossible because two people speak different languages. In this case it is necessary to obtain information through a third party, the interpreter. When an interpreter is used, the same guidelines for interviewing are employed.

The following principles apply primarily to the use of an adult interpreter (Kohut, 1975). Often no one other than an older child is available to help translate. In this situation it is important to stress *literal* translation of parent responses. To maximize correct translations, it may be necessary to interrupt the parent and ask the child to translate every few sentences. When children are used as interpreters, the nurse needs to ask questions directed at specific answers and must assess the interpreted translation in terms of nonverbal expressions of communication.

Role clarification and explanation of the interview. After introductions, the nurse should explain to the interpreter the reason for the interview and the type of questions that will be asked. An interpreter should know whether a detailed or brief answer is required and whether the translated response can be general or literal.

Introduction and preliminary acquaintance. The nurse should introduce the interpreter to each family member. Ideally the interpreter and parent are allowed some time together before the actual interview so that they can become acquainted.

Communicate directly with the parent. When asking questions, the nurse should address the parent directly in order to reinforce interest in the parent and observe carefully for nonverbal expressions, mentally noting to ask the interpreter about these later. It is important to refrain from interrupting the parent and interpreter while they are conversing. If the parent answers statements with lengthy discussions, it may be necessary to use more direct questions, rather than open-ended ones. If the translation is shorter than the actual answer, one should not assume that the interpreter is withholding information. He or she may have difficulty in understanding the explanation and need time for clarification.

The nurse should avoid commenting to the interpreter about the patient. It is best to presume that the parent understands some English.

Respect cultural differences. It is often best to pose questions about sex, marriage, or pregnancy indirectly. For example, it is best to ask about the child's "father" rather than the mother's "husband." The nurse must be aware of difficulty on the part of the interpreter in asking such questions.

Communicate directly with the interpreter. Following the interview, the nurse should allow time for the interpreter to share information in private. This is the time to ask about nonverbal clues to communication, to ask for personal interpretations of the parent's reliability or ease in revealing information, and to allow the interpreter an opportunity to share something that he or she felt could not be said earlier.

Continuity. Whenever possible, the nurse should arrange for the parent to speak with the same interpreter on subsequent visits. This helps all three parties feel more comfortable and facilitates effective translation of both words and feelings.

COMMUNICATING WITH CHILDREN

Although the greatest amount of verbal communication is usually carried out with the parent, the child should not be excluded during the interview. Periodic attention to infants and younger children through play or by occasionally directing questions or remarks to them makes children participants in the interview. Older children can be actively included as informants.

When relating with children of all ages, it is the nonverbal components of the communication process that convey the most significant messages to them. It is difficult to disguise feelings, attitudes, and anxiety when relating to children. They are very alert to surroundings and attach meaning to every gesture and move that is made. This is particularly true with very young children. It is best to avoid rushing in on a child with gestures or with words. The child should be allowed time to make the first move when possible. Sudden or rapid advances are frightening to a child, as are threatening gestures such as facial contortions, including very broad smiles. Although these are usually intended as friendly gestures, they frequently have the opposite effect.

Children are uncomfortable or even frightened when someone stares at them. It is best to refrain from extended eye contact with a child. Active attempts to make friends with children before they have had an opportunity to evaluate an unfamiliar person tend to increase their anxiety. A helpful tactic is to continue to talk to the child and parent but go about activities that do not involve the child directly, thus allowing him to carry out his observations from a safe position. If the child has a special toy or doll with him, it is helpful to "talk" to the doll first. Asking simple questions such as, "Does your teddy bear have a special name?" may ease the child into conversation.

Children should be met on their own eye level since communicating down to them emphasizes their smallness. Adults in strange places may assume overwhelming proportions to children who believe themselves to be in helpless positions. Sitting on a low chair, kneeling, squatting, or even sitting on the floor, if appropriate, places the nurse in a more favorable and less threatening position (Fig. 6-2). With very young children every effort should be made to preserve physical closeness with the parent. Consequently the entire interview may be done with the child sitting on the parent's lap. Giving the child a toy, bottle, or pacifier may help to quiet him.

At any age children respond best to a quiet, unhurried, and confident voice. Children attend to softly spoken words; they tend to withdraw when a voice is raised. Even a crying, distressed child is more apt to "hear" a voice that speaks quietly than one that is attempting to compete with the child's own volume. This is the most successful approach to calming even an uncooperative child.

When giving directions to or seeking cooperation from a child, the nurse should speak clearly, be specific, and use as few words as possible. Simple language is more easily understood. In addition, children's language comprehension precedes their use of words. Although they may not yet talk, it does not mean that they do not understand. The same concept applies when nurses and parents discuss children in their presence. It is more effective to use a positive approach in relating with children. Directions and suggestions are best stated in a *positive* way. An easy way to do this is to avoid using the word "don't." There is more likelihood

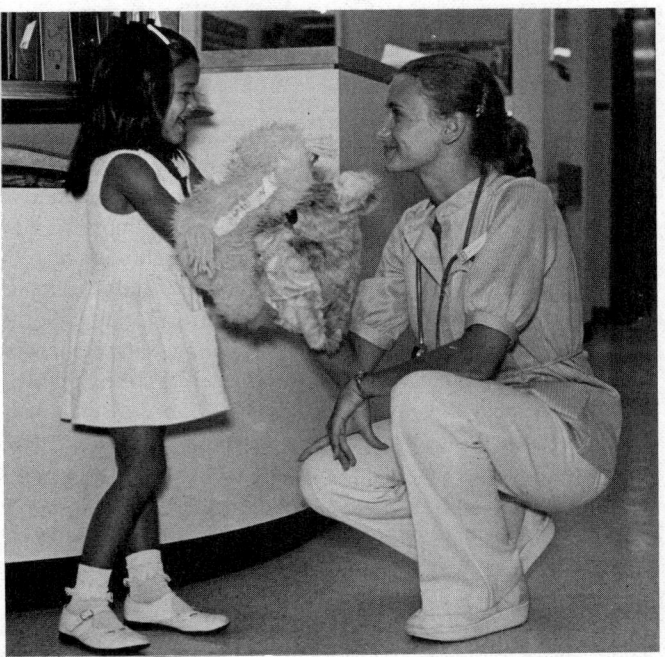

Fig. 6-2. Nurse talks to child using puppets and assumes position at child's level.

that a child's cooperation will be gained by saying, "The crayon is for writing" instead of "Don't eat the crayon."

The nurse should be honest with children and make no promises that are impossible to carry out. To assure them that a procedure, such as an injection, will not hurt is no measure of comfort to children who have either experienced the discomfort previously or who discover that indeed it *does* hurt. Any trust that has been built between the child and the nurse will be damaged by the deception, and the child will be justifiably angry.

Children should be told in advance what is going to happen to them. They are fearful of the unknown, and their active imaginations can fantasize images out of proportion to the actual event. The explanation or warning should immediately precede the action. Once the child has been told what to expect, the nurse should follow through without delay. Too much advance warning will be either nullified by intervening activities or will allow time for anxiety about the anticipated event to mount. When fearful procedures are being carried out, the child should be approached with confidence and the procedure executed swiftly and immediately following a brief warning. The child should be comforted with physical contact after a painful or stressful event. The parent who has always been the source of comfort to the child is an ideal person to provide consolation.

It is confusing to children if they are offered a choice when there actually is none. Again, a positive approach is most successful. For example, when clothes must be removed for an examination, the question "Would you like to take off your dress?" offers the child an alternative she in fact does not have. The statement "We need the dress off so that I can listen to your chest. Shall I help you take it off?" gives the child an explanation, a choice, and some measure of control in the situation.

Communication Related to Development of Thought Processes

The normal development of language and thought offers a frame of reference in knowing how to communicate with children. Thought processes progress from concrete to functional and finally to abstract, formal operations.

Infancy. Because they are unable to use words, infants primarily use and understand nonverbal communication. Infants communicate their needs and feelings through nonverbal behaviors and vocalizations that can be interpreted by someone who is around them for a sufficient amount of time. Infants smile and coo when content and cry when distressed. Crying is provoked by unpleasant stimuli from inside or outside, such as hunger, pain, body restraint, or loneliness. Adults interpret this to mean that an infant needs something and consequently try to alleviate the discomfort and reduce tension. Crying (or the desire to cry) persists as a part of everyone's communication repertoire.

Infants respond to adults' nonverbal behaviors. They become quiet when they are cuddled, patted, or receive other forms of gentle, physical contact. They derive comfort from the sound of a voice even though they do not understand the

words that are spoken. Until infants reach the age where they experience stranger anxiety, they readily respond to any firm, gentle handling and quiet, calm speech. Loud, harsh sounds and sudden movements are frightening.

Older infants' attentions are centered on themselves and their mothers; therefore, any stranger is a potential threat until proved otherwise. Holding out the hands and asking the child to "come" is seldom successful, especially if the infant is with the mother. If infants must be handled, the best approach is simply to pick them up firmly without gestures. It is helpful to observe the position in which the parent holds the infant. Most infants have learned to prefer a particular position and manner of handling. In general, infants are more at ease upright than horizontal. It is also best to hold infants in such a way that they can keep their parents in view. Until they have developed the understanding that an object (in this case the parent) removed from sight can still be present, they have no way of knowing that the object is still there.

Early childhood. Children under 5 years of age are almost completely egocentric. They see things only in relation to themselves and from their point of view. Therefore, any communication to them should be focused on *them*. They need to be told what they can do or how they will feel. Experiences of others are of no interest to them. It is futile to use another child's experience as an attempt to gain the cooperation of very small children. They should be allowed to touch, examine, and familiarize themselves with articles that will come in contact with them. A stethoscope bell will feel cold; palpating a neck might tickle. Although they have not yet acquired sufficient language skills to express their feelings and wants, toddlers are able to communicate effectively with their hands to transmit ideas without words. They push an unwanted object away, pull another person to show them something, point, and cover the mouth that is saying something they do not wish to hear.

Everything is direct and concrete to small children. They are unable to work with abstractions and base all deductions on literal formulations. Analogies escape them because they are unable to separate fact from fantasy. For example, they attach literal meaning to such common phrases as "two-faced," "sticky fingers," or "coughing your head off." Children who are told they will get "a little stick in the arm" may not be able to envision an injection (Fig. 6-3). Nurses must be aware of inadvertently using a phrase that might be misinterpreted by a small child.

Language should be used that is consistent with the child's developmental level. For example, in talking with a toddler, it is best to use simple, *short* sentences, repeat words that are *familiar* to the child, and limit descriptions to *concrete* explanations.

Children in this age category assign human attributes to inanimate objects. They endow mechanical devices and instruments with living characteristics. Consequently they fear that these objects may jump, bite, cut, or pinch all by themselves. Children do not know that these devices are unable to perform without human direction. Unfamiliar equipment

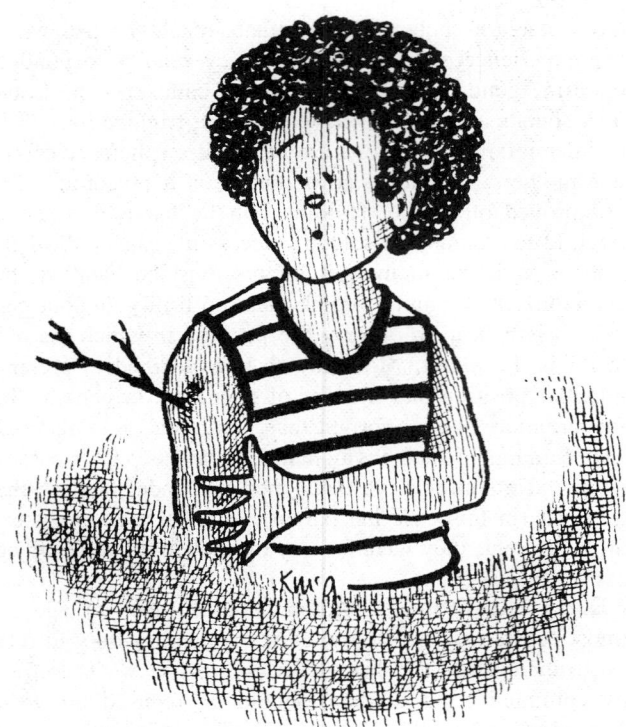

Fig. 6-3. To a young child the expression ''a little stick in the arm'' is taken literally.

needs to be simply explained without building the child's fantasies. Understanding comes slowly and is not usually achieved with one explanation, so things should be explained and described over and over again. If the child does understand, he may be seeking affirmation.

School-age years. Children aged 5 to 8 years rely less on what they see and more on what they know when faced with new problems. They want explanations and reasons for everything but require no verification beyond that. They are interested in the functional aspect of all procedures, objects, and activities. They want to know why an object exists, why it is used, how it works, and the intent and purpose of its user. They need to know what is going to take place and why it is being done to *them* specifically. For example, to explain a procedure such as taking a blood pressure, the nurse might show the child how squeezing the bulb pushes air into the cuff and makes the ''silver'' in the tube go up. The child should be permitted to operate the bulb. An explanation for the reason might be as simple as, ''I want to see how far the silver goes up when the cuff squeezes your arm.'' Consequently the child becomes an enthusiastic participant. Allowing children to ask questions about what is happening to them and maintaining a permissive atmosphere are conducive to questioning.

Children at this age have a heightened concern about body integrity. Because of the special importance and value they place on their body, they are overly sensitive to anything that constitutes a threat or suggestion of injury to it. This concern extends to their possessions also, so that they may appear to overreact to loss or threatened loss of trea-

sured objects. Helping children to voice their concerns enables the nurse to provide reassurance and to implement activities that reduce their anxiety. For example, if a reticent child fears being the single object of probing inquiry, the nurse can ignore that particular child by talking and relating to other children in the family or group. When the child no longer feels like a single target, he will usually interject his ideas, feelings, and interpretations of events.

Older children have an adequate and satisfactory use of language. They still require relatively simple explanations, but their ability to think concretely can facilitate communication and explanation. Commonly they have sufficient experience with health and health workers to understand what is transpiring and generally what is expected of them.

Adolescence. As children move into adolescence, they fluctuate between child and adult thinking and behavior. They are riding a current that is moving them rapidly toward a maturity that may be beyond their coping ability. Therefore, when tensions rise, they may seek the security of the more familiar and comfortable expectations of childhood. Anticipating these shifts in identity allows the nurse to adjust the course of interaction to meet the needs of the moment. No single approach can be relied on consistently, and one can expect to encounter hostility, anger, bravado, and a variety of other behaviors and attitudes. It is as much a mistake to regard the adolescent as an adult with an adult's wisdom and control as it is to confine to him the concerns and expectations of a child.

Frequently adolescents are more willing to discuss their concerns with an adult outside the family, and they often welcome the opportunity to interact with a nurse. They are extremely susceptible to the advances of anyone who displays a genuine interest in them. However adolescents are quick to reject persons who attempt to impose their values on them, whose interest is feigned, or who appear to have little respect for who they are and what they think or say.

As with all children, adolescents need to express their feelings. Generally they talk quite freely when given an opportunity. However, what adolescents say cannot always be taken at face value. When emotional factors are involved, the feelings that are interjected into words are as significant as the words that are used. The best way to give support is to be attentive, try not to interrupt, and avoid comments or expressions that convey disapproval or surprise. Prying and asking embarrassing questions should be avoided, and any impulse to give advice should be resisted. Frequently adolescents reveal their feelings or a source of concern or ask a question when they are involved in routine matters such as a physical assessment.

Teenagers characteristically have a language and culture all their own that further sets them apart from others. To avoid misinterpretation, frequent clarification of terms is advisable. Occasionally adolescents are reticent and answer only in monosyllables. Usually this happens when they are opposed to the contact with the nurse or do not yet feel safe enough to reveal themselves. In this instance the best approach is to confine discussions to irrelevant topics to re-

NEUROLINGUISTIC PROGRAMMING

Sensory mode communication
Visual mode: I can *see* that I do not *look* well.
Auditory mode: From what I *hear* the doctor *saying*, my child won't get better.
Kinesthetic mode: I *feel* that my child's prognosis is *weak*.

Appropriate response
Tell me what you *see*.
What have you *heard* that makes you *see* things this way?

Tell me more about *feeling* that her prognosis is *weak*.

duce the element of threat until such time as they feel more secure. The nurse must be alert for signals that indicate they are ready to talk. The major sources of concern for adolescents are attitudes and feelings toward sex, relationships with parents, peer group acceptance, and developing a sense of identity.

Interviewing the adolescent presents some special situations to the interviewer. The first may be whether to talk to the adolescent alone, with the parents, or to each individually. Of course, if the adolescent is alone, there is no question, except that the nurse might want to suggest to the teenager that she may talk with the parents at another time. If parents and teenager are together, talking with the adolescent first has the advantage of immediately identifying with the young person, thus fostering the interpersonal relationship. However, talking with the parents initially may provide insight into the family relationship. Whichever decision is made, both parties need an opportunity to be included in the interview. If time constraints are important, such as during history-taking, these need to be clarified at the onset to avoid appearing to "take sides" by talking more with one person than the other.

Confidentiality is of great importance when interviewing adolescents. The parents and the teenager need to know the limits of confidentiality, specifically that the young person's disclosures will be kept between him and the nurse. However, exceptions also must be clarified, such as breaking confidence if it is necessary for the welfare of the adolescent, as in the case of suicidal behavior.

Another dilemma in interviewing adolescents is that two views of a problem frequently exist—the teenager's and the parents'. Clarification of the problem is a major task. However, providing both parties with an opportunity to discuss their perceptions in an open and unbiased atmosphere can, by itself, be therapeutic. The nurse, by demonstrating positive communication skills, can help families communicate more effectively.

COMMUNICATION TECHNIQUES

In addition to such conventional interviewing methods as reflection, open-ended questions, and leading statements, there are a number of techniques that encourage family members to express their thoughts and feelings in a less directive and confrontational manner. The following verbal and nonverbal approaches can be helpful in a variety of instances. Throughout the book examples are given that use the techniques described here.

Verbal Techniques

A number of verbal techniques can be used to encourage communication. Several are techniques that the interviewer can employ to pose questions or concerns in a less threatening manner. Others can be presented as "word games" that are often well received by children.

Third-person technique. The third-person technique involves expressing a feeling in terms of a third person (he, she, they). This technique is less threatening than directly asking a child how he feels, because it gives him the opportunity to agree or disagree without being defensive. For example, the nurse may comment, "Sometimes when a person is sick a lot he feels angry and sad because he cannot do what others can," and either wait silently for a response or encourage a reply with a statement such as, "Did you ever feel that way?" This approach allows the child three choices: (1) to agree and, hopefully, express how he feels, (2) to disagree, or (3) to remain silent, in which case he probably has such feelings but is unable to express them at that time. Demonstrating to parents how useful such techniques are also helps them learn new ways of communicating with the child.

Neurolinguistic programming. A relatively new approach to understanding the communication process is neurolinguistic programming (NLP), which is concerned with the *manner* in which individuals access and understand information. Most people use one of three sensory modalities to communicate: visual, auditory, or kinesthetic. The specific sensory mode is identified by observing the type of verbs, adjectives, and adverbs the person uses. By using the same sensory mode, the nurse can enhance rapport and communicate information more effectively (see box above). Visual people also benefit from visual aids, such as diagrams and illustrations. The auditory person uses words or sounds. Children tend to use the kinesthetic mode and learn from manipulating objects (Knowles, 1983; Brockopp, 1983).

Facilitative responding. Facilitative responding is the careful listening and reflecting back to patients the feelings and content of their statements. Such responses are empathetic, nonjudgmental, and legitimize the person's feelings. The formula for facilitative responses is, "You feel _____ because _____." (Henrich and Bernheim, 1981). For example, if a child states, "I hate coming to the hospital and getting shots," a facilitative response is, "You feel unhappy because of all the things that are done to you."

Storytelling. Storytelling uses the language of the child

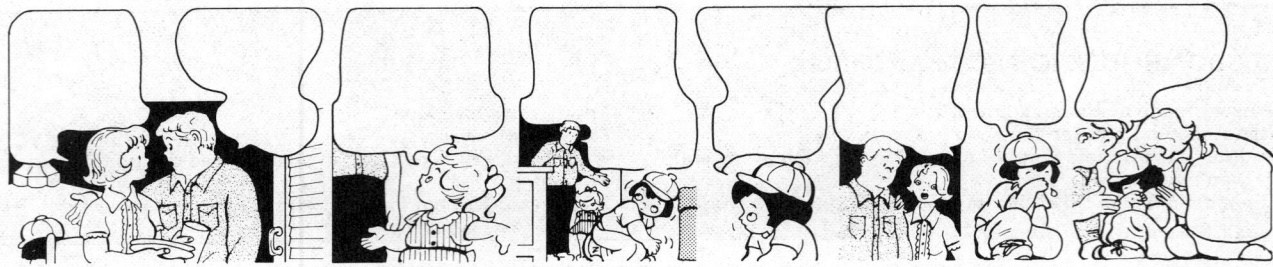

Fig. 6-4. Filling in the blanks on a comic strip is an effective communication technique with older children.

to probe into areas of his thinking while bypassing conscious inhibitions or fears. Children respond to a variety of storytelling techniques. The simplest is asking a child to relate a story about an event, such as "being in the hospital." Another approach involves showing him a picture of a particular event, such as a child in a hospital with other people in the room, and asking him to describe the scene. Comic strips cut from a newspaper with the words removed are excellent vehicles when the child ascribes his own statements to each comic scene (Epstein, 1975). If the child draws a family or hospital scene, he can fill in a short verbal communication above each person, similar to a comic strip theme (Fig. 6-4).

Mutual storytelling involves a more therapeutic approach. It not only serves to uncover the child's thinking but also attempts to change the child's perceptions or fears by retelling a somewhat different story. It is a powerful tool and must be used wisely. It begins by asking the child to tell a story about something, followed by another story told by the nurse that is similar to the child's tale but that has differences that help the child in problem areas. A typical example is the child's story of going to the hospital and never seeing his parents again. The nurse's story is also of a child (using different names but similar circumstances) in a hospital whose parents visit every day, but in the evening after coming home from work. In this way the child's fears of abandonment and separation are handled.

Sometimes children need help in beginning a story with encouragements, such as "Once upon a time . . ." or the use of a tape recorder. For a less verbal child, having him draw pictures or write about an event may help him relate stories.

Bibliotherapy. Bibliotherapy involves the use of books in a therapeutic and supportive process. Its goal is to help the child express feelings and concerns through the familiar activity of being read to or reading to himself. Although it incorporates an educational component, it involves more than using a book for its preparatory value, such as familiarizing a child with hospitalization or a procedure. It provides the child with an opportunity to explore an event that is similar to his own but sufficiently different to allow him to distance himself from it and remain in control. Since children tend to trust the characters in a book, they are able to feel familiar with the content even if they are suspicious of the nurse who reads the story. A book is essentially non-

threatening because the child can close it or stop reading it at any time.

Following are general guidelines for using bibliotherapy:

1. Assess the child's emotional and cognitive development.
2. Be familiar with the book's content and the appropriate age level for which it is written.
3. Share the book with the child, such as reading it to him.
4. Explore the meaning of the book with the child by having the child retell the story, reread a special section, draw a picture related to the story and discuss the drawing, talk about the characters, or summarize the moral or meaning of the story.

Several authors discuss bibliotherapy in more detail. Berg and associates (1980) present an annotated bibliography for children of different ages that deals with nondeath losses. Sources of books discussing loss from death are listed on p. 983. Fosson and Husband (1984) list books dealing with issues related to hospitalization.

Fantasy. A special type of bibliotherapy uses fantasy or fairy tales, such as *Hansel and Gretel*, *Cinderella*, or *Jack and the Beanstalk*. The figures and events of fairy tales personify and illustrate universal inner conflicts, such as the need to be loved, the fear that one is worthless, the love of life, and the fear of death. They subtly suggest how these conflicts may be solved and the endings give reassurance and hope for the future (Bettelheim, 1976). Without explanation children find meaning in the stories to meet their needs.

Dreams. Dreams often reveal unconscious and repressed thoughts and feelings. Although interpretation of dreams is a specialized area of psychotherapy, asking a child or parent to talk about a dream may uncover areas that were previously unknown to the nurse. For example, a mother whose child had been diagnosed with a life-threatening illness described dreams about her son's dying. As she relayed the dream, she also commented that she feared her dream would "cause" his death. Subsequently the nurse and mother were able to explore guilt feelings that were very disturbing to the parent.

Another approach toward using dreams is *guided imagery*. For example, a critically ill child dreamed that "the black angel" was in his room. When talking to the child about the nightmare, the nurse tried to have him imagine that he could tell the angel anything he wanted. He stated, "I would tell her to go away." They then talked about fears of being left alone or taken away. The nurse stressed that the child was safe and that no one would let anything happen to him. This calmed the child and the nightmare did not recur.

"What if" questions. "What if" questions encourage children to explore potential situations and to consider different problem-solving options. For example, the nurse can ask a child, "What if you got sick and had to go to the hospital?" The child's response reveals what he knows already and what he is curious about. His thoughts concerning a new experience are elicited in a nonthreatening manner. This type of communication is excellent for helping children learn coping skills, especially in potentially dangerous situations. For example, parents might ask, "What if a stranger comes to school to pick you up and tells you your mommy is sick?" to prepare a child for appropriate responses.

Three wishes. A strategy for engaging children in conversation is the "three wishes" technique. One simply asks, "If you could have any three things in the world, what would they be?" One child's answer to this was most revealing. He responded, "I don't want to be sick anymore." When asked about the other two wishes, he replied, "If that one came true, so would every other wish, so I don't have anymore." Following this the nurse and boy were able to talk about what being sick meant to him. Although the nurse could not make him better, she was able to make some of the other "wishes" come true. One of them was to arrange for school friends to visit the child during his hospitalization and convalescence at home. Before this conversation the youngster's desire for peer companionship had never been revealed.

Rating game. The rating game is particularly helpful in encouraging older children to talk. Instead of asking a youngster how he feels, the nurse asks him how his day has been "on a scale from 1 to 10, with 10 being the best." With a reply of "today is a 2," one can begin exploring why this day rates so poorly. An extension of this is to have the youngster keep a log of each day's rating and expand it into a diary. For children who are too young to understand the concept of numbers, a series of happy and sad faces can be used to rate feelings (see Faces rating scale, p. 1070).

Word association game. Another approach is the word association game. One can begin by having a list of key words and asking the child to say the first word that he thinks of when he hears the word. It is best to start with neutral words and then introduce more anxiety-producing words, such as illness, needles, hospitals, operation, and so on. The key words should be chosen to relate to some event in the child's life that is relevant.

Sentence completion. Without directly asking about feelings, one can probe into areas of concern by presenting a statement and having the child complete it. This is particularly useful with older school-age children and adolescents. Some sample statements are:

The thing I like best (least) about school is _____.
The best (worst) age to be is _____.
The most (least) fun thing I ever did was _____.

The thing I like most (least) about my parents is _____.
If I could change one thing about my family, it would be ____.
If I could be anything I wanted, I would be _____.
The thing I like most (least) about myself is _____.

The beginning statements are more neutral than the last ones, which center on feelings about oneself.

Pros and cons. A somewhat different approach to encouraging exploration of feelings is to select a topic, such as "being in the hospital," and have the child list "five good things and five bad things" about it. This is an exceptionally valuable technique when applied to relationships. For example, family members can be asked to write down five things they like and dislike about each other. In reviewing the lists, each member has the opportunity to discuss his or her feelings in a nonjudgmental atmosphere. However, when this technique is used, the nurse must be able to handle feelings that can surface unexpectedly.

Nonverbal Techniques

Many children and adults find talking about their feelings difficult. For them verbal communication may be more stressful than supportive. Several nonverbal techniques can be used to encourage communication, especially in young children.

Writing. Writing is an alternative communication approach for older children and adults. Specific suggestions include (1) keeping a journal or diary, (2) writing feelings or thoughts that are difficult to express, (3) writing "letters" that are never mailed (a variation is making up a "pen pal" to write to), or (4) keeping an account of the child's progress both from a physical and emotional viewpoint.

To initiate a conversation, the nurse can inquire about the writing, possibly even asking to read some of it. Frequently, as one writes down ideas, thoughts, or feelings, there is also an urge to discuss them. Once they are written, they are more real and tangible but often less frightening than when kept locked inside one's mind.

Writing can also have a long-term benefit. After the experience there can be growth in rereading about it. One mother used her journal to help her teenage daughter understand a serious childhood illness that had threatened the youngster's life. The adolescent had become resentful of comments about "when she was ill," but after reading the journal with the mother, she realized what a stressful time those earlier years had been and gained a deeper appreciation of her parents' continuing concern for her health.

Drawing. Drawing is one of the most valuable forms of communication—both nonverbal, from looking at the drawing, and verbal, from the child's story of the picture. Children's drawings tell a great deal about them because they are projections of their personality. A child's drawing is usually of himself, his experience, or those who are significant to him. Besides communicating about himself, art also provides the child with a natural activity that helps him deal with both conscious and unconscious feelings.

Drawing can be spontaneous or directed. *Spontaneous drawings* involve giving the child a variety of art supplies

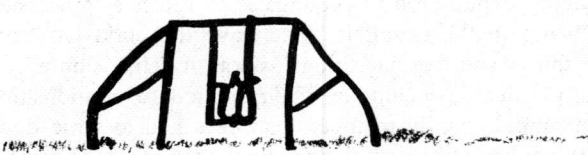

I Need A FRIEND

Fig. 6-5. With the three themes approach, this child chose the theme "the first day of school." The drawing and title reveal the child's loneliness and insecurity in a new setting.

(older children like felt-tipped pens) and providing the opportunity to draw. The only encouragement may be the statement, "Draw something for me." *Directed drawing* involves a more specific direction, such as "draw a person." In isolated figure drawings the child's response tends to be predominantly intellectual, in that he will produce a more complete picture with more parts than those he draws in a group picture. Figure drawings are the basis for certain intellectual tests (see p. 286).

If the child needs encouragement to draw, the "three themes" approach is helpful. This technique involves writing three statements about the child at the bottom of the paper and asking the child to choose one and draw a picture (Fig. 6-5).

The basic assumption in interpreting drawings is that the child is revealing something about himself. However, interpretation must be undertaken with an understanding of normal development in art expression (see p. 628). For example, it is normal for a 4-year-old to draw arms attached to a head but highly questionable in a 6-year-old. Understanding how to "read" and use drawings takes considerable time, experience, and study. It is just as dangerous to "read" too much into drawing and mislabel a person as it is to disregard a drawing as meaningless. When studying a drawing, every detail must be evaluated, as well as relationships of one part to another. It is helpful to label the characters (mother, father, and so on) and to denote the order in which each was drawn.

When evaluating a drawing the following features should be assessed:

1. Size of individual figures (expresses importance, power, authority)
2. Order in which figures are drawn (expresses priority in terms of importance)
3. Child's position to other family members (expresses feelings of status or alliance)
4. Exclusion of a member (may denote feeling of not belonging or desire to eliminate)

5. Accentuated parts (usually expresses concern for areas of special importance, for example, large hands may be sign of aggression)
6. Erasures, shadings, or cross-hatching (expresses ambivalence, concern, or anxiety with particular area)

These suggestions are by no means a complete inventory for analyzing drawing. However, they do provide initial guidelines that can offer much information about the child. One caution is that interpretation must be viewed in light of the child's particular circumstances. For example, while cross-hatching is generally a sign of anxiety, it can also be an attempt to reproduce a design in a particular artistic effect, in which case it has much less significance.

Kinetic family drawing. Group drawings are highly influenced by the child's feelings and the response is predominantly emotional. Consequently group drawings are valuable in disclosing what the child thinks about himself and others. The most valuable group drawing is of the family. A special type is the *kinetic family drawing* (Burns and Kaufman, 1970), in which the child is asked to "Draw your family doing something." In giving directions, one must be careful to offer only a general statement of encouragement and refrain from suggesting themes. Drawing the family is appropriate for children over 4 years of age.

Sociogram. Drawing need not be limited to children. Adults can be asked to draw, although they are much less likely to comply and may deliberately try to hide disclosures by drawing a very simple sketch. One type of drawing that is useful with adults and children as young as 5 years is the *sociogram (life-space drawing)* or *family circle*. For the sociogram or life-space drawing, the person is given blank paper and a pencil with the instructions: "Draw a circle to represent you. Around the circle draw circles to represent the most significant persons in your life and label each. Draw the circles in proximity to your circle to represent closeness. For example, the person who is most significant is the circle closest to you." In the family circle the directions differ slightly (Thrower, Bruce, and Walton, 1982): "Draw a circle to represent your family. Draw in smaller circles to represent you and the most significant persons in your life. People can be inside or outside the family circle. Draw the circles large or small depending on their significance or influence to you." Family members can label the relationships as supportive with a plus sign or negative with a minus sign.

The sociogram or family circle is an immediate portrait of significant persons in the individual's life. It is also a task that can uncover hidden or repressed relationships. For example, one mother drew a circle inside her circle to represent a severely retarded child who had been institutionalized for several years. She remarked that she had not realized how unresolved her feelings of attachment to this child were until she had to graphically place him in her life (Fig. 6-6).

After completing the sociogram or family circle, the family can be encouraged to explore their feelings further with questions such as the following:

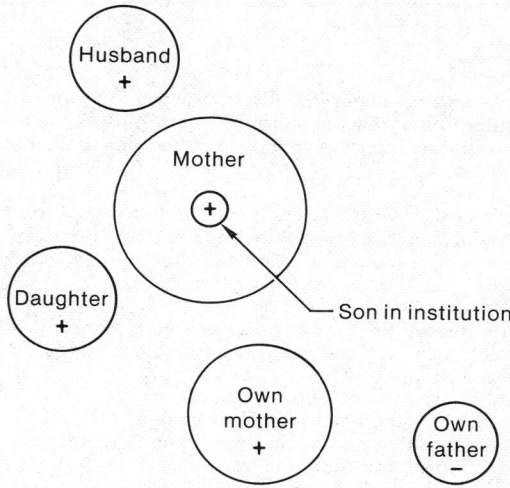

Fig. 6-6. Sociogram of mother with strong but unresolved feelings toward institutionalized son.

How would you change the circles to improve relationships?

How do you think you could accomplish these changes?

If one person in the circle were to change, what effect do you think that would have on others in the circle?

Conjoint family drawing. Another useful technique with children and adults is the *conjoint family drawing.* The family is given a large sheet of white paper and a box of colored pencils, pens, or crayons. Each member is asked to select a different color pen and not to exchange colors. They are instructed to work together on a drawing but without talking to each other. After the drawing is completed, each member is asked to discuss it. Emphasis is placed on "how" the drawing took place, rather than the symbolic meaning of each part. Suggestions for assessing the process include (Allmond, Buckman, and Gofman, 1979):

Who initiated the drawing?

Who uses the most or least space?

Does anyone infringe on another's "space"?

Do "subsystems" appear or is anyone deleted?

Does someone take the lead in organizing the drawing?

Who copies another's theme or draws something completely different?

The conjoint family drawing is a valuable tool in uncovering family dynamics and relationships. It can be used as a learning experience to help "well" families learn more about themselves. In a hospital setting it can be used with groups of children to discover their patterns of leadership and cooperation. When used with disturbed families, nurses must have sufficient skill in handling issues and feelings that may arise.

Play. Play is a universal language of children. It is one of the most important forms of communication and can be an effective technique in relating to them. Clues about physical, intellectual, and social developmental progress can often be gleaned from the form and complexity of a child's play behaviors. Play requires a minimum of equipment or none at all. Therapeutic play is often used to reduce the

trauma of illness and hospitalization (Chapter 26) and to prepare children for therapeutic procedures (Chapter 27).

Because their ability to perceive precedes their ability to transmit, small infants respond to activities that register on their senses. Patting, stroking, and other skin play convey messages. Repetitive actions such as stretching an infant's arms out to the side while he is lying on his back and then folding them across his chest or raising and revolving his legs in a bicycling motion will elicit pleasurable sounds. Colorful items to catch the eye or interesting sounds such as a ticking clock, chimes, bells, or singing can be used to attract the child's attention.

Older infants respond to simple games. The old game of peekaboo is an excellent means of initiating communication with infants while maintaining a "safe," nonthreatening distance. After this intermittent eye-to-eye contact, the nurse is no longer viewed as a stranger but as someone who is a friend. This can be followed by touch games. Clapping an infant's hands together for pat-a-cake or wiggling his toes for "this little piggy" delights an infant or small child. Much of the nursing assessment can be carried out with the use of games and simple play equipment while the infant remains in the safety of the mother's arms or lap. Talking to a foot or other part of the child's body is an effective tactic.

The nurse can capitalize on the natural curiosity of small children by playing games such as "Which hand do you take?" and "Guess what I have in my hand" or by manipulating items such as a flashlight or stethoscope. Finger games are very useful. More elaborate materials, such as puppets and replicas of familiar or unfamiliar items, serve as excellent means to communicate with small children (see Fig. 6-2). The variety and extent are limited only by the nurse's imagination.

Through play children reveal their perceptions of interpersonal relationships with their family, friends, or hospital personnel. Children may also reveal the wide scope of knowledge they have acquired from listening to others around them. For example, through needle play, children may disclose how carefully they have watched each procedure by precisely duplicating the technical skills. They may also reveal how well they remember those who performed procedures. One child who painstakingly reenacted every detail of a lymphangiogram also played the role of the physician who had continually shouted at her to be still for the entire 5-hour ordeal. Her anger at him was extremely evident during the play session and revealed the cause for her abrupt withdrawal and passive hostility toward the medical and nursing staff following this test.

Play sessions serve not only as assessment tools for determining children's awareness and perception of their illness but also as methods of intervention and evaluation. In the previous example, when the child revealed anger toward the physician, the nurse acted the part of the patient but this time did not accept the physician's harsh commands to stay still. Instead the nurse said to the physician all the things the child had wished she could say.

Subsequent play sessions can also be used for evaluation

OUTLINE OF A PEDIATRIC HEALTH HISTORY

Identifying information
1. Name
2. Address
3. Telephone
4. Birthdate and place
5. Race
6. Sex
7. Religion
8. Nationality
9. Date of interview
10. Informant

Chief complaint (CC): to establish the major *specific* reason for the child's and parents' seeking professional health attention

Present illness (PI): to obtain *all* details related to the chief complaint

Past history (PH): to elicit a profile of the child's previous illnesses, injuries, or operations
1. Birth history (pregnancy, labor, and delivery, perinatal history)
2. Previous illnesses, injuries, or operations
3. Allergies
4. Current medications
5. Immunizations
6. Growth and development
7. Habits

Review of systems (ROS): to elicit information concerning any potential health problem
1. General
2. Integument
3. Head
4. Eyes
5. Ears
6. Nose
7. Mouth
8. Throat
9. Neck
10. Chest
11. Respiratory
12. Cardiovascular
13. Gastrointestinal
14. Genitourinary
15. Gynecologic
16. Musculoskeletal
17. Neurologic
18. Endocrine

Family medical history (FMH): to identify the presence of genetic traits or diseases that have familial tendencies and to assess exposure to a communicable disease in a family member

Sexual history (SxH): to elicit information concerning the child's sexual concerns and/or activities and any pertinent data regarding adults' sexual activity that influence the child

Family history (FH): to develop an understanding of the child as an individual and as a member of a family and a community
1. Family composition
2. Home and community environment
3. Occupation and education of family members
4. Cultural and religious traditions
5. Family function and relationships

Nutritional assessment (NA): to elicit information on the adequacy of the child's nutritional intake and need
1. Dietary intake
2. Clinical examination

---

of the child's progress. A change in the type of drawing or the theme of the play may indicate progression toward or away from ability to deal with anxiety.

History-Taking

This section deals with interviewing as it relates to the health history. The precise depth and extent of a nursing history vary with its intended purpose. The nurse uses judgment in deciding what data are necessary and relevant for the identification of problems or concerns.

The format used resembles a medical history, but the objective of each assessment area is the identification of nursing diagnoses. The value in following the well-established medical approach is that it is systematic and familiar to members of the health team. The categories listed in the box above encompass the children's current and past health status and information about their psychosocial environment.

PERFORMING A HEALTH HISTORY

The methods used to perform a health history are innumerable. Each examiner will devise a unique approach. How-

ever, one important component of every history is organized and systematic data collection.

A systematic approach has several important functions: (1) it assures consistency and completeness, (2) it allows for individualized nursing care based on a comprehensive data base, (3) it maximizes the amount and quality of data for future evaluation of health status and efficacy of care, and (4) it provides an immediate basis for decision-making regarding the planning of nursing care.

The format used for history-taking may be (1) *direct*—the nurse asks for information via direct interview with the informant—or (2) *indirect*—the informant supplies the information by completing some type of questionnaire. The direct method is superior to the indirect approach or a combination of both. However, in view of time constraints, the direct approach is not always practical. If the direct approach cannot be used, it is important to review parents' written responses and question them regarding any unusual answers.

The direct method loses its value if the nurse asks questions directly from a form. In essence the parent is completing the form by listening to it rather than reading it. Using a systematic approach does not imply rote memory of a specific outline. Rather, it means using categories to define what areas of information are required. If nurses use as a model the basic categories outlined in the box and understand the objective of each, they can then obtain the required information as it arises during the course of the interview. However, the history is recorded using the established format.

Identifying Information

Much of the identifying information may already be available from other recorded sources. However, if the parent seems anxious, the nurse may use this opportunity to ask about such information to help the parent feel more comfortable.

Informant. One of the important areas under identifying information concerns the informant, the person(s) who furnished the information. The nurse should record certain data about the informant, such as (1) who he is (child, parent, and so on), (2) an impression of reliability and willingness to communicate, and (3) any special circumstances, such as the use of an interpreter or conflicting answers by more than one person.

Assessing reliability is one of the more important judgments to make. A totally reliable informant will always give the same answers to questions. Several generalizations are worthy in considering the parent's reliability (Hoekelman, Kelly, and Zimmer, 1976):

1. Concrete facts, such as birth weight, length, and date, are recalled most accurately.
2. Minor illnesses are forgotten more easily than major ones.
3. Mothers, particularly those of firstborns, tend to exaggerate the child's achievement of developmental skills.
4. Mothers of several children tend to be less accurate in their recall of most items than mothers of single children.
5. The mother's educational level is directly related to the accuracy of recall for some items, such as immunizations.
6. More specific and detailed questioning considerably increases the accuracy of recall.

The last generalization is particularly significant. Nurses who use these suggestions for approaches to history-taking are more likely to positively influence reliable parent recall than are those who fail to consider such factors.

An example of a statement that gives identifying information about an informant is: "Mother, reliability questionable, answers items with hesitation, speaks primarily Spanish, interpreter (Mrs. _____) present for history."

Chief Complaint

The chief complaint is the specific reason for the child's visit to the clinic, office, or hospital. Six guidelines determine appropriate recording of the chief complaint: it should (1) consist of a brief statement, (2) be restricted to one or two symptoms, (3) refer to a concrete complaint, (4) be recorded in the child's or parent's own words, (5) avoid the use of diagnostic terms or translations, and (6) state the duration of the symptoms.

The nurse elicits the chief complaint by asking open-ended, neutral questions such as, "Tell me what seems to be the matter," "How may I help you?" or "What brings you here?" Labeling-type questions such as, "How are you sick?" or "What is the problem?" should be avoided since the reason for the visit may not be an illness or a problem. For example, the visit may be for a routine health assessment, or the chief complaint may be of a nonphysical nature.

Examples of properly recorded chief complaints for a variety of situations may be: (1) ambulatory clinic—"My child has had a runny nose ·and sore throat for 4 days, but today it is worse"; (2) hospital admission—child states: "I need to have my tonsils fixed," has had sore throat and repeated earaches for 5 years; and (3) health center—"We are here for a routine checkup," last visit 1 year ago.

If the visit is for a well-child examination, one can ask, "Before we begin, is there anything of particular concern that you would like to discuss?" This type of statement encourages the parent (or child) to bring up an issue that may not surface during routine interviewing.

Occasionally it is difficult to isolate one symptom or problem as the chief complaint because the parent may identify many. In this situation it is important to be as specific as possible when asking questions. For example, asking informants to state which *one* problem or symptom caused them to seek help *now* may help them focus on the most immediate concern.

Present Illness

The history of the present illness* is a narrative of the chief complaint from its earliest onset through its progression to the present. The four major components are (1) details of *onset*, (2) complete *interval* history (from onset to present), (3) *present* status, and (4) reason for seeking help *now*. The focus of the present illness is on all factors that are relevant to the main problem, even if they have disappeared or changed during the onset, interval, and present status of the complaint.

Analyzing a symptom. Since pain is often the most characteristic symptom denoting onset of a physical problem, it is used as a prototype for analysis of a symptom. Assessment includes (1) type, (2) location, (3) severity, (4) duration, and (5) influencing factors.

The *type* or character of pain should be as specific as possible. However, for young children with limited verbal skills, describing the pain is difficult. Asking the parents how they know the child is in pain may help describe its type, location, and severity. For example, a mother stated, "My child must have a severe earache because she pulls at her ears, rolls her head on the floor, and screams. Nothing seems to help."

The nurse can help older children describe the pain or "hurt" by asking them if it is sharp, throbbing, dull, aching, stabbing, and so on. Whatever words they use should be recorded in quotes (see also p. 1068).

The *location* of the pain also must be specific. "Stomach pains" is too general a description. Older children can bet-

---

*NOTE: The term *illness* is used in its broadest sense to denote any problem or concern of a physical, emotional, or psychosocial nature. It is actually a history of the chief complaint.

ter localize the pain if the nurse asks them to "point with one finger to where it hurts." The nurse can also determine if the pain radiates by asking, "Does the pain stay there or move? Show me where it goes with your finger."

The *severity* of pain is best determined by finding out how it affects the child's usual behavior. Pain that prevents a child from playing, interacting with others, sleeping, and eating is most often severe.

Duration of pain includes the duration, onset, and frequency of attacks. It may be necessary to describe this in terms of activity and behavior, such as "pain lasted all night because child refused to sleep and cried intermittently."

Influencing factors are anything that causes a change in the type, location, severity, or duration of the pain. These include (1) precipitating events (those that cause or increase the pain), (2) relieving events (those that lessen the pain, such as medications), (3) temporal events (times when the pain is relieved or increased), (4) positional events (e.g., standing, sitting, and lying down), and (5) associated events (e.g., meals, stress, and coughing).

A standard method of analyzing a symptom is listed in the following outline. These three categories—onset, characteristics, and course since onset—comprise the essential data for the present illness. Although the analysis of a symptom has concentrated on discussion of physical complaints, the same process of description and investigation can be used for emotional or psychosocial problems.

Analysis of a Symptom

1. Onset
   a. Date of onset
   b. Manner of onset (gradual or sudden)
   c. Precipitating and predisposing factors related to onset (e.g., emotional disturbance, physical exertion, fatigue, bodily function, pregnancy, environment, injury, infection, toxins and allergens, therapeutic agents)
2. Characteristics
   a. Character (quality, quantity, consistency, or other)
   b. Location and radiation (of pain)
   c. Intensity or severity
   d. Timing (continuous or intermittent, duration of each, temporal relationship to other events)
   e. Aggravating and relieving factors
   f. Associated symptoms
3. Course since onset
   a. Incidence
      (1) Single acute attack
      (2) Recurrent acute attacks
      (3) Daily occurrences
      (4) Periodic occurrences
      (5) Continuous chronic episode
   b. Progress (better, worse, unchanged)
   c. Effect of therapy

Determining the reason for seeking help. The preceding discussion deals primarily with a description of the problem. However, since most chief complaints have a "duration," it follows that something significant must have occurred to motivate the person to seek help at this time.

Such factors may be a change in physical status, a change in behavioral reaction, or a result of social pressure. Eliciting such information may alter the possible nursing diagnosis and plan of care. The following example illustrates the potential significance of determining why a person seeks help at a particular time:

Chief complaint: "I can't control my son. It's been a problem, but for the past year and a half it has become worse."

Present history: Child has had temper tantrums since infancy. He "throws things, hits and kicks people, yells and screams." It occurs whenever he "doesn't get his way." They usually last "a minute or two" and occur at least weekly. Mother has responded to them in a variety of ways: hits him, ignores him, takes a special object or privilege away, insults him. Nothing seems to work. Mother admits that ignoring the behavior is the most difficult approach, and she rarely can do so without eventually hitting or scolding him. Mother is not able to identify why she sought help now.

Further physical history revealed nothing unusual. However, family history disclosed several significant facts, especially that (1) the father had died 2 months earlier, and (2) he had been ill for 1½ years before his death. The nurse focused the history on events that had occurred since the beginning of the father's illness, which coincided with the son's increased behavior problems. The mother revealed that during her husband's illness she had had too little time to concern herself with her son's behavior, other than realizing that it was a problem. However, after her husband's death, she could no longer ignore the severity of her son's behavior or its disruptive effect on the family. As she verbalized these thoughts, she began to identify the specific reason for seeking help now. She stated, "I used to wait for my husband to come home to take the children off my hands. When he was sick, I was too busy worrying about him. But now I am home all alone. When dinnertime comes, there is no one to relieve me."

Although the interventions included several approaches to managing the problem, one of them focused on providing the mother with some freedom from the responsibility of total parenting. Had the nurse not concentrated on uncovering the mother's reason for seeking help at this particular time, a very important clue in planning care might have been missed.

Past History

The past history contains information relating to all previous aspects of the child's health status and concentrates on several areas that are ordinarily deleted in the history of an adult, such as birth history, detailed feeding history, immunizations, and growth and development. Since much data are included in this section, it is more efficient for nurses to use a combination of open-ended and fact-finding questions. For example, the nurse may begin interviewing for each section with an open-ended statement, such as "Tell me about your child's birth," to provide informants with the opportunity to relate what they think is most important.

Fact-finding questions related to specific details are asked whenever necessary to focus the interview on certain topics.

Birth history. Birth history includes all data concerning (1) the mother's health during pregnancy, (2) the labor and delivery, and (3) the infant's condition immediately after birth. Since prenatal influences have significant effects on a child's physical and emotional development, a thorough investigation of birth history is essential. Since parents may question what relevance pregnancy and birth have on the child's present condition, particularly if the child is past infancy, it is best to explain why such questions are included. The nurse may state to the parents: "I will be asking you some questions about your pregnancy and _____'s (refer to child by name) birth. Your answers will give me a more complete picture of his overall health."

Pregnancy, labor, and delivery. An obstetric history should begin with an overview of the pregnancy, preferably by an open-ended question, such as, "How was your pregnancy?" This allows the mother to state what she thought was most significant. Most importantly the nurse should ask about the use of medications or other remedies that the mother used to relieve physical symptoms. For example, one mother, whose 3-year-old child had obviously discolored teeth, revealed that she had taken tetracycline during her pregnancy. She was unaware of the drug's effect on the formation of tooth enamel and thought that the child's brown teeth were the result of inadequate oral hygiene.

Basic information in an obstetric history includes maternal age, number of pregnancies (gravida), outcome of pregnancies (parity), length of gestation, and any complications. (For a more detailed obstetric history refer to maternity texts.)

Because emotional factors also affect the outcome of pregnancy and the subsequent parent-child relationship, it is important to investigate (1) concurrent crises during pregnancy and (2) prenatal attitudes toward the fetus.

It is best to approach the topic of parental acceptance of pregnancy through indirect questioning. Asking parents if the pregnancy was planned is a leading statement because they may respond affirmatively for fear of criticism if the pregnancy was unexpected. The nurse can encourage parents to disclose their true reactions by referring to specific facts relating to the pregnancy, such as the spacing between offspring, an extended or short interval between marriage and conception, or the concurrent experience of pregnancy and adolescence. The parent can choose to explore such statements with further explanations or, for the moment, may not be able to reveal such feelings. Silence should alert the nurse to the importance of refocusing on this topic later in the interview.

Perinatal history. The perinatal period refers to the first 28 days of extrauterine life, but the primary focus is on the immediate period after birth and during hospitalization. Specific data include (1) weight and length at birth; (2) loss of weight following delivery; (3) time of regaining birth weight; (4) condition of health immediately after birth, such

as quality of cry, level of activity (feeble or vigorous), and color of skin; (5) Apgar score (some mothers may be aware of this); and (6) possible problems, such as fever, convulsions, hemorrhage, snuffles, skin eruptions, desquamation, paralysis, birth injuries, deformities, or congenital anomalies.

Dietary history. The dietary history is discussed in detail at the end of this chapter under "Nutritional assessment."

Previous illnesses, injuries, and surgeries. When inquiring about past illnesses, the nurse can begin with a general statement, such as, "What other illness has your child had?" Since parents are most likely to recall serious health problems, it is important to specifically ask about colds, earaches, and common childhood diseases, such as measles, rubella (German measles), chickenpox, mumps, pertussis (whooping cough), diphtheria, scarlet fever, strep throat, tonsillitis, or allergic manifestations. It is best not to accept simple statements from the parents regarding the nature of the disease. Rather, encourage them to give onset, symptoms, course, and termination. For example, it is not uncommon for parents to confuse measles with rubella or strep throat with tonsillitis. Other important information concerning previous illnesses includes occurrence of similar symptoms in other children at the same time, course of convalescence with or without complications or sequelae, and geographic incidence of the disease.

In addition to illnesses, the nurse also questions the parent about injuries that required medical intervention, operations, and any other reason for hospitalization, including dates of each incident. It is important to focus on injuries such as falls, poisonings, choking, or burns since these may be potential areas for parental guidance. While obtaining a history of the injury, the nurse should ascertain what happened before the injury (who was the child with, where were the parents, had this ever happened before) as well as what immediate action the parent took.

The nurse should also inquire about the child's emotional reactions to each experience. For example, one mother stated that her 4-year-old daughter had recently been admitted to the hospital for respiratory distress and had become very afraid of medical personnel, procedures, and equipment. The nurse realized from this information that the child needed special preparation for the physical examination.

Allergies. The nurse should ask about commonly known allergic disorders, such as hay fever and asthma, as well as unusual reactions to food, drugs, or contact agents, such as poisonous plants, animals, household products, or fabrics. It is especially important to have the parent describe allergic reactions to drugs since a known side effect can be confused with an allergic reaction.

Current medications. In addition to any allergies to drugs, the nurse should ask about current drug regimens, including vitamins, aspirin, antibiotics, antihistamines, decongestants, or antitussives. All medications should be listed, including name, dose, schedule, duration, and reason for administration. Not infrequently parents are unaware of the actual name of the drug. Whenever possible, it is advisable to ask parents to bring the containers with them during the next visit. It is also possible to ask them for the name of the pharmacy and to call directly for a list of all the child's recent prescription medications. However, this approach does not reveal over-the-counter medications.

Immunizations. A record of all immunizations or "baby shots" is essential. Since many parents are unaware of the exact name and date of each immunization, the most reliable source of information is a hospital, clinic, or private physician's record. All immunizations and "boosters" should be listed, stating (1) name of the specific disease, (2) number of injections, (3) dosage if known (sometimes lesser amounts are given if a reaction is anticipated), (4) ages when administered, and (5) the occurrence of any reaction following the immunization. The nurse should also inquire about the child's attendance at a daycare center, the previous administration of any horse or other foreign serum, recent administration of gamma globulin or blood transfusion, or anaphylactoid reactions to neomycin or chicken eggs, and tuberculin testing. If testing was done, the child's positive or negative intradermal reaction should be recorded.

Growth and development. Parents' recall of physical growth and developmental milestones may be unreliable. Whenever possible, the responses should be compared to existing health records or to current evaluation of actual growth (height, weight, dentition) and developmental performance (screening tests such as Denver Developmental Screening Test, grades in school, scholastic achievement, play activities, social relationships).

The most important previous growth patterns to record are (1) approximate weight at 6 months, 1 year, 2 years, and 5 years of age; (2) approximate length at 1 and 4 years; and (3) dentition, including age of onset, number of teeth, and symptoms during teething. Developmental milestones include: (1) age of holding up head steadily, (2) age of sitting alone without support, (3) age of walking without assistance, and (4) age of saying first words with meaning.

Specific and detailed questions are essential when inquiring about developmental milestones. For example, "sitting up" can mean many different activities, such as sitting propped up, sitting in one's lap, sitting with support, sitting up alone but in a hyperflexed position for assisted balance, or sitting up unsupported with the back slightly rounded. The clue to misunderstanding of the requested activity is an unusually early age of achievement. For instance, one mother claimed that her daughter could sit up at 2 months of age. When the nurse asked her to describe what the child did, the mother explained that the infant "sat up" in a high chair, in a person's lap, or in the stroller. When the nurse inquired if the infant could sit without help, the mother quickly replied, "The baby would fall over unless we padded her in or supported her in our arms; she couldn't sit alone until 8 months!" Had the nurse clarified exactly which activity was asked for, the mother would have responded correctly.

Probing the area of developmental or intellectual performance can be a delicate one for parents, especially if there is a question concerning the child's progress. Therefore, it is best to approach such questioning with broad questions, such as, "How is Jimmy doing in school?" rather than with qualifying statements, such as, "Does Jimmy do well in school?" If the parents' response is vague and general, follow with questions such as, "How does he do in spelling, reading, or math?" Since these questions are appropriate for older children, they should be addressed directly to the child, as well as to the parent, for comparison of responses and increased reliability.

The importance of a school history cannot be overemphasized. It provides a general index of the child's functioning outside of the home. One can begin with a general question such as, "How's school?" followed by specific questions about present grade in school and scholastic achievement in various subjects. At this point the child may feel at ease to give opinions about such areas as the best and worst things at school, favorite teachers or subjects, or groups of friends. The nurse should also ask about after-school activities, such as hobbies and sports. (A school history may also be taken during the personal/social history.)

Habits. Habits are an important area to explore because numerous parental concerns may be uncovered. Habits include such items as:

1. Behavior patterns, such as nail biting, thumbsucking, pica (habitual ingestion of nonfood substances), rituals ("security" blanket or toy), and unusual movements (head-banging, rocking, overt masturbation, and walking on toes)
2. Activities of daily living, such as hour of sleep and arising, duration of nighttime sleep and naps, type and duration of exercise, regularity of stools and urination, age of toilet training, and occurrences of daytime or nighttime bed-wetting
3. Unusual disposition as well as response to frustration
4. Use or abuse of alcohol, drugs, coffee, and cigarettes

The last category is primarily applicable to adolescents, although nurses must be aware of increasing juvenile experimentation and the use of potentially harmful substances. If a youngster admits to smoking, drinking, or drug use, a specific average amount, such as one cigarette a week or two cans of beer on weekends, should be recorded. A statement such as, "I pop pills once in a while" has tremendously wide variations in meaning. Following this response with, "How many pills and when is once in a while?" may yield a measurable intake of drugs. If older children deny use of such substances, it is advisable to inquire about past experimentation. Asking, "You mean you never tried to smoke or drink?" implies that the nurse expects some such activity and consequently is likely to be nonjudgmental of an affirmative answer. One should also be aware of the confidential nature of such questioning and the adverse effect that the parents' presence may have on the adolescent's willingness to answer.

Review of Systems

Review of systems is exactly what the title implies—a specific review of each body system, similar to the order of the physical examination. Often the history of the present illness provides a complete review of the system involved in the chief complaint. Since asking questions about other body systems may appear unrelated and irrelevant to the parents or child, it is important to precede the questioning with an explanation of why the data are needed (similar to the explanation concerning relevance of birth history) and reassurance that the child's main problem has not been forgotten.

The review of a specific system is begun with a broad statement, such as, "How has your child's general health been?" or "Has your child had any problems with his eyes?" If the parent states that there have been past problems with some body function, this is pursued with an encouraging statement, such as, "Tell me more about that." If the parent denies any problems, it is best to query for specific symptoms, such as, "No headaches, bumping into objects, or squinting?" If the parent reconfirms the absence of such symptoms, positive statements to this effect are recorded in the history, such as, "Mother denies child's having headaches, bumping into objects, or squinting." In this way, anyone who reviews the health history is aware of exactly what symptoms were investigated.

The following is an outline of suggested areas for review of each body system. Although medical terminology may be used to record a symptom during the interview, only terms clearly understood by the parent or child should be used.

General Overall state of health, fatigue, recent and/or unexplained weight gain or loss (period of time for either), contributing factors (change of diet, illness, altered appetite), exercise tolerance, fevers (time of day), chills, night sweats (unrelated to climatic conditions), frequent infections, general ability to carry out activities of daily living

Integument Pruritus, pigment or other color changes, acne, eruptions, rashes (location), tendency to bruising, petechiae, excessive dryness, general texture, disorders or deformities of nails, hair growth or loss, hair color change (for adolescent, use of hair dyes or other potentially toxic substances, such as hair straighteners)

Head Headaches, dizziness, injury (specific details)

Eyes Visual problems (ask about behaviors indicative of blurred vision, such as bumping into objects, clumsiness, sitting very close to the television, holding a book close to the face, writing with head near desk, squinting, rubbing the eyes, bending the head in an awkward position), "cross-eye" (strabismus), eye infections, edema of lids, excessive tearing, use of glasses or contact lenses, date of last optic examination

Nose Nosebleeds (epistaxis), constant or frequent running or stuffy nose, nasal obstruction (difficulty in breathing), alteration or loss of sense of smell

Ears Earaches, discharge, evidence of hearing loss (ask about behaviors, such as need to repeat requests, loud speech, inattentive behavior), results of any previous auditory testing

Mouth Mouth-breathing, gum bleeding, toothaches, toothbrushing, use of fluoride, difficulty with teething (symptoms), last visit to dentist (especially if temporary dentition is complete), response to dentist

Throat Sore throats, difficulty in swallowing, choking (especially when chewing food—may be from poor chewing habits), hoarseness, or other voice irregularities

Neck Pain, limitation of movement, stiffness, difficulty in holding head straight (torticollis), thyroid enlargement, enlarged nodes or other masses

Chest Breast enlargement, discharge, masses, enlarged axillary nodes (for adolescent female, ask about breast self-examination)

Respiratory Chronic cough, frequent colds (number per year), wheezing, shortness of breath at rest or on exertion, difficulty in breathing, sputum production, infections (pneumonia, tuberculosis), date of last chest x-ray examination

Cardiovascular Cyanosis or fatigue on exertion, history of heart murmur or rheumatic fever, anemia, date of last blood count, blood type, recent transfusion

Gastrointestinal (Much of this in regard to appetite, food tolerance, and elimination habits has been asked elsewhere), nausea, vomiting (not associated with eating, may be indicative of brain tumor or increased intracranial pressure), jaundice or yellowing skin or sclera, belching, flatulence, recent change in bowel habits (blood in stools, change of color, diarrhea, or constipation)

Genitourinary Pain on urination, frequency, hesitancy, urgency, hematuria, nocturia, polyuria, unpleasant odor to urine, force of stream, discharge, change in size of scrotum, date of last urinalysis (for adolescent, sexually transmitted disease, type of treatment; for male adolescent, ask about testicular self-examination)

Gynecologic Menarche, date of last menstrual period, regularity or problems with menstruation, vaginal discharge, pruritus, date and result of last Pap smear (include obstetric history as discussed under birth history when applicable); if sexually active, type of contraception

Musculoskeletal Weakness, clumsiness, lack of coordination, unusual movements, back or joint stiffness, muscle pains or cramps, abnormal gait, deformity, fractures, serious sprains, activity level

Neurologic Seizures, tremors, dizziness, loss of memory, general affect, fears, nightmares, speech problems, any unusual habits

Endocrine Intolerance to weather changes, excessive thirst, excessive sweating, salty taste to skin, signs of early puberty

Family Medical History

The family medical history is used primarily for the purpose of discovering the potential existence of hereditary or familial diseases in the parents and child. In general it is confined to first-degree relatives (parents, siblings, and grandparents and their children) and is mose easily recorded using a pedigree chart or genogram (see p. 175). Information for each family member includes age, marital status, state of health if living, cause of death if deceased, and any evidence of the following conditions: heart disease, hypertension, cancer, diabetes mellitus, obesity, congenital anomalies, allergy, asthma, tuberculosis, sickle cell disease, mental retardation, convulsions, insanity or other emotional problems, syphilis, or rheumatic fever. In the case of genetic diseases a more in-depth inquiry into family transmission of the disorder is performed (see p. 174). The nurse confirms accuracy of the reported disorders by inquiring about the symptoms, course, treatment, and sequelae of each diagnosis.

Geographic location. One of the important areas to explore when assessing the family health history is geographic location, including birthplace and travel to different areas in or outside of the country for identification of possible exposure to endemic diseases. Although the primary interest focuses on the child's temporary residence in various localities, the nurse should also inquire about close family members' travel, especially during tours of military service or business trips. Children are especially susceptible to parasitic infestation in areas of poor sanitary conditions and to vector-borne diseases, such as those from mosquitoes or ticks in warm and humid or heavily wooded regions.

Sexual History

Sexual history is an essential component of each adolescent's health assessment. It is warranted regardless of the adolescent's degree of sexual activity since concerns about sexual matters can influence physical and psychologic well-being.

One way to initiate a conversation about sexual concerns is to begin with a history of peer interactions. Open-ended statements such as "Tell me about your social life," or "Who are your closest friends?" generally lead into a discussion of dating and sexual issues. Sometimes, to probe further, one can ask about the adolescent's attitudes on such topics as sex education, "going steady," "living together," and premarital sex. Questions should be phrased to reflect concern and not judgment and should not indicate any criticism of sexual practices.

In any conversation regarding sexual history, the nurse must be aware of the language that is used in either eliciting or conveying sexual information. For example, when asking if the adolescent is "sexually active" or "having sex," the exact meaning of either phrase needs to be clarified. To some it may signify foreplay, self-stimulation, erotic visual stimulation, or intercourse. Adolescents' fantasies and strong sexual desires are alone sufficient to cause them concern. Therefore the nurse not only wants to know the incidence of intimate sexual contacts but also looks for areas of sexual concern for the adolescent.

Since homosexual experimentation may occur during adolescence and can be a source of great concern and anxiety for the teenager, it is an important area to investigate. One approach is to use nonspecific questions and refer to all sexual contacts as "partners," not as "girlfriends" or "boyfriends." Applying a nongender label to an inferred

sexual partner indicates to the teenager that sexual preference is not being judged.

A detailed account of sexual partners is needed if the patient has a history of, displays any of the symptoms of, or asks for treatment of a sexually transmitted disease. A difficult but necessary part of the interview is to determine the sites of possible infection. Since sexual diseases can be contracted at any of the body orifices, the adolescent should be informed that a sexually transmitted disease can be acquired without visible signs of disease at nongenital sites.

The degree of inquiry into the parents' sexual activity depends on many factors. For example, it may be limited to a brief discussion of their plans regarding future children or contraception. In instances where overt adult sexual activity may be having an adverse effect on the children, a more detailed exploration of this area is warranted. The nurse must make this decision based on facts learned during the interview since this line of questioning should never be wanton prying. If parents ask the relevance of revealing such matters, the nurse must be prepared to offer a sound and logical explanation. It is every person's right to refuse to disclose personal information, especially if not informed of its significance or value.

Family Assessment

Assessment of the family, both its structure and function, is an essential component of the history-taking process. Numerous studies demonstrate that the quality of the functional relationship between the patient and family members is a major factor in emotional and physical health. Because of its significance in nursing of children, family assessment is discussed separately and in greater detail apart from the more traditional health history.

Family assessment is the collection of data about the composition of the family and the relationships among its members. In its broadest sense the family refers to all those individuals who are significant to the nuclear unit, including relatives, friends, and other social groups, such as the school and church. It differs from family therapy in several ways. First, the primary goal of family assessment is to collect information for planning care, intervention, evaluation, or referral. In family therapy, data collection is only the initial stage in the process of family counseling based on a "systems" model, which identifies the family as the patient (see Chapter 3). Second, the skills required for family therapy exceed those needed for assessment. Third, family assessment is a process often used with healthy families who may or may not be coping with stressful events. Family therapy is used primarily with families needing additional support to cope successfully with stress. Despite these differences, family assessment can and frequently is therapeutic. The mere act of involving family members in discussing family characteristics and activities often stimulates productive discussion and insight into family dynamics and relationships.

Because of the time involved in performing an in-depth family assessment as presented here, the nurse should be selective in deciding when knowledge of family function may facilitate nursing care. Indications for initiating a comprehensive family assessment include families with (Wright and Leahey, 1984; Smilkstein, 1984):

1. Children receiving comprehensive well child care
2. Children experiencing major stressful life events, such as chronic illness, disability, parental divorce, or death of a family member
3. Children requiring extensive home care
4. Children with developmental delays
5. Children with repeated accidental injuries and those with suspected child abuse
6. Children with behavioral or physical problems that suggest family dysfunction as the etiology

In addition to the discussion of family assessment presented here, assessment issues specific to the family of a child with a chronic illness or disability are included in Chapter 22, p. 938.

ASSESSMENT OF FAMILY STRUCTURE

Family structure refers to the composition of the family—who lives in the home and those social, cultural, religious, and economic characteristics that influence the child's and family's overall psychobiologic health (see also Chapter 2). Since the information elicited in this part of the history is often the most personal and confidential, it is left to the end of the interview, when the nurse-parent-child rapport is well established.

Structural Assessment Interview

The more traditional method of eliciting information on family structure is by interviewing family members. The principal areas of concern are (1) family composition, (2) home and community environment, (3) occupation and education of family members, and (4) cultural and religious traditions.

Family composition. Family composition is primarily concerned with the immediate members of the household, but should also include a review of the family's extended support system. For example, in a single-parent family, the household members may consist of the mother and two children, but the mother's parents may be very significant sources of childcare and financial support. Although the interview method can be used to collect information about household members—their relationship, ages, and roles within the family, as well as significant individuals outside the family unit—other efficient methods include those discussed under "Structural assessment tools" (p. 208).

In discussing family composition it is sometimes difficult to ascertain the status of the adult relationships. For example, the parent may fail to mention the other parent. In this case the nurse can then ask, "Where is the child's father (or mother)?" It is best to avoid the term *husband* or *wife* because that precludes the existence of nonmarital relationships. If the parent states that the child's father (or mother) is not part of the household, the nurse can explore this by inquiring about his or her continued relationship with the child and the presence of any other significant male (or female) within the home. The nurse should also inquire about previous marriages, separations, death of spouses, or divorces. It is important to ask about the children's reaction to any of these events, which usually have a tremendous effect on their general physical and emotional health.

Home and community environment. Information about the home environment includes (1) type of dwelling (private home, apartment, multiple dwelling, or trailer); (2) number of rooms, including sleeping arrangements, floors, and occupants; (3) accessibility of stairs or elevators; (4) adequacy of utilities; (5) safety features (fire escape, guardrails on high-rise windows, smoke detectors, and use of car restraints); and (6) housing problems (insects, poor sanitation, or flaking paint).

Recent stresses or changes in the home should be explored, such as relocation, change in employment status, marital discord or divorce, and addition of a new sibling. If any are identified, the nurse should inquire about the child's adjustment to the change.

Information regarding the community environment may vary according to geographic location, such as an urban or rural setting. It is the nurse's responsibility to have at least a general knowledge of the locality in order to focus questions on specific areas of significance. However, some general topics for investigation include (1) type of neighborhood (residential or industrial, relative age of neighboring families, willingness of neighbors to help one another, interracial or ethnic problems); (2) location of and distance to school; (3) usual transportation to school; (4) availability of age-mates for the child; and (5) available play areas. It is also important to focus on potential dangers in the community environment such as (1) proximity to industrial centers (for example, an asbestos or chemical factory); (2) incidence of crime; and (3) potential sources of injury such as a swimming pool, drainage ditch, or other adjacent body of water, steep hill or cliff, or heavy street traffic.

Occupation and education of family members. The occupational history of the parents consists of more than a listing of their career and place of employment. It should focus on (1) type of activity (manual or sedentary, individual-paced or highly pressured), (2) number of hours away from the home, (3) exposure to environmental hazards (chemicals, coal, radiation, lead, carbon monoxide, or fire), and (4) satisfaction associated with the employment.

The occupational history should also lead into a discussion of the family's financial status. Since some parents may resist disclosing their yearly income, the nurse can assess the adequacy of financial resources by inquiring about source of income when unemployed, usual housing expenses, and expenditures for food, shelter, clothing, and recreation. A general statement, such as, "The cost of living is certainly high today. How do you make ends meet?" may encourage parents to discuss any financial hardships without fear of criticism. The nurse also investigates the type of medical coverage or insurance the family has.

Ascertaining the parents' educational preparation usually follows a discussion of occupation. By the end of the interview the nurse has probably made some personal judgment regarding the parent's level of formal and/or informal education. However, since many people feel embarrassed to admit failure to complete the usual academic learning, it is best to approach the area of years in school indirectly whenever possible. For example, the nurse can ask about the type of training, education, or acquisition of special skills that may be required for the parents' vocation. This information is highly valuable in planning implementation of care (e.g., counseling, guidance, or teaching) and is another reason to refrain from actual intervention until the history (and physical examination whenever warranted) is completed.

Cultural and religious traditions. Knowledge of the family's cultural traditions and religious practices is essential in planning care. The influence of culture and religion on the family is discussed in Chapter 3. Cultural traditions and religious practices that should be assessed in the family history include childrearing beliefs, attitudes toward health care, and personal faith in a deity. Cultural practice in relation to nutrition is discussed on p. 39. The following questions encourage families to verbalize about their heritage:

How do your beliefs regarding _____ differ from those of your parents?
What special _____ (name of culture or nationality) traditions do you practice in your home?
What language do you speak in the home?
How are American children different from children in your country?
How is your religion a part of your life?

Structural Assessment Tools

Several structural assessment tools are valuable in collecting and recording data about family composition and environment. Like the interview method these tools also provide information about relationships, although several additional methods should be used to assess family function.

Tools that involve drawing have several advantages. They:

1. Provide an immediate visual presentation of the family tree and extended support systems
2. Yield extensive information in a short period of time
3. Are easily updated
4. May stimulate productive and meaningful communication among family members

Two tools involving drawing are presented below; the sociogram and kinetic family drawing are discussed on p. 198.

Genogram. The genogram (family tree, family diagram) involves the use of symbols to diagrammatically record data about family structure. It is a modification of the pedigree chart used in genetics to record the family medical history. Symbols often used in the genogram are presented

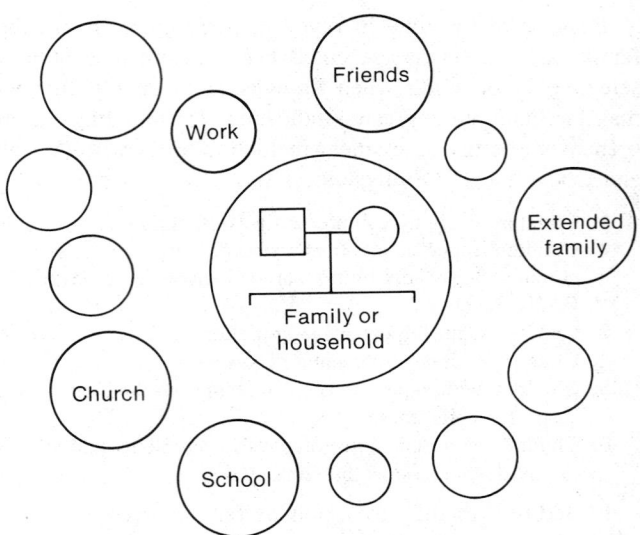

Fig. 6-7. Ecomap. Genogram is completed for immediate family members and circles are labeled as appropriate.

Modified from Hartman, A.: Finding families: an ecological approach to family assessment in adoption, Beverly Hills, CA, 1979, Sage Publications.

in Fig. 5-15, p. 174. Because there is no universal list of symbols, those used by other health professionals may differ. If in doubt regarding which symbol to use or if one does not exist, it is best to write in the word describing the relationship, such as *foster child*. Since the genogram is also concerned with the *strength* of family relationships, attachment symbols are often added as additional information on family functioning is obtained. Because a genogram can become complex, it is helpful to circle the nuclear family on the diagram. Instructions for beginning a genogram are similar to those for a pedigree (see p. 175).

Ecomap. The ecomap is a visual presentation of the family's support system outside the home. It begins with the genogram of the immediate family inside one circle and uses other smaller circles to represent each member's relationship with other significant people, agencies, or institutions (Hartman, 1979). A blank ecomap is shown is Fig. 6-7. The size of the circles is not important; rather, symbols of attachment (Fig. 6-8) are used to signify the type of relationship and arrows may be drawn along the connecting lines to denote flow of energy or resources.

ASSESSMENT OF FAMILY FUNCTION

Family function is concerned with how the family behaves toward one another and the quality of the relationships (see also p. 62). It is considered the most important component in determining "family health." Assessment of function requires more skill on the part of the interviewer than does assessment of structure and is best approached after structure is assessed.

Family Function Interview

As in assessment of family structure, the more traditional method of eliciting information on family function is by in-

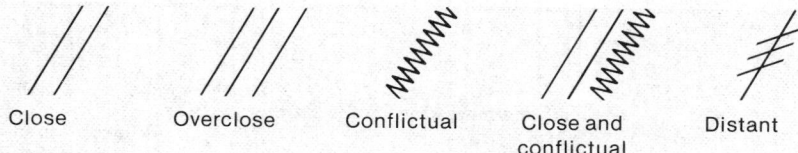

Fig. 6-8. Symbols of attachment or intensity of relationship.

terviewing family members. The principal areas of concern are the following characteristics, which are generally cited as significant variables in determining family health (Lewis and others, 1976; Wright and Leahey, 1984; Sargent, 1983; Phipps, 1980).

Family interaction and roles. Family interaction refers to the ways family members relate to each other. The chief concern is the amount of intimacy and closeness among the members, especially the spouses. Roles refer to the behaviors of people as they assume different statuses or positions. The more flexibility and sharing of roles, the better family members are able to meet each other's needs. In assessing interactions and roles, general observations are made about the family's response to each other (e.g., cordial, hostile, cool, loving, patient, or short-tempered), obvious roles of leadership versus submission, and support and attention shown to various members.

Asking questions concerning with whom the child shares a room, the child's household chores, and activities the family performs together gives some idea of how the family interacts. It is best to avoid direct questions such as, "How does your family get along with each other?" because the usual response is "OK." An effective way of approaching this topic, especially with adolescents, is use of the third-person technique (see p. 195). The nurse may say, for example, "Teenagers and parents have a way of seeing things differently, especially when it comes to money, dating, clothes, using the car, and curfew. Have you and your parents ever disagreed about such things?" The young person is then allowed an opportunity to present his views because he is aware that the nurse expects such events and is therefore less likely to judge or criticize his response. (For a more detailed discussion of family communication strategies, see pp. 188-199.)

Other assessment questions include:

Who do you talk to when something is bothering you?
Who usually oversees what is happening with the children, such as at school or concerning their health?
How easy or difficult is it for your family to change or accept new responsibilities for household tasks?

Power, decision-making, and problem-solving. Power and control in the family is a critical issue. Several family therapists conclude that clear boundaries of power, that is, shared power by the parents in rearing the children, is essential for family health (Lewis and others, 1979; Minuchin, 1974). Knowledge of who has power and how decisions are made usually offers clues to how problems are solved. One of the best methods of collecting data is to offer a hypothetical conflict or problem, such as a child with fail-

ing school grades, and ask the family how they would handle this situation. By observing the group dynamics, conclusions can be drawn about how the family typically deals with conflicts or problems.

Assessment questions include:

Who usually makes the decisions in your family?
(Directed to the child) If one parent makes a decision, can you appeal to the other parent to change it?
(Directed to the parents) What input do the children have in making decisions or discussing rules?
Who makes and enforces the rules?
What happens when a rule is broken?

Communication. In interviewing the family the nurse is concerned with the clarity and directness of communication patterns. Clear communication relays messages that are understood by all members. Direct communication is sent to the intended receiver. Assessments are made by observing who speaks to whom, if one person speaks for another or interrupts, if members appear disinterested when certain individuals speak, and if there is agreement between verbal and nonverbal messages. To further assess communication, the nurse can periodically ask family members if they understood what was just said and to repeat the message.

Expression of feelings and individuality. Healthy families allow expression of feelings and promote the development of individuality while encouraging family closeness. There is the space and freedom to grow with the limits and structure needed for guidance. Observing patterns of communication offers clues to how freely feelings are expressed.

Assessment questions include:

Is it OK to get angry or sad in your house?
Who gets angry most of the time? What do they do?
If you are upset, how do other family members try to comfort you?
Who comforts you?
When you want to do something new, such as try out for a new sport or get a job, what is the family's response (offer assistance, discourage you, or leave it to you to work out)?

Family Function Assessment Tools

In addition to observing and interviewing the family to assess family function, several other methods are available and should be used as needed to obtain a comprehensive assessment. The following section discusses selected instruments that are appropriate for the nurse to use. They are reliable and valid but require little formal training and minimal time to administer. The reader is referred to the conjoint family drawing on p. 199 and to reviews of other in-

FAMILY APGAR

Definition

Adaptation is the use of intrafamilial and extrafamilial resources for problem-solving when family equilibrium is stressed during a crisis.

Partnership is the sharing of decision-making and nurturing responsibilities by family members.

Growth is the physical and emotional maturation and self-fulfillment that is achieved by family members through mutual support and guidance.

Affection is the caring or loving relationship the exists among family members.

Resolve is the commitment to devote time to other members of the family for physical and emotional nurturing. It also usually involves a decision to share wealth and space.

Functions measured by the Family APGAR

How resources are shared, or the degree to which a member is satisfied with the assistance received when family resources are needed.

How decisions are shared, or the member's satisfaction with mutuality in family communication and problem-solving.

How nurturing is shared, or the member's satisfaction with the freedom available within the family to change roles and attain physical and emotional growth or maturation.

How emotional experiences are shared, or the member's satisfaction with the intimacy and emotional interaction that exists in the family.

How time (and space and money) is shared, or the member's satisfaction with the time commitment that has been made to the family by its members.

Relevant open-ended questions

How have family members aided each-other in time of need?

In what way have family members received help or assistance from friends and community agencies?

How do family members communicate with each other about such matters as vacations, finances, medical care, large purchases, and personal problems?

How have family members changed during the past years?

How has this change been accepted by family members?

In what ways have family members aided each other in growing or developing independent life-styles?

How have family members reacted to your desires for change?

How have members of your family responded to emotional expressions such as affection, love, sorrow, or anger?

How do members of your family share time, space, and money?

Modified from Smilkstein, G.: The Family APGAR: a proposal for a family function test and its use by physicians, J. Fam. Pract. **6**(6):1231-1239, 1978.

struments for further information (Humenick, 1982; Smilkstein, 1984; Speer and Sachs, 1985).

Family APGAR. The Family APGAR is a brief screening questionnaire designed to reflect a family member's satisfaction with the functional state of the family (Smilkstein, 1978) (see Appendix A). The acronym APGAR is for Adaptability, Partnership, Growth, Affection, and Resolve (commitment) (see box above). It bears no relationship with the Apgar scoring system for newborns, although the acronym was chosen because it is familiar to health professionals. It requires about 5 minutes to complete and can be used by nuclear families, as well as families with alternative lifestyles. The questions in the box can be used in the interview without the APGAR ratings to elicit similar types of information.

Family Functioning Index. The Family Functioning Index (FFI) is a simple, easily administered test designed to reflect the dynamics of family interaction in the areas of marital satisfaction, frequency of disagreement, communication, problem solving, and feelings of happiness and closeness (Pless and Satterwhite, 1973).* Administration time to answer the 15 questions is about 15 minutes.

Feetham Family Functioning Survey. The Feetham Family Functioning Survey was initially developed by a nurse to measure the effect of a child with spina bifida on families (Feetham and Humenick, 1982).* Although recommended primarily as a research instrument, it can provide the nurse with information about the family members' perception of the relationships that contribute to or are affected by family functioning.

The survey consists of 29 questions in the following areas of family functioning: household tasks; childcare; sexual and marital relationship; interaction with family, children, and friends; community involvement; and sources of emotional support. The questions are answered on a seven-point scale that rates "what is," "what should be," and "how important it is" (see box, p. 211). The discrepancy between the first two ratings, together with the degree of importance, contributes to the clinical assessment of family functioning. An advantage to the use of "discrepant scores" is that it controls for cultural and ethnic diversity, measuring the person's *perception* of the importance of an item, rather than the researcher's biased interpretation. The survey takes less than 10 minutes to complete, but persons with less than

*A copy of the FFI can be obtained from Betty Satterwhite, University of Rochester Medical Center, 601 Elm Avenue, Box 777, Rochester, NY 14642.

*The survey is available from Suzanne Feetham, Ph.D., F.A.A.N., Associate Director of Nursing for Education and Research, Children's Hospital National Medical Center, 111 Michigan Avenue, N.W., Washington, D.C. 20010. A check for $5.00 is appreciated to process the request.

a high school education may have some difficulty with the format.

Home Observation and Measurement of the Environment (HOME) and Home Screening Questionnaire (HSQ). Ideally a thorough assessment includes observing the child and family in a variety of settings. Undoubtedly the richest environment for observing a child's development and interactions with family members is the home. Two tools that can be used to assess the child's home environment are the Home Observation for Management of the Environment (HOME)* (Caldwell and Bradley, 1984) and the Home Screening Questionnaire (HSQ) (Frankenburg and Coons, 1986).† Both are divided into two age-groups—birth to 3 years of age and 3 to 6 years of age. HOME has an additional inventory for elementary age children. HOME (0 to 3 years) has 45 items in 6 major categories, the 3- to 6-year form consists of 55 items in 8 categories, and HOME (6 to 10 years) includes 59 items in 8 categories (see Appendix A). Some of the items require direct observation, whereas others necessitate questioning of the parents. Each item receives a "yes" or "no" response. The number of "yes" scores correlates with the amount of appropriate environmental stimulation. Any "no" scores indicate possible areas for intervention and counseling. Use of HOME requires about a 1-hour home visit with both the child and major caregiver.

The HSQ (Home Screening Questionaire) was developed using HOME as a guide. The 0- to 3-year form consists of 30 items plus a checklist of toys available to the child in the home. The 3- to 6-year form has 34 items and a similar toy checklist. The questions are written at approximately a third to sixth grade reading level and unlike the HOME can be completed by the parents in any setting in about 15 to 20 minutes. Scoring directions are detailed in the manual and are based on credits for different answers. For each age-group there is a minimum score for determining suspect or nonsuspect results.

In making a home or school visit, specific objectives for assessing the environment are listed on p. 940.

Nutritional Assessment

A nutritional assessment is an essential part of a complete health appraisal. Its purpose is to evaluate the child's nutritional status, the state of balance between nutrient intake and nutrient expenditure or need (Krause and Mahan, 1984). A thorough nutritional status assessment includes: (1) dietary intake, (2) clinical examination, and (3) biochemical analysis.

---

*The forms and a comprehensive manual are available for a fee of $12.00; the forms and an administration manual cost $6.00. Both are available from the Bureau of Educational Research, University of Arkansas, 33rd Street and University Avenue, Little Rock, AK 72204.
†The forms and manual are available for a fee from Denver Developmental Materials, Inc., P.O. Box 20037, Denver, CO 80220.

SAMPLE QUESTIONS FROM THE FEETHAM FAMILY FUNCTIONING SURVEY

1. The amount of talk with your *friends* regarding your concerns and problems.
   (15) a. How much is there now?

   LITTLE   MUCH
   1   2   3   4   5   6   7

   (16) b. How much should there be?

   LITTLE   MUCH
   1   2   3   4   5   6   7

   (17) c. How important is this to me?

   LITTLE   MUCH
   1   2   3   4   5   6   7

2. The amount of talk with your *relatives* (do not include your spouse) regarding your concerns and problems.
   (18) a. How much is there now?

   LITTLE   MUCH
   1   2   3   4   5   6   7

   (19) b. How much should there be?

   LITTLE   MUCH
   1   2   3   4   5   6   7

   (20) c. How important is this to me?

   LITTLE   MUCH
   1   2   3   4   5   6   7

3. The amount of time you spend with your *spouse*.
   (21) a. How much is there now?

   LITTLE   MUCH
   1   2   3   4   5   6   7

   (22) b. How much should there be?

   LITTLE   MUCH
   1   2   3   4   5   6   7

   (23) c. How important is this to me?

   LITTLE   MUCH
   1   2   3   4   5   6   7

Reproduced with the permission of Suzanne L. Feetham, Ph.D., R.N., F.A.A.N., Children's Hospital National Medical Center, Washington, DC. Developed from research funded by Division of Nursing, H.R.A., H.H.S., NU00632, Wayne State University, Detroit, MI, 1977–1980.

DIETARY INTAKE

Knowledge of the child's dietary intake is a useful and practical component of a nutritional assessment. However, it is also one of the most difficult factors to assess. Individuals' recall of food consumption, especially amounts eaten, is frequently unreliable. In addition people may be hesitant to reveal their eating patterns if they sense criticism from the

DIETARY HISTORY

What are the family's usual mealtimes?

Do family members eat together or at separate times?

Who does the family grocery shopping and meal preparation?

How much money is spent to buy food each week?

How are most foods prepared—baked, broiled, fried, other?

How often does the family or your child eat out?

    What kinds of restaurants do you go to?

    What kinds of food does your child typically eat at restaurants?

Does your child eat breakfast regularly?

Where does he eat lunch?

What are your child's favorite foods, beverages, and snacks?

    Average amounts consumed or usual size portions?

    Special cultural practices, such as family only eats ethnic food?

What foods and beverages does your child dislike?

How would you describe his usual appetite (hearty eater, picky eater)?

What are his feeding habits (breast, bottle, cup, spoon, eats by self, needs assistance, any special devices)?

Does he take vitamins or other supplements; do they contain iron or fluoride?

Are there any known or suspected food allergies; is your child on a special diet?

Has your child lost or gained weight recently?

Are there any feeding problems (excessive fussiness, spitting up, colic, difficulty sucking or swallowing); any dental problems or appliances, such as braces that affect eating?

What types of exercise does your child do regularly?

Is there a family history of cancer, diabetes, heart disease, high blood pressure, or obesity?

Additional questions for infants

What was the infant's birth weight; when did it double, triple?

Was the infant premature?

Are you breast-feeding or have you breast-fed your infant? For how long?

If you use a formula, what is the brand?

    How long has the infant been taking it?

    How many ounces does he drink a day?

Are you giving the infant cow's milk (whole, low-fat, skimmed)?

    When did you start?

    How many ounces does he drink a day?

Do you give your infant extra fluids (water, juice)?

If he takes a bottle to bed at nap or nighttime, what is in the bottle?

At what age did you start cereal, vegetables, meat or other protein sources, fruit/juice, finger food, table food?

Do you make your own baby food or use commercial foods, such as infant cereal?

Does the infant take a vitamin supplement? If so, what type?

Has the infant shown an allergic reaction to any food(s)? If so, list the foods and describe the reaction.

Does the infant spit up frequently, have unusually loose stools, or have hard, dry stools? If so, how often?

How often do you feed your infant?

How would you describe your infant's appetite?

---

nurse. People from different cultures may have difficulty adequately describing the types of food they eat. Despite these obstacles, however, a food intake record is essential. Several methods are available.

Dietary History

Regardless of the format used in recording food intake, every nutritional assessment should begin with a dietary history. The exact questions used to elicit a dietary history vary with the child's age. In general, the younger the child, the more specific and detailed the history should be. The box above provides a sample dietary history for children with additional questions regarding infant feeding.

The broad overview elicited from the dietary history can be helpful in evaluating food intake records (see box, p. 213). It also is concerned with financial and cultural factors that influence food selection and preparation. Because cultural practices are very prevalent in food preparation, it is important to consider carefully the kind of questions that are asked and the judgment made in regard to counseling. For example, some cultures, such as Hispanic, black, and American Indian, include many vegetables, legumes, and starches in their diet that together provide sufficient essential amino acids, even though the actual amount of meat or dairy protein is low. (See p. 39 for cultural food practices.)

Twenty-four-hour recall. The most common and probably easiest method of assessing daily intake is the 24-hour recall. The child or parent recalls every item eaten in the past 24 hours and the approximate amounts. The 24-hour recall is most beneficial when it is representative of a typical day's intake. Some of the difficulties with a daily recall are the family's inability to remember exactly what was eaten and inaccurate estimation of portion size. To increase accuracy of reporting portion sizes, the use of food models and additional questioning are recommended. In general this method is most useful in providing *qualitative* information about the child's diet.

Food diary. To improve the reliability of the daily recall, the family can complete a food diary by recording every food and liquid consumed for a certain number of days. A 3-day record consisting of 2 weekdays and 1 weekend day is representative for most people. Providing specific charts to record intake can improve compliance. The family should record items immediately after eating.

Food frequency record. A food frequency questionnaire or record provides information about the number of times in a day, week, or month a child consumes items from the four food groups (box, p. 213). In general, it provides more of a qualitative overview but has the advantage of avoiding recall based on a "typical" day. It can be especially useful when verifying a food history or diary.

FOOD FREQUENCY RECORD*

Food group	Number of servings (day, week)	Serving size (in cup, tablespoon, or ounce portions)	Food group	Number of servings (day, week)	Serving size (in cup, tablespoon, or ounce portions)
Milk/cheese Milk Cheese Yogurt Pudding Ice cream Other			*Fruits/juice* Citrus (orange, grapefruit, tangerine) Noncitrus Other		
Protein foods Meat Fish Poultry Egg Peanut butter Legumes (dried beans, peas) Nuts Other			*Fats* Butter, oil, margarine, mayonnaise, salad dress- ing		
Breads/cereals Bread, tortilla Cooked pasta, rice, hot cereal Dry cereal (not presweetened) Crackers Muffins Other			*Sweets* Soda, punch Cake/cookie, etc. Candy Presweetened cereal		
Vegetables Yellow or orange Green/leafy Other					

*For comparison of actual intake with recommended intake, see p. 611.

CLINICAL EXAMINATION

A significant amount of information regarding nutritional deficiencies is elicited from a clinical examination, especially from assessing the skin, hair, teeth, gums, lips, tongue, and eyes. Hair, skin, and mouth are vulnerable because of the rapid turnover of epithelial and mucosal tissue. Table 6-1 summarizes clinical signs of possible nutritional deficiency or excess. Few are diagnostic for a specific nutrient and if suspicious signs are found, they must be confirmed with dietary and biochemical data. Generally the clinical examination does not reveal children at risk for a deficiency or excess.

Anthropometry

An essential parameter of nutritional status is anthropometry, the measurement of height, weight, head circumference in young children, proportions, skinfold thickness, and arm circumference. Height and head circumference reflect past nutrition, while weight, skinfold thickness, and arm circum-

ference reflect present nutritional status, especially of protein and fat reserves. Skinfold thickness is a measurement of the body's fat content since approximately one half of the body's total fat stores are directly beneath the skin. The upper arm muscle circumference is correlated with measurements of total muscle mass. Since muscle serves as the body's major protein reserve, this measurement is considered an index of the body's protein stores (Gray and Gray, 1980). Ideally growth measurements are recorded over a period of time and comparisons made regarding the *velocity* of growth based on previous and present values. Techniques for anthropomorphic measurement are discussed in Chapter 7.

Biochemical Analysis

Numerous biochemical tests are available for assessing nutritional status and include analysis of plasma, blood cells, urine, or tissues from liver, bone, hair, and fingernails. Many of these tests are complicated and are not performed routinely. Common laboratory procedures for nutritional

Table 6-1   Clinical assessment of nutritional status

EVIDENCE OF ADEQUATE NUTRITION	EVIDENCE OF DEFICIENT OR EXCESS NUTRITION	DEFICIENCY/EXCESS*
General growth		
Within 5th and 95th percentiles for height, weight, and head circumference	Below 5th or above 95th percentiles for growth	Protein, calories, fats, and other essential nutrients, especially A, pyridoxine, niacin, calcium, iodine, manganese, zinc
Steady gain with expected growth spurts during infancy and adolescence	Absence of or delayed growth spurts; poor weight gain	
Sexual development appropriate for age	Delayed sexual development	Excess vitamin A, D
Skin		
Smooth, slightly dry to touch	Hardening and scaling	Vitamin A
Elastic and firm	Seborrheic dermatitis	Excess niacin
Absence of lesions	Dry, rough, petechiae	Riboflavin
Color appropriate to genetic background	Delayed wound healing	Vitamin C
	Scaly dermatitis on exposed surfaces	Riboflavin, vitamin C, zinc
	Wrinkled, flabby	Niacin
	Crusted lesions around orifices, especially nares	Protein and calories
	Pruritus	Zinc
	Poor turgor	Excess vitamin A, riboflavin, niacin
	Edema	Water, sodium
		Protein, thiamin
		Excess sodium
	Yellow tinge (jaundice)	Vitamin B$_{12}$
		Excess vitamin A, niacin
	Depigmentation	Protein, calories
	Pallor (anemia)	Pyridoxine, folic acid, vitamin B$_{12}$, C, E (in premature infants), iron
		Excess vitamin C, zinc
	Paresthesia	Excess riboflavin
Hair		
Lustrous, silky, strong, elastic	Stringy, friable, dull, dry, thin	Protein, calories
	Alopecia	Protein, calories, zinc
	Depigmentation	Protein, calories, copper
	Raised areas around hair follicles	Vitamin C
Head		
Even molding, occipital prominence, symmetric facial features	Softening of cranial bones, prominence of frontal bones, skull flat and depressed toward middle	Vitamin D
Fused sutures after 18 months	Delayed fusion of sutures	Vitamin D
	Hard tender lumps in occiput	Excess vitamin A
	Headache	Excess thiamin
Neck		
Thyroid not visible, palpable in midline	Thyroid enlarged; may be grossly visible	Iodine
Eyes		
Clear, bright	Hardening and scaling of cornea and conjunctiva	Vitamin A
Conjunctiva—pink, glossy	Night blindness	
Good night vision	Burning, itching, photophobia, cataracts, corneal vascularization	Riboflavin
Ears		
Tympanic membrane—pliable	Calcified (hearing loss)	Excess vitamin D
Nose		
Smooth, intact nasal angle	Irritation and cracks at nasal angle	Riboflavin
		Excess vitamin A

*Nutrients listed are deficient unless specified as excess.

Table 6-1 Clinical assessment of nutritional status—cont'd

EVIDENCE OF ADEQUATE NUTRITION	EVIDENCE OF DEFICIENT OR EXCESS NUTRITION	DEFICIENCY/EXCESS
Mouth		
Lips—smooth, moist, darker color than skin	Fissures and inflammation at corners	Riboflavin Excess vitamin A
Gums—firm, coral pink color, stippled	Spongy, friable, swollen, bluish-red or black color, bleed easily	Vitamin C
Mucous membranes—bright pink, smooth, moist	Stomatitis	Niacin
Tongue—rough texture, no lesions, taste sensation	Glossitis Diminished taste sensation	Niacin, riboflavin, folic acid Zinc
Teeth—uniform white color, smooth, intact	Brown mottling, pits, fissures Defective enamel Caries	Excess fluoride Vitamin A, C, D, calcium, phosphorus Excess carbohydrates
Chest		
In infants, shape is almost circular	Depressed lower portion of rib cage Sharp protrusion of sternum	Vitamin D
In children, lateral diameter increases in proportion to anteroposterior diameter		
Smooth costochondral junctions	Enlarged costochondral junctions	Vitamin C, D
Breast development—normal for age	Delayed development	See General growth, p. 214, especially zinc
Cardiovascular system		
Pulse and blood pressure (BP) within normal limits	Palpitations Rapid pulse	Thiamin Potassium Excess thiamin
	Arrhythmias	Magnesium, potassium Excess niacin, potassium
	Increased BP Decreased BP	Excess sodium Thiamin Excess niacin
Abdomen		
In young children, cylindric and prominent	Distended, flabby, poor musculature Prominent, large	Protein, calories Excess calories
Older children, flat	Potbelly, constipation	Vitamin D
Normal bowel habits	Diarrhea	Niacin Excess vitamin C
	Constipation	Excess calcium, potassium
Musculoskeletal system		
Muscles—firm, well-developed, equal strength bilaterally	Flabby, weak, generalized wasting Weakness, pain, cramps	Protein, calories Thiamin, sodium, chloride, potassium, phosphorus, magnesium Excess thiamin
	Muscle twitching, tremors Muscular paralysis	Magnesium Excess potassium
Spine—cervical and lumbar curves (double S curve)	Kyphosis, lordosis, scoliosis	Vitamin D
Extremities—symmetric; legs straight with minimum bowing	Bowing of extremities, knock-knees Epiphyseal enlargement Bleeding into joints and muscles, joint swelling, pain	Vitamin D, calcium, phosphorous Vitamin A, D Vitamin C
Joints—flexible, full range of motion, no pain or stiffness	Thickening of cortex of long bones with pain and fragility, hard tender lumps in extremities	Excess vitamin A
	Osteoporosis of long bones	Calcium Excess vitamin D

Continued.

Table 6-1 Clinical assessment of nutritional status—cont'd

EVIDENCE OF ADEQUATE NUTRITION	EVIDENCE OF DEFICIENT OR EXCESS NUTRITION	DEFICIENCY/EXCESS
Neurologic system *Behavior*—alert, responsive, emotionally stable	Listless, irritable, lethargic, apathetic (sometimes apprehensive, anxious, drowsy, mentally slow, confused)	Thiamin, niacin, pyridoxine, vitamin C, potassium, magnesium, iron, protein, calories Excess vitamin A, D, thiamin, folic acid, calcium
	Masklike facial expression, blurred speech, involuntary laughing	Excess manganese
Absence of tetany, convulsions	Convulsions	Thiamin, pyridoxine, vitamin D, calcium, magnesium Excess phosphorus (in relation to calcium)
Intact peripheral nervous system	Peripheral nervous system toxicity (unsteady gait, numb feet and hands, fine motor clumsiness)	Excess pyridoxine
Intact reflexes	Diminished or absent tendon reflexes	Thiamin

status include measurement of hemoglobin, hematocrit, albumin, creatinine, and nitrogen. Laboratory values for these tests and more specific nutrient measurements are given in Appendix D.

EVALUATION OF NUTRITIONAL ASSESSMENT

After collecting the data needed for a thorough nutritional assessment, the nurse should evaluate the findings to plan appropriate counseling. From the data, the child can be assessed as (1) malnourished, (2) at risk for becoming malnourished, or (3) well nourished with adequate reserves.

Often the majority of the findings are from dietary intake, anthropometry, and clinical examination. Singly neither of these measures nutritional status. For example, dietary intake is important in assessing the quality of nutrient consumption, in managing the child at risk of malnutrition, and in determining if the prescribed intake goals are being met.

The daily food diary is analyzed by comparing it to the four basic food groups. For example, if the list includes no vegetables, the nurse should ask the reason for this rather than assume that the child dislikes vegetables because it may be that the mother failed to serve any on that day. Based on the specific details of the nutrition history, appropriate counseling can be planned. More elaborate analysis can be done by calculating either by hand or with a computer the amounts of every nutrient in each food consumed.

Findings from clinical examination and anthropometry are evaluated with the data obtained from the dietary intake. For example, findings suggestive of anemia and a dietary record of iron poor foods necessitates laboratory analysis of hemoglobin. Any suspicious findings should be referred to the physician for further evaluation.

CONCEPT SUMMARIES

- Communication, the most important skill nurses must possess in the care of children, has verbal, nonverbal, and abstract components.

- To effectively establish a setting for communication, the nurse must make an appropriate introduction, clarify her role and the purpose of the interview, and ensure privacy and confidentiality.

- When communicating with parents, the nurse needs to encourage parental involvement, listen carefully, use silence, be empathic, and provide reassurance.

- Communication with children must reflect their development stage.

- Verbal communication techniques that have proved to be effective include the third-person technique, neurolinguistic programming, facilitative responding, storytelling, bibliotherapy, the use of "what if" questions, and other word games.

- Nonverbal communication with children may take the form of writing, drawing, and play.

- The objectives of performing a health history are to identify pertinent information, determine the chief complaint, analyze the present illness, secure the past history, and record a family and sexual history.

- Family assessment is the collection of data about family composition and relationships among its members and also focuses on home and community environment, occupation and education, and cultural and religious traditions.

- The family function interview examines interaction and roles, power, decision-making, problem-solving, communication, and expression of feelings and individuality.

- Nutritional assessment is performed by determination of dietary intake, clinical examination, and biochemical analysis.

REFERENCES

Allmond, B., Buckman, W., and Gofman, H.: The family is the patient: an approach to behavioral pediatrics for the clinician, St. Louis, 1979, The C.V. Mosby Co.

Berg, P.J., Devlin, M.K., and Gedaly-Duff, V.: Bibliotherapy with children experiencing loss, Issues Compr. Pediatr. Nurs. **4**:37-50, Aug. 1980.

Bettelheim, B.: The uses of enchantment: the meaning and importance of fairy tales, New York, 1976, Alfred A. Knopf, Inc.

Brockopp, D.Y.: What is NLP? Am. J. Nurs. **83**(7):1012-1014, 1983.

Burns, R.C., and Kaufman, S.H.: Kinetic family drawings, New York, 1970, Brunner/Mazel, Inc.

Caldwell, B., and Bradley, R.: Home Observation for Measurement of the Environment, Revised edition, Little Rock, AR, 1984.

Cassell, E.J.: Learning language skills: changing the words changes the world, Patient Care **14**:126-142, June 15, 1980a.

Cassell, E.J.: Learning language skills: untwisting the fibers of ''paralanguage,'' Patient Care **14**:186-204, Sept. 15, 1980b.

Epstein, C.: Nursing the dying patient, Reston, VA, 1975, Reston Publishing Co., Inc.

Feetham, S., and Humenick, S.: Feetham Family Functioning Survey. In Humenick, S., editor: Analysis of current assessment strategies in the health care of young children and childbearing families, Norwalk, CT, 1982, Appleton-Century-Crofts.

Fosson, A., and Husband, E.: Bibliotherapy for hospitalized children, South. Med. J. **77**(3):342-346, 1984.

Frankenburg, W., and Coons, C.: Home Screening Questionnaire: its validity in assessing home environment, J. Pediatr. **108**(4):624-626, 1986.

Gray, G.E., and Gray, L.K.: Anthropometric measurements and their interpretation: principles, practices, and problems, J. Am. Diet. Assoc. **77**(11):534-539, 1980.

Hartman, A.: Finding families: an ecological approach to family assessment in adoption, Beverly Hills, CA, 1979, Sage Publications, Inc.

Heineken, J., and Roberts, F.B.: Confirming, not disconfirming: communicating in a more positive manner, Am. J. Maternal Child. Nurs. **8**(1):78-80, 1983.

Henrich, A.P., and Bernheim, K.F.: Responding to patients' concerns, Nurs. Outlook **29**(7):428-433, 1981.

Hickson, G., and others: Concerns of mothers seeking care in private pediatric offices: opportunities for expanding services, Pediatrics **72**(5):619-624, 1983.

Hockelman, R.A., Kelly, J., and Zimmer, A.W.: The reliability of maternal recall, Clin. Pediatr. **15**(3):261-265, 1976.

Humenick, S., editor: Analysis of current assessment strategies in the health care of young children and childbearing families, Norwalk, CT, 1982, Appleton-Century-Crofts.

Knowles, R.D.: Building rapport through neuro-linguistic programming, Am. J. Nurs. **83**(7):1010-1014, 1983.

Kohut, S.A.: Guidelines for using interpreters, Hosp. Prog. **56**(4):39-40, 1975.

Krause, M.V., and Mahan, L.K.: Food, nutrition, and diet therapy, Philadelphia, 1984, W.B. Saunders Co.

Lewis, J., and others: No single thread: psychological health in family systems, New York, 1976, Brunner/Mazel, Inc.

Minuchin, S.: Families and family therapy, Cambridge, MA, 1974, Harvard University Press.

Phipps, L.: Theoretical frameworks applicable to family care. In Miller, J., and Janosik, E., editors: Family-focused care, New York, 1980, McGraw-Hill Book Co.

Pless, I., and Satterwhite, B.: A measure of family functioning and its application, Soc. Sci. Med. **7**:613-621, 1973.

Primeaux, M.: Caring for the American Indian patient, Am. J. Nurs. **77**:91-94, Jan. 1977.

Ryberg, J., and Merrifield, E.: Tuning in to parents' concerns, Child. Nurse **2**(2):1-4, 1984.

Sargent, A.J.: The family: a pediatric assessment, J. Pediatr. **102**(6):973-976, 1983.

Smilkstein, G.: The family APGAR: a proposal for a family function test and its use by physicians, J. Fam. Prac. **6**(6):1231-1239, 1978.

Smilkstein, G.: The physician and family function assessment, Fam. Systems Med. **2**(3):263-279, 1984.

Speer, J., and Sachs, B.: Selecting the appropriate family assessment tool, Pediatr. Nurs. **11**(5):349-355, 1985.

Thrower, S., Bruce, W., and Walton, R.: The Family Circle Method for integrating family systems concepts in family medicine, J. Fam. Pract. **15**(3):451-457, 1982.

Wasserman, R., and others: Pediatric clinicians' support for parents makes a difference: an outcome-based analysis of clinician-parent interaction, Pediatrics **74**(6):1047-1053, 1984.

Wright, L., and Leahey, M.: Nurses and families: a guide to family assessment and intervention, Philadelphia, 1984, F.A. Davis Co.

BIBLIOGRAPHY
Communication Strategies

Apley, J.: Listening and talking to patients: communicating with children, Part V, Br. Med. J. **281**:1116-1117, 1980.

Benjamin, A.: The helping interview, Boston, 1974, Houghton Mifflin Co.

Bentz, J.M.: Missed meanings in nurse/patient communication, Am. J. Maternal Child Nurs. **5**(1):55-57, 1980.

Burch, C.A.: Puppet play in a thirteen-year-old boy: remembering, repeating, and working through, Clin. Soc. Work J. **8**(2):79-89, 1980.

Cameron, C.O., Juszczak, L., and Wallace, N.: Using creative arts to help children cope with altered body image, Child. Health Care **12**(3):108-112, 1984.

Carek, D.J.: Focus on affect: the pediatrician and empathic confrontation, Clin. Pediatr. **17**:574-578, July 1978.

Cassell, E.J.: Learning language skills: hear what the patient means, say what you mean, Patient Care **14**:80-90, Jan. 15, 1980.

Cassell, E.J.: Learning language skills: listen: ''illogical'' patients often make sense, Patient Care **14**:91-106, Jan. 15, 1980.

Crews, N.E.: Developing empathy for effective communication, AORN J. **30**:536, 540, 542, 544-546, Sept. 1979.

DiLeo, J.H.: Interpreting children's drawings, New York, 1983, Brunner/Mazel, Inc.

DiLeo, J.H.: Children's drawings as diagnostic aids, New York, 1980, Brunner/Mazel, Inc.

Edwards, B.J., and Brilhart, J.K.: Communication in nursing practice, St. Louis, 1981, The C.V. Mosby Co.

Elmassian, B.J.: A practical approach to communicating with children through play, Am. J. Maternal Child Nurs. **4**(4):238-240, 1979.

Enzer, N.B.: Interviewing children and parents. In Enelow, A.J., and Swisher, S.N., editors: Interviewing and patient care, New York, 1979, Oxford University Press.

Farr, K.: Communication pitfalls in routine counseling, Pediatr. Nurs. **5**(1):55-57, 1979.

Fletcher, C.: Listening and talking to patients: some special problems, Part IV, Br. Med. J. **81**:1056-1058, 1980.

Forsyth, D.M.: Looking good to communicate better with patients, Nursing 83 **13**(7):34-37, 1983.

Fosson, A., and deQuan, M.M.: Reassuring and talking with hospitalized children, Child. Health Care **13**(1):37-44, 1984.

Furth, G.M.: The use of drawings made at significant times in one's life. In Kubler-Ross, E.: Living with death and dying, New York, 1981, Macmillan Publishing Co., Inc.

Gelhard, H.L.: Drawing and development, Pediatr. Nurs. **4**:23-25, Nov./Dec. 1978.

How should patients be addressed? AORN J. **31**:1142-1146, 1980.

Johnson, S.H.: Avoiding communication blocks with high-risk parents, Issues Compr. Pediatr. Nurs. **4**:61-72, Aug. 1980.

Jolly, J.D.: Through a child's eyes: the problems of communicating with sick children, Nursing (Oxford) **1**:1012-1014, 1981.

Kaufman, D.H.: An interview guide for helping children make health-care decisions, Pediatr. Nurs. **11**(5):365-367, 1985.

Kimball, A.J., and Campbell, M.M.: Psychologic aspects of adolescent patient health care, Clin. Pediatr. **18**:15-25, Jan. 1979.

Koppitz, E.M.: Psychological evaluation of children's human figure drawings, New York, 1968, Grune & Stratton, Inc.

Labarca, J.R.: Communication through art therapy, Perspect. Psychiatr. Care **17**:118-124, May/June 1979.

Langner, B.E.: Communication between children, Issues Compr. Pediatr. Nurs. **4**:1-15, Aug. 1980.

McLeavey, K.A.: Children's art as an assessment tool, Pediatr. Nurs. **5**(2):9-14, 1979.

Mengel, A.: Getting the most from patient interviews, Nursing 82 **12**(11):46-49, 1982.

Orndorf, R., and Deutch, J.A.: The power of positive suggestion: persuading patients to cooperate, Nursing 81 **11**:73, Aug. 1981.

O'Sullivan, A.L.: Privileged communication, Am. J. Nurs. **80**:947-950, May 1980.

Pederson, C.J., and Anderson, J.M.: Factors that impact data collection from children, Cancer Nurs. **3**(6):439-444, 1980.

Philbrick, M.: Developing your listening skills, Point View **23**(1):16-17, 1986.

Pidgeon, V.A.: Characteristics of children's thinking and implications for health teaching, Matern. Child Nurs. J. **6**:1-8, Spring 1977.

Pontious, S.L.: Practical Piaget: helping children understand, Am. J. Nurs. **82**(1):114-117, 1982.

Shufer, S.: Communicating with young children: teaching via the play-discussion group, Am. J. Nurs. **77**:1960-1962, 1977.

Smith, E.C.: Communicating with young children: are you really communicating? Am. J. Nurs. **77**:1966-1967, 1977.

Smith, J., and Felice, M.: Interviewing adolescent patients: some guidelines for the clinician, Pediatr. Ann. **9**:238-243, June 1980.

Snyder, J.C., and Wilson, M.F.: Elements of a psychological assessment, Am. J. Nurs. **77**(2):235-239, 1977.

Streff, M.B., and Streff, C.E.: The counselling dimension of the nurse practitioner, Pediatr. Nurs. **8**(1):9-13, 1982.

Wallace, N.E.: Special books for special children, Child. Health Care **12**(1):34-36, 1983.

Health Interview

Adams, G.: The sexual history as an integral part of the patient history, Am. J. Maternal Child Nurs. **1**(3):170-175, 1976.

Anderson, M.L.: Talking about sex—with less anxiety, J. Psychiatr. Nurs. **18**:10-15, June 1980.

Baer, E.D., McGowan, M.N., and McGivern, D.O.: Taking a health history, Am. J. Nurs. **77**(7):1190-1193, 1977.

Brown, M.S., and Murphy, M.A.: Ambulatory pediatrics for nurses, New York, 1979, McGraw-Hill Book Co.

Felman, Y.M., and Nikitas, J.A.: Obtaining history of patient's sexual activities, N.Y. State J. Med. **79**:1879-1881, 1979.

McBride, M.M.: Can you tell me where it hurts? Pediatr. Nurs. **3**(4):7-8, 1977.

Moss, M., and Schleutermann, J.: Assessment of the pediatric client. In Malasanos, L., and others, editors: Health assessment, ed. 3, St. Louis, 1986, The C.V. Mosby Co.

Pederson, C.J., and Anderson, J.M.: Factors that impact data collection from children, Cancer Nurs. **3**(6):439-444, 1980.

Prior, J.A., Silberstein, J.S., and Stang, J.M.: Physical diagnosis: the history and examination of the patient, ed. 6, St. Louis, 1981, The C.V. Mosby Co.

Roznoy, M.S.: How to take a sexual history, Am. J. Nurs. **76**(8):1279-1282, 1976.

Family Assessment

Bradley, R., and Caldwell, B.: Home Observation for Measurement of the Environment: a validation study of screening efficiency, Am. J. Ment. Defic. **81**(5):417-420, 1977.

Bradley, R., and Caldwell, B.: Home Observation for Measurement of the Environment: a revision of the preschool scale, Am. J. Ment. Defic. **84**(3):235-244, 1979.

Calloway, S.: Home Observation for Measurement of the Environment. In Humenick, S., editor: Analysis of current assessment strategies in the health care of young children and childbearing families, Norwalk, CT, 1982, Appleton-Century-Crofts.

Good, M.D., and others: The family APGAR index: a study of construct validity, J. Fam. Pract. **8**(3):577-582, 1979.

Hartman, A.: Diagrammatic assessment of family relationships, Soc. Casework **59**:465-476, 1978.

Holt, S.J., and Robinson, T.M.: The school nurse's "family assessment tool," Am. J. Nurs. **79**(5):950-953, 1979.

Hymovich, D.P.: The Chronicity Impact and Coping Instrument: Parent Questionnaire, Nurs. Res. **32**(5):275-281, 1983.

Jolly, W., Froom, J., and Rosen, M.G.: The genogram, J. Fam. Pract. **10**:251-255, Feb. 1980.

Lewis, J.M.: How's your family? New York, 1979, Brunner/Mazel, Inc.

Meister, S.B.: Charting a family's developmental status—for intervention and for the record, Am. J. Maternal Child Nurs. **2**(1):43-48, 1977.

Miller, J., and Janosik, E., editors: Family-focused care, New York, 1980, McGraw-Hill Book Co.

Roberts, C., and Feetham, S.: Assessing family functioning across three areas of relationships, Nurs. Res. **31**(4):321-325, 1982.

Rogers, J., and Durkin, M.: The semi-structured genogram interview: I. protocol, II. evaluation, Fam. Systems Med. **2**(2):176-187, 1984.

Rogers, R.R.: The assessment interview in parent-child relationships, Curr. Psychiatr. Ther. **20**:41-46, 1981.

Sargent, A.J.: Family therapy: a view for pediatricians, J. Pediatr. **102**(6):977-981, 1983.

Sargent, A.J.: The sick child and the family, J. Pediatr. **102**(6):982-987, 1983.

Satterwhite, B.B., and others: The Family Functioning Index—5-year test-retest reliability and implications for use, J. Comp. Fam. Stud. **7**:110-116, 1976.

Sedgwick, R., and Hildebrand, S.: Family health assessment, Nurse Pract. **6**(2):37-45, 1981.

Selig, A.L., and Selig, E.W.: The need for a family orientation. In Thornton, S.M., and Frankenburg, W.K., editors: Child health care communications, New Brunswick, NJ, 1983, Johnson & Johnson Baby Products Co.

Whall, A.L.: Nursing theory and the assessment of families, J. Psychiatr. Nurs. **19**(1):30-36, 1981.

Nutritional Assessment

American Academy of Pediatrics Committee on Nutrition: Assessment of nutritional status. In Pediatric nutrition handbook, ed. 2, Elk Grove Village, IL, 1985, The Academy.

Dansky, K.H.: Assessing children's nutrition, Am. J. Nurs. **77**(10):1610-1611, 1977.

Mahan, L.K., and Rees, J.M.: Nutrition in adolescence, St. Louis, 1984, Times Mirror/Mosby College Publishing.

Merritt, R.J., and Blackburn, G.L.: Nutritional assessment and metabolic response to illness of the hospitalized child. In Suskind, R.M., editor: Textbook of pediatric nutrition, New York, 1981, Raven Press.

Pipes, P.L.: Nutrition in infancy and childhood, St. Louis, 1985, The C.V. Mosby Co.

Slattery, J.S., Pearson, G.A., and Torre, C.T., editors: Maternal and child nutrition: assessment and counseling, New York, 1979, Appleton-Century-Crofts.

Solomons, N.W.: Assessment of nutritional status: functional indicators of pediatric nutriture, Pediatr. Clin. North Am. **32**(2):319-334, 1985.

Stuff, J.E., and others: A comparison of dietary methods in nutritional studies, Am. J. Clin. Nutr. **37**:300-306, Feb. 1983.

Todd, K.S., Hudes, M., and Calloway, D.H.: Food intake measurement: problems and approaches, Am. J. Clin. Nutr. **37**:139-146, Jan. 1983.

Walker, W., and Hendricks, K.: Manual of pediatric nutrition, Philadelphia, 1985, W.B. Saunders Co.

Williams, S.R.: Nutrition and diet therapy, ed. 4, St. Louis, 1985, Times Mirror/Mosby College Publishing.

Chapter 7

Physical and Developmental Assessment of the Child

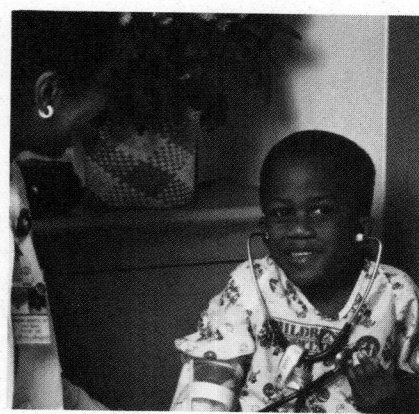

Preventive Child Health Services
General Approaches to Examining Children
Assessment Skills
    Inspection
    Palpation
    Percussion
    Auscultation

Physical Examination
    Growth measurements
        Length
        Height
        Weight
        Skinfold thickness and arm circumference
        Head circumference
    Physiologic measurements
        Temperature
        Pulse
        Respiration
        Blood pressure
    General appearance
        Physical appearance
        Nutrition
        Behavior
        Development
    Skin
        Physical factors influencing assessment
        Genetic factors influencing assessment of color

        Physiologic factors influencing assessment of color
        Reliable areas for assessment of color
        Variations in skin color
        Texture
        Temperature
        Turgor
        Accessory appendages
    Lymph nodes
    Head
    Neck
    Eyes
        Placement and alignment
        Inspection of external structures
        Inspection of internal structures
        Vision testing
    Ears
        Placement and alignment
        Inspection of external structures
        Inspection of internal structures
        Auditory testing
        Vestibular testing
    Nose
        Inspection of external structures
        Inspection of internal structures
    Mouth and throat
        Inspection of internal structures
    Chest
    Lungs
        Inspection
        Palpation
        Percussion
        Auscultation
    Heart
        Inspection
        Palpation
        Percussion
        Auscultation
    Abdomen
        Inspection
        Auscultation
        Percussion
        Palpation

    Genitalia
        Male genitalia
        Female genitalia
    Anus
    Back and extremities
        Spine
        Extremities
        Joints
        Muscles
    Neurologic assessment
        Behavior
        Cognitive-perceptual development
        Motor functioning
        Sensory functioning
        Cerebellar functioning
        Reflexes
        Cranial nerves
        "Soft" signs

Denver Developmental Screening Test
    Additional developmental screening tests
    Developmental screening and interpretation

Physical and developmental assessment is a continuous process that begins during the interview, primarily through inspection or observation, and continues to some degree throughout the professional relationship. Although the assessment resembles that of a medical physical examination, the objective of each assessment area is to formulate nursing diagnoses and evaluate the effectiveness of interventions.

This chapter discusses the influence of age on the preparation of children for physical examination, the tools used for assessment of health status, the performance of the examination, and methods of developmental assessment.

PREVENTIVE CHILD HEALTH SERVICES

The objectives of pediatric health care are maintenance of optimum health and prevention of illness. The concept of prevention necessitates an orderly and routine schedule of activities deliberately geared to these two objectives. The American Academy of Pediatrics (1985) has suggested the schedule shown in Table 7-1 for the care of well children who receive competent parenting and who have no serious health problems. Circumstances that may indicate the need for additional visits or procedures include families of diverse socioeconomic and cultural backgrounds, one-parent families, or those with children who have chronic illnesses or disabilities.

The services required by each child must be individualized by the health care provider. Nurses are in the best position to review children's previous schedule of health care and institute specific measures or referrals to update the health record. For example, during hospitalization children's overall record should be reviewed to ensure that they have had sensory screening, appropriate immunizations, and a yearly dental examination.

GENERAL APPROACHES TO EXAMINING CHILDREN

Ordinarily the examining sequence follows a head-to-toe direction to provide a general guideline for assessment of each body area in order to minimize omitting segments of the examination. The typical organization of a physical examination is listed in the chapter table of contents.

In examining children, this orderly sequence is frequently altered to accommodate the child's developmental needs, although written recording follows the traditional model. Using developmental and chronologic age as the main criteria for assessing each body system accomplishes several goals:

Table 7-1 Recommendations for preventive health care

ASSESSMENT AREA	_____ AGE* _____															
	2-4 WK	2 MO	4 MO	6 MO	9 MO	12 MO	15 MO	18 MO	24 MO	36 MO	4-6 YR	8 YR	10 YR	12 YR	14 YR	16-20 YR
History																
Initial						At first visit										
Interval						At each visit										
Measurements																
Height and weight						At each visit										
Weight for height			✓	✓	✓	✓	✓	✓	✓	✓	✓	✓	✓			
Skinfold														✓	✓	✓
Head circumference	✓	✓	✓	✓	✓	✓	✓	✓	✓							
Blood pressure										✓	✓	✓	✓	✓	✓	✓
Sensory screening																
Sight	✓		✓	✓		✓	✓				✓	✓	✓	✓	✓	✓
Hearing	✓			✓	✓				✓		✓	✓	✓	✓	✓	✓
Speech										✓	✓	✓				
Developmental appraisal						At each visit										
Physical examination						At each visit										
Immunization†		✓	✓	✓			✓	✓	✓		✓			✓	or	✓
Anticipatory guidance						At each visit										
Initial dentist's examination‡										✓						

Data from American Academy of Pediatrics: Health supervisor visits, Elk Grove Village, IL, 1985, The Academy.
Key: ✓ to be performed.
*If a child comes under care for the first time at any point on the schedule, or if any items are not accomplished at the suggested age, the schedule should be brought up to date at the earliest possible time.
†See also p. 526.
‡Subsequent examinations as prescribed by dentist.
Author's note: Change in schedule at 12 and 24 months made to accommodate most recent American Academy of Pediatrics' recommendations.

1. Minimizes stress and anxiety associated with assessment of various body parts.
2. Fosters a trusting nurse-child-parent relationship.
3. Allows for maximum preparation of the child.
4. Preserves the essential security of the parent-child relationship, especially with young children.
5. Maximizes the accuracy and reliability of assessment findings.

Most of the suggestions for performing a physical assessment according to different ages are based on logic and developmental principles. Since no child fits precisely into one age category, the guidelines for positioning, sequence, and preparation, as shown in Table 7-2, must be based on the preliminary assessment made by the nurse during the interview of the child's developmental achievements and needs. For example, even when the best approach is used, many toddlers are uncooperative and unable to be consoled for almost all of the physical examination. However, some seem intrigued by the new surroundings and unusual equipment and respond more like preschoolers than like toddlers. Likewise, some early preschoolers may require more of the "security measures" employed with younger children, such as continued mother-child contact, and less of the preparatory measures used with preschoolers, such as playing with

Table 7-2 Age-specific approaches to physical examination during childhood

AGE	POSITION	SEQUENCE	PREPARATION
Infant	Before sits alone: supine or prone, preferably in parent's lap; before 4 to 6 months: can place on examining table After sits alone: use this position whenever possible in parent's lap If on table, place with parent in full view	If quiet, auscultate heart, lungs, abdomen Record heart and respiratory rates Palpate and percuss same areas Proceed in usual head-toe direction Perform traumatic procedure last (eyes, ears, mouth [while crying], rectal temperature [if taken]) Elicit reflexes as body part examined Elicit Moro reflex last	Completely undress if room temperature permits Leave diaper on male Gain cooperation with distraction, bright objects, rattles, talking Smile at infant; use soft, gentle voice Pacify with bottle of sugar water or feeding Enlist parent's aid for restraining to examine ears, mouth Avoid abrupt, jerky movements
Toddler	Sitting or standing on/by parent Prone or supine in parent's lap	Inspect body area through play: "count fingers," "tickle toes" Use minimal physical contact initially Introduce equipment slowly Auscultate, percuss, palpate whenever quiet Perform traumatic procedures last (same as for infant)	Have parent remove outer clothing Remove underwear as body part examined Allow to inspect equipment; demonstrating use of equipment usually ineffective If uncooperative, perform procedures quickly Use restraint when appropriate; request parent's assistance Talk about examination if cooperative; use short phrases Praise for cooperative behavior
Preschool child	Prefer standing or sitting Usually cooperative prone/supine Prefer parent's closeness	If cooperative, proceed in head-toe direction If uncooperative, proceed as with toddler	Request self-undressing Allow to wear underpants if shy Offer equipment for inspection Briefly demonstrate use Make up "story" about procedure: "I'm taking blood pressure to see how strong muscles are" Use paper doll technique Give choices when possible Expect cooperation; use positive statements: "Open your mouth"
School-age child	Prefer sitting Cooperative in most positions Younger age prefer parent's presence Older age may prefer privacy	Proceed in head-toe direction May examine genitalia last in older child Respect need for privacy	Request self-undressing Allow to wear underpants Give gown to wear Explain purpose of equipment and significance of procedure, such as otoscope to see eardrum, which is necessary for hearing Teach about body functioning and care

Continued.

Table 7-2 Age-specific approaches to physical examination during childhood—cont'd

AGE	POSITION	SEQUENCE	PREPARATION
Adolescent	Same as for school-age child Offer option of parent's presence	Same as older school-age child	Allow to undress in private Give gown Expose only area to be examined Respect need for privacy Explain findings during examination: "'Your muscles are firm and strong" Matter-of-factly comment about sexual development: "Your breasts are developing as they should be" Emphasize normalcy of development Examine genitalia as any other body part; may leave to end

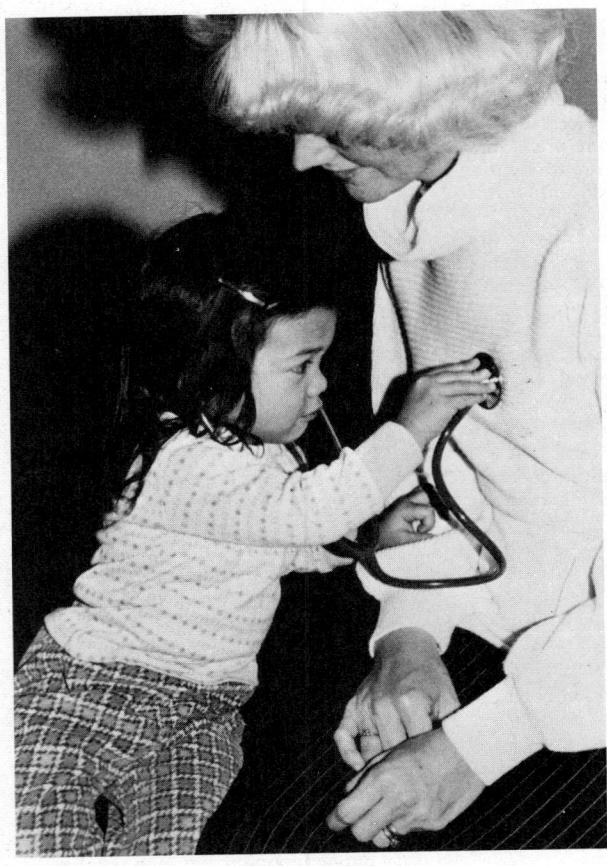

Fig. 7-1. Preparing child for physical examination.

the equipment before and during the actual examination (Fig. 7-1).

Some young children refuse to be examined for a variety of reasons, including fear of medical procedures, fear of separation from parents, and manipulative behavior. Some children may even fear the examiner because of prior physical abuse at home (Schmitt, 1984). Each of these situations requires individual attention. Fear of medical procedures and separation are managed effectively with the approaches in Table 7-2. Manipulative behavior requires a firm, direct approach in regard to what behavior is expected. It may be necessary to ask the parent to leave the room before the child's cooperation can be gained; the family also may benefit from discussion of more effective childrearing approaches. A child who is unduly afraid of the examiner, especially a male examiner, needs consideration of the possibility of previous traumatic experiences. When such situations are managed with sensitivity, they can promote the child's development by encouraging mastery of a difficult task (McClellan, 1984).

Certain behaviors signal readiness to cooperate, such as the child's willingness to talk to the nurse, make eye contact, accept the offered equipment, allow physical touching, smile, or choose to sit on the examining table rather than the parent's lap. Failure to observe these behaviors shows a need to delay the examination until the child "warms up." Several approaches can be used to facilitate this:

1. Talk to the parent while essentially "ignoring" the child and gradually focus on him or a favorite object, such as a doll.
2. Make complimentary remarks about the child's dress or appearance.
3. Tell a funny story or play a simple magic trick.
4. Have a nonthreatening "friend" available, such as a hand puppet to "talk" for the nurse.
5. Allow choices whenever possible, such as "Would you like to sit up on the table or in your mom's lap?"
6. Begin the examination with those activities that can be presented as games, such as tests for the cranial nerves (p. 282) or parts of the Denver Developmental Screening Test (DDST) (p. 283) and end with the more traumatic procedures, such as examining the ears and mouth.

Another approach that is effective in preparing the child for the examination is the "paper-doll technique." The child lies supine on the examining table, and his length is measured by marking the end points of the head and heels on the paper. When he sits up, the nurse asks him to look at the two marks and suggests that the rest of him be filled in to see "how big" he is. As the outline is completed, children are usually amazed to see their body take shape and quickly become absorbed in drawing more parts. Consequently, before areas of the body are assessed, they can be drawn on the "paper doll" and "examined." For example, before auscultating the heart, the nurse can draw in the heart, "listen" to it on the paper, and then say to the child, "Let's listen to your heart and see what sound it makes" (Fig. 7-2). With older children a more detailed drawing helps them learn about their bodies. At the conclusion of the visit the child can bring the paper doll home as a memento of his experience.

Whatever approach is used, statements should be made in a positive manner and in a tone of voice that says, "I expect you to cooperate." Suggestive statements, such as "I am going to feel your belly but it won't hurt," should be avoided, since the child immediately assumes it will hurt. Instead the nurse should state what is to be done and offer distractions, such as those suggested on pp. 224 and 271.

Although the variations in the general approaches are numerous, some of them are elaborated here because they are more common. For example, the suggested sequence may change considerably when the child is in pain or when obvious physical defects are present. In either situation it is preferable to examine the affected area last to minimize distress early in the examination and to focus on normal, healthy, or functioning body parts rather than defective ones.

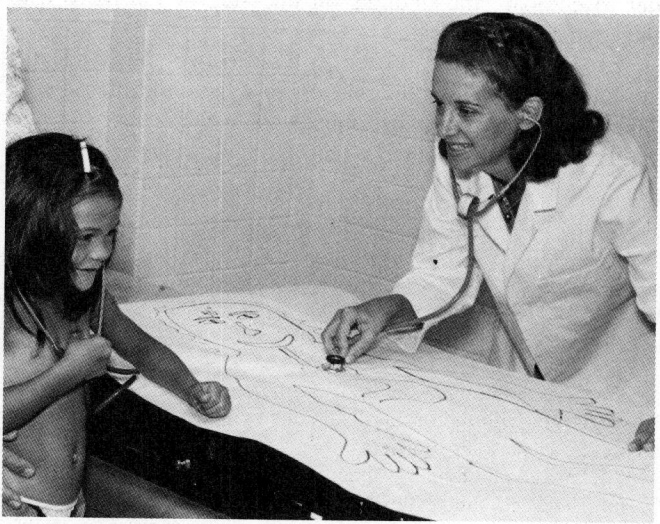

Fig. 7-2. Using paper-doll technique to prepare child for physical examination.

Positioning may also be altered because of physical distress. For example, the child who is having difficulty breathing may not be able to lie down; thus as much of the physical examination as possible should be performed in a sitting or slightly reclining position or the examination should be completed at another time.

With skill and the child's cooperation, the physical examination should be completed rapidly. The time consideration is important because an adequate initial interview may require as much as an hour, and a developmental screening test may take about 10 to 20 minutes. When combined with an unnecessarily prolonged physical assessment, the child and parent can become exhausted and less cooperative. Establishing one's own systematic sequence of performance for each age-group will greatly enhance one's ability to skillfully and thoroughly execute a complete physical appraisal.

ASSESSMENT SKILLS

The traditional four categories of assessment skills include inspection, palpation, percussion, and auscultation. Each involves a set of tools to facilitate its performance, usefulness, and accuracy. Although the trend has been to incorporate more specialized and technical equipment into nursing assessment, the nurse is equipped with all of the tools necessary for a fairly comprehensive and detailed physical examination. The use of the senses of sight, smell, hearing, and sometimes taste are necessary for inspection. The hands and fingers are the main tools of palpation and percussion, and the ear can be used for auscultation. Although several specific instruments refine the examination, it is important to remember that few of them can replace the human tools of skill, knowledge, and interpretation.

Inspection

Inspection is the most valuable, least mechanical, and most difficult skill to learn. It involves the use of the senses, primarily vision, to make judgments, comparisons, and decisions. Because inspection is a highly subjective process, it requires skill, repetition, and practice to establish reliable findings for distinguishing among ranges of normal, borderline, and abnormal.

Methods of inspection. One of the keys to competent inspection is the conscious, systematic, and active use of one's senses. As the nurse examines each body part, the visible areas are deliberately inspected for such factors as color, texture, firmness, hygiene, masses, hair distribution, tone, movement, behavior, tension, flaccidity, symmetry, location, position, and temperature. As each of these aspects is observed, it is compared to what constitutes normal anatomy and physiology. Although it is not the nurse's objective to "diagnose" an abnormality by labeling it as a specific disorder, defect, or disease, it is the nurse's responsibility to recognize and record its presence.

Inspection may be combined with specific instruments

for better visualization, such as the otoscope for the ear (p. 251), and with measurements to validate subjective impressions. For example, the nurse may observe that the child appears thin for his age; this impression is substantiated by recording height and weight on a growth chart, comparing the values, and judging those measurements in terms of genetic background, previous growth trends, physical status, and nutritional intake. After establishing a thorough data base, the nurse then proceeds to draw conclusions and formulate nursing diagnoses.

Frequently competent inspection involves intangible skills for which no yardstick exists. The most common example relates to measuring emotional state or behavior. An experienced nurse may look at a child and know that he is ill without any further assessment. Often, however, the nurse is unable to state specifically what behaviors have led to that conclusion. One way of developing assessment skills is to consciously analyze behaviors, such as appearance, movement, relationships, activity, verbal interaction, mood, and orientation and to record what is observed, not what is interpreted. For example, a *factual* statement is, "An 11-year-old Oriental male, color is pale, moves slowly, holds right lower quadrant of abdomen, occasional facial grimaces, answers questions slowly and briefly." An *interpretative* statement is, "An 11-year-old Oriental male in distress, pain in lower right abdomen, and refuses to talk." The latter statement is much more liable to erroneous or altered interpretations by others than the former statement, which is a list of what is observed.

Palpation

Palpation is primarily the use of touch or the tactile sense to detect both superficial and deeper characteristics of the body. It is combined with inspection, since in many instances it validates a visual impression, such as texture of the skin. Palpation uses touch to assess temperature, position, form, size, consistency, moisture, and movement, such as vibration or pulsation. It is used to examine all accessible parts of the body, such as organs, glands, blood vessels, bones, muscles, hair, skin, and mucosa. A thorough knowledge of anatomy is essential in differentiating palpation of normal body structures from abnormal ones, such as masses.

Methods of palpation. Palpation involves the use of the fingers and hands for superficial and deep examination of body parts. A general guide to palpating includes using:

Fingertips for small areas, such as the neck for lymph glands or the infant's skull for fontanels, or when fine tactile discriminations are made, such as texture of the skin

Fingertips and dorsa (back) of the hands for temperature differences

Palmar surfaces of the fingers and hand for detecting vibration, such as heart thrills or the point of maximum impulse of the heart on the chest wall

Grasping action of the fingers to evaluate consistency, position, and size of organs or masses

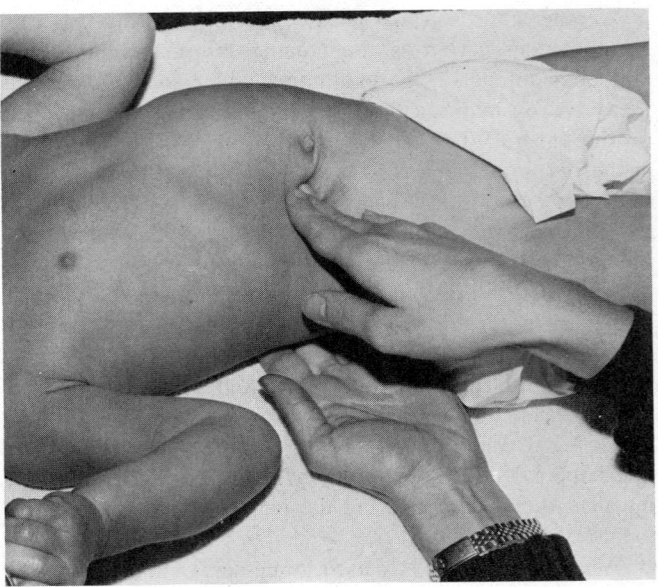

Fig. 7-3. Bimanual palpation.

When deeper organs are palpated, particularly those in the abdomen, a bimanual maneuver may be used. One hand is placed on the abdomen, and the other hand applies pressure to the first hand. Palpation is done with the cushions and palmar surfaces of the contact hand, not with the fingernails (which should be kept short and trimmed). In small children the distal palmar surfaces of the fingers are directly applied to the skin, and the other hand may or may not be used to apply pressure to the contact hand. Frequently the nonpalpating hand is placed against the child's back directly underneath the area to be palpated. In this way the organ is "caught" or felt between both hands (Fig. 7-3). Although the sequence generally follows suggestions in Table 7-2, the nurse should use a bilateral and symmetric approach in order to compare the findings on one side of the body with those on the other side.

For any type of palpation to be effective, but especially for deep palpation of internal organs, the child must be relaxed; otherwise the tense muscles act like a wall between the hand and the organ. To help the child relax:

1. Position him comfortably, such as in a semireclining position in a parent's lap.
2. Warm the hands before touching the skin.
3. Use distraction such as telling stories or talking to the child.
4. Teach the child to use deep breathing and concentrate on an object.
5. Give the infant a bottle or pacifier.
6. Begin with light superficial palpation and gradually progress to deeper palpation.
7. Palpate any tender or painful areas last.
8. Have the child hold the parent's hand and squeeze it if the palpation is uncomfortable.
9. Use the nonpalpating hand to comfort the child, such as placing the free hand on the child's shoulder while palpating the abdomen.

Percussion

Percussion is the striking or tapping of the body surface to produce sounds that correlate with the type of underlying tissue density. The principles of percussion are the same as those used to produce sounds in a musical instrument, such as the drum. For example, hollow, air-filled spaces, such as the lungs, create a low-pitched, well-sustained note called *resonance*. Dense, solid objects, such as organs or masses, create a high-pitched, short, thudding sound called *dullness*. Percussion sounds are described in terms of *tones* and *notes* (Table 7-3). Because sounds are difficult to describe in words, practice in percussing different areas of the body and comparing the emitted sounds is fundamental to developing skill and competence.

Methods of percussion. Techniques for percussion may be direct or indirect. *Direct* percussion is striking or tapping the body surface directly with the finger (Fig. 7-4, *A*). It is useful for percussing well-defined areas, such as a bone or the borders of an organ. It is also advantageous for greater accuracy when examining infants or small children, where body organs are in proximity.

In the *indirect* method the tapping is performed by striking a stationary finger positioned on the body. Some practitioners prefer this method because there is less perception by the patient of being hit or struck than in the direct approach. Indirect percussion is performed by (1) placing the index or middle finger against the body area to be percussed and (2) using the tip of the middle finger of the other hand to strike the base of the distal phalanx of the nonpercussing finger (Fig. 7-4, *B*). No other finger of the nonpercussing hand touches the chest wall. In order for the sound produced to be clear and not damped or muffled, quick, firm, sharp taps are necessary, similar to playing staccato notes on the piano. The nurse holds her forearm stationary and delivers the blows by using a loose hinge-joint action of the wrist. An excellent way of practicing correct percussion is by striking keys on a piano. If the blow is not sharp with a quick rebound of the finger, the note will be of a distinctly different sound than one that is staccato-like.

Auscultation

Auscultation is similar to percussion in that it involves evaluation of body sounds. It differs in that it concerns those sounds produced by the body, such as sounds arising from the heart, lungs, and abdomen. The characteristics of auscultatory sounds are the same as those used to describe percussion tones, that is, intensity, pitch, duration, and quality (see Table 7-3).

Methods of auscultation and types of stethoscopes. As with percussion, the direct or indirect method

---

Table 7-3 Definition of percussion sounds

PERCUSSION SOUNDS	EXAMPLES
Tones*	
Intensity—amplitude or loudness of tone	Loud tones—produced by more hollow, air-filled spaces, such as the lungs
	Soft tones—produced by more dense or solid masses, such as the heart
Pitch—frequency or number of vibrations per second; the greater the number of vibrations, the higher the pitch; the fewer the number, the lower the pitch	Low-pitched—air-filled lungs
	High-pitched—consolidated lung
Duration—time period of vibrations and length of time the sound lasts	Long duration—normal lungs
	Short duration—high-density organ, such as the heart
Quality or timbre—subjective evaluation that depends on the source of the sound	The same musical note from two different instruments produces a different quality or timbre of sound; for example, sounds of equal loudness and pitch from different organs, such as the lungs and heart, produce sounds of varying quality
Notes	
Resonance—clear hollow note, low pitch, long duration, relatively loud (heart with ease)	Normal lungs
Tympany—clear hollow note, higher pitched than resonance, musical with rich overtones (quality), long duration	Tympanic sound can be produced by lightly tapping an air-filled cheek with the finger; similar sound when percussing an airfilled stomach
Hyperresonance—cross between resonance and tympany; lower pitch than normal resonance, high intensity, and long duration	Usually indicates less density, such as increased amount of air or decreased amount of tissue; usually pathologic, such as pneumothorax or asthma
Dullness—high-pitched, short duration, soft (low intensity), and thudding	Related to increased density and solidity, such as the heart
Flatness—absolute dullness, high-pitched, very short, nonmusical in quality	Solid tissue, such as the thigh

*These same terms are used to describe any sound and are used in physical assessment to record auscultatory sounds.

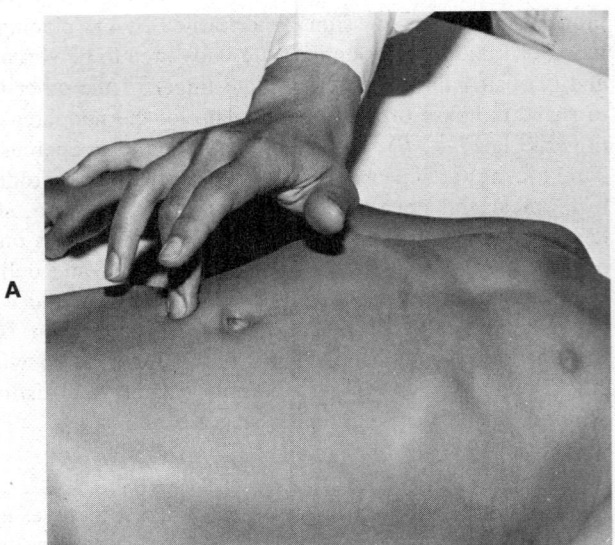
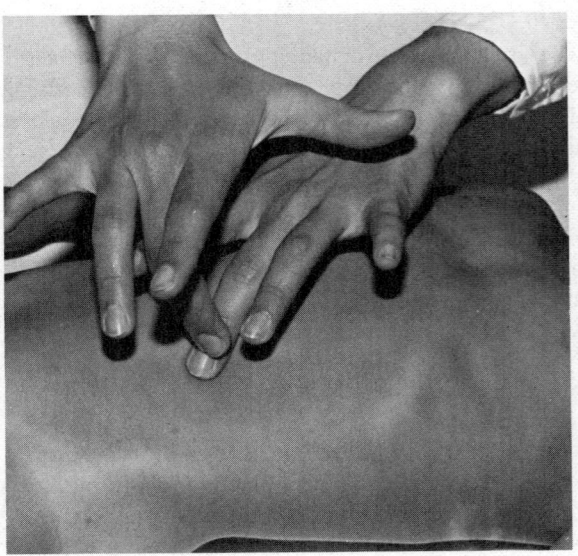

Fig. 7-4. Percussion. **A,** Direct. **B,** Indirect.

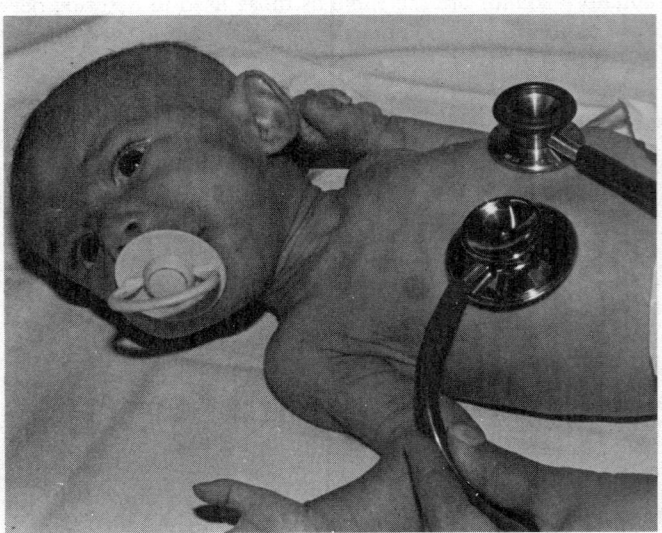

Fig. 7-5. Comparison of pediatric and adult-size stethoscopes on infant's chest. Closed-diaphragm chestpiece is against skin and open-bell chestpiece is facing upward.

of listening for sounds can be used. In the *direct* method the examiner's ear is applied directly to the body surface. In some instances loud sounds, such as grade VI murmurs or expiratory wheezes, can be heard by placing the ear close to the child, but not directly against the skin. The direct approach has disadvantages in terms of patient modesty, aversion to skin-to-skin contact, or possible infection to the examiner from skin lesions.

Indirect auscultation involves the use of a stethoscope to transmit internal body sounds to the ear. The main types of stethoscopes are the open bell and the closed diaphragm. The *open-bell,* or *Ford, chestpiece* consists of a short cone or funnel-shaped horn joined to a binaural headset and ear-

tips with flexible tubing. It has the advantage of conducting sounds with virtually no distortion of pitch or timbre and is better for the perception of certain low-pitched sounds, such as diastolic murmurs. However, it must be placed firmly against the body surface for an airtight seal. Normally the diameter of the bell does not exceed 2.5 cm (1 inch). A larger-width bell would not permit a tight seal on bony or small surfaces, thus resulting in admittance of ambient sounds. This restriction in size limits the volume of sound it can accumulate.

The larger, flatter, and less bulky *closed-diaphragm,* or *Bowles, chestpiece* is sealed by its own diaphragm. These features afford it several advantages. Its larger diaphragm admits a greater quantity of sound and is more sensitive to high-pitched sounds. The diaphragm filters out and suppresses low-frequency vibrations, so that sounds appear to be of higher pitch than when heard through the bell. The self-sealing diaphragm obviates the need for an airtight skin seal, so that a larger diaphragm is still accurate when placed on a bony or small chest. However, a close-fitting seal is still recommended in order to decrease the admittance of environmental sounds. In infants and small children, especially premature infants, the use of a specially sized pediatric diaphragm is recommended both to achieve sufficient skin contact and to localize sounds in segmented areas of the chest. For example, an adult-size diaphragm almost completely covers the landmarks used to localize heart sounds, whereas a smaller-size diaphragm permits placement of the stethoscope over appropriate thoracic sites, facilitating differentiation of heart sounds (Fig. 7-5).

The length of the flexible tubing may vary considerably without significantly affecting the transmission of sound. A sufficient length is about 50 cm (20 inches). The binaural headset should be light, flexible, and comfortable, and the earpieces should fit snugly to occlude the ear canals and prevent entry of extraneous noise. The ear tubes are inclined anteriorly in order to conform to the natural direction of the auditory canals. If they are positioned incorrectly, they are usually uncomfortable and decrease the perception of transmitted body sounds. The importance of comfortable, close-fitting earpieces cannot be overemphasized.

Use of the stethoscope. Using the stethoscope properly involves knowledge of how it works and factors that interfere with its performance. As with percussion, skill requires considerable practice, particularly in listening to normal body sounds. Although descriptions of auscultatory sounds are discussed in examination of the specific body system, general practical measures include the following:

1. Make sure the child is relaxed and not crying, talking, or laughing.
2. Check that the room is a comfortable temperature and as quiet as possible.
3. Warm the stethoscope before placing it against the skin.
4. Apply firm pressure on the chestpiece but not enough to prevent vibrations and transmission of sound.
5. Avoid placing the stethoscope over hair or clothing, moving it against the skin, breathing on the tubing, or sliding one's fingers over the chestpiece, which may cause sounds that falsely resemble pathologic findings.

Auscultation, like inspection, requires the mental discipline of concentrating on one aspect of many simultaneous stimuli. The nurse must consciously listen for one sound, such as breathing, while deliberately disregarding other sounds, such as the heartbeat or environmental noises. This is particularly important in children, whose thin chest wall effectively transmits sounds throughout the thoracic cavity. The nurse must also establish a systematic, symmetric approach to auscultation that proceeds from one area of the body to another. Because accurate auscultation requires additional time for the beginning practitioner, it is always thoughtful to explain to parents or older children why one is listening for so long, in order to allay their fears that some abnormality is suspected.

PHYSICAL EXAMINATION

Although the approach to and sequence of the physical examination differ according to the child's age, the following discussion outlines the traditional model for physical assessment. It emphasizes normal findings, variations from the norm that may cause parents or children concern but that require little or no intervention, and abnormalities that necessitate appropriate referral. Although the focus includes all age-groups, the reader is referred to Chapter 8 for a detailed discussion of a newborn assessment, since procedures or findings unique to the neonate are not included here.

Growth Measurements

Measurement of physical growth in children is a key element in evaluation of the health status of children. Physical growth parameters include weight, height (length), skinfold thickness, and head circumference.

Values for weight, length, and head circumference are plotted on growth charts, and the child's measurements in percentiles are compared to those of the general population.

The most commonly used growth charts in the United States are from the National Center for Health Statistics (NCHS) and are available for boys and girls ages:

1. **Birth to 36 months**—records weight by age, recumbent length by age, weight by length, and head circumference by age
2. **2 to 18 years**—records weight by age, stature by age
3. **Prepubescence**—records weight by stature

Two sets of charts include data for 2 to 3 years; one set (birth to 36 months) is based on recumbent length, and the other set (2 to 18 years) uses stature (standing height). Since these two modes of estimating length are not equivalent, the type of length measurement needs to be considered when selecting either chart.

These growth charts use the 5th and 95th percentiles as criteria for determining which children are outside the normal limits for growth. In general those whose height or weight falls below the 5th percentile are considered underweight or small in stature; those whose measurements are above the 95th percentile are considered overweight or large in stature. The use of standard growth charts for children from different ethnic groups is discussed below.

Questions and Controversies

How accurate are the United States growth charts for evaluating the growth of children from different ethnic and socioeconomic backgrounds?

A study by Habicht and others (1974) showed that differences in height and weight among well-nourished preschool children of different ethnic backgrounds were relatively small (3% for height and about 6% for weight), but the differences between these children and those of poorer socioeconomic level, regardless of ethnic background, were high (about 12% for height and 30% for weight). A more recent study found that 72% of elementary age Indochinese refugee children fell below the 10th percentile for weight for age and height for age on the United States (NCHS) growth charts. However, when weight-for-stature was compared, the results were within the normal range (Pickwell, 1982). Other studies have confirmed these findings. However, whether the differences are the result of nutritional factors or genetic background is still unclear. (Olness and others, 1984; Barry and others, 1983).

Such findings indicate that the present United States growth charts can serve as a *reference guide* for all racial or ethnic groups if used from the perspective that different groups of children have varying normal distributions on the growth curves. For example, the average weight and height for Chinese children based on standards from China (see Appendix C) falls on the 10th percentile, not the 50th percentile, on the NCHS growth charts. The NCHS charts can be used for United States black children because this group was included in the sample population (Moore and Roche, 1982).

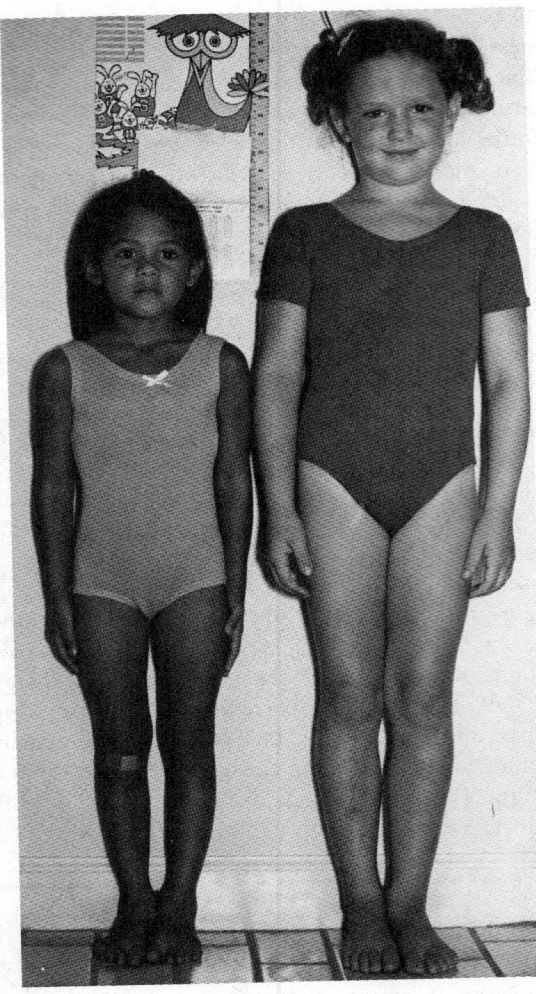

Fig. 7-6. These children of identical age (5 3/4 years) are markedly different in size. Child on left, of part Oriental descent, is at 5th percentile for height and weight. White child on right is above 95th percentile for height and weight. However, both children demonstrate normal growth patterns. (For growth measurements of Chinese children, see Appendix C.)

Overall evaluation of growth requires judgment in interpretation of growth percentiles. Generally, children whose height or weight falls below the 5th percentile or above the 95th percentile should be followed closely. However, small or large size may be genetic (Fig. 7-6). Comparing children's growth trends with those of their parents is essential in evaluating adequate growth. Special charts are available for parent-specific adjustments for evaluation of the child's height (Himes and others, 1985). Other children whose growth may be questionable include:

1. Children whose height and weight percentiles are widely disparate, for example, height in the 10th percentile and weight in the 90th percentile, especially with above average skinfold thickness
2. Children who fail to show the expected gain in height and weight, especially during the rapid growth periods of infancy and adolescence

3. Children who show a sudden increase, except during puberty, or decrease in a previously steady growth pattern

Since growth is a continuous but uneven process, the most reliable evaluation lies in comparison of growth measurements over a prolonged time.

Length. Until children are 24 months old (36 months if the child cannot stand unassisted), recumbent length is measured. Because of their normally flexed position during infancy, measuring length requires full extension of the body by (1) holding the head in midline, (2) grasping the knees together gently, and (3) pushing down on them until the legs are fully extended and flat against the table. If a measuring board is used, the head is placed firmly at the top of the board and the heels of the feet are placed firmly against the footboard.

If such a measuring device is not available, the child's length is measured by placing him on a paper-covered surface, marking the end points of the top of the head and heel of the feet, and measuring between these two points (see Fig. 7-9). Accurate measurement necessitates that the writing utensil be held at a right angle to the table when the cephalic point is marked and the feet be positioned with the toes pointing directly to the ceiling when the heel point is marked. Regardless of the method used, assistance in holding the child's head in midline is enlisted while the nurse extends the legs and takes the measurements.

Height. Recumbent or standing height (stature) may be taken in children who are over 24 to 36 months, although the latter is the usual procedure for those 3 years or older. Standing height is measured by having the child remove his shoes and stand as tall and straight as possible, with the head in midline and the line of vision parallel to the ceiling or floor. The child's back should be to the wall or other vertical flat surface, with the heels, buttocks, and back of the shoulders touching the wall. Any flexion of the knees, slumping of the shoulders, or raising of the heels of the feet are checked and corrected.

Height is measured by placing a firm, flat surface against the vertex or crown of the head. The movable measuring rod of platform scales is accurate only if it maintains a parallel position to the floor and rests securely on the topmost part of the crown. One way of improvising a flat surface for measuring length is to attach a paper or metal tape or yardstick to the wall, position the child adjacent to the tape, and place a three-dimensional object, such as a thick book or box, on his head. The side of the object must rest firmly against the wall to form a right angle. Length or stature is measured to the nearest 1 mm or 1/8 inch. It is essential to note the position of measurement since length can be up to 2 cm greater than stature.

Occasionally special length measurements are taken, such as *sitting height* or *crown-to-rump length* (see p. 306 for the newborn). In older infants and children, sitting height is most easily determined by having the child sit against the wall and measuring between the vertex of the head and the sitting surface. Although not a usual measurement, this method is used for children suspected of being dwarfs to help distinguish true dwarfism from small stature. Normally sitting height accounts for 70% of total body length at birth, 60% at 2 years, and about 52% at age 10 years.

Weight. Weight is measured with an appropriately sized beam balance scale, which measures weights to the nearest 10 g or ½ ounce for infants and 100 g or ¼ pound for children. Before the child is weighed, the scale is balanced by setting it at zero and noting if the balance registers exactly in the middle of the mark. If the end of the balance beam rises to the top or bottom of the mark, more or less weight, respectively, must be added. Some scales are designed to allow for self-correction, but others need to be recalibrated by the manufacturer.

Measurements are made in a comfortably warm room. Infants are weighed nude; older children are usually weighed while wearing their underpants or a light gown. It is essential to always respect their need for privacy. If the child must be weighed wearing some article of clothing or some type of special device, such as a prosthesis, this is noted when the weight is recorded. Children who are measured for recumbent length are usually weighed on a large platform type of infant scale and placed in a lying-down or sitting position. When weighing infants, the nurse places the hand lightly above the infant to prevent him from accidentally falling off the scale (Fig. 7-7, *A*). Once stature is taken, weight can also be measured on a standing type of upright platform scale. For maximum asepsis, either type of scale is covered with a clean sheet of paper that is changed between each child's measurement.

Skinfold thickness and arm circumference. Measures of relative weight and stature cannot distinguish between adiposity or muscularity. One convenient measure of body fat is skinfold thickness, which is increasingly recommended as a routine measurement (see also p. 213). Skinfold thickness is measured with special calipers, such as the Lange calipers. However, such instruments are costly and often are not available for general use. Plastic calipers, such as the Ross Adipometer (Fig. 7-8), are available at no cost from the manufacturer and have been shown to be an accurate substitute for the standard instruments (Jung and others, 1984; Ryan, 1985). The most common sites for measuring skinfold thickness are the triceps (most practical for routine clinical use), subscapula, suprailiac, abdomen, and upper thigh. For greatest reliability the exact procedure for measurement must be followed and the average of at least two measurements of one site recorded. Fig. 7-8 describes the procedure for measurement of triceps skinfold thickness.

Arm circumference is an indirect measure of muscle mass and is also recommended in the evaluation of nutritional status. Measurement of arm circumference follows the same procedure for skinfold thickness except the midpoint is measured with a paper or steel tape. Percentiles for triceps skinfold and arm circumference in children are listed in Appendix C.

Head circumference. Head circumference is usually taken in all children up to 36 months of age and in any child whose head size is questionable, such as a child with hydrocephalus. The head is measured at its greatest circumference, that is, slightly above the eyebrows and pinna of the ears and around the occipital prominence at the back of the skull (Fig. 7-9). A paper or metal tape is used because a cloth tape can stretch and give a falsely small measurement. The head size is plotted on the appropriate growth chart under head circumference. Generally head and chest circumference are equal at about 1 to 2 years of age. During

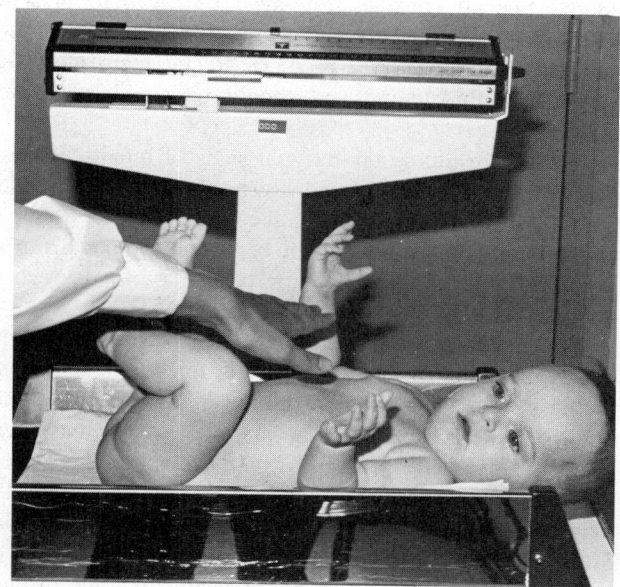
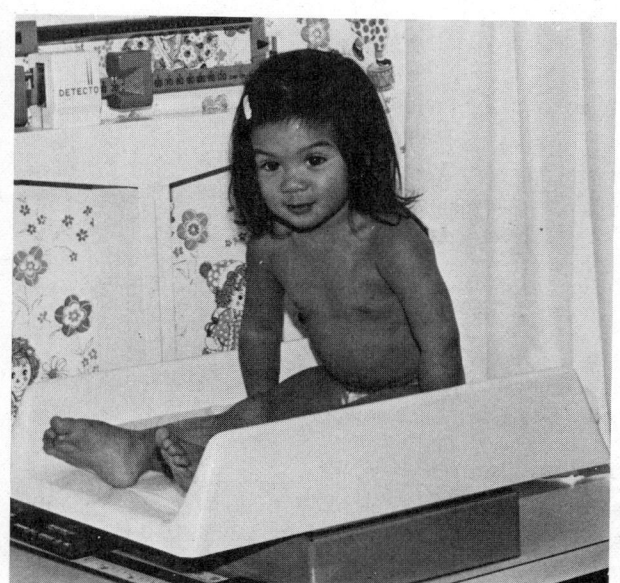

A   **B**

Fig. 7-7. A, Infant on scale. **B,** Toddler on scale.

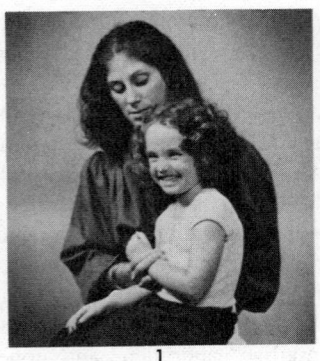
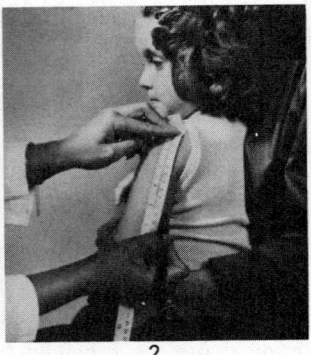
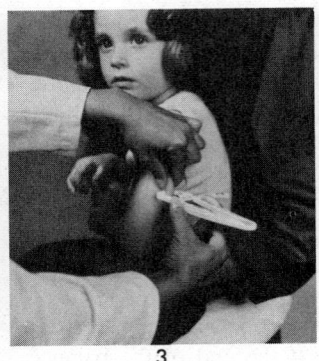
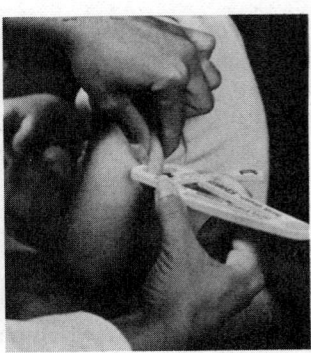

1 *For a child,* have an attendant hold the child's left hand or forearm with the elbow flexed to approximately 90 degrees and pressed gently against his or her abdomen. The child can be either standing or sitting.

For an infant, have an attendant (preferably the mother) hold the infant in a semi-upright position, with infant's right side next to but not touching mother's body, and with infant's head facing forward. Gently restrain the infant's left hand or forearm with the elbow flexed to approximately 90 degrees and pressed gently against his or her abdomen.

2 Marks are placed at the left acromion (shoulder) and olecranon (elbow). The distance between these marks is measured and the midpoint marked.

3 At a site 1 cm above midpoint, grasp a layer of skin and sub-cutaneous tissue with the first finger and thumb of one hand, gently pulling it away from the underlying muscle, and continue to hold until measurement is completed.

Place caliper jaws over the skinfold at the midpoint mark and apply pressure with the thumb to align the lines on the caliper. Do not apply excessive pressure.

4 Estimate reading to nearest 1.0 mm, 2 to 3 seconds after aligning lines. Three readings should be taken, averaged, and recorded. Compare present measurement with previous triceps skinfold measurement(s) to determine possible change.

Fig. 7-8. Measurement of triceps skinfold.
Reprinted with permission of Ross Laboratories, Columbus, OH 43216, from Adipometer Skinfold Caliper and Instruction Chart, 1978, Ross Laboratories.

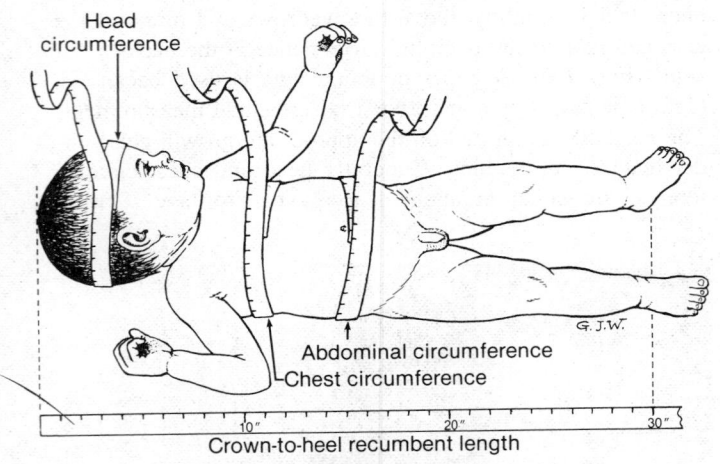

MEASUREMENTS

Fig. 7-9. Measurement of head, chest, and abdominal circumference and crown-to-heel (recumbent) length.

childhood chest circumference exceeds head size by about 5 to 7 cm (2 to 3 in). (For newborns see p. 305.)

Physiologic Measurements

Physiologic measurements, key elements in evaluating physical status of vital functions, include temperature, pulse, respiration, and blood pressure. Each physiologic recording is compared with normal values for that age-group (see inside front cover). In addition, the nurse compares the values taken on preceding health visits with present recordings. For example, a falsely elevated blood pressure reading may not indicate hypertension if previous recent readings have been within normal limits. The isolated recording may indicate some stressful event in the child's life.

As in most procedures carried out with children, older children and adolescents are treated much the same as are adults. Special consideration must be given to preschool children, whose fear of body mutilaton is intensified with any intrusive procedure (p. 632). Rectal temperatures are particularly threatening and should be avoided whenever possible.

For best results in taking vital signs of infants, the usual order of approach is reversed. Respirations are counted first, before the infant is disturbed, the pulse next, and temperature last. If vital signs cannot be taken without disturbing the child, the child's behavior (e.g., crying) is recorded with the measurement.

Temperature. Temperature can be taken by the oral, rectal, or axillary route. The only difference in selection of thermometers is that the rectal type has a more rounded blunt bulb as compared to the oral type, which has a more slender, elongated tip. *Oral temperatures* are taken in children who can be trusted to keep the thermometer under their tongue with their mouth closed without biting on the glass. Some institutions have a specific age for permitting oral temperatures, such as after 5 or 6 years. In some instances even younger children can cooperate. The newer electronic temperature-measuring equipment is ideally suited to pediatric use because the plastic sheath is unbreakable, the child's mouth can remain open, and the temperature registers within seconds. Electronic thermometer measurement is accurate for all three routes (Barrus, 1983). When used to take an axillary or oral temperature, electronic temperature equipment offers an ideal alternative to intrusive rectal procedures.

When an oral temperature is being taken, the thermometer is placed under the tongue in the right or left posterior sublingual pocket, not in the front of the tongue. Contrary to traditional belief, the sublingual site indicates rapid changes in core body temperature *better* than the rectum. The sublingual area has a rich blood supply derived from the carotid arteries, which are close to the temperature-regulating center in the brain and the central circulation at the heart (Erickson, 1980). However, several factors can affect the temperature of the mouth, such as hot beverages, smoking, and rapid breathing.

Rectal temperatures should be taken only when the oral or axillary route cannot be used. This includes children whose mental age or temperament precludes cooperation and understanding instructions, agitated children, and those who have had oral and axillary injuries or surgery. In some institutions rectal temperatures are taken after cardiac surgery. They are contraindicated in newborns and anyone who has had rectal surgery. One factor affecting the accuracy of rectal measurements is the presence of stool in the rectum.

To take a rectal temperature, children are placed in a side-lying, supine, or prone position. A convenient position for infants is supine with the knees flexed toward the abdomen. This position is maintained with one hand while the other hand is used to insert the lubricated bulb of the thermometer a maximum of 2.5 cm (1 inch) (Fig. 7-10, *A*). Further insertion increases the risk of perforation, because the colon curves at a depth of about 3 cm (1¼ inches). It is advisable to cover the penis because this procedure often stimulates urination.

An alternative position that works very well is for the parent to hold the child with his arms hugging the parent's neck and the legs wrapped around the parent's waist. With the child in this straddle position, the thermometer is gently inserted into the rectum. This approach is effective, especially with toddlers, because it preserves parental closeness and maintains an upright position.

Axillary temperatures are often recommended for children who object strongly to a rectal temperature but for whom an oral temperature is not feasible. Axillary temperatures have the advantage of avoiding an intrusive procedure and eliminating the risk of rectal perforation and possible peritonitis, especially in newborn and premature infants. To take an axillary temperature, the thermometer is placed in the axilla with the arm kept close to the child's side (Fig. 7-10, *B*).

A recent substitute for the mercury thermometer is the plastic strip thermometer, such as the Clinitemp Fever Detector. This device changes color in response to sensed temperature changes. Although it correlates fairly well with measurements taken with mercury thermometers, its readings are frequently lower than mercury readings. Consequently, the plastic strip thermometer may not predict a fever accurately (Lewit and others, 1982).

There is no universal agreement regarding the length of time mercury thermometers should be kept in place. Recommendations based on research are 7 minutes for an oral reading, 4 minutes for a rectal reading (Nichols and others, 1972), and 5 minutes for an axillary temperature (Eoff and Joyce, 1981). However, these times may vary widely within practice settings and may not represent *clinically significant* differences in temperature readings taken for shorter intervals. One of the advantages of electronic thermometers is their rapid response—under 60 seconds. Even axillary temperatures can be taken in about 20 to 30 seconds (Barrus, 1984).

Normal body temperature registers 37.0° C (98.6° F) via the oral route. Traditionally it has been assumed that rectal temperatures are 1° F higher and axillary temperatures 1° F lower than oral temperatures. However, it has been demonstrated that this difference may be considerably less, with axillary and rectal readings differing by an average of 0.49° C (0.9° F) (Eoff and Joyce, 1981). Because of these variations, the route is charted along with the recorded temperature reading.

A characteristic of some small children is the tendency toward a rapid temperature elevation with the associated risk of precipitating seizures. Whenever a child feels extra warm to the touch, his temperature should be taken, even if it was found to be normal only a short time before. Children under 3 years of age are especially vulnerable to febrile seizures.

Pulse. A satisfactory pulse can be taken radially in children over 2 years of age. However, in infants and young children the apical pulse (heard through a stethoscope held to the chest at the apex of the heart) is more reliable. (See Fig. 7-42 for location of the apex and Fig. 7-43 for location of pulses.) The pulse is counted for 1 full minute in infants and young children because of possible irregularities in rhythm. A comparison of radial and femoral pulses should be done at least once during early childhood to detect the presence of circulatory impairment, such as coarctation of the aorta. Because of the marked variability in heart rate with activity, the child's behavior is also recorded. (See inside front cover for normal rates for pediatric age-groups.)

Respiration. The respiratory rate is counted in the same manner as for the adult patient, except that in infants the movements are primarily diaphragmatic and therefore observed by abdominal movement. Since the movements are irregular, they should be counted for 1 full minute for accuracy (see also p. 261). (See inside front cover for normal respiratory rates in children.)

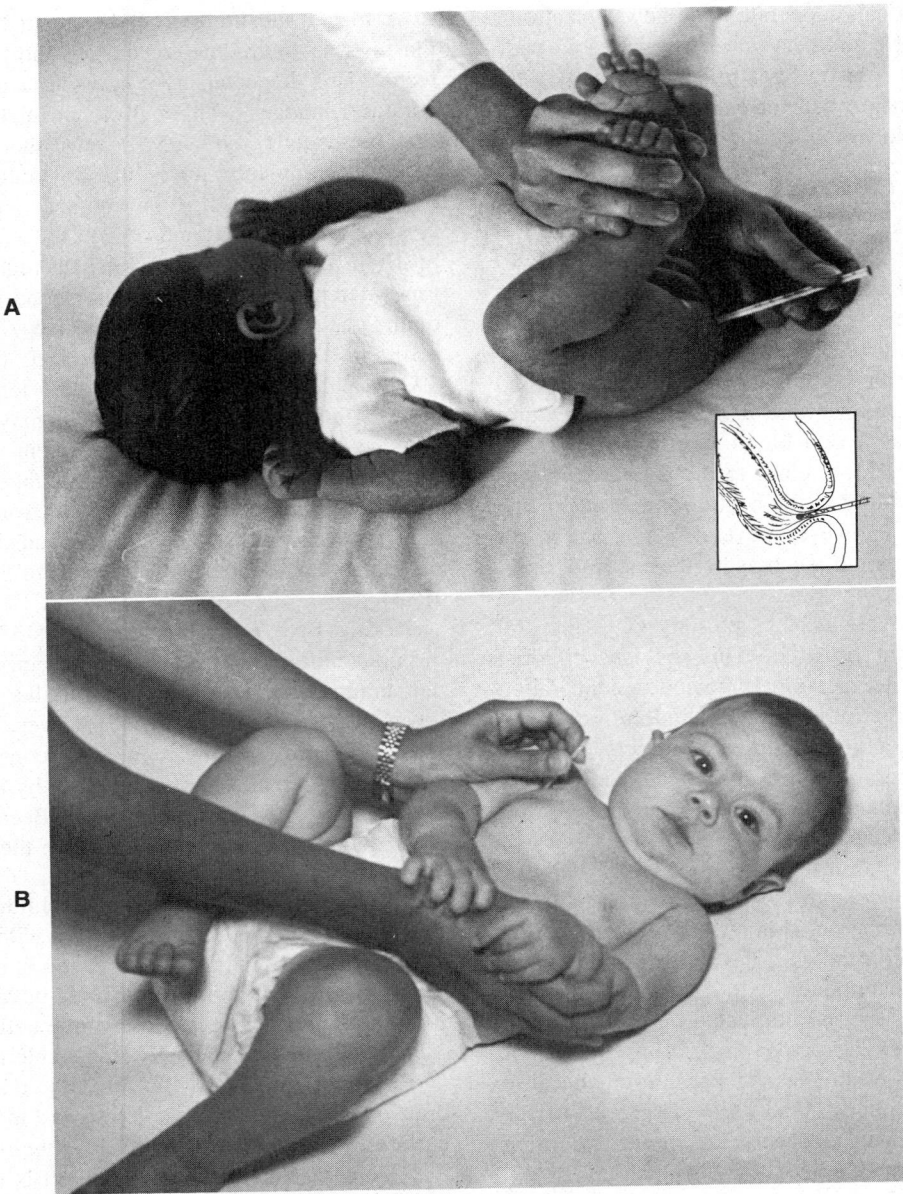

Fig. 7-10. A, Position for taking rectal temperature in infant. **B,** Position for taking axillary temperature. Insert of cross-section of rectum.illustrates curve at approximately 3 cm from anus.

Blood pressure. Blood pressure measurements are part of a routine vital sign determination in children 3 years of age and older. Several authorities recommend routine measurements from birth. Since the child should be quiet and relaxed during the procedure, blood pressure is measured before any anxiety-producing procedures are performed or injections given, and the nurse employs techniques for putting the child at ease. Infants and small children may be more quiet if the reading is taken while they are sitting in the parent's lap. Children's cooperation can be enlisted if the equipment and each step of the procedure are explained and if they are told how it will feel to them. Explanations

such as "I want to see how strong your muscle is" or "Let's watch the silver rise in the tube" are appealing to young children.

Studies of children demonstrate that blood pressure can vary significantly under different circumstances and that multiple measurements are needed, preferably on different days, for an accurate assessment (Cross, 1985b). For children with blood pressure in the high normal range or above, at least three different blood pressure measurements at separate visits are recommended (Blumenthal, 1977).

Selection of cuff. Accurate measurement requires the use of an appropriately sized cuff. The width of the cuff

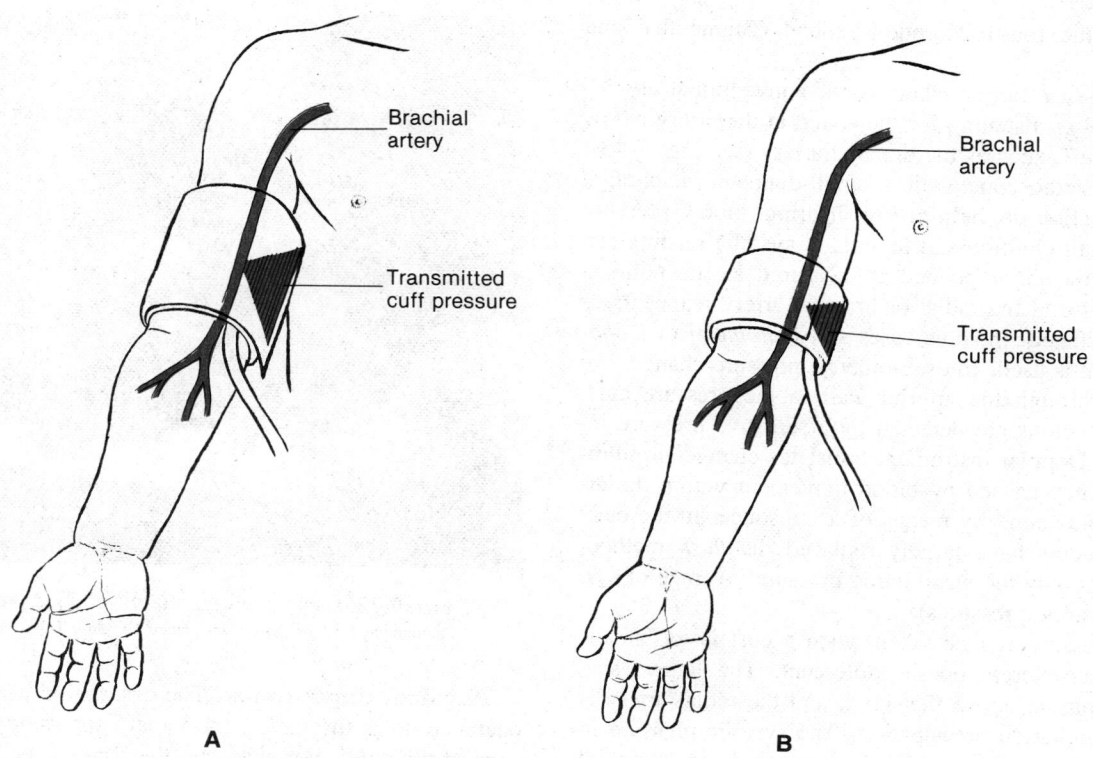

Fig. 7-11. Effect of cuff size on blood pressure measurement. **A,** Correct size cuff with adequate transmission of pressure to artery. **B,** Too small cuff with inadequate pressure to compress artery, resulting in falsely elevated reading.

should cover approximately two thirds of the upper arm (or thigh) or be 20% greater than the diameter of the extremity without causing pressure in the axilla or impinging on the antecubital fossa. In infants and young children a cuff width greater than two thirds the length of the upper arm is recommended (Steinfeld and others, 1978). The length of the inflatable bladder inside the cuff should be long enough to sufficiently encircle the extremity without overlapping.

Ill-fitting cuffs are a common cause of incorrect blood pressure readings. A small cuff causes a falsely elevated reading (Fig. 7-11). This may be a problem in the very obese child. Generally a large cuff results in a lower reading. Compression of the brachial artery in the axilla by clothing pushed up the arm may also produce a false low reading. However, wide cuffs apparently do not cause the low readings observed in adults (Steinfeld and others, 1978). Therefore in choosing cuff sizes, it is preferable to use an oversized cuff rather than an undersized one when the correct size is not available. Approximate guidelines for selection of cuff sizes are listed in the accompanying box, although the selection of a cuff must be individualized for the child. Guidelines are based on the range of cuff sizes sold by U.S. manufacturers. References to cuff size refer only to the inner inflatable bladder rather than to the cloth covering, which can be considerably wider and longer than the bladder (Blumenthal and others, 1977).

GUIDELINES FOR SELECTION OF BLOOD PRESSURE CUFFS

	Dimensions of bladder (cm)	
Age	**Width**	**Length**
Newborn	2.5-4	5-10
Infant	6-8	12-13.5
Child	9-10	17-22.5
Adult	12-13	22-23.5
Large adult arm	15.5	30
Adult thigh	18	36

Measurement. The technique of blood pressure measurement in children is generally the same as that used for adults. For greatest accuracy the same position and arm are used. Although there are no definite data to indicate that one position is superior to the other, the supine position can result in a higher systolic pressure than a sitting position (Hohn, Riopel, and Loadholt, 1984). The arm is positioned at the level of the heart. If the arm is positioned below this point, gravity will add its pressure to the brachial artery pressure, producing falsely high readings (Britton, 1981). Although there is controversy about the cut-off point for diastolic pressure in children, most authorities recommend the muffling of the fourth Korotkoff sound (Blumenthal and others, 1977).

Blood pressure can be taken by the conventional *auscultation* method by listening for the sound at the artery below the inflated cuff, such as the brachial artery (see Fig. 7-43). A pediatric stethoscope with a small-diameter diaphragm and amplification is helpful for hearing blood pressure sounds in small children and infants. A systolic reading can be obtained by *palpation* and is measured as the point at which the pulse at the radial or brachial artery reappears as the cuff is deflated. In some cases an *oscillometer* or *Doppler* instrument is used. In oscillometry, pressure changes are transmitted through the arterial wall to the pressure cuff, and the oscillations are detected by a sensitive pressure indicator. The Doppler instrument translates changes in ultrasound frequency caused by blood movement within the artery to audible sound by means of a transducer in the cuff. Such instruments have largely replaced the *flush* method, which reflects only the *mean* blood pressure (average of systolic and diastolic pressures).

Radial pressure can be taken when a cuff is too small, such as in a severely obese adolescent. The largest size arm cuff is placed above the wrist, and the radial artery is used for auscultation or palpation. The systolic pressure in the radial artery is 10 mm Hg lower than in the brachial artery.

Thigh blood pressure can be taken on small children when only large cuffs are available. The cuff is wrapped around the thigh just above the knee and the popliteal artery is auscultated or palpated (Fig. 7-12). Blood pressure in the thigh normally averages 10 mm Hg higher than the arm pressure. A lower pressure in the lower extremities may indicate some interference with circulation such as coarctation of the aorta. A comparison of blood pressure in the arm and leg should be done at least once during early childhood to detect circulatory impairment.

The average blood pressure readings at various ages throughout childhood are listed on the inside front cover. For quick reference the following formula gives an approximate average systolic blood pressure for females ages 5 to 16 and males ages 5 to 18 years:

$$83 + (2.5 \times \text{age in years})$$

For children ages 2 to 4 years, the blood pressure remains constant at the 5-year-old level.

General Appearance

The general appearance of the child is a cumulative, subjective impression of the child's physical appearance, state of nutrition, behavior, personality, interactions with parents and nurse (also siblings if present), posture, development, and speech. Although general appearance is recorded in the beginning of the physical examination, it encompasses all the observations of the child during the interview and physical assessment.

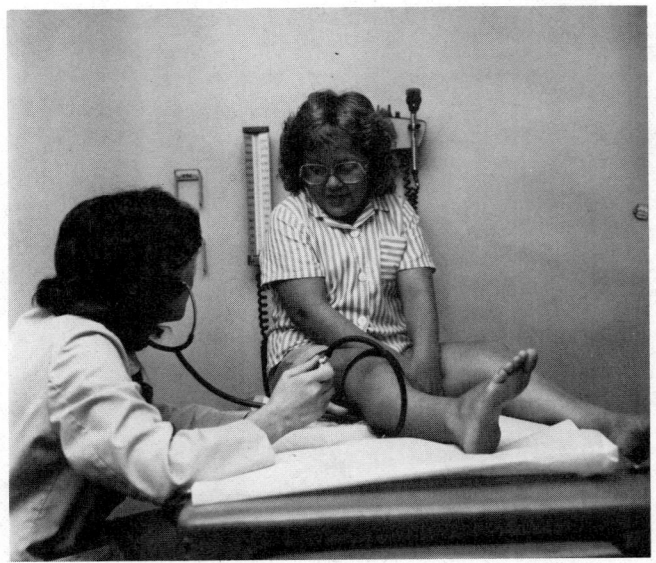

Fig. 7-12. Using popliteal artery for blood pressure.
Photography by John Roy, Saint Francis Hospital, Tulsa, OK.

Physical appearance. The description of physical appearance notes the *facies,* the facial expression and appearance of the child. For example, the facies may give clues to children who are in pain, have difficulty in breathing, feel frightened, discontent, or happy, are mentally deficient, or are acutely ill.

Posture, position, and types of *body movement* also are important in the overall assessment of physical appearance. The child with hearing or vision loss may characteristically tilt his head in an awkward position to facilitate perception of sound or sight. The child in pain may favor a body part. The child with low self-esteem or a feeling of rejection may assume a slumped, careless, and apathetic pose or posture. Likewise, a child with confidence, a feeling of self-worth, and a sense of security usually demonstrates a tall, straight, well-balanced posture. Although the nurse observes such "body language," it must not be interpreted too freely but rather recorded objectively.

Hygiene is noted in terms of the child's state of cleanliness, unusual body odor, the condition of the hair, neck, nails, teeth, and feet, and the condition of the clothing. Such observations give excellent clues to possible instances of neglect, inadequate financial resources, housing difficulties (e.g., no running water), or lack of knowledge of children's needs.

Nutrition. General appearance includes an overall impression of the child's state of nutrition. This impression is more than a statement describing body weight or stature, such as "slender and tall." It is an estimation of the quality, as well as quantity, of nutritional intake. For example, two children can be of the same height and weight, yet one can appear overweight because of flabby, loose skin, while the other child appears strong, robust, and well built because of firm, well-defined musculature. Likewise, a small, slender child may be well nourished with no signs of chronic undernutrition, such as bony prominences, protuberant abdomen, flat buttocks, gaunt facies, and poor muscle tone with evidence of wasting.

The nurse's impression of nutritional state is compared with the parents' history of feeding practices. Discrepancies between the two "impressions" may be a valuable area for nutritional counseling. For example, parents who believe that their child is too thin and eats too little, despite evidence of adequate growth and physical signs of proper nutrition, may find it helpful to keep a daily diary in order to calculate the child's cumulative food intake. Many parents are surprised at the quantity of food ingested, even though the amounts at each meal or snack are small.

Behavior. Behavior includes the child's personality, level of activity, reaction to stress, requests, or frustration, interactions with others, primarily the parent and nurse, degree of alertness, and response to stimuli. It is one of the most important observations that the nurse makes during a child's health assessment. (See also the Behavioral checklist, p. 278.)

Some mental questions that serve as reminders for observing behavior include:

1. What is the child's overall personality—calm, anxious, tense, content, outgoing, shy, talkative, aggressive, introverted, stable, or moody?
2. Is he active, sedentary, fidgety, or restless?
3. Does he have a long attention span or is he easily distracted?
4. Does he sit quietly on the examining table or parent's lap or does he climb, run, open doors, and otherwise explore his environment?
5. How does he react to commands—with fear or willingness to obey?
6. How advanced is his ability to follow requests? Can he follow two or three commands in succession without the need for repetition? Is he attentive to requests or must they be repeated several times?
7. Is he cooperative, belligerent, or argumentative?
8. What is his response to delayed gratification or frustration? Is he able to withstand momentary discomfort and wait for his requests to be met?
9. In what tone of voice does he make requests or talk to his parents?
10. Does he seek approval and gain satisfaction from it?
11. Does he use eye-to-eye contact during conversation?
12. Does he agree with his parents' answers or find reasons to disagree, interrupt, or argue? What is his reaction to the nurse—respectful, friendly, reserved, apprehensive, or uninterested?
13. Is he interested in his surroundings? Does he look around the room, ask questions about unfamiliar objects, seem to enjoy exploring them, or attempt to break or destroy them?
14. Can he follow directions for using the instruments or imitate their use? Is he quick or slow to grasp explanations?

Development. Although gross developmental achievement can usually be assessed from careful and detailed observation of the child, the impressions should be documented with screening tests, such as the Denver Develop-

mental Screening Test (DDST). Various tests for assessing development, speech, vision, and hearing are discussed later in this chapter and in Chapter 25.

An overall estimate of the child's speech development, motor skills, degree of coordination, and recent area of achievement is recorded under general appearance. For example, the following statement may apply to an 18-month-old child: "Motor development advanced for age, climbs, runs, jumps (most recent motor skill), manipulates small objects with ease, excellent coordination and balance, beginning to name many objects, uses two-word phrases, and enjoys 'talking' to self and others."

Skin

Skin is assessed for color, texture, temperature, moisture, and turgor. Hair is also inspected for color, texture, quality, distribution, and elasticity. Examination of the skin and its accessory organs primarily involves inspection and palpation.

Physical factors influencing assessment. Examination of the child is conducted in a well-illuminated room with nonglare lighting. Ideally the room should be neutral in color. Colors such as pink, blue, yellow, or orange cast deceiving glows on the skin. The room should also be comfortably warm, since air-conditioning can cause a cold-induced cyanosis and excessive heat can produce flushing. Poor hygiene and artificial paint on nails or lips also mask true determination of color. Sometimes it is necessary to clean the skin with soap and water and to remove cosmetics before beginning inspection. Although not a common situation in pediatrics, the nurse should remember that such factors can hide signs of ecchymoses, petechiae, pallor, or cyanosis.

Texture, temperature, moisture, and turgor can be subjectively inspected, but palpation must be done for greater accuracy. Clothing always interferes with palpation; thus the nurse needs to examine each area of the body nude, either as part of the general overall examination or combined with assessment of each body system. Since texture is affected by climatic exposure, such as cold, sun, and wind, the texture of protected areas of the body is compared to exposed areas.

Genetic factors influencing assessment of color. The normal color in light-skinned children varies from a milky-white and rosy color to a more deeply hued pink color. In general, cyanosis or bluish discolorations are not normal, except in the newborn (see p. 300). Dark-skinned children, such as those from American Indian, Hispanic, black, Latin, Mediterranean, or Oriental descent, have inherited various brown, red, yellow, olive-green, and bluish tones in their skin, which can falsely alter assessment. For example, some children of Mediterranean origin normally have bluish-tinged lips, suggestive of cyanosis. Oriental persons, whose skin is normally of a yellow tone, may appear to be jaundiced. Full-blooded black individuals often have normal bluish pigmentation of the gums, buccal cavity, borders of the tongue, and nail beds. The visible portion of their sclera may contain speckled deposits of brown melanin that resemble petechiae.

Physiologic factors influencing assessment of color. Edema of the skin affects color in all individuals because it increases the amount of interstitial fluid, thereby increasing the distance between the outermost layers of the epidermis and the pigmented and vascular layers. Edema decreases the intensity of skin color, sometimes producing a false pallor.

Exposure to sunlight, on the other hand, stimulates the melanocytes to produce more melanin, thereby increasing the color of the skin. Individuals who are deeply suntanned require as careful observation as those who are genetically dark skinned.

In general, the amount of adipose tissue does not markedly affect skin color because deposition of fat cells is below the pigmented layers of the skin. Overnutrition may not mean adequate nutrition, and pallor that may indicate nutritional-iron deficiency is carefully assessed.

Reliable areas for assessment of color. Color changes are most reliably assessed in those areas of the body where melanin production is least: sclera, conjunctiva, nail beds, lips, tongue, buccal mucosa, palms, and soles. These areas are rarely affected by edema or amount of adipose tissue but are sensitive to changes from physical factors, such as use of cosmetics, ingestion of colored food substances, or poor hygiene.

Variations in skin color. Many of the specific color changes peculiar to the newborn are described on p. 300. Differences in assessment of color changes in ethnic groups are presented in Table 7-4.

Pallor and cyanosis. The skin receives its pigmented color of yellow, brown, and black from melanin and its shades of red or blue from the color of hemoglobin. Oxygenated hemoglobin in the superficial capillaries of the dermis gives a rosy, pink glow. Reduced (deoxygenated) hemoglobin reflects a bluish tone through the skin, called *cyanosis*, which is evident when reduced hemoglobin levels reach 5 mg per dl of blood or more, regardless of the total hemoglobin. In general, the darker the skin pigmentation, the greater the amount of deoxygenated hemoglobin must be for cyanosis to be evident.

Pallor, or paleness, may be a sign of anemia, chronic disease, edema, or shock. However, it may be a normal complexion characteristic or an indication of indoor living.

Pallor or cyanosis can be compared to the color change normally produced by blanching. For example, in nonpigmented nails, pressing down on the free edge of the nail on the index or middle finger of a child with good skin color produces marked blanching or whitening as compared to the return blood flow. In a child with pallor the difference in color change will be slight. The blanching color change can be observed in dark-skinned individuals by gently applying pressure to their lips or gums.

Erythema. Erythema, or redness of the skin, may be the result of increased temperature from climatic conditions, local inflammation, or infection. It may also appear as a sign of skin irritation, allergy, or other dermatoses. The degree of redness reflects the amount of increased blood flow to the area. The nurse notes any reddening and describes its location, size, presence of warmth, itching, type of distribution (e.g., diffuse, clearly circumscribed, parallel to a vein), and the presence of characteristic lesions, such as macules, papules, or vesicles (see Chapter 18 for a description of skin lesions).

Plethora. Plethora is also redness of the skin but is caused by increased numbers of red blood cells as a compensatory response to chronic hypoxia. Intense redness of the lips or cheeks occurs.

Ecchymosis and petechiae. Ecchymosis and pete-

Table 7-4 Differences in color changes of racial groups

COLOR CHANGE	LIGHT SKIN	DARK SKIN
Cyanosis	Bluish tinge, especially in palpebral conjunctiva (lower eyelid), nail beds, earlobes, lips, oral membranes, soles, and palms	Ashen gray lips and tongue
Pallor	Loss of rosy glow in skin, especially face	Ashen-gray appearance in black skin More yellowish-brown color in brown skin
Erythema	Redness easily seen anywhere on body	Much more difficult to assess; rely on palpation for warmth or edema
Ecchymosis	Purplish to yellow-green areas; may be seen anywhere on skin	Very difficult to see unless in mouth or conjunctiva
Petechiae	Purplish pinpoints most easily seen on buttocks, abdomen, and inner surfaces of the arms or legs	Usually invisible except in oral mucosa, conjunctiva of eyelids, and conjunctiva covering eyeball
Jaundice	Yellow staining seen in sclera of eyes, skin, fingernails, soles, palms, and oral mucosa	Most reliably assessed in sclera, hard palate, palms, and soles

chiae are caused by extravasation or hemorrhage of blood into the skin; the only difference between the two is size. Ecchymoses are large, diffuse areas, usually black and blue in color, and are typically the result of accidental injuries in healthy, active children. Since ecchymotic areas may indicate systemic disorders or child maltreatment, the nurse should always investigate the reported cause of the bruises, especially when they are located in suspicious areas, such as the back or buttocks, rather than on the knees, shins, elbows, or forearms.

Petechiae are small, distinct pinpoint hemorrhages 2 mm or less in size, which can denote some type of blood disorder, such as decreased platelets in leukemia. Because of their size, ecchymoses are more readily observed than are petechiae, which may be visible only in areas of very light-colored skin. Areas of erythema can be distinguished from ecchymosis or petechiae by blanching the skin. Since erythema is a result of increased blood flow *to* the area, exerting pressure will momentarily empty the engorged vessels and produce blanching. Because the other discolorations are produced by blood leaking *into* tissue spaces, blanching will not occur.

Jaundice. Jaundice, a yellow staining of the skin usually caused by bile pigments, is always a significant finding. If a yellow-orange cast is noted in an otherwise healthy child, the nurse should inquire about the quantity of ingested yellow vegetables, such as carrots, which in excess produce a yellow-orange color from deposits of carotene in the skin, a condition called carotenemia.

Texture. The nurse palpates the skin for texture, noting moisture and temperature. Any marks or scars that are suggestive of healed injuries are noted, and inquiries are made about their origin. Normally the skin of young children is smooth, soft, and slightly dry to the touch, not oily or clammy. Any variations from these findings are noted, because they may indicate common problems of childhood such as cradle cap, eczema, diaper rash, or excessive dryness (xeroderma) all over the body from too frequent bathing, exposure to the weather, or vitamin A deficiency. Excessively moist, clammy skin may indicate serious health problems, particularly heart disease.

Temperature. Temperature is evaluated by symmetrically feeling each part of the body and comparing upper areas with lower ones. Any distinct difference in temperature is noted. Although not a common anomaly, one of the key signs for coarctation of the aorta is warm upper extremities and cool lower ones. The nurse also observes the skin temperature of the dressed child. Young children produce heat rapidly, and they quickly become overheated if dressed too warmly. Many parents do not realize this and fail to change the amount of clothing to accommodate climatic variations.

Turgor. Tissue turgor refers to the amount of elasticity in the skin. It is best determined by grasping the skin on the abdomen between the thumb and index finger, pulling it taut, and quickly releasing it. Elastic tissue immediately assumes its normal position without residual marks or creases. In children with poor skin turgor the skin remains suspended or tented for a few seconds before slowly falling back on the abdomen. Skin turgor is one of the best estimates of adequate hydration and nutrition.

While evaluating turgor, the nurse also inspects for signs of *edema,* normally evident as swelling or puffiness. Periorbital edema is a sign of several systemic disorders, such as kidney diseases, but may normally be evident in children who have been crying or sleeping or who have allergies. Edema is evaluated for change according to position, its specific location, and response to pressure. For example, in pitting edema, pressing a finger into the edematous area will cause a temporary indentation.

Accessory appendages. Inspection of the accessory organs of the skin, namely the hair, nails, and dermatoglyphics, may be performed while the skin is being examined or when the scalp and extremities are being assessed.

Hair. The hair is inspected for color, texture, quality, distribution, and elasticity. Children's scalp hair is usually lustrous, silky, strong, and elastic. Genetic factors affect the appearance of hair. For example, the hair of black children is usually curlier and coarser than that of white children. Hair that is stringy, dull, brittle, dry, friable, and depigmented may suggest poor nutrition. Any bald or thinning spots are recorded. Although alopecia can be a sign of various skin disorders, such as tinea capitis, loss of hair in infants is often the result of lying in the same position and may be a clue for counseling parents concerning the child's stimulation needs.

General cleanliness of the hair and scalp is noted. Various ethnic groups condition their hair with oils or lubricants, which, if not thoroughly washed from the scalp, clog the sebaceous glands, causing scalp infections. The nurse also inspects hair shafts for lice, whose ova appear as grayish translucent flakes. Ova or nits are distinguished from dandruff because the eggs adhere to the hair. If pediculosis capitis is suspected, the nurse should be careful to guard against self-infestation of the lice by wearing gloves and handwashing.

The scalp is also inspected for ticks, which appear as grayish or brown oval bodies. Although they can be found anywhere on the body, the most common sites are exposed parts, such as the head. Although not all dog or wood ticks transmit serious disease, a notation of removal is made on the child's chart in case symptoms appear.

Unusual hairiness anywhere on the body, such as arms, legs, trunk, or face, is noted. Tufts of hair anywhere along the spine, especially over the sacrum, are significant because they can mark the site of spina bifida occulta.

In older children who are approaching puberty, the nurse looks for growth of secondary hair as a sign of normally progressing pubertal changes (see p. 808). Precocious or delayed appearance of hair growth is noted because, although not always suggestive of hormonal dysfunction, it may be of great concern to the early- or late-maturing adolescent.

Nails. The nails are inspected for color, shape, texture, and quality. Normally the nails are pink, convex in shape, smooth, and hard but flexible, not brittle. The edges, which are usually white, should extend over the fingers. Dark-skinned individuals may have more deeply pigmented nail beds. Variation in color, such as blueness, is suggestive of cyanosis, and a yellow tint may indicate jaundice. Bluish-black discoloration usually indicates hemorrhage under the nail from trauma. Fungal infections cause the entire nail to become whitish with a pitting surface. Short, ragged nails are typical of habitual biting. Uncut nails with dirt accumulated under the edge sometimes indicate poor hygiene.

Changes in the shape of nails are also significant. For example, concave curves or "spoon nails," called *koilonychia,* are sometimes seen in iron-deficiency anemia, a common nutritional problem of children. Clubbing of the nails is always a significant finding and usually is associated with chronic cyanosis. In clubbing, the base of the nail becomes visibly swollen and feels springy when palpated, rather than firm as in the normal nail (see p. 1308).

Dermatoglyphics. Each individual has a distinct set of handprints and footprints. The patterns, or *dermatoglyphics,* are unique to the individual and vary a great deal in detail and complexity of patterns. Flexion creases also appear on the palm of the hand and the sole of the foot. The palm normally shows three flexion creases (Fig. 7-13, *A*). In some situations, such as Down syndrome, the two distal horizontal creases are fused to form a single horizontal crease called a *single palmar crease,* or *simian crease* (Fig. 7-13, *B*). If grossly abnormal lines or folds are observed, the nurse should sketch a picture to describe them and refer the finding to a specialist for further investigation.

Lymph Nodes

The body's extensive lymph system is usually assessed when examining the part of the body in which the glands are located. The usual sites for palpating accessible lymph nodes are shown in Fig. 7-14. Since the major function of lymph nodes is to collect and filter the lymph of bacteria and other foreign matter as it returns to the circulatory system, the nurse must have knowledge of the lymph's directional flow. Tender, enlarged warm lymph nodes are generally indicative of infection or inflammation *proximal* to

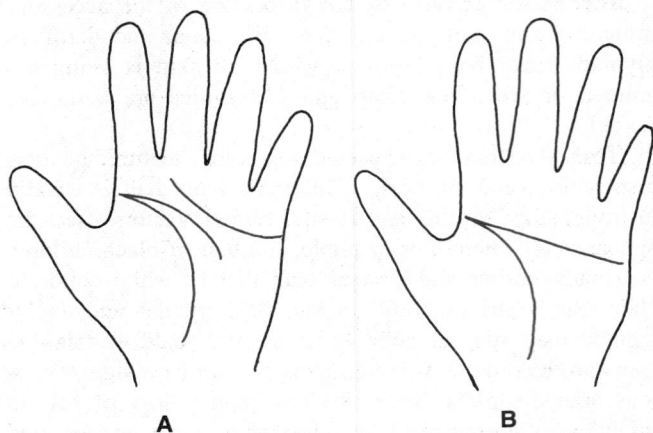

Fig. 7-13. Examples of flexion creases on palm. **A,** Normal. **B,** Simian crease.

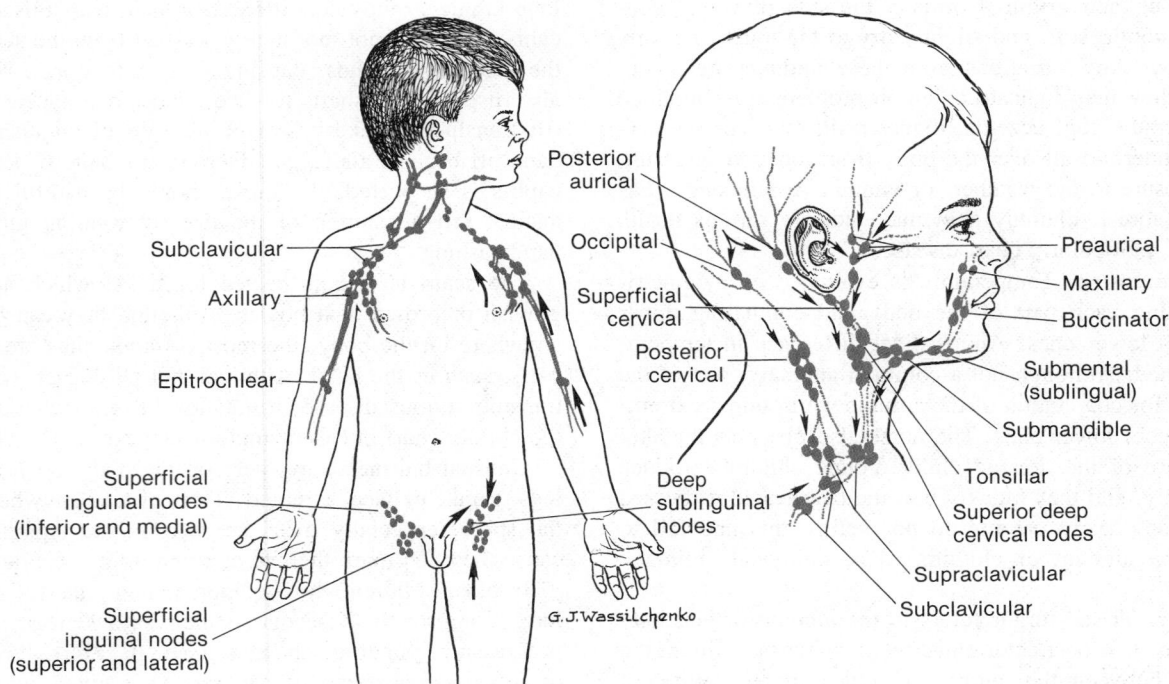

Fig. 7-14. Location of superficial lymph nodes. Arrows indicate directional flow of lymph.

their location. For example, occipital or postauricular aden-opathy is often seen in local scalp infection, such as pedi-culosis, tick bite, or external otitis. Cervical adenopathy usually accompanies acute infections in or around the mouth or throat. In children, however, small, nontender, movable nodes are frequently normal.

Nodes are palpated with the distal portion of the fingers by gently but firmly pressing in a circular motion along the regions where nodes are normally present. During assess-ment of the nodes in the head and neck, the child's head is tilted upward slightly but without tensing the sternocleido-mastoid or trapezius muscle. This position facilitates palpa-tion of the *submental, submaxillary, tonsillar,* and *cervical nodes*. The *axillary nodes* are palpated with the arms re-laxed at the side but slightly abducted. The *inguinal nodes* are best assessed with the child in the supine position. Size, mobility, temperature, and tenderness are noted, in addition to reports by the parents regarding any visible change of enlarged nodes.

Head

The head is inspected for general *shape* and *symmetry*. A flattening of one part of the head, such as the occiput, may indicate that the child continually lies in this position. Marked asymmetry is usually abnormal and may indicate premature closure of the sutures (craniosynostosis).

Head control in infants and head posture in older chil-dren are noted. Most infants by 4 months of age should be able to hold the head erect and in midline when in a vertical position. Significant head lag after 6 months of age strongly indicates cerebral injury.

Range of motion is evaluated by asking the older child to look in each direction (to either side, up, and down) or manually putting the younger child through each position. Limited range of motion may indicate wryneck, or *torticol-lis,* a result of injury to the sternocleidomastoid muscle, in

which the child holds the head to one side with the chin pointing toward the opposite side. Hyperextension of the head (opisthotonos) with pain on flexion is a serious indi-cation of meningeal irritation (see also Brudzinski sign, p. 282).

The *skull* is palpated for patent sutures, fontanels, frac-tures, and swellings. Normally the posterior fontanel closes by the second month of life and the anterior fontanel fuses between 12 and 18 months of age. Early or late closure is noted, since either may be a sign of a pathologic condition. For a more detailed discussion of the cranial bones, see p. 308.

While the head is being examined, the *face* is inspected for symmetry, movement, and general appearance. Asking the child to "make a face" assesses symmetric movement and discloses any degree of paralysis. Any unusual facial proportion is noted, such as unusually high or low forehead, wide or close-set eyes, or small, receding chin.

The nurse also notes any unusual swellings or sites of edema that may be associated with specific disorders, such as nephrosis, Cushing syndrome, or steroid therapy. Visible and palpable swelling anterior to the earlobe and above the angle of the jaw is characteristic of parotid gland enlarge-ment in mumps. It gives the child a characteristic "chip-munk" appearance.

Generally the head and face are not auscultated or per-cussed, with the exception of the sinuses. The *sinuses* are air cavities within certain bones adjacent to the nasal cavity (Fig. 7-15). The sinuses develop as the skull bones enlarge throughout childhood and adolescence. The maxillary sinus is usually present at birth but does not enlarge very much until after the teeth erupt. The frontal sinus begins to de-velop in early infancy, and the ethmoid and sphenoid si-nuses develop later in childhood. Normally the sinuses are not percussed, unless there are signs of an infection, such as headache and congestion.

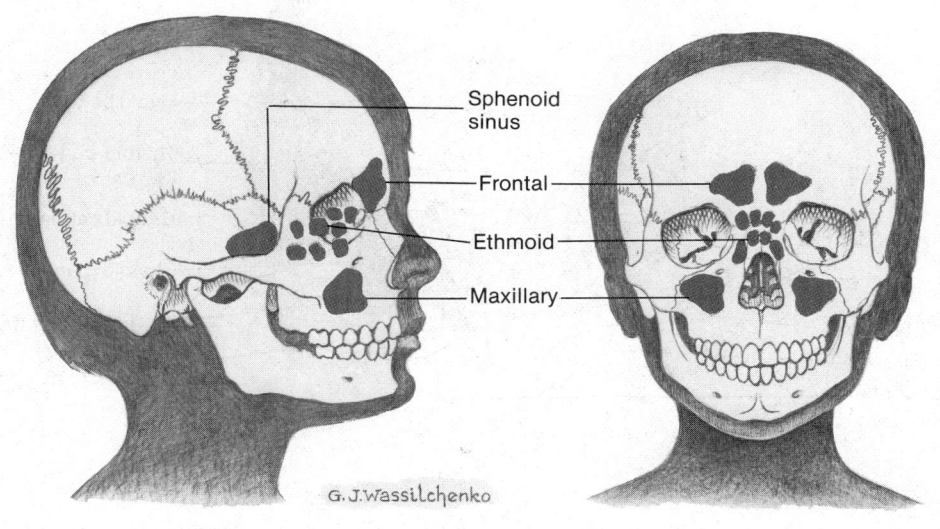

Sphenoid sinus

Frontal

Ethmoid

Maxillary

G. J. Wassilchenko

RIGHT LATERAL   FRONTAL

Fig. 7-15. Location of sinuses.

Neck

Besides assessing motility of the head and neck, the nurse also inspects the neck as to size and palpates it for associated structures. The neck is short with skin folds between the head and shoulders during infancy; however, it lengthens during the next 3 to 4 years. A short or webbed neck is associated with various anomalies, such as Turner syndrome. Marked edema of the neck may indicate mumps, local throat or mouth infections, or diphtheria. Distended neck veins often indicate difficulty on expiration, such as in asthma or cystic fibrosis.

The *trachea* is palpated by placing the thumb and index finger on each side and sliding them back and forth to note any masses. Normally the trachea is in the midline or slightly to the right of the midline. Any shift is noted since it can signify serious lung problems, such as a tumor or foreign body in the lung.

The *thyroid gland*, which is located at the base of the neck, is palpated. This butterfly-shaped gland straddles the trachea and has two lateral lobes connected by an isthmus or band of glandular tissue. The isthmus is the only portion of the thyroid that is usually palpable, because the lobes that curve posteriorly around the trachea are partially covered by the sternocleidomastoid muscle (Fig. 7-16). Normally the thyroid rises as the child swallows. However, palpating the thyroid takes considerable practice and is especially difficult in an infant, whose neck is short and thick. If any masses are detected in the neck, they are recorded and reported for further investigation.

Eyes

Examination of the eyes involves inspection of all exterior structures for size, symmetry, color, and motility, and inspection of the interior surfaces for examination of retinal structures. To examine each structure accurately requires an understanding of the anatomy of the eyeball (Fig. 7-17). The retinal examination requires the use of an ophthalmoscope and is a highly skilled procedure. Discussion of the funduscopic examination includes the basic normal findings that the nurse should be able to discern with some practice in using the ophthalmoscope. The third part of the examination involves vision testing.

Placement and alignment. The eyes are judged for relative placement on the face, symmetry of location, and general slant of the palpebral fissures or lids (Fig. 7-18). If any possible abnormality of placement is observed, these findings can be substantiated by measuring the interpupillary distance, which is approximately 4.5 to 5.5 cm (1¾ to 2¼ inches) or the inner canthal distance, which averages about 2.5 cm (1 inch) (Laestadius, Aase, and Smith, 1969). Large spacing between the eyes is called *hypertelorism*. Although a normal variant in some children, hypertelorism with other midfacial anomalies may suggest mental retardation.

Epicanthal folds, an excess fold of skin extending from the roof of the nose to the inner termination of the eyebrow and partially or completely overlapping the inner canthus of the eye, are frequently found in children of Asiatic descent (Fig. 7-18, *B*). They may be normally present in non-Ori-

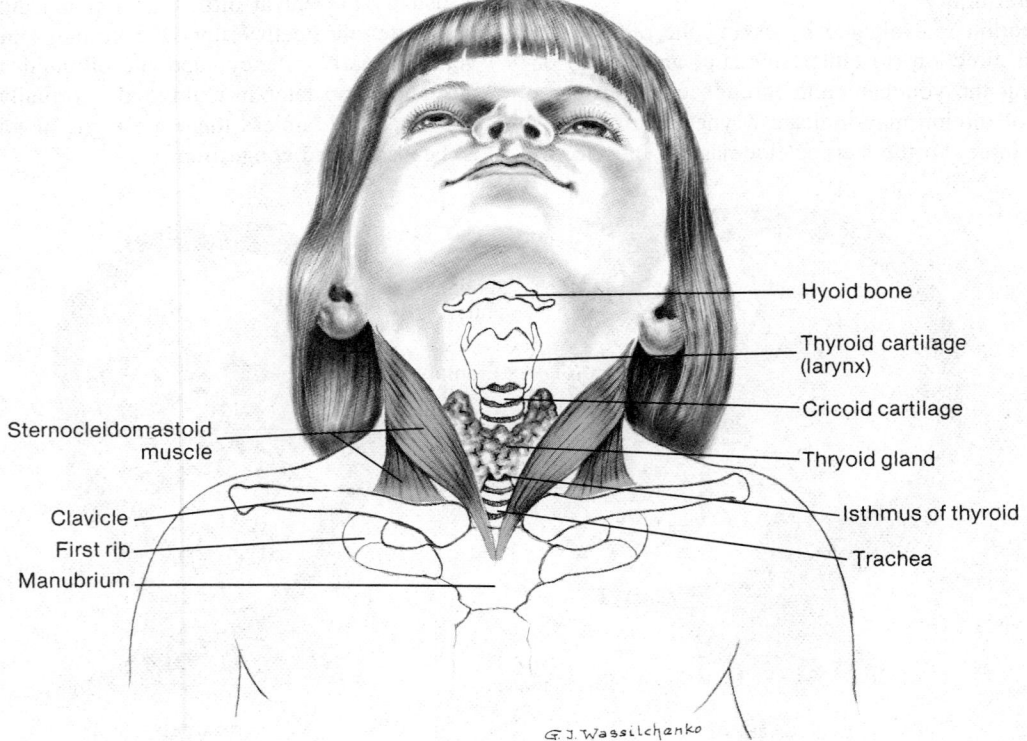

Sternocleidomastoid muscle

Clavicle

First rib

Manubrium

Hyoid bone

Thyroid cartilage (larynx)

Cricoid cartilage

Thryoid gland

Isthmus of thyroid

Trachea

G. J. Wassilchenko

Fig. 7-16. Anterior view of structures in neck.

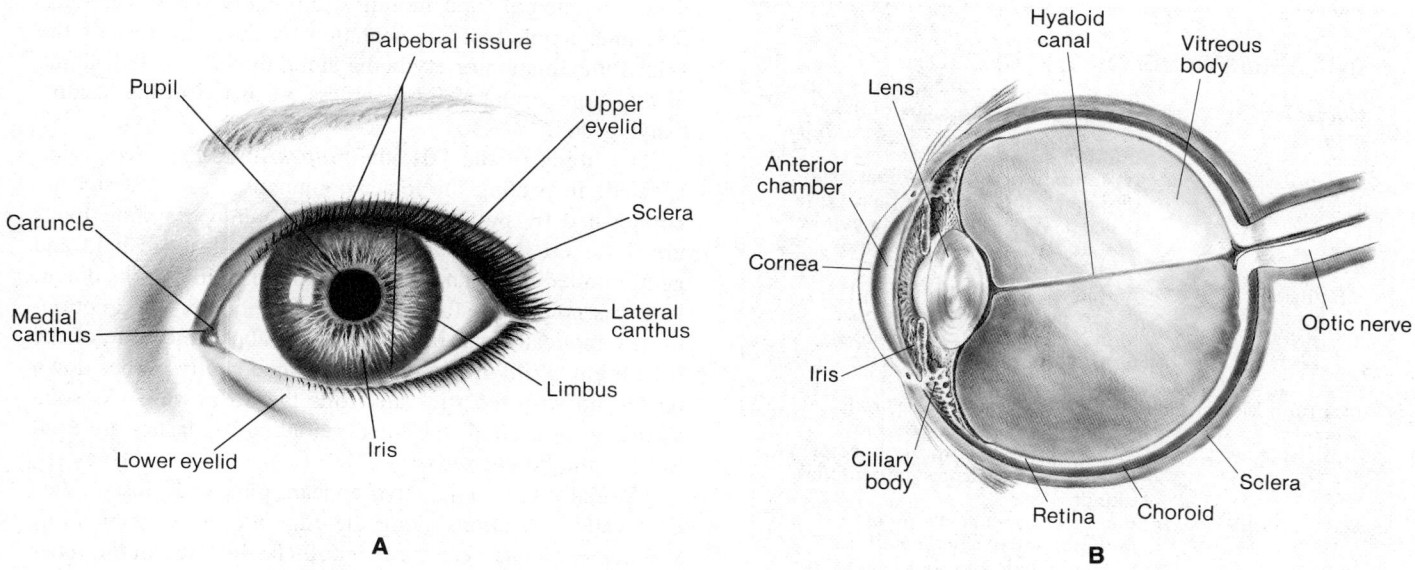

Fig. 7-17. Normal structure of eye. **A,** Anterior view. **B,** Cross-sectional view.

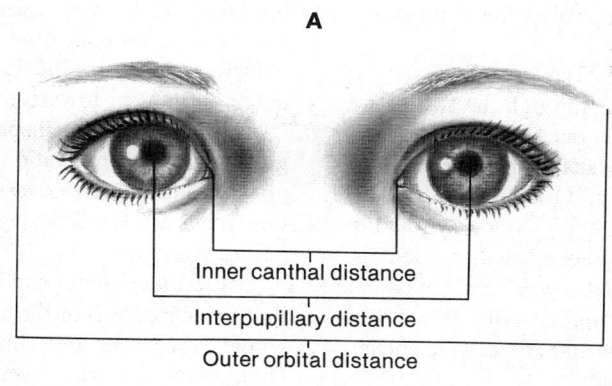

Inner canthal distance

Interpupillary distance

Outer orbital distance

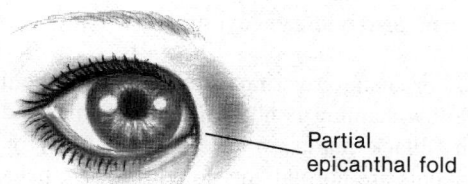

Partial epicanthal fold

Fig. 7-18. A, Anatomic landmarks of eye. **B,** Epicanthal folds. **C,** Upward palpebral slant.

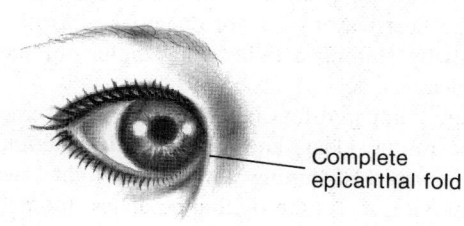

Complete epicanthal fold

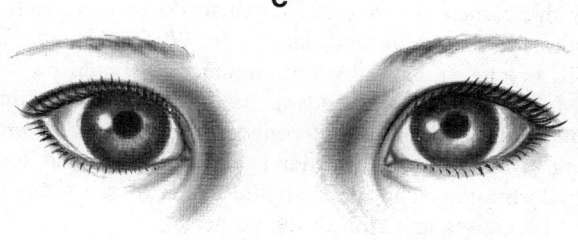

INFLAMMATIONS OF THE EYELID

Hordeolum or stye	Inflammation of sebaceous glands near lashes, usually on lower lid; painful, red, swollen areas
Internal stye	Acute inflammation of meibomian glands of upper lid; if upper lid is everted, stye appears as a yellow line across the tarsus (edge of eyelid)
Chalazion	Granulomas or cysts of internal sebaceous glands (meibomian glands); localized, nontender, firm, discrete swellings covered with freely movable skin
Marginal blepharitis	Inflammation of edge of lid; red, scaly, crusted lid edges; may include pustules around base of lashes and pus from meibomian glands
Dacryocytitis	Inflammation and blockage of lacrimal sac or duct; swelling, redness, and pain, below and to nasal side of inner canthus, with purulent discharge

ental infants, but they usually disappear as the child grows older.

The *palpebral slant* is inspected. The degree of slant is judged by drawing an imaginary line through the two points of the medial canthus and across the outer orbit of the eyes and aligning each eye on the line. Usually the palpebral fissures lie horizontally. However, in Oriental persons the slant is normally upward (Fig. 7-18, *C*). Since eye abnormalities are common in many chromosomal disorders, the nurse must be careful to observe and record any deviations from the expected. For example, children with Down syndrome characteristically demonstrate hypertelorism, epicanthal folds, and upward palpebral slant.

The *lids* are inspected for proper placement on the eye. When the eye is open, the upper lid should fall somewhere between the upper iris and upper rim of the pupil. *Ptosis* refers to a lid that covers part of the pupil or the lower part of the iris. The term *sunset eyes* or the *setting-sun sign* refers to an upper lid that covers no part of the iris, allowing some of the sclera or "white-of-the-eye" to show. Although either can be a normal variant of lid placement, it can also be a sign of several disorders.

When the eyes are closed, the lids should completely cover the cornea and sclera. Failure to do so can result in chronic eye irritation and infection. When the lids are opened or closed, no palpebral conjunctiva should be visible. Malposition of the eyelids includes *ectropion*, a rolling-out of the lids with exposed conjunctiva, and *entropion*, a turning-in of the lid. The latter is normally found in some Oriental children. The nurse should check to see if the in-turned lid causes irritation of the cornea.

Inspection of external structures. The lids are also observed for color (any sign of hemorrhage), size (any evi-

dence of edema), and mobility. Normally the lids contain the same amount of pigmentation as does the rest of the skin. Inflammation or erythema along the lid is noted. Some of the more common lid disorders are listed in the accompanying box.

The lining of the lids, the *palpebral conjunctiva*, is inspected. Inspecting the lower conjunctival sac is easily accomplished by pulling the lid down while the child looks up. To evert the upper lid, the upper lashes are held and gently pulled *down* and *forward* while the child looks down. If this is not successful, a tongue blade or stem of a cotton-tipped applicator can be placed 1 cm above the edge of the lid margin. With this in place, the nurse gently pushes down on the lid with the stick and rolls the lid upward. As soon as the lid is everted, the fingers holding the lashes are used to keep the lid everted.

Normally the conjunctiva appears pink and glossy. Vertical yellow striations along the edge are the *meibomian* or *sebaceous glands* near the hair follicle. Located in the inner or medial canthus and situated on the inner edge of the upper and lower lids is a tiny opening called the *lacrimal punctum*. Any excessive tearing or inflammation of the lacrimal apparatus is noted.

The lids are observed for blinking movement. Excessive blinking can indicate eyestrain or a nervous habit. Asymmetric or infrequent blinking can be a sign of paralysis or muscle weakness. The blink reflex is tested by making a quick movement toward the eye.

The *eyelashes* are inspected for distribution, direction of growth, and pigmentation. Normally the upper lashes curl upward and the lower lashes curve downward. Lashes that turn inward toward the eyeball can cause conjunctival irritation.

The *bulbar conjunctiva,* which covers the eye up to the limbus or junction of the cornea and sclera, should be transparent, revealing the white color of the underlying sclera. Dilation of the blood vessels in the conjunctiva makes it appear red. Although this redness is characteristic of many disorders, it can also indicate eyestrain, irritation, or fatigue.

The *sclera,* or white covering of the eyeball, should be clear. Any yellow staining is noted, since this may indicate jaundice. Tiny black marks in the sclera of heavily pigmented individuals are normal and do not indicate petechiae or the presence of a foreign body. A bluish tone may indicate disorders such as osteogenesis imperfecta or glaucoma.

The *cornea,* or covering of the iris and pupil, should be clear and transparent. Any opacities are recorded since they can be signs of scarring or ulceration, which can interfere with vision. The best way to test for opacities is to illuminate the eyeball by shining a light at an angle (obliquely) toward the cornea.

The *pupils* are compared for size, shape, and movement. They should be round, clear, and equal. Their *reaction to light* is tested by quickly shining a source of light toward the eye and removing it. As the light approaches, the pupils constrict; as the light fades, the pupils dilate. *Accommoda-*

tion, or the focusing ability of the eyes to produce clear vision at different distances, is tested by having the child look at a bright, shiny object at a distance and quickly moving the object toward his face. The pupils constrict as the object is brought near the eye. The normal findings when examining the pupil may be recorded as PERRLA, which means "pupil equal, round, reacts to light and accommodation."

The *iris* is inspected for size, color, and clarity. The iris should be perfectly round; a cleft or notch at its outer edge is called a *coloboma.* Since a visual field defect coincides with the coloboma, this finding warrants further ophthalmologic evaluation (Helveston and Ellis, 1980). Permanent eye color is usually established by 6 to 12 months of age. Lack of usual eye color and a pink glow to the iris is characteristic of albinism. The pink color is a reflection of the red reflex of the retina. Black-and-white speckling of the iris, known as *Brushfield spots,* is seen in Down syndrome.

As the iris and pupil are inspected, the *lens* is also examined. Normally the lens is not visible while looking into the pupil. White or gray spots usually indicate opacities or cataracts in the lens. Complete opacities prevent funduscopic examination of internal retinal structures.

Inspection of internal structures. Inspection of internal structures necessitates the use of a special instrument, the ophthalmoscope. The following discussion describes this instrument, outlines preparation of the child for the examination, and presents the major funduscopic findings.

Use of the ophthalmoscope. The ophthalmoscope permits visualization of the interior of the eyeball with a system of lenses and a high-intensity light. The "ophthalmic head" contains plus lenses (magnifiers), which are usually indicated by black numbers, and minus lenses (minifiers), which are indicated by red numbers. The lenses are changed by rotating a disk on the outside of the head. These lenses permit clear visualization of eye structures at different distances from the nurse's eye and correct visual acuity differences in the examiner and child.

If the nurse wears corrective lenses or glasses, they should be worn when the ophthalmoscope is being used. If the child wears glasses, these should be removed unless they are worn to correct severe astigmatism, which can cause distortion of the images. The lens of the ophthalmoscope can grossly detect visual acuity problems in the child if the nurse who has 20/20 vision is forced to use plus or minus lenses to see the retinal structures clearly. With hyperopia, or farsightedness, higher plus or convex lenses are needed; with myopia, or nearsightedness, more minus or concave lenses are used. Use of the ophthalmoscope requires practice to know which lens setting produces the clearest image.

The interior of the eye is illuminated by a light source within the ophthalmic head, which shines through the lens from a small window. There is also a light dial that changes the type of light emitted through the window. For general purposes the small, white circular light is used for the un-

dilated pupil and the larger white circular light is used for the dilated pupil.

Manipulating the ophthalmoscope. The nurse uses the ophthalmoscope by placing her hand around its body and resting the instrument against her nose and cheek so that the lens remains directly in front of the eye and the light shines toward the child's eye. With the instrument in position the nurse moves toward the child, approaching from the side at a 15-degree angle, not directly toward the eye. When examining the left eye, the nurse uses the left eye, and vice versa. This is to prevent eyestrain and to approach the child in the best juxtaposition. The nurse's free hand may be used to attract the child's attention away from the instrument's light source and toward a point directly in front of him or to help in guidance while moving as close as possible to the child. The examination should be done in a dimly lit, but not necessarily dark, room.

From a distance of about 1 foot, the examination of the cornea, iris, and lens begins with a lens setting of +8 to +2. Once near the child's face, the lens is changed to 0 or −2. Since the light source falls on only part of the retina at a time, the ophthalmoscope is systematically moved up and down and from side to side to visualize each structure within the fundus (Fig. 7-19).

Preparing the child. The nurse can prepare the child for the ophthalmic examination by showing him the instrument, demonstrating the light source and how it shines in the eye, and explaining the reason for darkening the room. For infants and young children who do not respond to such explanations, it is best to try to use distraction to encourage them to keep their eyes open. Forcibly parting the lids results in an uncooperative, watery-eyed child and a frustrated nurse. Usually, with some practice, the nurse can elicit a red reflex almost instantly while approaching the child and may also gain a momentary inspection of the blood vessels, macula, or optic disc.

Funduscopic examination. The illustration (Fig. 7-20) shows the structures of the back of the eyeball, or the *fundus.* The fundus is immediately apparent as the *red reflex.* The intensity of the color increases in darkly pigmented individuals. A brilliant, uniform red reflex is an important sign because it virtually rules out almost all serious defects of the cornea, aqueous chamber, lens, and vitreous chamber. Any dark shadows or opacities are recorded because they indicate some abnormality in any of these structures.

As the ophthalmoscope is brought closer to the eye, the most conspicuous feature of the fundus is the *optic disc,* the area where the blood vessels and optic nerve fibers enter and exit from the eye. The round or vertically oval disc is creamy pink but lighter than the surrounding fundus and derives its color from the rich capillary network. Its size is important because other structures of the fundus are measured in relationship to the disc diameter (DD). Most discs have a small, pale depression in their center, called the *physiologic cup* or *depression,* which represents the blind spot of the retina. It is not always visible but, when large

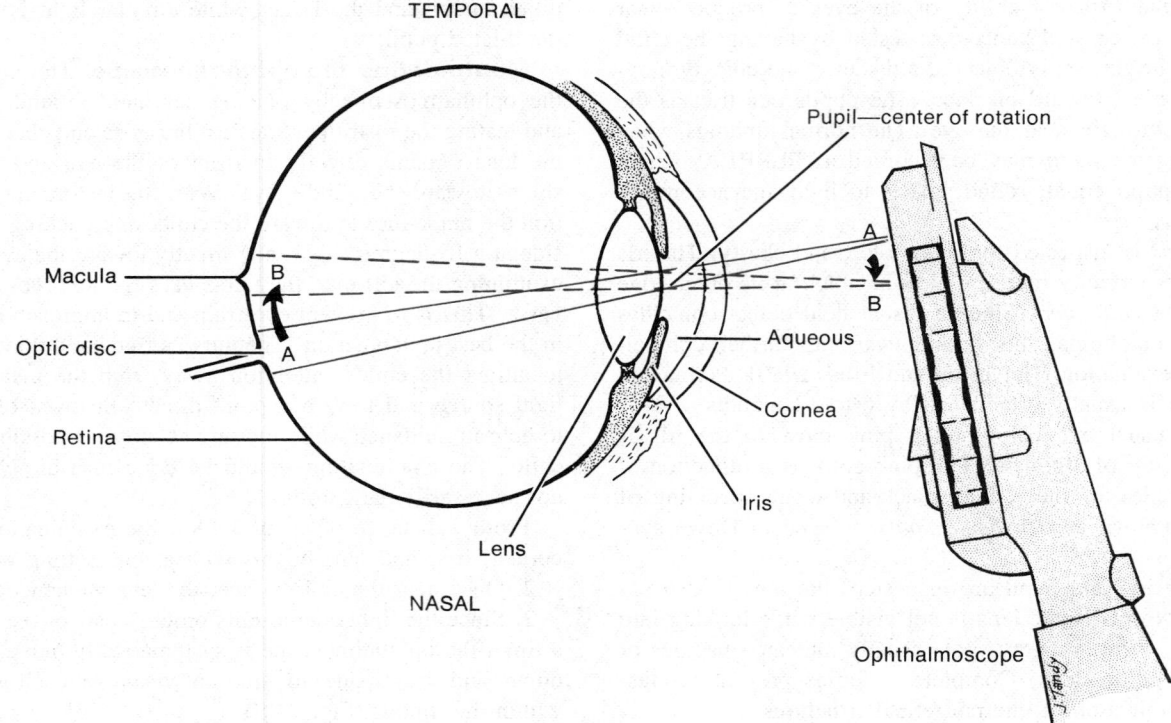

TEMPORAL

Pupil—center of rotation

A

B

Macula

Optic disc

Retina

A

Aqueous

Cornea

Iris

Lens

NASAL

Ophthalmoscope

J. Tandy

Fig. 7-19. Visual axis through ophthalmoscope. Beam of light (**A**) and its corresponding visual field is usual view when approaching child from side at 15-degree angle. **B** represents a direct visualization with child staring at light.

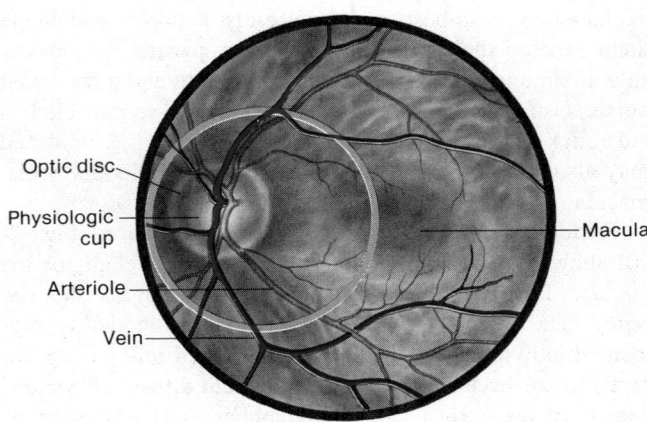

Optic disc

Physiologic cup

Arteriole

Vein

Macula

Fig. 7-20. Structures of fundus. Interior circle represents approximate size of area seen with ophthalmoscope.

enough to be seen, should not extend to the disc margin. Blurring of the disc margins, loss of the depression, and a bulging disc are important signs of papilledema or swelling of the optic nerve, which clinically indicates increased intracranial pressure.

After the optic disc is located, the area is inspected for *blood vessels.* The central retinal artery and vein appear in the depths of the disc and emanate outward with visible branching. The veins are darker in color and about one

fourth larger in size than the arteries. A narrow band of light, the *arteriolar light reflex,* is reflected from the center of an artery but does not appear in veins. Normally the branches of the arteries and veins cross each other. It is important to observe the pattern of branching for abnormalities such as notching or indenting at the crossings, tortuosity or dilation of the vessels, or small hemorrhages (dark areas) along the branches. Any of these findings are reported for further investigation.

About 2 DD temporal to the disc is the *macula,* the area of the fundus with the greatest concentration of visual receptors. It is about 1 DD in size and darker in color than the fundus (red reflex) or optic disc. The intensity of the color directly correlates with the individual's skin pigmentation; that is, the darker the skin, the darker the color of the macula. In the center of the macula is a minute glistening spot of reflected light called the *fovea centralis,* the area of most perfect vision.

Although abnormalities of the macula are usually not apparent unless the eye is dilated, permitting more detailed inspection, the nurse should at least note its presence. If locating the macula is difficult, the child is asked to look directly at the light. As Fig. 7-19 shows, a light shone directly into the eye falls on the fovea. However, since this is the most light-sensitive area of the retina, the nurse must be careful to focus on the macula only momentarily. If direct visualization does *not* cause the light to fall on the center of

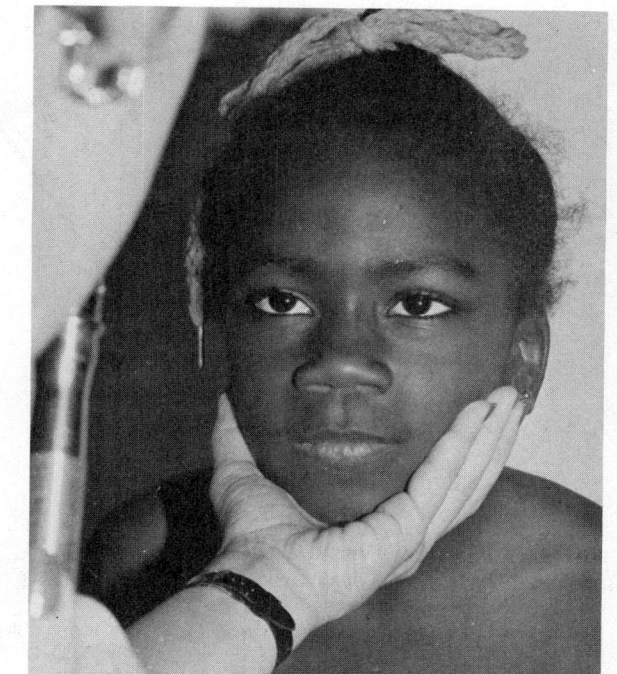
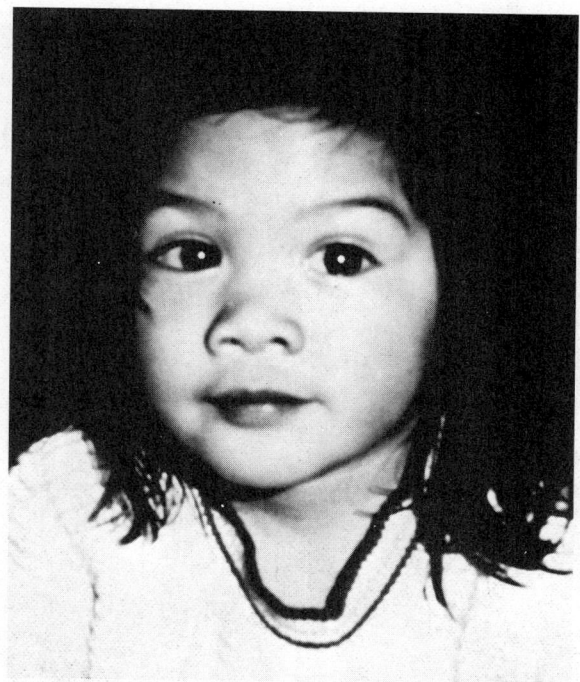

Fig. 7-21. A, Corneal light reflex test demonstrating orthophoric eyes. **B,** Pseudostrabismus. Inner epicanthal folds cause eyes to appear malaligned; however, corneal light reflexes fall symmetrically.

the fovea, strabismus may exist because fixation is occurring at a point other than the center of the macula. Recognition of this deviation is of great importance in determining the type of treatment for strabismus, because in this situation the usual regimen of occlusive therapy (covering the stronger eye to force the weaker or deviating eye to focus) will not benefit the child (Havener, 1984).

Vision testing. Several tests are available for assessing vision. This discussion focuses on four areas: (1) binocularity, (2) visual acuity, (3) peripheral vision, and (4) color vision. The reader is also referred to Chapter 25 for behavioral and physical signs that indicate visual impairment.

Binocularity. Normally, by the age of 3 to 4 months, children achieve the ability to fixate on one visual field with both eyes simultaneously (binocularity). One of the most important tests for binocularity is alignment of the eyes to detect nonbinocular vision or strabismus. In strabismus, or ''cross-eye,'' one eye deviates from the point of fixation. If the malalignment is constant, the weak eye becomes ''lazy'' and eventually the brain suppresses the image produced by that eye. If strabismus is not detected and corrected by age 4 to 6 years, a type of blindness, called *amblyopia,* may result.

Two tests commonly used to detect malalignment are the corneal light reflex or red reflex gemini test and the cover tests. In the corneal light reflex test, a flashlight or the light of the ophthalmoscope is shined directly into the eyes from a distance of about 40.5 cm (16 inches). If the eyes are orthophoric or normal, the light falls symmetrically within

each pupil (Fig. 7-21, *A*) or twin red reflexes are observed. If the light falls off center in one eye, the eyes are malaligned. Epicanthal folds may give a false impression of malalignment of the eyes (pseudostrabismus) (Fig. 7-21, *B*).

Terms for describing the types of strabismus are:

esotropia or **esophoria** Inward deviation of the eye (Fig. 25-3)

exotropia or **exophoria** Outward deviation of the eye

phoria Malalignment that is not obvious until fusion is disrupted

tropia Constant or intermittent malalignment of the eyes; more severe and more likely to result in amblyopia than phoria

In the *cover test,* one eye is covered and the movement of the *uncovered* eye is observed while the child gazes on a near (33 cm, or 13 inches) or distant (50 cm, or 20 inches) object. If the uncovered eye does not move, it is aligned. If the uncovered eye moves, a malalignment is present because when the stronger eye is temporarily covered, the weaker eye attempts to fixate on the object.

In the *uncover test,* occlusion is shifted back and forth from one eye to the other eye and movement of the *covered* eye is observed while the child is fixating at a point in front of him. If normal alignment is present, shifting the cover from one eye to the other eye will not cause movement of the covered eye. If malalignment is present, the covered eye will move from its position when covered to a straight position when uncovered. This test takes more practice than the other cover test because the occluder must be moved

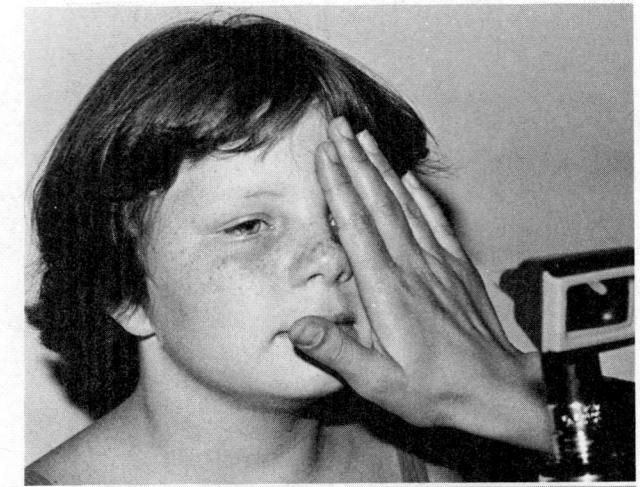

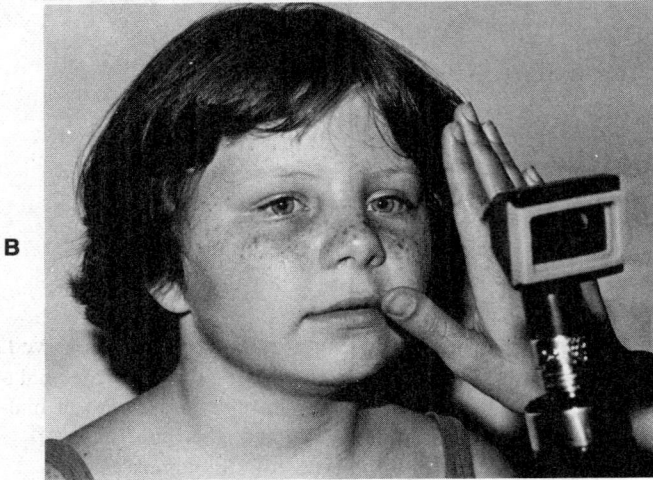

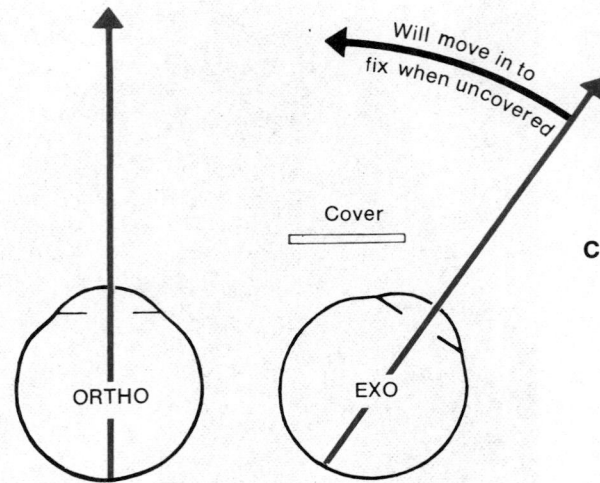

Fig. 7-22. Uncover test for strabismus. **A,** Eye is occluded, child is fixating on light source. **B,** If eye does not move when uncovered, eyes are aligned. **C,** Exophoria. As eye is uncovered, it shifts to fixate on object.

C from Prior, J.A., Silberstein, J.S., and Stang, J.M.: Physical diagnosis: the history and examination of the patient, ed. 6, St. Louis, 1981, The C.V. Mosby Co.

back and forth quickly and accurately in order to see the eye move. Usually it is easier to perform this test by using one's hand rather than a card or other object as the occluder (Fig. 7-22). Since deviations can occur at different ranges, particularly in the case of phorias, it is important to perform the cover tests at both near and far distances.

Visual acuity testing in young and school-age children. Visual acuity refers to the ability to see near and far objects clearly. The most common and accurate test for measuring acuity is the *Snellen letter chart* (Fig. 7-23, *A*). It consists of nine lines of letters in decreasing size. Each line is given a value, for example, line 8 is "20."

The person who is to be tested stands 20 feet from the chart and reads each line. If he can read line 8, he has 20/20 vision, the accepted standard for normal acuity. If the person can read only line 2, he has 20/100 vision. That means that what he is able to see at a distance of 20 feet, the person with 20/20 or normal eyesight can see at 100 feet.

Other letter or symbol screening tests are described in Table 7-5. Many of the tests that are suitable for preschoolers can also be used for difficult-to-test children, such as those with developmental delays. The Snellen symbol chart

is frequently used to screen preschool children (Fig. 7-23, *B*). However, many young children have difficulty because of confusion in identifying the direction of the **E**, rather than inability to see the symbol clearly. To avoid this problem, the Blackbird Vision Screening System was developed by a public health nurse (Fig. 7-24). The screening system uses a modified **E** that resembles a bird and a story about the Blackbird to help engage children's attention. Testing is done with flash cards and the children are instructed to indicate the direction of the bird's flight. With this test, 99% of 3- and 4-year-old children can be successfully tested, a rate considerably higher than the 15% to 80% rate using the Snellen **E** (Sato-Viacrucis, 1986).

Although most chart tests are designed for testing at 20 feet, modifications can be made for testing at closer ranges. Measurements at closer range are converted to the standard 20-foot scale by multiplying the two numbers by the number that converts the first one to 20. For example, 10/25 is equivalent to 20/50 (Holland, 1982). When closer ranges are used, proper positioning of the child is essential. Because young children are active, their tendency to move or lean forward can affect the testing more at close distances than farther ones.

The Snellen charts are usually used for testing far visual acuity to detect myopia (nearsightedness). However, in school-age children they can also be used to test for hyperopia (farsightedness). The *plus lens test for hyperopia* involves having the child wear a pair of convex or plus lenses. With these lenses the child should be *unable* to read the 20/20 or 20/30 line. Ability to see these lines clearly indicates excessive farsightedness and represents a need for referral.

Vision performance can also be measured using optical

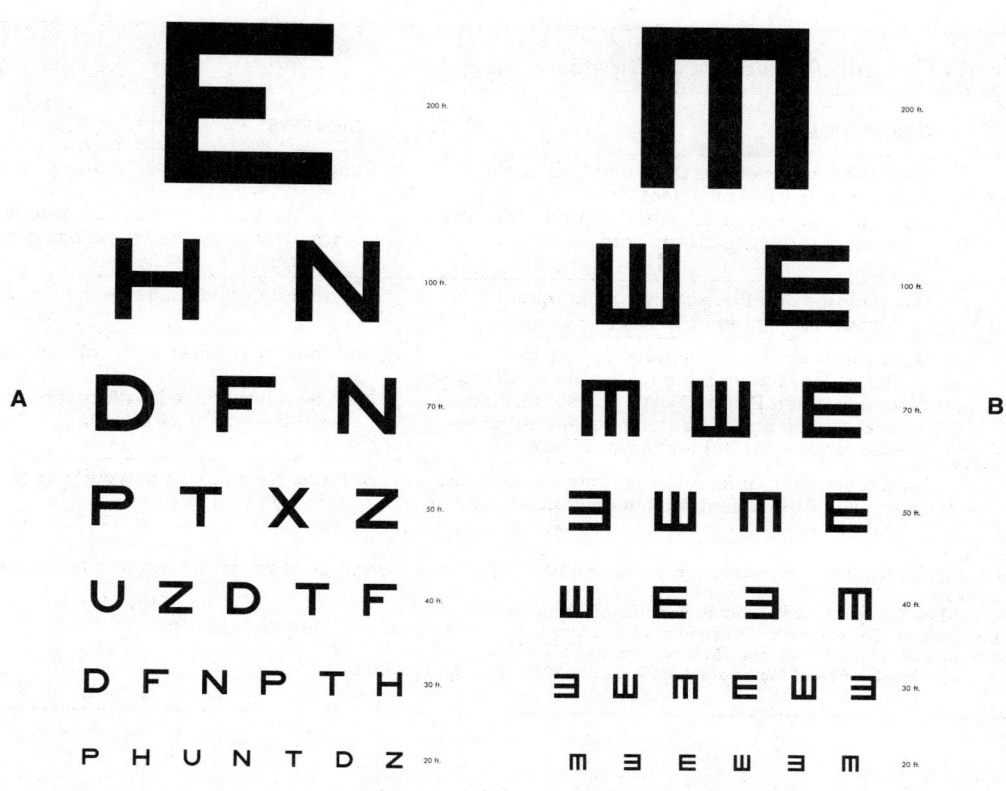

Fig. 7-23. Snellen Chart. **A**, Letter (alphabet) chart. **B**, Symbol E chart.
From National Society to Prevent Blindness, Inc., New York.

Table 7-5 Letter or symbol vision acuity tests

TEST	DESCRIPTION	COMMENTS*
Snellen Letter†	Uses letter of the English alphabet for testing at 20 feet	Suitable for most children above the second grade who are familiar with reading the alphabet
Snellen E†	Uses the capital letter E pointing in four directions; children "read" the chart by showing the direction of the letter E or using a large duplicate E to match the chart E at 20 feet	For illiterate or non-English speaking people and preschool children and grade 1 Preschool children often have difficulty with direction despite adequate vision
Home Eye Test for Preschoolers‡	Uses a large letter E for demonstration and an E chart for testing at 10 feet	Designed for use by parents for children 3 to 6 years
Blackbird Preschool Vision Screening System§	Uses a modified E to resemble a flying bird; children identify which way the bird is flying Uses flash cards, story-telling, and disposable cardboard eyeglass occluders	Designed for children as young as 3 years
Blackbird Storybook Home Eye Test§	Similar to above	Designed for use by parents for children as young as 2½ years

*Ages for testing are based on published reports. In actual practice only a small percentage of young children may be successfully screened with many of these tests.
†Available from Good-Lite Company, 1540 Hannah Ave., Forest Park, IL 60130.
‡Available from the National Society for the Prevention of Blindness, Inc., 79 Madison Ave., New York, NY 10016.
§Blackbird Vision Screening System, P.O. Box 7424, Sacramento, CA 95826.
‖ Available from Denver Developmental Materials, Inc., P.O. Box 20037, Denver, CO 80220.

Continued.

Table 7-5 Letter or symbol vision acuity tests—cont'd

TEST	DESCRIPTION	COMMENTS*
HOTV or Matching Symbol†	Uses the four letters H, O, T, and V on a chart for testing at 10 or 20 feet Child names the letters on the chart or matches them to a demonstration card	Suitable for children as young as 3 years Avoids the problem with image reversal and eye-hand coordination which can occur with the letter E
Faye Sumbol Chart†	Use pictures of a house, apple, and umbrella on a chart for testing at 10 feet	Suitable for children as young as 27 to 30 months
Denver Developmental Screening Test (DDST)‖	Uses single cards for the letter E, one for demonstration and one for testing at 15 feet Also uses Allen Picture Cards (a tree, birthday cake, horse and rider, telephone, car, house, and teddy bear) for testing at 15 feet	Suitable for children 2½ years and older May be reliably used with coooperative children from the age of 24 months
Dot Test†	Uses a series of different sized dots; child points to one of the nine dots randomly positioned on a disk	Suitable for children as young as 24 months

*Ages for testing are based on published reports. In actual practice only a small percentage of young children may be successfully screened with many of these tests.
†Available from Good-Lite Company, 1540 Hannah Ave., Forest Park, IL 60130.
‡Available from the National Society for the Prevention of Blindness, Inc., 79 Madison Ave., New York, NY 10016.
§Blackbird Vision Screening System, P.O. Box 7424, Sacramento, CA 95826.
‖ Available from Denver Developmental Materials, Inc., P.O. Box 20037, Denver, CO 80220.

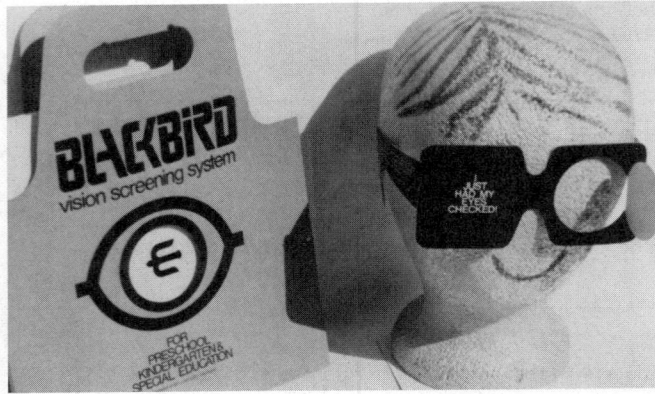

Fig. 7-24. Blackbird Vision Screening System. Note Blackbird symbol and special "eyeglass" occluder.
Courtesy Kiyo Sato-Viacrucis, Sacramento, CA.

instruments, such as the *Titmus Vision Tester.** Three sections of tests are available with the Professional Model Titmus Tester:

1. The Michigan Pre-School Test, which tests visual acuity and binocularity using the letter E in children from 3½ years of age through grade 1
2. The Massachusetts Vision Test, which tests visual acuity, hyperopia (plus lens test), and binocularity (both near and far) using the letter E in elementary school children
3. The Adult Series, which tests near and far visual acuity using the standard Snellen letters, binocularity, and color perception in secondary school children and adults

*Manufactured by Titmus Optical, Inc., Petersburg, VA 23804.

There are no universal criteria for referring children when using the Snellen charts. However, one widely accepted approach includes (National Society, 1982):

1. Three-year-old children with vision in either eye of 20/50 or less (inability to read the 40-foot line)
2. All other ages/grades with vision in either eye of 20/40 or less (inability to read the 30-foot line)
3. A two-line difference in visual acuity between the eyes in the passing range, for example, 20/20 in one eye and 20/40 in the other

Visual acuity testing in infants and difficult-to-test children. In newborns, vision is tested mainly by checking for *light perception* by shining a light into the eyes and noting responses such as pupillary constriction, blinking, following the light to midline, increased alertness, or refusal to open the eyes after exposure to the light. Although the simple maneuver of checking light perception and eliciting the pupillary light reflex indicates that the anterior half of the visual apparatus is intact, it does not confirm that the infant can see. In other words, this test does not assess whether the brain receives the visual message and interprets the signals.

Another test of visual acuity is the infant's ability to fix on and follow a target. Although any brightly colored or patterned object can be used, the human face is excellent. The infant is held upright while the nurse's face moves slowly from side to side. If visual fixation and following are not present by 3 to 4 months of age, further ophthalmologic evaluation is needed (Nelson and others, 1984).

Other signs that may indicate visual loss include fixed pupils, marked strabismus, constant nystagmus, setting-sun

Table 7-6 Special tests of visual acuity and estimated visual acuity at different ages

TEST	DESCRIPTION	BIRTH	4 MONTHS	1 YEAR	AGE OF 20/20 VISION
Optokinetic nystagmus	A striped drum is rotated or a striped tape is moved in front of infant's eyes. Presence of nystagmus indicates vision. Acuity is assessed by using progressively smaller stripes.	20/400	20/200	20/60	20-30 months
Forced choice preferential looking	Either a homogenous field or a striped field is presented to infant; an observer monitors the direction of the eyes during presentation of pattern. Acuity is assessed by using progressively smaller striped fields.	20/400	20/200	20/50	18-24 months
Visually evoked potentials	Eyes are stimulated with bright light or pattern, and electrical activity to visual cortex is recorded through scalp electrodes. Acuity is assessed by using progressively smaller patterns.	20/100 to 20/200	20/80	20/40	6-12 months

Data from Hoyt, C., Nickel, B., and Billson, F.: Ophthalmological examination of the infant: development aspects, Surv. Ophthalmol. **26:**177-189, 1982.

sign, and slow lateral movements. Unfortunately it is very difficult to test each eye separately; the presence of such signs in one eye could indicate unilateral blindness.

Special tests are available for testing infants and other difficult-to-test children to assess acuity and/or confirm blindness. These tests are presented in Table 7-6 with the estimated visual acuity at different ages. The discrepancy between the acuities obtained by the various techniques probably reflects the testing of different responses of the developing infant's brain (Hoyt, Nickel, and Billson, 1982).

Peripheral vision. In a child who is old enough to cooperate, peripheral vision, or the visual field of each eye, is estimated. The test is performed by having the child fixate on a specific point directly in front of him as an object, such as a finger or a pencil, is moved from beyond the field of vision into the range of peripheral vision. Each eye is checked separately and for each quadrant of vision. As soon as the child sees the object, he tells the nurse to stop moving it. At that point the angle from the anteroposterior axis of the eye (straight line of vision) to the peripheral axis (point at which the object is first seen) is measured. Normally the child sees about 50 degrees upward, 70 degrees downward, 60 degrees nasalward, and 90 degrees temporally. Limitations in peripheral vision may indicate blindness from damage to structures within the eye or to any of the visual pathways.

Color vision. Another important test is for color vision. It is estimated that from 8% to 10% of white males and less than half that percentage of black males have inherited the X-linked disorder known as *color vision deficit* (less acceptable term, *color blindness*). From 0.5% to 1% of white females are affected. Although the severity of impaired perception of color varies considerably, the two most common

types are *protanomaly,* in which the child confuses gray with pink or pale blue with green, and *deuteranomaly,* in which the child confuses gray with pale purple or green. In most of these individuals, the color vision deficit causes no major problems. However, some of the difficulties encountered by individuals with more severe deficits may be inability to distinguish amber or red traffic lights, failure to see a red brake light on the rear of a car, difficulty in distinguishing green traffic lights from certain types of incandescent street lamps, and a poor sense of color coordination of clothing. For school-age children the greatest difficulty lies in performance of academic skills that use color as a visual aid. Adolescents may be ineligible for certain vocational opportunities, such as electronics, photography, printing, interior decorating, pharmaceuticals, textiles, police work, and for several types of military service (Kovalesky, 1985).

The tests available for color vision include the *Ishihara test* and the *Hardy-Rand-Rittler* (HRR) *test.* Each consists of a series of cards (pseudoisochromatic) on which is printed a color field composed of spots of a certain ''confusion'' color. Against the field is a number or symbol similarly printed in dots but of a color likely to be confused with the field color by the person with a color vision deficit. As a result the figure or letter is invisible to an affected individual but is clearly seen by a person with normal vision. By using the HRR test, which uses symbols rather than numbers, reliable testing can be done on children as young as 3 years of age (Kovalesky, 1985). Nurses administering the test must be familiar with the testing materials and should be able to inform the parents of the disorder's effects on practical areas of living, its genetic transmission, and its irreversibility.

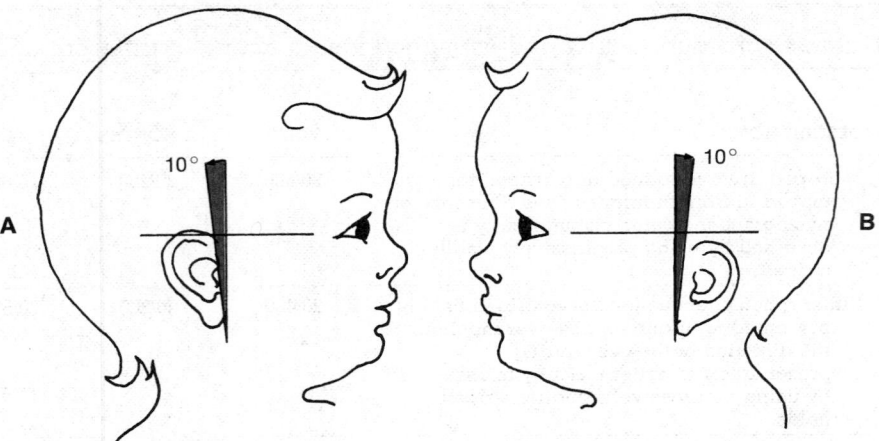

Fig. 7-25. Ear alignment. **A,** Normal. **B,** Abnormal.

Ears

Like the eyes, examination of the ears involves inspection of the external auditory structures, visualization of the internal landmarks using the otoscope, and screening for hearing ability.

Placement and alignment. The entire external earlobe is called the *pinna,* or *auricle,* and is located on each side of the head. The height alignment of the pinna is measured by drawing an imaginary line from the outer orbit of the eye to the occiput or most prominent protuberance of the skull. The top of the pinna should meet or cross this line (Fig. 7-25, *A*). Low-set ears (Fig. 7-25, *B*) are commonly associated with renal anomalies or mental retardation. The angle of the pinna is measured by drawing a perpendicular line from the imaginary horizontal line and aligning the pinna next to this mark. Normally the pinna lies within a 10-degree angle of the vertical line (Fig. 7-25, *A*). If it falls outside this area (Fig. 7-25, *B*), the nurse records the deviation and looks closely for other anomalies.

Normally the pinna extends slightly outward from the skull. Except in newborn infants, ears that are flat against the head or protruding away from the scalp may indicate problems. For example, masses or swelling make the pinna stand forward and may indicate mastoiditis, mumps, or postauricular abscesses. Flattened ears in infants may suggest a frequent side-lying position and may offer a clue to the parents' understanding of the child's stimulation needs.

Inspection of external structures. The pinna, or auricle, can be considered an ''oracle'' because deviations in structure can be a sign of possible middle ear anomalies and congenital conductive hearing loss (Jaffe, 1976). The illustration (Fig. 7-26) shows the usual landmarks of the pinna. The *helix* is the prominent outer rim of the pinna. The *antihelix* is a second curved rim that is adjacent and almost parallel to the helix. The *concha* is a deep cavity, within and partly surrounded by the antihelix, that leads into the external auditory canal. Lying anterior to the concha is a prominent protuberance called the *tragus,* and opposite to this is the *antitragus,* below which is the *lobule.* In some

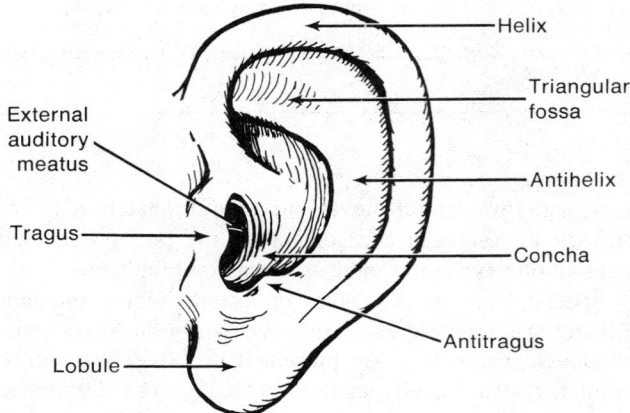

Fig. 7-26. Usual landmarks of pinna.

children the lobule is adherent with the helix in an upward and backward slant. An adherent lobule is considered a normal variation. Each of the major projections of the pinna form corresponding depressions. There is remarkable similarity among external pinnas; the nurse should be familiar with eminences and depressions in order to note deviations.

The skin surface around the ear is inspected for small openings, extra tags of skin, or sinuses. If a sinus is found, a special notation of this is made, since it may represent a fistula that drains into some area of the neck or ear. Cutaneous tags represent no pathologic process but may cause parents concern in terms of the child's appearance.

The ear is also inspected for general hygiene. An otoscope is not necessary to look into the external canal to note the presence of *cerumen,* a waxy substance produced by the ceruminous glands in the outer portion of the canal. If the ear canal appears totally free of cerumen, the nurse should inquire concerning how the ears are cleaned. Occasionally parents insert cotton-tipped swabs or thin objects, such as bobby pins, into the canal to remove wax. Deep insertion of such objects can damage the drum or walls of the canal, as well as push the wax against the tympanic membrane to form a plug. It is best to question parents about ear cleaning by remarking how clean the ears are and casually asking how they remove the wax. This approach is more likely to yield an honest answer than is direct questioning about the use of specific instruments.

In general, it is best to advise parents or children to clean the ears with a washcloth and, if they use a swab, to gently wipe only the outermost portion of the canal. They should always avoid using any sharp, hard object in the ear. If the cerumen is hard and dry (appears dark and crusted, rather than yellow-brown and soft), it can be softened and removed by instilling 2 or 3 drops of mineral oil into the ear for a few days and then rinsing the canal with an ear syringe. Commercial products (Cerumenex, Murine, Debrox) are also available without prescription to aid in removing desiccated cerumen.* Cerumen must be removed to adequately examine an ear if otitis media is suspected. Removal is most easily accomplished with irrigation, using normal saline and a WaterPik or rubber ball syringe (Watkins, Moore, and Phillips, l984).

The presence, color, and odor of any discharge from the aural canal is noted. If discharge is present in one canal, care is taken to prevent transmitting potentially infectious material to the other ear or to another child through handwashing and changing otic specula. Disposable specula are also available.

Inspection of internal structures. Inspection of internal structures necessitates the use of the otoscope. The following discussion describes the instrument and its use, outlines positioning and preparation of the child for the examination, and presents the major otoscopic findings.

Use of the otoscope. The otic head permits visualization of the tympanic membrane by use of a bright light, a magnifying glass, and a speculum. Some otoscopes have an attachment for a pneumonic device to insert air into the canal when a determination of membrane compliance (movement) is needed. The speculum comes in a variety of sizes (2, 3, 4, and 5 mm) to accommodate different canal widths. The largest speculum that fits comfortably into the ear should be used to achieve the greatest area of visualization. The lens or magnifying glass is movable, allowing the examiner to insert an object, such as a curette, into the ear canal through the speculum while still viewing the structures through the lens. The handle is the same as for the ophthalmic head and operates similarly. The nurse should become familiar with the instrument and practice attaching the speculum securely to the head.

Positioning the child. Before beginning the otoscopic examination, the child is positioned properly and restrained if necessary. Older children usually are cooperative and do not need restraint. However, the nurse should prepare them for the procedure by allowing them to play with the instrument, demonstrating how it works, and stressing the importance of remaining still. A helpful suggestion is letting them observe the nurse examining the parent's ear. Older children can view the inside of the ear. With younger children one can explain that he or she is looking for a "big elephant" in the ear. This kind of "fairy tale" is an absorbing distraction and usually elicits cooperation. After the ear has been examined, it is important to clarify that "looking for elephants" was only pretending.

As the speculum is inserted into the meatus, it is moved around the outer rim to accustom the child to the feel of something entering the ear. If examining a painful ear, it is helpful to touch some nonpainful part of the affected ear, then examine the unaffected ear, and finally return to the painful ear. By this time the child is usually less fearful of anything causing discomfort to the ear and will be more cooperative.

*A booklet for families regarding earcare is Caring for Your Ears, available from Ross Laboratories, 625 Cleveland Ave., Columbus, OH 43216.

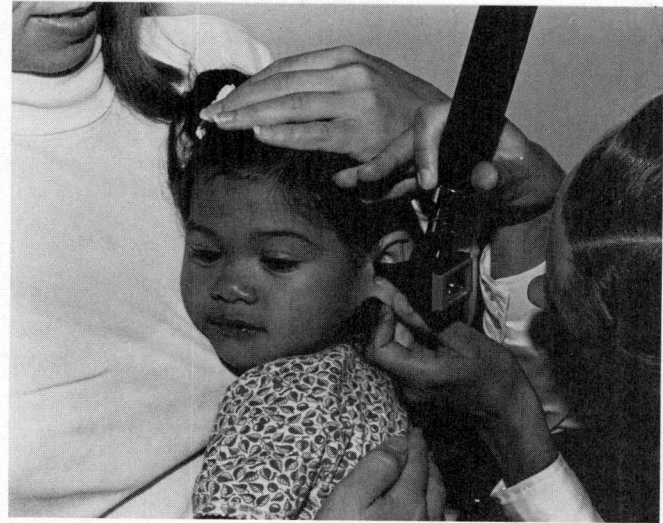 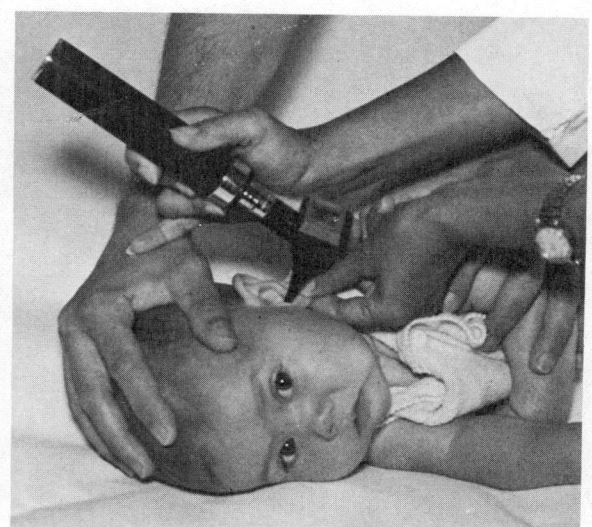

A   B

Fig. 7-27. Positions for restraint during otoscopic examination. **A,** Child. **B,** Infant.

For their protection and safety infants and toddlers must be restrained for the otoscopic exam. There are two general positions of restraint. In one the child is seated sideways in the parent's lap with one arm "hugging" the parent and the other arm at his side. The ear to be examined is toward the nurse. With one arm the parent holds the child's head firmly against his or her chest, and with the other arm "hugs" the child, thereby securing the child's free arm. The ear is examined using the same procedure for holding the otoscope as described later (Fig. 7-27, *A*).

The other position involves placing the child on the side or abdomen with the arms at the side and the head turned so that the ear to be examined points toward the ceiling. The nurse leans over the child and uses the upper part of the body to restrain the arms and upper trunk movements and the examining hand to stabilize the head. This position is practical for young infants or for older children who need minimum restraining, but it may not be feasible for other children who protest vigorously. For safety the nurse should enlist the parent's help in immobilizing the head by firmly placing one hand above the ear and the other on the child's back or side (Fig. 7-27, *B*).

With cooperative children the ear can be examined with the child in a side-lying, sitting, or standing position. One disadvantage to standing is that the child may "walk away" as the otoscope enters the canal. If the child is standing or sitting, proper positioning of the head is essential to achieve a full view of the membrane. The head is tilted slightly away from the nurse or toward the child's opposite shoulder to bring the drum to a 90-degree angle (Fig. 7-28).

Manipulating the otoscope. With the thumb and forefinger of the free (usually nondominant) hand, the nurse grasps the auricle. For the two positions of restraint, the otoscope is held upside down at the junction of its head and handle with the thumb and index finger. The other fingers are placed against the skull to allow the otoscope to move with the child in case he moves suddenly. In examining a cooperative child, the handle can be held with the otic head upright or upside down. The dominant hand can be used to examine both ears, as shown in Figs. 7-27 and 7-28, or reversed for each ear, whichever is more comfortable.

Entering the canal. Before the otoscope is introduced to the canal, the nurse visualizes the external ear and the tympanic membrane as superimposed on a clock (see Fig. 7-31). The numbers become important geographic landmarks. The speculum is introduced into the meatus between the 3 and 9 o'clock positions in a *downward* and *forward* position. Because the canal is curved, the speculum does not permit a panoramic view of the tympanic membrane unless the canal is straightened. In infants the canal curves

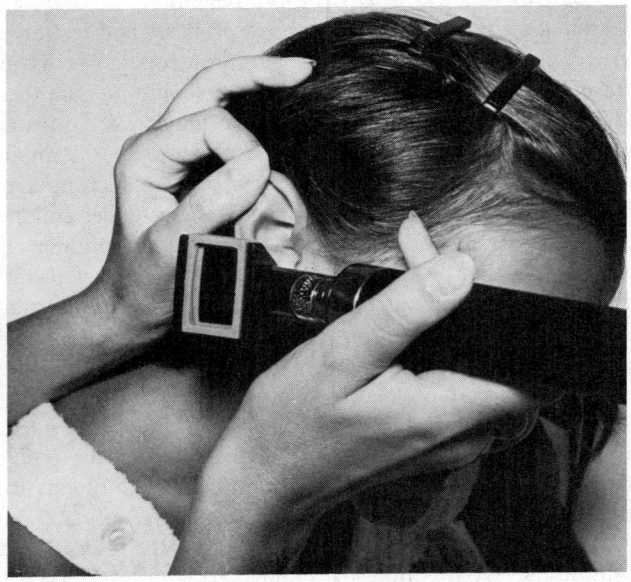

Fig. 7-28. Positioning head by tilting it toward opposite shoulder for full view of tympanic membrane.

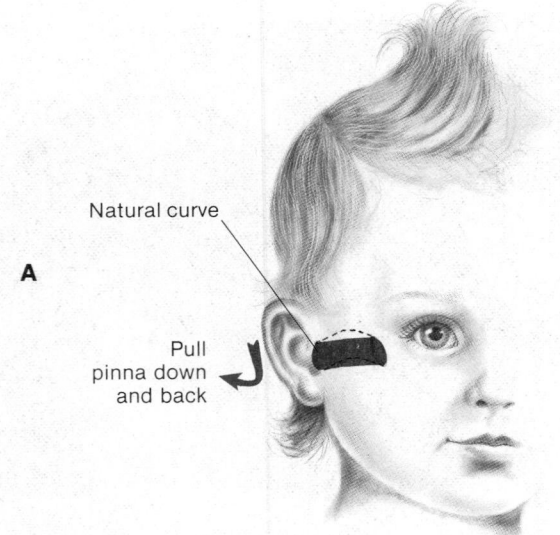

Natural curve

A

Pull pinna down and back

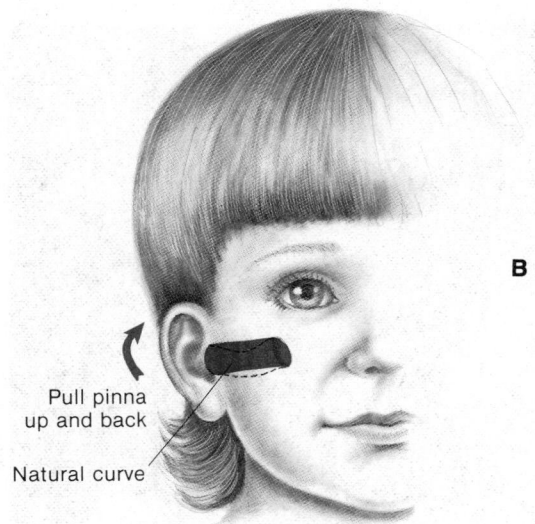

B

Pull pinna up and back

Natural curve

Fig. 7-29. Positioning of eardrum. **A,** Infant. **B,** Child older than 3 years of age.

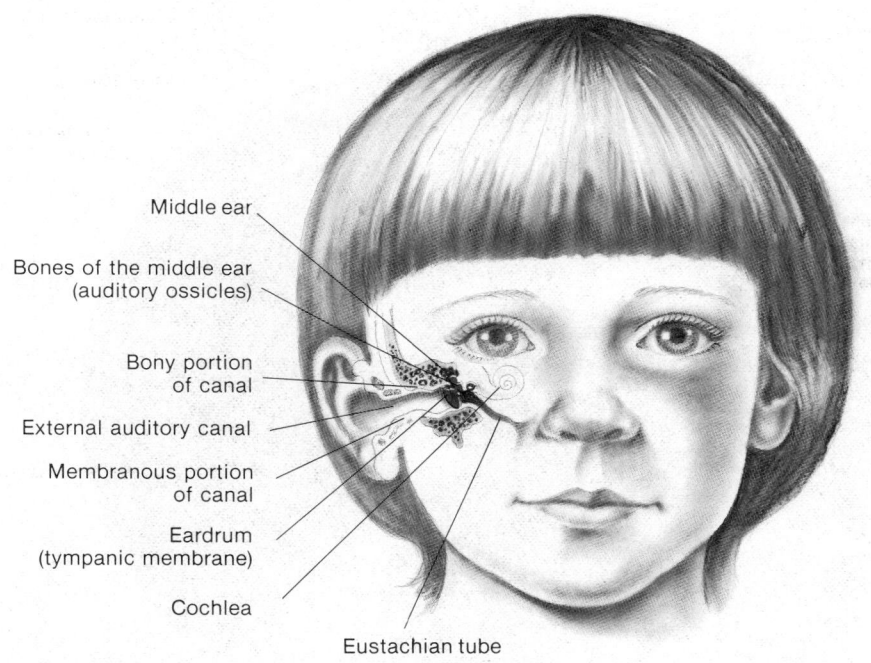

Middle ear

Bones of the middle ear
(auditory ossicles)

Bony portion
of canal

External auditory canal

Membranous portion
of canal

Eardrum
(tympanic membrane)

Cochlea

Eustachian tube

Fig. 7-30. Cross-section of external, middle, and parts of inner ear.

upward and the tympanic membrane lies almost horizontally along the upper wall of the canal. The pinna must be pulled *downward* and *backward* to the 6 to 9 o'clock range, which retracts the canal and the drum downward (Fig. 7-29, *A*).

With older children, usually those over 3 years of age, the canal curves downward and forward, and the drum, although more vertical, slopes inward and forward. Therefore the pinna is pulled *upward* and *back* toward a 10 o'clock position (Fig. 7-29, *B*). If there is difficulty in visualizing the membrane, it can be brought into view by repositioning the head, introducing the speculum at a different angle, and pulling the pinna in a slightly different direction.

In neonates and young infants the walls of the canal are pliable and floppy because of the underdeveloped cartilaginous and bony structures. Therefore the very small 2 mm speculum usually needs to be inserted deeper into the canal than in older children. Great care must be exercised not to damage the walls or drum. Because the small opening of the speculum permits a limited view, each quadrant of the membrane must be systematically inspected. In older children the speculum need not be inserted past the membranous portion of the canal, usually a distance of 0.60 to 1.25 cm (¼ to ½ inch). The entire canal is about 2.5 cm (1 inch) long. Insertion of the speculum into the posterior or bony portion of the canal causes pain (Fig. 7-30).

Otoscopic examination. As the speculum is introduced into the external canal, the walls of the canal, the color of the tympanic membrane, the light reflex, and the usual landmarks of the bony prominences of the middle ear are inspected. Fig. 7-31 illustrates the usual view of the tympanic membrane.

The *walls* of the external auditory canal are pink, although they are more pigmented in dark-skinned children. Minute hairs are evident in the outermost portion, where cerumen is produced. Signs of irritation, foreign bodies, or evidence of infection are noted.

Foreign bodies in the ear are not uncommon in children and range from erasers to beans. Symptoms may include pain, discharge, and affected hearing. Soft objects, such as paper or insects, can be removed with forceps. Small, hard objects, such as pebbles, can be removed with a suction tip or a hook. Irrigation may be used but is contraindicated if the object is vegetative matter, which swells when in contact with fluid. If there is any doubt about the ability to remove an object, referral is indicated (Harkess, 1982).

The *color* of the *tympanic membrane* is a translucent, light pearly pink or gray. Marked erythema (which may indicate suppurative otitis media), a dull nontransparent grayish color (sometimes suggestive of serous otitis media), or ashen gray areas (signs of scarring from a previous perforation) are noted. A black area usually suggests a perforation of the membrane that has not healed. Slight redness is normal in the newborn because of increased vascularity and is often evident in older infants and young children as a result of crying.

The characteristic tenseness and slope of the tympanic membrane cause the light of the otoscope to reflect at about the 5 or 7 o'clock position. The *light reflex* is a fairly well defined cone-shaped reflection, which normally points away from the face. Absence of the light reflex is always recorded, since it signifies bulging of the membrane and loss of its usual contours.

The *bony landmarks* of the drum are formed by the following structures. The *umbo,* or long arm of the malleus

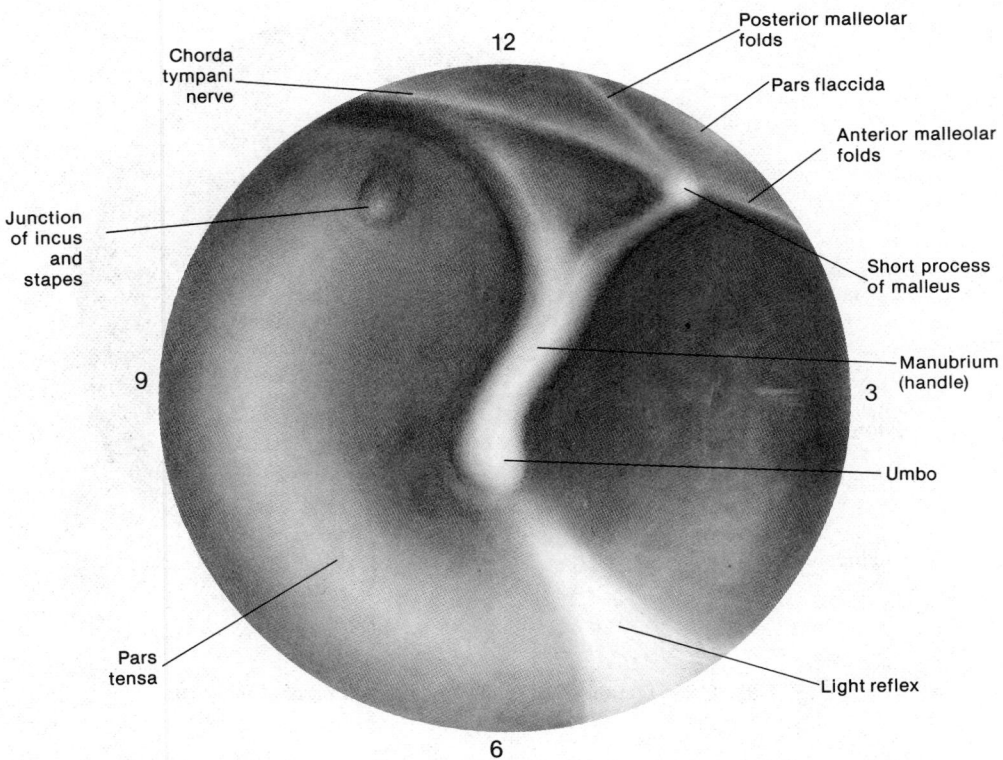

Chorda tympani nerve

Junction of incus and stapes

9

Pars tensa

12

Posterior malleolar folds

Pars flaccida

Anterior malleolar folds

Short process of malleus

Manubrium (handle)

3

Umbo

Light reflex

6

Fig. 7-31. Usual landmarks of right tympanic membrane with "clock" superimposed.

bone, appears as a small, round, opaque concave spot near the center of the drum. The *manubrium* (long process or handle) of the malleus appears to be a whitish line extending from the umbo upward to the margin of the membrane. At the upper end of the long process near the 1 o'clock position is a sharp knoblike protuberance, representing the *short process* of the malleus. Sometimes a shadow is seen at about the 10 or 11 o'clock position. This is the junction of the *incus* and the *stapes* bones.

The *anulus* is the fibrous ring surrounding the periphery of the membrane, except for an area of the anterior and posterior *malleolar folds*. The anulus is carefully inspected because it is a common location of perforations. Above the malleolar folds is a thin and slack membrane called the *pars flaccida*. The *chorda tympani nerve* is seen as a line running under the pars flaccida. The remainder of the membrane, such as the area of the light reflex, is taut and thus called the *pars tensa*. Loss of any of these landmarks is noted, since it is probably caused by the bulging of the membrane as a result of fluid accumulation in the middle ear. Retraction of the drum with abnormal prominence of the bony landmarks is suggestive of serious otitis media.

Auditory testing. Several types of hearing tests are available. Some of them, such as audiometric testing, involve specialized equipment that measures the degree of hearing loss. Others, such as tests for the startle reflex in neonates, are rough estimations of perception of sound. The nurse must operate under a high index of suspicion for those children who may have conditions associated with hearing loss and who may have developed behaviors indicative of

auditory impairment. Types of hearing loss, causes, clinical manifestations, and appropriate treatment are discussed in Chapter 25.

Audiometry. In audiometry an electrical audiometer measures the threshold of hearing for pure-tone frequencies and loudness. An audiogram is a record of the audiometric testing. A sound is transmitted to the child's ear and reduced until he indicates the sound is no longer heard. This procedure is repeated for several sounds covering the range found in conversation usually at a level of 20 or 25 decibels (dB) and for frequencies between 500 and 8000 Hz (Cross, 1985). In an air conduction audiogram the sounds are transmitted through earphones, which the nurse can describe to young children as part of a "space helmet." With bone conduction the sounds are passed through a plaque placed over the mastoid bone. Since the child is listening to very soft sounds, audiometry is performed in a soundproof room.

Pure-tone audiometry provides valuable information regarding the severity of the hearing loss, the sound cycles involved, and the possible location of the defect. However, it requires specialized training of personnel, expensive equipment, and cooperation from the child in terms of confirming the perception of sound. For children 24 months to about 5 years *play audiometry* can be implemented to increase cooperation. Based on behavior modification, it involves reinforcement for correct response. Also available is an Audioscope,* which incorporates hearing screening and otoscopy in a single instrument and has been shown to be

*Manufactured by Welch Allyn, Skaneateles Falls, NY 13153.

as accurate as traditional screening audiometry with children 3 years and older (Gershel and others, 1985).

Tympanometry. Acoustic impedance measurement, or *tympanometry*, measures tympanic membrane compliance (mobility) and estimates middle ear air pressure but does not measure perception of sound. A normal drum covering only air in the middle ear moves easily when negative or positive pressure is applied. Decreased or low compliance usually indicates middle ear effusion. This test aids in confirming the diagnosis of serous otitis media, a potential cause of conductive hearing loss. Measurements of compliance can also be done subjectively by blowing air gently into the ear with a pneumonic device attached to the otoscope.

Tympanometry is suitable for infants, young children, and those who are difficult to test by other methods, because little cooperation is necessary and the procedure is painless. A soft rubber cuff is pressed over the external canal, and when an airtight seal is achieved, an automatic reading of air pressure registers on an attached handheld probe. Visualization of the membrane, which frequently is very difficult if cerumen is present or if the child is in considerable discomfort, is not necessary. However, soft wax can occlude the probe tip, producing an abnormal tympanogram (Grimes, 1985).

Clinical hearing tests. In newborns hearing can be determined by eliciting the *startle reflex* (p. 314) and by observing other neonatal responses to loud noises, such as facial grimaces, blinking, gross motor movements, quieting if crying or crying if quiet, opening the eyes, or ceasing sucking activity. An objective sign may be a change in heart or respiratory rate because of a loud noise, usually a quickening of the rate. Absence of such alerting behaviors suggests a hearing loss.

During infancy the nurse can test for hearing loss by making a noise and noting the child's specific reaction to *localization of sound*. The nurse stands about 18 inches away from the child, to the side, and out of his peripheral field of vision. With the room silent and the child sitting contentedly in the parent's lap, distracted by a toy or other object, the nurse makes a voice sound, such as "ps" or "phth," which is high pitched, or "oo," which is low pitched, rings a bell or a rattle, or rustles tissue paper. The child's response in terms of localizing the sound is compared to the expected age response (see box, p. 496). This test is usually inadequate for toddlers and preschoolers because of their distractibility and lessened cooperation.

Brainstem auditory evoked potentials. In an attempt to objectively assess hearing in newborns and other hard-to-test children, a complex and expensive method called brainstem auditory evoked potentials has been developed. Through electrode wires attached to the infant's scalp, electrical or brain wave potentials generated within the auditory system are recorded into a computer. Following repetitive acoustic stimulation, the computer average waveforms from a normal sleeping or quiet infant consist of several peaks and valleys that reflect activations of neural structures of the brain. The recording is then analyzed by a specially trained technician to determine the threshold of hearing response.

Crib-o-gram. The Crib-o-gram,* a neonatal screening tool, analyzes hearing responses by comparing the infant's motor activity before, during, and after a sound is introduced. Both administration of the test and its scoring are totally automated. A motion-sensitive transducer is placed beneath the crib or Isolette mattress, and a microprocessor "reads" the infant's movement. A change in activity that coincides with the test sound is scored as a "pass." The sequence is repeated several times to ensure reliability.

Conduction tests. Two tests are also used to distinguish between air and bone conduction, the Rinne test and Weber test. In air conduction, sound is transmitted to the brain through the external, middle, and inner ear structures. In bone conduction the sound bypasses the external and middle ear and is transmitted to the brain through the mastoid bone to the inner ear structures and auditory nerve. Normally air conduction is considerably better than bone conduction.

In the *Rinne test* the stem of the tuning fork is placed against the mastoid bone until the sound ceases to be audible. It is moved so that the prongs are held near, but not touching, the auditory meatus. The child should again hear the sound (Rinne positive). If the sound is not again audible (Rinne negative), some abnormality is interfering with the conduction of air through the external and middle ear chambers. This test requires the cooperation and ability of the child to signal when the sound is no longer audible and when it is again heard. It is not useful for most children before preschool age.

In the *Weber test* the stem of the tuning fork is held in the midline of the head. The child should hear the sound equally in both ears (Weber positive). With air conductive loss he will hear the sound better in the *affected* ear (Weber negative). This test is frequently not suitable for young children because of their difficulty in discriminating between "better, more, or less." Any child who is suspected of a hearing loss because of poor performance using any of these tests is referred for special audiometric testing.

Vestibular testing. Vestibular testing for inner ear function concerning equilibrium is evaluated in young children by holding them at a 30-degree angle and rotating them in a complete circle in each direction. The normal response is nystagmus (movement of the eyes) in the direction of the rotation while being swung and in the opposite direction when the movement stops. This same procedure can be done by using a swivel chair for older children or by having them pivot quickly to one side, then the other.

Nose

The nose marks the beginning of the passageway through the respiratory tract. It is an important organ for filtration, temperature control, and humidification of inspired air, and a sensory organ for olfaction (smell). Each of these func-

---

*Manufactured by Telesensory Systems, Inc., Palo Alto, CA 94304.

tions depends on the patency of the passageways and the mucosal lining of the nasal cavity. Inspection is primarily used for assessing the external and internal structures.

Inspection of external structures. The nose is located in the middle of the face just below the eyes and above the lips. Its placement and alignment can be compared by drawing an imaginary vertical line from the center point between the eyes down to the notch of the upper lip. The nose should lie exactly vertical to this line, with each side exactly symmetric. Its location, any deviation to one side, and asymmetry in overall size and in diameter of the nares (nostrils) are noted. The bridge of the nose is sometimes flat in Oriental and black children. The alae nasi are noted for any sign of flaring, which indicates respiratory difficulty. Fig. 7-32 illustrates the usual landmarks used in describing the external structures of the nose.

Inspection of internal structures. The anterior vestibule of the nose is inspected by pushing the tip upward, tilting the head backward, and illuminating the cavity with a flashlight or otoscope without the attached ear speculum. For a deeper view of the inferior and middle turbinates and the middle meatus, a nasal speculum is used, such as a 9 mm speculum with a very short barrel that attaches to the otoscope head. Forceps specula are not routinely used in children. The short, wide speculum is inserted into the nares, slightly away from the septum, and the otoscope is tilted upward to straighten the passageway toward the posterior wall of the cavity. Pushing against the septum is avoided because it causes pain. Generally inspection is adequate without the speculum, unless one decides that a closer examination of the nasal membranes is warranted. If the nasal speculum is used, the process is explained to the child, similar to the type of preparation for using the otoscope.

The *color* of the *mucosal lining,* which is normally redder than the oral membranes, is noted, and any swelling, discharge, dryness, or bleeding. Nasal membranes that are abnormally pale, grayish pink, and swollen suggest nasal allergies. Red, swollen membranes are usually characteristic of the common cold. These differences in appearance are important diagnostic clues to distinguishing between allergy and cold symptoms.

Normally, there should be no discharge from the nose. However, if the child has been crying, a watery discharge is normal. At other times a thin, clear exudate may indicate allergies, chronic rhinitis, or sinusitis. Purulent discharge is caused by infection and can indicate upper respiratory tract infections resulting from either a viral or a bacterial agent. Discharge from one nostril may be caused by a foreign body. If possible, it is removed with forceps (tweezers). If it is deep in the cavity, the child is referred to a physician.

Looking deeper into the nose, the nurse inspects the *turbinates,* or *concha,* plates of bone enveloped by mucous membrane that jut into the nasal cavity. The turbinates greatly increase the surface area of the nasal cavity as air is inhaled. The spaces or channels between the turbinates are called the *meatus* and correspond to each of the three turbinates. Normally the front end of the inferior and middle turbinate and the middle meatus can be seen. They should be the same color as the lining of the vestibule. Enlarged, boggy, pale, grayish mucosa should be noted. Swollen turbinates greatly occlude the passageways for entry of air.

Inside the nose, the *septum,* which should equally divide the vestibules, is inspected. Any deviation is noted, especially if it causes an occlusion of one side of the nose. A perforation may be evident within the septum. If this is suspected, the nurse can shine the light of the otoscope into one naris and look for admittance of light through the perforation to the other nostril.

Since olfaction is an important function of the nose, testing for smell may be done at this point or as part of cranial nerve assessment (see p. 282).

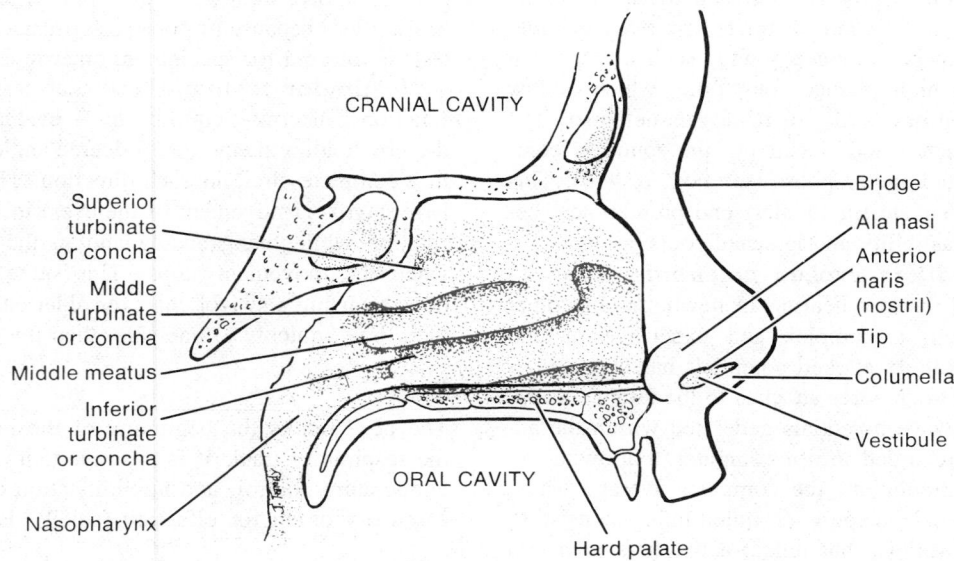

Fig. 7-32. External landmarks and internal structures of nose.

Mouth and Throat

The mouth is the beginning of the passageway to the digestive tract, but it also functions in the entry or exit of air. The major structure of the exterior of the mouth is the *lips*. Inspection of the lips for color has been discussed in the section on skin (p. 235). Any deviations are noted, such as *cheilitis*, the presence of painful, inflamed, and dried cracks or fissures of the lips. Cheilitis may be caused by exposure to harsh climatic conditions, habitual licking or biting of the

lips, mouth breathing from respiratory distress, or dehydration, particularly with fever in systemic disease. *Cheilosis*, or angular stomatitis, is fissuring at the angles or corners of the lips and may indicate deficiencies of riboflavin or niacin.

Any lesions on the lips are noted. The herpes simplex virus produces singular or clusters of vesicular eruptions on the lip, which are often called "cold sores." The lip may also be the site of a primary syphilitic chancre, which appears as a firm nodule that ulcerates and crusts. If one suspects a chancre, it is examined with a gloved hand for the nurse's protection.

Inspection of internal structures. The mouth and throat are divided into three areas: (1) the *oral cavity*, which extends from the lips to the palatopharyngeal arches, (2) the *oropharynx*, which extends from the epiglottis to the lower edge of the adenoids, and (3) the *nasopharynx*, which extends from above the lower edge of the adenoids to the nasal cavity. The major structures that are visible on examination within the oral cavity and oropharynx are the mucosal lining of the lips and cheeks, gums or gingiva, teeth, tongue, palate, uvula, tonsils, and posterior oropharynx (Fig. 7-33). Other pharyngeal structures that are not visible on examination are the epiglottis, lingual tonsils, and pharyngeal tonsils or adenoids.

With a cooperative child almost the entire examination can be done without the use of a tongue blade. The nurse asks the child to open his mouth wide, requests that he move his tongue in different directions for full visualization, and has him say "ahh" in order to depress the tongue for full view of the back of the mouth (tonsils, uvula, oropharynx). For a closer look at the buccal mucosa or lining of the cheeks, the nurse can ask the child to use his fingers to move the outer lip and cheek to one side. Performing the examination in front of a mirror is a great aid in enlisting the child's cooperation. Another approach is using a puppet and letting the child examine its wide-open mouth (Fig. 7-34, *A*).

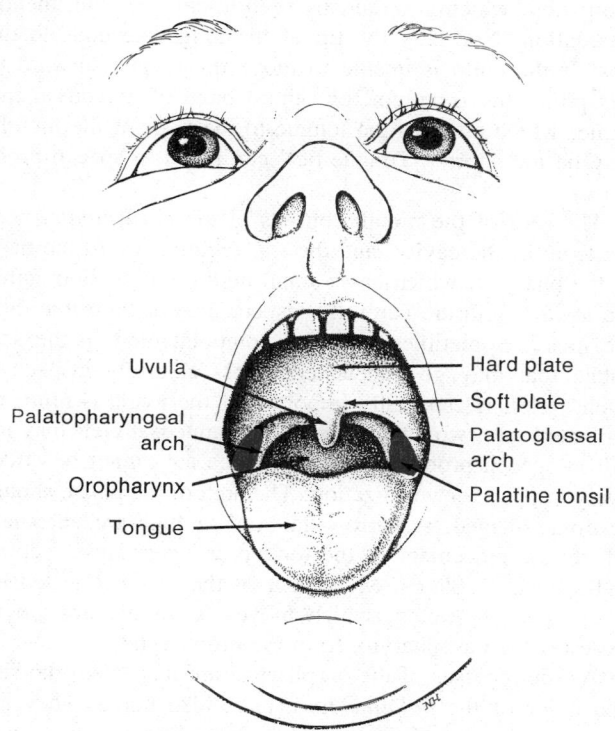

Uvula

Palatopharyngeal arch

Oropharynx

Tongue

Hard plate

Soft plate

Palatoglossal arch

Palatine tonsil

Fig. 7-33. Interior structures of mouth.

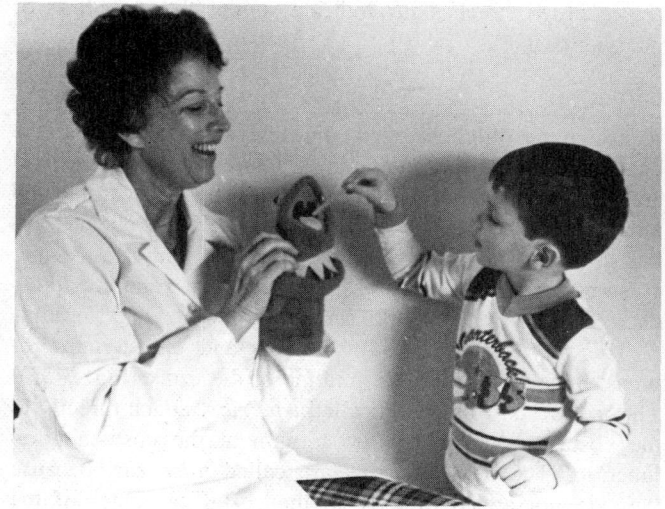

A

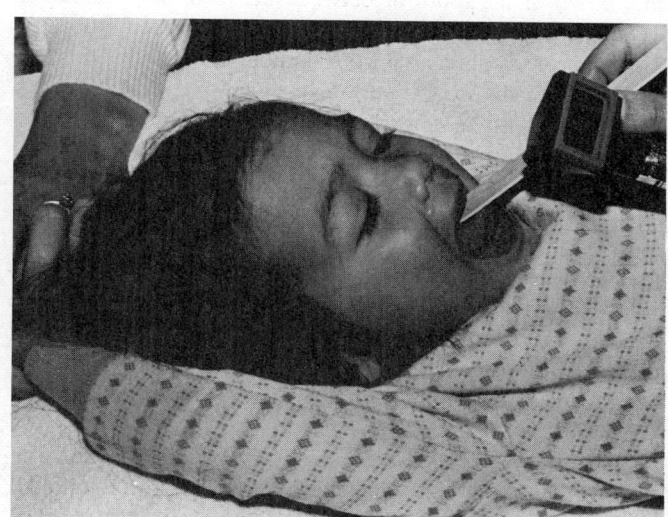

B

Fig. 7-34. A, Encouraging child to cooperate. **B,** Positioning child for examination of mouth.

Infants and toddlers, however, usually resist attempts to keep the mouth open. Because inspecting the mouth is an upsetting part of the examination, it is reserved until last (with examination of the ears) or performed during episodes of crying. However, the use of a tongue blade to depress the tongue is necessary. The tongue blade is placed along the *side* of the tongue, not the center back area where the gag reflex is elicited. Fig. 7-34, *B,* illustrates proper positioning of the child for oral examination. If the child resists in opening his mouth, pinching the nostrils closed forces the child to breathe by mouth and therefore open it.

All areas lined with *mucous membranes* (inside the lips and cheeks, gingiva, underside of tongue, palate, back of pharynx) are inspected. The membranes should be bright pink, smooth, glistening, uniform, and moist. Any deviations are noted, such as color, white patches or ulceration, bleeding, and sensitivity. For example, reddened areas with white ulcerated centers may be canker sores (aphthae), which may be caused by trauma to the gums during toothbrushing or chewing. White curdy plaques or patches anywhere on the oral mucosa, but particularly on the surface of the tongue and hard palate, that bleed when scraped are signs of moniliasis.

As the nurse observes the lining of the mouth, any odor (halitosis) is noted. Mouth odors are characteristic of a number of important health problems, such as poor dental hygiene, gingival disease, chronic constipation, dehydration, malnutrition, or systemic illness. A sudden, foul odor in the mouth may indicate a foreign body in the nose, particularly a bean or pea.

The *teeth* are inspected for number in each dental arch, hygiene, and occlusion or bite. The general rule for estimating the number of temporary teeth in children who are 2 years of age or younger is: *the child's age in months minus 6 months equals the number of teeth.* Discoloration of tooth enamel with obvious plaque (whitish coating on the surface of the teeth) is a sign of poor dental hygiene and indicates a need for dental counseling. Brown spots in the crevices of the crown of the tooth or between the teeth may be caries. Teeth that appear greenish black may be stained from oral ingestion of supplemental iron. Although unsightly, this disappears after the iron is no longer given.

Malocclusion or poor biting relationship of the teeth is evaluated in terms of (1) how the jaws relate to each other in vertical, transverse, and anteroposterior directions, for example, the "bucktoothed" appearance that results when the maxilla is forward in relation to the mandible, (2) how the teeth are aligned, and (3) how the teeth interdigitate when in occlusion. Although parents frequently express concern regarding thumb-sucking and the development of orthodontic problems, thumb-sucking that ceases before the age of 6 years probably does little harm (Starnbach and Gellin, 1977).

The *gums* surrounding the teeth are examined. The color is normally coral pink, and the surface texture is stippled, similar to the appearance of orange peel. In dark-skinned children the gums are more deeply colored and a brownish area is often observed along the gum line.

The *tongue* is inspected for the presence of papillae, small projections that contain several taste buds each and give the tongue its characteristic rough appearance. Changes in the surface texture are noted, such as (1) "geographic tongue," unusual patterns of papillae formation and denuded areas, (2) coated tongue, such as in thrush, or (3) an exceptionally beefy red and swollen tongue, which is a sign of various systemic diseases.

The size and mobility of the tongue are noted, especially protrusion, which is frequently seen in children with mental retardation. Normally the tip of the tongue extends to the lips. If the child is unable to move the tongue forward to this point, the frenulum, or central band of mucous membrane, which attaches the tongue to the floor of the mouth, may be too short. "Tongue-tie" can result in speech problems.

The roof of the mouth consists of the *hard palate,* near the front of the cavity, and the *soft palate,* toward the back of the pharynx, which has a small midline protrusion called the *uvula.* Both are carefully inspected to be sure that they are intact. Sometimes there is a pinpoint cleft in the soft palate that may go undetected unless carefully inspected. Such a cleft is especially important if the uvula is bifid, or separated into two appendages. A submucosal cleft may result in speech problems later on, since air cannot be effectively trapped for vocalization. The arch of the palate should be dome shaped. A narrow-flat roof or high-arched palate affects the placement of the tongue and can cause feeding and speech problems. Movement of the uvula is tested by eliciting a gag reflex, which moves the uvula upward to close off the nasopharynx from the oropharynx.

As the recesses of the oropharynx are inspected, the size and color of the *palatine tonsils* are also noted. They are normally the same color as the surrounding mucosa, glandular rather than smooth in appearance, and barely visible over the edge of the palatoglossal arches. Enlargement, redness, and white patches on the tonsils and surrounding area are recorded. Such signs indicate suppurative tonsillitis or pharyngitis.

Chest

Although the thoracic cavity houses two vital organs, the heart and lungs, the anatomic structures of the chest wall are important sources of information concerning cardiac and pulmonary function, skeletal formation, and secondary sexual development. The chest is inspected for size, shape, symmetry, movement, breast development, and the presence of the bony landmarks formed by the ribs and sternum.

The *rib cage* consists of 12 ribs and the sternum, or breast bone, located in the midline of the trunk (Fig. 7-35). The first seven ribs, often called *true ribs,* attach directly to the costal cartilages of the sternum at the costochondral junction. The next five ribs are called *false ribs* because they do not attach directly to the costal cartilages of the

Fig. 7-35. Rib cage.

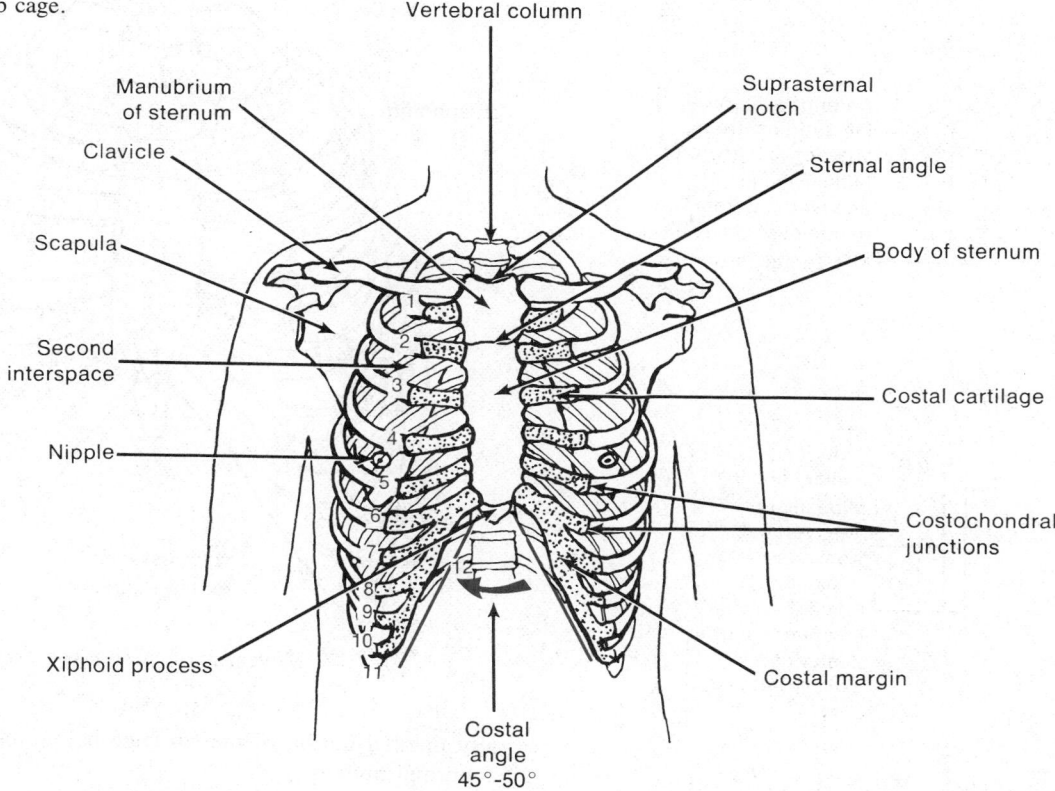

sternum. The eighth, ninth, and tenth ribs attach to the costal cartilages below the seventh rib, and the last two ribs, often called *floaters,* have no direct attachment to the sternum or anterior ribs, other than their posterior attachment to the vertebral column.

The *sternum* is composed of three main parts. The *manubrium,* the uppermost portion, can be felt at the base of the neck at the *suprasternal notch.* The largest segment of the sternum is the *body,* which forms the *sternal angle* as it articulates with the manubrium. At the end of the body is a small, movable process called the *xiphoid.* The angle of the costal margin as it attaches to the sternum is called the *costal angle* and is normally about 45 to 50 degrees. These bony structures are important landmarks in the location of ribs and intercostal spaces. The first rib attaches directly to the manubrium. The second rib attaches directly to the body of the sternum below the sternal angle. The sternal angle is felt as a ridge a few centimeters below the suprasternal notch. The space immediately below a rib is its corresponding *intercostal space.*

The nurse must become familiar with locating and properly numbering each rib, because ribs are geographic landmarks for palpating, percussing, and auscultating underlying organs. Normally all the ribs can be counted by palpating inferiorly from the second rib. The tip of the eleventh rib can be felt laterally, and the tip of the twelfth rib can be felt posteriorly. Other helpful landmarks include the nipples, which are usually located between the fourth and fifth ribs

or at the fourth interspace and, posteriorly, the tip of the scapula, which is located at the level of the eighth rib or interspace. In children with thin chest walls, correctly locating the ribs presents little difficulty.

The *thoracic cavity* is also divided into segments by drawing imaginary lines on the chest and back. Fig. 7-36 illustrates the anterior, lateral, and posterior divisions.

The *size* of the chest is measured by placing the tape around the rib cage at the nipple line (see Fig. 7-9). For greatest accuracy at least two measurements are taken, one during inspiration and the other during expiration, and the average recorded. Chest size is important mainly in comparison to its relationship with head circumference, which is discussed on p. 227. Marked disproportions are always recorded, because most are caused by abnormal head growth, although some may be the result of altered chest shape, such as barrel chest or pigeon chest.

During infancy the *shape* of the chest is almost circular, with the anteroposterior diameter equaling the transverse or lateral diameter. As the child grows, the chest normally increases in the transverse direction, causing the anteroposterior diameter to be less than the lateral diameter. In an older child the characteristic barrel shape of an infant's chest is a significant sign of chronic obstructive lung disease, such as asthma or cystic fibrosis. Other variations in shape that are usually variants of the normal configuration are *pigeon breast,* or *pectus carinatum,* in which the sternum protrudes outward, increasing the anteroposterior diameter, and *funnel*

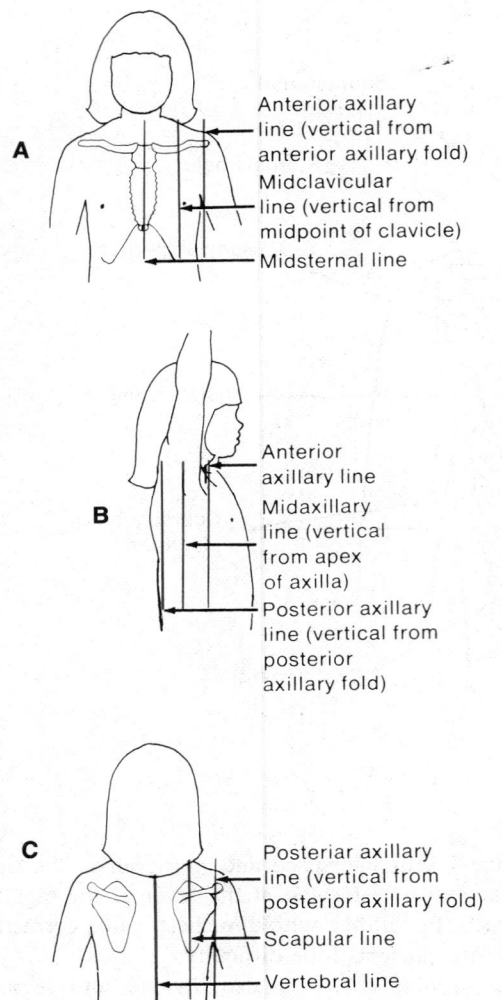

Fig. 7-36. Imaginary landmarks of chest. **A,** Anterior. **B,** Right lateral. **C,** Posterior.

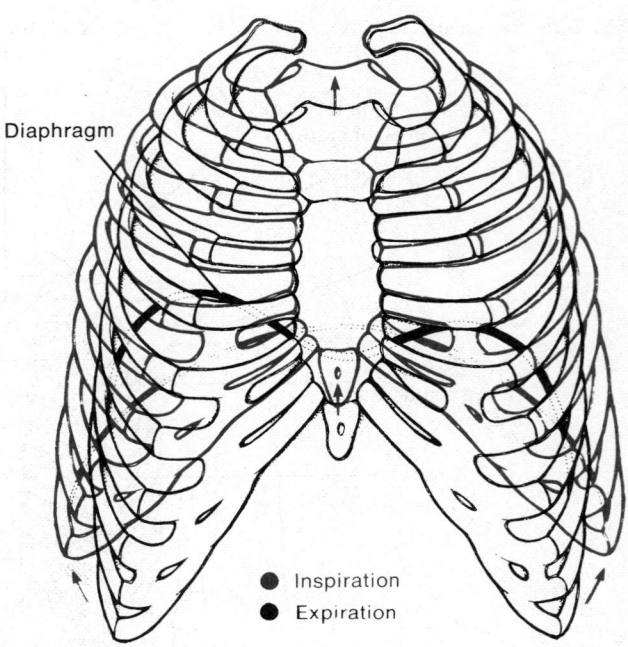

● Inspiration
● Expiration

Fig. 7-37. Movement of chest during respiration.

chest, or *pectus excavatum,* in which the lower portion of the sternum is depressed. A severe depression may impair cardiac function, but in general neither condition causes pathologic dysfunction. However, these conditions often cause parents and children concern regarding acceptable physical appearance.

The *angle* made by the lower costal margin and the sternum ordinarily is about 45 degrees. A larger angle is characteristic of lung diseases that also cause a barrel shape of the chest. A smaller angle may be a sign of malnutrition. As the rib cage is inspected, the junction of the ribs to the costal cartilage (costochondral junction) and sternum is noted. Normally the points of attachment are fairly smooth. Swellings or blunt knobs along either side of the sternum are known as the *rachitic rosary* and may indicate vitamin D deficiency. Another variation in shape that may either be normal or may suggest rickets (vitamin D deficiency) is *Harrison groove,* which appears as a depression or horizontal groove where the diaphragm leaves the chest wall. Usu-

ally marked flaring of the rib cage below the groove is an abnormal finding.

Body *symmetry* is always an important notation during inspection. Asymmetry in the chest may indicate serious underlying problems, such as cardiac enlargement (bulging on the left side of rib cage) or pulmonary dysfunction. However, asymmetry is most often a sign of scoliosis, lateral curvature of the spine. Asymmetry warrants further medical investigation.

Movement of the chest wall should be symmetric bilaterally and coordinated with breathing. During inspiration the chest rises and expands, the diaphragm descends, and the costal angle increases. During expiration the chest falls and decreases in size, the diaphragm rises, and the costal angle narrows (Fig. 7-37). In children under 6 or 7 years of age, respiratory movement is principally abdominal or diaphragmatic. In older children, particularly females, respirations are chiefly thoracic. In either type the chest and abdomen should rise and fall together.

Any asymmetry of movement is an important pathologic sign and must be reported. Decreased movement on one side of the chest may indicate pneumonia, pneumothorax, atelectasis, or an obstructive foreign body. Marked *retraction* of muscles either between the ribs (intercostal), above the sternum (suprasternal), or above the clavicles (supraclavicular) is always noted, because it is a sign of respiratory difficulty (see Fig. 31-6).

As the skin surface of the chest is inspected, the position of the *nipples* is observed as well as any evidence of *breast* development. Normally the nipples are located slightly lateral to the midclavicular line between the fourth and fifth ribs. Symmetry of nipple placement and normal configuration of a darker pigmented areola surrounding a flat nipple in the prepubertal child are noted.

Pubertal breast development usually begins in girls between 10 and 14 years of age (see p. 807). Precocious or delayed breast development is recorded, as well as evidence of any other secondary sexual characteristics. In males gynecomastia may be caused by hormonal or systemic disorders, but more commonly it is the result of adipose tissue from obesity or a transitory body change during early puberty. In either situation the nurse should investigate the child's feelings regarding breast enlargement.

In adolescent females who have achieved sexual maturity, the breasts are palpated for evidence of any masses or hard nodules. This opportunity should also be taken to discuss the importance of routine self-breast examination. Although carcinoma of the breast is rare in women under 20 years of age, it is advisable to stress the value of routine self-breast examination so that it becomes a practiced habit during later years. The vast majority of palpable masses are benign fibroadenomas (Sutow, Fernbach, and Vietti, 1984). This fact is emphasized to decrease any fear or concern that results when a mass is felt.

Lungs

The lungs are situated inside the thoracic cavity, with one lung on each side of the sternum. Each lung is divided into an *apex,* which is slightly pointed and rises above the first rib; a *base,* which is wide and concave and rides on the dome-shaped diaphragm; and a body, which is divided into *lobes.* The right lung has three lobes: the upper, middle, and lower. The left lobe has only two lobes, the upper and lower, because of the space occupied by the heart. The two surfaces of the lung are the *costal surface,* which faces the chest wall and backs up to the vertebral column, and the *mediastinal surface,* which faces the space lying between the lungs, the mediastinum. The center of the mediastinal surface is called the *hilus,* where the bronchus and blood vessels enter the lung (Fig. 7-38, *A*).

Examination of the lungs requires knowledge of their location and their relationship to the rib cage. The trachea bifurcates slightly below the level of the sternal angle. The apex of each lung rises about 2 to 4 cm above the inner third of the clavicles. The lower costal margin crosses the sixth rib at the midclavicular line and the eighth rib at the midaxillary line. The posterior base of the lungs crosses the eleventh rib at the vertebral line. The upper border of the right middle lobe parallels the inferior surface of the fourth rib. Fig. 7-38 illustrates the position of the lobes within the thoracic cavity during relaxation. Respiration causes displacement of the lobes upward (expiration) or downward (inspiration).

Inspection. Inspection of the lungs involves primarily observation of respiratory movements, which are discussed on p. 231. Respirations are evaluated for (1) rate (number per minute), (2) rhythm (regular, irregular, or periodic), (3) depth (deep or shallow), and (4) quality (effortless, auto-

matic, difficult, or labored). The nurse also notes the character of breath sounds based on inspection without the aid of auscultation, such as noisy, grunting, snoring, or heavy. Usual terms for describing various patterns of respiration are listed in Table 7-7.

Respiratory rate is always evaluated in relation to general physical status. For example, tachypnea is expected with fever, because for every degree Fahrenheit elevation in temperature, the respiratory rate increases four breaths per minute. The usual ratio of breaths to heartbeats is 1:4 (see inside front cover for normal respiratory rates at various ages).

Palpation. Respiratory movements are felt by placing each hand flat against the back or chest with the thumbs in midline along the lower costal margin of the lungs. The child should be sitting during this procedure and if cooperative should take several deep breaths. During respiration the hands will move with the chest wall. The amount of respiratory excursion is evaluated and any asymmetry of movement is noted. Normally in older children the posterior base of the lungs descends 5 to 6 cm (about 2 inches) during a deep inspiration.

The nurse also palpates for *vocal fremitus,* the conduction of voice sounds through the respiratory tract. With the palmar surfaces of the nurse's hands on the chest, the child repeats words, such as "ninety-nine," "one, two, three," or "eee-eee." Vibrations are felt as the hands move symmetrically on either side of the sternum and vertebral column. In general, vocal fremitus is most intense in the apex and least prominent at the base of the lungs. Decreased vocal fremitus in the upper airway may indicate several gross pulmonary changes. Absence of fremitus usually indicates obstruction of a major bronchus, which may occur as a result of aspiration of a foreign body. Decreased or absent fremitus is always recorded and reported for further investigation.

During palpation other vibrations that indicate pathologic conditions are noted. One is a *pleural friction rub,* which has a grating sensation. It is synchronous with respiratory movements and is the result of opposing surfaces of the inflamed pleural lining rubbing against one another.

Crepitation is felt as a coarse, cracking sensation as the hand presses over the affected area. It is the result of the escape of air from the lungs into the subcutaneous tissues caused by injury or surgical intervention. Both pleural friction rubs and crepitation can usually be both heard and felt.

Percussion. The lungs are percussed in order to evaluate the densities of the underlying organs. Fig. 7-39 illustrates the expected percussion sounds within the anterior thorax. *Resonance* is heard over all the lobes of the lungs that are not adjacent to other organs. *Dullness* is heard beginning at the fifth interspace in the right midclavicular line. Percussing downward to the end of the liver, a *flat* sound is heard because the liver no longer overlies the air-filled lung. *Cardiac dullness* is felt over the left sternal border from the second to the fifth interspace medially to the midclavicular

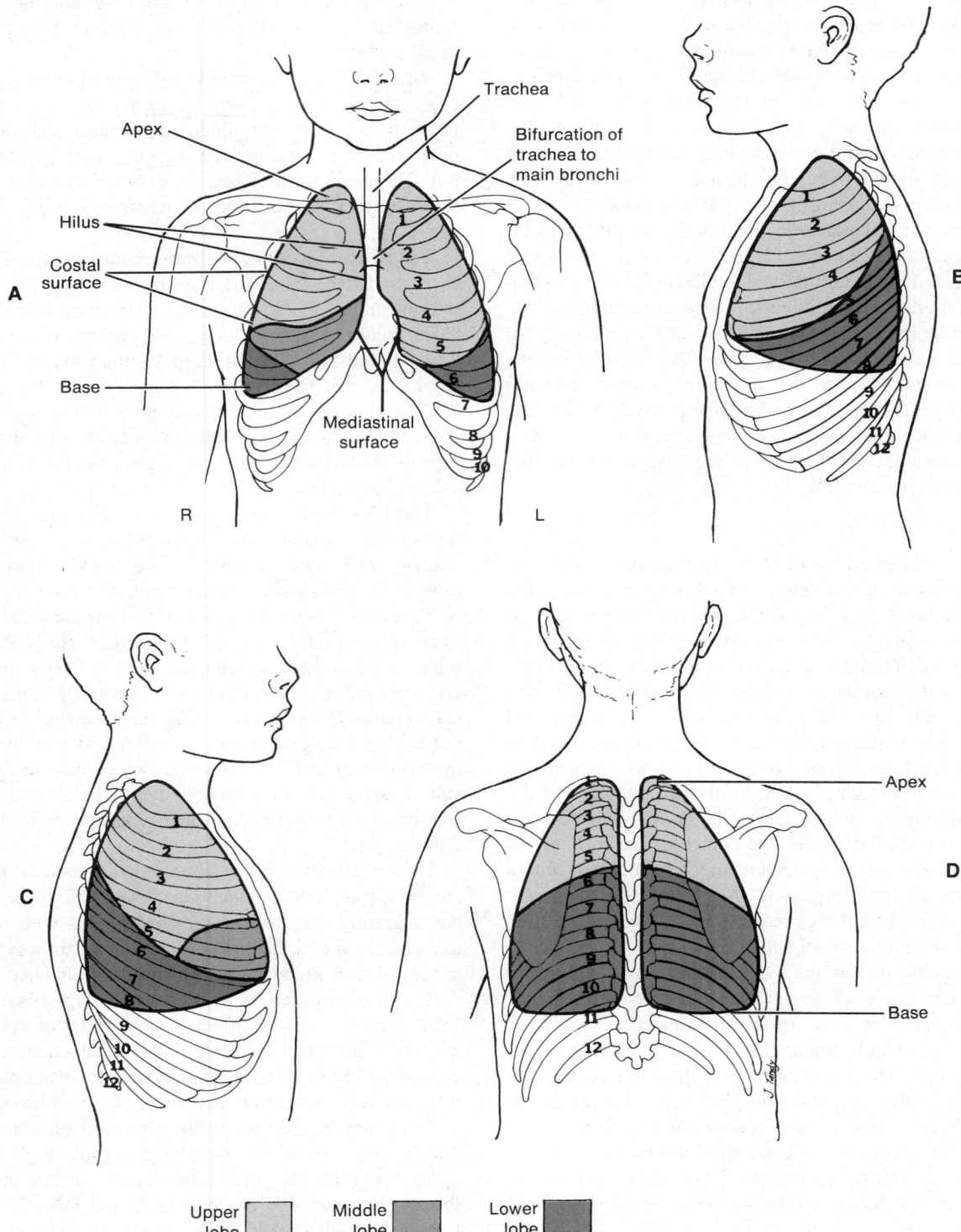

Fig. 7-38. Location of lobes of lungs within thoracic cavity. **A,** Anterior view. **B,** Left lateral view. **C,** Right lateral view. **D,** Posterior view.

Table 7-7 Various patterns of respiration

TERM	DESCRIPTION
Tachypnea	Increased rate
Bradypnea	Decreased rate
Dyspnea	Distress during breathing
Apnea	Cessation of breathing
Hyperpnea	Increased depth
Hypoventilation	Decreased depth (shallow) and irregular rhythm
Hyperventilation	Increased rate and depth
Kussmaul breathing	Hyperventilation, gasping and labored respiration, usually seen in diabetic coma or other states of respiratory acidosis
Cheyne-Stokes respirations	Gradually increasing rate and depth with periods of apnea
Biot breathing	Periods of hyperpnea alternating with apnea (similar to Cheyne-Stokes except that the depth remains constant)
Seesaw (paradoxic) respirations	Chest falls on inspiration and rises on expiration

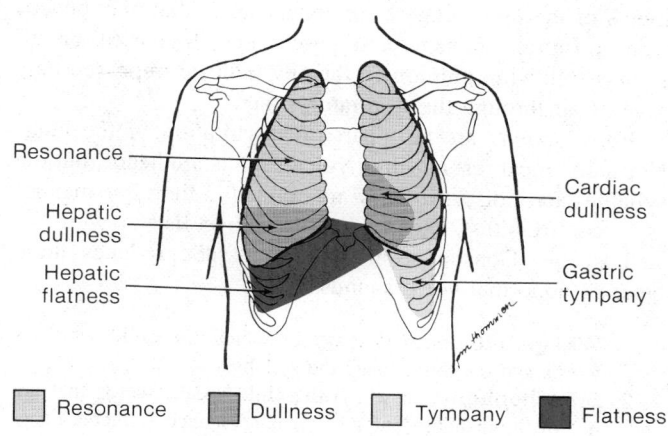

Fig. 7-39. Percussion sounds found in normal thorax.

line. Below the fifth interspace on the left side, *tympany* results from the air-filled stomach. Deviations from these expected sounds are always recorded and reported.

In percussing the chest, the anterior lung is percussed from apex to base, usually with the child in the supine or sitting position. Each side of the chest is percussed in sequence in order to compare the sounds, such as the dullness of the liver on the right side with the tympany of the stomach on the left side. When the posterior lung is percussed, the procedure and sequence are the same, although the child should be sitting. Normally only resonance is heard when percussing the posterior thorax from the shoulder to the eighth or tenth rib. At the base of the lungs dullness is heard as the diaphragm is percussed.

Auscultation. Auscultation involves using the stethoscope to evaluate breath and voice sounds. Breath sounds are best heard if the child inspires deeply. The child can be encouraged to "take a big breath" by following a demonstration of "breathing in through the nose and out through the mouth." Younger children respond well to activities such as making a pinwheel spin, "smelling" an artificial flower, or "blowing out" the light of the otoscope (Fig. 7-40).

In the lungs, breath sounds are classified as vesicular, bronchovesicular, or bronchial. They are described below:

Vesicular breath sounds, heard over entire surface of lungs, with exception of upper intrascapular area and area beneath manubrium; inspiration is louder, longer, and higher-pitched than expiration; sound is soft, swishing noise

Bronchovesicular breath sounds, normally heard over manubrium and in upper intrascapular regions where trachea and bronchi bifurcate; inspiration is louder and higher in pitch than in vesicular breathing

Bronchial breath sounds, heard only over trachea near suprasternal notch; almost reverse of vesicular sounds; inspiratory phase is short and expiratory phase is longer, louder, and of higher pitch

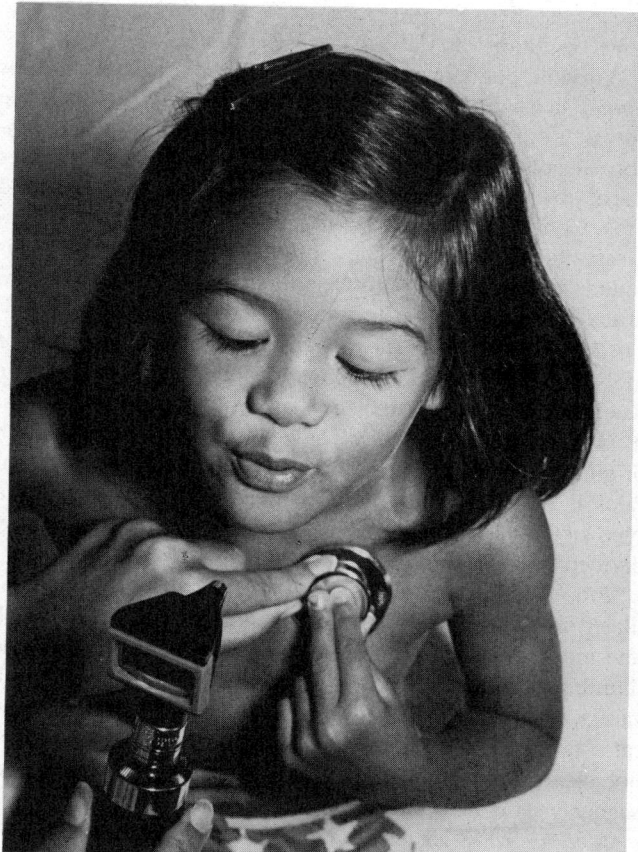

Fig. 7-40. Auscultating lungs while child "blows out" otoscope light.

Absent or *diminished breath sounds* are always an abnormal finding warranting investigation. Fluid, air, or solid masses in the pleural space all interfere with the conduction of breath sounds. Diminished breath sounds in certain segments of the lung suggest pulmonary areas that may benefit from postural drainage and percussion. Increased breath sounds following pulmonary therapy indicate improved passage of air through the respiratory tract.

Voice sounds are also part of auscultation of the lung. Normally vocal resonance or voice sounds are heard, but the syllables are indistinct. They are elicited in the same manner as vocal fremitus, except that the nurse listens with the stethoscope. Consolidation of lung tissue produces three types of abnormal voice sounds:

1. **Whispered pectoriloquy,** in which the child whispers words and the nurse hears the syllables
2. **Bronchophony,** in which the child speaks words that are not distinguishable but the vocal resonance is increased in intensity and clarity
3. **Egophony,** in which the child says "ee," which is heard as the nasal sound "ay" through the stethoscope

Decreased or absent vocal resonance is caused by the same conditions that affect vocal fremitus.

Various pulmonary abnormalities produce *adventitious sounds* that are not normally heard over the chest. They are not alterations of normal breath sounds but additional abnormal sounds often referred to as the three "R's": rales (from the French word meaning "rattle"), rhonchi, and rubs. Considerable practice with an experienced tutor is necessary to differentiate the various types of adventitious sounds. Often it is best to describe the type of sound heard in the lungs rather than to try and label it correctly.

Rales result from the passage of air through fluid or moisture. They are more pronounced when the child takes a deep breath. Even though the sound may seem continuous, it is actually composed of several discrete sounds, each originating from the rupture of a small bubble. The type of rales is determined by the size of the passageway and the type of exudate the air passes through. They are roughly divided into three categories: fine, medium, and coarse.

Fine rales (sometimes called *crepitant rales*) can be simulated by rubbing a few strands of hair between the thumb and index finger close to the ear or by slowly separating the thumb and index finger after they have been moistened with saliva. The result is a series of fine crackling sounds. Fine rales are most prominent at the end of inspiration and are not cleared by coughing. They occur in the smallest passageways, the alveoli and bronchioles.

Medium rales are not as delicate as fine rales and can be simulated by listening to the "fizz" from recently opened carbonated drinks or by rolling a dry cigar between the fingers. They are prominent earlier during inspiration and occur in the larger passages of the bronchioles and small bronchi.

Coarse rales are relatively loud, coarse, bubbling, gurgling sounds that occur in the large airways of the trachea, bronchi, and smaller bronchi. Often they clear partially during coughing. They are frequently heard in dying patients because the cough reflex is depressed, allowing thick secretions to accumulate in the trachea and major bronchi. Because they are so common when death is imminent, coarse rales are often called "the death rattle."

Rhonchi are sounds produced as air passes through narrowed passageways, regardless of the cause, such as exudate, inflammation, spasm, or tumor. Rhonchi are continuous, since sound is produced as long as air is being forced past an obstruction. Although they are often more prominent during expiration, they are usually present during both phases of respiration. Rhonchi are classified according to pitch as sibilant or sonorous.

Sibilant rhonchi are high pitched, musical, wheezing, or squeaking in character. The wheezing quality is often more pronounced on forced expiration. Sibilant rhonchi are produced in the smaller bronchi and bronchioles.

Sonorous rhonchi are low-pitched and often snoring or moaning in character. They are produced in the large passages of the trachea and bronchi. Like coarse rales, they can be partly cleared by coughing. Some clinicians classify sonorous rhonchi as coarse rales, or vice versa.

The other adventitious sound of importance is the *pleural friction rub,* discussed on p. 261. Its sound can be simulated by cupping one hand to the ear and rubbing a finger of the other hand across the cupped hand. The most common site for a friction rub to be heard is the lower anterolateral chest wall (between the midaxillary and midclavicular lines), the area of greatest thoracic mobility.

Heart

Knowledge of the anatomy and physiology of the normal heart is essential in order to properly evaluate the findings. In addition to the discussion below, the normal circulation of the blood through the heart chambers, major blood vessels, and valves is discussed in Chapter 34.

The heart is situated in the thoracic cavity between the lungs in the mediastinum and above the diaphragm (Fig. 7-41). About two thirds of the heart lies within the left side of the rib cage, with the other third on the right side as it crosses the sternum. Most of the anterior cardiac surface is occupied by the right ventricle. Part of the right atrium and left ventricle also faces anteriorly, whereas the left atrium lies primarily in a posterior position.

The heart is positioned in the thorax like a trapezoid:

Vertically along the right sternal border (RSB) from the second to the fifth rib

Horizontally (long side) from the lower right sternum to the fifth rib at the left midclavicular line (LMCL)

Diagonally from the left sternal border (LSB) at the second rib to the LMCL at the fifth rib

Horizontally (short side) from the RSB and LSB at the second intercostal space (ICS)

The *base* of the heart is actually the top of the trapezoid or the pulmonic and aortic areas. The *apex* is located at the

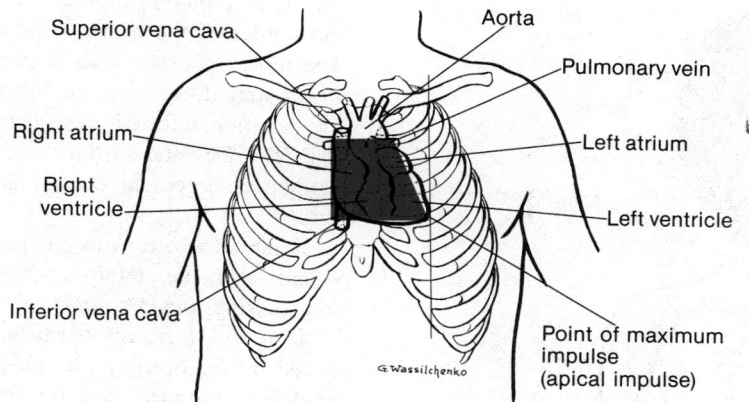

Fig. 7-41. Position of heart within thorax.

left midclavicular line and fifth intercostal space or mitral area. The heart of the infant is more horizontally positioned; therefore the apex is higher (third to fourth intercostal space) and to the left of the midclavicular line (Fig. 7-42). The apical impulse, or *point of maximum impulse* (PMI) (area where the heartbeat is loudest), is normally located at the apex.

Inspection. When the chest is examined, any obvious bulging is noted, especially on the left side, which may indicate cardiac enlargement. This is best done by observing the child sitting in a semi-Fowler position and looking at the anterior chest wall from an angle, comparing both sides of the rib cage to each other. Normally they should be symmetric. In children with thin chest walls, the PMI, or apical pulse, is sometimes apparent as a pulsation. Noting the location of the impulse may give some indication of the size and positioning of the heart, especially if it deviates from the expected apical site.

Since comprehensive evaluation of cardiac function is not limited to the heart, other findings are also considered, such as presence of all pulses (especially the femoral pulses) (Fig. 7-43), distended neck veins, clubbing of the fingers, peripheral cyanosis, edema, blood pressure, and respiratory status.

Palpation. Palpation is useful in determining the size of the heart by feeling for the PMI, which ordinarily corresponds to the apex. The apex is usually at a lower interspace and more lateral in a child with cardiac enlargement. The apex is felt by placing the fingertips or the palmar aspect of the fingers and the hand at the fifth intercostal space and left midclavicular line.

When the PMI is felt for, the presence of vibratory thrills and pericardial friction rubs is noted. *Thrills* are palpable vibrations most commonly produced by the flow of blood from one chamber of the heart to another through a narrowed or abnormal opening, such as a stenotic valve or a septal defect. They are best felt with the ball of the hand (palmar surface at the base of the fingers) and during expiration. Thrills feel similar to the placing of one's hand on a purring cat.

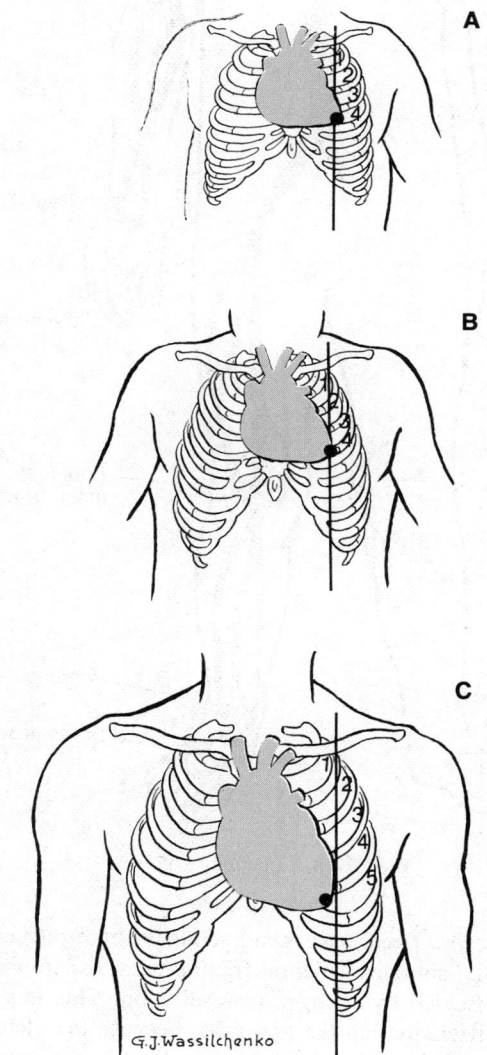

Fig. 7-42. Location of apex of heart. **A,** Infant. **B,** Child. **C,** Adult.

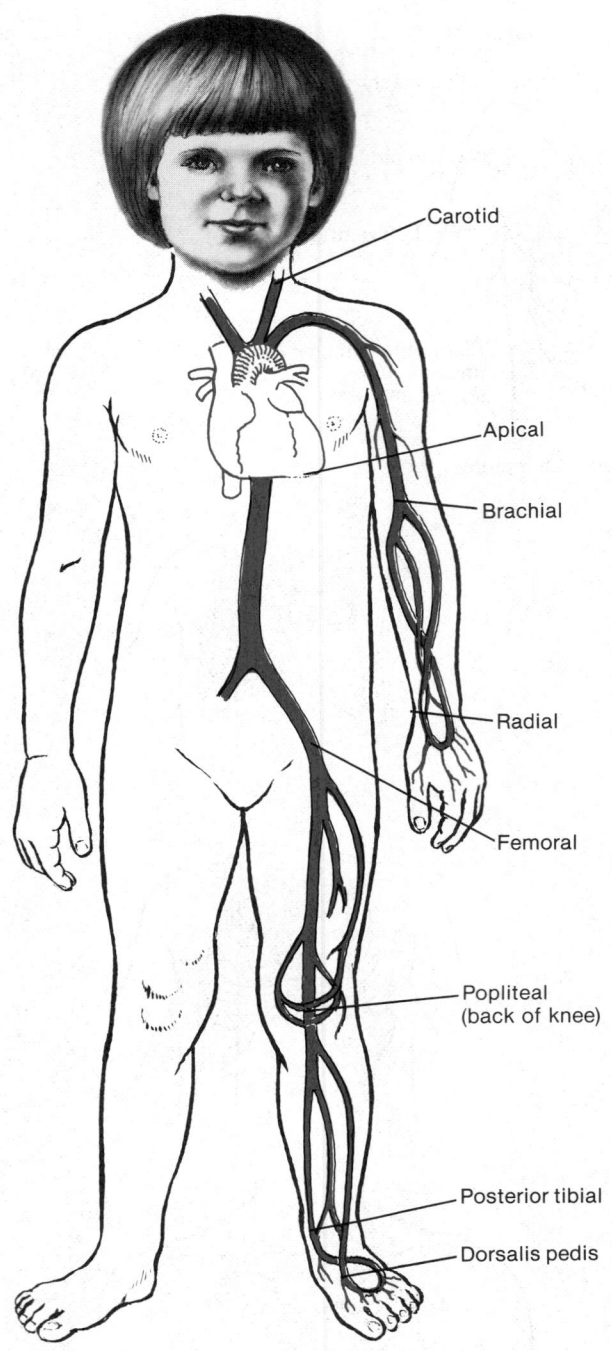

Fig. 7-43. Location of pulses.

Pericardial friction rubs are scratchy, high-pitched grating sounds, similar to pleural friction rubs, except that they are not affected by changes in respiration. This is a useful clue in differentiating the two rubs, because the pleural rub will cease if the child holds his breath, but the pericardial rub will not. Both thrills and rubs are abnormal and must be reported for further evaluation.

Percussion. Percussion is used mainly to determine the size of the heart by outlining its borders. Dullness is normally heard over the left area of the heart and partially over the right, although dullness on the right side descends past the border of the heart to the nearby liver (see Fig. 7-39). The most important area of percussion is dullness along the lower sternal border to the left midclavicular line. This finding is often referred to as *left border of cardiac dullness* (LBCD). Deviation from the expected finding may indicate cardiac enlargement or displacement and warrants further study.

Auscultation. Auscultation involves listening for heart sounds with the stethoscope, similar to the procedure used in assessing breath sounds.

Origin of heart sounds. The heart sounds are produced by the opening and closing of the valves and the vibration of blood against the walls of the heart and vessels. Normally two sounds—S_1 and S_2—are heard, which correspond respectively to the familiar "lub dub" often used to describe the sounds. S_1 is caused by the closure of the *tricuspid* and *mitral* valves (sometimes called the *atrioventricular* valves). Right ventricular contraction follows tricuspid valve closure, and left ventricular contraction follows mitral valve closure. The contractions (systole) occur almost simultaneously, although the mitral valve (left side) closes slightly before the tricuspid valve (right side). Normally this split of the sounds is so close that it is not audible, except occasionally at the apex of the heart.

S_2 is the result of the closure of the *pulmonic* and *aortic* valves (sometimes called *semilunar* valves). Aortic valve closing (left side) occurs slightly before pulmonic valve closing (right side). The flow of blood into the aorta and pulmonary artery occurs following closure of their respective valves. The interval between S_2 and S_1 is diastole, or relaxation, of the heart. Normally the split of the two sounds in S_2 is distinguishable and widens during inspiration, since inspiration prolongs right ventricular filling and delays pulmonic valve closure. "Physiologic splitting" is a significant normal finding that should be elicited. "Fixed splitting," in which the split in S_2 does not change during inspiration, is an important diagnostic sign of atrial septal defect.

The illustration (Fig. 7-44) shows the approximate anatomic position of the valves within the heart chambers and the auscultatory sites. The auscultatory sites, located in the direction of the blood flow through the valves, correspond to the area where the sounds are heard best.

Two other heart sounds—S_3 and S_4—may be produced. S_3 is the result of vibrations produced during ventricular filling. It is normally heard only in some children and young adults, but it is considered abnormal in older individuals. S_4 is caused by the recoil of vibrations between the atria and ventricles following atrial contraction at the end of diastole. It is rarely heard as a normal heart sound and indicates the need for further cardiac evaluation.

Another important category of heart sounds is *murmurs,* which are produced by vibrations within the heart chambers or in the major arteries from the back and forth flow of blood (see p. 1451 for a more detailed discussion). Murmurs are classified as:

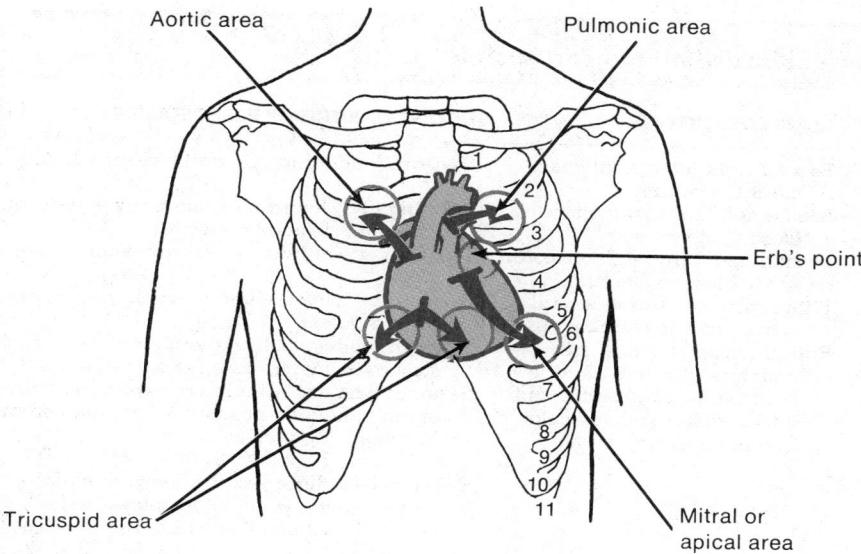

Fig. 7-44. Direction of heart sounds for anatomic valve sites and areas *(circled)* for auscultation.

1. **Innocent,** occurring in individuals with no anatomic or physiologic abnormality
2. **Functional,** found in individuals with no anatomic cardiac defect but with a physiologic abnormality such as anemia
3. **Organic,** occurring in individuals with a cardiac defect with or without a physiologic abnormality

The description and classification of murmurs are skills that require considerable practice and training. In general, the nurse should be able to recognize murmurs as distinct swishing sounds that occur in addition to the normal heart sounds and should record the following:

1. **Location** of the area of the heart where the murmur is heard best
2. **Time** of the occurrence of the murmur within the S_1S_2 cycle
3. **Intensity**—evaluation in relationship to the child's position
4. **Loudness**—estimation

The usual subjective method of grading the loudness or intensity of a murmur is listed in Table 7-8.

Although the nurse consults with a physician whenever a murmur is identified, the following guidelines can be used in distinguishing between innocent and organic murmurs. Innocent murmurs generally are:

1. Systolic, that is, they occur with or after S_1
2. Of short duration and have no transmission to other areas of the heart
3. Grade III or less in intensity and do not increase over time
4. Usually loudest in the pulmonic area (second or third intercostal space along the left sternal border)
5. Variable in relationship to position, respiration, and activity (e.g., audible in the supine position but absent in the sitting position; may be louder with exercise, fever, anxiety, or anemia)
6. Not associated with any physical signs of cardiac disease
7. Usually of a low-pitched, musical, or groaning quality

Table 7-8 Grading of the intensity of heart murmurs

GRADE	DESCRIPTION
I	Very faint, frequently not heard if child sits up
II	Usually readily heard, slightly louder than grade I, audible in all positions
III	Loud, but not accompanied by a thrill
IV	Loud, accompanied by a thrill
V	Loud enough to be heard with the stethoscope barely on the chest, accompanied by a thrill
VI	Loud enough to be heard with the stethoscope not touching the chest; often heard with the human ear close to the chest, accompanied by a thrill

There are a number of other abnormal sounds, such as ejection clicks, snaps, gallops, and hums. It is beyond the scope of this discussion to elaborate on such adventitious heart sounds. The best approach is to become familiar with normal heart sounds and to refer any questionable heart sound to a physician for further evaluation.

Differentiating normal heart sounds. In referring to Fig. 7-44, it is apparent that normally S_1 is louder at the apex of the heart in the mitral and tricuspid area and that S_2 is louder near the base of the heart in the pulmonic and aortic area. Each sound is auscultated by inching down the chest in the sequence outlined in Table 7-9. If there is difficulty in deciding which sound is S_1 or S_2, especially when the rate is rapid, the carotid pulse should be simultaneously palpated with the index and middle finger while the heart sounds are auscultated. S_1 is synchronous with the carotid pulse. In addition to the areas listed in Table 7-9, the following areas should be auscultated for sounds, such as mur-

Table 7-9 Sequence of auscultating heart sounds*

AUSCULTATORY SITE	CHEST LOCATION	CHARACTERISTICS OF HEART SOUNDS
Aortic area	Second right intercostal space close to sternum	S_2 heard louder than S_1; aortic closure heard loudest
Pulmonic area	Second left intercostal space close to sternum	Splitting of S_2 heard best, normally widens on inspiration; pulmonic closure heard best
Erb point	Second and third left intercostal space close to sternum	Frequent site of innocent murmurs and those of aortic or pulmonic origin
Tricuspid area	Fifth right and left intercostal space close to sternum	S_1 heard as louder sound preceding S_2 (S_1 synchronous with carotid pulse)
Mitral or apical area	Fifth intercostal space, left midclavicular line (third to fourth intercostal space and lateral to left midclavicular line in infants)	S_1 heard loudest; splitting of S_1 may be audible because mitral closure is louder than tricuspid closure S_3 heard best at beginning of expiration with child in recumbent or left side-lying position, occurs immediately after S_2, sounds like word "Ken-tuc-ky" S_1 S_2 S_3 S_4 heard best during expiration with child in recumbent position (left sidelying position decreases sound), occurs immediately before S_1, sounds like word "Ten-nes-see" S_4 S_1 S_2

*Use both diaphragm and bell chestpieces when auscultating heart sounds. Bell chestpiece is necessary for low-pitched sounds of murmurs, S_3, and S_4.

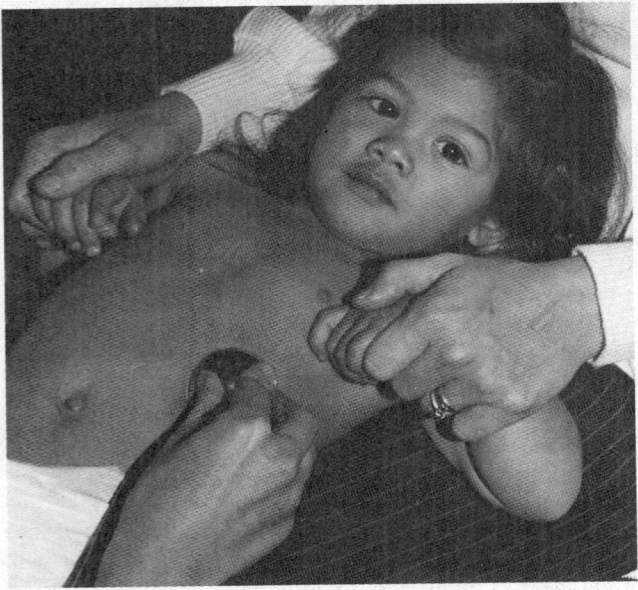

Fig. 7-45. Reclining position in parent's lap for auscultation of heart.

Table 7-10 Various patterns of heart rate or pulse

TERM	DESCRIPTION
Tachycardia	Increased rate
Bradycardia	Decreased rate
Pulsus alternans	Strong beat followed by weak beat
Pulsus bigeminus	Coupled rhythm in which beat is felt in pairs because of premature beat
Pulsus paradoxus	Intensity or force of pulse decreases with inspiration
Sinus arrhythmia	Rate increases with inspiration, decreases with expiration
Water-hammer or Corrigan pulse	Especially forceful beat caused by a very wide pulse pressure (systolic blood pressure minus diastolic blood pressure)
Dicrotic pulse	Double radial pulse for every apical beat
Thready pulse	Rapid, weak pulse that seems to appear and disappear

murs, which may radiate to these regions: the sternoclavicular area above the clavicles and manubrium, along the sternal border, along the left midaxillary line, and below the scapulae.

The heart is auscultated with the child in at least two positions, sitting and reclining (Fig. 7-45). If adventitious sounds are detected, they are further evaluated with the child standing, sitting and leaning forward, and lying on his left side. For example, atrial sounds such as S_4 are heard best with the person in a recumbent position and usually fade if the person sits or stands.

Heart sounds are evaluated for:

1. **Quality,** which should be clear and distinct, not muffled, diffuse, or distant
2. **Intensity,** especially in relation to location or auscultatory site
3. **Rate,** which should be the same as the radial pulse
4. **Rhythm,** which should be regular and even

A particular arrhythmia that occurs normally in many children is *sinus arrhythmia,* in which the heart rate increases with inspiration and decreases with expiration. This can be differentiated from a truly abnormal arrhythmia by

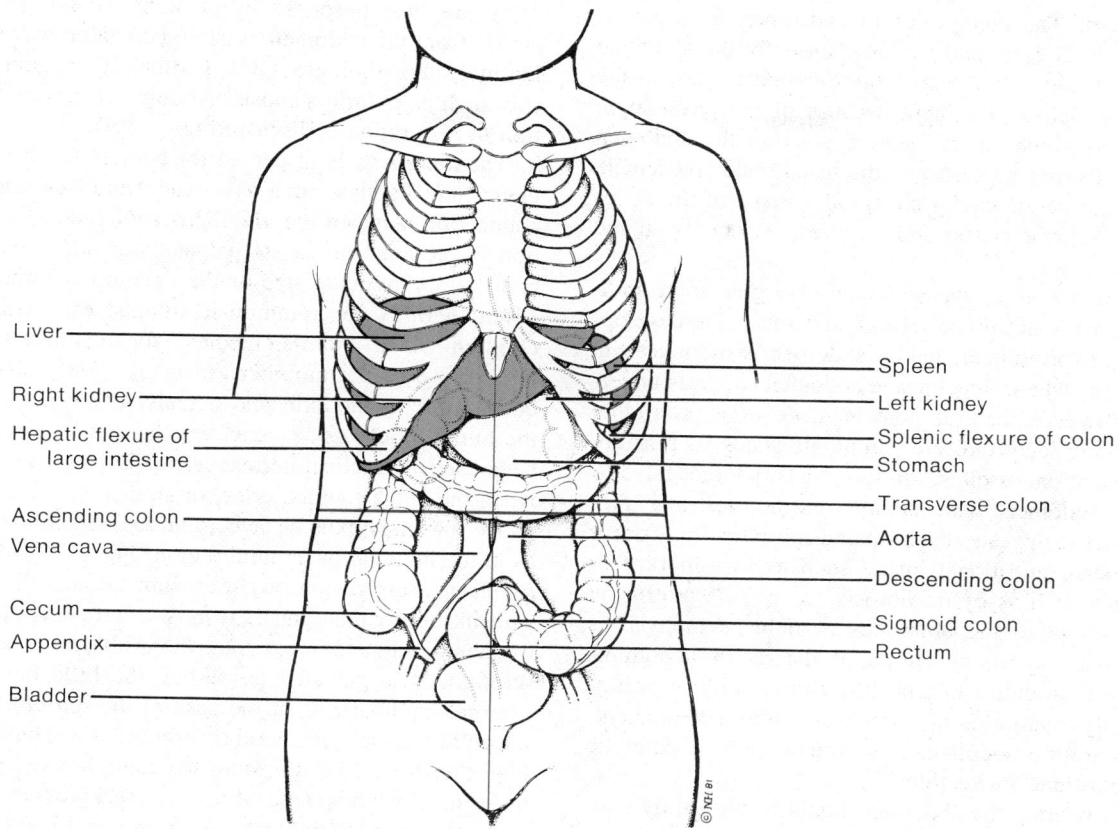

Fig. 7-46. Anatomy of major organs within abdominal cavity. (For illustrative purposes pancreas, small intestine, and gallbladder are not shown.) Color lines divide abdominal cavity into quadrants.

having the child hold his breath. In sinus arrhythmia, cessation of breathing causes the heart rate to remain steady. Table 7-10 lists variations in patterns of heart rate or pulse. Like respiratory rate, heart rate is always evaluated in relation to the child's general physical status. For example, the pulse rate is usually increased by 8 to 10 beats per minute for each degree Fahrenheit elevation in temperature. Athletic children occasionally have lowered heart rates that may even reach rates suggestive of bradycardia (below 60 beats per minute) but that represent a highly developed and efficient heart muscle (see inside front cover for normal heart rates at various ages).

Abdomen

Examination of the abdomen involves the usual four skills, except that the order is altered. Inspection is followed by auscultation, percussion, and palpation last because it may distort the normal abdominal sounds. The sequence of examination changes according to the age and cooperativeness of the child. Frequently all four types of assessment are performed at different times. For example, the nurse may auscultate for bowel sounds following evaluation of heart and lung sounds at the beginning of the examination when the child is quiet. Inspection may occur at any time during the

examination. Percussion usually follows lung percussion, and palpation may be done toward the end of the examination when the child is relaxed and more trusting.

Knowledge of the anatomic placement of the abdominal organs is essential to differentiate normal, expected findings from abnormal ones (Fig. 7-46). The *abdominal cavity* is the portion of the trunk from directly beneath the diaphragm and thoracic cavity to the region of the pelvic cavity. For descriptive purposes the abdominal cavity is divided into four quadrants by drawing a vertical line midway from the sternum to the pubic symphysis and a horizontal line across the abdomen through the umbilicus (Fig. 7-46). This method of division actually includes the pelvic cavity. Each section is designated as follows:

Right upper quadrant (RUQ)
Right lower quadrant (RLQ)
Left upper quadrant (LUQ)
Left lower quadrant (LLQ)

The abdominal cavity contains the major organs of digestion, and the pelvic cavity houses the internal reproductive organs, the lower parts of the digestive tract, and the urinary bladder. However, in infancy the bladder is an abdominal organ.

Inspection. The *contour* of the abdomen is inspected while the child is erect and supine. Normally the abdomen of infants and young children is quite cylindric and, in the erect position, fairly prominent because of the physiologic lordosis of the spine. In the supine position the abdomen appears flat. During adolescence the usual male and female contours of the pelvic cavity change the shape of the abdomen to form characteristic adult curves, especially in the female.

The *size* and *tone* of the abdomen also give some indication of general nutritional status and muscular development. A large, prominent, flabby abdomen is often seen in obese children, whereas a concave abdomen suggests undernutrition. However, careful note is made of a protruding abdomen, which may indicate pathologic states such as abdominal distention, ascites, tumors, or organomegaly. A protuberant abdomen with spindly extremities and flat, wasted buttocks suggests severe malnutrition that may occur from inadequate nutritional intake such as kwashiorkor or from diseases such as cystic fibrosis. A midline protrusion from the xiphoid to the umbilicus or pubic symphysis is usually *diastasis recti,* or failure of the rectus abdominis muscles to join in utero. In a healthy child a midline protrusion is usually a variation of normal muscular development. A tense, boardlike abdomen is a serious sign of paralytic ileus and intestinal obstruction.

The *skin* covering the abdomen should be uniformly taut, without wrinkles or creases. Sometimes silvery, whitish striae are seen, especially if the skin has been stretched as in obesity or with distention resulting from ascites. Any scars, ecchymotic areas, excessive hair distribution, or distended veins are noted.

Movement of the abdomen is observed. In infants and thin children *peristaltic waves* may be visible through the abdominal wall, and they always warrant careful evaluation.

They are best observed by standing at eye level to and across from the abdomen. Visible peristaltic waves most often indicate pathologic states, particularly intestinal obstruction such as pyloric stenosis. Abdominal movement in relation to respiration is discussed on p. 260.

The *umbilicus* is inspected for herniation, discharge, hygiene, and fistulas, such as a patent urachus (an abnormal connection between the umbilicus and bladder). If a herniation is present, the sac is palpated for abdominal contents and the approximate size of the opening is estimated. *Umbilical hernias* are common in infants, especially in black children. Since "home remedies" for treatment such as taping coins over the umbilicus or using "belly binders" may be harmful to the skin and actually delay natural closure, the nurse should ask parents whether such procedures have been used. Umbilical hernias normally protrude and expand when the child coughs, cries, or strains.

Hernias may exist elsewhere on the abdominal wall, such as in the inguinal or femoral region (Fig. 7-47). An *inguinal hernia* is a protrusion of peritoneum through the abdominal wall in the inguinal canal. It most often occurs in males, is frequently bilateral, and may be visible as a mass in the scrotum. It is palpated by sliding the little finger into the external inguinal ring at the base of the scrotum and asking the child to cough. If a hernia is present, it will hit the tip of the finger. If the child is too young to cough, he can try to inflate a balloon, which raises the intra-abdominal pressure sufficiently to demonstrate the presence of an inguinal hernia.

A *femoral hernia,* which occurs more frequently in girls, is felt or seen as a small mass on the anterior surface of the thigh just below the inguinal ligament in the femoral canal (a potential space medial to the femoral artery). Its location is estimated by placing the index finger of the right hand on the child's right femoral pulse (left hand for left pulse) and the middle ring finger flat against the skin toward the mid-

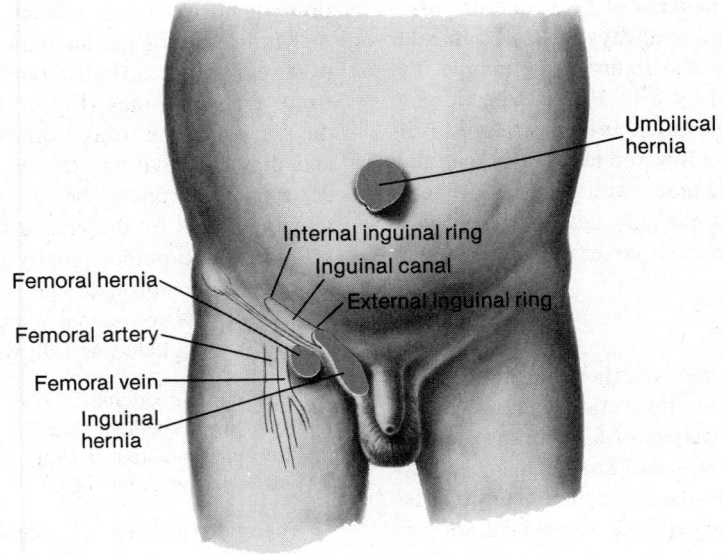

Fig. 7-47. Location of hernias.

line. The ring finger lies over the femoral canal, where the herniation occurs. Palpation of hernias in the pelvic region, particularly inguinal ones, is often part of the examination of genitalia.

Auscultation. Each of the four quadrants should be auscultated using the diaphragm and bell chestpieces. Unlike listening to the heart or lungs, in which the stethoscope rests gently on the skin, to hear bowel sounds the stethoscope must be pressed firmly against the abdominal surface. With the diaphragm chestpiece this usually presents no difficulty, but with the bell chestpiece, especially one with a short cone, the skin may occlude the opening and prevent transmission of sound.

The most important sound to listen for is *peristalsis,* or *bowel sounds,* which sound like short metallic clicks and gurgles. Loud grumbling noises, known as *borborygmi,* are the familiar "stomach growls" usually denoting hunger. Depending on when the child last ate, a sound may be heard every 10 to 30 seconds and its frequency per minute is recorded (e.g., 5 bowel sounds per minute). Bowel sounds may be stimulated by stroking the abdominal surface with a fingernail. Absence of bowel sounds or hyperperistalsis is recorded and reported, since either usually denotes abdominal disorder.

Various other sounds may be heard in the abdominal cavity. Normally the pulsation of the aorta is heard in the epigastrium. Sounds that resemble murmurs (called *bruits),* hums, or rubs are always referred for further evaluation.

Percussion. Percussion of the abdomen is performed in the same manner as percussion of the lungs and heart (see Fig. 7-39). Normally dullness or flatness is heard on the right side at the lower costal margin because of the location of the liver. Tympany is typically heard over the stomach on the left side and in the rest of the abdomen. An unusually tympanitic sound, like the beating of a tight drum, denotes air in the stomach, which is commonly caused by mouth breathing. However, it can also denote a pathologic condition such as low intestinal obstruction or paralytic ileus. Lack of tympany may occur normally when the stomach is full after a meal, but in other situations it may denote the presence of fluid or solid masses. Variation in percussion tones not explained by normal physiologic processes warrants referral for further investigation.

Palpation. Two types of palpation are performed, superficial and deep. In *superficial palpation* the hand is placed lightly against the skin and each quadrant is felt, noting any areas of tenderness, muscle tone, and superficial lesions, such as cysts. Skin turgor, discussed on p. 237, is also tested.

Since superficial palpation is often perceived as tickling, this problem can be minimized by (1) having children "help" with the palpation by placing their hand over the palpating hand, (2) having them place their hand on the abdomen with the fingers spread wide apart and palpating between the fingers, or (3) by distracting them with statements such as "I am trying to feel what you had for lunch." Ad-

monishing the child to stop laughing only draws attention to the sensation and decreases cooperation. Positioning the child supine with the legs flexed at the hips and knees helps relax the abdominal muscles. Other techniques for increasing relaxation and cooperation are discussed on p. 224.

Tenderness or pain anywhere in the abdomen during superficial palpation is always noted. There are two types of abdominal pain:

Visceral, which arises from the viscera or internal organs, such as the intestines, and is usually dull, poorly localized, and difficult for the patient to describe

Somatic, which arises from the walls or linings of the abdominal cavity such as the peritoneum, and is generally sharp, well localized, and more easily described

When assessing abdominal pain, it is important to remember that children often respond with an "all-or-none" reaction—either there is no pain or great pain. At times it is difficult to distinguish pain from fear. One approach is to ask children "how thin" and "how fat" they can make themselves. If this produces discomfort, then some degree of peritoneal irritation is probably present.

A special phenomenon called *rebound tenderness,* or *Blumberg sign,* may be performed if the child complains of abdominal pain. It is produced by pressing firmly over part of the abdomen distal to the area of tenderness. When the pressure is suddenly released, the child feels pain in the original area of tenderness. This response is found only when the peritoneum overlying a diseased organ is inflamed, such as in appendicitis.

Deep palpation is used for palpating organs and large blood vessels and for detecting masses and tenderness not discovered during superficial palpation. If the child complains of abdominal pain, that area of the abdomen is palpated *last.* Normally palpation of the midepigastrium causes pain as pressure is exerted over the aorta, but this should not be confused with visceral or somatic tenderness.

The abdominal organs are palpated by pressing them against the free hand, which is placed on the child's back (see Fig. 7-3). Palpation begins in the lower quadrants and proceeds upward. In this way the edge of an enlarged liver or spleen is not missed. Except for palpating the liver, successful identification of other organs, such as the spleen, kidney, and part of the colon, requires considerable practice with tutored supervision.

The lower edge of the *liver* is sometimes palpable in infants and young children as a superficial mass 1 to 2 cm (⅜ to ¾ inch) below the right costal margin (the distance is sometimes measured in fingerbreadths). If the liver is palpable 3 cm (1¼ inches) or 2 fingerbreadths below the costal margin, it is considered enlarged and this finding is referred to a physician. Normally the liver descends during inspiration as the diaphragm moves downward. This downward displacement should not be mistaken for a sign of hepatomegaly. In older children the liver frequently is not palpable.

The *spleen* is palpated by feeling it between the hand

placed against the back and the one palpating the left upper quadrant. The spleen is much smaller than the liver and positioned behind the fundus of the stomach. The tip of the spleen is normally felt during inspiration as it descends within the abdominal cavity. It is sometimes palpable 1 to 2 cm below the left costal margin in infants and young children. A spleen that is readily palpated more than 2 cm below the right costal margin is enlarged and is always reported for further medical investigation.

Other anatomic structures that are sometimes palpable in children include the kidney, bladder, cecum, and sigmoid colon. Palpation of the *kidney,* which is discussed under assessment of the neonate (p. 311), is quite difficult because of its deep position within the abdominal cavity. Normally only the tip of the right kidney is palpable because of its lower placement within the cavity and is best felt during inspiration. The *bladder* may be palpated slightly above the pubic symphysis in infants and young children. It descends deeper into the pelvic cavity during adolescence, when it is not palpable except if distended. Occasionally parts of the colon are palpable. The *cecum* is a soft, gas-filled mass in the right lower quadrant. The *sigmoid colon* is felt as a sausage-shaped mass that is freely movable over the pelvic brim in the left lower quadrant and is normally tender.

Although most of these structures are not routinely felt, awareness of their relative location and characteristics is necessary to avoid mistaking them for abnormal masses. The most common palpable mass in children is feces, which may be associated with pain in the right lower quadrant from a distended cecum. In sexually active pubescent females a palpable mass in the lower abdomen may be a pregnant uterus. Any questionable mass is referred to a physician before it is ruled out as benign.

During palpation of the abdomen the *femoral pulses* are felt by placing the tips of two or three fingers (index, middle, and/or ring) along the inguinal ligament about midway between the iliac crest and pubic symphysis. Both pulses are felt simultaneously to make certain that they are equal and strong (Fig. 7-48). Absence of femoral pulses is a significant sign of coarctation of the aorta.

When the abdomen is examined, *abdominal reflexes* are tested by scratching the skin toward the umbilicus. The normal response is for the umbilicus to move toward the stimulus or quadrant that was stroked. Normally the response may be absent in children under 1 year of age. Asymmetry or absence of response is noted and reported, although there is great variability in correctly eliciting a response.

Genitalia

Examination of genitalia conveniently follows assessment of the abdomen while the child is still supine. In adolescents, inspection of the genitalia may be left to the end of the examination. This part of the physical appraisal is usually uneventful for infants or toddlers but begins to be anxiety-producing for older preschoolers, school-age children, and adolescents, mainly because of their concern for modesty and privacy. The best approach is to examine the genitalia

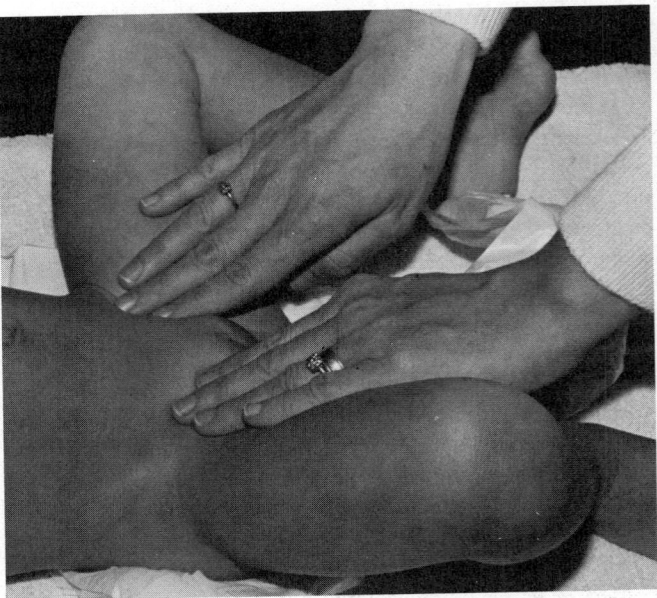

Fig. 7-48. Palpating for femoral pulses.

quickly, placing no more emphasis on this part of the assessment than on any other segment. It helps to relieve children's and parents' anxiety by stating the results of the findings, for example, "Everything looks fine here." If it is necessary to ask questions about deviations, such as about discharge or difficulty in urinating, consideration for the child's privacy is observed by covering the lower abdomen with the gown or underpants.

In examining the genitalia of adolescents it is sometimes advisable to wear gloves to guard against contamination from venereal disease. It might be helpful for the adolescent to know that this also prevents skin-to-skin contact. Each step of the examination is explained before it is performed, such as checking the scrotum for an inguinal hernia (discussed on p. 270) and the reason for asking the boy to cough. If the male adolescent does have an erection during the examination, the nurse assures him that this is a normal involuntary physiologic response to touch and proceeds with the remainder of the examination.

The examination of female genitalia is limited to inspection and palpation of external structures. If a vaginal examination is required, an appropriate referral is made unless the nurse is qualified to perform the procedure. Guidelines for performing a pelvic examination are outlined by Cavanaugh (1982) and NAACOG (1979). The adolescent female has the same needs for preparation, reassurance, and privacy as the male. For both sexes this part of the examination is an excellent time for eliciting questions of concern about body functioning or sexual activity. The nurse can also use this opportunity to increase or reinforce the child's knowledge of reproductive anatomy by naming each body part and explaining its function. For example, many females are unaware of the existence of two openings within the vulva. They assume that the passage of urine occurs from the vagina.

One of the most important factors in successfully performing the examination is that the nurse recognize any personal fears or anxieties and deal with them. Transfer of anxiety, especially in the beginning practitioner, can be the greatest deterrent to lessening the child's concern or fear.

Male genitalia. The external appearance of the glans and shaft of the penis, the prepuce, the urethral meatus, and the scrotum is noted (Fig. 7-49). The size of the *penis* is generally small in infants and young boys, until puberty, when it begins to increase in both length and width. A very small penis may actually be an enlarged clitoris in a genetically female child. In an obese child the penis often looks abnormally small because of the folds of skin partially covering it at the base. An enlarged penis in a young child may denote precocious puberty. One should be familiar with normal pubertal growth of the external male genitalia in order to compare the findings with the expected sequence of maturation (see p. 808).

The *glans* (head of the penis) and *shaft* (portion between the perineum and prepuce) are examined for signs of swelling, skin lesions, inflammation, or other irregularities. Any of these signs may denote underlying disorders. A *syphilitic chancre* appears as an oval or round, dark red, painless erosion or ulcer with an indurated base. Caution should be exercised in examining such lesions without gloves. Warts on the penis, perineum, or anal area, called *condylomata acuminata,* are infectious lesions, and like a chancre, should alert the nurse to the possibility of sexual abuse in young children (Seidel, Zonana, and Totten, 1979).

If the child is uncircumcised, the *prepuce* or foreskin covering the glans of the penis is inspected. In infants the prepuce is normally tight for the first several months of life and is not retracted for examination, since accidental tearing of the thin membrane may cause scarring and adhesion formation later on. In children the foreskin is gently retracted for examination of the glans and the meatus and then replaced. A tight foreskin that cannot be retracted is called *phimosis.*

The *urethral meatus* is carefully inspected for location and evidence of discharge. Normally it is centered at the tip of the shaft. If it opens on the ventral or underneath side of the glans or shaft, it is called *hypospadias.* An opening on the dorsal or top part of the penis is termed *epispadias.* If the urethral meatus opens into the perineum at the junction of the scrotum, the nurse carefully inspects for signs suggestive of ambiguous genitalia. If feasible during inspection, the strength and direction of the urinary stream during micturition are noted.

The size of the *scrotum* is noted. In infants the scrota appear large in relation to the rest of the genitalia. Normally, the left scrotum hangs lower than the right and both hang freely from the perineum behind the penis. Scrota that are small, close to the perineum, or with evidence of any midline separation, which could be enlarged labia, are noted. An abnormally large scrotal sac may indicate an inguinal hernia, a hydrocele, or inflammation of the internal reproductive structures, particularly the epididymis.

The skin of the scrotum is usually loose and highly rugated (wrinkled). During early adolescence the skin normally becomes redder and coarser. In dark-skinned children the scrota are more deeply pigmented. A smooth, shiny surface with pigmentation that varies markedly from the surrounding skin should be reported.

Hair distribution is also noted. Normally before puberty

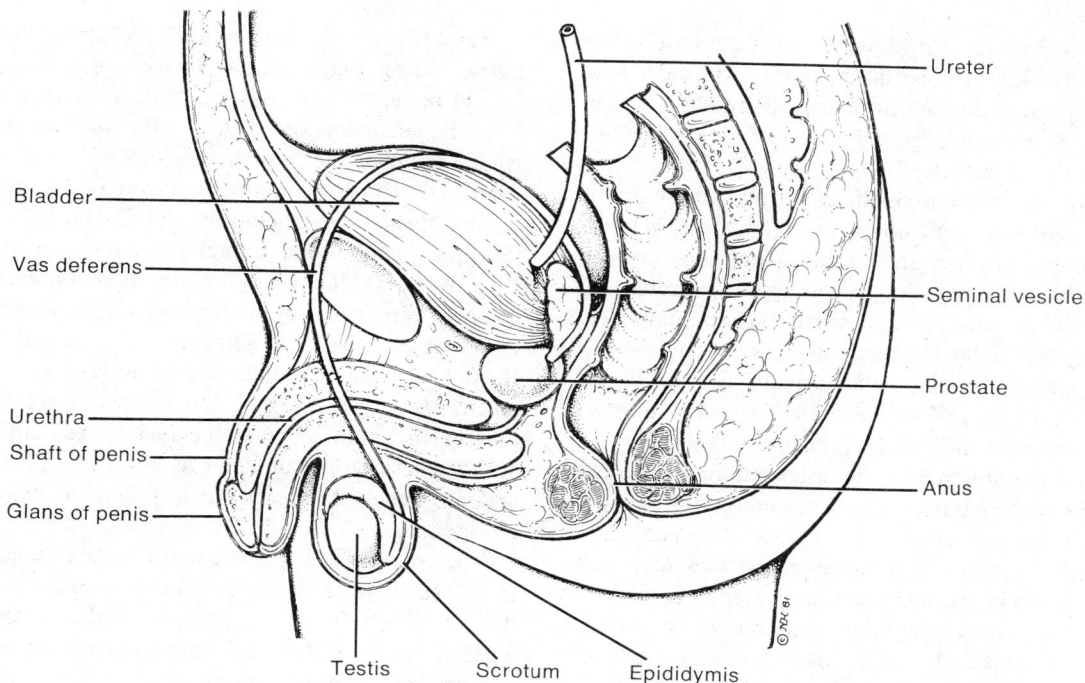

Fig. 7-49. Major structures of genitalia in circumcised prepubertal male.

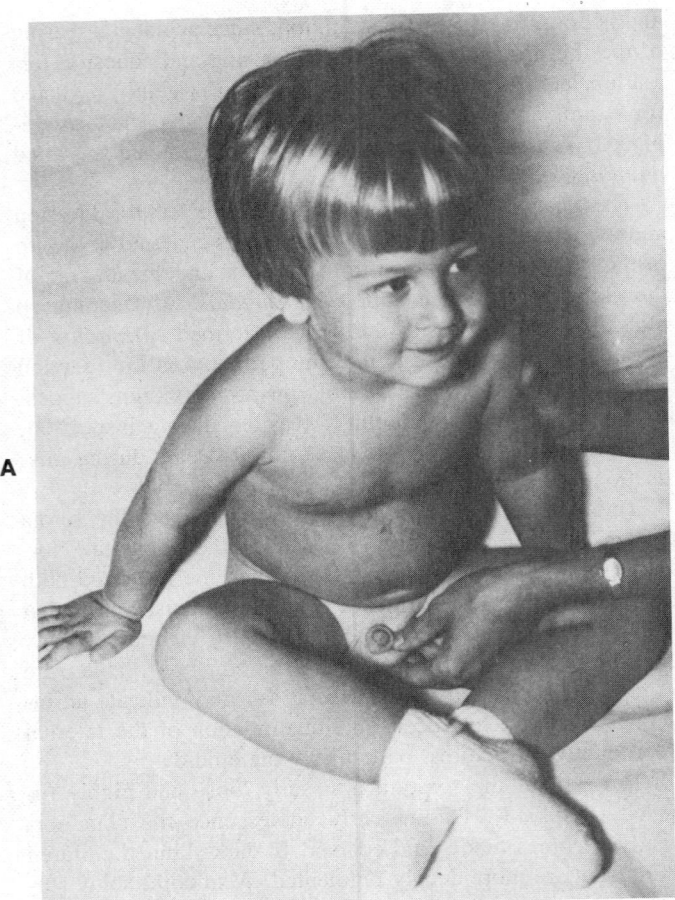

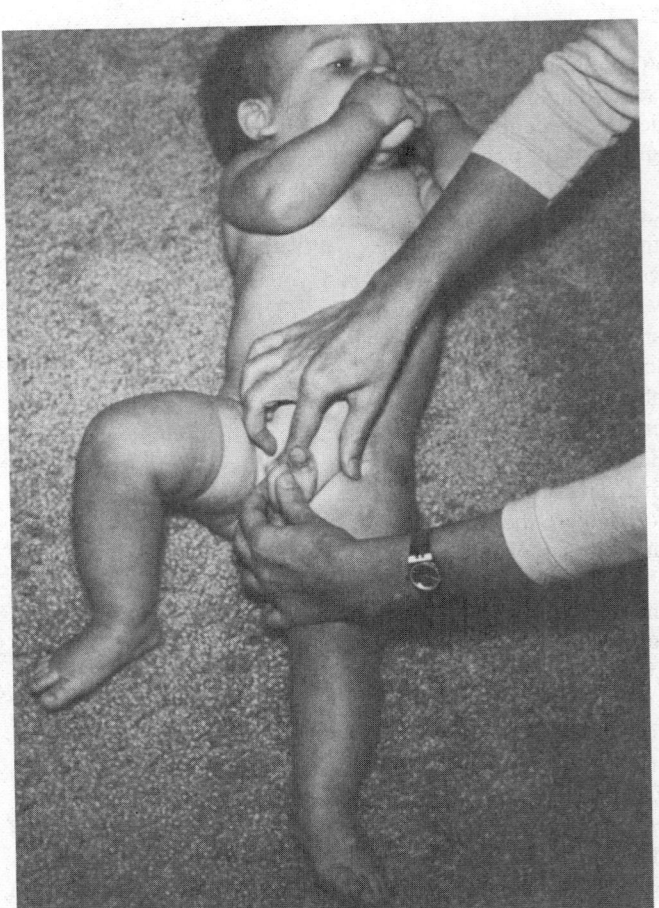

Fig. 7-50. A, Preventing cremasteric reflex by having child sit in "tailor" position. **B,** Blocking inguinal canal during palpation of scrotum for descended testes.

no pubic hair is present. Soft downy hair at the base of the penis is an early sign of pubertal maturation. In older adolescents the typical male pattern of hair distribution is usually triangular as it extends from the base of the penis along the midline to the umbilicus.

Palpation of the scrotum includes identification of the testes, epididymis, spermatic cords, and, if present, inguinal hernias. The two *testes* are felt as small ovoid bodies, about 1.5 to 2 cm (½ to ¾ inch) long—one in each scrotal sac. They do not enlarge until puberty, when they approximately double in size. Normally the testes descend during the last trimester of uterine development, usually by the eighth month of gestation. Therefore undescended testes *(cryptorchidism)* is a common finding in premature infants.

Palpating for the presence of the testes requires an understanding of the normal anatomy and physiology of the coverings of the testes and scrotal sac. The scrotum and testes are surrounded by fascia called the *cremaster muscle*, which attaches to a point in the abdomen and extends downward along the inner surface of the thigh. The muscle or *cremasteric reflex* is stimulated by cold, touch, emotional excitement, or exercise. It causes the skin of the scrotum to shrink and pulls the testes higher into the pelvic cavity.

Several measures are useful in preventing the cremasteric reflex during palpation of the scrotum. First, the hands should be warm, not cold. Second, if old enough, the child is examined while sitting in a tailor or "Indian" position, which stretches the muscle, preventing its contraction (Fig. 7-50, *A*). Third, the normal pathway of ascent of the testes can be blocked by placing the thumb and index finger over the upper part of the scrotal sac along the inguinal canal (Fig. 7-50, *B*). If there is any question concerning the existence of two testes, the index and middle fingers are placed in a scissors fashion to separate the right and left scrotum. If after using these techniques the testes have not been palpated, the inguinal canal and perineum are felt to locate masses that may be undescended testes. Although undescended testes may descend at any time during childhood and are checked at each visit, failure to palpate testes is reported.

The *epididymis* is palpated as a vertical ridge of soft nodular tissue behind the testes. The *spermatic cord* consists of the blood vessels, nerves, lymphatic glands, and the ductus deferens of the testes. Any masses, swelling, or tenderness is noted and reported.

Female genitalia. A convenient position for examination of the genitalia involves placing the young child supine on the examining table or in a semireclining position on the parent's lap with the feet supported on the nurse's knees as the nurse sits facing the child. The child's attention is diverted from the examination by instructing her to try to keep the soles of her feet pressed against each other. The labia majora (see below) are separated with the thumb and index finger and retracted outward in order to expose the labia minora, urethral meatus, and vaginal orifice. The child can use her hands "to help" (Fig. 7-51).

The genitalia are inspected for size and location of the structures of the *vulva* or *pudendum* (area of the external genital organs) (Fig. 7-52). The *mons pubis* is a pad of adipose tissue over the symphysis pubis. At puberty the mons is covered with hair, which extends along the labia. The

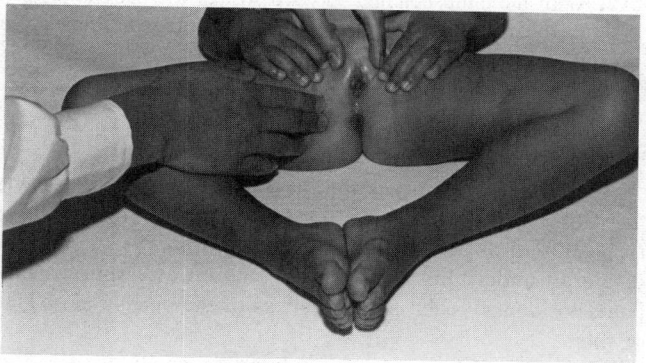

Fig. 7-51. Position for examining genitalia in female child.

usual pattern of female *hair distribution* is an inverted triangle. Any extension of hair along the linea alba to the umbilicus is noted. The appearance of soft downy hair along the labia majora is an early sign of sexual maturation.

The *clitoris* is an erectile organ located at the anterior end of the labia minora. It is covered by a small flap of skin, the *prepuce*. Its size is noted because, although variable, a large protruding clitoris may represent an underdeveloped phallus.

The *labia majora* are two thick folds of skin running posteriorly from the mons to the posterior commissure of the vagina. Internal to the labia majora are two folds of skin called the *labia minora*. Although the labia minora are prominent in the newborn, they gradually atrophy and are almost invisible until their enlargement during puberty.

The inner surface of the labia should be pink and moist. Any skin lesions such as chancres, blisters, or warts (condylomata acuminata) are noted and investigated since they may be sexually transmitted. The size of the labia and any evidence of fusion, which may suggest male scrota, are noted. Normally no masses are palpable within the labia. However, in genitalia of an ambiguous nature, palpable masses may represent descended testes.

The urethral meatus and vaginal orifice are located in the space between the labia, the *vestibule*. The *urethral meatus* is located posterior to the clitoris and is surrounded by Skene glands and ducts. Although not a prominent structure, the meatus can be more readily identified by wiping downward along the vestibule toward the perineum. It will appear as a small V-shaped slit. Its location is noted, espe-

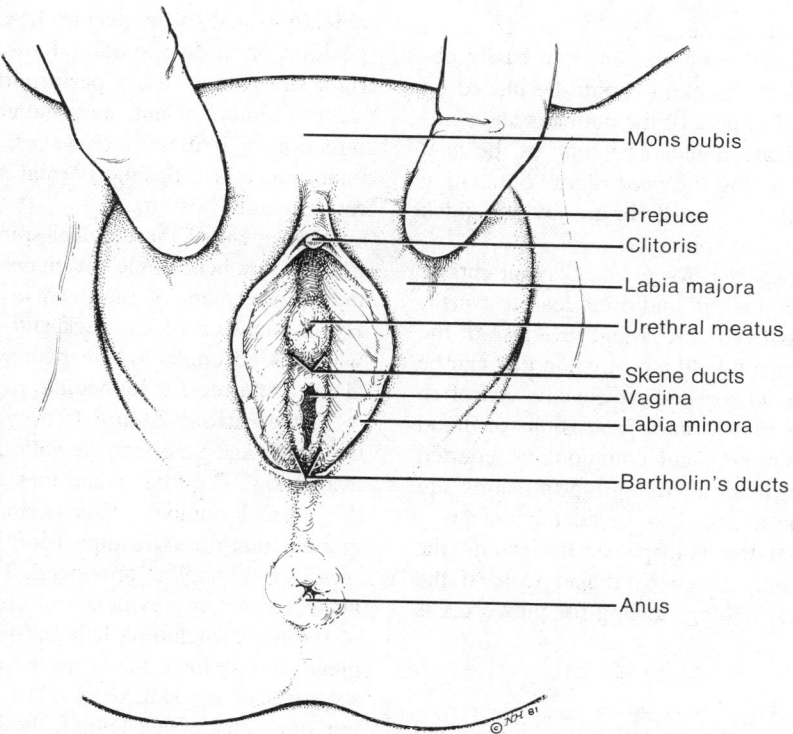

Fig. 7-52. External structures of genitalia in prepubertal female. Labia are spread to reveal deep structures.

cially if it opens from the clitoris or inside the vagina. The glands, which are common sites of cysts and venereal lesions, are gently palpated.

The *vaginal orifice* is located posterior to the urethral meatus. Its appearance is variable depending on individual anatomy and sexual activity. Ordinarily examination of the vagina is limited to inspection. However, in the presence of other signs suggestive of ambiguous genitalia, the nurse may decide to refer or perform a manual examination to determine if a vaginal vault exists.

In virgins a thin crescent-shaped or circular membrane, called the *hymen*, may cover part of the vaginal opening. In some instances, it completely occludes the orifice. After rupture, small rounded pieces of tissue called *caruncles* remain. Although an imperforate hymen denotes lack of penile intercourse, a perforate one does not necessarily indicate such activity.

Surrounding the vaginal opening are *Bartholin glands*, which secrete a clear, mucoid fluid into the vagina for lubrication during intercourse. The ducts are palpated for cysts. The discharge from the vagina is also noted, which is usually clear or whitish. Variations in the appearance, such as white and cheesy or yellow-greenish, and odor may indicate infection. Sudden, foul-smelling, and profuse discharge may suggest a foreign body inside the vaginal vault. The presence of feces or urine from the vagina usually suggests a fistula from the rectum or urethra. Any swelling, inflammation, or prolapsed area around the vagina is noted. Any such findings are referred for further gynecologic evaluation.

Anus

Following examination of the genitalia, one can easily observe the anal area, although the child should be placed on the abdomen. The general firmness of the buttocks and symmetry of the gluteal folds are noted. The tone of the anal sphincter is assessed by eliciting the *anal reflex*. Scratching or gently pricking the anal area results in an obvious quick contraction of the external anal sphincter.

The sphincter area is inspected for *fissures*, small cuts or tears in the mucosa that are painful and often lead to constipation as the child refrains from defecating; *prolapse* of the rectum, which is evident as a tubelike protrusion that can be retracted manually; *polyps*, cherry-red protrusions that often cause bleeding; and *hemorrhoids*, dark protrusions of blood vessels. Each of these, although not common, is reported for further medical investigation. Benign protrusions are small *mucosal tabs* of skin attached to the anal sphincter.

The skin around the anal area is inspected for lesions, the most common of which are caused by diaper rash. If the child complains of perianal itching, testing for pinworms is recommended.

Back and Extremities

While the child is prone, the spine, extremities, joints, and muscles are inspected. However, they are also observed with the child sitting and standing.

Spine. The general *curvature* of the spine is noted. Normally the back of a newborn is rounded or C-shaped from the thoracic and pelvic curves. The development of the cervical and lumbar curves approximates development of various motor skills, such as cervical curvature with head control, and gives the older child the typical double-S curve (see Fig. 4-5).

Marked curvatures in posture are abnormal (see Fig. 39-7). *Scoliosis,* lateral curvature of the spine, is an important childhood problem, especially in females. Although scoliosis may be palpated as one feels along the spine and notes a sideways displacement, more objective tests include:

1. With the child standing erect, clothed only in underpants (and bra if older girl), observe from behind, noting asymmetry of the shoulders and hips.
2. With the child bending forward so that the back is parallel to the floor, observe from the side, noting asymmetry or prominence of the rib cage.

A slight limp, a crooked hemline, or complaints of a sore back are other signs and symptoms of scoliosis.

The *back,* especially along the spine, is inspected for any tufts of hair, dimples, or discoloration. A small dimple (usually with a tuft of hair) called a *pilonidal cyst* may indicate an underlying spina bifida occulta. The spine is palpated to identify each spiny process of the vertebrae or lack of them.

Mobility of the vertebral column is easily assessed in most children because of their propensity for constant motion during the examination. However, mobility can be specifically tested for by asking the child to sit up from a prone position or to do a modified sit-up exercise. Maintaining a rigid straightness when performing these maneuvers is considered abnormal and may indicate central nervous system infection or irritation. However, some individuals who are unable to relax, despite normal skeletal function, may also retain a rigid posture.

Movement of the cervical spine is an important diagnostic sign for neurologic problems, such as meningitis. Normally movement of the head in all directions is effortless. Hyperextension of the neck and spine, called *opisthotonos*, which is accompanied by pain when the head is flexed, is always referred for immediate medical evaluation.

Extremities. Each extremity is inspected for symmetry of length and size; any deviation is referred for orthopedic evaluation. The fingers and toes are counted to be certain of the normal number. This normalcy is so often taken for granted that an extra digit (*polydactyly*) or fusion of digits (*syndactyly*) may go unnoticed. The fingers and toes are also inspected for any evidence of clubbing, cyanosis, disorders of the nails (including habitual nail biting), and general hygiene. These have been discussed in more detail under assessment of the skin (p. 235). If there is any doubt regarding symmetry of leg length, the legs are measured from the anterior iliac spine (felt as the point of the pelvis) to the medial malleolus (ankle bone).

The arms and legs are inspected for *temperature, color, tenderness,* and *masses*. Temperature in each extremity should be equal, although the feet may normally be colder than the hands. Coolness denotes decreased blood circulation, such as from occlusion of a blood vessel, whereas heat denotes increased blood flow, such as an infection or inflammation. Enlargement of bone, such as from swelling, with redness, heat, and tenderness needs further evaluation. It may signify trauma, infection, or an underlying disease process (e.g., sickle cell anemia). A solid mass palpable along a bone with or without pain may be a tumor. Although not all masses are malignant, they must be evaluated further.

Since accidental fractures are common in children, the nurse should be familiar with assessing orthopedic injuries. The five main criteria are (1) pain, (2) pulse, (3) paresthesia (abnormal sensation, such as numbness), (4) pallor, and (5) paralysis. Palpation over a possible fractured bone may elicit crepitation, a grating sound produced by movement of the broken ends of the bone.

The *shape* of bones is assessed. Several variations of bone shape may be observed in children. Although many of them cause parents concern, most are benign and require no treatment. *Bowleg,* or *genu varum,* is lateral bowing of the tibia. It is clinically present when the child stands with the medial malleoli (rounded prominence on either side of the ankle) in apposition and the space between the knees is greater than approximately 5 cm (2 inches) (Fig. 7-53). Toddlers are usually bowlegged after beginning to walk until all their lower back and leg muscles are well developed. Unilateral or asymmetric bowlegs that are present beyond the age of 2 to 3 years, particularly in black children, may represent pathologic conditions requiring further investigation.

Knock-knee, or *genu valgum,* appears as the opposite of bowleg, in that the knees are close together but the feet are

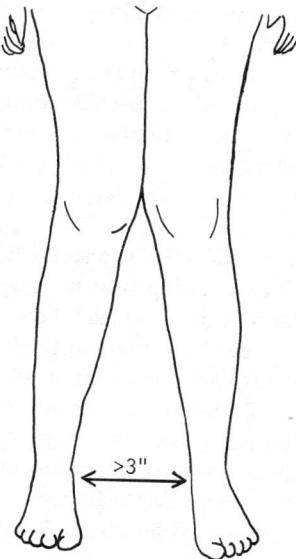

Fig. 7-54. Knock-knee.

spread apart. It is determined clinically by using the same method as for genu varum but by measuring the distance between the malleoli, which normally should be less than 7.5 cm (3 inches) (Fig. 7-54). Knock-knee is normally present in children from about 2 to 7 years of age. Knock-knee that is excessive (as measured roentgenographically by the tibiofemoral angle), asymmetric, accompanied by shortened stature, or evident in a child nearing puberty requires further evaluation (McDade, 1977).

The *feet* are observed for arch development and correct gait. Infants' and toddlers' feet appear flat because the foot is normally wide and the arch is covered by a fat pad. Development of the arch occurs naturally from the action of walking. Normally at birth the feet are held in a valgus (outward) or varus (inward) position. To determine whether a foot deformity at birth is the result of intrauterine position or development, the outer, then inner, side of the sole is scratched. If the foot position is self-correctable, it will assume a right angle to the leg.

Gait is assessed by having the child walk and estimating the angle of gait, which is the angle between the axis of the foot (imaginary line drawn through center of foot) and the line of progression (Fig. 7-55). Normally the feet turn outward less than 30 degrees and inward less than 10 degrees (Staheli, 1977). Variations in foot positions are described in Table 11-2.

Toddlers have a "toddling" or broad-based gait, which facilitates walking by lowering the center of gravity. As the child reaches preschool age, the legs are brought closer to-

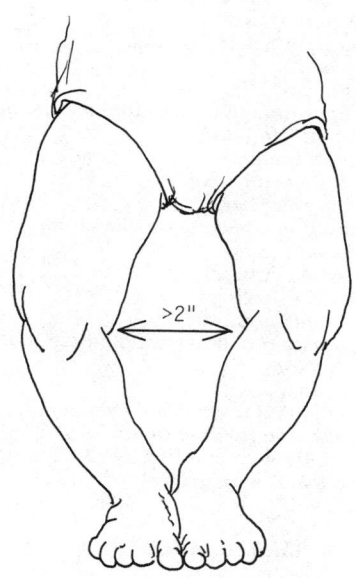

Fig. 7-53. Bowleg.

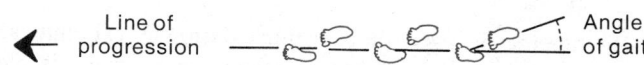

Fig. 7-55. Measurement of angle of gait.

gether. By school age the walking posture is much more graceful and balanced.

The most common gait problem in young children is pigeon toe or toeing in, which usually results from torsional deformities, such as internal tibial torsion (abnormal rotation or bowing of the tibia). Tests for tibial torsion include measuring the thigh-foot angle, which requires considerable practice for accuracy.

The *plantar* or *grasp reflex* is tested while examining the feet. It is elicited by exerting firm but gentle pressure with the tip of the thumb against the lateral sole of the foot from the heel upward to the little toe and then across to the big toe. The normal response in children who are walking is flexion of the toes. *Babinski sign,* dorsiflexion of the big toe and fanning of the other toes, is normal during infancy but abnormal after about 1 year or when locomotion begins (see Fig. 8-10, *B*). A positive Babinski sign after age 1 year is an indication of spinal cord lesions and requires further neurologic examination.

Joints. The joints are evaluated for *range of motion.* Normally this requires no specific testing if the nurse has been observant of the child's movements during the examination. However, the hips should be routinely investigated in infants for congenital dislocation. Signs of congenital hip dislocation are discussed on p. 452. Any evidence of joint immobility or hyperflexibility is reported.

The joints are routinely palpated for *heat, tenderness,* and *swelling.* These signs, as well as redness over the joint, may indicate infection or any of the collagen diseases. Such findings warrant further investigation.

Muscles. Much of the examination of the spine, extremities, and joints indicates muscular development, the shape and contour of the body both in a relaxed and tensed state. If there is asymmetry of development, the circumference of the muscle mass is measured with a tape measure and compared to the measurement of the contralateral muscle. Marked disparity between the two sizes is reported.

Development is closely associated with *tone* or the balance between the muscle mass and nervous stimulation. Tone is estimated by grasping the muscle and feeling its firmness when it is relaxed and contracted. A common site for testing tone is the biceps muscle of the arm. Children usually willingly "make a muscle" by clenching their fist.

Strength is estimated by having the child use an extremity to push or pull against resistance, as in the following example:

Arm strength: Child holds his arms outstretched in front of him and tries to raise the arms while downward pressure is applied.

Hand strength: Child shakes hands with nurse and squeezes one or two fingers of the nurse's hand.

Leg strength: Child sits on a table or chair with the legs dangling and tries to raise the legs while downward pressure is applied.

Symmetry of strength is estimated in the extremities, hands, and fingers. Evidence of paresis or weakness is reported.

Neurologic Assessment

The assessment of the nervous system is the broadest and most diverse, since every human function, both physical and emotional, is controlled by neurologic impulses. This discussion focuses primarily on a general appraisal of behavior, cognitive-perceptual development, sensory and cerebellar functioning, deep tendon reflexes, the cranial nerves, and "soft" signs.

Assessment of neurologic function requires the use of a few additional tools. A reflex hammer, which has a small rounded rubber head, is used to test deep tendon reflexes. A pin and cotton are useful when testing sensory function. For the assessment of the cranial nerves, some flavors to taste and some odors to smell are necessary, although nothing elaborate is required (see Table 7-11). Motor development is best evaluated with screening tests, such as the Denver Developmental Screening Test (DDST).

Behavior. There is no special testing for behavior. Rather, it is an overall impression of the child's personality, affect, level of activity, social interaction, and attention span. Some aspects of assessing behavior are discussed elsewhere (see p. 235). Difficulties at home, at school, and in social situations suggest the need for additional psychologic assessment.

Another approach toward assessing behavior is the use of a behavioral checklist (see box). It is designed for children 7 to 11 years old and focuses on five major areas: mood, play, school, friends, and family relations. Parents are asked these questions as part of the history. Scoring is based

---

BEHAVIORAL CHECKLIST

1. Prefers to play alone
2. Gets hurt in major accidents
3. Does he/she ever play with fire
4. Has difficulties with teachers
5. Gets poor grades in school
6. Is absent from school
7. Becomes angry easily
8. Daydreams
9. Feels unhappy
10. Acts younger than other children his/her age
11. Does not listen to parents
12. Does not tell the truth
13. Unsure of himself/herself
14. Has trouble sleeping
15. Seems afraid of someone or something
16. Is nervous and jumpy
17. Has a nervous habit
18. Does not show feelings
19. Fights with other children
20. Is understanding of other people's feelings
21. Refuses to share
22. Shows jealousy
23. Takes things that are not his/hers
24. Blames others for his/her troubles
25. Prefers to play with children not his/her age
26. Gets along well with grown-ups
27. Teases others

From Jellinek, M., Evans, N., and Knight, R.: J. Pediatr. **94**(1):156-158, 1979.

on a point system of 0 for "never," 1 for "sometimes," and 2 for "often." Because of the wording in items 20 and 26, the scoring is reversed. A score higher than 22 suggests the need for psychiatric evaluation and a score between 15 and 22 warrants closer observation of the child (Jellinek, Evans, and Knight, 1979).

State of consciousness is a specific area for behavior under neurologic assessment. Hyperirritability, hyporeactivity, lethargy, delirium, stupor, or coma requires immediate referral. Levels of consciousness are described on p. 1624. The nurse should always question parents' perceptions of change in behavior, which usually precedes an altered level of consciousness.

Cognitive-perceptual development. Cognitive-perceptual development is best assessed using a formal screening test such as the DDST. Adaptive and speech-comprehension development are significant indicators of intellectual functioning. If intellectual or perceptual impairment is suspected or learning difficulties exist, the child should be referred to an appropriate developmental study team for further evaluation. "Soft" signs that should suggest minimum or borderline brain dysfunction are discussed at the conclusion of assessment of the neurologic system (p. 283).

Motor functioning. Motor ability primarily involves assessment of voluntary muscle contraction and acquisition of age-specific developmental milestones for gross and fine motor skills (see DDST, p. 283). One of the most important milestones in motor development is head control. Since development proceeds in the cephalocaudal direction, head lag suggests early brain damage. Head control is usually acquired by 4 months of age, although even the newborn demonstrates some head control (see p. 309). Inability to hold the head erect and in midline while sitting or standing past 6 months of age requires immediate investigation.

Handedness is also observed. Infants and toddlers may show preference for one hand, but they usually do not display marked preference until the preschool years. Sole use of one hand may indicate paresis on the opposite side. Failure to demonstrate handedness by a school-age child suggests failure of the brain to develop dominance and is a frequent finding in children with minimum brain damage.

Sensory functioning. Sensory functioning is mainly assessed in terms of the sensory cranial nerves, in particular, vision and hearing and peripheral sensation. This discussion is devoted to testing of peripheral sensation. Testing of the cranial nerves is discussed on p. 282, and vision and auditory testing are on pp. 245 and 254, respectively.

Peripheral sensation. With children old enough to cooperate, *sensory discrimination* is assessed by performing the following with the child's eyes closed:

1. Touch the skin with a pin or piece of cotton and ask the child to describe the different sensations.
2. Place a cold or warm object on the skin (the rubber and metal heads of the reflex hammer work well) and have the child differentiate between them.
3. Touch different parts of the body simultaneously and see if the child can localize both points.

Because these tests are similar to playing a game, they may be performed at the beginning of the examination in order to decrease the child's anxiety and foster his trust. Decreased sensation or hyperesthesia (excessive sensation) are abnormal and must be referred for further neurologic evaluation.

Cerebellar functioning. The cerebellum mainly controls balance and coordination. Much of the assessment of cerebellar functioning involves observing the child's posture, body movements, gait, and development of fine and gross motor skills. Tests such as balancing on one foot and the heel-to-toe walk in the DDST also assess balance. Coordination is tested by asking the child to reach for a toy, button his clothes, tie his shoes, or draw a straight line on a piece of paper, provided he is old enough to accomplish these activities.

Several tests for cerebellar function that can be performed as games include:

1. **Finger-to-nose test:** With the child's arm extended, ask the child to touch his nose with the index finger with his eyes open and then closed.
2. **Heel-to-shin test:** With the child standing, have him run the heel of one foot down the shin or anterior aspect of the tibia of the other leg, both with his eyes opened and then closed.
3. **Romberg test:** With the eyes closed, have the child stand with his heels together; falling or leaning to one side is abnormal and is called *Romberg sign.* If there is any question of the child's ability to perform adequately, the nurse stands beside the child in case he falls.

School-age children should be able to perform these tests, although preschoolers normally can bring the finger only within 5 to 7.5 cm (2 to 3 inches) of their nose. Difficulty in performing these exercises indicates poor sense of position (especially with the eyes closed) and incoordination (especially with the eyes opened). Coordination can also be tested by any sequence of rapid successive movements, such as quickly touching each finger with the thumb of the same hand. Cerebellar testing is particularly significant in children with symptoms of hyperactivity or learning difficulty.

Reflexes. Testing reflexes is an important part of the neurologic examination. Persistence of primitive reflexes, loss of reflexes, or hyperactivity of deep tendon reflexes is usually the result of a cerebral insult. This discussion is primarily concerned with reflexes found in children past infancy. The primitive reflexes of the newborn are discussed in Chapter 8, pp. 314-315.

In eliciting reflexes, it is important to have some understanding of their basic physiology. A *reflex* is an involuntary response to a stimulus. However, three characteristics are unique: (1) the individual is aware of the movement, (2) he may be able to inhibit it, such as by tensing the muscle, but (3) when the activity occurs, it does so without the person's conscious assistance. Although reflexes are under the control of higher brain centers, they may continue to function even though the influence of the brain has been lost. This commonly occurs in spinal cord injury, when the child is unable to walk but still demonstrates the patellar reflex.

Reflexes can be elicited by using the rubber head of the reflex hammer, flat of the finger, or side of the hand. If the child is easily frightened by equipment, it is best to use one's hand or finger. Although testing reflexes is a simple procedure to perform, the child may inhibit the reflex by unconsciously tensing the muscle. The nurse should try to distract younger children with toys or by talking to them. Older children can concentrate on the exercise of grasping their two hands in front of them and trying to pull them apart to divert their attention from the testing and cause involuntary relaxation of the muscles.

Several *superficial reflexes* are present, such as the abdominal, cremasteric, anal, and plantar. These have already been discussed throughout the chapter. *Deep tendon reflexes* are stretch reflexes of a muscle. The most common deep tendon reflex is the *knee jerk,* or *patellar reflex* (sometimes called *quadriceps reflex*). The reflexes normally elicited are described in Figs. 7-56 through 7-60. Reflexes are evaluated by using the following grading system:

4+ extremely brisk, hyperactive
3+ brisker than normal
2+ average, normal
1+ diminished
0+ absent

Absent or hyperactive reflexes are reported for further evaluation.

Several other reflexes are normally present or absent but are not elicited unless specific indications exist. For example, in the presence of symptoms suggestive of meningeal irritation, the Kernig sign and the Brudzinski sign are elicited. To test for Kernig sign the child lies supine and the leg is flexed at the hip and knee. Resistance or pain on extending the leg at the knee is abnormal and is called a positive *Kernig sign* (Fig. 7-61). The test for Brudzinski sign

is performed by flexing the child's head while supine. If this causes pain or the knees and hips to flex involuntarily, *Brudzinski sign* is positive (Fig. 7-62).

Cranial nerves. The 12 cranial nerves arise directly from the brain and supply the structures of the head and neck. Parts of the tenth nerve, the vagus, branch off to supply structures of the trunk. Assessment of the cranial nerves is an important area of neurologic assessment (Table 7-11). With older children most of the tests can be presented as games and, because no traumatic equipment is used, may encourage trust and security at the beginning of the exami-

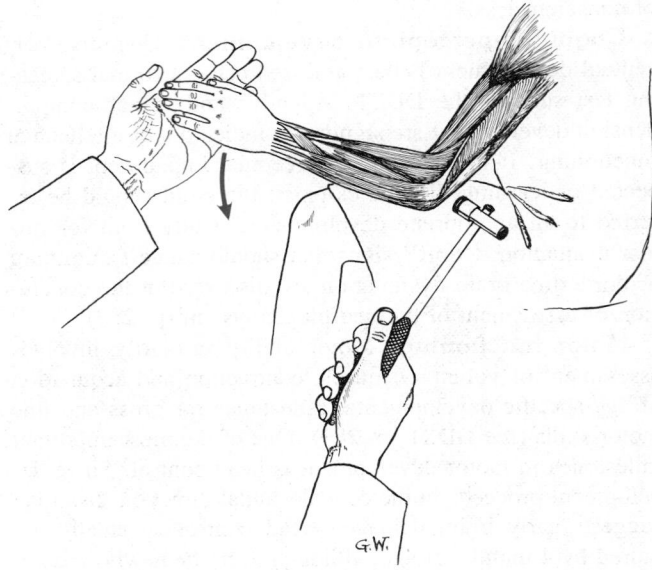

Fig. 7-57. Testing for triceps reflex. Child's arm is flexed at the elbow and child's hand is placed in examiner's palm. Triceps tendon is struck. Normal response is partial extension of forearm.

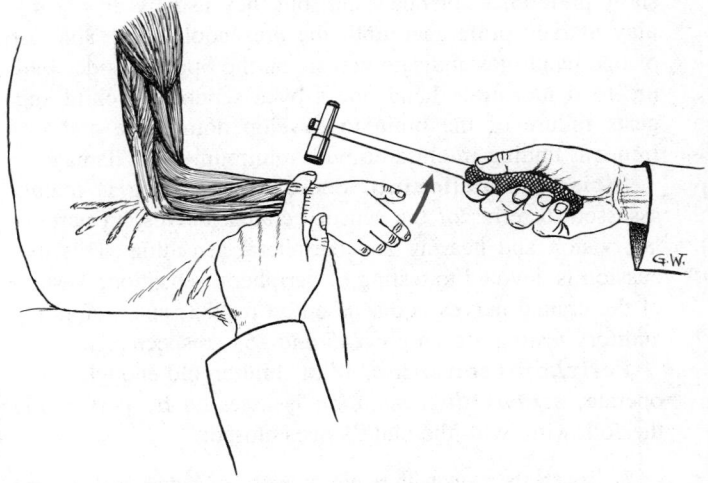

Fig. 7-58. Testing for brachioradialis reflex. Child's forearm is placed on his lap or abdomen with arm flexed at elbow and palm down. Radius is struck about 1 inch (depending on child's size) above wrist. Normal response is flexion of forearm and supination (turning upward) of palm.

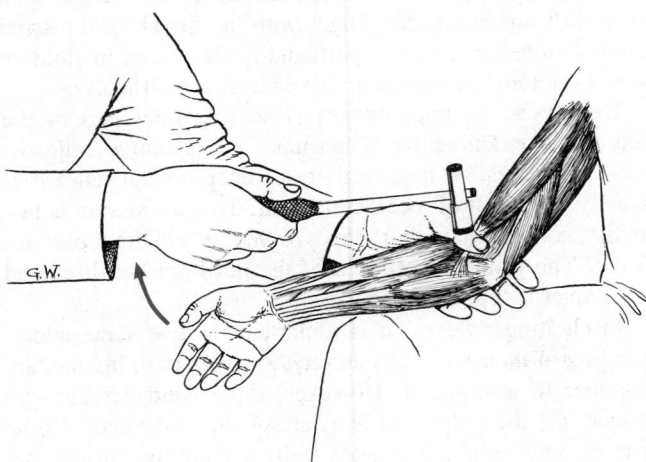

Fig. 7-56. Testing for biceps reflex. Child's arm is held by placing partially flexed elbow in examiner's hand with thumb over antecubital space. Examiner's thumbnail is struck with hammer. Normal response is partial flexion of forearm.

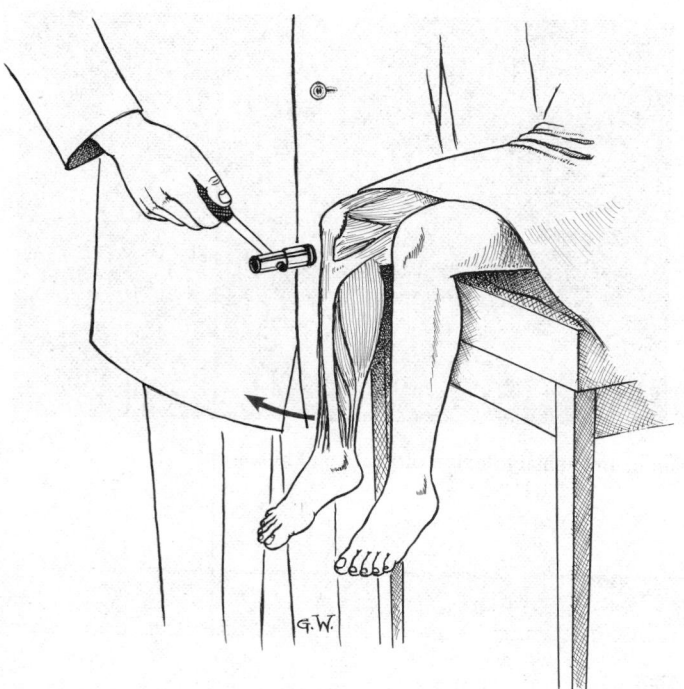

Fig. 7-59. Testing for patellar, or knee jerk, reflex. Child sits on edge of examining table (or on parent's lap) with lower legs flexed at knee and dangling freely. Patellar tendon is tapped just below kneecap. Normal response is partial extension of lower leg.

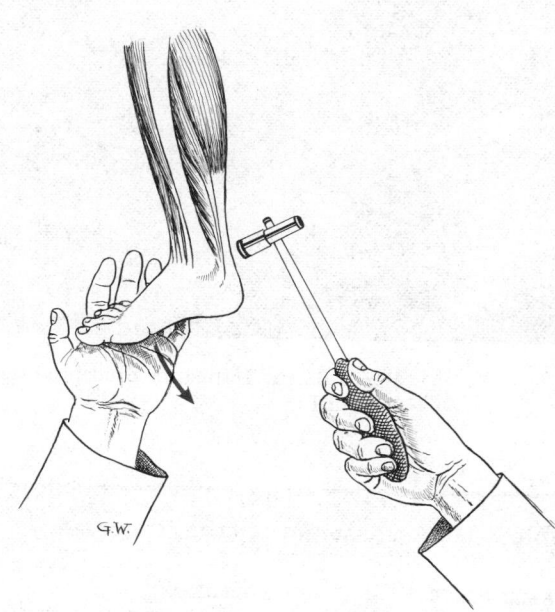

Fig. 7-60. Testing for Achilles reflex. Same position employed in eliciting knee jerk reflex is used. Foot is supported lightly in examiner's hand, and Achilles tendon is struck. Normal response is plantar flexion of foot (foot pointing downward).

A

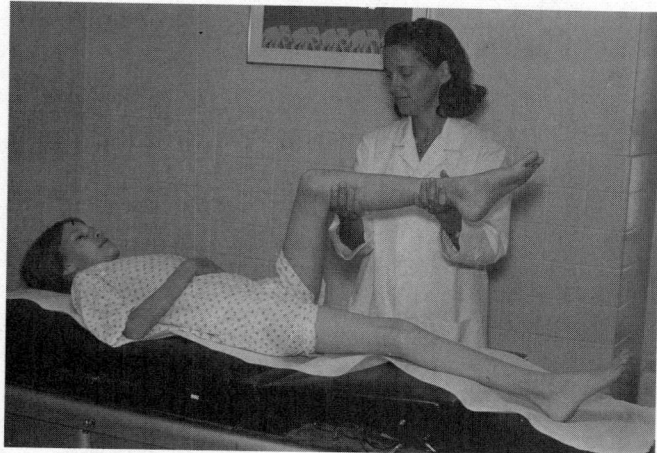

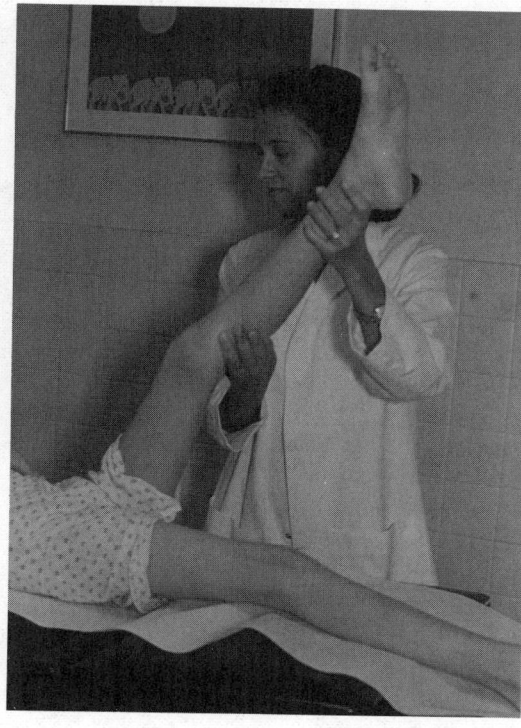

B

Fig. 7-61. A, Testing for Kernig sign. **B,** Pain or resistance on extension is abnormal.

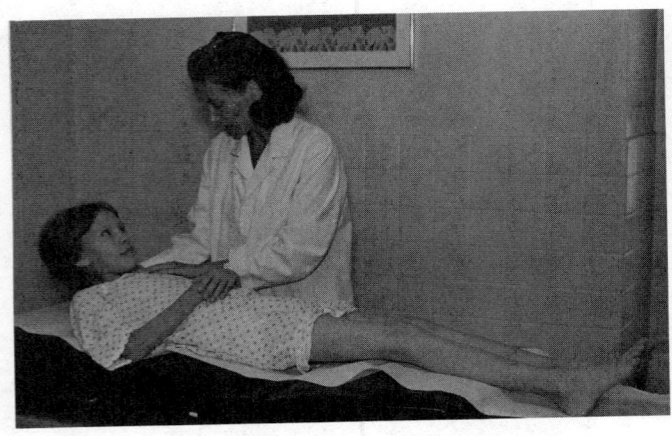
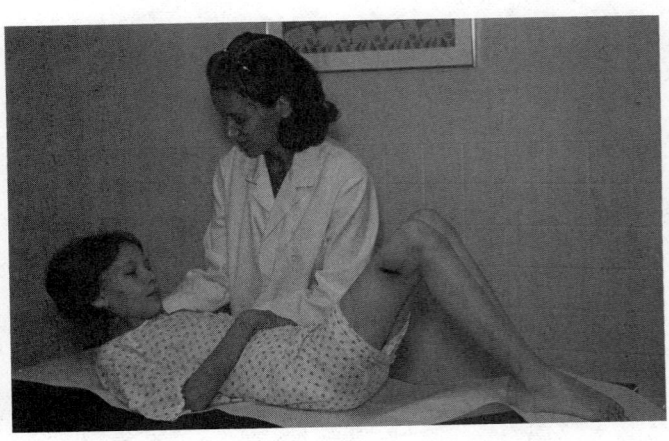

Fig. 7-62. **A,** Testing for Brudzinski sign. **B,** Pain or involuntary flexion of knees and hips is abnormal.

Table 7-11 Assessment of cranial nerves

CRANIAL NERVE	DISTRIBUTION	TEST
*I—Olfactory (S)**	Olfactory mucosal of nasal cavity	With his eyes closed, have child identify odors such as coffee, alcohol from a swab, or other smells; test each nostril separately
II—Optic (S)	Rods and cones of retina, optic nerve	Check for perception of light, visual acuity, peripheral vision, color vision, and normal optic disc
*III—Oculomotor (M)**	Extraocular muscles of eye. Superior rectus (SR)—moves eyeball up and in Inferior rectus (IR)—moves eyeball down and in Medial rectus (MR)—moves eyeball nasally Inferior oblique (IO)—moves eyeball up and out	Have child follow an object (toy) or light in the six cardinal positions of gaze (see Fig. 7-63)
	Pupil constriction and accommodation	Perform PERRLA (see p. 243)
	Eyelid opening	Check for proper placement of lid (see p. 242)
IV—Trochlear (M)	Superior oblique muscle (SO)—moves eye down and out	Have child look down and in (see Fig. 7-63)
V—Trigeminal (M, S)	Muscles of mastication	Have child bite down hard and open his jaw; test symmetry and strength
	Sensory: face, scalp, nasal and buccal mucosa	With his eyes closed, see if child can detect light touch in the mandibular and maxillary regions
		Test corneal and blink reflex by touching cornea lightly (approach child from the side so that he does not blink before cornea is touched)
VI—Abducens (M)	Lateral rectus (LR) muscle—moves eye temporally	Have child look toward temporal side (Fig. 7-63)

Fig. 7-63. Testing cardinal positions of gaze.

*S—sensory; M—motor.

Table 7-11 Assessment of cranial nerves—cont'd

CRANIAL NERVE	DISTRIBUTION	TEST
VII—Facial (M, S)	Muscles for facial expression	Have child smile, make funny face, or show his teeth to see symmetry of expression
	Anterior two thirds of tongue (sensory)	Have child identify a sweet, sour, or bitter solution; place each taste on anterior section and sides of protruding tongue; if child retracts tongue, solution will dissolve toward posterior part of tongue
	Nasal cavity and lacrimal gland, sublingual and submandibular salivary glands	Not tested
VIII—Auditory, acoustic, or vestibulochlear (S)	Internal ear	Test hearing; note any loss of equilibrium or presence of vertigo
IX—Glossopharyngeal (M, S)	Pharynx, tongue Posterior one third of tongue (sensory)	Stimulate the posterior pharynx with a tongue blade; the child should gag Test sense of taste on posterior segment of tongue
X—Vagus (M, S)	Muscles of larynx, pharynx, some organs of gastrointestinal system, sensory fibers of root of tongue, heart, lung, and some organs of gastrointestinal system	Note hoarseness of the voice, gag reflex, and ability to swallow Check that uvula is in midline; when stimulated with a tongue blade, should deviate upward and to the stimulated side
XI—Accessory (M)	Sternocleidomastoid and trapezius muscles of shoulder	Have child shrug his shoulders while applying mild pressure; with the hands placed on his shoulders, have child turn his head against opposing pressure on either side; note symmetry and strength
XII—Hypoglossal (M)	Muscles of tongue	Have child move tongue in all directions; have him protrude the tongue as far as possible; note any midline deviation Test strength by placing tongue blade on one side of tongue and having child move it away

nation. However, much of the testing can be included when each "system" is examined, such as tongue movement and strength, gag reflex, swallowing, and position of the uvula during examination of the mouth.

"Soft" signs. One of the difficulties in assessment of the nervous system is the clear-cut differentiation between normal and abnormal findings (sometimes referred to as "hard" signs). There is a gray area called "soft" signs, findings that are normal in a young child but that in the normal course of maturation disappear. They represent the persistence of a more primitive form of behavior or response and a failure to perform the age-specific activity. Although the list of soft signs is long and the controversy concerning their significance far from resolved, some of the classic signs are listed in the accompanying box.

DENVER DEVELOPMENTAL SCREENING TEST

One of the most widely used screening tests for assessing a young child's development is the *Denver Developmental Screening Test* (DDST) (see Appendix B). It is composed of four major categories: personal-social, fine motor–adaptive, language, and gross motor and is applicable for chil-

NEUROLOGIC "SOFT" SIGNS

Short attention span
Unusual body movements, such as mirroring
Poor coordination and sense of position
Excessive, sustained, and purposeless movement (hyperactivity)
Hypoactivity
Impulsiveness
Labile emotions
Distractibility
No established handedness
Language and articulation problems
Perceptual deficits (space, form, movement, time)
Problems with learning, especially reading, writing, and arithmetic

dren from birth through 6 years of age. The age divisions are monthly until 24 months and then every 6 months until 6 years of age. Allowances are made for infants who were born prematurely by subtracting the number of months of missed gestation from their present age and testing them at the adjusted age. For example, a 9-month-old infant who was born 1 month before the expected date of delivery is tested at an 8-month level.

The DDST and the revised DDST (DDST-R) have been subjected to several reliability and validity tests and have been found to yield normal, questionable, and abnormal results that correlate with psychometric tests, such as the Cattell Infant Intelligence Scale and the Revised Bayley Infant Scale. Studies have also shown a predictive correlation between results of the DDST and the later development of school problems. Results showed that children with questionable scores, as well as those with abnormal scores, are at risk for developing school problems despite adequate intelligence (Sturner, Green, and Funk, 1985). Such findings are extremely relevant to nurses, who are in an optimum position to identify high-risk children and refer them for further testing. One weakness of the DDST is its limitations in terms of predictive validity with lower socioeconomic groups (Frankenburg, Dick, and Carland, 1975) and children of different cultural backgrounds. For example, Southeast Asian children have demonstrated delays in the areas of personal-social development because of lack of familiarity with games like pat-a-cake and in language because of differences in word usage, such as absence of plurals (Miller, Onotera, and Deinard, 1984). The more protective parental attitude of Southeast Asians toward the young child may also prevent early learning of self-help skills (Fung and Lau, 1985). Several of these variations were noted also in native African children (Olade, 1984). Such cultural differences must be considered when administering the test to prevent erroneous labeling of the child as "developmentally delayed" (Fig. 7-64).

The major differences between the original DDST and the DDST-R are the arrangement of items on the form and the scoring. On the original form, items are scored as "P" for pass, "F" for fail, or "R" for refusal. On the DDST-R only the items passed are scored. The revised DDST-R has been found to have several advantages over the original form: (1) it is easier to use, especially for those not trained with DDST, (2) it facilitates using the short DDST (see p. 285), (3) it provides a more dynamic representation of the child's development because the form resembles a growth curve, and (4) subsequent testing of the child requires administering only those items not previously scored with a "P" that are to the left of the child's age line (Frankenburg and others, 1981). However, the instruction manual* uses the original form for training; therefore this form may be more familiar to practitioners.

The DDST is designed for administration by both professionals and paraprofessionals and takes about 15 to 20 minutes to complete. The kits for testing include a red wool "ball," raisins, a small clear bottle with a 5/8-inch opening, a rattle with a narrow handle, eight 1-inch square blocks in red, blue, yellow, and green colors, a small bell, a tennis ball, and a pencil.

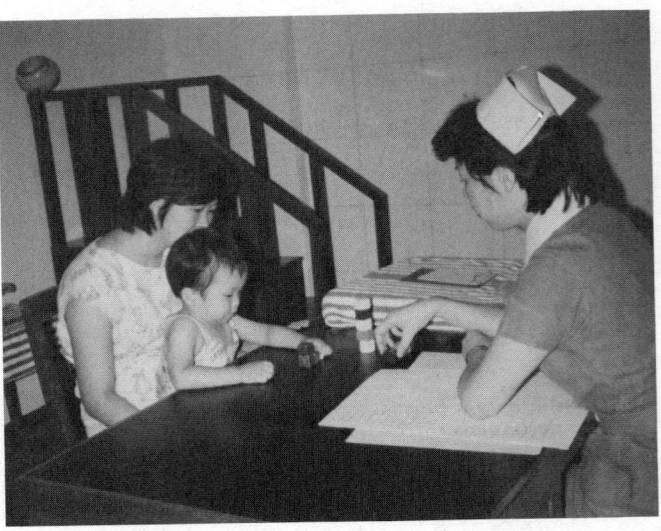

Fig. 7-64. When administering the DDST, the nurse must consider cultural variations that can erroneously label child delayed.
Courtesy T.K. Wong, Fanling Hospital, Kowloon, New Territories.

Each item is designated by a bar that represents the ages at which 25%, 50%, 70%, and 90% of the tested population could perform the particular item. Scoring is based on the number of *delays,* which are defined as "failure to perform an item which is passed by 90% of the children who are of the same age or any item which falls completely to the *left* of the age line." *Abnormal* is determined by either:

1. Two or more sectors with two or more delays
2. One sector with two or more delays plus one or more sectors with one delay and, in that same sector, no passes through the age line

Questionable is determined by either:

1. One sector with two or more delays
2. One or more sectors with one delay and in that same sector no passes through the age line

The child is considered *untestable* when the number of refusals is large enough to cause the test result to be questionable or abnormal *if* they were scored as failures. *Normal* is determined by any score that does not meet these three other criteria.

Although it is not the purpose of this discussion to detail the instruction manual, there are some points concerning preparation, administration, and interpretation of the DDST that necessitate emphasis. Before beginning the test, both the child and the parent need an explanation. For parents this means clarifying that the DDST is *not* an intelligence test but a method of helping the nurse observe what the child can do at a particular age. It is best to deemphasize the word *test* while emphasizing that the child is *not* expected to perform each item on the sheet.

The parent is told before the testing begins that the results of the child's performance will be explained after all the items have been concluded. It is the nurse's responsibil-

*Forms and instruction manual are available from Denver Developmental Materials, Inc., P.O. Box 20037, Denver, CO 80220.

ity to properly inform parents of any testing or screening procedure before its administration so that they are fully aware of its purpose and intent.

The nurse can prepare toddlers and preschoolers for the test by presenting it as a game. Frequently the DDST is an excellent way to begin a health appraisal because it is non-threatening, requires no painful or unfamiliar procedures, and capitalizes on the child's natural activity of play. Since children are easily distracted, it is best to perform the test quickly and to present only one toy from the kit at a time. After that toy's purpose is concluded, such as building a tower of blocks or identifying its color, the toy is replaced in the bag and another one is brought out for testing purposes. Other temporary factors that may interfere with the child's performance include fatigue, illness, fear, hospitalization, separation from the parent, or general unwillingness to perform activities asked of the child. In addition, undiagnosed mental retardation, hearing loss, vision loss, neurologic impairment, or a familial pattern of slow development greatly influences the child's performance.

Following completion of the DDST, the nurse asks the parent if the child's performance was typical of his behavior at other times. If the parent replies affirmatively and the child's cooperation was satisfactory, the results are explained, emphasizing all successful items first, then those items failed but which the child was not expected to pass, and finally those items that were delays.

In explaining a normal score, the nurse focuses on how well the child performed and reinforces the parents' efforts in satisfactorily stimulating their child. In addition to assessing the child's present developmental level, the DDST can be used to guide parents toward those activities that are appropriate, although not necessarily expected, for the child's age. Studies of parents' knowledge of developmental milestones indicate that parents have many misconceptions about normal development and either expect skills too early or fail to recognize delays (Shea and Fowler, 1983). By testing for items to the right of the age line (ones child is not expected to perform), children with advanced development, who may be gifted, can be identified (Fish and Burch, 1985).

In explaining delays, the parent's response is carefully noted, especially casual acceptance, such as "He'll catch up." Since all children with questionable or abnormal results should be rescreened before referral for diagnostic testing, some of the parents' more serious questions, such as "Does this mean my child is retarded?" can be deferred until the next screening session. The nurse must be aware of personal anxieties during these situations and refrain from giving glib reassurances, such as "I'm sure he will do better the next time." Rather, parents' questions are answered honestly yet with appropriate flexibility and concern by stating: "I need to observe your child again before I can give you any answers or even make assumptions concerning his developmental progress. I will retest him next week, and then possibly I will know more. What are your thoughts about how he performed the activities on the DDST?"

If the parents reply that the child's performance was not typical of his usual behavior, it is best to defer any scoring or discussion of the test results with the parents, especially if the refusals yield a questionable or abnormal rating. In this situation the DDST is rescheduled for a time when the child is more likely to cooperate.

Additional Developmental Screening Tests

Although the DDST is the most widely used screening test in the United States and many other countries, several other screening tests are available. Some of them are modifications of the DDST that require less time and training to administer. These are described below as well as selected others that are widely used and require self-training. Excellent reviews of additional tests are available (Castiglia and Petrini, 1985; Smith, 1984; Goldman, Stein, and Guerry, 1983).

Short form DDST. The short form DDST (DDST-S) uses the DDST or the DDST-R form, but only the three items immediately to the left but not intersecting the line in each of the four sectors are administered. If all 12 items are passed, the child receives no further testing until the next scheduled visit. However, if one or more items are failed or refused, then the full DDST is administered while the child is in the test setting. The major advantages of the DDST-S are that it takes less time (about 5 to 7 minutes) and the second stage testing can be done immediately if needed (Sturner and others, 1982).

Denver Prescreening Developmental Questionnaire. The Denver Prescreening Developmental Questionnaire (PDQ) is a prescreening test designed to identify children from 3 months to 6 years of age who require a more thorough screening with the DDST (Frankenburg and others, 1976). It is very easy and rapid to administer (it takes parents about 5 minutes to answer the questions). It consists of a total of 97 questions that focus on a child's current behavior, but only 10 questions must be answered for any one child. The questions are arranged in order according to the age at which 90% of children passed the corresponding DDST item. Scores of 9 or 10 are considered nonsuspect. Children with scores of 8 or below are retested with the PDQ in 2 to 4 weeks. Children with rescreening scores of 6 or below should be referred for diagnostic testing.

Developmental Profile. The Developmental Profile II is designed for use with children from birth through a functional age of 9½ years. With normal children it can be used appropriately from birth through 7 years. The following five scales are included: physical, self-help, social, academic, and communication. Administration time varies from 20 to 40 minutes depending on the child's age and the approach used, either interview, interview and direct testing, or self-interview. A detailed self-instructional manual is used for training (Alpern, Boll, and Shearer, 1985).*

McCarthy Scales of Children's Abilities. The McCarthy Scales of Children's Abilities (MSCA) is a de-

*The Developmental Profile II Manual is available from Western Psychological Services, 12031 Wilshire Blvd., Los Angeles, CA 90025.

METHOD OF SCORING GOODENOUGH DRAW-A-PERSON TEST*

1. Head present
2. Legs present
3. Arms present
4. Trunk present
5. Trunk longer than broad
6. Shoulder indicated
7. Both arms and legs attached to trunk
8. Legs and arms attached to trunk at proper level
9. Neck present
10. Outline of neck continuous with that of head or trunk or both
11. Eyes present
12. Nose present
13. Mouth present
14. Both nose and mouth in two dimensions; two lips shown
15. Nostrils indicated
16. Hair shown
17. Hair on more than circumference of head, nontransparent, better than scribble
18. Clothing present
19. Two articles of clothing, nontransparent
20. Entire clothing with sleeves and trousers shown, nontransparent
21. Four or more articles of clothing definitely indicated
22. Costume complete without incongruities
23. Fingers shown
24. Correct number of fingers
25. Fingers in two dimensions, length greater than breadth, angle subtended not greater than 180 degrees
26. Opposition of thumbs shown
27. Hands shown distinct from fingers and arms
28. Arm joints shown (elbow or shoulder or both)
29. Head in proportion
30. Arms in proportion
31. Legs in proportion
32. Feet in proportion
33. Arms and legs in two dimensions
34. Heel shown
35. Lines somewhat controlled
36. Lines well controlled
37. Head outline well controlled
38. Trunk outline well controlled
39. Outline of arms and legs well controlled
40. Outline of features well controlled
41. Ears present
42. Ears present in correct position
43. Eyebrows or lashes present
44. Pupil shown
45. Proportion of eyes correct
46. Glance directed to front in profile drawing
47. Both chin and forehead shown
48. Projection of shin shown
49. Profile with not more than one error
50. Correct profile

*In each item listed give the child 1 point. The number of points multiplied by 3 months plus 3 years equals the mental age.

with intelligence quotients from other accepted tests. It is a test that may be selected for follow-up when a child fails the DDST or is suspected to have retarded development (Hayes, 1981). A detailed self-instructional manual is used for training.*

Washington Guide to Promoting Development in the Young Child. The Washington Guide to Promoting Development in the Young Child provides a framework for developmental assessment based on direct observation of a child's specific behaviors in eight categories: feeding, sleep, play, language, motor activities, discipline, toilet training, and dressing. In each category developmental accomplishments that would be expected for age groups from birth to 5 years are grouped as "expected tasks" with an accompanying list of "suggested activities" for parental guidance. The Washington Guide differs from other developmental tools in that no score is obtained. It is used to observe the child on a systematic basis, to identify variations in development, and to provide suggestions regarding appropriate childrearing practices (Powell, 1981).

Preschool Readiness Experimental Screening Scale. Preschool Readiness Experimental Screening Scale (PRESS) is designed for screening 5-year-old children's readiness for school (Rogers and Rogers, 1972, 1975). It is a simple test that can be integrated into the physical examination or administered separately. Five areas are assessed: knowledge of numbers, general knowledge, drawing coordination, and an overall assessment of performance and maturity. The scoring system rates children for school readiness as (1) high to above average, (2) average, (3) borderline, or (4) insufficient. The last score indicates a need for referral to a school psychologist or diagnostic center for further evaluation.

Goodenough Draw-A-Person Test. A test that can be used to assess intellectual development is the Goodenough Draw-A-Person Test† (Goodenough, 1926). The child is given a pencil with an eraser and paper and simply asked to "draw a man or a person." No further directions are supplied regarding the drawing, other than he should draw the best picture of a person that he can. He should be left alone and given as much time as needed to finish the picture.

The scoring is determined by giving 1 point for each item included in the drawing (see box). Each point is equal to 3 months. The number of points are converted to months and/or years and added to the base age of 3 years. The final score in months/years is approximately equal to the child's mental age. The child's intelligence quotient (IQ) can be found by the ratio of mental age to chronologic age multiplied by 100. For example, if a 5-year-old child scores 12 points on the test, he has a mental age of 6 years (3 years + [12 × 3 months] = 6 years) and an IQ of 120.

Although reports concerning the reliability of the Good-

velopmental assessment tool for children 2½ to 8½ years old (McCarthy, 1972). It is based on six scales: verbal, perceptual-performance, quantitative, general cognition, memory, and motor. Administration time is from 45 minutes to 1 hour. Eighteen separate tests are administered to the child, and the scores from these tests contribute to one or more of the scores on the six scales. The final score correlates well

---

*The McCarthy Scales of Children's Abilities is available from Psychological Corporation, 7500 Old Oak Blvd., Cleveland, OH 44130.
†The Goodenough Draw-A-Person Test is available from Psychological Corporation, 7500 Old Oak Blvd., Cleveland, OH 44130.

enough test vary, it is a valuable procedure for assessing intellectual development in children 3 to 10 years of age, particularly in screening for children with low scores who may require further measurement of mental functioning.

Developmental Screening and Interpretation

Although screening tests are an effective method of applying the knowledge of children's expected rate of development to a large segment of the population, they are only as successful as the individual's expertise in administering them. Since many of the screening tests are devised to be used by paraprofessionals, there are inherent risks in screening if such individuals are not properly trained or supervised. For example, false-positives can label the child as developmentally delayed and cause problems that otherwise might not have existed. Nurses must ensure that screening tests are properly administered and the results correctly interpreted. The complexity of mental and physical health can never be measured by any one index. Evaluation of the child's total well-being is the result of evaluating data from a comprehensive history, physical examination, and developmental screening.

- The lungs are examined by methods of inspection, palpation, percussion, and auscultation.

- Heart murmurs are classified as innocent, functional, and organic and should be evaluated for location, time, intensity, and loudness.

- Abdominal assessment follows an orderly sequence of inspection, auscultation, percussion, and palpation, since the latter may distort normal abdominal sounds.

- Examination of the genitalia may be anxiety-provoking in the child, and the nurse must avoid any transference of anxiety.

- Neurologic assessment addresses behavior, cognitive-perceptual development, motor functioning, sensory and cerebellar functioning, reflexes, cranial nerves, and soft signs.

- The Denver Developmental Screening Test, one of the most widely used assessment tools, is composed of four categories: personal-social, fine motor–adaptive, language, and gross motor.

CONCEPT SUMMARIES

- The most common approach to examining children follows a head-to-toe sequence.

- The four categories of assessment are inspection, palpation, percussion, and auscultation.

- Growth measurements during the physical examination focus on length, height, weight, skinfold thickness, and arm and head circumference. Assessment of growth is measured against standard growth charts to determine a child's status in comparison with other children of his age.

- Measurements of temperature, pulse, respiration, and blood pressure constitute the physiologic approach to assessment.

- The general appearance of a child is a cumulative, subjective impression of physical appearance, state of nutrition, behavior, personality, interactions with parents and nurse, posture, development, and speech.

- Assessment of the skin, which primarily involves inspection and palpation, focuses on color, texture, temperature, moisture, and turgor. The nurse needs to be aware of both physiologic and ethnic factors that may affect these areas.

- In assessment of the lymph nodes, the nurse examines, by palpation, the part of the body in which the glands are located.

- The head is inspected for shape and symmetry.

- Assessment of the neck includes palpation of the trachea and thyroid gland.

- Examination of the eyes includes placement and alignment, inspection of external and internal structures, and vision testing.

- Ears are examined for placement and alignment, inspection of external and internal structures, and auditory testing.

REFERENCES

Alpern, G., Boll, T., and Shearer, M.: Developmental Profile II Manual, Los Angeles, CA, 1985, Western Psychological Services.

American Academy of Pediatrics: Guidelines for health supervision, Elk Grove, IL, 1985, The Academy.

Barrus, D.H.: A comparison of rectal and axillary temperatures by electronic thermometer measurement in preschool children, Pediatr. Nurs. 9(6):424-425, 1983.

Barrus, D.H.: Personal communication, January 12, 1984.

Barry, M., and others: Clinical findings in Southeast Asian refugees, JAMA 249(23):3200-3203, 1983.

Blumenthal, S., and others: Report of the task force on blood pressure control in children, Pediatrics 59(suppl.):797, 1977.

Britton, C.V.: Blood pressure measurement and hypertension in children, Pediatr. Nurs. 7:13-17, July/Aug. 1981.

Castiglia, P.T., and Petrini, M.A.: Selecting a developmental screening tool, Pediatr. Nurs. 11(1):8-17, 1985.

Cavanaugh, R.M., Jr.: Pelvic examination of adolescent girls, Am. Fam. Physician 26:105-108, Oct. 1982.

Cross, A.W.: Health screening in schools. Part I, J. Pediatr. 107(4):487-494, 1985a.

Cross, A.W.: Health screening in schools. Part II, J. Pediatr. 107(5):653-661, 1985b.

Eoff, M.J., and Joyce, B.: Temperature measurements in children, Am. J. Nurs. 81:1010-1011, May 1981.

Erickson, R.: Oral temperature differences in relation to thermometer and technique, Nurs. Res. 29(3):157-164, 1980.

Fish, L.J., and Burch, K.J.: Identifying gifted preschoolers, Pediatr. Nurs. 11(2):125-127, 1985.

Frankenburg, W.K., Dick, N.P., and Carland, J.: Development of preschool-aged children of different social and ethnic groups: implications for developmental screening, J. Pediatr. 87:125-232, July 1975.

Frankenburg, W.K., and others: The Denver Prescreening Developmental Questionnaire (PDQ), Pediatrics 57(5):744-753, 1976.

Frankenburg, W.K., and others: The newly abbreviated and revised Denver Developmental Screening Test, J. Pediatr. 99(6):995-999, 1981.

Fung, K., and Lau, S.: Denver Developmental Screening Test: cultural variables, J. Pediatr. 106(2):343, 1985.

Gershel, J., and others: Accuracy of the Welch Allyn AudioScope and traditional hearing screening for children with known hearing loss, J. Pediatr. 106(1):15-20, 1985.

Goldman, J., Stein, C.L., and Guerry, S.: Psychological methods of child assessment, New York, 1983, Brunner/Mazel, Inc.

Goodenough, F.L.: Measurement of intelligence by drawings, New York, 1926, World Book Co.

Grimes, C.T.: Audiologic evaluation in infancy and childhood, Pediatr. Ann. 14(3):211-219, 1985.

Habicht, J., and others: Height and weight standards for preschool children: how relevant are ethnic differences in growth potential? Lancet 1(7858):611-615, 1974.

Harkass, C.K.: Clearing the occluded auditory canal, Pediatr. Nurs. 8(1):23-25, 1982.

Havener, W.H.: Synopsis of ophthalmology, ed. 6, St. Louis, 1984, The C.V. Mosby Co.

Hayes, J.S.: The McCarthy scales of children's abilities: their usefulness in developmental assessment, Pediatr. Nurs. 7:35-37, July/Aug. 1981.

Helveston, E.M., and Ellis, F.D.: Pediatric ophthalmology practice, St. Louis, 1980, The C.V. Mosby Co.

Himes, J.H., and others: Parent-specific adjustments for evaluation of recumbent length and stature of children, Pediatrics 75(2):304-313, 1985.

Hohn, A., Riopel, D., and Loadholt, C.: Which blood pressure? J. Pediatr. 104(1):89-91, 1984.

Holland, S.H.: 20/20 vision screening, Pediatr. Nurs. 8(2):81-87, 1982.

Hoyt, C.S., Nickel, B.L., and Billson, F.A.: Ophthalmological examination of the infant: development aspects, Surv. Ophthalmol. 26(4):177-189, 1982.

Jaffe, B.F.: Pinna anomalies associated with congenital conductive hearing loss, Pediatrics 57(3):332-341, 1976.

Jellinek, M., Evans, N., and Knight, R.B.: Use of a behavior checklist on a pediatric inpatient unit, J. Pediatr. 94(1):156-158, 1979.

Jung, E., and others: Skinfold measurements in children: a comparison of Lange and McGaw calipers, Clin. Pediatr. 23(1):25-28, 1984.

Kovalesky, A: Nurses' guide to children's eyes, New York, 1985, Grune & Stratton, Inc.

Laestadius, N., Aase, J., and Smith, D.: Normal inner canthal and outer orbital dimensions, J. Pediatr. 74(3):465-468, 1969.

Lewit, E., and others: An evaluation of a plastic strip thermometer, JAMA 247:321-325, l982.

McCarthy, D.: Manual: McCarthy scales of children's abilities, New York, 1972, The Psychological Corp.

McClellan, M.A.: The use of the physical examination to promote development of the preschooler, Child. Health Care 12(4):174-178, 1984.

McDade, W.: Bow legs and knock knees, Pediatr. Clin. North Am. 24:825-839, Nov. 1977.

Miller, V., Onotera, R., and Deinard, A.: Denver Developmental Screening Test: cultural variations in Southeast Asian children, J. Pediatr. 104(3):481-482, 1984.

Moore, W., and Roche, A.: Pediatric anthropometry, Columbus, OH, 1982, Ross Laboratories.

NAACOG: Adolescent gynecology: the initial pelvic examination, NAACOG Technical Bulletin No. 5, Nov. 1979.

National Society for the Prevention of Blindness, Inc.: Children's eye health guide, New York, 1982, The Society.

Nelson, L.B., and others: Developmental aspects in the assessment of visual function in young children, Pediatrics 73(3):375-381, l984.

Nichols, G.A., and others: Measuring oral and rectal temperatures of febrile children, Nurs. Res. 21(3):261-264, 1972.

Olade, R.A.: Evaluation of the Denver Developmental Screening Test as applied to African children, Nurs. Res. 33(4):204-207, 1984.

Pickwell, S.: Primary health care of Indochinese refugee children, Pediatr. Nurs. 8(2):104,1982.

Powell, M.L.: Assessment and management of developmental changes and problems in children, ed. 2, St. Louis, 1981, The C.V. Mosby Co.

Rogers, W.B., and Rogers, R.A.: A new simplified preschool readiness experimental screening scale (The PRESS): a preliminary report, Clin. Pediatr. 11:558-562, Oct. 1972.

Rogers, W.B., and Rogers, R.A.: A follow-up study of the preschool readiness experimental screening scale (The PRESS), Clin. Pediatr. 14:253-256, March 1975.

Ryan, A.: The accuracy of the Ross Laboratories Adipometer skinfold caliper, Clin. Pediatr. 24(3):174, 1985.

Sato-Viacrucis, K.: Personal communication, January 8, l986.

Schmitt, B.D.: Preschoolers who refuse to be examined, Am. J. Dis. Child. 138:443-446, May 1984.

Seidel, J., Zonana, J., and Totten, E.: Condylomata acuminata as a sign of sexual abuse in children, J. Pediatr. 95(4):553-554, 1979.

Shea, V., and Fowler, M.G.: Parental and pediatric trainee knowledge of development, Dev. Behav. Pediatr. 4(1):21-25, 1983.

Smith, E.E.: Developmental assessment: office developmental screening. In Green, M., and Haggerty, R.J., editors: Ambulatory pediatrics III, Philadelphia, 1984, W.B. Saunders Co.

Staheli, L.T.: Torsional deformity, Pediatr. Clin. North Am. 24(4):799-811, 1977.

Starnbach, H.K., and Gellin, M.E.: What should the physician know about orthodontics? Clin. Pediatr. 16(6):552-555, 1977.

Steinfeld, L., and others: Sphygmomanometry in the pediatric patient, J. Pediatr. 92:934-938, June 1978.

Sturner, R.A., Green, J.A., and Funk, S.G.: Preschool Denver Development Screening Test as a predictor of later school problems, J. Pediatr. 107(4):615-621, 1985.

Sturner, R., and others: Adaptations of the Denver Developmental Screening Test: a study of preschool screening, Pediatrics 69(3):346-350, 1982.

Sutow, W.W., Fernbach, D.J., and Vietti, T.J.: Clinical pediatric oncology, ed. 3, St. Louis, 1984, The C.V. Mosby Co.

Watkins, S., Moore, T., and Phillips, J.: Clearing impacted ears, Am. J. Nurs. 84(9):1107, 1984.

BIBLIOGRAPHY
Physical Assessment

Abdulla, A.M., and Frank, M.J.: 'Abnormal' sounds in normal hearts, and what they mean, Consultant 22:163-165, 1982.

Adams, F.H.: Blood pressure of children in the United States, Pediatrics 61:931, June 1978.

Adams, F.H., and Landaw, E.M.: What are healthy blood pressures for children? Pediatrics 68:268-270, Aug. 1981.

Adler, J.: Patient assessment: abnormalities of the heartbeat, Am. J. Nurs. 77(4):647-673, 1977.

Alexander, M.M., and Brown, M.S.: Physical examination. Part 12. Examining the chest and lungs, Nursing 75 5(1):44-48, 1975.

Alexander, M.M., and Brown, M.S.: Physical examination. Part 13. Examining the abdomen, Nursing 76 6(1):65-70, 1976.

Alexander, M.M., and Brown, M.S.: Physical examination. Part 14. Male genitalia, Nursing 76 6(2):39-43, 1976.

Alexander, M.M., and Brown, M.S.: Physical examination. Part 16. The musculoskeletal system, Nursing 76 6(4):51-56, 1976.

Alexander, M.M., and Brown, M.S.: Physical examination. Part 17. Performing the neurological examination, Nursing 76 6(6):38-43, 1976.

Alexander, M.M., and Brown, M.S.: Physical examination. Part 18. Neurological examination, Nursing 76 6(7):50-55, 1976.

Ashcroft, M.T., and Deshi, P.P.: Ethnic differences in growth potential of children of African, Indian, Chinese and European origin, Trans. R. Soc. Trop. Med. Hyg. 70:5-6, l977.

Baker, N.C., and others: The effect of type of thermometer and length of time inserted on oral temperature measurements of afebrile subjects, Nurs. Res. 33(2):109-111, 1984.

Balk, S.J., Dreyfus, N.G., and Harris, P.: Examination of genitalia in children: 'the remaining taboo,' Pediatrics 70(5):751-753, 1982.

Barness, L.A.: Manual of pediatric physical diagnosis, ed. 5, Chicago, 1980, Year Book Medical Publishers, Inc.

Barry, M., and others: Clinical findings in Southeast Asian refugees, JAMA 249(23):3200-3203, 1983.

Baxter, P.: Association between use of cotton-tipped swabs and cerumen plugs, Br. Med. J. 287(6401):1260, 1983.

Birdsall, C.: How accurate are your blood pressures? Am. J. Nurs. 84(11):1414, 1984.

Blackburn, N.A., and Cebenka, D.L.: Honing your respiratory assessment technique, RN 43:28-33, May 1980.

Bloch, B., and Hunter, M.L.: Teaching physiological assessment of black persons, Nurse Educator 6:24-27, 1981.

Blumenthal, S., and others: Children's blood pressure in the United States, Pediatrics 66:328, 1980.

Borders, C.F.: Strabismus/amblyopia: when to refer, Patient Care 18:21-52, 1984.

Bowers, A., and Thompson, J.: Clinical manual of health assessment, ed. 2, St. Louis, 1984, The C.V. Mosby Co.

Brown, J.: Child health maintenance, Nurse Pract. 5:33-43, Jan./Feb. 1980.

Brown, M.S., and Alexander, M.M.: Physical examination. Part 15. Female genitalia, Nursing 76 6(3):39-41, 1976.

Brown, M.S., and Murphy, M.A.: Ambulatory pediatrics for nurses, ed. 2, New York, 1980, McGraw-Hill Book Co.

Cannon, C.: Hands on guide to palpation and auscultation, RN 43:20, 22-27, 76, March 1980.

Caufield, C.: A developmental approach to hearing screening in children, Pediatr. Nurs. 4(2):39-42, 1978.

Chard, M.: An approach to examining the adolescent male, Am. J. Maternal Child Nurs. 1(1):41-43, 1976.

Cohen, S.: Patient assessment: examination of the female pelvis. Part I, Am. J. Nurs. 78:1717-1746, 1978.

Cohen, S.: Patient assessment: examination of the male genitalia, Am. J. Nurs. 79:689-712, 1979.

Cohen, S.: Patient assessment: examining joints of the upper and lower extremities, Am. J. Nurs. 81:763-786, 1981.

DeAngelis, C., and others: Comparative values of school physical examinations and mass screening tests, J. Pediatr. 102(3):477-481, 1983.

Delancy, V.L., and North, C.: Skin assessment, Top. Clin. Nurs. 5(2):5-10, 1983.

Dessertine, P.S.: Those neglected heart sounds, Pediatr. Nurs. 3(1):18-20, 1977.

DiChiara, E.: A sound method for testing child's hearing, Am. J. Nurs. 84(9):1104-1106, 1984.

Dossey, B.: Perfecting your skills for systematic patient assessments, Nursing 79 9(2):42-45, 1979.

Dressler, D.K., Smejkal, C., and Ruffolo, M.L.: A comparision of oral and rectal temperature measurement on patients receiving oxygen by mask, Nurs. Res. 32(6):373-375, 1983.

Dunn, B.H.: Components of musculoskeletal examination, Orthop. Nurs. 1(6):33-36, 1982.

DuRant, R.H., and Linder, C.W.: An evaluation of five indexes of relative body weight for use with children, J. Am. Diet. Assoc. 78:35-41, Jan. 1981.

Egan, D., and Brown, R.: Vision testing of young children in the age range 18 months to 4-1/2 years, Child Care Health Dev. 10:381-390, 1984.

Eoff, M.J., Meier, R.S., and Miller, C.: Temperature measurement in infants, Nurs. Res. 23:457-460, Nov./Dec. 1974.

Erickson, B.: Detecting abnormal sounds, Nursing 86 16(1):58-63, 1986.

Folger, G.M.: The murmur in the well-appearing child—functional or organic? Pediatr. Basics 29:4-10, July 1981.

Freis, P.C.: Sounds of a healthy heart, Issues Compr. Pediatr. Nurs. 3:1-4, Dec. 1979.

Gammon, J.A.: Visual system screening in infants and young children, Pediatr. Rev. 4(3):71-73, 1982.

Gelfant, B.B.: Physical assessment skills: a necessity in nursing practice, Ethicon 22(1):18-19, 1985.

Goldring, D., and Hernandez, A.: Hypertension in children, Pediatr. Rev. 3(8):235-246, 1982.

Gryskiewicz, J.M., and Huseby, T.L.: Abdominal examination: techniques for the pediatrician, Pediatr. Basics 27(2):10-14, 1980.

Habicht, J.P., and others: Height and weight standards for preschool children: how relevant are ethnic differences in growth potential? Lancet 1(7858):611-614, 1974.

Hutchfield, K., and Crump, A.: Holding children for examination, Nursing (Oxford) 1:1003-1005, March 1981.

Johnson, J.L., and others: The school nurse's role in vision screening for the difficult-to-test student, J. School Health 53(6):345-349, 1983.

King, R.C.: Examining the thorax and respiratory system, RN 45:55-63, 1982.

Kirschen, D., Rosenbaum, A., and Ballard, E.: The dot visual acuity test—a new acuity test for children, J. Am. Optometr. Assoc. 54(12):1055-1059, 1983.

Koeckeritz, J.L.: Assessing the heart: what's normal and what's not, RN 45:59-63, 1982.

Kresch, M.: Axillary temperature as a screening test for fever in children, J. Pediatr. 104(4):596-599, 1984.

Leger, L., Lambert, J., and Martin, P.: Validity of plastic skinfold caliper measurements, Hum. Biol. 54(3):667-675, 1982.

Londe, S.: Fifth versus fourth Korotkoff phase, Pediatrics 76(3):460-461, 1985.

Longe, R.L., Taylor, A.T., and Calvert, J.C.: The thorax and the lungs, Drug Intell. Clin. Pharm. 15:166-174, March 1981.

Mancia, G., and others: Effects of blood pressure measurement by the doctor on patients' blood pressure and heart rate, Lancet 2(8352):695-698, 1983.

Marshall, W.A.: Geographical and ethnic variations in human growth, Br. Med. Bull. 37(3):273-279, 1981.

Mechner, F.: Patient assessment: examination of the eye. Part I, Am. J. Nurs. 74(11):1-24, 1974.

Mechner, F.: Patient assessment: examination of the eye. Part II, Am. J. Nurs. 75(1):1-24, 1975.

Mechner, F.: Patient assessment: examination of the ear, Am. J. Nurs. 75(3):1-24, 1975.

Mechner, F.: Patient assessment: examination of the head and neck, Am. J. Nurs. 75(5):1-24, 1975.

Mechner, F.: Patient assessment: neurological examination. Part III, Am. J. Nurs. 76(4):608-633, 1976.

Mechner, F.: Patient assessment: examination of the chest and lungs, Am. J. Nurs. 76(9):1453-1475, 1976.

Mechner, F.: Patient assessment: examination of the heart and great vessels. Part I, Am. J. Nurs. 76(11):1807-1830, 1976.

Mechner, F.: Patient assessment: auscultation of the heart. Part II, Am. J. Nurs. 77(2):275-298, 1977.

Michielutte, R., and others: The relationship between weight-height indices and the triceps skinfold measure among children 5 to 12, Am. J. Public Health 74(6):604-606, 1984.

Mitchell, J.R.: Male adolescents' concern about a physical examination conducted by a female, Nurs. Res. 29(3):165-169, 1980.

Mizrahi, E.M., and Dorfman, L.J.: Sensory evoked potentials: clinical applications in pediatrics, J. Pediatr. 97(1):1-10, 1980.

Moss, A.J.: Indirect methods of blood pressure measurement, Pediatr. Clin. North Am. 25(1):3-14, 1978.

Moss, J.R.: Helping young children cope with the physical examination, Pediatr. Nurs. 7(2):17-20, 1981.

Moss, J.R.: Predicting young children's cooperation with the physical examination, Pediatr. Nurs. 9(3):188-190, 1983.

Olness, K., and others: Height and weight status of Indochinese refugee children, Am. J. Dis. Child. 138:544-547, 1984.

Park, M.K., and Guntheroth, W.G.: Direct blood pressure measurements in brachial and femoral arteries in children, Circulation **41**:231-237, 1970.

Peltzman, P., and Lipson, E.: Infant hearing assessment: a new approach, Pediatr. Basics **28**:11-14, Jan. 1981.

Performing palpation, Nursing 83 **13**(1):68-69, 1983.

Performing percussion, Nursing 83 **13**(2):63-64, 1983.

Phillips, S., and others: Teenagers' preferences regarding the presence of family members, peers, and chaperones during examination of genitalia, Pediatrics **68**(5):665-669, 1981.

Pickwell, S.: Primary health care of Indochinese refugee children, Pediatr. Nurs. **8**(2):104, 1982.

Poland, R.M., Wells, D.H., and Ferlauto, J.J.: Methods for detecting hearing impairment in infancy, Pediatr. Ann. **9**:31-44, Jan. 1980.

Prior, J.A.: Analysis of breath sounds, Consultant **18**:112-115, April 1978.

Prior, J.A., Silberstein, J.S., and Stang, J.M.: Physical diagnosis: the history and examination of the patient, ed. 6, St. Louis, 1981, The C.V. Mosby Co.

Redman, J.F., and Bissada, N.K.: How to make a good examination of the genitalia in young girls, Clin. Pediatr. **15**(10):907-908, 1976.

Roach, L.B.: Color changes in dark skin, Nursing 77 **7**(1):48-51, 1977.

Roberts, A.: Systems and signs: digestive system—2. Abdomen inspection, Nurs. Times **77**:central pages, April 2, 1981.

Rodts, M.F.: An orthopedic assessment you can do in 15 minutes, Nursing 83 **13**(5):65-73, 1983.

Sato-Viacrucis, K.: The evolution of the Snellen E to the Blackbird, School Nurse, pp. 18-19, Spring 1985.

Saul, L.: For CE credit: heart sounds and common murmurs, Am. J. Nurs. **83**(12):1679-1689, 1983.

Schwartz, R.H., and others: Cerumen removal: how necessary is it to diagnosis outer otitis media, Am. J. Dis. Child. **137**(11):1064-1065, 1983.

Schweiger, J., Lang, J., and Schweiger, J.: Oral assessment: how to do it, Am. J. Nurs. **80**(4):654-663, 1980.

Shannon, D.A., and others: Hearing screening of high-risk newborns with brainstem auditory evoked potentials: a follow-up study, Pediatrics **73**(1):22-26, 1984.

Smith, C.E.: Abdominal assessment—a blending of science and art, Nursing 81 **11**:42-49, Feb. 1981.

Smith, C.E.: With good assessment skills you can construct a solid framework for patient care, Nursing 84 **14**(12):26-31, 1984.

Smith, C.E.: Assessing the liver, Nursing 85 **15**(7):36-37, 1985.

Solnit, A.J.: The risks of screening, Pediatrics **57**(5):646-647, 1976.

Stern, N., and Zaiken, H.: Assessing the child with short stature, Pediatr. Nurs. **11**(2):106-110, 1985.

Stool, S.E.: Otoscopy: how to improve your techniques, Consultant **23**(3):247-248, 1983.

Strain, J.E.: AAP periodicity guidelines: a framework for educating patients, Pediatrics **74** (suppl.):924-927, 1984.

Stright, P.A., and Soukup, M.: How to hear it right: evaluating and choosing a stethoscope, Am. J. Nurs. **77**(9):1477, 1977.

Swigarth, E., and Stool, S.E.: Hearing sensitivity and physical characteristics of the eardrum observed during otoscopic examination, Clin. Pediatr. **16**(6):556-560, 1977.

Tanner, J.M., and Davies, P.S.W.: Clinical longitudinal standards for height and height velocity for North American children, J. Pediatr. **107**(3):317-329, 1985.

Taylor, D.L.: Clinical applications: assessing heart sounds, Nursing 85 **15**:51-53, 1985.

Taylor, D.L.: Clinical applications: assessing breath sounds, Nursing 85 **15**(3):60-62, 1985.

Temperature-taking tips, Pediatr. Alert **8**(10):38-39, 1983.

Thomson, L.R.: Understanding tympanometry, Pediatr. Nurs. **8**(3):193-197, 1982.

Visich, M.A.: Knowing what you hear: a guide to assessing breath and heart sounds, Nursing 81 **11**(11):64-79, 1981.

Wagner, R.S.: Newer techniques in the evaluation of visual acuity in infants, J. Ophthalmic Nurs. Technol. **3**(6):233-236, 1984.

Walleck, C.: A neurological assessment procedure that won't make you nervous, Nursing 82 **12**(12):50-56, 1982.

Wong, D.L.: The paper-doll technique, Pediatr. Nurs. **7**(6):39-40, 1981.

Yoos, L.: A developmental approach to physical assessment, Am. J. Maternal Child Nurs. **6**(3):168-170, 1981.

Younger, J.: Detecting visual problems in children, Pediatr. Nurs. **5**:50-51, Nov./Dec. 1979.

Developmental Assessment

Bradshaw, M.M.: Denver Development Screening Test. In Humenick, S.S.: Analysis of current assessment strategies in the health care of young children and childbearing families, Norwalk, CT, 1982, Appleton-Century-Crofts.

Burgess, D., and others: Parent report as a means of administering the prescreening developmental questionnaire: an evaluation study, Dev. Behav. Pediatr. **5**(4):195-200, 1984.

Camp, B.W., and others: Preschool developmental testing in prediction of school problems, Clin. Pediatr. **16**(3):257-263, 1977.

Eyberg, S.M., and Ross, A.W.: Assessment of child behavior problems: the validation of a new inventory, J. Clin. Child Psychol. **16**:113-116, 1978.

Fandal, A.W., Kemper, M.B., and Frankenburg, W.K.: Needed: routine developmental screening for all children, Pediatr. Basics **24**:4-7, 1979.

Frankenburg, W.K.: Routine, periodic developmental screening: practical approaches for primary health care providers, Public Health Currents **24**(4):15-18, 1984.

Frankenburg, W.K., and Dodds, J.: The Denver Developmental Screening Test, J. Pediatr. **71**(2):181-191, 1967.

Frankenburg, W.K., and others: The reliability and stability of the Denver Developmental Screening Test, Child Dev. **42**:1315, 1971.

Frankenburg, W.K., and others: The revised Denver Developmental Screening Test: its accuracy as a screening instrument, J. Pediatr. **76**(6):988-995, 1971.

Frankenburg, W.K., and others: Validity of the Denver Developmental Screening Test, Child Dev. **42**:475, 1971.

Harris, C.: Assessment of children's behavior. In Hall, S., editor: Nursing assessment and strategies for the family at risk, ed. 2, Philadelphia, 1986, J.B. Lippincott Co.

Knobloch, H., and Pasamanick, B., editors: Gesell and Amatruda's developmental diagnosis: the evaluation and management of normal and abnormal neuropsychologic development in infancy and early childhood, New York, 1974, Harper & Row, Publishers, Inc.

Krajicek, M.J., and Tearney, A.I.: Detection of developmental problems in children: a reference guide for community nurses and other health care professionals, Baltimore, 1983, University Park Press.

Medenwald, N.A., and others: Is the DDST as good as you think it is? Pediatr. Nurs. **4**(5):53-55, 1978.

Metz, J.R., and others: A pediatric screening examination for psychosocial problems, Pediatrics **58**(4):595-606, 1976.

O'Pray, M.: Developmental screening tools: using them effectively, Am. J. Maternal Child Nurs. **5**(2):126-130, 1980.

Ulrey, G.: Psychological evaluation. In Frankenburg, W.K., Thornton, S.M., and Cohrs, M.E., editors: Pediatric developmental diagnosis, New York, 1981, Thieme-Stratton, Inc.

Unit Three

The Newborn

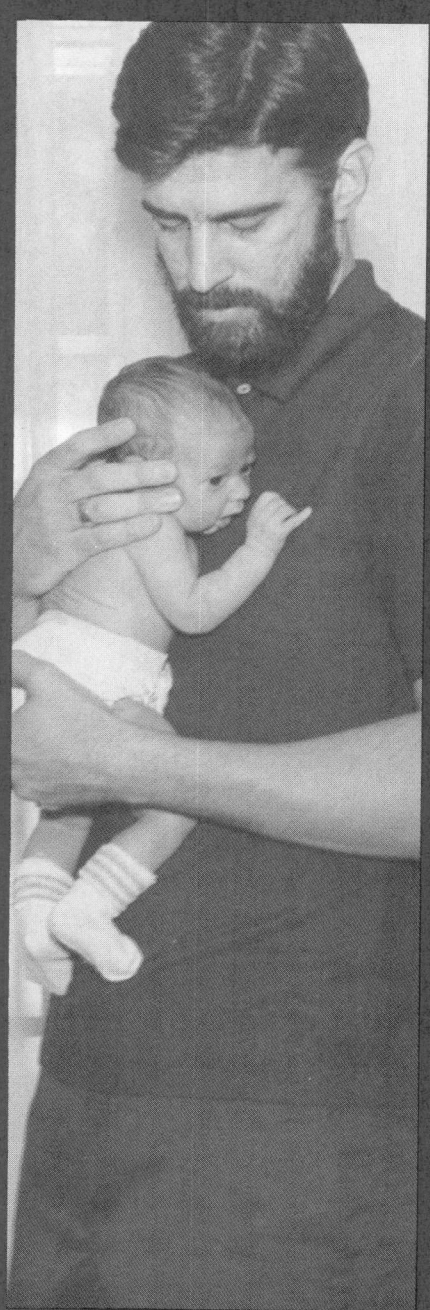

Probably no event is more dramatic or miraculous than the birth of a child. It is the culmination of a 9-month gestation period during which the fetus prepares for extrauterine existence and the parents prepare for the addition of a totally dependent member to their lives. At the time of delivery profound physiologic and psychologic reactions occur that further ready the child and parents for this experience.

In most instances the birth and the perinatal period are uneventful and infants return home with their parents to begin developing as vital, healthy, and loved children. Chapter 8, *Health Promotion of the Newborn and Family*, is concerned with infants' normal adjustment to extrauterine life, their physiologic status at birth, and the nursing knowledge required to care for them at and immediately following delivery, to perform a newborn assessment, and to promote parent-infant attachment. Chapter 9, *Health Problems of the Newborn*, deals with problems related to physical status, environmental agents, birth injury, or metabolic errors that may occur in normal newborns at or during the perinatal period. The emphasis is on the nurse's recognition of, prevention of, and intervention for each of these problems.

Unfortunately not all neonates are born fully matured or perfectly developed. Chapter 10, *The High-Risk Newborn and Family*, focuses on identification and assessment of high-risk neonates, problems common to them because of their high-risk status, physiologic conditions requiring medical and nursing intervention, and supportive care of the child and family throughout this ordeal. Chapter 11, *Conditions Caused by Problems in Physical Development*, discusses the more common defects requiring immediate, temporary, or permanent intervention. Emphasis is on recognition of the abnormality, prevention of complications before and after correction, and emotional support of the family grieving over the loss of the anticipated perfect child.

Chapter 8

Health Promotion of the Newborn and Family

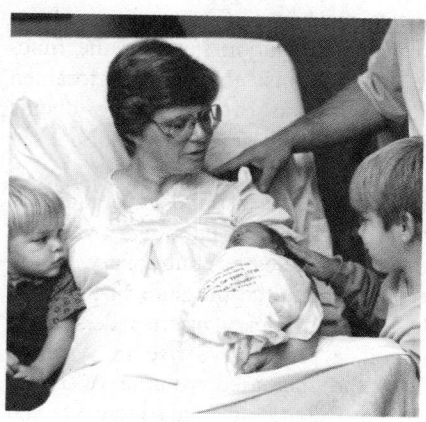

Adjustment to Extrauterine Life
    Immediate adjustments
        Respiratory system
        Circulatory system
    Physiologic status of other
    systems
        Thermoregulation
        Hemopoietic system
        Fluid and electrolyte balance
        Gastrointestinal system
        Renal system
        Integumentary system
        Musculoskeletal system
        Defenses against infection
        Endocrine system
        Neurologic system
        Sensory functions
Newborn Assessment
    Initial assessment: Apgar
    scoring
    Transitional assessment: periods
    of reactivity
        First period
        Second period

Physical assessment
    Assessment of clinical
        gestational age
    General measurements
    General appearance
    Skin
    Head
    Eyes
    Ears
    Nose
    Mouth and throat
    Neck
    Chest
    Lungs
    Heart
    Abdomen
    Female genitalia
    Male genitalia
    Back and anus
    Extremities
Neurologic assessment
Behavioral assessment
    Patterns of sleep and activity
    Cry
**Nursing Care of the Newborn
and Family**
    Provision of physical care
        Maintain a patent airway
        Maintain stable body
            temperature
        Protect from infection and
            injury
        Provide optimum nutrition
    Promotion of parent-infant
    bonding (attachment)
        Infant behavior
        Maternal attachment
        Paternal engrossment
        Siblings
        Assessment of attachment
            behaviors
    Discharge planning and care at
    home

Childbirth is an intense and exhausting physiologic and emotional experience for mothers and newborns (neonates). Even when this process progresses normally, neonates are required to withstand extreme changes as they leave a thermoconstant, aquatic, completely life-sustaining environment and enter a variable pressurized atmosphere that demands profound physiologic alteration for survival. The neonatal or perinatal period, the interval from viability until 28 days after birth, presents the greatest risk to newborns. In the United States, for example, about three quarters of all deaths during the first year of life occur during these 4 weeks.

The nurse's role is one of supporting the family and infant through the birth process, preventing physiologic complications in the neonate's adjustment to extrauterine life, and promoting the attachment process between child and parents. Expert technologic and psychologic nursing care during the immediate postpartum period lays a strong foundation for healthy parent-child development.

Adjustment to Extrauterine Life

The most profound physiologic change required of the newborn is transition from fetal or placental circulation to independent respiration. The loss of the placental connection means the loss of complete metabolic support, the most important and essential function being the supply of oxygen and the removal of carbon dioxide. The normal stresses of labor and delivery produce alterations of placental gas exchange patterns, acid-base balance in the blood, and cardiovascular activity in the neonate. Factors that interfere with this normal transition or increase fetal asphyxia (a condition of hypoxemia, hypercapnia, and acidosis) will affect the fetus's adjustment to extrauterine life. (Factors that influence neonatal adjustments are discussed in Chapter 5.)

IMMEDIATE ADJUSTMENTS

The newborn's adjustment to extrauterine life is a complex physiologic process. The first 24 hours are the most critical, since during this time respiratory distress and circulatory failure can occur rapidly and with little warning. There is a higher incidence of death during these initial 24 hours than during the entire succeeding perinatal period.

Respiratory System

The most critical and immediate physiologic change required of the newborn is the onset of breathing. The stimuli that help initiate the first respiration are primarily chemical and thermal. *Chemical* factors in the blood of low oxygen, high carbon dioxide, and low pH initiate impulses that excite the respiratory center in the medulla. The primary *thermal* stimulus is the sudden chilling of the infant who leaves a warm environment and enters a relatively cooler atmosphere. This abrupt change in temperature excites sensory impulses in the skin that are transmitted to the respiratory center.

The significance of *tactile* stimulation is questionable. Descent through the birth canal and normal handling during delivery, such as drying the skin, probably have some effect on initiation of respiration. Slapping the neonate's heel or buttocks has no beneficial effect; it can waste precious time in the event of respiratory difficulty and can cause additional damage if cerebral trauma has occurred.

The initial entry of air into the lungs is opposed by the surface tension of the fluid that filled the fetal lungs and alveoli. However, fetal lung fluid is removed by the pulmonary capillaries and lymphatic vessels. Some fluid is also removed during the normal forces of labor and delivery. As the chest emerges from the birth canal, fluid is squeezed from the lungs through the nose and mouth. Following complete emergence of the neonate's chest, a brisk recoil of the thorax occurs. Air enters the upper airway to replace the lost fluid. In cesarean birth the chest is not compressed and the newborn may need additional respiratory support.

In the alveoli the surface tension of the fluid is reduced by *surfactant,* a substance produced by the alveolar epithelium that coats the alveolar surface. The effect of surfactant in facilitating breathing is discussed in relation to respiratory distress syndrome (see p. 397).

Circulatory System

Equally important as the initiation of respiration are the circulatory changes that allow blood to flow through the lungs. These changes occur more gradually, and they are the result of shifts in pressure in the heart and major vessels from increased pulmonary and systemic blood volume secondary to decreased pulmonary vascular resistance and increased systemic vascular resistance. The transition from fetal circulation to postnatal circulation involves the functional closure of the fetal shunts: that is the foramen ovale, the ductus arteriosus, and eventually the ductus venosus. (For a brief review of fetal circulation, see Chapter 34.)

Once the lungs are expanded, the inspired oxygen dilates the pulmonary vessels, which decreases pulmonary vascular resistance and consequently increases pulmonary blood flow. As the lungs receive blood, the pressure in the right atrium, right ventricle, and pulmonary arteries decreases. At the same time there is a progressive rise in systemic vascular resistance from the increased volume of blood through the placenta at cord clamping. This increases the pressure in the left side of the heart. Since blood flows from an area of high pressure to one of low pressure, the circulation of blood through the fetal shunts is reversed (see Fig. 34-1).

The most important factor controlling ductal closure is the increased oxygen concentration of the blood. Secondary factors are the fall in endogenous prostaglandins and acidosis. The foramen ovale closes functionally at or soon after birth from compression of the two portions of the atrial septum. The ductus arteriosus is closed functionally by the fourth day. Anatomic closure from deposition of fibrin and cell products takes considerably longer. Failure of the ducts to close results in various types of congenital heart defects (see Chapter 34).

Because of the reversible flow of blood through the ducts during the early neonatal period, functional murmurs are occasionally heard. In conditions such as crying or straining the increased pressure shunts unoxygenated blood from the right side of the heart across the ductal opening, causing transient cyanosis.

PHYSIOLOGIC STATUS OF OTHER SYSTEMS

The major life-dependent physiologic changes in the cardiovascular and respiratory systems of the newborn have already been discussed. However, all of the body systems undergo some change, and most are immature at birth. Each should be observed closely for proper functioning and adjustment to extrauterine life.

Thermoregulation

Next to establishing respiration, heat regulation is most critical to the newborn's survival. Although the newborn's capacity for heat production is adequate, several factors predispose to excessive heat loss. First, the newborn's large surface area facilitates heat loss to the environment. The normal metabolic rate per unit weight of the newborn is about twice that of the adult, but the neonate's surface area per unit weight is about three times larger than that of the adult. Consequently, the infant produces only two thirds as much heat as an adult but loses twice as much heat per unit area. However, the large body surface is partially compensated by the newborn's usual position of flexion, which decreases the amount of surface area exposed to the environment.

The second factor that retards the conservation of body heat is the newborn's thin layer of subcutaneous fat. Since core body temperature is approximately 1° F higher than surface body temperature, this temperature gradient (difference) causes a heat transfer from a higher to lower temperature.

A third factor is the newborn's mechanism for producing heat. Unlike the adult, who can increase heat production through shivering, the chilled neonate cannot shiver but produces heat through nonshivering thermogenesis, which involves increased metabolism and oxygen consumption (see p. 377). The principal thermogenic sources are the heart, liver, and brain. However, there is an additional source unique to the newborn known as *brown adipose tissue* (BAT), or *brown fat*. Brown fat, which owes its name to its larger content of mitochondrial cytochromes, has a greater capacity for heat production through intensified metabolic activity than does ordinary adipose tissue. Heat generated in the brown fat is distributed to other parts of the body by the blood, which is warmed as it flows through the layers of this tissue. Superficial deposits of brown fat are located between the scapulae, around the neck, and behind the sternum. Deeper layers surround the kidneys, trachea, esophagus, some major arteries, and adrenals. The location of the brown fat may explain why the nape of the neck often feels warmer than the rest of the infant's body.

Although concern is usually for newborns' ability to conserve heat, they also can have difficulty dissipating heat in an overheated environment. This increases the risk of hyperthermia.

Hemopoietic System

The blood volume of the newborn depends on the amount of placental transfer of blood. The blood volume of the full-term infant is about 80 to 85 ml/kg of body weight. Immediately after birth the total blood volume averages 300 ml, but depending on how long the infant is attached to the placenta and whether the cord is stripped, as much as 100 ml can be added to the blood volume. However, cord stripping is not a routine procedure because it may cause hypervolemia. It is important that the delivery nurse take special note of the time interval between birth and cord clamping, since blood volume affects hematocrit values, initial blood pressure, and respiratory status. The blood values for the newborn are listed in Appendix D.

Fluid and Electrolyte Balance

Changes occur in the total body water volume, extracellular fluid volume, and intracellular fluid volume during transition from fetal to postnatal life. Early in gestation the fetus is composed almost entirely of water and at term is 73% fluid, as compared to 58% in the adult. There is a higher level of extracellular fluid than intracellular fluid in the fetus, but this shifts progressively throughout postnatal life, probably because of the growth of cells at the expense of extracellular fluid. The infant has a proportionately higher ratio of extracellular fluid than the adult and consequently has a higher level of total body sodium and chloride and a lower level of potassium, magnesium, and phosphate (see Chapter 28).

A very important aspect of fluid balance is its relationship to other systems. Besides the rate of fluid exchange being seven times greater in the infant than in the adult, the infant's rate of metabolism is twice as great in relation to body weight. As a result, twice as much acid is formed, leading to more rapid development of acidosis. In addition, the immature kidneys cannot sufficiently concentrate urine to conserve body water. These three factors make the infant more prone to problems of dehydration, acidosis, and possible overhydration.

Gastrointestinal System

The ability of the newborn to digest, absorb, and metabolize foodstuff is adequate but limited in certain functions. Enzymes are available to catalyze proteins and simple carbohydrates (monosaccharides and disaccharides), but deficient production of pancreatic amylase impairs utilization of complex carbohydrates (polysaccharides). Deficiency of pancreatic lipase limits the absorption of fats, especially with ingestion of foods that have a high saturated fatty acid content, such as cow's milk.

The liver is the most immature of the gastrointestinal organs. The activity of the enzyme *glucuronyl transferase* is reduced, affecting the conjugation of bilirubin with glucuronic acid, which contributes to the physiologic jaundice of the newborn. It is deficient in forming plasma proteins. The decreased plasma protein concentration probably plays a role in the edema usually seen at birth. Prothrombin and other coagulation factors are also low. The liver stores less glycogen at birth than later in life. Consequently the newborn is prone to hypoglycemia, which may be prevented by early and effective feeding, especially breast-feeding.

Some salivary glands are functioning at birth, but the majority do not begin to secrete saliva until about age 2 to 3 months, when drooling is common. The stomach capacity is limited to about 90 ml; thus the infant requires frequent small feedings. The emptying time is short, about 2½ to 3 hours, and peristalsis is rapid. These two factors increase the transit time of food passing through the stomach and colon. During the early weeks of life the newborn may have a bowel movement after each feeding.

The infant's intestine is longer in relation to body size than that in the adult. Therefore there are a larger number of secretory glands and a larger surface area for absorption as compared to the adult's intestine. There are rapid peristaltic waves and simultaneous nonperistaltic waves along the entire esophagus. These waves, combined with an immature relaxed cardiac sphincter, make regurgitation a common occurrence.

Progressive changes in the stooling pattern indicate a properly functioning gastrointestinal tract. The infant's first stool is *meconium,* which is sticky and greenish black. It is composed of intrauterine debris, such as bile pigments, epithelial cells, fatty acids, mucus, blood, and amniotic fluid. Passage of meconium should occur within the first 36 hours.

Usually by the third day after initiation of feedings, *transitional stools* appear. They are greenish brown to yellowish brown in color, thin, seeding, and less sticky than meconium, and may contain some milk curds. By the fourth day a typical *milk stool* is passed. In breast-fed infants the stools are yellow to golden in color and pasty in consistency. They have a peculiar odor, similar to that of sour milk. In infants fed cow's milk formula, the stools are pale yellow to light brown, are firmer in consistency, and have a more offensive odor.

Breast-fed infants usually have more stools than do bottle-fed infants. The stool pattern can vary widely; six stools a day may be normal for one infant, whereas a stool every other day may be normal for another.

Renal System

All structural components are present in the renal system, but there is a functional deficiency in the kidney's ability to concentrate urine and to cope with conditions of fluid and electrolyte fluctuations, such as dehydration or a concentrated solute load.

Total volume of urine per 24 hours is about 200 to 300 ml by the end of the first week. However, the bladder involuntarily empties when stretched by a volume of 15 ml, resulting in as many as 20 voidings per day. The first voiding should occur within 24 hours. The urine is colorless and odorless and has a specific gravity of 1.001 to 1.020.

Integumentary System

At birth all the structures within the skin are present, but many of the functions of the integument are immature. The two layers of the skin, the epidermis and dermis, are loosely bound to each other and are very thin. Slight friction across the epidermis, such as from rapid removal of adhesive tape, causes separation of these layers and blister formation. The transitional zone between the cornified and living layers of the epidermis is effective in preventing fluid from reaching the skin surface.

The *sebaceous glands* are very active late in fetal life and in early infancy because of high levels of maternal androgens. They are most densely located on the scalp, face, and genitalia and produce the greasy vernix caseosa that covers the infant at birth. Plugging of the sebaceous glands causes milia.

The *eccrine glands,* which produce sweat in response to heat or emotional stimuli, are functional at birth, and palmar sweating on crying reaches levels equivalent to anxious adults by 43 weeks of gestation. Observing palmar sweating is helpful in the assessment of pain (Harpin and Rutter, 1982). The eccrine glands produce sweat in response to higher temperatures than those required in adults, and the retention of sweat may result in miliaria.

The *apocrine glands* are another type of sweat gland that develop as an attachment to the hair follicle. They remain small and nonfunctional until puberty.

The growth phases of hair follicles usually occur simultaneously at birth. During the first few months the synchrony between hair loss and regrowth is disrupted, and there may be overgrowth of hair or temporary alopecia. Boys' hair grows faster than girls' hair, and in both sexes scalp hair growth is slower at the crown.

Because the amount of melanin is low at birth, newborns are lighter skinned than they will be as children. This also means that infants are more susceptible to the harmful effects of the sun.

Musculoskeletal System

At birth the skeletal system contains larger amounts of cartilage than ossified bone, although the process of ossification is fairly rapid during the first year. The nose, for example, is predominantly cartilage at birth and is frequently flattened by the force of delivery. The six skull bones are relatively soft and not yet joined. The sinuses are incompletely formed as well.

Unlike the skeletal system, the muscular system is almost completely formed at birth. Growth in the size of muscular tissue is caused by hypertrophy, rather than hyperplasia, of cells.

Defenses Against Infection

The infant is born with several defenses against infection. The first line of defense is the *skin* and *mucous membranes,* which protect the body from invading organisms. The second line of defense is the *reticuloendothelial system,* which produces several types of cells capable of attacking a pathogen. The neutrophils and monocytes are phagocytes, which means they can engulf, ingest, and destroy foreign agents. Eosinophils also probably have a phagocytic property, since in the presence of foreign protein they increase in number. The lymphocytes (T- and B-cells) are capable of being converted to other cell types, such as monocytes and antibodies. Although the phagocytic properties of the blood are present in the infant, the inflammatory response of the tissues to localize an infection is immature.

The third line of defense is the formation of specific *antibodies* to an antigen. This process requires exposure to various foreign agents for antibody production to occur. Infants are generally not capable of producing their own gamma globulins until the beginning of the second month of life, but they receive considerable passive immunity in the form of IgG from the maternal circulation and from human milk (see p. 321). They are protected against most major childhood diseases, including diphtheria, measles, poliomyelitis, infectious hepatitis, and rubella for about 3 months, provided the mother has developed antibodies to these illnesses.

Endocrine System

Ordinarily the endocrine system of the newborn is adequately developed, but its functions are immature. For example, the posterior lobe of the pituitary gland produces limited quantities of antidiuretic hormone (ADH), or vasopressin, which inhibits diuresis. This renders the newborn highly susceptible to dehydration.

The effect of maternal sex hormones is particularly evident in the newborn and it may cause a miniature puberty. The labia are hypertrophied, and the breasts may be engorged and secrete milk during the first few days of life. Female newborns may have pseudomenstruation (more often seen as a milky secretion than actual blood) from a sudden drop in progesterone and estrogen levels.

Neurologic System

At birth the nervous system is incompletely integrated but sufficiently developed to sustain extrauterine life. Most neurologic functions are primitive reflexes. The autonomic nervous system is crucial during transition because it stimulates initial respirations, helps maintain acid-base balance, and partially regulates temperature control.

Myelination of the nervous system follows the cephalo-caudal-proximodistal laws of development and is closely related to the observed mastery of fine and gross motor skills. Myelin is necessary for rapid and efficient transmission of nerve impulses along the neural pathway. Tracts that develop myelin earliest are the sensory, cerebellar, and extrapyramidal. This accounts for acute senses of taste, smell, and hearing in the newborn. All cranial nerves are present and myelinated except the optic and olfactory nerves.

Sensory Functions

The newborn's sensory functions are remarkably well developed and have a significant effect on growth and development, including the attachment process. Unfortunately, minimal research has been done on evaluating the senses, mainly because of difficulty in accurate assessment.

Vision. At birth the eye is structurally incomplete. The fovea centralis is not yet completely differentiated from the macula. The ciliary muscles are also immature, limiting the ability of the eyes to accommodate and fixate on an object for any length of time. The pupils react to light, the blink reflex is responsive to a minimal stimulus, and the corneal reflex is activated by a light touch. Tear glands usually do not begin to function until the infant is 2 to 4 weeks of age.

The newborn has the ability to momentarily fixate on a bright or moving object that is within 20 cm (8 inches) and in the midline of the visual field. In fact the infant's ability to fixate on coordinated movement is greater during the first hour of life than during the succeeding several days. Visual acuity is reported to be between 20/100 and 20/400, depending on the vision measurement techniques (see Table 7-6).

The infant also demonstrates visual preferences: medium colors (yellow, green, pink) over dim or bright colors (red, orange, blue); black and white contrasting patterns, especially geometric shapes and checkerboards; large objects with medium complexity rather than small, complex objects; and reflecting objects over dull ones (Ludington-Hoe, 1983).

Hearing. Once the amniotic fluid has drained from the ears, the infant probably has auditory acuity similar to that of an adult. The newborn is able to detect a loud sound of about 90 decibels and reacts with a startle reflex. The newborn's response to sounds of low frequency and high frequency differs; the former, such as a heartbeat, metronome, or lullaby, tends to decrease an infant's motor activity and crying, whereas the latter elicits an alerting reaction.

There also seems to be an early sensitivity to the sound of human voices, although not to specific speech sounds. One study found that infants younger than 3 days of age can discriminate the mother's voice from that of other females (DeCasper and Fifer, 1980). As early as age 2 weeks the newborn may stop crying to listen to the sound of a voice. The cortical activity associated with hearing or with any other sense is still incomplete at this age because of the immature myelination of the various neural pathways beyond the midbrain. This lack of cortical integration is responsible for the infant's response to sound.

The internal and middle ear are larger at birth, but the external canal is small. The mastoid process and the bony part of the external canal have not yet developed. Consequently, the tympanic membrane and facial nerve are very close to the surface and can be easily damaged.

Smell. Research conducted on newborns' ability to smell demonstrates that they respond differently to various odors. Newborns react to strong odors such as alcohol or vinegar by turning their heads away. Breast-fed infants are able to smell breast milk and will cry for their mothers when the breasts are engorged and leaking. Infants are also able to differentiate the breast milk from their mother or from other females by the smell (Macfarlane, 1977). Such maternal odors are believed to influence the attachment process (Porter, Cernock, and Perry, 1983).

Taste. The newborn is able to distinguish between tastes and various types of solutions elicit differing gustofacial reflexes. A tasteless solution elicits no facial expression, a sweet solution elicits an eager suck and a look of satisfaction, a sour solution causes the usual puckering of the lips, and a bitter liquid produces an angry, upset expression. During early childhood the taste buds are distributed mostly on the tip of the tongue.

Touch. At birth the infant is able to perceive tactile sensation in any part of the body, although the face (especially the mouth), hands, and soles of the feet seem to be most sensitive. There is increasing documentation that touch and motion are essential to normal growth and development. Gentle patting of the back or rubbing of the abdomen usually elicits a calming response from the infant. However, painful stimuli, such as a pinprick, will elicit an angry, upset response.

Newborn Assessment

The newborn requires thorough, skilled observation to ensure a satisfactory adjustment to extrauterine life. Assessment following delivery can be divided into three phases: (1) the initial assessment using the Apgar scoring system, (2) transitional assessment during the periods of reactivity, and (3) periodic assessment through systematic physical examination. Awareness of the expected normal findings during each assessment process helps the nurse recognize any deviation that may prevent the infant from progressing uneventfully through the early postnatal period.

INITIAL ASSESSMENT: APGAR SCORING

During the first seconds of the newborn's life, complex extensive physiologic changes occur. It is imperative that the nurse make astute observations during this time. One of the methods used to assess the newborn's immediate adjustment to extrauterine life is the Apgar scoring system, developed by Virginia Apgar in 1952. The score is based on observation of heart rate, respiratory effort, muscle tone, reflex irritability, and color (Table 8-1). Each item is given a score of 0, 1, or 2. Evaluations of all five categories are made 1 and 5 minutes after birth and are repeated until the infant's condition stabilizes. Total scores of 0 to 3 represent severe distress, scores of 4 to 6 signify moderate difficulty, and scores of 7 to 10 indicate absence of difficulty in adjusting to extrauterine life. Despite the severity of the distress with a score of 0 to 3, most survivors are neurologically intact and only a small minority have serious handicaps (Paneth and Fox, 1983).

The *heart rate* is the most evaluative of the five items. For accuracy, the heart rate is counted for 1 minute and correlated with the infant's activity. The apical pulse is taken with a stethoscope, although palpation of the umbilical cord at its junction with the abdomen is reliable, and visible pulsations of the cord may be counted.

A heart rate less than 100 beats/minute indicates severe asphyxia and usually means that some form of resuscitation is necessary. Tachycardia, or heart rate greater than 160 beats/minute, indicates moderate, but recent, asphyxia and usually means that resuscitation is necessary.

Respiratory effort is evaluated as an index of adequate ventilation. This is assessed by listening to the lungs with a stethoscope and counting the respiratory rate for a full minute. If the respirations are slow, shallow, irregular, or gasping, they are indicative of respiratory distress.

Muscle tone refers to the degree of flexion and resistance offered when the nurse attempts to extend the newborn's extremities. The normal infant's position is one of flexion—the extremities are flexed and close to the body and the fist is tightly clenched. Any attempt to alter this flexed position is met with resistance. At the other extreme, an asphyxiated infant is limp and offers no resistance to a change in position.

Reflex irritability is judged by the neonate's response to slapping the sole of the foot with the palm of the hand. The usual response from a healthy newborn is a loud, angry cry. A moderately depressed infant demonstrates annoyance by a facial grimace, but a severely depressed neonate has no behavioral response.

Color indicates central and peripheral tissue oxygenation. Few newborns are completely pink 1 minute after birth; most continue to have some blueness of the extremities, whereas the rest of the body is pink. Pallor and cyanosis all over the body indicate a severely asphyxiated neonate. In evaluating color, especially of dark-skinned newborns, it is important to inspect the color of the mucous membranes of mouth and conjunctiva as well as the color of the lips, palms of the hands, and soles of the feet.

TRANSITIONAL ASSESSMENT: PERIODS OF REACTIVITY

The newborn exhibits behavioral and physiologic characteristics that can at first appear to be signs of stress. However, during the initial 24 hours changes in heart rate, respiration, motor activity, color, mucous production, and bowel activity occur in an orderly, predictable sequence, which is normal and indicative of lack of stress. Distressed infants also progress through these stages but at a slower rate.

Table 8-1 Infant evaluation at birth—Apgar scoring system

	0	1	2
Heart rate	Absent	Slow (less than 100 beats/min)	Greater than 100 beats/min
Respiratory effort	Absent	Slow or irregular	Good; crying lustily
Muscle tone	Limp	Some flexion of extremities	Active motion; well flexed
Reflex irritability	No response	Grimace	Cough or sneeze; vigorous cry
Color	Blue or pale	Body pink, extremities blue	Completely pink

First Period

For 6 to 8 hours after birth the newborn is in the first period of reactivity. During the first 30 minutes the infant is very alert, cries vigorously, may suck a fist greedily, and appears very interested in the environment. At this time the neonate's eyes are usually open, suggesting that this is an excellent opportunity for mother, father, and child to see each other. Because the newborn has a vigorous suck reflex, this is an opportune time to begin breast-feeding. The newborn usually grasps the nipple quickly, satisfying both self and mother. This is particularly important for nurses to remember, since it is likely that after this initially highly active state the infant may be quite sleepy and uninterested in sucking. Physiologically the respiratory rate can be as high as 80 breaths/minute, rales may be heard, heart rate may reach 180 beats/minute, bowel sounds are active, mucous secretions are increased, and temperature may decrease slightly.

After this initial stage of alertness and activity the infant's responsiveness diminishes. Heart and respiratory rates decrease, temperature continues to fall, mucous production decreases, and urine or stool is usually not passed. The infant is in a state of sleep and relative calm. Any attempt at stimulation usually elicits a minimal response. This second stage of the first reactive period generally lasts 2 to 4 hours. Because of the decrease in body temperature, undressing or bathing the infant is avoided during this time.

Second Period

The second period of reactivity begins when the infant awakes from the deep sleep following the first period. The infant is again alert and responsive, heart and respiratory rates increase, the gag reflex is active, gastric and respiratory secretions are increased, and passage of meconium commonly occurs. This second period of reactivity lasts about 2 to 5 hours and provides another excellent opportunity for child and parents to interact. This period is usually over when the amount of respiratory mucus has decreased. Following this stage is a period of stabilization of physiologic systems and a vacillating pattern of sleep and activity.

After a discussion of the seemingly erratic patterns of behavior in the newborn, it is apparent that, in order to identify abnormalities or signs of distress in the respiratory, cardiovascular, or neurologic system, the nurse must thoroughly understand normal characteristics. Observation, not machinery, is the nurse's greatest tool for assessment, and the nursing goal is anticipation and prevention of neonatal stress. The timing of nursing care is based on observation of the neonate's physiologic status. For example, the infant should be dried immediately after delivery to minimize heat loss from evaporation; the initial bath should be postponed until after body temperature has stabilized; eye drops should be instilled after parents and child have established visual contact; and breast-feeding or bottle-feeding should be initiated during one of the two periods of reactivity.

PHYSICAL ASSESSMENT

An important aspect of the care of the newborn is a thorough physical assessment that includes estimation of gestational age and physical examination to identify normal characteristics and existing abnormalities. These initial and ongoing assessments are critical to establishing baseline data for planning, implementing, and evaluating care and should be one of the nurse's priorities in caring for the newborn. The discussion of physical examination focuses on normal findings, variations from the norm that require little or no intervention, and specific potential danger signs that require more careful observation. The reader is encouraged to review the material in Chapter 7 for further discussions of examination techniques. Table 8-2 summarizes physical examination of the newborn.

Table 8-2 Physical assessment of the newborn

AREA	USUAL FINDINGS	COMMON VARIATIONS/ MINOR ABNORMALITIES	POTENTIAL SIGNS OF DISTRESS/ MAJOR ABNORMALITIES
General measurements	Head circumference 33-35 cm (13-14 inches) Chest circumference 30.5-33 cm (12-13 inches) Head circumference should be about 2-3 cm (1 inch) larger than chest circumference Crown-to-rump length 31-35 cm (12.5-14 inches) Crown-to-rump length approximately equal to head circumference Head-to-heel length 48-53 cm (19-21 inches) Birth weight 2700-4000 g (6-9 pounds)	Molding after birth may decrease head circumference Head and chest circumferences may be equal for first 1-2 days after birth	Head circumference <10th or >90th percentile Birth weight <10th or >90th percentile

Continued.

Table 8-2 Physical assessment of the newborn—cont'd

AREA	USUAL FINDINGS	COMMON VARIATIONS/ MINOR ABNORMALITIES	POTENTIAL SIGNS OF DISTRESS/ MAJOR ABNORMALITIES
General appearance	Posture—flexion of head and extremities, which rest on chest and abdomen	Frank breech—extended legs, abducted and fully rotated thighs, flattened occiput, extended neck	Limp posture, extension of extremities
Skin	At birth, bright red, puffy, smooth Second to third day, pink, flaky, dry Vernix caseosa Lanugo Edema around eyes, face, legs, dorsa of hands, feet, and scrotum or labia Normal color changes: *Acrocyanosis*—Cyanosis of hands and feet *Cutis marmorata*—Transient mottling when infant is exposed to decreased temperature	Neonatal jaundice after first 24 hours Ecchymoses or petechiae caused by birth trauma Milia neonatorum Sudamina Normal, but less common color changes: *Erythema toxicum*—Pink papular rash with vesicles superimposed on thorax, back, buttocks, and abdomen; may appear in 2-8 hours and resolves after several days *Harlequin color change*—Clearly outlined color change as infant lies on side; lower half of body becomes pink and upper half is pale *Mongolian spots*—Irregular areas of deep blue pigmentation, usually in the sacral and gluteal regions; seen predominantly in newborns of African, Asian, or Hispanic descent *Telangiectatic nevi ("stork bites")*—Flat, deep pink localized areas usually seen in back of neck	Progressive jaundice, especially in first 24 hours Cracked or peeling skin Generalized cyanosis Pallor Grayness Hemorrhage, ecchymoses, or petechiae that persist Sclerema Poor skin turgor Rashes, pustules, or blisters
Head	Anterior fontanel—diamond-shaped, 4.0-5.0 cm (about 2 inches) at widest part Posterior fontanel—triangular-shaped 0.5-1 cm (0.2-0.4 inch) Fontanels should be flat, soft, and firm	Molding following vaginal delivery Third sagittal (parietal) fontanel Bulging fontanel because of crying or coughing Caput succedaneum Cephalhematoma	Fused sutures Bulging or depressed fontanels when quiet Widened sutures and fontanels Craniotabes
Eyes	Lids usually edematous Eyes usually closed Color—slate gray, dark blue, brown Absence of tears Presence of red reflex Corneal reflex in response to touch Pupillary reflex in response to light Blink reflex in response to light or touch Rudimentary fixation on objects and ability to follow to midline	Subconjunctival hemorrhages Retinal hemorrhages Searching nystagmus or strabismus	Pink color of iris Purulent discharge Mongoloid slant Hypertelorism (3 cm or greater) Congenital cataracts Constricted or dilated fixed pupil Absence of red reflex Absence of pupillary or corneal reflex Inability to follow object or bright light to midline
Ears	Position—top of pinna on horizontal line with outer canthus of eye Startle reflex elicited by a loud, sudden noise Pinna flexible, cartilage present	Inability to visualize tympanic membrane because of filled aural canals Pinna flat against head	Low placement of ears Absence of startle reflex in response to loud noise

Table 8-2 Physical assessment of the newborn—cont'd

AREA	USUAL FINDINGS	COMMON VARIATIONS/ MINOR ABNORMALITIES	POTENTIAL SIGNS OF DISTRESS/ MAJOR ABNORMALITIES
Nose	Nasal patency Nasal discharge—thin white mucus Sneezing	Flattened and bruised	Nonpatent canals Thick, bloody nasal discharge Flaring of nares (alae nasi)
Mouth and throat	Intact, high-arched palate Uvula in midline Frenulum of tongue Frenum of upper lip Sucking reflex—strong and coordinated Rooting reflex Gag reflex Extrusion reflex Absent or minimal salivation Vigorous cry	Precocious teeth Inclusion cysts Epstein pearls White patches (thrush)	Cleft lip Cleft palate Large, protruding tongue or posterior displacement of tongue Profuse salivation or drooling Inability to pass nasogastric tube Hoarse, high-pitched, or other abnormal cry
Neck	Short, thick, usually surrounded by skin folds Tonic neck reflex Neck-righting reflex Otolith-righting reflex	Torticollis	Excessive skin folds Resistance to flexion Absence of tonic neck, neck-righting, or otolith-righting reflex Fractured clavicle
Chest	Anteroposterior and lateral diameters equal Slight sternal retractions evident during inspiration Xiphoid process evident Breast enlargement	Funnel chest (pectus excavatum) Pigeon chest (pectus carinatum) Supernumerary nipples Secretion of milky substance from breasts	Depressed sternum Marked retractions of chin, chest, and intercostal spaces during respiration Asymmetric chest expansion or overexpansion Redness and firmness around nipples
Lungs	Rate—30-60 breaths/minute Respirations chiefly abdominal	Rate and depth of respirations may be irregular, periodic breathing	Apnea—> 20 seconds Dyspnea Tachypnea—rate above 60 breaths/minute
	Cough reflex absent at birth, present by 1-2 days Bilateral equal bronchial breath sounds	Rales shortly after birth	Persistent irregular breathing Periodic breathing with repeated apneic spells Grunting respirations Deep sighing respirations Seesaw respirations Unequal breath sounds Persistent fine rales Rhonchi Diminished breath sounds Peristaltic sounds on one side, with diminished breath sounds on same side
Heart	Rate—120-140 beats/minute and regular Apex—third to fourth intercostal space, lateral to midclavicular line S_2 slightly sharper and higher in pitch than S_1	Sinus arrhythmia Transient cyanosis on crying or straining	Dextrocardia Displacement of apex Cardiomegaly Abdominal shunts Murmurs Persistent cyanosis
Abdomen	Cylindric in shape Liver—palpable 3 cm below right costal margin Spleen—tip palpable < 1 cm below left costal margin Kidneys—palpable 1-2 cm above umbilicus Equal bilateral femoral pulses	Umbilical hernia Diastasis recti	Abdominal distention Localized bulging Distended veins Absent bowel sounds Enlarged liver and spleen Ascites Visible peristaltic waves Scaphoid or concave abdomen Palpable bladder distention following scanty voiding Absent femoral pulses

Continued.

Table 8-2 Physical assessment of the newborn—cont'd

AREA	USUAL FINDINGS	COMMON VARIATIONS/ MINOR ABNORMALITIES	POTENTIAL SIGNS OF DISTRESS/ MAJOR ABNORMALITIES
Female genitalia	Labia and clitoris usually edematous Labia minora larger than labia majora Urethral meatus behind clitoris Hymenal tag Vernix caseosa between labia Urinates within 24 hours	Blood-tinged discharge (pseudomenstruation)	Enlarged clitoris with urethral meatus at tip Fused labia Absence of vaginal opening Fecal discharge from vaginal opening No urination within 24 hours
Male genitalia	Urethral opening at tip of glans penis Testes palpable in each scrotum Scrotum usually large, edematous, and pendulous; usually deeply pigmented in dark-skinned ethnic groups Smegma Urinates within 24 hours	Urethral opening covered by prepuce Inability to retract foreskin Epithelial pearls Erection or priapism Testes palpable in inguinal canal Scrotum small Hydrocele	Hypospadias Epispadias Testes not palpable in scrotum or inguinal canal No urination within 24 hours Inguinal hernia Hypoplastic scrotum
Back and rectum	Spine intact, no openings, masses, or prominent curves Trunk incurvation reflex Patent anal opening Passage of meconium within 36 hours	Pilonidal cyst or sinus Anal fissures	Spina bifida Imperforate anus No meconium within 36 hours

Extremities	Ten fingers and toes
	Full range of motion
	Negative scarf sign—elbow does not reach midline
	Nail beds pink, with transient cyanosis immediately after birth
	Creases on anterior two thirds of sole
	Sole usually flat
	Symmetry of extremities
	Equal muscle tone bilaterally, especially resistance to opposing flexion
	Equal bilateral brachial pulses
		Partial syndactyly between second and third toes
		Clinodactyly of second toe with overlapping into third toe
		Wide gap between hallux and second toe
		Deep crease on plantar surface of foot between first and second toes
		Asymmetric length of toes
		Dorsiflexion and shortness of hallux
			Polydactyly
			Syndactyly
			Hyperflexibility of joints
			Persistent cyanosis of nail beds
			Yellowing of nail beds
			Sole covered with creases
			Fractures
			Dislocated or subluxated hip
			  Limitation in hip abduction
			  Unequal gluteal or leg folds
			  Unequal leg length (Allis sign)
			  Audible click on abduction (Ortolani sign)
			Asymmetry of extremities
			Unequal muscle tone or range of motion

Neuromuscular system	Extremities usually maintain some degree of felxion Extension of an extremity followed by previous position of flexion Head lag while sitting, but momentary ability to hold head erect Able to turn head from side to side when prone Able to hold head in horizontal line with back when prone	Quivering or momentary tremors	Limp extremities Straightening of extremities Paralysis Hypotonia Tremors, twitches, and myoclonic jerks Marked head lag in all positions

Examination of newborns generally presents few problems in terms of gaining their acceptance or cooperation. In general it is best to proceed in an orderly head-to-toe progression, with a few exceptions. Since exposing infants to the air when undressing them usually elicits crying, it is best to listen to the heart, lungs, and abdomen first. Head, chest, and length measurements are taken at the same time to record them accurately and to mentally note their relationship to each other. Weight should be taken with the infant fully undressed. If clothing is not removed, the scale is pre-balanced to adjust for the excess weight by weighing similar articles of clothing first. If irritability and crying occur during the examination, the newborn can be allowed to suck on a nipple or on one's gloved finger, which usually pacifies the child sufficiently to complete palpation and auscultation. Whether or not all these suggestions are followed is less important than establishing a routine that minimizes delay, haphazard organization, and omission of details.

Assessment of Clinical Gestational Age

Assessment of gestational age is an important criterion because perinatal morbidity and mortality are related to gestational age and birth weight. One of the most frequently used methods of determining gestational age is based on physical and neurologic findings. Although several scales are in current use, the one commonly used is the Simplified Assessment of Gestational Age by Ballard, Novack, and Driver (1979) (Fig. 8-1, *A*). The scale is an abbreviated version of

ESTIMATION OF GESTATIONAL AGE BY MATURITY RATING
Symbols: X - 1st Exam   O - 2nd Exam

NEUROMUSCULAR MATURITY

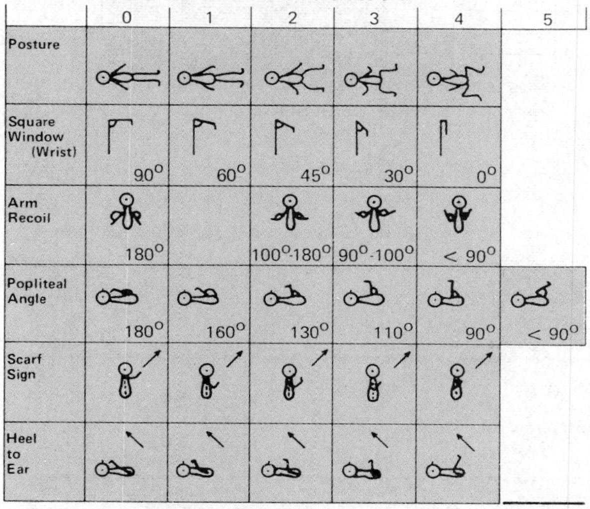

PHYSICAL MATURITY

	0	1	2	3	4	5
SKIN	gelatinous red, transparent	smooth pink, visible veins	superficial peeling &/or rash, few veins	cracking pale area, rare veins	parchment, deep cracking, no vessels	leathery, cracked, wrinkled
LANUGO	none	abundant	thinning	bald areas	mostly bald	
PLANTAR CREASES	no crease	faint red marks	anterior transverse crease only	creases ant. 2/3	creases cover entire sole	
BREAST	barely percept.	flat areola, no bud	stippled areola, 1–2 mm bud	raised areola, 3–4 mm bud	full areola, 5–10 mm bud	
EAR	pinna flat, stays folded	sl. curved pinna, soft with slow recoil	well-curv. pinna, soft but ready recoil	formed & firm with instant recoil	thick cartilage, ear stiff	
GENITALS Male	scrotum empty, no rugae		testes descending, few rugae	testes down, good rugae	testes pendulous, deep rugae	
GENITALS Female	prominent clitoris & labia minora		majora & minora equally prominent	majora large, minora small	clitoris & minora completely covered	

MATURITY RATING

Score	Wks
5	26
10	28
15	30
20	32
25	34
30	36
35	38
40	40
45	42
50	44

Gestation by Dates _____ wks

Birth Date _____ Hour _____ am / pm

APGAR _____ 1 min _____ 5 min

A

SCORING SECTION

	1st Exam=X	2nd Exam=O
Estimating Gest Age by Maturity Rating	_____ Weeks	_____ Weeks
Time of Exam	Date _____ am Hour _____ pm	Date _____ am Hour _____ pm
Age at Exam	_____ Hours	_____ Hours
Signature of Examiner	_____ M.D.	_____ M.D.

Continued.

Fig. 8-1. A, Newborn maturity rating.

Courtesy Mead Johnson & Co., Evansville, IN. A, Scoring section adapted from Ballard, J.L., and others: Pediatr. Res. **11:**374, 1977. Figures adapted from Sweet, A.Y.: Classification of the low-birth-weight infant. In Klaus, M.H., and Fanaroff, A.A.: Care of the high-risk infant, Philadelphia, 1977, W.B. Saunders Co.

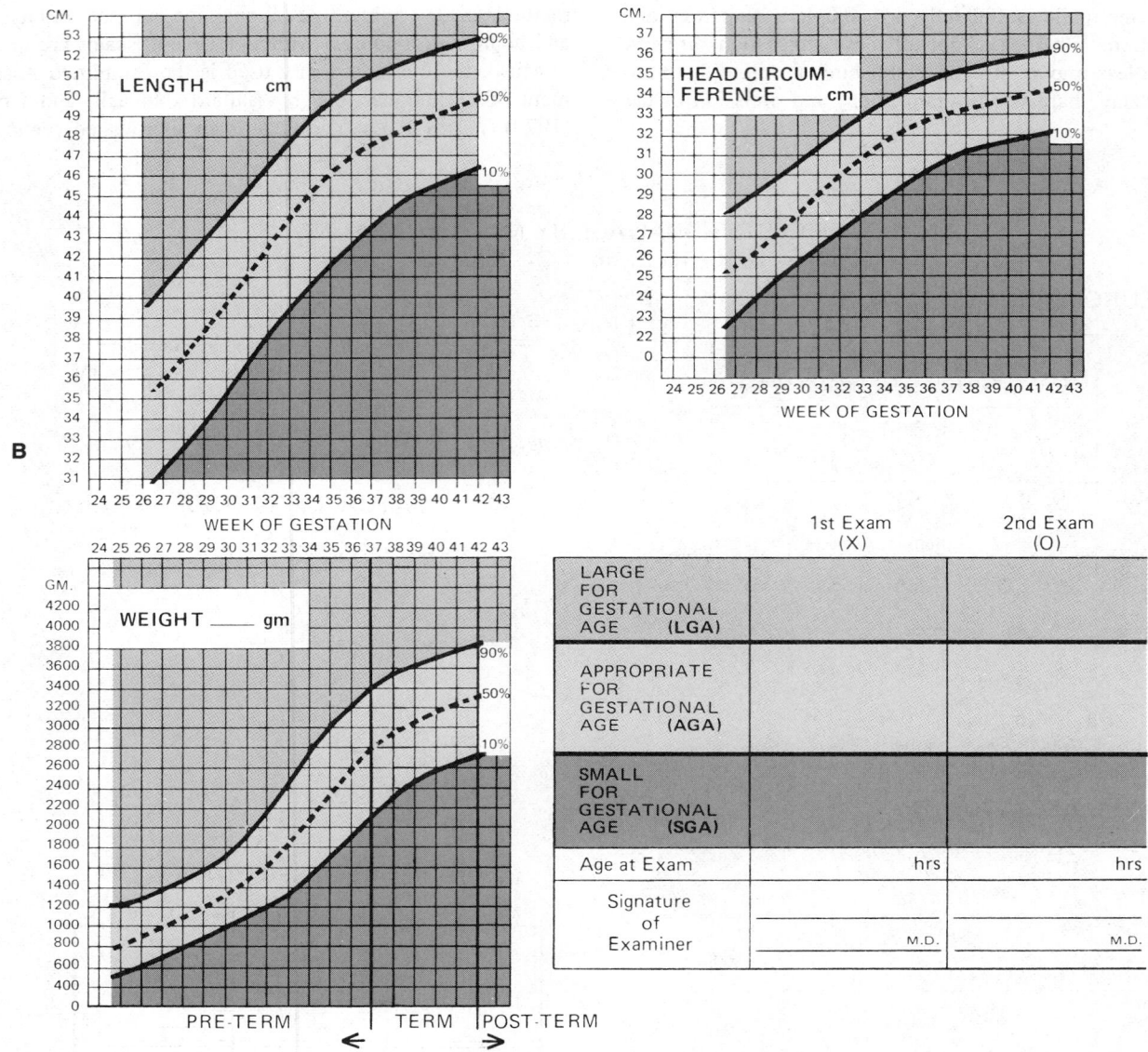

CLASSIFICATION OF NEWBORNS —
BASED ON MATURITY AND INTRAUTERINE GROWTH
Symbols: X - 1st Exam   O - 2nd Exam

Fig. 8-1, cont'd B, Newborn classification based on maturity and intrauterine growth.

B, Adapted from Lubchenko, L.C., Hansman, C., and Boyd, E.: J. Pediatr. **37:**403, 1966; Battagia, F.C., and Lubchenko, L.D.: J. Pediatr. **71:**159, 1967.

the assessment scale developed by Dubowitz, Dubowitz, and Goldberg (1970) and assesses six external physical and six neuromuscular signs. Each sign has a number score and the cumulative score correlates with a maturity rating from 26 to 44 weeks (see Maturity rating box on scale). The maturity rating is accurate within ±2 weeks of the infant's true age.

Assessments can be performed anytime from birth to 42 hours of age, but the greatest reliability is at 30 and 42 hours. By this time the infant has sufficiently stabilized and adjusted following birth, but changes resulting from rapid extrauterine maturation do not interfere with the findings. No matter what scale is used the infant should be examined when alert and with strict adherence to the directions described by the original authors.

In order to facilitate the use of the assessment chart, the following tests and relevant observations are further described:

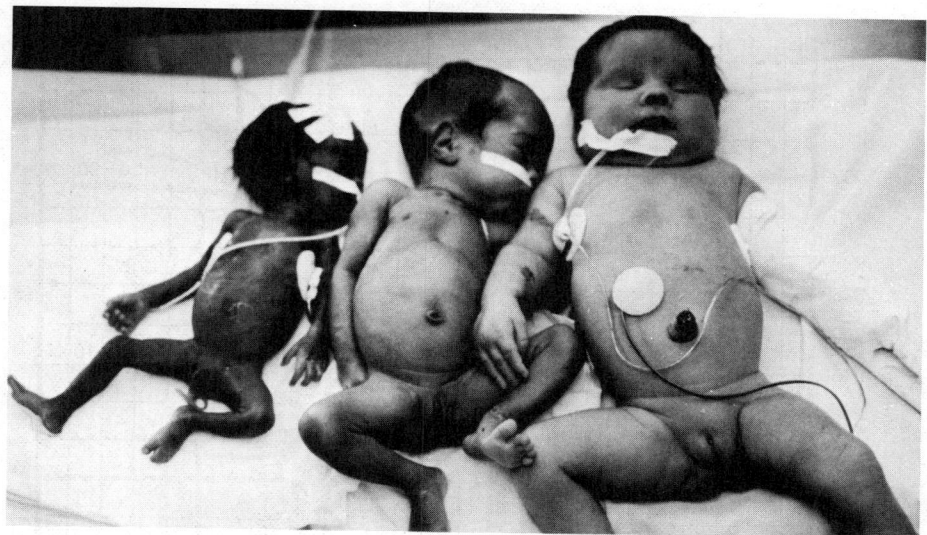

Fig. 8-2. Three babies, same gestational age, weight 600, 1400, and 2750 g, respectively, from left to right. They are plotted in Fig. 8-3 at points *A, B,* and *C.*

From Korones, S.B.: High-risk newborn infants: the basis for intensive nursing care, ed. 4, St. Louis, 1986, The C.V. Mosby Co., p. 118.

resting posture With the infant lying in a supine position, the degree of extension and flexion of arms and legs, knees and elbows, and adduction and abduction of hips are evaluated.

square window The examiner flexes the forearm with enough pressure applied to get as full a flexion as possible to measure the angle between the hypothenar eminence and the ventral aspect of the forearm.

recoil The arm is fully flexed for 5 seconds, then extended by traction on foot or hand, and the maximum response is noted. Full flexion is a maximum response. A brisk return to full flexion is characteristic of a full-term infant; the preterm infant displays sluggish return, only random movements, or no movement at all.

popliteal angle With the thigh in knee-chest position, the leg is extended by gentle pressure to measure the popliteal angle.

scarf sign The examiner attempts to place the infant's hand as far posteriorly around the neck as possible in the direction of the opposite shoulder.

heel-to-ear maneuver The infant's foot is drawn as near to the head as possible without force. The degree of extension and the distance between the foot and the head are noted.

Weight related to gestational age. The weight of the infant at birth also correlates with the incidence of perinatal morbidity and mortality. Since many infants who weigh less than 2500 g (5½ pounds) are not premature by gestational age, there is often confusion between the preterm and the small-for-gestational-age infants; fetal growth, gestational age, and fetal maturity are closely related but are not synonymous. Maturity implies functional capacity—the degree to which the neonate's organ systems are able to adapt to the requirements of extrauterine life. Therefore gestational age is more closely related to fetal maturity than is birth weight. Some infants' heredity influences their size at birth. Oriental and black infants tend to be smaller than white newborns. Small parents have smaller infants and vice versa; therefore it is important to note the size of other family members as part of the assessment process.

Classification of infants at birth by both weight and gestational age provides a more satisfactory method for predicting mortality risks and providing guidelines for management of the neonate. The infant's birth weight, length, and head circumference are plotted on standardized graphs that identify normal values for gestational age (Fig. 8-1, *B*). The infant whose weight is appropriate for gestational age (between tenth and ninetieth percentile) can be presumed to have grown at a normal rate regardless of the time of birth—preterm, term, or postterm. The infant who is large for gestational age (above ninetieth percentile) can be presumed to have grown at an accelerated rate during fetal life; the small-for-gestational-age infant (below tenth percentile) can be assumed to have grown at a retarded rate during intrauterine life. Fig. 8-2 illustrates the disparity between birth weights of three preterm infants of the same gestational age; Fig. 8-3 shows associated risks of mortality.

General Measurements

There are several important measurements of the newborn that have significance when compared to each other as well as when recorded over time on a graph. For the full-term infant, average *head circumference* is between 33 and 35.5 cm (13 to 14 inches). Head circumference may be somewhat less immediately after birth because of the molding process that occurs during a normal vaginal delivery. Usually by the second or third day the normal size and contour of the skull have replaced the molded one.

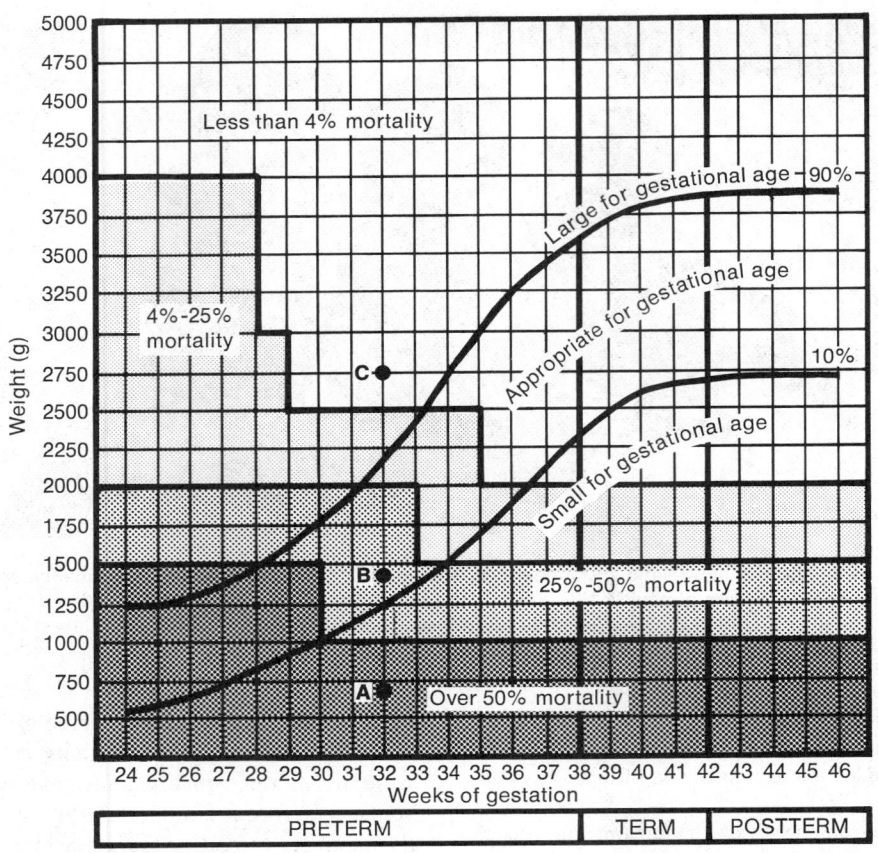

Fig. 8-3. Intrauterine growth status for gestational ages and according to appropriateness of growth.
Adapted from Battaglia, F.C., and Lubchenco, L.C.: J. Pediatr. **71:**159, 1967.

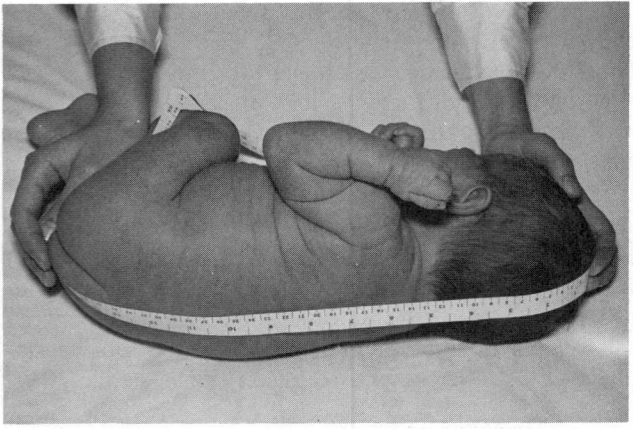

Fig. 8-4. Measurement of crown-to-rump length in newborn.

Chest circumference is 30.5 to 33 cm (12 to 13 inches). Head circumference is usually about 2 to 3 cm (about 1 inch) greater than chest circumference. Because of the molding of the head during delivery, these measurements may initially appear equal. However, if the head is significantly smaller than the chest, microcephaly or premature closure of the sutures (craniostenosis) should be suspected.

If the head is more than 4 cm (1¾ inches) larger than the chest in circumference and this relationship remains constant or increases over several days, then hydrocephalus must be considered. Other causes of increased head circumference are caput succedaneum, cephalhematoma, and subdural hematoma. Prematurity and malnutrition cause the head measurement to be significantly larger than the chest circumference, but this is because of decreased chest size, not increased head circumference.

Head circumference may also be compared with *crown-to-rump length,* or *sitting height* (Fig. 8-4). Crown-to-rump measurements are from 31 to 35 cm (12½ to 14 inches), approximately equal to head circumference. The relationship between the head and crown-to-rump measurements is more reliable than that between the head and chest.

Head-to-heel length is also measured. Because of the usual flexed position of the infant, the examiner must extend the leg completely when measuring total body length. The average length of the newborn is 48 to 53 cm (19 to 21 inches).

Body weight is taken soon after birth because weight loss occurs fairly rapidly. Normally the newborn loses about 10% of the birth weight by 3 to 4 days of age because of loss of excessive extracellular fluid and meconium, and lim-

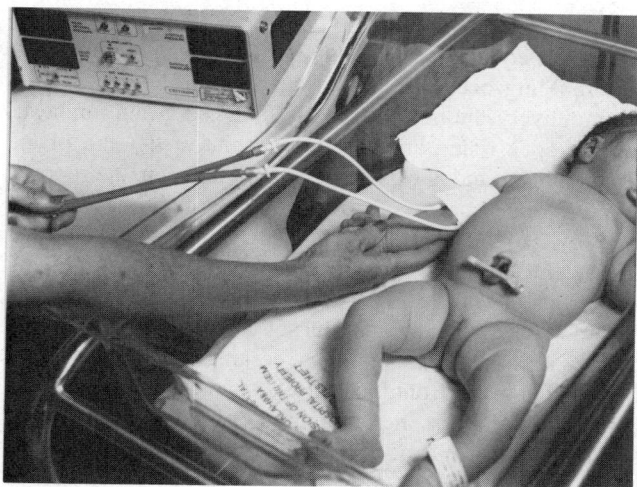

Fig. 8-5. Measurement of blood pressure.
Photography by John Roy, Saint Francis Hospital, Tulsa, OK.

ited food intake. The birth weight is regained by the tenth day of life. Most newborns weigh 2700 to 4000 g (6 to 9 pounds), the average weight being about 3400 g (7½ pounds). Accurate birth weights and lengths are important because they provide a baseline for assessment of risk status and future growth.

Another category of measurements is vital signs. *Axillary temperatures* are taken because insertion of a thermometer into the rectum can cause perforation of the mucosa. Core body temperature varies according to the periods of reactivity but should be 36.5° to 37.5° C (97.7° to 99.5° F). Skin temperature is slightly lower than core body temperature.

Pulse and *respirations* vary according to the periods of reactivity and to the infant's behaviors but are usually in the range of 120 to 140 beats per minute and 30 to 60 breaths per minute, respectively. Both are counted for a full 60 seconds to detect irregularities in rate, rhythm, and quality. Heart rate is taken apically with a stethoscope, although the brachial and femoral arteries are also palpated for equality of strength or fullness.

Blood pressure should be taken and is most accurately assessed using the Doppler method or oscillometry (Fig. 8-5). Comparisons should be made of the blood pressure in the upper and lower extremities and differences of more than 10 mm Hg reported. The average systolic blood pressure is 70 mm Hg at 2 days of age and 84 mm Hg at 2 weeks (Earley and others, 1980). Awake infants have blood pressures about 5 mm Hg higher than sleeping newborns (deSwiet, Fayers, and Shinebourne, 1980).

A suggested schedule for monitoring vital signs is at least once per hour until the infant's condition is stable for 2 hours and then once every 8 hours until discharge (American Academy of Pediatrics, 1983). However, this schedule may vary according to institutional policy. Any change in the infant, such as in color, muscle tone, or behavior, necessitates more frequent monitoring.

General Appearance

Before each body system is assessed, it is important to describe the general posture and behavior of the newborn. The overall appearance yields valuable clues to the physical status of the infant.

Posture. In the full-term newborn the posture is one of flexion, a result of in utero position (Fig. 8-6). Most infants are born in a vertex presentation and keep the head flexed, with the chin resting on the upper chest. The arms are flexed at the elbows and rest, folded, on the chest with hands clenched or fisted. The legs are flexed at the knees, the hips flexed with thighs resting on the abdomen, and the feet dorsiflexed against the anterior aspect of the legs. The vertebral column is also flexed.

Any deviation from this very characteristic fetal position must be recognized. For example, preterm as well as hypoxic infants do not assume an attitude of total flexion but rather one of limp extension. Nonvertex presentations also result in variations in posture. In breech presentations the posture will depend on the presenting part; for example, a frank breech presentation results in extended legs, abducted and fully rotated thighs, a flattened head on top, and a neck that appears elongated.

Behavior. The infant's behavior is carefully noted, especially the degree of alertness, drowsiness, and irritability, which are common signs of neurologic problems. Some questions to mentally ask when assessing behavior include:

- Is the infant awakened easily by a loud noise?
- Is the infant comforted by rocking, sucking, or cuddling?
- Do there seem to be periods of deep and light sleep?
- When awake, does the infant seem satisfied after a feeding?
- What stimuli elicit responses from him?
- When disturbed, how much does the infant protest?

Skin

The skin of the newborn is velvety smooth and puffy, especially about the eyes, the legs, the dorsal aspect of the hands and the feet, and the scrotum or labia.

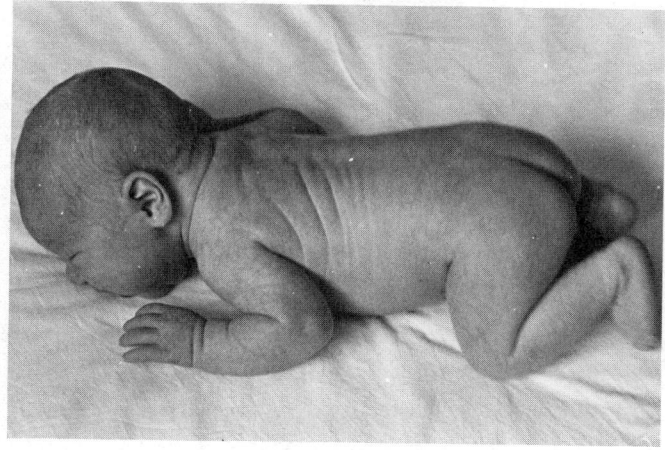

Fig. 8-6. Flexion position of neonate.

At birth the skin is covered with a grayish white, cheese-like substance called *vernix caseosa,* a mixture of sebum and desquamating cells. If it is not removed during the bath, it will dry and disappear by about 24 to 48 hours. A fine, downy hair called *lanugo* is present on the skin, especially on the forehead, cheeks, shoulders, and back. *Milia,* distended sebaceous glands, appear as tiny white papules on the cheeks, chin, and nose. They usually disappear spontaneously in a few weeks. *Sudamina* or *miliaria* are distended sweat (eccrine) glands that cause minute vesicles on the skin surface, especially on the face.

Skin color depends on racial and familial background and varies greatly among newborns. In general, the white infant is usually pink to red; the black newborn may appear a pinkish or yellowish brown. Infants of Hispanic descent may have an olive tint or a slight yellow cast to the skin. Infants of Oriental descent may be a rosy or yellowish tan. The color of American Indian newborns depends upon the tribe and can vary from a light pink to a dark, reddish brown. By the second or third day the skin turns to its more natural tone and is drier and flakier.

General observations are made about the color of the skin in relation to activity, position, and temperature changes. In general the infant becomes redder when crying and may demonstrate transient periods of cyanosis. Decreased temperature increases the degree of cyanosis because of vasoconstriction. Several other color changes that may be noted on the skin are described in Table 8-2.

Head

General observation of the contour of the head is important, since molding occurs in almost all vaginal deliveries. In a vertex delivery the head is usually flattened at the forehead, with the apex rising and forming a point at the end of the parietal bones and the posterior skull or occiput dropping abruptly. The usual, more oval contour of the head is apparent by 1 to 2 days after birth. The change in shape occurs because the bones of the cranium are not fused, allowing for overlapping of the edges of these bones to accommodate to the size of the birth canal during delivery. Such molding does not occur in infants born by cesarean section.

Six bones—the frontal, occipital, two parietals, and two temporals—comprise the cranium. Between the junction of these bones are bands of connective tissue called *sutures*. At the junction of the sutures are wider spaces of unossified membranous tissue called *fontanels*. The two most prominent fontanels are the *anterior fontanel,* formed by the junction of the sagittal, coronal, and frontal sutures, and the *posterior fontanel,* formed by the junction of the sagittal and lambdoidal sutures (Fig. 8-7, *A*). The location of the sutures can be easily remembered because the coronal suture "crowns" the head and the sagittal suture "separates" the head.

Two other fontanels—the *sphenoidal* and *mastoid*—are normally present but are not usually palpable. An additional third fontanel located between the anterior and posterior fontanels along the sagittal suture is found in some normal

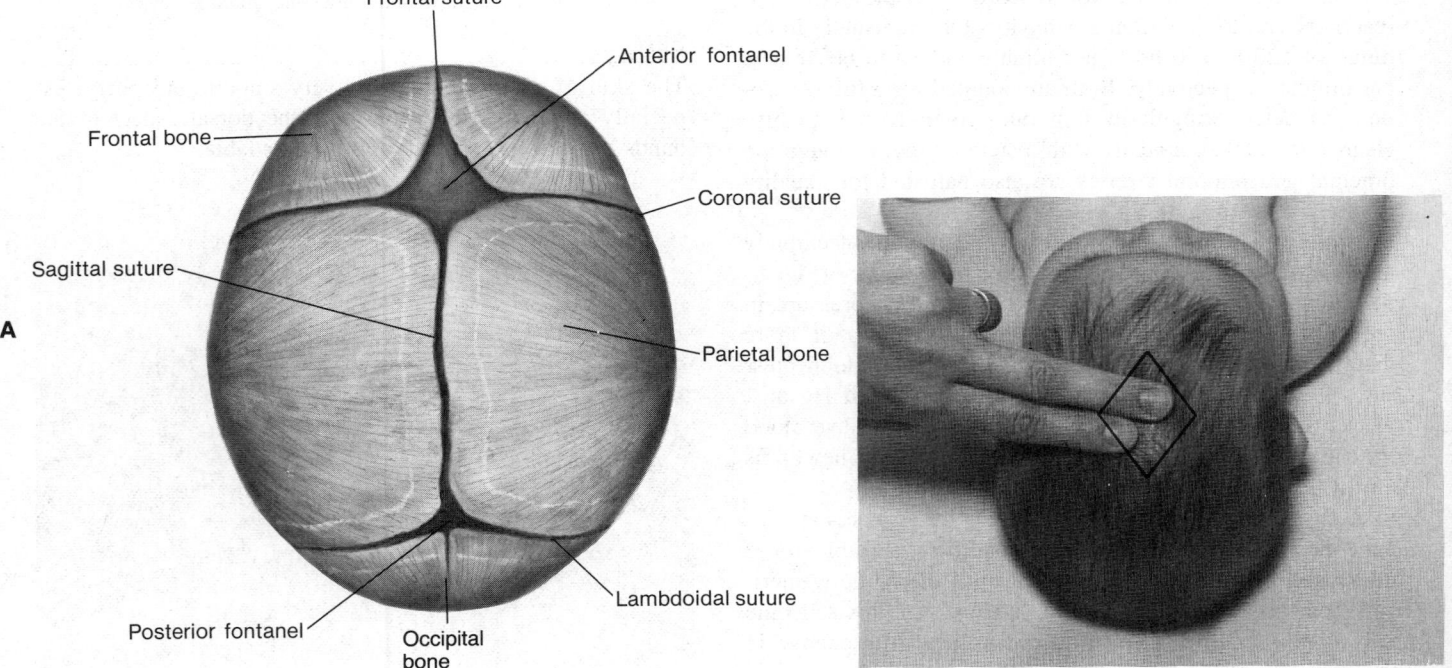

Fig. 8-7. A, Location of sutures and fontanels. **B,** Palpating anterior fontanel.

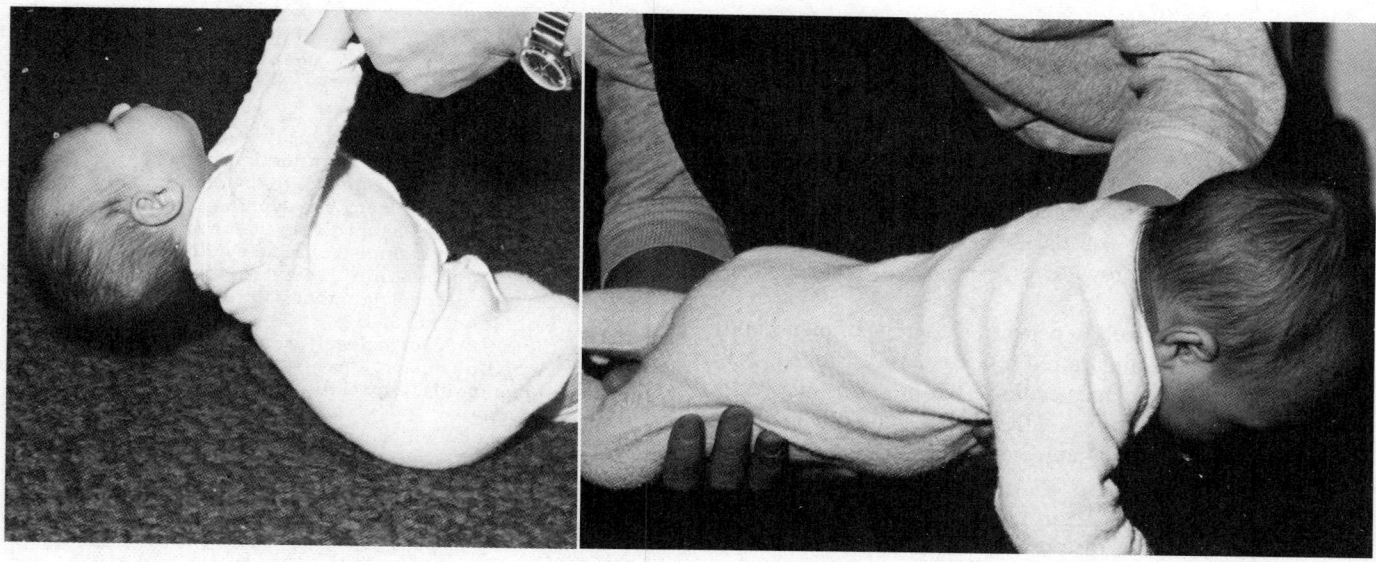

Fig. 8-8. Head control in infant. **A,** Inability to hold head erect when pulled to sitting position. **B,** Ability to hold head erect when placed in ventral suspension.

neonates but is also found in some infants with Down syndrome. The presence of this sagittal or parietal fontanel is always recorded.

The skull is palpated for all patent sutures and fontanels, noting size, shape, molding, or abnormal closure. Sutures are felt as cracks between the skull bones; fontanels are felt as wider "soft spots" at the junction of sutures. These are palpated by using the tip of the index finger and running it along the ends of the bones (Fig. 8-7, *B*).

The anterior fontanel is diamond shaped and measures 4 to 5 cm (about 2 inches) at its widest point (from bone to bone, rather than from suture to suture). The posterior fontanel is triangular shaped, measuring between 0.5 and 1 cm (less than ½ inch) at its widest part. It is easily located by following the sagittal suture toward the occiput.

The fontanels should feel flat, firm, and well demarcated against the bony edges of the skull. Frequently pulsations are visible at the anterior fontanel. Coughing, crying, or lying down may temporarily cause the fontanels to bulge and become more taut. However, a widened, tense, bulging fontanel is a sign of increased intracranial pressure. A markedly sunken, depressed fontanel is an indication of dehydration. Such findings are recorded and reported.

The skull is also palpated for any unusual masses or prominences, particularly those resulting from birth trauma, such as caput succedaneum or cephalhematoma (see p. 342). Because of the pliability of the skull, exerting pressure at the margin of the parietal and occipital bones along the lambdoid suture may produce a snapping sensation similar to the indentation of a Ping-Pong ball. This phenomenon, known as *physiologic craniotabes,* may be found normally, especially in newborns of breech birth, but also may indicate hydrocephalus or syphilis.

The degree of *head control* is assessed. Although *head lag* is normal in the newborn, the degree of ability to control

the head in certain positions should be recognized. If the supine infant is pulled from the arms into a semi-Fowler position, head lag and hyperextension are noted (Fig. 8-8, *A*). However, as infants are brought forward into a sitting position, they attempt to control their heads in an upright position. As the head falls forward onto the chest, many infants attempt to right it into the erect position. If they are held in ventral suspension—that is, held prone above and parallel to the examining surface—the head is held in a straight line with the spinal column (Fig. 8-8, *B*). When lying on the abdomen, newborns have the ability to lift the head slightly, turning it from side to side. Marked head lag is seen in Down syndrome, hypoxic infants, and newborns with brain damage.

Eyes

Since newborns tend to keep their eyes tightly closed, it is best to begin the examination of the eyes by observing the lids for edema, which is normally present for the first 2 days after delivery. A *mongoloid slant,* the lateral upward slope of the eyes with an inner epicanthal fold, may indicate Down syndrome. The eyes are observed for symmetry and for hypertelorism. The distance between the inner canthi is usually not measured unless there is cause for further investigation.

Tears may be present at birth, but purulent discharge from the eyes shortly after birth is abnormal. It may signify *ophthalmia neonatorum* and should be reported.

In order to visualize the surface structures of the eye, the the infant is held supine and the head gently lowered. The eyes will usually open, similar to the mechanism of a doll's eyes. The sclera should be white and clear.

The cornea is examined for the presence of any opacities or haziness. The *corneal reflex* is present at birth but is generally not elicited unless brain or eye damage is suspected.

The pupil usually responds to light by constricting. Absence of the *pupillary reflex,* particularly by 3 weeks of age, suggests blindness. A fixed, dilated, or constricted pupil may indicate anoxia or brain damage. A searching *nystagmus* is common after birth. *Strabismus* is a normal finding because of the lack of binocularity.

The color of the iris is noted. Most light-skinned newborns have slate gray or dark blue eyes, whereas dark-skinned infants have brown eyes. Absence of color is characteristic of albinism.

Although it is difficult to perform a complete funduscopic examination of the retina, a red reflex is easily elicited. Absence of the red reflex may indicate the presence of *retinal hemorrhages* or *congenital cataracts.* (Ocular findings resulting from birth trauma are discussed on p. 341.)

Ears

The ears are examined for position, structure, and auditory function. The pinna is often flattened against the side of the head from pressure in utero. An otoscopic examination is ordinarily not performed because the canals are filled with vernix caseosa and amniotic fluid, making visualization of the drum difficult.

Auditory ability is assessed by making a sharp, loud noise close to the infant's head and noting the presence of the *startle reflex* (see p. 314) or twitching of the eyelids. Absence of any behavioral response to a sudden noise may indicate congenital deafness and is always reported. In some nurseries hearing screening of newborns considered at risk for hearing loss may be performed (see box).

Nose

Patency of the nasal canals is assessed by holding the hand over the infant's mouth and one canal and noting the passage of air through the unobstructed opening. If nasal patency is questionable, it is reported because most newborns are obligatory nose breathers and are unable to breathe orally in response to nasal occlusion (Miller and others, 1985).

The nose is usually flattened after birth and bruises are common, especially if forceps were used. Thin white mucus is very common in the newborn, but a thick, bloody nasal discharge without sneezing may suggest the snuffles of congenital syphilis. *Sneezing* is very common. *Flaring* of the nares is always noted because it is a serious sign of air hunger from respiratory distress.

Mouth and Throat

The mouth is inspected for its existing structures. The palate is normally high arched and somewhat narrow. The hard and soft palates are inspected for any clefts, which warrant further investigation. A common finding is *Epstein pearls*—small, white, epithelial cysts along both sides of the midline of the hard palate. They are insignificant and disappear in several weeks.

The *frenulum* of the upper lip is a band of thick, pink tissue that lies under the inner surface of the upper lip and

---

INFANTS CONSIDERED AT RISK FOR HEARING LOSS

Family history of childhood hearing impairment
Congenital perinatal infection (e.g., cytomegalovirus, rubella, herpes, toxoplasmosis, syphilis)
Anatomic malformations involving the head or neck (e.g., dysmorphic appearance including syndromal and nonsyndromal abnormalities, overt or submucous cleft palate, and morphologic abnormalities of the pinna)
Birth weight less than 1500 g
Hyperbilirubinemia at a level exceeding indications for exchange transfusion
Bacterial meningitis, especially that caused by *Hemophilus influenzae*
Severe asphyxia, which may be exhibited by neonates who have Apgar scores of 0–3 or who fail to institute spontaneous respiration by 10 minutes of age, as well as by those with hypotonia persisting for 2 hours of age

From American Academy of Pediatrics and American College of Obstetricians and Gynecologists: Guidelines for perinatal care, Elk Grove Village, IL, 1983, The Academy, p. 102.

---

extends to the maxillary alveolar ridge. It usually disappears as the maxilla grows. It is particularly evident when the infant yawns or smiles.

The *sucking reflex* is elicited by placing a nipple or tongue blade in the infant's mouth. The infant should exhibit a strong, vigorous suck. The *rooting reflex* is obtained by stroking the cheek and noting the infant's response of turning toward the stimulated side and sucking (Fig. 8-9). The *gag reflex* is elicited when using a tongue blade to visualize the oropharynx.

The *uvula* can be inspected while the infant is crying and the chin is depressed. However, it may be retracted upward and backward during crying. Tonsillar tissue is generally not seen in the newborn. Natal teeth are seen infrequently and erupt chiefly at the position of the lower incisors. They are reported because most of them are loosely attached, increasing the risk of aspiration.

Neck

Since the newborn's neck is short and covered with folds of tissue, adequate assessment requires allowing the head to fall gently backward in hyperextension while the back is supported in a slightly raised position. The nurse observes for range of motion, shape, and any abnormal masses and palpates each clavicle for possible fractures.

Chest

The newborn's chest is almost circular because the anteroposterior and lateral diameters are equal. The ribs are very flexible, and slight intercostal retractions are normally seen on inspiration. The xiphoid process is commonly visible as a small protrusion at the end of the sternum. The sternum is generally raised and slightly curved.

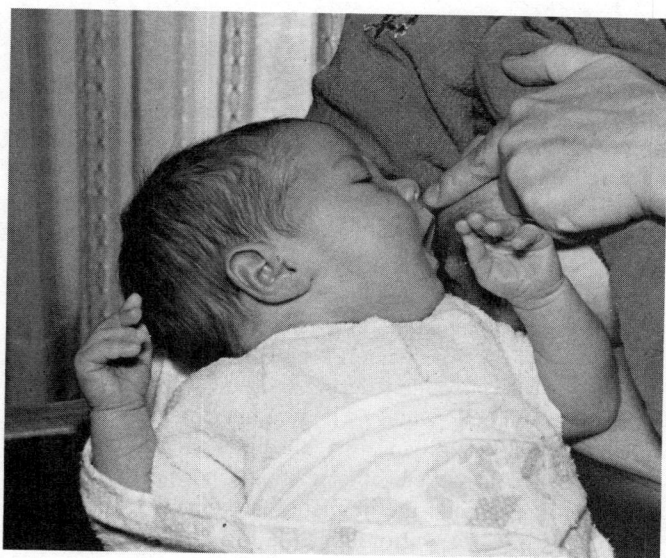

Fig. 8-9. Eliciting rooting reflex.

The breasts are inspected for size, shape, and nipple formation, location, and number. Breast enlargement appears in many newborns of either sex by the second or third day and is caused by maternal hormones. Occasionally a milky substance sometimes called "witch's milk" is secreted by the infant's breasts during the first week.

Lungs

The normal respirations of the newborn are irregular and abdominal, and the rate is between 30 and 60 breaths per minute. Periods of apnea lasting less than 15 seconds are considered normal. After the first forceful breaths required to initiate respiration, subsequent breaths should be easy and fairly regular in rhythm. Occasional irregularities occur in relation to crying, sleeping, and feeding.

Auscultation is best done when the infant is quiet. Bronchial breath sounds should be equal bilaterally. Any differences in auscultatory findings between symmetric sites is reported. *Rales* soon after birth indicate areas of atelectasis, which represent the normal transition of the lungs to extrauterine life. However, persistence of rales or presence of *rhonchi* is also reported.

Heart

Heart rate is auscultated and may range from 100 to 180 beats per minute shortly after birth and, when the infant's condition has stabilized, from 120 to 140 beats per minute. The location of the heart is determined by auscultation. The apex of the heart is usually at the third or fourth intercostal space, lateral to the midclavicular line, because of its more horizontal position in the newborn. Displacement of the apex is noted because it may indicate conditions such as diaphragmatic hernia or pneumothorax. If the heart is on the right side of the body, then *dextrocardia* exists and this is reported since the abdominal organs may also be reversed, with associated functional circulatory abnormalities.

Auscultation of the specific components of the heart sounds is difficult because of the rapid rate and effective transmission of respiratory sounds. However, the *first (S_1)* and *second (S_2) sounds* should be clear and well defined; the second sound is somewhat higher in pitch and sharper than the first. Murmurs are very frequently heard in the newborn, especially over the base of the heart or at the left sternal border in the third or fourth interspace. Ordinarily they are not associated with specific cardiac defects, since they more frequently represent the incomplete functional closure of fetal shunts. (Grading of heart murmurs is discussed in Chapter 7.) However, murmurs are always recorded and reported.

Abdomen

The normal contour of the abdomen is cylindric and usually prominent with visible veins. Bowel sounds are heard a few hours after birth. Visible peristaltic waves may be observed in thin newborns but should not be seen in well-nourished infants.

The umbilical cord is inspected to determine the presence of two arteries, which look like papular structures, and one vein, which has a larger lumen than the arteries and a thinner vessel wall. At birth the cord appears bluish white and moist. After clamping, it begins to dry and appears a dull, yellowish brown. It progressively shrivels in size and turns greenish black.

Palpation is done after inspection of the abdomen. The liver is normally palpable 3 cm (about 1 inch) below the right costal margin. The tip of the spleen can sometimes be felt, but a palpable spleen more than 1 cm below the left costal margin suggests enlargement and warrants further investigation.

Both kidneys should be palpated although they are difficult to locate. Failure to palpate these organs is significant because it generally indicates that no abnormal masses are present in the area. Palpation is best done soon after delivery, when muscle tone is least. Supporting the infant in a semi-Fowler position with one hand and palpating the abdomen with the other hand usually causes the abdominal muscles to relax. Flexing the infant's knees toward the abdomen while the infant is supine will also increase relaxation. Both hands are used to locate the kidneys. As one hand palpates the abdominal area, the other hand provides countertraction by pushing upward from the posterior flank area. The lower half of the right kidney and the tip of the left kidney may be felt 1 to 2 cm (about ½ inch) above the umbilicus. The kidney is felt as an oval structure between the fingers of each hand.

The suprapubic area should also be palpated for evidence of a *distended bladder*. The neonate should void during the first 24 hours after birth. A distended bladder following a scanty voiding may indicate urethral obstruction.

During examination of the lower abdomen, it is particularly important to palpate for femoral pulses, which should be strong and equal bilaterally. Absence of the femoral pulses may be a key indicator of coarctation of the aorta, a congenital heart defect.

Female Genitalia

Normally the labia minora and clitoris are edematous, especially following a breech delivery. However the labia and clitoris must be carefully inspected to identify any evidence of ambiguous genitalia or other abnormalities. Normally in a female the urethral opening is located behind the clitoris. Any deviation from this may suggest that the clitoris may mistakenly be identified as a small penis, which can occur in conditions such as adrenal hyperplasia.

A hymenal tag is occasionally visible from the posterior opening of the vagina. It is composed of tissue from the hymen and the labia minora. It usually disappears in several weeks. Generally the vaginal vault is not inspected. However, absence of the hymenal tag may indicate vaginal agenesis, and in this case further examination is warranted.

Vaginal discharge may be noted during the first week of life. This pseudomenstruation is a manifestation of the abrupt decrease of maternal hormones and usually disappears by 2 to 4 weeks. Fecal discharge from the vaginal opening indicates a rectovaginal fistula and is always reported. Vernix caseosa may be present in large amounts between the labia.

Male Genitalia

The penis is inspected for the urethral opening, which is located at the tip. However, the opening may be totally covered by the prepuce, or foreskin, which covers the glans penis. A tight prepuce is a very common finding in newborns and does not indicate phimosis. It should not be forcefully retracted. *Smegma,* a white cheesy substance, is commonly found around the glans penis, under the foreskin. An erection is not uncommon in the newborn. Small, white, firm lesions called *epithelial pearls* may be seen at the tip of the prepuce.

The scrotum may be large, edematous, and pendulous in the full-term neonate, especially in the infant born in breech position. It is more deeply pigmented in dark-skinned races. A noncommunicating *hydrocele* commonly occurs unilaterally and disappears within a few months. The scrotum should always be palpated for the presence of testes (see p. 274). In small newborns, particularly premature infants, the undescended testes may be palpable within the inguinal canal. Absence of the testes may also be a sign of ambiguous genitalia, especially when accompanied by a small scrotum and penis. *Inguinal hernias* may or may not be manifested immediately after birth. A hernia is more easily detected when the infant is crying.

Back and Anus

The spine is inspected with the infant prone. The shape of the spine should be gently rounded, with none of the characteristic S-shaped curves seen later in life. Any abnormal openings, masses, dimples, or soft areas are noted. A large, protruding sac anywhere along the spine, but most commonly in the sacral area, indicates some type of *spina bifida.* A small sinus, which may or may not be communicating with the spine, is a *pilonidal sinus.* It is frequently covered with a tuft of hair. Although it may have no pathologic significance, it may indicate the existence of spina bifida occulta or be a portal of entry into the spinal column. With the infant still prone, symmetry of the gluteal folds is carefully noted. Any evidence of asymmetry is reported, and tests for congenital hip dislocation are performed by trained (or skilled) examiners (see Chapter 11).

Passage of meconium during the first 24 to 48 hours of life indicates anal patency. If an imperforate anus is suspected and not readily visible, the little finger (gloved and lubricated) or a rubber catheter should be inserted into the anal opening. Rectal thermometers are not used because of the risk of mucosal perforation (see Fig. 7-10). In addition, the small diameter of the thermometer may pass through even a severely stenotic anus (El Haddad and Corkery, 1985).

With the infant still prone, the buttocks are gently separated to inspect the anal area for presence of *fissures,* or small cracks in the mucosa. Anal fissures are a common cause of constipation because the infant refuses to strain during defecation in order to avoid pain. Asymmetry of the mucosal folds around the sphincter also suggests fissures.

Extremities

The extremities are examined for symmetry, range of motion, and signs of malformation or trauma. The fingers and toes are counted, and supernumerary digits (*polydactyly*) or fusion of digits (*syndactyly*) is noted. A partial syndactyly between the second and third toes is a common variation seen in otherwise normal infants.

Range of motion of the extremities should be observed throughout the entire examination. *Hyperflexibility* of joints is characteristic of Down syndrome. Eliciting the *scarf sign* may be helpful in identifying abnormal flexion of joints (see p. 394).

The fingernails are examined; the nail beds should be pink, although slight blueness is evident in acrocyanosis. Persistent cyanosis of the nail beds indicates anoxia or vasoconstriction. Yellowing of the nail beds may indicate intrauterine distress, postmaturity, or hemolytic disease. Short or absent nails are seen in premature infants, whereas long nails, extending over the ends of the fingers, are characteristic of postmature newborns.

The palms of the hands should have the usual creases (see Fig. 7-13). A transverse palmar crease, called a *simian crease,* suggests Down syndrome. The full-term newborn usually has creases on the anterior two thirds of the sole of the foot. In postmature infants the sole is covered with deep creases, and in premature infants the creases are absent. The soles of the feet are flat with prominent fat pads. While examining the feet, the *grasp* and *Babinski reflexes* are elicited (see box on p. 314 and Fig. 8-10). Any foot abnormalities are reported.

The extremities are inspected for evidence of fractures from birth trauma. The humerus and femur are most commonly involved. Limitation of movement, visible deformity, asymmetry of reflexes, and malposition of the site suggest a fracture.

Muscle tone is also assessed. By attempting to extend a flexed extremity, the nurse determines if tone is equal bilaterally. Extension of any extremity is usually met with resistance, and, when released, the extremity will return to its previous flexed position. *Hypotonia* suggests some degree of hypoxia, neurologic disorder, or Down syndrome. Asymmetric muscle tone may indicate a degree of paralysis from brain damage. Failure to move the lower limbs suggests a spinal cord lesion or injury. *Tremors, twitches,* and *myoclonic jerks* characterize neonatal seizures or may indicate neonatal narcotic withdrawal syndrome. Quivering or momentary tremors are usually normal.

NEUROLOGIC ASSESSMENT

Assessing neurologic status is a critical part of the physical examination of the newborn. Much of the neurologic testing takes place during evaluation of body systems, such as eliciting localized reflexes and observing posture, muscle tone, head control, and movement. However, several important mass (total body) reflexes also need to be elicited. They are usually left until the end of the examination because they may disturb the infant and interfere with auscultation. These reflexes as well as several local reflexes are described in Table 8-3. Deviations are indicated by absence, asymmetry, persistence, or weakness of a reflex.

BEHAVIORAL ASSESSMENT

Only about a decade ago, newborns were described as primitive beings who reacted to the environment through reflexes and had little ability to influence the environment around them. Now studies are increasingly demonstrating newborns' ability to react to various stimuli willfully and to greatly affect how others relate to them. The ability to respond to stimulation of all the senses and integrate them is collectively termed *behavior.* The Brazelton Neonatal Behavioral Assessment Scale is an instrument designed to objectively and systematically record behavior responses of newborns (see p. 327). The principal areas of behavior for newborns are sleep, wakefulness, and activity, such as crying.

Patterns of Sleep and Activity

Newborns begin life with a systematic schedule of sleep and activity that is initially evident during the periods of reactivity. For the first hour infants born of unmedicated mothers spend 60% of the time in the quiet alert state and only 10% of the time in the irritable crying state (Saigal and others, 1981). They are intensely alert, the eyes are wide open, and sucking behavior is vigorous. They then become quiet and relatively unresponsive to either internal or external stimuli and fall asleep for a few minutes to 2 to 4 hours. On awakening, they may be hyperresponsive to stimuli. For the next 2 to 3 days it is not unusual for infants to sleep almost constantly in order to recover from the exhausting birth process.

Five distinct states comprise the infant's sleep and are summarized in Table 8-4. The cycle of these sleep states is highly variable and is based on the number of hours an infant sleeps per day, which may range anywhere from 10½

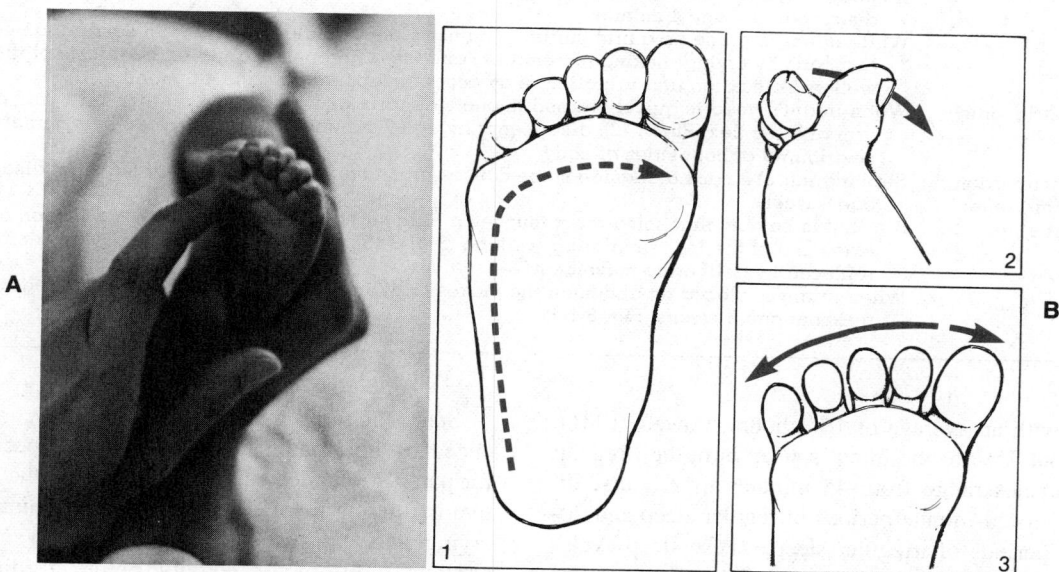

Fig. 8-10. A, Plantar or grasp reflex. **B,** Babinski reflex. *1,* Direction of stroke. *2,* Dorsiflexion of big toe. *3,* Fanning of toes.

Table 8-3 Assessment of reflexes in the newborn

REFLEXES	EXPECTED BEHAVIORAL RESPONSES
Localized	
Eyes	
Blinking or corneal reflex	Infant blinks at sudden appearance of a bright light or at approach of an object toward cornea; persists throughout life
Pupillary	Pupil constricts when a bright light shines toward it; persists throughout life
Doll's eye	As head is moved slowly to right or left, eyes lag behind and do not immediately adjust to new position of head; disappears as fixation develops; if persists, indicates neurologic damage
Nose	
Sneeze	Spontaneous response of nasal passages to irritation or obstruction; persists throughout life
Glabellar	Tapping briskly on glabella (bridge of nose) causes eyes to close tightly
Mouth and throat	
Sucking	Infant begins strong sucking movements of circumoral area in response to stimulation; persists throughout infancy, even without stimulation, such as during sleep
Gag	Stimulation of posterior pharynx by food, suction, or passage of a tube causes infant to gag; persists throughout life
Rooting	Touching or stroking the cheek along side of mouth causes infant to turn head toward that side and begin to suck; should disappear at about age 3-4 months, but may persist for up to 12 months (see Fig 8-9)
Extrusion	When tongue is touched or depressed, infant responds by forcing it outward; disappears by age 4 months
Yawn	Spontaneous response to decreased oxygen by increasing amount of inspired air; persists throughout life
Cough	Irritation of mucous membranes of larynx or tracheobronchial tree causes coughing; persists throughout life; usually present after first day of birth
Extremities	
Grasp	Touching palms of hands or soles of feet near base of digits causes flexion of hands and toes (see Fig. 8-10, *A*): palmar grasp lessens after age 3 months, to be replaced by voluntary movement; plantar grasp lessens by 8 months of age
Babinski	Stroking outer sole of foot upward from heel and across ball of foot causes toes to hyperextend and hallux to dorsiflex (see Fig. 8-10, *B*); disappears after age 1 year
Mass	
Moro	Sudden jarring or change in equilibrium causes sudden extension and abduction of extremities and fanning of fingers, with index finger and thumb forming a C shape, followed by flexion and adduction of extremities; legs may weakly flex; infant may cry (Fig. 8-11); disappears after age 3-4 months, usually strongest during first 2 months.
Startle	A sudden loud noise causes abduction of the arms with flexion of elbows; hands remain clenched; disappears by age 4 months
Perez	While infant is prone on a firm surface, thumb is pressed along spine from sacrum to neck; infant responds by crying, flexing extremities, and elevating pelvis and head; lordosis of the spine, as well as defecation and urination, may occur; disappears by age 4-6 months
Asymmetric tonic neck	When infant's head is quickly turned to one side, arm and leg extend on that side, and opposite arm and leg flex (Fig. 8-12); disappears by age 3-4 months, to be replaced by symmetric positioning of both sides of body
Trunk incurvation (Galant) reflex	Stroking infant's back alongside spine causes hips to move toward stimulated side; disappears by age 4 weeks
Dance or step	If infant is held so that sole of foot touches a hard surface, there is a reciprocal flexion and extension of the leg, simulating walking (Fig. 8-13); disappears after age 3-4 weeks, to be replaced by deliberate movement
Crawl	When infant is placed on abdomen, he makes crawling movements with arms and legs; disappears at about age 6 weeks (Fig. 8-14)

to 23 hours, with an average of 16½ hours (Powell, 1981). Generally about 75% of the infant's sleep is in the irregular state. Sleep cycles range from 45 minutes to 2 hours, divided into 10- to 20-minute periods of regular sleep and 20- to 45-minute periods of irregular sleep. These sleep cycles also roughly correlate with periods of REM and non–REM sleep (see p. 110).

States of sleep and periods of activity are highly influenced by environmental stimuli. It is especially important for parents to understand these states and the methods effective in altering them. Feeding usually terminates the state of crying when hunger is the cause. However, an awake infant exhibits more motor activity before feeding than after. Swaddling or wrapping an infant snugly in a blanket usually

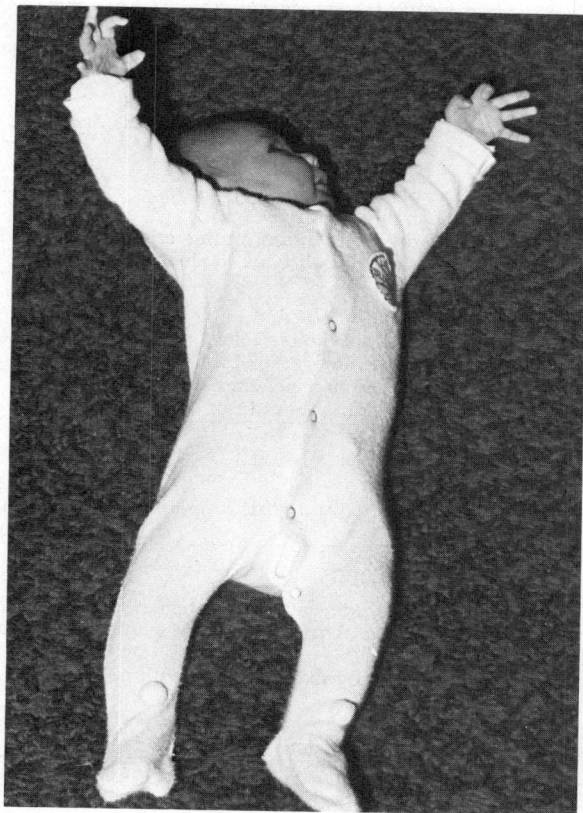

Fig. 8-11. Moro reflex.

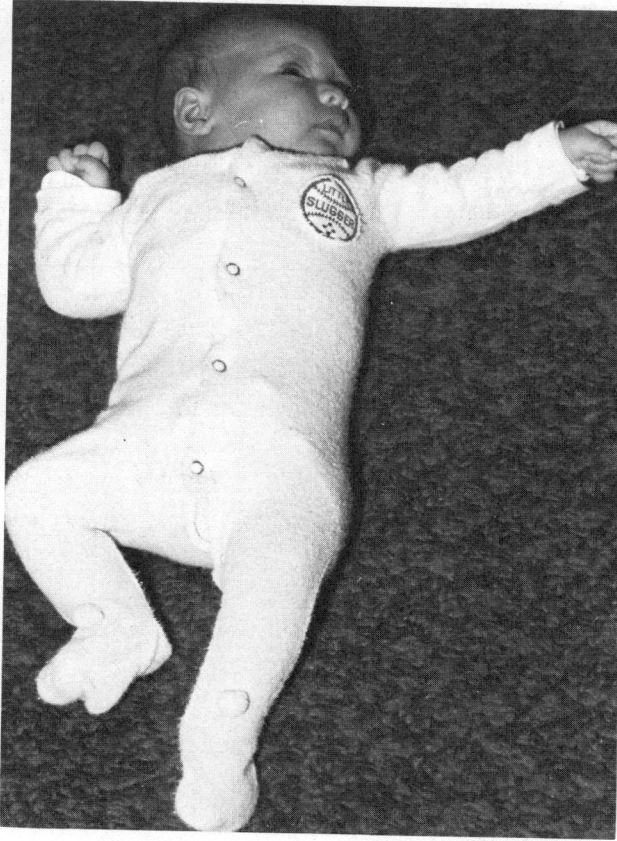

Fig. 8-12. Tonic neck reflex.

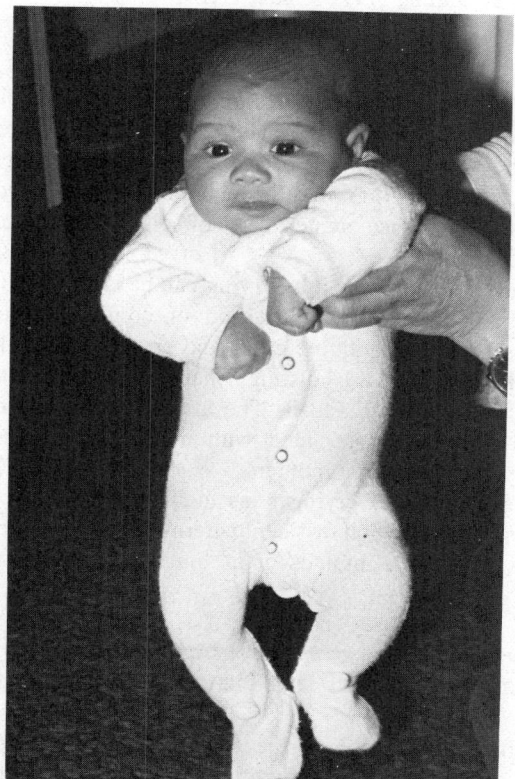

Fig. 8-13. Dance reflex.

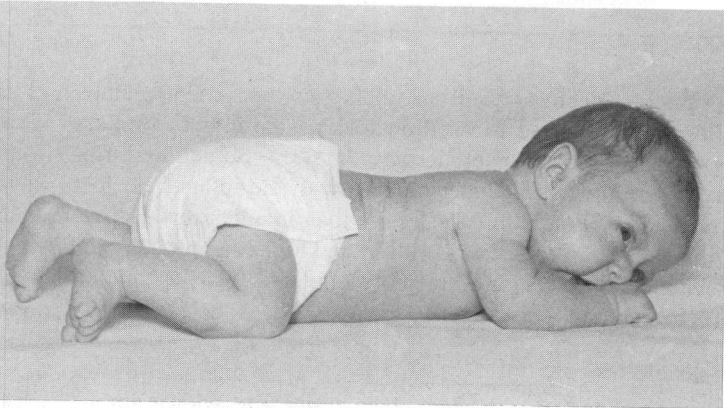

Fig. 8-14. Crawl reflex.

Table 8-4 States of sleep and activity

STATE/BEHAVIOR	DURATION	IMPLICATIONS FOR PARENTING
Regular sleep Closed eyes Regular breathing No movement except for sudden bodily jerks	4-5 hr/day, 10-20 min/sleep cycle	External stimuli do not arouse infant Usual house noises should continue If sudden loud noise awakens infant and he cries, he should be left alone; he will usually fall back to sleep
Irregular sleep Closed eyes Irregular breathing Slight muscular twitching of body	12-15 hr/day, 20-45 min/sleep cycle	External stimuli that did not arouse infant during regular sleep may minimally arouse him Periodic groaning or crying is usual and should not be interpreted as an indication of pain or discomfort
Drowsiness Eyes may be open Irregular breathing Active body movement	Variable	Most stimuli arouse infant Infant should be picked up during this time rather than left in crib
Alert inactivity Responds to environment by active body movement and staring at close-range objects	2-3 hr/day	Infant's needs such as hunger must be satisfied Infant should be placed in that part of home where activity is continuous Infant should not be left in crib or playpen with no stimuli nearby Objects should be within 17.5-20 cm (7-8 inches) of infant's view Constant stimulation initiates and prolongs this state
Waking and crying May begin with whimpering and slight body movement Progresses to strong, angry crying and uncoordinated thrashing of extremities	1-4 hr/day	Behavior provoked by intense internal or external stimuli; such stimuli must be removed for termination of this state Stimuli that were effective during alert inactivity are usually ineffective Rocking and swaddling may decrease crying

promotes sleep as well as maintains body temperature. Some studies have focused on rocking the infant to reduce crying and induce quiet alertness or sleep. Some interesting research findings include: rocking with the infant held in a vertical position is more effective than in a horizontal direction (Pedersen and others, 1969), and higher amplitudes and frequencies of rocking are more effective than lower ones (Pedersen and Ter Vrugt, 1973).

Cry

The newborn should begin extrauterine life with a strong, lusty cry. Variations in this initial cry can indicate abnormalities. A weak, groaning cry or grunt during expiration usually indicates severe respiratory disturbances. Absent, weak, or constant crying suggests brain damage. A high-pitched, shrill cry may be a sign of increased intracranial pressure. One study of newborns in the nursery found differences in the acoustic properties of the infant's cry. With the use of special equipment to analyze sound waves, it was possible to differentiate the normal infant from the abnormal infant, including infants at risk for sudden infant death syndrome (Golub and Corwin, 1982).

One study found that parents respond differently to the cry of normal and premature infants (Frodi and others,

1978). The cry of the premature neonate was perceived as more aversive than the normal infant, and parents reported that they were less eager to interact with the premature infant. Such findings may have important implications for understanding the greater risk of premature infants for abuse.

The sounds produced by crying can be classified into two groups, those of discomfort and of comfort. Discomfort sounds consist initially of gasps and cries in which the consonant ''H'' is clearly distinguishable. Later the sounds of ''W'' and ''L'' are added. The almost universal ''mama'' sound is usually associated with much discomfort and is readily recognized by mothers.

The duration of crying is as highly variable in each infant as is the duration of sleep patterns. Some newborns may cry as little as 5 minutes or as much as 2 hours or more daily.

Nursing Care of the Newborn and Family

The main nursing goal for newborns is provision of physical care, specifically the promotion and maintenance of homeostasis or body equilibrium. For the family the principal objective is promotion of psychologic care—in particular, the promotion of parent-infant attachment and integration of the newborn into the family system.

PROVISION OF PHYSICAL CARE

Physical care for newborn includes: (1) maintenance of a patent airway, (2) maintenance of a stable body temperature, (3) protection from infection and injury, and (4) provision of optimum nutrition. The focus of care is in the nursery rather than the delivery room. Readers who are interested in a more detailed discussion of the immediate care of the neonate are referred to the many excellent maternity texts.

Maintain a Patent Airway

Establishing a patent airway is a primary objective in the delivery room and is the responsibility of the attending physicians and obstetric nurses. However, maintaining a patent airway continues to be a priority goal in the nursery with attention to proper positioning of the infant to facilitate drainage of secretions, especially after feeding (see Fig. 8-18). A bulb syringe is kept near the infant and is used if suctioning is required. To avoid aspiration of amniotic fluid or mucus, the pharynx is cleared first, then the nasal passages. The bulb is compressed *before* insertion to prevent forcing secretions into the bronchi. If more forceful removal of secretions is required, mechanical suction is used. The use of the proper size catheter and correct suctioning technique is essential in order to prevent mucosal damage and edema. Gentle suctioning is necessary to prevent reflex bradycardia, laryngospasm, and cardiac arrhythmias from vagal stimulation. Suctioning is performed for 5 to 10 seconds to prevent depletion of the infant's oxygen supply.

In some nurseries the stomach is routinely lavaged to remove amniotic fluid that may cause abdominal distention and interfere with the establishment of respiration. Passing a catheter to the stomach also rules out esophageal atresia. Vital signs are closely monitored and any indication of respiratory distress is immediately reported.

Maintain Stable Body Temperature

Conserving the newborn's body heat is an essential nursing goal. It requires an understanding of the causes of heat loss—evaporation, radiation, conduction, and convection. Nursing care is based on preventing these.

At birth a major cause of heat loss is *evaporation,* the loss of heat through moisture. The amniotic fluid that bathes the infant's skin favors evaporation, especially when combined with the cool atmosphere of the delivery room. Heat loss through evaporation is minimized by rapidly drying the skin and hair with a warmed towel and placing the infant in a heated environment.

Another source of heat loss is by way of *radiation,* the loss of heat to cooler solid objects in the environment that are not in direct contact with the infant. Loss of heat through radiation increases as these solid objects become colder and closer to the infant. The temperature of ambient or surrounding air in the Isolette or incubator essentially has no effect on loss of heat through radiation. This is a critical point to remember when attempting to maintain a constant temperature for the infant because even though the temperature of the ambient air is optimum, the infant can be hypothermic.

An example of radiant heat loss is the placement of the incubator close to a cold window or air conditioning unit. The cold from either source will cool the walls of the incubator and subsequently the body of the neonate. To prevent this, the infant is placed as far away as possible from walls, windows, or ventilating units. If heat loss continues to be a problem, a radiant warmer may be placed over the infant or the infant and mother.

Heat loss can also occur through conduction and convection. *Conduction* involves loss of heat from the body from direct contact of skin with a cooler solid object; it is minimized by placing the infant on a padded, covered surface rather than directly on a hard table and by providing insulation through clothes and blankets. Placing the newborn very close to the mother, such as in her arms or on her abdomen immediately after delivery, is physically beneficial in terms of conserving heat as well as fostering maternal attachment.

Convection is similar to conduction, except that heat loss is aided by surrounding air currents. For example, placing the infant in the direct flow of air from a fan or air conditioner vent causes rapid heat loss through convection. Transporting the neonate in a crib with solid sides reduces airflow around the infant.

Protect from Infection and Injury

The most important practice for preventing cross-infection is through handwashing of all individuals involved in the infant's care. Several other procedures to prevent infection include eye care, bathing, and care of the circumcision or umbilical stump. Vitamin K is administered to protect against hemorrhage. In addition several safety measures are practiced, particularly in terms of proper identification, and screening tests are used to detect genetic disorders, such as phenylketonuria and hypothyroidism.

Identification. Proper identification of the newborn is the responsibility of the delivery room nurse. However, upon the infant's admission to the nursery the nursery nurse *must* check that two identifying bands are securely fastened, usually on the wrist and ankle, and verify the information (name, sex, mother's admission number, date, and time of birth) against the birth records and the child's actual sex. When the infant is brought to the mother, she should also be asked to verify the information on the identification bands and the child's sex.

Eye care. Prophylactic eye treatment against *ophthalmia neonatorum,* infectious conjunctivitis of the newborn, includes the use of (1) silver nitrate (1%) solution, (2) erythromycin (0.5%) ophthalmic ointment or drops, or (3) tetra-

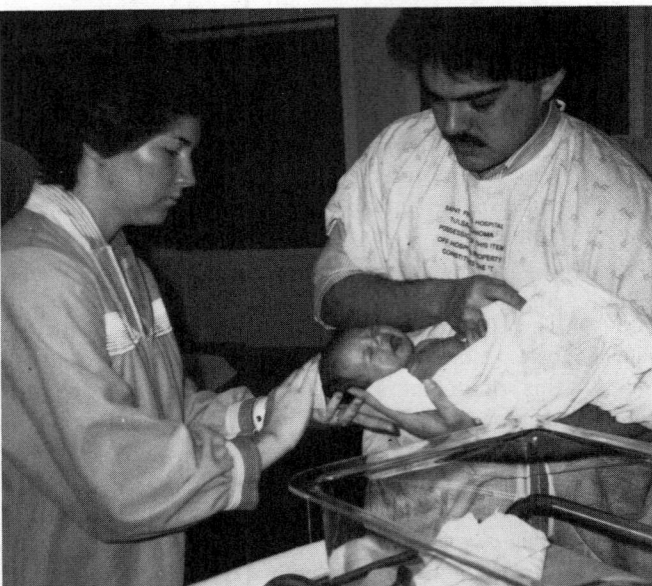

Fig. 8-15. Bath time is an excellent opportunity for parents to learn about their newborn.
Photography by John Roy, Saint Francis Hospital, Tulsa, OK.

cycline (1%) ophthalmic ointment or drops. The drug of choice is either erythromycin or tetracycline because both afford protection against *Chlamydia trachomatis,* a major cause of ophthalmia neonatorum. Silver nitrate is ineffective against this organism and can cause a severe chemical conjunctivitis.

Correct application of the drops or ointment is essential for optimum protection and includes (National Society, 1981):

1. Clean the eyelids with sterile cotton and sterile water if needed.
2. Separate lids and apply 2 drops or at least 1 to 2 cm (1/2 inch) of ointment to the conjunctival sac.
3. Manipulate lids to ensure spread of the medication.
4. Use 2 ampules, one for each eye, or one tube per infant, being careful not to touch eyelid or eyeball with the tip of the tube.
5. Wipe excess medication from eye 1 minute after application.
6. Do not rinse eyes with sterile normal saline.

Since studies on maternal attachment emphasize that in the first hour of life a newborn has a greater ability to focus on coordinated movement than at any other time during the next several days and since eye-to-eye contact is very important in the development of maternal-infant bonding, the routine administration of silver nitrate or antibiotics can be postponed up to 1 hour. However, there must be some kind of checklist to ensure that the drug is given as soon as possible.

Bathing. The bath time can be an opportunity for the nurse to accomplish much more than general hygiene. It is an excellent time for observations of the infant's behavior, such as irritability, state of arousal, alertness, and muscular activity.

In hospitals where there is rooming-in of infant and mother, the bath time provides an opportunity for the nurse to involve the parents in the care of their child and to learn about their infant's individual characteristics (Fig. 8-15). Parents are encouraged to examine every finger and toe of their infant. Frequently normal variations such as Epstein pearls, mongolian spots, or "stork bites" cause parents much worry because they are unaware of the insignificance of such findings. Minor birth injuries may appear as major defects to them. Explaining how these occurred and when they will disappear reassures parents of their infant's normalcy. Common variations are discussed further in Chapter 9.

One of the most important considerations in skin cleansing is preservation of the skin's "acid mantle," which is formed from the uppermost horny layer of the epidermis, sweat, superficial fat, metabolic products, and external substances such as amniotic fluid, microorganisms, and cosmetics. The infant's skin surface has a pH of about 4.9 soon after birth, and this offers important bacteriostatic effects. Consequently, only plain warm water should be used for the bath. Alkaline soaps such as Ivory, oils, powder, and lotions are not used because they alter the acid mantle, thus providing a medium for bacterial growth. Talcum has the added risk of aspiration if applied too close to the infant's face (see Questions and controversies, p. 573).

In the United States the sponging technique is generally used. However, bathing the newborn by immersion has been found to cause less heat loss and less crying (Henningsson and others, 1981).

Bathing is done in the nursery after the vital signs have stabilized. There is no need to immediately wash a newborn, except to remove blood from the face and head. In addition there may be some benefit to leaving the vernix on the skin. Proposed, but unproved, benefits include its insulating and lubricating properties.

Cleansing proceeds in the cephalocaudal direction. A washcloth is used and turned so that a clean part touches the skin with each stroke. The eyes are carefully wiped from the inner to the outer aspect of the lid. The face is cleansed next. The nares are carefully inspected for any crusted secretions. The scalp is usually wiped, although it is sometimes necessary to shampoo the hair. Shampooing is best accomplished by positioning the infant's head over a small basin, lathering the scalp with a mild soap, and rinsing by pouring water from a small vessel over the head into the basin. The rest of the body should be covered during the procedure. The head is dried quickly in order to prevent heat loss from evaporation. The ears are cleaned with the twisted end of a washcloth.

The rest of the body is washed in a similar manner. Although the infant's skin requires little rubbing for adequate cleansing, certain areas (e.g., folds of neck, axillae, and creases at joints) need special attention. The area around the neck is especially prone to a rash from regurgitation of feeding and should be thoroughly washed and dried.

The genitalia of both sexes require careful cleansing. Cleansing of the vulva is done in a front-to-back direction. The bath is a perfect opportunity to stress this part of hygiene to the mother, for both the infant's and her protection against urinary tract infection.

Cleansing the male genitalia involves washing the penis and scrotum. Sometimes smegma needs to be removed by wiping around the glans. The foreskin is not retracted because it is normally tight in newborns. If the infant is not to be circumcised, the parents are taught how to cleanse under and around the foreskin by retracting it gently only as far as it will go and returning it to its normal position. Leaving the prepuce in a retracted position constricts the blood vessels supplying the glans penis, causing edema.

The buttocks and anal area are thoroughly cleansed of any fecal material. As with the rest of the body, the area is dried to prevent a warm, moist environment that fosters growth of bacteria.

Diapers are applied after the bath. They should fit snugly around the thighs and abdomen to prevent urine from leaking. In males cloth diapers are folded with extra thickness in the front to provide greater absorbency. In females the placement of the extra fold depends on whether the infant is prone or supine. Diapers are fastened with the back side overlapping the front side to allow full flexion of the hips.

The nurse should discuss the choice of cloth or disposable diapers with parents. Using disposable diapers exclusively is the most expensive method, costing several times more than cloth diapers laundered at home. Diaper service costs vary but may be more than twice as much as the self-laundry method. Over 1 or 2 years the cost or savings can be considerable, particularly if more than one child is wearing diapers. However, some brands of disposable diapers may help prevent diaper dermatitis (see Questions and controversies, p. 573).

Care of the umbilicus. Because the umbilical stump is an excellent medium for bacterial growth, various methods of cord care are practiced. None has proved superior, although the topical application of triple dye (a solution of brilliant green, proflavine hemisulfate, and crystal violet) has been shown to be more effective than bacitracin ointment (Andrich and Golden, 1984). The dye is applied at the base of the cord with a cotton-tipped applicator and may be reapplied as prescribed by the physician. The diaper is placed below the cord to avoid irritation against the fabric.

Parents are instructed regarding stump deterioration and proper umbilical care. The stump deteriorates through the process of dry gangrene, and when triple dye is used, it falls off in 14 to 17 days (Wilson and others, 1985). The cord base takes a few more weeks to heal completely. During this time care consists of keeping the cord clean and dry and may include wiping the base with alcohol. Any signs of infection, such as presence of erythema and malodorous, purulent discharge, are reported.

Circumcision. Circumcision is the surgical removal of the foreskin on the glans penis. In the Jewish culture circumcision is performed during a highly significant ceremony called a berith, or brit, which takes place on the eighth day of life. A rabbi skilled in the procedure usually performs the circumcision. However, in most instances circumcision is routinely done in the hospital. Despite the frequency of the procedure in the United States, there is much controversy regarding the benefits and risks (see box on Questions and controversies).

In light of these arguments, parents must be allowed an *informed* consent regarding circumcision. Ideally prospective parents should have the opportunity to examine both sides of the question and to decide for themselves without unnecessary pressure from the educator or physician. Fact sheets can be useful in helping them decide (Boyer, 1980).

Circumcision is usually performed in the nursery. It should not be performed immediately after delivery because of the neonate's unstabilized physiologic status and increased susceptibility to stress. Preoperative nursing care includes allowing the infant nothing by mouth before the procedure to prevent aspiration of vomitus, checking for a

---

Questions and Controversies

What are the risks and benefits of neonatal circumcision?

According to the American Academy of Pediatrics (1975, 1983) there are no valid medical indications for circumcision of the newborn and a program of good personal hygiene offers all the advantages of circumcision without the attendant surgical risks. Complications of circumcision include hemorrhage, infection, dehiscence (separation of approximated skin edges), meatitis from loss of protective foreskin, adhesions, concealed penis, urethral fistula, and meatal stenosis (Gibbons, 1984).

Arguments for circumcision include prevention of penile cancer and posthitis (inflammation of prepuce), decreased incidence of balanitis (inflammation of glans), and prevention of complications associated with later circumcision (Boyce, 1983; Kochen and McCurdy, 1980). There is also some evidence that circumcision decreases the incidence of urinary tract infection in infant males (Wiswell and others, 1985). Another nonmedical consideration is preservation of a male's body image that is consistent with his peers, since circumcision is such a common practice in the United States.

Another adverse effect of circumcision that is less commonly considered is the pain inflicted on the infant. Recent studies on the use of regional anesthesia document the distress exhibited in unanesthetized infants, such as increased heart rate, prolonged crying, and decreased blood oxygenation (Holve and others, 1983; Kirya and Werthmann, 1978; Williamson and Williamson, 1983). In each of these studies the use of penile dorsal nerve block significantly reduced these signs of distress and produced no serious complications.

Since nonnutritive sucking has been shown to have a pacifying effect on term and preterm infants during heel-stick procedures (Field and Goldson, 1984), further nursing research could investigate if this nonpharmacologic intervention could reduce distress during circumcision.

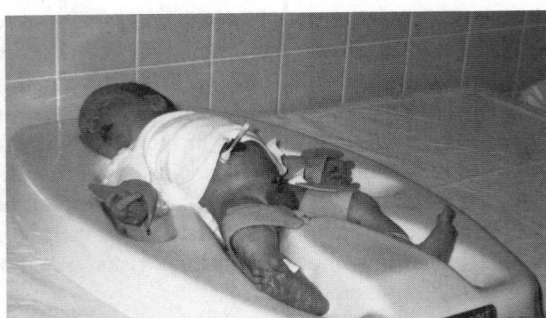

Fig. 8-16. Proper positioning of infant in circumstraint.

signed consent form, and adequately restraining the infant, usually on a special board (Fig. 8-16). All the equipment used for the procedure, such as gloves, instruments, alcohol wipes, dressings, and draping towels, must be sterile.

The procedure involves freeing the foreskin from the glans penis by using a scalpel, Gomco clamp, or Hollister Plastibell. In the Gomco technique the foreskin is clamped and removed; the clamp crushes the nerve endings and blood vessels, promoting hemostasis. In the Plastibell procedure the foreskin is removed using a plastic ring and a string tied around the foreskin like a tourniquet. The excess foreskin is trimmed. In about 5 to 8 days the plastic ring separates and falls off.

As soon as the procedure is completed, the infant is released from the restraints and comforted. Since parents are often concerned about the infant's well-being during this time, the nurse reassures them that the infant is recovering uneventfully. As soon as the infant is calmed and stabilized, he can be brought to the parents.

Care of the circumcision depends on the type of procedure. If a clamp was used, a petrolatum gauze dressing may be applied loosely to prevent adherence to the diaper. If the Plastibell was applied, no special dressing is required. Since the area is tender, the diaper is applied loosely to prevent friction against the penis. Normally on the second day a yellowish white exudate forms as part of the granulating process. This is not a sign of infection and should not be forcibly removed. As healing progresses, the exudate disappears. Parents are cautioned to report any evidence of bleeding or unusual swelling to the physician.

Vitamin K. Shortly after birth, vitamin K is administered intramuscularly to prevent hemorrhagic disease of the newborn (see p. 358). Normally, vitamin K is synthesized by the intestinal flora. However, since the infant's intestine is sterile at birth, and since breast milk contains low levels of vitamin K, the supply is inadequate for at least the first 3 to 4 days. The major function of vitamin K is to catalyze the synthesis of prothrombin in the liver, which is needed for blood clotting and coagulation. The vastus lateralis muscle is the preferred injection site because of the absence of other well-developed muscle masses.

Screening for metabolic disease. A number of genetic metabolic disorders can be detected in the newborn period. There is no national policy in the United States, therefore the extent of neonatal screening is determined by state laws and voluntary guidelines. Most states require screening for phenylketonuria (PKU) and hypothyroidism (see Chapter 9). Other genetic diseases that may be tested for include galactosemia, maple syrup urine disease, homocystinuria, and sickle cell anemia.

The nurse's responsibility is to educate parents regarding the importance of screening and to collect appropriate specimens at the recommended time. Follow-up of newborns discharged early or born at home is critical to prevent unidentified cases.

Transportation after discharge. An important area of counseling is the safe transportation of the newborn home from the hospital. Ideally this counseling should occur *before* delivery to allow parents an opportunity to purchase a suitable infant car restraint. Parents are more likely to use a restraint if the proper use of one is demonstrated and its necessity is stressed (Goodson, Buller, and Goodson, 1985). While federal safety standards do not specify the *minimum* weight of an infant and the appropriate type of restraint, newborns weighing 2.0 kg (4 pounds 8 ounces) receive relatively good support in convertible seats with seat back to crotch strap height of 14 cm (5½ inches) or less. Rolled blankets or towels may be needed under the crotch to prevent slouching. Seats with lap pads or shields are unacceptable because of their proximity to the infant's face (Bull and Stroup, 1985). (For a discussion of appropriate car restraints for infants, see p. 538.)

Provide Optimum Nutrition

Selection of a feeding method is one of the major decisions faced by parents. In general there are three acceptable choices: human milk, commercially prepared cow's milk formula, and modified cow's milk. There are significant nutritional, economic, and psychologic advantages and differences among these methods. Nurses need to be aware of the types of feeding to help parents choose the method that best meets their needs (see also Chapter 12).

Comparison of human milk and cow's milk. There are significant nutritional differences between human milk and whole cow's milk. Cow's milk contains much more available protein (3.5 g/dl) than human milk (0.7 g/dl), but more than the infant requires. The type of protein also differs. Human milk contains more whey proteins, especially lactalbumin, a more complete protein than casein protein. The higher percentage of casein in cow's milk results in formation of large, hard curds. Human milk is more easily digested because of the presence of soft, flocculent curds. Therefore, stomach emptying time is more rapid with human milk, necessitating more frequent feedings. Human milk also contains a higher amount of cystine, an amino acid essential during the first few weeks of life, because the enzyme cystathionase, which converts methionine to cystine, is very low in newborns.

Cow's milk and human milk both provide 20 kcal per

ounce, but human milk contains a higher amount of lactose, a disaccharide that is converted into the monosaccharides glucose and galactose. Galactose is essential for the formation of galactolipids, which are necessary for the growth of the central nervous system.

Although the amount of fat in both types of milk is similar, the type of fat differs. Human milk contains more monounsaturated fatty acids, especially linoleic acid, whereas cow's milk has more polysaturated fatty acids. Human milk has smaller fat globules than cow's milk, which enables the infant to absorb human milk fat more efficiently. In addition, the fat content of human milk varies during the feeding and with time of day. It is higher toward the end of feeding and in early morning.

The mineral content of cow's milk is considerably greater than that of human milk, with the exception of iron and fluoride. Although the amount of iron is low in both types of milk, the iron in human milk is much better absorbed by the infant. Another difference is the amount of calcium and phosphorus, minerals especially needed by the rapidly growing infant. Cow's milk contains more of these minerals but a lower calcium/phosphorus ratio (low calcium and high phosphorus). Because of the infant's immature regulatory mechanisms, calcium is excreted, resulting in tetany. Human milk contains a smaller but more balanced proportion of these minerals and a higher calcium/phosphorus ratio, which are adequate to meet the infant's needs. Both types of milk contain adequate amounts of zinc, a mineral identified as essential to the human. However, the zinc in human milk is more readily absorbed. Both types of milk are low in fluoride and supplementation is recommended (see p. 614).

Both human and cow's milk provide adequate amounts of vitamins A and B complex. Vitamin C is low in cow's milk but higher in human milk provided the mother's intake is adequate. Vitamin D is low in human milk but adequate depending on the mother's intake and the infant's exposure to sunlight. Cow's milk and its preparations are usually fortified with vitamin D. Human milk contains only one quarter the amount of vitamin K as cow's milk, requiring supplementation at birth.

In addition to the nutritional differences between the two types of milk, there exist other significant advantages to human milk. Recent evidence points to the presence of growth modulators, small molecules that modify growth or differentiation. They include taurine, ethanolamine, epidermal growth factor, nerve growth factor, enzymes, and interferons. Their role in human milk is still undefined but they probably act directly on the mammary gland; some may act on the gastrointestinal tract or be absorbed and exert their effect at another site (Gaull, Wright, and Isaacs, 1985). Human milk also offers some important immunologic advantages. It contains high levels of immunoglobin A (IgA) and affords protection against several bacterial and viral diseases, especially those of the respiratory and gastrointestinal systems. IgA also probably protects against development of food allergies. In addition human milk contains numerous

other host defense factors, such as macrophages, granulocytes, and T- and B-lymphocytes (Hanson and others, 1985). Other physiologic benefits of human milk are its laxative effect and less irritation of the skin from stools. Nonphysiologic advantages are discussed under Breast-feeding.

Evaporated milk and commercially prepared formulas. The analysis of human and cow's milk shows that whole cow's milk is unsuitable for infant nutrition. It must be diluted to meet the lowered protein requirement, but, when dilute, it does not meet the caloric or fat requirement. Modified evaporated milk or commercially prepared formula is chosen as a substitute.

In the United States only a very small percentage of infants are fed evaporated milk formula. However, it has many advantages over whole milk. It is readily available in cans, needs no refrigeration if unopened, is less expensive than commercial formula, provides a softer, more digestible curd, and contains more lactalbumin and a higher calcium/phosphorus ratio. A common rule for preparing evaporated milk formula is diluting the 13-ounce can of milk with 17 ounces of water and adding 1 to 2 tablespoons of sugar or corn syrup.

Evaporated milk must not be confused with condensed milk, which is a form of evaporated milk with 45% more sugar. Because of its high carbohydrate concentration and disproportionately low fat and protein content, condensed milk is not used for infant feeding. Likewise, skim milk should not be used because it is deficient in caloric concentration, significantly increases the renal solute load and water demands, and deprives the body of essential fatty acids.

Commercially prepared formulas are milk-based formulas that have been modified to closely resemble human milk (Table 8-5). Although they are not an exact substitute, they do provide an optimum source of nutrition. The formulas are available in three preparations: (1) a ready-to-use form in cans or bottles, (2) a concentrated liquid form that is diluted with an equal amount of water, and (3) a powdered form that must be prepared according to the manufacturer's directions. One consideration in the use of commercially prepared formulas is their cost. It is wise to advise parents to do comparison shopping since one preparation can be considerably more expensive than another.

Breast-feeding. Human milk is the preferred form of nutrition for the infant. In the United States about 60% of newborns in hospitals are breast-fed and about 25% are still breast-fed at 5 to 6 months. There is a continuing trend for more mothers from all socioeconomic levels to breast-feed and to continue breast-feeding longer, although the greatest incidence is among college-educated white women at upper income levels. More employed than unemployed mothers breast-feed but the trend is reversed when infants are 5 to 6 months of age (Martinez and Krieger, 1985). The American Academy of Pediatrics (1982) has repeatedly reaffirmed its recommendation of breast-feeding for full-term infants.

Besides the physiologic qualities of human milk, the most outstanding psychologic benefit of breast-feeding is

Table 8-5 Normal and special infant formulas

FORMULA (MANUFACTUER)	PROTEIN SOURCE	CARBOHYDRATE SOURCE	FAT SOURCE	INDICATIONS FOR USE	COMMENTS (NUTRITIONAL CONSIDERATIONS)
Milk and milk-based formulas					
Evaporated milk formulas Cow's milk	Milk protein; whey/casein ratio: 18:82	Lactose, sucrose	Butterfat	For full-term infants with no special nutritional requirements Undiluted cow's milk after 6 months only.	Supplement with iron and vitamin C; A and D if not fortified; fluoride if fluoridated water is not used for formula preparation.
Commercial infant formulas					
SMA (Wyeth)	Nonfat cow's milk, demineralized whey; whey/casein ratio: 60:40	Lactose	Oleo, coconut, oleic, and soy oils	Full-term and premature infants with no special nutritional requirements.	Supplemented with iron, 12 mg/L.
Enfamil (Mead Johnson)	Nonfat cow's milk, demineralized whey; whey/casein ratio: 60:40	Lactose	Soy, coconut oils	For full-term and premature infants with no special nutritional requirements.	Available fortified with iron, 12 mg/L.
Similac (Ross)	Nonfat cow's milk; whey/casein ratio: 18:82	Lactose	Soy and coconut oils, mono- and diglycerides	For full-term and premature infants with no special nutritional requirements.	Available fortified with iron, 12 mg/L.
Advance (Ross)	Nonfat cow's milk	Lactose	Corn	For feeding of older infants.	Lower caloric content; fortified with iron, 12 mg/L.
Products for premature infants					
"Preemie" SMA (Wyeth)	Milk protein, demineralized whey; whey/casein ratio: 60:40	Malto-dextrins, lactose	Oleo, coconut, oleic, and soy oils, MCT (coconut source)	For low-birth-weight infants.	Protein, 2.5 g/100 kcal. Calcium/phosphorus ratio: 1.9:1
Similac Special Care (Ross)	Nonfat cow's milk, demineralized whey solids: whey/casein ratio: 60:40	Corn syrup solids, lactose	MCT, corn and coconut oils	For low-birth-weight infants.	Calcium/phosphorus ratio: 2:1. Osmolality, 20 cal/oz: 250 mosm/kg water; 24 cal/oz: 290 mosm/kg water.
Enfamil Premature Formula (Mead Johnson)	Nonfat cow's milk, demineralized whey: whey/casein ratio :60: 40	Corn syrup solids	Corn oil, MCT (coconut source), coconut oil	For rapidly growing low-birth-weight infants and infants with special nutritional requirements.	Protein, 3 g/100 kcal. Calcium/phosphorus ratio: 2:1. Osmolality 300 mosm/kg water.
Similac 24 LBW (Ross)	Nonfat cow's milk	Corn syrup solids, lactose	MCT, coconut, and soy oils; mono- and diglycerides	For rapidly growing low-birth-weight infants and infants with special nutritional requirements.	Protein, 2.7 g/100 kcal. Osmolality 290 mosm/kg water.
Similac Natural Care (Ross)	Nonfat cow's milk; whey protein concentrate	Hydrolyzed corn starch, lactose	MCT, coconut and soy oils	For low-birth-weight infants. Fed mixed with human milk or fed alternately with human milk. Improves vitamin/mineral content of human milk.	Protein, 2.2 g/100 ml. Osmolality 300 mosm/kg water.

From Committee on Nutrition, American Academy of Pediatrics: Commentary on breast feeding and infant formulas including proposed standards for formulas. Pediatrics 1976; **57**:278. Committee on Nutrition, American Academy of Pediatrics: Nutritional needs of low-birth-weight infants. Pediatrics 1977; **60**:519. Modified from Kempe, C.H., Silver, H.K., and O'Brien, D., editors: Current pediatric diagnosis and treatment, ed. 8. Copyright 1984 by Lange Medical Publications, Los Altos, Calif.

Table 8-5 Normal and special infant formulas—cont'd

FORMULA (MANUFACTUER)	PROTEIN SOURCE	CARBOHYDRATE SOURCE	FAT SOURCE	INDICATIONS FOR USE	COMMENTS (NUTRITIONAL CONSIDERATIONS)
Products for milk protein–sensitive infants ("milk allergy")					
Prosobee (Mead Johnson)	Soy protein isolate	Corn syrup solids	Soy and coconut oils	With milk protein allergy, lactose intolerance, lactase deficiency, galactosemia.	Hypoallergenic, Zero band antigen. Lactose- and sucrose-free.
Isomil (Ross)	Soy protein isolate	Corn syrup, sucrose	Soy and coconut oils	With milk protein allergy, lactose intolerance, lactase deficiency, galactosemia.	Soy protein isolate. Lactose-free.
Isomil SF (Ross)	Soy protein isolate	Corn syrup solids	Soy and coconut oils	With milk protein allergy or sucrose intolerance.	Sucrose, free and lactose
Products for infants with malabsorption syndromes					
RCF (Ross)	Soy protein isolate		Soy and coconut oils	With carbohydrate intolerance.	Carbohydrate is added according to amount infant will tolerate.
Portagen (Mead Johnson)	Sodium caseinate	Corn syrup solids, sucrose	MCT (coconut source) and corn oil	For impaired fat absorption secondary to pancreatic insufficiency, bile acid deficiency, intestinal resection, lymphatic anomalies.	Fat: 87% MCT, 12% corn oil. Nutritionally complete.
Nutramigen (Mead Johnson)	Casein hydrolysate	Sucrose, modified tapioca starch	Corn oil	For infants and children intolerant to food proteins. Use in galactosemic patients.	Enzymatic hydrolysate of casein. Hypoallergenic formula. Nutritionally complete.
Pregestimil (Mead Johnson)	Casein hydrolysate and L-amino acids	Glucose polymerase, modified tapioca starch	Corn oil, MCT	Disaccharidase deficiencies, malabsorption syndromes, cystic fibrosis.	Nutritionally complete, easily digestible protein, carbohydrate, and fat.
Vital (Ross)	Partially hydrolyzed wheat, meat, and soy proteins; L-amino acids	Hydrolyzed corn starch and sucrose	Safflower oil, MCT (coconut source)	With impaired digestion or absorption, cystic fibrosis.	Nutritionally complete hydrolyzed diet. Osmolality 460 mosm/kg water at 1 kcal/ml.
Specialty formulas					
Lonalac (Mead Johnson) Powder	Casein	Lactose	Coconut	For children with congestive cardiac failure, who require reduced sodium intake.	For long-term management, additional sodium must be given. Supplement with vitamins C and D and iron. Na = 1 meq/L.
Similac PM 60/40 (Ross) Powder	Demineralized, delactosed whey	Lactose	Coconut, corn oils	For newborns predisposed to hypocalcemia and infants with impaired renal and cardiovascular functions.	Low phosphorus. Relatively low solute load. Na = 7 meq/L.

Continued.

Table 8-5 Normal and special infant formulas—cont'd

FORMULA (MANUFACTUER)	PROTEIN SOURCE	CARBOHYDRATE SOURCE	FAT SOURCE	INDICATIONS FOR USE	COMMENTS (NUTRITIONAL CONSIDERATIONS)
Modular formulas Polycose (Ross)		Glucose polymers		Used to increase calorie intake, as in failure-to-thrive infants.	Carbohydrate only. A powdered or liquid calorie supplement. Powder: 32 kcal/Tbsp.
MCT Oil (Mead Johnson)			90% MCT (coconut source)	With fat malabsorption.	Fat only, 8.3 kcal/g. 115 kcal/Tbsp (15 ml.).
For infants with inborn errors Lofenalac (Mead Johnson)	Casein hydrolysate, L-amino acids	Corn syrup solids, modified tapioca starch	Corn oil	For infants and children with phenylketonuria.	80 mg phenylalanine per 100 g. Must be supplemented with other foods to provide minimal phenylalanine.
Phenyl-free (Mead Johnson)	L-amino acids	Sucrose, corn syrup solids, modified tapioca starch	Corn oil	For children over 1 year of age with phenylketonuria.	Phenylalanine-free. Permits increased supplementation with normal foods.
PKU 1 (Milupa)	L-amino acids	Sucrose		For infants with phenylketonuria. (Available as PKU 2 for children over 1 year of age.)	Phenylalanine- and fat-free. Contains vitamins, minerals, and trace elements. Must be supplemented with phenylalanine/protein, carbohydrate, and fat.

the close maternal-child relationship. The infant is nestled very close to the mother's skin, can hear the rhythm of her heartbeat, feel the warmth of her body, and sense a peaceful security. The mother has a very close feeling of union with her child and feels a sense of accomplishment and satisfaction as the infant draws milk from her. Some mothers also experience a type of sensation similar to sexual excitement.

Breast-feeding is the most economical form of feeding, although it is not "free" milk because the lactating mother needs a high-protein, high-calorie diet. Breast milk is always available, ready to serve at room temperature, and free of contamination; there is no need to sterilize bottles. There is less chance of overfeeding and consequent obesity because the infant nurses until satisfied while bottle-fed infants are usually encouraged to finish all their formula. Consequently bottle-fed infants gain weight faster than do breast-fed infants.

The few contraindications to breast-feeding include any serious, debilitating maternal illness (such as severe heart disease or advanced cancer), maternal infections (such as sputum-positive tuberculosis or hepatitis B), and galactosemia in the infant (Miller and Chopra, 1984). Mastitis is usually not a contraindication if the discomfort is tolerable.

Rarely "breast milk jaundice" may require temporary cessation of breast-feeding (see p. 348).

The birth of twins need not create a breast-feeding problem. If both twins are full-term, they can begin feedings immediately after birth (Fig. 8-17).* Simultaneous feeding promotes the rapid production of milk needed for both infants and makes the milk that would normally be lost in the let-down reflex available to one of the twins. When only one infant is hungry, the mother should feed singly. She should also alternate breasts when feeding each infant and avoid favoring one breast for one infant. The sucking patterns of infants vary and each infant needs the visual stimulation and exercise that alternating breasts provides (Riordan, 1983).

Probably the greatest disadvantage of breast-feeding to many mothers is the perceived inconvenience of loss of freedom and independence. Being committed to feeding the infant every 2 to 3 hours can be overwhelming, especially to women with multiple responsibilities. Many women resume their careers shortly after their pregnancy and prefer to use bottle-feeding. However, breast-feeding and employ-

*A resource for mothers is *Breastfeeding Your Twins*, 1984, Health Education Associates, 520 School House Lane, Willow Grove, PA 09190.

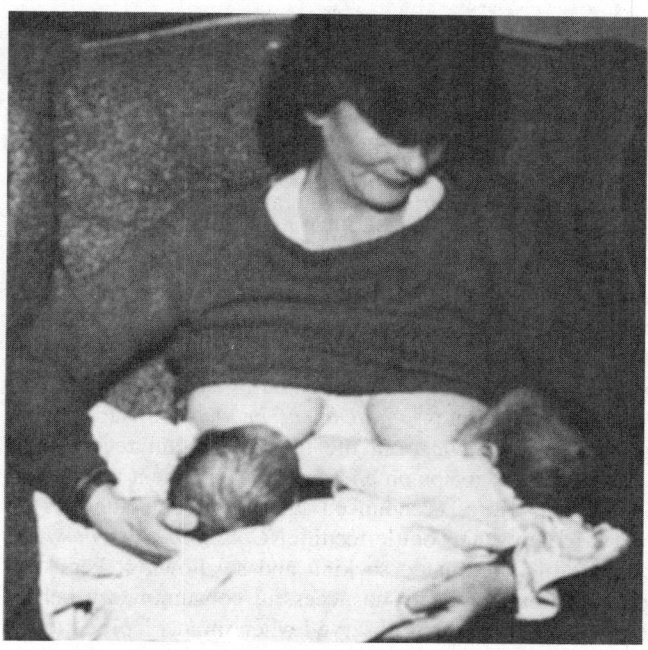

Fig. 8-17. Simultaneous breast-feeding of twins.

ment are possible and suggestions for the mother are discussed in Chapter 12. While breast-feeding is the preferred form of infant feeding, mothers' decision regarding their preferences must be supported and respected.

Successful breast-feeding probably depends more on the mother's desire to breast-feed, satisfaction with breast-feeding, and available support systems than on any other factors. Contrary to popular belief, breast-feeding is not instinctive. Mothers need support, encouragement, and assistance during their postpartum hospital stay to enhance their opportunities for success and satisfaction. Research increasingly supports the concept that the following hospital interventions promote breast-feeding (de Carvalho and others, 1983; Reiff and Essock-Vitale, 1985; Winikoff and Baer, 1980):

- Increased information and support to mothers
- Routines, such as frequent and early breast-feeding, especially during the first hour of life; immediate skin-to-skin contact, rooming-in, and careful control of drugs
- Direct modeling of the importance of breast-feeding by staff, such as implementing demand nursing with no supplemental bottles and decreased emphasis on infant formula products

Dissatisfaction and the perception of ''problems'' with breast-feeding within the first 2 weeks have been identified as predictors of early weaning (Humenick and Van Steenkiste, 1983). Possibly if these mothers were identified early and received additional nursing support and encouragement, breast-feeding might be encouraged for extended periods. Certainly, nurses play a very significant role in the breast-feeding decision and must make themselves available to families for guidance and support. Several excellent books

(Lawrence, 1985; Riordan, 1983) and organizations* are available as resources for professionals and breast-feeding mothers (see also Lawrence, 1985, p. 545).

Bottle-feeding. With commercial formulas that closely approximate human milk and with greatly improved conditions of sanitation, bottle-feeding is a perfectly acceptable method of feeding. However, nurses should not assume that new parents automatically know how to bottle-feed their infant. These parents also need support and assistance in meeting their infant's needs.

Providing newborns with nutrition is only one aspect of the feeding. Holding them close to the body and rocking or cuddling them help to ensure the emotional component of feeding. Like breast-fed infants, bottle-fed infants need to be held on either side of the lap to expose them to different stimuli. The feeding should not be hurried. Even though they may suck vigorously for the first 5 minutes and seem to be satisfied, they are allowed to continue sucking. Infants need at least 2 hours of sucking a day. If there are six feedings per day, then about 20 minutes of sucking at each feeding provides for oral gratification.

After feedings infants are positioned on the right side to permit the feeding to flow toward the lower end of the stomach and to allow any swallowed air to rise above the fluid and through the esophagus (Fig. 8-18). This position prevents regurgitation and distention. To maintain the side-lying position, a pillow can be placed snugly behind the back.

Propping the bottle is discouraged. Most importantly propping denies the infant the vital component of close human contact; feeding should be associated with socialization. Because infants do not have the motor control to voluntarily push the bottle away when finished, they may aspirate formula while sleeping. These infants also tend to contract more middle ear infections. As the infant lies flat

*La Leche League International, Inc., 9616 Minneapolis Ave., Franklin Park, IL 60131.

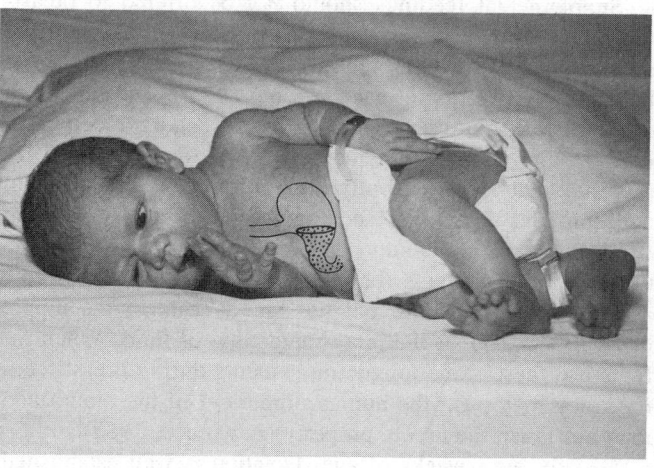

Fig. 8-18. Right-side-lying position after feeding.

and sucks, milk that has pooled in the pharynx becomes a suitable medium for bacterial growth. Bacteria then enter the eustachian tube, which leads to the middle ear, causing acute otitis media.

Preparation of formula. The two traditional ways of preparing formula are the terminal heat method and the aseptic method. In the terminal heat method all the utensils and formula are boiled together for 25 minutes. In the aseptic method the equipment is boiled separately, after which the formula is poured into the bottles.

Because of improved sanitary conditions, neither of these methods is essential. The clean technique is satisfactory. Persons preparing the formula should wash their hands well and then wash all the equipment used to prepare the formula, including the cans of formula or evaporated milk. The formula is prepared and bottled immediately before each feeding. Warming the formula is optional, although many parents prefer to warm it before feeding. Any milk remaining in the bottle after the feeding is discarded, since it is an excellent medium for bacterial growth. Opened cans of formula are covered and refrigerated until the next feeding.

Recent recommendations for labeling infant formulas require that the directions for preparation and use of the formula include pictures and symbols for nonreading individuals. In addition manufacturers are translating the directions into foreign languages, such as Spanish and Vietnamese, to prevent misunderstanding and errors in formula preparation. It is important to impress upon families that the proportions *must not be altered*—neither diluted to extend the amount of formula nor concentrated to provide more calories.

Feeding schedules. Ideally feeding schedules should be determined by the infant's hunger. Feeding infants when they signal readiness is called *demand feeding. Scheduled feedings* are arranged at predetermined intervals to meet family routines. Some hospitals routinely feed infants every 4 hours. Although this is satisfactory for bottle-fed infants, it hinders the breast-feeding process. Since breast-fed infants tend to be hungry every 2 to 3 hours, they should be fed on demand.

Supplemental feedings should *not* be offered to breast-fed infants in the nursery because, if satiated, they will not suck vigorously at the breast. Lactation depends on the breast being emptied at each feeding. If milk is allowed to accumulate in the ducts, causing breast engorgement, ischemia results, suppressing the activity of the acini or milk-secreting cells. Consequently milk production is reduced. In addition, the process of sucking from a bottle is different from breast-nipple compression. The relatively inflexible rubber nipple prevents the tongue from its usual rhythmic action. Infants learn to put the tongue against the nipple holes to slow down the more rapid flow of fluid. When infants use these same tongue movements during breast-feeding, they may push the human nipple out of the mouth and may not grasp the areola properly (Lawrence, 1985).

Usually by 3 weeks of age, lactation is well established and a feeding schedule has been formed. Bottle-fed infants retain about 2 to 3 ounces of formula at each feeding and are fed about six times a day. Breast-fed infants may feed as frequently as 10 to 12 times daily. Larger infants are able to retain increased amounts because of greater stomach capacity; as a result they generally sleep through the night sooner than smaller infants or breast-fed infants.

Feeding behavior. Five fairly distinct behavioral stages occur during successful feeding (O'Grady, 1971). Recognizing these steps can assist nurses in identifying potential feeding problems caused by improper feeding techniques. *Prefeeding behavior,* such as crying or fussing, demonstrates the infant's level of arousal and degree of hunger. *Approach behavior* is indicated by sucking movements or the rooting reflex. *Attachment behavior* includes those activities that occur from the time the infant receives the nipple until he grasps on and sucks. Attachment behavior is sometimes more pronounced during initial attempts at breast-feeding than bottle-feeding. *Consummatory behavior* consists of coordinated sucking and swallowing. Persistent gagging might indicate unsuccessful consummatory behavior. *Satiety behavior* is observed when infants let the mother know that they are satisfied. The most common expression of satiation is falling asleep.

PROMOTION OF PARENT-INFANT BONDING (ATTACHMENT)

The process of parenting is based on a mutual relationship between parent and infant. Much of past research on parent-child bonding has focused on the development of "mothering," or maternal attachment to the infant. Recently attention has focused on the infant's and father's role in this process. Although the words "bonding" and "attachment" are sometimes referred to as separate phenomena with bonding as the development of emotional ties from parent to infant and attachment representing the emotional ties from infant to parent, in this discussion the words are used interchangeably to denote both processes.

As more is learned of the complexity of neonates and of their potential for influencing and shaping their environments, particularly their interaction with significant others, one cannot help but realize that promoting positive parent-child relationships necessitates an understanding of factors involved in identifying behavioral steps in attachment, variables that enhance or hinder this process, and methods of teaching parents ways to develop a stronger relationship with their children, especially by recognizing potential problems.

Infant Behavior

Nurses must appreciate the individuality and uniqueness of each infant. According to the individual temperament, the infant will change and shape the environment, which will undoubtedly influence future development. Obviously an infant who sleeps 20 hours a day will be exposed to fewer stimuli than one who sleeps 16 hours a day. In turn, each infant will likely effect a different response from parents. The infant who is quiet, undemanding, and passive may receive much less attention than the infant who is responsive, alert, and active. Such behavioral characteristics as irritability and consolability have been shown to influence the ease of transition to parenthood and the parent's perception of the infant (Roberts, 1983).

One method of systematically assessing the infant's behavior is the use of the *Brazelton Neonatal Behavioral Assessment Scale* (Brazelton, 1973). The scale is designed to assess the infant's response to 27 items organized according to the following categories:

habituation How soon the infant diminishes response to stimuli.

orientation How much the infant responds to stimuli.

motor maturity The infant's motor coordination and control.

variation The infant's rate and amount of change during periods of alertness.

self-quieting abilities How much, how soon, and how effectively the infant quiets and consoles himself when upset.

social behaviors The infant's ability to smile and cuddle.

Besides its use as an initial and ongoing tool to assess neurologic and behavioral responses, the scale can be used as an assessor of initial parent-child relationships, as a preventive instrument that identifies the caregiver as one who may benefit from a role model, and as a guide for parents to help them focus on their infant's individuality and to develop a deeper attachment to their child. Studies have demonstrated that by showing parents the unique characteristics of their infant, there develops a more positive perception of the infant and increased interaction between infant and parent (Anderson, 1981; Liptak and others, 1983; Perry, 1983).

Nurses can intervene and positively influence the attachment of parent and child. The first step is recognizing individual differences and explaining to parents that such characteristics are normal. For example, most people believe that infants sleep throughout the day, except for a half-hour feeding. For some newborns this may be true, but for many it is not. Understanding that the infant's wakefulness is part of body rhythm and not a reflection of inadequate mothering can be crucial in promoting healthy parent-child relationships. Another aspect of helping parents concerns supplying guidelines on how to enhance the infant's development during awake periods. Placing the child in a crib to stare at the same mobile every day is not particularly exciting, but carrying the infant into each room as one does daily chores can be fascinating. A few simple suggestions can make life more stimulating for the infant and gratifying for the parents (see box above and box on p. 386).

Maternal Attachment

During pregnancy, and often even before conception occurs, parents develop an image of the "ideal or fantasy infant." The unborn child has an imagined appearance, pattern of behavior, expected accomplishments, and predetermined ef-

---

HOW TO MAKE THE INFANT'S WORLD MORE EXCITING*

Infant prefers animated and auditory objects.

Infant enjoys novelty, quickly tires of seeing same objects; mobile should be changed frequently.

Infant prefers to look at medium-intensity colors and contrasting colors, such as black and white.

Infant likes geometric shapes and checkerboards; prefers patterns over straight lines.

Contrasting lights and reflective surfaces such as mirrors are especially interesting.

But most of all, nothing is as fascinating as the human fact and voice!

*Objects should be placed about 20 cm (8 inches) away from infant.

---

fect on the life-style of the family. At birth the fantasy infant becomes the real infant. How closely the dream child resembles the real child influences the bonding process. Assessing such expectations during pregnancy and at the time of the infant's birth allows nurses to identify discrepancies in the parents' view of the fantasy vs real child syndrome.

The Neonatal Perception Inventory (NPI) (Broussard, 1979) is a screening tool that can be used to assess the mother's perception of her real infant as compared to her image of an "average" infant. It is hypothesized that for optimum mothering to occur the mother needs to see her infant as better than an "average" baby. Mothers who do not rate their infants as better than average may be at risk for developing parenting abilities that fail to meet the infant's needs. The NPI II (completed 4 weeks after delivery) was predictive of later childhood adjustment problems, whereas the NPI I (completed 1 to 2 days after infant's birth) was not (Broussard, 1976).

The labor process also significantly affects the immediate attachment of mothers to their newborn children. In general the mother's perception of maintaining control during the labor and birth process enhances the initial attachment, which ideally should take place during the first hour of life. A feeling of loss of control because of factors such as a long, difficult labor, excessive medication and sedation, or unwanted medical intervention hinders the initial bonding process. Encouraging mothers to talk about their feelings of loss of control, particularly about the specific event that they perceive caused the lack of self-control, allows them to dissipate the emotional energy invested in these feelings. It is not until such emotional tensions and anxieties are released that parents can attend to the emotional component of the attachment process.

It is believed that there is a *maternal sensitive period* immediately and for a short time after birth when parents have a unique ability to attach to their infants (Klaus and Kennell, 1982). During the development of the attachment process, Klaus and others (1972) found that mothers dem-

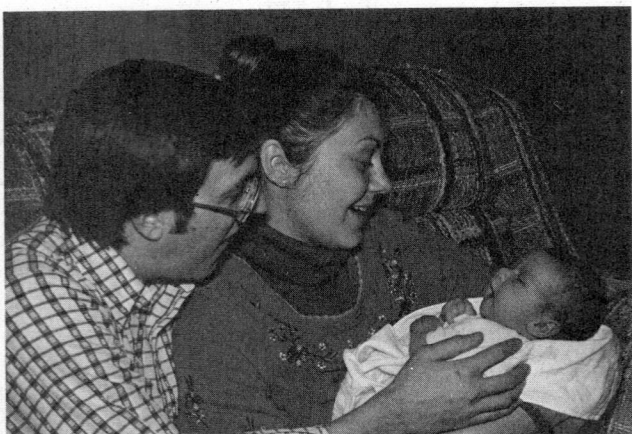

Fig. 8-19. En face position between parents and infant can be significant in attachment process.

onstrated a predictable and orderly pattern of behavior. When they were presented with their nude infants, they began examining the infant with their fingertips, concentrating on touching the extremities. In about 4 to 8 minutes they proceeded to massage and encompass the trunk with their entire hands. They also found that the *en face* position, a position in which the mother's and the infant's eyes meet in visual contact in the same vertical plane, was significant in the formation of affectional ties (Fig. 8-19).

Similar patterns of touching have been observed by others (Rubin, 1963), which has led many clinicians to use assessment of touch as an indicator of maternal-infant attachment. However, other studies demonstrate different patterns for mothers, as well as the same pattern for nonmaternal persons, such as male and female nurses. Therefore, caution must be exercised in rigidly applying this parameter in assessing maternal attachment (Tulman, 1985).

Additional studies have attempted to substantiate the long-term benefits of providing parents with opportunities to optimally bond with their infant during the initial postpartum period. There is considerable controversy over the validity of the findings and concern with the emphasis on a "critical" period for bonding. These issues are reviewed in the box Questions and controversies.

Another component of successful maternal attachment is the concept of *reciprocity* or reciprocal interaction. As the mother responds to the infant, the infant must respond to the mother by some signal such as sucking, cooing, eye contact, grasping, or molding (conforming to the other's body during close physical contact). Five steps are described in positive mother-infant reciprocity (Brazelton, 1974). The first step is *initiation*, in which interaction between infant and parent begins. Next is *orientation*, which establishes the partners' expectation of each other during the interaction. Following orientation is *acceleration* of the attention cycle to a peak of excitement. The infant reaches out and coos, both arms jerk forward, the head moves backward, the eyes dilate, and the face brightens. After a short time *deceleration* of the excitement and *turning away* occur,

Questions and Controversies

Does early and extended maternal-infant contact affect subsequent parenting and infant development?

Since Klaus and Kennell's initial research and postulation of a "maternal sensitive period," several investigators have sought to determine if early and extended maternal-infant contact has a significant influence on parenting and infant development. Among the more classic studies, researchers demonstrated that a total of 16 extra contact hours with their infant influenced mothers to be more reluctant to leave their infant with someone else, to show greater soothing behavior and fondling, and to engage in more eye-to-eye contact (Klaus and others, 1972; Kennell and others, 1974).

In a 2-year follow-up study the early contact group had better speech and communication patterns. In a 5-year follow-up, however, no differences were found between the groups in speech development, language comprehension, or intelligence. However, a correlation was noted in the early contact group between the mother's speech and communication patterns with the child at 2 years of age and the child's communication abilities at age 5 (Ringler and others, 1978).

There has been some evidence that increased parent-child contact at birth minimizes the risks of parenting disorders, such as abuse and neglect (O'Connor and others, 1980). However not all studies support these findings and when the influence of socioeconomic background variables are taken into consideration, they are more of a determinant of attachment than early and extended contact (Siegel and others, 1980). Another short-term benefit found by several investigators was prolonged breastfeeding (Goldberg, 1983).

In light of these conflicting reports and the concerns regarding study design, such as small sample sizes, lack of subject randomization, and different measures to assess attachment, some authorities claim that the emphasis on bonding has been unjustified and may lead to guilt and fear in those parents who did not receive early contact with their infant (Lamb, 1982; Tulman, 1981). There is also considerable concern over the literal interpretation of "sensitive" or "critical" to imply that without early contact, optimum bonding cannot occur or that early contact alone is sufficient to ensure competent parenting (Lamb, 1982; Mitchell and Mills, 1983).

While the answer to whether early contact does affect parenting and child development is inconclusive, it is well known that Klaus and Kennell's work has had a major impact on the "humanization" of obstetric practices (Goldberg, 1983; and McCall, 1982; Klaus and Kennell, 1983; Korsch, 1983). These alone have merit for creating a joyful and fulfilling experience for the family. Certainly it should be stressed to parents that while early bonding may be valuable, it does not represent an "all or none" phenomenon. Through the child's life there will be multiple opportunities for the development of parent-child attachment. Bonding is a complex process that develops gradually and is influenced by numerous factors, only one of which is the type of initial contact between the newborn and parent.

in which the infant's eyes shift away from the mother's and the child grasps his shirt. During this cycle of nonattention, repeated verbal or visual attempts to reinitiate the infant's attention are ineffective. This deceleration and turning away probably prevent the infant from being overwhelmed by excessive stimuli. In a good interaction both partners have synchronized their attention-nonattention cycles. Parents or other caregivers who do not allow the infant to turn away and who continually attempt to maintain visual contact encourage the infant to turn off the attention cycle and thus prolong the nonattention phase.

Although this description of reciprocal interacting behavior is usually observable in the infant by 2 to 3 weeks of age, nurses can use this information to teach parents how to interact with their infant. Recognizing the attention cycle vs nonattention cycle and understanding that the latter is not a rejection of the parent helps parents develop competence in parenting.

Monotropy is another component of attachment that has special meaning for health professionals. Monotropy refers to the principle that a person can become optimally attached to only one individual at a time (Klaus and Kennell, 1982). This is very significant in the attachment process that occurs in multiple births. If a parent can form only one attachment at a time, how then can all the siblings of a multiple birth receive optimum emotional care?

Minimal research is available on maternal-twin bonding and the conclusions of different authors vary. Some report that mothers bond equally to each twin at the time of birth, even if one twin is ill (Abbink, 1982). Others suggest that mothers of twins may take months or even years to form individual attachments to each child and even longer if the twins are identical. The mother's separation from a sick twin during the perinatal period can have devastating results, since attachment to the well child occurs quickly but may impede attachment to the other twin. Some authors offer practical suggestions for individualizing attachments to twins (Gromada, 1981).

Nurses can be instrumental in promoting bonding of twins. The most important principle is to assist the parents in recognizing the individuality of the children. The mother should visit with each newborn as much as possible after birth, including a sick infant. Rooming-in and breast-feeding are both feasible and should be encouraged. Any characteristics that are unique to each child are emphasized and each infant is called by name, rather than "the twins." Bonding behaviors are assessed and differences are noted, such as a parent's distinct preference for one twin over the other. In this situation the nurse can gently draw attention to these behaviors and encourage the parent to discuss feelings regarding a twin birth. The **National Organization of Mothers of Twins Club, Inc.***** can be a source of support to new parents.

Another area of attachment that has received minimal attention is maternal bonding of multiparous mothers. Research suggests that there are several additional tasks to "taking on" a second child. These include (Walz, 1983):

- Promoting acceptance and approval of the first child for the second
- Grieving and resolving the loss of an exclusive dyadic relationship with the first child

- Planning and coordinating family life to include a second child
- Reformulating a relationship with the first child
- Identifying with the second child by comparing with the first child for physical and psychologic characteristics
- Assessing one's affective capabilities in providing sufficient emotional support and nurturance simultaneously to two children

Spacing of children appears to influence maternal stress following birth of a second child. Those mothers with children less than 2 years apart may experience the most stress, followed by mothers with children greater than 6 years apart. The least stress is likely to be when children are spaced by 4 to 6 years (Lynch, 1982). Obviously multiparous mothers benefit from nursing support both in the hospital and at home. Unfortunately, they may be reluctant to admit concerns or problems because this is not a first-time experience. Providing sensitive care for their needs and fostering attachment behaviors, including in the siblings, is an essential component of nursing multiparous mothers.

Paternal Engrossment

Less attention and research have focused on father-infant bonding than on maternal bonding, although the important role fathers play in family development is being increasingly recognized. Like pregnant women, prospective fathers develop attachment behaviors to the fetus, such as talking to the unborn child, referring to the fetus by a nickname, and imagining caring for the newborn (Weaver and Cranley, 1983).

Fathers also show specific attachment behaviors to the newborn. This process of "engrossment," forming a sense of absorption, preoccupation, and interest in the infant, includes (1) visual awareness of the newborn, especially focusing on the beauty of the child, (2) tactile awareness, often expressed in a desire to hold the infant, (3) awareness of distinct characteristics with emphasis on those features of the infant that resemble the father, (4) perception of the infant as perfect, (5) development of a strong feeling of attraction to the child that leads to intense focusing of attention on the infant, (6) experiencing a feeling of extreme elation, and (7) feeling a sense of deep self-esteem and satisfaction. These responses are greatest during the early contacts with the infant and are intensified by the neonate's normal reflex activity, especially the grasp reflex and visual alertness (Greenberg and Morris, 1974).

The development of engrossment has significant implications for nurses. Initially it is imperative that nurses recognize the importance of early father-infant contact in releasing these behaviors. Fathers need to be encouraged to express their positive feelings, especially if such emotions are contrary to the cultural belief that fathers should remain stoic. If this is not clarified, fathers may feel confused and attempt to suppress the natural sensations of absorption, preoccupation, and interest in order to conform with societal expectations.

*5402 Amberwood Lane, Rockville, MD 20853.

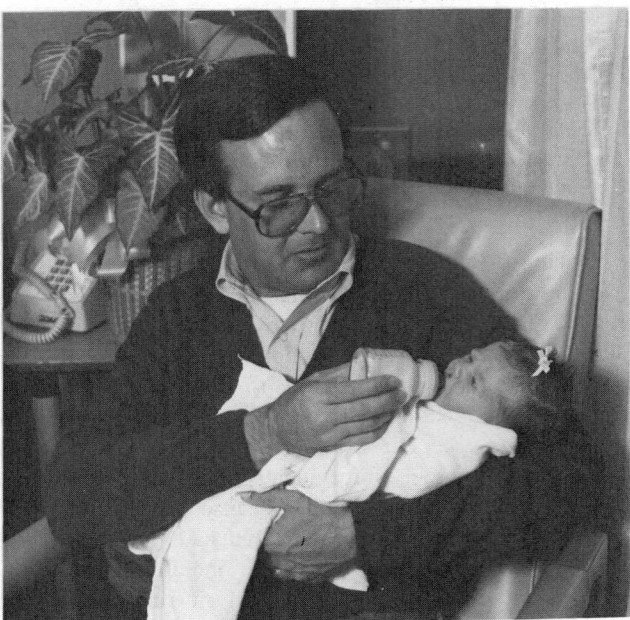

Fig. 8-20. A desire to hold the infant and participate in caregiving activities is an indication of paternal engrossment.
Photography by John Roy, Saint Francis Hospital, Tulsa, OK.

Mothers also need to be aware of the responses of the father toward the newborn, especially since one of the consequences of paternal preoccupation with the infant is less overt attention toward the mother. If both parents are able to share their feelings, each can appreciate the process of attachment toward their child and will avoid the unfortunate conflict of being insensitive and unaware of the other's needs. In addition, a father who is encouraged to form a relationship with his newborn is less likely to feel excluded and abandoned once the family returns home and the mother directs her attention toward caring for the infant.

Ideally the process of engrossment should be discussed with parents before the delivery, such as in prenatal classes, to reinforce the father's awareness of his natural feelings toward the expected child. Focusing on the future experience of seeing, touching, and holding one's newborn may also help expectant fathers become more comfortable in accepting their paternal feelings toward the unborn child. This in turn can assist them in being more supportive toward their wives, especially as the labor and delivery event draws near.

At the infant's birth the nurse can play a vital role in assisting the father to release or express engrossment by assessing the neonate in front of the couple; pointing out normal characteristics, especially the grasp reflex; encouraging identification through consistent referral to the child by name; encouraging the father to cuddle, hold, talk to, or feed the infant; and demonstrating whenever necessary the soothing powers of caressing, stroking, and rocking the child (Fig. 8-20). Fathers are encouraged to be with the mother during labor and delivery and to spend time alone with the mother and newborn after delivery. Whenever possible, the father should "room in" with the mother (Kunst-Wilson and Cronenwett, 1981).

The nurse observes for the same indication of affectional ties from the father as those expected in the mother, such as visual contact in the en face position and embracing the infant close to the body. When present, such behaviors are reinforced. If such responses are not obvious, the nurse needs to assess the father's feelings regarding this birth, cultural beliefs that may prevent his emotional expression, and other factors in order to help him facilitate a positive attachment during this critical period. Literature can also be given to the parents to help them understand the process of attachment and its importance in parent-infant bonding.

Siblings

Although the attachment process has been discussed almost exclusively in terms of the parents and infant, it is essential that nurses be aware of other family members, such as siblings and members of the extended family, who need preparation for the acceptance of this new child. Young children in particular need sensitive preparation for the birth to minimize sibling jealousy.

There is an increasing trend to allow siblings to visit the mother on the postpartum unit and to hold the newborn (Fig. 8-21). Research has demonstrated several benefits, such as more responsiveness of the visiting sibling to the mother and newborn (Schwab and others, 1983), less regressive behaviors after the birth (Kayiatos, Adams, and Gilman, 1984), and no adverse effects, such as increased bacterial infection of neonates (Kowba and others, 1985). In

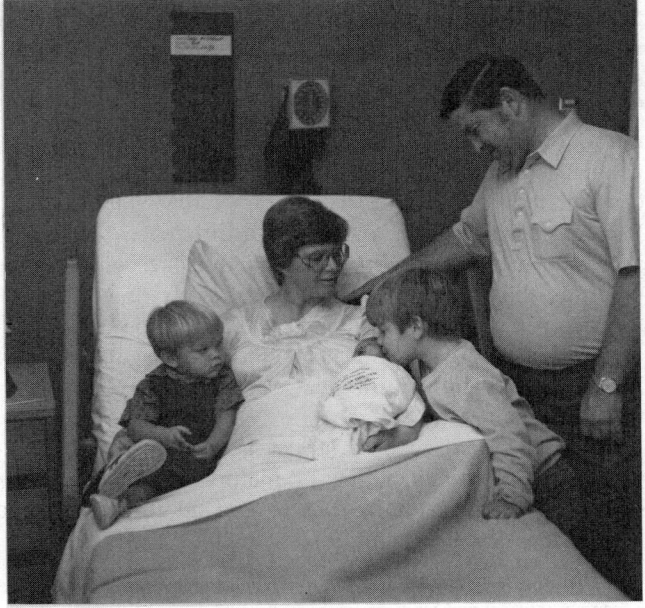

Fig. 8-21. Sibling visitation shortly after birth can be significant in the attachment process.
Photography by John Roy, Saint Francis Hospital, Tulsa, OK.

Questions and Controversies

What are the reactions and benefits/risks to sibling attendance at the birth?

Current research on sibling attendance at the labor and birth are preliminary and conflicting. Leonard and others (1979) reported on 40 children ages 3 to 14 years who attended the birth. Initially most children played or talked with the mother and some even timed the contractions. During late labor when the mother was absorbed in the labor process the children tended to withdraw by moving back in the room and watching; some of the children fell asleep. Most children observed the birth and became preoccupied with the infant so that few witnessed the delivery of the placenta or the episiotomy. The authors conclude that for the most part the experience was positive for the children, despite some concern from them regarding the mother's cries and episiotomy repair. However they also add that childbirth is primarily an adult event and that the presence of the siblings may be more to meet the parents' needs than the siblings' needs or wishes.

The findings from this study on the children's reactions are similar to those reported by others on observations from home births (Anderson, 1979; Mehl Brendsel, and Peterson, 1977). They found children also to be concerned with seeing blood and the mother's sounds during labor. An additional benefit was the children's greater knowledge of aspects related to the birth process (Daniels, 1983). Daniels also found that those children who were reared in a household where sexuality was openly discussed had the least difficulty during the experience.

The question remains regarding the benefits and ill effects on the siblings beyond the birth experience. While some studies demonstrate more regressive behaviors in those who did not attend the birth, this may be due to the longer separation from the mother (Trause and Irvin, 1982). Other researchers found no significant differences or ill effects (Lumley, 1983). It is probable that sibling attachment and adjustment to the newborn are complex processes that are influenced by a large number of variables, only one of which is related to witnessing the birth.

light of these findings, the American Academy of Pediatrics (1985) supports neonatal sibling visitation and has established guidelines for institutions.

Another trend has been siblings witnessing the birth. Unlike sibling visitation the evidence supporting this practice is much more controversial and conflicting (see the box Questions and controversies). As research mounts, birthing centers that allow siblings at the birth are developing more definitive guidelines, such as age requirement of at least 4 to 5 years, the presence of a supportive person for the sibling only, and an adequate sequence of preparation, in which parents explore all options for preparing their other children (Ballard and others, 1982; Daniels, 1983).

A film is available for preparing older preschool and school-age children for participation in the birth experience.*

Nicholas and the Baby (16 mm film or ¾-inch videocassette), Centre Productions, Inc., 1312 Pine St., Suite A, Boulder, CO 80302.

From preliminary observations during sibling visitation there is evidence that sibling attachment occurs and is not significantly affected by attendance at sibling preparation classes. The en face position is assumed much less often among the newborn and siblings than between mother and newborn, and when this position is used it is brief. Siblings focus more on the head or face than on touching or talking to the infant. The siblings' verbalizations are focused less on attracting the infant's attention and more on addressing the mother about the newborn (Marecki and others, 1985). Additional research is needed to establish theories on sibling bonding as have been constructed for parental bonding.

Assessment of Attachment Behaviors

Unlike physical assessment of the neonate, which has concrete guidelines to follow, assessment of parent-child attachment requires much more skill in terms of observation and interviewing. The assessment process is even more challenging when one considers that postpartum hospital recovery is shorter and shorter. However, rooming-in of mother and infant and liberal visiting privileges for father, siblings, and grandparents facilitate recognition of behaviors that demonstrate positive or negative attachment.

What should the nurse observe when with the parents and the infant? Probably the most important activities to observe include feeding, bathing, and comforting. The following questions serve as guidelines for assessment of bonding behaviors:

- When the infant is brought to the mother, does she reach out for the child, call the child by name, or involve the father in the greeting process?
- Do the parents speak about the child in terms of identification—whom the infant looks like; what appears special about their child over other infants; how "smart" they think their child is?
- When the mother or father is holding the infant, what kind of body contact is there—do parents feel at ease in changing the infant's position; are fingertips or whole hands used; are there parts of the body they avoid touching or parts of the body they investigate and scrutinize?
- When the infant is awake, what kinds of stimulation do the parents provide—do they talk to the infant, to each other, or to no one; how do they look at the infant—direct visual contact, avoidance of eye contact, or looking at other people or objects?

Talking to the parents uncovers many variables that will affect the development of attachment and parenting (see also p. 687). What expectations do they have for this child? In other words, how similar are their predictions of the fantasy child and their realizations about the real child? They should be encouraged to talk about their relationship with their own parents. Mothering and fathering of a child probably depend more on the type of parenting that parents received as a child than on any other variable. Is this a planned birth, how do they see the addition of a dependent family member affecting their life-style, and what arrangements have they

Nursing Care Summary: The Newborn and Family

NURSING GOALS	NURSING INTERVENTIONS	EXPECTED PATIENT/FAMILY OUTCOMES

HP-HMP   Infection, potential for
Risk factors: deficient immunologic defenses, environmental factors

NURSING GOALS	NURSING INTERVENTIONS	EXPECTED PATIENT/FAMILY OUTCOMES
	Transitional Care	
Protect from infection and trauma	Employ hand washing before and after caring for each infant Never leave infant unsupervised on a raised surface without sides Always close diaper pins and place them away from infant's body Keep pointed or sharp objects out of infant's reach Keep own fingernails short and trimmed; avoid jewelry that can scratch infant	Infant exhibits no evidence of infection or trauma
	Care in Nursery or Mother's Room	

	Check eyes daily for any discharge
	Ideally, involve mother and father in bathing of infant
	Clean vulva in posterior direction to prevent fecal contamination of vagina or urethra; stress this to parents
	While cleaning penis, do not retract foreskin; gently wipe away smegma
	Maintain asepsis during circumcision
	If infant has been circumcised, cover area with a petrolatum jelly gauze (if ordered)
	Keep umbilical stump clean and dry
	    Place diapers below umbilical stump
	    Assess cord daily for odor, color, and drainage
		Eyes remain clear with no evidence of irritation
		Genital area is free of irritation
		
		Cord appears dry, surrounding area free

N-MP   Thermoregulation: ineffective
Risk factor: immature temperature control

NURSING GOALS	NURSING INTERVENTIONS	EXPECTED PATIENT/FAMILY OUTCOMES
	Transitional Care	
Maintain stable body temperature	Wrap infant snugly in a warmed blanket Place infant in a preheated environment (under radiant warmer or next to mother) Place infant on a padded, covered surface Keep infant away from drafts, air conditioning vents, or fans Place infant in a recessed cubicle with walls high enough to shield from cross ventilation Warm all objects used to examine or cover infant, for example, place them under radiant warmer Uncover only one area of body for examination or procedures Monitor skin temperature and relate it to ambient air temperature; decreased skin temperature may indicate radiant heat loss Take axillary temperature according to institutional policy or until stable Be aware of signs of hypothermia or hyperthermia Postpone bath for first 4 to 6 hours until temperature stabilizes at 37°C Postpone circumcision until after postnatal recovery period	Infant's temperature remains at optimum level (36.5° to 37.5°C [97.7° to 99.5°F])
	Care in Nursery or Mother's Room	
	Take infant's temperature on arrival at nursery or mother's room and, if stable, proceed according to hospital policy Maintain room temperature between 24° and 25.5°C (75° to 78°F) and humidity about 40% to 50%	

*Nursing outcome.

Nursing Care Summary: The Newborn and Family —cont'd

NURSING GOALS	NURSING INTERVENTIONS	EXPECTED PATIENT/FAMILY OUTCOMES
	Dress infant in a shirt and diaper and swaddle in a blanket	
	Prevent chilling of infant during daily bath	
	If there is any question retarding stabilization of body temperature, postpone bath	
	Keep infant's head covered if heat loss is a problem	

N-MP   **Nutrition, alteration in: potential for less than body requirements**
Risk factors: immaturity, parental knowledge deficit

NURSING GOALS	NURSING INTERVENTIONS	EXPECTED PATIENT/FAMILY OUTCOMES
	Transitional Care	
Provide optimum nutrition	During first hour after delivery, put infant to mother's breast when possible	Infant demonstrates strong suck
	Postpone bottle-feeding of 5% glucose water until sucking and swallowing are well coordinated	
	Do not offer routine water or supplemental feedings to breast-feeding infants	
	Care in Nursery or Mother's Room	
	Assess strength of suck and coordination with swallowing	Infant receives an adequate amount of nutrients (specify amount and frequency of feedings)
	Bring breast-fed infants to mothers on demand during day and night	Infant loses 10% of birth weight or less
	Offer bottle-fed infants 2 to 3 ounces of formula after they have retained their glucose feeding	
	Support and assist breast-feeding mothers during initial feedings	
	Encourage father to remain with mother to help her and infant with positioning, relaxation, and reinforcement	
	Encourage father to participate in bottle-feeding	
	Place infant on right side after feeding to prevent regurgitation	Infant retains reedings
	Observe stool pattern	

A-EP   **Airway clearance, ineffective**
Etiology: excess mucus, improper positioning

NURSING GOALS	NURSING INTERVENTIONS	EXPECTED PATIENT/FAMILY OUTCOMES
	Transitional Care	
Establish and maintain patent airway	Suction mouth and nasopharynx with bulb syringe as needed	Breathing is regular and unlabored
	Lavage stomach of amniotic fluid and check for tracheoesophageal anomalies (not routinely done in all hospitals)	Respiratory rate is within normal limits (see inside front cover for normal variations)
	Position infant on side or abdomen with head slightly lower than chest (about 15 degrees) to facilitate drainage of secretions	Gastric aspirate is less than 20 ml (if performed)
	Perform as few procedures as possible on infant during first hour and have oxygen ready for use if respiratory distress should develop	
	Take vital signs according to institutional policy and more frequently if necessary	

Continued.

Nursing Care Summary: The Newborn and Family—cont'd

NURSING GOALS	NURSING INTERVENTIONS	EXPECTED PATIENT/FAMILY OUTCOMES
	Care in Nursery or Mother's Room	
	Position infant on right side or abdomen after feeding to prevent aspiration	Airway remains patent
	Keep diapers, clothing, and blankets loose enough to allow maximum lung (abdominal) expansion	
	Clean nares of any crusted secretions during bath or when necessary	
	Check for patent nares	

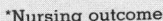 **RRP   Family process: alterations in**
Etiology: maturational crisis, birth of term infant, change in family unit

Facilitate siblings' adjustment to newborn	Allow to visit and touch newborn when feasible	Siblings express interest in newborn and realistic expectations for their age
	Explain physical differences in newborn, such as bald head, umbilical stump and clamp, circumcision	
	Explain to siblings realistic expectations regarding newborn abilities and needs	
	Requires complete care	
	Is not a playmate	
	Encourage siblings to participate in care at home	
	Encourage parents to spend individual time with other children at home	

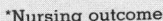 **RRP   Parenting: alterations in: potential**
Risk factors: knowledge deficit, lack of available role models

	Transitional Care	
Facilitate parent-infant attachment process	As soon after delivery as possible, allow parents to see and hold infant; place newborn close to face of parents so that visual contact can be established; ensure infant's identity	Parents establish contact with infant immediately or soon after birth
		*ID bracelet is in place
	Ideally, perform eye care after initial meeting of infant and parents, usually about 1 hour after birth	Parents demonstrate attachment behaviors, such as touch, eye contact, naming and calling infant by name, talking to infant, participating in caregiving activities
	Identify for parents specific behaviors manifested by infant, for example, alertness, ability to see, vigorous suck, rooting behavior, and attention to human voice	Family members avail themselves of needed services

	Care in Nursery or Mother's Room	
	Discuss with parents their expectations of fantasy child vs real child	Family discusses expectations for child and delivery experience
	Encourage parents to "talk out" their labor and delivery experience; identify any events that signify loss of control to either parent, especially mother	
	Identify behavioral steps in attachment process and evaluate those aspects that could be considered positive and those that may represent inadequate or delayed parenting	Parents demonstrate positive attachment behaviors
	Encourage family to call for infant frequently	Parents spend considerable time with infant (specified amount)
	Observe and assess the reciprocity of cues between infant and parent	
	Assist parents in recognizing attention-nonattention cycles and in understanding their significance	Parents recognize attention-nonattention cycles

*Nursing outcome.

Nursing Care Summary: The Newborn and Family—cont'd

NURSING GOALS	NURSING INTERVENTIONS	EXPECTED PATIENT/FAMILY OUTCOMES
	Assess variables affecting development of attachment through observing infant and parent and interviewing each parent or other significant caregiver	
	If parent-infant attachment is at risk, refer to appropriate agencies (social services, family and child services, at-risk programs)	*Appropriate referrals are made
Prepare for discharge	Instruct in newborn care Feeding (formula or breast) Bathing Umbilical and circumcision care	Family demonstrates ability to provide care for infant Infant rides home in federally approved car restraint
	Encourage participation in parenting classes, if offered	Family keeps appointments for follow-up care
	Discuss importance and proper use of federally approved car restraints	
	Refer to organizations that may rent car restraints	

Nursing Interventions Related to Medical Management

Protect from infection and injury
Instill prophylactic eye medication into conjunctival sac of each eye from inner canthus outward; do not irrigate eyes with sterile saline
Administer vitamin K intramuscularly, using vastus lateralis muscle as site of injection
Apply antibacterial agent or alcohol or both to cord as ordered
Assist in identifying congenital disorders
Collect blood specimens for required screening tests

made in terms of such changes in life-style? What "support system" or significant others are available for assistance? What are their views regarding childrearing?

Assessing the family's bonding to the newborn is a complex process. The above only serve as guidelines. Presently, there is no absolute instrument to measure successful attachment. Rather, one must be aware of expected behaviors and have a high index of suspicion for delayed bonding.

DISCHARGE PLANNING AND CARE AT HOME

With increasingly shorter postpartum admissions and home delivery, discharge planning, referral, and home visiting are important components of comprehensive care. First-time as well as "experienced" parents benefit from guidance and assistance with the infant's care, such as breast- or formula feeding, and with the family's integration of a new member, particularly sibling adjustment (see p. 330). To assess and meet these needs, discharge planning *must* begin immediately on admission to the hospital or birthing center. A nurs-

ing admission history assists in systematic collection of data to formulate nursing diagnoses and to plan care. This assessment continues throughout the admission and includes the family's support system. Nurses in the birthing, nursery, and postpartum units need to coordinate their assessments for the most effective interventions.

Ideally, the family should receive a home visit shortly after discharge. Some home care programs schedule three visits during the first 5 days if the mother is discharged the day of delivery and more frequently for families at risk, such as teenage parents. Common concerns or problems during this period are related to breast-feeding, maternal fatigue and depression, bonding, neonatal jaundice, and excessive infant crying (Jansson, 1985).

Professional support for the new family should be continued from the hospital to the home through community services as needed. The concept of family-centered care is practiced when the family receives consistent comprehensive care beginning with preventive prenatal care and continuing through child health maintenance.

CONCEPT SUMMARIES

- Transition from fetal or placental circulation to independent respiration is the most important physiologic change required of the newborn.

- Chemical and thermal factors help initiate the neonate's first respiration.

- Circulatory changes in the neonate result from shifts in pressure in the heart and major vessels and from functional closures of the fetal shunts.

- The newborn's large surface area, its thin layer of subcutaneous fat, and the newborn's unique mechanism for producing heat predipose the newborn to excessive heat loss.

- The infant's high rate of metabolism is closely correlated with the rate of fluid exchange, which is seven times greater in the infant than in the adult.

- The skin and mucous membranes, the reticuloendothelial system, and antibodies are the first, second, and third lines of defense against infection.

- Apgar scoring, the initial assessment of the newborn, focuses on heart rate, respiratory effort, muscle tone, reflex irritability, and color.

- Physical assessment of the newborn includes assessment of clinical gestational age, general measurements, general appearance, and head-to-toe assessment.

- Neurologic assessment focuses on localized reflexes and posture, muscle tone, head control, and movement and is best accomplished during the general physical examination.

- Behavioral assessment of newborns, with the Brazelton Neonatal Behavioral Assessment Scale, examines responses to 6 categories: habituation, orientation, motor maturity, variation, self-quieting abilities, and social behaviors.

- Physical care for the newborn includes maintaining a patent airway, maintaining stable body temperature, protecting from infection and injury, and providing optimum nutrition.

- Although the attachment, or bonding, process primarily affects infants and parents, siblings also play an important role.

REFERENCES

Abbink, C.: Bonding as perceived by mothers of twins, Pediatr. Nurs. 8(6):411-413, 1982.

American Academy of Pediatrics, Committee on Fetus and Newborn: Postpartum (neonatal) sibling visitation, Pediatrics 76(4):650, 1985.

American Academy of Pediatrics, Committee of Fetus and Newborn: Report of the Ad Hoc Task Force of Circumcision, Pediatrics 56:610-611, Oct. 1975.

American Academy of Pediatrics, Policy Statement Based on Task Force Report: The promotion of breast-feeding, Pediatrics 69(5):654-661, 1982.

American Academy of Pediatrics and American College of Obstetricians and Gynecologists: Guidelines for perinatal care, Elk Grove Village, IL, 1983, The Academy.

Anderson, C.J.: Enhancing reciprocity between mother and neonate, Nurs. Res. 30(2):89-93, 1981.

Anderson, S.: Siblings at birth: a survey and study, Birth Fam. J. 6:80-87, 1979.

Andrich, M.P., and Golden, S.M.: Umbilical cord care: a study of bacitracin ointment vs. triple dye, Clin. Pediatr. 23:342-344, 1984.

Ballard, J.L., Novak, K.K., and Driver, M.: A simplified score for assessment of fetal maturation of newly born infants, J. Pediatr. 95(5):769-774, 1979.

Ballard, R., and others: An alternative birth center in a hospital setting. In Klaus, M.H., and Kennell, J.H., editors: Maternal-infant bonding, ed. 2, St. Louis, 1982, The C.V. Mosby Co.

Boyce, W.T.: Care of the foreskin, Pediatr. Rev. 5(1):26-30, 1983.

Boyer, K.B.: Routine circumcision of the newborn: reasonable precaution or unnecessary risk? J. Nurs. Midwif. 25:27-31, Nov./Dec. 1980.

Brazelton, T.B.: Neonatal behavioral assessment scale, Philadelphia, 1973, J.B. Lippincott Co.

Brazelton, T.B.: Mother-infant reciprocity. In Klaus, M., and others, editors: Maternal attachment and mothering disorders, New Brunswick, NJ, 1974, Johnson & Johnson Baby Products Co.

Broussard, E.R.: Neonatal prediction and outcome at 10/11 years, Child Psychiatry Hum. Dev. 7(2):85-93, 1976.

Broussard, E.R.: Assessment of the adaptive potential of the mother-infant system: the Neonatal Perception Inventories, Semin. Perinatol. 3(1):91-100, 1979.

Bull, M.J., and Stroup, K.B.: Premature infants in car seats, Pediatrics 75(2):336-339, 1985.

Daniels, M.: The birth experience for the sibling: description and evaluation of a program, J. Nurs. Midwif. 28(5):15-22, 1983.

De Carvalho, M., and others: Effect of frequent breast-feeding on early milk production and infant weight gain, Pediatrics 72(3):307-311, 1983.

DeCasper, A.M., and Fifer, W.P.: Of human bonding: newborns prefer their mothers' voices, Science 208:1174-1176, June 1980.

DeSwiet, M., Fayers, P., and Shinebourne, E.A.: Systolic blood pressure in a population of infants in the first year of life: the Brompton study, Pediatrics 65(5):1028-1034, 1980.

Dubowitz, L.M.S., Dubowitz, V., and Goldberg, C.: Clinical assessment of gestational age in the newborn infant, J. Pediatr. 77(1):1-10, 1970.

Earley, A., and others: Blood pressure in the first 6 weeks of life, Arch. Dis. Child. 55:755-757, Oct. 1980.

El Haddad, M., and Corkery, J.J.: The anus in the newborn, Pediatrics 76(6):927-928, 1985.

Field, T., and Goldson, E.: Pacifying effects of nonnutritive sucking on term and preterm neonates during heelstick procedures, Pediatrics 74(6):1012-1015, 1984.

Frodi, A.M., and others: Fathers' and mothers' responses to the face and cries of normal and premature infants, Dev. Psychobiol. 14:490-498, 1978.

Gaull, G.E., Wright, C.E., and Isaacs, C.E.: Significance of growth modulators in human milk, Pediatrics 75(suppl.):142-145, 1985.

Gibbons, M.B.: Circumcision: the controversy continues, Pediatr. Nurs. 10(2):103-109, 1984.

Goldberg, S.: Parent-infant bonding: another look, Child Dev. 54:1355-1382, 1983.

Golub, H.L., and Corwin, M.J.: Infant cry: a clue to diagnosis, Pediatrics 69(2):197-201, 1982.

Goodson, J.G., Buller, C., and Goodson, W.H., III: Prenatal child safety education, Obstet. Gynecol. 65:312-315, 1985.

Greenberg, M., and Morris, N.: Engrossment: the newborn's impact upon the father, Am. J. Orthopsychiatry 44(4):520-531, 1974.

Gromada, K.: Maternal-infants attachment: the first step toward individualizing twins, Am. J. Maternal Child Nurs. 6(2):129-134, 1981.

Gulick, E.: Infant health and breast-feeding, Pediatr. Nurs. 9(5):359-362+, 1983.

Hanson, L.A., and others: Protective factors in milk and the development of the immune system, Pediatrics 75(suppl.):172-176, 1985.

Harpin, V.A., and Rutter, N.: Development of emotional sweating in the newborn infant, Arch. Dis. Child. 57:691-695, 1982.

Henningsson, A., and others: Bathing or washing babies after birth, Lancet 2:1401-1402, Dec. 1981.

Holve, R.L., and others: Regional anesthesia during newborn circumcision, Clin. Pediatr. 22:813-818, 1983.

Humenick, S.S., and Van Steenkiste, S.: Early indicators of breast-feeding progress, Issues Comp. Pediatr. Nurs. **6:**205-215, 1983.

Jansson, P.: Early postpartum discharge, Am. J. Nurs. **85**(5):547-550, 1985.

Kayiatos, R., Adams, J., and Gilman, B.: The arrival of a rival: maternal perceptions of toddlers' regressive behaviors after the birth of a sibling, J. Nurs. Midwif. **29**(3):205-213, 1984.

Kennell, J.H., and others: Maternal behavior one year after early and extended post-partum contact, Dev. Med. Child Neurol. **16:**172-179, April 1974.

Kirya, C., and Werthmann, M.W., Jr.: Neonatal circumcision and penile dorsal nerve block—a painless procedure, J. Pediatr. **92**(6):998-1000, 1978.

Klaus, M.H., and Kennell, J.H., editors: Maternal-infant bonding, ed. 2, St. Louis, 1982, The C.V. Mosby Co.

Klaus, M., and Kennell, J.: Parent to infant bonding: setting the record straight, J. Pediatr. **102**(4):575-576, 1983.

Klaus, M., and others: Maternal attachment—importance of the first postpartum days, N. Engl. J. Med. **286:**460, 1972.

Kochen, M., and McCurdy, S.: Circumcision and the risk of cancer of the penis, Am. J. Dis. Child. **134**(5):484-486, 1980.

Korsch, B.: More on parent-infant bonding, J. Pediatr. **102**(2):249-250, 1983.

Kowba, M., and others: Direct sibling contact and bacterial colonization in newborns, JOGN Nurs. **14**(5):412-417, 1985.

Kunst-Wilson, W., and Cronenwett, L.: Nursing care for the emerging family: promoting paternal behavior, Res. Nurs. Health **4:**201-211, 1981.

Lamb, M.E.: The bonding phenomenon: misinterpretations and their implications, J. Pediatr. **101**(4):555-557, 1982.

Lawrence, R.: Breast-feeding: a guide for the medical profession, ed. 2, St. Louis, 1985, The C.V. Mosby Co.

Leonard, C., and others: Preliminary observations on the behavior of children present at the birth of a sibling, Pediatrics **64:**949-951, 1979.

Liptak, G.S., and others: Enhancing infant development and parent-practitioner interaction with the Brazelton Neonatal Assessment Scale, Pediatrics **72**(1):71-78, 1983.

Ludington-Hoe, S.M.: What can newborns really see? Am. J. Nurs. **83**(9):1286-1289, 1983.

Lumley, J.: Preschool siblings at birth: short-term effects, Birth **10**(1):11-16, 1983.

Lynch, A.: Maternal stress following the birth of a second child. In Klaus, M.H., and Robertson, M.O., editors: Birth, interaction and attachment, Skillman, NJ, 1982, Johnson & Johnson Baby Products Co.

Macfarlane, A.: The psychology of childbirth, Cambridge, 1977, Harvard University Press.

Marecki, M., and others: Early sibling attachment, JOGN Nurs. **14**(5):418-423, 1985.

Martinez, G.A., and Dodd, D.A.: 1981 milk feeding patterns in the United States during the first 12 months of life, Pediatrics **71**(2):166-170, 1983.

Martinez, G.A., and Krieger, F.W.: 1984 milk-feeding patterns in the United States, Pediatrics **76**(6):1004-1008, 1985.

McCall, R.B.: A hard look at stimulating and predicting development: the cases of bonding and screening, Pediatr. Rev. **3**(7):205-212, 1982.

Mehl, L., Brendsel, C., and Peterson, G.: Children at birth: effects and implications, J. Sex Marital Ther. **3:**274-279, 1977.

Miller, M.J., and others: Oral breathing in newborn infants, J. Pediatr. **107**(3):465-469, 1985.

Miller, S.A., and Chopra, J.G.: Problems with human milk and infant formulas, Pediatrics **74**(suppl.):639-647, 1984.

Mitchell, K., and Mills, N.M.: Is the sensitive period in parent-infant bonding overrated? Ped. Nurs. **9**(2):91-94, 1983.

National Society to Prevent Blindness, Committee on Ophthalmia Neonatorum: Prevention and treatment of ophthalmia neonatorum, New York, 1981, The National Society.

O'Conner, S., and others: Reduced incidence of parenting inadequacy following rooming-in, Pediatrics **66:**176, 1980.

O'Grady, R.: Feeding behavior in infants, Am. J. Nurs. **71**(4):736-739, 1971.

Paneth, N., and Fox, H.E.: The relationship of Apgar score to neurologic handicap: a survey of clinicians, Obstet. Gynecol. **61:**547-550, 1983.

Pedersen, D.R., and Ter Vrugt, D.: The influence of amplitude and frequency of vestibular stimulation on the activity of two-month-old infants, Child Dev. **44:**122-128, March 1973.

Pedersen, D.R., and others: Relative soothing effects of vertical and horizontal rocking. Paper presented at the biennial meetings of the Society for Research in Child Development, Santa Monica, CA, March 1969.

Perry, S.E.: Parents' perceptions of their newborn following structured interactions, Nurs. Res. **32**(4):208-212, 1983.

Porter, R., Cernock, J., and Perry, S.: The importance of odors in mother-infant interactions, Maternal-Child Nurs. J. **12**(3):147-154, 1983.

Powell, M.: The Neonatal Behavioral Assessment Scale. In Powell, M.: Assessment and management of developmental changes and problems in children, ed. 2, St. Louis, 1981, The C.V. Mosby Co.

Reiff, M.I., and Essock-Vitale, S.M.: Hospital influences on early infant-feeding practices, Pediatrics **76**(6):872-879, 1985.

Ringler, N., and others: The effects of extra postpartum contact and maternal speech patterns on children's IQs, speech, and language comprehension at five, Child Dev. **49:**862-865, Sept. 1978.

Riordan, J.: A practical guide to breastfeeding, St. Louis, 1983, The C.V. Mosby Co.

Roberts, F.B.: Infant behavior and the transition to parenthood, Nurs. Res. **32**(4):213-217, 1983.

Rubin, R.: Maternal touch, Nurs. Outlook **11:**828-831, Nov. 1963.

Saigal, S., and others: Observations on the behavioral state of newborn infants during the first hour of life: a comparison of infants delivered by the Leboyer and conventional methods, Am. J. Obstet. Gynecol. **139:**715-719, March 1981.

Schwab, F., and others: Sibling visitation in neonatal intensive care unit, Pediatrics **71**(4):835-838, 1983.

Siegel, E., and others: Hospital and home support during infancy: impact on maternal attachment, child abuse and neglect, and health care utilization, Pediatrics **66**(2):183-190, 1980.

Trause, M., and Irvin, N.: Care of the sibling. In Klaus, M.H., and Kennell, J.H., editors: Maternal-infant bonding, ed. 2, St. Louis, 1982, The C.V. Mosby Co.

Tulman, L.J.: Theories of maternal attachment, Adv. Nurs. Sci. **3**(4):7-14, l981.

Tulman, L.J.: Mothers' and unrelated persons' initial handling of newborn infants, Nurs. Res. **34**(4):205-210, 1985.

Walz, B.L.: Maternal tasks of taking on a second child in the postpartum period, Maternal Child Nurs. J. **12**(3):185-216, 1983.

Weaver, R.H., and Cranley, M.S.: An exploration of paternal-fetal attachment behavior, Nurs. Res. **32**(2):68-72, 1983.

Williamson, P.S., and Williamson, M.L.: Physiologic stress reduction by a local anesthetic during newborn circumcision, Pediatrics **71**(1):36-40, 1983.

Wilson, C.B., and others: When is umbilical cord separation delayed? J. Pediatr. **107**(2):292-294, 1985.

Winikoff, B., and Baer, B.A.: The obstetrician's opportunity: translating "breast is best" from theory to practice, Am. J. Obstet. Gynecol. **138:**105-117, 1980.

Wiswell, T.E., and others: Decreased incidence of urinary tract infections in circumcised male infants, Pediatrics **75**(5):901-903, 1985.

BIBLIOGRAPHY
Physiologic Status of the Newborn/Assessment of the Neonate

Apgar, V.: The newborn (Apgar) scoring system, Pediatr. Clin. North Am. **13:**645, 1966.

Arnold, H.W., and others: The newborn: transition to extra-uterine life, Am. J. Nurs. **65:**77, 1965.

Arshavskii, I.A.: Physiological analysis of physical development with special reference to the newborn infant, Hum. Physiol. **5**(2):169-180, 1979.

Ashkenazi, S., and others: Size of liver edge in full-term, healthy infants, Am. J. Dis. Child. **138**:377-378, 1984.

Baron, M., and Tafuro, P.: The extremes of age: the newborn and the elderly, Nurs. Clin. North Am. **20**(1):181-190, 1985.

Binzley, V.A.: State: an overlooked factor in newborn nursing, Am. J. Nurs. **77**(1):102-103, 1977.

Clark, D.A.: Times of first void and first stool in 500 newborns, Pediatrics **60**(4):457-459, 1977.

Cloherty, J.P., and Stark, A.R., editors: Manual of neonatal care, ed. 2, Boston, 1985, Little, Brown & Co.

Davis, V.: The structure and function of brown adipose tissue in the neonate, J. Obstet. Gynecol. Neonatal Nurs. **9**(6):368-372, 1980.

Duara, S., and others: Neonatal screening with auditory brainstem responses: results of follow-up audiometry and risk factor evaluation, J. Pediatr. **108**(2):276-281, 1986.

Fanaroff, A., and Martin, R., editors: Behrman's neonatal-perinatal medicine, ed. 3, St. Louis, 1983, The C.V. Mosby Co.

The first six hours of life: assessment of risk in the newborn: evaluation during the transitional period, New York, 1980, March of Dimes—Birth Defects Foundation.

Graven, S.: Temperature control in newborn babies. In Neonatal thermoregulation, module 1, New York, 1976, The National Foundation—March of Dimes.

Greenberg, M.D.: Evaluating the newborn, Emergency **15**(6):22-25, 1983.

Harpin, V.A., and Rutter, N.: Barrier properties of the newborn infant's skin, J. Pediatr. **102**(3):419-425, 1983.

Johnson, T.R., and others: Children are different; developmental physiology, ed. 2, Columbus, Ohio, 1978, Ross Laboratories.

Judd, J.M.: Assessing the newborn from head to toe, Nursing 85 **15**(12):34-41, 1985.

Korones, S.B.: High-risk newborn infants: the basis for intensive nursing care, ed. 4, St. Louis, 1986, The C.V. Mosby Co.

Labson, L.H.: Newborn exam: evaluation in the nursery, Patient Care **17**(10):95-98, 1983.

Lebenthal, E., Lee, P.C., and Heitlinger, L.A.: Impact of development of the gastrointestinal tract on infant feeding, J. Pediatr. **102**(1):1-9, 1983.

Lubinsky, M.: Neonatal assessment for anomalies and syndromes, Pediatr. Basics **37**:4-7, 1984.

Marchbanks, P.: Newborn assessment: physical examination. In Humenick, S.S., editor: Analysis of current assessment strategies in the health care of young children and childbearing families, Norwalk, CT, 1982, Appleton-Century-Crofts.

Mimouni, F., and others: Occurrence of supernumerary nipples in newborns, Am. J. Dis. Child. **137**:952-953, 1983.

Moss, J.R.: Predicting young children's cooperation with the physical examination, Pediatr. Nurs. **9**(3):188-190, 1983.

Ruchala, P.: The effect of wearing headcoverings on the axillary temperatures of infants, Am. J. Maternal Child Nurs. **10**(4):240, 1985.

Scanlon, J.W., and others: A system of newborn physical examination, Baltimore, 1979, University Park Press.

Scharping, E.M.: Physiological measurements of the neonate, Am. J. Maternal Child Nurs. **8**(1):70-73, 1983.

Schiffman, R.F.: Temperature monitoring in the neonate: a comparison of axillary and rectal temperatures, Nurs. Res. **31**(5):274-277, 1982.

Taylor, K.M.: The Apgar scoring system. In Humenick, S.S., editor: Analysis of current assessment strategies in the health care of young children and childbearing families, Norwalk, CT, 1982, Appleton-Century-Crofts.

Taylor, K.M.: Gestational age assessment. In Humenick, S.S., editor: Analysis of current assessment strategies in the health care of young children and childbearing families, Norwalk, CT, 1982, Appleton-Century-Crofts.

Wilson, C.B.: Immunologic basis for increased susceptibility of the neonate to infection, J. Pediatr. **108**(1):1-12, 1986.

Nursing Care of the Neonate

Adam, H.M., Stern, E.K., and Stein, R.E.K.: Anticipatory guidance: a modest intervention in the nursery, Pediatrics **76**(5):781-786, 1985.

Callon, H.: Nursing responsibility in maintaining the body heat of the newborn infant. In Neonatal thermoregulation, module 1, New York, 1976, The National Foundation—March of Dimes.

Christophersen, E.R., and Sullivan, M.A.: Increasing the protection of newborn infants in cars, Pediatrics **70**(1):21-25, 1982.

Hammerschlag, M.R., and others: Enzyme immunoassay for diagnosis of neonatal chlamydial conjunctivitis, J. Pediatr. **107**(5):741-743, 1985.

Harris, C.C., and Stern, P.N.: Care of the prepuce in the uncircumcised child: reinforcing nature's laws of health, Issues Compr. Pediatr. Nurs. **5**:233-242, 1981.

Kuller, J.M., Lund, C., and Tobin, C.: Improved skin care for premature infants, Am. J. Maternal Child Nurs. **8**(3):200-203, 1983.

Lane, P.A., and Hathaway, W.E.: Vitamin K in infancy, J. Pediatr. **106**(3):351, 1985.

Lum, B., and Lortz, R.: Reappraising newborn eye care, Am. J. Nurs. **80**(9):1602-1603, 1980.

McCormack, M.: Screening for genetic traits and diseases, Am. Fam. Physician **24**(4):153-166, 1981.

McNinch, A.W., and others: Hemorrhaegic disease of the newborn returns, Lancet **1**:1089-1090, May 1983.

Porth, C., and Kaylor, L.: Temperature regulation in the newborn, Am. J. Nurs. **78**(10):1691-1693, 1978.

Principles of infant skin care: a current guide for the pediatric health care professional, Skillman, NJ, 1983, Johnson & Johnson Baby Products Co.

Rettig, P.: Chlamydial infections in pediatrics: not for babies only, J. Pediatr. **104**(1):82-83, 1984.

Sandstrom, K.I., and others: Microbial causes of neonatal conjunctivitis, J. Pediatr. **105**(5):706-711, 1984.

Sasso, S.C.: Erythromycin for eye prophylaxis, Am. J. Maternal Child Nurs. **9**:417, 1984.

Circumcision

Gibbons, M.B.: Why circumcise? Pediatr. Nurs. **5**:9-12, July/Aug. 1979.

Grimes, D.A.: Routine circumcision reconsidered, Am. J. Nurs. **1**(80):108-109, 1980.

Harris, C.C., and Stern, P.N.: Care of the prepuce in the uncircumcised child: reinforcing nature's laws of health, Issues Compr. Pediatr. Nurs. **5**:233-242, 1981.

Levine, I.: Circumcision: rite, rational, or both? Patient Care **12**:72-94, March 1978.

Lovell, J.E., and Cox, J.: Maternal attitudes toward circumcision, J. Fam. Pract. **9**:811-813, Nov. 1979.

McDermott, R.J., Wilson, D.D., and Marty, P.J.: Neonatal circumcision, Patient Counselling Health Ed. **3**(4):132-136, 1982.

Osborn, L.M., Metcalf, T.J., and Mariani, E.M.: Hygienic care in uncircumcised infants, Pediatrics **67**(3):365-367, 1981.

Warner, E., and Strashin, E.: Benefits and risks of circumcision, Can. Med. Assoc. J. **125**:967-976, Nov. 1981.

Wayland, J.R., and Higgins, P.G.: Newborn circumcision: father's involvement, Pediatr. Nurs. **9**(1):41-42, 1983.

Nutrition

Albers, R.M.: Emotional support for the breast-feeding mother, Issues Compr. Pediatr. Nurs. **5**:109-124, 1981.

American Academy of Pediatrics, Committee on Nutrition: Commentary on breast-feeding and infant formulas, including proposed standards for formulas, Pediatrics **57**(2):278-285, 1976.

American Academy of Pediatrics, Committee on Nutrition: Vitamin and mineral supplement needs in normal children in the United States, Pediatrics **66**(6):1015-1020, 1980.

American Academy of Pediatrics, Committee on Nutrition: Nutrition and lactation, Pediatrics **68**(3):435-441, 1981.

Anderson, G.H.: Human milk feeding, Pediatr. Clin. North Am. **32**(2):335-353, 1985.

Barness, L.A.: Nutritional requirements of the full-term neonate. In Suskind, R.M., editor: Textbook of pediatric nutrition, New York, 1981, Raven Press.

Berger, L.R.: When should one discourage breast-feeding? Pediatrics **67**(2):300-302, 1981.

Brostrom, K.: Human milk and infant formulas: nutritional and immunological characteristics. In Suskind, R.M., editor: Textbook of pediatric nutrition, New York, 1981, Raven Press.

Butler, J.E.: Immunologic aspects of breast feeding, antiinfectious activity of breast milk, Semin. Perinatol. **3**(3):255-270, 1979.

Current issues in feeding the normal infant, Pediatrics **75**(suppl.):135-215, 1985.

Cusson, R.M.: Attitudes toward breast-feeding among female high-school students, Pediatr. Nurs. **11**(3):189-191, 1985.

Eiger, M.S., Raursen, A.R., and Silverio, J.: Breast- vs. bottle-feeding: a study of morbidity in upper middle class infants, Clin. Pediatr. **23**(9):492-495, 1984.

Infant formula: labeling requirements, Fed. Register **48**:31880-31887, July 1983.

Jeffries, R.D.: A short course in breastfeeding, Issues Compr. Pediatr. Nurs. **5**:243-251, 1981.

Kemberling, S.R.: Supporting breast-feeding, Pediatrics **63**(1):60-63, 1979.

Myers, M.G., and others: Respiratory and gastrointestinal illnesses in breast- and formula-fed infants, Am. J. Dis. Child. **138**:629-632, 1984.

Pipes, P.L.: Nutrition in infancy and childhood, ed. 3, St. Louis, 1985, The C.V. Mosby Co.

Rassin, D.K., and others: Incidence of breast-feeding in a low socioeconomic group of mothers in the United States: ethnic patterns, Pediatrics **73**(2):132-137, 1984.

Report of the task force on the assessment of the scientific evidence relating to infant-feeding practices and infant health, Pediatrics **74**(suppl.):579-762, 1984.

Schlegel, A.M.: Observations on breast-feeding technique: facts and fallacies, Am. J. Maternal Child Nurs. **8**(3):204-208, 1983.

Taylor, L.S.: Newborn feeding behaviors and attaching, Am. J. Maternal Child Nurs. **6**(3):201-202, 1981.

Winikoff, B., and others: Dynamics of infant feeding: mothers, professionals, and the institutional context in a large urban hospital, Pediatrics **77**(3):357-365, 1986.

Wink, D.: Getting through the maze of infant formulas, Am. J. Nurs. **85**(4):388-392, 1985.

Parent-Infant Bonding (Attachment)

Anderson, C.J.: Enhancing reciprocity between mother and neonate, Nurs. Res. **30**(2):89-93, 1981.

Avant, P.K.: A maternal attachment assessment strategy. In Humenick, S.S., editor: Analysis of current assessment strategies in the health care of young children and childbearing families, Norwalk, CT, 1982, Appleton-Century-Crofts.

Avant, P.K.: Nursing diagnosis: maternal attachment, Adv. Nurs. Sci. **2**:45-55, Oct. 1979.

Brazelton, T.B.: On becoming a family: the growth of attachment, New York, 1981, Delta/Seymour Lawrence.

Bristor, M.W., Helfer, R.E., and Coy, K.B.: Effects of perinatal coaching on mother-infant interaction, Am. J. Dis. Child. **138**:254-257, 1984.

Buckner, E.B.: Use of Brazelton Neonatal Behavioral Assessment in planning care for parents and newborns, JOGN Nurs. **12**:26-30, 1983.

Cannon, R.B.: The development of maternal touch during early mother-infant interaction, J. Obstet. Gynecol. Neonatal Nurs. **6**(2):28-33, 1977.

Carter-Jessop, L.: Promoting maternal attachment through prenatal intervention, Am. J. Maternal Child Nurs. **6**(2):107-112, 1981.

Cronenwett, L.R., and Kunst-Wilson, W.: Stress, social support, and the transition to fatherhood, Nurs. Res. **30**(4):196-201, 1981.

Cropley, C.: Assessment of mothering behaviors. In Johnson, S.H., editor: Nursing assessment and strategies for the family at risk, ed. 2, 1986, Philadelphia, 1979, J.B. Lippincott Co., pp. 13-35.

Dean, P.G., Morgan, P., and Towle, J.M.: Making baby's acquaintance: a unique attachment strategy, Am. J. Maternal Child Nurs. **7**(1):37-41, 1982.

Dodge, J.: When childbirth is a family affair, RN **48**(12):20-21, 1985.

Fein, R.A.: Research on fathering: social policy and an emergent perspective, J. Soc. Issues **34**:122-135, 1978.

The first six hours of life: early parent-infant relationships, New York, 1978, The National Foundation—March of Dimes.

Foley, K.L.: Caring for the parents of newborn twins, Am. J. Maternal Child Nurs. **4**(4):221-226, 1979.

Freeman, M.H.: Giving family life a good start in the hospital, Am. J. Maternal Child Nurs. **4**(1):51-54, 1979.

Gibes, R.M.: Clinical uses of the Brazelton Neonatal Behavioral Assessment Scale in nursing practice, Pediatr. Nurs. **7**:23-26, May/June 1981.

Grace, J.T.: Does a mother's knowledge of fetal gender affect attachment? Am. J. Maternal Child Nurs. **9**:42-45, 1984.

Hale, N.: Birth of a family: the new role of the father in childbirth, New York, 1979, Anchor Books.

Heggenhougen, H.K.: Father and childbirth: an anthropological perspective, J. Nurse-Midwif. **25**:21-26, 1980.

Jenkins, R.L., and Westhus, N.K.: The nurse role in parent-infant bonding: overview, assessment, intervention, J. Obstet. Gynecol. Neonatal Nurs. **10**(2):114-118, 1981.

Klaus, M.H., and Robertson, M.O., editors: Birth, interaction and attachment, Skillman, NJ, 1982, Johnson & Johnson Baby Products Co.

Mercer, R.T.: The nurse and maternal tasks of early postpartum, Am. J. Maternal Child Nurs. **6**(5):341-345, 1981.

Murphy, C.M.: Assessment of fathering behaviors. In Johnson, S.H., editor: Nursing assessment and strategies for the family at risk, ed. 2, 1986 Philadelphia, 1979, J.B. Lippincott Co., pp. 36-49.

Nugent, J.K.: The Brazelton Neonatal Behavioral Assessment Scale: implications for intervention, Pediatr. Nurs. **7**:18-21, May/June 1981.

Parke, R.D., and others: The father's role in the family system, Semin. Perinatol. **3**(1):25-34, 1979.

Perez, P.: Nurturing children who attend the birth of a sibling, Am. J. Maternal Child Nurs. **4**(4):215-217, 1979.

Phillips, C.R., and Anzalone, J.T.: Fathering: participation in labor and birth, ed. 2, St. Louis, 1982, The C.V. Mosby Co.

Ricks, S.S.: Father-infant interactions: a review of empirical research, Family Relations **34**(4):505-511, 1985.

Toney, L.: The effects of holding the newborn at delivery on paternal bonding, Nurs. Res. **32**(1):16-19, 1983.

Trabert, C.: Prenatal tactile intervention can be encouraged, Am. J. Maternal Child Nurs. **6**(2):108-109, 1981.

Walker, L.O.: Brazelton Neonatal Behavioral Assessment Scale. In Humenick, S.S., editor: Analysis of current assessment strategies in the health care of young children and childbearing families, Norwalk, CT, 1982, Appleton-Century-Crofts.

Walker, L.O.: Neonatal Perception Inventories. In Humenick, S.S., editor: Analysis of current assessment strategies in the health care of young children and childbearing families, Norwalk, CT, 1982, Appleton-Century-Crofts.

Wieser, M.A., and Castiglia, P.T.: Assessing early father-infant attachment, Am. J. Maternal Child Nurs. **9**(2):104-106, 1984.

Chapter 9

Health Problems of the Newborn

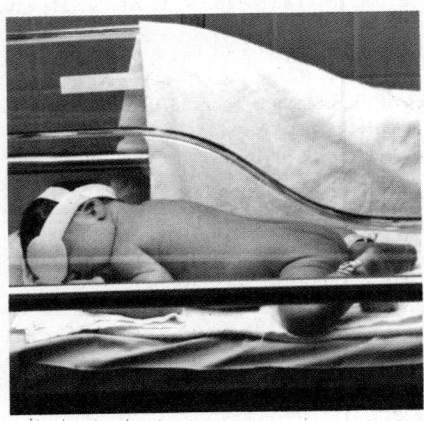

The newborn may experience a number of problems immediately or shortly after birth. Some, such as birth injuries, are caused by the forces of labor and delivery. Others, such as infections, are chiefly the result of environmental factors. Problems may also be related to the newborn's immature physiologic systems, particularly disorders related to jaundice. In addition, inborn errors of metabolism may be present at birth, and, if identified early, they can be successfully managed to prevent their deleterious effects.

Some conditions require no intervention other than careful assessment and continued observation to distinguish them from potential pathologic situations. Others require immediate identification and intervention to prevent future problems. The nurse's ability to recognize such conditions and institute appropriate care significantly affects newborns' immediate survival and later development.

Birth Injuries

Birth injuries are those injuries that occur during the birth process. The forces of labor and delivery may result in trauma, especially when the infant is large, the presentation is breech, forceful extraction is used, or inexperienced personnel are in attendance. Birth trauma ranks ninth as a cause of neonatal mortality. Birth injuries can be classified according to the type of body structure involved (see box).

Many injuries are minor and spontaneously resolve in a few days; others, although minor, require some degree of intervention. Still others can be serious and even fatal. Part of the nurse's responsibility is identification of such injuries in order that appropriate intervention can be initiated as soon as possible.

SOFT TISSUE INJURY

Various types of soft tissue injury may be sustained during the birth process, primarily in the form of bruises and/or abrasions secondary to dystocia. Soft tissue injury usually occurs when there is some degree of disproportion between the presenting part and the maternal pelvis (cephalopelvic disproportion). The following are common types of soft tissue injury:

erythema and abrasions Usually the result of the application of forceps; discoloration is the same configuration as the instrument.

petechiae Nonraised, pinpoint hemorrhages caused by a sudden increase and then release of pressure during passage through the birth canal; may be seen on the chest, face, and head.

ecchymoses Small hemorrhagic areas (larger than petechiae) that may occur after traumatic, rapid (or "precipitate"), or breech delivery.

subcutaneous fat necrosis Clearly outlined masses located in the subcutaneous tissues that are firm to the overlying skin but movable over the underlying tissue; most likely caused by traumatic manipulation during delivery.

subconjunctival (scleral) hemorrhages The result of rupture of capillaries in the sclera from pressure on the fetal head during delivery; most common location is the limbus of the iris.

retinal hemorrhages Flame-shaped, irregular, or round areas of bleeding in the retina from excessive pressure on the fetal head during delivery; extensive areas may indicate subdural hematoma or brain trauma.

These traumatic lesions generally fade spontaneously within a few days without treatment. However, petechiae may be a manifestation of some underlying bleeding disorder and should be evaluated.

Nursing Considerations

Nursing care is primarily directed toward assessing the injury, maintaining asepsis of the area to prevent breakdown and infection, and providing an explanation and reassurance

---

CLASSIFICATION OF NEONATAL BIRTH INJURY

Soft tissue
Erythema and abrasions
Petechiae
Ecchymoses
Subcutaneous fat necrosis
Subconjunctival (scleral) hemorrhages
Retinal hemorrhages
Hemorrhages into abdominal organs

Head
Caput succedaneum
Cephalhematoma

Bones
Skull molding
Skull fracture (depressed or linear)
Fractures of clavicle, humerus, or femur

Muscles and peripheral nerves
Facial paralysis
Brachial palsy (Erb-Duchenne paralysis, Klumpke palsy)
Phrenic nerve palsy (diaphragmatic paralysis)

Nervous system
Intracranial hemorrhage
Subdural hematoma
Spinal cord injury

---

to the parents. Regardless of how benign the injury, parents are concerned and mourn the loss of the expected "perfect" infant. Explanations of the cause and treatment, if any, need to be thorough and repeated frequently. If the injury is disfiguring, such as extensive facial bruising, the parental feelings of revulsion should be respected. Nurses can demonstrate acceptance of the child through their example of sensitive, personal care of the infant. Even if the injuries are temporary, the bonding process can be affected by the parents' initial feelings of shock, grief, and disappointment. Every effort should be made to facilitate bonding during the postpartum admission.

HEAD TRAUMA

Trauma to the head that occurs during the birth process is usually benign but occasionally results in more serious injury. The injuries that produce serious trauma, such as intraventricular hemorrhage and subdural hematoma, are discussed later in relation to neurologic disturbances (see Chapter 37). Skull fractures are discussed in association with other fractures sustained during the birth process. The common injuries, caput succedaneum and cephalhematoma, are discussed here and outlined in Table 9-1.

Caput Succedaneum

The most commonly observed scalp lesion is caput succedaneum, a vaguely outlined area of edematous tissue situated over the portion of the scalp that presents in a vertex

Table 9-1 Comparison of caput succedaneum and cephalhematoma

Injury
Caput succedaneum

Pathology
Edema of soft scalp tissue

Time of onset
Within 24 hours after birth

Clinical manifestations
Outline is ill defined
Mass is soft but not fluctuant
Pressure causes pitting of edema

Injury
Cephalhematoma

Pathology
Hematoma between periosteum and skull bone

Time of onset
After initial 24 to 48 hours after birth

Clinical manifestations
Outline is well defined against edge of bone margin
Mass is soft and fluctuant

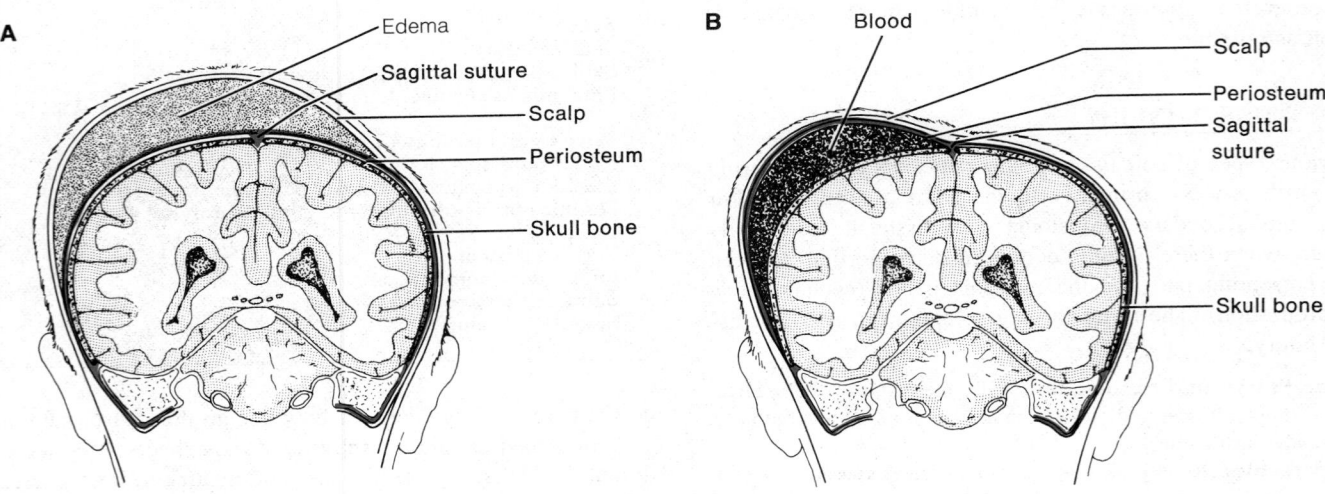

Fig. 9-1, A-B. From Jensen, M.D., and Bobak, I.M.: Maternity and gynecologic care: the nurse and the family, ed. 3, St. Louis, 1985, The C.V. Mosby Co.

delivery (Fig. 9-1, *A*). The swelling consists of serum and/or blood, which accumulate in the tissues above the bone. Typically, the swelling extends beyond the bone margins. The swelling may be associated with overlying petechiae or ecchymosis. It is present at or shortly after birth. No specific treatment is needed, and the swelling subsides within a few days.

Cephalhematoma

Infrequently a cephalhematoma is formed when blood vessels rupture during labor or delivery to produce bleeding into the area between the bone and its periosteum. Unlike caput succedaneum, the boundaries of the cephalhematoma are sharply demarcated and do not extend beyond the limits of the bone (Fig. 9-1, *B*). The cephalhematoma may involve one or both parietal bones. Less commonly the occipital and rarely the frontal bones are affected. The swelling is usually minimal at birth and increases in size on the second or third day.

No treatment is indicated for uncomplicated cephalhematoma. Most lesions are absorbed within 2 weeks to 3 months. Lesions that result in severe blood loss to the area or that involve an underlying fracture require further evaluation and appropriate therapy. A local infection can develop and is suspected when a sudden increase in swelling occurs.

Nursing Considerations

Nursing care is directed toward assessment and observation of the two common head injuries and vigilance in observing for possible associated complications such as infection, subdural hematoma, or intraventricular hemorrhage.

Because both of these visible injuries resolve spontaneously, parents need reassurance of their usual benign nature (see also earlier discussion of soft tissue injury).

FRACTURES

Fracture of the clavicle, or collarbone, is the most common birth injury. It is associated with difficult vertex or breech birth and delivery of infants of above average weight. The fracture may be detected during delivery by an audible click or snap, although the newborn may be asymptomatic. The problem should be suspected in infants who demonstrate limited use of the affected arm, a malposition of the arm, asymmetric Moro reflex, local swelling or tenderness, or who cry in pain when the arm is moved. Crepitus (the crackling sound produced by the rubbing together of fractured bone fragments) is often heard on further examination, and roentgenograms usually reveal a complete fracture with overriding of the fragments.

Fractures of long bones, such as the femur or humerus, may be undetected because the epiphysis is mostly cartilage, which is usually not dense enough to show clearly on radiographs.

Fractures of the neonatal skull are uncommon. The bones, which are less mineralized and more compressible, are separated by membranous seams that allow sufficient alteration in the head contour so that it can adjust to the birth canal during delivery. Skull fractures usually follow prolonged, difficult delivery or forceps extraction. Most fractures are linear, but some may be visible as depressed indentations resembling a ping-pong ball.

Nursing Considerations

Frequently no intervention may be prescribed other than proper body alignment, careful dressing and undressing of the infant, and handling and carrying that support the affected bone. For example, when picking up the infant who has a fractured clavicle, it is important to support the upper and lower back rather than pull the infant up from under the arms.

Occasionally, for immobilization and relief of pain, the arm on the side of the fractured clavicle is fixed on the body by pinning the sleeve to the shirt or by using a triangular sling or a figure-of-8 bandage. The family should be involved in caring for the infant during hospitalization, as part of discharge planning for care at home.

Linear skull fractures usually require no treatment. A "ping-pong" fracture usually can be decompressed by nonsurgical methods. The infant is carefully observed for signs of cerebral complications. The parents of an infant with a fracture of any bone should be involved in caring for the infant during hospitalization as part of discharge planning for care at home. Family support is similar to that discussed on p. 341 for soft tissue injury.

PARALYSES

Pressure exerted on nerves during a difficult labor can cause injury and paralysis of muscles that the nerves supply. The most frequently observed nerve injuries are those involving the facial nerve and the brachial plexus.

Facial Nerve Paralysis

Pressure on the facial nerve during delivery may result in injury to cranial nerve VII. Clinical manifestations are primarily loss of movement on the affected side, such as inability to completely close the eye, drooping of the corner of the mouth, and absence of wrinkling of the forehead and nasolabial fold (Fig. 9-2). The paralysis is most noticeable when the infant cries. The mouth is drawn to the unaffected side, the wrinkles are deeper on the normal side, and the eye on the involved side remains open.

No medical intervention is necessary. The paralysis usually disappears spontaneously in a few days but may take considerably longer.

Nursing considerations. Nursing care involves aiding the infant in sucking because part of the mouth cannot close tightly around the nipple. Using a soft rubber nipple with a large hole is often helpful. Sometimes the infant needs to be gavage-fed to prevent aspiration. Breast-feeding is not contraindicated, but the mother will need additional assistance in helping the infant to grasp on and compress the areolar area.

The eye on the affected side must be protected from injury to the cornea if the lid does not close completely. An eye patch may be applied, or artificial tears may need to be instilled daily to prevent drying of the conjunctiva, sclera, and cornea. If eye care is needed at home, the parents are taught the procedure for administration of eye drops before the infant's discharge from the nursery (see p. 1139).

Brachial Palsy

Plexus injury results from forces that alter the normal position and relationship of the arm, shoulder, and neck. *Erb palsy* (Erb-Duchenne paralysis), caused by damage to the upper plexus, is usually a result of stretching or pulling

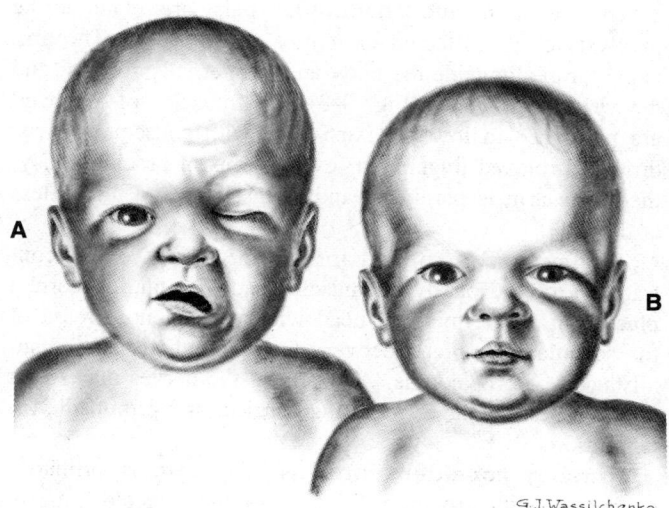

G.J.Wassilchenko

Fig. 9-2. A, Paralysis of right side of face 15 minutes after forceps delivery. Absence of movement on affected side is especially noticeable when infant cries. **B,** Same infant 24 hours later.

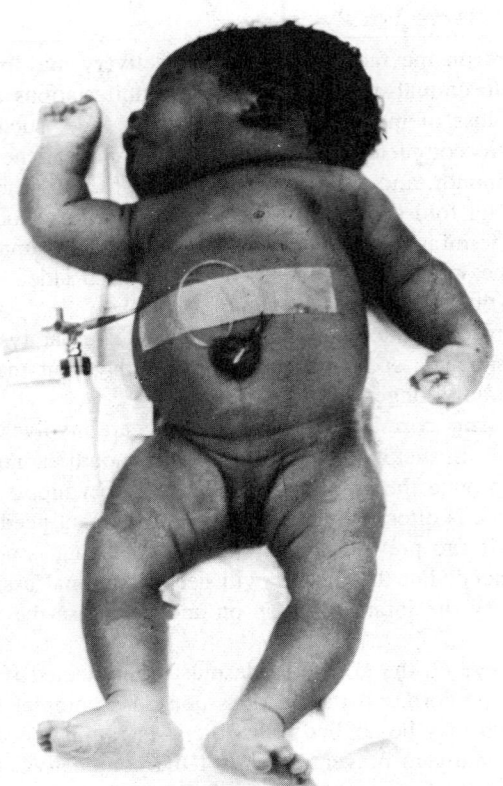

Fig. 9-3. Brachial plexus (Erb) palsy, left sided. Note extended, internally rotated arm and pronated wrist in affected side.
From Korones, S. B.: High-risk newborn infants: the basis for intensive nursing care, ed. 4, St. Louis, 1986, The C. V. Mosby Co.

away of the shoulder from the head. The less common lower plexus palsy, or *Klumpke palsy,* results from severe stretching of the upper extremity while the trunk is relatively less mobile.

The clinical manifestations of Erb palsy are related to the paralysis of the affected extremity and muscles. The arm hangs limp alongside the body and is internally rotated, and the wrist is pronated (Fig. 9-3). The muscles of the hand are paralyzed in lower plexus palsy with consequent wrist drop and relaxed fingers. In severe forms of brachial palsy, the entire arm is paralyzed and hangs limp and motionless at the side.

Treatment of an affected arm is aimed at preventing contractures of the paralyzed muscles and maintaining correct placement of the humeral head within the glenoid fossa of the scapula. Complete recovery from stretched nerves usually takes 3 to 6 months. Avulsion of the nerves may result in permanent damage, requiring surgical and orthopedic intervention.

Nursing considerations. Nursing care is primarily concerned with proper positioning of the affected arm. In upper arm paralysis the arm should be abducted 90 degrees with external rotation at the shoulder, 90-degrees flexion at the elbow, full supination of the forearm, and slight extension of the wrist so that the palm of the hand is turned to-

ward the face (Fanaroff and Martin, 1983). This position may be maintained with intermittent splinting.

The arm should also be put through complete passive range of motion exercises daily to maintain muscle tone and function. In dressing the infant, preference is given to the affected arm. Undressing begins with the unaffected arm, and redressing begins with the affected arm to prevent unnecessary manipulation and stress on the paralyzed muscles.

As with other birth injuries, family support is equally important (see discussion of soft tissue birth injury, p. 341). Also, because of the extended length of recovery, follow-up is essential.

Phrenic Nerve Paralysis

Phrenic nerve paralysis causes diaphragmatic paralysis and sometimes occurs in conjunction with brachial palsy. Respiratory distress is the most common and important sign of injury. Because injury to the phrenic nerve is usually unilateral, the lung on the affected side does not expand and respiratory efforts are ineffectual. To facilitate maximum expansion of the uninvolved lung, the infant is positioned on the affected side. Breathing is primarily thoracic, and cyanosis is a prominent sign. Pneumonia is a frequent complication.

Nursing care of the infant with phrenic nerve paralysis is the same as for any infant with respiratory distress, and the emotional needs of the family are similar to those discussed for soft tissue injury (see p. 341).

Common Problems in the Newborn

Numerous problems may be encountered in the newborn period. Many are innocuous conditions that are of concern only to the parents; others require intervention to prevent complications. Some are discussed elsewhere as appropriate throughout the book, for example, skin manifestations and color changes in the newborn (p. 300). One of the most common observations in the newborn period is jaundice. It is discussed later in this chapter (see Problems related to physiologic factors, p. 346).

ERYTHEMA TOXICUM

Erythema toxicum, also known as *flea bite dermatitis* or *newborn rash,* is a benign, self-limiting eruption that usually appears within the first 2 days of life. The lesions vary in character and number. They may be firm, pale yellow to white papules or pustules 1 to 3 mm in diameter on an erythematous base, erythematous macules, or simply blotchy erythema. The rash is most commonly located on the face, proximal extremities, trunk and buttocks and is more obvious during crying episodes. There are no systemic manifestations, and the cause is unknown. Although no treatment is necessary, parents are usually concerned about the rash and need to be reassured of its benign and transient nature.

CANDIDIASIS

Candida infections, also known as *moniliasis*, are not uncommon in the newborn. *Candida albicans*, the organism usually responsible, may cause disease in any organ system. It is a yeastlike fungus (producing yeast cells and spores) that can be acquired from a maternal vaginal infection during delivery, by person-to-person transmission (especially poor handwashing technique), or from contaminated hands, bottles, nipples, or other articles. Mucocutaneous, cutaneous, and disseminated candidiasis are all observed in this age-group. It is usually a benign disorder in the neonate, often confined to the oral and diaper regions.

Candidal Diaper Dermatitis

The warm, moist atmosphere created in the diaper area provides an optimum environment for candidal growth. The dermatitis appears in the perianal area, inguinal folds, and lower abdomen. The affected area is intensely erythematous with a sharply demarcated, scalloped edge, frequently with numerous satellite lesions that extend beyond the larger lesion. The usual source of infection is through the gastrointestinal tract when organisms are swallowed from the birth canal during delivery. It may also appear 2 to 3 days after an oral infection.

Therapy consists of applications of an anticandial ointment, such as nystatin, with each diaper change. The caregiver is taught to keep the diaper area as clean and dry as possible, and good hygienic care is essential to prevent spread. Sometimes the infant also is given an oral antifungal preparation to eliminate any gastrointestinal source of infection (see following discussion).

Oral Candidiasis

Oral candidiasis (thrush) is characterized by white adherent patches on the tongue, palate, and inner aspects of the cheeks. It is readily distinguished from coagulated milk when attempts to remove the patches are unsuccessful, usually resulting in bleeding from the scraped surfaces. The infant may refuse to suck because of pain in the mouth, but this is uncommon.

The condition tends to be acute in the newborn, chronic in infants and young children, and to appear when the oral flora are altered as a result of antibiotic therapy. Although the disorder is usually self-limiting, spontaneous resolution may take as long as 2 months, during which time lesions may spread to the larynx, trachea, bronchi, and lungs and along the gastrointestinal tract. The disease is treated with good hygiene, application of a fungicide, and correction of any underlying disturbance. The source of infection, usually the mother, should be treated to prevent reinfection.

Topical application of 1 ml nystatin (Mycostatin) over the surfaces of the oral cavity four times a day or every 6 hours is usually sufficient to prevent spread of the disease or prolongation of its course. Another effective therapy is application of 1% aqueous gentian violet three times a day.

For candidiasis that is unresponsive to conventional treatment, several other drugs may be used, including amphotericin B (Fungizone), clotrimazole (Lotrimin), or miconazole (Monistat, Micatin). Various preparations may be given intravenously or applied topically. Clotrimazole or nystatin suppositories can also be inserted tightly into the tip of a split pacifier and given to the infant to suck. In older children the suppositories can be used as oral "lozenges" (Mansour and Gelfand, 1981).

Nursing considerations. Nursing care is directed toward preventing spread of the infection and correct application of the prescribed topical medication. Mycostatin is applied after feedings. The medication is distributed to the surface of the oral mucosa and tongue with an applicator, and the remainder of the dose is deposited in the mouth to be swallowed in order to treat any gastrointestinal lesions. Therapy is continued for about 1 week, even when lesions have disappeared within a few days. The Mycostatin suspension is stable for only 1 week.

When gentian violet is used, the solution is applied directly to the patches. The infant is not allowed to swallow any excess because the medication is irritating to trachea, larynx, and esophagus. After application of the solution, the infant is placed prone for a short time to allow secretions to flow from the mouth. Special care is taken when administering this preparation because gentian violet stains skin, clothing, bed linens, and other objects.

Other measures to control thrush, in addition to good hygienic care, include rinsing the infant's mouth with plain water after each feeding before applying the medication and boiling reusable nipples and bottles for at least 20 minutes after thorough washing (spores are heat-resistant).

BULLOUS IMPETIGO (IMPETIGO NEONATORUM)

Bullous impetigo is an infectious skin condition caused by various strains of group A beta-hemolytic streptococci or coagulase-positive *Staphylococcus aureus*. It is characterized by vesicular lesions that vary in size from a few millimeters to several centimeters. The blebs usually occur in the axilla, in the groin, on the undersurface of the neck, and on the face. Once the vesicles rupture, reinfection occurs on other parts of the body, contributing to the contagious nature of this disease. Yellow crusts form over the lesions, which are surrounded by erythema. The lesions are pruritic, and scratching increases the chance of secondary infection.

Treatment of impetigo involves administration of systemic and local antibiotics. Isolation of the infant and initiation of meticulous handwashing techniques are essential because of the highly contagious nature of the disease.

Nursing Considerations

In caring for the infant with impetigo, wound and skin precautions are usually the isolation technique of choice. The infant may be placed in a private room. Gowns are worn when caring for the infant. Gloves are worn when directly caring for the infected lesion. Masks are not necessary. Articles that have been in contact with the infant are discarded separately.

The infant's arms may need to be restrained with elbow restraints or by pulling the undershirt sleeves over the hands and securing the openings with tape. If restraints of any kind are used, the infant is allowed freedom of movement at supervised times. Even though the infant is isolated, holding during feeding, rocking, and cuddling are essential components of care. Parents and other visitors are instructed regarding precautions for preventing spread of infection.

"BIRTHMARKS"

Discolorations of the skin are common findings in the newborn infant. (See Skin assessment of the newborn, p. 307.) Most, such as mongolian spots or telangiectatic nevi, involve no therapy other than reassurance to parents of the benign nature of these discolorations. Some can be a manifestation of a disease that suggests further examination of the child and other family members (e.g., the multiple light brown *cafe au lait spots* that often characterize the autosomal-dominant hereditary disorder neurofibromatosis and are common findings in Albright syndrome).

Darker and/or more extensive lesions demand further scrutiny, and excision of the lesion is recommended when feasible or excisional biopsy is performed. These lesions include the reddish-brown solitary nodule that appears on the face or upper arm and usually represents a spindle and epithelioid cell nevus (juvenile melanoma); a giant pigmented nevus (bathing trunk nevus); a dark-brown to black irregular plaque that is at risk of transformation to malignant melanoma; and the dark-brown or black macules that become more numerous with age (junctional or compound nevi).

Vascular birthmarks—orange or light-red (salmon patch) or dark-red or bluish-red (port wine stain) lesions—require no treatment during childhood, although good results have been obtained with the argon laser in postpubertal individuals (Dicken, 1985). Strawberry hemangiomas—red, rubbery nodules with a rough surface—may not be present at birth but may appear at 2 to 4 weeks of age. The parents can be reassured that these marks resolve spontaneously during childhood and usually require no treatment.

Nursing Considerations

Although most birthmarks are benign, they can cause parents a great deal of anxiety if they are located on highly visible areas, such as the face. A complete explanation of the type of birthmark and treatment options is given, and parents may need advice regarding the use of cosmetic coverings (such as Covermark) at a later time when they feel that the child may be adversely affected by the defect.

Problems Related to Physiologic Factors

Neonates are susceptible to a number of problems related to their immature physiologic status. Three of these—hyperbi-

lirubinemia, neonatal hypocalcemia, and neonatal hypoglycemia—are discussed here. Hyperglycemia resulting from maternal diabetes is discussed in Chapter 10.

HYPERBILIRUBINEMIA

The term *hyperbilirubinemia* refers to an excessive accumulation of bilirubin in the blood and is characterized by *jaundice,* or *icterus,* a yellowish discoloration of the skin and other organs. Hyperbilirubinemia is a common finding in the newborn and in most instances is relatively benign. However, it can also indicate a pathologic state. Following is a brief description of the classification of neonatal jaundice, pathophysiology of bilirubin production and excretion, complications of hyperbilirubinemia, and a discussion of several disorders that cause hyperbilirubinemia in the newborn.

Classification

Hyperbilirubinemia is classified according to the two types of bilirubin: unconjugated (indirect reacting) and conjugated (direct reacting). The determination of serum bilirubin as conjugated or unconjugated requires special testing that distinguishes between direct-reacting and indirect-reacting pigments.

Hyperbilirubinemia, characterized by elevation of *unconjugated* bilirubin, is the type most commonly seen in newborns, including "physiologic" jaundice and pathologic states resulting from increased production, decreased hepatic conjugation, or decreased hepatic uptake of bilirubin. Hyperbilirubinemia resulting from increased levels of *conjugated* bilirubin is rare in newborns. It implies a functioning liver but denotes serious hepatic problems, such as obstruction of bile into the biliary tree. The following discussion of hyperbilirubinemia is limited to the unconjugated type; disorders resulting in conjugated hyperbilirubinemia are discussed in Chapter 11.

Pathophysiology

Bilirubin is one of the breakdown products of hemoglobin from hemolyzed or dissolved red blood cells. As the cells reach the end of viability, they become too fragile to exist in the circulatory system, their cell membranes rupture, and the released hemoglobin is phagocytized by the reticuloendothelial cells, primarily in the liver and spleen. The hemoglobin is then split into heme and globin.

The exact pathway by which the heme complex is converted to bilirubin is not fully known. It is thought to be dependent on an enzyme, heme oxygenase, in the reticuloendothelial cells that transforms the heme molecule after loss of iron and globin to biliverdin. Biliverdin, a water-soluble green pigment, is rapidly reduced by the enzyme biliverdin reductase to form bilirubin.

The unconjugated (indirect) bilirubin, which is relatively insoluble in body fluids, is released by the reticuloendothelial cells and is rapidly bound to albumin. In the liver the bilirubin is detached from the plasma protein and in the

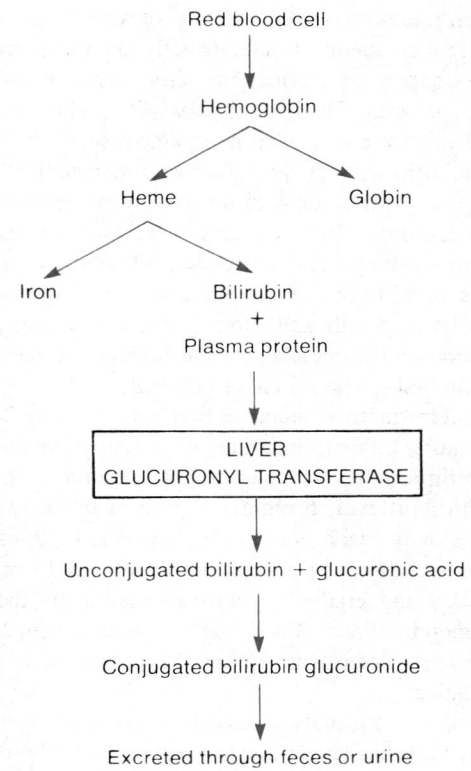

Fig. 9-4. Formation and excretion of bilirubin.

presence of the enzyme *glucuronyl transferase* is conjugated with glucuronic acid to produce a highly soluble form, bilirubin glucuronide, which is then excreted into the bile. The bile enters the intestine, where the action of the bacterial flora reduces the conjugated (direct) bilirubin to urobilinogen and stercobilin, the pigment that gives stool its characteristic color. Most of the reduced bilirubin is excreted through the feces, and a small amount is eliminated as urobilinogen in the urine (Fig. 9-4).

Normally the body is able to maintain a balance between the destruction of red blood cells and the utilization or excretion of by-products. When developmental limitations or a pathologic process interferes with this balance, bilirubin accumulates in the tissues to produce jaundice.

In the newborn, hyperbilirubinemia may be the result of (1) excess production of bilirubin, (2) disturbed capacity of the liver to conjugate bilirubin, or (3) bile duct obstruction resulting from biliary atresia (see p. 469). The most common cause is the relatively mild and self-limited *physiologic jaundice*. However, it may be the result of a disease process such as hemolytic disease of the newborn or infection. As a rule, jaundice that appears within the first 24 hours is caused by hemolytic disease of the newborn, sepsis, or one of the maternally derived diseases; jaundice that appears on the second or third day, peaks on the second to fourth days, and decreases between the fifth and seventh days is usually the result of physiologic jaundice; jaundice appearing after the third day but within the first week suggests sepsis.

Complications. The principal concern with elevated

levels of unconjugated bilirubin is its toxicity to neurons. The staining and necrosis of neurons results in *bilirubin encephalopathy* or *kernicterus*. The exact mechanisms responsible for brain damage are unknown. It is postulated that unconjugated bilirubin, which is lipid soluble, passes into the cell membrane of neurons and its various structures, blocking critical steps in the metabolism or transport of energy.

A direct relationship exists between the total serum bilirubin concentration and the risk of kernicterus. In general, a serum bilirubin level of 20 mg/dl in full-term infants is considered the maximum level before the development of brain damage. However, several factors affect this relationship. Normally only minute amounts of unconjugated bilirubin unbound to serum albumin enter the brain. Bound unconjugated bilirubin is unable to cross the protective blood-brain barrier. However, as conditions occur that lower the binding capacity of plasma, more free unconjugated bilirubin is available for cerebral entry. Factors that enhance the development of kernicterus include metabolic acidosis, lowered albumin levels, free fatty acids, and drugs such as salicylates or sulfonamides that compete for attachment to the plasma protein. In addition, any condition that increases the metabolic demands for oxygen or glucose, such as fetal distress or hypothermia, also increases the risk of brain damage despite lower serum levels of bilirubin.

The signs of kernicterus are those of central nervous system depression or excitation. Generally the clinical symptoms appear after the peak plasma bilirubin level has been established for several hours. Prodromal symptoms consist of decreased activity, lethargy, irritability, and a loss of interest in feeding. Within several hours these subtle findings are followed by rigid extension of all four extremities, opisthotonos, irritable cry, seizures, and gastric or pulmonary hemorrhage. Those who survive may eventually show evidence of neurologic damage, such as mental retardation, attention deficit disorder, delayed motor development or abnormal motor movement (especially ataxia or athetosis), behavior disorders, perceptual problems, or sensorineural hearing loss (Cashore and Stern, 1982).

Physiologic Jaundice

Physiologic jaundice *(icterus neonatorum)* is a result of the immaturity of hepatic functions in the newborn combined with an increased bilirubin load from increased hemolysis of red blood cells. It is not associated with any pathologic process, as in hemolytic disease of the newborn. Although almost all newborns experience elevated bilirubin levels, only about half demonstrate observable signs of jaundice.

The severity of physiologic jaundice differs markedly among different races. Infants of Oriental descent, including the American Indian and Eskimo, have mean bilirubin levels almost twice as high as those occurring in whites. In addition, newborns from certain geographic locations, particularly areas around Greece, demonstrate an increased incidence of hyperbilirubinemia. Black infants have a lower incidence than white newborns. The exact reasons for these differences are unclear but may include environmental factors, such as maternal ingestion of certain ethnic foods, or a genetic predisposition for decelerated hepatic maturation (Gartner and Lee, 1983; Linn and others, 1985).

Mechanisms involved in physiologic jaundice. The normal newborn produces an average of twice as much bilirubin as does an adult because of higher concentrations of circulating erythrocytes and a shorter life span of red blood cells (only 60 to 80 days in contrast to 120 days in the older child and adult). Polycythemia from delayed cord clamping or maternal-fetal transfusion, or extravasation of blood from birth injuries such as cephalhematoma, all increase the burden of red blood cell destruction. In addition, the liver's ability to conjugate bilirubin is impaired because of a deficiency of the enzyme glucuronyl transferase.

Other factors also contribute to the elevated bilirubin levels. Newborns have a lower plasma-binding capacity for bilirubin because of reduced albumin concentrations as compared to those of older children. The profound changes in hepatic circulation may represent a major hemodynamic shock, resulting in impaired liver function. At birth, closure of the ductus venosus deprives the liver of the richly oxygenated blood supplied by the umbilical vein and makes it dependent on the poorly oxygenated portal venous blood. Marked improvement in bilirubin excretion by the fourth day may represent hepatic adjustment to extrauterine circulatory changes.

Another cause of increased bilirubin load on the liver cells is the reabsorption of unconjugated bilirubin from the intestine. Normally conjugated bilirubin is reduced to urobilin by the intestinal flora and excreted in feces. However, the newborn's bowel is sterile, which prevents the conversion and excretion of bilirubin via this route. Consequently, some unconjugated bilirubin is reabsorbed by the intestine and circulated back to the liver (enterohepatic circulation). The beneficial effect of lowering bilirubin levels by introducing early feedings may be related to this mechanism because feeding stimulates peristalsis and produces more rapid passage of meconium, thus diminishing the amount of reabsorption of unconjugated bilirubin, and introduces bacteria to aid in reduction of bilirubin to urobilinogen. Rectal stimulation from rectal temperature measurement has also been shown to enhance intestinal bilirubin excretion because of more rapid passage of meconium (Cottrell and Anderson, 1984). However, this procedure has the attendant risk of rectal perforation.

Diagnostic evaluation. The first step in assessing jaundice is measuring the indirect and direct bilirubin levels in the blood. Normal values of unconjugated bilirubin are 0.2 to 1.4 mg/dl. Hyperbilirubinemia is defined as a serum bilirubin value greater than 12.9 mg/dl. In physiologic jaundice, bilirubin levels rarely reach this value. When blood samples are taken for bilirubin measurement, the phototherapy unit should be turned off to prevent a false reading from bilirubin destruction in the test tube.

For screening purposes, noninvasive procedures are available for measuring jaundice. The *transcutaneous bili-*

rubinometer measures the intensity of yellow color in the skin and subcutaneous tissue, usually on the forehead. A much less expensive device, the *icterometer*, consists of a strip of transparent Plexiglas that has five yellow transverse stripes of precise and graded hue painted on it. By pressing the plastic strip against the infant's skin, usually the nose, one compares skin color with the yellow stripes and assigns a jaundice score. These devices work well on dark- and light-skinned infants and correlate well with serum determinations of bilirubin level (Schumacher, Thornbery, and Gutcher, 1985; Smith and others, 1985). However, phototherapy reduces the accuracy of the instrument; therefore its value is limited to the initial assessment.

In full-term infants, jaundice first appears *after* 24 hours. (In premature infants, jaundice is initially evident by 48 hours.) Bilirubin levels peak by the second to third day (mean bilirubin level, 6 mg/dl), rapidly decline by the fifth day, and slowly reach normal levels by the tenth day. Bilirubin levels reach peak concentrations (10 to 12 mg/dl) by the fifth day and gradually return to normal by the end of the first month. Except for the icteric appearance, these infants are well. Postmature infants have little or no physiologic jaundice.

Skin color is routinely assessed for evidence of jaundice. However, bilirubin levels must exceed 5 mg/dl before jaundice is reflected in the sclera, nails, or skin. Once jaundice is observed, blood levels of bilirubin must be determined and monitored as necessary to establish the pattern of increase.

A careful history from the parents may reveal significant familial patterns of hyperbilirubinemia, especially those seen in various ethnic groups or during breast-feeding. Routinely, the maternal blood group and Rh type should be determined and compared to the infant's blood group and Rh type immediately after birth, and a direct Coomb test should be performed on cord blood to rule out hemolytic causes.

Jaundice in Breast-Fed Infants

Breast-feeding is associated with an increased incidence of jaundice. Early-onset breast-feeding jaundice (also referred to as jaundice "associated with breast-feeding") begins at 3 to 4 days of age and occurs in approximately 25% of breast-fed newborns. The late-onset type (also called "true breast-milk jaundice") begins at age 4 to 5 days and occurs in 2% to 30% of breast-fed infants (Maisels, 1985; Lascari, 1986). Despite rising levels of bilirubin that peak during the third week, then gradually diminish but may persist for 3 to 12 weeks, these infants are well.

The reason for the jaundice is unknown. The late-onset type may be caused by the presence of a factor in the breast milk of some women that reduces the bilirubin conjugation process by inhibiting the action of glucuronyl transferase in the infant liver. The early-onset jaundice may be related to the relatively fewer calories consumed by breast-fed vs bottle-fed infants before the milk supply is established, since fasting is associated with decreased hepatic clearance of bilirubin (Osborn, Reill, and Bolus, 1984).

Recommendations for prevention and management of breast-feeding jaundice, especially the early-onset type, include (Lascari, l986):

1. Encourage frequent breast-feeding, preferably every 2 hours, and avoid supplementation.
2. Monitor rising bilirubin levels on an outpatient basis.
3. Temporarily discontinue breast-feeding for 48 hours and use formula when bilirubin levels reach 15 to 16 mg/dl.
4. Resume breast-feeding after a decrease in bilirubin level, which confirms diagnosis.
5. When breast-feeding is temporarily discontinued, encourage use of breast pump to maintain lactation.

Nursing considerations. One of the most important nursing interventions is recognition of breast-feeding jaundice. Lack of familiarity among health professionals has caused many newborns prolonged hospitalization, termination of breast-feeding, and unnecessary phototherapy. Supportive care of the new mother can encourage successful and frequent breast-feeding. Parents also need reassurance of the benign nature of the jaundice and encouragement to resume breast-feeding if temporary cessation is prescribed.

Hemolytic Disease of the Newborn

Hyperbilirubinemia in the first 24 hours of life is most often the result of an abnormally rapid rate of red cell destruction. Rh incompatibility formerly was the major cause of hemolysis, but with the introduction of Rh-immune globulin (RhoGAM), the incidence of this disease has increased dramatically (see discussion below). The more common cause currently is ABO incompatibility.

The membranes of human blood cells contain a variety of antigens, also known as agglutinogens, which are substances capable of producing an immune response if recognized by the body as a foreign substance. It is the reciprocal relationship between the antigens in the red blood cells and the antibodies in the plasma that causes agglutination (clumping reaction) to take place. In other words, antibodies in the plasma of one blood group (except the AB group, which contains no antibodies) will produce agglutination when mixed with antigens of a different blood group. In the ABO blood group system, the antibodies occur naturally. In the Rh system, the person must be exposed to the Rh antigen before significant antibody formation takes place to cause a sensitivity response.

Rh incompatibility (isoimmunization). The Rh blood group, so named because of the experiments conducted on the rhesus monkey, consists of several antigens. The D antigen is the strongest and most common Rh antigen and the one implicated in Rh incompatibility. The D (dominant) and d (recessive; d represents the absence of D, not a separate antigen) alleles can genetically produce three genotypes—DD, Dd, and dd. The DD and Dd genotypes are Rh positive, which means that they contain D antigens; the dd genotype is Rh negative and therefore contains no antigens. In the white race 85% of the population are Rh positive and 15% are Rh negative. Only 5% to 7% of blacks

and less than 1% of Native Americans or other persons of the Mongoloid race are Rh negative.

Incompatibility results when the fetus's blood group is Rh positive and the mother's is Rh negative. Although the maternal and fetal circulations are distinctly separate, sometimes fetal red blood cells, with antigens foreign to the mother, gain access to the maternal circulation. The mother's natural defense mechanism responds by producing anti-Rh antibodies.

Ordinarily this process of isoimmunization does not affect the fetus during the first pregnancy because the initial sensitization to D antigens rarely occurs before the onset of labor. However, as larger amounts of fetal blood are transferred to the maternal circulation during placental separation, maternal antibody production is stimulated. Therefore during a second pregnancy maternal antibodies to the fetus's Rh-positive blood are present and, as they enter the circulation, cause destruction of fetal erythrocytes (Fig. 9-5). Since the disease begins in utero, the fetus attempts to compensate for the progressive hemolysis by accelerating the rate of erythropoiesis. As a result, immature red blood cells (erythroblasts) appear in the fetal circulation; hence the term *erythroblastosis fetalis.*

There is wide variability in the development of maternal sensitization to Rh-positive antigens. Sensitization may occur during the first pregnancy if the woman had previously received an Rh-positive blood transfusion, or it may result from small fetomaternal hemorrhages. No sensitization may occur in situations where a strong placental barrier prevents transfer of fetal blood into the maternal circulation. In about 10% to 15% of sensitized mothers there is no hemolytic reaction in the newborn.

The severest form of erythroblastosis fetalis results in *hydrops fetalis.* The progressive hemolysis causes fetal hypoxia, cardiac failure, generalized edema (anasarca), and effusions in the pericardial, pleural, and peritoneal spaces. The fetus may be delivered stillborn or in severe respiratory distress. Even with immediate exchange transfusions, few hydropic infants survive.

Diagnostic evaluation. Diagnosis of Rh incompatibility before delivery is confirmed through amniocentesis and analysis of bilirubin levels in amniotic fluid. Increasing bilirubin levels represent progressive fetal hemolysis and may indicate the need for an intrauterine transfusion or immediate termination of the pregnancy.

Erythroblastosis fetalis can also be assessed by evaluating rising anti-D antibody titers in the maternal circulation (indirect Coombs test). The disease can be confirmed postnatally by detecting antibodies attached to the circulating erythrocytes of affected infants (direct Coombs test).

Prevention. The administration of Rho-immune globulin (RhoGAM*) to all unsensitized Rh-negative mothers after delivery or abortion of an Rh-positive infant or fetus prevents the development of maternal sensitization to the Rh factor. When RhoGAM is given to unsensitized mothers

---

*Orthodiagnostics, Raritan, NJ.

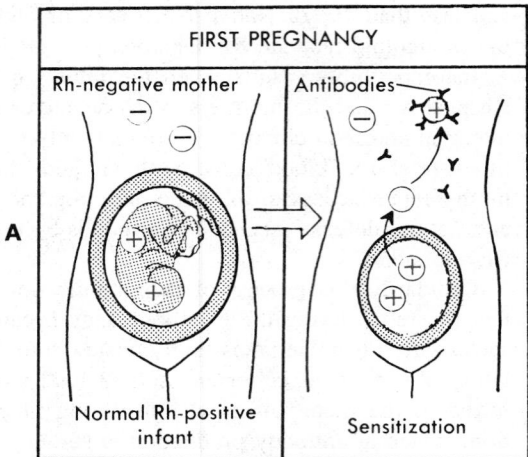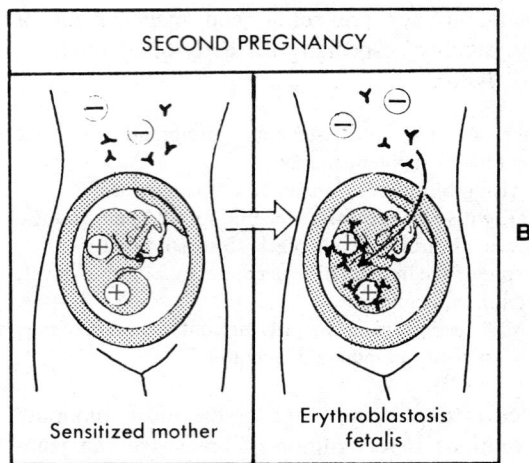

Fig. 9-5. Development of maternal sensitization to Rh antigens. **A,** Fetal Rh-positive erythrocytes enter maternal system. Maternal anti-Rh antibodies are formed. **B,** Anti-Rh antibodies cross placental barrier and attack fetal erythrocytes.

within 72 hours (but possibly as long as 3 to 4 weeks) after delivery or abortion, injected anti-Rh antibodies destroy the fetal erythrocytes passing into the maternal circulation before they are able to exert their immunogenic effect. To be effective, RhoGAM must be administered after the first delivery and repeated after subsequent ones. There is some evidence that prophylactic use of RhoGAM at 28 weeks of gestation further reduces the incidence of isoimmunization in those women sensitized during the first pregnancy (Hammer, Bower, and Messina, 1984; Bowman, 1985). Although prenatal use of Rh-immune globulin is common practice in countries such as Canada, it is controversial in the United States. Major arguments against the practice are the relative scarcity of the product and the increased cost. RhoGAM is not effective against existing Rh-positive antibodies in the maternal circulation.

ABO incompatibility. Hemolytic disease can also occur when the major blood group antigens of the fetus are different from those of the mother. The major blood groups are A, B, AB, and O. The incidence of these blood groups varies according to race and geographic location. In the North American white population, 46% have O blood group, 42% have A blood group, 9% have B blood group, and 3% have AB blood group.

The presence or absence of antibodies and antigens determines whether agglutination will occur (Table 9-2). Antibodies in the plasma of one blood group (except the AB group, which contains no antibodies) will produce an agglutination or clumping reaction when mixed with antigens of a different blood group. For example, if an individual with type-A blood receives type-B blood, the donor's antibodies (anti-A) are diluted in the recipient's circulation and cause little harm. However, the naturally occurring anti-B antibodies in the recipient's blood cause agglutination of the donor's red blood cells. The agglutinated donor cells become trapped in the recipient's peripheral blood vessels. The cells then hemolyze, releasing large amounts of biliru-

bin into the circulation. Clinical manifestations of transfusion reaction represent the pathophysiology of blocked blood vessels or released toxins into the vascular system. Renal shutdown is the most significant response and can cause death from kidney failure.

The most common blood group incompatibility in the neonate is between a mother with O blood group and an infant with A or B blood group. (Other possible ABO incompatibilities are listed in Table 9-3.) The naturally occurring anti-A or anti-B antibodies already present in the maternal circulation cross the placenta and attack the fetal red blood cells, causing hemolysis. Usually the hemolytic reaction is less severe than in Rh incompatibility, and severe anemia is rare. Although the traditional thinking has been that the number of pregnancies is insignificant in the severity of ABO incompatibility, newer evidence suggests that the risk of hyperbilirubinemia is greater for subsequent offspring, especially if the first newborn had hyperbilirubinemia (Plotz, 1985).

Laboratory evaluation and treatment of ABO reactions are also similar to those for Rh incompatibility.

Clinical manifestations. The clinical manifestations of blood incompatibility result from the hemolysis of large numbers of erythrocytes (anemia) and the liver's inability to conjugate and excrete the excess bilirubin (hyperbilirubinemia and jaundice). Most erythroblastotic newborns are not jaundiced at birth. However, shortly after birth (during the initial 24 hours), jaundice is evident and unconjugated bilirubin levels rise rapidly. Hepatosplenomegaly may be evident. If the fetus is severely affected, signs of anemia—notably, marked pallor—are seen in the newborn.

Therapeutic Management

The aims of therapy for hyperbilirubinemia are to prevent kernicterus and, in any blood group incompatibility, to reverse the hemolytic process. The main forms of treatment involve phototherapy, exchange transfusion, and pharmacologic management.

Table 9-2 ABO relationships of antigens/antibodies and donor-recipient compatibility

BLOOD GROUP (PHENOTYPE)	GENOTYPE	RED CELL ANTIGENS	PLASMA ANTIBODIES	RED CELL COMPATIBILITY	
				AS DONOR TO TYPE	AS RECIPIENT FROM TYPE
A	AA,AO	A	B	AB,A	O,A
B	BB,BO	B	A	AB,B	O,B
AB	AB	A and B	None	AB	O,A,B,AB
O	OO	None	A and B	AB,A,B,O	O

Table 9-3 Potential maternal-fetal ABO incompatibilities

MATERNAL BLOOD GROUP	INCOMPATIBLE FETAL BLOOD GROUP
O	A or B
B	A or AB
A	B or AB

Phototherapy. Phototherapy involves the application of intense fluorescent light on the infant's exposed skin. Light in the blue range enhances bilirubin excretion by the process of photoisomerization, which produces a structural change in the bilirubin to form a more soluble form, lumirubin (McDonagh and Lightner, 1985). Because blue light alters the appearance of the infant and is distressing to staff, the normal light of full-spectrum fluorescent bulbs is preferred. However, there is evidence that light in the green spectrum enhances the formation of lumirubin and is more effective in treating neonatal jaundice (Vechi and others, 1986). It is possible that bililights will use green lights in the near future. Although the value of phototherapy in effectively reducing or preventing rising bilirubin levels is well documented, its long-term effects are unclear.

No universally accepted protocols exist for recommended uses of phototherapy. However, studies from the National Institute of Child Health and Human Development (NICHHD) demonstrated that phototherapy was most effective in the following situations (Brown and others, 1985):

1. Low-birth-weight infants (<2,000 g) who received phototherapy at 24 ± 12 hours of life for 96 hours, regardless of bilirubin concentration. In addition, the rate of exchange transfusion was significantly lower in these infants than in control infants.
2. Infants of birth weight from 2,000 to 2,499 g who received phototherapy after serum bilirubin concentration had risen above 10 mg/dl and infants of birth weight >2,500 g who received phototherapy after serum bilirubin concentration had risen above 13 mg/dl, provided there was no hemolytic disorder. If hemolysis was present, phototherapy was not effective in controlling the hyperbilirubinemia.

Other findings showed that black infants responded as well to phototherapy as white infants and that phototherapy was most effective in the first 24 to 48 hours of its application.

The effectiveness of phototherapy is determined by a decrease in bilirubin levels, usually a fall of 3 to 4 mg/dl after 8 to 12 hours of therapy. Concurrently, the infant's total physical status is assessed because the suppression of jaundice may mask signs of sepsis, hemolytic disease, or hepatitis. Although the bilirubin levels may be controlled in mild erythroblastosis fetalis, the hemolysis may continue, causing severe anemia.

A recent trend in phototherapy is its use in the home to treat some types of neonatal hyperbilirubinemia. The controversy surrounding home phototherapy, especially its benefits and risks, is discussed in Questions and controversies.

Questions and Controversies

What are the benefits and risks of home phototherapy?

Because jaundice is such a common occurrence among newborns, home phototherapy has been recommended as an alternative means of providing care. Studies of its benefits cite cost savings from what otherwise would be prolonged hospitalizations and prevention of parent-infant separation (Eggert and others, 1985; Slater and Brewer, 1984). Depending on the geographic location, savings are about 75% of the cost of hospitalization. Both studies demonstrated that the treatment was safe and effective.

However, home phototherapy is not universally endorsed. The American Academy of Pediatrics (1985) considers the available data on safety and efficacy inadequate. As guidelines for eligibility for home phototherapy, the Academy suggests considering as candidates only term infants who (1) are older than 48 hours; (2) are otherwise healthy as evidenced by the history, physical examination, and various blood and urine tests; and (3) have a serum bilirubin concentration greater than 14 mg/dl but less than 18 mg/dl with no elevation in conjugated bilirubin levels. In addition, the caretakers must be willing to assume the responsibilities and be capable of implementing the care. Risks, such as the possibility that a displaced eye patch may occlude the infant's airway, must be explained. Once serum bilirubin levels fall below 14 mg/dl, therapy should be discontinued with appropriate follow-up.

Nurses will obviously play an important role in establishing the risks and benefits of home phototherapy as they participate in the preparation, teaching, and supervision of these families.

Exchange transfusion. Exchange transfusion, in which the infant's blood is removed in small amounts and replaced with compatible blood (such as Rh-negative blood), is a standard mode of therapy for treatment of severe hyperbilirubinemia and is the treatment of choice for hyperbilirubinemia caused by Rh incompatibility. Exchange transfusion removes the sensitized erythrocytes, lowers the serum bilirubin level to prevent kernicterus, corrects the anemia, and prevents cardiac failure.

The principal indication for exchange transfusion is an indirect serum bilirubin level of 20 mg/dl in full-term infants, 15 mg/dl in high-risk infants weighing 1500 g, and approximately 10 mg/dl for infants weighing 1000 g or less (Cashore and Stern, 1982). These guidelines may vary according to institutional practice and the newborn's gestational age and condition. Therapy may begin earlier when asphyxia, acidosis, hypothermia, hypoalbuminemia, sepsis, hemolysis, or hypoglycemia are present. An infant born with hydrops fetalis or signs of cardiac failure is a candidate for immediate exchange transfusion.

In exchange transfusion, fresh whole blood is typed and cross-matched to the mother's serum. The amount of donor blood used is usually double the blood volume of the infant, which is about 85 mg/kg body weight but is limited to no more than 500 ml. The two-volume exchange transfusion replaces approximately 85% of the neonate's blood.

An exchange transfusion is a sterile surgical procedure and requires 1 to 2 hours to complete. The umbilicus is cut, and a catheter is inserted into the umbilical vein and threaded into the inferior vena cava. Depending on the infant's weight, 5 to 20 ml of blood is withdrawn within 15 to 20 seconds, and the same volume of donor blood is infused over 60 to 90 seconds.

Pharmacologic management. Pharmacologic treatment of hyperbilirubinemia has focused mainly on the use of barbiturates, such as phenobarbital, which stimulate protein synthesis (increasing available albumin for binding with unconjugated bilirubin) and promote hepatic glucuronyl transferase synthesis (increasing conjugation of bilirubin and hepatic clearance of the pigment in bile). The best results are observed when the drug is given to the mother 1 to 2 weeks before delivery. This therapy has not gained widespread acceptance because when given to an infant with hyperbilirubinemia, treatment is not rapid enough to be effective.

Nursing Considerations

The primary nursing consideration is recognition of jaundice and differentiation of the physiologic type from pathologic causes. The routine physical assessment includes observing for evidence of jaundice at regular intervals. Jaundice is most reliably assessed by observing the color of the sclera, nails, and skin, including palms, soles, and mucous membranes. Applying direct pressure to the skin, especially over bony prominences such as the tip of the nose or the sternum, causes blanching and allows the yellow stain to be more pronounced. For dark-skinned infants, the color of gums is the most reliable indicator. The nurse observes the infant in natural daylight for a true assessment of color. Any neonate who becomes icteric during the first 24 hours of life and has rapidly rising bilirubin levels is referred to the physician for immediate evaluation.

Supportive care. Prevention of physiologic and breast-feeding jaundice may be possible with early introduction of feedings and frequent nursing. Every effort is made to provide an optimum thermal environment to reduce metabolic needs. In instances in which blood incompatibility is suspected, the cord is kept moist with a sterile saline-soaked dressing to preserve the umbilical vein for possible exchange transfusion.

Phototherapy. Several precautions are instituted to protect the infant during phototherapy. The infant's eyes are shielded by an opaque mask to prevent exposure to the light (Fig. 9-6). The eye shield should be properly sized and correctly positioned to prevent any occlusion of the nares. The infant's eyelids are closed before the mask is applied, since the corneas may become excoriated if they come in contact with the dressing. On each nursing shift the eyes are checked for evidence of discharge, excessive pressure on the lids, or corneal irritation. If the shield allows light to enter, the area of jaundice around the eyes will begin disappearing, indicating the need for better eye protection.

The infant is placed nude under the fluorescent light and turned frequently, since phototherapy must come in contact with the skin surfaces to be effective. Areas that are protected from the light retain their jaundiced appearance and indicate the need for repositioning.

The phototherapy unit is often combined with a radiant heat warmer or servocontrolled incubator to provide an op-

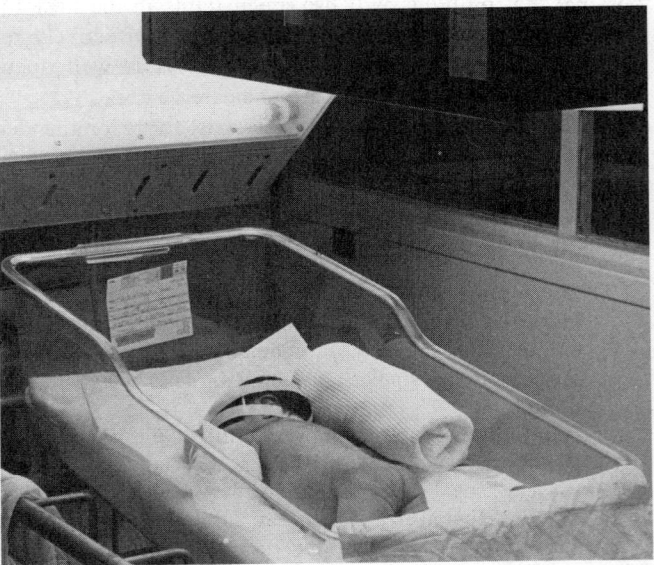

Fig. 9-6. Infant under phototherapy units. Note that the eyes are shielded and the skin is exposed for maximum safety and therapeutic effect.

timally regulated thermal environment. The thermistor should be attached to the infant or covered with opaque tape so that it is not exposed to direct radiation. This may require changing the sensor from the abdomen to the back according to the infant's position. Vital signs are taken at least every 4 hours to ensure that the infant's body temperature is normothermic. Sometimes it is necessary to regulate the temperature in the Isolette to maintain proper body heat.

Infants who are in an open crib must have a protective Plexiglas shield between them and the fluorescent lights to minimize the amount of undesirable ultraviolet light reaching their skin and to protect them from accidental bulb breakage. Their temperature is closely monitored to prevent hyperthermia and, less often, hypothermia.

Accurate charting is another important nursing responsibility and includes (1) times that phototherapy is started and stopped, including intervals when no light was applied, (2) proper shielding of the eyes, (3) type of fluorescent lamp (by manufacturer), (4) number of lamps, (5) distance between surface of lamps and infant, (6) use of phototherapy in combination with an Isolette or open bassinet, (7) photometer measurement of light intensity, and (8) occurrence of side effects.

At present the long-term risks from phototherapy are not known. Although some minor side effects occur, there appears to be no increased mortality in infants treated with phototherapy (Lipsitz, Gartner, and Bryla, 1985). Minor side effects, which the nurse should be alert for, include loose, greenish stools, hyperthermia, increased metabolic rate, increased water loss, electrolyte disturbances, such as hypocalcemia, and priapism. Although the effect of phototherapy on the eyes is uncertain, animal studies indicate that retinal degeneration may occur after several days of continuous exposure.

To prevent or minimize these effects, the temperature is closely monitored to detect early signs of hyperthermia and the skin is observed for evidence of dehydration and drying, which can lead to excoriation and breakdown. Oily lubricants or lotions are not used on the skin in order to prevent increased tanning, or a "frying" effect. Infants receiving phototherapy require up to 25% additional fluid volume to compensate for insensible and intestinal fluid loss. There is some evidence that the use of stockinette caps to cover the head prevents phototherapy-induced hypocalcemia in premature infants 37 gestational weeks or younger (Bergstrom and Hakanson, 1980; Blake, 1983).

Another reaction to phototherapy is the *bronze-baby syndrome,* in which the serum, urine, and skin become blackish-brown in color several hours after the infant is placed under the light. The cause of this reaction is not known; it may represent a benign cosmetic response, a sign of hepatocellular disease, an inborn error of metabolism, or an unusual toxic effect of phototherapy. Since this syndrome almost always occurs in infants who have elevated conjugated hyperbilirubinemia, it is essential that the direct-reacting bil-

irubin level be determined. If the direct-reacting pigment is increased, phototherapy should not be instituted (Gartner and Lee, 1983).

Exchange transfusions. Besides assisting the physician during the initial stages of this procedure, the nurse keeps accurate records of blood volumes exchanged, including amounts of blood withdrawn and infused, time of each procedure, and cumulative record of the total volume exchanged. Vital signs that are monitored electronically are evaluated frequently and correlated with removal and infusion of blood. If signs of restlessness or cardiac arrhythmias occur, rate of infusion is slowed.

Throughout the procedure the nurse attends to the infant's thermoregulation needs. The procedure is done under a radiant warmer, and the blood is warmed before infusion. Hypothermia increases oxygen and glucose consumption, causing metabolic acidosis. Not only do these consequences hinder the infant's overall physical ability to withstand the long procedure, but they also inhibit the binding capacity of albumin and bilirubin and the hepatic enzymatic reactions, thus increasing the risk of kernicterus. Conversely, hyperthermia damages the donor erythrocytes, elevating the free potassium content and predisposing the infant to cardiac arrest.

Exchange transfusion can cause several complications that are related to the actual procedure, to the blood transfusion. Although it is a relatively safe procedure, reported mortality is from 0.5% to 3% (Keenan and others, 1985). Therefore conscientious care of the newborn is essential, such as attention to asepsis to prevent infection and observation for signs of transfusion reactions (see Table 35-2, p. 1537). After the procedure is completed, the umbilical site is inspected for evidence of bleeding. The catheter may remain in place for use during repeated exchanges.

Family support. Parents need constant reassurance concerning their infant's progress. All the procedures are explained to familiarize them with the benefits and risks.* For example, they need to be reassured that the naked infant who is under the bilirubin light is warm and comfortable. Parents may be concerned about the blindfolds, since "blindness" is a frightening experience. Blindfolds are removed when the parents are visiting to facilitate the attachment process, and the parents can be reassured that the neonate is accustomed to darkness after months of intrauterine existence and benefits a great deal from auditory and tactile stimulation. If bronzing occurs, parents are informed that the discoloration disappears within 2 to 3 months.

Parents frequently feel guilty because they think they have caused the blood incompatibility. Parents should never be made to feel responsible or negligent. They are encouraged to express their thoughts. Actions they took to prevent problems, such as frequent antepartum examinations and blood tests, are to be emphasized and praised.

---

*A short description of "Jaundice in Newborns" is available from Wyeth Laboratories, Philadelphia, PA 19101.

Nursing Care Summary: The Newborn with Hyperbilirubinemia

NURSING GOALS	NURSING INTERVENTIONS	EXPECTED PATIENT/FAMILY OUTCOMES

MP-HMP   **Injury: potential for tissue damage**
Risk factors: breakdown products of red blood cells in greater than normal amounts, immature blood-brain barrier, exposure to phototherapy

NURSING GOALS	NURSING INTERVENTIONS	EXPECTED PATIENT/FAMILY OUTCOMES
Identify infants at risk for hyperbilirubinemia	Observe for evidence of jaundice, anemia, and central nervous system irritability Refer infant with signs of jaundice and rising bilirubin levels during first 24 hours to physician Be aware of conditions (acidosis, hypoxia, hypothermia, and so on) that increase the risk of kernicterus at lower bilirubin levels Encourage early and frequent breast-feeding	*Signs of hyperbilirubinemia are detected early and appropriate interventions implemented
Protect infant during phototherapy	Shield infant's eyes 　　Make certain that lids are closed before applying shield 　　Check eyes each shift for drainage or irritation Place infant nude under light Change position frequently Monitor body temperature 　　Check axillary temperature with reading on servocontrolled unit Ensure that protective Plexiglas shield separates infant from lights Chart duration of therapy, type of lights, distance of lights to infant, use of open or closed bassinet, and shielding of infant's eyes Avoid the use of oily applications on the skin Observe for hyperthermia, signs of dehydration, loose stools Monitor hydration and ensure an adequate fluid intake	Infant's eyes show no evidence of irritation Infant exhibits no signs of adverse effects of phototherapy Infant's position is changed q 2 hrs Infant's temperature remains below 38° C (100.4° F) Infant exhibits no signs of dehydration
Prevent adverse effects from exchange transfusion	Give infant nothing by mouth prior to procedure (usually for 3-4 hours) Check donor blood with physician for correct blood group and Rh type Assist physician during procedure; ensure asepsis Keep accurate records of amounts of blood infused and withdrawn Monitor vital signs Maintain optimum body temperature of infant during procedure Observe for signs of exchange transfusion reactions Have resuscitative equipment (supplemental oxygen, airway, AMBU bag, endotracheal tube, and laryngoscope) at bedside Check umbilical site for bleeding or infection Monitor vital signs following transfusion	Infant exhibits no signs of adverse effects from transfusion Vital signs remain within normal limits (see inside front cover for normal variations) There is no evidence of infection or bleeding at infusion site
Prevent complications from hyperbilirubinemia	Observe for signs of central nervous system depression (lethargy, diminished or absent reflexes, hypotonia, poor sucking reflex) or excitation (irritability, tremors, convulsions, high-pitched cry, opisthotonos)	*Signs of complications are detected early and appropriate intervention initiated

*Nursing outcome.

Nursing Care Summary: The Newborn with Hyperbilirubinemia—cont'd

NURSING GOALS	NURSING INTERVENTIONS	EXPECTED PATIENT/FAMILY OUTCOMES
RRP Family process, alteration in **Etiology: situational crisis (child with an adverse physiologic response)**		
Provide emotional support to family	Explain reason for jaundice Discontinue phototherapy during family visiting; remove infant's eye shields Emphasize benign nature of physiologic jaundice Assure family that skin will regain normal pigmentation Advise breast-feeding mothers of possibility of prolonged jaundice Encourage continued breast-feeding if temporary cessation is prescribed Explain to family the therapies for hyperbilirubinemia Educate regarding therapies required in home phototherapy Reassure parents during various procedures	Family demonstrates an understanding of the disease process, therapies, and prognosis
	Allow family to express any feelings regarding their "causing" a blood incompatibility Reinforce family's previous attempts to provide optimum care for their infant, such as frequent antepartal checkups	Family verbalizes feelings and concerns
Plan for follow-up, especially if bilirubin levels approached 20 mg/100 ml in full-term neonate	Encourage family to report the perinatal history during subsequent infant assessments, especially when the child is seen by unfamiliar health personnel Plan for early developmental and hearing assessment See also Family of the hospitalized child, p. 1081	Family complies with follow-up care

Nursing Interventions Related to Medical Management

Monitor progress of therapy
   Collect specimens for serum bilirubin levels
Prevent hyperbilirubinemia and kernicterus
   Determine blood group and Rh type of pregnant women
   Follow all Rh-negative pregnant women with possibility of Rh-positive fetus for rising bilirubin levels (amniocentesis, indirect Coombs test)
   Administer Rho(D) immune globulin (RhoGAM) to Rh-negative women at delivery or time of abortion as prescribed

Discharge planning and home care. Discharge planning and home care depend on the type of jaundice and the treatment instituted. Most newborns are discharged after the bilirubin levels are near normal and no special care is needed. In jaundice associated with breast-feeding, follow-up blood studies are usually required to assess the progress of the jaundice. If temporary cessation of breast-feeding is prescribed, every effort is made to teach the mother breast pumping to facilitate lactation. Most mothers, if supported during this brief time, resume breast-feeding.

If home phototherapy is instituted, the nurse is usually responsible for teaching the family and assessing their ability to implement the treatment safely. General guidelines for home care preparation and education are discussed on p. 1094. Written instructions and supervision of care, especially application of eye shields, are essential. The minor side effects of phototherapy are reviewed, and parents may need instruction in taking axillary temperature. One significant factor for the postpartal couple is the small amount of time before discharge for adequate teaching. These families require continued surveillance in the home, usually through referral to home care nursing agencies. Regardless of how benign the disorder or the therapy, these parents need support and understanding. Siblings also benefit from an explanation of the therapy to allay fears or misconceptions.

Unless kernicterus develops, most infants recover satis-

factorily after hemolytic disease. If kernicterus has occurred, the family is apprised of the need for periodic assessments to detect sensorineural hearing loss, cerebral
damage, or developmental lag in the child.

HYPOGLYCEMIA

Hypoglycemia is said to be present when the infant's blood
glucose concentration is significantly lower than that of the
majority of infants of the same age and weight. In the full-
term newborn, hypoglycemia is defined as plasma glucose
concentrations of less than 35 mg/100 ml in the first 72
hours and 45 mg/100 ml thereafter; in low-birth-weight infants it is less than 25 mg/100 ml (Pildes and Lilien, 1983).

After birth the infant must supply his own nutrients to
meet his energy requirements for maintaining body temperature, respiration, muscular activity, and regulation of blood
glucose. At birth he relies on the glycogen stores deposited
in the liver, heart, and skeletal muscles during the last
trimester of pregnancy, and the full-term infant, under normal circumstances, usually has sufficient sources for the
first 2 or 3 days. However, any condition that causes increased energy requirements can rapidly deplete these
stores. Four categories of neonatal hypoglycemia have been
described:

early transitional adaptive hypoglycemia These are
large infants or infants of normal size for their gestational
age, including infants of mothers with diabetes mellitus or
gestational diabetes and erythroblastotic infants. These infants appear to be suffering from hyperinsulinism and are
otherwise asymptomatic. The hypoglycemia responds readily to intravenous glucose infusions.

classical transient neonatal hypoglycemia This group
consists of infants who have suffered intrauterine malnutrition that has reduced hepatic glycogen stores and body fat.
In this category are infants who are small for their gestational age, small twins, infants of preeclamptic mothers, and
infants with abnormalities of the placenta. Males appear to
be affected more frequently than females. Cardiomegaly and
polycythemia may be present in addition to the hypoglycemia. This type of hypoglycemia may be more severe than
other categories and is likely to recur.

secondary hypoglycemia This type of hypoglycemia occurs
as a response to a variety of perinatal stresses that have increased the infant's metabolic needs relative to the glycogen
stores available. Stresses include asphyxia, respiratory distress syndrome, pathologic conditions of the central nervous
system, sepsis, hemorrhage, drug withdrawal, and iatrogenic events such as interruption of glucose infusions. This
type of hypoglycemia responds to glucose administration
and rarely recurs.

recurrent, severe hypoglycemia This category consists of
infants who have hypoglycemia secondary to an enzymatic
or a metabolic-endocrine defect such as galactosemia, hypothyroidism, hypopituitarism, and any number of the inborn errors of metabolism. Diagnosis of the disorder determines the therapy.

Clinical Manifestations

The signs of hypoglycemia are usually vague and often indistinguishable from those observed in other conditions,
such as hypocalcemia, septicemia, central nervous system
disorders, or cardiorespiratory problems. Because the brain
depends on glucose for energy, cerebral signs such as jitteriness, tremors, twitching, weak or high-pitched cry, lethargy, limpness, apathy, convulsions, and coma are prominent. Other clinical manifestations are cyanosis, apnea,
rapid and irregular respirations, sweating, eye rolling, and
refusal to feed. Frequently the symptoms are transient but
recurrent.

Diagnostic Evaluation

Diagnosis must be confirmed by direct analysis of blood
glucose concentration. Two specimens of blood should be
analyzed because of the many factors that can affect correct
readings. Proper handling of the specimen is essential, since
storage at room temperature increases glycolysis. Accurate
readings can be facilitated by storing the blood sample in
ice or removing the red blood cells by centrifugation.

Blood sugar level may also be determined with a drop of
blood placed on a reagent strip such as Dextrostix or Chem-
strip-BG and read either manually or with a glucose reflec-
tance meter. Although simple procedures, the tests are very
sensitive and must be performed correctly to prevent false
readings. For example, the blood must remain on the Dextrostix for exactly 1 minute and then be compared to the
color chart. Inaccurate timing will produce varying stages of
the reaction. Color changes that indicate a blood glucose
level of less than 45 mg/100 ml should be confirmed by a
laboratory analysis of whole blood.

Therapeutic Management

Intravenous infusion of glucose is the therapy for hypoglycemia. Infants who are at increased risk for developing hypoglycemia should have their blood glucose measured
within 1 hour after birth. The procedure should be repeated
every 1 to 2 hours for the first 6 to 8 hours, then every 4 to
6 hours for 2 days.

Oral glucose feedings are ineffective as a treatment for
hypoglycemia, and in high concentrations can cause gastric
irritation and asmotic diarrhea. Hypoglycemia can be prevented in most instances by the initiation of early feeding in
normoglycemic newborns. Breast-fed infants should be put
to breast as soon as possible after delivery. If feedings are
poorly tolerated, intravenous glucose may be administered
to these infants if they develop hypoglycemia.

Nursing Considerations

Much of the nursing responsibility for the hypoglycemic infant involves identification of the problem through careful
observation of physical status. Another concern is to reduce
environmental factors that predispose the infant to the development of a decreased blood glucose level, such as cold

stress and respiratory difficulty. Use of proper feeding techniques with the breast-fed or bottle-fed infant promotes adequate ingestion of nutrients, particularly carbohydrates.

Preventing, anticipating, and recognizing potential dangers of concentrated dextrose infusion are also major nursing objectives. Too rapid infusion of the hypertonic solution can cause circulatory overload, hyperglycemia, and intracellular dehydration. Maintaining the ordered flow rate decreases the chance of such hazards. If the intravenous transfusion has been temporarily discontinued, nurses should not try to "catch up" by increasing the rate to make up for the fluid lost during the interruption.

The infusion is administered through a large peripheral vein to increase hemodilution of the concentrated solution and to prevent irritation of the vessel walls. Extravasation of the fluid into the surrounding area can cause sloughing of the tissues. Termination of the glucose solution must be gradual in order to prevent hypoglycemia caused by hyperinsulinism.

Because hypoglycemia is frequently a symptom of some other underlying pathophysiologic process, parents are usually very concerned about their infant's progress, particularly since these infants do not feed well or behave responsively. Nurses need to be aware of parents' thoughts, to allow them to express their feelings, and to keep parents aware of the infant's progress.

HYPOCALCEMIA

Hypocalcemia, like many conditions in the neonate, is difficult to differentiate from other disorders, and the etiology is ill defined. There are two times during the neonatal period when the incidence is highest. *Early-onset hypocalcemia,* which appears within the first 48 hours, is the more common form and typically affects the premature or small-for-date infant who has experienced perinatal hypoxia. Symptoms include jitteriness, apnea, cyanotic episodes, edema, a high-pitched cry, and abdominal distention.

Late-onset hypocalcemia, which is not apparent until after the first 3 to 4 days of life, is commonly referred to as cow's milk–induced hypocalcemia or *neonatal tetany.* It is observed in well-nourished infants who are fed unmodified cow's milk. Cow's milk with a high phosphorus-to-calcium ratio depresses parathyroid activity, resulting in diminished serum calcium levels. The manifestations of neonatal tetany reflect neuromuscular irritation—twitching, tremors, and focal or generalized convulsive seizures that can be triggered by even minor stimuli and that vary in duration from a few seconds to 10 minutes. Neonatal tetany is rarely seen because of the prevalent use of commercial formula or human milk as the newborn's primary nutrition.

Diagnostic Evaluation

Diagnosis of hypocalcemia is confirmed with serum electrolyte determinations. Normal serum calcium values are between 8 and 10 mg/dl (4 to 5 mEq/L). Hypocalcemia is indicated at levels below 8 mg/dl in full-term neonates and levels under 7 mg/dl in premature infants during the first 3 days of life.

Therapeutic Management

In most instances early-onset hypocalcemia is temporary and reverses itself in 1 to 3 days. Restoration of a normal calcium level is facilitated by early feedings, physiologic correction of the hypoparathyroidism, and sometimes administration of calcium supplements. Because of the tendency for the condition to correct itself, even in sick infants, intravenous calcium supplementation should be reserved for infants with persistent hypocalcemia, tetany, or a seizure disorder.

Treatment of hypocalcemia involves intravenous administration of 10% calcium gluconate. Administration must be slow, usually over a period of 10 minutes, to prevent nausea, vomiting, bradycardia, and circulatory collapse. It is advisable to monitor the heart rate and blood pressure electronically. Care must be taken to ascertain that the needle is positioned within the vein because extravasation into surrounding tissue causes local calcification and sloughing. Intramuscular administration of calcium gluconate is contraindicated because it precipitates in the tissue, causing necrosis. If the infant can tolerate oral fluids, oral doses of calcium are given.

Nursing Considerations

Nursing care of the infant with hypocalcemia is directed toward identifying the cause of the manifestations observed and administration of calcium. The infant is monitored continuously during intravenous infusions. Calcium gluconate can cause tissue necrosis and scar formation; therefore it is recommended that the scalp veins be avoided. Calcium gluconate is also incompatible with a number of drugs, most notably sodium bicarbonate ($NaHCO_3$), which is often given for acidosis. To prevent tissue necrosis, the infusion site should be changed frequently (ideally every 12 hours), the needle should be firmly secured by tape to the skin, and during removal gentle pressure should be applied at the puncture site for at least 1 minute.

The nurse also observes for signs of acute hypercalcemia (nausea, vomiting, bradycardia). If such symptoms occur, the injection or infusion is discontinued and the physician is notified. Since convulsions are common, seizure precautions are instituted. Minor stimuli, such as picking the infant up for a feeding or a sudden jarring of the crib, can provoke tremors or seizures. During the acute phase the environment is manipulated to allow for maximum rest and minimum activity around the infant to prevent tiring him.

The restlessness, irritability, and convulsive activity of the infant are of much concern to the parents. The nurse supports them during the hospitalization and emphasizes that the condition will subside rapidly with no subsequent ill effects. During the acute phase parents are advised to disturb the infant as little as possible. However, as soon as the calcium level rises, they are encouraged to hold and feed the infant in order to reestablish parent-child attachment.

If the infant is discharged on formula feedings supplemented with calcium salts, the parents are taught the correct procedure for diluting the mineral in the formula and are advised to use only commercially prepared or modified evaporated milk formulas. The parents should be told that oral calcium may result in more frequent bowel movements so they will not associate this change with diarrhea or another gastrointestinal disorder.

HEMORRHAGIC DISEASE OF THE NEWBORN

Hemorrhagic disease of the newborn is a bleeding disorder that may appear within 1 to 5 days of life as a result of a deficiency of vitamin K. Vitamin K stores are virtually absent in the newborn. Consequently, vitamin K–dependent coagulation factors (II, VII, IX, X) are significantly reduced.

In addition, the newborn's sterile intestinal tract is unable to synthesize the vitamin until feedings have begun. Breast-fed infants are particularly at risk because human milk is a poor source of vitamin K. Hemorrhagic manifestations rarely occur in infants fed cow's milk on the first day of life because it is an adequate source of the vitamin.

Signs and symptoms of hemorrhagic disease typically occur on the second or third day and include (1) oozing from the umbilicus or circumcision site, (2) bloody or black stools, (3) hematuria, (4) ecchymosis on skin and scalp, and (5) epistaxis.

Diagnosis can be confirmed in the presence of prolonged prothrombin time (PT) and partial thromboplastin time (PTT) but normal platelet count and fibrinogen levels.

Therapeutic Management

The goal is prevention of hemorrhagic disease of the newborn with prophylactic administration of vitamin K. In the United States, intramuscular administration of vitamin K (Aquamephyton, Mephyton) in a dose of 0.5 to 1 mg once during the first 24 hours of life is a standard practice. However, the use of prophylactic vitamin K is not routine treatment in all countries.

In newborns with the disease, treatment is the same as the preventive measures, except that the vitamin may be given intravenously to prevent a hematoma at an intramuscular site. Bleeding usually ceases within 2 to 4 hours of vitamin K administration.

Nursing Considerations

Nursing care is primarily directed toward prevention and involves careful administration of the vitamin into the vastus lateralis muscle because of the absence of other well-developed muscle masses. In instances when this procedure is not routinely done (e.g., home births or emergency deliveries),

the nurse observes for signs of the disorder and notifies the physician for appropriate diagnosis and treatment.

Inborn Errors of Metabolism

Inborn errors of metabolism is a term applied to a large number of inherited diseases caused by the absence or deficiency of a substance essential to cellular metabolism, usually an enzyme, and most are characterized by abnormal protein, carbohydrate, or fat metabolism.

All biochemical processes are under genetic control, and each consists of a complex sequence of reactions. Fig. 9-7, *A*, schematically represents a portion of a normal metabolic pathway. A substrate (the substance on which an enzyme acts) is converted to a product through the action of a specific enzyme. A metabolic pathway consists of many such reactions, or steps, each depending on the previous reaction and each catalyzed by a specific enzyme. Fig. 9-7, *B*, illustrates how a change in a gene that interferes with the synthesis of an essential enzyme interrupts this process. A block in the normal pathway can produce an accumulation of the substances preceding the block, such as galactose in galactosemia or phenylalanine in phenylketonuria, or might create a deficiency in the product, such as thyroxine in familial hypothyroidism. Sometimes alternate pathways are used and there is an increase in the products of these processes, such as the production of phenylketones in phenylketonuria. These effects of defective gene action are observable in the individual as diseases.

Most of the diseases are rare, and the mode of inheritance is almost always autosomal recessive. This is best understood by considering the "double-dose effect" as it relates to the concept that one gene is responsible for one enzyme. If a specific gene controls the formation of an essential enzyme and each individual has two such genes (the normal homozygote), then the enzyme is produced in normal amounts. The heterozygote, having one gene with a normal effect, is still able to produce the enzyme in sufficient amounts to carry out the metabolic function under normal circumstances. Therefore the heterozygote does not exhibit symptoms of the disorder. However, the abnormal homozygote, who inherits a defective gene from both parents, has no functioning enzyme and thus is clinically affected.

It is becoming possible to detect and screen for an increasing number of inborn errors of metabolism—to detect the presence of the disease in the heterozygote, the newborn, and the fetus before birth. Some of the more significant inborn errors of metabolism and related nursing responsibilities are discussed below.

CONGENITAL HYPOTHYROIDISM

Congenital hypothyroidism (CH) (sometimes called by the undesirable term *cretinism*) has a number of etiologic fac-

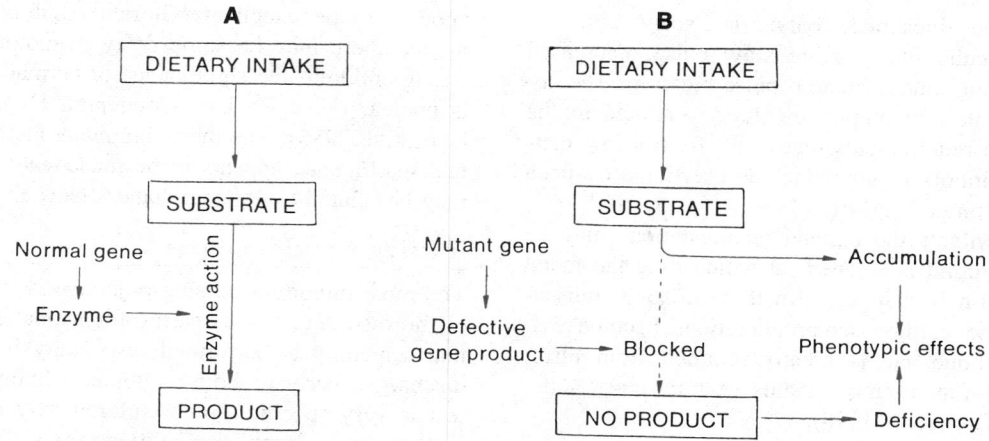

Fig. 9-7. Metabolic pathway. **A,** Normal metabolic pathway. **B,** Effect of defective gene action.

tors and may be permanent or transient. Permanent CH may result from failure of embryonic development of the thyroid gland, from an inborn enzymatic defect in the synthesis of thyroxine, or, rarely, from pituitary dysfunction. In the transient type intrauterine transfer of goitrogens (substances that can induce a goiter), such as the antithyroid drugs phenylbutazone, paraaminosalicylic acid, and cobalt, may inhibit thyroid secretion, resulting in congenital cretinism. Although this type is self-limiting, it is a potentially fatal condition because once the maternal supply is terminated the infant's thyroid is unable to produce its own hormones. In addition, a large goiter in a neonate may cause total obstruction of the airway.

Results of screening tests in the United States show that CH occurs in one of every 4000 to 5000 births, an incidence almost twice that of phenylketonuria (Levy and Mitchell, 1982). Infants with Down syndrome have a much higher rate of either permanent or transient forms of the disorder (Fort and others, 1984).

Clinical Manifestations

The severity of the disorder depends on the amount of thyroid tissue present. Usually the newborn does not exhibit obvious signs of hypothyroidism, probably because of the exogenous source of thyroid hormone supplied by means of the maternal circulation. Manifestations are delayed in breast-fed infants because breast milk contains suboptimum amounts of thyroid hormone. Table 9-4 summarizes possible indications of CH at birth and those that may become apparent by 3 months of age.

If CH is untreated, further changes become evident. Impaired development of the nervous system leads to severe mental retardation. The severity of the intellectual deficit is related to the degree of hypothyroidism and the duration of the condition before treatment. Other nervous system manifestations include slow, awkward movements and abnormal deep tendon reflexes (often referred to as ''hung-up'' because the relaxation phase after the contraction is slow).

Table 9-4 Possible indications of congenital hypothyroidism

AT BIRTH	BEFORE 3 MONTHS OF AGE
Gestation >42 weeks	Umbilical hernia
Birth weight >4 kg (8.8 lb)	Mottled and dry skin
Widened posterior fontanelle	Constipation
Hypothermia, 95° F or less	Large tongue
Peripheral cyanosis	Hoarse
Respiratory distress	Cold to touch
Edema	Excessive sleepiness
Prolonged physiologic jaundice	Difficulty feeding related to lethargy
Abdominal distention	Minimum crying
Vomiting	
Delayed passage of meconium	
Feeding difficulties	
Hypoactivity	

Modified from Smith, D., and others: Congenital hypothyroidism—signs and symptoms in the newborn period, J. Pediatr. 87(6):958-962, 1975.

Because skeletal growth is severely stunted, the child is short and infantile proportions persist in that the length of the trunk remains long in relation to the legs. The decreased metabolic rate results in weight gain and often leads to obesity. Characteristic infantile facial features from myxedema include a short forehead; wide, puffy eyes; wrinkled eyelids; broad, short, upturned nose; and a large, protruding tongue. The hair is often dry, brittle, or lusterless and follows a low hairline. Dentition is delayed and usually defective. Such facial features give the child a characteristic dull expression.

The skin is yellowish from carotenemia as a result of the depressed hepatic conversion of carotene to vitamin A. The loss of heat from reduced metabolism is reflected in a cool skin. Cold intolerance is another common consequence. Anemia results in pallor, fatigue, and lethargy, and vitamin

A deficiency causes thickened, coarse, dry, scaly skin.

The cardiovascular changes are slow pulse, decreased circulation, mottling, and decreased pulse pressure. The decreased cardiac rate and output are directly related to the decreased oxygen requirements that result from a low metabolic rate. Respiratory changes include exertional dyspnea and decreased respiratory effort.

In breast-fed infants the clinical manifestations may be delayed until the child is weaned, at which time the facial features, skin and hair changes, growth retardation, muscular hypotonia, and cardiovascular alterations become evident. However, bone age is greatly retarded from birth, while intellectual functioning remains near normal (Bode, Vanjonack, and Crawford, 1978).

Diagnostic Evaluation

Diagnosis is aimed at early identification of the disorder to prevent the serious effects on mental development resulting from delayed treatment. Neonatal screening employs filter-paper blood specimens and radioimmunoassay for thyroxine (T_4) and thyroid-stimulating factor (TSH). Although the heel-stick blood sample can be obtained at any time soon after birth, specimens are usually taken after 24 hours because the test is usually part of a concurrent screen for other metabolic defects, such as phenylketonuria (see discussion on p. 362).

Screening results that show a low level of T_4 and a high level of TSH indicate CH and the need for further tests to confirm the exact cause of the diagnosis. Additional tests include serum measurement of thyroxine, triiodothyronine (T_3), protein-bound iodine (PBI), and thyrotropin-releasing factor to ascertain the amount of thyroid hormone secreted and the intactness of the homeostatic mechanisms. Tests of thyroid gland function (thyroid scan and uptake) usually involve an oral infusion of a radioactive isotope of iodine (^{131}I) and measurement of the iodine uptake by the thyroid, usually within 24 hours. In CH, protein-bound iodine, thyroxine, triiodothyronine, and free thyroxine levels are low and thyroid uptake of ^{131}I is decreased. Roentgenography is employed to assess bone age.

Therapeutic Management

Treatment involves life-long replacement therapy with a thyroid hormone preparation as soon as possible after diagnosis to abolish all signs of hypothyroidism and reestablish normal physical and mental development. A number of oral thyroid preparations are available, including dessicated thyroid U.S.P., thyroglobulin, and synthetic forms of T_4 and T_3. The drug of choice is synthetic levothyroxine sodium (Na T_4), which is commercially available as Synthroid or Levothroid (American Academy of Pediatrics, 1978). To prevent the risk of overdosage of thyroid hormones, thyroxine and triiodothyronine levels are measured regularly. Bone age surveys are also performed to ensure optimum growth.

If adequate thyroid hormone replacement is begun shortly after birth, the chance for normal growth and intelligence appears to be excellent (Glorieux and others, 1985). Although there may be some delay in motor development in young children, the significance or permanence of the delay is unclear (New England Congenital Hypothyroidism Collaborative, 1985). The most significant factor affecting eventual intelligence appears to be inadequate treatment, which may be related to noncompliance (New England, 1984).

Nursing Considerations

The most important nursing objective is early identification of the disorder. Nurses caring for neonates must be certain that screening is performed, especially in infants who are discharged early or born at home. Although the screening test is very specific, some children may not be identified, and nurses in ambulatory settings for well-infant care need to be aware of the earliest signs of the disorder. Parental remarks about an unusually "quiet and good" baby coupled with any of the early physical manifestations should lead the nurse to suspect hypothyroidism and refer the child for specific tests. Unfortunately, many parents harbor guilt about their impressions of the infant before the diagnosis because the child's inactivity may not have alerted them to a problem, with the result that treatment is delayed.

Once the diagnosis is confirmed, parents need an explanation of the disorder and the necessity of life-long treatment. The importance of compliance with the drug regimen must be stressed. Since the drug is tasteless, it can be crushed and added to formula, water, or food. If a dose is missed, twice the dose should be given the next day (Coody, 1984). Parents also need to be aware of signs indicating overdose, namely, rapid pulse, dyspnea, irritability, insomnia, fever, sweating, and weight loss. Ideally they should know how to count the pulse and be instructed to withhold a dose and consult the physician if the pulse rate is above a certain value. Signs of inadequate treatment are fatigue, sleepiness, decreased appetite, and constipation.

If the diagnosis was delayed past early infancy, the chance of permanent mental retardation is great. Parents need the same guidance in caring for their child as do others who have an offspring with cognitive impairment (Chapter 24). They need an opportunity to discuss their feelings regarding late recognition of the disorder. Although treatment will not reverse the intellectual deficit, it may prevent further damage. Genetic counseling is important, especially if the disorder is caused by an inborn error of thyroid hormone synthesis, which is autosomal recessive. (For a discussion of genetic counseling, see p. 172.)

PHENYLKETONURIA

Phenylketonuria (PKU) is a genetic disease, inherited as an autosomal-recessive trait, that results in the body's inability to metabolize the essential amino acid phenylalanine. It is not a common inborn error of metabolism, affecting 1:10,000 to 15,000 live births. PKU primarily affects whites, with the incidence being highest in people living in the United States or Northern Europe. It is very rare in the African, Jewish, and Japanese populations.

In recent years it has become apparent that severe, classic PKU is at one end of a spectrum of conditions now known as *hyperphenylalaninemia.* At the other end are rarer forms that are referred to as *variants* of hyperphenylalaninemia. Unlike classic PKU, the variant forms are caused by defects in the phenylalanine hydroxylase system rather than in phenylalanine hydroxylase itself. They are the result of a deficiency of enzymes, such as *dihydropteridine reductase* (DHPR) or *dihydrobiopterin synthetase* (DHBS). These defects are responsible for a lack of *tetrahydrobiopterin synthesis,* also referred to as BH_4 deficiency. These variant forms are diagnosed and treated differently from classic PKU. Although the phenylalanine levels exceed the normal range, restriction of phenylalanine is not sufficient to prevent neurologic damage. Treatment involves the replacement of the neurotransmitters dopamine and serotonin with L-dopa and 5-hydroxytryptophan (Dhondt, 1984). The following discussion of PKU is limited to the severe, classic form.

Pathophysiology

The hepatic enzyme *phenylalanine hydroxylase,* which normally controls the conversion of phenylalanine to tyrosine, is absent in PKU. This results in the accumulation of phe-

nylalanine in the bloodstream and urinary excretion of its abnormal metabolites, the phenyl acids (Fig. 9-8). One of these phenyl ketones, *phenylpyruvic acid,* which gives urine the characteristic musty odor associated with this disease, is responsible for the term *phenylketonuria.*

Accumulation of phenylalanine, and presumably the decreased levels of the neurotransmitters dopamine and tryptophan, affect the normal development of the brain and central nervous system, resulting in defective myelinization, cystic degeneration of the gray and white matter, and disturbances in cortical lamination. Mental retardation occurs *before* the metabolites are detected in the urine and will progress if ingested phenylalanine levels are not lowered.

Besides the accumulating phenylalanine, there is also an absence of the amino acid tyrosine, which is needed for the formation of the pigment melanin and the hormones epinephrine and thyroxin. Decreased melanin production results in similar phenotypes of most children with phenylketonuria. Typically they have blonde hair, blue eyes, and fair skin that is particularly susceptible to eczema and other dermatologic problems. Children of genetically darker skin color may be red-haired or brunette.

Clinical Manifestations

Clinical manifestations of PKU include failure to thrive, frequent vomiting, irritability, hyperactivity, and unpredicta-

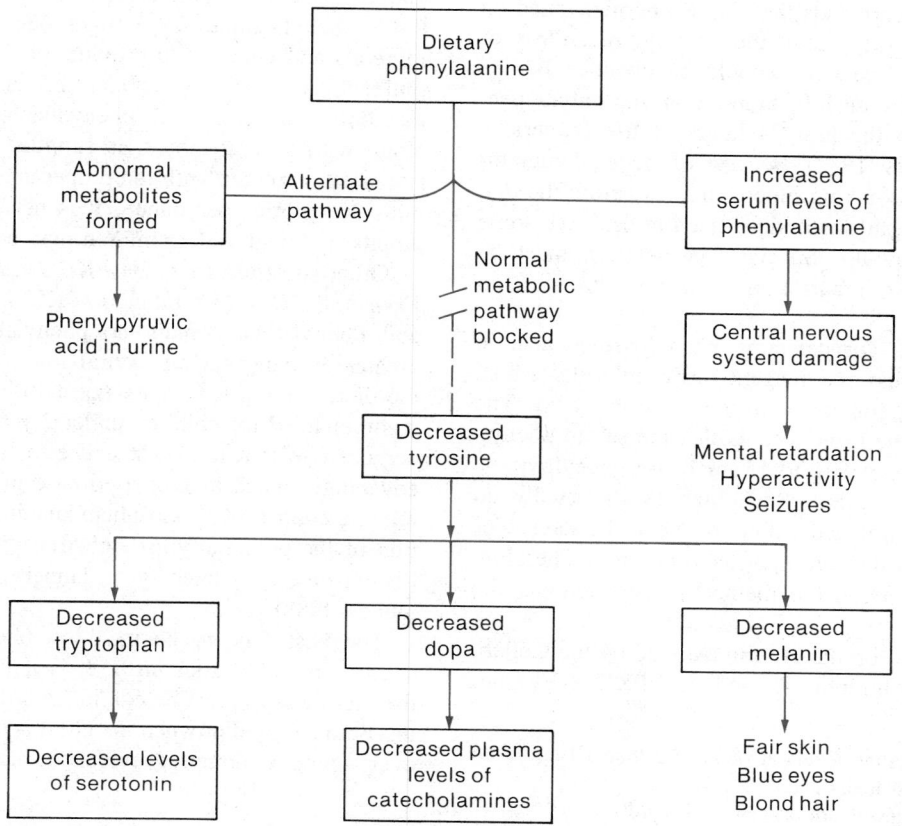

Fig. 9-8. Metabolic errors and consequences in phenylketonuria.

ble, erratic behavior. Bizarre or schizoid behavior patterns are common, such as fright reactions, screaming episodes, head banging, arm biting, disorientation, failure to respond to strong stimuli, and catatonia-like positions. Many of the severely retarded children have convulsions, and about 80% of untreated persons with PKU demonstrate abnormal electroencephalographs, regardless of whether overt seizures occur.

Diagnostic Evaluation

The objective in diagnosing or treating the disorder is to prevent mental retardation. The most commonly used test for screening newborns is the *Guthrie blood test,* which is mandatory for all newborns in most states. If properly done, it detects serum phenylalanine levels greater than 4 mg/dl (normal value is 2 mg/dl). The Guthrie test is a bacterial inhibition procedure. *Bacillus subtilis,* which is present in the culture medium, requires a sufficient amount of phenylalanine in order to grow. If a drop of blood that contains abnormal quantities of phenylalanine is placed on the culture medium and the bacteria grow, PKU is suspected. Only fresh heel blood, not cord blood, can be used for the test. Since this test provides a qualitative analysis, serum phenylalanine and tyrosine levels should be taken.

The screening test is most reliable if the blood sample is taken after the infant has ingested a source of protein. However, because of early discharge, the American Academy of Pediatrics (1982) recommends that the test be performed on all newborns before they leave the nursery, regardless of age. A repeat blood specimen should be obtained by the third week of life from all infants in whom the initial specimen is taken within the first 24 hours of life (American Academy of Pediatrics, 1982). Because of the legal and ethical issues involved in taking blood samples before the disease can be detected, all institutions need to establish some mechanism for follow-up. Special consideration must be given to screening of infants born at home who have no hospital contact.

Several tests exist for detecting phenylpyruvic acid in urine. All of them use the reagent ferric chloride, which turns green when in contact with phenylpyruvic acid. The main problem with the urine tests is that the serum phenylalanine level must exceed 10 to 15 mg/dl for phenylpyruvic acid to be present in urine. Such high levels usually do not occur until the affected infant is 10 to 14 days old, by which time brain damage may have ocurred. Therefore urine testing is not a reliable method of screening in the neonate.

Diagnosis is based on the criteria adopted by the Collaborative Study of Children Treated for PKU (O'Flynn, 1980):

1. Serum phenylalanine levels at or greater than 20 mg/dl on two occasions 24 hours apart
2. Serum tyrosine levels not exceeding 5 mg/dl
3. Urinary metabolites found in classic PKU, such as o-HPAA and phenylalanine, present in excess

Because of the possibility of variant forms of hyperphenylalaninemia, a natural protein challenge test is recommended after about 3 months of dietary treatment to confirm the diagnosis of classic PKU.

Therapeutic Management

Treatment of PKU is dietary. Since the genetic enzyme is intracellular, systemic administration of phenylalanine hydroxylase is of no value. Phenylalanine cannot be eliminated because it is an essential amino acid in tissue growth. Therefore dietary management must meet two criteria:

1. It must meet the child's nutritional need for optimum growth.
2. It must maintain phenylalanine levels within a safe range.

The diet is calculated to allow 20 to 30 mg per kg of body weight per day of phenylalanine, which should maintain blood levels between 3 and 10 mg/dl. Significant brain damage usually occurs when levels are greater than 10 to 15 mg/dl. At levels less than 2 mg/dl the body begins to catabolize its protein stores, resulting in growth retardation.

Since all natural food proteins contain about 15% phenylalanine, specially prepared milk substitutes, such as *Lofenalac,* * are given to the infant. Total or partial breastfeeding, because of the low phenylalanine content of breast milk, may be possible with close monitoring of phenylalanine levels (Lawrence, 1985). Lofenalac is made from specially treated enzymatic casein hydrolysate, which provides 0.4% phenylalanine (28.5 mg/8 ounces). It also contains minerals and vitamins to provide a balanced nutritional formula. Since tyrosine is deficient because of the block in the metabolic conversion of phenylalanine, this amino acid, along with several others, is supplied to the infant. When Lofenalac is mixed with the proper amount of water, it supplies 20 calories per ounce. It is usually well accepted by infants, although older children may not find it palatable.

Other substitutes include *PKU 1*†, *PKU 2*†, and *Phenyl-Free* *. PKU 1 (for infants), PKU 2 (for older children), and Phenyl-Free contain no phenylalanine and allow for greater exchanges with natural low-phenylalanine foods in the diet, leading to a more normal diet. Phenyl-Free is not recommended for children under 2 years of age, but studies demonstrate that it is safe and effective and offers several advantages, such as increased ease of breast-feeding, more reliable control of serum phenylalanine levels, and elimination of the potentially difficult transition from Lofenalac to Phenyl-Free at a later age (Flannery, Hitchcock, and Mamunes, 1983).

The best time to begin a low-phenylalanine diet is as soon as possible after birth. It is not yet known how long the diet therapy must be continued. At present many centers discontinue the diet when the child is 6 to 8 years old. However, there is mounting evidence that increased phenylala-

---

*Mead Johnson & Co., Evansville, IN.
†Milupa Corp., Darien, CT.

nine levels beyond this age have neuropsychologic sequelae, such as lowered intelligence quotient, attentional and academic difficulties, especially in arithmetic, and visual-spatial problems (Seashore and others, 1985; Brunner, Jordan, and Berry, 1983). There is also the difficulty of compliance in resuming the diet, such as during pregnancy (Michals and others, 1985).

To evaluate the effectiveness of dietary treatment, frequent monitoring of blood phenylalanine levels is necessary. Phenylalanine deficiency is associated with acidosis, hypoglycemia, extensive skin rash, anemia, and fulminating infection. Suboptimum phenylalanine levels will cause retarded growth in height and weight.

With improved dietary control of PKU, the increased life span of individuals with this disorder presents additional concerns. High phenylalanine blood levels in mothers with PKU affect the normal embryologic development of the fetus, leading to growth retardation, congenital malformations, microcephaly, and/or mental retardation in the infant (Lipson and others, 1984). For this reason the low-phenylalanine diet should be resumed *prior to* pregnancy, although dietary therapy is not yet of proven efficacy in preventing these fetal effects (Lenke and Levy, 1982).

Nursing Considerations

The principal nursing considerations involve family teaching regarding the dietary restrictions. Although the treatment may sound simple, the task of maintaining such a strict dietary regimen is very demanding. Foods with low phenylalanine levels, such as vegetables, fruits, juices, and some cereals, breads, and starches, must be measured to provide the prescribed amount of phenylalanine. Most high-protein foods, such as meat and dairy products, are either eliminated or restricted to small amounts. The sweetener aspartame (NutraSweet) must be avoided because it is converted to phenylalanine in the body. Also, the substitutes are quite expensive, adding financial burdens.

During infancy, Lofenalac or PKU 1 is used as a formula and presents few problems. Solid foods, such as cereal, fruits, and vegetables, are introduced as usual to the infant. As the child gets older, more difficulties can arise. Decreased appetite and refusal to eat may reduce consumption of the calculated phenylalanine requirement. The child's increasing independence may inhibit absolute control of what he eats. Either factor can result in decreased or increased phenylalanine levels. During the school years, peer pressure becomes a major force in deterring the child from consuming the substitutes or abstaining from high-protein foods such as milkshakes or ice cream. It is easy to understand the limitations in the diet when one considers that a quarter-pound hamburger may be equal to a 2-day phenylalanine allowance for a school-age child (Wyatt, 1978). In addition, illness and growth spurts will increase the body's need for this essential amino acid.

The assistance of a well-qualified nutritionist is essential. Parents need a basic understanding of the disorder and prac-

tical suggestions regarding food selection and preparation.* Meal planning is based on an exchange list, and as soon as children are old enough, usually by early preschool, they should be involved in the daily calculation, menu planning, and formula preparation. Using a musical or voice-synthesizer calculator, colored beads, or an abacus can help children keep track of the daily allowance of phenylalanine foods (Messer, 1985).

Preparation of Lofenalac can present some difficulties because it tends to be lumpy and has a distinctive odor and taste that has been described as similar to potato but more bitter. A blender or mixer dissolves the powder more easily, but this is inconvenient when traveling. Although the taste is virtually impossible to camouflage, adding orange Tang, fruit-flavored powdered punch, or strawberry or chocolate Quik helps vary the flavor somewhat without greatly altering the phenylalanine content. The chocolate-flavored formula can be heated and served as hot cocoa or frozen into popsicles. Fortunately, Phenyl-Free is more easily flavored to produce a fairly pleasant drink.

Family support. As with the birth of any child with a permanent disorder, parents of children with PKU first mourn the loss of a perfect son or daughter. These parents have the extra burden of knowing that they are carriers of the defect and must make serious decisions regarding future children, since there is no prenatal screening test to detect homozygotes. Genetic counseling is especially important for an affected child, who theoretically has a 50% chance of bearing an affected offspring, in addition to offspring without the disorder who may have numerous other defects. (For a discussion of genetic counseling, see p. 172.)

GALACTOSEMIA

Galactosemia is a rare autosomal-recessive disorder affecting approximately 1:50,000 births. It involves an inborn error of carbohydrate metabolism in which the hepatic enzyme *galactose-1-phosphate uridine transferase (UDP-galactose transferase)* is absent. The enzyme is one of three needed for the conversion of galactose to glucose (Fig. 9-9). As galactose accumulates in the blood, several organs are affected. Hepatic dysfunction leads to cirrhosis, resulting in jaundice in the infant by the second week of life. The spleen subsequently becomes enlarged as a result of portal hypertension. Cataracts are usually recognizable by 1 or 2 months of age; cerebral damage is detectable soon afterward, evidenced by the symptoms of lethargy and hypotonia.

Infants with this disorder appear normal at birth but within a few days after ingesting milk, which has a high lactose content, begin to vomit and lose weight. Drowsi-

---

*A helpful book is by Schuett, V., editor: Low-protein cookery for phenylketonuria, 1977, University of Wisconsin Press, 114 N. Murray St., Madison, WI 53715. For mothers who are breast-feeding, detailed information is presented by Ernest, A., and others: Guide to feeding the infant with PKU, Superintendent of Documents, U.S. Government Printing Office, Washington, DC 20402.

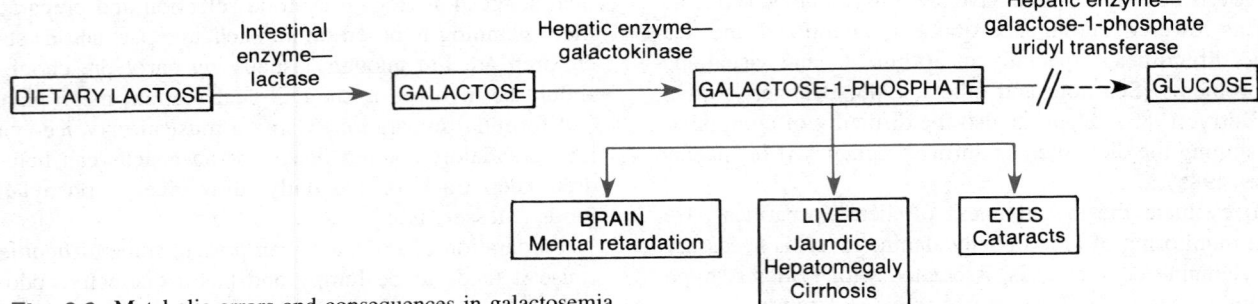

Fig. 9-9. Metabolic errors and consequences in galactosemia.

ness, jaundice, nausea, and diarrhea also occur, and death during the first month of life is not uncommon in infants with untreated galactosemia.

Diagnostic Evaluation

Diagnosis is made on the basis of galactosuria, increased levels of galactose in the blood, or decreased levels of UDP-galactose transferase activity in erythrocytes (normal range: 2.5 to 9 units of enzyme per g of hemoglobin). Cord blood can be analyzed at birth to establish a diagnosis in suspected infants; carriers can also be identified by this test, since heterozygotic individuals have significantly lower levels of the enzyme. Although asymptomatic, such individuals have been noted to spontaneously dislike and therefore limit ingestion of galactose-containing foods.

Several screening tests are available for use in newborns, including the *Beutler test,* which employs a procedure similar to the Guthrie blood test for PKU (Levy and Hammersen, 1978). Mass screening is done in several states but has been an issue of controversy because of the rarity of the disorder and the expense of screening.

Therapeutic Management

Treatment of galactosemia is dietary and consists of eliminating all milk and lactose-containing foods, including breast milk. During infancy, lactose-free formulas are used, with soy-protein formula being the feeding of choice (American Academy of Pediatrics, 1983).

Follow-up studies of children treated from birth or within the first month demonstrate that most of them have normal growth and intellectual functioning. However, these children may have speech and language deficits (Waisbren and others, 1983), and some develop neurologic sequelae, such as mental retardation, tremors, and ataxia (Lo and others, 1984). Children treated later tend to have mental scores from normal to mildly retarded, but most have some degree of visual-perceptual handicap (Fishler and others, 1980).

Nursing Considerations

Nursing interventions are similar to those for PKU, except that the dietary restrictions are easier to maintain because many more foods are allowed. However, reading food labels very carefully for the addition of any form of lactose, especially dairy products, is mandatory. Many drugs, such as penicillin, contain lactose as filler and must also be avoided. Unfortunately, lactose is an unlabeled ingredient in pharmaceuticals. Strict adherence to the diet is necessary for the first 7 to 8 years, followed by a modified regimen throughout life.

CONCEPT SUMMARIES

- Problems of the newborn may be attributed to birth injuries, infections, inborn errors of metabolism, and immature physiologic systems.

- The forces of labor and delivery may cause soft tissue injury, head trauma, fractures, and paralysis.

- The most common forms of paralysis in the newborn are facial nerve, brachial plexus, and phrenic nerve palsies.

- Common problems of the newborn include erythema toxicum, candidiasis, bullous impetigo, and discolorations of the skin.

- Because of immature physiologic status, infants may be predisposed to hyperbilirubinemia, neonatal hypocalcemia, and neonatal hypoglycemia.

- Hyperbilirubinemia is classified according to the two types of bilirubin: unconjugated and conjugated. In the newborn it may result from excess production of bilirubin, disturbed capacity of the liver to conjugate bilirubin, or bile duct obstruction resulting from biliary atresia.

- Treatment of unconjugated hyperbilirubinemia includes phototherapy, exchange transfusion, and pharmacologic management.

- Four categories of hypoglycemia are early transitional adaptive, classical transient neonatal, secondary, and recurrent severe.

- Hemorrhagic disease of the newborn is characterized by oozing from the umbilicus or circumcision site, bloody or black stools, hematuria, ecchymosis on skin and scalp, and epistaxis.

- The most significant inborn errors of metabolism are congenital hypothyroidism, phenylketonuria, and galactosemia.

- Dietary control is the treatment of choice for phenylketonuria and galactosemia.

- Thyroid replacement is required to treat congenital hypothyroidism.

REFERENCES

American Academy of Pediatrics, Committee on Drugs: Treatment of congenital hypothyroidism, Pediatrics 62(3):413-417, 1978.

American Academy of Pediatrics, Committee on Fetus and Newborn: Home phototherapy, Pediatrics 76(1):136-137, 1985.

American Academy of Pediatrics, Committee on Genetics: New issues in newborn screening for phenylketonuria and congenital hypothyroidism, Pediatrics 69(1):104-106, 1982.

American Academy of Pediatrics, Committee on Nutrition: Soy-protein formulas: recommendations for use in infant feeding, Pediatrics 72(3):359-363, 1983.

Bergstrom, W.H., and Hakanson, D.O.: Phototherapy-induced hypocalcemia: prevention by caps in human infants and newborn rats, Pediatr. Research 14(4):572, 1980.

Blake, S.J.: The bright side of phototherapy, Am. J. Maternal Child Nurs. 8(1):23, 1983.

Bode, H.H., Vanjonack, W.J., and Crawford, J.D.: Mitigation of cretinism by breast-feeding, Pediatrics 62(1):13-16, 1978.

Bowman, J.M.: Controversies in Rh prophylaxis, Am. J. Obstet. Gynecol. 151:289-294, 1985.

Brown, A.K., and others: Efficacy of phototherapy in prevention and management of neonatal hyperbilirubinemia, Pediatrics 75(2)(suppl.):393-400, 1985.

Brunner, R.L., Jordan, M.K., and Berry, H.K.: Early-treated phenylketonuria: neuropsychologic consequences, J. Pediatr. 102(6):831-835, 1983.

Cashore, W.J., and Stern, L.: Neonatal hyperbilirubinemia, Pediatr. Clin. North Am. 29(5):1191-1203, 1982.

Coody, D.: Congenital hypothyroidism, Pediatr. Nurs. 10(5):342-345, 1984.

Cottrell, B.H., and Anderson, G.C.: Rectal or axillary temperature measurement: effect on plasma bilirubin and intestinal transit of meconium, J. Pediatr. Gastroenterol. Nutr. 3:734-739, 1984.

Dhondt, J.: Tetrahydrobiopterin deficiencies: preliminary analysis from an international survey, J. Pediatr. 104(4):501-508, 1984.

Dicken, C.H.: More on the treatment of port-wine stains with the argon laser, Mayo Clin. Proc. 60:115-117, 1985.

Eggert, L., and others: Home phototherapy treatment of neonatal jaundice, Pediatrics 76(4):579-584, 1985.

Fanaroff, A., and Martin, R., editors: Behrman's neonatal-perinatal medicine, ed.3, St. Louis, 1983, The C.V. Mosby Co.

Fishler, K., and others: Developmental aspects of galactosemia from infancy to childhood, Clin. Pediatr. 19:38-44, Jan. 1980.

Flannery, D.B., Hitchcock, E., and Mamunes, P.: Dietary management of phenylketonuria from birth using a phenylalanine-free product, J. Pediatr. 103(2):247-249, 1983.

Fort, P., and others: Abnormalities of thyroid function in infants with Down syndrome, J. Pediatr. 104(4):545-549, 1984.

Gartner, L.M., and Lee, K.: Jaundice and liver disease. I. Unconjugated hyperbilirubinemia. In Fanaroff, A., and Martin, R., editors: Behrman's neonatal-perinatal medicine, ed. 3, St. Louis, 1983, The C.V. Mosby Co.

Glorieux, J., and others: Follow-up at ages 5 and 7 years on mental development in children with hypothyroidism detected by Quebec Screening Program, J. Pediatr. 107(6):913-914, 1985.

Hammer, R.M., Bower, E.J., and Messina, L.J.: The prenatal use of Rho(D) immune globulin, Am. J. Maternal Child Nurs. 9:29-31, 1984.

Keenan, W.J., and others: Morbidity and mortality associated with exchange transfusion, Pediatrics 75(2)(suppl.):417-421, 1985.

Lascari, A.D.: "Early" breast-feeding jaundice: clinical significance, J. Pediatr. 108(1):156-158, 1986.

Lawrence, R.A.: Breastfeeding: a guide for the medical profession, ed. 2, St. Louis, 1985, The C.V. Mosby Co.

Lenke, R.R., and Levy, H.L.: Maternal phenylketonuria—results of dietary therapy, Am. J. Obstet. Gynecol. 142:584-593, March 1982.

Levy, H.L., and Hammersen, G.: Newborn screening for galactosemia and other galactose metabolic defects, J. Pediatr. 92:871-877, June 1978.

Levy, H.L., and Mitchell, M.L.: The current status of newborn screening, Hospital Practice 17:89-97, 1982.

Linn, S., and others: Epidemiology of neonatal hyperbilirubinemia, Pediatrics 75(4):770-774, 1985.

Lipsitz, P.J., Gartner, L.M., and Bryla, D.A.: Neonatal and infant mortality in relation to phototherapy, Pediatrics 75(2)(suppl.):422-426, 1985.

Lipson, A., and others: Maternal hyperphenylalaninemia fetal effects, J. Pediatr. 104(2):216-220, 1984.

Lo, W., and others: Curious neurologic sequelae in galactosemia, Pediatrics 73(3):309-312, 1984.

Maisels, M.: Hyperbilirubinemia. In Nelson, N.M., editor: Current therapy in neonatal-perinatal medicine, St. Louis, 1985, The C.V. Mosby Co.

Mansour, A., and Gelfand, E.W.: A new approach to the use of antifungal agents in infants with persistent oral candidiasis, J. Pediatr. 98:161-162, Jan. 1981.

McDonagh, A.F., and Lightner, D.A.: 'Like a shrivelled blood orange'—bilirubin, jaundice, and phototherapy, Pediatrics 75(3):443-455, 1985.

Messer, S.S.: PKU: a mother's perspective, Pediatr. Nurs. 11(2):121-123, 1985.

Michals, K., and others: Return to diet therapy in patients with phenylketonuria, J. Pediatr. 106(6):933-936, 1985.

New England Congenital Hypothyroidism Collaborative: Neonatal hypothyroidism screening: status of patients at 6 years of age, J. Pediatr. 107(6):915-918, 1985.

New England Congenital Hypothyroidism Collaborative: Characteristics of infantile hypothyroidism discovered on neonatal screening, J. Pediatr. 104(4):539-544, 1984.

O'Flynn, M.E., and others: The diagnosis of phenylketonuria: a report from the Collaborative Study of Children treated for Phenylketonuria, Am. J. Dis. Child. 134:769-774, Aug. 1980.

Osborn, L.M., Reiff, M.I., and Bolus, R.: Jaundice in the full-term neonate, Pediatrics 73(4):520-525, 1984.

Pildes, R.S., and Lilien, L.D.: Carbohydrate metabolism in the fetus and neonate. In Fanaroff, A., and Martin, R., editors: Behrman's neonatal-perinatal medicine, ed. 3, St. Louis, 1983, The C.V. Mosby Co.

Plotz, R.D.: Familial occurrence of hemolytic disease of the newborn due to AO blood group incompatibility, Human Path. 16:113-116, 1985.

Schumacher, R.E., Thornbery, J.M., and Gutcher, G.R.: Transcutaneous bilirubinometry: a comparison of old and new methods, Pediatrics 76(1):10-14, 1985.

Seashore, M.R., and others: Loss of intellectual function in children with phenylketonuria after relaxation of dietary phenylalanine restriction, Pediatrics 75(2):226-232, 1985.

Slater, L., and Brewer, M.: Home versus hospital phototherapy for term infants with hyperbilirubinemia: a comparative study, Pediatrics 73(4):515-519, 1984.

Smith, D., and others: Use of noninvasive tests to predict significant jaundice in full-term infants: preliminary studies, Pediatrics 75(2):278-280, 1985.

Vechi, C., and others: Phototherapy for neonatal jaundice: clinical equivalence of fluorescent green and "special" blue lamps, J. Pediatr. 108(3):452-456, 1986.

Waisbren, S.E., and others: Speech and language deficits in early-treated children with galactosemia, J. Pediatr. 102(1):75-77, 1983.

Wyatt, D.S.: Phenylketonuria: the problems vary during different developmental stages, Am. J. Maternal Child Nurs. 3(5):296-302, 1978.

BIBLIOGRAPHY
Birth Injuries

Cohen, A.W., and Otto, S.R.: Obstetric clavicular fractures: a three-year analysis, J. Reprod. Med. 25:119-122, Sept. 1980.

Cumming, W.A.: Neonatal skeletal fractures, birth trauma or child abuse? J. Can. Assoc. Radiol. 30:30-33, March 1979.

Greenwald, A.G., and others: Brachial plexus birth palsy: a ten year report on incidence and prognosis, J. Pediatr. Orthoped. 4:689-692, 1984.

Gresham, E.L.: Birth trauma, Pediatr. Clin. North Am. 22(2):317-328, 1975.

Ingardia, C.J., and Cetrulo, C.L.: Forceps—use and abuse, Clin. Perinatol. **8**:63-66, Feb. 1981.

Jain, I.S., and others: Ocular hazards during birth, J. Pediatr. Ophthalmol. Strabismus **17**:14-16, Jan./Feb. 1980.

Mangurten, H.H.: Birth injuries. In Fanaroff, A., and Martin, R., editors: Behrman's neonatal-perinatal medicine, ed. 3, St. Louis, 1983, The C.V. Mosby Co.

Common Problems

Abramovits, W.: Resistant oral candidiasis in an infant due to pacifier contamination, Clin. Pediatr. **20**:393, June 1981.

Casneuf, J., and others: Oral thrush in children treated with miconazole gel, Mykosen **23**:75-78, Sept. 1979.

Chetty, G.N., and others: Candidiasis in mother and child, Mykosen **23**:580-582, Dec. 1979.

Daftary, S.S., and others: Oral thrush in the new-born, Indian Pediatr. **17**:287-288, March 1980.

Feigin, F.D.: Postnatally acquired infections. In Fanaroff, A., and Martin, R., editors: Behrman's neonatal-perinatal medicine, ed. 3, St. Louis, 1983, The C.V. Mosby Co.

Finn, M.C., Glowacki, J., and Mulliken, J.B.: Congenital vascular lesions: clinical application of a new classification, J. Pediatr. Surg. **18**(6):894-900, 1983.

The first six hours of life: assessment of risk in the newborn: birth injuries, module 4, New York, 1982, March of Dimes–Birth Defects Foundation.

Montello, J.M., and others: Clotrimazole by thumb, N. Engl. J. Med. **301**(18):1005, 1979.

Hyperbilirubinemia

Adams, J.A., Hey, D.J., and Hall, R.T.: Incidence of hyperbilirubinemia in breast- vs. formula-fed infants, Clin. Pediatr. **24**(2):69-73, 1985.

Beal, R.W.: Non-rhesus (D) blood group isoimmunization in obstetrics, Clin. Obstet. Gynecol. **6**:493-508, Dec. 1979.

Bibeau, P., and Perez, R.H.: Care of the patient with hyperbilirubinemia. In Perez, R.H.: Protocols for perinatal nursing practice, St. Louis, 1981, The C.V. Mosby Co.

Costarino, A.T., and others: Bilirubin photoisomerization in premature neonates under low- and high-dose phototherapy, Pediatrics **75**(3):519-522, 1985.

Costarino, A.T., Jr., and others: Effect of spectral distribution on isomerization of bilirubin in vivo, J. Pediatr. **107**(1):125-128, 1985.

Curtis-Cohen, M., and others: Randomized trial of prophylactic phototherapy in the infant with very low birth weight, J. Pediatr. **107**(1):121-124, 1985.

D'Epiro, P.: Neonatal jaundice: knowing when to treat, Patient Care **19**(14):140-143, 1985.

Davey, M.: The prevention of rhesus-isoimmunization, Clin. Obstet. Gynecol. **6**:509-530, Dec. 1979.

deVries, L.S., Lary, L., and Dubowitz, L.M.S.: Relationship of serum bilirubin levels to ototoxicity and deafness in high-risk low-birth-weight infants, Pediatrics **76**(3):351-354, 1985.

Gannon, R.B., and Pickett, K.: Jaundice, Am. J. Nurs. **83**(3):404-407, 1983.

Gitzelmann-Cumarasamy, N., and Kuenzle, C.C.: Bilirubin binding tests: living up to expectations? Pediatrics **64**:375-378, Sept. 1979.

Hensleigh, P.A.: Preventing Rhesus isoimmunization, Am. J. Obstet. Gynecol. **146**:749-755, 1983.

Hensleigh, P.A.: Further prevention of RH immunization, Perinatal Press **5**:19-2, March 1981.

Jaundiced babies bloom with home phototherapy, Am. J. Nurs. **84**(7):871, 1984.

Kasprisin, D.O., and Kasprisin, C.A.: Introduction to transfusion therapy: a programmed text, New York, 1980, Medical Examination Publishing Co., Inc.

Kivlahan, C., and James, E.J.P.: The natural history of neonatal jaundice, Pediatrics **74**(3):364-370, 1984.

Levine, D.H., and Meyer, H.B.P.: Newborn screening for ABO hemolytic disease, Clin. Pediatr. **24**:391-394, 1985.

Maisels, M.J.: Jaundice in the newborn, Pediatr. Review **3**(10):305-320, 1982.

Matulich, N.: Jaundice in the neonate: theory and practice, Curr. Pract. Pediatr. Nurs. **3**:85-97, 1980.

Mauer, H.M., and others: Phototherapy for hyperbilirubinemia of hemolytic disease of the newborn, Pediatrics **75**(2)(suppl.):407-412, 1985.

Morrison, J.C.: The use of Rho immune globulin: review of ACOG Technical Bulletin, Perinatal Press **5**:67-68, June 1981.

Onishi, S., and others: Mechanism of development of bronze baby syndrome in neonates treated with phototherapy, Pediatrics **69**(3):273-276, 1982.

Osborn, L.M., and others: Phototherapy in full-term infants with hemolytic disease secondary to ABO incompatibility, Pediatrics **74**(3):371-374, 1984.

Poland, R.L.: Breast milk jaundice, J. Pediatr. **99**(1):86-87, 1981.

Rosenthal, P., Ramos, A., and Mungo, R.: Management of children with hyperbilirubinemia and green teeth, J. Pediatr. **108**(1):103-105, 1986.

Slater, L., and Brewer, M.: Home versus hospital phototherapy for term infants with hyperbilirubinemia: a comparative study, Pediatrics **73**(4):515-519, 1984.

Tufts, F., and Johnson, F.: Neonatal jaundice and phototherapy, Can. Nurse **75**:45-47, Dec. 1979.

Walther, F.J., Wu, P.Y.K., and Siassi, B.: Cardiac output changes in newborns with hyperbilirubinemia treated with phototherapy, Pediatrics **76**(6):918-921, 1985.

Wu, P.Y.K., and others: Metabolic aspects of phototherapy, Pediatrics **75**(2)(suppl.):427-433, 1985.

Hypoglycemia and Hypocalcemia

Brown, D.R., Steranka, B.H., and Taylor, F.H.: Treatment of early-onset neonatal hypocalcemia, Am. J. Dis. Child. **135**:24-28, Jan. 1981.

The first six hours of life: hypoglycemia in the newborn, module 2, New York, 1977, The National Foundation/March of Dimes.

Lilien, L.D., and others: Treatment of neonatal hypoglycemia with minibolus and intravenous glucose infusions, J. Pediatr. **97**(2):295-298, 1980.

McFadden, E.A., Zaloga, G.P., and Chernow, B.: Hypocalcemia: a medical emergency, Am. J. Nurs. **83**:227-230, 1983.

Romagnoli, C., and others: Phototherapy-induced hypocalcemia, J. Pediatr. **94**(5):815-816, 1979.

Salsbury, D.J., and Brown, D.R.: Effect of parenteral calcium treatment on blood pressure and heart rate in neonatal hypocalcemia, Pediatrics **69**(5):605-609, 1982.

Schedewie, H.K., and others: Parathormone and perinatal calcium homeostasis, Pediatr. Res. **13**:1-6, Jan. 1979.

Scott, S.M., and others: Effect of calcium therapy in the sick premature infant with early neonatal hypocalcemia, J. Pediatr. **104**(5):747-751, 1984.

Sexson, W.R.: Incidence of neonatal hypoglycemia: a matter of definition, J. Pediatr. **105**(1):149-150, 1984.

Taur, K.M.: Physiologic mechanisms in childhood hypoglycemia, Pediatr. Nurs. **9**(5):341-344, 1983.

Tripp, A.: Hyper and hypocalcemia, Am. J. Nurs. **76**(7):1142-1145, 1976.

Varma, S.K.: Hypoglycemia in infancy and childhood, South. Med. J. **72**:57-64, Jan. 1979.

Weiss, Y., Ackerman, C., and Shmilovitz, L.: Localized necrosis of scalp in neonates due to calcium gluconate infusions: a cautionary note, Pediatrics **56**(6):1084-1086, 1975.

Hemorrhagic Disease of the Newborn

American Academy of Pediatrics, Committee on Nutrition: Vitamin K supplementation for infants receiving milk substitute infant formulas and for those with fat malabsorption, Pediatrics **48**:483-487, 1971.

Behrmann, B.A., and others: Resurgence of hemorrhagic disease of the newborn: a report of three cases, Can. Med. Assoc. J. **133**(9):884-885, 1985.

Chaou, W., Chou, M., and Eitzman, D.V.: Intracranial hemorrhage and vitamin K deficiency in early infancy, J. Pediatr. **105**(6):880-884, 1984.

Lane, P.A., and Hathaway, W.E.: Vitamin K in infancy, J. Pediatr. **106**(3):351-359, 1985.

McNinch, A.W., and others: Hemorrhagic disease of the newborn returns, Lancet **1**:1089-1090, 1983.

Motohara, K., and others: Severe vitamin K deficiency in breast-fed infants, J. Pediatr. **105**(6):943-945, 1984.

Shearer, M.J., and others: Plasma vitamin K_1 in mothers and their newborn babies, Lancet **2**:460-463, 1982.

Congenital Hypothyroidism

Abassi, V., and Steinour, T.A.: Successful diagnosis of congenital hypothyroidism in four breast-fed neonates, J. Pediatr. **97**:259-261, 1980.

Brown, A.L., and others: Racial differences in the incidence of congenital hypothyroidism, J. Pediatr. **9**(6):934-936, 1981.

Delange, F., and others: Transient hypothyroidism in the newborn infant, J. Pediatr. **92**(6):974-976, 1978.

LaFranchi, S.H., and others: Screening for congenital hypothyroidism with specimen collection at two time periods: results of the Northwest Regional Screening Program, Pediatrics **76**(5):734-740, 1985.

Novogoder, M.: Neonatal screening for congenital hypothyroidism, Pediatr. Clin. North Am. **27**:881-890, 1980.

Smith, D., and others: Congenital hypothyroidism—signs and symptoms in the newborn period, part 1, J. Pediatr. **87**(6):958-962, 1975.

Phenylketonuria

American Academy of Pediatrics, Committee on Genetics: Maternal phenylketonuria, Pediatrics **76**(2):313-314, 1985.

American Academy of Pediatrics, Committee on Nutrition: New developments in hyperphenylalaninemia, Pediatrics **65**(4):844-846, 1980.

Barnico, L.M., and Cullinane, M.M.: Maternal phenylketonuria: an unexpected challenge, Am. J. Maternal Child Nurs. **10**:108-110, 1985.

Berry, H.: The diagnosis of phenylketonuria: a commentary, Am. J. Dis. Child. **135**:211-213, March 1981.

Binder, J., and others: Delayed elevation of serum phenylalanine level in a breast-fed child, Pediatrics **63**:334-336, Feb. 1979.

Cederbaum, S.D., Koch, R., and Donnell, G.N.: Symposium on genetic engineering and phenylketonuria, Pediatrics **74**(3):406-407, 1984.

Holm, V.A., and others: Physical growth in phenylketonuria. II. Growth of treated children in the PKU Collaborative Study from birth to 4 years of age, Pediatrics **63**:700-707, May 1979.

Holtzman, N.A.: Ethical issues in the prenatal diagnosis of phenylketonuria, Pediatrics **74**(3):424-427, 1984.

Johnson, C.F.: Phenylketonuria: a diagnosis that affects the entire family, Med. Times **107**:27-40, April 1979.

Kaufman, S.: Differential diagnosis of variant forms of hyperphenylalaninemia, Pediatrics **65**:840-842, April 1980.

Koch, R., and Friedman, E.G.: Accuracy of newborn screening programs for phenylketonuria, J. Pediatr. **98**:267-269, Feb. 1981.

Lenke, R.R., and others: Maternal phenylketonuria and hyperphenylalaninemia: an international survey of the outcome of untreated and treated pregnancies, N. Engl. J. Med. **303**:1202-1208, 1980.

Levy, H.L., and Waisbren, S.E.: Effects of untreated maternal phenylketonuria and hyperphenylalaninemia, New Engl. J. Med. **309**:1269-1274, 1983.

Matalon, R.: Current status of biopterin screening, J. Pediatr. **104**(4):579-581, 1984.

Meryash, D.L.: Prospective study of early neonatal screening for phenylketonuria, N. Engl. J. Med. **304**:294-296, Jan. 1981.

O'Flynn, M.E., and others: The diagnosis of phenylketonuria, Am. J. Dis. Child. **134**:769-774, Aug. 1980.

Reyzer, N.: Diagnosis: PKU, Am. J. Nurs. **78**:1895-1898, 1978.

Sbravati, C., and Fischer, R.G.: What sugar substitutes are available and are there any differences between them? Pediatr. Nurs. **9**(2):138, 1983.

Schor, D.P.: Phenylketonuria and temperament in middle childhood, Children's Health Care **14**(3):163-167, 1986.

Sepe, S.J., Levy, H.L., and Mount, F.W.: An evaluation of routine follow-up blood screening of infants for phenylketonuria, N. Engl. J. Med. **300**:600-609, March 1979.

Sturtevant, F.M.: Use of aspartame in pregnancy, Int. J. Fertil. **30**(1):85-87, 1985.

Williamson, M.L., and others: Correlates of intelligence test results in treated phenylketonuric children, Pediatrics **68**:161-167, Aug. 1981.

Woo, S.L.C.: Prenatal diagnosis and carrier detection of classic phenylketonuria by gene analysis, Pediatrics **74**(3):412-423, 1984.

Galactosemia

American Academy of Pediatrics, Committee on Drugs: "Inactive" ingredients in pharmaceutical products, Pediatrics **76**(4):635-643, 1985.

Berger, L.R.: When should one discourage breast-feeding? Pediatrics **67**:300-302, Feb. 1981.

Brown, J.: The health hazard of unlabeled ingredients in pharmaceuticals, Pediatrics **73**(3):402-404, 1984.

Komrower, G.: Inborn errors of metabolism, Pediatr. Rev. **2**:175-181, Dec. 1980.

Lechter, M.: "Hidden" lactose a source of GI distress, Patient Care **16**(8):122, 1982.

Levy, H.L., and Hammersen, G.: Newborn screening for galactosemia and other galactose metabolic defects, J. Pediatr. **92**(6):871-877, 1978.

Segal, S., Rutman, J.Y., and Frimpter, G.W.: Galactokinase deficiency and mental retardation, J. Pediatr. **95**:750-752, Nov. 1979.

Smith, E.J.: Galactosemia: an inborn error of metabolism, Nurse Pract. **5**:8-9, March/April 1980.

Chapter 10

The High-Risk Newborn and Family

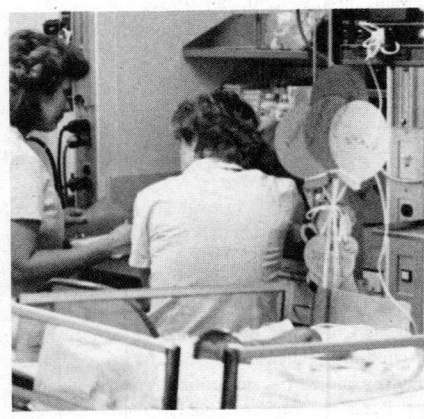

General Management of High-Risk Newborns
Identification of high-risk newborns
Anticipation of problems
Classification of high-risk newborns
Intensive care facilities
Organization of services
Transporting high-risk newborns

Nursing Care of High-Risk Newborns
General nursing management and care
Immediate care
Protection from infection
Monitoring physiologic data
Systematic assessment of the high-risk infant
Thermoregulation
Hydration
Skin care
Administration of medications

Meeting nutritional needs of high-risk neonates
Physiologic characteristics
Nutritional needs
Feeding methods
Supportive care of high-risk neonates and their families
Developmental correlates
Infant stimulation
Parental involvement
Facilitating parent-infant relationships
Discharge planning and home care
Neonatal loss

High-Risk Conditions Related to Dysmaturity
Preterm infants
Etiology
Characteristics
Therapeutic management
Nursing considerations
Postmature infants

High Risk Related to Disturbed Respiratory Function
Apnea of prematurity
Respiratory distress syndrome
Meconium aspiration syndrome
Extraneous air syndromes (air leaks)
Bronchopulmonary dysplasia

High Risk Related to Infectious Processes
Sepsis
Necrotizing enterocolitis

High Risk Related to Cardiovascular Complications
Persistent patent ductus arteriosus
Persistent pulmonary hypertension of the newborn
Anemia

Polycythemia/hyperviscosity syndrome
Retinopathy of prematurity

High Risk Related to Neurologic Disturbance
Perinatal hypoxic-ischemic brain injury
Periventricular-intraventricular hemorrhage
Intracranial hemorrhage
Subdural hematomas
Subarachnoid hemorrhage
Intracerebellar hemorrhage
Neonatal seizures

High Risk Related to Maternal Conditions
Infants of diabetic mothers
Maternal management
Effects of diabetes on the fetus
Drug-addicted infants
Infant of the mother who smokes

High-risk neonates can be defined as newborns, regardless of gestational age or birth weight, who have a greater than average chance of morbidity or mortality because of conditions or circumstances that are superimposed on the normal course of events associated with birth and the adjustment to extrauterine existence. This includes the periods in human growth and development from the time of viability until 28 days following birth and involves threats to life and health that occur during the prenatal, perinatal, and postnatal periods.

General Management of High-Risk Newborns

In recent years there has been an increase in the survival rate of newborns that has coincided with the establishment of programs to improve the health of mothers and the timing of their pregnancies, and the introduction of important new techniques in neonatal care (David and Siegel, 1983). This decreased neonatal mortality and the survival of low-birth-weight newborns has generated considerable debate and concern regarding the possibility of increased disability of survivors that might place additional demands on societal resources. Results of studies are variable and subject to interpretation, but there is evidence to suggest that the decline in mortality is not necessarily accompanied by increased morbidity (Starfield and others, 1982; Shapiro and others, 1983). However, there is an inverse relationship between the rate of survival and the incidence of newborns of very low birth weight (Kwang-sun and others, 1980). When problems are anticipated, preparations can be made for intensive care during the periods of greatest threat; through this care the incidence of fetal and neonatal mortality can be significantly reduced.

IDENTIFICATION OF HIGH-RISK NEWBORNS

Nurses in a variety of settings play an important role in detection and intervention where high-risk factors are most likely to occur. This care begins in the preconception period when parents at risk for problems associated with procreation (usually genetic defects) are provided with information to make a judicious decision regarding childbearing. In the prenatal period the most important aspect in anticipating or averting problems is early and consistent prenatal care. Nurses in the community are in a position to detect families in need and to arrange for ongoing prenatal observation. During labor and delivery the obstetric nurse alert to signs of fetal distress and maternal conditions that contribute to neonatal morbidity can avert numerous problems. Assessment and prompt intervention in life-threatening emergencies often make the difference between a favorable outcome and a lifetime of disability. The nurse in the newborn nursery is familiar with the characteristics of neonates and recognizes the significance of benign and serious deviations from expected observations.

It is estimated that 5% of newborns require care in special, intensive care nurseries and that only approximately half of the infants with potentially serious problems are identified at birth. Therefore the nurse is in the crucial position to identify those subtle signs that indicate impending difficulties—color changes, lethargy, poor feeding, altered vital signs, and other unusual behavior. When the need for specialized care can be anticipated and planned for, the probability of successful outcome is increased.

Anticipation of Problems

Many of the factors that influence the outcome of these vulnerable periods occur simultaneously and in combination. For example, infants born prematurely often suffer from perinatal asphyxia, have cerebral hemorrhage during delivery, have associated congenital anomalies, and develop hyaline membrane disease. The list of factors associated with increased risk in the neonatal period continues to grow as applied research in the fields of perinatology and neonatology adds new data. The major situations that contribute to perinatal morbidity, mortality in infancy, and possibly the future physical and intellectual qualities of the child, or that warn of impending difficulties include the following:

Preconceptual

Hereditary diseases or abnormalities—inborn errors of metabolism, anomalies of heart and central nervous system, sickle cell anemia, and many others

Socioeconomic factors—poor nutrition and general health of mother; frequently teenage pregnancy

High altitude—associated with low-birth-weight infants

Parental age
  Maternal—over 35 or under 16 years of age
  Paternal—over 40 years of age

Maternal size—less than 5 feet; prepregnant weight greater than 20% over or under standards for height and weight

Grand multiparity—more than five, especially when the mother is over 35 years of age

History of obstetric complications—prolonged period of infertility, spontaneous abortion, placental accidents, previous larger-than-average or small-for-date newborns, eclampsia, isoimmunization, multiple pregnancies, previous birth of abnormal infant

Uterine abnormality—tumors (fibroid, myoma), developmental anomalies (uterus bicornis), incompetent cervix

Prenatal

Maternal disease—preeclampsia, hypertension, malignancy, heart disease, hemoglobinopathy, renal diseases, endocrine diseases (thyroid, diabetes)

Maternal infection—bacterial, viral, spirochetal, protozoal

Maternal disorders associated with pregnancy—preeclampsia, placental abnormalities, hyperemesis gravidarum

Socioeconomic problems—malnutrition, long-delayed or absent prenatal care

Maternal addiction—narcotics, barbiturates, amphetamines, hallucinogens

Maternal medication—no drug is absolutely safe

Gases—maternal smoking, anesthesia

Multiple pregnancy—smaller fetal size and premature delivery

Isoimmunization—Rh or ABO blood incompatibility

Uterine accidents—abruptio placentae, placenta previa, ruptured uterus, trauma

Fetal size—larger or smaller than expected for age; over or under normal gestational age (preterm, postterm); cephalopelvic disproportion

Polyhydramnios or oligohydramnios—often associated with fetal anomalies

Diagnostic procedures—x-ray films or treatment, amniocentesis

Surgical procedures—incidental operation during course of pregnancy

Natal (Intrapartum)

Fever—may indicate maternal infection

Premature labor—preterm infant is at greater risk

Premature rupture of fetal membranes—associated with intrauterine infection and prolapse of umbilical cord

Fetal distress—tachycardia (fetal heart rate above 180 beats per minute), bradycardia (fetal heart rate below 120 beats per minute), irregular heart rate, meconium-stained amniotic fluid (in vertex presentation), abnormal deceleration curve (monitored), scalp vein pH 7.2 or less

Abnormalities of fetal position—transverse, breech, unengaged presenting part

Cesarean section—associated with higher neonatal morbidity; often performed because of adverse prenatal or natal conditions

Abnormal labor and/or delivery—precipitous, prolonged, breech, assisted (forceps), other complications

Uterine accidents—rupture, abruptio placentae

Cord accidents—knots, tight nuchal cord, prolapse

Maternal analgesia or anesthesia—may cause depression in fetus and newborn

Postnatal (Immediate)

Single umbilical artery—may be associated with fetal anomalies

Low Apgar score—especially 5-minute test

Abnormal placenta—massive infarction, evidence of separation, amnionitis

Prematurity—newborn less able to withstand rigors of birth and transition

Multiple birth—newborns usually small and immature at birth

Disproportion between weight or length and gestational age—may indicate intrauterine growth retardation, intrauterine malnutrition, concomitant disorders e.g., infant of diabetic mother)

Depression—may indicate central nervous system damage, hypoxia, maternal oversedation

Birth trauma—head injury, fractures, nerve damage

Presence of congenital anomalies—cleft palate, imperforate anus, choanal atresia, omphalocele, diaphragmatic hernia, tracheoesophageal fistula, cardiovascular defect

Severe blood loss, sepsis, meconium aspiration—adversely influence adjustment

Postnatal (Warning Signs)

Abnormal respiration—may indicate congenital anomalies, lung syndromes, acidosis

Apneic episodes—may be caused by such factors as central nervous system disturbance, immaturity of regulatory mechanisms, congestion, obstruction, drugs, cardiac anomalies, hypoglycemia, hypocalcemia

Tremor and/or seizures—may indicate hypoglycemia, hypocalcemia, narcotic addiction, central nervous system hemorrhage or infection, postasphyxia, depression

Limpness and/or lethargy—may be the result of sepsis, central nervous system damage, hypoxia, Down syndrome, hypothyroidism

Vomiting or difficulty in swallowing—central nervous system damage, immature reflexes, congenital defects

Abdominal distention—may indicate congenital anomalies

Failure to void or pass meconium in first 24 hours—associated with congenital anomalies

Pallor—may indicate anemia, hemorrhage, or cold stress

Jaundice—especially serious when appears in first 24 hours

Petechiae—a sign of thrombocytopenia

Thermal instability—iatrogenic factors, central nervous system damage, immaturity, environmental factors

Failure to regain birth weight by 10 days of age—congenital anomalies, metabolic disorders, central nervous system damage, sepsis, feeding difficulties

Cyanosis—respiratory or cardiac disorders, apnea

Although not considered high-risk situations in the usual sense, difficulties in the ability of the mother to properly care for the child or disturbances in the mother-child relationship can have serious consequences—both immediate and long term—for the infant. These difficulties may be caused by neurologic, malignant, rheumatic, or other disorders that impair the mother's ability to physically care for her infant by psychologic illness that interferes with her ability to provide proper care for the child. These situations are not discussed in depth here; however, nurses must be alert to indications of these special problems that may profoundly influence the well-being of the infant and place the infant at risk.

Classification of High-Risk Newborns

High-risk infants are most often classified according to size, gestational age, and predominant pathophysiologic problems. The more common problems related to physiologic status are closely associated with the state of maturity of the infant and usually involve chemical disturbances (e.g., hypoglycemia, hypocalcemia) and consequences of immature functioning organs and systems (e.g., hyperbilirubinemia, respiratory distress, hypothermia). Since high-risk factors are common to several specialty areas, particularly obstetrics, pediatrics, and neonatology, specific terminology is needed to describe the developmental status of the newborn.

Formerly, weight at birth was considered to reflect a reasonably accurate estimation of gestational age. That is, if infants' birth weights exceeded 2500 g (5½ pounds), they were considered to be mature. However, accumulated data have shown that intrauterine growth rates are not the same for all infants and that other factors (e.g., heredity, placental insufficiency, and maternal disease) influence intrauterine growth and birth weight of the infant. From these data a more definitive and meaningful classification system that encompasses size, gestational age, and fetal outcome has been developed. It has also been determined that the lowest perinatal mortality is found in the full-term infant who weighs between 3500 and 4000 g.

Classification According to Size

low-birth-weight (LBW) infant An infant whose birth weight is less than 2500 g regardless of gestational age

very-low-birth-weight (VLBW) infant An infant whose weight is less than 1500 g

appropriate-for-gestational-age (AGA) infant An infant whose intrauterine growth was normal at the moment of birth

small-for-date (SFD) or small-for-gestational-age (SGA) infant An infant whose rate of intrauterine growth was slowed and who was delivered at or later than term; these infants are usually 2 standard deviations below the mean for infants of appropriate weight at birth, and their birth weight falls below the 10th percentile on intrauterine growth curves

intrauterine growth retardation (IUGR) Found in infants whose intrauterine growth is retarded (sometimes used as a more descriptive term for the SGA infant)

large-for-gestational-age (LGA) infant An infant whose birth weight falls above the 90th percentile on intrauterine growth curves

Classification According to Gestational Age

premature (preterm) infant An infant born before completion of the 37 weeks of gestation, regardless of birth weight

term infant An infant born between the beginning of the 38 weeks and the completion of the 42 weeks of gestation, regardless of birth weight

postmature (postterm) infant An infant born after 42 weeks of gestational age, regardless of birth weight

Classification According to Mortality

live birth Birth in which the neonate manifests any heartbeat, breathes, or displays voluntary movement, regardless of gestational age

fetal death Death of the fetus after 20 weeks of gestation and before delivery, regardless of gestational age and with absence of any signs of life following birth

neonatal death Death that occurs in the first 28 days of life; early neonatal or postnatal deaths occur in the first week of life

perinatal mortality Describes the total number of fetal and early neonatal deaths per 1000 births

Many problems can be anticipated before delivery. Prenatal testing and labor monitoring have reduced the incidence of perinatal mortality, and specialized care of the distressed newborn is improving the survival rate. If the infant is likely to require special therapy at or soon after birth, plans can be made for the delivery to take place at or near a hospital that has the facilities to provide such care. In this way there is no delay in initiating needed care, and some of the hazards associated with transporting the sick newborn are averted.

INTENSIVE CARE FACILITIES

Awareness of the unique characteristics of perinatal disorders has generated the provision of special care units in major medical facilities. Rapid advances in the understanding of the pathophysiology of the neonate and the increased ca-

pacity to apply this knowledge have emphasized the need for appropriate settings in which to care for the seriously ill infant. Much of the impetus for special care units arose in response to advancements in electronics and biochemistry and to the emergence of neonatology and perinatology as separate disciplines of medicine and nursing. New methods for monitoring cardiorespiratory function, microtechniques for biochemical determination from minute quantities of blood, and new methods for assisted ventilation and conservation of body heat have made it possible to effectively manage the newborn with serious illness.

Intensive care of the ill and immature newborn requires specialized knowledge and skill in a number of areas of expertise. Much of the equipment long used in the care of the critically ill adult is unsuited to the singular needs of the very small infant; therefore commonplace apparatus has been modified to meet these needs. Examples of modifications include respirators that deliver small volumes of oxygen in the proper concentration and pressure, infusion pumps that deliver very small amounts accurately, and crib units that provide a constant source of warmth and at the same time allow maximum access to the infant. Most important, intensive care has created a need for highly skilled personnel specially trained in the art of neonatal intensive care.

Special care units are designed to meet a wide range of special needs, from the observation of apparently well infants who have been determined to be at risk of serious illness to the intensive treatment of acutely ill infants whose survival is in doubt. This diversity requires that the unit be arranged for graduated care for the infant population. There should be adequate facilities and skilled personnel to provide one-to-one nursing care for each seriously ill infant in addition to a means for graduation to one-to-four or one-to-five nursing care in a convalescent area where the infants require less intensive care until they are ready to leave the unit.

Nurses in the neonatal intensive care unit (NICU) are highly trained in the management of a variety of sophisticated mechanical devices and educated in the art of recognizing subtle changes in infants' behavior, interpreting observations of others, and timing interventions appropriately. Proficiency is developed through daily observation and practice under the guidance of a skilled practitioner; in-service education is one of the prime objectives in the ongoing management of a successful NICU. The teaching activities of nurses in the NICU are extended to include not only new nurses but also residents, interns, and parents.

Organization of Services

It is not economically feasible for every institution to have a functioning neonatal intensive care facility; therefore most services of this kind are organized on a regional basis. A regionalized system consists of facilities within a designated geographic area that provide three prescribed levels of care with special equipment, skilled personnel, and ancillary services concentrated in a centralized institution. The characteristics of these facilities are:

Level I—a facility designed to provide management of normal maternal and newborn care but able to identify high-risk pregnancies and/or high-risk neonates early and implement emergency care in the event of complications. These are usually small community hospitals removed from urban areas but vital to health care in the area.

Level II—a facility that serves larger communities, usually is located in urban or suburban areas, and provides a full range of maternity and newborn care. It is equipped to manage the majority of maternal and neonatal complications, depending on the resources available.

Level III—a facility that offers the full range of maternal and newborn services of a level II facility. In addition, it has the capacity to provide care for the most complex neonatal complications. At least one full-time neonatologist is on the staff as well as an impressive complement of pediatric subspecialists, including pediatric surgeons, geneticists, radiologists, anesthesiologists, and hospital epidemiologists who are at the disposal of the unit. All but some highly specialized types of cases are managed in a level III facility. Occasionally an infant requires specialized services not provided by all units, such as the infant with congenital heart disease or some other complex congenital anomaly.

Transporting High-Risk Newborns

When the infant at risk is identified or anticipated, arrangements are made for care in the intensive care facility. There is no question that the uterus is the ideal transport unit for the infant with anticipated difficulties; therefore whenever possible the mother is taken where special care is available for her delivery.

However, many infants develop difficulties after a seemingly normal pregnancy and uncomplicated labor. Since it is impossible to predict when infants will require intensive care, a coordinated system is needed to ensure them an optimum opportunity for survival. Each hospital that delivers infants should be able to provide for appropriate stabilization and arrange for transport to a centralized facility. The infant must be warm, well-oxygenated (including intubation if indicated), and when possible, receiving an intravenous infusion. It may be up to 4 hours before the infant is sufficiently stabilized for transfer.

Communication is the key to the success of a transport system. The neonatologist in the intensive care facility controls and directs the operation, which must be available on a 24-hour basis. The transfer is initiated by the referring physician, who communicates the problem to the neonatologist. The neonatologist in turn notifies the transport team and alerts the intensive care unit to the nature of the problem so that preparations can be made to receive the infant. The transport unit is dispatched to the referring institution. The infant is transported in a specially designed incubator unit, containing a complete life-support system that can be carried by ambulance, van, or helicopter (Fig. 10-1). The

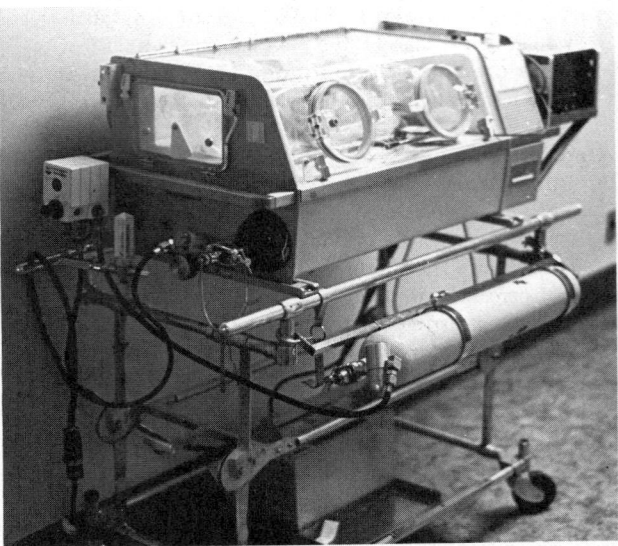

Fig. 10-1. Self-sustained infant transport unit.

team also takes along a monitor and an assortment of emergency equipment.

The transport team may consist of one or more of the highly trained persons from the NICU: a neonatologist (or a Fellow in Neonatology), a respiratory therapist, and one or more nurses. When complex problems are anticipated, the neonatologist or Fellow accompanies the infant; in relatively uncomplicated cases a nurse may go alone. The person assigned to accompany the infant must be constantly alert to every change in the infant's condition and be able to intervene appropriately. The neonate who must be moved from one place to another within the hospital (e.g., to surgery, from delivery room to nursery) is transported in an incubator or radiant warmer accompanied by necessary personnel and equipment.

Nursing Care of High-Risk Newborns

Nurses in an NICU are vital to the successful operation of the unit and the ultimate outcome of infant therapy. Neonatal intensive care nursing is a highly specialized area of knowledge and practice that requires lengthy supervised experience to reach a level of competence that permits independent nursing care. It involves an understanding of neonatal physiology and characteristics, a knowledge of the function and management of a number of mechanical devices and apparatus, the ability to recognize very subtle deviations from the expected, and the ability to implement a judicious course of action.

Nurses working in NICUs are subject to stresses not found in most nursing units. The critical nature of their patients' conditions generates a stressful atmosphere. The care demands constant observation with rapid evaluation and intervention. The infants are unresponsive, physical eye contact is impossible or minimum at best, and even during the recovery phase the infant is unable to provide any positive reinforcement because of his developmental level. Parents may be able to supply some encouragement but their own concerns and anxieties impede such responses and more often place additional obligations on nurses (see p. 387). In addition, although the environment with large expanses of glass and counters allows for maximum visibility of the infants, staff members are placed under constant observation as well.

GENERAL NURSING MANAGEMENT AND CARE

Since the majority of infants who are admitted to intensive care facilities are born before the estimated date of delivery, the major discussion of problems related to the high-risk neonate will be directed toward the preterm infant. Prematurity is generally accepted as the single largest factor contributing to infant mortality (see p. 393 for a description of the characteristics of preterm infants). The incidence of neonatal complications, (e.g., hyperbilirubinemia, and hyaline membrane disease) is highest in this group, and often other high-risk factors (e.g., severe congenital malformations) are found in association with prematurity.

Many of the components of care and observation that apply to the nursing of the high-risk newborn are discussed in Chapters 8 and 9. Particularly relevant are: Assessment of gestational age (p. 303), Hyperbilirubinemia (p. 346), Hypoglycemia (p. 356), and Hypocalcemia (p. 357). Other factors are considered throughout the remainder of this chapter and summarized in relation to specific patient problems. Nursing problems encountered in the intensive care nursery are discussed, followed by a consideration of common complications. Nursing care of high-risk infants with more serious disorders is examined in relation to specific high-risk conditions.

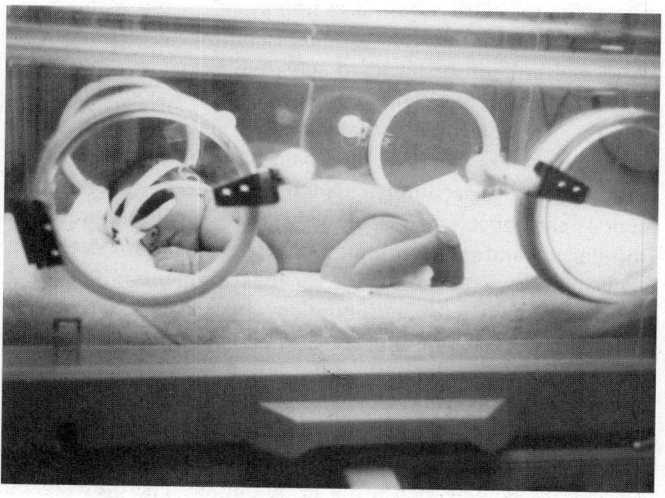

Fig. 10-2. Infant in Isolette.

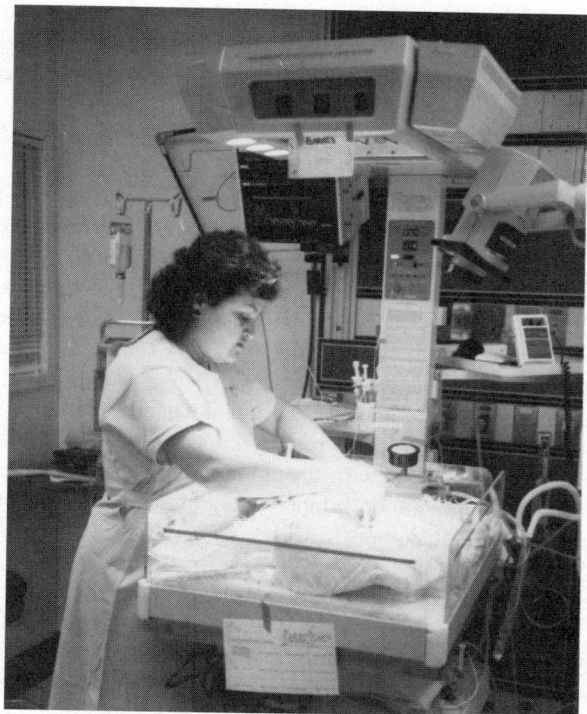

Fig. 10-3. Infant under overhead warming unit.

Immediate Care

At birth the newborn is given a rapid assessment to determine any apparent problems and identify those that demand immediate attention. This examination is primarily concerned with the evaluation of cardiopulmonary and neurologic functions. The assessment includes the assignment of an Apgar score (see p. 298) and an evaluation for pallor, cyanosis, prematurity, any obvious congenital anomalies, or evidence of neonatal disease. Delivery rooms are equipped with a special resuscitation area where infants with a low Apgar score or other evidence of distress are resuscitated and evaluated before being transported to the NICU for initiation of therapy and more extensive assessment. During all activities a prime consideration is the conservation of body heat.

The naked infant is placed in the controlled microenvironment of an Isolette. A Plexiglas top affords a clear view of the infant from all aspects. Easy access through portholes minimizes temperature and oxygen loss, and a large door provides a more extensive approach (Fig. 10-2). Maximum accessibility is provided by an open unit with an overhead radiant warming system. These units are employed for distressed infants who require a wide range of mechanical instrumentation, such as a ventilator, monitors, and intravenous infusions, and frequent manipulation, such as vital signs, suctioning, and chest percussion (Fig. 10-3).

Maintaining detailed, ongoing records of all activities and observations is an important responsibility of nurses in the intensive care setting. Knowledge and operation of complex pieces of equipment and mechanical devices are inherent in the care of the ill neonate. However, sophisticated monitoring and life-support systems cannot replace the vigilance and constant scrutiny of the infants by experienced personnel.

Protection from Infection

The life saving attributes of the neonatal intensive care facility do not obviate the need for ongoing measures to avoid the imposition of additional hazards on the infant who is already at risk. Protection from infection is an integral part of all newborn care. Preterm and sick neonates are particularly susceptible; therefore care must be exercised to avoid their contact with contaminants.

Thorough, meticulous, and frequent handwashing is the foundation of a preventive program and includes all persons who come in contact with the infants and their equipment. After handling another infant or equipment, no one ever touches an infant without washing hands first.

Special clothing furnished by the institution is worn by everyone working in the unit. Fresh scrub dresses or suits are put on before entering the unit and are changed any time they become contaminated. When personnel leave the unit, the clothing is protected by a cover gown that is removed and discarded in the laundry hamper when reentering. Anyone entering the unit for a short time, whether or not they provide any care, must scrub thoroughly and either change to appropriate clothing or wear a cover gown. Parents are taught these precautionary measures and become willing and cooperative allies in protecting their infants from infection.

The sources of infection rise in direct relationship to the number of persons and pieces of equipment coming in contact with the infants. All linen and equipment used in the care of the infants is either sterile or scrupulously clean, and nondisposable items are cultured regularly for the presence of infectious organisms; protocol is established by each institution. Since organisms thrive best in water, plumbing and humidifying equipment are particularly hazardous. Disposable equipment used for water-related therapies, such as nebulizers and tubing, is changed regularly. For example, plastic tubes are discarded after 24 hours and water in humidifiers is changed every 8 hours.

Personnel with infectious disorders either are barred from the unit until they can no longer transmit the disease to the infants and other personnel or are required to wear suitable shields, such as masks or gloves, to reduce the likelihood of contamination. Most of the infants are effectively isolated from airborne infective agents in the protective environment of the Isolette. However, the Isolette must be cleaned regularly as part of the infection control measures.

Monitoring Physiologic Data

Most neonates under intensive observation are placed in a controlled thermal environment and monitored for heart rate, respiratory activity, and temperature. Routine monitoring of heart rate consists of a pulse rate indicator that signals each ventricular contraction by an audible beep and flashing light. The indicator is integrated with an alarm system so that a pulse rate above or below predetermined limits triggers the alarm. When the heart rate falls below or rises above the preset rate, both audio and visual alarms alert the nurse. The limits for cardiac monitors are determined by the condition of the individual infant and the philosophy of the special care unit, but they are usually set to activate when below 100 beats per minute and above 180 beats per minute. Each alarm requires the nurse to observe, assess the situation, and make a decision regarding the infant's status. Factors other than altered infant condition may trigger the alarm, for example, poor contact between the infant and the electrodes, loose connections, poor placement, inadequate grounding, soiled electrodes, or movement. Cardiac monitors with the sensitivity set too high sometimes register more than one point of the QRS complex in the cardiac cycle, giving a falsely high pulse reading. Therefore it is essential to check the heartbeat and compare it with the monitor reading. Proper placement and maintenance of electrodes and their connections are nursing responsibilities. Electrodes are either attached topically to the outer aspects of the chest wall, one on each side, by special electrode paste or jelly and adhesive disks or by needle electrodes inserted intradermally and anchored with transpore tape.

Respiratory activity is also monitored because the heart rate does not always drop with apnea, although bradycardia frequently follows an apneic spell. Apnea monitors consist of an impedance monitor that measures the electrical resistance across the chest as it changes with respiration. The alarm works in the same manner as the cardiac monitor. It is usually set at a 10- to 15-second delay for apnea. This involves electrode placement as in cardiac monitoring, and the two are often combined in the same monitoring equipment.

The placement of electrodes is a continual nursing problem because of the lack of flat areas on the neonate's chest and the limited space for alternating sites, the size of the electrodes, and irritation from the paste or tape. Electrodes for monitors can often be applied to the upper arms to provide relief for chest areas. It is important to follow the manufacturer's directions for care and handling of electrodes to avoid malfunction or burns to sensitive skin.

Blood pressure is monitored routinely in the sick neonate by either internal or external means. Direct recording with arterial catheters is often employed but carries the risks inherent in any procedure in which a needle or other implement is introduced into a blood vessel. The transcutaneous Doppler apparatus is a simple, effective means for detecting weak impulses (see Fig. 10-4 for measurements).

In the NICU, frequent laboratory examinations are an integral part of the ongoing assessment of infants' progress. Accurate intake and output records are kept on all infants. An accurate output can be obtained by collection of urine in a plastic urine collection bag (see p. 1127) or by weighing the diapers. Weighing the diapers is the simplest and least traumatic means of measuring urine output. The preweighed wet diaper is weighed on a gram scale, and the gram weight of the urine is converted directly to milliliters, for example,

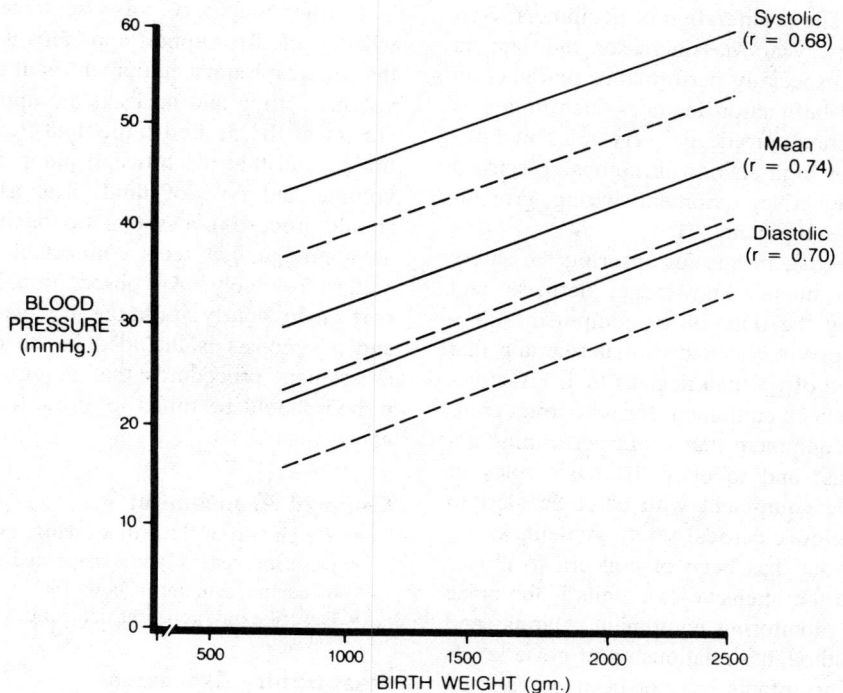

Fig. 10-4. Linear regression of systolic, mean, and diastolic blood pressure vs. birth weights during the first 24 hours of life in 59 premature infants (n = 120). The dotted lines represent lowest systolic, diastolic, and mean pressures at 90% confidence level.

From Fanaroff, A.A., and Martin, R.J., editors: Neonatal-perinatal medicine, St. Louis, 1983, The C.V. Mosby Co., p. 128.

25 g = 25 ml. Cotton balls inside the diaper next to the perineum absorb moisture that can be easily extracted with a syringe or weighed. Plastic collecting devices can be used when it is necessary to collect urine for laboratory examination. Specific gravity is often measured as a screening for renal function and adequacy of hydration. Since the volume normally voided is insufficient to float the standard urometer, a refractometer requiring only a single drop of urine is standard equipment in the NICU. A drop of urine can be easily aspirated from the wet diaper or cotton balls with a syringe.

Blood examinations are a necessary part of the ongoing assessment and monitoring of the sick neonate's progress. The tests performed most often are blood glucose, bilirubin, calcium, hematocrit, and blood gases. Samples may be obtained by taking blood from the heel, by venipuncture, or by an indwelling catheter in an umbilical vein, umbilical artery, or peripheral artery. The indwelling catheter is usually connected to a heparin lock system in order to prevent clotting of blood in the needle. When the specimen is being collected, it is important to relate the type of test to the treatment the infant is receiving. For example, when an infant is receiving an intravenous infusion of glucose solution, collecting a sample of blood from the heel would provide a more accurate picture of the blood glucose level than would a sample from the intravenous catheter, and phototherapy must be discontinued when a blood sample is drawn for a bilirubin level test because the light will alter the bilirubin in the sample.

Capillary samples are usually collected from the heel after the foot has been warmed to approximately 45.5° C (110° F), which takes 5 to 10 minutes. Wrapping the foot in a warm washcloth is simple way to create adequate vasodilation (see p. 1129 for procedure). This is a stress-producing procedure, but research has indicated that nonnutritive sucking during the procedure produces a pacifying effect on the infant (Field and Goldson, 1984). When numerous samples must be drawn, it is important to keep a record of the amount of blood removed, since a tiny infant's blood supply can be seriously depleted over a period of time.

To secure frequent samples for monitoring arterial blood gas levels, it is preferable to use transcutaneous oxygen measurements in order to avoid repeated arterial punctures. Continuous readings of oxygen tensions can be obtained from transcutaneous sensors secured to the skin by electrodes. The device provides PO_2 values from warmed skin that closely correlate with arterial PO_2 values. The nurse must note any changes associated with handling to take advantage of optimum position based on interpretation of readings. Hourly readings are recorded with vital signs. Other monitoring devices may be employed in the care of the high-risk neonate, such as transcutaneous bilirubinometry (p. 348).

Safety measures. The proliferation of equipment technology over the past few years has increased the dangers associated with its use, especially performance malfunction and electrical hazards. Malfunction includes such things as inaccurate monitor function, erratic delivery rates in infusion devices, and low or high suction in pumps. Electrical hazards are related to defective equipment, wiring, grounding, or improper use of equipment.

One of the most effective means for ensuring the safety of infant and staff is the nurse's knowledge, alertness, and common sense regarding the function of equipment. Electronic monitoring devices are checked to make certain that the alarms are not turned off, which negates their effectiveness. It is important to check equipment for all correct component parts, to report equipment that is not performing according to specifications, and to obey the basic rules of electrical safety—handle equipment with care, be alert to signs of trouble, and follow electrical safety guidelines.

A hazard to infants that has been of concern to nurses and others who work in the intensive care units is the noise level that results from monitoring equipment, alarms, and general unit activity. Although a relationship of noise levels and deafness in surviving infants has not been proven and risk criteria have not been established, personnel are cautioned to reduce noise-generating activities such as closing doors, loud radios and conversation, and handling equipment (e.g., trash containers) (Hansen, 1982). Noise levels have been correlated with the incidence of intracranial hemorrhage, especially in the very low-birth-weight infant, as determined by auditory brainstem potentials (Marshall and others, 1980).

Parents need to be instructed regarding safety precautions and observations. They are usually uncomfortable around the equipment and atmosphere of an intensive care unit and therefore appreciate an explanation of the purposes and functions of the devices and pertinent safety aspects.

Systematic Assessment of the High-Risk Infant

Subtle changes not apparent through the mechanical devices can be detected by alert nurses, for example, changes in color and regurgitated formula, which will not register on a monitor until aspiration produces an apneic spell. Some of the crucial factors in observation of ill newborns cannot be detected by monitors, including feeding behaviors, abdominal distention and stool characteristics, behavior, skin manifestations, character and location of heart sounds, and respiratory data such as retractions, flaring nares, and grunting.

Nurses are usually responsible for the same infants each day, which allows for more accurate determination of day-to-day progress. During the course of daily care the nurse makes frequent systematic assessments of physical status, since vital signs of small infants change several times in the period of a very few hours. It has been said that the newborn undergoes as many changes in 4 to 6 hours as an adult does in 24 hours.

In the course of an assessment the nurse ascertains whether the life-support apparatus is functioning properly—that the respiratory equipment is at the correct pressure and volume setting and no leaks are apparent, that the monitors are set at the desired limits and tracings are within normal limits, and that the infusion pump is delivering the correct volume and type of fluid. The assessment of the infant should proceed in a systematic manner. Each nurse develops an approach that feels comfortable and follows the same pattern routinely. An observational assessment is usually performed hourly, or more frequently on very ill infants, and a synopsis is included in the charting. However, any assessment procedures that require that the infant be disturbed should be timed to allow for sufficient rest between assessments.

General Assessment

- Weigh two or three times daily, as ordered.
- Describe general body shape and size, presence and location of edema, amount of body fat.
- Describe any apparent deformities.

Respiratory Assessment

- Describe shape of chest (barrel, concave), symmetry, presence of incisions, chest tubes, or other deviations.
- Describe use of accessory muscles: nasal flaring or substernal, intercostal, or subclavicular retractions.
- Determine respiratory rate and regularity.
- Describe breath sounds: rales, rhonchi, wheezing, wet diminished sounds, areas of absence of sound, grunting.
- Determine whether suctioning is needed.
- Describe cry.
- Describe ambient oxygen and method of delivery; if intubated, describe size of tube, type of ventilator, and settings.

Cardiovascular Assessment

- Determine heart rate and rhythm.
- Describe heart sounds, including any suspected murmurs.
- Determine the point of maximum intensity (PMI), the point where the heartbeat sounds loudest (a change in the point of maximum intensity may indicate a mediastinal shift).
- Describe infant's color (may be of cardiac, respiratory, or hematopoietic origin): cyanosis, pallor, plethora, jaundice.
- Determine blood pressure (see Fig. 10-4). Indicate extremity used.
- Describe peripheral pulses.
- Determine central venous pressure (if central venous pressure line is part of infant's apparatus).
- Describe monitors and their parameters.

Gastrointestinal Assessment

- Determine presence of any indication of abdominal distention: increase in circumference, shiny skin.
- Determine any signs of regurgitation, especially following feeding; character and amount of residual if gavage-fed; if nasogastric tube in place, describe type of suction, drainage (color, consistency, pH, guaiac).
- Describe amount, color, consistency, and odor of any emesis.

- Describe amount, color, and consistency of stools; check for occult blood if indicated by physician's order or appearance of stool.
- Describe bowel sounds: presence or absence.

Genitourinary Assessment

- Describe any abnormalities of genitalia.
- Describe amount (as determined by weight), color, pH, lab-stick findings, and specific gravity of urine (to screen for adequacy of hydration).
- Check weight (the most accurate measure for assessment of hydration).

Neurologic-Musculoskeletal Assessment

- Describe infant's movements: random, purposeful, jittery, twitching, spontaneous, elicited.
- Describe infant's position or attitude: flexed, extended.
- Describe reflexes observed: Moro, sucking, Babinski, and other expected reflexes.
- Determine level of response.
- Determine changes in head circumference (if indicated).
- Determine pupillary responses.

Temperature

- Determine axillary temperature.
- Determine relationship to environmental temperature.

Skin Assessment

- Describe any discoloration, reddened area, or signs of irritation, especially where monitoring equipment, infusions, or other apparatus comes in contact with skin; also check and note any skin preparation used (e.g., povodine-iodine).
- Determine texture and turgor of skin: dry, smooth, flaky, peeling, etc.
- Describe any rash or skin lesion.
- Determine whether intravenous infusion catheter or needle is in place and observe for signs of infiltration.
- Describe parenteral infusion lines: location, type (arterial, venous, hyperalimentation, central venous pressure); type of infusion and relevant information; type of infusion pump and rate of flow; type of needle (butterfly, Quik-Cath); appearance of insertion site.

The infant's position is changed every 1 to 2 hours, and any significant reaction to the changing process or to a specific position is noted. To conserve the infant's energy, the position changing and periodic treatments should be timed to coincide with an assessment. Much of the assessment can be accomplished without moving the child, but necessary handling is minimum and as atraumatic as possible.

Thermoregulation

After the establishment of respiration, the most crucial need of the LBW infant is application of external warmth. Prevention of heat loss in the distressed infant is absolutely essential for survival, and maintaining a neutral thermal environment is a challenging aspect of neonatal intensive nursing care. Heat production is a complicated process that involves the cardiovascular, neurologic, and metabolic systems, and the immature neonate has all the problems related to heat production that are faced by the full-term infant (see p. 295). However, LBW infants are placed at further disadvantage by a number of additional problems. They have an even smaller muscle mass for producing heat, lack insulating subcutaneous fat, and have poor reflex control of skin capillaries.

Pathophysiology. The immature neonate, unable to increase activity and lacking a shivering response, produces heat primarily through increased metabolic processes. Some heat continues to be generated by liver, heart, brain, and skeletal muscles, but the major source of increased production of heat during cold stress is *nonshivering thermogenesis*. Norepinephrine, secreted by the sympathetic nerve endings in response to chilling, stimulates fat metabolism in the richly vascularized brown adipose tissue to produce internal heat, which is then conducted through the blood to surface tissues. Significantly an increase in metabolism requires an increase in oxygen consumption.

The consequences of cold stress that produce additional hazards to the neonate are hypoxia, metabolic acidosis, and hypoglycemia. Increased metabolism in response to chilling creates a compensatory increase in oxygen and calorie consumption. If available oxygen is not increased to accommodate this need, arterial oxygen tension is decreased. This is further complicated by a smaller lung volume in relation to metabolic rate that creates diminished oxygen in the blood. There is a small advantage gained by the persistence of fetal hemoglobin (HgF) because its increased capacity to carry oxygen allows the infant to exist for longer periods in conditions of lowered oxygen tension.

It also appears that norepinephrine, released in response to cold stress, causes pulmonary vasoconstriction, which further reduces the effectiveness of pulmonary ventilation. This decrease in oxygen diminishes the supply available for glucose metabolism. As a result, glucose is broken down by an alternate, hypoxic pathway (anaerobic glycolysis) that generates increased lactic acid formation. This, together with acid end-products of brown fat metabolism, contributes to the acidotic state. Anaerobic metabolism dissipates glycogen at a greatly increased rate over aerobic metabolism, thus precipitating hypoglycemia. This condition is especially marked when glycogen stores are diminished at birth and when there is inadequate caloric intake after birth.

Maintaining thermoneutrality. To delay or prevent the effects of cold stress, newborns at risk are placed in a heated environment immediately following birth where they remain until they are able to maintain *thermal stability*, the capacity to balance heat production and conservation and heat dissipation. Since overheating produces an increase in oxygen and calorie consumption, the infant is also jeopardized in a hyperthermic environment. A *neutral thermal environment* is one that permits the infant to maintain a normal core temperature with minimum oxygen consumption and calorie expenditure.

The VLBW infant, with thin skin and almost no subcutaneous fat, can control body heat loss or gain only within a very limited range of environmental temperature. In these infants evaporative heat loss is three to five times greater than in larger infants, and a decrease in body temperature is associated with an increase in mortality (Saur and Visser, 1984).

The three methods for maintaining a neutral thermal environment are by the use of a radiant warming panel, an Isolette, and an open bassinet with cotton blankets. The dressed infant under blankets can maintain a temperature within a wider range of environmental temperatures; however, the close observations required by a high-risk infant are best accomplished if the infant remains unclothed. The use of double-walled Isolettes significantly improves the infant's ability to maintain a desirable temperature and reduce energy expenditure related to heat regulation. When the infant is removed from the warm environment of the Isolette for feeding or cuddling, he is clothed and wrapped warmly in blankets. To prevent undue heat loss from the head, a small stocking cap can be fashioned from stockinette for the infant to wear outside the enclosed crib or Isolette (Fig. 10-5).

The most effective means for maintaining the desired range of temperature in the naked infant is by way of a manually adjusted or automatically controlled (servocontrolled) heat panel. The latter mechanism, when set at the upper and lower limits of the desired circulating air temperature range, adjusts automatically in response to signals from a thermal sensor attached to the abdominal skin. If the infant's temperature drops, the warming device is triggered to increase heat output.

There are always disadvantages inherent in any mechanical device; therefore an important part of nursing assessment is to compare the infant's temperature with the temperature in the Isolette. For example, if the infant's temperature fluctuates in response to sepsis or intracranial hemorrhage, the servocontrolled mechanism would respond by decreasing or increasing the ambient air temperature. Therefore a critical observation could be easily overlooked. A heat-sensing probe attached to the abdomen registers a false high temperature when the infant is in the prone position. Either the probe should be moved to the flank area of the back when the infant is placed in the prone position or the infant should remain on the back or side or in a partial side-lying position.

Body temperature regulation can also be influenced by thermal sensors located in the trigeminal area of the face and on the forehead. When the infant's face is exposed to a cool environmental temperature, even though the body is adequately warmed, these temperature-stimulation zones respond as though the infant is cold stressed. For this reason oxygen or any source of air, such as an oxygen mask or tube, should not blow directly on the infant's face. Oxygen concentrated around the head, such as that supplied to a hood, must be warmed.

Because of their relative lack of thermal insulation by body fat, preterm infants have temperatures that vary less

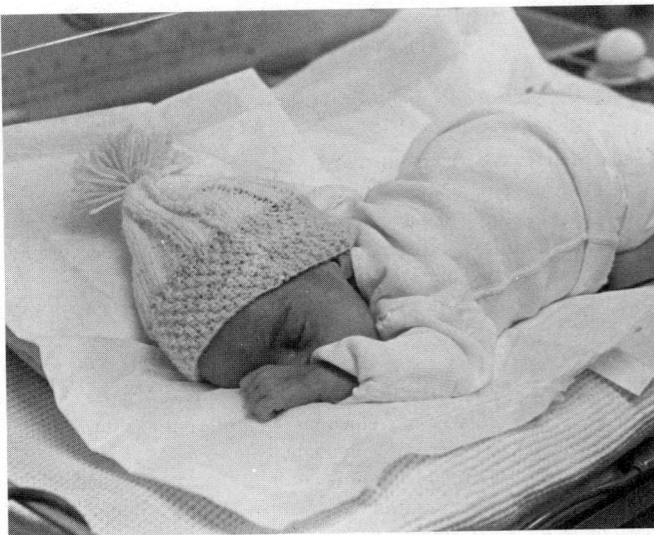

Fig. 10-5. Infant wearing cap knit for him by his mother. A satisfactory substitute can be fashioned from piece of stockinette.

with the site of measurement than full-term infants. The axillary temperature provides the best indication of an infant's temperature. Rectal temperature, in addition to the possibility of producing injury and vagal stimulation, is often misleading, since it registers core temperature. Heat production is activated by a lowered skin temperature; therefore core temperature drops only after body heat cannot be maintained by increased metabolic activity.

The physical factors that effect temperature regulation operate to influence temperature regulation in Isolettes and radiant heat units. Loss of heat by convection is a constant problem in the open units, and the skin probe should be covered with a small foam or felt disk to avoid the effect of radiant heat acting directly on the sensor itself. Otherwise the heated sensor discontinues the heat source, and the infant remains cold.

Radiant heat loss is one of the greatest threats to temperature regulation in the Isolette, since the temperature of circulating air within has no influence on heat loss to cooler surfaces without, such as windows, walls, or a lower nursery temperature. Some nurses have found that lining the inside of the Isolette with aluminum foil may help prevent heat loss caused by radiation, but it must not extend so high that the view of the infant is obscured.

A high-humidity atmosphere contributes to body temperature maintenance by reducing *evaporative* heat loss. Humidity is provided in some Isolettes by air circulating over a heated water reservoir, which has the additional advantage of decreasing heat loss by convection as the air flows over the infant. Since stagnant, warm water provides an excellent breeding medium for microorganisms, the reservoir is emptied every 8 to 24 hours and replaced with sterile distilled water. The recommended humidity is 50% to 65%; higher humidity and a warmer environment are recommended for VLBW infants. Because of the ever-present danger of infection, most nurseries no longer use water in Isolettes. Humidity is provided from an external source such as humidified oxygen or air.

Conductive heat loss can be reduced by warming all items that come in direct contact with the infant, such as scales, radiographic film, blankets, and the hands of caregivers. Warming the items before use can reduce this source of heat loss, for example, storing blankets in a warming unit ready for use, placing a free-standing warming unit or a gooseneck lamp over a scale before weighing an infant. Some units place the infants on a water-heated pad in the crib to reduce heat transfer (Topper and Stewart, 1984).

Two simple methods have been employed to reduce oxygen consumption, insensible water loss, and radiant heat demand, especially in VLBW infants under open radiant warmers. The most widely used approach is a thin plastic heat shield that reduces evaporative, convective, and radiant heat loss. This consists of plastic wrap (such as Saran Wrap) stretched across the crib to produce a microenvironment around an infant (Fig. 10-6) (Baumgart and others, 1981; Baumgart, 1981). A plastic bubble wrap, or body hood (similar to that used as a packing material), is sometimes used as a blanket to help preserve heat and prevent insensible fluid loss, especially in infants under the radiant warmer. Although the body hood reduces evaporative loss, it tends to interfere with radiant heat delivery (Baumgart, Fox, and Polin, 1982).

Hydration

It is not uncommon for high-risk infants to receive supplemental parenteral fluids to supply additional calories, electrolytes, or water. Adequate hydration is particularly important in premature infants because extracellular water content is higher than that of a full-term infant (70% in full-term infants and up to 90% in preterm infants), and the capacity

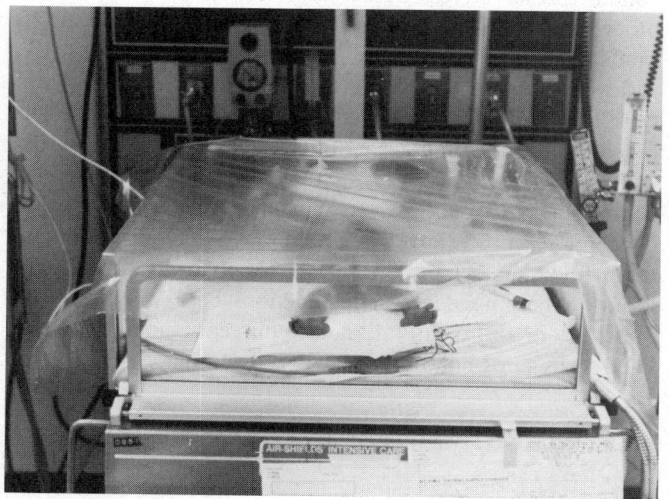

Fig. 10-6. Infant under plastic wrap, which produces a draft-free environment.
Photography by Anne Kunke, San Jose, CA.

for osmotic diuresis is limited in premature infants' underdeveloped kidneys. Nephrogenesis is still taking place at a rapid rate during the later weeks of gestation, and early birth implies less than a full complement of functioning nephrons. As a result, preterm infants are highly vulnerable to water depletion, especially when there are increased losses through the gastrointestinal tract, lungs, and skin.

The preferred sites for intravenous (IV) infusions in neonates are peripheral veins on the dorsal surfaces of hands or feet and umbilical vessels; alternative, but less frequently used, sites are scalp veins and antecubital veins. Contraindications to the use of peripheral lines are administration of very hypertonic solutions and hyperalimentation. The peripheral sites allow for maximum infant mobility except for the restrained IV site. If these sites are exhausted by long-term therapy, a venous cutdown (usually inserted in the saphenous vein) may be employed. However, the increased use of small-gauge percutaneous catheters has reduced the need for this option.

In most facilities the intensive care nurses are able to insert IV needles and catheters as well as maintain the infusions. The IV is most often delivered by way of continuous infusion pumps (volumetric) that deliver minute volumes at a preset flow rate. Less often the peristaltic infusion pump is employed (see p. 1175 for a discussion of IV infusion). The needle is secured to the skin with tape, preferably transparent tape, with care not to cause undue pressure from the needle hub and tubing. Since very small infants are highly vulnerable to fluid shifts, the rates are very slow, carefully regulated, and checked hourly to prevent dehydration and avoid rapid development of congestive heart failure, pulmonary edema, or intraventricular hemorrhage.

The very small, fragile blood vessels (unless an umbilical vessel is used) are subject to rupture and subsequent infiltration. The situation is compounded by the consistent use of pump type of infusion apparatus that continues to pump fluid into tissues following infiltration. Consequently nurses are constantly on the alert for signs of infiltration, which are very difficult to ascertain, especially in preterm infants. Nurses must be alert for signs of infiltration, since many infusions contain drugs that can cause severe tissue damage, and for signs of overhydration (see p. 1161). The restraints are assessed frequently for tightness and to ascertain that they are accomplishing their purpose.

There is a great deal of heat and moisture lost in rapid breathing, and infants under a radiant warmer or phototherapy lights must be closely watched for signs of dehydration. It is important to obtain frequent weights (often every 4 hours), accurately measure intake and output, and determine serum electrolyte levels to maintain fluid and electrolyte balance.

A common problem observed in infants who have umbilical or peripheral catheters in place is a reflex vasoconstriction of peripheral vessels, known as "cath toes," that can seriously impair circulation. The response is triggered by irritation at the end of the catheter as a result of alteration in pressure or osmolality, such as injection of medication. Circulatory effects are observed first in the middle three toes of the foot but may extend to include the buttocks. The toes first flush, then turn a mulberry color, and, if the condition is not corrected, blanch. The problem can usually be corrected by warming the foot on the unaffected extremity. Reflex vasodilation relaxes the vessels in the affected extremity. If this treatment is ineffective, the catheter is removed to relieve the circulatory occlusion.

Skin Care

The skin of premature infants is characteristically immature relative to that of full-term infants. Because of the increased sensitivity and fragility of premature skin, it is recommended that no alkaline-base soap or detergent be used that might destroy the "acid mantle" of the skin. The skin is cleansed with plain, clear water or mild, nonalkaline cleanser only two to three times per week. Any topical preparation (including creams, lotions, or medicated ointments) should be carefully assessed for possible toxic effects before application. The increased permeability of the skin facilitates absorption of ingredients. Hexachlorophene has been discontinued as a cleansing agent because of its proven toxic effect. Other germicides (e.g., alcohol or povidone-iodine) are used with caution, and the skin is rinsed after their use (Kuller, Lund, and Tobin, 1983). These substances may cause severe irritation in VLBW infants.

The skin is easily excoriated and denuded; therefore care must be taken to avoid damage to the delicate structure. The total thickness of the skin is less than that of full-term infants and has fewer elastic fibers, and there is less cohesion between the thinner skin layers. Adhesives used after heel sticks or to secure monitoring equipment or intravenous infusions may excoriate the skin or adhere to the skin surface so well that the skin can be separated from understructures and pulled away with the tape. Transpore tape is the only safe tape to apply directly to the skin of small infants. It is best to first apply a coating of a protective substance to which the adhesive tape is attached. When correctly applied, the polyurethane elastic film Hollihesive has been used with success in many units. The film serves as a protective layer on which adhesive can be attached and serves as a protective layer over abrasions and excoriations. Another product, Op-Site, is effective for protecting wounds, damaged skin, and IV sites (Kuller, Lund, and Tobin, 1983). Eucerin cream creates a satisfactory moisture barrier and is frequently used under tape and applied to denuded areas. Many NICUs now use limb bands rather than adhesive-backed electrodes for attaching monitor equipment. These consist of wires encased in plastic tubing with saline or other electrolyte solution used to activate the connection. This eliminates the need for adhesives.

When dressings or adhesive tape is removed from the extremities of very small and immature infants, it is unsafe to use scissors because it is easy to snip off tiny extremities or nick loosely attached skin. Adhesive tape is best removed by applying water-soaked cotton balls to the tape, then lifting the tape *carefully* while applying pressure on the skin directly beneath the tape. Solvents used to remove tape tend to dry and burn the delicate skin.

During skin assessment of preterm infants, nurses are also alert to the subtle signs that indicate zinc deficiency, a common problem in these infants. Breakdown usually occurs in the areas around the mouth, buttocks, fingers, and toes. In VLBW infants it may also occur in the creases of the neck, wrists, ankles, and around wounds. Zinc deficiency is most likely to appear in infants with sepsis, those experiencing nasogastric losses, or those who had surgery. Any suspicious lesions are reported to the physician so that zinc supplements can be prescribed.

Administration of Medications

Administration of therapeutic agents, such as drugs, ointments, intravenous infusions, and oxygen, requires judicious handling and meticulous attention to details. The computation, preparation, and administration of drugs in minute amounts often requires collaboration between nurses to reduce the chance of error. In addition, the immaturity of an infant's detoxification mechanisms and inability to demonstrate symptoms of toxicity (e.g., signs of auditory nerve involvement from ototoxic drugs such as kanamycin) complicate drug therapy and require that nurses be particularly alert for signs of adverse reaction. (See section on Administration of medications in Chapter 27, p. 1129.)

Recently warnings have been issued regarding the hazards of bacteriostatic and hyperosmolar solutions to infants. Benzyl alcohol, a common preservative in bacteriostatic water and saline, has been shown to be toxic to newborns and should not be used to flush intravenous catheters or to dilute or reconstitute medications. It is recommended that medications with preservatives be avoided whenever possible (Food and Drug Administration, 1982; Committee on Fetus and Newborn, 1983). Because a number of medications contain preservatives, nurses must read labels carefully in order to detect their presence in any medication to be administered to an infant.

Hyperosmolar solutions present a potential danger to preterm infants. It has been found that hyperosmolar solutions given orally to infants can produce clinical, physiologic, and morphologic alterations, the most serious of which is necrotizing enterocolitis (Atakent and others, 1984). More concentrated doses have been administered to ensure that all the medication is ingested, but the practice is questioned. It is now recommended that medications be administered parenterally or sufficiently diluted to prevent complications related to hyperosmolality.

MEETING NUTRITIONAL NEEDS OF HIGH-RISK NEONATES

Optimum nutrition is critical in the management of LBW preterm infants, but there are difficulties in providing for their nutritional needs. The various mechanisms for ingestion and digestion of foods are not fully developed, and the younger the infant, the greater the problem. In addition, the nutritional requirements for this group of infants are not known with certainty. It is known that all preterm infants are at risk because of poor nutritional stores and several physical and developmental characteristics.

Physiologic Characteristics

An infant's need for rapid growth and daily maintenance must be met in the presence of several anatomic and physiologic disabilities. Although some sucking and swallowing activities are demonstrated before birth and in premature infants, coordination of these mechanisms does not occur until approximately 32 to 34 weeks of gestation, and they are not fully developed until after birth. Initial sucking is not accompanied by swallowing, and esophageal contractions are uncoordinated. Consequently infants are highly prone to aspiration and its attendant dangers. As infants mature, the suck-swallow pattern develops but is slow and ineffectual, and these reflexes may also become easily exhausted.

As with most full-term infants, preterm infants have poor muscle tone in the area of the inferior esophageal (cardiac) sphincter. This causes milk in the stomach to be easily regurgitated into the esophagus, where it can interfere with diaphragmatic movement. As a consequence, infants breathe more rapidly, there may be vagal stimulation, and again there is the ever-present danger of aspi-

ration. The stomach has a very limited capacity in preterm infants and is easily overdistended, further compromising respiration.

Physiologically preterm infants have approximately the same capacity to digest and absorb protein as full-term infants. However, carbohydrates and fats are less well tolerated. The secretion of lactase, a late developing enzyme, is low in infants born before 34 weeks of gestation; therefore formulas containing lactose are inadvisable for these infants. Although amylase is deficient in preterm infants, an alternative enzyme (glucoamylase) is able to compensate in most neonates so that they are able to tolerate moderate amounts of starch (Lebenthal, 1982). Preterm infants are inefficient in digesting and absorbing lipids, especially the saturated triglycerides of cow's milk, because they have low levels of pancreatic lipase and low bile acid. Table 10-1 summarizes the characteristics and problems related to immaturity.

Nutritional Needs

The demand for nutrients in LBW infants is much higher compared to that of larger infants, and individual infants vary in activity level, ease of achieving basal energy expenditure, thermoneutrality, condition, and efficacy of nutrient absorption. The estimated maintenance requirements for LBW infants in a thermoneutral environment is approximately 50 kcal per kg per day by 2 to 3 weeks of age

Table 10-1 Characteristics, problems, and management related to selected nutriments for the preterm infant

CHARACTERISTIC	PROBLEM	MANAGEMENT
Deficiency of proteolytic enzymes	Difficulty digesting casein protein	Feed whey-predominant formula or human milk
Low lactase activity	Poor digestion of lactose providing substrate for bacterial growth in lower intestinal tract; distention from osmotic effect of lactose	Provide low lactose; feed glucose polymers
Pancreatic lipase; low bile salt levels	Unable to digest and absorb saturated triglycerides	Feed unsaturated medium-chain triglycerides, human milk; provide supplemental vitamin E
Poor sodium conservation	Hyponatremia	Feedings higher in sodium
Rapid bone growth and mineralization	Osteopenia; rickets	Feedings higher in calcium and phosphorus; supplemental vitamin D
Negative zinc balance	Skin lesions Related to poor fat absorption	Feed easily digested fats Feedings with zinc supplementation
Low iron	Anemia	Provide supplemental iron
Poor muscle tone of cardiac sphincter	Regurgitation: interference with diaphragm excursion; vagal stimulation (bradycardia)	Semi-upright position during feeding; feed small amounts
Limited stomach capacity	Inadequate intake Distention	Small frequent feedings; continuous drip gavage feeding Nutrient supplementation
Noncoordination of suck/swallow reflexes	Aspiration Inadequate intake	Alternative feeding methods
Muscle weakness	Exhaustion	Alternative feeding methods

(Brooke, Alvear, and Arnold, 1979). In addition, each gram of weight gain requires 5 to 6 kcal. The Committee on Nutrition of the American Academy of Pediatrics (1985) supports the caloric requirements of preterm infants shown in Table 10-2. Since most of the nutritional stores are accumulated in the final months of gestation, preterm infants are also hampered by low stores of calcium, iron, phosphorus, proteins, and vitamins A and C.

Nutrition can be provided by either the parenteral or the enteral routes or by a combination of the two, but there is still some controversy regarding the type of enteral feeding that best meets the nutritional needs of LBW infants. The predominant view supports the use of milk from an infant's own mother or modified infant formulas. Commercial formulas have been designed specifically to meet the needs of small preterm infants (see Table 8-0) and provide for adequate growth and metabolic stability (studies reported by Committee on Nutrition, 1985). Prepared formulas have the added advantage of allowing more concentrated feedings.

Evidence indicates that milk produced by mothers whose infants are born before term contains higher concentrations of protein, sodium, and chloride (Gross and others, 1980; Anderson, Atkinson, and Bryan, 1981) and immunoglobulin A. Thus mothers appear to be the preferred source of milk for their preterm infants. The milk produced by mothers for their infants changes in content as the infants grow, so milk provided by mothers of older infants may not be appropriate for premature infants. Infants fed with their own mother's milk displayed a more rapid rate of growth in all parameters and a shorter length of time to regain birth weight (Gross, Oehler, and Eckerman, 1983). Supplements have been recommended for some infants who require additional calories and nutrients (Schanler, Garza, and Nichols, 1985)

The antiinfectious attributes of human milk provide additional advantages for preterm infants. Secretory immunoglobulin A (IgA) concentration is higher in the milk from mothers of preterm infants than from mothers of full-term infants. Immunoglobulin A is important in the control of bacteria in the intestinal tract, where it inhibits adherence and proliferation of bacteria at epithelial surfaces (Gross

and others, 1981). Finally, the psychologic advantages of using the milk from an infant's own mother cannot be overlooked.

Pooled human milk is less favored for preterm infants than it was previously. The composition of pooled milk does not meet all the nutritional requirements of preterm infants, resulting in a slower rate of growth than is achieved with the milk of the premature newborn's mother or commercial formula (Tyson and others, 1983). Also, breast milk contributed by donors is essentially raw milk and as such is a potential source of infection, especially for the transmission of cytomegalovirus (Dworsky and others, 1983).

Feeding Methods

The amount and method of feeding are determined by the size and condition of the infant. Very small or ill infants are fed by the parenteral route until their condition is stabilized and their neurologic and physical state permits enteral feedings. Often enteral feedings must be supplemented by parenteral infusions to ensure an adequate intake of carbohydrates and water.

Although the timing of the first feeding has been a matter of controversy, most authorities now believe that early feeding, usually within 3 to 6 hours, after birth reduces the incidence of complicating factors such as hypoglycemia, dehydration, and the degree of hyperbilirubinemia. The feeding regimen employed varies from institution to institution. However, the initial enteral feeding is not attempted until infants have adapted to extrauterine existence as evidenced by temperature neutrality, normal breathing, and good color, tone, and cry.

Nipple feeding. Vigorous infants can be fed from a soft nipple with little difficulty (Fig. 10-7), whereas weaker infants will require alternative methods. Sterile water is offered first, the same as for any newborn, because it causes no pulmonary reaction if aspirated as has been found with both milk and glucose water. The amount to be fed is determined largely by the infant's weight and is gradually and cautiously increased by increments of 1 to 2 ml per feeding each day, regulated by each infant's tolerance, until a satisfactory caloric intake is ensured. Sometimes supplementary calories are needed in the form of dietary additives, such as Lipomul-Oral,[*] which provides vegetable fat and carbohydrates, and MCT oil,[†] which provides fat in the form of medium-chain triglycerides.

Bottle-feedings are continued if infants are able to tolerate the feedings and take the required amount. The rate of increase that is well tolerated varies from one infant to another and is often a nursing responsibility to determine. It is important not to tire the infants or overtax their capacity to retain the feedings. For example, infants with stomach capacities of 5 ml are unable to take enough formula to meet even the minimum daily requirements. When infants require more than 30 minutes to complete a feeding, the next one

Table 10-2 Estimated caloric requirement in typical, growing premature infants	
CALORIC EXPENDITURE	**Kcal/kg/d**
Resting caloric expenditure	50
Intermittent activity	15
Occasional cold stress	10
Specific dynamic action	8
Fecal loss of calories	12
Growth allowance	25
TOTAL	120

From Committee on Nutrition, American Academy of Pediatrics: Nutritional needs of low-birth-weight infants, Pediatrics **75:**976-986, 1985.

[*]The Upjohn Co., Kalamazoo, MI.
[†]Mead Johnson & Co., Evansville, IN.

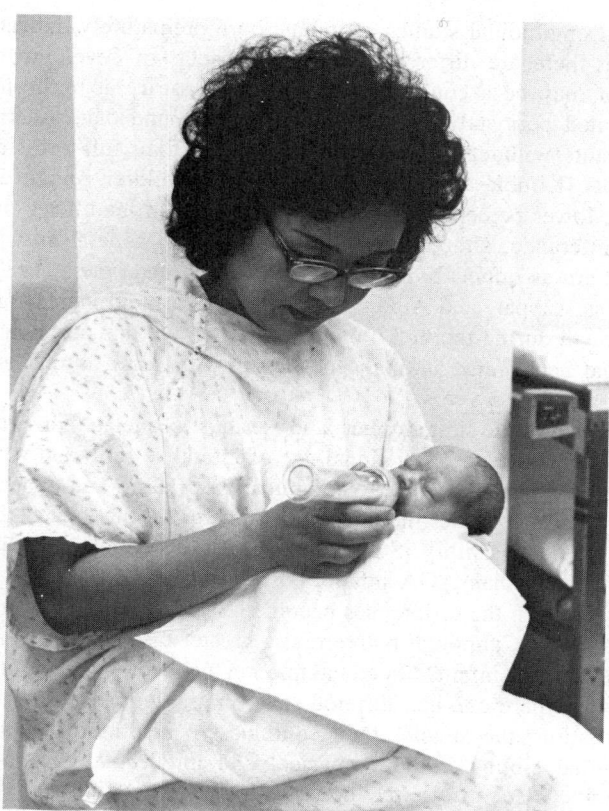

Fig. 10-7. Position for nipple-feeding premature infant.

should be given by gavage. When infants are unable to tolerate bottle-feedings, intermittent feedings by gavage are instituted until they gain enough strength and coordination to use the nipple. Poor sucking in infants who have been feeding well may indicate serious illness and should be reported to the physician.

It is believed that many digestive powers require signal stimulation to respond. Some premature infants respond more slowly than full-term infants; therefore the feeding interval as well as the amount of the feeding is individualized. Some investigators find that premature neonates thrive well on demand rather than scheduled feedings and on the average can be discharged earlier (Collinge and others, 1982).

The complications of aspiration make it important that infants are not overfed. If infants take very little and appear to be tired, their feedings may have to be repeated in a short while and then at more frequent intervals. Preterm infants are often slow feeders and require periods of rest and frequent bubbling. To determine how well infants tolerate feedings, stomach contents may be aspirated before each feeding and the residual fluid recorded and replaced as part of the feeding. If more than 5 ml is aspirated for two successive feedings, or if residual is persistent, this should be called to the attention of the physician.

Breast-feeding. Mothers who wish to breast-feed their preterm infants are encouraged to pump their breasts until

their infants are sufficiently stable to tolerate breast-feeding. Before premature infants are allowed to breast-feed, they must (Boggs and Rau, 1983):

Weigh at least 1500 g
Experience short wakeful periods
Exhibit a sucking reflex
Tolerate a gavage feeding
No longer require oxygen or ventilatory support

It requires more time, patience, and dedication on the part of the mother and the staff to help infants with breast-feeding. The process is begun slowly—feeding once daily and gradually increased when infants are able to nurse steadily for 10 minutes. Because teaching infants to breast-feed after they are accustomed to nipple feeding is difficult, these infants are given supplementary gavage feedings until they are breast-feeding and gaining weight satisfactorily (Boggs and Rau, 1983).

Gavage feeding. Gavage feeding is one of the safest means for meeting the nutritional requirements of infants who are less than 32 weeks of gestation or infants who weigh less than 1650 g. These infants are usually too weak to suck effectively and are unable to coordinate swallowing. The predominant philosophy is to provide the feedings by continuous drip regulated via infusion pump rather than by a bolus of formula at prescribed intervals. For larger infants who become excessively tired, are listless, or become cyanotic, intermittent gavage feeding is used as an energy-conserving technique.

A 15-inch (37.5 cm) size 5 or 8 French polyethylene feeding tube is used to instill the formula, and the usual methods for determining correct placement are employed (see p. 1141 for technique). Although the more relaxed cardiac sphincter makes passage of the tube easier, there may be changes in heart rate and blood pressure in response to vagal stimulation. The procedure is best accomplished when an infant is in a prone or a right side-lying position with the head slightly elevated. It is preferable to insert the tube through the mouth rather than the nares. Nasal insertion obstructs nose breathing and may irritate the delicate nasal mucosa. Passage through the mouth also provides an opportunity to observe the sucking response.

The stomach is aspirated, the contents measured, and the aspirant returned as part of the feeding. The amount of the aspirant depends on the length of time since the previous feeding or concurrent illness. Whether or not the amount of the aspirant is deducted from the total feeding varies among units. Some advocate deducting to avoid overdistending the stomach. For example, if a feeding is 25 ml and the aspirant is 5 ml, the aspirant is returned plus 20 ml of feeding for a total of 25 ml. In other units the amount is determined on an individual basis.

The formula is allowed to flow by gravity, and the length of time should approximate the time required for a nipple-feeding. This procedure is not used as a time-saving method for the nurse. The tube is rarely left in place between feedings because of complications such as obstructed nares, mucous plugs, purulent rhinitis, epistaxis, and possible stomach perforation that sometimes occur with indwelling catheters. This method is reserved for infants who cannot tolerate the intubation process.

The intermittent method of gavage feeding stimulates the infant to begin making attempts at sucking and swallowing. The nurse needs to observe premature infants closely for behaviors that indicate readiness to handle bottle-feedings. These include: (1) a strong, vigorous suck, (2) coordination of sucking and swallowing, (3) sucking in response to the gavage tube or other objects placed near the mouth, and (4) wakefulness before and sleeping after feedings. When these behaviors are noted, infants can be challengd with nipple-feedings introduced slowly.

Nonnutritive sucking (NNS) on a pacifier by infants during gavage feedings has been shown to be beneficial. It helps nurses assess the sucking ability of the infants and helps them to associate the sucking with the feeling of food in the stomach. When compared with other LBW infants, those who are allowed NNS are ready for bottle-feeding earlier, require fewer tube feedings, demonstrate better weight gain, are discharged earlier, and have fewer complications (Measel and Anderson, 1979; Field and others, 1982; Bernbaum and others, 1983). NNS has also been found to increase oxygen tension when measured during tube feeding (Bernbaum and others, 1983; Paludetto and others, 1984).

SUPPORTIVE CARE OF HIGH-RISK NEONATES AND THEIR FAMILIES

Often professional health workers are so absorbed in the life-saving physical aspects of care that the emotional needs of infants and their families are ignored. The significance of early parent-child interaction and infant stimulation has been documented by reliable research, and nurses, aware of these infant and family needs, must incorporate activities that facilitate family interaction into the nursing care plan.

Developmental Correlates

Some physiologic systems in preterm infants mature earlier than they would if the infants had remained within the uterus, for example, the function of some enzyme and immunologic systems and organs, such as kidney and gastrointestinal efficiency; others slow down, such as growth in height and weight; still others keep pace with the development of those of their counterparts still in utero, for example, reflex behaviors. The factors that affect the growth and development of preterm infants are:

Past history
Gestational age at birth
Head circumference, weight, and length at birth
Length of growth delay
Days necessary to regain birth weight
Measurements at term date
Head circumference, weight, length at discharge from hospital

Longitudinal studies of infants born prematurely indicate that there are differences in many aspects of development that may be a consequence of the immaturity at birth and related perinatal problems. It has been found that preterm infants without sequelae remain smaller than full-term infants (Kimble and others, 1982). These children remain in the lower percentile range for height, weight, and head circumference, although they follow the same general growth pattern as infants born at term (Westwood and others, 1983; Ross, Lipper, and Auld, 1985). There is a rapid increase in growth during the first 6 months, and growth remains somewhat accelerated until the normal growth curve is reached by age 2 to 3 years.

Neurologic impairment and serious sequelae correlate with the size and gestational age of infants at birth and with the severity of neonatal complications (Hack and others, 1984). The greater the degree of immaturity, the greater the degree of disability. SGA infants appear to be less at a disadvantage than AGA infants born preterm until age 4 to 5 years when the differences become less divergent (Vohr and Oh, 1983), although both are at a greater disadvantage than are normal infants. For example, in pairs of monozygotic twins where one has suffered severe intrauterine growth retardation, the smaller twin continues to be inferior to the normal sibling in both physical and intellectual development. Also, full-term, nonasphyxiated SGA infants, although physically growth-impaired, have an encouraging prognosis for neurologic and cognitive development (Westwood and others, 1983).

There is an increase in the incidence of neurologic sequelae in preterm infants, such as cerebral palsy, attention deficit disorder, visual-motor deficits, and altered intellectual functioning. The highest incidence of neurologic disability is found in infants who are born before 38 weeks of gestation but who weigh more than 2500 g. Also, postnatal head growth is a better predictor of developmental outcome than head circumference at birth (Gross, Oehler, and Eckerman, 1983). All infants at risk seem to benefit from special care, since undesirable sequelae appear to be decreased in infants who receive intensive medical and nursing care as opposed to those who receive routine care. Although the risk of perinatal complications is highest in VLBW infants and the mortality is higher, a positive outcome is believed to be possible even for these survivors of extremely low birth weight (Bennett, Robinson, and Sells, 1983).

A concern of personnel in NICUs is the incidence of sensory impairment in surviving premature infants. Retinopathy of prematurity, a dreaded complication of oxygen therapy, is discussed on p. 413. More difficult to anticipate and detect is a hearing deficit. Because LBW infants show significant visual-motor deficits compared to full-term infants at a later time, many NICUs routinely screen infants for hearing acuity. Two methods have proven valuable in testing very small infants. The Crib-o-gram employs a motion-sensing transducer placed beneath the infant's mattress that detects changes in motor activity coincident with the introduction of a calibrated sound stimulus. The brainstem evoked response

(BSER) is one of several electrophysiologic methods for screening purposes. It monitors stimulus-related changes in the electrical activity of the auditory pathway by way of noninvasive electrodes applied to the scalp. Follow-up testing is a vital part of prenatal screening.

Infant Stimulation

Recently attention has been focused on the effects of early stimulation, or its lack, on both normal and preterm infants. Findings indicate that infants are able to respond to a greater variety of stimuli than was previously thought. Numerous studies have been based on the assumption that premature infants receive inadequate stimulation. Others have observed that the atmosphere and activities of the NICU are overstimulating. More current studies suggest that infants are not necessarily understimulated but instead are subjected to *inappropriate* stimulation (Barnard and Bee, 1983; VandenBerg, 1985).

The present approach to infant stimulation is one of tailoring the stimulation program to the developmental level and tolerance of each infant. Three stages of organization have been identified for premature infants (Gorski, Davison, and Brazelton, 1979):

1. Physiologic organization (infants less than 33 weeks of gestation)—the primary need of infants is for stabilization and integration of autonomic functions, such as respiration, heart rate, and temperature.
2. Coming out (between 34 and 36 weeks of gestation)—development of motor systems; infants are able to respond to visual and auditory stimuli if interaction begins when they are in an alert state.
3. Reciprocity (36 to 40 weeks of gestation and beyond)—emergence of defined states of consciousness, such as sleeping, waking, crying, and alertness; infants can benefit from individualized stimulation programs.

During the early stages of development, stimulation produces uncoordinated, random activity, such as jerky limb extension, hyperflexion, and irregular vital signs. At this stage infants need to have minimum stimulation. They are handled with slow, controlled movements (some infants are unstable if moved abruptly), and their random movements are controlled with limbs held close to their bodies during turning or other position changes. This containment prevents or diminishes motor disorganization and reduces stress (VandenBerg, 1985). Additional containment measures include support with blanket rolls, if medically feasible. A nest constructed by placing blanket rolls underneath the bed sheet assists infants in maintaining an attitude of flexion when prone or side-lying (Cole and Frappier, 1985). This is believed to approximate the normal intrauterine position in which preterm infants would lie at this stage of gestation. The flexed position is believed to facilitate hand-to-mouth ability (McCrae, 1982).

The prone position has been found to be the optimum position for many preterm infants and appears to result in improved oxygenation, better tolerated feedings, and more organized sleep-rest patterns (Martin and others, 1979; Wa-

gaman and others, 1979). Others appear to prefer a side-lying posture. Supine positioning for preterm infants is not desirable because they appear to lose their sense of equilibrium when supine and use up vital energy in attempts to recover balance by postural changes (Cole and Frappier, 1985).

When infants have reached sufficient developmental organization and stability, interventions are designed and implemented to support their growing abilities. Nurses become adept at learning to read infants' behavioral clues and supplying appropriate stimulation. Behavioral clues include both approach and avoidance behaviors (Cole, 1985). Approach behaviors that should be supported and enhanced are positive movements, such as tongue extension, handclasp, hand-to-mouth movements, sucking, looking, and cooing. Avoidance behaviors that signal for "time-out" include spitting up, gagging, arching, finger splaying, yawning, frowning, and averting a gaze.

It must be emphasized that any intervention program for premature infants must be individualized. When infants are free of support systems, medically stable, and on room air, they are assessed with a tool such as Brazelton's Assessment of Preterm Infant Behavior Scale, a modification of the Brazelton Neonatal Behavioral Assessment Scale (see p. 327), to document their behavioral styles. An effective program may be designed to provide limited sensory stimulation that involves one or two senses or multisensory stimulation that includes tactile, visual, auditory, vestibular, olfactory, and gustatory stimulation. The objective of any stimulation program is to avoid stressing infants—overstimulation is as detrimental as understimulation.

Twenty-four-hour surveillance of sick infants implies maximum visibility. However, many units have instigated a program to help establish a night-day sleep pattern by either darkening the room, if the infants' condition allows, covering cribs with blankets, or placing eye patches over the infants' eyes at night. Others believe that rest for these infants is so vital to their growth that they are provided with one hour of every three for total rest. The cribs or Isolettes are covered with blankets and the infants are not disturbed for handling of any kind during this rest period (Brazelton, 1984).

When the condition of an infant is sufficiently advanced to begin a stimulation program, some activities are individualized according to each infant's cues, temperament, state, behavioral organization, and particular needs. Stimulation periods are short, for example, 1 to 2 minutes for visual stimulation, 2 to 3 minutes of voices, and 5 minutes for quiet music. Some suggested activities are outlined in the box. When a stimulation program is implemented, the parents should be involved as early as possible. See the discussion that follows for further suggestions.

Parental Involvement

The birth of a preterm infant is usually an unexpected and stressful event for which families are emotionally unprepared. They find themselves simultaneously coping with their own needs, the needs of their infants, and the needs of their families (especially when there are other children). To compound the situation, the precarious nature of their infant's condition engenders an atmosphere of apprehension and uncertainty. They are faced with multiple crises and overwhelming feelings of responsibility, expense, and frustration.

INTERVENTIONS FOR INFANT STIMULATION

General guidelines
Offer stimulation only during periods of alertness.
Limit stimulation to one or two types of stimulus per session.
Provide stimulation for short periods.
Space stimulation periods according to infant's tolerance.

Visual stimulation
Place magazine photographs (black and white schematic faces) in visual range (19 to 22 cm) in "en face" position.
Cover mattress with black and white patterned material for length of stimulation period.
Provide black and white mobiles with varied hanging shapes.
Initiate eye-to-eye contact repeatedly.
Alternate holding black and white pattern still and moving it across the infant's visual field.

Tactile stimulation
Stroke skin slowly and gently in head-to-toe direction.
Provide alternate textures, e.g., sheepskin, satin, velvet.

Auditory stimulation
Play tape of parents' voices.
Play classical music recording or music box (jazz or rock are less effective).
Speak with a variety of voice inflections; alternate adult and baby talk.
Call infant by name at each interaction.

Vestibular stimulation
Place on waterbed with oscillations and waves per minute determined on an individual basis; alternate oscillation with rest periods.
Rock in chair.
Place in sling and rock.
Provide passive range-of-motion exercise to knee and hip joints.
Close infant's fist around cloth toy.
Lift head to upright position, tip to right and then to left, stopping at midline.

Olfactory stimulation
Pass open breast milk or formula container under nose.
Pass various sweet smelling items under nose, e.g., cherry syrup, cinnamon, nutmeg, strawberry extract.

Gustatory stimulation
Place infant's hand or pacifier in mouth when sucking movements are observed or during gavage feeding.
Place 2 drops of milk in infant's mouth with each tube feeding.

Derived extensively from Chaze, B.A., and Ludington-Hoe, S.M.: Sensory stimulation in the NICU, Am. J. Nurs. **84**:68-71, January 1984.

All parents have some anxieties about the outcome of a pregnancy, but following a premature birth the concern is heightened about both the viability and the intactness of their infant. Mothers see their infant only briefly before the newborn is removed to the intensive care unit or even to another hospital, leaving mothers with just the recollection of their infant's very small size and unusual appearance. They usually feel alone or lost in the maternity ward, belonging neither with mothers who have lost their infants nor with those who delivered healthy, full-term infants. The staff and physicians are often guarded in discussing the infant's condition; mothers are continually expecting to hear that their infant has died, and they are sensitive to the anxieties of other mothers and staff members. Leaving their infant and going home empty-handed only serves to compound their feelings of disappointment, failure, and deprivation.

When an infant is to be transported from the hospital, the parents need a description of the facility where the infant is going. They need to know the location, reputation, and nature of the facility and the care that the infant is expected to receive. The name of the infant's physician and the telephone number of the nursery should be given to them, and unfamiliar terms should be explained to them, such as neonatologist, ventilator, infusion, and Isolette. Explanations should be simple, and parents should be given the opportunity to ask questions. If booklets are available that describe the facility, they should be given to the family.

Perhaps most important of all, the parents, especially the mother, should be allowed some contact with the infant before the transport. To be able to see, touch, and (if possible) hold their infant facilitates the attachment process. Often a photograph, or even a videotape, of their infant can serve as a bond until the parents are able to travel to the regional facility. When possible, it is often advisable to transfer the mother to the same institution as her infant.

Parents need to be informed of their infant's progress and reassured that he is receiving proper care. They need to understand the smallest aspects of the infant's condition and treatment. Although details are comforting to parents, it is not necessary to share too much information, such as very technical facts that do not contribute to their understanding. Considering the parents' fears, the nurse can be truthful without being unduly candid regarding the more negative aspects of their child's condition. Most infants survive despite early, worrisome problems.

Nursing interventions relative to the needs of parents are directed toward assisting them with tasks that must be accomplished during their infant's care. Parents need to (Grant, 1978):

Realistically perceive their infant's medical condition and needs
Adapt to the infant's hospital environment
Assume the primary caregiving role
Assume total responsibility for care upon discharge
For some families, cope with death of an infant

Facilitating Parent-Infant Relationships

Because of their insecure status, the infants are separated from their mothers immediately and surrounded by a complex, impenetrable barrier of glass windows, mechanical equipment, and special caregivers. There is increasing evidence to indicate that the emotional separation that accompanies the physical separation of mothers and infants interferes with the normal maternal-infant attachment process (see p. 330). Maternal attachment is a cumulative process that begins before conception, is strengthened by significant events during pregnancy, and matures through maternal-infant contact during the neonatal period.

When an infant is sick, the necessary physical separation appears to be accompanied by an emotional estrangement on the part of parents that may seriously damage the capacity for parenting their infant. This detachment is further hampered by the tenuous nature of the infant's condition. When their infant's survival is in doubt, parents may be reluctant to establish a relationship with him. They prepare themselves for the death of the infant while continuing to hope for his recovery. This anticipatory grief (see p. 970) and hesitancy to embark on a relationship are evidenced by behaviors such as delay in giving the infant a name, reluctance in visiting the nursery, or when they do visit, focusing on equipment and treatments rather than on their infant, and hesitancy to touch or handle the infant when they are provided the opportunity.

The present concept in the comprehensive management of high-risk newborns is to encourage parental involvement rather than to isolate the parents from their infant and his care. This is particularly important in relation to mothers, and to reduce the effects of physical separation, mothers are united with their newborn at the earliest opportunity. Preparing the parents to see their infant for the first time is a nursing responsibility. Before the first visit the parents should be prepared for their infant's appearance, the equipment that is attached to him, and some indication of the general atmosphere of the unit. The initial encounter with the intensive care unit is a stressful experience, and the frightening array of people, equipment, and activity is likely to be overwhelming. A book of photographs that shows infants in Isolettes or under radiant warmers, monitors, mechanical ventilators, and intravenous equipment provides a useful and nonthreatening introduction to the NICU.

Parents should be allowed to visit their infant as soon as possible. Even if they saw the infant at the time of transport or shortly after birth, the infant may have changed considerably, especially if there are a number of medical and equipment requirements associated with their immediate environment. At the bedside the nurse should explain the function of each piece of equipment and the role it plays in facilitating recovery. When possible, some items related to therapy can be removed, for example, phototherapy can be temporarily discontinued and eye patches removed to permit eye-to-eye contact.

Parents appreciate the support of a nurse during the initial visit with their infant, but they should be left alone with the infant for a short while. It is important during the early visits to emphasize positive aspects of their infant's behavior to help the parents focus on their infant as an individual rather than on the equipment that surrounds him. For example, the nurse may describe the infant's spontaneous behaviors during care, such as grasp, swallowing, and movement, or make comments about the infant's biologic functions. Most institutions allow parents to visit their infant as often as they wish and encourage them to do so.

Parents vary greatly in the degree to which they are able to interact with their infant. Some may wish to touch or hold their infant during the first visit, whereas others may not feel comfortable enough even to enter the nursery. These reactions depend on a variety of prenatal and postnatal factors, such as the parity of the mothers and their preparation before birth, the size, condition, and physical appearance of the infant, and the type of treatment he is receiving. It is essential to recognize that the individualized pacing and quality of the interactions are more important than early onset of these interactions. Parents may not be receptive to early and extended infant contact, since they need time to adjust to the impact of an infant with birth problems and should be allowed a grieving period before acceptance of their infant can take place (Ross, 1980).

The parents' inability to focus on their infant is a clue for the nurse to concentrate on the parents and allow them to express their feelings of guilt, anxiety, helplessness, inadequacy, anger, and ambivalence. Nurses can help parents deal with these distressing feelings and recognize that they are normal responses shared by other parents. It is important to point out and reinforce the positive aspects of parents' behavior and interactions with their infant.

Most parents feel shaky and insecure about initiating interaction with their infant. Nurses can sense parents' level of readiness and offer encouragement in these initial efforts. Parents of premature infants follow the same acquaintance process as do parents of normal infants. They may quickly proceed through the process or may require several days or even weeks to complete the process. Parents begin by touching their infant's extremities with their fingertips and poking the infant tenderly, then proceed to caresses and fondling (Fig. 10-8). Touching is the first act of communication between parents and their child. Parents need to be prepared for their infant's exaggerated and generalized startle responses to a touch so that they will not interpret these as negative reactions to their overtures.

Eventually parents begin to endow their infant with an identity—a part of the family. When an infant no longer resembles "chicken" or other nonhuman counterparts and begins to take on aspects of family members, such as the father's chin or the sister's nose, nurses can facilitate this incorporation. Parents are encouraged to bring in clothes and toys for their infant, and the nurse can help parents set goals for themselves and for the infant. Feeding schedules are discussed, and parents are encouraged to visit at times when they can become involved in the care of their infant (Fig. 10-9).

Throughout the parental-infant acquaintance process, the nurse listens carefully to what the parents say in order to assess their concerns and their progress toward incorporating their infant into their lives. The manner in which parents refer to their infant and the questions they ask reveal their worries and feelings and can serve as valuable clues to future relationships with the infant. The alert nurse is attuned to these subtle indications of parents' needs that provide guidelines for nursing intervention. Often all that parents need is reassurance that the behaviors about which they are concerned are normal reactions and will disappear as the infant matures (e.g., an exaggerated Moro reflex or inability to coordinate swallowing) and that they will have the support of the nurse during caregiving activities.

Parents need guidance in their relationships with their infant and assistance in their efforts to meet their infant's physical and developmental needs. The nursing staff must help parents understand that their preterm infant offers few behavioral rewards and show them how to accept small rewards from their infant. The infant's reactions and behaviors are explained to parents, who take their infant's jerky, rejective behavior personally. They need reassurance that these behaviors are not a reflection on their parenting skills. Parents are taught to recognize their infant's cues regarding stimulation, handling, and other interaction, especially aversive behaviors that indicate a need for rest. Nurses need to include parents in planning their infant's care and selecting stimulation materials, such as a music box or recording.

Above all, nurses must encourage and reinforce parents during their caregiving activities and interactions with their infant in order to promote healthy parent-child relationships. The importance of facilitating the parental-infant attachment process cannot be overemphasized, since studies indicate

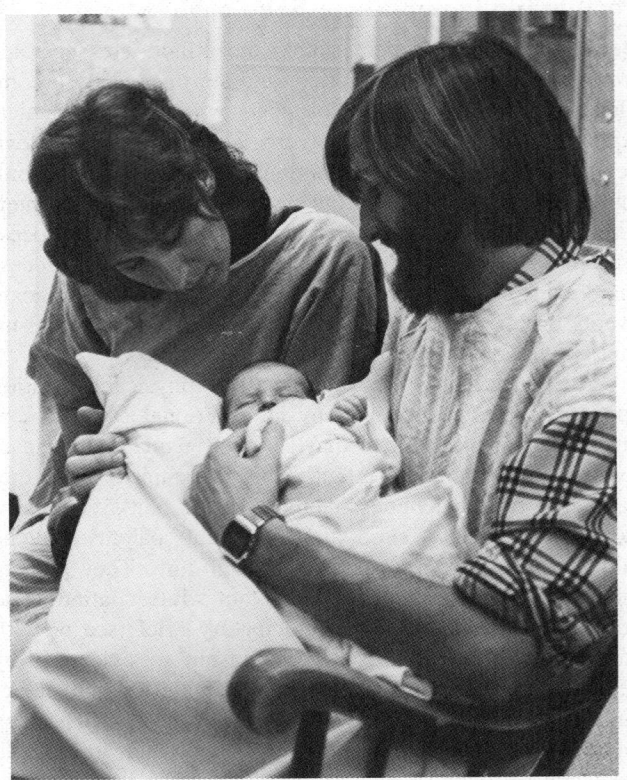

Fig. 10-9. Mother and father visit their newborn infant.

that lack of early attachment in premature infants may contribute to the high incidence of child abuse that occurs later to these infants (Fomufod, 1976).

Although the primary emphasis is directed toward the parents, other members of the family should not be ignored. Siblings are often bewildered about the newborn and the anxiety he generates. The advisability of sibling visitation continues to be a matter of controversy. In some units siblings are allowed into the unit as soon as infants are transferred to the transitional care or extended care unit or section (Fig. 10-10).

Support groups. Parents need to feel that they are not alone. Parent support groups have been of immeasurable value to families of infants in the NICU. Some groups consist of parents who have infants in the hospital who share the same anxieties and concerns. Other groups include parents who have had infants in the NICU and who have dealt with the crisis effectively. The groups are usually under the leadership of a staff person and involve physicians, nurses, and social workers, but it is the parents who can offer other parents something that no one else can provide.

A relatively new national organization evolved from a local parents group. **Parent Care**[*] provides information, referrals, and support to parents and professionals concerned with the care of high-risk infants. It also publishes a na-

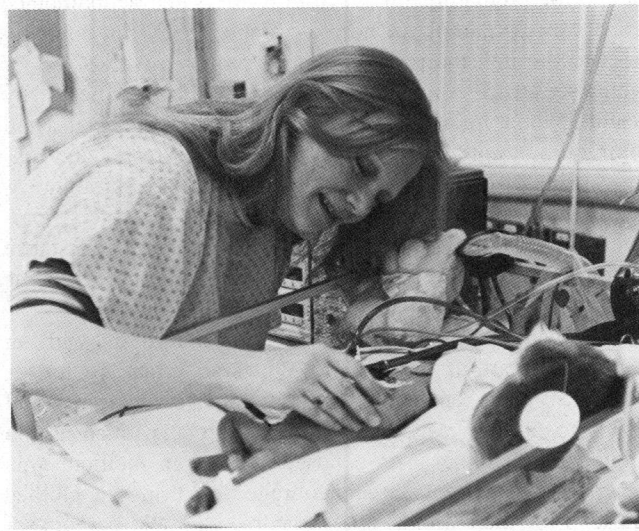

Fig. 10-8. Encouraging interaction of mother and her premature infant in intensive care unit facilitates mother-infant attachment process.

---

*University of Utah Medical Center, 50 North Medical Drive, Room 2A210, Salt Lake City, UT 84132.

tional newsletter and a resource directory that provide information on items useful to parents, such as "preemie" clothing. Information can be obtained by contacting or forming a local group.

Discharge Planning and Home Care

Parents become very apprehensive and excited as time for discharge approaches. They have many concerns and insecurities regarding the care of their infant. They fear the child may still be in danger, that they will be unable to recognize signs of distress or illness in their infant, and that the infant may not yet be ready for discharge. Nurses need to begin early to assist parents in acquiring or increasing their skills in the care of their infant. Appropriate instruction must be provided and sufficient time allowed for the family to assimilate the information and learn the continuing special care requirements. Where rooming-in or other live-in arrangements are available, parents can stay for a few days and assume the care of their infant under the supervision and support of the nursery staff.

There should be appropriate medical and nursing follow-up and referrals to services that can benefit the family. Public health agencies provide nursing supervision and counseling. Organized support groups are part of many communities, including those discussed previously and those designed for parents of infants who require special care, because of specific defects or disabilities, and those for parents of multiple births (see p. 70). Some manufacturers provide for the special needs of such infants. For example, premature size disposable diapers are available from the manufacturers of Pampers.*

At this writing there are no car seats designed especially for very small infants. There are several models that can be adapted for small infants with the placement of blanket rolls on each side of an infant to support the head and trunk. For adequate support without slumping the seat-back-to-crotch strap distance must be 14 cm or less (Bull and Stroup, 1985). See p. 538 for a discussion of infant car restraints.

Knowing that members of the staff are available for telephone or personal contact when the parents take the infant home provides a measure of security to anxious parents. Most NICU facilities maintain a policy of open communication between staff and parents both during the infant's hospitalization and following discharge. It is the responsibility of the NICU staff to make certain that parents are prepared to care for their infant—emotionally and physically.

Neonatal Loss

The precarious nature of many high-risk infants makes death a very real and ever-present possibility. Although infant mortality has been reduced sharply with improved technology, the mortality rate is still greatest in the neonatal period of life. Nurses in the NICU are the persons who must pre-

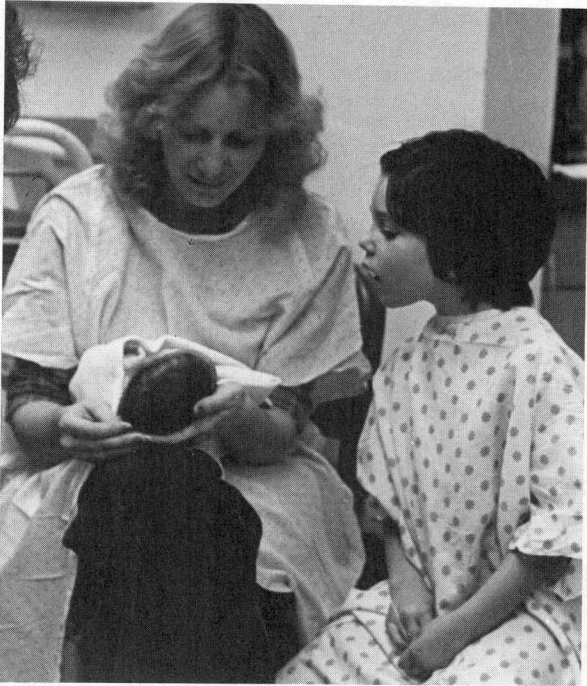

Fig. 10-10. Big sister gets acquainted with the new baby.

Questions and Controversies

Should children be allowed to visit high-risk siblings?

The advisability of sibling visitation is still a matter of controversy in neonatal care. Most units are reluctant to allow even scheduled sibling visits. However, in many areas the trend is toward allowing siblings into the unit as soon as the infant can be transferred to a transitional care unit. The primary concerns appear to be fear of infection and disruption of nursing routines. These fears have not been substantiated (Umphenour, 1980; Wranesh, 1982; Kowba and Schwirian, 1985; Scrimshaw and March, 1984).

Birth of a preterm infant is a difficult time for siblings who rely on the support of understanding parents. When the happy anticipation is changed to sadness, worry, and altered routines, siblings are deprived of their parents' attention and they are bewildered. They know something is wrong, but they have only a dim understanding of what it is (Klaus and Kennell, 1982). Concern regarding the effect of the ill newborn on visiting siblings has not been substantiated. Children did not hesitate to approach or touch the infant, and children less than 5 years of age were less reluctant than older children (Schwab and others, 1983), and there was no measurable differences between previsit and postvisit behaviors (Trause and others, 1981).

The potential benefits of sibling visits are weighed against the harmful effects of infection and exposure of the child to the environment of the intensive care unit. Unfortunately data are inadequate, but contact with the infant appears to have a positive effect on the siblings in helping them to deal with the reality rather than the bizarre fantasies that are characteristic of young children. It also helps to bond the family as a unit.

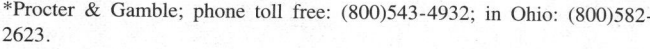

*Procter & Gamble; phone toll free: (800)543-4932; in Ohio: (800)582-2623.

Nursing Care Summary: The Low-Birth-Weight Infant

NURSING GOALS	NURSING INTERVENTIONS	EXPECTED PATIENT/FAMILY OUTCOMES

 All **Growth and development, altered**
Etiology: preterm birth

NURSING GOALS	NURSING INTERVENTIONS	EXPECTED PATIENT/FAMILY OUTCOMES
Facilitate physical adjustments	Assess physiologic status Provide appropriate physiologic support as outlined in appropriate nursing diagnoses	*Physiologic status is determined
Determine physiologic status	Measure infant Assess gestational age based on external characteristics and neurologic signs Weigh daily	Gestational age of infant is recorded at birth *Any deviation from baseline information is detected early and appropriate action implemented

 HP-HMP **Infection, potential for**
Etiology: deficient immunologic defenses

Prevent infection	Carry out meticulous handwashing before handling infant Ensure that all equipment in contact with infant is scrupulously clean or sterile Prevent personnel with infections from coming into direct contact with infant Isolate other infants who have infections	Infant exhibits no evidence of infection

 N-MP **Thermoregulation, ineffective**
Etiology: immature temperature control

Provide neutral thermal environment	Place infant in humidified Isolette, radiant warmer, or warmly clothed in open crib Monitor temperature hourly in unstable infants (take axillary temperature; check function of servocontrolled mechanism when used) Check temperature of infant in relation to temperature of heating unit Avoid situations that might predispose infant to chilling, such as exposure to cool air	Infant's temperature remains at optimum level

 N-MP **Fluid volume deficit, potential**
Risk factors: physiologic characteristics of preterm infant

Maintain hydration	Monitor therapies that increase insensible water loss, e.g., phototherapy Ensure adequate intake Assess state of hydration, e.g., skin turgor, temperature, weight, urine specific gravity	Infant exhibits no evidence of dehydration

 N-MP **Nutrition, alteration in: less than body requirements**
Etiology: inability to ingest nutrients because of weakness

Provide nutrition	Bottle-feed infant if strong sucking and swallowing reflexes are present Gavage feed if infant tires easily or has weak sucking, gag, or swallowing reflexes Assist mothers with breast-feeding if feasible and desirable	Infant receives an adequate amount of nutrients Infant demonstrates a steady weight gain

 N-MP **Skin integrity, impairment of: potential**
Risk factors: immature skin structure, immobility

Prevent skin breakdown	Cleanse skin with clear water or approved cleanser Avoid use of alkaline-based or hexachlorophene cleansing products or lotions	Skin remains clean and intact with no evidence of irritation

*Nursing outcome.

NURSING GOALS	NURSING INTERVENTIONS	EXPECTED PATIENT/FAMILY OUTCOMES
	Use transpore tape only to secure items to the skin Apply protective covering to skin on which tape or adhesive-backed items, e.g., electrodes, may be attached Exert extreme care when performing activities involving skin, e.g., removing dressings, electrodes, tape Place infant on water pillow or fleece Turn at least every 2 hours	

N.D. A-EP Breathing pattern, ineffective
Etiology: neuromuscular impairment (immature respiratory center), decreased energy, and fatigue

Support respiratory efforts	Position for optimum air exchange (head supported when on side) Observe for deviations from desired functioning; recognize signs of distress Suction as necessary to remove accumulated mucus from nasopharynx, trachea, and (where necessary) endotracheal tube Carry out percussion, vibration, and postural drainage to loosen secretions in respiratory tree Prevent aspiration Observe for signs of respiratory distress—nasal flaring, retractions, tachypnea	Breathing is regular and unlabored Respiratory rate is within normal limits (specify)

N.D. A-EP Activity intolerance
Etiology: imbalance between oxygen supply and demand

Conserve energy	Maintain neutral thermal environment Concentrate activites to allow for longer periods of rest Administer gavage feeding when infant tires easily Ensure minimum handling of infant	Infant rests 1 hour (uninterrupted) at regularly scheduled intervals (specify)

N.D. CPP Sensory-perceptual alteration: visual, auditory, kinesthetic, gustatory, tactile, olfactory
Etiology: therapeutically restricted environment

Provide sensory stimulation	Tactile
	  Caress, fondle, and otherwise provide skin contact; hold and cuddle infant if condition permits
	Auditory
	  Talk to infant during care
	  Encourage parents and others to talk to infant
	  Allow parents to provide musical toys
	Visual
	  Place colorful mobiles and toys within visual field
	  Hold face within 9 to 12 inches of infant's face and stimulate infant to follow head movements
	Kinesthetic
	  Rock infant
	  Alter position periodically
	  Move extremeities periodically
	Gustatory
	  Encourage mouthing activity
	  Provide for nonnutritive sucking, expecially during gavage feeding, painful procedures
		Infant responds to stimuli

N.D. RRP Family process, alteration in
Etiology: situational/maturational crisis, knowledge deficit (birth of a preterm infant)

Keep parents informed of infant's progress	Answer questions, allow expression of concern regarding care and prognosis Encourage mother and father to visit and/or call unit Emphasize positive aspects of infant status Be honest but not overly candid or overly optimistic	Parents express feelings and concerns regarding the infant and his prognosis

NURSING GOALS	NURSING INTERVENTIONS	EXPECTED PATIENT/FAMILY OUTCOMES
Facilitate sibling-infant attachment	Allow siblings to visit infant when feasible Explain environment, events, and strange appearance of infant, e.g., why infant cannot come home, "special" bed Provide photos of infant or other items if siblings unable to visit	Siblings visit infant in nursery Siblings exhibit an understanding of explanations (specify) Siblings receive infant-related items (specify)
Prepare for infant's discharge	Assess readiness of family (especially mother) to care for infant Teach necessary techniques and observations Arrange for public health referral if indicated Reinforce follow-up care Refer to appropriate agencies or services for needed assistance Encourage and facilitate involvement with parent group Teach family infant cardiopulmonary resuscitation technique and response to choking incident	Family demonstrates the ability to provide care for the infant Family members take advantage of available services Family members keep appointments for follow-up care

RRP   **Parenting, alteration in**
       Etiology: interruption of bonding process

Facilitate parent-infant attachment process	Initiate parents' visit as soon as possible
	Encourage parents to
	  Visit infant frequently
	  Touch, fondle, and caress infant
	  Become actively involved in infant's care
	  Bring clothing to dress up infant as soon as condition permits
	Reinforce parents' endeavors
	Be alert to signs of tension in parents
	Allow parents to spend time alone with infant
	Help parents interpret infant responses; comment regarding any positive infant response
	Help parents by demonstrating techniques and offer support
		Parents visit infant soon after birth and at frequent intervals
		Parents relate positively with infant
		Parents provide care for the infant and demonstrate an attitude of comfort in relationships with the infant

Nursing Interventions Related to Medical Management

Support respiratory efforts
  Maintain ambient oxygen at level to ensure satisfactory skin color with minimum respiratory effort and energy expenditure
  Carry out regimen prescribed for supplemental oxygen therapy (maintain ambient oxygen concentration at minimum Fio_2 level to maintain good color and energy expenditure)
  Apply and manage monitoring equipment correctly
  Understand functioning of respiratory support apparatus
    Assisted ventilation apparatus
    Controlled ventilation apparatus
    Insufflation bags with masks and/or endotracheal adaptor
    Oxygen hoods
    Humidifier warmers
Provide nutrition
  Maintain parenteral fluid or hyperalimentation therapy as ordered
Maintain hydration
  Regulate parenteral fluids
  Avoid administering hypertonic fluids, e.g., undiluted medications
Monitor physiologic data
  Understand proper function and use of monitoring equipment and maintain at desired settings
    Apnea monitor
    Heart rate monitor, including oscilloscope and electrocardiograph printout units

    Temperature monitor, usually with skin probe
    Oxygen analyzers
    Transcutaneous monitors
  Collect specimens
    Blood for glucose, bilirubin, electrolytes, and pH determinations
    Blood for hemoglobin, hematocrit, microscopic examination, and culture
    Urine for laboratory examination
  Take vital signs as ordered (axillary temperature, apical pulse)
Prevent or control infection
  Administer prophylactic antibiotics as ordered
Assist in specific therapies
  Phototherapy—implement and maintain protective measures
  Administer medications as ordered
    Antibiotics prophylactically or therapeutically
    Vitamin K to prevent hemorrhage
    Sedatives, etc., for withdrawal symptoms, seizures, irritability
    Electrolyte replacement
    Alkali therapy in acidosis
  Avoid use of substances known to be toxic to premature infants, e.g., benzyl alcohol or other preservatives
  Provide assisted ventilation and therapeutic measures as indicated

pare the parents for an inevitable death and facilitate a family's grieving process after an expected or an unexpected death.

The loss of an infant has special meaning for the grieving parents. It represents a loss of a part of themselves (especially for mothers), a loss of the potential for immortality that offspring represent, and the loss of the dream child that has been fantasized throughout the pregnancy. There is a sense of emptiness and failure. In addition, when an infant has lived for such a short time, there are few, if any, pleasant memories to serve as a basis for identification and idealization that are part of the resolution of a loss.

To help the parents understand that the death is a reality, it is important that the parents are allowed to hold their infant before death and if possible be present at the time of death so that their infant can die in their arms if they choose (Wooten, 1981). Parents should be provided with an opportunity to see, touch, hold, caress, examine, and talk to their infant privately after death and to bathe their infant if they desire as a final act to perform. If parents are hesitant about seeing their dead infant, it is advisable to keep the body in the unit for a few hours, since many parents change their minds after the initial shock of the death. The nurse should remain available and stay with the parents if they desire.

Some units have implemented a hospice approach for families with infants for whom the decision has been made not to prolong life and who are receiving only palliative care. A special "family" room is set aside that contains all supportive equipment needed for the care of the infant and also provides a homelike atmosphere for the family. All hospice services are available to the family, and the infant remains under the care and supervision of the NICU staff (Whitfield and others, 1982). (See p. 967 for further discussion of hospice care.)

A photograph of the infant taken before or after death is highly desirable. The parents may not wish to see the photograph at the time of death, but the chance to refer to it later will help make their infant seem more real, which is a part of the normal grief process (Mahan and Schreiner, 1980; Speck and Kennell, 1980; Wooten, 1981). A photograph of their infant being held by the hand or touched by an adult offers a more positive image than a morgue type of photograph. Other tangible remembrances of the child can be provided, such as name tags, armbands, and locks of hair shaved for intravenous insertion or other procedures. If the parents have not done so, they should be encouraged to name their infant.

At least one nurse who is familiar to the family should be present during the discussion about a dead or dying infant. The nurse should talk with parents openly and honestly about funeral arrangements, since few of them have had experience with this aspect of death. Many funeral homes now offer inexpensive arrangements for these special cases. Someone from the NICU should take the responsibility for acquiring this type of information. Families need to be informed of options available, but it is preferable to encourage a funeral because the ritual provides an opportunity for parents to feel the support of friends and relatives. A clergyman of the appropriate faith is offered if available.

Before the parents leave the hospital, they are given the telephone number of the unit (if they do not have it) and invited to call any time they have any further questions. Many intensive care units make it a point to contact the parents following a neonatal death to assess parents' coping mechanisms and evaluate the grieving process. (See Chapter 23 for further discussion of the family and the grief process.)

Baptism. Since most Christian parents wish to have their child baptized if death is anticipated or a decided possibility, this becomes a nursing responsibility. Whenever possible, it is most desirable that a representative of the parents' faith—that is, a Roman Catholic priest or a Protestant minister—perform such a ritual. When death is imminent, a nurse or a physician can perform the baptism by simply pouring water on the infant's forehead (a medicine dropper is a convenient means) while repeating the words, "I baptize you in the name of the Father and of the Son and of the Holy Spirit." This includes a birth of any gestational age, particularly when the parents are of the Roman Catholic faith.

When the faith of the parents is uncertain, a conditional baptism can be carried out by saying, "If you are capable of receiving baptism, I baptize you in the name of the Father and of the Son and of the Holy Spirit." The fact of the baptism is recorded in the infant's chart and a notice placed on the crib or Isolette. Parents are informed at the first opportunity.

High-Risk Conditions Related to Dysmaturity

In any newborn, various disease states and congenital abnormalities are associated with increased risk in the neonatal period and may or may not be related to the state of maturity. This segment of the chapter is devoted to a description of the dysmature states, prematurity and postmaturity. Although prematurity is encountered more frequently and is a greater threat to life, postmaturity is not without problems.

PRETERM INFANTS

Prematurity accounts for the largest number of admissions to an NICU. Not only does the immaturity of these infants place them at risk for neonatal complications (e.g., hyperbilirubinemia and hyaline membrane disease, which is highest in the preterm infant), but also other high-risk factors (e.g., congenital abnormalities in association with prematurity). Prematurity is generally accepted as the single greatest factor contributing to infant mortality.

Etiology

Most of the aspects concerning high-risk neonates listed on pp. 369 to 371 are related to the incidence of prematurity;

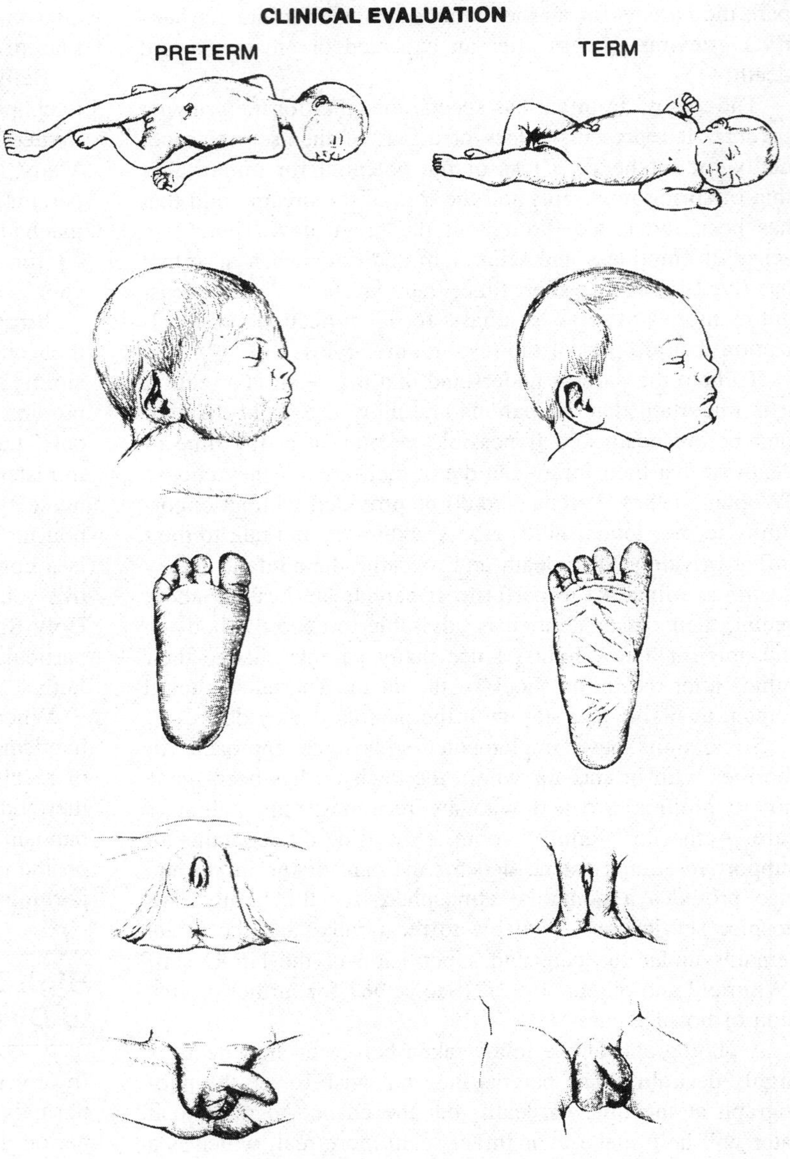

The preterm infant lies in a "relaxed attitude," limbs more extended; his body size is small, and his head may appear somewhat larger in proportion to the body size. The term infant has more subcutaneous fat tissue and rests in a more flexed attitude.

The preterm infant's ear cartilages are poorly developed, and the ear may fold easily; the hair is fine and feathery, and lanugo may cover the back and face. The mature infant's ear cartilages are well formed, and the hair is more likely to form firm separate strands.

The sole of the foot of the preterm infant appears more turgid and may have only fine wrinkles. The mature infant's sole (foot) is well and deeply creased.

The preterm female infant's clitoris is prominent, and labia majora are poorly developed and gaping. The mature female infant's labia majora are fully developed, and the clitoris is not as prominent.

The preterm male infant's scrotum is undeveloped and not pendulous; minimal rugae are present, and the testes may be in the inguinal canals or in the abdominal cavity. The term male infant's scrotum is well developed, pendulous, and rugated, and the testes are well down in the scrotal sac.

CLINICAL EVALUATION

PRETERM   TERM

Fig. 10-11. Clinical and neurologic examinations comparing preterm and full-term infants. Adapted from Pierog, S.H., and Ferrara, A.: Medical care of the sick newborn, ed. 2, St. Louis, 1976, The C.V. Mosby Co.

however, the actual cause of prematurity is not known in most instances. The incidence of prematurity is lowest in the middle to high socioeconomic classes, in which pregnant women are generally in good health, are well nourished, and receive prompt and comprehensive prenatal care; the incidence is highest in the low socioeconomic class, in which a combination of deleterious circumstances is present. Other factors, such as multiple pregnancies, preeclampsia, and placental accidents that interrupt the normal course of gestation prior to completion of fetal development, are responsible for a large number of premature births.

The outlook for premature infants is largely, but not entirely, related to the state of physiologic and anatomic immaturity of the various organs and systems at the time of birth. Infants at term have advanced to a state of maturity

sufficient to allow a successful transition to the extrauterine environment. Infants born prematurely must make the same adjustments but with functional immaturity proportional to the stage of development reached at the time of birth. The degree to which infants are prepared for extrauterine life can be predicted to some extent by weight and estimated gestational age (see p. 303). The landmarks of prenatal development in Table 5-6 provide some concept of the status of the systems at various stages of development that must cope with the functional changes that occur with birth.

Characteristics

Preterm infants have a number of characteristics that are distinctive at various stages of development. Identification of these characteristics provides valuable clues to the gesta-

NEUROLOGIC EVALUATION

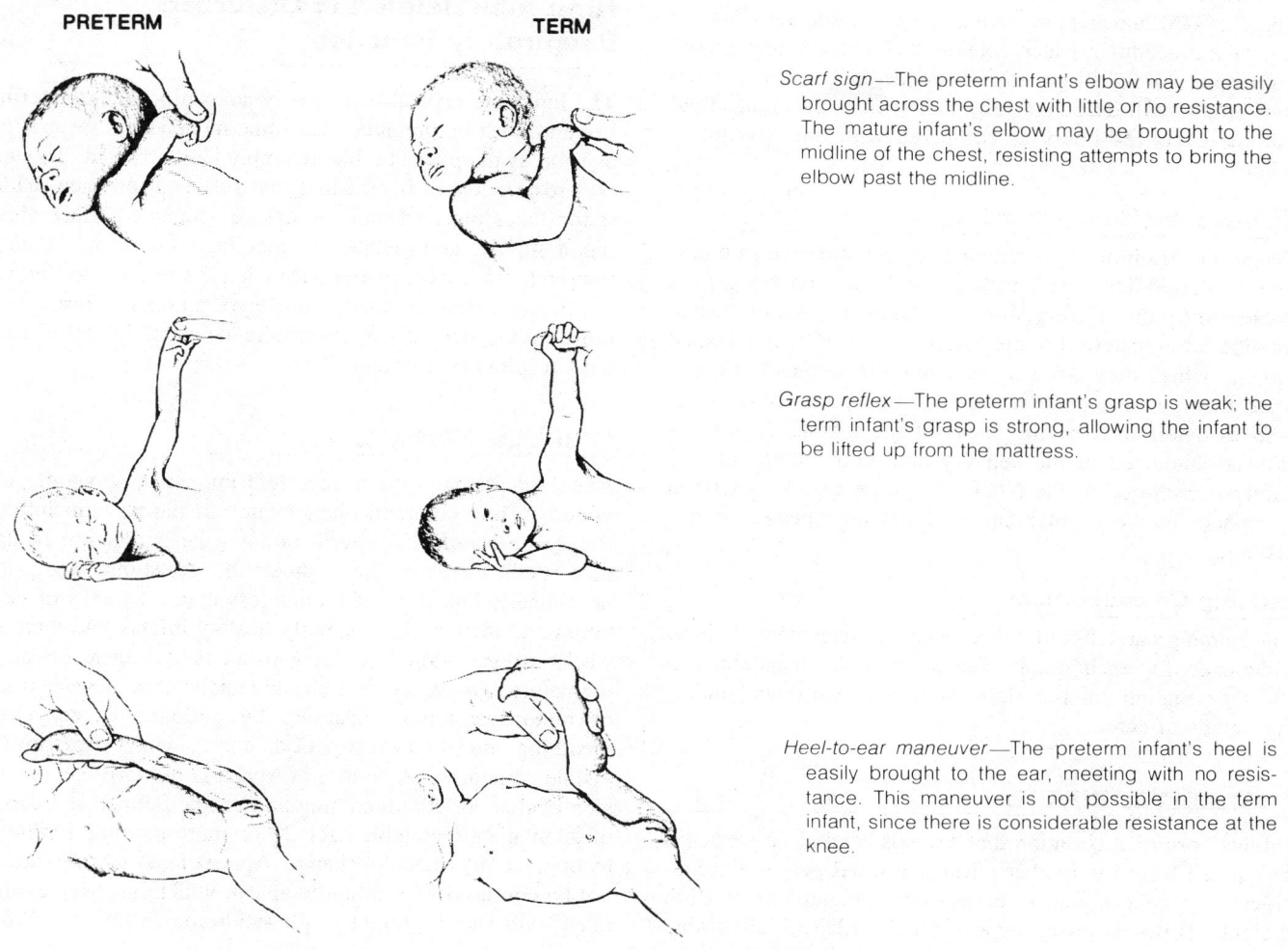

PRETERM

TERM

Scarf sign—The preterm infant's elbow may be easily brought across the chest with little or no resistance. The mature infant's elbow may be brought to the midline of the chest, resisting attempts to bring the elbow past the midline.

Grasp reflex—The preterm infant's grasp is weak; the term infant's grasp is strong, allowing the infant to be lifted up from the mattress.

Heel-to-ear maneuver—The preterm infant's heel is easily brought to the ear, meeting with no resistance. This maneuver is not possible in the term infant, since there is considerable resistance at the knee.

Fig. 10-11, cont'd. For legend see opposite page.

tional age and hence to the physiologic capabilities of infants. The general, outward physical appearance changes as the fetus progresses to maturity. Characteristics of skin, general attitude when supine, appearance of hair, and amount of subcutaneous fat provide cues to a newborn's physical development. Observation of spontaneous, active movements and response to stimulation and passive movement contributes to the assessment of neurologic status. The appraisal is made as soon as possible after admission to the nursery, since much of the observation and management of infants depends on this information.

On inspection premature infants are very small and appear scrawny because they lack or have only minimum subcutaneous fat deposits, with a proportionately large head in relation to the body, which reflects the cephalocaudal direction of growth. Of all the body measurements, the head is reduced least, and sucking pads in the cheeks are strikingly prominent. The skin is bright pink, smooth, and shiny (may be edematous) with small blood vessels clearly visible underneath the thin, transparent epidermis. The fine lanugo hair is abundant over the body but is sparse, fine, and fuzzy

on the head. The ear cartilage is soft and pliable, and the soles and palms have minimum creases, resulting in a smooth appearance. The bones of the skull and the ribs feel soft, and the prominent eyes are closed. Male infants have few scrotal rugae, and the testes are undescended; labia and clitoris are prominent in females. (See Fig. 10-11 for a comparison of the features of normal and premature infants.)

In contrast to full-term infants' overall attitude of flexion and continuous activity, premature infants are inactive and torpid. The extremities maintain an attitude of extension and remain in any position in which they are placed. Reflex activity is only partially developed—sucking is absent, weak, or ineffectual; swallowing, gag, and cough reflexes are weak; and other neurologic signs are absent or diminished. Physiologically immature, preterm infants are unable to maintain body temperature, have limited ability to excrete solutes in the urine, and have increased susceptibility to infection. A pliable thorax along with immature lung tissue and regulatory center lead to periodic breathing, hypoventilation, and frequent periods of apnea. They are more susceptible to biochemical alterations such as hyperbilirubinemia (p. 346) and hypoglycemia (p. 356), and they have a higher extracellular water content that renders them more vulnerable to fluid and electrolyte derangements. Premature infants will exchange fully half their extracellular fluid volume every 24 hours as compared with one seventh in adults.

Therapeutic Management

When preterm infants are anticipated, the intensive care nursery is alerted and a pediatrician, ideally a neonatologist, is present for their delivery. Infants who do not require resuscitation are transferred immediately to the NICU in a heated Isolette where they are weighed, and intravenous lines, oxygen therapy, and other therapeutic interventions are initiated as determined by the needs of the infants. Resuscitation is conducted in the delivery area until infants can be safely transported to the NICU. Ongoing care is described elsewhere in the chapter and will not be repeated in this section.

Nursing Considerations

The nursing care, like the therapeutic management, is individualized for each infant. See appropriate discussions in the segments on nursing high-risk infants and their families for details of care.

POSTMATURE INFANTS

Infants born of a gestation that extends beyond 42 weeks as calculated from the mother's last menstrual period are considered to be postmature or postterm, regardless of birth weight. This comprises approximately 12% of all births. The cause of delayed birth is unknown. Some infants are appropriate for gestational age, but many show the characteristics of progressive placental dysfunction. Others—often called postmature infants—display the characteristics of infants who are 1 to 3 weeks of age, such as absence of lanugo, little if any vernix caseosa, abundant scalp hair, long fingernails, and whiter skin than term newborns. Frequently the skin is cracked, parchmentlike, and desquamating. A common finding in postmature infants is a wasted physical appearance that reflects intrauterine impoverishment. There is a depletion of subcutaneous fat that gives them a thin, long appearance. The little vernix caseosa that remains in the skin folds is usually stained a deep yellow or green.

There is a significant increase in fetal and neonatal mortality in postterm infants compared to those born at term. They are especially prone to intrauterine hypoxia associated with the decreasing efficiency of the placenta and to the meconium aspiration syndrome. The greatest risk occurs during the stresses of labor and delivery, particularly in infants of *primigravidas,* women delivering their first child. Cesarean section or induction of labor is usually recommended when infants are significantly overdue.

High Risk Related to Disturbed Respiratory Function

The lungs are critical to the early adaptation to extrauterine life and must be prepared to assume independent respiration as soon as the placental blood supply is interrupted. To support respiration, it is essential that sufficient prenatal maturation takes place in order to ensure adequate surface area, blood supply, and metabolic capability to maintain ventilation and tissue oxygenation. Deficiencies relative to this vital function can seriously impair respiratory efforts, and most of the neonates who require neonatal intensive care have respiratory problems.

APNEA OF PREMATURITY

Apnea of prematurity, or recurrent idiopathic apnea of prematurity, is a common phenomenon in the preterm infant. Rarely observed in full-term infants, the prevalence of apneic spells increases the younger the gestational age. Approximately one third of infants less than 32 weeks of gestation and almost all apparently healthy infants less than 30 weeks of gestation have apneic spells. Characteristically, premature infants are periodic breathers; they have periods of rapid respiration separated by periods of very slow breathing and often short periods during which there are no visible or audible respirations. Apnea is primarily an extension of this periodic breathing and can be defined as a lapse of spontaneous breathing for 20 or more seconds followed by bradycardia and color change. Apnea of prematurity should not be confused with infantile apnea, which has been associated with sudden infant death syndrome (SIDS) (p. 578).

Pathophysiology

Although the cause of apnea of prematurity is unknown, it probably reflects the immature and poorly refined neurologic and chemical respiratory control mechanisms. These infants are not as responsive to oxygen and carbon dioxide, and their neurons have fewer dendritic associations than the more mature infant. The respiratory reflexes of these infants are significantly more immature, which may be a contributing factor in the etiology (Gerhardt and Bancalari, 1984). In addition, apnea is characteristically observed during periods of rapid eye movement in sleep.

Clinical Manifestations

A number of factors that appear to promote the incidence of apnea in preterm neonates can be treated. Apnea can be anticipated in infants with any of the circumstances listed below; conversely one of these disorders may be suspected in infants with persistent apneic spells. Although apnea is an expected event in preterm neonates, it should not be designated as such until all other causes are ruled out. The observation of apnea is cause to screen for any of the following possible causes:

Airway obstruction with mucus or poor position

Anemia

Dehydration

Cooling

Overheating

Hypercapnia

Hypocapnia

Hypoglycemia

Hypocalcemia

Sepsis, meningitis

Seizures

Increased vagal tone (frequently observed in infants with very full stomachs after eating)

Prolonged periodic breathing

Central nervous system depression from pharmacologic agents

Intracranial hemorrhage

Heart failure

Depression following maternal obstetric sedation

Respiratory-distressed infants who are tiring

Therapeutic Management

It has been found that oral administration of theophylline is often effective in reducing the frequency of primary apnea-bradycardia spells in newborns. Theophylline appears to act centrally by increasing infants' sensitivity to carbon dioxide. Neonates who receive the drug must be closely observed for tachycardia; a rate greater than 180 to 190 beats per minute indicates a need to reduce the dosage (Myers and others, 1980; Roberts, Mathew, and Thach, 1982). Caffeine (Murat and others, 1981) and doxapram (Eyal and others, 1985; Barrington and others, 1986) have been found to be effective also.

Nursing Considerations

Management of periodic apnea consists of monitoring respiration and heart rate routinely in all small preterm infants and prevention of conditions that might precipitate it. Mechanical apnea monitors provide a means to alert the staff to cessation of respiration according to a preset delay time, usually 10 to 15 seconds. Effective monitoring devices do not make alert nursing observation unnecessary. Any mechanical device is subject to malfunction. When the alarm sounds, infants are first assessed for color and for presence of respiration. If they display the usual color and respirations, the nurse should investigate possible causes of a false alarm, such as faulty lead placement, detached or disconnected leads, improper alarm setting, or mechanical failure. Without close observation, even of monitored infants, many unidentified episodes of prolonged apnea and severe bradycardia occur (Southall and others, 1983).

Gentle tactile stimulation will stop most apneic spells if it is begun early. If stimulation fails to reinstitute respiration, nose and oropharynx are suctioned, and if breathing does not begin, the chin is raised gently and sufficient pressure applied with mask and Ambu bag to lift the rib cage. After breathing is restored, infants are assessed for possible precipitating factors, such as temperature, humidity, distention (if not observed earlier), and ambient oxygen content

of Isolette. It is important for nurses to document episodes of apnea. A careful record is maintained of the number of apneic spells, the appearance of infants during and after attacks, and whether the infants self-stimulate or if exogenous stimulation is needed to restore breathing. Persistent and repeated periods of apnea are treated by mechanical ventilation with the respirator set at low pressure and rate.

Various methods devised to provide an intermittent stimulus for breathing have achieved variable success, such as oscillating water beds. A water bed providing continuous, gentle, irregular, head-to-foot oscillations by way of a small, inflatable bladder connected to an electronic oscillator supplies very subtle vestibular-proprioceptive stimulation for breathing. Although in one study LBW infants on water beds were found to sleep more, to be less restless during sleep, and to display fewer jittery or unsmooth movements, the incidence of apnea was not affected (Korner, Ruppel, and Rho, 1982). VLBW infants were more distressed on water beds than were larger LBW infants.

RESPIRATORY DISTRESS SYNDROME

Respiratory distress is a name applied to respiratory dysfunction in neonates and is primarily a disease related to developmental delay in lung maturation. The terms *respiratory distress syndrome* (RDS), *idiopathic respiratory distress syndrome* (IRDS), and *hyaline membrane disease* (HMD) are most often applied to the severe lung disorder that is not only responsible for more infant deaths than any other disease but also carries the highest risk in terms of long-term neurologic complications (see p. 1373 for a discussion of adult RDS). It is seen almost exclusively in preterm infants. The disorder is rare in infants of narcotic-addicted mothers or infants who have been subjected to intrauterine stress (e.g., maternal preeclampsia or hypertension) and is seldom seen in black female infants.

Pneumonia in the neonatal period is respiratory distress caused by pathogenic organisms. The disease may occur alone or as a complication of HMD. However, because so many of the terms are used interchangeably, for this discussion the more general term RDS will be used except where HMD is particularly applicable.

Pathophysiology

Preterm infants are born before the lungs are fully prepared to serve as efficient organs for gas exchange. This appears to be a critical factor in the development of respiratory distress syndrome. Although the precise cause is still undetermined, several features in the development of the disorder are established and there are a number of interdependent relationships that complicate the situation.

Before birth there is evidence of fetal respiratory activity. The lungs make feeble respiratory movements, and fluid is excreted through the alveoli. Since the final unfolding of the alveolar septa, which increases the surface area of the lungs, takes place during the last trimester of pregnancy, premature infants are born with numerous underdeveloped and many uninflatable alveoli. There is limited pulmonary blood flow resulting from the collapsed state of the fetal lungs and from poor vascular development in general and an immature capillary network in particular. Because of the increased pulmonary vascular resistance, the major portion of fetal blood is shunted from the lungs by way of the ductus arteriosus and foramen ovale (see p. 1449).

At the time of birth, infants must initiate breathing and then keep the previously fluid-filled lungs inflated with air. At the same time the pulmonary capillary blood flow must be increased approximately tenfold to provide for adequate lung perfusion and to alter the intracardiac pressure that closes the fetal cardiac structures. Most full-term infants successfully accomplish these adjustments; preterm infants with respiratory distress are unable to do so. Although numerous factors are involved, most authorities believe that the central factor responsible for this adaptation is normal development of the surfactant system.

Surfactant is a surface-active phospholipid secreted by the alveolar epithelium. Acting much like a detergent, this substance reduces surface tension of fluids that line the alveoli and respiratory passages, resulting in uniform expansion and maintenance of lung expansion at low intraalveolar pressure. Immature development of these functions produces consequences that seriously compromise respiratory efficiency. Deficient surfactant production causes unequal inflation of alveoli on inspiration and collapse of alveoli on end expiration. Without surfactant, infants are unable to keep their lungs inflated and therefore exert a great deal of effort to reexpand the alveoli with each breath. It has been estimated that each breath requires as much negative pressure (60 to 75 cm H_2O) as the initial lung expansion at birth. As a result, infants use more oxygen to expend this energy than they take in, which rapidly leads to exhaustion. With increasing exhaustion they are able to open fewer and fewer alveoli. This inability to maintain lung expansion produces widespread atelectasis.

In the absence of alveolar stability (normal functional residual capacity) and with progressive atelectasis, the pulmonary vascular resistance increases, whereas with normal lung expansion it would decrease. Consequently there is hypoperfusion to the lung tissue with a decrease in effective pulmonary blood flow. The increase in pulmonary vascular resistance causes partial reversion to the fetal circulation with a right-to-left shunting of blood through the persisting fetal communications—the ductus arteriosus and foramen ovale. Inadequate pulmonary perfusion and ventilation produce hypoxemia and hypercapnia. Pulmonary arterioles, with their thick muscular layer, are markedly reactive to diminished oxygen concentration. Thus a decrease in oxygen tension causes vasospasm in the pulmonary arterioles that is further enhanced by a decrease in blood pH. This vasoconstriction contributes to a marked increase in pulmonary vascular resistance. In normal ventilation with increased oxy-

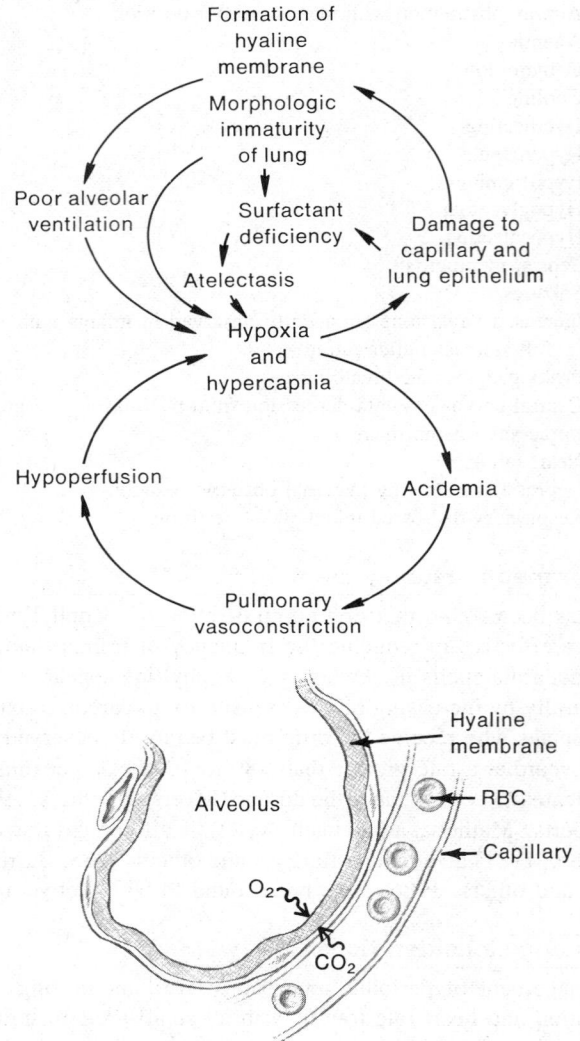

Fig. 10-12. Interdependent relationship of factors involved in pathology of respiratory distress syndrome.
From Pierog, S.H., and Ferrara, A.: Medical care of the sick newborn, ed. 2, St. Louis, 1976, The C.V. Mosby Co.

gen concentration, the ductus arteriosus constricts and the pulmonary vessels dilate to decrease pulmonary vascular resistance (Fig. 10-12).

To compound this situation, prolonged hypoxemia activates the anaerobic glycolysis that produces increased amounts of lactic acid. An increase in lactic acid causes metabolic acidosis; inability of the atelectatic lungs to blow off excess carbon dioxide produces respiratory acidosis. Lowered pH causes further vasoconstriction. With deficient pulmonary circulation and alveolar perfusion, the blood oxygen concentration continues to fall, the pH falls, and materials needed for surfactant production are not circulated to the alveoli.

Pulmonary edema observed in the early stages of IRDS also contributes to impaired gas exchange. Factors believed to facilitate this fluid accumulation in the lungs include renal immaturity or insufficiency resulting from hypoxemia, high fluid intake and patent ductus arteriosus, left ventricular dysfunction associated with papillary muscle necrosis, low serum protein concentration and low colloid osmotic pressure, increased alveolar surface tension that enhances the shift of interstitial fluid to alveolar spaces, oxygen toxicity, and high plasma vasopressin (summarized by Yeh and others, 1982). Spontaneous diuresis usually occurs after approximately 72 hours.

Deficiencies in other systems contribute to respiratory distress. For example, a high threshold of the respiratory center to afferent stimuli and weak gag and cough reflexes reflect the immaturity of the nervous system. In addition, the persistence of fetal hemoglobin, so beneficial in prenatal existence, may place the infant at a disadvantage during respiratory distress. Although the binding power of fetal hemoglobin for oxygen is much greater than in adult hemoglobin, this increased affinity also causes less oxygen to be released to the tissues at normal oxygen tension. In the newborn the arterial oxygen concentration must fall to a lower level for bound oxygen to be released from fetal hemoglobin.

The hyaline membrane, pathognomonic of HMD, is formed as hypoxemia and the increased pulmonary vascular pressure cause transudation of fluid into the alveoli. Necrotic cells from damaged alveoli plus the fibrin in the transudate form a membranous layer that lines the alveoli and inhibits gas exchange. Presence of the membrane contributes to respiratory difficulties by greatly diminishing lung distensibility, or *compliance,* the elastic quality of lung tissue that permits expansion in response to a given amount of applied pressure during inspiration. Affected lungs are stiffer and require far more pressure than do normal lungs to achieve an equal amount of expansion. The major factors that produce respiratory distress in immature infants are summarized in Table 10-3.

HMD is a self-limiting disease, and following a period of deterioration (approximately 48 hours) and in the absence of complications, the affected infants begin to improve by 72 hours, often heralded by the onset of diuresis. The improvement has been attributed primarily to increased production and greater availability of surface-active material.

Clinical Manifestations

Infants with RDS can develop respiratory insufficiency either acutely or over a period of hours. Usually the observable signs produced by the pulmonary changes begin to appear in infants who apparently achieve normal breathing and color soon after birth. In 30 minutes to 2 hours breathing gradually becomes more difficult and the infants display substernal retractions. Retractions, a prominent feature of pulmonary difficulties in preterm infants, are the result of a compliant chest wall. Weak chest wall muscles and the highly cartilaginous nature of the rib structure produce an abnormally elastic rib cage. Thus considerable negative pressure is wasted as the infant attempts to produce higher

Table 10-3 Major factors in respiratory distress

CAUSE	EFFECT
Increased surface tension of alveoli (surfactant deficiency)	Alveolar collapse; atelectasis; increased difficulty of breathing
Impaired gas exchange	Hypoxemia and hypercapnia with respiratory acidosis
Increased pulmonary vascular resistance	Hypoperfusion of pulmonary circulation
Hypoperfusion (with hypoxemia)	Tissue hypoxia and metabolic acidosis
Increased transudation of fluid into lungs	Hyaline membrane formation; impaired gas exchange

intrathoracic pressure changes. During this early period infants' color remains satisfactory and auscultation reveals good air entry. Some of the criteria for evaluating respiratory distress in infants are illustrated in Fig. 10-13.

Within a few hours, respiratory distress becomes more obvious. The respiratory rate increases (to 80 to 120 breaths per minute), and breathing becomes more labored. It is significant to note that infants will increase the *rate* rather than the *depth* of respiration when in distress. Substernal retractions become more pronounced as the diaphragm works hard in an attempt to fill collapsed air sacs. Fine inspiratory rales can be heard over both lungs, and there is an audible expiratory grunt. This grunt, a useful mechanism observed in the earlier stages of RDS, serves to increase end-expiratory pressure in the lungs, thus maintaining alveolar expansion and allowing gas exchange for an additional brief period. Flaring of the nares is also a sign that accompanies tachypnea, grunting, and retractions in respiratory distress. Cyanosis appears but can usually be abolished by increasing the ambient oxygen so the infant obtains pink skin.

At this point the respiratory distress may gradually decrease over 12 to 24 hours with eventual recovery, or it may increase in severity. In distressed infants cyanosis becomes more marked despite increases in ambient oxygen concentration. Often there is pallor caused by peripheral vasoconstriction, but it is frequently masked by cyanosis. The infants become flaccid and unresponsive and begin to display frequent apneic episodes. Chest auscultation reveals diminished breath sounds. The chances of recovery without assisted ventilation are then very small. Severe hyaline membrane disease is often associated with a shocklike state, as manifested by diminished cardiac inflow and low arterial blood pressure.

Infants with RDS who survive the first 96 hours have a reasonable chance of recovery. Complications of RDS include those described as complications of oxygen therapy (p. 1314), patent ductus arteriosus and congestive heart failure, persistent pulmonary hypertension, intraventricular hemorrhage, and necrotizing enterocolitis.

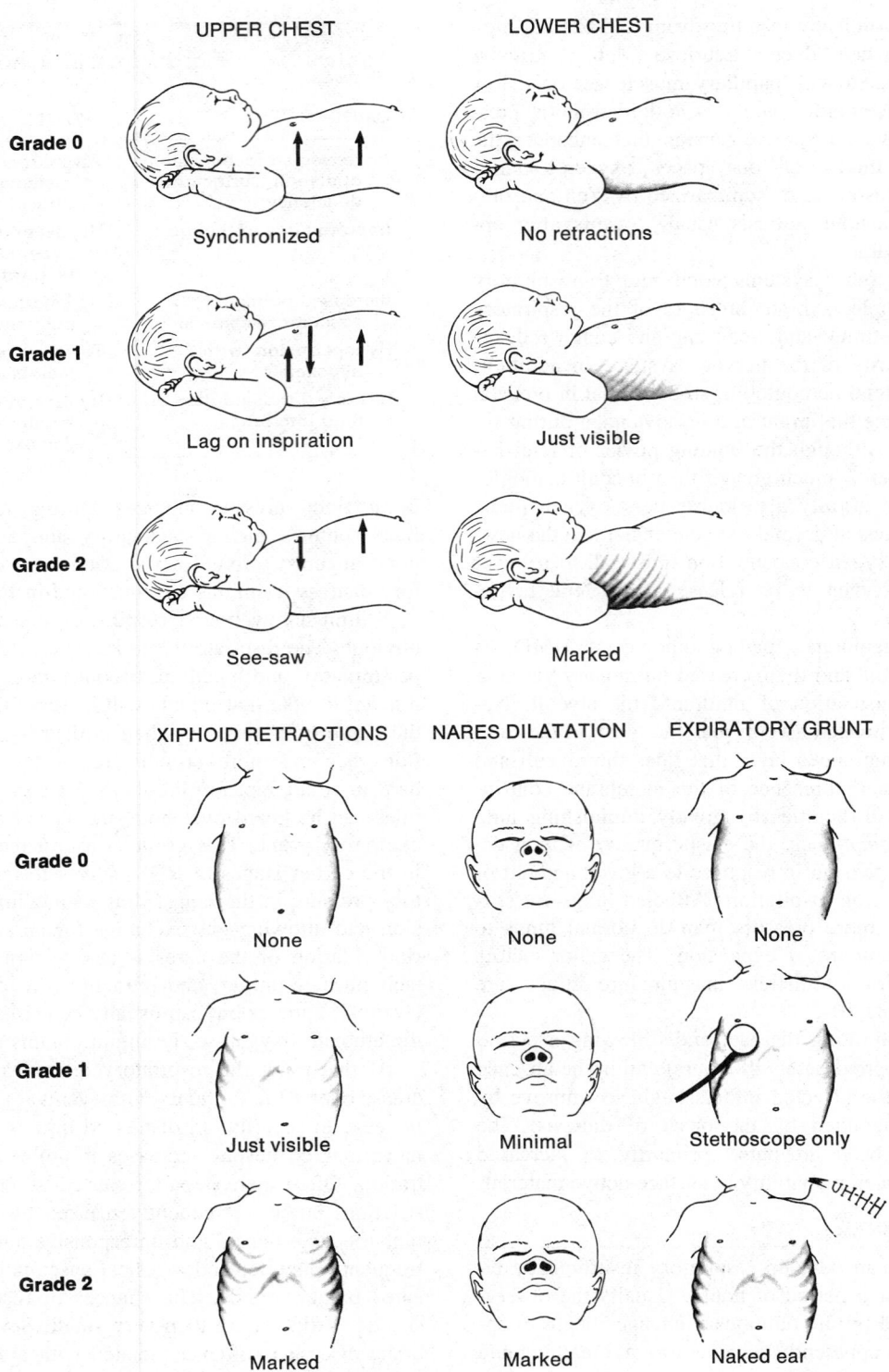

Fig. 10-13. Criteria for evaluating respiratory distress.
Adapted from Silverman, W.A., and Anderson, D.H.: Pediatrics **17**:1, 1956. Copyright American Academy of Pediatrics, 1956.

Diagnostic Evaluation

Laboratory data are nonspecific, and abnormalities observed are identical to those observed in numerous biochemical abnormalities of the newborn, that is, the findings of hypoxemia, hypercapnia, and acidosis. To determine complicating factors, specific tests are carried out, such as blood, urine, and spinal fluid cultures (to rule out sepsis), blood glucose (to test for hypoglycemia), serum calcium (for hypocalcemia), and blood gas measurements for serum pH (for presence of acidosis). Other special examinations may be employed to diagnose or rule out complications.

Radiographic findings characteristic of hyaline membrane disease include: (1) a diffuse granular pattern over both lung fields closely resembling ground glass that represents alveolar atelectasis, and (2) dark streaks, or bronchograms, within the ground glass areas that represent dilated air-filled bronchioles (Fig. 10-14). It is important to distinguish between HMD and pneumonia in infants with respiratory distress.

Prenatal diagnosis. Fetal lung maturity depends on gestational age, except in some specific instances that may not be known until the time of labor or delivery. Functional maturity of the fetal lung can be determined by using surfactant phospholipids in amniotic fluid as indicators of maturity. The most commonly tested is the lecithin/sphingomyelin (L/S) ratio, which measures the relationship between these two lipids during gestation. Phospholipids are synthesized by fetal alveolar cells and the concentrations in amniotic fluid change during gestation. Initially there is more sphingomyelin, but at about 32 to 33 weeks the concentrations become equal, and then sphingomyelin diminishes and lecithin increases significantly until the fetus has developed sufficient surface-active material to maintain alveolar stability at about 35 weeks.

Other key surfactant compounds (also phospholipids) that are needed to stabilize surfactant are phosphatidylinositol (PI) and phosphatidylglycerol (PG). Without these compounds lecithin is not functional as a surfactant. Concentrations of PI parallel those of lecithin, peaking at 35 weeks and gradually decreasing. At 36 weeks PG appears in amniotic fluid and increases until term. By measuring these phospholipids—L/A ratio, PI, and PG—the maturity of the lungs can be estimated with a high degree of accuracy. Abnormal pregnancies may be associated with acceleration (before 33 weeks) or delay (later than 37 weeks) in fetal lung maturation.

Other, but less frequently employed, methods have been devised to provide rapid, inexpensive, and accurate measures of lung maturity. These include the "shake" or "bubble" test, in which stable foam or bubbles form when amniotic fluid is shaken in the presence of ethanol, and the tap tests, in which abundant bubbles appear in a test tube of amniotic fluid with 6N hydrochloric acid and diethyl ether (Socol, Sing, and Depp, 1984).

Therapeutic Management

The treatment of RDS is largely supportive and includes all the general measures required for any premature infant as well as those instituted to correct imbalances. The supportive measures that are most crucial to a favorable outcome are: (1) correct metabolic acidosis by intravenous administration of sodium bicarbonate, which also dilates pulmonary vessels and reduces the constriction response, (2) maintain neutral temperature environment to conserve utilization of oxygen, (3) prevent hypotension and hypovolemia, and (4) provide additional fractional inspired oxygen (FiO_2) content by increasing ambient oxygen concentration or by assisted ventilation. Nipple feedings are contraindicated in any situation that creates a marked increase in respiratory rate because of the greater hazards of aspiration. Nutrition is provided by gavage and/or parenteral feedings.

Oxygen therapy. The goals of oxygen therapy are to provide adequate oxygen to the tissues, prevent lactic acid accumulation resulting from hypoxia, and at the same time avoid the toxic effects of oxygen. Numerous methods have been devised to improve oxygenation (Table 10-4). All require that the gas be warmed and humidified before entering the respiratory tract. If the infant does not require mechanical ventilation, oxygen supplied to the Isolette or a plastic hood placed over affected infant's head supplies variable concentrations of humidified oxygen (see p. 1313). A widely used method is assisted ventilation, in which continuous positive pressure of 3 to 10 cm H_2O is supplied and the infant must breathe against it. This method, known as *continuous positive airway pressure* (CPAP) or *continuous positive pressure breathing* (CPPB), takes advantage of an

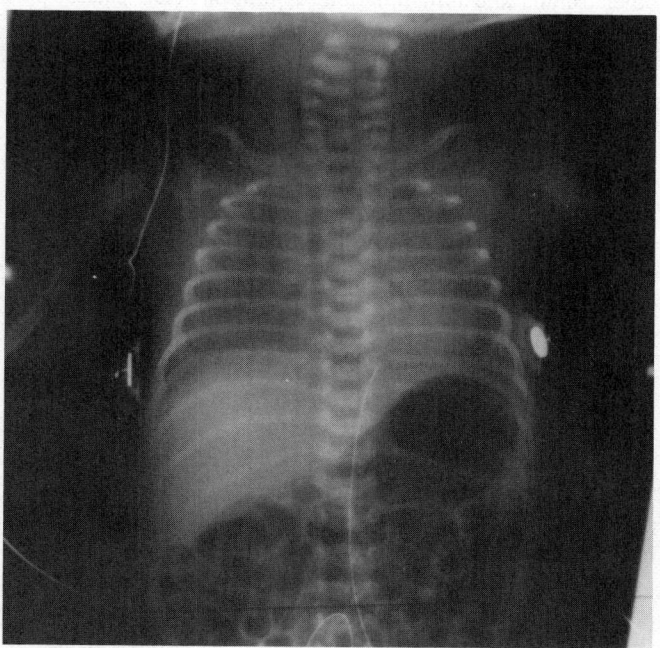

Fig. 10-14. Reticulogranular infiltrate and air bronchogram in hyaline membrane disease. Note air in stomach.
Photography by Anne Kunke, San Jose, CA.

Table 10-4 Common methods for assisted and controlled ventilation in respiratory distress syndrome

METHOD	DESCRIPTION	HOW PROVIDED
Continuous positive airway pressure (CPAP) or continuous positive pressure breathing (CPPB)	Provides constant distending pressure to airway in spontaneously breathing infant	Mask Head box or hood Nasal prongs Endotracheal tube
Positive end-expiratory pressure (PEEP)	Provides increased end-expiratory transpulmonary pressure that prevents alveolar collapse during controlled ventilation	Endotracheal intubation
Continuous positive pressure ventilation (CPPV)	Maintains continuous positive pressure to airways in the infant attached to ventilator	Endotracheal intubation and either volume- or pressure-controlled ventilators
Intermittent mandatory ventilation (IMV)	Allows infant to breathe spontaneously at own rate but provides hyperinflation at regular preset intervals	Endotracheal intubation and ventilator
High-frequency ventilation (HFV): High-frequency positive pressure ventilation (HFPPV)	Low-compliant circuit provides high gas flow through the circuit; operates at rates between 60 and 150 breaths/minute	Conventional infant ventilators; endotracheal tube
High-frequency oscillation (HFO)	Application of high-frequency, low-volume, sine-wave flow oscillations to the airway at rates between 480 to 1200 breaths/minute	Variable-speed piston pump (or loudspeaker, fluidic oscillator); endotracheal tube
High-frequency jet ventilation (HFJV)	Uses a separate, parallel, low-compliant circuit and injector port to deliver small pulses or jets of fresh gas deep into airway at rates between 250 and 900 breaths/minute	May be used alone or with low-rate IMV

infant's spontaneous respiration. *Intermittent mandatory ventilation* (IMV) allows infants to breathe spontaneously at their own rate but provides hyperinflation at regular preset intervals. The objective of CPAP and IMV is to apply just enough pressure to open and keep open most of the alveoli and yet avoid overdistending the already expanded alveoli.

If oxygen saturation (PO_2) of the blood cannot be maintained at a satisfactory level and the carbon dioxide level (PCO_2) rises, the infant will require controlled ventilation, usually positive end-expiratory pressure (PEEP) or one of the three *high-frequency ventilation* (HFV) modalities. HFV delivers gas at very rapid rates to provide adequate minute volumes using lower proximal airway pressures by way of *high-frequency positive-pressure ventilation* (HFPPV), *high-frequency oscillation* (HFO), or *high-frequency jet ventilation* (HFJV). HFV is recommended for intractable respiratory failure, especially for infants with pulmonary air leaks. It is primarily a short-term therapy, and it is believed to reduce the incidence of barotrauma, which frequently complicates oxygen therapy (Boros and others, 1985; Pokora and others, 1983; Carlo and others, 1984).

Complications of oxygen therapy. Although life-saving, oxygen therapy is not without hazards. Positive pressure introduced by mechanical apparatus has caused an increased incidence of air leaks that produce complications, such as *pneumothorax* and *pneumomediastinum* (see discussion on p. 405). Other complications directly related to oxygen therapy include *retinopathy of prematurity* (p. 413),

bronchopulmonary dysplasia (p. 406), and various problems, including nasal, tracheal, or pharyngeal perforation or other trauma and inflammation, aspiration, cleft palate, palatal grooves, and subglottic stenosis.

Medical therapies. In addition to the establishment of one or more intravenous lines to maintain hydration and nutrition, infants with respiratory distress syndrome receive a variety of medications. Those that are usually administered are outlined in Table 10-5.

A relatively recent addition to the medical therapies for RDS is the administration of artificial surfactant or surfactant obtained from exogenous sources, such as human amniotic fluid (Hallman and others, 1983), human pulmonary lavage (Sherman, Shelly, and Balis, 1985), and animal lungs (Kwong and others, 1985; Shapiro and others, 1985). The surfactant is given at birth or on diagnosis of RDS to prevent atelectasis and contribute to fluid clearance from alveoli, thereby increasing compliance and decreasing the work of breathing. In addition, the patent alveoli decrease pulmonary vascular resistance and increase blood flow to improve gas exchange.

An even newer approach to management of infants with RDS is the use of *extracorporeal membrane oxygenation* (ECMO) with a modified heart-lung machine. Blood is shunted from the right atrium to a servoregulated roller pump, pumped through a membrane lung, and a small heat exchanger, and returned to the systemic circulation via the aorta. The ECMO provides oxygen to the circulation and allows the lungs to rest (Bartlett and others, 1985). The therapy has had very limited use but is a promising substitute for conventional ventilator therapy.

Prevention. Since idiopathic respiratory distress syndrome (RDS) appears to be a maturational disorder primarily related to the production of pulmonary surfactant, one approach to prevention is through stimulation of surfactant production. Some experiments with administration of corticosteroids to mothers from 24 hours to 7 days before delivery have demonstrated a significant reduction in the incidence of hyaline membrane disease in their infants when compared with controls (Collaborative Group on Antenatal Steroid Therapy, 1981). The practice is controversial, and more conclusive evidence on a broader scale will be needed before this will be accepted as common practice. There have been no beneficial effects in prevention of hyaline membrane disease by administration of corticosteroids to infants after birth.

The most successful approach to prevention of hyaline membrane disease is prevention of premature delivery, especially in elective early delivery and cesarean section. Improved methods for assessing the maturity of the fetal lung by amniocentesis, although not a routine procedure, allow a reasonable prediction of adequate surfactant formation (see Diagnostic evaluation). Since estimation of a date of delivery can be miscalculated by as much as 1 month, these tests are particularly valuable when scheduling elective cesarean section.

Nursing Considerations

Care of infants with RDS involves all the observations and interventions described for high-risk infants. In addition, the nurse is concerned with the complex problems related to respiratory therapy and the constant threat of hypoxemia and acidosis that complicates the care of patients in respiratory difficulty.

A respiratory therapist, an important member of the neo-

Questions and Controversies

Should procedures be "clustered" to allow sufficient time for rest between disturbances or should procedures be scattered to reduce the time spent at each disturbance?

The environment of the NICU has been shown to be highly disturbing and stress producing to infants (Gorski, 1985). In an effort to reduce the number of times an infant is disturbed, nurses have been performing a number of procedures (clustering) at one time. A number of authorities are advocating lengthy periods of rest without disturbance for these infants (Brazelton, 1986).

Researchers have found that many routine nursing procedures, especially tracheal suctioning, are highly stressful to vulnerable infants. Norris, Campbell, and Brenkert (1982) demonstrated that infants with RDS reacted to nursing procedures with decreased tcPO₂ measurements, and the longer the disturbance the sharper was the decrease and the longer the recovery time. Perlman and Volpe (1983) also noted a marked increase in blood pressure following suctioning, which places vulnerable infants at risk for intraventricular hemorrhage.

natal intensive care team, is responsible for the maintenance of respiratory equipment. However, it is a nursing responsibility to regulate and understand the function of the apparatus and to recognize when it is not functioning correctly according to the physician's specifications. The most essential nursing function is to observe and assess the infant's response to therapy. Since oxygen concentration and continuous positive airway pressure are prescribed according to the infant's color and blood gas measurements and because an infant's status can change rapidly, frequent monitoring and close observation are mandatory.

Changes in oxygen concentration are based on these observations. The amount of oxygen administered, expressed as the fraction of inspired air (FiO_2), is determined on an

---

Table 10-5   Medications used in the treatment of respiratory distress syndrome

MEDICATION	PURPOSE	COMMENTS
Antibiotics	Treat pneumonia Pneumonia prophylaxis	Observe for adverse response
Aminoglycosides	Therapy for sepsis	Ototoxic; test for possible hearing impairment
Pancuronium	Muscle relaxant to prevent additive pressures generated during mechanical ventilation and, thus, air leaks	A controversial therapy Close observation of infant for signs of respiratory dysfunction
Furosemide	Facilitates renal excretion of fluid; reduces pulmonary edema Especially valuable when spontaneous diuresis does not occur	Observe for onset of diuresis Requires observation and fluid regulation to prevent dehydration
Vitamin E	Decreases oxygen-derived free radical production Given prophylactically to infants on oxygen therapy to prevent or reduce the severity of ROP, IVH, and BPD	Oxygen-free radicals believed to cause oxidative damage to tissues Use of drug is controversial

individual basis according to transcutaneous oxygen measurements ($tcPO_2$), arterial oxygen concentration, or capillary blood samples. Transcutaneous oxygen measurements are obtained with a sensor applied to the skin which dilates the blood vessels in the capillary bed. The sensor reads the amount of O_2 diffusing through the skin, converts the reading to oxygen tension, and then displays the value in mm Hg. Arterial samples (PaO_2) are drawn from an umbilical artery catheter or percutaneous arterial catheter, primarily from the radial or posterior tibial arteries. For capillary samples, blood is most often collected from the heel (see p. 1129 for the procedure). These nursing activities are frequently carried out at least every 4 hours on sick infants and as often as every 15 minutes on acutely ill infants.

Infants receiving assisted or controlled ventilation are subject to problems associated with the therapy. Thick, tenacious mucus frequently forms in the respiratory tract, interferes with gas flow, and predisposes the infant to obstruction of the passages, including the endotracheal tube. Routine suctioning may be required every 2 hours or as needed based on assessment. Care must be exercised because the procedure may cause bronchospasm or vagal nerve stimulation that can produce bradycardia. When the nasopharyngeal passages, trachea, or endotracheal tube is being suctioned, the catheter should be inserted gently but quickly, then intermittent suction applied as the catheter is withdrawn. It is imperative that the time the airway is obstructed by the catheter be limited to no more than 5 to 10 seconds because continuous suction removes air from the lungs along with the mucus. The transcutaneous PO_2 monitor is observed before and during the suctioning to provide an ongoing assessment of blood gas measurements to prevent hypoxemia. The infant may require "bagging" following suctioning to restore oxygen levels rapidly. Instillation of 0.25 to 0.5 ml of sterile normal saline in the endotracheal tube before insertion of the suction catheter aids in loosening mucus and removing secretions.

Removal of secretions can be further facilitated by positioning and application of percussion and vibration to the thoracic wall. The technique and positioning for postural drainage, percussion, and vibration are outlined in Chapter 31. The principles are the same, but the cupped hand is much too large to be used on very small infants. An effective way to provide percussion is to use small plastic cups with padded rims or a small face mask with the airway opening occluded (Fig. 10-15). Vibration is even more difficult to accomplish on infants whose respiratory rate is 60 to 80 breaths per minute. Some units have found an electric toothbrush with foam padding placed over the handle to be a helpful aid. When applied to the chest, this instrument provides effective vibrations. Percussion and vibration are performed every 2 hours, with rotation of segments of the lungs that are percussed. Preterm infants are unable to tolerate a full regimen each time. The length of time allotted to any given segment is also subject to the individual infant's tolerance and the degree of lobar involvement, which is best determined through radiologic evaluation.

The most advantageous positions for facilitating an infant's open airway are on the side with the head supported in alignment by a small folded towel or, when on the back, positioned to keep the neck slightly extended. With the head in the "sniffing" position, the trachea is opened at its maximum; hyperextension reduces the tracheal diameter in neonates.

Inspection of the skin is part of routine infant assessment. Position changes and use of water pillows or fleece are helpful in guarding against skin breakdown.

Mouth care is especially important when infants are receiving nothing by mouth, and the problem is often aggravated by the drying effect of oxygen therapy. Drying and cracking can be prevented by good oral hygiene using saline swabs. Irritation to the nares or mouth that occurs from appliances used to administer oxygen may be reduced by the use of a water-soluble ointment.

MECONIUM ASPIRATION SYNDROME

Meconium aspiration is a serious condition that accounts for a substantial number of neonatal fatalities. It occurs when fetuses have been subjected to fetal asphyxia or other intrauterine stress that causes increasing peristalsis, relaxing of the anal sphincter, and passage of meconium into the amniotic fluid. Aspiration of meconium takes place either in utero or with the first breath. During normal fetal breathing and gasping associated with asphyxia, the amniotic fluid and meconium are inhaled into the fetal trachea. When infants are born and begin air breathing, the fluid and meconium are inhaled.

Pathophysiology

The nature of the meconium significantly affects the degree to which aspiration is deleterious. Amniotic fluid that is stained the color of "old gold" represents meconium that

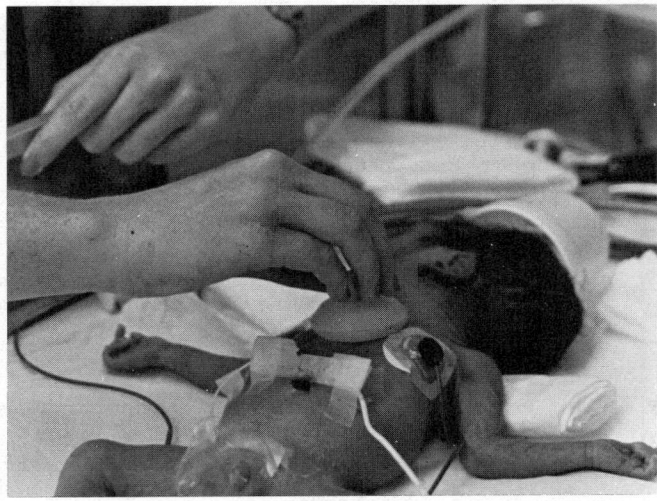

Fig. 10-15. Use of face mask for percussion of infant.

has been passed 4 to 6 hours previous to inhalation. It is less sticky and can be removed with relative ease. Older "tea-colored" fluid represents thin meconium, which usually does not cause any difficulty. Pea-colored particulate matter produces disease. Fresh meconium is very sticky and tenacious and, when inhaled, adheres to airways and alveoli, producing uneven obstruction and inhibiting normal air flow to and from gas-exchanging surfaces. This uneven ventilation, perfusion, and decreased lung compliance result in respiratory distress.

Affected infants increase respiratory efforts in order to create greater negative intrathoracic pressures and improve gas flow into the lungs. Hyperinflation plus hypoxemia and acidemia cause increased pulmonary vascular resistance. Right-to-left shunting (intrapulmonary, atrial, or ductus arteriosus) often follows. Air trapping associated with meconium obstructions of multiple airways causes overdistention of portions of the lungs and contributes to air leaks, which are common.

Clinical Manifestations

Affected infants are meconium stained, tachypneic, hypoxic, and depressed at birth. They develop expiratory grunting and retractions similar to those experienced by infants with HMD. Infants usually hyperventilate early in the course of the disease; later hypoventilation is noted. Cardiovascular hypoxemia, acidemia, hyperinflation, and pulmonary cardiovascular involvement contribute to cyanosis. The infants are often stressed, hypothermic, hypoglycemic, and hypocalcemic. The disease progressed to respiratory failure in several cases.

Diagnostic Evaluation

At birth, meconium can often be visualized in the respiratory passages and vocal cords. Chest radiographs show uneven distribution of patchy infiltrates and increased lung fluid, which usually clears in the first 24 hours.

Therapeutic Management

Immediate treatment for meconium aspiration is vigorous suctioning of the hypopharynx before delivery of the shoulders and immediate on visualization of the vocal cords. If meconium is in the vocal cords, endotracheal suction is applied with the largest catheter that can be accommodated. The suctioning is repeated until no more meconium is obtained, then resuscitation is initiated and maintained until the infant is breathing spontaneously and has good color.

Infants with respiratory distress are admitted to the NICU. Management of chemical pneumonitis consists of ventilatory support, intravenous fluids, and chest percussion and postural drainage (this is not unanimously supported). These infants are prone to develop persistent pulmonary hypertension; therefore the tendency is to keep them somewhat hyperoxic as a precautionary measure. Complications are managed symptomatically or as described under the specific disorder.

Nursing Considerations

Nursing considerations are the same as for any neonates. See nursing care in oxygen therapy, persistent pulmonary hypertension, and other complications.

EXTRANEOUS AIR SYNDROMES (AIR LEAKS)

Extraneous air syndromes, extraalveolar air accumulation, and *air leaks* are names applied to various clinically recognized disorders produced as a result of alveolar rupture and subsequent escape of air to tissues in which air is not normally present (Korones, 1986). Extraneous air collection (1) may occur spontaneously in normal neonates, (2) can result from congenital renal/pulmonary malformations, and (3) often complicates underlying respiratory disease and its therapy.

Following alveolar rupture, air often vents directly into the pleural space to create *pneumothorax*. It may vent into the perivascular interstitium, the *perivascular emphysema* space, where it can dissect along the perivascular sheaths to eventually enter the mediastinum and cause *pneumomediastinum*. More extensive leaks involve the pericardium, manifested as *pneumopericardium*, or emphysema in the cervical, subcutaneous, or retroperitoneal soft tissues.

Clinical Manifestations

Spontaneous pneumothorax usually occurs during the first few breaths after birth primarily in term or postterm infants and is evident by the gradual onset of symptoms of respiratory distress after arrival in the nursery. Positive pressure introduced by mechanical apparatus has created an increase in the incidence of ruptured alveoli. Early manifestations include restlessness and irritability, lethargy, tachypnea, grunting, flaring nares, and retractions. It can be suspected on the basis of absent or diminished breath sounds and a shift in location of maximum intensity of heart sounds. These may proceed to the more severe signs described next.

Pneumothorax during ventilatory assistance is common— predominantly tension pneumothorax, which is evident from abrupt and profound duskiness or cyanosis, and significant declines of heart rate, arterial blood pressure, pulse pressure, and poor peripheral perfusion. There is also chest asymmetry, altered cardiac sounds (diminished, shifted, or muffled), palpable liver and spleen, and subcutaneous emphysema.

Therapeutic Management

Diagnosis is confirmed by transillumination of the chest with a fiberoptic probe and/or radiographic examination. Treatment is urgent. Evacuation of trapped air is accomplished by chest tube insertion into the pleural space through a small chest incision that is then attached to continuous suction via water-seal drainage. Sometimes a needle aspiration serves as an emergency measure until chest tubes can be inserted. Pneumomediastinum seldom requires treatment but pneumopericardium is managed by needle aspiration or tube drainage.

Nursing Considerations

The most important nursing function is close vigilance for the possibility of air leak in susceptible infants, which is most effective for early detection. Nurses maintain a high level of suspicion in (1) infants with RDS with or without positive pressure ventilation, (2) infants with meconium-stained amniotic fluid, (3) infants with radiographic evidence of interstitial or lobar emphysema, (4) infants who required resuscitation at birth, or (4) infants receiving CPAP or positive-pressure ventilation.

The general nursing care of the infant with an exogenous air syndrome is the same as that for all high-risk neonates. Respiratory management is similar to that for infants with RDS. Frequent assessment of breath sounds, monitoring efficacy of gas exchange, and regulating oxygen therapy according to the needs of the infants are vital nursing functions. Care of chest tubes is an additional responsibility and is not significantly different from observations in older children and adults.

BRONCHOPULMONARY DYSPLASIA

Bronchopulmonary dysplasia (BPD), also known as *chronic or respiratory lung disease,* is a pathologic process that may develop in the lungs of infants, primarily VLBW infants, with lung disorders (e.g., hyaline membrane disease, meconium aspiration, and persistent pulmonary hypertension). The etiology of bronchopulmonary dysplasia is unknown. However, its development appears to be related to several factors: alveolar damage caused by lung disease, exposure to high oxygen concentrations, use of positive-pressure ventilation (CPAP or PEEP), endotracheal intubation, and prolonged use of these therapies. The reported incidence of the disorder in survivors of HMD is between 10% and 20%, and the incidence of infants surviving with milder forms of chronic lung disease is much higher (Bancalari and Gerhardt, 1986). The infants who survive are at risk for frequent hospitalization because of their borderline respiratory reserve, hyperactive airway, and increased susceptibility to respiratory infection.

Pathophysiology

The pulmonary changes are characterized by interstitial edema and epithelial swelling followed by thickening and fibrotic proliferation of the alveolar walls and squamous metaplasia of the bronchiolar epithelium. Areas of atelectasis and cystlike foci of hyperaeration are visible on radiographs between 10 and 20 days of life and persist for weeks; however, some infants may not demonstrate cystic foci. In addition, the ciliary activity is paralyzed by high oxygen concentrations that interfere with the ability to clear the lung of mucus, thus aggravating airway obstruction and atelectasis.

To date there is no evidence to indicate a relationship between the incidence of bronchopulmonary dysplasia and the increased survival rate of infants with severe HMD. The marked similarity between bronchopulmonary dysplasia and the *Wilson-Mikity syndrome,* in which the lungs of premature infants exhibit alveolar thickening and cystlike patterns of hyperventilation, has led some investigators to theorize that the two disorders may be part of a continuous spectrum of the same lung disease. Other diseases associated with similar radiographic findings include congenital heart disease, viral pneumonia caused by cytomegalovirus, and pulmonary interstitial emphysema. There are no specific clinical signs or laboratory alterations that confirm a diagnosis, which is made on the basis of radiographic findings.

Therapeutic Management

The first approach to management is prevention of the disorder in susceptible infants. When mechanical ventilation is being used, the lowest peak airway pressure necessary to obtain adequate ventilation is maintained and the duration of oxygen therapy is limited as much as possible to reduce the risk of barotrauma and infection. Fluid administration is carefully controlled and restricted. Drug or surgical intervention is indicated when there is a patent ductus arteriosus.

There is no specific treatment for bronchopulmonary dysplasia except to maintain adequate arterial blood gases with the administration of oxygen and avoid progression of the disease. Weaning infants from the ventilator is difficult and must be accomplished gradually. These infants do not tolerate excessive or even normal amounts of fluid well and have a tendency to accumulate interstitial fluid in the lungs, which aggravates the condition.

Some success has been reported with oral diuretics in controlling interstitial fluid. Bronchodilators may be effective before the development of significant fibrosis, and although dexamethasone has proven of short-term value, the protective value of vitamin E has not been confirmed (Hodgmen, 1986).

Reports vary regarding the mortality rate for this disorder. The hospital stay is frequently long because of the infant's need for supplemental oxygen, although home oxygen therapy has provided selected infants the opportunity for discharge. However, a significant proportion of deaths occur after discharge from the hospital. Growth and development are delayed in some infants with BPD, related in part to the difficulties in providing adequate nutrition and in part to the lack of normal sensory stimulation, since many of the infants spend extended periods in oxygen tents isolated from their environment (Bancalari and Gerhardt, 1986). A large percentage of survivors have significant disabilities, such as cerebral palsy, mental retardation, deafness, and blindness, which is consistent with the VLBW infant population and probably unrelated to the BPD.

Nursing Considerations

Infants with BPD expend considerable energy in their efforts to breathe; therefore it is important that they receive plenty of opportunities for rest and additional fluids and calories. Growth records provide clues to the need for change in their diets, and some infants require nutritional supplements. Since they tire easily and large quantities of formula might compromise respiration, small frequent feedings are better tolerated. Adequate hydration is extremely important because greater amounts of fluid are lost through respiration, and secretions must be thinned sufficiently to facilitate removal by coughing and suctioning. However, since BPD increases lung permeability, some infants are subject to pulmonary edema. Therefore nurses must be alert to signs of both overhydration and underhydration, such as weight changes, skin turgor, output measurements, urine specific gravity, and signs of edema.

Parents are extremely anxious regarding the prognosis when their infant has BPD. In addition, the lengthy hospitalization interferes with parent-child relationships and deprives the infant of parental stimulation. The nurses should encourage the parents to visit the infant and become involved in the routine care. The parents need to be informed regarding medical care, equipment, and procedures related to their infant and taught procedures, such as suctioning and chest physiotherapy.

Home care. Since the availability of home cardiac/apnea monitors and home oxygen therapy has increased, many of these infants can be discharged at approximately 3 months of age. Home care is desirable to promote parent-infant bonding, minimize health care costs, and prevent nosocomial infections. Preparation for home care requires education and considerable reassurance. Management of home monitoring equipment and home oxygen therapy is stress-provoking, but most families become comfortable with the machinery while their infant is still in the hospital. Families must be reminded about their infant's increased risk of infection and cautioned regarding contact with persons who have respiratory infections. Because of their minimum respiratory reserve, these infants can be threatened by even a minor illness.

Because of the high mortality rate in the first year, parents are taught cardiopulmonary resuscitation and how to manage any other emergency that might be anticipated for their infant. Helping families cope with their anxieties and reassuring them of their ability to manage the care of their infant are important nursing functions. Parents need follow-up in the home and the comfort of knowing that help is only a telephone call away.

High Risk Related to Infectious Processes

Newborns are highly susceptible to infection. Their immature immune systems and their inability to localize infection render them especially vulnerable to infectious organisms. Prevention of infection in neonates, particularly in infants who are already compromised by physiologic or structural disorders, is a primary nursing function. The nurse must be aware of potential sources of transmission and recognize those infants who are at risk.

SEPSIS

Sepsis, or *septicemia,* refers to a generalized bacterial infection in the bloodstream. Neonates are highly susceptible to infection as a result of diminished nonspecific (inflammatory) and specific (humoral) immunity, such as impaired phagocytosis, delayed chemotactic response, minimum or absent IgA and IgM, and decreased complement levels. Because of the infant's poor response to pathogenic agents, there is usually no local inflammatory reaction at the portal of entry to signal an infection and the resulting symptoms tend to be vague and nonspecific. Consequently diagnosis and treatment may be delayed.

Before the introduction of antibiotics, mortality approached 90% from sepsis. With the use of antibiotics, mortality has decreased considerably and presently is in the range of 13% to 45%, depending on the infecting organism. However, the incidence of septicemia has not diminished. Nursery epidemics are not infrequent, and the high-risk infant has a four times greater chance of developing septicemia than does the normal neonate. The frequency of infection is almost twice as great in male infants as in females and carries a higher mortality for males as well. Other factors increasing the risk of infection are prematurity and bottle-feeding. Bottle-feeding can introduce pathogens from environmental contamination of formula or equipment.

Breast-feeding has a protective benefit against infection. Colostrum contains agglutinins that are effective against gram-negative bacteria. Human milk contains large quantities of IgA and iron-binding protein that exert a bacteriostatic effect on *Escherichia coli.* Human milk also contains macrophages and lymphocytes that promote a local inflammatory reaction.

Pathophysiology

The premature withdrawal of the placental barrier leaves infants vulnerable to most common viral, bacterial, fungal, and parasitic infections. Normally, immune substances, primarily immunoglobulin G (IgG), are acquired from the maternal system and stored in fetal tissues during the final weeks of gestation to provide newborns with passive immunity to a variety of infectious agents. Early birth interrupts this transplacental transmission; thus preterm infants have a low level of circulating IgG; the concentrations of immune substances directly relate to the length of gestation. Immunoglobulin A (IgA), which plays a role in defense against viral infections, and immunoglobulin M (IgM), with properties that are most efficient in dealing with gram-negative organisms, are not transferred to fetuses, leaving infants highly vulnerable to invasion by these organisms.

Defense mechanisms of neonates are further hampered by a low level of complement, diminished opsonic ability, monocyte dysfunction, and reduced number and inefficient functioning of circulating leukocytes. Furthermore, these leukocytes, with diminished motility and phagocytic capacity, are unable to concentrate their limited numbers selectively at the site of infection. In addition, a hypofunctioning adrenal gland contributes only a meager antiinflammatory response. Consequently these deficiencies permit rapid invasion, spread, and multiplication of organisms.

Sources of Infection

Sepsis in the neonatal period can be acquired prenatally across the placenta from the maternal bloodstream or during labor from ingestion or aspiration of infected amniotic fluid. Prolonged rupture of the membranes always presents a risk of this type from maternal-fetal transfer of pathogenic organisms. In utero transplacental transfer of organisms can occur, such as *Treponema pallidum* (syphilis), which crosses the placental barrier during the latter half of pregnancy.

During birth, infection can occur from direct contact with maternal tissues during passage through the birth canal. The most common infecting organism is *E. coli,* which may be present in the vagina from fecal contamination. *E. coli* accounts for about two thirds of all cases of sepsis caused by gram-negative organisms. Proper hygiene of the perineum is one method of preventing this mode of transmission. Other pathogens that are harbored in the vagina and that may infect the infant include gonococci, *Candida albicans,* herpes simplex virus (type II), *Listeria* organisms, and β-hemolytic streptococci.

The infant is at risk for self-infection because of the proximity of the umbilical wound to the perineum. Bacterial invasion can also occur through sites other than the umbilical stump, such as the skin, mucous membranes of the eye, nose, pharynx, and ear, and internal systems such as respiratory, nervous, urinary, and gastrointestinal systems.

Postnatal infection is acquired by cross-contamination from other infants, personnel, or objects in the environment. Bacteria that are frequently called ''water bugs'' (because they are able to grow in water) are found in water supplies, humidifying apparatus, sink drains, suction machines, most respiratory equipment, and indwelling venous and arterial catheters used for infusions, blood sampling, and monitoring vital signs. Neonatal sepsis is most common in the infant at risk, particularly the preterm infant or the infant born following a difficult or traumatic labor and delivery, who is least capable of resisting such bacterial invasion. Frequently these organisms are transmitted by the personnel from person to person or object to person by poor handwashing and inadequate housecleaning.

Clinical Manifestations

A few neonatal infections (e.g., pyoderma, conjunctivitis, omphalitis, and mastitis) are easily recognized. However, systemic infections are characterized by subtle, vague, nonspecific, and almost imperceptible physical signs. Often the only complaint concerning an infant's progress is ''failure to do well,'' not looking ''right,'' or nonspecific respiratory distress. Rarely is there any indication of a local inflammatory response, which would suggest the portal of entry into the bloodstream. The presence of some bacteria is indicated by a specific characteristic, for example, *Pseudomonas* organisms, which produce necrotic purplish skin lesions, or group B β-hemolytic streptococci, which usually result in severe respiratory distress and periods of apnea.

All body systems tend to show some indication of sepsis, although often there is little correlation between the manifestations and the etiologic factors involved. For example, convulsions may not represent central nervous system infection, and fever, a universal feature of infection in older children, may be absent in neonates. It is usually nursing observation of subtle changes in the appearance and behavior of infants that leads to the detection of infection. The nonspecific, early signs are hypothermia and changes in color, tone, activity, and feeding resulting in unabsorbed formula with abdominal distention, jaundice, lethargy, and apnea. Significantly, similar signs may be manifestations of a number of clinical conditions unrelated to sepsis, such as hypoglycemia, hypocalcemia, heroin withdrawal, or central nervous system disorders. Since meningitis is a frequent sequela of sepsis, signs of increased intracranial pressure may also be evident.

Clinical signs that may indicate possible neonatal sepsis are listed in the accompanying box. Because sepsis is so easily confused with other neonatal disorders, the definitive diagnosis is established by laboratory and roentgenographic examination.

Diagnostic Evaluation

Isolation of the specific organism is always attempted through cultures of blood, urine, and cerebrospinal fluid. Direct (conjugated) hyperbilirubinemia often occurs in infants with sepsis, particularly sepsis of gram-negative origin. Blood studies may show signs of anemia, leukocytosis, or leukopenia. Leukopenia is usually an ominous sign because of its frequent association with high mortality.

Therapeutic Management

Early recognition and diagnosis with institution of vigorous therapeutic measures are essential to increase the infant's chance for survival and reduce the likelihood of permanent neurologic damage. Often diagnosis of sepsis is based on suspicion, and antibiotic therapy is initiated before laboratory results are available for confirmation and identification of the exact organism. Treatment consists of aggressive administration of antibiotics, such as ampicillin, and an aminoglycoside, such as gentamicin, to provide a broad-spectrum antibiotic therapy that is effective against approximately 90% of all potential organisms. Drug therapy is continued for 7 to 10 days and is most often administered via intravenous infusion.

Recently transfusions with polymorphonuclear leukocytes obtained from adult donors by continuous-flow centrifugation leukapheresis have been introduced as therapy for bacterial sepsis (Cairo and others, 1984). The results have proven to be highly effective in lowering mortality from this disease.

MANIFESTATIONS OBSERVED IN NEONATAL SEPSIS

General signs
Infant generally "not doing well"
Poor temperature control—hyperthermia, hypothermia

Circulatory system
Pallor, cyanosis, or mottling
Cold, clammy skin
Hypotension
Edema
Abnormal heartbeat—arrhythmia, tachycardia

Respiratory system
Irregular respirations, apnea, or tachypnea
Cyanosis
Grunting
Dyspnea
Retractions

Central nervous system
Diminished activity—lethargy, hyporeflexia, coma
Increased activity—irritability, tremors, seizures
Full fontanel
Increased or decreased tone
Abnormal eye movements

Gastrointestinal system
Poor feeding
Vomiting
Diarrhea or decreased stool
Abdominal distention
Hepatomegaly

Hematopoietic system
Jaundice
Pallor
Purpura, petechiae, ecchymosis
Splenomegaly
Bleeding

Supportive therapy usually involves administration of oxygen if respiratory distress or cyanosis is evident, careful regulation of fluids and correction of electrolyte or acid-base imbalance, and temporary discontinuation of oral feedings. Blood transfusions may be needed to correct anemia and shock, and electronic monitoring of vital signs and regulation of the thermal environment are mandatory. Affected infants are isolated from other infants.

Prognosis is variable. Before the discovery of antibiotics the mortality from bacterial sepsis was 95% to 100%, but early recognition, antibiotics, and supportive therapy have reduced mortality to less than 50% (Bruhn and Jones, 1985). However, mental retardation can occur with late diagnosis of meningitis.

Nursing Considerations

Nursing care of the infant with sepsis involves observation and assessment as outlined for any high-risk infant. Recognition of the existing problem is of paramount importance; it is usually the nurse who observes and assesses infants and who identifies that "something is wrong" with them. Aware-

ness of the potential modes of infection transmission also helps the nurse identify those at risk for developing sepsis.

Much of the care of infants with sepsis involves the medical treatment of the illness. Knowledge of the side effects of the specific antibiotic and proper regulation and administration of the drug are vital. Because the volume of fluid required to administer antibiotics via Soluset would seriously compromise a small infant, antibiotics are usually administered via a heparin lock system or special injection cap near the infusion site. The medication is administered slowly by mechanical pump.

Prolonged antibiotic therapy poses additional hazards for affected infants. Oral antibiotics destroy intestinal flora responsible for synthesis of vitamin K, which can reduce blood coagulability. In addition, it predisposes the infants to growth of resistant organisms and infection from fungal or mycotic agents, such as *Candida albicans*. Nurses must be alert for evidence of such complications.

A number of specimens may be needed to help identify the cause and source of the infection. For obtaining spinal fluid for examination, the time-honored positioning in the side-lying, flexed posture has been recently challenged (Gleason and others, 1983). The investigators found that although Po_2 decreased and heart rate increased with infants in any of three positions (lateral recumbent with full flexion, lateral recumbent with partial neck extension, and sitting with head support and spine flexion), the Pco_2 increased only in the fully flexed position. It is recommended that the fully flexed position be avoided and that the side-lying position (modified with neck extension) or the sitting position be used for obtaining spinal fluid specimens.

Part of the total care of infants with sepsis is to decrease any additional physiologic or environmental stress. This includes providing an optimum thermoregulated environment and anticipating potential problems, such as dehydration or hypoxia. Isolation of affected infants prevents spread of infection to other newborns, but to be effective, isolation must be carried out by all caregivers. Proper handwashing, use of disposable equipment (e.g., linens, catheters, feeding utensils, and intravenous equipment), disposing of excretions (e.g., vomitus and stool), and adequate housekeeping of the environment and equipment are essential. Since nurses are the most consistent caregivers involved with sick infants, it is usually their responsibility to oversee that all phases of isolation are maintained.

Another aspect of caring for infants with sepsis involves observation for signs of meningitis, including a full or bulging anterior fontanel; opisthotonos is rare. Usually the infectious agent is the same for both conditions; however, antibiotic therapy chosen for treatment of sepsis may not diffuse into spinal fluid, so intrathecal administration of appropriate drugs may be required.

Other complications of sepsis include pyarthrosis (which may affect any joint but most commonly localizes in the hip) and osteomyelitis. Local inflammation of the involved area is again uncommon, so identification is difficult. Limited movement of the affected joint and/or extremity may be one of the few indications of infection.

A severe complication of sepsis is shock, caused by the release of toxins into the bloodstream. Signs of shock are often difficult to distinguish from those of sepsis, such as rapid, irregular respirations and pulse. However, blood pressure usually falls when an infant is in shock, and therefore this measurement should be a part of the monitoring of all infants' routine vital signs.

NECROTIZING ENTEROCOLITIS

Necrotizing enterocolitis (NEC) is a disease with increased incidence in preterm and other high-risk infants, but it is most common in those who weigh less than 2000 g. Three factors appear to play an important role in its development: intestinal ischemia, colonization by pathogenic bacteria, and excess substrate (formula feeding) in the intestinal lumen.

Pathophysiology

The precise cause of the disorder is still uncertain, although it appears to occur in infants whose gastrointestinal tract has suffered vascular compromise. Intestinal ischemia in fetuses is most commonly a consequence of decreased cardiac output as a result of asphyxia. In newborns enteric vascular ischemia is an effect of an earlier oxygen depletion in the brain and heart that triggered the "diving reflex." To meet the oxygen needs of these vital organs, blood is shunted away from the organs that are better able to withstand prolonged anoxia, such as the intestines. As a result of this circulatory shunting, there is convulsive vasoconstriction of the mesenteric vessels with a severe reduction of blood supply to the intestines.

The damage to mucosal cells lining the bowel wall is great—diminished blood supply to these cells causes their death in large numbers, they stop secreting protective, lubricating mucus, and the thin, unprotected bowel wall is attacked by proteolytic enzymes. Thus the bowel wall continues to swell and break down. In addition, it is unable to synthesize protective immunoglobulin M (IgM), and the mucosa is permeable to macromolecules, such as exotoxins, which further hampers intestinal defenses. Gas-forming bacteria invade the damaged areas to produce *pneumatosis intestinales*, the presence of air in the submucosal or subserosal surfaces of the colon.

A consistent relationship has been observed between the development of necrotizing enterocolitis and enteric feeding of hypertonic substances, for example, formula and hyperosmolar medications. Although not unheard of, NEC in unfed infants is rare (Kosloske, 1984). It is unclear whether this connection is the result of the formula imposing a stress on an ischemic bowel or serving as a substrate for bacterial growth.

Clinical Manifestations

The prominent clinical signs of necrotizing enterocolitis are a distended (often shining) abdomen, gastric retention, and blood in the stools or gastric contents. Nonspecific signs include lethargy, poor feeding, hypotension, apnea, vomiting (often bile-stained), decreased urine output, and unstable temperature. The onset is usually between 4 and 10 days, but signs may be evident as early as 4 hours and as late as 30 days. NEC in full-term infants almost always occurs in the first 10 days when the gut is least mature; late-onset NEC is confined primarily to preterm infants (Wilson and others, 1982).

Diagnostic Evaluation

Radiographic studies show a sausage-shaped dilation of the intestine that progresses to marked distention and the characteristic pneumatosis intestinales. There may be air in the portal circulation or free air observed in the abdomen indicating perforation. Laboratory findings may include anemia, leukopenia, leukocytosis, and electrolyte imbalance. In severe cases coagulopathy and/or thrombocytopenia may be evident. Organisms are often cultured from blood, although bacteremia or septicemia may not be prominent early in the course of the disease.

Therapeutic Management

Treatment of NEC begins with prevention. Oral feedings are withheld for at least 24 to 48 hours from infants who are believed to have suffered birth asphyxia and as long as deemed necessary from VLBW infants. Breast milk is the preferred enteral nutrient because it confers some passive immunity (IgA), macrophages, and lysozymes. It has been suggested that prenatal administration of glucocorticoids may protect against NEC (Bauer and others, 1984).

Treatment of confirmed NEC consists of discontinuation of all oral feedings, institution of abdominal decompression via nasogastric suction, administration of intravenous antibiotics (ampicillin and aminoglycosides), and correction of extravascular volume depletion, electrolyte abnormalities, and acid-base imbalances. Replacing oral feedings with parenteral fluids decreases the need for oxygen and circulation to the bowel.

With early recognition and treatment, medical management is increasingly successful. If there is progressive deterioration under medical management or evidence of perforation, surgical resection and anastomosis are carried out. Extensive involvement may necessitate establishment of an ileostomy or colostomy. Sequelae in surviving infants include short-gut syndrome, colonic stricture with obstruction, fat malabsorption, and failure to thrive secondary to intestinal dysfunction.

Nursing Considerations

Nursing responsibilities begin with early recognition. Because the signs are similar to those observed in many other disorders of the newborn, nurses must constantly be aware of the possibility of this disease and be alert to indications of its early development. Checking the abdomen frequently for distention, measuring residual gastric contents before feedings, listening for presence of bowel sounds, and performing all routine assessments for high-risk neonates (p. 376) are especially important in detecting the early signs of necrotizing enterocolitis.

When the disease is suspected, the nurse assists with diagnostic procedures and implements the therapeutic regimen. Vital signs, including blood pressure, are monitored for changes that might indicate impending sepsis or cardiovascular shock, and measures are instituted to prevent transmission to other infants. It is especially important to avoid rectal temperatures because of the increased danger of perforation. To avoid pressure on the distended abdomen, infants are not diapered or positioned on the abdomen.

Conscientious attention to nutritional and hydration needs is essential, and antibiotics are administered as prescribed. The time at which oral feedings are reinstituted varies considerably but is usually at least 7 days following diagnosis. Plain water or electrolyte solution is given for two feedings; this is followed by dilute human milk formula. The concentration is gradually increased over a 2- to 3-week period until the infant is again taking full-strength feedings.

Since NEC is an infectious disease, one of the most important nursing functions is control of infection. Strict handwashing is the primary barrier to spread, and confirmed cases are isolated with the use of cohort nursing, the same nurses caring for the infected infants. No one with gastrointestinal disorder symptoms should care for these infants, and all linen is given separate handling.

The infant who requires surgery requires the same careful attention and observation as any infant with abdominal surgery, including ostomy care. This disorder is one of the most frequent reasons for performing ileostomies on newborns. Throughout the medical and surgical management of infants with NEC, the nurse is continually alert to signs of complications, such as sepsis, disseminated intravascular coagulation, hypoglycemia, and other metabolic derangements.

High Risk Related to Cardiovascular Complications

LBW infants and those who are otherwise physically compromised are subject to complications in all major systems. This segment is not concerned with congenital cardiac anomalies or the complications that result from these lesions (see Chapter 34). The disorders described here are observed in the neonatal period, usually as complications of pulmonary dysfunction and respiratory therapy.

PERSISTENT PATENT DUCTUS ARTERIOSUS

A common complication of severe respiratory disease in preterm infants is persistent patent ductus arteriosus (PDA). It occurs in the majority of preterm infants under 1200 g, and the incidence diminishes in direct relationship to in-creasing birth weight. During fetal life the ductus remains patent through the vasodilatory action of prostaglandins within its tissues. Postnatally the increase in oxygen tension has a constricting effect on the ductus, but it may reopen in these small infants in response to the lowered oxygen tension associated with respiratory impairment. It is still unknown whether PDA is a contributing factor in the development of respiratory distress or whether respiratory distress contributes to the development of PDA.

Clinical Manifestations

Signs of PDA appear at approximately 5 to 10 days of age when respiratory support for respiratory distress is being gradually withdrawn. Spontaneous closure usually takes place within 12 weeks, but in infants with severe lung involvement the left-to-right shunting of blood leads to life-threatening pulmonary insufficiency. Early signs of PDA are increased PCO_2 and recurrent apnea. Other signs include bounding peripheral pulses, pericardial hyperactivity, cardiomegaly, and a systolic or continuous murmur. Confirmation of the diagnosis may be determined by echocardiography or, less frequently, by contrast studies via an umbilical catheter.

Therapeutic Management

Therapy consists of careful fluid regulation, respiratory support, and administration of indomethacin, a prostaglandin synthetase inhibitor that has been successful in constricting the ductus in critically ill, preterm infants. If a ductus reopens following cessation of therapy, reinstitution of the medication usually produces a favorable response. Other therapies might include furosemide to prevent renal complications of indomethacin and digoxin. Surgical ligation may be necessary if medical therapy is unsuccessful after 48 hours, although this remains controversial.

Nursing Considerations

Nursing observations are important in the recognition and management of PDA. Assisting in early detection, assessing cardiovascular status carefully, and monitoring for complications following implementation of therapy are nursing responsibilities. The focus of activities related to therapy include collection of specimens for laboratory examination, continued assessment of renal function (adequate urine output, any abnormal laboratory findings), and observation for any bleeding tendencies (hematest-positive stools or gastric aspirate, oozing from heelsticks or venipuncture sites, and laboratory evidence of clotting abnormalities) (Cohen, 1983).

Other nursing observations and management are the same as for high-risk infant and the infant with PDA (p. 1463).

PERSISTENT PULMONARY HYPERTENSION OF THE NEWBORN

Persistent pulmonary hypertension of the newborn (PPHN), or *persistent pulmonary hypertension* (PPH), formerly known as *persistent fetal circulation* (PFC), is a condition in which affected infants display severe pulmonary hypertension, with pulmonary artery pressure levels equal to or greater than systemic pressure, and large right-to-left shunts through both the foramen ovale and ductus arteriosus. Since full development of pulmonary arterial musculature occurs late in gestation, PPHN is primarily a condition of full-term or postterm infants, many of whom were products of complicated pregnancies or deliveries. The condition is often associated with massive aspiration, cold stress, and/or respiratory distress (e.g., hyaline membrane disease or pneumonia) and is believed to be precipitated by perinatal factors, such as perinatal asphyxia, that cause or contribute to vasospasm.

PPHN can be either primary or secondary: primary PPHN occurs when the pulmonary vascular system fails to open with the initial respiration at birth; secondary PPHN results from stress that increases pulmonary vascular resistance and causes a return to fetal cardiopulmonary circulation. Secondary PPHN is more common than primary PPHN and is more frequently observed in infants at 35 to 44 weeks of gestation who have a history of perinatal asphyxia and respiratory distress within the first 24 hours. The infants become hypoxic when agitated and display marked cyanosis, tachypnea with grunting and retractions, and decreased peripheral perfusion. A loud pulmonary component of the second heart sound and sometimes a systolic ejection murmur are present. Mild cases may display only minimum tachypnea and cyanosis during stressful episodes, such as crying or feeding.

Diagnosis is established from clinical signs and diagnostic tests including chest radiography, electrocardiography, echocardiography, and sometimes cardiac catheterization.

Therapeutic Management

Treatment includes careful fluid regulation and evaluation of intravascular fluid volume. Supplemental oxygen is administered to reduce hypoxia and decrease pulmonary vasoconstriction. Assisted ventilation may be needed if hypoxia is not corrected by noninvasive methods, often accompanied by paralysis with pancuronium to minimize opposition to the respirator (Fox and Duara, 1983). Tolazoline, a potent vasodilator, may be administered through a separate peripheral intravenous infusion.

Nursing Considerations

The nursing care is the same as for infants with respiratory difficulties and infants supported by mechanical respirators. Because handling for any reason causes a decrease in arterial oxygen concentration, the stresses imposed by routine care must be weighed against the risk of iatrogenic hypoxia. It is important to decrease noxious stimuli that cause crying and struggling and to employ nursing interventions, such as giving pacifiers, that keep nonsedated infants calm. Continuous monitoring of central venous pressure, vital signs, and blood pressure and transcutaneous monitoring of blood gases decrease the need for physical manipulation and dis-

turbance. Infants receiving tolazoline are assessed for pulmonary vascular response, for example, increased PaO_2 and signs of systemic hypotension, gastrointestinal bleeding, or pulmonary hemorrhage.

ANEMIA

Preterm infants tend to develop anemia that is more severe and appears earlier than in more mature infants. It may be the result of hemorrhage during the course of labor and delivery (into brain, liver, spleen, or kidneys), blood disorders (hemolytic disease, thrombocytopenia), or conditions that produce swelling or distention of abdominal organs. Physiologic characteristics of prematurity tend to contribute to development of anemia, that is, a drop in the production of fetal hemoglobin and shortened survival time of the red blood cells. This lag in hematopoiesis during continued growth results in physiologic anemia, probably as a consequence of diminished erythropoietin values (Stockman and others, 1984).

Fortunately even VLBW infants are able to accommodate the gastrointestinal absorption of iron required for their high needs. Iron is supplied in iron-fortified formulas or iron supplements as both a preventive and therapeutic measure. Transfusions with packed red blood cells are often required for severe anemia, usually for replacement of blood loss resulting from iatrogenic measures. At 4 to 12 weeks of age a "physiologic anemia" reaches a peak at which time infants sometimes display signs that suggest true anemia.

Nursing Considerations

In addition to the routine care of preterm infants, one of the most common causes of anemia in preterm infants is blood loss associated with frequent sampling for blood gas and metabolic analyses. Therefore an important nursing responsibility is careful monitoring of all blood drawn for tests. It is surprising how easily and rapidly the small total blood volume of premature infants is depleted by repeated withdrawals.

Observation for signs of anemia is a vital nursing function. The traditional signs of anemia in the child are often observed in the preterm infant: feeding difficulties, dyspnea, tachycardia, tachypnea, diminished activity, and pallor. However, some infants may not display all these signs. Poor weight gain may be an indication of a lowered hemoglobin level. Nursing precautions and observations during blood transfusion for the preterm infant are similar to those for any child (see p. 1536).

POLYCYTHEMIA/HYPERVISCOSITY SYNDROME

Polycythemia is a physiologic adaptation to advancing gestational age of the fetus but is now considered to be a complicating factor in neonatal management. The current definition of polycythemia is a venous hematocrit of 65% or more. Polycythemia is a result of in utero twin-to-twin transfusion and maternal-fetal transfusion, prolonged emptying of placental blood to the infant at birth, or increased red cell production after birth. Among infants with polycythemia a high incidence of cardiopulmonary distress symptoms (persistent fetal circulation, cyanosis, and apnea), seizures, hyperbilirubinemia, and gastrointestinal abnormalities exists. However, there is confusion regarding which infants will display neonatal symptoms, which infants will have persistent neurologic and developmental abnormalities, and whether treatment affects the clinical course.

The therapy is equally controversial. However, appropriate therapy for correcting metabolic disturbances (e.g., hypoxia, hypoglycemia, and hyperbilirubinemia) is implemented, and lowering blood viscosity by partial plasma exchange transfusion may be considered in some cases.

Nursing Considerations

Nursing care involves watching for signs of polycythemia and assisting with diagnostic tests and therapeutic procedures. Care of the infant with hyperbilirubinemia is discussed on p. 346.

RETINOPATHY OF PREMATURITY

Retinopathy of prematurity (ROP) is a term used to describe all phases of retinal changes observed in preterm infants. The older term, *retrolental fibroplasia* (RLF), describes the cicatricial changes that characterize the later stages in the most severely affected infants. It is a disease of unknown origin that occurs primarily, but not exclusively, in premature infants, and the incidence of the disease correlates with the degree of the infant's maturity—the younger the gestational age, the greater the likelihood of the development of ROP.

Numerous factors have been implicated in the cause of ROP in addition to immaturity, including hyperoxemia and hypoxemia, hypercarbia and hypocarbia, patent ductus arteriosus, prostaglandin synthetase inhibitors, apnea, intraventricular hemorrhage, infection, vitamin E deficiency, lactic acidosis, maternal diabetes, prenatal complications, and genetic factors. Previously considered to be an iatrogenic disease related to hyperoxia, ROP is now believed to be a complex disease of prematurity with multiple causes and therefore difficult to manage.

Pathophysiology

The disorder is characterized by severe vascular constriction in the immature retinal vasculature followed by hypoxia in those areas. This appears to stimulate vascular proliferation of retinal capillaries into the hypoxic areas where veins become numerous and dilate. As new vessels proliferate toward the lens, the aqueous humor then the vitreous humor become turbid. The retina becomes edematous, and hemorrhages separate the retina from its attachment. Advanced scarring occurs from the retina to the lens, destroying the normal architecture of the eye. This extensive retinal detachment and scarring result in irreversible blindness.

Diagnostic Evaluation

A system of classification has been established to describe the location and extent of the developing vasculature involved. Normal vascular growth proceeds in an orderly fashion from the disc toward the *ora serrata,* the irregular anterior margin of the retina. The four stages of retinopathy are (An international classification, 1984):

1. A demarcation line (separates the avascular retina anteriorly from the vascularized retina posteriorly)
2. A ridge (formed from the demarcation line with height and width, occupies volume, and extends beyond the plane of the retina)
3. A ridge with extraretinal fibrovascular proliferation
4. Retinal detachment

Therapeutic Management

Although judicious use and careful monitoring of supplemental oxygen have reduced the incidence of ROP, the disease has not been eradicated. Prophylactic administration of vitamin E has been used in some units but is considered to be an experimental drug by the Committee on Fetus and Newborn (1985); its use is not without complications.

Although prevention is the primary goal of therapeutic management, treatment of retinal pathology is directed toward arresting the proliferation process. Cryotherapy has been used with some success and photocoagulation has been advocated.

Nursing Considerations

There is no definitive nursing care other than careful monitoring of gas studies during oxygen administration and adherence to standards of drug administration when these therapies are employed. Constant assessment and vigilance are necessary just as for any high-risk neonate. When the infant suffers partial or complete visual impairment, the parents will need a considerable amount of support and assistance in meeting the special developmental needs of the infant (see Chapter 25).

High Risk Related to Neurologic Disturbance

Neurologic complications are observed with increased frequency in preterm infants and in infants born following a difficult labor and delivery. A disproportionately high incidence of perinatal encephalopathy, or cerebral palsy, and psychomotor retardation is found in the high-risk infant population, especially the VLBW infants. Preterm infants are also more vulnerable to cerebral insults, such as hypoxia and chemical alterations. In addition, fragility and increased permeability of capillaries and prolonged prothrombin time predispose the brain of the preterm infant to trauma when delicate structures are subjected to increased pressure, such as the forces of labor, high mechanical ventilatory pressures, and seizure activity. All of these factors contribute to intracranial insults including traumatic bleeding in the newborn, which consists of four major types: intraventricular, subdural, primary subarachnoid, and intracerebellar.

PERINATAL HYPOXIC-ISCHEMIC BRAIN INJURY

Hypoxic-ischemic brain injury is the most common cause of neurologic impairment of a nonprogressive type observed in infants and children. The brain damage usually results from intrauterine asphyxia, either before or during delivery, but it can happen postnatally as well. Ischemia and hypoxemia occur together, although one or the other predominates. The major causes of serious hypoxemia in the perinatal period are (Hill and Volpe, 1981):

1. Intrauterine asphyxia with respiratory failure at the time of birth
2. Postnatal respiratory insufficiency secondary to severe hyaline membrane disease or recurrent apnea
3. Severe cyanotic heart defects (right-to-left shunts) or persistent fetal circulation

The primary causes of cerebral ischemia are (Hill and Volpe, 1981):

1. Intrauterine asphyxia with cardiac insufficiency
2. Postnatal cardiac insufficiency secondary to severe congenital heart disease or recurrent apnea
3. Postnatal cardiovascular collapse secondary to sepsis

Newborns are particularly vulnerable to ischemic injury caused by decreased cerebral blood flow following asphyxia. Most infants who have suffered intrauterine oxygen deprivation have low Apgar scores; thus postnatal hypoxia is superimposed on an already existing problem.

Clinical Manifestations

The neurologic signs that indicate encephalopathy appear within the first hours after the hypoxic episode with manifestations of bilateral cerebral dysfunction. The infant is stuporous or comatose. Seizures begin after 6 to 12 hours in about 50% the infants, and they become more frequent and severe by 12 to 24 hours. Between 24 and 72 hours there may be deterioration in the level of consciousness, and after 72 hours persistent stupor, abnormal tone (usually hypotonia), and disturbances of sucking and swallowing are evident. Muscular weakness of the hips and shoulders is observed in full-term infants, and lower limb weakness occurs in premature infants. Apneic episodes are seen in approximately 50% of the affected infants.

Improvement in the neurologic deficiencies is highly variable and difficult to predict, although infants who demonstrate the most rapid initial improvement appear to have the best prognosis. Myocardial failure and acute tubular necrosis are frequent complications. The major long-term sequelae of hypoxic-ischemic injury are mental retardation, seizures, and cerebral palsy.

Therapeutic Management

Treatment involves vigorous supportive care to provide adequate ventilation to prevent aggravating the existing hypoxia and measures to maintain cerebral perfusion and prevent cerebral edema. Seizures are managed as described in the discussion on p. 416. Prevention is the most important therapy, however, and every effort should be made to recognize high-risk pregnancies, monitor the fetuses, and initiate appropriate therapy early.

Nursing Considerations

Nursing care is primarily the same as for any high-risk infant: careful assessment and observation for signs that might indicate cerebral hypoxia or ischemia, monitoring of ventilatory and intravenous therapy, observation and management of seizures, and general supportive care to infants and parents, including guidelines for management in the event of permanent neurologic damage (see Chapter 24). These infants are usually on intravenous alimentation.

PERIVENTRICULAR-INTRAVENTRICULAR HEMORRHAGE

Periventricular-intraventricular hemorrhage (PVH/IVH) is known by a variety of terms according to the locus of bleeding: *periventricular hemorrhage* (PVH), *intraventricular hemorrhage* (IVH), *general matrix hemorrhage-intraventricular hemorrhage* (GMH/IVH), and *subependymal-intraventricular hemorrhage* (SE/IVH). Most authorities use the term IVH to describe this disorder, which is responsible for a significant percentage of seriously ill infants and neonatal mortality. IVH is extremely common in preterm infants, especially the very small birth-weight infants.

Pathophysiology

During the early months of prenatal development there is an extensive but fragile vascular network in the region of the ventricles that receives a disproportionately large amount of cerebral blood flow. Toward term, more blood is directed to the germinal matrix located in the periventricular region near the caudate nuclei of the cerebrum. Therefore premature infants are subject to rupture in this heavily vascularized region, especially during an event that is likely to increase cerebral blood flow such as hypoxic episodes and the associated increased venous pressure. In PVH the bleeding originates in these capillaries. The blood may rupture through the ependymal lining of the ventricles and fill all or part of the ventricular system. Under pressure the ventricular system can dilate and cause acute hydrocephalus. Eventually obliterative arachnoiditis may develop and obstruct the flow of cerebrospinal fluid. In severe cases the hemorrhage extends into the cerebral parenchyma.

There are several clinical features that are associated with IVH, such as birth asphyxia, early gestational age, low birth weight, respiratory distress, metabolic derangements, and hypertension. An abnormal platelet aggregation related to maternal ingestion of aspirin has also been linked to IVH (Rumack and others, 1981).

Clinical Manifestations

An increase in intracranial pressure (ICP) from hemorrhage is manifested by a tense, bulging anterior fontanel, separated sutures, and neurologic signs, such as twitching, stupor, apnea, and convulsions. Consumption of clotting factors during PVH may contribute to further bleeding and ventriclar hemorrhage. Survivors of IVH may develop hydrocephalus, a variety of motor deficits, and mental retardation.

Diagnostic Evaluation

When intracranial hemorrhage is suspected, studies of intracranial stuctures are performed by ultrasonography or computed tomography. A classification based on the extent of germinal matrix hemorrhage:

0 -no bleeding
1 -germinal matrix only
2 -germinal matrix with blood in the ventricles and hydrocephalus
3 -germinal matrix with blood in the ventricles and hydrocephalus
4 -intraventricular and parenchymal bleeding (other than germinal matrix)

Therapeutic Management

Treatment of IVH is confined to supportive care, including ventilatory support, maintenance of oxygenation, regulation of fluid and acid-base balance, suppression of seizures, and any attendant complications. Although a number of therapies have been proposed, including spinal and ventricular taps, diuretics, phenobarbital, vitamin E, and steroids, none have maintained the medical community's support.

Nursing Considerations

In addition to the routine observations and management, nursing care is directed toward prevention of increased cerebral blood pressure. It has been observed that some nursing procedures increase (ICP). For example, there is a marked increase in blood pressure during suctioning (Perlman and Volpe, 1983), and head positioning produces measurable changes in ICP. It has been found that ICP is highest when infants are in the dependent position and decreases when the head is elevated 30 degrees (Emery and Peabody, 1983). However, this finding is not universally supported.

Cerebral pressure is lower when infants are in a midline position as opposed to a right side-lying position. When the head is turned to the right without body alignment, the resulting venous congestion creates hydrostatic pressure fluctuations that increase ICP (Goldberg and others, 1983). Infants encumbered with tubes and monitoring equipment are more difficult to turn while maintaining head-body alignment.

INTRACRANIAL HEMORRHAGE

Intracranial hemorrhage (ICH) in neonates, although manifested as the same types as those described in older children occurs with different frequencies and different degrees of severity.

Subdural Hematomas

Subdural hematomas, life-threatening collections of blood in the subdural space, are most often produced by the stretching and tearing of the large veins in the *tentorium cerebelli*, the dural membrane that separates the cerebrum from the cerebellum. With improved obstetric care these have become relatively uncommon; however, they are especially serious because of the inaccessibility of the hematoma to aspiration by subdural tap. Less frequently, hemorrhage occurs when veins in the subdural space over the surface of the brain are torn (see also p. 1643).

Subarachnoid Hemorrhage

Subarachnoid hemorrhage, although very common and a frequent cause of neonatal seizures, is of venous origin, usually self-limited, and seldom of major importance.

Intracerebellar Hemorrhage

Intracerebellar hemorrhage is a common finding on postmortem examination of the premature infant and can be a primary hemorrhage in the cerebellum associated with skull compression during abrupt, precipitous delivery, or it may occur secondary to extravasation of blood into the cerebellum from a ventricular hemorrhage. In the full-term infant the bleeding may follow a difficult delivery.

Nursing Considerations

Nursing care is the same as care of the infant with periventricular-intraventricular hemorrhage or with perinatal hypoxic-ischemic brain injury.

NEONATAL SEIZURES

Seizures in the neonatal period are usually the clinical manifestation of a serious underlying disease. Although not life threatening as an isolated entity, seizures constitute a medical emergency because they signal a disease process that may produce irreversible brain damage. Consequently it is imperative to recognize a seizure and its significance so that the cause as well as the seizure can be treated (see box).

Pathophysiology

The features of neonatal seizures are different from those observed in the older infant or child. For example, the well-organized, generalized tonic-clonic seizures seen in older children are rare in infants, especially preterm infants. The newborn brain, with its immature anatomic and physiologic status and less cortical organization and myelination, is insufficient to allow ready development and maintenance of a generalized seizure. The advanced degree of development of limbic structures with connections to the diencephalon and brainstem probably accounts for the higher frequency of seizure manifestations that originate in these structures, such as oral movements, oculomotor deviations, and apnea.

Clinical Manifestations

Seizures in newborns may be subtle and barely discernible or grossly apparent. Since most neonatal seizures are subcortical, they do not have the etiologic and prognostic significance of seizures in children. The type of seizure is seldom important since one may produce any of a variety of manifestations. Neonatal seizures can be divided into five major types. In order of frequency, these classifications are: subtle, generalized tonic, multifocal clonic, focal clonic, and myoclonic.

Subtle seizures may develop in either full-term or preterm infants and are often overlooked by the inexperienced observer. The clinical manifestations include clonic horizontal eye deviation, repetitive blinking or fluttering of the eyelids, drooling, sucking or other oral-buccal-lingual movements, arm movements resembling rowing or swimming, leg movements described as pedaling or bicycling, and apnea. These signs may appear alone or in combination with other signs, especially apnea, a common phenomenon in premature infants that in isolation almost always results from other causes.

Generalized tonic seizures are usually manifested as extensions of all four limbs similar to decerebrate rigidity, or occasionally the upper limbs are maintained in a stiffly flexed position resembling decorticate rigidity (p. 1629). Tonic seizures appear more frequently in premature infants. *Multifocal clonic* seizures consist of rhythmic jerking movements, about 1 to 3 per second, which may migrate randomly from one part of the body to another. Simultaneous involvement of separate areas often occurs, and the convulsive movements may start at different times and at different rates. *Focal clonic* seizures are usually well localized and frequently accompany other seizure types. *Myoclonic* seizures consist of single or multiple flexion jerks of the limbs. These last two types are relatively uncommon or rare in newborns.

Jitteriness or tremulousness in the newborn is a repetitive shaking of an extremity or extremities that may be observed with crying, may occur with changes in sleeping state, or may be elicited with stimulation. Jitteriness is relatively common in newborns and in a mild degree may be considered normal during the first 4 days of life. It can be distinguished from seizures by several characteristics: jitteriness is not accompanied by ocular movement as are seizures; the dominant movement in jitteriness is tremor, and seizure movement is clonic jerking that cannot be stopped by flexion of the affected limb; and jitteriness is highly sensitive to stimulation whereas seizures are not. If jittery movements persist beyond the fourth day, if the movements are persistent and prolonged after a stimulus, or if they are easily elicited with minimum stimulus, further evaluation is indicated.

Diagnostic Evaluation

Early evaluation and diagnosis of seizures are urgent. In addition to a careful physical examination, the pregnancy and family histories are investigated for familial and prenatal causes. Blood is drawn for glucose and electrolyte examination, and cerebrospinal fluid is obtained for examination for gross blood, cell count, protein, glucose, and culture. Electroencephalography may help identify subtle seizures but is less helpful in establishing a diagnosis. Other diagnostic procedures, such as computed tomography and echoencephalography, may be indicated.

Therapeutic Management

Treatment is directed toward prevention of cerebral damage and involves correction of metabolic derangements, respiratory and cardiovascular support, and suppression of the seizure activity. The underlying cause is treated, for example, glucose infusion for hypoglycemia, calcium for hypocalcemia, and antibiotics for infection. If needed, respiratory support is provided for hypoxia, and anticonvulsants may be administered, especially when the other measures fail to control the seizures. Phenobarbital is the drug of choice given orally or intramuscularly, but the intravenous

---

CAUSES OF NEONATAL SEIZURES

Metabolic
Hypoglycemia
Hypocalcemia
Hypomagnesemia
Pyridoxine deficiency
Aminoacidurias (e.g., phenylketonuria, maple syrup urine disease)

Toxic and electrolyte
Hypernatremia
Hyponatremia
Narcotic withdrawal
Uremia
Bilirubin encephalopathy (kernicterus)

Infections
Bacterial meningitis
Viral meningoencephalitis
Toxoplasmosis
Syphilis
Cytomegalic inclusion disease
Herpes simplex

Trauma at birth
Hypoxic encephalopathy
Intracranial hemorrhage

Malformations
Central nervous system agenesis
Hydroencephalopathy
Parencephalopathy
Tuberous sclerosis

Miscellaneous
Degenerative disease
Benign familial neonatal seizures

Table 10-6 White's classification of diabetes in pregnancy (modified)

Gestational diabetes	Abnormal GTT, but euglycemia maintained by diet alone; or diet alone insufficient, insulin required
Class A	Diet alone, any duration or onset age
Class B	Onset age 20 yrs or older and duration less than 10 yrs
Class C	Onset age 10 to 19 yrs or duration 10 to 19 yrs
Class D	Onset age under 10 yrs, duration over 20 yrs, background retinopathy, or hypertension (not eclampsia)
Class R	Proliferative retinopathy or vitreous hemorrhage
Class F	Nephropathy with over 500 mg/day proteinuria
Class RF	Criterial for both R and F coexist
Class H	Arteriosclerotic heart disease clinically evident
Class T	Prior renal transplantation

From Hare, J.W., and White, P.: Gestational diabetes and the White classification, Diabetes Care **3:**394-397, 1980.

route is used if seizures are severe and persistent. Other drugs that may be employed are phenytoin (Dilantin), paraldehyde, and diazepam (Valium).

Nursing Considerations

The major nursing responsibilities in the care of infants with seizures are to recognize when the infant is having a seizure so that therapy can be instituted, to carry out the therapeutic regimen, and to observe the response to the therapy and any further evidence of seizures or other symptomatology. Assessment and other aspects of care are the same as for all high-risk infants. Parents need to be informed of their infant's status, and the nurse should reinforce and clarify the explanations of the attending physician. The infant's behaviors need to be interpreted for the parents, and the significance of the infant's responses to the treatment must be anticipated and explained. Parents are encouraged to visit their infant and perform the parenting activities consistent with the plan of care. Seizures are a frightening phenomenon and generate a great deal of anxiety and fear, which is easily compounded by the justifiable concern of the staff. Providing support and guidance is an important nursing function.

High Risk Related to Maternal Conditions

Conditions in the maternal system can have a significant effect on the fetus that extends into the postnatal period. A number of these conditions that are congenital malformations and disorders and can cause permanent disability are discussed in Chapter 11. Maternal diabetes and drug addiction are presented in the following section.

INFANTS OF DIABETIC MOTHERS

Before insulin therapy, few diabetic women were able to conceive; for those who did, the mortality rate for both mother and infant was high. As a result of effective control of maternal diabetes and an increased understanding of fetal disorders, the morbidity and mortality of infants of diabetic mothers (IDM) have been significantly reduced.

Maternal Management

The severity of the maternal diabetes affects infant survival. There is a higher incidence of stillborn infants in the more severe, insulin-dependent diabetic women, and their liveborn infants appear to be more at risk than those born to mothers with less severe diabetic involvement. Severity of maternal diabetes is classified according to the duration of the disease before pregnancy, the age of onset, and the extent of vascular complications (Table 10-6). Another classification system is determined by abnormalities of the current pregnancy, or "prognostically bad signs of pregnancy," which are designated as: chemical pyelonephritis, precoma or severe acidosis, toxemia, or as mothers who are "neglectors," those women who do not maintain a prescribed regimen of care (Pederson, 1976).

The single most important factor influencing fetal well-being is the euglycemic status of the mother. It has been found that reasonable metabolic control started before conception and continued during the first weeks of pregnancy can prevent malformations in infants of diabetic mothers (Fuhrmann and others, 1983). To achieve the ideal state, the diabetic woman contemplating pregnancy should:

1. Have a thorough examination to detect any signs of diabetic complications.
2. Bring blood glucose into the normal range and maintain strict control before and during pregnancy. Poor control during early pregnancy can cause abnormalities in the developing fetal organs; later, poor control can cause macrosomia in the fetus.
3. Monitor blood glucose levels several times daily during pregnancy to keep track of the body's insulin needs.

Effects of Diabetes on the Fetus

Hypoglycemia, defined as a blood sugar level below 30 mg per dl for normal newborns and below 20 mg per dl for premature infants, appears a short time after birth and is associated with increased insulin activity in the blood. It has been demonstrated that infants of diabetic mothers have hypertrophy and hyperplasia of the pancreatic islet cells and that they are actually in a state of hyperinsulinism. It is generally agreed that during fetal life high maternal blood sugar levels provide a continual stimulus to the fetal islet cells for insulin production. This sustained state of hyperglycemia promotes fetal insulin secretion that ultimately leads to excessive growth and deposition of fat, which probably accounts for the infants who are large for gestational age. When the glucose supply is removed abruptly at the time of birth, the continued production of insulin soon depletes the blood of circulating glucose, creating a state of hyperinsulinism within 2 to 4 hours, especially in infants of mothers with class C diabetes or beyond. Precipitous drops in blood glucose levels can cause serious neurologic damage or death.

Tests of fetal well-being are performed routinely during pregnancy. Ultrasonography is performed at 18 to 20 weeks to determine fetal size and to rule out the presence of fetal anomalies. It may be repeated periodically during the course of fetal development. Urinary estriol, protein, and creatinine are measured weekly after 30 weeks of gestation, and nonstress or oxytoxin challenge tests for assessment of fetal and placental function are performed after 33 weeks. Before delivery, fetal lung maturation tests via amniocentesis are carried out, including lecithin/sphingomyelin ratio, phosphatidylglycerol, and disaturated phosphatidylcholine measurements.

Some mothers are hospitalized at 36 to 37 weeks of gestation for management. Insulin and dietary alterations are made in accordance with blood glucose determinations. Techniques such as closed- or open-loop continuous insulin infusion devices may be employed to maintain a satisfactory blood glucose concentration.

Clinical Manifestations

Infants of well-controlled diabetic mothers are essentially no different from other infants, but infants of poorly controlled diabetic mothers have a characteristic appearance. They are usually macrosomic for their gestational age, very plump and full-faced, liberally coated with vernix caseosa, and plethoric. The placenta and umbilical cord are also larger than average. However, infants of mothers with advanced diabetes, such as Class C and D or more, may be small for gestational age because of the maternal vascular involvement. There is an increase in congenital anomalies in this group in addition to a high susceptibility to hypoglycemia, hypocalcemia, hyperbilirubinemia, and hyaline membrane disease. No satisfactory explanation has been accepted for all the abnormalities in these infants, although complications may be related to the prematurity factor in a number of cases (e.g., hyaline membrane disease). Although they are large, these infants are often prematurely born in an elective early delivery or because of complications.

Therapeutic Management

The most effective management appears to be careful observation of all infants of diabetic mothers, often in the special care nursery. The infants are examined for the presence of any anomalies or birth injuries, and blood studies for initial determinations of glucose, calcium, hematocrit, and bilirubin are obtained on a regular basis.

Feedings of 5% to 10% glucose are begun 1 hour after birth and followed by formula, if tolerated. Some pediatricians prefer early feedings of nonglucose carbohydrates, such as invert sugar or galactose, because they are less insulinogenic. Critically ill infants require intravenous infusions. Approximately half of these infants do very well and adjust without complications. However, since the hypertrophied pancreas is so sensitive to blood glucose concentrations, the administration of glucose may trigger a massive insulin release resulting in rebound hypoglycemia. Therefore frequent blood glucose determinations are needed for the first 2 days of life to assess the degree of hypoglycemia present at any given time. Testing blood taken from the heel with reagent strips is a simple and effective screening evaluation which can then be confirmed by laboratory examinations several times a day.

Nursing Considerations

In addition to the routine care of the newborn, the infant of the diabetic mother requires observation for signs of complications, such as hypoglycemia (p. 356), hyperbilirubinemia (p. 346), and respiratory distress (p. 397). Because some are born prematurely, these infants are subject to the problems discussed in relation to the preterm infant.

DRUG-ADDICTED INFANTS

Narcotics, which have a low molecular weight, readily cross the placental membrane and enter the fetal system. When the mother is a habitual user of narcotics, especially heroin or methadone, the unborn child also becomes passively addicted to the drug, which places such infants at risk during the early neonatal period.

Clinical Manifestations

Most passively addicted infants of drug-dependent mothers appear normal at birth but begin to exhibit signs of drug withdrawal within 12 to 24 hours if the mother has been taking heroin by itself. If mothers have been taking methadone, the signs appear somewhat later, anywhere from 1 or 2 days to a week or more after birth. The manifestations become most pronounced between 48 and 72 hours of age and may last anywhere from 6 days to 8 weeks, depending on the severity of the withdrawal (see box).

The clinical manifestations of withdrawal in neonates, which are predominantly those of autonomic nervous system hyperirritability, may persist for 3 or 4 months. The most common acute signs are tremors, restlessness, hyperactive reflexes, increased muscle tone, sneezing, tachypnea, and a high-pitched, shrill cry. Although these infants suck avidly on fists and display an exaggerated rooting reflex, they are poor feeders with uncoordinated and ineffectual sucking and swallowing reflexes. Regurgitation and vomiting after feedings are common, and diarrhea is a later manifestation. An unusual observation in a large percentage of these infants is generalized sweating, the incidence of which is double that in normal newborns who display sweating. It is significant that although passively addicted infants have some tachypnea, cyanosis, and/or apnea, they rarely develop respiratory distress syndrome. Apparently heroin or stress factors in the intrauterine environment cause accelerated lung maturation even with a high incidence of prematurity.

Not all infants of heroin-addicted mothers will show signs of withdrawal. Because of irregular and varying degrees of drug use, quality of drug, and mixed drug usage by the mother, some infants display mild or variable manifestations. Most manifestations are the vague nonspecific signs characteristic of all infants in general; therefore it is important to differentiate between drug withdrawal and other disorders before specific therapy is instituted. Often other states, for example, hypocalcemia, hypoglycemia, or sepsis, coexist with the drug withdrawal.

Infants who do not display the signs of fetal alcohol syndrome but are born to mothers who are heavy alcohol drinkers have significantly more tremors, hypertonia, restlessness, excessive mouthing movements, crying, and inconsolability than infants of mothers who do not drink (Coles and others, 1984). An added concern regarding drug users is that many of the mothers often use other drugs, such as tranquilizers, sedatives, narcotics, amphetamines, phencyclidine (PCP), and other psychotropic agents.

Therapeutic Management

The treatment of the passively addicted infant initially consists of intramuscular administration of chlorpromazine or phenobarbital followed by oral administration individualized in amount and frequency. Diazepam has proven effective for selected infants. If there are gastrointestinal symptoms such as diarrhea, paregoric may be the drug of choice.

Nursing Considerations

When possible, the nursery personnel are alerted to the likelihood of drug-addicted infants. If the mothers have had

---

SIGNS OF NARCOTIC WITHDRAWAL IN THE NEONATE

Irritability
Tremors
Shrill cry
Hypertonicity of muscles
Frantic sucking of hands
Poor feeding
Hyperactivity
Little sleeping
Sweating
Tachypnea (>60/min)
Excoriations (knees, face)
Frequent sneezing
Frequent yawning
Vomiting
Low-grade fever
Diarrhea
Convulsions

---

good prenatal care, the physician is aware of the problem and therapy has been instituted before delivery. However, a number of mothers deliver their infants without the benefit of adequate care, and the addiction is unknown to health care personnel at the time of delivery. The degree of narcosis or withdrawal is closely related to the amount of drug the mother has habitually taken, the length of time she has been taking the drug, and the drug level of the mother at the time of delivery. The most severe symptoms are observed in the infants of mothers who have taken large amounts of drugs over a long period. In addition, the nearer to the time of delivery that the mother takes the drug, the longer it takes for the child to develop withdrawal and the more severe are the manifestations.

Once the presence of withdrawal is identified in an infant, nursing care is directed toward reducing the stimuli that might trigger hyperactivity and irritability, providing adequate nutrition and hydration, and promoting maternal-infant relationships. Irritable and hyperactive infants have been found to respond to comforting, movement, and close contact. Wrapping infants snugly and holding them tightly limits their ability to self-stimulate. Arranging nursing activities to reduce the amount of disturbance helps to decrease exogenous stimulation.

Loose stools and poor intake and regurgitation following feeding predispose the infants to malnutrition, dehydration, and electrolyte imbalance that can progress to shock and coma. Frequent weighing, careful monitoring of intake and output, and supplemental parenteral fluids may be necessary. In addition, they burn up energy with continual activity and increase oxygen consumption at the cellular level. It takes considerable time and patience to ensure that the infants receive a sufficient calorie and fluid intake.

Hyperactive infants must be protected from skin abrasions on the knees, toes, and cheeks that are caused by rubbing on bed linens when lying on their abdomens. Monitoring and recording activity level and its relationship to other activities, such as feeding and preventing complications, are important nursing functions.

A valuable aid to anticipating problems in newborns is recognizing drug addiction in the mothers. Unless the mothers are enrolled in a methadone rehabilitation program, they seldom risk calling attention to their habit by seeking prenatal care. Consequently infants and mothers are exposed to the additional hazards of obstetric and medical complications. Moreover, the nature of heroin addiction makes the user susceptible to disorders such as infection, hepatitis, foreign body reaction, and the hazards of inadequate nutrition and premature birth. Methadone treatment does not prevent withdrawal reaction in neonates, but the clinical course may be modified. Also, the intensive psychologic support of mothers is a factor in the treatment and the reduction of perinatal mortality. Experience has indicated that mothers are usually anxious and depressed, lack confidence, have poor self-images, and have difficulty with interpersonal relationships. They have a psychologic need for the pregnancy and an infant.

Recurrence of withdrawal symptoms may develop after discharge from the hospital; therefore it is important to establish rapport and maintain contact with the family so that they will return for treatment if this occurs. Long-term follow-up to evaluate the status of the infant and the family is very important. Sudden infant death syndrome (SIDS) and acquired immune deficiency syndrome (AIDS) are observed more frequently in infants born to users of methadone and heroin (Oleske and others, 1983).

There are many problems in relation to the disposition of infants of drug-dependent mothers. Those who advocate separation of mothers and children argue that the mothers are not capable of assuming responsibility for their infant's care, that child care is frustrating to them, and that their existence is too disorganized and chaotic. Others encourage the maternal-infant bond and recommend a protected environment such as a therapeutic community, a halfway house, or continuous, ongoing, supportive services in the home after discharge. Each situation requires careful evaluation and the cooperative efforts of a variety of health professionals, whether the choice is foster home placement or supportive follow-up care of mothers who keep their infants.

INFANT OF THE MOTHER WHO SMOKES

Cigarette smoking during pregnancy is clearly associated with birth weight deficits up to 250 g for full-term newborns (Stein and Susser, 1984). Studies show a definite dose-response relationship between the number of cigarettes smoked by the mother and birth weight deficits in the newborn. Light and heavy smokers have 54% to 130% increases in the prevalence of newborns who weigh less than 2500 g (Meyer, Jonas, and Tonascia, 1976). This dose-related response also affects the Apgar scores—the number of infants with low Apgar scores (mothers smoked three packs per day) is nearly four times that of infants whose mothers smoked none or only one pack per day (Garn and others, 1981). Also, reviews of large studies indicate that 21% to 39% of the incidence of low birth weight is attributable to maternal cigarette smoking (Department of Health and Human Services [DHHS], 1983).

The rate of preterm births is increased in mothers who smoke, but the infants are smaller at *all* stages of gestation. They show fetal growth retardation in length, weight, and chest and head circumference, and these deficits are not related to maternal appetite or weight gain (DHHS, 1983). Concentrations of two pharmacologically active substances found in tobacco, nicotine and cotinine, have been found to be higher in newborns of mothers who smoke than in their mothers. In addition, these substances secreted in breast milk have a half-life of 70 to 80 minutes (Luck and others, 1982). It has also been shown that cigarette smoking has detrimental effects beyond the neonatal period with deficits in growth, intellectual and emotional development, and behavior (DHHS, 1983; Naeye and Peters, 1984). (See also Effects of passive smoking, p. 1375.)

The overwhelming evidence of the detrimental effects of maternal cigarette smoking on newborns has led some investigators to suggest the diagnostic term *fetal tobacco syndrome* for infants who fit the following key features (Nieburg and others, 1985):

1. The mother smoked five or more cigarettes a day throughout pregnancy.
2. The mother had no evidence of hypertension during pregnancy, specifically: (a) no preeclampsia, and (b) documentation of normal blood pressure at least once after the first trimester.
3. The newborn has symmetrical growth retardation at term (up to or greater than 37 weeks), defined as: (a) a birth weight less than 2500 g, and (b) a ponderal index ([weight in g] / [length in m^3]) greater than 2.32.
4. There is no other obvious cause of intrauterine growth retardation (e.g., congenital infection or anomaly).

The purpose of this suggestion is to focus attention on this important health problem that is directly related to maternal behavior.

Nursing Considerations

Nurses are prime candidates for disseminating information to expectant mothers about the risks related to smoking. Mothers who stop or substantially reduce smoking during pregnancy improve the quality of life for their unborn infants. In one study, infants of expectant mothers who were given information, support, encouragement, practical guidance, and behavior modification during pregnancy delivered infants with significantly higher birth weights than controls (Sexton and Hebel, 1984). If mothers continue to smoke while breast-feeding, they should be told to do so *immediately after* breast-feeding to reduce the amount of nicotine and cotinine in the breast milk (Luck and others, 1982).

CONCEPT SUMMARIES

- High-risk neonates may be defined as newborns, regardless of gestational age or birth weight, who have a greater than average chance of morbidity or mortality because of conditions or circumstances superimposed on the normal course of events associated with birth and adjustment to extrauterine existence.

- Identification of high-risk newborns may occur during any one of the following stages: preconceptual, prenatal, natal, postnatal.

- High-risk infants may be classified according to size, gestational age, and mortality.

- Newborn intensive care units are categorized according to population served and degree of treatment.

- General management of the newborn entails immediate care; protection from infection; monitoring physiologic data, including heart rate, respiratory activity and temperature, blood pressure; laboratory date, and systematic assessment of the high-risk infant.

- Assessment of the newborn includes a general assessment, respiratory assessment, cardiovascular assessment, gastrointestinal assessment, genitourinary assessment, neurologic-musculoskeletal assessment, skin assessment, and temperature.

- Because their metabolic processes are immature, newborns are placed in a heated environment to help control thermoneutrality.

- Because of the immature, fragile skin of premature infants, the nurse should use caution when applying topical preparations and when removing bandages or dressings.

- Meeting the high-risk infant's nutritional needs requires specific knowledge of physiologic characteristics, the infant's particular needs, and methods of feeding.

- Delayed development in high-risk neonates is a concern; infant stimulation techniques are used to minimize the effects.

- Parental involvement in the care of high-risk infants is important, and nurses should help to facilitate parent-infant relationships by guiding them to support groups and home health teaching.

- Prematurity accounts for the largest number of admissions to a neonatal ICU.

- Several severe respiratory conditions place the infant at high risk: apnea of prematurity, respiratory distress syndrome, meconium aspiration syndrome, extraneous air syndromes, bronchopulmonary dysplasia. Therapeutic management of respiratory distress syndromes includes oxygen therapy and assisted ventialtion.

- Newborns are highly susceptible to infection, particularly sepsis.

- Cardiovascular complications in the high-risk infant may include persistent patent ductus arteriosus, persistent pulmonary hypertension, anemia, and polycythemia/hyperviscosity syndrome.

- Neurologic disturbances in the high-risk newborn may include perinatal hypoxic-ischemic brain injury, periventricular-intraventricular hemorrhage, intracranial hemorrhage, and neonatal seizures.

- Maternal conditions that pose a threat to the newborn include diabetes, drug addiction, and smoking.

REFERENCES

An international classification of retinopathy of prematurity, Pediatrics **74**:127-133, 1984.

Anderson, G.C., and others: Effects of time-controlled non-nutritive sucking opportunities, Nurs. Res. **31**:63, 1982.

Anderson, G.H., Atkinson, S.A., and Bryan, M.H.: Energy and macronutrient content of human milk during early lactation from mothers giving birth prematurely and at term, Am. J. Clin. Nutr. **34**:258-265, 1981.

Atakent, Y., and others: The adverse effects of high oral osmolal mixtures in neonates, Clin. Pediatr. **23**:487-490, September 1984.

Bancalari, E., and Gerhardt, T.: Bronchopulmonary dysplasia, Pediatr. Clin. North Am. **33**:1-23, 1986.

Barnard, K.E., and Bee, H.L.: The impact of temporally patterned stimulation on the development of preterm infants, Child Dev. **54**:1156-1167, 1983.

Barrington, K.J., and others: Physiologic effects of doxapram in idiopathic apnea of prematurity, J. Pediatr. **108**:124-129, 1986.

Bartlett, R.H., and others: Extracorporeal circulation in neonatal respiratory failure: a prospective randomized study, Pediatrics **76**:479-487, 1985.

Bauer, C.R., and others: A decreased incidence of necrotizing enterocolitis after prenatal glucocorticoid therapy, Pediatrics **73**:682-688, 1984.

Baumgart, S.: Reduction of oxygen consumption, insensible water loss, and radiant heat demand with use of a plastic blanket for low-birth-weight infants under radiant warmers, Pediatrics **74**:1022-1028, 1984.

Baumgart, S., Fox, W.W., and Polin, R.A.: Physiologic implications of two different heat shields for infants under radiant warmers, J. Pediatr. **100**:787-790, 1982.

Baumgart, S., and others: Radiant warmer power and body size as determinants of insensible water loss in the critically ill neonate, Pediatr. Res. **15**:1495-1498, 1981.

Bennett, F.C., Robinson, N.M., and Sells, C.J.: Growth and development of infants weighing less than 800 grams at birth, Pediatrics **71**:319-323, 1983.

Bernbaum, J.C., and others: Nonnutritive sucking during gavage feeding enhances growth and maturation in premature infants, Pediatrics **71**:41-45, 1983.

Boggs, K.R., and Rau, P.K.: Breastfeeding the premature infant, Am. J. Nurs. **83**:1437-1439, 1983.

Boros, S.J., and others: Neonatal high-frequency jet ventilation: four years' experience, Pediatrics **75**:657-663, 1985.

Brazelton, T.B.: Personal communication, 1984.

Brooke, O.G., Alvear, J., and Arnold, M.: Energy retention, energy expenditure, and growth in healthy immature infants, Pediatr. Res. **13**:215-220, 1979.

Bruhn, F.W., and Jones, B.: Infection in the neonate. In Merenstein, G.B., and Gardner, S.L.: Handbook of neonatal intensive care, St. Louis, 1985, The C.V. Mosby Co.

Bull, M.J., and Stroup, K.B.: Premature infants in car seats, Pediatrics **75**:336-339, 1985.

Cairo, M.S., and others: Improved survival of newborns receiving leukocyte transfusions for sepsis, Pediatrics **74**:887-888, 1984.

Carlo, W.A., and others: Decrease in airway pressure during high-frequency jet ventilation in infants with respiratory distress syndrome, J. Pediatr. **104**:101-105, January 1984.

Cohen, M.A.: The use of prostaglandins and prostaglandin inhibitors in critically ill neonates, Am. J. Maternal Child Nurs. **8**:194-199, 1983.

Collaborative Group on Antenatal Steroid Therapy: Effect of antenatal dexamethasone administration on the prevention of respiratory distress syndrome, Am. J. Obstet. Gynecol. **141**:276, 1981.

Cole, J.G.: Infant stimulation reexamined: an environmental- and behavioral-based approach, Neonatal Network **3**(5):24-31, 1985.

Cole, J.G., and Frappier, P.A.: Infant stimulation reassessed. A new approach to providing care for the preterm infant, JOGN Nurs. **14**:471-477, 1985.

Coles, C.D., and others: Neonatal ethanol withdrawal: characteristics in critically normal nondysmorphic neonates, J. Pediatr. **105**:445-451, 1984.

Collinge, J.M., and others: Demand vs. scheduled feedings for premature infants, JOGN Nurs. **11**:362-367, 1982.

Committee on Fetus and Newborn: Vitamin E and the prevention of retinopathy of prematurity, Pediatrics **76**:315-316, 1985.

Committee on Fetus and Newborn, Committee on Drugs: Benzyl alcohol: toxic agent in neonatal units, Pediatrics **72**:356-358, 1983.

Committee on Nutrition: Nutritional needs of low-birth-weight infants, Pediatrics **75**:976-986, 1985.

Curran, J.S., and others: Results of feeding a special formula to very low-birth-weight infants, J. Pediatr. **100**:327-332, 1982.

David, R.J., and Siegel, E.: Decline in neonatal mortality, 1968 to 1977: better babies or better care? Pediatrics **71**:531-540, 1983.

Department of Health and Human Services: The health consequences of smoking for women: a report of the surgeon general, Washington, D.C., 1983, publication 410-889/1284.

Dworsky, M., and others: Cytomegalovirus infection of breast milk and transmission in infancy, Pediatrics **72**:295-299, 1983.

Emery, J.R., and Peabody, J.L.: Head position affects intracranial pressure in newborn infants, J. Pediatr. **103**:950-953, 1983.

Eyal, F., and others: Aminophylline versus doxapram in idiopathic apnea of prematurity: a double-blind controlled study, Pediatrics **75**:709-713,1985.

FDA Drug Bulletin: Benzyl alcohol may be toxic to newborns, **12**:10-11, 1982.

Field, T., and Goldson, E.: Pacifying effects of nonnutritive sucking on term and preterm neonates during heelstick procedures, Pediatrics **74**:1012-1015, 1984.

Field, T., and others: Nonnutritive sucking during tube feedings: effects on preterm neonates in an intensive care unit, Pediatrics **70**:381-384, 1982.

Fomufod, A.K.: Low birthweight and early neonatal separation as factors in child abuse, J. Natl. Med. Assoc. **68**:106-109, 1976.

Fox, W.W., and Duara, S.: Persistent pulmonary hypertension in the neonate: diagnosis and management, J. Pediatr. **103**:505-514, 1983.

Fuhrmann, K., and others: Prevention of congenital malformations in infants of insulin-dependent diabetic mothers, Diabetes Care **6**:219-223, 1983.

Garn, S.M., and others: Effect of maternal cigarette smoking on Apgar scores, Am. J. Dis. Child **135**:503-506, 1981.

Gerhardt, T., and Bancalari, E.: Apnea of prematurity: I. Lung function and regulation of breathing, Pediatrics **74**:58-59, 1984.

Gerhardt, T., and Bancalari, E.: Apnea of prematurity: II. Respiratory reflexes, Pediatrics **74**:63-64, 1984.

Gleason, C.A., and others: Optimal position for a spinal tap in preterm infants, Pediatrics **71**:31-35, 1983.

Goldberg, R.N., and others: The effect of head position on intracranial pressure in the neonate, Crit. Care Med. **11**:428-430, 1983.

Gorski, P.A., Davison, M.F., and Brazelton, T.B.: Stages of behavioral organization in the high-risk neonate: theoretical and clinical considerations, Semin. Perinatol. **3**:61-72, 1979.

Grant, P.: Psychosocial needs of families of high-risk infants, Fam. Com. Health **1**(3):91-102, 1978.

Gross, S.J., Oehler, J.M., and Eckerman, C.O.: Head growth and developmental outcome in very-low-birth-weight infants, Pediatrics **71**:70-75, 1983.

Gross, S.J., and others: Nutritional composition of milk produced by mothers delivering preterm, J. Pediatr. **96**:641-644, 1980.

Gross, S.J., and others: Elevated IgA concentration in milk produced by mothers delivered of preterm infants, J. Pediatr. **99**:389-393, 1981.

Hack, M., and others: Catch-up growth in very-low-birth-weight infants, Am. J. Dis. Child. **138**:370-375, 1984.

Hallman, M., and others: Exogenous human surfactant for treatment of severe respiratory distress syndrome: a randomized prospective clinical trial, J. Pediatr. **106**:963-969, 1983.

Hansen, F.H.: Nursing care in the neonatal intensive care unit, JOGN Nurs. **11**:17-20, 1982.

Hill, A., and Volpe, J.J.: Seizures, hypoxic-ischemic brain injury, and intraventricular hemorrhage in the newborn, Ann. Neurol. **10**:109-121, 1981.

Hodgman, J.E.: Bronchopulmonary dysplasia. In Gellis, S.S., and Kagan, B.M.: Current pediatric therapy 12, Philadelphia, 1986, W.B. Saunders Co.

Kimble, D.J., and others: Growth to age 3 years among very-low-birth-weight sequelae-free survivors of modern neonatal intensive care, J. Pediatr. **100**:622-624, 1982.

Klaus, M.H., and Kennell, J.H.: Maternal infant bonding, ed. 2, St. Louis, 1982, The C.V. Mosby Co.

Korner, A.F., Ruppel, E.M., and Rho, J.M.: Effects of water beds on the sleep and motility of theophylline-treated preterm infants, Pediatrics **70**:864-869, 1982.

Korones, S.B.: High-risk newborn infants: the basis for intensive nursing care, ed. 4, St. Louis, 1986, The C.V. Mosby Co.

Kosloske, A.M.: Pathogenesis and prevention of necrotizing enterocolitis: a hypothesis based on personal observation and a review of the literature, Pediatrics **74**:1086-1092, 1984.

Kowba, M.D., and Schwirian, P.M.: Direct sibling contact and bacterial colonization in newborns, JOGN Nurs. **14**:412-417, 1985.

Kuller, J.M., Lund, C., and Tobin, C.: Improved skin care for premature infants, Am. J. Matern. Child Nurs. **8**:200-203, 1983.

Kwang-sun, L., and others: The very low-birth-weight rate: principal predictor of neonatal mortality in industrialized populations, J. Pediatr. **97**:795-764, 1980.

Kwong, M.S., and others: Double-blind clinical trial of calf lung surfactant extract for the prevention of hyaline membrane disease in extremely premature infants, Pediatrics **76**:585-592, 1985.

Lebenthal, E.: Physiologic considerations in the feeding of the premature and compromised infant, Child Care Newsletter **1**(3):5-8, 1982.

Lee, K., and others: The very low-birth-weight rate: principal predictor of neonatal mortality in industrialized populations, J. Pediatr. **97**:759-764, 1980.

Luck, W., and others: Nicotine and cotinine—two pharmacologically active substances as parameters for the strain on fetuses and babies of mothers who smoke, J. Perinat. Med. **10**:107-108, 1982.

Mahan, C.K., and Schreiner, R.L.: Care for the family mourning a perinatal death. In Schreiner, R.L., editor: Care of the newborn, New York, 1980, Raven Press.

Marshall, R.E., and others: Auditory function in newborn intensive care unit patients revealed by auditory brain-stem potentials, J. Pediatr. **96**:731-735, 1980.

Martin, R.J., and others: Effect of supine/prone position on arterial oxygen tension in the preterm infant, Pediatrics **63**:528-531, 1979.

McCrae, M.: Medical perspectives on brain damage and development. Family centered resource project, Reading, PA, 1982, Albright College.

Measel, C.P., and Anderson, G.C.: Nonnutritive sucking during tube feedings: effect on clinical course in premature infants, JOGN Nurs. **8**:265-272, 1979.

Meyer, J., Jonas, B.S., and Tonascia, J.A.: Perinatal events associated with maternal smoking during pregnancy, Am. J. Epidemiol. **103**:464-476, 1976.

Murat, I., and others: The efficacy of caffeine in the treatment of recurrent idiopathic apnea in premature infants, J. Pediatr. **99**:984-989, 1981.

Myers, T.F., and others: Low-dose theophylline therapy in idiopathic apnea of prematurity, J. Pediatr. **96**:99-103, 1980.

Naeye, R.L., and Peters, E.C.: Mental development of children whose mothers smoked during pregnancy, Obstet. Gynecol. **64**:60-107, 1984.

Nieburg, P., and others: The fetal tobacco syndrome (Commentary), JAMA **253**:2998-2999, 1985.

Norris, S., Campbell, L.A., and Brenkert, S.: Nursing procedures and alterations in transcutaneous oxygen tension in premature infants, Nurs. Res. **31**:330-336, 1982.

Oleske, J., and others: Immune deficiency syndrome in children, JAMA **249**:2345-2347, 1983.

Paludetto, R., and others: Transcutaneous oxygen tension during nonnutritive sucking in preterm infants, Pediatrics **74**:539-542, 1984.

Pederson, J.: The pregnant diabetic and her newborn, Baltimore, 1976, Williams & Wilkins.

Perlman, J.M., and Volpe, J.J.: Suctioning in the preterm infant: effects on cerebral blood flow velocity, intracranial pressure, and arterial blood pressure, Pediatrics **72**:329-334, 1983.

Pokora, T., and others: Neonatal high-frequency jet ventilation, Pediatrics **72**:27-32, 1983.

Roberts, J.L., Mathew, O.P., and Thach, B.T.: The efficacy of theophylline in premature infants with mixed and obstructive apnea and apnea associated with pulmonary and neurologic disease, J. Pediatr. **100**:968-970, 1982.

Ross, G.S.: Parental responses to infants in intensive care: the separation issue reevaluated, Clin. Perinatol. **7**(1):47-60, 1980.

Ross, G., Lipper, E.G., and Auld, P.A.M.: Physical growth and developmental outcome in very low birth weight premature infants at 3 years of age, J. Pediatr. **107**:284-286, 1985.

Rumack, C.M., and others: Neonatal intracranial hemorrhage and maternal use of aspirin, Obstet. Gynecol. Suppl. **58**:52-56, 1981.

Sauer, P.J.J., and Visser, H.K.A.: The neutral temperature of very low-birth-weight infants, Pediatrics **74**:288-289, 1984.

Schanler, R.J., Garza, C., and Nichols, B.L.: Fortified mothers' milk for very low birth weight infants: results of growth and nutrient balance studies, J. Pediatr. **107**:437-445, 1985.

Schwab, F., and others: Sibling visiting in a neonatal intensive care unit, Pediatrics **71**:835-838, 1983.

Scrimshaw, S.C.M., and March, D.M.: I had a baby sister but she only lasted one day, JAMA **251**:732-733, 1984.

Sexton, M., and Hebel, J.R.: A clinical trial of change in maternal smoking and its effect on birth weight, JAMA **251**:911-915, 1984.

Shapiro, D.L., and others: Double-blind, randomized trial of a calf lung surfactant extract administered at birth to very premature infants for prevention of respiratory distress syndrome, Pediatrics **76**:593-599, 1985.

Shapiro, S., and others: Changes in infant morbidity associated with decreases in neonatal mortality, Pediatrics **72**:408-415, 1983.

Sherman, J.M., Shelly, S.A., and Balis, J.U.: Pulmonary lavage as a source of human surfactant, J. Pediatr. **106**:126-127, 1985.

Socol, M.L., Sing, E., and Depp, O.R.: The tap test: a rapid indicator of fetal pulmonary maturity, Am. J. Obstet. Gynecol. **148**:445-450, 1984.

Southall, D.P., and others: Undetected episodes of prolonged apnea and severe bradycardia in preterm infants, Pediatrics **72**:541-551, 1983.

Speck, W.T., and Kennell, J.H.: Management of perinatal death, Pediatr. Rev. **2**(2):59-62, 1980.

Starfield, B., and others: Mortality and morbidity in infants with intrauterine growth retardation, J. Pediatr. **101**:978-983, 1982.

Stein, Z.A., and Susser, M.: Intrauterine growth retardation: epidemiological issues and public health significance, Semin. Perinatol. **8**:5-14, 1984.

Stockman, J.A., and others: Anemia of prematurity: determinants of the erythropoietin response, J. Pediatr. **105**:786-795, 1984.

Topper, W.H., and Stewart, T.P.: Thermal support for the very-low-birth-weight infant: role of supplemental conductive heat, J. Pediatr. **105**:810-814, 1984.

Trause, M.A., and others: Separation for childbirth: the effect on the sibling, Child Psychiatry Hum. Dev. **12**:32-35, 1981.

Tyson, J.E., and others: Growth, metabolic response, and development in very-low-birth-weight infants fed banked human milk or enriched formula. I. Neonatal findings, J. Pediatr. **103**:95-104, 1983.

Umphenour, J.H.: Bacterial colonization in neonates with sibling visitation, JOGN Nurs. **9**:73-75, 1980.

VandenBerg, K.A.: Revising the traditional model: an individualized approach to developmental interventions in the intensive care nursery, Neonatal Network **3**(5):32-38, 1985.

Vohr, B.R., and Oh, W.: Growth and development in preterm infants small for gestational age, J. Pediatr. **103**:941-945, 1983.

Wagaman, M.J., and others: Improved oxygenation and lung compliance with prone positioning of neonates, J. Pediatr. **94**:787-791, 1979.

Westwood, M., and others: Growth and development of full-term nonasphyxiated small-for-gestational-age newborns: follow-up through adolescence, Pediatrics **71**:376-382, 1983.

Whitfield, J.M., and others: The application of hospice concepts to neonatal care, Am. J. Dis. Child **136**:421-424, 1982.

Wilson, R., and others: Age onset of necrotizing enterocolitis: an epidemiologic analysis, Pediatr. Res. **12**:82-84, 1982.

Wooten, B.: Death of an infant, Am. J. Maternal Child Nurs. **6**:257-260, 1981.

Wranesh, B.L.: The effect of sibling visitation on bacterial colonization rate in neonates, JOGN Nurs. **11**:211-213, 1982.

Yeh, T.F., and others: Furosemide prevents the renal side effects of indomethacin therapy in premature infants with patent ductus arteriosus, J. Pediatr. **101**:433-437, 1982.

BIBLIOGRAPHY
General

Beaton, J.F.: A systems model of premature birth: implications for neonatal intensive care, JOGN Nurs. **13**:173-177, 1984.

Bergman, I., and others: Cause of hearing loss in the high-risk premature infant, J. Pediatr. **106**:95-101, 1985.

Bethea, S.W.: Primary nursing in the infant special care unit, JOGN Nurs. **14**:202-208, 1985.

Cole, C.H.: Prevention of prematurity: can we do it in American Pediatrics **76**:310-312, 1985.

Curran, C.L., and Kachoyeanos, M.K.: The effects on neonates of two methods of chest physical therapy, Am. J. Maternal Child Nurs. **4**:309-313, 1979.

Dingle, R.E., and others: Continuous transcutaneous O_2 monitoring in the neonate, Am. J. Nurs. **80**:890-893, 1980.

Duara, S., and others: Neonatal screening with auditory brainstem responses: results of follow-up audiometry and risk factor evaluation, J. Pediatr. **108**:276-281, 1986.

Earley, A., and others: Blood pressure in the first 6 weeks of life, Arch. Dis. Child. **55**:755-757, 1980.

Ernst, J.A., and others: Osmolality of substances used in the intensive care nursery, Pediatrics **72**:347-352, 1983.

Fanaroff, A., and Martin, R.J.: Behrman's neonatal-perinatal medicine, ed. 3, St. Louis, 1983, The C.V. Mosby Co.

Finer, N.N.: Newer trends in continuous monitoring of critically ill infants and children, Pediatr. Clin. North Am. **27**:553-566, 1980.

Gatch, G.: Care of the infant requiring surgery, Crit. Care Update **6**(1):8-18, 1979.

Glasgow, A.M., and others: Hyperosmolality in small infants due to propylene glycol, Pediatrics **72**:353-355, 1983.

Gunn, S.: Critical care concepts related to maturational problems, Crit. Care Q. **4**(1):1-7, 1981.

Haddock, N.: Blood pressure monitoring in neonates, Am. J. Maternal Child Nurs. **5**:131-135, 1980.

Hyde, B.B., and McCown, D.E.: Classical conditioning in neonatal intensive care nurseries, Pediatr. Nurs. **12**:11-14, 1986.

Jensen, M., Benson, R.C., and Bobak, I.M.: Maternity care: the nurse and the family, ed. 2, St. Louis, 1981, The C.V. Mosby Co.

LaRossa, M.M., and Brown, J.V.: Foster grandmothers in the premature nursery, Am. J. Nurs. **82**:1834-1835, 1982.

Levin, D.L., Morriss, F.C., and Moore, G.C.: A practical guide to pediatric intensive care, ed. 2, St. Louis, 1984, The C.V. Mosby Co.

Lund, C., and others: Evaluation of a pectin-based barrier under tape to protect neonatal skin, JOGN Nurs. **15**:39-44, 1986.

MacDonald, H.M., and others: Neonatal asphyxia: I. Relationship of obstetric and neonatal complications to neonatal mortality in 38,405 consecutive deliveries, J. Pediatr. **96**:898-902, 1980.

Merenstein, G.B., and Gardner, S.L.: Handbook of neonatal intensive care, St. Louis, 1985, The C.V. Mosby Co.

Miller, H.X.A.: A model for studying the pathogenesis and incidence of low-birth-weight infants, Am. J. Dis. Child. **134**:323-327, 1983.

Mulligan, J.C., and others: Neonatal asphyxia: II. Neonatal mortality and long-term sequelae, J. Pediatr. **96**:903-907, 1980.

Penticuff, J.H.: Psychologic implications in high-risk pregnancy, Nurs. Clin. North Am. **17**:69-78, 1982.

Perez, R.H.: Protocols for perinatal nursing practice, St. Louis, 1981, The C.V. Mosby Co.

Sammons, W.A.H., and Lewis, J.M.: Premature babies: a different beginning, St. Louis, 1985, The C.V. Mosby Co.

Intensive Care Facilities

Bellig, L.L., and Tomasulo-Roborecky, F.: The expanded neonatal nursing role and the high-risk family, Neonatal Network 2:20-24, 1983.

Blackburn, S.: The neonatal ICU: a high-risk environment, Am. J. Nurs. 82:1708-1712, 1982.

Buxton, A.E.: Nosocomial infection in the intensive care unit, Crit. Care Update 9:32-37, 1982.

Chaze, B.A., and Ludington-Hoe, S.M.: Sensory stimulation in the ICU, Am. J. Nurs. 84:68-71, 1984.

Committee on Environmental Hazards, American Academy of Pediatrics: Infant radiant warmers, Pediatrics 61:113, 1978.

Donowitz, L.G.: Failure of the overgrown to prevent nosocomial infection in a pediatric intensive care unit, Pediatrics 77:35-38, 1986.

Endo, A.S.: Using computers in newborn intensive care settings, Am. J. Nurs. 81:1336-1337, 1981.

Harper, R.G., Little, G.A., and Sia, C.G.: The scope of nursing practice in level III neonatal intensive care units, Pediatrics 70:875-878, 1982.

Jacobson, G., and others: Handwashing: ring-wearing and number of microorganisms, Nurs. Res. 34:186-188, 1985.

Kavalhuna, R., and Malnight, M.: Meeting the needs of the extended care NICU patient, Neonatal Network 2:19-25, 1984.

Kennedy, J.: Evacuation of a neonatal unit, Can. Nurse 79:26-29, 1983.

Magnuson, P.E., and Pederson, N.L.: Regionalization of perinatal care: a cooperative community program, J. Maternal Child Nurs. 7:355-358, 1982.

Marshall, R.E., and Kasman, C.: Burnout in the neonatal intensive care unit, Pediatrics 65:1161-1165, 1980.

Murrow, M.E.: Managing stress in critical care nursing, Crit. Care Update 9(5):39-42, 1982.

Philip, A.G.S.: Noninvasive diagnostic techniques in newborn infants, Pediatr. Clin. North Am. 29:1275-1298, 1982.

Reedy, N.J., and others: Maternal fetal transport: a nurse team, JOGN Nurs. 13:91-100, 1984.

Ruegsegger, D.R., Jr.: Radiation exposure levels in an intensive care nursery, Pediatr. Nurs. 8:244-247, 1982.

Sande, D.: Preventing burnout in intensive care nurseries, Pediatr. Nurs. 9:364-366, 394, 1983.

Sandelowski, M.: Perinatal nursing: whose specialty is it anyway? J. Maternal Child Nurs. 8:317-322, 1983.

Seaman, C.K.: Monitoring the critically ill neonate, Crit. Care Q. 4(1):9-17, 1981.

Weeks, H.: Bioinstrumentation in the care of the neonate, Nurs. Clin. North Am. 13:597-609, 1978.

White, P.L., Fomufod, A.K., and Mamidanna, S.R.: Comparative accuracy of recent abbreviated methods of gestational age determination, Clin. Pediatr. 19:319-321, 1980.

Thermoregulation

Baumgart, S., and others: Effect of heat shielding on convective and evaporative heat losses and on radiant heat transfer in the premature infant, J. Pediatr. 99:948-956, 1981.

Bell, E.F., and others: The effects of thermal environment on heat balance and insensible water loss in low-birth-weight infants, J. Pediatr. 96:452-459, 1980.

Capobianco, J.A.: How to safeguard the infant against life-threatening heat loss, Nursing 80 10(5):64-67, 1980.

Engle, W.D., and others: Insensible water loss in the critically ill neonate, Am. J. Dis. Child. 135:516-520, 1981.

Kaplan, M., and Eidelman, A.I.: Improved prognosis in severely hypothermic newborn infants treated by rapid rewarming, J. Pediatr. 105:468-469, 1984.

Marks, K.H., and others: Thermal head wrap for infants, J. Pediatr. 107:956-959, 1985.

Mayfield, S.R., and others: Temperature measurement in term and preterm neonates, J. Pediatr. 104:271-275, 1984.

Ruchala, P.: The effect of wearing headcoverings on the axillary temperatures of infants, J. Maternal Child Nurs. 10:240, 1985.

Schiffman, R.F.: Temperature monitoring in the neonate: a comparison of axillary and rectal temperatures, Nurs. Res. 31:274-278, 1982.

Warshaw, J.B.: Intrauterine growth retardation: adaptation or pathology? Pediatrics 76:998-999, 1985.

Weldon, A.C., and Rutter, N.: The heat balance of small babies nursed in incubators and under radiant warmers, Early Hum. Dev. 6:131-135, 1982.

Yeh, T.F., and others: Oxygen consumption and insensible water loss in premature infants in single- versus double-walled incubators, J. Pediatr. 101:387-390, 1982.

Hydration

Arant, B.S.: Fluid therapy in the neonate—concepts in transition, J. Pediatr. 101:387-390, 1982.

Costarino, A., and Baumgart, S.: Modern fluid and electrolyte management of the critically ill premature infant, Pediatr. Clin. North Am. 33:153-178, 1986.

Lorenz, J.M., and others: Water balance in very low-birth-weight infants: relationship to water and sodium intake and effect on outcome, J. Pediatr. 101:423-432, 1982.

Oelerich, W.J., and Dombrowski, J.M.: Mini IV patients . . . maximum precautions, RN 44:43-47, 1981.

Feeding and Nutrition

Atkinson, S.A., Bryan, M.H., and Anderson, G.H.: Human milk feeding in premature infants: protein, fat, and carbohydrate balances in the first two weeks of life, J. Pediatr. 99:617-624, 1981.

Atkinson, S.A., and others: Macromineral balances in premature infants fed their own mothers' milk or formula, J. Pediatr. 102:99-106, 1983.

Chessex, P., and others: Influence of postnatal age, energy intake, and weight gain on energy metabolism in the very low-birth-weight infant, J. Pediatr. 99:761-766, 1981.

Churella, H.R., Bachhuber, W.L., and MacLean, W.C.: Survey: methods of feeding low-birth-weight infants, Pediatrics 76:243-249, 1985.

Cooke, R.J., and Nicholalds, G.: Nutrient retention in preterm infants fed standard formulas, J. Pediatr. 108:448-451, 1986.

Goldblum, R.M., and others: Rapid high-temperature treatment of human milk, J. Pediatr. 104:380-385, 1984.

Goldman, A.S., and others: Effects of prematurity on the immunologic system in human milk, J. Pediatr. 101:901-905, 1982.

Gross, S.J., and others: Nutritional composition of milk produced by mothers delivering preterm, J. Pediatr. 96:641, 1980.

Gross, S.J., and others: Elevated IgA concentration in milk produced by mothers delivered of preterm infants, J. Pediatr. 99:389-393, 1981.

Guilleminault, C., and Coons, S.: Apnea and bradycardia during feeding in infants weighting more than 2000 gm, J. Pediatr. 104:932-935, 1984.

Hay, W.W.: Nurtritional requirements and recommended feeding for premature infants, Pediatr. Basics 42:4-11, 1985.

Lebenthal, E., Lee, P.C., and Heitlinger, L.A.: Impact of development of the gastrointestinal tract on infant feeding, J. Pediatr. 102:1-9, 1983.

Measel, C.P.: A practical popular pacifier, Pediatr. Nurs. 8(3):199-200, 1982.

Meier, P., and Pugh, E.J.: Breast-feeding behavior of small preterm infants, J. Maternal Child Nurs. 10:396-401, 1985.

Moran, J.R., and others: Epidermal growth factor in human milk: daily production and diurnal variation during early lactation in mothers delivering at term and at premature gestation, J. Pediatr. 103:402-405, 1983.

Narayanan, I., Prakash, K., and Gujral, V.V.: The value of human milk in the prevention of infection in the high-risk low-birth-weight infant, J. Pediatr. 99:496-498, 1981.

Pereira, G.R., and Barbosa, M.M.: Controversies in neonatal nutrition, Pediatr. Clin. North Am. 33:65-89, 1986.

Putet, G., and others: Nutrient balance, energy utilization, and composition of weight gain in very-low-birth-weight infants fed pooled human milk or a preterm formula, J. Pediatr. 105:79-82, 1984.

Rönnholm, K.A.R., Sipilä, I., and Siimes, M.A.: Human milk protein supplementation for the prevention of hypoproteinemia without metabolic imbalance in breast milk-fed, very low-birth-weight infants, J. Pediatr. **101**:243-247, 1982.

Savilahti, E., Järvenpää, A., and Räihä, N.C.R.: Serum immunoglobulins in preterm infants: comparison of human milk and formula feeding, Pediatrics **72**:312-316, 1983.

Schanler, R.J., Garza, C., and Nichols, B.L.: Fortified mothers' milk for very low birth weight infants: results of growth and nutrient balance studies, J. Pediatr. **107**:437-445, 1985.

Schanler, R.J., Garza, C., and Smith, E.O.: Fortified mothers' milk for very low birth weight infants: results of macromineral balance studies, J. Pediatr. **107**:767-774, 1985.

Volz, V.R., Book, L.S., and Churella, H.R.: Growth and plasma amino acid concentrations in term infants fed either whey-predominant formula or human milk, J. Pediatr. **102**:27-31, 1983.

Developmental Correlates

Escalona, S.K.: Babies at double hazard: early development of infants at biologic and social risk, Pediatrics **70**:670-676, 1982.

Fria, T.J.: Assessment of hearing, Pediatr. Clin. North Am. **28**:757-775, 1981.

Gross, S.J., and Eckerman, C.O.: Normative early head growth in very-low-birth-weight infants, J. Pediatr. **103**:946-949, 1983.

Harvey, D., and others: Abilities of children who were small-for-gestational-age babies, Pediatrics **69**:296-300, 1982.

Hirata, T., and others: Survival and outcome of infants 501 to 750 gm: a six-year experience, J. Pediatr. **102**:741-748, 1983.

Manser, J.I.: Growth in the high-risk infant, Clin. Perinatol. **11**:19-22, 1984.

Rice, B.R., and Feeg, V.D.: First-year developmental outcomes for multiple-risk premature infants, Pediatr. Nurs. **11**(1):30-35, 1985.

Ross, G., Krauss, A.N., and Auld, P.A.M.: Growth achievement in low-birth-weight premature infants: relationship to neurobehavioral outcome at one year, J. Pediatr. **103**:105-108, 1983.

Shannon, D.A., and others: Hearing screening of high-risk newborns with brainstem auditory evoked potentials: a follow-up study, Pediatrics **73**:22-26, 1984.

Villar, J., and others: Heterogeneous growth and mental development of intrauterine growth-retarded infants during the first 3 years of life, Pediatrics **74**:783-791, 1984.

Vohr, B.R., and Coll, C.T.G.: Neurodevelopmental and school performance of very low-birth-weight infants: a seven-year longitudinal study, Pediatrics **76**:345-350, 1985.

Vohr, B.R., and Hack, M.: Developmental follow-up of low-birth-weight infants, Pediatr. Clin. North Am. **29**:1441-1454, 1982.

Infant Stimulation

Gorski, P.A., and others: Direct computer recording of premature infants and nursery care: distress following two interventions, Pediatrics **72**:198-202, 1983.

Gottfried, A.W., and Hodgman, J.E.: How intensive is newborn intensive care? An environmental analysis, Pediatrics **74**:292-294, 1984.

Leib, S.A., Benfield, D.G., and Guidubaldi, J.: Effects of early intervention and stimulation on the preterm infant, Pediatrics **64**:83-90, 1980.

Supportive Care

Campbell, L.A.: The very low birth weight infant: sensory experience and development, Top. Clin. Nurs. **6**(4):19-33, 1985.

Chitwood, L.: A lesson in living, Nursing 84 **14**(1):55-56, 1984.

Donnelly, G.F., and Conroy, N.: Parent-neonate communication in the care-giving system, Top. Clin. Nurs. **1**(3):1-9, 1979.

Eager, M., and Exoo, R.: Parents visiting parents for unequaled support, Am. J. Maternal Child Nurs. **5**:35-36, 1980.

Gennaro, S.: Maternal anxiety, problem-solving ability, and adaptation to the premature infant, Pediatr. Nurs. **11**:343-348, 1985.

Hawkins-Walsh, E.: Diminishing anxiety in parents of sick newborns, Am. J. Maternal Child Nurs. **5**:30-34, 1980.

Jacknik, M., Gumerman, S., and Parker, C.: Evaluating public health nursing follow-up of the high-risk infant, Am. J. Maternal Child Nurs. **8**:251-256, 1983.

Jenkins, R.L., and Tock, M.K.S.: Helping parents bond to their premature infant, Am. J. Maternal Child Nurs. **11**:32-34, 1986.

Johnson, S.H.: The premature infant. In Johnson, S.H., editor: Nursing assessment and strategies for the family at risk, ed. 2, Philadelphia, 1986, J.B. Lippincott Co.

Klaus, M., and Kennell, J.: Interventions in the premature nursery: impact on development, Pediatr. Clin. North Am. **29**:1263-1273, 1982.

Leib, S.A., Benfield, D.G., and Guidubaldi, J.: Effects of early intervention and stimulation on the preterm infant, Pediatrics 83-90, 1980.

Magyary, D.: Early social interactions: preterm infant-parent dyads, Issues Compr. Pediatr. Nurs. **7**:233-254, 1984.

Mahan, C.K.: Care of the family of the critically ill neonate, Crit. Care Q. **4**:89-103, 1981.

Mahan, C.K.: The family of the critically ill neonate, Crit. Care Update **10**(6):24-35, 1983.

Marino, B.L.: When nurses compete with parents, J. Assoc. Care Child. Health **8**:94-98, 1980.

Miles, M.S., and Carter, M.C.: Assessing parental stress in intensive care units, Am. J. Maternal Child Nurs. **8**:354-359, 1983.

Minde, K., and others: Self-help groups in a premature nursery—a controlled evaluation, J. Pediatr. **96**:933-940, 1980.

Paludetto, R., and others: Reactions of sixty parents allowed unrestricted contact with infants in a neonatal ICU, Early Hum. Dev. **5**(4):401-409, 1981.

Schraeder, B.D.: Attachment and parenting despite lengthy intensive care, Am. J. Maternal Child Nurs. **5**:37-41, 1980.

Stengel, T.J.: Infant behavior, maternal psychological reaction, and mother-infant interactional issues associated with the crises of prematurity: a selected review of the literature, Phys. Occup. Ther. Pediatr. **2**(2/3):3-25, 1982.

Thornton, J., Berry, J., and Dal Santo, J.: Neonatal intensive care: the nurse's role in supporting the family, Nurs. Clin. North Am. **19**:125-137, 1984.

Turley, M.A.: A meta-analysis of informing mothers concerning the sensory and perceptual capabilities of their infants: the effects on maternal-infant interaction, Matern. Child Nurs. J. **14**(3):183-198, 1985.

Varner, B., Ossenkop, D., and Lyon, J.: Prematures, too, need rooming-in and care-by-parent programs, Am. J. Maternal Child Nurs. **5**:431-432, 1980.

Yu, V., Jamieson, J., and Astbury, J.: Parents' reactions to unrestricted parental contact with infants in the intensive care nursery, Med. J. Aust. **1**:294-296, 1981.

Discharge and Follow-up

Cassady, G., and Setzer, E.: Impact of neonatal intensive care on quality of life. In Aladjem, S., Brown, A.K., and Sureau, C., editors: Clinical perinatology, ed. 2, St. Louis, 1980, The C.V. Mosby Co.

Desmond, M.M., and others: The very low birth weight infant after discharge from intensive care: anticipatory health care and developmental course, Curr. Probl. Pediatr. **10**(6):3-56, 1980.

Hayes, J.S.: Premature infant development; the relationship of neonatal stimulation, birth condition, and home environment, Pediatr. Nurs. **6**(6):33-36, 1980.

Sibling Visitation

Klaus, M.H., and Kennell, J.H.: Parent-infant bonding, ed. 2, St. Louis, 1982, The C.V. Mosby Co.

Kowba, M.D., and Schwirian, P.M.: Direct sibling contact and bacterial colonization in newborns, JOGN Nurs. **14**:412-417, 1985.

Maloney, M., and others: A prospective controlled study of scheduled sibling visits to a newborn intensive care unit, J. Am. Acad. Child Psychiatry **22**:565-568, 1983.

Schwab, F., and others: Sibling visiting in a neonatal intensive care unit, Pediatrics **71**:835-838, 1983.

Trause, M.A., and others: Separation for childbirth: the effect on the sibling, Child Psychiatry Hum. Dev. **12**:32-36, 1981.

Umphenour, J.E.: Bacterial colonization in neonates with sibling visiting, JOGN Nurs. **9**:73-75, 1980.

Wranesh, B.L.: The effect of sibling visitation on bacterial colonization rate in neonates, JOGN Nurs. **11**:211-213, 1982.

Neonatal Loss

Adolf, A., and Patt, R.: Neonatal death: the family is the patient, J. Fam. Pract. **10**:317-321, 1980.

Beckey, R.D., and others: Development of a perinatal grief checklist, JOGN Nurs. **14**:194-199, 1985.

Bryan, E.M.: When a twin dies, Nurs. Times **80**(10):24-26, 1984.

Estok, P. and Lehman, A.: Perinatal death: grief support for families, Birth **10**(1):17-25, 1983.

Forrest, G.C., and others: Support after perinatal death: a study of support and counseling after perinatal bereavement, Br. Med. J. **285**:1475-1479, 1982.

Furlong, R.M., and Hobbins, J.C.: Grief in the perinatal period, Obstet. Gynecol. **61**:497-500, 1983.

Glassman-Feibusch, B.: Extremely uncaring (Letters to the editor), Am. J. Maternal Child Nurs. **8**:442, 1983.

Kennell, J.H., and Klaus, M.H.: Caring for the parents of a stillborn or an infant who dies. In Klaus, M.H., and Kennell, J.H., editors: Parent-infant bonding, ed. 2, St. Louis, 1982, The C.V. Mosby Co.

Mahan, C.K.: Care of the family of the critically ill neonate, Crit. Care Q. **4**:89-103, 1981.

Mahan, C.K., Schreiner, R.L., and Green, M.P.: Bibliotherapy: a tool to help parents mourn their infant's death, Health Soc. Work **8**:126-132, 1983.

Mahan, C.K., and others: Neonatal death: parental evaluation of the NICU experience, Issues Compr. Pediatr. Nurs. **5**:279-292, 1981.

Mina, C.: A program for helping grieving parents, Am. J. Maternal Child Nurs. **10**:118-121, 1985.

Peppers, L., and Knapp, R.: Maternal reactions to involuntary fetal/infant death, Psychiatry **43**:155-159, 1980.

Peppers, L., and Knapp, R.: Motherhood and mourning—perinatal death, New York, 1980, Praeger Publishers.

Rappaport, C.: Helping parents when their newborn infants die: social work implications, Soc. Work Health Care **6**(3):57-67, 1981.

Sahu, S.: Coping with perinatal death, J. Reprod. Med. **26**:129-132, 1981.

Shwartz, D.: When the baby doesn't come home, Child. Today **13**:21-24, 1984.

Taylor, P., and Gideon, M.: Crisis counseling following the death of a baby, J. Reprod. Med. **24**:208-211, 1980.

Thomas, N., and Cordell, A.: The dying infant: aiding parents in the detachment process, Pediatr. Nurs. **9**:355-357, 1983.

Walker, L.J., and McDonough-Tuccillo, C.A.: Family support following infant death, Neonatal Network **2**:41-43, 1983.

Wilson, A.L., and others: The death of a newborn twin: an analysis of parental bereavement, Pediatrics **70**:587-591, 1982.

Work, R.B.: When we cannot cure, care, (Letters to the editor), Am. J. Maternal Child Nurs. **8**:111-112, 1983.

Apnea of Prematurity

Aranda, J.V., Grondin, D., and Sasyniuk, B.I.: Pharmacologic considerations in the therapy of neonatal apnea, Pediatr. Clin. North Am. **28**:113-133, 1981.

Banagale, R.C., and others: Apnea in newborn infants: approach to management, Resuscitation **11**(½):9-20, 1984.

Barrinton, K.J., and others: Physiologic effects of doxapram in idiopathic apnea of prematurity, J. Pediatr. **108**:125-129, 1986.

Behrman, R.E.: Preventing low birth weight: a pediatric perspective, J. Pediatr. **107**:842-854, 1985.

Brouard, C., and others: Comparative efficacy of theophylline and caffeine in the treatment of idiopathic apnea in premature infants, Am. J. Dis. Child. **139**:698-701, 1985.

Dulock, H.L.: Monitoring apnea in premature newborns: how effective are conventional techniques? Focus Crit. Care **10**(6):30-32, 1983.

Mathew, O.P., Roberts, J.L., and Thach, B.T.: Pharyngeal airway obstruction in preterm infants during mixed and obstructive apnea, J. Pediatr. **100**:964-968, 1982.

Miller, M.J., and others: Continuous positive airway pressure selectively reduces obstructive apnea in preterm infants, J. Pediatr. **106**:91, 1985.

Rigatto, H.: Apnea, Pediatr. Clin. North Am. **29**:1105-1116, 1982.

Respiratory Distress Syndrome

Avery, M.E.: The argument for prenatal administration of dexamethasone to prevent respiratory distress syndrome, J. Pediatr. **104**:240, 1984.

Boros, S.J., and others: Using conventional infant ventilators at unconventional rates, Pediatrics **74**:487-492, 1984.

Boynton, B.R., and others: Combined high-frequency oscillatory ventilation and intermittent mandatory ventilation in critically ill neonates, J. Pediatr. **105**:297-300, 1984.

Cassady, G.: Transcutaneous monitoring in the newborn infant, J. Pediatr. **103**:837-848, 1983.

Cohen, M.A.: Transcutaneous oxygen monitoring for sick neonates, Am. J. Maternal Child Nurs. **9**:324-330, 1984.

Collaborative Group on Antenatal Steroid Therapy: Effects of antenatal dexamethasone administration in the infant: long-term follow-up, J. Pediatr. **104**:259-267, 1984.

Crone, R.K., and Favorito, J.: The effects of pancuronium bromide on infants with hyaline membrane disease, J. Pediatr. **97**:991-993, 1980.

Curet, L., and others: Maternal smoking and respiratory distress syndrome, Am. J. Obstet. Gynecol. **147**:446-450, 1983.

Doyle, L.W., and others: Effects of antenatal steroid therapy on mortality and morbidity in very low birth weight infants, J. Pediatr. **108**:287-292, 1986.

Engle, W.D., and others: Diuresis and respiratory distress syndrome: physiologic mechanisms and therapeutic implications, J. Pediatr. **102**:912-917, 1983.

Enhorning, G., and others: Prevention of neonatal respiratory distress syndrome by tracheal instillation of surfactant: a randomized clinical trial, Pediatrics **76**:145-153, 1985.

Erenberg, A., and Nowak, A.J.: Palatal groove formation in neonates with orotracheal tubes, Am. J. Dis. Child. **134**:974, 1984.

Garland, J.S., and others: Increased risk of gastrointestinal perforations in neonates mechanically ventilated with either face mask or nasal prongs, Pediatrics **76**:406-410, 1985.

Goodwin, S.R., Graves, S.A., and Haberkern, C.M.: Aspiration in intubated premature infants, Pediatrics **75**:85-88, 1985.

Gruden, M.: High-frequency ventilation: an overview, Crit. Care Nurs. **5**:36-40, 1985.

Have ECMO, will travel, Am. J. Nurs. **86**:117, 1986.

Heldt, G.P., and others: Exercise performance of the survivors of hyaline membrane disease, J. Pediatr. **96**:995-999, 1980.

Kaplow, R., and Fromme, L.R.: Nursing care plan for the patient receiving high-frequency jet ventilation, Crit. Care Nurs. **5**:25-27, 1985.

Kirkpatrick, B.V., and others: Use of extracorporeal membrane oxygenation for respiratory failure in term infants, Pediatrics **72**:872-876, 1983.

Langman, C.B., and others: The diuretic phase of respiratory distress syndrome and its relationship to oxygenation, J. Pediatr. **98**:462-466, 1981.

Mason, T.N.: A hand ventilation technique for neonates, Am. J. Maternal Child Nurs. **7:**366-369, 1982.

McCann, E.M., and others: Controlled trial of furosemide therapy in infants with chronic lung disease, J. Pediatr. **106:**957-960, 1985.

McFadden, R.: Decreasing respiratory compromise during infant suctioning, Am. J. Nurs. **81:**2158-2161, 1981.

McMillan, D.D., and others: Benefits of orotracheal and nasotracheal intubation in neonates requiring ventilatory assistance, Pediatrics **77:**39-44, 1986.

Oellrich, R.G.: Pneumothorax, chest tubes, and the neonate, Am. J. Maternal Child Nurs. **10:**29-35, 1985.

Peevy, K.J., and Hall, M.W.: Transcutaneous oxygen monitoring: economic impact on neonatal care, Pediatrics **75:**1065-1067, 1985.

Phelps, D.L.: Neonatal oxygen toxicity—is it preventable? Pediatr. Clin. North Am. **29:**1233-1240, 1982.

Reid, T.J.: Newborn cyanosis, Am. J. Nurs. **83:**1230-1234, 1983.

Runkle, B., and Bancalari, E.: Acute cardiopulmonary effects of pancuronium bromide in mechanically ventilated newborn infants, J. Pediatr. **104:**614-617, 1984.

Schreiner, R.L., and others: Improved survival of ventilated neonates with modern intensive care, Pediatrics **66:**985-988, 1980.

Special conference report: High frequency ventilation for immature infants, Pediatrics **71:**280-287, 1983.

Meconium Aspiration

Levin, D.L.: Meconium inhalation syndrome. In Levin, D.L., Morriss, F.C., and Moore, G.C., editors: A practical guide to pediatric intensive care, St. Louis, 1984, The C.V. Mosby Co.

Mammel, M.D., and others: Comparison of high-frequency jet ventilation and conventional mechanical ventilation in a meconium aspiration model, J. Pediatr. **103:**630-634, 1983.

Murphy, J.D., Vawter, G.F., and Reid, L.M.: Pulmonary vascular disease in fetal meconium aspiration, J. Pediatr. **104:**785-789, 1984.

Bronchopulmonary Dysplasia

Abman, S.H., Accurso, F.J., and Koops, B.L.: Experience with home oxygen in the management of infants with bronchopulmonary dysplasia, Clin. Pediatr. **23:**471-474, 1984.

Avery, G.B., and others: Controlled trial of dexamethasone in respirator-dependent infants with bronchopulmonary dysplasia, Pediatrics **75:**106-107, 1985.

Kao, L.C., and others: Effect of oral diuretics on pulmonary mechanics in infants with chronic bronchopulmonary dysplasia: results of a double-blind crossover sequential trial, Pediatrics **74:**37-40, 1984.

Markestad, T., and Fitzhardinge, P.M.: Growth and development in children recovering from bronchopulmonary dysplasia, J. Pediatr. **98:**597-602, 1981.

Schick, J.B., and Goetzman, B.W.: Chronic lung disease of prematurity, Pediatrics **76:**652, 1985.

Workshop on bronchopulmonary dysplasia, J. Pediatr., **85:**815-920, 1979.

Sepsis

Starr, S.E.: Antimicrobial therapy of bacterial sepsis in the newborn infant, J. Pediatr. **106:**1043-1048, 1985.

Stegagno, M., and others: Immunologic follow-up of infants treated with granulocyte transfusion for neonatal sepsis, Pediatrics **76:**508-511, 1985.

Strodtbeck, F.: Critical care concepts related to neonatal septicemia and septic shock, Crit. Care. Q. **4**(1):71-77, 1981.

Necrotizing Enterocolitis

Brown, E.G., and Sweet, A.Y.: Neonatal necrotizing enterocolitis, Pediatr. Clin. North Am. **29:**1149-1170, 1982.

Dammert, W.: Necrotizing enterocolitis. In Levin, D.L., Morriss, F.G., and Moore, G.C., editors: A practical guide for pediatric intensive care, ed. 2, St. Louis, 1984, The C.V. Mosby Co.

Gaines, R.P., and others: The role of host factors in an outbreak of necrotizing enterocolitis, Am. J. Dis. Child. **138:**1118-1120, 1984.

Kliegman, R.M., and Fanaroff, A.A.: Neonatal necrotizing enterocolitis: a 9-year experience: I. Epidemiology and uncommon observations, Am. J. Dis. Child. **135:**603-607, 1981.

Kliegman, R.M., and Fanaroff, A.A.: Neonatal necrotizing enterocolitis: a 9-year experience: II. Outcome assessment, Am. J. Dis. Child. **135:**608-611, 1981.

Kliegman, R.M., and others: Epidemiologic study of necrotizing enterocolitis among low-birth-weight infants, J. Pediatr. **100:**440-444, 1982.

Plapp, P.R.: Nursing implications in the early recognition of necrotizing enterocolitis, Issues Compr. Pediatr. Nurs. **4**(2):77-81, 1980.

Schullinger, J.N., and others: Neonatal necrotizing enterocolitis: survival, management, and complications: a 25-year study, Am. J. Dis. Child. **135:**612-614, 1981.

Stoll, B.J., and others: Epidemiology of necrotizing enterocolitis: a case control study, J. Pediatr. **96:**447-451, 1980.

Walsh, M., and Kliegman, R.M.: Necrotizing enterocolitis: treatment based on staging criteria, Pediatr. Clin. North Am. **33:**179-201, 1986.

Whiteman, L., Wuethrick, M., and Egan, E.: Infants who survive necrotizing enterocolitis, Matern. Child. Nurs. J. **14**(3):123-134, 1985.

Patent Ductus Arteriosus

Bhat, R., and others: Patent ductus arteriosis: recent advances in diagnosis and management, Pediatr. Clin. North Am. **29:**1117-1136, 1982.

Clyman, R.I., and Heymann, M.A.: Pharmacology of the ductus arteriosus, Pediatr. Clin. North Am. **28:**77-94, 1981.

Dooley, K.J.: Management of the premature infant with a patent ductus arteriosus, Pediatr. Clin. North Am. **31:**1159-1174, 1984.

Dudell, G.G., and Gersony, W.M.: Patent ductus arteriosus in neonates with severe respiratory disease, J. Pediatr. **104:**915-919, 1984.

Foster, S.D.: Indomethacin: pharmacologic closure of the ductus arteriosus, Am. J. Matern. Child Nurs. **7:**171, 1982.

Gersony, W.M., and others: Effects on indomethacin in premature infants with patent ductus arteriosus: results of a national collaborative study, J. Pediatr. **102:**895-906, 1983.

Merritt, T.A., and others: Early closure of the patent ductus arteriosus in very low-birth-weight infants: a controlled trial, J. Pediatr. **99:**281-286, 1981.

Persistent Pulmonary Hypertension

Hageman, J., Adams, A., and Gardner, T.: Persistent pulmonary hypertension of the newborn, Am. J. Dis. Child. **138:**627-695, 1984.

Henry, G.W.: Noninvasive assessment of PPHN, Clin. Perinatol. **2:**627-639, 1984.

Sell, E., and others: Persistent fetal circulation—neurodevelopment outcome, Am. J. Dis. Child. **139:**25-28, 1985.

Anemia of Prematurity

Black, V.D., and Lubchenco, L.O.: Neonatal polycythemia and hyperviscosity, Pediatr. Clin. North Am. **29:**1137-1148, 1982.

Brown, M.S., and others: Decreased response of plasma immunoreactive erythropoietin to "available oxygen" in anemia of prematurity, J. Pediatr. **105:**793-797, 1984.

Dallman, P.R.: Erythropoietin and the anemia of prematurity, J. Pediatr. **105:**756-757, 1984.

Siimes, M.A., and Järvenpää, A.: Prevention of anemia and iron deficiency in very low-birth-weight infants, J. Pediatr. **101:**277-280, 1982.

Stockman, J.A.: Anemia of prematurity, Pediatr. Clin. North Am. **33:**111-128, 1986.

Retinopathy of Prematurity

Lucey, J.F., and Dangman, B.: A reexamination of the role of oxygen in retrolental fibroplasia, Pediatrics **73:**82-96, 1984.

Purohit, D.M., and others: Risk factors for retrolental fibroplasia: experience with 3,025 premature infants, Pediatrics **76:**339-344, 1985.

Shohat, M., and others: Retinopathy of prematurity: incidence and risk factors, Pediatrics **72:**159-162, 1983.

Neurologic Disturbances

Allan, W.C., and Volpe, J.J.: Periventricular-intraventricular hemorrhage, Pediatr. Clin. North Am. **33:**47-63, 1986.

Clark, C.E., and others: Risk factor analysis of intraventricular hemorrhage in low-birth-weight infants, J. Pediatr. **99:**625-628, 1981.

Kuban, K., and Teele, R.L.: Rationale for grading intracranial hemorrhage in premature infants, Pediatrics **74:**358-363, 1984.

MacDonald, H.M., and others: Neonatal asphyxia: I. Relationship of obstetric and neonatal complications to neonatal mortality in 38,405 consecutive deliveries, J. Pediatr. **96:**898-902, 1980.

Mulligan, J.C., and others: Neonatal asphyxia: II. Neonatal mortality and long-term sequelae, J. Pediatr. **96:**903-907, 1980.

Papile, L., Munsick-Bruno, G., and Schaefer, A.: Relationship of cerebral intraventricular hemorrhage and early childhood neurologic handicaps, J. Pediatr. **103:**273-277, 1983.

Perlman, J.M., and Volpe, J.J.: Episodes of apnea and bradycardia in the preterm newborn: impact on cerebral circulation, Pediatrics **76:**333-338, 1985.

Tarby, T.J., and Volpe, J.J.: Intraventricular hemorrhage in the premature infant, Pediatr. Clin. North Am. **29:**1077-1104, 1982.

Neonatal Seizures

Ellison, P.H., Largent, J.A., and Bahr, J.P.: A scoring system to predict outcome following neonatal seizures, J. Pediatr. **99:**455-459, 1981.

Painter, M.J., Bergman, I., and Crumrine, P.: Neonatal seizures, Pediatr. Clin. North Am. **33:**91-109, 1986.

Perlman, J.M., and Volpe, J.J.: Seizures in the preterm infant: effect on cerebral blood flow velocity, intracranial pressure, and arterial blood pressure, J. Pediatr. **102:**288-293, 1983.

Torrence, C.: Neonatal seizures: Part I. A developmental and clinical understanding, Neonat. Network **4**(8)9-15, 1985.

Infants of Diabetic Mothers

Burns, E.M.: Diabetes mellitus and pregnancy, Nurs. Clin. N. Am. **18:**673-685, 1983.

Cowett, R.M., and Schwartz, R.: The infant of the diabetic mother, Pediatr. Clin. North Am. **29:**1213-1231, 1982.

Perlman, R.H.: The infant of the diabetic mother: pathophysiology and management, Primary Care **10:**751-760, 1983.

Riblett, B.: Insuring a safe pregnancy for your diabetic patient, RN **46**(2):50-56, 1983.

Drug-Addicted Infants

Committee on Drugs, Neonatal drug withdrawal, Pediatrics **102:**895-902, 1983.

Green, M., and Suffett, F.: The neonatal narcotic withdrawal index: a device for the improvement of care in the abstinence syndrome, Am. J. Drug Alcohol Abuse **8:**203-208, 1981.

Householder, J., and others: Infants born to narcotic-addicted mothers, Psychol. Bull. **92:**383-391, 1980.

Lemons, P.M.: Prenatal addiction: a dual tragedy, Crit. Care Q. **4**(1):79-88, 1981.

Lemons, P.K.M.: Victims of addiction. Crit. Care Update **10**(5):12-17, 1983.

Merker, L., Higgins, P., and Kinnard, E.: Assessing narcotic addiction in neonates, Pediatr. Nurs. **11:**177-181, 1985.

Sweet, A.Y.: Narcotic withdrawal syndrome in the newborn, Pediatr. Rev. **3:**285-291, 1982.

Infant of Smoking Mother

Berman, S.M., Hogue, C.J.R., and Marks, J.S.: Maternal cigarette smoking: effect on infant birth weight (Letter), JAMA **253:**911-915, 1984.

Bureau, M.A., and others: Maternal cigarette smoking and fetal oxygen transport: a study of P50, 2,3-diphosphoglycerate, total hemoglobin, hematocrit, and type F hemoglobin in fetal blood, Pediatrics **72:**22-26, 1983.

Etzel, R.A., and others: Urine cotinine excretion in neonates exposed to tobacco smoke products in utero, J. Pediatr. **107:**146-148, 1985.

Streissguth, A.P., Barr, H.M., and Martin, D.C.: Effects of maternal alcohol, nicotine and caffeine use during pregnancy on infant development at eight months, Alcoholism **4:**152-157, 1980.

Wilcox, A.J.: Intrauterine growth retardation: beyond birth weight criteria, Early Hum. Dev. **8:**189-193, 1983.

Chapter 11

Conditions Caused by Problems in Physical Development

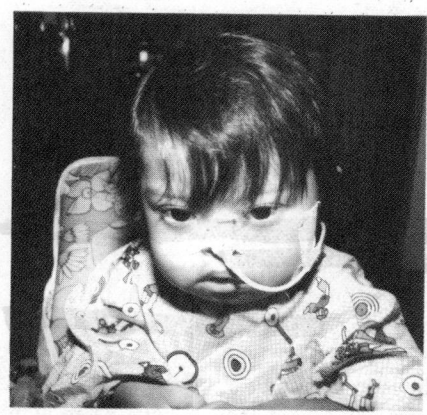

Congenital malformations constitute a large percentage of the health problems of infants and children, and although many severe disorders of childhood can be either prevented or effectively treated, very little progress has been achieved in prevention of congenital defects. It is calculated that approximately one third of hospitalized children suffer from a congenital abnormality or its sequelae. Not all congenital defects are considered to be malformations—for example, inborn errors of metabolism and mental retardation. However, this chapter is primarily concerned with structural abnormalities, most of which are apparent at birth, and with the impact on the family of the birth of a child with a physical defect.

BIRTH OF A CHILD WITH A PHYSICAL DEFECT

The parents are the most significant influences in the life of the child, and the initial parent-infant attachment is the relationship on which future interactions are based. The birth of any child is considered by some to constitute a crisis situation, but when the newborn suffers from a physical or mental defect, the parents' need for understanding and supportive care from health professionals is magnified. The manner in which nurses and other health personnel work with the parents immediately after the birth profoundly influences the situation for all persons concerned.

Parental Responses

Part of the preparation for childbirth involves fantasies and images of the expected infant. Normally every parent wishes for a perfect child, but at the same time they fear that the infant will be abnormal. This fear is often expressed by the expectant parents when they state that their concern is not whether the child is to be a girl or a boy, just that the infant is healthy. One of the first things the mother wishes confirmed at the time of birth is: "Is my baby all right?" In many instances there is some discrepancy between the parents' idealized child and the infant the mother delivers, as, for example, the birth of a boy when they had hoped for a girl. Resolution of this discrepancy is a developmental task of parenthood and is essential to the establishment of a healthy parent-child relationship. If this discrepancy is too great, as with the birth of an infant with a gross defect, or when the wishes of the parents are unrealistic, the resulting emotional stress may be overwhelming.

The more severe the defect, the greater the impact of the experience, especially for the mother. The birth of a child with a physical defect abruptly ends the psychologic attachment the mother has formed during pregnancy with the idealized child. She and the father must now deal with loss of this wished-for, healthy child while they face meeting the demands of the abnormal child for care and affection. The birth of an infant with a defect evokes the same psychologic reaction as the death of a child. The need for the parents to grieve for the loss of the expected child while adapting to the care of the child with a disability places overwhelming demands on them at a time when their own psychologic and physiologic resources have been depleted by the birth experience (Solnit and Stark, 1963). The impact of this new and unexpected burden inhibits the accomplishment of the grief work that normally follows a loss.

The grief reaction experienced by parents at the birth of a child with a physical disability is the same as the response that follows the loss of any valued or significant object. The parents experience shock, frustration, and anger at what has happened to them, and they ask themselves, "Why? Why me?" Parents may feel shame and embarrassment, often with feelings of personal failure and guilt. Frequently the mother believes that she might have caused harm to the unborn child, and she may associate the condition with wrongdoing or evil thoughts, especially if the pregnancy was unwanted initially. She may believe the defect to be the result of passive or active attempts to terminate the pregnancy, such as deliberate attempts to induce abortion or failure to obtain prenatal care or comply with the physician's instructions.

There is a phase of overwhelming *shock*, accompanied by weeping and feelings of helplessness. To deal with stress and anxiety, parents use defense mechanisms that have provided protection in their past. A very common response is *disbelief* and *denial*, which may be short-lived or may last for many months. They do not appear to "hear" what is told to them about their child, and they behave as though nothing is wrong with the child. However, denial during the shock phase of the grief process can serve as a constructive means for parents to deal with the sudden and profound impact of the initial stress until they are better able to cope with the situation.

When parents are unable to face the reality of the infant's condition, they *withdraw* from the situation either physically or emotionally. They frequently become incapacitated and unable to function in their usual manner. They avoid interpersonal contacts. Unable to face relatives and friends for fear of the reactions they may encounter, parents choose the protection of isolation. They feel as though they are alone in a world all their own. Avoidance behaviors on the part of others, including health workers, contribute to this withdrawal and compound the feelings of loneliness that are so common in parents of an abnormal infant.

Parents often extend this avoidance behavior to include the infant. They seem to be unable to face the infant and do not visit the child in the nursery or the pediatric unit. Sometimes it takes time for the parents to master their own feelings before they are able to deal constructively with the situation. A more subtle form of isolation is seen in parents who are very objective in their behavior toward the infant and his defect. They are intellectually concerned with their infant's medical care but display no emotional involvement. Their attention is focused on the abnormality, not on the infant.

Parental reactions may be quite varied, including guilt, anger, anxiety, and sadness, which often extend for years

Questions and Controversies

Are there times or circumstances under which certain infants should be denied medical care?

One of the most painful dilemmas faced by families and health professionals is the decision regarding the care of children with severe defects, including decisions for life or death. In most cases there is no problem; infants are treated and deformities corrected as early as possible. The ethical, moral, and legal dilemmas are encountered when decisions must be made for children with lethal or borderline prognoses. Most parents and professionals resist keeping children alive who have universally fatal disorders, such as anencephaly or trisomy 13. The usual management is sedation and skilled nursing and parental care. No heroic measures are attempted. With infants who are borderline—that is, those for whom the quality of life may be questionable—the problem becomes more complex. These are infants with conditions such as severe prematurity, brain damage, and severe spina bifida.

As knowledge and technology continue to advance, more and more high-risk and borderline children are surviving neonatal hazards. With the increased survival rate the incidence of severe developmental defects and chronic sequelae also increases (Britton, Fitzhardinge, and Ashby, 1981; Christianson and others, 1981). The prevailing philosophy is to treat these children. However, the reasons are varied: it is morally right; to treat is best because the outcome is uncertain; it is hospital or nursery policy; it is a way to learn about treatment; to allow a child to die sets a poor example for staff; and it avoids legal entanglements. Most of the reasons have little to do with the interests of the child (Duff, 1981). The wisdom of these rescue efforts is being questioned. Likewise, the question has arisen regarding who has the right to deny treatment for severely afflicted children. All too often health professionals, oriented toward aggressive treatment and saving lives, impose their values on families who are aware of the long-term implications but who are made to feel guilty if they resist therapeutic efforts on the child's behalf. Many times salvaging the lethally impaired or marginally viable child places such an emotional and financial burden on the family that both the child and the family suffer.

The Committee on Bioethics of the American Academy of Pediatrics (1983) has stated that "while the needs and interests of parents, as well as the larger society, are proper concerns . . . (the) primary moral and legal obligation is to the child-patient. Withholding or withdrawing life-sustaining treatment is justified only if such a course serves the interests of the patient." The Academy (1984) has provided some principles on which care and treatment of disabled infants can be based. Both the Academy and the President's Commission for the Study of Ethical Problems in Medicine and Biomedical and Behavioral Research (1983) recommend establishment of infant bioethics committees to aid parents and treating physicians in making ethical decisions.

Ideally decisions regarding care of a child who is severely disabled should be shared by both family and health professionals. Parents need to know the long-term personal and social implications of the decision, and, even when greatly stressed, the parents are capable of sharing these difficult decisions (Benfield, Lieb, and Vollman, 1978). When families are forced into a position of helplessness and professionals are unable to assume the responsibility, the ultimate decision is turned over to a committee or to the courts. It is becoming increasingly important for families of children who are severely disabled

to "have a major voice in deciding what constitutes practical, sensible help and minimal tyranny" (Duff, 1981).

The controversy will not be resolved to the satisfaction of all, and each situation must be determined by the principal persons involved. Unfortunately, the person central to the issues (the child) is unable to have a voice in the matter. Whether later repercussions, such as lawsuits related to right to a life of questionable quality, become a reality, is only hinted at presently. The debate will undoubtedly continue for some time. However, "physicians, parents, hospital bioethical review committees, and society as a whole must deal realistically, and compassionately, with the complex issues at hand to provide the proper treatment for affected infants (Strain, 1983)."

and which depend to a large extent on the type and severity of the defect. A gross, visible anomaly, especially one involving the face, elicits a more intense emotional response than one that is less apparent, such as a heart defect. The extent of the impairment cannot be used as a criterion to determine the degree of parental depressive reactions. Because of their limited contact with congenital defects, parents' perception of the abnormality and its implications may be distorted, and much depends on previous feelings they may have experienced with a similar abnormality. Therefore their reactions may seem out of proportion to the actual extent and severity of the impairment as viewed by health professionals.

Nursing Considerations

The attitudes and behaviors of nurses and other health personnel at the birth of a child with a defect significantly influence the effect that the situation has on the parents. During this time parents are particularly sensitive and responsive to the behaviors of those with whom they are in contact. Therefore the reactions of health professionals toward the infant and the parents provide cues to the parents that can affect their feelings toward the infant and themselves. Parents are the persons who exert the greatest influence on the growth and development of the child, and the initial relationship with the child significantly affects the subsequent course of interaction.

Initial contact. The first indication that all is not well occurs at the time of delivery. The atmosphere of happy anticipation suddenly changes to one laden with anxiety. Even when the mother is unable to see the infant, she may sense with terrifying awareness the heightened and prolonged tension in the room, which conveys to her that something is seriously wrong. Personnel, unprepared for this disturbing experience, find it difficult to cope with their own feelings and react with frustration and resentment toward a situation that they are powerless to change. As a result they may forget about or retreat from the parents, who at this moment are suffering the most.

Most physicians believe that it is their responsibility to inform the parents of a congenital anomaly. At the time of delivery, unless a pediatrician is in attendance, there is a

Questions and Controversies

Should the government, representing society, determine the type and extent of care for disabled infants?

The "Baby Doe" legislation and subsequent controversies have engendered considerable reaction from health professionals and the public. The controversy arose from the case of an infant born with Down syndrome and severe congenital anomaly. The infant was denied definitive treatment and died a short time after birth. The resultant complaints of pro-life groups and others prompted the Department of Health and Human Services to add a provision to the Child Abuse Prevention and Treatment Act that gives federal investigators power to intervene directly in decisions about treatment of infants who are severely disabled. The wording of the legislation continues to be modified, but the issues still generate considerable debate, regulatory action and reaction, and medical, legal, and social debate.

delay while the physician is involved with the mother's care. During this period the mother, unable to see her child and feeling the tense atmosphere, will believe either that the child is normal but that others do not share her enthusiasm or that the child is so terrible that the professional people in the room are unable to talk about it. A nurse, the person who is most likely to be free to support the mother and who is familiar with most common congenital anomalies, can make truthful statements about the defect.

The manner in which nurses present the infant to the parents may well set the tone for the early parent-child relationship. It is probably best to explain briefly in simple language what the defect is and something concerning the prognosis before the infant is shown to them, when they are more apt to "hear" what is said. Parents attach a great deal of meaning to the behavior of others during this critical period and will watch the facial expressions of others closely for signs of revulsion or rejection. Presenting the infant as something precious, although incomplete, and emphasizing the well-formed aspects of the infant's body provide some reassurance to parents in this crisis period. It is important to allow time and opportunity for the parents to express their initial response to the situation. They need to be encouraged to ask questions and to receive honest, straightforward answers without undue optimism or pessimism.

Family support. Parents must be allowed ample time to grieve for the loss of the expected child before they are able to form an emotional attachment to the child they have. However, as long as the disabled child remains a living reminder of their loss, parents may never be able to totally resolve their grief. It is a nursing responsibility to help parents with their grief work and to facilitate the formation of a satisfactory adjustment to the child with a defect. They need help to see their infant as a *person,* support in coping with their situation, and guidance in physical care of the child.

Nurses who understand the grief response will be prepared to support the parents through this necessary process.

This is particularly important with the birth of a child with a defect because the parents cannot begin to invest any feeling for the child until they are able to talk about and work through their feelings of disappointment, resentment, guilt, and helplessness. Parents need to talk, and the supportive nurse is one who creates and maintains an atmosphere that encourages expression of feelings. Open expression is difficult for many people, and the parent(s) may hesitate to display intense feelings. Containing those feelings burns a great deal of energy that would be better used later on to develop a relationship with the infant. Nurses, therefore, need to listen closely for cues that indicate areas of discomfort or readiness to talk.

Parents may not be ready to talk about their feelings during the first few days following the birth. Their dream has vanished and when others avoid them it is often interpreted as another abandonment. Staying near and available tells them that they are not alone and that someone cares about them and their feelings. What is said to them is also important. Cliches such as "You will be able to have more children" or "It could be a lot worse" are not a comfort to the parents. Such behavior implies that this infant is not important, and this behavior may lose the parents' trust (Paparella, 1982).

It is sometimes useful to initiate a discussion about matters that were of concern to others in a similar situation and help the parents to know that their feelings are natural. Parents need to be allowed silence and solitude if this is their wish. The parents are likely to be angry and will often direct this anger at any one at hand—doctors, nurses, friends, and families who have normal children. Serving as a nonjudgmental target for their frustrations helps parents to relieve some of their distress. Nurses must be prepared to accept any or all of the parental reactions and defenses—anger, hostility, rejection, dependency—without anger and without withdrawing from the situation. If nurses make themselves available to the parents for support, they can often find nonthreatening ways to help, comfort, and support. Most importantly, nurses need to promote communication and understanding within the family and help strengthen family interpersonal relationships. Family disintegration is a sequel that is all too common to the birth of a child with a physical disability.

Care of the infant. Parents are very uneasy about handling their infant and require support and encouragement in their caregiving tasks. A longer period of dependency is needed by these parents to regroup their resources for coping. Although they should not feel forced to care for the infant until they are ready for the responsibility, they can be given opportunities to assume care of the infant as soon as possible to help them deal with the reality of the infant's condition. Parent's responses are highly individual and must be evaluated on this premise. However, all parents need sympathetic, patient, and understanding help to gain feelings of adequacy in the care of their child and to facilitate development of a positive relationship with the infant later on. As anxiety and the intensity of emotional responses abate, parents begin to feel more comfortable with the infant and more confidence in their ability to provide needed care.

Supplying information. Parents need to have accurate, up-to-date information given to them early and in language they can understand. Since they do not hear all that is said the first time it is told to them, they want careful explanations about the child's defect, the treatments outlined, and what will be expected of them. Parents often misinterpret information and therefore require repeated explanations. Often the nurse's responsibility is to explain, interpret, and clarify information that has been given by the physician and to answer questions. Following basic concepts of interviewing, the nurse determines what the parents know and proceeds from that point. One cannot assume that the parents' failure to ask questions means they understand. Most parents have little or no knowledge of basic anatomy or physiology; therefore, pictures and other visual aids can be used effectively to explain both normal and deviant structures.

Teaching the parents to provide the special care that is frequently required for an infant with a physical defect is an important nursing responsibility. Special feeding, holding, and positioning techniques need to be explained and demonstrated. Anticipatory guidance regarding problems that are peculiar to each abnormality reduces apprehension and stimulates the parents to institute preventive measures and to make alert observations.

Numerous agencies and organizations offer services to families of children with congenital defects. Some provide services for a variety of defects; others are devoted to specific disorders. They help families with ongoing problems and with anticipating problems they will encounter in raising a child with a defect, including financial burdens. All have unique and specialized services designed to help support the family and aid parents in their problem solving. Among those that include most types of defects and diseases are the **National Easter Seal Society for Crippled Children and Adults,** * the **March of Dimes–Birth Defects Foundation,** † and the **Association of Birth Defects in Children,** ‡ most of which have branches in all major cities and communities. The state **Crippled Children's Services** of the Public Health System is also a prime source of assistance.

Malformations of the Central Nervous System

Defects of the central nervous system are usually the result of embryologic developmental failures. Some can be attributed to genetic factors; others may be a result of postnatal infections. However, in most cases the etiology is obscure.

---

*2023 West Ogden Ave., Chicago, IL 60612.
†1275 Mamaroneck Ave., White Plains, NY 10605.
‡3526 Emerywood Lane, Orlando, FL 32806.

The defects that will be discussed are abnormalities of neural tube closure and hydrocephalus, characterized by an increase of free fluid in the cranial cavity.

DEFECTS OF NEURAL TUBE CLOSURE

Abnormalities that are derived from the embryonic neural tube (neural tube defects, or NTD) constitute the largest group of congenital anomalies that is consistent with multifactorial inheritance. Normally the spinal cord and cauda equina are encased in a protective sheath of bone and meninges (Fig. 11-1, *A*). Failure of neural tube closure produces defects of varying degrees. They may involve the entire length of the neural tube or may be restricted to a small area only. Terms applied to these abnormalities are as follows:

myelodysplasia All-inclusive term that refers to defective development of any part of the spinal cord; usually used to describe abnormalities without gross superficial defects

rachischisis Fissure in the spinal column that leaves the meninges and spinal cord exposed

spinal dysrhaphia Defect in closure of the vertebral column with varying degrees of tissue protrusion through the bony cleft

spina bifida Synonymous with spinal dysraphia

spina bifida occulta Fusion failure of posterior vertebral arches without accompanying herniation of spinal cord or meninges; usually not visible externally (Fig. 11-1, *B*)

spina bifida cystica Defect in closure with external saccular protrusion through the bony spine with varying degrees of nerve involvement

meningocele Form of spina bifida; consists of a saclike cyst of meninges filled with spinal fluid (Fig. 11-1, *C*)

myelomeningocele (meningomyelocele) Hernial protrusion of a saclike cyst containing meninges, spinal fluid, and a portion of the spinal cord with its nerves (Fig. 11-1, *D*)

encephalocele Herniation of brain and meninges through a defect in the skull producing a fluid-filled sac in the occipital region

anencephaly Absent brain; this anomaly consists of only an exposed vascular mass with no bony covering; incompatible with life

Etiology

Two of the defects, anencephaly and spina bifida, occur in association with one another more often than would be expected by chance, suggesting a common origin. The central nervous system defects may alternate in siblings, which also tends to support the theory of a common origin. In a family who has had a child with either anencephaly or spina bifida, the possibility of having a subsequent child with either anomaly is higher than in the general population. There is some speculation regarding a viral cause of spina bifida, since there appears to be an increased incidence of the defects in fetuses conceived in the early winter months. Radiation and other environmental influences have also been implicated, based on animal experiments.

The discussion of neural tube defects is limited to the two most common types, spina bifida occulta and myelomenin-

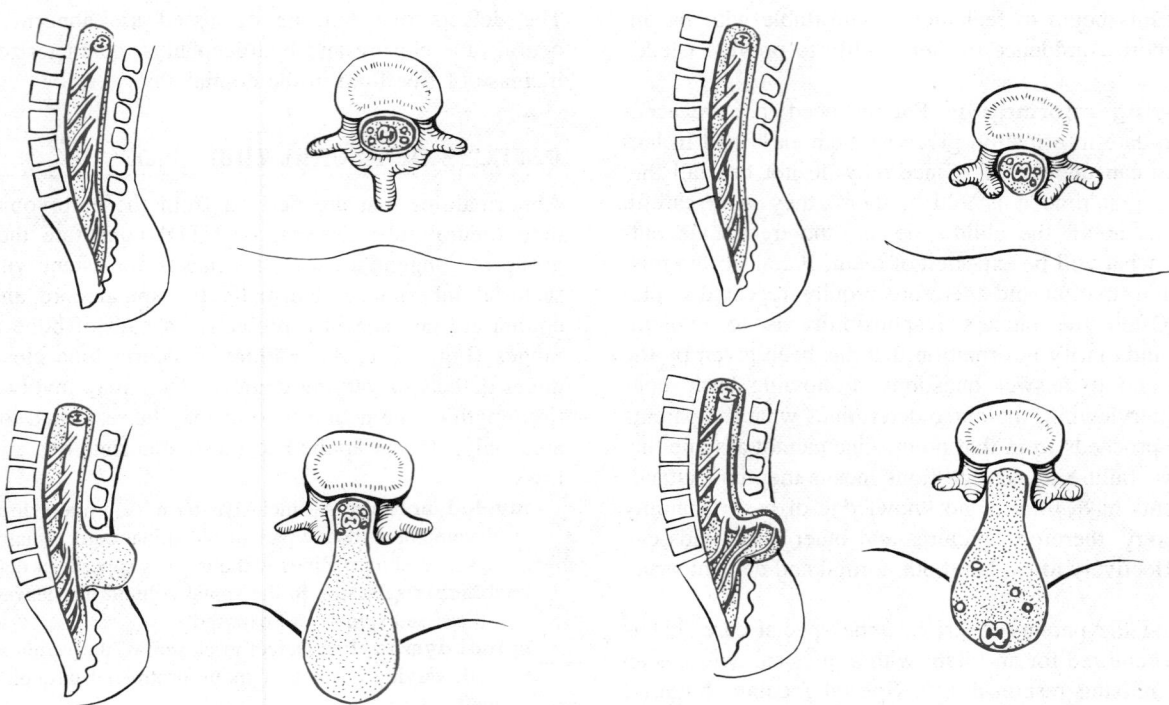

Fig. 11-1. Midline defects of osseous spine with varying degrees of neural herniations.

gocele, an abnormality that causes significant childhood disability.

SPINA BIFIDA OCCULTA

Noncystic spina bifida is failure of the spinous processes to join posteriorly in the lumbosacral area (L5 and S1). Routine radiographic examinations indicate that the disorder is quite common, but it may not be apparent unless there are associated cutaneous manifestations or neuromuscular disturbances. The incidence is estimated to occur in up to 25% of younger children, in whom there is eventual fusion of the vertebral arches, and in approximately 5% to 10% of all individuals (Scarff and Fronczak, 1981). Superficial indications include a skin depression or dimple (which may also mark the outlet of a dermal sinus tract that extends to the subarachnoid space), port-wine angiomatous nevi, dark tufts of hair, or soft, subcutaneous lipomas. These signs may be absent, appear singly, or be present in combination. Neuromuscular disturbances usually consist of progressive disturbance of gait with foot weakness and/or bowel and bladder sphincter disturbances caused by abnormal adhesion of the spinal cord to the area of the malformation, resulting in traction on the spinal cord and cauda equina with growth. (See Fig. 40-37 for areas innervated by specific spinal nerves.)

MYELOMENINGOCELE (MENINGOMYELOCELE)

The cystic defect myelomeningocele affects about 1 of every 1000 live births (Khoury, Erickson, and James, 1982) but may be as high as 4.2 per 1000 live births in some parts of the world (Owens and others, 1981). It is detected at birth, accounts for 90% of spinal cord lesions, and may be located at any point along the spinal column. Usually the sac is encased in a fine membrane that is prone to tears through which cerebrospinal fluid leaks. In other instances the sac may be covered by dura, meninges, or skin, in which instances there is rapid and spontaneous epithelialization. Since the lumbar segment is the last portion of the neural tube to close, the largest number of myelomeningoceles are found in the lumbar or lumbosacral area (Fig. 11-2). When the defect is located below the second lumbar vertebra, the nerves of the cauda equina are involved, giving rise to symptoms such as flaccid, areflexic partial paralysis of the lower extremities and varying degrees of sensory deficit.

The anomaly most frequently associated with myelomeningocele is hydrocephalus, and 75% of infants with the defect require shunt procedures (McLone, Raimondi, and Sommers, 1981, cited in Myers, 1984). This is usually some form of the defect involving the downward displacement of the brainstem and cerebellum through the foramen magnum, known as the *Arnold-Chiari malformation* (p.

442). In most cases hydrocephalus is apparent at birth; in other children it appears shortly thereafter, evidenced by increasing occipitofrontal circumference measurements (see p. 441 for a discussion of hydrocephalus).

Pathophysiology

The pathophysiology of spina bifida is best understood when related to the normal formative stages of the nervous system. At approximately 20 days of gestation a decided depression, the neural groove, appears in the dorsal ectoderm of the embryo. During the fourth week of gestation the groove deepens rapidly and its elevated margins develop laterally and then fuse dorsally to form the neural tube. Neural tube formation begins in the cervical region near the center of the embryo and advances in both directions—caudally and cephalically—until by the end of the fourth week of gestation the ends of the neural tube, the anterior and posterior neuropores, are closed. The primary defect in neural tube malformations is believed by most authorities to be a failure of neural tube closure. However, there is evidence to indicate that the defects are a result of splitting of the already closed neural tube as a result of an abnormal increase in cerebrospinal fluid pressure during the first trimester.

Clinical Manifestations

The manifestations of spina bifida vary widely according to the degree of the spinal defect. The defect is readily apparent on inspection. The degree of neurologic dysfunction is directly related to the anatomic level of the defect and thus the nerves involved. Sensory disturbances usually parallel motor dysfunction. The upper level of sensory and motor

impairment can be determined by observation of the infant's response to a pinprick over the legs and trunk. The infant will respond to the sensory stimulus with limb movement, arousal, and crying. When withdrawal activity is used to determine the lowest level of spinal cord function, the response to pinprick should begin above the lesion. It is important to observe the infant's behavior in conjunction with the stimulus, since limb movements can be induced in response to spinal cord reflex activity that has no connection with the higher centers. Defective nerve supply to the bladder affects both sphincter and detrusor tone to produce overflow incontinence with constant dribbling of urine. Often there is poor anal sphincter tone and poor anal skin reflex, which result in lack of bowel control and sometimes rectal prolapse. If the defect is located below the third sacral vertebra, there is no motor impairment but there may be saddle anesthesia with bladder and anal sphincter paralysis.

Sometimes the denervation to the muscles of the lower extremities will produce joint deformities in utero. These are primarily flexion or extension contractures, talipes valgus or varus contractures, kyphosis, lumbosacral scoliosis, and hip dislocations. The extent and severity of these associated deformities again depend on the degree of nerve involvement. Most flexion deformities result from the pull of stronger, fully innervated muscles acting without the counterpull of their nonfunctioning paralyzed antagonists.

Diagnostic Evaluation

The diagnosis is made on the basis of clinical manifestations and examination of the meningeal sac. If the mass can be transilluminated (that is, becomes translucent when a light is held behind it), the defect is probably a meningocele. In

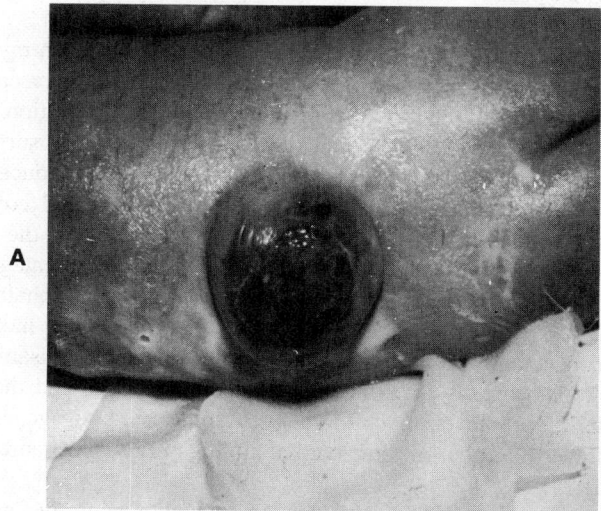
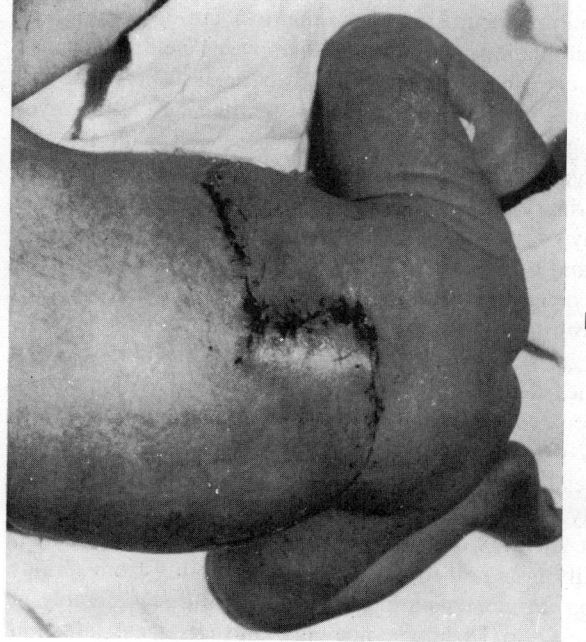

Fig. 11-2. A, Meningomyelocele before surgery. (An antibacterial dressing was used.) **B,** Repair of same patient.
Courtesy M.C. Gleason, M.D., San Diego, CA. From Ingalls, A.J., and Salerno, M.C.: Maternal and child health nursing, ed. 4, St. Louis, 1979, The C.V. Mosby Co.

these cases neurologic function is rarely disturbed even though the nerve roots are somewhat displaced. If the mass does not transilluminate, it is more likely a myelomeningocele. Supplementary diagnostic measures include plain radiography to disclose the precise bony defect in symptomatic lesion and to establish the diagnosis in the suspected, nonsymptomatic occult variety. Other spinal tomograms and myelography are used to differentiate between spina bifida occulta and other spinal disorders. Skull tomography helps to establish the presence or absence of hydrocephalus.

Laboratory examinations are used primarily to determine causative organisms in the major complications of myelomeningocele—meningitis and urinary tract infections. Children with urinary tract incontinence require urinalysis, culture, blood urea nitrogen (BUN) evaluation, and creatinine clearance evaluation.

Prenatal detection. It is possible to determine the presence of some major open neural tube defects prenatally. Ultrasonic scanning of the uterus and elevated concentrations of alpha-fetoprotein (AFP), a fetal-specific gamma-1 globulin, in amniotic fluid can indicate the presence of anencephaly or myelomeningocele. The optimum time for performing these diagnostic tests is between the fourteenth and sixteenth weeks of gestation, before AFP concentrations normally diminish and in sufficient time to permit a therapeutic abortion. It is recommended that such diagnostic procedures be considered for all mothers who have borne an affected child. Only 5% are detected in this manner; 95% of affected children are born to parents anticipating a normal child (Myers, 1984).

Therapeutic Management

Management of the child who has a myelomeningocele requires a multidisciplinary approach involving the specialties of neurology, neurosurgery, pediatrics, urology, orthopedics, rehabilitation, and physical therapy, as well as intensive nursing care in a variety of specialty areas. The collaborative efforts of these specialists are focused on (1) the myelomeningocele and the problems associated with the defect—hydrocephalus, paralysis, orthopedic deformities, genitourinary abnormalities, (2) possible acquired problems that may or may not be associated, such as meningitis, hypoxia, and hemorrhage, and (3) other abnormalities, such as cardiac or gastrointestinal malformations.

Infancy. Initial care involves prevention of infection, neurologic assessment, including observation for associated anomalies, and dealing with the impact of the anomaly on the parents. Although meningoceles are repaired early, especially if there is danger of rupture of the sac, the philosophy regarding skin closure of myelomeningocele varies radically. Most authorities believe that early closure, within the first 24 to 48 hours, offers the most favorable outcome, especially in regard to morbidity and mortality from serious infection. Proponents argue that early closure, preferably in the first 12 to 18 hours, not only prevents local infection and trauma to the exposed tissues but also avoids stretching

of other nerve roots, which may occur as the meningeal sac expands during the first 24 hours after birth, thus preventing further motor impairment (Reigel, 1982).

There are those who recommend that surgical repair is best delayed for further assessment of neurologic function, intellectual potential, and extent of complications (Charney and others, 1985). They believe that, in addition to increased ability of the infant to tolerate the surgical procedure, delay allows for better epithelialization of the sac (thus reducing the risk of infection) and permits easier mobilization of skin for closure. Delay is also thought to be beneficial by some because early closure contributes to the development of hydrocephalus by reducing the absorptive surface provided by the meningocele (Linder and others, 1984). It is also argued that delay frees the family from immediate decision making and allows time to hear all the facts and weigh the consequences of decisions.

A variety of plastic surgical procedures are employed for skin closure without disturbing the neural elements or removing any portion of the sac (for example, Fig. 11-2, *B*). The objective is satisfactory skin coverage of the lesion and meticulous closure. Wide excision of the large membranous covering may damage functioning neural tissue. Where the skin over the defect is intact, as often occurs with meningocele, surgical intervention may be performed for cosmetic reasons.

Associated problems are assessed and managed by appropriate surgical and supportive measures. Shunt procedures provide relief from imminent or progressive hydrocephalus (see p. 445). Often, in instances where a shunt procedure is performed before closure of the spinal defect, relief of the hydrocephalus also produces a collapse of the myelomeningocele with subsequent epithelialization of the sac. Meningitis, urinary tract infection, and pneumonia are treated with vigorous antibiotic therapy and supportive measures.

Outcome. The early prognosis for the child with myelomeningocele depends on the neurologic deficit present at birth, including motor ability and bladder innervation and the presence of associated cerebral anomalies. Early surgical repair of the spinal defect, antibiotic therapy to reduce the incidence of total meningitis and ventriculitis, and correction of hydrocephalus have significantly increased the survival rate. However, in addition to the high percentage of children who require shunt procedures for hydrocephalus, a large percentage are left with total paralysis and incontinence, and the remainder have significant motor disability. Approximately one third are mentally retarded, and the intelligence level in children with spina bifida is generally lower than that of their normal siblings (Tew and Laurence, 1973).

There are those who question whether operative procedures should be considered for children with overwhelming neurologic deficit or whether the disorder should be allowed to assume its natural course. Considerable research is directed toward selection of infants for surgical repair and infants for supportive care only (Gross and others, 1983; Lorber and Salfield, 1981). There are supporters and critics of this philosophy (Letters to the editors, 1984). Criteria for selection or nonselection are based on prognosis for quality of life. Such controversies present serious ethical problems (see p. 431).

Improved surgical techniques do not alter the major physical disability and deformity, retardation, and chronic urinary tract and pulmonary infections that affect the quality of life for these children. Superimposed on these physical problems are the effects that the disorder has on family life and finances and on school and hospital services.

Orthopedic considerations. According to most orthopedists, musculoskeletal problems that will affect later locomotion should be evaluated early, and treatment, where indicated, should be instituted without delay. In collaboration with appropriate members of the team, the child is evaluated in regard to the true level of neurologic functioning and corrective measures are carried out in coordination with the activities of the neurosurgeon. Casting, bracing, traction, and surgical techniques for correction of hip, knee, and foot deformities are employed when they may aid later ambulation. The minimum degree of future disability can usually be ascertained, although the maximum degree of disability is impossible to predict.

There is great diversity in individual patterns of musculoskeletal involvement. The hip flexors and adductors are innervated by L1 to L3, while extensors and abductors are innervated by L5 to S1. Consequently there is often an imbalance in muscle pull around a joint. Since most myelomeningoceles involve the midlumbar region, there are often or spastic abnormalities of muscles innervated by the upper lumbar cord and flaccidity or spasticity of muscles innervated from lower cord levels. Children with lesions at L2 or above have some hip flexion and are usually confined to a wheelchair for mobility. Children with lesions at L2 to L5 have strong hip flexors and are candidates for crutches and braces, although the majority use a wheelchair most of the time. At levels L3 and L4 there is usually an imbalance between sensory and motor nerve involvement and hip dislocation is often a problem. Children with sacral lesions are able to walk but some require ankle bracing.

A variety of devices are available to provide mobility to children with spinal cord lesions, including lightweight braces, special "walking" devices, and custom-built wheelchairs (see also p. 1794). Corrective procedures, when indicated, are best initiated at an early age so that the child will not lag significantly behind age-mates in developmental progress. Where there is little hope for lower extremity functioning, surgery is seldom recommended.

Management of genitourinary function. Myelomeningocele is one of the most common causes of neurogenic bladder dysfunction in childhood, and the prognosis for children who survive the early hazards of meningitis and hydrocephalus ultimately depends on the severity of their renal disease. Not only does renal failure pose a threat to life, but the lack of bladder control is important to the de-

velopment of self-image and the social acceptability of the child. Ongoing assessment and monitoring of urologic status are lifelong problems in management of the myelodysplastic child with or without surgical repair of the spinal defect. Since the majority of these children suffer from incontinence and are subject to recurrent or persistent pyuria, prevention and treatment of renal complications are a constant goal.

There are two types of bladder abnormalities. The *flaccid* bladder has incomplete emptying and normal vesicoureteral closure is not maintained. A *spastic* bladder is one in which coordination between the detrusor muscle and the outlet muscle is faulty, creating high intravesical pressure with decreased drainage from the ureters and incomplete emptying. The residual urine predisposes to infection and the vesicoureteral reflux can lead to hydronephrosis, both of which can cause progressive renal deterioration and eventual renal failure.

Treatment of renal problems includes regular urologic care with prompt and vigorous treatment of infections. Some type of regular emptying of the bladder is established without causing retrograde ureteral reflux. Intermittent clean catheterization (ICC) is the most popular option for facilitated drainage. It can be performed easily by parents, even in neonates, and self-catheterization can be successfully taught to children as young as 4 to 6 years of age. It is particularly valuable when urinary retention, overflow incontinence, and reflux are problems (Shoenberg and Meador, 1982). Although many children achieve dryness for 2 hours or more with ICC, the technique is not successful for others.

Medications are often used to improve bladder storage and continence, including bethanechol (Urecholine), propantheline (Pro-Banthine), phenoxybenzamine (Dibenzyline), and ephedrine; these prove useful in some cases. In many areas the surgically implanted artificial urinary sphincter and bladder pacemaker procedures are used. In cases of intractable severe hydronephrosis or incontinence, urinary diversion such as a ureteroileostomy, ureterostomy, or cystostomy may be necessay.

Bowel control. Some degree of fecal continence can usually be achieved in most children with myelomeningocele with diet modification, regular toilet habits, and prevention of constipation and impaction. It is frequently a lengthy process, but biofeedback training is proving to be effective in helping some children to gain control more quickly (Whitehead, Parker, and Masek, 1981).

Nursing Considerations

Care of the infant and child with myelomeningocele requires both immediate and long-term nursing and medical supervision. At the time of delivery an examination is performed to assess the intactness of the membranous cyst, and every effort is made to prevent trauma to this protective covering. In the newborn period nursing responsibilities are directed toward preventing infection of and trauma to the fragile cyst, observing for complications, and providing support for and education of parents. Long-term management involves an interdisciplinary team effort to help the child and family with the multitude of problems associated with this disability.

Care of myelomeningocele sac. The infant is usually placed in an Isolette or warmer so that temperature can be maintained without clothing or covers that might irritate the delicate lesion. When an overhead warmer is used, the dressings over the defect require more frequent moistening because of the dehydrating effect of the dry heat.

Before surgical closure the myelomeningocele is prevented from drying by the application of a sterile, moist, nonadherent dressing over the defect. The moistening solution is usually sterile normal saline, although soaks with antibacterial drugs such as silver nitrate or bacitracin are also advocated. Dressings are changed frequently (every 2 to 4 hours), and the sac is closely inspected for leaks, abrasions, irritation, or any signs of infection. It must be carefully cleansed if it becomes soiled or contaminated. Any opening in the sac greatly increases the risk of infection to the central nervous system. If surgical closure is to be delayed, measures are directed toward facilitating the drying, granulation, and eventual epithelialization of the sac. In this instance the sac is usually left exposed to the air or covered with a dry gauze or nonadherent dressing.

Special measures to toughen the skin or membrane, such as application of benzoin tincture, may be indicated, but care must be taken to prevent a dressing from adhering to and damaging the sac. Prolonged use of ointments or moist dressings is usually contraindicated to avoid maceration and breakdown of the tissues. A large doughnut-shaped piece of foam rubber or other spongy material can be fashioned to provide a protective shield for the sac. The edges should be left sufficiently wide to allow for adequate anchoring with strips of bandage or paper tape. A sterile drape, gauze, or other protective cover can form a roof over the opening but should not come in contact with the sac.

Positioning. One of the most difficult, important, and challenging aspects in the early care of the infant with myelomeningocele is positioning. Before surgery the infant is kept in the prone position to minimize tension on the sac and the risk of trauma. The prone position allows for optimum positioning of legs, especially in cases of associated hip dysplasia. Ideally the infant is placed in a low Trendelenburg position to reduce spinal fluid pressure in the sac, with the hips only slightly flexed to reduce tension on the defect. The legs are maintained in abduction with a pad between the knees to counteract hip subluxation, and a small roll is placed under the ankles to maintain a neutral foot position. A variety of aids, including diaper rolls, pads, small sandbags, or specially designed frames and appliances, can be used to maintain the desired position.

The prone position affects other aspects of the infant's care. For example, in this position the infant is more difficult to keep clean, pressure areas are a constant threat, and feeding becomes a problem. The infant's head is turned to one side for feeding. Fortunately most defects are repaired early and the infant can be held for feeding as soon as the surgical site is sufficiently healed to permit handling.

General care. Diapering the infant is contraindicated until the defect has been repaired and healing is well advanced or epithelialization has taken place. The padding beneath the diaper area is changed as needed to keep the skin dry and free of irritation. When urinary retention is present, gentle pressure applied to the suprapubic area will facilitate emptying of the bladder, which is still an abdominal organ in early infancy. Since the bowel sphincter is frequently affected, there is continual passage of stool, often misinterpreted as diarrhea, which is a constant irritant to the skin and a source of infection to the spinal lesion. This provides another rationale for closure before the infant's first feeding while the meconium is still free of organisms.

Areas of sensory and motor impairment are subject to skin breakdown and therefore require meticulous care. Placing the infant on a soft foam or fleece pad reduces pressure on the knees and ankles. Periodic cleansing, application of lotion, and gentle massage aid circulation. Changing linen is best accomplished by two persons—one changes the linen while the other holds the infant, assuring that the spine is maintained in good alignment without tension in the area of the defect.

Gentle range of motion exercises are sometimes carried out to prevent contractures, and stretching of contractures is performed when indicated. However, these exercises may be restricted to the foot, ankle, and knee joint. Where the hip joints are unstable, stretching against tight hip flexors or adductor muscles, which act much like bowstrings, may aggravate a tendency toward subluxation. In addition, the bones of these infants tend to be fragile and subject to fractures.

Since infants with unrepaired myelomeningocele are unable to be held in the arms and cuddled as unaffected infants are, their need for tactile stimulation is met by fondling, stroking, and other comfort measures. Bright mobiles or other objects can be placed within the infant's view, and other stimulating activities usually provided for infants are appropriate. All infants respond to pleasant sounds (see Table 10-3).

Postoperative care. Postoperative care of the infant with myelomeningocele involves the same basic care as that of any postsurgical infant—monitoring vital signs, monitoring intake and output, nourishment, and observation for signs of infection. Wound management is carried out according to the directions of the surgeon, and general care is continued as preoperatively.

The prone position is maintained after operative closure, although may neurosurgeons allow a side-lying or partial side-lying position unless it aggravates a coexisting hip dysplasia or permits undesirable hip flexion. This offers an opportunity for position changes, which reduces the risk of pressure sores and facilitates feeding. If permitted by the

Nursing Care Summary: The Infant with Myelomeningocele

NURSING GOALS	NURSING INTERVENTIONS	EXPECTED PATIENT/FAMILY OUTCOMES

HP-HMP **Injury: potential for infection, trauma**
Risk factors: presence of meningeal sac

NURSING GOALS	NURSING INTERVENTIONS	EXPECTED PATIENT/FAMILY OUTCOMES
Prevent local infection	Inspect meningomyelocele for any changes in appearance, for example, abrasions, tears, signs of infection, drainage Report any change in appearance Position infant to prevent contamination from urine and stool Wear sterile gloves and mask when changing dressings	Meningeal sac remains clean, intact, and exhibits no evidence of infection
Prevent local trauma	Handle infant carefully Place infant in prone or side-lying position, if permitted Apply protective devices Avoid adherent dressings Modify routine nursing activities, for example, feeding, making bed, comforting activities	Meningeal sac remains intact
Identify impending complications	Observe for signs of hydrocephalus 　Measure head circumference daily 　Check fontanels for tenseness or bulging 　Note irritability, lethargy, difficulty in feeding, high-pitched cry Observe for signs of meningeal irritation and inflammation, for example, fever, nuchal rigidity, irritability Check all drainage from meningeal sac for glucose	*Signs of developing hydrocephalus are detected early and appropriate interventions implemented
Prevent urinary infection	Avoid contamination with stool Observe for signs of urinary tract infection	Infant remains free of infection

N-MP **Skin integrity, impairment of: potential**
Risk factors: skin insensitivity

NURSING GOALS	NURSING INTERVENTIONS	EXPECTED PATIENT/FAMILY OUTCOMES
Prevent skin breakdown	Change position frequently Place soft foam or fleece pad under infant Apply gentle massage to skin periodically to stimulate circulation Maintain meticulous skin cleanliness Maintain acid skin mantle, avoid soap Avoid pressure to prominent points such as knees and ankles Position side-to-side as soon as allowed Apply protective lotion to areas where excoriation is most likely—anal and perineal areas, knees, elbows, ankles, chin, and so on Change diapers as soon as soiled Keep perianal area clean and dry	Infant's position is changed at least every 2 hours Skin remains clean and intact Perianal area remains clean and dry; no evidence of irritation

A-EP **Mobility, impaired physical**
Etiology: neuromuscular impairment

NURSING GOALS	NURSING INTERVENTIONS	EXPECTED PATIENT/FAMILY OUTCOMES
Prevent or minimize hip and lower extremity deformity	Carry out passive range-of-motion exercises Do not push past point of resistance Carry out muscle stretching when indicated Carry out exercises with care to avoid fracturing fragile bones Maintain hips in slight to moderate abduction to prevent dislocation; feet in neutral position	Lower extremities maintain flexibility
Facilitate ambulation	Teach use and care of mobilizing devices when appropriate (braces, crutches, wheelchair)	Child moves about with minimum or no assistance

*Nursing outcome.

Continued.

Nursing Care Summary: The Infant with Myelomeningocele—cont'd

NURSING GOALS	NURSING INTERVENTIONS	EXPECTED PATIENT/FAMILY OUTCOMES
RRP Family process, alteration in **Etiology: situational crisis (child with a physical defect)**		
Deal with family's anxiety about recurrence in future children	Encourage expression of feelings Refer to genetic counseling service	Family discusses feelings and concerns regarding child's condition

Prepare family for discharge of child	Assess ability of family to care for infant
	Teach family essential aspects of infant's physical care
	  Allow ample time for preparation
	  Encourage questions and expression of feelings
	  Allow for supervised practice in care
	Refer for evaluation of foster-care placement when family is unable or unwilling to care for child
	Encourage family to take an active role in infant's care
		Family demonstrates skills and knowledge needed to carry out home care of infant (specify learning and manner of demonstration)
		Child is placed in foster care if indicated
		Family provides care for the infant at their own rate and abilities

Provide anticipatory guidance	Discuss developmental expectations
	Teach family to observe for signs of complications
	  Signs of infection
	  Signs of possible shunt failure (when shunt procedure has been performed for hydrocephalus)
	Provide and reinforce information, listen to family concerns, correct misconceptions
		Family demonstrates an understanding of developmental accomplishments and signs of complications (specify)

Facilitate developmental progress	Help parents plan activities appropriate to developmental level	Infant engages in appropriate activities (specify)
Support parents	Provide or arrange for ongoing contact with family Refer to parent groups and organizations such as the Spina Bifida Association of America	Family makes appropriate contacts
Coordinate services	Plan for home visits where needed Maintain contact with family Make appointments for follow-up care Make referrals to special agencies as needed Act as liaison between inpatient and outpatient services	Child and family are not lost to health agencies

Nursing Interventions Related to Medical Management

Prevent infection
  Cleanse myelomeningocele carefully with sterile saline
  Apply sterile dressings; moisten with sterile solution as ordered (saline, silver nitrate, antibiotic)
    Administer antibiotics as ordered
    Administer similar care of operative site postoperatively

physician, the infant can be held upright against the body, with care to avoid pressure on the operative site.

The nurse is in a position to aid the physician in determining the extent of neuromuscular involvement. Movement of the extremities or skin response, especially an anal reflex, that might provide cues to the degree of motor or sensory status is noted. The head circumference is measured daily (see p. 229), and the fontanels are examined for signs of tension or bulging. The nurse is also alert to early signs of infection, such as elevated temperature (axillary), irritability, lethargy, and nuchal rigidity, and to signs of increased intracranial pressure.

Family support and home care. As soon as the parents are able to cope with the infant's condition, they are encouraged to become involved in care. They need to learn how to continue at home the care that has been initiated in the hospital—positioning, feeding, skin care, and range of motion exercises when appropriate. Parents are taught clean catheterization technique when prescribed. The family needs to know the signs of complications and how to reach assistance when needed. In cases in which the defect has not been repaired, they are taught to care for the lesion.

As the child grows and develops, it is important that the parents encourage and stimulate the infant to accomplish age-appropriate developmental tasks within the limits imposed by the disabilities. Upper limb movement can be stimulated early by placing the infant on the floor in a prone position with toys within reach. Activities that encourage body consciousness, such as rolling over and pulling to a sitting position, should be encouraged at the appropriate times. Creeping and crawling, even in a limited way, help the child to explore the environment. The parents may need help to modify appliances and activities normally expected of a growing child. For example, the paraplegic infant should be encouraged to use arms and shoulders as much as possible. When sitting in an infant seat, stroller, high chair, or feeding table, the infant's hips can be supported, a footrest provided, and hard-soled shoes worn to maintain the feet in correct alignment and to protect the insensitive feet from trauma. A standing table is helpful for a variety of activities, and it is best for the child to begin supported weight bearing and standing as close as possible to the time expected for normal children.

It is important for the family to understand the nature of sensory deficit in a child with a spinal defect. The child will be insensitive to pressure or other sources of tissue injury. Therefore the family must be alert to hot or cold items that could cause thermal injury to tissues and to inspect the skin regularly for signs of pressure, especially over bony prominences. Because of sensory impairment, the child is unaware of bladder discomfort; therefore signs of urinary tract infections may be easily overlooked. Urinary tract infection is often considered when the child becomes ill.

The long-range planning with and support of parents and child begin in the hospital and extend throughout childhood and even beyond. Long-term care of these children is of uncertain length. Nurses assume an important role as a central member of the health team. As a coordinator the nurse reviews information with the family, takes responsibility for family teaching, and acts as liaison between inpatient and outpatient services. The child will need numerous hospitalizations over the years, and each one will be a source of stress to which the younger child is especially vulnerable.

Habilitation involves not only solving problems of self-help and locomotion but also the most distressing problem of incontinence, which threatens the child's social acceptability. Assistance with placement in schools designed to accommodate the deficiencies and special needs of children with disabilities helps provide a better initial adjustment to broader social experiences. It would be difficult to enumerate all that the condition entails in terms of suffering, frustration, family stress, and economic burden. Numerous organizations and agencies are able to offer assistance and support to children and families. The **Spina Bifida Association of America*** is organized to provide services and support for families of children with spinal lesions. Other organizations whose services extend to all children with physical disabilities are listed in Appendix E.

---

*343 S. Dearborn #310, Chicago, IL 60604.

The multiple aspects in care of the child with a disability are discussed in Chapter 22 and need not be elaborated here, nor will the complex problems associated with partial or complete lower extremity paralysis, which are discussed in Chapter 40. These include bowel and bladder control, orthopedic appliances, and the observation and management of complications, especially urinary tract infections and pressure necrosis.

HYDROCEPHALUS

Hydrocephalus is a condition caused by an imbalance in the production and absorption of cerebrospinal fluid (CSF) in the ventricular system. When production is greater than absorption, CSF accumulates within the ventricular system, usually under increased pressure, producing passive dilation of the ventricles.

Pathophysiology

In order to understand the condition, the dynamics of CSF and the relationship between the various structures that make up the ventricular and subarachnoid spaces is necessary (Fig. 11-3). The primary site of CSF formation is believed to be the choroid plexuses of the lateral ventricles, although it is also believed to be produced by the brain parenchyma.

Ventricular circulation. The fluid flows from the lateral ventricles through the *foramen of Monro* to the third ventricle, where it combines with fluid secreted into the third ventricle. From there it flows through the *aqueduct of Sylvius* into the fourth ventricle, where more fluid is formed; it then leaves the fourth ventricle by way of the lateral *foramen of Luschka* and the midline *foramen of Magendie* into the *cisterna magna*. From there it flows to the cerebral and cerebellar subarachnoid spaces where it is absorbed by some mechanism that is not entirely clear. A large portion is absorbed through the arachnoid villi, but the sinuses, veins, brain substance, and dura also participate in absorption.

Mechanisms of fluid imbalance. The causes of hydrocephalus are varied but the result is either (1) impaired absorption of CSF fluid within the subarachnoid space *(communicating hydrocephalus)* or (2) obstruction to the flow of CSF within the ventricles *(noncommunicating hydrocephalus)*. Rarely, a tumor of the choroid plexus causes increased CSF secretion. Any imbalance of secretion and absorption causes an increased accumulation of CSF in the ventricles, which become dilated and compress the brain substance against the surrounding rigid bony cranium. When this occurs before fusion of the cranial sutures, it produces enlargement of the skull as well as dilation of the ventricles.

Most cases of noncommunicating hydrocephalus are a result of developmental malformations. Although the defect usually is apparent in early infancy, it may become evident at any time from the prenatal period to late childhood or early adulthood. Other causes include neoplasms, infections, and trauma. An obstruction to the normal flow can

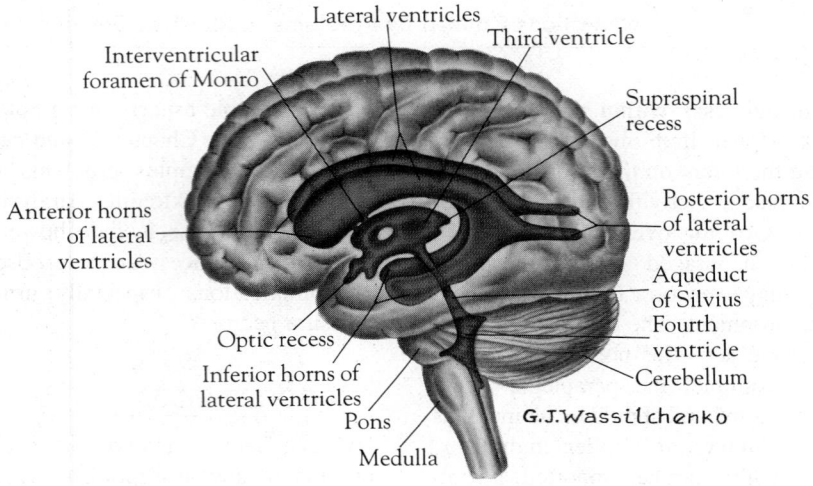

Fig. 11-3. Cerebral ventricular system.

From Thompson, J., and others: Clinical nursing, St. Louis, 1986, The C.V. Mosby Co., p. 294.

Table 11-1 Sites and types of hydrocephalus

SITE AND TYPE	CAUSES AND COMMENTS
Noncommunicating hydrocephalus	
Site: Aqueduct of Sylvius	Accounts for 20% of hydrocephalus
Type: Stenosis or atresia	Congenital (X-linked recessive in small number) Insidious onset of symptoms from birth to adulthood
Gliosis	Postinflammatory, usually secondary to perinatal infection or hemorrhage Prenatal maternal infection (toxoplasmosis)
Obstructive	Tumors of third ventricle or midbrain Ependymitis from maternal toxoplasmosis Congenital aneurysm of vein of Galen
Site: Fourth ventricle and foramen magnum	Accounts for 50% of all hydrocephalus
Type: Chiari malformations	Account for 40% of fourth ventricle obstructions
Type I	A neural tube defect with herniation of medulla through foramen magnum; may be asymptomatic
Type II (Arnold-Chiari malformation)	A more severe defect; downward displacement of brainstem, fourth ventricle, and lower parts of cerebellum through foramen magnum with fixed attachment of spinal cord at site of a myelomeningocele
Type III	High cervical or occipitocervical myelomeningocele with cervical herniation through body defect
Absence or occulsion of ventricles	Congenital (Dandy-Walker syndrome) caused by obstruction of foramina of Luschka and Magendie Tumors of posterior fossa (e.g., medulloblastoma) cause pressure on surrounding tissues to produce obstruction Less often: subdural hematoma, bacterial or granulomatous meningitis
Communicating hydrocephalus	
Site: Arachnoid villi and cisterna magna	Obstruction by thick arachnoid membrane or meninges
Type: Meningitis	Bacterial or granulomatous Acute phase: clumping of purulent fluid in drainage channels Chronic phase: organization of blood and exudate that results in fibrosis of subarachnoid spaces
Prenatal maternal infections	Toxoplasmosis, cytomegalic inclusion disease, mumps
Meningeal malignancy	Secondary to leukemia or lymphoma
Arachnoid cyst	Located in basal cistern or (uncommon) over cerebral cortex
Tuberculosis, fungal, or parasitic infection	More common in children age 2 to 10 years

occur at any point in the CSF pathway to produce increased pressure and dilation of the pathways proximal to the site of obstruction. Table 11-1 describes the most frequent sites of obstruction and the consequences.

Developmental defects—for example, Arnold-Chiari malformations, aqueduct stenosis, and aqueduct gliosis—account for most cases of hydrocephalus from birth to 2 years of age. Hydrocephalus is so often associated with myelomeningocele that all such infants should be observed for its development. In the remainder of cases there is a history of intrauterine infection, perinatal hemorrhage (anoxic or traumatic), and neonatal meningoencephalitis (bacterial or viral). In older children hydrocephalus is most often the result of space-occupying lesions, preexisting developmental defects (aqueduct stenosis, Arnold-Chiari malformations),

intracranial infections, or hemorrhage. The sites and types of hydrocephalus are outlined in Table 11-1.

Clinical Manifestations

The two factors that influence the clinical picture in hydrocephalus are the time of onset and the presence of preexisting structural lesions. In infancy before closure of the cranial sutures, head enlargement is the predominant sign, whereas in older infants and children the lesions responsible for hydrocephalus produce other neurologic signs through pressure on adjacent structures before causing cerebrospinal fluid obstruction.

Infancy. In infants the head grows at an abnormal rate, although the first signs may be bulging fontanels without head enlargement (Figs. 11-4 and 11-5). The anterior fon-

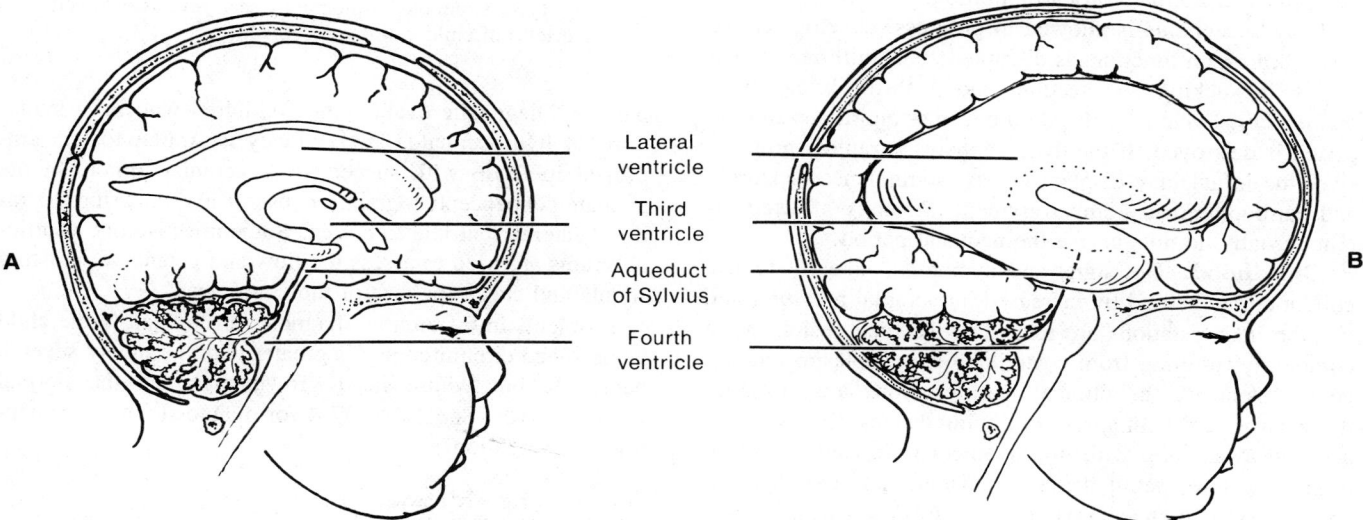

Lateral ventricle

Third ventricle

Aqueduct of Sylvius

Fourth ventricle

Fig. 11-4. Hydrocephalus: a block in flow of cerebrospinal fluid. **A,** Patent cerebrospinal fluid circulation. **B,** Enlarged lateral and third ventricles caused by obstruction of circulation—stenosis of aqueduct of Sylvius.

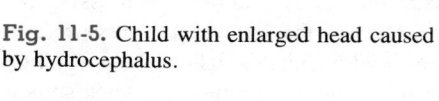

Fig. 11-5. Child with enlarged head caused by hydrocephalus.

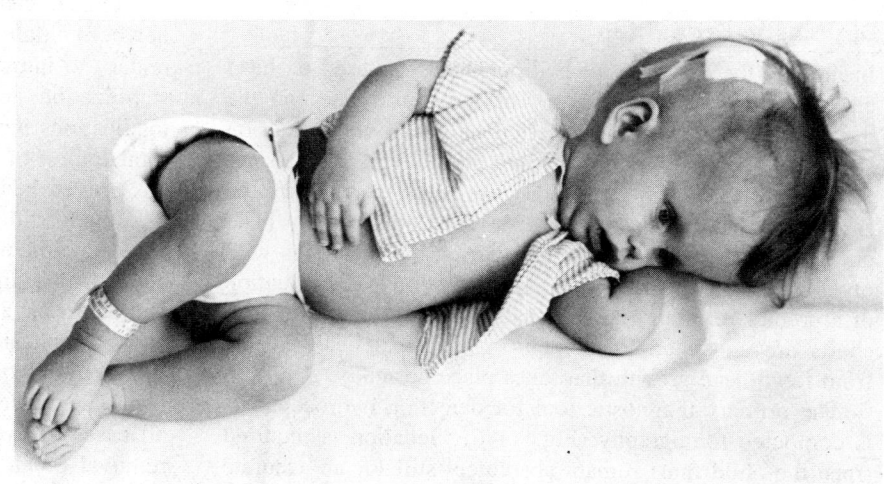

tanel is tense, often bulging, and nonpulsatile. Scalp veins are dilated and markedly so when the infant cries. With the increase in intracranial volume the bones of the skull become thin and the sutures become palpably separated to produce the "cracked-pot" sound (Macewen sign) on percussion of the skull. There may be frontal enlargement or "bossing" with depressed eyes and a "setting-sun" sign, in which the sclera is visible above the iris because of pressure on a thinned orbital roof or the third ventricle on the tectum of the mesencephalon. Pupils are sluggish with unequal response to light.

The infant is irritable and lethargic and may display changes in level of consciousness, opisthotonos (often extreme), and lower extremity spasticity. The infant will cry when picked up or rocked and quiet when allowed to lie still. Early infantile reflex acts may persist and normally expected responses fail to appear, indicating failure in the development of normal cortical inhibition.

If hydrocephalus is allowed to progress, development of lower brainstem functions is disrupted, as manifested by difficulty in sucking and feeding and a shrill, brief, high-pitched cry. Eventually the skull becomes enormous and the cortex is destroyed. If the hydrocephalus is rapidly progressive, the infant may display emesis, somnolence, seizures, and cardiopulmonary embarrassment. Severely affected infants usually do not survive the neonatal period.

Childhood. The signs and symptoms in early to late childhood are caused by increased intracranial pressure, and specific manifestations are related to the focal lesion. Most commonly resulting from posterior fossa neoplasms and aqueduct stenosis, the clinical manifestations are primarily those associated with space-occupying lesions, that is, headache on awakening with improvement following emesis or upright posture, papilledema, strabismus, and extrapyramidal tract signs such as ataxia (see p. 1624). As with infants, the child will be irritable, lethargic, apathetic, and confused and often incoherent. In one of the congenital defects with later onset, the Dandy-Walker syndrome, characteristic manifestations are bulging occiput, nystagmus, ataxia, and cranial nerve palsies.

Diagnostic Evaluation

In infancy the diagnosis of hydrocephalus is based on head circumference that crosses one or more grid lines on the measurement chart within a period of 2 to 4 weeks and on associated neurologic signs that are present and progressive. However, other diagnostic studies are needed to localize the site of cerebrospinal fluid obstruction. Routine daily head circumference measurements are carried out in infants with myelomeningocele and intracranial infections. In evaluation of a premature infant, specially adapted head circumference charts are consulted to distinguish abnormal head growth from rapid head growth that takes place normally.

The primary diagnostic tool for detecting hydrocephalus is computed tomography (Fig. 11-6). Sedation is required since the child must remain absolutely still for an accurate

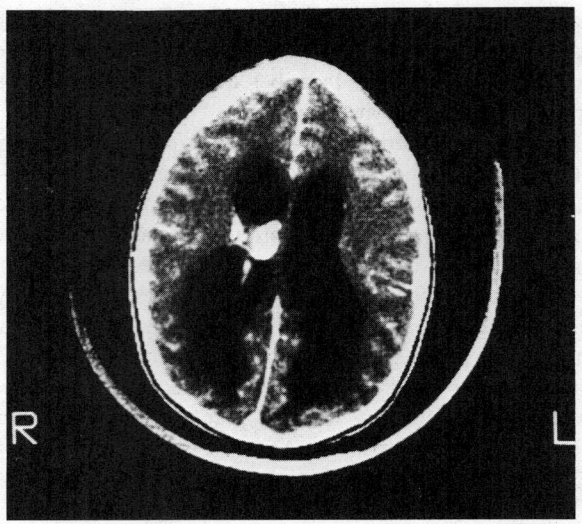

Fig. 11-6. Computed tomography scan reveals enlarged ventricles of child with hydrocephalus.

picture. Diagnostic evaluation of children who have symptoms of hydrocephalus after infancy is similar to that employed in those with suspected intracranial tumor. In the neonate echoencephalography is useful in comparing the ratio of lateral ventricle to cortex. Sometimes isotope ventriculograms are used to assess the flow and patency of existing shunts and check the size of the ventricles.

Problems in differential diagnosis are related to the child whose head circumference is greater than the ninety-seventh percentile but whose head growth parallels the normal growth curve. (See Table 37-4 for diagnostic tests for neurologic evaluation.)

Therapeutic Management

The treatment of hydrocephalus is directed toward (1) relief of the hydrocephalus, (2) treatment of complications, and (3) management of problems related to the effect of the disorder on psychomotor development. The treatment is, with few exceptions, surgical.

Medical therapy has been largely disappointing. Many newborn infants with progressive cranial enlargement secondary to intracranial hemorrhage demonstrate spontaneous stabilization and resolution. Serial lumbar punctures and medications have been used with varying success. The administration of acetazolamide and isosorbide or furosemide has proved beneficial in decreasing the production of cerebrospinal fluid in selected cases of slowly progressive disease. The medication reduces the intracranial pressure until spontaneous arrest of hydrocephalus takes place (Shinnar and others, 1985) or as a temporizing measure when surgery is contraindicated.

Surgical treatment. Improved techniques have established surgical treatment as the therapy of choice in almost all cases of hydrocephalus. This is accomplished by direct removal of an obstruction, for example, resection of neoplasm, cyst, or hematoma or, in rare instances of fluid over-production, by choroid plexus extirpation (plexectomy or electric coagulation). However, most children require a shunt procedure that provides primary drainage of the CSF from the ventricles to an extracranial compartment, usually the peritoneum.

Most shunt systems consist of a ventricular catheter, a flush pump, a unidirectional flow valve, and a distal catheter. All are radiopaque for easy visualization after placement, and all are tested for accuracy before insertion. A reservoir is frequently added to allow direct access to the ventricular system for administration of medications and removal of fluid. In all models the valves are designed to open at a predetermined intraventricular pressure and close when the pressure falls below that level, thus preventing backflow of secretions. High-pressure valves are used to prevent complications from rapid decompression of the ventricles. Medium-pressure valves are used in most children, especially those with long-standing hydrocephalus. Low-pressure valves are used in small infants.

The preferred procedure is the ventriculoperitoneal (VP) shunt, especially in neonates and young infants (Fig. 11-7). There is greater allowance for excess tubing, which minimizes the number of revisions needed as the child grows. Since it requires repeated lengthening, the ventriculoatrial (VA) shunt (ventricle to right atrium) is reserved for older children who have attained most of their somatic growth and children with abdominal pathology. The VA shunt is contraindicated in children with cardiopulmonary disease or elevated cerebrospinal fluid protein.

A ventricular bypass into intracranial channels may be used in older children with noncommunicating hydrocephalus caused by aqueduct stenosis or posterior fossa masses (e.g., medulloblastoma). Technical difficulties preclude its use in infants, since these spaces are poorly developed in the infant.

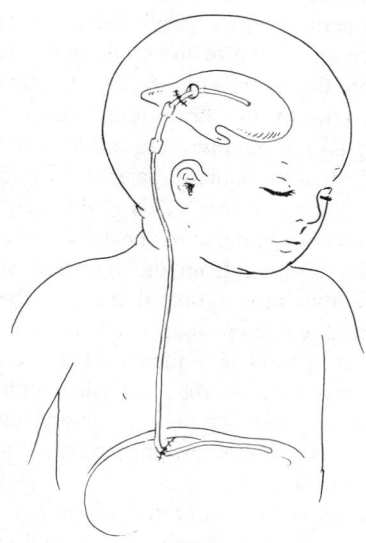

Fig. 11-7. Ventriculoperitoneal shunt.

The initial shunt is placed at about 3 to 4 months of age and, although there is wide variation, revisions are ordinarily planned for 18 to 24 months, 4 to 6 years, and when approximately 80% of adult height has been attained (usually 10 to 12 years of age) (Noetzel, 1986). In all mechanisms the initial success rate is relatively high; however, shunts are associated with complications that interfere with continued shunt function or that threaten the life of the child.

Complications. The major complications of VP shunts are infection and malfunction. All shunts are subject to mechanical difficulties, such as kinking, plugging, or separation or migration of the tubing. Malfunction is most often caused by mechanical obstruction either within the ventricles from particulate matter (tissue or exudate) or at the distal end from thrombosis or displacement as a result of growth. The child with a shunt obstruction often presents as an emergency with clinical manifestations of increased intracranial pressure, frequently accompanied by worsening neurologic status.

The most serious complication, shunt infection, can occur at any time but the period of greatest risk is 1 to 2 months following placement. The infection is generally the result of intercurrent infections at the time of shunt placement. Infections include septicemia, bacterial endocarditis, wound infection, shunt nephritis, meningitis, and ventriculitis. Meningitis and ventriculitis are of greatest concern since any complicating central nervous system infection is a significant predictor of intellectual outcome. Infection is treated with massive doses of antibiotics administered by the intravenous route or directly into the ventricles via the shunt reservoir. A persistent infection requires removal of the shunt until the infection is controlled.

A serious shunt-related complication is subdural hematoma caused by too rapid reduction of intracranial pressure and size. This usually can be averted by careful assessment of intracranial pressure prior to insertion of the shunt and use of correct valvular pressure. Other complications that may occur include peritonitis, abdominal abscesses, perforation of abdominal organs by catheter or trochar (at time of insertion), fistulas, hernias, and ileus.

Prognosis. Untreated, hydrocephalus has a 50% to 60% mortality rate caused by the disorder or intercurrent illnesses. Of the survivors, very few (less than 10%) are intellectually normal, and a large majority have major physical and/or disabling neurologic handicaps such as ataxia, spastic diplegia, poor fine motor coordination, and perceptual deficits. Spontaneous arrest occurs occasionally in approximately 40% of those with near-normal intelligence.

The prognosis of children with treated hydrocephalus depends largely on the rate at which hydrocephalus develops, the duration of raised intracranial pressure, the frequency of complications, and the cause of the condition. For example, malignant tumors may have a high mortality regardless of other complicating factors.

Surgically treated hydrocephalus with continued neurosurgical and medical management has a survival rate of about 80%, with the highest incidence of mortality occurring within the first year of treatment. Of the surviving children approximately one third are both intellectually and neurologically normal and one half have neurologic disabilities. However, the intelligence is in the lower ranges of normal, with deficits more pronounced in nonverbal intellectual skills. These children are also at greater risk for developing an emotional problem, such as anxiety neurosis or antisocial-conduct disorder (Noetzel, 1986).

Hydrocephalus complicating a meningomyelocele carries a less favorable prognosis. In some children irreversible damage may have been produced by the hydrocephalus or from the original infection; in addition, there are sometimes coincidental cerebral defects. Generally noninfective hydrocephalus appears to carry the best prognosis.

Nursing Considerations

Preoperatively the infant with diagnosed or suspected hydrocephalus is observed carefully for signs of increasing intracranial pressure. In infants the head is measured daily at the point of largest measurement—the occipitofrontal circumference (OFC) (see p. 229 for technique). To avoid the likelihood of wide discrepancies the point at which the measurements are taken is indicated on the head with a marking pen. Fontanels and suture lines are gently palpated for size, signs of bulging, tenseness, and separation. However, an infant with normal intracranial pressure will display bulging under certain circumstances such as straining or crying; therefore such accompanying behavior should be noted. Irritability, lethargy, or seizure activity as well as altered vital signs and feeding behavior may indicate advancing pathology.

General nursing care of the infant with hydrocephalus may present special problems. Maintaining adequate nutrition often requires flexible feeding schedules to accommodate diagnostic procedures since feeding before or after handling can precipitate an episode of vomiting. Small feedings at more frequent intervals are often better tolerated than are larger ones spaced farther apart. These infants are often difficult to feed and require extra time and innovation.

In older children, who are usually admitted to the hospital for elective or emergency shunt revision, the most valuable indicator of increasing intracranial pressure is an alteration in the child's level of consciousness and the way in which the child interacts with the environment. Changes are identified by observation and by comparing present behavior with customary behavior, sleep patterns, developmental capabilities, and habits obtained through a detailed history and a baseline assessment. This baseline information serves as a guide for postoperative assessment and evaluation of shunt function (Jackson, 1980).

In addition to measuring head circumference and observation of neurologic signs, the nurse is responsible for preparation of the child for diagnostic tests such as tomography and for assisting the physician with procedures such as a ventricular tap, which is often performed to relieve excessive pressure during the preoperative period, and cerebrospinal fluid examination. (See Chapter 27 for preparing children for procedures.)

Fortunately, almost all children are recognized and treatment is begun early. For those children with significant head enlargement care must be exercised to see that the head is well supported when the infant is fed or moved to prevent extra strain on the infant's neck, and measures must be taken to prevent development of pressure areas. As the hydrocephalus progresses, untreated children become increasingly helpless and prone to the multiple problems of immobility, for example, pressure sores and contracture deformities. Not infrequently infants with irreversible brain damage or with severe developmental defects such as hydranencephaly, in which both cerebral hemispheres fail to develop and are replaced with a membranous sac filled with cerebrospinal fluid, are placed in long-term institutions specially designed for care of these infants.

Postoperative care. In addition to routine postoperative care and observation, the infant or child is positioned carefully on the unoperated side to prevent pressure on the shunt valve and pressure areas. The child is kept flat to help avert complications resulting from too rapid reduction of intracranial fluid. When the ventricular size is reduced too rapidly, the cerebral cortex may pull away from the dura and tear the small interlacing veins, producing a subdural hematoma. This is not a problem in children with elective shunt revision, since their intraventricular size and pressure have been normal. The surgeon indicates the position to be maintained and the extent of activity allowed. If there is increased intracranial pressure, the surgeon will prescribe the head of the bed to be elevated and/or allow the child to sit up to enhance gravity flow through the shunt. Sedation is avoided because the level of consciousness is an important observation.

Observation for signs of increased intracranial pressure, which indicate obstruction of the shunt, is continued. Neurologic assessment includes pupil dilation (pressure causes compression or stretching of the oculomotor nerve, producing dilation on the same side as the pressure) and blood pressure (hypoxia to the brainstem causes variability in these vital signs). Sometimes the valve can be tested for patency and flushed to maintain patency by pumping several times to relieve the pressure. This is done by compressing the reservoir or antechamber of the valve mechanism, thus forcing a bolus of fluid from the reservoir into the distal catheter. Fluid that moves out of the chamber indicates a patent peritoneal catheter; ready refilling of the chamber with cerebrospinal fluid is evidence of a patent ventricular catheter. The procedure is repeated when indicated or routinely (a prescribed number of times every hour or two) as ordered. If these measures are unsuccessful, the shunt may require replacement.

Intake and output are carefully monitored. Children are often placed on fluid restriction with nothing by mouth (NPO) for 24 to 48 hours. The intravenous infusion is closely monitored to prevent fluid overload. Routine feeding is resumed after the prescribed NPO period, but the presence of bowel sounds is determined before feeding children with VP shunts.

Since infection is the greatest hazard of the postoperative period, nurses are continually on the alert for the usual manifestations of cerebrospinal fluid infection, which may include elevated vital signs, poor feeding, vomiting, decreased responsiveness, and seizure activity. There may be signs of local inflammation at the operative sites and along the shunt tract. Antibiotics are administered by the intravenous route as ordered, and the nurse may also need to assist the physician with intraventricular instillation. The incision site is inspected for leakage and any suspected drainage is tested for glucose, an indication of cerebrospinal fluid.

Meticulous skin care is continued postoperatively with extra care to prevent tissue damage from pressure. A sheepskin pad underneath the child and a doughnut for the head help prevent pressure on prominent areas. Skin is inspected regularly for any signs of pressure, irritation, or infection.

Family support. Specific needs and concerns of parents during periods of hospitalization are related to the reason for the child's hospitalization (shunt revision, infection, diagnosis) and the diagnostic and/or surgical procedures to which the child must be subjected. Often parents have very little understanding of anatomy; therefore they need further exploration and reinforcement of information that was given to them by the physician and neurosurgeon as well as information about what they can expect. They are especially frightened of any procedure that involves the brain, and the fear of retardation or brain damage is very real and pervasive. Nurses can do much to allay their anxiety with explanations of the rationale underlying the various nursing and medical activities such as positioning or testing and by simply being available and willing to listen to their concerns.

To prepare for the child's discharge and home care, the parents are instructed how to recognize signs that indicate shunt malfunction or infection and how to pump the shunt, if necessary. Active children may have accidents, such as a fall, that can damage the shunt, and the tubing may pull out of the distal insertion site or become disconnected during normal growth.

The management of hydrocephalus in a child is a demanding task for both family and health professionals, and helping a family cope with the child is an important nursing responsibility. It is important to emphasize that hydrocephalus is a life-long problem and that the child will require evaluation on a regular basis. The overall aim is to establish realistic goals and an appropriate educational program that will assist the child to achieve the optimum potential.

Anticipatory guidance will prepare parents for possible problems and help them to avoid being overprotective of the child. There need be few restrictions placed on the child's activities (mainly contact sports), and the child should be encouraged to live as would any other of the same age and abilities. Parents need support and encouragement in coping with the child and problems he may encounter in relationships with peers and others. Reactions of other children when the child has a noticeably enlarged head or requires shaving at the times of revision are stress situations for both child and parents (see Chapter 22 for problems and coping with the child with a disability).

Cranial Deformities

In the normal newborn the cranial sutures are separated by membranous seams several millimeters wide. For the first few hours to 1 to 2 days after birth, the cranial bones are highly mobile, which allows the cranial bones to mold and slide over one another, adjusting the circumference of the head to accommodate to the changing shape and character of the birth canal. The principal sutures in the infant's skull are the sagittal, coronal, and lambdoidal sutures, and the major soft areas at the juncture of these sutures are the anterior and posterior fontanels (see Fig. 8-7).

Following birth, growth of the skull bones occurs in a direction *perpendicular* to the line of the suture and normal closure occurs in a regular and predictable order. Although there are wide variations in the age at which closure takes place in individual children, normally all sutures and fontanels are ossified by the following ages:

8 weeks: posterior fontanel closed
6 months: fibrous union of suture lines and interlocking of serrated edges
18 months: anterior fontanel closed
12 years: sutures unable to be separated by increased intracranial pressure

Solid union of all sutures is not completed until very late childhood.

Closure of a suture before the expected time inhibits the perpendicular growth. Since normal increase in brain volume requires expansion, the skull is forced to grow in a direction *parallel* to the fused suture. This alteration in skull growth always produces a distortion of the head shape when the underlying brain growth is normal. The small head with closed and normal shape is the result of deficient brain growth; the suture closure is secondary to this brain growth failure. Failure of brain growth is not secondary to suture closure.

Various types of cranial deformities are encountered in early infancy. These include the enlarged head with frontal protrusion, or bossing, characteristic of hydrocephalus, the parietal bossing that is seen in chronic subdural hematoma, the small head, and a variety of skull deformities (Fig. 11-8). Some occur during prenatal development; in others, head circumference is usually within normal limits at birth and the deviation from normal development becomes apparent with advancing age.

MICROCEPHALY

Primary microcephaly reflects a small brain and may be caused by an autosomal-recessive disorder, a chromosomal

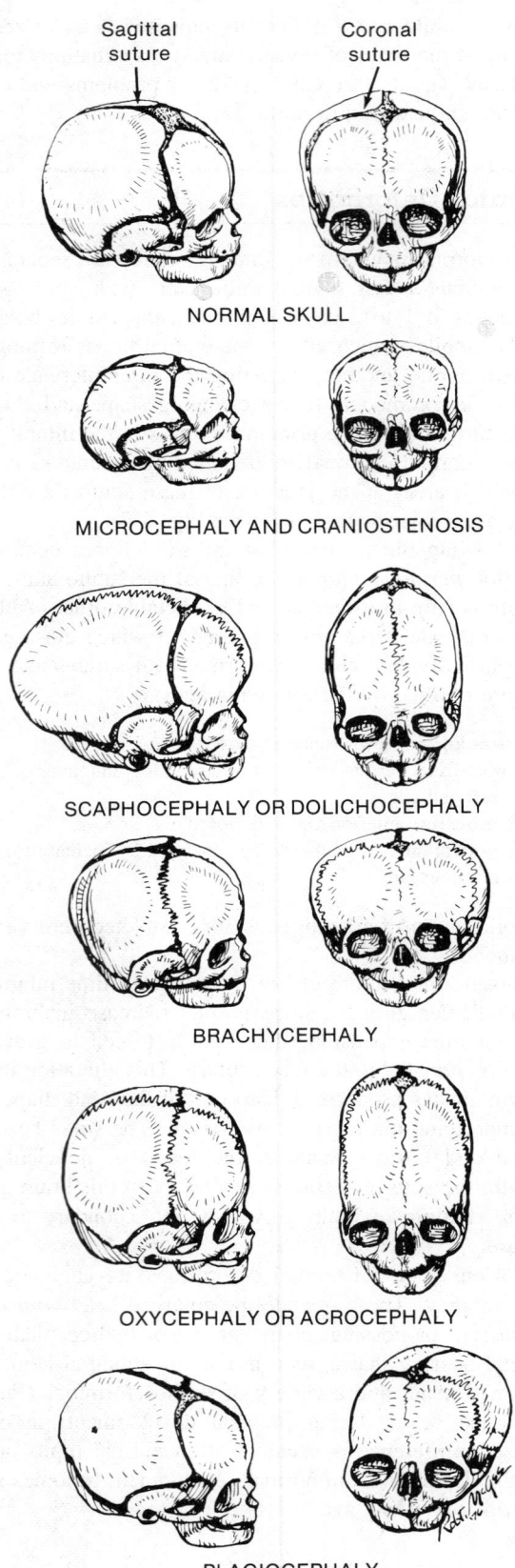

Sagittal suture

Coronal suture

NORMAL SKULL

MICROCEPHALY AND CRANIOSTENOSIS

SCAPHOCEPHALY OR DOLICHOCEPHALY

BRACHYCEPHALY

OXYCEPHALY OR ACROCEPHALY

PLAGIOCEPHALY

Fig. 11-8. Craniostenosis. Abnormal head configuration resulting from premature closing of cranial sutures.

abnormality, or application of a toxic stimulus during the period of induction and major cell migration in prenatal development. These stimuli may be irradiation (especially between 4 and 20 weeks of gestation), maternal infection (notably toxoplasmosis, rubella, or cytomegalovirus), or chemical agents. *Secondary microcephaly* can result from a variety of insults that occur during the third trimester of pregnancy, the perinatal period, or early infancy. Infection, trauma, metabolic disorders, and anoxia are all capable of causing decreased brain growth and early closure of cranial sutures.

In both types the neurologic manifestations range from decerebration, complete unresponsiveness, and/or autistic behavior to mild motor impairment, educable mental retardation, and/or mild hyperkinesis. There appears to be a decided relationship between microcephaly and mental retardation of varying degrees.

Nursing Considerations

There is no treatment. Nursing care is directed toward helping parents adjust to rearing a brain-damaged child (see Chapter 23).

CRANIOSYNOSTOSIS (CRANIOSTENOSIS)

In craniosynostosis, contrasted with microcephaly, suture closure is the primary defect and is not the result of impaired brain growth. As a consequence brain growth continues and the clinical picture depends on which sutures close, the duration of the closure process, and the success or failure of the other sutures to compensate by expansion. Usually the skull growth is inhibited in a direction at right angles to the closed sutures (see Fig. 11-8).

The most common form is premature closure of the sagittal suture with resulting elongation of the skull in the anteroposterior direction. (A similar head shape is seen as a result of postnatal position maintenance in some premature infants.) All degrees of craniosynostosis cause an increase in intracranial pressure, which may or may not cause mental retardation but can result in progressive papilledema, optic atrophy, and eventual blindness.

Therapeutic Management

Treatment, if any, involves surgical excision of long bars of bone along or parallel to the fused suture. Various surgical procedures are employed in an effort to release the fused suture and direct growth. Lining the bony margins of the suture with silicone to delay closure is infrequently used. Surgery is performed to achieve the best possible cosmetic effect and, in severe cases, to relieve cerebral pressure symptoms and complications. The advised timing of suture release is at 3 months of age (Jackson, 1986).

Nursing Considerations

Nursing care is primarily observation for signs of hemorrhage or infection. Following cranial surgery pressure bandages are applied and carefully maintained to reduce swelling. Providing emotional support to families is an important nursing function.

CRANIOFACIAL ABNORMALITIES

Craniofacial abnormalities are those deformities involving the skull and facial bones. They have a low incidence rate in the population but their effects can be psychologically devastating to affected children and their families. Abnormal growth of bones can produce a variety of deformities including:

hypertelorism Wide spacing between the eyes

Crouzon disease Craniofacial dysostosis (abnormal ossification of fetal cartilages) with shallow orbits and underdevelopment of the middle third of the face

Apert syndrome Craniostenosis resulting in a pointed head; may be extracranial abnormalities, such as syndactyly (webbing) of fingers and toes and cardiac defects

Treacher Collins syndrome Asymmetric facial deformity including absent cheekbones, underslung jaw, and small chin; there is also antimongoloid slant of the eyes and other minor defects

Pierre Robin syndrome Displacement of the chin as a result of micrognathia (mandibular hypoplasia) or retrognathia (normal sized mandible positioned posteriorly); there is also glossoptosis with obstruction of the airway, and a cleft palate may be present

The disorders are compatible with life; therefore unless they are corrected or modified, affected children go through their growing period under the burden of a grotesque, freaklike appearance often so severe that parents keep their children away from school, playmates, and sometimes even siblings (Koop, 1981).

Therapeutic Management

Surgical correction of defects involves peeling the patient's face away from the skull and remolding the understructures. Parts can be brought together, the skull reshaped, and pieces removed. The procedures are performed at various ages, depending on the anomaly, in centers specializing in this pediatric problem. The timing of surgery is determined on an individual basis to ensure normal growth and before school entry. Depending on the abnormality, other surgeries are performed, such as mandibular and digit correction. Following surgery, continued growth conforming to the inborn abnormality is unlikely.

Nursing Considerations

Nursing efforts are directed toward preparation for surgery (there may be several surgical procedures over a period of time), postoperative care similar to care of any child with cranial surgery, and support of the child and family. There is frequently adjustment to the unfamiliar body image, which may be as traumatic as the previous deformity. A

helmet is worn to protect the operative site and bone grafts for varying lengths of time, from 6 months to 2 years. Follow-up care is very important.

PLAGIOCEPHALY

Plagiocephaly is a rhomboid-shaped deformity that occurs in at least 1:300 live births and is rarely caused by brain malformation or unilateral suture stenosis (Clarren, 1981). The rapidly growing infant head is easily molded by continued pressure against a surface, such as the uterine wall or a mattress. As a result the skull is progressively flattened. There is usually a history of the infant lying on the flattened aspect of the head with limited head movement when lying down.

Therapeutic Management

Surgical correction of cosmetically disfiguring plagiocephaly is performed according to the nature and extent of the deformity. A recent innovation involves application of a helmet constructed of polypropylene shaped normally but large enough to fit the largest diameter of the head. Treatment is begun at 4 to 10 months of age, and the helmet is worn until the head conforms to the shape of the helmet.

Nursing Considerations

An important nursing function is helping to identify children with significant deformity and referring for evaluation. Nursing care of the surgical patient is the same as that for other children with similar surgery. Care of the child with helmet therapy involves teaching parents the importance of making certain that the child wears the device as prescribed. Mild unpleasant scalp odors that develop are controlled by daily washing of both scalp and helmet (Clarren, 1981).

Skeletal Defects

The types and variations of deformity in developmental skeletal defects are numerous and display an equally diverse spectrum of physical disability. Some skeletal deformities constitute one or more of the manifestations associated with a syndrome, for example, the short extremities of the various forms of dwarfism, the long, thin extremities and sternal deformities of arachnodactyly (Marfan syndrome), and somatic defects in chromosomal aberrations. Many are isolated defects with hereditary (clawhand, polydactyly), environmental (thalidomide phocomelia or amelia), or multifactorial (congenital hip dysplasia) etiology. This discussion is limited to those defects in development that are most common, that are amenable to therapy, and that involve nurses to a considerable extent. Less common defects and disorders are listed in Table 11-2.

Table 11-2 Congenital defects involving the skeleton

DISORDER	DESCRIPTION AND ANATOMIC VARIATION	THERAPY
Achondroplasia	Inherited (autosomal dominant) Defect in ossification at the epiphyseal plate, resulting in very short limbs, large head, and lordosis	None
Osteogenesis imperfecta	Inherited (autosomal dominant, autosomal recessive) Characterized by brittle, fragile, and easily fractured bones Intrauterine fractures may produce congenital deformities	Reduction of fractures Careful handling of extremities
Pes planus (flatfoot)	Normal finding in infancy May be result of muscular weakness in older child	Rarely indicated Wedge on inner side of heel and sole for persistent or severe cases
Pes valgus	Eversion of entire foot but sole rests on ground	Exercises
Pes varus	Inversion of entire foot but sole rests on ground	Exercises
Metatarsus valgus	Eversion of forefoot while heel remains straight Also called toeing out or duck walk	Passive exercises
Talipes* valgus	Eversion (turning outward) of foot so that only inner side of foot rests on ground	Passive exercises
Talipes varus	Inversion (turning inward) of foot so that only outer sole of foot rests on ground	Passive exercises May require casting
Talipes equinus	Extension or plantar flexion of foot so that only ball and toes rest on ground; commonly combined with talipes varus (most common of clubfoot deformities)	Repeated casting Exercises
Talipes calcaneus	Dorsal flexion of foot so that only heel rests on ground	Exercises
Supernumerary digits (polydactyly)	Excessive number of fingers, toes, or both; usually inherited (autosomal dominant)	No treatment, or amputation of extra digits to improve function or for cosmetic reasons
Genu varum (bowleg)	May be congenital, result of rickets, or caused by osteochondrosis of proximal tibial epiphysis	Corrective splinting Osteotomy in severe or neglected cases
Genu recurvatum (back knee)	Congenital, result of prenatal developmental defect or abnormal intrauterine position Developmental, result of postnatal trauma or infection	Repeated corrective casting Exercises
Klippel-Feil syndrome	Absence of one or more cervical vertebrae and two or more fused together Neck short and limited in motion Sometimes kyphosis and scoliosis	Rarely indicated Scapula brought down and fixed if marked deformity or loss of function Bracing of spinal deformities
Arachnodactyly (Marfan syndrome)	Inherited (autosomal dominant) Abnormal length of fingers, toes, and extremities; hypermobility of joints; defects of spine and chest (pigeon breast); other associated abnormalities	Supportive measures
Congenital spine deformities	Kyphosis, scoliosis, lordosis, or a combination of these	Prevention of progression of defect with growth Casting and/or bracing Operative stabilization of affected vertebrae
Arthrogryposis multiplex congenita	Incomplete fibrous ankylosis of many or all joints (except spine and jaw) associated with hypoplasia of attached muscles Contracture deformities—some extension, others flexion	Bracing, splinting, correcting surgery, and rehabilitation efforts

CONGENITAL HIP DYSPLASIA

The broad term *congenital hip dysplasia* describes imperfect development of the hip that can affect the femoral head, the acetabulum, or both. More commonly known as congenital hip dislocation (CHD) or congenital dislocated hip (CDH), the disorder is apparent at birth and displays various degrees of deformity. The condition is reversible with early treatment but can rapidly progress to dislocation as the child begins to walk. The cause of hip dysplasia is unknown, but it is one of the most common congenital defects, with an incidence of about 1:500 to 1:1000 births.

The disorder occurs more frequently in females than in

males (7:1) and occurs 25 to 30 times more often in first-degree relatives than in the general population. The concordance in monozygotic twins is 40% but only 3% in dizygotic twins, which suggests that genetic factors play a role in the etiology. One fourth of cases involve both hips, and when only one hip is involved the left hip is affected three times more often than the right. Congenital hip dysplasia is frequently associated with other conditions, such as spina bifida.

Pathophysiology

Three degrees of congenital dysplasia can be identified (Fig. 11-9):

acetabular dysplasia (or preluxation) The mildest form, in which there is neither subluxation nor dislocation. The dysplasia reflects an apparent delay in acetabular development evidenced by osseous hypoplasia of the acetabular roof that is oblique and shallow although the cartilaginous roof is comparatively intact. The femoral head remains in the acetabulum.

subluxation Accounts for the largest percentage of congenital hip dysplasias. Subluxation implies incomplete dislocation or dislocatable hip and is sometimes regarded as an intermediate state in the development from primary dysplasia to complete dislocation. The femoral head remains in contact with the acetabulum, but a stretched capsule and ligamentum teres cause the head of the femur to be partially displaced. Pressure on the cartilaginous roof inhibits ossification and produces a flattening of the socket.

dislocation The femoral head loses contact with the acetabulum and is displaced posteriorly and superiorly over the fibrocartilaginous rim. The ligamentum teres is elongated and taut.

There appear to be intrauterine, racial, and cultural factors associated with congenital hip disorders. There appears to be a striking relationship between the development of dislocation and methods of handling infants. Among the cultures with the highest incidence of dislocation, that is, Navajo Indians and Canadian Eskimos, newly born infants are tightly wrapped in blankets or other swaddling material or are strapped to cradle boards. In cultures where mothers traditionally carry infants on their backs or hips in the widely abducted straddle position, for example the Far East, the disorder is virtually unknown.

Prenatal factors that are considered to influence development of hip abnormalities are maternal hormone secretion and mechanical factors of intrauterine posture. Toward the end of pregnancy there is increased maternal pelvic laxity mediated by maternal hormone secretion (principally estrogen), which affects the fetal joints as well. All joints are more lax in the newborn period, and the greater incidence of hip dislocation in females may be explained by their greater reactivity to the maternal hormones. In addition, there is reliable evidence of an association between a higher incidence of congenital hip deformities and breech presentations and cesarean section (often necessitated by abnormal intrauterine position). The position of the legs in frank breech position—that is, with the hips acutely flexed and knees extended—is an important factor in the etiology of hip dislocation. The excess of firstborn children may be related to this factor, since the breech position in first deliveries is nearly always a frank breech. Other prenatal factors that contribute to hip dysplasia include twinning and large infant size.

Clinical Manifestations

The diagnosis of congenital hip dysplasia should be made in the newborn period if possible, since treatment initiated before 2 months of age achieves the highest rate of success. In the newborn period dysplasia usually appears as hip joint laxity rather than as outright dislocation. Subluxation and the tendency to dislocate can be demonstrated by the Ortolani or Barlow tests. With the infant relaxed in the supine position and the legs facing the examiner, the hips are flexed at right angles and the knees are flexed. The examiner places the middle finger of each hand over the greater trochanter and the thumbs on the inner side of the thigh at a point opposite the lesser trochanter. The knees are carried to midabduction and each hip joint in turn is submitted first to forward pressure exerted behind the trochanter and second to backward pressure exerted from the thumbs in front as the opposite joint is held steady. If the femoral head can be felt to slip forward into the acetabulum on pressure from

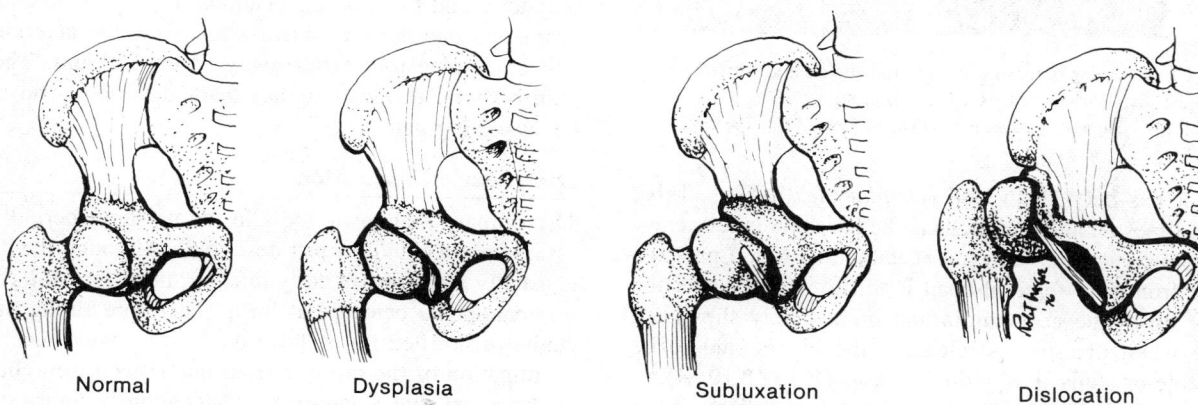

Normal   Dysplasia   Subluxation   Dislocation

Fig. 11-9. Configuration and relationship of structures in congenital hip deformities.

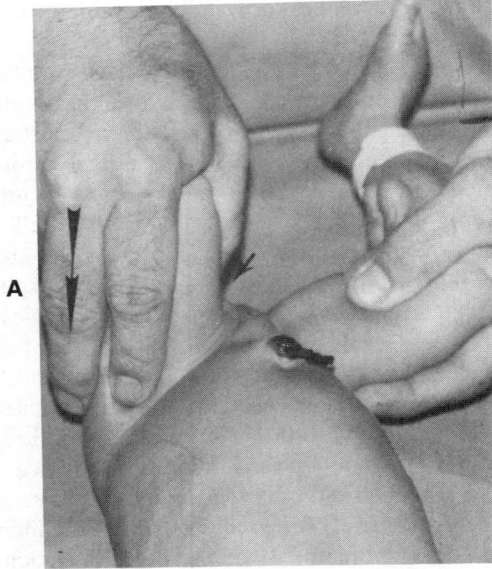

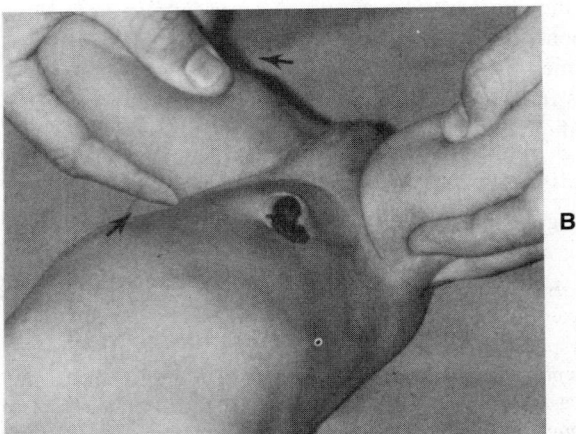

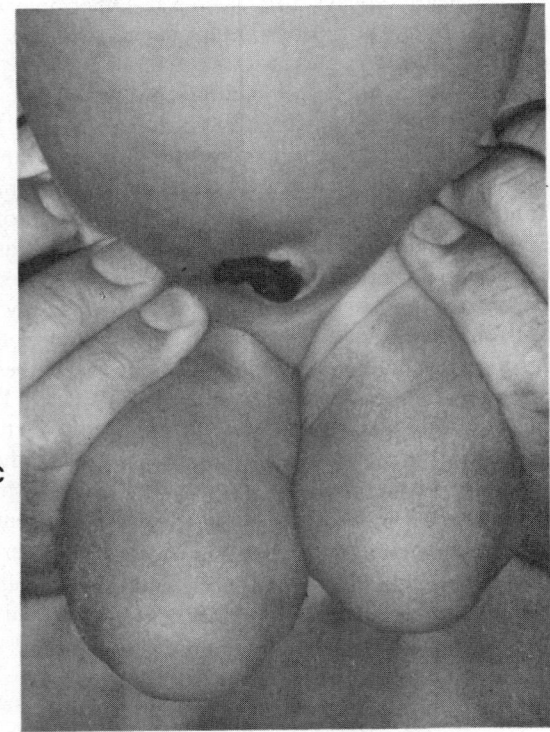

Fig. 11-10. Tests for detecting congenital dislocated hip. **A,** Ortolani test. **B,** Barlow test. **C,** Galleazzi sign.

From Filston, H.C.: Surgical problems in children, St. Louis, 1982, The C.V. Mosby Co.

behind, it has been dislocated *(Ortolani test)* (Fig. 11-10, *B*). Sometimes an audible click can be heard on exit or entry of the femur out of or into the acetabulum. If, on pressure from the front, the femoral head is felt to slip out over the posterior lip of the acetabulum and immediately slips back in place when pressure is released, the hip is said to be dislocatable or "unstable" *(Barlow test)* (Fig. 11-10, *A*).

The Ortolani and Barlow tests are most reliable from birth to 2 months of age and must be performed by experienced operators to prevent fracture or other damage to the hip. For example, when performed too vigorously in the first 2 days of life, when the hip subluxes freely, persistent dislocation may occur (Cheetham and others, 1983). Adduction contractures develop at about 6 to 10 weeks and the Ortolani sign disappears. After this time the most sensitive test is limited abduction. Other signs are shortening of the limb on the affected side *(Galleazzi sign)* (Fig. 11-10,*C*), asymmetric thigh and gluteal folds, and broadening of the perineum (in bilateral dislocation). Weight bearing may precipitate a transition from subluxation to dislocation in unrecognized cases. Often the disorder is not apparent at birth.

In the older infant and child the affected leg will be shorter than the other with telescoping or piston mobility, that is, the head of the femur can be felt to move up and down in the buttock when the extended thigh is pushed first toward the child's head and then pulled distally. Instability of the hip on weight bearing delays walking and produces a characteristic limp. When the child stands first on one foot and then on the other (holding onto a chair, rail, or someone's hands) bearing weight on the affected hip, the pelvis tilts downward on the normal side instead of upward as it would with normal stability *(Trendelenburg sign)*. In both unilateral and bilateral dislocations the greater trochanter is prominent and appears above a line from the anterior superior iliac spine to the tuberosity of the ischium. The child with bilateral dislocations has marked lordosis and a peculiar waddling gait.

Diagnostic Evaluation

The primary diagnostic tools in the newborn period are the assessment techniques just described. Although the disorder is usually identified in early infancy, there is also a category that cannot be detected at birth. Therefore ruling out congenital dislocated hip at birth does not provide security and examination of the hip is carried out at each well-child visit in the event that a late-onset dislocation becomes evident. In older infants and children radiographic examination is useful in confirming the diagnosis. An upward slope in the roof of the acetabulum (the acetabular angle) greater than 40 degrees with upward and outward displacement of the femoral head is a frequent finding in older children. Radiographic examination in early infancy is not reliable because ossification of the femoral head does not normally take place until the third to sixth month of life. However, the cartilaginous head can be visualized directly with real-time high-resolution ultrasonography.

Therapeutic Management

Treatment is begun as soon as the condition is recognized, since early intervention is more favorable to the restoration of normal bony architecture and function. The longer treatment is delayed, the more severe the deformity, the more difficult the treatment, and the less favorable the prognosis. The treatment varies with the age of the child and the extent of the dysplasia.

Newborn to six months. The hip joint is maintained by dynamic splinting in a safe position with the proximal femur centered in the acetabulum in an attitude of flexion. A variety of abduction devices are available for maintaining the femur in the acetabulum. Of these the Pavlik harness is the most widely used device, and with time, motion, and gravity the hip works into a more abducted, reduced position (Fig. 11-11). The harness is worn full time until the hip

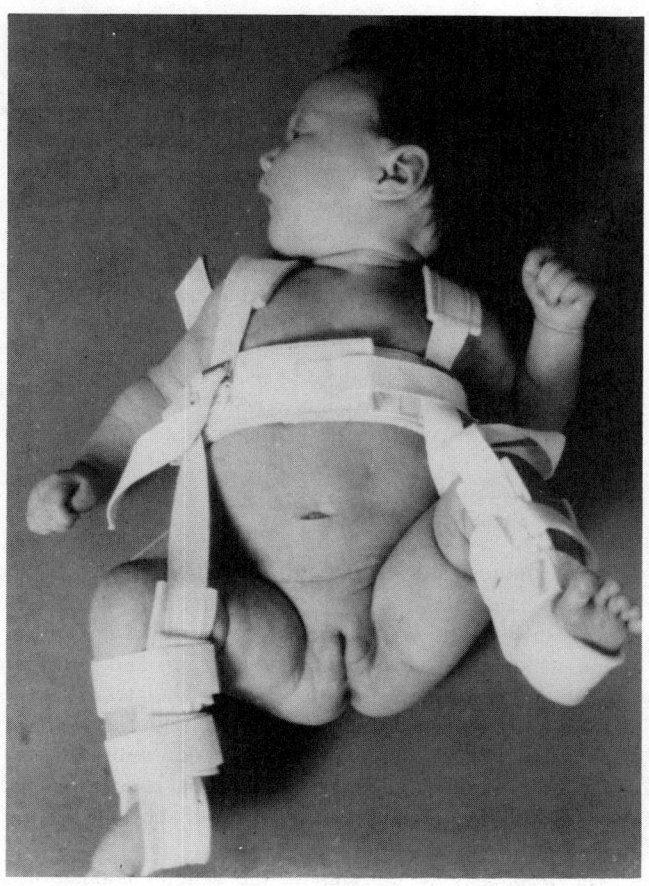

Fig. 11-11. Child in Pavlik harness.
Courtesy Dr. Mark Capehart, Tulsa, OK.

is clinically and radiographically stable, usually about 3 to 6 months. It is highly effective when the device is well constructed, follow-up care is adequate, and the parents follow instructions in its use.

When adduction contracture is present, other devices are employed to slowly and gently stretch the hip to full abduction, after which wide abduction is maintained until stability is attained. When there is difficulty in maintaining stable reduction, a plaster hip spica cast is applied and changed periodically to accommodate the child's growth. After 3 to 6 months, sufficient stability is acquired to allow transfer to a removable protective abduction brace. The duration of treatment depends on development of the acetabulum but is usually accomplished within the first year.

Six to eighteen months. In this age-group the dislocation is not recognized until the child begins to stand and walk, when attendant shortening of the limb and contractures of hip adductor and flexor muscles become apparent. Gradual reduction by traction is followed by plaster cast immobilization, which is maintained until radiographic examination confirms a stable joint. Often soft tissue may obstruct and complicate reduction and subsequent joint development. In this case open reduction is performed to remove the obstruction with postoperative spica cast immobilization and, after 4 to 6 months, replacement with an abduction splint.

Older child. Correction of the hip deformity in the older child is inherently more difficult than in the preceding age-groups because secondary adaptive changes complicate the condition. Operative reduction, which may involve preoperative traction, tenotomy of contracted muscles, and any one of several innominate osteotomy procedures designed to construct an acetabular roof, is usually required. After cast removal and before weight bearing is permitted, range of motion exercises help restore movement. Next, rehabilitative measures are instituted. Successful reduction and reconstruction become increasingly difficult after the age of 4 years and are usually impossible or inadvisable after age 6 because of severe shortening and contracture of muscles and deformity of the femoral and acetabular structures.

Nursing Considerations

Nurses are in a unique position to detect congenital dislocation of the hip in the newborn. During the infant assessment process and routine nurturing activities the hips and extremities are inspected for any deviations from normal. Usually only nurses specially trained in the technique are permitted to perform Ortolani and Barlow tests, but any nurse can be alert to other signs such as leg shortening, gluteal folds, and limited abduction. Diapering, for example, provides an excellent opportunity to observe for limited movement and a wide perineum. These observations are reported to the attending physician, and the ambulatory child who displays a limp or an unusual gait should be referred for evaluation. This may indicate an orthopedic or neurologic problem.

Care of the child in a reduction device. The major nursing problems in the care of an infant or child in a cast or other device are related to maintenance of the device and adapting nurturing activities to meet the needs of the infant or child. Generally treatment and follow-up care of these children are carried out in a clinic, physician's office, or outpatient unit. Hospitalization may be necessary for cast application or brace fitting but seldom exceeds 24 to 48 hours. Longer hospitalization is required for open reduction or if the child is hospitalized for a concurrent illness.

The major nursing function is teaching parents to apply and maintain the reduction device. The Pavlik harness allows for easy handling of the infant and usually produces less apprehension in the parent than heavy braces and casts. It is important that parents understand the correct use of the appliance, which may or may not allow for its removal during bathing. When the infant has a harness that is not removed, a sponge bath is recommended and the skin beneath the harness is assessed daily for irritation. Powders and lotions are not used because they tend to cake or "ball" underneath straps or clothing.

The parents are permitted to pad shoulder straps at pressure points if desired, but unbuckling or removal is determined individually based on the family's level of understanding and the degree of deformity in the hip. If allowed, the family needs to know how to adjust the harness if buckles become loose. Many physicians prefer to see the child before any adjustment is attempted to make certain the hips are in correct placement before the harness is resecured (Mulley, 1984).

Casts and braces offer more challenging nursing problems since they cannot be removed for routine care, although sometimes the physician allows a brace to be removed for bathing. Care of an infant or small child with a cast requires nursing innovation to reduce irritation and to maintain cleanliness of both the child and the cast, particularly in the diaper area. Cast care and observation are discussed in Chapter 40 and therefore are not elaborated here. However, inasmuch as congenital dislocated hip is almost the exclusive reason for application of casts in early infancy, some of the problems specific to that age-group are mentioned.

Parents are taught the proper care of the cast (or brace) and are helped to devise means for maintaining cleanliness. A disposable diaper (newborn size) is tucked beneath the entire perineal opening of the cast. A larger (toddler size) diaper can be applied and fastened over the small diaper and cast (Holland, 1983). For heavy wetters or for night use, a sanitary napkin can be placed inside the small diaper for added absorbency. Both diapers are changed at each wetting.

For tightly fitting casts the Op-Site sheeting can be cut into strips as for petalling (p. 1805) and one edge applied to the cast edge and the other directly to the perineum; this forms a continuous waterproof bridge between the perineum and the cast to prevent leakage. An additional advantage to the use of this transparent dressing material is that it keeps both the skin and cast dry while allowing for observation of skin beneath the dressing.

Older infants and small children may stuff bits of food, small toys, or other items under the cast; parents should be alerted to this possibility so that suitable preventive measures can be instigated.

Feeding the infant in a hip spica cast or brace offers problems of positioning. Very young infants can be fed in the supine position with head elevated, and, with the infant's hips and legs supported on a pillow at her side, the mother can cuddle the infant in her arms during feeding. A somewhat similar position can be used for breast-feeding, that is, with the infant supported on pillows or held in a "football" hold facing the mother with the legs behind her. An alternate position is to hold the infant upright on the mother's lap with the legs of the infant astride the mother's leg. Infants who are able to sit up can be fed in a feeding table or modified high chair. Parents may be able to fashion a tilt board with padded seat or an adjustable chair.

It is important for nurses, parents, and other caregivers to understand that these children need to be involved in all the activities of any child in the same age-group. Toys are chosen that can be used in a prone position on the floor or in the seats devised for feeding and other activities. Confinement in a cast or appliance should not exclude children from family (or unit) activities. They can be held astride a lap for comfort and transported to areas of activity. The child may be allowed to walk in a cast or brace. See Chapter 40 for further discussion of care of a child in a spica cast.

CONGENITAL CLUBFOOT

Clubfoot is a general term used to describe a common deformity in which the foot is twisted out of its normal shape or position. Any foot deformity involving the ankle is called *talipes,* derived from *talus,* meaning ankle, and *pes,* meaning foot. Deformities of foot and ankle are conveniently described according to the position of the ankle and foot. The more common positions involve the following variations:

talipes varus An inversion or a bending inward
talipes valgus An eversion or bending outward
talipes equinus Plantar flexion in which the toes are lower than the heel
talipes calcaneus Dorsiflexion, in which the toes are higher than the heel

Most clubfeet are a combination of these positions, and the most frequently occurring type of clubfoot (approximately 95%) is the composite deformity *talipes equinovarus,* in which the foot is pointed downward and inward in varying degrees of severity (Fig. 11-12). Unilateral clubfoot is somewhat more common than bilateral clubfoot and may occur as an isolated defect or in association with other disorders or syndromes such as chromosomal aberrations, arthrogryposis (a generalized immobility of the joints), cerebral palsy, or spina bifida.

The frequency of clubfoot in the general population is 1:700 to 1:1000 live births, with boys affected twice as of-

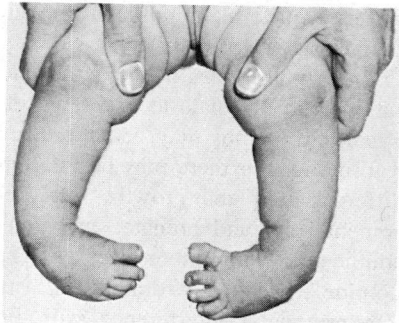

Fig. 11-12. Bilateral congenital talipes equinovarus (congenital clubfoot) in 2-month-old infant.

From Brashear, H.R., Jr., and Raney, R.B.: Shands' handbook of orthopaedic surgery, ed. 9, St. Louis, 1978, The C.V. Mosby Co.

ten as girls. There is a 35% concordance in monozygotic twins as opposed to a 3% concordance in dizygotic twins, which indicates a hereditary component.

Pathophysiology

The precise cause is unknown. There are those who attribute the defect to abnormal positioning and restricted movement in utero, although the evidence is not conclusive. Others implicate arrested or anomalous embryonic development, since the foot normally goes through flexion and eversion during early development and gradually assumes a normal attitude by the seventh month. Arrested development during this early stage tends to result in a rigid deformity, whereas mechanical pressures from intrauterine position are more likely to be operating in the more flexible deformities. Embryologists are divided in acceptance of the embryonic arrest theory.

Diagnostic Evaluation

The deformity is readily apparent and easily detected at birth. However, it must be differentiated from some positional deformities that can be passively corrected or overcorrected. The true clubfoot is fixed. Paralytic changes in the lower extremity of children with neuromuscular involvement often produce equinovarus deformity.

Therapeutic Management

The rapid growth during infancy is a potent remodeling force. When treatment is indicated, this rapid growth will improve the result, facilitate the quality of correction, and decrease the time required for treatment (Bunch, 1979). Treatment is begun as soon as the deformity is recognized and involves three stages: (1) correction of the deformity, (2) maintenance of the correction until normal muscle balance is regained, and (3) follow-up observation to avert possible recurrence of the deformity. Some feet respond to treatment readily, some respond only to prolonged, vigorous, and sustained efforts, and the improvement in others remains disappointing even with maximal effort on the part of all concerned.

Correction of talipes equinovarus is most reliably accomplished by manipulation and the application of a series of casts begun immediately or shortly after birth and continued until marked overcorrection is reached (Fig. 11-13). Successive casts allow for gradual stretching of tight structures on the medial side and gradual contraction of lax structures on the lateral side of the foot. Manipulation and casting are repeated frequently (every few days for 1 to 2 weeks then at 1- to 2-week intervals) in order to accommodate the rapid growth of early infancy. Because of strong, thickened ligaments, cartilaginous anlages of the bone may become distorted. If manipulation is ineffective, surgical correction is performed to correct bony deformity, release tight ligaments, or lengthen or transplant tendons. The extremity or extremities are casted until the desired result is achieved.

Nursing Considerations

Nursing care of the child with nonsurgical correction of clubfoot is the same as it is for any child who has a cast (p. 1805). The child will spend a considerable time in a corrective device; therefore, nursing care plans include both long-term and short-term goals. Conscientious observation of skin and circulation is particularly important in young infants because of their normally rapid growth rate. Since treatment and follow-up care are handled in the orthopedist's office, clinic, or outpatient department, parent education and support are important in nursing care of these children.

Parents need to understand the overall treatment program, the importance of regular cast changes, and the role they play in the long-term effectiveness of the therapy. Reinforcing and clarifying the orthopedist's explanations and instructions, teaching parents about care of cast or appliance, including vigilant observation for potential problems, and encouraging parents to facilitate normal development within the limitations imposed by the deformity or therapy are all part of nursing responsibilities.

METATARSUS ADDUCTUS (VARUS)

Metatarsus adductus, or metatarsus varus, is probably the most common congenital foot deformity. In most instances it is the result of abnormal intrauterine positioning and is usually detected at birth. The deformity is characterized by

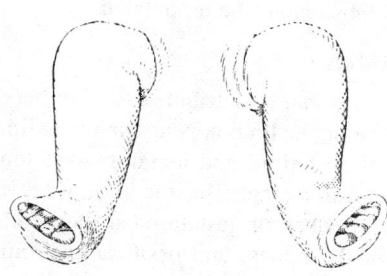

Fig. 11-13. Feet casted for correction of bilateral congenital talipes equinovarus.

From Brashear, H.R., Jr., and Raney, R.B.: Shands' handbook of orthopaedic surgery, ed. 9, St. Louis, 1978, The C.V. Mosby Co.

medial adduction of the toes and forefoot, frequently associated with inversion, and convexity of the lateral border of the foot. Unlike talipes equinovarus, with which it is often confused, the angulation occurs at the tarsometatarsal joint while the heel and ankle remain in a neutral position. This deformity often causes a pigeon-toed gait in the child.

Management depends on the rigidity of the deformity. Correction can usually be accomplished by gentle manipulation and passive stretching of the foot, which the parent is taught to perform. Repeated and consistent stretching is continued for the first 6 weeks, after which the treatment is based on the flexibility of the foot. Those feet that do not respond to the manipulation require orthopedic therapy. If the child is able to actively overcorrect the deformity voluntarily on stimulation, continued stretching is generally sufficient. If the foot cannot be actively or passively overcorrected, the feet are stretched and manipulated and held with casts.

Nursing Considerations

The nursing role primarily involves identifying the defect, so that early therapy can be instigated, and parent teaching. The nurse teaches the parents how to hold the heel firmly and to stretch only the forefoot, otherwise undue force on the heel may produce a valgus deformity. If casting is needed, the nurse instructs the parents in cast care and observation (see p. 1807).

SKELETAL LIMB DEFICIENCY

Congenital limb deficiencies, or reduction malformations, are manifest by a variety of degree of loss of functional capacity. They are characterized by underdevelopment of skeletal elements of the extremities. The range of malformation can extend from minor defects of the digits to serious abnormalities such as *amelia,* absence of an entire extremity, or *meromelia,* partial absence of an extremity that includes *phocomelia* (seal limbs), an intercalary deficiency of long bones with relatively good development of hands and feet attached at or near the shoulder or the hips.

In rare instances prenatal destruction of limbs has been reported, but most reduction deformities are primary defects of development (agenesis, aplasia). Therefore, congenital amputations, in the literal sense, are not amputations, since nonexistent limbs cannot be amputated.

Pathophysiology

Limb deficiencies can be attributed to both heredity and environment. The upper limb appears first as a limb bud in the fourth week of gestation, and its entire skeleton can be recognized in its early stages by the fifth week of gestation. During the sixth week of gestation cartilage forms the structural model of the bones, and ossification from humerus to phalanges begins between the sixth and seventh weeks of gestation. The development of the upper limbs precedes that of the lower limbs slightly, and the cartilaginous structure appears in a proximodistal sequence. By 8 weeks of gesta-

tion the digits are well formed and their number determined; by 12 weeks of gestation primary centers of ossification can be detected in nearly all bones of the extremities.

Malformations can originate at any stage of limb development. Formation of limbs may be suppressed at the time of limb bud formation, or there may be interference in later stages of differentiation and growth. Heredity appears to play a prominent role, and prenatal environmental insults have been implicated in a number of cases. The well-publicized thalidomide tragedy is a dramatic illustration of the effects of environmental interference with limb development. Children damaged by maternal ingestion of the drug displayed a variety of serious limb anomalies that demonstrated a clear relationship between the time of exposure and the presence and type of limb deformity.

Therapeutic Management

It is generally agreed that children with congenital limb deficiencies should be fitted with prosthetic devices whenever possible and that such a functional replacement should be applied at the earliest possible stage of development in an attempt to match the motor readiness of the infant. This favors natural progression of prosthetic use. For example, an infant with an upper extremity deficiency is fitted with a simple passive device, such as a mitten prosthesis, between 3 and 6 months of age when limb exploration is active, sitting is beginning with the extremities needed for support, and bilateral hand activities are to be encouraged. Lower limb prostheses are applied when the infant is ready to pull to a standing position. In preparation for prosthetic devices surgical modification is often necessary to ensure the most favorable use of the device, since severe deformity can interfere with its effective use. Phocomelic digits are preserved for controlling switches of externally powered appliances in upper extremities. Digits (in both upper and lower extremities) provide the child with surfaces for tactile exploration and stimulation. Prostheses are replaced to accommodate growth and increasing capabilities of the child.

Nursing Considerations

Prosthetic application training and habilitation are most successfully carried out in a center that specializes in meeting the special needs of these children, especially the very young children and those with multiple amputations. It involves a team of health professionals including the parents, who must encourage the child in making age-commensurate adjustments to the environment. Although these children need assistance, excessive overprotection may produce overdependency with later maladjustment to school and other situations.

Disorders of the Gastrointestinal Tract

Congenital defects of the gastrointestinal (GI) tract can involve any portion from the mouth to the anus. Most are apparent at birth or shortly after and are anomalies in which normal growth ceased at a crucial stage of embryonic development, leaving the structure in an embryonic form or only partially completed. The result may be atresia, malposition, nonclosure, or any number of variations.

Atresia is absence or closure of a normal body orifice. Closure at any point along the length of the GI tract creates an obstruction to the normal progress of nutrients and secretions. Most common anomalies are atresias of the esophagus, intestine, and anus, requiring surgical intervention.

Other defects of development include *annular pancreas,* in which the head of the pancreas surrounds and constricts the second segment of duodenum, and *malrotation of the colon,* in which associated structures remain in abnormal positions. For example, the cecum remains in the upper right quadrant and the posterior fixation of the mesentery is inadequate and allows twisting of the small intestine, or *volvulus,* to create an obstruction.

Obstruction can also be caused by *peritoneal bands* or *folds* that cross the duodenum as they attach the abnormally placed cecum to the right peritoneum. Thus the duodenum is partially obstructed by the external pressure of the bands. In *meconium ileus* the intestine becomes obstructed by thick, inspissated, impacted meconium—the earliest manifestation of cystic fibrosis. *Congenital megacolon (Hirschsprung disease)* is caused by the absence or deficiency of innervation to the musculature of the rectum and distal colon, which inhibits propulsive peristalsis and creates a functional obstruction.

The diagnosis and management of most intestinal atresias and obstructions are similar to that of intestinal obstruction from other factors, most of which are discussed in Chapter 33. The congenital defects considered in this chapter include abnormalities of the lip and palate, esophagus, anus, and biliary tree. Biliary atresia is also considered here because the liver is part of the digestive system, although the condition does not interfere with the passage of food. Some malformations of the gastrointestinal tract are considered here since they are identified at birth and are cause for considerable parental concern.

CLEFT LIP AND/OR PALATE

Clefts of the lip and palate are facial malformations that are common to all human populations and constitute a severe handicap to the affected individual. The defects are classified into two major groups. The first includes those clefts that involve the lip and anterior maxilla regardless of whether the defect involves the remaining portions of the hard and soft palate (sometimes called harelip). The second group consists of those clefts that involve only the hard and soft palate. Although there are differences in the severity and extent of deformities within each category, the terms and their abbreviations associated with these groups are:

CL Clefts that involve the lip
CLP Clefts that involve the lip and palate
CL(P) Clefts that involve the lip with or without cleft palate

CP Clefts that involve the hard and soft palate only
CL/P All types of clefts that involve the lip and/or palate

The term *complete cleft* indicates the maximum degree of clefting.

Etiology

Many factors appear to be involved in the etiology of cleft of the lip and/or palate, and evidence indicates that cleft lip with or without cleft palate is developmentally and genetically different from cleft palate. Defective development of the embryonic *primary* palate may result in clefts of the lip and anterior maxilla; clefts of the hard and soft palate are caused by defective development of the embryonic *secondary* palate and often appear in persons with cleft lip. There are no less than 50 recognized syndromes that include cleft lip and/or palate as a feature: some are caused by mutant genes, others result from chromosomal abnormalities, and teratogens have been implicated in a very small number.

The great majority of cases appear to be consistent with the concept of multifactorial inheritance as evidenced by an increased incidence in relatives and a higher concordance in monozygotic than in dizygotic twins. However, there is apparently no relationship between the incidence of cleft lip with or without cleft palate and the incidence of cleft palate among relatives; that is, relatives of persons with cleft palate have an increased incidence of cleft palate but not cleft lip with or without cleft palate and vice versa.

The overall incidence of cleft lip and/or cleft palate is 1:750 to 1:1000 births (American Cleft Palate Education Foundation, undated) and shows a wide variation in races. The defect appears more often in Orientals and certain tribes of American Indians than in whites and less frequently in American blacks. There is less racial difference in the specific defects. More males than females have cleft lip with or without cleft palate, particularly the more severe defects, but cleft palate occurs more often in females. Cleft lip and palate are the most common of the facial malformations (40%) (March of Dimes–Birth Defects Foundation, undated).

Pathophysiology

Development of the primary and secondary palates takes place at different times and involves different developmental processes. Cleft lip with or without cleft palate results from failure of the maxillary processes to fuse with the nasal elevations on the frontal prominence, which normally occurs during the sixth week of gestation (Fig. 11-14, *A*). Merging of the upper lip at the midline is completed between the seventh and eighth weeks of gestation. There is evidence that in some cases separation may be the result of rupture subsequent to fusion, however.

Fusion of the secondary palate (hard and soft palate) takes place later in development, between the seventh and twelfth weeks of gestation (Fig. 11-14, *B* to *D*). At the time the primary palate is completed, the two lateral palatine processes are situated in a vertical position at the side of the tongue. In the process of migrating to a horizontal position they are, for a short time, separated by the tongue. With

to the floor of the nose. Where the cleft is unilateral, about two thirds is on the left side, and an associated cleft palate is found more often with bilateral than with unilateral cleft lip. Varying degrees of nasal distortion usually accompany cleft lip, and the defect frequently involves supernumerary, deformed, or absent teeth.

Clefts of the palate may occur as an isolated defect or in association with cleft lip. Less obvious than cleft lip, the defect may not be detected without a thorough assessment of the mouth. The deformity can be identified by placing the examiner's fingers directly on the palate. Without a proper evaluation, the defect may not be detected until the infant has difficulty with initial feedings. As with cleft lip, the degree of deformity varies and may involve only the uvula or may extend through both the soft and hard palates to the incisive foramen. The isolated cleft palate occurs in the midline, but, when associated with cleft lip, it may involve the midline of the soft palate and extend into the hard palate on the side of the lip cleft or on both sides in bilateral clefts. Clefts of the hard palate form a continuous opening between the mouth and the nasal cavity. This creates special feeding problems. The infant is unable to develop suction because of the defect and has difficulty in swallowing. The open pathway must be closed in order to provide sufficient pressure for the swallowing sequence.

Therapeutic Management

Treatment of the child with cleft lip and palate involves the cooperative efforts of a number of specialists—pediatrician, nurses, plastic surgeon, orthodontist, prosthodontist, otolaryngologist, speech therapist, and sometimes a psychiatrist. Treatment continues over a long time, but even after completion of a program of health care the child will probably retain defects of speech, facial appearance, or other problems related to the cleft. Management is directed toward closure of the cleft(s), prevention of complications, habilitation, and facilitation of normal growth and development of the child.

Surgical correction: cleft lip. Closure of the lip defect precedes that of the palate, although the optimum times for surgery are still being debated. Those who favor immediate repair of the lip argue that it makes the infant more acceptable to the parents before discharge from the hospital, thereby improving establishment of satisfactory parent-child relationships. Others prefer to wait until the infant shows a steady weight gain and a satisfactory hemoglobin level. They believe that the delay helps the infant better withstand the surgery, offers time to detect any associated serious anomalies unrecognized at birth, and reduces parental disappointment with surgical repair. That is, parents ordinarily adjust to the defect during this time and more fully appreciate the cosmetic effects of the surgical correction. Technical repair of the cleft lip and/or palate can be done quite successfully at any age.

The method of repair of the lip cleft involves one of several staggered suture lines to minimize notching of the lip from retraction of scar tissue. Postoperatively the suture line

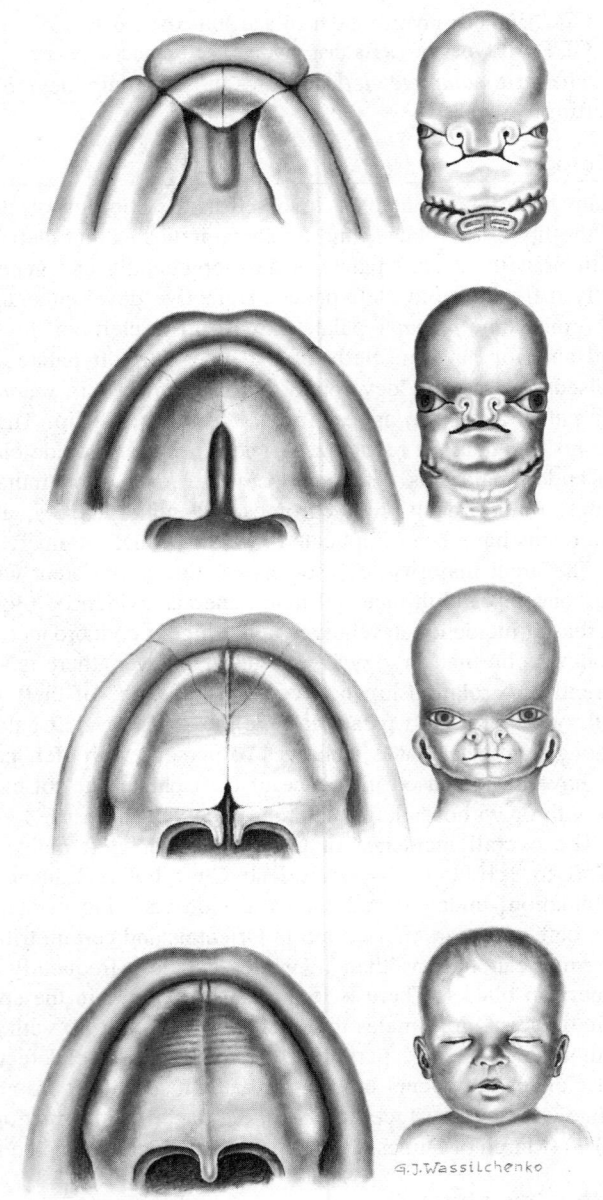

Fig. 11-14. Stages in palatine development.

development of the neck and jaws, the tongue moves downward, allowing the palatine processes to fuse with each other and with the primary palate to form the roof of the mouth. If there is delay in this movement or if the tongue fails to descend soon enough, the remainder of development proceeds but the palate never fuses.

Diagnostic Evaluation

The cleft that involves the lip with or without cleft palate is readily apparent at birth and is one of the defects that elicits the most severe emotional reactions in parents. Incomplete fusion of the primary palate produces a variation in the degree of malformation (Fig. 11-15). Clefts of the lip may be unilateral or bilateral and may range from a notch in the vermilion border of the lip to complete separation extending

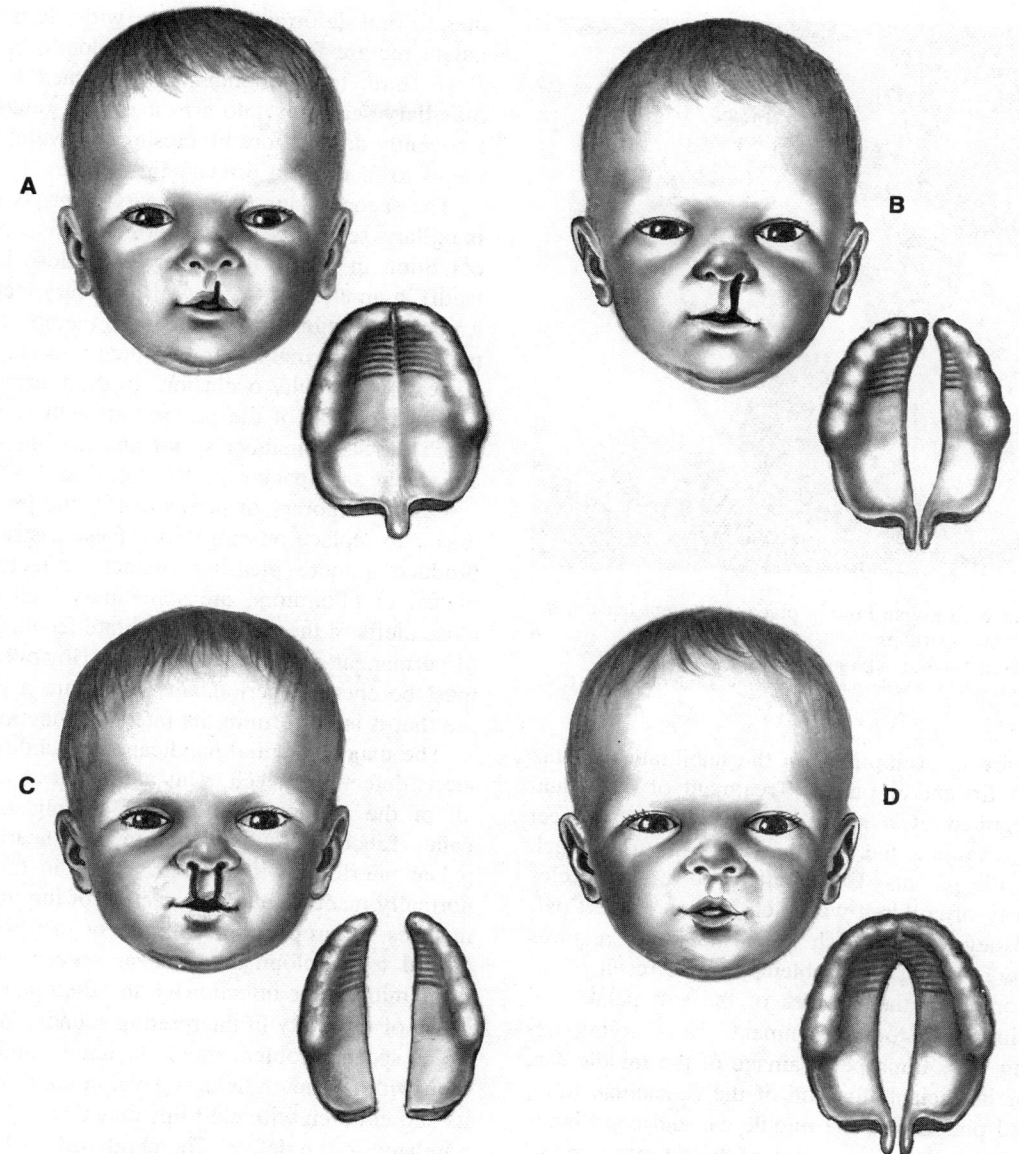

Fig. 11-15. Variations in clefts of lip and palate at birth. **A,** Notch in vermilion border; **B,** unilateral cleft lip and palate; **C,** bilateral cleft lip and cleft palate; **D,** cleft palate.

is protected from tension by a thin, arched metal device (the Logan bow) (Fig. 11-16) taped to the cheeks or a butterfly-type adhesive restraint, and the arms are restrained at the elbows to prevent the infant's hands from rubbing the incision.

Improved surgical techniques have minimized deformity related to scar retraction, but good cosmetic results are difficult to obtain in defects that are more severe initially. In the absence of infection or trauma, healing takes place with little scar formation; however, in some instances the results are less than satisfactory from the parents' (and, later, the child's) viewpoint. Undesirable physical characteristics of the older child are residual nasal deformity, mildly protruding lower lip, and a somewhat flattened lower third of the upper lip usually with an abnormally shaped red lip margin. Not infrequently revisions may be required at a later age.

Surgical correction: cleft palate. Cleft palate repair is generally postponed until a later age than repair of the cleft lip in order to take advantage of palatal changes that occur with normal growth. Since clefts vary considerably in size, shape, and degree of deformity, the timing of repair is individualized but is usually performed sometime between the ages of 6 months and 5 years. Most surgeons prefer to close the cleft between 1 and 2 years of age, before the child develops faulty speech habits. Others believe that best results are obtained when surgery is delayed until 4 years of age. If surgery is delayed beyond 3 years of age, a special denture plate helps occlude the cleft to assist in development of normal speech patterns. In addition, it is inadvisable to remove the tonsils because they trap air and thus allow for better speech.

Long-term problems. The team concept in the deliv-

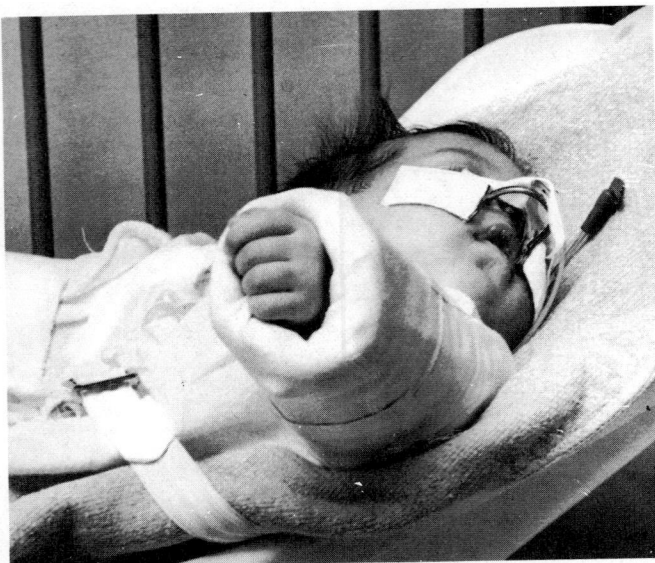

Fig. 11-16. Infant with Logan bow in place to prevent tension on suture line and elbow restraints.

Courtesy Children's Health Center, San Diego, CA. From Ingalls, A.J., and Salerno, M.C.: Maternal and child health nursing, ed. 4, St. Louis, 1979, The C.V. Mosby Co.

ery of health care is exemplified in the habilitation of the child with cleft lip and/or palate. Treatment of individual patients is integrated by a group of specialists who meet periodically to examine the child and consult with each other and with the parents. Even with good anatomic closure, the majority of children with cleft lip and/or cleft palate have some degree of speech impairment that requires speech therapy. The physical problems are the result of inefficient functioning of the muscles of the soft palate and nasopharynx, improper tooth alignment, and varying degrees of hearing loss. Improper drainage of the middle ear, as the result of inefficient function of the eustachian tube, causes increased pressure in the middle ear and contributes to recurrent otitis media with scarring of the tympanic membrane. This scarring plus the additional accumulation of fluid under pressure hampers the movement of the eardrum and the small bone of the middle ear, which leads to hearing impairment in a large proportion of children with palatal clefts. The problem may be easily overlooked in the infant and young child, thereby contributing to permanent impairment. Upper respiratory infections require immediate and meticulous attention, and pressure-equalizing drainage tubes may be inserted to facilitate drainage in chronic serous otitis media.

Extensive orthodontics and prosthodontics are usually needed to correct problems of malposition of teeth and maxillary arches. Changes take place in the structures of the teeth next to the cleft. There may be extra teeth present, or the teeth may be malformed or malpositioned, which can interfere with feeding. In addition a significant number of these children have an inadequate nasal airway that forces them to breathe through their mouths, which also contrib-

utes to oral deformity. Children with clefts of both lip and palate require four stages of orthodontic therapy. The first stage (birth to 18 months) is concerned with aligning the maxillary segments into a near-normal relationship. This is frequently done before lip closure in severely expanded segments to facilitate a primary lip closure.

The second stage (2 to 5 years) consists of repositioning maxillary segments and/or correcting a dental crossbite (a condition in which the upper teeth close inside the lower teeth) in an attempt to allow the primary teeth to develop in a normal relationship. Third stage therapy (10 to 11 years) takes place during the mixed dentition stage and involves correction of faulty occlusion. In the fourth stage (12 to 18 years) treatment of the permanent teeth is accomplished in much the same manner as for any teenage child except for alignment and spacing in the cleft area.

Often temporary or permanent dental prostheses are necessary to replace missing teeth; these assist in chewing and produce a more pleasing cosmetic effect. Special dental plates, or obturators, are sometimes used to mechanically close clefts in the palate to facilitate feeding and speech until permanent closure is attempted. However, any appliance must be checked periodically to ensure a proper fit and to see that it is performing its intended function.

The major potential handicap for a child with a cleft palate is defective speech. This can occur as a result of any or all of the previously discussed complications: insufficient palate function, faulty dentition, and hearing loss. A cleft palate interferes with speech sounds in the mouth that are normally made through interaction of the throat and palatine muscles. Improper tooth alignment can pose a mechanical hazard to development of clear speech, and hearing loss from middle ear infection is an additional impediment because of difficulty in interpreting sounds. With isolated cleft lip no speech problem should be anticipated. However, children without mouth defects develop undesirable speech habits and children with cleft lips may develop speech problems unrelated to the defect. The child with a cleft palate usually requires the services of a competent speech therapist.

Some of the more difficult long-term problems are related to social adjustment of the child. The better the physical habilitation, the better the chance for emotional and social adjustment, although the presence of the defect and the degree of residual disability are not directly related to a satisfactory adjustment. Physical defects are always a threat to the self-image, and abnormal speech quality is an impediment to social expression.

Nursing Considerations

The immediate nursing problems in the care of an infant with cleft lip and palate deformities are related to feeding the infant and dealing with the severe parental reaction to the defect. Facial deformities are particularly disturbing to parents. A cleft lip is the most disfiguring of the visible defects and generates strong negative responses in both nurses and parents. It is especially important for nurses to emphasize the positive aspects of the infant's physical appearance and optimism regarding surgical correction. The manner of the nurse in handling the infant should convey to the parents that the infant is indeed a precious human being.

Unless there are associated complicating anomalies, other aspects of nursing care of these children offer no significant differences from that of any newborn except in modification of feeding techniques.

Feeding. Feeding the infant offers a special challenge to nurses. The process is often time consuming and laborious. Clefts of lip or palate reduce the infant's ability to suck, which interferes with compression of the areola or nipple and usually renders both breast-feeding and bottle-feeding difficult. Liquid taken into the mouth has a tendency to escape via the cleft through the nose. Feeding is usually best accomplished with the infant's head in an upright position, either held in the nurse's hand or cradled in the arm. The type of feeding equipment and rate of feeding must be individualized for each infant.

Normal nipples are often unsuitable for these infants, who are unable to generate the suction required; therefore special nipples or other feeding devices are needed. A variety of special "cleft palate" nipples have been devised and used with some success. However, large, soft nipples with large holes, Nursettes, or the long, soft lamb's nipples appear to offer the best means for nipple feeding (Fig. 11-17). Plastic bottles aid the feeding process. Compressing the bottle sides facilitates flow and reduces the amount of negative

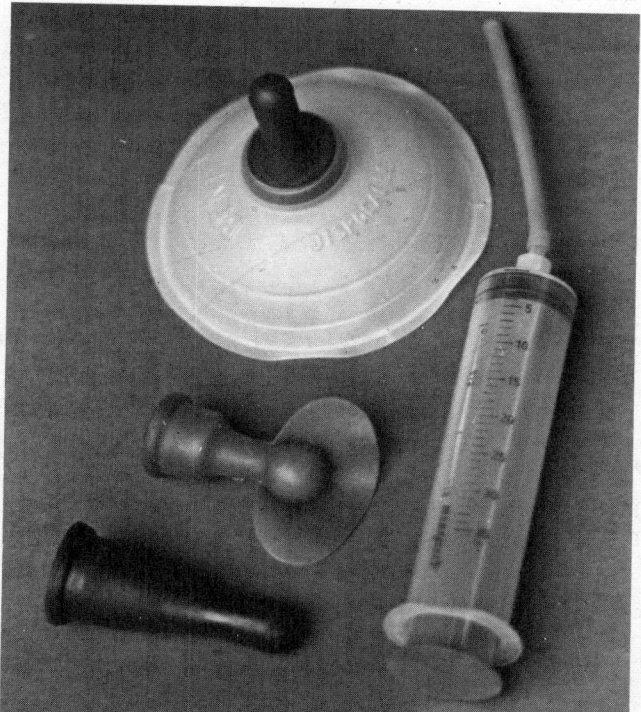

Fig. 11-17. Some devices used to feed infant with cleft palate. Clockwise, lamb's nipple, flanged nipple, special nurser, and syringe with rubber tubing (Breck feeder).

pressure exerted by the infant, which frequently increases the amount of ingested air.

Success has also been achieved by the modification of a standard nipple. A single small slit or a crosscut is made in the end of the nipple with a sharp surgical blade or a pair of scissors with sharp, thin blades. This allows the infant to express the formula readily. The size of the slit is adjusted to the needs of the infant. If the formula dribbles from the sides of the nipple or the nostrils during the feeding, the slit is too long; if it takes longer than 30 minutes to feed, the slit is too short.

Using these various types of nipples for feeding also has the advantage of helping to meet the infant's sucking needs and, when placed in the normal sucking position (not through the cleft), encouraging use of the sucking muscles. Muscle development is especially important for later development of speech. The nipple should be positioned in such a way that it is compressed by the infant's tongue and existing palate. If a single-slit nipple is used, the slit should be placed vertically so that the infant will be able to produce and stop a flow of milk by alternately opening and closing the opening. No matter which type of nipple is used, gentle, steady pressure on the base of the bottle reduces the chance of choking or coughing, and the person feeding should resist the temptation to remove the nipple frequently because of the noise the infant makes or for fear that the infant will choke.

When the infant has trouble with nipple feeding, either a rubber-tipped medicine dropper, Asepto syringe, or the plastic bottle described already often provides an efficient, safe feeding device. The rubber extension or thin nipple should be sufficiently long to extend well back into the mouth to reduce the likelihood of regurgitation through the nose. The formula is deposited on the back of the tongue and the flow controlled by bulb compression that is adjusted to the infant's capacity to handle it.

Success has been reported with the use of a specially made plastic palate constructed of rapid setting acrylic from a mold of the infant's mouth. With the device the infant is able to feed more normally, including breast-feeding. The device has an added advantage of allowing for more normal "speech" sounds, which is reassuring to the parents (Learning to close the cleft, 1982).

Because of their difficulty generating suction and occluding the oral cavity, these infants have a tendency to swallow more air than infants with normal oral cavities. Consequently, the infant must be fed slowly and bubbled more frequently and may require more frequent feedings.

With some infants, spoon feeding of formula works best. The parents should begin to feed the infant as soon as possible, preferably after the initial nursery feeding. In this way they are able to help determine the method best suited to them and the infant and to become adept in the technique before the infant is discharged from the hospital.

Preoperative care. In preparation for surgical repair, the parents are frequently instructed to accustom the infant

Postoperative Hospital Nursing Care Summary: The Infant with Cleft Lip Repair

NURSING GOALS	NURSING INTERVENTIONS	EXPECTED PATIENT/FAMILY OUTCOMES
HP-HMP Injury: potential for trauma, aspiration **Risk factors: fresh operative site, immature reasoning**		
Prevent trauma to suture line	Position on back or side (cleft lip) Use nontraumatic feeding techniques Restrain arms to prevent access to operative site Use jacket restraints on older infant Avoid placing objects in the mouth following palate repair (suction catheter, tongue depressor, straw, pacifier, small spoon)	Operative site remains undamaged
Prevent aspiration of secretions	Position to allow for mucus drainage (partial side-lying position)	Secretions are managed without aspiration
N-MP Nutrition, alteration in: less than body requirements **Etiology: difficulty eating**		
Provide adequate nutritional intake	Administer diet appropriate for age Modify feeding techniques to adjust to defect Feed in sitting position Use special appliances Encourage frequent bubbling Assist with breast-feeding if method of choice	Infant consumes an adequate amount of nutrients (specify amounts)
N-MP Skin integrity, impairment of: potential **Risk factors: mouth secretions, application of restraining devices**		
Prevent tissue infection and breakdown	Keep suture line dry	Skin remains clean and free of irritation
CPP Sensory-perceptual alterations: gustatory, tactile **Etiology: feeding methods (some), arm restraints**		
Provide comfort measures	Remove restraints periodically Provide cuddling and tactile stimulation Involve parents in infant's care	Infant rests quietly, is not irritable
RRP Family process, alteration in **Etiology: situational crisis (child with a physical defect)**		
Facilitate family's acceptance of infant	Allow expression of feelings Convey attitude of acceptance of infant and family Indicate by behavior that infant is a valuable human being	Family discusses feelings and concerns regarding the infant's defect, its repair, and future prospects
Educate family	Describe surgical results Use photographs of satisfactory results Involve family in determining best feeding methods Teach feeding and suctioning techniques Teach cleansing and restraining procedures, especially when infant will be discharged before suture removal	Family demonstrates ability to carry out postoperative care
Meet parents' concerns about recurrence in future children	Refer to genetic counseling services if family requests Reinforce and/or clarify information from genetic counseling	Parents avail themselves of services

Postoperative Hospital Nursing Care Summary: The Infant with Cleft Lip Repair—cont'd

NURSING GOALS	NURSING INTERVENTIONS	EXPECTED PATIENT/FAMILY OUTCOMES
Provide for continued support	Refer to public health agency for continuity of care Refer to social service Refer to Crippled Children's Services for financial assistance Refer to local cleft palate parent group and other agencies Ensure follow-up care and management See also The family of the hospitalized child, p. 1081	Family uses appropriate resources

Nursing Interventions Related to Medical Management

Prevent trauma to operative site Maintain lip protective device	**Prevent tissue damage** Cleanse suture line gently after feeding and as necessary in manner ordered by surgeon

to some of the needs of the early postoperative period, particularly if surgery is delayed several months. Since it is mandatory for the infant to avoid prone positioning postoperatively, it is helpful to accustom the infant to lie on the back or side to reduce the irritability and resistance associated with any change in routine. It is also helpful to place the infant or child in arm restraints periodically before admission and, after admission, to feed the infant in the manner to be used postoperatively. No special formula is required, and the infant is usually allowed to eat up to about 6 hours preoperatively. Preoperative preparation, including medication, is determined by the surgeon and anesthesiologist.

Postoperative care: cleft lip. The major efforts in the postoperative period are directed toward protecting the operative site. Before the infant leaves the operating room the metal appliance (if used) or the butterfly closure is taped securely to the cheeks to relax the operative site and prevent tension on the suture line caused by crying or other facial movement. Arm restraints are applied to prevent the infant from rubbing or otherwise disturbing the suture line and are ready at the bedside for immediate application on arrival at the unit. It is advisable to pin the cuff of the restraints to the infant's clothing or bed to prevent rubbing the face with the upper arms.

An older infant who is able to roll over will require a jacket restraint in addition to arm restrints, to prevent rolling on the abdomen and rubbing the face on the sheet. It is important to remove the restraints periodically to allow for exercising the arms, to provide relief from restrictions, and to observe the skin for signs of irritation. It is advisable to release the restraints one at a time, especially in a very vigorous, active infant or child. Removing restraints also offers an opportunity for cuddling and body contact. Sitting the child in an infant seat provides a change of position and a different perspective of the environment. Sedation is sometimes needed for a very restless, anxious infant.

Feeding is essentially the same as previous to surgery. It is safe to offer clear liquids when the infant has fully recovered from the anesthesia, and formula feeding is usually resumed when tolerated. The surgeon will specify any preferences or restrictions in feeding method. The mouth should be rinsed with water before and after each feeding.

The suture site is carefully cleansed of formula or serosanguineous drainage as needed with a gauze- or cotton-tipped swab dipped in saline or other solution, depending on the preference of the surgeon. Meticulous care of the suture line is a nursing responsibility, since inflammation or sloughing will interfere with optimum healing and the ultimate cosmetic effect of the surgical repair. The area is carefully inspected at each feeding.

Gentle aspiration of mouth and nasopharynx secretions is necessary to prevent aspiration and minimize the chances of respiratory complications. A side-lying or partial side-lying position is helpful for the infant in the immediate postoperative period and for one who has difficulty in handling secretions. As with any infant, the child with cleft lip repair is placed on the right side after feedings to reduce the chance of aspirating regurgitated formula.

Preparation for discharge and home care. Parents are encouraged to participate in the care of the infant as soon as feasible following surgery. They can resume the preoperative feeding method with the infant in a sitting position. The infant should be fed slowly and carefully and bubbled at frequent intervals. Parents are taught to follow each feeding with water (in the same manner as the feeding) and to cleanse the suture line to free any crusts that might form. This promotes healing and helps prevent undue scarring. If the surgeon approves, ointment (such as A and D Ointment) or mineral oil may be applied to keep the area lubricated.

Parents are cautioned to continue with elbow restraints until the suture line is well healed. The infant should not be allowed to cry, if possible, to prevent undue stress on the suture line. Cuddling, holding, and other comfort measures usually are effective, in addition to the time spent during feedings.

Postoperative care: cleft palate. The child with a cleft palate repair is allowed to lie on the abdomen, especially immediately postoperatively. The nurse avoids the use of suction or other objects in the mouth, such as a tongue depressor when the suture lines are being checked or straws when the child is given liquids. The child with a cleft palate repair may be fed with a wide-bowl spoon (such as a soup spoon) or from the side of the spoon, with the nurse or parent taking care not to insert the spoon into the mouth where it might damage the suture line. Forks are contraindicated and thermometers are not placed in the mouth. Fluids are best taken from a cup.

Sometimes the child will have difficulty breathing following surgery, since it is often necessary to alter an established pattern of breathing and adjust to breathing through the nose. This is frustrating but seldom requires more than positioning and support. Sometimes the infant or child is placed in a mist tent for a short period after surgery. Some surgeons place a single suture at the end of the tongue to facilitate extending the tongue if the airway should become obstructed. It is usually removed after the first 24 hours.

The elbows are restrained to keep the hands away from the mouth, and the parents are instructed to maintain this precaution at home until the palate is healed. They should be instructed to remove the restraints (usually one at a time) at frequent intervals to allow the child to exercise the arms. As with the infant with a cleft lip, the child should be kept from crying if possible by giving attention and affection and providing diversional activities.

The child is usually discharged on a soft diet, which parents are instructed to continue until the surgeon directs them otherwise. They should be cautioned against allowing the child to eat hard items such as toast, hard cookies, and potato chips, which could damage the newly repaired palate. The nurse might suggest that the parents not offer the child any food harder than mashed potatoes.

Long-Term Parental Guidance

The problems of parents and the child with a cleft palate extend beyond the initial adjustment to the defect, acceptance of the child, and surgical correction of the defect. These families need support and encouragement by health professionals and guidance in activities that facilitate the most normal outcome for the child. With the combined efforts of family and the health team the majority of these children achieve a satisfactory habilitation. Parents need to understand the function of therapy and the purpose of any appliance. They are taught proper care and placement of any device, and establishing good mouth care and proper brushing habits is especially important for these children.

Because of the increased risk of middle ear infection, the ears are examined regularly and hearing tests are scheduled early and repeated periodically throughout childhood. It is particularly important to emphasize the need for an ear ex-amination when the child has a cold in nose, throat, or chest. When treatment can be implemented early, the chances are greater that permanent changes in the ear can be avoided. Parents can be alert to signs of any hearing impairment in the child in order to obtain needed help and prevent progression of any deficit (see p. 1017).

The parents are also provided with guidance in helping the child to develop normal speech. They should encourage the child's early attempts to make sounds. Some parents erroneously believe that the child may form poor speech habits if he tries to speak before the palate is repaired. Attempting to delay speech further hampers its development. Activities that encourage the child to use the natural inclination to imitate sounds, including his own, are valuable aids; these include singing, repeating rhymes, and speaking games such as "patty cake." The child with a cleft palate is able to produce many sounds clearly, and parents should try to understand what the child is saying without correcting the speech during these early attempts. As with any toddler who is learning to use speech communication, "baby talk" is discouraged. Parents can use simple speech with short two- to three-word sentences. Parents should also understand that normal children at this age often leave out final sounds of words and should not attribute this characteristic to the defect.

Following surgery parents can assist palatal function by stimulating the child to use simple words that require coordination of the speech apparatus, encouraging chewing and frequent swallowing to exercise throat and palatine muscles, and engaging in blowing games to help close off the posterior palate. The speech therapist evaluates the individual needs of the child and directs the parents in specific activities to facilitate speech development. The more the child is encouraged to use speech, the sooner he will gain self-confidence and assurance in social situations. Some children may require additional surgery to correct defective speech that cannot be managed with speech therapy alone.

Throughout the child's habilitation the ultimate goal should be the development of a healthy personality and self-esteem. Several agencies provide services for children with cleft lips and/or palate and their families. These include the **American Cleft Palate Education Foundation, Inc.,*** the **National Institute of Dental Research,† March of Dimes–Birth Defects Foundation;‡, Canadian Cleft Lip and Palate Family Association,§** and state **Crippled Children's Services**.

ESOPHAGEAL ATRESIA WITH TRACHEOESOPHAGEAL FISTULA

Congenital atresia of the esophagus and tracheoesophageal (T-E) fistula (TEF) are rare malformations that represent a failure of the esophagus to develop as a continuous passage.

---

*331 Salk Hall, University of Pittsburgh, Pittsburgh, PA 15261.
†Westwood Building, 5333 Westbard Ave., Bethesda, MD 20205.
‡1275 Mamaroneck Ave., White Plains, NY 10605.
§170 Elizabeth St., Toronto, Ontario, Canada M5G1E8.

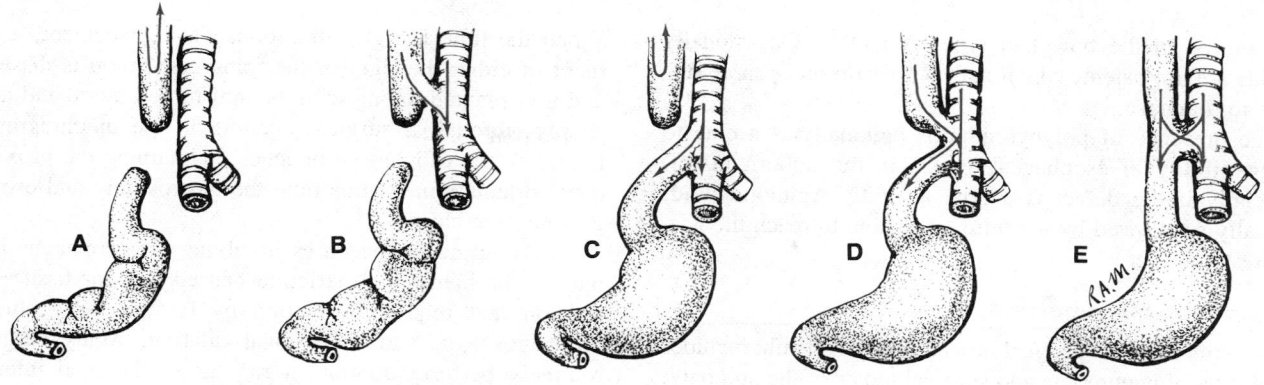

Fig. 11-18. Five most common types of esophageal atresia and tracheoesophageal fistula.

These defects may occur as separate entities or in combination (Fig. 11-18) and without early diagnosis and treatment they are rapidly fatal.

The incidence of esophageal atresia and T-E fistula is not known. Various authorities have estimated the incidence to be from 1:800 to 1:5000 live births. There appear to be no sex differences, but the birth weight of most affected infants is significantly lower than average and there is an unusually high percentage of prematurity. A history of maternal hydramnios is common, and approximately half the infants with esophageal defects have associated anomalies, especially congenital heart disease, anorectal malformations, and genitourinary anomalies. There is little evidence to implicate heredity as a factor.

Pathophysiology

The esophagus develops from the first segment of the embryonic gut. During the fourth and fifth weeks of gestation, this foregut normally lengthens and separates longitudinally and each longitudinal portion fuses to form two parallel channels (the esophagus and the trachea) that are joined only at the larynx. Anomalies involving the trachea and esophagus are caused by defective separation, incomplete fusion of the tracheal folds following this separation, or altered cellular growth during the process. The resulting esophageal defect may consist merely of two blind pouches, one at the pharyngeal end and one at the gastric end. More often one portion ends in a blind pouch and the other is connected to the trachea by way of a fistula.

The most commonly encountered form of esophageal atresia and T-E fistula (80% to 95% of cases) is one in which the proximal esophageal segment terminates in a blind pouch and the distal segment is connected to the trachea or primary bronchus by a short fistula at or near the bifurcation (Fig. 11-18, *C*). The second most common type (5% to 8%) consists of a blind pouch at each end, widely separated and with no communication to the trachea (Fig. 11-18, *A*). Less frequently an otherwise normal trachea and esophagus are connected by a fistula (Fig. 11-18, *E*). Extremely rare anomalies involve a fistula from the trachea to the upper esophageal segment (Fig. 11-18, *B*) or to both the upper and lower segments (Fig. 11-18, *D*).

Clinical Manifestations

The presence of esophageal atresia is suspected in an infant with excessive salivation and in a newborn with drooling that is frequently accompanied by choking, coughing, and sneezing. If fed, the infant swallows normally but suddenly coughs and struggles and the fluid returns through the nose and mouth. The infant becomes cyanotic and may stop breathing as the overflow of fluid from the blind pouch is aspirated into the trachea or bronchus. The cyanosis is the result of laryngospasm, the protective mechanism that operates to prevent aspiration into the trachea.

In the infant with type C malformation the stomach becomes distended with air, and thoracic and abdominal compression (especially during crying) cause the gastric contents to be regurgitated through the fistula into the trachea, producing a chemical pneumonitis. When the upper segment of the esophagus opens directly into the trachea (types B and D), the infant is in danger of drowning immediately from any swallowed material. Cyanosis or choking during feeding may be the only symptom of type E fistula.

Diagnostic Evaluation

To establish a diagnosis of esophageal atresia, a catheter is gently passed into the esophagus. It will meet with resistance if the lumen is blocked but will pass unobstructed if the lumen is patent. A moderately stiff catheter is used to avoid coiling in the esophageal pouch. Aspiration of stomach contents or auscultation over the stomach as air is introduced through the catheter confirms a patent esophagus. Gastric lavage immediately after delivery, although not a universal practice, offers earlier diagnosis of esophageal atresia.

Although the diagnosis is established on the basis of clinical signs and symptoms, the exact type of anomaly is determined by roentgenographic studies. A radiopaque catheter is inserted into the hypopharynx and advanced until it encounters an obstruction. Chest films are taken to ascertain whether the tube reaches the stomach and whether it appears to pass through the normal or abnormal channels. Films that show air in the stomach indicate a connection between the trachea and the distal esophagus in types C and D. No gas is observed in the bowel in types A and B. Occasionally fistulas are not patent, which makes their presence more difficult to diagnose.

The presence of polyhydramnios prenatally is a clue to the possibility of esophageal atresia in the unborn infant, especially if the defect is a type A or C. Amniotic fluid, normally swallowed by the fetus, is unable to reach the gastrointestinal tract.

Therapeutic Management

The treatment of esophageal atresia and T-E fistula includes prevention of pneumonia and surgical repair of the anomaly. Since type C is the most common, the discussion is directed primarily toward that anomaly.

When a T-E fistula is suspected, the infant is immediately deprived of oral intake, started on intravenous fluids, and placed in the most advantageous position to decrease the likelihood of aspiration, that is, head elevated for a type C anomaly (head down would be indicated for type A or B). Accumulated secretions are suctioned frequently from the mouth and pharynx. A catheter is placed into the upper esophageal pouch, and the infant's head is kept in an upright position so that fluid collected in the pouch is easily removed and to prevent aspiration of gastric contents. A gastrostomy is usually performed to decompress the stomach and prevent further aspiration of gastric contents by way of the fistula. Since aspiration pneumonia is almost inevitable and appears early, broad-spectrum antibiotic therapy is instituted.

Surgical correction. Most malformations can be corrected surgically in one operation or staged with two or more procedures. The success depends on early diagnosis before complicating factors (pneumonia, dehydration, and inanition) have progressed to an irreversible stage, skilled nursing care, and the technical skill and judgment of the surgeon. With measures instituted to prevent aspiration pneumonia and to ensure adequate hydration and nutrition, surgery can be postponed to allow for more effective treatment of pneumonia so that the infant can better withstand the complex surgery. The delay also offers an opportunity for further evaluation and assessment to rule out any associated anomalies.

The surgery consists of a thoracotomy with division and ligation of the T-E fistula and an end-to-end anastomosis of the esophagus. For infants who are premature, have multiple anomalies, or are in very poor condition, a staged operation is preferred that involves palliative measures, including gastrostomy, ligation of the T-E fistula, and provision of constant drainage of the esophageal pouch.

There are rare instances in which a primary anastomosis cannot be accomplished because of insufficient length of the two segments of esophagus. In these cases the defect must be bridged with a segment of intestine. This esophageal replacement is usually deferred until the child is 18 to 24 months old. In the meantime the fistula is closed and the child fed directly by gastrostomy, and the upper esophageal segment is drained by means of a cervical esophagostomy.

When the time is right for esophageal replacement, a segment of either the right or the transverse colon is dissected and transplanted, along with its undisturbed blood and nerve supply, through a surgical opening in the diaphragm and ligated to the esophageal pouches maintaining the proximodistal orientation. At this time the gastrostomy and esophagostomy are closed.

In all surgical procedures involving the esophagus there may be problems with stricture caused by scar tissue contraction that require evaluation by barium x-ray studies, esophagoscopy, and mechanical dilation. Many surgeons routinely perform dilation at regularly scheduled intervals for some time after surgery. The procedure may need to be repeated several times during growth. Strictures that do not respond to dilation require surgical intervention.

Nursing Considerations

Nursing responsibility for detection of this serious malformation begins *immediately* after birth. The defect is suspected in any infant who has an excessive amount of mucus or difficulty with secretions and unexplained episodes of cyanosis—the three Cs of T-E fistula: coughing, choking, and cyanosis. Ideally the condition is diagnosed before the initial feeding, but often it is not. Poor handling of mucus is characteristic of other problems, for example, the infant with central nervous system damage and the preterm infant with weak or absent cough and swallowing reflexes. This is often a cause of confusion, especially with the premature infant who may also have a T-E fistula. Cyanosis is usually the result of laryngospasm caused by overflow of saliva into the larynx from the proximal esophageal pouch, and it normally clears after removal of the secretions from the oropharynx by suctioning. Any suspicion of a T-E fistula or esophageal atresia is reported to the physician immediately.

The infant is placed in an Isolette or under a radiant warmer, and oxygen is administered to help relieve respiratory distress. Positive pressure is contraindicated because it may add to air pressure in the stomach and compound the distress.

Preoperative care. The mouth and nasopharynx are carefully suctioned, and the infant is placed in an optimum position to facilitate drainage. It is common practice to place an infant who appears to have difficulty with secretions in the head-down position to facilitate drainage. Without a fistulous communication to the stomach (as in type A or B), this would be of benefit, but since the majority are type C anomalies, the head-down position could have adverse effects. The most desirable position for a newborn who is suspected of having a T-E fistula is supine with the head elevated on an inclined plane of at least 30 degrees. This positioning serves to minimize the reflux of gastric secretions up the distal esophagus into the trachea and bronchi, especially when intraabdominal pressure is elevated during episodes of crying.

It is imperative that any secretions that can be a source of aspiration be removed at once. Until surgery the blind pouch is kept empty by intermittent or continuous suction through an indwelling nasal catheter that extends to the end of the pouch. The catheter has a tendency to become clogged with mucus; therefore it is usually replaced daily by the physician. On diagnosis the gastrostomy tube is inserted and left open so that any air that enters the stomach through the fistula can escape, thus minimizing the danger that gastric contents will be regurgitated into the trachea. The tube empties by gravity drainage. Feedings through the gastrostomy tube and irrigations with fluid are contraindicated before surgery.

Often the infant must be transferred to a hospital with specialized care units. Care is exercised to maintain the desired position and continue suctioning during transport. Specially designed units are equipped for transporting infants to critical care facilities. During transport the infant is accompanied by a physician, nurse, or a physician/nurse team.

Postoperative care. Postoperative care for these infants is essentially the same as for any high-risk newborn. The infant is returned to the warm, high-humidity atmosphere of the Isolette, and the gastrostomy tube is returned to gravity drainage until the infant can tolerate feedings, usually the second or third postoperative day. At this time the tube is elevated and secured at a point above the level of the stomach. This allows gastric secretions to pass to the duodenum, while swallowed air can escape through the open tube. If tolerated, gastrostomy feedings are continued until the esophagus anastomosis is healed, about the tenth to fourteenth day, after which oral feedings are initiated.

The initial attempt at oral feeding must be carefully observed to make certain that the infant is able to swallow without choking. Oral feedings are begun with glucose water followed by frequent, small feedings of formula. Until the infant is able to take a sufficient amount by mouth, oral intake may need to be supplemented by gastrostomy feedings. Ordinarily the infant is not discharged until he is taking oral fluids well and the gastrostomy tube has been removed. However, the infant who has undergone palliative surgery will be discharged with the gastrostomy tube in place. The nurse is responsible for making certain that the caregiver is educated and practiced in the care of the gastrostomy.

Special problems. Upper respiratory complications are a threat to life in both the preoperative and the postoperative periods. In addition to pneumonia, there is a constant danger of respiratory embarrassment resulting from atelectasis, pneumothorax, and laryngeal edema. Any persistent respiratory difficulty after removal of secretions is reported to the surgeon immediately.

In the infant awaiting esophageal replacement surgery, the catheter is removed and the upper esophageal segment is drained by means of an artificial opening in the neck (cervical esophagostomy), which allows escape of the swallowed saliva. This is a source of annoyance, since the skin may become irritated by moisture from the continual discharge of saliva. Frequent removal of drainage and application of a thin layer of protective ointment are usually sufficient treatment.

Meeting the oral needs of infants who are unable to suck on a bottle should not be overlooked. A pacifier offered periodically is an acceptable substitute until oral feedings are instituted. The child who has corrective surgery delayed until 18 to 24 months of age may have a different problem. Some children who have not been able to go through the processes of eating in the normal manner have difficulty with this new task and require patient, firm guidance in learning the techniques of taking food into the mouth and swallowing.

Discharge planning and home care. Preparing parents for discharge of their infant involves teaching the techniques that will be continued in home care, such as careful suctioning, gastrostomy feeding, and skin care. The parents are taught child or infant behaviors that might be expected after corrective surgery, such as those that indicate that the child needs to be suctioned, signs of respiratory difficulty, and signs that indicate constriction of the esophagus. They are reminded that it is particularly important to guard against the child swallowing foreign objects. With a child in any of the stages of locomotion this is no simple problem. Parents will also need help in acquiring needed equipment, such as a suction machine, and special services.

ANORECTAL MALFORMATIONS

Malformations in the anorectal region of the GI tract are manifest in several variations, all classified as *imperforate anus*. They are among the more common congenital malformations caused by abnormal development (approximately 1:5000). A large number of infants with anorectal defects will have another serious associated congenital anomaly, the most common of which are those involving the genitourinary tract, heart, and esophagus.

Clinically anorectal malformations can be divided into three categories according to the relationship of the rectum to the puborectalis muscle. Distinction between these categories is important for planning therapy and determining a prognosis (Seashore, 1986). Anorectal anomalies are classified as follows:

low anomalies Rectum has descended normally through the puborectalis muscle, the internal and external sphincters are present and well developed with normal function, and there is no connection to the gastrointestinal tract. These may be anal stenosis with or without an obstructive membrane (Fig. 11-19, *A* or *B*), frequently with an external fistula to the perineum or vestibule through which meconium is passed.

intermediate anomalies Rectum is at or below the level of the puborectalis muscle, the anal dimple and external sphincter are positioned normally, but the anal opening is located anteriorly in the perineum. There may be a persistent connection to the gastrointestinal tract.

high anomalies Rectum ends above the puborectalis muscle. There is absence of internal and external sphincters and the puborectalis muscle is relatively ineffectual. These anomalies occur almost exclusively in males where there is usually a rectourethral fistula; a rectovaginal communication is

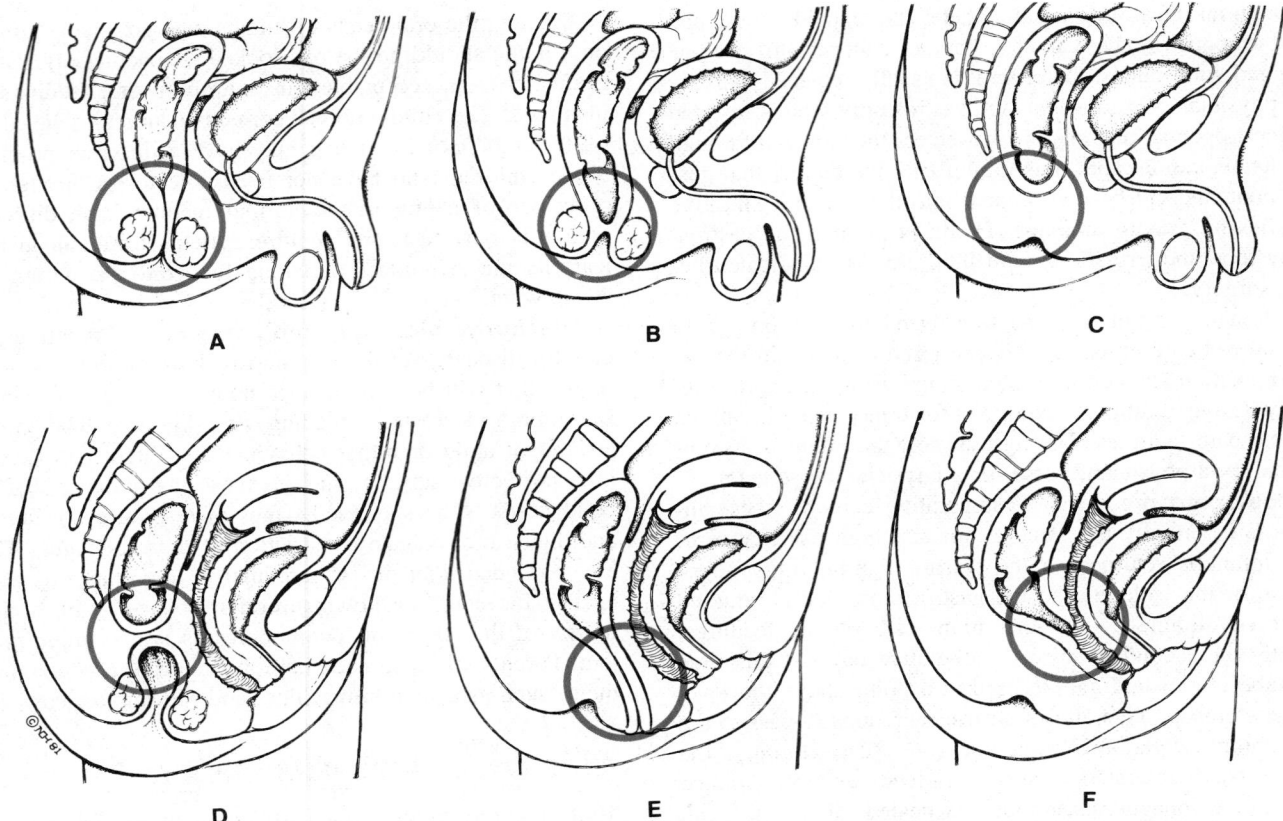

Fig. 11-19. Anorectal stenosis and imperforate anus. **A,** Congenital anal stenosis; **B,** anal membrane atresia; **C,** anal agenesis; **D,** rectal atresia; **E,** rectoperoneal fistula; **F,** rectovaginal fistula.

found in females (Fig. 11-19, *F*). Wide variations are found in high anomalies and they are often associated with maldevelopment of the sacrum, which interferes with innervation to anal and urethral musculature.

Pathophysiology

About the seventh week of gestation the future rectum and anus develop from an expanded portion of the caudal hindgut, the *cloaca*, which is subsequently divided by downward growth of a urorectal septum into a urogenital sinus and a rectum. At about the same time the lower urogenital portion has acquired an external opening, whereas the rectum is separated from the exterior by the *anal membrane*. This membrane breaks down by the beginning of the eighth week of gestation to form a continuous patent communication between the outside and the remainder of the gut. Most anorectal malformations result from abnormal partitioning of the cloaca by the urorectal septum.

Diagnostic Evaluation

Checking for patency of the anus and rectum is a routine part of the newborn assessment and includes observation or inquiries regarding the passage of meconium. Inspection of the perineal area reveals absence of an anal opening or the thin translucent membrane of anal membrane atresia. Digital

and endoscopic examination identify constriction or the blind pouch of rectal atresia. Stenosis may not become apparent until 1 year of age or older when the child has a history of difficult defecation, abdominal distention, and ribbonlike stools. Fistulas may not be apparent at birth, but as peristalsis gradually forces the meconium through the fistula they can be identified by careful examination. A rectourinary fistula is suspected on the basis of meconium in the urine and confirmed by radiographs of contrast media injected through a tiny catheter into the fistula.

Definitive diagnosis of the extent and location of the high lesion is made by radiographic examination. With the infant inverted and an opaque marker at the anal dimple, air ascending into the rectum and lower bowel will outline the location of the pouch in relation to the anal depression. Renal ultrasound is recommended before discharge of the infant with a high lesion to identify or rule out the possibility of associated anomalies of the urinary tract. Further examination is also indicated if there is evidence of urinary tract infection or other symptoms.

Therapeutic Management

Successful treatment for anal stenosis is generally accomplished by manual dilations. The procedure, begun by the physician, is repeated on a regular basis by the nurses in the hospital and continued at home by the parents, after they are carefully instructed in the technique. An imperforate anal membrane is excised and followed by daily anal dilations.

Reconstruction of an anus in the proper position is the goal of surgical treatment of intermediate anorectal malformations. The most important consideration in the probable success of reconstruction is the level at which the rectum terminates, especially in its relationship to the puborectalis sling of the levator ani muscle. Where the bowel has come through this structure, surgical correction often can be accomplished in the neonatal period by way of an abdominal-perineal pull-through procedure and/or anoplasty.

Infants with high anomalies require a divided sigmoid colostomy in the newborn period. This allows time for the infant to gain weight, a more leisurely evaluation of the anomaly, and protection of the genitourinary tract from fecal contamination from a fistula. Antibiotics are usually administered prophylactically. Final correction of higher defects is usually postponed for a year. A permanent colostomy is sometimes the best solution for children who fail to achieve bowel control at a reasonable age.

Nursing Considerations

The first nursing responsibility is identification of undetected anorectal malformations. A poorly developed anal dimple, a rounded perineum, or vertebral abnormality suggests a high lesion. A newborn who does not pass a stool within 24 hours of birth requires further assessment, and meconium that appears at an inappropriate orifice is reported.

Postoperative nursing care ordinarily presents few problems and is primarily directed toward healing of the anoplasty without infection or other complications. Where the infant has undergone a pull-through procedure with anoplasty, special nursing care involves maintaining the anal area as clean as possible with scrupulous perineal care. There may or may not be a temporary dressing and drain, but when the infant is passing stool, dressings are of little value. The preferred placement is a side-lying prone position with the hips elevated or a supine position with the legs suspended at a 90-degree angle to the trunk to prevent pressure on perineal sutures. Periodic application of a heat lamp facilitates healing.

The infant is given regular infant formula as soon as peristalsis returns. In the meantime there may be a nasogastric tube for abdominal decompression and intravenous feedings. Care of the infant with a colostomy involves frequent dressing changes, meticulous skin care, and correct application of a collection device.

Family support. Long-term follow-up is essential for children with high lesions. Toilet training is difficult and complete continence is seldom achieved at the usual ages of 3 to 4 years. Bowel habit training, diet modification, and administration of stool softeners help children slowly improve bowel management, but optimum results may not be achieved until adolescence. Support and reassurance during the slow progression to normal function are essential and any type of coercive toilet training is discouraged. Approximately 80% will ultimately achieve normal or at least socially acceptable continence (Seashore, 1986).

Nursing care of children with permanent colostomies is the same as for any child with a colostomy (see p. 1145).

BILIARY ATRESIA

Biliary atresia is the obstruction or absence of a portion of the bile ducts. Blockage may be either *intrahepatic,* the absence of bile ducts within the liver, or *extrahepatic,* in which there is absence or obstruction of the main bile passages outside the liver. Numerous variations are encountered, but the most common abnormality is complete atresia of the extrahepatic structures. The cause is unknown. It is generally considered to be a developmental anomaly, but recent evidence implicates a viral infection before or shortly after birth (Glaser, Balistreri, and Morecki, 1984). The predictable course of the disease terminates in irreversible obliteration of the extrahepatic bile ducts.

Clinical Manifestations

Jaundice is usually the earliest evidence of biliary atresia and is the most striking feature of the disorder. It is first observed in the sclera. It may be present at birth but is not usually apparent until the child is 2 to 3 weeks of age. The urine becomes dark and stains the diaper, and the stools are lighter than expected. Hepatomegaly and abdominal distention are common, and splenomegaly occurs later. Poor fat metabolism results in poor weight gain and general failure to thrive. As the disease progresses, the child becomes irritable and difficult to comfort.

Diagnostic Evaluation

No single test or combination of tests is diagnostic. The disease is suspected on the basis of clinical signs, including a steady increase in *conjugated* hyperbilirubinemia. Percutaneous liver biopsy is performed to identify the presence or absence of intrahepatic bile ducts. Presence of bile ducts indicates that the atresia is of extrahepatic origin and amenable to surgical exploration.

Therapeutic Management

The major hope in care of these children is that the condition will benefit from surgery. Surgical reconstruction is possible in about 10% of extrahepatic atresia when the lesion is either a distal atresia with patent proximal hepatic duct or a cystic dilation of ducts adjacent to the hilum of the liver. Surgery is most successful when performed early; therefore diagnosis is urgent.

In the more common atresias there are no patent extrahepatic ducts. In these cases the Kasai procedure is employed, in which a substitute duct is formed from a segment of jejunum if there are any hepatic duct remnants.

Liver transplantation has recently become a more encouraging alternative for children with uncorrectable atresia. The

1-year survival rate has improved from 25% to 75% with the use of the newer immunosuppressive agent, cyclosporine, and low doses of steroids (Iwatsuki and Starzl, 1986). Pettitt, Zitelli, and Rowe (1984) report 84% survival. As a result, liver transplant is rapidly becoming the surgical treatment of choice, although the Kasai procedure is often performed in these children to provide relief and prevent nutritional deficiencies while they are awaiting a donor liver.

Medical management is primarily supportive. It is the method of choice for intrahepatic atresia and supplemental to surgical therapy in extrahepatic atresia. Medical management consists of a high-calorie formula containing fats that can be digested without bile (Pregestimil, Portagen) and water-miscible vitamins. The bile acid–binding drug cholestyramine is sometimes useful to prevent reabsorption of bile from the intestines. However it is not effective where bile is not excreted into the intestines. Phenobarbital helps reduce irritability. A low-salt diet and diuretics may reduce ascites formation.

Nursing Considerations

Nursing care of the infant with biliary atresia is primarily supportive. Initially the infant is not uncomfortable and requires care suited to any infant of the same age. As the disease progresses, the accumulation of toxic products causes the child to become irritable, restless, and difficult to comfort. Efforts are extended to allow as much sleep and rest as possible. The child is cared for on awakening and given sedatives and comforting measures as tolerated.

During the diagnostic phase of the illness the nurse assists with tests and procedures as ordered. The child who has undergone exploratory or corrective surgery is given the same care as any infant following abdominal surgery. Infants with the Kasai operation require care of the double stoma and collection, measurement, and replacement of bile via the stomal openings. Parental teaching includes this practice, administration of medications, and observation for signs of cholangitis.

The child who is selected for transplantation is transferred to an institution where the procedure is to be performed. It is an anxious period as well as one of hope. Families need a great deal of support. The **Children's Liver Foundation*** provides educational materials, programs, and support systems for parents of children with liver disease. Other agencies that provide services for children with congenital disabilities are listed in Appendix E.

Hernias

A hernia is a protrusion of a portion of an organ or organs through an abnormal opening. The danger from herniation arises when the organ protruding through the opening is

*28 Highland Ave., Maplewood, NJ 07040 or 139 S. Beverly Drive #312, Beverly Hills, CA 90212.

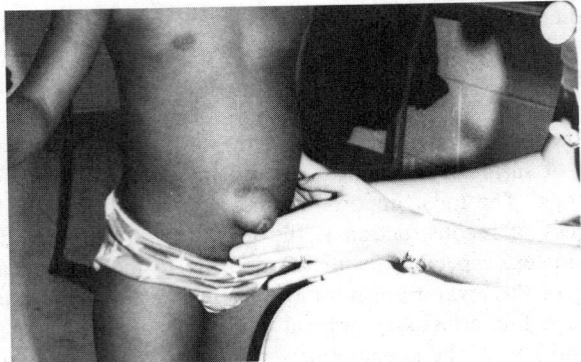

Fig. 11-20. Child with an umbilical hernia.
Photography by Kristie Nix, Tulsa, OK.

constricted to the extent that circulation is impaired or when the protruding organs encroach upon and impair the function of other structures. The herniations of concern here are those that protrude through the diaphragm, the abdominal wall, or the inguinal canal. Because they involve the genitourinary tract, inguinal and femoral hernias are discussed in the next section.

UMBILICAL HERNIA

Ordinarily the umbilical ring, through which the umbilical blood vessels provide essential elements to the developing fetus, undergoes spontaneous, gradual closure after birth. Incomplete closure of this fascial ring results in the protrusion of portions of omentum and intestine through the opening. The size of the defect varies from less than 1 cm (½ inch) to 4 or 5 cm (about 2 inches) (Fig. 11-20). The hernias are seen as soft swellings or protrusions covered by skin that are readily reducible with the finger, and small defects usually close spontaneously by 3 to 4 years of age. However very large hernias often persist. Those that have not disappeared by school age require surgical closure. Strangulation or incarceration of herniated bowel is rare but requires immediate surgical intervention.

Nursing Considerations

Because the sight of an umbilical hernia is very disconcerting to parents, they need reassurance regarding the innocuous nature of the defect. Taping or strapping appears to be of no value in expediting closure and may even retard it. The application can also cause troublesome skin irritation; when done improperly, it may cause strangulation.

DIAPHRAGMATIC HERNIA

In congenital diaphragmatic hernia (CDH) the abdominal contents herniate through the diaphragm into the pleural cavity, seriously compromising respiration. The defect is associated with an exceptionally high mortality and constitutes a surgical emergency in the immediate newborn period.

Pathophysiology

The herniation represents failure of the pleuroperitoneal canal to close completely during embryonic development, which allows various degrees of protrusion of abdominal viscera through the defect into the thoracic cavity. It is not unusual to find most of the abdominal organs (stomach, small intestine, spleen, left lobe of liver, left kidney, and all but the descending colon) in the thorax. The more severe defects occur with herniation through the foramen of Bochdalek; less severe are herniations through the foramen of Morgagni.

Respiration is compromised by hypoplasia and compression of the lung, including airways and blood vessels, on the affected side. Ineffective motion of the leaf of the diaphragm on the affected side interferes with the normal diaphragmatic breathing of the neonate. Respiration is further compromised when the stomach and intestine (generally found within the chest) rapidly become distended with swallowed air as the result of crying. Negative thoracic pressure from crying tends to pull the intestines into the chest and further distends those already there. This increased volume in the chest cavity displaces the mediastinum to the unaffected side to produce a partial collapse of the opposite lung.

Clinical Manifestations

Severe respiratory distress, including dyspnea and cyanosis, is often present at birth, but signs may appear at any time in the neonatal period or even later. There is a 50% to 70% mortality when the signs of the defect are evident at delivery, 40% when identified within 24 hours, and approach 0% when signs appear after 24 hours (Ramenofsky, 1986). In addition to dyspnea the infant may display vomiting, signs of severe colicky pain, discomfort after feeding, and constipation. The chest is barrel shaped and the abdomen markedly scaphoid (sunken). Less frequently the defect is asymptomatic and is discovered by radiographic examination.

Diagnostic Evaluation

The diagnosis is usually established by radiographic examination, which shows fluid and air-filled loops of intestine in the affected side of the chest (80% are present on the left side). The mediastinum is shifted to the unaffected side, causing a similar shift in the point of maximum intensity on auscultation. Auscultation also reveals absence of breath sounds on the affected side of the thorax, and bowel sounds may be present. Blood gas and pH determinations are made to assess the status of oxygenation and acidosis.

Therapeutic Management

The affected infant requires immediate respiratory support, which includes positioning with the head and thorax higher than the abdomen and feet to facilitate downward displacement of abdominal organs, nasogastric suction for decompression of the stomach, and conscientious efforts to prevent the infant from crying. Oxygen is provided but positive pressure ventilation, if needed, is administered cautiously by endotracheal tube to prevent pneumothorax, a constant danger because of the uneven distribution of intrapulmonary pressures in the hypoplastic, atelectatic, and compressed lung tissue (Behrman and Speck, 1983). Low ventilatory pressure with rapid ventilatory rate is preferred; positive end-expiratory pressure is contraindicated (Ramenofsky, 1986).

Intravenous fluids are begun by way of an umbilical artery catheter, metabolic and respiratory acidosis are corrected, and antibiotics are usually administered prophylactically. Following these and other preparations, the infant is taken for surgical repair of the defect. If the infant is to be transported to a special facility, stabilization and transport are accomplished as quickly as possible.

Postoperative management involves continuation of ventilatory therapy, acid-base stabilization, and attention to pulmonary arterial pressure and mediastinal positioning. Right-to-left shunting frequently occurs in these infants through the foramen ovale, through the ductus arteriosus, or within the lung, and all are associated with development of pulmonary hypertension. These complications are managed symptomatically.

Following surgery for severe defects there is usually a period of relative pulmonary stability that lasts up to 18 hours. After this "honeymoon" period the infant often develops progressive pulmonary insufficiency. The deterioration is the result of several factors, one of which is overexpansion of the normal lungs into the empty space on the affected side created by the undeveloped lung. This causes a shift in the mediastinum, which is mobile in the neonate. Additional factors include circulatory problems secondary to a mediastinal shift and pulmonary infection.

Nursing Considerations

Preoperative nursing care is primarily supportive. Upright positioning is maintained and measures are implemented to decrease crying, such as performing distressing procedures at one time. Oxygen therapy, abdominal decompression, and intravenous fluids are maintained and the infant prepared for surgery.

Postoperative care includes the routine observations discussed in the care of the high-risk infant. The infant should be positioned on the affected side to take advantage of gravity, which facilitates expansion of the unaffected lung and reduces the likelihood of overexpansion into the unaffected side. Close observation to detect signs of respiratory embarrassment or fluid and electrolyte imbalances are crucial. The infant is closely monitored for signs of mediastinal shift, pulmonary hypertension, and infection.

Because of the serious nature of the condition and urgency of treatment, the parents are in great need of support and guidance. Because the condition is one of high risk, the interventions outlined for the high-risk infant are appropriate here.

HIATAL HERNIA

Congenital herniations through the normal esophageal hiatus in the newborn are usually of the sliding type. Because the muscular ring of the hiatus is not snug, it permits the cardiac end of the stomach to slide above the diaphragm and back into the abdomen. This produces the symptoms seen with associated incompetent or relaxed cardiac sphincter *(chalasia)*, that is, reflux of gastric contents into the esophagus with subsequent regurgitation.

Therapeutic management is directed toward treatment of the esophageal reflux. When conservative management, such as upright posture and feeding modification, is disappointing, the defect is repaired surgically.

Nursing considerations are the same as for gastrointestinal reflux (p. 1424).

OMPHALOCELE AND GASTROSCHISIS

Omphalocele and gastroschisis have been considered to be embryologically distinct disorders for quite some time. The distinction at birth has been that an omphalocele is a covered defect of the umbilical cord whereas an uncovered defect with a normally inserted umbilical cord is a gastroschisis. This distinction is being questioned (Glick and others, 1985). Because the controversy is unresolved the two disorders are considered separately in this discussion.

Omphalocele

Omphalocele is a serious congenital malformation in which a variable amount of the abdominal contents protrudes into the base of the umbilical cord. As the embryonic midgut grows and elongates, it projects from the abdomen, which is too small to contain it, into the umbilical cord. This migration takes place from the sixth to the tenth week of fetal life. Normally the intestines return rapidly into the abdomen by the eleventh week of gestation; failure to return produces an omphalocele. In contrast to an umbilical hernia, the omphalocele is covered only by a translucent sac of amnion to which the umbilical cord inserts. The sac may contain only a small loop of bowel or most of the bowel and other abdominal viscera. If the sac ruptures, the abdominal contents eviscerate through the opening in the abdominal wall. The abdomen is smaller than usual, making replacement of the bowel more difficult. The anomaly is associated with other anomalies (such as trisomies 13 and 18) in the majority of cases.

Since the advent of ultrasonography, an increasing number of these defects are detected before birth. This has created a debate regarding the optimum mode of delivery—vaginal vs surgical. At present the majority favor surgical delivery especially when the defect is a large one (Pomerance, 1986).

The omphalocele is covered immediately with moist gauze and kept moist until the infant is taken to the operating room. The moist dressing is covered with plastic wrap to avoid loss of heat and moisture. Small lesions are repaired as soon as possible to prevent infection or tissue damage. Larger lesions may require gradual reduction by way of plastic material sewn to the margins of the defect and pulled together at the top to form a chimney and steady pressure applied to the protruding mass over a course of days to gradually enlarge the intraabdominal space to accommodate the intestinal contents. Rarely nonoperative treatment, consisting of repeated application of a cicatrizing or toughening solution to the sac, is used with excessively large omphaloceles; surgical repair is postponed for 6 to 12 months. Management of ruptured omphalocele is similar to that for gastroschisis. Complications include infection, rupture, and intestinal obstruction. The defect is often associated with other malformations.

Gastroschisis

Gastroschisis is herniation through a defect of the abdominal wall that permits extrusion of abdominal contents without involving the umbilical cord. The defect is usually located to the right of the intact umbilicus and is not encased in a protective sac. Herniation through the defect can take place prenatally or perinatally. If the evisceration is of long standing, the abdominal cavity will be small and the protruding bowel is thickened as a result of poor blood return and irritation from amniotic fluid. The bowel is almost normal and the abdominal cavity adequate in eviscerations that take place just before birth.

Therapy is directed toward prevention of infection, nutrition, and surgical closure of the defect. A primary closure is preferred but is not always possible. When the abdomen is too small to accommodate the extruded contents, a Silastic pouch is placed over the herniated viscera to contain the bowel and to aid in reduction until surgical closure is attempted (Fig. 11-21). When the bowel has returned to the abdominal cavity with the aid of gravity, the opening is surgically closed. The return may take a few hours to a few days, depending on the size of the abdominal cavity relative to the amount of viscera.

Some of the problems that may be encountered postsurgically when the abdomen is unable to accommodate the viscera are respiratory embarrassment caused by the increased pressure on the diaphragm, decreased venous return to the heart because of pressure on the vena cava, and possible bowel necrosis from excessive crowding. If the infant develops respiratory distress, the sutures may need to be released and the pouch replaced until adequate respiratory function can be reinstated. However, the longer the bowel remains outside, the more difficult the reduction becomes, because of growth.

Nursing Considerations

Nursing care is the same as for any high-risk infant. Infection is a constant threat before surgery, and careful positioning and handling are needed to prevent rupture of the intact omphalocele sac or disturbance of the Silastic bag for reduction of a gastroschisis. Postsurgical care includes particular

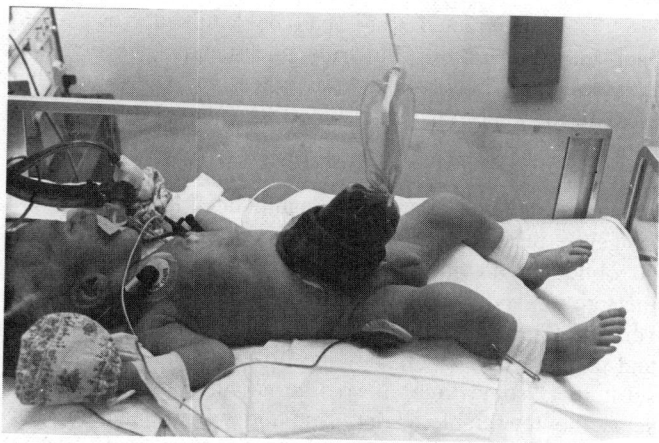

Fig. 11-21. Gastroschisis enclosed in a Silastic pouch.

attention to observation for signs of complications and assessment to detect indications that the replaced bowel is functioning.

Defects of the Genitourinary Tract

External defects of the genitourinary tract are usually obvious at birth. Several, such as hypospadias, epispadias, and undescended testes (cryptorchidism), do not necessitate immediate repair but may require one or more staged repairs during early childhood. Others, such as exstrophy of the bladder, require initial intervention at birth with repeated medical and surgical treatment for several years. The anatomic location of these defects frequently causes more psychologic concern to children and parents than does the actual condition or treatment. Hernias are common in young children and are usually repaired as soon as diagnosis is established.

Psychologic Problems Related to Genital Surgery

It has long been observed that hospitalization and separation can have a traumatic effect on children. Also the location and site of the defect and the need for repeated surgery cause some children more emotional concern than does the actual defect. Observations have also shown that the timing of medical and surgical procedures has wide-ranging effects on later adult behavior. Surgery involving sexual organs can be particularly disruptive to children, especially preschoolers fearing punishment, retaliation, body mutilation, or castration. More emotional disturbances have been noted in children who had genitourinary surgery than those who had ear, nose, or throat surgery (Blotcky and Grossman, 1978), and profound problems with concepts of body image and sexuality have developed.

There are four areas that appear to influence the reaction of children to genital surgery (Manley, 1982): (1) separation anxiety, (2) the hospital experience, (3) the anxiety of the

parents, and (4) body image and castration anxiety. The problem of separation anxiety has been diminished through short-term hospitalization, ambulatory surgery, and unrestricted visiting by parents. The same practices have also reduced the effects of the hospital experience (see Chapter 26). It is the presence of the attachment object(s) that is most important for reducing anxiety. Children are less distressed in a strange environment when a familiar person is present to provide a secure base for their adaptive responses. The child is particularly vulnerable at approximately 15 to 22 months of age, when separation is incomplete and the child requires frequent reunion with a parent.

The body image of a child is largely derived as a result of feedback from the primary caregivers, and parental anxiety regarding an acceptable physical appearance and adequate future sexual competency is readily communicated to the affected child. Therefore children with birth defects are at risk for developing a distorted body image that reflects the caregivers' subtly communicated evaluation of their bodies (Schultz, Klykylo, and Wacksman, 1983). The trend toward repair of visible genital defects is based in large part on these psychologic variables. The earlier a repair can be achieved, the more likely the development of a normal body image. Also, the earlier the repair, the shorter the time that the parents must look at the defect and risk transferring their anxiety and concern to the child.

During the years from 3 to 6, the phallico-oedipal period, children show a strong interest and concern about the genital area, sex differences, and genital normality or its lack. This is especially true if there is an older male sibling or playmate with whom to make comparisons. It is also a time when children are frightened of what they perceive to be threats to their body, especially the sex organs. They also view any untoward happening as a punishment for real or imagined wrongdoing or unacceptable sexual feelings, such as masturbation, sex play, or erotic feelings. Surgical repair is recommended before the development of these fears and anxieties. Postoperative withdrawal and aggressive behavior have been observed in 2- to 6-year-old boys who had hypospadias repair (Lepore and Kessler, 1979).

PHIMOSIS

Phimosis is a narrowing or stenosis of the preputial opening of the foreskin that prevents retraction of the foreskin over the glans penis. It is a normal finding in infants and very young boys and usually disappears as the child grows and the distal prepuce dilates. Occasionally the narrowing obstructs the flow of urine, resulting in a dribbling stream or even ballooning of the foreskin with accumulated urine during voiding.

Treatment of mild cases includes manual retraction of the foreskin and proper cleansing of the area. Severe phimosis is treated surgically by circumcision or the Heineke-Mikulicz procedure in which the constricting preputial skin is divided vertically and sutured transversely.

Nursing Considerations

If manual retraction is recommended, it is best accomplished during the child's bath. However, caution must be exercised in instructing parents to replace the foreskin over the glans penis. If left retracted, the tight band of skin constricts the blood vessels, causing edema, bluish discoloration, pain, dysuria, and eventually necrosis. The resulting edema and pain further complicate attempts to replace the foreskin in its normal position. Local applications of cold compresses and use of analgesics may help, but a physician should always evaluate the condition.

CRYPTORCHIDISM (CRYPTORCHISM)

Cryptorchidism is failure of one or both testes to descend normally through the inguinal canal. Absence of testes within the scrotum can be the result of (1) undescended testes, (2) retractable testes, (3) ectopic testes, or (4) anorchia (absence of testes).

Pathophysiology

Normally the testes descend from the abdomen, where they develop, into the scrotum during the seventh to ninth month of gestation. The progress is aided by the gubernaculum, a mass of tissue containing smooth muscle that is attached to the lower pole of the testes. The process is poorly understood and the role of hormones in facilitating and/or initiating the descent is also unclear. The testes descend to the scrotum behind the processus vaginalis, a peritoneal outpocketing that retains a communication with the peritoneal cavity and projects down through various muscle and fascial planes before the testes enter the inguinal canal (see Fig. 11-22, A to D).

Normally the upper part of the processus vaginalis atrophies and closes and the lower part is pinched off to form the tunica vaginalis of the testes. Cryptorchidism occurs when one or both testes fail to descend through the inguinal canal. The descent can be arrested at any point along its normal path. Congenital inguinal hernias frequently accompany the defect. *Ectopic testis* is a testis that has progressed normally through the inguinal canal but, after passing through the external inguinal ring, has become lodged in superficial tissue of abdominal wall, upper thigh, or perineum.

Clinical Manifestations

Undescended testes are rarely a cause of discomfort. The entire scrotum, or one side of it, is smaller than normal and appears incompletely developed, an observation made by concerned parents who often bring the child for medical evaluation. Diagnosis of undescended testes is complicated by the normal retraction of testes by the cremasteric reflex, the so-called retractable, migratory, or "yo-yo" testes. This reflex is particularly sensitive to touch and cold. However, it can be obviated by placing the child in a squatting or tailorlike position or by applying firm finger pressure on the external ring before palpating the abdomen or genitalia (see

Fig. 7-50). Retracted testes can be "milked" or pushed back into the scrotum, but truly undescended ones cannot. Ectopic testes may be felt along the inguinal canal, but those in the abdominal cavity usually cannot.

Therapeutic Management

A retractable testis that can be manipulated into the scrotum by gentle pressure on the upper lateral edge of the testis in an obliquely downward direction will eventually lodge in the scrotum spontaneously without medical or surgical intervention. The diagnosis is not made at a single examination and parents are asked if they have observed the testes in the scrotum at some time. If so, the anomaly probably represents the retractable variety and the parents can be reassured. By 1 year of age the cryptorchid testes will descend spontaneously in approximately 75% in both term and preterm infants (Penny, 1986).

Most authorities favor a trial of human chorionic gonadotropin therapy in older children. This is not a valuable means of obtaining descent before age 3 years and of limited usefulness at age 3 or 4 (Garagorri and others, 1982). Testes below the external ring may descend by the treatment, but those lodged inside the inguinal canal or fixed in an abnormal position usually require surgical intervention (orchiopexy).

If the testes do not descend spontaneously, orchiopexy is performed before the child's third birthday, preferably between 1 and 3 years of age (Penny, 1986). Surgical repair is done to (1) prevent damage to the undescended testicle by the higher degree of body heat, (2) decrease the incidence of tumor formation, which is higher in undescended testicles, (3) avoid trauma and torsion, (4) close the processus vaginalis, and (4) prevent the cosmetic and psychologic handicap of an empty scrotum. Because of increased propensity toward neoplastic changes (even after orchiopexy), cryptorchid testes are better observed in scrotal position.

The timing of the surgery is important, as it is in any genital surgery. The repair is not attempted in the first year unless there is an accompanying hernia. Fewer psychologic effects and a higher rate of fertility are reported in adults who had their repair at an early age. Having both testes in the scrotum by school age prevents psychologic problems related to body image and peer group embarrassment, since the empty scrotum is smaller in size and altered in shape.

In the routine procedure for undescended testes, the testes are brought down into the scrotum and secured in that position without tension or torsion. A simple orchiopexy for a palpable testis can usually be performed in an outpatient surgical unit without the need for overnight hospitalization. More complex disorder requires considerable surgical skill because of technical problems resulting from variations in the length of the spermatic cord.

Nursing Considerations

The postoperative nursing care is directed toward prevention of infection and instructing parents in home care of the child. Infection is prevented by carefully cleansing the operative site of stool and urine. Parents are concerned about the future fertility of the child. Therefore the prognosis for fertility is determined and the family is counseled regarding this eventuality and the optimum time for discussing the probabilities with the child—ideally as a part of sex education.

INGUINAL HERNIA

Inguinal hernias account for approximately 80% of all hernias and are the most common surgical procedures performed in infancy (with the possible exception of circumcision). Inguinal hernias occur more frequently in boys (90%) than in girls; femoral hernias occur more often in females but are uncommon in children.

Pathophysiology

Inguinal hernia is derived from persistence of all or part of the processus vaginalis, the tube of peritoneum that precedes the testicle through the inguinal canal into the scrotum during the eighth month of gestation. Following descent of the testicle, the proximal portion of the processus vaginalis normally atrophies and closes, whereas the distal portion forms the tunica vaginalis, which envelopes the testicle in the scrotum. When the upper portion fails to atrophy, the abdominal fluid or an abdominal structure can be forced into

it, creating a palpable bulge or mass. The persistent sac may end at any point along the inguinal canal; it may stop at the inguinal ring or extend all the way into the scrotum (Fig. 11-22). The hernial sac is present at birth but does not usually become apparent until the infant is able to build up sufficient intraabdominal pressure to open the sac, usually 2 to 3 months of age. Since the inguinal canal is short, hernias occur relatively early.

Clinical Manifestations

This very common defect is asymptomatic unless the abdominal contents are forced into the patent sac. Most often it appears as a painless inguinal swelling that varies in size. It disappears during periods of rest or is reducible by gentle compression; it appears when the infant cries or strains or when the older child strains, coughs, or stands for a long period. The defect can be palpated as a thickening of the cord in the groin, and the "silk glove" sign can be elicited by rubbing together the sides of the empty hernial sac.

Sometimes the herniated loop of intestine becomes partially obstructed, producing variable symptoms that may include fretfulness and irritability, tenderness, anorexia, abdominal distention, and difficulty in defecating. Occasionally the loop of bowel becomes incarcerated (irreducible), with symptoms of complete intestinal obstruction that, left untreated, will progress to strangulation and gangrene.

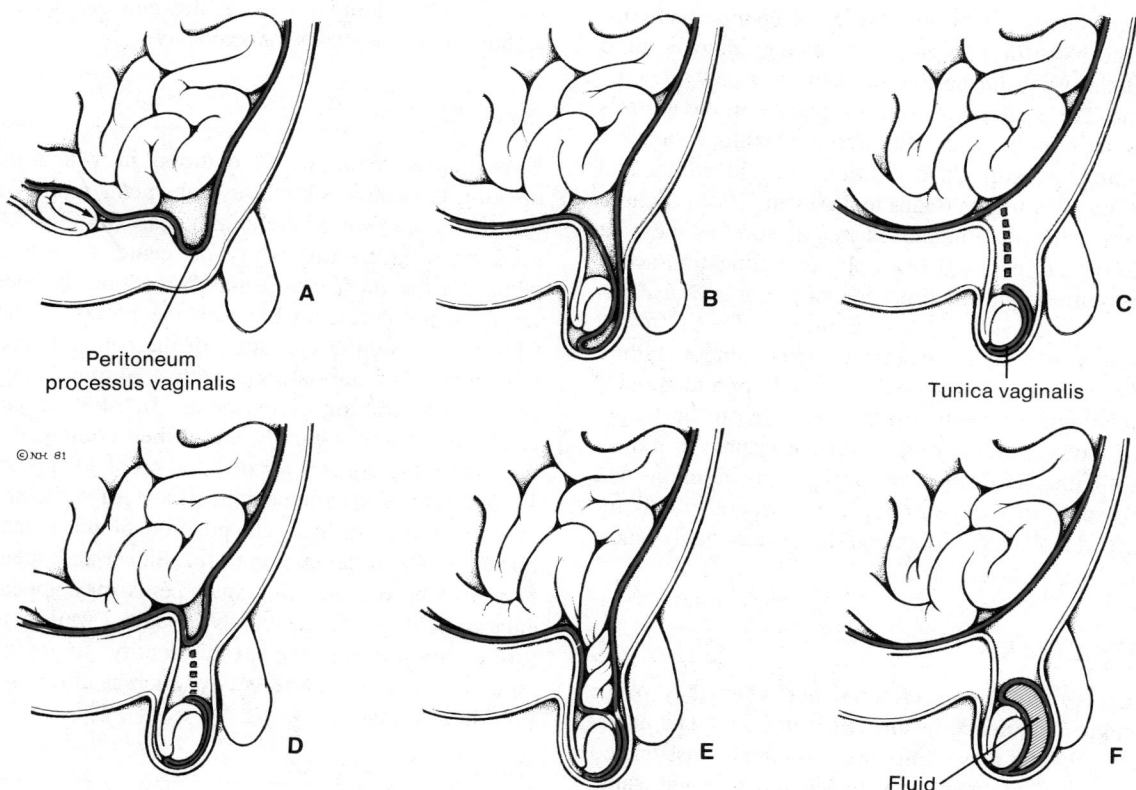

Peritoneum
processus vaginalis

Tunica vaginalis

©NK 81

Fluid

Fig. 11-22. Development of inguinal hernias. **A** and **B,** Prenatal migration of processus vaginalis. **C,** Normal. **D,** Partially obliterated processus vaginalis. **E,** Hernia. **F,** Hydrocele. (See also Fig. 7-47.)

Incarceration occurs more often in infants under 10 months of age and is more common in girls.

Therapeutic Management

The treatment for hernias is prompt, elective surgical repair in healthy infants and children as soon as the defect is diagnosed. Many physicians advocate exploration of both sides, since there is a high incidence of recurrence on the contralateral side. This practice of exploration remains controversial, however. It is preferable to attempt reduction of a recently incarcerated hernia in order that surgery can be delayed to allow the injured tissues to recover somewhat, but irreducible or strangulated hernias are treated as emergencies.

Nursing Considerations

Both infants and children tolerate surgery very well. There is usually no restriction placed on their activities, and it is not uncommon for the child to be discharged from the hospital on the day of surgery. Every attempt is made to keep the wound clean and reasonably dry. With infants and small children who are not yet toilet trained, the wound is left without a dressing. Changing diapers as soon as they become damp helps reduce the chance of irritation or infection of the incision, or the child may be left undiapered. It is seldom necessary to apply a urine-collecting device; in doing so, it is often difficult or impossible to avoid the incision.

Parents are instructed to give the child sponge baths instead of a tub bath for 1 week and to change diapers more frequently than usual during the day and once or twice during the night. There are no restrictions placed on the infant's or toddler's activity, but older children are cautioned against lifting, pushing, wrestling and fighting, bicycle riding, and athletics for about 3 weeks (Gans and Austin, 1986). School children are permitted to attend classes as soon as they are comfortable but are excused from physical education activities for the same length of time described for physical activity.

If surgery is postponed because of acute illness, failure to thrive, exposure to communicable disease, or a temporary family psychologic problem, the parents need to be taught the signs of incarcerated hernia, simple measures to reduce it (a warm bath, avoidance of upright positioning, and comfort measures to reduce crying), and where to call for assistance if relief is not obtained in a reasonably short time.

FEMORAL HERNIA

Femoral hernias are rare in children but when they occur there is a higher incidence in girls than in boys. The disorder is suspected from a swelling in the groin area associated with severe pain. Treatment and management are the same as for inguinal hernia. Strangulation is a frequent complication.

HYDROCELE

Hydrocele is the presence of fluid in the persistent processus vaginalis and is the result of the same developmental process as inguinal hernia (Fig. 11-22, *F*). When the upper segment of the processus vaginalis has been obliterated but the tunica vaginalis still contains peritoneal fluid, this is called a *noncommunicating hydrocele.* This type of hydrocele is common in newborns and often subsides spontaneously as fluid is gradually absorbed.

A *communicating hydrocele* is one in which the processus vaginalis remains open and into which peritoneal fluid may be forced by intraabdominal pressure and gravity. The length of the hydrocele depends on the length of the processus vaginalis and may extend into the tunica vaginalis within the scrotum. The hydrocele is asymptomatic except for a palpable bulge in the inguinal or scrotal areas. Unlike a hernia, the hydrocele is unable to be reduced and cannot be produced by a sudden increase in intraabdomnal pressure (such as straining). The scrotum appears to be larger after an active day and smaller in the morning. Since a hydrocele represents a patent processus vaginalis, it can predispose to herniation; therefore, surgical repair is indicated if spontaneous resolution does not take place by 1 year of age.

Nursing Considerations

The nursing care of the infant with a hydrocele is essentially the same as that for inguinal hernia. Parents are advised that there is often temporary swelling and discoloration of the scrotum that resolves spontaneously.

HYPOSPADIAS

Hypospadias refers to a condition in which the urethral opening is located behind the glans penis or anywhere along the ventral surface of the penile shaft (Fig. 11-23). In very mild cases the meatus is just off center from the tip of the penis. In the most severe malformations the meatus is located on the perineum between the halves of the scrotum. Chordee, or ventral curvature of the penis, results from the replacement of normal skin with a fibrous band of tissue, causing constriction of the penis. In addition, the foreskin is usually absent ventrally and, when combined with chordee, gives the organ a hooded and crooked appearance (Fig. 11-24). The altered appearance may leave the sex in doubt at birth, since the perineal position of the meatus may be mistaken for a female urethra. Since undescended testes may also be present, the small penis may appear to be an enlarged clitoris. Occasionally a vaginal vault is also found, further complicating the sexual identity. In any case of ambiguous genitalia, further study, such as chromosomal analysis, is essential.

Surgical Correction

The principal objectives in surgical correction are (1) to enable the child to void in the standing position by voluntarily

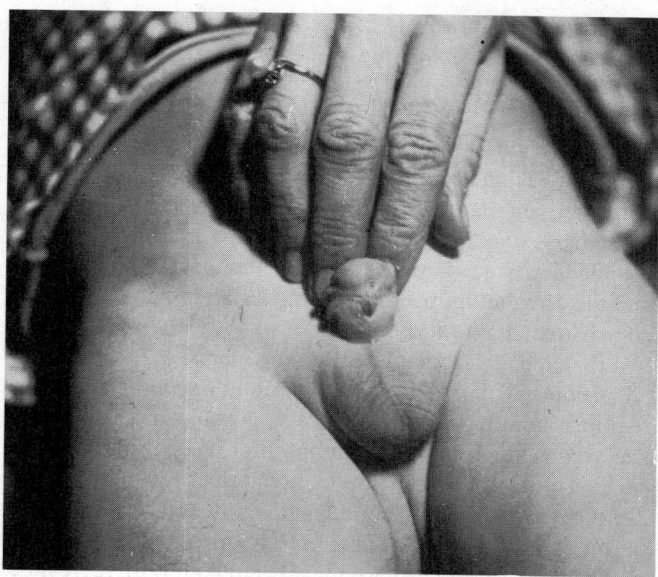

Fig. 11-23. Hypospadias.

Courtesy M.C. Gleason, M.D., San Diego, CA. From Ingalls, A.J., and Salerno, M.C.: Maternal and child health nursing, ed. 4, St. Louis, 1979, The C.V. Mosby Co.

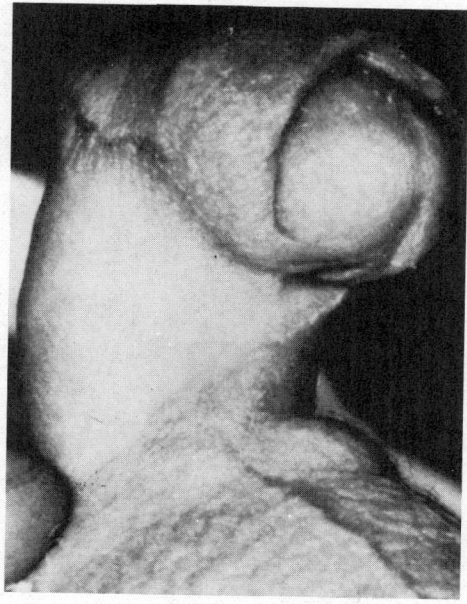

Fig. 11-24. Hypospadias with significant chordee.

From Shirkey, H.C.: Pediatric therapy, ed. 6, St. Louis, 1980, The C.V. Mosby Co.

directing the stream in the usual manner, (2) to improve the physical appearance of the genitalia for psychologic reasons, and (3) to produce a sexually adequate organ. The procedure involves releasing the chordee, extending the length of the urethra, and constructing a new meatal opening. Since the prepuce is valuable skin for the reconstructive surgery, circumcision should not be done on these infants.

A minimum defect without chordee usually requires no treatment except perhaps for cosmetic reasons; when the meatus is located on the glans penis, no intervention may be required except to release the chordee. In most instances the surgical repair can be accomplished with one-stage procedures, even as outpatient surgery. When hypospadias is more severe, repair often requires more than one surgical procedure to progressively extend the length of the urethra.

The preferred time for surgical repair is 6 to 18 months, before the child has developed body image and castration anxiety. Occasionally a short course of testosterone is administered preoperatively to achieve additional penile size to facilitate the surgery. Microscopic optical magnification and delicate instruments are used during surgery. Sometimes repairs for more severe cases of hypospadias may result in fistulas and strictures, necessitating additional surgical intervention.

Nursing Considerations

Preparation of parents and child for the type of procedure to be done and the expected cosmetic result helps avert later problems. Frequently parents are informed of what is to be surgically corrected but are not advised of what to expect as a reasonable consequence. As a result they are greatly disappointed to see a physically imperfect penis. If the child is

old enough to understand what is occurring, he is also prepared for the operation and the expected outcome.

Urethroplasty usually requires some type of urinary diversion to promote optimum healing and to maintain the position and patency of the newly formed urethra. The child is often placed under a bed cradle and immobilized with arm and leg restraints. Restraints can be removed periodically when the child is awake and under supervision and appropriate diversional activities provided. Sedation may be required for the excessively irritable or restless child. Parental rooming-in is recommended to reduce the child's anxiety.

Parents are taught to care for the indwelling catheter and irrigation technique. They need to know when and how to empty the urine bag and how to avoid kinking, twisting, or blockage of the catheter. They are taught how to tape the drainage bag to the leg to allow the child to be mobile and to *never* clamp off a catheter. An extra bag is sent home with the family in case of tears or leakage. The family is advised to encourage the child to increase fluid intake. Twice daily bathing is recommended, as is loose clothing. Straddle toys, sandboxes, swimming, and rough activities are avoided until allowed by the surgeon.

EPISPADIAS

Epispadias is a rare defect in which the meatal opening is located on the dorsal surface of the penis. As in hypospadias, the defect can occur in differing degrees of severity. The treatment is surgical and usually includes penile and urethral lengthening plus bladder neck reconstruction when necessary. The nursing considerations are similar to those discussed for hypospadias.

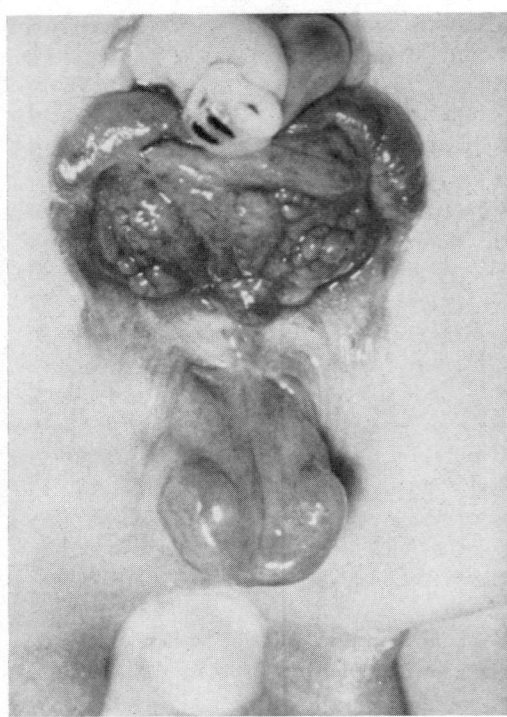

Fig. 11-25. Exstrophy of bladder.

Courtesy E.S. Tank, M.D., Division of Urology, University of Oregon Health Sciences Center, Portland, OR.

EXSTROPHY OF BLADDER

Exstrophy of the bladder is an obvious and serious congenital defect that occurs three times more frequently in males than in females (Fig. 11-25). There is no familial tendency, but it rarely occurs in siblings. There are varying degrees of the defect, ranging from an abdominal opening (epispadias) to vestiges of the primitive cloaca, embryonic endodermal tissue from which the bladder is eventually derived. Incontinence accompanies all degrees of the anomaly.

Pathophysiology

Exstrophy results from failure of the abdominal wall and underlying structures, such as the ventral wall of the bladder, to fuse in utero. As a result the lower urinary tract is exposed and the everted bladder appears bright red through the abdominal opening. Abnormal ureteral outlets and the external urethral meatus cause a constant seepage of urine, making the area malodorous and highly susceptible to infection. The constant accumulation of urine on the surrounding skin produces tissue ulceration and further infection. Progressive renal damage from infection and obstruction may terminate in renal failure.

In males the defect is almost always associated with epispadias and may include other problems, such as undescended testes, a short penis, or inguinal hernia. The sexual handicap in males may be severe because the penis protrudes inadequately. In females the genitalia may be affected, with a cleft clitoris, completely separated labia, and

absent vagina. In either sex, separation of the pubic bones causes difficulty in walking, such as a waddling gait.

Therapeutic Management

The objectives of treatment include (1) preservation of renal function, (2) attainment of urinary control, (3) adequate reconstructive repair for psychologic benefit, and (4) improvement of sexual function, particularly in males. Closure of the bladder is accomplished within the first 48 hours of life and the circulating maternal hormones allow the pelvis to be approximated anteriorly.

Final repair is completed before school age. Essentially all patients with exstrophy have vesiculoureteral reflux that requires antireflux surgery, usually accompanied by vesical neck reconstruction in an attempt to produce urinary continence. These initial procedures are ordinarily performed at 2½ to 3 years of age, penile lengthening and release of dorsal chordee at 4 years of age, and urethral construction with advancement of the urinary meatus at about 6 to 12 years of age (Kramer and Kelalis, 1986).

In females the urethroplasty and other reconstruction are performed at the same time as the anti-incontinence procedure but vaginoplasty is delayed until puberty. Both boys and girls in whom surgery is delayed may require a temporary urinary diversion procedure. Those with complications or continued problems with continence are candidates for an artificial genitourinary sphincter or antirefluxing intestinal diversion, such as ureteral sigmoid implant, bilateral ureterostomy, or ileal conduit.

Nursing Considerations

One of the most devastating aspects of exstrophy of the bladder is its gross appearance. Although the actual procedures are not difficult, it is not easy for parents to assume responsibility for what to them seems an enormous task because of the emotional impact of the defect.

Physical care of the unrepaired defect includes meticulous hygiene of the bladder area to prevent infection and excoriation of the surrounding tissue. A sterile nonadherent dressing is placed over the exposed bladder area to prevent infection and to keep the diaper from adhering to the mucosa. An ointment may be prescribed for the surrounding skin to protect it from the constantly draining urine.

Ordinarily diapers are placed over the defect in the usual manner, although an additional cloth diaper wrapped around the lower abdomen can give added absorbency. Diapers are changed frequently to prevent infection, ulceration, and odor and immediately after a bowel movement to prevent contamination of the exposed area. General infant care remains unchanged except for sponge baths rather than immersion in water. A public health referral is an important component of discharge planning, and ideally home visits should begin immediately after the infant's release from the hospital.

Parents and child should be instructed regarding realistic outcome of surgery, since unrealistic expectations of the cosmetic result may leave them very disappointed and discouraged. Continuous care by one nurse helps the family adjust to all aspects of recovery. As difficult as it was for parents to adjust to the defect at the time of the child's birth, it may be equally disturbing for them to accept the fact that surgical closure does not ensure normal urination and that urinary diversion is necessary. The prospect of a permanent ileal conduit or other similar procedure provokes powerful emotional responses. Parents often worry about the child's sexual adjustment, even though they may not voice such thoughts.

Part of the nursing admission history is directed toward evaluating the parents' and child's expectation of the surgical repair, knowledge of the possibility of eventual ileostomy appliance for an ileal conduit or urinary control with a sigmoid implant, and feelings concerning this permanent change in body function.

It is not unusual for parents to be ambivalent in their feelings toward surgical creation of a urinary diversion, especially if they have become accustomed to the general care, which for infants differs little from diapering an unaffected child. In such situations it is good to discuss the long-range advantages of a permanent urinary diversion in contrast to the ever-present danger of infection and kidney damage and the constant inconvenience of seeping urine. A well-fitting ileostomy bag allows the child almost unrestricted freedom in activities enjoyed by other children and results in no major alteration in toileting, except emptying the bag at periodic intervals. This is extremely important to older children and adolescents, who want to be accepted as one of the group and deplore any stigma of being different.

Other aspects of preoperative care are similar to those for any major abdominal surgery. Since a routine urinalysis is part of most admission procedures, a urine specimen can be obtained by allowing urine to drip into a container by holding the child prone over a basin or by aspirating some urine directly from the bladder area into a medicine dropper or syringe. If a sterile specimen is needed for evaluation of existing infection, the former procedure is preferable, but a sterile container must be used.

Postoperative care differs little from that of any surgical patient. An abdominal dressing is placed over the closure site and is kept clean and checked for any presence of urine. If an ileal conduit or ureterostomy was performed, a separate absorbent dressing is placed over the stoma to collect the urine and prevent contamination of the other dressing. An appliance is usually fitted as soon as possible to allow the child and parents adequate time to learn its proper use and adjust to the change in body image.

Even with improved reconstructive surgery for these patients, substantial psychologic support and guidance are needed to help them adjust to their fears of inadequate penile size, ugliness of genitalia, potential inability to procreate, and rejection by peers, especially the opposite sex. Ongoing discussion groups for parents and children are particularly useful in promoting resolution of these fears and allowing for optimum psychologic adjustment, particularly during adolescence.

ABERRANT SEXUAL DEVELOPMENT

The birth of a child with ambiguous genitalia is a situation that constitutes a crisis quite different from that of many other congenital anomalies. Uncertain sex is no threat to life in a physical sense but is a potential lifetime social tragedy for the child and family. The problem of appropriate sex must be solved quickly and accurately and requires no less speed and skill than life-threatening anomalies such as tracheoesophageal fistula. There are studies that can be carried out during the first few days of life that help guide those involved in making a correct gender choice. Even a brief delay in gender assignment can generate rumors that can be a source of distress to a child and family for years.

Etiology

Genetic sex is determined at the time of conception and depends on whether the ovum is fertilized by a sperm bearing an X chromosome or one bearing a Y chromosome. The phenotypic evidence of sex depends on whether subsequent processes proceed normally: differentiation of primitive gonads, differentiation and development of internal duct systems, and differentiation and development of external genitalia. The normal order of events can be altered by abnormalities of the chromosomal complement, defects of embryogenesis, or biochemical (hormonal) abnormalities. Disturbances in any of these processes will lead to abnormal sexual development evidenced by the presence of ambiguous genitalia at birth.

Normal sexual development. For the first 6 weeks of life the developing embryo is morphologically neutral, neither male nor female. The primitive, bipotential (able to form either a testicle or an ovary) gonad consists of an outer layer, the cortex, and an inner medulla. Differentiation into testes and ovary takes place during the seventh and eighth weeks of gestation. At this time, in the male the medullary portion develops and the cortical zone regresses; in the female the cortex is preserved while the medulla regresses. It appears that without the presence of a masculine inductor stimulus determined by the Y chromosome the primitive gonad has an inherent tendency to feminize. The embryonic ovary develops in the absence of stimulation.

In the 7-week-old embryo the internal genital ducts of the bipotential embryo consist of both wolffian and müllerian duct systems. Differentiation of these duct systems depends on the presence or absence of locally acting male organizer substances secreted by Leydig cells of the testes. One, an androgen, stimulates development of the wolffian duct system into epididymis, vas deferens, and seminal vesicles; another, not an androgen, actively inhibits the müllerian duct system, which subsequently regresses. In the absence of a testis the müllerian system is preserved to give rise to the uterine tubes, uterus, and upper vagina, whereas the wolffian system passively regresses (Fig. 11-26).

The final stage of sex development is differentiation of the external genitalia, which in the early embryo consists of a urogenital sinus, two lateral labioscrotal swellings, and an

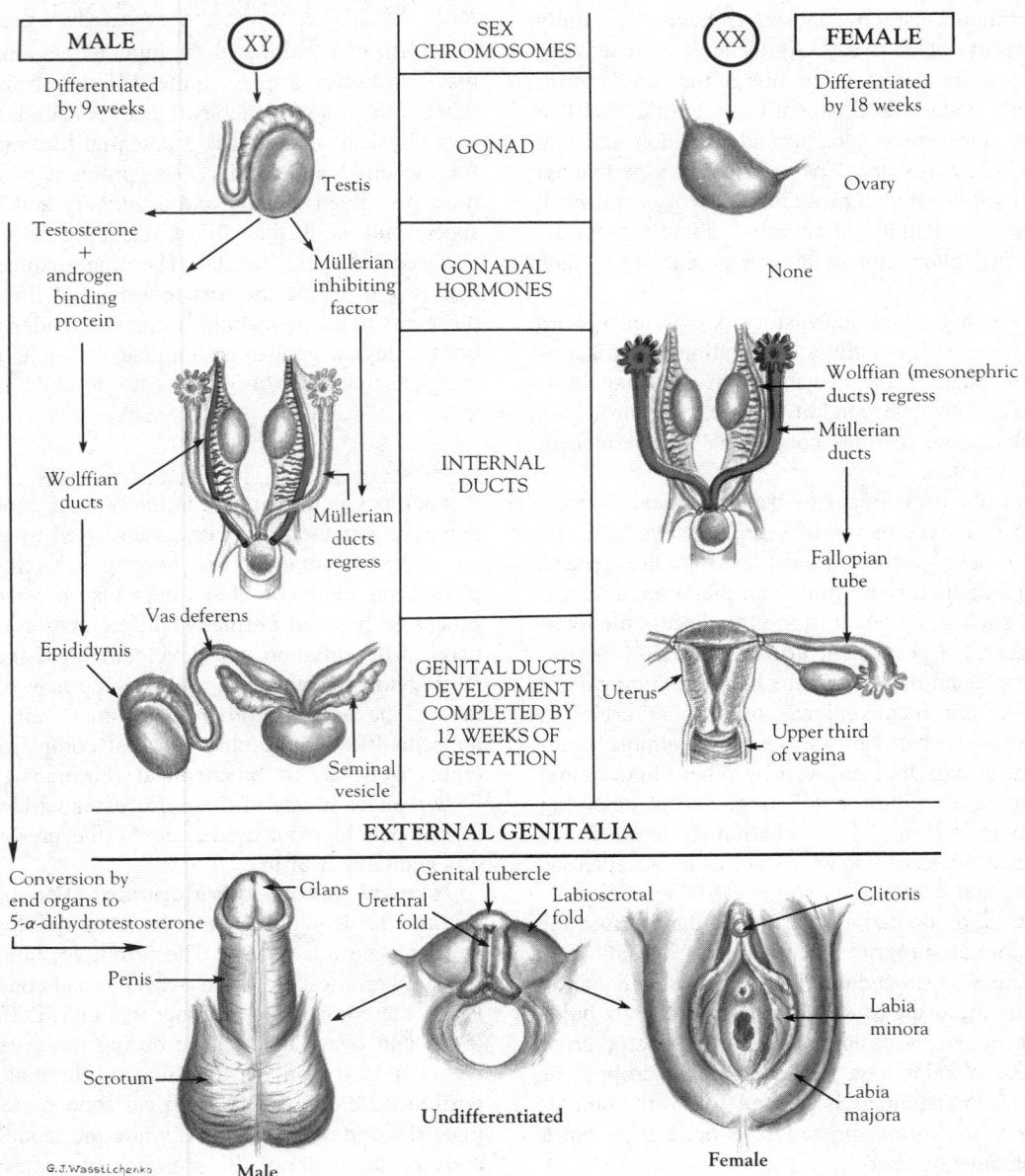

Fig. 11-26. Sex differentiation in male and female.
From Thompson, J. and others: Clinical nursing, St. Louis, 1986, The C.V. Mosby Co.

anteriorly situated genital tubercle. Depending on the presence or absence of male hormones, the genital tubercle differentiates into a penis or a clitoris. In response to testicular androgens, the labiosacral folds fuse to form a scrotum and ventral skin of the penis; the urethral folds form the perineal and penile urethra. Without the influence of masculinizing secretions, the urethral folds do not fuse and instead become the labia minora, the labiosacral folds remain unfused to separate into the labia majora, and the urogenital sinus differentiates into a lower vagina and the vaginal and urethral openings (see Fig. 11-26).

Abnormal sexual development. Disturbances in the normal order of events in sex determination will produce abnormal sex development with the presence of ambiguous or inappropriate external genitalia at birth. Ambiguous gen-

italia can be variable and often closely conform to one sex or the other. In some forms the external sexual structures represent those of a perfectly normal male or female, whereas the genetic sex is the direct opposite. A situation in which the phenotypic sex differs from the chromosomal sex is often termed *intersex*.

A failure or abnormality in any of the four steps of sexual development can lead to abnormal development in subsequent stages. The mechanisms and site of defective development are summarized below.

abnormal sex determination Chromosomal abnormalities that result in disturbance of sexual development are discussed on p. 148 and in relation to delayed development in Chapter 20.

abnormal differentiation of gonads When induction of the bipotential gonad fails, sex differentiation proceeds in the direction of the female phenotype, regardless of the genetic sex.

abnormal differentiation of ductal systems Biologic inactivity of androgenic male organizer substance or insensitivity of ductal tissue to its action results in deficient wolffian duct differentiation, whereas normal secretion of the second male organizer produces normal regression of the müllerian duct system (seen in testicular feminization syndrome). Defective function of the second male organizer substance causes persistence of the müllerian duct system, which leads to the presence of a uterus and uterine tubes, whereas the normal androgenic substance stimulates normal male differentiation (uterine hernia syndrome).

abnormal secretion of or tissue insensitivity to testicular androgen Complete failure of male hormone secretion produces female external genitalia in a genetic male. Partial or incomplete failure results in incomplete masculinization with ambiguity of external genitalia. The genetic female fetus exposed to large amounts of androgenic hormone (from maternal hyperproduction, fetal adrenal hyperplasia, or maternal ingestion of androgenic steroid substances) may exhibit varying degrees of masculinization of the external genitalia (congenital adrenal hyperplasia).

Types of Abnormalities

Some disorders with abnormal sexual development are not characterized by ambiguous genitalia in the newborn period. For example, the most common sex chromosomal disorders do not become apparent until later childhood, adolescence, or even young adulthood when the individual seeks medical attention because of problems of delayed development or infertility. The four conditions producing ambiguous genitalia in the newborn that require prompt and accurate evaluation are: the masculinized female (female pseudohermaphrodite), the incompletely masculinized male (male pseudohermaphrodite), the true hermaphrodite, and mixed gonadal dysgenesis.

The most common condition that produces ambiguous genitalia in the newborn is the masculinized female as the result of virilization by adrenal androgens after the time of early differentiation of gonadal tissues. The most common type, congenital adrenal hyperplasia, is caused by an inherited deficiency in the enzymes of adrenal corticoid synthesis. The resulting decrease in cortisol stimulates pituitary secretion of corticotropin (ACTH), which causes the adrenal cortex to respond with increased production of other adrenal hormones, including the androgens. Since the adrenal gland differentiates later than the gonadal duct systems but before differentiation of the external genitalia, the masculinization of the external genitalia is the predominant feature. The internal female anatomy is normal. This inherited disorder is the only intersex problem that is life-threatening, and it should be considered in any situation where sex is doubtful. Congenital adrenal hyperplasia is discussed further in Chapter 38.

In the incompletely masculinized male the external structures may be incompletely masculine, ambiguous, or completely female. The complex nature of virilization offers numerous opportunities for disturbance in the process. In some disorders there is deficient production of fetal androgen, in others there is deficiency in any of the enzymes needed in the numerous steps of testosterone biosynthesis, or more commonly there is unresponsiveness or subresponsiveness of genital structures to testosterone. True hermaphrodites are rare and may be either genetic males or females with *both* ovarian and testicular tissues, with an ovary on one side and a testis on the other, or a combination of ovotestis. The external genitalia may be male, usually cryptorchid, or normal female, but in the majority of cases are ambiguous.

The second most commonly seen disorder is mixed gonadal dysgenesis in which affected infants are sex chromosomal mosaics (see p. 147). Genitalia vary greatly, but in those who appear predominantly female, the dysplastic testis may cause masculinization at puberty. Some defects in sexual development are outlined in Table 11-3. External appearance of genitalia is described in Table 11-4.

Diagnostic Evaluation

Diagnostic tools and their significant findings that help determine sex and assist in making a gender assignment include:

1. **History.** Previous abortions may help identify chromosomal aberrations; ingestion of steroids; relatives with ambiguous genitalia or who died in the first weeks of life.
2. **Physical examination.** Seldom of significant value.
3. **Buccal smear.** Detects presence or absence of sex chromatin; results available within 24 hours.
4. **Chromosomal analysis.** Detects chromosomal abnormalities and precise genetic sex; results available in 2 to 3 days.
5. **Endoscopy and x-ray contrast studies.** Reveal presence, absence, or nature of internal genital structures.
6. **Biochemical tests.** Urinary steroid excretion patterns help detect several of the adrenal cortical syndromes. Tests include 17-ketosteroids, 17-hydroxycorticoids, and urinary pregnanediol.
7. **Laparotomy or gonad biopsy.** In some instances this is the only way to arrive at a definitive diagnosis.

Therapeutic Management

The assignment of a gender sex to the infant whose sex is doubtful constitutes a social emergency. The long-term implications are such that a hasty decision based on appearance alone may be disastrous, and the optimum sex of rearing may not be the same as the genetic or gonadal sex. The infant's anatomy rather than genetic sex is the primary criterion on which the choice of gender should be based. An incomplete female is better able to adjust than is an inadequate male. A functional vagina can be constructed surgically, and with appropriate administration of hormones the anatomically incomplete female can lead a relatively normal life, but it is as yet impossible to construct a satisfactory penis from an inadequate phallus for an equally satisfactory adjustment of the incomplete male.

In most instances of ambiguous genitalia it is recom-

Table 11-3 Abnormalities of sexual development

ABNORMALITY	INTERNAL/EXTERNAL STRUCTURES	COMMENTS AND MANAGEMENT

Masculinized female
Congenital adrenal hyperplasia
	XX, chromation positive
	Genitalia: female
	    Enlarged clitoris; varying degrees of labial fusion
	Often indistinguishable from cryptorchid male
	Female pseudohermaphrodite
	Internal: ovaries, female duct system present
		Caused by adrenal androgens
		    Autosomal-recessive inheritance
		    Maternal virilizing adrenal tumor
		    Maternal ingestion of steroids or progestinal agents
		Fertile at maturity if course arrested
		Endogenous: hydrocortisone for life; progressive virilization if untreated
		Exogenous: not progressive after birth
		Surgical correction if needed, e.g., clitoral recession, vaginoplasty
		Gender assignment: female

Incompletely masculinized male Complete testicular femininization	Male pseudohermaphrodite XY, chromatin negative Genitalia: female with blind vaginal pouch Internal: testes in abdomen, inguinal canal, or labia Duct systems present Germ cells absent or early forms	 Inherited: autosomal-dominant? X-linked? Develop female secondary sex characteristics Gender assignment: female
Incomplete testicular femininization	XY, chromatin negative Genitalia: ambiguous with blind vaginal pouch Internal: testes in abdomen, inguinal canal, or labia Duct systems present Germ cells absent or early forms	Inherited: autosomal-dominant? X-linked? Develop female secondary sex characteristics; may be minimum Gender assignment: female
Pseudovaginal perineoscrotal hypospadias	XY, chromatin negative Genitalia: ambiguous, severe hypospadias; blind vaginal pouch Internal: testes in labial folds, inguinal canal, or abdomen Duct systems and sperm cells (immature forms) present	Inherited: autosomal-recessive Masculinized at puberty Gender assignment: usually male
Uterine hernia syndrome	XY, chromatin negative Genitalia: male; often cryptorchid Normal duct system and germ cells Hernia containing müllerian structures	Cause unknown Normal masculinization at puberty Gender assignment: male
Anorchism	XY, chromatin negative Genitalia: male, small Internal: absent internal genital structures and germ cells	Cause unclear No secondary sex characteristics Androgen therapy at puberty Gender assignment: male
True hermaphrodite	XY, XX, or XX/XY, chromatin variable Genitalia: male, female, or ambiguous Internal: ovary and testes or ovotestes present Germ cells present Internal structures present and correspond to adjacent gonads	Cause unknown Gender assignment: depends on predominant characteristics
Mixed gonadal dysgenesis	X/XY Genitalia: male, female, or ambiguous Internal: infantile uterus, vagina, and fallopian tubes present; usually unilateral testis with streak gonad contralateral	Cause unknown Gender assignment: depends on predominant characteristics Masculinization at puberty
Turner syndrome (p. 856)	X, chromatin negative Genitalia: female Internal: absent or mere vestiges	Cause: chromosomal aberration May develop varying degrees of secondary sex characteristics
Klinefelter syndrome (p. 857)	XXY, chromatin positive Genitalia: male Internal: dysgenic duct system present; small testes present; germ cells absent	Cause: chromosomal aberration Deficient masculinization at puberty Gynecomastia common

Table 11-4 Ambiguous genitalia

NORMAL FINDINGS	AMBIGUOUS FINDINGS
Male	
Penile shaft protrudes from perineum and hangs freely	Small penis (less than 2 to 3 cm [0.8 to 1.2 inches] in newborn) may be enlarged clitoris
Urethral meatus centered at tip of glans penis	Urethral meatus anywhere along dorsal or ventral surface of penis, especially on perineum
Two scrotal sacs hang freely, covered with loose, wrinkled skin	Small scrotum with smooth, tight skin and any degree of separation in midline may be enlarged labia
Palpable testes in each scrotum	Absent testes may be undescended: if combined with small scrotum, may be evidence of enlarged labia
Female	
Small clitoris at anterior end of labia	Enlarged clitoris that protrudes from labia may be small penis
Urethral meatus located between clitoris and vagina	Urethral meatus located in clitoris may suggest small penis
Labia minora prominent in newborn but atrophied and almost absent in prepubertal female; completely separated from clitoris to posterior vault of vagina; on palpation, no masses in labia	Prominent labia, partially or completely fused with palpable masses on each side, may be small scrotum with testes

mended that the infant be reared as a female. Genetic males with a phallus of adequate size that will respond to testosterone at the time of puberty can be considered for male rearing. Adequate studies should be carried out early to assist in gender selection, even though they may delay final sex assignment for several days or even weeks. Supportive measures, such as appropriate surgical reconstruction techniques, that provide normal-appearing external structures are carried out. Removal of inappropriate internal structures and dysgenic gonads is recommended.

Nursing Considerations

Families need a great deal of support and encouragement from nurses and other members of the health team to cope with this emotionally charged situation. Parents are confused, anxious, and overwhelmed by feelings of guilt and shame. They may pressure for immediate sex assignment because they are concerned about the child and the child's future, and because they must face questioning relatives and friends. The best approach is honesty. The disorder should be treated as any other disorder and no attempt should be

made to camouflage the problem. The sequence of embryologic events leading to the defect can be explained using correct terminology to describe sexual deviations. An understanding of the anomaly assists parents in explaining the defect to others just as with any other physical defect. It requires sympathy and understanding to deal with parental anxiety during this trying period and to guide them throughout the long-term management (see also Chapter 22).

Congenital Defects Caused by Prenatal Factors

Several syndromes involving a variety of malformations have been attributed to an adverse prenatal environment. Crowding in the uterus and pressure of one fetal part against another produce limb and facial deformities of greater or lesser consequence, and amniotic bands can constrict blood supply to limbs to alter their configuration. There are also several syndromes or neonatal infections caused by maternal infections or ingestion of teratogenic drugs during a sensitive period of development.

DEFECTS CAUSED BY INFECTIOUS AGENTS

The clinical picture of disorders caused by transplacental transfer of infectious agents is not always well defined. One group of microbial agents can cause remarkably similar manifestations, and it is not uncommon to test for all when a prenatal infection is suspected. This is the so-called TORCH complex, an acronym that represents the following infections:

T Toxoplasmosis
O Other (e.g., hepatitis)
R Rubella
C Cytomegalovirus infection
H Herpes simplex

To determine the causative agent in a symptomatic infant, tests are carried out to rule out each of these infections. The "O" category may involve testing for several viral infections (e.g., hepatitis, varicella zoster, measles, mumps) as well as testing for syphilis and listeriosis. Bacterial infections are not included in the TORCH workup because they are usually identified by clinical manifestations and readily available laboratory tests. Gonococcal conjunctivitis (ophthalmia neonatorum) and chlamydia conjunctivitis have been virtually eliminated by prophylactic measures at birth and are discussed in Chapter 8 and Table 11-5.

Nursing Considerations

One of the major goals in care of infants suspected of having an infectious disease is identification of the causative organism. Until diagnosis is established, the infant is isolated from contact with other infants. In suspected cytomegalovirus and rubella infections, pregnant personnel are cautioned to avoid contact with the infant. Herpes simplex is easily transmitted from one infant to another; therefore risk of cross-contamination is reduced or eliminated by wearing gloves and gowns for patient contact. Masks may be required for personnel when caring for infants with an infection such as congenital rubella. The hospital infection control department provides guidelines for the type and duration of precautions. Careful handwashing is always an important nursing intervention in reducing spread of any infection.

Infants with feeding difficulties will require special feeding techniques, and those subject to seizures are protected from adverse environmental stimuli. When possible, long-term disabilities are prevented by early evaluation and implementation of therapy. The family is taught any special handling techniques needed for the care of their infant and signs of complications or possible sequelae. If sequelae are inevitable, the family will need assistance in determining how they can best cope with the problems, such as assis-

tance with home care, referral to appropriate agencies, or placement in an institution for care.

The major goal of nursing care is prevention of these disorders with provision of adequate prenatal care for the expectant mother and precautions regarding exposure to teratogenic infections (Table 11-5) (Fig. 11-27).

DEFECTS CAUSED BY CHEMICAL AGENTS

In the wake of the thalidomide tragedy of the early 1960s, in which hundreds of malformed children were born, chemical agents have been implicated in a number of congenital defects. Consequently expectant mothers are cautioned against ingesting any medication without first consulting their physicians. The common "social" drug, alcohol, is associated with lower birth weight and other defined characteristics in the infant. It is also believed that even moderate use of alcohol during pregnancy may impair the mother/

Table 11-5 Congenital disorders acquired from maternal infections

FETAL OR NEWBORN EFFECT	COMMENTS AND NURSING CONSIDERATIONS
Coxsackie virus (Group B) Poor feeding, vomiting, diarrhea, fever; cardiac enlargement, arrhythmias, congestive heart failure; lethargy, seizures, meningeal involvement	Transmitted: first trimester or late in pregnancy Wear gloves for direct care of infant
Chlamydia infection (Chlamydia trachomatis) Conjunctivitis, pneumonia	Transmitted: last trimester or intrapartum Apply prophylactic medication to eyes at time of birth Wear gloves for direct care of infant Treatment: antibiotics
Cytomegalic inclusion disease—CMD (Cytomegalovirus [CMV]) Microcephaly, cerebral calcifications, chorioretinitis Jaundice, hepatosplenomegaly Petechial or purpuric rash Neurologic sequelae: seizure disorders, sensorimotor deafness, mental retardation	Transmitted: throughout pregnancy Affected individuals excrete the virus Virus detected in the urine by electron microscopy Avoid kissing affected child Pregnant women should avoid close contact with those who have known cases • Treatment: antimetabolites, antiviral agent
Gonococcal disease (Neisseria gonorrhoeae) Ophthalmitis Neonatal gonococcal arthritis, septicemia, meningitis	Transmitted: last trimester or intrapartum Apply prophylactic medication to eyes at time of birth Isolate suspected cases; obtain smears for culture Treatment: penicillin
Hepatitis B (virus) May be asymptomatic Acute hepatitis, changes in liver function	Transmitted: transplacental, contaminated maternal secretions during delivery Treatment: hepatitis B immune globulin to all infants of HBsAg-positive mothers
Herpes, neonatal (herpes simplex virus) Cutaneous lesions: vesicles at 6 to 10 days of age, may be no lesions Disseminated disease: resembles sepsis Visceral involvement: granulomas Early nonspecific signs: fever, lethargy, poor feeding, irritability, vomiting May include hyperbilirubinemia, seizures, flaccid or spastic paralysis, apneic episodes, respiratory distress, lethargy, or coma	History of genital infection in mother/partner in 50% of cases Transmitted: intrapartum either ascending and/or direct contact Incubation period 6 to 10 days Rarely acquired as intrauterine infection during first trimester and intrapartum Cesarean section a frequent preventive measure Isolate suspected infant until disease determined by blood cultures Strict isolation of confirmed cases until illness ends

Table 11-5 Congenital disorders acquired from maternal infections—cont'd

FETAL OR NEWBORN EFFECT	COMMENTS AND NURSING CONSIDERATIONS
Listeriosis (Listeria) Acquired in late pregnancy: stillborn or acutely ill; may die within an hour after birth Late onset: septicemia; meningitis	Transmitted: transplacentally or by aspiration of secretions at birth Segregate infants until cultures negative
Rubella, congenital (rubella virus) Eye defects: cataracts (unilateral or bilateral), microphthalmia, retinitis, glaucoma Central nervous system signs: microcephaly, seizures, severe mental retardation Congenital heart defects: patent ductus arteriosus Auditory: high incidence of delayed hearing loss Intrauterine growth retardation Hyperbilirubinemia, spinal fluid abnormalities, thrombocytopenia, hepatomegaly	Transmitted: first trimester; early second trimester Pregnant women should avoid contact with all affected persons, including infants with rubella syndrome Emphasize vaccination of all unimmunized prepubertal children, susceptible adolescents, and adult females of childbearing age Caution women against pregnancy for at least 3 months following vaccination Strict isolation of affected infant
Syphilis, congenital (Treponema pallidum) Copper-colored maculopapular cutaneous lesions (after 7th day), mucous membrane patches, hair loss, nail exfoliation, snuffles (syphilitic rhinitis), profound anemia, poor feeding, pseudoparalysis of one or more limbs	Transmitted: transplacental, usually after 18th week of pregnancy Most severe form of syphilis Strict isolation of infant Treatment: penicillin
Toxoplasmosis (Toxoplasma gondii) Hydrocephaly, cerebral calcifications, chorioretinitis (classic triad) Microcephaly Encephalitis, myocarditis, hepatosplenomegaly, anemia, jaundice, diarrhea, vomiting, seizures, pupura	Transmitted: throughout pregnancy Predominant host for organism is cats May be transmitted through cat feces, poorly cooked or raw infected meat Caution pregnant women to avoid contact with cat feces, e.g., emptying cat litter boxes Treatment: sulfonamides, pyrimethamine
Varicella (chickenpox) (varicella virus) Skin lesions, microcephaly, limb deformities, encephalomyocarditis, visceral involvement	Transmitted: first trimester or intrapartum Isolate infant

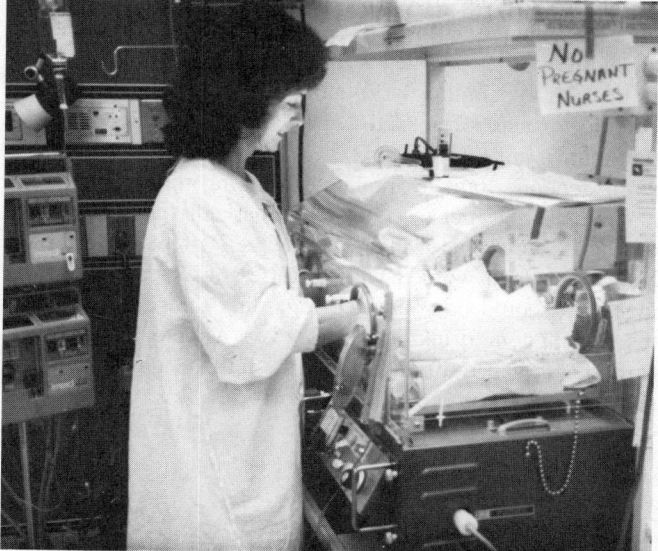

Fig. 11-27. Hospital personnel practice preventive measures when caring for affected infants.

Photography by Anne Kunke, San Jose, CA.

child bonding process. Observers have concluded that there is no safe level of alcohol consumption in pregnancy (Davis, Partridge, and Storrs, 1982) and that women who plan to become pregnant should stop consuming alcohol at least 3 months before they plan to become pregnant.

FETAL ALCOHOL SYNDROME

The term *fetal alcohol syndrome* is now widely used to describe infants with characteristic facial and associated features attributed to excessive ingestion of alcohol by the mother during pregnancy. It is now known that alcohol (ethanol and ethyl alcohol) definitely interferes with normal pregnancy, that the effects on the fetus are permanent, and that the disorder may be more prevalent in western society than is now recognized (Iber, 1980).

The teratogenesis of fetal alcohol syndrome is only beginning to be understood. It is unclear to what extent the defects are related to the amount of alcohol consumed. It is not the degree of alcoholism in the mother that is related to the presence of abnormalities in the fetus; rather, it is the amount consumed in excess of the liver's ability to detoxify that places the fetus at risk. The liver's capacity to detoxify

Major features of fetal alcohol syndrome

Facial features
Short palpebral fissures
Hypoplastic philtrum (vertical ridge in upper lip)
Thinned upper lip
Short, upturned nose
Hypoplastic maxilla
Micrognathia or prognathia in adolescence
Retrognathia in infancy

Neurologic
Mental retardation
Motor retardation
Microcephaly
Poor coordination
Hypotonia

Behavior
Irritability (infancy)
Hyperactivity (child)

Growth
Prenatal growth retardation
Persistent postnatal growth lag

is limited and inflexible—when the liver receives more alcohol than it is able to handle, the excess is continually recirculated until the organ is able to reduce it to carbon dioxide and water. This circulating alcohol has a special affinity for brain tissue. Other factors that contribute to the teratogenic effects include toxic acetyl aldehyde (a degradation by-product of ethanol) and other substances that may be added to the alcohol. The poor nutritional state of the alcoholic mother further compromises the fetus.

The effects on the fetal brain are reflected in the central nervous system manifestations of fetal alcohol syndrome. The major features of fetal alcohol syndrome are outlined in the boxed material. Mental retardation and a variety of defects in craniofacial development are prominent features. (Fig. 11-28). Affected infants display the physical features of the syndrome and the characteristic behaviors beginning in the first 24 hours of life (Lemons, 1983). These include difficulty in establishing respirations, irritability, lethargy, seizure activity, tremulousness, opisthotonos, poor suck reflex, and abdominal distention. Affected infants frequently develop metabolic problems.

The initial difficulties in the newborn period are managed by preventing excess stimulation that might precipitate seizures, sedation and/or anticonvulsant therapy, and general supportive measures. However, the defects and their effects are irreversible, so the major emphasis must be aimed at prevention.

Nursing Considerations

The nursing care of affected infants involves the same assessment and observations that are employed for any high-risk infant (see Chapter 10). Poor feeding is characteristic of infants with FAS and can be a significant problem throughout infancy. Special emphasis should be placed on monitoring weight gain, analyzing feeding behaviors, and devising strategies to promote nutritional intake.

Identifying and treating the alcoholic mother provide a greater challenge. As with all pregnant women, the pregnant alcoholic mother is urged to obtain prenatal care and to abstain from consuming large amounts of alcohol. The exact quantity of alcohol needed to produce teratogenic effects in the fetus is not known.

In general, light to moderate drinking throughout pregnancy does not appear to have any markedly adverse effects on the offspring. However, the dangers of heavy drinking are known, and women with histories of excessive alcohol ingestion should be counseled regarding the risks to the fetus. Change in drinking habits even as late as the third trimester (when brain growth in the fetus is greatest) is associated with improved fetal outcome.

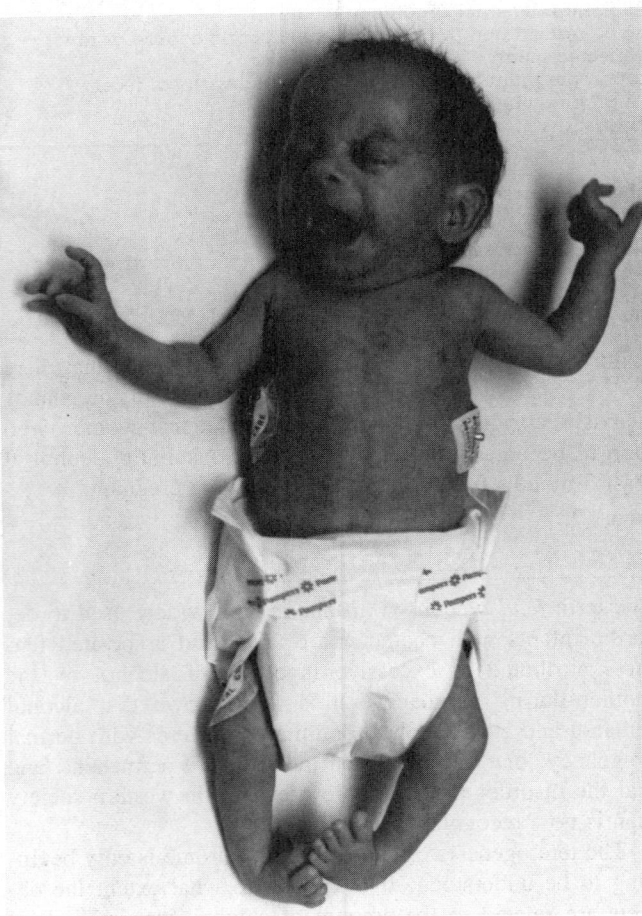

Fig. 11-28. Infant with fetal alcohol syndrome.
Photography by Anne Kunke, San Jose, CA.

CONCEPT SUMMARIES

- Approximately one third of hospitalized children suffer from a congenital abnormality or its sequelae.

- Typical reactions from parents to children with physical defects include grief over "loss" of a perfect child, shock, and withdrawal.

- The nurse's primary roles include caregiver, provider of family support, and supplier of information.

- One of the largest groups of congenital anomalies include those associated with the embryonic neural tube. The most common of these are spina bifida occulta and myelomeningocele.

- Care of the infant and child with myelomeningocele requires both immediate and long-term nursing and medical supervision. Associated problems are infection, neurologic damage, impaired renal function, and musculoskeletal damage.

- Therapeutic management of hydrocephalus focuses on relief of the condition, treatment of complications, and management of problems related to the effect of the disorder on psychomotor development.

- Positioning, prevention of infection, and emotional support of the family are the hallmarks of nursing care for the child with hydrocephalus.

- More common forms of craniofacial abnormalities include hypertelorism, Crouzon disease, Apert syndrome, Treacher-Collins syndrome, and Pierre Robin syndrome.

- The most common types of skeletal defects include congenital hip dysplasia, congenital clubfoot, metatarsus adductus, and skeletal limb deficiency.

- The three degrees of congenital dysplasia are acetabular dysplasia, subluxation, and dislocation.

- Congenital hip disorders may display intrauterine, racial, and cultural predisposition.

- Treatment of clubfoot involves surgical correction of the deformity, maintenance of the correction until normal muscle balance is regained, and follow-up observation to avert possible recurrence of the deformity.

- Common disorders of the gastrointestinal tract include cleft lip, cleft palate, esophageal atresia with tracheoesophageal fistula, anorectal malformations, and biliary atresia.

- Cleft lip and palate, the most common of the facial malformations, may involve nutritional, dental, and speech problems.

- Anorectal defects commonly display associated congenital anomalies, such as those involving the genitourinary tract, heart, and esophagus.

- Separation anxiety, hospitalization, parental anxiety, and body image and castration anxiety are four areas that influence the child's reaction to genital surgery.

- Common defects of the genitourinary tract include phimosis, cryptorchidism, inguinal hernia, hydrocele, hypospadias, epispadias, exstrophy of the bladder, and aberrant sexual development.

- The TORCH complex represents the following infections that may lead to defects: toxoplasmosis, other (e.g., hepatitis), rubella, cytomegalovirus infection, and herpes simplex.

REFERENCES

American Academy of Pediatrics, Infant Bioethics Task Force and Consultants: Guidelines for infant bioethics committees, Pediatrics **74**:306-310, 1984.

American Cleft Palate Education Association: Information about cleft lip and palate, undated material.

Benfield, D.G., Lieb, S.A., and Vollman, J.H.: Grief responses of parents to neonatal death and parent participation in deciding care, Pediatrics **62**:171, 1978.

Blotcky, M.J., and Grossman, I.: Psychological implications of childhood genitourinary surgery, J. Am. Acad. Child Psychiatry **17**:488-492, 1978.

Britton, S.B., Fitzhardinge, P.M., and Ashby, S.: Is intensive care justified for infants weighing less than 801 gm at birth? J. Pediatr. **99**:937-943, 1981.

Bunch, W.H.: Common deformities of the lower limb, Pediatr. Nurs. **5**(4):18-22, 1979.

Charney, E.B., and others: Management of the newborn with myelomeningocele: time for a decision-making process, Pediatrics **75**:58-64, 1985.

Cheetham, C.H., and others: Congenital dislocation of the hip (letter), Bri. Med. J. **286**:277, 1983.

Clarren, S.K.: Plagiocephaly and torticollis: etiology, natural history, and helmet treatment, J. Pediatr. **98**:92-95, 1981.

Committee on Bioethics: Treatment of critically ill newborns, Pediatrics **72**:565-566, 1983.

Davis, P.J.M., Partridge, J.W., and Storrs, C.N.: Alcohol consumption in pregnancy: how much is safe? Arch. Dis. Child. **57**:940-943, 1982.

Duff, R.S.: Counseling families and deciding care of severely defective children: a way of coping with "medical Vietman," Pediatrics **67**:315-320, 1981.

Gans, S.L., and Austin, E.: Hernias and hydroceles. In Gennis, S.S., and Kagan, B.M.: Current pediatric therapy 12, Philadelphia, 1986, W.B. Saunders Co.

Garagorri, J., and others: Results of early treatment of cryptorchidism with human chorionic gonadotropin, J. Pediatr. **101**: 923-927, 1982.

Glaser, J.H., Balistreri, W.F., and Morecki, R.: Role of reovirus type 3 in persistent infantile cholestasis, J. Pediatr. **105**:912-915, 1984.

Glick, P.L., and others: The missing link in the pathogenesis of gastroschisis, J. Pediatr. Surg. **20**:406-409, 1985.

Gross, R.H., and others: Early management and decision making for the treatment of myelomeningocele, Pediatrics **72**:450-458, 1983.

Holland, S.H.: Up-to-date home care of a baby in a hip spica cast, Pediatr. Nurs. **9**(2):114-115, 1983.

Iber, F.L.: Fetal alcohol syndrome, Nutr. Today, Sept./Oct., 1980, pp. 4-11.

Iwatsuki, S., and Starzl, T.E.: Disorders of the biliary tree. In Gellis, S.S., and Kagan, B.M.: Current pediatric therapy 12, Philadelphia, 1986, W.B. Saunders Co.

Jackson, I.T.: Craniofacial malformations. In Gellis, S.S., and Kagan, B.M.: Current pediatric therapy 12, Philadelphia, 1986, W.B. Saunders Co.

Jackson, P.L.: Ventriculoperitoneal shunts, Am. J. Nurs. **80**:1104-1109, 1980.

Khoury, M.J., Erickson, J.D., and James, L.M.: Etiologic heterogeneity of neural tube defects: clues from epidemiology, Am. J. Epidemiol. **115**:538-548, 1982.

Koop, C.E.: The most important advances of the last 10 years, Pediatr. Consult. **12**(1):1-6, 1981.

Kramer, S.A., and Kelalis, P.P.: Exstrophy of the bladder. In Gellis, S.S., and Kagan, B.M.: Current pediatric theraphy 12, Philadelphia, 1986, W.B. Saunders Co.

Learning to close the cleft, Time Magazine, April 12, 1982.

Lemons, P.K.M.: The sequelae to addiction, Crit. Care Update **10**(6):7-10, 1983.

Lepore, A.G., and Kesler, R.W.: Behavior of children undergoing hypospadias repair, J. Urol. **122**:68-72, 1979.

Letters to the editors: Care of the child with myelomeningocele, Pediatrics **74**:162-167, 1984.

Linder, M., and others: Effects of meningomyelocele closure on the intracranial pulse pressure, Child's Brain **11**:176-182, 1984.

Manley, C.B.: Elective genital surgery at one year of age: psychological and surgical considerations, Surg. Clin. North Am. **62**(6):941-953, 1982.

March of Dimes–Birth Defects Foundation: Public health information sheet: cleft lip and palate, White Plains, NY, undated material, March of Dimes–Birth Defects Foundation.

Mulley, D.A.: Harnessing babies' dysplastic hips, Am. J. Nurs. **84**:1006-1008, 1984.

Myers, G.J.: Myelomeningocele: the medical aspects, Pediatr. Clin. North Am. **31**:165-175, 1984.

Noetzel, M.J.: Hydrocephalus. In Gellis, S.S., and Kagan, B.M.: Current pediatric therapy 12, Philadelphia, 1986, W.B. Saunders Co.

Owens, J.R., and others: 19-year incidence of neural tube defects in area under constant surveillance, Lancet, Nov. 7, 1981, pp. 1032-1035.

Paparella, B.H.: Caring for the severely handicapped newborn, Nursing 82 **12**(12):61-64, 1982.

Penny, R.: Undescended testes. In Gellis, S.S., and Kagan, B.M.: Current pediatric therapy 12, Philadelphia, 1986, W.B. Saunders Co.

Pettitt, B.J., Zitelli, B.J., and Rowe, M.I.: Patients with biliary atresia coming to liver transplantation, J. Pediatr. Surg. **19**:779-785, 1984.

Pomerance, J.J.: Disorders of the umbilicus. In Gellis, S.S., and Kagan, B.M.: Current pediatric therapy 12, Philadelphia, 1986, W.B. Saunders Co.

President's Commission for the Study of Ethical Problems in Medicine and Biomedical and Behavior Research. Deciding to forego life-sustaining treatment, Bethesda, MD, 1983, U.S. Government Printing Office.

Ramenofsky, M.L.: Congenital diapragmatic hernia. In Gellis, S.S., and Kagan, B.M.: Current pediatric therapy 12, Philadelphia, 1986, W.B. Saunders Co.

Reigel, D.H.: Spina bifida. In McLauren, R.L.: Pediatric psychology, New York, 1982, Grune & Stratton, Inc.

Ryberg, J.W., and Maryfield, F.B.: What parents want to know, Nurs Pract. **9**(6):24-32, 1984.

Scarff, T.B., and Fronczak, S.: Myelomeningocele: a review and update, Rehab. Lit. **42**(5-6):143-146, 192, 1981.

Schultz, J.R., Klykylo, W.M., and Wacksman, J.: Timing of elective hypospadias repair in children, Pediatrics **71**:342-351, 1983.

Seashore, J.H.: Disorders of the anus and rectum. In Gellis, S.S., and Kagan, B.M.: Current pediatric therapy 12, Philadelphia, 1986, W.B. Saunders Co.

Shinnar, S., and others: Management of hydrocephalus in infancy: use of acetazolamide and furosemide to avoid cerebrospinal fluid shunts, J. Pediatr. **107**:31-37, 1985.

Shoenberg, W.H., and Meador, M.: Analysis of 48 children with myelodysplasia, J. Urol. **127**:749-750, 1982.

Solnit, A., and Stark, M.: Mourning and the birth of a defective child, Psychoanal. Study Child. **16**:523-537, 1963.

Strain, J.E.: The decision to forgo life-sustaining treatment for seriously ill newborns, Pediatrics **72**:572-573, 1983.

Tew, T., and Laurence, K.M.: Mothers, brothers, and sisters of patients with spina bifida, Dev. Med. Child. Neurol. **15** (Suppl. 29):69-76, 1973.

Whitehead, W.E., Parker, L.H., and Masek, B.J.: Biofeedback treatment of fecal incontinence in patients with myelomeningocele, Dev. Med. Child. Neurol. **23**:313-322, 1981.

BIBLIOGRAPHY
General

Darling, R.J., and Darling, J.: Birth defects in society: helping families with children who are different, St. Louis, 1982, The C.V. Mosby Co.

Darling, R.J., and Darling, J.: Children who are different: meeting the challenge of birth defects in society, St. Louis, 1982, The C.V. Mosby Co.

Davidson, B., and Dosser, D.: A support system for families with developmentally disabled infants, Fam. Rel. **31**:295-299, 1983.

Downey, J.A., and Low, N.L., editors: The child with disabling illness, principles of rehabilitation, ed. 2, Philadelphia, 1984, W.B. Saunders Co.

Garner, J.S., and Simmons, B.P.: Guideline for isolation precautions in hospitals, Infect. Control **4**(suppl.):245-325, 1983.

Heller, A., and others: Birth defects and psychosocial adjustment, Am. J. Dis. Child **139**:257-263, 1985.

Kalter, H., and Warkany, J.: Congenital malformations. Part 1, N. Engl. J. Med. **308**:424-431, 1983.

Kalter, H., and Warkany, J.: Congenital malformations. Part 2, N. Engl. J. Med. **308**:491-497, 1983.

Lubinsky, M.: Neonatal assessment for anomalies and syndromes, Pediatr. Basics **37**:407, 1984.

Smith, D.W.: Recognizable patterns of human malformation: genetic, embryologic, and clinical aspects, ed. 3, Philadelphia, 1981, W.B. Saunders Co.

Williams, J.K.: Evaluating the dysorphic child, Pediatr. Nurs. **9**(4):241-248, 1983.

Birth of a Child with a Defect

Chitwood, L.: A lesson in living, Nursing 84 **14**(1):55-56, 1984.

Davidhizar, R.M., and Monhaut, N.: Giving bad news by phone, Nursing 85 **15**(4):58-59, 1985.

Drane, J.F.: The defective child: ethical guidelines for painful dilemmas, JOGN Nurs. **13**:42-48, 1984.

Fost, N.: Ethical issues in the treatment of critically ill newborns, Pediatr. Ann. **10**:16-22, 1981.

Fost, N.: Counseling families who have a child with a severe congenital anomaly, Pediatrics **67**:321-324, 1981.

Hall, L.F., and Stoops, P.M.: Acquainting a new mother with her less-than-perfect baby, Am. J. Maternal Child Nurs. **9**:136, 1984.

Horan, M.L.: Parental reaction to the birth of an infant with a defect: an attributional approach, Adv. Nurs. Sci. **4**(1):57-68, 1982.

Irvin, N.A., Kennell, J.H., and Klaus, M.H.: Caring for the parents of an infant with a congenital malformation. In Klaus M.H., and Kennell, J.H.: Parent-infant bonding, ed. 2, St. Louis, 1982, The C.V. Mosby Co.

Jackson, P.L.: When the baby isn't "perfect," Am. J. Nurs. **85**:396-399, 1985.

Kikuchi, J.: Assimilative and accommodative responses of mothers to their newborn infants with congenital defects, Maternal Child Nurs. J. **9**:141-219, 1980.

McCollum, A.T.: Grieving over the lost dream, Exceptional Parent, Feb. 1984.

Pi, E.H.: Congenitally handicapped children and their families: early crisis intervention. Postgrad. Med. **68**(2):157-160, 1980.

Romney, M.C.: Congenital defects: implications on family development and parenting, Issues Compr. Pediatr. Nurs. **7**:1-15, 1984.

West, M.: The mother, the developmentally disabled child and the nurse, Topics Clin. Nurs. **6**(3):19-29, 1984.

Young, R.K.: Chronic sorrow: parent's response to the birth of a child with a defect, Am. J. Maternal Child Nurs. **2**(1):38-42, 1977.

Decisions Regarding Care

Angell, M.: Handicapped children: Baby Doe and Uncle Sam, N. Engl. J. Med. **309**:659-661, 1983.

Bandman, E.L., and Bandman, B.: The nurse's role in protecting the patient's right to live or die. In Chinn, P.L., editor: Ethical issues in nursing, Rockville, MD, 1986, Aspen Systems Corp.

Bator, A.: Subjectively speaking . . . , Am. J. Nurs. **84**:883, 1984.

Commentaries: The "Baby Doe" rule: is it all bad? Pediatrics **73**:729-730, 1984.

Cushing, M.: Do not feed . . . , Am. J. Nurs. **83**:602-604, 1983.

Cushing, M.: The implications of withdrawing nutritional devices, Am. J. Nurs. **84**:191-192, 1984.

Davis, A.J.: A newborn's right to life vs. death, Am. J. Nurs. **81**:1035, 1981.

Davis, P.S.: Medico-legal considerations and the quality of life, Clin. Nurs. **3**(3):79-85, 1981.

Dolan, M.B.: Where do you stand on the coding question, Nursing 84 **14**(3):42-48, 1984.

Duff, R.S.: Guidelines for deciding care of critically ill or dying patients, Pediatrics **64**:17, 1979.

Elsea, S.B.: Ethics in maternal-child nursing, Am. J. Maternal Child Nurs. **10**:303-308, 1985.

Fotion, N.C.: Ethics and the afflicted child, Crit. Care Q. **8**(12):75-83, 1985.

Fromer, M.J.: Solving ethical dilemmas in nursing practice. In Chinn, P.L., editor: Ethical issues in nursing, Rockville, MD, 1986, Aspen Systems Corp.

Healy, A.: Treatment of disabled infants, Pediatrics **73**:563-564, 1984.

Homer, M.B.: Selective treatment, Am. J. Nurs. **84**:309-312, 1984.

Joint Policy Statement: Principles of treatment of disabled infants, Pediatrics **73**:559-560, 1984.

Rhodes, A.M.: ''Baby Doe'' rules: implications for nurses, Am. J. Maternal Child Nurs. **10**:405, 1985.

Sachs, B.: Update on ''Baby Doe'' legislation, regs, In Touch **3**(1):1, 1985.

Shufer, S.: What's best for Willie? Am. J. Nurs. **12**:470-472, 1982.

The right to die, Nursing Life **4**(2):45-52, 1984.

Verzemnieks, I.L., and Nash, D.: Ethical issues related to pediatric care, Nurs. Clin. North Am. **19**:319-328, 1984.

Watchko, J.F.: Decision making on critically ill infants by parents, Am. J. Dis. Child. **137**:795-798, 1983.

Defects of Neural Tube Closure

Campbell, J.A.: Catheterizing prone female infants: how can you see what you're doing? Am. J. Maternal Child Nurs. **4**:376-377, 1979.

Clark, L.W.: The importance of touch with an anencephalic baby, Am. J. Maternal Child Nurs. **7**:336-337, 1982.

Colgan, M.T.: The child with spina bifida, Am. J. Dis. Child. **135**:854-858, 1981.

Crooks, K.K., and Enrile, B.G.: Comparison of the ileal conduit and clean intermittent catheterization for myelomeningocele, Pediatrics **72**:203-206, 1983.

James, H.E., and Walsh, J.W.: Spinal dysraphism, Curr. Probl. Pediatr. **11**(8):1-25, 1981.

Jeffries, J.S., Killam, P.E., and Varni, J.W.: Behavioral management of fecal incontinence in a child with myelomeningocele, Pediatr. Nurs. **8**:267-270, 1982.

Killam, P.E., and others: Behavioral pediatric weight rehabilitation for children with myelomeningocele, Am. J. Maternal Child Nurs. **8**:280-286, 1983.

Letters to the editors: Early management and decision making for the treatment of myelomeningocele: a critique, Pediatrics **74**:564-566, 1984.

Macbriar, B.R.: Self-concept of preadolescent and adolescent children with a meningomyelocele, Issues Compr. Pediatr. Nurs. **6**:1-11, 1983.

Pinyerd, B.J.: Siblings of children with myelomeningocele: examining their perceptions, Am. J. Maternal Child Nurs. **12**(1):61-70, 1983.

Richardson, K., and others: Biofeedback therapy for managing bowel incontinence caused by meningomyelocele, Am. J. Maternal Child Nurs. **10**:388-392, 1985.

Shurtleff, D.B.: Myelodysplasia: management and treatment, Curr. Probl. Pediatr. **10**(3):1-56, 1980.

Vigliaroto, D.: Managing bowel incontinence in children with meningomyelocele, Am. J. Nurs. **80**:105-107, 1980.

Hydrocephalus

Arsenault, L.: Delayed onset symptomatic hydrocephalus related to aqueductal stenosis, J. Neurosurg. Nurs. **15**(5):291-297, 1983.

Bernardo, M.L.: When your caseload includes a hydrocephalic child, Pediatr. Nurs. **5**(3):27-29, 1979.

Conway-Rutkowski, B.L.: Carini and Owens' neurological and neurosurgical nursing, ed. 8, St. Louis, 1982, The C.V. Mosby Co.

Grant, L.: Hydrocephalus: an overview and update, J. Neurosurg. Nurs. **16**(6):313-318, 1984.

Graziani, L., and others: Ultrasound studies in preterm infants with hydrocephalus, J. Pediatr. **97**:624-631, 1980.

Icenogle, D.A., and Kaplan, A.M.: A review of congenital neurologic malformations, Clin. Pediatr. **20**:565-576, 1981.

Jackson, P.L.: Peritoneal shunting for hydrocephalus, Crit. Care Update **10**(4):33-39, 1983.

Odio, C., McCracken, G.H., and Nelson, J.D.: CSF shunt infections in pediatrics, Am. J. Dis. Child **138**:1103-1108, 1984.

Craniofacial Deformities

Bernardo, M.L.: Craniosynostosis: the child's care from detection through correction, Am. J. Maternal Child Nurs. **4**:234-237, 1979.

Graham, J.M.: Craniostenosis: a new approach to management, Pediatr. Ann. **10**:258-264, 1981.

Graham, J.M., deSaxe, M., and Smith, D.W.: Sagittal craniostenosis: fetal head constraint as one possible cause, J. Pediatr. **95**:747-750, 1979.

Hanus, S.H., Bernstein, N.R., and Kapp, K.A.: Immigrants into society: children with craniofacial anomalies, Clin. Pediatr. **20**(1):37-41, 1981.

Humphrey, P.A., Britt, P.H., and Peters, C.R.: Craniofacial malformations, Am. J. Nurs. **79**:1230-1234, 1979.

Pleet, H., Graham, J.M., and Smith, D.W.: Central nervous system and facial defects associated with maternal hyperthermia at four to 14 weeks' gestation, Pediatrics **67**:785-789, 1981.

Skeletal Defects

Coleman, S.S.: When a child is born with hip problems, Patient Care **17**(14):68-98, 1983.

Eilert, R.E., Locke, R.K., and Smith, E.: Foot care for the very young patient, Patient Care, May 15, 1979, pp. 108-140.

Hirsch, P.J., and others: Treatment of hip dysplasia in the first nine months, Orthop. Clin. North Am. **13**(3):605-618, 1982.

Sherk, H.H., Pasquariello, P.S., and Watters, W.C., III: Congenital dislocation of the hip: a review, Clin. Pediatr. **20**:513-523, 1981.

Swagman, A.: Caring for limb-deficient children and their families, Am. J. Maternal Child Nurs. **11**:46-52, 1986.

Swanson, A.B.: Congenital limb deformities: classification and treatment, Clin. Symp. **33**(3):3-32, 1981.

Trott, A.W.: Children's foot problems, Orthop. Clin. North Am. **13**:641-655, 1982.

Cleft Lip and/or Palate

Colburn, N., and Cherry, R.S.: Community-based team approach to the management of children with cleft palate, Child. Health Care **13**:122-128, 1985.

Heller, A., Tidmarsh, W., and Pless, I.B.: The psychosocial functioning of young adults born with cleft lip or palate, Clin. Pediatr. **20**:459-465, 1981.

Pashayan, H.M., and McNab, M.: Simplified method of feeding infants born with cleft palate with or without cleft lip, Am. J. Dis. Child. **133**:145-147, 1979.

Styer, G.W., and Freeh, K.: Feeding infants with cleft lip and/or palate, JOGN Nurs. **10**:329-331, 1981.

Biliary Atresia

Altman, R.P., Lilly, J.R., and Smith, E.I.: When an infant needs bile duct surgery, Patient Care **13**(6):156-163, 1979.

Barkin, R.M., and Lilly, J.R.: Biliary atresia and the Kasai operation: continuing care, J. Pediatr. **96**:1015-1019, 1980.

Barss, V.A., Benacerraf, B.R., and Frigoletto, F.D.: Antenatal sonographic diagnosis of fetal gastrointestinal malformations, Pediatrics **76**:445-450, 1985.

Burgess, D.B., Martin, H.P., and Lilly, J.R.: The developmental status of children undergoing the Kasai procedure for biliary atresia, Pediatrics **70**:624-629, 1982.

Ghishan, F.K., and others: The evolving nature of ''infantile obstructive cholangiopathy,'' J. Pediatr. **97**:27-32, 1980.

Karrer, F.M., and Lilly, J.R.: Corticosteroid therapy in biliary atresia, J. Pediatr. Surg. **20**:693-695, 1985.

Kobayashi, A., Itabashi, F., and Ohbe, Y.: Long-term prognosis in biliary atresia after hepatic portoenterostomy: analysis of 35 patients who survived beyond 5 years of age, J. Pediatr. **105**:243-246, 1984.

Lilly, J.R.: Biliary atresia and liver transplantation: the National Institutes of Health point of view, Pediatrics **74**:159-160, 1984.

Lilly, J.R., and Karrer, F.M.: Contemporary surgery of biliary atresia, Pediatr. Clin. North Am. **32**:1233-1246, 1985.

Stevens, M.S., and Reinitz, M.: Nursing a child through exstrophic bladder reconstruction surgery, Am. J. Maternal Child Nurs. **5**:265-270, 1980.

Williams, L.: Care of the pediatric liver transplant patient in the ICU, Crit. Care Q. **8**(1):13-25, 1985.

Hernias

Aaronson, I., and Eckstein, H.: Role of Silastic prosthesis in the management of gastroschisis, Arch. Surg. **11**:297-302, 1977.

Geggel, R.L., and others: Congenital diaphragmatic hernia: arterial structural changes and persistent pulmonary hypertension after surgical repair, J. Pediatr. **107**:457-464, 1985.

Hall, D.E., Roberts, K.B., and Charney, E.: Umbilical hernia: what happens after age 5 years? J. Pediatr. **99**:415-417, 1981.

Hazle, N.: An infant who survived gastroschisis, Am. J. Maternal Child Nurs. **6**:35-40, 1981.

Moynihan, P., and Gerraughty, A.: Diaphragmatic hernia: low stress = higher survival, Am. J. Nurs. **85**:662-665, 1985.

Defects of the Genitourinary Tract

Marshall, D.G.: Femoral hernias in children, J. Pediatr. Surg. **18**:160-162, 1983.

Peevy, K.J., Speed, F.A., and Hoff, C.J.: Epidemiology of inguinal hernia in preterm neonates, Pediatrics **77**:246-247, 1986.

Ambiguous Genitalia

DiGrande, A.: The child born with ambiguous genitalia: family assessment and nursing intervention, Issues Compr. Pediatr. Nurs. **7**:307-318, 1984.

Mazur, T.: Ambiguous genitalia: detection and counseling, Pediatr. Nurs. **9**:417-422, 1983.

Saenger, P.: Abnormal sex differentiation, J. Pediatr. **104**:1-17, 1984.

Prenatal Influences: Maternal Infections

Adler, S.P., and others: Cytomegalovirus infections in neonates due to blood transfusions, Pediatr. Infect. Dis. **2**:114-118, 1983.

Beasley, R.P., and others: Prevention of perinatally transmitted hepatitis B virus infections with hepatitis B immune globulin and hepatitis B vaccine, Lancet **2**:1099-1102, 1983.

Brown, S.G.: The devastating effects of congenital rubella, Am. J. Maternal Child Nurs. **4**:171-173, 1979.

Butt, W., and others: Intracranial lesions of congenital cytomegalovirus infection detected by ultrasound scanning, Pediatrics **73**:611-614, 1984.

Committee on Fetus and Newborn, Committee on Infectious Diseases: Perinatal herpes simplex virus infections, Pediatrics **68**:147-148, 1980.

Delaplane, D., and others: Fatal hepatitis B in early infancy: the importance of identifying HB$_s$Ag-positive pregnant women and providing immunoprophylaxis to their newborns, Pediatrics **72**:176-180, 1983.

DeVore, N.E., Jackson, V.M., and Piening, S.L.: TORCH infections, Am. J. Nurs. **83**:1660-1665, 1983.

Dworsky, M.E., and others: Cytomegalovirus infection of breast milk and transmission in infancy, Pediatrics **72**:295-299, 1983.

Dworsky, M.E., and others: Occupational risk for primary cytomegalovirus infection among pediatric health-care workers, N. Engl. J. Med. **309**:950, 1983.

Faix, R.G.: Survival of cytomegalovirus on environmental surfaces, J. Pediatr. **106**:649-652, 1985.

Frinkel, J.K.: Toxoplasmosis, Pediatr. Clin. North Am. **32**:917-932, 1985.

Gauntt, C.J., and others: Coxsackievirus Group B antibodies in the ventricular fluid of infants with severe anatomic defects in the central nervous system, Pediatrics **76**:64-68, 1985.

Hanshaw, J.B.: Cytomegalovirus infections, Pediatr. Rev. **2**:245-251, 1981.

Hayden, G.F., and others: Subclinical congenital rubella infection associated with maternal rubella vaccination in early pregnancy, J. Pediatr. **96**:869-872, 1980.

Hinman, A.R.: Prevention of congenital rubella infection: symposium summary, Pediatrics **75**:1162-1165, 1985.

Jemison-Smith, P., and Hamm, P.: Rubella, Crit. Care Update **9**(12):34-36, 1982.

Kumar, M.L., and others: Congenital and postnatally acquired cytomegalovirus infections: long term follow-up, J. Pediatr. **104**:674-679, 1984.

Kumar, M.L., and others: Postnatally acquired cytomegalovirus infection in infants of CMV-excreting mothers, J. Pediatr. **104**:669-679, 1984.

Mascola, L., and others: Congenital syphilis, JAMA **252**:1719-1722, 1984.

Nankervis, G.A., and others: A prospective study of maternal cytomegalovirus infection and its effect on the fetus, Am. J. Obstet. Gynecol. **149**:435-440, 1984.

Paryani, S.G., and others: Sequelae of acquired cytomegalovirus infection in premature and sick term infants, J. Pediatr. **107**:451-456, 1985.

Ritter, S.E., and Vermund, S.H.: Congenital toxoplasmosis, JOGN Nurs. **14**:435-439, 1985.

Stagno, S.: Toxoplasmosis, Am. J. Nurs. **80**:720-722, 1980.

Whitley, R.J., and others: Neonatal herpes simplex virus infection: follow up evaluation of vidarabine therapy, Pediatrics **72**:778-785, 1983.

Yeager, A.S., Ashley, R.L., and Corey, L.: Transmission of herpes simplex virus from father to neonate, J. Pediatr. **103**:905-907, 1983.

Fetal Alcohol Syndrome

Enloe, C.F.: How alcohol affects the developing fetus, Nutr. Today, Sept./Oct. 1980, pp. 12-15.

Frias, J.L., and others: A cephalometric study of fetal alcohol syndrome, J. Pediatr. **101**:870-873, 1982.

Golden, N.L., and others: Maternal alcohol use and infant development, Pediatrics **70**:931-934, 1982.

Hingson, R., and others: Effects of maternal drinking and marijuana use on fetal growth and development, Pediatrics **70**:539-546, 1982.

Iosub, S., and others: Fetal alcohol syndrome revisited, Pediatrics **68**:475-479, 1981.

Leland, D., and others: The use of TORCH titers, Pediatrics **72**:41-43, 1983.

Little, R.E., and others: Decreased birth weight in infants of alcoholic women who abstained during pregnancy, J. Pediatr. **96**:974-977, 1980.

Mills, J., and others: Maternal alcohol consumption and birth weight: how much drinking during pregnancy is safe? JAMA **252**:1875-1879, 1984.

Ouellette, E.M.: The fetal alcohol syndrome, Contemp. Nutr. **9**(3):1-2, 1984.

Rosett, H.L., and others: Patterns of alcohol consumption and fetal development, Obstet. Gynecol. **61**:539-546, 1983.

Rosett, H.L., and others: Strategies for prevention of fetal alcohol effects, Obstet. Gynecol. **57**(1):1-7, 1981.

Stephens, C.J.: The fetal alcohol syndrome: cause for concern, Am. J. Maternal Child Nurs. **6**:251-256, 1981.

Tennes, K., and Blackard, C.: Maternal alcohol consumption, birth weight, and minor physical anomalies, Am. J. Obstet. Gynecol. **138**(7):774-780, 1980.

Unit Four

Infancy

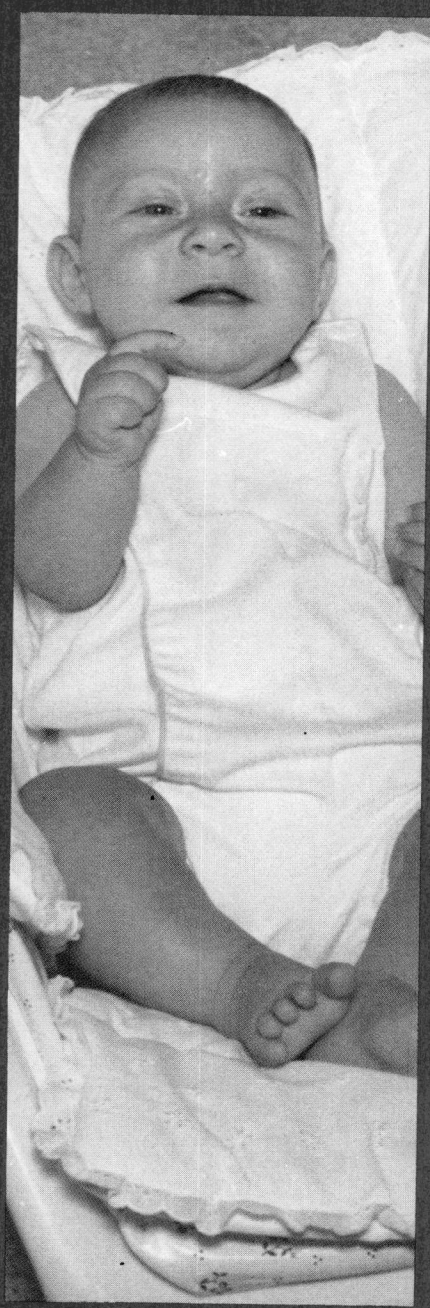

The first 12 months of childhood is the period of most rapid gain in physical size and most dramatic achievement of developmental milestones in an individual's entire life. It is marked by an orderly progression of physical, intellectual, and social maturation. It is also a highly vulnerable period for both positive and negative influences governing optimum growth and development.

Chapter 12, *Health Promotion of the Infant and Family*, investigates the infant's biologic, psychosocial, cognitive, and social development. It is concerned with fostering optimum health through anticipatory guidance regarding nutrition, prevention of disease and injury, and promotion of parent-child attachment. Chapter 13, *Health Problems During Infancy*, deals with health problems that commonly occur during the first year, usually as a result of environmental rather than pathologic processes, and that therefore can be prevented. It is also concerned with conditions of unknown cause, such as sudden infant death syndrome, which has profound emotional consequences on the developing family.

Chapter 12

Health Promotion of the Infant and Family

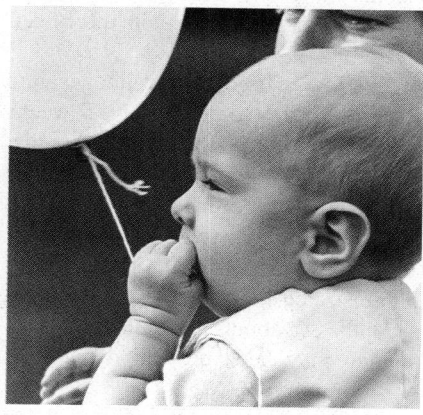

Promoting Optimum Growth and Development

Biologic development
    Proportional changes
    Sensory changes
    Maturation of systems
    Fine motor development
    Gross motor development
Psychosocial development
    Erikson: Developing a sense of
        trust
    Freud: The oral stage
Cognitive development
    Piaget: The sensorimotor
        phase
Development of body image
Social development
    Attachment
    Language development
    Personal-social behavior
    Play

Temperament
    Childrearing practices related
        to temperament
Summary of growth and
    development during infancy
Coping with concerns related
    to normal growth and
    development
    Fears
    Daycare
    Limit-setting and discipline
    Thumb-sucking and use of
        pacifier
    Teething
    Infant shoes

Promoting Optimum Health During Infancy

Nutrition
    Infant feeding
    Selection of foods
    Food preparation
    Food storage
    Method of introduction
    Weaning
    Nutritional counseling
Sleep and activity
    Sleep disturbances
Dental health
Immunizations
    Current status of
        immunizations
    Schedule for immunizations
    Recommendations for routine
        immunizations
    Recommendations for selected
        immunizations
    Reactions
    Contraindications
    Administration/precautions

Injury prevention
    Aspiration of foreign objects
    Suffocation
    Falls
    Poisoning
    Burns
    Motor vehicle injuries
    Bodily damage
    Nurse's role in injury
        prevention
Anticipatory guidance—care of
    families

The miracle of birth is surpassed only by the wonder of growth and development unfolding over the succeeding months and years. The biologic growth and developmental maturation of the infant are a study of perfection in nature. The nurse's understanding of these processes is essential to the optimum care of the child and family. To present relevant data for appreciation of growth and development, it is necessary to systematize and categorize the facts into various levels of maturation and age groups. However, we must always bear in mind that no child will be represented in any one table or chart, because each child is as much an individual as the number of variables that influence his or her existence.

Promoting Optimum Growth and Development

General concepts of growth and development, such as stages and patterns of development and individual differences, are discussed extensively in Chapter 4. This chapter is primarily concerned with biologic, psychosocial, cognitive, and social development of the child from 1 to 12 months of age. It also includes a discussion of common parental concerns that are typical of the developmental characteristics of this age group.

BIOLOGIC DEVELOPMENT

At no other time in life are physical changes and developmental achievements so dramatic as during infancy. All major body systems undergo progressive maturation, and there is concurrent development of skills that increasingly allows infants to respond to and cope with the environment. Acquisition of these fine and gross motor skills occurs in an orderly sequence, following usual cephalocaudal-proximodistal laws.

Proportional Changes

During the first year growth is very rapid, especially during the initial 6 months. Infants gain 680 g (1½ pounds) per month until age 6 months, when the birth weight has at least doubled. An average weight for a 6-month-old child is 7.26 kg (16 pounds). Weight gain decreases by half that amount during the second 6 months. By 1 year of age the infant's birth weight has tripled, with an average weight of 9.75 kg (21½ pounds).

Height increases by 2.5 cm (1 inch) during the first 6 months, and by half that amount during the second 6 months. Average height is 65 cm (25½ inches) at 6 months and 74 cm (29 inches) at 12 months. By 1 year the birth length has increased by almost 50%. The increase in length occurs mainly in the trunk, rather than in the legs, and contributes to the characteristic physique of the older infant (see Fig. 12-9, A).

Head growth is also rapid. During the first 6 months head circumference increases approximately 1.5 cm (½ inches) per month, but decreases to only 0.5 cm (¼ inches) during the second 6 months. The average size is 43 cm (17 inches) at 6 months and 46 cm (18 inches) at 12 months. By 1 year head size has increased by almost 33%. Closure of the cranial sutures occurs, with the posterior fontanel fusing by 6 to 8 weeks of age and the anterior fontanel closing by 12 to 18 months of age.

Expanding head size reflects the growth and differentiation of the nervous system. By the end of the first year the brain has increased in weight about two and one half times. The maturation of the brain is exhibited in the dramatic developmental achievements of infancy (see Table 12-3). The primitive reflexes (see p. 314) are replaced by voluntary, purposeful movement, and new reflexes that influence motor development appear (see box).

The chest assumes a more adult contour, with the lateral diameter becoming larger than the anteroposterior diameter. The chest circumference approximately equals head circumference by the end of the first year. The heart grows less rapidly than does the rest of the body. Its weight is usually doubled by 1 year of age, in comparison with body weight, which triples during the same period. The size of the heart is still large in relation to the chest cavity; its width is about 55% of the width of the chest (see Fig. 7-42).

Sensory Changes

During infancy visual acuity gradually improves and binocular fixation is established. The major developmental characteristics of vision during infancy are listed in the boxed material.

Binocularity, or the fixation of two ocular images into one cerebral picture (fusion), begins to develop by 6 weeks of age and should be well established by age 4 months. Lack of binocular vision results in strabismus and must be detected early to prevent permanent blindness (see p. 1027).

Depth perception (stereopsis) begins to develop by age 7 to 9 months but may exist earlier as an innate safety mechanism. Studies have demonstrated that even 2- to 3-month-old infants distinguish depth. At about 7 months the parachute reflex appears, which may be a protective response during a fall (Fig. 12-1 and box on p. 495).

Infants also have a *visual preference* for looking at the

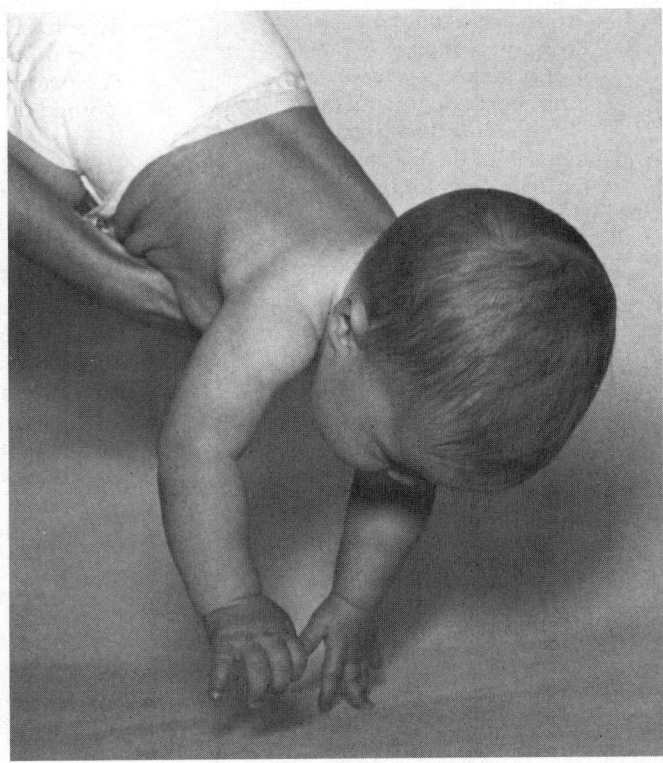

Fig. 12-1. Parachute reflex.

NEUROLOGIC REFLEXES THAT APPEAR DURING INFANCY

Reflex	Expected behavioral response	Age of appearance (months)
Labyrinth-righting	Infant in prone or supine position is able to raise head	2, strongest at 10
Neck-righting	While infant is supine, head is turned to one side; shoulder, trunk, and finally pelvis will turn toward that side	3, until 24-36
Body-righting	A modification of the neck-righting reflex in which turning hips and shoulders to one side causes all other body parts to follow	6, until 24-36
Otolith-righting	When body of an erect infant is tilted, head is returned to upright, erect position	7-12, persists indefinitely
Landau	When infant is suspended in a horizontal prone position, the head is raised, legs and spine are extended	6-8, until 12-24
Parachute	When infant is suspended in a horizontal prone position and suddenly thrust downward, hands and fingers extend forward as if to protect himself from falling (Fig. 12-1)	7-9, persists indefinitely

human face, which also has a developmental sequence. For example, at age 6 weeks they show more interest in a picture of a face with eyes than without. By 10 weeks of age a picture with both eyes and eyebrows elicits more response, and by 20 weeks of age the mouth is also necessary. By age 6 months infants respond to facial expressions and can distinguish between familiar and strange faces. This is about the same time as stranger anxiety is manifested (see p. 506).

With progressive myelination of the auditory pathway, the specific responses of locating sound replace the generalized response of the neonate. (Fig. 12-2). The major developmental characteristics of hearing are listed in the box. (For a further discussion of hearing and the senses of smell, taste, and touch, see Chapter 8.)

Maturation of Systems

Other organ systems also change and grow during infancy. The respiratory rate slows somewhat (see inside front cover) and is relatively stable. Respiratory movements continue to be abdominal. Growth of the respiratory tract is gradual. Several factors predispose the infant to more severe and acute respiratory problems. The close proximity of the trachea to the bronchi and its branching structures rapidly transmits an infectious agent from one anatomic location to another. The short, straight eustachian tube closely communicates with the ear, allowing infection to ascend from the pharynx to the middle ear. In addition, the immunologic ability of the mucosal lining provides less protection against infection in infancy than during later childhood.

Although the lumen of the trachea and bronchi enlarges during infancy, it remains small in comparison with the total size of the lung, maintaining low resistance to the volume of air inspired. The ability of the entire respiratory tract to produce mucus is diminished, decreasing the humidification of the large volume of inspired air. In addition, the volume of dead space, that amount of air needed to fill the respiratory passages with each breath, is large, requiring the infant to breath about twice as fast as the adult to provide the body with the needed amount of oxygen.

MAJOR DEVELOPMENTAL CHARACTERISTICS OF VISION

Age (weeks)	Development
Birth	Visual acuity 20/100-20/400*
	Pupillary and corneal (blink) reflexes present
	Able to fixate on moving object in range of 45 degrees when held 20-25 cm (8-10 inches) away
	Cannot integrate head and eye movements well (doll's eye reflex—eyes lag behind if head is rotated to one side)
4	Can follow in range of 90 degrees
	Can watch parent intently as he or she speaks to infant
	Tear glands begin to function
	Visual acuity is hyperopic because of less spheric eyeball than in adult
6-12	Has peripheral vision to 180 degrees
	Binocular vision begins at age 6 weeks, is well established by age 4 months
	Convergence on near objects begins by age 6 weeks, is well developed by age 3 months
	Doll's eye reflex disappears
12-20	Recognizes feeding bottle
	Able to fixate on a 1.25 cm (½ inch) block
	Looks at hand while sitting or lying on back
	Looks at mirror image
	Able to accommodate to near objects
20-28	Adjusts posture to see an object
	Able to rescue a dropped toy
	Develops color preference for yellow and red
	Able to discriminate between simple geometric forms
	Prefers more complex visual stimuli
	Develops hand-eye coordination
	Pats image of self in mirror
28-44	Can fixate on very small objects
	Depth perception begins to develop
	Lack of binocular vision indicates strabismus
44-52	Visual acuity, 20/40-20/60
	Visual loss may develop if strabismus is present
	Can follow rapidly moving objects

*Measurement of visual acuity differs according to testing procedures (see also Table 7-6, p. 249).

MAJOR DEVELOPMENTAL CHARACTERISTICS OF HEARING

Age (weeks)	Development
Birth	Responds to loud noise by startle reflex Responds to sound of human voice more readily than to any other sound Low-pitched sounds, such as lullaby, metronome, or heartbeat, have quieting effect
8-12	Turns head to side when sound is made at level of ear
12-16	Locates sound by turning head to side and looking in same direction (Fig. 12-2)
16-24	Can localize sounds made below ear, which is followed by localization of sound made above ear; will turn head to the side and then look up or down Begins to imitate sounds
24-32	Locates sounds by turning head in a curving arc Responds to own name
32-40	Localizes sounds by turning head diagonally and directly toward sound
40-52	Knows several words and their meaning, such as "no," and names of members of the family Learns to control and adjust own response to sound, such as listening for the sound to occur again

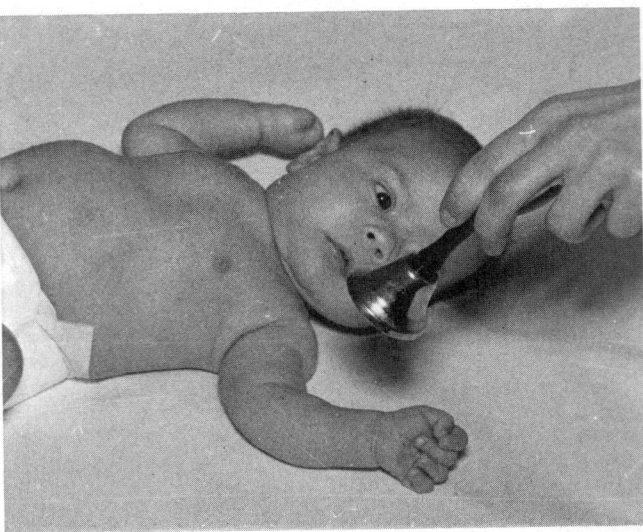

Fig. 12-2. Three-month-old infant locates sound by turning head to side and looking in direction of the sound.

The heart rate slows (see inside front cover), and the rhythm is frequently sinus arrhythmia (rate increases with inspiration and decreases with expiration). Blood pressure also changes during infancy (see inside front cover). The rising systolic pressure is a result of the increasing ability of the left ventricle to pump blood into the systemic circulation. Fluctuations in blood pressure occur during varying states of activity and emotion.

Significant hemopoietic changes occur during the first year (see Appendix A). Fetal hemoglobin is present for the first 5 months, with adult hemoglobin forming at about 13 weeks of age. Maternal iron stores are present for the first 5 to 6 months in full-term newborns, and then gradually diminish, which partially accounts for lowered hemoglobin levels toward the end of the first 6 months.

Physiologic anemia is seen at 2 to 3 months of age because of the decreasing number of red blood cells. This phenomenon is thought to be caused by the depression of the hemopoietic system because of the high level of fetal hemoglobin, which suppresses the production of erythropoietin, a hormone released by the kidney. The occurrence of physiologic anemia is not affected by an adequate supply of iron. However, when erythropoiesis is stimulated, iron supplies are then necessary for formation of hemoglobin.

The digestive processes are immature at birth. Saliva is secreted in small amounts, but the majority of the digestive processes do not begin functioning until age 3 months, when drooling is common because of the poorly coordinated swallowing reflex. The enzyme *ptyalin* (also called amylase) is present in small amounts but usually has little effect on the foodstuff because of the small amount of time the food stays in the mouth. Gastric digestion in the stomach consists primarily of the action of hydrochloric acid and rennin, an enzyme that acts specifically on the casein in milk to cause the formation of curds, coagulated semisolid particles of milk. The curds cause the milk to be retained in the stomach long enough for digestion to occur. The amount of rennin decreases throughout life. This enzyme functions best in a moderately acidic medium; the child's stomach has less acidity than the adult's, which enhances the action of rennin.

Digestion also takes place in the duodenum, where pancreatic enzymes and bile begin to break down protein and fat. Secretion of the pancreatic enzyme *amylase,* which is needed for digestion of complex carbohydrates, is deficient until about the fourth to sixth month of life. *Lipase* is also limited, and infants do not achieve adult levels of fat absorption until 4 to 5 months of age. *Trypsin* is secreted in sufficient quantities to catabolize protein into polypeptides and some amino acids.

The immaturity of the digestive processes is evident in the appearance of stools. During infancy solid foods, such as peas, carrots, corn, and raisins, are passed incompletely broken down in the feces. An excess quantity of fiber easily disposes the child to loose, bulky stools.

The rapid peristaltic activity of the gastrointestinal tract slows down throughout infancy, and the stomach enlarges to accommodate a greater volume of food. By the end of the first year the infant is able to tolerate three meals a day and an evening bottle and may have one or two bowel movements daily. However, with any type of gastric irritation the transit time is increased above its already rapid rate, making the infant vulnerable to diarrhea, vomiting, and dehydration (see Chapter 29).

The liver is the most immature of all the gastrointestinal organs throughout infancy. The ability to conjugate bilirubin and to secrete bile is achieved after the first couple of weeks of life. However, the capacities for gluconeogenesis, formation of plasma protein and ketones, storage of vitamins, and deaminization of amino acids remain relatively immature for the first year of life.

Maturation of suckling, sucking, and swallowing reflexes parallel the changes in the gastrointestinal tract and prepare the infant for the introduction of solid foods. *Suckling,* which is first seen at birth, denotes extension and a pulling-in pattern of tongue movements as in licking. During breast-feeding the lips gently clamp the areola in place as the mandible and tongue thrust forward to grasp the nipple and areola. The sucking fat pads in the cheeks fill the mouth and help maintain negative pressure. The tongue then moves rhythmically forward to the gums and lips and back toward the hard palate, compressing the areola between itself and the palate to "milk" the collecting ductules. As milk flows from the nipple, it stimulates the swallowing reflex and is ejected into the esophagus.

In bottle-feeding the *sucking* action is different. Consequently breast-fed infants may become confused. The relatively inflexible rubber nipple may prevent the tongue from moving rhythmically forward and backward. In addition, the flow of milk may be too rapid, causing choking. The infant learns to control the stream of milk by pushing the tongue against the rubber nipple holes. When given the breast again, he may use the same action and push the human nipple out of the mouth (Lawrence, 1985).

Swallowing (deglutition) is the ability to collect the food (bolus) and propel it into the esophagus. Mature sucking and swallowing are acquired with development of the orofacial muscles. During the *infantile (visceral) swallow reflex* (Fig. 12-3, *A*) food lies in a shallow groove on the dorsum of the tongue. As the tongue is pressed upward toward the palate, the milk flows by gravity down the sloping tongue to the pharynx. The milk also flows along the sides of the mouth in lateral furrows between the tongue and cheek pads. As the bolus moves downward, the posterior wall of the pharynx comes forward to displace the soft palate. The larynx is then elevated, and the epiglottis diverts the flow to either side of the pharnyx so that the food passes around, but not over, the larynx and into the laryngopharynx. The bolus is then propelled by pharyngeal peristaltic movement into the esophagus (Pipes, 1985).

As the infant grows, the tongue becomes smaller in proportion to the oral cavity and attains greater motility. Consequently the *mature (somatic) swallow reflex* (Fig. 12-3, *B*) is significantly different. The tongue remains behind the central incisors, and the mandible no longer thrusts forward. The dorsum of the tongue is less concave, remains higher and parallel, not inclined, against the palate, and the lateral furrows are absent because of tooth eruption. Tongue pressure and movement against the hard palate pushes the bolus back into the pharynx, where the food is passed over the epiglottis to enter the laryngopharynx and esophagus. The development of mature sucking is thought to develop after the first 6 months.

The immunologic system undergoes numerous changes during the first year. The newborn receives significant amounts of maternal IgG, which confers immunity for about 3 months against antigens to which the mother was exposed. During this time the infant begins to synthesize IgG, and about 40% of adult levels are reached by 1 year of age. Significant amounts of IgM are produced at birth, and adult levels are reached by 9 months of age. The production of IgA, IgD, and IgE is much more gradual, and maximum levels are not attained until early childhood.

During infancy the ability of the skin to contract and shiver in response to cold increases. The peripheral capillaries respond to change in ambient temperature to regulate heat loss. In response to cold, the capillaries constrict, conserving core body temperature and decreasing potential evaporative heat loss from the skin surface. In response to heat the capillaries dilate, decreasing internal body temperature through evaporation, conduction, and convection. Shivering causes the muscles and muscle fibers to contract, generating metabolic heat, which is distributed throughout the body. Accumulation of adipose tissue during the first 6 months serves to insulate the body against heat loss.

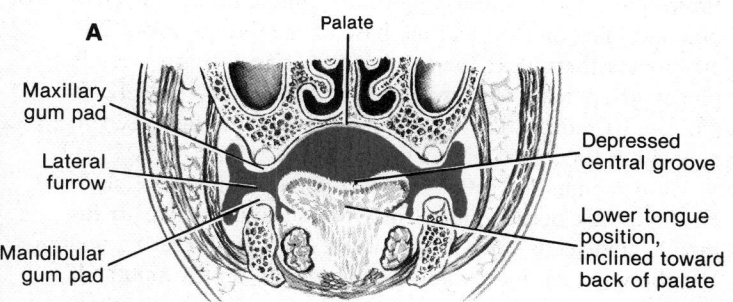

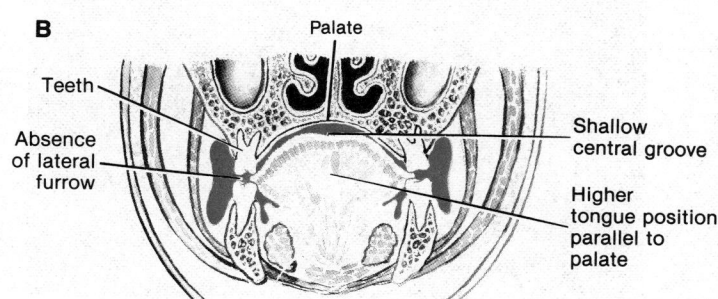

Fig. 12-3. Comparison of **A,** infantile (visceral) swallow reflex, and **B,** mature (somatic) swallow reflex.

The shift in the total body fluid at birth—from a higher level of intracellular fluid to extracellular fluid—continues during the first year, resulting in about 35% extracellular fluid and 40% intracellular fluid, or a total body fluid of 75%. The proportionally higher ratio of extracellular fluid, which is composed of blood plasma, interstitial fluid, and lymph, predisposes the infant to a more rapid loss of total body fluid and consequently dehydration.

The immaturity of the renal structures also predisposes the infant to dehydration. Complete maturity of the kidney occurs during the latter half of the second year, when the cuboidal epithelium of the glomeruli becomes flattened. Before this time the filtration capacity of the glomeruli is reduced.

The endocrine system is adequately developed at birth, but its functions are immature. The interrelatedness of all the endocrine organs has a major effect on the function of any one gland. The lack of homeostatic control because of various functional deficiencies renders the infant especially vulnerable to imbalances in fluid and electrolytes, glucose concentration, and amino acid metabolism.

For example, corticotropin (ACTH) is produced in limited quantities during infancy. ACTH acts on the adrenal cortices to produce their hormones, particularly the glucocorticoids and aldosterone. Because the feedback mechanism between ACTH and the adrenal cortex is immature during infancy, there is much less tolerance for stressful conditions, which affect fluid and electrolytes and the metabolism of fats, proteins, and carbohydrates. In addition, although the islets of Langerhans produce insulin and glucagon during fetal life and early infancy, blood sugar levels tend to remain labile, particularly under conditions of stress.

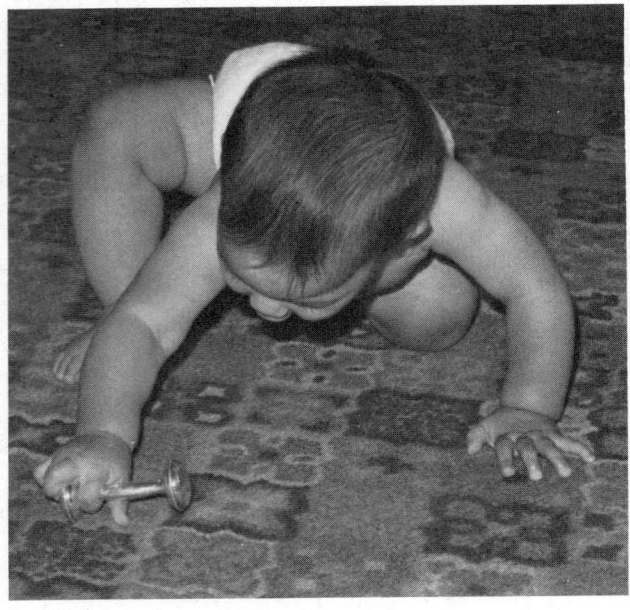

Fig. 12-4. Crude pincer grasp.

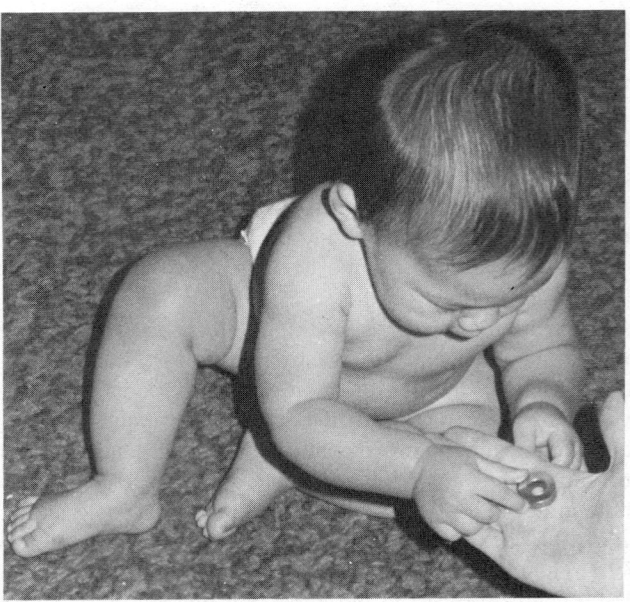

Fig. 12-5. Neat pincer grasp.

Fine Motor Development

Fine motor behavior includes the use of the hands and fingers in the prehension of an object. Grasping occurs during the first 2 to 3 months as a reflex and gradually becomes voluntary. At 1 month the hands are predominantly closed, and by 3 months are mostly open. By this time the infant demonstrates a desire to grasp an object, but "grasps" more with the eyes than with the hands. By 4 months he regards a small pellet and his hands and looks from the object to the hands and back again. Hand regard is common at this age because of the limitation of symmetric positioning, which prevents the infant from exploring the periphery. Hand regard occurs in children who are blind, because it is a developmental process that occurs without visual stimulation. The fingering usually includes pulling at blankets and clothes and sucking on the fists or fingers.

By 5 months the infant is able to voluntarily grasp an object, but prehension is two-handed. The palmar grasp begins with grasping the object in the ulnar side of the palm (toward the fourth and fifth fingers) for the first 6 months. From 6 to 8 months, grasping occurs on the radial side (second and third fingers) and the base of the thumb. From 8 to 10 months the index, fourth, and fifth fingers form a crude pincer grasp with the lower part of the thumb (Fig. 12-4, A). By 10 months the index finger and thumb are used in apposition for a neat pincer grasp (Fig. 12-5).

By 6 months the infant has increased manipulative skill. He holds his bottle, grasps his feet and pulls them to his mouth, and feeds himself a cracker. He enjoys tearing and crumbling paper and explores it thoroughly in his mouth. If he is given two objects, he will hold one and drop the other. By 7 months he transfers objects from one hand to the other (see Fig. 12-8, *E*) and employs one hand for grasping. He enjoys banging objects and explores movable parts in a toy.

By 10 months pincer grasp is established and the infant is able to pick up a raisin and other finger foods. He can deliberately let go of an object and will offer it to someone, but true casting, deliberate throwing of objects, one after the other, is not evident until 12 to 15 months of age. By 11 months he puts objects into a container and likes to remove them. By 1 year of age the infant tries to build a tower of two blocks, but fails. Deliberately releasing an object has advanced; he now releases a cube into a cup following a demonstration.

Gross Motor Development

Gross motor behavior includes developmental maturation in posture, head balance, sitting, creeping, standing, and walking. The full-term neonate is born with some ability to hold the head erect and reflexly assumes the postural tonic neck position when supine. Several of the primitive reflexes have significance in terms of development of later gross motor skills. The *righting reflexes* elicit certain postural responses, particularly of flexion or extension. They are responsible for certain motor activities, such as rolling over, assuming the crawl position, and maintaining normal head-trunk-limb alignment during all activities. The neck-righting reflex, which turns the body to the same side as the head, enables the child to roll over from supine to prone. Other reflexes, such as the otolith-righting and labyrinth-righting reflexes,

enable the infant to raise the head (see box, p. 495.)

The asymmetric tonic neck reflex, which persists from birth to 3 months, prevents the infant from rolling over. The symmetric tonic neck reflex, which is evoked by flexing or extending the neck, helps the infant to assume the crawl position. When the head and neck are extended, the extensor tone of the upper extremities and the flexor tone of the lower extremities increase. The child extends the arms and bends the knees. Because of the strong flexor tone of the lower extremities, the infant may initially crawl backward before forward. This reflex disappears when neurologic maturity allows actual crawling to occur because independent limb movement is required.

Head control. The full-term newborn can momentarily hold the head in midline and parallel when the body is suspended ventrally and can lift and turn the head from side to side when prone. However, marked head lag is evident when the infant is pulled from a lying to a sitting position. By 3 months the infant can hold his head well beyond the plane of his body, and by 4 months he can lift the head and front portion of the chest about 90 degrees above the table, bearing his weight on the forearms. Only slight head lag is evident when the infant is pulled from a lying to a sitting position. By 6 months he can raise the chest and upper part of the abdomen off the table, maintaining his weight on the hands. By 7 months he can bear weight on one hand while exploring with the other. Figs. 12-6 and 12-7 illustrate development of head control.

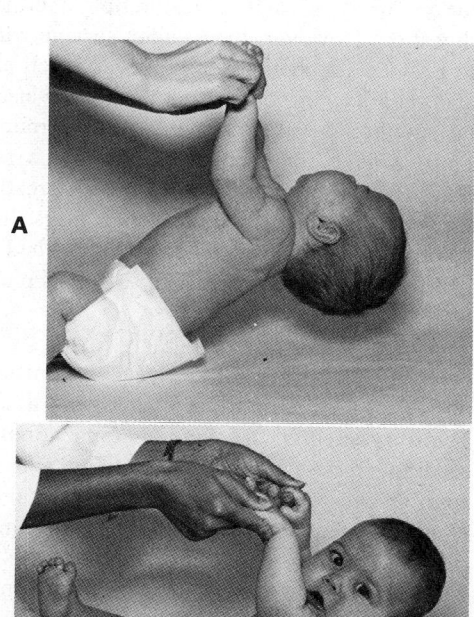
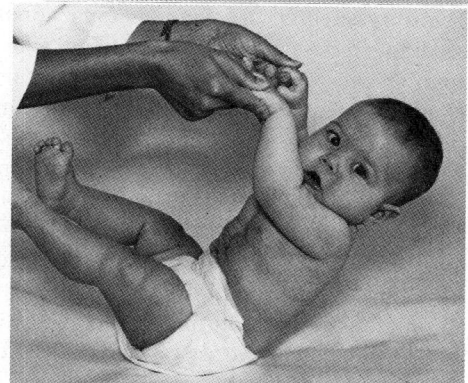
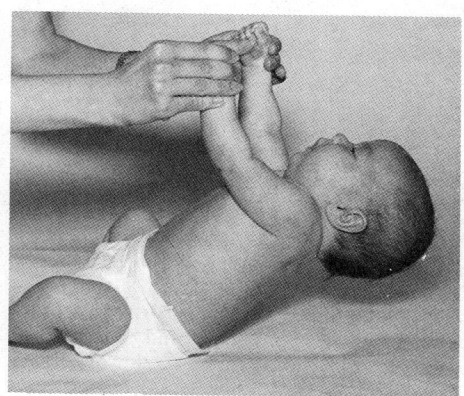

Fig. 12-6. Head control while pulled to sitting position. **A,** Complete head lag at 1 month. **B,** Partial head lag at 2 months. **C,** Almost no head lag at 4 months.

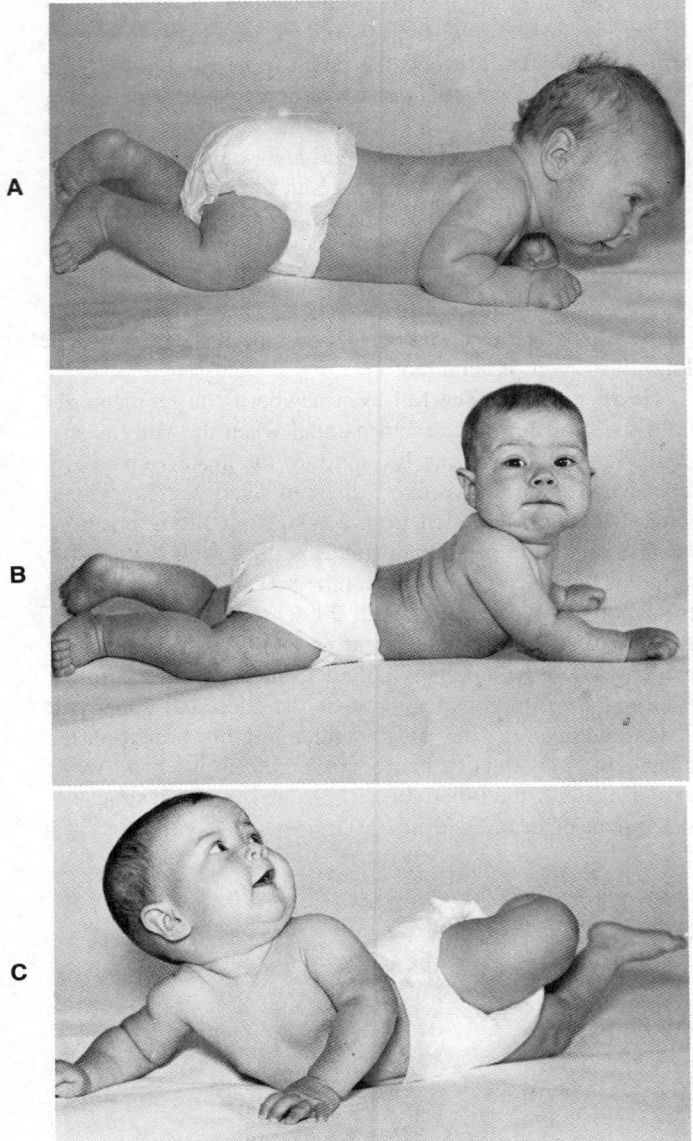

Fig. 12-7. Head control while prone. **A,** Momentarily lifts head at 1 month. **B,** Lifts head and chest 90 degrees and bears weight on forearms at 4 months. **C,** Lifts head, chest, and upper abdomen and can bear weight on hands at 6 months. Note how this position facilitates turning from abdomen to back.

Rolling over. The newborn may accidentally roll over because of his rounded back. The neck-righting reflex enables him to roll from back to side at 4 months. The ability to willfully turn from the abdomen to the back occurs at 5 months, and from the back to the abdomen at 6 months. It is noteworthy that the parachute reflex, which elicits a protective response to falling, appears at 7 months.

Sitting. The ability to sit follows progressive head control and straightening of the back, as shown in Fig. 12-8. Although there is marked head lag in the sitting position at birth, the infant contracts the neck, shoulder, and arm muscles, enabling him to raise the head when pulled halfway to

a sitting position. He will make attempts to lift the chin and right the head while sitting. At 3 months head lag is slight; at 4 months it is absent; by 6 months the infant lifts the head when he is about to be pulled in sitting. By the next month he spontaneously raises the head in an attempt to sit up by himself.

For the first couple of months the back is uniformly rounded. As the spinal column straightens, the infant is able to be propped in a sitting position. By 7 months he can sit alone, leaning forward on his hands for support. By 8 months he can sit well unsupported and begins to explore his surroundings in this position rather than in a lying position. By 10 months he can maneuver from a prone to a sitting position.

Locomotion. If the young infant is placed in a standing position, the body is usually limp at the hips and knees. By 6 to 7 months the infant is able to bear all his weight. By 9 months he stands holding onto furniture and can pull himself to the standing position but is unable to maneuver himself back down, except by falling. At 10 months he can step with one foot and crawls well. At 11 months he can creep and cruise or walk while holding onto furniture or with both hands held. By 52 weeks he is able to walk with one hand held. Fig. 12-9 illustrates development of locomotion.

PSYCHOSOCIAL DEVELOPMENT

Infants are born with the basic abilities needed for extrauterine survival, such as respiration, thermoregulation, and digestion. However, they cannot survive without a caregiver to provide for their essential needs, such as food, warmth, and security. In addition to their basic needs, which must be supplied for them, infants have certain tasks that they must achieve for themselves during the first year of life. How their needs are met by others greatly determines to what degree they accomplish their tasks. The stages of development have been studied and described by several noted psychoanalysts, including Erikson and Freud.

Erikson: Developing a Sense of Trust

Erikson's phase I (birth to 1 year) is concerned with *acquiring a sense of trust* while overcoming a sense of *mistrust.* The trust acquired in infancy is foundational for all the succeeding phases. It allows the infant a feeling of physical comfort and security, which assists him in experiencing unfamiliar, unknown situations with a minimum of fear. The crucial element for the achievement of this task is the *quality* of the mother (caregiver)-child relationship. The provision of food, warmth, and shelter are alone inadequate for the development of a strong ego. The infant and mother must jointly learn to satisfactorily meet their needs in order for mutual regulation of frustration to occur. When this synchrony fails to develop, mistrust is the eventual outcome.

The acquisition of trust involves the libidinal or psychologic energy of the erotic centers of the body, namely the mouth. Erikson has described particular stages in the oral

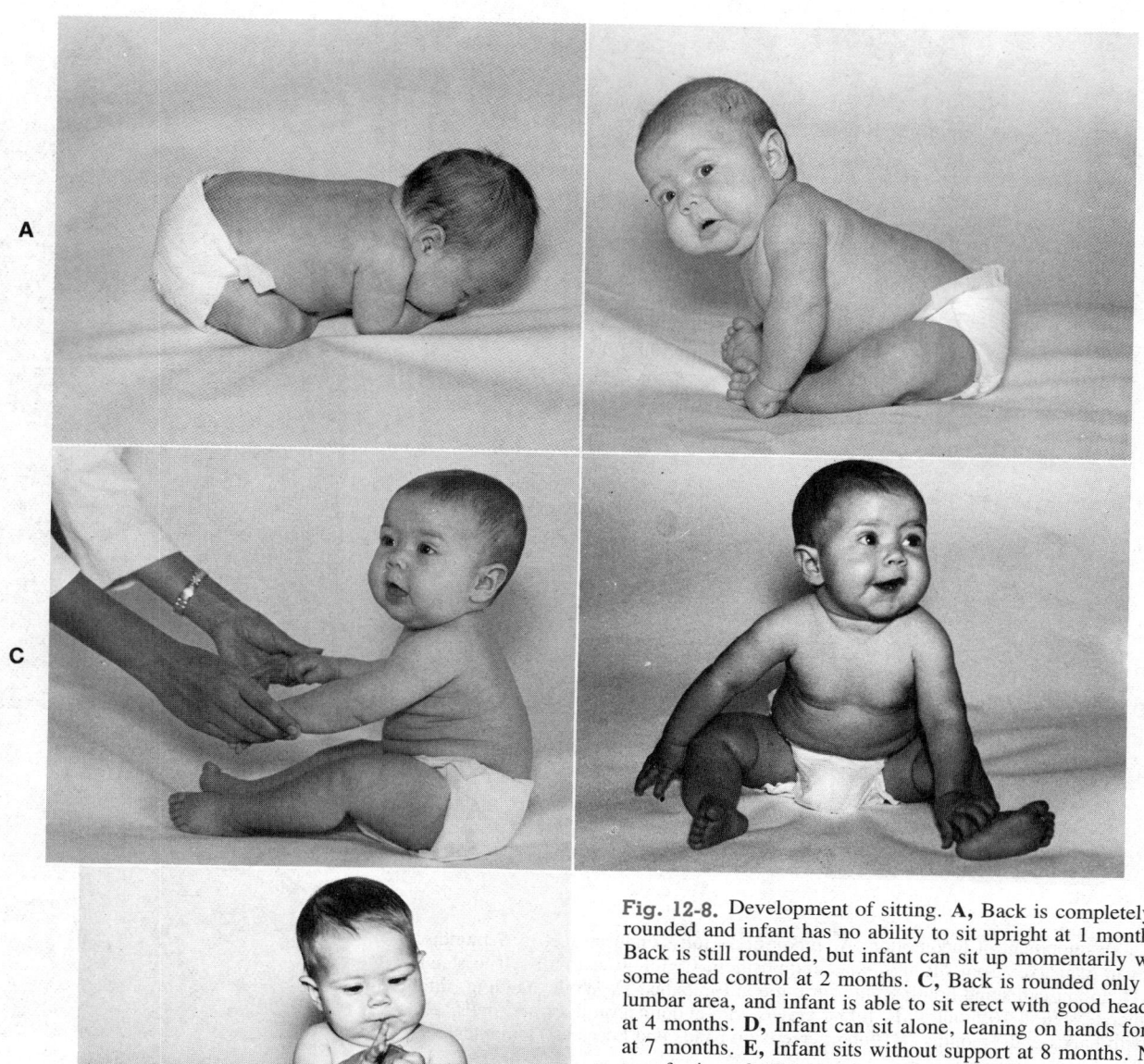

Fig. 12-8. Development of sitting. **A,** Back is completely rounded and infant has no ability to sit upright at 1 month. **B,** Back is still rounded, but infant can sit up momentarily with some head control at 2 months. **C,** Back is rounded only in lumbar area, and infant is able to sit erect with good head control at 4 months. **D,** Infant can sit alone, leaning on hands for support at 7 months. **E,** Infant sits without support at 8 months. Note transferring of objects that occurs at 7 months.

phase. The first social modality is primarily *oral*. During the first 3 to 4 months food intake is the most important social activity in which the infant engages. The id processes are most evident; the newborn can tolerate little frustration or delay of gratification. Primary *narcissism* is at its height. However, as bodily processes such as vision, motor movements, and vocalization are more cortically controlled, the id processes, which operate on the *pleasure principle,* become a component of the ego structure, which operates on

the *reality principle*. The infant gradually learns to accept delayed gratification and alternative methods of eliciting a positive response from the environment.

Either extreme in terms of ''delayed gratification'' leads to mistrust. If the mother or caregiver always meets the child's needs before he signals his readiness, the infant will never learn to test his ability to control the environment. If the delay is prolonged, the infant will experience constant frustration and eventually mistrust others in their efforts to satisfy him.

The next social modality involves an incorporative mode of reaching out to others through *grasping*. Initially grasping is reflexive, but it has a powerful social meaning to the parents. The reciprocal response of the infant's grasping is the parents' holding on and touching.

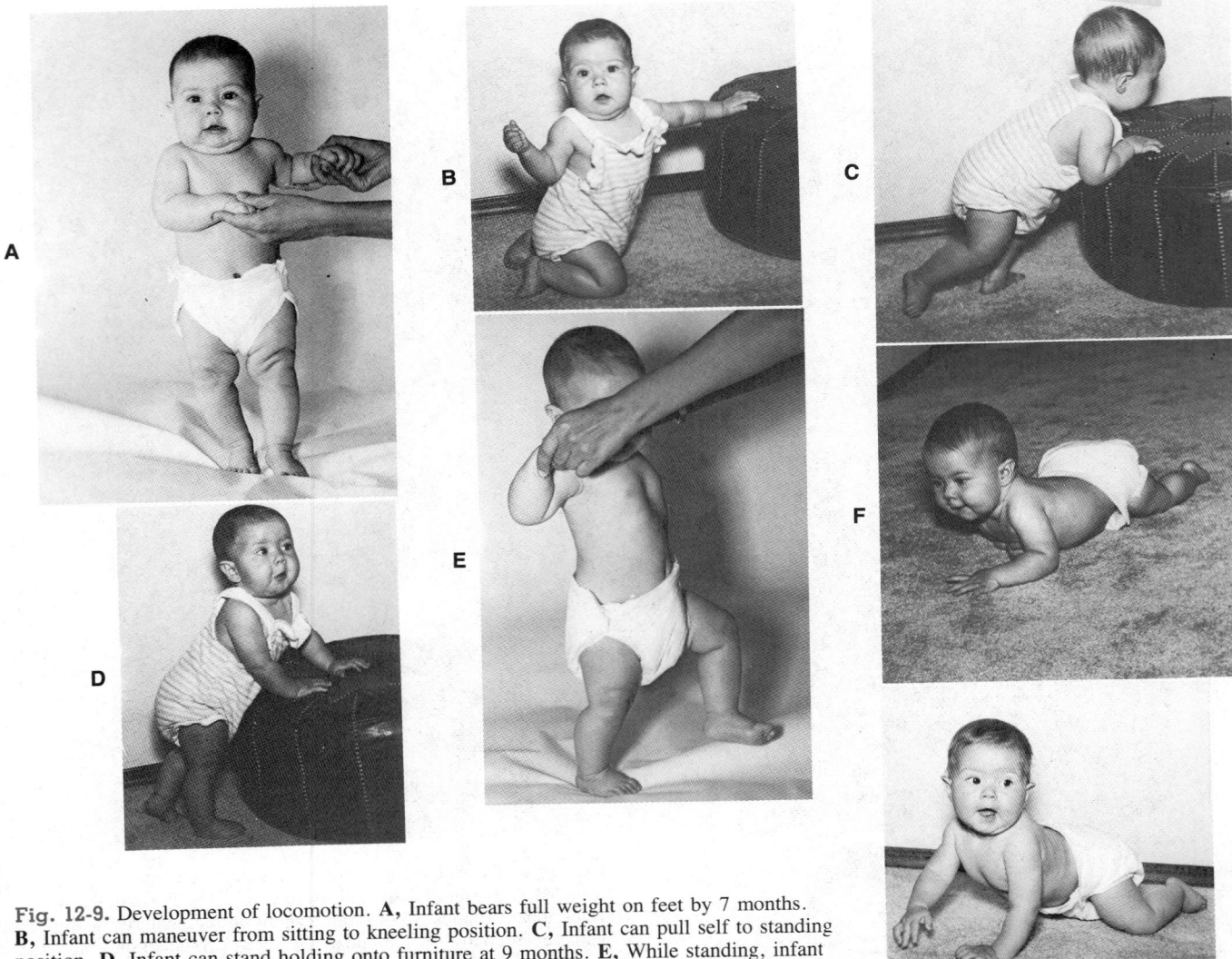

Fig. 12-9. Development of locomotion. **A,** Infant bears full weight on feet by 7 months. **B,** Infant can maneuver from sitting to kneeling position. **C,** Infant can pull self to standing position. **D,** Infant can stand holding onto furniture at 9 months. **E,** While standing, infant takes deliberate step at 10 months. **F,** Infant crawls with abdomen on floor and pulls self forward with hands at 10 months. **G,** Infant creeps on hands and knees at 11 months.

Tactile stimulation is significant in the total process of acquiring trust. During the newborn period the parent's exploration of the infant's body is considered an important aspect of bonding. Continued physical contact becomes an important (if not crucial) determinant of attachment of the caregivers. Rejection of physical contact by *attachment figures,* not mere acquaintances or strangers, eventually leads to anger and conflict in the child (Biggar, 1984). Therefore the degree of mothering skill, the quantity of food, or the length of sucking does not determine the quality of the experience; rather, it is the total nature of the interpersonal relationship, including the component of touch, that regulates the infant's formulation of trust.

During the second incorporative stage, the more active and aggressive modality of *biting* occurs. The infant learns that he can hold on to what is his own and can more fully control his environment. During this stage the infant is confronted with one of his first conflicts of breast-feeding as he quickly learns that biting causes withdrawal of the nipple and anxiety in the mother. Yet biting also brings internal relief from teething discomfort and a sense of power or control. The successful resolution of this conflict strengthens the mother-child relationship at a time when the infant is recognizing her as the most significant person in his life.

At about the same time (6 months of age), stranger anxiety is evident. The infant has formed strong attachments to the most significant people in his world, his parents. Separation can be devastating and, if prolonged, can affect future personality development. Athough unpleasant to experience, demonstration of stranger anxiety is an important component of parent-infant attachment.

Freud: The Oral Stage

Freud's oral stage during infancy involves id gratification through oral satisfaction. Before the teeth erupt, usually during the first 6 months of life, the infant is in the *oral-passive,* or *oral-dependent, stage.* Pleasure is derived through sucking, eating, and rooting. During and after teething the infant is in the *oral-aggressive stage* and can bite as well as suck for gratification.

The erogenous zones are the mouth and lips; any object that comes in contact with this zone is potentially pleasurable. The "mouthing activity" of the infant is very evident during the first year, when everything is explored by sucking or biting. The sucking needs of infants vary, just as the "oral needs" of adults differ. Some infants are satisfied by the amount of sucking supplied through feeding, whereas others require additional opportunities for sucking pleasure, such as the use of a pacifier.

COGNITIVE DEVELOPMENT

Intellectual development is concurrent with biologic, motor, language, and personal-social achievements, many of which must occur before learning can take place. For example, visual ability must be sufficient for the infant to see objects clearly before associations about the object can be made. Learning occurs when behavior changes as a result of experience or growth. As motor function progresses, learning occurs through the infant's more active participation in the environment. The theory most frequently quoted to explain cognition, or the ability to know, is that of Piaget.

Piaget: The Sensorimotor Phase

The period of birth to 24 months is termed the sensorimotor phase and is composed of six stages; however, inasmuch as this discussion is concerned with ages birth to 12 months, only the first four stages are discussed (Table 12-1; see Table 14-1 for the stages from 12 to 24 months).

During the sensorimotor phase the infant progresses from reflex behavior to simple repetitive acts to imitative activity. Three crucial events take place during this phase. First, the infant learns to separate himself from other objects in the environment. He realizes that others besides himself control the environment and that certain readjustments must take place for mutual satisfaction to occur. This coincides with Erikson's concept of the formation of trust and mutual regulation of frustration. Piaget also believes in a "conflict" during each phase. The goal during one phase is to establish a balance between the desire to function at a higher level while recognizing the limitations created by the environment. He believes that achieving a near equilibrium in a constantly changing environment is the goal of biologic, affective (emotional), and mental functions.

The second major achievement is the concept of *permanency,* or the realization that objects that leave the visual field still exist. A typical example of the development of object permanency is the infant's ability to separate from his parents at bedtime because of his realization that they will be present when he awakens. Eventually he broadens this concept to tolerate brief periods of separation with a different caregiver.

The last major intellectual achievement of this period is the ability to use *symbols* or "mental representation." The use of symbols allows the infant to think of an object or situation without actually experiencing it. The recognition of symbols is the beginning of understanding of time and space.

Use of reflexes. The first stage, from birth to 1 month, is identified by the infant's use of reflexes. At birth the in-

Table 12-1 Sensorimotor phase during infancy*

STAGE	AGE (MONTHS)	COGNITIVE DEVELOPMENT	BEHAVIOR
I. Use of reflexes	Birth-1	Repetitious use of reflexes establishes a pattern of experiences Totally autistic (self-centered) being	Mostly reflexive (sucking, swallowing, rooting, grasping, crying) Little or no tolerance for frustration or delayed gratification
II. Primary circular reactions	1-4	Use of reflexes is gradually replaced by voluntary activity Recognition of causality occurs when repetition of events causes one stimulus to produce a consistent response Beginning notion of temporal space or time occurs as infant realizes the progression of an orderly sequence of events Beginning separation of self from others Learns from type of interaction between object or individual rather than from object itself Engages in an activity for the pleasure of the activity more than for its result	Recognizes familiar faces and objects (for example, bottle) Shows anticipation before feeding Awareness of strange surroundings indicates memory Discovers parts of own body—plays with hands, fingers, feet Becomes bored when left alone Shows no stranger anxiety unless caregiver's skill differs from usual routine

*For phases during toddlerhood see Table 14-1.

Continued.

Table 12-1 Sensorimotor phase during infancy—cont'd

STAGE	AGE (MONTHS)	COGNITIVE DEVELOPMENT	BEHAVIOR
III. Secondary circular reactions	4-8	Intentional activity replaces repetitious activity that did not produce a desired result Beginning of object permanency when object is beyond perceptual range Progressive idea of time, awareness of before and after in a sequence of events Able to imitate selective activity from several events Further separation of self from environment Idea of quality and quantity Beginning recognition of symbols as type of communication	Secures objects by pulling on a string Searches for objects that have fallen Shows stranger anxiety Able to tolerate some frustration and delayed gratification Imitates sounds and simple gestures Great interest in mirror image (Fig. 12-4) Beginning independence in self-feeding Shows displeasure if activity is inhibited Language development, attracts attention by methods other than crying Realizes that parents are present even if not in visual field
IV. Coordination of secondary schemata and its application to new situations	9-12	Concept of object permanence advances, beginning of intellectual reasoning Associates symbols with events, but classification is based on own experience Distinguishes objects from the related activity and perceives them as objects Distinguishes end products from their means, attempts to remove barriers to achieve the end	Actively searches for a hidden object (Fig. 12-10) Comprehends meanings of words and simple commands Knows that gestures (bye-bye, kiss) have certain meanings Is able to put objects in a container Works to get toy that is out of reach Ventures away from mother to explore surroundings

fant's individuality and temperament are expressed through the physiologic reflexes of sucking, rooting, grasping, and crying. The repetitious nature of the reflexes is the beginning of associations between an act and a sequential response. When the infant cries because he is hungry, a nipple is put in his mouth, and he sucks, feels satisfaction, and sleeps. He is assimilating this experience while perceiving auditory, tactile, and visual cues. This experience of perceiving certain patterns, or "ordering," is foundational for the subsequent stages.

Primary circular reactions. This stage marks the beginning of the replacement of reflexive behavior with voluntary acts. During the period from 1 to 4 months, activities such as sucking or grasping become deliberate acts that elicit certain responses. The beginning of accommodation is evident. The infant incorporates and adapts his reactions to the environment and recognizes the stimulus that produced a response. Previously the infant would cry until the nipple was brought to his mouth. Now he associates the nipple with the sound of the mother's voice. He accommodates this new piece of information and adapts by ceasing to cry when he hears her voice, before he receives the nipple. A realization of causality and a recognition of an orderly sequence of events is taking place. The environment is taken in with all the senses and with whatever motor ability is present.

Secondary circular reactions. The secondary circular reaction stage is a continuation of primary circular reactions and lasts until 8 months of age. In this stage the pri-

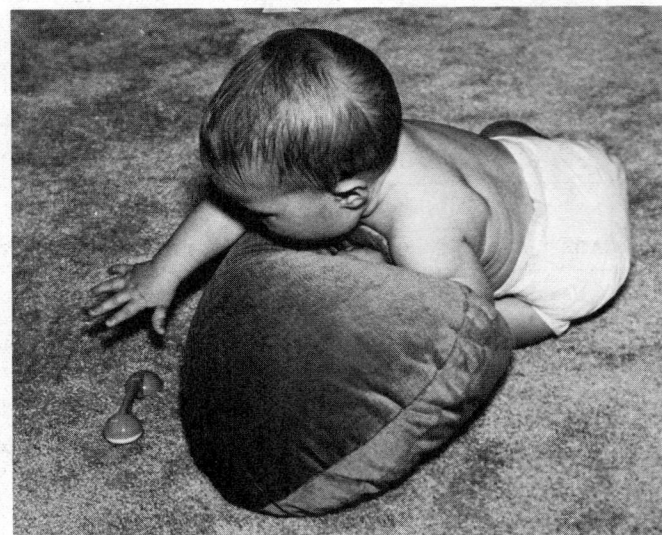

Fig. 12-10. Nine-month-old infant actively searches for object hidden behind pillow.

mary circular reactions are repeated and prolonged for the response that results. Grasping and holding now become shaking, banging, and pulling. Shaking is performed to hear a noise, not solely for the pleasure of shaking. Quality and quantity of an act become evident. "More" or "less" shaking produces different responses. Causality, time, deliberate intention, and separateness from the environment begin to develop.

Three new processes of human behavior—imitation, play, and affect—occur. *Imitation* requires the differentiation of selected acts from several events. By the second half of the first year the infant can imitate sounds and simple gestures. *Play* becomes evident as the infant takes pleasure in performing an act after he has mastered it. Much of the infant's waking hours are absorbed in sensorimotor play. *Affect* is seen as the infant begins to develop a sense of permanency. During the first 6 months the infant believes that an object exists only for as long as he can visually perceive it. In other words, out of sight—out of mind. When the object continues to be present or remembered even though it is beyond the range of perception, affect to external objects is evident. Object permanence is a critical component of parent-child attachment (p. 506) and is seen in the development of stranger anxiety at 6 to 8 months of age (p. 506). Another is the game of peekaboo, in which the child tests out the reality of being and not being. Some theorists postulate that this type of activity represents the beginning development of the concept of death.

Coordination of secondary schemata and their application to new situations. During the fourth sensorimotor stage, the infant uses previous behavioral achievements primarily as the foundation for adding new intellectual skills to his expanding repertoire. This stage is largely transitional. Increasing motor skills allow for greater exploration of the environment. He begins to discover that hiding an object does not mean that it is gone but that removing an obstacle will reveal the object. This marks the beginning of intellectual reasoning. Furthermore, he can experience an event by *observing* it, and he begins to associate symbols with events, such as "bye-bye" with "Daddy goes to work," but the classification is purely his own. Unlike the second stage, where the infant learned from the type of interaction between objects or individuals, in this stage the

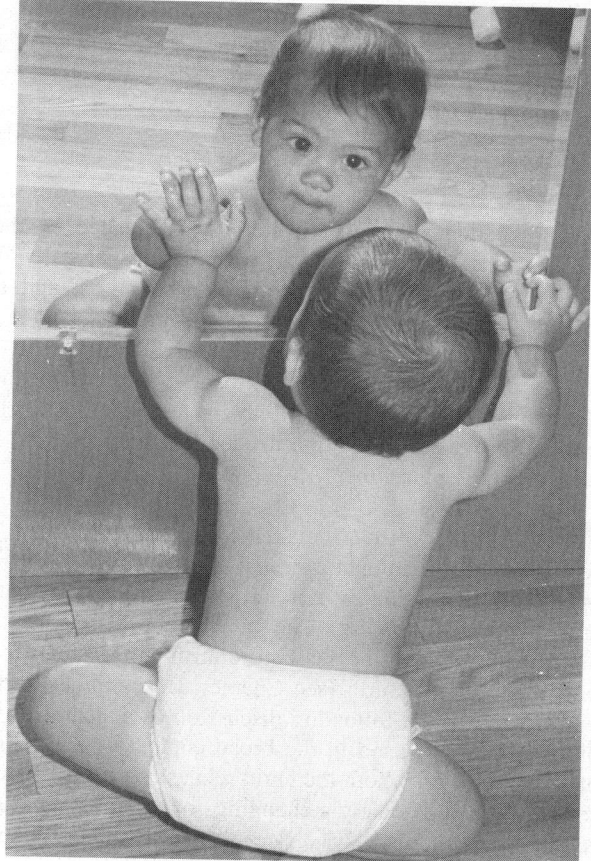

Fig. 12-12. Eight-month-old infant enjoying her image in mirror.

child learns from the object itself. Intentionality is further developed in that now the infant will actively attempt to remove a barrier to his desired (or undesired) action (Fig. 12-10). If something is in his way, he will attempt to climb over it or push it away. Previously an obstacle would cause him to give up any further attempt to achieve his desired goal.

DEVELOPMENT OF BODY IMAGE

The development of body image parallels sensorimotor development. Infants' kinesthetic and tactile experiences are the first perceptions of their body and the mouth is the principal area of pleasurable sensations. Other parts of the body are primarily objects of pleasure—the hands and fingers to suck and the feet to play with (Fig. 12-11). As physical needs are met, they feel comfort and satisfaction with their body. Messages conveyed by the caregivers reinforce these feelings. For example, when infants smile, they receive emotional satisfaction from others who smile back.

Achieving the concept of object permanence is basic to the development of self-image. By the end of the first year infants recognize that they are distinct from their parents. At the same time there is increasing interest in their image, especially in the mirror (Fig. 12-12). As motor skills de-

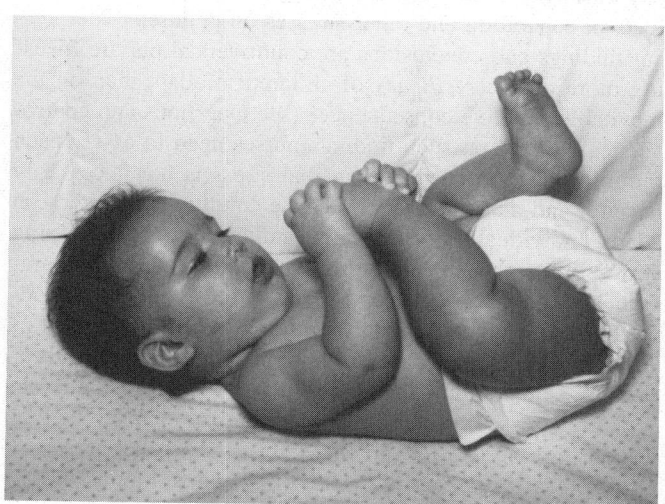

Fig. 12-11. During early infancy, body parts are primarily objects of pleasure for the child.

velop, they learn that parts of the body are useful; for example, the hands bring objects to the mouth and the legs help them move to different locations. All of these achievements transmit messages to them.

SOCIAL DEVELOPMENT

Infants' social development is initially influenced by their reflexive behavior, such as the grasp, and eventually depends primarily on the interaction between them and the principal caregivers. Attachment to the parent is increasingly evident during the second half of the first year. In addition, tremendous strides are made in communication and personal-social behavior. Play is a major socializing agent and provides stimulation needed to learn from and interact with the environment.

Attachment

The importance of human physical contact cannot be overemphasized. Parenting is not an instinctual ability but a learned acquired process. The attachment of parent and child, which probably begins before birth and assumes even more importance at birth (see Chapter 8), continues during the first year. In the following discussion of attachment, the word "mother" is used in the broad context of the consistent caregiver with whom the child relates more than anyone else. However, in society's changing social climate and sex role stereotypes, this may very well be the father. Studies on father-child attachment demonstrate that similar stages occur as with mother attachment (Lincoln, 1984).

During infancy attachment progresses with the child assuming an increasingly significant role. Two components of cognitive development are required for attachment: (1) the ability to discriminate the mother from other individuals and (2) the achievement of object permanence. Both of these processes prepare the infant for an equally important aspect of attachment—separation from the parent. Separation-individuation should occur as a harmonious, parallel process with emotional attachment (Sherwen, 1983).

During the formation of attachment to the parent the infant progresses through four distinct but overlapping stages. For the first few weeks the infant responds indiscriminately to anyone. Beginning at about 8 to 12 weeks of age, the infant cries, smiles, and vocalizes more to the mother than to anyone else but continues to respond to others, whether familiar or not. At age 6 months or so the infant shows a distinct preference for the mother. He follows her more, cries when she leaves, enjoys playing with her more, and feels most secure in her arms. About 1 month after showing attachment to the mother, many infants begin attaching to other members of the family, most often the father.

Infants acquire other developmental behaviors that influence the attachment process. These include (1) differential crying, smiling, and vocalization (more to mother than to anyone else), (2) visual-motor orientation (looking more at mother even if she is not close), (3) crying when mother leaves the room, (4) approach through locomotion (crawl-

ing, creeping, or walking), (5) clinging (especially in presence of a stranger), and (6) exploring away from mother while using her as a secure base.

Effects of prolonged separation. Attachment is considered so critical to optimum child development that many researchers have documented the effects of prolonged and early separation on infants in the absence of quality mother substitutes. Some of the most famous research on emotional deprivation has been done by John Bowlby, John Robertson, and René Spitz. Bowlby (1956) studied the effects of the infant's separation from the mother and noted severe mental and physical retardation, particularly if emotional deprivation occurred during the first 3 years of life. He observed that the progressive retardation could be arrested or reversed if no further emotional deprivation occurred after the first 2 years but that prolonged severe deprivation beginning early in the first year and lasting for 3 years led to severe permanent effects. Among these were the inability to form trusting, intimate interpersonal relationships, language impairment, and deficiency in abstract thinking. Bowlby and Robertson found typical behavioral reactions of infants who were hospitalized and separated from their mothers (Chapter 26).

Spitz (1945) studied the effects of emotional deprivation of children raised in foundling homes or institutions. The infants were cared for by one nurse who had responsibility for eight children. Although the caregiver might be a loving, motherly person, she lacked the time necessary to devote individual attention and stimulation to each child. As a result the children were retarded in physical growth, were more susceptible to disease, and demonstrated decreasing developmental quotients over a 2-year period. Spitz found that children who were given one-to-one attention by a mother substitute developed normally.

Although these studies represent extreme examples of young children reared in environments essentially devoid of quality mothering, rather than temporary separation, such as day care, the question remains regarding the long-term effects of separation and other stresses on children. The present findings and conclusions are controversial but are focusing more on the *resiliency* of children to adapt than on the inevitable negative consequences (see Questions and controversies). Based on such findings nurses need to assess each family with the understanding that stress is not necessarily harmful and that even under adverse conditions children can adapt. Individual risk factors that influence a child's coping ability are evaluated, and tools such as the Infant Temperament Questionnaire (see p. 510) are used to assess "goodness of fit." When parental separation occurs, every effort is made to help the family provide suitable mothering substitutes for the child. The child's plasticity and resiliency to cope are stressed to the family to minimize their feelings of responsibility and guilt (Nelms, 1985).

Separation anxiety. Between 4 and 8 months the infant progresses through the first stage of separation-individuation and begins to have some awareness of self and mother as separate individuals. At the same time object per-

Questions and Controversies

How detrimental and permanent are stressful events, such as maternal deprivation, during infancy?

Much of the present research on the effects of stress during childhood demonstrates that children have an incredible ability to adapt despite adversity. Thomas and Chess (1984) revealed a very high rate of recovery in children with adjustment problems and found that neither parent separation, divorce, nor death was predictive of early adult status. Extensive reviews of research regarding the effects of stress on children, such as maternal deprivation, hospitalization, birth of a sibling, and parental death, confirmed similar findings (Rutter, 1979, 1981). Such studies have identified risk factors that increase children's vulnerability to stress, such as "difficult" temperament, lack of "fit" between child and parent, age (especially between 6 months and 5 years), male gender, genetics, below-average intelligence, multiple and continuing stresses such as frequent hospital admissions or foster care placements and homes marked by discord or divorce, and lack of social supports.

However, the basic conclusion is that stress alone does not dictate inevitable negative consequences. Rather, emphasis must be placed on individual differences in vulnerability to deprivation and stress. Significant separation or lack of attachment to the mother figure must be viewed in light of other substitutes in the child's life, such as fathers, siblings, relatives, neighbors, and teachers, who also can significantly influence development (Garmezy and Rutter, 1983).

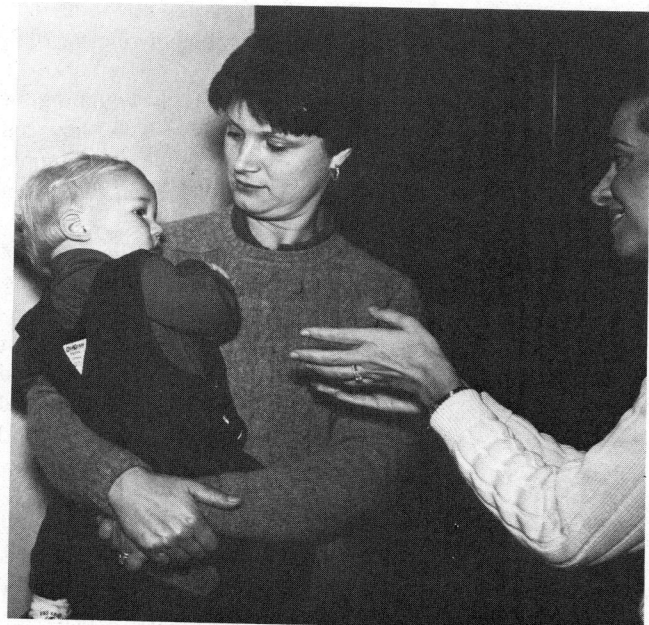

Fig. 12-13. Stranger fear behaviors include clinging to the parent and turning away from a stranger.

manence is developing and the infant is aware that the parent can be absent. Consequently, separation anxiety develops and is manifest through a predictable sequence of behaviors.

During the early second half of the first year the infant protests when placed in his crib, and a short time later objects when his mother leaves the room. Subsequently the infant may not notice the mother's absence if he is absorbed in an activity. However, when he realizes her absence, he protests. From this point onward he becomes very alert to her activities and whereabouts. By 11 to 12 months he is able to anticipate her imminent departure by watching her behaviors and begins to protest *before* she leaves. At this point many parents learn to postpone alerting the child to their departure until just before leaving (Bowlby, 1969).

Stranger fear. As the infant demonstrates attachment to one person, he correspondingly exhibits less friendliness to others. Between ages 6 and 8 months fear of strangers and stranger anxiety become most prominent and are related to the infant's ability to discriminate between familiar and nonfamiliar people. Such behaviors as clinging to the parent, crying, and turning away from the stranger are common (Fig. 12-13). Suggestions for coping with stranger fear and separation anxiety are discussed on p. 516.

Language Development

The infant's first means of verbal communication is crying. Crying as a biologic sign conveys a message of urgency and

signals displeasure, such as hunger. However, crying is also a social event that affects the development of the parent-infant relationship, either by its absence, which usually has a positive effect on parents, or its presence, which may evoke a negative response or persuade parents to minister to the child's physical or emotional needs.

In the first few weeks of life crying has reflexive quality and is mostly related to physiologic needs. Crying is also a mechanism for discharging energy or tension and can occur in response to too much stimulation. The increase in crying during the first few months for no apparent reason may be related to the discharge of energy and the maturational changes in the central nervous system. During the end of the first year infants cry for attention, from fear, especially stranger fear, and from frustration, usually in response to their developing but inadequate motor skills (Lester, 1983).

Many parents state that they can distinguish between different types of cry and from these messages are able to interpret the infant's needs. However, crying can be a source of acute distress for parents, especially the unconsolable crying of colic (see p. 565). Parents benefit from an explanation of the variability of crying among infants and assurance that periods of "unexplained fussiness" are normal. Some parents may need guidance in consoling techniques, such as holding, swaddling, massaging, caressing, rocking, walking, or stimulating sucking.

Vocalizations heard during crying eventually become some syllables and the words, for example, the "mama" heard during vigorous crying. Infants vocalize as early as 5 to 6 weeks by making small throaty sounds. By 2 months they make single vowel sounds, such as *ah*, *eh*, and *uh*. By 3 to 4 months the consonants *n, k, g, p*, and *b* are added and infants coo, gurgle, and laugh aloud. By 8 months they add the consonants *t, d,* and *w* and combine syllables, such as "dada," but do not ascribe meaning to the word until 11 to 12 months. They make sounds, such as coughing or snorting, to attract attention. By 9 to 10 months they can comprehend the meaning of the word "no," obey simple commands, and respond to their name. By 1 year they can say two to three words with meaning.

During the acquisition of new language skills it is not unlikely for the child to temporarily give up other recently learned sounds or words. This is often distressing for parents after waiting in anticipation for the words "dada" or "mama." However, these sounds are frequently abandoned for other vocalizations and may not be repeated for several weeks. It is reassuring for parents to know that the child will again say these words, probably with meaning.

Personal-Social Behavior

Personal-social behavior includes the child's personal responses to the environment. It is the area most influenced by external stimuli but, as in the other fields of behavior, follows certain developmental laws. Personal-social behavior implies communication with one's self and with others. It is foundational for the successful mastery of skills such as feeding, control of bodily functions, independence, and cooperativeness in play.

Infants have the ability to shape their environment and to elicit certain responses. The newborn shows visual preference for the human face and, as early as 1 week of age, begins to watch his mother intently as she speaks to him. As he regards her face his activity diminishes, his head bobs up and down, and his mouth moves almost as if trying to say something.

By 6 to 8 weeks a social smile in response to pleasurable stimuli is present. This has a profound effect on family members and is a tremendous stimulus for evoking continued responses from others. By 3 months the infant shows considerable interest in the environment: excitement when a toy is presented, refusal to be left alone, recognition of mother, and demonstration of pleasure by squealing. By 4 months he laughs aloud and enjoys strange, novel stimuli.

By 6 months the infant is a very personable child. He plays games such as peekaboo when his head is hidden in a towel, he signals his desire to be picked up by extending his arms, and he shows displeasure when a toy is removed or his face is washed. There is increasing demonstration of his ability to control his environment. The acquisition of fine and gross motor skills allows much more independence in movement.

By the second half of the first year the infant understands simple discipline, such as the meaning of the word "no" or a scolding remark. He comprehends different facial expressions and is sensitive to emotional changes in others. Imitation is developing during this time. By 7 months he imitates acts and noises, by 8 months, sounds, and by 10 months games such as pat-a-cake and peekaboo.

From 11 months onward he is increasingly independent. He is learning to feed himself and use a spoon and cup and can help with dressing by putting his foot out for a shoe or pushing his arm through the sleeve. He not only comprehends the meaning of "no," but shakes his head to signal his understanding. He can follow simple directions and will gladly perform for others to attract and prolong attention.

Play

Play during infancy is representative of the various social modalities observed during cognitive development. The infant's activity is primarily narcissistic, revolving around his own body. As discussed under development of body image, parts of the body are primarily play and pleasure objects.

During the first year play becomes more sophisticated and interdependent. From birth to 3 months the infant's response to the environment is global and largely undifferentiated. Play is dependent; pleasure is demonstrated by a quieting attitude (1 month), later by a smile (2 months), and then by a squeal (3 months). From 3 to 6 months the infant shows more discriminate interest in the stimuli presented to him and begins to play alone with a rattle or soft stuffed toy or to play with someone else. There is much more interaction during play. By 4 months of age he laughs aloud, shows preference for certain toys, and becomes excited when food or a favorite object is brought to him. He recognizes an image in a mirror, smiles at it, and vocalizes to it.

By 6 months to 1 year play involves sensorimotor skills. Actual games are played, such as peekaboo, pat-a-cake, verbal repetition, and imitation of simple gestures in response to demonstration. Play is much more selective, not only in terms of specific toys but also in terms of "playmates." Although play is solitary or one-sided, the infant chooses with whom he will interact. At 6 to 8 months he usually refuses to play with strangers until he begins to know them. Parents are definite favorites, and he knows how to attract their attention. At 6 months he extends his arms to be picked up, at 7 months he coughs to make his presence known, at 10 months he pulls the parent's clothing, and at 12 months he calls them by name. This represents a tremendous advance from the newborn who signaled biologic needs by crying to express displeasure.

Stimulation is as important for psychosocial growth as food is for physical growth. Knowledge of developmental milestones allows nurses to guide parents regarding proper play for infants. It is not sufficient to place a mobile over a crib and toys in a playpen for a child's optimum social, emotional, and intellectual development. Play must provide interpersonal contact as well as recreational and educational stimulation. Infants need to be *played with,* not merely *allowed to play.* Although the type of play infants engage in is called *solitary,* this is only a figurative, not literal, term to denote one-sided play. The kind of toys given to the child is much less important then the quality of personal interaction that occurs.

Table 12-2 Play during infancy

AGE (MONTHS)	VISUAL STIMULATION	AUDITORY STIMULATION	TACTILE STIMULATION	KINETIC STIMULATION
Suggested activities				
Birth-1	Look at infant at close range Hang bright, shiny object within 20-25 cm (8-10 in) of infant's face and in midline	Talk to infant, sing in soft voice Play music box, radio, television Have ticking clock or metronome nearby	Hold, caress, cuddle Keep infant warm May like to be swaddled	Rock infant, place in cradle Use carriage for walks
2-3	Provide bright objects Make room bright with pictures or mirrors on walls Take infant to various rooms while doing chores Place him in infant seat for vertical view of environment	Talk to infant Include in family gatherings Expose to various environmental noises other than those of home Use rattles, wind chimes	Caress infant while bathing, at diaper change Comb hair with a soft brush	Use swing Take in car for rides Exercise body by moving extremities in swimming motion
4-6	Place infant so that he can look in mirror Place in front of television with family Give brightly colored toys to hold (small enough to grasp)	Talk to infant, repeat sounds he makes Laugh when he laughs Call him by name Crinkle different papers by his ear Place rattle or bell in hand, show him how to shake them	Give infant soft squeeze toys of various textures Allow to splash in bath Place nude on soft furry rug and move extremities	Use swing or stroller Bounce infant in lap while holding him in standing position Help him roll over Support him in sitting position, let him lean forward to balance himself Put him in an open box and tilt gently
Suggested toys				
	Nursery mobiles Unbreakable mirrors See-through crib bumpers Contrasting colored sheets *Tracking tube *Visual panels	Music boxes Musical mobiles Crib dangle bells Small-handled clear rattle *Spin-a-round	Stuffed animals Soft clothes Soft or furry quilt Soft mobiles	Rocking crib/cradle Weighted or suction toy
Suggested activities				
6-9	Give infant large toys with bright colors, movable parts, and noisemakers Infant enjoys mirror, pats it, talks to image Infant enjoys peekaboo, especially hiding his face in a towel Make funny faces to encourage imitation Give infant paper to tear, crumple Give ball of yarn or string to pull apart	Call infant by name Repeat simple words such as "dada," "mama," "bye-bye" Speak clearly Name parts of body, people, and foods Tell him what you are doing Use "no" only when necessary Give simple commands Show how to clap hands, bang a drum	Let infant play with fabrics of various textures Have bowl with foods of different size and textures to feel Let him "catch" running water Encourage "swimming" in large bathtub or shallow pool Give wad of sticky tape to manipulate	Place infant on floor to crawl, roll over, sit Hold upright to bear weight and bounce Pick up, say "up" Put down, say "down" Place toys out of reach; encourage infant to get them Play pat-a-cake

*These toys, from a specially designed series called Playpath Playthings produced as part of the Johnson & Johnson Baby Products Child Development Program, are available for purchase; information can be obtained by writing to Johnson & Johnson, Grandview Rd., Skillman, NJ 08558.

Continued.

Table 12-2 Play during infancy—cont'd

AGE (MONTHS)	VISUAL STIMULATION	AUDITORY STIMULATION	TACTILE STIMULATION	KINETIC STIMULATION
9-12	Show infant large pictures in books Take him to places where there are animals, many people, different objects (shopping center) Play ball by rolling it to child, demonstrate "throwing" it back Demonstrate building a two-block tower	Read infant simple nursery rhymes Point to body parts and name each one Imitate sounds of animals	Give infant finger foods of different textures Let infant mess and squash food Let him feel cold (ice cube) or warm objects, say what temperature each is Let him feel a breeze (fan blowing)	Give large push-pull toys to encourage walking Place furniture in a circle to encourage cruising Encourage "roughhouse" play, turn in different positions
Suggested toys	Various colored blocks Nested boxes or cups Books with rhymes and bright pictures Strings of big beads and snap beads Simple take-apart toys Large ball Cup and spoon *Fitting forms Large puzzles	Rattles of different sizes, shapes, tones, and bright colors Squeaky animals and dolls Records with light, rhythmic music *Balls in a bowl	Soft, different textured animals and dolls Sponge toys, floating toys Squeeze toys Teething toys Books with textures and objects, such as fur and zipper	Push-pull toys Baby swing

*These toys, from a specially designed series called Playpath Playthings produced as part of the Johnson & Johnson Baby Products Child Development Program, are available for purchase; information can be obtained by writing to Johnson & Johnson, Grandview Rd., Skillman, NJ 08558.

Table 12-2 lists play activities that are appropriate for the developmental level of the infant in view of motor, language, and personal-social achievements. Although the activities are grouped according to the major mode of stimulation provided, there is overlap in many instances. In addition, play activities suggested for one age group may be appropriate for older infants but inappropriate for younger infants.

TEMPERAMENT

The infant's temperament or behavioral style influences the kind of interaction that occurs between the child and parents, and other family members (see general discussion of Temperament on p. 110 and Questions and controversies). In assessing a child's temperament, it is the parents' perception of the child and the degree of *fit* between their expectations and the child's actual temperament that is important. The more dissonance or lack of harmony between the child's temperament and the parent's ability to accept and deal with the behavior, the more risk for subsequent parent-child conflicts.

The Infant Temperament Questionnaire (ITQ) (Carey and McDevitt, 1978) can be used as a screening tool with parents. The questionnaire focuses on nine temperament variables, but the questions relate specifically to activities such as sleep, feeding, play, diapering, and dressing. The scores from the ITQ help identify the child's temperamental style. Use of the ITQ is well accepted by parents and should be accompanied by an adequate explanation of the results (Little, 1983, 1985). In discussing the results it is best to avoid terms such as "difficult" and describe the child's temperament in terms of characteristics, such as intense or irregular.

With knowledge of the infant's temperament, nurses are better able to (1) provide parents with background information that will help them see their child in a better perspective, (2) offer a more organized picture of their child's behavior and possibly reveal distortions in their perceptions of the behavior, and (3) guide parents regarding appropriate childrearing techniques (Blosser, 1979; Carey, 1981; Chess and Thomas, 1985.)

Childrearing Practices Related to Temperament

Most parents realize that their infant is born with unique characteristics, and few parents of difficult infants need to be told of the challenge of caring for them. However, very few parents are aware of the significance of the temperamental characteristics and of constructive approaches to dealing with them. The following are examples of interventions that promote more positive parenting of infants with different temperament styles.

"Difficult" children may respond better to scheduled feedings and structured care-giving routines than demand feedings and frequent changes in daily routines. These children sleep less and may need more structured approaches to bedtime to prevent bedtime problems. "Highly distractible children" may require additional soothing measures such as swinging, rocking, or being carried in a pack that the parent wears across the chest or back. Children with "high activ-

ity" levels require vigilant watching, and parents need to take extra precautions in safeguarding the home. These children benefit from increased opportunities for gross motor activity to constructively channel their energy.

The child who is "slow to warm up" may demonstrate more stranger fear than other children and may require more gradual and frequent preparation for new situations, such as substitute mother care. Even the "easy child" can present problems in that the parents may need reminders to feed the child who sleeps for prolonged intervals and rarely signals needs by crying. They may have to "retrain" the child because of the ease of developing troublesome habits, such as keeping the child up late or allowing frequent television watching.

Appropriate counseling based on awareness of the child's temperament can greatly enhance the quality of interaction between parents and infant. Even just letting parents know that "difficult" traits are innate can greatly relieve feelings of guilt and incompetence.

SUMMARY OF GROWTH AND DEVELOPMENT DURING INFANCY

Knowledge of the developmental sequence allows the nurse to assess normal growth and minor or abnormal deviations, helps parents gain realistic expectations of their child's ability, and provides guidelines for suitable play and stimulation. Several studies document that parents lack knowledge of child growth and development, are apt to set inappropriate behavioral expectations for their children, and desire information about developmental landmarks (Shea and Fowler, 1983; Kliman and Vukelich, 1985). Emphasizing the child's *developmental age* rather than chronologic age strengthens the parent-child relationship by fostering trust and lessening frustration. Therefore, the importance of a thorough understanding and appreciation of the growth and development of children cannot be overemphasized.

Because of the complexity of the developmental process during the first 12 months, Table 12-3 is presented to help organize and clarify the data already discussed. Although all milestones are important, some represent essential integrative aspects of development that lay the foundation for the achievement of more advanced skills. These essential milestones are designated by a bullet (●) in the chart. The table represents the *average* monthly age at which various skills are attained. It must be remembered that although the sequence is the same, the rate will vary among children.

COPING WITH CONCERNS RELATED TO NORMAL GROWTH AND DEVELOPMENT

New parents, and some who are experienced, have many concerns about childrearing during the first year. Fears, day care, discipline, thumb or pacifier sucking, and teething are just a sampling of topics that parents have questions about.

Text continued on p. 516.

Questions and Controversies

What effect does infant temperament have on parenting?

Although the importance of temperament is generally acknowledged, its influence on parenting is less clear. Numerous studies have sought to establish the influence of infant temperament on the family, but much of the results are confounded by the use of different measurement scales and other variables. However, there is evidence that infant temperament does affect parenting, at least in terms of parents' perception of their parenting role.

An "easy" child is apt to make parents feel more thankful and content in their parenting role, whereas a less soothable, more fussy infant may cause parents to be depressed and anxious (Ventura, 1982). Infants who are less predictable in their behavior, such as sleeping, feeding, and general satisfaction, cause parents to feel less competent and to experience less ease in transition to parenthood (Roberts, 1983). Mothers have been noted to react less and be less responsive to infants who demonstrate "difficult" behavior (Campbell, 1979). Mothers, especially of first-born children, report having major concerns regarding the behavior of "difficult" infants and of having to make large family adjustments because of their infants (Kronstadt and others, 1979).

Infants with "difficult" temperament also tend to have more colic, injuries, and night waking (Carey, 1972, 1974). These children sleep about 2 hours less a night and 1 hour less during the day than the "easy" child (Weissbluth, 1981). Exactly what effect these variables have on parenting is unclear, but it is not unlikely for parents to feel overwhelmed by the increased incidence of problems such as colic and night waking.

Table 12-3 Summary of growth and development during infancy

AGE (MONTHS)	PHYSICAL	GROSS MOTOR	FINE MOTOR
1	Weight gain of 150 to 210 g (5 to 7 oz) weekly for first 6 months Height gain of 2.5 cm (1 in) monthly for first 6 months Head circumference increases by 1.5 cm (½ in) monthly for first 6 months Primitive reflexes present and strong Doll's eye reflex and dance reflex fading Obligatory nose breathing (in most infants)	●Assumes flexed position with pelvis high but knees not under abdomen when prone (at birth, knees flexed under abdomen) ●Can turn head from side to side when prone, lifts head momentarily from bed (Fig. 12-7, A) Marked head lag, especially when pulled from lying to sitting position (Fig. 12-6, A) Holds head momentarily parallel and in midline when suspended in prone position Assumes asymmetric tonic neck reflex position when supine Makes crawling movements when prone When held in standing position, body limp at knees and hips In sitting position back is uniformly rounded, absence of head control (Fig. 12-8, A)	Hands predominantly closed Grasp reflex strong Hand clenches on contact with rattle
2	Posterior fontanel closed Crawling reflex disappears	●Assumes less flexed position when prone—hips flat, legs extended, arms flexed, head to side Less head lag when pulled to sitting position (Fig. 12-6, B) Can maintain head in some plane as rest of body when held in ventral suspension When prone, can lift head almost 45 degrees off table When held in sitting position, head is held up but bobs forward (Fig. 12-8, B) Assumes asymmetric tonic neck reflex position intermittently	Hands frequently open Grasp reflex fading
3	Primitive reflexes fading	Able to hold head more erect when sitting, but still bobs forward Only slight head lag when pulled to sitting Assumes symmetric body positioning Able to raise head and shoulders from prone position to a 45- to 90-degree angle from table; bears weight on forearms When held in standing position, able to bear slight fraction of weight on legs Regards own hand	●Actively holds rattle but will not reach for it Grasp reflex absent Hands kept loosely open Clutches own hand, pulls at blankets and clothes
4	Drooling begins Moro, tonic neck, rooting, and Perez reflexes have disappeared	●Almost no head lag when pulled to sitting position (Fig. 12-6, C) *Balances head well in sitting position (Fig. 12-8, C) Back less rounded, curved only in lumbar area Able to sit erect if propped up Able to raise head and chest off couch to angle of 90 degrees (Fig. 12-7, B) Assumes predominant symmetric position Rolls from back to side	●Inspects and plays with hands, pulls clothing or blanket over face in play Tries to reach objects with hand but overshoots Grasps object with both hands Plays with rattle placed in hand, shakes it, but cannot pick it up if dropped Can carry objects to mouth
5	Growth rate may begin to decline Beginning signs of tooth eruption	No head lag when pulled to sitting position When sitting, able to hold head erect and steady Able to sit for longer periods when back is well supported Back straight When prone, assumes symmetric positioning with arms extended When held in standing position, able to bear most of weight Can turn over from abdomen to back When supine, puts feet to mouth	●Able to grasp objects voluntarily Uses palmar grasp, bidextrous approach Plays with toes Takes objects directly to mouth Holds one cube while regarding a second

●Milestone that represents essential integrative aspects of development that lay the foundation for the achievement of more advanced skills.

SENSORY	VOCALIZATION	SOCIALIZATION
• Able to fixate on moving object Follows light to midline Quiets when hears a voice	Cries to express displeasure Makes small throaty sounds Makes comfort sounds during feeding	Watches parent's face intently as she or he talks to infant
Binocular fixation and convergence to near objects beginning When supine, follows dangling toy from side to point beyond midline Visually searches to locate sounds Turns head to side when sound is made at level of ear	• Vocalizes, distinct from crying Crying becomes differentiated Coos Vocalizes to familiar voice	• Social smile in response to various stimuli
• Follows object to periphery (180 degrees) • Locates sound by turning head to side and looking in same direction (Fig. 12-2) Begins to have ability to coordinate stimuli from various sense organs	• Squeals aloud to show pleasure Coos, babbles, chuckles Vocalizes when smiling "Talks" a great deal when spoken to Less crying during periods of wakefulness	Much interest in surroundings Ceases crying when parent enters room Can recognize familiar faces and objects, such as feeding bottle Shows awareness of strange situations
Able to accommodate to near objects Binocular vision fairly will established Can focus on a 1.25 cm (½-in) block Beginning eye-hand coordination	Makes consonant sounds n, k, g, p, b Laughs aloud Vocalization changes according to mood	Demands attention by fussing; becomes bored if left alone Enjoys social interaction with people Anticipates feeding when sees bottle Shows excitement with whole body, squeals, breathes heavy Shows interest in strange stimuli
Visually pursues a dropped object Able to sustain visual inspection of an object Can localize sounds made below the ear	• Squeals Vowel cooing sounds interspersed with consonant sounds (for example, ah-goo)	Smiles at mirror image Pats bottle with both hands More enthusiastically playful, but may have rapid mood swings Able to discriminate strangers from family Vocalizes displeasure when object taken away

Continued.

Table 12-3 Summary of growth and development during infancy—cont'd

AGE (MONTHS)	PHYSICAL	GROSS MOTOR	FINE MOTOR
6	Birth weight doubled Weight gain of 90 to 150 g (3 to 5 oz) weekly for next 6 months Height gain of 1.25 cm (½ in) monthly for next 6 months Teething may begin with eruption of two lower central incisors ●Chewing and biting occur	When prone, can lift chest and upper abdomen off table, bearing weight on hands (Fig. 12-7, C) When about to be pulled to a sitting position, lifts head Sits in high chair with back straight Rolls from back to abdomen When held in standing position, bears almost all of weight Hand regard absent	Resecures a dropped object Drops one cube when another is given Grasps and manipulates small objects Holds bottle Grasps feet and pulls to mouth
7	Eruption of upper central incisors	●When supine, spontaneously lifts head off table ●Sits, leaning forward on both hands (Fig. 12-8, D) When prone, bears weight on one hand Sits erect momentarily Bears full weight on feet (Fig. 12-9, A) When held in standing position, bounces actively	●Transfers objects from one hand to the other (Fig. 12-8, E) Unidextrous approach and grasp Holds two cubes more than momentarily Bangs cube on table Rakes at a small object
8	Begins to show regular patterns in bladder and bowel elimination Parachute reflex appears (Fig. 12-1)	●Sits steadily unsupported (Fig. 12-8, E) Readily bears weight on legs when supported, may stand holding on to furniture Adjusts posture to reach an object	Beginning pincer grasp using the index, fourth, and fifth fingers against the lower part of the thumb Releases objects at will Rings bell purposely Retains two cubes while regarding the third cube Secures an object by pulling on a string Reaches persistently for toys out of reach
9	Eruption of upper lateral incisor may begin	Crawls, may progress backward at first Sits steadily on floor for prolonged time (10 minutes) Recovers balance when leans forward but cannot do so when leaning sideways Pulls self to standing position and stands holding onto furniture (Fig. 12-9, B, C, D)	●Ability to use thumb and index finger in crude pincer grasp (Fig. 12-4) Preference for use of dominant hand now evident Grasps third cube Compares two cubes by bringing them together
10	Labyrinth-righting reflex is strongest	Crawls by pulling self forward with hands (Fig. 12-9, F) Can change from prone to sitting position Pulls self to sitting position Stands while holding onto furniture, sits by falling down Recovers balance easily while sitting While standing, lifts one foot to take a step (Fig. 12-9, E)	Crude release of an object beginning Grasps bell by handle

●Milestone that represents essential integrative aspects of development that lay the foundation for the achievement of more advanced skills.

SENSORY	VOCALIZATION	SOCIALIZATION
Adjusts posture to see an object Prefers more complex visual stimuli Can localize sounds made above the ear Will turn head to the side, then look up or down	●Begins to imitate sounds ●Babbling resembles one-syllable utterances—ma, mu, da, di, hi Vocalizes to toys, mirror image Laughs aloud Takes pleasure in hearing own sounds (self-reinforcement)	Recognizes parents; begins to fear strangers Holds arms out to be picked up Has definite likes and dislikes Beginning of imitation (cough, protrusion of tongue) Excites on hearing footsteps Laughs when head is hidden in a towel Briefly searches for a dropped object (object permanence beginning) Frequent mood swings—from crying to laughing with little or no provocation
●Can fixate on very small objects Responds to own name Localizes sound by turning head in a curving arch Beginning awareness of depth and space Has taste preferences	●Produces vowel sounds and chained syllables—baba, dada, kaka Vocalizes four distinct vowel sounds "Talks" when others are talking	●Increasing fear of strangers; shows signs of fretfulness when mother disappears Imitates simple acts and noises Tries to attract attention by coughing or snorting Plays peekaboo Demonstrates dislike of food by keeping lips closed Exhibits oral aggressiveness in biting and mouthing Demonstrates expectation in response to repetition of stimuli
	Makes consonant sounds t, d, and w Listens selectively to familiar words Utterances signal emphasis and emotion Combines syllables, such as dada, but does not ascribe meaning to them	Increasing anxiety over loss of parent, particularly mother, and fear of strangers Responds to word "no" Dislikes dressing, diaper change
Localizes sounds by turning head diagonally and directly toward sound Depth perception increasing	Responds to simple verbal commands Comprehends "no-no"	Parent (mother) is increasingly important for own sake Increasing interest in pleasing mother Begins to show fears of going to bed and being left alone Puts arms in front of face to avoid having it washed
	●Says dada, mama with meaning Comprehends "bye-bye" May say one word (for example, hi, bye, what, no)	Inhibits behavior to verbal command of "no-no" or own name Imitates facial expressions, waves bye-bye Extends toy to another person but will not release it Looks around a corner or under a pillow for an object Repeats actions that attract attention and cause laughter Pulls clothes of another to attract attention Plays interactive games such as pat-a-cake Reacts to adult anger, cries when scolded Demonstrates independence in dressing, feeding, locomotive skills, and testing of parents Looks at and follows pictures in a book

Continued.

Table 12-3 Summary of growth and development during infancy—cont'd

AGE (MONTHS)	PHYSICAL	GROSS MOTOR	FINE MOTOR
11	Eruption of lower lateral incisors may begin	•Creeps with abdomen off floor (Fig. 12-9, G) When sitting, pivots to reach toward back to pick up an object Cruises or walks holding onto furniture or with both hands held	Can hold crayon to make a mark on paper Explores objects more thoroughly (for example, clapper inside bell) Neat pincer grasp (Fig. 12-5) Drops object deliberately for it to be picked up Puts one object after another into a container (sequential play) Able to manipulate an object to remove it from tight-fitting enclosure
12	Birth weight tripled Birth length increased by 50% Head and chest circumference equal (head circumference 46.5 cm [18½ in]) Has total of six to eight deciduous teeth Anterior fontanel almost closed Landau reflex fading Babinski reflex disappears Lumbar curve develops, lordosis evident during walking	Walks with one hand held Cruises well May attempt to stand alone momentarily Can sit down from standing position without help	Releases cube in cup Attempts to build two-block tower but fails Tries to insert a pellet into a narrow-neck bottle but fails Can turn pages in a book, many at a time

•Milestone that represents essential integrative aspects of development that lay the foundation for the achievement of more advanced skills.

Nurses must be aware of these concerns and provide answers that give guidance and help decrease anxiety.

Fears

During infancy a number of fears can appear. Some of these are innate, such as fear of loud noises, which elicits a startle reflex in young infants. Overstimulation may be frightening, such as sudden moves, fast-approaching objects, and intense sounds (including excited conversation). As in any other age group, acquired fears can develop in response to some traumatic or frightening event. However, the fear that causes parents most concern is fear related to strangers and separation.

Although erroneously interpreted by some as a sign of undesirable, antisocial behavior, stranger fear and separation anxiety are important components of a strong, healthy parent-child attachment. However, this period can present difficulties for parent and child. Parents may be more confined to the home because baby-sitters are violently protested by the infant. To accustom the infant to new people, parents are encouraged to have close friends or relatives visit often. This provides for other persons with whom the child is comfortable and who can give parents time for themselves.

Infants also need opportunities to safely experience strangers. Usually toward the end of the first year infants begin to venture away from the parent and demonstrate curiosity about strangers. If allowed to explore at their own rate, many infants will eventually "warm up." If parents hold the child away from their face, the infant can observe while maintaining close physical contact. The best approach for the stranger (who may be the nurse) is to talk to the parent, maintain a safe distance from the infant, and avoid gestures, such as holding the arms out and smiling broadly.

Parents also may wonder whether they should encourage the child's clinging, dependent behavior, especially if there is pressure from others who view this as "spoiling" (see Questions and controversies). Parents need to be reassured

SENSORY	VOCALIZATION	SOCIALIZATION
	Imitates definite speech sounds Uses jargon	Experiences joy and satisfaction when a task is mastered Reacts to restrictions with frustration Rolls ball to another on request Anticipates body gestures when a familiar nursery rhyme or story is being told (for example, holds toes and feet in response to "This little piggy went to market") Plays game up-down, "so big," or peekaboo Shakes head for "no"
Discriminates simple geometric forms (for example, circle) Amblyopia may develop with lack of binocularity Can follow rapidly moving object Controls and adjusts response to sound; listens for sound to recur	●Says two or more words besides dada, mama Comprehends meaning of several words (comprehension always precedes verbalization) Recognizes objects by name Imitates animal sounds Understands simple verbal commands (for example, "Give it to me," "Show me your eyes")	Shows emotions such as jealousy, affection (may give hug or kiss on request), anger, fear Enjoys familiar surroundings and explores away from mother Fearful in strange situation, clings to mother May develop habit of "security blanket" or favorite toy Uncreasing determination to practice locomotor skills

Questions and Controversies

Does fostering attachment behaviors lead to "spoiling" the child?

A common concern of parents is that too much attention can "spoil" a child. However, many of the recommendations for promoting attachment, such as attending to the infant's needs to establish trust, accepting fear of strangers and separation from parent, and holding and rocking the crying child, are described by parents as methods of spoiling (Wilson, Witzke, and Volin, 1981). Parents also contend that spoiled children are "difficult to control, demanding, and obnoxious" rather than "happy, alert, sociable, or content." Unfortunately, research is lacking to document whether "spoiled" infants are actually demonstrating temperamental characteristics or behaviors encouraged by well-meaning but indulgent parents.

Research on parents' response to crying during early infancy does not support the contention that "picking up a crying baby" leads to spoiling. Ainsworth (1982) found that the amount an infant cried during the first 3 months had no correlation with the frequency of crying during the rest of the first year. However, the degree of maternal responsiveness to crying did. Mothers who were less responsive, such as not picking up the infant immediately on crying, had infants who cried *more* than mothers who responded promptly to crying. The infants who cried less also demonstrated less separation anxiety. It is postulated that responding to crying fosters infants' trust and expectations that the mother will be responsive. Consequently, these infants are more secure in their attachment to their mothers.

Obviously, parental concern for spoiling can affect the type of responses toward infants and needs to be considered when counseling parents. It is necessary to investigate the parents' definition of "spoiling" and how the parents deal with behaviors, such as fear of strangers (Nelms, 1983). Future research regarding the temperamental characteristics of infants labeled as "spoiled" may help clarify the origin of the behaviors (innate vs acquired). Also, parents' perception of "giving into the child" may need to be balanced with appropriate limit setting toward the end of the first year.

that such behavior is healthy, desirable, and necessary for the child's optimum emotional development. If parents can reassure the infant of their presence, the infant will learn to realize that they are still there even if not physically present. Talking to infants when leaving the room, allowing them to hear one's voice on the telephone, and using transitional objects, such as a favorite blanket or "mommy's purse," reassures them of the parent's continued presence.

This is a no less trying but necessary time for infants, because parents cannot always be with the child. An excellent example of necessary separation is bedtime. Fear of going to bed or being left alone in the dark commonly occurs during the second half of the first year. Fear at bedtime is only one of the many bedtime problems that can occur in young children, and is discussed on p. 647.

Daycare

For many parents, especially working mothers, the need for locating safe and competent daycare facilities for the infant is an increasingly difficult problem—one that is compounded by the number of women with children working outside the home. Over the past 25 years there has been a marked shift in child care arrangements, with fewer children cared for at home and more children cared for in group centers or other settings.

Types of child care. The basic types of care are in-home care, either in the parent's or caregiver's home, and center-based care, usually in a daycare center. In-home care may consist of a full-time baby-sitter who lives in the home, a full-time baby-sitter who comes to the home, cooperative arrangements such as exchange baby-sitting, and family daycare. A family daycare home typically provides care and protection for up to five children for part of a 24-hour day and does not include informal arrangements such as exchange baby-sitting or caregivers in the child's own home. The five children include the family daycare parents' own children younger than 5 years of age living in the home.

Center-based care usually refers to a daycare facility that provides care for six or more children, for 6 or more hours in a 24-hour day. Work-based group care is another option that is becoming increasingly popular as employers recognize the benefit of quality and convenient child care to their employees (Chabin, 1983).

Nurses have an important role in providing guidance to parents in selecting suitable, well-qualified facilities or individuals to care for their child. The decision to leave an infant in another's care often engenders doubt and guilt in the parent, despite reassurance that the provision of competent, loving care by someone other than the parent is not detrimental to the child's future development (see p. 92). Therefore any assistance is often appreciated.

Guidelines for selecting daycare facilities are discussed in Chapter 15. The same conscientious attention should be applied to locating competent baby-sitters. References from other employers are essential, and there is no substitute for observing the interaction between the individual and the child. Although very young infants need little if any preparation for the introduction of a new caregiver, older infants may benefit from a gradual placement to reduce stranger fear. At all times the parent should have the right to visit the child, and regular conferences should be established to review the child's progress. The American Academy of Pediatrics (1984a) also recommends that health professionals expand their role to include establishing a system for exchanging information about the child with the daycare provider as well as with the parent.

Limit-Setting and Discipline

As infants' motor skills advance and mobility increases, parents are faced with the need to set safe limits (see discussion of nurse's role in injury prevention on p. 540). Although there are numerous disciplinary techniques, some are more appropriate for this age than others. Parents can begin discipline using a negative voice and stern eye-to-eye contact. When more definitive measures must be used, one of the most effective approaches is time-out. The basic principles are the same as those discussed in Chapter 14, except the place for time-out needs to be commensurate with the child's abilities. For example, the playpen is better for most infants than a chair. Although corporal punishment is not recommended, at times *one* slap on the hand or buttocks may be effective in conveying the message that a behavior is unacceptable, especially when time-out is impractical or the child insists on performing a dangerous activity. Although parents may be concerned with instituting discipline during infancy, it is important to stress that the earlier effective disciplinary methods are employed, the easier it is to continue these approaches.

Thumb-Sucking and Use of Pacifier

Sucking is the infant's chief pleasure, and it may not be satisfied by breast- or bottle-feeding. It is such a strong need that infants who are deprived of sucking, such as those with a cleft lip repair, will suck on their tongue. Some newborns are born with sucking pads on their fingers from in utero sucking activity. Several benefits of nonnutritive sucking have been documented, such as increased weight gain in premature infants and decreased crying (Anderson, 1986).

Problems arise when parents are concerned about sucking of fingers, thumb, or pacifier and attempt to restrain this natural tendency. Before giving advice, nurses should investigate the parents' feelings and base guidance on this information. For example, some parents may see no problem with the use of a pacifier but may find the use of a finger repulsive.

In general, there is no need to restrain either. Malocclusion may occur if thumb sucking persists past 4 years of age or when the permanent teeth erupt. There is probably less dental displacement with the use of pacifier than with the use of a hard, rigid finger. Pacifiers may be relinquished earlier than thumbs because they are less readily available. The effect of continual use of a pacifier on early speech and language development is unknown, but it is possible that the pacifier may decrease the child's desire to imitate sounds and affect intelligibility. Parents need to be alerted that continual dependency on a pacifier may influence speech development (Merrifield and Ryberg, 1985). If the child uses a pacifier, safety considerations in purchasing one must be stressed (see p. 534).

To decrease dependence on nonnutritive sucking, sucking pleasure can be increased by prolonging feeding time. A small-holed, firm nipple causes stronger sucking and slower feeding. Also the parent's excessive use of the pacifier to calm the child should be explored. It is not unusual for parents to place a pacifier in the infant's mouth as soon as crying begins, thus reinforcing a pattern of distress-relief.

Thumb-sucking reaches its peak at ages 18 to 20 months and is most prevalent when the child is hungry or tired. Persistent thumb-sucking in a listless, apathetic child always warrants investigation. It may be a sign of an emotional problem between parent and child or of boredom, isolation, and lack of stimulation.

Teething

One of the more difficult periods in the infant's (and parents') life is the eruption of the deciduous (primary) teeth, often referred to as teething. The age of tooth eruption shows considerable variation among children, but the order of their appearance is fairly regular and predictable (Fig. 12-14). The first primary teeth to erupt are the lower central incisors, which appear at approximately 6 to 8 months of age. These are followed closely by the upper central incisors. A quick guide to assessment of deciduous teeth during the first 2 years is: *age of the child in months − 6 = number of teeth.*

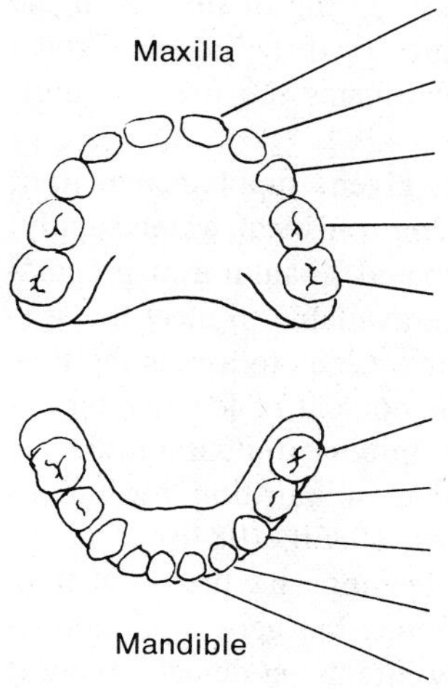

	Average age of eruption (mo)	Average age of shedding (yr)
	9.6	7.5
	12.4	8
	18.3	11.5
	15.7	10.5
	26.2	10.5
	26.0	11
	15.1	10
	18.2	9.5
	11.5	7
	7.8	6

Fig. 12-14. Sequence of eruption and shedding of primary teeth.

The exact mechanisms responsible for the eruption of teeth are not fully understood. The growth of the root, dentin, and pulp of the tooth, the pressure exerted against the periodontal tissue, and hormonal control of pituitary growth hormone and thyroid hormone are some of the theories under investigation.

Teething is a physiologic process, and as the crown of the tooth breaks through the periodontal membrane, some discomfort may be experienced. Some children show minimum evidence of teething, such as drooling, increased finger-sucking, or biting on hard objects. Others are very irritable, have difficulty sleeping, and refuse to eat. Generally signs of illness such as fever, vomiting, or diarrhea are not symptoms of teething but of illness. Continued irritability may be a clue to disturbances other than teething and warrants further investigation.

Inasmuch as teething pain is a result of inflammation, cold is soothing. Giving the child a cold metal spoon, a frozen teething ring, or an ice cube wrapped in a washcloth helps relieve the inflammation. Several nonprescription topical analgesics are available, such as Anbesol or Baby Ora-Jel. The active ingredient in most of them is benzocaine. If these are used, parents are advised to apply them correctly.

In the event of persistent irritability that affects sleeping and feeding, systemic analgesics, preferably nonaspirin compounds such as acetaminophen, can be given judiciously. Parents should know that this is a temporary measure. The use of teething powders or procedures such as cutting or rubbing the gums with aspirin are discouraged, because ingestion of the powder, infection or irritation of the tissue, or aspiration of the aspirin can occur.

Infant Shoes

Many parents are unaware of the type of shoes that are appropriate for the older infant and buy expensive infant shoes because of misleading advertising claims. Inflexible shoes that have hard soles can be detrimental by delaying walking, aggravating intoeing and outtoeing, and impeding the development of supportive foot muscles. Therefore counseling parents regarding footwear should begin when the infant is 5 to 6 months old (Weiss and others, 1981).

It is helpful to begin by explaining to parents that changes in the feet occur during infancy and early childhood as locomotion and weight bearing progress. At birth the feet are flat because the arches are protected by fat pads on the soles of the feet. As the bones in the arches develop, the pads disappear and the feet begin to assume a mature shape. A normal arch is determined by proper alignment of all the bones and development of the surrounding musculature, not by the height of the arch.

When children begin walking, the main reason for shoes is *protection*. To provide protection, the shoe should retain its fit, be made of durable material with a smooth interior and few construction seams to irritate the skin, and be soft and flexible, especially in the toe area. The sole should be approximately 0.6 cm (¼-inch) thick and may have a 0.6 to

0.9 cm (¼- to ⅜-inch) heel. A high-top shoe is not necessary for support but may be helpful in keeping the foot in the shoe.

The shape of the shoe should conform to the anatomic shape of the foot. In particular, the toe area should be rounded and have sufficient room. When bearing weight, there should be at least the space of half the width of the thumbnail, or 1.25 cm (½ inch), between the end of the longest toe and the shoe. Socks should also be roomy and square-toed to allow for proper growth and alignment. Inexpensive but well-constructed sneakers or soft-leather moccasin-type shoes are suggested as adequate footgear for walking infants (Weiss and others, 1981).

Even if the shoes are fitted properly, frequent changes are needed to accommodate the infant's rapidly growing feet. Shoe size changes at approximately 3-month intervals during the first year and a half; during this time the child's foot should be measured every 2 months (Wenger, 1983). Curled toes when shoes are removed and redness and irritation of the skin on the bottom of the toes indicate the need for a larger size.

Promoting Optimum Health During Infancy

The infant's first year is a time of monumental change and achievement, and the rapidity of the changes can easily overwhelm parents. Each month and phase of development have implications for care of the child. Health promotion during this time involves nutritional guidance, appropriate sleep and activity, proper dental care, prevention of disease through immunization, and provision of a safe environment.

NUTRITION

Ideally, discussion of optimum nutrition should begin prenatally with the decision to breast- or bottle-feed the infant. The choice for either is highly individual, and is discussed in Chapter 8. This section is primarily concerned with infant nutrition during the next 12 months, when growth needs and developmental milestones ready the child for introduction of solid foods. Frequently the nurse is asked when to begin feeding solid foods, how to introduce new foods, and what foods are best. A thorough understanding of each of these areas prepares the nurse to answer these questions so that the nutritional needs of each child are met.

Infant Feeding

A great deal of controversy has existed regarding infant feeding and the need for solid foods. Before 1920 solid foods were seldom offered until 1 year of age. Yet, after that time there was a trend to add solid foods at increasingly earlier ages. However, clinical studies have not offered substantial proof of superior nutritional states over breast milk, commerically prepared formula, or modified cow's milk

when solids are fed to infants younger than 4 months of age. Except for deficiencies in some types of infant formulas, there is little need to supplement additional foods for the first several months. There may, however, be some hazards to introducing foods too early, although nutritional research is still not complete.

The first 6 months. Human milk is the most desirable complete diet for the infant for the first 6 months. The normal infant receiving breast milk from a well-nourished mother needs no specific vitamin and mineral supplements, with the exceptions of fluoride in a dose of 0.25 mg daily (regardless of the fluoride content of the local water supply) and iron by 6 months of age (when fetal iron stores are depleted). Supplements of 400 IU of vitamin D daily may be indicated if the mother's vitamin D intake is inadequate or if the infant does not benefit from adequate ultraviolet light because of dark skin color or little exposure to light (American Academy of Pediatrics, 1980a).

Employed mothers can continue breast-feeding with guidance and encouragement. Most mothers find that a program of breast-pumping when away from home and bottle-feeding of breast milk, with or without supplemental formula feedings, is successful. Milk can be expressed by hand or pump and safely stored at room temperature for up to 6 hours (Pittard and others, 1985). After that time refrigeration is required, and freezing is suggested for storing milk longer than 24 hours (Ballard, 1983). However, in addition to efficient breast-pumping, these mothers also cite the need for child care by a trusted agency or individual and support and assistance from significant others (MacLaughlin and Strelnick, 1984; Reifsnider and Myers, 1985). Like all breast-feeding mothers, these women must have proper nutrition and rest for lactation. With a schedule of work and child care, careful planning is required to successfully manage the demands of both responsibilities.

An acceptable alternative to breast-feeding is commercial iron-fortified formula. Like human milk, it supplies all the nutrients needed by the infant for the first 6 months. The only supplementation required is 0.25 mg of fluoride if the local water supply is not fluoridated or if the infant is given ready-to-feed formula, which eliminates the use of fluoridated tap water.

If evaporated milk formula is given, supplemental iron, vitamin C, and fluoride (depending on local water supply) are required. Commercially prepared vitamin/iron preparations with or without fluoride are available to meet the specific needs of the infant. The nurse needs to assess the type of formula given and the fluoride content of local water before advising the parent. Low-fat milk or imitation milks are not acceptable as a major source of nutrition for infants (American Academy of Pediatrics, 1983b, 1984b).

The amount of formula per feeding, and the number of feedings per day vary among infants, but general guidelines are given in Table 12-4. Usually infants on demand feeding determine their own feeding schedule, but some infants, especially those with "easy" temperaments, may need a more

Table 12-4　Volume of formula per feeding and number of feedings per day*

AGE IN MONTHS (MIDPOINT)	FORMULA VOLUME PER FEEDING		FEEDINGS PER DAY
	(ML)	(OZ)	
1	126	4.1	6
2	142	4.6	5
3	161	5.2	5
4	168	5.4	5
5	191	6.2	4
6	179	5.8	5
7-9	131	4.2	5
10	136	4.4	5
11	125	4.0	5
12	141	4.5	4

Data analysis performed by Alan S. Ryan, Ph.D., 1985, Ross Laboratories, Columbus, Ohio 43216. (Reproduced with permission of Ross Laboratories.)

*Infants fed human milk or a combination of cow's milk, human milk, and formula excluded.

planned schedule based on average feeding patterns to ensure sufficient nutrients.

The addition of solid foods before 5 to 6 months of age is not recommended. Solid foods during the early months are not yet compatible with the ability of the gastrointestinal tract and nutritional needs of the infant. For example, feeding solids to the infant exposes him to food antigens that may produce food protein allergy, because the gastrointestinal tract is still permeable to macromolecules.

Developmentally the infant is not ready for solid food. The extrusion (protrusion) reflex is strong, and often pushes food out of the mouth. The infant may also instinctively suck when given food. Because of his limited range of motor abilities, the infant is unable to deliberately push food away or avoid feeding. Therefore, early introduction of solids can be viewed as a type of forced feeding.

The second 6 months. During the second half of the first year human milk or formula continues to be the primary source of nutrition. If breast-feeding is discontinued, commercial iron-fortified formula should be substituted. Whole cow's milk can be given if the infant is consuming one third of the calories as supplemental foods consisting of a balanced mixture of cereal, vegetables, fruits, and other foods to ensure adequate sources of iron and vitamin C (American Academy of Pediatrics, 1983a). However, a large proportion of infants who receive a diet of solid food and cow's milk do not consume adequate amounts of iron, but excessive amounts of sodium, potassium, chloride, and protein (Montalto, Benson, and Martinez, 1985).

The major change in feeding habits is the addition of solid foods to the infant's diet. Physiologically and developmentally the infant 5 to 6 months of age is in a transition period. By this time the gastrointestinal tract has matured sufficiently to handle more complex nutrients and is less sensitive to potentially allergenic foods. Tooth eruption is beginning and facilitates biting and chewing. The extrusion reflex has disappeared, and swallowing is more coordinated to allow the infant to easily accept solids. Head control is well developed, permitting the infant to sit with support and purposely turn his head away to communicate disinterest in food. Voluntary grasping and improved eye-hand coordination gradually allow the infant to pick up "finger" foods and feed himself. His increasing sense of independence is evident in his desire to hold his own bottle and try to "help" during feeding. The major developmental milestones associated with feeding are listed in the accompanying box.

Selection of Foods

The choice of foods to introduce first is variable but should meet the reasons for feeding, such as supplying nutrients not found in formula or breast milk. Cereal is generally introduced first because of its high iron content (7 mg/3 tablespoons of dry cereal). There are several types of commercially prepared ready-to-serve dry cereals, such as rice, barley, oatmeal, and high-protein cereals, but rice is usually suggested as an initial food because of its easy digestibility and low allergenic potential. Cereal such as Cream of Farina should not be used because infant commercial cereals are a superior source of iron. Some of the commercial baby cereals are combined with fruit. There is little nutritional ben-

---

DEVELOPMENTAL MILESTONES ASSOCIATED WITH FEEDING

Age (months)	Behavior
Birth	Sucking, rooting, and swallowing reflexes
	Feels hunger and indicates desire for food by crying; expresses satiety by falling asleep
	Extrusion reflex is strong
3-4	Extrusion reflex is fading
	Beginning eye-hand coordination
4-5	Can approximate lips to the rim of a cup
5-6	Can use fingers to feed self a cracker
6-7	Chews and bites
	May hold own bottle, but may not drink from it (prefers for it to be held)
7-9	Refuses food by keeping lips closed; has preferences
	Holds a spoon and plays with it during feeding
	May drink from a straw
	Drinks from a cup with assistance
9-12	Picks up small morsels of food (finger foods) and feeds self
	Holds own bottle and drinks from it
	Drinks from a cup but spills some of the contents
	Uses a spoon with much spilling

SUMMARY OF METHOD OF INTRODUCING SOLID FOODS TO INFANTS

1. Introduce solids when infant is hungry.
2. Begin spoon feeding by pushing food to back of tongue because of infant's natural tendency to thrust tongue forward.
3. Use a small spoon with straight handle; begin with 1 or 2 teaspoons of food; gradually increase to a couple of tablespoons per feeding.
4. Introduce one food at a time, usually at intervals of 4 to 7 days to allow for identification of food allergies.
5. As the amount of solid food increases, decrease the quantity of milk to prevent overfeeding.
6. Do not introduce foods by mixing them with formula in the bottle.

efit from this preparation, and it is also more expensive. Inasmuch as all new foods should be added one at a time, mothers should avoid this type of cereal when beginning a new grain.

Cereal is mixed with formula until whole milk is given. If the infant is breast-fed, the cereal is mixed with expressed breast milk or water rather than with cow's milk because the child may be sensitive to cow's milk. If fruit juices have been started, they can be mixed with the dry cereal. The vitamin C content of the juice enhances the absorption of iron in the cereal. Because of their benefit as a source of iron, infant cereals should be continued until the child is 18 months of age.

The addition of other foods is arbitrary. A common sequence is strained fruits followed by vegetables and finally meats. At 6 months foods such as a cracker or zwieback can

Table 12-5 Guidelines for feeding during the first year

AGE	TYPE OF FEEDING	SPECIFIC RECOMMENDATIONS
Birth-6 months	Breast-feeding	Most desirable complete diet for first half of year Requires supplements of flouride (0.25 mg) regardless of the fluoride content of the local water supply, and iron by 6 months of age Requires supplements of vitamin D (400 units) if mother's diet is inadequate or if infant is not exposed to sufficient sunlight
	Formula	Iron-fortified commercial formula is a complete food for the first half of the year Requires fluoride supplements (0.25 mg) when the concentration of fluoride in the drinking water is below 0.3 parts per million (ppm) Evaporated milk formula requires supplements of vitamin C, iron, and fluoride (in accordance with the fluoride content of the local water supply)
6-12 months	Solid foods	May begin to add solids by 5 to 6 months of age; earlier introduction tends to contribute to overfeeding First foods are strained, pureed, or finely mashed "Finger foods" such as teething crackers, raw fruit, or vegetables can be introduced by 6 to 7 months Chopped table food or commercially prepared junior foods can be started by 9 to 12 months With the exception of cereal, the order of introducing foods is variable; a recommended sequence is weekly introduction of other foods, beginning with fruit, followed by vegetables, and then meat Breast-fed infants require more high-protein foods than formula-fed children As the quantity of solids increases, the amount of formula should be limited to approximately 900 ml (30 oz) daily
	Cereal	Introduce commercially prepared iron-fortified infant cereals, and administer daily until 18 months of age Rice cereal is usually introduced first because of its low allergenic potential Can discontinue supplemental iron once cereal is given
	Fruits and vegetables	Applesauce, bananas, and pears are usually well tolerated Avoid fruits and vegetables marketed in cans that are not specifically designed for infants, because of variable and sometimes high lead content and addition of salt, sugar, or preservatives Offer fruit juice only from a cup, not a bottle, to reduce the development of "nursing bottle caries"
	Meat, fish, and poultry	Avoid fatty meats Prepare by baking, broiling, boiling, steaming, or poaching Include organ meats such as liver, which has a high iron, vitamin A, and vitamin B complex content If soup is given, be sure all ingredients are familiar in child's diet
	Eggs and cheese	Serve egg yolk hard boiled and mashed, soft cooked, or poached Introduce egg white in small quantities (1 tsp) toward end of first year to detect any allergic manifestation Use cheese as a substitute for meat and as "finger food"

be offered as a type of finger and teething food. By 8 to 9 months junior foods and nutritious finger foods such as a firmly cooked vegetable, raw pieces of fruit, or cheese can be given. By 1 year well-cooked table foods are served. General guidelines for feeding and introducing solid foods to infants are listed in the box and in Table 12-5.

Food Preparation

Commercially prepared baby foods are the most commonly used types of food served to infants in the United States. They are convenient, contain no added salt or sugar, and are relatively expensive. An alternative is preparing baby foods at home, which is a simple and inexpensive process. Fruits and vegetables can be steamed in a small amount of water and pureed in a blender or food processor. Many of them can be mashed fine with a fork, such as ripe banana. Fruits such as apples or pears require little or no water in the cooking process. Vegetables such as carrots, potatoes, or string beans require additional water in the cooking and blending process.

No water used in cooking should be discarded, because the water-soluble vitamins will be lost. Vitamin C is naturally destroyed by heat; therefore cooked fruits or vegetables do not supply this essential nutrient. Orange juice should not be warmed for this reason. Vitamin C is also destroyed by oxidation and alkaline solutions. Containers used for juice should always be light-resistant, kept covered, and refrigerated to prevent oxidative loss.

Meats can easily be prepared by steaming, boiling, baking, or poaching but not by frying. Meat should be lean, because the infant's ability to handle saturated fats is limited. Meat can be pureed in a blender with liquid, such as leftover vegetable broth or meat broth. Baby food grinders are also available that finely grind small portions of cooked table food. Inasmuch as the food is ground dry, some type of liquid or other pureed ingredient, such as mashed potatoes, squash, carrots, or other vegetable to which the infant has already been introduced, must be added. When chewing is fairly well established, table food can be chopped finely and placed on the high-chair tray for the child to pick up and eat.

Generally any foods served in the home can be given to an infant. However, because the precise relationship between salt intake and high blood pressure has not been established and the safety of "extremes" in children's diets is unknown, it is recommended that salt or sugar be used in moderation in preparing food (American Academy of Pediatrics, 1983b). If sweetening is needed, refined sugar or corn syrup can be used, but honey is avoided because of the risk of infant botulism (Long, 1985). Preferably, foods prepared for the infant should be fresh or frozen, because canned foods other than those prepared for infants may have excessive sodium or sugar or be a source of lead from the container.

Food Storage

Storage of commercial baby food requires a few simple rules. Unopened jars can remain on the shelf indefinitely. Opened jars are refrigerated and can be used for a couple of days. If the infant does not finish a jar of food at one time, a portion of the food is removed from the jar using a clean spoon. If this is not done, bacteria are introduced and the salivary enzymes on the feeding spoon begin to digest unused portions of the food. The dried baby foods (manufactured by Heinz) are prepared in individual portions, thus eliminating storage problems and waste of unused food.

For convenience home-prepared baby foods can be made in advance and frozen in small jars or in special plastic bags that are sealed by heat and can be reheated by placing them in boiling water or a microwave oven. If microwave heating is used, the food is mixed thoroughly and checked to ensure a safe temperature before feeding. Individual portions of food can be frozen in ice cube trays, transferred to a large container, and individually defrosted as needed. With reasonable care in the preparation and storing of foods there is little need to worry about bacterial contamination.

Method of Introduction

When the spoon is first introduced to the infant, the likelihood is that he will push it away and appear dissatisfied. Some patience and skill are required to overcome this initial response. A small-bowled, straight, long-handled spoon, similar to a demitasse spoon, allows a small portion of food to be placed toward the back of the tongue. If food is placed on the front of the tongue, it will be pushed out. It is simply scooped up and refed. As the child becomes accustomed to the spoon, he will more eagerly accept the food and will eventually open his mouth in anticipation (or keep it closed in dislike). Inasmuch as the first introduction of food is a new experience, spoon feeding should be attempted after ingestion of some breast milk or formula to associate this new experience with a pleasurable and satisfying experience. Trying to introduce a food *after* the entire milk feeding is usually useless because the infant is satiated and has no inclination to try something new.

After several spoon feedings, food can be introduced at the beginning of a meal. It is best to introduce many foods during the first year when the infant is more likely to eat them because of a hearty appetite resulting from a rapid growth rate. During the toddler years eating becomes less of an adventure and strong food preferences become evident.

Each new food is introduced alone and at intervals of 4 to 7 days to allow for identification of food allergies. New foods are fed in small amounts, from 1 teaspoon to a few tablespoons. As the amount of solid food increases, the quantity of milk is decreased to less than 1 L daily to prevent overfeeding.

Because feeding is a learning process as well as a means of nutrition, new foods are given alone to allow the child to learn new tastes and textures. Sometimes it is necessary to camouflage a new food by mixing it with another favorite food to encourage the child to try it, although this should not become a routine. Food should not be mixed in the bottle and fed through a nipple with a large hole. This deprives the child of the pleasure of learning new tastes and developing a discriminating palate. It can also cause problems with poor chewing of food later in life because this experience is lacking. A summary of the principles that govern the introduction of new foods is given in the box, p. 522.

Introducing solid foods can be an exciting time for parent and child. Most infants are good eaters and enjoy eating from a spoon and later feeding themselves. However, the transition from "mother doing it" to "baby doing it" can be a trying experience, particularly for those who value a clean house or who view cleaning up the mess as a waste of time. The infant's first, second, and often twentieth try at self-feeding or cup feeding is a sloppy experience. Finger foods such as soft fruits or vegetables are just as good playthings as food; they can be squeezed, smeared, squashed, and thoroughly painted on oneself, others, and the surrounding environment. However, all of this is part of learning, and mastery follows many accidents.

If parents find this experience distressing, a few suggestions may prove helpful. They should designate as a feeding area a section that has a floor that can be easily wiped (not a rug) and is relatively far from walls, upholstered furniture, or drapes. A hand-held portable vacuum is helpful in cleaning up crumbs. Messes are confined to one area if the child is seated in a high chair rather than allowed to crawl or walk around while drinking or eating. The infant should be expected to get himself covered with food; therefore a large bib (plastic can be wiped easily but needs to be removed after feeding) should be used, and washable clothes that are easily removed. Outdoor dining provides an excellent opportunity for practicing with a cup, spoon, or fingers because accidents are simple to hose or sweep away. Children cannot be pressured into eating neatly or developing table manners before manipulative skill is acquired.

If a young child suddenly refuses to eat, the feeding process should be investigated. It is not unusual for an 11-month-old infant to become stubborn, push the spoon away, and refuse to open his mouth. He may not be content with having his own spoon to play with while someone else feeds him; he probably wants to do it himself, even though others can do it so much better. Helping parents understand this may prevent many temper tantrums and power struggles later on.

Weaning

Weaning, the process of giving up one method of feeding for another, usually refers to relinquishing the breast or bottle for a cup. In Western societies this is generally regarded as a major task for infants and is frequently seen as a potentially traumatic experience. It is psychologically significant because the infant is required to give up a major source of oral pleasure and gratification.

There is no one time for weaning that is best for every child, but generally most infants show signs of readiness during the second half of the first year. They have learned that good things come from a spoon. Their increasing desire for freedom of movement may lessen their desire to be held

close for feedings. They are acquiring more control over their actions and can easily manipulate a cup to their lips (even if it is held upside down!). Imitation becomes a powerful motivator by age 8 or 9 months, and they enjoy using a cup or glass like others do. Because most children can approximate the rim of a cup to their lips by 4 or 5 months of age, this is not too early to introduce a cup.

Weaning should be gradual by replacing one bottle- or breast-feeding at a time. The last feeding to be discontinued is usually the nighttime feeding. It is advisable to never begin allowing a child to take a bottle of milk to bed, because this is a major cause of dental caries in deciduous teeth. If breast-feeding must be terminated before 5 or 6 months of age, weaning should be to a bottle to provide for the infant's continued sucking needs. If discontinued later, weaning can be directly to a cup.

Nutritional Counseling

The addition of solid foods during the first year should provide a nutritionally sound diet and teach good eating habits. Often both objectives are influenced by the sociocultural background of the family rather than by knowledge of well-balanced nutrition. Inasmuch as "we are what we eat," nurses have a great responsibility for teaching optimum nutrition as early as possible. Common myths such as "a fat baby is a healthy baby" are difficult to dispel. In some cultures overweight infants are regarded as a sign of good mothering and any suggestion regarding altering the child's weight is threatening to the parent. Because obesity in infancy may predispose the individual to obesity in later life, rectifying this problem as early as possible is essential.

A thorough nutritional history is a prerequisite for counseling. Asking questions such as, "Does your child drink too much milk?" yields little reliable information. Phrasing the question by saying, "Your child certainly looks well nourished (or well fed); how many bottles of milk a day does he drink?" lessens parents' defensiveness and offers an objective number of ounces. (See also Chapter 6 for a discussion of nutritional assessment.)

Frequently the problem of overfeeding stems from the fact that as solid foods are added milk is not decreased. Baby foods contain different caloric contents, and knowing which foods are less fattening can provide satisfactory substitutions without greatly altering feeding habits. Calculating the caloric density of the infant's diet is very important, because commercially strained foods can yield greater or lesser concentrations of calories compared with formula, which yields 67 kcal per dl. About 20% of commercial baby foods yield less than 50 kcal per 100 g, whereas 20% have greater than 100 kcal per 100 g. This is a considerable difference when one considers the total daily calorie consumption from formula or from solid foods. For the child who is underweight, selecting foods with higher caloric density may be beneficial. The caloric and nutritive contents of the food are listed on the package, and parents should be encouraged to do "comparison" shopping for baby foods that add or subtract calories.

SLEEP AND ACTIVITY

Sleep patterns vary among infants, and active infants typically sleep less than placid children. Generally by 3 to 4 months of age most infants have developed a nocturnal pattern of sleep lasting from 8 to 10 hours. The total daily sleep is 13 to 15 hours. The number of naps per day varies, but by the end of the year infants may take one or two naps. Breast-fed infants usually sleep for less prolonged periods, with frequent waking, especially during the night, than do bottle-fed infants. Because of the trend toward breast-feeding, sleep norms such as those described above, which were based primarily on bottle-fed infants, may no longer be relevant (Elias and others, 1986).

Most infants are naturally active and need no encouragement to be mobile. However, problems can arise when devices such as playpens, strollers, commercial swings, and walkers are used excessively. These restrict movement and prevent infants from exploring and developing gross motor skills. Contrary to popular belief, walkers do not enhance coordination and have inherent hazards (Stoffman and others, 1984).

Sleep Disturbances

Concerns regarding sleep are common during infancy. Sometimes they are as basic as parents' questioning the infant's need for additional sleep. In this case it is best to investigate the reason for their concern, stressing the individual needs of each child. Infants who are active during wakeful periods and who are growing normally are sleeping a sufficient amount of time.

However, there are a number of more serious concerns that require intervention. Sleep disturbances caused by organic dysfunction are rare with the exception of colic, which is discussed in Chapter 13. The more common sleep disturbances that are a learned pattern or developmentally characteristic of some infants are summarized in Table 12-6 with suggested management (Ferber, 1984; Schmitt, 1981). Although many families may report sleep problems that are typical of these patterns, interventions should be offered only when the pattern is disruptive to the family. For example, co-sleeping or the "family bed," in which parents allow the children to sleep with them, is a relatively common and accepted practice, especially among black, Hispanic, and Asian families (Lozoff, Wolf, and Davis, 1984).

However, when a sleeping problem is presented, a careful assessment is warranted. Questions regarding the frequency and duration of waking, the usual bedtime routine, the number of nighttime feedings, the perceived problem (e.g., how much disruption does the behavior generate), and the attempted interventions are important in planning effective approaches. A common suggestion to parents is to "let the child cry until falling asleep," but this is very difficult to implement. Once the parents relent and console the child, they have only reinforced the crying. An equally effective but more practical approach is to let the child cry for progressively longer times between *brief* parental interventions that consist only of reassurance, not rocking, holding, or using the bottle or pacifier. For example, the parents may check on the child every 5 minutes during the first night, and progressively extend this interval by 5 minutes on successive nights (Ferber, 1984).

Table 12-6 Sleep disturbances during infancy

DISORDER	DESCRIPTION	MANAGEMENT
Night feeding	Child has a prolonged need for middle-of-night bottle- or breast-feeding Crying occurs nightly, usually after age 4 months	Increase daytime feeding intervals to 4 hours or more (may need to be gradual) Offer last feeding as late as possible at night; may need to gradually reduce amount of formula or duration of breast-feeding Offer no bottles in bed Put to bed *awake* When crying, check at progressively longer intervals each night; reassure child but do not hold, rock, take to own bed, or give bottle or pacifier
Night crying	Child typically falls asleep in place other than own bed, such as on rocking chair or parents' bed, and is brought to own bed while asleep; on awakening, cries until usual routine is instituted, such as rocking Usually over age 4 months	Put child in own bed when *awake* If possible, arrange sleeping area separate from other family members When crying, check at progressively longer intervals each night; reassure child but do not resume usual routine that led to night crying
Developmental night crying/nightmares	Child aged 6-12 months with previously undisturbed nighttime sleep awakes abruptly; may be accompanied by nightmares	Reassure parents that this is temporary phase Enter room immediately to check on child but keep reassurances *brief* Avoid feeding, rocking, taking to own bed, or any other routine that may initiate trained night crying

The best way to prevent sleep problems is to encourage parents to establish bedtime rituals that do not foster problematic patterns. One of the most constructive is placing infants *awake* in their own crib. When infants are accustomed to falling asleep somewhere else, such as their parent's arms, and then being transferred to their crib, they awaken in unfamiliar surroundings and are unable to fall asleep until the routine is repeated. Also, the bed should be used for sleeping only—not as a playpen. It is advisable not to hang playthings over or on the bed; in this way the child associates the bed with sleep—not with activity. Although these interventions described above and in Table 12-6 are usually successful, it is much easier to prevent the problem with appropriate counseling during the early months of the infant's life*.

DENTAL HEALTH

Good dental hygiene begins as soon as the primary teeth erupt. During infancy the teeth are cleaned by wiping them with a damp cloth; toothbrushing is too harsh for the tender gingiva. Fluoride supplements, an essential mineral for building caries-resistant teeth, are prescribed as appropriate for:

- All infants 2 weeks of age or older who live in areas with suboptimum levels of fluoride in the local water supply
- Exclusively breast-fed infants regardless of the fluoride content of the local water supply
- Infants who consume relatively little fluoridated tap water, such as those receiving ready-to-serve formula

Dietary considerations are also important because habits begun during infancy tend to continue into later years. Foods with concentrated sugar should be used sparingly (if at all) in the infant's diet. The practice of coating pacifiers with honey or using commercially available hard-candy pacifiers is discouraged. Besides being cariogenic, honey also may cause infant botulism. Parents need to be counseled regarding the detrimental effects of frequent and prolonged bottle- or breast-feeding during sleep, when the sweet milk or other fluid, such as juice, bathes the teeth, producing *nursing-bottle caries*. (See also Chapter 14 for a more extensive discussion of dental care, including nursing-bottle caries.)

IMMUNIZATIONS

One of the most dramatic advances in pediatrics has been the decline of infectious diseases over the past 40 years because of the widespread use of immunization for preventable diseases. Although many of the presently available immunizations can be given to individuals of any age, the recommended primary schedule begins during infancy and, with the exception of boosters, is completed during early childhood. Therefore the discussion of childhood immuni-

zations for diphtheria, tetanus, pertussis, polio, measles, mumps, rubella, and *Haemophilus influenzae* type b is included under health promotion during the first year. Selected vaccines that are generally reserved for children considered at high risk for the disease are discussed on p. 530 and as appropriate throughout the text.

To facilitate the understanding of immunization, the following terms are defined for reference throughout the next section:

immunity An inherited or acquired state in which an individual is resistant to the occurrence or the effects of a specific disease, particularly an infectious agent.

natural immunity Innate immunity or resistance to infection or toxicity.

acquired immunity Immunity from exposure to the invading agent, either bacteria, virus, or toxin.

active immunity Immune bodies are actively formed against specific antigens, either *naturally* by having had the disease clinically or subclinically or *artificially* by introducing the antigen (vaccine) into the individual.

passive immunity Temporary immunity by transfusing plasma proteins either *artificially* from another human or an animal that has been actively immunized against an antigen or *naturally* from the mother to the fetus via the placenta.

antibody A protein, found mostly in serum, that is formed in response to exposure to a specific antigen.

antigen A variety of foreign substances, including bacteria, viruses, toxins, and foreign proteins that stimulate the formation of antibodies.

antitoxin Antibody formed in response to a toxin (antigen).

toxin A poisonous substance, usually produced by the invading microorganism.

toxoid A toxin that has been treated to destroy its toxic properties but retain its antigenic quality.

vaccine Collectively, a term to denote any type of active immunization agent, such as toxoids or attenuated live viruses; specifically, a suspension of disease-causing bacteria or viruses that acts like an antigen, stimulates antibody production, and produces active acquired immunity.

attenuate Reduce the virulence (infectiousness) of a pathogenic microorganism by such measures as treating it with heat or chemicals or cultivating it on a certain medium.

Current Status of Immunizations

The routine use of immunizations has dramatically altered the morbidity and mortality from once common and feared childhood diseases. At one time diphtheria occurred in more than 200,000 children, with a mortality rate of 5% to 10%. From 1980 to 1983 only 15 cases were reported, and 11 were among persons 20 years of age or older. Substantial reductions have also occurred with tetanus and pertussis (Recommendation of ACIP, 1985a).

Before the measles vaccine became available in 1963 the average annual incidence rate of measles was 315 cases per 100,000 population; in 1983 the rate was 0.6 per 100,000—a 99.8% decrease (Bloch and others, 1985). However, even with such impressive statistics there is cause for concern. Outbreaks of measles, especially among college students, continue to occur, and some authorities suggest the routine

---

*An excellent resource for parents is Ferber, R.: Solve your child's sleep problems, New York, 1985, Simon & Schuster.

revaccination of children born before 1972 who received live measles virus vaccine at or before 12 months of age (Yeager and others, 1983). The consequences of only a few unimmunized individuals is readily apparent from current experiences with diseases such as measles.

The impact of rubella vaccination is still under investigation. The benefit is prevention of congenital rubella syndrome, and it is estimated that the current program in the United States will have a tremendous impact on the pattern of rubella and congenital rubella syndrome (Hinman, 1985). The use of mumps vaccine has been less successful than measles or rubella vaccine, probably because of the perceived mildness of the disease and concerns about the vaccine's effectiveness. However, studies on the costs of the mumps document the benefits of routine immunization (Sullivan and others, 1985).

Another major change has been the routine discontinuation of smallpox vaccination because the risks from receiving the vaccine became greater than the chance of contracting the disease. In 1980 the World Health Organization announced the worldwide eradication of smallpox (Recommendation of ACIP, 1980).

Several advances in the area of vaccines have also been significant, especially the introduction of *Haemophilus influenzae* type b (Hib) vaccine (see discussion on p. 529) and the current development of the varicella (chicken pox) vaccine. At this writing the varicella vaccine is under investigation for use in immunization of high-risk children, such as those who are immunosuppressed. Findings demonstrate that the vaccine is effective, is well tolerated, produces few reactions, and does not result in viral spread to siblings (Weibel and others, 1984).

Public concern and education. Unfortunately, public concern for the safety of vaccines, especially pertussis, has led to serious consequences. In the United Kingdom and Japan public concern regarding the dangers of the vaccine prompted the termination of routine immunization against pertussis—a decision that led to major epidemics of the disease (Hinman and Koplan, 1984). Companies in the United States that manufacture vaccines curtailed or stopped production in 1985 because of lawsuits. This situation was resolved, but controversy regarding the risks and benefits of vaccines continues despite evidence supporting the overall safety and medical benefits of immunization.

Health professionals need to be aware of these controversies and of the importance of education in dispelling fears. Inasmuch as nurses frequently administer vaccines during well-child care, they may have the responsibility for adequately informing parents of the nature, prevalence, and risks of the disease; the type of immunization product to be used; expected benefits; risk of side effects; and need for accurate immunization records (Fulginiti, 1984). Referring to immunizations as "baby shots" and limiting the discussion to a vague statement about their benefit are unacceptable.

Most state health departments have materials designed for patient education, which are available by writing to their immunization coordinator. These information sheets typically include a section that the parents sign in order to confirm their understanding of the benefits and risks of the vaccine. In essence the sheet is a signed informed consent that the drug can be given. Although this procedure is not always practiced, it does emphasize the need for health professionals to adequately inform parents before administering immunizations, both as a professional obligation and a personal legal safeguard.

Schedule for Immunizations

Two organizations—The Advisory Committee on Immunization Practices (ACIP) of the U.S. Public Health Service and the Committee on Infectious Diseases of the American Academy of Pediatrics (AAP)—govern the recommendations for immunization policies and procedures. Because The Advisory Committee on Immunization Practices is concerned primarily with national health issues and the Committee on Infectious Diseases formulates its recommendations for infants and children who receive regular health care, there are occasionally different perspectives in each group's recommendations. The policies of each committee are recommendations, not rules, and they change as a result of advances in the field of immunology. Nurses need to realize the purpose of each committee, to view immunization practices in light of the needs of an individual child as well as of a community, and to keep informed of the latest advances and changes in policy.

The recommended age for beginning primary immunizations of normal infants is 2 months (Table 12-7). Recommended schedules for children not immunized during infancy are included in Table 12-8. Children who began primary immunization at the recommended age but who fail to receive all the doses do not have to begin the series again, but receive only the missed doses.

Certain combinations of simultaneously administered vaccines have been shown to be satisfactory. These include diphtheria-tetanus-pertussis (DTP) and oral poliovirus (OPV), DTP and measles-mumps-rubella (MMR), and MMR and the third or fourth dose of OPV. Although all possible combinations have not been tested, in situations when there is doubt that the child will return for immunization according to the optimum schedule, DTP, OPV, and MMR can be administered simultaneously. DTP and MMR are given in separate syringes in different injection sites (Recommendation of ACIP, 1985a).

Recommendations for Routine Immunizations

Several vaccines are administered to all children in the United States according to the schedules listed in Tables 12-7 and 12-8. The following is a brief description of the immunizations.

Diphtheria. Diphtheria vaccine is commonly administered (1) in combination with tetanus and pertussis vaccines (DTP) for normal children younger than 7 years of age, (2) in a combined vaccine with tetanus (DT) for children younger than 7 years of age who have some contraindication for

Table 12-7 Recommended schedule for active immunization of normal infants and children

RECOMMENDED AGE	IMMUNIZATION(S)	COMMENTS
2 mo	DTP, OPV	Can be initiated as early as 2 weeks of age in areas of high endemicity or during epidemics
4 mo	DTP, OPV	2-months interval desired for OPV to avoid interference from previous dose
6 mo	DTP (OPV)	OPV is optional (may be given in areas with increased risk of polio exposure)
15 mo	Measles, mumps, rubella, (MMR)	MMR preferred to individual vaccines; tuberculin testing may be done
18 mo	DTP,*† OPV†	
24 mo	HBPV	
4-6 yr‡	DTP, OPV	At or before school entry
14-16 yr	Td	Repeat every 10 years throughout life

DTP, diphtheria and tetanus toxoids with pertussis vaccine; *HBPV*, *Haemophilus influenzae* type b polysaccharide vaccine; *MMR*, live measles, mumps, and rubella viruses in a combined vaccine; *OPV*, oral poliovirus vaccine containing attenuated poliovirus types 1, 2, and 3; *Td*, adult tetanus toxoid (full dose) and diphtheria toxoid (reduced dose) in combination.
*Should be given 6 to 12 months after the third dose.
†May be given simultaneously with MMR at 15 months of age.
‡Up to the seventh birthday.
From American Academy of Pediatrics: Report of the Committee on Infectious Diseases, ed. 20, Elk Grove Village, IL, 1986. Copyright American Academy of Pediatrics, 1986.

Table 12-8 Recommended immunization schedules for children not immunized in first year of life

RECOMMENDED TIME	IMMUNIZATION(S)	COMMENTS
Younger than 7 years old		
First visit	DTP, OPV, MMR	MMR if child ≥15 months old; tuberculin testing may be done
Interval after first visit		
1 mo	HBPV*	For children 24-60 months
2 mo	DTP, OPV	
4 mo	DTP (OPV)	OPV is optional (may be given in areas with increased risk of poliovirus exposure)
10-16 mo	DTP, OPV	OPV is not given if third dose was given earlier
4-6 yr (at or before school entry)	DTP, OPV	DTP is not necessary if the fourth dose was given after the fourth birthday; OPV is not necessary if recommended OPV dose at 10-16 months following first visit was given after the fourth birthday
Age 14-16 yr	Td	Repeat every 10 years throughout life
7 years old and older		
First visit	Td, OPV, MMR	
Interval after first visit		
2 mo	Td, OPV	
8-14 mo	Td, OPV	
Age 14-16 yr	Td	Repeat every 10 years throughout life

DTP, diphtheria and tetanus toxoids with pertussis vaccine; *HBPV*, *Haemophilus influenzae* type b polysaccharide vaccine; *MMR*, live measles, mumps, and rubella viruses in combined vaccine; *OPV*, oral poliovirus vaccine; *Td*, tetanus toxoid and diphtheria toxoid.
Haemophilus influenzae type b polysaccharide vaccine can be given, if necessary, simultaneously with DTP (at separate sites). The initial three doses of DTP can be given at 1- to 2-month intervals; so, for the child in whom immunization is initiated at 24 months old or older, one visit could be eliminated by giving DTP, OPV, MMR at the first visit; DTP and HBPV at the second visit (1 month later); and DTP and OPV at the third visit (2 months after the first visit). Subsequent DTP and OPV 10 to 16 months after the first visit are still indicated.
From American Academy of Pediatrics: Report of the Committee on Infectious Diseases, ed. 20, Elk Grove Village, IL, 1986. Copyright American Academy of Pediatrics, 1986.

receiving pertussis vaccine, (3) in smaller doses (15% to 20% of that in DTP or DT) with tetanus vacine (Td) for use in children age 7 years and older, or (4) as a single antigen when combined antigen preparations are not indicated. Although the diphtheria vaccine does not produce absolute immunity, when given according to the recommended schedule protective antitoxin persists for 10 years or more.

Tetanus. Three forms of tetanus vaccine—tetanus toxoid, tetanus immune globulin (TIG) (human), and tetanus antitoxin (usually horse serum)—are available. Tetanus toxoid is used for routine primary immunization, usually in one of the combinations listed above, and provides protective antitoxin levels for 10 years or more.

For wound management, passive immunity is available with TIG or animal-source antitoxin. However, because the risk of severe reaction, such as anaphylactic shock or serum sickness, is always greater to the foreign substances of animal serum, the choice should be TIG. In persons with a history of two previous doses of tetanus toxoid, a booster dose of the toxoid can be given. When tetanus toxoid and TIG are given concurrently, separate syringes and different sites are used. Table 12-9 presents a summary of the recommended procedure for tetanus prophylaxis in wound management.

Pertussis. Pertussis is recommended for all children 6 weeks through 6 years of age (up to the seventh birthday) who have no neurologic contraindications to its use. It is not given to children 7 years or older because the risk of receiving the vaccine increases as the incidence, severity, and fatality of the disease decrease.

Polio. The trivalent oral form of poliovirus (TOPV) (developed by Sabin) is recommended for all children younger than 18 years of age who have no specific contraindications to its use, regardless of the number of administrations of inactivated poliovirus vaccine (IPV) (developed by Salk) they have received. For infants and children with immune deficiency diseases and for their siblings, IPV is the vaccine of choice because it has no reported history of causing vaccine-associated paralysis. However, it has the disadvantages of being given by subcutaneous injection and requiring periodic boosters to maintain immunity.

Measles. Because of the presence of maternal antibodies, measles virus vaccine should be delayed until 15 months of age for infants who live in communities where the disease is not prevalent. However, during the course of measles outbreaks, the vaccine can be given any time after 6 months of age, followed by a second inoculation after age 15 months.

Mumps. Mumps virus vaccine may be given at any time to children between 15 months and 12 years of age who have not had the disease.

Rubella. Rubella is a relatively mild infection in children, but in a pregnant woman it presents serious risks to the developing fetus. Therefore the aim of rubella immunization is actually protection of the unborn child rather than the recipient of the immunization.

Table 12-9 Guide to tetanus prophylaxis in routine wound management

HISTORY OF ABSORBED TETANUS TOXOID (DOSES)	CLEAN, MINOR WOUNDS		ALL OTHER WOUNDS*	
	Td†	TIG	Td†	TIG
Unknown or < three	Yes	No	Yes	Yes
≥ three‡	No§	No	No‖	No

Recommendation of the Immunization Practices Advisory Committee (ACIP): Diphtheria, tetanus, and pertussis: guidelines for vaccine prophylaxis and other preventive measures, MMWR **34**(27):405-426, 1985.

*Including but not limited to wounds contaminated with dirt, feces, soil, saliva, etc.; puncture wounds; avulsions; and wounds resulting from missiles, crushing, burns, and frostbite.

†For children younger than 7 years old; DTP (DT, if pertussis vaccine is contraindicated) is preferred to tetanus toxoid alone. For persons 7 years old and older, Td is preferred to tetanus toxoid alone.

‡If only three doses of *fluid* toxoid have been received, a fourth dose of toxoid, preferably an adsorbed toxoid, should be given.

§Yes, if more than 10 years since last dose.

‖Yes, if more than 5 years since last dose. (More frequent boosters are not needed and can accentuate side effects.)

Rubella immunization is recommended for all children at 12 months of age or older. If administered in a combined form with measles vaccine, it should be given to children at about 15 months of age. Increased emphasis should also be placed on vaccinating all unimmunized prepubertal children and susceptible adolescents and adult women in the childbearing age group.

Because the live attenuated virus may cross the placenta and present a risk to the developing fetus, rubella vaccine is not given to any pregnant woman or to any woman who may become pregnant in the 3 months following the immunization. Although the precaution of maintaining adequate contraception for this 3-month period following the vaccination is standard practice, current evidence from women who received the vaccine while pregnant and delivered unaffected offspring indicates that the risk to the fetus is negligible (Hinman, 1985). In addition, there is no reported danger of administering rubella vaccine to a child if the mother is pregnant.

***Haemophilus influenzae* type b.** *Haemophilus influenzae* type b (Hib) polysaccharide vaccine was licensed in 1985 and provides protection against a number of serious infections caused by Hib, especially bacterial meningitis, epiglottitis, bacterial pneumonia, septic arthritis, and sepsis. Current recommendations include its use in (Recommendation of ACIP, 1985c):

- All children at 24 months of age
- Children at 18 months of age with increased risk of Hib infection, such as those attending daycare facilities, with anatomic or functional asplenia such as sickle cell disease, and with malignancies associated with immunosuppression

- Children older than 24 months of age who are at increased risk as above

There is controversy regarding the use of Hib vaccine in children 18 to 24 months because the effectiveness of the vaccine is considerably less than in children 24 months of age or older. Consequently these children may require re-vaccination after 24 months of age to ensure immunity. Hib and DTP vaccines can be administered simultaneously at different sites.

Tuberculin testing. Tuberculin testing is included as part of the immunization schedule to permit systematic screening of the population for exposure to tuberculosis. However, it is not an immunization.

Two types of tuberculin preparations are used for skin tests: *old tuberculin (OT)* and *purified protein derivative (PPD)* of tuberculin. The PPD is used most widely, and the standard dose is 5 tuberculin units (TU) in 0.1 ml of solution, injected intradermally. Common techniques for injection are (1) the *Mantoux test,* in which 0.1 ml of PPD is injected directly into the dermis, and (2) the *multiple-puncture tests* (Tine, Heaf, SclavoTest, Sterneedle, Mono-Vac), which may contain OT or PPD.

A positive reaction indicates that the person has been infected and developed a sensitivity to the protein of the tubercle bacillus. However, it does not confirm the presence of active disease. Once individuals react positively, they will continue to react positively. A previously negative result that becomes positive indicates that the person has been infected since the last test. Test results are read according to instructions provided by the manufacturer.

In theory tuberculin testing should be done before or at the same time as measles immunization. Exacerbation of tuberculosis is known to occur with natural measles infection and could result from the live attenuated measles virus vaccine. In addition, viral interference from the vaccine may cause a false-negative reaction. However, in actual practice neither of these two possibilities is considered a contraindication to measles immunization, especially in the event of an epidemic.

Recommendations for Selected Immunizations

A number of vaccines are available for immunization of selected individuals. The following discussion is limited to those that may be administered to children but are not recommended for mass immunization. Other vaccines may be indicated in special circumstances, such as to prevent rabies (see p. 1654) or during travel to areas of endemic disease.

Influenza virus vaccine. The influenza virus vaccine is used for the control of various strains of influenza and is not be confused with the Hib vaccine. It is recommended for children ages 6 months and older with chronic disorders of the cardiovascular or pulmonary systems whose severity warranted regular medical care or hospitalization during the preceding year. Other children that may be eligible include those with diabetes mellitus, renal dysfunction, anemia, such as sickle cell disease, immunosuppression, or asthma.

The vaccine is administered in the fall and is associated with mild flulike symptoms for 1 to 2 days (Recommendation of ACIP, 1985b).

Pneumococcal polysaccharide vaccine. The pneumococcal vaccine (Pneumovax; Pnu-Immune) affords protection against 23 types of *Streptococcus pneumoniae,* which frequently causes otitis media, bacterial pneumonia, bacterial meningitis, and sinusitis in children. Children who should be vaccinated include those aged 2 years and older with sickle cell disease, functional or anatomic asplenia, nephrotic syndrome, and Hodgkin disease prior to beginning cytoreduction therapy (American Academy of Pediatrics, 1985c).

Hepatitis B vaccine. Hepatitis B vaccine (Heptavax-B), which confers immunity against hepatitis B virus (HBV), is recommended for several high-risk groups, especially adults who are at risk for infection from contaminated blood products. Among children, however, the greatest concern is with prevention of HBV in infants born to mothers who are hepatitis B surface antigen (HBsAg) positive. Without prophylaxis about 90% of these infants will become infected, and most will become permanent carriers of HBV. About 25% of the carriers will eventually die from some form of liver disease, and all will be a source of infection for their intimate contacts and future offspring.

To confer the greatest degree of protection a combined regimen of hepatitis B immune globulin (HBIG) and hepatitis B vaccine is recommended at birth, with two additional doses of the vaccine at 1 and 6 months of age (American Academy of Pediatrics, 1985b). Both preparations are given intramuscularly at separate sites, preferably in the vastus lateralis muscle. In older individuals improved effectiveness is achieved when the vaccine is injected into the deltoid muscle rather than the gluteal site (Hepatitis B vaccine, 1985).

Reactions

Vaccines for routine immunizations are among the safest and most reliable drugs available. However, minor side effects do occur following many of the immunizations, and rarely a serious reaction may result from the vaccine (Table 12-10).

With inactivated antigens, such as DTP, side effects are most likely to occur within a few hours or days of administration and are usually limited to local tenderness, erythema, and swelling at the injection site; low-grade fever; and irritability. Local reactions tend to be less severe when the dorsogluteal site is used rather than the vastus lateralis muscle (Baraff, Cody, and Cherry, 1984), but the gluteal site is not recommended for infants. Rarely more severe reactions may occur, especially with pertussis (see Table 12-10). Reactions to DTP tend to be more severe if they occurred with a previous immunization.

Hib vaccine is one of the safest vaccines available but may be associated with low-grade fever and mild local reactions at the site of subcutaneous injection, which resolve rapidly. Fever (temperature more than 38.5° C) may rarely occur (American Academy of Pediatrics, 1985a).

Unlike the inactivated antigens, live attenuated virus vaccines such as measles, mumps, rubella, and oral poliovirus multiply for days or weeks, and unfavorable reactions and "vaccine associated" disorders can occur for a period of 30 to 60 days. However, they are usually mild, although reactions to rubella tend to be more troublesome in older children and adults.

Contraindications

The general contraindication for all immunizations is a severe febrile illness. This precaution is to avoid adding the risk of adverse side effects from the vaccine on an already ill child or mistakenly identifying a symptom of the disease as having been caused by the vaccine. The presence of minor illnesses such as the common cold is *not* a contraindication.

Live virus vaccines are not administered to anyone with an altered immune system, because multiplication of the virus may be enhanced, causing a severe vaccine-induced illness. Such children include (1) those with immunologic deficiency disease, such as leukemia, lymphoma, or generalized malignancy, and (2) those receiving immunosuppressive therapy, such as steroids, chemotherapy, or radiation. In addition, household contacts of such children should not receive oral poliovirus because the virus multiplies in the gastrointestinal tract and excreted virus in the stool can be communicated to the immunosuppressed child.

Another contraindication to live virus vaccines is the presence of recently acquired passive immunity through blood transfusions, immunoglobulin, or maternal antibodies. Administration of such vaccines should be postponed until 3 months after passive immunization with immune serum globulin.

Table 12-10 Possible side effects of recommended childhood immunizations and nursing responsibilities*

IMMUNIZATION	REACTION	NURSING RESPONSIBILITIES
Diphtheria	Fever usually within 24-48 hours Soreness, redness, and swelling at injection site	Instructions for DTP: advise parents of possible side effects
Tetanus	Same as for diphtheria but may include urticaria and malaise All may have delayed onset and last several days Lump at injection site may last for weeks, even months, but gradually disappears	May recommend prophylactic use of acetaminophen if fever occurred following previous DTP immunization Recommend use of antipyretics if fever occurs following present immunization Advise parents to notify physician *immediately* of any unusual side effects, such as those listed under pertussis
Pertussis	Same as for tetanus but may include loss of consciousness, convulsions, persistent inconsolable crying episodes, generalized or focal neurologic signs, fever (temperature at or above 40.5° C (10.5° F), systemic allergic reaction	Before administering next dose of DTP, inquire about reactions, especially those listed under pertussis on p. 532
Poliovirus (TOPV)	Essentially no immediate side effects Vaccine-associated paralysis rarely occurs within 2 months of immunization (estimated risk 1:10 million doses)	Assess presence of family members at risk from TOPV because of immune deficiency states
Measles	Anorexia, malaise, rash, and fever may occur 7 to 10 days after immunization Rarely (estimated risk 1:1 million doses) encephalitis may occur	Advise parents of more common side effects and use of antipyretics for fever If a persistent fever with other obvious signs of illness occurs, have them notify physician immediately
Mumps	Essentially no side effects other than a brief, mild fever	See general comment to parents*
Rubella	Fever, lymphadenopathy, or mild rash that lasts 1 or 2 days within a few days after immunization Arthralgia, arthritis, or paresthesia of the hands and fingers may occur about 2 weeks after vaccination and is more common in older children and adults	Advise parents of side effects, especially of time delay before joint swelling and pain; assure them that these symptoms will disappear May recommend use of mild analgesics for pain
Haemophilus influenzae type B (Hib)	Low-grade fever Mild local reactions at injection site Rarely fever above 40° C (105°F)	Advise parents of possible mild side effects

*General comment to parents regarding each immunization: the benefit of being protected by the immunization is believed to greatly outweigh the risk from the disease.

Pregnancy is a known contraindication to mumps, measles, and rubella vaccines. In addition, these vaccines should not be given to women who are likely to become pregnant within 3 months after vaccination. Oral poliovirus may also be withheld unless there is risk of exposure during an outbreak of polio.

A final contraindication is a known allergic response to a previously administered vaccine or a substance in the vaccine. If any of the following adverse events occur after combined DTP or single-antigen pertussis vaccination, further immunization with pertussis vaccine is contraindicated: (1) allergic hypersensitivity, (2) fever (temperature 40.5° C [105° F] or greater) within 48 hours, (3) collapse or shock-like state within 48 hours, (4) persistent, inconsolable crying lasting 3 hours or longer or an unusual, high-pitched cry occurring within 48 hours, (5) convulsions within 3 days, or (6) encephalopathy (alterations in consciousnesss with generalized or focal neurologic signs) within 7 days (Recommendation of ACIP, 1985a).

Measles, mumps, and rubella virus vaccines contain minute amounts of neomycin, and measles and mumps vaccines, which are grown on chick embryo tissue cultures, may contain substances allergenic to egg-sensitive individuals. However, only a history of anaphylactoid reaction to the antibiotic or to egg is considered a contraindication to their use. To identify the rare child who may not be able to receive the vaccines, a careful allergy history is taken. If the child has a history of anaphylaxis, it is reported to the physician before administering the vaccine. Although rare, severe reactions to measles vaccine have occurred in children with egg allergy, and as a precaution such children should be skin tested for sensitivity and given incremental doses of vaccine (Herman, Radin, and Schneiderman, 1983).

Administration/Precautions

The principal precautions in administering immunizations include proper storage of the vaccine to protect its potency and institution of recommended procedures for injection. The nurse must be familiar with the manufacturer's directions for storage and reconstitution of the vaccine. For example, if the vaccine is to be refrigerated it should be stored on a center shelf, not on the door where frequent temperature increases from opening the refrigerator can alter the vaccine's potency. Faulty refrigeration and excess exposure to light are major causes of primary vaccine failure (Hayden, 1979). For protection against light the vial can be wrapped in aluminum foil. Periodic checks should be established to ensure that no vaccine is used after its expiration date.

The DTP vaccines contain an adjuvant aluminum compound that is used to retain the antigen at the depot site and prolong the stimulatory effect. Because subcutaneous or intracutaneous injection of the substance can cause local irritation, inflammation, or abscess formation (Bernier, Frank, and Nolan, 1981), a needle of adequate length to deposit the antigen deep in the muscle mass is selected. To prevent tracking the fluid through the skin the immunizing needle should be changed after withdrawing the vaccine into the syringe and an air bubble used to clear the needle after injecting the fluid. The total series requires a number of injections, and every attempt is made to administer them as painlessly as possible (see Chapter 27). Freezing the site with Frigiderm (an aerosol coolant) has been shown to significantly reduce the perception of pain (Eland, 1981).

INJURY PREVENTION

Injuries are a major cause of death during infancy, especially for children 6 to 12 months old. Constant vigilance, awareness, and supervision are essential as the child gains increased locomotor and manipulative skills that are coupled with an insatiable curiosity about the environment. Injuries can be grouped into the following categories: aspiration of foreign objects, suffocation, falls, poisoning, burns, motor vehicle injuries, and bodily damage. Table 12-11 lists the major developmental achievements of each period during infancy and the appropriate injury prevention plan.

Aspiration of Foreign Objects

Asphyxiation by foreign material in the respiratory tract is the leading cause of fatal injury in children younger than 1 year of age. The size, shape, and consistency of foods or objects are important determinants of fatal obstruction. For example, small objects (less than 3.2 cm, or 1¼ inches) are more likely to completely obstruct the airway. A spheric or cylindric object is likely to plug the airway more completely than any other shaped object. Pliable objects are less likely to be expelled than rigid ones (Baker and Fisher, 1980). Unfortunately, common household items can be deadly to infants.

Nonfood items cause the majority of deaths in young children. Balloons, whether partially inflated, uninflated, or popped, cause more deaths in children than any other kind of small object and should be kept from infants and young children (Baker and Fisher, 1980). Another hazard is plastic lining from diapers; with the present interest in baby dolls, such as Cabbage Patch dolls, the accessibility of the plastic diaper lining is especially dangerous to young children.

As soon as the infant has the ability to find his mouth, he is vulnerable to aspiration of small objects, such as those left within reach or removable parts of objects that may on initial inspection appear safe. Rattles, for example, have small beads in them to produce noise. A broken or cracked rattle can be dangerous because the beads can easily be swallowed while the infant has the toy in his mouth. Stuffed animals are another potentially dangerous toy if any of the parts, such as the eyes or nose, are removable buttons or plastic pieces.

All toys must be carefully inspected for potential danger. An active infant can grab a low-hanging mobile and quickly chew off a small piece. As soon as the infant crawls or plays on the floor, the floor must be kept free of any small articles that can be picked up and swallowed, such as coins.

Table 12-11 Injury prevention during infancy

AGE: BIRTH-4 MONTHS

Major developmental accomplishments

Involuntary reflexes, such as the crawling reflex, may propel infant forward

May roll over

Increasing eye-hand coordination and voluntary grasp reflex

Injury prevention

Aspiration

Not as great a danger to this age group, but should begin practicing safeguarding early (see under 4-7 months)

Never shake baby powder directly on infant; place powder in hand and then on infant's skin; store container closed and out of infant's reach

Suffocation

Keep all plastic bags stored out of infant's reach; discard large plastic garment bags after tying in a knot

Do not cover mattress or pillows with plastic

Use a firm mattress, no pillows, and loose blankets

Make sure crib design follows federal regulations and mattress fits snugly

Position crib away from other furniture

Avoid sleeping in bed with infant

Do not tie pacifier on a string around infant's neck

Remove bibs at bedtime

Drowning—never leave infant alone in bath

Falls

Always raise crib rails; tie them to crib if malfunctioning

Never leave infant on a raised, unguarded surface

When in doubt where to place child, use the floor

Restrain child in the infant seat and never leave him unattended while the seat is resting on a raised surface

Avoid using a high chair until child is old enough to sit well

Poisoning

Not as great a danger to this age group, but should begin practicing safeguarding early (see under 4-7 months)

Burns

Install smoke detectors in home

Use caution when warming formula in microwave oven; always check temperature of liquid before feeding

Check bath water

Do not pour hot liquids when infant is close by, such as sitting on lap

Beware of cigarette ashes that may fall on infant

Do not leave infant in the sun for more than a few minutes

Wash flame-retardant clothes according to label directions

Use cool-mist vaporizers

Do not leave child in parked car

Check surface heat of car restraint before placing child in seat

Motor vehicles

Transport infant in federally approved rear-facing car seat*

Do not place infant on the seat or in lap

Do not place child in a carriage or stroller behind a parked car

Bodily damage

Avoid sharp, jagged objects

Keep diaper pins closed and away from infant

AGE: 4-7 MONTHS

Major developmental accomplishments

Rolls over

Sits momentarily

Grasps and manipulates small objects

Resecures a dropped object

Has well-developed eye-hand coordination

Can focus on and locate very small objects

Mouthing very prominent

Injury prevention

Aspiration

Keep buttons, beads, and other small objects out of infant's reach

Use pacifier with one-piece construction and loop handle

Keep floor free of any small objects

Do not feed infant hard candy, nuts, food with pits or seeds, or whole hot dogs

Do not feed infant while he is lying down

Inspect toys for removable parts

Avoid balloons as playthings

Discard used button-size batteries; store new batteries in safe area

Keep baby powder, if used, out of reach

Suffocation

May begin to teach swimming as part of water safety

Do not tie toys across crib rails

Falls

Restrain in a high chair

Keep crib rails raised to full height

Poisoning

Make sure that paint for furniture or toys does not contain lead

Place toxic substances on a high shelf or in locked cabinet

Hang plants or place on high surface rather than on floor

Avoid storing large quantities of cleaning fluid, paints, pesticides, and other toxic substances

Discard used containers of poisonous substances

Do not store toxic substances in food containers

Know telephone number of local poison control center (usually listed in front of telephone directory)

Burns

Keep faucets out of reach

Place hot objects (cigarettes, candles, incense) on high surface

Motor vehicles

(See under Birth-4 months)

Bodily damage

Give toys that are smooth and rounded, preferably made of wood or plastic

Avoid long, pointed objects as toys

Avoid toys that are excessively loud

Keep sharp objects out of infant's reach

*Car safety instructions for families are available in Wong, D., and Whaley, L.: Clinical handbook of pediatric nursing, ed. 2, Copyright © 1986, The C.V. Mosby Co., St. Louis.

Continued.

Table 12-11   Injury prevention during infancy—cont'd

AGE: 8-12 MONTHS

Major developmental accomplishments

Crawls

Stands, holding onto furniture

Stands alone

Cruises around furniture

Walks

Climbs

Pulls on objects

Throws objects

Able to pick up small objects

Explores by putting objects in mouth

Dislikes being restrained

Explores away from parent

Increasing understanding of simple commands and phrases

Helpless in water

Injury prevention

Aspiration

(See under 4-7 months)

Suffocation

Keep doors of ovens, dishwashers, refrigerators, and frontloading clothes washers and dryers closed at all times

If storing an unused appliance, such as a refrigerator, remove the door

Fence swimming pools; always supervise when near any source of water, such as cleaning buckets

Keep bathroom doors closed

Falls

Fence stairways at top and bottom if child has access to either end

Dress infant in safe shoes and clothing

Avoid walkers, especially near stairs

Poisoning

Administer medications as a drug, not as a candy

Do not administer medications unless so prescribed by a physician

Replace medications and poisons immediately after use; replace caps properly if a child-protector cap is used

Have syrup of ipecac in home; use only if advised

Burns

Place guards in front of or around any heating appliance, fireplace, or furnace

Keep electrical wires hidden or out of reach

Place plastic guards over electrical outlets; place furniture in front of outlets

Keep hanging tablecloths out of reach

Do not allow infant to play with electrical appliance

Apply a sunscreen when infant is exposed to sunlight

Motor vehicles

Do not use adult seat or shoulder belt without federally approved infant car seat

Do not allow to crawl behind a parked car

If infant plays in a yard, have the yard fenced or use a playpen

Bodily damage

Do not allow infant to use a fork for self-feeding

Use plastic cups or dishes

Check safety of toys and toy box

Protect from young children and animals, especially dogs

A previously unrecognized danger is ingestion of button-size batteries that are used in devices such as hearing aids, calculators, watches, and cameras. Because they are bright and shiny they are attractive to children. However, they can cause severe morbidity, even death, if lodged in the esophagus (Litovitz, 1985). As a precaution small batteries must be safely stored and discarded where young children cannot easily retrieve them.

When infant clothes are purchased, the type of closure used should be considered. A front button can easily be pulled off and swallowed. Safety pins for diapers should be kept closed and away from the dressing table. Even though a young infant may not search for them, practicing this good habit from the beginning prevents future injuries.

Food items are the second most common cause of aspiration, and the most frequent offenders are hot dogs, candy, nuts, and grapes (Harris and others, 1984). When new foods are given to the child, nuts, hard candies, or fruits with pits or seeds should be avoided. When traveling, especially in airplanes, or entertaining, snack foods such as peanuts and popcorn should be kept away from young children. If given

to young children, hot dogs must be cut into small, irregular pieces rather than served whole or sliced into sections, because their size (diameter), round shape, and consistency allow for complete occlusion of the airway.

Pacifiers can also be dangerous because the entire object may be aspirated if it is small or the nipple and shield may become detached from the handle and become lodged in the pharynx. Improvised pacifiers, such as those commonly made in hospitals from a padded nipple, also present dangers. The nipple may separate from the plastic collar and be aspirated (Millunchick and McArtor, 1986). In addition, parents may continue to offer this pacifier to the infant at home. Safe pacifiers should be of one-piece construction, have a shield or flange that is large enough to prevent entry into the mouth, and have a handle that can be grasped (Fig. 12-15). To prevent the hazards of improvised pacifiers, hospitals should use only safe commercial types.

Another commonly aspirated substance is baby powder, which is usually a mixture of talc (hydrous magnesium silicate) and other silicates. Although the use of talc has been discouraged, it is a common baby care product and can

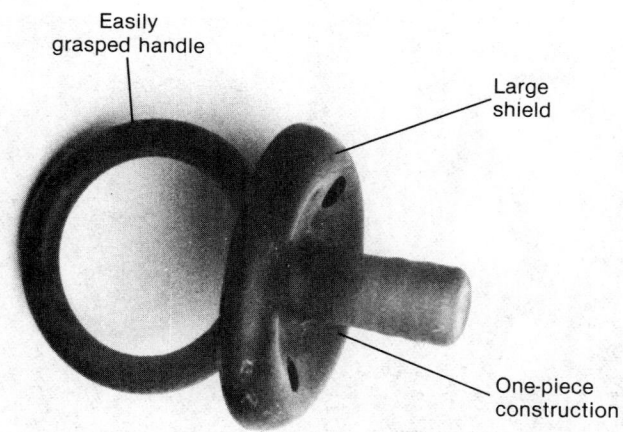

Easily
grasped handle

Large
shield

One-piece
construction

Fig. 12-15. Design of a safe pacifier.

cause severe and often fatal aspiration pneumonia. One of the factors involved in talc aspiration is the similar appearance of baby powder containers and nursing bottles. Talc containers often become favorite playthings and are placed in the mouth (Mofenson and others, 1981). Improper use of powder by sprinkling it directly on the skin creates a cloud of talc dust that is easily inhaled. Parents are advised of the danger of baby powder and discouraged from using it. If they prefer to use a powder, a cornstarch preparation can be substituted (see Questions and controversies, p. 573). Whenever a powder is used, it should be placed in the hand and then applied to the skin, never shaken directly from the container to the skin. The container is kept closed and immediately stored in a safe place, especially away from curious toddlers who often imitate caregiving activities and may accidentally shake it on the infant.

Suffocation

Mechanical suffocation is another important cause of death by asphyxiation and includes asphyxiation by covering the mouth and nose, by pressure on the throat and chest, and by exclusion of air, such as by refrigerator entrapment.

An infant who is placed in a bed under blankets and sheets that are tucked in can be caught under them and be unable to wriggle free. There are potential dangers in adults sleeping with a small infant because of the possibility of their rolling over and smothering the child. Even though this possibility is slight, the consequent parental guilt if it happens can be devastating.

Another cause of suffocation is plastic bags. Large plastic bags used over garments are very lightweight and can easily and quickly be wrapped around the head of an active infant or pressed against his face. Pillows and mattresses should not be covered with plastic for this reason. Older infants may play with a plastic bag and accidentally pull it over their heads. Because plastic is nonporous, suffocation takes place in a matter of minutes.

Anything tied around the infant's neck can potentially cause strangulation. Bibs should be removed at bedtime,

and objects such as pacifiers should never be hung on a string around the infant's neck. This is a common practice in some cultures, and can be remedied by attaching a short string tied to a pacifier and pinning the string on the child's shirt.

Toys that have strings attached, such as a telephone, or toys that are tied to cribs or playpens can be hazards because the string can become wrapped around the child's neck or the child can become entrapped in the toy. As a precaution all cords should be less than 30 cm (12 inches) long. Crib toys should be hung high enough that the infant cannot become entangled in them or avoided once the child is able to reach them.

Restraining straps, if applied too loosely or left unfastened, can be a hazard. For example, a child may slide off a high chair beneath the tray and strangle himself on the loose strap. All straps should be fastened securely.

Infant strangulation may occur if the infant's head becomes caught between the crib slats and mattress or objects close to the crib. According to federal regulation the distance between crib slats should not be more than 2⅜ inches (about 6 cm), roughly the width of three adult fingers. Mattresses and bumper pads should fit snugly against the slats. A general rule is that if two adult fingers can be placed between the mattress and crib side, the mattress is too small. A temporary solution is to place large, rolled towels in the space to create a snug fit. Ideally, information regarding correct crib design should be given prenatally before parents have purchased or borrowed a crib.*

Mesh-sided playpens and cribs can result in death if the sides are left in the lowered position. Infants have suffocated when they fell off the edge of the mattress and the head or chest was compressed between the floorboard and mesh side. Parents should be advised of this danger and encouraged to *always* keep the sides locked securely in the up position whenever the child is in the playpen or crib.

The crib should be positioned away from large furniture, because children who crawl out of the crib may become caught between the two objects. Cribs should also be located away from windows, where drape cords can become wrapped around the infant's neck.

Drowning is another cause of asphyxiation. Infants should never be left unsupervised in a bathtub, hot tub, or near a source of water such as a swimming pool, toilet, or bucket. One way to stress water safety is to teach infants to swim. Infants younger than 6 months of age have two reflexes that enhance swimming. The crawl reflex causes a swimming motion strong enough to propel the infant through water for a short distance. The dive reflex inhibits breathing when the infant is submerged. Most infants, if introduced to the water properly, will not be afraid and can be taught to float and to swim underwater for a few feet. Not until they are 3 or 4

*The booklet *It Hurts When They Cry* gives basic information on hazards, safety features, and proper use of nursery furniture and equipment. It is available at no charge from U.S. Consumer Product Safety Commission, Washington, DC 20207.

years old can they swim above water for longer distances, because of the proportionately heavy weight of the head. Regardless of swimming instructions, no infant can be expected to learn the elements of water safety or to react appropriately in an emergency. Therefore all young children need to be considered at risk when near water.

Falls

Falls are most common after 4 months of age when the infant has learned to roll over, but they can occur at any age. Newborns are normally active, assume a flexed position, and have crawling and Moro reflexes that can propel them forward. The best advice is never to place a child unattended on a raised surface that has no type of guardrails. When in doubt, the safest place is the floor. Even though young infants cannot climb over a partially raised crib rail, it is best to form a habit of raising the side rail all the way, because someday that infant will be able to climb out. Crib sides should have a latching device that cannot be easily released. Ideally cribs should be placed on carpeted, not hard, floors.

Another danger area for falling is a changing table, which is usually high and narrow. Although these tables have a restraining belt, it is unwise to leave the child unattended even when so restrained. The best way to avoid having to leave is to arrange the area with all necessary articles within easy reach so the child is always in full sight of the caregiver. It only takes a fraction of a second for an infant to fall off. During the latter half of the first year, infants usually resist dressing and diapering and may be difficult to manage. If there is danger that the child is strong enough to resist restraining, he should be changed on the floor.

Infant seats, high chairs, walkers, and swings present additional opportunities for falls. If the infant seat is placed on a table where he has an excellent panorama of his environment, he should never be left unrestrained or unattended. The same rule is essential for other baby equipment, particularly when the child has learned to crawl and to stand up. Small infants can slip through a high chair if a protective harness is not used. High chairs are designed for older infants who can sit well and who are tall enough to have the tray at the level of their chest or abdomen. Walkers are responsible for a number of different types of injuries that occur because the walker tipped over or fell down stairs. Parents need to be warned of these dangers and encouraged to keep a constant vigil on their child's activities.

Although the infant begins to develop depth perception by age 9 months, that is no guarantee of his ability to perceive danger. His curiosity may still propel him forward and over, or his immature locomotor skills may be inadequate to keep him from falling even though he is aware of the danger. Infants should not be allowed to crawl unsupervised on any raised surface, near stairs, or near any water reservoir. Gates should be used at the bottom and top of stairs, because both present dangers to the crawling and climbing infant. However, certain types of gates can present hazards.

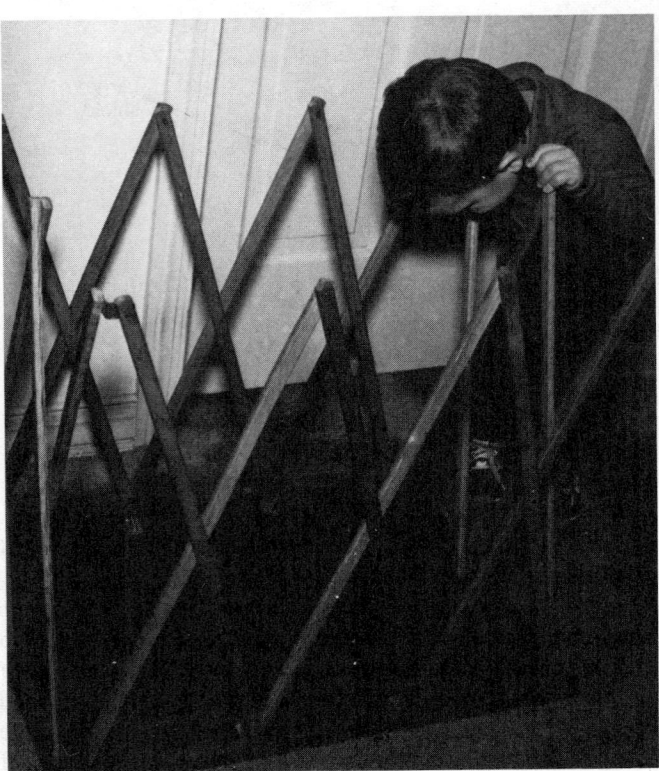

Fig. 12-16. Free-standing enclosures can cause head entrapment, but when secured to the floor they provide a protective barrier from heaters such as this floor furnace.

Free-standing enclosures constructed of criss-crossed wood slats that expand and contract can trap the head or neck when children attempt to climb over them (Fig. 12-16). If these types of gates are used, they must be securely fastened to prevent mobility of the slats.

Sometimes even when the environment is made safe infants may literally trip over their own feet. Slippery socks; hard, slick soles on shoes or rubber soles that can catch, especially on a carpet; and long pants or pajama bottoms can easily upset a child's balance. Such dangers need to be pointed out to parents, especially when the infant is taking his first steps.

Poisoning

Poisoning is one of the major causes of death in children younger than 5 years of age. The highest incidence occurs in those in the 2-year-old group, with the second highest incidence in 1-year-old children. The infant who has not learned to crawl is relatively free from danger of poisonous agents by virtue of his confinement. However, once locomotion begins, danger from poisoning is present almost everywhere. There are more than 500 toxic substances in the average home, and about 34% of all poisonings occur in the kitchen.

The major reason for ingestion of poisons is improper storage. To protect the infant, avoid placing toxic agents on a low shelf, table, or floor. Drugs that are kept in a purse pose additional dangers; if the purse is given to the infant to play with, he may open it and ingest the drug. Another unrecognized hazard is during diaper changes when infants are near many toxic substances such as ointments, creams, oils, and talc. Parents may even hand the infant a potentially poisonous object to quiet him. Such dangers need to be stressed to parents and toys kept at diapering areas to minimize risks.

Poisoning is almost always the result of inadequate supervision, but it may not represent neglect. Children are very fast, and it takes only seconds to eat a bar of soap, or a handful of cleanser or detergent. Although infants usually do not possess the manipulative skill to open closed jars, they are amazingly persistent and inventive. For example, an ant trap placed in an out-of-the-way corner is easy for a crawling infant to find.

Plants are another source of poisoning for infants. Plants are frequently placed on the floor, and the leaves or flowers are attractive and easy to pull off. More than 700 species of plants are known to have caused illness or death.

The only sure way to prevent poisoning is to remove toxic agents, which means placing them high out of the infant's reach. However, because crawling infants soon become climbing toddlers, it is best to keep all toxic agents, especially drugs, in a locked cabinet. Special plastic hooks can be attached to the inside of cabinet doors to keep them securely closed (see Fig. 12-19). Firm thumb pressure is required to unlatch the hook, and small children are usually unable to manipulate them. Locks are best, but for cleaning agents frequently used, such as under a kitchen sink, hooks are a practical alternative. Impractical suggestions are usually ignored, and some protection is better than none.

With several hundred toxic substances in each house, locking up all potentially toxic substances could present a problem; however, careful planning can help. A large surplus of cleaning agents, furniture polishes, laundry additives, paints, insecticides, and solvents should be avoided. Used poison containers should be promptly discarded and not used to store another poison without adequately marking the package. Inasmuch as young children cannot read, any potentially hazardous substance should not be stored in any type of food container. A popular container used to store toxic liquids is a soda bottle. A child who is unaware of the dangerous contents is a vulnerable victim for poisoning. Parents should know the location of local poison control centers and call them in the event of a suspected poisoning. Emergency measures for poisoning are discussed in Chapter 16.

Burns

Burns are generally not thought of as a particular danger to infants, but several important hazards exist, such as scalding from water that is too hot, excessive sunburn, and burns from electrical wires, sockets, and heating elements such as radiators, registers, and floor furnaces. The infant's skin is particularly sensitive to irritation, and the mechanisms for temperature perception are not completely developed. As a general precaution all homes should have smoke alarms installed near the bedroom areas.

Scald burns from hot tap water can be prevented by lowering the hot water heater to a safe temperature of between 49° and 52° C (120° to 125° F). In addition, the bathwater should be checked before the infant is immersed. If formula or food is warmed in a microwave oven, it must be checked before feeding because the container may remain cool while the contents are hot (Sando, Gallaher, and Rodgers, 1984). The handles of cooking utensils should be turned toward the back of the stove. When the infant is underfoot, pouring hot liquids and cooking with hot oil are avoided. Hanging tablecloths are also placed out of the infant's reach.

Sunburn can be a source of a first- or second-degree burn. Exposure to direct sunlight or filtered light through a window should be gradual, about 5 minutes initially. The infant's head should be covered because it represents a large proportion of body surface. Sunscreen agents may be helpful and should be applied 20 to 30 minutes before swimming or sweating. Although black-skinned infants burn less readily, their thin skin can become sunburned also.

Electrical outlets should be covered with protective plastic caps that prevent the child from sucking on the outlet or putting objects such as hairpins into it (see Fig. 12-19). Live wires are placed out of reach so that curious infants cannot chew on them and break the rubber coating (Fig. 12-17). Infants should not be allowed to play near television sets, stereo units, or other appliances, whether these units are on or off; infants cannot determine when the appliance is safe.

Any heat-producing element should have a guard placed in front of it. Fireplaces should be well screened because they are very appealing and within easy access. Small portable heaters should be placed on a high surface. Floor furnaces should have barrier gates to prevent children from crawling or walking over them (see Fig. 12-16). Burning cigarettes, candles, and incense are kept out of reach, and infants should not be held by a smoking adult, because fall-

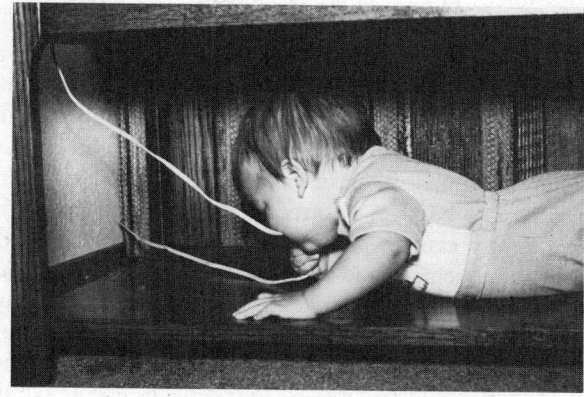

Fig. 12-17. Crawling infants can find hazardous electric wires even in "hidden" areas.

ing ashes are a hazard, especially to the eyes. Heated-mist vaporizers are a source of burns and should not be used. If humidity is needed, only cool-mist vaporizers are safe.

By law all infant sleepwear must be flame retardant. Unfortunately this does not apply to all infant clothing. Flame-retardant fabric must never be viewed as the ultimate protection against burns. Repeated washing reduces the flame-retardant properties, and the use of soap or bleach destroys the protection. Inasmuch as detergent should be used for washing flame-retardant clothing, infants who are sensitive to such wash agents are unprotected when their clothing is washed even with a mild soap. If sleepwear is home sewn, mothers should be advised to look for specially treated flame-retardant fabric.

Another type of thermal injury occurs when children are exposed to excessive heat during confinement in poorly ventilated cars. The practice of leaving the windows open a couple of inches does not appear to be protective. The nurse should caution parents never to leave children in parked cars, especially when the automobile is in direct sunlight.

Children can also be burned by overheated metal hardware and vinyl seats in cars parked in the sun. As a precaution the surface heat of car restraints should be determined before placing children in them. Covering the restraints and hardware (such as metal latches on seat belts) may be necessary to prevent skin burns. An additional safeguard is buying a light-colored restraint, which absorbs less heat.

Motor Vehicle Injuries

Automobile injuries are the leading cause of accidental death in children older than 1 year of age. However, a significant number of infants die mainly from improper restraint within the vehicle. It is recommended that all infants, newborns included, be secured in a special car restraint rather than held or placed on the seat of the car.

A variety of car seats are available for young children. For infants up to 9 kg (20 pounds) the recommended type is a rear-facing molded plastic shell seat or convertible infant-toddler seat that includes a shoulder restraint and uses the car seat belt (Fig. 12-18). In this position the most dangerous forces in a crash are absorbed by the infant's back.

Generally the middle of the back seat is considered the safest area of the car. However, with an infant restraint it is preferable to position the child in the front seat, where the driver can observe the infant without having to turn around.

For restraints to be effective they must be used properly. Dressing the infant in an outfit with sleeves and legs allows the harness to be placed correctly. A small blanket or towel rolled tightly can be placed on either side of the head to minimize movement and increase comfort. Although many infant restraints can be recliners, they should only be used in the car in the position specified by the manufacturer. Many of the infant car restraints also serve as baby carriers, a point that should be stressed to parents to encourage their purchasing a suitable restraint. (For further discussion of restraints see Chapter 14.)

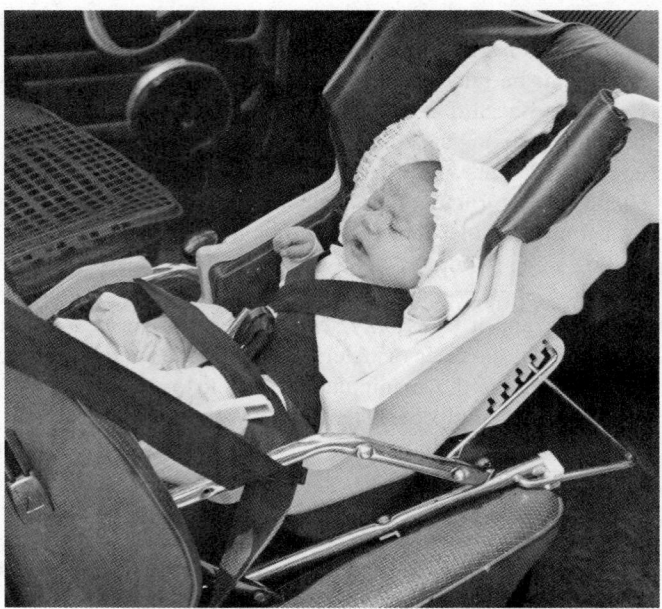

Fig. 12-18. Infant car restraint. Child's clothing allows proper placement of harness, and rolled blankets on either side of head facilitate proper positioning of child.

Another potential vehicular injury is caused by placing a carriage or stroller behind a car, particularly a car parked in a garage or driveway. It is possible that the driver may not see the small stroller and, while driving in reverse, run over the child. Once the child crawls, he should not be allowed to play in areas where vehicles can be a hazard.

Bodily Damage

Injuries can occur in numerous ways. Sharp, jagged-edged objects can cause wounds in the skin. Long, pointed articles, such as the common toothpick or fork, can be poked into the eye or ear, causing serious damage (Budnick, 1984). Such articles should be safely stored away from the infant's reach; forks are best avoided for self-feeding until the child has mastered the spoon, usually by age 18 months.

In addition to hazards such as aspiration from toys, small articles can be placed in the ear or nose, and excessive noise from toys can result in sensorineural hearing loss. Although toys with the highest noise levels are model airplanes, air guns, toy cap guns, and firecrackers, even common squeaking toys used by young children may be harmful if placed close to the ear (Axelsson and Herson, 1985).

Even clothes can present dangers to infants who cannot call attention to the problem. For example, excessively tight bands on socks can cause constriction injuries (Rosen, 1983). Another frequently unrecognized danger to infants is dog attacks. Helpless infants, as newcomers to the home, can provoke jealousy in the animal (Pinckney and Kennedy, 1982). Parents must be constantly vigilant of protecting the child from household pets.

CHILD SAFETY HOME INVENTORY

Safety: Fire, electrical, burns
*Guards in front of or around any heating appliance, fireplace, or furnace
*Electrical wires hidden or out of reach
 No frayed or broken wires
*Plastic guards or caps over electrical outlets, furniture in front of outlets
*Hanging tablecloths out of reach and away from open fires
 Smoke detectors tested and operating properly
*Kitchen matches stored out of child's reach
 Large, deep ashtrays throughout house (if used)
 Small stoves, heaters, and other hot objects (cigarettes, candles, coffee pots) placed where they cannot be tipped over or reached by children
 Hot water heater set to 125° F or lower
 Pot handles turned toward back of stove
 No loose clothing worn near stove
 No cooking or eating with child nearby or in lap
 All small appliances, such as iron, turned off and disconnected when not in use
 Cool, not hot, mist vaporizer used
 Fire extinguisher available and checked periodically
 Electrical fuse box and gas outlet accessible
 Family escape plan in case of a fire, and practiced periodically
 Telephone number of fire or rescue squad posted near phone

Safety: Poisoning
 Toxic substances placed on a high shelf or in locked cabinet
*Toxic plants hung or placed on high surface rather than on floor
 Excess quantities of cleaning fluid, paints, pesticides, drugs, and other toxic substances not stored in home
 Used containers of poisonous substances discarded where child cannot obtain access
 Telephone number of local poison control center posted near phone
 Syrup of ipecac in home, with two doses per child
 Medicines clearly labeled in childproof containers and stored out of reach; old medicines discarded
 Household cleaners, disinfectants, and insecticides kept in their original containers, separate from food and out of reach
 Alcoholic beverages stored out of reach
 Ashtrays empty or kept out of reach

Safety: Suffocation and aspiration
*Small objects stored out of reach
*Toys inspected for small removable parts or long strings
*Plastic bags stored away from young child's reach; large plastic garment bags discarded after tying in a knot
*Mattress or pillow not covered with plastic
*Crib design according to federal regulations with snug-fitting mattress

*Crib positioned away from other furniture or windows
*Button-size batteries stored safely and discarded properly, where child will not have access
*Bathroom doors kept closed and toilet seats down
*Faucets turned off firmly
 Pool fenced, with locked gate
 Proper safety equipment at poolside
 Electric garage door openers stored safely and adjusted to raise when door strikes object
*Doors of ovens, trunks, dishwashers, refrigerators, and front-loading clothes washers and dryers closed at all times
*Unused appliance, such as a refrigerator, securely closed with lock or doors removed
*Food served in small noncylindric pieces to young children
*Toy chests with lids that securely lock in open position
*Pails and buckets kept empty
 Clothesline above head level

Safety: Bodily injury
 Knives, power tools, and unloaded firearms stored safely or placed in locked cabinet
 Garden tools returned to storage racks after use
 Pets properly restrained and immunized for rabies
 Swings, slides, and other outdoor play equipment kept in safe condition
 Yard clear of broken glass, nail-studded boards, and other litter

Safety: Falls
 Nonskid mats, abrasive strips, or textured surfaces in tubs and showers
 Exits, halls, and passageways in rooms kept clear of toys, furniture, boxes, or other items that could be obstructive
 Stairs and halls well lighted, with switches at both top and bottom
 Sturdy handrails for all steps and stairways
 Nothing stored on stairways
 Treads, risers, and carpeting in good repair
 Glass doors and walls marked with decals
 Safety glass used in doors, windows, and walls
*Gates on top and bottom of staircases
*Guardrails on upstairs windows with locks that limit window opening
*Crib siderails raised to full height; mattress lowered as child grows
*Restraints used in high chairs, walkers, or other baby furniture
 Scatter rugs secured in place or used with nonskid backing
 Walks, patios, and driveways in good repair

*Safety measures are specific for homes with young children. All safety measures should be implemented in homes where children reside and visit frequently, such as those of grandparents or babysitters.

Nurse's Role in Injury Prevention

When the potential environmental dangers to which infants are vulnerable are considered, the task of preventing these injuries only begins to be appreciated. Nurses must be aware of the possible causes of injury in each age group in order for *anticipatory* preventive teaching to occur. For example, the guidelines for injury prevention during infancy presented in Table 12-10 should be discussed before the child reaches the susceptible age group. Preventive teaching ideally occurs during pregnancy. Inasmuch as two thirds of all injuries to children occur in the home, the importance of safety cannot be overemphasized. The box on p. 539 summarizes a home safety inventory plan that can be presented to parents to increase their awareness of danger areas in the home and assist them in implementing safety devices and practices *before* their absence can inflict injury on infants. In addition, displays such as a safety demonstration board (Fig. 12-19) can be helpful in familiarizing parents with inexpensive, commercial devices that can be used in the home to prevent injuries.

Injury prevention requires *protection* of the child and *education* of the parents or caregiver. Nurses in ambulatory care settings, health maintenance centers, or visiting nurse agencies are in a most favorable position for injury education. This does not exclude nurses in inpatient facilities, who could use visiting times as an excellent opportunity for discussing this topic.

One approach to teaching injury prevention is to relate why children in various age groups are prone to specific types of injuries. Stressing prevention is just as important as emphasizing the *why* of the injury. However, injury prevention must also be practical. For example, suggesting that *all* potentially toxic substances be locked in a cabinet or placed on a high shelf may be so impractical that no change will occur. Asking parents for their ideas leads to realistic suggestions that can be followed. For instance, bathroom cleaning agents, cosmetics, and personal care items can be placed on a top shelf in the linen closet, and towels or sheets can be stored on the lower shelves and floor.

If an injury has occurred, the nurse should not be too quick to admonish the parent. Injuries do not always indicate neglect. It is a difficult task to watch children carefully without overprotecting or unnecessarily confining them. Small falls help children learn the dangers of heights. Touching a hot object once can emphasize to the child the pain of a burn. Allowing children to explore while maintaining *consistent, age-appropriate limits* is sound advice.

Parents need to remember that infants and young children cannot anticipate danger or understand when it is or is not present. A dead electrical wire may present no actual harm, but if the child is allowed to play with it a poor behavior is enforced and will be practiced when the child encounters a live wire. Although it is always wise to explain why something is dangerous, it must be remembered that small children need to be physically removed from the situation.

It is not easy to teach safety, supervise closely, and re-

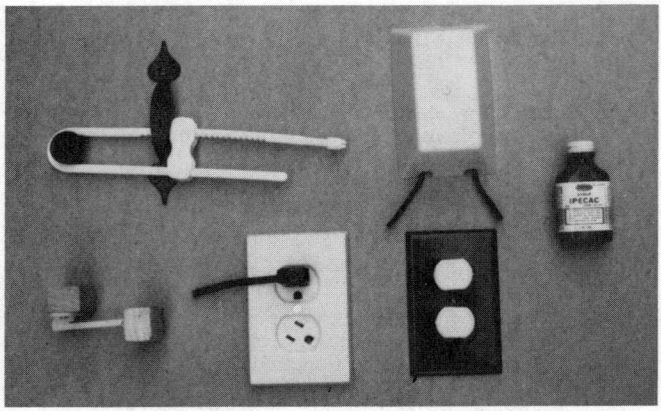

Fig. 12-19. Safety demonstration board (clockwise from lower left): cabinet latch, cabinet lock, shock guard for electric outlet, syrup of ipecac, and two types of outlet covers (white cover is passive device that automatically covers outlet when plug is removed).

frain from saying "no" a hundred times a day. Parents become acutely aware of this dilemma as soon as the infant learns to crawl. Preventing injuries to children is usually the first reason for limit setting and discipline, but also to prevent damage to valuable household objects. When small children are in the home dangerous objects must be removed or guarded and valuable articles placed out of reach. Children, even the youngest crawling infant, will almost always test their parents. It is better to learn a lesson from breaking an inexpensive ashtray than a valuable crystal decanter or by falling off a step stool rather than down a flight of stairs. In either case the lesson is similar, but the price is different.

When children are taught the meaning of "no," they should also be taught what "yes" means. Children should be praised for playing with suitable toys, their efforts at behaving or listening should be reinforced, and recreational toys that are innovative and creative should be provided for them. Infants love to tear paper, and avidly pursue books, magazines, or newspapers left on the floor. Instead of always scolding them for destroying a valued book, old, discarded reading material should be kept available for them to play with. If they enjoy pots and pans, a cabinet can be arranged with safe utensils for them to explore.

One additional factor must be stressed concerning injury prevention and education. Children are imitators; they copy what they see and hear. *Practicing safety teaches safety,* which applies to parents and their children and to nurses and their clients. Saying one thing but doing another confuses children and can lead to difficulties as the child grows older.

ANTICIPATORY GUIDANCE—CARE OF FAMILIES

Childrearing is no easy task; it presents challenges to new parents as well as to "seasoned" parents. With society's changing roles and mores, combined with a highly mobile population, there is little stability for traditional role models

PARENTAL GUIDANCE DURING INFANT'S FIRST YEAR

First 6 months

Understand each parent's adjustment to newborn, especially mother's postpartal emotional needs

Teach care of infant and assist parents to understand his individual needs and temperament and that he expresses his wants through crying

Reassure that infant cannot be spoiled by too much attention during the first 4 to 6 months

Encourage parents to establish a schedule that meets needs of child and themselves

Help parents understand infant's need for stimulation in environment

Support parents' pleasure in seeing child's growing friendliness and social response, especially smiling

Plan anticipatory guidance for safety

Stress need for artificial immunization

Prepare for introduction of solid foods

Second 6 months

Prepare parents for child's "stranger anxiety"

Encourage parents to allow child to cling to mother or father and avoid long separation from either

Guide parents concerning discipline because of infant's increasing mobility

Encourage use of negative voice and eye contact rather than physical punishment as a means of discipline; if unsuccessful, use one slap on the hand

Encourage showing most attention when infant is behaving well, rather than when crying

Teach accident prevention because of child's advancing motor skills and curiosity

Encourage parents to leave child with suitable mother substitute to allow some free time

Discuss readiness for weaning

Explore parents' feelings regarding infant's sleep patterns

infant's habits, sleep routine, and waking activities will yield invaluable information concerning the mother's feelings of caring for her child. This is also the time to begin discussing introduction of new foods and potential sources of injuries in the home.

During the second 6 months the child's increasing dependence on mother and increasing independence through locomotion present major challenges. Preparing parents for the child's fear of strangers and encouraging them to allow the clinging dependent behavior helps minimize potential conflicts. Stressing that such behavior indicates a strong parental attachment focuses on the *positive* aspects of stranger anxiety. Encouraging parents to find a suitable baby-sitter, particularly someone who can visit often, allows them freedom and enjoyment together without feelings of guilt. This is important not only for the child, who learns how to adjust to a crisis, but also for the parents, who need to spend time alone with each other to communicate, to love, and to enjoy one another's company. Time for one another can easily be lost in the responsibilities of raising a family.

As the infant achieves greater skill in all areas of development, safety becomes a major problem. Helping parents *anticipate* potential dangers in the home decreases the possibility of injuries occurring. Limit setting is part of teaching safety, and establishing certain "rules" early helps children learn what is acceptable behavior. Neither a laissez-faire nor a dictator approach to discipline is advisable. A commonsense approach that incorporates understanding, firmness, and consistency by both parents usually yields the best results.

and time-honored methods of raising children. As a result parents look more to professionals for guidance. Nurses are in an advantageous position to render assistance and suggestions. Every phase of a child's life has its particular traumas—toilet training for toddlers, unexplained fears for preschoolers, or identity crises for adolescents. For parents of an infant some challenges center around dependency, discipline, increased mobility, and safety. Major areas for parental guidance during the first year are listed in the box above.

At birth the major task for parents and infant is attachment. Nursing interventions to promote parent attachment to the infant are discussed in Chapter 8. In addition, during the first 6 months there are several important areas of teaching. Parents may not realize the infant's need for stimulation or be aware of how to provide it, and suggestions for suitable toys may be needed (see Table 12-2).

During the early months the infant's social responses, such as smiling, grasping, and vocalizing, should be supported. It is most important that during these first few months parent and child develop reciprocal relationships and meet each other's needs. It may very well be that problems such as maternal deprivation or child abuse begin when two individuals are relating on different levels. Investigating the

CONCEPT SUMMARIES

- Biologic development of the child encompasses proportional changes; sensory changes, including binocularity, depth perception, and visual preference; maturation of biologic systems, fine motor development, and gross motor development.

- Erikson's theory of psychosocial development (birth to 1 year) is concerned with acquiring a sense of trust while overcoming a sense of mistrust.

- Freud's oral stage during infancy involves gratification of the id through oral satisfaction.

- Piaget's theory of cognitive development, as it applies to the infant, focuses on the sensorimotor phase, which includes the use of reflexes, primary circular reactions, secondary circular reactions, and coordination of secondary schemata and their application to new situations.

- Development of body image begins in infancy; by 1 year of age infants recognize that they are distinct from their parents.

- Social development of the infant is guided by attachment, language development, personal-social behavior, and participation in play.

- Temperament is an important indicator of the kind of interaction that occurs between the child and parents and siblings.

- Parents are faced with many concerns, including infant fears, daycare, limit-setting and discipline, thumb-sucking and pacifier use, teething, and choice of infant shoes.

- Breast milk or formula is the most desirable food for the infant during the first 6 months, followed by gradual introduction of solid food during the second 6 months.

- Infants may be prone to sleep disturbances, and the nurse should instruct the parents, after careful assessment, in adjusting the infant's schedule.

- Fluoride supplements and dietary intake promote good dental hygiene.

- Recommended routine immunizations include those for diphtheria, tetanus, pertussis, polio, measles, mumps, rubella, and *Haemophilus influenzae* type B.

- Recommended immunizations for selected groups of children are influenza virus, pneumococcal polysaccharide, and hepatitis B vaccines.

- Because injuries are a major cause of death during infancy, parents should be alerted to aspiration of foreign objects, suffocation, falls, poisoning, burns, motor vehicle injuries, and bodily damage, and preventive actions needed to be taken to make the environment safe for infants.

REFERENCES

Ainsworth, M.: Early caregiving and later patterns of attachment. In Klaus, M., and Robertson, M., editors: Birth, interaction, and attachment, Skillman, N.J., 1982, Johnson & Johnson Baby Products Co.

American Academy of Pediatrics, Committee on Early Childhood, Adoption, and Dependent Care: The pediatrician's role in promoting the health of a patient in day care, Pediatrics 74(1):157-158, 1984a.

American Academy of Pediatrics, Committee on Infectious Diseases: *Haemophilus* type b polysaccharide vaccine, Pediatrics 76(2):322-323, 1985a.

American Academy of Pediatrics, Committee on Infectious Diseases: Prevention of hepatitis B virus infections, Pediatrics 75(2):362-364, 1985b.

American Academy of Pediatrics, Committee on Infectious Diseases: Recommendations for using pneumococcal vaccine in children, Pediatrics 75(6):1153-1158, 1985c.

American Academy of Pediatrics, Committee on Nutrition: Vitamin and mineral supplement needs in normal children in the United States, Pediatrics 66(6):1015-1020, 1980a.

American Academy of Pediatrics, Committee on Nutrition: On the feeding of supplemental foods to infants, Pediatrics 65(6):1178-1181, 1980b.

American Academy of Pediatrics, Committee on Nutrition: The use of whole cow's milk in infancy, Pediatrics 72(2):253-255, 1983a.

American Academy of Pediatrics, Committee on Nutrition: Toward a prudent diet for children, Pediatrics 71(1):78-80, 1983b.

American Academy of Pediatrics, Committee on Nutrition: Imitation and substitute milks, Pediatrics 73(6):876, 1984b.

Anderson, G.: Pacifiers: the positive side, Am. J. Maternal Child Nurs. 11(2):122-124, 1986.

Axelsson, A., and Jerson, T.: Noisy toys: a possible source of sensorineural hearing loss, Pediatrics 76(4):574-578, 1985.

Baker, S.P., and Fisher, R.S.: Childhood asphyxiation by choking or suffocation, JAMA 244(12):1343-1346, 1980.

Ballard, P.: Breast-feeding for the working mother, Issues Compr. Pediatr. Nurs. 6:249-259, 1983.

Baraff, L.J., Cody, C.L., and Cherry, J.D.: DTP-associated reactions: an analysis by injection site, manufacturer, prior reactions, and dose, Pediatrics 73(1):31-36, 1984.

Bernier, R.H., Frank, J.A., and Nolan, T.F.: Abscesses complicating DTP vaccination, Am. J. Dis. Child. 135:826-828, Sept. 1981.

Biggar, M.: Maternal aversion to mother-infant contact. In Brown, C., editor: The many facets of touch, 1984, Skillman, N.J., Johnson & Johnson Baby Products Co.

Bloch, A.B., and others: Health impact of measles vaccination in the United States, Pediatrics 76(4):524-532, 1985.

Blosser, C.: Avoiding potential behavior problems in children, Pediatr. Nurs. 5(3):11-15, 1979.

Bowlby, J.: Attachment and loss, vol. 1, Attachment, New York, 1969, Basic Books, Inc.

Budnick, L.D.: Toothpick-related injuries in the United States, 1979 through 1982, JAMA 252(6):796-797, 1984.

Campbell, S.B.G.: Mother-infant interaction as a function of maternal ratings of temperament, Child Psychiatry Human Dev. 10(2):67-76, 1979.

Carey, W.: Intervention strategies using temperament data. In Brown, C.C., editor: Infants at risk: assessment and intervention, Skillman, N.J., 1981, Johnson & Johnson Baby Products Co.

Carey, W.B.: Clinical applications of infant temperament measurements, J. Pediatr. 81(4):823-828, 1972.

Carey, W.B.: Night waking and temperament in infancy, J. Pediatr. 84(5):756-758, 1974.

Carey, W.B., and McDevitt, S.C.: Revision of the infant temperament questionnaire, Pediatrics 61(5):735-739, 1978.

Chabin, M.: Hospital-supported child care, Am. J. Nurs. 83(4):548-551, 1983.

Chess, S., and Thomas, A.: Temperamental differences: a critical concept in child health care, Pediatr. Nurs. 11(3):167-171, 1985.

Eland, J.: Minimizing pain associated with prekindergarten intramuscular injections, Issues Compr. Pediatr. Nurs. 5:361-372, 1981.

Elias, M., and others: Sleep/wake patterns of breast-fed infants in the first 2 years of life, Pediatrics 77(3):322-329, 1986.

Ferber, R.: Diagnosis and treatment of sleep disorders in childhood, Pediatr. Basics 39:7-14, 1984.

Fulginiti, V.A.: Patient education for immunizations, Pediatrics (suppl.) 74(5):961-963, 1984.

Garmezy, N., and Rutter, M., editors: Stress, coping, and development in children, New York, 1983, McGraw-Hill Book Co.

Harris, C.S., and others: Childhood asphyxiation by food, JAMA 251:2231-2235, 1984.

Hayden, G.F.: Measles vaccine failure, Clin. Pediatr. 18(3):155-167, 1979.

Hepatitis B vaccine: where to inject it, Am. J. Nurs. 85(11):1268, 1985.

Herman, J.J., Radin, R., and Schneiderman, R.: Allergic reactions to measles (rubeola) vaccine in patients hypersensitive to egg protein, J. Pediatr. 102(2):196-199, 1983.

Hinman, A.R.: Prevention of congenital rubella infection: symposium summary, Pediatrics 75(6):1162-1165, 1985.

Hinman, A.R., and Koplan, J.P.: Pertussis and pertussis vaccine, JAMA 251(23):3109-3113, 1984.

Kliman, D.S., and Vukelich, C.: Mothers and fathers: expectations for infants, Fam. Rel. 34:305-313, 1985.

Kronstadt, D., and others: Infant behavior and maternal adaptations in the first six months of life, Am. J. Orthopsychiatry 49(3):454-464, 1979.

Lawrence, R.A.: Breast-feeding, ed. 2, St. Louis, 1985, The C.V. Mosby Co.

Lester, B.M.: There's more to crying than meets the ear, Child Care Newsletter 2(2):1-4, 1983.

Lincoln, L.M.: Fathering and the separation-individuation process, Maternal Child Nurs. J. 13(2):103-111, 1984.

Little, D.L.: Parent acceptance of routine use of the Carey and McDevitt Infant Temperament Questionnaire, Pediatrics 71:104-106, 1983.

Little, D.L.: Written explanation of temperament scores, Pediatrics **75**(2):275-277, 1985.

Litovitz, T.L.: Battery ingestions: product accessibility and clinical course, Pediatrics **75**(3):469-476, 1985.

Long, S.S.: Epidemiologic study of infant botulism in Pennsylvania: report of the Infant Botulism Study Group, Pediatrics **75**(5):928-934, 1985.

Lozoff, B., Wolf, A.W., and Davis, N.S.: Cosleeping in urban families with young children in the United States, Pediatrics **74**(2):171-182, 1984.

MacLaughlin, S., and Strelnick, E.G.: Breast-feeding and working outside the home, Issues Compr. Pediatr. Nurs. **7**(1):67-81, 1984.

Merrifield, E.B., and Ryberg, J.W.: What parents should know about pacifiers, Child. Nurse **3**(4):1-3, 1985.

Millunchick, E., and McArtor, R.: Fatal aspiration of a makeshift pacifier, Pediatrics **77**(3):369-370, l986.

Mofenson, H.C., and others: Baby powder—a hazard! Pediatrics **68**(2):265-266, 1981.

Montalto, M.B., Benson, J.D., and Martinez, G.A.: Nutrient intakes of formula-fed infants and infants fed cow's milk, Pediatrics **75**(2):343-351, 1985.

Nelms, B.C.: Attachment versus spoiling, Pediatr. Nurs. **9**(1):49-51, 1983.

Nelms, B.C.: Stress during childhood: long-lasting effects? Pediatr. Nurs. **11**(2):95-98, 1985.

Pinckney, L.E., and Kennedy, L.A.: Traumatic deaths from dog attacks in the United States, Pediatrics **69**(2):193-196, 1982.

Pipes, P.L.: Nutrition in infancy and childhood, ed. 3, St. Louis, 1985, The C.V. Mosby Co.

Pittard, W.B., III, and others: Bacteriostatic qualities of human milk, J. Pediatr. **107**(2):240-243, 1985.

Recommendation of the Advisory Committee on Immunization Practices (ACIP): Smallpox vaccine, MMWR **29**(35):417, 1980.

Recommendation of the Immunization Practices Advisory Committee (ACIP): Diphtheria, tetanus, and pertussis: guidelines for vaccine prophylaxis and other preventive measures, MMWR **34**(27):405-426, 1985a.

Recommendation of the Immunization Practices Advisory Committee (ACIP): Influenza virus vaccine, MMWR **34**:261-275, 1985b.

Recommendation of the Immunization Practices Advisory Committee (ACIP): Polysaccharide vaccine for prevention of *Haemophilus influenzae* type b disease, MMWR **34**(15):201-205, 1985c.

Reifsnider, E., and Myers, S.T.: Employed mothers can breast-feed, too! Am. J. Maternal Child Nurs. **10**:256-259, 1985.

Roberts, F.B.: Infant behavior and the transition to parenthood, Nurs Res. **32**(4):213-217, 1983.

Robertson, J.: Young children in hospitals, New York, 1958, Basic Books, Inc.

Rosen, R.: Stocking constriction injuries, J. Pediatr. **103**(6):937, 1983.

Rutter, M.: Stress, coping and development: some issues and some questions, J. Child Psychol. Psychiatry **22**(4):323-356, 1981.

Sando, W.C., Gallaher, K.J., and Rodgers, B.M.: Risk factors for microwave scald injuries in infants, J. Pediatr. **105**(6):864, 1984.

Schmitt, B.D.: Infants who do not sleep through the night, Dev. Behav. Pediatr. **2**(1):20-23, 1981.

Shea, V., and Fowler, M.G.: Parental and pediatric trainee knowledge of development, Dev. Behav. Pediatr. **4**(1):21-25, 1983.

Sherwen, L.N.: Separation: the forgotten phenomenon of child development, Topics Clin. Nurs. **5**(1):1-11, 1983.

Spitz, R.A.: Hospitalism: an inquiry into the genesis of psychiatric conditioning in early childhood. In Fenechel, D., and others, editors: Psychoanalytic studies of the child, vol. 1, New York, 1945, International University Press.

Stafford, E.M.: Flying, peanuts, and crying babies, Pediatrics **76**(6):1018, 1985.

Stoffman, J.M., and others: Injuries to children from vehicles with wheels: baby walkers . . ., Can. Med. Assoc. J. **131**:573-575, 1984.

Sullivan, K.M., and others: Mumps disease and its health impact: an outbreak-based report, Pediatrics **76**(4):533-536, 1985.

Thomas, A., and Chess, S.: Genesis and evolution of behavioral disorders: from infancy to early adult life, Am. J. Psychiatry **141**(1):1-9, 1984.

Ventura, J.N.: Parent coping behaviors, parent functioning, and infant temperament characteristics, Nurs. Res. **31**(5):269-273, 1982.

Wagner, T.J., and Hindi-Alexander, M.: Hazards of baby powder?, Pediatr. Nurs. **10**(2):124-125, 1984.

Weibel, R.E., and others: Live attenuated varicella virus vaccine, N. Engl. J. Med. **310**(22):1409-1415, 1984.

Weiss, J., and others: Purchasing infant shoes: attitudes of parents, pediatricians, and store managers, Pediatrics **67**(5):718-720, 1981.

Weissbluth, M.: Sleep duration and infant temperament, J. Pediatr. **99**(5):817-819, 1981.

Wenger, D.R.: Baby needs shoes! Foot Ankle **3**:207, 1983.

Wilson, A.L., Witzke, D.B., and Volin, A.: What it means to "spoil" a baby: parents' perception, Clin. Pediatr. **20**(12):798-802, 1981.

Yeager, A.S., and others: Need for measles revaccination in adolescents: correlation with birth date prior to 1972, J. Pediatr. **102**(2):191-195, 1983.

BIBLIOGRAPHY
Growth and Development

Baumann, S.: Physical aspects of the self: a review of some aspects of body image development in childhood, Psychiatr. Clin. North Am. **4**(3):455-470, 1981.

Belfer, M., and Lukens, P.: Body image: impacts and distortions. In Levine, M., and others, editors: Developmental-behavioral pediatrics, Philadelphia, l983, W.B. Saunders Co.

Brown, M., and Murphy, M.: A child grows, Pediatr. Nurs. **1**(1):9, 1975.

Brown, M., and Murphy, M.: A child grows. Part II. How the child grows and develops psychologically, socially, and culturally, Pediatr. Nurs. **1**(2):22-30, 1975.

Brown, M., and Murphy, M.: A child grows. Part III. The child's cognitive development, Pediatr. Nurs. **1**(3):7-12, 1975.

Brown, M., and Murphy, M.: A child grows. Part IV. The child's perceptual and linguistic development, Pediatr. Nurs. **9**(4):15, 1975.

Buckler, J.M.: A reference manual of growth and development, London, 1978, Blackwell Scientific Publications.

Carey, W.B.: A simplified method for measuring infant temperament, J. Pediatr. **77**(2):188-194, 1970.

Chance, P.: Learning through play, Skillman, N.J., 1979, Johnson & Johnson Baby Products Co.

Chase, R.A., and Rubin, R.R.: The first wondrous year, New York, 1979, Macmillan Publishing Co., Inc.

Coley, I.L.: Pediatric assessment of self-care activities, St. Louis, 1978, The C.V. Mosby Co.

Erikson, E.: Childhood and society, ed. 2, New York, 1963, W.W. Norton & Co., Inc.

Filer, L.J.: Studies of taste preference in infancy and childhood, Pediatr. Basics **12**:5-9, 1975.

Fraiberg, S.: The magic years, New York, 1968, Charles Scribner's Sons.

Illingworth, R.S.: Development of the infant and young child, ed. 7, New York, 1980, Churchill Livingstone, Inc.

Kaluger, G., and Kaluger, M.F.: Human development: the span of life, ed. 2, St. Louis, 1979, The C.V. Mosby Co.

Knobloch, H., and Pasamanick, B.: Gesell and Amatruda's developmental diagnosis, New York, 1974, Harper & Row, Publishers, Inc.

Lowrey, G.H.: Growth and development of children, ed. 7, Chicago, 1978, Year Book Medical Publishers, Inc.

Maier, H.: Three theories of child development, ed. 3, New York, 1978, Harper & Row, Publishers, Inc.

Newman, B., and Newman, P.: Development through life: a psychosocial approach, Homewood, IL, 1984, The Dorsey Press.

Papalia, D., and Olds, S.: A child's world, infancy through adolescence, New York, 1979, McGraw-Hill Book Co.

Piaget, J.: The construction of reality in the child, New York, 1975, Ballantine Books, Inc.

Reilly, A.P., editor: The communication game, Skillman, N.J., 1980, Johnson & Johnson Baby Products Co.

Stern, D.: Play and learning in the first year: new insights, Pediatr. Nurs. 5(5):37, 1979.

Taft, L.T., and Cohen, H.J.: Neonatal and infant reflexology. In Hellmuth, J., editor: Exceptional infant, vol. 1. The normal infant, Seattle, 1976, Special Child Publishers.

Thomas, E.B., and Trotter, S.: Social responsiveness of infants, Skillman, N.J., 1978, Johnson & Johnson Baby Products Co.

Zigler, E., and Lang, M.E.: The emergence of ''superbaby'': a good thing? Pediatr. Nurs. 11(5):337-342, 1985.

Attachment/Temperament

Als, H.: Assessing infant individuality. In Brown, C.C., editor: Infants at risk, Skillman, N.J., 1981, Johnson & Johnson Baby Products Co.

Bird, H.R.: Stranger reaction versus stranger anxiety, J. Am. Acad. Psychoanal. 8(4):555-563, 1980.

Blank, D.M.: Development of the infant tenderness scale, Nurs. Res. 34(4):211-216, 1985.

Brewer, J.M.H.: The revised infant temperament scale. In Humenick, S.S., editor: Analysis of current assessment strategies in the health care of young children and childbearing families, Norwalk, CT, 1982, Appleton-Century-Crofts.

Campbell, S.B.: Mother-infant interaction as a function of maternal ratings of temperament, Child Psychiatry Human Dev. 10(2):67-76, 1979.

Carey, W.B.: Measuring infant temperament, J. Pediatr. 96(3):423-425, 1980.

Carey, W.B., and McDevitt, S.C.: Stability and change in individual temperament diagnoses from infancy to early childhood, Am. Acad. Child Psychiatry 17:331-337, Spring 1978.

Chamberlin, R.: Behavioral problems and their prevention, Pediatr. Rev. 2(1):13-18, 1980.

Harris, C.H.: Assessment of children's behavior. In Johnson, S.M., editor: Nursing assessment and strategies for the family at risk, New York, 1986, J.B. Lippincott Co.

Harris, F.G.: Strategies for parenting during the early stages of a child's life, Issues Ment. Health Nurs. 2(3):71-84, 1980.

Klaus, M., and Kennell, J.: Parent-infant bonding, ed. 2, St. Louis, 1982, The C.V. Mosby Co.

Kronstadt, D., and others: Infant behavior and maternal adaptations in the first six months of life, Am. J. Orthopsychiatry 49(3):454-464, 1979.

Persson-Blennow, I., and McNeil, T.F.: A questionnaire for measurement of temperament in six-month-old infants: development and standardization, J. Child Psychol. Psychiatry 20:1-13, 1979.

Powell, M.L.: Assessment of infant temperament. In Powell, M.L., editor: Assessment and management of developmental changes and problems in children, ed. 2, St. Louis, 1981, The C.V. Mosby Co.

Scholom, A., Zucker, R.A., and Stollak, G.E.: Relating early child adjustment to infant and parent temperament, J. Abnorm. Child Psychol. 7(3):297-308, 1979.

Skerrett, K., Hardin, S.B., and Puskar, K.R.: Infant anxiety, Maternal Child Nurs. J. 12(1):51-59, 1983.

Snyder, C., Eyres, S.J., and Barnard, K.: New findings about mothers' antenatal expectations and their relationship to infant development, Am. J. Maternal Child Nurs. 4(6):354-357, 1979.

Thomas, A., and Chess, S.: Temperament and development, New York, 1977, Brunner/Mazel, Inc.

Vaughn, B., Deinard, A., and Egeland, B.: Measuring temperament in pediatric practice, J. Pediatr. 96(3):510-514, 1980.

Wolman, B.B.: Children's fears, New York, 1978, Grosset & Dunlap.

Concerns Related to Growth and Development

For bibliography on daycare, see Chapter 15.

Bradshaw, T.W.: Teething, Pediatr. Nurs. 7(3):41-42, 1981.

Cowell, H.R.: Shoes and shoe corrections, Pediatr. Clin. North Am. 24(4):719-720, 1977.

Fletcher, B.T.: Etiology of fingersucking: review of literature, J. Dent. Child 42:293-298, 1975.

Hawkins, A.C.: A constructive approach to thumbsucking habit, J. Clin. Orthod. 12:846-848, 1978.

McDonald, R.: Dentistry for the child and adolescent, ed. 3, St. Louis, 1978, The C.V. Mosby Co.

Musselman, R.J.: Oral facial development and oral habits, Pediatr. Basics 30:12-14, 1981.

Paynter, A.S., and Alexander, F.W.: Salicylate intoxication caused by teething ointment, Lancet 2(8152):1132, 1979.

Swann, I.L.: Teething complications, a persisting misconception, Postgrad. Med. J. 55:24-25, Jan. 1979.

Nutrition

American Academy of Pediatrics and American Academy of Pedodontics: Juice in ready-to-use bottles and nursing bottle caries, News Comment 29(1):11, 1978.

American Academy of Pediatrics, Committee on Infectious Diseases: Raw milk, News Comment 31(3):9, 1980.

American Academy of Pediatrics, Committee on Nutrition: Iron supplementation for infants, Pediatrics 58(5):765, 1976.

American Academy of Pediatrics, Committee on Nutrition: Fluoride supplementation: Pediatrics 77(5):758-761, 1986.

American Academy of Pediatrics, Committee on Nutrition: Sodium intake of infants in the U.S., Pediatrics 68(3):444-445, 1981.

American Academy of Pediatrics, Committee on Nutrition: Pediatric nutrition handbook, ed. 2, Elk Grove Village, IL, 1985, The Academy.

Andrew, E.M., Clancy, K.L., and Katz, M.G.: Infant feeding practices of families belonging to a prepaid group practice health care plan, Pediatrics 65(5):978-988, 1980.

Anholm, P.C.H.: Breastfeeding: a preventive approach to health care in infancy, Issues Compr. Pediatr. Nurs. 9(1):1-10, 1986.

Barness, L.A.: Infant feeding: formula, solids, Pediatr. Clin. North Am. 32(2):355-362, 1985.

Beaton, G.H.: Nutritional needs during the first year of life: some concepts and perspectives, Pediatr. Clin. North Am. 32(2):275-288, 1985.

Bishop, W.S.: Weaning the breast-fed toddler or preschooler, Pediatr. Nurs. 11(3):211-214, 1985.

Butte, N.F., and others: Human milk intake and growth in exclusively breast-fed infants, J. Pediatr. 104(2):187-195, 1984.

Crummette, B., and Munton, M.: Mothers' decisions about infant nutrition, Pediatr. Nurs. 6(6):16-19, 1980.

Current issues in feeding the normal infant, Pediatrics (suppl.) 75(1):135-181, 1985.

Dusdieker, L.B., and others: Effect of supplemental fluids on human milk production, J. Pediatr. 106(2):207-211, 1985.

Finberg, L.: Human milk feeding and vitamin D supplementation, J. Pediatr. 99(2):228-229, 1981.

Fomon, S.J., and others: Recommendations for feeding normal infants, Pediatrics 63(1):52-59, 1979.

Fried, R.I.: One hundred years of infant feeding, Clin. Pediatr. 16(3):215-218, 1977.

Humphrey, N.: Common questions about breast-feeding, Child. Nurse 3(2):1-3, 1985.

Katcher, A.L., and Lanese, M.G.: Breast-feeding by employed mothers: a reasonable accommodation in the work place, Pediatrics 75(4):644-647, 1985.

Lawrence, R.A.: Breast-feeding, ed. 2, St. Louis, 1985, The C.V. Mosby Co.

Lieberman, E.: Hypertension and infant feeding, Dialogues Infant Nutr. 1(7):1-4, 1978.

Lindquist, B.: Recent views on infant nutrition, Paediatrician 8(suppl. 1): 37-47, 1979.

Martinez, G.A., and Ryan, A.S.: Nutrient intake in the United States during the first 12 months of life, J. Am. Diet. Assoc. 85(7):826-830, 1985.

Martinez, G.A., Ryan, A.S., and Malec, D.J.: Nutrient intakes of American infants and children fed cow's milk or infant formula, Am. J. Dis. Child. 139:1010-1018, 1985.

Mittleman, R.: Need for iron supplementation in infants on prolonged breast feeding, J. Pediatr. **94**(2):346, 1979.

Morse, W., Sims, L.S., and Guthrie, H.A.: Mothers' compliance with physicians' recommendations on infant feeding, J. Am. Diet. Assoc. **75**:140-148, Aug. 1979.

Report of the Task Force on the Assessment of the Scientific Evidence Relating to Infant-Feeding Practices and Infant Health, Pediatrics (suppl.) **74**(4):579-762, 1984.

Ross, L.: Weaning practices, J. Nurse-Midwifery **26**(1):9-14, 1981.

Saarinen, U.M.: Need for iron supplementation in infants on prolonged breast feeding, J. Pediatr. **93**(2):177-180, 1978.

Satter, E.: Developmental guidelines for feeding infants and young children, Food Nutr. News **56**(4):21-26, 1984.

Shulman, R.J., and others: Utilization of dietary cereal by young infants, J. Pediatr. **103**(1):23-28, 1983.

Siimes, M.A., Salmenpera, L., and Perheentupa, J.: Exclusive breast-feeding for 9 months: risk of iron deficiency, J. Pediatr. **104**(2):196-199, 1984.

Singer, L., and Ophaug, R.: Total fluoride intake of infants, Pediatrics **63**(3):460-466, 1979.

Sleep and Activity

Anders, T., and Keener, M.: Sleep-wake development and disorders of sleep. In Levine, M., and others, editors: Developmental-behavioral pediatrics, Philadelphia, 1983, W.B. Saunders Co.

Christophersen, E.R.: Incorporating behavioral pediatrics into primary care, Pediatr. Clin. North Am. **29**(2):261-296, 1982.

Clark, M.K.: Exercise and physical fitness for good health in children, Child. Nurse **4**(1):1-3, 1986.

Edgil, A.E., Wood, K.R., and Smith, D.P.: Sleep problems of older infants and preschool children, Pediatr. Nurs. **11**(2):87-89, 1985.

Lozoff, B., Wolf, A.W., and Davis, N.S.: Sleep problems seen in pediatric practice, Pediatrics **75**(3):477-483, 1985.

Osterholm, P., Lindeke, L.L., and Amidon, D.: Sleep disturbance in infants aged 6 to 12 months, Pediatr. Nurs. **9**(4):269-271, 1983.

Powell, M.L.: Sleep. In Powell, M.L., editor: Assessment and management of developmental changes and problems in children, ed. 2, St. Louis, 1981, The C.V. Mosby Co.

Romanko, M.V., and Brost, B.A.: Swaddling: an effective invention for pacifying infants, Pediatr. Nurs. **8**(4):259-261, 1982.

Weissbluth, M., Davis, A.T., and Poncher, J.: Night waking in 4- to 8-month-old infants, J. Pediatr. **104**(3):477-480, 1984.

Younger, J.B.: The management of night waking in older infants, Pediatr. Nurs. **8**(3):155-158, 1982.

Dental Health

For bibliography, see Chapter 14.

Immunizations

American Academy of Pediatrics, Committee on Infectious Diseases: Revised recommendations on rubella vaccine, Pediatrics **65**(6):1182-1184, 1980.

American Academy of Pediatrics, Committee on Infectious Diseases: Screening tests for tuberculosis, News Comment **30**(1):7, 1979.

American Academy of Pediatrics: Report of the Committee on Infectious Diseases, ed. 20, Elk Grove Village, IL, 1986, The Academy.

Baraff, L.J., and others: Immunologic response to early and routine DTP immunization in infants, Pediatrics **73**(1):37-42, 1984.

Barkin, R.M., and others: Pediatric diphtheria and tetanus toxoids vaccine: clinical and immunologic response when administered as the primary series, J. Pediatr. **106**(5):779-781, 1985.

Bindler, R.M.: Truths and trends in immunization, Child. Nurse **2**(1):1-4, 1984.

Butler, A.B., and others: The immunoglobulin response to reimmunization with rubella vaccine, J. Pediatr. **99**(4):531-534, 1981.

Chilton, L.A.: Inexpensive method of increasing immunization rates, Pediatrics **66**(5):800-801, 1980.

Chin, J.: Prevention of chronic hepatitis B virus infection from mothers to infants in the United States, Pediatrics **71**(2):289-292, 1983.

Choices in polio immunization, Emerg. Med. **14**(9):97-103, 1982.

Church, J., and Richards, W.: Recurrent abscess formation following DTP immunizations: association with hypersensitivity to tetanus toxoid, Pediatrics **75**(5):899-900, 1985.

Claypool, J.M.: Rubella protection for maternal child health care providers, Am. J. Maternal Child Nurs. **6**(1):53-56, 1981.

Cody, C.C., and others: Nature and rates of adverse reactions associated with DTP and DT immunizations in infants and children, Pediatrics **68**(5):650-660, 1981.

English, P.C.: Diphtheria and theories of infectious disease: centennial appreciation of the critical role of diphtheria in the history of medicine, Pediatrics **76**(1):1-9, 1985.

Fulginiti, V.: Curent topics in immunization, Pediatr. Consult. **4**(2):1-8, 1985.

Granoff, D.M., and Cates, K.L.: *Haemophilus influenzae* type b polysaccharide vaccines, J. Pediatr. **107**(3):330-336, 1985.

Henderson, D.A.: The saga of smallpox eradication: an end and a beginning, Can. J. Public Health **70**:21-27, Jan./Feb. 1979.

Hull, H.F., and others: Risk factors for measles vaccine failure among immunized students, Pediatrics **76**(4):518-523, 1985.

Mansell, K.A.: New immunization against *H. influenzae* type b, Pediatr. Nurs. **11**:433-435, 1985.

Marcuse, E.K.: Pediatricians' immunization consent practice, Washington State, Pediatrics **63**(3):419-422, 1979.

Marshall, G., and others: Diffuse retinopathy following measles, mumps, and rubella vaccination, Pediatrics **76**(6):989-991, 1985.

McGraw, T.T.: Reimmunization following early immunization with measles vaccine: a prospective study, Pediatrics **77**(1):45-48, 1986.

Moxon, R.: *Haemophilus influenzae* vaccine, Pediatrics **77**(2):258-260, 1986.

Pajares, K.F., Parks, B.R., Jr., and Fischer, R.G.: Rubella vaccination, Pediatr. Nurs. **10**(1):72, 1984.

Recommendation of the Immunization Practices Advisory Committee (ACIP): Postexposure prophylaxis of hepatitis B, MMWR **33**:285-287, 1984.

Recommendation of the Immunization Practices Advisory Committee (ACIP): Inactivated hepatitis B virus vaccine, MMWR **31**(24):317-328, 1982.

Reichman, L.B.: Tuberculin skin testing: the state of the art, Chest **76**(suppl.):764-770, 1979.

Sabin, A.B.: Immunization: evaluation of some currently available and prospective vaccines, JAMA **246**(3):236-241, 1981.

Scott, R.M., and others: Ineffectiveness of historical data in predicting measles susceptibility, Pediatrics **73**(6):777-780, 1984.

Sherrod, J.L., and others: Effect of timing of measles vaccination on compliance with immunizations during the second year of life, J. Pediatr. **102**(2):186-190, 1983.

Smolen, P., and others: Antibody response to oral polio vaccine in premature infants, J. Pediatr. **103**(6):917-919, 1983.

Stetler, H.C., and others: History of convulsions and use of pertussis vaccine, J. Pediatr. **107**(2):175-179, 1985.

Tafuro, P., and Gurevich, I.: Prevention and management of varicella in high-risk individuals, Am. J. Maternal Child Nurs. **9**(5):314-317, 1984.

Injury Prevention

For additional citations, see bibliography Chapters 1 and 14.

American Academy of Pediatrics, Committee on Pediatric Aspects of Physical Fitness, Recreation, and Sports: Swimming instruction for infants, Pediatrics 65(4):847, 1980.

Bass, J.L., and others: Educating parents about injury prevention, Pediatr. Clin. North Am. 32(1):233-243, 1985.

Bausell, R.B.: A national survey assessing pediatric preventive behaviors, Pediatr. Nurs. 11:438-442, 1985.

Berger, L.R., and others: Promoting the use of car safety devices for infants: an intensive health education approach, Pediatrics 74(1):16-19, 1984.

Berger, L.R., and Kalishman, S.: Floor furnace burns to children, Pediatrics 71(1):97-99, 1983.

Bergeson, P.S., Hernreid, C.S., and Sonntag, P.L.: Infant strangulation, Pediatrics 59(6):1043-1045, 1977.

Bergman, A.: Use of education in preventing injuries, Pediatr. Clin. North Am. 29(2):331-338, 1982.

Cotton, W.H., and Davidson, P.J.: Aspiration of baby powder, N. Engl. J. Med. 313:1662, 1985.

Dershewitz, R.A., and Christophersen, E.R.: Childhood household safety, Am. J. Dis. Child. 138:85-88, 1984.

DeSwarte, J.: Nursing's responsibility in promoting the use of car safety seats for children, Home Health Care 2(1):23-25, 1984.

Feldman, K.W.: Prevention of childhood accidents: recent progress, Pediatr. Rev. 2(3):75-82, 1980.

Feldman, K.W., and Simms, R.J.: Strangulation in childhood: epidemiology and clinical course, Pediatrics 65(6):1079-1085, 1980.

Feldman, K.W., and others: Tap water scald burns in children, Pediatrics 62(1):1-7, 1978.

Gallagher, S.S., Hunter, P., and Guyer, B.: A home injury prevention program for children, Pediatr. Clin. North Am. 32(1):95-112, 1985.

Geddis, D.C., and Appleton, I.C.: Establishment and evaluation of a pilot child car seat rental scheme in New Zealand, Pediatrics 77(2):167-172, 1986.

Greensher, J., and Mofenson, H.C.: Injuries at play, Pediatr. Clin. North Am. 32(1):127-139, 1985.

Greensher, J., and Mofenson, H.C.: Aspiration accidents: choking and drowning, Pediatr. Ann. 12(10):747-750, 1983.

Holland, S.H.: Car safety for infants, Child. Nurse 2(5):1-3, 1984.

Johnson, N.: Pacifiers: safety and security, Pediatr. Nurs. 4(6):58-60, 1978.

Kavanagh, C.A., and Banco, L.: The infant walker: a previously unrecognized health hazard, Am. J. Dis. Child. 136:205-206, March 1982.

King, K., Negus, K., and Vance, J.C.: Heat stress in motor vehicles: a problem in infancy, Pediatrics 68(4):579-582, 1981.

Krassner, L.S.: Child restraint devices, Pediatr. Ann. 12(10):733-736, 1983.

Kravath, R.E.: A lethal pacifier, Pediatrics 58(6):853-855, 1976.

Kravath, R.E., and others: Prevention of childhood accidents by eliminating the agent of injury, J. Pediatr. 99(4):575-576, 1981.

Lipe, H.P.: Prevention of nervous system trauma from travel in motor vehicles, J. Neurosurg. Nurs. 17(2):77-82, 1985.

Marcus, D.F.: Child car seats: a must for safety, Pediatr. Nurs. 7(3):13-17, 1981.

Miller, R.E., and others: Pediatric counseling and subsequent use of smoke detectors, Am. J. Public Health 72:392-393, 1982.

Mofenson, H.C., and Greensher, J.: Management of the choking child, Pediatr. Clin. North Am. 32(1):183-192, 1985.

Nachem, B., and Bass, R.A.: Children still aren't being buckled up, Am. J. Maternal Child Nurs. 9(5):320-323, 1984.

Post, C., and Robinson, J.: A "good beginning" for families, Pediatr. Nurs. 6(4):32-36, 1980.

Puczynski, M., Rademaker, D., and Gatson, R.L.: Burn injury related to the improper use of a microwave oven, Pediatrics 72:714-715, 1983.

Reinhard, S.C.: Nursing responsibility in infant car safety, Am. J. Maternal Child Nurs. 5(1):26, 1980.

Roberts, K.B., and Roberts, E.C.: The automobile and heat stress, Pediatrics 58(1):101-104, 1976.

Rumack, B.H.: Diapers and poisons, JAMA 248:2164, 1982.

Shelness, A., and Charles, S.: Children and car seats, Pediatrics 77(2):256-258, 1986.

Sinal, S.H., and Stanton, W.A.: Infant strangulation in a mesh portable crib, Pediatrics 63(4):669-670, 1979.

Surveyer, J.A., and Halpern, J.: Age-related burn injuries and their prevention, Pediatr. Nurs. 7(5):29-34, 1981.

Temple, D.M., and McNeese, M.C.: Hazards of battery ingestion, Pediatrics 71(1):100-103, Jan. 1983.

Toy Safety—United States, 1984, MMWR 34:755-756, 1985.

Tron, V.A., Baldwin, V.J., and Pirie, G.E.: Hot tub drownings, Pediatrics 74(4):789-790, 1985.

Wagner, T.J., and Hindi-Alexander, M.: Hazards of baby powder? Pediatr. Nurs. 10(2):124-125, 1984.

Walker, S., and Middelkamp, J.N.: Pail immersion accidents, Clin. Pediatr. 20(5):341-343, 1981.

Yamamoto, L.G., and Wiebe, R.A.: Survey of childhood burns in Hawaii, Pediatr. Emerg. Care 1(3):120-122, 1985.

Yanofsky, N.N., and Morain, W.D.: Upper extremity burns from woodstoves, Pediatrics 73(5):722-726, 1984.

Chapter 13

Health Problems During Infancy

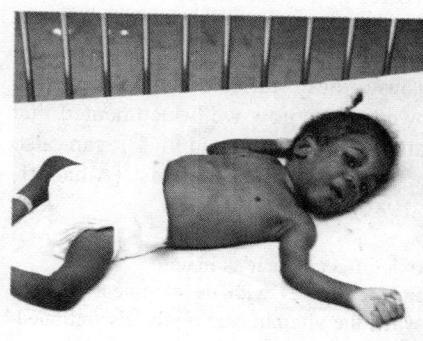

The infant's immature physiologic system predisposes to several potential health problems during the first year. This chapter deals primarily with health problems that are influenced by environmental factors affecting the physical or psychologic development of the child. Some of the problems, such as nutritional disturbances, have special implications for nurses because they are preventable. Others, such as sudden infant death syndrome (SIDS), are uncontrollable and unpredictable, but the intervention needed after the death of the child is crucial for the reintegration of the family. Although several of the topics discussed here can occur in age-groups other than infancy, the greatest significance of these disorders is evident during the early months and years of life. Prompt awareness and identification of health problems hopefully will avert complications in later life. Prevention, whenever possible, rather than treatment should be every health professional's goal in the care of children.

Nutritional Disturbances

Malnutrition is a general term that refers to poor or inadequate nutrition. Although it is generally thought of in terms of undernutrition, it also includes overnutrition, which may be manifested as obesity or hypervitaminosis. Inadequate nutrition is most commonly seen as iron-deficiency anemia (see Chapter 35), vitamin deficiencies, or failure to thrive. The most severe states of malnutrition, involving protein and calorie deficiencies, are kwashiorkor and marasmus. Each of these are related to a wide variety of factors—economic, social, and cultural. While poverty is the economic precursor of malnutrition, it is usually when certain cultural and social factors coincide with poverty that malnutrition becomes a threat. Culture influences food selection and may limit certain nutritious foods because of preference, not availability. Social factors include a detached parenting style, such as that seen in nonorganic failure to thrive, and an inability of the family to independently take advantage of food assistance programs (Karp, Scholl, and Greene, 1985).

Since all of these nutritional disturbances are amenable to some degree of alteration through intervention, the nutritional disturbances to be discussed could potentially be eliminated. However adequate food supplies alone are not the answer, especially when sociocultural factors that affect food consumption are considered. Therefore nutritional counseling becomes a complex process that must take into account all the variables affecting the physical and psychologic makeup of the family.

VITAMIN DISTURBANCES

Vitamins are an essential food element, and function in small quantities by regulating specific metabolic activity, usually by acting as *coenzymes*. When vitamin coenzymes enter the body, they are combined with a protein *apoenzyme* that has been synthesized within the cell to form a *holoenzyme*. The quantity of apoenzymes any cell can produce limits the body's ability to make use of excessive vitamins (Jarvis, 1984). A deficiency of the vitamin directly affects the metabolic activity it regulates. However regular ingestion of excessive amounts of vitamins may produce a toxic effect.

True vitamin disturbances are rare in the United States, but subclinical deficiencies are commonly seen, especially in lower socioeconomic groups where proper dietary intake may be unbalanced. In a study of children ages 7 to 18 years, approximately a third of the children and two thirds of adolescent girls consumed less than the recommended amount of vitamin B_6 (Study of calcium intake, 1984). Vitamin D–deficient rickets, once rarely seen because of vitamin-D fortified milk, has increased. Populations at risk include (1) children born of mothers who are vitamin D deficient, (2) individuals who are exposed to minimal sunlight because of distinctive clothing, housing in areas of

high pollution, or dark skin pigmentation, (3) adherence to vegetarian diets that are low in sources of vitamin D, and (4) use of milk products, such as yogurt or raw cow's milk, as the primary source of milk (Bachrach, Fisher, and Parks, 1979; Saal and others, 1985). Children may also be at risk secondary to disorders or their treatment. For example, vitamin deficiencies of the fat-soluble vitamins A and D may occur in malabsorptive disorders. Children on high-dose salicylate levels, such as for rheumatoid arthritis, may have impaired vitamin C storage (Olness, 1985).

Of equal, if not greater concern, is the overuse of vitamins. With the addition of vitamins to commercially packaged foods, the potential for hypervitaminosis has escalated, especially when combined with the injudicious use of vitamin supplements. Hypervitaminosis of A and D present the greatest problems because these fat-soluble vitamins are stored in the body. However it is now well-documented that the water-soluble vitamins (B complex and C) can also cause toxicity by the following mechanisms (Alhadeff, Gualtieri, and Lipton, 1984):

1. May have direct toxic effects, such as niacin
2. May lead to dependency states with development of deficiency symptoms when the vitamin is abruptly discontinued, such as ascorbic acid
3. May mask signs of a disease, such as vitamin C and interference with Clinitest results (common test used to detect glucose or acetone in urine) in diabetes
4. May interact with drugs or other vitamins, such as folic acid's effect on reducing serum phenytoin levels
5. May be combined with high doses of fat-soluble vitamins, such as high-dose multisupplement preparation.

Deficiencies and excesses of vitamins A, B complex, C, D, E, and K are summarized in Table 13-1. General nursing considerations are discussed below and specific interventions are presented in Table 13-1.

MINERAL DISTURBANCES

A number of minerals are essential nutrients. The *macrominerals* refer to those with daily requirements greater than 100 mg and include calcium, phosphorus, magnesium, sodium, potassium, chloride, and sulfur. *Microminerals* or *trace elements* have daily requirements less than 100 mg and include several essential minerals and those whose exact role in nutrition is still unclear. The greatest concern with minerals is deficiency, especially iron-deficiency anemia (see Chapter 35). However, other minerals that may be inadequate in children's diets include calcium, magnesium, and zinc (Study of calcium intake, 1984).

The regulation of mineral balance in the body is a complex process. Dietary extremes of mineral intake can cause a number of mineral-mineral interactions that could result in unexpected deficiencies or excesses. For example, excessive amounts of one mineral, such as zinc, can result in a deficiency of another mineral, such as copper, even if sufficient amounts of copper are ingested. This is thought to be the

Text continued on p. 553.

Table 13-1 Vitamins and their nutritional significance

PHYSIOLOGIC FUNCTIONS/SOURCES	RESULTS OF DEFICIENCY OR EXCESS	NURSING CONSIDERATIONS

Vitamin A (retinol)*
 	
 Functions
 Necessary component in formation of pigment rhodopsin (visual purple)
 Formation and maintenance of epithelial tissue
 Normal bone growth and tooth development
 Needed for growth and spermatogenesis
 Involved in thyroxine formation
 	
 Sources
 Natural form—liver, kidney, fish oils, milk and nonskimmed milk products, egg yolk
 Provitamin A (carotene)—carrots, sweet potatoes, squash, apricots, spinach, collards, broccoli, cabbage, artichokes
	Deficiency
	 Night blindness
	 Keratinization (hardening and scaling) of epithelium
	   Xerophthalmia (hardening and scaling of cornea and conjunctiva)
	   Phrynoderma (toadskin)
	   Drying of respiratory, gastrointestinal, and genitourinary tracts
	 Defective tooth enamel
	 Retarded growth
	 Impaired bone formation
	 Decreased thyroxine formation
	
	 Excess
	 Early signs—irritability, anorexia, pruritus, fissures at corners of nose and lips
	 Later signs—hepatomegaly, jaundice, retarded growth, poor weight gain, thickening of the cortex of long bones with pain and fragility, hard tender lumps in extremities and occiput of the skull
	 NOTE: Overdose only results from ingestion of large quantities of the vitamin, not the provitamin; large amounts of carotene (carotenemia) cause yellow or orange discoloration of the skin (not the sclera urine, or feces as in jaundice), but none of the above symptoms
		Encourage foods rich in vitamin A, such as whole cow's milk
		 As milk consumption decreases, encourage foods rich in vitamin A
		
		 Emphasize correct use of vitamin supplements and potential hazards of excess
		 Investigate child's dietary habits to calculate approximate intake; if excessive, remove supplemental source
		
		 Advise parents of the benign nature of carotenemia; treatment is avoidance of excess pigmented fruits or vegetables, especially carrots; skin color returns to normal in 2 to 6 weeks

Vitamin B₁ (thiamine)† **Functions** Coenzyme (with phosphorus) in carbohydrate metabolism Needed for healthy nervous system **Sources** Pork, beef, liver, legumes, nuts, whole or enriched grains	**Deficiency** BERIBERI Gastrointestinal—anorexia, constipation, indigestion Neurologic—apathy, fatigue, emotional instability, polyneuritis, tenderness of calf muscles, partial anesthesia, muscle weakness, paresthesia, hyperesthesia, decreased or absent tendon reflexes), convulsions and coma (in infants) Cardiovascular—palpitations, cardiac failure, peripheral vasodilation, edema **Excess** Headache Irritability Insomnia Rapid pulse Weakness	VITAMIN B COMPLEX Encourage foods rich in B vitamins Stress proper cooking and storage techniques to preserve potency, such as minimal cooking of vegetables in small amount of liquid; storage of milk in opaque container Advise against fad diets that severely restrict groups of food, such as vegetarianism Explore need for vitamin supplements when dieting or when using goat milk exclusively for infant feeding (deficient in folic acid) Emphasize correct use of vitamin supplements and potential hazards of excesses
Vitamin B₂ (riboflavin)† **Functions** Coenzyme (with phosphorus) in carbohydrate, protein, and fat metabolism Maintains healthy skin especially around mouth, nose, and eyes	**Deficiency** ARIBOFLAVINOSIS Lips—cheilosis (fissures at corners of lips), prelèche (inflammation at corners of lips) Tongue—glossitis Nose—irritation and cracks at nasal angle	Same as above

*Fat soluble.
†Water soluble.

Continued.

Table 13-1 Vitamins and their nutritional significance—cont'd

PHYSIOLOGIC FUNCTIONS/SOURCES	RESULTS OF DEFICIENCY OR EXCESS	NURSING CONSIDERATIONS
Vitamin B₂—cont'd **Sources** Milk and its products, eggs, organ meats (liver, kidney, and heart), enriched cereals, some green leafy vegetables, legumes	Eyes—burning, itching, tearing, photophobia, corneal vascularization, cataracts Skin—seborrheic dermatitis, delayed wound healing and tissue repair **Excess** Paresthesis, pruritus	Same as vitamin B complex
Niacin (nicotinic acid, nicotinamide)† **Functions** Coenzyme (with riboflavin) in protein and fat metabolism Needed for healthy nervous system, skin, and normal digestion **Sources** Meat, poultry, fish, peanuts, beans, peas, whole or enriched grains except corn and rice Milk and its products are sources of tryptophan (60 mg of tryptophan = 1 mg of niacin)	**Deficiency** PELLAGRA Oral—stomatitis, glossitis Cutaneous—scaly dermatitis on exposed areas Gastrointestinal—anorexia, weight loss, diarrhea, fatigue Neurologic—apathy, anxiety, confusion, depression, dementia Death **Excess** Release of vasodilator, histamine (flushing, decreased blood pressure, increased cerebral bloodflow; aggravates asthma) Dermatologic problems (pruritus, rash, hyperkeratosis, acanthosis nigricans) Increased gastric acidity (aggravates peptic ulcer disease) Hepatotoxicity Increased serum uric acid levels (increased incidence of gouty arthritis) Elevated plasma glucose levels Certain cardiac arrhthymias	Same as vitamin B complex
Vitamin B₆ (pyridoxine)† **Functions** Coenzyme in protein and fat metabolism Needed for formation of antibodies, hemoglobin Needed for utilization of copper and iron Aids in conversion of tryptophan to niacin **Sources** Meats, especially liver and kidney, cereal grains (wheat and corn), yeast, soybeans, peanuts	**Deficiency** Scaly dermatitis, weight loss, anemia, retarded growth, irritability, convulsions, peripheral neuritis **Excess** Peripheral nervous system toxicity (unsteady gait, numb feet and hands, clumsiness of hands, sometimes perioral numbness) May cause peptic ulcer disease or seizures	Same as vitamin B complex
Folic acid (folacin; reduced form is called folinic acid or citrovorum factor)† **Functions** Coenzyme for single-carbon transfer (purines, thymine, hemoglobin) Necessary for formation of red blood cells	**Deficiency** Macrocytic anemia, bone marrow depression, glossitis, intestinal malabsorption	Same as vitamin B complex

*Fat soluble.
†Water soluble.

Table 13-1 Vitamins and their nutritional significance—cont'd

PHYSIOLOGIC FUNCTIONS/SOURCES	RESULTS OF DEFICIENCY OR EXCESS	NURSING CONSIDERATIONS
Folic acid—cont'd **Sources** Green leafy vegetables (spinach), asparagus, liver, kidney, nuts, eggs, whole grain cereals	**Excess** Rare because megadoses not available over the counter May cause insomnia and irritability	
Vitamin B₁₂ (cobalamin)† **Functions** Coenzyme in protein synthesis; indirect effect on formation of red blood cells (particularly on formation of nucleic acids and folic acid metabolism) Needed for normal functioning of nervous tissue **Sources** Meat liver, kidney, fish, milk, eggs, cheese (no vegetable source is known)	**Deficiency** PERNICIOUS ANEMIA General signs of severe anemia Lemon yellow tinge to skin Spinal cord degeneration **Excess** Excess is rare because oral form is ineffective	Same as vitamin B complex
Biotin **Functions** Coenzyme in carbohydrate, protein, and fat metabolism Interrelated with functions of other B vitamins **Sources** Liver, kidney, egg yolk, tomatoes, legumes, nuts	**Deficiency** Deficiency is uncommon because synthesized by bacterial flora **Excess** Unknown	Same as vitamin B complex
Pantothenic acid† **Functions** Coenzyme in carbohydrate, protein, and fat metabolism Synthesis of amino acids, fatty acids, and steroids **Sources** Liver, kidney, heart, salmon, eggs, vegetables, legumes, whole grains	**Deficiency** Deficiency is uncommon because of its multiple food sources and synthesis by bacterial flora **Excess** Minimum toxicity (occasional diarrhea and water retention)	Same as vitamin B complex
Vitamin C (ascorbic acid)† **Functions** Essential for collagen formation Increases absorption of iron for hemoglobin formation Enhances conversion of folic to folinic acid Affects cholesterol synthesis and conversion of proline to hydroxyproline Probably a coenzyme in metabolism of tyrosine and phenylalanine May play role in hydroxylation of adrenal steroids May have stimulating effect on phagocytic activity of leukocytes and formation of antibodies Antioxidant agent (spares other vitamins from oxidation)	**Deficiency** SCURVY Skin—dry, rough, petechiae, perifollicular hyperkeratotic papules (raised areas around hair follicles) Musculoskeletal—bleeding into muscles and joints, pseudoparalysis from pain, swelling of joints, costochondral beading (scorbutic rosary) Gums—spongy, friable, swollen, bleed easily, bluish red or black color, teeth loosen and fall out General disposition—irritable, anorexic, apprehensive, in pain, refuses to move, assumes semi-froglike position when supine (scorbutic pose) Signs of anemia Decreased wound healing	Encourage foods rich in vitamin C Investigate infant's diet for sources of vitamin, especially when cow's milk is principal source of nutrition Stress proper cooking and storing techniques to preserve potency Wash vegetables quickly; do not soak in water Cook vegetables in covered pot with minimal water and for short time; avoid copper or cast iron cookware Do not add baking soda to cooking water Use fresh fruits and vegetables as soon as possible; store in refrigerator Store juice in airtight opaque container

*Fat soluble.
†Water soluble.

Continued.

Table 13-1 Vitamins and their nutritional significance—cont'd

PHYSIOLOGIC FUNCTIONS/SOURCES	RESULTS OF DEFICIENCY OR EXCESS	NURSING CONSIDERATIONS

Vitamin C—cont'd
Sources
Citrus fruits, strawberries, tomatoes, potatoes, melon, cabbage, broccoli, papaya, mango
	Increased susceptibility to infection	In caring for child with scurvy:
		  Position for comfort and rest
		  Handle very gently and minimally
		  Administer analgesics as needed
		  Prevent infection
		  Provide good oral care
		  Provide soft, bland diet
		  Emphasize rapid recovery when vitamin is replaced

	Excess Diarrhea Increased excretion of uric acid and acidification of urine (may cause urate precipitation and formation of oxalate stones in those with abnormal renal function) Hemolysis Impaired leukocytosis activity Damage to beta cells of pancreas and decreased insulin production Reproductive failure "Rebound scurvy" from withdrawal of large amounts	Emphasize correct use of vitamin supplement and potential hazards of excess Identify groups at risk for vitamin C supplements; those with thalassenia; those on anticoagulant or aminoglycoside antibiotic therapy

Vitamin D₂ (ergocalciferol) and D₃ (cholecalciferol)*
 	
Functions
Absorption of calcium and phosphorus and decreased renal excretion of phosphorus
 	
Sources
Direct sunlight
Cod liver oil, herring, mackerel, salmon, tuna, sardines
Enriched food sources—milk, milk products, cereals, margarine, breads, many breakfast drinks
	Deficiency
	
	RICKETS
	Head—craniotabes (softening of cranial bones, prominence of frontal bones) deformed shape (skull flat and depressed toward middle), delayed closure of fontanels
	Chest—rachitic rosary (enlargement of costochondral junction of ribs), Harrison groove (horizontal depression in lower portion of rib cage), pigeon chest (sharp protrusion of sternum)
	Spine—kyphosis, scoliosis, lordosis
	Abdomen—potbelly, constipation
	Extremities—bowing of arms and legs, knock-knee, saber shins, instability of hip joints, pelvic deformity, enlargement of epiphysis at ends of long bones
	Teeth—delayed calcification, especially of permanent teeth
	Rachitic tetany—seizures
		Encourage foods rich in vitamin D, especially fortified cow's milk
		In breast-fed infants encourage use of vitamin D, especially fortified cow's milk
		In breast-fed infants encourage use of vitamin D supplements if maternal diet inadequate or infant exposed to minimal sunlight
		Emphasize importance of exposure to sun as source of vitamin
		In caring for child with rickets:
		  Maintain good body alignment
		  Reposition frequently to prevent decubiti and respiratory infection
		  Handle very gently and minimally
		  Prevent infection
		  Institute seizure precautions
		  Have 10% calcium gluconate available in case of tetany
		  Observe for possibility of overdose from supplements
		  If prescribed, supervise proper use of orthopedic splints or braces

	Excess Acute—vomiting, dehydration, fever, abdominal cramps, bone pain, convulsions, and coma Chronic—lassitude, mental slowness, anorexia, failure to thrive, thirst, urinary urgency, polyuria, vomiting, diarrhea, abdominal cramps, bone pain, pathologic fractures	Same as vitamin A; may include low-calcium diet during initial therapy

*Fat soluble.
†Water soluble.

Table 13-1   Vitamins and their nutritional significance—cont'd

PHYSIOLOGIC FUNCTIONS/SOURCES	RESULTS OF DEFICIENCY OR EXCESS	NURSING CONSIDERATIONS
Vitamin D—cont'd	Calcification of soft tissue—kidneys, lungs, adrenal glands, vessels (hypertension), heart, gastric lining, tympanic membrane (deafness) Osteoporosis of long bones Elevated serum levels of calcium and phosphorus	
Vitamin E (tocopherol)* **Functions** Production of red blood cells Muscle and liver integrity Coenzyme factor in tissue respiration Minimizes oxidation of polyunsaturated fatty acids and vitamins A and C in intestinal tract and tissues **Sources** Vegetable oils, wheat germ oil, milk, egg yolk, muscle meats, fish, whole grains, nuts, legumes, spinach, broccoli	**Deficiency** Hemolytic anemia from hemolysis caused by shortened life of red blood cells, especially in premature infants, and focal necrosis of tissues Causes infertility in rats, but not in humans (does *not* increase human male virility or potency) **Excess** Little is known: less toxic than other fat-soluble vitamins but excess of water-soluble preparations has been fatal in premature infants	Initiate early feeding in premature infants; may need supplementation
Vitamin K* **Functions** Catalyst for production of prothrombin and blood clotting factors II, VII, IX, and X by the liver **Sources** Pork, liver, green leafy vegetables (spinach, kale, cabbage), tomatoes, egg yolk, cheese	**Deficiency** Hemorrhage **Excess** Hyperbilirubinemia in infants Hemolytic anemia in individuals who are deficient in glucose-6-phosphate dehydrogenase	Administer prophylactically to newborns Other indications include intestinal disease, lack of bile, prolonged antibiotic therapy, or use of anticoagulants such as heparin or dicumarol (bishydroxycoumarin), which are vitamin K antagonists

result of competition in the process of absorption because of (1) displacement of one mineral by another on the molecule necessary for their uptake from the lumen in the intestinal cell or (2) competition for pathways through the intestinal wall or into the bloodstream. Therefore megadose therapy with one mineral may not cause toxicity from an excess but rather from a deficiency in a competing mineral.

Deficiencies can also occur when various substances in the diet interact with minerals. For example, both zinc and calcium are capable of forming insoluble complexes with phytates (found in plant proteins), which can cause a zinc or calcium deficiency (Solomons, 1982a). This type of interaction is particularly significant in vegetarian diets.

Deficiencies and excesses of the essential macro- and microminerals are summarized in Table 13-2. General nursing considerations are discussed below and specific interventions are presented in the table.

VEGETARIAN DIETS

The importance of vegetarian diets and their relationship to potential nutritional deficiencies in children cannot be over-emphasized. The stricter the vegetarian diet, the more difficult it becomes to ensure adequate nutrition for infants and children. The major types of vegetarianism are (MacLean and Graham, 1980):

lactoovovegetarians exclude meat from their diet but eat milk and eggs and sometimes fish

lactovegetarians exclude meat and eggs but drink milk

pure vegetarians (vegans) eliminate any food of animal origin, including milk and eggs

zen macrobiotics are even more restrictive than pure vegetarians in that cereals, especially brown rice, are the mainstay of the diet

Many individuals who are concerned about healthful diets subscribe to vegetarian diets that are not typified by

Text continued on p. 558.

Table 13-2 Minerals and their nutritional significance

PHYSIOLOGIC FUNCTIONS/SOURCES	RESULTS OF DEFICIENCY OR EXCESS	NURSING CONSIDERATIONS

Calcium
Functions
Bone and tooth development and maintenance (in combination with phosphorus)
Muscle contractions, especially the heart
Blood clotting
Absorption of vitamin B_{12}
Enzyme activation
Nerve conduction
Integrity of intracellular cement substances and various membranes
 	
Sources
Dairy products, egg yolk, sardines, canned salmon with bones, dark-green leafy vegetables, soybeans, dried beans and peas
	Deficiency
	Rickets
	    Tetany
	Impaired growth, especially of bones and teeth
	
	Excess
	Drowsiness, extreme lethargy
	    Impaired absorption of other minerals (iron, zinc, manganese)
	    Calcium deposits in tissues (renal failure)
		Encourage foods rich in calcium, especially dairy products
		Caution that phytates in leafy vegetables, oxalates in chocolates, and a high phosphorus intake (especially from carbonated beverages) can decrease calcium absorption
		
		Discourage use of whole cow's milk in newborns because the high phosphorus-to-calcium ratio favors excretion of calcium
		Advise against fad diets, especially those that restrict dairy products
		Emphasize correct use of calcium supplement, especially the possible interaction between megadoses of calcium and resulting deficiency states of other minerals

Chloride **Functions** Acid-base and fluid balance Enzyme activation in saliva Component of hydrochloric acid in stomach **Sources** Salt, meat, eggs, dairy products, many prepared and preserved foods	**Deficiency** Acid-base disturbances (hypochloremic alkalosis, dehydration); occurs mostly in combination with sodium loss **Excess** Acid-base disturbance	Deficiency and excess is unusual; most diets supply adequate chloride (usually in combination with sodium) Disease states such as excessive vomiting can necessitate chloride replacement
Chromium **Functions** Involved in glucose metabolism and energy production **Sources** Meat, cheese, whole grain breads and cereals, legumes, peanuts, brewer's yeast, vegetable oils	**Deficiency** Possible abnormal glucose metabolism **Excess** Unknown	No specific recommendations are needed
Copper **Functions** Production of hemoglobin Essential component of several enzyme systems **Sources** Organ meats, oysters, nuts, seeds, legumes, corn oil margarine	**Deficiency** Anemia, leukopenia, neutropenia **Excess** Severe vomiting and diarrhea Hemolytic anemia	Deficiency from inadequate food sources is less likely than from excess intake of other minerals, especially zinc and possibly iron; therefore emphasize the correct use of any vitamin supplement Caution against cooking acid foods in unlined copper pots, which can lead to chronic and toxic accumulation of copper
Fluorine **Functions** Formation of caries-resistant teeth Strong bone development	**Deficiency** Increased susceptibility to tooth decay	In areas with optimally fluoridated water, encourage sufficient intake to supply recommended amount of fluoride (see p. 614)

Table 13-2 Minerals and their nutritional significance—cont'd

PHYSIOLOGIC FUNCTIONS/SOURCES	RESULTS OF DEFICIENCY OR EXCESS	NURSING CONSIDERATIONS
Flourine—cont'd **Sources** Fluoridated water and foods or beverages prepared with fluoridated water; fish, tea, commercially prepared chicken for infants	**Excess** Fluorosis (mottling and/or pitting of enamel) Severe bone deformities	In areas of unfluoridated water, stress the importance of fluoride supplements In areas with excess fluoride in the water, consider the use of bottled water in drinking and possibly cooking to reduce the fluoride intake to safe levels Fluorine has the narrowest range of safe and adequate intake; therefore, stress the importance of storing supplements in a safe area
Iodine **Functions** Production of thyroid hormone Normal reproduction **Sources** Seafood, kelp, iodized salt, sea salt	**Deficiency** Goiter (enlarged thyroid from decreased thyroxine formation) **Excess** Unknown from food sources; may occur from ingestion of iodine preparations, such as saturated solutions of potassium iodide (SSKI)	Encourage use of iodized salt for individuals living far from the sea If iodine preparations are in the home, stress the importance of safe storage
Iron **Functions** Formations of hemoglobin and myoglobin Essential part of several enzymes and proteins **Sources** Liver, especially pork, followed by calf, beef, and chicken; kidney, red meat, poultry, shellfish, egg yolk, whole grains, enriched cereals and bread, legumes, nuts, green leafy vegetables, dried fruits, potatoes, molasses	**Deficiency** Anemia (see box below) **Excess** Hemosiderosis (excess iron storage in various tissues of the body, especially the spleen, liver, lymph glands, heart, and pancreas) Hemochromatosis (excess iron storage with cellular damage)	Encourage foods rich in iron, especially liver, meat, and egg yolk Discourage excessive milk consumption, especially more than 1 liter per day (milk is a very poor source of iron) If iron supplements are prescribed, teach parents factors that affect absorption (see box below) Stress the importance of storing iron supplements in a safe area

---

FACTORS THAT AFFECT IRON ABSORPTION

Increase	*Decrease*
Acidity (low pH)—administer iron between meals (gastric hydrochloric acid) Ascorbic acid (vitamin C)—administer iron with juice, fruit, or multivitamin preparation Calcium Tissue need Meat, fish, poultry	Alkalinity (high pH)—avoid any antacid preparation Phosphates—milk is unfavorable vehicle for iron administration Phytates—found in cereals Oxalates—found in many fruits and vegetables (plums, currants, green beans, spinach, sweet potatoes, tomatoes) Tannins—found in tea Tissue saturation Malabsorptive disorders Disturbances that cause diarrhea or steatorrhea

Continued.

Table 13-2 Minerals and their nutritional significance—cont'd

PHYSIOLOGIC FUNCTIONS/SOURCES	RESULTS OF DEFICIENCY OR EXCESS	NURSING CONSIDERATIONS
Magnesium **Functions** Bone and tooth formation Production of proteins Nerve conduction to muscles Activation of enzymes needed for carbohydrate and protein metabolism **Sources** Whole grains, nuts, soybeans, meat, green leafy vegetables (uncooked), tea, cocoa, raisins	**Deficiency** Tremors, spasm Irregular heartbeat Muscular weakness Lower extremity cramps Convulsions, delirium **Excess** Nervous system disturbances due to imbalance in calcium to magnesium ratio	Deficiency and excess are unusual, except in disease states such as prolonged vomiting or diarrhea or kidney dysfunction, where replacement may be needed
Manganese **Functions** Activation of enzymes involved in reproduction, growth, and fat metabolism Normal bone structure Nervous system functioning **Sources** Nuts, whole grains, legumes, green vegetables, fruit	**Deficiency** Unknown **Excess** Unknown	No specific recommendations are needed
Molybdenum **Functions** Essential component of several oxidative enzymes **Sources** Legumes, whole grains, organ meats, some dark green vegetables	**Deficiency** Very rare; diagnosed in patients on complete total parenteral alimentation **Excess** Produces secondary copper deficiency (growth failure, anemia, and disturbed bone development)	No specific recommendations are needed
Phosphorus **Functions** Bone and tooth development (in combination with calcium) Involved in numerous chemical reactions, including protein, carbohydrate, and fat metabolism Acid-base balance **Sources** Dairy products, eggs, meat, poultry, legumes, carbonated beverages	**Deficiency** Weakness, anorexia, malaise, bone pain **Excess** Produces secondary calcium deficiency from disturbed calcium-to-phosphorus ratio	Dietary deficiency is uncommon, although prolonged use of antacids can produce deficiency, in which case supplementation is recommended To preserve calcium-to-phosphorus ratio in newborns, discourage use of whole cow's milk
Potassium **Functions** Acid-base and fluid balance (major extracellular fluid areas) Nerve conduction Muscular contraction, especially the heart Release of energy **Sources** Bananas, citrus fruit, dried fruits, meat, fish, bran, legumes, peanut butter, potatoes, coffee, tea, cocoa	**Deficiency** Cardiac arrhythmias Muscular weakness Lethargy Kidney and respiratory failure Heart failure **Excess** Cardiac arrhythmias Respiratory failure Mental confusion Numbness of extremities	Dietary deficiency and excess are unlikely, although disease states such as prolonged nausea and vomiting, or the use of diuretics can result in hypokalemia; in such instances, encourage replacement with supplements of rich food sources such as bananas

Table 13-2 Minerals and their nutritional significance—cont'd

PHYSIOLOGIC FUNCTIONS/SOURCES	RESULTS OF DEFICIENCY OR EXCESS	NURSING CONSIDERATIONS
Selenium	**Deficiency**	
Functions	Keshan disease—cardiomyopathy in children (found in China)	Deficiency and excess are uncommon in North America, although selenium deficiency can occur in patients on prolonged total parenteral alimentation; in these instances supplementation is required
Antioxident, especially protective of vitamin E		
Protects against toxicity of heavy metals		
Associated with fat metabolism		
Sources	**Excess**	
Seafood, organ meats, egg yolk, whole grain, chicken, meat, tomatoes, cabbage, garlic, mushrooms, milk	Eye, nose, and throat irritation Increased dental caries Liver and kidney degeneration	
Sodium	**Deficiency**	
Functions	Dehydration Hypotension Convulsions Muscle cramps	Deficient intake is very rare, although losses secondary to nausea, vomiting, excessive sweating, and use of diuretics can occur and require replacement
Acid-base and fluid balance (major extracellular fluid cation)		
Cell permeability; absorption of glucose		
Muscle contraction		
Sources	**Excess**	
Table salt, seafood, meat, poultry, numerous prepared foods	Edema Hypertension Intracranial hemorrhage	Encourage parents to limit excessive use of salt in preparing foods and commercial foods with high sodium content, such as smoked meats
Sulfur	**Deficiency**	
Functions	Unknown	No specific recommendations are needed
Essential component of cell protein, especially of hair and skin	**Excess**	
Enzyme activation	Unknown	
Associated with energy metabolism		
Detoxification of certain chemical reactions		
Sources		
Dairy products, eggs, meat, fish, nuts, legumes		
Zinc	**Deficiency**	
Functions	Loss of appetite Diminished taste sensation Delayed healing Skin lesions—erythematous, crusted lesions around body orifices Alopechia Growth failure Retarded sexual maturity	Encourage food sources rich in zinc, especially protein Caution that fiber, phytates, oxalates, tannins (in tea or coffee), and calcium adversely affect zinc absorption Recognize groups at risk for zinc deficiency, such as vegetarians and Mexican-Americans, whose diets may have restricted or low meat content and high fiber, phytate content
Component of about 100 enzymes		
Synthesis of nucleic acids and protein in immune system and coagulation		
Release of vitamin A from liver		
Improved wound healing with vitamin C		
Sources	**Excess**	
Seafood (especially oysters), meat, poultry, eggs, wheat, legumes	Vomiting and diarrhea Malaise, dizziness Anemia, gastric bleeding Impaired absorption of calcium and copper	Emphasize correct use of zinc supplements and the possible interaction with other minerals

the above categories. Therefore during nutritional assessment it is necessary to clearly list exactly what the diet includes and excludes.

The lactoovovegetarian diet is associated with the least deficiencies, although protein intake needs to be monitored. The lactovegetarian diet may be low in protein, as well as iron. The major deficiencies in the stricter vegetarian diets are inadequate protein for growth, inadequate calories for energy and growth, poor digestibility of many of the natural, unprocessed foods, especially for infants, and deficiencies of vitamin B_{12}, niacin, thiamine, riboflavin, vitamin D, iron, calcium, and zinc. In the United States vegetarian diets are common among members of Black Muslim or Seventh Day Adventist faiths.

Because vegetarian diets eliminate the major sources of complete proteins (those proteins with all the essential amino acids in amounts needed to support physiologic functions), protein deficiency can occur. Fortunately, this problem is easily remedied by selecting foods with complementary amino acids and consuming them at the same meal. The three basic combinations of foods consumed by vegetarians that generally provide the appropriate amounts of essential amino acids are (Fanelli and Kuczmarski, 1983):

> **grains** (cereal, rice, pasta) and **legumes** (beans, peas, lentils, peanuts)
> **grains** and **milk products** (milk, cheese, yogurt)
> **seeds** (sesame, sunflower) and **legumes**

Achieving a nutritionally adequate vegetarian diet is not difficult, but it requires careful planning and knowledge of nutrient sources. For children, the lactoovovegetarian diet is nutritionally adequate; however, the vegan diet requires supplementation with vitamins D and B_{12}, particularly for children ages 2 to 12 years. Infants on a vegan diet should be breast-fed for the first 6 months and preferably for 1 year, fed solid foods after about 4 months, and receive iron-fortified cereal for at least 18 months. The use of vitamin C juices with foods high in iron will further improve iron absorption. If cow's or human milk is not given, fortified soy milk is recommended (Fannelli and Kuczmarski, 1983). When solid foods are introduced, the safety and digestibility of the selections must be considered. Raw fruits with seeds, vegetables, and nuts are hazardous for young children because of the danger of aspiration. Beans, grain cereals, and vegetables should be served well-cooked and mashed during infancy. A variety of foods should be introduced during the early years to ensure a more well-balanced intake.

NURSING CONSIDERATIONS

Identification of nutrient imbalance is the initial nursing goal and requires assessment, based on a dietary history and physical examination, for signs of deficiency or excess (pp. 212-216). Once assessment data is collected it should be evaluated against standard intakes to identify areas of concern. The most widely used standard is the Recommended Dietary Allowances (RDA), developed by the National Academy of Sciences, Food and Nutrition Board. The RDA are not average requirements but recommendations intended to meet the physiologic needs of almost every healthy person. To meet the needs of those with the highest requirements, the RDA will exceed most people's requirements. Therefore children consuming less than the RDA are not necessarily consuming an inadequate diet but are more likely at risk for deficiency than those who are consuming nutrients in amounts equal to the RDA.

The RDA are used primarily by professionals involved in nutrition. To provide consumers with reliable information about the nutrient content of the foods they purchase, the U.S. Recommended Daily Allowances (U.S. RDA) were developed and provide information about nutrition on package labels. Eight nutrients must be listed—protein, vitamin A, vitamin C, thiamin, riboflavin, niacin, calcium, and iron, as well as caloric density. Listing of other minerals and vitamins is optional unless they are added to a food. Since the U.S. RDA are based on the RDA, they also include a margin of safety and are generally higher than the needs of most people. In counseling families regarding selection of nutrients to provide a balanced intake, the use of U.S. RDA on food labels should be explained. Since children are learning food habits during infancy, it is not too early to expose families to information that may prevent the development of nutritional disturbances.

Unfortunately there are no restrictions on the availability of toxic doses of vitamins or minerals. With the unsubstantiated claims for megadose therapy in curing ailments from the common cold to cancer, many individuals consume large amounts of nutrients. Nurses need to inform families of the potential dangers from excess vitamins or minerals. The idea that "more is better" is incorrect and is probably best dispelled by a simple explanation of the body's inability to use more than the needed requirement.

PROTEIN AND CALORIE MALNUTRITION

Hunger is one of the world's gravest and most prevalent health problems. Three fourths of the world population suffers some form of malnutrition. Mortality and morbidity among children in underdeveloped countries illustrate the severity of this problem where in the 1- to 4-year-old age-group the death rate may be 20 to 50 times higher than in the United States.

Even in the United States, the protein and energy malnutrition (PEM) diseases of kwashiorkor and marasmus are reported in hospitals each year. They occur primarily as (1) a complication of an underlying disease process, (2) a result of fad diets, such as some types of vegetarianism, (3) because of lack of parental education regarding infant nutrition, (4) because of incorrect preparation of formula, such as adding extra water out of ignorance or economic need, or (5) inappropriate management of food allergy (e.g., the use of high-fat, low-protein, nondairy creamer as a substitute for milk) (Sinatra and Merritt, 1981).

Kwashiorkor

Kwashiorkor is a deficiency of protein with an adequate supply of calories. The word comes from the Ghan language and means "the sickness the older child gets when the next baby is born." It is an appropriate name because it is a syndrome that develops in the first child, usually between 1 and 4 years of age, when he is weaned from the breast once the second child is born and fed a diet consisting mainly of starch grains or tubers. Such a diet provides adequate calories in the form of carbohydrates but an inadequate amount of high-quality proteins.

Pathophysiology and clinical manifestations.
The pathophysiology of kwashiorkor results from protein deficiency, both in quantity and quality. Since protein is essential for tissue growth and cell repair, all body systems are affected, but rapidly growing cells, such as those of the epithelium and mucosa, are most severely damaged. The skin is scaly and dry and has areas of depigmentation. Several dermatoses may be evident, partly resulting from the vitamin deficiencies. Permanent blindness results from the severe lack of vitamin A. Immunity is severely affected and is of considerable importance in the development of infections.

Mineral deficiencies are common, especially iron, calcium, and zinc. Acute zinc deficiency is a common complication of severe PEM and results in skin rashes, loss of hair, impaired immune response and susceptibility to infections,

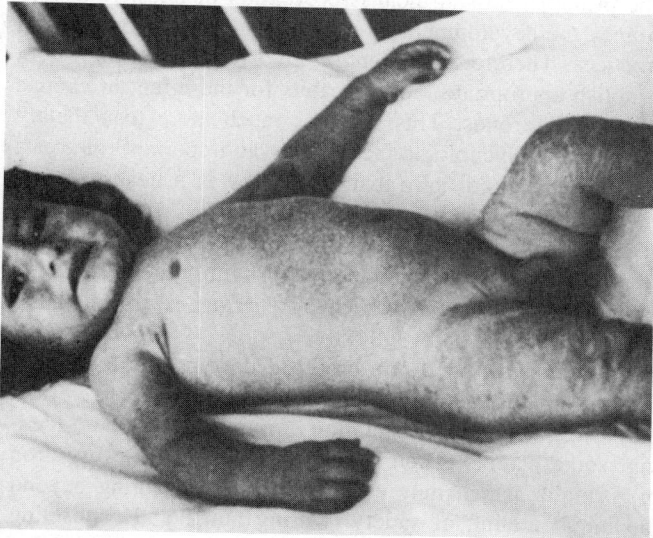

Fig. 13-1. Child with kwashiorkor. Note the edema, which masks muscle wasting.

From Guthrie, H.A.: Introductory nutrition, ed. 6, St. Louis, 1986, The C.V. Mosby Co. Courtesy Dr. John Beard, Pennsylvania State University.

digestive problems, night blindness, changes in affective behavior, defective wound healing, and impaired growth. Its depressant effect on appetite further limits food intake (Solomons, 1982a).

With kwashiorkor the hair is thin, dry, coarse, and dull. Depigmentation is common, and patchy alopecia may occur. There is loss of weight in conjunction with edema (ascites) from the hypoalbuminemia. The edema often masks the severe muscular atrophy, making the child appear less debilitated than he actually is (Fig. 13-1). Total body water increases, but total body potassium decreases with retention of sodium, causing signs of hypokalemia and hypernatremia.

Diarrhea frequently occurs from a lowered resistance to infection and further complicates the electrolyte imbalance. Gastrointestinal disturbances occur, such as fatty infiltration of the liver and atrophy of the acini cells of the pancreas. Behavioral changes are evident as the child grows progressively more irritable, lethargic, withdrawn, and apathetic. Fatal deterioration may be caused by diarrhea and infection or as the result of circulatory failure.

Marasmus

Marasmus is the result of general malnutrition of both calories and protein. It is a common occurrence in underdeveloped countries during times of drought, such as Ethiopia. Because children are fed last in these cultures, there is seldom enough food remaining for the younger ones.

Marasmus is usually a syndrome of physical and emotional deprivation and is not confined to geographic areas where food supplies are inadequate. It may be seen in failure-to-thrive children, where the cause is not solely nutritional but primarily emotional.

Pathophysiology and clinical manifestations.
Marasmus is characterized by gradual wasting and atrophy of body tissues, especially subcutaneous fat (Fig. 13-2). Children with the condition appear to be very old; their skin is flabby and wrinkled, unlike children with kwashiorkor, who appear more rounded from the edema. Fat metabolism is less impaired than in kwashiorkor, so that vitamin A deficiency is usually minimal or absent.

In general, the clinical manifestations of marasmus are similar to those seen in kwashiorkor with the following exceptions: no edema from hypoalbuminemia or sodium retention, which contributes to a severely emaciated appearance; no dermatoses caused by vitamin deficiencies; little or no depigmentation of hair or skin; more normal fat metabolism and lipid absorption; and smaller head size and slower recovery following treatment.

As in kwashiorkor, body metabolism is minimal, and maintaining body temperature is complicated by lack of subcutaneous fat. The child is fretful, apathetic, withdrawn, and so lethargic that prostration frequently occurs. Intercurrent infection with debilitating diseases such as tuberculosis, parasitosis, and dysentery is common. Severe, chronic mal-

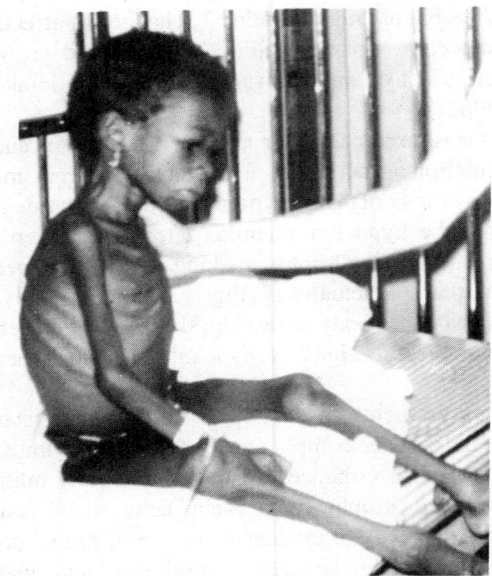

Fig. 13-2. Child with marasmus.
Courtesy Donald Anderson, M.D., Travis Air Force Base, CA. From Dodge, P.R., Prensky, A.L., and Feigin, R.D.: Nutrition and the developing nervous system, St. Louis, 1975, The C.V. Mosby Co.

nutrition in infancy results in decreased brain growth and has implications for the child's future mental capacity.

Therapeutic Management

Treatment includes providing a diet high in quality proteins and/or carbohydrates as well as vitamins and minerals. Electrolyte imbalance requires immediate attention, and parenteral fluid replacement may be necessary initially to correct the dehydration and restore renal function. Occasionally oral fluids are not tolerated, necessitating the use of hyperalimentation. Coexisting problems such as infection, diarrhea, parasitic infestation, and anemia necessitate prompt attention for optimum recovery.

A recent recommendation is the addition of psychosocial stimulation to the treatment of severely malnourished children. A long-term structured play program involving parents has been shown to result in marked developmental improvements. However these children continued to be behind in nutritional status and locomotor development (Grantham-McGregor and others, 1983).

Nursing Considerations

Provision of essential physiologic needs such as rest, individually tailored activity, and protection from infection is paramount. Since the child is usually weak and withdrawn, he is dependent on others to feed him. Hygiene may be distressing because of the poor integrity of the skin, and decubiti are a constant threat. Appropriate developmental stimulation should also be provided.

A larger problem is prevention of these conditions through education concerning the importance of high-quality proteins and adequate carbohydrates. Since children with marasmus may suffer from emotional starvation as well,

care should be consistent with care of the failure-to-thrive child (p. 567).

OBESITY

Obesity is a complex condition that may or may not be related to the chronic ingestion of more calories than are needed to supply the body's energy requirement. Genetic factors play a significant role since there is a strong correlation of obesity among biologic family members that is not evident among parents and adopted children (Stunkard and others, 1986). For example, obese infants have a two to three times greater risk of being obese in childhood, although the obesity may not persist into adulthood (Dine and others, 1979). Also the type of feeding may play a role. Breast-feeding may have a protective effect against the development of obesity, although present information only supports a short-term benefit (Kramer and others, 1985b). Other factors that may influence infant obesity include birth weight, sex (especially male), age at introduction of solid foods, and activity level (Kramer and others, 1985a; Berkowitz and others, 1985).

Despite the current controversy on exactly what causes obesity, all authorities agree that *prevention* holds greater promise than treatment. Besides the physiologic component of increased numbers of fat cells, there are also the psychologic disadvantages of firmly entrenched food habits and dependency on food. Consequently evaluation of overnutrition *early* in life is essential, with attention to those factors that may prevent obesity. (For a more extensive discussion of obesity beyond infancy, see p. 889.)

Nursing Considerations

The principal nursing goal is prevention of obesity. During infancy the development of obesity is influenced by parental practices. Therefore intervention involves helping the parent establish appropriate feeding habits for the infant or change inappropriate ones. This involves much more than dietary counseling. Psychologic factors play an important role, particularly the philosophy that a fat baby is a healthy baby, or, more subconsciously, that a fat "healthy" baby is a sign of good mothering. Such beliefs are difficult to dispel and counseling may need to include other family members, such as grandmothers, who can greatly influence the mother's practices (Winkelstein, 1984).

Although the exact role breast-feeding has on the development of subsequent obesity is unclear, its protective effect may be related to self-regulation of intake. With bottle-feeding, some parents encourage the infant to finish every drop of formula, which may establish a habit of eating beyond the initial feeling of satiety. During nutritional counseling the nurse should discuss with parents appropriate feeding habits, such as allowing the child to regulate the need for formula and solid food. With proper education parents can come to understand that a "good eater" is not a big eater but one who eats moderately without necessarily "cleaning the plate."

The addition of solid foods is another important aspect of nutritional counseling. When solid foods are added, the quantity of milk should be decreased to less than 1 L to maintain the proper caloric balance. If the infant seems unsatisfied with fewer bottle feedings and refuses water, the milk or formula can be diluted to yield fewer calories per ounce. Other alternatives are substituting water for a bottle of formula or using a smaller-hole nipple to prolong sucking with less intake. A commercial formula, Advance, is also available and provides 20% less calories than regular formula or whole cow's milk. Substituting skim or low-fat milk for whole milk or formula is unacceptable. Although they contain a significant reduction in calories, they are not nutritionally sound for infants. Their low fat content deprives the infant of essential fatty acids, significantly increased amounts of solids and electrolytes elevate the renal solute load and water demands, and their vitamin A content is reduced. A comparison of whole, nonfat (skimmed) and low-fat (partially skimmed) milk is presented in Table 13-3.

The selection of solid foods should also be considered. Approximately 20% of commercial baby foods contain less than 50 kcal/100 g, whereas another 20% contain more than 100 kcal/100 g. Choosing low-calorie foods can significantly lower the daily calorie intake without actually decreasing the total quantity of food. Food charts can be used to familiarize parents with the calorie content of foods, as well as encouraging reading of food labels (Markesbery and Wong, 1979). Sweet foods should be kept to a minimum. This includes not adding additional sugar to the formula or cereal and avoiding finger foods such as cookies. Other foods rich in calories that should be restricted in serving size rather than eliminated include butter, cream, ice cream, pudding, and chocolate.

Parents are also encouraged to interpret the infant's signals of discomfort and intervene in ways other than through feeding. Crying, fussiness, or sucking do not necessarily indicate hunger. Rocking, stroking, holding, and offering a pacifier may be more appropriate than automatically responding with food (Wishon and Kinneck, 1986).

FOOD INTOLERANCE

Food intolerance is a broad term that includes any adverse response to food. Although there is no general agreement regarding specific terms, the following categories of food intolerance are recognized (McCarty and Frick, 1983):

food allergy Generally limited to IgE-mediated, immediate-onset food sensitivity (reaginic type); the most common food antigens producing reaginic reactions are peanuts, eggs, cow's milk, seafood, and nuts

food sensitivity Includes both reaginic and nonreaginic immune responses to ingested antigens; this category includes a diverse set of disorders, such as gluten-sensitive enteropathy (celiac disease), milk-induced acute gastroenteropathy, and lactose intolerance

Nutritional intolerance can occur in anyone at any age, and frequently the allergic response is exhibited after the food has been ingested one or more times. Food allergies are common during infancy because the child is exposed to many new food antigens. Physiologically the intestinal tract is immature and is permeable to many more inadequately catabolized proteins, which, unlike the amino acids, are capable of producing an allergic response. As the intestinal tract matures, many food allergies disappear. The chief offenders are cow's milk, eggs, and wheat. Sensitivity to fish and nuts is also likely but is less often outgrown than allergy to the other substances.

There is some evidence that nutritional allergies can be delayed and possibly prevented. Exclusive breast-feeding for 6 months or longer reduces the chances of developing antibodies to cow's milk protein. However mothers with allergies or a family history of allergy must also avoid ingesting all milk products while breastfeeding and possibly even prenatally. In a child with a strong family history for allergy, certain foods should be avoided during the first year. Table 13-4 lists common foods that are potentially allergenic. Soy-based formula is recommended as a substitute for cow's milk formulas in these infants. In addition, following careful schedules for introducing new foods can quickly identify the offending agent. If any local inflammation occurs, such as swelling of the lip or urticaria around the mouth, the food must be avoided and is usually not reintroduced for a period of 6 or more months.

Cow's Milk Sensitivity

Cow's milk sensitivity (milk allergy, milk intolerance) is a multifaceted disorder representing adverse systemic and local gastrointestinal reactions to cow's milk protein. Several clinical syndromes of milk sensitivity have been described, including milk-induced acute gastroenteropathy, protein-losing enteropathy, malabsorption syndrome, and chronic

Table 13-3 Nutritive values of milk (per 8 oz)*

	WHOLE MILK	NONFAT OR SKIM MILK	LOW-FAT OR PARTIALLY SKIM MILK
Calories	150	86	121
Protein (g)	8	8	8
Fat (g)	8	0.5	5
% milk fat	3.25 (min.)	0.5 (max.)	2 (avg.)
Carbohydrates (g)	11	12	12
Calcium (mg)	291	302	297
Iron (mg)	0.12	0.10	0.12
Vitamin A (IU)	307	500	500
Thiamine (mg)	0.09	0.09	0.10
Riboflavin (mg)	0.4	0.3	0.4
Niacin (mg)	0.2	0.2	0.2
Vitamin C (mg)	2	2	2

*Data from Newer knowledge of milk and other fluid dairy products, Rosemont, IL, 1979, National Dairy Council.

blood loss in the gastrointestinal tract. The latter, a common cause of anemia in infancy, can occur without symptoms.

Milk intolerance is the most common nutritional allergy during infancy, affecting 0.3% to 7% of all infants. It usually presents within the first 2 months of life following cow's milk feeding. Some newborns and exclusively breast-fed infants may be symptomatic following their first exposure to cow's milk, suggesting placental sensitization in utero or sensitization by cow's milk protein in breast milk from maternal ingestion of milk. Many children who are initially sensitive to cow's milk can tolerate it by 2 years of age.

Table 13-4   Hyperallergenic foods

FOOD	SOURCES
Milk	Ice cream, butter, margarine, yogurt, cheese, pudding, baked goods, wieners, bologna, canned creamed soups, instant breakfast drinks, powdered milk drinks, milk chocolate
Eggs	Mayonnaise, creamy salad dressing, baked goods, egg noodles, some cake icing, meringue, custard, pancakes, french toast, root beer
Wheat	Almost all baked goods, wieners, bologna, pressed or chopped cold cuts, gravy, pasta, some canned soups
Peanuts, legumes	Peanut butter or oil; legumes, such as beans, peas, lentils (peanuts are a legume, not a nut)
Nuts	Chocolate, baked goods, cherry soda (may be flavored with a nut extract)
Fish or shellfish	Cod liver oil, pizza with anchovies, Caesar salad dressing, any food fried in same oil as fish
Chocolate	Cola beverages, cocoa, chocolate-flavored drinks
Buckwheat	Some cereals, pancakes
Pork, chicken	Bacon, wieners, sausage, pork fat, chicken broth
Strawberries, melon, pineapple	Gelatin, syrups
Corn	Popcorn, cereal, muffins, cornstarch, corn meal
Citrus fruits	Orange, lemon, lime, grapefruit; any of these in drinks, gelatin, juice, or medicines
Tomatoes	Juice, some vegetable soups, spaghetti, pizza sauce, and catsup
Spices	Chili, pepper, vinegar, cinnamon

Cow's milk sensitivity can present with a variety of clinical manifestations (Table 13-5). Health professionals must have a high index of suspicion for milk allergy because frequently the symptoms appear to be unrelated to milk ingestion.

Lactose Intolerance

Lactose intolerance refers to at least two different entities that involve a deficiency of the enzyme lactase, which is needed for the digestion of lactose. *Congenital lactose intolerance* appears soon after birth when the diet contains lactose from milk. *Late-onset lactose intolerance* is similar to the congenital type but manifests later in life. Ethnic groups with a high incidence of lactose intolerance include Orientals, southern Europeans, Arabs, Jews, and blacks. The principal manifestations include diarrhea, abdominal pain, distension, and flatus shortly after ingesting milk products.

Diagnostic Evaluation

The diagnosis of milk intolerance is initially made from the findings of the history. Preliminary tests include stool analysis for blood, white blood cells, and sugar. To detect sugar (lactose), the stool is tested with Clinitest. A number of other tests may be performed, such as skin-prick testing and the radioallergosorbent test (RAST) for a specific antigen or the lactose tolerance test or hydrogen breath test for lactase activity. However the simplest and most frequently used approach is an elimination diet followed by challenge testing, in which the suspect food is ingested in measured amounts to detect resurgence of symptoms. Careful observation of the child is required during a challenge test because of the possibility of anaphylactic shock.

Therapeutic Management

Management of milk allergy involves elimination of cow's milk. The main difficulty is identification of the sensitivity and selection of an acceptable substitution. The initial alternative is soy milk, although approximately 1:5 children who are allergic to cow's milk are also sensitive to soy milk. Commercially available soy formulas include Prosobee and Isomil. Commercial formulas that are suitable cow's and soy milk substitutes include Nutramigen, Pregestimil, and Vivonex, which contain hydrolyzed protein or amino acid mixtures. Goat's milk is not an acceptable substitute because it cross-reacts with cow's milk protein and is deficient in folic acid. Lactose-intolerant individuals are usually able to tolerate dairy products in which lactose has been fermented, such as yogurt, buttermilk, and cheese. Small amounts of cow's milk may also be consumed with meals without causing symptoms. When milk products are limited, the child's intake of vitamin D and calcium must be monitored to avoid deficiencies.

Infants who are milk sensitive are maintained on the diet until after 1 year of age. At this time very small quantities of milk are gradually reintroduced. Children with eczema or other allergic disorders may not be given milk for a considerably longer period of time.

Table 13-5   Signs and symptoms of cow's milk sensitivity

SYSTEM AFFECTED	SIGNS/SYMPTOMS
Gastrointestinal	*Diarrhea *Vomiting *Colic *Abdominal pain Malabsorption Enteropathy Constipation Anorexia Colitis
Respiratory	*Rhinitis *Bronchitis *Asthma *Sneezing *Coughing *Chronic nasal discharge Recurrent croup Serous otitis media
Dermatologic	*Eczema Urticaria Hives
Central nervous and behavioral	Excessive night waking *Excessive crying Excessive sweating Headache Hyperirritability Hyperactivity Lethargy
Vascular	Facial pallor Infraorbital edema (swelling under eyes)
Constitutional	Failure to thrive Retarded growth Malnutrition

*Most common.

Nursing Considerations

The principal nursing objectives are identification of potential milk sensitivity and appropriate counseling of parents regarding substitute formulas. If milk sensitivity is suspected, finding acceptable substitutions is frequently time-consuming, frustrating, and expensive. Parents are advised to purchase small quantities of the formula and to ask if unused portions can be returned.

The protein hydrolysate formulas are less palatable than milk-based formulas. Consequently reluctance to accept the new formula may be a problem. This can be overcome by introducing the formula gradually over a few days using 1 ounce of new formula to 7 ounces of old formula, then 2 to 6 ounces, 3 to 4, and as needed. Parents also need to be reassured that the infant will receive complete nutrition from the new formula and will suffer no ill effects from the absence of cow's milk.

Parents need guidance in avoiding all associated milk products (see Table 13-4). This requires carefully reading all food labels to avoid potential addition of milk products to the prepared food. If the infant is sensitive to soy, parents should be advised that it is commonly found in baby junior foods and cereals. In addition, some medications, such as penicillin, vitamins, and diaper ointment, contain lactose as a filler or bulk agent. Parents should be advised to check with the pharmacist regarding this possibility when obtaining drugs. Since allergy to one protein may mean allergy to other proteins, particularly egg albumin and wheat, such hyperallergenic foods should be restricted from the infant's diet for the first 9 to 12 months of life.

Feeding Difficulties

A number of feeding difficulties can occur during the infant's first year. Minor breast-feeding problems are common and often cause mothers considerable concern and discomfort. Some, such as spitting up, require little more than parental reassurance. Others, such as colic, can tremendously disrupt a family, although the problem resolves spontaneously. Still other disorders, such as rumination, can be fatal even though there is no organic cause.

BREAST-FEEDING PROBLEMS

Many mothers have concerns regarding breast-feeding and with earlier discharge from postpartum units, common problems, such as engorgement and painful nipples, may occur after the mother is at home. New mothers are often concerned about their milk supply and excessive anxiety can affect successful lactation. There is also increasing evidence that some completely breast-fed infants gain weight more slowly than expected, especially after the first 3 months. Whether this is because of insufficient nutrition from human milk to support adequate growth or a reflection of present growth charts whose standards are based on primarily formula-fed infants is unknown (Duncan and others, 1984; Stahl and Guida, 1984). However, vigilant observation of growth during the first year is required, and the situation may necessitate intervention to increase the frequency and amount of breast-feeding and/or supplementation.

The more common breast-feeding problems and their interventions are summarized in Table 13-6. Most of them are easily remedied, provided the mother receives the attention needed to identify the concern. Assessment includes a detailed history of the complaint, examination of the breasts, and observation of breast-feeding. When observing the breast-feeding couple, the following should be noted (Lawrence, 1985):

1. Position of mother, her body language, and tension
2. Position of infant: child's ventral surface should be next to mother's ventral surface with the face directly in front of the breast; infant cannot swallow if head has to turn to breast

3. Position of mother's hand on breast: using two fingers to compress areola and support breast facilitates infant's ability to grasp areola properly
4. Position of infant's lips on areola: lips should gently clamp the *entire* areola; lower lip should not be folded in so infant sucks lip
5. Use of alternate breasts and feeding time on each breast
6. Technique to break suction: should release suction using fingers between areola and lips, not pull infant from breast

Many breast-feeding problems respond rapidly to simple interventions, such as correcting the infant's feeding position. However the mother needs continual reassurance of success and support that allow her the needed rest and relaxation to nurse her infant. Referral to supportive agencies, such as La Leche League, may be beneficial (p. 325).

REGURGITATION AND "SPITTING UP"

The return of small amounts of food after a feeding is a common occurrence during infancy. It should not be confused with actual vomiting, which can be associated with a number of disturbances that may be insignificant or serious. It is usually benign, although persistent regurgitation necessitates medical evaluation to rule out gastroesophageal re-

---

Table 13-6 Common breast-feeding problems

PROBLEM	COMMENTS/INTERVENTIONS

Engorgement	Best intervention is prevention with frequent nursing on both breasts for complete emptying of ducts
	If engorgement occurs, infant is unable to properly grasp the distended areola
	Interventions:
	    Express manually small amount of milk; electric pump may be beneficial for some
	    Use warm compresses or a warm shower; for severely engorged breasts, cold compresses may be helpful to reduce vascularity
	    Compress areola with fingers to facilitate infant's grasp
	    Use well-fitting nursing brassiere and wear 24 hours a day
	    For excessive discomfort, take aspirin or acetaminophen 30 minutes before feeding

Painful nipples	Most common causes are poor feeding technique, improper care of breasts, excessive moisture from milk leaking
	If left untreated, discomfort may cause mother to terminate breast-feeding
	Interventions for care of breasts:
	    Avoid soaps, oils, or self-prescribed treatments
	    Can apply hydrous lanolin or A and D ointment, which do not need to be removed for nursing
	    Apply small amount of breast milk to areola after feeding and let dry
	    Air nipples as much as possible; use heat (60-watt bulb placed 18 inches away or hair dryer on low setting)
	Interventions related to feeding:
	    Begin nursing with less affected breast, then nurse on affected side
	    Position infant properly at breast; check that entire areola is grasped
	    Change infant's position; use football hold
	    May need to use nipple shield temporarily
	    For excessive discomfort, take aspirin or acetaminophen 30 minutes before feeding

Let-down reflex	Let-down (ejection) reflex is essential to delivery of milk from alveoli and smaller milk ducts into larger lactiferous ducts and sinuses
	Controlled primarily by release of prolactin and oxytocin
	Pain, stress, and anxiety can interfere with reflex
	Interventions:
	    Provide quiet, relaxing atmosphere for nursing; for example, soothing music, privacy, pillows for positioning, decreased distractions
	    Stroke the breast gently
	    Apply warmth to the breast
	    May need to use oxytocin nasal spray to induce a reflex

Inadequate milk supply	Production of milk depends on supply and demand
	Rarely is related to organic causes, such as decreased glandular tissue
	Interventions:
	    Reassure mother that her milk supply is probably adequate and depends on frequent nursing
	    Encourage more frequent nursing (at least six times daily at both breasts)
	    Encourage adequate rest, nutrition, and fluids (increased fluids, however, have not been shown to increase milk production)
	    Avoid use of supplemental formula feedings before breast-feeding is well established to prevent nipple confusion
	    Monitor the infant's growth; in some cases formula supplementation may be indicated; an alternative to bottle-feeding is the use of Lact-Aid, a device consisting of a plastic bag for formula and a thin feeding tube which is placed next to the mother's nipple during nursing

flux. For clarification the following terms are defined:

regurgitation Return of undigested food from the stomach, usually accompanied by burping

spitting up Dribbling of unswallowed formula from the infant's mouth immediately after a feeding

The insignificance of regurgitation or spitting up should be explained to parents, especially to those who are unduly concerned about it. It can be reduced by some simple measures, such as frequent burping during and after feeding, minimal handling at feeding and after, and positioning the child on the right side with the head slightly elevated after feeding. A test to check if the infant has burped involves placing one hand on the infant's abdomen and the other on the back and gently jiggling the child. If a splashing sound is heard, the infant has not burped (Temple and Farley, 1983). The inconvenience of spitting up can be managed with the use of absorbent bibs on the infant and protective cloths on the parent.

Sometimes frequent dribbling of formula causes excoriation of the corners of the mouth, chin, and neck. Keeping the area dry promotes healing but can be difficult to maintain. Helpful suggestions include applying a thin film of petrolatum jelly or A and D ointment to the affected areas after cleansing and using absorbent nonplastic-lined terry-cloth bibs, which are changed frequently.

PAROXYSMAL ABDOMINAL PAIN (COLIC)

Colic is generally described as paroxysmal abdominal pain or cramping that is manifested by loud crying and drawing the legs up to the abdomen. It is more common in young infants under the age of 3 months than in older infants, and infants with "difficult" temperaments are more likely to be colicky (Weissbluth, Christoffel, and Davis, 1984). Despite the obvious behavioral indications of pain, the child tolerates the formula well, gains weight, and thrives.

Many theories have been investigated as potential causative factors but currently no one theory is supported universally. In fact, much controversy exists over the etiology of the condition, and some authorities question if colic merely represents a maturational stage (see Questions and Controversies).

While colic is considered a minor ailment, the presence of a colicky, crying, irritable infant can have an intense emotional impact on parent-child attachment and family relationships. Mothers often relate histories of a daily routine that is laden with feelings of frustration, anger, despair, and helplessness. A vicious cycle ensues in which the parent's own anxiety may be transferred to the infant, further increasing the tension, irritability, and crying.

Therapeutic Management

Management of colic should begin with an investigation of diagnosable causes, such as cow's milk sensitivity. If a sensitivity to cow's milk is strongly suspected, a trial substitu-

Questions and Controversies

What are the causes of colic?

Among the theories that have been investigated as potential causes are too rapid feeding, overeating, swallowing excessive air, improper feeding technique (especially in positioning and burping), and emotional stress or tension between parent and child. While all of these may occur, there is no evidence that one factor is consistently present. Recent research indicates that colic may be a sign of cow's milk sensitivity and that eliminating cow's milk products from the diet of lactating mothers can reduce the symptoms (Jakobsson and Lindbery, 1983). Parental smoking has also been associated with colic and it is hypothesized that gastrointestinal contractions are triggered by olfactory or gustatory stimulation through a vagal reflex mechanism (Said, Patois, and Lellouch, 1984).

Some investigators discount the physical aspects of colic and attribute the problem to parents' ineffective responses to the infant's crying (Taubman, 1984). It is of interest that the incidence of colic differs markedly among social classes—with more parents from a higher socioeconomic status reporting colic. A possible explanation may be greater acceptance of an infant's crying behavior among lower social groups (Hide and Guyer, 1982). Increase in crying over the first several weeks is normal and is thought to represent maturation of the nervous system. It may be that some parents are particularly sensitive to crying, particularly if it occurs in infants who also demonstrate difficult temperament. One of the difficulties with the emotional theories of colic is whether or not the parents' concern with crying caused the colic or resulted from it. When one considers that children's cries can reach sound levels of 116 decibels, which is roughly equivalent to a pneumatic hammer, it is quite reasonable for parents to react inappropriately and become anxious (Bostrom and others, 1983).

tion of another formula, such as a casein hydrolysate (Nutramigen), is warranted. Soy formulas should be avoided because of the possibility of sensitivity to soy protein as well. When no specific inciting agent can be found, the supportive measures discussed under Nursing considerations are employed. In some instances drug therapy may be instigated with agents such as phenobarbitol elixir or dicyclomine hydrochloride (Bentyl syrup) (Carey, 1984; Weissbluth, Christoffel, and Davis, 1984).

Nursing Considerations

The initial step in managing colic is to take a thorough, detailed history of the usual daily events. Areas that should be stressed include (1) diet of the breast-feeding mother, (2) time of day when attacks occur, (3) relationship of the attacks to feeding time, (4) presence of specific family members during attacks, (5) activity of the mother or usual caregiver before, during, and after the crying, and (6) measures used to relieve the crying. Of special emphasis is a careful assessment of the feeding process via *demonstration* by the parent.

In breast-feeding mothers a milk-free diet (see Table 13-4) should be followed for a minimum of 5 days in an attempt to reduce symptoms in the infant. Mothers need to be cautioned that some nondairy creamers may contain calcium caseinate, a cow's milk protein. If this approach is helpful, lactating mothers may need calcium supplements to meet the body's requirement.

More often than not, no change is required in feeding practices. When no cause can be identified, it is preferable to determine the time of the onset of crying and attempt to manipulate the circumstances associated with it. For example, some infants have episodes of colic around the family's dinner time, when all household members are home and the mother is preoccupied with cooking. The overstimulating, more tense atmosphere may upset the infant. Encouraging someone else to prepare dinner or the mother to prepare dinner earlier in the day and feed the infant in a more quiet area of the house may help reverse the environmental conditions that may have provoked the attack of colic. Other approaches for relieving colic are listed opposite. Parents are encouraged to try as many of them as possible because not all are effective for every infant.*

One of the most important areas of nursing concern is the support of parents during the colic period. It should be stressed that despite the crying and obvious pain, the infant is doing well. Colic disappears spontaneously, usually by 3 months of age, although guarantees should never be given because it may continue for much longer. The parent, especially the mother, should be encouraged to leave the house and arrange for some free time. Most importantly, it should be emphasized that colic does not indicate poor or inadequate parenting. The mother's negative feelings toward the infant and her insecurities regarding her mothering abilities are normal. She should be encouraged to talk about them, since active listening may do more to relieve the colic syndrome than offering stereotyped advice, remedies, and glib statements such as, ''Don't worry about it; your child will eventually outgrow the colicky spells.''

RUMINATION

Rumination is the active, voluntary return of swallowed food into the mouth. The food is then rechewed, partially or completely reswallowed, or expelled. Technically, this is not a feeding problem since infant ruminators usually have hearty appetites. However in some instances rumination may lead to progressive malnutrition and even death, since considerable food and fluid loss can occur.

Rumination differs from regurgitation, which is involuntary. The ruminating infant makes purposeful movements of the mouth, tongue, and stomach in an attempt to force food back into the oropharynx. On successful regurgitation the infant is obviously satisfied with the activity.

Organic causes for rumination are rarely found, although the possibility of gastroesophageal reflux should be investigated in the differential diagnosis. It may also be seen in profoundly retarded children. However it is most often considered a result of a disturbance in the parent-child relationship. The factors culminating in the disorder are similar to those described in nonorganic failure to thrive. Some authorities believe it is a conditioned behavioral response to an increased need for self-stimulation or parental attention (Linscheid, 1985).

Treatment typically involves psychotherapy to improve parenting ability or behavior modification techniques to modify eating patterns. Behavioral approaches vary, but may include increased attention, such as holding before, during, and after meals, or aversive techniques, such as electric shock or the use of time-out (Whitehead and others, 1985).

Nursing Considerations

The primary objective is to terminate the ruminating behavior and restore normal feeding patterns. This is accomplished through a structured feeding plan. Generally the same guidelines apply to feeding the ruminating child as apply to feeding the failure-to-thrive child (see p. 569). In addition, emphasis should be placed on the following areas:

1. Have the same person feed the child as often as possible. This is even more critical than in failure to thrive.
2. Continue *positive* attention immediately after the feeding, since ruminating infants often vomit after a feeding once they are left unattended.

> ### SUGGESTIONS FOR RELIEVING COLIC
>
> Place infant prone over a hot-water bottle, heated towel, or covered heating pad.
> Massage abdomen.
> If the infant seems to be straining during bowel movements, use a glycerine suppository (child-size only) or administer a 1- or 2-ounce warm-water enema; peristalsis may also be stimulated by gently dilating the infant's anal sphincter with a well-lubricated little finger.
> Change the infant's position frequently; walk with him face down with his body across the parent's arm and hand under the abdomen applying gentle pressure.
> Use a front carrier for transporting the infant.
> Swaddle tightly with a soft, stretchy blanket.
> Place in a wind-up swing.
> Take for car rides or outside for a change in environment.
> Provide smaller, frequent feedings; burp during and after feedings using the shoulder position, and place in an upright seat after feedings.
> Introduce a pacifier for added sucking.
> Try giving warm, dilute herbal teas using one teaspoon fennel chamomile or anise.
> In breast-fed infants, have mother avoid all milk products for a trial period.
> If household members smoke, avoid smoking near infant; preferably confine smoking activity to outside of home.
> If nothing reduces the crying, place infant in crib and allow to cry; periodically hold and comfort child and put down again.

---

*A booklet that may be helpful is *Coping with Infant Colic: A Guide for Parents*, Columbus, OH, 1982, Ross Laboratories.

3. Introduce new foods, with emphasis on texture, consistency, and flavor. These children are often "picky eaters," and new foods introduced too quickly can increase rumination.
4. If acceptance of solids is a problem, give the child a small quantity of milk (or juice), immediately followed by 1 teaspoon of solid food. Begin with pureed food, and once accepted advance to junior and adult foods. Gradually give fewer sips of milk and more spoonfuls of food until a regular diet for the child's age is achieved.

These children may require prolonged inpatient intervention to reduce their rumination. Positive stimulation programs must accompany the feeding plan as loneliness has been known to trigger ruminating episodes (Fleisher, 1979). Parents need to be included in learning how to feed the child, and follow-up after discharge is essential to prevent a recurrence of the behavior.

FAILURE TO THRIVE

The term *failure to thrive* (FTT) is used to describe infants and children whose weight and sometimes height fall below the fifth percentile for their age. Beyond this definition there are several suggested subcategories of FTT. Generally the following two categories are recognized:

Organic failure to thrive (OFTT) is the result of a physical cause, such as congenital heart defects, neurologic lesions, microcephaly, chronic urinary tract infection, gastroesophageal reflux, renal insufficiency, malabsorption syndrome, endocrine dysfunction, or cystic fibrosis.

Nonorganic failure to thrive (NFTT or NOFTT) is caused by factors unrelated to organic dysfunction and is most often the result of psychosocial factors, the problem being between the child and primary caregiver, usually the mother. However NFTT may also occur when parents are uncertain of childrearing practices and infrequently feed the child. As many as one third of the cases may be described as "unexplained" by the usual organic and environmental etiologies (Berwick, Levy, and Kleinerman, 1982).

CHARACTERISTICS OF CHILDREN WITH NFTT

Growth failure—below fifth percentile in height and weight
Developmental retardation—social, motor, adaptive, language
Apathy
Poor hygiene
Withdrawn behavior
Feeding or eating disorders, such as vomiting, anorexia, voracious appetite, pica, rumination
No fear of strangers (at age when stranger anxiety is normal)
Avoidance of eye-to-eye contact
Wide-eyed gaze and continual scan of the environment ("radar gaze")
Stiff and unyielding or flaccid and unresponsive
Minimum smiling

NFTT has been described under a variety of names, including maternal deprivation, environmental deprivation, and deprivation dwarfism. *Psychosocial dwarfism (PSD)* refers to children who have physical characteristics and endocrine function tests similar to those found in the clinical state of hypopituitarism but who improve in response to environmental change without hormonal therapy. Some authors use PSD to refer to children with NFTT who are at least 18 months of age (Thompson, 1981) (see also p. 859).

Regardless of the classification, a minority of children (20% to 30%) are found to have organic causes and the diagnosis of NFTT is usually made on the basis of exclusion of pathophysiologic findings. Unfortunately many of these children are unnecessarily subjected to exhausting, traumatic, and expensive diagnostic procedures. To prevent this, NFTT should be considered *early* in the differential diagnosis, when a careful history and physical examination rule out a gross medical cause. Clinical criteria that can be used to diagnose NFTT include (Barbero, 1974):

1. Weight below the fifth percentile with subsequent weight gain in the presence of adequate nurturing or mothering
2. No evidence of systemic disease or congenital abnormality that explains the growth failure
3. Developmental retardation with subsequent improvement following appropriate stimulation
4. Clinical signs of deprivation that decrease in a more nurturing environment
5. Presence of significant environmental psychosocial interruption

NFTT has traditionally been referred to as *maternal deprivation syndrome* because of the findings that mothers of FTT children have difficulty relating to and perceiving the needs of these children. However the disturbance in the relationship involves at least two individuals: the child and the primary caregiver. Because complex physical, psychosocial, and emotional variables affect this relationship, it is more correct to refer to the problem as one of *parent-child attachment*. This broader interactional view permits an understanding of the characteristics of the child, parent, and environment important in preventing, diagnosing, and treating NFTT.

Characteristics of Failure-to-Thrive Children and Their Families

The child. Besides the obvious signs of malnutrition and delayed development, these children interact differently from children with OFTT (see box). They display intense interest in inanimate objects, such as a toy, but less interest in social interactions. They are vigilant of people at a distance but become increasingly distressed as they come closer. They dislike being touched and avoid face-to-face contact. However, when held, they protest on being put down. The protest is not sustained and the infants are apathetic when left alone. These characteristics of approach and withdrawal behavior can be used with infants ages 6 to 16 months to differentiate types of FTT (Rosenn, Loeb, and Jura, 1980).

Frequently there is a history of difficult feeding, vomiting, sleep disturbance, and excessive irritability. Difficulties in infant feeding may include poor appetite, poor suck, crying during feedings, vomiting, hoarding food in the mouth, ruminating after feeding, refusal to switch from liquids to solids, and aversion behavior such as turning from food or spitting food. Ultimately these habit patterns become attention-seeking mechanisms to prolong the attention received at mealtime. In addition, chronic reduction in calories can lead to appetite depression, which compounds the problem.

An outstanding feature of FTT children is their irregularity (low rhythmicity) in activities of daily living. Some of these children typify the "difficult" temperament pattern. However another type are the passive, sleepy, lethargic infants who do not wake up for feedings. Parents who have been advised of "demand feeding schedules" may be unsure of whether to wake the child or let him sleep. Because of their inexperience and lack of guidance, they may develop a pattern of infrequent feeding that is inadequate to meet the infant's nutritional needs. Such a pattern is particularly devastating with the breast-feeding infant, where frequent nursing is essential to an adequate milk supply.

It cannot be assumed that such characteristics in a child result in FTT. Rather, there is probably a complex set of variables that are significant. One may be the degree of *fit* between the child's temperament and that of the parents. Since the personalities of infants can have definite effects on the parent-child attachment process, identifying situations of disharmony between the mother's expectations of the average child vs her child by using such tools as the Neonatal Perception Inventory (p. 327) may be one approach toward prevention and anticipatory guidance.

The parents. Some parents are at increased risk for attachment problems because of (1) isolation and social crisis, (2) inadequate support systems, and (3) receiving poor parenting themselves as children. Other factors that should be considered are lack of education; physical and mental health problems, such as retardation, depression, or drug dependence; immaturity, especially in adolescent parents; and lack of commitment to parenting, such as giving higher priority to career goals.

Frequently these parents and their families are under stress and in multiple chronic emotional, social, and financial crises. Of particular significance is the prevalence of marital discord, including frequent arguments, separations, and reconciliations (Altemeier and others, 1985).

Many of these parents display negative maladaptive feelings toward the infant (see box). Inadequate feeding and caring may be part of an abuse cycle. Ambivalence toward pregnancy can be an early clue when combined with other characteristics of high-risk parents. Being alert to such clues may avert a potential FTT situation by identifying these parents prenatally and planning interventions aimed at increasing satisfying parenting skills (see also p. 686).

FTT children are not limited to lower socioeconomic groups. Although financial crisis generally means "poor," families with adequate monetary resources can be in chronic financial stress if their standard of living exceeds their income. Emotional deprivation, a kind of rejection, can also occur in financially stable homes where all childrearing responsibilities are left to others. Although this is less visible and frequently produces emotionally neglected children, such families can include children who are physically and emotionally starved. Refusal to eat may be the child's response to an uncaring environment. It is essential for nurses to set aside stereotypes and prejudices in order to be aware of the potential for existence of such children in *any* family situation.

Prognosis

The prognosis for FTT is uncertain. The question of whether helping the parent learn new ways of relating to and caring for the child can permanently change behavior in conflict-laden, stressful situations always remains. Many of these children are below normal in intellectual development,

---

PARENTAL MALADAPTIVE BEHAVIORS TOWARD INFANT

Persistent ambivalence or negative feelings about the fetus and the pregnancy during the prenatal period

Makes no plans for obtaining basic infant supplies

Appears indifferent to infant at time of delivery; may appear sad or angry; is expressionless

Makes no effort to establish eye-to-eye contact with infant

Handles infant only when necessary

Does not talk to infant

Makes few or no spontaneous movements with infant

Asks few questions about care

Sees infant as ugly, fat, or unattractive

Displays disgust with infant's drooling and sucking sounds; is revolted by infant's body fluids

Annoyed with diaper changing

Perceives infant's odor as revolting

Holds infant with little support to head and body

Holds infant away from body during feeding or props bottle for feeding; seldom cuddles infant

Does not coo or talk to infant

Refers to infant in an impersonal manner

Develops inappropriate responses to infant's needs, such as leaving infant in one place for long periods, leaving him alone in room, overfeeding or underfeeding, overstimulating or understimulating infant, forcing or refusing eye contact, bouncing or tickling infant when he is fatigued

Cannot discriminate between infant's signals for hunger, comfort, rest, body contact

Is convinced the infant has a defect or disease even when reassured to the contrary

Makes negative statements regarding mothering role

Believes the infant is judging her and her efforts as an adult

Believes the infant does not love her and exposes her as an unlovable and unloving mother

Develops paradoxical attitudes and behaviors toward the infant

have poorer language development and less well-developed reading skills, attain lower social maturity, and have a higher incidence of behavioral disturbances (Oates, Peacock, and Forrest, 1985). Such findings support the contention that a long-term plan is needed for the optimum development of these children.

Nursing Considerations

The priority nursing goal is providing the infant with sufficient nutrients for growth. More specific nursing care depends on identifying the cause of FTT. If an organic etiology is confirmed, care is primarily related to management of the disorder. If the problem is one of inadequate knowledge regarding child-feeding, parental education is required. When serious psychosocial factors are involved, hospitalization is needed and additional interventions are required to structure the environment for positive interactions. The following discussion is concerned with hospitalization of the child with NFTT.

Since part of the difficulty between parent and child is dissatisfaction and frustration, the NFTT child should have a consistent primary nurse for all three shifts. Only the same nurse caring for the child over a period of time can learn to perceive the child's cues and reverse the cycle of dissatisfaction, especially in the area of feeding. Since these children are not ill with any physical disorder but debilitated from general malnutrition, they should be placed in a room with noninfectious children of a similar age.

Each child with NFTT is responding to stimuli that have led to negative feeding patterns. The first goal of care is to assess those patterns and tailor the feeding process so that negative habits can be changed and replaced with positive ones. Several general guidelines can be established for the feeding interaction:

1. **Provide a quiet, unstimulating atmosphere.** A number of these children are very distractible and their attention can be diverted with minimal stimuli. Older children do well at a feeding table; younger children should always be held. A single adult in the feeding situation is recommended.
2. **Maintain a calm, even temperament throughout the meal.** Negative outbursts may be commonplace in this child's habit formation. Limits on eating behavior definitely need to be provided, but they should be stated in a firm, calm tone. If the nurse is hurried or anxious, the feeding process will not be optimized.
3. **Talk to the child by giving directions about eating.** "Take a bite, Lisa" is appropriate and directive. The more distractible the child, the more directive the nurse should be to refocus attention on feeding. Positive comments about feeding should be actively given.
4. **Follow the child's rhythm of feeding.** The child will set a rhythm when the previous conditions are met.
5. **Develop a structured routine.** NFTT children are in particular need of routine feeding patterns. Disruption in their other activities of daily living have great impact on feeding responses, so these should also be structured. The same nurse should feed the child in the same way and place as often as possible. The length of the feeding should also be established (usually 30 minutes).
6. **Be persistent.** This is perhaps one of the most important guidelines. Parents often give up when the child begins negative feeding behavior. Calm perseverance through 10 to 15

Nursing Care Summary: The Child with Nonorganic Failure to Thrive

NURSING GOALS	NURSING INTERVENTIONS	EXPECTED PATIENT/FAMILY OUTCOMES
HP-HMP	**Injury: potential for trauma, neglect** **Risk factors: mothering failure**	
Identify mothers (and fathers) at risk	Be alert to parental maladaptive behaviors toward the infant (see box, p. 569) Determine extent and quality of mother's mothering Determine if pregnancy was planned or unplanned Determine if there were any disturbing events associated with pregnancy or delivery of the child	*High-risk parents are identified early and appropriate intervention is initiated
Recognize characteristics of parents of failure-to-thrive children	Be alert to the following History of maternal deprivation as a child Low self-esteem; feelings of inadequacy Desire for dependency Loneliness, isolation Limited support system Multiple life crises and stress	Same as above
Identify children who fail to thrive	Suspect nonorganic failure to thrive in infants and young children who display typical characteristics (see box, p. 567)	*Children are identified and appropriate care is implemented

*Nursing outcome.

Continued.

Nursing Care Summary: The Child with Nonorganic Failure to Thrive—cont'd

NURSING GOALS	NURSING INTERVENTIONS	EXPECTED PATIENT/FAMILY OUTCOMES

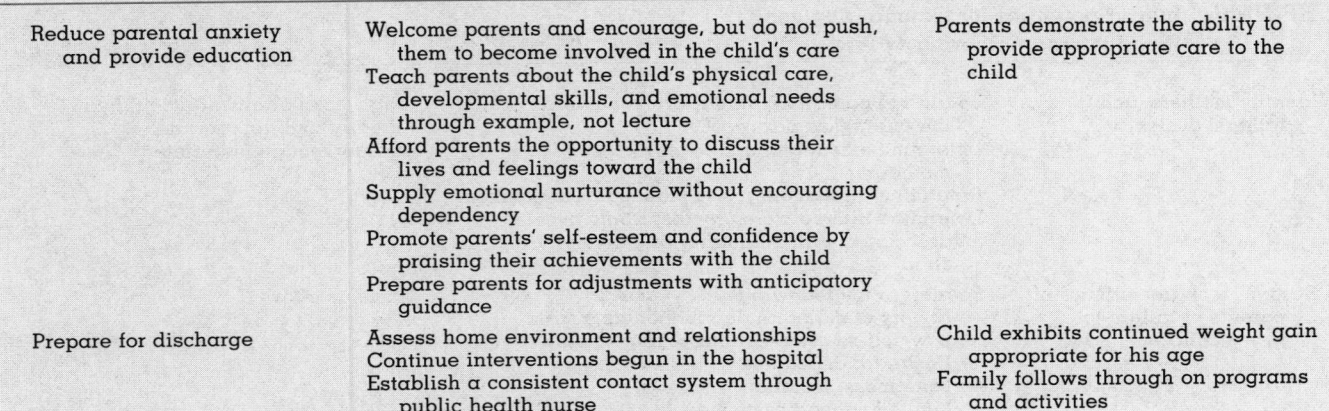

N-MP   Nutrition, alteration in: less than body requirements
Etiology: deprivation of necessities, emotional deprivation

NURSING GOALS	NURSING INTERVENTIONS	EXPECTED PATIENT/FAMILY OUTCOMES
Make feeding a priority goal	Provide unlimited feedings of a regular diet for the age of the child (preferably foods to which the child is accustomed) Avoid interruption of feedings with other activities, such as laboratory examinations or radiography Keep accurate record of intake to ensure ingestion of calculated daily calories Weigh daily and record to ascertain weight gain	Child gains 1 to 2 ounces per day (minimum)
Introduce a positive feeding environment	Assign one nurse for feeding Maintain calm, even temperament; be persistent Provide a quiet, unstimulating environment Hold young child for feeding Maintain eye-to-eye contact with child Talk to child by giving appropriate directions and praise for eating Follow the child's rhythm of feeding Establish a structured routine and follow it consistently	Infant responds positively to feeding practices (specify)

CPP   Sensory-perceptual alteration: visual, auditory, kinesthetic, gustatory, tactile, olfactory
Etiology: socially restricted environment (infant deprivation)

NURSING GOALS	NURSING INTERVENTIONS	EXPECTED PATIENT/FAMILY OUTCOMES
Provide a nurturing environment for the hospitalized child	Assess child's developmental age Apply primary care concepts to ensure continuity of care with a minimum number of caregivers Provide gentle, sure, and loving handling Perform physical care with as much holding, rocking, and cuddling as the child will respond to Encourage eye-to-eye contact Employ consistent schedule in meeting child's needs for food, hygiene, care, and rest Assign a foster grandparent or child life specialist to child Provide sensory stimulation and play appropriate to the child's developmental level	Infant displays a positive response to interventions e.g., social smile

RRP   Parenting, alteration in: actual
Etiology: specify (knowledge deficit, poverty, neglect, etc.)

NURSING GOALS	NURSING INTERVENTIONS	EXPECTED PATIENT/FAMILY OUTCOMES
Reduce parental anxiety and provide education	Welcome parents and encourage, but do not push, them to become involved in the child's care Teach parents about the child's physical care, developmental skills, and emotional needs through example, not lecture Afford parents the opportunity to discuss their lives and feelings toward the child Supply emotional nurturance without encouraging dependency Promote parents' self-esteem and confidence by praising their achievements with the child Prepare parents for adjustments with anticipatory guidance	Parents demonstrate the ability to provide appropriate care to the child
Prepare for discharge	Assess home environment and relationships Continue interventions begun in the hospital Establish a consistent contact system through public health nurse Establish an infant stimulation program Provide for stress-relieving services to the family Refer to appropriate agencies for assistance with financial, social, mental health, or other family needs	Child exhibits continued weight gain appropriate for his age Family follows through on programs and activities

minutes of food refusal will eventually diminish negative behavior. Although forced feeding should be avoided, ''strictly encouraged'' feeding is essential.

7. **Maintain a face-to-face posture with the child when possible.** Encourage eye contact and remain with the child throughout the meal.

The optimum method for changing feeding habit patterns negative to growth is to stop the feeding interaction between parent and child. It is recommended that staff members feed these children. Initially parents should be encouraged to visit often but not at mealtime until caloric intake and weight gain are adequate. With toddlers, role-modeling and play activities, such as feeding dolls or stuffed animals, may be helpful and less distractible children may benefit from observing the eating behavior of other children.

Foods appropriate to the child's age should be selected. To increase caloric intake, supplements, such as Polycose, can be added to foods. Often, NFTT children have been exclusively bottle-fed and refuse all solids. In these situations, introduction of solids begins with pureed foods, then junior foods, finger foods, and finally regular table food.

Besides attending to the physical needs of the child, the nurse must plan care for appropriate developmental stimulation. The word ''appropriate'' is emphasized because it refers to the child's developmental, not chronologic, age. Assessing the developmental age should be done on admission by administering the Denver Developmental Screening Test (DDST) or another psychometric test. The DDST gives an approximate age for the child's present achievement in gross/fine motor, social-adaptive, and language skills. Only after objective measurements are available can a plan of care for stimulation be organized. Periodic testing is an excellent tool for evaluation of the child's developmental progress.

Nursing care of NFTT children involves a systems approach. In other words, for the entire family to become healthy, each member must be helped to change. To nurture the child back to physical, developmental, and emotional health during hospitalization while neglecting the emotional needs of the parents does not solve the problem. Therefore the nursing care plan must also include the parents and siblings. Other significant persons, who can be helped to be more emotionally, physically, and financially supportive to the family unit, can become the emotional reservoir needed by parents to give nurturance to their child. Some hospitals have child-life specialists or volunteer foster grandparents who spend scheduled, consistent periods of time with the infant as a kind of surrogate mother.

Mental health services, such as individual or group therapy, may also be beneficial. Care of the mother is aimed at helping her increase her feelings of self-esteem through positive, successful mothering skills. Initially this necessitates providing an environment in which she feels welcomed and accepted. Because these women are often distrustful of authority figures, it may take some time before the mother develops any trust toward the nurse. One approach is to empathize with the parent about the difficulties of child-rearing. For example, the nurse may state that many parents find adjusting to parenthood a trying time or that the demands of caring for an infant can become overwhelming.

Once the mother feels comfortable enough to visit with her infant, infant care techniques should be taught through *example* and *demonstration,* not by lecturing. As the nurse perceives the infant's cues, these are emphasized to the mother. For example, during a feeding the nurse might comment that the infant is still hungry because he sucks vigorously and looks at her. When he is satisfied, the nurse points out that the infant is signaling this by releasing the strong suck, closing his eyes, and breathing deeply and more slowly. By example, the child is then gently placed in the crib for a nap.

At the same time the mother is offered an opportunity to care for the infant without making demands on her. For example, the nurse suggests that at the next feeding the mother offer her child the bottle. Whenever the mother participates, she is praised for her efforts and encouraged to continue caring for the child.

Before discharge, plans should be made to continue these interventions at home. A public health referral is made, and if a foster grandparent was included, this person should also visit the family. Social agencies that can provide financial or housing assistance to lessen the stress of everyday life should also be contacted.

Skin Disorders

A number of skin problems manifest themselves during infancy. The most common is diaper dermatitis; others that occur during infancy are seborrheic dermatitis or eczema. While these conditions can be benign, they are often of considerable concern to parents. The nurse is in an advantageous position to counsel parents regarding care of these common skin problems.

DIAPER DERMATITIS

Dermatitis in the diaper area is encountered frequently by nurses in all pediatric settings. Approximately 50% of young children demonstrate some degree of diaper dermatitis and about 5% have severe rash (intense erythema, scaling, papules, and ulcerations). The peak age for diaper dermatitis is 9 to 12 months and may be associated with decreased frequency of diaper changes and modifications in diet, such as change from breast milk to formula and introduction of solids. The incidence is greater in bottle-fed than in breast-fed infants (Jordan and others, 1986).

Pathophysiology and Clinical Manifestations

Diaper dermatitis is caused by prolonged and repetitive contact with an irritant, principally urine, feces, soaps, detergents, ointments, and friction. Although the obvious irritant

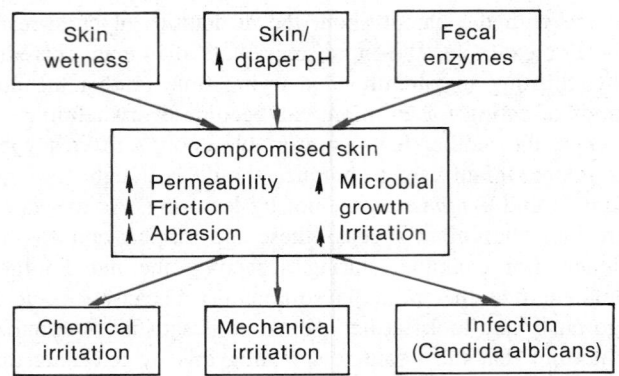

Fig. 13-3. Principal factors involved in development of diaper dermatitis.
Modified from a model developed by L. Benjamin, R.W. Berg, W.E. Jordan, A.M. Marrer, and R.E. Zimmerer. Reproduced with permission of the Procter & Gamble Co.

in the majority of incidences is urine and feces, the specific components that contribute to irritation are poorly understood. Current research, however, supports the following model (Fig. 13-3).

Prolonged contact of the skin with diaper wetness affects several skin properties. It produces higher friction, greater abrasion damage, increased transepidermal permeability, and increased microbial counts (Zimmerer, Lawson, and Calvert, 1986). Therefore healthy skin becomes less resistant to potential irritants.

While ammonia has long been thought to cause diaper rash because of the association between the strong odor on diapers and dermatitis, this alone is not sufficient. The important function of urine is related to an increase in pH from the breakdown of urea in the presence of fecal urease. The increased pH promotes the activity of fecal enzymes, principally proteases and lipases, which act as irritants. Fecal enzymes also increase the permeability of skin to bile salts, another potential irritant in feces. The decreased incidence of diaper dermatitis in breast-fed infants is felt to be related to this interaction between pH and fecal enzymes, since feces from breast-fed infants have lower fecal enzyme activity and lower pH (Berg, Buckingham, and Stewart, 1986; Buckingham and Berg, 1986).

The eruption of diaper dermatitis can be manifested primarily on convex surfaces or in the folds, and the lesions can represent a variety of types and configurations (Table 13-7). Eruptions involving the skin in most intimate contact with the diaper (e.g., the convex surfaces of buttocks, inner thighs, mons pubis, and scrotum) but sparing the folds are likely to be caused by chemical irritants, especially from urine and feces. Other causes are detergents or soaps from inadequately rinsed cloth diapers or the fragrance added to some diapers.

Perianal involvement is usually the result of chemical irritation from feces, especially diarrheal stools. *Candida albicans* infection produces perianal inflammation with satellite lesions; whether *C. albicans* initiates diaper dermatitis or aggravates an existing rash is not known.

Therapeutic Management

Treatment is primarily related to the measures discussed under Nursing considerations. For stubborn inflammations that do not respond to these interventions, topical glucocorticoid preparations are sometimes required. If steroids are prescribed, their use should be limited to low-potency preparations such as 1% hydrocortisone cream. Potent fluorinated steroids should be avoided because of the potential side effects of striae, epidermal atrophy, suppression of the pituitary-adrenal axis, cessation of longitudinal growth, and frank Cushing syndrome (Weston, Lane, and Weston, 1980). The common use of triamcinolone-containing preparations combined with antiyeast and antibacterial agents such as Mycolog is not recommended.

Candida infections are treated with nystatin ointment. Where *Candida* is the causative agent, oral administration of a fungicide is advised because the gastrointestinal tract is usually the source of infection (see p. 345).

Nursing Considerations

Nursing interventions are aimed at altering the three factors considered to produce dermatitis—wetness, pH, and fecal irritants. The most significant factor amenable to interven-

Table 13-7 Skin eruptions in the diaper area*

AREA INVOLVED	USUAL DIAGNOSIS/CAUSE
Convex surfaces involved; folds spared	Contact dermatitis Allergic or irritant dermatitis/Chemical irritants (urine, feces, detergents, soaps)
Folds involved, sharply demarcated	Intertrigo/Heat, moisture, and sweat retention Seborrheic dermatitis/Inborn trait
Folds involved with satellite lesions	Seborrheic dermatitis with secondary candidiasis/Inborn trait plus *Candida albicans* infection
Perianal	Chemical and mechanical irritation/Chemical irritants (fecal enzymes)
Perianal with satellite lesions	Primary candidiasis/*C. albicans* infection
Band of erythema at diaper margins	"Tide mark" dermatitis/Plastic or rubber border on diaper and sweat retention
Small, sterile vesicopustules	Miliaria "Heat rash," "prickly heat"/Hot, humid climate in diaper area
Vesicles of bullae	Bullous impetigo Herpes (less common)/*Staphylococcus aureus* Herpes simplex

*Modified from Jacobs, A.H.: Pediatr. Clin. North Am. **25**(2):209-224, 1978.

tion is the moist environment created in the diaper area. Changing the diaper as soon as it becomes wet eliminates a large part of the problem, and removing the diaper entirely for extended periods to expose the area to light and air facilitates drying and healing. Occlusive diaper coverings, such as plastic pants, prevent evaporation and should not be used except for brief social occasions. During the nighttime the diaper should be changed at least once, such as before the parents retire. Double diapering, the use of two cotton or disposable diapers *without* the plastic lining, or the use of disposable diapers with absorbent gelling material, increases absorbency and draws wetness away from the skin.

After soiling, the perineal area should be cleansed. Wiping with a wet cloth is usually sufficient to remove urine. However, after stooling, the area, especially the skin folds, needs to be thoroughly cleansed, rinsed, and dried. In some instances, especially with diarrheal stools and irritated skin, a sponge bath may be given. Exposing the skin to warm, dry air for a few minutes before applying the diaper is helpful. Parents should be advised that the use of disposable wet towels can aggravate the problem because the child may be sensitive to one or more agents in the product.

Occasionally applying an occlusive ointment, such as zinc oxide or petrolatum, to noninflamed skin can prevent

Questions and Controversies

What are the benefits and risks of talc vs cornstarch?

Talc and cornstarch are common ingredients in baby powders and the majority of parents routinely use such products to keep the diapered area dry, to make the baby smell nice, and to prevent or treat diaper rash (Hayden and Sproul, 1984). However there is considerable concern with the safety of using talc and cornstarch and controversy regarding their benefits.

Talc is a soft, flexible, crystalline magnesium-silicate that is chemically related to several asbestos group minerals (Lockey and Parry, 1984). Mined talc is seldom pure and may contain several other mineral fibers, including asbestos. Epidemiologic studies have clearly linked lung cancer and other pleural disorders to asbestos exposure, including the amount found in talc. There is also evidence that talc may be linked to ovarian cancer (Cramer and others, 1982). However the greatest risk among young children is aspiration pneumonia from accidental inhalation (see p. 534).

Cornstarch is an absorbable starch. Unlike talc it is not associated with pulmonary complications. However, traditionally, it has been assumed that cornstarch promotes the growth of *Candida albicans*. A study comparing cornstarch and talc found that neither product supports growth of the fungi under conditions normally found in the diaper area (Leyden, 1984).

The benefits of both products are related to their ability to absorb moisture and reduce friction. Cornstarch is somewhat more effective in reducing friction and tends to cake less than talc when the skin is wet. (Leyden, 1984). Based on these properties and its safety in terms of inhalation injury, cornstarch is the preferred product if the parents choose to apply a powder.

Questions and Controversies

Can the type of diaper influence the development of diaper dermatitis?

The type of diapers commonly used in the United States are disposable and home-laundered or commercially laundered cloth diapers. The majority of infants wear disposable diapers. Studies comparing the incidence of diaper dermatitis generally support the finding of decreased rash in infants wearing disposable or commercially laundered cloth diapers as compared with the home-laundered type (Jordan and others, 1986; Grant, Street, and Fearnow, 1973; Stein, 1982). Although the reasons for this are not clear, one explanation is the reduced wetness against the skin from disposable versus cloth diapers (Zimmerer, Lawson, and Calvert, 1986).

There is also evidence that the type of disposable diaper can affect the incidence of dermatitis. Based on the theory that diaper dermatitis is related to interaction among skin wetness, pH, and fecal enzymes, manufacturers of one disposable diaper (Ultra Pampers*) have added absorbent gelling material (AGM) to the cellulose core of the diaper. When in contact with fluid, the AGM forms a gel which traps wetness away from the skin and helps separate the deposition of urine and feces on the diaper. Less mixing of these substances decreases the effect of urine pH on the fecal enzymes. AGM also has a buffering ability toward the acidic side, which further weakens the pH and enzymatic interaction (Campbell, 1986).

*Manufactured by Procter & Gamble, Cincinnati, OH.

the development of diaper dermatitis, provided good hygiene is also practiced. During cleansing, the ointment is removed and then reapplied. Zinc oxide is most easily removed with mineral oil. These ointments should not be applied to inflamed areas because they tend to contribute to sweat retention. The use of talcum powder is of questionable benefit and poses the hazard of accidental aspiration (see Questions and controversies). Despite the known risks of talc it is a common baby care product. The majority of parents are likely to receive a free sample of the product in the nursery and to continue using that brand (Hayden and Sproul, 1984). While no known research exists to substantiate if this practice influences the incidence of inhalation injury, nurses have a responsibility to inform parents of the risks and to instruct them in the correct application and safe storage of powders (see p. 535).

The selection and care of diapers are very important aspects in preventing inflammation or further irritation. There is also evidence that the type of diaper can influence the development of dermatitis (see Questions and controversies).* If diapers are laundered at home, they should be soaked in a quaternary ammonium compound (such as Dia-

*A pamphlet, *Diaper Rash*, which describes the development of diaper rash related to kinds of diapers, is available from the American Academy of Pediatrics, 141 Northwest Point Blvd., P.O. Box 927, Elk Grove Village, IL 60007 (1-800-433-9016).

parene) or dilute hypochlorite (bleach), washed in hot water with a simple laundry soap (such as Ivory), and run through the rinse cycle twice.

SEBORRHEIC DERMATITIS

Seborrheic dermatitis is a chronic, recurrent, inflammatory reaction of the skin, that occurs most commonly on the scalp (cradle cap), but may involve the eyelids (blepharitis), external ear canal (otitis externa), nasolabial folds, and inguinal region. The cause is unknown, although it is more common in early infancy when sebum production is increased. The lesions are characteristically thick, adherent, yellowish, scaly, oily patches that may or may not be mildly pruritic. Unlike eczema, seborrheic dermatitis is not associated with a positive family history for allergy and is very common in infants shortly after birth. Diagnosis is made primarily by the appearance and location of the crusts.

Nursing Considerations

Cradle cap may be prevented with adequate scalp hygiene. Not infrequently parents omit shampooing the infant's hair from fear of damaging the "soft spots" or fontanels. The nurse should discuss how to shampoo the infant's hair and emphasize that the fontanel is like skin anywhere else on the body—it does not puncture or tear with mild pressure.

When seborrheic lesions are present, the treatment is mainly directed at removing the crusts. Parents should be taught the appropriate procedure to clean the scalp, which may necessitate a demonstration. Shampooing should be done daily with a mild soap or commercial baby shampoo. If an oil such as baby oil is applied, it should be massaged into the scalp and allowed to penetrate and soften the crusts and then thoroughly washed out. Using a fine-tooth comb or a small toothbrush after shampooing helps remove the loosened crusts from the strands of hair. Topical preparations are usually not necessary but if prescribed require the same teaching as discussed for atopic dermatitis.

ATOPIC DERMATITIS (ECZEMA)

Atopic dermatitis is a common dermatologic condition that presents in three distinct forms:

Infantile, which usually begins between 2 and 6 months of age
Childhood, which may follow the infantile phase and occurs by 2 to 3 years of age
Adolescent and adult, which begins at about 12 years of age and frequently continues into the early twenties

Infantile eczema usually undergoes spontaneous and permanent remission by 3 years of age. However, because the disease occurs predominantly in infancy, this discussion is restricted to the infantile form.

The cause of eczema is unknown. However several factors support a role for IgE-mediated hypersensitivity: (1) approximately two thirds of children have a positive family history for atopic disease; (2) 50% to 80% of children with eczema develop asthma or allergic rhinitis; (3) serum IgE concentrations are usually elevated; and (4) most children have positive skin tests to a variety of allergens, especially eggs, peanuts, and cow's milk (Sampson and McCaskill, 1985).

There is much controversy regarding prevention of eczema. Some studies suggest that infants are less likely to develop atopic dermatitis if given breast milk or if introduction of hyperallergenic foods is delayed until the latter half of the first year. It is also suggested that lactating mothers of infants with a family history of allergy avoid hyperallergenic foods during the breast-feeding period. Although conclusive evidence is lacking, these practices should be recommended because they may be beneficial to some infants at risk for eczema.

Clinical Manifestations

The lesions are characteristic in appearance and location, depending on age. In infants the lesions are erythematous, papulovesicular, exudative, and highly pruritic. The affected areas include the cheeks and extensor surfaces of the arms, legs, and wrists. In childhood and beyond the lesions are dry and lichenification (thickening of the epidermis) occurs; the distribution favors the flexor surfaces, especially the antecubital, popliteal, and collar regions, and spares the face. The intense itching associated with the rash may result in secondary infection if the lesions are scratched. The child is usually very irritable, fretful, and unable to sleep because of the persistent pruritus.

The unaffected areas of the body tend to be dry and rough. Lymphadenopathy, particularly near affected sites such as the cervical area, is common. Other systemic manifestations are rare.

Therapeutic Management

Treatment of eczema is primarily supportive. The first objective is removal of specific allergens. The onset of eczema is frequently associated with the introduction of cow's milk or new foods, particularly egg white, to infants. The child is placed on a hypoallergenic diet that typically restricts the foods listed in Table 13-4.

A hypoallergenic diet for an infant might include a milk substitute such as soy formula, rice cereal, apples, apricots, carrots, string beans, beef, and aqueous multiple-vitamin supplements. The diet is followed for 10 days; if remission occurs, each food from the restricted list is added one at a time at weekly intervals to identify specific food allergens. Milk and then wheat are usually the first two foods added for suspected sensitivity. Even if all foods can be accepted, eggs are usually not permitted. If response to the hypoallergenic diet is unsuccessful, environmental control is attempted to lessen the amount of inhalants.

Pruritus is the most difficult medical and nursing problem. Itching and scratching lead to infection, which in turn results in loss of the stratum corneum or lichenification. Measures that reduce skin irritation are discussed under Nursing considerations. Not infrequently the itching and irritability warrant the judicious use of medication, such as chloral hydrate, diphenhydramine (Benadryl), hydroxyzine hydrochloride (Atarax or Vistaril), or cyproheptadine (Periactin).

Since the use of hot water and soap intensifies skin drying and irritation, baths are either avoided or given with plain, tepid water. Nonlipid, hydrophilic agents, such as Cetaphil lotion, are useful cleansing and lubricating solutions. Colloid baths, such as the addition of 2 cups of cornstarch to a tub of warm water, temporarily relieves itching and may help the child sleep if given before bedtime. Wet soaks or dressings are soothing to the skin and provide antiseptic protection.

Nursing Care Summary: The Child with Eczema

NURSING GOALS	NURSING INTERVENTIONS	EXPECTED PATIENT/FAMILY OUTCOMES
N-MP Skin integrity: impairment of **Etiology: immunologic deficit**		
Prevent or minimize scratching	Keep fingernails and toenails short and clean Wrap hands in soft cotton gloves or stockings; pin to shirt cuff Avoid overheating, high humidity, and perspiration Use elbow restraints when absolutely necessary, but allow supervised periods of unrestricted movement Encourage exposure to ultraviolet light, but avoid sunburn	Affected areas remain unirritated
A-EP Diversional activity, deficit **Etiology: restricted movement, restraining devices**		
Encourage play activities that are suitable to skin condition and child's developmental age	Avoid any furry, hairy stuffed toys or dolls Provide kinesthetic, moving toys, large toys, which require less fine motor skills if hands are covered, and quiet musical or visual toys	Child engages in activities appropriate for age
SRP Sleep pattern disturbance **Etiology: discomfort and restlessness**		
Promote rest	Plan meals, baths, medications, and treatments around nap or bedtime Make child as comfortable as possible before sleep to enhance restfulness (for example, give sedation and then bath before bedtime)	Child receives an adequate amount of rest for age
CPP Sensory-perceptual alteration: tactile **Etiology: skin lesions, dressings, and/or restraining devices**		
Provide tactile contact	Hold child Remember that there is no substitute for the stimulation and comfort of human contact Touch and caress unaffected area	Child exhibits signs of comfort Child responds positively to tactile stimulation
SP-SCP Self-care deficit: feeding, bathing/hygiene, dressing/grooming, toileting (specify level) **Etiology: developmental level, special needs**		
Promote nutrition	Provide nutritious meals within limitations of food restrictions Feed child when he is well rested Do not force or introduce a restricted food to encourage eating	Child consumes an appropriate amount of nutrients (specify) Restricted foods are eliminated Child assists with feeding within his capabilities

Continued.

Nursing Care Summary: The Child with Eczema—cont'd

NURSING GOALS	NURSING INTERVENTIONS	EXPECTED PATIENT/FAMILY OUTCOMES
Promote nutrition—cont'd.	Stress need for vitamin and mineral supplements Allow child to feed himself if that is usual routine	
Provide hygienic care without aggravating lesions	Administer good personal hygiene—baths with tepid water, little or no soap (using only mild, unperfumed product), and no bubble bath, bath oil, perfume, or powder Dress in loose-fitting, one-piece, long-sleeve and long-pants outfit (if appropriate for weather conditions) Eliminate any woolen or rough garment or furry stuffed toys; nylon garments promote sweating Launder all clothes or bedsheets in mild detergent and rinse very well	Child is clean, well groomed, and exhibits no evidence of irritation

N **RRP** **Family process, alteration in**
D **Etiology: situational crisis (child with a chronic skin disorder)**

NURSING GOALS	NURSING INTERVENTIONS	EXPECTED PATIENT/FAMILY OUTCOMES
Assist parents in avoiding causative allergens	Stress reason for hypoallergenic diet or removal of inhalants, especially that positive results are not immediate Give written list of foods restricted as well as those allowed Identify hidden sources of allergenic foods, such as milk, wheat, and eggs Assess home environment *before* suggesting ways to eliminate inhalants Make public health referral for long-term home care follow-up	Family eliminates irritating substances from diet and environment of child
Prepare family for home care	Demonstrate proper procedure for dilution of soaks and applying wet dressings Suggest applying dressings at quiet times when child is well rested and after he has received medication for itching Schedule times for administering oral antibiotics that maintain continuous high blood levels of the drug, if ordered	Family demonstrates correct performance of procedures (specify procedures)
Provide emotional support for child and family	Encourage family to play with child and to realize that irritable behavior is directly related to physical discomfort Stress to family that child still needs limit-setting and discipline Be aware of overprotectiveness and restrictiveness, which can stifle child's emotional growth Allow and encourage family members, particularly the one who cares for the child most of the time to express negative feelings, such as anger, frustration, and perhaps guilt Stress that negative feelings are normal, acceptable, and expected but that they must have an outlet in order for family members to remain healthy	Family demonstrates positive interaction with child Family expresses feelings of frustration and concern

Nursing Interventions Related to Medical Management

Determine cause of eczema
  Assist with allergy testing
  Supervise elimination diet

Treat skin lesions
Carry out prescribed therapeutic regimen
Administer topical treatments and applications
Administer systemic medications, if ordered
Prevent lesions
Provide hypoallergenic diet as prescribed

Topical steroids in strengths of 0.01% to 1% are the most effective local treatment because of their potent antiinflammatory effect. One important consideration concerning the use of steroids is that signs of infection will be masked. In addition, prolonged use of steroids must be carefully evaluated because, following discontinuance of the drug, the lesions often exacerbate in a more severe form than before treatment was begun.

In cases of chronic eczema in which lichenification has occurred, keratolytic agents, such as coal tar or salicylic acid-sulfur preparations may be used to produce a mild irritation, which promotes granulation and healing. However, with the effective use of topical steriods, these are employed less frequently.

Nursing Considerations

Long-term treatment of eczema is usually established on an outpatient basis. As a result, the major burden of responsibility and physical care rests on the parents in the home. A vicious cycle of exacerbation—scratching, infection, irritability, and frustration—is the usual course unless the initial phase can be altered. The primary objective is to identify the allergen or allergens to which the child is sensitive. When a hypoallergenic diet is prescribed, parents need help in understanding the reason for the diet and guidelines for following it. Eliminating such foods (see Table 13-4) becomes more of a problem when the child eats table food than during early infancy. Since hypoallergenic diets take time before visible effects are observed, parents need reassurance that this is not an immediate cure.

Eliminating environmental allergens is another time-consuming and tedious task. Often the financial resources are not sufficient to make optimum adjustments, and improvisation is essential. Referral to a public health nursing agency and educational material* can assist the family in coping with the difficulties of following a special diet and "allergyproofing" the home.

Probably the most difficult problem in caring for the child with eczema is controlling the intense pruritus. To prevent infection, the child must be restricted from scratching. Fingernails and toenails should be cut short, kept clean, and filed frequently to prevent sharp edges. Gloves or cotton stockings may have to be placed over the hands and pinned to shirt-sleeves. To prevent any contact with the skin, elbow restraints are sometimes necessary. One-piece outfits with long sleeves and long pants also decrease direct contact with the skin. Whether gloves or restraints are used, the child needs time when he is free from such restrictions. An excellent time to remove any protective devices is during the bath or after receiving sedative or antipruritic medication. Restraints should not be removed during sleep because of the likelihood of the child scratching while asleep.

Conditions that increase itching should be eliminated when possible. Woolen clothes or blankets, rough fabrics, and furry stuffed animals should be removed. During cold months, synthetic—not wool—fabrics should be used for overcoats, hats, gloves, and snowsuits. Since heat and humidity cause perspiration, which intensifies itching, proper dress for climatic conditions is essential. Exposure to sunlight, which has a beneficial drying effect on weeping lesions, is encouraged but monitored carefully to prevent burning. Any topical beauty aid, such as perfumes, powder, or oils, should be avoided. Clothes and sheets should be laundered in a mild detergent and rinsed thoroughly, preferably by using a second complete wash cycle without detergent.

Preventing infection is usually secondary to preventing scratching. Personal hygiene must be accomplished without the liberal use of soap. Baths are to be given as prescribed, the water kept tepid, and bubble baths as well as oils or powder avoided. Hot tubs pose special hazards because of the risk of herpes infection. Skin folds and diaper areas need frequent cleansing with plain water.

If antiseptic soaks are prescribed, they should be applied as directed. Demonstrating the technique is preferable to explaining it. For example, children have great difficulty in remaining still for a 10- or 15-minute wet soak. One suggestion is to apply the wet dressing at naptime or when the child is watching television or listening to a story. If the soaking solution is to be diluted at home, explicit instructions should be given. For example, if 1 part of solution is mixed with 20 parts of water, it is preferable to express the ratio as 1 cup of solution mixed with 20 cups of water.

If topical ointments are prescribed, adequate instruction should be given to ensure correct application. Parents are advised that one thick application is *not* equivalent to several thin applications and excessive use of an agent, particularly steroids, can be hazardous.

Since adequate rest is also important for these children, planning meals, baths, medications, and treatments during awake periods is paramount. Sleepy, tired children are normally cranky, and such behavior only intensifies the urge to scratch. During periods of irritability, these children tend to be anorectic, which is worsened by restriction of their usual foods. Forcing them to eat should be avoided; it is better to be lenient about food consumption than to allow them to have a potentially allergic food. Multiple-vitamin and mineral supplements may be needed during these times, particularly to prevent iron, calcium, and vitamin C deficiencies.

When management at home becomes impossible, hospitalization is required. Since one of the risks during hospitalization (and at home) is contraction of a pyogenic or viral infection, particularly herpes simplex or varicella (chicken pox), the child should be placed in a room with children of similar ages who are noninfectious. Hospitalization may dramatically improve the child's condition because environmental agents can be more carefully controlled and the component of constant parental frustration is lessened.

---

*A booklet about allergies for parents and children is *Sneezing, Wheezing, and Scratching* by D. Rapp, available from the ECR collection, P.O. Box 615, Los Altos, CA 94022.

Family support. Perhaps it is because the physical problems seem insurmountable during periods of acute exacerbation that the emotional stress becomes so intense for the family. Parents are told, "Don't let the child scratch," but the child scratches, the lesions worsen, infection begins, and the parents are overwhelmed with feelings of helplessness, frustration, anger, and guilt. They need time to discuss such negative feelings and to be reassured that these feelings are expected, normal, acceptable, and healthy provided there is an emotional outlet to dissipate the invested energy. Parents should be informed that the lesions will not produce scarring (unless secondarily infected) and that the disease is not contagious.

Supporting parents through the initial phase of identifying the specific allergens is crucial because improvement is not immediate, although dramatic recovery can occur once the sensitizing agents are completely removed. During acute phases, relieving as much anxiety as possible in both parents and child has a beneficial emotional and physical effect, since stress tends to aggravate the severity of eczema.

Disorders of Unknown Etiology

A number of disorders may occur during early childhood in which the etiology is unknown or speculative. However two of the disorders, sudden infant death syndrome and autism, occur almost exclusively during infancy and generate tremendous stress for the family. In one, the family must cope with the loss of an infant; in the other the family must deal with the stresses of caring for a severely disturbed child. Competent and sensitive nursing care can relieve some of the emotional burden.

SUDDEN INFANT DEATH SYNDROME

Sudden infant death syndrome (SIDS, cot, or crib death) is defined as "the sudden death of any infant or young child, which is unexpected by history, and in which a thorough postmortem examination fails to demonstrate an adequate cause for death" (Beckwith, 1970). It is the leading cause of death in children between the ages of 1 week and 1 year and claims the lives of nearly 8000 infants annually. Table 13-8 summarizes the major characteristics of SIDS.

Etiology

Numerous theories have been proposed regarding the etiology of SIDS; however, the cause is unknown. Of the leading hypotheses, two are strongly supported by evidence found in many, but not all, SIDS victims. The *hypoxemia hypothesis* suggests that SIDS occurs because of damage to the respiratory control centers in the brainstem as a result of chronic hypoxemia. The *apnea theory* proposes that SIDS victims experience periods of prolonged apnea during sleep and eventually die during one of these episodes because of a failure in the autonomic regulation of breathing (D'Epiro, 1984). However infantile apnea (IA) does not cause SIDS. The vast majority of infants with apnea do not die and only a minority of SIDS victims have documented life-threatening episodes of apnea (see discussion of infantile apnea, p. 580). Theories that have been disproven include SIDS association with diptheria, tetanus, and pertussis vaccines.

Although the etiology is unknown, autopsies reveal consistent pathologic findings, such as pulmonary edema and intrathoracic hemorrhages, that confirm the diagnosis of SIDS. Consequently all infants with suspected SIDS deaths should be autopsied and these findings shared with the parents as soon as possible after the death.

Children at Risk for SIDS

Certain groups of children are at increased risk for SIDS. One is the "near-miss" infant, which refers to a child who has ceased breathing and seems to have died suddenly and unexpectedly but whose life is apparently saved by timely intervention, usually by a parent or baby-sitter (Valdés-Dapena, 1980). Another group includes infants with infantile apnea (IA). While they are often referred to as "near-miss SIDS," IA is not always part of the initial presentation.

Whether subsequent siblings of the SIDS infant are at increased risk is unclear. Some studies report a tenfold greater risk (Brooks, 1982), while others report that the risk in the SIDS family is virtually the same as that among families of like size and maternal age (Peterson, Sabotta, and Daling, 1986).

Table 13-8 Characteristics of SIDS

FACTORS	OCCURRENCE
Incidence	2:1000 live births
Peak age	2 to 4 months; 90% occur by 6 months
Sex	Higher percentage of males affected
Time of death	During sleep
Time of year	Increased incidence in winter; peak in January
Racial	Greater incidence in blacks
Socioeconomic	Increased occurrence in lower socioeconomic class
Birth	Higher incidence in: Premature infants, especially infants of low birth weight Multiple births Neonates with low Apgar scores Infants with central nervous system disturbances
Feeding habits	Not significant; breast-feeding does not prevent SIDS
Siblings	May have greater incidence
Maternal	Younger age Cigarette smoking Methadone use

Studies conducted on these children demonstrate differences in physiologic function from that of normal infants, especially cardiac and respiratory functions. However heart and respiratory rate patterns do not predict SIDS (Wilson and others, 1985). Consequently there is much concern for the survival of these children. Many of them undergo home apnea monitoring until they are past the age of vulnerability and demonstrate normal pneumograms (see discussion of home monitoring, p. 581).

Nursing Considerations

Loss of a child from SIDS presents several crises with which the parents must cope. In addition to grief and mourning for the death of their child, the parents must face a tragedy that was extremely sudden, unexpected, and unexplained. The psychologic intervention for the family must deal with these additional variables. This discussion focuses primarily on the objectives of care for families experiencing SIDS, rather than on the process of grief and mourning, which is explored in Chapter 23.

One approach toward delineating the nursing care plan for these families is to base it on the usual sequence of events that occurs after the infant is found. This approach encompasses the different areas in which nurses may be involved with the family.

Finding the infant. Usually it is the mother who finds the child dead in the crib. Typically the child is in a disheveled bed, with blankets over his head, and huddled into a corner. Frothy, blood-tinged fluid fills the mouth and nostrils, and the infant may be lying face down in the secretions, suggesting that he bled to death. The diaper is wet and full of stool, which is consistent with a cataclysmic type of death. The hands may be clutching the sheets, as if the child were in distress before he died. The initial appearance of the child combined with the shock of such an unexpected event adds to the horror that the parents must face.

Frequently the mother is alone and must deal with her initial shock, panic, grief, questions of the other siblings, and the decision of where to find help. The first persons to arrive may be the police and ambulance attendants. Hopefully they will handle the situation by asking few questions, giving *no* indication of wrongdoing, abuse, or neglect, making sensitive judgments concerning the resuscitation efforts for the child, and comforting the members of the family as much as possible. These individuals should be properly informed about SIDS in order to recognize its characteristic signs and tell parents that their child probably died from a disease called sudden infant death syndrome, which cannot be predicted or prevented. A compassionate, sensitive approach to the family during the very first few minutes can help spare them some of the overwhelming guilt and anguish that frequently follow this type of death.

Arriving at the emergency room. The first contact that nurses typically have with these families is in the emergency room, when the infant is seen by a physician in order

to be pronounced dead. Usually there is no attempt at resuscitation. During the time in the emergency room several aspects warrant special consideration. Parents are asked only factual questions, such as when they found the infant, how he looked, and who they called for help. Any remarks that may suggest responsibility, such as why didn't they go in earlier, didn't they hear him cry out, was his head buried in a blanket, or were the other siblings jealous of this child, should be avoided.

The events that took place when help arrived are discussed. If resuscitation was attempted, the infant may have fractured ribs, internal bleeding, and traumatic bruising, which can simulate physical abuse. Also if statements were made that were misguided, such as, "This looks like suffocation," they can be corrected before parents harbor them in their minds as indications of their guilt. The discussion of an autopsy should be presented at this time, especially if it is not state mandated.

Another very important aspect of compassionate care toward these parents is allowing them to say good-bye to their child. A happy, beautiful, living part of themselves has suddenly been snatched from them forever. Before they go into the examining room, any blood or emesis is removed from the child, he is covered partially with a sheet or blanket, and the room is put in order, especially if instruments and equipment were used. These are the parents' last moments with their child, and they should be as quiet, meaningful, peaceful, and undisturbed as possible. The child's belongings are packaged for the parents to take home if they wish. Nothing involved in the care of these grief-stricken people should be complicated, difficult, or time-consuming; it only involves being human.

Returning home. When the parents return home, they should be visited by a competent, qualified professional as soon after the death as possible. A referral should also be made to the local **Foundation of Sudden Infant Death**. Printed material that contains excellent information about SIDS (available from the national* or local organizations*) should be provided.

During the initial home visit one of the nursing objectives is to assess what the parents have been told, what they think happened, and how they have explained this to the other siblings. If parents have been told about SIDS, they may answer the questions factually and seem to understand and accept the diagnosis. Although this might be so, it is unusual for parents not to have second thoughts, doubts, and feelings of guilt. It may also be intellectualization, a type of denial that can be erroneously misjudged as positive coping.

*National Foundation for Sudden Infant Death, Inc., 2 Metro Plaza, Suite 205, 8240 Professional Place, Landover, MD 20785; Sudden Infant Death Syndrome Clearinghouse, 8201 Greensboro Drive, Suite 600, McLean, VA 22102; American Sudden Infant Death Syndrome Institute, 275 Carpenter Dr., Suite 100, Atlanta, GA 30328, 1-800-232-SIDS (in Georgia, 1-800-847-SIDS); Council of Guilds for Infant Survival, P.O. Box 3841, Davenport, IA 52808.

Pursuing the factual answer by asking about feelings or emotions may uncover repressed thoughts that, when once said aloud, can be dealt with.

The nurse cannot deal with all the issues related to the child's death in one visit. During the initial visit the nurse may be doing most of the talking, as the parents are helped to gain an understanding of the disease. If the visit is made within a day or two of the death, the parents are in the impact phase of crisis, in which their thinking abilities are disorganized and distracted. It is difficult for them to deal with the crisis in concrete terms, especially in exploring problem-solving approaches. During the turmoil phase, which is usually the first week following the death, there is more structured thinking, although it is global rather than specific.

During the second visit the goal is to help the parents bring their feelings out into the open. This may require "precipitating" emotions by asking about crying and feeling sad, angry, or guilty. It is an attempt to provoke a display of emotions, not just an admission of a feeling. During this session the parents should be helped to explore their usual coping mechanisms and, if these are ineffectual, to investigate new approaches. It may be a time when parents are making rash decisions such as moving away to avoid questions or deciding never to have another child. This is not the time to decide these issues rationally and logically but rather to acknowledge that they are unable to deal with them.

Because questions like these do arise and must be answered eventually, the number of visits and plan for intervention must be flexible. For example, the needs of the siblings must be considered. Although they may initially appear accepting of the explanation and well-adjusted, subsequent problems are common and may include (1) changes in the parent-child interaction, such as increased anger toward the parent or increased discipline probems; (2) altered sleep patterns, including resistance to going to bed and bedtime fears; and (3) changes in social patterns, from withdrawn to aggressive behavior (Mandell, McAnulty, and Carlson, 1983). Children need an opportunity to talk about their perception of the death. With young children, the use of stories about death, drawing, or play is recommended (see Chapter 6 for communication techniques). Even if they express no concerns, their safety and the inability to have predicted, prevented, or caused the death *must* be emphasized.

One of the distressing dilemmas for many parents is the question of a subsequent pregnancy and their concern regarding recurrent SIDS. If another pregnancy occurs before both parents are ready, they may be forced to deal with an additional crisis before resolution of the first. One of the dangers of having another child soon after the other's death is that this infant may become a "replacement" child. Even when parents are well-prepared for the birth of a subsequent child, they may have difficulty conceiving, have doubts about his well-being, be overprotective, especially near the age of the other infant's death, and need support that these responses are normal. Because of increased risk of SIDS in siblings, home monitoring is recommended.

INFANTILE APNEA

Infantile apnea (IA) or apnea of infancy (AI) is defined as cessation of breathing for at least 20 seconds or a briefer apneic episode with bradycardia, cyanosis, or pallor (American Academy of Pediatrics, 1985). While most young infants experience periods of apnea, prolonged apnea can occasionally be fatal. Although the term, "near-miss SIDS," is often applied to children with IA, this is an unfortunate choice because it assumes an unproven cause and effect relationship between IA and SIDS. It also produces anxiety in the parents, who are now dealing with a child that they perceive may be in imminent danger of sudden death.

Diagnostic Evaluation

No universal agreement exists regarding the evaluation necessary for confirmation of the diagnosis. However, diagnostic procedures generally include a number of tests (blood chemistry, chest roentgenogram, electrocardiography, and electroencephalography) to rule out specific, sometimes treatable causes, such as seizures. The most widely used test, however, is continuous recording of cardiorespiratory patterns (cardiopneumogram). A more sophisticated test, polysomnography ("sleep test") also records brainwaves, eye and body movements, and oxygen measurements. Yet none of these tests is predictive of risk. Some children with normal results may still have subsequent apneic episodes.

Therapeutic Management

Treatment is also controversial but usually involves continuous home monitoring of cardiorespiratory rhythms and/or the use of respiratory stimulant drugs, such as theophylline. Guidelines for instituting home monitoring vary, especially in the child with essentially normal findings, but generally include (Spitzer and Fox, 1986):

1. History of severe apneic episodes
2. Documentation of apnea
3. Sibling who died of SIDS
4. Severe feeding difficulties with apnea and bradycardia
5. Some pulmonary, cardiac, or neurologic problems

The duration for home monitoring also varies. The trend is to continue monitoring only for as long as it is needed because of the family stress it generates. General guidelines include cessation after 2 months of no recorded apneic activity and a normal pneumogram. There is usually a minimum age of 6 months or 1 month older than the age of death of a SIDS sibling (Spitzer and Fox, 1986). However, all children should be evaluated individually for optimum benefit of the family.

Nursing Considerations

The diagnosis of IA engenders great anxiety and concern in parents and the institution of home monitoring presents additional physical and emotional burdens. If monitoring is required, the nurse can be a major source of support to the family in terms of education about the equipment, observation of the infant's status, and immediate intervention during apneic episodes, including cardiorespiratory resuscitation (CPR). To help the family cope with the numerous procedures they must learn, adequate preparation before discharge and written instructions are essential.*

Before the actual teaching begins parents need an opportunity to discuss their feelings about the diagnosis, especially if another child has died from SIDS. Excessive fears and concerns, especially since monitoring offers no guarantees of survival, can block their readiness to learn (Duncan and Webb, 1983). When explaining about the disorder, the term "near-miss SIDS" should be avoided and any misconceptions between IA and SIDS should be clarified.

Several types of home monitors are available and most hospitals select the model that the infant will use at home. Nurses, especially those involved in the care at home, must become familiar with the equipment, including its advantages and disadvantages (Webb and Duncan, 1983). Safety is a major concern since monitors can cause electical burns and electrocution. The following precautions are recommended (Center for Devices, 1985):

1. Remove leads when infant is not attached to monitor.
2. Unplug power cord from electrical outlet when cord is not plugged into monitor.
3. Use safety covers on electrical outlets to discourage children from inserting objects into a socket.

Siblings should also be supervised when near the infant and taught that the monitor is not a play object. Other safety practices include informing local utility and rescue squads of the home monitoring in case of an emergency. Telephone numbers for these services should be posted near all telephones in the home. In addition families are usually taught cardiopulmonary resuscitation in the event of severe apnea.

Family support. Although IA is not a chronic illness, many of the stresses observed during the monitoring period are characteristic of those families with chronically ill children. Parents report increased stress, anxiety, and fatigue, especially mothers who typically have to respond 24-hours a day and feel responsible for the infant's survival (DiMaggio and Sheetz, 1983). There are disturbing reports that some couples divorce after the monitoring is discontinued and implicate the monitoring as a factor in the decision

*Home care instructions for apnea monitoring and CPR are available in Wong, D., and Whaley, L.: Clinical handbook of pediatric nursing, ed. 2, St. Louis, 1986, The C.V. Mosby Co. Educational materials may also be obtained from the National Foundation of Sudden Infant Death and the American Sudden Infant Death Syndrome Institute.

(Wasserman, 1984). Siblings are also affected and behavioral problems, regression, or anxiety are not uncommon. Apnea and/or the monitoring can be detrimental to the affected child, who may be characterized as "spoiled" and have developmental delays, decreased attention span, or hyperactivity (Wasserman, 1984; Deykin and others, 1984). To deal with these potential effects, nurses need to employ the same interventions as those discussed for chronically ill children (see Chapter 22) and be aware of the need for referral when difficulties are suspected.

To lessen the continuous responsibility of monitoring, other family members such as grandparents should be taught how to manipulate the equipment, read and interpret the signals, and administer CPR. They are encouraged to stay with the infant for regular periods to allow parents respite. Support groups of other families who have successfully completed monitoring can also be of benefit. Since babysitters are difficult to locate, support group members or nursing students may be potential sources of qualified caregivers.

INFANTILE AUTISM

Autism is a complex developmental disorder accompanied by severe and usually permanent intellectual and behavioral deficits. It occurs in about 4 to 5:10,000 children under age 15 years and is 4 times more common in males than females. Over the years the definition and diagnostic criteria for determining autism have been controversial and conflicting. Currently the diagnostic criteria from the Diagnostic and Statistical Manual of Mental Disorders (DSM-III, 1980) are generally accepted and include the following:

1. Onset before age 30 months
2. Serious lack of social response
3. Language deficit—gross
4. Speech peculiar, if present
5. No delusions/hallucinations

Under the DSM-III classification system, infantile autism is considered a pervasive developmental disorder and is differentiated from childhood schizophrenia by age of onset, which is under 30 months.

Origins of Infantile Autism

The etiology of autism is still an unsolved and controversial question. Basically three theories have been proposed. The *psychogenic* or *nurture* theory proposes that the disorder has its pathology in the parent-child relationship. In the *nature-nurture* theory the infants are viewed as biologically impaired whose parents enhance the problem because of emotional inadequacies in dealing with a "vulnerable" child. The *biogenic* or *organic theory* places no blame on the parents but considers the disorder basically an expression of a biologic abnormality.

Currently there is little support for the first two theories and strong evidence for the theory that autism results from damage to the central nervous system, although the exact defect is unknown. For example, autistic children experience more prenatal and perinatal complications as compared with unaffected children. These include breech delivery, the presence of amniotic meconium, low birth weight, low Apgar scores, elevated bilirubin levels, hemolytic disease, and respiratory distress syndrome (Finegan and Quarrington, 1978).

There is also evidence for a genetic basis. Nontwin siblings have an increased incidence of autism and many of the unaffected siblings demonstrate subnormal intellectual functioning, especially in verbal skills (Minton and others, l982). A possible association also exists between fragile X syndrome and autism (Fisch and others, l986).

Characteristics of Autistic Children

Children with autism demonstrate several peculiar and bizarre characteristics, primarily in social relations, behavior, language, and sensory/perceptual processes. Intellectual functioning is impaired, usually in the severe range.

Social relations. The most prominent characteristics of infantile autism are extreme interpersonal isolation and intense, abnormal concern for preservation of sameness. The social development of these children is retarded to the point that there is no advancement from the typical behavior of a 1-month-old child. They fail to develop a smiling response to others or the usual anticipatory movements, such as putting their arms out to be picked up. They are unyielding to cuddling and holding and fail to show any signs of satisfaction or pleasure in tactile contact. They have a blank, detached look in their eyes and do not respond to verbal stimulation, which may lead others to suspect deafness. Most notably they fail to demonstrate the usual 6- to 8-month stranger anxiety and fear of separation from mother. In fact, they have no difficulty in tolerating separation and seem unaware of the parent's absence. Autistic children are content to be left alone and provide no satisfaction or feedback to the parent for any type of nurturing.

Behavior. Autistic children engage in peculiar and bizarre behaviors, usually demonstrated in their intense preoccupation with the preservation of sameness and their attachment to mechanical objects. Typically during their second year they become engrossed in odd repetitive behaviors, such as flicking a light switch on and off, passing a toy back and forth from one hand to other, or walking around a room feeling the walls. Other self-stimulatory behaviors include rocking, twirling, flapping of arms, or flicking of hands and fingers before their eyes while staring at bright lights. If they are interrupted while engaged in these activities or if their environment is disturbed, they will react with a violent temper tantrum.

Language. Recognition of autism usually follows the appearance of the typical language and communication defects of this disorder, such as *echolalia* or *parrot speech*—the automatic repetition of words spoken to them; *pronominal reversal*—the tendency to use ''you'' for ''I'' and the striking absence of the first person to refer to oneself; and literal, concrete use of words, for example, ''in'' to mean ''door.'' Although their phonation and articulation of sounds are clear, their highly individualized and specialized speech makes communication with others almost impossible.

Sensory/perceptual processes. Sensory deficits are common in autistic children, even though vision and hearing are usually intact. Autistic children often act as if they are deaf, yet a moment later may be overly sensitive to the same sound. They cover their ears and cringe from certain sounds but emit piercing noises when annoyed. They are fascinated by music, light patterns, different textures, and sometimes offensive tastes and odors. They often appear to be ''looking through'' people and eye-to-eye contact is lacking. They may be hyposensitive or hypersensitive to pain and have an aversion to touch.

These children have severe perceptual problems, most characteristically ''stimulus overselectivity,'' which refers to the ability to respond only to a few cues from a larger range of available cues in a learning task (DeMyer, Hingtgen, and Jackson, l981). Therefore multiple and complex cues pose special problems for these children and greatly affect their learning ability.

Intellectual functioning. Occasionally an autistic child may excel in one area, such as motor ability, or may demonstrate unusual musical talent. Such instances of normal to exceptional ability have called into question the child's overall mental ability. However it is now well documented that almost all of these children are retarded and the majority have IQs of less than 52. Mental functioning is an important prognostic factor, since children with IQs above 60 or 70 have a better outcome in terms of intellectual progress and social adjustment (DeMyer, Hingtgen, and Jackson, 1981).

Nursing Considerations

Therapeutic intervention for the autistic child is a specialized area, involving professionals with advanced training. While numerous therapies have been employed, the most promising results have been from highly structured and intensive behavioral modification programs. In general the objective is to increase social awareness of others, teach verbal communication, and decrease unacceptable behavior. However about 1% to 2% achieve independent living, with the vast majority needing assistance and supervision throughout adulthood.

Autism, like so many other chronic conditions, becomes a "family disease." Unfortunately the psychogenetic theory is well-known and, although unsupported by current findings, greatly multiplies the parents' guilt. Stressing what is known about the disorder from a biologic standpoint as well as how little is known can help lessen guilt and shame. Carefully questioning parents about the infant's very early behavior usually yields evidence of autistic tendencies before significant parental or environmental factors could have negatively influenced the child.

Parents need expert counseling early in the course of the disorder and should be referred to the **National Society for Autistic Children (NSAC)**.* NSAC is the most efficient clearinghouse for information about education, treatment programs and techniques, and specialized facilities such as camps and group homes. There is also a siblings group called SHARE (Siblings Helping Persons with Autism Through Resources and Energy).

When these children are hospitalized, they usually present many management problems. Decreasing stimulation by using a private or semiprivate room, avoiding extraneous auditory and visual distraction, and encouraging parents to bring in possessions the child is attached to may lessen the disruptiveness of hospitalization. Since physical contact frequently upsets these children, minimum holding and physical care may be necessary to prevent temper tantrums. A thorough assessment of the child's usual routine and activities helps maintain an environment that is manageable and conducive to physical recovery.

A key principle in caring for these children is not assuming that they can name, define, or locate even ordinary experiences. For example, if another child is crying, it is necessary to point out to the autistic child that *he* is not crying. In the hospital setting the nurse needs to define for the child what is happening in the environment, such as clarifying what sounds are being heard (Harris, 1978).

Because autistic children have difficulty organizing their behavior and redirecting their energy, they need to be told directly what to do. For example, if they are throwing toys, they should be told to stop throwing them on the floor and should be instructed to drop them into a container. Moralizing about "breaking toys" or "hurting someone" is useless and only serves to confuse the child. Directions need to be precise and concrete. As much as possible the parents are involved in the child's care and effective approaches used by the family in dealing with disruptive behavior should be employed.

*1234 Massachusetts Avenue, NW, Washington, DC 20005.

CONCEPT SUMMARIES

- Common nutritional disturbances of infancy include vitamin and mineral disturbances, some types of vegetarian diets, protein and calorie malnutrition, obesity, and food intolerance.

- Malnutrition refers to poor or inadequate nutrition, and may result from undernutrition or overnutrition. Common manifestations of undernutrition in the infant include iron-deficiency anemia, vitamin deficiencies, and failure to thrive. Manifestations of overnutrition are hypervitaminosis and obesity.

- Mineral disturbances may be caused by mineral-mineral interactions and mineral-diet interactions.

- Vegetarians may be classified into four groups: lacto-ovovegetarians, lactovegetarians, pure vegetarians, and zen macrobiotics.

- Protein and energy malnutrition may occur as a complication of underlying disease, result of fad diets, lack of parental education about infant nutrition, inappropriate management of food allergy, and incorrect preparation of formula.

- Calorie consumption, method of feeding, birth weight, sex, age at introduction of solid foods, and activity level all play a part in infant obesity.

- Food intolerance encompasses food allergies and food sensitivities, the most serious of which are cow's milk sensitivity and lactose intolerance.

- Common feeding difficulties in the infant include breast-feeding problems, regurgitation and "spitting up," paroxysmal abdominal pain (colic). Less frequent but serious feeding problems include rumination and failure to thrive.

- Treatment of colic may involve change in feeding practices, correction of stressful environment, and support of parent.

- Failure to thrive may be classified as organic, resulting from some physical cause, and nonorganic, resulting from psychosocial factors involving the child and caregiver (e.g., maternal deprivation), environmental causes (e.g., inadequate parental knowledge of child feeding), or unexplained causes.

- Common skin disorders of infancy are diaper dermatitis, seborrheic dermatitis, and atopic dermatitis.

- Disorders of unknown etiology include sudden infant death syndrome (SIDS), infantile apnea, and infantile autism.

- Sudden infant death syndrome is the leading cause of death in children between the ages of 1 week and 1 year. Two theories point to hypoxemia and apnea as the leading causes.

- The primary nursing responsibility in care associated with SIDS and other conditions of unknown etiology is emotional support of the family.

REFERENCES

Alhadeff, L., Gualtieri, T., and Lipton, M.: Toxic effects of water-soluble vitamins, Nutr. Rev. **42**(2):33-40, 1984.

Altemeier, W.A. III, and others: Prospective study of antecedents for non-organic failure to thrive, J. Pediatr. **106**(3):360-365, 1985.

American Academy of Pediatrics, Task Force on Prolonged Infantile Apnea: Prolonged infantile apnea: 1985, Pediatrics **76**(1):129-131, 1985.

Bachrach, S., Fisher, J., and Parks, J.S.: An outbreak of vitamin D deficiency rickets in a susceptible population, Pediatrics **64**(6):871-877, 1979.

Barbero, G.: Failure to thrive. In Klaus, M., and others, editors: Maternal attachment and mothering disorders, New York, 1974, Johnson & Johnson Baby Products Co.

Beckwith, J.: Discussion of terminology and definition of sudden infant death syndrome. In Bergman, A., and others, editors: Proceedings of the Second International Conference on Causes of Sudden Death in Infants, Seattle, 1970, University of Washington Press.

Berg, R.W., Buckingham, K.W., and Steward, R.L.: Etiologic factors in diaper dermatitis: the role of urine, Pediatr. Derm. **3**(2):102-106, 1986.

Berkowitz, R.I., and others: Physical activity and adiposity: a longitudinal study from birth to childhood, J. Pediatr. **106**(5):734-738, 1985.

Berwick, D.M., Levy, J.C., and Kleinerman, R.: Failure to thrive: diagnostic yield of hospitalisation, Arch. Dis. Child. **57**:347-351, 1982.

Bostrom, B., and others: Listen! N. Engl. J. Med. **309**:1194, 1983.

Brooks, J.G.: Apnea of infancy and sudden infant death syndrome, Am. J. Dis. Child. **136**:1012-1023, 1982.

Buckingham, K.W., and Berg, R.W.: Etiologic factors in diaper dermatitis: the role of feces, Pediatr. Derm. **3**(2):107-112, 1986.

Campbell, R.L., Paper Product Development, Procter & Gamble, Cincinnati, OH, Personal communication, March 13, l986.

Cant, A., Marsden, R.A., and Kilshaw, P.J.: Egg and cow's milk hypersensitivity in exclusively breastfed infants with eczema and detection of egg protein in breast milk, Br. Med. J. **291**:932-935, 1985.

Carey, W.B.: ''Colic''—primary excessive crying as an infant-environment interaction, Pediatr. Clin. N. Am. **31**(5):993-1005, 1984.

Center for Devices and Radiological Health warns of hazard with apnea monitors, Med. Devices Bull. **3**(4):1-3, 1985.

Cramer, D.W., and others: Ovarian cancer and talc, Cancer **50**:372-376, 1982.

DeMyer, M.K., Hingtgen, J.N., and Jackson, R.K.: Infantile autism reviewed: a decade of research, Schizophr. Bull. **7**(3):388-451, 1981.

D'Epiro, P.: When sudden infant death strikes, Patient Care **18**(5):18-37, 1984.

Deykin, E., and others: Apnea of infancy and subsequent neurologic, cognitive, and behavioral status, Pediatrics **73**(5):638-645, 1984.

Diagnostic and statistical manual of mental disorders (DSM-III), ed. 3, Washington, DC, 1980, American Psychological Association.

DiMaggio, G.T., and Sheetz, A.H.: The concerns of mothers caring for an infant on an apnea monitor, Am. J. Maternal Child Nurs. **8**(4):294-297, 1983.

Dine, M.S., and others: Where do the heaviest children come from? A prospective study of white children from birth to 5 years of age, Pediatrics **63**(1):1-7, 1979.

Duncan, J.A., and Webb, L.Z.: Teaching families home apnea monitoring, Pediatr. Nurs. **9**(3):171-175, 1983.

Duncan, B., and others: Reduced growth velocity in exclusively breast-fed infants, Am. J. Dis. Child. **138**:309-313, 1984.

Fanelli, M.T., and Kuczmarski, R.J.: Food selection for vegetarians, Diet. Curr. **10**(1):1-6, 1983.

Finegan, J., and Quarrington, B.: Pre-, peri-, and neonatal factors and infantile autism, J. Child Psychol. Psychiatry **20**:119-128, July 1978.

Fisch, G.S., and others: Autism and the fragile X syndrome, Am. J. Psychiatry **143**:71-73, 1986.

Fleisher, D.R.: Infant rumination syndrome, Am. J. Dis. Child. **133**:266-269, March 1979.

Grant, W., Street, L., and Fearnow, R.: Diaper rashes in infancy: Studies on the effects of various methods of laundering, Clin. Pediatr. **12**:714-716, 1973.

Grantham-McGregor, S., Schofield, W., and Harris, L.: Effect of psychosocial stimulation on mental development of severely malnourished children: an interim report, Pediatrics **72**(2):239-243, 1983.

Harris, M.: Understanding the autistic child, Am. J. Nurs. **78**(10):1682-1685, 1978.

Hayden, G.F., and Sproul, G.T.: Baby powder use in infant skin care: parental knowledge and determinants of powder usage, Clin. Pediatr. **23**:163-165, 1984.

Hide, D.W., and Guyer, B.M.: Prevalence of infant colic, Arch. Dis. Child. **57**:559-560, 1982.

Jakobsson, I., and Lindberg, T.: Cow's milk proteins cause infantile colic in breast-fed infants: a double-blind crossover study, Pediatrics **71**(2):268-271, 1983.

Jarvis, W.T.: Vitamin use and abuse, Contemporary Nutrition **9**(10):1-2, 1984.

Jordan, W.E., and others: Diaper dermatitis: frequency and severity among a general infant population, Pediatr. Derm., **3**(3):198-207, 1986.

Karp, R.J., Scholl, T.O., and Greene, G.W.: Precursors of malnutrition in children, Public Health Curr. **25**(3):11-14, 1985.

Kramer, M.S.: Determinants of weight and adiposity in the first year of life, J. Pediatr. **106**(1):10-14, 1985a.

Kramer, M.S., and others: Infant determinants of childhood weight and adiposity, J. Pediatr. **107**(1):104-107, 1985b.

Lawrence, R.A.: Breastfeeding: a guide for the medical profession, ed. 2, St. Louis, 1985, The C.V. Mosby Co.

Leyden, J.J.: Cornstarch, Candida albicans, and diaper rash, Pediatr. Derm. **1**(4):322-325, 1984.

Linscheid, T.R.: Feeding disorders during infancy and early childhood, Feelings and Their Medical Significance **27**(3):11-14, 1985.

Lockey, J.E., and Parry, W.T.: Health implications of naturally occurring mineral fibers, Fam. Commun. Health **7**(3):1-7, 1984.

MacLean, W.C., and Graham, G.G.: Vegetarianism in children, Am. J. Dis. Child. **134**:513-519, May 1980.

Mandell, F., McAnulty, E.H., and Carlson, A.: Unexpected death of an infant sibling, Pediatrics **72**(5):652-657, 1983.

Markesbery, B.A., and Wong, W.M.: Watching baby's diet: a professional and parental guide, Am. J. Maternal Child Nurs. **4**(3):177-180, 1979.

McCarty, E.P., and Frick, O.L.: Food sensitivity: keys to diagnosis, J. Pediatr. **102**(5):645-652, 1983.

Minton, J., and others: Cognitive assessment of siblings of autistic children, J. Am. Acad. Child Psychiatr. **21**(3):256-261, 1982.

Oates, R.K., Peacock, A., and Forrest, D.: Long-term effects of nonorganic failure to thrive, Pediatrics **75**(1):36-40, 1985.

Olness, K.N.: Nutritional consequences of drugs used in pediatrics, Clin. Pediatr. **24**(8):417-420, 1985.

Peterson, D., Sabotta, E., and Daling, J.: Infant mortality among subsequent siblings of infants who died of sudden infant death syndrome, J. Pediatr. **108**(6):911-914, 1986.

Rosenn, D., Loeb, L., and Jura, M.: Differentiation of organic from non-organic failure-to-thrive syndrome in infancy, Pediatrics **66**(5):698-704, 1980.

Saal, H.M., Ratzan, S.K., and Carey, D.E.: Yogurt: contributory factor in development of nutritional rickets, Clin. Pediatr. **24**:452-454, 1985.

Said, G., Patois, E., and Lellouch, J.: Infantile colic and parental smoking, Br. Med. J. **289**(6446):660, 1984.

Sampson, H.A., and McCaskill, C.C.: Food hypersensitivity and atopic dermatitis: evaluation of 113 patients, J. Pediatr. **107**(5):669-675, 1985.

Sinatra, F., and Merritt, R.: Iatrogenic kwashiokor in infants, Am. J. Dis. Child. **135**(1):21-23, 1981.

Solomons, N.W.: Mineral interactions in the diet, Contemp. Nutr. **7**(7):1-2, 1982a.

Solomons, N.W.: Zinc bioavailability: implications for pediatric nutrition, Pediatr. Basics **33**:4-11, 1982b.

Spitzer, A.R., and Fox, W.W.: Infant apnea, Pediatr. Clin. North Am. **33**(3):561-581,1986.

Stahl, M.D., and Guida, D.A.: Slow weight gain in the breast-fed infant: management options, Pediatr. Nurs. **10**(2):117-120, 1984.

Stein, H.: Incidence of diaper rash when using cloth and disposable diapers, J. Pediatr. **101**(5):721-723, 1982.

A study of the calcium intake of children and teenagers, Minneapolis, MN, 1984, General Mills, Inc.

Stunkard, A., and others: An adoption study of human obesity, N. Engl. J. Med. **314**(4):193-198, 1986.

Taubman, B.: Clinical trial of the treatment of colic by modification of parent-infant interaction, Pediatrics **74**(6):998-1003, 1984.

Temple, W.J., and Farley, D.H.: The succussion splash as an infant "burp" sign, N. Engl. J. Med. **308**(26):1604, 1983.

Thompson, R.G.: Nutritional considerations in the development and treatment of psychosocial dwarfism. In Suskind, R.M., editor: Textbook of pediatric nutrition, New York, 1981, Raven Press.

Valdés-Dapena, M.A.: Sudden infant death syndrome: a review of the medical literature, 1974-1979, Pediatrics **66**(4):597-614, 1980.

Wasserman, A.L.: A prospective study of the impact of home monitoring on the family, Pediatrics **74**(3):323-329, 1984.

Webb, L.Z., and Duncan, J.A.: Selecting the right home apnea monitor, Pediatr. Nurs. **9**(3):179-182, 1983.

Weissbluth, M., Christoffel, K.K., and Davis, A.T.: Treatment of infantile colic with dicyclomine hydrochloride, J. Pediatr. **104**(6):951-955, 1984.

Weston, W.L., Lane, A.T., and Weston, J.A.: Diaper dermatitis: current concepts, Pediatrics **66**(4):532-536, 1980.

Whitehead, W.E., and others: Rumination syndrome in children treated by increased holding, J. Pediatr. Gastroenterol. Nutr. **4**:550-556, 1985.

Wilson, A.J., and others: Respiratory and heart rate patterns in infants destined to be victims of sudden infant death syndrome, Br. Med. J. **290**:497-501, 1985.

Winkelstein, M.L.: Overfeeding in infancy: the early introduction of solid foods, Pediatr. Nurs. **10**(3):205-208, 1984.

Wishon, P.M., and Kinnick, V.G.: Helping infants overcome the problem of obesity, Am. J. Maternal Child Nurs. **11**(2):118-121, 1986.

Zimmerer, R.E., Lawson, K.D., and Calvert, C.J.: The effects of wearing diapers on skin, Pediatr. Derm. **3**(2):95-101, 1986.

BIBLIOGRAPHY
Vitamin and Mineral Disturbances

American Academy of Pediatrics, Committee on Nutrition: Vitamin and mineral supplement needs in normal children in the United States, Pediatrics **66**(6):1015-1020, 1980.

Cerrato, P.L.: Vitamin C: who needs it? and when?, RN **48**(8):59-60, 1985.

Cerrato, P.L.: When to worry about vitamin overdose, RN **48**(10):69-70, 1985.

Ehrenkranz, R.A.: Vitamin E and the neonate, Am. J. Dis. Child. **134**(12):1157-1166, 1980.

Gibson, R.S.: Dietary intakes of trace elements in infants during their first year, Food Nutr. News **57**(10):1-6, 1985.

Goel, K.: Rickets: an old enemy returns, Nurs. Mirror **152**(13):16-18, 1981.

Golden, N.H.N.: Trace elements in human nutrition, Human Nutr. Clin. Nutr. **36C**:185-202, 1982.

Harper, A.: Recommended dietary allowances in perspective, Food. Nutr. News **58**(2):7-10, 1986.

Lippe, B., and others: Chronic vitamin A intoxication, Am. J. Dis. Child. **135**(7):634-636, 1981.

Mahoney, C.P., and others: Chronic vitamin A intoxication in infants fed chicken liver, Pediatrics **65**(5):893-896, 1980.

Mertz, W.: The significance of trace elements for health, Nutr. Today **18**(5):26-31, 1983.

Mertz, W.: The essential elements: nutritional aspects, Nutr. Today **19**(1):22-30, 1984.

Nurses's quick guide to nutritional disorders, Nursing 83 **13**(4):56-57, 1983.

Purvis, G.A.: Carotenemia, Pediatr. Basics **41**:1, 1985.

Purvis, G.A.: Vegetarian nutrition in infancy, Pediatr. Basics **34**:1, 1982.

Sorenson, A.W., and Butrum, R.R.: Zinc and copper in infant diets, J. Am. Diet. Assoc. **83**(3):291-297, 1983.

Thomas, K.: Folic acid deficiency related to the use of goat milk for infant feeding, Issues Compr. Pediatr. Nurs. **4**:37-43, 1980.

Vilter, R.W.: Nutritional aspects of ascorbic acid uses and abuses, West. J. Med. **133**(6):485-492, 1980.

Walker, W.A., and Hendricks, K.M.: Manual of pediatric nutrition, Philadelphia, 1985, W.B. Saunders Co.

Williams, S.R.: Nutrition and diet therapy, ed. 5, St. Louis, 1985, The C.V. Mosby Co.

Vegetarian Diets

Dietz, W.H., and Dwyer, J.T.: Nutritional implications of vegetarianism for children. In Suskind, R.M., editor: Textbook of pediatric nutrition, New York, 1981, Raven Press.

Dwyer, J.T., and others: Risk of nutritional rickets among vegetarian children, Am. J. Dis. Child. **133**:134-140, Feb. 1979.

Hanning, R.M., and Zlotkin, S.H.: Unconventional eating practices and their health implications, Pediatr. Clin. N. Am. **32**(2):429-445, 1985.

Johnston, P.K.: Getting enough to grow on, Am. J. Nurs. **84**(3):336-339, 1984.

Purvis, G.A.: Vegetarian nutrition in infancy, Pediatr. Basics **34**:1, 1982.

Rudy, C.A.: Vegetarian diets for children, Pediatr. Nurs. **10**(5):329-333, 1984.

Rudy, C.A.: Teaching families about the well-balanced vegetarian diet, Child. Nurse **3**(5):1-3, 1985.

Zmora, E., Gorodischer, R., and Bar-Ziv, J.: Multiple nutritional deficiencies in infants from a strict vegetarian community, Am. J. Dis. Child. **133**:141–144, Feb. 1979.

Protein and Calorie Malnutrition

Goodall, J.: Malnutrition and the family: deprivation in kwashiorkor, Proc. Nutr. Soc. **38**(1):17-27, 1979.

Hoorweg, J., and Stanfield, J.P.: The effects of protein energy malnutrition in early childhood on intellectual and motor abilities in later childhood and adolescence, Dev. Med. Child. Neurol. **18**:330-350, 1976.

Keusch, G.T., and others: Impairment of hemolytic complement activation by both classical and alternative pathways in serum from patients with kwashiorkor, J. Pediatr. **105**(3):434-436, 1984.

Steginak, L.: Current concepts of protein digestion and absorption, Pediatr. Basics **15**:9-13, July/Aug. 1976.

Viteri, F.E.: Primary protein-energy malnutrition: clinical, biochemical, and metabolic changes. In Suskind, R.M., editor: Textbook of pediatric nutrition, New York, 1981, Raven Press.

Obesity

American Academy of Pediatrics, Committee on Nutrition: Nutritional aspects of obesity in infancy and childhood, Pediatrics **68**(6):880-883, 1981.

Charney, E., and others: Childhood antecedents of adult obesity: do chubby infants become obese adults? N. Engl. J. Med. **295**(1):6-9, 1976.

Dietz, W.H., Jr.: Childhood obesity: susceptibility, cause, and management, J. Pediatr. **103**(5):676-686, 1983.

Epstein, L.H., Wing, R.R., and Valoski, A.: Childhood obesity, Pediatr. Clin. N. Am. **32**(2):363-379, 1985.

Knittle, J.L., and others: Childhood obesity. In Suskind, R.M., editor: Textbook of pediatric nutrition, New York, 1981, Raven Press.

Kramer, M.S.: Breast-feeding, solid foods and subsequent obesity, J. Pediatr. **98**:883-887, June 1981.

Morgan, J.: Prevention of childhood obesity, Issues Compr. Pediatr. Nurs. **9**(1):33-38, 1986.

Newmann, C.: Obesity in childhood. In Levine, M.D., and others, editors: Developmental-behavioral pediatrics, Philadelphia, 1983, W.B. Saunders Co.

Udall, J.N., and others: Interaction of maternal and neonatal obesity, Pediatrics **62**(1):17-19, 1978.

Van Itallie, T.: Bad news and good news about obesity, N. Engl. J. Med. **314**(4):239-240, 1986.

Food Intolerance

American Academy of Pediatrics, Committee on Nutrition: Soy-protein formulas: recommendations for use in infant feeding, Pediatrics **72**(3):359-363, 1983.

American Academy of Pediatrics, Committee on Nutrition: The practical significance of lactose intolerance in children, Pediatrics **62**(2):240-245, 1978.

Anderson, J.A.: Food allergy and food intolerance, Contemp. Nutr. **9**(9):1-2, 1984.

Bierman, C.W., and Furukawa, C.T.: Food allergy, Pediatr. Rev. **3**(7):213-220, 1982.

Bock, S.A.: Food sensitivity, a critical review and practical approach, Am. J. Dis. Child. **134**:973-982, Oct. 1980.

Brockwell, C.: Cow's milk allergy in babies—a review, Health Visitor **54**:236-237, June 1981.

Butler, H.L.: Pediatric review: cow's milk intolerance, J. Arkansas Med. Soc. **77**(8):329-333, 1981.

Deamer, W.C., Gerrard, J.W., and Speer, F.: Cow's milk allergy: a critical review, J. Fam. Pract. **9**(2):223-232, 1979.

Eastham, E.J., and Walker, W.A.: Adverse effects of milk formula ingestion on the gastrointestinal tract: an update, Gastroenterology **76**(2):365-374, 1979.

Fomon, S.S., and others: Cow's milk feeding in infancy: gastrointestinal blood loss and iron nutritional status, J. Pediatr. **98**:540-545, April 1981.

Institute of Food Technologists' Expert Panel on Food Safety and Nutrition: Food allergies and other food sensitivities, Contemp. Nutr. **10**(11):1-2, 1985.

Kahn, A., and others: Insomnia and cow's milk allergy in infants, Pediatrics **76**(6):880-884, 1985.

Powell, G.K.: Milk- and soy-induced enterocolitis of infancy, J. Pediatr. **93**(4):553-560, 1978.

Purvis, G.A.: Food sensitivity—Part II, Pediatr. Basics **29**:3, July 1981.

Questions and answers about food allergy, Patient Care **19**(3):178-182, 1985.

Sampson, H.A., and Albergo, R.: Comparison of results of skin tests, RAST, and double-blind, placebo-controlled food challenges in children with atopic dermatitis, J. Allergy Clin. Immunol. **74**:26-33, 1984.

Savilahti, E.: Cow's milk allergy, Allergy **36**(2):73-88, 1981.

Stern, M., and Walker, W.A.: Food allergy and intolerance, Pediatr. Clin. N. Am. **32**(2):471-492, 1985.

White, J.E., and Owsley, V.B.: Helping families cope with milk, wheat, and soy allergies, Am. J. Maternal Child Nurs. **8**:423-428, 1983.

Whitington, P.F., and others: Soy protein intolerance: four patients with concomitant cow's milk intolerance, Pediatrics **59**:730, 1977.

Feeding Difficulties

Carey, W.B.: "Colic" or excessive crying in young infants. In Levine, M.D., and others, editors: Developmental-behavioral pediatrics, Philadelphia, 1983, W.B. Saunders Co.

Dixie, M.: Maternal food allergy as a cause of infantile colic in the breast-fed baby, Health Visitor **54**(6):240-241, 1981.

Evans, R.W., and others: Maternal diet and infantile colic in breast-fed infants, Lancet **2**:1340-1342, June 1981.

Griffin, J.B.: Rumination in a 7-year-old child, South. Med. J. **70**(2):243-245, 1977.

Humphrey, N.M.: Minor breast-feeding problems, Child. Nurse **3**(7):1-4, 1985.

Imber, J.H.: Living and coping with colic, Am. Baby **42**:29, Dec. 1980.

Loughlin, H.H., and others: Early termination of breast-feeding: identifying those at risk, Pediatrics **75**(3):508-513, 1985.

Murray, M.E., Doman, K.K., and McCarver, J.W.: Behavioral treatment of rumination—a case study, Clin. Pediatr. **15**(7):591-596, 1976.

Neifert, M.R., Seacat, J.M., and Jobe, W.E.: Lactation failure due to insufficient glandular development of the breast, Pediatrics **76**(5):823-828, 1985.

O'Donovan, J.C., and others: The failure of conventional drug therapy in the management of infantile colic, Am. J. Dis. Child. **133**(10):999-1001, 1979.

Pittard, W.: Practical advice for the nursing mother, Pediatr. Basics, **43**:10-15, 1986.

Romanko, M.V., and Brost, B.A.: Swaddling: an effective invention for pacifying infants, Pediatr. Nurs. **8**:259-261, 1982.

Rowell, P.A.: Infantile colic: reviewing the situation, Pediatr. Nurs. **4**(3):20-21, 1978.

Waldman, W.H., and Sarsgard, D.: Helping parents to cope with colic, Pediatr. Basics **33**:12-14, 1982.

Wichelow, M.J., and others: Coping with colic in the breast-fed baby, Health Visitor **53**(1):6–7, 1980

Failure to Thrive

Ayoub, C., Pfeifer, D., and Leichtman, L.: Treatment of infants with non-organic failure to thrive, Child Abuse Neglect **3**:937-941, 1979.

Bithoney, W., and Rathbun, J.: Failure to thrive. In Levine, M.D., and others, editors: Developmental-behavioral pediatrics, Philadelphia, 1983, W.B. Saunders Co.

Casey, P.H., Bradley, R., and Wortham, B.: Social and nonsocial home environments of infants with nonorganic failure to thrive, Pediatrics **73**(3):348-353, 1984.

Corcoran, M.: Nursing role and management of failure-to-thrive clients, Issues Compr. Pediatr. Nurs. **3**:29-40, Oct. 1978.

Drotar, D., and Malone, C.: Family-oriented intervention with the failure-to-thrive infant. In Klaus, M.H., and Robertson, M.O., editors: Birth, interaction and attachment, Skillman, NJ, 1982, Johnson & Johnson Baby Products Co.

Funke-Furber, J., and Roemer, C.: Failure to thrive, Can. Nurse **74**:30-34, Dec. 1978.

Gordon, A.H., and Jameson, J.C.: Infant-mother attachment in patients with nonorganic failure to thrive syndrome, J. Am. Acad. Child Psychiatry **18**(2):251-259, 1979.

Gottsacker, J.: Maternal attachment in relation to failure to thrive. In Brandt, P.A., and others, editors: Current practice in pediatric nursing, vol. I, St. Louis, 1976, The C. V. Mosby Co.

Harrison, L.: The failure-to-thrive child. In Johnson, S., editor: Nursing assessment and strategies for the family at risk, ed. 2, Philadelphia, 1986, J.B. Lippincott Co.

Harrison, L.: Nursing intervention with the failure-to-thrive family, Am. J. Maternal Child Nurs. **1**(2):111-116, 1976.

Holmes, G.I.: Evaluation and prognosis in nonorganic failure to thrive, South. Med. J. **72**(6):693-695, 1979.

Homer, C., and Ludwig, S.: Categorization of etiology of failure to thrive, Am. J. Dis. Child. **135**:848-851, Sept. 1981.

Hufton, I.W., and Oates, R.K.: Nonorganic failure to thrive: a long-term follow-up, Pediatrics **59**(1):73-77, 1977.

Koepke, J.M., and Thyer, B.A.: Behavioral treatment of failure to thrive in a two-year-old, Child Welfare **64**(5):511-516, 1985.

Mira, M., and Cairns, G.: Intervention in the interaction of a mother and child with nonorganic failure to thrive, Pediatr. Nurs. **8**(2):41-46, 1981.

Mitchell, W.G., Gorrell, R.W., and Greenberg, R.A.: Failure to thrive: a study in primary care setting, epidemiology, and follow-up, Pediatrics **65**(5):971-977, 1980.

Norris, T.N., and Anderson, A.S.: Failure to thrive in infants and very young children, Pediatr. Basics **26**:4-7, March 1981.

Pollitt, E., and Eichler, A.: Behavioral disturbances among failure-to-thrive children, Am. J. Dis. Child. **130**:24-29, Jan. 1976.

Roper, K., and others: Failure to thrive: an opportunity for innovative nursing, Pediatr. Nurs. **2**(5):43-45, 1976.

Rosenn, D.W., Loeb, L.S., and Jura, M.B.: Differentiation of organic from nonorganic failure-to-thrive syndrome in infancy, Pediatrics **66**(5):698-704, 1980.

Sills, R.H.: Failure to thrive: the role of clinical and laboratory evaluation, Am. J. Dis. Child. **132**:967-969, 1978.

Steele, S.: Nonorganic failure to thrive: a pediatric social illness, Issues Compr. Pediatr. Nurs. **9**(1):47-58, 1986.

Stickler, G.B.: 'Failure to thrive' or failure to define, Pediatrics **74**(4):559, 1984.

Whitten, C.F.: Growth failure. In Ellerstein, N.S., editor: Child abuse and neglect: a medical reference, New York, 1981, John Wiley & Sons.

Yoos, L.: Taking another look at failure to thrive, Am. J. Maternal Child Nurs. **9**(1):32–36, 1984.

Skin Disorders

Buckley, R.H., and Mathews, K.P.: Common 'allergic' skin diseases, JAMA **248**(2):2611-2622, 1982.

David, T.J., and Longson, M.: Eczema and herpes simplex infection, Arch. Dis. Child. **60**:338-343, 1985.

Esterly, N.B.: Atopic dermatitis: the challenge of effective management, Child Care Newsletter **1**(2):1-4, 1982.

Fritz, G.K.: Psychological aspects of atopic dermatitis, Clin. Pediatr. **18**(6):360-364, 1979.

Gonzalez, J., and Hogg, R.J.: Metabolic alkalosis secondary to baking soda treatment of a diaper rash, Pediatrics **67**(6):820-822, 1981.

Hide, D., and Guyer, B.: Clinical manifestations of allergy related to breast- and cow's milk-feeding, Pediatrics **76**(6):973-975, 1985.

Hurwitz, S.: Eczematous eruptions in childhood, Pediatr. Rev. **3**(1):23-30, 1981.

Jacobs, A.H.: Eruptions in the diaper area, Pediatr. Clin. North Am. **25**(2):209-224, 1978.

Jordan, W.E.: Relationship of diapers to diaper rashes, J. Pediatr. **96**(5):957-958, 1980.

Koblenzer, P.J.: Diaper dermatitis: diagnosis and treatment, Child Care Newsletter **1**(3):1-4, 1982.

Kramer, M.S., and Moroz, B.: Do breast-feeding and delayed introduction of solid foods protect against subsequent atopic eczema? J. Pediatr. **98**(4):546-550, 1981.

Leyden, J.J.: Diaper dermatitis, Child Care Newsletter **4**(1):1-3, 1985.

MacKie, R.M., and Scott, E.: Topical miconazole cream in infantile napkin dermatitis, Practitioner **222**:124-126, Jan. 1979.

Margileth, A.M.: Allergic dermatoses in children, Pediatr. Ann. **8**(8):495-506, 1979.

Munz, D., Powell, K.R., and Pai, C.H.: Treatment of candidal diaper dermatitis: a double-blind placebo-controlled comparison of topical nystatin with topical plus oral nystatin, J. Pediatr. **101**(6):1022-1025, 1982.

Rasmussen, J.E.: Diseases of the scalp, Pediatr. Rev. **7**(4):109-116, 1985.

Saarinen, U.M., and others: Prolonged breast-feeding as prophylaxis for atopic disease, Lancet **2**:163-166, July 1979.

Sampson, H.A., and Jolie, P.L.: Increased plasma histamine concentrations after food challenges in children with atopic dermatitis, N. Engl. J. Med. **311**(6):372-376, 1984.

Schamberg, I.L.: Dermatoses of the groin, J. Fam. Pract. **8**(4):825-833, 1979.

Tunnessen, W.W.: Common skin problems in children, Del. Med. J. **52**(10):533-536, 1980.

Wiener, F.: The relationship of diapers to diaper rashes in the 1-month-old infant, J. Pediatr. **95**(3):422,424, 1979.

Sudden Infant Death Syndrome/Infantile Apnea

Bakke, K., and Dougherty, J.: Sudden infant death syndrome and infant apnea: current questions, clinical management, and research directions, Issues Compr. Pediatr. Nurs., **5**:77-88, 1981.

Black, L., and others: Effects of birth weight and ethnicity on incidence of sudden infant death syndrome, J. Pediatr. **108**(2):209-214, 1986.

Black, L., Hersher, L., and Steinschneider, A.: Impact of the apnea monitor on family life, Pediatrics **62**(5):681-685, 1978.

Brady, J.P., McCann, E.M.: Control of ventilation in subsequent siblings of victims of sudden infant death syndrome, J. Pediatr. **212**(2):212-217, 1985.

Cain, L.P., Kelly, D.H., and Shannon, D.C.: Parents' perceptions of the psychological and social impact of home monitoring, Pediatrics **66**(1):37-41, 1980.

Cepeda, M.L.: Sudden infant death syndrome: helping bereaved parents talk with children, South. Med. J. **74**(1):9-10, 1981.

Clapp, L., and Price, J.H.: Sudden infant death syndrome, J. Nurs. Care **13**(3):13-17, 1980.

Coons, S., and Guilleminault, C.: Motility and arousal in near-miss sudden infant death syndrome, J. Pediatr. 107(5):728-732, 1985.

Cordell, A.S., and Apolito, R.: Family support in infant death, JOGN Nurs. 10(4):281-285, 1981.

Couriel, J.M., and Olinsky, A.: Response to acute hypercapnia in the parents of victims of sudden infant death syndrome, Pediatrics 73(5):652-655, 1984.

Deal, A., and Bordeaux, B.: The phenomenon of SIDS, Pediatr. Nurs. 5(1):48-50, 1980.

DeFrain, J.D., and Ernst, L.: The psychological effects of sudden infant death syndrome on surviving family members, J. Fam. Pract. 6(5):985-989, 1978.

Gould, J.B., and James, O.: Management of the near-miss infant: a personal perspective, Pediatr. Clin. N. Am. 26(4):857-865, 1979.

Graber, H.P., and Balas-Stevens, S.: A discharge tool for teaching parents to monitor infant apnea at home, Am. J. Maternal Child Nurs. 9(3):178, 1984.

Guilleminault, C., and others: Sleep parameters and respiratory variables in 'near miss' sudden death syndrome infants, Pediatrics 68(3):354-360, 1981.

Guilleminault, C., and others: Five cases of near-miss sudden infant death syndrome and development of obstructive sleep apnea syndrome, Pediatrics 73(1):71-78, 1984.

Guilleminault, C., and others: Near-miss sudden infant death syndrome in eight infants with sleep apnea-related cardiac arrhythmias, Pediatrics 76(2):236-242, 1985.

Hartsell, M.: Selecting home monitors, J. Pediatr. Nurs. 1(1):54-57, l986.

Hunt, C.E., and others: Home pneumograms in normal infants, J. Pediatr. 106(4):551-555, 1985.

Kaplan, D.W., Bauman, A.E., and Krous, H.F.: Epidemiology of sudden infant death syndrome in American Indians, Pediatrics 74(6):1041-1046, 1984.

Kotsubo, C.Z.: Helping families survive SIDS, Nursing '83 13(5):94-96, 1983.

Krein, N.: Sudden infant death syndrome: acute loss and grief reactions, Clin. Pediatr. 18(7):414-416, 1979.

Lewak, N., Zebal, B.H., and Friedman, S.B.: Management of infants with apnea and potential apnea, Clin. Pediatr. 23(7):369-373, 1984.

Lewak, N., van den Berg, B.J., and Beckwith, J.B.: Sudden infant death syndrome risk factors, Clin. Pediatr. 18(7):404-411, 1979.

Longo, A.: Teaching parents CPR, Pediatr. Nurs. 9(6):445-447, 1983.

Lundeen, K.W.: When baby makes three . . . challenges, Nursing 82 12(3):74-75, 1982.

Nikolaisen, S.: The impact of sudden infant death on the family: nursing intervention, Top. Clin. Nurs. 3(3):45-53, 1981.

Nikolaisen, S.M., and Williams, R.A.: Parent's view of support following the loss of their infant to sudden infant death syndrome, West. J. Nurs. Res. 2(3):593-601, 1980.

Orr, W.C., and others: Effect of sleep state and position on the incidence of obstructive and central apnea in infants, Pediatrics 75(5):832-835, 1985.

Perrin, D.G., and others: Ultrastructure of carotid bodies in sudden infant death syndrome, Pediatrics 73(5):646-651, 1984.

Price, M., and others: Maternal perceptions of sudden infant death syndrome, Child. Health Care 14(1):22-31, 1985.

Rehm, R.S.: Teaching cardiopulmonary resuscitation to parents, Am. J. Maternal Child Nurs. 8(6):411-414, 1983.

SIDS Clearinghouse, Am. J. Maternal Child Nurs. 7(1):68, 1982.

Swoiskin, S.: Sudden infant death: nursing care for the survivors, J. Pediatr. Nurs. 1(1):33-39, 1986.

Webb, L.Z., and Duncan, J.A.: Selecting the right home apnea monitor, Pediatr. Nurs. 9(3):179-182, 1983.

Weissbluth, M., and others: Respiratory patterns during sleep and temperament ratings in normal infants, J. Pediatr. 106(4):688-690, 1985.

Williams, R.A., and Nikolaisen, S.M.: Sudden infant death syndrome: parents' perceptions and responses to the loss of their infant, Res. Nurs. Health 5:55-61, 1982.

Infantile Autism

Christian, W.P.: Childhood autism. In Levine, M., and others, editors: Developmental-behavioral pediatrics, Philadelphia, 1983, W.B. Saunders Co.

Cruz, V.K., Andron, L., and Sammons, C.: Cookie monster is autistic . . . help younger children with developmentally disabled siblings cope, Child. Today 13(2):18-20, 1984.

Cullinan, D., Epstein, M.H., and Lloyd, J.W.: Behavior disorders of children and adolescents, Englewood Cliffs, NJ, 1983, Prentice-Hall, Inc.

Dudziak, D.: Parenting the autistic child, J. Psychosoc. Nurs. Mental Health Services 20(1):11-16, 1982.

Gualtieri, C.: Fenfluramine and autism: careful reappraisal is in order, J. Pediatr. 108(3):417-419, 1986.

Ho, H.H., and others: Blood serotonin concentrations and fenfluramine therapy in autistic children, J. Pediatr. 108(3):465-469, 1986.

Killion, S., and McCarthy, S., Hospitalization of the autistic child, Part I—Assessment, Part II—Autistic children, intervention, Am. J. Maternal Child Nurs. 5(6):412-423, 1980.

Lewis, M.: Gifted or dysfunctional: the child savant, Pediatr. Ann. 14(10):733-742, 1985.

Lovaas, O.I., Koegel, R.L., and Shreibman, L.: Stimulus overselectivity in autism: a review of research, Psychol. Bull. 86(6):1236-1254, 1979.

Moss, B.K.: When autism threatens family balance, Patient Care 15:15-33, April 1981.

Ney, P.G.: A psychopathogenesis of autism, Child Psychiatry Hum. Dev. 9(4):195-205, 1979.

Zoltak, B.: Autism: recognition and management, Pediatric Nurs. 12(2):90-94, 1986.

Unit Five

Early Childhood

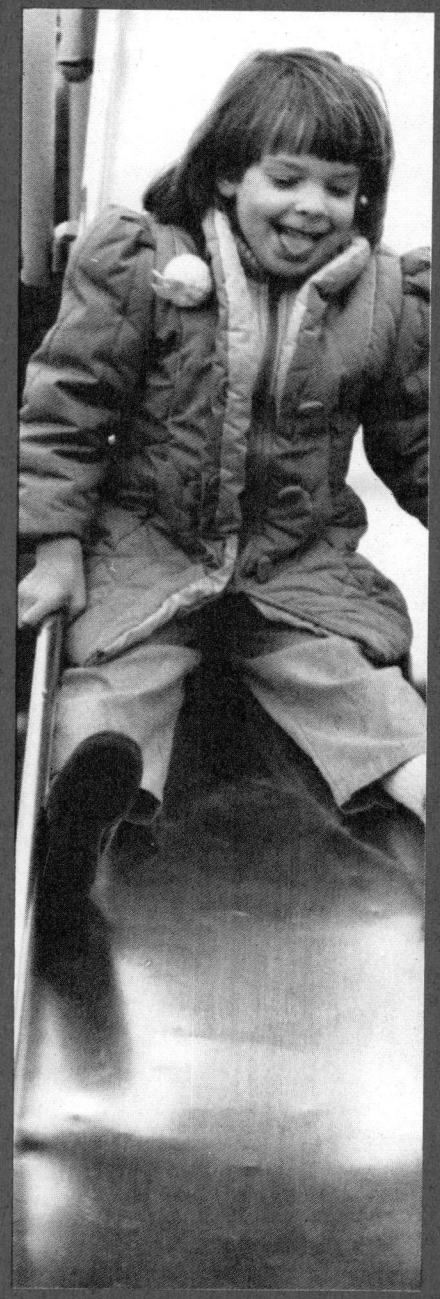

Early childhood comprises the period of toddlerhood and the preschool years. It is primarily a time of physical development and refinement, attainment of social skills, and achievement of independent behavior. Dramatic changes occur in the child as he leaves the dependent world of infancy and readies himself for the self-sufficient life of a school-age child. Chapters 14 and 15, *Health Promotion of the Toddler and Family* and *Health Promotion of the Preschooler and Family*, are concerned with the biologic growth and psychologic development of the toddler and preschooler. However, the family is the focus of nursing care to provide for the child an environment that fosters mental and physical health. Emphasis is placed on promoting optimum development during each phase of early childhood, especially through anticipatory guidance regarding nutrition, achievement of self-care activities, prevention of injury, and specific parental concerns.

Chapter 16, *Health Problems of Early Childhood*, deals with health problems that commonly occur during early childhood. Although many of the disorders typical of this period are caused by infectious processes, most of the child's care is implemented in the home, necessitating nursing guidance rather than direct intervention. The other conditions discussed are environmental and social factors to which toddlers and preschoolers are especially vulnerable or by which they are greatly influenced. In the discussion of each of these health problems, emphasis is placed on prevention, recognition, and nursing interventions that return the child to an optimum physical and mental status following recovery.

Chapter 14

Health Promotion of the Toddler and Family

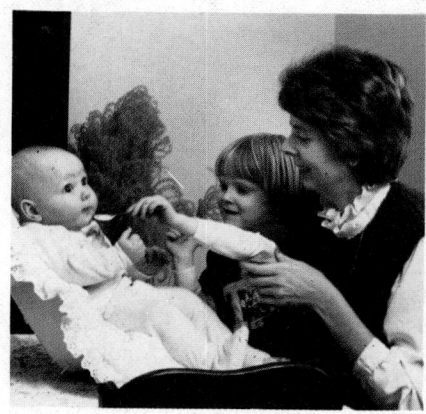

The *terrible twos* has often been used to describe the toddler years, a period from 12 months to 2 years of age. It is a time of intense exploration of the environment as children attempt to find out how things work, what the word *no* means, and how to control others with temper tantrums, negativism, and obstinacy. The phrase "he gets into everything" actually underestimates the toddler's voracity for adventure, but the very adventure of getting into things is the means of acquisition of learning and knowledge.

Although this can be a difficult time for parents and child as each learns to know the other better, it is also an extremely important period for developmental achievement and intellectual growth. Successful mastery of the tasks of this age requires a strong foundation of trust during infancy and frequently necessitates guidance from others when parent and toddler face the struggles of toilet training, limit-setting and discipline, and sibling rivalry. Nurses who understand the dynamics of growth and development of the toddler can help families deal effectively with the developmental needs of this age.

Promoting Optimum Growth and Development

General concepts of growth and development, such as stages and patterns of development and individual differences, have been extensively discussed in Chapter 4. This chapter is primarily concerned with biologic, psychosocial, cognitive, and social development of toddlers. It also includes a discussion of common parental concerns typical of the developmental characteristics of this age-group.

BIOLOGIC DEVELOPMENT

Biologic development and maturation of body systems is less dramatic during early childhood than infancy. However, maturation of body systems continues and many organs achieve mature functioning. The acquisition of fine and gross motor skills is dramatic and allows toddlers to master a wide variety of activities.

Proportional Changes

Growth slows considerably during toddlerhood. The average weight gain is 1.8 to 2.7 kg (4 to 6 pounds) per year. The average weight at 2 years is 12 kg (27 pounds). The birth weight is quadrupled by 2½ years of age. The rate of increase in height also slows. The usual increment is an addition of 7.5 cm (3 inches) per year and occurs mainly in elongation of the legs rather than the trunk. The average height of a 2-year-old is 86.6 cm (34 inches). In general, adult height is about twice the child's height at 2 years of age. Accurate measurement of height and weight during the toddler years should reveal a steady growth curve that is *steplike* in nature rather than linear (straight), which is characteristic of the growth spurts during the early childhood years.

The rate of increase in head circumference slows somewhat by the end of infancy and head circumference is usually equal to chest circumference by 1 to 2 years of age. The usual total increase in head circumference during the second year is 2.5 cm (1 inch). Then the rate of increase slows until at age 5 years the increase is less than 1.25 cm (½ inch) per year. The anterior fontanel closes between 12 and 18 months.

Chest circumference continues to increase in size and exceeds head circumference during the toddler years. Its shape also changes as the transverse or lateral diameter exceeds the anteroposterior diameter. After the second year the chest circumference exceeds the abdominal measurement, which, in addition to the growth of the lower extremities, gives the child a taller, leaner appearance. However, the toddler retains a squat, "pot-bellied" appearance because of the less well-developed abdominal musculature and short legs (Fig. 14-1). The legs retain a slightly bowed or curved appearance during the second year from the weight of the relatively large trunk.

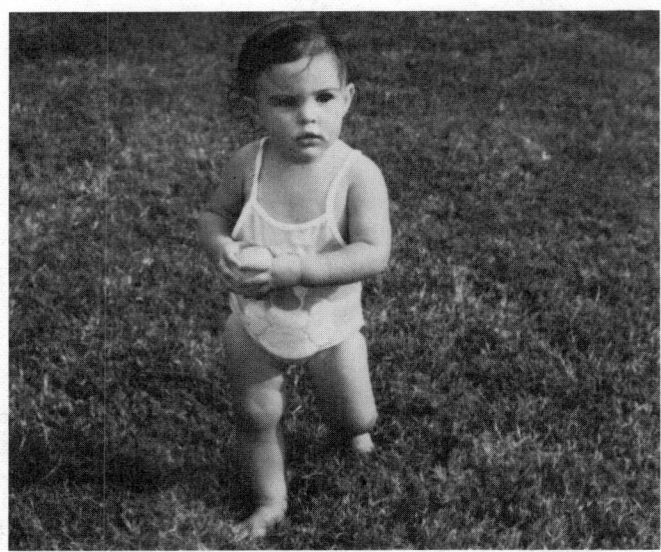

Fig. 14-1. Typical toddling gait.

Sensory Changes

Visual acuity of 20/20 is achieved during the toddler years, although 20/40 is considered acceptable. Full binocular vision is well developed by 12 months of age, and any evidence of persistent strabismus should receive professional attention as early as possible to prevent amblyopia. Depth perception continues to develop but, because of the child's lack of motor coordination, falls from heights continue to be a persistent danger.

The senses of hearing, smell, taste, and touch become increasingly well developed, coordinated with each other, and associated with other experiences. All of the senses are used to explore the environment. The toddler will visually inspect an object by turning it over; he may taste it, smell it, and touch it several times before he is satisfied with his investigation. He will shake it to see if it makes noise and vigorously test its durability.

Another example of the integrated function of the senses is the toddler's development of specific taste preferences. The child is much less likely than infants to try a new food because of its appearance or smell, not only its taste. Nonsensory associations with objects also take on significance. For example, if parents refuse a particular food because of their dislike, they will transfer this negative connotation to the child before the child has had an opportunity to taste it. Awareness of these factors is important in several areas of childrearing, such as feeding, teaching socially acceptable habits, and reinforcing appropriate behavioral responses to various situations.

Touch continues to be important to the toddler. Descending development of the spinal tract is evidenced by increased sensation in the lower extremities, such as tickling the feet. Pleasant tactile sensations soothe and comfort the toddler, especially in times of stress or fatigue.

Maturation of Systems

Most of the physiologic systems are relatively mature by the end of toddlerhood. By the end of the first year all the brain cells are present but continue to increase in size. Myelination of the spinal cord is almost complete by 2 years of age, which parallels the completion of most of the gross motor skills associated with locomotion. Brain growth is 75% completed by the end of 2 years.

Development of various areas of the brain seems to correspond with the progressive intellectual capacity of the child. Various areas of the cerebral cortex undergo specific changes as developmental progress occurs, such as Broca area for speech and cortical areas for control of the legs, hands, feet, and sphincters. Because this neuromotor organization is so inclusive, complex, and intricate, the child is limited in his ability to attend to any one aspect of behavior for more than a few minutes.

Between 2 and 3 years of age coordination and consolidation of these voluntary functions allows the toddler to listen better, look longer, and have an extended span of attention. Although postural control is increasingly developed as myelination of the spinal cord advances, the immaturity of this control, combined with the child's limited experiences and the lack of visual perception makes simple acts such as seating oneself in a chair or climbing down stairs difficult tasks.

Volume of the respiratory tract and growth of associated structures continues to increase during early childhood, lessening some of the factors that predisposed the child to frequent and serious infections during infancy. However, the internal structures of the ear and throat continue to be short and straight, and the lymphoid tissue of the tonsils and adenoids continues to be large. As a result, otitis media, tonsillitis, and upper respiratory infections are common. The respiratory and heart rates slow and the blood pressure increases (see inside front cover). Respirations continue to be abdominal.

The digestive processes are fairly complete by the beginning of toddlerhood. The acidity of the gastric contents continues to increase and has a protective function, since it is capable of destroying many types of bacteria. Transit time slows and stomach capacity increases to allow for the usual schedule of three meals a day. The slower transit time results in somewhat less vulnerability to dehydration from diarrhea.

One of the more prominent changes of the gastrointestinal system is the voluntary control of elimination. With complete myelination of the spinal cord, control of anal and urethral sphincters is gradually achieved. Urination and defecation is controlled by a visceral reflex. For example, as urine accumulates in the bladder, the proprioceptors within the muscle tissues are activated by the stretching of the walls. Impulses are sent by the visceral afferent fibers to the spinal cord and then to the autonomic nervous system, which in turn causes the smooth muscle of the bladder wall to contract and expel the urine. The physical ability to control the sphincters probably occurs somewhere between ages 18 and 24 months. Bladder capacity also increases considerably. By 14 to 18 months of age the child is able to retain urine for up to 2 hours or longer.

The skin functionally matures during early childhood. The epidermis and dermis are more tightly bound together, increasing their resistance to infection and irritation and creating a more effective barrier against fluid loss. Production of sebum is minimum, which contributes to the development of dry skin. The eccrine glands are functional during early childhood and react to changes in temperature, but they produce very minimal amounts of sweat. Hair grows thicker and coarser and usually darkens and loses some curliness. Fine hair is evident on the lower arms and legs. Production of adipose tissue declines as hyperplasia of muscle cells increases. With the concurrent growth of the lower extremities, the child assumes more adultlike proportions.

Under conditions of moderate variation in temperature, the toddler rarely has the difficulties of the young infant in maintaining body temperature. The capillaries are able to conserve core body temperature by constricting in response to cold and dilating in response to heat. Shivering is much more effective as a source of thermogenesis. Shivering is an involuntary act that results in rhythmic muscle contraction, which increases cellular metabolism, producing heat. The child also learns mechanisms to control body temperature, by putting on clothing when cold or removing it when warm.

The defense mechanisms of the tissues and blood, particularly phagocytosis, are much more efficient in the toddler than in the infant. The production of antibodies is well established. Immunoglobulin G (IgG), which neutralizes microbial toxins, reaches adult levels by the end of the second year of life. Passive immunity from maternal transfer during fetal life disappears by the beginning of toddlerhood. Immunoglobulin M (IgM), which responds to artificial immunizing techniques and combats serious infection, attains adult levels during late infancy. Immunoglobulins A, D, and E increase gradually, not reaching eventual adult levels until later childhood. Many young children demonstrate a sudden increase in colds and minor infections when entering nursery school because of the exposure to new antigens.

Gross and Fine Motor Development

The major gross motor skill during the toddler years is the development of locomotion. By 15 months toddlers walk alone, by age 18 months they try to run but fall easily, and by 2 years they walk well and run fairly well, using a wide stance for extra balance. Between 2 and 3 years refinement of the upright, biped position is evident in improved coordination and equilibrium. By 2 years toddlers can walk up and down stairs, and by age 2½ years they jump, using both feet, stand on one foot for a second or two, and manage a few steps on tiptoe. By the end of the second year they stand on one foot, walk on tiptoe, and climb stairs with alternate footing.

Fine motor development is demonstrated in increasingly skillful manual dexterity. Once the pincer grasp is achieved, usually at 9 to 10 months of age, toddlers combine this skill with other developing sensory and cognitive abilities. For example, by age 12 months they are able to grasp a very small object but are unable to release it at will. At 15 months they can drop a pellet into a narrow-necked bottle. Casting, or voluntarily throwing objects, and retrieving them become almost obsessive activities around 15 months of age. By 18 months they can throw a ball overhand without losing their balance.

Visual perception of geometric shapes is also evident at this time. At age 12 months children selectively look at a round hole in a special form board but are unable to insert a round object. By age 15 months they promptly place the round object in the hole, even if the board is reversed or turned upside down. Spatial relations also are evident in their ability to build a tower with blocks. By age 15 months they can build a tower of two blocks; by age 18 months, a tower of three to four blocks; by age 24 months, a tower of six to seven blocks; and by age 30 months, a tower of eight blocks or more.

Fine motor skill and visual ability are demonstrated in toddlers' progressive adeptness in manipulating a pencil. By age 15 months they will scribble spontaneously and by 24 months of age will imitate a circular stroke and a vertical line. By the end of the toddler period copying a circle and imitating a cross is possible.

Mastery of gross and fine motor skills is evident in all phases of the child's activity, such as play, dressing, language comprehension, response to discipline, social interaction, and proneness to injuries. Activities occur less in isolation and more in conjunction with other physical and mental abilities to produce a purposeful result. For example, the toddler walks to reach a new location, releases a toy to pick it up or to choose a new one, and scribbles to look at the image produced. The possibilities of the exploration, investigation, and manipulation mastery of the environment—and its hazards—are endless.

PSYCHOSOCIAL DEVELOPMENT

The toddler is faced with the mastery of several important tasks. If the need for basic trust has been satisfied, he is ready to give up dependence for control, independence, and autonomy. Some of the specific tasks to be dealt with include (1) differentiation of self from others, particularly the mother; (2) toleration of separation from parent; (3) ability to withstand delayed gratification; (4) control over bodily functions; (5) acquisition of socially acceptable behavior; (6) verbal means of communication; and (7) ability to interact with others in a less egocentric manner. Mastery of these goals is only begun during late infancy and toddler years, and such tasks as developing interpersonal relationships with others may not be completed until adolescence. However, crucial foundations for successful completion of such developmental tasks are laid during these early formative years.

Erikson: Developing a Sense of Autonomy

According to Erikson, the developmental task of toddlerhood is acquiring a sense of *autonomy* while overcoming a sense of *doubt* and *shame*. As the infant gains trust in the predictability and reliability of his parents, his environment, and his interaction with others, he begins to discover that his behavior is his own and that it has a predictable, reliable effect on others. However, although he realizes his will and control over others, he is confronted with the conflict of exerting his autonomy and relinquishing his much enjoyed dependence on others. Exerting his will has definite negative consequences, whereas retaining dependent, submissive behavior is generally rewarded with affection and approval. However, continued dependency creates a sense of doubt regarding his potential capacity to control his actions. This doubt is compounded by a sense of shame for feeling this urge to revolt against others' will and a fear that he will exceed his own capacity for manipulating his environment. The latter fear is a basis for instituting limit-setting and consistent discipline at this age. Without appropriate limits on what is acceptable vs nonacceptable behavior, the child has no guidelines for establishing the end points of his ability to control.

Just as the infant has the social modalities of grasping and biting, the toddler has the newly gained modality of holding on and letting go. To hold on and let go is evident with the use of the hands, mouth, eyes, and, eventually, the sphincters, when toilet training is begun. These social modalities are expressed constantly in the child's play activities, such as casting or throwing objects away, taking objects out of boxes, drawers, or cabinets, holding on tighter when someone says, "No, don't touch," and spitting out food as taste preferences become very strong.

Several characteristics, especially negativism and ritualism, are typical of toddlers in their quest for autonomy. As the toddler attempts to express his will, he often acts contrary to everything around him. The words "no" or "me do" can be the sole vocabulary. Emotions become very strongly expressed, usually in rapid mood swings. One minute the toddler can be engrossed in an activity, and the next minute he might be violently angry because he was unable to manipulate a toy or open a door. If scolded for doing something wrong, he can have a temper tantrum and almost instantaneously pull at his mother's legs to be picked up and comforted. Often these swift changes are difficult for parents to understand and cope with. Many parents find the negativism exasperating and, instead of dealing constructively with it, give into it, which further threatens the child in his search for learning acceptable methods of interacting with others (see p. 609).

In contrast to negativism, which frequently disrupts the environment, ritualism becomes the needed buffer to maintain sameness and reliability. The toddler can venture out with security when he knows that there still exist familiar people, places, and routines. One can easily understand why change, such as hospitalization, represents such a threat to these children. Without the comfortable rituals, there is little opportunity to exert autonomy. Consequently dependency and regression occur (see p. 610).

Erikson focuses on the development of the *ego* during this phase of psychosocial development. There is a struggle as the child deals with the impulses of the id and attempts to tolerate frustration and learns socially acceptable ways of interacting with the environment. The ego, which may be thought of as reason or common sense, is evident as the child is able to tolerate delayed gratification. It operates on the *reality principle,* whereas the id operates on the *pleasure principle.*

There is also a rudimentary beginning of the *superego,* or conscience, which is the incorporation of the morals of society and the process of acculturation. With the development of the ego the child further differentiates himself from others and expands his sense of trust within himself. But as he begins to develop awareness of his own will and capacity to achieve, he also becomes aware of his ability to fail. This ever-present awareness of potential failure creates fear of doubt and shame. Successful mastery of the task of autonomy necessitates opportunities for self-mastery while withstanding the frustration of necessary limit-setting and delayed gratification. Opportunities for self-mastery are present in appropriate play activities, toilet training, the cri-sis of sibling rivalry, and successful interactions with significant others.

Freud: The Anal Stage

Freud's anal stage roughly corresponds with Erikson's stage of autonomy, or the period from 18 months to 3 years of age. Within this psychosexual framework the anal zone becomes the center of the child's physical, emotional, and psychologic efforts. Pleasure comes from moving his bowels, but the child is also met with the conflict of gaining physical satisfaction from involuntary evacuation vs gaining emotional reinforcement by holding on and letting go at mother's will. The process of toilet training is regarded as the resolution of this conflict.

COGNITIVE DEVELOPMENT

By the beginning of the second year it is quite clear that the toddler "thinks" and "reasons" things out. There is deliberate trial-and-error experimentation to produce certain results. The mental abstracts of time, space, and causality begin to have meaning, but the child's conception of each is different from that of the adult's. The main cognitive achievement of early childhood is the acquisition of language, which represents mental symbolism.

Piaget: The Sensorimotor and Preconceptual Phase

The period of 12 to 24 months of age is a continuation of the final two stages of the sensorimotor phase (Table 14-1). During this time the cognitive processes develop rapidly and at times seem similar to mature thinking. However, reasoning skills are still quite primitive and need to be understood

---

Table 14-1 Sensorimotor and preconceptual phases during toddlerhood*

STAGE	AGE	COGNITIVE DEVELOPMENT	BEHAVIOR
Sensorimotor V. Tertiary circular reactions	13-18 months	Active experimentation to achieve previously unattainable goals Increased concept of object permanence Differentiation of oneself from objects Early traces of memory Beginning awareness of spatial, causal, and temporal relationships Able to enter into an action at any point without reproducing the entire sequence	Insatiable curiosity about the environment Uses all sensory cues for exploration Ventures away from mother for longer periods Uses physical skills to achieve a particular goal Can find hidden objects, but only in first location Able to insert a round object into a hole Fits smaller objects into each other (nesting) Gestures "up" and "down" Puts objects into a container and takes them out Realizes that "out of sight" is not out of reach; opens doors and drawers to find objects Gains comfort from parent's voice even if the parent is not visually present

*For the previous four stages during early infancy see Table 12-1.

Continued.

Table 14-1 Sensorimotor and preconceptual phases during toddlerhood—cont'd

STAGE	AGE	COGNITIVE DEVELOPMENT	BEHAVIOR
VI. Invention of new means through mental combinations	19-24 months	Awareness of object permanence regardless of the number of invisible displacements Can infer a cause while only experiencing the effect Imitation is increasingly symbolic Beginning sense of time in terms of anticipation, memory, and ability to wait Egocentricism in thought and behavior Global organization of thought	Searches for an object through several hiding places Will infer a cause by associating two or more experiences (such as candy missing, sister smiling) Imitates words and sounds of animals Imitates adult behavior (domestic mimicry) Follows directions and understands requests Uses words "up," "down," "come," and "go" with meaning Has some sense of time; waits in response to "just a minute"; may use word "now" May sit and wait for meals at the table for short period of time Refers to self by name Engages in parallel play; demonstrates awareness of ownership Very concerned with ritualistic, routinized schedule
Preconceptual	2-4 years†	Increased use of language as mental symbolization Egocentricism still present in thought, play, and behavior Increased sense of time, space, causality Global organization of thought Transductive reasoning Concept of animism Unable to conceptualize two aspects of one object Magical thinking	Uses two- to three-word phrases Increased vocabulary Refers to self by pronoun Possessive of own toys, uses word "mine" Begins to use past tense of verbs Uses phrases "going to," "in a minute," "today," "all done" Uses many future-oriented words, such as "tomorrow," "next day," "afternoon," but poor conception of passage of time Follows directions using prepositions—up, behind, under, in back of, and so on Transfers knowledge of one object to same object in another location (for example, electrical outlet) Very traditional and ritualistic, small change in routine represents a drastic change in entire schedule Reasoning of causal relationships is directed by proximity of two or more events

*Cognitive development and behavior apply primarily to ages 24 to 36 months.

to effectively deal with the typical behaviors of this age child.

Tertiary circular reactions. In the fifth stage (from 13 to 18 months), the child uses active experimentation to achieve previously unattainable goals. Newly acquired physical skills are increasingly important for the function they serve rather than for the acts themselves. The child incorporates the old learning of secondary circular reactions and applies the combined knowledge to new situations, with emphasis on the results of the experimentation. In this way there is the beginning of rational judgment and intellectual reasoning. During this stage there is further differentiation of oneself from objects. This is evident in the child's increasing ability to venture away from his mother and to tolerate longer periods of separation.

Awareness of a causal relationship between two events is apparent. As the child flips a light switch, he is aware that a reciprocal response occurs. However, he is not able to transfer that knowledge to new situations. Therefore every time he sees what appears to be a light switch, he must

reinvestigate its function. Such behavior demonstrates the beginning of categorizing data into distinct classes, subclasses, and so on. There are innumerable examples of this type of behavior as toddlers continuously explore the same object each time it appears in a new place. A classic example is their curiosity about electrical outlets. Even if they receive a shock from one of them, they will adamantly poke, taste, and inspect every other outlet. This inability to transfer information leaves toddlers particularly vulnerable to accidents. However, traces of memory are evident because they will usually avoid the outlet where the shock occurred.

Since classification of objects is still rudimentary, the appearance of an object denotes its function. For example, if the child's toys are stored in a paper bag or large container, that toy receptacle is no different than the garbage pail or laundry basket. If the child is allowed to turn over the toy receptacle, he will just as quickly do the same to other similar objects because, for him, there is no difference. Expecting the child to judge which receptacles are permissible to explore and which are not is inappropriate for this age-group. Instead, the forbidden object such as the garbage pail should be placed out of reach.

The discovery of objects as objects leads to the awareness of their spatial relationships. The child is able to recognize different shapes and their relationship to each other. For example, he can fit slightly smaller boxes into each other (nesting) and can place a round object into a hole, even if the board is turned around, upside down, or reversed. However, not until 2 years of age can he do the same thing with a square. He is also aware of space and the relationship of his body to dimensions such as height. He will stretch, stand on a low stair or stool, and pull a string to reach an object.

Object permanence has also advanced. Although he still cannot find an object that has been invisibly displaced or moved from under one pillow to another pillow without his seeing the change, the toddler is increasingly aware of the existence of objects behind closed doors, in drawers, and under tables. Parents are usually acutely aware of this developmental achievement because they find high places and locked cabinets the only areas inaccessible to toddlers. Parents also experience the child's protest behavior when they leave, since the toddler is aware that his parents are absent when he cannot see them.

Invention of new means through mental combinations. During ages 19 to 24 months the child is in the final sensorimotor stage. This stage completes the more primitive, autistic thought processes of infancy and prepares the way for more complex mental operations during the phase of preoperational thought. One of the most dramatic achievements of this stage is in the area of object permanence. The child will now actively search for an object in several potential hiding places. In addition, he can infer a cause when only experiencing the effect. He can infer that an object was hidden in any number of places even if he only saw the original hiding place.

Imitation displays deeper meaning and understanding. Earlier, imitation was very concrete and action oriented. For example, "bye-bye" was a behavioral response more than a conceptual gesture of departure. Now it has a broader meaning, such as Daddy is going to work, it is time for a walk, or something is no longer present. There is greater symbolization to imitation.

One type of symbolic imitation is domestic mimicry, the imitation of household activity. Toddlers are acutely aware of others' actions and attempt to copy them in gestures and in words. They can imitate the parents' performance of a household task both physically and verbally. Parents often remark how accurately they see themselves in their child when the child engages in domestic mimicry. Such activity is part of the child's learning sex-role behavior.

The conception of time is still embryonic, but the child has some sense of timing in terms of anticipation, memory, and the limited ability to wait. He may listen to the command, "Just a minute," and behave appropriately. However, his sense of timing is exaggerated; for him 1 minute can last

an hour. The toddler's limited attention span also indicates his sense of immediacy and concern for the present.

Egocentrism, or the inability to envision situations from perspectives other than one's own, is evident in all aspects of toddlers' behavior. They see, experience, and live every event in reference to themselves. For example, if a person is positioned between the toddler and another child, the toddler will explain that both children can see the middle person's face. The young child is unable to realize that the other person views the middle person from a different perspective, the back. A common example of egocentric behavior is the toddler who takes a toy away from another child. The child is concerned only with playing with the toy and is unable to conceptualize that taking the toy away will make the other child unhappy.

Preconceptual phase. At approximately 2 years of age the child enters the preconceptual phase of cognitive development, which lasts until about 4 years. The preconceptual phase is a subdivision of the *preoperational phase,* which spans ages 2 to 7 years. The preconceptual phase is primarily one of transition, which bridges the purely self-satisfying behavior of infancy and the rudimentary socialized behavior of latency. The principal characteristics of this stage are egocentric use of language and dependence on perception in problem-solving (Thomas, 1985).

During 2 to 4 years children learn a variety of words and there is an increasing use of language. In fact, toddlers talk a lot. Speech is primarily of two types—egocentric or socialized. *Egocentric speech* consists of repeating words and sounds for the pleasure of hearing oneself and is not intended to communicate. This *collective monologue* reflects the child's lingering self-centeredness.

Socialized speech is for communication; however, it is still egocentric in that children communicate about themselves to others. Before age 3 most speech is directed at self-fulfillment or self-reference, such as, "Want drink," or "I do," and is directed mostly to adults. Since children think that everyone else's world is the same as theirs, they expect others to understand their verbal messages even when limited information is conveyed.

Preoperational thinking implies that children cannot think in terms of "operations"—the ability to manipulate objects in relation to each other in a logical fashion. Rather, toddlers think primarily based on their perception of an event. Problem-solving is based on what they see or hear directly rather than on what they recall about objects and events. Critical to this type of thought is the concept of *centration*—the tendency to focus on one aspect rather than consider all the possible alternatives. Another aspect of their thinking relates to reasoning. Toddlers' reasoning is neither deductive, from the general to the specific, or inductive, from the specific to the general, but *transductive,* from the particular to the particular. For example, if they did not like one food on the table, they may not like any other food. This prelogic is often very difficult to understand and confusing for parents, who will respond to the previous example by stating,

"What does this food have to do with that food?" As far as toddlers are concerned, the decision is logical because it is based on their frame of reference. No amount of "reasoning" will reverse this logic.

Typical of toddlers' thinking is *global organization* of thought processes, or the idea that changing any part of the whole changes the entire whole. Behaviorally this is repeatedly demonstrated in the toddler's ritualistic and rigidly traditional world. Everything must remain the same for the entire event to remain constant. Changing the smallest detail disrupts the entire experience. For example, moving the crib a few inches upsets the entire room. Substituting a new dish for the usual one spoils the entire meal. Rescheduling one part of the day's activity ruins the whole day. Such preoccupation with sameness is usually not evident in every phase of the child's life. It may center around a "security blanket" or a favorite teddy bear, but the ritualism represents a secure and reassuring foundation. When one realizes the importance of tradition and routine, the great disruption that illness and hospitalization represent to toddlers can be appreciated.

Another peculiarity of preconceptual thought is the concept of *animism,* in which the child attributes to inanimate objects lifelike qualities. For example, if the child falls down the stairs, he blames the stairs for causing the accident and will frequently "scold" the stairs. Cause and effect is more related to proximity of events than to anything else. In some instances this is a correct assumption, such as flicking the light switch turns the lamp on. But in other circumstances two simultaneous events do not cause each other, such as turning the light off at bedtime and the parent leaving the room. Fears of darkness are not unlikely when in the child's mind darkness is the "cause" of separation. Being aware of this type of causal thinking is especially important when young children are subjected to painful or frightening procedures. For example, when lights are turned off in a radiology room, the x-ray machine is turned on. The sudden darkness and loud noise can be frightening even though no pain is inflicted. Explaining the procedures by turning the machine and lights on with people present will help the child disassociate the two events of darkness and loud noise.

Another significant cognitive characteristic is *irreversibility*—the child is unable to undo or reverse mentally the actions he initiates physically. Therefore when told to stop doing something, the child is unable to conceive of the opposite behavior. Consequently, directions should be phrased *positively,* such as "Put the toy down," rather than "Don't throw the toy."

Within the second year the child increasingly uses language symbolically and is concerned with the "why" and "how" of things. For example, a pencil is "something to write with" and food is "something to eat." However, such mental symbolization is closely associated with prelogical reasoning. For instance, a needle is "something that hurts." Such painful experiences take on new significance, since memory is associated with the specific event and fears are likely to develop, such as resistance to people who wear white uniforms or rooms that look like the physician's office. Sometimes the child's ability to recall events is underestimated, and little thought is given to his preparation for visits to a hospital or other health facility, resulting in fears that can last a lifetime. Because of the vulnerability of these early years, it is essential to prepare children for new experiences, whether it is a new baby-sitter or a visit to the dentist.

MORAL DEVELOPMENT

Moral development is usually viewed as one aspect of socialization, as children learn to conform to the expectations of their culture. Several theorists incorporate moral development into their theoretical frameworks and most view its progress as paralleling that of cognitive development. One of the more prominent theories is that of Lawrence Kohlberg.

Kohlberg: Preconventional or Premoral Level

Toddlers' development of moral judgment is at the most basic level. There is little, if any, concern for why something is wrong. Young children behave because of the freedom or restriction that is placed on actions. In the *punishment and obedience orientation* whether an action is good or bad depends on whether it results in reward or punishment. If children are punished for it, the action is bad. If they are not punished, the action is good, regardless of the meaning of the act. For example, if parents allow hitting, the child will perceive that hitting is good because it is not associated with punishment (Thomas, 1985).

Type of discipline also affects children's moral development. When parents use power to control behavior, such as physical punishment or withholding privileges, children receive a negative view of morals, especially toward authority figures, such as law enforcement agencies. When parents withdraw love or attention, children behave primarily because of guilt, rather than from an internalization of morals. However, when parents give explanations for the misbehavior and try to help children change through positive approaches, such as consequences or rewards, children feel less hostility and are more likely to base their actions on an analysis of why an act may be wrong (Schuster and Ashburn, 1986). Of course, the effect of discipline is not limited to the toddler years and the sole use of explanation is inappropriate. However, parents usually establish discipline techniques at this time and the use of constructive approaches should begin early (see p. 607).

SPIRITUAL DEVELOPMENT

Because of their immature cognitive processes, toddlers have only a vague idea of God and religious teachings. However, routines, such as saying prayers before or at bedtime, can be very important and comforting. Toward the end of toddlerhood, when children are in preoperational thought, there is some advancement of their understanding of God. Religious teachings may influence their behavior, such as reward or fear of punishment (heaven or hell) and moral development (see also discussion in Chapter 15.)

DEVELOPMENT OF BODY IMAGE

As in infancy, the development of body image closely parallels cognitive development. With increasing motor ability toddlers recognize the usefulness of body parts and gradually learn their respective names. They also learn that certain parts of the body have various meanings: for example, during toilet training the genitals become significant and cleanliness is emphasized. This is consistent with Freud's psychosexual reference to this period as the anal stage. By 2 years there is recognition of sexual differences and reference to self by name and then by pronoun.

Once they begin preoperational thought, toddlers can use symbols to represent objects but their thinking may lead to inaccuracies. For example, if someone who is pregnant is called "fat," they will describe all "fat" ladies as having babies. There is probably some recognition of words used to describe physical appearance, such as "pretty," "handsome," or "big boy." Such expressions eventually influence how children view their own bodies.

Although there has been little research done on body image development in young children, it is evident that body integrity is poorly understood and that intrusive experiences are threatening. For example, during a physical assessment toddlers forcefully resist procedures such as examining the ear or mouth and taking a rectal temperature. Toddlers also have unclear body boundaries and may associate nonviable parts, such as feces, with essential body parts. This can be seen in the toddler who is upset by flushing the toilet and watching the stool disappear (Griffiths, 1983).

SOCIAL DEVELOPMENT

Toddlers are very social beings. As they begin to develop a sense of separateness, they are increasingly able to explore away from the parent, although anxiety related to imposed separations and strangers is at a peak. Major advances occur in language ability and personal-social behavior, although social skills, such as waiting a turn or manners, are extremely rudimentary. Play continues to be a major socializing agent and provides toddlers with invaluable opportunities to learn about the environment.

Individuation-Separation

A major task of the toddler period is differentiation of self from significant others, usually the mother. The differentiation process consists of two phases: *separation*, the children's emergence from a symbiotic fusion with the mother, and *individuation*, those achievements that mark children's assumption of their own individual characteristics in the environment (Mahler, Pine, and Bergman, 1975). Although the process begins during the latter half of infancy, the major achievements occur during the toddler years.

Toddlers have an increased understanding and awareness of object permanence and some ability to withstand delayed gratification and tolerate moderate frustration. They begin to lose some of the previous resistance to separation, yet appear to become even more concerned about the parent's whereabouts. They have learned from experience that parents exist when physically absent. Repetition of events such as going to bed without the parents but waking to find them again reinforces the reliability of such brief separations. Consequently toddlers are able to venture away from their parents for brief periods because of the security of knowing that the parent will be there when they return. Verbal and visual reassurance from the parent gradually replace some of the previous need to be physically close for comfort.

Toddlers also show less fear of strangers, but only when their parents are present. When left alone with a stranger, they are very fearful; acutely anxious; manifest depressive behavior, such as crying and withdrawal; and may become restless, hyperactive, or passive, reverting to regressive behaviors. Such reactions may be evident when a child is left with a baby-sitter or during the first day of nursery school.

These behaviors are not pathologic or harmful if parents realize how desperately their children need them. In fact, indiscriminate friendliness toward strangers and lack of anxiety during separation from parents is reason for concern. Sensitive, perceptive parents will be aware of the child's need for increased love, affection, and attention when they are together. An attitude such as "They will get used to the baby-sitter" will not help young children positively tolerate separation.

Parents often need help in realizing the necessity of preparing children for an inevitable separation. Particularly with the firstborn, parents tend to overprotect children, shield them from any anxiety-producing experience, and insulate them from less than immediate gratification. Although this is not necessarily harmful, especially if opportunities for independence are allowed later, it does not prepare children for unexpected events. A typical example is the birth of a sibling. The child is faced with the crisis of sibling rivalry as well as separation from the parent. No wonder the child will not welcome the infant; in his mind the intruder caused his mother to leave him. Allowing children to experience brief periods of separation early during infancy prepares them for such experiences later. Indeed they may still manifest the typical behaviors of protest, but they will also have learned that mother or father always returns. Therefore it is easy to appreciate the tremendous loss that the death of a parent represents for young children; unlike their other experiences with separation, this time the parent will not return. (For a discussion of the controversy regarding long-term consequences of separation, see Questions and controversies, p. 507.)

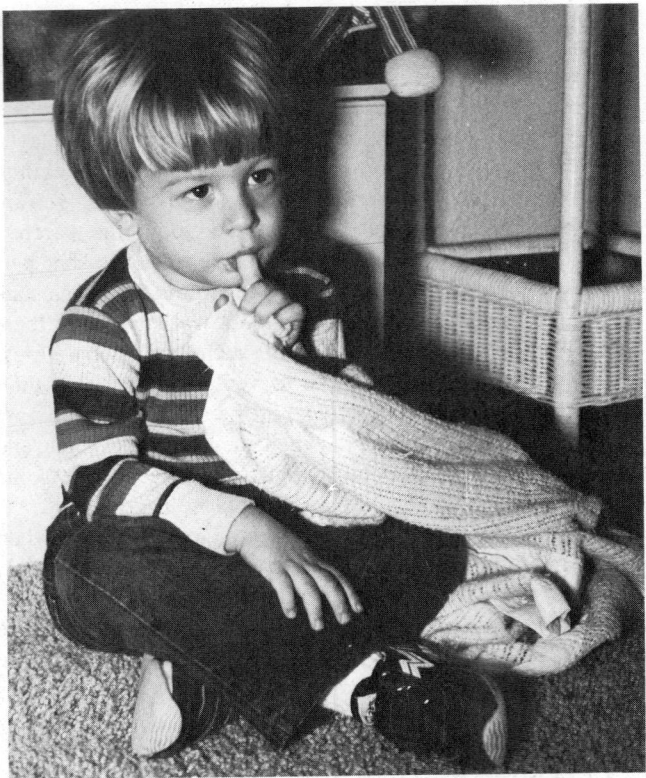

Fig. 14-2. Transitional objects, such as a warm and fuzzy blanket and a finger, are sources of security to toddlers.

Transitional objects, such as a favorite blanket or toy, provide security for the child, especially when he is separated from parents, dealing with a new stress, or just fatigued (Fig. 14-2). Security objects often become so important to toddlers that they refuse to have them taken away. Such behavior is normal; there is no need to discourage this tendency. During separations, such as daycare, hospitalization, or even overnight with a relative, transitional objects should be provided to minimize any feelings of fear or loneliness.

Learning to tolerate and master brief periods of separation is an important developmental task of children in this age-group. In addition, it is a necessary component of parenting, since brief periods of separation allow parents to recoup their energy and patience and to minimize directing their irritations and frustrations at the children.

Language Development

The most striking characteristic of language development during early childhood is the increasing level of comprehension. Although the number of words acquired—from about four at 1 year of age to approximately 300 at age 2 years—is notable, the ability to comprehend and understand speech is much greater than the number of words the child can say. This is particularly evident in bilingual families where the vocabulary may be delayed, but comprehension in either language is appropriate.

At age 1 year the child uses one-word sentences or holophrases. The word "up" can mean "pick me up" or "look up there." For the child the one word conveys the meaning of a sentence, but to others it may mean many things or nothing. During this age about 25% of the vocalizations are intelligible. By the age of 2 years the child uses multiword sentences by stringing together two or three words, such as the phrases, "mama go bye-bye" or "all gone," and approximately 66% of the speech is understandable.

Personal-Social Behavior

One of the most dramatic aspects of development in the toddler is his personal-social interaction. Parents frequently wonder why their manageable, docile, lovable infant has turned into a determined, strong-willed, volatile-tempered little tyrant. In addition the tyrant of the terrible twos can swiftly and unpredictably revert back to the adorable infant. All of this is part of his "growing up" and is evident in such areas as dressing, feeding, playing, and establishing self-control.

The toddler is developing skills of independence, which are evident in all areas of behavior. The 15-month-old child feeds himself, drinks well from a cup, and manages a spoon, with considerable spilling. By 18 months he uses a spoon well and may be using a fork. Between ages 2 and 3 years he eats with the family, likes to help with chores such as setting the table or removing dishes from the dishwasher, but lacks table manners and may find it difficult to sit through the family's entire meal.

In dressing, the toddler also demonstrates strides in independence. The 15-month-old child helps his mother by putting his arm or foot out for dressing and pulls his shoes and socks off. The 18-month-old child removes his own gloves, helps with pullover shirts, and may be able to unzip. By age 2 years he removes most of his clothing and puts on his socks, shoes, and pants without regard for right or left and back or front.

Play

Play magnifies the toddler's physical and psychosocial development. Interaction with people becomes increasingly important. The solitary play of infancy progresses to *parallel* play. The toddler plays alongside, not with, other children. Although sensorimotor play is still prominent, there is much less emphasis on the exclusive use of one sensory modality. The toddler inspects the toy, talks to the toy, tests its strength and durability, and invents several uses for it.

Play assumes many forms and serves several functions (Table 14-2). Imitation is one of the most distinguishing characteristics of play and enriches children's opportunity to engage in fantasy. With less emphasis on sex-stereotyped toys, play objects such as dolls, carriages, dollhouses, dishes, cooking utensils, child-sized furniture, trucks, and dress-up clothes are suitable for both sexes (Fig. 14-3).

Table 14-2 Play during toddlerhood

PHYSICAL DEVELOPMENT	SOCIAL DEVELOPMENT	MENTAL DEVELOPMENT AND CREATIVITY
Suggested activities		
Provide space in which to encourage physical activity	Provide replicas of adult tools and equipment for imitative play	Provide for water play
Provide sandbox, swing, and other scaled-down playground equipment	Permit child to "help" with adult tasks	Encourage building, drawing, and coloring
	Encourage imitative play	Provide various textures in objects for play
	Provide toys and activities that allow for expression of feelings	Provide large boxes and other safe containers for imaginative play
	Allow child to play with some actual items used in the adult world, for example, let him help wash dishes or play with pots and pans and other utensils (check for safety)	Read stories appropriate to age
		Monitor television viewing
Suggested toys		
Push-pull toys	Music and a phonograph	Wooden puzzles
Rocking horse, stick horse	Purse	Cloth picture books
Balls	Housekeeping toys (broom, dishes)	Paper, finger paint, thick crayons
Blocks (unpainted)	Toy telephone	Blocks
Pounding board	Dishes, stove, table and chairs	Large beads to string
Low gym and slide	Mirror	Wooden shoe for lacing
Pail and shovel		Appropriate TV programs
Containers		
Play dough		

Increased locomotive skills make push-pull toys, stick horses, straddle trucks or cycles, a small, low gym and slide, varied size balls, and rocking horses appropriate for the energetic toddler. Finger paints, thick crayons, chalk, blackboard, paper, and puzzles with large simple pieces use the child's developing fine motor skills. Interlocking blocks in varied sizes and shapes provide hours of fun and, during later years, are useful objects for creative and imaginative play.

Talking is a form of play for the toddler, who enjoys musical toys such as play phonographs, "talking" dolls and animals, and play telephones. Appropriate children's television programs are excellent for children in this age-group who learn to associate words with visual images. Toddlers also enjoy "reading" stories from a picture book and imitating the sounds of animals.

Tactile play is also important for the exploring toddler. Water toys, a sandbox with pail and shovel, finger paints, soap bubbles, and clay provide excellent opportunities for free creative and manipulative recreation. Parents sometimes forget the fascination of feeling slippery cream, catching airy bubbles, squeezing and reshaping clay, or smearing paints. These types of unstructured activities are as important as educational play to allow children freedom of expression.

Selection of appropriate toys must involve safety factors, especially in relation to size and sturdiness. The oral activity of toddlers makes them at risk for aspirating small objects. Parents need to be especially vigilant of toys played with in other children's homes or those of older siblings. Toys are a potential source of serious bodily damage to toddlers, who

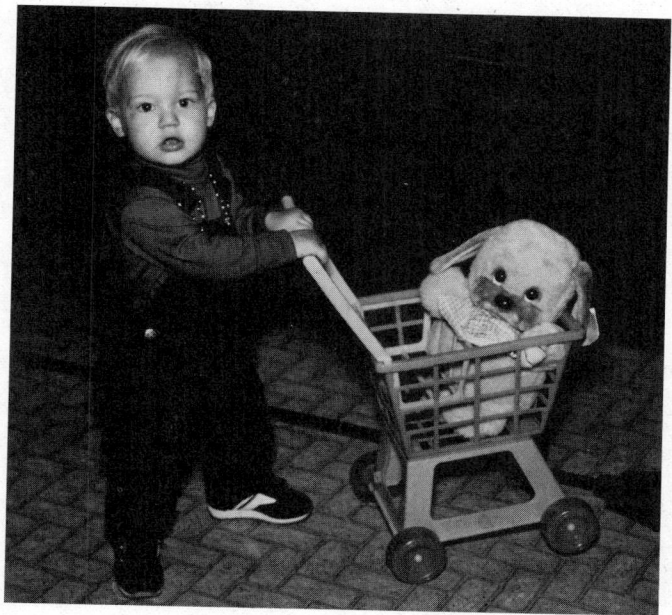

Fig. 14-3. Imitative play is common during toddler years.

may have the physical strength to manipulate them but not the knowledge to appreciate their danger (see Guidelines for toy safety on p. 137).

TEMPERAMENT

Temperamental characteristics of children during infancy tend to predominate during toddlerhood. Most difficult infants remain difficult during early childhood, but the easy infants also become less easy (Carey and McDevitt, 1978). In addition, mothers are more likely to rate children as difficult at 1 to 3 years than earlier (McDevitt and Carey, 1981). It is not surprising for parents to see toddlers as more challenging, especially considering the typical negativistic traits of this age-group. Parents of easy infants may be particularly distressed by the behavior change, whereas parents of difficult children may be more prepared, because of a previously troublesome year, or be overwhelmed by the additional behaviors. The use of the Toddler Temperament Scale can assist in identifying temperamental characteristics that benefit from individualized approaches to childrearing (Fullard, McDevitt, and Carey, 1984).

While temper tantrums are common in toddlers, certain temperament characteristics make some children more prone to such outbursts. Active, intensely responding children are apt to have yelling, screaming, and flinging behavior during tantrums. Parents benefit from forewarning of extreme outbursts and the knowledge that the intensely negative behavior is not abnormal and is tempered by the child's intensely happy moods (Zuckerman and Frank, 1983).

Discipline is also influenced by temperament. Easy children generally respond well to mild forms of discipline, including a stern voice and sustained eye contact. However, difficult children often need more structured types of discipline such as time-out or rewards and the effectiveness of one approach may be shortlived. Efforts at preventing misbehavior are especially important with children who have persistent natures (see box, p. 607). Without "friendly warnings" such children often have difficulty terminating an activity. These children may be punished for behavior that

is merely typical of their temperament, and if allowed to continue, the pattern can develop into a behavior problem (Chess and Thomas, 1985). Slow-to-warm-up children may also present challenges, especially when combined with toddlers' usual fear of strangers. These children require gradual introduction to new situations, such as daycare and babysitters.

SUMMARY OF GROWTH AND DEVELOPMENT DURING TODDLERHOOD

Developmental achievements during the toddler years occur in physical, gross and fine motor, language, and social areas. The key developmental ages are 18 and 24 months, although the chronologic ages of 15 and 30 months are also significant. Fifteen months of age is a particularly integrative period of developmental achievement, since it represents the completion or fruition of many skills that were unperfected at 1 year of age. Table 14-3 presents a summary of the major features of growth and development for the age-groups of 15, 18, 24, and 30 months.

COPING WITH CONCERNS RELATED TO NORMAL GROWTH AND DEVELOPMENT

The toddler years can be one of the most trying and confusing periods for parents. Behaviorally the toddler can be described as untiringly energetic, insatiably inquisitive, annoyingly negative, and obstinately ritualistic. Understanding these behaviors helps parents realize their necessity and allows them to effectively deal with the developmental tasks of children in this age-group.

Table 14-3 Summary of growth and development during the toddler years

AGE (MONTHS)	PHYSICAL	GROSS MOTOR	FINE MOTOR
15	Steady growth in height and weight Head circumference 48 cm (19 inches) Weight 11 kg (24 pounds) Height 78.7 cm (31 inches)	Walks without help (usually since age 13 months) Creeps up stairs Kneels without support Cannot walk around corners or stop suddenly without losing balance Assumes standing position without support Cannot throw ball without falling	Constantly casting objects to floor Builds tower of two cubes Holds two cubes in one hand Releases a pellet into a narrow-necked bottle Scribbles spontaneously Uses cup well but rotates spoon
18	Physiologic anorexia from decreased growth needs Anterior fontanel closed Physiologically able to control sphincters	Runs clumsily, falls often Walks up stairs with one hand held Pulls and pushes toys Jumps in place with both feet Seats self on chair Throws ball overhand without falling	Builds tower of three to four cubes Release, prehension, and reach well developed Turns pages in a book two or three at a time In drawing, makes stroke imitatively Manages spoon without rotation

Toilet Training

One of the major tasks of toddlerhood is toilet training. Voluntary control of the anal and urethral sphincters is achieved sometime after the child is walking, probably between ages 18 and 24 months. However, complex psychophysiologic factors are required for readiness. The child must be able to recognize the urge to let go and hold on and be able to communicate this sensation to the parent. In addition, there is probably some necessary motivation in the desire to please the parent by holding on, rather than pleasing oneself by letting go.

Usually physical and psychologic readiness is not complete until the latter half of the second year. By this time the child has mastered the majority of essential gross motor skills, can communicate intelligibly, is less in conflict with self-assertion and negativism, and is aware of his ability to control his body and please his parent. One of the most important responsibilities of nurses is to help parents identify the readiness signs in their child. These are summarized in Table 14-4.

A number of techniques can be helpful when initiating training. One is the selection of a potty chair and/or use of the toilet. A free-standing potty chair allows children a feeling of security (Fig. 14-4). Planting the feet firmly on the floor also facilitates defecation. Another option is a portable seat attached to the regular toilet, which may ease the transition from potty chair to regular toilet. Placing a small bench under the feet helps to stabilize the child's position. It is probably best to keep the potty in the bathroom and to let the child observe the excreta flushed down the toilet to associate these activities with usual practices. If a potty-seat is not available, having the child sit *facing* the toilet tank

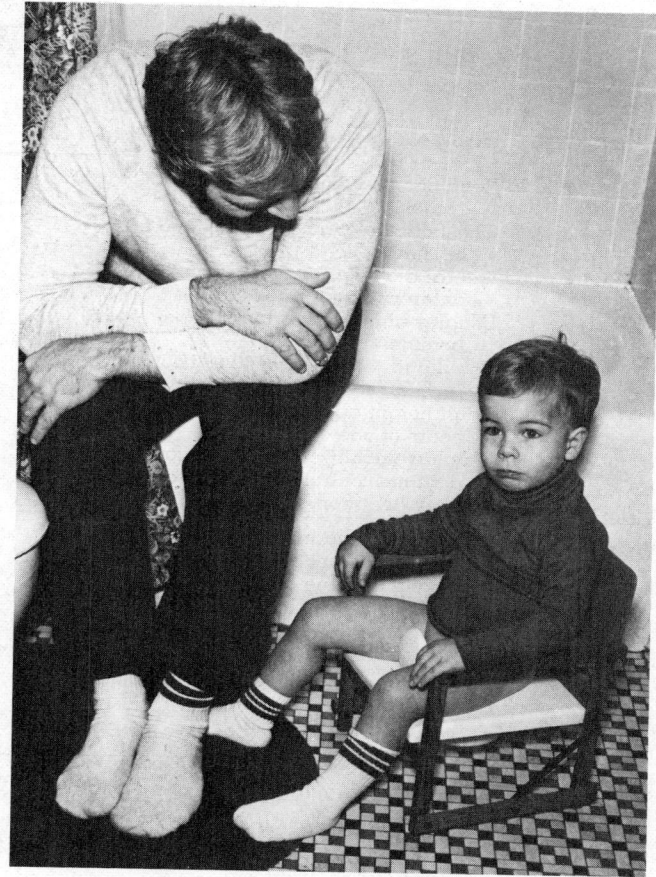

Fig. 14-4. Toddler on free-standing potty chair.

SENSORY	VOCALIZATION	SOCIALIZATION
Able to identify geometric forms; places round object into appropriate hole Binocular vision well developed Displays an intense and prolonged interest in pictures	Uses expressive jargon Says four to six words, including names "Asks" for objects by pointing Understands simple commands May use head-shaking gesture to denote "no" Uses "no" even while agreeing to the request	Tolerates some separation from mother Less likely to fear strangers Beginning to imitate parents, such as cleaning house (sweeping, dusting), folding clothes Feeds self using cup with little spilling May discard bottle Manages spoon but rotates it near mouth Kisses and hugs parents, may kiss pictures in a book Expressive of emotions, has temper tantrums
	Says 10 or more words Points to a common object, such as shoe or ball, and to two or three body parts	Great imitator ("domestic mimicry") Manages spoon well Takes off gloves, socks, and shoes and unzips Temper tantrums may be more evident Beginning awareness of ownership ("my toy") May develop dependency on transitional objects, such as "security blanket"

Continued.

Table 14-3 Summary of growth and development during the toddler years—cont'd

AGE (MONTHS)	PHYSICAL	GROSS MOTOR	FINE MOTOR
24	Head circumference 49 to 50 cm (19.5 to 20 inches) Chest circumference exceeds head circumference Lateral diameter of chest exceeds anteroposterior diameter Usual weight gain of 1.8 to 2.7 kg (4 to 6 pounds) Usual gain in height of 10 to 12.5 cm (4 to 5 inches) Adult height approximately double height at 2 years of age May have achieved readiness for beginning daytime control of bowel and bladder Primary dentition of 16 teeth	Goes up and down stairs alone with two feet on each step Runs fairly well, with wide stance Picks up object without falling Kicks ball forward without overbalancing	Builds tower of six to seven cubes Aligns two or more cubes like a train Turns pages of book one at a time In drawing, imitates vertical and circular strokes Turns doorknob, unscrews lid
30	Birth weight quadrupled Primary dentition (20 teeth) completed May have daytime bowel and bladder control	Jumps with both feet Jumps from chair or step Stands on one foot momentarily Takes a few steps on tiptoe	Builds tower of eight cubes Adds chimney to train of cubes Good hand-finger coordination; holds crayon with fingers rather than fist Moves fingers independently In drawing, imitates vertical and horizontal strokes, makes two or more strokes for cross

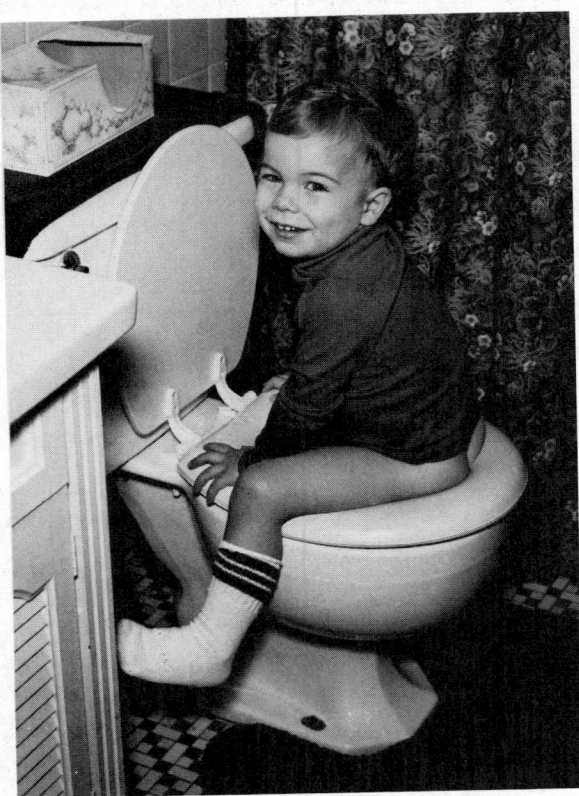

Fig. 14-5. Sitting in reverse fashion on regular toilet provides additional security to young child.

provides added support (Fig. 14-5). Practice sessions should be limited to 5 or 10 minutes, a parent should stay with the child, and sanitary habits should be employed after every session. Children should be praised for cooperative behavior and/or successful evacuation. Dressing children in easily removed clothing, using training pants or fancy panties and encouraging imitation by watching others are other helpful suggestions. Forcing children to sit on the potty for long periods, spanking them for having accidents, or other methods of negative control should be avoided.

Parents need to be very clear in the instructions given to toddlers to encourage elimination. For example, one mother used the phrase "Put pee in potty," when the child sat on the toilet. Several hours later, the child brought the potty to the mother with plastic letters of "P" in it. Also it may be helpful to stress to children that when they feel the urge to eliminate, they have the time to get to the toilet and then urinate or defecate. The entire process of elimination is new to toddlers and relationships between body functions and habits that adults take for granted may not be clear to children.

Bowel training is usually accomplished before bladder training because of its greater regularity and predictability. There is a stronger sensation for defecation than urination, which can be brought to the child's attention. In fact, nighttime bladder training may not be completed until 4 or 5 years of age, and even later training generally does not indicate pathology. Limiting fluid intake before the children's

SENSORY	VOCALIZATION	SOCIALIZATION
Accommodation well developed In geometric discrimination, able to insert square block into oblong space	Has vocabulary of approximately 300 words Uses two- to three-word phrases Uses pronouns I, me, you Understands directional commands Gives first name; refers to self by name Verbalizes need for toileting, food, or drink Talks incessantly	Stage of parallel play Has sustained attention span Temper tantrums decreasing Pulls people to show them something Increased independence from mother Dresses self in simple clothing
	Gives first and last name Refers to self by appropriate pronoun Uses plurals Names one color	Separates more easily from mother In play, helps put things away, can carry breakable objects, pushes with good steering Begins to notice sex differences; knows own sex May attend to toilet needs without help except for wiping

Table 14-4 Indications of readiness for toilet training

PHYSICAL READINESS	MENTAL READINESS	PSYCHOLOGICAL READINESS	PARENTAL READINESS
Voluntary control of anal and urethral sphincters, usually by 18 to 24 months Ability to stay dry for 2 hours; decreased number of wet diapers; waking dry from nap Regular bowel movements Gross motor skills of sitting, walking, and squatting Fine motor skills to remove clothing	Recognizes urge to defecate or urinate Verbal or nonverbal communicative skills to indicate when wet or has urge to defecate or urinate Cognitive skills to imitate appropriate behavior and follow directions	Expresses willingness to please parent Able to sit on toilet for 5 to 10 minutes without fussing or getting off Curiosity about adults' or older sibling's toilet habits Impatience with soiled or wet diapers; desire to be changed immediately	Recognizes child's level of readiness Willing to invest the time required for toilet training Absence of family stress or change, such as a divorce, moving, new sibling, or imminent vacation

hour of sleep and waking them once around midnight may help decrease the incidence of bed-wetting but do not teach voluntary control. Boys may begin toilet training in the stand-up position or by sitting on a potty chair or toilet. Imitating father during the preschool years is a powerful motivating force.

Daytime accidents are also common, particularly during periods of intense activity. Young children become so engrossed in play activity that if they are not reminded they will wait until it is too late to make it to the bathroom. The following example illustrates appropriate intervention:

Three-year-old Susan had been toilet-trained during the day for the last 4 months. Occasional accidents had decreased to almost zero. Now that the weather was warmer, her mother had been allowing her to play outside for a few hours each afternoon, but she noticed that Susan's pants were wet each time. She did not scold Susan for the accidents but reminded herself to bring the child into the house every hour and to show her how to open the door and call for her mother. She also brought the potty-chair downstairs where Susan could reach it quickly. After the first day of the hourly reminders, Susan called her mother and came in on her own. She still needed to be reminded, at least once during the afternoon, but the accidents were few. (For other suggestions regarding toilet training, refer to Chapter 24.)

Sibling Rivalry

The arrival of a new infant into the family represents a crisis for even the best prepared toddler. The toddler does not hate or resent the infant but despises the change that this additional sibling produces. Mother and father now share their love and attention with someone else, the usual routine is disrupted, and the toddler may lose his crib—all at a time when he thought he was in control of his world. It is not so difficult to understand the child's unwelcomed feelings toward this intruder when one considers the kinds of ambivalent feelings that surround the experience of parenting. Parents will ventilate feelings of jealousy concerning loss of independence and freedom. The difference between both types of jealousy is that the adult can rationalize and understand the change, but toddlers cannot.

Sibling rivalry tends to be most pronounced in the firstborn, who experiences "dethronement," loss of sole parental attention. It also seems to be most difficult for children under 2 years old, particularly in terms of mother-child interaction (Feiring, Lewis, and Jaskir, 1983). Three- and 4-year-old children are more secure within themselves and have other interpersonal attachments besides their mother. They have achieved a greater degree of independence in dressing, feeding, toileting, and playing; therefore they are less dependent on the parent for physical comfort and psychologic fulfillment. Five-year-olds may again have difficulty in accepting a new sibling because they are adjusting to the separation from home imposed by entering school.

Preparation of children for the birth of a sibling is quite individual, but age dictates some important considerations. Time for toddlers is a vague concept. Tomorrow could be yesterday or next week, and a month from now could be never. Preparing children too soon for the birth may lessen their interest by the time the event occurs. Toddlers are aware of something when mother's belly gets large and changes have taken place within the house. A month or two in advance is ample time for preparing the child.

Older children need to be prepared earlier because frequently they are aware of the expected sibling from overhearing adults' conversation. Jealousy can develop from feeling left out, and, since fantasy dictates reality, fear of the unknown can lead to fear of abandonment, separation anxiety, and insecurity.

Children can benefit from "siblings'" classes that may be part of prenatal sessions. They learn about the characteristics of infants and are taught simple tasks of caring for the new baby (Honig, 1986; MacLaughlin and Johnston, 1984). Books can help children prepare for birth and cope with sibling rivalry (Gates, 1979; Grossman, 1982; Honig, 1986).*

The toddler also needs to have a realistic idea of what the newborn will be like. Telling him that a new playmate will come home soon is foolish, since it is untrue and sets

up unrealistic expectations. Rather parents should stress the activities that will take place when the baby arrives home, such as diapering, bottle- or breast-feeding, bathing, and dressing. At the same time parents should emphasize which routines will stay the same, such as reading stories or going to the park. If the toddler has had no contact with an infant, it is a good idea to introduce him to one, if feasible. Providing a doll on which toddlers can imitate parental behaviors is another excellent strategy. They can tend to the doll's needs (diapering, feeding) at the same time the parent is performing similar activities for the infant (Fig. 14-6). Frequently other preparations, such as introducing the toddler to a regular bed or moving him to a different room, should be made earlier. If these changes are done well in advance, they will not be associated with the infant's arrival.

It helps to show favoritism to the child whenever possible, since this reinforces his acceptance and importance within the family. Visitors may initiate problems when they inadvertently shower the infant with attention and presents while neglecting the older child. Parents can minimize this by having small presents on hand for the toddler and including him in the visit as much as possible.

How children exhibit jealousy is complex. Some will overtly hit the infant, push him off mother's lap, or pull the bottle or breast from his mouth. More often the expressions of hostility and resentment are much more subtle and covert. Toddlers may verbally express a wish that the infant "go back inside mommy," or they will revert to more infantile forms of behavior, such as demanding a bottle, soiling their diaper, clinging for attention, using baby talk, or aggressively acting out toward others. The latter is particularly common in preschoolers who may seem accepting of the new sibling at home but behave poorly in nursery school. This is a form of displacement that says, "I can't

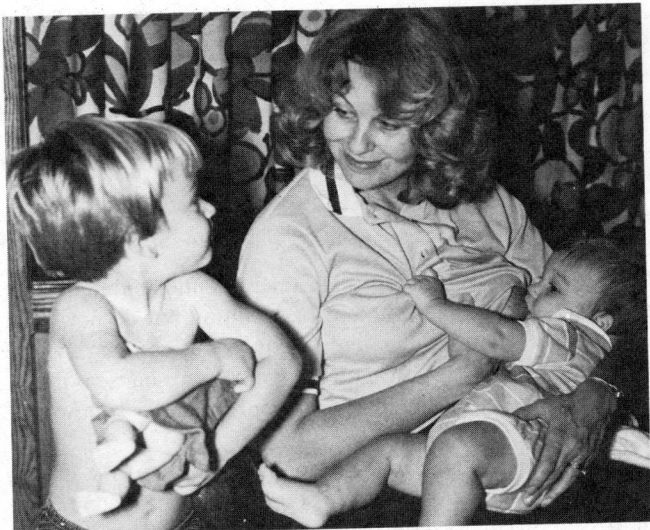

Fig. 14-6. Toddlers enjoy participating in caregiving activities for new sibling, such as this toddler who is "breast-feeding" his doll.

---

*Another excellent book is *The New Baby* by Fred Rogers, New York, 1985, G.P. Putnam's Sons.

let my parents know how I feel, so I will tell you.'' Encouraging parents to explore how their older child is acting with other caregivers is an important aspect of intervention.

Regardless of how well adjusted and accepting toddlers or preschoolers appear, infants must be protected by supervising the interaction between siblings. Other safety considerations are ''baby-proofing'' the house and instructing children regarding the dangers of small, sharp, or pointed objects to infants. Side rails on cribs should be kept fully raised and the mattress lowered to discourage toddlers from picking up the infant. Infant seats or bassinets should be placed on the floor so that young children cannot pull them off a raised surface ''to see the baby'' (MacLaughlin and Johnston, 1984).

The first few weeks at home with a newborn and sullen toddler are difficult for parents. Assuring them that this period will pass, that the toddler will learn to accept the changes in his life-style, and that the newborn will sleep through the night is part of the intervention. Allowing parents to talk about their feelings of ambivalence and frustration and suggesting ways of dealing with the jealousy help all members of the family survive this experience.

Limit-Setting and Discipline

In its broadest sense, discipline means to teach or refers to a set of rules governing conduct and may be used interchangeably with limit-setting. However, they can also refer to different concepts: *limit-setting* referring to establishing the rules or guidelines for behavior, and *discipline* being the action taken to enforce the rules following noncompliance. Generally the clearer the limits are set and consistently enforced, the less need there is for discipline.

Therefore the initial nursing goal is to help parents establish realistic and concrete ''rules.'' Limit-setting and discipline are positive, necessary components of childrearing and serve several useful functions as they help children:

1. Test their limits of control.
2. Achieve in areas appropriate for mastery at their level.
3. Channel undesirable feelings into constructive activity.
4. Protect themselves from danger.
5. Teach socially acceptable behavior.

Children want and need limits. Unrestricted freedom is a tremendous threat to their security and safety. Through testing the limits imposed on them, they learn the extent to which they can manipulate their environment as well as gain reassurance from knowing that others will be there to protect them from potential harm.

Minimizing misbehavior. The best approach toward discipline is to structure interactions with children so that unacceptable behavior is prevented or minimized. While many parents devise strategies that are most effective for their child, general guidelines include those listed in the above box.

General guidelines for implementing discipline. Regardless of the type of discipline used, certain principles

---

APPROACHES TOWARD MINIMIZING MISBEHAVIOR

Praise children for desirable behavior with attention and verbal approval.

Structure the environment to prevent unnecessary difficulties; for example, place fragile objects in inaccessible area.

Set clear and reasonable rules; expect the same behavior regardless of the circumstances and if exceptions are made, clarify that the change is for one time only.

Teach desirable behavior through own example, such as using a quiet, calm voice rather than screaming.

Review expected behavior before special or unusual events, such as visiting a relative or dinner in a restaurant.

Phrase requests for appropriate behavior positively, such as "Put the book down," rather than "Don't touch the book."

Call attention to unacceptable behavior as soon as it begins; use distraction to change the behavior or offer alternatives to annoying actions, such as a quiet toy for one that is excessively noisy.

Give "friendly warnings" such as "When the TV program is over, it is time for dinner" or "I'll give you to the count of three and then we have to go."

Be attentive to situations that increase the likelihood of misbehaving, such as overexcitement or fatigue, or decreased personal tolerance to minor infractions.

Offer sympathetic explanations for not granting a request, such as "I am sorry I can't read you a story now, but I have to finish dinner. Then we can spend time together."

Keep any promises made to children.

Avoid outright conflicts; temper discussions with statements like "Let's talk about it and see what we can decide together" or "I have to think about it first."

---

are essential in ensuring the efficacy of the approach (see box on p. 608). Many strategies, such as behavior modification, can only be implemented effectively when principles of consistency and timing are followed. A pattern of intermittent or occasional enforcement of limits actually prolongs the undesired behavior because toddlers learn that if they are persistent, the behavior is permitted eventually. Delaying punishment weakens its intent and practices such as telling the child, ''Wait until your father comes home,'' are not only ineffectual, but also convey negative connotations about the other parent.

Types of discipline. To deal with misbehavior, parents need to implement appropriate disciplinary action. Numerous approaches are available and some have definite advantages over others. The following discussion presents the more common strategies.

Corporal punishment. Corporal punishment most often takes the form of spanking. Based on the principles of aversive therapy, inflicting pain through spanking causes a dramatic decrease in the behavior. However, there are some serious flaws in this approach: (1) it teaches children that violence is acceptable; (2) many times the spanking is the result of parental rage and may physically harm the child;

GENERAL GUIDELINES FOR IMPLEMENTING DISCIPLINE

Consistency—implement disciplinary action exactly as agreed on and for each infraction

Timing—initiate discipline as soon as the child misbehaves; if delays are necessary, such as to avoid embarrassment, verbally disapprove of the behavior and state that disciplinary action will be implemented

Committment—follow through with the details of the discipline, such as timing of minutes; avoid distractions that may interfere with the plan, such as telephone calls

Unity—make certain that all caregivers agree on plan and are familiar with the details to prevent confusion and alliances between child and one parent

Flexibility—choose disciplinary strategies that are appropriate to the child's temperament and the severity of the misbehavior

Planning—plan discipline strategies in advance and prepare child if feasible, for example, explaining the use of time-out; for unexpected misbehavior, try to discipline when calm

Behavior-orientation—always disapprove of the behavior, not the child, with such statements as "That was a wrong thing to do. I am unhappy when I see behavior like that."

Privacy—administer discipline in private, especially with older children who may feel ashamed in front of others

Understanding—follow discipline with concern for children's feelings, such as "I am sad that you had to stay at home because you were grounded for breaking the rules"; avoid lecturing or bringing up the infraction once discipline has been implemented

Termination—once the discipline is administered, consider the child as having a "clean slate" and avoid bringing up the incident or lecturing

and (3) children become "accustomed" to spanking, requiring more severe corporal punishment each time. Consequently parents may use paddles, whips, or other objects, or they may eliminate a spanking because of their unwillingness to "hit the child harder," a practice that may prolong the behavior.

Although there is controversy regarding the use and abuse of corporal punishment, there are some instances when it is effective, especially in children who refuse to listen to verbal commands. For example, slapping the child's hand while saying, "No, don't touch," reinforces the meaning of the statement. A good rule when using mild physical punishment is that only one slap is given because the first slap is for the child; additional slaps are for the punisher.

Reasoning and scolding. Reasoning involves explaining why an act is wrong and is usually appropriate for older children, especially when moral issues are involved. However, young children cannot be expected to "see the other side" because of their egocentricity. Sometimes children use the "reasoning" as a way of gaining attention. For example, they may misbehave in order for the parents to give them a lengthy explanation of the wrongdoing because

negative attention is better than none. When children use this technique, parents may have to end the explanation with a statement of, "This is the rule and this is how I expect you to behave. I won't explain it any further."

Unfortunately reasoning is frequently combined with scolding, which sometimes takes the form of shame or criticism. For example, the parent may state, "You are a bad boy for hitting your brother." Unfortunately children take such remarks seriously and personally, believing that *they* are bad. It is important to focus only on the misbehavior not on the child (see box, Behavior orientation). Use of "I" messages rather than "you" messages expresses personal feelings without accusation or ridicule. For example, an "I" message attacks the behavior—"I am upset when Johnny is punched. I don't like to see him hurt"—not the child.

Reward. Reward is based on behavior modification theory—if an act is consistently rewarded, the desired behavior will be strengthened. Using rewards is a positive approach; by encouraging children to behave in specified ways, the tendency to misbehave is lessened. With young children using stars is a very effective method. For older children, the "token system" is appropriate, especially if a certain number yields a special reward, such as a trip to the movies or a new book. In planning a reward system, the expected behaviors must be clearly explained to the child and the rewards must be reinforcing. A chart should be used to record the stars or tokens and every earned reward promptly given. Verbal approval should always accompany extrinsic rewards.

Ignoring or extinction. Ignoring also uses behavior modification theory—if an act is consistently ignored, the unreinforced behavior will eventually be extinguished. Although this approach sounds very simple, it is often difficult to implement consistently. Parents frequently "give in" and resort to previous patterns of discipline. Consequently the behavior is actually reinforced because the child learns that persistence gains parental attention.

For this approach to be effective, health professionals must devote a fair amount of time toward (1) explaining the approach in detail, (2) recording behavior before the extinction process is instituted to see if a problem exists and to compare results after ignoring is begun, (3) making certain that the parent's attention is the reinforcer, and (4) warning parents of a phenomenon called "response burst," which refers to an *increase* in the child's behavior soon after initiating the process because the child is "testing" the parents to see if they are serious about the plan.

Time-out. Time-out is actually a refinement of the common practice of "sending the child to his room." It is also based on the premise of removing the reinforcer, that is, the satisfaction or attention the child is receiving from the activity. With the child placed in an unstimulating and isolated place, he becomes bored and consequently agrees to behave in order to reenter the family group. Time-out avoids many of the problems of the other disciplinary approaches because no physical punishment is involved, no reasoning or scolding is given, and the parent is usually not present for all of the time-out, facilitating his ability to consistently apply the punishment. It also offers both the child and parent a "cooling off" time.

To be effective, time-out must be planned in advance. The basic components include:

1. Select an area for time-out that is safe, convenient, and unstimulating, but where the parent can monitor the child, such as the bathroom, hallway, or laundry room.
2. Determine what behaviors warrant a time-out.
3. Make sure the child understands the "rules" and how he is expected to behave.
4. Explain to him the process of time-out:
   a. When he misbehaves, he will be given *one* warning.
   b. If he does not obey, he will be sent to the place designated for time-out.
   c. He is to sit there for a specified period of time.
   d. If he cries, refuses, or displays any disruptive behavior, the time-out period will begin *after* he quiets down.
   e. When he is quiet for the duration of the time, he can then leave the room.
5. A rule for the length of time-out is *1 minute per year of age;* a kitchen timer with an audible bell should be used to record the time rather than a watch.
6. Implement time-out in a public place by selecting a suitable area or explain to the child that time-out will be spent immediately upon returning home and mark the child's hand with a felt-tip pen as a reminder.

Consequences. The strategy of consequences involves allowing children to experience the results of their misbehavior and includes three types:

natural Those that occur without any intervention, such as being late and missing dinner

logical Those that are directly related to the rule, such as not being allowed to play with another toy until the used ones are put away

unrelated Those that are imposed deliberately, such as no playing until homework is completed

Natural or logical consequences are preferred but are effective only when they are meaningful to children. For example, the natural consequence of living in a messy room may do little to encourage cleaning up, but no friends over until the room is neat can be very motivating! The use of withdrawing privileges is often a form of unrelated consequences. After the child experiences the consequence, the parent should refrain from any comment, because the usual tendency is for the child to try and place blame for imposing the rule.

Temper Tantrums

Toddlers may assert their independence by violently objecting to attempts at restricting their behavior. They may lie down on the floor, kick their feet, and scream at the top of their lungs. Head-banging, head-rolling, and breath-holding are other behaviors some children use. While these mannerisms are very disturbing to observe, they usually do not become behavior problems (Abe, Oda, and Amatomi, 1984).

Breath-holding and fainting from lack of oxygen causes no physical harm because the accumulation of carbon dioxide stimulates the respiratory control center to initiate breathing. However, head-banging results in self-inflicted injury and the child requires protection, such as a padded crib.

The best approach toward extinguishing attention-seeking behavior is to ignore it (no verbal or eye contact with the child), provided the behavior is not inflicting injury. The parent should remain close by and after the tantrum has subsided offer a toy or a favorite activity to substitute for the ungranted request and to reward the post-tantrum behavior. When tantrums do occur, it is important to intervene *immediately* to prevent feeling angry and being unable to calmly ignore the behavior. Frequently temper tantrums can be avoided using the approaches on p. 607.

Negativism

One of the more difficult aspects of rearing toddlers is their persistent negative "no" response to every request. The negativism is not an expression of being fresh or insolent, but a necessary assertion of self-control. One method of dealing with the negativism is reducing the opportunities for a "no" answer. Asking the child, "Do you want to go to sleep now?" is almost certain to be met with an emphatic "no." A more appropriate approach is to tell the child that it is time to go to sleep and proceed accordingly.

In their attempt to exert control, children like to make choices. When confronted with appropriate choices, such as, "You can have a peanut butter and jelly sandwich or chicken noodle soup for lunch," they are more likely to choose one than automatically say no. However if their response is negative, parents should make the choice for the child.

Coping with Stress

Adults rarely think of young children as being exposed to stress or suffering its consequences. However the normal demands of growing-up coupled with the usual pressures most families experience mean that few, if any, young children are reared "stress free." Minimum amounts of stress are beneficial during the early years to help children develop effective coping skills. However, excessive stress is destructive, and young children are especially vulnerable because of their limited capacity to cope.

To help parents deal with stress in their children's life, they must be aware of signs suggestive of stress (see p. 128) and be helped to identify the source. The normal stresses during toddlerhood are listed in the box on p. 610. In addition any number of other stresses may be imposed on children, such as alternate caregiving arrangements, birth of a sibling, marital discord, relocation, or illness. Watching children at play can identify stressors. For example, one child was seen pounding on his doll, yelling "Go away! Go away!" The parent was quick to observe that the child's recent irritability was probably caused by the stress of a new sibling.

SOURCES OF STRESS IN TODDLERS

Negativism—does not like to take orders; may be down-right contrary

Rigidity—wants own way; is upset when rituals are disrupted; dislikes interference

Lack of sociability—engages in solitary or parallel play but is generally disinterested in socializing

Self-centeredness—believes the world revolves around her or him; does not want to share; may dawdle

Separation anxiety—fears loss of parents

Stranger anxiety—fears strangers; is shy

Toilet training

Bedtime—dislikes being ordered to bed; may fear bedwetting or separation from parents; may have terrifying dreams

Tantrums—may revert to temper tantrums or destructive behavior; may hit or bite

Security object—may have a security object that, if lost or misplaced, leads to great emotional upset

Overdoing—may become overstimulated or overtired

Fears—in particular, may include animals or anything that makes a loud noise

Doctors—visits to the pediatrician may prove extremely stressful

From Kuczen, B.: Childhood stress: don't let your child be a victim, New York, 1982, Delacorte Press, p. 15.

The best approach to dealing with stress is prevention—monitoring the amount of stress in children's lives so that levels exceeding their coping ability do not occur. In many instances this is as simple as increasing the child's rest periods to allow for quiet recovery time. Often it involves adequately preparing the child for change, such as daycare or a new sibling. It also requires helping the child cope with stress. Play is an excellent vehicle for venting anger or frustration and toys such as drums, play nails and hammer, clay, and Play-Doh provide alternative methods of dissipating anxiety. They also begin to teach socially acceptable ways of dealing with such feelings. Another approach is the use of relaxation and imagery. Even young children can learn to "let their bodies go limp like a rag doll" or "imagine floating on a cloud."

Regression. Regression is a retreat from a present pattern of functioning to past levels of behavior. It usually occurs in instances of stress, when one attempts to cope by reverting to patterns of behavior that were successful in earlier stages of development. Regression is common in toddlers because almost any additional stress lessens their ability to master present developmental tasks. At first such regression appears acceptable and comfortable for children, but on closer inspection it becomes evident that the loss of newly acquired achievements is frightening and threatening, since children are aware of their total helplessness in the recent past. Parents, too, become concerned about regressive behavior and frequently in their efforts to deal with it force the child to cope with an additional source of stress—the pressure to live up to expected standards.

When regression does occur, the best approach is to ig-nore it, while praising existing patterns of appropriate behavior. The child is saying, "I can't cope with this present stress and perfect this new skill as well, but I will if given patience and understanding." For this reason it is not advisable to attempt new areas of learning when an additional crisis is present or expected, such as beginning toilet training shortly before a sibling is born or attempting new areas of learning during a brief period of hospitalization.

Fears. Fears are very common during this age and include fear of annihilation, going to sleep, animals, and engines, especially the vacuum cleaner, with the greatest fear continuing to be fear of strangers and separation. Because fear of strangers and separation begins in infancy, it is discussed in Chapter 12. The other fears often escalate in the preschool period and consequently are discussed in Chapter 15.

Promoting Optimum Health During Toddlerhood

Physical and psychosocial changes in toddlers affect several areas of health maintenance and promotion, namely, nutrition, sleep and activity, dental health, and injury prevention. Nursing intervention, especially anticipatory guidance, can positively affect the optimal development of the child and family during this exciting, but often troublesome, period of childhood.

NUTRITION

During the period from 12 to 18 months of age the growth rate slows, resulting in an adjustment from a previous caloric requirement of about 110 kcal/kg (50 kcal/pound) of body weight during infancy to 100 kcal/kg (45 kcal/pound) during the next 2 years. Protein requirements also decrease slightly from 2.2 to 2.0 g/kg for infants to 1.8 g/kg for toddlers but are still higher than at succeeding ages to meet the demands of muscle tissue growth. Fluid needs drop from an infant requirement of approximately 140 ml/kg to a toddler requirement of 115 ml/kg. The reduced fluid requirement represents a decrease in the total body water and an increase in fluid within the cells (intracellular fluid).

The requirements for most vitamins and minerals increase slightly during toddlerhood. The need for minerals such as iron, calcium, and phosphorus may be difficult to meet considering the characteristic food habits of children in this age-group. Milk intake, the chief source of calcium and phosphorus, should average 3 cups a day. More than a quart of milk consumption daily considerably limits the intake of solid foods, resulting in deficient dietary iron as well other nutrients.

At approximately 18 months of age most toddlers manifest this decreased nutritional need in a phenomenon known as *physiologic anorexia*. They become picky, fussy eaters with strong taste preferences. They may eat voraciously one day and almost nothing the next. They are increasingly aware of the nonnutritive function of food: the pleasure of eating, the social aspect of mealtime, and the control of refusing food. They are influenced by factors other than taste when choosing food. If a family member refuses to eat something, the child is likely to imitate that response. If the plate is overfilled, he is likely to push it away, overwhelmed by its size. If food does not appear or smell appetizing, he will probably not agree to try it. In essence mealtime is more closely associated with psychologic components than nutritional ones and nutritional counseling must address the characteristics of this age-group.

Nutritional Counseling

Eating habits established in the first 2 or 3 years of life tend to have lasting effects on subsequent years. If food is used as a reward or sign of approval, a child may overeat for nonnutritive reasons. If food is forced and mealtime is consistently unpleasant, the usual pleasure associated with eating may not develop. Mealtimes should be enjoyable rather than times for discipline or family arguments. The social aspect of mealtime may be distracting for young children; therefore an earlier feeding hour may be appropriate. Young children are unable to sit through a long meal and become fidgety and disruptive. This is particularly common when children are brought to the table just after active play. Calling them in from play 15 minutes before mealtime allows them ample opportunity to get ready for eating while settling down their active minds and bodies.

The method of serving food also takes on more importance during this period. Toddlers need to feel control and achievement in their abilities. Giving them large, adult-size portions contributes to their feeling overwhelmed. In general what is eaten is much more significant than how much is consumed. Small amounts of meat and vegetables supply greater food value than a large consumption of bread or potato. Serving sizes need to be appropriate for age (Table 14-5). A general guide to serving size is: 1 tablespoon of solid food per year of age. Young children tend to like less spicy, bland food, although this is a culturally determined preference. Substitutions should be provided for foods that they do not enjoy.

The ritualism of this age also dictates certain principles in feeding practices. Toddlers like the same dish, cup, or spoon every time they eat. They may reject a favorite food simply because it is served in a different utensil. If one food touches another, they often refuse to eat it. Mixed foods, such as stews or casseroles, are also rarely favorites. Since toddlers are unpredictable in their table manners, it is best to use plastic dishes and cups, both for economic and safety reasons. A regular mealtime schedule also contributes to their desire and need for predictability and ritualism.

Appetite and food preferences are sporadic during these years. A child may enjoy one food for 3 days in a row and then suddenly refuse to eat it again for days. Such food fads or "jags" do not ensure a well-balanced diet, but attempts

Table 14-5 Servings per day for children based on basic four food groups

FOOD GROUP	SERVINGS PER DAY

Milk or equivalent
½ cup whole milk equals:
   ¾ ounce cheese
   ½ cup yogurt, milk pudding
   1 cup cottage cheese
   ¾-1 cup ice cream
	3 for child
	4 for adolescent
	Usual serving:
	   Toddler and
	      preschooler—½
	      to ¾ cup
	   School-age and
	      older—1 cup

Meat, fish, poultry, or equivalent
1 ounce meat equals:
   1 egg
   1 ounce cheese
   2 tablespoons peanut butter
   ¼ cup tuna fish
   ½ cup cooked legumes
	2 for child and
	adolescent
	Usual serving:
	   Toddler and
	      preschooler—
	      1 egg, 1 to 2 ounces
	      meat
	   School-age and
	      older—1 egg,
	      3 ounces meat

Vegetables and fruits
Citrus equivalents:
   1 orange or tomato
   ½ cup orange or grapefruit
      juice
   ¾ cup strawberries
	4 for child and
	adolescent
	1 citrus daily; 1
	yellow or dark green
	vegetable
	3 to 4 times
	weekly
	Usual serving:
	   Toddler and
	      preschooler—2
	      tablespoons
	      to ¼ cup
	   School-age and
	      older—½ cup

Breads and cereals
1 slice enriched bread equals:
   ¾ cup dry cereal
   ½ cup cooked pasta, rice, or
      cereal
   ½ hamburger bun
   1 small muffin or biscuit
	4 for child and
	adolescent
	Usual serving:
	   Toddler and
	      preschooler—
	      ½ slice bread
	   School-age and
	      older—1 slice
	      bread

to alter them are met with bitter resentment and unwavering obstinacy. It is preferable to accept such extremes and offer other foods in small portions. Generally the child will choose another "favorite food" that may compensate for the nutritional inadequacy. Introducing at least three items from the basic four food groups at each meal helps develop a variety of taste preferences and well-balanced habits (see Table 14-5). The box on p. 612 suggests sample menus for toddlers.*

Developmentally most children by 12 months of age are

---

*A helpful resource for parents is *Food before six: a feeding guide for parents of young children,* available from the National Dairy Council, 6300 North River Road, Rosemont, IL 60018-4233.

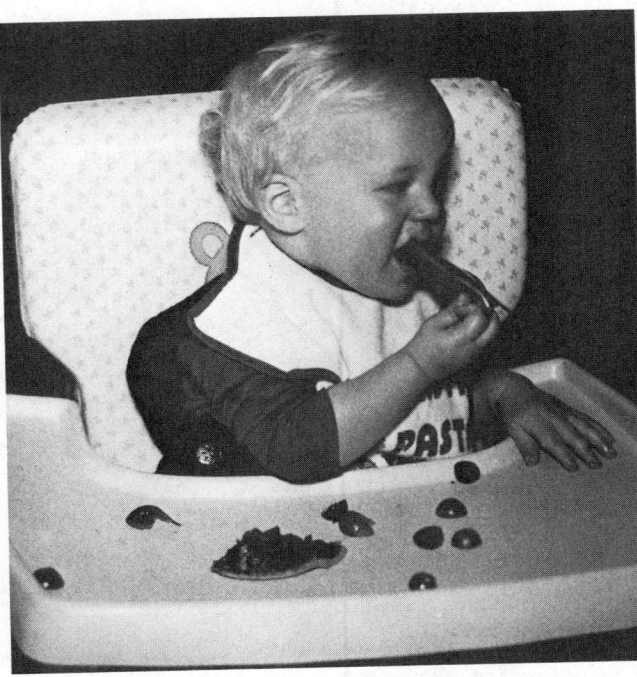

Fig. 14-7. Toddlers enjoy "finger feeding."

Table 14-6 Developmental milestones associated with feeding

AGE (MONTHS)	DEVELOPMENT
12-18	Drools less Drinks well from a household cup but may drop it when finished Holds cup with both hands Begins to use a spoon but turns it before reaching mouth
24	Can use a straw Chews food with mouth closed and shifts food in mouth Distinguishes between finger and spoon foods Holds small glass in one hand; replaces glass without dropping Uses spoon correctly but with some spilling
36	Spills small amount from spoon Begins to use fork; holds it in fist Uses adult pattern of chewing, which involves rotary action of jaw

---

SAMPLE MENU FOR TODDLERS BASED ON BASIC FOOD GROUPS

Breakfast
½ cup orange juice
1 poached egg
½ slice enriched toast with 1 teaspoon butter
½ cup milk

Lunch
½ cup cooked peas and carrots
2 tablespoons chopped roasted chicken
½ banana or apple
½ cup milk

Dinner
½ cup baked macaroni with 1 ounce cheese*
½ cup string beans
½ slice bread
½ cup pudding
½ cup milk (after dinner or before bed)

Snack during day
½ apple
½ cup milk or juice
⅓ cup ice cream†
1 blueberry muffin

*Used as a meat substitute.
†Concentrated sweets and empty calories should be avoided.

---

eating the same food prepared for the rest of the family. Some may have mastered using a cup with occasional spilling, although most cannot adeptly use a spoon until 18 months of age or later (Table 14-6) and generally prefer using their fingers (Fig. 14-7). Some children find weaning easy and voluntarily relinquish the bottle by the first birthday. Others are unable to sacrifice that pleasure and require a bottle at nighttime or occasionally during the day. Allowing the child to give up the bottle when he is ready is preferable to forcing the issue.

Some toddlers reject all solid food in preference for the bottle, a practice that can be discouraged by gradually diluting the milk with water to make it less satisfying and introducing foods at times when the child is most likely to be hungry, such as on awakening. Occasionally it may be necessary to withhold bottle feedings until the child is hungry enough to eat solid foods. Forcing the child to eat solid foods usually results in conflicts and does little to establish healthy eating habits.

SLEEP AND ACTIVITY

Total sleep decreases only slightly during the second year and averages about 12 hours. Most children take one nap a day and by the end of the third year many relinquish this habit. The activity level is high and there is rarely a problem with too little physical exercise, provided inappropriate restrictions are not instituted. With increasing numbers of young children cared for outside the home, attention to the kinds of activity provided is important. For example, children with high activity levels may benefit from an environment in which outdoor play is encouraged.

Sleep problems are common, especially going to bed and falling asleep, and are probably related to fears of separation. Bedtime rituals (same hour of sleep, snack, quiet activity) are helpful and transitional objects, such as a favorite stuffed animal or blanket, can help ease the insecurity at bedtime. For problems that persist, the interventions outlined in Table 12-6 should be employed.

DENTAL HEALTH

The importance of oral hygiene in preserving the teeth and maintaining healthy gums cannot be overemphasized or begun too early. Nurses are in an optimum position to promote dental hygiene both in their care of well children and ill children during hospitalization.

Regular Dental Examinations

Ideally the child should see a dentist (or pedodontist) soon after the first teeth erupt and no later than by 2½ years when primary dentition is completed. During these visits the dentist can begin to develop a relationship with the child, assess oral health, teach parents correct methods of dental hygiene, and provide nutritional counseling, especially in relation to preventing nursing bottle caries.

Initial visits to the dentist should be nontraumatizing. Since toddlers react negatively to new and potentially frightening experiences, the initial visit can center around meeting the dentist, seeing the equipment, and sitting in the chair. If the child is cooperative, the dentist may just look at the teeth but reserve a more thorough examination for another visit. Modeling can also be effective—the child can observe procedures performed on the parent or a cooperative sibling. This type of conditioning is very important in preparing the child for future experiences.*

Removal of Plaque

The objective of oral hygiene is removal of *plaque,* soft bacterial deposits that adhere to the teeth and cause dental caries (decay) and periodontal (gum) disease. The most effective methods for plaque removal are brushing and flossing. Several brushing techniques exist although there is no universal agreement regarding the best method. One that is suitable for cleaning the primary teeth is the *scrub* method. The tips of the bristles are placed firmly at a 45-degree angle against the teeth and gums and moved back and forth in a vibratory motion. The ends of the bristles should be wiggling but not moving forcefully back and forth, which can damage the gums and enamel. All the surfaces of the teeth are cleaned in this manner except the lingual (inner) surfaces of the anterior teeth. To clean these surfaces, the toothbrush is placed vertical to the teeth and moved up and down. Only a few teeth are brushed at one time, using six to eight strokes for each section. A systematic approach is used so that all surfaces are thoroughly cleaned.

For young children the most effective cleaning is done by parents. Several positions can be used that facilitate access to the mouth and help stabilize the head for comfort, such as sitting on a couch or bed with the child's head in the parent's lap or sitting on a floor or stool with the child's head straddled by the parent's thighs (Fig. 14-8). The latter position is advantageous because the child can be kept

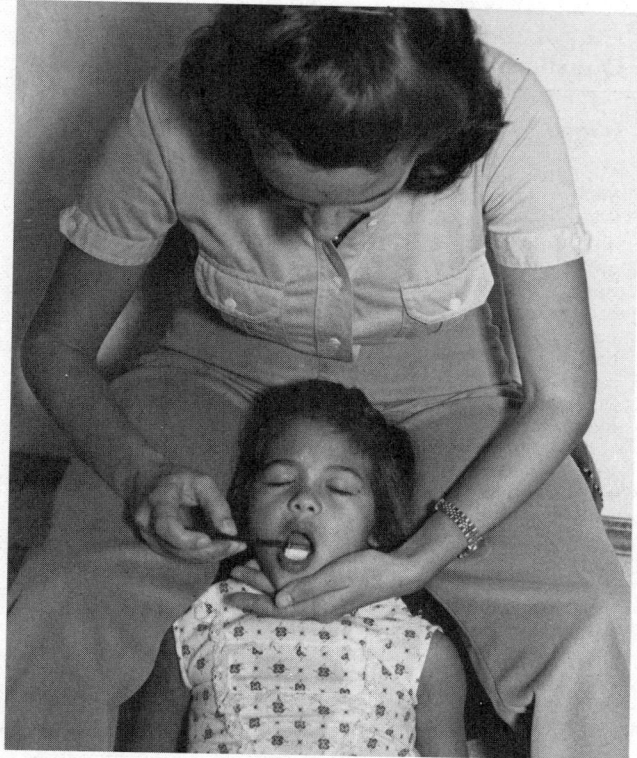

Fig. 14-8. Position that facilitates parent's brushing of child's teeth.

amused watching television during the brushing, provided there is a receptacle for the child to spit out toothpaste. For easier access to back teeth the mouth is held partially open; fully opening the mouth causes the masseter muscle to contract, narrowing the space near the back molars.

For effective cleaning, a small toothbrush with soft, rounded, multitufted nylon bristles that are short and uniform in length is recommended. Nylon bristles dry more rapidly after use and retain their shape better than natural bristles. Children should have at least two toothbrushes, which are used alternately to allow them to dry thoroughly. Wet bristles are less resilient and consequently less effective in removing plaque. Toothbrushes are replaced as soon as the bristles are frayed or bent. With young children brushing may be more easily accomplished using only water, since many children dislike the foam from toothpaste and the foam interferes with visibilty. There is also the danger of swallowing fluoridated toothpaste (see following discussion under Fluoride). When using toothpaste, children should select the flavor they like to encourage the brushing habit.

After the teeth have been cleaned, flossing with dental floss is done to remove plaque and debris from between the teeth and below the gum margin where brushing is ineffective. Since young children do not have the dexterity to manipulate the floss, parents are taught the procedure. A length of dental floss about 45 cm (18 inches) can either be tied in a circle or wrapped around the fingers. The circle method may be easier for children to learn. With about 2.5 cm (1 inch) of floss held tautly against the thumbs, the floss is

*A book to help parents prepare the child is *When your child goes to the dentist,* by Fred Rogers, Family Communications, 4802 Fifth Avenue, Pittsburgh, PA 15213.

Questions and Controversies

Is mass fluoridation harmful?

Among the arguments against mass fluoridation the following have generated the most public concern: increased incidence of cancer, Down syndrome, and allergies among those living in fluoridated areas (Margolis and Cohen, 1985). However, none of these claims has been substantiated. Researchers have found that the rate of cancer is no greater in fluoridated areas than in comparable locations without fluoridation (Hoover, McKay, and Fraumeni, 1976). The same conclusion was reached regarding Down syndrome (Needleman, Pueschel, and Rothman, 1974). The American Academy of Allergy's statement (1971) on allergy and fluoride concludes that there is no evidence to support this association.

The one well-known effect of excessive fluoride ingestion is fluorosis, which can cause staining (chalky white to yellow or brown) of the teeth and in more severe forms, loss and decreased resistance of the enamel to decay. Very mild fluorosis is not a public health hazard, nor a major cosmetic concern for affected children. Moderate and severe fluorosis is directly related to the fluoride dosage and occurs predominately in areas with high levels of natural fluoridation, not in areas of artificial fluoridation where optimal fluoride levels are provided. Ingesting excessive fluoride after age 5 or 6 years does not result in fluorosis because of complete calcification of the permanent teeth, except the third-year molars. Like any drug, acute toxicity can occur from ingestion of large quantities of the mineral. A lethal dose for children is estimated to be 32 to 64 mg/kg (Heifetz and Horowitz, 1986). However, this is not a contraindication to its use. The same precautions must be practiced as with any drug—store out of reach of children and avoid large supplies of the drug in the home (Hess and others, 1984).

gently inserted between two teeth and wrapped around the base of the tooth in a C shape and is directed *below* the gingival margin to remove plaque. The floss is then moved toward the occlusal (biting) surface of the tooth to remove plaque between the teeth as well. This sweeping motion is repeated a few times on every tooth surface, using a clean segment of floss.

A disclosing agent is helpful in identifying those areas of the teeth where plaque accumulates. It also helps motivate children to clean their teeth because plaque is difficult to see. After cleaning, the mouth is inspected to ensure that all traces of plaque have been removed.

Ideally the teeth should be cleaned after each meal and especially before bedtime and the child given nothing to eat or drink after the night brushing except water. At those times when brushing is impractical, the ''swish-and-swallow'' method of cleaning the mouth is taught: with a mouthful of water the child rinses the mouth and swallows, repeating the procedure three or four times.

Fluoride

Several studies have documented the effectiveness of fluoride in reducing the incidence of tooth decay. Children who drink water containing 1 part per million (ppm) fluoride when their teeth are forming may have a 50% to 70% decrease in caries (Horowitz, 1981). When adequate amounts of fluoride are ingested before eruption of the teeth and to a lesser extent after tooth eruption, the enamel is more resistant to caries. Fluoride replaces the hydroxyl ion in the calcium hydroxyapatite molecule to form calcium fluorapatite, which alters the crystal of the tooth, making it more resistant to acid solubility. The changes in crystalline structure also affect the anatomy of the tooth—the cusps are shorter and the crevices smaller—thus facilitating plaque removal (Kula and Tinanoff, 1982).

Despite the proven benefits of fluoride, only about half of the population in the United States have naturally or artificially fluoridated water (Crall, 1985). Numerous controversies exist regarding the proposed dangers of mass fluoridation and antifluoridationists have been successful in preventing communities from instituting this public health benefit (see Questions and controversies).

In communities where the water supply is not fluoridated, oral fluoride supplements are recommended (Table 14-7). Nurses have a responsibility to ensure an optimal fluoride regimen for children and to counsel families regarding correct use of supplements (see box on p. 615). One advantage of supplements is that the child receives a known quantity of fluoride daily. This is in contrast to fluoridated water, where the supply depends on the amount of water consumed and where parents need to be encouraged to use water to prepare drinks and foods. A major disadvantage of supplementation is compliance and cost. The supplements are considerably more expensive than community fluoridation and adhering to a daily administration schedule for 16 years is difficult for many families.

Another consideration is the brand of toothpaste. A fluoride dentifrice reduces caries even further when the water supply is fluoridated. However, a concern with fluoride toothpaste is excess ingestion by young children and the possibility of fluorosis, a condition characterized by an increase in the degree and extent of the enamel's porosity. As

Table 14-7 Supplemental fluoride dosage schedule (mg/day*)

AGE	CONCENTRATION OF FLUORIDE IN DRINKING WATER (PPM)		
	<0.3	0.3-0.7	>0.7
2 weeks-2 years	0.25	0	0
2-3 years	0.50	0.25	0
3-16 years	1.00	0.50	0

From American Academy of Pediatrics, Committee on Nutrition: Fluoride supplementation, Pediatrics **77**(5):758-761,1986.
*2.2 mg sodium fluoride contains 1 mg fluoride.

GUIDELINES FOR AN OPTIMUM FLUORIDE REGIMEN

Base recommendations on the fluoride content of the drinking water, including well water, with the exception of amounts for breast-feeding infants, who should receive fluoride supplements regardless of fluoride content of the water supply.

If the water is fluoridated, encourage consumption of tap water either through supplemental feedings to infants or through preparation of frozen-concentrated juice, powdered drinks, soup, gelatin or other foods made with fluoridated water.

If impractical and the child ordinarily drinks little tap water, consider a fluoride supplement.

In areas with excessive fluoride levels, suggest the use of bottled unfluoridated water.

Encourage parents to supervise the young child's toothbrushing, to use a minute amount of fluoridated toothpaste or to substitute a nonfluoridated brand, and to teach children not to eat toothpaste.

If the water is unfluoridated, instruct in proper administration of supplements:

Place drops directly on the tongue to allow it to mix with saliva and come in contact with the teeth.

Encourage older children to chew the tablet and swish it in the mouth for 30 seconds before swallowing.

Give nothing to eat or drink afterward for 30 minutes.

Administer supplements on an empty stomach without calcium-rich products, such as milk.

Recommend the daily use of a fluoridated mouthrinse in children 4 years and older and instruct in proper technique:

Use only the recommended amount.

Expectorate after a timed 1-minute rinse.

Avoid food or fluid for 30 minutes afterward.

Advise parents to store fluoridated dentifrice, mouthrinse, and supplements in a safe place away from small children and to keep no more than a 4-month supply of supplements in the home.

Encourage compliance by administering the supplement at same time each day and posting reminders, such as fluoride sticker on bathroom mirror.

Modified from Hess, C., and others: Fluoride: too much or too little, Pediatr. Nurs. **10**(6):397-403, 1984.

---

a safeguard the child's use of toothpaste should be supervised to prevent swallowing of excessive amounts. Fluoride rinses, which also offer topical benefits, are not recommended for children under 5 years of age because of their likelihood of swallowing the liquid.

Low-Cariogenic Diet

Diet is critical to developing good teeth because the carious process depends primarily on fermentable sugars, especially sucrose. Refined table sugar is not the only concentrated sweet food that is cariogenic. Natural foods, including honey, molasses, corn syrup, and dried fruits such as raisins, are highly cariogenic.

Ideally such foods should be eliminated. However, since this is impractical, some suggestions can be helpful. The first is that *the frequency with which sugar is consumed is more important than the total amount eaten.* Therefore when sweets are eaten, they are less damaging if consumed immediately after a meal rather than as a snack between meals. When sweets are served as the dessert, the teeth can be cleaned afterward, decreasing the amount of time the sugar is in the mouth.

The form of sugar is also important. The more cariogenic foods are those that are sticky or hard, since they remain in the mouth longer. Consequently sucking on lollipops or chewing gum is more cariogenic than eating a chocolate bar.

These suggestions can help parents plan "treats" in a way that is less damaging to the teeth. In addition, parents should be aware of foods that are good snacks without con-

Table 14-8 Low-cariogenic snack foods

BASIC FOOD GROUP	GOOD SNACKS EATEN ALONE	SNACKS BETTER SERVED WITH MEALS
Bread and cereal	Popcorn and other seeds	Bread and cereals, crackers, pretzels, all sweet baked goods
Fruit and vegetable	All raw, fresh, frozen or waterpack fruit or vegetables or their juices prepared without addition of sugars*	All items prepared or used with the addition of sugars,* dried fruits such as raisins, catsup, gelatin†
Meat	Meat of all kinds including luncheon meats, leftovers and smoked meat; nuts of all kinds; peanut butter*; bean dips*	Meats prepared with sugars,* candy-coated nuts
Dairy	Milk—whole, low-fat, skim, or buttermilk; all cheeses including cottage; plain yogurt; dips and spreads*; flavored drinks*; hard-boiled eggs	Chocolate milk, malts, shakes, cocoa, ice cream, ice milk, sherbet, other dairy desserts, flavored yogurt

Adapted from Madsen, K.O.: Advances in dietary counseling for the prevention of dental caries. In Wei, S.H.: National symposium on dental nutrition, Iowa City, 1978, University of Iowa.
*Check labels for added sugars. Look for (cane, maple, brown) sugar (sucrose), molasses, invert sugar, honey, dextrose (glucose), (modified) corn (sugar, syrup, sweetener, solids), lactose, levulose (fructose), and carob.
†A low-sugar gelatin can be made with unsweetened fruit juice and unflavored gelatin.

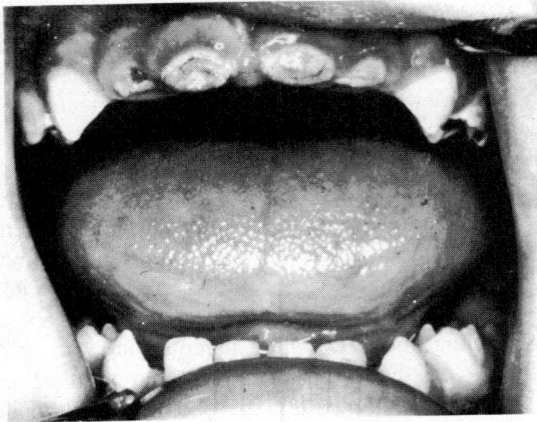

Fig. 14-9. Nursing bottle caries. Note the extensive carious involvement of maxillary primary incisors.

From McDonald, R., and Avery D.: Dentistry for the child and adolescent, ed. 4, St. Louis, 1983, The C.V. Mosby Co.

Table 14-9 Sucrose content of selected cereals

CEREAL (1-OUNCE SERVING)	SUCROSE (GRAMS/ 1-OUNCE SERVING)
Shredded Wheat	0
Cheerios	1
Cornflakes	2
Total	3
Rice Krispies	3
Quaker 100% Natural Cereal	6
Raisin Bran	9*
Honey Nut Cheerios	10
Frosted Flakes	11
Frosted Rice	11
Fruit Loops	13
Apple Jacks	14

*4 g occur naturally in raisins.

tributing to tooth decay (Table 14-8). Substitutes for cariogenic sweets can also include sugarless gum and candy. Likewise, parents should know about hidden sources of sugar, contained in many popular cereals, including the "all-natural" variety (Table 14-9). Reading food labels is essential in eliminating sources of sucrose.

A special form of tooth decay in children between 18 months and 3 years of age is *nursing bottle caries* (also called *bottle-mouth caries*), which occurs when the child is routinely given a bottle of milk or juice at nap or bedtime. Frequent nocturnal breast-feeding for prolonged periods also leads to extensive destruction of the teeth (Brahms and Maloney, 1983). The practice of coating pacifiers in honey can also contribute to caries and may be a potential source of botulism poisoning. As the sweet liquid pools in the mouth, the teeth are bathed for several hours in this cariogenic environment. The maxillary (upper) incisors and molars are affected most, since the mandibular (lower) incisors are thought to be protected by the lower lip and tongue (Fig. 14-9). Severely decayed teeth may require the application of stainless steel bands to preserve the spacing until the permanent teeth erupt.

Prevention involves eliminating the bedtime bottle completely, feeding the last bottle before bedtime, substituting a bottle of water for milk or juice, and never coating pacifiers in sweet substances. Juice in bottles, especially commercially available ready-to-use bottles, should be discouraged, since the beverage is especially damaging because the sugar is more readily converted to acid. Juice should always be offered in a cup in order to avoid prolonging the bottle-feeding habit.

Nurses are in an excellent position to counsel parents regarding this habit, especially if it occurs during a hospitalization. Although the child may need the comfort of the bottle at this stressful time, parents can be shown photographs depicting the typical tooth destruction and given literature about the condition.* Over an extended hospital stay children can be gradually weaned from the bedtime bottle or given a bottle of water. It is hoped that health professionals never contribute to the habit by propping bottles for convenience during feedings.

INJURY PREVENTION

Injuries cause more deaths in children 1 to 4 years than in any other childhood period except adolescence. In addition, the injury death rate has remained relatively unchanged during the past decade, whereas the corresponding rates from all other causes of death combined have declined significantly. Injury's prominence as the leading cause of death among toddlers and preschoolers underscores the need to emphasize safety awareness among parents. Child protection and parent education are key determinants in injury prevention.

A major factor in the critical increase of injuries during early childhood is the unrestricted freedom achieved through locomotion combined with an unawareness of danger within the environment. Specific categories of injuries and appropriate prevention are best understood by associating them with the major developmental achievements of young children (Table 14-10). The discussion of injuries in Chapters 1 and 12 are also relevant to safety concerns at this age.

*Sources of information about nursing bottle caries and other aspects of child dental health include: National Institute of Dental Research, Westwood Building, 5333 Westbard Ave., Bethesda, MD 20205; American Society of Dentistry for Children, 211 E. Chicago Ave., Suite 920, Chicago, IL 60611; and American Dental Association, 211 E. Chicago Ave., Chicago, IL 60611. Guidelines for children's dental care are available in Wong, D., and Whaley, L.: Clinical handbook of pediatric nursing, ed. 2, St. Louis, 1986, The C.V. Mosby Co.

Table 14-10 Injury prevention during early childhood

MAJOR DEVELOPMENTAL ACCOMPLISHMENTS	INJURY PREVENTION
Walks, runs, and climbs Able to open doors and gates Can ride tricycle Can throw ball and other objects	**Motor vehicles** Use federally-approved car restraint; if restraint is not available, use lap belt Supervise children while playing outside Do not allow to play on curb or behind a parked car Do not permit to play in pile of leaves, snow, or large cardboard container in trafficked area Supervise tricycle riding Lock fences and doors if not directly supervising children Teach children to obey pedestrian safety rules 　Obey traffic regulations; cross only at crosswalks and only when the traffic signal indicates it is safe to cross 　Stand back a step from the curb until it is time to cross 　Look left, right, and left again and check for turning cars before crossing the street 　Use sidewalks; when there is no sidewalk, walk on the left, facing the traffic 　Wear light colors at night, and attach fluorescent material to clothing
Able to explore if left unsupervised Has great curiosity Helpless in water; unaware of its danger; depth of water has no significance	**Drowning** Supervise closely when near *any* source of water Keep bathroom doors closed Have fence around swimming pool and lock gate Teach swimming and water safety
Able to reach heights by climbing, stretching, and standing on toes Pulls objects Explores any holes or opening Can open drawers and closets Unaware of potential sources of heat or fire Plays with mechanical objects	**Burns** Turn pot handles toward back of stove Place guard rails in front of radiators, fireplaces, or other heating elements Store matches and cigarette lighters in locked or inaccessible area Place burning candles, incense, hot foods, and cigarettes out of reach Do not let tablecloth hang within child's reach Do not let electric cord from iron or other appliance hang within child's reach Cover electrical outlets with protective plastic caps Keep electrical wires hidden or out of reach Do not allow child to play with electrical appliance Stress danger of open flames; teach what "hot" means Always check bathwater; adjust hot-water temperature to 52° C (125° F) or lower; do not allow to play with faucets
Explores by putting objects in mouth Can open drawers, closets, and most containers Climbs	**Poisoning** Place all potentially toxic agents out of reach or in a locked cabinet Caution against eating nonedible items, such as plants Replace medications and poisons immediately; replace child-protector caps properly
Cannot read labels	Administer medications as a drug, not as a candy Do not store large surplus of toxic agents Promptly discard empty poison containers; never reuse to store a food item or other poison Never remove labels from containers of toxic substances Have syrup of ipecac in home; use only if advised Know number and location of nearest poison control center (usually listed in front of telephone directory)
Able to open doors and some windows Goes up and down stairs Depth perception unrefined	**Falls** Keep screen in window, nail securely, and use guard rail Place gates at top and bottom of stairs Keep doors locked when there is danger of falls (stairwells, porches) Keep crib rails fully raised and mattress at lowest level Place carpeting under crib and in bathroom Keep child restrained in vehicles; never leave unattended in shopping cart Supervise at playgrounds; select safe play areas with soft ground cover Check child's shoes and trousers

Continued.

Table 14-10 Injury prevention during early childhood—cont'd	

MAJOR DEVELOPMENTAL ACCOMPLISHMENTS	INJURY PREVENTION
Puts things in mouth May swallow hard or nonedible pieces of food	***Choking and suffocation*** Avoid large chunks of meat, such as whole hot dogs Avoid fruit with pits, fish with bones, dried beans, hard candy, chewing gum, and nuts Choose large sturdy toys without sharp edges or small removable parts Discard old refrigerators, ovens, and so on If storing an old appliance, remove the doors Keep automatic garage door transmitter in inaccessible place Select safe toy boxes or chests without heavy, hinged lids
Still clumsy in many skills	***Bodily damage*** Avoid giving sharp or pointed objects—such as knives, scissors, or toothpicks—especially when walking or running Do not allow lollipops or similar objects in mouth when walking or running Teach safety precautions, for example, to carry knife or scissors with pointed end away from face Store all dangerous tools, garden equipment, and firearms in locked cabinet Be alert to danger of unsupervised animals and household pets Have identification on child, such as plastic "shoe pocket" attached to shoelaces Use safety glass and decals on large glassed areas, especially sliding glass doors

Motor Vehicle Injuries

Motor vehicle injuries cause more accidental deaths in all pediatric age-groups after age 1 year than any other type of injury or disease and are responsible for almost one half of all accidental deaths among children ages 1 to 4 years. Many of the deaths are caused by injuries within the car when restraints have not been used or have been used improperly. Approved restraints properly installed and applied can reduce fatalities by 90% and injuries by 69% (Shurtz, 1981).

Nurses have a responsibility for educating parents regarding the importance of car restraints and their proper use. Three basic types of federally-approved restraints are available: (1) infant-only device, (2) convertible models for both infants and toddlers, and (3) toddler-only restraints. Since the infant-type restraints are discussed in Chapter 12, the other types are included here.

Toddler restraints are designed for children who can sit by themselves and are over 7.7 to 9 kg (17 to 20 pounds). Both convertible models and toddler-only models are available. The convertible type is suitable for infants in the rearward facing position and for toddlers in the forward-facing position (Fig. 14-10). Toddler-only models provide protection only in the forward-facing position and may consist of a shell or a raised booster seat. The shell restraints consist of a molded hard plastic or metal frame with energy-absorbing padding and a special harness system designed to maximize pressure over the pelvic bones rather than the more vulnerable abdomen. Booster seats are made of similar material but lack the side protection afforded by the shell (Fig. 14-11). The restraint is held in place by the car lap-belt. The shoulder strap on the seat-belt system is either placed behind the restraint or with the lap belt but never in front of the child's face or neck, which can cause strangulation in the event of a crash. Cars with inertia-type seat belts that move except on impact require the use of a metal locking clip to keep the belt in a tight-holding position. The locking clip is threaded onto the belt above the metal insert piece (Marcus, 1981).

Some older model restraints require the use of a top anchor (tether) strap to prevent the child from pitching forward in a crash. If the tether strap is not used, up to 90% of the restraint's protection is lost. Instructions for proper installation of the tether strap and permanent bracket are included with the car restraint. If parents object to drilling holes in the car to install the bracket, they should select a model without this feature. Car restraints that do not require a top anchor strap have the lap-belt placement arched midway through the back of the car seat to hold the restraint against the back of the vehicle seat.

Children should use their restraints until they have outgrown them. The "rule of fours" serves as a guide: if the child either weighs about 40 pounds (18 kg), is 40 inches (100 cm) tall, or is 4 years old, then the restraint can be replaced by a lap belt. Children who outgrow the toddler shell seat may still be able to ride safely in a booster seat. If the car's restraint system is used, only the lap belt is applied until the child is 55 inches (123 cm) tall. Once the

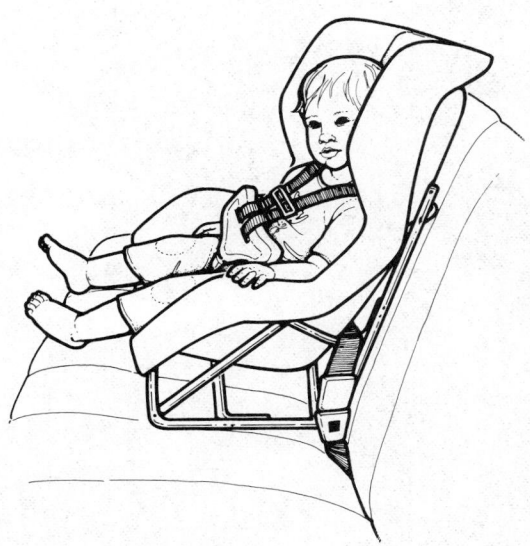

Fig. 14-10. Convertible seat in foward-facing position for older infants and children.

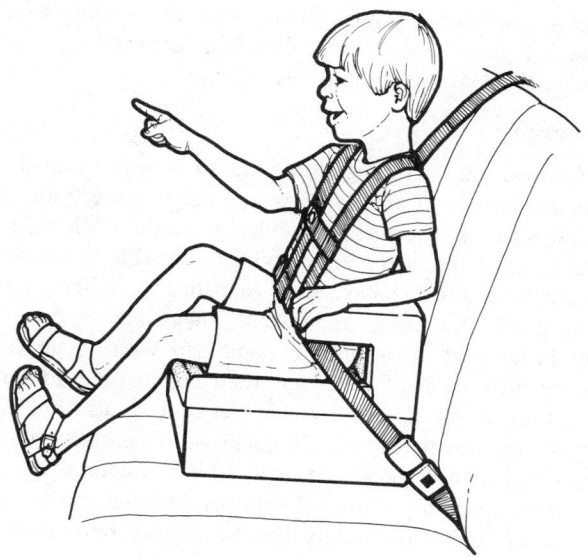

Fig. 14-11. Automobile booster seat. Model uses harness attached to auto seat belt; harness held in place by tether strap.

child is over 55 inches, the seat belt/shoulder harness system is used (Policastro, 1979). Regardless of the child's age, the lap belt provides more protection than no restraint. The safest area of the car for children is the middle of the back seat.

When purchasing a restraint, parents should consider cost and convenience. The convertible-type seats are more expensive initially but cost less than two separate systems. Convenience is a major factor because a cumbersome restraint may be used less and improperly. Before buying a restraint, it is best to try out different models. For example, some types are too large for subcompact cars. Asking neighbors about the advantages and disadvantages of their restraints is helpful. Some service clubs and hospitals have loan programs for restraints. Information about approved models and other aspects of car restraints is available from several organizations and sources.*

For any restraint to be effective it must be used consistently and properly. Reasons for decreased compliance during the toddler years include: removal of straps by the child; inability to attach straps over heavy winter clothing; and child's crying, fussing, and boredom (Arneson and others, 1985). To ensure compliance, these concerns must be addressed and certain "rules of riding" should be practiced:

1. Do not start the car until *everyone* is properly restrained.
2. *Always* use the restraint, even for short trips.
3. If the child begins to climb out or undo the harness, firmly

say, "No." It may be necessary to stop the car to reinforce the expected behavior. The use of rewards, such as stars, for cooperative behavior is very effective.
4. Encourage the child to help attach buckles and straps.
5. Decrease boredom on long trips. Keep special toys in the car for quiet play; talk to the child; point out objects and teach the child about them. Stop periodically. If the child wishes to sleep, make sure he stays in the restraint.

Children riding in car seats are generally much better behaved than children left unrestrained, which can be a major benefit to parents and should be stressed as an additional advantage of safety restraints (Christophersen, 1977).

Children over 3 years of age are often involved in pedestrian traffic injuries, with the majority occurring between noon and 6 PM (Guyer, Talbot, and Pless, 1985). Because of their gross motor skills of walking, running, and climbing and their fine motor skills of opening doors and fence gates, they are able to leave most restricted areas when unsupervised. Unaware of danger and unable to approximate the speed of a car, they are hit by moving vehicles. Running after a ball, playing in a pile of leaves or snow or inside a cardboard box, riding a tricycle, and playing behind a parked car or near the curb are common activities that may result in a vehicular tragedy. A precaution when children are playing in driveways is attaching to the tricycle a pole with a bright flag that is high enough to be visible through an automobile's back window.

Preventing vehicular injuries involves protecting and educating children about the danger from moving or parked vehicles. Although preschool children are too young to be trusted to always obey, emphasis on looking for moving vehicles before crossing the street, recognizing the color of traffic lights for stop and go, and following traffic officers'

---

*Physicians for Automotive Safety, 50 Union Ave., Irvington, NJ 07111; American Academy of Pediatrics, Division of Health Education, 141 Northwest point Rd., Elk Grove, IL 60007; and National Child Passenger Safety Association, P.O. Box 841, Ardmore, PA 19003. Guidelines for car seat safety are available in Wong, D., and Whaley, L.: Clinical handbook of pediatric nursing, ed. 2, St. Louis, 1986, The C.V. Mosby Co.

signals emphasizes a good habit. Most importantly what is preached must be practiced. Children learn through imitation, and consistency reinforces learning.

Drowning

Drowning, not including drowning from water transportation, ranks second among boys and third among girls ages 1 to 4 years as a cause of accidental death. With well-developed skills of locomotion, toddlers are able to reach potentially dangerous areas, such as bathtubs, toilets, swimming pools, hot tubs, and lakes. Their intense drive for exploration and investigation, combined with an unawareness of the danger of water and their helplessness in water, makes drowning always a viable threat. It is also one category of injuries that results in death within minutes, diminishing the chance for rescue and survival. Supervising children when near any source of water is essential and teaching swimming and water safety can be helpful but cannot be regarded as sufficient protection.

Burns

Burns rank second to motor vehicle injuries among girls and third among boys in this age-group as a cause of accidental death. A major contributing factor to the sex difference is that girls tend to play indoors and imitate sex-related functions, such as cooking at the stove. Their ability to climb, stretch, and reach objects above their head makes any hot surface a potential source of danger. Scalds from pulling pots on top of themselves are a major source of burns. As a precaution, pot handles should be turned toward the back of the stove. Ideally the knobs for controlling the range burners should be out of reach, not on the front panel where nimble fingers can turn them on and accidentally touch the hot burner. Oven doors should be closed whenever the oven is turned on or when it is cooling. The outside of doors of automatic self-cleaning ovens may become hot and, if touched, could cause a burn. Other sources of heat, such as radiators, fireplaces, accessible furnaces, kerosene heaters, or wood-burning stoves, should have guards placed in front of them. The tops of some of these heaters are designed to become hot enough to boil water to provide humidity. They are hazardous if touched or if the pan of water is spilled (Rissmiller, 1983). Portable electric heaters must be placed in a high area, well out of reach of climbing young children.

Hot objects such as candles, incense, cigarettes, pots of tea or coffee, or irons must be placed away from children. The flame of a candle and the smoke of a cigarette invite investigation. Ashtrays with a center well are preferred to prevent the cigarette from falling off the rim and adults should try not to smoke, cook, or drink hot liquids when children are physically close. If tablecloths are used, the edges should be placed out of reach to prevent injuries from both burns and falling objects.

Flame burns represent one of the most fatal types of burns and commonly occur when children play with matches and accidentally set themselves (and the home) on

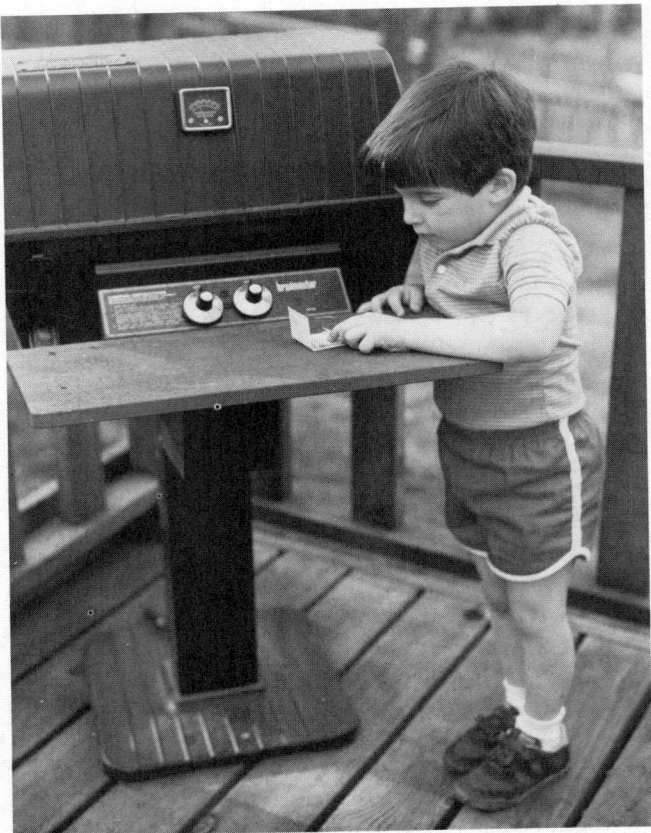

Fig. 14-12. Matches are potentially deadly hazard for young children.

fire (Fig. 14-12). All matches must be stored safely away from children and parents need to teach children the dangers of playing with matches. In addition, all homes should have smoke detectors, installed to alert the occupants to fire, and a safety plan for immediate escape.

Electrical burns also represent an immediate danger to children. With preschoolers' ability to manipulate small, thin objects, they are able to insert hairpins or other conductive articles into electrical sockets. Young toddlers may explore outlets and wires by mouthing them. Since water is an excellent conductor, the chance for a severe circumoral electrical burn is great. Electrical outlets should have protective guards plugged into them when not in use or made inaccessible by placing furniture in front of them when feasible. Children should not be allowed to play with electrical cords or appliances, which should be kept out of reach as much as possible.

An example of an appliance that interests children and can present a hazard is an electric popcorn popper. Children can become so excited by the popping that they may inadvertently pull the electric cord and popper off the table, resulting in a burn from contact with the hot oil, corn, or appliance.

Scald burns are the most common type of thermal injury

in children. Among young children a significant type of scalding burn is caused by high-temperature tap water, which children come in contact with either as a result of turning on the hot-water faucet, falling into a bathtub of hot water, or deliberate abuse. Besides the obvious prevention of always supervising youngsters when they are near tap water and checking bathwater temperatures, a recommended passive prevention is to limit household water temperatures to less than 52° C (125° F). At this temperature it takes 2 minutes for exposure to the water to cause a full-thickness burn. Setting the temperature only 3° C lower than 52° C raises the time necessary for a third-degree burn to 10 minutes. Conversely water temperatures of 54° C (130° F), the usual setting of most water heaters, expose household members to the risk of full-thickness burns within 30 seconds (Feldman and others, 1978). Nurses can help prevent such burns by advising parents of this common household danger and recommending that they readjust the water heater to a safe temperature of between 49° and 52° C (120° to 125° F). A meat or candy thermometer is a convenient way to measure water temperature. A special "Frog Prince" thermometer, which changes color to show water temperature, is also available at nominal cost.*

Poisoning

Ingestion of toxic agents is extremely common during early childhood. The highest incidence occurs in children in the 2-year-old group. Although in many instances poisoning does not result in mortality, it may cause significant morbidity, such as esophageal stricture from lye ingestion. Although mouthing activity decreases after 1 year of age, exploring objects by tasting them is part of children's curious investigation. Young children's taste is not refined and discriminating. Children under 6 years of age are more likely to eat "disgusting" substances (Rozin and others, 1985). While young children may be able to identify some items as poisonous, they do not understand the toxic effects of ingesting excessive amounts of a familiar drug, such as vitamins. In addition, the apparent safety of such drugs is reinforced by their daily administration (Osborne and Garrettson, 1985). Almost every nonfood substance is potentially harmful, including many house plants, and by 2 years of age toddlers are able to climb most heights, open most drawers or closets, and unscrew most lids. By trial and error younger children also manage to undo tops of bottles, plastic containers, aerosol cans, and jars.

However, they are most likely to ingest substances that are on their level, such as plants, cleaning agents stored under sinks, rat poison, or diaper pail deodorizers. Childguard tops are required on some substances, such as prescription drugs, but many young children have outwitted such "safe" caps. In addition, pharmacists often transfer drugs to regular containers for the elderly, who may have difficulty with child-guard closures. Therefore such drugs

*Clinitemp, Inc., PO Box 40273, Indianapolis, IN 46240.

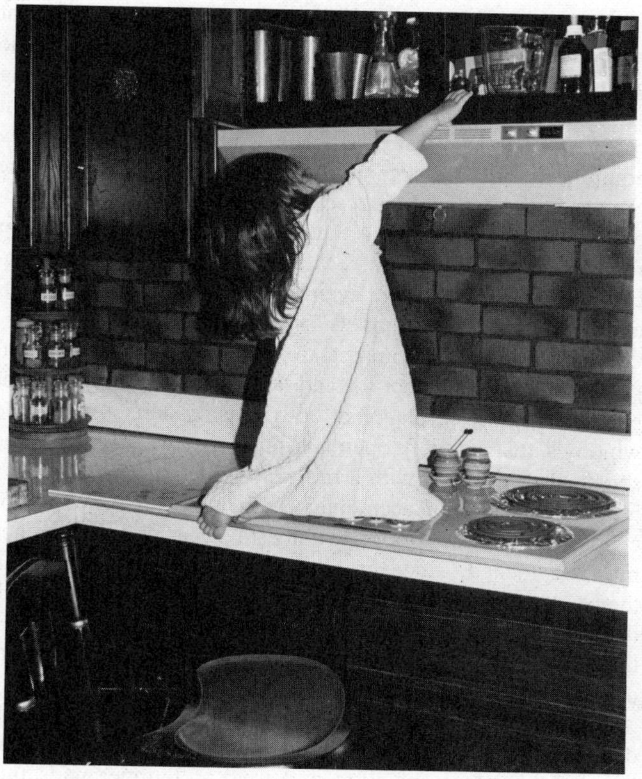

Fig. 14-13. No unlocked cabinet can be considered safe with young children. This 3-year-old child used her high chair to climb onto the counter to open high storage area. Note additional danger of stepping on stove, where accidental burns can occur.

can be hazardous if accessible to young children. Many potentially toxic substances are not protected with safety caps and must be stored properly. Even common household items, such as mouthwash that contains ethanol (alcohol), can be toxic to young children (Weller-Fahy, Berger, and Troutman, 1980).

The major reason for poisoning is improper storage. The guidelines suggested in Chapter 12 are applicable to children in this age-group as well. However, unlike the infant who was confined to certain heights and unable to unlatch inventive locks, preschoolers manage to find access to many high-level, tight-security places. Sometimes it is necessary to test a lock or high shelf by challenging the child to undo or reach it to prevent tragedies later on (Fig. 14-13).

Parents should have two doses of ipecac syrup for each child in the home, know its proper use and administration, and have the phone number and location of the nearest poison control center. Emergency and preventive measures for accidental poisoning are discussed in Chapter 16.

Falls

Falls are still a hazard to children in this age-group, although by the later part of early childhood gross and fine motor skills are well developed, decreasing the incidence of falls down stairs or from chairs. However, playground injuries become common. Children need to be taught safety at play areas, such as no horseplay on high slides or jungle gyms, *sitting* on swings, and staying away from moving swings. Passive prevention includes the use of a resilient surface, such as grass, sand, or wood chips, under play equipment. If loose organic material is used, it will require replacement as it pulverizes. Swing seats made of plastic, canvas, or rubber, rather than wood and with smooth or rounded edges are safest. Slides should not exceed an incline of 30 degrees, have evenly spaced rungs for climbing, and have protective "tunnels" (McAtee, 1982).

The climbing and running of the typical toddler is complicated by total neglect for and lack of appreciation of danger. Gates must be placed at both ends of stairs. Accessible windows that are left open during warm weather must be screened or guarded with a rail. Falling from open windows is a major cause of accidental death in urban lower socioeconomic groups. Doors leading to stairwells or porches must be locked, since preschool children can easily open them. A convenient type of lock is a sliding bar or hook that can be attached to the door and frame at a level higher than the child can reach, provided that inventive youngsters do not pull a chair over to unlatch the hook or bar.

Another source of falls is from cribs and vehicles. In addition to crib rails being fully raised, the mattress should be kept at the lowest position and toys or bumper pads that may be used as steps to climb out should be removed. Ideally the floor should be carpeted. Once the child reaches a height of 89 cm (35 inches), he should sleep in a bed rather than a crib.

To prevent falls from vehicles, children must always be properly restrained. They should never ride in the open back of a truck; the danger of falls can be compounded by another vehicle striking the child. An unrecognized hazard is grocery shopping carts. Children left unattended can easily fall out.

Clothing can also increase the chance of falling. Slippery shoes or socks, rubber-soled shoes that "catch" on the floor and rug, and loose or cuffed pants can easily make a child fall. Simple safety measures, such as checking clothing and shoes, keeping shoelaces tied with double knots, or using Velcro closures, can prevent such needless injuries.

Aspiration and Suffocation

Usually by 1 year of age children chew well, but they may have difficulty with large pieces of food such as meat or whole hot dogs and with hard foods such as nuts or dried beans. Young children cannot discard pits from fruit or bones from fish like older children. It takes practice to learn how to chew gum without swallowing it. Therefore the same precautions as discussed for infants regarding food selection must be implemented. Play objects for toddlers must still be chosen with an awareness of the danger of small parts. Large, sturdy toys without sharp edges or removable parts are safest. Coins, paper clips, pull-tabs on cans, thumbtacks, nails, screws, jewelry, and all types of pins are common household objects that can cause significant harm

if swallowed. Because of the danger of aspiration, parents should be taught emergency procedures for choking (p. 1331).

Another cause of death by traumatic asphyxiation is from electrically operated garage doors (Satran, 1981). Young children playing in the garage may become trapped under the door. Although the automatic doors should reverse when striking an object, they may not do so when hitting a flexible object or one that is very close to the ground. Precautions include placing controls where they are inaccessible to children, such as high on a wall and in a locked car, and instructing children that the transmitter is not a toy. Periodically the door should be checked to be certain it returns when striking an object.

Suffocation is less frequent from causes seen during infancy but is an ever-present threat from old refrigerators, ovens, and other large appliances. Toddlers can climb inside these appliances and if they close the door behind them will be trapped inside. Discarding old appliances and removing all doors during storage prevent such tragic injuries.

Bodily Damage

Toddlers are still clumsy in many of their skills and can seriously harm themselves when walking while holding a sharp or pointed object or having food or objects such as spoons in their mouths. Preventing such occurrences is the best approach with toddlers. With preschoolers teaching safety is most important. The child should be taught that when walking with a pointed object such as a knife or scissors, the pointed end is held away from the face. Dangerous garden or workshop equipment and all firearms should be stored in a locked cabinet. Power lawn mowers are especially dangerous and young children should not be allowed in an area where a mower is being used; nor should they be taken for a ride on a mower. Safety education should include respect for firearms and their proper and appropriate use. In addition, the child should be warned of and protected against potential danger from animals, including household pets, such as dogs and cats. Child education regarding safety from animals includes: avoiding all strange animals, not disturbing animals who are sleeping or eating, and not overexciting or teasing an animal.

Toys can be a source of danger, and safety must be a prime consideration when selecting toys (see Guidelines for toy safety, p. 137). Most toys have age ranges written on them to designate their safety, but this must be tempered with knowledge of the specific child's readiness.

Household safety should be practiced and includes the usual precautions recommended for any age-group (see Child safety home inventory, p. 539). An additional safeguard for young children is the use of safety glass in doors and windows and the application of decals on glassed areas to lessen the likelihood of running through glass.

ANTICIPATORY GUIDANCE—CARE OF FAMILIES

Understanding toddlers is fundamental to successful child-rearing, regardless of the approach used. Nurses, particu-

PARENTAL GUIDANCE DURING TODDLER YEARS

Age (months)	Guidance
12-18	Prepare parents for expected behavioral changes of toddler, especially negativism and ritualism
	Assess present feeding habits and encourage gradual weaning from bottle and increased intake of solid foods
	Stress expected feeding changes of physiologic anorexia, presence of food fads and strong taste preferences, need for scheduled routine at mealtimes, inability to sit through an entire meal, and lack of table manners
	Assess sleep patterns at night, particularly habit of a bedtime bottle, which is a major cause of dental caries, and procrastination behaviors that delay hour of sleep
	Prepare parents for potential dangers of the home, particularly motor vehicular, poisoning, and falling injuries; give appropriate suggestions for safeproofing the home
	Discuss need for firm but gentle discipline and ways in which to deal with negativism and temper tantrums; stress positive benefits of appropriate discipline
	Emphasize importance for both child and parents of brief, periodic separations
	Discuss new toys that use developing gross and fine motor, language, cognitive, and social skills
18-24	Emphasize need for dental supervision, types of basic dental hygiene at home, and food habits that predispose to caries; stress importance of supplemental fluoride
	Stress importance of peer companionship in play
	Explore need for preparation for additional sibling; stress importance of preparing child for new experiences
	Discuss present discipline methods, their effectiveness, and parents' feelings about child's negativism; stress that negativism is important aspect of developing self-assertion and independence and is not a sign of spoiling

Age (months)	Guidance
18-24	Discuss signs of readiness for toilet training; emphasize importance of waiting for physical and psychologic readiness
	Discuss development of fears, such as darkness or loud noises, and of habits, such as security blanket or thumbsucking; stress normalcy of these transient behaviors
	Prepare parents for signs of regression in times of stress
	Assess child's ability to separate easily from parents for brief periods of separation under familiar circumstances
	Allow parents opportunity to express their feelings of weariness, frustration, and exasperation; be aware that it is often difficult to love toddlers at times when they are not asleep!
	Point out some of the expected changes of the next year, such as longer attention span, somewhat less negativism, and increased concern for pleasing others
24-36	Discuss importance of imitation and domestic mimicry and need to include child in activities
	Discuss approaches toward toilet training, particularly realistic expectations and attitude toward accidents
	Stress uniqueness of toddlers' thought processes, especially through their use of language, poor understanding of time, causal relationships in terms of proximity of events, and inability to see events from another's perspective
	Stress that discipline still must be quite structured and concrete and that relying solely on verbal reasoning and explanation leads to injuries, confusion, and misunderstanding
	Discuss investigation of nursery school or daycare center toward completion of second year

larly those in ambulatory or child health centers, are in a most favorable position to assist parents in meeting the tasks and needs of children in this age-group. It seems to be an almost universal phenomenon that prevention yields better results than treatment. Anticipatory guidance in each of the areas presented in the box above is paramount if one wishes to prevent future problems. Advice is sometimes not the sole answer. Actual assistance, such as being available for home visiting or telephone consulting, should be part of the nurse's flexible repertoire of interventions. Whether parents are experiencing the rearing dilemmas of a first or a subsequent child, they benefit from sharing their feelings, frustrations, and satisfactions. They need adult companionship, freedom from childrearing responsibilities, and periodic separations from their children. Sometimes they lose perspective of the needs of each other in the marital relationship and fail to communicate effectively. Part of a nurse's responsibility is to provide opportunities for ventilation of parents' feelings and guidance in areas such as marital needs, career fulfillment, and peer companionship.

CONCEPT SUMMARIES

- The toddler stage, extending from 12 months to 36 months, is a period of intense exploration of the environment.

- Biologic development during the toddler years is characterized by the acquisition of fine and gross motor skills that allow children to master a wide variety of activities.

- Although most of the physiologic systems are mature by the end of toddlerhood, development of certain areas of the brain is still occurring, allowing for greater intellectual capacity.

- Locomotion is the major gross motor skill acquired during toddlerhood, followed by increased eye-hand coordination.

- Specific tasks in the psychosocial development of a toddler include differentiating self from others, tolerating separation from parent, coping with delayed gratification, controlling bodily functions, acquiring socially acceptable behavior, verbally communicating, and interacting with others in a less egocentric manner.

- According to Erikson, the major developmental task of toddlerhood is acquiring a sense of autonomy while overcoming a sense of doubt and shame.

- Language is the major cognitive achievement in toddlerhood.

- In Piaget's sensorimotor and preconceptual phases of development, the toddler experiments by incorporating the old learning of secondary circular reactions with new skills and applies this knowledge to new situations. There is the beginning of rational judgment, an understanding of causal relationships, discovery of objects as objects, imitation, and egocentrism.

- Preconceptual thought is characterized by global organization of thought processes, animism, and irreversibility.

- Discipline, or a punishment-obedience orientation, aids in children's moral development.

- Development of body image occurs with increasing motor ability, at which point toddlers recognize the importance and capacity of body parts.

- The two phases of differentiation of self from significant others are separation and individuation.

- The most striking characteristic of language development during early childhood is the increasing level of comprehension.

- Parental concerns during the toddler years include toilet training, coping with sibling rivalry, limit-setting and discipline, dealing with temper tantrums, negativism, and coping with stress.

- Effective discipline techniques for toddlers include reward, ignoring or extinction, and time-out.

- Nutrition is important at this stage because eating habits established in toddlerhood tend to have lasting effects on subsequent years.

- Regular dental examinations, fluoride supplementation, removal of plaque, and provision of a low-cariogenic diet promote optimum dental health.

- Because of increased locomotion, toddlers are at high risk for sustaining injuries. Fatal injuries are primarily the result of motor vehicle accidents, drownings, and burns.

REFERENCES

Abe, K., Oda, N., and Amatomi, M.: Natural history and predictive significance of head-banging, head-rolling, and breath-holding spells, Dev. Med. Child Neurol. 26 (5):644-648, 1984.

American Academy of Allergy: A statement of the question of allergy to fluoride as used in the fluoridation of community water supplies, J. Allergy 45:347-348, 1971.

Arneson, S., and others: Factors affecting parental use of child automobile safety restraints, J. Assoc. Care Child. Health 13(4):181-186, 1985.

Brahms, M., and Maloney, J.: "Nursing bottle caries" in breast-fed children, J. Pediatr. 103(3):415-416, 1983.

Carey, W.B., and McDevitt, S.: Stability and change in individual temperament diagnoses from infancy to early childhood, Am. Acad. Child Psychiatr. 17(2):331-337, 1978.

Chess, S., and Thomas, A.: Temperamental differences: a critical concept in child health care, Pediatr. Nurs. 11(3): 167-171, 1985.

Christophersen, E.R.: Children's behavior during automobile rides: do car seats make a difference? Pediatrics 60(1):69-74, 1977.

Crall, J.J.: Prevention of oral disease in children: concepts and practices, Pediatr. Ann. 14(2):140-147, 1985.

Feiring, C., Lewis, M., and Jaskir, J.: Birth of a sibling: effect on mother–firstborn child interaction, J. Dev. Behav. Psychol. 4:190-195, 1983.

Feldman, K.W., and others: Tap water scald burns in children, Pediatrics 62(1):1-7, 1978.

Fullard, W., McDevitt, S., and Carey, W.: Assessing temperament in one- to three-year-old children, J. Pediatr. Psychol. 9: 205-217, 1984.

Gates, S.: Children's literature: it can help children cope with sibling rivalry, Am. J. Maternal Child Nurs. 5(5):351-352, 1979.

Griffiths, S.S.: The role of the pediatric nurse clinician in promoting the development of body image in children. In Beal, J.A., editor: Issues and advanced practice in pediatric nursing, Reston, VA, 1983, Reston Publishing Company, Inc.

Grossman, C.S.: Using children's books to foster acceptance of a new sibling into a one-child family, Clin. Pediatr. 21(8):502, 1982.

Guyer, B., Talbot, A.M., and Pless, I.B.: Pedestrian injuries to children and youth, Pediatr. Clin. N. Am. 32(1):163-174, 1985.

Heifetz, S., and Horowitz, H.: Amounts of fluoride in self-administered dental products: safety considerations for children, Pediatrics 77(6): 876-882, 1986.

Honig, J.C.: Preparing preschool-aged children to be siblings, Am. J. Maternal Child Nurs. 11(1):37-43, 1986.

Hoover, N., McKay, F., and Fraumeni, J.: Fluoridated drinking water and the occurrence of cancer, J. Natl. Cancer Inst. 57(4):757-768, 1976.

Horowitz, H.S.: Community water fluoridation. In Forrester, D.J., Wagner, M.L., and Fleming, J., editors: Pediatric dental medicine, Philadelphia, 1981, Lea & Febiger.

Kula, K., and Tinanoff, N.: Fluoride therapy for the pediatric patient, Pediatr. Clin. N. Am. 29:669-680, 1982.

MacLaughlin, S.M., and Johnston, K.B.: The preparation of young children for the birth of a sibling, J. Nurs.-Midwif. 29(6):371-376, 1984.

Mahler, M.S., Pine, F., and Bergman, A.: The psychological birth of the human infant: symbiosis and individuation, New York, 1975, Basic Books.

Marcus, D.F.: Child car seats: a must for safety, Pediatr. Nurs. 7(3):13-17, 1981.

Margolis, F.J., and Cohen, S.N.: Successful and unsuccessful experiences in combating the antifluoridationists, Pediatrics 76(1):113-118, 1985.

McAtee, J.M.: How to help your kids play it safe, Fam. Safety 41(2):12-13, 1982.

McDevitt, S., and Carey, W.: Stability of ratings vs. perceptions of temperament from early infancy to 1-3 years, Am. J. Orthopsychiatry 51(2):342-345, 1981.

Needleman, H., Pueschel, S., and Rothman, K.: Fluoridation and occurrence of Down's syndrome, N. Engl. J. Med. 291:821-823, 1974.

Osborne, S., and Garrettson, L.: Perception of toxicity and dose by 3- and 4-year-old children, Am. J. Dis. Child. 139(8):790-792, 1985.

Policastro, A.M.: Childhood automotive safety, Am. Fam. Physician 20(4):139-142, 1979.

Rissmiller, R.: Kerosene heaters—a new burn threat to children, Clin. Pediatrics **22**(3):203, 1983.

Rozin, P., and others: Children's concept of food; the development of contamination sensitivity to disgusting substances, Devel. Psychol. **21**(6):1075-1079, 1985.

Satran, L.: Fatalities caused by electrically operated garage doors, Pediatrics **68**(3):422-42, 1981.

Schuster, C.S., and Ashburn, S.S.: The process of human development: a holistic approach, ed. 2, Boston, 1986, Little, Brown and Co.

Shurtz, R.G.: Fatal motor vehicle accidents of child passengers from birth through 4 years of age in Washington state, Pediatrics **68**(4):572-575, 1981.

Thomas, R.M.: Comparing theories of child development, ed. 2, Belmont, CA, 1985, Wadsworth Publishing Co.

Weller-Fahy, E., Berger, L., and Troutman, W.: Mouthwash: a source of acute ethanol intoxication, Pediatrics **66**(2):302-304, 1980.

Zuckerman, B.S., and Frank, D.A.: Infancy. In Levine, M.D., and others, editors: Developmental-behavioral pediatrics, Philadelphia, 1983, W.B. Saunders Co.

BIBLIOGRAPHY

For additional citations relevant to toddlerhood, refer to Chapter 12.

Growth and Development

Ames, L.B., and Ilg, F.L.: Your two-year-old: terrible or tender, New York, 1979, Delacorte Press.

Lincoln, L.M.: Fathering and the separation-individuation process, Maternal Child Nurs. J. **13**(2):103-111, 1984.

Pontious, S.L.: Practical Piaget: helping children understand, Am. J. Nurs. **82**(1):114-117, 1982.

Selekman, J.: The development of body image in the child: a learned response, Top. Clin. Nurs. **5**(1):12-21, 1983.

Shelly, J.A., and others: The spiritual needs of children, Downers Grove, IL, 1982, Inter-Varsity Press.

Toilet Training

Carlson, S., and Asnes, R.: Maternal expectations and attitudes toward toilet training: a comparison between clinic mothers and private practice mothers, J. Pediatr. **84**(1):148-151, 1974.

Euler, M.M., and McClellan, M.A.: Toilet training: ready or not? Pediatr. Nurs. **7**(1):15-20, 1981.

Euler-Horner, M.M.: The challenge of toilet training—bowel management for the child with psychogenic encopresis or neurogenic deficit, Pediatr. Basics **32**:4-10, 1982.

Sibling Rivalry

Bahr, J.E.: Canine and feline rivalry: another form of sibling rivalry, Pediatr. Nurs. **7**(4):14-15, 1981.

Dunn, J., Kendrick, C., and MacNamee, R.: The reaction of first-born children to the birth of a sibling: mothers' reports, J. Child Psychol. Psychiatry **22**(1):1-18, 1981.

Fine, L.L., and Friedman, M.S.: The sibling experience: developmental considerations. In Children are different: behavioral development monograph series, Number 11, Columbus, OH, 1984, Ross Laboratories.

Malinowski, J.S.: Answering a child's questions about sex and a new baby, Am. J. Nurs. **79**:1965-1968, Nov. 1979.

Riley H.D., and others: Meeting the new arrival: how to arm yourself for the potential battles between siblings, Am. Baby **42**:56-57, Oct. 1980.

Sweet, P.T.: Helping children to accept and welcome a new baby, Am. J. Maternal Child Nurs. **4**(2):82-83, 1979.

Swingle, M.H.: How to prepare the family for sibling rivalry, Child. Nurse **2**(2):1-3, 1984.

Vestal, K.W.: Siblings: adapting to accommodate the neonate, Issues Health Care Women **1**:13-25, 1979.

Limit-Setting and Discipline

American Academy of Pediatrics, Committee on Psychosocial Aspects of Child and Family Health: The pediatrician's role in discipline, Pediatrics **72**(3): 373-374, 1983.

Briggs, D.C.: Your child's self-esteem: the key to his life, Garden City, NY, 1970, Doubleday & Co., Inc.

Campbell, S.B., and others: A multidimensional assessment of parent-identified behavior problem toddlers, J. Abnorm. Child Psychol. **10**(4):569-592, 1982.

Christophersen, E.R.: The pediatrician and parental discipline, Pediatrics **66**(4):641-642, 1980.

Christophersen, E.R.: Incorporating behavioral pediatrics into primary care, Pediatr. Clin. N. Am. **29**(2):261-296, 1982.

Drabman, R.S., and Jarvie, G.: Counseling parents of children with behavior problems: the use of extinction and time-out techniques, Pediatrics **59**(1):78-85, 1977.

Farber, J.M.: Mild 'punishment' works, Pediatrics **68**(2):298, 1981.

Gonzalez-Mena, J.: A positive approach to discipline, Twins **1**(5):44-45, 1985.

Hammer, D., and Drabman, R.S.: Child discipline: what we know and what we can recommend, Pediatr. Nurs. **7**(3):31-35, 1981.

Hirsch, D.L.O., and Russo, D.C.: Behavior management. In Levine, M.D., and others, editors: Developmental-behavioral pediatrics, Philadelphia, 1983, W.B. Saunders Co.

Kvols-Riedler, K., and Kvols-Riedler, B.: Redirecting children's misbehavior, Pediatrics: Nursing Update **1**(3), Princeton, NJ, 1985, Continuing Professional Education Center.

Melichar, M.M.: Using crisis theory to help parents cope with a child's temper tantrums, Am. J. Maternal Child Nurs. **5**(3):181-185, 1980.

Murphy, M.: When parents ask about discipline, Pediatr. Nurs. **2**(6):28-32, 1976.

Schaefer, C.E.: Raising children by old-fashioned parent sense, Child. Today **7**:7-9, 1978.

Wessel, M.A.: The pediatrician and corporal punishment, Pediatrics **66**(4):639-640, 1980.

Stress

Garmezy, N., and Rutter, M., editors: Stress, coping, and development in children, New York, 1983, McGraw-Hill, Inc.

Kuczen, B.: Childhood stress: don't let your child be a victim, New York, 1982, Delacorte Press.

Lamontagne, L.L., Mason, K.R., and Hepworth, J.T.: Effects of relaxation on anxiety in children: implications for coping with stress, Nurs. Res. **34**:289-292, 1985.

Medeiros, D.C., Porter, B.J., and Welch, I.O.: Children under stress, Englewood Cliffs, NJ, 1983, Spectrum Books.

Saunders, A., and Remsberg, B.: The stress-proof child: a loving parent's guide, New York, 1984, Holt, Rinehart & Winston.

Scandrett, S., and Uecker, S.: Relaxation training. In Bulechek, G.M., and McCloskey, J.C., editors: Nursing interventions: treatments for nursing diagnoses, Philadelphia, 1985, W.B. Saunders Co.

Nutrition

American Academy of Pediatrics, Committee on Nutrition: Pediatric nutrition handbook, ed. 2, Elk Grove Village, IL, 1985, The Academy of Pediatrics.

Brock, D.T.: Decreasing toddlers' sodium intake, Pediatr. Nurs. **11**(1):47-50, 1985.

Dwyer, J.: Diets for children and adolescents that meet the dietary goals, Am. J. Dis. Child. **134**:1073-1080, Nov. 1980.

Eden, A.N.: Toddler diet, Pediatr. Basics **39**:4-6, 1984.

Henneman, A., and Koziol, J.: Preschool feeding problems: it's not nutritious unless they eat it, Issues Compr. Pediatr. Nurs. **4**:7-12, Dec. 1980.

Lucas, B.: Nutrition in childhood. In Krause, M.V., and Mahan, L.K.: Food, nutrition, and diet therapy, ed. 7, Philadelphia, 1984, W.B. Saunders Co.

Pipes, P.: Nutrition in infancy and childhood, ed. 3, St. Louis, 1985, The C.V. Mosby Co.

Satter, E.: Developmental guidelines for feeding infants and young children, Food & Nutr. News **56**(4):21-26, 1984.

Wurtman, J.J.: What do children eat? Eating styles of the preschool, elementary school, and adolescent child. In Suskind, R.M., editor: Textbook of pediatric nutrition, New York, 1981, Raven Press.

Dental Health

American Academy of Pediatrics: Juice in ready-to-use bottles and nursing bottles caries, News Comment **29**(1):11, 1978.

American Academy of Pediatrics, Committee on Nutrition: Fluoride supplementation, Pediatrics **77**(5):758-761, 1986.

Carey, W.B.: Swallowed toothpaste—a danger or not, Pediatrics **67**(6):938, 1981.

Coll, J.A., and Conlan, J.G.: The pediatric dental office, Pediatr. Clin. North Am. **29**(3):743-759, 1982.

Current preventive concepts. In Council on Dental Therapeutics: accepted dental therapeutics, ed. 39, Chicago, 1982, American Dental Association.

Coutts, L.: Dental health education for mothers of pre-school children, Midwif. Health Visit Comm. Nurse **16**(8): 328-331, 1980.

Feigal, R.J.: Common oral diseases of children, Pediatr. Ann. **14**(2):133-138, 1985.

Forrester, D.J., Wagner, M.L., and Fleming, J., editors: Pediatric dental medicine, Philadelphia, 1981, Lea & Febiger.

Hess, C., and others: Fluoride and caries prevention, Children's/Nurse **4**(2):1-4, 1986.

Hess, C.S., and others: Fluoride: too much or too little, Pediatr. Nurs. **10**(6):397-403, 1984.

Horowitz, A.M, and Frazier, P.J.: Effective public education for achieving oral health, Fam. Comm. Health, J. Health Promo. Maint. **3**:91-101, Nov. 1980.

Jolley, H.M., and Pless, I.B.: Dental health and pediatrics, Pediatr. Rev. **3**(1):13-22, 1981.

Kilmon, F.C., and Helpin, M.L.: Update on dentistry for children, Pediatr. Nurs. **7**(5):41-44, 1981.

Kronmiller, J.E., and Nirschl, R.F.: Preventive dentistry for children, Pediatr. Nurs. **11**:446-449, 1985.

Kuster, C.G.: The modern pediatric dental office experience, Pediatr. Ann. **14**(2):148-158, 1985.

Livingston, J.F., and Muirden, D.M.: Supervised toothbrush instruction for pre-school children, Aust. Nurs. J. **9**(8):44-46, 1980.

Margolis, F.J., and others: Fluoride supplements for children, Am. J. Dis. Child. **134**:865-868, 1980.

McDonald, R.E., and Avery, D.R.: Dentistry for the child and adolescent, ed. 4, St. Louis, 1983, The C.V. Mosby Co.

Nizel, A.E.: Nutritional support for optimizing children's dental health. In Suskind, R.M., editor: Textbook for pediatric nutrition, New York, 1981, Raven Press.

Pinkman, J.: Dental health examination techniques for the pediatrician, Pediatr. Basics **23**:10-14, 1979.

Ripa, L.W.: Nursing habits and dental decay in infants: "nursing bottle caries," Contemp. Nutr. **3**(5), 1978.

Wei, S.H.: Nutrition, diet, fluoride, and dental health, Pediatr. Basics **30**:4-7, 1981.

Injury Prevention

Agran, P.F., Dunkle, D.E., and Winn, D.G.: Motor vehicle accident trauma and restraint usage patterns in children less than 4 years of age, Pediatrics **76**(3):382-386, 1985.

Agran, P.F.: Motor vehicle occupant injuries in noncrash events, Pediatrics **67**(6):838-840, 1981.

American Academy of Pediatrics, Committee on Accident and Poison Prevention: Automatic passenger protection systems, Pediatrics **74**(1):146-147, 1984.

Baptiste, M.S., and others: Preventing tap water burns, Am. J. Public Health **70**:272, 1980.

Chang, A., and others: Teaching car passenger safety to preschool children, Pediatrics **76**(3):425-428, 1985.

Chun, Y., Berkelhamer, J.E., and Herold, T.E.: Dog bites in children less than 4 years old, Pediatrics **69**:119-120, 1982.

Colombo, J.L., Hopkins, R.L., and Waring, W.W.: Steam vaporizer injuries, Pediatrics **67**(5):661-663, 1981.

D'Epiro, P.: Teaching parents about car seats, Patient Care **18**(17):166-180, 1984.

DeWitt, D.E.: Traveling with children, Pediatr. Basics **40**:10-14, 1985.

Elfert, H.: Helping preschool children learn to be safe, Can. Nurse **75**:26-29, Dec. 1979.

Faber, M.M., Hoppe, S.K., and Diehl, A.K.: Physician knowledge and clinical behavior regarding automobile safety for children, Pediatrics **75**(2):248-253, 1985.

Hall, M.H.: Road traffic accidents, Practitioner **222**:754-764, June 1979.

Hot water frogs, Am. J. Maternal Child Nurs. **6**:213, May/June 1981.

Jeffers, R., and others: Pull-tab—the foreign body sleeper, J. Pediatr. **92**(6):1023-1024, 1978.

Krassner, L.S.: Child restraint devices, Pediatr. Ann. **12**(10):733-736, 1983.

Macknin, M.L.: Dog and cat bites, Pediatr. Basics **35**:7-11, 1983.

Meyer, R.J.: Save that child: children and automobile restraints, Public Health **71**(2):122-123, 1981.

Nachem, B., and Bass, R.A.: Children still aren't being buckled up, Am. J. Maternal Child Nurs. **9**(5):320-323, 1984.

Questions and answers about child safety seats, Patient Care **18**(17):196-198, 1984.

Righi, F.C., and Krozy, R.E.: The child in the car: what every nurse should know about safety, Am. J. Nurs. **83**(10): 1421-1424, 1983.

Smith, R.G., and Berkline, R.R.: The use of infants' and children's occupant safety devices in motor vehicles: an observation study, Hawaii Med. J. **39**(11):282-285, 1980.

Southard, S.C., and Arena, J.M.: A comprehensive protocol for evaluating the safety of toys for preschool children, Clin. Pediatr. **15**(12):1107-1109, 1976.

Surveyer, J.A., and Halpern, J.: Age-related burn injuries and their prevention, Pediatr. Nurs. **7**(5):29-34, 1981.

Tanz, R., Christoffel, K.K., and Sagerman, S.: Are toy guns too dangerous? Pediatrics **75**(2):265-268, 1985.

Tron, V.A., Baldwin, V.J., and Pirie, G.E.: Hot tub drownings, Pediatrics **75**:789-790, 1985.

Williams, A.F.: Children killed in falls from motor vehicles, Pediatrics **68**(4):576-578, 1981.

Wright, J.C.: Severe attacks by dogs: characteristics of the dogs, the victims, and the attack settings, Public Health Rep. **100**:55-61, 1985.

Chapter 15

Health Promotion of the Preschooler and Family

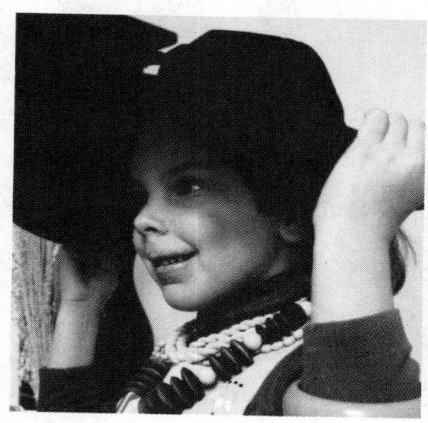

Promoting Optimum Growth and Development
Biologic development
    Gross and fine motor behavior
Psychosocial development
    Erikson: developing a sense of initiative
    Freud: the oedipal stage
Cognitive development
    Piaget: the preoperational phase
Moral development
    Kohlberg: preconventional or premoral level
Spiritual development

Development of body image
Social development
    Individuation-separation
    Language
    Personal-social behavior
    Play
Temperament
Summary of growth and development during the preschool years
Coping with concerns related to normal growth and development
    Preschool or daycare experience
    Guiding parents in selecting a preschool program
    Preparing the child
    Sex education
    Gifted children
    Aggression
    Speech problems
    Coping with stress
    Fears

Promoting Optimum Health During the Preschool Years
Nutrition
Sleep and activity
    Sleep disturbances
Dental health
Injury prevention
Anticipatory guidance—care of families

The preschool years, a period from 3 to 5 years of age, comprise the end of early childhood. This is an age of discovery, inventiveness, curiosity, and developing sociocultural patterns of behavior. In some ways it is a time of ease and comfort for parents, particularly when many of the childrearing tasks, such as toileting, independence, and self-caring abilities, have been mastered.

The years from birth until the child enters school are considered the most critical period for emotional and psychologic development. It is also the time of greatest parental influence on the formation of the child. Once children enter school, their environment widens beyond the home. School becomes a major contributing factor, and peers, teachers, and other authority figures, as well as selected "idols" from the mass media, greatly influence their thinking and behavior. Helping families realize and understand the pliability and malleability of young children as early as possible is an important nursing responsibility.

Promoting Optimum Growth and Development

The combined biologic, psychosocial, cognitive, spiritual, and social achievements of children in this age-group prepare preschoolers for their most significant change in lifestyle—entrance into school. Their control of bodily systems, experience of brief and prolonged periods of separation, ability to interact cooperatively with other children and adults, use of language for mental symbolization, and increased attention span and memory ready them for the next major period—the school years. Successful achievement of previous levels of growth and development is essential for preschoolers to refine many of the tasks that were mastered during the toddler years.

BIOLOGIC DEVELOPMENT

The rate of physical growth slows and stabilizes during the preschool years. Average weight gain remains about 2.3 kg (5 pounds) per year. The average weight at 3 years is 14.6 kg (32 pounds), at 4 years 16.7 kg (36.75 pounds), and at 5 years 18.7 kg (41.25 pounds).

Growth in height also remains steady at a yearly increase of 6.75 to 7.5 cm (2.5 to 3 inches) and generally occurs in elongation of the legs rather than of the trunk. The average height at 3 years is 95 cm (37.25 inches), at 4 years 103 cm (40.5 inches), and at 5 years 110 cm (43.25 inches).

Physical proportions no longer resemble those of the squat, potbellied toddler. The preschooler is slender but sturdy, graceful, agile, and posturally erect. There is little difference in physical characteristics according to sex, except as dictated by such factors as dress and hairstyle.

Most bodily systems are mature and stable and can adjust to moderate stress and change. Motor development consists for the most part of increases in strength and refinement of previously learned skills, such as walking, running, and jumping. However, muscle development and bone growth are still far from mature. Excessive activity and overexertion can injure delicate tissues. Properly fitted shoes, good posture, appropriate exercise, and adequate rest are essential for optimum development of the musculoskeletal system.

Gross and Fine Motor Behavior

Walking, running, climbing, and jumping are well-established by 36 months. Refinement in eye-hand and muscle coordination is evident in several areas. At age 3 the preschooler rides a tricycle, walks on tiptoe, balances on one foot for a few seconds, and broad jumps. By age 4 he skips and hops proficiently on one foot (Fig. 15-1) and catches a ball reliably. By the time the child is 5, he skips on alternate feet, jumps rope, and begins to skate and swim.

Drawing. Drawing shows several advancements in perception of shape and development of fine muscle coordina-

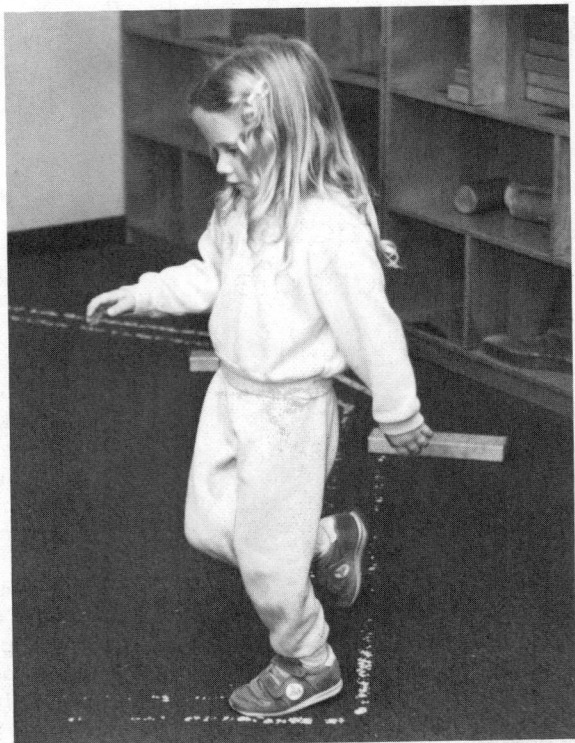

Fig. 15-1. A 4-year-old child has sufficient balance to walk or hop on one foot.
Photography by John Roy, Saint Francis Hospital, Tulsa, OK.

tion. The 3-year-old child copies a circle and imitates a cross and vertical and horizontal lines. He holds the crayon with his fingers rather than in his fist. He scribbles or scrawls but names what he has drawn. He is not able to draw a complete stick figure but draws a round circle, later adds facial features, and by age 5 or 6 can draw several parts (head, arms, legs, body, and facial features). Between 4 and 5 years he can trace a cross and copy a square. The triangle and diamond are usually the last geometric figures to be mastered, sometime between 5 and 6 years.

Children's drawings have been studied extensively. As children progress from scribbling to picture making, they advance through four distinguishable stages (Kellogg, 1969). In the *placement stage* the 15-month-old child places his very earliest spontaneous scribblings on the paper in a specific placement pattern, such as in the center, all over, across the lower half, or across the page in a diagonal direction (Fig. 15-2). Approximately 17 different placement patterns appear by age 2 years and once developed are never lost.

By 3 years of age, children are in the *shape stage*. They draw single-line outline forms, such as rectangles, circles, ovals, crosses, and other odd shapes. As soon as they draw diagrams, they almost immediately progress to the *design stage*, in which simple forms are drawn together to make structured designs. When two diagrams are united, the resulting design is called a *combine*. Three or more united diagrams produce an *aggregate*. Between the ages of 4 and 5 most children enter the *pictorial stage,* in which their designs are recognizable as familiar objects. Early pictorial drawings are suggestive of such things as human figures, houses, animals, and trees. Later pictorial drawings are more clearly defined and recognizable; they are not representations of the actual object but esthetically satisfying structures that *resemble* familiar objects. For example, the initial human figure drawing is a circle with arms attached to the head. It is more an aggregate drawing than any attempt to copy a human figure. Drawings of animals follow the human figure drawing but are only a slight modification, such as attaching ears to the top of the head.

Children's drawings before age 6 are strikingly similar from country to country, culture to culture, and past to present. This suggests that there are some inherent neurologic mechanisms that influence the type of self-taught art forms. After age 6 environmental influence, particularly from parents and teachers, shapes much of what children draw. Kellogg suggests that uninhibited scribbling and drawing are necessary for children to learn to read, and that children who have been free to experiment and produce abstract forms have developed the mental set required for learning symbolic language. Scribbling and drawing also help develop the fine muscle skills and eye-hand coordination eventually required for making precise letters and numbers.

Drawing is also a tool used for assessing intelligence, personality development, and psychosocial adjustment. The precise value of using drawing to measure such concepts is still an inexact science. However, children do reveal thoughts about themselves in their drawings, especially school-age children. It is generally not necessary to have in-depth knowledge of children's drawings to make assumptions about their significance. Being receptive to all the clues, both verbal and nonverbal, is essential to understand how and what children are communicating to others. (For further discussion of children's drawing, see pp. 198 and 286.)

PSYCHOSOCIAL DEVELOPMENT

By the time children reach 3 years of age their gross and fine motor abilities are sufficiently developed to enable them to pursue almost limitless activities. If they have been allowed to express their independence and negativism constructively, they are ready to direct their energy toward new learning. They learn how to interact and relate to other children and adults; they learn appropriate sex-role functions and socially acceptable behavior; they learn right and wrong and the types of reward or punishment associated with each. However, learning does not necessarily imply success. Without appropriate guidance and reinforcement, children can learn unacceptable behavior and instead of feeling accomplishment will feel inadequacy, guilt, and inferiority.

Erikson: Developing a Sense of Initiative

If preschoolers have mastered the tasks of the toddler period, they are ready to face the developmental endeavors of this stage. Erikson maintains that the chief psychosocial task of the preschool period is acquiring a sense of initiative. The child is in a stage of energetic learning. He plays, works, and lives to the fullest and feels a real sense of accomplishment and satisfaction in his activities. Conflict arises when the child oversteps the limits of his ability and inquiry and experiences a sense of *guilt* for not having behaved or acted appropriately. Feelings of guilt, anxiety, and fear may also result from thoughts that differ from expected behavior.

A particularly stressful thought is wishing one's parent dead. As a sense of rivalry or competition develops between the same-sex child and parent, the child may think of ways to get rid of the interfering parent. In most situations this contest is resolved when the child strongly identifies with the same-sex parent and peers during the school years. However, if that same-sex parent dies before the identification process is completed, the preschooler can be overwhelmed with feelings of guilt for having wished and therefore causing (he thinks) the death. Clarifying for children

SEQUENTIAL DEVELOPMENT IN SELF-TAUGHT ART

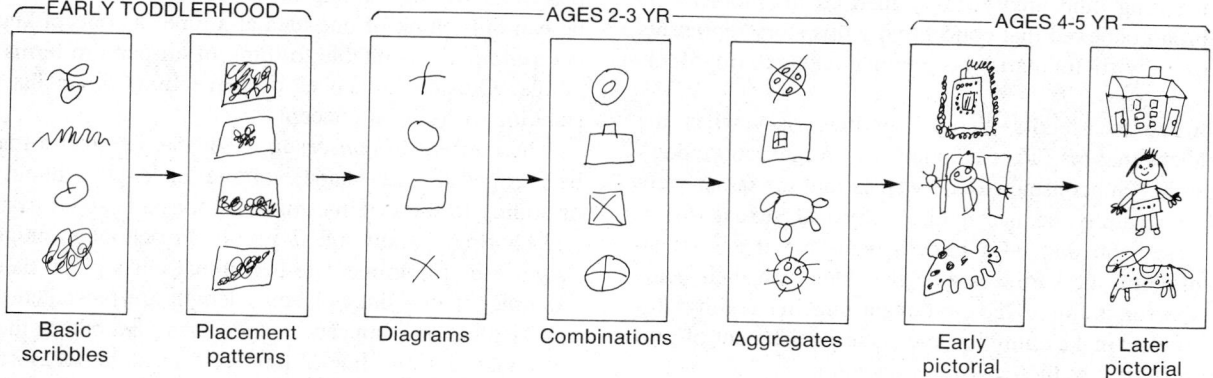

Fig. 15-2. Sequential development in self-taught art.
From Kellogg, R.: Understanding children's art. In Readings in Psychology Today, Del Mar, CA, 1969, Communications/Research/Machines/Inc.

that wishes cannot and do not make events occur is essential in helping them overcome their guilt and anxiety.

Development of the *superego,* or *conscience,* starts toward the end of the toddler years and is a major task for preschoolers. Learning right from wrong and good from bad is the beginning of morality. Children in this age-group are generally unable to understand the reasons why something is acceptable or unacceptable. They are aware of appropriate behavior primarily through punishment or reward and rely almost completely on parental principles for developing their own moral judgment. However, verbal enforcement of limits is much more effective. For example, in order to prevent accidents, parents need to supervise the toddler, keep him fenced in, and tell him not to run into the street. The preschooler is much more aware of danger and can be relied on to listen and obey in most instances. If allowed to disagree and question, he will develop socially acceptable behavior and independence in thought and action.

Developing a conscience implies learning the *sociocultural mores* of the family's heritage. Depending on the type of attitudes conveyed, the child will learn not only appropriate behaviors but also tolerant, biased, or prejudiced values concerning his ethnic, religious, and social background and those of other groups. Much of this influence may remain dormant until he associates with children or adults of a different heritage. Then depending on the particular group, he may be accepted or ostracized for his attitudes.

Freud: The Oedipal Stage

As soon as children comprehend their separateness as persons, they begin to realize that there are categories of objects, such as things, people, males, females, children, and adults. One of the principal goals in further differentiation of oneself from others is learning sex differences and sexually appropriate behavior.

Freud has long recognized this task by describing the period as the *oedipal,* or *phallic* stage. The Oedipus complex is based on the Greek mythology concerning Oedipus, the king's son who had been raised in a foster family since infancy. When he grew to manhood, he accidentally killed his father, the king, and unknowingly married his mother, the queen. Freud believed that conceptually this story represents every boy's wish to marry his mother and get rid of his father.

According to Freud's theory, conflict arises when the child realizes that his father is much stronger and more powerful than he. Subconsciously he wishes that his father were dead. Concurrently he has noticed physical sexual differences, in specific that boys have a penis but that girls do not. In his mind he surmises that girls have lost their penis for some wrongdoing. His guilt regarding his feelings toward his father makes him fear the same punishment of mutilation, resulting in the *castration complex.*

Girls have similar wishes to marry their father and kill their mother, a phenomenon sometimes called the *Electra complex,* named after the female counterpart of Oedipus. However, females do not fear castration because they have no penis to be removed; rather they experience *penis envy* (desire to have a penis). Freud has developed the female role in the phallic stage less fully than the male's role.

The resolution of the Oedipus or Electra complex is identification with the same-sex parent. *Sex typing,* or the process by which an individual develops the behavior, personality, attitudes, and beliefs that are appropriate for his or her culture and sex, occurs through several mechanisms during this period. Probably the most powerful are childrearing practices and imitation. The ways in which parents dress, hold, cuddle, caress, discipline, and talk to their child all express some aspect of sexually oriented behavior. Studies increasingly demonstrate that gender identification is not solely biologic or genetic but primarily a result of complex postnatal psychologic factors and that most children are aware of their sex and the expected set of related behaviors by 1½ to 2½ years of age. Although toddlers might be aware of their particular sex, they do not possess the language and cognitive skills to investigate sexual identity as fully as preschoolers.

COGNITIVE DEVELOPMENT

One of the tasks related to the preschool period is readiness for school and scholastic learning. Many of the thought processes of this period are crucial for achieving such readiness, and it is intentional that the child begins school when 5 to 6 years old rather than at an earlier age.

Piaget: The Preoperational Phase

Piaget's cognitive theory actually does not include a period specifically for children 3 to 5 years old. The preoperational phase comprises the age span from 2 to 7 years and is divided into two stages, the *preconceptual phase,* ages 2 to 4, and the phase of *intuitive thought,* ages 4 to 7.

One of the main transitions during these two phases is the shift from totally egocentric thought to social awareness and the ability to consider other viewpoints. This transition is very closely associated with the development of the superego. The child is able to think and verbalize his mental processes without having to act out his thinking. However, he can only think of one idea at a time, a concept known as *centration.* He is unable to think of all parts in terms of the whole. Outside influences or perceptions direct his understanding of a visual concept.

The concept of *conservation,* or the idea that a mass can be changed in size, shape, volume, or length without losing or adding to the original mass, is not understood by prelogical children (below age 7 years). Preschoolers judge what they see by the immediate perceptual clues given them. For example, if two lines of equal length are presented in such a way that one appears longer than the other, the child will state that one line is longer, even if he measures both lines with a ruler or yardstick and finds that each has the same length. The child therefore judges experiences by outside appearances and results, not by intrinsic, logical indicators.

Understanding this prelogical thinking in young children can help nurses interact with them in an efficacious manner. One example of how the manipulation of matter according to the child's understanding can facilitate the performance of an activity concerns the administration of drugs. If the child is to receive 5 ml of liquid medication, it is advisable to give it in a small medicine cup rather than a large cup, since the child will imagine that the large vessel contains more liquid. Since he is unable to perceive the two dimensions of height and width simultaneously, the child will choose one dimension and measure the amount according to that standard. If the child refuses the medicine in the small cup, he may accept it once it is poured into a large cup because the liquid will appear less in a tall, wide container.

There are many everyday examples of how the young child's inability to understand conservation of matter influences his behavior. Probably one of the most common situations involves eating and the amount of food placed on a dish. If the same amount of food is placed on a small and a large plate, the child may state that the large plate contains more food and may feel overwhelmed by the apparently large quantity. Parents are usually "taught" this by their children and "learn" ways to use this thinking to delude the child. Meat that is cut thin and flat appears to be more in quantity than the same amount of meat that is cut thick, and the child will generally consume more of the thicker portion. The opposite also has its advantages. Giving a child a large, flat cookie will please and satisfy him more than a small, thick one.

Children develop logical thought processes and understanding of conservation of numbers, substance, and length during the school-age years (Chapter 17). It is no accident that learning subjects such as mathematics or science is begun at age 6 and later. Although some younger children might comprehend the meaning, reversibility, and symbolization of numbers, most do not until age 6 or 7.

Language continues to develop during the preschool period. Speech remains primarily a vehicle of egocentric communication. The child assumes that everyone thinks as he does and that a brief explanation of his thinking makes his meaning understood by others. Because of this self-referenced, egocentric verbal communication, it is frequently necessary to explore and understand the young child's thinking through other, nonverbal approaches. For children in this age-group, the most enlightening and effective method is *play*. Play becomes the child's work of understanding, adjusting to, and working out his life's experiences. Because of the child's rich imagination and unlimited ability to invent and imitate, all kinds of play hold therapeutic and communicative value. At this age the child's egocentricity dominates his interaction. Expressions about others, such as a doll, puppet, truck, and dog, are actually descriptions of himself. To know what a child is really thinking demands skill, time, and patience of those willing to learn to look beyond the words and into the hearts and minds of children.

Preschoolers afford adults, particularly parents, teachers, and nurses, the richest opportunity for comprehending the uniqueness, innocence, and genuineness of children. Children's conversation with their toys can tell more in a few minutes than many long hours of conversation between two adults, which is illustrated in the following example:

> Five-year-old Ann is playing mommy and has her family of dolls nearby. She is "talking" on her telephone, exclaiming to her doll children, "Be quiet! Can't you see that I am busy? This is an important business call. Go away and play somewhere else." She hangs up the phone and becomes the little girl at whom she had just yelled. She pretends she is crying and says, "I always do bad things. I wish Mommy wouldn't yell at me all the time."
>
> Ann's mother has overheard this play conversation and is acutely aware of the similarity between the play session and real-life experiences in the home. She had never before realized how the child must have felt when she was preoccupied with other business. She had always been irritated by her daughter's inconsiderateness. As she analyzed the example more closely, she realized that this was happening a few times a day and that, with her working part-time, she never really gave the child her undivided attention. She planned to set aside 1 hour every morning before leaving for work to play or read to Ann and to confine her business telephone calls to the evening when Ann's father was home.

This mother was perceptive to clues regarding the child's feelings. However, not all parents are as aware and frequently negate what they hear, believing it to be unimportant or irrelevant. To understand children is to listen to their spoken and nonspoken language. Communicating messages to them may also necessitate using their methods, such as play, imitation, and role-playing. Unlike toddlers who respond less favorably to anticipatory explanation or preparation for a potentially frightening experience, preschoolers have the ability to comprehend simple explanations, can enjoy preparation such as seeing or playing with equipment, and can relate how they feel and think by using puppets or dolls.

Preschoolers increasingly use language without comprehending the meaning of words, particularly concepts of right or left, time, and causality. The child may use the concepts correctly but only in the circumstances he has learned them. For example, he may know how to put on his shoes by remembering that the buckle is always on the outside of the foot. However, if different shoes have no buckles, he cannot reason which shoe fits which foot. Any experience is judged by its end product. For example, the child who wins the race is the "fastest," even if he ran a shorter distance or started before the others. Rules of the game are only governing statements that can be changed and altered according to the specific events. To return to the preceding example, the school-age child will state that the child who ran a shorter distance or started before the others did not play fairly and therefore did not win and is not the fastest. This difference in thinking often complicates play activity between children in these two age-groups because each judges the situation by different standards.

Superficially *causality* resembles logical thought. The child explains a concept as he heard it described by others, but his understanding is limited. The concept of death illustrates this type of thinking. The adult concept of death implies inevitability and irreversibility. The preschooler may state that when a person dies it is forever. When asked what forever means, he may explain that the person has gone away, but that he may return someday. Some of the explanations offered to children about death support this idea of reversibility, such as ''He has gone on a trip and will not be back for a very long time.'' Since *time* is still incompletely understood, the child interprets this according to his own frame of reference, such as ''A long time means until Christmas.'' Explaining life events accurately and honestly helps children form correct concepts and leaves them with fewer self-interpreted meanings.

Time is best explained in relationship to an event, such as ''Your mother will visit you after you finish your lunch.'' Avoiding terms such as *yesterday, tomorrow, next week,* and *Tuesday* to express when an event is expected to occur and associating time with usual expected daily occurrences help children learn about temporal relationships and increase their trust in others' predictions. Children are usually not able to tell time on a clock until 7 or 8 years of age.

Age is another concept that is judged by one set of criteria, such as size or physical appearance. A 5-year-old child's question, ''Was the baby just born?'' illustrates that the small 10-month-old infant could be a newborn to the preschooler. Children gradually develop the ability to judge age based on multiple factors other than size when they are approximately 8 years old.

Preschoolers' thinking is often described as *magical*. Because of their egocentrism and transductive reasoning (association of one event with a simultaneous event), they believe that thoughts are all-powerful. Such thinking places them in the vulnerable position of feeling guilty and responsible for bad thoughts, which may coincide with the occurrence of a wished event. A typical example is wishing a new sibling dead. If that sibling does die, young children think their wish caused the death. Their inability to logically reason the cause and effect of illness or an accident makes it especially difficult for them to understand such events.

Preschoolers believe in the power of words and accept their meaning literally. A significant example of this type of thinking is calling the child ''bad'' because he did something wrong. In the child's mind telling him that he is bad means that he is bad. For this reason it is better to relate such words to the act by saying, for example, ''That was a bad thing to do.''

MORAL DEVELOPMENT

Moral development continues to advance and is influenced by the cognitive processes typical of the preschool years. While many theorists incorporate moral development within their theoretic framework, one of the more prominent theorists whose work deals primarily with moral development is Lawrence Kohlberg.

Kohlberg: Preconventional or Premoral Level

Moral issues are based on preschoolers' egocentric, limited, and cognitively biased considerations. Three-year-old children continue to behave according to the punishment-obedience orientation typical of toddlers. From approximately 4 to 7 years of age children are in the stage of *naive instrumental orientation,* in which actions are directed toward satisfying their needs and less frequently the needs of others. There is a very concrete sense of justice. Reciprocity or fairness involves the philosophy of ''You scratch my back and I'll scratch yours,'' with no thought of loyalty or gratitude (Thomas, 1985).

SPIRITUAL DEVELOPMENT

Children's knowledge of faith and religion is learned from significant others in their environment, usually from the parents and their religious practices. However, young children's understanding of spirituality is influenced by their cognitive level. Preschoolers have a concrete conception of a God with physical characteristics who is often like an imaginary friend. They understand simple Bible stories and memorize short prayers, but their understanding of the meaning of these rituals is limited. They benefit from concrete representations of religious practices, such as picture Bible books, and small statues, such as those of the Nativity scene (Shelley and others, 1982).

Development of the conscience is strongly linked to spiritual development. At this age children are learning right from wrong and behave correctly to avoid punishment. Wrongdoing provokes feelings of guilt, and preschoolers often misinterpret illness as a punishment for real or imagined transgressions. It is important that children view God as one who bestows unconditional love, rather than as a judge of good or bad behavior. Praying to God and observing religious traditions, for example, prayers before meals or bedtime, can help children through stressful periods, such as hospitalization.

DEVELOPMENT OF BODY IMAGE

The preschool years play a significant role in the development of body image. With increasing comprehension of language, preschoolers recognize that individuals have undesirable and desirable appearances. They recognize differences in skin color and racial identity and are vulnerable to learning prejudices and biases. They are aware of the meaning of words, such as *pretty* or *ugly,* and reflect the opinions of others regarding their own appearance. For example, by 5 years of age children compare their size to their peers' and can become conscious of being large or short, especially if others refer to tnem as ''so big'' or ''so little'' for their age.

Despite the advances in body image development, preschoolers have poorly defined body boundaries and little knowledge of their internal anatomy. Intrusive experiences are frightening, especially those that disrupt the integrity of the skin, such as injections and surgery. There is a fear that if the skin is "broken" all their blood and "insides" can leak out. Therefore, bandages are critical to "keeping everything from coming out."

Sexual identity is developing beyond gender recognition, and modesty may become a concern, as well as fears of mutilation. There is sex-role imitation, and "dressing up" like Mommy or Daddy is an important activity. Attitudes and responses of others to role-playing can condition the child to views of self or others. For example, comments such as "Boys shouldn't play with dolls" can influence a boy's self-concept of masculinity. This may be a time when children begin forming ideal images of how they would want to look as adults (Selekman, 1983).

SOCIAL DEVELOPMENT

Dramatic advancements in social development occur during the preschool period. The individuation-separation process is complete. Language allows for greater verbal communication of needs and feelings, and personal-social skills are improving to the point of almost complete independence.

Individuation-Separation

Preschoolers have relinquished much of the anxiety with strangers and the fear of separation of earlier years. They relate to unfamiliar people easily and tolerate brief separations from parents with little or no protest. However, they still need parental security, reassurance, guidance, and approval, especially when entering nursery school or elementary school. Prolonged separation, such as that imposed by illness and hospitalization, is difficult, but preschoolers respond very well to anticipatory preparation and concrete explanation. They can cope with changes in daily routine much better than toddlers; however, they may develop more imaginary fears. They gain security and comfort from familiar objects, such as toys, dolls, or photographs of family members. They are able to work through many of their unresolved fears, fantasies, and anxieties through play, especially if guided with appropriate play objects, for example, dolls or puppets, that represent family members, medical and nursing staff, and other children.

Language

Language during the preschool years is quite sophisticated and complex. It also becomes a major mode of communication and social interaction. Vocabulary increases dramatically, from 300 words at age 2 to over 2100 words at the end of 5 years. Sentence structure, grammatical usage, and intelligibility also advance to a more adult level (Lowrey, 1986).

Children between the ages of 3 and 4 form sentences of about three to four words and include only the most essential words to convey a meaning. Such speech is often termed *telegraphic* for its brevity in length. Three-year-old children ask many questions and use plurals, correct pronouns, and the past tense of verbs. They name familiar objects, such as animals, parts of the body, relatives, and friends. They can give and follow simple commands. They talk incessantly, regardless of whether anyone is listening or answering them. They enjoy musical or talking toys or dolls and imitate new words proficiently.

From ages 4 to 5 preschoolers use longer sentences of four to five words and use more words to convey a message, such as prepositions, adjectives, and a variety of verbs. They follow simple directional commands, such as "Put the ball on the chair," but can carry out only one request at a time. They answer questions, such as "What do you do when you are hungry?" by describing the appropriate action. The pattern of asking questions is at its peak, and children usually repeat the question until they receive an answer.

By the end of age 5 children use all parts of speech correctly, except for deviations from the rule. They can define simple words by describing their use, shape, or general category of classification, not only by stating their outward appearance. For example, they define a ball as "round, something you bounce, or a toy," rather than by its color. They can give some opposites, such as "If Mommy is a woman, Daddy is a man." By the time they are 6 years old, they can describe an object according to its composition, such as "A spoon is made of metal."

Personal-Social Behavior

The pervasive ritualism and negativism of toddlerhood gradually diminish during the preschool years. Although self-assertion is still a major theme, preschoolers demonstrate their sense of autonomy differently. They are able to verbalize their request for independence and perform independently because of their much refined physical and cognitive development. They fully care for themselves by 4 or 5 years of age, needing little if any assistance with dressing, eating, or toileting (Fig. 15-3). They can also be trusted to obey warnings of danger, although 3- or 4-year-old children may exceed their boundaries at times.

They are also much more sociable and willing to please. They have internalized many of the standards and values of the family, and their conscience dictates many of their actions. By the end of early childhood they begin to question parental values and compare them to those of their peer group and other authority figures; as a result, they may be less willing to abide by the family's code of conduct. Preschoolers become increasingly aware of their position and role within the family. Although this is a more secure age for experiencing the addition of another sibling, relinquishing the position of first or youngest is still difficult and requires appropriate preparation (see Chapter 14).

Play

Various types of play are typical of this period, but preschoolers especially enjoy associative play—group play in similar or identical activities but without rigid organization

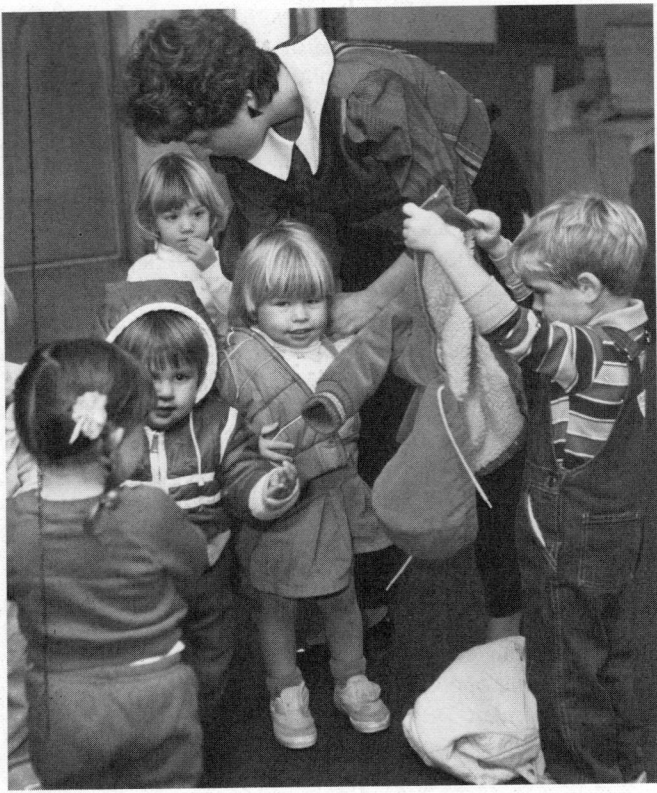

Fig. 15-3. Most preschoolers are able to dress themselves, needing help only for more difficult items of clothing.
Photography by John Roy, Saint Francis Hospital, Tulsa, OK.

or rules. Play should provide for physical, social, and mental development (Table 15-1).

Play activities for physical growth and refinement of motor skills include jumping, running, and climbing. Tricycles, trucks, wagons, gym and sports equipment, sandboxes, wading pools, and winter sleds can help develop muscles and coordination. Activities such as swimming, ice skating, and skiing teach safety as well as muscle development and coordination.

Manipulative, constructive, creative, and educational toys provide for quiet activities, fine motor development, and self-expression. Easy construction sets, large blocks of various sizes and shapes, a counting frame, alphabet or number flash cards, paints, crayons, simple carpentry tools, musical toys, illustrated books, simple sewing or handicraft sets, large puzzles, and clay are suitable toys. Electronic games, such as Speak & Spell* and educational computer programs for television, are especially valuable in helping children learn basic skills, such as letters and simple words. Although their attention span is still short, preschoolers are beginning to enjoy crafts, especially with the guidance and assistance of adults (Fig. 15-4). A helpful rule in planning creative activities is one simple project per year of age. For example, 3-year-old children usually have the patience to decorate three eggs, but become bored and restless with more.

Probably the most characteristic and pervasive pre-

*Texas Instruments, Dallas, TX 75243-1108.

Table 15-1 Play during preschool years

PHYSICAL DEVELOPMENT	SOCIAL DEVELOPMENT	MENTAL DEVELOPMENT AND CREATIVITY
Suggested activities Provide space for the child to run, jump, and climb Teach child to swim Teach simple sports and activities	Encourage interaction with neighborhood children Intervene when children become destructive Enroll child in nursery school	Encourage creative efforts with raw materials Read stories Monitor television viewing Attend theater and other cultural events appropriate to child's age Take short excursions to park, seashore, museums
Suggested toys Seesaw Medium-height slide Adjustable swing Vehicles to ride Tricycle Wading pool Wheelbarrow Sled Wagon Roller skates, speed-graded to skill	Sailboat Cash register, toy typewriter Child-size playhouse Dolls, stuffed toys Dishes, table Ironing board and iron Trucks, cars, trains, airplanes Play clothes for dress-up Doll carriage, bed, high chair Doctor and nurse kits Nails, hammer, saw Grooming aids, makeup or shaving kits	Books Jigsaw puzzles Musical toys (xylophone, toy piano, drum, horns) Picture games Blunt scissors, paper, paste Newsprint, crayons, poster paint, large brushes, easel, finger paint Musical and rhythmic toys Flannel board and pieces of felt in colors and shapes Pregummed geometric shapes (colored) Records, tapes Blackboard and chalk (colored and white) Wooden and plastic construction sets Magnifying glass, magnet

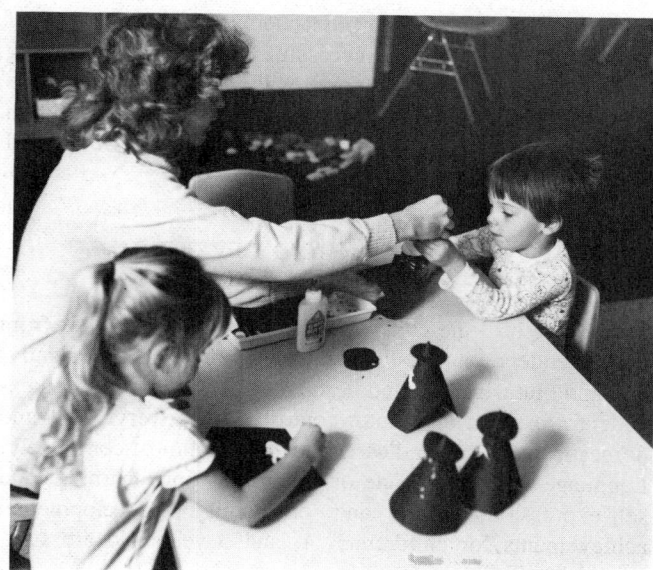

Fig. 15-4. Preschoolers are beginning to enjoy creative activities and appreciate the attention and assistance of adults.
Photography by John Roy, Saint Francis Hospital, Tulsa, OK.

schooler activity is *imitative, imaginative,* and *dramatic play*. Dress-up clothes, dolls, housekeeping toys, dollhouses, play-store toys, telephones, farm animals and equipment, village sets, trains, trucks, cars, planes, hand puppets, and doctor and nurse kits provide hours of self-expression. Probably at no other time is the reproduction of the behavior of significant adults so faithful and absorbing as in 4- and 5-year-old children. Toward the end of the preschool period, children are less satisfied with make-believe or pretend objects and enjoy actually doing the activity, such as cooking and carpentry.

Television and video also have their places in children's play, although each should only be one part of children's total repertoire of social and recreational activities. In counseling parents regarding the effect of television on children, the nurse should explain some of the negative effects of excessive watching, such as aggressive behavior, decreased school performance, and poorer health habits (Palumbo and Dietz, 1985; Zuckerman and Zuckerman, 1985). Parents are encouraged to supervise selection of programs, preview programs for appropriateness, and schedule hours for television viewing. Children enjoy and learn from educational children's programs, which are purposely shown before dinner or after meals to provide a quiet activity. Television can become an interactive activity when parents view programs with children and discuss program content.

Imaginary playmates. Play is so much a part of the young child's life that reality and fantasy become blurred. The make-believe is reality during play and only becomes fantasy when the toys are put away or the dress-up clothes are removed. It is no wonder that imaginary playmates are so much a part of this age period. The appearance of imaginary companions usually occurs between the ages of 2½

and 3 years, and for the most part such playmates are relinquished when the child enters school. There seems to be a relationship between the level of intelligence and the presence of the imaginary companion. The more intelligent children tend to have the most vivid and complex pretend playmates (Fish and Burch, 1985).

Imaginary companions serve many purposes—they become friends in times of loneliness, they accomplish what the child is still attempting, and they experience what the child wants to forget or remember. It is not unusual for the "friend" to have a myriad of vices and to be blamed for wrongdoing. Sometimes the child hopes to escape punishment by saying, "My friend George broke the glass." At other times the preschooler may fantasize that the "companion" misbehaved and the child plays the role of parent. This becomes a way of assuming control and authority in a safe situation.

Parents often worry about their child having imaginary playmates, not realizing how normal and useful they are. They need to be reassured that children's fantasy is a sign of health that helps them differentiate between make-believe and reality. Parents can acknowledge the presence of imaginary companions by calling them by name and even agreeing to simple requests such as setting an extra place at the table, but they should not allow the child to use the playmate to avoid punishment or responsibility. For example,

Questions and Controversies

What are the long-term consequences of temperamental characteristics in young children?

The long-term consequences of temperamental characteristics are of concern because recognition of characteristics associated with later difficulties may be amenable to early intervention. Of the different types of temperament, children with the difficult pattern are most vulnerable to the development of behavior problems, especially between 3 and 5 years old. Their intense negative withdrawal reactions to new situations, slow adaptability, and biological irregularity make the demands of early socialization especially stressful. Although the difficult pattern accounts for only 10% of the children studied, 70% of this group developed behavior disorders (Chess and Thomas, 1983). However, by adolescence more than half had recovered and almost all were either recovered or improved by adulthood (Thomas and Chess, 1984).

Several studies have established that scholastic adjustment is affected by temperament. In particular, low adaptability has been related to teachers' assessments of children's intelligence and adjustment, to neurological referrals, and to scores on academic achievement tests. Difficult children may be labeled as immature and held back in school and slow-to-warm-up children are frequently described as insecure. There is also concern that difficult children will be erroneously labeled as minimum brain dysfunction upon entering school because of their high activity level (Carey, 1981). Most authorities contend that such problems are not necessarily due to temperament, but occur when the demands for change and adaptation exceed the child's capacities and therefore become stressful.

if the child blames the companion for upsetting the room, the parents need to state clearly that the child is the only person they see and therefore the child is responsible for cleaning up.

TEMPERAMENT

Temperament influences children's social development and interactions. In Chapters 8, 12, and 14 the importance of temperament during early childhood has been discussed. Since temperamental characteristics tend to remain stable, the same considerations in terms of childrearing apply during the preschool years. One major concern in this age-group is the effect of temperament on adjustment in group situations, especially school, and the long-term consequences of temperamental characteristics (see Questions and controversies). In particular the degree of adaptability to new situations, intensity of response, distractibility, amount of persistence, mood, and activity level may influence a child's chances for success in school (Schor, 1985). Consequently parents can benefit from suggestions that can promote preschoolers' adjustment. For example, slow-to-warm-up children need gradual introduction to new situations and may benefit from the parent's presence until they have settled in. Children with high activity levels tend to adjust better to environments that allow freedom of movement, rather than a structured or regimented classroom. The more awareness parents have of their children's unique behaviors, the

better able they are to inform teachers or other caregivers of the children's needs and successful approaches to handling the youngsters. The Behavioral Style Questionnaire can be used to identify temperamental characteristics in children who are in the age range of 3 to 7 years (McDevitt and Carey, 1978).

SUMMARY OF GROWTH AND DEVELOPMENT DURING THE PRESCHOOL YEARS

By the age of 3 the child has made tremendous strides from the dependency and callowness of infancy and the negativism and clumsiness of toddlerhood. The preschooler has excellent gross and fine motor control. He is a very social and domesticated being and cares for himself almost completely. Language use is a vehicle of communication, learning, and self-expression. These and other major developmental achievements for children 3, 4, and 5 years old are summarized in Table 15-2.

COPING WITH CONCERNS RELATED TO NORMAL GROWTH AND DEVELOPMENT

In many respects the preschool years present few childrearing problems. However, there are special situations during this period that require parental guidance. They include preschool or daycare experience, sex education, speech problems, and stress. In addition, parents may need counseling

Table 15-2 Growth and development during preschool years

AGE (YEARS)	PHYSICAL	GROSS MOTOR	FINE MOTOR	LANGUAGE
3	Usual weight gain of 1.8 to 2.7 kg (4 to 6 pounds) Average weight of 14.6 kg (32 pounds) Usual gain in height of 7.5 cm (3 inches) Average height of 95 cm (37.25 inches) May have achieved nighttime control of bowel and bladder	Rides tricycle Jumps off bottom step Stands on one foot for a few seconds Goes up stairs using alternate feet, may still come down using both feet on step Broad jumps May try to dance, but balance may not be adequate	Builds tower of nine or ten cubes Builds bridge with three cubes Adeptly places small pellets in narrow-necked bottle In drawing, copies a circle, imitates a cross, names what he has drawn, cannot draw stickman but may make circle with facial features	Has vocabulary of about 900 words Uses primarily "telegraphic" speech Uses complete sentences of three to four words Talks incessantly regardless of whether anyone is paying attention Repeats sentence of six syllables Constantly asks questions

regarding children who exhibit signs of giftedness or aggressive behavior. The issue of divorce, which has a significant impact on preschoolers, is discussed in Chapter 3.

Preschool or Daycare Experience

During the preschool years many children attend some type of early childhood program, usually nursery school or a daycare center. Group care has become commonplace with the large number of mothers presently employed outside the home. The effects of early education and stimulation on children have increasingly gained recognition and importance (for a discussion of the effects of daycare on young children, see p. 92). Since social development widens to include age-mates and other significant adults, preschool provides an excellent vehicle for expanding children's experiences with others.

In nursery school or daycare centers children are exposed to opportunities for learning group cooperation, adjusting to various sociocultural differences, and coping with frustration, dissatisfaction, and anger. If activities are tailored to provide mastery and achievement, children increasingly feel success, self-confidence, and personal competence. Whether or not structured learning is imposed is less important than the social climate, type of guidance, and attitude toward the children that is fostered by the teacher or leader. With a teacher who is aware of preschoolers' developmental abilities and needs, the children will learn from any activity that is provided. Most nursery schools incorporate a similar daily schedule of quiet play, active outdoor activity, group activities such as games and projects, creative or free play, and snack and rest periods.

Nursery school is particularly beneficial for children who lack a peer group experience, such as an only child, and for children from culturally deprived homes. Nursery school provides extensive stimulation for language, physical, and social development. It also is an excellent preparation for entrance into elementary school. For a child from a poor home, elementary school can be so overwhelming that all learning is impeded by the sensory overload. Regular school places many more demands on children for prolonged attention, self-disciplined behavior, and demonstrated progress in performance and achievement than the less-structured atmosphere of preschool. Nursery school and kindergarten are a transitional preparation for the demands of academic learning in later years.

Guiding Parents in Selecting a Preschool Program

A major nursing responsibility is guiding parents in locating suitable facilities with a well-qualified staff. State licensing agencies can help parents identify daycare centers that accept children of specific age-groups and are conveniently located to home and work. Their records are available to the public and provide reports from the health, safety, and fire departments, periodic evaluations from the licensing agency, complaints filed against the center, and qualifications of the center's employees. State-licensed programs are

SOCIALIZATION	COGNITION	FAMILY RELATIONSHIPS
Dresses self almost completely if helped with back buttons and told which shoe is right or left	Is in preconceptual phase	Attempts to please parents and conform to their expectations
Buttons/unbuttons accessible buttons	Is egocentric in thought and behavior	Is less jealous of younger sibling; may be opportune time for birth of additional sibling
Pulls on shoes	Has beginning understanding of time; uses many time-oriented expressions, talks about past and future as much as about present, pretends to tell time	Is aware of family relationships and sex-role functions
Has increased attention span		
Feeds self completely		Boys tend to identify more with father or other male figure
Pours from a bottle or pitcher	Has improved concept of space as demonstrated in understanding of prepositions and ability to follow directional command	Has increased ability to separate easily and comfortably from parents for short periods
Can prepare simple meals, such as cold cereal and milk		
Can help to set table; can dry dishes without breaking any	Has beginning ability to view concepts from another perspective	
Likes to "help" entertain by passing food		
May have fears, especially of dark and going to bed		
Knows own sex and appropriate sex of others		
In play, parallel and associative phase		
Begins to learn simple games and meaning of rules, but follows them according to self-interpretation		
Speaks to toys, such as doll, animal, truck		
Begins to work out social interaction through play		
Able to share toys, although expresses idea of "mine" frequently		

Continued.

Table 15-2 Growth and development during preschool years—cont'd

AGE (YEARS)	PHYSICAL	GROSS MOTOR	FINE MOTOR	LANGUAGE
4	Pulse and respiration rates decrease slightly Growth rate is similar to that of previous year Average weight of 16.7 kg (36.75 pounds) Average height of 103 cm (40.5 inches) Length at birth is doubled Maximum potential for development of amblyopia	Skips and hops on one foot Catches ball reliably Throws ball overhand Walks downstairs using alternate footing	Uses scissors successfully to cut out picture following outline Can lace shoes, but may not be able to tie bow In drawing, copies a square, traces a cross and diamond, adds three parts to stick figure	Has vocabulary of 1500 words or more Uses sentences of four to five words Questioning is at peak Tells exaggerated stories Knows simple songs May be mildly profane if he associates with older children Obeys four prepositional phrases, such as "under," "on top of," "beside," "in back of" or "in front of" Names one or more colors Comprehends analogies, such as, "If ice is cold, fire is __" Repeats four digits Uses words liberally but frequently does not comprehend meaning
5	Pulse, respiration, and blood pressure rates decrease slightly Average weight of 18.7 kg (41.25 pounds) Average height of 110 cm (43.25 inches) Eruption of permanent dentition may begin, especially if deciduous tooth eruption was early (before age 6 months) First permanent teeth to erupt are four molars, which come in behind last temporary teeth (often mistaken for temporary molars) Handedness is established (about 90% are right-handed)	Skips and hops on alternate feet Throws and catches ball well Jumps rope Skates with good balance Walks backward with heel to toe Jumps from height of 12 inches, lands on toes Balances on alternate feet with eyes closed	Ties shoelaces Uses scissors, simple tools, or pencil very well In drawing, copies a diamond and triangle, adds seven to nine parts to stickman, prints a few letters, numbers, or words, such as his first name	Has vocabulary of about 2100 words Uses sentences of six to eight words, with all parts of speech Names coins (e.g., nickel, dime) Names four or more colors Describes drawing or pictures with much comment and enumeration Asks meaning of words Asks inquisitive questions Can repeat sentence of 10 syllables or more Knows names of days of week, months, and other time-associated words Defines words using action as well as description Knows composition of articles, such as, "A shoe is made of _____" Can follow three demands in succession

SOCIALIZATION	COGNITION	FAMILY RELATIONSHIPS
Very independent	Is in phase of intuitive thought	Rebels if parents expect too much, such as impeccable table manners
Tends to be selfish and impatient	Causality still related to proximity of events	Takes aggression and frustration out on parents or siblings
Aggressive physically as well as verbally	Understands time better, especially in terms of sequence of daily events	Do's and don'ts become important
Takes pride in accomplishments	Unable to conserve matter	May have rivalry with older or younger siblings, may resent older's privileges and younger's invasion of privacy and possessions
Has mood swings	Judges everything according to one dimension, such as height, width, or order	
Boasts and tattles	Immediate perceptual clues dominate judgment	May run away from home
Shows off dramatically, enjoys entertaining others	Can choose longer of two lines or heavier of two objects	Identifies strongly with parent of opposite sex
Tells family tales to others with no restraint	Is beginning to develop less egocentrism and more social awareness	Is able to run errands outside the home
Still has many fears	May count correctly but has poor mathematic concept of numbers	
Play is associative	Still believes that thoughts cause events	
Imaginary playmates common	Obeys because parents have set limits, not because of understanding of reason behind right or wrong	
Uses dramatic, imaginative, and imitative devices		
Works through unresolved conflicts, such as jealousy toward sibling, anger toward parent, or unconquered fear in himself		
Sexual exploration and curiosity demonstrated through play, such as being "doctor" or "nurse"		

Less rebellious and quarrelsome than at age 4 years	Begins to question what parents think by comparing them to age-mates and other adults	Gets along well with parents
More settled and eager to get down to business	May notice prejudice and bias in outside world	Does not try to run away from home
Not as open and accessible in thoughts and behavior as in earlier years	Is more able to view other's perspective, but tolerates differences rather than understands them	May seek out mother more often than at age 4 years for reassurance and security, especially when entering school
Independent but trustworthy, not foolhardy, more responsible	Tends to be matter-of-fact about differences in others	Is upset not to find parent, for example, when he comes home from school
Has fewer fears; relies on outer authority to control world	May begin to show understanding of conservation of numbers through counting objects regardless of arrangement	Tolerates siblings, but finds 3-year-old children a special nuisance
Eager to do things right and to please; tries to "live by the rules"	Uses time-oriented words with increased understanding	Begins to question parents' thinking and principles
Acts "manly" or "womanly"	Very curious about factual information regarding world	Strongly identifies with parent of same sex, especially boys with their fathers
Has fairly consistent and polished manners		Enjoys doing activities, such as sports, cooking, shopping with parent of same sex
Cares for self totally, occasionally needing supervision in dress or hygiene		
May complain over minor injuries but tries to be brave for major pain		
Play is associative		
Likes rules and tries to follow them but may cheat to avoid losing		
Begins to notice group conformity and sense of belonging		
Very industrious, tries to accomplish a goal and feels pride and satisfaction, as well as unhappiness and discontent		
May demand to watch television more now that he understands programs better		
Not ready for concentrated close work or small print because of slight farsightedness and still unrefined eye-hand coordination		
Imitative play mimics the portrayed adult like a mirror image		
Wants to use real objects during play, such as actual ingredients to make cookies rather than sand or mud		

supposed to abide by established standards, which represent the *minimum* requirements and safeguards. However, enforcement of the standards is sometimes inadequate. Early childhood programs may also belong to a voluntary accreditation system, the National Academy of Early Childhood Programs, which serves as a model for *optimum* care.* References from other parents are also helpful provided they have investigated the center carefully and have remained involved with the agency's activities.

Other areas for parents to evaluate are the center's daily program, teacher qualifications, student-to-staff ratio, environmental safety precautions, provision of meals, sanitary conditions, adequate indoor/outdoor space per child, and fee schedule. Although fees vary considerably, it is well to point out that a program that charges a minimum fee may also be providing minimum services. In terms of an overall evaluation there is *no substitute for a personal observation of the facility*. Parents should arrange to meet the director and some of the employees, especially those who would be caring for the child. Checklists are helpful to systematically evaluate the center and make comparisons with other facilities (Soderman and Whiren, 1980; Wong, 1986). Several resources are also available to familiarize parents with characteristics of quality child care.

One of the areas that is increasingly important in selecting child care centers is the agency's sanitary practices. Centers that care for infants and young children, who are not toilet-trained can pose an increased risk of infection among children. Outbreaks of a number of organisms have be reported, including *Shigella* organisms, *Giardia lamblia,* rotavirus, cryptosporidiosis, *Campylobacter jejuni, Hemophilus influenzae* type B, cytomegalovirus, and hepatitis A (Bartlett and others, 1985; Pass and others, 1984; Alpert and others, 1986; Smith, 1986a). Nurses play an important role in infection control. Not only can they advise parents regarding the evaluation of a center's sanitary practices, they can also take an active part in educating staff in measures to minimize transmission by stressing the importance of (1) handwashing of children and employees (Fig. 15-5), (2) changing diapers as soon as they are soiled, (3) proper disposal of diapers, preferably placed in a plastic bag and discarded in a closed container stored away from children, and (4) proper cleaning of the diaper changing surface and accessory items that may become contaminated during a diaper change. In addition, staff who care for children should not prepare food, and children who are ill should be excluded from school or cared for in a separate area.

Preparing the Child

Children need preparation for the preschool experience, whether it is a formal nursery school, organized daycare

*Information about the accreditation criteria and procedures of the National Academy of Early Childhood Programs is available from the National Association for the Education of Young Children, 1834 Connecticut Avenue, N.W., Washington, DC 20009. These criteria are excellent guidelines for evaluating nursery or daycare centers.

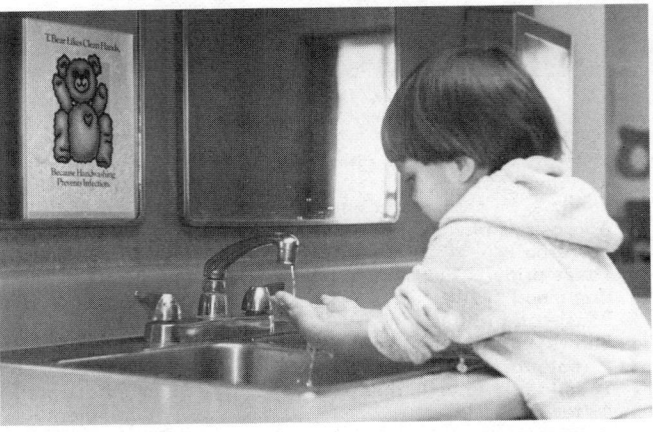

Fig. 15-5. Thorough handwashing is the single most effective method of preventing infection. Note the poster on the mirror; the T. Bear symbol is part of the national infection control campaign sponsored by U.S. Department of Health and Human Services. Photography by John Roy, Saint Francis Hospital, Tulsa, OK.

center, or casual gathering in a neighbor's home. The following suggestions are also appropriate for children entering kindergarten. For young children these programs represent a change from their usual home environment and prolonged separation from parents. Even if children have been cared for by a baby-sitter, preschool or daycare differs because the individualized attention is not as intense or sustained.

The nurse helps the parents assess the children's readiness in terms of age, physical ability, and social development. For example, a group experience may be difficult for young children with short attention spans. These children may require a different type of preschool experience that provides for more individualized attention.

Before children begin the school experience, the parents should present the idea as exciting and pleasurable. Talking to them about activities such as painting, building with blocks, or enjoying swings and other outdoor equipment allows the children to fantasize about the forthcoming event in a positive manner. When the day arrives to begin school, the parents should behave confidently. Such behavior requires the parents to have resolved their own feelings regarding the nursery or daycare experience.

Parents should introduce their child to the teacher and familiarize him with the school. In some instances it is helpful to remain for at least some part of the first day until the child is comfortable and at ease. If parents do stay, they should be available to the child but inconspicuous. Frequently a full-day routine is too overwhelming for a child and needs to be shortened to a morning or afternoon session. This is particularly important to remember for children beginning in a daycare center. Another action that can facilitate children's adjustment is providing the school with detailed information about the home environment, such as familiar routines, favorite activities, food preferences, names of siblings or pets, and personal habits. Such information helps the child feel familiar in the strange surroundings.

When schools automatically request this information, the parent has a valuable clue to evaluating the quality of the program, since it represents the staff's awareness of each child's needs. Transitional objects, such as a favorite toy or blanket, may also help the child bridge the gap from home to school.

The nurse should also encourage parents to discuss their feelings regarding the child's separation from home, particularly guilt about leaving the child in someone else's care when the parent returns to work. Practical ways of alleviating anxiety and improving the quality of time spent with the child include planning a household schedule that divides major chores into smaller ones, combining household duties with a childcare activity, such as cleaning the bathroom while the child is bathing, and providing time for relaxation and activity with the child.

Sex Education

Preschoolers have absorbed a tremendous amount of information and experienced many things during their short lifetimes. Although their thinking may not be adultlike, they search constantly for explanations and reasons that are logical and reasonable to them. The word *why* seems to supplant the word *no,* which was common in toddlerhood. One of their major developmental achievements has been severing the psychologic "placenta" from their mother as they discover their sense of self apart from others. It is only natural that as they learn about "me," they will also want to know such things as "why me," and "how me." Questions such as "Where do babies come from?" are sexual in content but informational in intent. Such inquiries are as casual as "Why is the sky blue?" "What makes it rain?" or "Who is that?" It is the *way* in which questions about procreation are answered that conditions even the youngest children to separate these questions from others about their world. If these questions are answered honestly and as matter-of-factly as any other inquiry, children will continue to search for answers. If they are answered with a "tall tale" or an anxious "You are too young to know about that," children will learn to keep such questions to themselves. Unfortunately as they harbor these silent mysteries, they are formulating their own theories to explain birth. Since magical thinking need not be based on logic or fact, any fantastic, often terrifying explanation can substitute for truth.

Regardless of whether children are given sex education, they will engage in games of sexual curiosity and exploration. At about 3 years of age children are aware of the anatomic differences between the sexes and are very concerned with how the other sex "works." This is not really "sexual" curiosity, because many children are still unaware of the reproductive function of the genitals. Their curiosity concerns the eliminative function of the anatomy. Boys watch girls urinate because they wonder how they can without a penis. Since they cannot see anything but a stream coming out, they want to observe further for where it comes out. "Doctor play" is often a game invented for just such

investigation. Girls are no less curious about boys' anatomy. It is intriguing to have a closer inspection of this "thing" that girls do not have.

Even if children's curiosity is satisfied about the eliminative differences, once they are told about the "special place where babies come out," they are more mystified and determined to find that opening. Unfortunately investigation often yields even fewer answers and may result in anxiety and shame if they are caught and scolded for their behavior. When considering the facts of reproduction and viewing them in terms of the young child's thinking processes, it becomes clear how absurd and incredible the "facts of life" really are. Think about the "special place where the baby grows," "the seed or egg that grows when the father's seed or sperm meets it," and "the special opening" that is so small it cannot be found but through which a fairly large person emerges. And most fantastic of all is how the father's sperm meets the mother's egg! Surely this is more preposterous than any fairy tale about witches, princesses, or monsters!

As children absorb these facts, no matter how expertly they are explained, they will form their own theories. Since the only framework they have for "special place," "growing," "seed or egg," and "opening" is eating and eliminating, they fit all the new information into this understandable explanation. Children need the correct information repeated several times as they attempt to assimilate it as logical and reasonable.

Parents' role in sex education. Preschoolers do not have the benefit of potential sex education in school or from their peer group as older children do. They rely on parental information or misinformation in their search for "how me" (how they came to be). Although sexual mores have seen a kind of liberation movement in the past several decades, parents still may feel uncomfortable when faced with their child's probing questions. Usually overanxious parents react in one of two ways: they close communication either by giving no answers or by giving too much information. The latter approach temporarily ends further inquiry because children can become so overwhelmed with "illogical, incredible" answers that they need time to ponder them before asking more questions.

Two rules govern answering questions about sex or other sensitive issues, such as death, divorce, or adoption. The first is to *find out what the child thinks.* By investigating the theories he has conjured in his mind as a reasonable explanation, parents can not only give correct information but also help the child understand why his explanation is inaccurate. For example, before children ever ask about where babies come from, they usually have imagined that the mother "ate" something, which made the baby grow in her stomach. Therefore the baby will come out like a bowel movement. When parents give the appropriate information, they can also correct this "eating-elimination" theory. The following example illustrates how uncorrected misconceptions can lead to unexpected problems:

Five-year-old John knew his mother was to have a baby soon. He saw how large her abdomen was becoming and, when he asked why, was told that the baby was growing inside mother's stomach. At about the same time, John began eating excessively and became extremely constipated. He would violently object to any measures directed at relieving the constipation and if he evacuated, he would become very upset. During a visit to a nurse friend's home, his mother related these events. The nurse asked about John's understanding of the baby's conception and birth. Mother offered the same limited explanation that she had given her son. The nurse pointed out that based on the information that the "baby grows in the stomach," John probably thought he did understand. According to his logic, he was having a baby by eating a lot and did not want it to come out in the only way he knew body products to exit. Mother saw the logic behind this theory and agreed that they should explore it with John.

John related almost precisely the story as predicted by the nurse. If his mother could have a baby, so could he by eating so much that his belly would enlarge. As he saw himself grow bigger, he was sure that he was pregnant, and he greatly feared that the baby would come out "prematurely" (as he had overheard) if he had a bowel movement. When the nurse explained the correct facts, John was relieved, although somewhat disappointed to learn of his inability to bear children. He asked about the father's role and was given the appropriate explanation. He wondered about "Daddy entering Mommy in a special place and giving her a sperm that made the egg grow," and stated, "I guess for now I won't make any babies. Can I go out and play?" The overeating and constipation resolved without any further intervention.

Another reason for ascertaining what the child thinks before offering any information is that the "unasked for" answer may be given. For example, 4-year-old Sally asked her father, "Where did I come from?" Both parents quickly took this inquiry as a clue for offering sex education. After the explanation, the child exclaimed, "I don't want to know about all that! All I know is Mary came from New York and I want to know where I was born."

The second rule for giving information is *honesty*. It is true that much of the correct information will be forgotten or misunderstood by the preschooler, but what is more important is that the correct information be restated until the child absorbs and comprehends the facts. Even though the correct anatomic words may be hard to pronounce or even more difficult to remember, they become foundational content for explaining other concepts later on. They also reinforce the fact that procreation is not associated with ingestion or elimination but that it occurs in a place that is near but not the same as where the child urinates or defecates. Parental honesty also shows children that parents will be truthful in other phases of inquiry and learning. This approach avoids the establishment of a "double standard," whereby parents can tell "little white lies" but children must always be straightforward.

Honesty does not imply imparting to children every fact of life or allowing excessive permissiveness in sexual curiosity. When children ask one question, they are looking for one answer, not the entire procreation cycle. When they are

ready, they will ask about the other "unfinished" parts of the story. Sooner or later they will wonder how the "sperm meets the egg" and "how the baby gets out," but it is best to wait until they ask.

When children do not ask questions, parents should take advantage of natural opportunities to discuss reproduction, such as talking about someone who is pregnant or discussing a television program or movie about biologic aspects. Observing or explaining how animals procreate is also helpful. Many excellent books on sex education are available for preschool children and the **Sex Information and Education Council of the United States (SIECUS)*** and local chapters of **Planned Parenthood Federation of America†** have bibliographies of suggested reading material.

The question usually arises of how much sexual curiosity should be satisfied? Developmentally, children progress through different stages of sexual exploration. The infant who finds his genitals is not really masturbating but is exploring another pleasurable part of his body. The 3-year-old child who peeks into the bathroom to watch his sister urinate is not perverted but is finding out how she urinates without a penis. Five-year-old children engaged in doctor play are not promiscuous but are trying to find concrete evidence to support explanations about birth. Regardless of how normal these activities are, many parents are confused and bewildered by them and do not know what to say or do when confronted with such behavior.

One positive approach is neither to condone nor condemn the sexual curiosity but to express that if the child has questions he should ask his parents, and then encourage the child to engage in some other activity. In this way children can be helped to understand that there are ways other than through playing investigative games that their sexual curiosity can be satisfied. This in no way condemns the activity but stresses alternative methods to seek solutions and answers. Allowing children unrestricted permissiveness only intensifies their anxiety and concern, since exploring and searching usually yield little evidence to satisfy their sexual curiosity.

Occasionally parents are faced with special dilemmas, for example, when children ask to see "how Mommy and Daddy do it" or accidentally witness lovemaking. When such events occur, parents must remember that sex education is much more than textbook facts. It is part of a greater concept called *sexuality*. Two people unite intimately because of the special relationship they have together. Intercourse is not a physical act apart from feeling or emotion but a private act that two people share in caring and pleasure. Such an explanation does not deny children's right to be curious, nor does it deny them the request because their wish is bad or dangerous. On the contrary, it teaches appropriate social behavior and in particular stresses the meaningful, intimate relationship between man and woman. When children witness sexual acts, parents should use the oppor-

---

*80 Fifth Avenue, New York, NY 10011.
†National office: 810 Seventh Avenue, New York, NY 10019.

tunity (even if days or weeks later) to communicate that sex is healthy and natural. However, to prevent subsequent interruptions, children are cautioned to always knock first or if they are too young to understand or comply, a lock on the door is appropriate (Goldsmith, 1986).

Masturbation. Parents' attitudes toward masturbation closely parallel their view toward sex education for their children. Much of what has been discussed under sexual curiosity applies to masturbation as well. Masturbation, or self-stimulation of the genitals, occurs at any age for a variety of reasons and if not excessive is normal and healthy. For preschoolers it is a part of sexual curiosity and exploration.

Many individuals have certain beliefs about masturbation. Traditionally people have believed it to be sinful and harmful to health. A common myth was that masturbation led to insanity, probably from the observation that mentally ill people masturbate excessively. However, this behavior is a symptom—not a cause—of mental illness. Some people with strong religious beliefs think that masturbation distracts people from the true ideal of sexuality: primarily procreation within a marital relationship. Others who think of themselves as neutral regard masturbation as a subject that requires further study, but they do not encourage it as something positive or healthy. Finally those who take a liberal or permissive view hold that it is not only harmless but positively good, healthy, and at times necessary. They believe that it helps young people grow up sexually in a natural way.

If parents are concerned with masturbation by their children, it is essential for nurses to assess which belief the parents hold as doctrine for acceptable moral conduct. Individuals who view any form of masturbation as negative and unacceptable will need more help in understanding it as a natural, healthy expression of sexual development. In all cases it is advisable to investigate the circumstances associated with so-called masturbation, because all genital stimulation is not masturbation for sexual stimulation but may be an expression of anxiety, boredom, or unresolved conflicts. For example, a boy who repeatedly touches his penis all day is not masturbating for pleasure but may be reassuring himself that it is intact. This may be an expression of castration anxiety and should be investigated further. Children who openly and publicly masturbate are inviting a reaction, such as discipline, punishment, or criticism. They may be overwhelmed by their sexual feelings and asking others to help them channel their emotions into more constructive outlets. Masturbation may be considered excessive when it interferes with children's regular activities or causes soreness, pain, or sufficient tissue damage to create a potential for infections. As part of teaching their children socially acceptable behavior, parents should emphasize that masturbation, like other forms of sex play, is a private act.

Gifted Children

The importance of the identification of gifted children and their needs is increasingly being recognized. While the def-

---

CHARACTERISTICS OF GIFTED CHILDREN

Birth weight and head circumference above 50th percentile

Early developmental milestones, especially walking

Early development of language and complex usage of speech

Temperamental characteristics of persistence, intensity, extreme self-confidence, sensitivity, and responsiveness to stimulation

Constant questioning and curiosity

Rich fantasy, such as imaginary playmates

Highly developed sense of humor

Strong interest in special areas, such as music, science, or mechanical skills

Modified from Fish, L., and Burch, K.: Identifying gifted preschoolers, Pediatr. Nurs. 1(2):125-127, 1985; Goldsmith, L.T., and Feldman, D.H.: Identifying gifted children: the state of the art, Pediatr. Ann. 14(10):709-716, 1985.

---

inition of *gifted* varies, the most widely used criterion is superior intelligence—usually defined as an intelligence quotient of 130 or above, although this depends on the test. A broader view considers specific academic aptitude, creative or productive thinking, leadership ability, visual and performing arts, and psychomotor ability either singly or in combination as signs of giftedness (Goldsmith and Feldman, 1985; Landesman, 1985). Most children are identified as gifted when they enter school and receive IQ tests. However, not all children are so fortunate, and the tragic loss of the opportunity to develop their potential may result. Consequently nurses who are aware of the behavioral and developmental characteristics of giftedness can assess children's mental and physical capabilities and assist in early identification (Fish and Burch, 1985). The accompanying box lists those characteristics frequently observed in gifted children.

Gifted children can present unique challenges to parents. They often demand increased stimulation as infants and continue to seek a great deal of attention from their parents. Their high energy level and persistence can lead to discipline problems similar to those seen in children with difficult temperaments. Parents may be intimidated by having a child smarter than themselves and be hesitant to set limits. However, gifted children are children first and have the same needs for love, security, and consistent controls as other youngsters. Sometimes children's above average skills in one area cause adults to exaggerate their abilities in all areas and thus expect excessively mature behavior. Parents may mislabel slower achievement in a particular skill as lack of trying, when it really represents children's natural progression of abilities (McGuffog, 1985). These children also benefit from academic settings that provide enrichment and accelerated learning commensurate with their capabilties (Robinson, 1985). Consequently early identification of giftedness and appropriate parental guidance can be critical to the optimum development of giftedness and the children's emotional adjustment. A number of organizations provide information, testing, and other services to families with gifted children and to professionals.*

Aggression

Aggression refers to behavior that attempts to hurt a person or destroy property. It differs from anger, which is a temporary emotional state, but anger may be expressed through aggression. Aggression is influenced by a complex set of biologic, sociocultural, and familial variables. There is evidence that gender differences exist and that males are more aggressive than females (Maccoby and Jacklin, 1980). Preschool children are most often aggressive to peers (Fig. 15-6). Other factors that tend to increase aggressive behavior are frustration, modeling, and reinforcement.

Frustration, or the continual thwarting of self-satisfaction by parental disapproval, humiliation, punishment, and insults, can lead children to act out their frustration on others as a means of release. Especially if they fear their parents, these children will displace their anger on others, particularly peers and other authority figures. This type of aggression frequently applies to the ''well-behaved child'' at home who is a discipline problem at school or a ''bully'' among his playmates.

Modeling, or imitating behavior of significant others, is a powerful influencing force in preschoolers and may explain why aggressive behavior in children from disturbed or broken homes is usually greater than in children from harmonious families. Children who see their parents fighting, both physically or verbally, are observing behavior that they come to know as acceptable. Another aspect of modeling is establishing a double standard for acceptable conduct. For example, in some families aggression is synonymous with masculinity and boys are encouraged to defend themselves. Although defending one's rights is to be encouraged for both sexes, at times the principle of ''toughness'' or ''standing up for yourself'' is not tempered with judgment, fairness, or equality but becomes an excuse for ruling and dominating others. Such permissive aggression can be extremely anxiety-producing for children because it makes them feel out of control, even though they outwardly may appear the ''boss'' or ''leader.''

Another significant source for modeling is television. Numerous studies have found a positive correlation between viewing violent programs and immediate aggression (Singer, 1985). These findings received widespread attention when the National Institute of Mental Health concluded that violence on television does lead to aggression by children who watch the programs (Pearl, 1982). Consequently parents need encouragement to supervise programming, especially for those children with aggressive tendencies (see discussion under Play).

*The Association of the Gifted, 140 Ruffner Hall, University of Virginia, 405 Emmet St., Charlottesville, VA 22903; Foundation for Gifted and Creative Children, 395 Diamond Hill Rd., Warwick, RI 02886; Gifted Child Society, P.O. Box 120, Oakland, NJ 07436; National Association for Gifted Children, 2070 County Rd. H, St. Paul, MN 55112.

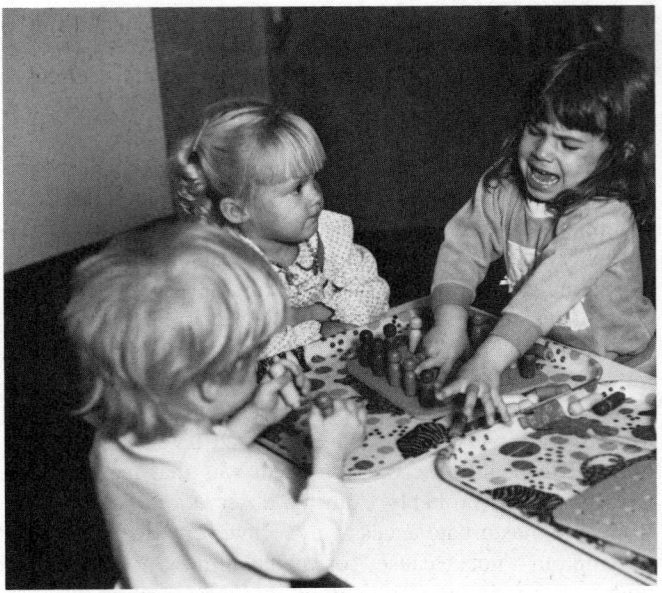

Fig. 15-6. Preschoolers generally direct their aggression toward peers, especially when their desires are frustrated.
Photography by John Roy, Saint Francis Hospital, Tulsa, OK.

Reinforcement can also shape aggressive behavior and is closely associated with modeling ''masculine'' behavior. Sometimes the reward for aggressive behavior is negative, such as punishment or disapproval, but is reinforcing because it represents attention. For example, the child who is ignored by his parents until he hits his brother or sister learns that such acts are forceful attention mechanisms. In addition, parents who permit aggressive behavior by not interfering communicate silent, implicit approval of such acts.

One of the tasks of preschoolers is learning socially acceptable behavior and the ability to control and redirect aggression toward the appropriate source. Parents can help children by modeling appropriate behavior and encouraging children to express themselves verbally. For example, rather than hitting another child for taking a toy, parents can suggest that the child state how he feels, such as ''I am angry when you take my ball. Give it back.''

Children should not be made to feel guilty or ashamed for being angry or frustrated. When they recognize these feelings, they are better able to channel them into constructive, not destructive, outlets. One of the earliest demonstrations of aggression is temper tantrums. If parents handle them constructively by not attending to or reinforcing them and by helping children find control through appropriate play situations, young children will learn to acknowledge such feelings and express them in alternative ways, such as pounding on clay or hitting a punching bag. When children are out of control, they may need to be physically restrained or removed from the scene to prevent them from hurting themselves or others. Such actions should not be seen as punishment but as clear messages that such behavior is not tolerated (Anderson, 1978).

Sometimes the type of discipline employed to extinguish other forms of unacceptable behavior actually promotes aggressive behavior. For example, if the child is spanked for the act, aggression is employed to "teach" a lesson against aggression! Parental permissiveness and lack of discipline may also foster aggressiveness (Shonkoff, 1983). The combined use of time-out and reinforcement for solitary play has been found to be an effective intervention for aggression (Wahler and Fox, 1980). In addition, approaches to minimizing anger and frustration can lead to fewer opportunities for acting out behavior (see box, p. 607).

When extreme behaviors, such as aggression, are present in children, parents are often concerned about the need for professional help. Generally, the difference between "normal" and "problematic" behavior is not the actual behavior, but the *quantity* (number of occurrences), *severity* (interfering with social or cognitive functioning), *distribution* (different manifestations), and *duration* (at least 4 weeks) of the activity. In addition, any *sudden change* in behavior should be taken seriously (Phillips, Sarles, and Friedman, 1980). When aggressive tendencies are evaluated, these factors are assessed to distinguish between behaviors typically seen at various ages and those that may represent an underlying problem.

Speech Problems

The most critical period for speech development occurs between 2 and 4 years of age. During this period the child is using his rapidly growing vocabulary to interact with the environment. However, the rate of vocabulary acquisition does not parallel the advancing mental ability or the degree of comprehnsion. This failure to master sensorimotor integrations results in the child's stuttering or stammering as he tries to say the word he is already thinking about. This hesitancy or nonfluency in speech pattern is a *normal* characteristic of language development. However, when parents or other significant caregivers place undue emphasis or stress on this pattern, a real speech problem can occur. Children who are pressured into producing sounds ahead of schedule may cope by reverting to baby speech or stuttering.

The best therapy for speech problems is prevention and early detection. One of the most essential factors involves anticipatory preparation of parents for the expected hesitation in speech during the preschool period and discussion of developmental achievements characteristic of children in each age-group. Each of these is discussed in Chapter 25 and should be included in the health promotion of preschoolers.

Coping with Stress

Although the preschool years generally are less troublesome than toddlerhood for parents, this period of life presents children with many unique stresses. Many are innate and stem from their unique understanding of the world, such as fears. Others are imposed, such as beginning school. Although minimum amounts of stress are beneficial during the

SOURCES OF STRESS IN PRESCHOOLERS

Three-year-old:

Infantile behavior—reverts to babyish ways; can't completely let go of babyhood

Stubbornness—although the child is developing an interest in social relationships and a concept of "we," the child may lapse into uncooperative behavior

Possessiveness—guards belongings and may be bossy about them

Jealousy—particularly when it comes to parents' love

Separation anxiety

Stranger anxiety

Confusion—can't always discriminate between fantasy and reality

White lies—may result from wishful thinking, fantasy, and desire to please or impress

Imaginary playmate—often blamed in the white lies

Fears—may be precipitated by imagination; may also fear dogs or other animals

Speech—may stutter or stumble over words

Activity level—seems to be in perpetual motion; may exhaust himself or herself

Eating—may forget to eat or lose interest in food

Nap or bedtime—may fear bad dreams, the dark, or missing out on some fun while asleep

Destructiveness—may enjoy wrecking or destroying

Questions—continually asks "why," and is upset if trusted adults do not respond or do not know the answer

Four-year-old:

Insecurity—may develop nervous habits such as nail biting, facial tic, thumb-sucking, genital manipulation, eye-blinking, or nose-picking; may insist on bringing a familiar item from home to preschool

Exaggerations—may attempt to boost self-image with boasts

Companionship—enjoys interacting with friends, although there may be many quarrels

Silliness—tends to engage in rambunctious, silly play; likes words and is fascinated by rhyming syllables or foul language; is disciplined for lack of control

Property rights—protects belongings; may become bossy

Sex—interested in the human body; may engage in exhibitionism

Activity level—enjoys running, jumping, and slamming doors; may be punished for disruptive behavior

Fears—picks up fears from adults; may fear dark room, snakes and lizards, or anything perceived as "creepy"

Attention—likes to talk and is frustrated if ignored or put off; whines to get own way

Five-year-old:

Approval—parents' love and acceptance are vital; seeks praise

School—may have difficulty adjusting to kindergarten

Separation anxiety—particularly fears loss of mother

Infantile behavior—may occasionally lapse into babyish behavior as a result of realizing that babyhood is ended

Worrying—may develop irrational fears, take information out of context, or fret over a misinterpreted, overheard conversation

Masturbation—is concerned about being "bad"

Belongings—protects possessions

Showing off—performs in order to gain praise

Procrastination—may dillydally now and then

Name calling—insults others to boost self-image, but is upset when she or he is the victim of mockery

From Kuczen, B.: Childhood stress: don't let your child be a victim, New York, 1982, Delacorte Press, pp. 15-17.

early years to help children develop effective coping skills, excessive stress is harmful, and young children are especially vulnerable because of their limited capacity to cope.

To help parents deal with stress in their child's life, they must be aware of signs of stress (see p. 128) and be helped to identify the source (see box, p. 645). In addition, any number of other stresses may be present, such as the birth of a sibling, marital discord, relocation, or illness. The best approach to dealing with stress is prevention—monitoring the amount of stress in children's lives so that levels exceeding their coping ability do not occur. In many instances structuring children's schedules to allow rest and preparing them for change, such as entering school, are sufficient measures. Because stress is such a constant aspect of daily living, the preschool years are not too young to help children learn to cope with stress. They can learn the meaning of the word *stress* and recognize physical signs of stress reaction, such as rapid pulse, pounding heart, or fatigue. Teaching children relaxation and imagery is very effective. Young children can learn to ''let their bodies go limp like a rag doll'' or ''imagine flying like bird.'' Parents can use stories to help children imagine pleasurable events. As language skills improve, preschoolers should be encouraged to talk about their feelings and to explore other ways of expressing emotions. Play is an excellent vehicle for venting anger or frustration, and toys such as drums, clay, and punching bags provide alternative methods of dissipating anxiety. Toys also begin to teach socially acceptable ways of dealing with such feelings.

Fears

The greatest number and variety of real and imagined fears are present during the preschool years and include fear of the dark, being left alone (especially at bedtime), animals (particularly large dogs and snakes), ghosts, sexual matters (castration), and objects or persons associated with pain. The exact cause of children's fears is unknown. Freudians believe that the upsurge of fears during the preschool years results from the anxiety of being injured and mutilated (castration complex). Piaget views fears as a product of the type of thinking of children in this age-group. Preschoolers are caught between the egocentric thinking of infants, which protects them from imagined fears, and the more logical thought processes of school-age children, which help explain and dispel potential fears. Children in the preconceptual stage still engage in egocentric thought but are now able to imagine an event without actually experiencing it. For example, seeing someone hurt is sufficient for realizing what the hurt must be like and for consequently fearing that hurt. In medical practice this is frequently observed. If a young child witnesses another child getting an injection, he becomes very upset, almost as if he himself had received the injection. The concept of animism (ascribing lifelike qualities to inanimate objects) explains why children fear objects. For example, hearing the noise of a vacuum cleaner *means* it is ''noisy,'' ''angry,'' and ''mean.''

A fear that is peculiar to this age is fear of annihilation. Because of poorly defined body boundaries and improved cognitive abilities, toddlers develop concerns related to loss of body parts, such as feces being flushed away or bath water going down the drain. Although they are now aware that objects can disappear, preschool children cannot understand concepts of size, for example, that they cannot disappear down the drain because they are too large.

Preschoolers are also likely to develop parent-induced fears—fears that stem from imitating their parents. When parents demonstrate their fears, the concerns are communicated to the children. Such fears tend to be long-lasting and difficult to dispel (Wolman, 1978).

The best way to help children overcome their fears is by actively involving them in finding practical methods to deal with experiences that frighten them. This may be as simple as keeping a dim night-light on in the child's bedroom to assure him that no monsters lurk in the dark or letting the child bathe a doll or play with toys in a tub of water and then opening the drain with the toys still in the tub to demonstrate that large objects cannot go down the drain. In this way the experience that created the fear in the child can be reconstructed without involving the child directly as the victim. The child is allowed alternative methods to feel in control and powerful while overcoming his fear.

Exposing children to the feared object in a safe situation provides a type of conditioning or desensitization. For instance, children who are afraid of dogs should never be forced to approach or touch one, but they may be gradually introduced to the experience by watching other children play with the animal. This type of modeling, demonstrating fearlessness in others, can be very effective if the child is allowed to progress at his own rate.

Sometimes fears do not subside with simple measures or developmental maturation. When children experience severe fears that disrupt family life, professional help is required. Successful training programs may include (1) muscle relaxation, (2) imagining a pleasant scene, and (3) reciting brave statements. Rewards or ''tokens'' may be given for ''bravery'' and not being afraid (Graziano and Mooney, 1980). Such interventions can be applied in clinical settings to reduce fears (e.g., of being alone or of painful procedures).

Promoting Optimum Health During the Preschool Years

Health promotion mainly involves guidance regarding nutrition, sleep, dental health, and injury prevention. A brief discussion of each subject is presented to emphasize the particular needs or differences of preschoolers vs toddlers. (For a more comprehensive understanding the reader is urged to also review the material presented in Chapter 14 under Promoting optimum health during the toddler years.)

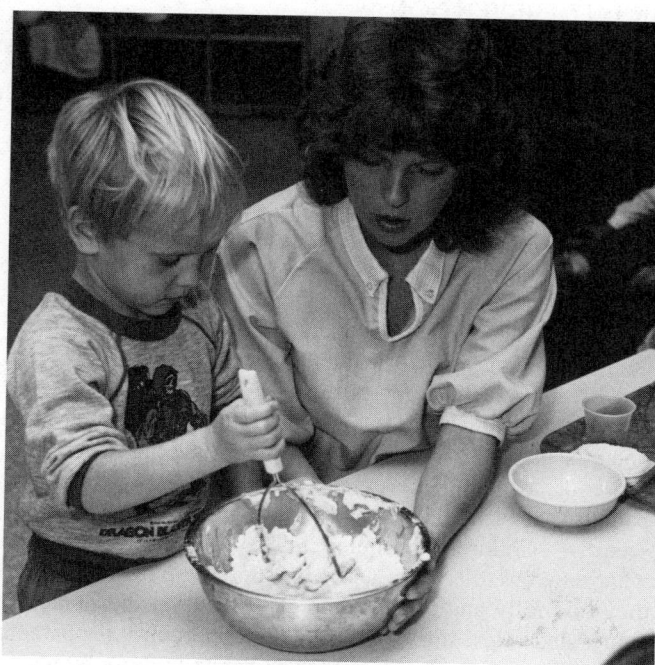

Fig. 15-7. Preschool children enjoy helping adults and are more likely to try new foods if they can assist in the preparation. Photography by John Roy, Saint Francis Hospital, Tulsa, OK.

NUTRITION

Nutritional requirements for preschoolers are fairly similar to those for toddlers. The requirement for calories per unit of body weight continues to decrease slightly to 85 kcal per kg for an average daily intake of 1700 calories. Fluid requirements may also decrease slightly to about 100 ml per kg daily but depend on activity level, climatic conditions, and state of health. Protein requirements are 1.5 g per kg for an average daily consumption of 30 g.

Some preschoolers still have food habits that are typical of toddlers, such as food fads and strong taste preferences. When children reach 4 years of age, they seem to enter another period of finicky eating, which is generally characteristic of the more rebellious and rowdy behavior of children in this age-group. By age 5 years children are greatly influenced by the food habits of others and are more agreeable to try new foods, especially if encouraged by an adult who allows the child to help with food preparation or experiments with a new taste or different dish (Fig. 15-7). Mealtimes can become battlegrounds if parents expect impeccable table manners. Usually the 5-year-old child is ready for the "social" side of eating, but the 3- or 4-year-old child still has difficulty sitting quietly through a long family meal.

Parents sometimes worry about the quantity of food preschoolers consume. In general, the quality is much more important than the quantity, a fact that should be stressed during nutritional counseling. Young children often consume more food than parents realize. One approach toward lessening this parental concern is advising parents to keep a weekly record of everything the child eats. In particular, the need for measuring the amount of food, such as setting aside ½ cup of vegetables, and serving the child from this premeasured amount should be stressed. In this way there is a more accurate estimate of food intake at each meal. Usually by the end of the week when they look at the food chart parents are amazed at how much the child has consumed, even though at each meal the amount seemed minimum. In general, preschoolers consume only slightly more than toddlers, or about half of an adult's portion.

SLEEP AND ACTIVITY

Sleep patterns vary widely, but the average preschooler sleeps about 12 hours a night and infrequently takes daytime naps. Children with reported sleep problems sleep less than those without sleeping difficulties (Edgil, Wood, and Smith, 1985; Smith, 1986b). Activity levels continue to be high, although quiet activities, such as television, are increasingly appealing and can become an unhealthy substitute for active play. Preschoolers' increased gross motor abilities and coordination provide them the opportunity to engage in many sports, if only at a novice level. Whether young children should begin formalized training in an activity at this early age is controversial. The consensus is to expose children to a wide variety of physical activities rather than concentrate on one area. However, children's interest in specific events should be respected, since early training can be advantageous.

Sleep Disturbances

The preschool years are a prime time for sleep disturbances. Young children sometimes have trouble going to sleep, especially after so much activity and stimulation during the day. Others may develop bedtime fears, wake during the night, or have nightmares. Still others may prolong the inevitable through elaborate rituals.

After a careful assessment of the events surrounding the problem, a recommended approach involves counseling parents about the importance of a consistent bedtime ritual and emphasizing the normalcy of this type of behavior in young children. Attention-seeking behavior should be ignored, and the child should not be taken into the parents' bed or allowed to stay up past a reasonable hour. If nightmares occur, the child should be comforted but left in his own bed. Sometimes the child's door must be locked in order to enforce the limits, although the safety of this procedure in case of a fire must always be considered. Other measures that may be helpful include keeping a light on in the room, providing transitional objects, such as a favorite toy, or leaving a drink of water by the bed. (For a further discussion of sleep problems and interventions, see p. 525.)

Helping children slow down before bedtime also contributes to less resistance to going to bed. One approach is to establish limited rituals that signal readiness for bed, such as a bath or story. Parents can reinforce the pattern by stating, "After this story it is bedtime," and consistently carrying through the routine. If extra stimulation such as having visitors arrive at bedtime is disruptive to children's routine, it is advisable to settle children in bed beforehand.

For some children a change in eating habits may be helpful, such as increasing the protein intake with snacks of peanut butter, cheese, or nuts (Morris and Lubin, 1985). L-Tryptophan, an amino acid, has been shown to be an effective sleeping aid.

Children with sleeping problems resistant to these approaches may benefit from a program of neuromuscular relaxation (Schumann, 1981). Helping children learn head-to-toe relaxation may facilitate falling asleep at bedtime and on nighttime awakening.

DENTAL HEALTH

By the beginning of the preschool period, the eruption of the deciduous teeth is complete. Dental care is essential to preserve these temporary teeth and to teach good dental habits (see Chapter 14). Although preschoolers' fine motor control is improved, they still require assistance and supervision with brushing, and flossing should be done by parents. For children cared for away from home, parents are encouraged to monitor the dental care provided by others, including the diet to keep cariogenic foods to a minimum.

INJURY PREVENTION

Because of improved gross and fine motor skills, coordination, and balance, preschoolers are less prone to falls than toddlers. They tend to be less reckless, listen more to parental rules, and are aware of potential danger, such as hot objects, sharp instruments, and dangerous heights. Putting objects in the mouth as part of exploration has all but ceased, although poisoning is still a danger. Pedestrian motor vehicle injuries increase from activities such as playing in the street, riding tricycles, running after balls, or forgetting safety regulations when crossing streets. In general, the guidelines suggested for injury prevention in Table 14-10, p. 617, apply to children in this age-group as well.

However, emphasis is now on *education* for safety and potential hazards, in addition to appropriate protection. Because preschoolers are great imitators, it is essential that parents set a good example by "practicing what they preach." Children are quick to observe discrepancies in what they are told to do and what they see others do. Since they faithfully and unquestioningly believe in their parents' values and rules, this is an excellent opportunity for parents to practice and teach safe, cautious habits in daily living.

ANTICIPATORY GUIDANCE—CARE OF FAMILIES

Although the preschool years present fewer childrearing difficulties than earlier years, this stage of development is facili-

---

Table 15-3 Parental guidance during preschool years

AGE (YEARS)	GUIDANCE	AGE (YEARS)	GUIDANCE
3	Prepare parents for child's increasing interest in widening relationships	4	Prepare for more aggressive behavior including motor activity and shocking language
	Encourage enrollment in nursery school		Expect resistance to parental authority
	Emphasize importance of setting limits		Explore parental feelings regarding child's behavior
	Prepare parents to expect exaggerated tension-reduction behaviors, such as need for "security blanket"		Suggest some kind of respite for primary caregiver such as placing child in nursery school for part of day
	Encourage parents to offer child choices when child vacillates		Prepare for increasing sexual curiosity
	Expect marked changes at 3½ years when child becomes less coordinated (in motor and emotional control), becomes insecure, exhibits emotional extremes, and develops behaviors such as stuttering		Emphasize importance of realistic limit-setting on behavior and appropriate discipline techniques
			Prepare parents for the highly imaginary 4-year-old who indulges in "tall tales" (to be differentiated from lies) and for child's acquisition of imaginary playmates
	Prepare parents to expect extra demands on their attention as a reflection of child's emotional insecurity and fear of loss of love		Suggest swimming lessons if not begun earlier
	Warn parents that the equilibrium of the 3-year-old will change to the aggressive out-of-bounds behavior of the 4-year-old		Explain Oedipus feelings and reactions
			Expect nightmares or an increase in them and suggest parents make certain the child is fully awakened from a frightening dream
	Anticipate a more stable appetite with more expansive food selection		Provide reassurance that a period of calm begins at 5 years of age
	Stress needs for protection and education of child to prevent injury		
		5	Expect a tranquil period at 5 years
			Prepare and assist child through initial entrance into school environment
			Make certain immunizations are up-to-date before entering school

tated by appropriate anticipatory guidance in the areas already discussed (Table 15-3). There is also a shift in childrearing practices from one mainly of protection to one primarily of education, especially in terms of injury prevention.

During this period an emotional transition between parent and child occurs. Although children are still attached to their parents and accept all their values and beliefs, they are nearing the period of life when they will question previous teachings and prefer the companionship of peers. Entry into school marks a separation for parents, as well as for children. Parents need help in adjusting to this change, particularly if the mother has focused her daily activity on home responsibilities. As preschoolers begin nursery or elementary school, mothers may need to seek activities beyond the family, such as community involvement or pursuing a career. In this way all family members are adjusting to change, which is part of the process of growing and developing.

- In selecting a daycare facility parents should inquire about daily programs, teacher qualifications, accreditation, student-to-staff ratio, safety, meals, fees, and sanitary conditions.

- Two rules that govern answering questions about sex and other sensitive issues are to find out what the child thinks and to be honest.

- Preschool aggression may result from frustration, modeling behavior, and reinforcement.

- Fears constitute a great part of preschool period; objects, potential annihilation, and parent-induced fears are common sources.

CONCEPT SUMMARIES

- The preschool years comprise the period from 3 to 5 years of age, a time that is considered critical for emotional and psychologic development.

- Biologic development in the preschool period is characterized by mature body systems and refinement in gross and fine motor behavior, as evidenced by participation in activities such as running, riding a bicycle, and drawing.

- According to Erikson, acquiring a sense of initiative is the chief psychosocial task of the preschooler. Development of the superego occurs during this period, and conscience begins to emerge.

- In Freudian theory, preschoolers are in the oedipal stage. Resolution of this stage occurs when children strongly identify with their parent of the same sex.

- According to Piaget, the preschool age is characterized by intuitive or prelogical thinking and a move toward logical thought processes through advanced, complex learning, language, and understanding of causality.

- The seeds of moral development are planted during the preschool period. According to Kohlberg, children are in the stage of naive instrumental orientation, in which they are concerned with satisfying their own needs and, less frequently, the needs of others.

- Social development booms in this period with individuation-separation, more sophisticated language, greater independence, and more complex, imaginative forms of play.

- A major concern in the preschool period is the effect of temperament on adjustment in group situations and the long-term consequences of temperamental characteristics.

- Four areas of special concern to parents during the preschool period are preschool or daycare experience, sex education, speech problems, and stress.

REFERENCES

Alpert, G., and others: Outbreak of cryptosporidiosis in a day-care center, Pediatrics **77**(2):152-157, 1986.

Anderson, L.S.: The aggressive child, Children Today **7**(1):11-14, 1978.

Bartlett, A.V., and others: Diarrheal illness among infants and toddlers in day care centers, part I, epidemiology and pathogens, J. Pediatr. **107**(4):495-502, 1985.

Carey, W.: Intervention strategies using temperament data. In Brown, C., editor: Infants at risk: assessment and intervention, Skillman, NJ, 1981, Johnson & Johnson Baby Products Co.

Chess, S., and Thomas, A.: Dynamics of individual behavioral development. In Levine, M.D., and others, editors: Developmental-behavioral pediatrics, Philadelphia, 1983, W.B. Saunders Co.

Edgil, A., Wood, K., and Smith, D.: Sleep problems of older infants and preschool children, Pediatr. Nurs. **11**(2):87-89, 1985.

Fish, L., and Burch, K.: Identifying gifted preschoolers, Pediatr. Nurs. **1**(2):125-127, 1985.

Goldsmith, L.T., and Feldman, D.H.: Identifying gifted children: the state of the art, Pediatr. Ann. **14**(10):709-716, 1985.

Goldsmith, S.: Human sexuality: the family source book, St. Louis, 1986, The C.V. Mosby Co.

Graziano, A.M., and Mooney, K.C.: Family self-control instruction for children's nighttime fear reduction, J. Consult. Clin. Psychol. **48**(2):206-213, 1980.

Kellogg, R.: Understanding children's art. In Readings in Psychology Today, Del Mar, CA, 1969, Communications/Research/Machines/Inc.

Landesman, S.: Defining giftedness, Pediatr. Ann. **14**(10):698-706, 1985.

Lowrey, G.: Growth and development of children, ed. 8, Chicago, 1986, Year Book Medical Publishers.

Maccoby, E.E., and Jacklin, C.N.: Sex differences in aggression: a rejoinder and reprise, Child Dev. **51**:964-980, 1980.

McDevitt, S., and Carey, W.: The measurement of temperament in 3-7 year old children, J. Child Psychol. Psychiatry **19**:245-253, 1978.

McGuffog, C.: Problems of gifted children, Pediatr. Ann. **14**(10):719-726, 1985.

Morris, D., and Lubin, A.: A review of the symposium: "diet and behavior—a multidisciplinary evaluation," Contemp. Nutr. **10**(5):1-2, 1985.

Palumbo, F.M., and Dietz, W.H., Jr.: Children's television: its effect on nutrition and cognitive development, Pediatr. Ann. **14**(12):793-801, 1985.

Pass, R., and others: Increased frequency of cytomegalovirus infection in children in group day care, Pediatrics **74**(1):121-126, 1984.

Pearl, D., editor: Television and behavior: ten years of scientific progress and implications for the eighties I. U.S. Department of Health and Human Services, No. ADH82-1195, 1982.

Phillips, S., Sarles, R., and Friedman, S.: Consultation and referral: when, why, and how, Pediatr. Ann. **9**(7):36-45, 1980.

Robinson, N.M.: Educational options for gifted children, Pediatr. Ann. **14**(10):745-756, 1985.

Schor, D.P.: Temperament and the initial school experience, Child. Health Care **13**(3):129-134, 1985.

Schumann, M.J.: A method for inducing sleep in young children, Pediatr. Nurs. **7**(5):9-13, 1981.

Selekman, J.: The development of body image in the child: a learned response, Top. Clin. Nurs. 5(1):12-21, 1983.

Shelly, J., and others: The spiritual needs of children, Downer's Grove, IL, 1982, Inter-Varsity Press.

Shonkoff, J.P.: Preschool. In Levine, M.D., and others, editors: Developmental-behavioral pediatrics, Philadelphia, 1983, W.B. Saunders Co.

Singer, D.G.: Does violent television produce aggressive children? Pediatr. Ann. 14(12):804-810, 1985.

Smith, D.: Common diseases children contract in day care: patterns and prevention, Pediatr. Nurs. 12(3):175-179, 1986a.

Smith, D.: Sleep problems in children, Child Care Newsletter 5(1):4-6, 1986b.

Soderman, A., and Whiren, A.: Assessing quality day care: a checklist, Day Care Early Educ. 8:9-12, 1980.

Thomas, A., and Chess, S.: Genesis and evolution of behavioral disorders: from infancy to early adult life, Am. J. Psychiatry 141:1-9, 1984.

Thomas, R.M.: Comparing theories of child development, ed. 2, Belmont, CA, 1985, Wadsworth Publishing Co.

Wahler, R.G., and Fox, J.J.: Solitary toy play and time out: a family treatment package for children with aggressive and oppositional behavior, J. Appl. Behav. Anal. 13(1):23-39, 1980.

Wolman, B.B.: Children's fears, New York, 1978, Grossett & Dunlap.

Wong, D.: Guiding parents in selecting day-care centers, Pediatr. Nurs. 12(3):181-187, 1986.

Zuckerman, D.M., and Zuckerman, B.S.: Television's impact on children, Pediatrics 75(2):233-240, 1985.

BIBLIOGRAPHY

References specific to preschoolers are included here; additional references can be found in Chapters 12 and 14.

Growth and Development

American Academy of Pediatrics, Committee on Pediatric Aspects of Physical Education, Recreation, and Sports: Fitness in the preschool child, Pediatrics 58(1):88-89, 1976.

Ames, L.B., and Ilg, F.I.: Your three-year-old: friend or enemy, New York, 1980, Delacorte Press.

Ames, L.B., and Ilg, F.I.: Your four-year-old: wild and wonderful, New York, 1981, Delacorte Press.

Ames, L.B., and Ilg, F.I.: Your five-year-old: sunny and serene, New York, 1981, Delacorte Press.

Betz, C.: Faith development in children, Pediatr. Nurs. 7(2):22-25, 1981.

Dietz, W.H., Jr., and Gortmaker, S.L.: Do we fatten our children at the television set? Obesity and television viewing in children and adolescents, Pediatrics 75(5):807-812, 1985.

Kay, P.: The imaginary companion: review of the literature, Matern. Child Nurs. J. 9:8-11, 1980.

Mitchell, S.: Imaginary companions: friend or foe? Pediatr. Nurs. 6(6):29-30, 1980.

Murray, J.P.: Television & youth: 25 years of research & controversy, Boys Town, NE, 1980, The Boys Town Center for the Study of Youth Development.

Palumbo, F.M.: Television: effects on the development of children. In Children are different: behavioral development monograph series: Number 14, Columbus, OH, 1985, Ross Laboratories.

Rothenberg, M.B.: Role of television in shaping the attitudes of children, Child. Health Care 13(4):148-149, 1985.

Sahler, O.J., and McAnarney, E.R.: The child from three to eighteen, St. Louis, 1981, The C.V. Mosby Co.

Schickendanz, J., and Schickendanz, D.: Toward understanding children, Boston, 1983, Little, Brown & Co., Inc.

Preschool or Daycare Experience

American Academy of Pediatrics, Committee on Early Childhood, Adoption, and Dependent Care: The pediatrician's role in promoting the health of a patient in day care, Pediatrics 74(1):157-158, 1984.

American Academy of Pediatrics, Committee on Psychosocial Aspects of Child and Family Health: The mother working outside the home, Pediatrics 73(6):874-875, 1984.

Baker, J., and Proett, P.: One hospital's response: a child care referral service, Am. J. Nurs. 83(4):550-551, 1983.

Ballard, P.: Selecting child care, Issues Compr. Pediatr. Nurs. 5:219-231, 1981.

Bartlett, A.V., and others: Diarrheal illness among infants and toddlers in day care centers. Part II. Comparison with day care homes and households, J. Pediatr. 107(4):503-509, 1985.

Berkseth, J.: Assisting clients with day care decisions, Nurs. Practitioner 5(4):12-16, 1980.

Chabin, M.: Hospital-supported child care, Am. J. Nurs. 83(4):548-551, 1983.

Chang, A., and others: Care of mildly ill children enrolled in day-care centers, West. J. Med. 134(2):181-185, 1981.

Child Day Care Infectious Disease Study Group: Infectious diseases in day care centers, J. Pediatr. 105(5):683-701, 1984.

Child Welfare League of America, Standards for Day Care Service, New York, 1984, The League.

Clore, E.: The working mother with young children, Child Care Newsletter 4(1):4-6, 1985.

Crowther, J.H., Bond, L.A., and Rolf, J.E.: The incidence, prevalence, and severity of behavior disorders among preschool-aged children in day care, J. Abnorm. Child Psychol. 9(1):23-42, 1981.

Goodman, N., and Andrews, J.: Cognitive development of children in family and group day care, Am. J. Orthopsychiatry 51(2):271-284, 1981.

Goodman, R., and others: Infectious diseases and child day care, Pediatrics 74(1):134-139, 1984.

Hadler, S.C., and others: Risk factors for hepatitis A in day care centers, J. Infect. Dis. 145(2):255-261, 1982.

Hadler, S.C., and others: Do day-care centers pose excessive health risks to children? JAMA 249(1):48-53, 1983.

Istre, G.R., and others: Risk factors for primary invasive *Haemophilus influenzae* disease: increased risk from day care attendance and school-aged household members, J. Pediatr. 106(2):190-195, 1985.

Jordan-March, M.: Factors in the delivery of comprehensive services through child care programs, West. J. Nurs. Res. 5(4):337-353, 1983.

Mayer, G.: Choosing daycare, Am. J. Nurs. 81(2):346-348, 1981.

Nahata, M.C.: Prevention of infection by handwashing, Child Care Newsletter 5(1):6-8, 1986.

Ogden, L.: Day-care diseases, Home Healthcare Nurs. 2(1):48-49, 1984.

Payne, P.A.: Day care and its impact on parenting, Nurs. Clin. North Am. 12(3):525-533, 1977.

Pickering, L.K., and others: Occurrence of *Giardia lamblia* in children in day care centers, J. Pediatr. 104(4):522-526, 1984.

Richardson, J.: Nursery schools, Midwife Health Visit Community Nurse 16(6):256, 1980.

Rutter, M.: Social-emotional consequences of day care for preschool children, Am. J. Orthopsychiatry 51(1):4-28, 1981.

Smith, D.: Myths about day care: fact or fantasy? Pediatr. Nurs. 10(4):278-280, 1984.

Solomons, H.: Accidents in day-care centers, Child. Nurse 3(6):1-4, 1985.

Solomons, H., and others: Is day care safe for children? Accident records reviewed, Child. Health Care 10(3):90-93, 1982.

Trumpp, C.E., and Karasic, R.: Management of communicable diseases in day care centers, Pediatr. Ann. 12(3):219-229, 1983.

Watkins, S.: The day care decision, Pediatr. Nurs. 4(3):9-11, 1978.

Sex Education

Aquilino, M.L., and Ely, J.: Parents and the sexuality of preschool children, Pediatr. Nurs. 11(1):41-46, 1985.

Bullough, V., and Bullough, B.: PNPs, patients, parents, and sexuality, Pediatr. Nurs. 8(3):177-182, 1982.

Calderone, M.S.: Sexual health and the child, Compr. Ther. 6(12):3-7, 1980.

Calderone, M.S.: Adolescent sexuality: elements and genesis, Pediatrics (suppl.) 76(4):699-703, 1985.

Children's books on sex and siblings, Am. J. Nurs. **79**(11):1968, 1979.

Gallo, A.: Early childhood masturbation, Pediatr. Nurs. **5**(5):47-49, 1979.

Greydanus, D.E., and Geller, B.: Masturbation, N.Y. State J. Med. **80**(12):1892-1896, 1980.

Malinowski, J.S.: Answering a child's questions about sex and a new baby, Am. J. Nurs. **79**(11):1965-1968, 1979.

Aggression

Bloomfield, I.: Psychological aspects of violence and aggression, Int. J. Soc. Psychiatry **26**(3):218-221, 1980.

Hayes, S.C., Rincover, A., and Volosin, D.: Variables influencing the acquisition and maintenance of aggressive behavior: modeling versus sensory reinforcement, J. Abnorm. Psychol. **89**(2):254-262, 1980.

Jacklin, C.N., and Maccoby, E.E.: Issues of gender differentiation. In Levine, M.D., and others, editors: Developmental-behavioral pediatrics, Philadelphia, 1983, W.B. Saunders Co.

Penalver, M.: Helping the child handle his aggression, Am. J. Nurs. **73**(9):1554-1555, 1973.

Sleep Problems

Anders, T.F., Carskadon, M.A., and Dement, W.C.: Sleep and sleepiness in children and adolescents, Pediatr. Clin. North Am. **27**(1):29-43, 1980.

Hewitt, K.E.: Sleeping problems in pre-school children: what to ask and what to do, Health Visitor **54**:100-101, March 1980.

Inglis, S.: The nocturnal frustration of sleep disturbance, Am. J. Matern. Child Nurs. **1**(5):280-287, 1976.

Jones, D.P.H., and Verduyn, C.M.: Behavioural management of sleep problems, Arch. Dis. Child. **58**:442-444, 1983.

Prescott-Day, S.: Sleep variations of the pre-school child, Health Visitor **52**:465-468, Nov. 1979.

Schowalter, J.E.: Emotional disorders in children. In Children are different: behavioral development monograph series: Number 4, Columbus, OH, 1983, Ross Laboratories.

Siegel, F.: Eating and sleeping difficulties in young children, Consultant **22**(10):95-107, 1982.

Fears

Derevensky, J.L.: Children's fears: a developmental comparison of normal and exceptional children, J. Genetic Psychol. **135**:11-21, 1979.

DuPont, R.L.: Phobias in children, J. Pediatr. **102**(6):999-1002, 1983.

Graziano, A.M., Degiovanni, I.S., and Garcia, K.A.: Behavioral treatment of children's fears: a review, Psychol. Bull. **86**(4):804-830, 1979.

Miller, S.R.: Children's fears: a review of the literature with implications for nursing research and practice, Nurs. Res. **28**(4):217-223, 1979.

SUGGESTED READINGS FOR PARENTS ON DAYCARE

Child sexual abuse prevention: tips to parents, U.S. DHHS, National Center on Child Abuse and Neglect, 1984. (Includes an excellent section on choosing a child care center; copies are free from NCCAN Clearinghouse, P.O. Box 1182, Washington, DC 20013.)

Clark-Stewart, A.: Daycare, Cambridge, MA, 1982, Harvard University Press.

Coleman, M., and Priner, P.: What about day care? Columbia, MO, 1980, Missouri Cooperative Extension Service, University of Missouri-Lincoln University. (Single copies are $1.00 and may be ordered from Cooperative Extension Service, 1408 I. 70 Drive, S.W., Columbia, MO 65203.)

Endsley, R.G., and Bradbard, M.: Quality day care: a handbook of choices for parents and caregivers, Englewood Cliffs, NJ, 1981, Prentice-Hall, Inc.

How to choose a good early childhood program, Washington, DC, 1984, National Association for the Education of Young Children. (Single copies are free with a self-addressed, stamped, business-size envelope from NAEYC, 1834 Connecticut Avenue, N.W., Washington, DC 20009.)

Mitchell, G.: The day care book, Briarcliff Manor, NY, 1979, Stein & Day Publishers, Scarborough House.

Plain talk about when your child starts school, Rockville, MD, 1980, National Institute of Mental Health, US DHHS Pub. No. (ADM)80-1021.

Rogers, F.: Going to day care, New York, 1985, G.P. Putnam's Sons. (Recommended for preparing young children for day care.)

Rogers, F.: When your child goes to school, Pittsburgh, Family Communications, Inc.

Rogers, F.: When you have a child in day care, Pittsburgh, Family Communications, Inc.

Scarr, S.: Mother care/other care, New York, 1984, Basic Books, Inc., Publishers.

Seigel-Gorelick, B: The working parent's guide to child care, Boston, 1983, Little, Brown & Co., Inc.

Tips on selecting the ''right'' day care facility, Elk Grove Village, IL, 1985, American Academy of Pediatrics. (Single copies are $.50 and may be ordered from the Academy, P.O. Box 927, Elk Grove Village, IL 60007.)

Chapter 16

Health Problems of Early Childhood

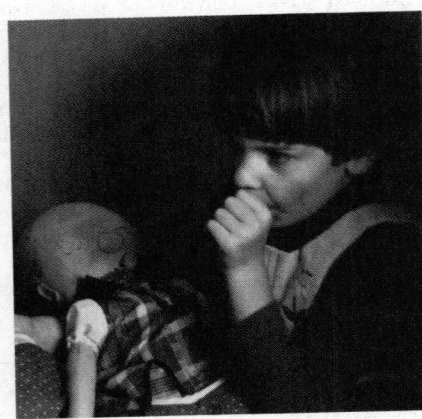

Disorders Related to Infectious Processes
　Communicable diseases
　　Nursing considerations
　Conjunctivitis
　　Clinical manifestations
　　Therapeutic management
　　Nursing considerations

Parasitic Intestinal Infections
　General nursing considerations
　Giardiasis
　　Life cycle, pathogenesis, and transmission
　　Clinical manifestations
　　Diagnostic evaluation
　　Therapeutic management
　　Nursing considerations
　Enterobiasis (pinworms)
　　Life cycle, pathogenesis, and transmission

　　Clinical manifestations
　　Diagnostic evaluation
　　Therapeutic management
　　Nursing considerations

Ingestion of Injurious Agents
　Principles of emergency treatment
　　Assessment
　　Gastric decontamination
　　Family support
　　Prevention of recurrence
　Plants
　Salicylate poisoning
　　Pathophysiology and clinical manifestations
　　Diagnostic evaluation
　　Therapeutic management
　　Nursing considerations
　Acetaminophen poisoning
　　Pathophysiology
　　Clinical manifestations
　　Diagnostic evaluation
　　Therapeutic management
　　Nursing considerations
　Heavy metal poisoning
　Iron poisoning
　　Clinical manifestations
　　Diagnostic evaluation
　　Therapeutic management
　　Nursing considerations
　Lead poisoning (plumbism)
　　Factors related to lead ingestion
　　Pathophysiology and clinical manifestations
　　Diagnostic evaluation
　　Therapeutic management
　　Nursing considerations

Child Maltreatment
　Child neglect
　　Types of neglect
　　Identification of neglect
　　Nursing considerations
　Physical abuse
　　Factors predisposing to physical abuse
　　Identification of physical abuse
　　Nursing considerations
　Sexual abuse
　　Characteristics of abusers and victims
　　Initiation and perpetuation of sexual abuse
　　Identification of sexual abuse
　　Nursing considerations

This chapter is concerned with health problems that occur most frequently during the early childhood years, such as poisoning and child abuse, and with disease or illness that requires intervention, such as communicable disease. The influence of growth and development on each health problem is of special concern, since the etiology or the treatment may be directly affected by the child's age. Optimum care includes knowledge of the pathologic, psychologic, developmental, and familial variables of the health problem in order to plan and provide care that is individualized to meet each child's particular needs.

Disorders Related to Infectious Processes

Young children are especially susceptible to infectious disease, and a number of disorders occur predominantly during these early years. At this age their resistance to infectious agents may still be low, but their exposure to such agents is beginning to increase as a result of social involvement outside the home. These disorders include the typical childhood communicable diseases, intestinal parasitic infections, and conjunctivitis. Other common infectious diseases, such as otitis media, are discussed in those chapters devoted to specific biologic system disorders.

COMMUNICABLE DISEASES

The incidence of common childhood communicable diseases has declined tremendously since the advent of immunizations. Serious complications resulting from such infections have been further reduced through the use of antibiotics and antitoxins. However, infectious diseases do occur, and nurses must be familiar with the infectious agent in order to recognize the disease and institute appropriate preventive and nursing interventions. In order to facilitate understanding of communicable diseases, the following terms are defined (Benenson, 1985):

communicable disease An illness caused by a specific infectious agent or its toxic products through a direct or indirect mode of transmission of that agent from a reservoir.

epidemic A disease occurring in a greater than the expected number of cases in a community.

endemic A disease occurring regularly within a geographic location.

pandemic A disease affecting large portions of the population throughout the world.

infectious agent An organism, such as bacteria or virus, that is capable of producing infection or infectious disease.

reservoir The environment in which an infectious agent lives and multiplies and on which it depends for survival; man is the most frequent reservoir of infections that are capable of producing disease in other humans.

host A person, or other living animal, that affords subsistence or lodgment to an infectious agent under natural conditions.

source of infection The person, object, or substance from which an infectious agent passes immediately to the host; may be the reservoir (e.g., man) or any one of the several modes of transmission (e.g., contaminated water).

carrier A person or animal that harbors an infectious agent without apparent clinical disease and serves as a potential source of infection.

contact A person or animal that has been in association with an infected person, animal, or a contaminated environment that might provide an infective agent.

mode of transmission The mechanism by which an infectious agent is transported from the reservoir to a susceptible human host. Types of transmission include the following:

direct Direct and immediate transfer of infectious agents either by direct contact (touching, biting, kissing, or sexual intercourse) or droplet spread usually limited to a distance of about 1 meter or less (sneezing, coughing, spitting, singing, or talking).

indirect Contact with contaminated objects or other infected source.

vehicle Any object serving as an intermediate means by which an infectious agent is transported from the reservoir to the host, usually objects (fomites), water, soil, food, or biologic products such as plasma.

vector Arthropods or other invertebrates that transmit infection by inoculation or deposition of infectious agents on skin, food, or other objects.

airborne The dissemination of microbial aerosols usually into the respiratory tract; may be droplet nuclei or dust (e.g., fungus spores separated from dry soil by wind).

incubation period Time interval between infection or exposure to disease and appearance of initial symptoms.

period of communicability Time or times during which infectious agent may be transferred directly or indirectly from infected person to another person.

prodromal period Interval between time when early manifestations of disease appear to time when overt clinical syndrome is evident.

control measures Methods used to prevent spread of the organism; most common methods are immunizations, health education, medical treatment of infected person, and isolation or quarantine.

isolation Separation of infected persons from noninfected persons for the period of communicability under conditions that will prevent the transmission of the etiologic agent.

quarantine Restriction of activities of persons who have been exposed to a communicable disease until the incubation period has expired.

Nursing Considerations

The principal nursing goals are (1) identification of the communicable disease, (2) provision of comfort, (3) prevention of spread to others, and (4) prevention of complications. For most of the diseases, care is chiefly symptomatic and the nursing intervention is to help parents provide care for the child at home.

Identification. Identification of the infectious agent is of primary importance in order to prevent exposure to susceptible individuals. Nurses in ambulatory care settings, such as emergency rooms, health maintenance centers, nursery or elementary schools, and physicians' offices, are often the first persons to see signs of a communicable disease, such as a rash or sore throat. The nurse must operate under a high index of suspicion for common childhood diseases in order to identify potentially infectious cases and to recognize diseases that require medical intervention. An illustrative example is the common complaint of sore throat. Although most often a symptom of a minor viral infection, it can signal diphtheria or a streptococcal infection, such as scarlet

Text continued on p. 660.

Table 16-1 Infectious diseases that occur during early childhood

DISEASE

Chicken pox (Fig. 16-1)

Agent: varicella zoster

Source: primary secretions of respiratory tract of infected persons; to a lesser degree skin lesions (scabs not infectious)

Transmission: direct contact, droplet spread, and contaminated objects

Incubation period: 2 to 3 weeks, commonly 13 to 17 days

Period of communicability: probably 1 day before eruption of lesions (prodromal period to 6 days after first crop of vesicles when crusts have formed)

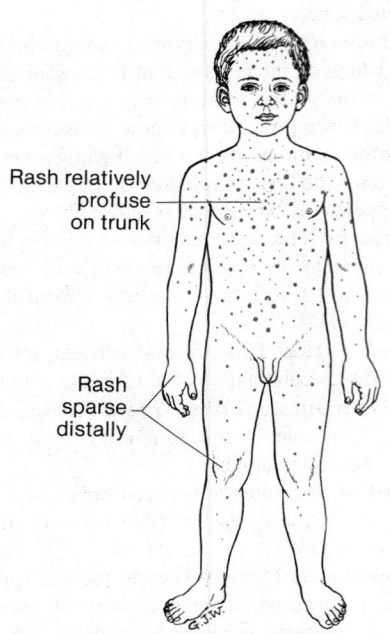

Fig. 16-1. Chicken pox.

Rash relatively profuse on trunk

Rash sparse distally

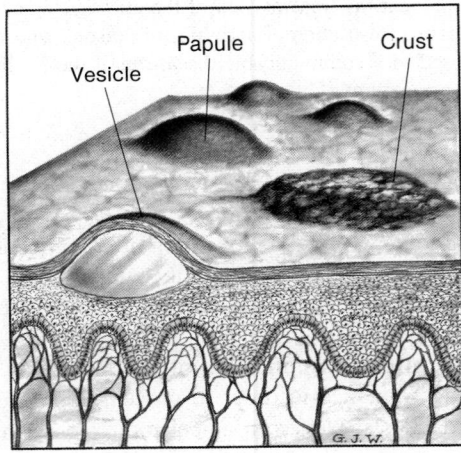

Vesicle

Papule

Crust

Diphtheria

Agent: Corynebacterium diphtheriae

Source: discharges from mucous membranes of nose and nasopharynx, skin, and other lesions of infected person

Transmission: direct contact with infected person, a carrier, or contaminated articles

Incubation period: usually 2 to 5 days, possibly longer

Period of communicability: variable; until virulent bacilli are no longer present (identified by three negative cultures); usually 2 weeks but as long as 4 weeks

Erythema infectiosum (fifth disease)

Agent: probably virus

Source: infected persons

Transmission: presumably direct contact by droplet infection

Incubation period: 6 to 14 days

Period of communicability: uncertain; most outbreaks subside in 1 to 2 months

Exanthema subitum (roseola)

Agent: probably virus

Source: unknown

Transmission: unknown (virtually limited to children between 6 months and 2 years of age)

Incubation period: unknown

Period of communicability: unknown

CLINICAL MANIFESTATIONS	THERAPEUTIC MANAGEMENT/COMPLICATIONS	NURSING CONSIDERATIONS
Prodromal stage: slight fever, malaise, and anorexia for first 24 hours; rash highly pruritic; begins as macule, rapidly progresses to papule and then vesicle (surrounded by erythematous base, becomes umbilicated and cloudy, breaks easily and forms crusts); all three stages (papule, vesicle, crust) present in varying degrees at one time (Fig. 16-1) *Distribution:* centripetal, spreading to face and proximal extremities but sparse on distal limbs *Constitutional signs and symptoms:* elevated temperature from lymphadenopathy, irritability from pruritus	*Specific:* none *Supportive:* Diphenhydramine hydrochloride or antihistamines to relieve itching; skin care to prevent secondary bacterial infection *Complications:* 　Secondary bacterial infections (abscesses, cellulitis, pneumonia, sepsis) 　Encephalitis 　Varicella pneumonia 　Hemorrhagic varicella (tiny hemorrhages in the vesicles and numerous petechiae in the skin) 　Reye syndrome (possibly related to aspirin)	Isolation of child in home until vesicles have dried (usually 1 week after onset of disease) and isolation of high-risk children Administer skin care: give bath and change clothes and linens daily; administer topical aplication of calamine lotion or paste of baking soda and water; keep child's fingernails short and clean; apply mittens if child scratches Lessen pruritus; keep child occupied Remove loose crusts that rub and irritate skin Teach child to apply pressure to pruritic area rather than scratch it If older child, reason with him regarding danger of scar formation from scratching Avoid use of aspirin
Varies according to anatomic location of pseudomembrane *Nasal:* resembles common cold, serosanguineous mucopurulent nasal discharge without constitutional symptoms; may be frank epistaxis *Tonsillar/pharyngeal:* malaise; anorexia; sore throat; low-grade fever; pulse increased above expected for temperature within 24 hours; smooth, adherent, white or gray membrane; lymphadenitis possibly pronounced (bull's neck); in severe cases, toxemia, septic shock, and death within 6 to 10 days *Laryngeal:* fever, hoarseness, cough, with or without previous signs listed; potential airway obstruction, apprehensive, dyspneic retractions, cyanosis	Antitoxin (usually intravenously); preceded by skin or conjunctival test to rule out sensitivity to horse serum Antibiotics (pencillin or erythromycin) Complete bed rest (prevention of myocarditis) Tracheostomy for airway obstruction Treatment of infected contacts and carriers *Complications:* 　Myocarditis (second week) 　Neuritis	Maintain *strict* isolation Participate in sensitivity testing; have epinephrine available Administer antibiotics; observe for signs of sensitivity to penicillin Administer *complete* care to maintain bed rest Use suctioning as needed Regulate humidity for optimum liquefaction of secretions Observe respirations for signs of obstruction
Rash appears in three stages: *I*—erythema on face, chiefly on cheeks, "slapped face" appearance; disappears by 1 to 4 days *II*—about 1 day after rash appears on face, maculopapular red spots appear, symmetrically distributed on upper and lower extremities; rash progresses from proximal to distal surfaces and may last a week or more *III*—rash subsides but reappears if skin is irritated or traumatized (sun, heat, cold, friction)	None necessary *Complications:* 　Self-limited arthritis and arthralgia	Reassure parents regarding benign nature of condition
Persistent high fever for 3 to 4 days in child who appears well Precipitious drop in fever to normal with appearance of rash *Rash:* discrete rose-pink macules or maculopapules appearing first on trunk, then spreading to neck, face, and extremities; nonpruritic, fades on pressure, lasts 1 to 2 days *Associated signs and symptoms:* cervical/postauricular lymphadenopathy, injected pharynx, occasionally catarthal otitis media	None specific Antipyretics to control fever Anticonvulsives for child with history of febrile seizures *Complications:* 　Febrile seizures	Teach parents measures for lowering temperature (antipyretic drugs) If child is prone to seizures, discuss appropriate precautions Reassure parents regarding benign nature of illness

Continued.

DISEASE

Measles (rubeola) (Fig. 16-2)

Agent: virus

Source: respiratory tract secretions, blood, and urine of infected person

Transmission: usually by direct contact with droplets of infected person

Incubation period: 10 to 20 days

Period of communicability: from 4 days before to 5 days after rash appears but mainly during prodromal (catarrhal) stage

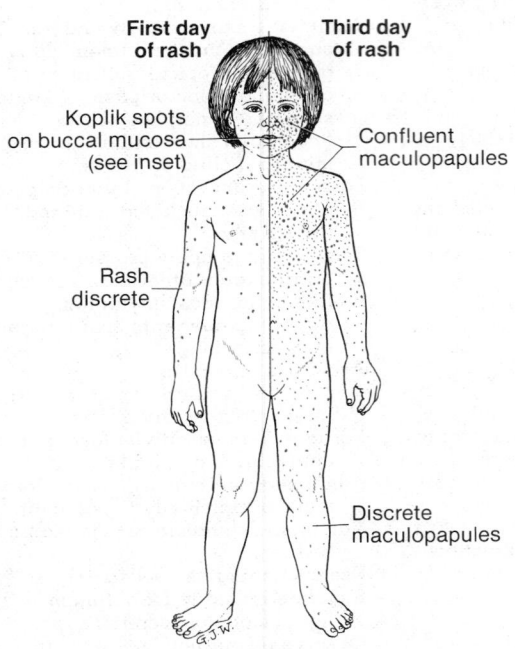

First day of rash   **Third day of rash**

Koplik spots on buccal mucosa (see inset)

Confluent maculopapules

Rash discrete

Discrete maculopapules

Fig. 16-2. Measles (rubeola).

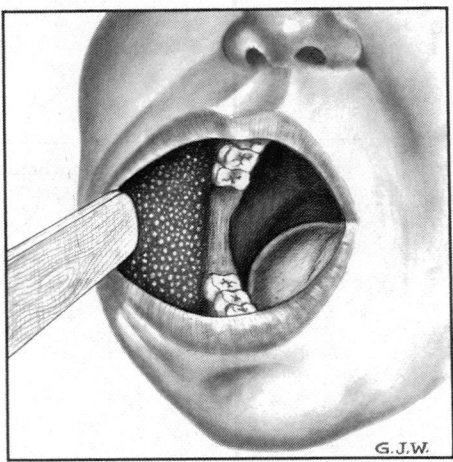

Koplik spots

Mumps

Agent: virus

Source: saliva of infected persons

Transmission: direct contact with or droplet spread from an infected person

Incubation period: 14 to 21 days

Period of communicability: most communicable immediately before and after swelling begins

Pertussis (whooping cough)

Agent: *Bordetella pertussis*

Source: discharge from respiratory tract of infected persons

Transmission: direct contact or droplet spread from infected person; indirect contact with freshly contaminated articles

Incubation period: 5 to 21 days, usually 10

Period of communicability: greatest during catarrhal stage before onset of paroxysms and may extend to fourth week after onset of paroxysms

CLINICAL MANIFESTATIONS	THERAPEUTIC MANAGEMENT/COMPLICATIONS	NURSING CONSIDERATIONS
Prodromal (catarrhal) stage: fever and malaise, followed in 24 hours by coryza, cough, conjunctivitis, Koplik spots (small, irregular red spots with a minute, bluish white center first seen on the buccal mucosa opposite the molars [Fig. 16-2]) 2 days before rash; symptoms gradually increase in severity until second day after rash appears, when they begin to subside *Rash:* appears 3 to 4 days after onset of prodromal stage, begins as erythematous maculopapular eruption on face and gradually spreads downward; more severe in earlier sites (appears confluent) and less intense in later sites (appears discrete); after 3 to 4 days assumes brownish appearance, and fine desquamation occurs over areas of extensive involvement *Constitutional signs and symptoms:* anorexia, malaise, generalized lymphadenopathy	*Supportive:* bed rest during febrile period; antipyretics Antibiotics to prevent secondary bacterial infection in high-risk children *Complications:* Otitis media Pneumonia Bronchiolitis Obstructive laryngitis and laryngotracheitis Encephalitis	Isolation until fifth day of rash; if hospitalized, institute respiratory precautions Maintain bed rest during prodromal stage; provide quiet activity *Fever:* instruct parents to administer antipyretics; avoid chilling; if child is prone to seizures, institute appropriate precautions (fever spikes to 40°C [104°F] between fourth and fifth days) *Eye care:* dim lights if photophobia present; clean eyelids with warm saline solution to remove secretions or crusts; keep child from rubbing his eyes; examine cornea for signs of ulceration *Coryza/cough:* use cool mist vaporizer; protect skin around nares with layer of petrolatum; encourage fluids and soft bland foods *Skin care:* keep skin clean; use tepid baths as necessary
Prodromal stage: fever, headache, malaise, and anorexia for 24 hours, followed by "earache" that is aggravated by chewing *Parotitis:* by third day, parotid gland(s) (either unilateral or bilateral) enlarges and reaches maximum size in 1 to 3 days; accompanied by pain and tenderness *Other manifestations:* submaxillary and sublingual infection, orchitis, and meningoencephalitis	*Symptomatic and supportive:* analgesics for pain and antipyretics for fever Intravenous fluid may be necessary for child who refuses to drink or vomits because of meningoencephalitis *Complications:* Sensorineural deafness Postinfectious encephalitis Myocarditis Arthritis Hepatitis Epididymo-orchitis Sterility (extremely rare in adult males)	Isolation during period of communicability; institute respiratory isolation during hospitalization Maintain bed rest during prodromal phase until swelling subsides Give analgesics for pain; if child is unwilling to chew medication, use elixir form Encourage fluids and soft, bland foods; avoid foods requiring chewing Apply hot or cold compresses to neck, whichever is more comforting To relieve orchitis, provide warmth and local support by means of tight-fitting underpants (stretch bathing suit works well)
Catarrhal stage: begins with symptoms of upper respiratory infection, such as coryza, sneezing, lacrimation, cough, and low-grade fever; symptoms continue for 1 to 2 weeks, when dry, hacking cough becomes more severe *Paroxysmal stage:* cough that most commonly occurs at night consists of a series of short, rapid coughs followed by a sudden inspiration that is associated with a high-pitched crowing sound or "whoop"; during paroxysms cheeks become flushed or cyanotic, eyes bulge, and tongue protrudes; paroxysm may continue until a thick mucous plug is dislodged; vomiting frequently follows an attack; stage generally lasts 4 to 6 weeks, followed by convalescent stage	Antimicrobial therapy (such as erythromycin) Administration of pertussis-immune globulin *Supportive treatment:* hospitalization required for infants, children who are dehydrated, or those who have complications Bed rest Increased oxygen intake and humidity Adequate fluids Intubation possibly necessary *Complications:* Pneumonia (usual cause of death) Atelectasis Otitis media Convulsions Hemorrhage (subarachnoid, subconjunctival, epistaxis) Weight loss and dehydration Hernia Prolapsed rectum	Isolation during catarrhal stage; if hospitalized, institute respiratory isolation Maintain bed rest as long as fever is present Keep child occupied during the day (interest in play is associated with fewer paroxysms) Reassure parents during frightening episodes of whooping cough Provide restful environment and reduce factors that promote paroxysms (dust, smoke, sudden change in temperature, chilling, activity, excitement); keep room well ventilated Encourage fluids; offer small amount of fluids frequently; refeed child after vomiting Keep child in Croupette with high humidity; suction gently but often to prevent choking on secretions Observe for signs of airway obstruction (increased restlessness, apprehension, retractions, cyanosis) Involve public health nurse if child is cared for at home

Continued.

DISEASE

Poliomyelitis

Agent: enteroviruses, 3 types; type 1—most frequent cause of paralysis, both epidemic and endemic, type 2—least frequently associated with paralysis, type 3—second most frequent in association with paralysis

Source: feces and oropharyngeal secretions of infected persons, especially young children

Transmission: direct contact with persons with apparent or inapparent active infection; spread is via fecal-oral and pharyngeal-oropharyngeal routes

Incubation period: usually 7 to 14 days, with range of 5 to 35 days

Period of communicability: not exactly known; virus is present in throat and feces shortly after infection and persists for about 1 week in throat and 4 to 6 weeks in feces

Rubella (German measles) (Fig. 16-3)

Agent: virus

Source: primarily nasopharyngeal secretions of persons with apparent or inapparent infection; virus also present in blood, stool, and urine

Transmission: direct contact and spread via infected person; indirectly via articles freshly contaminated with nasopharyngeal secretions, feces, or urine

Incubation period: 14 to 21 days

Period of communicability: 7 days before to about 5 days after appearance of rash

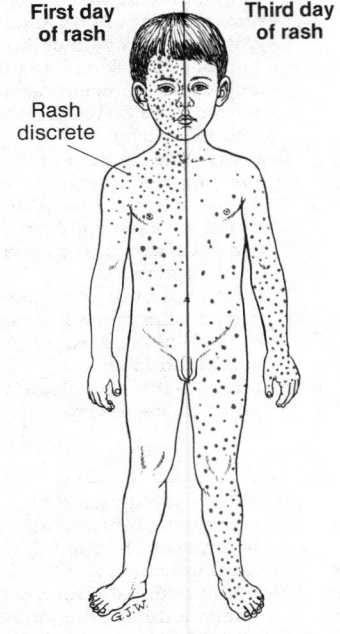

First day of rash   Third day of rash

Rash discrete

Fig. 16-3. Rubella (German measles).

Scarlet fever (Fig. 16-4)

Agent: group A β-hemolytic streptococci

Source: usually from nasopharyngeal secretions of infected persons and carriers

Transmission: direct contact with infected person or droplet spread; indirectly by contact with contaminated articles, ingestion of contaminated milk or other food

Incubation period: 2 to 4 days, with range of 1 to 7 days

Period of communicability: during incubation period and clinical illness approximately 10 days; during first 2 weeks of carrier phase, although may persist for months

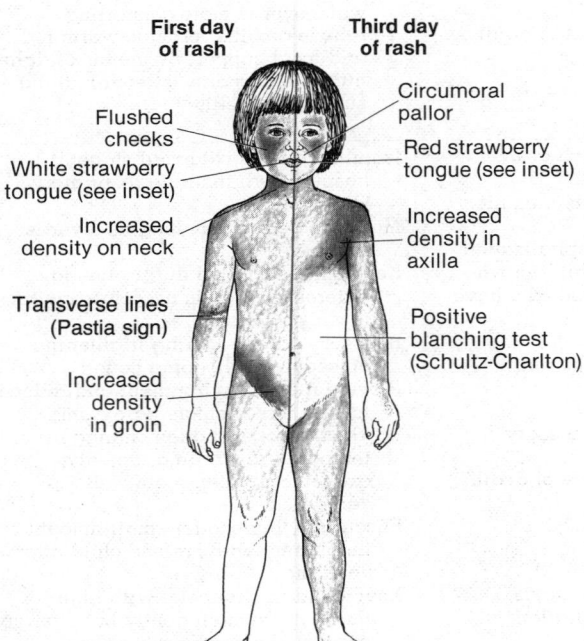

First day of rash   Third day of rash

Flushed cheeks
White strawberry tongue (see inset)
Increased density on neck
Transverse lines (Pastia sign)
Increased density in groin

Circumoral pallor
Red strawberry tongue (see inset)
Increased density in axilla
Positive blanching test (Schultz-Charlton)

Fig. 16-4. Scarlet fever.

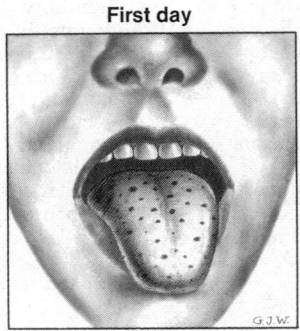

First day

White strawberry tongue

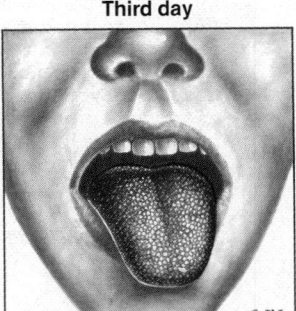

Third day

Red strawberry tongue

CLINICAL MANIFESTATIONS	THERAPEUTIC MANAGEMENT/COMPLICATIONS	NURSING CONSIDERATIONS

May be manifest in three different forms:
Abortive or inapparent—fever, uneasiness, sore throat, headache, anorexia, vomiting, abdominal pain; lasts a few hours to a few days
Nonparalytic—same manifestations as abortive but more severe, with pain and stiffness in neck, back, and legs
Paralytic—initial course similar to nonparalytic type, followed by recovery and then signs of central nervous system paralysis
	No specific treatment, including antimicrobials or gamma globulin
	Complete bed rest during acute phase
	Assisted respiratory ventilation in case of respiratory paralysis
	Physical therapy for muscles following acute stage
	Complications:
	  Permanent paralysis
	  Respiratory arrest
	  Hypertension
	  Kidney stones from demineralization of bone during prolonged immobility
		Maintain complete bed rest
		Administer mild sedatives as necessary to relieve anxiety and promote rest
		Participate in physiotherapy procedures (use of moist hot packs and range of motion exercises)
		Position child to maintain body alignment and prevent contractures or decubiti; use footboard
		Encourage child to move; administer analgesics for maximum comfort during physical activity
		Observe for respiratory paralysis (difficulty in talking, ineffective cough, inability to hold breath, shallow and rapid respirations); report such signs and symptoms to physician; have tracheostomy tray at bedside

Prodromal stage: absent in children, present in adults and adolescents; consists of low-grade fever, headache, malaise, anorexia, mild conjunctivitis, coryza, sore throat, cough, and lymphadenopathy; lasts for 1 to 5 days, subsides 1 day after appearance of rash **Rash:** first appears on face and rapidly spreads downward to neck, arms, trunk, and legs; by end of first day body is covered with a discrete, pinkish red maculopapular exanthema; disappears in same order as it began and is usually gone by third day **Constitutional signs and symptoms:** occasionally low-grade fever, headache, malaise, and lymphadenopathy	No treatment necessary other than antipyretics for low-grade fever and analgesics for discomfort **Complications:** Rare (arthritis, encephalitis, or purpura); most benign of all childhood communicable diseases; greatest danger is teratogenic effect on fetus	Reassure parents of benign nature of illness Employ comfort measures as necessary Isolate child from pregnant women

Prodromal stage: abrupt high fever, pulse increased out of proportion to fever, vomiting, headache, chills, malaise, abdominal pain
Enanthema: tonsils enlarged, edematous, reddened, and covered with patches of exudate; in severe cases appearance resembles membrane seen in diphtheria; pharynx is edematous and beefy red; during first 1 or 2 days tongue is coated and papillae become red and swollen (white strawberry tongue [Fig. 16-4]); by the fourth or fifth day white coat sloughs off, leaving prominent papillae (red strawberry tongue [Fig. 16-4]); palate is covered with erythematous punctate lesions
Exanthema: rash appears within 12 hours after prodromal signs; red pinhead-sized punctate lesions rapidly become generalized but are absent on the face, which becomes flushed; rash is more intense in folds of joints; by end of the first week desquamation begins, which may be complete by 3 weeks or longer
	Treatment of choice is a full course of penicillin (or erythromycin in penicillin-sensitive children); fever should subside 24 hours after beginning therapy
	Antibiotic therapy for newly diagnosed carriers (nose or throat cultures positive for streptococci)
	Supportive measures: bed rest during febrile phase, analgesics for sore throat
	Complications:
	  Otitis media
	  Peritonsillar abscess
	  Sinusitis
	  Rheumatic fever
	  Glomerulonephritis
		Institute respiratory isolation until 24 hours after initiation of treatment
		Ensure compliance with oral antibiotic therapy (intramuscular benzathine penicillin G [Bicillin] may be given if parents' reliability in giving oral drugs is questionable)
		Maintain bed rest during febrile phase; provide quiet activity during convalescent period
		Relieve discomfort of sore throat with analgesics, gargles, lozenges, antiseptic throat sprays (Chloraseptic), and inhalation of cool mist
		Encourage fluids during febrile phase; avoid irritating liquids (citrus juices) or rough foods; when child is able to eat, begin with soft diet
		Advise parents to consult physician if fever persists after beginning therapy
		Discuss procedures for preventing spread of infection

fever. Each of these conditions requires appropriate medical treatment to prevent serious sequelae.

Several important factors are helpful in identifying potentially communicable diseases: (1) recent exposure to a known case, (2) history of prodromal symptoms or evidence of constitutional symptoms, such as a fever or rash (Table 16-1; see also Fig. 18-3), (3) history of previous immunizations, and (4) previous history of having the disease. Since immunizations are available for several of the diseases and in almost every situation an attack confers lifelong immunity, the possibility of many infectious agents can be ruled out based on these last two criteria.

The nurse should also be familiar with tests commonly used to confirm or rule out the diagnosis of infectious diseases. Specific tests for scarlet fever include a throat culture and the anti-streptolysin O, which detects rising antibody titer to streptolysin O. A test for diagnosing diphtheria is the Schick test, which detects a reaction to inoculation with diphtheria toxin. Knowledge of test results allows for appropriate decision making regarding the need for treatment or isolation. For example, rubella is a benign childhood disease that requires no special intervention. Ordinarily the recommendation is to confine the child to the home for about 7 days after the appearance of the rash. However, if the mother is in the first trimester of pregnancy, immediate steps need to be taken to isolate the child from her if her antibody titer is low. In addition, any visitors who are pregnant should avoid close contact with the child.

Provision of comfort. Most communicable diseases require only supportive measures until the illness subsides. Children are usually cared for at home until the disease is no longer communicable and they feel well enough to resume normal activity. The chief discomfort from most of the rashes is itching, and measures such as cool baths (usually without soap) and lotions, such as calamine, are helpful. To avoid overheating, which increases itching, children should wear lightweight, loose, nonirritating clothing and keep out of the sun. If the child persists in scratching, the nails are kept short and smooth; mittens and clothes with long sleeves or legs may be needed. For severe itching, antipruritic medication, such as diphenhydramine (Benadryl) or hydroxyzine (Atarax), may be required, especially when the child tries to sleep.

An elevated temperature is common, and both antipyretic medication and environmental manipulation are implemented (see p. 1116). Aspirin is not given if chicken pox is present because of its association with Reye syndrome. A sore throat, another frequent symptom, is managed with lozenges, saline rinses (if the child is old enough to cooperate), and analgesics. Since most children are anorectic during an illness, bland foods and increased liquids are usually preferred. During the early stages of the disease children voluntarily curtail their activity, and while bed rest is beneficial, it should not be imposed. During periods of irritability, quiet activity, for example, reading, music, television, puzzles, and coloring, helps distract children from the discomfort.

Prevention of spread. Prevention consists of two components: prevention of the disease and control of the spread of the disease to others. Primary prevention rests almost exclusively on immunization (see Chapter 12). Identification of a household member with a communicable disease should alert the nurse to investigate the possibility of contact with nonimmunized persons. Other measures (available to prevent the occurrence of scarlet fever) include screening for streptococcal throat infections and administration of penicillin therapy. Nurses in school systems or public health agencies are frequently involved in such programs and need to be aware of the importance of adequate follow-up of children with positive cultures.

Control measures to prevent spread of the disease include appropriate isolation and early definitive treatment when necessary. Since most children are cared for at home, the nurse is responsible for instructing parents regarding isolation techniques. The most important procedure to stress is handwashing. Persons providing direct care or handling contaminated articles must wash their hands before and after caring for the child. Children are instructed to practice good handwashing technique after toileting and before eating. They may be confined to their room (preferably alone, but not necessarily so) until the specified period of communicability is over. It is important to remember that many of the diseases are not infectious even if a rash is still present. For example, the scabs that form with chicken pox are not a source of the virus. Children can return to school in about 1 week even if healing is not complete.

With the exception of those diseases requiring strict isolation, no special precautions need to be observed in cleaning the child's room, intimate articles, or clothing. However, the child should use disposable tissues that are discarded in a plastic, sealed bag. Eating and drinking utensils should not be shared by others unless washed thoroughly beforehand. The room is aired out and cleaned without spraying dust in the air. Vacuuming is preferable to using a dust mop, and sheets should be collected and placed in a receptacle, not shaken in the room. For those diseases spread by droplets, the parents are instructed in measures aimed at reducing airborne transmission, such as covering the child's face with a tissue when the child is coughing or sneezing. Persons who are susceptible to the disease should not come in close contact with the child.

Whenever the child is hospitalized, rigid adherence to appropriate isolation procedures is required. It is the nurse's responsibility to ensure that correct isolation procedures are instituted and properly implemented. In the instance of a child who is admitted with an undiagnosed exanthema, strict isolation is instituted until a diagnosis is established. To facilitate nursing care and minimize the possibility of spread of infection, nursing activities are organized to allow for the least number of trips in and out of the room. Parents and other visitors are taught isolation protocol. Suggestions for preparing the child for isolation are discussed in Chapter 26.

In suggesting isolation procedures for the home, the family's cultural and socioeconomic background is considered.

Nursing Care Summary: The Child with Communicable Disease

NURSING GOALS	NURSING INTERVENTIONS	EXPECTED PATIENT/FAMILY OUTCOMES

HP-HMP   Infection, potential for
Risk factors: susceptible host, infectious agents

NURSING GOALS	NURSING INTERVENTIONS	EXPECTED PATIENT/FAMILY OUTCOMES
Assist in identifying etiologic agent	Recognize exanthema associated with communicable diseases Operate under a high index of suspicion for children who are susceptible to infectious diseases Identify high-risk children to whom communicable disease may be fatal; in case of an outbreak, advise parents to confine child to the home Assist in performing tests used to identify the organism, such as collection of specimens for culture Be aware of significance of test results in terms of the etiologic agent and child's level of immunity	*Disease is recognized early and appropriate interventions implemented
Prevent occurrence of the disease	Participate in public education regarding prophylactic immunizations and method of spread of communicable diseases Participate in immunization programs or screening programs to identify streptococcal infections	*Disease is prevented
Prevent spread of the disease	Institute appropriate isolation procedures Post isolation procedures on door to child's room Make referral to public health nurse when necessary to ensure appropriate isolation procedures in the home Work with families to ensure compliance with therapeutic regimens Identify close contacts who may require prophylactic treatment (specific immune globulin or antibiotics) Report disease to local health department	Infection remains confined to original source
Prevent complications	Ensure compliance with therapeutic regimen (bed rest, antibiotics, adequate hydration) Institute seizure precautions if febrile convulsions are a possibility Monitor temperature; unexpected elevations may signal an infection Attend to good body hygiene Ensure adequate hydration with small frequent sips of water or favorite drinks and soft, bland foods (gelatin, pudding, ice cream, soups); feed again after vomiting; observe for signs of hydration	Child exhibits no evidence of complications such as infection or dehydration

N-MP   Skin integrity, impairment of: potential
Risk factors: child's propensity to scratch

NURSING GOALS	NURSING INTERVENTIONS	EXPECTED PATIENT/FAMILY OUTCOMES
Prevent child from scratching the skin	Keep nails short and clean Apply mittens or elbow restraints Dress in lightweight, loose, and nonirritating clothing Cover affected areas (long sleeves, pants) Bath in cool water with no soap Apply soothing lotions Avoid exposure to heat or sun	Skin remains intact

A-EP   Self-care deficit: feeding, bathing/hygiene, dressing/grooming, toileting (specify level)
Etiology: decreased strength and endurance

NURSING GOALS	NURSING INTERVENTIONS	EXPECTED PATIENT/FAMILY OUTCOMES
Provide or assist with basic care	Maintain bed rest; administer complete care as needed	Child is clean, groomed, and assists in care according to his capabilities

*Nursing outcome.

Continued.

Nursing Care Summary: The Child with Communicable Disease—cont'd

NURSING GOALS	NURSING INTERVENTIONS	EXPECTED PATIENT/FAMILY OUTCOMES

CPP   Sensory-perceptual alteration: visual, auditory, tactile
Etiology: isolation

| Prepare child for isolation | Explain reason for confinement and use of any special precautions
Allow child to play with gloves, mask, and gown
Always introduce yourself to child and allow him to see your face before donning protective clothing
Provide diversionary activity
Encourage parents to remain with child during hospitalization
Help child view isolation experience as challenging rather than solely negative
Discontinue isolation as soon as period of communicability is over; discuss this with family if child is at home
Recognize loneliness imposed by isolation; encourage contact with friends via telephone (in hospital can use intercom between room and nurse's station) | Child engages in suitable activities |

CPP   Comfort, alteration in: pain
Etiology: skin lesions, malaise

| Relieve discomfort | Keep mucous membranes moist with use of cool-mist vaporizer, gargles, and lozenges
Apply petrolatum to chapped lips or nares
Cleanse eyes with physiologic saline solution
Keep skin clean (change bedclothes and linens at least daily)
Administer oral hygiene
Assess need for pain or antipyactic medication
Employ nonpharmacologic pain reduction techniques, such as distraction through quiet play | Skin and mucous membranes are clean and free of irritants
Child exhibits minimum evidence of discomfort (specify) |

RRP   Family process, alteration in
Etiology: situational crisis (child with an acute illness)

| Provide emotional support | Reinforce family's effort to carry out plan of care
Provide assistance when necessary, such as visiting nurse to help with home care
Keep family aware of child's progress; stress rapidity of recovery in most cases | Family continues to comply with expectations |

Nursing Interventions Related to Medical Management

Relieve discomfort
Schedule analgesics, antipyretics and antipruritic medication for maximum relief of discomfort

For example, it is useless to recommend confining the child to his own room if the entire family sleeps together. A more appropriate suggestion would be to select for the child a sleeping area, such as a couch or one end of the bed, that is not in direct contact with the other members. Ideally, the best approach is to make a home visit and suggest practical measures based on the family's living situation. During a visit the nurse also questions other family members about symptoms suggestive of the child's disease.

Prevention of complications. Most children recover uneventfully from communicable diseases. However, there are groups of children who are at risk for serious, even fatal, complications, especially those diseases of viral etiology. This includes children who are undergoing steroid or other immunosuppressive therapy, those who have a generalized malignancy, such as leukemia or lymphoma, or those who have an immunologic disorder. The nurse should immediately refer children who have signs of a communicable disease to a physician. School nurses who are aware of such children who are susceptible have the responsibility of warning the parents of recent outbreaks of a communicable disease in order to prevent their exposure to children with the disease. In most instances the child is kept out of school until the outbreak is over. At the present time chicken pox is the disease most frequently requiring isolation of high-risk children because no immunization is available.

Prevention of complications with diseases such as diphtheria and scarlet fever necessitates parental compliance with antibiotic therapy. Whenever possible, oral preparations are prescribed to prevent the trauma of an injection. However, if there is serious question regarding compliance with the full 10-day schedule, one injection of benzathine penicillin G (Bicillin) is given. As in any other situation, the nurse prepares the child beforehand for the procedure. Discomfort from the injection can be reduced if the drug is allowed to warm to room temperature before administration.

Nursing care of the child with a communicable disease is summarized in the accompanying box; since most of the diseases are associated with skin manifestations, the reader is also referred to Chapter 18 for a discussion of nursing care in dermatologic conditions.

CONJUNCTIVITIS

Acute conjunctivitis, inflammation of the conjunctiva, is a common condition in children. It develops from a variety of causes that are typically age-related. In infants recurrent conjunctivitis may be a sign of nasolacrimal duct obstruction. In children the usual sources are bacterial, viral, allergic, or a foreign body. Bacterial infection accounts for most instances of acute conjunctivitis in children and *Haemophilus influenzae* is the most prevalent infectious agent, followed by *Streptococcus pneumoniae* (Gigliotti and others, 1981).

Clinical Manifestations

Clinical manifestations depend primarily on the cause and are usually diagnostic. The distinguishing symptom of bacterial conjunctivitis (often called "pink eye") is purulent drainage, causing crusting of the eyelids when the child awakens. The conjunctiva is inflamed and the lids are swollen. Frequently both eyes are infected.

Viral conjunctivitis usually occurs in association with an upper respiratory infection. The eyes appear swollen and red, and there is serous (watery) drainage. Acute hemorrhagic conjunctivitis is caused by a specific virus, enterovirus 70, and is characterized by severe inflammation, subconjunctival hemorrhage, and photophobia. Epidemics usually occur in densely populated coastal communities in tropical regions, such as Florida. The cardinal symptom of allergic conjunctivitis is itching; other manifestations include watery to viscous stringy discharge, lid redness, and swelling. The chief sign of conjunctivitis caused by a foreign body is the presence of symptoms, such as tearing, pain, and inflammation, in only *one* eye. In this instance, the eye is carefully examined for evidence of an object.

Therapeutic Management

Treatment of conjunctivitis depends on the cause. Viral conjunctivitis and bacterial conjunctivitis are self-limited. However, bacterial conjunctivitis is usually treated with topical antibacterial agents such as polymyxin and bacitracin (Polysporin), which shorten the duration of clinical disease and enhance eradication of the organism (Gigliotti and others, 1984). Drops may be used during the day and an ointment at bedtime because the ointment preparation remains in the eye longer. Ointments are usually not used in the daytime because they blur vision. Corticosteroids are avoided because they reduce ocular resistance to bacteria. Supportive treatment includes removal of the accumulated secretions.

Nursing Considerations

Nursing goals include keeping the eye clean and properly administering ophthalmic medication. Accumulated secretions are always removed by wiping from the inner canthus downward and outward, away from the opposite eye. Warm, moist compresses, such as a clean washcloth wrung out with hot tap water, are helpful in removing the crusts. Compresses are *not* kept on the eye because an occlusive covering promotes bacterial growth. Medication should be instilled immediately after the eyes have been cleaned and according to correct procedure (see p. 1139).

Prevention of infection in other family members is an important consideration with bacterial conjunctivitis. The child's washcloth and towel are kept separate from those used by others. Tissues used to clean the eye are disposed of properly. The child should refrain from rubbing the eyes and is instructed in correct handwashing technique.

Table 16-2 Common intestinal parasites

LIFE CYCLE, PATHOGENESIS, TRANSMISSION	CLINICAL MANIFESTATIONS	COMMENTS
Ascariasis—*Ascaris lumbricoides* (common roundworm) Adult lays eggs in small intestine; eggs deposited in stool; incubation in soil 2-3 weeks; swallowed eggs hatch in small intestine, larvae penetrate intestinal villi, enter portal vein to liver, proceed to lungs, rupture capillaries into respiratory system, ascend to upper passages to be swallowed, proceed to small intestine, and mature into adult worms (total time 2-3 months) Transferred to mouth by way of contaminated food, fingers, toys, etc.	Light infections: asymptomatic Heavy infections: anorexia, irritability, nervousness, enlarged abdomen, weight loss, fever, intestinal colic Severe infections: intestinal obstruction, appendicitis, perforation of intestine with peritonitis, obstructive jaundice, lung involvement—pneumonitis	Largest of the intestinal helminths Affects principally young children 1-4 years of age Prevalent in warm climates
Hookworm disease—*Necator americanus* Worms live in small intestine and feed on villi; process of attachment produces bleeding; ova deposited in bowel, expelled in feces; hatch in damp, shaded soil; larvae attach to skin, penetrate and enter bloodstream, migrate to lungs, exit into alveoli, migrate to upper passages to be swallowed; develop in upper intestine Transmitted by discharging eggs on the soil and in turn pick up infection from direct skin contact with contaminated soil	Light infections in well-nourished individuals; no problems Heavier infections: mild to severe anemia, malnutrition May be itching and burning ("ground itch") followed by erythema and a papular eruption in areas to which the organism migrates	Wearing shoes is recommended, although children playing in contaminated soil expose many skin surfaces
Strongyloidiasis—*Strongyloides stercoralis* (threadworm) Life cycle similar to that of hookworm, except that worm is not attached to intestinal mucosa and feeding larvae (not eggs) may be deposited in soil; also sometimes penetrate colonic mucosa and enter systemic circulation, migrate to respiratory structures, and are subsequently swallowed Transmission is same as for hookworm except autoinfection common	Light infection: asymptomatic Heavy infection: respiratory signs and symptoms; abdominal pain, distention; nausea and vomiting; diarrhea—large, pale stools, often with mucus Threat to life in children with weakened immunologic defenses	Older children and adults affected more often than young children Severe infections may lead to severe nutritional deficiency
Visceral larva migrans—*Toxocara canis* (dogs) **Intestinal toxocariasis—*Toxocara cati* (cats)** In natural host (dog or cat), larvae migrate to liver and lungs and reach maturity in intestines; when ingested by immature host (man), larvae migrate aimlessly to become encapsulated in muscles and organs such as liver, lungs, kidney, eye, and brain; most serious are those in eye and central nervous system Transmitted by direct contamination of hands from contact with dog, cat, or objects or ingestion of soil	Depends on reactivity of infected individual May be asymptomatic except for eosinophila Specific diagnosis difficult	Dogs and cats should be kept away from areas where children play; sandboxes especially important transmission areas Periodic deworming of diagnosed dogs and cats Control of dog population Continued education and laws to prevent indiscriminate canine defecation
Trichuriasis—*Trichuris trichura* (whipworm) Adult worms live in the cecum; in heavy infections, also in the colon and rectum; passed in feces, slow development in soil (3-4 weeks); eggs swallowed, larvae hatch in small intestine, penetrate villi and mature; return to lumen and migrate to cecum Transmitted from contaminated soil, vegetables, toys, and other objects	Light infections: asymptomatic Heavy infections; abdominal pain and distention; diarrhea	Most frequent in warm, moist climates Occurs most often in undernourished children living in unsanitary conditions

Parasitic Intestinal Infections

Intestinal parasitic diseases, including helminths (worms) and protozoa, constitute the most frequent infections in the world, and although many are concentrated in the tropical regions, others are not. A number of these infections are encountered with relative frequency in the United States and are of importance in children in the pediatric age-groups. Young children are especially at risk because of typical hand-mouth activity and uncontrolled fecal habits. Recently the incidence of intestinal parasitic disease, especially giardiasis, has increased among young children who are attending day-care centers.

The structure of helminths is biologically adapted to a parasitic existence. With a ready supply of predigested nutrients and the ability to live under conditions that are essentially anaerobic, the systems of most parasitic worms are reduced or absent, with the exception of the reproductive system, which is greatly elaborated and can produce enormous amount of ova.

The integument, or outer covering, of the parasite is designed to provide protection for the organism. It may be hardened, tough, elastic, or relatively delicate, but in most instances it is highly resistant to digestion while the organism is alive. It is often equipped with spines, hooks, cutting plates, stylets, or other armature for attachment to, penetration of, or abrasion of the host's tissues. Many are provided with secretory glands near the mouth that secrete a lytic substance to digest the tissues of the host for food or enable the parasite to migrate through the host to the optimum site for maturation.

Depending on the organism, the life cycle of the parasite may or may not require an intermediate host, such as an animal (e.g., dog). An understanding of the life cycle of the infecting parasite, its mode of transmission, the site in the body where it becomes established, the symptomatology displayed by the host, and the habits of the host is essential in planning the eradication of the organism and/or prevention of infection. Most infections result from ingestion of parasite eggs (ova) that hatch within the host environment. Depending on the organism, the eggs may continue to mature in the gastrointestinal tract; the hatched larvae may burrow through the intestinal lining to the bloodstream, where they are carried to the lungs (usually) or other organs; or the organisms may make their way through ducts and passages to other areas where they produce symptoms associated with the affected organs. Light infections may be asymptomatic, but all infections produce symptoms and pathologic conditions when the organism is present in large numbers.

Parasitic intestinal infections in man are caused by a number of infecting organisms. This discussion is limited to the two most common parasitic infections among children in the United States—giardiasis and pinworms. Table 16-2 describes the outstanding features of other helminths that belong to the family of nematodes. Most nematodes, with the exception of threadworm and *Toxocara,* are effectively treated with mebendazole, pyrantel pamoate, or piperazine citrate (Table 16-3).

GENERAL NURSING CONSIDERATIONS

Nursing responsibilities related to parasitic intestinal infections are identification of the parasite, treatment of the in-

Table 16-3 Drugs used to treat intestinal parasitic infections

DRUG/PEDIATRIC DOSAGE	SIDE EFFECTS	COMMENTS
Furazolidone (Furoxone) 1.25 mg/kg q.i.d. × 7 days (maximum 100 mg q.i.d.)	Nausea Vomiting Headache Hemolysis possible in glucose-6-phosphate dehydrogenase (G-6-PD) deficiency	Drug of choice for giardiasis if cost is not a factor Contraindicated during pregnancy
Mebendazole (Vermox) 100 mg b.i.d. × 3 days 100 mg × 1; repeat in 2 weeks for pinworm	Occasional, transient abdominal pain Diarrhea in massive infection with expulsion of worms	Drug of choice of hookworm, roundworm, pinworm, and whipworm Tablets may be chewed, crushed, or mixed with food Not recommended during pregnancy Recommended for children over 2 years
Metronidazole (Flagyl) 15 mg/kg/day (maximum 750 mg) t.i.d. × 5 days	Nausea Diarrhea Vomiting Metallic taste Abdominal cramps Headache	Maybe ineffective in children on phenobarbital Not recommended during pregnancy

Continued.

Table 16-3 Drugs used to treat intestinal parasitic infections—cont'd

DRUG/PEDIATRIC DOSAGE	SIDE EFFECTS	COMMENTS
Piperazine citrate (Antepar) 75 mg/kg/day (maximum 3.5 g) × 2 (repeat in 2 weeks for pinworm)	Nausea Vomiting Diarrhea Abdominal cramping Urticaria	Side effects are rare with recommended dose May exacerbate seizures in children with seizure disorders
Pyrantel pamoate (Antiminth) 11 mg/kg × 1 (maximum 1 g) (repeat in 2 weeks for pinworm)	Nausea Vomiting Diarrhea Abdominal cramps Tenesmus	Side effects are rare with recommended dose Little published data on safety in pregnant women and children under 2 years of age Protect drug from light
Pyrvinium pamoate (Povan) 5 mg/kg × 1 (maximum 350 mg) (repeat in 2 weeks for pinworm)	Nausea Vomiting Diarrhea Abdominal cramping	Alternative drug for pinworms Warn parents that drug stains stool and vomitus bright red, as well as clothing or skin if in contact with drug Swallow tablets whole to avoid staining teeth
Quinacrine (Atabrine) 6 mg/kg/day (maximum 300 mg) × 7 days	Nausea Vomiting Temporary discoloration of skin and urine	Highest frequency of side effects Take with meals to decrease gastric upset Advise parents of benign discoloration which may take 3 months to fade Crush tablets and mix with strong flavoring (e.g., jam) to disguise bitter taste
Thiabendazole (Mintezol) 25 mg/kg b.i.d. (maximum 3 g/day) × 2 days	Drowsiness Dizziness Giddiness Headache Impaired alertness and coordination	Treatment for severe cases of *Toxocara*; also used for threadworm Use with caution in patients with renal or hepatic dysfunction Warn parents of drowsiness and dizziness in child Administer after meals

fection, and prevention of initial infection or reinfection. Identification of the organism is accomplished by laboratory examination of substances containing the worm, its larvae, or embryonated ova. Most are identified by examining feces smears from the stools of persons suspected of harboring the parasite. Stool specimens should be large enough to obtain an ample sampling, not merely a fecal fragment. Specimens are easily obtained from diapers, although the stool should not be contaminated with urine. For toilet-trained children, a simple procedure for collecting a specimen is placing plastic wrap over the toilet bowl to catch the stool. Fresh specimens are best for revealing parasites or larvae; therefore collected specimens should be taken directly to the laboratory for examination. If this is not feasible, the specimen is placed in a container with a preservative. Parents need clear instructions on obtaining an adequate sample and the number of samples required.*

In most parasitic infections, examination of other family members, especially children, may be carried out to identify those who are similarly affected. Nurses are frequently the persons who assume the responsibility for directing and instructing the families in the collection and disposition of specimens. The treatment regimen may need further explanation and reinforcement, particularly when it involves other members of the household and care of clothing and bed linen. When other members are treated, the family needs to understand the nature of transmission and that in some cases the medication must be repeated in 2 weeks to 1 month to kill organisms hatched since initial treatment.

The nurse's most important function in relation to these parasites is preventive education of children and families regarding good hygiene and health habits. Careful handwashing before eating or handling food and after using the toilet is the most important precautionary method. Other preventive practices are listed in the box on p. 667.

In areas where infections are endemic or where conditions are conducive to infection and reinfection, nurses can become involved in working with public health officials for provision of better living conditions, such as reduction of overcrowding in living accommodations and provision of adequate, sanitary disposal systems for human feces.

*The patient education aid, Stool specimen collection, is available in Patient Care **17**(14):277, 1983.

GIARDIASIS

Giardiasis is caused by the protozoan, *Giardia lamblia* (also called *G. intestinalis*, *G. duodenalis*, and *Lamblia intestinalis*). It is the most common intestinal parasitic pathogen in the United States, and its prevalence among children in daycare centers may range from 9% to 38% (Keystone and others, 1984). Breast milk may play a protective role in infants exposed to these organisms (Gillin and Reiner, 1983), and this area needs further research.

Life Cycle, Pathogenesis, and Transmission

Infection begins with ingestion of the cysts, the nonmotile stage of the protozoa. The stomach acid activates the cysts, which then pass into the duodenum. Following completion of excystation, trophozoites (parasites in their active feeding stage) emerge and colonize the distal duodenum and proximal jejunum. As the cycle continues, cysts are passed in feces; they are not infective initially but must complete a process of maturation requiring hours to days. Cysts can survive in the environment for months (Craft, 1985). The mechanism of pathogenesis is not known.

Chief modes of transmission are person-to-person; water, especially mountain lakes, streams, and pools frequented by diapered infants; food; and animals, especially puppies. In children, person-to-person transmission is the most likely cause.

Clinical Manifestations

Although individuals infected with giardiasis may be asymptomatic, young children, especially infants, usually manifest symptoms such as diarrhea, vomiting, anorexia, and failure to thrive. Children over 5 years of age most often complain of abdominal cramps with intermittent loose stools and constipation. The stools may be malodorous, watery, pale, and greasy. Most infections resolve spontaneously in 4 to 6 weeks, except in rare instances in which the infection becomes chronic and may last for months or years. The chronic form is usually associated with intermittent loose, foul-smelling stools with or without abdominal bloating, flatulence, sulfur-tasting belches, epigastric pain, vomiting, headache, and weight loss (Craft, 1985).

Diagnostic Evaluation

Unlike most other intestinal parasites, *G. lamblia* is not easily diagnosed from stool specimens. Since *Giardia* organisms are excreted in a highly variable pattern, 6 or more stool specimens collected over several weeks may be necessary to identify the trophozoites or cysts. Other tests that appear promising for rapid and accurate diagnosis involve detecting *Giardia* antigen in the stool by counterimmunoelectrophoresis (CIE) or enzyme-linked immunosorbent assay (ELISA).

Therapeutic Management

Three drugs are available for treatment of giardiasis (see Table 16-3). The drug of choice is quinacrine based on economics (it is less than one tenth the cost of furazolidone) and inadequate knowledge of the long-term safety of metronidazole. Unfortunately, quinacrine has the highest frequency of side effects, especially nausea and vomiting, causes temporary yellow staining of the skin, sclera, and urine, and has a very bitter taste (Turner, 1985).

Nursing Considerations

The most important nursing consideration is prevention of giardiasis, especially among children attending daycare centers and the staff. Attention to meticulous sanitary practices, especially during diaper changes, is essential (see box below and Fig. 16-5 on p. 668). Nurses can play an important role in educating daycare staff regarding appropriate sanitation.

Once children are infected, compliance with the treatment is essential and the interventions suggested in Table 16-3 for the administration of quinacrine are given to parents. If other household members are infected, the nurse should inquire about any pregnant members, since treatment for giardiasis is contraindicated during pregnancy.

ENTEROBIASIS (PINWORMS)

Enterobiasis, or pinworms, caused by the nematode *Enterobius vermicularis,* is the most common helminthic infection in the United States. It is universally present in temperate climatic zones, and may infect 20% of all children at any one time (Borgatti, 1983). Crowded conditions, such as in classrooms and daycare centers, favor transmission.

Life Cycle, Pathogenesis, and Transmission

Infection begins when the eggs are ingested or inhaled. The eggs hatch in the upper intestine, mature in 2 to 4 weeks, and migrate to the cecal area. The females then mate, mi-

---

SUGGESTIONS FOR PREVENTING PARASITIC INTESTINAL DISEASE

Always wash hands and fingernails with soap and water before eating and handling food and after toileting.

Avoid placing fingers in mouth and biting nails.

Discourage children from scratching bare anal area.

Change diapers as soon as soiled and dispose of in plastic bags in closed receptable out of children's reach.

Disinfect toilet seats and diaper changing areas; use dilute household bleach (10% solution) or Lysol and wipe clean with paper towels.

Drink water that is specially treated, especially if camping.

Wash all raw fruits and vegetables or food that has fallen on the floor.

Avoid growing foods in soil fertilized with human excreta.

Teach children to defecate only in a toilet, not on the ground.

Keep dogs and cats away from playgrounds or sandboxes.

Avoid swimming in pools frequented by diapered children.

Wear shoes outside.

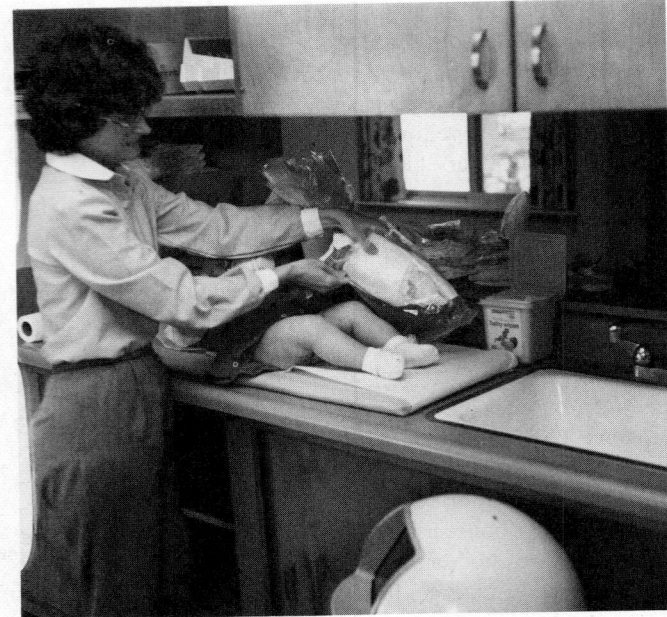
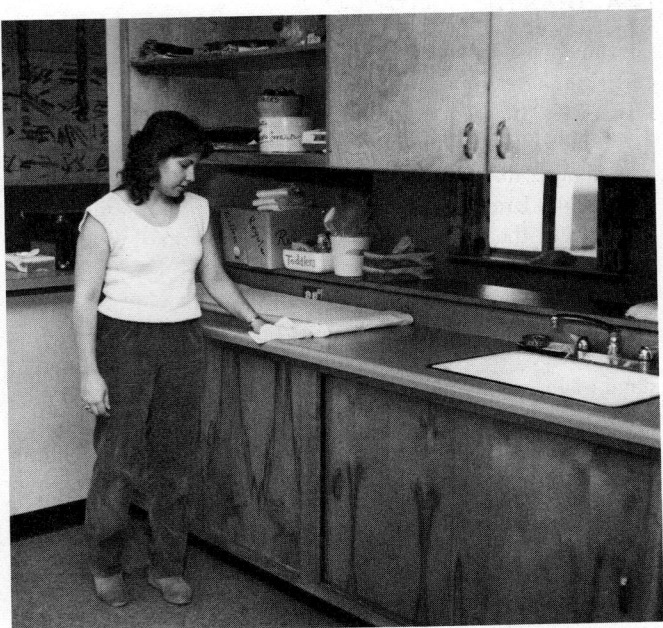

Fig. 16-5. Prevention of giardiasis, especially in daycare centers, requires sanitary practices during diaper changes such as **A,** wrapping diapers in plastic bags and discarding in a covered receptacle; **B,** cleaning diaper changing surfaces; and **C,** handwashing after diaper changing.
Photography by John Roy, Saint Francis Hospital, Tulsa, OK.

grate out the anus, and lay up to 17,000 eggs (Jones, 1983). The movement of the worms on skin and mucous membrane surfaces causes intense itching, and since the surface of the eggs is durable and adhesive, they easily adhere to almost any surface. As the child scratches, eggs are deposited on the hands and under the fingernails. The typical hand-to-mouth activity of youngsters makes them especially prone to continual reinfection. Pinworm eggs also persist in the home to contaminate anything they contact, such as toilet seats, doorknobs, bed linen, underwear, and food. Since they float in the air, they are also easily inhaled.

Clinical Manifestations

The principal symptom of pinworms is intense perianal itching. However, in young children who have difficulty verbalizing this discomfort, general irritability, restlessness, poor sleep, bed-wetting, distractibility, and short attention span should arouse suspicion that the disorder is present. In females the worms may migrate to the vagina and urethra to cause infection.

Diagnostic Evaluation

The most common test for diagnosing pinworms is the tape test (see discussion under Nursing considerations). The worms may also be identified by using a flashlight to inspect the anal area while the child sleeps. The room must remain dark and it is best not to place underpants on the child. If worms are found, this can be very upsetting to parents, a fact that should be considered before recommending this procedure.

Therapeutic Management

Four drugs are available for treatment of pinworms (see Table 16-3). The drug of choice is mebendazole, which is safe, effective, convenient, and has few side effects. However, it is not recommended for children under 2 years of age or for pregnant women. Since pinworms are easily transmitted, all household members are treated. Any of the drugs is repeated in 2 weeks to prevent reinfection.

Nursing Considerations

Nursing care is directed at identifying the parasite, eradicating the organism, and preventing reinfection. Parents need clear, detailed instructions for the tape test. A loop of transparent (not "frosted") tape, sticky side out, is placed around the end of a tongue depressor, which is then firmly pressed against the child's perianal area. A convenient commercially prepared tape is also available for this purpose. Pinworm specimens are collected in the morning as soon as the child awakens and *before* the child has a bowel movement or bathes. The procedure may need to be repeated more than once before eggs are collected. Parents are instructed to place the tongue blade in a glass jar or loosely in a plastic bag so that it can be brought in for microscopic examination.* For specimens collected in the hospital, physician's office, or clinic, the tape is placed smoothly on a glass slide, sticky side down, for examination.

---

*The patient education aid, Pinworm egg collection, is available in Patient Care **17**(14):273, 1983.

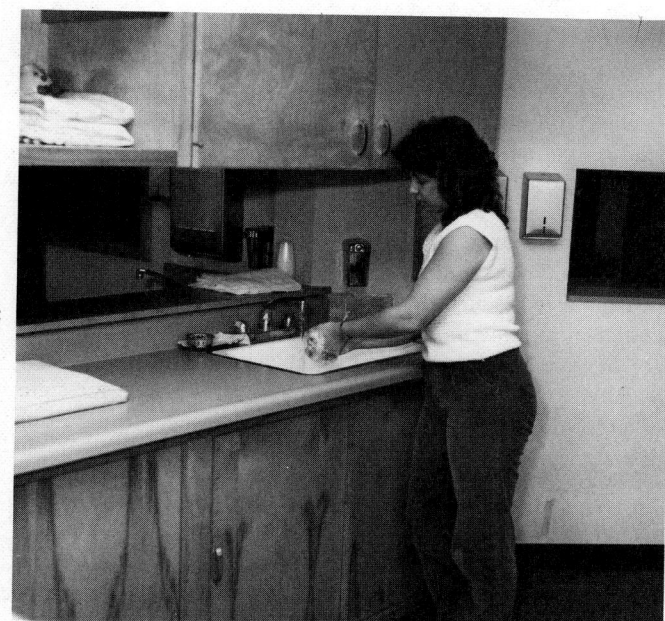

c

Compliance with the drug regime is usually excellent because the duration of treatment is typically only one dose. However, the family is reminded of the need to take a second dose in 2 weeks. Posting a reminder on the refrigerator door or bathroom mirror is helpful.

To prevent reinfection, certain housecleaning practices are recommended, although there is little documentation on their effectiveness, since pinworms survive on so many surfaces. In addition, pinworms are not necessarily associated with poor housekeeping. Parents are instructed to wash all bedding and underwear in hot water immediately after treatment. Bed linen and clothing are handled carefully to avoid scattering eggs into the air and on the floor. Family members should wear a clean pair of long pajamas to sleep and underclothing that fits snugly and is changed daily. Bedrooms and bathrooms are vacuumed or damp-mopped and all washable surfaces, especially the toilet seat, are cleaned with a disinfectant (see box, p. 667). The child's fingernails are cut short to minimize the chance of ova collecting under the nails, and all family members are encouraged to practice handwashing after toileting and before eating.

Ingestion of Injurious Agents

Since the passage of the Poison Prevention Packaging Act of 1970, which provides that certain potentially hazardous drugs and household products be sold in child-resistant containers, the incidence of poisonings in children has decreased dramatically (Unintentional poisoning, 1983). However, despite these advances, poisoning remains a significant health concern with nearly two thirds of the cases occurring in children under 6 years of age. Children are poisoned by a variety of substances (see box, above) although

not all common household items are toxic (see box, above and Table 16-5). Knowledge of nontoxic substances prevents unnecessary crises in the family and overtreatment. Over 90% of poisonings occur in the home (Veltri and Litovitz, 1984), although a significant number take place elsewhere, especially in a grandparent's or friend's home (Polakoff and others, 1984).

The developmental characteristics of young children predispose them to poisoning by ingestion. Infants and toddlers explore their environment through oral experimentation. Since the sense of taste is less discriminatory at this age, many unpalatable substances are ingested. In addition, toddlers and preschoolers are developing autonomy and intiative, which increase their curiosity and exploration. Imita-

Table 16-4   Common signs of poisoning

GENERAL SIGNS	SPECIFIC SIGNS
Gastrointestinal system	*Hydrocarbons*
Abdominal pain	Gagging, choking, and
Vomiting	coughing
Diarrhea	Nausea
Anorexia	Vomiting
	Alterations in
	sensorium,
	such as lethargy
	Weakness
	Respiratory symptoms
	of pulmonary involve-
	ment
	Tachypnea
	Cyanosis
	Retractions
	Grunting
Respiratory/circulatory	*Corrosives*
system	Severe burning pain
Depressed respirations	in mouth, throat
Labored respirations	and stomach
Unexplained cyanosis	White, swollen mucous
Signs of shock—increased,	membranes, edema of
weak pulse; decreased	lips, tongue,
blood pressure; increased,	and pharynx
shallow respiration; pallor;	(respiratory obstruction)
cool, clammy skin	Violent vomiting
	(hemoptysis)
	Drooling and inability
	to clear secretions
	Signs of shock
	Anxiety and agitation
Central nervous system	*Salicylates*
Convulsions	Nausea
Overstimulation	Disorientation
Sudden loss of conscious-	Vomiting
ness	Dehydration
Dizziness	Diaphoresis
Stupor, lethargy	Hyperpnea
Coma	Hyperpyrexia
	Oliguria
	Tinnitus
	Coma
	Convulsions

tion is also a powerful motivator, especially when combined with lack of awareness of danger.

This section is primarily concerned with the immediate emergency treatment of ingestion of injurious agents and the specific management of plant, salicylate, acetaminophen, iron, and lead poisoning. Appropriate suggestions for prevention are discussed in Chapter 14.

PRINCIPLES OF EMERGENCY TREATMENT

A poisoning may or may not require emergency intervention, but in every instance medical evaluation is necessary to initate appropriate action. Parents are advised to call the Poison Control Center (PCC) *before* initiating any intervention, since instructions on labels of many household prod-

ucts are not correct treatment measures. The local PCC telephone number (usually listed in the front of the telephone directory*) should be posted near each phone in the house.

Based on the initial telephone assessment, the PCC counsels the parents to begin treatment at home and/or to bring the child to an emergency facility. When a call is taken, the name and telephone number of the caller is recorded to reestablish contact if the connection is interrupted. Since the majority of poisonings are managed outside health care facilities, usually at the patient's home, expert advice is essential in minimizing adverse effects. When the exact quantity or type of ingested toxin is not known, admission to a hospital for laboratory evaluation and surveillance for signs of poisonings (Table 16-4) is critical during postingestion period.

General guidelines for the emergency home treatment for poisoning are listed in the box, p. 671; selected interventions, especially those that require professional intervention, are discussed below.

Assessment

The first and most important principle in dealing with a poisoning is to treat the child first, not the poison. This necessitates an immediate concern for life support; vital signs are taken and respiratory and/or circulatory support instituted as needed. The victim's condition is routinely reevaluated. The increased recovery rate from acute poisonings is largely attributable to vigorous use of supportive measures after symptoms appear. Since shock is a complication of several types of household poisons, particularly corrosives, measures to reduce the effects of shock, such as elevation of legs and head to the level of the heart to promote venous drainage and provision of warmth and rest, are important. Maintenance of respiratory function may require mouth-to-mouth resuscitation or insertion of an airway and/or mechanical ventilation.

The emergency room nurse's responsibility is to be prepared for immediate intervention with any of the necessary equipment. Since time and speed are critical factors in recovery from serious poisonings, anticipation of potential problems and complications may mean the difference between life and death.

Gastric Decontamination

In general, the immediate treatment is to remove the ingested poison by inducing vomiting. The preferred method for use at home is to administer ipecac syrup, an emetic that exerts its action by direct stimulation of the vomiting center and an irritant effect on the gastric mucosa. The use of an emetic is generally contraindicated in conditions that increase the risk of aspiration and when emesis of the poison, such as corrosives, redamages the mucosa of the esophagus and pharynx.

Proper administration of ipecac is essential (see box on

---

*Also available by calling 1-800-555-1212 for any state.

Emergency treatment). Ipecac is available in 1-ounce (30 ml) vials. However, the label information does not include directions for a second dose. Therefore parents need clear instructions for proper use and dose. Drinking tepid water after the administration of ipecac is believed to increase the local irritant effect. Large amounts of water are not given because they may enhance gastric emptying, and milk is contraindicated because it delays emesis. Increasing the child's activity is not effective in promoting vomiting (Boehnert and others, 1985; Rodgers and Matyunas, 1986).

As a precaution, parents are advised to have one full dose of ipecac for *each child* in the home, to carry the emetic when traveling, and to be certain that other caregivers (baby-sitters or relatives) have the emetic available. Because children share activities, it is not uncommon for more than one child to ingest the toxic substance. In an emergency ipecac can be obtained from an all-night pharmacy, convenience store, emergency squad, or emergency department. It is inexpensive and has a shelf life of 5 years (Boehnert and others, 1985). Despite the fact that ipecac is highly effective, its use as a home emetic is a source of dispute (see Questions and controversies).

If the child is admitted to an emergency facility, gastric lavage may also be done to empty the stomach of the toxic agent. Indications for lavage include: young infants for whom ipecac is contraindicated; the patient is comatose, convulsing, or requires a protected airway; or the ingested poison is one that is rapidly absorbed (strychnine or cya-

Questions and Controversies

How safe is ipecac and should it be recommended for home use?

Ipecac is considered the emetic of choice for removal of toxic substances from the stomach. However, there is concern over its safety and its abuse by individuals with anorexia nervosa and bulimia. In some countries other than the United States ipecac is available only with a prescription. This practice, however, severely limits its timely use during home management of poisonings.

Reports of adverse effects from ipecac include lethargy, diarrhea, and protracted vomiting (Czajka and Russell, 1985); however, it is not possible to distinguish if these effects are solely caused by the ipecac or the poison. Isolated deaths have occurred from excessive amounts of ipecac to treat poisonings, and health care professionals are concerned about chronic abuse by those with eating disorders, in which peripheral myopathies and often fatal cardiomyopathies can occur (Friedman, 1984). Other studies demonstrate that ipecac is very safe, even when used without appropriate consultation (Chafee-Bahamon, Lacouture, and Lovejoy, 1985). Consequently, most authorities continue to support its use in the home (Mofenson and Caraccio, 1986), even to infants 6 to 11 months of age (Litovitz and others, 1985). Health education has been shown to be effective in educating parents on home use of ipecac (Dershewitz, Posner, and Paichel, 1983).

Emergency Treatment: *Poisoning*

1. Assess the victim:
   (a) take vital signs; re-evaluate routinely
   (b) initiate cardiorespiratory support if needed
   (c) treat other symptoms, such as seizures

2. Terminate exposure:
   (a) empty mouth of pills, plant parts, or other material
   (b) flush thoroughly eyes and/or skin with tap water if involved
   (c) remove contaminated clothing (e.g., if gasoline has spilled)
   (d) bring victim of an inhalation poisoning into fresh air
   (e) give water to dilute ingested poison

3. Identify the poison:
   (a) question the victim and witnesses
   (b) save all evidence of poison (empty bottle, opened container, vomitus, urine)
   (c) be alert to signs/symptoms of potential poisoning in absence of other evidence (see Table 16-4)
   (d) call Poison Control Center or other competent emergency facility for immediate advice regarding treatment

4. Remove poison/prevent absorption:
   (a) induce vomiting; administer ipecac*
      —9 to 12 months: 10 ml; do not repeat
      —1 to 12 years: 15 ml repeat dosage once if vomiting
      —over 12 years: 30 ml has not occurred within 30 minutes
      —give 10 to 20 ml/kg of clear fluids after ipecac
   (b) do not induce vomiting if:
      —victim is comatose, in severe shock, or convulsing, or has lost the gag reflex
      —poison is a low-viscosity hydrocarbon (mineral seal oil) or a strong corrosive (acid or alkali)
   (c) place child in side-lying, sitting, or kneeling position with head below chest to prevent aspiration
   (d) administer activated charcoal (15 to 30 g for children under 12 years and 50 to 100 g for those over 12)† 30 to 60 minutes *after* inducing vomiting with ipecac, if ordered

*Dosage recommendations from Boehnert and others, 1985.
†Dosage recommendations from Rodgers and Matyunas, 1986.

---

nide). The use of lavage in petroleum distillate poisoning is controversial because of the danger of aspiration. When lavage is performed, the largest diameter tube that can be inserted is used to facilitate passage of gastric contents.

Another method of decontaminating the stomach is the use of activated charcoal, an odorless, tasteless, fine black powder that adsorbs many compounds, creating a stable complex. It is used within 1 hour of the poisoning but *after* giving an emetic, to avoid the charcoal also adsorbing the emetic and preventing its pharmacologic effect. It is mixed with water or saline cathartic to form a slurry. Slurries are neither gritty nor distasteful but look like black mud. They are often accepted more readily if mixed with flavoring and served through a straw and opaque glass with a cover, such as a disposable coffee cup and lid. Sorbitol, an artificial sweetener, has been used successfully as a flavoring in slurries and also acts as a cathartic. Cathartics, such as sodium or magnesium, may be administered to stimulate evacuation of the bowel, thus decreasing systemic absorption of the poison and aiding in removal of charcoal.

In a minority of poisonings specific antidotes are available to counteract the poison. They are highly effective and should be available in all emergency facilities. The supply of antidotes should be checked routinely and replaced as used or according to expiration dates. Among the more commonly employed antidotes are N-acetylcysteine for acetaminophen poisoning, oxygen for carbon monoxide inhalation, naloxone for narcotic overdose, and antivenin for certain poisonous bites.

Corrosives. Corrosive or caustic substances include strong acids or alkalis that cause chemical burns of mucosal surfaces (see Table 16-4 for signs of poisoning). Numerous household products are corrosive, including drain, toilet, or oven cleaners, electric dishwasher detergent, some detergents or cleansers, mildew remover, batteries, Clinitest tablets, and denture cleaners. Household bleach, which is moderately alkaline, is perhaps the most frequent corrosive material ingested. Although it may induce mucosal burns and edema, extensive necrosis and subsequent stricture formation do not occur, as is typical of the other substances (Wasserman and Ginsburg, 1985). Liquid products cause more damage than granular substances because they are swallowed and can damage the mucosa as far down as the duodenum, whereas granular material adheres to the oral mucosa and causes burns limited to that area (Moore, 1986).

Vomiting is contraindicated in the treatment of corrosives, since emesis can cause repeated damage to the mucosal wall. Emergency care is aimed at preventing further damage by diluting the corrosive agent with water. Milk is not recommended by some authorities because it coats the mucous membranes and may obscure the surface for evaluation of burns. Neutralization with vinegar or lemon juice is contraindicated because the neutralizing reaction may produce heat, thus causing a thermal burn in addition to the chemical burn. Other aspects of care include providing a patent airway if necessary, administering analgesics for pain, and giving the child either nothing by mouth or only a liquid diet if tolerated. Long-term care may involve surgery to correct an esophageal stricture. A potential sequelae is the development in adulthood of squamous cell carcinoma at the site of the stenosis (Benirschke, 1981). These children need to be instructed as young adults to immediately seek medical advice if dysphagia develops.

Hydrocarbons. Hydrocarbons refer to organic compounds that contain carbon and hydrogen; many, but not all, hydrocarbons are distillates of petroleum. Hydrocarbons of concern if ingested include gasoline, kerosene, lamp oil, mineral seal oil (a product found in furniture polish), lighter fluid, turpentine, many paint thinners and removers, and certain furniture polishes and cleaning agents—all products

---

QUESTIONNAIRE FOR POISON PREVENTION

1. Where do I store cleaning products, medicines, laundry aids, and garden supplies?
2. What do I keep under the sink in the kitchen and bathroom?
3. Do I have any medicines (e.g., aspirin, tranquilizers, birth control pills, antacids) in my purse?
4. Are all the medicines and household products clearly labeled and in their original container?
5. Do I refer to medicine as candy to encourage my child to take it?
6. Are any medications left on the table or kitchen counter for handy use?
7. Do I keep drugs prescribed for previous illnesses?
8. Is my child out of sight when I take medicine?
9. When using any medicine or household product, do I put it away immediately after use, keep my eye on it at all times, or put it down where my child cannot get it?
10. Are any of my garden plants or houseplants poisonous?
11. Do all cabinets have a lock on them?
12. What is stored in the garage or basement?
13. Are paints, gasoline, solvents, insecticides, poisons, and fertilizers either on a high shelf or locked in a cabinet?
14. Do I teach my child never to touch any nonfood item without asking me first?

---

that may be found in the home and garage. Because they are frequently stored incorrectly in unmarked containers and may have a pleasant aroma, they are often ingested by young children (Klein and Simon, 1986).

The immediate danger from most hydrocarbons is aspiration, since even small amounts aspirated into the lungs can cause severe, sometimes fatal, chemical pneumonitis (see Table 16-4 for signs of poisoning). However, adverse systemic effects from gastrointestinal absorption are usually mild. High viscosity (thick) hydrocarbons, such as Vaseline, vegetable oil, or mineral oil, are nontoxic and may have a laxative effect if large amounts are ingested. Distillates having high volatility (evaporate quickly), low viscosity, and low surface tension, such as gasoline, kerosene, lighter fluid, mineral seal oil, or turpentine, cause the most severe pneumonitis because they tend to spread easily over a large surface area. The following conservative approach serves as a general guide for dealing with the ingestion of toxic hydrocarbons (Anas, Namasonthi, and Ginsburg, 1981):

1. Asymptomatic children with initial normal or abnormal chest roentgenograms and symptomatic children with normal chest roentgenograms are observed for 6 hours and are admitted if their symptoms persist or worsen.
2. Symptomatic children with abnormal roentgenograms are admitted at the initial evaluation.
3. Emesis is induced only if the child ingested more than 1 ml of the substance/kg of body weight or if the hydrocarbon contains a potentially toxic substance (insecticide, heavy metal, camphor). Emesis is not induced if central nervous system depression is present.

Family Support

A poisoning is more than a physical emergency for the child. It usually represents an emotional crisis for the parents, particularly in terms of guilt, self-reproach, and insecurity in the parenting role. The emergency room is no place to admonish the parents for negligence, lack of appropriate supervision, or failure to safe-proof the home. Rather it is a time to calm and support the child and parents, while unaccusingly exploring the circumstances of the accident. If the nurse prematurely attempts to discuss ways of preventing such an accident from recurring, the parents' anxiety will block out any suggestions or offered guidance. Therefore it is preferable for the nurse to delay the discussion until the child's condition is stabilized or, if the child is discharged immediately after emergency treatment, to make a public health referral.

TEACHING STRATEGY FOR PARENT EDUCATION AND PREPARATION IN CASE OF AN ACCIDENTAL POISONING

Question	Intervention
If you suspected that your child had ingested (eaten) a poison, what would you do first?	If answer is correct, ask for more specifics, such as number of local poison control center If answer does not include knowledge of local poison control center, supply information Stress necessity of not wasting time and need to save all evidence of poisoning
Do you have ipecac syrup in your home?	If answer is yes, ask for specific directions concerning its dosage and readministration If answer is no, supply correct information
Should you always make the child vomit?	If answer is no, ask for specific poisons that are treated differently, such as turpentine and drain cleaner If answer is yes, supply correct information Emphasize that instructions on container of household products are minimum and sometimes inaccurate emergency treatment; medical advice should *always* be sought before relying on that information alone
If you suspected that your child had taken a poison, but there were no signs of illness and the child denied doing so, what would you do?	Emphasize need to always seek medical advice rather than waiting for signs or believing the child

Prevention of Recurrence

The ultimate objective is to prevent poisonings from occurring or recurring. One effective counseling method is first to discuss the difficulties of constantly watching and safeguarding young children. In this way the monumental task of raising children is shared as a common problem, with injury prevention as one part of the parental role, not as the central issue. This approach also incorporates other contributory causes for the incident, such as inadequate support systems, marital discord, discipline techniques (especially use of physical punishment), and maternal distress (Bithoney and others, 1985). A visit to the home, especially after a repeat poisoning situation, is recommended as part of the follow-up care to assess hazards, including family factors, and to evaluate appropriate safe-proofing measures. One method of identifying risk areas is to ask specific questions or to have the parent complete a questionnaire designed to isolate factors that predispose children to poisoning.

The box on p. 672 is a sample questionnaire of items that may determine what environmental manipulation is needed to "poison-proof" homes. The box opposite is a teaching plan designed to assess parents' preparedness in case of an accidental poisoning and to supply appropriate strategy and instruction where necessary. Such tools enable nurses to systematically and efficiently counsel families in the area of injury prevention.

Passive measures (those that do not require active participation) have been the most successful in preventing poisoning and include child-resistant closures and limited number of tablets in one container, such as bottles of baby aspirin. Other methods include the use of warning labels to alert children to potential dangers. However, the effectiveness of such labels is questionable (see Questions and controversies). If labeling is used, it must be combined with parental counseling and emphasis on proper storage of poisonous agents. Poison-warning stickers with information about the local PCC can also be placed on the telephone.

Questions and Controversies

How effective are poison-warning stickers in preventing ingestions?

Although programs advocating the use of poison-warning labels, such as Mr. Yuk, Officer Ugg, or a skull and crossbones, have been popular, studies to determine their effectiveness have not supported the belief that supplying such stickers to families reduces risks of accidental poisoning. Vernberg, Culver-Dickinson, and Spyker (1984) found that children actually preferred to touch labeled containers after undergoing education incorporating Mr. Yuk stickers. Reasons for the failure of warning labels include inadequate labeling of all poisons in the home and poisoning by substances that cannot be labeled, such as plants (Fergusson and others, 1982). Despite these findings it may be possible that warning labels are an important *adjunct* to an integrated poisoning prevention campaign or are effective for older children.

Table 16-6 Poisonous and nonpoisonous plants

POISONOUS PLANTS	TOXIC PARTS	NONPOISONOUS PLANTS
Apricot	Leaves, stem, seed pits	African violet
Azalea	Foliage and flowers	Aluminum plant
		Asparagus fern
Buttercup	All parts	Begonia
Cherry (wild or cultivated)	Twigs and foliage	Boston fern
		Christmas cactus
Chrysanthemum	All parts	Coleus
Daffodil	Bulbs	Gardenia
Dumb cane, Dieffenbachia	All parts	Grape ivy
		Jade plant
Elephant ear	All parts	Piggyback begonia
English ivy	All parts	Piggyback plant
Foxglove	Leaves, seeds, flowers	Prayer plant
		Rubber tree
Holly, mistletoe	Berries	Snake plant
Honeysuckle	All parts	Spider plant
Hyacinth	Bulbs	Swedish ivy
Ivy	Leaves	Wax plant
Oak tree	Acorn, foliage	Weeping fig
Philodendron	All parts	Zebra plant
Plum	Pit	
Poinsettia	Leaves	
Poison ivy, poison oak	Leaves, fruit, stems, smoke from burning plants	
Pothos	All parts	
Rhubarb	Leaves	
Tulip	Bulbs	
Water hemlock	All parts	
Wisteria	Seeds, pods	
Yew	All parts	

PLANTS

Ingestion of plant parts is the most common cause of childhood poisoning. Fortunately, most of these children are not seriously affected and do not require hospitalization. However, some are severely, even fatally, poisoned. Given the abundance of plants both in and outside the home, it is essential that parents be advised of this danger. Table 16-5 lists some of the more common poisonous plants as well as nontoxic varieties that can be safely grown. Preventive measures include (1) placing houseplants out of young children's reach, such as on high shelves or in hanging baskets, (2) teaching children *never* to eat anything without parental permission, and (3) avoiding making teas or homemade medicines from plants. Treatment is usually symptomatic and supportive. If the plant ingested cannot be identified, careful observation without aggressive intervention is recommended (McGuigan, 1984).

SALICYLATE POISONING

Aspirin (acetylsalicylic acid), the most common salicylate, is a drug frequently ingested by children. However, in recent years the incidence of acute salicylate poisoning has declined, primarily due to child-resistant closures and limited quantity of the drug per container (Snodgrass, 1986). The association of Reye syndrome with aspirin ingestion has also probably led to less use of the drug (Barrett and others, 1986). Unfortunately, the incidence of chronic poisoning (salicylism) has not decreased. The most common reasons for misuse of aspirin are parents' misunderstanding of health professional's instructions, incorrect dosage information from health professionals, use of aspirin without medical supervision, and use of several aspirin-containing products simultaneously (McGuigan, 1983).

Despite the decline in acute ingestions, they still do occur. Of particular concern are adult-strength aspirin, since the 5-grain tablets are four times stronger than the children's preparation, and time-released aspirin, which causes symptoms to be delayed for several hours. In addition, time-released preparations are frequently used by people with arthritis who find the safety caps very difficult to open. As a result, they may transfer the drug to an ordinary container or incorrectly replace the safety cap. Either of these possibilities increases the chance of young children gaining access to the drug and accidentally ingesting it.

Another source of acute salicylate intoxication is methyl salicylate, which is commercially available in oil of wintergreen, a flavoring agent. One teaspoon of oil of wintergreen, which is about one ''swallow,'' contains the equivalent of 5 g of salicylate or 21.7 adult aspirin tablets—an amount that can be fatal to a child (Howrie, Moriarty, and Breit, 1985). Toxicity occurs more rapidly due to increased absorption.

Salicylate toxicity is dose related. Acute ingestions of less than 150 mg/kg (2 gr/kg) are mildly toxic; ingestion of 150 to 300 mg/kg (2 to 4 gr/kg) constitutes moderate toxicity. Severe toxicity results when 300 to 500 mg/kg (4 to 7 gr/kg) or more is ingested (Temple, 1981). For a child who weighs 20 pounds (9 kg), severe toxicity occurs with the ingestion of 7 adult aspirin or 28 baby aspirin (1.25 grains). Chronic ingestions of more than 100 mg/kg/day for 2 days or more may produce toxicity (the usual therapeutic dose of aspirin is 65 mg/kg/day) (McGuigan, 1983).

Pathophysiology and Clinical Manifestations

Toxic amounts of salicylates directly affect the respiratory system. Hyperventilation, the most obvious clinical manifestation of salicylate overdose, causes loss of carbon dioxide and respiratory alkalosis. Signs of respiratory alkalosis include confusion, loss of consciousness, and, if not treated, coma and death from respiratory failure. Salicylates also increase metabolism, resulting in greater oxygen consumption, carbon dioxide production, and heat production, which is manifest as hyperpyrexia. Metabolic acidosis occurs from the accumulation of ketones and other organic acids and results in symptoms of anorexia, vomiting, and diaphoresis.

In a chronic overdose, salicylates can cause bleeding tendencies because aspirin inhibits platelet aggregation and prothrombin production. The other symptoms of chronic poisoning are similar to acute overdose but are more subtle during onset, tend to be more severe, especially dehydration, coma, and/or seizures (Gaudreault, Temple, and Lovejoy, 1982), and may be confused with the illness being treated. Therefore chronic poisoning is considered a more serious intoxication than acute ingestions.

Diagnostic Evaluation

Aspirin exerts its peak effect in 2 to 4 hours, and its effects may last for as long as 18 hours. There is usually a delay of up to 6 hours before evidence of toxicity is noted. This delay represents a serious diagnostic problem, because by the time symptoms are evident, pathophysiologic disturbances are fairly advanced. Since there is a delay in the manifestation of symptoms, laboratory tests to determine serum salicylate levels are essential. These levels are compared to a special chart (nomogram) that determines the degree of toxicity from the time of ingestion.

Therapeutic Management

Treatment depends on the amount of the drug ingested. Salicylate ingestions of less than 300 mg/kg can be managed at home by inducing vomiting if there is no delay in treatment. In instances where there is a substantial amount of time between ingestion and initiation of treatment, the child should be brought to a health care facility.

Severe intoxications are managed in a health care facility. The immediate treatment is removal of the drug from the stomach either by forced emesis or gastric lavage, followed by the administration of activated charcoal and a cathartic. Further therapy depends on serum salicylate levels and clinical manifestations. The acid-base disturbances are treated with appropriate electrolyte transfusions. Intravenous administration of sodium bicarbonate facilitates salicylate excretion. Calories and fluids are supplied to meet the increased metabolic rate. The hyperpyrexia is controlled with cool sponges and hypothermia blankets to reduce the possibility of convulsions. Vitamin K may be administered to decrease bleeding tendencies. In extreme cases of salicylate poisoning, external removal of the drug may be attempted through peritoneal dialysis or hemodialysis, but such intervention is usually reserved for situations of life-threatening intoxication.

A major problem exists after accidental ingestion of time-released aspirin, since symptoms may not arise until 6 to 16 hours have elapsed. Cathartics and colonic irrigations are helpful in removing the unabsorbed drug, and in severe cases dialysis may be necessary.

Nursing Considerations

The major nursing objectives are removal of the poison, observation of latent effects from the overdose, assistance with any medical treatments of the complications, prevention of recurrence of the poisoning, and emotional support of the child and parents. Relevant interventions are discussed under Principles of emergency treatment and in the box on p. 671.

Prevention of acute ingestion involves the same precautions as recommended for any toxic substance. However,

many parents are unaware of the danger of methyl salicylate, especially since oil of wintergreen is sold as a food additive and may not be perceived as potentially toxic. Therefore public education is essential to prevent this uncommon but life-threatening poisoning.

Of special concern is prevention of chronic salicylate poisoning. Parents need education regarding correct dosage of aspirin (see Table 27-2) and the potential danger in giving too much, especially from multiple drug preparations, such as cold medication. They are advised to call a physician if symptoms such as fever or pain persist, rather than continuing to treat the child with multiple doses of aspirin.

ACETAMINOPHEN POISONING

Acetaminophen is increasingly used as a mild analgesic/antipyretic drug, especially as a substitute for aspirin, and is the most common source of drug poisoning among children. Like aspirin, acetaminophen is available in many palatable forms that are well accepted by youngsters.

Acetaminophen poisoning occurs primarily from acute overdose. Toxicity from chronic therapeutic use has been documented in adults, especially in individuals who abuse alcohol (Benson, 1983), but it is not known to occur in children (Rumack, 1983, 1984; McGuigan, 1983). The recommended dosages for children are listed in Table 27-3. The precise toxic dose is uncertain, although ingestions of 140 mg/kg have produced liver injury.

Pathophysiology

Acute overdose of acetaminophen results in hepatic damage. The damage is not from the drug itself but from one of its metabolites, which in large quantities is toxic to the liver cells. Normally the liver produces the substance glutathione, which combines with the metabolite to negate its toxic effect; the detoxified combination is excreted through the kidneys. However, large doses of acetaminophen exceed the liver's supply of glutathione, allowing the metabolite to cause hepatic necrosis.

Clinical Manifestations

Signs and symptoms occur in four stages if the poisoning is untreated. In the first stage, 2 to 24 hours after ingestion, there are signs of nausea, vomiting, anorexia, sweating, and pallor. Some patients recover completely at this point, but others experience a latent period (the second stage) of 24 to 36 hours, which occurs between ingestion and onset of hepatic symptoms. The latent period is significant because many individuals who have ingested a toxic dose may feel better after the initial symptoms and may not seek medical care. Pain in the upper right quadrant followed by signs of hepatic damage (jaundice, confusion, stupor, and coagulation abnormalities) comprise the third stage. In most patients the third stage lasts no more than 7 to 8 days. Those patients who do not die as a result of hepatic failure enter a fourth stage, in which the liver enzyme SGOT (serum glutamic-oxaloacetic transaminase) begins to drop and recovery occurs.

Diagnostic Evaluation

Because of the initially mild symptoms, diagnosis is confirmed by serum acetaminophen levels drawn at least 4 hours after ingestion. Liver and renal function tests are performed to assess the pathologic effect of toxicity on the liver and kidneys.

Therapeutic Management

Initial management is induced emesis or lavage if the ingested dose is greater than 140 mg/kg. If the child arrives at the health care facility within 2 hours of the ingestion or if other toxins were ingested, activated charcoal may be used. If charcoal is used and the antidote N-acetylcysteine (Mucomyst) is to be given, the charcoal is removed by lavage before administering the antidote. If treatment is delayed longer than 2 hours, N-acetylcysteine is administered after emesis or lavage and activated charcoal is not given. N-acetylcysteine functions as a glutathionine substitute and binds with the metabolite so that the liver is protected. It is given orally (mixed with cola or fruit juice) or via nasogastric tube. Because of its offensive odor (similar to rotten eggs), it may be accepted more readily if given by the latter route. If vomiting occurs within 1 hour of administration of acetylcysteine, the dose is repeated.

Nursing Considerations

Nursing goals are essentially the same as those discussed for salicylate poisoning. The nurse needs to be familiar with acetaminophen preparations, such as cold remedies, to identify possible instance of ingestion. As with any poisoning, the primary goal is prevention. With the present emphasis on acetaminophen as a "safe" substitute for aspirin, it is important to stress that in excess this drug, like any other, is capable of toxic and lethal side effects.

HEAVY METAL POISONING

Heavy metal poisoning can occur from the ingestion of a variety of substances, the most common being lead. Other sources are iron from medicinal supplement preparations and mercury, most often found in excessive quantities in seafood harvested from polluted waters. Another source of mercury poisoning is the elemental form found in thermometers. Elemental mercury is nontoxic when ingested but poisonous when inhaled.

Heavy metals have an affinity for certain essential tissue chemicals, which must remain free for adequate cell functioning. When metals are bound to these substances, cellular enzyme systems are inactivated. Consequently the pathologic effects and treatment are similar to those for lead poisoning. Differences do occur in terms of the body systems involved and the choice of chelating agent.

IRON POISONING

Of all classes of pharmaceutical preparations ingested by young children, vitamins rank second (see box, p. 669),

and 35% of vitamin ingestions involve vitamins containing iron. Factors thought to be responsible for the frequency of iron ingestions include widespread availability, large number of tablets prescribed and packaged, failure of parents to recognize the potential lethality of iron, and failure of safety closures (Banner and Tong, 1986). The similarity between enteric-coated iron tablets and candy-coated chocolate, such as M&Ms, contributes to their attractiveness to children.

The toxic dose of an iron ingestion is based on the amount of elemental iron in various salts (sulfate, gluconate, fumarate), which ranges from 20% to 33%. Ingestions of 20 to 60 mg/kg can be potentially dangerous and above 60 mg/kg can be severe, even fatal (Banner and Tong, 1986).

Clinical Manifestations

Iron is toxic to several body systems, and intoxication produces five distinct stages of clinical manifestations that are related to the amount of iron ingested and the response to treatment (Barkin and Rosen, 1984):

1. Initial period (1/2 to 6 hours after ingestion). Gastrointestinal symptoms of vomiting, hematemesis, diarrhea, hematochezia (bloody stools), and gastric pain occur.
2. Latency (2 to 12 hours). The patient improves.
3. Systemic toxicity (4 to 24 hours after ingestion). Metabolic acidosis, fever, hyperglycemia, bleeding, shock, and death may occur.
4. Hepatic injury (48 to 96 hours). Seizures and coma are present, and the prognosis is poor.
5. In rare situations late sequelae of pyloric stenosis develops at 2 to 5 weeks.

Diagnostic Evaluation

Diagnosis is based on the calculation of ingested elemental iron and the child's clinical status, especially presence of spontaneous vomiting, diarrhea, and epigastric pain. Specific tests include serum iron, total iron-binding capacity (TIBC), blood glucose, and abdominal radiographs for presence of iron masses. A serum concentration of greater than 500 μg/dl strongly supports the need for aggressive therapy.

Therapeutic Management

Initial management consists of forced emesis or lavage. The administration of oral sodium bicarbonate or phosphate solution to form a nonabsorbable complex of iron is controversial. For severe intoxication, chelation therapy with deferoxamine is instituted. In rare instances surgical removal of large amounts of iron tablets may be warranted. Supportive care includes preventing shock and maintaining adequate renal function by correcting plasma and volume deficiencies, since blood and fluid losses in the gastrointestinal tract caused by mucosal injury from the corrosive effects of iron can rapidly progress to life-threatening hypovolemia.

Nursing Considerations

Nursing interventions are similar to those for any drug ingestion (see Salicylate poisoning) with the main emphasis on supportive care during the critical stages of the intoxication and family counseling to prevent recurrence.

LEAD POISONING (PLUMBISM)

Lead poisoning is a prevalent pediatric problem. An estimated 4%, or approximately 675,000, of children 6 months to 5 years of age in the United States show evidence of excessive amounts of lead in their blood. Black children have a six times greater incidence than white children (Annest and others, 1982). The peak age is from 2 to 3 years, and most poisoning occurs in warm weather months.

Factors Related to Lead Ingestion

Several factors influence the ingestion of lead-containing substances, and successful long-term cure and prevention of lead poisoning involves change in all the variables.

Environmental characteristics. The first contributing factor is the availability of lead in the environment. Lead enters the system either by ingestion or inhalation; the accompanying box lists the more common sources. Lead-based paint from dilapidated housing remains the most frequent high-dose source of lead. A few chips of paint may contain several hundred times the usual safe daily ingestion of lead.

It was not until the late 1970s that the U.S. Consumer Product Safety Commission finally banned the addition of lead to paints for residential use. Consequently substantial amounts of lead remain on the painted interior and exterior surfaces of homes. Although the child's immediate environment is usually the source of lead, other living conditions should be investigated, such as nursery or daycare centers.

POTENTIAL SOURCES OF LEAD

Ingested
Lead-based paint
  Interior: walls, windowsills, floors, furniture
  Exterior: door frames, fences, porches, siding
Plaster, caulking
Unglazed pottery
Colored newsprint
Painted food wrappers
Cigarette butts and ashes
Water from leaded pipes
Foods or liquids from cans soldered with lead
Household dust
Soil, especially along heavily trafficked roadways
Food grown in contaminated soil
Urban playgrounds
Folk remedies

Inhaled
Burning of leaded objects
  Automobile batteries
  Newspaper logs of colored paper
Sanding and scraping of lead-based painted surfaces
Automobile exhaust
Cigarette smoke
Sniffing leaded gasoline
Dust
  Poorly cleaned urban housing
Contaminated clothing and skin of household members working in smelting factories or working as urban policemen

---

Other sources of lead often are related to isolated occupations, such as lead smelter workers or urban policemen, or practices, including folk remedies that contain lead (Mexican *azarcon* or *greta* and Oriental *paylooah*—fine powders that are fed to young children as a cure for fever or rash) (Centers for Disease Control, 1983a, 1983b). There is increasing concern about lead levels in soils of urban areas and foods cultivated in these areas (Mielke and others, 1983).

Characteristics of the child. Developmentally young children are at risk for lead poisoning because of their high level of oral activity. Particularly during late infancy and toddlerhood, children explore their environment by putting objects in their mouth. This normal hand-to-mouth activity contributes to the amount of lead they ingest in dust and dirt. By virtue of their size, young children inhale air that is closer to the ground, which is more heavily contaminated with lead. In addition, the child who ingests lead often practices *pica*, the habitual, purposeful, and compulsive ingestion of nonfood substances.

To add to the risk is the fact that three times more lead is absorbed in children than in adults. Absorption is also enhanced by dietary deficiencies of iron and calcium, common conditions among youngsters already living in lead-burdened environments (Pearce and Burg, 1982).

Lead poisoning is not confined to the young child who ingests the substance. It can also occur in older children who habitually sniff leaded gasoline. The nurse must be aware of children experimenting with drugs or other psychotropic substances and the possibility of gasoline sniffing, which is especially prevalent among American Indian children on reservations (Coulehan and others, 1983).

Parental characteristics. Parent-child interaction is another significant variable in the ingestion of lead. Children with lead poisoning generally receive less adequate child care than children without plumbism, including poor hygienic practices, insufficient feeding to promote adequate nutrition, infrequent use of medical facilities, and insufficient rest. Parents use few resources to stimulate the child, tend to be less affectionate, and have an immature attitude toward maintaining discipline. These findings are not related to differences in income, educational level, age of parents, or number of household occupants—factors commonly felt to be associated with lead poisoning (Hunt, Hepner, Seaton, 1982). The correlation between parental behavior and lead levels is significant after children are 6 months of age, when their mobility and oral activity make lead accessible (Dietrich and others, 1985).

Pathophysiology and Clinical Manifestations

Normally, lead ingested within the safe daily range of 300 μg is very slowly excreted via the kidneys, alimentary tract, and, to a small extent, sweat. Retained lead is stored chiefly in the bone, where it is inert. However, under conditions of chronic ingestion the rate of absorption exceeds the rate of excretion, and excess lead is deposited in the tissues and circulatory system with about 90% attached to the erythrocytes. Even when the chronic ingestion stops, it takes the body twice as long to excrete the stored lead as it did to accumulate it. As a result, several body systems continue to be affected after the environmental removal of the poison (Fig. 16-6).

Hematologic system. Lead is extremely toxic to the biosynthesis of heme, preventing the formation of hemoglobin and causing its precursors, especially erythrocyte protoporphyrin (EP), coproporphyrin, and delta-aminolevulinic acid (ALA), to increase in the body. EP is elevated in the blood when the blood-lead concentration is only minimally increased and is a sensitive, but not specific, indicator of abnormal lead levels. The latter two intermediary metabolites are found in the urine in excessive amounts when the blood-lead concentration reaches 80 µg/dl of whole blood. Reduction of the heme molecule in the red blood cell results in anemia, one of the initial signs of the disease.

Renal system. Lead damages the cells of the proximal tubules, resulting in abnormal excretion of glucose, protein, amino acids, and phosphate. With adequate treatment kidney damage is usually reversible. Severe irreversible lead nephropathy is probably limited to protracted childhood plumbism.

Central nervous system. The most serious and irreversible side effects of lead intoxication are on the nervous system. Initially there is an increase in membrane permeability, with a shift of fluid into the interstitial spaces of the brain. As a result, increased intracranial pressure causes cortical atrophy and lead encephalopathy—convulsions, mental retardation, paralysis, blindness, and ultimately coma and death. Lead encephalopathy is almost always associated with a blood-lead concentration greater than 100 µg/dl.

However, before lead encephalopathy occurs, behavioral changes indicate lead toxicity. Hyperactivity, aggression, impulsiveness, decreased interest in play, lethargy, irritability, delay or reversal in verbal maturation, loss of newly acquired motor skills, clumsiness, deficits in sensory perception, learning difficulties, short attention span, and distractibility are common signs of asymptomatic or borderline poisoning. Studies also demonstrate that as lead levels increase, the child's intelligence quotient decreases (Bellinger and Needleman, 1983). Such manifestations of behavioral disturbance are important clues to the identification of children with early poisoning.

Prominent clinical signs of gasoline sniffing are mainly those of central nervous system toxicity: irritability, tremor, hallucinations, confusion, lack of impulse control, depression, delirium, chorea, ataxia, and sleep disturbances.

Other manifestations. Other vague symptoms of plumbism, including that caused by inhalation, are acute crampy abdominal pain, vomiting, constipation, anorexia, headache, and fever, which are sequelae of increasing toxicity. Short stature from impaired growth is also seen in children with asymptomatic plumbism (Schwartz, Angle, and Pitcher, 1986).

Diagnostic Evaluation

Several tests are available to detect the presence of toxic amounts of lead in the body. The most frequently used pro-

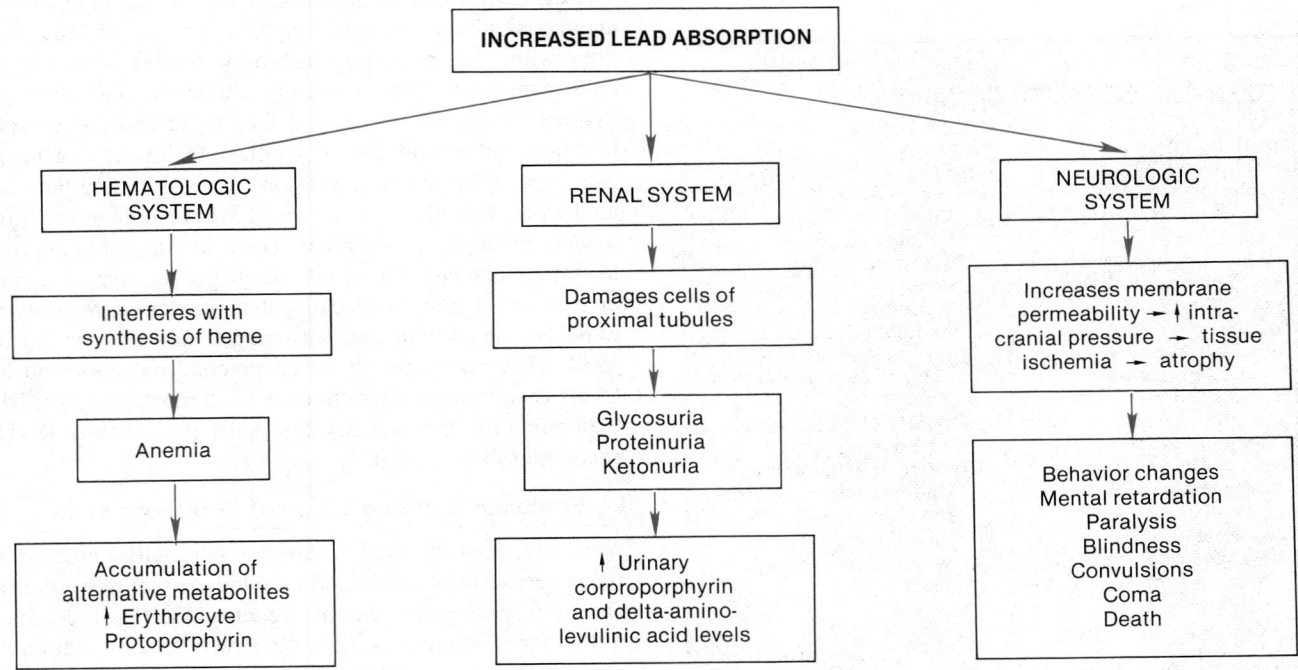

Fig. 16-6. Main effects of lead on body systems.

Table 16-6 Classification of lead poisoning according to blood-lead and erythrocyte-protoporphyrin levels

BLOOD LEAD (μg/dl)	ERYTHROCYTE PROTOPORPHYRIN (μg/dl WHOLE BLOOD)			
	$\leq$49	50-109	110-249	$\geq$250
Not done	I*	†	†	†
$\leq$29	I	Iα	Iα	EPP‡
30-49	Ib	II	III	III
50-69	§	III	III	IV
$\geq$70	§	§	IV	IV

Adapted from Centers for Disease Control: J. Pediatr. **93**(4):709-720, 1978.
*See text for classification.
†Blood lead necessary to estimate risk.
‡Erythropoietic protoporphyria; although rarely iron deficiency may cause EP elevations to 300 μg/dl.
§Combination of results generally not observed in practice; if observed, retest with venous blood immediately.

cedures for routine screening are the blood-lead concentration and the erythrocyte-protoporphyrin (EP) level. Blood lead levels reflect absorption from recent exposure to lead, while EP determinations measure the adverse metabolic effect of lead on heme synthesis. Screening is recommended at least yearly for children from 1 to 6 years of age who live in or frequently visit poorly maintained housing units constructed before the 1960s or who are exposed to other hazardous lead sources, such as heavily trafficked roadways. Ideally, children 12 to 36 months of age who are at risk should be screened every 2 to 3 months during the peak season of May through October (Centers for Disease Control, 1978).

Based on the results of these screening tests, the Centers for Disease Control (1978) have established a classification of *risk* (Table 16-6) to determine priority for further testing. For example, class IV children are at urgent risk and require immediate medical evaluation. Children in class II and III are at moderate and high risk respectively and need to receive further diagnostic tests but are not in immediate danger. Children in class I are at low risk and are usually not given diagnostic tests.

The diagnosis of lead poisoning is based on a number of laboratory tests, as well as findings from the history and physical examination. Such tests include radiographic evidence of "lead lines" in long bones or lead deposits in the abdomen, increased levels of urinary coproporphyrin and delta-aminolevulinic acid, and evidence of anemia (not a specific finding). A calcium disodium edetate mobilization test may also be performed to document increasing levels of lead in the urine. In addition, lead poisoning is defined by several criteria, including (1) two successive blood lead levels of 70 μg/dl or greater, or (2) a blood lead level of 50 μg/dl or greater and an EP level equal to or greater than 250 μg/dl, either with or without symptoms.

Therapeutic Management

The objective of treatment is to mobilize the lead from the blood and soft tissues by enhancing its deposition in bones and its excretion in the urine. Chelation therapy involves the removal of the metal by combining it with another substance. Calcium disodium edetate (CaNa$_2$EDTA) is the chelating agent of choice; disodium edetate (Na$_2$EDTA) is not used because of the risk of tetany from loss of calcium. Calcium disodium edetate forms a fairly stable, highly soluble compound that causes free lead to be readily excreted in the urine. It increases the urinary excretion of lead by 20 to 50 times, thereby relieving the symptoms of lead intoxication. It is usually used in combination with the chelating drug dimercaprol, also called BAL (British anti-lewisite). A combination of the drugs is thought to result in less saturation of each (therefore fewer side effects) and better removal of lead from the brain. Although calcium disodium edetate results in lower lead levels in general, it is less effective than BAL in removing lead from the nervous system because of its failure to penetrate the cerebral spinal fluid. Because of the rapid rise in serum lead once it is mobilized from the bone, initial treatment with CaNa$_2$EDTA can precipitate severe, even fatal, seizures. Consequently BAL is administered first (Pearce and Burg, 1982). Success of treatment is measured by urinary excretion of lead.

D-Penicillamine (Cuprimine, Depen) is the only commercially available oral chelating drug, although others are under investigation. It enhances urinary excretion of lead, but less effectively than CaNa$_2$EDTA. It is sometimes used on an outpatient basis, but patients must be carefully monitored for side effects and reactions. It is contraindicated in anyone with a history of penicillin allergy.

The exact course of therapy depends on the determination of risk from the diagnostic evaluation and includes (Centers of Disease, 1978):

Urgent risk—children with confirmed lead poisoning require inpatient chelation therapy

High risk—children whose repeat screening tests fall in class II and III but who also have positive confirmatory diagnostic tests may receive inpatient or outpatient chelation therapy

Moderate risk—children whose repeat screening tests fall in class II but who have negative diagnostic tests do not require chelation therapy but removal of lead sources and careful follow-up

Low risk—children in class I require periodic rescreening until they are 6 years old

The exact protocol for chelation therapy differs according to physician preference, but it generally includes a schedule of CaNa$_2$EDTA and BAL 6 times a day for 5 days. If encephalopathy is present, fluid volume is restricted to prevent additional cerebral edema and the drugs are administered intramuscularly. Children without encephalopathy can receive the drugs intravenously.

Symptomatic treatment largely involves controlling seizures, which are often severe and protracted, since the anoxia that accompanies the convulsions compounds the brain damage from lead. Hepatic and renal function is carefully monitored; nephrotoxicity is a side effect of plumbism and $CaNa_2EDTA$. Daily serum electrolyte levels should be taken. Cleansing enemas are ordered for episodes of acute lead ingestion or when lead is visible on radiologic examination in the gastrointestinal tract. Every effort is made to prevent infection and maintain adequate hydration. If iron deficiency anemia coexists with plumbism, it is treated after chelation therapy.

Nursing Considerations

The goals of nursing care are many when dealing with plumbism. The first is primary prevention of lead poisoning. However, this is an objective that cannot be accomplished by one person. It involves a multidisciplinary approach that combines efforts of pediatrician, nurse, social worker, and social services to deal with all three factors involved in lead poisoning—the child, the parent, and the environment.

As has been discussed previously, identification of the child at risk in terms of all three causative factors is essential. Besides the laboratory screening procedures to isolate borderline or asymptomatic cases, careful history-taking is one of the most useful and valuable tools and should concentrate on the following areas:

1. Sources of lead in the child's environment
2. History of pica or evidence of this behavior during the interview
3. Recent change in behavior, particularly disinterest in play
4. Developmental delay or recent loss of acquired skills, especially speech
5. Behavior problems such as aggression or hyperirritability

Parental characteristics, such as those discussed under Factors related to lead ingestion, are important contributing factors to high-risk situations. The value of a home visit, using such tools as the Home Observation and Measurement of the Environment (HOME) (see p. 211 and Appendix A), to evaluate the social and physical surroundings cannot be overestimated in the overall plan for diagnosis and prevention.

For the child who must undergo chelation therapy, the nurse has several priorities of care. One of the most significant is preparing of children for the number of injections they will receive. For example, if $CaNa_2EDTA$ and BAL are to be administered as separate injections every 4 hours for 5 days, the child will receive a total of 60 injections. The nurse prepares children through needle play on a doll or stuffed toy before the therapy begins and after they receive each injection (see Chapter 27). It is important to allow them an outlet for the pain and anger they typically feel and to emphasize the reason for the treatment, particularly that it is not a punishment for eating lead or paint. Children deserve an explanation, such as "This is to take the lead (paint) out of your body so that your tummy (or other physical discomfort) feels better." The parents are also prepared for the child's drug treatment and forewarned of possible psychologic and physical reactions.

Since $CaNa_2EDTA$ and BAL are both viscous solutions, they must be administered deeply into a different large muscle mass. Sometimes a local anesthetic such as procaine is injected simultaneously with the $CaNa_2EDTA$ or BAL to help lessen the pain during administration. If this is done, the chelating agent is drawn into the syringe, followed by the anesthetic. In this way the anesthetic is the first medication to be injected into the tissue. It is introduced slowly in order to allow some time for it to exert its deadening effect. An air bubble at the top of the syringe flushes the needle of any remaining medication, thereby decreasing the chance of tracking the drug through the layers of the skin on withdrawal of the syringe.

Planning a rotation schedule for each series of injections is essential to prevent tissue damage and to ensure maximum tissue absorption. Since the peak incidence of lead poisoning is during the toddler years, the vastus lateralis, ventrogluteal, and gluteal sites are satisfactory available areas for rotation of multiple injections.

A complication of multiple injections in one site is the development of hard, painful areas of fibrotic tissue. The nodules feel firm and almost circular when palpated. It is advisable to routinely feel the muscle mass before preparing the injection site to avoid administering additional medication into the same area. A systematic approach should be used to specify the sequence of injection sites (e.g., right vastus lateralis, upper left corner) so that each site is used as few times as possible. Local application of warm soaks or insulated hot packs to fibrotic areas helps relieve the discomfort, although the pain may persist and be severe enough to limit movement.

Since $CaNa_2EDTA$ and lead are toxic to the kidneys, records are kept of intake and output and frequent urinalysis is performed to evaluate renal functioning. Urine and blood specimens are routinely collected to measure lead levels and assess the efficacy of treatment.

Comprehensive management of the child with lead poisoning involves "treating" the environment to prevent recurrence after hospital discharge. However, this is not part of discharge planning, but rather a priority objective as soon as diagnosis of lead poisoning is made. When it is not possible for the family to move to better housing or expensively refurbish their present home, some simple, inexpensive measures can be instituted. As much of the old flaking paint as possible is scraped from the walls, ceilings, and floors. However, when sanding or burning is employed, children and pregnant women must not remain in the home (day or night) until the process is completed (Piomelli and others, 1984). Since a new coating of lead-free paint does not prevent additional chips from falling away from the plaster, the walls are covered with wallpaper, contact paper, fabric, or burlap.

Other sources of lead can be minimized by meticulous housecleaning, including wet mopping (Charney and others,

1983); frequent handwashing, especially after outdoor play; and elimination of contaminated clothing. Workers, such as lead smelters or urban policeman, should change into clean clothing before leaving work. Members of cultures using folk remedies that contain lead must be advised of the danger and encouraged to avoid such products.

In addition, the children must be supervised and guided toward activity other than pica. Helping parents learn methods of stimulating their children, locating preschool or day-care centers, or helping parents organize a play group are methods of improving parenting and consequently lessening those factors that contribute to plumbism.

Health professionals have an even broader responsibility in terms of educating the public regarding the signs and symptoms of the disease, especially in children with lead levels that are clinically borderline. The most frequent behavior deviations of extreme negativism, distractibility, and constant need for attention may well be mistakenly diagnosed as other behavior problems, with labels such as learning disorder, delinquency, emotional disturbance, or hyperactivity, when in reality the child is suffering from the physical effects of a toxic substance. If such children were detected and treated earlier, the chance for optimum development would probably be greater. However, until lead poisoning is attacked as a social problem as well as a physical problem, its high incidence, rate of recurrence, and serious irreversible sequelae may not be significantly altered.

Child Maltreatment

Child maltreatment is a broad term that includes intentional physical abuse or neglect, emotional abuse or neglect, or sexual abuse of children usually by adults. It is one of the most significant social problems affecting children. Although statistics only partially reflect the true incidence of child maltreatment, it is estimated that over 1.7 million children are reported yearly to child protective services in the United States (Highlights, 1986).

CHILD NEGLECT

Child neglect involves more children than any other form of maltreatment—58% of children are reported for neglect and 44% of all maltreatment-related fatalities are associated with deprivation of necessities (Highlights, 1986). Neglect is generally considered an omission, rather than a commission, of a direct act or behavior that has a detrimental effect on the child's psychologic development. Polansky and others (1977) offer this working definition of *child neglect:*

> A condition in which a caretaker responsible for the child either deliberately or by extraordinary inattentiveness permits the child to experience avoidable present suffering and/or fails to provide one or more of the ingredients generally deemed essential for developing a person's physical, intellectual, and emotional capacities.

Unlike the study of physical abuse, relatively little research has been done on the etiology of neglect, although it appears that many of the risk factors identified in physical abuse apply to neglect as well (see discussion on p. 683). For example, neglectful parents often demonstrate a lack of knowledge of parenting skills. They may be unaware that an infant needs to be fed every 3 to 4 hours, be unable to cook a meal, or not know what constitutes a nutritious meal. The most serious lack of knowledge is failure to recognize emotional nurturing as an essential need of children. Instead, emotional nurturing is viewed as spoiling the child by giving him attention. The reader is also encouraged to review the discussion of Failure to thrive (p. 567), which may be due to physical or emotional neglect.

Types of Neglect

Neglect takes many forms and can be classified broadly as physical or emotional maltreatment. *Physical neglect* involves the deprivation of necessities, such as food, clothing, shelter, supervision, medical care, and education. *Emotional neglect* generally refers to the failure to meet the child's needs for affection, attention, and emotional nurturance. It may also include lack of intervention for or fostering maladaptive behavior, such as delinquency or substance abuse. Overprotection may also be included, as it deprives children of the opportunity to develop to their maximum potential (Snyder, Hampton, and Newberger, 1983). *Emotional abuse* is an even more difficult aspect of maltreatment to define but refers to the deliberate attempt to destroy or significantly impair a child's self-esteem or competence. Verbal abuse is probably the most common form and includes scapegoating, put-downs, humiliation, labeling, and unrealistic expectations (Garbarino, 1978).

Identification of Neglect

Neglect from deprivation of necessities is easier to identify than emotional neglect or abuse, because physical signs are usually evident (Table 16-7). While emotional maltreatment may be readily suspected, it is very difficult to substantiate. Physical signs are often nonspecific, and nurses must rely on behavioral indicators, which range from depression to acting-out behavior, to help identify a possible abuse situation. Although primary caregivers are generally responsible for instances of emotional maltreatment, this is not always the case. School teachers can inflict emotional abuse on students; indications in children of teacher abuse include excessive worry about school performance; expressed fear of the teacher; negative perception of self and of school; excessive crying, nightmares, headaches, and stomachaches; and decreased attendance (Krugman and Krugman, 1984).

Nursing Considerations

Nursing goals are similar to those discussed under physical abuse with identification and prevention as priorities (see p. 687). All professionals working with children must have a

Table 16-7 Potential signs of child maltreatment

I. Physical neglect
A. Physical indicators
1. Failure to thrive
2. Signs of malnutrition, such as thin extremities, abdominal distention, lack of subcutaneous fat
3. Poor personal hygiene, especially of teeth
4. Unclean and/or inappropriate dress
5. Evidence of poor health care, such as nonimmunized status, untreated infections, frequent colds
6. Frequent injuries from lack of supervision
B. Behavioral indicators
1. Dull and inactive; excessively passive or sleepy
2. Self-stimulatory behaviors, such as finger sucking or rocking
3. Begging or stealing food
4. Absenteeism from school ⎫ in older child
5. Drug or alcohol addiction ⎬
6. Vandalism or shoplifting ⎭

II. Emotional abuse and neglect
A. Physical indicators
1. Failure to thrive
2. Feeding disorders, such as rumination
3. Enuresis
4. Sleep disorders
B. Behavioral indicators
1. Self-stimulatory behaviors, such as biting, rocking, sucking
2. During infancy, lack of social smile and stranger anxiety
3. Withdrawal
4. Unusual fearfulness
5. Antisocial behavior, such as destructiveness, stealing, cruelty
6. Extremes of behavior, such as overcompliant and passive or aggressive and demanding
7. Lags in emotional and intellectual development, especially language
8. Suicide attempts

III. Physical abuse
A. Physical indicators
1. Bruises and welts
   (a) On face, lips, mouth, back, buttocks, thighs, or areas of torso
   (b) Regular patterns descriptive of object used, such as belt buckle, hand, wire hanger, chain, wooden spoon, squeeze or pinch marks
   (c) May be present in various stages of healing
2. Burns
   (a) On soles of feet, palms of hands, back, or buttocks
   (b) Patterns descriptive of object used, such as round cigar or cigarette burns, "glovelike" sharply demarcated areas from immersion in scalding water, rope burns on wrists or ankles from being bound, burns in the shape of an iron, radiator, or electric stove burner
   (c) Absence of "splash" marks and presence of symmetric burns
3. Fractures and dislocations
   (a) Skull, nose, or facial structures
   (b) Injury may denote type of abuse, such as spiral fracture or dislocation from twisting of an extremity or whiplash from shaking the child
   (c) Multiple new or old fractures in various stages of healing
4. Lacerations and abrasions
   (a) On backs of arms, legs, torso, face, or external genitalia
   (b) Unusual symptoms, such as abdominal swelling, pain, and vomiting from punching
   (c) Descriptive marks such as from human bites or pulling the hair out
5. Chemical
   (a) Unexplained repeated poisoning, especially drug overdose
   (b) Unexplained sudden illness, such as hypoglycemia from insulin administration
B. Behavioral indicators
1. Wary of physical contact with adults
2. Apparent fear of parents or going home
3. Lying very still while surveying environment
4. Inappropriate reaction to injury, such as failure to cry from pain
5. Lack of reaction to frightening events
6. Apprehensive when hearing other children cry
7. Indiscriminate friendliness and displays of affection
8. Superficial relationships
9. Acting-out behavior, such as aggression, to seek attention
10. Withdrawal behavior

Table 16-7   Potential signs of child maltreatment—cont'd

IV. Sexual abuse
  A. Physical indicators
    1. Bruises, bleeding, lacerations or irritation of external genitalia, anus, mouth, or throat
    2. Torn, stained, or bloody underclothing
    3. Pain on urination or pain, swelling, and itching of genital area
    4. Penile discharge
    5. Sexually transmitted disease, nonspecific vaginitis, or venereal warts
    6. Difficulty in walking or sitting
    7. Unusual odor in the genital area
    8. Recurrent urinary tract infections
    9. Pregnancy in young adolescent
  B. Behavioral indicators
    1. Withdrawn, excessive daydreaming
    2. Preoccupied with fantasies, especially in play
    3. Poor relationships with peers
    4. Sudden changes, such as anxiety, loss or gain of weight, clinging behavior
    5. In incestuous relationships, excessive anger at mother for not protecting daughter
    6. Regressive behavior, such as bed-wetting or thumb-sucking
    7. Sudden onset of phobias or fears, particularly fears of the dark, men, strangers, or particular settings or situations (e.g., undue fear of leaving the house or staying at the daycare center or the baby-sitter's house)
    8. Running away from home
    9. Sudden emergence of sexually-related problems, including excessive or public masturbation, age-inappropriate sexual play, promiscuity, or overtly seductive behavior
    10. Substance abuse, particularly of alcohol or mood-elevating drugs
    11. Profound and rapid personality changes, especially extreme depression, hostility, and aggression (often accompanied by social withdrawal); rapidly declining school performance; and suicidal attempts or ideation

high index of suspicion regarding evidence of maltreatment. Often neglect is due to ignorance, and early education of caregivers regarding children's basic physical and emotional needs can avert serious problems. Parents must also be aware that emotional abuse can occur outside the home, such as in substitute care facilities or school. Any persistent change in children's behavior is a clue to unsatisfactory situations and must be taken seriously. Nurses can be alert to such problems by routinely incorporating questions about children's activities into their assessment and investigating directly or through referral any suspicious complaints.

PHYSICAL ABUSE

Physical abuse has received more attention than any other type of child maltreatment and is reported in about 50% of all cases. Major physical abuse accounts for 47% of all fatalities from abuse (Highlights, 1986).

As pervasive as the problem is, not one definition of child abuse is universally accepted. Kempe and others (1962) coined the term *battered child syndrome* (BCS) to refer to:

A clinical condition in young children who have received serious physical abuse, generally from a parent or foster parent.

However, this definition restricts abuse to the most severe forms and is less appropriate than broader definitions that include the spectrum of abuse. Currently each state in the United States defines abuse according to its individual reporting laws.

Factors Predisposing to Physical Abuse

The exact cause of child abuse is not known, but three major criteria—parental characteristics, characteristics of the child, and environmental characteristics—seem to predispose children to physical injury by their parents or other caregivers. These are discussed below.

Parental characteristics. In order to abuse, the parents must have the potential to abuse, which is believed to be the result of specific life experiences in their childhood. Although no two abusing individuals are exactly alike, there are several common factors that help identify potential abusers. It is important to remember that only about 10% of child abusers have a history of mental or psychotic disorders and these families require different treatment approaches.

One of the most significant factors is the type of parenting they received as a child. Most abusing parents were themselves abused as children, and if abuse was not overt, they typically recall their punishment as unfair and severe (Altemeier and others, 1982). Their relationship with their parents is viewed as negative (Oates, Forrest, and Peacock, 1985). Some studies suggest that living in this kind of environment conditions people to consider violence acceptable (Gelles and Cornell, 1985). Abusing parents tend to have difficulty controlling aggressive impulses, and the free expression of violence is one of the most consistent qualities of these families (Altemeier and others, 1982). In addition, abusing parents have low self-esteem and more distrust of others than nonabusing parents.

Another characteristic is that abusing parents may have inadequate knowledge of normal developmental expectations. Thus they expect their children to nurture and parent them, in the same way their parents demanded similar behavior. This concept of *role reversal,* or the parent acting as the child and expecting the child to become the parent, is an important reason why some children escape abuse, whereas others become the victims.

Often the precipitating factor for the abuse is not a stressful event for most parents; but to the potentially abusing parent, episodes of crying and ordinary tasks of childrearing, such as toilet training, speech development, or self-help skills, trigger uncontrollable battering. With no realistic knowledge of children's age-appropriate capabilities, the parent may expect learning to take place automatically. For example, the parent may decide that the 1-year-old child is ready for toilet training and expect that once the child is put on the potty-chair he will immediately learn to control elimination. When the child fails, the parent punishes him for not complying with the expected behavior. This partially explains why most physical injury occurs during usual child-caring activities, (e.g., bathing, dressing, and feeding) and why most abused children are under school age.

Another consequence of role reversal is the expectation that children have the maturity and responsibility of an adult. For example, very young children may be left alone with a 4- or 5-year-old child because the parent assumes that the preschooler is capable of looking after them. Another instance is the parent who fails to safeguard the house because of the belief that ''warning the child about the danger'' is sufficient. This lack of parental judgment often leads to serious or fatal injuries.

Abusing parents often live in social isolation and find little pleasure and satisfaction from interpersonal relationships. With such needs unmet, they may seek gratification in a marriage partner, who may be the same type of person. If this is the situation, either parent may be the abuser. The marriage partner may also be a passive, dependent individual who condones the abuse by not interfering with it. In either situation, marital discord is common and further adds to the stress within the family. With no available support system and the presence of concurrent stresses imposed by the child or environment, these parents are extremely vulnerable to additional crises of any nature and literally strike out at the child as a method of releasing their increasing frustration and anxiety. Some studies suggest that the level of social support is an important factor in identifying potential abusers, and that enhancement of the person's support system may be a strategy for prevention or intervention of abuse (Turner and Avison, 1985).

Characteristics of the child. The child also unintentionally contributes to the abusing situation. In families of two or more children it is usual to find only one child as the victim of abuse. This child's temperament, position in the family, additional physical needs if ill, activity level, or sensitivity to parental needs all in some way contribute to

why he escapes or fosters physical abuse. For example, the firstborn may not be abused if he fits into the ''easy-child pattern,'' and demands little other than routine feeding and diapering. As he grows older, the docile child may learn how to meet the parent's needs by being quiet, playing alone, showing the parent affection, and acting as grown up and self-sufficient as possible. However, this situation is never safe for the child. Any added stress, such as illness, pregnancy, birth of a sibling, or financial need, can upset this precarious balance between parent-child role reversal.

Not infrequently the abused child is illegitimate, unwanted, brain damaged (especially in situations where the parents cannot accept the retardation), hyperkinetic, physi-

---

Questions and Controversies

How serious is the problem of "mistaken" diagnosis of child abuse?

Although most of the concern among health professionals is to detect child abuse early and to protect the child from further abuse, there must also be recognition of the possibility of mistaken diagnosis of child maltreatment. Incidence data indicates that approximately 60% of the 1.7 million reports in 1984 were unsubstantiated for child abuse and neglect by child protective services (Highlights, 1986). Although some degree of overreporting is to be expected because the law requires the reporting of suspected maltreatment, the present level of overreporting is considered unreasonably high. Some of the increase is most likely due to the practice of "defensive" medicine—health professionals are legally required to report suspected maltreatment but there is no penalty for reporting unsubstantiated cases. Therefore playing it "safe" is preferable to failing to report and facing criminal prosecution. Another negative effect of the overreporting is that the protective child services are so overburdened with minor cases that children in real danger of serious maltreatment may be poorly investigated (Besharov, 1985).

There are numerous reports of mistaken diagnosis in the literature. Some of them involve lack of understanding of cultural traditions, such as the Oriental practices of coin rubbing and cupping, which produce welts or bruises (Saulsbury and Hayden, 1985; Asnes and Wisotsky, 1981) or the use of heat (moxibustion), which causes circular burns (Feldman, 1984). Several diseases may be erroneously attributed to abuse, such as hemophilia, meningitis, sudden infant death syndrome, osteogenesis imperfecta, and erythema multiforme (Kirschner and Stein, 1985; Adler and Kane-Nussen, 1983). Nonintentional injuries may also be wrongly diagnosed as abuse, such as burns from metal buckles on car seats (Schmitt, Gray, and Britton, 1978) or lacerations from seat belts (Baker, 1986). Such wrongful accusations can cause families tremendous grief* and can be minimized with meticulous attention to history taking and physical examination. The parents must be given every opportunity to present their account, and it is suggested that they be involved in every phase of the investigative process, such as the initial proceedings of hospital-suspected child abuse and neglect (SCAN) temas (Reid, 1985).

*An organization of victims wrongfully accused of abuse is Victims of Child Abuse Laws (VOCAL), P.O. Box 11335, Minneapolis, MN 55411 (612-521-9714).

cally disabled, or from a broken home. Sometimes the child is abused because he reminds the parent of someone the parent dislikes, for example, a younger brother or sister who received all the attention from their own parents. Premature infants may be at risk for maltreatment because of the failure of parent-child bonding during early infancy. Often a difficult pregnancy, labor, or delivery is a predisposing factor in abuse, especially when the infant is born prematurely or with congenital anomalies.

Although one child is usually the victim in an abusing family, if that child is removed for his own protection, the parents quickly replace him with another victim. Child abuse is not confined to one child because of a disturbed parent-child relationship but is the result of dysfunctioning parenting, which can involve any child. Therefore no child is safe if left in the abusing environment unless the parents can be helped in some way to learn new parenting skills and to meet their needs and release their frustration through alternatives other than attacking their children.

Environmental characteristics. The environment is an integral part of the potential abusing situation. Typically the environment is one of chronic stress, including problems of divorce, extramarital relations, financial deficit, unemployment, poor housing, alcoholism, and drug addiction.

The social milieu of the abusive family is one devoid of adequate support systems. The environment becomes a trap from which there is no emotional exit except to direct the anger and frustration toward a helpless victim, the child.

Although most reporting of abuse has been from lower socioeconomic populations, child abuse is by no means a problem of any one societal group. It spans all educational, social, and economic levels. Certainly stresses imposed by poverty predispose lower socioeconomic families to abusive situations, and abuse in these groups is more apt to be reported. However, concealed crises can also be present in upper class families. For example, a wealthy family experiencing major life changes, such as rehousing, the birth of an additional child, or marital discord, may have sufficient environmental stressors imposed on them to produce a potentially abusing situation. Wealthy families may be so overinvolved with commitments outside the home that abuse may be inflicted by substitute caregivers. Nurses need to be cognizant of such factors in order to identify the hidden sources of child abuse and neglect.

Identification of Physical Abuse

One of the most critical responsibilities of health professionals is identifying abusive situations as early as possible. The characteristics discussed above can serve as a framework for assessing the vulnerability of families to abuse but are never predictive of actual abuse. Rather a thorough physical examination and a careful, detailed history are the diagnostic tools to identify abuse. Nurses have a very special role because they may be the first person to see the child and parent, and be the consistent caregiver if the child is hospitalized.

Evidence of maltreatment. Recognition of abuse or neglect necessitates a familiarity with both physical and be-

---

INDEX OF SUSPICION OF ABUSE

Physical evidence of abuse and/or neglect, including old injuries

Conflicting stories about the "accident" or injury from the parents or others

Cause of injury blamed on sibling or other party

An injury inconsistent with the history, such as a concussion and broken arm from falling off a bed

History inconsistent with child's developmental level; such as a 6-month-old turning on the hot water

A complaint other than the one associated with signs of abuse; for example, a chief complaint of a cold when there is evidence of first- and second-degree burns

Inappropriate parental concern for the degree of the injury, such as an exaggerated or absent emotional response

Refusal of the parents to sign for additional tests or agree to necessary treatment

Excessive delay in seeking treatment

Absence of the parents for questioning

Inappropriate response of child, such as little or no response to pain, fear of being touched, excessive or lack of separation anxiety, indiscriminate friendliness to strangers

Previous reports of abuse in the family

Repeated visits to emergency facilities with injuries

---

havioral signs suggestive of maltreatment (see Table 16-7). No one indicator is exclusively diagnostic of maltreatment; rather it is a pattern or combination of indicators that should arouse suspicion and further investigation. In addition, signs of possible abuse must be coupled with an understanding of cultural practices, such as cupping or coin rubbing (see p. 43), to avoid mistaken diagnosis of abuse (see Questions and controversies, p. 684).

Evidence of physical abuse is not always obvious. One of the more unusual and perplexing types of physical abuse is the *Munchausen syndrome by proxy,* which refers to illness that is fabricated or induced by one person in another. In children it is usually the mother who fabricates signs and symptoms in her child (Meadow and Lennert, 1984). It can take many forms, such as adding maternal blood to the child's urine to simulate hematuria (Outwater and others, 1981), presenting a fictitious medical history (Guandolo, 1985), or chronic poisoning of the child (Shnaps and others, 1981).

Such cases are often very difficult to confirm and require a high index of suspicion to protect the child from numerous unnecessary and painful diagnostic procedures. A number of warning signals are significant, including discrepancies between clinical findings and the history, clinical manifestations that occur primarily in the mother's presence, and the child's lack of response to the treatment (Meadow, 1982).

History pertaining to the incident. Besides observable evidence of abuse, the type of history revealed by the parents or other caregiver, such as the baby-sitter or mother's boyfriend, is a significant diagnostic factor. Those areas of the history that should arouse suspicion of abuse are summarized in the box above.

Incompatibility between the history and the injury is probably the most important criterion on which to base the decision to report suspected abuse (Solomons, 1980). However, an important point to remember is that maltreated children rarely betray their parents by confessing to the abuse they received. If questioned, they will repeat the same story as the parents and try to defend their parents' actions. If the interviewer directly accuses the parents of abuse, the child may accept responsibility for the act in an attempt to vindicate the parents from the accusation. Whether children respond in this way out of fear is uncertain. However, children do fear losing whatever security and love they have. Between abusive acts children may receive some measure of attention and love from the parents. If they betray the parents, they may lose this and be uncertain or fearful of the consequences, such as foster care. Preserving the present situation may be less frightening than the unknown future.

Parental behaviors. Certain behavioral responses of the parents to their child and to the interviewer should alert the nurse to the possibility of maltreatment. Typically the parents have difficulty in showing concern toward their child. They are unable to comfort him and give no indication of realizing how the child may feel, physically or emotionally. Instead they are critical of the child and angry with him for being injured. They maintain that the child injured himself, and if asked any question regarding their responsibility of protecting or supervising the child, they become hostile and aggressive. They act as if the child's injury is an assault on them. Their entire perception of the incident is in terms of how it affects them, not the child, which is an indication of their preoccupation with their own needs and their inability to give any support to others.

During the child's hospitalization they may not become involved in the child's care and may show little concern for his progress, eventual discharge, or need for follow-up care. However, if they are pressured during interrogation, they immediately demand to take the child home, regardless of the child's readiness for discharge.

If the interviewer avoids judging the parent and attempts to ask questions directed at the parent's history, the parent will usually reveal feelings about his childhood, particularly of loneliness, longing for a loving mother, and overwhelming feelings of worthlessness and dependency. As the interviewer shifts the focus from the child's ''injury'' to the parent's life, there is usually a marked transition in the parent's attitude, from one of distrust, suspicion, and hostility to one of attentiveness, heightened interest, and security.

Child behaviors. Abused children's response to their parents or the injury may also support the suspicion of abuse. Although no one pattern is typical, extremes of behavior may be observed. Children may be very unresponsive to the parent or excessively clinging and intolerant of separation. There may be over-attachment to the abusing parent, possibly in the hope of preventing any upset that may precipitate anger and another attack. During care of the injury children may be passive and accepting of the discom-

---

OBSERVATIONS OF PARENTS-TO-BE DURING PRENATAL CARE

1. Are the parents overconcerned with the baby's sex?
2. Are the parents overconcerned with the baby's performance? Do they worry that he will not meet the standard?
3. Is there an attempt to deny that there is a pregnancy (mother not willing to gain weight, no plans whatsoever, refusal to talk about the situation)?
4. Is this child going to be one child too many? Could he be the "last straw"?
5. Is there great depression over this pregnancy?
6. Is the mother alone and frightened, especially by the physical changes caused by the pregnancy? Do careful explanations fail to dissipate these fears?
7. Is support lacking from husband and/or family?
8. Where are the parents living? Do they have a listed telephone number? Are their relatives and friends nearby?
9. Did the mother and/or father formerly want an abortion but not go through with it or wait until it was too late?
10. Have the parents considered relinquishment of their child? Why did they change their minds?

From Kempe, C.N.: Approaches to preventing child abuse, Am. J. Dis. Child. **130**:941-947, Sept. 1976. Copyright 1976, American Medical Association.

---

fort or uncooperative and fearful of any physical contact. While some children shy away from strangers as if frightened, others are unusually affectionate and outgoing.

Nursing Considerations

Nursing care involves several important areas, ideally beginning with prevention of abuse and, following an abusive act, the identification and protection of the child from further abuse.

Prevention. Prevention involves identifying potential abusers and instituting supportive intervention before the occurrence of an abusive act. Frequently there are clues that point to potentially abusive parents before the birth of a child (see box on observing parents-to-be). Nurses in prenatal health centers need to be attuned to parents who are at risk by specifically questioning them regarding their attitude toward the pregnancy, future expectations for the child, and available support systems to help them adjust to parenthood. Of significance is information about the parents' own child-rearing and incidents of physical or emotional abuse during their childhood.

As soon as the infant is born, the nurse assesses the parent-child attachment process and notes behaviors that signal lack of understanding of the infant's needs, disappointment in the child, little identification with him, lack of support from the father or other family members, and additional environmental stressors (see box on postpartum observations, p. 687). Behaviors that signify positive adjustment to parenthood that offset the pressure of negative factors are also observed (see box on positive family characteristics, p. 687).

Once high-risk families have been identified, they need to be involved in a plan to promote the parent-child relationship. This involves helping the parents identify with the child, teaching them effective childrearing practices, and promoting their self-esteem. Nurses in a variety of settings can implement these goals. Nurses in prenatal clinics can prepare expectant families for the adjustment of parenthood. Nursery and postpartum nurses can foster the attachment process by encouraging parents to hold and look at their infant. In neonatal intensive care units nurses can minimize the effects of separation by encouraging parents to visit and help them become comfortable in the child's care. Those in

---

OBSERVATIONS TO BE MADE AT POSTPARTUM AND PEDIATRIC CHECKUPS

1. Does the mother have fun with the baby?
2. Does the mother establish eye contact (direct en face position) with the baby?
3. How does the mother talk to the baby? Is everything she expresses a demand?
4. Are most of her verbalizations about the child negative?
5. Does she remain disappointed over the child's sex?
6. What is the child's name? Where did it come from? When was the child named?
7. Are the mother's expectations for the child's development far beyond the child's capabilities?
8. Is the mother very bothered by the baby's crying? How does she feel about the crying?
9. Does the mother see the baby as too demanding during feedings? Is she repulsed by the messiness? Does she ignore the baby's demands to be fed?
10. What is the mother's reaction to the task of changing diapers?
11. When the baby cries, does she or can she comfort him?
12. What was/is the husband's and/or family's reaction to the baby?
13. What kinds of support is the mother receiving?
14. Are there sibling rivalry problems?
15. Is the husband jealous of the baby's drain on the mother's time and affection?
16. When the mother brings the child to the physician's office, does she get involved and take control over the baby's needs and what's going to happen (during the examination and while in the waiting room) or does she relinquish control to the physician or nurse (e.g., undressing the child, holding him, allowing him to express his fears)?
17. Can attention be focused on the child in the mother's presence? Can the mother see something positive for her in that?
18. Does the mother make nonexistent complaints about the baby? Does she describe to you a child that you do not see there at all? Does she call with strange stories that the child has, for example, stopped breathing, turned color, or is doing something "on purpose" to aggravate the parent?
19. Does the mother make emergency calls for very small things, not major things?

From Kempe, C.N.: Approaches to preventing child abuse, Am. J. Dis. Child. **130:**941-947, Sept. 1976. Copyright 1976, American Medical Association.

POSITIVE FAMILY CHARACTERISTICS

1. The parents see likable attributes in the baby and perceive him as an individual.
2. The baby is healthy and not disruptive to the parents' life-style.
3. Either parent can rescue the child or relieve one another in a crisis.
4. The parents' marriage is stable.
5. The parents have a good friend or relative to turn to, a sound "need-meeting" system.
6. The parents exhibit coping abilities, such as capacity to plan, and understand the need for adjustments because of the new baby.
7. The mother is intelligent and her health is good.
8. The parents had helpful role models when they grew up.
9. The parents can have fun together and with their personal interests and hobbies.
10. The parents practice birth control; the baby was planned or wanted.
11. The father has a steady job. The family has its own home, and living conditions are stable.
12. The father is supportive of the mother and involved in the care of the baby.

From Kempe, C.N.: Approaches to preventing child abuse, Am. J. Dis. Child. **130:**941-947, Sept. 1976. Copyright 1976, American Medical Association.

---

ambulatory settings can teach parents appropriate methods of bathing, feeding, toileting, disciplining, and preventing accidents, while stressing the normal needs and developmental characteristics of children. Nurses need to be sensitive to the parents' needs for attention, reassurance, and reinforcement. Ideally community nurses should visit these families to ensure that adequate support and help are available.

Identification and protection from further abuse. Initially, identification of instances of suspected abuse or neglect is essential. The nurse may come in contact with abused children in an emergency room, physician's office, or school. Signs that indicate possible abuse (see Table 16-10) must be recognized. *The priority is to remove the child from the abusive situation to prevent further injury.*

All states and provinces in North America have laws for mandatory reporting of child maltreatment. Suspected child abuse is reported to the local authorities.* Referrals usually come to the Bureau of Child Welfare and are assigned to a caseworker in an agency such as the Child Protective Services (CPS). In most states, once a referral has been made, there is an automatic court order, which gives the agency the right to keep the child in protective custody for 72 hours. This allows the caseworker sufficient time to investigate the report in the event of intervening holidays or weekends. If the caseworker finds no justification for the

---

*Telephone numbers are usually listed under "Child abuse" in the business white pages of the local directory, or call the emergency child abuse hotline: 1-800-422-4453 (1-800-4-A-CHILD).

charge, the child is returned to the home. If there is evidence of abuse, further action is taken against the parents.

A court proceeding may be necessary before the child can be placed outside the home or when parental rights may be terminated. When the courts are involved, they usually require firsthand testimony by the referring parties. This may mean that nurses in the school, hospital, or public health agency are subpoenaed or that their records are introduced as evidence. In either situation nurses have a great responsibility in reporting facts, not hearsay or subjective opinion, to present evidence of abuse or to vindicate individuals wrongfully accused of abuse. (see Questions and controversies, p. 684.)

Accurate nurses' notes are critical in any suspected abuse situation. A suggested outline for recording pertinent assessment data is presented in the box below. In addition, color photographs should be taken. Behaviors are described, not interpreted, and are recorded daily to establish a progress record. Conversations between the nurse, child, and parent are recorded in quotation form as much as possible. The nurse must bear in mind that the record of the hospital admission or home visit may be the most supporting evidence available. Nurses must be willing to take an active, responsible part in reporting and testifying to child abuse. Part of the long-term plan is help for parents, but the priority must be protection of the child.

Care of child. Frequently children suspected of abuse are hospitalized for medical management of their injuries.

GUIDELINES FOR ASSESSMENT DATA IN SUSPECTED ABUSE

History of injury
1. Date, time, and place of occurrence
2. Sequence of events with recorded times
3. Presence of witnesses
4. Time lapse between injury's occurrence and initiation of treatment
5. Interview with child when appropriate, including verbal quotations and information from drawing or other play activities
6. Interview with parent, witnesses, or other significant persons, including verbal quotations
7. Description of parent-child interactions (verbal interactions, eye contact, touching, parental concern)

Physical examination
1. Location, size, shape, and color of bruises; approximate location, size, and shape on drawing of body outline
2. Distinguishing characteristics, such as a bruise in the shape of a hand; round burn (possibly caused by cigarette)
3. Symmetry or asymmetry of injury; presence of other injuries
4. Degree of pain (see p. 1070); any bone tenderness
5. Evidence of old injuries; general state of health and hygiene
6. Developmental level of child; perform screening test such as Denver Developmental Screening Test (see p. 283)

Their needs are the same as those of any hospitalized child but are multiplied by their situation. Even though they tend to adjust easily to their new environment and make friends quickly, they need a consistent caregiver. At times the child's indiscriminate affection for any adult seems to diminish the necessity of consistency. However, such behavior is a learned response from previous relationships with others. The child wants to love and attach himself to one special person, but his efforts to do so with his parents, especially his mother, often were met with frustration and physical punishment or neglect. Therefore the child is no longer inclined to assume the same risk, unless the effort comes from the other person.

The nurse has the obligation of demonstrating acceptance and affection for the child, while not expecting the same in return, until the child begins to trust that the nurse will not turn against him for not meeting the nurse's needs. This can be made very difficult by the child's behavior, such as clinging for attention.

The nurse is placed in the position of showing the child acceptance while attempting to modify the negative behavior. Using anger or any aggressive act is avoided. Instead, a program of attention based on play, group interaction with other children, and quiet time with the child is planned. Behavior modification is employed to foster positive behavior and may include praise or tokens for rewards. Through such modeling, alternate ways of interacting and disciplining their child can be demonstrated to parents.

Hospitalization is often extended as eventual placement is arranged. Frequently this is longer than necessary for recovery from the injury or neglect. The child must be guided toward physical and mental wellness during this period. He is treated as a child with the usual physical needs, developmental tasks, and play interests—not as a dramatic victim of abuse. The nurse is his advocate in this goal. Others who want to question the child without justified reason are intercepted by the nurse, who also encourages the child in his continuing relationship with his parents. The nurse does not become a substitute parent to the exclusion of the child's natural parents. Such an intent only intensifies the parents' feelings of inadequacy, worthlessness, and isolation. It in no way helps them understand their child or promotes their trust in health professionals. The goal of the consistent nurse-child relationship is to provide a role model for the parents in helping them to relate positively and constructively to their child and to foster a therapeutic environment for the child in his reprieve from the abusing situation.

Discharge planning should begin as soon as the legal disposition for placement has been decided, which may be temporary foster home placement, return to the parents, or permanent termination of parental rights. The latter is the most drastic resolution, but it is necessary in situations of repeated abuse. Whenever children are remanded to a foster home or juvenile institution, they must be allowed the opportunity to express their feelings. No matter how severe the abuse, they usually mourn the loss of their parents. They need help to understand why they must not return home and that this new home is in no way a punishment. Whenever possible, foster parents should be encouraged to visit, and the nurse should take an active role in helping these parents understand the child. It is unfortunate that some abused children live in torment as they are sent from one foster home to another, sometimes enduring worse circumstances than existed in their original home. Only through constant evaluation of the placement residence and the child's adjustment to a new environment can the vicious cycle of abuse, abandonment, and neglect be stopped.

Care of family. One of the most difficult, yet essential, components of success with abusing parents is the quality of the therapeutic relationship. It must be one of genuine concern and treatment, not one of accusation and punishment. Nurses must examine their personal feelings toward these parents, particularly when sexual abuse is present. Some see the act of abuse as disgusting and totally without justification, whereas others can identify with it, at least in the sense of realizing the exasperation and frustration occasionally felt toward their own children. In some way, such as group discussion, nurses must come to an understanding of their feelings to be effective with abusing parents. For example, viewing the parent as the patient and the child as the victim of abuse places the emphasis on "treatment" rather than "punishment." Unless the nurse's attitude is positive, abusing parents will not be motivated to change, since they will not be working with a trusting person who demonstrates the kind of behavior that is being asked of them.

These parents cannot be fooled. Their survival as a child depended on their perception of other peoples' needs, and they are very skillful at saying what is expected of them while not making any attempts to change. Possibly it is for this reason that self-help groups, such as **Parents Anonymous*** (a group for parents who have abused or fear that they may abuse their child, but only in terms of physical abuse, not sexual abuse), are so successful, since the members cannot be deluded because they know the "game" so well. Such groups also are very accepting and nonjudgmental, because everyone has been in the same position. Group peer pressure and commitment are important motivating factors that keep parents from reverting to previous behaviors. The group also provides a release mechanism because, when parents are angry, they can call a fellow member and vent their feelings over the phone rather than on the child.

Since these parents have unrealistic expectations of children's capabilities, the nurse also fosters knowledge and understanding of normal growth and development. The nurse demonstrates how to handle children, how to teach them at their age level, and what realistically to expect from them. Since these parents are very sensitive to criticism or domination and already possess a very low self-esteem, teaching is implemented through demonstration and example rather

than through lecturing. Any competent parenting abilities they demonstrate are praised in an attempt to promote their sense of parental adequacy. Abusing parents desperately need "mothering" in order to be able to mother or father their own children. The nurse attends to their needs for security, trust, and release from responsibility. Home visits may be planned at times when the children are at school, with a friend, or asleep to allow maximum attention to the parent.

The solution to child abuse is not an easy one. Success is never certain, and the penalty for failure may well be a child's life. For those children who do survive, there is the possibility of their becoming abusive parents and consequently continuing the pattern of maltreatment, the threat of institutionalization because of retardation resulting from brain damage, and the risk of becoming juvenile offenders. It has been reported that almost 80% of adolescent delinquents incarcerated for serious, violent offenses have been abused during their childhood (Lewis and others, 1979).

However, services are available, such as Parents Anonymous, psychiatric or mental health intervention, and group therapy sessions, that help parents achieve major changes within themselves. Nurses have a responsibility to work individually with those families they care for in the hospital or community to establish a supportive and trusting relationship and to refer parents for additional help whenever possible.*

SEXUAL ABUSE

Sexual abuse is one of the most devastating types of child maltreatment, and current estimates indicate that it has increased tremendously during the past decade. This is not only because of growing public awareness, but is also associated with the expansion of definitions to include extrafamilial abuse, increase in the numbers of programs to treat sexual abusers and victims, and shifts in state and local policy to increase emphasis on reporting and investigating sexual maltreatment. The number of reported occurrences was approximately 13% of all child maltreatment cases in 1984 (Highlights, 1986), but is probably a small percentage of the actual incidence, since many instances are never reported because the victim, female or male, is afraid, feels guilty or ashamed, thinks he or she will not be believed, or fears the loss of love from someone, such as a parent.

As with all forms of child maltreatment, no universal definition for sexual abuse exists. The National Center on Child Abuse and Neglect (NCCAN) defines it as:

---

*7120 Franklin Ave., Los Angeles, CA 90046; call 1-800-421-0353.

*The National Directory of Children & Youth Services contains information for every social services agency, health department and juvenile court/youth agency at the state level and in all counties and independent cities, as well as licensed private providers of services for the victims of child abuse and neglect. It is available for purchase from the American Association for Protecting Children, American Humane Association, 9725 East Hampden Ave., Denver, CO 80231; information on referral services is also available from the child abuse hotline: 1-800-4-A-CHILD.

Contacts or interactions between a child and an adult when the child is being used for the sexual stimulation of that adult or another person. Sexual abuse may also be committed by a person under age 18.

Sexual abuse includes several types of sexual maltreatment, including the following (definitions of rape are presented on p. 875) (Kempe and Kempe, 1984):

incest Any physical sexual activity between family members; blood relationship is not required and abusers can include stepparents, nonrelated siblings, grandparents, uncles, and aunts.

molestation A vague term which includes "indecent liberties" such as touching, fondling, kissing, single or mutual masturbation, or oral-genital contact

exhibitionism Indecent exposure, usually exposure of the genitals by an adult male to children or female adults

child pornography Arranging and photographing in any media sexual acts including children, adults, or animals, regardless of consent by the child's legal guardian; the distribution of such material in any form with or without profit

child prostitution Involving children in sex acts for profit and usually with changing partners

pedophilia Literally means "love of child" and does not denote a type of sexual activity but the preference of an adult for prepubertal children as the means of achieving sexual excitement

Characteristics of Abusers and Victims

Much less is known about the characteristics of sexual abusers and their victims than in any other type of child maltreatment. However, there are some significant differences depending on whether the abuse occurs outside or within the family context.

Extrafamilial sexual abuse. In the majority of incidences of extrafamilial sexual abuse the offender is known to the victims or their families and is often a friend, neighbor, or someone in a position of authority. In a significant number of situations the sexual abuse has taken place repeatedly over weeks or months. Families are often ambivalent about reporting abuse to avoid disgrace, or they may not believe the victim. Offenders come from all levels of society and may even be prominent persons in the community.

Exhibitionists are usually younger men from late adolescents through their 20s and 30s. Unlike the sterotype of "dirty old men," their numbers decline after the age of 40. They usually have normal intelligence, a good work history, and may appear socially intact. They are often described as shy and immature but may be married and have children. They prefer younger girls as victims because of their more frightened response. Rarely does exhibitionism include actual sex acts or violence, but the potential does exist (Kempe and Kempe, 1984).

Pedophiliacs are often called "child molesters" but actually they may force a child to engage in any number of different sex acts or may love the child without any actual contact. The principal characteristic of these individuals is that they prefer children to adults as sex objects. The sexual activity tends to be a fairly immature form of sexual gratification (undressing and looking at the child, touching, kissing, and fondling, and perhaps masturbation) and reveals a desire to dominate the sexual activity. Pedophiliacs may be men or women and their preference may be the same- or the opposite-sex child. Most prefer children in certain age groups. Pedophilia, like homosexuality, is a way of life; most pedophiliacs see no harm in what they are doing, since they do have a genuine love of children. They are usually involved in careers that cater to children, such as coaching or teaching, and may be known and respected by the community. They tend to frequent child-oriented places, such as skating rinks, video arcades, or amusement parks. They are very sensitive to identifying youngsters in need of love and attention, such as those from unhappy homes, runaways, and missing children. The sexual activity may begin after a rather lengthy relationship with the offender that has engendered the child's trust. Children are pressured to participate in sexual activity and to keep it a secret by many of the same ploys used by most offenders (see Initiation and perpetuation of sexual abuse, p. 691).

Pornography and prostitution may involve strangers as well as the children's own parents. There are no typical characteristics of these offenders, although the abused children tend to be runaways—young adolescents who engage in these activities to provide money for food, shelter, drugs, and alcohol.

Intrafamilial sexual abuse. About three fourths of all reported instances of incest occurs between father or stepfather and daughter. Mother-son, mother-daughter, and sibling incest account for most of the remaining cases. Sexual play or experimentation is common among young siblings and usually stops as the children become older. In most instances sibling abuse has less disturbing emotional consequences for the victims than other types of incestuous relationships, but this is not always so, especially when the victim is forced to submit. However, these cases are less likely to come to the attention of authorities.

Incestuous relationships between father and daughter are generally prolonged, and the victims are usually reluctant to report the situation because of fear of retaliation and fear that they will not be believed. Typically, incestuous relationships begin later than other forms of child abuse, and the average age of the victim is 9.3 years (Highlights, 1986). The eldest daughter is usually abused, but in her absence another sister is substituted.

Sexual abuse is not limited to girls. Boys are also victims of both intrafamiliar and extrafamilial abuse. Incidence rates are at best inaccurate and range from conservative estimates of 5 to 6:1000 to 1:10 (Zaphiris, 1986). Males are much less likely to report abuse, and available research indicates that they suffer much greater emotional harm from incestuous relationships, especially between mother-son, than female victims. The reason for the greater emotional damage is not known but may be related to the lack of opportunity for identification with the father. Boys are more likely than girls to be subjected to oral-genital contact, to have fewer observable effects, and to be abused outdoors. No significant differences tend to be found in the race of the abuser, the relationship of the abuser to the victim, the number of abusers and times of abuse, or the use of bribes, threats, and physical violence (Farber and others, 1984).

Initiation and Perpetuation of Sexual Abuse

The cycle of sexual abuse often starts innocently, unless it involves an isolated attack, such as rape. Often offenders spend time with the victims to gain their trust before initiating any sexual contact. Most victims are then pressured into being an accessory to the sexual activity through various means. The methods of pressure are such that the child may be totally unaware that sexual activity is part of the offer. Frequently used methods include the following:

1. The child is offered material goods, such as special favors or privileges.
2. The adult misrepresents moral standards by telling the child that it is "okay to do." Children grow up believing that if an adult tells them to do something they should do it.
3. Isolated and emotionally and socially impoverished children are enticed by adult males who meet their needs for warmth and human contact.
4. The successful sex offender pressures the victim into secrecy regarding the activity by describing it as a "secret between us" that other people may take away if they found out.
5. The offender also plays on the child's fears, including fear of punishment by the offender, fear of repercussions if the child tells, and fear of abandonment or rejection by the family.

It is not uncommon for children to reveal the fear that their parents would not believe them if they told—especially if the offender is a trusted member of the family. Some fear they will be blamed for the situation, and many young children with limited vocabulary have difficulty in describing the activity when they do have the courage or opportunity to complain. Consequently the abuse is perpetuated over a prolonged period.

Seductiveness by the child does not initiate incest. Most young females experiment in seduction, especially during the preschool years, but the father's response is normally one that differentiates this playfulness from overt sexual invitation. While the reasons for incest are complicated and can occur in any number of family types, it does not occur in healthy families (Kempe and Kempe, 1984). Most relationships are directly related to sexual maladjustment and estrangement between husband and wife and begin following the cessation of sexual relationships with the usual partner. Most fathers experience little guilt, and the wives almost invariably are aware of the incestuous affair. The wife reacts by tolerating the situation or resorts to the obvious

use of denial (Hogan and Juhasz, 1984). Consequently the home offers little protection to young victims, since abusers have easy access to their victims and the children feel they cannot reveal their secret to other family members.

Identification of Sexual Abuse

Unlike physical abuse or neglect, sexual abuse may occur with few if any obvious physical indications of the activity. Also, many individuals are hesitant to believe children and unwilling to report incidents. Even health professionals are sometimes at fault when they perform cursory physical examinations of the genitalia and ignore behavior or verbal comments that suggest abuse. When sexual abuse is suspected, other children in the family should also be checked, since multiple victims are not uncommon.

Unfortunately, there is no typical profile of the victim and there must be a high index of suspicion to identify these children. Physical signs vary and may include any of those listed in Table 16-7 for sexual abuse. Every effort is made to thoroughly examine children for physical clues. Most authorities agree that in any young child with a sexually transmitted disease, nonspecific vaginitis, or venereal warts (condylomata acuminata), a thorough medical and social evaluation is essential to rule out sexual abuse (Neinstein, Goldenring, and Carpenter, 1984; Hammerschlag and others, 1985; DeJong, Weiss, and Brent, 1982). However, the presence of such diseases does not automatically confirm sexual transmission.

Numerous behavioral manifestations may be exhibited by the victim, but unfortunately they may be considered insignificant or attributed to the normal stresses of childhood, especially in older school-age children or adolescents. However, serious manifestations that should alert the health professional to investigate further are chronic depression, isolation from peers, apathy, and eventually suicide attempts (Sarles, 1980).

The disclosure of the secret comes about in a variety of ways—the act is observed by others, resulting in a direct confrontation; the child tells someone, such as a parent of a friend; visible clues of the relationship are observed, such as an accumulation of coins, gifts, or candy; or more obvious clues are seen, such as a child coming home disheveled or becoming pregnant; and physical or behavioral signs and symptoms are observed. Children usually describe the experience in terms of whether it was unpleasant or hurt or was pleasurable (usually a response to hand-genital contact); some indicate no reaction. Young children often feel no guilt or shame because the act is pleasurable and they are unaware of its inappropriateness.

Response of families. Families respond to sexual abuse with a wide variety of emotional reactions that may be as intense and disruptive as they are for the victim, regardless of the type of abuse. The immediate reactions range from emotional shock to near hysteria on the part of one or both of the parents, which may interfere with care of the victim. In incestuous abuse the most common reaction

ACTION SUGGESTIONS FOR PARENTS

Sexual assault of children is much more common than most of us realize. It may be preventable if children have good preparation. *To provide protection and preparation, as parents we can:*

Pay carefull attention to who is around our children. (Unwanted touch *may* come from someone we like and trust.)

Back up a child's right to say "No."

Encourage communication by taking seriously what our children *say.*

Take a second look at signals of potential danger.

Refuse to leave our children in the company of those we do not trust.

Include information about sexual assault when teaching about safety.

Provide specific definitions and examples of sexual assault.

Remind children that even "nice" people sometimes do mean things.

Urge children to tell us about *anybody* who causes them to be uncomfortable.

Prepare children to deal with bribes and threats, as well as possible physical force.

Virtually eliminate secrets between us and our children.

Teach children how to say "No," ask for help, and control who touches them and how.

Model self-protective and limit-setting behavior for our children.

Should it ever become necessary *to help a child recover from a sexual assault,* as parents we can:

Listen carefully and understand how children tell us.

Support the child for telling by praise, belief, sympathy, lack of blame.

Know local resources, and choose help carefully.

Provide opportunities to talk about the assault.

Provide opportunities for the entire fmaily to go through a recovery process.

Sexual assault affects all of us, whether or not our own children are assaulted. *To help deal with this social problem,* all of us can:

Provide sympathetic care and support to those who have been victimized.

Recognize that offenders do not change without intervention.

Organize neighborhood programs to support each other's efforts to protect children.

Encourage schools to provide information about sexual assault as a problem of health and safety.

Organize community groups to support educational, treatment, and law enforcement programs.

From Adams, C., and Fay, J.: *No more secrets: protecting your child from sexual assault,* San Luis Obispo, Calif., 1981, Impact Publishers, Inc.

the child, and themselves. The parents commonly express anger at the child for "stupid" behavior and may even restrict the child's privileges as punishment. When the victim is a female, the parents may question her sexual provocation of the event. Self-blaming parents assume full responsibility, believing that they have been inadequate parents or should not have allowed the child to go out. When a baby-sitter or trusted relative is involved in the assault and the child's complaint has not been believed until gross evidence is presented, the parents are often devastated by guilt.

Nursing Considerations

Nursing care of sexually abused children involves the same objectives as those discussed for physically maltreated victims: prevention, identification, and protection from further abuse. Many of the interventions are identical, such as reporting the abuse and caring for the child in the hospital if admission is required, and are discussed on p. 687. Because evidence of sexual maltreatment may be less obvious than in other types of abuse, nurses must have a high index of suspicion and be aware of clues to sexual abuse (see Table 16-7). When the child has sustained physical harm, the care is consistent with that provided a rape victim, with the same considerations for the child's preparation and psychologic needs during the examination (see p. 876).

Prevention. One aspect of sexual abuse that is receiving increasing attention is prevention. Ideally, educating children regarding "anyone touching them in private parts of their body" should be as commonplace as the admonition "Don't go with strangers" and should be included in sex education. One must remember that children, especially preschoolers and school-age children, have little concept of sexual activities and easily succumb to statements such as "I just want to be nice to you," "This is our little secret," "If you tell your mommy, she will be angry with you." Bewildered, the child agrees to the act, often with familiar "nice" people, and remains secretive, sometimes for years, especially in incestuous relationships.

The box at left includes several suggestions for protecting and educating children against possible molestation. The nurse is frequently in a position to discuss this topic with parents as part of health maintenance and to provide guidelines. Books are available for parents that describe sexual abuse and its prevention.* Helpful games such as "What if the baby-sitter wants to wrestle and hug but tells you to keep it a secret?" can be used to explore dangerous situ-

is denial of the child's accusation. There may be surprising inability on the part of the parents to provide adequate emotional support to the child at this time, even when their attitude toward the child has been supportive in the past.

Parents and other family members may display the same type of emotional responses as the victim, such as inability to eat or sleep and somatic complaints of headache or backache. In the acute emotional phase, parents have a need to blame someone. The three common targets are the offender,

*A comprehensive listing of Child Sexual Abuse Prevention Resources is available for a fee of $2.00 from the National Committee for Prevention of Child Abuse, Publishing Dept., 332 S. Michigan Ave., Suite 950, Chicago, IL 60604-4357; additional informational resources are the National Center on Child Abuse and Neglect, P.O. Box 1182, Washington, DC; C. Henry Kempe National Center for the Prevention and Treatment of Child Abuse and Neglect, 1205 Oneida St., Denver, CO 80220; American Association for Protecting Children, American Humane Association, 9725 East Hampden Ave., Denver, CO 80231; Family Life Education Publishing Cooperative, Network Publications, 1700 Mission St., Dept. P, P.O. Box 8506, Santa Cruz, CA 95061-8506.

ations in advance and help children learn the importance of saying ''No.'' They need reassurance that no matter what the other person says or does, the parents want to know and will not punish the child. Even if the child does participate in the activity before telling the parents, he must be reassured that it was not his fault.

In addition, parents need to be made aware that ''nice'' people, including friends and relatives, can be offenders; parents should carefully observe how others act toward the child. A sudden change in the child's behavior and a response such as ''I don't like uncle anymore'' are clues to investigate the relationship. In the event of any doubt, further solitary encounters with this person and the child should be prevented. It is sometimes to the child's great misfortune that parents do not take certain comments seriously, such as ''He hugs me too tight'' or ''I don't want to go with him.'' Casual parental statements such as ''He just loves you'' or ''You do whatever adults tell you to do'' can place children in jeopardy. Health professionals can alert parents to such dangers and guide them toward an appreciation of the problem, providing concrete guidelines toward child education and protection.

Care of child. The type of care needed by the child depends on the circumstances of the sexual abuse and varies from reassurance and support when the act involves exhibitionism to long-term counseling in incestuous situations. The precise role nurses play in abusive cases also varies but several interventions are standard. First, *children who report abuse must be believed*. Children do not have sufficient experience with sexual activity to fabricate stories. While their stories may sound contradictory, this may reflect the child's experiences in several instances of abuse. In fact, children who repeatedly tell identical facts may have been prompted to do so (Kempe and Kempe, 1984).

Since nurses are often the first professionals to interview these children, there must be an awareness of the need for sensitivity and discretion. Every effort is made to make the child feel comfortable with appropriate introductions and to avoid duplicating the behaviors typically used by offenders, such as touching the child without permission. The interview is conducted in a quiet and private location, preferably a neutral place, such as a school playroom, or office, and not where the abuse occurred. Neutral questions are asked first, such as the child's reaction to the hospital (if appropriate) and then to a discussion of the incident in general terms. The interview should include such questions as ''Do you know why you were brought to the hospital?'' ''Do you know what will happen here?'' or ''How do you feel about being here?'' Later the question ''Can you tell me what happened?'' and other questions may then elicit an account of the incident. Sometimes the parents are able to help the child to describe the incident, and questions can become directed to the circumstances of the assault. Questions should progress chronologically and proceed from the nonsexual to the more sexual content. If the child shows evidence of becoming too upset, the focus can be redirected toward more neutral and less emotionally charged areas.

Children are given the opportunity to ask questions but if they are reticent, they are never pressured into talking. Young children in particular lack the verbal skills to adequately describe body parts. These children benefit from play situations that provide opportunities for disclosure, such as drawing, using puppets or anatomically correct dolls, and doll houses. For example, the nurse can encourage the child to draw a picture ''of what happened'' or ''of what you remember.'' Drawings can reveal a number of details, such as shading of body parts, emphasis on genitals, or gender confusion, that support the occurrence of abuse (Kelley, 1985).

Anatomically correct male and female dolls can be used to encourage children to reenact the events. The nurse can also play a game by pointing to various body parts and asking the child to name them. Neutral parts are presented first, following by the genitals. As the child learns the names of the parts these are used throughout the conversation. Gradually the child is asked to describe what happened using the dolls. If the child is still reluctant, the nurse can talk for the ''victim'' doll and interact with it as if it were the child, asking open-ended questions, such as ''I wonder if Mary has a secret someone told her not to tell anyone about.'' Often the child will begin to talk for the doll and reveal the events of the abuse (Miller, 1985).

In interviewing the victim, every effort is made to coordinate the number of interviewees and to assign a primary professional to work with the child. Videotaping or audiotaping is ideal for limiting the number of traumatic events for the victim. If nurses are not the primary professional, they can serve as the child's advocate to prevent excessive questioning and embarrassment by others.

Care of family. Care of the family also depends on the circumstances of the sexual abuse. In the situation of a nonparent offender the family may be more able to support the child than if incest was involved. Family members are encouraged to express their feelings of anger, guilt, shame, and/or embarrassment, but are also cautioned to avoid displacing such feelings on the child. For example, it is easy for parents to admonish the child with statements, such as ''We told you never to go with strangers,'' which makes the child feel responsible.

Family members are advised to encourage the child to resume normal activities and to observe the child for signs of distress. Children express their feelings primarily through behavior. Parents should be alert for changes in behavior that indicate distress resulting from the incident, such as remaining in the house, refusing to go to school, changes in sleeping patterns, and frequency of dreams and nightmares. The child is encouraged to talk about these feelings and nightmares, since the more the child can talk about the experience, the more he will be able to gain control over it.

In incestuous relationships, the goal is to protect the child and the preferred approach is to remove the offender, not the victim, from the home. However, this is not always pos-

Nursing Care Summary: The Maltreated Child

NURSING GOALS	NURSING INTERVENTIONS	EXPECTED PATIENT/FAMILY OUTCOMES
HP-HMP	**Injury: potential for (trauma)**	
	Risk factors: characteristics of child, characteristics of caregiver(s), environmental characteristics	

Protect from further abuse	Perform physical assessment
	Assess emotional state and evaluate behaviors
	Implement measures to prevent abuse
	   Report suspicions to appropriate authorities
	   Assist in removing child from unsafe environment and establishing in a safe environment
	   Establish protective measures for the hospitalized child as indicated
	Keep factual, objective records of:
	   The child's physical condition
	   The child's behavioral response to parents, others, and environment
	   Interviews with family members
	Report suspected child abuse to local authorities
		Suspected child abuse victim is removed from abusive environment

Prevent recurrence	Collaborate efforts of multidisciplinary team to continually evaluate progress of child in foster home or in return to own family Be alert for signs of continued abuse or neglect Help parents identify those circumstances that precipitate an abusive act and ways in which to deal with the release of anger in ways other than attacking child Refer for alternative placement when indicated	Families avoid precipitating situations Signs of abuse or neglect are detected early and the child referred for appropriate intervention
SP-SCP	**Powerlessness**	
	Etiology: interpersonal interaction	
Provide consistent caregiver and therapeutic environment during hospitalization	Demonstrate acceptance of child while not expecting same in return Show attention while not reinforcing inappropriate behavior Plan appropriate activities for attention with nurse, other adults, and other children; use play to work through relationships Avoid displacing anger on child, such as shouting or yelling, as method of dealing with own frustration toward child's negative behavior Praise child's abilities in order to promote his self-esteem	Child exhibits evidence of distress
Relieve anxiety in child	Treat child as one who has a specific physical problem for hospitalization, not as "abused" victim Avoid asking too many questions Use play, especially family or doll house activity, to investigate kinds of relationships perceived by child Provide one consistent person to whom child relates regarding events of abuse	Child appears calm and engages in positive relationships with caregivers
RRP	**Parenting, alteration in: actual or potential**	
	Etiology: child, caregiver, or situational characteristics that precipitate abusive behavior	
Prevent abuse	Identify families at risk for potential abuse Promote parental attachment to child Emphasize childrearing practices, especially effective methods of discipline Increase parents' feeling of adequacy and self-esteem	Families exhibit evidence of positive interaction with children Parents keep important phone numbers easily accessible

Nursing Care Summary: The Maltreated Child—cont'd

NURSING GOALS	NURSING INTERVENTIONS	EXPECTED PATIENT/FAMILY OUTCOMES
Support parents	Encourage support systems that lessen stress and total responsibility of child care on one or both parents Be available for assistance Give parents the number of local Parents Anonymous Provide "mothering" by directing attention to parents, taking over child care responsibilities until parents feel ready to participate, and focusing on parents' needs Refer parents to Parents Anonymous (initially may need to attend with parents as their advocate) or Parents United Help identify a support group for parents, such as extended family or nearby neighbors; help these significant others understand their important role in also preventing further abuse	Parents demonstrate appropriate parenting activities Parents seek group and individual support
Teach parents	Teach realistic expectations of child's behavior and capabilities Emphasize alternate methods of discipline, such as reward and verbal disapproval Suggest methods of handling developmental problems or goals, such as toddler negativism, toilet training, and independence Teach through demonstration and role modeling, rather than lecture; avoid authoritarian approach	Parents dmeonstrate an understanding of noraml expectations for their child
Lessen environmental crises	Refer to social agencies that can provide assistance in areas such as financial support, adequate housing, and employment	Parents receive assistance with problems
Promote a sense of parental adequacy during child's hospitalization	Orient parents to hospital unit and help them feel welcomed and an important part of child's care and recovery Reinforce competent child care activities Focus on the abuse as a problem that requires therapeutic intervention, not as a behavior characteristic or deficiency of the parents Empathize with difficulties of rearing children, especially with additional life crises, while not condoning the act of abuse or neglect Foster healthy aspects of parent-child relationship	Parents demonstrate an attitude of concern for and ability to care for the child

Plan for discharge	Prepare for discharge as soon as disposition is finalized
	Home placement:
	  Encourage parents to visit as much as possible during hospitalization
	  Plan for close supervision and counseling of family
	Foster home placement:
	  Encourage foster family members to visit child before discharge
	  Stress to them child's need to regress in order to complete missed stages of development
	  Help child grieve this loss, if parents' rights are being terminated permanently, especially if it entails separation from siblings (long-term counseling is optimum goal)
		Parents demonstrate ability and desire to care for child
		Child is placed in appropriate environment

Nursing Interventions Related to Medical Management

Determine extent of injuries
Assist with diagnostic procedures

sible, especially when the offender refuses to admit responsibility or the other parent, usually the mother, sides with the father and prefers that the child leave the home. If the child is placed in a foster home, the same interventions are appropriate as those discussed under physical abuse (p. 688). However, the child may feel even more responsible for the family break-up than in other situations of maltreatment because of the intimate part he played in the abuse.

Numerous treatment programs exist for sex offenders but currently no one approach has proven successful. Research indicates that a combination of individual and group therapy for at least 2 years is needed for treatment of incest; even less is known about treatment of other types of perpetrators. Self-help groups such as **Parents United** and its adjunct, **Daughters and Sons United*** have been successful in helping sexually abused families, and nurses can be instrumental in making referrals to local chapters. There is no way to predict which families will be successfully rehabilitated, although the best results occur when the offender accepts full responsibility for the act, the victim's mother acknowledges her role in failing to protect the child, and the victim is able to understand and forgive the parents and develop a positive self-image despite the traumatic experience (Kempe and Kempe, 1984).

*P.O. Box 952, San Jose, CA 95108; call 1-408-280-5055.

CONCEPT SUMMARIES

- Common disorders during early childhood include communicable diseases, intestinal parasitic infections, and conjunctivitis.

- Nursing goals in the treatment of a communicable disease are identification, provision of comfort, prevention of spread to others, and prevention of complications.

- Intestinal parasitic diseases constitute the most common infections in the world, giardiasis and enterobiasis being the most widespread parasitic infections among children in the United States.

- Although the incidence of poisoning has decreased in the last 15 years as a result of more stringent packaging regulations, childhood poisoning remains a serious health concern.

- The major principles of emergency treatment for poisoning are assessment, supportive measures, gastric decontamination, family support, and prevention of recurrence.

- Ingestion of plant parts is the most common childhood poisoning, and parents should be advised to place houseplants out of young children's reach, to teach children not to eat anything without permission, and to avoid making teas or homemade medicines from plants.

- Aspirin is a frequently ingested drug among children; however, the limitation of the quantity per container and the creation of child-resistant caps have reduced acute poisoning by this salicylate.

- Acetaminophen is the most common drug poisoning among children and occurs from acute, not chronic, overdose.

- Potential sources of heavy metal poisoning are lead, iron from medicinal supplements, and mercury from seafood and thermometers (only inhaled).

- Lead ingestion may be attributed to environmental factors, specific characteristics of the child, and parental characteristics. Health professionals have a major responsibility to educate parents regarding these factors.

- Child maltreatment may take the form of physical abuse or neglect, emotional abuse or neglect, and sexual abuse.

- Parental, child, and environmental characteristics are criteria that singly or together predispose children to physical abuse.

- Identification of physical abuse entails securing evidence of maltreatment, taking a history pertaining to the incident, and assessing parental and child behaviors.

- Sexual abuse has soared in the last decade; common forms are incest, molestation, rape, exhibitionism, child pornography, child prostitution, and pedophilia.

REFERENCES

Adler, R., and Kane-Nussen, B.: Erythema multiforme: confusion with child battering syndrome, Pediatrics **72**(5):718-720, 1983.

Altemeier, W.A., III, and others: Antecedents of child abuse, J. Pediatr. **100**(5):823-829, 1982.

Anas, N., Namasonthi, V., and Ginsburg, C.M.: Criteria for hospitalizing children who have ingested products containing hydrocarbons, JAMA **246**(8):840-843, 1981.

Annest, J.L., and others: Blood lead level for persons 6 months-74 years of age: U.S., 1976-80, Vital and health statistics, National Center for Health Statistics, Advance Data **79**: 1-24, May 12, 1982.

Asnes, R.S., and Wisotsky, D.H.: Cupping lesions simulating child abuse, J. Pediatr. **99**:267-268, 1981.

Baker, R.B.: Seat belt injury masquerading as sexual abuse, Pediatrics **77**(3):435, 1986.

Banner, W., Jr., and Tong, T.G.: Iron poisoning, Pediatr. Clin. North Am. **33**(2):393-409, 1986.

Barkin, R.M., and Rosen, P., editors: Emergency pediatrics, St. Louis, 1984, The C.V. Mosby Co.

Barrett, M.J., and others: Changing epidemiology of Reye syndrome in the United States, Pediatrics **77**(4):598-602, 1986.

Bellinger, D.C., and Needleman, H.L.: Lead and the relationship between maternal and child intelligence, J. Pediatr. **102** (4):523-528, 1983.

Benenson, A.S., editor: Control of communicable diseases in man, ed. 14, Washington, DC, 1985, The Amerian Public Health Association.

Benirschke, K.: Time bomb of lye ingestion? Am. J. Dis. Child. **135**(1):17-18, 1981.

Benson, G.D.: Hepatotoxicity following the therapeutic use of antipyretic analgesics, Am. J. Med. **75**(5A):85-93, 1983.

Besharov, D.J.: "Doing something" about child abuse: the need to narrow the grounds for state intervention, Harvard J. Law and Pub. Policy **8**(3):539-589, 1985.

Bithoney, W.G., and others: Childhood ingestions as symptoms of family distress, Am. J. Dis. Child. **139**(3):456-459, 1985.

Boehnert, M.T., and others: Advances in clinical toxicology, Pediatr. Clin. North Am. **32**(1):193-211, 1985.

Borgatti, R.: When worms cause intestinal infection, Patient Care **17**(14):257-281, 1983.

Centers for Disease Control: Preventing lead poisoning in young children, J. Pediatr. **93**(4):709-720, 1978.

Centers for Disease Control: Folk remedy-associated lead poisoning in Hmong children—Minnesota, Morbid. Mortal. Weekly Report **32**(42):555-556, 1983a.

Centers for Disease Control: Lead poisoning from Mexican folk remedies—California, Morbid. Mortal. Weekly Report **32** (42):554-555, 1983b.

Chafee-Bahamon, C., Lacouture, P., and Lovejoy, F.: Risk assessment of ipecac in the home, Pediatrics **75**(6):1105-1109, 1985.

Charney, E., and others: Childhood lead poisoning: a controlled trial of the effect of dust, N. Engl. J. Med. **309**(18): 1089-1093, 1983.

Coulehan, J.L. and others: Gasoline sniffing and lead toxicity in Navajo adolescents, Pediatrics **71**(1):113-117, 1983.

Craft, J.C.: Giardiasis in childhood. In Nelson, J.D., and McCracken, G.H., editors: Clinical reviews in pediatric infectious disease, St. Louis, 1985, The C.V. Mosby Co.

Czajka, P.A., and Russell, S.L.: Nonemetic effect of ipecac syrup, Pediatrics **75**(6):1101-1104, 1985.

DeJong, A., Weiss, J., and Brent, R.: Condyloma acuminata in children, Am. J. Dis. Child. **136**(8):704-706, 1982.

Dershewitz, R.A., Posner, M.K., and Paichel, W.: The effectiveness of health education on home use of ipecac, Clin. Pediatr. **22**:268-270, 1983.

Dietrich, K.N., and others: Contribution of social and developmental factors to lead exposure during the first year of life, Pediatrics **75**(6):1114-1119, 1985.

Farber, E.D., and others: Boy victims of sexual abuse, J. Clin. Child Psychology **13**:294-297, 1984.

Feldman, K.W.: Pseudoabusive burns in Asian refugees, Am. J. Dis. Child. **138**(8):768-769, 1984.

Fergusson, D.M., and others: A controlled field trial of a poisoning prevention method, Pediatrics **69**(5):515-520, 1982.

Friedman, E.J.: Death from ipecac intoxication in a patient with anorexia nervosa, Am. J. Psychiatry **141**:702-703, 1984.

Garbarino, J.: The elusive 'crime' of emotional abuse, Child Abuse Neglect **2**:89-99, 1978.

Gaudreault, P., Temple, A.R., and Lovejoy, F.H.: The relative severity of acute versus chronic salicylate poisoning in children: a clinical comparison, Pediatrics **70**(4): 566-569, 1982.

Gelles, R.J., and Cornell, C.P.: Intimate violence in families, Beverly Hills, CA, 1985, Sage Publications, Inc.

Gigliotti, F., and others: Etiology of acute conjunctivitis in children, J. Pediatr. **98**(4):531-536, 1981.

Gigliotti, F., and others: Efficacy of topical antibiotic therapy in acute conjunctivitis in children, J. Pediatr. **104**(4):623-626, 1984.

Gillin, F.D., and Reiner, D.S.: Human milk kills parasitic intestinal protozoa, Science **221**(4617):1290-1292, 1983.

Guandolo, V.L.: Munchausen syndrome by proxy: an outpatient challenge, Pediatrics **75**(3):526-530, 1985.

Hammerschlag, M.R., and others: Nonspecific vaginitis following sexual abuse in children, Pediatrics **75**(6):1028-1031, 1985.

Highlights of official child neglect and abuse reporting 1984, Denver, 1986, The American Humane Assoc.

Hogan, N.S., and Juhasz, A.M.: The detection of incest, Home Healthcare Nurse **2**(4):20-26, 1984.

Howrie, D.L., Moriarty, R., and Breit, R.: Candy flavoring as a source of salicylate poisoning, Pediatrics **75**(5):869-871, 1985.

Hunt, T.J., Hepner, R., and Seaton, K.W.: Childhood lead poisoning and inadequate child care, Am. J. Dis. Child. **136**:538-542, 1982.

Jones, J.E.: Common intestinal parasites of children, Pediatr. Basics **36**:7-14, 1983.

Kelley, S.J.: Drawings: critical communications for sexually abused children, Pediatr. Nurs. **11**(6):421-426, 1985.

Kempe, C.H., and others: The battered child syndrome, JAMA **181**:17-24, 1962.

Kempe, R.S., and Kempe, C.H.: The common secret: sexual abuse of children and adolescents, New York, 1984, W.H. Freeman and Co. Publishers.

Keystone, J.S., and others: Intestinal parasites in metropolitan Toronto day-care centres, Can. Med. Assoc. J. **131**(7): 733-736, 1984.

Kirschner, R.H., and Stein, R.J.: The mistaken diagnosis of child abuse: a form of medical abuse? Am. J. Dis. Child. **139**:873-875, 1985.

Klein, B.L., and Simon, J.E.: Hydrocarbon poisonings, Pediatr. Clin. North Am. **33**(2):411-419, 1986.

Krugman, R.D., and Krugman, M.K.: Emotional abuse in the classroom, Am. J. Dis. Child. **138**(3):284-286, 1984.

Lewis, D.O., and others: Violent juvenile delinquents: psychiatric, neurological, psychological, and abuse factors, J. Am. Acad. Child Psychiatry **18**:307-319, 1979.

Litovitz, T.L., and others: Ipecac administration in children younger than 1 year of age, Pediatrics **76**(5):761-764, 1985.

McGuigan, M.A.: Chronic salicylate poisoning: when therapy turns into intoxication, Pediatr. Consult **2**(3):1-8, 1983.

McGuigan, M.A.: Treatment of poisoning, Clinical Symposia **36**(5):1-32, 1984.

Meadow, R.: Muchausen syndrome by proxy, Arch. Dis. Child. **57**:92-98, 1982.

Meadow, R., and Lennert, T.: Munchausen by proxy or Polle syndrome: which term is correct? Pediatrics **74**(4): 554-556, 1984.

Mielke, H.W., and others: Lead concentrations in inner-city soils as a factor in the child lead problem, Am. J. Public Health **73**(12):1366-1369, 1983.

Miller, E.L.: Interviewing the sexually abused child, Am. J. Maternal Child Nurs. **10**:103-105, 1985.

Mofenson, H.C., and Caraccio, T.R.: Benefits/risks of syrup of ipecac, Pediatrics **77**(4):551-552, 1986.

Moore, W.: Caustic ingestions: pathophysiology, diagnosis, and treatment, Clin. Pediatr. **25**(4):192-196, 1986.

Neinstein, L.S., Goldenring, J., and Carpenter, S.: Nonsexual transmission of sexually transmitted diseases: an infrequent occurrence, Pediatrics **74**(1):67-76, 1984.

Oates, R.K., Forrest, D., and Peacock, A.: Mothers of abused children: a comparison study, Clin. Pediatr. **24**(1):9-13, 1985.

Outwater, K.M., and others: Factitious hematuria: diagnosis by minor blood group typing, J. Pediatr. **98**(1):95-97, 1981.

Pearce, J., and Burg, F.D.: Lead poisoning in children, Drug Therapy **12**(5):87-102, 1982.

Piomelli, S., and others: Management of childhood lead poisoning, J. Pediatr. **105**(4):523-532, 1984.

Polakoff, J., and others: The environment away from home as a source of potential poisoning, Am. J. Dis. Child. **138**: 1014-1017, 1984.

Polansky, N.A., and others: Profile of neglect: a survey of the state of knowledge, U.S. Department of Health, Education and Welfare, Office of Human Development Services, Administration for Public Services, (OHDS) 77-02004, 1977.

Reid, D.: Pitfalls in determining child abuse, Lancet **1**(8441):1316-1317, 1985.

Rodgers, G.C., Jr., and Matyunas, N.J.: Gastrointestinal decontamination for acute poisoning, Pediatr. Clin. North Am. **33**(2):261-285, 1986.

Rumack, B.: Acetaminophen overdose in young children, Am. J. Dis. Child. **138**(5):428-433, 1984.

Rumack, B.H.: Aspirin and acetaminophen, Clin. Toxicol. **15**(3):313-340, 1979.

Rumack, B.H.: Acetaminophen overdose, Am. J. Med. **75** (5A):104-112, 1983.

Sarles, R.M.: Incest, Pediatr. Rev. **2**(2):51-54, 1980.

Saulsbury, F.T., and Hayden, G.F.: Skin conditions simulating child abuse, Pediatr. Emer. Care **1**(3):147-150, 1985.

Schmitt, B., Gray, J., and Britton, H.: Car seat burns in infants: avoiding confusion with inflicted burns, Pediatrics **62**(4):607-609, 1978.

Shnaps, Y., and others: The chemically abused child, Pediatrics **68**(1):119-121, 1981.

Snodgrass, W.R.: Salicylate toxicity, Pediatr. Clin. North Am. **33**(2):381-391, 1986.

Snyder, J.C., Hampton, R., and Newberger, E.H.: Family dysfunction: violence, neglect, and sexual misuse. In Levine, M.D., and others, editors: Developmental-behavioral pediatrics, Philadelphia, 1983, W.B. Saunders Co.

Solomons, G.: Trauma and child abuse, Am. J. Dis. Child. **134**:503-505, May 1980.

Schwartz, J., Angle, C., and Pitcher, H.: Relationship between childhood blood lead levels and stature, Pediatrics **77** (3):281-288, 1986.

Temple, A.R.: Acute and chronic effect of aspirin toxicity and their treatment, Arch. Intern. Med. **141**:364-369, 1981.

Turner, J.A.: Giardiasis and infections with Dientamoeba fragilis, Pediatr. Clin. North Am. **32**(4):865-880, 1985.

Turner, R.J., and Avison, W.R.: Assessing risk factors for problem parenting: the significance of social support, J. Marriage and Fam. **47**(4):881-892, 1985.

Unintentional poisoning among young children—United States, JAMA **249**(13):1700, 1983.

Veltri, J., and Litovitz, T.: 1983 annual report of the American Association of Poison Control Centers National Data Collection System, Am. J. Emer. Med. **2**:420-443, 1984.

Vernberg, K., Culver-Dickinson, P., and Spyker, D.A.: The deterrent effect of poison-warning stickers, Am. J. Dis. Child. **138**:1018-1020, 1984.

Wasserman, R.L., and Ginsburg, C.M.: Caustic substance injuries, J. Pediatr. **107**(2):169-174, 1985.

Zaphiris, A.G.: The sexually abused boy, Preventing Sexual Abuse **1**(1):1-4, 1986.

BIBLIOGRAPHY

Communicable Diseases

American Academy of Pediatrics: Report of the Committee on Infectious Diseases, ed. 20, Elk Grove Village, IL, 1986, The Academy.

Casano, K.: Rates of most infectious diseases in children hitting all time lows, Pediatr. News **15**(2):1, 1981.

English, P.C.: Diphtheria and theories of infectious disease: centennial appreciation of the critical role of diphtheria in the history of medicine, Pediatrics **76**(1):1-9, 1985.

Fleisher, G., and others: Life-threatening complications of varicella, Am. J. Dis. Child. **135**:896-899, Oct., 1981.

Fleming, J.W.: How to differentiate dermatologic conditions—often confusing and difficult—in infants and school-age children, Am. J. Maternal Child Nurs. **6**(5):346-354, 1981.

Hayman, L.L.: Varicella, Nursing 83 **13**(4):41, 1983.

Krugman, S., Katz, S., Gershon, A., and Wilfert, C.: Infectious diseases of children, ed. 8, St. Louis, 1985, The C.V. Mosby Co.

Holderman, M.: Skin problems: a guide for making "rash" decisions, Nursing 84 **14**(11):22-23, 1984.

Jackson, M.M., and Lynch, P.: Infection control: too much or too little? Am. J. Nurs. **84**(2):208-210, 1984.

Labson, L.H.: Doctor, I can't stand this itching! Patient Care **18**(17):89-121, 1984.

Miller, D.L., Alderslade, R., and Ross, E.M.: Whooping cough and whooping cough vaccine: the risks and benefits debate, Epidemiol. Rev. **4**:1-24, 1982.

Moree, N.A., and Garner, J.S.: New infection control guideline, Am. J. Nurs. **84**(2):210-211, 1984.

Preblud, S.R.: Age-specific risks of varicella complications, Pediatrics **68**(1):14-17, 1981.

Relief for that persistent itch, Patient Care **18**(17):185, 1984.

Scott, R.M., and others: Ineffectiveness of historical data in predicting measles susceptibility, Pediatrics **73**(6): 777-780, 1984.

Shahan, M.R.: Mumps, Nursing 83 **13**(2):43, 1983.

Sullivan, J.L., Herrod, H.G., and Levine, L.: The Schick test, Am. J. Dis. Child. **135**(7)618-620, 1981.

Sullivan-Bolyai, J.Z., and Smith, A.L.: Varicella, Am. J. Dis. Child. **135**(10)895, 1981.

Wiswall, J.: Update on common exanthematous communicable diseases, Pediatr. Nurs. **4**(5):50-51, 1978.

Intestinal Parasitic Infection

Borgatti, R.: When protozoa invade the GI tract, Patient Care **17**(14):226-253, 1983.

Carroll, M.J.: Routine procedures for examination of stool and blood for parasites, Pediatr. Clin. North Am. **32**(4): 1041-1046, 1985.

Flores, E.C., Plumb, S.C., and McNeese, M.C.: Intestinal parasitosis in an urban pediatric clinic population, Am. J. Dis. Child. **137**(8):754-756, 1983.

Getting rid of pinworms, roundworms, scabies mites, or lice, Patient Care **18**(17):189-190, 1984.

Gupte, S.: Phenobarbital and metabolism of metronidazole, N. Engl. J. Med. **308**:529, 1983.

Harter, L., and others: Giardiasis in an infant and toddler swim class, Am. J. Pub. Health **74**(2):155-156, 1984.

Henley, M., and Sears, J.R.: Pinworms: a persistent pediatric problem, Am. J. Maternal Child Nurs. **10**(6):111-113, 1985.

Kuntz, R.E.: Parasites of children in the United States, Pediatr. Nurs. **5**(6):12-17, 1979.

Malarkay, L.M.: Ridding schoolchildren of parasites—a community approach, Am. J. Maternal Child Nurs. **4**:363-366, 1979.

Markell, E.K.: Intestinal nematode infections, Pediatr. Clin. North Am. **32**(4):971-986, 1985.

Sears, J.R.: To prevent reinfestation (letters to the editor), Am. J. Maternal Child Nurs. **10**(6):377, 1985.

Seidel, J.S.: Treatment of parasitic infections, Pediatr. Clin. North Am. **32**(4):1077-1095, 1985.

Silverman, A., and Roy, C.: Pediatric clinical gastroenterology, ed. 3, St. Louis, 1983, The C.V. Mosby Co.

Sokol, R., Lichtenstein, P., and Farrell, M.: Quinacrine hydrochloride-induced yellow discoloration of the skin in children, Pediatrics **69**(2):232-233, 1982.

Unger, B., and others: Enzyme-linked immunosorbent assay for the detection of giardia lamblia in fecal specimens, J. Infec. Dis. **149**(1):90-97, 1984.

Vinayak, V.K., and others: Detection of *Giardia lamblia* antigen in the feces by counterimmunoelectrophoresis, Ped. Infect. Dis. **4**(4): 383-386, 1985.

Wolfe, M.S.: Giardiasis, Pediatr. Clin. North Am. **26**: 295-304, 1979.

Worley, G., and others: Toxocara canis infection: clinical and epidemiological associations with seropositivity, J. Infec. Dis. **149**(4):591-597, 1984.

Conjunctivitis

Acute hemorrhagic conjunctivitis—Florida, North Carolina, Morbid. Mortal. Weekly Report **30**(40):501-502, 1981.

Bodor, F.F., and others: Bacterial etiology of conjunctivitis-otitis media syndrome, Pediatrics **76** (1):26-28, 1985.

Friedlaender, M.H., Okumoto, M., and Kelley, J.: Diagnosis of allergic conjunctivitis, Arch. Ophthalmol. **102**:1198-1199, 1984.

Hammerschlag, M.: Conjunctivitis in infancy and childhood, Pediatr. Rev. **5**(9):285-290, 1984.

Havener, W.: Synopsis of ophthalmology, St. Louis, ed. 6, 1984, The C.V. Mosby Co.

Helveston, E.M., and Ellis, F.D.: Pediatric ophthalmology practice, ed. 2, St. Louis, 1984, The C.V. Mosby Co.

Moore, R., and Schmitt, B.: Conjunctivitis in children, Clin. Pediatr. **18**(1):26-32, 1979.

Ingestion of Injurious Agents

Arena, J.M.: Prevention of poisoning in children, Public Health Curr. **23**(1):1-4, 1983.

Bayer, M.J., and Rumack, B.H.: Poisoning and overdose, Rockville, MD, 1983, Aspen Systems Corp.

Benson, B.E., and others: Warning labels: a source of toxicity information for parents, Clin. Pediatr. **23**(8):441-444, 1983.

Driggers, D.A., and Johnson, R.: Initial management of pediatric poisoning, Pediatr. Basics **35**:4-6, 1983.

Fazen, L.E., III, Lovejoy, F.H., Jr., and Crone, R.K.: Acute poisoning in a children's hospital: a 2-year experience, Pediatrics **77**(2):144-151, 1986.

Foster, S.D.: In case of an emergency: ipecac syrup, Am. J. Maternal Child Nurs. **7**(4):227, 1982.

Gillies, C.: Management of pediatric poisoning, role of the nurse practitioner, Pediatr. Nurs. **6**(5):33-35, 1980.

Holbrook, M.L.: Child poisonings, Pediatr. Basics **41:** 13-15, 1985.

King, R.C.: Dealing with poisonings, RN **47**(12):45-48, 1984.

Krenzelok, E.P., and Garber, R.J.: Teaching poison prevention to pre-school children, their parents, and professional educators through child care centers, Am. J. Public Health **71**(7):750-752, 1981.

Lovejoy, F.: Management of pediatric poisoning. Part I. Pediatr. Nurs. **6**(5):37-39, 1980.

Lybarger, P.M.: Accidental poisoning in childhood: an ongoing problem, Issues Compr. Pediatr. Nurs. **1**(6):30-39, 1977.

Manoguerra, A.S.: Assessment and management of poisonings, Emer. Nurs. Update Series **2**(3), Princeton, NJ, 1981, Continuing Professional Education Center.

Mofenson, H., and Greensher, J.: Poisonings—an update, Clin. Pediatr. **18**(3):144-146, 1979.

Moulin, D., and others: Upper airway lesions in children after accidental ingestion of caustic substances, J. Pediatr. **106**(3):408-410, 1985.

Saracino, M., Flowers, J., and Lovejoy, F.H.: The epidemiology of poisoning from drug products, Am. J. Dis. Child. **134**(8):763-765, 1980.

Shinn, A.F.: Poison control potpourri, Critical Care Update, **10**(6):11, 1983.

Steel, P., and Spyker, D.A.: Poisonings, Pediatr. Clin. North Am. **32**(1):77-86, 1985.

Survey points up poison dangers, Am. J. Nurs. **85**(3):235, 1985.

Temple, A.: Management of pediatric poisoning. Part II. Pediatr. Nurs. **6**(5):40-43, 1980.

Walton, W.W.: An evaluation of the poison prevention packaging act, Pediatrics **69**(3):363-370, 1982.

Zieserl, E.: Hydrocarbon ingestion and poisoning, Compr. Ther. **5**(6):35-42, 1979.

Plant Poisoning

Edwards, N.: Local toxicity from a poinsettia plant: a case report, J. Pediatr. **102**(3):404-405, 1983.

Frazier, C.A.: Children and poisonous plants, Pediatr. Basics **22:**10-14, 1978.

Keim, K.A.: Preventing and treating plant poisonings in young children, Am. J. Maternal Child Nurs. **8**(4):287-289, 1983.

Salicylate/Acetaminophen Poisoning

Atwood, S.J.: The laboratory in the diagnosis and management of acetaminophen and salicylate intoxications, Pediatr. Clin. North Am. **27**(4):871-879, 1980.

Barber, J.M.: Acute salicylate poisoning, Emer. Nurs. Update Series **1**(22), Princeton, NJ, 1982, Continuing Professional Education Center.

Benson, G.D.: Hepatotoxicity following the therapeutic use of antipyretic analgesics, Am. J. Med. **75**(5A):85-93, 1983.

Leoni, M.P.: Management of acetaminophen overdose, Crit. Care Nurse **5**(4):44-47, 1985.

Lieh-Lai, M.W., and others: Metabolism and pharmacokinetics of acetaminophen in a severely poisoned young child, J. Pediatr. **105**(1):125-128, 1984.

Mitchell, A.A., and others: Acetaminophen and aspirin: prescription, use, and accidental ingestion among children, Am. J. Dis. Child. **136**(11):976-979, 1982.

Robinson, L.A., Roper, K.E., and Fisher, R.E.: Nursing considerations in the use of non-prescription analgesic-antipyretic aspirin and acetaminophen, Pediatr. Nurs. **3**(4):18-24, 1977.

Rumack, B.H., and Peterson, R.G.: Acetaminophen toxicity, West J. Med. **132**(1):61, 1980.

Swetnam, S.M., and Florman, A.L.: Probable acetaminophen toxicity in an 18-month-old infant due to repeated overdosing, Clin. Pediatr. **23**(2):104-105, 1984.

Wall, C.: The real risk of acetaminophen overdose, RN **48**(8):35-38, 1985.

Heavy Metal Poisoning

Adler, R., and others: Metallic mercury vapor poisoning simulating mucocutaneous lymph node syndrome, J. Pediatr. **101** (6):967-968, 1982.

Bellinger, D.C., and Needleman, H.L.: Lead and the relationship between maternal and child intelligence, J. Pediatr. **102** (4):528-528, 1983.

Burdick, M.P., and Harris, V.G.: Prevention of lead poisoning in children, Public Health Curr. **24**(3):11-14, 1984.

Chisolm, J.: Poisoning from heavy metals (mercury, lead, and cadmium), Pediatr. Ann. **9**(12):28-42, 1980.

Colliver, J.A., Kolm, P., and Verhulst, S.J.: Dentine lead and IQ: interpretation of results of residuals analysis, J. Pediatr. **102**(4):573-574, 1983.

Dolcourt, J.L., and others: Hazard of lead exposure in the home from recycled automobile storage batteries, Pediatrics **68**(2):225-230, 1981.

Drummond, A.H., Jr.: Lead poisoning in children, J. School Health **51**(1):43-47, 1981.

Erler, M.: Iron poisoning, J. Emer. Nurs. **6**(2):40-42, 1980.

Ernhart, C.B., and others: Subclinical levels of lead and developmental deficit: a multivariate follow-up reassessment, Pediatrics **67**(6):911-919, 1981.

Galazka, S.S.: Lead poisoning in children: a multidimensional hazard, Pediatr. Basics **36:**4-6, 1983.

Krenzelok, E.D., and Hoff, J.V.: Accidental childhood iron poisoning: a problem of marketing and labeling, Pediatrics **63**(4):591-596, 1979.

Lacouture, P.G., and others: Emergency assessment of severity in iron overdose by clinical and laboratory methods, J. Pediatr. **99**(1):89-91, 1981.

Langner, B., and Modrcin-McCarthy, M.A.: Lead poisoning: an ongoing pediatric nursing concern, Issues Compr. Pediatr. Nurs. **4**(3):23-36, 1980.

Lee, J.S.: Cadmium, mercury, and lead—the heavy metal gang, Fam. Comm. Health **7**(3):8-14, 1984.

Markowitz, M.E., and Rosen, J.F.: Assessment of lead stores in children: validation of an 8-hour CaNa$_2$EDTA provocative test, J. Pediatr. **104**(3):337-341, 1984.

Miller, S.J.: Nursing care of the lead-burdened child: a problem oriented approach, Pediatr. Nurs. **7**(5):47-52, 1981.

Moutinho, M., and others: Acute mercury vapor poisoning, Am. J. Dis. Child. **135**(1):42-44, 1981.

Needleman, H., and others: Deficits in psychologic and classroom performance of children with elevated dentine lead levels, N. Engl. J. Med. **300:**689, 1979.

Ng, R.C.W., Perry, K., and Martin, D.J.: Iron poisoning, Clin. Pediatr. **18**(10):614-616, 1979.

Pearce, J., and Burg, F.D.: Lead poisoning in children, Drug Ther. **12**(5):87-102, 1982.

Robotham, J.L., and Lietman, P.S.: Acute iron poisoning: a review, Am. J. Dis. Child. **134**(9):875-879, 1980.

Venturelli, J., and others: Gastrotomy in the management of acute iron poisoning, J. Pediatr. **100**(5):768-769, 1982.

Yip, R., and Dallman, P.R.: Developmental changes in erythrocyte protoporphyrin: roles of iron deficiency and lead toxicity, J. Pediatr. **104**(5):710-713, 1984.

Child Abuse and Neglect

Altemeier, W.A., and others: Prediction of child maltreatment during pregnancy, J. Am. Acad. Child Psychiatry **18:**205-228, 1979.

Ayoub, C., and Pfeifer, D.: Burns as a manifestation of child abuse and neglect, Am. J. Dis. Child. **133**(9):910-914, 1979.

Behling, D.W.: Alcohol abuse as encountered in 51 instances of reported child abuse, Clin. Pediatr. **18**(2):87-91, 1979.

Berger, D.: Child abuse simulating ''near-miss'' sudden infant death syndrome, J. Pediatr. **95**(4):554-556, 1979.

Bergman, A.B., Larsen, R.M., and Mueller, B.A.: Changing spectrum of serious child abuse, Pediatrics **77**(1):113-116, 1986.

Billmire, M.E., and Myers, P.A.: Serious head injury in infants: accident or abuse? Pediatrics **75**(2):340-342, 1985.

Bittner, S., and Newberger, E.H.: Pediatric understanding of child abuse and neglect, Pediatr. Rev. **2**(7):197-207, 1981.

Bottom, W., and Lancaster, J.: An ecological orientation toward human abuse, Fam. Comm. Health **4**(2):1-10, 1981.

Carley, L.: Helping the helpless: the abused child, Nursing 85 **15**(11):34-38, 1985.

Christensen, M.L., Schommer, B.L., and Velasquez, J.: An interdisciplinary approach to preventing child abuse, Am. J. Maternal Child Nurs. **9**(2):108-112, 1984.

Council on Scientific Affairs: AMA diagnostic and treatment guidelines concerning child abuse and neglect, JAMA **254** (6):796-800, 1985.

Deitch, E.A., and Staats, M.: Child abuse through burning, J. Burn Care and Rehabil. **3**(2):89-94, 1982.

Dietrich, K.N., Starr, R.H., and Weisfeld, G.E.: Infant maltreatment: caretaker-infant interaction and developmental consequences at different levels of parenting failure, Pediatrics **72**(4):532-540, 1983.

Dine, M.S., and McGovern, M.E.: Intentional poisoning of children—an overlooked category of child abuse: report of seven cases and review of the literature, Pediatrics **70** (1):32-35, 1982.

Ellerstein, N.S., editor: Child abuse and neglect: a medical reference, New York, 1981, John Wiley & Sons, Inc.

English, P.C.: Pediatrics and the unwanted child in history: foundling homes, disease, and the origins of foster care in New York City, 1860 to 1920, Pediatrics **73**(5):699-711, 1984.

Fontana, V.J.: The maltreated child, ed. 4, Springfield, IL, 1979, Charles C Thomas, Publisher.

Fontana, V.J., and Robison, E.: Observing child abuse, J. Pediatr. **105**(4):655-660, 1984.

Gray, J.D., and others: Prediction and prevention of child abuse, Semin. Perinatol. **3**:85-88, 1979.

Hampton, R.L., and Newberger, E.H.: Child abuse incidence and reporting by hospitals: significance of severity, class, and race, Am. J. Public Health **75**(1):56-60, 1985.

Heindl, M.C., editor: Child abuse and neglect, Nurs. Clin. North Am. **16**(1):101-188, 1981.

Helberg, J.L.: Documentation in child abuse, Am. J. Nurs. **83**(2):238-239, 1983.

Helfer, R.: Where to now, Henry? a commentary on the battered child syndrome, Pediatrics **76**(6):993-997, 1985.

Helfer, R.E.: Preventing the abuse and neglect of children, Pediatr. Basics **23**:4-7, April 1979.

Helfer, R.E., and others: Trauma to the bones of small infants from passive exercise: a factor in the etiology of child abuse, J. Pediatr. **104**(1):47-50, 1984.

Helfer, R.E., and Kempe, C.H.: The battered child, ed. 3, Chicago, 1980, University of Chicago Press.

Hight, D.W., Bakalar, H.R., and Lloyd, J.R.: Inflicted burns in children: recognition and treatment, JAMA **242**(6):517-520, 1979.

Holder, W.M., and Schene, P.: Understanding child neglect and abuse, Denver, 1981, The American Humane Assoc.

Holter, J.C.: Child abuse, Nurs. Clin. North Am. **14**(3):417-427, 1979.

Hurwitz, S.: Child abuse: the signs may be only skin deep, Child Care Newsletter **4**(2):1-3, 1985.

Josten, L.: Prenatal assessment guide for illuminating possible problems with parenting, Am. J. Maternal Child Nurs. **6**(2):113-117, 1981.

Kanter, R.K.: Retinal hemorrhage after cardiopulmonary resuscitation or child abuse, J. Pediatr. **108**(3):430-432, 1986.

Kauffman, C.K., Neill, M.K., and Thomas, J.N.: The abusive parent. In Johnson, S.J., editor: Nursing assessment and strategies for the family at risk, ed. 2 Philadelphia, 1986, J.B. Lippincott Co.

Kempe, C.H., and Helfer, R.E., editors: The battered child, ed. 3, Chicago, 1982, University of Chicago Press.

Malatack, J.J., and others: Munchausen syndrome by proxy: a new complication of central venous catheterization, Pediatrics **75**(3):523-525, 1985.

McKittrick, C.A.: Child abuse: recognition and reporting by health professionals, Nurs. Clin. North Am. **16**(1):103-115, 1981.

Murphy, J.F., and others: Objective birth data and the prediction of child abuse, Arch. Dis. Child. **56**:295-297, 1981.

Nalepka, C., O'Toole, R., and Turbett, J.P.: Nurses' and physicians' recognition and reporting of child abuse, Issues Compr. Pediatr. Nurs. **5**:33-44, 1981.

Ortman, E.: Attachment behaviors in abused children, Pediatr. Nurs. **5**(4):25-29, 1979.

Peterman, P.J.: Parenting and environmental considerations, Am. J. Orthopsychiatry **51**(2):351-355, 1981.

Reece, R.M., and Grodin, M.A.: Recognition of nonaccidental injury, Pediatr. Clin. North Am. **32**(1):41-60, 1985.

Rosen, B., and Stein, M.T.: Women who abuse their children: implications for pediatric practice, Am. J. Dis. Child. **134**(10):947-950, 1980.

Rosenthal, P.A., and Doherty, M.B.: Serious sibling abuse by preschool children, J. Am. Acad. Child Psychiatry **23**(2):186-190, 1984.

Runyan, D.K., and Gould, C.L.: Foster care for child maltreatment. I. Impact on delinquent behavior, Pediatrics **75**(3):562-568, 1985.

Runyan, D.K., and Gould, C.L.: Foster care for child maltreatment, II. Impact on school performance, Pediatrics **76**(5):841-847, 1985.

Saulsbury, F., Chobanian, M., and Wilson, W.: Child abuse: parenteral hydrocarbon administration, Pediatrics **73**(5):719-722, 1984.

Scharer, K.M.: Rescue fantasies: professional impediments in working with abused families, Am. J. Nurs. **78**:1483-1484, 1978.

Starr, R.H., Jr., editor: Child abuse prediction: policy implications, Cambridge, MA, 1982, Ballinger Publishing Co.

Subramanian, K.: Reducing child abuse through respite center intervention, Child Welfare **64**(5):501-509, 1985.

Velasquez, J., Christensen, M.L., and Schommer, B.L.: Intensive services help prevent child abuse, Am. J. Maternal Child Nurs. **9**(2):113-117, 1984.

Sexual Abuse

Alexander, P.C.: A systems theory conceptualization of incest, Fam. Proc. **24**:79-88, 1985.

Browning, D.G., and Boatman, B.: Incest: children at risk, Am. J. Psychiatry **134**:69-72, 1977.

Cline, F.: Dealing with sexual abuse of children, Nurs. Pract. **5**(3):52-54, 1980.

Ellerstein, N.S., and Canavan, J.W.: Sexual abuse of boys, Am. J. Dis. Child. **134**:255-257, 1980.

Fore, C.V., and Holmes, S.S.: Sexual abuse of children, Nurs. Clin. North Am. **19**(2):329-340, 1984.

Funk, J.B.: Management of sexual molestation in preschoolers, Clin. Pediatr. **19**:686-688, 1980.

Gorline, L.L., and Roy, M.M.: Examining and caring for the child who has been sexually assaulted, Am. J. Maternal Child Nurs. **4**:110-113, 1979.

Krugman, R.: Preventing sexual abuse of children in day care: whose problem is it anyway? Pediatrics **75**(6):1150-1151, 1985.

Ledray, L.: Victims of incest, Am. J. Nurs. **84**(8):1010-1014, 1984.

Pascoe, D.J.: Management of sexually abused children, Pediatr. Ann. **8**:309-316, 1979.

Rimsza, M.E., and Niggemann, E.H.: Medical evaluation of sexually abused children: a review of 311 cases, Pediatrics **69**(1):8-14, 1982.

Robertson, K.E., and Wilson-Walker, J.A.: A program for preventing sexual abuse of children, Am. J. Maternal Child Nurs. **10**(2):100-102, 1985.

Ryan, M.T.: Identifying the sexually abused child, Pediatr. Nurs. **10**(6):419-421, 1984.

Scherzer, L.N., and Lala, P.: Sexual offenses committed against children, Clin. Pediatr. **19**:679-685, 1980.

Sullivan, R.A., Schaefer, J.L., and Goldstein, F.L.: Child molestation, Am. Fam. Physician **19**(3):127-132, 1979.

Summit, R.C.: The child sexual abuse accommodation syndrome, Child Abuse & Neglect **7**:177-193, 1983.

Thomas, J.N., and Rogers, C.M.: Sexual abuse of children: case finding and clinical assessment, Nurs. Clin. North Am. **16**:179-188, 1981.

Weitzel, W.D., and others: Clinical management of father-daughter incest, Am. J. Dis. Child. **132**:127, 1978.

White, S., and others: Sexually transmitted diseases in sexually abused children, Pediatrics **72**(1):16-21, 1983.

Unit Six

Middle Childhood

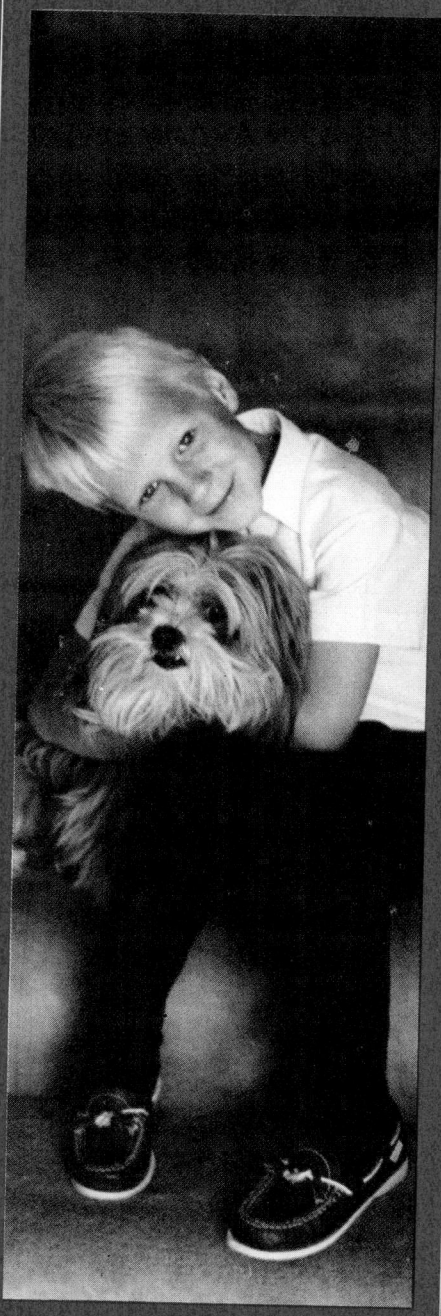

Children in the middle childhood years enjoy a relatively stable period of slow but steady growth and maturation with few physical or emotional stresses. It is a comfortable period of adjustment with a developmental pace sufficiently slow to meet the physical and psychologic demands placed on them. It becomes a period of broadening horizons as children encounter a wider sphere of influence—school, peers, and multiple opportunities for social interaction. During this period children learn the fundamental skills of their culture and develop inner resources for coping with larger social units. The emphasis during this period is on competence in physical and mental tasks and on equally important changes in social relationships.

Chapter 17, *Health Promotion of the School-Age Child and Family*, provides a brief overview of the developmental changes that take place in middle childhood, including a lengthy summary of the major characteristics of each age within the period of middle childhood. Chapter 18, *Health Problems of Middle Childhood*, outlines the more common health problems encountered during these years. Few major illnesses are associated with middle childhood, although children during this time are still subject to many of the problems that characterize the earlier childhood years, such as injuries, and, with wider social relationships, communicable diseases that continue to be prevalent.

Chapter 17

Health Promotion of the School-Age Child and Family

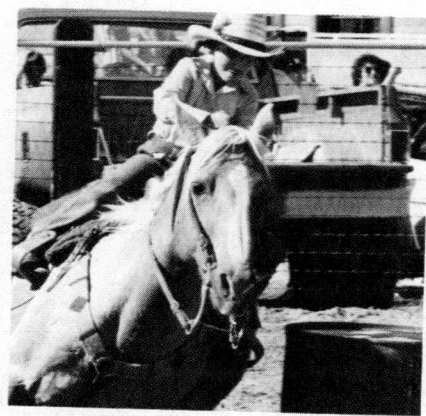

The segment of the life span that extends from age 6 to approximately age 12 has been endowed with a variety of labels, each of which describes an important characteristic of the period. The middle years are most often referred to as *school-age* or the *school years*. This period begins with entrance into the wider sphere of influence represented by the school environment, which has a significant impact on development and relationships. The term *gang age* describes children's affiliation with age-mates and with learning the culture of childhood. Within peer groups children establish the first close relationships outside the family group.

From a psychoanalytic point of view this is the period of *latency*, which has been considered to be a time of sexual tranquility between the oedipal phase of early childhood and the eroticism of adolescence. It is during this time that children experience the intimacy of relationships with same-sex peers following the indifference of earlier years and preceding the heterosexual fascination that accompanies the changes of puberty. However, the concept of sexual latency is now being questioned in the light of early sexual exploration and the exploitation of sex in the media.

Promoting Optimum Growth and Development

Physiologically the middle years begin with shedding the first deciduous tooth and end at puberty with the acquisition of final permanent teeth (with the exception of the wisdom teeth). During the preceding 5 to 6 years, children have progressed from helpless infants to sturdy, complicated individuals with the capacity to communicate, conceptualize in a limited way, and become involved in complex social and motor behavior. Physical growth has been equally rapid. In contrast, the period of middle childhood, between the rapid growth of early childhood and the turmoil of the prepubescent growth spurt, is a time of gradual growth and development with steadier and more even progress in both its physical and emotional aspects.

Children's physical health is generally good, and it is a comfortable period of physical adjustment. Physiologic processes in general have developed to the point that they can be maintained at stable levels under ordinary conditions or can be readily adjusted to meet changing needs and stresses. Under normal circumstances these children are usually well able to meet the physical and psychologic demands that are placed on them.

There is a special quality about the middle childhood years. This is the period of childhood the adult remembers with fond recollection. School-age children like this age period, and it is the one that preschoolers eagerly look forward to and for which adolescents yearn. In the Western world school-age children have a good deal of freedom and few responsibilities.

With a firm foundation of trust, autonomy, and initiative, school-age children are ready and eager for the wider world of learning and competition associated with developing a sense of industry and the successful acquisition of earlier, simpler skills. These skills are accompanied by the mild but persistent expectations of the society in which the children live, which serve as guidelines for behavior. Children who succeed in achieving the tasks of early childhood are able to move into middle childhood with the skills of locomotion, language, and control of body functions. They move from the egocentricity of early childhood to the subperiod of cognitive domain described as *concrete operations* and are now ready to undertake the tasks associated with the school experience. These tasks are characterized by three outward thrusts: the interpersonal push from home and family into the peer group, the physical thrust into the world of active games and work that requires neuromuscular skills, and the mental thrust into the world of mature concepts, logic, symbolism, and communication.

Until recently middle childhood generated the least interest and preoccupation among psychologists and others concerned with the effects of childhood experiences on later adjustments. However, it has been found that this period makes an important contribution to children's learning the fundamental skills of their culture and developing competence and self-esteem. It is a time of intellectual growth, investment in work, and the first real commitment to a social unit outside of and larger than the family.

BIOLOGIC DEVELOPMENT

During middle childhood, growth in height and weight assume a slower but steady pace as compared with the earlier years and the years immediately ahead. Between ages 6 and 12, children will grow an average of 5 cm (2 inches) per year to gain 30 to 60 cm (1 to 2 feet) in height and will almost double in weight, increasing 2 to 3 kg (4 ½ to 6 ½ pounds) per year. The average 6-year-old child is about 116 cm (45 inches) tall and weighs about 21 kg (46 pounds); the average 12-year-old child stands about 150 cm (59 inches) tall and weighs approximately 40 kg (88 pounds). During this age period girls and boys differ very little in size, although boys tend to be slightly taller and somewhat heavier than girls. Toward the end of the school-age years both boys and girls begin to increase in size, although most girls begin to surpass boys in both height and weight, to the acute discomfort of both.

Proportional Changes

School-age children are more graceful than they were as preschoolers, and they are steadier on their feet. Their body proportions take on a slimmer look with longer legs, varying body proportion, and a lower center of gravity. Posture improves over that of the peschool period to facilitate locomotion and efficiency in using the arms and trunk. These proportions make climbing, bicycle riding, and other activities much easier. Fat gradually diminishes and its distribution patterns change, contributing to the thinner appearance of children during the middle years.

Accompanying the skeletal lengthening and fat diminution is an increase in the percentage of body weight represented by muscle tissue. By the end of this age period both boys and girls will double their strength and physical capabilities, and their steady and relatively consistent acquisition of refined coordination will increase their poise and skill. However, this increased strength can be misleading. Although strength increases, muscles are still functionally immature when compared with those of the adolescent and are more readily damaged by muscular injury caused by overuse.

The most pronounced changes and those that seem best to indicate increasing maturity in children are a decrease in head circumference in relation to standing height, a decrease in waist circumference in relation to height, and an increase in leg length related to height. These observations often provide a clue to a child's degree of maturity that has proved useful in predicting readiness for meeting the demands of school. There appears to be a correlation between physical indications of maturity and success in school.

Certain physiologic and anatomic characteristics are typical of children in the years of middle childhood. Facial proportions change as the face grows faster in relation to the

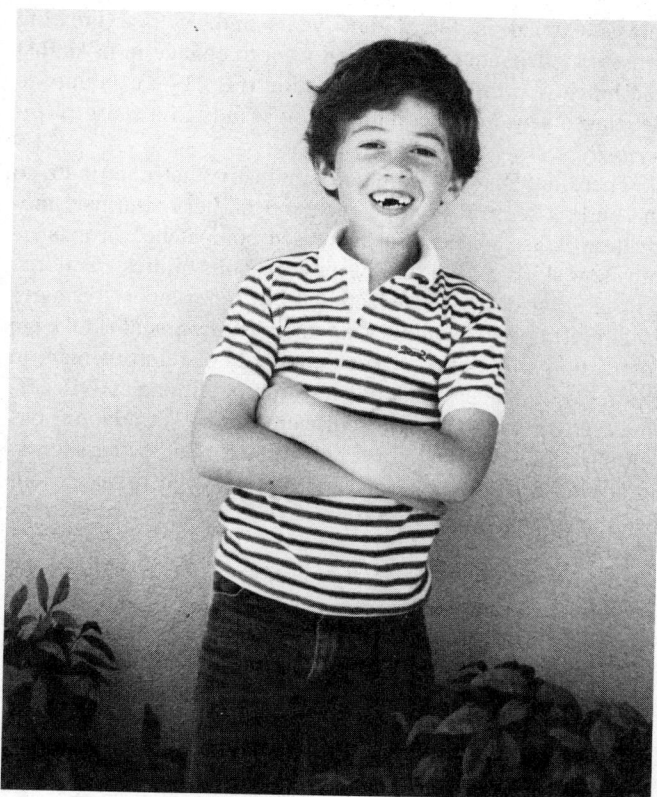

Fig. 17-1. Middle childhood is the stage of development when deciduous teeth are shed.

remainder of the cranium. The skull and brain grow very slowly during this period and increase little in size thereafter. Since all of the primary (deciduous) teeth are lost during this age span, middle childhood is sometimes known as the *age of the loose tooth* (Fig. 17-1) and the early years of middle childhood as the *ugly duckling stage,* when the new secondary (permanent) teeth appear to be much too large for the smaller face.

Maturation of Systems

Maturity of the gastrointestinal system is reflected in fewer stomach upsets, better maintenance of blood sugar levels, and an increased stomach capacity, which permits retention of food for longer periods. The school-age child does not need to be fed as carefully, as promptly, or as frequently as before. Caloric needs in relation to stomach size are less than they were in the preschool years and less than they will be during the coming adolescent growth spurt.

Physical maturation is evidenced in other body tissues and organs. Bladder capacity, although differing widely among individual children, is generally greater in girls than in boys. There are individual variations in frequency of urination and differences in one child according to circumstances such as temperature, humidity, time of day, amount of fluids ingested, and emotional state.

The heart grows more slowly during the middle years and is smaller in relation to the rest of the body than at any other period of life. Consequently many believe that strongly competitive sports with prolonged, intense physical exertion may be damaging to school-age children. The heart and respiratory rates steadily decrease and the blood pressure increases during ages 6 to 12 (see inside front cover).

Bones continue to ossify throughout childhood, but, since mineralization is not completed until maturity, children's bones resist pressure and muscle pull less than mature bones. Consequently care must be taken to prevent alterations in bone structure and children should be provided with well-fitted shoes and chairs and desks that allow correct sitting posture with the feet able to reach the floor and the hips able to fit well back in the seat. Children should have ample opportunity to move around and should observe appropriate caution in carrying heavy loads. For example, they should shift books from one arm to the other, and newspaper carriers who transport heavy bundles slung from the shoulders should alternate the load from one shoulder to the other to avoid developing a low shoulder or spine curvature.

There are wider differences between children at the end of middle childhood than at the beginning—and the differences are sometimes striking. These differences become increasingly apparent and, if extreme or unique, may create emotional problems unless the associated characteristics of height and weight relationships, rapid or slow growth, and other important features of development are recognized and explained to the children and their families. In addition, physical maturity is not necessarily correlated with emotional and social maturity. Seven-year-old children who look like 10-year-old children will, in fact, think and act like 7-year-old children. To expect behavior appropriate for 10-year-old children from them is unrealistic and can be detrimental to their development of competence and self-esteem. Conversely, to treat 10-year-old children as though they were 7 years old is an equal disservice to them.

Prepubescence

The preadolescent years, roughly ages 10 to 13, are years of transition. Soon the child will leave childhood behind forever and move on to adolescence. Preadolescence is childhood at its highest form of development. This is a healthy period of childhood—the period between childhood diseases and the diseases of adulthood. Preadolescence is, for some, a period of rapid growth, especially for girls; for others, mostly boys, it is generally a period of steady growth in height and weight.

There is no universal age at which children assume the characteristics of preadolescence. The first physiologic signs begin to appear at about 9 years (particularly in girls) and are usually clearly evident in 11- to 12-year-old children. Although preadolescent children do not want to be different, at this age the variability in physical growth and physiologic changes between children of the same sex, between the two sexes, and even within each individual child is often striking. This variability, especially in relation to the onset of secondary sex characteristics, is of utmost concern to the preadolescent. Either early or late appearance of these characteristics is a source of embarrassment and uneasiness to both sexes.

Preadolescence is a time when there is considerable overlapping of developmental characteristics with elements of both middle childhood and early adolescence. However, there are sufficient unique characteristics to set this period apart as an age category, even with the wide range of variability in ages 11 and 12 (or even 9 to 13) in some children. Generally the earliest age at which puberty begins is 10 years in girls and 12 years in boys, although there has been an increase in the number of girls reaching puberty at age 9. The average age of puberty in girls is 12, and in boys it is 14. Boys experience little sexual maturation during preadolescence.

PSYCHOSOCIAL DEVELOPMENT

There is no concept more difficult to assess or more elusive than that of the personality or the ''self.'' Most persons draw inferences regarding children's personalities from observation of their behaviors. These behaviors are based on many different innate and acquired characteristics, the way in which these characteristics are organized, and the manner in which each characteristic modifies or alters the other to contribute to the unique quality of each child. Personality is reflected in the way in which children react to themselves and others, the way in which others react to them, and the way in which they adjust to their environment. Evolution of the personality involves a number of different types of development—physical, intellectual, social, and emotional— all of which are profoundly influenced by the environment in which children grow and develop.

Erikson: Developing a Sense of Industry

Successful mastery of Erikson's first three stages of psychosocial development is probably the most important accomplishment in terms of development of a healthy personality (Erikson, 1963). With a foundation of trust, autonomy, and initiative, children are fairly certain to progress through subsequent stages with relative ease. Successful completion of these stages implies confidence in an environment of loving relationships within a stable family unit that has prepared the child to engage in experiences and relationships beyond these intimate groups. It has been suggested that the individual's fundamental attitude toward work is established during middle childhood. It is during this time that children receive the systematic instruction prescribed by their individual cultures and develop the skills needed to become useful, contributing members of their social communities.

A sense of industry, for which a more descriptive term is the *stage of accomplishment,* is achieved somewhere between age 6 and adolescence. The goal of this stage of development is to achieve a sense of personal and interpersonal competence by the acquisition of technologic and social skills. School-age children are eager to build skills and participate in meaningful and socially useful work. Interests expand in the middle years and, with a growing sense of independence, children want to engage in tasks that can be carried through to completion (Fig. 17-2). Failure to develop a sense of accomplishment results in a sense of *inferiority.*

There are many attributes of industry that contribute to the child's sense of competence and mastery. Intrinsic motivation is associated with increased competence in mastering new skills and assuming new responsibilities. Children gain a great deal of satisfaction from independent behavior in exploring and manipulating their environment and from interaction with peers. Extrinsic sources of reinforcement in the form of grades, material rewards, additional privileges, and recognition provide encouragement and stimulation. Often the acquisition of skills is a means for achieving success in special activities such as athletics or social organizations such as scouting. Peer approval is a strong motivating power.

The danger inherent in this period of personality development is the imposition of situations that might result in a sense of inadequacy or inferiority. This may happen if the previous stages have not been successfully achieved or if a child is incapable of or unprepared for assuming the responsibilities associated with developing a sense of accomplishment. Feelings of inferiority or lack of worth can be derived from children themselves or from the social environment. Children with physical or mental limitations are at a disadvantage for acquisition of certain skills, and, when the reward structure is based on evidence of mastery, children who are incapable of developing these skills are bound to feel inadequate and inferior.

Even children without chronic disabilities represent such a wide range of individual differences in capabilities and preferences that they will experience feelings of inadequacy in some areas. No child is able to do well in everything, and children must learn that they will not be able to master each skill that they attempt. All children, even children who in most instances have positive attitudes toward work and their own capabilities, will feel some degree of inferiority in regard to a specific skill that they cannot master.

To some extent, success or aptitude in one area may compensate for failure or ineptitude in another. However, differences in reinforcement provided for success in various areas have a very significant effect on feelings of adequacy. For example, in the United States reading proficiency is more highly rewarded than mechanical aptitude such as tinkering with broken automobile engines. A higher social value is placed on success in team sports than on success in operating a ham radio. However, compensating for the inability to excel in more socially valued skills through mastery of other less valued skills is difficult for the child. Also, as a corollary to this, the social environment places a negative value on any kind of failure and this serves to further stimulate feelings of inferiority in the less capable child. Repeated failures often generate such strong feelings in the child that eventually he is reluctant to attempt any new task that may bring failure or is fearful that he will not be able

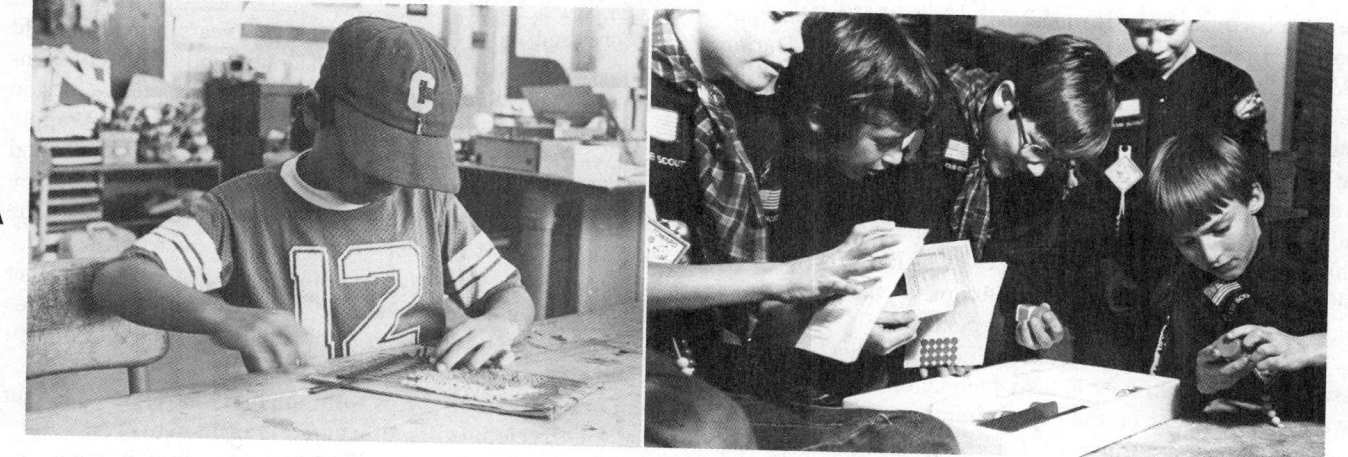

Fig. 17-2. School-age children are motivated to complete tasks. **A,** Working alone. **B,** Working with others.

to perform as well as his peers. Thus intrinsic motivation toward engaging in a task for the pleasure of the challenge conflicts with the external forces that cause feelings of doubt and inferiority. Consequently the child may no longer try.

Much depends on the child's concept of success or failure. Children who aspire for more than they are capable of will usually experience failure. In contrast, children who set their aspirations lower than their level of achievement are more likely to experience success. Most accomplishments during the school years are very public. Success or failure in school is known to family, teachers, peers, and others. In the social environment of school and sometimes at home, feelings of inferiority may be produced through comparison with others, suggesting that the child is not as good as some peer, sibling, or another subcultural group. This inadequacy becomes a source of embarrassment. The child may even be shamed for his failure. These earlier conflicts of doubt and guilt are very closely associated with feelings of inferiority.

A sense of accomplishment also involves the ability to cooperate and to compete with others—to cope more effectively with people. Middle childhood is the time when children learn the value of doing things alongside and with others and the benefits derived from division of labor in the accomplishment of goals. Children need and want real achievement. When they have access to tasks that need to be done, that they are able to do well despite individual differences in their innate capacities and emotional development and that they are suitably rewarded for, children will be able to achieve a sense of industry and accomplishment that prepares them for establishing a stable identity later in life.

Freud: Latency Period

Middle childhood is the period in psychosexual development that Freud has described as the *latency period*. He maintains that this time of life involves consolidation and elaboration of previously acquired traits and skills with the

assumption that no new significant conflicts or impulses will arise. Growth and development patterns follow the lines established in earlier stages. The primary personality development is that of the superego. It is a time of preparation for the important and dramatic psychosexual changes that take place during the genital stage of adolescence.

Developing Self-Esteem

Closely associated with developing a sense of industry is developing a concept of one's value and worth. With the emphasis on skill building and broadened social relationships, children are continually occupied in the process of self-evaluation. If they regard themselves as worthwhile or satisfactory persons, they are considered to have self-esteem, self-confidence, or a positive self-image. If they view themselves as worthless, they are said to have poor or low self-esteem.

In the process of self-evaluation, children actively strive to come up to internalized goals or levels of attainment that they hope to achieve. At the same time they continually receive feedback on the quality of their performance from those whom they consider to be authorities. By the time they reach school age, children have already received messages regarding the extent to which they are able to accomplish tasks that have been delegated to them. For example, one child may have been given prestigious responsibilities at home or at school or received special commendation for an achievement. On the other hand, another child may have been sent to a special class for slow learners or may have been the last person chosen when children choose sides for a game. These and other signs serve as clues to social evaluation that children then incorporate as part of their self-evaluation.

Children approach the process of self-evaluation from a framework of either self-confidence or self-doubt. Children, who during the preschool years have mastered the maturational crises of autonomy and initiative, are able to face the world with feelings of pride rather than shame. At first children's self-concepts are formed exclusively from what they perceive to be their parents' evaluation of them. During middle childhood the opinions of peers and teachers further complicate the process. The criticisms and peer approval are sources of data for evaluation. Now parents and other adults are not the only persons who respond to their skills, talents, and abilities. Peers also identify skills and capabilities, and each child soon begins to internalize these outside opinions. Children's self-concepts are composed of their own critical self-assessment plus what they interpret as the opinions of family members and outside social contacts.

The difficulty that children encounter in the attempt to assess their own abilities is their inclination to rely on their own expectations or on the expectations expressed by others regarding their performance. They depend almost entirely on external evidence of worth, such as school grades, teachers' comments, and parental and peer approval. Children do not yet have the capacity to develop their own, independent criteria by which they can evaluate their own accomplishments, and it is especially difficult for them to assess their achievement in abstract skills.

Nothing succeeds like success. The significant adults in children's lives can often manage, unseen, to manipulate their environment so that they meet with success. Each small success increases a child's self-image a little. The more positive children feel about themselves, the more confident they feel in trying again for success. All children profit from feelings that they are in some way special to significant adults. A positive self-concept makes them feel likable, worthwhile, and persons with a valuable contribution to make in their world. Such feelings lead to self-respect, self-confidence, and a general feeling of happiness. Parents can assist their school-age children to develop self-esteem by helping to increase their self-confidence, by being honest, providing opportunities for creativity, helping them succeed in activities, and providing positive reinforcement.

COGNITIVE DEVELOPMENT

Somewhere around the beginning of the school years, children begin to acquire the ability to relate a series of events and actions to mental representations that can be expressed both verbally and symbolically. This is the stage in development that Piaget describes as *concrete operations,* wherein children are able to use their thought processes to experience events and actions. Since the word *operation* implies an action that is performed on an object or set of objects, a mental operation is an alteration or transformation that is carried out in thought rather than in action. Toddlers or preschool children can perform acts that involve ordering, such as correctly arranging a graduated set of circles from largest to smallest on a stick, or they can find their way to a friend's house, but they are unable to verbalize the action or actions involved in the process. School-age children are able to articulate the process and can perform the action mentally without the need to carry out the behaviors.

Piaget: Developing Concrete Operations

As children move from the preschool years into the world of wider relationships, their conceptual abilities become increasingly flexible. During the *concrete-operational* period children rapidly acquire cognitive operations and apply these new skills when thinking about objects, situations, and events. Their rigid, egocentric outlook is replaced by thought processes that allow them to see things from the point of view of another. They become aware of a variety of perspectives and become more sensitive to the fact that others do not always perceive events exactly as they do. They are able to delay an action until they have evaluated alternative responses to situations, and their steady reduction in egocentricity helps form the basis for logical thought and the development and maturation of morality.

The concrete-operational stage takes place between the years 7 and 11. During this stage children develop an understanding of and use for relationships between things and ideas. They progress from making judgments based on what they see (perceptual) to making judgments based on what they reason (conceptual). They are increasingly able to master symbols and to use their memory store of past experiences in evaluating and interpreting the present. They gain insight into the basic components of concrete operational thought: conservation, classification, and combinational skills.

Conservation. One of the major cognitive tasks of school-age children is learning that physical matter does not appear and disappear by magic. They learn that certain properties of the environment are not changed simply by altering their disposition in space. They are able to resist perceptual cues that suggest such alterations in the physical state of an object.

Conservation of mass is usually demonstrated by the use of two soft clay balls of the same size and shape. When children have determined to their satisfaction that the balls are identical, one is flattened into a pancake-shaped mass. A child is asked to tell which has more clay or if the masses are the same: the child who is still in the preoperational phase of cognitive thought, relying on personal perceptions to make the judgment, will say that the pancake-shaped mass has more clay because it is wider or larger around. The child who is able to conserve will insist that the masses still contain the same amount of clay. To explain the observations that the mass has been unaltered, the child may use one of the following three concepts:

1. The concept of *identity*—since nothing has been added and nothing has been taken away, the pancake is still the same clay with nothing changed but the shape.
2. The concept of *reversibility*—the clay can be reshaped into its original form, that of a ball.
3. The concept of *reciprocity*—although the pancake appears larger in circumference, the ball is much thicker. In this instance the child demonstrates the ability to deal with two dimensions at the same time and comprehend that a change in one dimension compensates for a change in another.

When children are able to use the concepts of identity, reversibility, and reciprocity, they can conserve along any physical dimension. They no longer perceive a tall, thin glass of water as containing a greater volume than an equal amount in a short, wide glass; they can distinguish between the weight of items regardless of their size. They recognize that size is not necessarily related to weight or volume. They can solve concrete problems that they are able to manipulate or "see" in a concrete manner. They recognize that logical operations move in two directions, such as addition and subtraction or multiplication and division. They learn that certain properties are invariant; for example, 7 remains 7 whether it is represented by 3 + 4, 2 + 5, or seven buttons, seven stars, or seven boys.

Children learn that a given number of objects such as pennies will remain the same no matter how far apart they are spaced. Younger school-age children, when presented with two rows of pennies, will declare that a row of six pennies closely aligned is not equivalent to a row of six pennies spaced apart (conservation of length). As they advance in development, they see that the numbers remain the same no matter how they are related to one another in space.

There appears to be a developmental sequence in children's capacity to conserve matter. Children usually grasp conservation of numbers (ages 5 to 6) before conservation of substance. Conservation of liquids, mass, and length usually is accomplished at about age 6 to 7, weight sometime later (ages 9 to 10), and volume displacement last (ages 9 to 12).

Reversibility is used by children in selecting a course of action, thus providing greater control over themselves and their environment. They have the ability to think through an action sequence, anticipate the consequences, and, if needed, return to the beginning and rethink the action in a different direction. They no longer need to experience an action before they can anticipate the results. Reversibility allows mental action to replace physical action and provides the children with the ability to disassemble and reassemble certain kinds of things in their thoughts.

Classification. Classification skills involve the ability to group objects according to the attributes that they share in common. School-age children now have the ability to place things in a sensible and logical order, to group and sort, and, in doing so, to hold a concept in their minds while they make decisions based on that concept. It is characteristic of middle childhood that children derive a great deal of enjoyment from classifying and ordering their environment. They become occupied with numerous and varied collections of objects, such as wrappers, stamps, shells, dolls, cars, stones, and anything that is classifiable. They even begin to order friends and relationships, such as first best friend, second best friend, and so on.

As children mature, they progress from collecting simply for the sake of collecting and become more selective and discriminating. Their classification systems become more complex and are based on abstract ideas rather than on perception and experience. Much of the pleasure of collections is the appraising, ordering, and reordering of the parts.

School children are able to *serialize,* that is, to arrange objects according to some ordinal scale or quantified dimension such as size, weight, or color. They develop the ability to understand relational terms and concepts, such as bigger and smaller; darker and paler; heavier and lighter; to the right of and to the left of; first, last, and intermediate relationships (e.g., fourth, second); and more than and less than. They can see family relationships in terms of reciprocal roles; for example, in order to be a brother, one must have a sibling. It is common for a preschool child to refer to the adult female in a family as "your mother" even when discussing the relationship with the woman's husband.

Combinational skills. It is during the school-age years that children develop the ability to manipulate numbers and to learn the skills of addition, subtraction, multiplication, and division. They learn to apply the basic operations to any object or quantity. They learn the alphabet and the ever-widening world of symbols called words that can be arranged in terms of structure and their relationship to the alphabet. They learn to tell time, to see the relationship of events in time (history) and places in space (geography), and to combine time and space relationships (geology and astronomy).

School-age children are able to entertain a hypothesis through use of conceptual principles and perceived events and to evaluate evidence that might support or disprove a hypothesis. These capabilities allow them to expand beyond the limits of their own experience and to consider events that happened before, will happen in the future, and are hypothesized to be happening in the present.

The most significant skill, the ability to read, is acquired during the school years and becomes the most valuable tool for independent inquiry. Children's capacity for exploration, imagination, and expansion of knowledge is enhanced with the ability to read as they progress from the repetition and confusion of early efforts to increasing facility and comprehension.

It is through no accident that the schools are prepared to meet the essentials of children's intellectual capabilities at the time that their cognitive processes are ready to assume appropriate intellectual achievements. The increase in capacity for logical thinking during this stage of concrete operations is based on the sensorimotor schemes of infancy and the representational abilities of preschool children. Children are now able to move into the formal operations that characterize the period of adolescence.

BODY IMAGE DEVELOPMENT

School-age children are quite knowledgeable about the human body, and social development during this period focuses to a large extent on the body and its capabilites. School-age children are able to draw a recognizable human figure although, individually, their portrayal of body parts may vary considerably. They are acutely aware of bodies—their own, those of their peers, and those of adults.

Social development during the school years, with the emphasis on peer relationships, prescribes that children conform to group norms. They evaluate themselves to determine how their physical appearance, body configuration, and coordination compare to those of their peers. They also model themselves after their parents and compare themselves to favored peers and images observed in the media.

It is not unusual for children in middle childhood to be curious about their own bodies and the bodies of other children. They often experiment with their own bodies and it is a common occurrence for two or more children to unclothe (to varying degrees) and play "doctor." Such experimentations and explorations allow children to pursue an investigation of similarities and differences as one means for acquiring norms. Fortunately such self-investigations are not observed by others, but if children are surprised in the act, the best approach is to provide reassurance that the behavior is normal, thus relieving any anguish or guilt they may feel. It is only when these activities are carried to the extreme or when parents over-react to them that they become clinical problems (Levine, 1983).

Children are acutely aware of physical disabilites in others and it is not unusual for them to believe that their own bodies are not all right, are not the right size or the right shape, or that they are in some way defective. They respond to such concerns in a variety of ways. For example, they will conceal perceived shortcomings of body or performance, such as the obese child who refrains from going swimming, the child who conveniently forgets a gym suit, the child who conceals an imagined defect, or the child with enuresis who declines invitations to slumber parties. Children seldom express these concerns to families. However, they need to be reassured about both the uniqueness and the sameness of their bodies while respecting their privacy and allowing them appropriate protective strategies. Children who are different become acutely aware of the differences and may find themselves excluded from the "gang." When children are teased or criticized about being different, the effect will be lasting. They remember the teasing well into adulthood.

MORAL DEVELOPMENT (KOHLBERG)

As children move from egocentrism to more logical patterns of thought, they also move through stages in the development of conscience and moral standards. The beginning of this development is evident during the preschool years when children, to some extent, adopt and internalize the moral values of their parents and their standards for evaluating the behavior of themselves and others. Adopting parental standards makes children feel similar to the parents, thereby strengthening their identification.

Growth in moral thought and judgment progresses be-

tween ages 6 and 12. Young children do not believe that standards of behavior come from within themselves but that rules are established and set down by others. At first rules are perceived as definite, covering limited situations, and requiring no reason or explanation. Children learn the standards for acceptable behavior, act according to these standards, and feel guilty when they violate the standards. Although children 6 or 7 years old know the rules and what they are supposed to do, they do not understand the reasons behind them. Young children usually judge an act by its consequences. Rewards and punishment guide their judgment; a "bad act" is one that breaks a rule or does harm. When a child and an adult conflict in judging an act, the adult is right. Children may believe that what other people tell them to do is right and that what they think themselves is wrong. Consequently children 6 or 7 years old are more likely to interpret accidents and misfortunes as punishment for misdeeds.

Older school-age children are able to judge an act by the intentions that prompted it rather than just by the consequences. Rules and judgments become less absolute and authoritarian and begin to be founded more on the needs and desires of others. Rules of conduct are more readily considered in terms of mutual agreement and based on cooperation and respect for others. For older children a rule violation is apt to be viewed in relation to the total context in which it appears; reactions are influenced by the situation as well as by the morality of the rule itself. However, it is not until adolescence or beyond that children are able to view morality on an abstract basis with sound reasoning and principled thinking. Whereas a younger child can judge an act only according to whether it is right or wrong, older children will take into account a different point of view to make a judgment. They are able to understand and accept the concept of doing as they would have others do to them.

SPIRITUAL DEVELOPMENT

Children at this age think in very concrete terms but are avid learners and have a great desire to learn about their God. They picture God as human and tend to describe him in terms of character traits such as loving and helping. He is a very important person in the lives of many children. They are fascinated by heaven and hell and, with a developing conscience and concern about rules, they fear going to hell for misbehavior. School-age children want and expect to be punished for misbehavior but, if given the option, tend to choose a punishment that "fits the crime." Often they view illness or injury as a punishment for a real or imagined misdeed. The beliefs and ideals of family and religious personages are more influential than their peers in matters of faith.

School-age children begin to learn the difference between the natural and the supernatural but have difficulty understanding symbols. Consequently religious concepts must be presented to them in concrete terms. They try to relate phenomena in the world in a logical, systemic manner, which

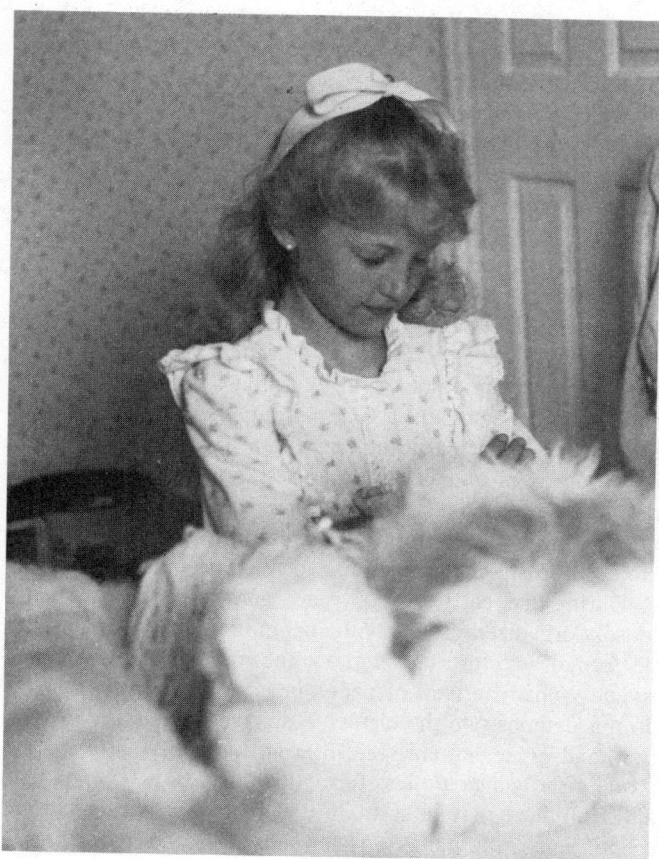

Fig. 17-3. Children are comforted by prayer or other religious rituals.

Photography by Earl Fillmore, Salt Lake City, UT.

is at once both satisfying and occasionally disheartening. Religion affords a means whereby children can relate themselves to their deity in a direct and personal way.

Children are comforted by prayer or other religious rituals and, if this is a part of their daily lives, these activities can help them cope with threatening situations (Fig. 17-3). Their petitions to their God in prayers tend to be for very tangible rewards and, although younger children expect their prayers to be answered, as they get older they begin to recognize that this does not always occur and become less concerned when prayers are not answered. They are able to discuss their feelings about their faith and how it relates to their lives.

SOCIAL DEVELOPMENT

Children at the beginning of the middle childhood years normally enter a period of less intense emotions, secure in their dependency on their parents and family and with self-confidence tempered by a more realistic perspective. Their energies are now available to explore the environment beyond the family, to gradually increase the scope of interpersonal interactions, and to invest their curiosity in a greater understanding of the world.

Identification with peers appears to be a strong influence in children's gaining independence from parents. The aid and support of the group provide children with enough security to risk the moderate parental rejection brought about by each small victory in their development of independence.

Questions of masculinity and femininity take on importance as sex-role learning assumes more prominence. Boys associate with boys and girls with girls, each pursuing their own interests, with communication between the sexes confined to that which is necessary. Much of the child's concept of the appropriate sex role is acquired through relationships with peers. During the early school years there is little difference relative to sex in the play experiences of children. Games and many other activities are shared by both girls and boys. However, in the later school years the differences become marked. Boys and girls grow more intolerant of each other, especially on the surface.

Social Relationships and Cooperation

Daily relationships with age-mates provide the most important social interactions in the life of school-age children. For the first time children are able to join in group activities with unrestrained enthusiasm and steady participation, when formerly interactions had been limited to short periods under considerable adult supervision. With increased skills and wider opportunities, children are able to become involved with one or several peer groups in which they can gain status as respected members.

There are valuable lessons to be learned from daily interaction with age-mates. First, children learn to appreciate the numerous and varied points of view that are represented in the peer group. As they play together, children discover that there are numerous occupations for fathers and mothers, perhaps more than one version of the same song, different rules for the same game, and different customs for celebrating the same holiday. As children interact with peers who see the world in ways that are somewhat different from the way they see it, they become aware of the limits of their own point of view. Because age-mates are peers and are not forced to accept one another's ideas as they are expected to accept those of adults, other children have a significant influence on decreasing the egocentric outlook of the individual child. Consequently they learn to argue, persuade, bargain, cooperate, and compromise in order to maintain friendships.

Second, children become increasingly sensitive to the social norms and pressures of the peer group. The peer group establishes standards for acceptance and rejection, and children may be willing to modify their behavior in order to be accepted by the group. They are judged by the physical impression they convey, the skills they can perform, and other abilities they can demonstrate. This need for peer approval becomes a powerful influence toward conformity. The child learns to dress, talk, and otherwise behave in a manner acceptable to the group. A variety of roles, such as class joker or class hero, may be assumed by the individual

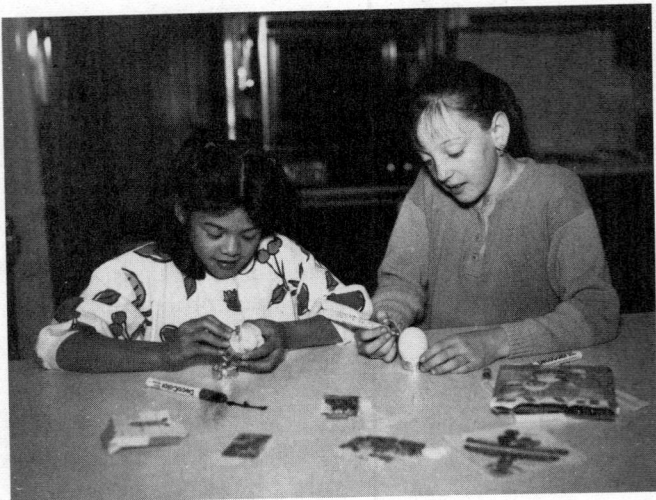

Fig. 17-4. School-age children enjoy engaging in activities with a "best friend."

child in order to gain approval from the group. However, no child will be able to adapt perfectly to all the requirements made by the peer group. If some children find the discrepancies between the values of the peer group and the values of their families are too great, they may be forced to relinquish the pleasure of interaction with the group in order to abide by the regulations established in the home. Thus, to diminish conflict within the family, some children may be forced into a position outside the peer group.

Third, the interaction among peers leads to the formation of intimate friendships between same-sex peers (Fig. 17-4). School age is the time when children have "best friends" with whom they share secrets, private jokes, adventures, and come to one another's aid in times of trouble. In the course of these friendships children also fight, threaten, break up, and reunite. These dyadic relationships, in which children experience love and closeness for a peer, seem to be important as a foundation for heterosexual relationships in adulthood. The conflicts encountered in the relationship are usually resolved in terms that the children are able to control. Since neither child has authority over the other, as in an adult-child relationship, the children must work through their differences within the framework of their commitment to one another.

Gangs. One of the outstanding characteristics of middle childhood is the formation of formalized groups, or gangs. Initially children in the early middle years merely hang around the periphery of the formalized group watching, learning, practicing various skills, and participating in group activities whenever the members of the gang allow them to do so. In a year or two, as they advance in age, children eventually take their places as full-fledged participating members. The process is facilitated if they have a buddy.

One of the prominent features of middle childhood gangs is the code of rigid rules imposed on the members. There is an exclusiveness in the selection of persons who have the privilege of joining. Acceptance in the group is often deter-

mined on a pass-fail basis that is based on social or behavioral criteria. Conformity is the core of the gang structure. There are often secret codes, shared interests, and special modes of dress, and each child must abide by a standard of behavior established by the group. Understanding of and conformity to the rules provide children with feelings of security and relieve them of the responsibility of making decisions.

Membership in the gang provides children with a comfortable place in society. Many of the values of the gang, such as physical strength, daring, ingenuity, and comradeship, have not been stressed in the family group, but these, too, are worthy values and contribute to an individual child's total personality. By merging their identities with that of their peers, children are able to move from the family group to an outside group as a step toward seeking further independence. They substitute conformity to a peer-group pattern for conformity to a family pattern while they are still too shaky and insecure to function independently.

During the early school years gangs are rather small, loosely organized groups with changing membership and little formal structure and without the more prolonged cohesiveness characteristic of gangs in later school years. They do not demonstrate the elements of give-and-take, cooperation, and order that are seen in groups of older children. As a rule girls' gangs are less formalized than boys' gangs, and although there may be a mixture of both sexes in the earlier school years, the gangs of later school years are composed predominantly of children of the same sex. Common interests are a frequent basis around which a gang is structured.

Children's strong desire not to be different creates problems for those who are for various reasons unable to meet the accepted standards of the peer group. Children with disabilities or those who are in some way so deprived that they are unable to compete have a difficult time. Self-consciousness results when children are unable to dress as other children dress, do not have spending money like other children, or appear different from other children, such as the child who has numerous freckles, red hair, or such minor physical defects as strabismus. Any of these differences will set a child apart from the group and often make him a target for the criticism and ridicule of the peer group.

Although peer group identification and association are essential to a child's emergence into the world, there can be dangers inherent in strong peer-group attachment. Peer pressures may force children into taking risks, even against their better judgment. Minor infractions and immoralities, such as stealing apples from the neighbor's tree, smoking, or sexual exposure, are disturbing to adults but seem to be a normal part of gang activity. However, acts of violence or destruction and foolhardy risks to safety are sometimes the outgrowth of overzealous gang cohesiveness.

Relationships with Families

Although the peer group is highly influential and necessary to normal child development, parents are still the primary influence in shaping children's personalities, setting standards for behavior, and establishing value systems. It is the family values that usually predominate when parental and peer value systems come into conflict. Although children may appear to reject parental values while testing the new values of the peer group, ultimately they will retain and incorporate into their own value systems the parental values they have found to be of worth. Peer associations seem to remain within a social class system; there may be discriminate membership on the basis of ethnic or racial origin.

As children move into the wider world of peer-group relationships, parents are faced with the task of relinquishing their hold. They may find it difficult to face the rejection that is demonstrated as their children stand solidly with the peer group. During this time children will want to spend more time in the company of their peers and may seem anxious to leave the house; they will often prefer activities of the gang to family activities. This can be very disturbing to parents. During this time parents can best serve the interests of their children through tolerant understanding and support even when their children become intolerant and critical of the parents and their ways when those ways deviate from that of the gang. In the child's eyes the parents no longer assume the stature they previously enjoyed. Children discover that parents can be wrong, and they begin to question the knowledge and authority of the parents who previously were considered to be all-knowing and all-powerful.

Although increased independence is the goal of middle childhood, children are not yet prepared to reject parental control. Children need and want restrictions placed on their behavior; they are not yet prepared to cope with all the problems of their expanding environment. They feel more secure knowing that there is an authority greater than themselves to implement such controls and restrictions. Children may complain loudly about the restrictions and try their best to break down parental barriers, but they are uneasy if they can succeed in doing so. Children feel secure with reasonable, consistent controls. They respect the adults on whom they can rely to prevent them from acting on each and every urge. Children sense in this behavior an expression of love and concern for their welfare.

Children also need their parents as adults, not as pals. Sometimes parents, hurt at their children's rejection, attempt to maintain their love and gratitude by assuming the role of "pals." Children need the stable, secure strength provided by mature adults to whom they can turn during troubled relationships with peers or stressful changes in their world. During a disruption in their lives, such as times of failure, periods of illness, or a move that separates them from the security of friends, children need the firm, secure anchor of parental interest and concern. With a secure base in a loving family, children are able to develop confidence in themselves and the maturity needed to break loose from the gang and stand independently.

Play

As children enter the school years, their play takes on new dimensions that reflect a new stage of development. Not only does play involve increased physical skill, intellectual ability, and fantasy, but, as they form gangs and cliques, children begin to evolve a sense of team or club. To belong to a group is of vital importance. Each individual child must abide by the rules of the group, which may be extremely rigid, and energy is devoted to team success as well as personal success.

Rules and ritual. The need for conformity in middle childhood is strongly manifested in the activities and games so important in the life of school-age children. Up to this point they have either played games they have invented themselves or have played in the company of a friend or an adult when rules more or less evolved with the game. Now they begin to see the need for rules, and the games they play have fixed and unvarying rules that may be bizarre and extraordinarily rigid (especially those made up by the group). But part of the enjoyment of the game is to know the rules, since knowing means belonging. Once the rules are established and agreed on, the demand for conformity is vigorous. A child who does not conform to the rules is excluded because individuality is not tolerated by the group. Clubs and secret societies are an integral part of the culture of childhood (Fig. 17-5).

Conformity and ritual permeate the play of school-age children. Not only do they dominate in games, but they are also evident in much of the children's behavior and language. Childhood is full of chants and taunts such as, "Eeny, meeny, miney, mo," "Johnny's mad and I'm glad," "Last one is a rotten egg," and "Step on a crack, break your mother's back." Children derive a great deal of pleasure from such sayings that have been handed down with few changes through generation after generation of children. Sometimes these sayings are elaborated on with particular variations to meet the special attributes of a particular group. The undeviating ritual frequently is invested with some magical quality that serves to give the children involved a sense of power over the unconquerable world about them.

Team play. A more complex form of group play that evolves from group games is the team game and those sports that form part of the life of the early school years. The rules of such games may even require the presence of a referee, umpire, or person of authority in order that they can be followed more accurately. Team membership has three significant characteristics that promote child development during the middle years (Newman and Newman, 1984).

First, children learn to subordinate personal goals to group goals. Team membership means that each child is accountable to the other team members and carries with it the responsibility that each member's acts may affect the success or failure of the entire group. Each member's behavior is open to public evaluation, and children risk ostracism or ridicule if they contribute to a team loss. Team accomplishments reflect on all the players. Although individual skills are recognized, team successes and failures are shared by all members—the best and the poorest alike. In this way chil-

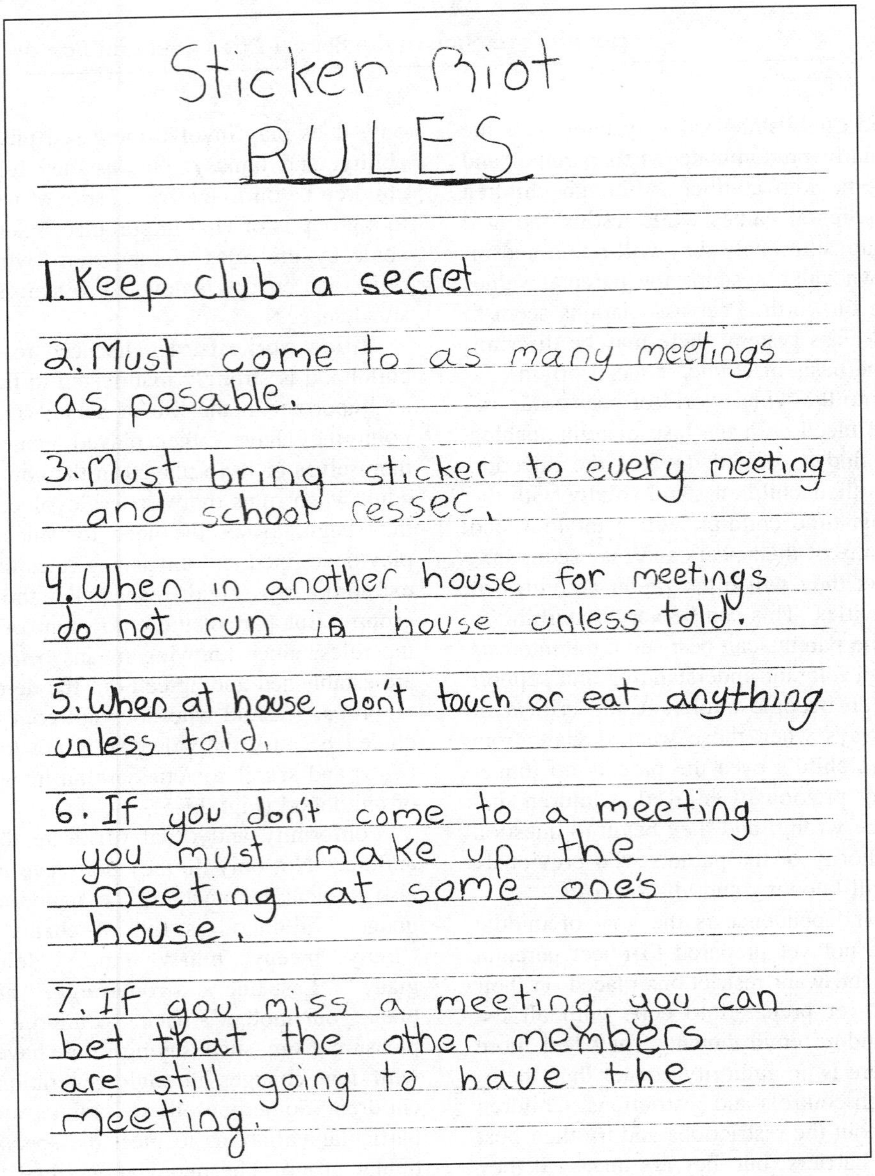

Sticker Riot
RULES

1. Keep club a secret

2. Must come to as many meetings as posable.

3. Must bring sticker to every meeting and school ressec.

4. When in another house for meetings do not run in house unless told.

5. When at house don't touch or eat anything unless told.

6. If you don't come to a meeting you must make up the meeting at some one's house.

7. If you miss a meeting you can bet that the other members are still going to have the meeting.

Fig. 17-5. A list of club rules compiled by a group of nine-year-old children.

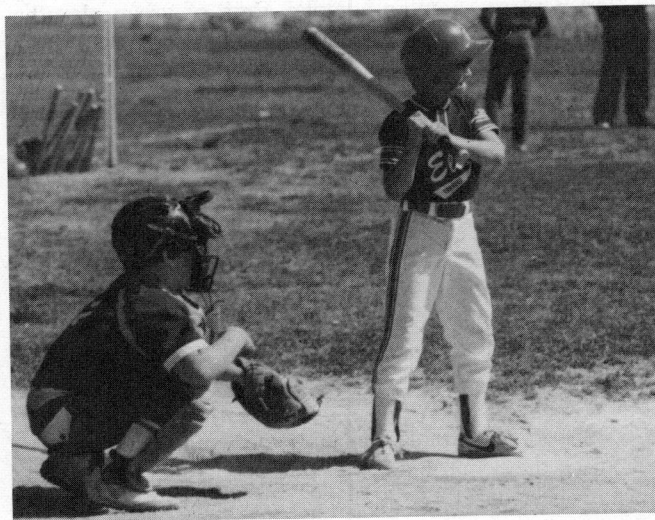

Fig. 17-6. Activities engaged in by school-age children, such as Little League baseball, vary according to the child's interest and opportunity.

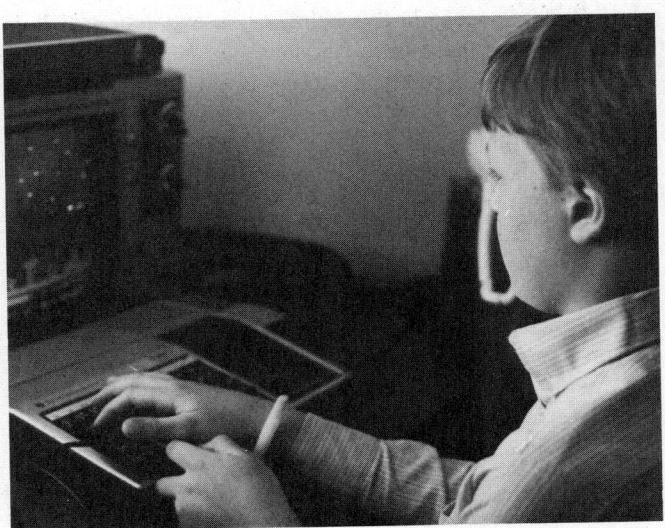

Fig. 17-7. A home computer provides educational and recreational activity.
Photography by Earl Fillmore, Salt Lake City, UT.

dren learn the concept of interdependence, that all players must rely on one another. Unfortunately instead of the better members helping the weaker members to improve, all too often the poorer members are scorned and scapegoated, especially when the team loses.

Second, children learn about division of labor as an effective strategy for the attainment of a goal. They learn that each position on a team has a specific function and that the team has a greater chance of winning if each person performs a specific function instead of the work of all the other members. Once children learn this concept in team play, they can transfer the knowledge to other aspects of life. Once they learn that certain goals are best accomplished by dividing tasks among several individuals, they begin to see a relationship to principles of organization in other social structures. A corollary to this is the concept that some children are best equipped to perform one part of the task, whereas other children are best suited to another aspect of the task.

Third, team play helps children to learn about the nature of competition and the importance of winning—an attribute highly valued in the United States. In all team play there is a winning and losing side. Since losing is often interpreted as failure, children will go to great lengths to avoid the public embarassment and personal shame that accompany failure. The more a child identifies with the team and values the membership in the group, the more distasteful losing becomes. Fear of losing and the failure it implies are strong incentives for group commitment. The importance of winning is not universally valued however. Some cultures and subcultures place emphasis on the game and consideration for one's companions rather than on the outcome.

Team play can also contribute to children's social, intellectual, and skill growth. Children will work hard to develop the skills needed to become members of a team, to improve their contribution to the group effort, and to anticipate the consequences of their behavior for the group. Team play helps stimulate cognitive growth as children are called on to learn many complex rules, make judgments about those rules, plan strategies, and assess the strengths and weaknesses of members of their own team and the opposing team (Fig. 17-6).

Quiet games and activities. Although the play of school-age children is highly active, they also enjoy many quiet and solitary activities (Fig. 17-7). The middle childhood years are the time for collections, which constitute another ritual. Young school-age children's collections are an odd assortment of unrelated objects in messy, disorganized piles. Collections of later years are more orderly and selective, and they are organized neatly in scrapbooks, on shelves, or in boxes.

School-age children become fascinated with increasingly complex board or card games, such as Monopoly and rummy, that they can play with a best friend or a group. As in all games, their adherence to rules is fanatic. There is usually much discussion and argument, but the disagree-

ment is easily resolved through reading the appropriate rule of the game.

The newly acquired skill of reading becomes increasingly satisfying as school-age children begin to expand their knowledge of the world through books. School-age children never tire of stories and, just as preschool children, they love to have stories read aloud. Sewing, cooking, carpentry, gardening, and creative endeavors such as painting are other activities children enjoy. Many of these creative skills, as well as athletic skills such as swimming, riding, hiking, dancing, and skating that are acquired and delighted in during childhood continue to be enjoyed into adolescence and adulthood.

Hero worship is another characteristic of children and adolescents. The object of the adoration can be any of a variety of persons, such as a friend, relative, teacher, or national sports or entertainment figure (Fig. 17-8). The difficulty arises when the idol provides an inappropriate role model.

Ego mastery. Play also affords children the means to acquire representational mastery over themselves, their environment, and other persons. Through play children can feel as big, as powerful, and as skillful as their imaginations will allow, and they can attain vicarious mastery and power over whomever and whatever they choose. They need to feel in control in their play. School children still need the opportunity to use large muscles in exuberant outdoor play and the freedom to exert their newfound autonomy and initiative. They need space in which to exercise large muscles and to work off tensions, frustrations, and hostility. Physical skills practiced and mastered in play help them develop a feeling of personal competence, which contributes to a sense of accomplishment and helps provide a place of status in the peer group.

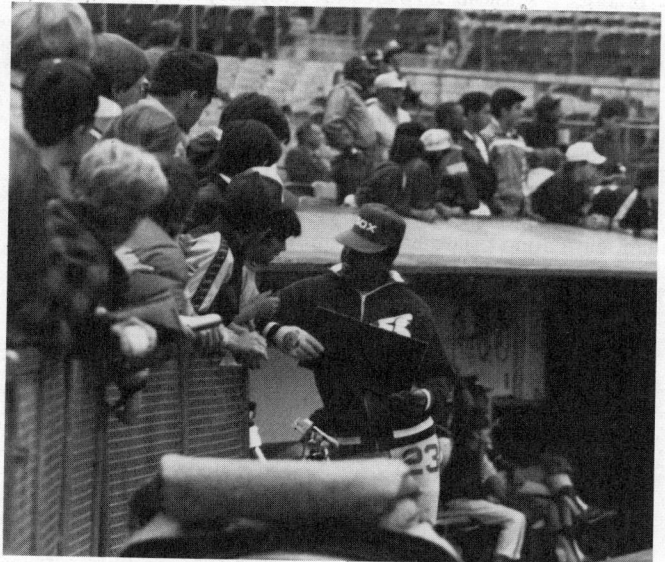

Fig. 17-8. Hero worship is a characteristic of middle childhood.

TEMPERAMENT

The enduring reactivity patterns or temperamental traits identified in infancy continue to be important in middle childhood as determinants of some aspects of behavior. Analyzing behavioral patterns observed in past situations can provide clues to the way that a child may react to new situations, although long-range projections are not always successful. Through interaction with environment, experiences, motives, and abilities, many children change. Major temperamental characteristics persist into adolescence in many children; in others they do not.

Parents and teachers are persons who are in the best position to assess a child's behavioral style and try to make their demands and expectations consonant with the individual child's temperamental characteristics. With easy children this rarely poses a problem. They adapt readily to almost any child-rearing program and new situation. School entry or other experiences are usually smooth and accomplished with minimum stress. Problems arise with difficult, slow-to-warm-up children, and children who are easily distracted.

Slow-to-warm-up children who usually exhibit discomfort when introduced to new situations need time to become accustomed to a new environment, authority figures, and expectations. These children may respond with tears, somatic complaints, or other maneuvers to avoid the event. They should be encouraged to try new experiences but also should be allowed to adapt to their surroundings at their own speed. Pressure to move quickly into new situations only strengthens the tendency to withdraw. Even after-school activities can be cause for reaction, but attending with a friend or contracting for permission to withdraw after a trial of a specified number of times may provide them with sufficient incentive to try.

Difficult or easily distracted children may benefit from "practice" sessions in which they are prepared for the event by role-playing, visiting the site, stories, or other methods of getting them acquainted with what to expect. Children who are very persistent need to know when they are expected to stop what they are doing so that the signal to stop will not come as a surprise, thus triggering a reaction. Children with difficult temperaments need to be handled with exceptional patience, firmness, and understanding so they can learn appropriate behavior in their interactions with others. It is important for teachers to be matched to the temperament of children whenever possible to ensure a "good fit." Although teachers should be sensitive and understanding of children with all temperaments, there are some who are better able to cope with difficult children.

SUMMARY OF GROWTH AND DEVELOPMENT IN MIDDLE CHILDHOOD

The preceding stages of child development increasingly demonstrate individuality in the patterns of development. As children grow and mature, these differences become more pronounced. Although the rate generally slows, develop-ment continues to be uneven, with periods of acceleration in some areas followed by a leveling-off period. At the same time other areas progress normally. In addition, each child has a unique developmental pattern; therefore, any attempt to describe the typical child of any age-group can only represent an average and should not be considered as absolute criteria for any given child (Table 17-1, p. 718).

COPING WITH CONCERNS RELATED TO NORMAL GROWTH AND DEVELOPMENT

Middle childhood is not a period of latent development. It is a period of searching, goal-directed exploration, and increasingly complex decision-making. It is a time of preparation, trying new experiences, testing abilities, and refining performance. When difficult problems arise most school-age children have developed sufficient coping skills to be ready to confront them and to persevere until they are solved.

School Experience

The school serves as the agent for transmitting the values of the society to each succeeding generation of children and as the setting for much of their relationship with peers. As a socializing agent second only to the family, the school exerts a profound influence on the social development of children. Until school entrance at approximately 5 or 6 years, the primary sphere of influence over children is the family, in which their major interactions are with parents and siblings. Neighborhood children, daycare, and nursery school provide broader relationships, but parents serve as the only continuous adult contact for most children—those with whom they are most intimately involved and who set the pattern of their daily lifes. School entrance marks a sharp change in the children's experiences. Their world at once becomes more complex, requiring adjustments to a new set of expectations.

School entrance constitutes a sharp break in the structure of a child's world. For some children it is their first experience in conforming to a group pattern imposed by an adult who is not a parent and who has responsibility for too many children to be constantly aware of each child as an individual (Fig. 17-9). Children want to go to school and usually adapt to the new condition with little difficulty. Successful adjustment is directly related to the child's physical and emotional maturity and the parent's readiness to accept the separation associated with school entrance. Unfortunately some parent's express their unconscious attempts to delay their child's maturity by clinging behavior, particularly with their youngest child.

Anticipatory socialization. By the time they enter school, the majority of children have a fairly realistic concept of what school involves. They receive information regarding the role of pupil from parents, playmates, and the communication media. In addition, most children have had some experience with kindergarten and with nursery school as well.

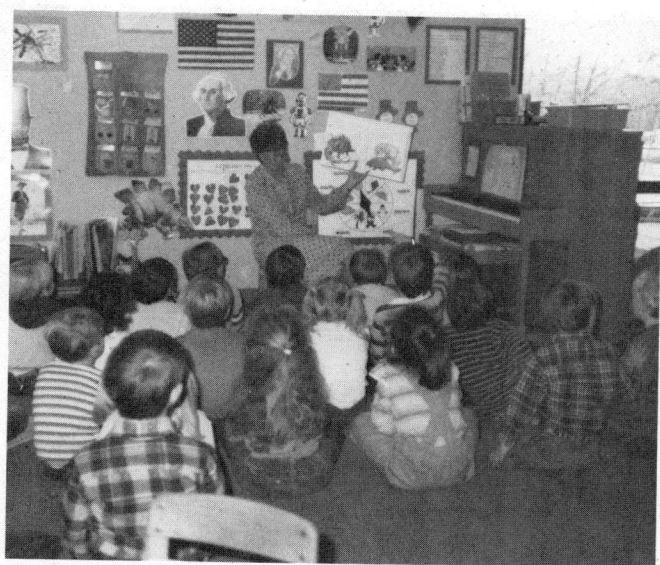

Fig. 17-9. School represents an important change in a child's life, and teachers exert a significant influence on the child.

Children's attitudes toward school and the extent of their adjustment is strongly influenced by the attitudes of their parents. Middle-class children have fewer adjustments to make and less to learn about expected behavior since the school tends to reflect dominant middle-class customs and values. Parents who view school as a place that they have helped to create and support and that is directed toward the same objectives for socialization as their own usually prepare their children with useful anticipatory socialization and furnish them with confidence to meet the challenge. Parents who view the school as an agency of an alien culture and one that they have little, if any, power to affect may unknowingly teach their children to be fearful of school, even though they agree with its purposes and objectives.

Anticipatory socialization is also provided by television, whose power cannot be overestimated in the acquisition of information and attitudes. Whether programming has socialization as the primary objective (such as the children's program, "Sesame Street") or general entertainment (including commercials), most observers believe that television viewing increases a child's vocabulary, extends the child's horizons, and helps pave the way for the school experience. This is particularly true among children in poorer families.

Although most children have had some experience with schooling before they enter first grade, the extent to which early childhood education prepares children for primary school varies. Some preschool programs merely provide custodial care; others emphasize emotional, social, and intellectual development as well. Early childhood programming that stresses a cognitive over a social emphasis appears to be more effective in facilitating later academic performance, particularly in children from low-income families.

Role of the teacher. The transition from home to school is usually accomplished with little disturbance. To facilitate the process, educators select teachers with personality characteristics that allow them to deal with potential problems of young children. Children react to the teacher on the basis of past experience; therefore they respond best to teachers with attributes that they would desire in a warm, loving parent. As a parent surrogate the teacher in the early grades performs many of the activities formerly assumed by the parents (usually the mother), such as recognizing the children's personal needs (such as a need to go to the bathroom or for help with clothing) and helping to develop their social behavior (such as manners).

Teachers, like parents, are concerned about the psychologic and emotional welfare of children. Although the functions of teachers and parents differ, both place constraints on behavior and both are in a position to enforce standards of conduct. However, the teacher's primary responsibility is stimulating and guiding children's intellectual development but not their physical welfare beyond the school setting. The teacher shares the parental influence in shaping a child's attitudes and values. Teachers serve as models with whom children can identify and whom they try to emulate. Teacher approval is sought; teacher disapproval is avoided. The teacher is a very significant person in the life of a child during the early school years, and hero worship of a teacher may extend into late childhood and preadolescence. It is not uncommon for the first or second grader to be heartbroken and tearful at leaving a familiar teacher at the end of the school term or to be upset when faced with a substitute teacher for even a short period.

Children's interest in school and learning and much of their social interaction and self-concept are related to interactions with the teacher. The differential systems of reward and punishment administered by the teachers affect the emotional adjustment and self-concept of children as well as how they respond to school in general. The interaction between the teacher and individual pupils affects the pupil's acceptance by other children, which in turn affects the child's self-concept. Behaviors praised by the teacher usually acquire a positive value, whereas those viewed negatively by the teacher are similarly devalued by the children. In this way the teacher exerts considerable influence in a number of areas, such as attitudes toward minority groups, the disabled, or less favorably endowed children. Teacher approval of and self-acceptance in children are very closely related.

The teacher sets the emotional tone of the classroom. Teachers who are able to establish a positive social climate are usually concerned about the mental health and social dynamics of the children. Feeling a responsibility for personality development in their pupils, they are alert and sensitive to a child's anxieties, peer-group relationships, self-concepts, and general attitudes toward school. Learner-centered behaviors, such as supportive statements that reassure or commend children, accepting and clarifying statements that help them refine ideas and feelings to provide a sense of being understood, and constructive assistance that assists them with their own problem-solving, all contribute to the expansion and development of a positive self-concept.

Text continued on p. 730.

Table 17-1　Age profiles of school-age children

PROFILE AREA	6 YEARS	7 YEARS	8 YEARS
General characteristics	Is full of surprises Is egocentric; center of his world Wants to be best or first Is eager to begin a project but has difficulty in completing it Has prodigious appetite for new experiences Is easily distracted by environment Is expansive; ready for anything Is eager to try anything new Meets new situations head-on Has rapid mood swings Is quarrelsome, argumentative When all goes well, is delightful; when things go badly, resorts to tears and tantrums Finds that backyard can no longer contain him; needs room Dawdles much of the time	Is less of a problem than at 6 years of age Is more quiet and withdrawn, introspective, pensive Likes to be alone; wants a room of his own At times feels that everyone is against him and picks on him Demands much of himself; needs help to define stopping point May lack confidence to the point of not trying Has intense but short-lived interests Is conscientious; tries to take responsibilities seriously, but is too young to be completely reliable Can be reasoned with Has good days and bad days; high-learning and "forget-everything" days Is generally less happy and satisfied with life than younger children	Is exuberant—ready for anything Has insatiable curiosity Is always in a hurry Is concerned about relationships with others Thinks that nothing is too difficult—in his estimation Begins activities with a burst of energy and enthusiasm that may be followed by failure, discouragement, and tears May need to be protected from trying too much and self-criticism that is too excessive Tends to be dramatic Enjoys taking trips and visiting new places Is usually punctual
Motor behavior	Has boundless energy Is excited by speed and motion Runs, jumps, climbs, hops, skips Is unable to sit still for any length of time; wriggles in chair, sits on the edge, bangs and thumps; may fall off chair Is clumsy and awkward Has much oral activity, that is blowing, extending tongue, various mouthing noises Can use scissors Enjoys fine motor activity but becomes restless after a short time; has imprecise small-muscle coordination—a frequent cause of frustration	Has eye-hand coordination that is still not fully developed Has cautious but not fearful gross motor actions Is more cautious in approaches to new performances Repeats performances to master them Although more quiet, still displays spurts of energy and activity Has usually learned to swim and ride a bicycle	Has increased smoothness and speed in fine motor control Is always on the go; jumps, chases, skips Is fluid, almost graceful, in his movements Is apt to overdo; is often hard to quiet down after recess
Personal care and responsibility	Can dress and undress but may need help with dressing Usually requires, but resists, help with bathing Needs reminding to wash before meals Plays exuberantly in bath tub but needs help to get clean Leaves clothes wherever they are removed	Needs reminding to wash hands before meals Dawdles in bath and self-care activities May dislike baths; can get fairly clean without help Prefers old clothes but accepts whatever is selected for him Still drops clothes on floor or chair	Dresses self completely Is careless, messy, impatient Enjoys selecting own clothes Needs reminding to go to bed Likes to be tucked in Sleeps well

9 YEARS	10 YEARS	11 YEARS	12 YEARS
Is more quiet and inward directed Is independent, self-reliant, capable, and trustworthy Is peer-oriented Has more confidence in contacts with the world Works hard and plays hard Finishes jobs that he starts Makes decisions quickly and easily Is motivated by own interests more than by obligations Is anxious; worries; takes things hard Complains; often copes with an unpleasant situation with a physical complaint Is concerned about his relationship with others Rebels against authority—usually by complaining or passively by withdrawal	Is relatively predictable Is in a comfortable equilibrium; is sincere, happy, relaxed, confident, congenial Has gradual, smooth transition from 9 to 10 years of age Is generally content with self Is oblivious Is in one of the happiest ages Is highly competitive Has mainly superficial feelings	Is filled with conflict, turmoil, and stormy behavior; is paradoxical Is sulky, fidgety, restless, resentful Is gay, kind to friends, eager, pleasant Is relatively independent and tolerant Assumes much responsibility for self Has strengthened superego and greater self-control Is full of energy and activity Is interested in exploration and adventure Is a clown; enjoys slap-stick humor and puns; can get silly over anything Is unpredictable Is interested in money—allowance or earning	Is more companionable, reasonable, tolerant Is less insistent Is even-tempered, happy, good natured Is adjustable Has a charming sense of humor Is self-reliant Is fairly satisfied with self and world Appears to be trying to "grow up" Becomes more calm and relaxed Has enthusiasm as a prime characteristic (boys—enthusiasm for sports; girls—enthusiasm for child care) Likes variety and change
Has fully developed hand-eye coordination that still needs refinement May work hard to perfect a skill Develops good timing and skillful control in motor activities Has apparent individual skills	Develops greater strength and coordination in all motor skills Delights in physical activity—running, skating, sliding, climbing, jumping, cycling Has greater stamina	Has increased motor and mental activity Is less poised Bounces and jerks more; acts more clumsily	Takes part in intense activity; suddenly reaches saturation point and collapses Is capable of more refined motor activities Still enjoys gross motor activity
Often rests in strange, awkward positions Needs no help in bathing or dressing Is unaware of dirty clothes Girls discover an interest in clothes; are more fastidious than boys Needs to be reminded to brush teeth Keeps room and personal effects reasonably tidy	May wear same thing continually Cannot be bothered with personal hygiene; needs constant reminding Has positive antipathy for water and heroically resists bathing but in bath will play for long periods Keeps room in constant disarray Leaves clothes wherever they fall	Is rebellious in relation to parental standards for mealtimes, washing, dressing Has self-awareness in terms of grooming—especially girls Has less resistance to bathing; still has trouble cleaning back of neck and ears Has difficulty in keeping hair clean and combed Is dissatisfied with earliness of bedtime; needs prodding	Continues to be more concerned about personal cleanliness and appearance Bathes frequently; prefers showers May still need help with shampoo Has difficulty with bedtime; is more easily roused in the morning Is concerned about wearing clothes that are in vogue, that fit well, and that match

Continued.

Table 17-1 Age profiles of school-age children—cont'd

PROFILE AREA	6 YEARS	7 YEARS	8 YEARS
Personal care and responsibility—cont'd	Takes responsibility for toileting, but may have to dash; accidents are rare, but disturbing, and are usually related to overexcitement Wants help but refuses to accept it	May need encouragement to go to bed; may still take favorite toy to bed Can brush and comb hair acceptably without help of "going over"	
Social behavior and manners	Experiences rapid expansion of social environment Centers life around school Has unpredictable behaviors—is agreeable, loving, and cooperative one minute; dislikes everything and everybody the next Is unaware of ethnic identity of playmates Is demanding of others; rigid in his demands Must have things his way; he cannot adapt—others are expected to do adapting Does not yet know how to speak or act properly; often forgets to say "Please" or "Thank you" Is ritualistic about food preferences Has frequent "accidents" at mealtime: spilled milk, food on clothes Usually has "eyes that are bigger than his stomach"	Likes to help and have a choice Is less resistant and stubborn; is more polite, responsible, and sensitive than at 6 years of age Enjoys teasing Is very talkative; fights verbally rather than physically Is more cooperative Must be called at least twice for meals Hastens through meals so that he can return to activities Likes to eat in front of television Enjoys family conversation at meals	Is more sociable Is expansive, gregarious Is constantly busy and active Enjoys new experiences, new friends Is better behaved Responds to reward system Runs useful errands Is silly; laughs and giggles Prefers companionship to solitude; hates to do things alone Is alert, friendly, interested in people Is sensitive to criticism Is first to finish a meal Gobbles food down Has social manners that are generally better than at 7 years of age but that still need improvement Verbalizes proper greetings
Relationships with family	Experiences sibling jealousy Enjoys hearing about when he was a baby Has worst relationship so far with mother; loves her one minute and hates her the next, with little provocation Blames mother for all that goes wrong At times is very close with parents	Feels constantly mistreated; may threaten to run away Complains about parents If has vigorous imagination, may believe that he is adopted Desires family approval Admires older sibling Looks after younger sibling, but fights with him a good deal; jealousy still occurs at times	Is easy to get along with at home Wants a close, understanding relationship with mother—sometimes to her puzzlement and concern Is sensitive to parental approval/disapproval Has more to give to others; expects more in return Competes with siblings

9 YEARS	10 YEARS	11 YEARS	12 YEARS
Is frank about food likes and dislikes Still needs to be reminded to go to bed Often gets up early to have time to "mess around" before school	Is not always aware when tired and ready for bed Boys go to bed more easily and rapidly than girls Has poor posture at meals	Has difficulty in getting up in the morning Girls highly interested in clothes and "what to wear" but hang up only best clothes Often has small job after school and during summer Needs reminding and prefers to have a choice in whatever is demanded of him	Rapid growth often necessitates new wardrobes Girls may try to look glamorous; want to wear lipstick for special occasions Enjoys shopping for clothes; choice of clothes better than care of clothes Needs reminding about care of clothes Spends time decorating room, less on keeping it tidy Has less interest in money, but manages money well Is helpful with tasks but often "in a couple of minutes" Is able to assume more complex chores Is motivated by earning money
Is more sociable Is easy to discipline Has strong social feelings; shows empathy and sympathy Begins hero worship and prejudices Has greater refinement in behavior Is aware of appropriate sex roles Understands explanations and tries to do things well Has acceptable manners when guests are present; less so when family is alone Chews with mouth closed when reminded	Experiences sharp outbursts of anger; tends to be brief, explosive, and shallow Cries when angry but does not bear a grudge or nurse hurt feelings Experiences outbursts of happiness and demonstrations of affection Is able to tolerate frustration Has huge appetite Has acceptable manners	Loves conversation Resists imposed tasks and proprieties Strives hard for conformity Has little interest in adults May have increased shyness but hates to be alone Rarely chooses to be alone; elects to be involved in family group or peer group Is often at his best behavior away from home	Is excellent conversational company Boys becoming more interested in attending social gatherings, such as dancing, school parties, and so on Enjoys group activities involving both sexes Has better control of emotions, especially anger Is more capable of give-and-take Is more aware of others' feelings Seldom gets in conflict with others Is diplomatic in his actions Has fairly accurate assessment of others
Resists too much bossing by parents Considers opinions of parents less important than opinions of friends Is less interested in relationships with parents, but enjoys going places with them Rebels against parental oversolicitousness Takes part in family decisions Enjoys running errands, helping when mother is busy or ill	Is fond of home and loyal to it Has closer attachment to family than at 9 years of age Has better mother-child relationship Respects parents and their role Gets along well with father and enjoys his companionship Readily participates in family activities Gets along least well with siblings ages 6 to 9 years of age	Is constantly present in family circle Can be a pleasant companion Enjoys family group activities Has worst relationship with siblings Is rebellious with parents Argues about everything; is aware of parents' fallibilities and does not hesitate to point them out	Is less demonstrative about affection than at 11 years of age Gets along better with parents and argues less; demands less from them Recognizes changes of behavior with fatigue Has less fighting with siblings near his age; young siblings may bother him, but he relates well with preschoolers

Continued.

Table 17-1 Age profiles of school-age children—cont'd

PROFILE AREA	6 YEARS	7 YEARS	8 YEARS
Relationships with family— cont'd		Gets along better with mother Is developing closer relationship with father	Is very strict when tending younger siblings Shows preference for mother, but father gets increased share of affection
Relationships with peers	Rarely appears in public singly; when 6-year-old children appear, they soon move together No longer waits for others to come to him but goes where he can find the company of others Is found in groups that are loosely organized and flexible; there is much coming and going Each child within group goes his own way; there is little visible cooperation Is anxious to be with peers; fears he will lose his place in group if not there physically Has simple group rules, for example, must not cry when hurt; must act, look, and talk like the others	Seeks approval of peers Sex discrimination appearing in play groups Begins to have boyfriends and girlfriends Becomes more concerned about his place in the group and being liked May develop "love affairs" Is in a "for-or-against" age; an age of cliques and outsiders	Has usually completed transition to peer culture Shows preference in friends and groups; ready for and wants a two-way relationship Values best friends Plays mostly with groups of own sex Is interested in boy-girl relationship, but will not admit overtly Begins to be interested in clubs and gangs, especially secret clubs Gives allegiance to peers rather than to adults in case of conflict Argues, plans, makes deals Gains security through group membership
Health	Is more susceptible to diseases Communicable diseases increased on school entry Has frequent sore throats, colds, often with complications Has somatic complaints related to going to school Has hypersensitivity of face and neck to washing Is more apt to break arm if falls	Has fewer illnesses than at 6 years of age Is subject to communicable diseases, which are still prevalent Is subject to frequent colds Complains of headache with fatigue or excitement; muscular pain Tends to have minor accidents to eyes Becomes fatigued often	Has improving health Has fewer illnesses; shorter duration Has increase in allergies Has frequent accidents— falls, automobile accidents, bicycle accidents Is more apt to break leg if falls

9 YEARS	10 YEARS	11 YEARS	12 YEARS
Willingly responds to parental demands—if he hears them Has better relationship with siblings	Is nurturing to younger (preschool) children and animals	Usually gets along better with one parent than with the other Boys embarrassed if mothers kiss them in front of friends Wishes to become somewhat financially independent from parents Family tensions may develop over parents' "nagging" to eat better, stand up straight, and so on Is critical and resistant to mother; is more tolerant of father	Responds especially well to sympathetic older sibling Expects parents to respect need for privacy Still wants limits set on his behavior
Is loyal to friends Values "special" friends Still determines friendship on basis of sex Enjoys chatting with groups of friends Boys chase girls	Is fond of his friends; extols their virtues to family Is apt to be cliquey Clubs (for example, Cub Scouts) have great appeal Is serious about organized group life; avidly forms clubs, which are often short-lived Joins informal, temporary groups as well as established gangs and organized groups Girls prefer small, more intimate groups Most girls have a "best friend" for an extended period Still separate by choice into like-sex groups for group games and activities Experiences hero worship Wants to measure up to a challenge as defined by peer group Can subordinate own desires for good of the group	Is more intense, emotional, and complicated Chooses friends more selectively Values membership in clubs and community activities Boys often in friendship groups of three to five with whom they shift; girls more apt to have single "best friend" "Detests" opposite sex, but girls enjoy being teased by boys Is often jealous of peers Demonstrates friendship—girls put arms around each other; boys punch each other Boys may get into fist fights Likes to stay overnight with a friend May be strongly influenced by best friend	Has easy relationship with peers May rotate among several friends; rarely at a loss for friends Prefers small groups May join larger groups for athletic activities Most large, spontaneous clubs begin to break up Girls are more prone to segregate into twosomes Has interest in the opposite sex For many, is an age of considerable boy-girl interest and activity during school Shifts interest from one friend to another Girls enjoy talking about boys
Has improved health, few illnesses Has minor complaints—usually related to a task, for example, eyes burn when studying, hands hurt when practicing piano, stomach hurts when doing dishes	Has, on the whole, good to excellent health Has lessening somatic complaints Has big appetite; has more food likes than dislikes	Has generally good health but has frequent colds Is hypochondriacal; has many somatic complaints such as feet hurt, has a headache, is tired Has good appetite Understands rationale behind health and hygiene practices, such as covering mouth and nose when coughing or sneezing	May suffer extreme fatigue, especially after intense activity May require a day or two of rest Has good health but less consistent May still have sudden, unexpected, sharp but short-lived pains, frequently in head or abdomen Is concerned about vision

Continued.

Table 17-1 Age profiles of school-age children—cont'd

PROFILE AREA	6 YEARS	7 YEARS	8 YEARS
Play activities	Likes rough-and-tumble play Values wind, speed, and coordination Loves active games Insists on a bicycle Is not ready for competitive sports, especially those that demand coordination; must learn to work with others before he can work against them; best suited are those with simple rules, for example, relay races Likes group games (for example, London Bridge, tag, hide and seek) that do not demand special skills Delights in tricks and stunts Likes table games, for example, checkers, simple card games Paints, colors, draws Uses clay Collects odds and ends Enjoys stories, including at bedtime	Is more careful with toys Occupies himself alone for long periods Likes to play alone, but prefers group play Has more intense interest in some activities, fewer new ventures Has "mania" for certain activities Enjoys magic tricks, collecting in quantity, puzzles, "swapping"	Has variety of interests; prefers companionship in play Likes to compete and play games Enjoys books, comics, television, movies; may retire early in order to read Requires supervision in play—unsupervised play frequently ends in brawl Has collections that reflect quality as well as quantity Likes making things Enjoys quiet play Loves prizes in cereal boxes, Cracker Jack Likes to put on dramatic shows Begins to be interested in group games
Fears	Is very fearful Fears loud noises—doorbell; telephone; ugly voice tones; animal, bird, or insect noises; static Fears supernatural, that is, witches, ghosts, goblins Fears large animals Fears imagined unseen persons, that is, under bed, inside closet, in cellar Fears elements—fire, thunder, lightning, water Fears being lost Fears being hurt, that is, that others will hit him Fears that mother will not be home when he arrives; that something may happen to her; that she may die	Has many fears Fears visual things, such as the dark, attics, cellars; interprets shadows as ghosts, witches Fears imaginary things, such as war, burglars, spies, persons hiding under the bed or in closets Is stimulated by mass media Worries about self—that things will be too difficult; that second grade will be too hard; that people may not like him; that something may happen to him; that he will be late for school Fears trying something new on his own	Has fewer fears Worries less Is able to evaluate fears; has reasonable fears, for example, personal failings Has less fear of the dark

9 YEARS	10 YEARS	11 YEARS	12 YEARS
Develops "crazes" for certain activities	Enjoys just "fooling around" with neighborhood children	Considers play not as important as formerly	Enjoys collections; new dimension—mementos such as ticket stubs, clippings, photographs
Has variety of play interests	Loves large-muscle activity and gross motor games out-of-doors	Considers people more important than play	Needs bulletin board for display
Works hard at play	Enjoys collections	Is active; team games are very popular	Enjoys parties, but requires supervision, otherwise may get out of hand
Enjoys more complicated table games	Enjoys reading	Has impulse to be out-of-doors	Likes games involving close, accidental contact with opposite sex
Takes part in organized play—group rewards are powerful incentives	Especially enjoys bicycle riding	Although clumsy in the home, is agile in sports	Likes group activities but can enjoy solitude
Loves stunts of all sorts	Likes noise and makes a great deal of it	Enjoys taking walks	Is seldom bored
Continues collections, some of which develop into organized hobbies		Still maintains collections, especially for purpose of trading	Has wide range of interests
Loves making things		Enjoys comic books	Segregates into athletic and nonathletic groups
Participates in outdoor sports of the large-muscle, rough-and-tumble variety		Loves to construct a tree house, including the problems of construction, membership, and so on	Likes athletic sports in season
Enjoys sports such as baseball, skating, and swimming		Is less interested in television; leans toward teen-age interest in popular music; has more interest in movies	Likes swimming; girls like horseback riding
Individual differences in play become more apparent		Enjoys humor, puns, corny jokes	Enjoys some sort of organization in activities
Delights in legends; this is the age of stories			Reads less
Girls enjoy dancing school; boys have little interest in dancing			
Loves to read			
Spends much time in solitary activities			
Has high interest in competitive sports			
Has fewer fears; has reasonable fears	Has many fears, but fewer than in preadolescence to come	Is in one of the most worried and fearful ages	Is less fearful than at 11 years of age
Worries less	Fears animals, especially snakes and wild animals, high places, fires, criminals, the dark, blood, ghosts	Is mainly afraid to be alone	Is still uncomfortable in the dark; hears creaky noises at night; fears an intruder
Has fears that relate to personal ineptitudes	Has fewer worries than fears	Worries about school, money, parents' welfare, his own health	
Fears failure in school	Worries about school—homework, grades, being late	Afraid of physical pain, infection, and that something might happen to his mother	
Has scary dreams, but quiets easily		Is afraid that no one— especially girls—likes him	
		Fears strange animals	

Continued.

Table 17-1   Age profiles of school-age children—cont'd

PROFILE AREA	6 YEARS	7 YEARS	8 YEARS
Tension-stress behaviors	Bites nails Bites lower lip Taps foot May return to temper tantrums Stutters If history of thumb-sucking, may increase	Has very few tension outlets Fidgets Wriggles loose teeth Blinks Scowls Decreases old tension-reducing habits; attempts to control, those that remain	Cries with fatigue May return to earlier patterns such as blinking or rubbing eyes or biting nails Picks at fingers
Mental activity and school	Is in first grade Knows right from left and morning from afternoon Can describe objects in a picture; defines objects in terms of their use Has not firmly established concept of "cause and effect" Can see differences more easily than similarities Has difficulty in making decisions Memory: can repeat sentences of ten or twelve words; repeats four digits in order Knows number combinations up to 10 Is easily distracted at school Loves "show and tell" Recognizes simple words and phrases and "sounds out" words to pronounce them Draws a man, including neck, hands, and clothes Has somewhat clumsy pencil manipulation Prints capital letters, some of which may be uneven or reversed Uses every form of sentence structure Is ready to learn to read May find lengthy school sessions too fatiguing, half-day may be best	Is in second grade Is more aware of consequences and cause and effect Begins to be able to put himself in another's place; moved by sad stories Can tell time and make small purchases Can name day, month, and season Has speech that is no longer egocentric but sociocentric (other-centered) Begins to use elementary logic Can count by multiple of 2, 5, and 10 Grasps basic idea of addition and subtraction Enjoys school and learning with others Fears being late for school Is more dependent on teacher as a person Has strong emotional responses to teacher; may believe that teacher is unfair Notices that certain parts are missing from pictures Can copy a diamond shape	Is in third grade Shows interest in causal relationships Develops through experience Has increasing memory span Has increased vocabulary; can give more precise definitions Finds school a source of social activity Likes school; does not like to miss any Is afraid of failing a grade; is ashamed of bad grades Often finds need to communicate with his neighbor a source of difficulty Talks about school more than previously Evaluates his work in relation to others

9 YEARS	10 YEARS	11 YEARS	12 YEARS
Stamps feet Fiddles Picks at self Drops and breaks things Taps pencil Grumbles and mutters Feels dizzy; has other somatic complaints Draws in lips	May increase finger-to-mouth activity May increase fidgeting and other motor activity at middle of tenth year; more common in girls	Often expresses frustrations by withdrawal May snuggle up to mother in private Uses tension outlets that involve increased motor activity, such as blinking, snuffing, and grimaces Displays sudden, uncontrolled outbursts of anger, frequently ending in tears; expresses anger in yelling, sometimes hitting May revert to falling down or dropping and breaking things	Has nervous mannerisms that may appear when tired
Is in fourth grade Understands explanations and tries to do things well Has somewhat longer attention span than at 8 years of age Is intellectually more stimulating As a group, girls are superior to boys Good grades are standard achievement, excellent grades less so Exceptionally bright children may become outcasts Is ashamed of failure; competes for pride Is more concerned with subjects than with teacher Is interested in schoolwork	Is in the fifth grade Manages time fairly well Enjoys learning Begins to handle simple fractions and numbers better Begins to think of social problems in terms of cause and effect; still has problem combining facts and seeing relationships May have difficulty in combining time and space to arrive at a place at a specified time Has short interest span Loves to memorize Likes school Likes to talk and listen rather than work, but may like to be motivated to work difficult problems Is more aware of teacher's appearance and manner Needs schedules—is unable to plan Has difficulty in connecting facts	Is in sixth grade Can define increasingly abstract terms, such as "justice" Is still excited about learning Often has trouble over homework Is interested in the "why" and "how" of things Begins to understand workings of simple machines Is more critical in evaluating own work Likes a teacher who provides a challenge Takes part in a great deal of note passing Will enjoy reading more if it was enjoyed before Attends school primarily for peer association Loves competition, especially, boys against girls Works for good grades, pleased when doing well Begins to think realistically about career and/or marriage	Is in seventh grade Has wide variety of interests in schoolwork but prefers sports Eagerly absorbs information and accumulates ideas Asks many questions Is interested in scientific matters and social studies Seeks reality in social and physical relationships Collects facts; enjoys hearing about faraway places and distant times Has less interest in and time for books Tends to like teacher; wants one who knows and who demands decorum Is concerned with schoolwork and being well liked Competes less intensely; prefers to be even with friends Boys excel at number manipulation; girls excel at language, rote memory, and writing skills Likes to be involved in dramatics Is open and uninhibited in the classroom

Continued.

Table 17-1 Age profiles of school-age children—cont'd

PROFILE AREA	6 YEARS	7 YEARS	8 YEARS
Ethical sense and morality	Is unable to put rules of the game above need to win; therefore may break rules—even those he made himself Is too uncertain of himself to lose gracefully Tattles on others who cheat	Has good intentions, but may become distracted Lies less—still concerned about other's wrongdoing Makes alibis Has more abstract and generalized concept of good or bad; outside influences are seen as "luck" or "fairness" Is becoming conscious of right or wrong in self and others	Prefers to work for immediate reward (preferably cash) Will carry out a request if it is insisted on Considers money of utmost importance Has more advanced concept of goodness and badness Is essentially truthful
Sexuality	Has increased interest in opposite sex Has strong interest in origin of babies; will accept idea that baby grows from seed inside mother's stomach; vague idea that babies follow marriage Is interested to know how baby gets out and if it hurts Giggles at sound of urine stream; name calling involves words dealing with elimination Has marked interest in and awareness of sex differences Mutual investigation by both sexes Takes part in mild sex play or exhibitionism Plays hospital	Wants a new baby in family Knows that having babies can be repeated Knows that older women do not have babies Is interested in pregnancies Is satisfied to know that babies come from two seeds Has less interest in sex Takes part in some exploration, experimentation, and sex play, but less than at 6 years of age Tends to be modest in front of opposite sex	Understands growth of baby inside mother Wants more exact information Asks very searching questions Has rather high interest in sex Girls more curious than boys regarding conception, pregnancy, birth, and menstruation Decreases exploration and sex play Has interest in smutty jokes, peeping

9 YEARS	10 YEARS	11 YEARS	12 YEARS
Evaluates self and family	Is concrete in matters of conscience	Can extract the meaning or moral from stories	Is level-headed
Recognizes his own weaknesses; often makes self-effacing remarks	Is seriously opposed to cheating; wants stern codes against dishonesty	Is keenly aware of how people treat one another	Makes decisions based on considered thinking, past experience, and analysis of consequences—less on feeling
Can accept blame for his actions	May defer to parent in solving ethical problems	Is concerned about fairness	
Is more willing to interrupt own activity in response to a request or demand from an adult—if he hears them	Has a conscience that is still relatively immature	Knows what is right but does not always do what is right	
Is less interested in money; works for service	Is more preoccupied with wrong than right	May not always tell the truth or accept blame; is more concerned about self-protection than truthfulness	
Is honest, fair; feels guilty when "bad"	Believes in justice and fair play	May cheat or steal	
		Is too often influenced by feelings rather than established dogma	
		Has fairly good controls through conscience	

Is sexually modest	Expresses disinterest or disrelish of opposite sex, but not too vehemently	Begins to comprehend prenatal growth	Is aware that intercourse occurs apart from conception
Has increased awareness of sexuality	Most know about sexual intercourse	Is interested to know how "seed is planted from father to mother," but has difficulty in comprehending	Views sex as less "dirty"
Majority know about menstruation	Is interested in smutty jokes	Is apt to consider intercourse as "nasty"	**Girls**
Has mild interest in father's part in reproduction	May begin to see discrepant growth between sexes	Boys are interested in smutty jokes and in observing animal copulation	Are less self-conscious about development; may even flaunt their developing form
May discuss sex information with friends	Girls begin to show unmistakable signs of approaching adolescence during the tenth year—slight projection of nipples, rounding of contours	Few boys are willing to discuss sex matters with parents	Are usually more cognizant of sex matters in general than boys
Is interested in details of own organs and functions	No sexual maturation apparent in boys	Frequent erections occur in many boys	Are fairly comfortable in discussing sex with mother
Begins sex swearing; sex poems	Girls more aware of sex than boys, although less outspoken	Boys are becoming more aware of girls as girls	Few show any of the premenstrual behavior changes associated with later years
Some 9-year-old girls begin pubertal changes		Girls have absorbed interest in their own body changes, which may be a source of pride or of embarrassment	**Boys**
Boys hesitant to ask questions of parents		Girls are interested in imminent onset of menstruation	Become more interested in sex than previously; may seek information from magazines, books, and dictionaries
			Are usually less interested in sex activity of grown-ups; are more absorbed with own sex interest
			Have frequent bull sessions about sex
			Have erections frequently
			Masturbation common

WAYS IN WHICH PARENTS CAN HELP CHILDREN IN SCHOOL

General guidelines
Be supportive—through companionship share ideas and thoughts

Be positive—every child should experience some success each day

Share an interest in reading—use the library, discuss books they are reading

Support and encourage activity rather than passivity

Encourage originality—help children make their own projects from discarded articles or other available materials

Foster the development of hobbies and collections

Encourage children to wonder and reflect during free time

Encourage family experiences and trips to places of interest

Encourage questions—help children discover sources for information or places in which to explore and investigate

Stimulate creative thinking and problem-solving—help children try out new solutions to problems without fear of making mistakes

Use rewards rather than punishment

Specific guidelines
Meet the teacher at the beginning of school and plan to visit the school to see what is taught and expected

Send the child to school every day—teachers are concerned when parents make other plans for their children; it conveys the impression that school is unimportant

Demonstrate an interest in what the child is learning

Demonstrate an interest in content and growth more than in grades

Set goals that the child can achieve

Take advantage of situations that support and reinforce school learning

Share information with teachers that will help them understand the child better

Communicate with the teacher if there appears to be a problem—avoid waiting for a scheduled conference

Provide a quiet, well-lighted area for study that is safe from interruption; do not allow television, radio

Enforce regular study time—some children can do their work at a single session; others do best in 20- to 30-minute sessions with breaks between study times

Support the child in home study; offer guidance for finding the answers but do not give the answers; before providing explanations, determine what the child understands about the problem, read the material aloud, and discuss it briefly with the child

Teach the child to break large tasks (such as a report) into smaller manageable tasks spread over the allotted time rather than attempt the entire project the night before it is to be completed.

Role of the parents. Parents share responsibility with the schools for helping children achieve their maximum potential. There are numerous ways in which parents can supplement the school program. Some general and specific suggestions are outlined in the box above.

Limit-Setting and Discipline

Numerous factors influence the amount and manner of discipline and limit-setting imposed on school-age children: the psychosocial maturity of the parents, childhood childrearing experiences of the parents, temperament of the children, context of the children's misconduct, and response of the children to rewards and punishments. The purpose of discipline is (1) to help the child interrupt or inhibit a forbidden action, (2) to point out a more acceptable form of behavior so that the child knows what is right in a future situation, (3) to provide some reason, understandable to the child, that explains why one action is inappropriate and another action is more desirable, and (4) to stimulate the child's ability to empathize with the victim of a misdeed (Newman and Newman, 1984).

As children are increasingly able to see a situation from the point of view of another, they are able to understand the effects of their reactions on others and themselves. Disciplinary techniques should help children control their own behavior. Reasoning is an effective technique for this age-group. With advancing cognitive skills they are able to benefit from more complex types of disciplinary strategies. For example, withholding privileges, requiring recompense, imposing penalties, and contracting can be used with great success. Problem-solving is the best approach to limit-setting, and children themselves can be included in the process of determining appropriate disciplinary measures.

Dishonest Behavior

During middle childhood it is not uncommon for children to engage in what is considered to be antisocial behavior. Lying, stealing, and cheating may become manifest in previously well-behaved children. It is especially disturbing to parents who may have difficulty coping with this behavior.

Lying. Preschool children often have difficulty distinguishing between fact and fantasy. They do not as yet have the cognitive capacity to deliberately mislead. Sometimes they misperceive or fail to remember an event. By the time they reach school age they still tell stories but can distinguish between what is real and what is make-believe. If not, they need to be taught to distinguish between fantasy and reality. Often children will exaggerate a story or situation as a means to impress their family or friends.

Young children will lie to escape punishment or get out of some difficulty even when the evidence of their misbehavior is before their eyes. Lying is more common in families where punishment is severe. Also, the honesty and veracity modeled by the parents is repeated in the children. If parents lie, the children will emulate their behavior. Older children may lie in order to meet expectations set by others to which they have been unable to measure up. They may lie because of a low self-esteem, as a means for getting ahead or acquiring something with little effort, or for a variety of other reasons. However, most children are very concerned with the wrongness of lying and cheating—especially in their friends. They are quick to tell on others when they detect them in the act of cheating.

Parents need to be reassured that all children lie sometimes and that they often have difficulty separating fantasy from reality. Parents should be helped to understand the importance of their own behavior as role models and being truthful in their relationships with children. The issue can be discussed with the children directly to impress upon them how much of their own security and respect is lost when they are not believed (Schowalter, 1983).

Cheating. Cheating is most common in young children, aged 5 to 6. They find it difficult to lose at a game or contest and cheat in order to win. They have not yet acquired the full realization of the wrongness of this behavior and do it almost automatically. It usually disappears as they mature. However, when children observe parental behaviors, such as boasting about cheating on income taxes or some transaction, they assume this to be appropriate behavior. Parents need to be aware of the types of behaviors they model for their children. When they set examples of honesty, children are more likely to conform to these standards.

Stealing. Like other ethically related behavior, stealing is not an unexpected event in the younger child. Between 5 and 8 years children's sense of property rights is limited and they tend to take something simply because they are attracted to it or to take money for what it will buy. They are equally likely to give away something valuable that belongs to them. When young children are caught and punished they are penitent—"didn't mean to," and promise "never to do it again," but it is quite likely that they will repeat the performance the following day. Often they not only steal but will lie about it as well or attempt to justify the act with excuses. It is seldom helpful to trap children into admission by asking directly if they did the offensive thing. Children do not take on such responsibility until nearer the end of middle childhood.

There are several reasons why children steal: lack of a sense of property rights, trying to acquire the means with which to bribe favors from other children, a strong desire to own the coveted item, or as a means for revenge in order to "get back at someone" (usually a parent) for what they consider to be unfair treatment. Older children may steal to supplement an inadequate income from other sources. Sometimes stealing is an indication that something is seriously wrong or lacking in the child's life. For example, a child may steal to make up for love or another satisfaction that he feels is lacking.

In the lower socioeconomic levels where living arrangements are crowded and children have little privacy and much of the family property is communal, children may fail to develop a sense of property rights. Also, sometimes parents unintentionally confuse children with seemingly conflicting values. In the attempt to teach unselfishness and forcing children to share belongings with others they may fail to develop a true sense of property rights.

If children are told not to take money from their mother's purse or their father's pocket but observe the parents doing the same thing, they receive conflicting messages. Parents may go through a child's pockets or other private areas at night, and even discard, without explanation, items of which they do not approve. Children should have some place that is private to them alone and is respected by other family members. If children's personal rights are respected, they are more likely to respect the rights of others.

It is difficult for many parents to cope with stealing in their children. However, in most situations it is best not to attempt to find a hidden or deep meaning to the stealing. An admonition together with an appropriate and reasonable punishment, such as having the older child pay back the money or return the stolen items, will ordinarily take care of the majority of cases. Most children can be taught to respect the property rights of others with little difficulty despite the temptations and opportunities presented to them. Some children simply need more time to learn the importance of the culture's rules regarding private property.

Coping with Stress

Children of today are under a tremendous amount of stress, and they are pressured from a variety of directions. It is impossible to describe all the stressors to which children are subjected. Some are discussed elsewhere in this book under specific types of stresses, especially those in which nurses assume a major role, such as hospitalization, illness, abuse, crippling injuries, and death or the threat of death.

In the normal course of growing up children are pressured by their peers to identify with their friends; to eat, dress, and look like their friends; to talk about the same things that their friends talk about; to engage in the same activities as their friends and yet to compete with them. They are pressured by parents to excel in school, in athletics, or other activities, and socially at ever younger ages. Children in middle-class America today face more stresses in their effort to live up to greater expectations than have children in previous generations. They are overprogrammed with activities such as ballet lessons, music lessons, athletics, and other activities until the cumulative effect is overwhelming.

Although children receive better treatment than in earlier times when beatings and child labor were commonplace, their physical and emotional well-being is threatened by different stresses. Children are stressed by conflict within the home and are in constant anxiety regarding separation that these disruptions can engender. The divorce rate and the number of single-parent families is higher than ever before, resulting in altered relationships and increasing responsibilities. The stress of the arms race and the impact of the nuclear threat on children is beginning to be investigated; even very young children know about the threat and fear a nuclear disaster (Beardslee and Mack, 1982).

Although beatings at school are no longer permitted, the school environment is often a stressful experience for some children and a threat to their self-image. A recent report (Krugman and Krugman, 1984) describes a number of children who were emotionally abused by an elementary school teacher whose behavior included harassment, labeling ("stupid"), screaming at the children until they cried, inappropriate threats to obtain class control, unrealistic academic goals, fear-inducing techniques, and physical punishments. The students displayed behaviors noticeably different

POTENTIAL SOURCES OF STRESS IN MIDDLE CHILDHOOD

Sources of stress for the six-year-old:

Expectations—parents, teachers, and other adults begin to demand more

School—first grade introduces the child to the more formal, academic setting; it may be the child's first experience away from home all day

Activity level—may find it difficult to sit still for long periods of time; may have frequent accidents, such as spilling milk

Competition—the child wants to be "first" or best

Shyness—may initially be shy in a new situation, but usually recovers quickly

Aggression—may become hostile or aggressive; temper tantrums peak

Sensitivity—begins to read body language or facial expressions and becomes upset when disapproval is sensed

Teasing—engages in teasing, but becomes upset when on the receiving end

Decisions—has difficulty coping with increasing independence

Jealousy—sibling rivalry is common

Fears—usually center around newly found independence and might include fear of getting lost or fear of making an embarrassing social blunder

Sources of stress for the seven-year-old:

Moodiness—is often moody, unhappy, or pensive

Approval—continues to need praise and approval from peer group and parents

Modesty—demands privacy when in the bathroom or dressing

Organization—is comfortable with rules, regulations, routines, and order; becomes upset when they are disrupted

Interruptions—hates to be disturbed when intensely involved in an activity

Idols—has a desire to be more like an admired idol

Friendship—becomes more selective about playmates

Sources of stress for the eight-year-old:

Self-criticism—is very critical of personal ability and performance

Parental authority—is beginning to resent parental authority

Loneliness—likes frequent interaction with friends; may hate to miss school

Praise—continues to seek approval but can identify when praise is not genuine

Independence—may begin to stay alone for brief periods of time while parents run errands, with resulting feelings of uneasiness

Sources of stress for the nine-year-old:

Rebelliousness—occasionally tests independence by rebelling

Opposite sex—engages in sex-segregated play; expresses an aversion to the opposite sex

Fair play—has a keen sense of what is fair and is vehement in demanding personal rights when a situation is perceived as unfair

Interruptions—continues to dislike interruptions but will usually resume an activity after an interruption

Propriety—has a sense of propriety and will often be upset if siblings or parents offend the child's notion of decorum or dignity

Sources of stress for the ten- to twelve-year-olds:

Sexual maturation—girls, in particular, may become self-conscious regarding obvious signs of development

Social issues—a new level of awareness can generate concern regarding pressing societal problems

Size—both boys and girls may be upset by the fact that the girls are taller; the extremely small or extremely large child may be concerned about his or her size

Shyness—if the child already has a problem in this area, it is likely to become more pronounced at this stage

Opposite sex—may become interested, yet shy, around members of the opposite sex

Confusion—too much freedom can cause the child to flounder

Health—it is not uncommon for a child to become a hypochondriac during this period of development

Money—child is anxious to earn and handle money, but often uses poor judgment

Competition—continues to be highly competitive and looks to peer group for prestige

Burnout—child may become vigorously involved in so many activities that he or she finally becomes exhausted

Self-concept—may engage in teasing, scapegoating, or vicious attacks to temporarily boost his or her self-image; guilt often ensues; may be self-conscious about attempting a new skill

Parents—often becomes highly critical or intolerant of parents

Idols—continues hero-worshipping

Fair-play—continues to have a highly developed sense of fair play

Drugs and sex—may be tempted to experiment with drugs or sex because everyone is doing it

Peer pressure—becomes a powerful motivating force

Self-criticism—child may be highly critical of personal performance

From Kuczen, B.: Childhood stress: don't let your child be a victim, New York, 1982, Delacorte Press.

from previous school years, symptoms of stress, expressions of excessive worry about school, change from positive to negative self-perception, and verbalizations of fear of physical harm from the teacher. Although parents and nurses should be cautious in attempts to interpret such behaviors (they are in many ways similar to school phobia, p. 793), a high degree of suspicion might be justified if the symptoms are not explained by other factors or represent a marked change from previous patterns.

Children are also being encouraged to feel, think, and behave at a level of maturity far beyond what could reasonably be expected of persons their age (Elkind, 1981). They are expected to take on many adult-type responsibilities, to make decisions they are not really able to make, and to achieve more. They have little time for being *children*. Children need time for the spontaneous activities of childhood.

The sources of such problems can be categorized as (1)

inner feelings, such as being angry, embarrassed, feeling jealous, or being unable to fall asleep; (2) the behavior of others, such as fights with friends, being teased, being ignored, not being listened to, parents traveling or fighting, teachers getting angry; and (3) objective situations, such as school, moving, hospitalization, auditions, sports, being left alone (Saunders and Remsberg, 1984). The responses are those observed in any stress situation: doing nothing, acting impulsively without thought, or problem-solving. For sources of stress see the box on p. 732.

To help children cope with the stresses in their lives the parent, teacher, or health worker must be able to recognize signs that indicate a child is undergoing stress (see Signs of stress, p. 128) and identify the source promptly. Children need to be taught how to recognize signs of stress in themselves, such as a pounding heart, rapid breathing, or butterflies in the stomach. Once they are able to recognize that they are stressed, they can employ techniques for managing their stress. Probably the most useful technique is to help them plan a means for dealing with any stress through problem-solving (Kuczen, 1982).

First, they need to learn relaxation techniques such as deep breathing exercises, progressive relaxation of muscle groups, and positive imagery (see p. 1071). Encouraging them to "blow off steam" through physical activity reduces tension and anxiety. Second, they must identify the problem. Those involving situations or actions of others are relatively simple to identify. Feelings within themselves are sometimes more difficult. Third, alternative actions must be explored. Children should list all possibilities, including those that they know will not work. Fourth, they need to examine what might happen as a consequence of each alternative they have listed. By this time they are relaxed and ready for the final step, to select what they perceive to be the best option. It is sometimes helpful to have children model their behavior after someone they know who has successfully coped with a similar problem. When children are assisted with the process a few times, they are able to apply problem-solving automatically.

Fears. School-age children are afraid of a number of things. They are less fearful of body safety than they were as preschoolers although they still fear being hurt, poisoned, kidnapped, or having to undergo surgery. There is also a lessening of the fear of noises, darkness, storms, and dogs. Most of the new fears that trouble school-age children are related to school and family—for example, fear of failing, of teachers, and bullies. There are some differences between the sexes in fears. Girls are proportionately more fearful than boys of bugs, snakes, cemeteries, tornadoes and strong winds, strangers, getting lost, war, and something bad happening to their parents (Moracco and Camilleri, 1983).

Parents and other persons involved with children should discuss children's fears with them individually or through group activities. Their viewpoints must be respected and their need to communicate their concerns recognized. Sometimes children of this age are often inclined to hide their fears to avoid being ridiculed or labeled "a baby" or "chicken." Hiding fears does not end them; therefore children who are afraid to communicate them may develop displaced fears, or phobias. Children need to know that their concerns are listened to and understood. Parents who convey this to their children without becoming overprotective will help them feel less lonely and, therefore, less frightened.

Latchkey Children

The term *latchkey children* is used to describe children who are left to care for themselves or whose care arrangements are so loose that they are ineffective (Long and Long, 1982). The increasing numbers of single-parent families and working mothers together with the lack of available child care has created a stress-provoking situation for as many as 10 million school-age children in the United States (McClellan, 1984).

Inadequate adult supervision after school leaves children at greater risk for injury and delinquent behavior. Latchkey children feel more lonely, isolated, and fearful than children who have someone to care for them—fully one fourth of children interviewed in one study lived in constant fear, some to the point of absolute terror (Long and Long, 1982). To cope with their fears and anxieties while alone, these children devised several strategies—hiding (in a bathroom, closet, shower, or under a bed), playing the television at loud volume as a distraction to drown out noises and indicate that someone was at home, and using pets as a comfort.

Many communities and persons concerned about their welfare are trying to help children and their parents deal with this potentially serious problem. School-age care programs have been implemented by some communities and employers. Other types of programs include those designed to teach self-help skills to children and those that provide telephone check-in and reassurance programs for children. Some topics that are appropriate for presentation to parents and/or children to help alleviate their stress and increase the children's safety are listed in the box on p. 734.

Promoting Optimum Health During the School Years

Health supervision of children, begun in early childhood, is continued in middle childhood; it includes the periodic ongoing health assessment and guidance advised for children 6 to 12 years of age. Since regular health checkups and prophylactic measures such as immunizations are a routine function of health supervision, this need not be reiterated. The frequency of checkups is usually reduced to yearly assessment of growth progress and screening for vision, hearing, posture, and general health status.

When children enter school, they leave the relatively protected environment of home and neighborhood and experience interpersonal contacts with a larger number of children. Although the incidence of childhood disease has declined significantly in recent times, some diseases are not as yet controlled. Many childhood illnesses can be pre-

SUGGESTIONS FOR LATCHKEY CHILDREN

Safety

Teach the child not to display keys and to always lock doors.

Tell the child not to enter the house after school if the door is ajar, a window is open, or if anything appears unusual.

Walk through the after-school routine with the child.

Consult with public safety officials about burglar-proofing and fireproofing the home.

Teach the child first-aid procedures.

Teach safety rules to the child who is expected to cook (microwave ovens are safest).

Emphasize fire safety rules and conduct practice fire drills.

Teach and reinforce traffic and bicycle safety.

Teach the child weather-related safety (e.g., stay inside but do not take a bath during an electrical storm, go to and stay in a storm cellar during a tornado warning).

Teach and reinforce water safety practices (e.g., do not go swimming alone, caution about safe bathing methods and keeping the toilet lid down when infants or toddlers are in their care).

Keep firearms securely locked away and teach the child that they are for adult use only.

Telephone use

Be certain that the child knows home telephone number, address, and the parents' names.

Teach the child to tell callers that the parents are "busy"; do not tell a caller that parents are not at home.

Keep a list of emergency numbers by the telephone. Make certain the child knows how to report emergencies.

Have a list of telephone numbers of friends or neighbors who will be at home and available for help with emergencies.

Ask public safety officials to offer classes about when and how to call them.

If a "telephone hotline" for latchkey children exists, teach the child how to use it.

After-school activities

Arrange for the child to spend some afternoons with friends.

Provide structured activities for the child.

Have the child attend a public library–sponsored activity rather than watch television at home.

Discuss with the child things to do after school.

Emphasize the positive aspects of independence and resourcefulness but do not demand too much from the child.

Help the child feel successful in self-care.

Counsel parents to consider the potential problems of an older child assuming care of younger ones before the child is developmentally ready.

Loneliness

Help the child talk about experiences and feelings about being alone after school.

Consider a pet to help comfort and provide company for the child.

Be punctual in arriving home. A child's anxiety level accelerates when parents are not home when expected.

Call the child if there is to be a delay in arriving home.

Leave a tape-recorded message for the child to play on arrival home from school.

Form a group of parents with flex-time so that their children can be cared for by one of the group after school.

Modified from McClellan, M.A.: On their own: latchkey children, Pediatr. Nurs. **10**:198-202, 1983.

vented by careful health supervision. For example, most of the communicable diseases, formerly a cause of high morbidity in school children, can be prevented by immunization (see p. 526). The body's natural defenses against illness should be supported through careful attention to diet, rest, exercise, and protection from extreme mental and physical stress.

It is not uncommon for school-age children to complain of assorted physical symptoms that are particularly apparent at age 9 and during preadolescence. The more common somatic complaints are headaches, dizziness, or sudden, unexpected pains in various part of the body, most often localized in the head or stomach but occasionally in the leg. Sometimes the discomfort can be directly related to an unpleasant situation at school or a distasteful task at home, but often the desire for play overpowers the demands of the symptoms. In the preadolescent period children may suffer periods of extreme fatigue when they are so "out of sorts" that they hate everything and everybody. At this time they may benefit from a day home from school in which to rest

and recoup their resources. When school officials are aware of this need, they are ready to cooperate and allow absence when it is desirable. Children of this age do not like to miss school and usually will not take undue advantage of the situation.

HEALTH BEHAVIORS

Children should begin to learn good health practices at an early age and be able to actively and responsibly participate in their health care. With increased cognitive skills they become more self-reliant in making decisions and selecting from alternatives. They are capable of making decisions about what health behavior they will pursue.

Health education is a primary element in comprehensive health care and programs should be designed to promote desired health behavior through guided learning and modeling. Essential elements of an optimum program that helps children to accept personal responsibility for health are (Lasky, Gulbrandsen, and Scoblic, 1981):

1. Health education must be provided that allows children to:
   a. Learn about their bodies
   b. Learn how their behavior affects their health
   c. Recognize that adaptation may be needed to protect health
2. Health services are needed that focus on health rather than illness.
3. A delivery system that enables children to understand how their behavior impacts on both health and illness responses is essential.

By the end of middle childhood, children should be able to assume responsibility for self-care in the areas of nutrition, exercise and recreation, sleep, and safety. Competence involves the ability to make decisions based on evaluation of internal strengths and weaknesses and external environmental influences. Children need education, involvement, and reinforcement from caregivers and health professionals who support and encourage positive health behaviors (Koster, 1983).

NUTRITION

Although calorie needs are diminished in relation to body size during middle childhood, resources are being laid down for the increased growth needs of the adolescent period. It is important to impress on children and their parents the value of a diet balanced to promote growth. When children enter school, they develop an eating style that is increasingly independent of parental influence and scrutiny. Parents do not know what their children eat when they are away from home. A parent may pack a lunch to be eaten at school but be unaware of how much is eaten, traded, sold, or thrown away.

Influenced by the mass media and the temptation of an immense variety of "junk food," it is all too easy for children to fill up on empty calories—foods that do not promote growth, such as sugars, starches, and excess fats. They have more freedom to move without parental supervision and often have small amounts of money to spend on candy, soft drinks, and other easily accessible treats. Midafternoon snacks are common, and it is wise to encourage fruit, nuts, and other wholesome finger foods to meet this need.

Mealtime continues to be a central issue in most families. Although it should be a pleasant part of a child's day, parents' concern and emphasis on manners often make it a battleground. Likes and dislikes established at an early age continue in middle childhood, although the propensity for single food preferences begins to end and children acquire a taste for an increasing variety of foods. Since children usually eat as the family does, the quality of their diet depends to a large extent on their family's pattern of eating. Other interests and participation in outside activities often compete with mealtime.

Working parents, assuming their children to be sufficiently mature, frequently leave the responsibility for preparation of meals to them. Although most older school-age children are capable of preparing simple fare, all too often breakfast and/or lunch may be inadequate, makeshift, or nonexistent. In recognition of this problem the federal government has established the National School Lunch Program (NSLP) and more recently the School Breakfast Program (SBP) in many areas. These meals must meet specified nutritional requirements and furnish one third of the daily recommended dietary allowance for children in the United States. Most schools subscribe to the programs, and although it is difficult to measure directly, it is believed that these school feeding programs positively influence the behavior and learning capacity of children. However, children who purchase school lunches often select only the items they want or, if they must take all the items in the lunch, no one insists that they eat them.

The threat of childhood obesity is an increasingly prevalent health problem in school-age children today in the United States. The easy availability of high-calorie foods combined with the tendency toward more sedentary activities such as watching television and the trend away from walking or cycling and toward transportation by automobile and bus have reduced the caloric expenditure. The problem of childhood obesity is discussed further in Chapter 21. Given the threat of obesity and a diet-conscious society, however, many school-age children attempt to diet in an effort to prevent obesity or to reduce because of imagined overweight or to conform to peer behaviors and pressures. Children need to be educated about food selection and the importance of body building nutrients as opposed to empty caloric intake.

Nutrition is a joint responsibility of both the child and the family. Nutrition education can and should be integrated throughout a child's school years as part of classroom learning. In school the basic food groups, serving sizes, and the elements of a wholesome diet can be taught, as well as how food products are grown, processed, and prepared. School projects often include growing vegetables in the classroom or at home, and science projects in the more advanced grades might include some simple animal experiments. The school nurse can take an active role in nutrition education by working with teachers to plan and implement units of nutrition instruction and with parents and children to give nutritional guidance (see Servings per day for the average child, p. 611).

SLEEP AND REST

The amount of sleep and rest required during middle childhood is a highly individual matter. There is no specific amount needed by a child at any given age. The amount depends rather on the child's age, activity level, and other factors such as health status. The growth rate has slowed; therefore less energy is expended in growth than was expended during the preceding periods and than will be required during the adolescent growth spurt.

During the school years children usually do not require a

nap, but they sleep an average of 11 to 12 hours nightly at age 6 and 9 to 10 hours a night at age 11 or 12 (see p. 110). Although there are fewer bedtime problems with advancing years, there are still occasional difficulties associated with the necessary bedtime ritual. Usually there is little problem for children 6 and 7 years old, and the task of going to bed can be facilitated by encouraging quiet activity before bedtime, such as coloring and reading. For many children bedtime is improved considerably by allowing them a small radio to which they can listen for a specified time.

Although most children in middle childhood must frequently be reminded to go to bed, 8- to 9-year-old children and 11-year-old children are particularly resistant. Often children are unaware that they are tired; if they are allowed to remain up later than usual, they are fatigued the following day. Sometimes bedtime resistance can be resolved by allowing a later bedtime in deference to their advancing age. However, it should be made clear that this privilege depends on compliance—going to bed without stalling and without complaints. A firm approach to bedtime is usually the most successful. Parents can help children by giving them a little advance warning, but they should realize that when the final bedtime is announced they really mean it. Twelve-year-old children usually offer no difficulty in relation to bedtime. Some even retire early in order to enjoy slow preparations for bed, to read, or to listen to their radio or tape recorder.

The cause of bedtime resistance is not always clear. For some children it is related to normal fears of their age, such as fear of the dark, strange noises, intruders, or other imagined phenomena. Children who are subject to frightening dreams are hesitant to retire, and their sleep is more apt to be disturbed following emotional stimulation before bedtime. Sometimes children are loathe to give up some exciting or interesting activity in which they are involved, or they are reluctant to leave the protective social circle of the family. Another factor associated with time for retirement is related to status. For example, older children are given the privilege of a later bedtime than younger children. Promotion to a later bedtime is highly prestigious, and age-mates compare their bedtimes. This may explain why parental decisions are often hotly contested by children who believe that playmates enjoy a more privileged position in this area. In some situations going to bed is used as a method of control. When going to bed early is imposed as a punishment or staying up a little longer is a reward, children may view bedtime as punitive or status-degrading.

Sleep Disorders

During middle childhood the night terrors of preschool children are replaced by sleepwalking (somnambulism) and sleeptalking. Like night terrors, sleepwalking is associated with a prolonged stage 3 to 4 non–REM sleep and occurs approximately 90 to 120 minutes following the onset of sleep. The phenomenon is more common in boys than in girls and there is evidence to indicate that there may be a hereditary basis to its occurrence (Abe and others, 1984). The episodes begin when the child sits up abruptly.

During sleepwalking, movements are clumsy and repetitive; finger and hand movements are often observed. Most commonly children move about restlessly then lie down and return to sleep. However, they may get out of bed and engage in nonpurposeful walking. They rarely perform purposeful acts during sleepwalking. Any attempts to communicate with a child elicit only mumbled and slurred responses. Sleeptalking, like sleepwalking, is not purposeful and speech is usually incomprehensible and monosyllabic (Anders and Keener, 1983)

The best approach is to leave sleepwalking children alone unless they are in danger or may endanger others. However, clumsiness and stereotyped movements can make sleepwalking very dangerous. If the environment is not safe, a child can get hurt. Usually children complete their mission and return quietly to bed. If they must be wakened, it is best to call them by name slowly and softly, orient them to where they are, explain that they were walking in their sleep, and assure them that it will not happen when they are more relaxed. Preventive measures include avoiding overfatigue, getting adequate rest, and relieving any stress the children may be experiencing.

Approximately 15% of children between ages 5 and 12 walk at least once (Anders and Keener, 1983). Persistent sleepwalking occurs in only a small percentage of children. The problem is usually self-limited and requires no treatment. Children who sleepwalk persistently must be protected from harm during their wandering, and some troublesome cases may require low-dose sedation, such as diazepam before retiring.

PHYSICAL ACTIVITY

Exercise is essential for developmental progress in a number of areas, including muscle development and tone, refinement of balance and coordination, gaining strength and endurance, and stimulating body functions and metabolic processes. Throughout middle childhood children's increasing capabilities and adaptability permit greater speed and effort in motor activities, and larger, stronger muscles with greater efficiency and skill permit longer and increasingly strenuous play without exhaustion. During this age period children acquire the necessary coordination, timing, and concentration that are required to participate in adult-type activities, even though they may lack the strength, stamina, and control of the adolescent and adult. Consequently a larger amount of physical activity should be expected and encouraged during the school years.

Children should be afforded opportunities of various kinds that provide satisfying experiences to meet individual likes and dislikes. Children need ample space in which to run, jump, skip, and climb and safe facilities and equipment to use both inside and outside. Appropriate activities that promote coordination and development during the school-age years include running, skipping rope, swimming, roller skating, ice skating, and bicycle riding. Positive reinforcement achieved by experiencing increasingly smooth, rhythmic, and efficient use of the body conditions the child toward regular physical activity. It must be kept in mind, however, that although school-age children are large and appear to be strong, they may not be prepared yet for strenuous competitive athletics.

Most children need little encouragement to engage in physical activity. They have so much energy that they seldom know when to stop. However, children with disabilities or those who hesitate to become involved in active play, such as obese children, require special assessment and help in determining activities that will appeal to them, that are compatible with their limitations, and that at the same time meet their developmental needs. Also parents need to limit television viewing to encourage outside activities.

Sports. A great deal of controversy has surrounded the trend toward earlier participation in competitive athletics and determining the amount and type of competitive sports that are appropriate for children in the elementary grades. The current view is that virtually every child is suited for some type of sport, and authorities do not discourage participation if children are matched to the type of sport appropriate to their abilities and to their physical and emotional constitution. School-age children enjoy competition and, when those involved with children in this age-group understand each child's physical limitations and teach them the proper techniques and safety to avoid injury to developing bones and muscles, a safe and appropriate sport can be found for even the most unskilled and nonaggressive child.

During middle childhood girls have the same basic structure as boys and thus have a similar response to systematic exercise training. At puberty, when boys become larger and have more muscle mass, it is usually recommended that girls compete only against other girls. Before puberty there is no essential difference in strength and size between girls and boys, making these precautions unnecessary (Shaffer, 1980).

The American Association for Health, Physical Education, and Recreation; the American Academy of Pediatrics, the American Medical Association Committee of the Medical Aspects of Sports; and the Society of State Directors of Health, Physical Education, and Recreation issued a joint statement setting forth guidelines in sports for children and younger adolescents (Magill, Ash, and Smoll, 1978). These guidelines stress the importance of:

1. Proper physical conditioning for children entering competition
2. Proper grouping of young athletes according to body size, skill, and maturation
3. Good protective equipment
4. Periodic health appraisals of participants
5. Availability of a physician during games and practice sessions

The American Academy of Pediatrics in their guidelines for age-specific sports for children (1978) recommend noncombat sports that focus on individual skills for young children (age 6 years). Approved sports include swimming, gymnastics, track and field, martial arts, tennis, and skating. Additional sports approved for children around 8 years of age are basketball, volleyball, soccer, and wrestling. Participation in collision sports is best deferred until children are 10 to 12 years of age. These could include football, rugby, and hockey (Martins and Seefeldt, 1979).

In addition to ensuring the interest, suitability, and safety of the sport, parents must make certain that coaches (if involved in the sport) are skillful in managing children and do not engage abusive types of behavior. Any sport for children should emphasize the pleasure of the activity, which more often involves individual rather than team sports. It is wise to expose children to a variety of individual sports. The overall emphasis of both team and individual sports should be on playing and learning, not on winning. Parents who pressure their children to perform beyond their capabilities run the risk of injury to the child and developing a distaste for the activity as well as contributing to a lowered self-image (Committee on School Health, 1983).

The same principles described above apply to children with chronic illnesses such as diabetes, epilepsy, asthma, or allergies if the disorder is mild and can be controlled with medication. Mentally retarded children need not be excluded from sports competition if they are matched evenly against other children of equal abilities and provided with skilled supervision and coaching. Sometimes the activities need to be modified to accommodate the limitations of these children.

Acquisition of Skills

School-age children also demonstrate increasing capacity in fine muscle facility and complex artistic skills. Handedness is well established by the beginning of the school years, and the child makes great strides in writing and drawing during this age period. It is a period of energetic and vibrant creative productivity. With the tools of language and reading, children can create poems, stories, and plays. With more advanced fine motor skills, they are able to master an unlimited variety of handicrafts, such as ceramics, needlework, wood carving, and beadwork. They avidly pursue these skills in solitude, with a friend, or in programs offered through organizations such as boys' or girls' clubs, scouting, or the YWCA and YMCA, which use crafts as a means to occupy, entertain, and educate children.

Music is a favorite form of expression in middle childhood (Fig. 17-10). School-age children are stimulated and invigorated by music. They can sing in harmony, play instruments in orchestras and bands, and otherwise manage music at a more complex level. They can compose original songs, learn lyrics almost effortlessly, and turn any empty moment into an occasion for singing to which any family, bus driver, or group leader can attest.

School-age children are capable of assuming responsibility for their own needs, although their distaste for soap and water and ''dress'' clothes is legendary. School-age children can and want to assume their share of household tasks, which usually are related to the male and female roles that have been defined by their culture, and many assume re-

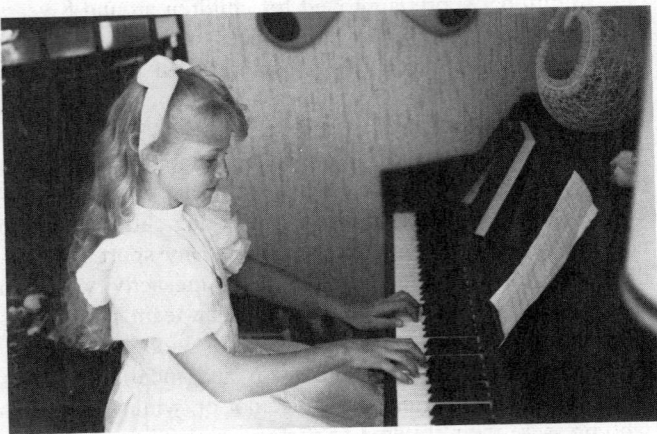

Fig. 17-10. Music is a favorite form of expression for school-age children.
Photography by Earl Fillmore, Salt Lake City, UT.

sponsibility for tasks outside the home, such as babysitting, yard tending, or paper routes (Fig. 17-11).

Television

For some time child development specialists and parents have been concerned about the effect that television has on child development and behavior. There is no doubt that children learn from television, but the values and attitudes are not always realistically displayed and often conflict with those they have been taught. School-age children are better able to distinguish fantasy from reality and some have had sufficient life experience to be able to view much of television fare with skepticism. However, television rarely depicts the reality of day-to-day situations that confront children. For example, the concept of work is distorted. Children on television do not perform household tasks; frequently there is no evidence of work in the television family. Sex roles and those of minorities are usually not depicted realistically on television—adult, white males predominate, and they are shown as dominant, authoritative, and the main source of financial support (McCown, 1979).

The greatest criticism of television, however, centers around violence. Studies have found that children become desensitized to real life aggression after viewing violence on the screen. Children imitate the behavior of role models and may eventually incorporate the observed aggressive behavior into their own behavior unless it is tempered by the presence of a calm adult to point out the inappropriateness and consequences of undesirable behaviors. Otherwise the child may become more willing to harm others, become more aggressive in play, and select aggression as a response to conflict situations (see also p. 130).

A relationship has also been observed between television watching and obesity in children. It is unclear whether the obesity is a result of decreased physical activity or other factors associated with the viewing, such as snacking, observing food advertisements (children often influence food purchases), and imitating the eating behavior of family members during viewing (Dietz and Gortmaker, 1985).

DENTAL HEALTH

The first permanent (secondary) teeth erupt at about 6 years of age. Before their appearance they have been developing in the jaw beneath the deciduous (primary) teeth. Meanwhile, the roots of the latter are gradually being absorbed so that at the time a deciduous tooth is shed, only the crown remains. At 6 years of age all the primary teeth are present and those of the secondary dentition are relatively well formed. At this time eruption of the permanent teeth begins, usually starting with the 6-year molar, which erupts posterior to the deciduous molars. The others appear in approximately the same order as eruption of the primary teeth and follow shedding of the deciduous teeth (Fig. 17-12).

The pattern of shedding primary teeth and the eruption of secondary teeth are subject to wide variation among children. To allow the larger permanent teeth to occupy the limited space left by shed primary teeth, a series of complicated changes must take place in the jaws. It is at this time that many of the difficulties created by crowding of teeth become apparent. With the appearance of the second permanent (12-year) molar, most of the permanent teeth are present. The third permanent molars, or wisdom teeth, may erupt from 18 to 25 years of age or later. Permanent dentition, as in other aspects of development, is somewhat more advanced in girls than it is in boys.

Since it is during the school-age years that the permanent teeth erupt, good dental hygiene and regular attention to dental caries are a vital part of health supervision during this period (see p. 739). Correct brushing and flossing techniques should be taught or reinforced, and the role that fermentable carbohydrates play in production of dental caries should be emphasized. It is also important to be alert to possible malocclusion problems that may result from irregular eruption of permanent teeth and that may impair function.

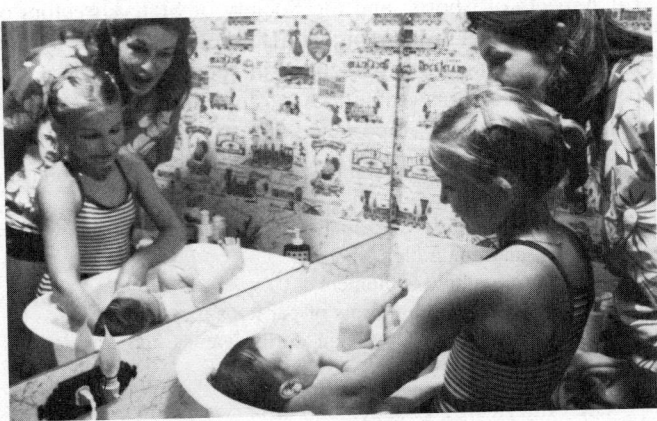

Fig. 17-11. Children can assume responsibility for a variety of household tasks.
Photography by Wayne Kunke, San Jose, CA.

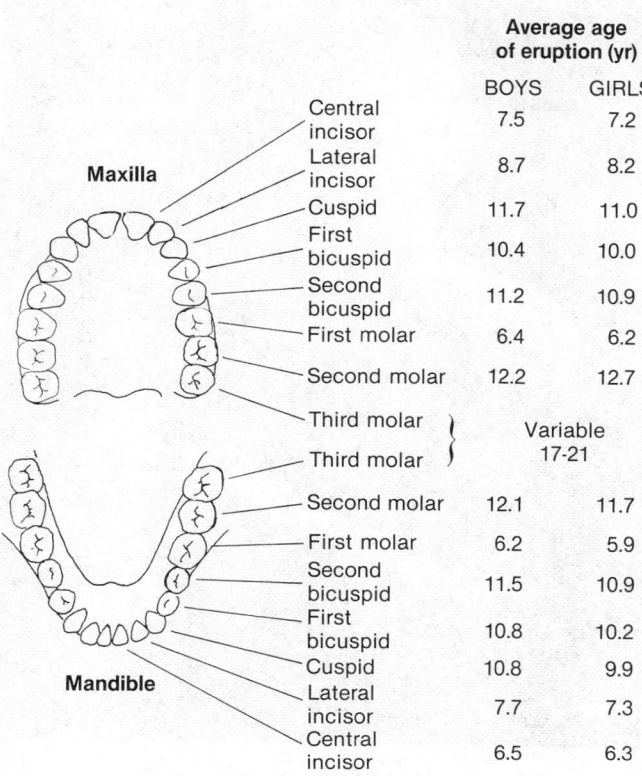

		Average age of eruption (yr)	
		BOYS	GIRLS
Maxilla	Central incisor	7.5	7.2
	Lateral incisor	8.7	8.2
	Cuspid	11.7	11.0
	First bicuspid	10.4	10.0
	Second bicuspid	11.2	10.9
	First molar	6.4	6.2
	Second molar	12.2	12.7
	Third molar	Variable 17-21	
	Third molar		
	Second molar	12.1	11.7
	First molar	6.2	5.9
	Second bicuspid	11.5	10.9
	First bicuspid	10.8	10.2
	Cuspid	10.8	9.9
Mandible	Lateral incisor	7.7	7.3
	Central incisor	6.5	6.3

Fig. 17-12. Sequence of eruption of secondary teeth.

Regular dental supervision is as essential as regular medical supervision and should be an integral part of the overall health maintenance program. Dental prophylaxis (teeth cleaning) and fluoride application are continued to decrease the susceptibility of the tooth enamel to acid breakdown (see p. 613 for discussion of fluoride and other aspects of dental care).

Brushing

One of the most effective means of preventing dental caries is a regimen of proper oral hygiene tailored to the individual child by the dentist. Children should be taught to carry out their own dental care under the supervision and guidance of parents. Parents should learn proper brushing technique along with their children and should inspect their children's efforts until the children can assume full responsibility for their own care. Most practitioners believe that the majority of children do not possess the fine motor skills needed to brush their teeth properly until they are able to write in script—at approximately 7 years (Boraz, 1981). Teeth should be brushed after meals, after snacks, and at bedtime. The bedtime brushing is especially important because there is more time for interaction between oral bacteria and unremoved substrate on the tooth substance. Children who brush their teeth frequently and become accustomed to the feel of a clean mouth at an early age usually maintain the habit throughout life.

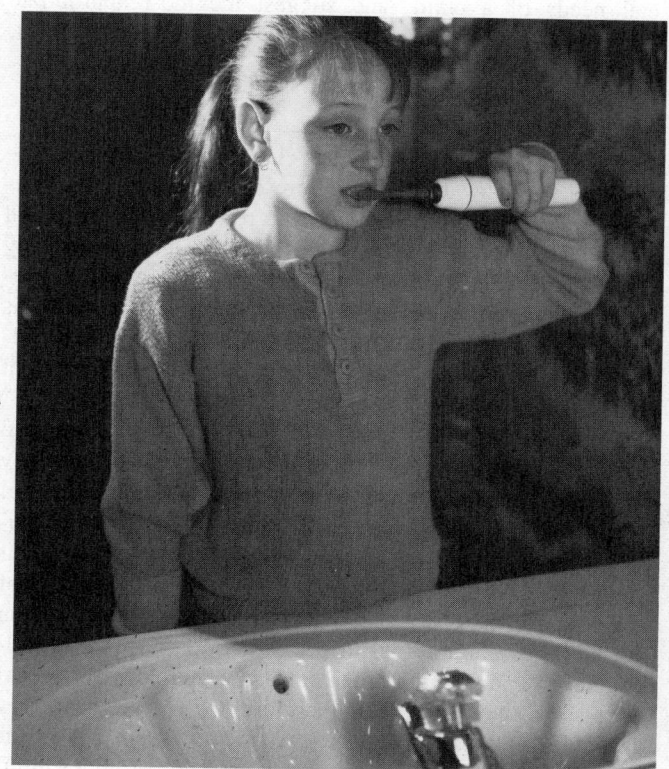

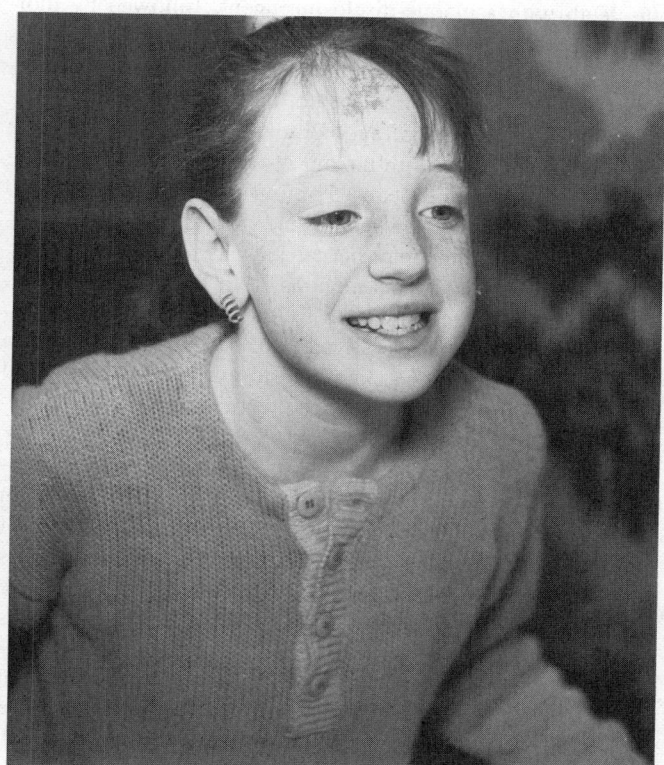

Fig. 17-13. Brushing teeth. **A,** Brushing. **B,** Inspection after using a disclosing tablet.
Continued.

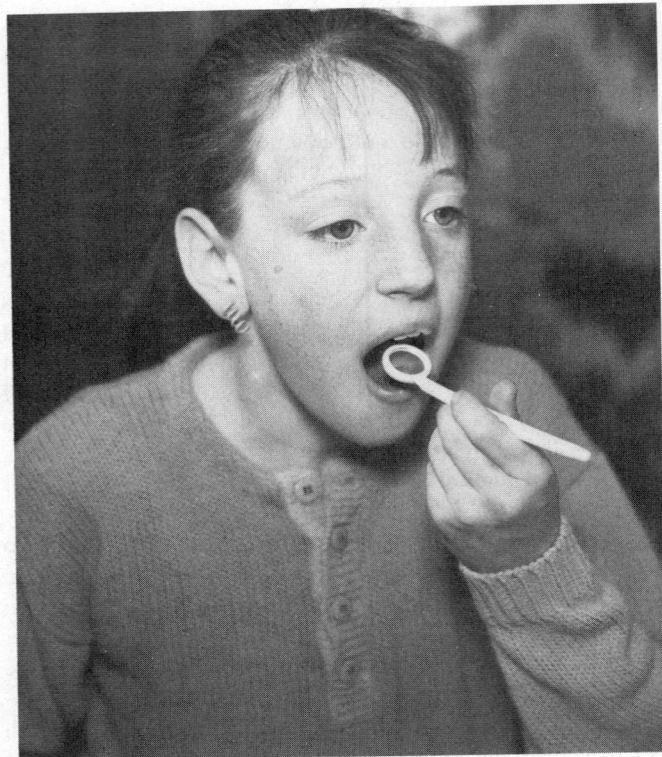

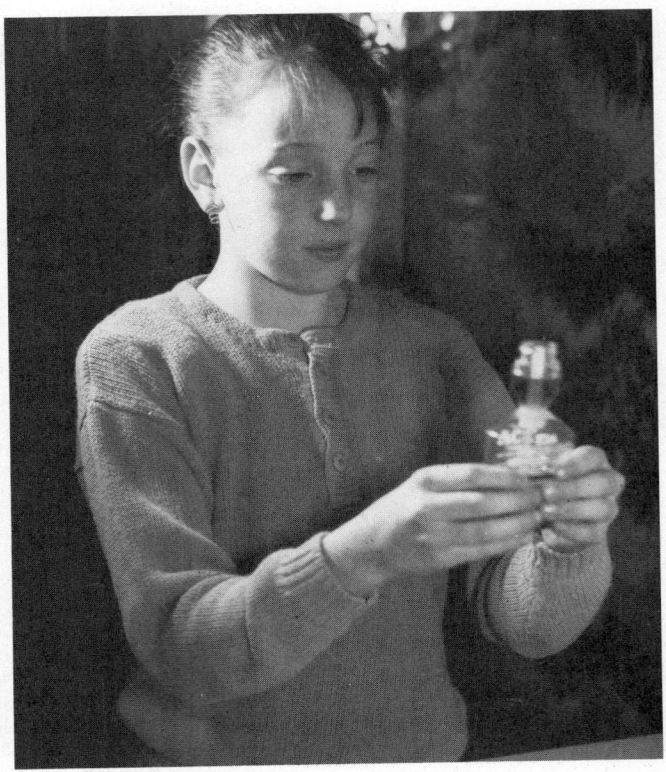

Fig. 17-13, cont'd. C, Continued inspection. **D,** Using fluoride rinse.

One regimen advocated by authorities includes staining the teeth with a plaque-disclosing agent, followed by thorough brushing with plain water and flossing. Flossing is done by the parents until children aquire the manual dexterity needed. Most children are not able to floss properly until about 8 or 9 years of age (Boraz, 1981). After the teeth have been inspected with the aid of a mirror under adequate light, they are again cleansed, this time with a fluoridated dentifrice to freshen the mouth and provide further protection. This procedure may be carried out regularly or occasionally, according to instructions from the child's dentist. The toothpastes recommended by the American Dental Association are Crest*, Colgate†, Macleans‡, and Ultra Brite†. They have been submitted to exhaustive testing and demonstrate the ability to reduce the incidence of dental caries when used correctly (Boraz, 1981).

For school-age children with mixed and permanent dentition the best toothbrush is one of soft nylon bristles with an overall length of about 21 cm (6 inches). The design of the brush is of little importance; it is usually left to a child's preference. Numerous methods of brushing the teeth have been described and recommended for children but there is no conclusive evidence that one method is superior over another. The thoroughness of the cleaning is more important than the specific technique used (Fig. 17-13). The dentist will assess all factors, such as manipulative skills and special needs of a child, and suggest the most appropriate brushing technique and regimen (Shelton and Ferretti, 1982).

SEX EDUCATION

Evidence indicates that many children experience some form of sex play during or before preadolescence as a response to normal curiosity, not as a result of love or sexual urge. Children are experimentalists by nature, and this play is incidental and transitory. Any adverse emotional consequences or guilt feelings depend on how the behavior is managed by the parents, if it is discovered, or whether children view their actions as wrong in the eyes of significant persons, particularly the parents.

Much of children's attitude toward sex that is acquired indirectly at a very early age affects the way in which they respond to sexual information presented at a later time. With few exceptions, parents discourage sex exploration either through subtle substitution of activities that divert their children's attention from the genitalia or by expressions of anger or disgust at their behavior. These tactics set limits on their curiosity and ability to learn. In addition, parents seldom teach young children the correct terminology for sexual organs or sexual feeling; therefore the only vocabulary available to them is the one that identifies sexual organs with excretory functions. Thus these parental attitudes influence the children's perception of the cleanliness of their genitalia in relation to their actual function.

---

*Proctor & Gamble, Cincinnati, OH 45202.
†Colgate-Palmolive, New York, NY 10022.
‡Beecham Products, Pittsburgh, PA 15230.

Because parents often either repress or avoid their children's sexual curiosity, the sexual information that they receive in childhood is acquired almost entirely from their peers. When peers are the primary source of sexual information, it is transmitted and exchanged in secret, clandestine conversation and contains a large amount of misinformation. The context in which these communications take place creates anxiety in children and barriers to trust; therefore they continue to keep sexuality a secret. These reactions inhibit spontaneous expressions or questioning of the parents.

The subject of where sex education should be taught and by whom arouses a good deal of controversy. Many individuals and groups are unconditionally opposed to the inclusion of sex education in the schools. Others believe that sex information should not be taught separately from other information but should be presented as naturally as information about other body functions and natural phenomena such as the solar system, the changing seasons, and the migratory habits of birds. Children's questions about sex should be answered to the same extent as their questions about any other topic—honestly and at their level of understanding. During the preschool years children will be satisfied with simple answers, but as they gain more knowledge and understanding of the world, their curiosity about everything will be deeper. When sex is treated as though it is a normal part of growth and development and questions are answered matter-of-factly, parental responses are less apt to contain overtones of guilt and anxiety that in turn produce anxiety in children.

Middle childhood appears to be an ideal time for formal sex education, and many authorities believe that the topic is best presented from a life-span approach. Initial curiosity about differences in body structure between boys and girls and between children and adults occurrs in the preschool years, and the next stage, adolescence, arouses both anxiety and excitement about sexual encounters. Information about sexual maturation and the process of reproduction presented during middle childhood helps to minimize a child's uncertainty, embarrassment, and feelings of isolation that often accompany the events of puberty.

Although sex education programs are not universally a part of the elementary school curriculum, some progressive educators have successfully incorporated sex education into a number of school programs. Because of the natural social orientation of this period of development, structured group learning situations can be successfully used for discussion of sexuality. An ideal approach that has been advanced suggests that sexuality can best be presented in the context of its central role as a biologic mechanism for the survival of the culture. This allows children to approach the topic at a distance, with sexual maturation and reproduction as each individual's contribution to the natural order of things. It then provides a natural entry into discussion of sexuality as a basis for family units, marriage, and attitudes toward children as well as into a presentation of the biologic facts of sexuality. More difficult, but equally important, is for children to view sexual intimacy as a close, personal relationship and a means of conveying love as well as a means for ensuring the survival of the species.

Nurse's Role in Sex Education

No matter where nurses practice, they can provide information on human sexuality to both parents and children. Nurses can help parents by first becoming knowledgeable about human sexuality themselves, including the common myths and misconceptions associated with sex and the reproductive process. They need to know their own attitudes and feelings toward sexuality and to feel comfortable with these feelings.

During encounters with parents, nurses can be open and available for questions and discussion. They can set an example by the language they use in discussing body parts and their function and by the way in which they deal with problems that have emotional overtones, such as exploratory sex play and masturbation. Parents need to be helped to understand normal behaviors and to view sexual curiosity in their children as a part of the developmental process. Assessing the parent's level of knowledge and understanding of sexuality provides cues to their need for supplemental information that will better prepare them for the increasingly complex explanations that will be needed as their children grow older.

Sometimes short classes or group discussions for parents are helpful for discussing disturbing behaviors and anticipating the questions and forthcoming learning needs of the children. When possible it is wise to include both parents. Sex education in the home should be assumed by both parents so that the children will not acquire a distorted view of either the male or the female role that may alter relationships with the opposite sex in later life. Most importantly nurses should take an active role in encouraging, developing, and providing sex education to children at all levels as an integral part of their learning.

SCHOOL HEALTH

Child health maintenance is ultimately the responsibility of parents; however, public schools and health departments in the United States have contributed to the improvement of child health by providing a healthful school environment, health services, and health education functions that emphasize sound health practices. Most of these constitute major components of community health services and involve large amounts of public funds and large numbers of health professionals, including nurses, on either a full-time or part-time basis. School health programs contribute to the goals of the community toward education and the development of children.

A safe and healthful school environment is the first essential element of any school health program. Conditions within the school setting should make a positive contribution to the physical, mental, and social development of the children. Factors that contribute to healthful school living include the following:

1. A clean, safe, and wholesome school and classroom environment that provides suitable lighting, seating, heating, ventilation, furniture, equipment, and a safe play area
2. A health program that is concerned about the physical and mental health of children, teachers, and other staff members involved in the school operation
3. A schedule of activities that is suited to the capabilities and maturational level of each child
4. A regular physical education program
5. A planned food service program that provides both meal services and an example of good nutrition practices

A school health program should also be involved in ongoing health maintenance through assessment, screening, and referral activities. Routine health services provided by most schools include the following:

1. Health appraisal—screening tests (vision, hearing), measurements (height, weight), and medical, dental, and psychologic examinations
2. Emergency care and safety—emergency treatment (first aid), notification of parents, and transportation of the ill or injured child to home or hospital
3. Communicable disease control—detection and exclusion of affected children and policies for readmission and attendance at school (immunizations required in most states before school entry)
4. Counseling and guidance—health guidance, referral, and follow-up for parents and children with special health needs
5. Adjustment to individual student needs

Health Education

Health education of school children is primarily directed toward providing knowledge of health and influencing habits, attitudes, and conduct in relation to health and accident prevention. The Committee on School Health of the American Academy of Pediatrics believes that community health programs can be instrumental in changing poor health practices and makes the following recommendations (Committee on School Health, 1985):

1. Health education is a subject that should be taught as part of basic education and deserves the same priority in the curriculum as traditional subjects.
2. Planned integrated programs of comprehensive health education should be a requirement for students from kindergarten through grade 12 and should be taught by specially qualified teachers or those certified to teach health education.
3. Health education should include the active participation of students for the most effective learning of sound health concepts.
4. Financial support for health education programs must be ensured. Proper funding is critical to the development of effective programs, and the agencies responsible must be convinced to continue or increase funding.
5. Comprehensive health education programs should be directed by qualified health educators who function in consultation and cooperation with school personnel and administrators.

6. The programs should be monitored by a well-organized school health committee composed of representative parents, students, pediatricians, and health agencies (e.g., public health nurses) in the community.
7. Health education should be a part of every elementary school and secondary school teachers' training program.
8. School districts, other public agencies, the medical community, and private agencies should intensify their health education program for adults as part of a coordinated community health education effort, and pediatricians should make health education a regular component of the child health supervision and routine illness visit.
9. Research studies to evaluate the impact of such programs on students must be carried out at local and national levels.

A viable health education program is based on sound health concepts but should be adjusted to meet specific local needs, objectives, and legal requirements. Parents must understand and approve the health education curriculum so that its teaching will be reinforced at home. A comprehensive approach to health education is more successful in developing positive health practices than one in which the subjects are taught in isolation. The Committee on School Health (1985) recommends integration of health subjects appropriate to the age and maturity of children at each level. There are some topics that may be associated with differing social and cultural attitudes and should be presented accurately but with sensitivity to those attitudes.

School Nursing Services

School nurses are in a position to assume a major role in the school health program. Working in collaboration with others in the school and community, their service consists of three interrelated aspects of child health care: health supervision, health counseling, and health education. These functions are not necessarily limited to the confines of the school environment but also extend into the community in which the students live. As a health practitioner the school nurse is in a position to promote and evaluate health services throughout the community as they affect children and to collaborate with agencies in planning for health and safety.

Traditionally school nurses have been viewed from a limited perspective that placed them in the role of disease detector, applier of Band-Aids, and official caregiver in cases of illness and injury. Although these are still important functions and their importance should not be minimized, this traditional role has acquired much broader dimensions. School nurses are being prepared to provide primary health care on a broader scale that includes assessment of physical, psychomedical, psychoeducational, behavioral, and learning disorder problems and to provide comprehensive well-child care. The school nurse practitioner is also concerned with development, implementation, and evaluation of health care plans and programs.

Since the passage of Public Law 94 requiring the integration of chronically ill or disabled children into the regular classrooms, school nurses are responsible for the medical and nursing needs of these children in the school setting. School nurses assess and monitor all health problems that come into the school and compile a health care list of all such problems and their associated therapies. Nurses usually call the parent of the child and arrange for a visit to the home, made by either themselves or a public health nurse, where they gather information and determine if a nursing care plan is needed at the school. They collaborate with the family, including their suggestions in the care plan. The plan is discussed with the child's teachers and any needed education provided. School nurses are the only ones in the school system qualified to deal with medical problems.

Sometimes all that is required is an assessment and making the teacher aware that the child has a health problem. In other cases more complex teaching is needed, such as how to observe for certain signs (e.g., insulin reaction), techniques that must be learned (e.g., tracheostomy suctioning, gastrostomy or nasogastric tube feedings), and management of emergencies (care of a child during a seizure). Teachers are taught the necessary procedures and the school nurse reviews their performance approximately every 4 weeks. Most teachers are required to demonstrate competence in cardiopulmonary resuscitation.

Children who must take medications at school need written authorization from the child's attending physician and/ or written permission from the parents allowing the nurse to administer or supervise the administration of the medication. The medication must be brought to the school in a container appropriately labeled by the pharmacist or physician (Committee on School Health, 1984). Medications are kept locked up in the nurse's office; the child is not allowed to carry them at school. This may vary in some school districts or situations involving children who usually have the responsibility for taking their own medications. The children are allowed to do so provided the physician and a parent provide the required authorization. Guidelines for administration of medications in schools can also be obtained from the **National Association of School Nurses, Inc.***

The preparation, qualifications, and utilization of school nurses and school nurse practitioners vary throughout the United States. Some communities consider the school nurse an essential member of the school organization with a full-time school commitment; in other communities school health practice is merely a part of the total community health program assumed by the health department. The relative merits of the two types of services are a matter of controversy. It has been shown that screening programs and physical examinations by a competent nurse practitioner maximize the identification and resolution of health problems (DeAngelis and others, 1983; Oda and others, 1985).

INJURY PREVENTION

Because school-age children have developed more refined muscular coordination and control and can apply their cog-

nitive capacities to a more judicious course of action, the incidence of unintentional injury is diminished in children in this age-group when compared with the incidence in early childhood. As previously described, the type of injuries most prevalent in children in any age-group largely reflects the child's developmental stage. The box on p. 745 outlines some of the developmental characteristics and accomplishments of middle childhood that predispose such children to physical injury.

Achieving social acceptance is a primary objective for school-age children and they will often attempt dangerous acts (sometimes extreme behaviors) to prove themselves worthy of acceptance and improve their status in the peer group (Levine, 1983). Peer pressure is a normal part of psychologic development but at the same time it is a major contributor to risk-taking behaviors. In one study approximately 50% of peer challenges encouraged problem behavior that placed children at risk for injury or hazardous habits (Lewis and Lewis, 1984). School-age children are in the process of moving from preoperational to concrete operational thinking and are only beginning to understand causal relationships. Therefore they may attempt certain activities without planning or evaluating the consequences.

The incidence of injury during middle childhood is significantly higher in school-age boys than in school-age girls, and their death rate is twice that of girls (Greensher, 1984). Most injuries occur in or near the home or school. The prevalence of injury depends on the dangers present in the environment, protection offered by adults, and the behavior patterns of the children. Also school-age children, although conscious of rules and frequently imposing them in relationships with peers, tend to challenge established rules. It is often difficult to maintain a balance between the level of supervision and restriction needed by children and the children's need for freedom and independence.

The incidence of transportation-related injuries in school-age children is twice that of younger children, and in this age-group the rate of bicycle injuries not involving motor vehicles is twice that of teenagers and four times that of preschool children (Guyer and Gallagher, 1985). The rate of injuries from burns and poisonings are lowest in school-age children. However, physically active school-age children are highly susceptible to cuts and abrasions, and the incidence of childhood fractures, strains, and sprains is impressive.

Children at Increased Risk

There is some controversy regarding whether or not there is an entity that has been labeled the "accident-prone child." The temperament of some children seems to render them at increased risk for injury. This includes children who are stubborn, easily frustrated, overreactive, restless, careless, overly aggressive, or lacking in self-control. Some children, in situations of stress, become increasingly impulsive and disorganized to the point that they are unable to recognize or heed danger signals. The resentful, hostile child and the immature or mentally subnormal child who attempts to com-

*Lamplighter Lane, P.O. Box 1300, Scarborough, ME 04074.

BICYCLE SAFETY

Ride bicycles with traffic and away from parked cars
Ride single file
Walk bicycles through busy intersections
Give hand signals well in advance of turning or stopping
Keep as close to the curb as practical
Watch for drain grates, potholes, soft shoulders, and
    loose dirt or gravel
Keep both hands on handlebars, except when signaling
Never ride double on a bicycle
Do not carry packages that interfere with vision or control
Watch for and yield to pedestrians
Watch for cars backing up or pulling out of driveways
Be especially careful at intersections
Never hitch a ride on a truck or other vehicle
Learn rules of the road and respect for traffic officers
Obey all local ordinances
Wear well-fitted helmet
Wear shoes while riding
Wear light colors at night and attach fluorescent material
    to clothing and bicycle
Be certain the bicycle is the correct size for rider
Equip bicycle with proper lights and reflectors
Have the bicycle inspected to ensure good mechanical
    condition

pete with others beyond his capacity in a hazardous environment represent other types of children who have many injuries.

It is not established to what extent these injuries may be self-motivated. Certainly with the overreactive and impulsive child, whose characteristics are those of a child with an attention deficit disorder (p. 786), and with the immature child, this is doubtful. It has also been shown that children undergoing stressful changes in their lives are more susceptible to accidents. There is concern regarding some accidental injuries in school children, such as poisoning, that are considered to be nonaccidental unless specifically reported otherwise. The "accident" may be a manifestation of a significant mental health problem (see Suicide, p. 905).

Motor Vehicle Injury

As in all other age-groups, the most common cause of severe accidental injury and death in school-age children is motor vehicle accidents—either as pedestrian or passenger. Pedestrian fatalities are two and a half times more frequent than occupant deaths in school-age children and the peak incidence is in the 5- to 9-year-old age-group (Rivara and Barber, 1985). Half occur at night. Most of the injuries are caused by children who misinterpret traffic signs or disobey common traffic safety regulations, and cross the street against a red light, cross in other than designated crosswalks, dart into the street, and walk in the same direction as the traffic. Teaching and modeling correct pedestrian behavior can reduce the incidence of these injuries.

Use of restraint systems, door-lock mechanisms, and appropriate passenger seating and behavior are simple but effective measures for eliminating noncrash injuries and reducing the severity of crash injuries. The importance of emphasizing the correct use of seat restraints cannot be overemphasized. Children in this age-group do not usually require special car seats but parents should make certain that the restraints are fitted to their children and fastened correctly (see p. 618 for further discussion of safety restraints).

Bicycle Injury

The majority of school-age children have bicycles and their penchant for riding them increases the risk of injury on streets and byways. Each year bicycles lead to 1 million injuries and 372,000 visits to emergency rooms, and the bicycle leads the Consumer Product Safety Commission's list of causes of product-related injuries (Greensher, 1984). Seventy percent of bicycle injuries are related to violations of traffic laws by the bicyclist, including wrong-way riding (facing traffic), failure to yield right-of-way, and turning violations (Paulson, 1983). Half of all bicycle accidents are of the "dashing out" type (Pless and Stulginskas, 1982). Deaths are usually caused by head injuries and almost always are the result of bicycle/motor vehicle collision (Friede and others, 1985). Much of the difficulties of school-age

Questions and Controversies

Is playing video games bad for school-age children?

Video games have been criticized and supported in relation to their effect on children and adolescents. They have been reputed to keep children from school and to cause tension, sleeplessness, and violence. Others support the activity as a means for improving eye-hand coordination and as a substitute for the inactivity of passive television viewing. Other benefits include development of inductive reasoning (drawing generalizations from specific observations), improving spatial perception, and learning to handle multiple variables that interact simultaneously.

Parents and educators have expressed concern regarding the effects of video games on children and complain that games are addictive, distract students from homework, reduce involvement in sports, provide less opportunity to develop social skills, and promote criminal activity (Soper and Miller, 1983). There has been no confirmation of these suggested effects. At least one observer finds that relatively few children are led to deviant behavior by playing video games, even in arcades (Ellis, 1984). Other researchers found support, on a short-term basis, for the notion that playing video games affects children's aggression fantasies (Graybill and others, 1985). Although there are some compulsive aspects in the play, no identifiable problems were correlated with the amount of time spent playing (Egli and Meyers, 1984).

At least one researcher suggests that the ability to suspend reality in video games dissipates the dilemmas and conflicts of everyday existence (Klein, 1984). There is interest among educators concerning the use of video games as a means of improving reading speed as well as skimming and scanning skills, but the habitual use of short, incomplete sentences without punctuation does not provide positive writing models (Radencich, 1984).

In some instances children play video games in arcades for much the same reason that they watch television: escape, a sense of personal involvement in the action, and a source of (or substitute for) companionship (Selnow, 1984).

children can be attributed to the developmentally related limited range of vision and the inability to process their perceptions of road situations sufficiently well and quickly enough to ride safely in traffic.

To prevent bicycle injuries both parents and children should learn and periodically review bicycle safety. Children need bicycles that are suited to their size and age—they should be able to stand with the balls of both feet on the ground when seated on the bicycle, be able to place both feet flat on the ground when straddling the center bar, and be able to grasp the brake lever comfortably and easily enough to apply sufficient pressure to brake the bicycle (American Academy of Pediatrics, 1978). Children should be able to demonstrate to parents a basic competence in handling themselves on the bicycle before they are allowed to use it without supervision (Betz, 1983). Other suggestions for bicycle safety are listed in the box on p. 744.

Other Injuries

Serious injuries are associated with other moving conveyances, including injuries on skateboards, roller skates, skis, and other sports equipment (see also p. 737 and Sports injuries, p. 843). Falls are still a source of injury but less so than in preschool children and toddlers. Injuries at public playgrounds, amusement parks (especially water slides), injuries around the home (power tools, power mowers, ladders, fireworks), and at school are ongoing concerns of parents and health care providers. Sharp missiles (including toothpicks) must be handled with care to prevent puncture wounds.

MAJOR DEVELOPMENTAL ACCOMPLISHMENTS OF MIDDLE CHILDHOOD RELATED TO PHYSICAL INJURY

Developing increasing independence
Increased physical skills
Growth in height exceeds muscular growth and coordination
Needs strenuous physical activity
Delights in physical activity
Interested in acquiring new skills and perfecting attained skills
Daring and adventurous
Attempts hazardous feats
Frequently plays in hazardous places
Desires group loyalty; strong need for approval of friends
Accompanies friends to potentially hazardous facilities
Confidence often exceeds physical capacity
Likely to overdo

INJURY PREVENTION DURING SCHOOL-AGE YEARS

Motor vehicles
Educate regarding proper use of seat belts while a passenger in a vehicle
Maintain discipline while a passenger in a vehicle, for example, keep arms inside, do not lean against doors or interfere with driver
Emphasize safe pedestrian behavior
Teach safety and maintenance of two-wheeled vehicles, such as bicycles (see box, p. 744)
Insist on wearing of safety apparel (e.g., helmet) where applicable, such as riding motorcycle

Drowning
Teach to swim
Teach basic water safety, especially swimming with a buddy

Burns
Instruct in behavior in the areas involving contact with potential burn hazards, for example, gasoline, matches, bonfires or barbecues, firecrackers, lighters, cooking utensils, chemistry sets; avoid climbing around high-tension wires
Instruct in proper behavior in the event of fire (e.g., fire drills at home or school)
Teach proper behavior if clothing becomes ignited
Advise regarding excessive exposure to sunlight (ultraviolet burn)

Poisoning
Educate regarding hazards of taking nonprescription drugs and chemicals, including aspirin and alcohol
Keep potentially dangerous products in properly labeled receptacles—preferably out of reach

Falls
Instruct in proper use of playground equipment
Instruct in proper use and care of sports equipment, especially the more hazardous devices (e.g., skateboards, trampolines, skis)
Emphasize use of protective equipment when engaged in individual activities such as skateboarding and cycling and team sports such as soccer or hockey

Bodily damage
Help provide facilities for supervised activities
Encourage playing in safe places
Keep firearms safely locked up except during adult supervision
Teach proper care of, use of, and respect for devices with potential danger (e.g., power tools, firecrackers)
Stress eye protection when using potentially hazardous objects or devices or when engaged in potentially hazardous sports
Teach safety regarding use of corrective devices (glasses); if child wears contact lenses, monitor duration of wear to prevent corneal damage
Stress careful selection and maintenance of sport and recreation equipment
Emphasize proper conditioning for sports or other recreational activities
Caution against engaging in hazardous sports, such as those involving trampolines
Have identification on child, such as plastic "shoe pocket" attached to shoe laces

PARENTAL GUIDANCE DURING MIDDLE CHILDHOOD

Age (years)	Guidance
6	Expect strong food preferences and frequent refusals of specific food items
	Expect increasingly ravenous appetite
	Prepare parents for emotionality as child experiences erratic mood changes
	Anticipate increase in susceptibility to illness and more sickness than at previous ages
	Teach injury prevention and safety, especially bicycle safety
	Respect the child's need for privacy; provide a room of his own if possible
	Prepare for increasing interests outside the home
	Encourage interaction with peers
7-10	Expect improvement in health with fewer illnesses; however, allergies may increase or become apparent
	Prepare for increase in minor injuries
	Emphasize caution in selection and maintenance of sports equipment and re-emphasize teaching safety
	Expect increased involvement with peers and interest in activities outside the home
	Encourage independence but maintain limit-setting and discipline
	Expect more demands upon mother at 8 years
	Expect increasing admiration for father at 10 years; encourage father-child activities
	Prepare for prepubescent changes in girls
11-12	Prepare child for body changes of pubescence
	Expect a growth spurt in girls
	Make certain the child's sex education is adequate with accurate information
	Expect energetic but stormy behavior at 11 to become more even-tempered at 12
	Encourage child's desire to "grow up" but allow regressive behavior when needed
	Expect an increase in masturbation
	Child may need increased amount of rest
	Educate child regarding experimentation with potentially harmful activities

Health guidance
Provide for regular health and dental care
Teach and model sound health practices—including diet, rest, activity
Encourage children to engage in appropriate physical activities
Provide a safe physical and emotional environment
Teach and model safety practices

Recently, attention has been focused on injuries related to farm animals, equipment, and structures (Cogbill, Busch, and Stiers, 1985; Rivara, 1985). Agriculture is reported as the second most dangerous occupation in the United States (underground mining is first) (National Safety Council, 1983), and school-age children are involved in most of the farm activities and play in the farm environment. Many, including children of migrant workers, constitute a significant proportion of agricultural workers. Health facilities are also more scattered and less accessible for emergency treatment than they are in urban areas.

Injuries to eyes are a constant threat to school-age children involved in rough play (see Prevention, p. 1030). The normally shallow bony orbit of children in this age group make them particularly vulnerable to eye trauma, especially during contact sports or activities.

Nurse's Role in Injury Prevention

Nurses are primary advocates for preventive care and guidance. Safety education can be incorporated in all aspects of nursing care and anticipatory guidance for both parents and school-age children are part of nursing interventions. The most effective means of prevention is education of the child and family regarding the hazards of risk-taking and improper use of equipment. No piece of equipment is safe unless a child is physically and mentally equipped to use it. A careful history and a knowledge of normal growth and development serve as guidelines for both planned and impromptu consultation.

It is especially important for nurses to be conscientious regarding preventive teaching and guidance. Parents are often unaware of hazards to their children at various ages, especially those related to normal developmental progress. Primary physicians vary considerably in the efforts they expend in educating parents regarding preventive care. In one study related to automobile safety, it was found that only 29% of physicians always or usually ask if child restraints are used (Faber, Hoppe, and Diehl, 1985).

A major function of school nurses is preventive education and safety. They should be alert to hazards in the school and instrumental in evaluating safety risks and implementing safety programs. Preventive education for children, parents, and school personnel is an ongoing part of the school nurse's responsibility. Characteristics of the school-age child and preventive measures are listed on p. 745.

ANTICIPATORY GUIDANCE—CARE OF FAMILIES

The parents of the school-age child find themselves in the position of sharing their child's time and interests with the increasingly important peer group. As a child feels the need to fit into a peer group and gain a sense of industry through individual and cooperative production and performance, he moves away from the close, familiar relationships of the family group. It is through these early peer relationships that children begin to prepare for moving from narrow, sheltered family relationships to a broader world of relationships and increased independence. Parents must learn to provide support as unobtrusively as possible without feeling rejected, hurt, or angry. The nurse can help parents of the school-age child by providing anticipatory guidance and reassurance throughout this period of child development and maturation (see box).

CONCEPT SUMMARIES

- Middle childhood, ages 6 to 12 years, is a period when the school environment exercises a profound influence on development and relationships. It is an important period when children venture outside the family group, learn about their culture, and develop feelings of competence and self-esteem.

- Skeletal lengthening, higher ratio of muscle mass to fat, and maturation of the gastrointestinal system are major components in biologic development during middle childhood.

- Erikson's sense of industry, or stage of accomplishment, is a major task during the middle years.

- Freud described middle childhood as a latency period, a period of consolidation and elaboration of previously acquired traits and skills and development of the superego.

- Piaget's theory of concrete operations refers to the school-age period, when children are able to use their thought processes to experience events and actions and make judgments based on what they reason.

- Through identity, reversibility, and reciprocity, children master the cognitive task of conservation.

- Moral development progresses with the move to more logical thought, although much is still attributed to parental influence and standards.

- Spiritual development entails a curiosity about deities, a knowledge of the difference between the natural and supernatural, and reliance on prayers or other religious rituals.

- Entertaining different points of view, becoming sensitive to social norms of peers, and forming peer friendships are the most important features of social development in the middle years.

- Play takes the form of rules and ritual, team activity, quiet games and activities, and ego mastery.

- Typical parental concerns during middle childhood include dishonest behavior, lying, cheating, stealing, and school-related stress.

- Providing optimum nutrition may be hampered by availability of junk foods and coordinating meal schedules with working parents.

- Because of advanced intellectual activity, middle childhood may be the ideal time for formal sex education.

- School health programs commonly offer health appraisal, emergency care and safety, communicable disease control, counseling and guidance, adjustment to individual student needs, and health education.

REFERENCES

Abe, K., and others: Sleepwalking and recurrent sleeptalking in children of children sleepwalkers, Am. J. Psychiatry **141**:800-801, 1984.

American Academy of Pediatrics: Child safety suggestions: choosing the right size bicycle for your child, 1978, Evansville, IL.

Anders, T.F., and Keener, M.A.: Sleep-wake state development and disorders of sleep in infants, children, and adolescents. In Levine, M.D., and others: Developmental-behavioral pediatrics, Philadelphia, 1983, W.B. Saunders Co.

Beardslee, W., and Mack, J.: The impact of nuclear developments on children and adolescents. In Task Force Report No. 20, Washington, DC, 1982, American Psychological Association.

Betz, C.L.: Bicycle safety: opportunities for family education, Pediatr. Nurs. **9**:109-111, 1983.

Boraz, R.A.: Preventive dentistry for the pediatric patient, Issues Compr. Pediatr. Nurs. **5**:89-97, 1981.

Cogbill, T.H., Busch, H.M., and Stiers, G.R.: Farm accidents in children, Pediatrics **76**:562-566, 1985.

Committee on School Health: Administration of medication in school, Pediatrics **74**:433, 1984.

Committee on School Health: Health education and schools, Pediatrics **75**:1160-1161, 1985.

Committee on School Health: Sports medicine: health care for young athletes, Evanston, IL, 1983, American Academy of Pediatrics.

DeAngelis, C., and others: Comparative values of school physical examinations and mass screening tests, J. Pediatr. **102**:477-481, 1983.

Dietz, W.H., Jr., and Gortmaker, S.L.: Do we fatten our children at the television set? Obesity and television viewing in children and adolescents, Pediatrics **75**:807-812, 1985.

Egli, E.A., and Meyers, L.S.: Bull. Psychonomic Soc. **22**:309-312, 1984.

Elkind, D.: The hurried child. growing up too fast too soon, Menlo Park, CA, 1981, Addison-Wesley Publishing Co. Inc.

Ellis, D.: Video arcades, youth, and trouble, Youth Soc. **16**(1):47-65, 1984.

Erikson, E.H.: Childhood and society, ed. 2, New York, 1963, W.W. Norton & Co. Inc.

Faber, M.M., Hoppe, S.K., and Diehl, A.K.: Physician knowledge and clinical behavior regarding automobile safety for children, Pediatrics **75**:248-253, 1985.

Friede, A.M., and others: The epidemiology of injuries to bicycle riders, Pediatr. Clin. North Am. **32**:141-151, 1985.

Graybill, D., and others: Effects of playing violent versus nonviolent video games on the aggressive ideation of aggressive and nonaggressive children, Child Study J. **15**:199-205, 1985.

Greensher, J.: Prevention of childhood injuries, Pediatrics **74**(suppl.):970-975, 1984.

Guyer, B., and Gallagher, S.S.: An approach to the epidemiology of childhood injuries, Pediatr. Clin. North Am. **32**:5-15, 1985.

Klein, M.H.: The bite of Pac-Man, J. Psychohistory **11**:395-401, 1984.

Koster, M.K.: Self-care: health behavior for the school-age child, Top. Clin. Nurs. **5**(1):29-40, 1983.

Krugman, R.D., and Krugman, M.K.: Emotional abuse in the classroom, Am. J. Dis. Child. **138**:284-286, 1984.

Kuczen, B.: Childhood stress, New York, 1982, Delacorte Press.

Lasky, P.A., Gulbrandsen, M., and Scoblic, M.: Health education translated into health behavior, Issues Compr. Pediatr. Nurs. **5**:167-175, 1981.

Levine, M.D.: Middle childhood. In Levine, M.D., and others: Developmental-behavioral pediatrics, Philadelphia, 1983, W.B. Saunders Co.

Lewis, C.E., and Lewis, M.A.: Peer pressure and risk-taking behaviors in children, Am. J. Publ. Health **74**:580-584, 1984.

Long, T.J., and Long, L.: Latchkey children: the child's view of self care, U.S. Educational Resources Information Center, ERIC Document ED 214 666, 1982.

Magill, R.A., Ash, M.J., and Smoll, F.L., editors: Children in sport: a contemporary anthology, Champaign, IL, 1978, Human Kinetics Publishers.

Martens, R., and Seefeldt, V., editors: Guidelines for children's sports, The American Alliance for Health, Physical Education, Recreation, and Dance, 1979.

McClellan, M.A.: On their own: latchkey children, Pediatr. Nurs. **10**:198-202, 1984.

McCown, D.: TV: its problems for children, Pediatr. Nurs. **5**(2):17-19, 1979.

Moracco, J.C., and Camilleri, J.: A study of fears in elementary school children, Elementary Sch. Guid. Counsel. **18**:82-87, 1983.

National Safety Council: Accident facts, Chicago, 1983, National Safety Council.

Newman, B.M., and Newman, P.R.: Development through life: a psychosocial approach, ed. 3, Homewood, IL, 1984, Dorsey Press.

Oda, D.S., and others: Nurse practitioners and primary care in schools, J. Maternal Child Nurs. **10:**127-131, 1985.

Paulson, J.A.: Accidental injuries. In Behrman, R.E., and Vaughan, V.C., III: Textbook of pediatrics, ed. 12, Philadelphia, 1983, W.B. Saunders Co.

Pless, I.B., and Stulginskas, J.: Accidents and violence as a cause of morbidity and mortality in childhood, Adv. Pediatr. **29:**471-495, 1982.

Radencich, M.C.: From Dick and Jane to Tron? Reading World **24**(2):1-3, 1984.

Rivara, F.P., and Barber, M.: Demographic analysis of childhood pedestrian injuries, Pediatrics **76:**375-381, 1985.

Saunders, A., and Remsberg, B.: The stress-proof child, New York, 1984, Holt, Rinehart, and Winston.

Schowalter, J.E.: Common topics of parental concern: developmental considerations, Columbus, OH, 1983, Ross Laboratories.

Selnow, G.W.: Playing videogames: the electronic friend, J. Communic. **34:**148-156, 1984.

Shaffer, T.E.: The young athlete: new guidelines in sports medicine, Pediatr. Consult. **1**(5):1-12, 1980.

Shelton, P.G., and Ferretti, G.A.: Maintaining oral health, Pediatr. Clin. North Am. **29:**653-668, 1982.

Soper, W.B., and Miller, M.J.: Junk-time junkies: an emerging addiction among students, Sch. Counselor **31:**40-43, 1983.

BIBLIOGRAPHY
General

Allen, M.T.: An overview of the type A behavior pattern in children and adolescents, Pediatr. Nurs. **9:**407-412, 1983.

Belkengren, R.B., and Sapala, S.: Physical fitness from infancy through adolescence, Pediatr. Nurs. **8:**A-I, 1982.

Betz, C.L.: Faith development in children, Pediatr. Nurs. **7**(2):22-25, 1981.

Chess, S., and Thomas, A.: Temperamental differences: a critical concept in child health care, Pediatr. Nurs. **11:**167-171, 1985.

Committee on School Health: School health: a guide for health professionals, 1981, Evanston, IL, 1981, American Academy of Pediatrics.

DeAngelis, C.: Health care for the elementary school age child. In Green, M., and Haggerty, R.J.: Ambulatory pediatrics, Philadelphia, 1984, W.B. Saunders Co.

DuPont, R.L.: Phobias in children, Pediatrics **102:** 999-1002, 1983.

Elkind, D.: The child and society, New York, 1979, Oxford University Press, Inc.

Flavell, J.H.: Cognitive development, ed. 2, Englewood Cliffs, NJ, 1985, Prentice-Hall, Inc.

Garmezy, N.: Stressors of childhood. In Garmezy, N., and Rutter, M.: Stress, coping, and development in children, New York, 1983, McGraw-Hill, Inc.

Goldsmith, H.H., and Gottesman, I.I.: Origins of variation in behavioral style: a longitudinal study of temperament in young twins, Child Dev. **2:**91-99, 1981.

Hegvik, R.L., McDevitt, S.C., and Carey, W.B.: The middle childhood temperament questionnaire, Dev. Behav. Pediatr. **3**(6):197-200, 1982.

Kaluger, G., and Kaluger, M.F.: Human development: the span of life, ed. 3, St. Louis, 1984, The C.V. Mosby Co.

LaMontagne, L.L.: Three coping strategies used by school-age children, Pediatr. Nurs. **10:**25-28, 1984.

Lewis, C.E., Siegel, J.M., and Lewis, M.A.: Feeling bad: exploring sources of stress among pre-adolescent children, Am. J. Public Health **74:**117-122, 1984.

Maccoby, E.E.: Social development: psychological growth and the parent-child relationship, New York, 1980, Harcourt Brace Jovanovich, Inc.

McCown, D.E.: Moral development in children, Pediatr. Nurs. **10:**42-44, 1984.

Reasoner, R.W.: Enhancement of self-esteem in children and adolescents, Fam. Comm. Health **5**(2):51-64, 1983.

Schor, D.P.: Temperament and the initial school experience, Child Health Care **13:**129-134, 1985.

Selekman, J.: The development of body image in the child: a learned response, Top. Clin. Nurs. **5**(1):12-21, 1983.

Shaffer, D.R.: Developmental psychology: theory, research, and applications, Monterey, CA, 1985, Brooks/Cole Publishing Co.

Shelly, J.A.: The spiritual needs of children, Downers Grove, IL, 1982, Inter-Varsity Press.

Sherwin, L.N.: Separation: the forgotten phenonmenon of child development, Top. Clin. Nurs. **5**(1):1-11, 1983.

Southall, C.: Family life and sex education, Am. J. Nurs. **77:**1473-1476, 1977.

Stanwyck, D.J.: Self-esteem through the life span, Family Comm. Health **6**(2):11-28, 1983.

Stone, L.J., and Church, J.: Childhood and adolescence, ed. 5, New York, 1983, Random House, Inc.

Sutterly, D.C., and Donnelly, G.F.: Perspectives in human development, ed. 2, Philadelphia, 1980, J.B. Lippincott Co.

Switzer, K.H., and Kelly, J.T.: The nurse: a member of the school team, Am. J. Maternal Child Nurs. **6:**289-293, 1981.

Valenti, S.M.: Stressors at school age, Fam. Comm. Health **2**(4):15-29, 1980.

Williams, R.E., and Ceen, R.F.: Craniofacial growth and the dentition, Pedatr. Clin. North Am. **29**(3):503-522, 1982.

Wold, S.J.: School nursing: a framework for practice, St. Louis, 1981, The C.V. Mosby Co.

Zaichkowsky, L.D., Zaichkowsky, L.B., and Martinek, T.J.: Growth and development: the child and physical activity, St. Louis, 1980, The C.V. Mosby Co.

Health Promotion

Bausell, R.B.: A national survey assessing pediatric preventive behaviors, Pediatr. Nurs. **11:**438-444, 1985.

Bruhn, J.G., and Nader, P.R.: The school as a setting for health education, health promotion, and health care, Fam. Comm. Health **4**(1):57-69, 1982.

Courtnage, L.: The use of prescribed medication in the schools: a status report on the state policies and guidelines, J. Sch. Health **52:**543-548, 1982.

Cross, A.W.: Health screening in schools, Part I, J. Pediatr. **107:**487-494, 1985.

Cross, A.W.: Health screening in schools, Part II, J. Pediatr. **107:**653-661, 1985.

Czupryna, L.: Primary prevention in a camp setting, J. Maternal Child Nurs. **9:**197-199, 1984.

Dailey, C.P.: Teaching parents and children preventive health behaviors, Fam. Comm. Health **7**(1):34-43, 1985.

DeAngelis, C., and others: Achieving optimal immunization levels in school-age children, J. Pediatr. **103**(5):811-814, 1983.

Denehy, J.: What do school-age children know about their bodies? Pediatr. Nurs. **10:**290-292, 1984.

Gulbrandsen, M., Lasky, P.A., and Scoblic, M.: Translating health knowledge into health behavior, Issues Compr. Pediatr. Nurs. **5:**177-184, 1981.

Hull, H.F., and others: Risk factors for measles vaccine failure among immunized students, Pediatrics **76:**518-523, 1985.

Hussey, C.G., and Hirsh, A.M.: Health education for children, Top. Clin. Nurs. **5**(1):22-28, 1983.

Kaufman, D.H.: An interview guide for helping children make health-care decisions, Pediatr. Nurs. **11:**365-367, 1985.

Lasky, P.A., and Eichelberger, K.M.: Health-related views and self-care behaviors of young children, Fam. Rel. **34:**13-18, 1985.

Lewis, C.E., and Lewis, M.A.: Determinants of children's health-related beliefs and behaviors, Fam. Comm. Health **4** (4):85-97, 1982.

Lindsey, C.N., and others: Children on medication: a guide for teachers, Rehab. Lit. **41**(5-6):124-126, 1980.

Morris, N.M.: Pediatric health promotion through risk reduction, Fam. Comm. Health 3(1):63-76, 1980.

Murray, R., and Zentner, J.: Nursing assessment and health promotion through the life span, ed. 2, Englewood Cliffs, NJ, 1980, Prentice-Hall, Inc.

Oda, D.: A viewpoint on school nursing, Am. J. Nurs. **81**:1677-1678, 1981.

Otto, J.: Be prepared for camp nursing, Am. J. Nurs. **80**:906-907, 1980.

Perrin, E.C., and Perrin, J.M.: Clinician's assessments of children's understanding of illness, Am. J. Dis. Child. **13**:874-878, 1983.

Robinson, T.: School nurse practitioners on the job, Am. J. Nurs. **81**:1674-1676, 1981.

Seybold, S.A., and Klisch, M.L.: Preparing grade school faculty to teach family life education, J. Maternal Child Nurs. **7**:50-54, 1982.

Smith, N.J.: Sports participation: current developmental considerations in childhood and adolescence, Columbus, OH, 1985, Ross Laboratories.

Wold, L.J.: School nursing: problems and prospects. In Reinhardt, A.M., and Quinn, M.D., editors: Family centered community nursing, Vol. II, St. Louis, 1980, The C.V. Mosby Co.

Wood, S.P.: School aged children's perceptions of the causes of illness, Pediatr. Nurs. **9**:101-104, 1983.

Nutrition

Lowenberg, M.E.: The development of food patterns in young children. In Pipes, P.L.: Nutrition in infancy and childhood, ed. 3, St. Louis, 1985, The C.V. Mosby Co.

Williams, S.R.: Nutrition and diet therapy, ed. 5, St. Louis, 1985, Times Mirror/Mosby College Publishing.

Wurthman, J.J.: What do children eat? Eating styles of the preschool, elementary school, and adolescent child. In Suskind, R.M., editor: Textbook of pediatric nutrition, New York, 1981, Raven Press.

Injury Prevention

Agran, P.A., and Dunkle, D.E.: Motor vehicle occupant injuries to children in crash and noncrash events, Pediatrics **70**:993-996, 1982.

American Academy of Pediatrics: Child safety suggestions: safe bicycling, Evanston, IL, 1978, American Academy of Pediatrics.

Arenson, S., and others: Factors affecting parental use of child automobile safety restraints, Children's Health Care **13**(4):181-186, 1985.

Berger, L.R., Kaishman, S., and Rivara, F.P.: Injuries from fireworks, Pediatrics **75**:877-882, 1985.

Bergman, A.B.: Use of education in preventing injuries, Pediatr. Clin. North Am. **29**:331-338, 1982.

Committee on Accident and Poison Prevention: Automatic passenger protection systems, Pediatrics **74**:146-147, 1984.

Committee on Research, and Committee on Accident and Poison Prevention: Reducing the toll of injuries in childhood requires support for a focused research effort, Pediatrics **72**:736-737, 1983.

Greensher, J.: How anticipatory guidance can improve control of childhood "accidents," Pediatr. Consult. **3**(2):1-5, 1984.

Greensher, J., and Mofenson, H.C.: Injuries at play, Pediatr. Clin. North Am. **32**:127-139, 1985.

Guyer, B., Talbot, A.M., and Pless, I.B.: Pedestrian injuries to children and youth, Pediatr. Clin. North Am. **32**:163-174, 1985.

Micik, S., and Miclette, M.: Injury prevention in the community: a systems approach, Pediatr. Clin. North Am. **32**:251-265, 1985.

Power mower injuries: is there lack of anticipatory guidance? Wellcome Trends, March 1985.

Righi, F.C., and Krozy, R.E.: The child in the car: what every nurse should know about safety, Am. J. Nurs. **83**: 1421-1424, 1983.

Rivara, F.P.: Traumatic deaths of children in the United States: currently available prevention strategies, Pediatrics **75**:456-462, 1985.

Rivara, F.P.: Fatal and nonfatal farm injuries to children and adolescents in the United States, Pediatrics **76**:567-573, 1985.

Westman, J.A., and Morrow, G.: Moped injuries in children, Pediatrics **74**:820-822, 1984.

Zuckerman, B.S., and Duby, J.C.: Developmental approach to injury prevention, Pediatr. Clin. North Am. **32**:17-29, 1985.

Chapter 18

Health Problems of Middle Childhood

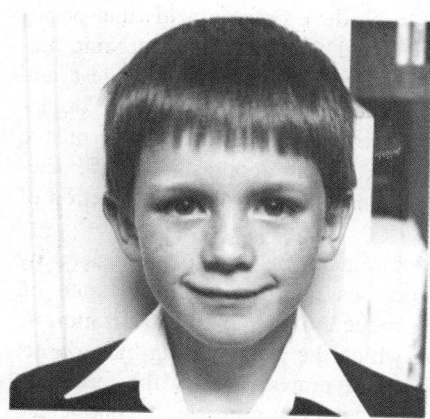

As a group, school-age children are fairly healthy when compared with children in infancy and early childhood, and ages 9 to 12 are usually the healthiest years. As would be expected, respiratory illnesses (the leading cause of morbidity) and gastrointestinal upsets are most common. A factor contributing to this overall health state is the quantity of lymphoid tissue, at its height during this stage, which helps to fight infection and ward off disease. An eleven-year-old child has almost twice the amount of a young adult.

Most children in this age-group have either contracted the communicable diseases of childhood or have been immunized against them. Their excellent appetites, adequate rest, and sufficient physical exercise further contribute to their general good health. The common health problems of school-age children are not illnesses of serious import as individual entities and all are amenable to therapy. Conditions that are not uncommon in middle childhood are dental problems and emotional or behavior disorders. Allergic manifestations, especially asthma, may reach a peak during the middle childhood years, and a variety of other serious disorders make a significant contribution to childhood morbidity. These will be considered as appropriate in relation to ill children.

Dental Problems

Since all of the permanent teeth (except the wisdom teeth) erupt during middle childhood, dental health is of particular importance. Ideally children should receive regular preventive dental care and supervision in daily hygienic care from the time the teeth begin to erupt (see pp. 613 and 726). The importance of dental care is undisputed; however, limited or inadequate dental care results in the most prevalent of all childhood health problems, chiefly dental caries, malocclusion, peridontal disease, and trauma. Although these conditions are not considered illnesses, they have harmful long-range effects on children's health.

DENTAL CARIES

Dental caries is one of the most common chronic diseases that affect individuals at all ages. Although 100% preventable, dental caries is the principal oral problem in children and adolescents. While the overall incidence of dental caries in children has decreased since the introduction of fluoridation, it is still an important health problem. Reducing the incidence and consequences of the disorder is of primary importance in childhood because dental caries, if untreated, results in total destruction of involved teeth. The ages of greatest vulnerability are 4 to 8 years for the primary dentition and 12 to 18 years for the secondary or permanent dentition (see pp. 519 and 727 for sequence of tooth eruption).

Pathophysiology

Dental caries is a multifactorial disease. The incidence of lesions and the likelihood of progressive invasion vary considerably and depend on a number of factors being present in the right combination: (1) the host, (2) microorganisms, (3) substrate, and (4) time.

Host. The prevalence of caries is directly related to the tooth size and morphology and to the consistency, composition, and amount of saliva. Improperly developed, crowded, or deeply fissured teeth increase the incidence of caries. The areas most subject to attack by bacteria are (in order of difficulty of complete cleansing) grooves and fis-sures, interdermal areas, gum margins, and other smooth surfaces. Newly erupted teeth that have not yet acquired sufficient surface minerals are more susceptible to decay than those that have been erupted for 2 or more years. Undoubtedly hereditary factors influence resistance and susceptibility, since similar patterns and anatomic characteristics are seen in successive generations. Salivary flow can mechanically clean away bacteria and food debris. It also contains buffering systems, lysozymes, peroxidases, and immunoglobulins that influence the development of caries.

Microorganisms. Three types of microflora that produce different effects contribute to the formation of dental caries. Acidogenic bacteria act on fermentable carbohydrates in dental plaque to produce organic acids that decalcify hard surface tooth enamel. With the inner organic matrix exposed, proteolytic organisms and acids digest and destroy the inner tooth structure. These destructive organisms are harbored and protected in a gelatinous plaque formed on the tooth surface by still another group of bacteria that are thought to play no primary role in production of decay.

Substrates. Caries formation is strongly influenced by the two concurrent processes that continually operate on enamel surfaces—acid production and acid neutralization by saliva. The material on which the acid-forming bacteria act consists essentially of carbohydrates. Among the fermentable carbohydrates, sucrose has been consistently implicated as the most cariogenic. Sucrose-containing substances, especially in tenacious forms that cling (such as chewy candy) or that promote prolonged contact with the teeth (such as chewing gum, hard candy, and lollipops), when ingested between meals, contribute markedly to the development of dental caries. Saliva and other foods that are ingested at mealtime tend to help neutralize much of the acid formed from sucrose.

Time and other factors. Bacterial enzymes act on salivary glycoproteins to produce a tenacious protein matrix on the tooth surface. This substance along with the microorganisms forms *dental plaque*. If plaque removal is inadequate or nonexistent for a significant length of time (a few days), the plaque is metabolized by the bacteria to form acid, which initiates the demineralization of enamel (Rule, 1982).

Other factors that contribute to caries formation are heredity, the amount of fluoride in drinking water, lack of or ineffectual oral hygiene, and the child's general state of health. Hereditary factors appear to influence both resistance and susceptibility to dental caries. For example, structural defects, such as deep fissures on occlusive surfaces, predispose to decay, and persons in whom acid formation exceeds neutralization are more prone to caries. The effectiveness of the buffering action of saliva is highly variable among individuals.

Fluoride incorporated into the crystallites of the surface enamel increases the resistance to acid dissolution. Poor oral hygiene that permits the accumulation of food debris on tooth surfaces provides for proliferation of acid-forming bacteria that thrive in this environment. Removal of food particles and bacteria-laden plaque inhibits destructive acid formation.

The susceptibility to dental decay may be influenced by the general health of the child. Children who suffer from chronic debilitating disease show increased caries activity, as do children with systemic conditions that alter the quality and quantity of saliva produced.

Diagnostic Evaluation

Because the permanent teeth erupt during middle childhood, children are more susceptible to development of dental caries during this time than at any other age. Caries penetrate the vulnerable teeth rapidly at this age, as opposed to the slower, intermittent activity characteristic at later ages.

Caries on visible surfaces are easily detected by oral inspection. Large, extensive caries are apparent even to the untrained eye, but small, beginning lesions are best identified by trained professionals. Caries between the teeth may not be located without x-ray examination.

Therapeutic Management

Dental caries can usually be controlled by the following measures:

1. Frequent, regular observation by a dentist beginning when all primary teeth have erupted but at least by 3 years of age. The recommended frequency is usually twice yearly, but this depends on the individual child. Deep fissures and grooves of susceptible teeth are covered with a plasticized sealant, which is effective in blocking cavity formation.
2. Surgical removal of all carious portions of teeth as soon as detected, preparation of a retentive cavity, and replacement of the lost portion of the tooth with a material that is durable in the mouth environment. This restoration of involved teeth not only prevents progression of established caries but also reduces the number of bacteria in the oral cavity to decrease the danger to uninvolved teeth.
3. Oral hygiene that emphasizes thorough mechanical removal of plaque and other material from tooth surfaces by brushing, rinsing, and the use of dental floss. Cleansing is most effective when carried out after meals and snacks.
4. Elimination of concentrated sugars between meals and reducing the mealtime ingestion of sweets to a minimum. This includes excessive ingestion of sweetened soft drinks and juices.
5. Sound nutrition practices including an adequate intake of building materials, such as protein, calcium, fluoride, and vitamin D, to help form teeth that resist caries and build healthy supporting structures.
6. Systemic administration and topical application of fluoride to the teeth. Increase in the concentration of fluoride in the surface enamel is believed to be the most effective preventive measure against dental caries in young children. Many pedodontists also advocate the use of fluoridated toothpaste for dental hygiene.

Nursing Considerations

Oral inspection is an integral part of the nursing assessment of the child in any setting. If there is any evidence of dental caries or other unhealthy state, the child is referred for dental services. The family may have a family dentist or a pedodontist who can provide needed care. An alarming number of children do not receive regular dental supervision, and a significant number reach adulthood without having been examined or treated by a dentist. Nurses can be active members of preventive educational programs and serve as counselors to families regarding the importance of regular dental care, oral hygiene, and dietary management.

Nurses can encourage good oral hygiene by teaching correct tooth cleaning to both children and their parents. The random brushing allowed during the early childhood years should be replaced by more careful and methodical cleansing techniques. Children are taught to brush the teeth according to the method recommended by the dentist and the proper use of dental floss (p. 613). The importance of regular administration of fluoride is emphasized (see p. 614). School-age children can usually manage the chewable tablets, which have both a topical and a systemic effect. It is often difficult for parents to give medications on a daily basis over a period of years; therefore the children are taught to assume responsibility for taking fluoride as part of their daily dental hygiene.

Restriction of cariogenic foods is also important in the preventive management of dental caries, but this should be viewed as an activity in which all family members are involved and not simply a directive for the child to obey. It should not be communicated in such a way that the child interprets the withholding of sweets as a punishment. Children with chronic illness who regularly take medications containing sugar are cautioned to brush their teeth after taking the medication just as they would after eating any carbohydrate substance. Children taking tricyclic antidepressants are more prone to develop dental caries.

Sometimes the greatest task for nurses is not the teaching aspect of dental care but counseling children and families for motivation to develop sound dental hygiene and nutritional practices. Children should be prepared for dental services in such a way that visits to the dentist are a positive experience. Keeping appointments and following through on recommended treatments and practices are habits that extend beyond childhood.

PERIODONTAL DISEASE

Periodontal disease, inflammatory and degenerative conditions involving the gums and tissues supporting the teeth, often begins in childhood and accounts for a significant amount of tooth loss in adulthood. The more common periodontal problems are *gingivitis* (simple inflammation of the gums) and *periodontitis* (inflammation of the gums and loss of connective tissue and bone in the supporting structures of the teeth). An uncommon condition is *acute necrotizing ulcerative gingivitis* ("trench mouth").

The most prevalent periodontal disease, gingivitis, begins very early in many children and is associated with the buildup of plaque on the teeth. Changes take place in the plaque bacteria, in both type and number of organisms,

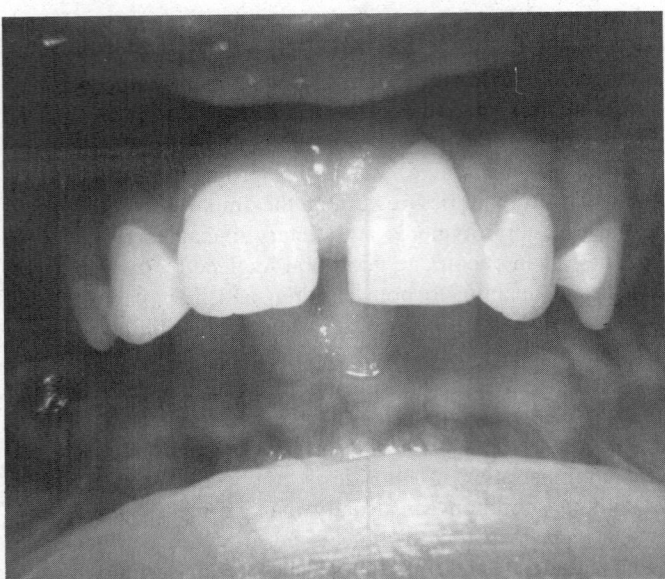

Fig. 18-1. Malocclusion in a school-age child.
Courtesy Dr. Frank Sommer, Tulsa, OK.

causing them to release a variety of destructive exotoxins, enzymes, and other noxious agents. They act to produce an inflammatory reaction in the gingival tissues, causing the gums to become red, edematous, tender, and subject to bleeding at the slightest irritation.

Management is directed toward prevention by conscientious brushing and flossing and by depriving the bacteria of the substrates required to produce the disease. The implementation and maintenance of preventive dental practice plus good dental hygiene are effective in preventing both caries and periodontal disease.

Nursing Considerations

Nursing care for the child with periodontal disease is primarily preventive; it includes education regarding dental hygiene and regular inspection of the gingival tissues for signs of early inflammation. The child should be directed to see the dentist at any signs of inflammation or irritation.

MALOCCLUSION

When teeth of the upper and lower dental arches approximate in the proper relationships, the physiologic function of mastication is more effective and the cosmetic effect is more pleasing. Teeth that are uneven, crowded, or overlapping or that otherwise interfere with their ability to meet their opponents in the opposite jaw in the appropriate relationships may be predisposed to dental disease (Fig. 18-1). More than half of children 12 to 17 years of age suffer from malocclusions that could be corrected (Guide to Dental Health, 1985).

The most common cause of malocclusion is hereditary factors, but abnormal growth and habits such as thumb-sucking and tongue thrusting also contribute to the disordered alignment and occlusion of the teeth. The important aspects in treatment of malocclusion are elimination of habits that aggravate the deformity and corrective therapy at the optimum time. Orthodontic treatment is usually most successful when it is started in the later school-age years or the early adolescent years, after the last primary teeth have been shed and before growth ceases. However, the trend is toward early correction to prevent problems if the irregularity interferes with normal function and speech; therefore referral should be made as soon as malocclusion is evident. For example, removal of extra teeth, impacted teeth, or prosthetic replacement of missing teeth can prevent problems from developing.

Nursing Considerations

The nurse who detects evidence of malocclusion in a child is obligated to recommend that the teeth be examined by a dentist for possible orthodontia. With the trend toward earlier correction, the sooner the child is evaluated the better will be the chance for receiving needed treatment. Dealing with habits that predispose to malocclusion, such as thumb or finger sucking, is more difficult to manage.

Although orofacial appearance is a subjective phenomenon, there may be a risk of adverse effect on a child's self-esteem and body image. Poorly aligned teeth can be a source of psychologic as well as physical stress to affected children. Many children with malocclusion suffer from teasing from peers or siblings if the irregularities are severe enough (Graber and Lucher, 1980). However, it is usually the parents who initiate an orthodontic examination.

After fixed appliances, or braces, have been applied, the child is advised that there will be some discomfort for a few days. During the orthodontic treatments, which average 18 to 30 months, proper oral hygiene is vital. Although the bands or brackets protect the teeth they cover, plaque can collect on the unprotected surfaces or under loose-fitting bands. The teeth are to be brushed with a fluoride toothpaste after every meal and snack and at bedtime, using the method recommended by the dentist. Some orthodontists recommend using an oral irrigating device to remove food from between the teeth and around the braces. However, the device does not remove plaque and is not a substitute for thorough brushing. The orthodontist cautions the child about foods that should not be eaten. Some can damage the braces; others may be difficult to remove from the teeth during cleaning. Forbidden items include chewing gum, ice, nuts, toffee, hard candy, corn-on-the-cob, uncut apples, hard taco shells, and nachos.

Occasionally tooth movement or poking at braces with a pencil or other object may cause an arch wire to break or protrude. If this happens the child is instructed to cover the broken portion with a special wax provided by the dentist and schedule an appointment as soon as possible. Regular visits are usually scheduled every 3 to 6 weeks.

TRAUMA

Injury to the teeth is not an uncommon occurrence in childhood. This includes fractures of varying degrees of severity, dislocation, or evulsion. All tooth injuries require prompt treatment by a competent dentist in order to prevent permanent displacement or loss. Delayed examination and diagnosis of tooth damage all too frequently result in infection or pulp involvement that can be avoided by early attention.

There are three periods during childhood when children experience an increased frequency of dental trauma (Berkowitz, Ludwig, and Johnson, 1980):

1. Preschool (1 to 3 years): injury is usually secondary to falls or child abuse
2. School age (7 to 10 years): injury is more often subsequent to bicycle and playground accidents
3. Adolescence (16 to 18 years): injury is generally sustained secondary to fights, athletic injury, and automobile accidents

Boys experience injury to permanent teeth much more frequently than girls, although this observation is not supported in all studies. Trauma usually involves the maxillary incisors, and children with protruding teeth, craniofacial abnormalities, or neuromuscular disorders are more likely to sustain dental injuries.

Nursing Considerations: Tooth Evulsion

A tooth that is evulsed (avulsed, exarticulated, or "knocked out") should be replanted by the child, parent, or nurse and stabilized as soon as possible. If the tooth is replaced within 30 minutes, there is a 70% chance that it will become reattached and roots will not resorb or the crown exfoliate.

Before reimplantation it is important to carefully rinse a dirty tooth under running water to avoid disturbing the adhering periodontal membrane, which is essential to the success of the reimplantation. The tooth is held by the crown, not the root, while rinsing, with the drain plugged. The tooth is then gently replaced in the socket and held in place by the child during transportation to a dentist. Care is taken to avoid sudden stops or turns that might cause the child to swallow or aspirate the loose tooth.

If the child or parents are reluctant to reimplant the tooth, the next best alternative is to place the tooth in cold milk for transport to the dentist. The cold milk has precisely the osmolality to maintain fluid balance within the tissues surrounding the tooth. The third best means of transport is under the child's tongue, or under the parent's tongue if the child is too young or too anxious. After implantation the tooth will usually become firmly attached, although endodontic therapy is always required and the tooth is eventually replaced by a prosthetic device. The reimplanted tooth may be retained anywhere from 6 months to 12 years and serves to facilitate normal development and occlusion, since loss of teeth during the period of permanent tooth eruption may adversely affect such development.

Emergency Treatment: *Evulsed Tooth*

Recover tooth
Hold tooth by crown; avoid touching root area
If tooth is dirty, rinse it gently under running water or saline; be sure to insert drain in sink or basin (to avoid tooth loss)
Insert tooth into socket
Have child maintain tooth in place
Transport child to dentist immediately
Avoid sudden stops or sharp turns to prevent dislodging tooth

---

If reluctant to reimplant tooth:
Place evulsed tooth in suitable medium for transport
  a. Cold milk
  b. Saliva—under the child's or parent's tongue
If child is holding tooth in, avoid sudden stops to prevent swallowing tooth

DON'T FORGET TO TAKE TOOTH

Disorders Affecting the Skin

Skin disorders are common at all ages; therefore many skin disorders that are usually limited to a specific age-group are discussed in relation to children in that age category, for example, birthmarks in the newborn, diaper rash and eczema in infancy, and acne during adolescence. Chemical dermatitis caused by poisons is included in the discussion of poisoning in Chapter 16.

THE SKIN

The skin and its component and associated structures constitute the integumentary system. The largest organ in the body, the skin is a thin structure (only about 1 mm thick at birth, increasing to approximately twice that thickness at maturity) that serves primarily as an insulator, not as an organ of exchange.

Anatomically and physiologically the skin differs markedly in various areas of the body, and each variation is adapted to meet special stresses. Regions such as the soles of the feet, the eyelids, and the back vary in skin thickness and looseness and in the kinds and quantities of appendages they contain, such as sweat glands and hair follicles. These variations are the basis for the localization of many disorders to specific areas and for the distribution of certain eruptions in characteristic patterns.

Purposes of the Skin

This functionally simple but morphologically complex structure serves several physical functions essential to life.

Protection. The skin serves as a protection against trauma, including mechanical, thermal, chemical, and ra-

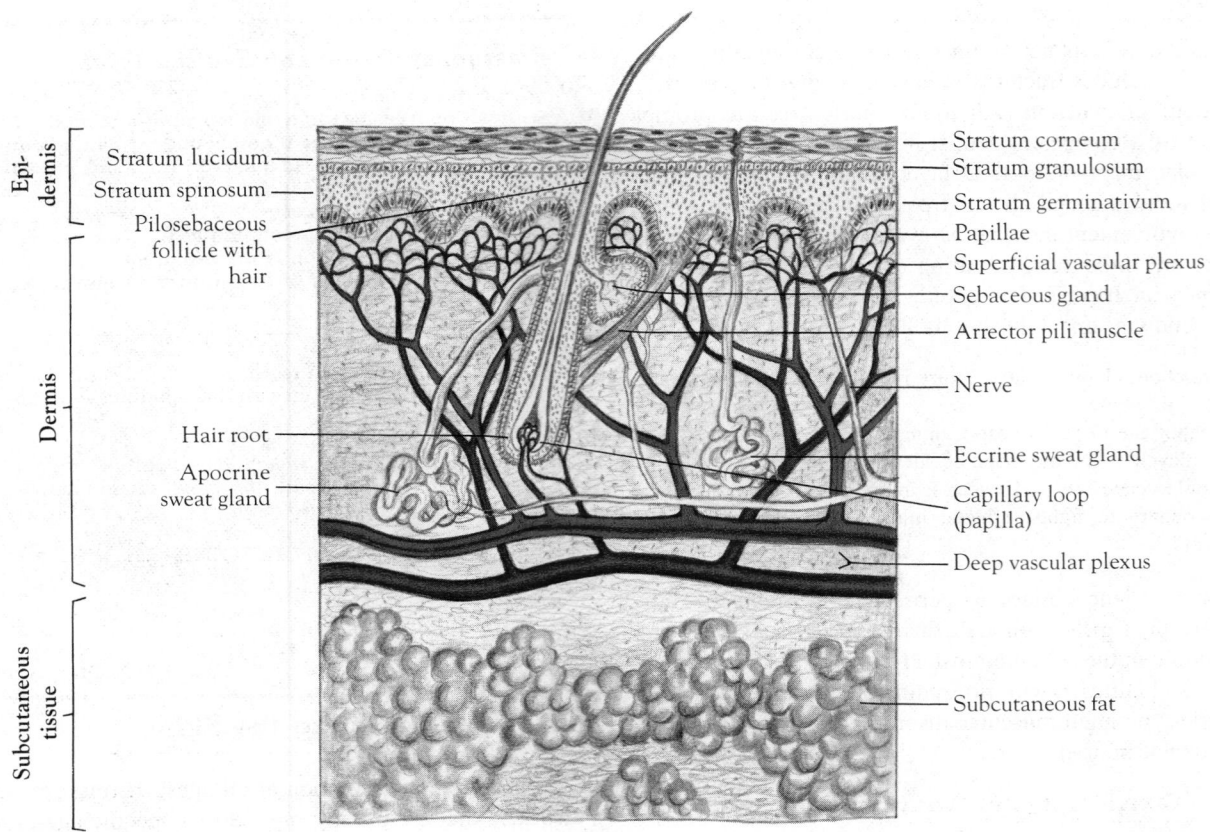

Fig. 18-2. Cross-section of normal skin.

From Thompson, J.M., and others: Clinical nursing, St. Louis, 1986, The C.V. Mosby Co., p. 544.

diant. The intact tough outer layer is a mechanical barrier. Organisms and chemicals penetrate it with difficulty, and it is further protected by the oily and slightly acid secretions of its sebaceous glands, which limit the growth of bacteria.

Impermeability. Very few substances are able to penetrate the skin with ease. It seals the body from the environment. The outer side of the upper layer, with its low water content, is in equilibrium with the viable cells underneath. It protects against loss of essential body constituents to the environment. The effectiveness of this impermeable membrane is demonstrated by the profuse fluid loss that follows damage to the epidermis by superficial burns, injury, poison ivy, or other agents. Loss of water and some electrolytes takes place only through pores in this effective barrier.

Heat regulation. The skin also adjusts heat loss to heat production to maintain the thermal balance of the body. This is accomplished primarily through functioning of cutaneous blood vessels and sweat glands. The vascular supply to the skin, much more extensive than needed for tissue nourishment, is regulated by way of central and local neural and hormonal processes.

Sensation. As a sensory organ, perceptions (touch, pain, heat, and cold) are registered through the nerves that permeate the skin. To some extent, skin is also an organ of

expression that betrays strong feelings: blushing (shame or embarrassment), redness (anger), blanching (fear), and sweating (anxiety).

Skin Structure

The skin consists of three layers: the epidermis, the corium or dermis, and an inner layer composed of fatty tissue of varying thickness that separates the skin from the subcutaneous tissues. The activity of the skin is controlled by the autonomic nervous system and the endocrine glands (Fig. 18-2).

The efficiency with which the skin layers prevent evaporative loss of water (independent of sweat) increases with development. A transitional zone between the epidermal layers allows more of the larger fluid content (70%) of the lower layers to enter the outer, drier layers (15% water), where it is lost in greater or lesser amounts depending on environmental temperature and humidity. In the young child the transitional zone is less effective than that in an older child or adult. The fluid loss is most marked in the prematurely born infant.

Epidermis. The epidermis, the outermost layer of relatively uniform thickness, is separated from the dermis by a layer of specialized cells called basal cells that are continually replacing the cell population. As they multiply, the older cells are displaced outwardly by the constant stream of new cells. The older cells progressively flatten and alter until they form dead, scalelike, or horny flakes with no cellular details and composed of *keratin*. These flakes are constantly sloughed off the surface of the body. This continual epidermal renewal is nourished by fluid from blood vessels in the dermis. The intact epidermis provides a relatively impenetrable barrier to the loss of body contents and the entrance of environmental hazards.

Elaborating this outer layer are specialized cellular invaginations of epidermal origin, the glandular appendages and hair follicles. Although they are situated mainly in the dermis, these structures are lined with epithelial cells and are derived from the epithelial skin layer. This has significance when a large area of epidermis is damaged. It is from the cells lining these structures that new epithelium is derived.

Diseases of the skin focus sharply on the epidermis, which is the site of many distinctive patterns ranging from the vesiculation of contact dermatitis to common superficial tumors. Clearly visible, these morphologic changes produce the varied patterns on which a dermatologic diagnosis is made.

Dermis. The dermis, or *corium,* constitutes the bulk of the skin. It is a firm, fibrous, and elastic connective tissue network containing an elaborate system of blood vessels, lymphatics, and nerves and varies throughout the body from 1 to 4 mm in thickness. In addition, it is invaded by the epidermal downgrowth of hair follicles and glands. Functionally the corium has a major protective role for these varied essential components of the skin.

More hidden than the epidermis, changes in the corium are more difficult to interpret on inspection. Biopsy and histologic studies are more often needed to confirm a diagnosis based on manifestations in the corium. Since it is composed predominantly of connective tissue, the dermis frequently permits an awareness and observation of many diffuse systemic disorders of connective tissue—the "collagen" diseases.

Subcutaneous tissue. A thick layer of subcutaneous tissue lies beneath the dermis and is composed of a looser type of connective tissue that varies greatly in extent in various parts of the body. In addition to larger blood vessels, lymph channels, and nerve trunks, the subcutaneous tissue serves as a depot for the storage of fat that acts as a cushion, insulates the body against cold, and largely determines its contours.

Hair. The various skin appendages develop at different times and at different rates. An extensive growth of fine body hair, lanugo, begins to appear at the end of the second intrauterine month, reaches its maximum development between the seventh and eighth months of fetal life, and begins to decrease before birth. It continues to regress steadily during early infancy and is replaced by a less extensive distribution of hair. Hair follicles are fully developed at birth but the amount and texture of scalp hair vary between individual infants. The scalp hair is lost during the first few months after birth, then is slowly replaced by permanent hair, which gradually thickens and often darkens as the child grows.

At puberty the secretion of androgenic hormones stimulates an increase in the thickening and darkening of scalp hair, the growth of hair in the axilla and pubic regions of both sexes, and the growth of facial hair in boys. Late in adolescence some boys acquire additional amounts and distribution of body hair, such as on the chest.

Sebaceous glands. The sebaceous glands form in connection with hair follicles. Their function is to produce a fatty secretion called sebum that helps keep the skin supple by decreasing water loss. The sebaceous activity is maintained at a relatively constant rate by the secretion of androgens; an increase in androgens causes an increase in sebum production. Sebaceous glands have a regional distribution and are most abundant on the scalp, the face, and the genitals; are less numerous on the trunk; are sparse on the extremities; and do not appear on the palms and soles.

Sebaceous glands begin to form during the fifth month of fetal life and are very active during the month before birth, when they produce the protective vernix caseosa observed on newborn infants. The sebaceous activity slowly subsides after birth and continues to decrease throughout infancy. In the newborn period and early infancy sebaceous secretion may cause minor problems such as "cradle cap" in some infants. The secretion remains low during early childhood, which contributes to dryness and susceptibility to chapping, especially during the winter months. Sebaceous secretion gradually rises in childhood to increase markedly at puberty, where it remains constant and contributes greatly to the disturbing skin problems of adolescence.

Sweat glands. The sweat glands, both eccrine and apocrine, are present at birth. They appear between the fifth and seventh months of fetal life, but their activity is scant. The eccrine sweat glands function primarily as part of the body heat–regulating mechanism and to some extent in maintaining electrolyte balance. At birth the density of the eccrine glands is greater than at any time of life (because of the smaller skin surface area) because no new glands are formed after birth. The sweat glands are equivalent in size, structural maturity, and position within the dermis in the full-term newborn and the adult (Shalita, 1981). They function poorly at birth but produce more sweat as childhood advances, to reach full potential at puberty. There are individual differences in the amount of sweat produced, and there are no sex differences until after puberty, when males sweat more than females. Numerous factors influence the amount and chemical content of the sweat, for example, emotions and some disease states such as congestive heart failure in infancy and cystic fibrosis. The apocrine sweat glands are located primarily in the axilla and the genital and anal areas. They are inactive throughout infancy and childhood and mature during puberty.

Skin of younger children. The major skin layers arise from different embryologic origins. Early in the embryonic period, a single layer of epithelium forms from the ectoderm, while simultaneously the corium develops from the mesenchyme. In the infant and small child the epidermis is still loosely bound to the corium. This poor adherence causes the layers to separate readily during an inflammatory process to form blisters. This is especially true in preterm infants, who have an even greater propensity to blister formation and separation during careless handling (such as removal of adhesive tape). The skin is thinner than in older children and the cells of all strata are more compressed.

Several characteristics influence skin responses in infants and young children. Their skin is far more susceptible to superficial bacterial infection. They are more likely to have associated systemic symptoms with some infections and are more apt to react to a primary irritant than to a sensitizing allergen. Infants and young children are more frequently affected by chronic atopic dermatitis (eczema). The infant's skin is much more prone to develop a toxic erythema as a result of skin eruptions or drug reactions and is subject to maceration, infection, and the sweat retention associated with diaper rash.

Pathophysiology

Lesions of the skin can be a result of a wide variety of specific etiologic factors. In general skin lesions originate from (1) contact with injurious agents such as infectious organisms, toxic chemicals, and physical trauma, (2) hereditary factors, (3) some external factor that produces a reaction in the skin (for example, allergens), or (4) a systemic disease of which the lesions are a cutaneous manifestation (e.g., measles, lupus erythematosus, nutritional deficiency diseases). Such responses are highly individual. An agent that may be harmless to one individual may be damaging to another, and a single agent may produce various types of responses in different individuals.

Among other factors involved in the etiology of skin manifestations is the age of the child. For example, infants are subject to "birthmark" malformations and atopic dermatitis that appears early in life, the school-age child is susceptible to ringworm of the scalp, and acne is a characteristic skin disorder of puberty. Contact dermatitis, such as poison ivy, is seen only where the noxious agent is a feature of the area. Similarly, reactions to animal bites are associated with life cycle and seasonal activities. Although less common in children, tension and anxiety may produce, modify, or prolong many skin conditions.

Over half of dermatologic problems are various forms of dermatitis. This implies a sequence of inflammatory changes in the skin that are grossly and microscopically similar but that are diverse in course and causation. Acute responses produce intercellular and intracellular edema, the formation of intradermal vesicles, and an initial minimum infiltration of inflammatory cells into the epidermis. In the dermis there is edema, vascular dilation, and early perivascular cellular infiltration. The location and manner of these reactions produce the lesions characteristic of each disorder. The changes are reversible, and the skin ordinarily recovers without blemish, completely intact, unless complicating factors such as ulceration from the primary irritant, scratching, and infection are introduced or if underlying vascular disease develops. In chronic conditions more permanent effects are seen that vary according to the disorder, the general condition of the affected individual, and available therapy.

Clinical Manifestations

One of the advantages of skin disorders is that often the diagnosis is readily established after simple, careful inspection. Much can be determined by the distribution, size, and arrangement of the components of the lesions and by the morphology of individual lesions. In addition, intrinsic causes must be distinguished from extrinsic causes. Extrinsic causes usually result from physical, chemical, or allergic irritants or from an infectious agent such as bacteria, fungi, viruses, or animal parasites. Skin manifestations can be produced by such intrinsic causes as a specific infection, drug sensitization, or other allergic phenomena.

Lesion. According to the nature of the pathologic process, lesions assume more or less distinct characteristics. They are usually the result of disturbance of function, inflammation, or growth. Although the names that have been applied to these lesions are of little value in themselves, they are important for descriptive purposes in the processes of record keeping and communication. To examine the various aspects of the lesion requires that the inspection take place under natural or adequate artificial light. A low-powered magnifying lens serves as a useful adjunct and, in diseases with abnormalities of pigmentation or those associated with fluorescence, a Wood light is useful.

Nurses should become familiar with the more common terms used to describe the following skin lesions seen in dermatologic conditions:

erythema A reddened area caused by increased amounts of oxygenated blood in the dermal vasculature

ecchymoses (bruises) Localized red or purple discolorations caused by extravasation of blood into dermis and subcutaneous tissues

petechiae Pinpoint tiny and sharply circumscribed spots in the superficial layers of the epidermis

primary lesions Skin changes produced by some causative factor (Fig. 18-3)

secondary lesions Changes that result from alteration in the primary lesions, such as those caused by rubbing, scratching, medication, or involution and healing (Fig. 18-4)

Distribution pattern. How lesions are distributed over the body is a useful aid in diagnosis. Local processes are distinguished from generalized ones. Many lesions are primarily associated with specific areas, such as extensor areas in atopic dermatitis or uncovered areas that allow exposure to sun or noxious agents such as poison ivy; others are related to location of specific cutaneous appendages, such as the unique sebaceous gland distribution of acne.

Fig. 18-3. Primary skin lesions.

Flat circumscribed area of color changes less than 1 cm in diameter, neither elevated nor depressed and with no alteration in skin texture

Example: Freckle, nevus, measles

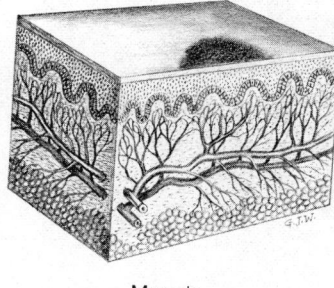

Macule

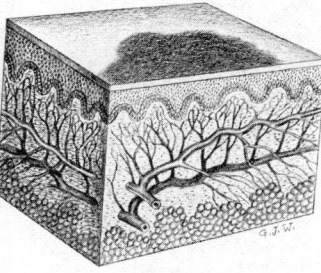

Patch

Flat circumscribed discoloration of skin greater than 1 cm in diameter

Example: Mongolian spot, vitiligo

Small, circumscribed solid elevation of the skin, less than 1 cm in diameter; exists mostly above the plane of the skin surface, and the more superficial it is, the more distinct are the borders

Example: Wart, ringworm

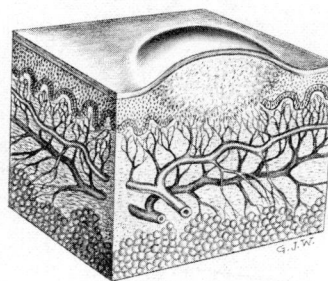

Papule

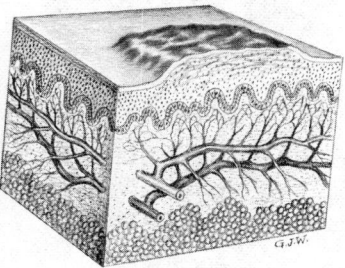

Plaque

Flattened, raised lesion in which the surface area involved is relatively large in relation to its height

Example: Psoriasis

Solid circumscribed elevation, round or ellipsoid, located deep in dermis or subcutaneous tissue

Example: Dermatofibroma

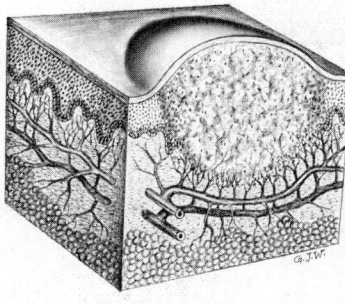

Nodule

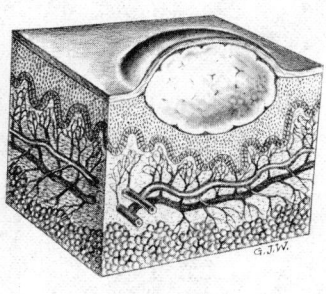

Tumor

Circumscribed infiltration of skin or subcutaneous tissue that is larger (greater than 1 cm in diameter) and deeper than nodule

Example: Cavernous hemangioma

Encapsulated semisolid or fluid-filled mass in dermis or subcutaneous tissue

Example: Epidermoid cyst

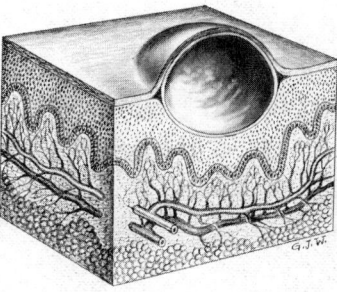

Cyst

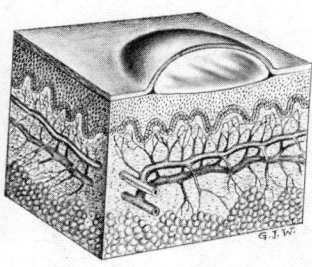

Vesicle

Small (less than 1 cm in diameter), superficial circumscribed elevation of the skin containing serous or blood-tinged fluid

Example: Chickenpox, herpes, poison ivy, dermatitis

Continued.

Fig. 18-3, cont'd. Primary skin lesions.

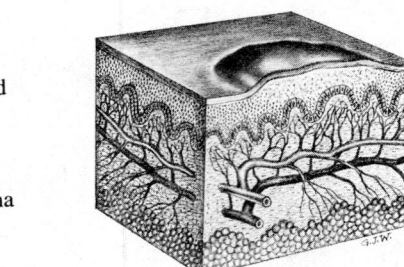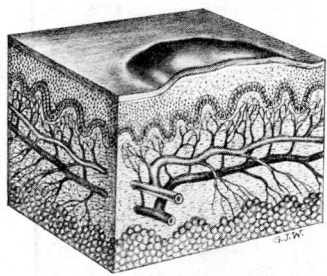

Vesicle filled with pus that may or may not be caused by infection

Example: Acne, impetigo, folliculitis

Pustule

Bulla

Fluid-filled vesicle greater than 1 cm in diameter; a large vesicle; bleb; blister

Example: Second-degree burn

Round or flat-topped and irregularly shaped, evanescent lesions resulting from acute accumulation of edema fluid in upper dermis

Example: Mosquito bites, urticaria

Wheal

Fig. 18-4. Secondary skin lesions.

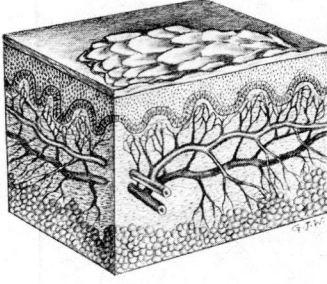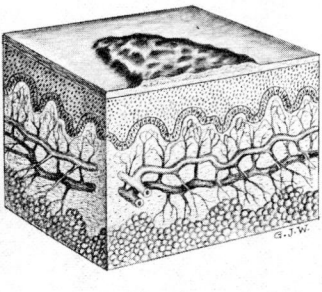

Flakes of dead, cornified tissue being shed from skin

Example: Psoriasis, ringworm

Scale

Crust

Dried masses of serum, pus, dead skin, and debris that can be found surmounting any lesion

Example: Impetigo, other infectious dermatitis

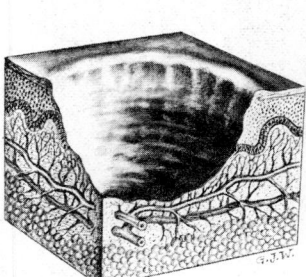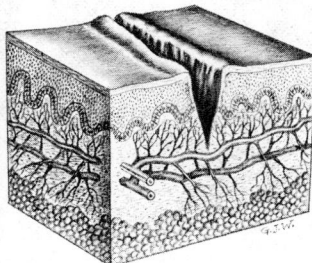

Irregularly shaped excavation caused by loss of substance with gradual disintegration and necrosis of tissue

Example: Decubiti

Ulcer

Fissure

Deep linear split through epidermis into dermis

Example: Chapping

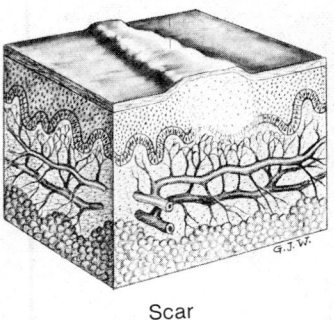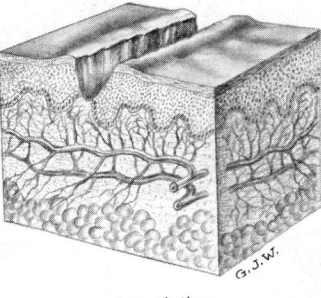

Permanent dermal changes with production of excess collagen following damage to corium

Example: Vaccination, burns, deep scratches

Scar

Excoriation

Superficial excavation of the epidermis that may be linear or punctate produced by mechanical means

Example: scratch, abrasion

Configuration and arrangement. The size, shape, and arrangement of a lesion or groups of lesions assist in diagnosis. Discrete lesions are distinguished from clustered, diffuse, or confluent configurations. Grouped or clustered lesions are characteristic in herpes eruptions; annular (ringed) or arciform lesions are typical of ringworm and diseases resulting from vascular reactions, such as urticaria or drug reaction; linear arrangements usually represent an exogenous influence that has either caused the process or contributed to its spread, such as scratching.

Subjective symptoms. Many cutaneous lesions are associated with local symptoms, the most common being itching, which varies in kind and intensity. Pain or tenderness often accompanies some skin lesions, and other sensations may be described as burning, prickling, stinging, or crawling. Alterations in local feeling or sensation include anesthesia (absence of sensation), hyperesthesia (excessive sensitivity), and hypesthesia or hypoesthesia (diminished or lessening of sensaton). These symptoms may remain localized or may migrate, may be constant or intermittent, and may be aggravated by a specific activity or circumstance, such as exposure to sunlight.

Diagnostic Evaluation

It is important to determine whether the child has had an allergic condition such as asthma or hay fever or has had previous skin disease. Eczema, often associated with allergies, frequently begins in infancy. When the lesion or symptom first became apparent should be determined, as well as whether it is related to ingestion of a food or other substance, including any medication the child might be taking. It should be kept in mind that it may be related to some activity, such as contact with plants, insects, or chemicals.

When it is suspected that a skin problem might be related to a systemic disease, such as one of the collagen diseases or immune deficiency disease, studies to rule out these possibilities are carried out. Diagnostic modalities include microscopic examination, cultures, skin biopsy, cytodiagnosis, patch testing and examination under Wood light. Allergic skin testing, and various other laboratory tests (blood count, sedimentation rate) are employed when indicated.

Therapeutic Management

The human body tends to heal, therefore treatment is directed toward eliminating or ameliorating influences that interfere with normal healing processes. Some disorders may demand aggressive therapy, but by and large the major aim of any treatment is to prevent further damage, eliminate the cause, prevent complications, and provide relief from discomfort while tissues undergo healing. Factors that contribute to the dermatitis and prolong the course of the disease must be eliminated where possible. The most common offenders in pediatrics are environmental factors (such as soaps, bubble baths, shampoos, rough or tight clothing, blankets, and toys) and the natural elements (such as dirt, sand, heat, cold, moisture, and wind). Dermatitis can also be aggravated by home remedies and medications.

Most skin disorders will respond to topical therapy, that is, application of an active ingredient directly to the affected areas. This is applied by way of a pharmacologically inert vehicle that contributes to the therapy with physical properties that protect, soothe, or cleanse. However, there are occasions when systemic administration of therapeutic agents is employed. Since the type of medication and the active ingredient vary with the preference of individual practitioners, in the discussions of the various types of skin disorders only a representative example of some of the preferred therapeutic regimens are included.

Topical applications. A variety of agents and methods are available for treatment of dermatologic problems. In selecting a therapeutic program, the following are considered:

1. The active ingredient of choice must be safe and suited to the specific disorder.
2. The proper vehicle must be used to apply the active ingredient to the area. It must reach and maintain sufficient contact with the affected area; it must be nonirritating to affected and healthy skin.
3. The cosmetic effect of the preparation should not be more unsightly than the lesion.
4. The cost must be maintained within the means of the family.
5. Instructions for use of the preparation must be clear.

In addition, several basic concepts are kept in mind. Overtreatment should be avoided. For example, when the dermatitis is acute, the applications should be mild and bland to avoid further irritation. Broken or inflamed skin, especially in children, is more absorbent than intact skin, and chemicals that are nonirritating to intact skin may be quite irritating to inflamed skin. The dermatitic skin is also more likely to develop allergic contact-type sensitization to substances applied as medication or base. Infants and small children are particularly sensitive to topical antihistamines and the "caine" type of anesthetics, both of which are potent allergic sensitizers. Phenol, often incorporated into medications as an antipruritic, is avoided with children.

Topical applications may be applied to treat the disorder, reduce the itching associated with many diseases, decrease external stimuli, or apply external heat or cold. The emollient action of soaks, baths, and lotions provides a soothing film over the skin surface that reduces external stimuli. Application of heat tends to aggravate most conditions, and its use is usually reserved for reducing specific inflammatory processes, such as folliculitis and cellulitis. Ordinarily applications offer most relief when they are lukewarm, tepid, or cool.

The most frequent means for topical treatment of skin disorders are wet dressings, soaks, lotions and shake solutions, baths, creams and ointments, sprays and aerosols, pastes, powders, occlusive dressings, soaps and shampoos, other topical treatments, and topical glucocorticoid therapy.

Topical corticosteroid therapy. The glucocorticoids are the therapeutic agents used most widely for skin disorders. Their local anti-inflammatory effects are merely palliative so that the medication must be applied until the disease state undergoes a remission or the causative agent is eliminated. Corticosteroids are applied directly to the affected area, and, because they are essentially nonsensitizing and have only minor side effects, they can be applied over prolonged periods with continuing effectiveness. As with the use of any steroids, in large amounts they may mask signs of infection and there may be exacerbation of symptoms following termination of the drug.

Hydrocortisone preparations are available in sprays, lotions, creams, ointment, gels, suspension, and powders. Many can be purchased without a prescription. Families should be cautioned that the medication cannot be used for all skin disorders. The concentrations available without prescription are not adequate for some stubborn conditions (e.g., psoriasis) and may cause worsening of inflammation caused by fungus or bacteria. It has also been found that users apply too much topical hydrocortisone; therefore they should be counseled that it is both effective and economical to apply only a thin film and massage it into the skin.

Other topical therapies. Other topical treatments include chemical cautery (especially useful for warts), cryosurgery, electrodesiccation (chiefly used for warts, granulomas, and nevi), ultraviolet therapy (primarily used in psoriasis and acne), and special acne therapies such as dermabrasion and acne "surgery."

Systemic therapy. Therapeutic agents are often used as an adjunct to topical therapy in dermatologic disorders, and those most frequently used therapeutically are the corticosteroids and the antibiotics. The corticosteroid hormones with their capacity to inhibit inflammatory and allergic reactions are valuable in the treatment of severe skin disorders. Dosage is carefully adjusted and gradually tapered to the minimum that is effective and tolerated. In infants and children, dosage is larger than is usually calculated from body-weight ratios. Protracted use may temporarily suppress growth, however.

Antibiotics, which interfere with the growth of microorganisms, are used in severe or widespread skin infections. The danger inherent in the use of antibiotics is their tendency to produce a hypersensitivity in the patient; therefore they are used with caution. Antifungal agents are the only means for treating systemic fungal infections.

Nursing Considerations

Skin disorders present nurses with some of their most challenging problems. In children the identification of skin disorders requires a familiarity with various type of lesions in order to accurately describe them and to advise parents regarding medical consultation. Removal of foreign objects (such as small splinters), mild sunburn, and scratches pose no problem, but lesions, lacerations, and bites need careful evaluation and referral.

Identification of skin disorders. To assist in establishing a diagnosis, it is important for nurses to accurately describe any deviation in the character of the skin, using both inspection and palpation. The color, shape, and distribution of the lesions are noted, including absence of pigment (vitiligo). The individual lesions are described according to the accepted terminology and may involve more than one type, such as a maculopapular rash.

To confirm or amplify the findings made by inspection, the skin is gently palpated to detect characteristics such as temperature, moisture, texture, elasticity, and the presence of edema. It should be indicated whether the findings are restricted to the area of the lesion(s) or are generalized.

The child's subjective symptoms provide additional information. Older children are able to describe the condition as painful, itching, tingling, or other descriptive terms. However, much can be determined by observation of the child's behavior and the parents' account of these reactions. Does he scratch? Is he restless or irritable? Does the child favor or avoid using a body part? A careful history may provide clues. Has the child had access to chemicals? Has he been in the woods or around a woodpile? Has he eaten a new food? Is he taking medication? Has he any known allergy? Do any playmates have a similar lesion? A doubtful diagnosis is frequently confirmed on the basis of history.

Nurse's role in therapy. Since only a few skin diseases are contagious, it is usually not necessary to isolate the affected child unless there is a danger of acquiring a secondary infection. This is usually the child who is receiving large doses of corticosteroids or other immunosuppressant drugs or the child with an immunologic deficiency disorder. If the skin manifestation is caused by a viral exanthem, such as measles or chicken pox, the child should be prevented from exposing other susceptible children.

Autoinoculation is a constant hazard in some disorders such as impetigo or (to a lesser extent) warts. The cooperation of older children can be obtained, although they may need reminding to stop scratching or rubbing, but smaller and uncooperative children require the use of techniques and devices such as mittens, restraints, or special coverings. These methods, along with general cleanliness and hygiene, also serve to reduce the likelihood of secondary infection of a primary lesion.

Therapeutic programs are usually designed to provide general measures such as rest, protection, and relief of discomfort and specific treatments such as a definitive medication or physical technique. They usually involve some type of topical treatment, and the mode of application depends on the nature and location of the lesion being treated. For example, soothing lotions, creams, and intermittent wet dressings or soaks help cool and dry; ointments, lotions, and creams soften and lubricate dry, scaling areas. Most of the therapeutic regimens are directed toward relief of pruritus, the most common subjective complaint. Cooling applications that reduce external stimuli to the part are highly beneficial together with maintenance of cleanliness and good aeration. Clothing and bed linen should be soft and lightweight to decrease the irritation from friction and stimulation. During any type of treatment both affected and unaffected skin is protected from damage and secondary infection.

Nurses and parents are responsible for the application of topical therapeutic agents and the administration of systemic

Nursing Care Summary: The Child with Disorders of the Skin

NURSING GOALS	NURSING INTERVENTIONS	EXPECTED PATIENT/FAMILY OUTCOMES
HP-HMP Infection, potential for **Etiology: infectious agents**		
Prevent spread of infection to self and others	Isolate affected child from susceptible individuals if indicated Maintain careful handwashing after caring for child Avoid unnecessary close contact with affected child during infective stage of disease Use correct technique for disposal of dressings, solutions, and other fomites in contact with lesion(s) Teach and reinforce positive habits of hygienic care	Infection remains confined to primary site Child and family comply with preventive measures
N-MP Skin integrity, impairment of: actual **Etiology: environmental agents, somatic factors**		
Identify lesion and its cause	Describe skin lesion accurately; use descriptive terminology for type, configuration, and distribution of lesion(s) Describe any associated characteristics such as temperature, moisture, texture, elasticity, and hardness of skin in general or in area of lesion(s) Obtain history of onset, possible precipitating events, and course of development Determine any symptoms associated with disorder such as itching, pain, and fever	*Lesion(s) is accurately described *Associated factors are enumerated
Promote healing	Carry out therapeutic regimens as prescribed or support and assist parents in carrying out treatment plan Prevent secondary infection and autoinoculation Encourage rest Reduce external stimuli that aggravate condition Encourage well-balanced diet	Affected area exhibits signs of healing
N-MP Skin integrity, impairment of: potential **Risk factors: communicability of skin disorder, mechanical trauma, depressed defense** **mechanisms**		
Prevent secondary infection	Maintain careful handwashing before handling affected child Wear surgical gloves when handling or dressing affected parts if indicated by nature of lesion Teach child and family hygienic care and medical asepsis Devise methods to prevent secondary infection of lesion in small or uncooperative children	Infection remains confined to primary lesions
Protect healthy skin surface	Teach and impress on child importance of keeping hands away from lesion(s) Help child determine ways of preventing autoinoculation Devise means for keeping small or uncooperative children from spreading infection to other areas Protect healthy skin from maceration by keeping it dry	Skin lesions remain confined to primary sites
Prevent occurrence and/or recurrence	Avoid or reduce contact with agents or circumstances known to precipitate skin reaction Teach child to recognize agents or circumstances that produce reaction	Child avoids precipitating agents

*Nursing outcome.

Continued.

Nursing Care Summary: The Child with Disorders of the Skin—cont'd

NURSING GOALS	NURSING INTERVENTIONS	EXPECTED PATIENT/FAMILY OUTCOMES
CPP **Comfort, alteration in: pain** **Etiology: skin lesions**		
Relieve discomfort	Assess need for pain medication (p. 1068) Avoid or reduce external stimuli that aggravate discomfort, such as clothing and bed linen Implement other appropriate nonpharmacologic pain reduction techniques (p. 1071)	Child remains calm and exhibits no evidence of discomfort
SP-SCP **Self-concept, disturbance in: body image** **Etiology: perception of appearance**		
Promote a positive self-image	Encourage child to express feelings about his appearance and the way he thinks others view him	Child verbalizes feelings and concerns
Support child	Teach self-care where appropriate Involve child in planning treatment schedules Support and encourage child in efforts to deal with multiple problems that may be associated with disorder, including discomfort, rejection, discouragement, and feelings of self-revulsion Encourage child to maintain usual activities	Child collaborates in determining means for improving appearance Child maintains customary activities and relationships
RRP **Family process, alteration in** **Etiology: situational crisis (child with a skin condition)**		
Support family	Teach family skills needed to carry out therapeutic program Inform family of expected and unexpected results of therapy and a course of action to follow Help devise special techniques to carry out therapy Encourage family in efforts to carry out plan of care Provide assistance when appropriate Refer to agencies and services that assist with social, financial, and medical problems	Family demonstrates necessary skills (specify) Family contacts appropriate agencies (specify)

Nursing Interventions Related to Medical Management

Assist with diagnosis
    Participate in special tests such as collection of specimens for laboratory examination, use of Wood light, or elimination diet
Promote healing
    Carry out therapeutic regimen
        Topical treatments and applications
    Administer systemic medications as prescribed
Relieve discomfort
    Apply soothing treatments and topical applications as ordered
    Administer medications to relieve discomfort and/or restlessness and irritability

medications. Therefore an understanding of the various methods of application, the type and consistency of the preparation, and their purposes and uses is needed for effective application. Most topical preparations are applied systematically with the contour of the body surface (not simply up and down) with the bare hands, unless the patient has open, draining lesions or the topical medication is irritating to the applicator's skin. The use of bare hands has the added advantage of communicating an attitude of acceptance to the child and the family.

It is especially important to wash the hands before and after application of topical therapies. The skin is assessed before the treatment or application of medication and reassessed after the treatment is completed. Any observed changes are noted and described. Nursing responsibilities related to specific disorders are discussed in relation to those disorders.

Wet dressings. Open wet dressings and compresses are probably the mildest form of topical therapy. They cool the skin by evaporation, relieve itching and inflammation, and cleanse the area by loosening and removing crusts and debris. Any of a variety of ingredients, such as the time-honored Burow solution (available without a prescription), can be applied on Kerlix gauze, plain gauze, or (preferably) soft cotton cloths such as freshly laundered handkerchiefs or strips from diaper, sheeting, or pillowcase material.

Dressings immersed in the desired solution are wrung out slightly and applied to the affected area wet but not dripping. They are applied flat and smooth and in such a way that motion is not totally restricted—fingers are wrapped separately and arms and legs are wrapped so that elbows and knees can bend. Dressings are kept in place by Kerlix or other cotton wrap, tubular stockinette, mittens, and socks (two pair—one to hold the dressings in place, the other to take up movement) but are left uncovered. When evaporation begins to dry them, the dressings are removed, rewet in the solution, and reapplied to the area using aseptic technique. The solution is not poured or syringed directly over the dressings. As fluid evaporates, the solution becomes increasingly concentrated, altering the strength of the solution, which may be damaging to sensitive lesions.

Water is the most important ingredient in wet dressings and evaporation is primarily responsible for the symptomatic relief experienced by the patient. The most common solutions used for wet dressings are aluminum acetate (Burow solution) and normal saline, which are applied to cleanse and disinfect open, oozing, crusting, and/or secondarily infected lesions. Sometimes fresh warm or tepid tap water is used alone or in conjunction with topical steroids.

Fresh solution at room temperature is applied at 2-, 3-, or 4-hour intervals and is allowed to remain on the lesion from 30 minutes to 1½ hours. Wet dressings are seldom continued after about 48 hours. The child must be guarded against chilling during treatment, and no more than one third of the body should be covered at one time. After treatment the skin is dried thoroughly by patting with a towel. Application of lotion or other medication may be ordered at this time.

Occlusive dressings. Used primarily in association with topical steroids, occlusive dressings are usually restricted to treatment of chronic dermatoses. A thin application of ointment or cream is covered with a thin, transparent, pliable plastic film anchored with adhesive. Occlusive dressings promote moisture retention, nonevaporation of the vehicle, and maceration of the epidermis, all of which increase the penetration of medications. Although of value in certain situations, the dangers are bacterial and candidal infections, sweat retention, and increased likelihood of side effects from the medication used. The treatment consists of an 8- to 10-hour period, usually overnight, and covers no greater than 10% of the body.

Small children may need some type of restraint, depending on the location of the dressing. Often clothing can be worn that covers the area; for example, leg dressings are covered with pants legs. If the child attempts to remove or disturb the dressings, elbow restraints may be needed. Diversional activities are always a useful nursing tool.

Soaks. When young children are uncooperative in the use of wet dressings, soaks are often employed for removal of crusts and for their mild astringent action, using the same solution employed for wet compresses. Gaining young children's cooperation for hand or foot soaks is difficult unless the procedure is made attractive to them through play. Older infants and toddlers delight in playing with brightly colored objects or poker chips scattered over the bottom of the receptacle, and preschoolers can be challenged to hold a floating item beneath the water surface. These activities require supervision; infant and small children will often place items in their mouths and children can easily lose control with water play. Washing dishes, cars, dolls, or doll clothes will occupy many children for quite some time. The older child is able to cooperate but may need something to do during the procedure such as listening to music, a story, or watching television.

Soaking a single extremity (a foot or a hand) can be easily accomplished by placing the solution and the extremity in a plastic Ziploc* bag. The closure is then zipped snugly around the limb. This method for soaking fingers or toes can be highly entertaining to young children (Perelson and Seyler, 1985).

Baths. Baths are especially useful in the treatment of widespread dermatitis by evenly distributing the soothing antipruritic and anti-inflammatory effects of the solution, usually oatmeal or mineral oil preparations. The solution is added to a tub of lukewarm water. The temperature of the bath is tepid and the duration of treatment is usually 15 to 30 minutes. Therapeutic baths are always more interesting when the child is accompanied by toy boats or other items for water play.

Lotions. Lotions are preparations of powder suspended in solution; the container must be well shaken before application. As the liquid evaporates, it cools the skin and provides it with a coating of soothing, lubricating, protective, and drying powder. Lotions are applied evenly over the skin with the hands or gauze or are painted on with an ordinary paintbrush (children love to be ''painted''), frequently after wet dressings or soaks. Lotions are not applied to oozing surfaces. They are not ordinarily washed off between applications but may be removed by soaking with the solution used for soaks or dressings. An emulsion can be formed by the addition of an oil and a dispersant.

Creams and gels. Creams and gels are easily and evenly spread over the skin. Both tend to disappear when rubbed into the skin, are less occlusive, and are esthetically more pleasing. Gels are clear and range in consistency from a firm jelly to a thinner lotion. Creams are light and opaque

---

*The Dow Chemical Company, Indianapolis, IN 46268.

and can be either a thick liquid or a soft solid. Creams contain an oil with a high melting point. Both creams and gels are nongreasy, easily applied, and readily removed with soap and water. They are applied by placing a teaspoonful in the palm of the hand, rubbing the preparation briskly between the hands, and applying to the skin area when the consistency is thin and smooth.

Ointments. The major constituent of ointments is oil. The lipid component may consist of animal fats, such as lard or wool fat (lanolin), petrolatum, or vegetable oils. Ointments (such as cold cream and Eucerin) that contain 20% to 50% water vanish on application and are removable with water but leave a greasy sensation to the skin. Absorbent ointments contain no water but will absorb water and are more lubricating than water in oil preparations. They have a greasy sensation and are difficult to remove with soap and water. Water-repellent ointments, such as petrolatum, retain heat for increased absorption of medications but are difficult to remove and can cause maceration when used with an occlusive dressing. If ointment is not absorbed but remains on the skin, too much is being applied. Ointments are not used in hairy, intertriginous, or macerated areas.

Pastes. Pastes are powders mixed with an ointment base. More porous and less occlusive than ointments, they absorb moisture and produce a drying effect, and medications incorporated into pastes are released more slowly than from creams and ointments. Because they are difficult to apply and must be removed from the skin with mineral oil, pastes are used less frequently than other preparations. They are most easily applied with a tongue depressor and "buttered" on.

Powders. Powders have a controversial use in pediatrics. They are very effective for soothing, absorbing moisture, and protecting the skin by reducing friction. Chemically inert, their chief use is prophylactic when applied to intertriginous areas. However, powder must be applied in a fine film that does not cake or form lumps when wet, and care must be exerted to prevent the child from inhaling the powder, especially one containing talc or kaolin. To reduce the risk of inhalation, powder is sprinkled in the palm of the hand and then applied to the skin surface. Powder is never sprinkled directly onto the patient's skin, and the container is placed well out of reach of the child.

Sprays and aerosols. Many active agents are now available suspended in an alcohol-based spray. It serves as an alternative method of delivering a solution to the skin when direct application is difficult or uncomfortable for the patient. The container must be shaken thoroughly before application and the child's face shielded from the spray to avoid inhalation.

Soaps and shampoos. Germicidal soaps are useful adjunctive therapy for skin infections. Bactericidal agents incorporated in soaps include hexachlorophene and the halogenated salicylanilides and carbanilides, one or more of which are found in many of the well-known soaps. Soaps containing hexachlorophene are used with caution to reduce the risk of absorption, especially on broken or denuded areas. When absorbed, large amounts of the drug can cause central nervous system symptoms. Another effective topical microbicide is povidone-iodine (Betadine) skin cleanser, which contains a detergent mixture with iodine and polyvinyl pyrrolidone that assists in disinfecting the skin and is effective in eliminating common pathogens, including *Staphylococcus aureus.*

Shampoos that are used in dermatologic skin conditions include tar shampoos for resistant scalp seborrhea and psoriasis and antiparasitic shampoos such as gamma benzene hexachloride (Kwell) for pediculosis capitis and scabies (see pp. 778 and 779).

Sunscreening agents. Some chemicals have the capacity to absorb certain wavelengths of light and thus provide protection to the cutaneous surface when applied to the skin. They are especially useful in dermatoses in which light plays an important causative role. They are applied to light-exposed areas and provide protection for hours under ordinary circumstances. (For further discussion of sunscreening agents, see Sunburn, p. 775.)

Discharge planning and family support. Childhood dermatologic conditions always involve the parents. Since few situations require hospitalization and children who do require hospitalization will complete a therapy program at home, the parents are the persons who must carry out the treatment plan; therefore their cooperation is essential. Child and parents are more apt to be motivated if they are told why something is being done in a certain way. Success of treatment depends on the correct interpretation of instructions, and it is often the nurse's responsibility to teach the parent how to carry out the instructions and offer encouragement, support, and assistance with problem solving.

Regimens that are simple to accomplish in the hospital or office situation may be frustrating and baffling at home. Parents often need assistance in adapting equipment available in the home to the therapy, for example, dressings from scraps and rags and the use of utensils for soaks. One of the most difficult areas to deal with is the child's irritability and tendency to disturb dressings and scratch or pick at lesions. Here nurses can help parents devise protective restraining devices and distracting activities for the child. Treatments at home, in the clinics, or in the clinician's office that are scheduled and arranged to accommodate the child's schooling as well as the parents' affairs are more apt to be carried out.

It is important that parents and child be given as much explanation as possible about both the expected and the unexpected results of treatment, including any ill effects that might occur. Although a treatment plan is chosen for its probability of being beneficial without doing harm, using medications that contain the fewest and safest ingredients, persons with skin disorders are highly susceptible to irritation. They are directed to discontinue treatment and report any unexpected reactions to the appropriate person(s). Skin changes bother people so that they often try anything, including home remedies and patent medicines. The use of patent medicines is discouraged unless this has first been discussed with the attending physician and has received approval.

Since the skin is the most visible portion of the body, defects in its surface that alter its appearance are sometimes an additional source of distress to the affected child and the family. Unsightly lesions or medicinal preparations applied to the skin are often sources of revulsion and rejection by others. Other children will proffer derogatory comments and may even reject the affected child. Parents of other children may fear that their children will "catch" the disorder. Occasionally the affected child's own family will reduce their interaction with him, especially close physical contact, or otherwise demonstrate a distaste for the condition that the child may interpret as rejection. This is seldom a difficulty with dermatitis of short duration, but chronic conditions can create problems in development of a positive self-concept.

Infections of the Skin

Dermatologic infections and other disorders of the skin constitute a significant portion of children's visits to offices and clinics. Most are troublesome ailments and are the source of considerable physical and emotional discomfort. For most of the disorders the diagnosis and treatment are relatively simple; for others the management is more complex and puzzling.

BACTERIAL INFECTIONS

Normally the skin harbors a variety of bacterial flora, including the major pathogenic varieties of staphylococci and streptococci. The degree of their pathogenicity depends on the specific organism's invasiveness and toxigenicity, the integrity of the skin, the barrier of the host, and the immune and cellular defenses of the host. Children with immune deficiency states are highly susceptible to bacterial invasion. This includes infants, children with congenital immune deficiency disorders, children in a debilitated condition, those on immunosuppressive therapy, and those with a generalized malignancy such as leukemia or lymphoma.

Because of the characteristic "walling-off" process of the inflammatory reaction (abscess formation), staphylococci are more difficult to attack and the local infected area is associated with an increase in numbers of bacteria all over the skin surface that serves as a source of continuing infection. Staphylococcal infections occur most often in children in the younger age-groups, and the incidence decreases with advancing age. All of these factors emphasize the importance of careful handwashing and cleanliness when caring for infected children and their lesions to prevent spread of the infection and as an essential prophylactic measure when caring for infants and small children. Common bacterial skin disorders are outlined in Table 18-1.

Table 18-1 Bacterial infections

DISORDER/ORGANISM	MANIFESTATIONS	TREATMENT	COMMENTS
Impetigo contagiosa (Fig. 18-5)— *Streptococcus, Staphylococcus*	Begins as a reddish macule Becomes vesicular Ruptures easily, leaving superficial, moist erosion Tends to spread peripherally in sharply marginated irregular outlines Exudate dries to form heavy, honey-colored crusts Pruritus common Systemic effects: minimal or asymptomatic	Careful removal of undermined skin, crusts, and debris by softening with 1:20 Burow solution compresses Topical application of bactericidal ointment Systemic administration of oral or parenteral antibiotics (pencillin) in severe or extensive lesions	Tends to heal without scarring unless secondary infection Autoinoculable and contagious Very common in toddler, preschooler
Pyoderma— *Staphylococcus, Streptococcus*	Deeper extension of infection into dermis Tissue reaction more severe Systemic effects: fever, lymphangitis	Soap and water cleansing Wet compresses Bathing with antibacterial soap as prescribed	Autoinoculable and contagious May heal with or without scarring
Folliculitis (pimple), furuncle (boil), carbuncle (multiple boils)— *Staphylococcus aureus*	Folliculitis: infection of hair follicle Furuncle: larger lesion with more redness and swelling at a single follicle Carbuncle: more extensive lesion with widespread inflammation and "pointing" at several follicular orifices Systemic effects: malaise, if severe	Skin cleanliness Local warm moist compresses Topical application of antibiotic agents Systemic antibiotics in severe cases Incision and drainage of severe lesions, followed by wound irrigations with antibiotics or suitable drain implantation	Autoinoculable and contagious Furuncle and carbuncle tend to heal with scar formation A lesion should *never* be squeezed

Continued.

Table 18-1 Bacterial infections—cont'd

DISORDER/ORGANISM	MANIFESTATIONS	TREATMENT	COMMENTS
Cellulitis— *Streptococcus, Haemophilus influenzae*	Inflammation of skin and subcutaneous tissues with intense redness, swelling, and firm infiltration Lymphangitis "streaking" frequently seen Involvement of regional lymph nodes common May progress to abscess formation Systemic effects: fever, malaise	Oral or parenteral penicillin Rest and immobilization of both affected area and child Hot moist compresses to area	Hospitalization may be necessary for child with systemic symptoms

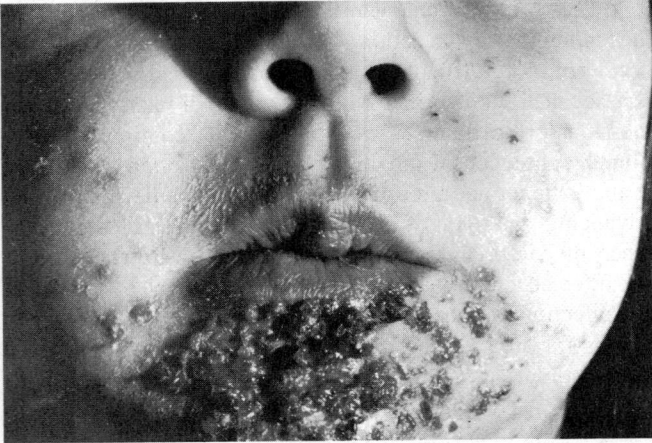

Fig. 18-5. Impetigo contagiosa.
From Stewart, W.D., Danto, J.L., and Maddin, S.: Dermatology: diagnosis and treatment of cutaneous disorders, ed. 4, St. Louis, 1978, The C.V. Mosby Co.

Nursing Considerations

The major nursing functions related to bacterial skin infections are to prevent the spread of infection and to prevent complications. Handwashing is mandatory before and after contact with an affected child. Handwashing is also emphasized to both the child and the family, and the child should be provided with towels separate from other family members. Impetigo contagiosa is easily spread by self-inoculation; therefore the child must be cautioned against touching the involved area. This is difficult to accomplish. Distraction or reminders are useful but are not helpful when the child is alone, such as bedtime.

Children and parents are often tempted to squeeze follicular lesions. They must be warned that squeezing will not hasten the resolution of the infection and that there is a risk of making the lesion worse or spreading the infection. No attempt should be made to puncture the surface of the pustule with a needle or sharp instrument. A child with a sty may waken with the eyelids of the affected eye sealed shut with exudate. The child or the parents are instructed to gently wipe the lid with clear warm water and a clean washcloth until the exudate has been removed.

The child with limited cellulitis of an extremity is usually managed at home on oral antibiotics and warm compresses. The parents are taught the procedures and instructed in administration of the medication. Children with more extensive cellulitis, especially around a joint with lymphadenitis or on the face, are usually admitted to the hospital for parenteral antibiotics. Nurses are responsible for administering the medication, applying compresses, and maintaining the intravenous infusion.

VIRAL INFECTIONS

Viruses are intracellular parasites that produce their effect by using the intracellular substances of the host cells. Composed of only a DNA or RNA core enclosed in an antigenic protein shell, viruses are unable to provide for their own metabolic needs or to reproduce themselves. After a virus penetrates a cell of the host organism, it sheds the outer shell and disappears within the cell, where the nucleic acid core stimulates the host cell to form more virus material from its intracellular substance. In a viral infection the epidermal cells react with inflammation and vesiculation (as in herpes simplex) or by proliferating to form growths (warts).

Most of the communicable diseases of childhood are associated with rashes, and each rash is characteristic. The type of lesion and the configuration of the viral exanthems of rubeola, rubella, scarlet fever, and chicken pox are described in Table 16-1. Other common viral disorders of the skin are outlined in Table 18-2.

DERMATOPHYTOSES (FUNGAL INFECTIONS)

The dermatophytoses (ringworm) are infections caused by a group of closely related filamentous fungi that invade primarily the stratum corneum, hair, and nails. These are superficial infections that live on, not in, the skin. They are confined to the dead keratin layers but are unable to survive in the deeper layers. Since the keratin is being desquamated

Table 18-2 Viral infections

DISEASE	MANIFESTATIONS	TREATMENT	COMMENTS
Verruca (warts)	Small, benign tumors Usually well-circumscribed, gray or brown, elevated firm papules with a roughened, finely papillomatous texture Occur anywhere but usually appear on exposed areas such as fingers, hands, face, and soles	Not uniformly successful Local destructuve therapy, individualized according to location, type, and number—surgical removal, electrocautery, curettage, cryotherapy (liquid nitrogen), caustic solutions (lactic acid and salicylic acid in flexible collodion, retinoic acid, salicylic acid plasters), x-ray treatment Hypnotherapy may be effective	Common in children Tend to disappear spontaneously Course unpredictable Most destructive techniques tend to leave scars Autoinoculable Repeated irritation will cause to enlarge
Variants: Verruca vulgaris (common wart)	A skin-colored to brown, rough-surfaced epithelial growth May be single or multiple Asymptomatic Most frequent sites are dorsal and palmar surfaces of hands, fingers, and around nails		
Verruca plana juvenilis (juvenile wart)	Flat, skin-colored to brown, slightly raised, smooth lesion Asymptomatic Lesions multiple Commonly located on face and dorsum of hands		
Verruca plantaris (plantar wart)	Located on plantar surface of feet and, because of pressure, are practically flat; may be surrounded by a collar of hyperkeratosis	Apply caustic solution to wart, wear foam insole with hole cut to relieve pressure on wart; soak 20 min after 2-3 days. Repeat until wart comes out	
Herpes simplex virus type I (cold sore, fever blister)	Grouped, burning, and itching vesicles on inflammatory base, usually on or near mucocutaneous junctions (lips, nose, genitals, buttocks) Vesicles dry, forming a crust, followed by exfoliation and spontaneous healing in 8-10 days May be accompanied by regional lymphadenopathy	Avoidance of secondary infection Burow solution compresses during weeping stages No topical therapy has proved to be effective	Heal without scarring unless secondary infection Aggravated by corticosteroids Positive psychologic effect from treatment
Herpes zoster (shingles)	Caused by same virus that causes varicella (chicken pox) Virus has affinity for posterior root ganglia, posterior horn of spinal cord, and skin; crops of vesicles usually confined to dermatome following along course of affected nerve Usually preceded by neuralgic pain, hyperesthesias, or itching May be accompanied by constitutional symptoms	Symptomatic Salicylates for pain Mild sedation sometimes helpful Local moist compresses Drying lotions may be helpful Ophthalmic variety: systemic corticotropin (ACTH) and/or corticosteroids	Pain in children usually minimal Postherpetic pain does not occur in children Chicken pox may follow exposure; isolate affected child from other children in a hospital May occur in children with depressed immunity; can be fatal
Molluscum contagiosum	Caused by a pox virus Flesh-colored papules with a central caseous plug Usually asymptomatic	Cases in well children resolve spontaneously in about 18 months Treatment reserved for troublesome cases	Common in schoolage children Spread by person-to-person contact and by autoinoculation

Table 18-3   Dermatophytoses (ringworm)

DISEASE/ORGANISM	MANIFESTATIONS	TREATMENT	COMMENTS
Tinea capitis—*Microsporum audouini, M. canis* (see Fig. 18-6, *A*)	Lesions in scalp but may extend to hairline or neck Characteristic configuration of scaly, circumscribed patches and/or patchy, scaling areas of alopecia Generally asymptomatic, but severe, deep inflammatory reaction may occur that manifests as boggy, encrusted lesions (kerions) Pruritic Diagnosis: fluoresce green under Wood light; check at 2-week intervals Direct examination of scales and culture if doubtful	Oral griseofulvin Oral ketoconazole for difficult cases Selenium sulfide shampoos Topical antifungal agents, e.g., clotrimazole, haloprogin, miconazole	Person-to-person transmission Animal-to-person transmission Rarely, permanent loss of hair *M. audouini* transmitted from one human being to another directly or from personal items; *M. canis* usually contracted from household pets
Tinea corporis—*Trichophyton, Microsporum* (see Fig. 18-6, *B*)	Generally round or oval, erythematous scaling patch that spreads peripherally and clears centrally; may involve nails (tinea unguium) Diagnosis: direct microscopic examination of scales	Oral griseofulvin Local application of antifungal preparation such as tolnaftate, haloprogin, miconazole, clotrimazole	Usually of animal origin from infected pets Majority of infections in children caused by *M. canis* and *M. audouini*
Tinea cruris ("jock itch")—*Epidermophyton floccosum, T. rubrum*	Skin response similar to tinea corporis Localized to medial proximal aspect of thigh and crural fold; may involve scrotum in males Pruritic Diagnosis: same as for tinea corporis	Local application of tolnaftate liquid Wet compresses or sitz baths may be soothing	Rare in preadolescent children Health education regarding personal hygiene
Tinea pedis (athlete's foot)—*E. floccosum, T. rubrum, T. interdigitale*	On intertriginous areas between toes or on plantar surface of feet Lesions vary: Maceration and fissuring between toes Patches with pinhead-sized vesicles on plantar surface Pruritic Diagnosis: direct microscopic examination of scrapings	Oral griseofulvin Local applications of tolnaftate liquid and antifungal powder containing tolnaftate Acute infections: compresses or soaks followed by application of glucocorticoid cream Elimination of conditions of heat and perspiration by clean, light socks and well-ventilated shoes; avoidance of occlusive shoes	Most frequent in adolescents and adults; rare in children Transmission to other individuals rare despite general opinion to contrary Ointments not successful

constantly, the fungus must multiply at a rate that equals the rate of keratin production to maintain itself; otherwise the infection would be shed with the discarded skin cells. Common dermatophytoses are outlined in Table 18-3.

Three principal types of fungi are responsible for dermatophyte infections: *Trichophyton, Microsporum,* and *Epidermophyton.* They are designated by the Latin word *tinea,* with further designation related to the area of the body where they are found, for example, tinea capitis (ringworm of the scalp) (Fig. 18-6, *A*). Dermatophyte infections are most often transmitted from one person to another or from infected animals to humans. They exert their effect by means of an enzyme that digests and hydrolyzes the keratin of hair, nails, and the stratum corneum. Dissolved hair breaks off to produce the bald spots characteristic of tinea capitis. In the annular lesions the fungi are found principally in the edge of the inflamed border as they move outward from the inflammation. Nurses who suspect ringworm in school children are able to identify the organism by means of a Wood light, under which the fungus is fluorescent.

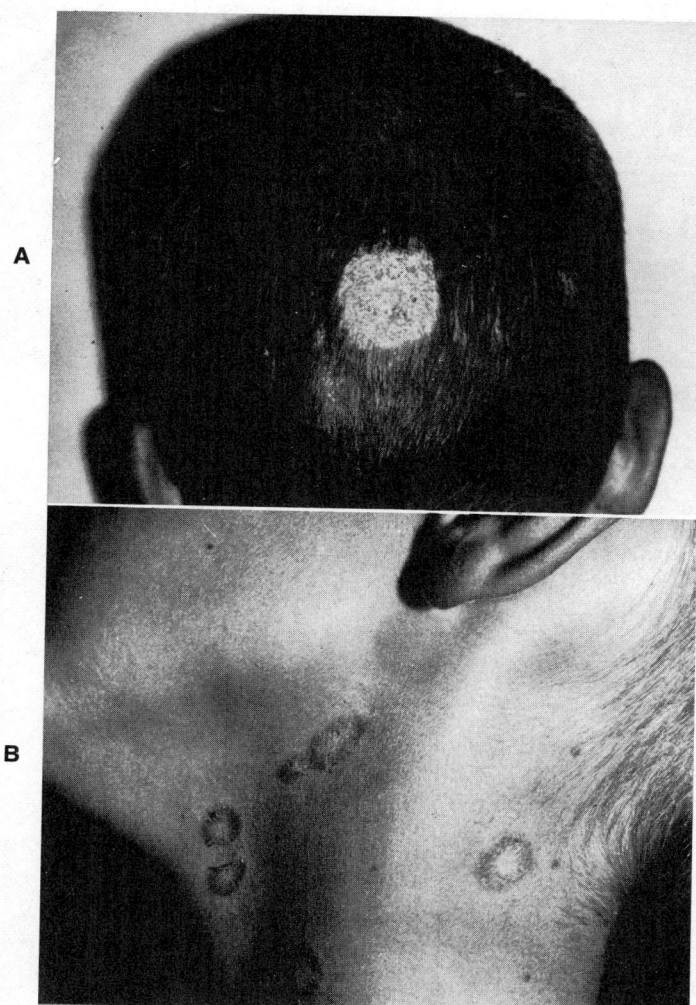

Fig. 18-6. A, Tinea capitis. **B,** Tinea corporis. Both infections caused by *Microsporum canis,* the "kitten" or "puppy" fungus. From Stewart, W.D., Danto, J.L., and Maddin, S.: Dermatology: diagnosis and treatment of cutaneous disorders, ed.. 4, St. Louis, 1978, The C.V. Mosby Co.

Nursing Considerations

When teaching families regarding the care of children with ringworm, it is important to emphasize good health and hygiene. Because of the infectious nature of the disease, several basic hygienic measures are particularly pertinent. Affected children are not to exchange with other children any grooming items, headgear, scarves, or other articles of apparel that have been in proximity to the infected area. Affected children are provided with their own towel and directed to wear a protective cap at night to avoid transmitting the fungus to bedding, especially if they sleep with another person. Since the infection can be acquired by animal-to-human transmission, all household pets should be examined for the presence of the disorder. Other sources of infection are seats with head rests, such as theater seats or seats in public transportation.

Treatment with the drug griseofulvin frequently lasts for weeks or months, and because subjective symptoms subside, children or parents may be tempted to decrease or discontinue the drug. The nurse should impress on members of the family the importance of maintaining the prescribed dosage schedule. They are also instructed regarding the possibility of side effects from the drug such as headache, gastrointestinal upset, fatigue, insomnia, and photosensitivity. For children who take the drug over many months, periodic testing is required to monitor leukopenia and assess liver and renal function.

SYSTEMIC MYCOTIC (FUNGAL) INFECTIONS

Mycotic (systemic or deep fungal) infections have the capacity to invade the viscera as well as the skin. The best known of these are primarily lung diseases, which are usually acquired by inhalation. They produce a variable spectrum of disease, and some are quite common in certain geographic areas. They are not transmitted from person to person but appear to reside in the soil, from which their spores are airborne. The cutaneous lesions are granulomatous and appear as ulcers, plaques, nodules, fungating mosses, and abscesses. The course of deep fungal diseases is chronic with slow progression that favors sensitization (Table 18-4).

RICKETTSIAL INFECTIONS

Rickettsiae are intracellular parasites, similar in size to bacteria, that inhabit the alimentary tract of a wide range of natural hosts. With the exception of Q fever, mammals become infected only through the bites of infected insects (lice and fleas) or arachnids (ticks and mites), which serve as both infectors and reservoirs. Rickettsial diseases are more common in temperate and tropical climates and in areas where humans live in association with arthropods. Infection in humans is incidental (except epidemic typhus) and not necessary for the survival of the rickettsial species. However, once the organism invades a human it causes a disease that varies in intensity from a benign self-limiting illness to a fulminating and frequently fatal one. (Some rickettsial infections are outlined in Table 18-5.)

Skin Disorders Related to Chemical or Physical Contacts

Children come in contact with an endless variety of substances and objects in day-to-day activities, including sunshine. Some children are troubled very little by these encounters; others are sensitive to many commonplace substances. The following discussion is restricted to the more frequently observed dermatides or reactions.

Table 18-4 Systemic mycoses

DISORDER/ ORGANISM	SKIN MANIFESTATIONS	SYSTEMIC MANIFESTATIONS	TREATMENT	COMMENTS
Actinomycosis— *Actinomyces israelii*	Deep-seated granulomatous nodules and subcutaneous abscesses that drain as chronic fistulas, especially in jaw or neck	General health not affected	Penicillin or other antibiotics Incision and wide debridement of lesions	Access frequently through a carious tooth or mucous membranes of mouth Uncommon in children Noninfectious
North American blastomycosis— *Blastomyces dermatitidis*	Chronic granulomatous lesions and microabscesses in any part of body Initial lesion is a papule; undergoes ulceration and peripheral spread	Pulmonary symptoms such as cough, chest pain, weakness, and weight loss May have skeletal involvement, with bone destruction and formation of cutaneous abscesses	Intravenous administration of amphotericin B	Usual portal of entry is lungs Source of infection unknown Noninfectious Pulmonary infections may be mild and self-limiting and require no treatment Progressive disease often fatal
Cryptococcosis— *Cryptococcus neoformans (Torula histolytica)*	Usually on face; acneiform, firm, nodular, painless eruption	Central nervous system (CNS) manifestations; headache, dizziness, stiff neck, and signs of increased intracranial pressure Low-grade fever, mild cough, lung infiltration	Intravenous amphotericin B; may be administered intrathecally for CNS involvement 5-Flurocytosine for meningitis Excision and drainage of local lesions	Acquired by inhalation of dust, but may enter through skin Prognosis serious Noninfectious Increased incidence in persons receiving corticosteroids with lymphoreticular malignancies, or type II diabetes
Histoplasmosis— *Histoplasma capsulatum*	Not distinctive or uniform but most appear as punched-out or granulomatous ulcers	General systemic symptoms may include pallor, diarrhea, vomiting, irregular spiking temperature, hepatosplenomegaly, and pulmonary symptoms Any tissue of body may be involved with related symptoms	Intravenous amphotericin B for severe cases Oral ketoconazole	Organism cultured from soil, especially where contaminated with fowl droppings Fungus enters through skin or mucous membranes of mouth and respiratory tract Endemic in Mississippi and Ohio River valleys Disseminated diseases most common in infants and children
Coccidioidomycosis (valley fever)— *Coccidiodes immitis*	Erythema nodosum	Primary lung disease usually asymptomatic May be sign of acute febrile illness Disseminated disease is very serious	Intravenous amphotericin B Intravenous miconazole (synthetic imidazole) Intraventricular miconazole plus oral ketoconazole for CNS involvement Surgical resection of persistent pulmonary cavities	Inhalation of aerospores from soil Endemic in southwestern United States Usually resolves spontaneously Increased incidence in dark-skinned races (Filipino, black, Mexican, Asian)

Table 18-5 Eruptions caused by rickettsiae

DISORDER/ORGANISM/HOST	MANIFESTATIONS	TREATMENT	COMMENTS
Rocky Mountain spotted fever—*R. rickettsii* Arthropod: tick Transmission: tick bite Mammal source: wild rodents; dogs	Gradual onset: fever, malaise, anorexia, myalgia Abrupt onset: rapid temperature elevation, chills, vomiting, myalgia, severe headache Maculopapular or petechial rash primarily on extremities (ankles and wrists) but may spread to other areas	Control: protection from tick bite by proper wearing apparel, tick repellent Tetracycline or chloramphenicol Vigorous supportive therapy	Usually self-limited in children Onset in children may resemble any infectious disease Severe disease rare in children Children and dogs should be inspected regularly if they play in wooded areas See Table 27-6 for management of ticks
Epidemic typhus—*R. prowazekii* Arthropod: body louse Transmission: infected feces into broken skin Mammal source: humans	Abrupt onset of chills, fever, diffuse myalgia, headache, malaise Maculopapular rash 4 to 7 days later spreading from trunk outward	Control: immediate destruction of vectors Tetracycline or chloramphenicol	Patient should be isolated until deloused See discussion on p. 778 for management of pediculosis Excreta from infected lice also in dust—disinfect patient's clothing, bedding, and possessions with DDT and wash in hot water
Endemic typhus—*R. mooseri* Arthropod: rat fleas, or lice Transmission: flea bite; inhaling or ingesting flea excreta Mammal source: rats	Headache, arthralgia, backache followed by fever; may last 9-14 days Maculopapular rash after 1-8 days of fever begins in trunk and spreads to periphery; rarely involves face, palms, soles	Control; eliminate rat reservoir, insect vectors, or both Supportive treatment	Fairly common in U.S. Shorter duration than epidemic typhus A mild, seldom fatal illness Difficult to distinguish from epidemic typhus
Rickettsialpox—*R. akari* Arthropod: mouse mite Transmission: mite Mammal source: house mouse	Maculopapular rash following primary lesion at site of bite, fever, chills, headache	Control: eradication of rodent reservoir and mite vector Tetracycline or chloramphenecol Supportive treatment	Self-limited nonfatal disease Endemic in New York City Found in many cities in U.S.
Q fever—*Coxiella burnetti* Arthropod: tick Transmission: inhalation of dried, infected material Mammal source: domestic farm animals (cattle, sheep, goats)	Abrupt onset of chills, fever, weakness, and nonspecific symptoms Severe frontal headache often associated with pain upon eye movement After 1 week—cough and chest pains	Control: impossible; exact mode of spread unknown Tetracycline or chloramphenicol Supportive treatment	Usually a mild disease Duration 2-3 weeks Endemic in California Milk should be pasteurized Persons who work around farm animals are at risk

CONTACT DERMATITIS

Contact dermatitis is an inflammatory reaction of the skin to chemical substances, natural or synthetic, that evoke a hypersensitivity response or to those agents that cause direct irritation. The initial reaction occurs in an exposed region, most commonly the face and neck, backs of the hands, forearms, male genitalia, and lower legs. There is characteristically a sharp delineation between inflamed and normal skin early in the reaction that ranges from a faint, transient ery-

thema to massive bullae on an erythematous swollen base. Itching is a constant symptom.

The cause may be a *primary irritant* or a *sensitizing agent*. A primary irritant is one that irritates any skin; a sensitizer irritates in relatively low concentrations only persons who are allergic to it, that is, those who have met something chemically related to it, have undergone an immunologic change, and have become sensitized. Prior exposure is not a factor in the reaction. The course is relatively short (1 to 4 weeks) if the causative agent is eliminated, and it depends on the severity of the original reaction whether or not there are complications from secondary invasion or reactions to topical therapy.

Sensitizing reactions are acquired by repeated exposure or prolonged exposure, and the sensitizing capacity of different substances varies widely. Strong sensitizers require only one or two exposures and occur in a higher percentage of individuals; weak sensitizers require numerous exposures, and a smaller percentage of those exposed will be sensitized. The length of time from exposure to development of sensitivity varies considerably and may be as short as a week or much longer. Sometimes with repeated exposure and reactions the skin loses its capacity to return to normal or secondary factors become predominant to produce a chronic inflammatory process.

The major goal in treatment is to prevent further exposure of the skin to the offending substance. Providing there is not further irritation, the normal recuperative powers of the skin will produce satisfactory results without treatment. The most frequent offenders are plant and animal irritants, the prototype of which is poison ivy (see separate discussion).

The most common contact dermatitis in infants occurs on the convex surfaces of the diaper area as a result of chemical irritation from ammonia, putrefactive enzymes acting on urinary amino acids, or, less often, laundry products (see p. 571). Other agents that frequently produce dermatologic responses from contact are animal irritants such as wool, feathers, and furs; vegetable irritants such as oleoresins, oils, and turpentine; and chemicals of all kinds, including synthetic fabrics (including shoe components), dyes, metals, cosmetics, perfumes, and soaps (including bubble baths). The list is endless.

Several cosmetic products advertised as safe for children may be responsible for skin irritation in children. These include a cream hair relaxer marketed especially for children that contains lye and must be used with extreme care. Because children's hair is more resistant to artificial curling or straightening, pediatric preparations contain chemicals as strong or stronger than those intended for use on adults.

Nursing Considerations

Nurses frequently detect evidence of contact dermatitis during routine physical assessments. Skin manifestations in specific areas suggest limited contact, such as around the eyes (mascara), areas of the body covered by clothing but not protected by undergarments (wool), or areas of the body not covered by clothing (ultraviolet injury). Generalized involvement is more likely to be bubble bath or soap. Often nurses are able to elicit the offending agent and counsel families regarding management. If the lesions persist, are extensive, or show evidence of infection medical evaluation is indicated.

POISON IVY, OAK, AND SUMAC

Contact with the dry or succulent portions of any of three poisonous plants produces localized, streaked or spotty, oozing, and painful impetiginous lesions. Poison ivy grows almost everywhere east of the Rockies, poison oak is mainly found west of the Rockies, and poison sumac is usually restricted to swamp areas of the Southeast. Only Nevada, Hawaii, and Alaska (and regions above 4000 feet) appear to be free of the plants (Fig. 18-7).

The offending substance in these plants is an oil, urushiol, that is extremely potent. Sensitivity to urushiol is not inborn but is developed after one or two exposures and may change over a lifetime. Repeated exposures appear to lower the reaction; exposure after long periods away from it may elicit a heightened response. Some highly sensitive persons may suddenly become resistant and vice versa. All parts of the plants contain urushiol, so dried leaves and stems contain the irritant. Even smoke from burning brush piles can produce a reaction. There is widespread contact with the skin from the smoke of burning plants and lung reactions from smoke inhalation can be life-threatening.

Animals do not seem to be affected by the oil; dogs or other animals who have run or played in the plants may carry the sap on their fur and animals who eat the plants can transfer the oil in saliva. Shoes, tools, and toys can transfer the oil. Golf balls that have been in the rough are sources of contact.

Clinical Manifestations

The substance begins to take effect as soon as it touches the skin. It penetrates through the epidermis and bonds with the

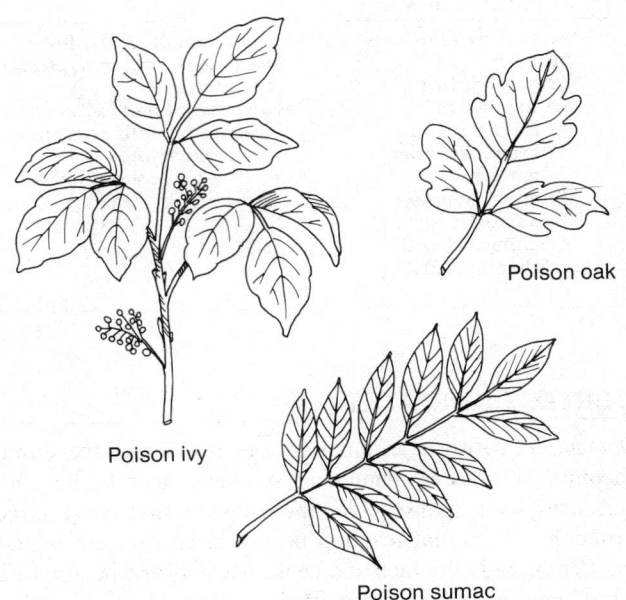

Poison ivy

Poison oak

Poison sumac

Fig. 18-7. Poison ivy, poison oak, and poison sumac.

dermal layer where it initiates an immune response. The full-blown reaction is evident after about 2 days with redness, swelling, and itching at the site of contact. Several days later streaked or spotty blisters oozing serum from damaged cells produce the characteristic impetiginous lesions. The lesions dry and heal spontaneously and itching stops by 10 to 14 days.

Therapeutic Management

Treatment of the lesions include calamine lotion, soothing Burow solution compresses, and/or Aveeno baths to relieve discomfort. Topical corticosteroid gel is very effective for prevention or relief of inflammation, especially when applied before formation of blisters. Oral corticosteroids may be needed for severe reactions, and a sedative such as diphenhydramine (Benadryl) may be ordered.

Nursing Considerations

When it is known that the child has made contact with the plant the area is immediately flushed (within 15 minutes) with *cold* running water to neutralize the urushiol not yet bonded to the skin. If there is a stream nearby an effective method is to have the child enter the water (clothes and all) and allow the water to rinse the oil from both skin and clothing. Soap is contraindicated because it removes protective skin oils and dilutes the urushiol, allowing it to spread, and hard scrubbing irritates the skin. All clothing that has come in contact with the plant is removed with care and thoroughly laundered in hot water and detergent. Every effort should be made to prevent the child from scratching the lesions. Although the lesions do not spread by contact with the blister serum or from scratching, the lesions can become secondarily infected.

Prevention. Prevention is best accomplished by avoidance of contact and removal of the plant from the environment when feasible. All children, especially those known to be sensitive, should be taught to recognize the plant. Information about means for destroying plants can be obtained from the U.S. Departments of Agriculture or Forestry.

DRUG REACTIONS

Adverse reactions to drugs are seen more often in the skin than in any other organ. Cutaneous manifestations can resemble almost any skin disease and can be seen in almost any degree of severity. With few exceptions, the distribution of a drug eruption is widespread, since it results from a circulating agent, appears as an inflammatory response with itching, is sudden in onset, and may be associated with constitutional symptoms such as fever, malaise, gastrointestinal upsets, anemia, or liver and kidney damage.

Although any drug is capable of producing almost any form of reaction in the susceptible individual, some of them have a tendency to produce a particular reaction consistently, and some drugs are more likely than others to pro-

duce an untoward effect. Many are allergenic responses following a prior administration of the drug, even a topical application. Other factors influence a drug response in a particular individual. For example, drug eruptions occur with less frequency in children than in adults, climate may be a factor when light sensitivity produces a response on sun-exposed surfaces, and it is well known that there are genetic factors that affect the way in which some individuals are able to metabolize specific drugs.

Individual drug reactions may vary from a single lesion to extensive, generalized epidermal necrosis. Drug reactions are also related to the amount of drug administered and the route of administration. For example, larger amounts precipitate a more severe response than a small amount, and drugs taken orally are less sensitizing than those administered intravenously. Another common response is a fixed eruption, that is, a recurrent eruption at the same site with each readministration of the drug. The lesion, a purplish red round or oval plaque with a sharp border seen most frequently on the extremities, disappears slowly, and the pigmentation deepens with each episode.

Treatment for cutaneous reactions consists of discontinuation of the drug. In urticarial-type eruptions antihistamines may be ordered, and for widespread and severe lesions corticosteroids are beneficial. Severe anaphylactic reactions are a medical emergency.

Nursing Considerations

Nurses who suspect that a rash is caused by a medication should withhold any further dose and report the eruption to the attending physician. The most frequent offenders in drug reactions are penicillin and sulfonamides, and nurses must be alert to this possibility. However, even commonplace drugs, including aspirin, barbiturates, and chemical agents in a number of foods, flavoring agents, and preservatives, are capable of producing an undesired response. Persons who have severe reactions are reminded to obtain and wear an identifying bracelet or chain in case of emergency or inadvertent administration of the offending drug.

SUNBURN

Sunburn is a very common skin injury caused by overexposure to ultraviolet light waves—either sunlight or artificial light in the ultraviolet range. The sun emits a continuous sectrum of visible and nonvisible light rays that range in length from very short to very long. The shorter higher frequency waves are more damaging than longer wavelengths, but much of the light is filtered out as it travels through the atmosphere. Of the light that does filter through, ultraviolet A (UVA) waves are the longest and cause only minimum burning but play a significant role in photosensitive and photoallergic reactions. Ultraviolet B (UVB) waves are shorter and responsible for tanning, burning, and most of the harmful effects attributed to sunlight.

Numerous factors influence the amount of UVB exposure. Maximum exposure occurs at midday (11 AM to 3 PM), when the distance from the sun to a given spot on the earth is shortest. There is more exposure at higher altitudes, less when the sky is hazy (although its effect is easily underestimated). Window glass effectively screens out UVB but not UVA. Fresh snow and water reflect ultraviolet rays, especially when the sun is directly overhead; some is reflected by sand.

Some persons are more susceptible to sunburn than others. Protection from effects of the sun is provided by the fibrous keratin of the outer epidermis and the pigment melanin, produced by the melanocytes of the innermost, or basal, layer of the epidermis. Areas of the body with thick keratin layers (palms and soles) offer the greatest protection. The protective pigment layer decreases the intensity of all ultraviolet light by physically blocking and scattering the radiation. Ultraviolet rays stimulate the melanocytes to produce more melanin, turning the skin darker. After several days of exposure, the dark melanin is able to absorb most of the incoming ultraviolet radiation before the rays can cause further damage.

Persons with light skin and eyes produce melanin slowly and are more prone to burn, while very dark-skinned people are able to tolerate more rays without damage. Other factors can play a role in sensitivity to ultraviolet rays. People with certain diseases (e.g., porphyria, lupus erythematosus) are more sensitive to the sun's rays. Some substances increase the skin's sensitivity, for example, numerous medications (e.g., barbiturates, oral contraceptives, sulfonamides, anticonvulsants), topical products (e.g., antiseptic soap, aftershave lotions, colognes), and certain foods containing photosensitizing chemicals (e.g., carrots, parsley, limes).

The ultraviolet rays penetrate the skin surface where they precipitate a chemical change in the cell molecules, producing toxic by-products that irritate surrounding tissues. The result is redness, tissue swelling, increased capillary permeability, and the tenderness characteristic of superficial (first-degree) burns and the coagulation, necrosis, and blistering of partial thickness (second-degree) burns (see Burns, p. 1218). Sunburned skin is exquisitely sensitive, and severe sunburn may be accompanied by nausea, chills, fever, abdominal cramping, and headache. Dehydration may occur.

Nursing Considerations

Treatment involves stopping the burning process, decreasing the inflammatory response, and rehydrating the skin. Local application of cool tap water soaks or immersion in a tepid water bath for 20 minutes or until the skin is cool limits tissue destruction and relieves the discomfort. After the cool applications, an oil-in-water moisturizing lotion can be applied, but petrolatum-based products that trap radiant heat in the tissues are avoided (Anders and Leach, 1983). Aspirin is recommended for relief of discomfort in the first 24 to 48 hours because of its prostaglandin-inhibiting properties.

Partial thickness burns are treated the same as those from any heat source.

Prevention. Protection from sunburn is the major goal management, and the harmful effects of the sun on the delicate skin of infants and children is receiving increased attention. The safest time to sunbathe is when the sun is nearest the horizon (before 9 or 10 AM and after 3 or 4 PM), when rays must travel the greatest distance. The skin needs time to build up protection; one should begin sunning slowly, approximately 10 to 20 minutes each day, and gradually extend the exposure time until tolerance develops. When skin is exposed to the sun for extended periods a protective covering is advised.

Two types of products are available for sun protection: topical sunscreens, which partially absorb ultraviolet light, and sun blockers, which block out ultraviolet rays by reflecting sunlight. The most frequently recommended sun blockers are zinc oxide and titanium dioxide ointments. Sunscreens are products containing a sun protective factor (SPF) based on evaluation of effectiveness against ultraviolet rays. The SPF is indicated by number with an SPF of 22 providing the maximum protection. The most effective sunscreens are para-aminobenzoic acid (PABA) and PABA-esters. PABA is more effective but may stain clothing; PABA-esters are less likely to stain clothing but are less effective than PABA. Benzophenones also offer protection but are less effective than the PABA preparations and wash off easily.

Sunscreens are applied evenly to all exposed areas with special attention to skin folds and areas that might become exposed as clothing shifts. For the best effect, sunscreens are applied about 45 minutes before exposure and should be reapplied in 4 to 6 hours and after swimming or perspiring. Parents are directed to read labels of sunscreen products carefully for the SPF.

COLD INJURY

Cold injuries are most commonly seen in very cold regions. The nature of the heat regulating mechanisms of the body are such that the inner portion of the body, or core, produces heat and the periphery, or outer area, conserves or dissipates the heat. When the body attempts to conserve heat the outer tissues are subjected to low temperatures, and local trauma may result.

Chilblain occurs when extremities, usually the hands, are exposed intermittently to temperatures 30° to 60° F. The response may vary but is characterized by intense vasodilation that increases the temperature of involved tissues above unaffected tissue and produces edematous, reddish-blue patches that itch and burn. As warming takes place the sensations become more intense but ordinarily subside in a few days.

Frostbite results from sufficient exposure to cool the tissues to the point that small ice crystals form in interstitial spaces of superficial and deep structures, resulting in variable degrees of tissue loss and function. The frostbitten part appears white or blanched, feels solid, and is without sensation. Rapid rewarming produces a flush (sometimes deep purple) and a return of sensation, which is extremely painful. Large blisters appear 24 to 48 hours after rewarming, which begin to reabsorb within 5 to 10 days followed by formation of a hard black eschar. Superficial injury often heals without incident. Rewarming is accomplished by immersing the part in well-agitated water at 100° to 108° F. Discomfort is managed with analgesics and sedatives. Care of blistered skin is similar to that described for burns. It is seldom possible to estimate the extent of tissue loss until new skin layers are revealed after the eschar layer separates.

TRAUMA AND FOREIGN BODIES

Cuts, scratches, scrapes, and abrasions are all part of growing up. No child escapes them. Small injuries are managed by the parents at home with only a few simple guidelines. Cuts on the face, a gaping cut longer than ¼ inch, or one that bleeds persistently should be evaluated for possible suturing. To prevent possible tatooing, an abrasion from which the dirt cannot be removed will require abrading under topical anesthesia and those covering a very large area (over 15% of the body) will need medical attention. There is also a high risk of contamination from wounds sustained in a bicycle injury. Since abrasions are often painful, analgesics such as acetaminophen are advised.

Nursing Considerations

Advice to parents regarding management of small wounds to the skin is often assumed by nurses. Parents are instructed to wash their hands, then wash the wound vigorously but gently with soap and water for at least 5 minutes, and rinse the wound well. If possible the wound is left exposed to air since wounds heal faster without a dressing. However, if the area is one that will probably get dirty, it can be covered with a Band-Aid sterile dressing. Ointments, sprays, alcohol, or Merthiolate are not needed; some sting and can damage normal tissue.

Abrasions are cleaned in the same manner as wounds except that any foreign matter must be removed with clean tweezers and loose skin cut off with sterile scissors. Small abrasions are left exposed; larger ones are covered with Telfa or other nonstick dressing that is changed in 12 hours and left uncovered after 24 hours. Bruises are managed with ice applications for 20 to 30 minutes.

Puncture wounds that do not require a tetanus booster are soaked in hot water and soap for 15 minutes. Causing the wound to rebleed may be helpful. A Band-Aid can be applied if desired. Puncture wounds of the head, chest, or abdomen or those that could still contain a portion of the puncturing object need to be evaluated.

Parents are cautioned against opening blood blisters and against kissing the wound "to make it better." The wound can easily become contaminated from germs in the human mouth. Also, scabs would be allowed to slough off without assistance; picking or early removal may cause scarring. Parents are advised to seek medical help if there is evidence of infection.

Foreign Bodies

Small wooden splinters can be removed by parents with a needle and tweezers that have been sterilized with alcohol or a flame. The area around the sliver is washed with soap and water before attempting the removal. The sliver is exposed with the needle, then grasped firmly by the tweezers and pulled in the same direction in which it entered. Some foreign bodies should have medical evaluation; these include a fishhook, a glass or other difficult-to-see object, or a deeply imbedded object such as a needle in a foot or near a joint.

Cactus prickles or spines are readily removed by one of several methods. Wax from a lighted candle dripped over the affected area (from a sufficient height to avoid burning the skin), then cooled by immersion in cold water and lifted off will bring the foreign bodies with it. Another method is to apply a thin coat of white woodworking or household glue to the area, allow to dry about 10 minutes, and apply a second coat. When this coat becomes dry the sheet of glue along with the cactus pines is peeled from the skin. A layer of facial gel is equally efficient (Gelbard, 1984; Putnam and Lawton, 1985).

Skin Disorders Related to Insect and Animal Contacts

Children come in contact with a variety of animal species. Usually the contact is of no consequence, but children might be injured by the encounter and receive a physical injury (such as an animal bite or insect sting), or they can provide a host for a parasite (such as lice or mites). A parasitic relationship involves a one-sided nutritive association between two organisms of different species in which one (the parasite) derives physical protection and nourishment from the other (the host) without reciprocation. Although this relationship can be fatal to the host, it is to the advantage of the parasite that the host not be destroyed. The effect on the host may be negligible or, with heavy infections, fatal. A parasitic relationship in which the parasite lives within the body of the host *(endoparasite)* is designated as an *infection.* An example of endoparasite infections is the helminths (p. 665). Parasites that are attached to the skin or temporarily invade the superficial tissues *(ectoparasites)* produce an *infestation.*

School children's social nature and proximity to other children render them highly susceptible to communicable diseases, including those caused by parasites. Because they spend considerable time outdoors and in fields and vacant lots, children often come in contact with insects. Consequently children are frequently the victims of insects that puncture the skin for the purpose of sucking blood, injecting venom, or laying their eggs. In the process of these activities, substances foreign to the victim may create an allergic sensitivity in that individual to produce pruritus, urticaria, or systemic reactions of greater or lesser degree depending on the child's sensitivity.

Ordinarily insect bites are of little significance and cause only minor inconvenience. However, they can attain importance if:

1. They cause symptoms that interfere with the child's normal activities, such as the effects of a spider bite.
2. They signify the presence of a contagious skin disease, such as scabies.
3. The parasite is able to transmit other diseases, for example, ticks that transmit Rocky Mountain spotted fever.
4. The venom causes an immune response that can be life-threatening, such as bee stings.

Infestations with insect parasites are more prevalent in nonhygienic environmental conditions but are also encountered in scrupulously clean persons. The infestations encountered most frequently in childhood are scabies and pediculosis capitis. Body lice infestations are rarely seen in the United States, and pubic lice (pediculosis pubis, or "crabs") are rare in childhood. They can be a problem in adolescence, however.

SCABIES

Scabies is an endemic infestation that becomes pandemic at 15-year cyclic intervals, with each incidence lasting approximately 15 years. The current pandemic is nearing completion. Lesions are created as the impregnated female scabies mite burrows into the stratum corneum of the epidermis (never into living tissue) where she deposits her eggs and fecal material. These burrows form minute, linear, grayish-brown threadlike lesions that are often difficult to see.

Clinical Manifestations

The reaction causes intense pruritus that leads to punctate discrete excoriations secondary to the itching. Maculopapular lesions are characteristically distributed in intertriginous areas: interdigital surfaces, axillary-cubital area, popliteal folds, and inguinal region. However, there is large variability in type of lesions. Infants often develop an eczematous eruption; therefore the observer must look for discrete papules, burrows, or vesicles. A mite is identified as a black dot at the end of a burrow. In children over 2 years of age the largest percentage of eruptions are found in the hands and wrists and, in children less than 2 years, on feet and ankles. Children with Down syndrome do not complain of itching and therefore they can get a severe infestation before it is recognized.

The inflammatory response and itching occur after the host becomes sensitized to the mite, approximately 30 to 60 days following initial contact. After this time, anywhere the mite has traveled will begin to itch and develop the characteristic eruption. Consequently mites will not necessarily be located at all sites of eruption. Also, a person needs prolonged contact with the mite to become infested; transient body contact is less likely to cause transfer of the mite.

Therapeutic Management

The diagnosis is made by microscopic identification from scrapings of the burrow. Treatment is application of 1% lindane (Kwell) in a vanishing cream base. Because of the length of time between infestation and the physical symptoms (30 to 60 days), all persons who were in close physical contact with the affected child will need treatment. This may include persons such as boy friends, baby sitters, and grandparents, as well as immediate family members. The objective is to treat as thoroughly as possible the first time.

Nursing Considerations

Nurses instructing families in use of the scabicide should emphasize the importance of following the directions accurately. The lotion is applied to cool dry, skin—not following a hot bath. It is applied over the entire cutaneous surface from the neck down and left on for the recommended time, usually 4 hours for infants and 6 hours for older children and adults. Since it is a superficial skin disorder penetration need not be promoted. One liberal application is sufficient. The physician usually prescribes enough medication for the entire family, allowing 2 ounces for adults and 1 ounce for each child.

Touching and holding contacts with the affected child should be reduced until treatment is completed. Nurses in hospitals are to wear gloves when caring for the child. Following treatment freshly laundered bed linen and underclothing are used and previously worn clothing is washed in very hot water and ironed. Parents need to know that although the mite will be killed, the rash and the itch will not be eliminated until the stratum corneum is replaced, which takes approximately 2 to 3 weeks. Soothing ointments or lotions can be used for pruritus.

PEDICULOSIS CAPITIS

Pediculosis capitis (head lice, or "cooties") is an infestation of the scalp by *Pediculus humanus capitis,* a very common parasite, especially in school-age children. Lice infestations are not a major health threat but they are highly communicable and create embarrassment and a panic reaction in the family and community. They can also cause a child to be ridiculed by other children.

The louse is a blood-sucking organism that requires approximately five meals a day. The adult louse lives only about 48 hours when away from a human host and the life span of the average female is only 1 month. The female lays her eggs at night at the junction of a hair shaft and close to the skin, because the eggs need a warm environment. The eggs hatch in approximately 7 to 10 days; the egg is thus about 4 mm from the scalp at the time of hatching (McLaury, 1983). It has been commonly believed that nits more than ¼ inch from the scalp are incapable of hatching; however, new evidence suggests that viable nits can be found at any distance from the scalp (Taplin and others, 1982).

Clinical Manifestations

Itching, caused by the crawling insect and insect saliva on the skin, is usually the only symptom. The most common sites of involvement are the occipital area, behind the ears, at the nape of the neck, and (occasionally) the eyebrows and eyelashes. Diagnosis is made by observation of the white eggs (nits) firmly attached to the base of the hair shafts. Because of their brief life span and mobility, adult lice are more difficult to locate. Nits must be differentiated from dandruff, lint, hair spray, and other items of similar size and shape. The nits will fluoresce white under Wood light. Scratch marks and/or inflammatory papules, caused by secondary infection, may also found on the scalp in the vulnerable areas.

Therapeutic Management

Treatment consists of the application of pediculocidal shampoos and manual removal of nit cases. A number of shampoos are available that are highly effective. One of the leading therapies is 1% lindane shampoo (gamma benzene hexachloride—Kwell, Kwellada) applied as prescribed and repeated in 7 to 10 days to kill the hatching nymphs. However, lindane is not effective against nits and, if not used properly, is potentially toxic, especially in infants. Equally effective against adult lice and lethal to nits as well is 0.5% malathion (Prioderm*) lotion applied as directed. Preparations of pyrethrin with piperonyl butoxide (RID, A-200 pyrinate, Nix, and Triple X) can be obtained without a prescription and appear to be as effective as lindane.

Recent studies comparing the effectiveness of the various pediculocides report that lindane shampoo is the slowest acting preparation, requiring 3 hours to kill lice and 30% of the eggs hatched after treatment. The pyrethrin products killed lice in 10 to 23 minutes and 23% to 32% of eggs survived to hatch. Malathion killed lice within 5 minutes with only 5% of eggs hatching (Altschuler and Kenney, 1986, Meinking and others, 1986). However, no treatment can be effective unless it is accompanied by an educational and reinfestation-prevention program.

Nursing Considerations

There are several things that nurses should be aware of in order to successfully manage or to assist parents in coping with the problem. It should be emphasized that *anyone* can

---

*Prioderm lotion has been removed from the market by the manufacturer, Purdue-Fredrick Company of Norwalk, CT, who finds it no longer profitable to manufacture (Clore, 1985).

get pediculosis. It has no respect for age, socioeconomic level, or cleanliness. The louse does not jump or fly but it can be transmitted from one person to another on personal items. Therefore children are cautioned against sharing combs, hats, caps, scarves, coats, and other items used on or near the hair. Children who share lockers are more likely to contract an infestation, and slumber parties place children at risk. Lice are not carried or transmitted by household pets.

Parents should carefully inspect the head of a child who scratches the head more than usual for bite marks, redness, and nits. The hair is systematically spread with two Popsicle sticks or tongue depressors and the scalp observed for any movement that indicates a louse. Lice are visible to the naked eye. The nits, or eggs, appear as tiny whitish oval specks adhering to the hair shaft about ¼ inch from the scalp. The adherent nature of the nits distinguish them from dandruff, which falls off readily. Empty nit cases, indicating hatched lice, are translucent rather than white and are located more than ¼ inch from the scalp.

If evidence of infestation is found it is important to perform the treatment according to the directions described on the label of the pediculocide. Parents are advised to read the directions several times in a quiet room before beginning treatment (McLaury, 1983). For example, lindane is applied to *wet* hair, lathered generously, and left on for 4 to 5 minutes before rinsing. Pyrethrin is applied to *dry* hair, gently rubbed until the scalp is completely wet, and allowed to remain on the hair for at least 10 minutes. The hair is then washed with regular shampoo. Instructions on the labels indicate that dead lice and remaining nits are removed with an extra-fine-tooth comb. However, most combs are not fine enough to dislodge the firmly adhered nits. Although it can be a tedious process, the most effective approach is to remove the nit cases between fingernails or tweezers. A dilute vinegar rinse may help to loosen the nits for easier removal.

The child should be made as comfortable as possible during the application process because the pediculocide must remain on the scalp and hair for several minutes. Playing "beauty parlor" is a useful strategy. The child lies supine with the head over a sink or basin and covers the eyes with a dry towel or washcloth during the shampoo to protect them from splashing medication into the eyes, which can cause a chemical conjunctivitis. If eye irritation occurs, the operator must flush the eyes well with tepid water.

Washable items of clothing and bed linen are laundered in hot water and dried in a hot drier. Combs, brushes, and other items can be soaked in the louse shampoo or lotion for an hour or in very hot water (105° F) for 5 to 10 minutes. All mattresses and upholstered furniture should be vacuumed carefully to remove any living lice or nits that may be attached to fallen hair. Spraying with insecticide is not recommended because of the danger to children and animals. Some advocate placing nonwashable, noncleanable items in a tightly closed plastic bag that remains sealed for 14 days. Ova are able to lie dormant for this length of time.

Families should also be advised that the pediculocide is relatively costly, especially when several members of the household require treatment.

The psychologic effects of lice infestations can be highly stressful to children. They are influenced by the reactions of others, including their parents, and may be made to feel ashamed or guilty. Parents are strongly cautioned against cutting a child's hair or, worse, shaving a child's head. Lice infest short hair as readily as long hair, and these actions only compound the child's distress and serve as a continual reminder to peers, who are always ready to taunt another with something out of the ordinary (McLaury, 1983).

Prevention. The increasing incidence of pediculosis in school children has become a serious concern for school nurses, parents, and community health agencies. School nurses are constantly on the alert for evidence of infestation. **The National Pediculosis Association*** has been organized by a group of parents frustrated by repeated infestations of their children. They have developed an approach to the problem that offers hope that vigorous effort on the part of parents and the community will reduce the epidemics in children. Some of their suggestions include encouraging parents to notify others if a child becomes infected and preventing children from re-entering school until they are completely free of nits.

*P.O. Box 149, Newton, MA 02161.

INSECT STINGS

Children come in contact with a variety of insects during their play. Some of the stinging or biting insects (such as mosquitoes, fleas, and gnats) are found almost everywhere; others seem to be more common to specific areas. For example, honey bees are more prevalent in suburbs and rural areas. Hornets, wasps, and yellow jackets are more often found in the cities. Being scavengers, they often feed on garbage. The fire ant is located predominantly in the Southeast. Insect bites are high morbidity but, fortunately, low mortality disorders.

The more common classes of insects, their method of producing a reaction, and the management are outlined in Table 18-6. Most bites are managed by simple symptomatic measures such as cool compresses, calamine lotion, and prevention of secondary infection. Children are taught to wear shoes when playing out-of-doors, especially in areas that may harbor crawling insects. The emergency treatment or specific suggestions for some of their bites or stings are discussed briefly.

Hymenoptera Stings

When an insect stings, its stinger often remains imbedded in the skin. Since bees have barbed stingers that penetrate the skin, any pressure on the venom sac at the tip of the barb pushes more venom into the skin. The best approach is to flick the stinger off with the fingernail or knife blade—

Table 18-6 Skin lesions caused by insect bites and stings

MECHANISM/MANIFESTATIONS	TREATMENT	COMMENTS
Insect bites—flies, gnats, mosquitoes, fleas		
Mechanism:	Antipruritic agents and baths	Hypersensitivity reaction
Foreign protein in insects' saliva introduced when skin penetrated for a blood-sucking meal	Antihistamines	Little or no reaction in nonsensitized person
	Prevent secondary infection	Avoidance of contact
Manifestations:		Remove focus such as treating furniture, mattresses, carpets, and pets, where insects may live
Papular urticaria		
Firm papules; may be capped by vesicles or excoriated		Apply insect repellant when exposure is anticipated
Hymenopters stings—bees, wasps, hornets, yellow jackets, fire ants		
Mechanism:	Carefully scrape off stinger if present	Severe reactions caused by hypersensitivity and/or multiple stings
Injection of venom through stinging apparatus;	Cleanse with soap and water	
Venom contains histamine, allergenic proteins, and often a spreading factor, hyaluronidase	Apply cool compresses or ice packs	Child taught to wear shoes, to avoid wearing bright clothing or perfumed grooming products that might attract the insect, and to avoid places where the insect may be contacted
	Elevate involved extremity	
	Antihistamines	
Manifestations:	Severe reactions: administer epinephrine, corticosteroids; treat for shock	
Local reaction: small red area, wheal, itching, and heat		Hypersensitive children should wear identifying tag to indicate allergy and therapy needed; parents should keep emergency medication and be taught its administration
Systemic reactions: may be mild to severe, including generalized edema, pain, nausea and vomiting, confusion, respiratory embarrassment, and shock		

never squeeze the area. Another method is to cover the area with transparent tape, then peel the tape off. The stinger should come off with the tape (Gorrell, 1985).

The usual response to a sting is sharp pain, a local wheal, and erythema accompanied by intense itching at the site. Emergency treatment consists of applications of a substance that relieves the swelling and discomfort. Direct applications made from readily available common household products have proved to be effective. These include aspirin (or liquid aspirin), baking soda, or Adolph's meat tenderizer mixed with water to make a paste and placed directly on the bite or sting. Some proteins are species specific, others are common to a number of species; therefore crossover reactivity is common.

Children are taught to avoid contact with bees and to recognize the insect (it is not part of the flower). Wearing appropriate clothing and shoes and avoiding substances that might attract bees (perfumes, jelly, ice cream) when they may be encountered are good prophylactic practices.

Children who have become sensitized to hymenoptera bites may demonstrate a severe systemic response that can be life threatening. One sting can produce generalized urticaria, respiratory difficulty (from laryngeal edema), hypotension, and death within 1 hour. Intramuscular administration of epinephrine provides immediate relief and must be available for emergency use. Hypersensitive children need a kit available that contains epinephrine, a hypodermic syringe, and perhaps ephedrine and an antihistamine preparation (a tourniquet is included in the kit but its use is not recommended). Hypersensitive children should wear a Medic Alert bracelet and the families are reminded to check the expiration date on the kit and replace an outdated one. Families should determine if a school nurse is available at the school; if not someone at the school should be designated to inject the epinephrine in case of an emergency.

Some authorities recommend that children with a history of generalized reactivity to an insect sting undertake a program of skin testing and desensitization to prevent serious or fatal reactions. Others believe that the risk of systemic reactions is so low that it does not justify subjecting these children to a protracted and expensive treatment regimen.

Arachnid Bites

Most arachnids in the United States are relatively harmless, including tarantulas. All spiders produce venom that is injected via fangs. Some are unable to pierce skin; in others the venom is insufficiently toxic. There is a local tissue reaction that is relieved by cool compresses or the methods described for hymenoptera stings.

Only scorpions and two spiders—the brown recluse and black widow—inject venom deadly enough to require immediate attention. Children bitten by any of these arachnids must receive medical attention as soon as possible. Antivenin is available for the black widow spider and scorpions but not for the brown recluse spider. More definitive description and therapies are listed in Table 18-7.

Table 18-7 Skin lesions caused by arachnids

MECHANISM/MANIFESTATIONS	TREATMENT	COMMENTS

Black widow spider
Mechanism:
  Venom injected through a clawlike appendage; has neurotoxic action
Manifestations:
  Mild sting at time of bite
  Area becomes swollen, painful, and erythematous
  Dizziness, weakness, and abdominal pain
  May produce delirium, paralysis, convulsions, and (if large amount of venom absorbed) death
	Cleanse wound with antiseptic
	Apply ice packs
	Antivenin
	Muscle relaxant such as calcium gluconate
	Analgesics and/or sedatives
		Spider is recognized by red or orange hourglass-shaped marking on underside
		Avoids light and bites in self-defense
		Teach children to avoid places that harbor the spider, e.g., woodpiles

Brown recluse spider
Mechanism:
  Venom injected via fangs
  Venom contains powerful necrotoxin
Manifestations:
  Mild sting at time of bite
  Transient erythema followed by bleb or blister; mild to severe pain in 2-8 hours; purple, star-shaped area in 3-4 days; necrotic ulceration in 7-14 days
  Systemic reactions may include fever, malaise, restlessness, nausea and vomiting, and joint pain
  Generalized petechial eruption
	Local application of cool compresses
	Antibiotics
	Corticosteroids
	Relief of pain
	Wound may require skin graft
	Some advocate early excision of necrotic area and surrounding tissue
		Spider is fawn to dark brown and recognized by fiddle-shaped mark on head
		Shy; bites only when annoyed or surprised
		Prefers dark areas where seldom disturbed
		Teach children to avoid possible nesting sites
		Wound heals with scar formation

Continued.

Table 18-7 Skin lesions caused by arachnids—cont'd

MECHANISM/MANIFESTATIONS	TREATMENT	COMMENTS

Scorpions
Mechanism:
    Sting by means of a hooked caudal stinger that discharges venom
    Venom of more venomous species contains hemolysins, endotheliolysins, and neurotoxins
Manifestations:
    Intense local pain, erythema, numbness, burning, restlessness, vomiting
    Ascending motor paralysis with convulsions, weakness, rapid pulse, excessive salivation, thirst, dysuria, pulmonary edema, coma, and death
	Delay absorption of venom by application of tourniquets for 10-15 minutes apply cold with ice packs or submerge in cold water
	Administration of antivenin
	Surveillance in PICU
		Some species produce only local tissue reaction with swelling at puncture site (distinctive)
		Usual habitat is southwestern United States
		Symptoms subside in a few hours
		Deaths occur among children under 4 years of age, usually in first 24 hours

Ticks
Mechanism:
    In process of sucking blood, head and mouth parts are buried in skin
Manifestations:
    Produce firm, discrete, intensely pruritic nodules at site of attachment
    May cause urticaria or persistent localized edema
	See text for removal
	If bare hands touch tick during removal wash hands thoroughly with soap and water
		Feed on blood of mammals
		Significant in humans because of pathologic organism carried
		May be vectors of various infectious diseases such as Rocky Mountain spotted fever, Q fever, tularemia, relapsing fever, lyme disease, tick paralysis
		Must attach and feed 1-2 hours to transmit disease
		Usual habitat is very wooded area

Ticks

Ticks are troublesome creatures since they become partially imbedded in the skin as they feed. Numerous methods have been suggested for their removal but the only really effective method is to grasp the tick with curved forceps (or fingers protected with tissue) as close as possible to the point of attachment and pull straight up with a steady, even pressure (Needham, 1985). If a portion of the body (e.g., the head) remains, it can be removed with a sterile needle in the same manner as a sliver. The bite is cleansed with soap and a disinfectant after removal. If the hands have touched the tick they are washed thoroughly with soap and water.

ANIMAL BITES

Animal bites are common injuries and include those caused by both wild and domestic animals. Wild animal bites are discussed in relation to rabies and the local wounds are treated the same as with domestic animals, such as dogs, cats, hamsters, and mice; therefore this discussion is directed primarily toward dog bites.

Over 1 million persons are bitten by dogs each year, and children are the most frequent victims (Chun, Berkelhamer, and Herold, 1982). Younger children are more defenseless and more vulnerable. Over half the victims are less than 4 years of age, and boys are bitten more frequently than girls. Contrary to accepted belief, stray dogs are seldom involved in the attacks; most of the dogs are owned by the family of the victim or a neighbor (Lauer, White, and Lauer, 1982; Pinckney and Kennedy, 1982). Bites from cats are fewer than those of dogs but cat scratches are extremely common (see Cat scratch fever, p. 784). Most dog or cat injuries are to the upper extremities. However, small children are more likely to receive bites or scratches to the head, face, and neck because of their tendency to put their heads near the animal's head and flail their arms rather than protecting their heads.

Most dog attacks occur in or adjacent to the owners' yards, and the attack is usually preceded by verbal or physical contact with the animal (Wright, 1985). The injuries vary from small puncture wounds to complete evulsion of tissue and can be associated with significant crush injury. German shepherds account for a disproportionate number of severe attacks.

Therapeutic Management

General wound care consists of rinsing the wound with copious amounts of water or saline under pressure (syringe) and washing the surrounding skin with mild soap. A clean pressure dressing is applied and the extremity elevated if the wound is bleeding. Medical evaluation is advised since there is danger of tetanus and rabies, although dogs in most urban areas are required to be immunized against rabies. Bites from wild animals, such as squirrels, bats, and raccoons, are potentially dangerous.

Prophylactic antibiotics are indicated for puncture wounds and wounds in areas that may prove to be cosmetically or functionally impaired if infected. Extensive lacerations are sutured. Tetanus toxoid is administered according to standard guidelines (p. 529) and rabies protocol followed (p. 1655). Cat bites become infected more easily than dog bites but no more than lacerations from other causes. Injuries to poorly vascularized areas such as the hands are more likely to become infected than those in more vascularized areas such as the face; puncture wounds are more apt to become infected than lacerations.

Nursing Considerations

The most important aspect related to animal bites is prevention. It is important that children understand animal behavior and develop an honest respect for all animals. It is vital that they learn how to treat animals and how to react to them. Suggestions about what families can do and tell children about animals is outlined in the box. Meeting a strange dog can be both frightening and a danger to a child (Fig.

18-8). The child should remain calm and follow the suggestions outlined.

Parents who are contemplating buying a pet, especially a dog, for themselves or their children should receive some advice about the dog that is least likely to be a danger to

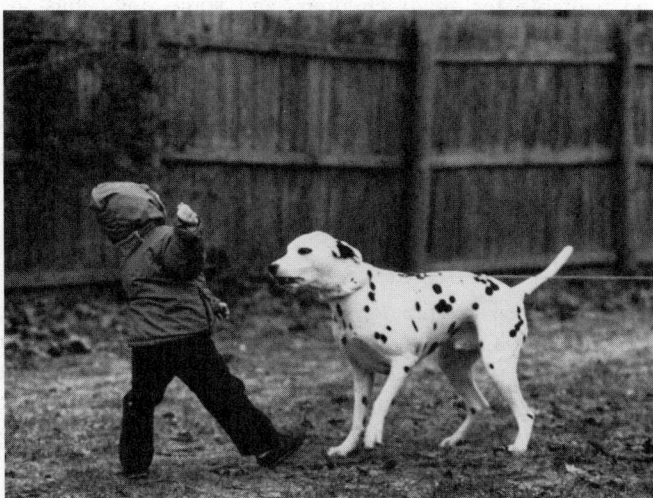

Fig. 18-8. Children need to be taught how to behave around both strange and familiar dogs.
Photography by G. Robert Bishop.

WHAT TO TELL CHILDREN ABOUT ANIMALS

Avoid all strange animals, especially wild, sick, or injured ones. The same techniques employed in teaching children not to talk to strangers should be used to teach them not to approach strange animals.

Notify the Health Department or police of any wild, sick, or injured animals.

Never permit a child to break up an animal fight, even when his own pet is involved. Use a rake, broom, or garden hose to separate the animals.

Become aware, and make children aware, of the danger of mistreating or teasing pets. Pets are not toys, but living creatures who will bite if mauled, annoyed, or frightened.

Alert your child to dangerous and nervous animals in your neighborhood and do not permit him to enter yards or houses that harbor them.

Do not allow a child to disturb an animal that is eating or sleeping. Set a good example by your own behavior.

Do not let your pet come into indiscriminate contact with other animals.

Avoid the indiscriminate contact between your pet and human beings.

Do **not** purchase or obtain pets for your children until such time as they demonstrate their maturity and ability to handle and care for the pets. This ability is rare in a child under 4 years of age and unusual in a child under 6. Factors to be considered at any age are the maturity and disposition of the child and the animal. Some people never develop this maturity.

Stress to children the importance of avoiding routes, when riding bicycles of tricycles, where dogs are known to chase vehicles.

Teach children that each animal has the right to a free existence and freedom from man-inflicted pain. Set a good example by your own behavior.

Under your supervision or that of some other adult, have children make friends with pets, in the immediate neighborhood, with which the children will be in contact.

Never hold your face close to an animal.

Do not permit a child or young person to lead a large dog.

Never tease, pull the tail, or take away food, bone, or toy with which an animal is playing.

Do not run, ride a bicycle, or skate in front of a dog. It will startle him.

Do not touch a dog while he is asleep or unaware of your presence. Always speak to any dog that has not seen you approach so that he becomes aware of your presence and will not be startled.

Avoid all unnecessary contact with wild animals—now an important spreader of rabies.

Do not overexcite an animal, even in play.

Do not keep animals confined with short ropes or chains. This may make them aggressive and vicious, especially when teased.

Have children avoid dogs raised in a home without children. Such animals may resent children.

Do not allow an inexperienced child or adult to feed a dog. Such persons may pull back when the animal moves to take the food, frightening the animal. This practice is dangerous.

From Mofenson, H.C., Greensher, J., and Teitelbaum, H.: How to avoid animal bites, Med. Times **100:**92, 1972.

their children. The level of sociability with children is the key to a selection, and dogs range from dangerous, bad, and unsuitable to tolerant of children to exceptionally good with children—some under certain conditions. For example, dogs that are too clumsy, impetuous, or vigorous are not suitable for small children, and some dogs must be raised with the children. Small dogs are usually recommended for children but if a large dog is desired, a Labrador retriever is a good choice (Lauer, White, and Lauer, 1982). A categorization of dogs related to their potential interaction with children can be found in the publication "The right dog for you."*

HUMAN BITES

Children often acquire lacerations from the teeth of other humans in rough play, during fights, or as victims of child abuse. Many preschool children bite others out of frustration or anger. Because human dental plaque and gingiva harbor pathogenic bacteria, all human bites should receive attention.

If the laceration is less than ¼ inch in length the wound can be treated at home. The wound is washed vigorously with soap and water and a pressure dressing applied to stop bleeding. Ice applications minimize discomfort and swelling. Increased pain or redness at the wound site is an indication that the child should receive medical attention for antibiotic therapy. Tetanus toxoid is needed if more than 5 years has elapsed since the last immunization. Wounds greater than ¼ inch should receive medical attention.

CAT SCRATCH DISEASE

Cat scratch disease (CSD) is described as a subacute regional adenitis that follows the scratch or bite of an animal, especially a cat (99% of cases). The disease is usually a benign, self-limiting illness that resolves spontaneously in about 2 to 4 months. The disease is believed to be caused by a bacillus (Margileth & others, 1984).

The usual manifestations are a painless, nonpruritic erythematous papule at the site of inoculation followed by regional lymphadenitis. The disease may persist for several months before gradual resolution. In some children the adenitis progresses to suppuration, and a few children may be very ill with various symptoms, including a prolonged high temperature. The diagnosis is made on the basis of three of the following: (1) cat contact (usually a kitten), (2) lymphadenopathy, (3) an inoculation site, and (4) a positive CSD skin test (Carithers, 1985).

The treatment is primarily supportive. Antibiotics do not appear to shorten the duration or prevent progression to suppuration. Activity is limited to prevent trauma to the large lymph nodes and bed rest is indicated for children who have fevers. Analgesics may be needed for discomfort and fever.

*Tortora, D.F.: The right dog for you, New York, 1980, Simon & Schuster.

Most children can continue normal activities during the course of the disease. The animals are not ill during the time they transmit the disease, and most authorities do not recommend disposal of a cherished pet.

Miscellaneous Skin Disorders

There are a number of skin lesions caused by extrinsic or intrinsic factors. Some of these are listed in Table 18-8. Some are discussed briefly in the following discussion and elsewhere in the book as appropriate.

NEUROFIBROMATOSIS

Neurofibromatosis (NF), or von Recklinghausen disease, is a relatively common genetic disorder with an autosomal dominant inheritance pattern. It occurs in 1:3000 persons and has one of the highest mutation rates known (Cohen, 1984). The manifestaions are highly variable and appear to result from some defect that alters peripheral nerve differentiation and growth.

There is marked clinical variability in manifestations that first appear as small, discrete, pigmented skin lesions (café-au-lait spots, pigmented nevi) and/or axillary freckling that develop in early infancy or childhood. Slow-growing cutaneous and subcutaneous neurofibromas that grow along the course of a peripheral nerve may appear in later childhood or adolescence. Other characteristics may include developmental delay or retardation, seizures, scoliosis or kyphosis, short stature, macrocephaly, speech defects, learning disabilities, or a variety of congenital malformations. The severity varies considerably and can vary within the same family. One member may have only café-au-lait spots or axillary freckling while another has more severe manifestations.

The diagnosis is established by physical findings observed or, in doubtful cases, nodule biopsy. Six or more café-au-lait spots (0.5 cm in diameter in children) are considered to be diagnostic, although there is some debate. A family history is elicited to determine if the specific case is inherited or if it represents a new mutation. The risk of transmitting the disorder to offspring is 50%. Therapy is limited to excisions of tumors, which produce pain or impair function, and symptomatic management of other manifestations.

Nursing Considerations

Nursing care is primarily recognition of signs that indicate a possibility of the disease, referral for diagnosis, and family counseling and support. It is important that a diagnosis be made, even when the only manifestations are a few café-au-lait spots. The family will need to know the genetic implications and to be alert for any signs that indicate the child is developing any of the more serious characteristics at a

Table 18-8   Miscellaneous skin disorders

DISEASE/CAUSATIVE AGENT	LOCAL MANIFESTATIONS	TREATMENT	COMMENTS
Urticaria—usually allergic response to drugs or infection	Development of wheals Vary in size and configuration and tend to appear quickly, spread irregularly, and fade within a few hours May be constant or intermittent, sparse or profuse, small or large, discrete or confluent May be acute, chronic, or recurrent in acute attacks	Local soothing and antipruritic applications Antihistamines Epinephrine or ephedrine Cortisone or corticotropin (ACTH) in severe cases Severe upper respiratory involvement may require tracheostomy	Known etiologic agents should be avoided May be accompanied by malaise, fever, lymphadenopathy Severe cases may involve mucous membranes, internal organs, and joints Obstruction to air passages constitutes medical emergency (see p. 1213)
Psoriasis—unknown; hereditary predisposition	Round, thick, dry, reddish patches covered with coarse, silvery scales over trunk and extremities; first lesions commonly appear in scalp; facial lesions more common in children than adults Affected cells proliferate at a much more rapid rate than normal cells	Exposure to sunlight, ultraviolet light Topical corticosteroids Tar derivatives Trihydroxyanthracine Keratolytic agents (salicylic acid) Psoralin—ultraviolet A (PUVA)*	Uncommon in children under age 6 Persons are otherwise healthy individuals Coal tar and psoralin act synergistically with ultraviolet light Keratolytic agents enhance absorption of corticosteroids
Alopecia Alopecia areata	Sudden onset of asymptomatic, noninflammatory, round, bald patches in hairy parts of body	Psychologic support Inducement of allergic contact dermatitis to stimulate growth of hair Minoxidil (peripheral vasodilator)	Family history in 10%-26% of cases Some concern regarding drug therapy safety Refer to support groups†
Traumatic alopecia	Traction alopecia around scalp margins from tight hair styles (e.g., braids, pony tails, corn rows)	Counseling regarding hair styling, use of hair cosmetics, hot combs, rollers	More prevalent in black children and adolescents Prolonged traction can produce fibrosis of hair root and permanent loss
	Compulsive hair pulling	Determine and treat cause	Chronic hair pulling may require psychologic therapy
Tinea capitis	See Table 18-3	See Table 18-3	See Table 18-3

*Still considered investigational.
†National Alopecia Areata Foundation, P.O. Box 5027, Mill Valley, CA 94941.

later time. Other members of the family should be assessed for possible signs of the disorder.

Families can be referred to the **National Neurofibromatosis Foundation***, an organization whose purpose is to increase public awareness of neurofibromatosis, to provide help and support to families affected by the disorder, and to stimulate research.

LYME DISEASE

Lyme disease is a relatively recently recognized disorder caused by a spirochete transmitted by ticks. The disease may present in three stages: (1) the tick bite at the time of inoculation; (2) development of erythema chronicum migrans (EMC) at the site of the bite, which begins as a small erythematous papule that enlarges radially, resulting in a large circumferential ring with a raised, edematous doughnut-like border; and, (3) the most serious stage of the disease, systemic involvement of neurologic, cardiac, and musculoskeletal systems that appears several weeks after the cutaneous phase is completed. Cases seen at the second stage are treated with appropriate antibiotics. The treatment is effective in preventing third stage manifestations in most cases.

Neurologic manifestations include meningoencephalitis, cranial neuritides, and radiculoneuritis; these are managed with a short course of oral prednisone if symptoms have been present less than 24 hours and with antibiotics. Cardiac manifestations, commonly atrioventricular conduction abnormalities that may result in severe heart block, are treated

*141 Fifth Ave., 7-S, New York, NY 10010.

the same as neurologic symptoms with the addition of acetylsalicylic acid (aspirin) and daily prednisone.

Musculoskeletal pains that involve the tendons, bursae, muscles, and synovia can begin at the same time as the cutaneous EMC, but the pauciarticular arthritis usually does not develop for 1 to 4 months. In children the arthritis is characterized by intermittently painful swollen joints (primarily the knees), with spontaneous remissions and exacerbations. Symptomatic relief is attained with aspirin or prednisone. Oral penicillin is prescribed if not begun earlier (Anderson, 1986).

Prevention of the disorder is educating parents to examine their children carefully for signs of the skin lesion if they are known to have been exposed to the tick vector. Parents should always examine their children for the presence of ticks if they have been in areas where ticks are likely to be found.

CONGENITAL SKIN DISORDERS

There are a number of congenital skin disorders, usually inherited as an autosomal dominant trait. Psoriasis in children less than 16 years of age is common (see Table 18-8), and photosensitivity eruptions associated with some inherited diseases appear early in childhood. Ichthyoses are a heterogenous group of disorders characterized by scaling that create a challenging problem in treatment. Because of wide variability, these disorders are not discussed in detail.

Behavioral Disorders in School-Age Children

A number of classification systems have been employed to outline the various problems of middle childhood that interfere with development, learning, and social relationships. Although there is no universal categorization, most authorities seem to broadly classify behavioral disorders in some manner that identifies mental subnormality, learning disabilities, neuroses, psychoses, and antisocial behavior. Many disorders have a major organic or developmental component, whereas others are seen almost exclusively in children of school age. Still others are primarily problems of adolescence, and many extend throughout the course of childhood. Very often a change in behavior is one of the manifestations of an organic disease; at other times emotional problems produce somatic symptoms of greater or lesser seriousness.

The variety and extent of emotional and behavioral disorders of childhood are much too numerous to be considered here; some are discussed elsewhere (e.g., mental retardation in Chapter 23 and sensory impairment in Chapter 24).

ATTENTION DEFICIT DISORDER

Attention deficit disorder (ADD) is the term applied to various behavior problems that in some way impair the child's capacity to profit from new experiences. The syndrome of manifestations affects a significant number of children and is 10 times more frequent in boys than in girls. The difficulties are most often school-related, behavioral or academic, and difficulties with social relationships in general often manifest by aggressive behavior and mood lability that interferes with peer relationships and difficulty with discipline.

Considerable confusion and disagreement exist regarding ADD, but the disorder is delineated into two subtypes: *ADD with hyperactivity* and *ADD without hyperactivity*. Presently it is unclear whether these are two forms of a single disorder or whether they represent two distinct disorders. In addition, there are individuals who evidenced attention deficit disorder with hyperactivity at an earlier age but who no longer demonstrate the hyperactivity.

Early identification of affected children is needed, since the characteristics of the disorder significantly interfere with the normal course of emotional and psychologic development. Many of these children, in the attempt to cope with attention deficit, develop maladaptive behavior patterns that are a deterrent to psychosocial adjustment. Their behavior evokes negative responses from others, and repeated exposure to negative feedback adversely affects the child's self-concept.

The term *specific learning disabilities* refers to the behavioral outcomes of impaired functioning in central processing such as dyslexia, dysphasia, and inability to calculate or draw. It is primarily an educational concern and mentioned briefly at the conclusion of this segment.

Etiology

The etiology of attention deficit disorder is uncertain, obscure, and often speculative. As the definition implies, it may be related to virtually any illness or trauma affecting the brain that occurs at any stage of development—before, during, or after birth. Multiple causes, including psychosocial factors, are probably involved.

Behavioral and learning disorders have been noted in children with some of the sex chromosomal abnormalities. For example, in girls with Turner syndrome there is a high incidence of impaired spatial abilities and right-left directional sense, and a large number of boys with Klinefelter syndrome have learning, behavioral, or peer problems. A sex-linked factor may be operating because the hyperkinetic syndrome is much more common in boys than in girls.

A popular theory is the concept of a developmental lag. Distractibility, short attention span, and impulsiveness are all normal characteristics of children at a much younger developmental level. Since the symptoms tend to diminish with age, it is postulated that this may have an anatomic basis, that is, a maturational lag in myelination of the prefrontal cortex that takes place through adolescence. In addition, hyperactivity may be merely a normal variant of innate temperament in some children who represent the extreme end of the normal distribution curve for activity.

Support for a biochemical etiology is suggested by the way in which a majority of hyperactive children respond to central nervous system stimulant drugs. In these hyperactive children there appears to be an absence or insufficiency of norepinephrine, a neurotransmitter that normally appears in high concentrations in areas of the brain that have much to do with activity level, mood, and awareness. Another theory suggests some alteration in the reticular activating system of the midbrain, a key area for controlling consciousness and attention, that interferes with its function of filtering out extraneous stimuli. Consequently these children are unable to focus on one stimulus but are compelled to respond to every stimulus in the environment. Central nervous system stimulants that increase the level of norepinephrine and/or activate the reticular activating system cause a reduction in the undesired behavior. The fact that these children show few, if any, symptoms in a stress situation (such as the clinician's or principal's office) provides additional support to this hypothesis, because stress increases the level of norepinephrine.

In the past there has been interest in diet and hyperkinesis. There are those who believe that the observed behavioral patterns are related to an innate sensitivity to certain food items and/or food additives. Although this theory does not have wholehearted support, some children do show improvement when certain foods are eliminated from their diet, particularly those containing salicylates and those with specific additives such as artificial coloring, sweetening, and preservatives.

Clinical Manifestations

The behaviors exhibited by the child with attention deficit disorder are not unusual aspects of child behavior. The difference lies in the quality of motor activity and developmentally inappropriate inattention, impulsivity, and hyperactivity the child displays. The manifestations may be numerous or few, mild or severe, and will vary with the developmental level of the child. Any given child will not have every manifestation that is characteristic of a syndrome, and the degree of severity is highly variable. Mild manifestations of the symptoms may not be apparent in a good educational and family environment, whereas severe symptomatology will be recognizable even in the most healthy and accommodating environment. Every dysfunctional child is, in some respects, different from all other children with attention deficit disorder.

Most of the behavioral manifestations are apparent at an early age, but the learning disabilities may not become evident until the child enters school. The symptoms are more prominent before age 10, after which they become more subtle, tending to diminish with advancing age. The disorder is unpredictable; it may remit spontaneously at any age, and the number of years a child will need medication is unknown. Although it appears that most characteristics of attention deficit disorder do not extend into adolescence, increasing evidence indicates that hyperactive children do not necessarily outgrow their symptoms (Brown, 1986). Con-

comitant emotional difficulties are frequent, and there are indications of continued difficulties in school, difficulties with peers and authority figures, and continued aggressive behavior.

As adults there is an increased incidence of alcoholism, personality and affective disorders, and psychoses in a significant number of these children. It is questionable how many of these persistent behavioral problems may be caused by the cerebral dysfunction and how many by the undesirable effects of childhood experiences. Children who are unable to function normally in their home and school environment will meet with constant failure and rejection and will react with hostility or other inappropriate behaviors. Their frequent recognition that they are "bad" or are not "right inside" will produce a negative self-concept and reactive hostility. A problem facing families of persons with ADD is finding health professionals who are willing to continue therapy in the adult years (Huessy, 1985).

The basic characteristics outlined in the accompanying boxes reflect disturbances in central processing. These criteria are the basis for establishing a diagnosis of ADD. Research has found that children with ADD with hyperactivity

---

ATTENTION DEFICIT DISORDER: DIAGNOSTIC CRITERIA

Diagnostic criteria for attention deficit disorder with hyperactivity

The number of symptoms specified is for children between the ages of 8 and 10, the peak age range for referral. In younger children, more severe forms of the symptoms and a greater number of symptoms are usually present. The opposite is true of older children.
A. **Inattention.** At least three of the following:
  1. Often fails to finish things he or she starts
  2. Often doesn't seem to listen
  3. Easily distracted
  4. Has difficulty concentrating on schoolwork or other tasks requiring sustained attention
  5. Has difficulty sticking to a play activity
B. **Impulsivity.** At least three of the following:
  1. Often acts before thinking
  2. Shifts excessively from one activity to another
  3. Has difficulty organizing work (this not being due to cognitive impairment)
  4. Needs a lot of supervision
  5. Frequently calls out in class
  6. Has difficulty awaiting turn in games or group situations
C. **Hyperactivity.** At least two of the following:
  1. Runs about or climbs on things excessively
  2. Has difficulty sitting still or fidgets excessively
  3. Has difficulty staying seated
  4. Moves about excessively during sleep
  5. Is always "on the go" or acts as if "driven by a motor"
D. Onset before the age of 7.
E. Duration of at least 6 months.
F. Not due to schizophrenia, affective disorder, or severe or profound mental retardation.

From Diagnostic and statistical manual of mental disorders, ed. 3 (DSM-III), Washington, DC, 1980, American Psychiatric Association.

exhibit attention, behavioral, and cognitive impairments whereas children with ADD without hyperactivity show deficits in an attention/cognitive dimension (Berry, Shaywitz, and Shaywitz, 1985). Management problems and antisocial behavior are associated with hyperactivity; increased impulsivity is not associated with attention deficits in the absence of hyperactivity.

The same researchers found that there are sex differences in children with ADD. Disruptive, uncontrolled behaviors are more frequent among boys; girls with ADD without hyperactivity display poor self-esteem and are significantly older than boys with the same type of ADD. Girls with ADD with or without hyperactivity are more likely to suffer peer rejection than boys. Girls may not be diagnosed as readily as boys and cognitive deficits play a more prominent role with girls; behavioral disturbances increase the likelihood of identification for boys.

Diagnostic Evaluation

The most significant and essential tool for diagnosis is a thorough history. Neurologic and psychologic examinations are useful in detecting specific defects, and observations made in a familiar environment may help confirm suspicions. However, it is the history that ultimately determines the diagnosis. The child seldom displays symptoms in the practitioner's office and acts reasonably normal in a one-to-one relationship.

A history, both medical and developmental, and description of the child's behavior should be obtained from as many observers of the child as possible, especially parents and teachers, as well as the observations of the health professionals involved. It should include descriptions of the child's behavior in home and school situations. In obtaining descriptive material, the interviewer must question the observers carefully because some persons, especially parents, may be so concerned with gross behaviors that they often overlook less distressing but equally important symptoms. For example, parents may report a "colicky" infant, a child who began to run as soon as he walked, a toddler who was compelled to touch everything he saw, and a child who resisted sleep until exhausted. A history of delayed or atypical language development is associated with specific learning disabilities. A pregnancy and birth history may provide clues to a situation that might have produced an episode of hypoxia.

A physical examination including a detailed neurologic evaluation will help rule out any severe neurologic disorders. Psychologic testing, especially projective tests, is valuable in determining visual-perceptual difficulties, problems with spatial organization, and other phenomena that suggest cortical or diencephalic involvement and helps to identify the child's intelligence and achievement levels. Psychiatric disorders need to be ruled out. Other causes of hyperactivity that may need to be excluded include lead poisoning, petit mal seizures, partial hearing loss, psychosis, and witnessing sexual activity (common in children in lower socioeconomic groups). An electroencephalogram may be of value in differentiation of other disorders, such as a temporal lobe seizure disorder or "absence spells."

Therapeutic Management

Management of the child with attention deficit disorder usually involves a multiple approach that includes family education and counseling, medication, remedial education, environmental manipulation, and sometimes psychotherapy for the child.

Behavioral therapy and psychotherapy. Behavioral therapy is often successful for the child whose behavior, mood, and reality-perception disturbances are not severe. This consists of a relatively controlled environment in conjunction with behavior modification techniques, family counseling, and/or psychotherapy (see Nursing considerations). Diet modification has proved effective for some children but is not a standard therapeutic modality.

Pharmacologic therapy. Many drugs have been advocated for management of the symptoms of ADD. The most frequently prescribed medications are the sympathomimetic amines methylphenidate (Ritalin) or dextroamphetamine (Dexedrine). They produce strong effects on central nervous system dopamine and norepinephrine. Methylphenidate is preferred because its effect on prolactin and growth hormone is less marked than dextroamphetamine. The child is begun on a small dose that is gradually increased until the desired response is achieved.

Drugs that are less often prescribed are magnesium pemoline (Cylert) and the tricyclic antidepressants. Pemoline is a mild central nervous system stimulant with a slower onset and its effect appears less marked. Tricyclic antidepressants, principally imipramine (Tofranil), have proved to be effective in some children, but cardiac side effects must be monitored. Other pharmacologic agents that have been employed with variable degrees of success are the major tranquilizers (phenothiazines and haloperidol), lithium carbonate, and the antihistamine diphenhydramine hydrochloride (Benadryl).

Nursing Considerations

Nurses are active participants in all aspects of management of the child with attention deficit disorder, especially school nurses. Nurses in the community setting work with families in the home on a long-term basis to help plan and implement therapeutic regimens and to evaluate the effectiveness of therapy. They are in the best position to coordinate services and serve as liaison between other health and education professionals directly involved in a child's therapy program. The nurse in the school who has an understanding of the child's special needs can work with teachers. The nurse in any setting (community, school, hospital, clinician's office) can provide support and guidance to children and families during the difficult tasks associated with growing up with a disabling condition.

The management of the child with attention deficit disorder begins with an explanation to the parents and the child about the diagnosis, including the nature of the problem and the clinician's concept of the underlying central nervous system basis for the disorder. Most parents are confused and feel some measure of guilt. To some it is confirmation of the fear that the child may be "crazy" or has something irrevocably bad; to others it is a relief. They need the opportunity to ventilate their feelings and suspicions. A common complaint of parents is that health professionals have not listened to what they have to say about their child.

The parents need information about the prognosis and an understanding of the treatment plan. The greater their understanding of the disorder and its effects, the more likely they will be to carry out the recommended program of therapy. It is important that they understand that the therapy is not necessarily a panacea and that it will extend over a long period. This has particular significance for changes they need to make in environmental management.

Medication. Parents are reminded that some medications (pemoline) require 2 to 3 weeks to achieve an effect. Others are begun at low dosage and increased until the desired affect is attained. When evaluating the child's response to the medication, it is helpful to obtain reports from the teacher as well as from the parents, since the parents may see the child when the effects of the drug are wearing off. Observing the child's behavior through visits to home and school is useful for assessing attention span, interactional patterns with others at school, and behaviors with academic tasks. The nurse can consult with the teacher about the child's behavior in general. This provides data needed to regulate dosage based on recorded, systematic observations of the child's behaviors in at least two settings.

Parents need to be informed of the possible side effects of the medication—anorexia, blurred vision, and sleeplessness—which usually disappear after several weeks. A common complaint is that the child becomes quiet and very sensitive, crying at the slightest provocation. Sleeplessness is reduced by administering the medication early in the day. It has also been found that the absorption of methylphenidate is accelerated when administered with meals and impeded when given before meals (Chan and others, 1983). Another troublesome side effect is depressed growth, probably caused by interference with the release of growth hormone; therefore the physician may sometimes discontinue the drug on weekends or on vacations to allow for some catch-up growth, although some believe there is no theoretic or practical advantage to the practice (Brown, 1986).

Children on tricyclic antidepressants display a dramatic increase in the incidence of dental caries (Slome, 1984). The marked anticholinergic action of the drugs increases saliva viscosity and produces a dry mouth. Emphasis on rigorous dental hygiene, conscientious home fluoride treatment, regular visits to the dentist, limited intake of refined carbohydrates, and artificial saliva is an important nursing function. The child should be kept well hydrated.

Parents may express concern that the child may become addicted to antidepressant drugs. There is always the possibility of abuse, including suicide attempts; however, usually the child is no longer interested in the drug once the need is past—particularly since the effect of the drug in these children is opposite that produced in normal individuals. However, parents are cautioned to keep the drugs safely stored away from children who may inadvertently ingest them.

In those children in whom a salicylate-free diet relieves the disordered behavior, which is caused by an allergic reaction to food additives, the parents may need help with the child's diet; for example, it is the nurse's responsibility to find out what the child *can eat* and help the parents find sources for the proper foods, especially if the child is on a special metabolic diet.

Environmental manipulation. The child's environment is simplified by decreasing external stimuli, reducing alternatives, encouraging desired patterns of behavior, and sometimes diet control. The parents may need assistance to determine firm but reasonable limits and support in their efforts to provide a stable and predictable environment with regular routines of sleeping, eating, working, and playing. The child needs an environment in which distractions are reduced to a minimum and that is relatively free of external stimuli. In addition, the more the environment is controlled, the less medication is required.

Remedial education. Special training activities in the schools are designed to offer a direct attack on such areas of deficit as visual perception, auditory perception, and other areas involving integration and coordination. These may be accomplished in self-contained classes with a limit of six to eight children, special resource rooms with equipment and teaching teams, mobile consultants who move from room to room to provide assistance to teachers and children, and special first-grade programs in which high-risk children receive special attention to prevent or reduce the need for services as they progress. The purpose of programs for children with special learning disabilities is to assist them toward more successful achievement, personal adjustment, and eventual retention in the regular classroom. However, because a true perceptual problem exists, improvement is noted by an increased attention span, allowing the child to focus on one stimulus while blocking out others; refinement of fine motor control; and advancement in other areas of disability.

Psychiatric, psychologic, and social therapies. On the whole, psychotherapy is relatively unsuccessful in the treatment of the basic characteristics of attention deficit disorder. However, psychotherapy is sometimes useful in children who have experienced negative experiences to the extent that their self-image is threatened. Often children with this disorder describe themselves as stupid or "mentally retarded." They are different from the other children, and they know it. Although they have strengths, they do not get an opportunity to demonstrate them. Consequently they develop coping mechanisms to deal with their negative self-image. They are restless and disruptive, resort to clowning, and develop somatic symptoms. They may become apathetic, resort to daydreaming, appear "not to care," or display perfectionistic perseverance in the attempt to do well. Shy children may withdraw. The child with behavior problems is the one who will get help earlier than the quiet child. Therefore the quiet child may not receive help until the problem is well advanced, which is a disadvantage because remediation takes longer when it is begun with older children. Both child and family may need help during certain periods of stress. Professionals who serve as consultants to health professionals, schools, and families include education specialists, language specialists, and behavior technologists, as well as psychologists, social workers, and physician specialists.

SPECIFIC LEARNING DISABILITY

Learning-disabled children are those who exhibit a disorder in one or more of the basic psychologic processes involved in understanding or in using spoken or written language. The disability may be manifested in disorders of listening, thinking, talking, reading, writing, spelling, or calculating. They include conditions that have been referred to as perceptual disabilities and developmental aphasia. They do not include learning problems, which result primarily from visual, hearing, or motor disabilities, mental retardation, emotional disturbances, or environmental disadvantage.

These learning disabilities occur frequently in children diagnosed with attention deficit disorder with or without hyperactivity. *Learning disability* is an educational term, and schools, recognizing this disability, provide services for affected children. The types of disabilities include dyslexia (difficulty with reading), dysgraphia (difficulty with writing), dyscalculia (difficulty with calculation), right-left confusion, and short attention span. Most affected children are hypoactive, and their needs are frequently overlooked or their behavior is mistaken for retardation. Special education classes offer help and encouragement for these children and their parents, and early recognition facilitates the process of gaining the special assistance needed to function in the school situation. The **Association for Children and Adults with Learning Disabilities*** provides information and support to families with a learning disabled child.

ENURESIS

Enuresis is a common and troublesome disorder that is difficult to define because of the variable ages at which children achieve bladder control. Bladder control depends on a number of factors, including the individual child's developmental tempo, the manner in which training is carried out, the personality makeup of the child, and the emotional climate of the home environment. In a broad sense enuresis can be defined as repeated involuntary urination (usually nocturnal) in children who are beyond the age when voluntary bladder control should normally have been acquired. Some authorities place 4 years as an arbitrary age by which diurnal and nocturnal bladder control is normally accomplished, although 5 years of age is probably more accurate.

Enuresis can also be defined as *primary,* wherein there has never been a long dry or symptom-free period, or *secondary* or *acquired,* in which the enuresis occurs after a dry period of at least a year, and as nighttime *(nocturnal),* daytime *(diurnal),* or both. The incidence is approximately 5% to 17% in otherwise normal children between 3 and 15 years of age.

There is no clear-cut etiology for enuresis as a distinct entity. Some observers have established a hereditary basis in a number of instances. There appears to be a history of high frequency of bed-wetting in parents, siblings, and other near relatives of symptomatic children, and these observations are supported by a high concordance rate in enuretic monozygotic twins. Family studies indicate that the closer the relationship, the higher the incidence of enuresis. It appears that these persons have difficulty in inhibiting the mechanisms that regulate the emptying of the bladder.

Enuresis is more common in boys than in girls, although the reason for this higher frequency is not altogether clear. Some authorities believe that it may be related to the fact

---

*4156 Library Road, Pittsburgh, PA 15234.

that girls are usually neater and more conscious of cleanliness than boys and that they more readily respond to training procedures. There is a high frequency in children in the lower socioeconomic groups, and a higher frequency has been observed in black children than in white children. It has also been observed that there is an increased prevalence of enuresis among late maturing adolescents, both male and female, than early or midmaturers, and the children describe themselves as tense, having difficulty sleeping, and having bad dreams. Children ages 6 through 11 had temperaments described as high strung and lost their temper easily (Levine, 1983). Enuretic children are more likely to be afraid of the dark.

Socioeconomic differences are probably related to a number of incidental factors. Bed-wetting is less frequent in homes where cleanliness is prized, a toilet is nearby, bedtime fluid intake is regulated, the mother makes a special effort with toilet training, and the child is taken from the bed to empty his bladder during the night. Bed-wetting is more apt to be increased in children who live in homes in which poor habits of cleanliness are practiced, toilet facilities are not readily accessible, and the temperature is cold at night and in children who sleep with a bed-wetting sibling.

Pathophysiology

Enuresis is primarily a problem of delayed or incomplete neuromuscular maturation of the bladder and as such is benign and self-limiting. There are children who exhibit temporary regressive behavior after the birth of a sibling or who have occasional "accidents" when they become involved in play to such an extent that they are unaware of a full bladder, become excited, or "forget" to empty the bladder. In other children enuresis may be caused by problems associated with toilet training that are related to the age at which training is begun, the emotional atmosphere that surrounds the training situation, or an excessive amount of emotional dependence on the mother. In some children enuresis is one behavioral manifestation of a personality disorder. However, behavioral problems associated with enuresis are probably a result rather than a cause of the enuresis.

A significant number of nocturnal enuretic episodes are related to deep sleep. These children seem to sleep more soundly than others and to waken from either external or internal stimuli. Many of these children demonstrate increased frequency and magnitude of spontaneous bladder contractions during the non-rapid-eye-movement (N-REM) stage of sleep preceding bed-wetting. Bed-wetting appears to occur as the child moves from the deeper stages of non-REM sleep into the REM stage.

Enuresis has a strong familial tendency and seems to be associated with a developmental delay that causes such intense urgency that the child is unable to inhibit bladder contraction after the bladder is distended beyond a certain volume. Such children acquire bladder control with difficulty and, even after control, are more prone to enuresis when

subjected to stress than are other children. In addition, most enuretic children have a borderline functional bladder capacity. The small bladder is unable to hold a full night's urine excretion.

Clinical Manifestations

The predominant symptom is urgency that is immediate and accompanied by acute discomfort, restlessness, and sometimes urinary frequency. Nocturnal enuresis is most common and is occasionally accompanied by diurnal wetting; diurnal bed-wetting without nocturnal bed-wetting is unusual. In most enuretic children nocturnal bed-wetting is a primary maturational problem and usually ceases between ages 6 and 8, although it may continue into adolescence.

Diagnostic Evaluation

Organic causes that may be related to enuresis should be ruled out before psychogenic factors are considered. These include structural disorders of the urinary tract, urinary tract infection, major neurologic deficits, nocturnal epilepsy, disorders such as diabetes mellitus and diabetes insipidus that increase the normal output of urine, and disorders such as chronic renal failure or sickle cell disease that impair the concentrating ability of the kidneys. In other cases the enuresis is influenced by emotional factors, although it is doubtful that they are etiologic factors.

In older children routine examinations are carried out to rule out infection, and bladder capacity is determined by having the child hold off voiding until he feels urgency, at which time he voids into a measured container. A bladder volume of 300 to 350 ml is sufficient to hold a night's urine.

Therapeutic Management

Enuresis not resulting from organic causes can be approached in several ways. No method is so successful as to achieve universal endorsement; however, some have proved helpful in keeping the child dry during the night. Frequently more than one technique is employed.

Conditioning devices. A number of electrical devices are available that are based on the conditioned reflex response. These consist of a wire pad attached to a bell or buzzer that wakens the child as soon as the first drops of urine create a closed circuit. The child is thus conditioned to waken at the initiation of micturition or to the stimulus of the bell or buzzer. Most have reported a substantial success rate with the device. There appear to be no undesirable emotional effects, although this is debatable.

There are disadvantages to the use of electrical devices. A practical problem is the disturbance it may create when other children sleep in the same room or in the same bed. The child may be too sleepy or forget to reset the alarm following its activation to render it effective for the remainder of the night. There may be a risk of ulceration and scarring caused by slow electrolysis of tissue cells when the child does not hear the alarm or turns the alarm off without waking while the current continues to flow or when the batteries have run down to a feeble point where the alarm is insufficiently loud.

Drug therapy. A number of pharmacologic agents can be used in the treatment of enuresis, either alone or in combination with other techniques. The selection depends on the interpretation of the cause. The drug used most frequently is the tricyclic antidepressant drug imipramine (Tofranil), which exerts an anticholinergic action on the bladder to inhibit urination. The dosage and time of administration are individualized, and the drug is given in amounts sufficient to lighten sleep but not to cause wakefulness. The suggested length of treatment is 6 to 8 weeks, followed by gradual withdrawal over 4 weeks. Since this drug is dangerous in overdosage, parents must be cautioned about judicious use and keeping supplies of the drug far from the reach of younger siblings.

Bladder training. It has been known for some time that enuretic children have smaller functional bladder capacities. Bladder training is aimed at stretching the bladder to accommodate increasingly larger volumes of urine. After forcing fluids the child is instructed to postpone voiding as long as can be tolerated before emptying the bladder. The heightened threshold for retention allows the child to remain dry throughout the night.

Withholding fluids. Restricting or eliminating fluids after the evening meal is aimed at decreasing the output of urine during the night. This method has proved to be of questionable value.

Sleep interruption. Having the child void before retiring and then wakened and taken to the bathroom has met with limited success. Favorable responses are probably a result of the focused concern by both parents and child and of the positive behavioral reinforcement it provides. For this to be effective, the parent should be sure that the child is fully awake when the bladder is emptied.

Nursing Considerations

No matter what techniques are employed, the nurse can help both children and parents to understand the problem of enuresis, the treatment plan, and the probable difficulties they may encounter in the process. Essential to the success of any method is the supportive management of parents and their children. Both need encouragement and patience. The problem is discussed with the parents and, since any treatment involves and requires the child's active participation, children are included as well. The most important predictor for the outcome of treatment is family difficulties. Family disturbances influence the initial arrest of the enuresis, the relapse rate, and the long-term success rate (Dische and others, 1983).

Many parents believe that enuresis is caused by an emotional disturbance and fear that they have somehow produced the situation by imprudent child-rearing practices. They need reassurance that the bed-wetting is not a manifestation of emotional disturbance nor does it represent willful misbehavior. They should be informed about the nature of enuresis and cautioned against scolding, shaming, threat-

ening, and punishing a child, which are useless and harmful. Communication with children is directed toward eliminating the emotional impact of the problem by relieving them of feelings of shame, guilt, and the burden of parental disapproval and toward building up their self-confidence and motivating them toward independent control. More importantly the nurse can provide consistent support and encouragement to help sustain them through the inconsistent and unpredictable treatment process. Children need to believe that they are helping themselves and to sustain feelings of confidence and hope.

ENCOPRESIS

Encopresis is the repeated voluntary or involuntary passage of feces of normal or near-normal consistency into places not appropriate for that purpose in the individual's own sociocultural setting; it is not the result of any physical disorder (American Psychiatric Association, 1980). The disorder is less common than enuresis, but the two may coexist. It is seldom an isolated symptom and is commonly clustered with other somatic symptoms—social withdrawal, antisocial-aggressive behaviors, affective-dependent behaviors, and somatic manifestations.

Primary, or *continuous,* encopresis is identified by age 4 when the child has not achieved fecal continence for at least a year. This type is more frequently observed as a result of neglect, lax training methods, mental subnormalities, and familial causes. *Secondary,* or *discontinuous,* encopresis is fecal incontinence occurring between ages 4 and 8 that has been preceded by a period of fecal continence. Predisposing factors seem to be inadequate, inconsistent toilet training and psychosocial stress, such as entering school or the birth of a sibling. The disorder is more common in males than in females. When incontinence is involuntary, it frequently occurs secondary to constipation, impaction, or retention of feces with subsequent overflow. It is not unusual for soiling to take place after bathing because of reflex stimulation.

School performance and attendance are affected as the child's offensive odor becomes a target for scorn and derision from classmates. The child is not well liked by peers because of it and may be severely rejected by the parents as a result of the symptom. The rejection by peers and parents causes further withdrawal and other behavioral manifestations.

Etiology

One of the most common causes of encopresis is constipation, which is often precipitated by environmental change, such as birth of a new sibling, moving to a new house, changing schools, or even having to use new or unfamiliar toilet facilities (Johns, 1985). Voluntary retention usually follows a painful incident with voluntary suppression of defecation (e.g., a child with anal fissures). Involuntary retention may be produced by emotional problems caused by the encopresis that sets up a fear-pain cycle and results in a learned process of abnormal defecation patterns. Psychogenic encopresis, in which the soiling is caused by the emotional problems, is often related to a disturbed mother-child relationship.

Clinical Manifestations

The manifestation of simple constipation is painful expulsion of hard, pellet-like stools. Voluntary retention is usually temporary and there is a history of a painful precipitating episode and blood-streaked stools. Involuntary retention is associated with a history of abdominal pain, distention, moodiness, poor appetite, and accumulation of stools with periodic passage of voluminous stools. Children display a characteristic posturing during suppression of colonic signals to defecate—stiffening, "doing a little dance," "crawling," or hiding behind furniture or a tree when playing outdoors (Younger and Hughes, 1983). They typically hide soiled underwear. Children are usually nonchalant about their soiling (Johns, 1985).

Therapeutic Management

Treatment is directed toward the cause of the soiling. Diet, lubricants, and a toilet ritual that encourages the child to establish normal defecation are used (Younger and Hughes, 1983). Fecal impaction is relieved by catharsis, suppositories, and/or mineral oil. Usual dosages are usually insufficient. Dietary changes may be helpful, such as elimination of milk and dairy products and increased amounts of high-fiber foods, such as fruits, vegetables, and cereals, and increased fluids. Behavior therapy may be indicated to eliminate any fear that has developed as a result of painful defecation. Frequently psychotherapeutic intervention with the child and the family becomes necessary.

Nursing Considerations

The prevailing attitude of nurses toward the family of a child with encopresis is one of no-fault, thus relieving the guilt of both parents and child. Education regarding the physiology of normal defecation, toilet training as a developmental process, and the treatment outlined for the particular family is prerequisite to a successful outcome. Parents are relieved to know that other parents share this problem and are surprised to know that functional changes that take place as the condition develops make control of seepage impossible.

The regimen prescribed for stimulating elimination is outlined and explained to parents. Sitting the child on the toilet at routine intervals is not recommended because it may intensify parent-child conflict and result in a power play. Enemas may be needed for impactions but long-term use prevents the child from assuming responsibility for defecation (Johns, 1985). Initially, lubricants are given liberally but stimulant cathartics often cause abdominal cramps that can be a frightening experience for a child.

Family counseling is directed toward reassurance that most problems resolve successfully, although the child may have relapses during periods of stress, such as vacation or illness. If encopresis persists beyond occasional relapses the condition will need to be reevaluated. Behavior modification techniques are explained and the family assisted with a plan suited to their particular situation.

SCHOOL PHOBIA

School phobia is a term used to describe children, other than beginning students, who resist going to school because of dread of the school situation, concerns with leaving home, or both. Anxiety that frequently verges on panic is a constant manifestation, and children can develop symptoms as a protective mechanism to keep them from facing the situation that distresses them. Physical symptoms are prominent and may affect any part of the body—for example, anorexia, nausea, vomiting, diarrhea, dizziness, headache, leg pains, or abdominal pains. They may even develop a low-grade fever. A striking feature of school phobia is the prompt subsiding of symptoms when it is evident that the child can remain at home. Another significant observation is absence of symptoms on weekends and holidays, unless they are related to other places such as Sunday school or parties. Occasional mild reluctance is not uncommon among school children, but if the fear continues for longer than a few days, it must be considered as a serious problem—a warning of an important personality problem.

Unlike most other behavior problems of children, school phobia is more common in girls than in boys, there is no relationship to socioeconomic status, ethnic origin, or other subcultural affiliation, and no particular age predominates. The onset is usually sudden and precipitated by a school-related incident. A poor attendance record for trivial reasons can be elicited by a careful history.

Etiology

School phobia can be caused by a number of factors. Sometimes the complaints can be related to a transient, specific cause such as fear of a mismatched or overcritical teacher, fear of failing an examination or giving an oral recitation for a painfully shy child, or discrimination based on race, dress, or physical defect. Sometimes it may be related to a school bully or threatening gang. An insecure home situation in which the child fears that he may be deserted by a parent while he is gone may be the basis of anxiety, especially if the parent has previously threatened to leave for some reason.

A frequent source of fear is separation anxiety based on a strong dependent relationship between the mother and child in which the child is reluctant to leave the mother and she is equally reluctant (even though this may be unconscious) to have him leave her. The intense need for closeness between mother and child is normal in infancy, but the persistence of this type of relationship into childhood is totally inappropriate. Characteristically these children are not afraid to go to school, but rather they are afraid to leave home. The symptoms may be precipitated by any situation that intensifies the mutual dependency between the mother and the child, such as illness, arrival of a new baby, move to a strange neighborhood or a new school, or parental discord.

In some instances children have an unrealistic, exaggerated view of their abilities and achievements. When they feel threatened by incidents that challenge their estimate of themselves, such as a minor episode that leads to embarrassment, return to school after an absence, transfer to another class, or even imagined social or academic failure, they become anxious and withdraw, frequently seeking proximity to the mother. Sometimes the step-up in expectations at school is a contributing factor or change of important personnel at school (e.g., teacher or principal). Occasionally the child may be suffering from an undiagnosed learning disability.

Therapeutic Management

The treatment for school phobia depends on the cause. The children really *want* to go to school but just cannot force themselves to do so; they are not delinquent children. They are anxious, tense, and distressed because they are unable to muster enough courage to attend school. If the cause of the problem is an examination, relationships with a bully, or a mismatch between teacher and child, it can be dealt with accordingly. When the child is helped to understand and cope with the fear, the symptoms usually disappear spontaneously. In severe cases when returning to school is unsuccessful, professional psychiatric consultation is usually desirable to help identify possible distorted family relationships or a personality disturbance in the child and to help both child and family to understand the sources of the problem.

Nursing Considerations

The primary goal for the child with school phobia is to *return the child to school*. The longer the child is permitted to stay out of school, the more difficult it is to reenter. Well-meaning parents or others who permit the child to stay away from school and support any efforts with written excuses only confirm the child's feelings of worthlessness and inability to cope. Parents must be convinced gently but firmly that *immediate* return is essential and that they, the parents, are the ones who must insist upon the child's return for it to be effective.

For the child with severe symptoms it may be necessary to make some modifications in school attendance. The child who is unable to return to the regular classes may be allowed to go to school on a part-time basis, spending the time in the counselor's office or nurse's office and getting homework from the teacher after class. It may be necessary to transport the child to and from school or even have a parent attend class with the child. However, this practice is not allowed to continue for an unlimited time, and the time limit should be agreed on beforehand. The essential factor is that the child must return to school right away, maintain the pattern of going, and remain there even while a solution is being worked out. The school nurse can provide both

teacher and parents with support in carrying out this plan.

Prevention. Prevention of school phobia as well as other dependency problems can be developed by the encouragement of independence at appropriate times during infancy and early childhood. For example, by 6 months of age children are left with a baby-sitter during a parents' night out. Two-year-olds can be left home (while awake) with a sitter. By 3 years of age children should experience being left somewhere other than their home (e.g., grandparents' home). As soon as they are able they are allowed to feed, dress, and wash themselves. By 3 to 4 years of age children can be allowed to play in the yard by themselves, and later they should be allowed to play in the neighborhood by themselves. It is also helpful if the parents plan for and discuss with the child the separation of going to school.

RECURRENT ABDOMINAL PAIN

Recurrent abdominal pain (RAP) is one of the somatic complaints of childhood that is almost always attributed to a psychogenic etiology, although it can be a symptom of either psychosomatic or organic disease. RAP is traditionally defined as three or more separate episodes of abdominal pain during a 3-month period. Similar to the "spastic" or "irritable colon syndrome" of adulthood, the disorder affects 10% to 20% of school-age children at some time in their childhood. In 90% to 95% no organic cause can be found (Farrell, 1984; Poole, 1984).

Etiology

Support for the psychologic aspects of this disorder is based on observations of aggravation of symptoms during times of tension or stress. The common sources of stress and concern in children of this age-group are:

Home: Parental arguments, separation or divorce; illness or abdominal pain in family member; loss of family member; change of residence; frightening event; excessively rigid parental style

Peers: Teasing; scapegoating; loss of friends; pressure

School: Pressures associated with school teacher-pupil disharmony; test; changing schools; feelings of inadequacy in the face of academic challenges

Antecedent event: Illness with abdominal pain (especially attention-getting type)

Children at risk for RAP tend to be high achievers who have great personal goals or whose parents have unusually high expectations. They are described as more mature and sensitive than others or as worriers. At risk are children who are overly concerned about what others think about them but have difficulty meeting the expectations of parents, teachers, and others. They are uncomfortable with expressions of anger or argument, especially in those persons who are significant in their lives. School attendance is adversely affected, and these children generally exhibit poor learning performance. It is not uncommon for symptoms to be aggravated during school days.

Clinical Manifestations

Children with RAP have real pain that is usually located in the periumbilical and/or epigastric area. However, on palpation the pain is more likely to be experienced in the epigastric area or in the lower right or left quadrant and is accompanied by vague tenderness without muscle guarding. Other symptoms that may accompany the abdominal pain are headache, flushing, pallor, dizziness, and fatigue. Nausea, vomiting, and diarrhea are sometimes part of the syndrome. The symptoms reflect the heightened intensity of response to stimulation of the autonomic bowel sites. The loose stools are the result of the exaggerated propulsive motility, and the pain is caused by the sharply increased mechanical tension in the gut.

Diagnostic Evaluation

Psychophysiologic RAP is diagnosed when (1) symptoms can be related to specific stresses, concerns, or events in a patient's life, (2) other pathologic processes are ruled out, (3) physical examination reveals no organic disease, and (4) stool tests for blood, complete blood count, sedimentation rate, urinalysis, and urine culture are normal (Poole, 1984).

Therapeutic Management

Treatment is difficult. Hospitalization may be necessary, and the child frequently shows improvement in the hospital environment. Initial efforts are directed toward ruling out organic causes of the pain, relieving discomfort, and attempting to determine the situations that precipitate attacks. Some advocate adding fiber in the diet in the form of fiber-containing cookies (Feldman and others, 1985). When simple measures are ineffective, an antispasmodic drug such as propantheline bromide may be prescribed to relieve the muscle spasm, and psychotherapy may be recommended.

Nursing Considerations

The nurse can be instrumental in assessment and management of recurrent abdominal pain in children. Many of the techniques employed in a routine assessment can elicit information that might help identify those factors that contribute to the child's symptomatology. Questions that provide clues to parent-child relationships and how the family deals with angry feelings provide useful information for diagnosis and management. Relationships with peers, school problems, and other concerns of the child need to be explored, and any evidence of depression should be noted. It is also significant that psychogenic somatic symptoms generally do not awaken the child from sleep.

Once the diagnosis has been established, the parents and the child need an explanation of the pain, which can be compared to a skeletal muscle cramp or ''charley horse'' for easier comprehension. Reassurance that the symptoms are not unique to their child and that the pain can be expected to subside is helpful in relieving parental fears and anxieties. When parents are reassured that there is no organic cause of the pain, they will need some guidance regarding what they can do during a pain episode. All too often they feel helpless and anxious, which tends to compound the child's distress. The simple expedient of putting the child at rest by having him lie down in a peaceful, quiet environment and providing comfort will often relieve the symptoms in a short time. A heating pad may also help ease the discomfort. If pain is not relieved by these simple measures, the parents are taught how to administer antispasmodics. For example, if pain is precipitated by meals, having the child take the medication 20 to 30 minutes before mealtime may prevent an episode.

The most valuable measures that the nurse can provide are support and reassurance to the family. One of the most difficult aspects of therapy is helping parents and child understand the cause of the pain. When open communication is established and families are able to see a relationship between stress-provoking situations and the child's symptoms, the chance for remedial action is enhanced. Follow-up care and continued support are essential because the symptoms tend to remit and exacerbate; therefore the availability of a supportive health professional can be a source of comfort to the child and family.

CONVERSION REACTION

Conversion reaction, also known as hysteria, hysterical conversion reaction, conversion symptoms, and childhood hysteria, is a psychophysiologic disorder with a sudden onset that can usually be traced to a precipitating environmental event. The manifestations involve primarily the voluntary musculature and special senses and include abdominal pain, fainting, pseudoseizures, paralysis, headaches, and visual field restriction. Once considered rare in childhood, the diagnosis occurs more frequently than has generally been acknowledged. In childhood the disorder is observed with equal frequency in both sexes, but girls outnumber boys during adolescence. The most commonly observed symptom is seizure activity, which can be differentiated from those of neurogenic origin by formal tests, the most useful of which is the finding of a normal electroencephalogram.

It has been observed that nearly all children with conversion reaction have experienced a major family crisis before the onset of symptoms. Particularly traumatic is an unresolved grief reaction in the child, such as loss of a parent or other significant person through death, divorce, or moving (Maloney, 1980). It is not uncommon for the child to exhibit symptoms of the lost person. The families of children with conversion reaction characteristically display problems in communication, and depression or hypochondriasis in a parent is a common finding.

Discussions about underlying emotional stresses or feelings may alleviate the child's symptoms, although families are not always receptive to the intervention. If deep personality problems are evident, psychiatric consultation is usually indicated. Nursing care is similar to that for the child with recurrent abdominal pain.

DIAGNOSTIC CRITERIA FOR MAJOR DEPRESSION

Dysphoric mood
At least four of the following present ≥2 weeks
    Poor appetite/weight loss; weight gain
    Insomnia/hypersomnia
    Psychomotor agitation or retardation
    Apathy
    Loss of energy/fatigue
    Feelings of worthlessness, self-reproach, guilt
    Diminished ability to think or concentrate
    Recurrent thoughts of death, suicidal ideation, suicide attempt

From Aylward, G.P.: Understanding and treatment of childhood depression, J. Pediatr. **107**:1-9, 1985; as modified from Diagnostic and statistical manual of mental disorders, ed. 3 (DSM-III), Washington, DC, 1980, American Psychiatric Association.

CHILDHOOD DEPRESSION

Depression in childhood is often difficult to detect because children may be unable to express their feelings and tend to act out their problems and concerns. Authorities agree that childhood depression exists but they do not agree whether or not it is the same as adult depression. The characteristics of depression are largely determined by parallel developments in symbolism, language, and cognitive development (Aylward, 1985). Younger children demonstrate a more cause-and-effect relationship between the stressors and the depressive manifestations, which are primarily the biologic, deprivation syndromes. As children develop, the relationships between stressful events and depression are less clear. Their reactions are less physiologic and more cognitively complex and the observed behaviors tend to be age specific (Herzog and Rathburn, 1982).

Some states of depression are of a temporary nature, for example, acute depression precipitated by a traumatic event. This might include a period of hospitalization, loss of a parent through death or separation, or loss of a significant relationship with something (a pet), someone (a friend or family member), or a place (move from a familiar home, neighborhood, or city). The easily identified manifestations include a sad, downcast face, tearfulness, irritability, and withdrawal from previously enjoyed activities and relationships. The child tends to spend more time in solitary activities, especially television viewing, and schoolwork is impaired. Some children become more dependent and clinging; others become more aggressive and disruptive. Sleeplessness and/or loss of appetite are not common reactions. Responses are not sustained and can be modified with social and family support.

More serious and less common are depressive responses to more chronic stress and loss; these are frequently observed in children with chronic illness or disability. There is no apparent precipitating event but there is often a history of frequent disruptions in important relationships. Commonly there is also a history of depressive illness in one or both parents during the child's lifetime. The manifestations are similar to responses to acute reactions. Some of the primary and associated symptoms that are observed in depressed children, the DSM-III criteria currently used for establishing a diagnosis of major depression, and the symptoms designated as "dysthymic disorder" in the DSM-III are outlined in the boxes. There are a number of similarities among major depressive disorders in childhood and several other psychologic disorders.

The management of childhood depression is usually psychotherapeutic and highly individualized. Nurses should be aware that depression is a problem that can easily be overlooked in the school-age child and one that can interrupt normal growth and development. Recognizing depression and making appropriate referrals is an important nursing function. Identification of the depressed child requires a careful history (health, growth and development, social, and family health), interviews with the child, and observations by the nurse, parents, and teachers. See Chapter 21 for a more definitive discussion of depression and suicide.

DIAGNOSTIC CRITERIA FOR DYSTHYMIC DISORDER

For the past 2 years, depressive symptoms of insufficient intensity and duration to meet criteria for major depression
Depressive symptoms *may* be intermittent
Prominent depressed mood or loss of interest in usual activities during depressed periods
At least three of the following present during depressed periods:
    Insomnia/hypersomnia
    Low energy level, chronic tiredness
    Feelings of inadequacy, loss of self-esteem, self-depreciation
    Decreased effectiveness or productivity at school or home
    Decreased attention, concentration, or ability to think clearly
    Social withdrawal
    Loss of interest in or enjoyment of pleasurable activities
    Irritability or excessive anger (in children, expressed toward parents or caretakers)
    Inability to respond with apparent pleasure to praise or rewards
    Less active or talkative than usual, feels slowed down, restless
    Pessimistic attitude toward the future; brooding about past events
    Tearfulness or crying
    Recurrent thoughts of death or suicide

From Aylward, G.P.: Understanding and treatment of childhood depression, J. Pediatr. **107**:1-9, 1985; as modified from Diagnostic and statistical manual of mental disorders, ed. 3 (DSM-III), Washington, DC, 1980, American Psychiatric Association.

PRIMARY AND ASSOCIATED SYMPTOMS OF DEPRESSION IN CHILDREN

Primary symptoms
Depressed affect (dysphoric mood)
Anhedonia (loss of pleasure)
Self-deprecatory ideation
Tearfulness
Low sense of self-worth/self-esteem
Social withdrawal
Impairment of schoolwork
Psychomotor retardation
Difficulty with biologic functions (sleeping, eating)
Morbid ideation/suicide attempts
Associated symptoms
Irritability
Moodiness
Social interactive difficulties
Pathologic guilt
Fatigue
Somatic complaints
Anxiety, decreased concentration
Obsessive rumination and thoughts
Attention deficit
Feelings of helplessness/hopelessness
Enuresis/encopresis
Aggressive and explosive behaviors

From Aylward, G.P.: Understanding and treatment of childhood depression, J. Pediatr. **107:**1-9, 1985; as modified from Diagnostic and statistical manual of mental disorders, ed. 3 (DSM-III), Washington, DC, 1980, American Psychiatric Association.

CHILDHOOD SCHIZOPHRENIA

There is considerable disagreement regarding the cause of schizophrenia, both adult and childhood onset. Some authorities favor a biochemical basis, whereas others support the theory of a complex combination of psychosocial and environmental stresses. Support for an interpersonal theory of schizophrenia comes from a number of sources. The major theories point to disturbed family or parent-child relationships as an etiologic basis. There is evidence to indicate that genetic factors contribute significantly to its development. The likelihood of children born to a schizophrenic parent to develop the disorder is 15 times greater than for children in the general population—even when they are separated from the parent at an early age. There is also a high concordance rate (40% to 60%) in monozygotic (identical) twins.

The symptomatology among children shows wide variation according to each affected child's developmental level, the age of onset, the nature of early childhood experiences, and the type of defense mechanisms used. However, the basic core disturbance is a lack of contact with reality and the subsequent development of a world of the child's own. Unlike the abrupt onset of the adult disorder, childhood schizophrenia is characterized by a gradual onset of neurotic symptoms followed by any of more than 100 different abnormal manifestations, including the following:

Bizarre behavioral patterns and stereotyped movements such as robot like walking, whirling, or graceful gyrations
Periods of hypoactivity alternating with periods of hyperactivity
Inappropriate affect that ranges from flatness to explosiveness
Common occurrences of temper tantrums
Language disturbances such as speaking in fragmented sentences, parrotlike repetition of words, development of a private language, and altered tone of voice; some schizophrenic children are mute or will only utter a single word on rare occasions
Distorted time orientation with a blending of past, present, and future
Distorted sense of and use of their bodies
Apparent denial of the human quality in people, such as attempting to use a person as a step stool to reach an object
Conveying a nonhuman identity by action, sounds, or posture, such as barking or calling himself a vacuum cleaner
Frequent occurrences of compulsive behavior and phobias

Nursing Considerations

Nursing care is directed toward identifying children and referral for specialized care. Consistent application of a therapeutic plan is mandatory for a successful program of care, and nurses with special skills work with these children on a long-term basis. Since it is a specialized area of nursing practice, the reader is directed to seek further information from textbooks on child psychiatry.

CONCEPT SUMMARIES

- Middle childhood is a relatively healthy period, and most problems encountered are not considered serious.
- Dental care is of extreme importance during middle childhood; common problems that arise are dental caries, periodontal disease, malocclusion, and trauma.
- Control of dental caries includes frequent dental examinations, proper dental procedures, good oral hygiene, reduction of sugar intake, sound nutrition practices, and administration of fluoride.
- Periodontal disease that is prevalent during middle childhood includes gigngivitis, periodontitis, and acute necrotizing ulcerative gingivitis.
- Common skin disorders of middle childhood include contact dermatitis; scabies, pediculosis, ringworm; sunburn; bites and stings; trauma; and foreign body injury.
- The skin, composed of the epidermis, dermis, subcutaneous tissue, hair, and sebaceous and sweat glands, serves several important functions: protection, impermeability, heat regulation, and sensation.
- Skin lesions result from contact with injurious agents, hereditary factors, external factors producing a reaction, or systemic disease.
- Infections of the skin are categorized as bacterial, viral, fungal, systemic, mycotic, and rickettsial.

- Contact dermatitis may involve a primary irritant or a sensitizing agent.

- Adverse reactions to drugs occur more often in the skin than in any other organ.

- Common skin disorders related to insect and animal contact include scabies, pediculosis capitis, insect stings, animal bites, human bites, and cat scratch fever.

- Broad classification of behavioral disorders in children identifies mental subnormality, learning disabilities, neuroses, psychoses, and antisocial behavior.

- Behavioral problems in middle childhood include attention deficit disorders, enuresis, encopresis, school phobia, recurrent abdominal pain, childhood depression, conversion reaction, and childhood schizophrenia.

- Effective treatment of attention deficit disorder usually involves a multiple approach: family education and counseling, medication, remedial education, environmental manipulation, and psychotherapy.

REFERENCES

Altschuler, D.X., and Kenney, L.R.: Pediculocide performance, profit, and the public health, Arch. Dermatol. **122:**259-261, 1986.

American Psychiatric Association: Diagnostic and statistical manual of mental disorders, ed. 3 (DSM-III), Washington, DC, 1980, American Psychiatric Association.

Anders, J.E., and Leach, E.E.: Sun versus skin, Am. J. Nurs. **83:**1015-1020, 1983.

Anderson, F.P.: Lyme disease. In Gellis, S.S., and Kagan, B.M.: Current pediatric therapy 12, Philadelphia, 1986, W.B. Saunders Co.

Aylward, G.P.: Understanding and treatment of childhood depression, J. Pediatr. **107:**1-9, 1985.

Berkowitz, R., Ludwig, S., and Johnson, R.: Dental trauma in children and adolescents. J. Pediatr. **19:**166-171, 1980.

Berry, C.A., Shaywitz, S.E., and Shaywitz, B.A.: Girls with attention deficit disorder: a silent minority? A report on behavioral and cognitive characteristics, Pediatrics **76:**801-809, 1985.

Brown, G.L.: Attention deficit disorder. In Gellis, S.S., and Kagan, B.M.: Current pediatric therapy 12, Philadelphia, 1986, W.B. Saunders Co.

Carithers, H.A.: Cat-scratch disease—an overview based on a study of 1,200 patients, Am. J. Dis. Child **139:**1124-1133, 1985.

Chan, Y-P.M., and others: Methylphenidate hydrochloride given with or before breakfast: II. Effects on plasma concentration of methylphenidate and ritalinic acid, Pediatrics **72:**56-59, 1983.

Chun, Y-T., Berkelhamer, J.E., and Herold, T.E.: Dog bites in children less than 4 years old, Pediatrics **69:**119-120, 1982.

Clore, E.: Prioderm and permethrin: product update, Progress, **1**(2):1, 1985.

Cohen, F.L.: Clinical genetics in nursing practice, Philadelphia, 1984, J.B. Lippincott Co.

Dische, S., and others: Childhood nocturnal enuresis: factors associated with outcome of treatment with an enuresis alarm, Dev. Med. Child Neurol. **25:**67-80, 1983.

Editorial comment: Pediatric Alert **9:**22, 1984.

Farrell, M.K.: Abdominal pain, Pediatrics **74**(Suppl.):955-957, 1984.

Feldman, W., and others: The use of dietary fiber in the management of simple, childhood, idiopathic, recurrent, abdominal pain: results in a prospective double-blind, randomized, controlled trial, Am. J. Dis. Child.:1216-1218, 1985.

Gelbard, M.K.: Removal of small cactus spines from the skin, JAMA **252:**3368, 1984.

Gorrell, R.: Practical pointers, Consultant **25:**154, 1985.

Graber, L.W., and Lucher, G.W.: Dental esthetic self-evaluation and satisfaction, Am. J. Orthod. **77:**163, 1980.

Guide to dental health, J. Am. Dent. Assoc. Suppl., 1985, pp. 37-46.

Herzog, G.B., and Rathburn, J.M.: Childhood depression, Am. J. Dis. Child **136:**115-119, 1982.

Huessy, H.R.: Adolescents and ritalin, Pediatrics **75:**614, 1985.

Johns, C.: Encopresis, Am. J. Nurs. **85:**153-156, 1985.

Lauer, E.A., White, W.C., and Lauer, B.A.: Dog bites—a neglected problem in accident prevention, Am. J. Dis. Child **136:**202-204, 1982.

Levine, M.D.: Disordered processes of elimination. In Levine, M.D., and others: Developmental-behavioral pediatrics, Philadelphia, 1983, W.B. Saunders Co.

Maloney, M.J.: Diagnosing hysterical conversion reactions in children, J. Pediatr. **97:**1016-1020, 1980.

Margileth, A.W., and others: Cat-scratch disease, JAMA **252:**928-931, 1984.

McLaury, P.: Head lice—pediatric social disease, Am. J. Nurs. **83:**1300-1303, 1983.

Meinking, T.L., and others: Comparative efficacy of treatments for pediculosis capitis infestations, Arch. Dermatol. **122:**267-271, 1986.

Needham, G.R.: Evaluation of five popular methods for tick removal, Pediatrics **75:**997-1002, 1985.

Perelson, A.M., and Seyler, M.F.: First aid: soaking an injured finger or toe, Emerg. Med. **16:**158, 1985.

Pinckney, L.E., and Kennedy, L.A.: Traumatic deaths from dog attacks in the United States, Pediatrics **69:**193-197, 1982.

Poole, S.R.: Recurrent abdominal pain in childhood and adolescence, Am. Fam. Physician **30:**131-137, 1984.

Putnam, M.H., and Lawton, M.B.: Resourceful women unmask cactus spines, JAMA **253:**2830, 1985.

Rule, J.T.D: Recognition of dental caries, Pediatr. Clin. North Am. **29:**439-456, 1982.

Shalita, A.R.: Principles of infant skin care, Skillman, NJ, 1981, Johnson & Johnson Baby Products Co.

Slome, B.: Rampant caries: a side effect of tricyclic antidepressant therapy, Gen. Dent. **32:**494-496, 1984.

Taplin, D., and others: Malathion for treatment of pediculus humanus var capitis infestation, JAMA **247:**3103-3105, 1982.

Wright, J.C.: Severe attacks by dogs: characteristics of the dogs, the victims, and the attack settings, Public Health Rep. **100:**55-61, 1985.

Younger, J.B., and Hughes, L.S.: No-fault management of encopresis, Pediatr. Nurs. **9:**185-187, 1983.

BIBLIOGRAPHY
Dental Problems

Babington, M.A., and Spadaro, D.C.: Cariogenic medications, Pediatr. Nurs. **8:**165-171, 1982.

Cormier, J.F., and Trammel, H.: Fight tooth decay: the fluoride plan, Pediatr. Nurs. **5**(3):18-22, 1979.

Heifetz, S.B., and Horowitz, H.S.: Fluorides and sealants for the prevention of dental caries, Fam. Comm. Health **3**(3):23-32, 1980.

Hess, C.S., and others: Fluoride: too much to too little? Pediatr. Nurs. **10:**397-403, 1984.

Jenkins, N.: Diet and dental caries, Food Nutr. News **56:**29-32, 1984.

Jolley, H.M., and Pless, I.B.: Dental health and pediatrics, Pediatr. Rev. **3:**13-22, 1981.

Josell, S.D., and Abrams, R.G.: Traumatic injuries to the dentition and its supporting structures, Pediatr. Clin. North Am. **29:**717-741, 1982.

Kilmon, C., and Helpin, M.L.: Update on dentistry for children, Pediatr. Nurs. **7**(5):41-44, 1981.

Kilmon, C., and Helpin, M.L.: Recognizing dental malocclusion in children, Pediatr. Nurs. **9:**204-208, 1983.

Kronmiller, K.E., and Nirschl, R.F.: Preventive dentistry for children, Pediatr. Nurs. **11:**446-449, 1985.

Kula, K., and Tinanoff, N.: Fluoride therapy for the pediatric patient, Pediatr. Clin. North Am. **29:**669-680, 1982.

Mertz-Fairhurst, E.J.: Current status of sealant retention and caries prevention, J. Dent. Educ. **48**(Suppl. 2):80-85, 1984.

Miller, R.E., and Rosenstein, D.I.: Childrens' dental health: overview for the physician, Pediatr. Clin. North Am. **29:**429-438, 1982.

Stamm, J.W.: Causes of oral diseases and general approaches to their prevention, Fam. Comm. Health **3**(3):13-21, 1980.

Starr, R.M., and Gravitz, R.F.: Pit and fissure sealants in the prevention of tooth decay, Pediatr. Nurs. **11:**289-291, 1985.

Suomi, J.D.: Methods for the prevention of periodontal diseases, Fam. Comm. Health **3**(3):41-49, 1980.

Sweeny, E.A.: Pediatric dentistry, Curr. Probl. Pediatr. **11**(4):1-51, 1981.

Disorders Affecting the Skin: General

Akers, W.A.: Urticaria—finding the cause is the toughest part, Mod. Med. **49:**38, 1981.

Anders, J.E.: Topicals: a welter of options calls for refined application techniques, RN **45**(9):33-42, 1982.

Brown, J.L.: Telephone medicine: a practical guide to pediatric telephone advice, St. Louis, 1980, The C.V. Mosby Co.

Caputo, R.V.: Recent advances in pediatric dermatology, Pediatr. Clin. North Am. **30:**735-747, 1983.

Cohen, B.A.: Common dermatoses of childhood, Am. Fam. Physician **32**(4):186-203, 1985.

Fleming, J.W.: Common dermatologic conditions in children, Am. J. Maternal Child Nurs. **6:**346-354, 1981.

Hawkins, K.: Wet dressings, Crit. Care Update **9**(11): 24-26, 1982.

Lester, R.S.: Topical formulary for the pediatrician, Pediatr. Clin. North Am. **30:**749-765, 1983.

McBurney, E.I.: Diagnostic dermatologic methods, Pediatr. Clin. North Am. **30:**419-434, 1983.

Norins, A.L., and Treadwell, P.A.: The management of persistent pediatric skin problems, Pediatr. Clin. North Am. **29:**37-53, 1982.

Rasmussen, J.E.: Psoriasis in childhood, Dermatol Clin. North Am. **4:**99-106, 1986.

Riccardi, V.M.: The multiple forms of neurofibromatosis, Pediatr. Rev. **3:**293-298, 1982.

Rosen, T., Lanning, M.B., and Hill, M.J.: The nurse's atlas of dermatology, Boston, 1983, Little, Brown & Co.

Schachner, L., and others: A therapeutic update of superficial skin infections, Pediatr. Clin. North Am. **30:**397-404, 1983.

Stroud, J.D.: Hair loss in children, Pediatr. Clin. North Am. **30:**641-657, 1983.

Twarog, F.J.: Urticaria in childhood: pathogenesis and management, Pediatr. Clin. North Am. **30:**887-897, 1983.

Weston, J.A., Hawkins, K., and Weston, W.L.: Foot dermatitis in children, Pediatrics **72:**824-827, 1983.

Bacterial and Viral Infections

Carter, S.: Etiology and treatment of facial cellulitis in pediatric patients, Pediatr. Infect. Dis. **2:**222, 1983.

Fleisher, G., Ludwig, S., and Compos, J.: Cellulitis: bacterial etiology, clinical features, and laboratory findings, J. Pediatr. **97:**591-593, 1980.

Guess, H.A., and others: Epidemiology of herpes zoster in children and adolescents: a population-based study, Pediatrics **76:**512-517, 1985.

Heckman, B.H.: Jeans folliculitis, N. Engl. J. Med. **305:**524, 1981.

Krugman, S., and others: Infectious diseases of children, ed. 8, St. Louis, 1985, The C.V. Mosby Co.

Middleton D.B., and Ferrante, J.A.: Periorbital and facial cellulitis, Am. Fam. Physician **21:**98, 1980.

Rasmussen, J.E.: Warts and what to do about them, Drug Therapy **11:**65-73, 1981.

Tunnessen, W.W.: Cutaneous infections, Pediatr. Clin. North Am. **30:**515-532, 1983.

Fungal Infections

Allen, H., and others: Selenium sulfide: adjunctive therapy for tinea capitis, Pediatrics **69:**81-83, 1982.

Caputo, R.V.: Fungal infections in children, Dermatol. Clin. North Am. **4:**137-150, 1986.

Kafka, J.A., and Catanzaro, A.: Disseminated coccidioidomycosis in children, J.Pediatr. **98:**355-361, 1981.

Krowchuk, D.P., and others: Current status of the identification and management of tinea capitis, Pediatrics **72:**625-631, 1983.

Notarangelo, P.R., and Dixon, D.M.: Opportunistic systemic mycoses and the critical care patient, Crit. Care Update **10:**7-11, 1983.

Rees, P.L., and Dixon, D.M.: Opportunistic mycoses, Am. J. Nurs. **81:**1160-1165, 1981.

Stein, D.H.: Superficial fungal infections, Pediatr. Clin. North Am. **30:**545-561, 1983.

Rickettsial Diseases

Helmick, C.: Incidence of Rocky Mountain spotted fever rises in young, Pediatr. News **15:**12, 1981.

Riley, H.D.: Rickettsial diseases and Rocky Mountain spotted fever, part I, Curr. Probl. Pediatr. **11**(5):1-46, 1981.

Riley, H.D.: Rickettsial diseases and Rocky Mountain spotted fever, part II, Curr. Probl. Pediatr. **11**(6):1-38, 1981.

Thompson, S.: Summertime and ticks, Am. J. Nurs. **83:**768-769, 1983.

Woodward, W.E.: What clinicians should know about Rocky Mountain spotted fever, Drug Ther. **12:**106-114, 1982.

Chemical and Physical Injuries

Brown, F.E., and others: Frostbite: long term effects on bone growth, Pediatrics **71:**955-959, 1983.

DeLapp, T.D.: Taking the bite out of frostbite and other cold-weather injuries, Am. J. Nurs. **80:**56-60, 1980.

Gedrose, J.: When cold can be a killer: prevention and treatment of hypothermia and frostbite, Nursing 80 **10**(2):34-36, 1980.

LaVoy, K.: Dealing with hypothermia and frostbite, RN **48**(1):53-56, 1985.

Pathak, M.A.: Sunscreens: topical and systemic approaches for protection of human skin against harmful effect of solar radiation, J. Am. Acad. Dermatol. **7:**285-312, 1982.

Plein, E.M.: Sunscreens, Nurse Pract. **6:**35, 1981.

Ramsay, C.A.: Photosensitivity in children, Pediatr. Clin. North Am. **30:**687-699, 1983.

Robinson, L.A.: Sun exposure and sun protection, Pediatr. Nurs. **8:**272-273, 1982.

Warshauer, D.M., and Steinbaugh, J.R.: Sunlight and protection of the skin, Am. Fam. Physician **27**(6):109-115, 1983.

Wingate, E.: A nursing perspective on frostbite, Crit. Care Update **10:**8-15, 1983.

Infestations

Clore, E.R.: Lice: ancient pest with new resistance, Pediatr. Nurs. **9:**347-350, 1983.

Hepatotoxic potential of ketoconazole under investigation, FDA Drug Bull. **12**(2):11-12, 1982.

Shacter, B.: Treatment of scabies and pediculosis with lindane preparations: an evaluation, J. Am. Acad. Dermatol. **5:**517-527, 1981.

Insect and Animal Injuries

Amitai Y., and others: Scorpion sting in children, Clin. Pediatr. **24:**136-140, 1985.

Baker, S.F.: What to do about animal and insect bites, Mod. Med. **48:**26, June 15, 1980.

Callahan, M.: Prophylactic antibiotics in common dog bite wounds: a controlled study, Ann. Emerg. Med. **9:**410-414, 1980.

Cardoni, A.A.: Meat tenderizer and bee stings (letter), Pediatrics **74:**447, 1984.

Chipps, B.E., and others: Diagnosis and treatment of anaphylactic reactions to hymenoptera stings in children, J. Pediatr. **97:**177-184, 1980.

Elliot, D.L., and others: Pet-associated illness, N. Engl. J. Med. **313:**985-995, 1985.

Frazier, C.A.: Severe toxic and allergic reactions to insect bites and stings, Crit. Care Update **8**(9):17-24, 1981.

Ginsburg, C.M.: Cat-scratch adenitis, Pediatr. Infect. Dis. **3**(5):437-438, 1984.

Ginsburg, C.M.: Fire ant envenomation in children, Pediatrics **73**:689-692, 1984.

Graft, D.F., and Schuberth, K.C.: Hymenoptera allergy in children, Pediatr. Clin. North Am. **30**:873-886, 1983.

Honig, P.J.: Bites and parasites, Pediatr. Clin. North Am. **30**:563-581, 1983.

Jaffe, A.C.: Animal bites, Pediatr. Clin. North Am. **30**:405-413, 1983.

King, R.C., and Giles, J.: Dealing with insect bites, RN **47**(5):53-55, 1984.

Margileth, A.M.: Cat-scratch disease update, Am. J. Dis. Child. **138**:711-713, 1984.

Patterson, R.: Anaphylaxis and related allergic emergencies including reactions due to insect stings, JAMA **248**: 2632-2636, 1982.

Schuberth, K.C., and others: An epidemiologic study of insect allergy in children. I. Characteristics of the disease, J. Pediatr. **100**:546-551, 1982.

Toewe, C.H.: Bug bites and stings, Am. Fam. Physician **21**(5):90-95, 1980.

Wear, D.J., and others: Cat scratch disease: a bacterial infection, Science **221**:1403-1408, 1983.

Zook, E.G., and others: Successful treatment protocol for canine fang injuries, J. Trauma **20**:243, 1980.

Attention Deficit Disorder

Brown, R.T., and Wynne, M.E.: Sustained attention in boys with attention deficit disorder and the effect of methylphenidate, Pediatr. Nurs. **10**:35-39, 1984.

Dulcan, M.K.: Attention deficit disorder: evaluation and treatment, Pediatr. Ann. **14**:383-398, 1985.

Eichlseder, W.: Ten years of experience with 1,000 hyperactive children in a private practice, Pediatrics **76**:176-184, 1985.

Erb, L., and Andresen, B.D.: Hyperactivity: a possible consequence of maternal alcohol consumption, Pediatr. Nurs. **7**(4):30-33, 1981.

Howell, D.C., Huessy, H.R., and Hassuk, B.: Fifteen-year follow-up of a behavioral history of attention deficit disorder, Pediatrics **76**:185-190, 1985.

Jellinek, M.S.: Current perspectives on hyperactivity, Drug Ther. **11**:77-81, 1981.

Jellinek, M.S.: Hyperactivity: separating fact from fiction, Drug Ther. **11**:83-86, 1981.

Levine, M.D., and Melmed, R.D.: The unhappy wanderers: children with attention deficits, Pediatr. Clin. North Am. **29**: 105-120, 1982.

Palfrey, J., and others: An analysis of observed attention and activity patterns in preschool children, J. Pediatr. **98**:1006, 1981.

Robinson, L.A.: Food allergies, food additives, and the Feingold diet, Pediatr. Nurs. **6**(6):38-39, 1980.

Safer, D.J., and Krager, J.M.: Trends in medication treatment of hyperactive school children, Clin. Pediatr. **22**:500-503, 1983.

Schultz, F.R., and others: Methylphenidate treatment of hyperactive children: effects of the hypothalamic-pituitary-somatomedin axis, Pediatrics **70**:987-992, 1982.

Sleator, E.K., and others: Can the physician diagnose hyperactivity in the office? Pediatrics **67**:13-17, 1981.

Varley, C.K.: A clinical nurse specialist's role in the comprehensive management of attention deficit disorder, Child. Health Care **13**:139-142, 1985.

Specific Learning Disability

Bassett, L.B., Gudas, L.J., and McAnulty, E.H.: The learning-disabled child: recognition, evaluation, and management, Pediatr. Nurs. **8**:325-329, 1982.

Feagans, L.: A current view of learning disabilities, J. Pediatr. **102**:487-494, 1983.

Shaywitz, S.E., Grossman, H.J., and Shaywitz, B.A., editors: Symposium on learning disorders, Pediatr. Clin. North Am. **31**:1, 1984.

Shaywitz, S.E., and others: Current status of the neuromaturational examination as an index of learning disability, J. Pediatr. **104**:819-823, 1984.

Silverstein, R.A.: Learning problems as a symptom of family dysfunction, J. Assoc. Care Child Health **9**(4):122-125, 1981.

White, J.E.: Special nursing needs of hospitalized children with learning disabilities, Am. J. Maternal Child Nurs. **8**:209-212, 1983.

Enuresis and Encopresis

Crowley, A.A.: A comprehensive strategy for managing encopresis, Am. J. Maternal Child Nurs. **9**:395-400, 1984.

Hague, M., and others: Parental perceptions of enuresis, Am. J. Dis. Child. **135**:809-811, 1981.

Levine, M.D.: Encopresis: its potentiation, evaluation, and alleviation, Pediatr. Clin. North Am. **29**:315-330, 1982.

Levine, M.D., Mazonson, P., and Bakow, H.: Behavioral symptom substitution in children cured of encopresis, Am. J. Dis. Child. **134**:663-667, 1980.

Olness, K., McParland, F.A., and Piper, J.: Biofeedback: a new modality in the management of children with fecal soiling, J. Pediatr. **96**:505-509, 1980.

O'Regan, S., and others: Constipation: a commonly unrecognized cause of enuresis, Am. J. Dis. Child **140**:260-261, 1986.

Ruble, J.A.: Childhood nocturnal enuresis, Am. J. Maternal Child Nurs. **6**:26-31, 1981.

Schmitt, B.D.: Nocturnal enuresis: an update on treatment, Pediatr. Clin. North Am. **29**:21-35, 1982.

Schmitt, B.D.: Encopresis, Primary Care **11**:497-511, 1984.

Schmitt, B.D.: Nocturnal enuresis, Primary Care **11**: 485-495, 1984.

Shapiro, S.R.: Enuresis: treatment and overtreatment, Pediatr. Nurs. **11**(3):203-207, 1985.

Emotional Problems

American Psychiatric Association: Diagnostic and statistical manual of mental disorders, ed. 3 (DSM-III), Washington, DC, 1980, American Psychiatric Association.

Brady, M.A., and others: Childhood depression: development of a screening tool, Pediatr. Nurs. **10**:222-227, 1984.

Bumbalo, J.A., and Siemon, M.K.: Nursing assessment and diagnosis: mental health problems of children, Topics Clin. Nurs. **5**(1):41-54, 1983.

Child, A.A., Murphy, C.M., and Rhyne, M.C.: Depression in children: reasons and risks, Pediatr. Nurs. **6**(4):9-13, 1980.

Extended sleep (hypersomnia) in young depressed patients, Am. J. Psychiatry **142**:905-910, 1985.

Fond, K., and Brosnan, J.: School phobia: the school anxiety syndrome, Pediatr. Nurs. **6**(5):9-13, 1980.

Freedman, A.M., Kaplan, H.I., and Sadock, B.J.: Comprehensive textbook of psychiatry II, vol. II, ed. 3, Baltimore, 1980, The Williams & Wilkins Co.

Herman, S.P., and Schowalter, J.E.: Depression, suicide, and the young child, Emerg. Med. **13**(16):61-68, 1981.

Lebenthal, E.: Recurrent abdominal pain in childhood, Am. J. Dis. Child. **134**:347-348, 1980.

Levine, M.D., and Rappaport, L.A.: Recurrent abdominal pain in school children: the loneliness of the long-distance physician, Pediatr. Clin. North Am. **31**:969-991, 1984.

McConville, B.J.: The causes and treatment of depression in young children, J. Child Contemp. Soc. **15**(6):61-68, 1982.

Nelms, B.C.: Assessing childhood depression: do parents and children agree? Pediatr. Nurs. **12**:23-26, 1986.

Nelms, B.C., and Brady, M.A.: Assessment and intervention: the depressed school-age child, Pediatr. Nurs. **6**(4):15-19, 1980.

Rutter, M.: Prevention of children's psychosocial disorders: myth and substance, Pediatrics **70**:883-894, 1982.

Ryan, N.M.: Recurrent abdominal pain among school-age children, Am. J. Maternal Child Nurs. **11**:102-106, 1986.

Unit Seven

Adolescence

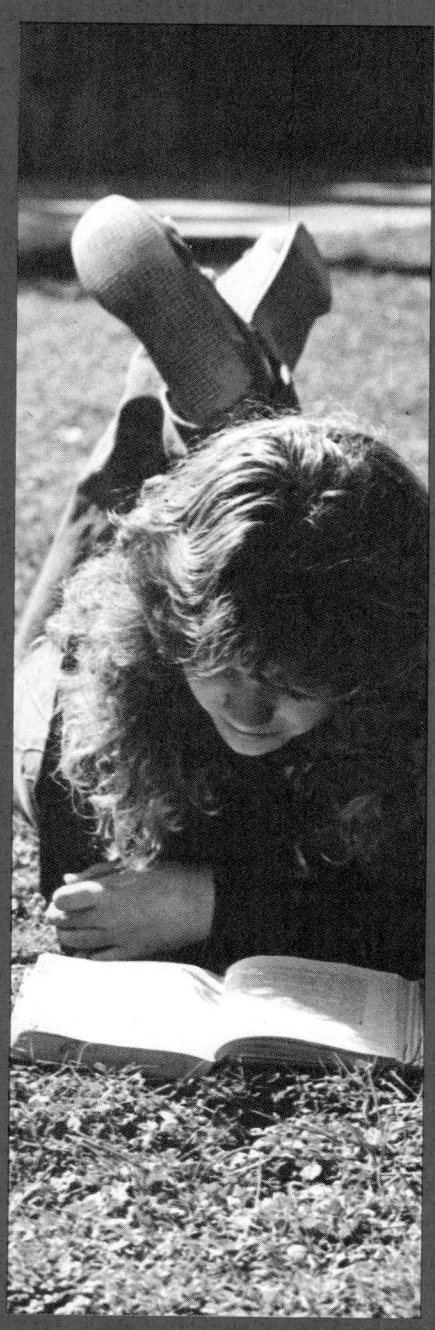

Adolescence is a period of transition that is based on childhood experiences and accomplishments and ultimately aspires to mature, independent, and responsible functioning. This transition is a biologic, emotional, and social process, a preparatory period requiring the accomplishment of defined developmental tasks in order to attain satisfactory adjustment to adulthood. The early years of adolescence are concerned with individuation from previous dependency roles and a gradual movement toward peer-group identity. The focus of an adolescent's world is the peer group—the persons they know who are going through the same transition and who understand the problems and frustrations they are experiencing. Later years of adolescence are centered around acquiring a personal identity, completing the separation process from family, and career-directed activity.

The physiologic changes that take place during puberty have both psychologic and social significance for adolescent boys and girls, and the rate and degree of equanimity with which adolescents grow and mature varies widely among individuals. Although it is a relatively healthy period of life, most of the health and emotional problems of teenagers are directly related to the biologic alterations and the emotional responses associated with this tumultuous period of life.

Chapter 19, *Health Promotion of the Adolescent and Family*, provides an overview of the transitional adolescent period during which youth must adjust to rapid body changes, establish a personal identity, gain emotional and (for some) economic freedom from their parents, and evolve a set of values uniquely their own. Chapters 20 and 21 are concerned with some of the health problems associated with adolescence as a result of either the changes related to biologic maturation or the psychologic adjustments imposed by these changes and societal expectations of society. Chapter 20, *Physical Health Problems of Adolescence*, is devoted primarily to physical problems of this age-group including problems related to sexuality; Chapter 21, *Behavioral Health Problems of Adolescence*, focuses on health problems that are related to the multiple changes of adolescence and that impose a serious threat to health and well-being.

Chapter 19

Health Promotion of the Adolescent and Family

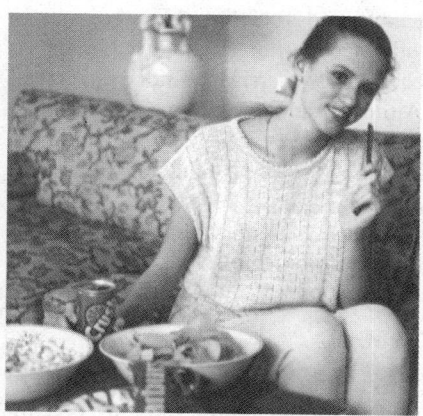

Adolescence begins at puberty and accompanying the pubertal changes there are corresponding changes in the personality. There is considerable variation in the time of the onset of puberty and in the manner different individuals cope with the multiple developmental events associated with pubertal changes. Adolescence is a period of transition and a time of physical, social, and emotional maturing as the girl prepares for womanhood and the boy readies for manhood. During this period of development the individual makes the most significant progress in learning to live effectively in society.

Promoting Optimum Growth and Development

The precise boundaries of adolescence are difficult to define, but this period is customarily viewed as beginning with the gradual appearance of secondary sex characteristics at about 11 or 12 years of age and ending with cessation of somatic growth at 18 to 20 years. However, there are such wide individual and cultural variations that, more than any other age category, no sharp age delineation can be made. Adolescence tends to begin and end earlier in girls than in boys.

There are several terms that are commonly used in reference to this particular stage of growth and development. *Puberty* primarily refers to the maturational, hormonal, and growth process that occurs when the reproductive organs begin to function and the secondary sex characteristics develop. This process is sometimes further delineated as *pubescence,* the period of about 2 years immediately before puberty characterized by the prepubertal growth spurts, when the child is developing preliminary physical changes that herald sexual maturity; *puberty,* the point at which sexual maturity is achieved, marked by the first menstrual flow in girls and by less obvious indications in boys; and *postpubescence,* a 1- to 2-year period following puberty during which skeletal growth is completed and reproductive functions become fairly well established. Puberty ends with the ability to reproduce, which in girls is soon after the onset of menstruation with the establishment of regular ovulation and in boys is soon after the first nocturnal emission when spermatogenesis is established. *Adolescence,* less firmly fixed, literally means ''to grow into maturity'' and is generally regarded as the psychologic, social, and maturational process initiated by pubertal changes. The term *teenage years* is used synonymously with *adolescence* to describe the years between ages 13 and 19.

Although the changes that take place during adolescence are primarily those affecting the body and personality, children in this period are highly influenced by the culture in which they grow and develop. In some of the more primitive societies the transition to adulthood is recognized soon after or simultaneously with puberty. The event is solemnized by some type of ritual, ceremony, or other ''rite of passage.'' From that point on the young people assume the privileges, responsibilities, and status accorded adults in the society. Decisions regarding the future are made when they are young, and the psychologic stage is relatively brief. The youngsters know from early childhood what is expected; prepared for their roles in adult activities, they slip easily into the new position accepted by parents, society, and themselves.

In more complex societies this transition is less clearly delineated, and society is equally vague about attainment of adult status. School years are legally over at 16 to 18 years but may continue to age 25 or beyond for many young people. Adolescents are legally permitted to drive as young as age 14 in some states and at a later age in others, but adult insurance premiums are not granted until age 25. In many states adolescents are not allowed to gamble or purchase liquor until age 21. Many activities in which young people are allowed to participate are considered to be those of adults, such as wars, voting, marriage, and childbearing, whereas at the same time they are considered youngsters in relation to social status and control of resources in the adult community. This ambiguity of society and parents contributes to the adolescents' own confusion and uncertainty about themselves.

In addition to this prolonged period of cultural maturation, adolescents' ultimate goals and adult roles are less defined and clear-cut in advanced societies than they are in primitive societies. In advanced cultures there are choices to be made regarding occupation, marriage, and even social and religious values. Although adolescents want to achieve adult status and privileges, they are faced with so many possibilities and choices that they are often reluctant to assume the associated responsibilities. They are eager to grow up yet fearful of the implications. It is no wonder that adolescence is a time of confusion and turmoil.

BIOLOGIC DEVELOPMENT

The physical changes of puberty are primarily the result of hormonal activity influenced by the central nervous system, although all aspects of physiologic functioning are mutually interacting. Growth and change are more dramatically and visibly demonstrated at this time than at any other period in life. The very obvious physical changes are noted in increased physical growth and the appearance and development of secondary sex characteristics; less obvious are physiologic alterations and neurogonadal maturity accompanied by the ability to procreate. Physical distinction between the sexes is determined on the basis of differential characteristics: *primary sex characteristics* are the external and internal organs that carry on the reproductive functions; *secondary sex characteristics* are the characteristics that distinguish the sexes from each other but play no direct part in reproduction. Because most of the physical changes that take place during adolescence are directly related to the hormonal changes of that period, a discussion of these changes is first, followed by a consideration of general growth trends and development of secondary sex characteristics.

Hormonal Changes of Puberty

It is generally accepted that the events of puberty are caused by hormonal influences and are controlled by the anterior pituitary gland (adenohypophysis) in response to a stimulus from the hypothalamus. Probably in some way related to brain maturation, hypothalamic stimulation causes the anterior pituitary to release gonadotropins that in turn stimulate the gonads. Stimulation to the gonads results in fulfillment of a dual function: (1) production and release of gametes—production of sperm in the male and maturation and release of ova in the female—and (2) secretion of sex-appropriate hormones—estrogen and progesterone from the female ovaries and testosterone from the male testes.

The dynamics of the reproductive hormone system include both neural and endocrine functions involving principally the hypothalamus, the adenohypophysis, and the gonads. The chain of reactions that causes ripening of the ovum in the female and production of sperm in the male begins in the region of the hypothalamus. Neurosecretory hormones, the *gonadotropin-releasing factors (GnRF),* synthesized and discharged by the hypothalamus, are carried via the hypophyseal portal vessels to the adenohypophysis, where they trigger the release of the gonadotropins *follicle-stimulating hormone* (FSH) and *luteinizing hormone* (LH), also known in the male as *interstitial cell–stimulating hormone* (ICSH). Increasing levels of these gonadotropic hormones in the blood stimulate the appropriate responses in the gonads.

Inhibition, or *negative feedback,* in the reproductive endocrine system refers to diminished gonadotropin secretion as a result of increasing serum levels of sex hormones. When sex hormone levels increase, GnRF secretion is diminished; when sex hormone levels decrease, the hypothalamus is stimulated to release GnRF, again initiating the sequence that produces the appropriate gonadal responses (Fig. 19-1).

Initiation of puberty. The precise mechanism that institutes the changes at puberty is not completely understood. Evidence suggests that bone age is the somatic marker that best correlates with readiness to initiate puberty (Kaplan, 1982). Although the pituitary and gonads are capable of mature function and can respond to stimuli at any age, the hypothalamic-pituitary-gonadal system is maintained in a dormant state throughout prepubescent childhood by some central nervous system inhibitory factor in the region of the hypothalamus. It is believed that the receptor sites in the hypothalamus are so highly sensitive that the most minute quantities of circulating sex hormones are sufficient to inhibit the secretion of GnRF during childhood. The hypothalamus loses this negative sensitivity at puberty and allows the hypothalamic-pituitary-gonadal mechanism to attain full secretory function. As puberty progresses, a powerful amplification process causes the pituitary and gonads to become increasingly sensitive to positive stimulation.

Sex hormones. Sex hormones are secreted by the ovaries, testes, and adrenal glands; they are produced in varying amounts in both sexes throughout life. The adrenal cortex is responsible for the small amounts secreted during the prepubescent years, but the sex hormone production that accompanies maturation of the gonads is responsible for the variety of biologic changes observed during pubescence and puberty. (See Table 38-1 for the major somatic effects produced by the sex hormones.)

Estrogen, the feminizing hormone, is found in low quantities during childhood and is secreted in slowly increasing amounts until about age 11. In males this gradual increase continues through maturation. In females the onset of estrogen production in the ovaries causes a pronounced estrogen

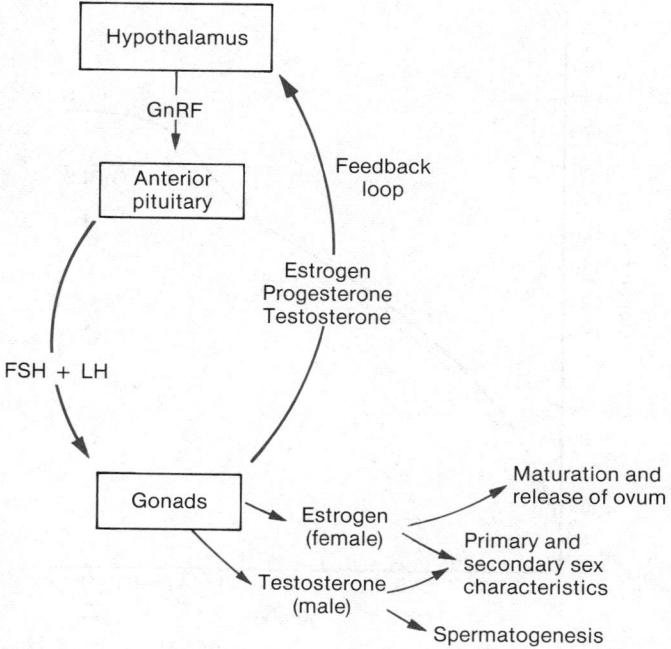

Fig. 19-1. Hormonal interaction between hypothalamus, pituitary, and gonads.

increase that continues to rise until about 3 years after the onset of menstruation, at which time it reaches a maximum level that is then maintained throughout the reproductive life of the female.

Androgens, the masculinizing hormones, are also secreted in small and gradually increasing amounts until approximately age 7 to 9, when there is a rapid increase in output in both sexes, especially boys, until about age 15. These hormones appear to be responsible for most of the rapid growth changes of early adolescence. With onset of testicular function, the level of androgens (principally testosterone) in males increases over that in females and continues to increase until a maximum is attained at maturity.

Pubertal Growth Spurt

A constant phenomenon associated with sexual maturation is a dramatic increase in growth. The relatively uniform physical growth of childhood shifts to markedly diverse rates of growth in adolescence. The final 20% to 25% of linear growth is achieved during puberty, and most (but not all) of this growth occurs during a 24- to 36-month period—the adolescent *growth spurt* (Figs. 19-2 and 19-3). This accelerated growth occurs in all children but as in other areas of development is highly variable in age of onset, duration, and extent. Visible signs of puberty are the development of secondary sex characteristics.

Puberty in girls can begin any time between 8 and 14 years of age and once initiated usually is completed within 3 years. The average girl, in whom the growth spurt is slower and less extensive than in boys, will gain 5 to 20 cm (2 to 8 inches) in height and 7 to 25 kg (15 to 55 pounds) in weight. Menarche, the onset of menstruation, occurs

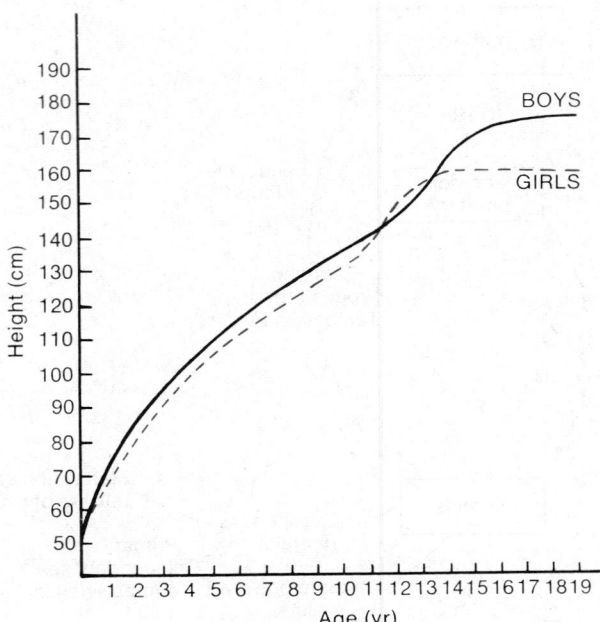

Fig. 19-2. Linear growth throughout childhood.

From Tanner, J.M., Whitehouse, R.H., and Takaishi, M.: Arch. Dis. Child. **41:**454-471, 1966.

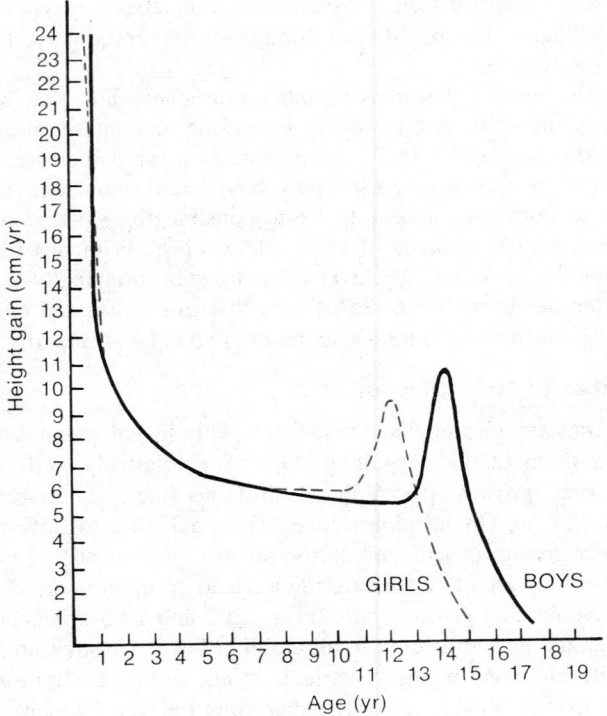

Fig. 19-3. Linear growth in centimeters per year.

From Tanner, J.M., Whitehouse, R.H., and Takaishi, M.: Arch. Dis. Child. **41:**454-471, 1966.

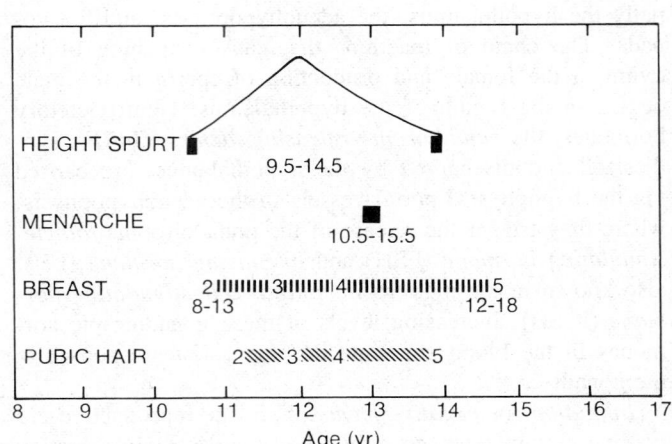

Fig. 19-4. Approximate timing of developmental changes in girls. Numbers indicate stages of development. Range of ages during which some of the changes occur is indicated by inclusive numbers below them. See Figs. 19-6 and 19-7 for explanation.

From Marshall, W.A., and Tanner, J.M.: Arch. Dis. Child. **44:**291, 1969.

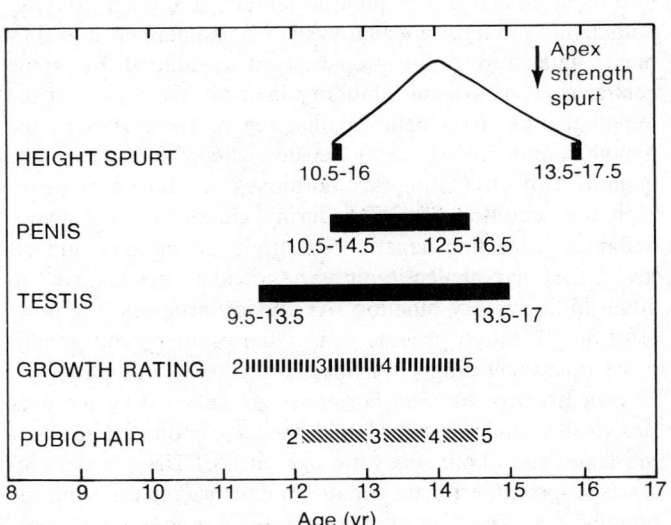

Fig. 19-5. Approximate timing of developmental changes in boys. Numbers indicate stages of development. Range of ages during which some of the changes occur is indicated by inclusive numbers below them. See Fig. 19-8 for explanation.

From Marshall, W.A., and Tanner, J.M.: Arch. Dis. Child. **45:**13, 1970.

about 2½ years after the onset of puberty. At this time girls will have achieved 90% to 95% of adult height. Growth in height ceases in girls at 16 or 17 years of age (Fig. 19-4).

On the average, puberty begins about 1½ to 2 years later in boys—between 9½ and 16 years of age. During this period the average boy will gain 10 to 30 cm (4 to 12 inches) in height and 7 to 30 kg (15 to 65 pounds) in weight. In boys growth in height commonly ceases at 18 or 20 years of age. The major developmental changes of puberty are the growth and maturation of the gonads and the appearance of secondary sex characteristics (Fig. 19-5).

Sexual Maturation

The visual evidence of sexual maturation is achieved in orderly sequence, and the state of maturity can be estimated on the basis of the appearance of these external manifestations. The age at which the changes are observed and the time required to progress from one stage to another may vary considerably between individual children.

Sexual maturation in girls. In most girls the initial indication of puberty is a broadening of the pelvic girdle. A benign physiologic leukorrhea occurs as the vaginal and uterine tissues begin to mature and expand. However, the most dramatic evidence of pubertal development is the appearance of breast buds, an event known as *thelarche* (Fig. 19-6). This is followed in approximately 2 to 6 months by growth of pubic hair on the mons pubis (Fig. 19-7).

The initial appearance of menstruation, or *(menarche)*, occurs about 2 years after the appearance of the first pubescent changes, approximately 1 year after attainment of peak height velocity and 6 months after attainment of peak weight velocity. Menarche has been related to a critical gain in body fat content although this is controversial (Garn, LaVelle, and Pilkington, 1983) (see p. 849). The normal age range of menarche is usually considered to be 10 to 15 years, with the average age being 12½ years for North American girls. During the establishment of the ovarian cycle, the menstrual periods are usually scanty and irregular

Stage 2
(pubertal)

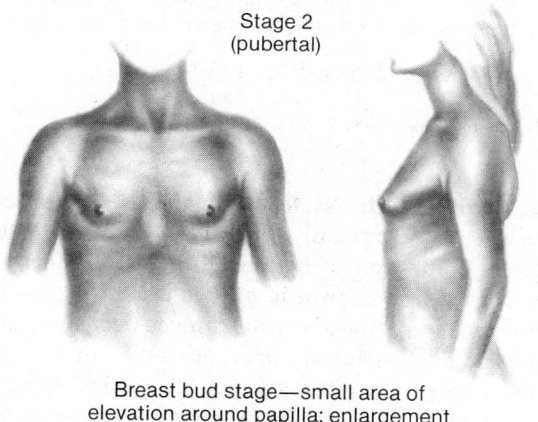

Breast bud stage—small area of
elevation around papilla; enlargement
of areolar diameter

Stage 4

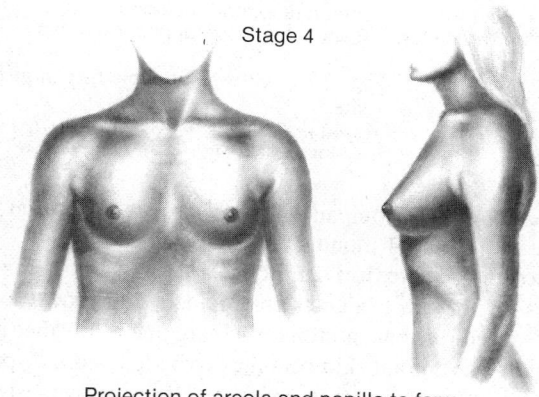

Projection of areola and papilla to form
a secondary mound (may not occur
in all girls)

Stage 3

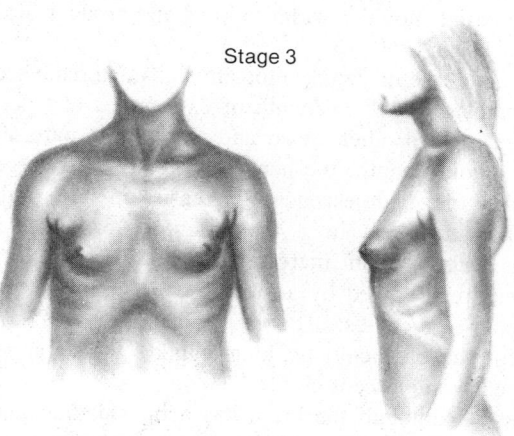

Further enlargement of breast and areola
with no separation of their contours

Stage 5

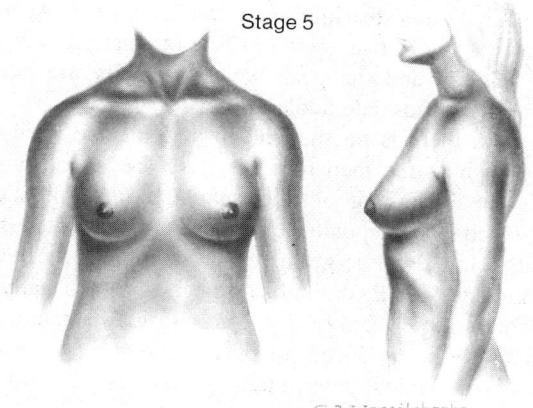

Mature configuration; projection of papilla
only caused by recession of areola
into general contour

Fig. 19-6. Development of the breast in girls—average age span, 11 to 13 years. Stage 1 (prepubertal—elevation of papilla only) is not shown.

Adapted from Marshall, W.A., and Tanner, J.M.: Arch. Dis. Child. **44:**291, 1969; and Daniel, W.A., and Paulshock, B.Z.: Patient Care, May 13, 1979, pp. 122-124.

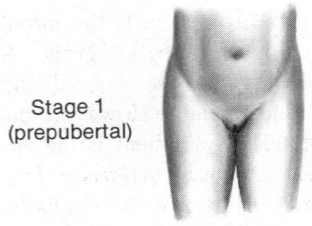

Stage 1
(prepubertal)

No pubic hair; essentially the same as
during childhood; no distinction between hair
on pubis and over the abdomen

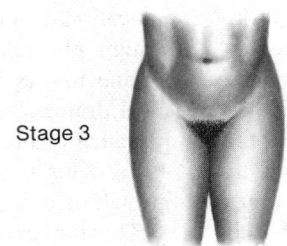

Stage 3

Hair darker, coarser, and curly and spread sparsely
over entire pubis in the typical female triangle

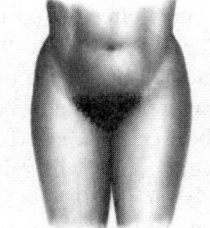

Stage 5

Hair adult in quantity, type, and pattern
with spread to inner aspect of thighs

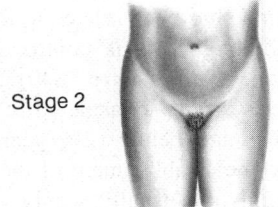

Stage 2

Sparse growth of long, straight, downy, and
slightly pigmented hair extending along labia;
between stages 2 and 3 begins to appear on pubis

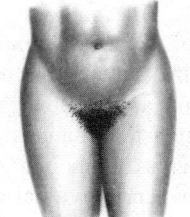

Stage 4

Pubic hair denser, curled, and adult in distribution
but less abundant and restricted to the pubic area

Fig. 19-7. Growth in pubic hair in girls—average age span for stages 2 through 5, 11 to 14 years.
Adapted from Marshall, W.A., and Tanner, J.M.: Arch. Dis. Chilld. **44**:291, 1969; and Daniel, W.A., and Paulshock, B.Z.: Patient Care, May 13, 1979, pp. 122-124.

and may not be accompanied by ovulation. Ovulation usually occurs 12 to 24 months after menarche.

Sexual maturation in boys. Early pubertal changes in boys begin with testicular enlargement and growth of internal structures but minimum enlargement of the penis (phallus). The scrotal skin becomes wrinkled and red, penile and testicular enlargement continues, spermatogenesis begins, and pubic hair growth starts (Fig. 19-8). As puberty advances there is an increase in length and width of the penis, scrotal skin becomes darkly pigmented, and the characteristic male hair distribution pattern is evident. As serum testosterone levels rise over a 12-month period, the peak height velocity and the peak weight velocity are attained concurrently during late adolescence.

For boys there is no sudden physical change to indicate puberty such as the menarche in girls. The overt signal in boys is the beginning of nocturnal emissions of seminal fluid, which occur spontaneously during sleep at periodic intervals. Unlike cyclic germ cell production in the female, spermatogenesis is a continuous process that is usually well established by 17 years of age. As with girls, mature germ cells may not be produced for several months. The average age range at which boys attain puberty is 12½ to 16½ years, with a mean of 14 years.

Changes in Body Systems

Concurrent with pubertal changes, other organ systems are altered through the influence of hormone secretion and growth. Almost every system is affected, some strikingly so, and the changes differ between boys and girls.

Skeletal growth. Skeletal growth differences between boys and girls are primarily reflected in limb length and are apparently a function of hormonal effects at puberty. The earlier cessation of growth in girls is caused by epiphyseal unity under the potent effect of estrogen secretion, and the hormonal effect on female bone growth is much stronger than the similar effect of testosterone in males. In boys the prolonged growth period before puberty and the less rapid epiphyseal closure are reflected in their greater overall height and longer arms and legs. Other skeletal differences are increased shoulder width in boys and broader hip development in girls.

This increase in size develops in a characteristic sequence of changes. Growth in length of extremities and neck precedes growth in other areas, and since these parts are first to reach adult length, the hands and feet appear larger than normal during adolescence. Increases in hip and chest breadth take place in a few months, followed several months later by an increase in shoulder width. These changes are followed by an increase in length of the trunk and depth of the chest. This sequence of changes is responsible for the characteristic long-legged, gawky appearance of the early adolescent child.

Head. Although the brain has achieved the major portion of its growth before adolescence, proportional changes in the skull occur as the face lengthens concurrently with other body alterations. A disproportion is noted in the facial features as the forehead becomes higher and wider, and the nose appears large as it lengthens before puberty. Later the mouth and lips become fuller, and last the jaw reaches adult

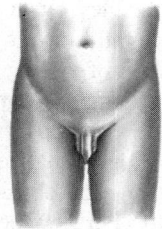

Stage 1 (prepubertal)

No pubic hair; essentially the same as during childhood; no distinction between hair on pubis and over the abdomen

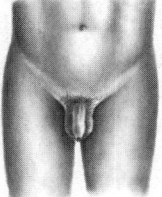

Stage 2 (pubertal)

Initial enlargement of scrotum and testes; reddening and textural changes of scrotal skin; sparse growth of long, straight, downy, and slightly pigmented hair at base of penis

Fig. 19-8. Developmental stages of secondary sex characteristics and genital development in boys—average age span, 12 to 16 years.

Adapted from Marshall, W.A., and Tanner, J.M.: Arch. Dis. Child. **45**:13, 1970; and Daniel, W.A., and Paulshock, B.Z.: Patient Care, May 13, 1979, pp. 122-124.

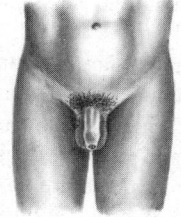

Stage 3

Initial enlargement of penis, mainly in length; testes and scrotum further enlarged; hair darker, coarser, and curly and spread sparsely over entire pubis

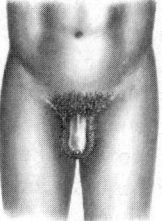

Stage 4

Increased size of penis with growth in diameter and development of glans; glans larger and broader; scrotum darker; pubic hair more abundant with curling but restricted to pubic area

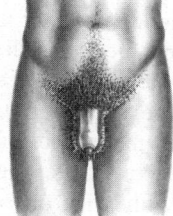

Stage 5

Testes, scrotum, and penis adult in size and shape; hair adult in quantity and type with spread to inner surface of thighs

size and configuration. The baby face of childhood disappears and the large head, characteristic of childhood, becomes smaller in relation to the total body size.

Hypertrophy of the laryngeal mucosa and enlargement of the larynx and vocal cords occur in both boys and girls to produce voice changes. Girls' voices become slightly deeper and considerably fuller, but the effect in boys is striking. The "change of voice" in adolescent boys is one of the most noticeable traits of puberty, causing the voice to shift uncontrollably from deep to high tones in the middle of a sentence.

Body mass. Growth of lean body mass, principally muscle, tends to occur during adolescence after the bone growth spurt and is both quantitatively and qualitatively greater in males than in females at comparable stages of pubertal development. Muscle development, under the influence of androgenic hormones, increases steadily. Muscles become very well developed in boys, but in girls muscle mass increase is proportionate to general tissue growth.

Nonlean mass, primarily fat, also increases but follows a less orderly pattern of growth. There may be a transient increase in subcutaneous fat just before the skeletal growth spurt, especially noted in boys, followed 1 to 2 years later by a modest to marked decrease, again more noticeable in boys. Variable amounts of fat are then deposited to fill out and contour the mature physique in patterns characteristic of the adult of the appropriate sex. In both sexes, fat on the trunk increases at a fairly steady rate, but under the influence of ovarian hormones, the overall fatty tissue deposition in girls is more pronounced. Adipose tissue is distributed over the entire body, particularly in the regions over the

thighs, hips, and buttocks and around the breast tissue, altering the angular childhood figure to the smoother, rounded body contours of the mature female.

Skin changes. Hormonal influences in puberty cause acceleration in growth and maturation of the skin and its structural appendages. Secretion of estrogen causes the skin of the female to develop a soft, smooth, but thicker texture with increased vascularity; androgenic hormones produce increased thickness and some darkening of the skin. *Sebaceous* glands are extremely active at this time, especially on genitals and in "flush areas" of the body (face, neck, shoulders, and upper back and chest). This increased activity and the structural nature of the glands are important in pathogenesis of a common problem of puberty, acne (p. 836).

Eccrine sweat glands, present almost everywhere on the human skin, become fully functional during puberty. Under sympathetic control these glands produce sweat over the entire body where evaporation helps eliminate body heat. The eccrine glands respond to emotional as well as thermal stimulation. Heavy sweating appears to be more pronounced in boys than in girls. The palms and soles ordinarily produce sweat on emotional stimulation but may cause sweating with more intense thermal heating. This also applies to the forehead and axillae.

Apocrine sweat glands, larger than eccrine glands and nonfunctional in childhood, reach secretory capacity during puberty. Unlike the eccrine glands, the apocrine glands are limited in distribution and grow in conjunction with hair follicles in the axillae, around the areola of the breast, around the umbilicus, on the external auditory canal, and in the genital and anal regions. Apocrine glands release a thick secretion as a result of emotional stimulation that, when acted on by surface bacteria, becomes highly odoriferous. The pH of the axillae, acid during childhood, shows a progressive rise to a distinctly alkaline level during adolescence when the apocrine glands begin to function.

Body hair assumes characteristic distribution patterns and texture changes during puberty. Some are common to both boys and girls; others appear to be related entirely to male androgen secretion. Estrogens seem to produce no consistent effect. Under the influence of gonadal and adrenal androgens, hair coarsens, darkens, and lengthens at sites related to secondary sex characteristics. Pubic and axillary hair appears in both sexes, although pubic hair is more extensive in males than in females. Beard and mustache hair normally depends on testicular androgens but can be increased in hirsute women. Body hair that usually appears on the chest, upward along the linea alba, and sometimes on other areas (such as the back and shoulders) appears in males and is androgen dependent. Extremity hair appears in varying amounts in both males and females but is also more prolific in the male. There is a strong genetic influence on the degree of extremity hirsutism in both sexes.

Cardiopulmonary system. The size and strength of the heart, blood volume, and systolic blood pressure increase, whereas the pulse rate and basal heat production decrease (see inside front cover). Consistent with the general developmental timetable, these changes appear earlier in girls, who establish a slightly higher pulse rate and a slightly lower systolic blood pressure than boys. Blood volume, which has increased steadily during childhood, reaches a higher value in boys than in girls, a fact that may be related to the increased muscle mass in pubertal boys. Adult values are reached for all formed elements of the blood, but hematocrit levels are higher in boys, platelet count and sedimentation rate are increased in girls, and white blood cell numbers are decreased in both boys and girls.

Respiratory rate, decreasing steadily throughout childhood, reaches the adult rate in adolescence. However, respiratory volume, vital capacity, and other physiologic properties related to respiratory function are increased, and to a far greater extent in males than in females. The differences between the sexes are a result of the greater lung growth associated with the increased shoulder and chest size in boys.

Other changes. Other changes relative to the attainment of mature physiologic capacity are evident in body fluid volume and composition and in basal metabolic rate; declining throughout life, they reach adult levels during the adolescent years. The slightly higher metabolic rate in boys is thought to be a function of androgenic hormones.

Through progressive maturation of the body as it reaches adult size, the adolescent develops the ability to respond to physical stresses and strains equal to or in excess of adult competence. During this period physiologic responses to exercise change drastically: performance improves, especially in boys, and the body is able to make the physiologic adjustments needed for normal function after exercise is completed. These capabilities are a result of the increased size and strength of muscles and the increased level of cardiac, respiratory, and metabolic functioning. Adolescents enjoy physical activity, and there appears to be a positive relationship between regular exercise and physical conditioning activities and improved general health, endurance, and appearance.

PSYCHOSOCIAL DEVELOPMENT

Adolescence is a time when young people are learning how to use their developing mental capacities. Their ability to reason, to assess and evaluate, and to use divergent thinking to come up with new ideas increases during this period of life. The adolescent begins to think beyond the present and into the future. However, these capacities and the ability to make good judgments are still limited by inexperience and as yet insufficient knowledge from which to gain an adequate perspective for problem solving.

Whereas the changes that take place during the middle childhood years are relatively gradual and regular, during early adolescence the alterations occur quickly. Adolescents experience rapid body changes, a shift from the homogeneous uniformity of grade school to the heterogeneous world of classmates, teachers, and courses in high schools, and expanding relationships and expectations for behavior. These fast-paced changes undoubtedly are responsible for much of the inner turmoil that finds external expression in the adolescent.

Erikson: Developing a Sense of Identity

The traditional psychosocial theory identifies the developmental crisis of adolescence as establishing a sense of identity (Erikson, 1963). Throughout childhood, individuals go through the process of identification as they concentrate on various parts of the body at specific times. During infancy children identify themselves as separate from the mother, during early childhood they establish a gender role identification with the appropriate sex parent, and in later childhood they establish who they are in relation to others. In adolescence they come to see themselves as distinct individuals, somehow unique and separate from every other individual.

The early period of adolescence with its rapid physical growth and maturational changes causes the youngsters to experience new and unfamiliar feelings and a heightened sensitivity to peer approval. During this time the adolescent

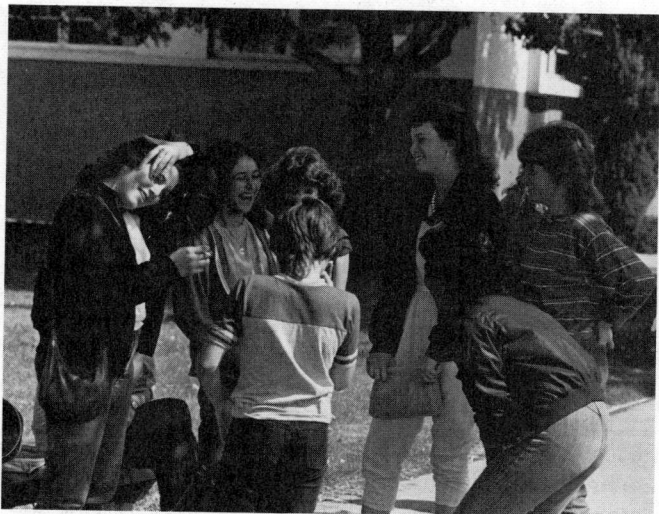

Fig. 19-9. The peer group is a major influence in adolescent development.
Photography by Garibaldi, San Lorenzo, CA.

is faced with the crisis of *group identity* vs alienation. In the period that follows, the individual hopes to attain autonomy from the family and develop a sense of *personal identity* as opposed to role diffusion. A sense of group identity appears to be essential as a prelude to a sense of personal identity. Young adolescents must resolve questions concerning relationships with a peer group before they are able to resolve questions about who they are in relation to family and society.

Group identity. During the early stage of adolescence the pressure to belong to a group is intensified (Fig. 19-9). For teenagers it is essential to find a group to which they feel that they can belong and that provides them with status. Belonging to a crowd helps adolescents to define the differences between themselves and their parents. They dress as the group dresses and wear makeup and hairstyles according to group criteria—all of which are different from those of the parental generation. Language, music, and dancing reflect a culture that belongs exclusively to the adolescent. When adults begin to emulate these fashions and interests, the style changes immediately. Evidence of adolescent conformity to the peer group and nonconformity to the adult group provides teenagers with a frame of reference in which they can display their own self-assertion while they reject their identity with their parents' generation.

The peer group offers an identity to the young adolescent in terms of acceptance and of the roles it defines. Within the group the young person can try out and experiment with a variety of roles while surrounded by the security and warmth of those who face the same problems, feel the same way, behave the same way, and wear the same symbols of belonging. There is comfort in standing together against those who do not understand—to giggle, shout, and act silly in the company of those with whom they share an emotional attachment. To be different is to be unaccepted and alienated from the group.

Individual identity. The quest for personal identity is part of the ongoing identification process. As youngsters establish an identity within a group, they are also attempting to incorporate multiple body changes into a concept of the self. Body awareness is part of self-awareness, and for some time the adolescent will engage in assimilating the self represented by this physical dimension. In this search for identity, adolescents take into consideration the relationships that have developed between themselves and others in the past as well as the directions they hope to be able to take in the future.

Significant others hold certain expectations for the behavior of the adolescent. Often these expectations or demands are persistent enough to induce certain decisions that might be made differently or not at all if the individual could be solely responsible for identity formation. It is all too easy to slip into the roles that are expected by these external influences without incorporating personal goals or questioning these decisions in relation to the developing personality. Thus the individual becomes what parents or others wish him to be based on these premature decisions. In addition, a young person might form a negative identity when society or his culture provides him with a self-image that is contrary to the values of the community. Labels such as ''juvenile delinquent,'' ''hood,'' or ''failure'' are applied to certain adolescents who then accept and live up to these labels with behaviors that validate and strengthen them.

The process of evolving a personal identity is time-consuming and fraught with periods of confusion, depression, and discouragement. To determine an identity and a place in the world is a critical and perilous feature of adolescence. However, as the pieces gradually shift and settle into place, a positive identity will eventually emerge from the confusion. *Role diffusion* results when the individual is unable to formulate a satisfactory identity from the multiplicity of aspirations, roles, and identifications.

Sex-role identity. Adolescence is the time for consolidation of a sex-role identity. In the preschool and early school years children learn to apply an appropriate gender label to themselves, they acquire information about sex-associated expectations, and they develop a sex-role preference. The establishment of close relationships with same-sex peers, which begins in later childhood, is intensified during early adolescence. Through these relationships children learn about the possibility of intimacy between equals and are exposed to peer standards for appropriate sex-role behavior. In early adolescence the peer group begins to communicate some expectations regarding heterosexual relationships, and as development progresses, adolescents encounter expectations for mature sex-role behavior from both peers and adults. Expectations such as these vary from culture to culture, between geographic areas, and between socioeconomic groups.

Adolescents are urged to make a career choice, and the decision about an occupation has important implications for their sex-role identity. Although most occupations or careers are now viewed as appropriate for either sex, some members of society still categorize jobs according to how they relate to sex-role expression. If the choice is considered ''sex appropriate,'' the work environment will support the sex-role identity. To enter a career that is not generally selected by one's own sex may lead to constant tension as a result of challenges directed toward the individual's competence and sex-role identity. The trend toward equalizing career opportunities and minimizing the sex-role connotations of many occupations ideally will eliminate much of this source of antagonism.

Freud: The Genital Stage

The genital period, the longest and last of Freud's psychosexual stages, begins with puberty and extends to old age. It is the stage in which the individual arrives at full sexual potency. Throughout adolescence and young adulthood the libido is invested in activities that prepare the individual to satisfy the mature sex instinct through procreation. The activities are primarily those of forming friendships, preparing for a career, courting, and marriage.

Unlike the phallic stage of early childhood when sexuality is primitive and mainly self-centered, sexuality in the genital stage is heterosexual. Sexual interests increase markedly in vigor and intensity and are focused on members of the opposite sex. New problems arise as adolescents find social disapproval and prohibitions of their own consciences conflicting with intense heterosexual desires.

COGNITIVE DEVELOPMENT

In the final stage of cognitive development the child is no longer limited to the concrete or the observable. Like the preceding stages the advanced stage of cognitive development determines what young people learn when they interact with other people and how they will behave toward others.

Piaget: Developing Formal Operations

Progression in the realm of cognitive thinking culminates with the capacity for abstract thinking. This stage, the period of *formal operations,* is Piaget's fourth and last stage and is attained at different ages, depending on the individual child's motivation, practice, opportunities, and cultural differences.

Young people can begin thinking about the world in new ways. Living in the nonpresent as well as the present, they are no longer concerned with and restricted to the real and actual, which was typical of the period of concrete thought, but they are also concerned with the possible. They now think beyond the present. At this time their thoughts can be influenced more by logical principles than by their own perceptions and experiences. They become capable of scientific reasoning and formal logic. Without having to center attention on the immediate situation, they can imagine the possible—a sequence of events that might occur, such as college and occupational possibilities, how things might change in the future, such as relationships with parents, and

the consequences of their actions, such as dropping out of school.

They are capable of mentally manipulating more than two categories of variables at the same time. For example, they can consider the relationship between speed, distance, and time in planning a trip. They can detect logical consistency or inconsistency in a set of statements and evaluate a system or set of values in a more analytic manner. For instance, they question the parent who insists on honesty in the youngster but at the same time cheats on an income tax report or expense account.

Young people can consider their own thinking and the thinking of others. They wonder what opinion others have of them, and they are increasingly able to imagine the thoughts of others. With this capacity comes the ability to differentiate between others' thoughts and their own and to interpret the thoughts of others more accurately. Thus they see themselves and the world in more relativistic ways. As they come to know that other cultures and communities have different norms and standards from their own, it becomes easier to accept members of these other cultures, and the decision to behave in their own culture in an accepted manner becomes a more conscious commitment to that culture.

Idealism

With the capacity for abstract thinking and the use of deductive reasoning, youth are concerned about gaining a clear understanding of life and its purpose. They often become disillusioned with the world they see and search for an ideal and decent world to which their ideal and decent selves can respond. This part of the self is hidden from view and may not be revealed to any but closest friends. Adolescents are continually discarding old illusions and constructing new ones to take their place. Consequently they may embrace idealistic movements and causes. Many turn to religion—their own or a new one—as a source of comfort and reassurance.

Most adolescents accept society as it exists and attempt to adjust as best they can to things as they are. Some devote themselves to a life of pleasure and seek to extend this existence as long as they possibly can. Others, convinced that injustice and repression have reached an intolerable point, become revolutionaries or radical reformers in an attempt to create a better place in which to live. A highly visible few resort to psychopathic behavior as they seek gratification by an exploitative and sometimes brutal approach to others.

As a whole, adolescents are able to maintain the conviction that virtue and decency are possible, and they are seldom totally disillusioned. They are able to discern in others the idealism that they feel. They are prone to setbacks with feelings of helplessness and depression, and few are able to carry their idealism beyond adolescence in careers and organizational activities. By late adolescence most have come to terms with things as they are. They have evaluated their capabilities in relation to their ambitions and economic realities and have either entered the work force or the armed forces or embarked on the pursuit of an educational goal. Very few are able to hold fast to their ideals in the face of the pressures and stress associated with the turbulent transition to adulthood.

BODY IMAGE DEVELOPMENT

Physical growth and maturation during adolescence occur so rapidly that young people have difficulty adjusting to the changes, which creates feelings of confusion about their bodies. They have lost the security of a familiar body and feel a strangeness about their altered bodies. Consequently they may try either to hide them or to advertise them, or they may alternate between the two extremes. Teenagers are acutely aware of their appearance as they begin to acquire an image of themselves as adults, but they see discrepancies between their ideal and their actual skills and abilities.

Strange and unfamiliar feelings press on them as inner urges announce a sexual awakening. These feelings must also be integrated into the self-image. Sexuality is not the same for boys as it is for girls, and it has different psychic overtones that influence behavior and adaptation. Although it appears that the intensity of the sexual drive is different in adolescent boys and girls, this has not been conclusively demonstrated. Current findings indicate that the difference may be related to the physiologic nature of the sex drive rather than to its intensity. Sexual arousal in males is very direct and centered in the genitalia, whereas in females it is more vague, diffuse, and closely linked to their total personality.

Adolescents are continually comparing themselves to their peers and making judgments of their own normality based on these observations. Pubertal children feel most comfortable when they are just like their friends and agemates. Perceived defects or deviations from the group average are threatening to their idealized image. Any blemish is likely to be magnified out of proportion, and any delay of the visible evidence of maturity is cause for worry. Unfortunately this is also the time when the hormonal effect of the sebaceous glands produces acne that creates problems for many youngsters. To the adolescent even the most insignificant pimple may be viewed as a colossal disfigurement; every blemish is a major catastrophe. The advent of chronic disease or a permanent physical disability has very special significance during adolescence and creates additional stresses for both the affected youngster and health workers.

It has been determined that the body image established during adolescence is the one that individuals retain throughout life. Much of adolescents' search for identity takes place before a mirror as they try to read from the reflected features just who they are and what they look like to other people. Adolescents practice facial expressions and postures, try out hair arrangements, worry about a pimple, and in other ways attempt to assess the best means to achieve a maximum effect—to reveal the "true self."

Although many of the changes of puberty have features common to both girls and boys, the implications and responses are different in the two sexes, and many of these adjustments are influenced by the values and prohibitions of the culture. Often the body changes per se may be less significant than the meaning and importance that these changes have for adolescents and other persons in their lives.

Boys' Responses to Puberty

The early adolescent increases in height and muscle mass are welcomed by the adolescent boy whose growth for several months has lagged significantly behind that of his female agemates. Although his more mature physique brings highly valued increase in strength and greater athletic skills, this rapid growth is uneven, and therefore he has some trouble adjusting. When bones grow faster than muscles, muscles are taut and respond with quick, jerky movements; when muscles grow faster than bones, they become somewhat loose and sluggish. For a time he is awkward and uncoordinated. Often his size outstrips his strength and he tires more easily. Fatigue, lack of coordination, and appearing "funny" and "out of shape" are sources of embarrassment, selfconsciousness, and feelings of inadequacy. He has difficulty in accepting his new body image at first, and accusations of clumsiness, laziness, or stupidity do little to strengthen his self-concept during a time that offers such strong challenges to his self-esteem.

The development of secondary sex characteristics, especially the growth of facial and body hair, has psychologic and social meaning to the adolescent boy. This, more than any other secondary characteristic, is associated with the masculine sex role, and the ritual act of shaving at the slightest evidence of growth is a means for the young boy to validate his identification with this role (Fig. 19-10). Shaving also provides a legitimate excuse to gaze at and admire the broadening shoulders and altered features of his changing body image. Unfortunately with many adolescent boys the appearance of acne and an awkward appearance when assuming adult poses often interfere with the pleasure of this experience.

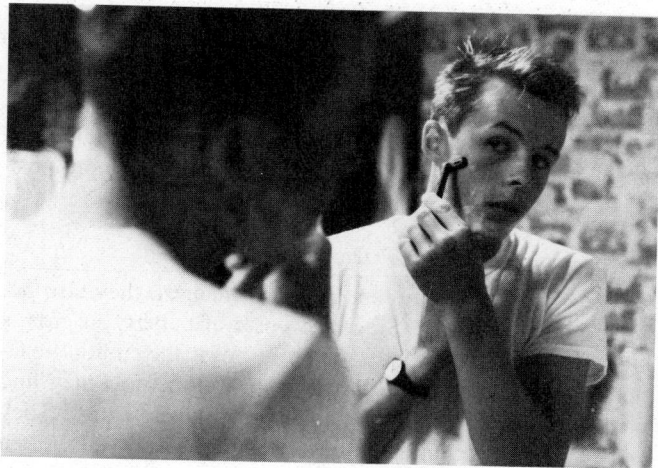

Fig. 19-10. The act of shaving offers the adolescent male the opportunity to study his changing appearance.
Photography by Anne Kunke, San Jose, CA.

The growth of the penis and testes creates some important problems for the adolescent male. Unlike the reproductive organs in the female, the male reproductive organs are readily visible and provide the boy with concrete evidence of his masculine character. He knows by the sensations localized within these organs that he is now a man. His reproductive organs become very sensitive to sexual stimulation. Sexual feelings are directly related to the genitalia, desire is urgent, and he seeks rapid relief from pressure and tension through ejaculation. Sexual needs in the pubertal boy are a highly specific physical phenomenon, centered around the sex act itself, and are initially quite separate from ideas of love. These sexual cravings appear to reach a peak in the 1 to 2 years after puberty.

Adolescent boys are generally not well prepared for the maturation of the reproductive organs. Spontaneous ejaculations are frequently puzzling, troublesome, and embarrassing events. Unless he has been prepared in advance for this eventuality, the boy often finds it difficult to seek an explanation from his parents; therefore he turns to friends or reading material to gain information or he may puzzle about the meaning in his own mind.

The opportunity for gratification of these genital urges through heterosexual expression is denied to the adolescent by Western cultural standards. Premarital sexual involvement is fraught with many problems and conflicts, and homosexual activities are generally condemned by society. As a consequence the teenage boy may masturbate. It is a normal activity, and almost every boy masturbates alone or in relation to sexual experimentation with others of the same sex. However, this too is often associated with guilt and anxiety. Misconceptions still dominate the feelings of many people who believe masturbation to be evil, unmanly, or "not nice" and who attribute a wide assortment of ills to the practice. Current enlightenment accepts that to engage in the practice from time to time is normal and temporarily helps provide the young man with important information about how his body works and how adult physical sexuality and reproduction are accomplished. He learns that organ responses to sexual excitement can be initiated at will and that orgasmic climax with a predictable release of tension, or repeatedly deferred at will, contributes to a developing sense of mastery over sexual impulses and new sexual capacities. Without guilt and worry, the adolescent boy can incorporate this aspect of his masculinity into a more positive self-concept.

Girls' Responses to Puberty

As girls begin to experience pubertal changes, they also become body conscious. Since the onset of puberty in girls is almost 2 years in advance of that in boys, their initial reaction to increased height may be embarrassment as they find themselves towering above their male classmates. They worry about becoming too tall. Adolescent girls often slouch or adopt a hunched posture in an attempt to minimize this increased height, especially early-maturing girls who are normally of above-average height. The increase in weight and the normal plumping of features with fat deposition are predominant concerns of pubescent girls. They often perceive these changes as evidence of a tendency toward obesity, and many attempt to avoid such alterations by strict and faddish dieting. This ill-timed strategy can deprive their bodies of essential nutrients during a period of rapid body development.

The young girl is interested in her changing form and feminine curves. The average girl looks on her budding breasts with pleasure as a sign of approaching maturity and evidence of her femininity. She observes and may even measure the growth of her developing breasts and continually compares her own progress with that of her friends and classmates. She begins to wear a brassiere. Some girls are sensitive about their breast development and attempt to hide it, whereas others are delighted with their new figures and wear tight sweaters and clothes that accentuate their curves.

Development of some of the secondary sex characteristics may be less pleasing to girls than they are to boys, particularly the growth of body hair. A culture in which smooth-skinned females are preferred makes it necessary for the girl to shave her underarms and legs regularly to meet the standards for feminine appearance. Although this practice is another indication of maturity, it does not have the same sex-role significance as face shaving for the adolescent boy. The girl becomes increasingly conscious of the feminine ideal, and in an effort to approach this standard, she experiments with a variety of cosmetics and hairstyles. Alone and together, she and her friends spend endless hours before the mirror posing, applying cosmetics, and combing their hair. This practice provides the same narcissistic outlet for the girl that is available to the boy through shaving.

The advent of menstruation, that exclusive feature of female puberty, provides the greatest impetus toward full realization and acceptance of female sexuality. Menstruation is positive evidence of womanhood and the potential for pregnancy and childbearing. Most girls are adequately prepared for the event and take this new function in stride, looking forward to menstruation, feeling satisfaction at its onset, and seeing it as the symbol of their passage from childhood to womanhood. Others find it distressing, frightening, and difficult to accept. In some it reawakens old fears of body injury and castration. Still others accept it matter-of-factly. Because of its sudden onset, the first menstruation can be a traumatic experience for the girl who has not been taught what to expect. As a rule, if the young girl has established a positive gender role during childhood, the transition to womanhood, with all its ramifications, is accepted as the normal phenomenon that it is.

Unlike the adolescent boy, strong sexual feelings in the adolescent girl are not usually centered in the genital region but are more generalized and ill defined. Her reproductive apparatus, less obvious than that of the boy, contributes in only a vague way to sexual awareness. The girl in early adolescence may experience pleasant sensations and even tingling in the genital area, but these feelings are diffuse and difficult to separate from other body sensations. In the adolescent girl the urge for self-stimulation is not as strong as it is in the male. Although many girls handle the genitalia for the pleasant sensation that is evoked, not all carry the activity to a climax. Her sexual feelings are centered less on the genitalia and erotic gratification with release of tension than on the manipulation of a pleasant state with romantic feelings about love. However, with the more open, liberal views regarding female sexual responses, it is being revealed that much of the nature of the adolescent girl's sexual arousal may have more of a cultural rather than a biologic basis.

A difficulty faced by the pubescent girl is related to the discrepancy in the onset of puberty in girls and in boys. She is often placed in the position where she must explain or hide the fact of her own body changes from her male peers. The dissemination of information to boys about these changes lags significantly behind; therefore the girl finds it difficult to accept the changes she is experiencing while attempting to hide or mask them from the boys whose attention and approval she is seeking.

MORAL DEVELOPMENT

As children move through the stages of cognition and logical thought, they also progress through sequential stages of moral development. As with other developmental processes, moral development approaches or achieves adult levels during adolescence.

Kohlberg: Conventional and Postconventional Levels

Kohlberg's theory of development of moral judgment and thought (1975) proposes that at the conventional level, which includes youngsters of preadolescence and adolescence, ages 10 to 16, the major concern is to act or behave in a way that will gain or maintain the approval of others. There are obedience of rules and respect for authority.

The shift from conventional to postconventional morality that takes place during late adolescence is characterized by serious questioning of existing moral values and their relevance to society and the individual. Adolescents can easily appreciate the thoughts and feelings of another. They understand duty and obligation based on reciprocal rights of others as well as the concept of justice that is founded on making amends for misdeeds and repairing or replacing what has been spoiled by wrongdoing. However, they seriously question established moral codes, often as a result of observing that adults verbally ascribe to a code but do not adhere to it. Their advanced cognitive development makes adolescents more aware of moral questions and values and closely parallels the general process of identity formation. Coincident with these advancements are rapidly changing social demands that require continual reappraisal of these values and

beliefs. They are aware of the contradictions in the existing social and value structures in which they participate.

Adolescent boys and girls must make choices. They are changing as is their social world. They find that there are many ways to live their lives, their behavioral domain is expanded, and they encounter situations that they have never before faced that require decisions about actions to be taken and decisions based on moral evaluation and judgment. Whereas the younger child merely accepts the decisions or point of view of adults, the adolescent must substitute his own set of morals and values in order to gain autonomy from adults. When old principles are challenged but new and independent values have not yet emerged to take their place, young people search for a moral code that preserves their personal integrity and guides their behavior, especially in the face of strong pressure to violate the old values. Their decisions involving moral dilemmas must be based on an internalized set of principles that provides them with the resources to evaluate the demands of the situation and to plan a course of action consistent with their ideals.

SPIRITUAL DEVELOPMENT

As youngsters move toward independence from parents and other authorities, some begin to question the values and ideals of their families. Others cling to these values as a stable element in their lives as they struggle with the conflicts of this turbulent period. Adolescents need to work out these conflicts for themselves, but they also need support from authority figures and peers for their resolution. Often the peer group is more influential than parents, although values acquired during the formative years are usually maintained.

Adolescents are capable of understanding abstract concepts and interpreting analogies and symbols. They are able to empathize, philosophize, and think logically. Most are searching for ideals and speculate about illogical statements and conflicting ideologies. Their tendency toward introspection and emotional intensity at this age often makes it difficult for others to know what they are thinking. They tend to keep their thoughts private, fearing that no one will understand these feelings that they perceive to be unique and special. Young people may reject the formal worship service but engage in individual worship in the privacy of their rooms. It is not uncommon for them to reveal deep spiritual concerns and then act silly and deny these feelings (Shelly, 1982). They need support and encouragement in their struggle for understanding and the freedom to question without censure.

Youth today appear to be placing more emphasis on personal than on institutionalized religion (Dickinson, 1982). This is consistent with the greater stress young people place on personal values, relationships, and moral standards and their lessening reliance on traditional social beliefs and institutions. Evangelistic types of worship are increasingly attractive to younger persons. Many adolescents are attracted to the new religious sects (e.g., the so-called Jesus Movement, Hare Krishna, and Children of God) (Galanter, 1980). These affiliations may be a response to disillusionment with conventional religious structures, an anchor following a period of rootlessness and identity confusion, or a source of satisfying values in a chaotic society. For some, joining a particular movement represents a fad with the adventure of confounding conventional parents (Conger and Petersen, 1984).

SOCIAL RELATIONSHIPS

To achieve full maturity, adolescents must free themselves from family domination and define an identity independent of parental authority. However, this process is fraught with ambivalence on the part of both teenagers and their parents. Adolescents want to grow up and be free of parental restraints, yet they are fearful as they try to comprehend the responsibilities that are linked with independence. A predominant theme of discussions with teenagers involves the escape from parental dominance. However, this is usually an attempt to conceal the feelings of dependence and anxiety that are generated by the preparation for leaving the sanctuary of the family—the final separation-individuation process of childhood.

Part of this emancipation process involves developing social relationships outside the family that help teenagers identify their role in society. Increasing absence from home through frequent contacts with peers is essential to this socialization process. Adolescence is a time of intense sociability and often a time of equally intense loneliness. Acceptance by peers, a few close friends, and the secure love of a supportive family are requisites for the interpersonal maturation process.

Relationships with Parents

During adolescence the parent-child relationship changes from one of protection-dependency to one of mutual affection and equality. The process of achieving independence often involves turmoil and ambiguity as both parent and adolescent learn to play new roles and work toward this end while at the same time resolving the often painful series of rifts essential to establishing the ultimate relationships.

Most of the behavior observed in adolescents is related to the external restrictions and checks that are placed on this spontaneous maturation process. On one hand, adolescents are accepted as maturing preadults. They are allowed privileges formerly denied, and they are provided with increasing responsibilities. On the other hand, because of their unpredictability and insecurity in evaluating situations and making sound judgments, they must conform to regulations and restrictions set by adults. This state of affairs is particularly exemplified by the struggle between parents and adolescents concerning the hour of curfew.

During adolescence the behavior observed in the toddler is relived as the individual again seeks autonomy. If what occurred during the toddler period is known, it is possible to make some predictions regarding the probable behavior of the adolescent (Blos, 1979). The teenager's earliest attempts to achieve emancipation from parental controls are manifested in a period of rejection of the parents. Adolescents are critical, argumentative, and generally remote with both parents. They are frequently absent from home and family activities and spend an increasing amount of time with the peer group. They are less close and confiding in relationships with parents. This rejection is not consistent, however, and varies with mood changes. At times young teenagers feel highly competent and demand their "rights"; at other times, after being hurt in battles with the world, they may accept parental guidance and security.

As teenagers assert their rights for grown-up privileges, they frequently create tensions within the home. They resist parental control, and conflicts can arise from almost any situation or any subject. Some of the favorite topics of dispute include use of the telephone, manners, dress, chores and duties, homework, disrespectful behavior, friendships, dating, money, automobiles, and time schedules. Present in these areas of conflict are the overriding argument that "Everyone else has one" or is allowed the desired item or privilege and the ever-present assertion that "You don't understand me" and "You always treat me like a baby." Spoken or unspoken, parents' reactions consist of "Is this all the thanks I get for what I have done, or am doing, for you?"

With advancing adolescence, teenagers become more competent, and with this competence comes a need for more autonomy. However, although they are psychologically better prepared for independence, they are often thwarted in their efforts by lack of money or by other parental barriers. Much conflict arises from the teenager's outside activities and the elements of privacy and trust. Too many parents believe that they must know all of their adolescent's activities and feelings; they may go through the teenager's belongings in an attempt to find out what he is doing. To gain the respect and trust of their adolescent, parents must respect his privacy and show an honest and sincere interest in what he believes and feels. Teenagers need not only guidance and support from their parents but also enough leeway to establish their own individuality.

Sometimes teenagers prove to be a source of pleasure and fulfillment beyond the parents' expectations. The adolescent may be one who is of a particularly happy disposition or one whose talents and abilities in areas such as music, art, scholastic achievement, or athletics provide the parents with pleasure and gratification. Most parental disappointments in their adolescent children are related to their own expectations for success or failure.

The recent trends in society in terms of equality and relaxation of previous moral standards have made the adjustments of teenagers and parents increasingly difficult. The so-called generation gap is widening in relation to a number of attitudes, values, and beliefs. Parents can no longer find guidance from their own experiences in understanding the needs of today's teenager. Consequently in their frustration, bewilderment, and disappointment, they are forced to undertake a painful reevaluation of a number of their previously held attitudes and beliefs.

Peer Relationships and Influence

Although parents remain the primary influence in the lives of adolescents, most adolescents find that peers assume a more significant role at this time than they did during childhood. The peer group serves as a strong support to teenagers, individually and collectively providing them with a sense of belonging and a feeling of strength and power. It forms that transitional world between dependence and autonomy. As adolescents spend increasing amounts of time among their peers and have less contact with their parents, the peer group becomes an important socializing agent. It acts as is a support for conformity and for questioning and challenging adult values and societal institutions; the peer group is a new frame of reference from which to reject the old.

Peer group. Adolescents have always been social, gregarious, and group-minded. Although there are a few who remain outside either from preference or rejection, the majority seek the safety, companionship, and reciprocal reinforcement of a group. The peer group has an intense influence on the adolescent's self-evaluation and behavior. In order to gain acceptance by a group, the early teenager tends to conform completely in such things as modes of dress, hairstyle, taste in music, and vocabulary, often at the expense of individuality and self-assertion. The teenager's entire being is measured by the reaction of his peers. Since most teenagers are still insecure and lacking in confidence, they are unable to tolerate differences between themselves and their peers; therefore conformity is the rule within primary friendship groups. To belong is of utmost importance; thus adolescents behave in a way that will ensure their establishment in a group. Adolescents are highly susceptible to social approval, acceptance, and demands. To be ignored or criticized by peers creates feelings of inferiority, inadequacy, and incompetence.

Except in a few small, homogeneous high schools, teenagers distribute themselves into a relatively predictable social hierarchy. The largest social division is the *set*. Both boys and girls can be members of a set, but for some occasions and activities they separate into like-sex crowds. The adolescents know to which set they and others belong, although in large schools they may not all know each other. Thus the circle of acquaintances is broadened, and within their set adolescents develop the adult social skill of exchanging breezy, pert greetings with people they know only slightly.

Based on common tastes, interests, and background, smaller, distinct, and rather exclusive crowds or cliques of selected close friends, who are emotionally attached to each other, exist within the set. Although cliques may become formalized, most remain informal and small. Each clique has an identifying feature that proclaims its difference from others and its solidarity within itself in much the same way the adolescent generation as a whole sets itself apart from the adult generation. Although the criteria for membership may not be publicly voiced, the groups tend to include or exclude persons according to consistent standards. Cliques are usually made up of one sex, and girls tend to be more cliquish than boys and to have a greater need for close friendships (Kaluger and Kaluger, 1984). Groups congregate at lunch, at a favorite hangout, or in the intimacy of someone's bedroom to talk about things that are of utmost concern to teenage girls, such as clothes, makeup, and especially boys. Boys' groups tend to revolve around sports, hobby activities, and rough games, although they too gossip and discuss the opposite sex. Within the intimacy of the group, adolescents gain support in learning about themselves, consideration for the feelings of others, and increased ego development and self-reliance.

The school is psychologically important to adolescents as a focus of social life, a setting in which to define and elaborate relationships with peers. In addition, most teenagers have a selected gathering place or hangout to which they can go alone or preferably with others of the same sex to mingle with a group of persons from the opposite sex without the formalities or financial obligations of a date.

Best friends. Personal friendships of the one-to-one variety usually develop between like-sex adolescents. This relationship is closer and more stable than it is in middle childhood, and it is important in the quest for identity. A best friend is the best audience on whom to try out possible roles and identities that the adolescent wants to test. Best friends may try a role together, each providing support for the other. Each cares about what the other thinks and feels. Since a sense of intimacy grows within a permanent relationship, the stability of this like-sex friendship is an important link in the progress toward an intimate heterosexual relationship in young adulthood.

Heterosexual Relationships

During adolescence, relationships with members of the opposite sex take on new importance. The increased interest in heterosexual relationships is a natural outgrowth of the physical maturation of the reproductive organs that is taking place at this time. The interaction between body development and cultural expectations helps adolescents incorporate ideas about mature sexuality. As they begin to assimilate and integrate the changes of puberty, adolescents turn with increasing frequency toward the opposite sex, not motivated by a need to find a permanent partner but rather as a means to enhance their own sex-role identity. Early dating is usually closely related to peer-group membership and social status and like other phases of development follows a predictable, sequential pattern. However, the time and rapidity of progress are influenced by many cultural factors, such as the philosophy of the community, traditions, parents' wishes, and the teenagers themselves.

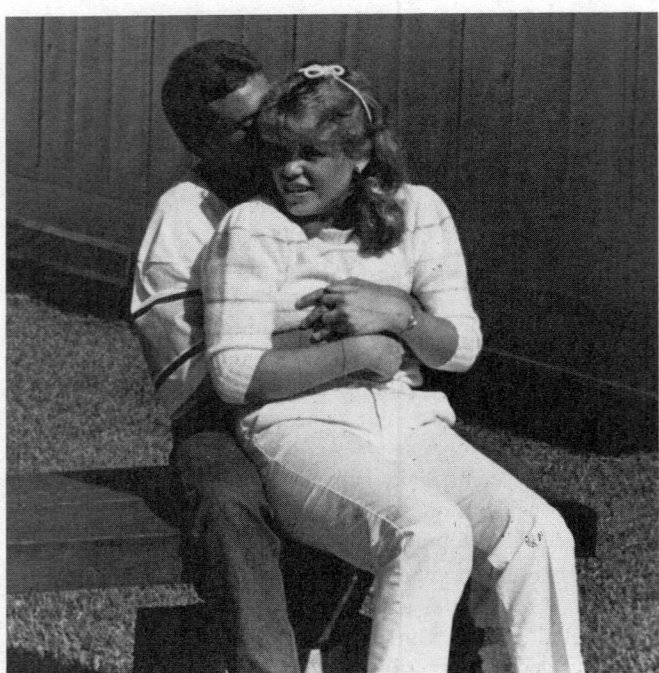

Fig. 19-11. Heterosexual relationships are an important part of adolescence.

Photography by Garibaldi, San Lorenzo, CA.

Typically, 12-year-old children still maintain same-sex friendships, although there are increasing opportunities for mixed-group activities. Although there seems to be a trend toward earlier dating, on the *average,* dating activities begin in the seventh and eighth grades and are usually "crowd" dates at organized school functions. For example, a group of girls just happens to be around a certain group of boys at most activities. There is seldom pairing off within the group, although a few boys and girls may see each other on a paired-off basis. By the ninth grade crowd dates are still popular, but now there is more pairing off of couples. In the tenth grade paired crowd dates, in which some boys and girls come as couples and join the crowd consisting of several couples and perhaps a few unattached friends, are the rule (Kaluger and Kaluger, 1984).

Double-dating follows group dating and is the more common practice in the eleventh grade; both double-dating and single-pair dating are common by the twelfth grade. Most adolescents are dating to some degree by the time they leave high school. The group dating patterns provide a means whereby the potential stress and anxiety associated with heterosexual relationships are buffered by the peer group. When the focus is on group activities rather than on dyadic contacts, heterosexual friendships are less threatening.

The type and degree of seriousness of heterosexual relationships vary. The initial stage is usually noncommittal, extremely mobile, and seldom characterized by any deep romantic attachments. Crushes, those strong feelings of attachment to an important or well-liked adult in the youngster's life who embodies the qualities considered most valuable by the adolescent, are common in early adolescence; they constitute one of the earliest "love" attachments. During early midadolescence as their sexual capacity is evolving, young boys frequently feel the need to test out the power of their sexuality by numerous exploits and conquests. It may be a response to inner sexual pressures or a need to conform to group expectations. With advancing adolescence and more firm sexual identities, steady dating and boy-girl love relationships with deeper commitment become more numerous among teenage youngsters.

Steady dating is evidence of adolescent insecurity and uncertainty—an escape from loneliness and being left out—and provides a sense of belonging (Fig. 19-11). The relationship continues until misunderstanding or boredom ends the association, and the process is often repeated with another partner. During this time the relationship between love and sexuality is brought into focus. Boys and girls in the middle teens find it hard to believe that sex can exist without love; therefore each boy-girl attachment is viewed as real love. Parental attempts to break up these early heterosexual relationships may only cause the youngsters to prolong the attachments as a further expression of defiance. Hasty marriages based on such rebellion are therefore usually doomed to failure.

Authorities disagree regarding the value of early opposite sex relationships in the development of a sexual identity. Some believe that longer like-sex relationships are necessary to fully develop the characteristics of their own sex, whereas others believe that dating provides adolescents with experience in human relationships, promotes social skills, and enhances their ability to choose a mate wisely. A variety of dating partners and experiences undoubtedly promotes a wiser mate selection and favors earlier and longer dating practices; however, early dating can involve an adolescent pair in a close sexual relationship before they are ready for intimacy. The sense of intimacy, the developmental crisis of early adulthood, must be built on a firm sense of identity which early adolescents lack.

Sexual codes. Heterosexual codes among teenage youngsters have undergone a notable change in recent years. The extent to which adolescents engage in intimate sexual relationships is not known precisely. Studies indicate that casual sexual relationships are generally not acceptable. Some degree of permanent commitment is needed before sexual intimacy is considered appropriate. Most adolescents have indulged in petting, including transient, exploratory homosexual petting, and petting is generally more acceptable than intercourse as a form of sexual expression. However, available information indicates that 22% of young women 15 years and under and 42% of those 16 to 18 have engaged in sexual intercourse (Teenage pregnancy, 1981).

In general, males experience sexual relationships with a number of females, whereas most females restrict their experiences to steady boyfriends, most often their future mates. For girls such intimacy is closely allied to an affectionate commitment. The overall major sexual codes in adolescence appear to be (1) petting with affection, in which the couple stops short of full sexual intercourse; (2) permissiveness with affection, which permits coitus in a stable relationship, usually between a steady-dating pair of older adolescents; and (3) the double standard of male sexual behavior, in which the majority of boys feel justified to engage in coitus with other girls to demonstrate and enhance their virility while expecting abstinence from the girl to whom they are romantically committed.

Adolescents engage in sexual relationships to experience pleasurable sensations, to satisfy sexual drives, to satisfy curiosity, to achieve conquests, to express some degree of affection, or to conform. Often the urge to belong and gain reassurance and the wish to really belong to someone provoke a series of increasingly intimate physical contacts with a favored boyfriend or girlfriend, with each contact being more sexually provocative than the last. Eventually sexual intercourse can become established as a behavior pattern and a method for ensuring social participation or even as an end in itself.

Society places the responsibility on the girl for inhibiting

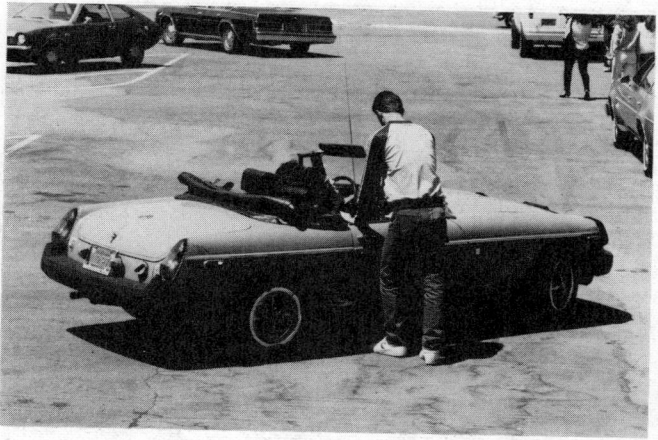

Fig. 19-13. The automobile becomes an important status symbol of adolescence.
Photography by Garibaldi, San Lorenzo, CA.

the boy's sexual advances; therefore if she concedes through a need to conform or for acceptance, she is faced with fears of disease, pregnancy, and being labeled "fast" or "bad." Often the experience can be psychologically harmful, especially when it produces a conflict of values, resulting in feelings of guilt and worthlessness. The increasing incidence of sexual activity among teenagers has important implications for health professionals because of the associated health-related problems.

The current trend toward greater permissiveness regarding adolescent sexual behavior will undoubtedly have an effect on the adolescent developmental experience. It is likely that young people will be accorded progressively more decision-making authority concerning control over their bodies. These alterations in the attitudes and value systems toward sex will have important implications for health professionals. It has been predicted that attitudes toward sex will shift from a moral context to a predominantly health context within a few years.

Interests and Activities

During early adolescence the interests and activities of girls and boys are in sharp contrast. Boys spend a great deal of time in active outdoor sports or "just going out with the guys." They enjoy hobbies and clubs, television takes up a good part of their time, and school-related activities are increasingly important (Fig. 19-12). Girls and mixed-sex activities occupy the interest and concern of boys, but they do not become prominent concerns until their development more nearly approaches that of the more rapidly maturing girls. As their bodies gain strength and size, "making the team" is a major concern for many youths, and a boy may spend an excessive amount of time in attempting to perfect athletic skills. The essential bicycle of middle childhood is replaced by the automobile, the symbol of status to the adolescent (Fig. 19-13). If a car cannot be acquired, a motorcycle or motor bike is preferable to walking, riding the bus,

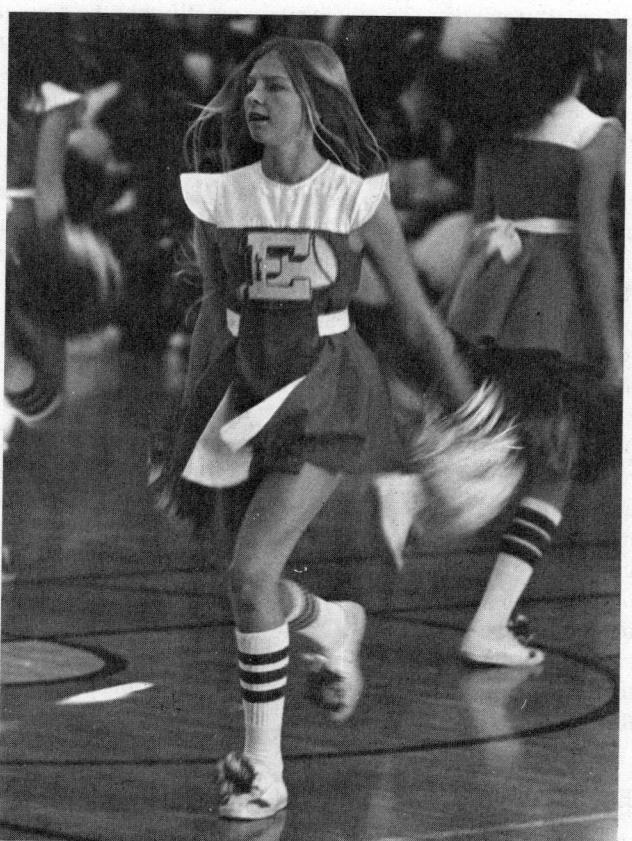

Fig. 19-12. School-related activities occupy an important role in early adolescence.

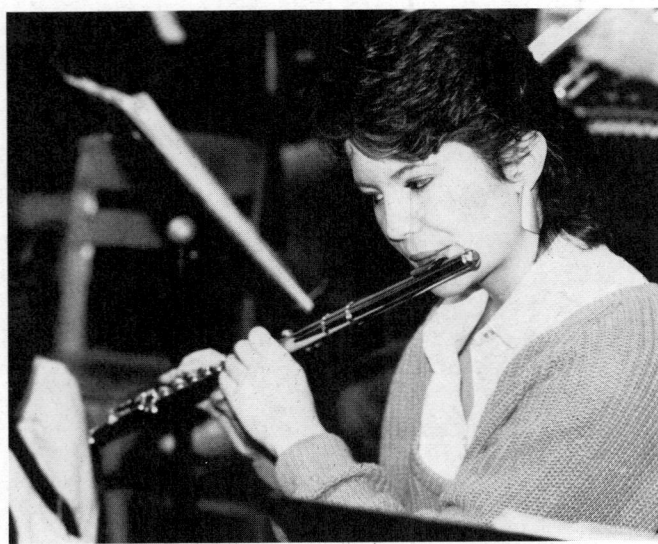

Fig. 19-14. Developing skills and abilities is a prime interest of the young adolescent.
Photography by Garibaldi, San Lorenzo, CA.

or the humiliation of being chauffeured by a parent or sibling. Most boys avidly seek part-time employment, many because of economic necessity.

Although girls' leisure interests involve many outdoor activities, a greater interest in parties and social activities is evident. They are interested in hobbies, self-improvement (Fig. 19-14), and volunteer activities, and many seek part-time jobs out of economic need or in order to purchase more clothes and other teenage "necessities." A large number of girls, and some boys, assume the responsibility for the care of small children as baby-sitters, a common means of earning money during adolescence. However, teenage baby-sitters need some basic guidelines (see box).

Teenagers are avid conversationalists and spend much of their time in the company of other girls talking, listening to records, and experimenting with makeup, hairstyles, and clothes. They enjoy shopping for clothes, but there is seldom agreement between mother and daughter regarding types and styles of clothing. Many of their thoughts and feelings are confessed in a diary. Daydreaming is a prominent characteristic of the adolescent.

Members of both sexes enjoy movies, rock concerts, dancing, and other communal activities and entertainment. Girls seem to prefer sentimental, romantic films when they are available, whereas boys would rather see sports, mystery, or action films. X-rated movies are crowded with adolescents. With the availability of a variety of video films adolescents are congregating in small groups to watch on home video recorders. However, there is little research on the types of video films teenagers watch. Teenage girls and boys begin to appreciate and enjoy the theater and to share in the experience of audience reaction to the performance. They increasingly progress toward enjoyment of more adult activities and interests, and their developing social competence makes them more willing to accompany adults on occasion to share in the fun and activity.

Reading is still a favorite occupation of teenagers and may serve to satisfy some of their needs for vicarious experiences. Reading is more purposeful at this stage than at earlier ages, and most adolescents prefer to read magazines rather than books. The avid interest in collections that was so prominent in middle childhood declines during adolescence to be replaced by individual hobbies in the areas of the arts and sciences.

Teenagers have an affinity for stereo tape players, which assume an important role in their lives, and they are avidly addicted to transistor radios that accompany many of their other activities, such as studying, walking, or working. Much of their money is spent on records and tapes, which are collected in much the same way as books are. Often a favorite recording is regarded with the feeling accorded a well-loved book and is played over and over again.

When not engaged in other activities, they are probably participating in "rap sessions" or in endless telephone conversations. The telephone provides that essential link between peers when they are physically removed from one another. It is a way to fulfill the need for flight from parents to peers without leaving the home. The conversations may consist of gossip, plans, experiences, or an account of the activities of the day. The topics vary greatly, but the amount of time so engaged is often measured in hours. For boy-girl conversations, the telephone provides a means for closeness without fear of complications that physical proximity may engender.

Teenage interests and activities are subject to rapid change. Each succeeding generation of teenagers has its own peculiar characteristics evidenced by their behavior, vocabulary, dress, and other external manifestations that reflect and establish a clear line of separateness, although superficial, between the peer and the adult cultures. The rapidity with which these external trappings change is often astonishing.

The adolescent age-group is a major force in the economic marketplace. Today's adolescents have more money to spend than any previous generation of teenagers, and the advent of television and movies for some ethnic groups has made adolescents a much more visible and identifiable group. Symbols of their identity are brought to their attention through the media by advertisers of cosmetics, radios, records, and fad clothing. Members of this easily impressionable group are readily persuaded to part with money in their ever-present quest for acceptance and popularity, even though based on superficial values.

EMOTIONALITY

The pubertal changes in physical appearance are accompanied by alterations in emotional control and response. The stability of the prepubescent period is replaced by the turmoil precipitated by the physical and psychologic changes

GUIDELINES FOR THE FIRST-TIME BABY SITTER

Before baby-sitting:

Get to know family before planning to baby-sit; telephone and then visit family

Try to meet child(ren) so you will not be a stranger

Learn about family routines that relate to your baby-sitting

Discuss pay, responsibilities, and transportation home; baby-sitter should always be accompanied home by one parent even if only across the street

Baby-sitter must be in good health when expected to baby-sit; job should not be accepted if ill or have something contagious

Before parents leave, find out:

Location of second exit or fire escape

Location of fire extinguisher if any and how to use it

Where they will be and phone number where they can be reached

What time they plan to return

Name and number of nearby neighbor or relative

Emergency numbers for police, fire department, family doctor, hospital, rescue squad, and poison control center—keep list by phone

Rules about baby-sitter's eating, TV watching, friends coming to visit

Names and times of special medicines to be given if any

Location of first aid supplies

While baby-sitting:

Remain awake; when feeling drowsy, walk around, splash face with cool water

Keep doors locked when inside and never open to strangers

Telephone messages for parents should be written down, but telephone number, address, or fact that baby-sitter is alone should not be divulged to caller

Unnecessary calls should be kept short in case parents are trying to call home

Watch child(ren) at all times unless he/she (they) are asleep; check sleeping children at least every half hour

A basic first aid course is a valuable asset in case of emergency

Be prepared to handle minor emergencies and know how to reach help in case of major difficulties

Carry out basic injury prevention:

Keep stairways blocked to avoid falls

Do not leave an infant or small child on a piece of furniture from which he/she might fall

Keep child away from items that might cause injury, e.g., matches, stoves, hot water, sharp items

Know how to call the poison control center

Keep away items from child that might be swallowed, aspirated, or cause suffocation

When a situation is frightening to baby-sitter or child, a call to parents or neighbor can usually help solve problem

A serious situation may merit a call to public safety department

If child is taken outside:

Dress child appropriately according to weather

Discuss with parents where child is allowed to play

Be cautious around driveways, roads, swimming pools, garages, and strange animals

Be prepared for routines and management:

Bedtime rituals and behavior

Mealtime—know how to feed infants and toddlers

Baths

Dressing, including diapering

Learn about appropriate play activities and toys for children of various ages

Abridged and outlined from *Guide for the First-Time Baby Sitter*, available from Johnson & Johnson, Grandview Rd., Skillman, NJ 08558.

---

that teenagers experience. They are deluged with new sensations and feelings they cannot understand. The behavior of adolescents is bewildering to others and often to the adolescents themselves. They are frequently labeled as unstable, inconsistent, and unpredictable. The behaviors they exhibit have even been described as pseudopathologic or as representing a normal psychosis. It is true that many of the transient symptoms that are relatively common in adolescence resemble pathologic syndromes in the adult, such as mood swings, depression, periodic regression to childhood, and mild antisocial behavior.

Most feelings in early adolescence seem to originate from within the individual rather than from the environment. Adolescents characteristically exhibit alternating and recurrent episodes of disturbed behavior with periods of relative tranquility. There is an increase in moods and sentiments. They vacillate between emotional ups and downs and between considerable maturity and childlike behavior. One minute they are exuberant and enthusiastic; the next minute they are depressed and withdrawn. Unpredictable but essentially normal outbursts of primitive behavior appear as the teenager loses control over instinctual drives.

Little things can cause an emotional upheaval and, depending on the teenager's interpretation, can mean a great deal. As the tension is relieved, emotion is brought under control and the individual retreats in order to work over what has happened, to attempt to master his anger, and in the overall process to grow in his ability to control his emotions and gain from the new experience. These emotional outbursts and ensuing periods of calm may last only a few minutes or hours or may extend over a period of weeks. Adolescents are given to extensive daydreaming that may be so intense that they do not hear another person speaking to them. On the other hand, they may become hostile or ready to fight, complain, or resist everything.

The cyclic pattern that has been apparent throughout childhood continues in adolescence (p. 101). The outgoing, balanced child is replaced by the withdrawn, pensive, and

Table 19-1 Growth and development during adolescence

DIMENSION	EARLY ADOLESCENCE 11-14 YEARS	MIDDLE ADOLESCENCE 14-17 YEARS	LATE ADOLESCENCE 17-20 YEARS
Growth	Rapidly accelerating growth Reaches peak velocity Secondary sex characteristics appear	Growth decelerating Stature reaches 95% of adult height Secondary sex characteristics well advanced	Physically mature Structure and reproductive growth almost complete
Cognition	Limited ability for abstract thinking Explores newfound ability for abstract thought Clumsy groping for new values and energies Comparison of "normality" with peers of same sex	Developing capacity for abstract thinking Enjoys intellectual powers, often in idealistic, altruistic terms Concern with philosophic, political, and social problems	Established abstract thought Can perceive and act on long-range options Able to view problems comprehensively Intellectual and functional identity established
Identity	Preoccupied with rapid body changes Trying out of various roles Measurement of attractiveness by acceptance or rejection of peers Conformity to group norms	Reestablishes body image as growth decelerates Very self-centered; increased narcissism Tendency toward inner experience and self-discovery Has a rich fantasy life Idealistic Able to perceive future implications of current behavior and decisions; variable application	Body image and gender role definition nearly secured Irreversible sexual identity Phase of consolidation of identity Stability of self-esteem Comfortable with physical growth Social roles defined and articulated
Relationships with parents	Defining independence-dependence boundaries Strong desire to remain dependent on parents while trying to detach No major conflicts over parental control	Major conflicts over independence and control Low point in parent-child relationship Greatest push for emancipation; disengagement Final and irreversible emotional detachment from parents; mourning	Emotional and physical separation from parents completed Independence from family and less conflict Emancipation nearly secured Extension of independence without conflict
Relationships with peers	Seeks peer affiliations to counter instability generated by rapid change Upsurge of close idealized friendships with members of the same sex Struggle for mastery takes place within peer group	Strong need for identify to affirm self-image Behavioral standards set by peer group Acceptance by peers extremely important—fear of rejection Exploration of ability to attract the opposite sex	Recedes in importance in favor of individual friendship Testing of male-female relationships against possibility of permanent alliance Relationships characterized by giving and sharing
Sexuality	Self-exploration and evaluation Limited dating Limited intimacy	Multiple plural relationships Decisive turn toward heterosexuality (if is homosexual, know by this time) Exploration of "sex appeal" Feeling of "being in love" Tentative establishment of relationships	Forms stable relationships and attachment to another Growing capacity for mutuality and reciprocity Preeminence of individual as dating partner Intimacy involves commitment rather than exploration and romanticism
Emotionality	Most ambivalence Wide mood swings Intense daydreaming Anger outwardly expressed with moodiness, temper outbursts, and verbal insults and name-calling	Tendency toward inner experiences; more introspective Tendency to withdraw when upset or feelings are hurt Vacillation of emotions in time and range Feelings of inadequacy common; difficulty in asking for help	More constancy of emotion Anger more apt to be concealed

moody early adolescent child who is often unhappy and humorless. Adolescents again shift to a more vigorous, expansive state during the middle teens. They are less apt to have their feelings hurt and are less inclined to cry at the least provocation as was evident earlier. Teenagers again retreat into a phase of withdrawal, moodiness, and introspection. They often feel excessively tired. For many it is a troubled time. Teenagers are better able to control their emotions in later adolescence. They can approach problems more calmly and rationally, and although they are still subject to periods of depression, their feelings are less vulnerable, and they are beginning to demonstrate the more mature emotions of later adolescence.

In later adolescence sources of emotion are more apt to come from the external environment than from within. Anger is the most disruptive emotion, often a consequence of interruption or restriction of activities. However, whereas early adolescents react immediately and emotionally, older adolescents can control their emotions until they can be expressed in a socially acceptable time and place. They are still subject to heightened emotion, and when it is expressed, their behavior reflects feelings of insecurity, tension, and indecision.

SUMMARY OF GROWTH AND DEVELOPMENT

Growth and development during adolescence is both physically and psychologically rapid and dramatic. At the end of this turbulent period young people are able to verbalize conceptually, establish independence, become comfortable with their bodies, build new and meaningful relationships, seek economic and social stability, and develop a workable value system (Adams and others, 1976).

The characteristics described throughout the chapter are summarized as *early adolescence* during which youngsters cast off childhood, emerge as adolescents, and find a new self; *middle (or mid) adolescence* when teenagers belong to an adolescent subculture and begin to find a place in the large community; and *late adolescence* when the youngsters crystallize an identity and emerge as adults. These periods represent an *average* pattern and may not necessarily apply to any single individual (Table 19-1).

COPING WITH CONCERNS RELATED TO NORMAL GROWTH AND DEVELOPMENT

The stresses encountered during adolescence are continual and affect almost every aspect of a youngster's daily life. Normal body changes in relation to attainment of sexual maturity and the process of adjustment to an altered body image are prime sources of stress and anxiety. Late-maturing children are especially sensitive to the stresses of being different from their peers. Many feel intense anxiety over their sense of self and identity. The major areas of stress during adolescence are listed in the accompanying box.

Coping with Stress

A common stress of adolescence is the "cultural shock" of the high school milieu. The youngster moves from the familiar and relatively narrow sphere of relationships with neighborhood children and homogeneous subgroups to a wider representation of peers. The peer group now represents geographic, cultural, and socioeconomic groups different from those with which the youngster is familiar. The teenager is confronted with behaviors and conduct of other adolescents that are entirely unanticipated. The structure of social relationships is different. Whereas school-age relationships are determined mainly by who lives nearby, in the high school setting the groups are often determined by ethnic background, intelligence, or social status. The members of these groups organize themselves into clubs or exclusive groups that emphasize likenesses and exclude those who do not meet the criteria for inclusion. Thus young people who have felt accepted in groups in the past are now faced with the impact of social prejudice and the shock of *exclusion* (Elkind, 1984).

Unlike the socialization of school-age children that consists of cooperative activities centered on a common goal, the new relationships and social interactions of teenagers are based on mutual trust and loyalty. Inexperienced youth now encounter complex and multilayered relationships. When they find their loyalty used and exploited, they experience another form of shock, *betrayal*. Youngsters also discover that the objects of their idealization, that is, persons whom they admire or on whom they develop "crushes," are merely human which produces another type of shock, *disillusionment* (Elkind, 1984). The accompanying box lists the areas of greatest stress in the adolescent's life.

The adolescent is faced with pressures from his peers to conform, which often involves flaunting adult authority and even serious health risks. Health risks include pressures for sexual experimentation and use of hard drugs, alcohol, and cigarettes, as well as potentially dangerous physical activities (see Chapter 21 and Injury prevention, p. 830). The likelihood of incestual relationships is greatest at this time (for further information, see Sexual abuse, p. 689 and Rape, p. 875).

AREAS OF STRESS IN ADOLESCENCE

Body image
Sexuality conflicts
Scholastic pressures
Competitive pressures
Relationships with parents
Relationships with siblings
Relationships with peers
Finances
Decisions about present and future roles
Career planning
Ideologic conflicts

Fears

Teenagers are not afraid of darkness, loud noises, bogey-men, or separation, but they are fearful that they may not be able to live up to what they believe to be their roles and responsibilities as adults. The intense adolescent sexual urge generates fear and anxieties about the size and appearance of primary and secondary sexual characteristics and the ability to perform. Many adolescents fear relationships with persons of the opposite sex. Youngsters who are shy and afraid to relate to persons of the opposite sex may develop a hatred to compensate for the craving they are unable to satisfy. Some fear losing self-control.

Many young people are worried about homosexuality. Most teenagers go through a brief phase, usually during early adolescence, when they are attracted to members of the same sex. Sexual experimentation commonly occurs between same sex individuals or groups and is a temporary defense against the fears associated with full heterosexual relationships. For most youngsters the phase passes with only the temporary concerns regarding the possible implications, but in some instances the attraction may be a permanent one that is accompanied by the associated stigma.

Teenagers are fearful regarding their ability to assume the responsibilities expected of an adult. They worry that they will be unable to make a living and to cope with the independence that adulthood implies. All teenagers live with the fear of nuclear war and the possible end of existence as they know it. Boys especially are worried about having to serve in the armed forces.

Limit-Setting and Discipline

Adolescence is probably the most difficult period of development for both the child and the parents. Parents are confused about how much freedom to allow their teenager, and the youngster is torn between the desire for independence and the security of dependence. Conflicts between parents and teenagers are not unexpected (see Relationships with parents, p. 816). Teenagers need firm but reasonable limitations to protect them from behaviors that place them in jeopardy.

With their capacity for abstract thought and reasoning, teenagers are able to understand limits imposed by parents. They often rebel against restrictions but feel more secure with the protection they afford, especially when a parental mandate provides a face-saving means for avoiding a situation they do not feel competent to manage. It is much easier for an adolescent to place the onus on parents rather than on themselves when they decline to engage in an activity with peers in which they may feel insecure or fearful.

Teenagers need firm limits in areas such as curfews, minimum activities on school nights, and chaperoned activities. Privileges should balance limitations, and teenagers should be allowed increasing privileges as they demonstrate mature behavior worthy of more freedom. Discipline, as always, must be fair and suitable to the offense. Unusually harsh limitations only serve to stimulate rebellion. Many of the strategies employed earlier are appropriate for this age-group, such as withholding privileges, contracting, and negotiation. Also it is vitally important that a youngster is not chastised in the presence of peers.

Promoting Optimum Health During Adolescence

Adolescents are on the whole healthy individuals. The disease level is low during this age period, but there is heightened concern about the body. Most of the health problems and the more common illnesses are in some way related to the physical changes of puberty. The disorders associated with adolescent development are discussed in Chapter 20; health promotion in persons in this age-group is primarily one of health teaching and guidance.

Adolescents as a group are eager to learn about themselves, and nurses who are truly interested in them, who respect them as persons, and who are willing to listen to them will be able to gain their confidence and trust. It is important to establish rapport with the adolescent, at the first interview if possible. Overidentification with the adolescent should be avoided. Relating naturally and honestly, acting neither as a young person nor as a parent, is the best approach. Nurses should be prepared to talk to parents following the time spent with the youngster, and the young person should be invited to stay during the discussion.

During this period of gaining independence from families and the strong peer-group influences, teenagers are vulnerable to practices that may be hazardous to their health and well-being. They need someone to whom they can turn for guidance, with whom they can test out ideas, and with whom they feel free to express their fears and feelings. Nurses as health professionals and respected adults have the opportunity to provide adolescents with factual information about what is taking place in their bodies and to clarify misconceptions about menstruation, nocturnal emissions, pregnancy, and other physical changes of puberty.

Both individual and group conferences with teenagers provide excellent opportunities to discuss actual or potential health problems, such as pregnancy, sexually transmitted disease, the hazards of smoking, and experimenting with drugs, including alcohol. Adolescents are frequently confused about the information they receive from parents, friends, and written material to which they have access. Very often teenagers feel more comfortable in a group situation. With peer support they are better able to explore ideas that they may not be able to express individually. Individual counseling provides adolescents with a knowledgeable adult in whom they can confide without the threat of an intimate relationship.

Adolescents are able to assume the major responsibility for their own health, including maintaining health practices (e.g., tooth brushing, caring for appliances), taking prescribed medications, keeping appointments, and performing procedures when necessary. Laws and practices regarding medical care of adolescents without consent of their parents varies (see Consent, p. 1103). This is especially relevant in relation to the youngster seeking guidance regarding possible sexually transmitted diseases, contraception, and pregnancy (see Chapter 20).

NUTRITION

The rapid and extensive development in height, weight, muscle mass, and sexual maturity of adolescence is accompanied by new and greater nutritional requirements. Since nutritional needs are closely related to the increase in body mass, the peak requirements occur in the year of maximum growth, during which time the body mass almost doubles. This period occurs between the tenth and twelfth years in girls and about 2 years later in boys. The calorie and protein requirements during this year are higher than at almost any other time of life. As a result of this increased anabolic need, the adolescent is highly sensitive to caloric restrictions. Adolescents want food, their appetites soar, and their capacity to consume food is often awe-inspiring, as any parent of a teenage boy can attest. A fast-growing boy may never get enough. His stomach may be too small to accommodate the amount of food he requires to meet his growth needs unless he eats at very frequent intervals. Failure to consume an adequate diet at this time can potentially retard growth and delay sexual maturation.

Not only do teenagers eat at every pause in the day's activities, but they enjoy food and the pleasures related to its consumption. Food is part of the attraction of the "hangouts" and gathering places that teenagers frequent. For example, the corner deli or fast-food diner provides such favored items as hamburgers, ice cream, soft drinks, and the company of their equally hungry peers. Large bags of assorted snacks are an essential part of beach gatherings, rock concerts, and other outdoor get-togethers.

The nutritional needs of adolescents are difficult to determine because of the meager nutritional information on members of this age-group. Defining dietary requirements is further complicated by the influence of emotional and other stress factors that affect nutrient utilization and the psychologic factors that influence adolescent eating habits. In addition, the diverse variations in growth rates during adolescence and the equally wide range in ages at which these changes take place complicate any attempt to set minimum dietary standards for this age-group. Consequently the recommended dietary allowances for teenagers include a safety factor that attempts to allow for these differences under average circumstances. Energy needs are highly variable; nutrition should be adjusted to meet increased energy requirements during physical activity. Inactive teenagers are subject to obesity even though their energy intake is below the recommended level, whereas extremely active youngsters will require more than the recommended amounts. Therefore food required for energy must be balanced with energy expenditure.

Protein intake remains a constant need throughout childhood and adolescence to meet continual growth needs. There is usually sufficient intake well above the recom-

mended dietary allowance, except in those young people who limit their food intake because of economic problems or in an attempt to lose weight. When the supply is limited, dietary protein will be used to meet energy requirements at the expense of new tissue synthesis. Consequently a reduction in the growth rate can occur despite what appears to be an adequate protein intake.

Minerals that are most likely to be deficient in the adolescent diet are calcium, iron, and zinc. There is a substantial increase in the need for these minerals during the period of rapid growth—calcium for skeletal growth, iron for expansion of muscle mass and blood volume, and zinc for the generation of both skeletal and muscle tissue (Marino and King, 1980). Calcium retention varies considerably with the growth rate of the adolescent. On the average, boys accumulate a greater amount during peak periods of growth than girls, and fast-growing youngsters retain more than slow-growing youngsters. Increased amounts of milk are usually required to supplement an average diet to ensure an adequate calcium intake during this time. Evidence indicates that boys are more likely than girls to eat foods that meet calcium requirements (Marino and King, 1980).

Iron is essential for meeting the needs of the increased muscle and soft tissue growth and the rapid growth demands of an expanding red cell mass. Although this expansion occurs more quickly in adolescent boys, adolescent girls have an additional iron loss from menstruation. Consequently the need is probably equivalent in both sexes. An inadequate iron intake is reflected in the high incidence of anemia in the adolescent population at all socioeconomic levels. Few adolescents consume sufficient amounts of iron and therefore should be advised to include good sources of iron in their diet, such as red meats, dried beans, green vegetables, iron-fortified cereals, and snacks that include peanuts, raisins, and other dried fruits. It has also been determined that ascorbic acid improves the absorption of iron from nonheme iron sources. Zinc is now recognized as essential for growth and sexual maturation of the adolescent. American adolescents tend to consume less than the recommended intake of this mineral. Sources rich in zinc include animal products such as meat, seafood, eggs, and milk.

Eating Habits and Behaviors

Eating and behavior toward food are primarily family-centered during early and middle childhood, and food habits are largely related to cultural and individual family preferences and patterns. With adolescence and the move toward independence, family influences on the child change. Teenagers' interests, attitudes, and routines are altered as an increasing number of meals are eaten away from home. These changes are largely a result of the high value that teenagers place on peer acceptability and sociability; therefore their eating habits are easily influenced by their associates. In addition, family criticism about food habits tends to have a negative effect on a wise selection of an adequate diet.

Omitting breakfast or eating a breakfast that is nutritionally poor in quality is frequently a problem. Often adolescent youngsters are sleepy in the morning, hate to get up, and delay getting up as long as possible; consequently they have no time to eat. Many do not like breakfast food items. Other reasons for skipping breakfast are that they are not hungry, there is no one with whom to eat, or no breakfast is prepared for them. The youngster who dislikes traditional breakfast fare may react favorably to a peanut butter sandwich or a hamburger, both of which are nutritionally good and often more acceptable to the teenager. The goal of an adequate, good-tasting breakfast requires that someone prepare it and that the youngster arrange the time to eat it.

Pressure for time and their commitments to activities adversely affect teenagers' eating habits. Snacks, usually selected on the basis of accessibility rather than nutritional merit, become more and more a part of the habitual eating pattern during adolescence. Adolescents characteristically reject or only infrequently eat a sufficient amount of fresh fruits and vegetables, especially those that are rich in ascorbic acid. Fast-food items, to which they are especially attracted, contain few fruits and vegetables, thus contributing to a low dietary intake of vitamins C, A, and folic acid. Fast foods are also high in energy, fat, and sodium but low in fiber, all of which have been implicated in the etiology of degenerative diseases in later life (Marino and King, 1980). Milk is usually passed over in favor of soft drinks, the appropriate social drink of the peer culture.

Overeating or undereating during adolescence presents special problems. As they experience the normal increase in weight and fat deposition of the growth spurt, teenage girls often resort to dieting. The desire for the admired slim figure and a fear of becoming ''fat'' prompt teenage girls to embark on nutritionally inadequate reducing regimens that sap their energy and deprive their growing bodies of essential nutrients. They resort to diets on their own or with peers in an effort to conform. Many adopt the current fad diets and are victims of food misinformation. Vegetarian diets are becoming increasingly popular among teenagers and are a source of concern; unless they are carefully planned to provide sufficient dairy products and eggs, optimum growth and development may be compromised. Boys are less inclined to undereat. They are more concerned about gaining in size and strength. However, they tend to eat foods high in calories but low in other essential nutrients.

Iron-deficiency anemia is relatively common in undernourished teenage girls, and the severe form of malnutrition, anorexia nervosa, occurs most frequently during adolescence when the girl becomes obsessed with self-denial of eating pleasures. Obesity from either overeating or underactivity is another form of inadequate nutrition that occurs often in adolescence.

Nursing Considerations

Nothing can *make* adolescents eat wisely. Since their food habits reflect many influences and conditions, these must be considered when planning nutritional education and guidance. Food habits begun in early childhood are difficult to break. In some families, failure to develop the habits of eat-ing nutritious foods and a habitual lack of variety in a family's diet contribute to a lack of adequate nutrition. The quality of a diet is related to the number of different food items eaten in a day, and consistently skipped meals are associated with a poor diet.

When helping teenagers select a nutritious diet, the nurse should begin with their present diet and actively involve them in the process. It is important to remember that there are many ways to achieve an adequate diet, and that no pattern should be prejudged as inadequate until it is determined that it is indeed deficient in essential nutrients. Adolescents do not respond well to judgmental attitudes. It is not unusual to discover that their diet patterns, although unusual by adult standards, are actually satisfactory. Teenagers dislike being talked down to or preached at, but they do respond when their independence is respected and they are given the opportunity to make their own decisions regarding food choices.

In general, adolescents are body-conscious and concerned about their appearance. When diet is associated with clear skin, firm flesh, and glossy hair, the teenager is more likely to be receptive to nutritional education. However, helping young persons arrive at a decision for change is more difficult than providing information. They respond best when the counselor provides straightforward information, talks with them and not at them, and listens to what they have to say. Listening objectively to their ideas, clarifying misconceptions without ridicule, and involving them in diet planning are necessary if essential knowledge is to be translated into action. It is best to begin at the nutritional level where the individual is. A current food fad may be a good point from which to build a nutritious diet, taking into consideration other factors (cultural, social, economic) without prohibitions or declaring any food to be ''bad.''

As snacks become more a part of adolescents' eating patterns, it is important that they contribute something other than calories to their diet. Although ''empty calorie'' snacks are not a desirable substitute for nutritious foods, because adolescents' energy requirements are so high, they are able to consume some of these foods without compromising their nutrition, provided high-quality foods are eaten the rest of the day (Gregor, Devibliss, and Aschenbeck, 1979). More often than not, what adolescents eat is determined by what is available. When made readily accessible, items such as fruits, vegetables, and dairy products are excellent and nutritious snack foods. A refrigerator shelf stocked by parents with good-tasting snack items especially for their youngsters can contribute significantly to improving adolescents' diets and giving them a feeling that they are important and worthwhile persons. Similarly schools might provide nutritious snack foods in cafeterias and on-campus vending machines to encourage the purchase of these items by the teenage population.

It is often necessary to work with parents to help them understand the dietary needs and eating behavior of their teenagers. Many are conscious of their responsibility for the nutrition of their children, whereas others are indifferent.

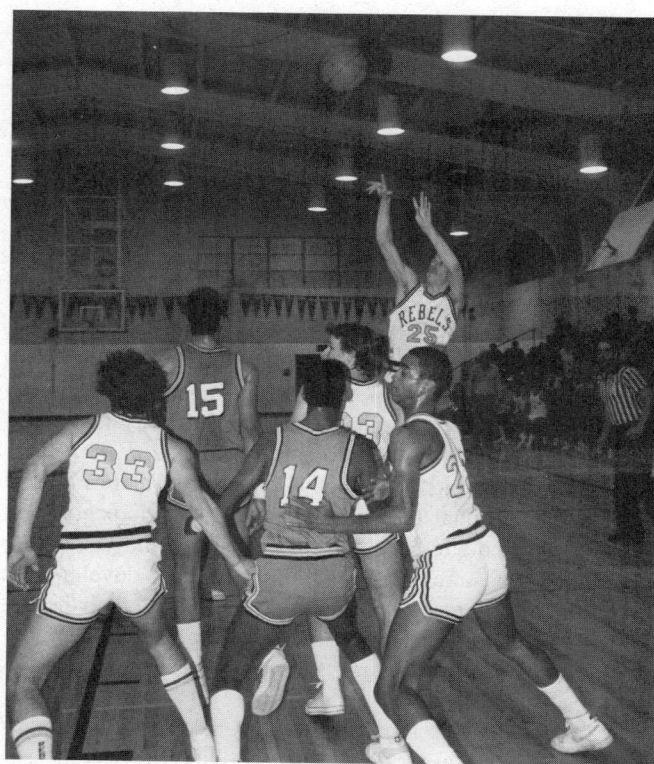

Fig. 19-15. Most adolescents aspire to become a member of a school athletic team.
Photography by Garibaldi, San Lorenzo, CA.

Family influence on adolescents is likely to change as the teenagers move toward independence and the peer group exerts a greater influence. Poorer food practices appear to result when status, sociability, independence, and enjoyment are predominant influences. Diets tend to be better when adolescents consider health to be an important factor. Good family relationships, emotional stability, and adjustment to reality are also characteristics associated with better food habits.

SLEEP AND REST

Teenagers vary in their need for sleep and rest. Rapid physical growth, the tendency toward overexertion, and the overall increased activity of this age contribute to fatigue in adolescents. Their propensity for staying up late makes it very difficult to get out of bed in the mornings, and they sleep late at every opportunity. Adequate sleep and rest at this time are important to a total health regimen.

EXERCISE AND ACTIVITY

Adolescents probably spend more time and energy practicing and participating in sports activities than members of any other age-group. The practice of sports and games contributes significantly to growth and development, the education process, and better health. It provides exercise for growing muscles, interactions with peers, and a socially ac-

ceptable means to enjoy stimulation and conflict. In addition, competitive activities help the teenager in the process of self-appraisal, development of self-respect, and concern for others (Fig. 19-19). Sports for young people are discussed further in relation to sports injuries (p. 843).

Dancing has always occupied a central place in the customs of many cultures. There is delight in physical movement and a feeling of relief that comes from release of tension in activity. Dancing can also serve as a means of expressing specific sexual and aggressive urges in symbolic form and action. Many of the popular dances have decided sexual overtones and erotic movements. At the same time the structure of the dance is such that dancers seldom touch one another. In this way the urges can be expressed without the danger of close physical contact (Fig. 19-16).

DENTAL HEALTH

Dental health should not be neglected during adolescence, although the rate of caries formation is not as great as it was in childhood. Early adolescence is usually the time when corrective orthodontic appliances are worn, and these are frequently a source of embarrassment and concern to the youngster. Reassurance regarding the temporary nature of the annoyance and anticipation of an improved appearance help to make the inconvenience tolerable. It is also important to reinforce the orthodontist's directions regarding use and care of the appliances and to emphasize careful attention to toothbrushing during this time.

PERSONAL CARE

The body-conscious teenager is highly receptive to discussion and counseling about personal care and hygiene. Body changes associated with puberty bring with them special needs for cleanliness. The hyperactive sebaceous glands and newly functioning apocrine glands make the daily bath im-

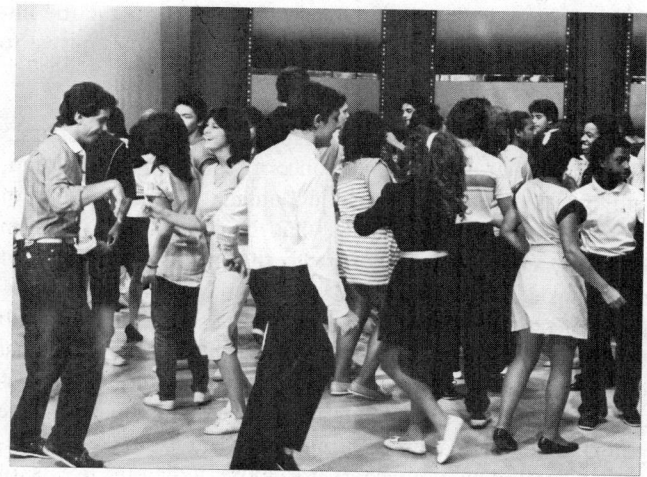

Fig. 19-16. Adolescents enjoy the activity and social aspects of dancing.
Photography by Garibaldi, San Lorenzo, CA.

perative, and underarm deodorants assume an important place in personal care. The adolescent will find that hair requires more frequent shampooing, and girls will have questions about hair removal, use of cosmetics, and menstrual hygiene. Many group discussions center around the virtues of particular products or methods. Adolescents are continually bombarded with messages from the media regarding the best means to enhance their popularity and appeal to the opposite sex. Nurses are in a position to help them evaluate the relative merits of commercial products.

Ear Piercing

The popular trend of ear piercing may sometimes create a health problem for the uninformed teenager. It is a nursing responsibility to caution girls or boys against the practice of having their ears pierced by friends, mothers, or themselves. Although in most cases there are few if any serious side effects, there is always a danger of such complications as infection, cyst or keloid formation, bleeding, dermatitis, or metal allergy. Therefore the procedure should be performed by a physician or qualified nurse using proper sterile technique. This is especially important if the youngster has a history of diabetes, allergies, or skin disorders. Teenagers are prone to the development of keloids, particularly if there is a history of keloid formation in the family.

Vision

Regular vision testing is a vital part of health care and supervision during adolescence. At this time the incidence of visual refractive difficulties reaches a peak that is not exceeded until the fifth decade of life. Adolescents may not have poorer vision than children or adults, but the increased demands of schoolwork make good vision important for academic success. Consequently teenagers are more likely to be referred for visual evaluation. The need for corrective lenses can create psychologic problems for teenagers if they believe that glasses spoil their appearance or do not fit their body image. For those who are able to tolerate and afford them, contact lenses are a happy solution. For some the impact of a visual defect, no matter how slight, may prove to be a great personal concern.

Hearing

There has been considerable concern regarding current teenage practices causing possible damage to the hearing of youngsters. Cochlear damage has been documented from relatively continuous exposure to the loud sound levels of rock music, especially from stereos and radios. The popularity of portable FM radios and stereo cassette players with lightweight earphones, which enable the listener to adjust the volume, are of particular concern to health care professionals. When these units are used for extended periods, the potential for permanent hearing loss is undisputed. Appealing to individual youngsters for more judicious use is of doubtful benefit, although they should be informed of the risk. Efforts directed toward legislating legal limits to the noise exposure that can be achieved through the sets and

widespread education may be possible solutions. (See p. 1013 for a discussion of noise related hearing loss.)

Posture

The process of normal development during adolescence does little to promote good posture in the teenage girl or boy. The rapid skeletal growth that is usually associated with a significant lag in muscular growth leads to weakness, easy fatigability, and awkwardness. These characteristics predispose youngsters to slumping and make them less inclined to stand or sit erectly. A relative reduction in physical activity, which often accompanies rapid skeletal growth, aggravates the situation, especially in teenage girls. The adolescent who is routinely engaged in vigorous physical activity appears to have fewer problems with posture.

Many adolescents, especially those early-maturing few who gain additional height in advance of their peers, feel conspicuous and attempt to disguise their height by adopting a slouching posture. Early pubescent breast development may cause shy girls to hunch forward and drop their heads. This is usually a transient phase that disappears as they develop confidence and maturity. Most of these postural problems resolve as the adolescent matures.

A few preexisting musculoskeletal problems, such as lateral spine deviation, or scoliosis, are likely to become exaggerated during the growth spurt and require treatment. However, most postural problems do not require special attention and treatment, and poor posture is not a source of pain. Actually the teenager's posture is primarily of concern to the parents, who continually admonish the youngster to "sit up" or "stand up straight." The teenager, unaware of any postural defect, fails to see or understand the problem. Consequently parental nagging only creates additional hostility and resistance on the part of the adolescent.

The best approach to counseling teenagers about posture is to show, not tell, them and to serve as a proper model. Good posture can be demonstrated best when the adolescent stands before a full-length mirror. Postural defects and desired alterations can be pointed out in full view of both the young person and the nurse. A sunken chest, winged scapulas, a swayback, protuberant abdomen, and drooping head and shoulders are clearly visible, and the nurse can demonstrate the simple corrections that can transform the youngster into a more attractive and ultimately healthier person. Adolescents will need reassurance that the fatigue they feel when attempting to maintain correct posture is a transient effect caused by weak muscles, especially those of the back, and that they will soon acquire the strength and endurance to maintain the desired posture. If they concentrate on assuming correct positioning several times each day, with regular practice it will eventually become a permanent aspect of their person.

Serious postural defects detected in the process of a physical assessment will require early medical intervention. Scoliosis is usually intensified during adolescence, and tight muscles often produce postural problems that need special attention. Nurses can refer the youngster to the appropriate source, such as the family physician, pediatrician, or health clinic, for evaluation and implementation of corrective therapy. Nurses are important sources of support and reassurance to the teenager and the parents throughout lengthy bracing, casting, and exercise programs.

Slow Maturation

Both early- and late-maturing children feel out of place among their classmates, but the slow-maturing children appear to suffer the most pronounced inner turmoil and may be hesitant to voice their concerns. The rate of maturation is important during the school years, but at puberty it assumes gigantic proportions to these children and often to their parents. Late-maturing youngsters are painfully aware of their shortcomings and find themselves being left out of private discussions about body changes experienced by the group, some to the point of ostracism or, especially among boys, an object of scorn and ridicule. They feel cheated and may well believe that they are doomed to a permanent position outside the group. Such fears and failures only serve to accentuate the normal doubts and concerns about the self that are part of this critical age period.

The girl feels out of place among her companions whose hips and bosoms are developing, feels cheated because she has not yet menstruated, and feels that she is not a part of the giggling and boy-talk of her friends. The boy feels weak and small compared with his muscular companions with whom he can no longer compete, and his high voice sounds childish compared to the deep tones around him. Slow-maturing youngsters need support and reassurance that they are not abnormal and need only to be patient until the time comes when they too will develop the characteristics for which they yearn. Early-maturing boys are less at a disadvantage than early-maturing girls or late-maturing boys. Late-maturing boys usually suffer most. The child with endocrine or genetic disorders that interfere with the maturation process needs special help (see Chapter 20).

SEX EDUCATION AND GUIDANCE

Contemporary adolescents are constantly exposed to sexual symbolism and erotic stimulation from the mass media. At the same time the development of primary and secondary sex characteristics and the increased sensitivity of the genitalia generate thoughts and fantasies about heterosexual relationships. In addition, the culture expects that adolescents will date, flirt, and experience tender feelings. As a result, teenagers are often confused and ambivalent about sexuality and heterosexual relationships. Although many adolescents have received sex education from parents and school throughout childhood, they are not always adequately prepared for the impact of puberty. A large portion of their knowledge is acquired from peers, provocative illustrations, and graffiti on the walls of public restrooms. Consequently much of the sex information they accumulate is incomplete, inaccurate, riddled with cultural and moral issues, and usually not very helpful.

The questions of who is responsible for teaching and how the teaching can be best accomplished must be considered. Sex education is and has been assumed by parents, schools, churches, community agencies such as **Planned Parenthood Federation of America, Inc.,*** and health professionals. Among this last group, nurses should —and many do— take an active role in talking to young people about their sexuality. To be able to discuss the topic with teenagers adequately, nurses must have not only an understanding of the physiologic aspects of sexuality and a knowledge of cultural and societal values but also an awareness of their own attitudes, feelings, and biases about sexuality. One cannot give information without simultaneously conveying attitudes. These attitudes in turn influence the behavior of young people.

The most comprehensive approach to sex education is offered by the **Sex Information and Education Council of the United States (SIECUS),**† an interdisciplinary organization founded to establish sexuality as a health entity and to dignify it by openness of approach, study, and scientific research. SIECUS maintains that every sex education program should present the topic from six aspects: biologic, social, health, personal adjustments and attitudes, interpersonal associations, and the establishment of values.

Whether nurses counsel young people on an individual basis, in mixed groups, or in groups segregated by sex makes little difference. Some nurses and teenagers are uneasy in mixed groups for discussions of sexuality, and no hard-and-fast rule prevails. Ideally boys and girls should be able to discuss sex objectively with one another and in groups, but this is not always possible. The difference in the rate of maturation between boys and girls and between different members of the same sex often makes it desirable to discuss certain aspects of sexuality in segregated groups. Sometimes individuals or small groups will deliberately seek the opportunity to talk over some subjects in the security of unmixed company. As a general rule, the need for separate discussion groups diminishes as young people progress toward maturity.

Sex education should consist of instructions concerning normal body function and associated feelings and emotions. Information should be presented in a straightforward manner using correct terminology. When discussing sex and sexual activities, nurses should use simple but correct language— not street language, highly scientific terminology, or evasive jargon. For example, the term *sexual intercourse* is usually understood by teenagers, whereas few are familiar with the terms *coitus* or *copulation;* the term *sexual relationships* is too vague, and the four-letter street terms are inappropriate. Once the meaning of biologic terms such as *uterus, testicles,* and *vagina* is understood, teenagers prefer to use them in their discussions.

Both boys and girls need to know more about what is going on in their bodies than they are able to see. Although

---

*810 Seventh Ave., New York, NY 10019.
†80 Fifth Ave., Suite 801-2, New York, NY 10011.

most girls are adequately prepared for menstruation, they do not always understand its relationship to the total process of reproduction. Many are under the erroneous impression that the "safe" time for sexual intercourse is midway between menstrual periods. Whether they are sexually active or not, adolescents should receive accurate information about pregnancy, including when and how it occurs and ways by which it can be avoided. They need to know about sexually transmitted diseases, how they are transmitted, symptoms, and how to get treatment if anyone becomes infected.

Teenagers as a whole are limited in their knowledge and understanding of the sexuality of the opposite sex. Unless they are taught differently, each assumes that members of the other sex feel as they do. When girls understand the directness of the drive for sexual release that is experienced by young boys, they are better able to conduct themselves appropriately. This same knowledge will help boys to understand that girls do not feel the same urges as they do. Both need to recognize that they have a responsibility for their own behavior.

It is also important for teenagers to know that the thoughts and fantasies that may be disturbing to them are a normal part of the developmental process and should not be a source of guilt feelings. Adolescents, girls in particular, will want answers to questions such as, "What is it like?" "Does it hurt?" "What happens when ...?" and "Is it all right if you ...?" Boys are often concerned about the fallacy that there is a relationship between penis size and sexual function. They need reassurance that masturbation is a normal and common practice, that pornography is not harmful, that some degree of homosexuality is not unusual in early adolescence, and that oral-genital relations are normal substitutes for intercourse in certain situations.

Young people are at the stage of life when the sexual aspects of interpersonal relationships become particularly important. Societal expectations push them toward dating, and their own inner sex drive urges them toward exploration. Teenagers' curiosity and desire for information extend beyond the need for anatomic and physiologic knowledge. They need to know more than the mechanics of conception, gestation, and birth. They need to know about the sexuality of the opposite sex and to be helped to view the nature of sex as a powerful life force—a force to be used as an intense, vital human experience that is earned by maturity— and not as a childhood game at which to play.

An excellent resource for sex education is *Sex Education for Adolescents: A Bibliography of Low-Cost Materials* available from the Committee on Adolescence of the Academy of Pediatrics.*

INJURY PREVENTION

Physical injuries are the greatest single cause of death in the adolescent age-group and claim more lives than all other

*141 Northwest Point Rd, P.O. Box 927, Elk Grove Village, IL 60007.

causes combined. Motor vehicle collisions account for nearly half of the deaths of adolescents between the ages of 16 and 19 and are a major cause of death in the younger age-groups (see p. 7). The tragedy of this is that the figures remain fairly constant from year to year, and almost all fatal injuries are preventable. The next most frequent causes of death are homicide, suicide, drowning, and firearms.

As in all age-groups, injury is closely related to the developmental characteristics associated with normal growth and maturation. During adolescence, peak physical, sensory, and psychomotor function gives teenagers a feeling of strength and confidence that they have never experienced before, and the physiologic changes of puberty give impetus to many basic instinctual forces. One manifestation of this is an increase in energy that simply must be discharged through action, often at the expense of logical thinking and other control mechanisms. Because of this need for action, adolescents are prone to act impulsively. Their propensity for risk-taking behavior plus a feeling of indestructibility make adolescents especially prone to injury (Fig. 19-17).

The care and management of specific types of injuries are discussed where appropriate throughout the book and are not considered here. These include head injuries, spinal cord injuries, burns, near drowning, and fractures.

Motor Vehicle Related Injuries

Teenage drivers contribute substantially to vehicular fatalities, both their own and those of others. Almost half the fatalities in the adolescent age-group are related to motor vehicles. The adolescent's newly acquired ability to drive and the normal developmental need for independence and freedom make the automobile an attractive if not necessary part of adolescent life. They love to be propelled through space at a rapid pace. A significant number of fatal teenage injuries involve vehicles that were being driven too fast for the existing conditions. Almost all are related to the actions of the driver and the number is disproportionately high among young drivers—often caused by ignorance of or disregard for sound and defensive driving principles. Most fatal injuries involving adolescent drivers occur because of improper driving or poor judgment on the part of the driver. These young people, delighted with the freedom that a driver's license affords them, are less concerned about the new responsibilities associated with this freedom. They have yet to learn behavioral patterns that are gained with experience and maturity.

The use of drugs, including alcohol and marijuana, by adolescents has further compounded the problem of motor vehicle injuries involving youth. Overindulgence in alcohol is known to impair the ability of the best driver. Adolescents are not only learning to drive but learning to use intoxicants at the same time (Brown, Sanders, and Schonberg, 1986). The combination of inexperience, lack of defensive driving skills, and inexperience with drinking is a lethal one, and the unfortunate consequences are predictable.

Motor vehicle injuries are preventable, but although the

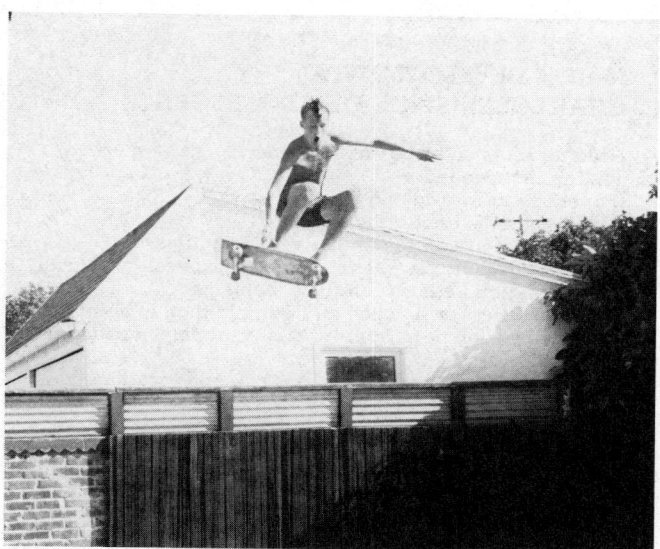

Fig. 19-17. Teenager riding a skateboard from the roof of a neighbor's house into a backyard swimming pool.
Photography by Anne Kunke, San Jose, CA.

implications for prevention are obvious, the preventive measures are not always easy to implement, especially when behavioral characteristics such as poor impulse control, recklessness, and hostility are also involved. A degree of social experimentation is involved in much of adolescents' behavior. Young men feel pressured to be brave and exhibit a "macho" image, which often involves disregarding speed limits and other safety laws as well as intentional failure to use passenger restraints (Brown, Sanders, and Schonberg, 1986). Teenagers use seat belts only half as often as adults (Williams, Wells, and Lund, 1983). Young drivers are also encouraged by peers to speed, overcrowd the vehicle, and drink.

The role that nurses can play in prevention of motor vehicle injuries is to become active proponents of driver education and safety programs in the school and community that emphasize the use of good driving habits and judgment. They can encourage teenagers to obtain such instruction and encourage parents to determine the quality of this instruction and to take measures to improve the quality if it is found lacking.

Moped injuries. The increasing use of other motorized vehicles, such as mopeds and snowmobiles, has caused an increase in injuries related to these vehicles, especially among youngsters below the legal age for driving automobiles. The mean age of children sustaining moped injuries is 12.8 years (Westman and Morrow, 1984). The injuries are more serious than bicycle injuries, although mopeds are often considered to be deluxe bicycles rather than motorized vehicles. Consequently little driver preparation and instruction are required. The majority of injuries involve the moped and another vehicle but burn injuries have been reported from contact with the hot muffler, especially when youngsters are riding double (Bantz and Auerbach, 1982).

It has been recommended that moped use be regulated, including minimum age for driving, mandatory use of helmets, riding within prescribed limits (within 3 feet of the right side of the road), and providing safety equipment on the moped (e.g., rearview mirror, turning signals).

Firearms

Improper use of firearms continues to be one of the leading causes of death in the adolescent age-group, occurring mainly in or on home premises. The natural interest in gun-related activities is accelerated in this age-group, when almost half the victims of firearm fatalities are between ages 15 and 24. Instruction in the use of firearms should be taught at an appropriate age by parents and is probably best accomplished in cooperation with a youth organization or professional association. Most injuries from firearms can be prevented when proper safety precautions are taken in the use and storage of firearms. For example, loaded guns should never be permitted in or around the home, and guns and ammunition must be stored where only appropriate adults have access to them.

Nonpowder firearms. Nonpowder guns (air rifles, BB guns), although viewed as toys by many, account for almost as many injuries as powder guns. Among children ages 5 to 14 the incidence of injury is three times that of powder guns (Christoffel and others, 1984). The regulations regarding nonpowder guns are relaxed; they can be purchased legally by youngsters and are labeled as suitable for children as young as 8 years. Few states regulate their use. As child advocates, nurses can push for legislation to regulate the sale of these potentially dangerous "toys."

Nursing Considerations

Injury prevention is an ongoing part of nursing responsibility throughout the childhood years. Anticipatory guidance to parents regarding the expected problems and hazards related to growth and development does not end as the child nears maturity. However, adolescent health and safety education and guidance are more effective when the young people are involved directly. Parents can emphasize the importance of safety in the execution of activities and skills and the proper use of equipment. They can encourage the proper conditioning and preparation for sports, including rest, nutrition, and the activity best suited to the individual youngster's physical and emotional capabilities.

School nurses, in cooperation with other persons involved with youth, such as teachers, activity leaders, and parent groups, can help to evaluate sports and athletic programs, assess environmental conditions, and institute changes that emphasize prevention of injury. They can help to assess the needs for emergency services, institute such services, and provide care and guidance when needed. The boxes on p. 832 list the developmental characteristics of adolescents that predispose them to injury and suggestions for injury prevention related to these developmental expectations.

ACCIDENT PREVENTION

Motor vehicles
Pedestrian—emphasize and encourage safe pedestrian behavior
Passenger—promote appropriate behavior while riding in a motor vehicle
Driver—provide competent driver education; encourage judicious use of vehicle, discourage drag racing, "chicken"; maintain vehicle in proper condition (brakes, tires, etc.)
Teach and promote safety and maintenance of two-wheeled vehicles
Promote and encourage wearing of safety apparel such as helmet, long trousers
Reinforce the dangers of drugs (including alcohol) when operating a motor vehicle

Drowning
Teach to swim (if adolescent unable to do so)
Teach basic rules of water safety
   Judicious selection of places to swim
   Sufficient water depth for diving
   Swimming with companion

Burns
Reinforce proper behavior in areas involving contact with burn hazards (gasoline, electric wires, fires)
Advise regarding excessive exposure to sunlight (ultraviolet burn)
Discourage smoking
Encourage use of sunscreen

Poisoning
Educate in hazards of drug use, including alcohol

Falls
Teach and encourage general safety measures in all activities

Bodily damage
Promote acquisition of proper instruction in sports and use of sports equipment
Promote use of appropriate arena for sports activities
Instruct in safe use of and respect for firearms and other devices with potential danger (e.g., power tools, firecrackers)
Provide and encourage use of protective equipment when using potentially hazardous devices
Promote access to and/or provision of safe sports and recreational facilities
Be alert for signs of depression (potential suicide)
Discourage use of and/or availability of hazardous sports equipment (trampoline, surfboards)
Instruct regarding proper use of corrective devices such as glasses, contact lenses, hearing aids
Encourage and foster judicious application of safety principles and prevention

MAJOR DEVELOPMENTAL CHARACTERISTICS OF ADOLESCENTS

Need for independence and freedom
Testing independence
Propensity for risk-taking
Feeling of indestructibility
Age permitted to drive a motor vehicle (varies)
Need for discharging energy, often at expense of logical thinking and other control mechanisms
Peak incidence for practice and participation in sports
Strong need for peer approval; may attempt hazardous feats
Access to more complex tools, objects, and locations
Can assume responsibility for own actions

PARENTAL GUIDANCE DURING ADOLESCENCE

Accept adolescent as a human being
Respect adolescent's ideas, likes and dislikes, wishes
Provide opportunity for choosing options and accept natural consequences of these choices
Allow youngster to learn by doing, even when choices and methods differ from those of adults
Provide adolescent with clear, reasonable limits
Allow increasing independence within limitations of safety and well-being
Be available but avoid pressing youngster too far
Respect adolescent's privacy
Try to share adolescent's feelings of joy or sorrow
Respond to feelings as well as words
Be available to answer questions, give information, and provide companionship
Listen and try to be open to youngster's views, even when they disagree with parental views
Try to make communication clear
Assist adolescent in selecting appropriate career goals and preparing for adult role
Provide undemanding love

Be aware that:
Adolescent is subject to turbulent, unpredictable behavior
Adolescent is struggling for independence
Adolescent is extraordinarily sensitive to feelings and behavior that affect him or her
Message given to adolescent may not be message received
Friends are extremely important to adolescent
Adolescent has a strong need "to belong"
Adolescent sees things in black or white, good or bad

ANTICIPATORY GUIDANCE—CARE OF FAMILIES

The parents of the adolescent are usually as confused and perplexed as the youngster is about the changes and behavior of this stage of development. They also need support and guidance to help them through this trying time. They need to understand the changes taking place and to understand and accept the expected behaviors that accompany the process of detachment, to be prepared to "let go," and to promote the changed relationship from one of dependence to one of mutuality. The accompanying box lists suggestions for anticipatory guidance of parents with an adolescent.

CONCEPT SUMMARIES

- Adolescence is an important period of development in which significant psychologic, social, and maturational adjustments are made in the move toward adulthood.

- Biologic development during puberty is characterized primarily by hormonal activity in which sexual maturation and skin changes take place.

- According to Erikson, the major developmental crisis of adolescence is establishing a sense of identity.

- In Freudian terms, adolescence marks the beginning of the genital period, in which sexual maturation prepares the individual to satisfy the sex instinct through procreation.

- Cognitive development in adolescence is revealed through thinking beyond the present, logical thought, and a sense of idealism.

- Development of body image is closely tied to sexual awareness, as adolescents cope with sexual maturation.

- According to Kohlberg's theory of moral development, adolescents begin to question existing moral values and learn to make choices.

- Spiritual development is characterized by the questioning of family values and ideals, a move to more philosophical thinking, and emphasis on personal religion.

- Adolescent relationships with parents may be strained, while the influence of the peer group and heterosexual relationships increases.

- Emotionality in adolescence fluctuates between periods of stability and periods of instability.

- Nutritional needs for protein, minerals, and iron may be impaired by adolescents' eating habits of snacking and irregular mealtimes.

- Motor vehicle injuries and drowning are the greatest causes of mortality from injuries in this age-group.

REFERENCES

Adams, B.N., and others: The pregnant adolescent—a group approach, Adolescence **11**:467-485, 1976.

Bantz, E., and Auerbach, J.: Leg burns from mopeds, Pediatrics **70**:304-305, 1982.

Blos, P.: The adolescent passage: developmental issues, New York, 1979, International Universities Press, Inc.

Brown, R.C., Sanders, J.M., and Schonberg, S.K.: Driving safety and adolescent behavior, Pediatrics **77**:603-607, 1986.

Christoffel, K.K., and others: Childhood injuries caused by nonpowder firearms, Am. J. Dis. Child. **138**:557-561, 1984.

Conger, J.J., and Petersen, A.C.: Adolescence and youth; psychologic development in a changing world, ed. 3, New York, 1984, Harper & Row, Publishers.

Dickinson, G.E.: Changing religious behavior of adolescents 1964-1979, Youth Soc. **13**:283-288, 1982.

Elkind, D.: All grown up and no place to go: teenagers in crisis, Menlo Park, CA, 1984, Addison-Wesley Publishing Co., Inc.

Erikson, E.H.: Childhood and society, ed. 2, New York, 1963, W.W. Norton & Co., Inc.

Galanter, M.: Psychological induction into the large group: findings from a contemporary religious sect, Am. J. Psychiatry **137**:157-159, 1980.

Garn, S.M., LaVelle, M., and Pilkington, J.J.: Comparisons of fatness in premenarcheal and postmenarcheal girls of the same age, J. Pediatr. **103**:328-331, 1983.

Gregor, J.L., Devibliss, L., and Aschenbeck, S.K.: Dietary habits of adolescent females, Ecol. Food Nutr. **7**:213-220, 1979.

Kaluger, G., and Kaluger, M.F.: Human development: the span of life, ed. 3, St. Louis, 1984, The C.V. Mosby Co.

Kaplan, S.A.: Clinical pediatric and adolescent endocrinology, Philadelphia, 1982, W.B. Saunders Co.

Marino, D.D., and King, J.C.: Nutritional concerns during adolescence, Pediatr. Clin. North Am. **27**:125-140, 1980.

Shelly, J.A.: The spiritual needs of children, Downers Grove, IL, 1982, Inter-Varsity Press.

Teenage pregnancy: the problem that hasn't gone away, New York, 1981, The Alan Guttmacher Institute.

Westman, J.A., and Morrow, G., III: Moped injuries in children, Pediatrics **74**:820-822, 1984.

Williams, A.F., Wells, J.K., and Lund, A.K.: Seat belt use among American high school students, Accid. Anal. Prev. **15**:161-165, 1983.

BIBLIOGRAPHY
General

Berzonsky, M.D.: Inter- and intra-individual differences in adolescent storm and stress: a life-span developmental view, J. Early Adoles. **2**(3):211-217, 1982.

Cohen, M.T.: The process of adolescence: its psychologic and physiologic basis, Pediatr. Nurs. **4**(6):27-29, 1978.

DeMaio-Esteves, M., and Shuzman, E.: Technological society: its impact on youth, Topics Clin. Nurs. **10**:55-65, 1983.

DiCaprio, N.S.: Personality theories: a guide to human nature, ed. 2, New York, 1983, CBS Publishing.

Erikson, E.H.: Identity: youth and crisis, New York, 1968, W.W. Norton & Co., Inc.

Erikson, E.H.: Dimensions of a new identity, New York, 1974, W.W. Norton & Co., Inc.

Finkelstein, J.W.: The endocrinology of adolescence, Pediatr. Clin. North Am. **27**:53-69, 1980.

Grady, K., Gersick, K.E., and Boratynski, M.: Preparing parents for teenagers: a step in the prevention of adolescent substance abuse, Fam. Rel. **34**:541-549, 1985.

Gross, R.T., and Duke, P.M.: The effects of early versus late physical maturation on adolescent behavior, Pediatr. Clin. North Am. **27**:71-77, 1980.

Guyton, A.C.: Textbook of medical physiology, ed. 6, Philadelphia, 1981, W.B. Saunders Co.

Harlan, W.R., Harlan, E.A., and Grillo, G.P.: Secondary sex characteristics of girls 12 to 17 years of age: the U.S. Health Examination Survey, J. Pediatr. **96**:1074-1078, 1980.

Hoffman, A.D., editor: Adolescent medicine, Menlo Park, CA, 1983, Addison-Wesley Publishing Co., Inc.

Kerrins, K.M.: Comparing the self-image of prepubescent girls before and after four sessions on body awareness, J. School Health **53**:541-543, 1983.

Long, T.J., and others: Basic issues in adolescent medicine, Curr. Probl. Pediatr. **14**(10):3-49, 1984.

Lowery, G.H.: Growth and development of children, ed. 8, Chicago, 1986, Year Book Medical Publishers, Inc.

Mahon, N.E.: Developmental changes and loneliness during adolescence, Topics Clin. Nurs. **5**(1):66-76, 1983.

Mercer, R.T.: Perspectives in health care, Philadelphia, 1979, J.B. Lippincott Co.

Nelms, B.C.: What is a normal adolescent? Am. J. Maternal Child Nurs. **6:**402-406, 1981.

Piaget, J.: The theory of stages in cognitive development, New York, 1969, McGraw-Hill Book Co.

Reres, M.E.: Stressors in adolescence, Fam. Comm. Health **2**(4):31-41, 1980.

Rosenberg, M.S.: The nurse and the adolescent in today's changing social structure. In Reinhardt, A.M., and Quinn, M.D., editors: Family-centered community nursing, vol. 2, St. Louis, 1980, The C.V. Mosby Co.

Sapala, S., and Strokosch, G.: Adolescent sexuality: use of a questionnaire for health teaching and counseling, Pediatr. Nurs. **7**(6):33-35, 1981.

Shaffer, D.R.: Developmental psychology: theory, research, and applications, Monterey, CA, 1985, Brooks/Cole Publishing Co.

Stone, L.J., and Church, J.: Childhood and adolescence, ed. 5, New York, 1983, Random House, Inc.

Sutterly, D.C., and Donnelly, G.F.: Perspectives in human development, ed. 2, Philadelphia, 1981, J.B. Lippincott Co.

Wolman, B.B.: Children's fears, New York, 1978, Grosset & Dunlap.

Health Promotion During Adolescence

Adams, B.N.: Adolescent health care: needs, priorities and services, Nurs. Clin. North Am. **18:**237-248, 1983.

Anders, T.F., Carskadon, M.A., and Dement, W.C.: Sleep and sleepiness in children and adolescents, Nurs. Clin. North Am. **27:**29-43, 1980.

Bradley, J.M.: Do adolescents practice what they preach about health? Pediatr. Nurs. **10:**285-289, 1984.

Casamassimo, P.S., and Castaldi, C.R.: Considerations in the dental management of the adolescent, Pediatr. Clin. North Am. **29:**631-651, 1982.

Durfee, M.F., and Badger, D.W.: Adolescent health care: sharing the responsibility, Fam. Comm. Health **4:**43-55, 1982.

Elkind, D.: Teenage thinking: implications for health care, Pediatr. Nurs. **10:**383-385, 1984.

Fisher, M., and others: Are adolescents able and willing to pay the fee for confidential health care? J. Pediatr. **170:**480-483, 1985.

Greene, J.W., and others: Stressful life events and somatic complaints in adolescents, Pediatrics **75:**19-22, 1985.

Hofmann, A.: Adolescent medicine, Menlo Park, CA, 1983, Addison-Wesley Publishing Co., Inc.

Irwin, C.E., Millstein, S.G., and Shafer, M.B.: Appointment-keeping behavior in adolescents, J. Pediatr. **99:**799-802, 1981.

Jordan, D., and Kelfer, L.S.: Adolescent potential for participation in health care, Issues Compr. Pediatr. Nurs. **6:**147-156, 1983.

Kimball, A.J., and Campbell, M.M.: Psychologic aspects of adolescent patient health care, Clin. Pediatr. **18:**15-24, 1979.

Kovar, M.G.: Some indicators of health-related behavior among adolescents in the United States, Public Health Rep. **94:**109-118, 1979.

Leiman, A.H., and Strasburger, V.C.: Counseling parents of adolescents, Pediatrics **76:**664-667, 1985.

Litt, I.F.: Know thyself—adolescents' self-assessment of compliance behavior, Pediatrics **75:**693-696, 1985.

Litt, I.F., and Cuskey, W.R.: Compliance with medical regimens during adolescence, Pediatr. Clin. North Am. **27:**3-15, 1980.

Marks, A.: Health screening of the adolescent, Pediatr. Nurs. **4**(4):37-41, 1978.

Marks, A.: Aspects of biosocial screening and health maintenance in adolescents, Pediatr. Clin. North Am. **27:**153-161, 1980.

Perry, C.L., and Murray, D.M.: Enhancing the transition years: the challenge of adolescent health promotion, J. School Health **52:**307-311, 1982.

Surgeon General's Report on Health Promotion and Disease Prevention: Healthy people, Department of Health, Education and Welfare, (DHEW) (PHS) Pub. No. 79-55071A, Washington, DC, 1979, U.S. Government Printing Office.

Nutrition

Food and Nutrition Board, National Research Council: Recommended dietary allowances, ed. 9, Washington, DC, 1980, National Academy of Sciences.

Forbes, G.B.: Nutritional requirements in adolescence. In Suskind, R.M., editor: Textbook of pediatric nutrition, New York, 1981, Raven Press.

Gutierrez, Y.: Nutrition and the adolescent. In Mercer, R.T., editor: Perspectives on adolescent health care, Philadelphia, 1979, J.B. Lippincott Co.

Lucas, B., Rees, J.M., and Mahan, L.K.: Nutrition and the adolescent. In Pipes, P.L.: Nutrition in infancy and childhood, ed. 3, St. Louis, 1985, The C.V. Mosby Co.

Mahan, L.K., and Rees, J.M.: Nutrition in adolescence, St. Louis, 1984, The C.V. Mosby Co.

Williams, S.R.: Nutrition and diet therapy, ed. 5, St. Louis, 1985, The C.V. Mosby Co.

Wurtman, J.J.: What do children eat? Styles of the preschool, elementary school, and adolescent child. In Suskind, R.M., editor: Textbook of pediatric nutrition, New York, 1981, Raven Press.

Injury Prevention

Bass, J.L., Gallagher, S.S., and Mehta, K.A.: Injuries to adolescents and young adults, Pediatr. Clin. North Am. **32:**31-39, 1985.

Blocker, S., Coln, D., and Chang, J.H.T.: Serious air rifle injuries in children, Pediatrics **9:**751-754, 1982.

Chistoffel, K.K., and Tanz, R.: Motor vehicle injury in childhood, Pediatr. Rev. **4:**247-250, 1983.

Litt, I.F., and Steinerman, P.R.: Compliance with automotive safety devices among adolescents, J. Pediatr. **98:**484-486, 1981.

Osguthorpe, N.C., and Osguthorpe, J.D.: Scuba diving hazards: emergency management, Am. J. Nurs. **81:**1456-1458, 1981.

Schetky, D.H.: Children and handguns, Am. J. Dis. Child. **139:**229-231, 1985.

Shaffer, T.E.: New guidelines in sports medicine, Pediatr. Consult. **1**(5):1-12, 1980.

Tanz, R., Christoffel, K.K., and Sagerman, S.: Are toy guns too dangerous? Pediatrics **75:**265-268, 1985.

Sex Education and Guidance

Bullough, V., and Bullough, B.: PMPs patients, parents, and sexuality, Pediatr. Nurs. **8:**A-I, 1982.

Burke, R.J.: Sex differences in adolescent life; stress, social support, and well-being, J. Psychol. **98**(2):277-288, 1978.

Calderone, M.S.: Adolescent sexuality: elements and genesis, Pediatrics **76:**699-703, 1985.

Committee on Adolescence: Homosexuality and adolescence, Pediatrics **72:**249-250, 1983.

Duke, P.M.: Adolescent sexuality, Pediatr. Rev. **4:**44-52, 1982.

Katchadourian, H.: Adolescent sexuality, Pediatr. Clin. North Am. **27:**17-28, 1980.

Kuhnen, K.K., and others: Barny: a computer for teaching sex education, Am. J. Maternal Child Nurs. **8:**350-353, 1983.

Parcel, G.S., and others: Sex concerns of young adolescents, Birth Fam. J. **6**(1):43-47, 1979.

Powell, L.H., and Jorgensen, S.R.: Evaluation of church-based sexuality education program for adolescents, Fam. Rel. **34:**475-482, 1985.

Sapala, S., and Strokosch, G.: Adolescent sexuality: use of a questionnaire for health teaching and counseling, Pediatr. Nurs. **7:**33-34, 52, 1981.

Sheehan, M.K., Ostwald, S.K., and Rothenberger, J.: Perceptions of sexual responsibility: do young men and women agree? Pediatr. Nurs. **12:**17-21, 1986.

Woods, N.F.: Human sexuality: in health and illness, ed. 3, St. Louis, 1984, The C.V. Mosby Co.

Chapter 20

Physical Health Problems of Adolescence

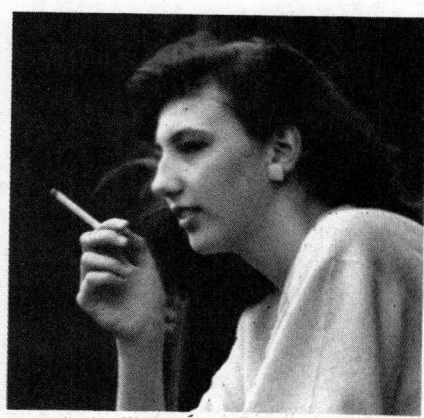

Common Problems of Adolescence
    Acne
    Smoking
    Infectious mononucleosis

Health Problems Related to Sports Participation
    Preparation for sports
    Types of injury
    Acute injuries
    Overuse syndromes
    Underwater sports–related injuries
    Health concerns associated with sports
    Nurse's role in children's sports

Alterations in Growth and Maturation
    Assessment
    Short stature
    Tall stature
    Precocious puberty
    Turner syndrome
    Klinefelter syndrome

    Delayed development caused by pathologic conditions
    Psychosocial dwarfism

Health Problems of the Male Reproductive System
    Health problems related to urinary function
    Penile problems
    Testicular tumors
    Varicocele
    Testicular torsion
    Other disorders of the scrotum and testes
    Gynecomastia

Health Problems of the Female Reproductive System
    The gynecologic examination
    Amenorrhea/delayed menarche
    Dysmenorrhea
    Premenstrual tension syndrome
    Endometriosis
    Pelvic inflammatory disease
    Dysfunctional uterine bleeding
    Vaginitis and vulvitis (vulvovaginitis)
    Exposure to diethylstilbestrol

Health Problems Related to Sexuality
    Adolescent pregnancy
    Contraception
    Rape

Sexually Transmitted Diseases
    Gonorrhea
    Chlamydial infection
    Herpes genitalis
    Trichomoniasis
    Candidiasis (moniliasis)
    Syphilis
    Nursing considerations

In many ways the health problems of adolescents are very different from those of either children or adults. Because adolescence is a healthy period of life, teenagers' contacts with health professionals vary considerably from routine health checkups to treatment of serious illness or injury. Most health problems are related to the physical changes taking place in their bodies and the crucial psychosocial crises of identity formation. The usual motives for which adolescents seek medical attention are skin problems, obesity, headaches, abdominal discomfort, menstrual symptoms, and anxieties about physical development and sexual changes. Major diseases are at a relatively low incidence, but when they do occur, they have unusual significance for the adolescent.

The increase in numbers of teenagers, their earlier maturation, plus a more mobile, permissive, and contraceptive-conscious society allow more adolescents the opportunity to become sexually active at an increasingly younger age. Sexual involvement has attendant problems; and consequently health professionals are seeing more and more health problems related to adolescent sexuality. Those of major importance are sexually acquired diseases and teenage pregnancies.

The multiple aspects of adolescence, both physiologic and psychologic, influence the evaluation and care of members of this age-group. It is characteristic of adolescents that the very nature of their health problems is a deterrent to seeking health care. For most problems related to developmental changes the youngster can be reassured regarding the source of his anxiety. Contacts with the health professional afford an excellent opportunity for health teaching and anticipatory guidance.

Common Health Problems of Adolescence

There are a number of health problems that have their onset in adolescence or are more prominent at this stage of development than at earlier or subsequent ages. Most are not life-threatening but may create psychologic problems that influence the establishment of a positive identity.

ACNE

Adolescents are subject to the same skin conditions that affect the school-age child, such as bacterial, viral, and fungal infection, contact dermatitis, and drug reactions. However, there is one skin disorder that, although not limited to the adolescent age-group, appears predominantly at this time—acne vulgaris. Acne is an almost universal occurrence during these years and involves anatomic, physiologic, biochemical, genetic, immunologic, and psychologic factors of significant import.

It is estimated that about 70% of the population will have had acne by the end of the teenage years, and as many as 25% to 50% of children before the age of 10 have evidence of the disorder. However, the peak incidence is in late adolescence, at about age 16 to 17 in girls and 17 to 18 years in boys, and the disorder is more common in males than in females (Yonkosky and Pochi, 1986). After this, the disease usually slackens off, but it may persist well into adulthood. The degree to which an individual is affected may range from nothing more than a few isolated comedones to a severe inflammatory reaction. Although the disease is self-limited and is not life-threatening, its significance to the affected adolescent is great, and it is a mistake to underestimate the impact that it can have on young persons.

Etiology

The etiology of acne is still unclear, although a number of factors appear to be related to its development. Its distribution in families and a high degree of concordance in identical twins suggest that hereditary factors predispose to susceptibility to acne. Androgens are implicated, since observations indicate a diminished effect on acne during pregnancy, its virtual absence in castrated males and young children, and its higher incidence in adolescent males. The disease seems to be aggravated by emotional stress, winter weather, some stimulant drugs, and the premenstrual period. There is no positive evidence that any specific foods are factors, except perhaps with individual youngsters. Corticosteroids administered systemically over a period of weeks may produce a form of acne with typical lesions that does not appear to be associated with sebaceous hyperplasia and that slowly subsides after the steroids have been discontinued.

Pathophysiology

Acne is a disease that involves the pilosebaceous follicles (the hair follicle and sebaceous gland complex) of the face, neck, shoulders, back, and upper chest—the so-called flush areas of the skin. However, there is no abnormality of the gland; it is the glandular secretion, sebum, initiated by androgenic hormones, that is involved in the pathogenesis of this disease. Increased sebum production begins at the time of adrenocortical maturation (adrenarche) and slowly continues to increase until the late teens.

There are two basic types of lesions seen in acne: (1) *noninflamed* lesions called *comedones,* consisting of compact masses of keratin, lipids, fatty acids, and bacteria that dilate the follicular duct, which may be plugged (closed comedones, or whiteheads with no visible opening) or open (blackheads, with visible dilated openings that are discolored as fatty acids are oxidated by air) and (2) *inflamed* lesions that result when the follicular wall ruptures to produce papules, pustules, nodules, and cysts (Fig. 20-1). The inflammatory acne is responsible for the destructiveness and propensity for scarring.

The maturation of the sebaceous glands begins as an early pubertal occurrence, and the development of acne as adolescence progresses appears to be the result of a sequence of events. Under the influence of the accelerated androgen secretion from the adrenal glands and gonads, the sebaceous gland increases in size, secretory productivity, and turnover of the follicular epithelium. These changes are accompanied by an alteration in the follicular lining that allows the accumulation and stagnation of sebum and keratinized material derived from the lining cells. Normally the growing hair shaft prevents this accumulation by functioning as a "pipe cleaner" and moving the material out of the follicle. In acne the small, fine, vellus hairs occupying sebaceous follicles are unable to move the fixed material and the acne lesion develops. The noninflammatory comedones may resolve or become infected pustules.

A normally harmless bacterium, *Corynebacterium acnes,* is attracted to the sebum, which it hydrolyzes into fatty acids. These fatty acids are the major tissue irritants in the sebum and initiate the inflammatory response. Inflammation is preceded by rupture of the distended follicles, which allows the follicular contents to leak into the dermis. The resultant damage causes a further wall-rupturing effect from leukocytes that invade the dermis. Those that become cystic are likely to form scars when they heal.

Secondary invasion by *Staphylococcus albus* can complicate the acne lesion, and adolescents' concern about their

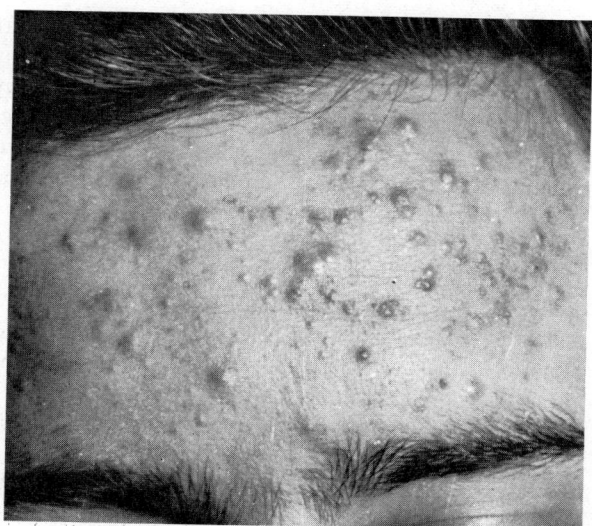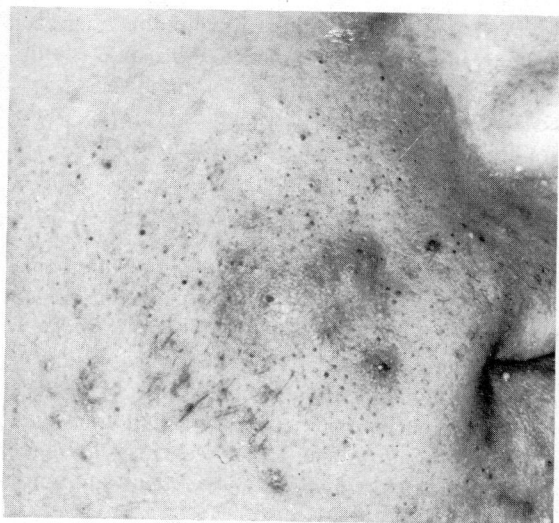

Fig. 20-1. Acne vulgaris. Papular pustules and comedones.
From Stewart, W.D., Danto, J.L., and Maddin, S.: Dermatology: diagnosis and treatment of cutaneous disorders, ed. 4, St. Louis, 1978, The C.V. Mosby Co.

appearance tempts them to pick, finger, squeeze, and otherwise manipulate the lesions, which plays an important role in the perpetuation of acne. In addition to the precipitating factors mentioned previously, the application of creams, oils, and some cosmetics that add to the plugging of the follicles may aggravate acne; therefore cosmetic agents should be selected to avoid those with greasy or occlusive bases. It has also been shown that iodides markedly increase the cellular phase of inflammation.

Exposure to oily substances, chlorinated hydrocarbons, and coal tar distillates profoundly exaggerates acne, which may influence the choice of occupation among adolescents. Exposure to excessive warmth and humidity may cause marked exacerbations in adolescents with more severe types of acne. It appears that sweating decreases the openings of the pilosebaceous ducts. This may necessitate discontinuing some active sports, such as football or wrestling, or employment in a hot, humid environment, for example, working as a cook. Local increases in heat produced by occlusive clothing or mechanical irritation by wool and other rough textures may also produce exacerbations.

Therapeutic Management

There is little evidence that treatment shortens the duration of the entire course of the disease. However, much can be done to control acne, reduce the inflammatory process and scarring, and improve the appearance. All too often parents and health professionals have a tendency to dismiss acne as a normal part of growing up.

The treatment of acne requires long-term management with patience and perseverance on the part of patient, family, and health professionals. Unlike many dermatologic conditions the acne lesions resolve slowly, and improvement may not be apparent for many weeks. Also, in early stages of treatment the persistent postinflammatory erythem-

atous macules may lead the patient to believe the therapy has been ineffective. In addition, there is no uniform treatment that can be applied to every case; therefore in many instances inadequate or inappropriate treatment may have damaging consequences for the emotional health of the affected youngster.

No single therapeutic agent is effective in the management of acne except in a few mild cases. It is usually more effective to employ a combination of therapies. The treatment most commonly consists of measures directed toward improving the general health of the youngster, removing comedones, preventing their formation, controlling excessive sebaceous gland activity, controlling infection, and preventing scar formation. The treatment consists of some general measures of care and specific treatments largely determined by the type of lesions involved and the preference of the dermatologist. Although the combination of therapies and brands selected vary, the objectives are similar.

General measures. A general explanation of the disease process and the plan of care is given to the youngster with emphasis on his responsibility to faithfully carry out the program for as long as the process persists. It is also important to obtain the cooperation and understanding of the parents; therefore they should be present at the initial discussion.

Improvement of the adolescent's overall health status is part of the general management. Adequate rest, moderate exercise, a well-balanced diet, reduction of emotional stress, elimination of any foci of infection, and correction of constipation (if it exists) are all part of general health promotion. There is no convincing evidence to implicate any single dietary item or combination of foods in the exacerbation of acne, with the possible exception of iodides and bromide in therapeutic amounts. Occasionally a youngster will demonstrate an aggravation of symptoms after each ingestion of a given food. In such instances the food is eliminated for a time to assess its influence on the disease.

Medications. There is a wide range of types and combinations of topical agents for the treatment of acne, with selection depending on the type and severity of the lesions. Tretinoin (retinoic acid) is the only drug that effectively interrupts abnormal follicular keratinization that produces microcomedones, the invisible precursors of the visible comedones. Tretinoin alone is usually sufficient for management of comedonal acne (Shalita, 1986).

Since most patients also have some inflammatory lesions accompanying the comedones, a topical antibacterial agent is prescribed. Benzoyl peroxide, clindamycin, tetracycline, erythromycin, and minocycline are the agents of choice. Benzoyl peroxide also functions as an exfoliant and comedolytic.

The most effective therapy involves the use of benzoyl peroxide, tretinoin, or a combination of these. Both agents can cause redness and peeling early in their use; therefore the treatment usually begins with graded increases in concentration and/or frequency of application according to the patient's tolerance. Both are available in cream or gel preparations. Creams are less irritating, but the gels, which offer more efficient penetration, are favored as the most effective vehicle (Melski and Arndt, 1980; Tunnessen, 1984). The usual regimen is to apply one medication in the morning and the other at night. They should not be applied together, since the benzoyl peroxide may oxidize the retinoic acid and render it impotent (Tunnessen, 1984).

Systemic antibiotic therapy may be needed for some patients who do not respond to topical therapy for inflammatory acne. Isotretinoin, 13-*cis* retinoic acid (Accutane), a very potent and effective topical agent, is reserved for severe cystic acne. The use of isotretinoin is limited as a universal treatment of inflammatory acne because of its side effects, which include dryness of skin and mucous membranes, musculoskeletal symptoms, and premature epiphyseal closure. The drug has also been found to be teratogenic and therefore unsuitable for pregnant women (Benke, 1984). All sexually active teenagers should be identified before treatment and the drug given only if they use an effective form of contraception during and for 3 to 4 months after completion of treatment (Committee on Drugs, 1983).

Intralesional injections of steroids can hasten the resolution of inflammatory nodules, which decrease in size in about 48 hours (Yonkosky and Pochi, 1986). However, systemic corticosteroids, because of their acneogenic properties, are not used in the treatment of acne. Estrogen-progestin therapy in a cyclic routine has produced good responses in carefully selected older teenage females.

Other topical agents for treatment of acne include sulfur, resorcin, and salicylic acid. Although their beneficial effects have been proved over the years, they now have only a minor place in acne management.

Cleansing. Gentle cleansing with a mild cleanser once or twice daily is usually sufficient. Harsh, rough soaps and excessive scrubbing may irritate the skin and cause rupture of the pilosebaceous ducts, thus enhancing papulopustule formation (Tunnessen, 1984). For some adolescents hygiene of the hair and scalp appears to be related to the clinical activity of acne. In these persons acne of the forehead can be improved by brushing the hair away form the forehead and more frequent shampooing.

Nursing Considerations

As in many long-term problems of adolescence, nurses are involved in the assessment and therapy of the teenager with acne on a sustained basis. Often it is the nurse who establishes the initial contact with the affected adolescent and is instrumental in the youngster's seeking medical advice and embarking on a course of treatment. Teenagers do not always seek advice on their own; therefore the nurse will need to ferret out their concerns about facial blemishes. During professional contact with an adolescent, such as a routine physical assessment or incidental visit for another problem, nurses can ask the youngster if he or she would like them to do something about "those few pimples (or 'zits')." It is not uncommon for troubled teenagers to deliberately seek advice on another matter in hopes that they may get the opportunity to discuss the skin condition without revealing the extent of their concern. To the adolescent even a minor facial blemish can assume monumental proportions. In addition, adolescents may have unspoken concerns about the relationship of acne to sexual feelings, sexual intercourse or lack of it, masturbation, venereal disease, contagion, being unclean, and a myriad of myths that surround acne. Voluntary reassurance can do much to relieve these unspoken fears.

The adolescent should be encouraged to seek medical treatment for the skin lesions by a sympathetic and understanding dermatologist; however, the extent of physician involvement varies. Self-treatment is extremely common and associated with the many myths related to the cause and treatment of acne. During conversations with teenagers the nurse can dispel the common myths often associated with acne and allow them to discuss any feelings related to the disorder, such as self-consciousness and anxieties regarding relationships with others, and sometimes help them explore job or other after-school interests. The acne lesions need not become an excuse to avoid social contacts and activities after school.

Teenagers need a supportive, caring individual to help them maintain the persistence required to deal with the disorder over such an extended period of time. The condition is a chronic one and treatment is needed until the condition subsides spontaneously. They should not expect to see a change in the lesions for 4 to 6 weeks after beginning therapy. If they have no unrealistic expectations and disappointments concerning the progress of therapy, they are more likely to comply with instructions for personal hygiene and management. However, it is essential that the youngster with inflammatory lesions obtain medical treatment in order to control the process and reduce the incidence of scarring.

Teenagers are subject to the influence of commercial advertising in many media concerning acne care and have ready access to a variety of over-the-counter preparations. Therefore it is important that affected adolescents receive an explanation of the disease so that they have some knowledge of its causes and the rationale underlying the prescribed treatment. An instruction sheet that describes the etiology and therapeutic regimen is often helpful, and parents should be cautioned against nagging. Adolescents should assume responsibility for following through on the instructions. The importance of using only those preparations prescribed for their particular needs and applying medication to the entire face, not to lesions alone, is emphasized. They are advised that the medications often cause erythema, peeling, itching, and burning, especially if applied immediately after face washing. The irritative effects are also aggravated by factors that dry the skin, for example, wind, low humidity, and low temperature. Over-the-counter preparations of benzoyl peroxide have a short shelf life, some more so than others. Therefore a youngster who is using one of these preparations and appears to get poor results should be advised to change to a different brand and to check dates on packages to be sure of purchasing the most recent preparation.

Some researchers have found that water avoidance is effective in reducing skin lesions. They recommend cleansing the skin with lipid-free cleanser (for example, Cetaphil) applied with the fingers and gently removed with a soft cotton towel after cleansing. An emollient cream (Eucerin) applied to the face before showering, bathing, swimming, or shampooing and removed afterward offers protection against the drying effect of water (Swinyer, Swinyer, and Britt, 1980).

Teenagers need to be cautioned against damaging the skin through too vigorous scrubbing. Picking, squeezing, and manual expression with fingernails break down ductal walls and cause the acne to worsen. Other factors that exacerbate the lesions are wearing hair over the face and maintaining hand contact with the face, for example, resting the chin on the palms or sleeping on an arm. Nurses can help girls select proper water-base cosmetic preparations. If the makeup comes in a tube, jar, stick, or cake, it is too thick. Those best suited to acne are liquid and should shake easily in the bottle. Oil-base and water-base cosmetics can be differentiated by placing a small amount on the tip of the fingers, rinsing under running water for 10 seconds, then blotting fingertip with a tissue. Oil-base preparations do not rinse off. Cosmetics should not be left on overnight. Teenagers are also cautioned against using any suntan-promoting products, since they are predominantly oily preparations and many sunscreens are prepared in an oil-base vehicle.

Expression of comedones. The nontraumatic removal of comedones serves two purposes. It reduces the risk of future inflammatory lesions and scarring, and produces a prompt improvement in the youngster's appearance. Blackheads, which have open communication with the skin surface, can be effectively expressed with a comedo extractor, a small metal scoop with a hole in the center. The hole is placed directly over the blackhead and pressure applied against the skin with a slight sliding movement across the skin. Initially the procedures are carried out in the physician's office by the physician or nurse, but the adolescent or the parents can be taught to remove comedones with the extractor. Whiteheads, which do not have open communication with the skin surface, cannot be removed easily with the extractor alone. The epidermal covering of the whitehead must be gently and superficially nicked with a No. 11 Bard-Parker scalpel blade point before extrusion with the comedo extractor. Some extractors are constructed with a blade attached to the end opposite the loop.

The face should be cleansed before and after extraction, and the instrument cleaned and cared for in the manner directed by the individual physician. The instrument usually is cleaned with soap and water and then either stored in alcohol or wiped with alcohol and stored in a receptacle such as a clean, dry envelope.

The parents and adolescent are cautioned against excessive pressure that might bruise the skin. A blackhead that cannot be removed readily should be left until another time. Some dermatologists limit home treatment to removal of blackheads only. Satisfactory results can be obtained by the removal of a small number (five or 10) each day on a regular basis, thus minimizing family friction. Although the comedones tend to recur in the same follicle, periodic removal properly carried out by this procedure will produce no scarring and will reduce the likelihood of follicular rupture and subsequent inflammation with possible scar formation.

SMOKING

The problem of smoking among teenagers is becoming increasingly serious. The habit appears to be spreading among teenagers even as the evidence of the relationship between smoking and health problems increases. Smoking is considered to be a dependence disorder and is formally included in the diagnostic nomenclature of the American Psychiatric Association (1980). Statistics indicate that not only has the incidence of smoking among teenagers increased but the age of onset has decreased (U.S. Public Health Service, 1979). A recent finding in one area disclosed that 22% of the girls were smoking and 11% of the boys. However, 35% of the boys admit using smokeless tobacco (Guggenheimer and others, 1986); another study reported 37% of males and 2.2% of females using smokeless tobacco (Marty and others, 1986).

The hazards of smoking at any age are undisputed (U.S. Public Health Service, 1981); however, a preventive approach to teenage smoking is especially important for several reasons. There is high probability that regular smoking in childhood leads to a lifetime habit with concomitant increases in morbidity and mortality. Smoking has been linked to respiratory disorders in teenagers (Harrison and others, 1979), and in later years the mortality of those who smoked since they were 15 years of age has been found to be 50% higher than that of those who started smoking in early adulthood (U.S. Public Health Service, 1979).

Etiology

In most instances the smoking habit begins in adolescence, and there are a variety of reasons why teenagers begin smoking. The significant factors related to onset of smoking can be categorized as social, sociodemographic, psychosocial, and biologic. Once smoking behavior is established, smoking itself is thought to produce enough reinforcement to sustain the practice without the initial pressure (Bragg and Hughes, 1984).

Social factors. Social pressures to smoke include imitation of the smoking behavior and attitudes of parents and other adults, the association of smoking with maturity or as representative of "mature" behavior, pressures from peers who view smoking as the popular thing to do, and the use of smoking as an outlet for real or imagined school, social, or home pressures. Other pressures come from advertisers who aim directly at members of this vulnerable age-group.

Parental approval or disapproval of their children's smoking is an important force in predicting teenage smoking. In one study 34% of teenage smokers had smoked at least one cigarette in their homes, implying that smoking was accepted by the parents (Biglan and others, 1984). The social influence of same-sex family members or peers is an important factor, and the number of smokers in the immediate environment increases the probability of subsequent smoking by a youngster. The social nature of smoking is also significant (Flay and others, 1983), as well as anticipation of enjoyment. However, the influence of friends on beliefs and behavior depends in part on the adolescent's tendencies toward rebelliousness and disobedience (McAlister, Krosnick, and Milburn, 1984).

The mass media have contributed to the incidence of smoking in easily influenced adolescents. In advertisements smokers are engaged in activities and dressed in clothes suitable for adolescents, and the ads associate smoking with fun, risk taking, and sexual adventure as well as a sign of maturity and autonomy. It also implies "youthful vigor, good health, good looks, and personal, social, and professional acceptance and success" (Staff Report on the Cigarette Advertising Investigation, 1981).

Sociodemographic factors. Sociodemographic factors include socioeconomic status, sex, and performance in school. A consistent, negative association has been observed between socioeconomic status and smoking (especially among boys) and there is a consistent correlation between low academic goals and performance and smoking (cited in Flay and others, 1983). Smokers have been found to be from families of lower socioeconomic levels and do not participate in school activities. Adolescents who participate in and dominate school activities tend to come from the upper end of the social continuum (Eckert, 1983).

Psychosocial factors. A primary feature of early adolescence is development of an identity, an autonomous self-concept. During this time the self-conscious young adoles-

cent endeavors to alter the real self-image to approximate the ideal self-image (Chassin and others, 1981). It appears that adolescents who are performing well academically and in school-related activities, especially athletics, derive their status through seniority in the system; the significant minority who are failing place a premium on status that can be achieved through voluntary group associations. Cigarette smoking may be an attempt on the part of these youngsters to emulate the personality traits of toughness, friendliness, confidence, attractiveness, and enthusiasm, traits that are popularly attributed to smokers. They feel a need for social skills that make them appear to be adroit, fluent, authoritative, and worthwhile persons who are sufficiently attractive to warrant inclusion in significant peer groups. Smoking is an easily mastered vehicle with motor activities that convey an air of ease and social adeptness (Wong-McCarthy and Gritz, 1982).

Biologic factors. Biologic factors serve to both encourage and deter further experimentation of would-be smokers. Initial harshness, nausea, and irritation are sufficient to influence many youngsters not to try smoking again; to others it may represent a challenge to overcome (Jarvik, 1979). Smoking has been found to lower endurance by decreasing breathing capacity or ventilatory muscle endurance (Dessendorfer, Amsterdam, and Odland, 1983). Dependence is thought to be the result of nicotine, the primary alkaloid in tobacco. Nicotine exerts both stimulating and sedating affects on central and peripheral nervous systems and several organ systems. Attempts at stopping the smoking habit are accompanied by severe craving and withdrawal symptoms.

Process of Becoming a Smoker

Researchers have identified three stages in the process: trying the first cigarette, experimental smoking (less than weekly), and regular smoking (at least weekly) (Flay and others, 1983). Some recognize a preparation or initiation stage in which psychosocial, environmental, and possibly biologic factors prepare certain youngsters to be smokers (Leventhal and Cleary, 1981). Characteristics of the four stages are:

Preparation—early learning experiences provided in the environment, for example, parent or sibling smokers in the family

Initiation—trying the first cigarette; peer influences are more important than family influences in determining when cigarettes are first tried

Experimentation—learning to smoke by repeated experimentation; decision to quit or continue

Regular smoking—smoke sufficiently often to be considered a regular smoker

Smokeless Tobacco

The term *smokeless tobacco* refers to tobacco products that are placed in the mouth but not ignited, for example, snuff and chewing tobacco. This increasingly popular substitute for cigarettes is now posing a serious hazard to children and adolescents as well as young adults. These products are proved to be carcinogenic, and regular use has been reported to cause dental diseases including foul-smelling breath, periodontal disease, erosion of teeth, and tooth loss (Greer, 1983). The American Academy of Pediatrics (Committee on Environmental Hazards, 1985) states that "for the protection of the present and future health of the children of this nation, the selling and advertising of all forms of smokeless tobacco must be controlled without delay."

Nursing Considerations

Prevention of regular smoking in teenagers appears to be the most effective way to reduce the overall incidence of smoking. Obviously, early education is the ideal approach, but most school-based or large-scale public information campaigns have had no significant impact on smoking habits. A variety of methods has been employed to deal with the problem. Communication through posters, charts, displays, statistics, and the use of examples of actual damaged lungs all have their supporters and doubters. While some believe that these are a waste of time, others give evidence that many children are influenced by these "scare tactics." Presentation of films and demonstrations in science classes have proved to be of value in some schools.

RECOMMENDED NONSMOKING STRATEGIES

Provide only a cursory mention of long-term health consequences (e.g., cardiovascular and cancer risks)

Discuss immediate physiologic consequences in some detail (e.g., changes in heart rate and blood pressure, minor respiratory symptoms, and blood carbon monoxide concentrations)

Mention alternatives to smoking for establishing a self-image that appears tough, independent, mature, or sophisticated (e.g., establishing a weight-lifting regimen, jogging and dancing, joining a Boys' Club or a Girls' Club, engaging in volunteer work for a hospital or political or religious group)

Mention the negative effects of smoking (e.g., earlier wrinkling of skin, yellow stains on teeth and fingers, tobacco odor on breath and clothing)

Mention the increasing ostracism of smokers by nonsmokers, both legal and informal, in places of work and public places

Mention the increasing evidence that second-hand smoke is injurious to the health of nonsmokers who are regularly exposed, especially small children

Acknowledge that many adults once believed that important social benefits were associated with smoking; but point out that the vast majority of adult smokers would now quit smoking if they could

Arm the cooperative adolescent with arguments for dealing with peer pressure (e.g., by not smoking, a teenager demonstrates independence and nonconformity, traits normally prized by youth)

Request posters and pamphlets from local voluntary agencies (e.g., American Cancer Society, American Heart Association, and American Lung Association) to display prominently

Modified from Wong-McCarthy, W.J., and Gritz, E.R.: Preventing regular teenage cigarette smoking, Pediatr. Ann. **11**:683-689, 1982.

Questions and Controversies

Does the smoking behavior of health professionals influence antismoking health teaching of teenagers?

It is known that smoking by adults, especially parents, is influential in some teenagers' decision to begin smoking (see discussion). Role models are extremely important influences on growth and development of children at any age. Some of the influential adults are teachers, coaches, physicians, and nurses. It has been found that about 36% of all nurses smoke, which is higher than the average for all men and 10% higher than for women in general (U.S. Department of Health and Human Services, 1980). At the same time, the percentage of physicians who smoke has been reduced from 45% to 20% in the past 20 years (U.S. Public Health Service, 1979).

For the most part smoking-prevention programs that focus on negative long-term effects of smoking on health have been uniformly ineffective. Those emphasizing immediate effects and youth-to-youth programs have been somewhat more effective, but primarily in improving the teenagers' attitudes toward smoking (Leventhal and Cleary, 1980; Evans and others, 1981). Because smoking and smoking-related behavior function as a key social symbol, antismoking campaigns must be addressed to the norms of the potential smokers, and anything that ridicules or threatens the social norms of the group can be unproductive or counterproductive (Eckert, 1983).

Two areas of focus are gaining interest among health advocates: peer-led programming and use of media in smoking prevention, that is, videotapes and films. Peer-led programs emphasizing social consequences of not smoking have proved most successful. If a significant number of influential peers can "sell" their classmates on the idea that the habit is not popular, the followers will imitate their behavior. Short-term rather than long-term consequences are emphasized, for example, the effects of smoking on personal appearance, such as the unattractive stains on teeth and hands and the unpleasant odor that smoking gives to the breath and clothing.

Nurses in schools and other agencies of the community are in a position to implement and reinforce teaching, to serve as consultants and counselors to student, teacher, and parent groups, and to be advocates in all areas in which antismoking campaigns might be effective. Several strategies are recommended (see box at left). (See also Questions and controversies, above, for a discussion of whether the smoking behavior of health professionals influences antismoking health teaching of teenagers.)

INFECTIOUS MONONUCLEOSIS

Infectious mononucleosis (IM) is an acute, self-limiting infectious disease that is relatively common among young persons between 12 and 25 years of age. However, recent evidence indicates that the disease is more common in younger children than previously thought (Sumaya and Ench, 1985). The disease is characterized by an increase in the mononuclear elements of the blood and general symptoms of an infectious process. The course is usually mild but occasionally can be severe or, rarely, accompanied by serious complications.

Pathophysiology

Recent evidence establishes the herpes-like Epstein-Barr virus (EBV) as the principal cause of infectious mononucleosis. The disease appears in both sporadic and epidemic forms, the sporadic cases being more common. The mechanism of spread has not been conclusively established, although the disease is believed to be transmitted by direct intimate contact. It also appears to be only mildly contagious, and the period of communicability is unknown. The incubation period after exposure is 2 to 6 weeks. There are enlargement of lymph nodes from mononuclear infiltration and variable infiltration of most of the body tissues.

Clinical Manifestations

The onset of symptoms of infectious mononucleosis appears anywhere from 10 days to 6 weeks after exposure and may be acute or insidious. The common presenting symptoms vary greatly in type, severity, and duration. The characteristics of the disease are malaise, sore throat, and fever with generalized lymphadenopathy and splenomegaly that may persist for several months. Most often the symptoms appear insidiously with fatigue, lack of energy, and sore throat that may not become prominent. The youngster's chief complaint is difficulty in maintaining his usual level of activity. This is often attributed to lack of sleep, an upper respiratory infection, or both. In many instances the manifestations never arouse enough concern to bring the affected individual to medical attention. Many cases of infectious mononucleosis are no doubt never recognized as such. Many young children do not develop all the expected clinical and laboratory findings; often a complication is the only or presenting symptom (Alpert and Fleisher, 1984).

A skin rash is present in a few cases, most often a discrete macular eruption most prominent over the trunk. More young children have rashes, and older children have abdominal pain. Other symptoms may include headache and epistaxis. The tonsils may be enlarged, reddened, and sometimes covered with a diphtheria-like membrane. Failure to thrive, otitis media, and episodes of recurrent tonsillopharyngitis are more closely associated with childhood disease. Hepatic involvement to some degree is almost always present, often associated with jaundice, which may cause the disease to be confused with infectious hepatitis. The extensive mononuclear infiltration produces symptoms related to any body tissue so that the clinical picture can resemble that of many conditions, including neurologic manifestations and cardiac involvement.

The clinical manifestations of infectious mononucleosis are usually less severe (often subclinical or unapparent) and the convalescent phase is shorter in younger children than in older children and young adults. There is a decided relationship between early-acquired disease and poor economic and hygienic conditions. Children in lower socioeconomic levels acquire the virus at a younger age than middle-class children, who remain susceptible well into adolescence. This probably accounts for the higher incidence of the illness among young people in colleges and universities.

Diagnostic Evaluation

The diagnosis is established on the basis of clinical manifestations, absolute increase in atypical leukocytes in a peripheral blood smear, and a positive heterophil agglutination test. Differential diagnosis depends on the clinical symptoms present. For example, the pharyngitis may simulate symptoms of other diseases such as diphtheria and streptococcal pharyngitis. Lymphadenopathy, fever, and malaise are all characteristic of numerous disorders. Jaundice, nervous system manifestations, and skin eruptions each similarly indicate a variety of conditions. The leukocyte count may be normal or low, but usually lymphocyte leukocytosis develops; of these, approximately 10% are atypical lymphocytes.

The heterophil antibody test determines the extent to which the patient's serum will agglutinate sheep red blood cells. In infectious mononucleosis a titer of 1:160 is considered diagnostic, although a rising titer during the earlier stages is the best indicator. Because young children have a lower rate of heterophil antibody responses, the diagnosis may be overlooked in this group (Sumaya and Ench, 1985).

The "spot test" (Monospot), a slide test of high specificity, has been developed for the diagnosis of infectious mononucleosis. It is rapid, sensitive, inexpensive, and easy to perform, and it has the advantage that it can detect significant agglutinins at lower levels, thus permitting earlier diagnosis.

Therapeutic Management

The course of infectious mononucleosis is self-limiting and usually uncomplicated. Contrary to popular belief, mononucleosis is not necessarily a difficult, prolonged, disabling disease, and the prognosis is generally good. Acute symptoms usually disappear within 7 to 10 days, and the persistent fatigue subsides within 2 to 4 weeks. A number of affected youngsters may need to restrict activities for 2 to 3 months; the disease rarely extends for longer periods.

There is no specific treatment for infectious mononucleosis. Common symptoms are ordinarily relieved by simple remedies. A mild analgesic is usually sufficient to relieve the bothersome symptoms of headache, fever, and malaise. Bed rest is encouraged for fatigue but is not imposed for any specified period of time. Affected youngsters are instructed to regulate activities according to their own tolerance, unless complicating factors are present. If the spleen is enlarged, for example, activities in which they might receive a blow to the abdomen or chest should be avoided.

A short course of oral penicillin is sometimes prescribed for sore throat, especially if β-hemolytic streptococci are present. Administration of ampicillin frequently precipitates a maculopapular rash in affected persons; therefore its use is contraindicated. Sore throat can be relieved by gargles, hot drinks, analgesic troches, or analgesics. Some physicians favor the use of corticosteroids for suppression of high fever and/or severe sore throat but usually limit their use to the period of more intense symptoms or if the youngster is severely ill. Complications are uncommon but can be serious and require appropriate management. Liver involvement is present to some degree in almost all cases and may become chronic. Neurologic complications are seen in some outbreaks and vary in severity and outcome. Other complications include pneumonitis, myocarditis, hemolytic anemia, thrombocytopenia, and ruptured spleen. There is also some evidence to indicate a depressed cellular immune reactivity during the course of the disease and for some time afterward so that live vaccines are best avoided until several months after recovery.

Nursing Considerations

Nursing responsibilities are directed toward comfort measures to relieve the symptoms and helping the affected youngster and his family determine appropriate activities according to the stage of the disease and his interests. They may need diet counseling to select foods that contain sufficient calories to meet growth and energy needs and yet are easy to swallow. Every effort should be made to prevent a secondary infection; therefore the adolescent is counseled to limit contact with persons outside the family, especially during the acute phase of the illness.

The protracted nature of the illness and its associated weakness and fatigue frequently cause depression and resentment on the part of the usually vigorous, active teenager. It is important to spend time with the youngster to listen to his concerns and to allow him to express his feelings and vent his anger. The adolescent needs to be reassured that the limitations are only temporary and that social activities, so essential at this stage of development, can be resumed after the acute phase and that he will have sufficient autonomy to determine the extent of his capabilities and the rate of resumption of activities.

Health Problems Related to Sports Participation

Adolescents probably spend more time and energy practicing and participating in sports activities than members of any other age-group. The practice of sports and games contributes significantly to growth and development, to the education process, and to better health. It provides exercise for growing muscles, interactions with peers, and a socially

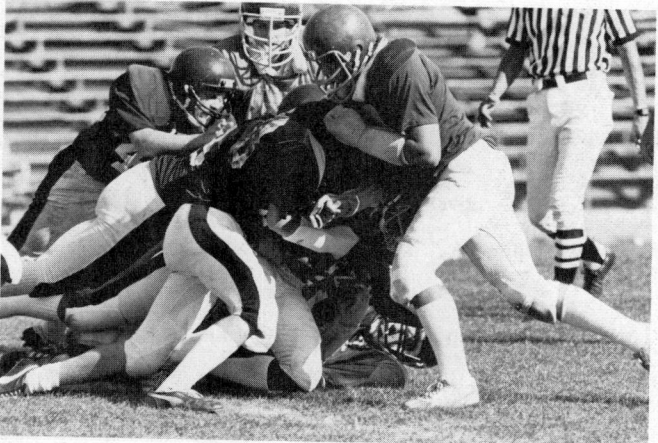

Fig. 20-2. Football is an example of a strenuous collision sport. Photography by Garibaldi, San Lorenzo, CA.

acceptable means to enjoy stimulation and conflict. In addition, competitive activities help the teenager in the process of self-appraisal, development of self-respect, and concern for others.

Every sport has some potential for injury to the participant—whether the youngster engages in serious competition or participates for pure enjoyment. Serious injury is not limited to the athlete who competes in rough contact sports; a large number of severe or fatal injuries occur to persons who are not physically prepared for the activity. For example, a body build may not be suited to the sport, muscles and support systems (respiratory and cardiovascular) may not have not been sufficiently conditioned to withstand the rigors of the physical stress, or a youngster may not possess insight and judgment to recognize when an activity is beyond his capabilities. Rapidly growing bones, muscles, joints, and tendons are especially vulnerable to unusual strain.

The awkward and inexperienced youngster suffers more injury than the more skilled and experienced one; strong muscles are less easily damaged than weak ones and will provide better protection to the joints they cross, and fatigue significantly impairs muscle function and judgment. More injuries occur during recreational sports participation than in organized athletic competition. The increase in strength and vigor in adolescence may tempt youngsters to overextend themselves, especially boys who are egged on by teammates or are stimulated by the admiration of female observers.

Not only does the activity itself pose a hazard of greater or lesser degree (Fig. 20-2), but the environment and the sports or recreational equipment present additional risks. Adolescents participate in physical activity in a variety of environments, both indoors and outdoors, on floors, on the ground, on snow, on or beneath water surfaces, and sometimes in free air space. These activities frequently involve equipment that intensifies the risk factor. (See box, p. 844, and Fig. 20-3.)

CLASSIFICATION OF SPORTS

Strenuous
Collision
Football
Ice hockey
Lacrosse (boys)
Rugby
Wrestling
Diving

Contact
Team basketball
Basketball
Field hockey
Lacrosse (girls)
Soccer
Team volleyball

Noncontact
Crew
Cross-country
Fencing
Gymnastics
Skiing
Competitive swimming
Tennis
Track and field
Water polo
Weight lifting
Cycling

Moderately strenuous
Contact
Baseball
Recreational basketball
Recreational volleyball

Noncontact
Tournament golf
Noncompetitive swimming
Badminton
Table tennis
Curling

Minimally strenuous
Archery
Riflery
Bowling
Recreational swimming
Recreational golf

From Micheli, L.J., and Yost, J.G.: Preparticipation evaluation and first aid for sports. In Micheli, L.J., editor: Pediatric and adolescent sports medicine, Boston, 1984, Little, Brown & Co., p. 40, and Smith, N.J.: Checkout for the would-be athlete, Emerg. Med. **12**:65-79, 1980.

PREPARATION FOR SPORTS

The degree of physical maturation varies greatly among adolescents of the same age, and many of the physical characteristics important in sports are related to hormone production. Consequently physical strength, coordination, endurance, and size vary considerably among adolescents who wish to compete against each other. Sports competition between young people who differ markedly in strength and agility is unfair and hazardous. Matching of candidates for sports should be made relative to physical maturity, height, weight, and physical fitness and skills, particularly in a sport involving rigorous body contact. Age is a less important consideration.

The role of health professionals in relation to sports injuries is directed toward prevention, treatment, and rehabilitation. Of these, the area of prevention is perhaps the most important. To this end, those youth who are actively involved in athletic programs need medical evaluation as a prerequisite to participation; education in sports skills with correct training and conditioning methods; omission of those tactics that are dangerous beyond the ordinary risk associated with the specific sport; use of appropriate protective equipment, properly maintained and suited to the individual; and an environment with maximum provision for safety and availability of first-aid and medical services.

The same protective principles apply to noncompetitive sports enthusiasts. They need the same education in basic safety precautions, encouragement to acquire proper instruction in the skills required for performance of the activity (instruction in water safety, skiing techniques, and so on), and proper maintenance of equipment.

TYPES OF INJURY

The injuries sustained in sports or recreational activities can involve any part of the body and extend from relatively minor cuts, bruises, and abrasions to totally incapacitating central nervous system injuries or death. Some of these injuries are discussed in chapters devoted to the major topic, for example, fractures and spinal cord injuries (Chapter 40), and head injuries (Chapter 37).

There are some sports that are particularly dangerous for children. The Academy of Pediatrics (Committee on Accident and Poison Prevention, 1977) issued a statement calling for a ban on the use of trampolines in schools because

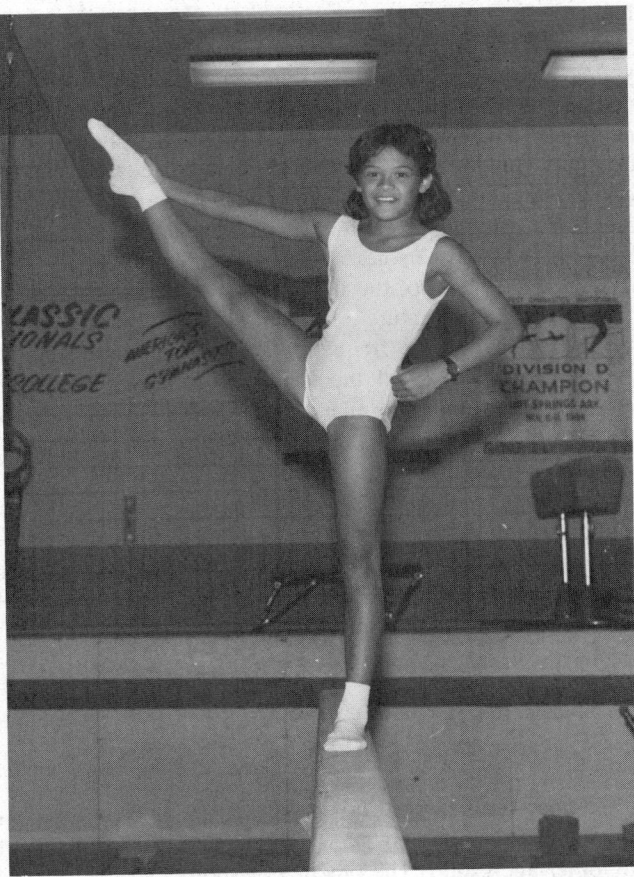

Fig. 20-3. Gymnastics is an example of a strenuous noncontact sport.

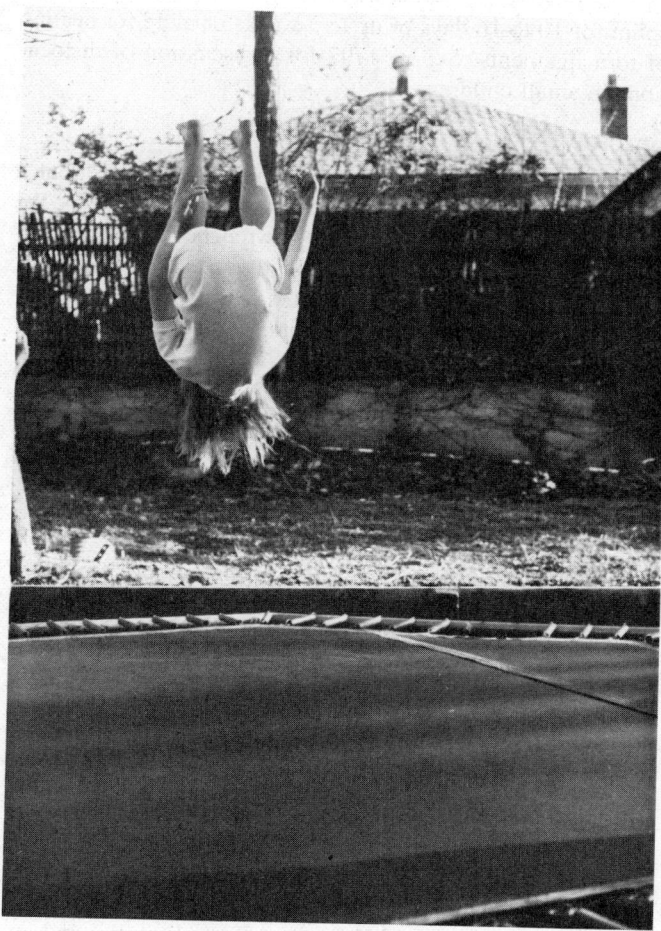

Fig. 20-4. Trampolines are not recommended for home or recreation use.
Photography by Earl Fillmore, Salt Lake City, UT.

of the high incidence of quadriplegic injuries caused by the apparatus but has since modified the statement to allow some controlled use (Committee on Accident and Poison Prevention and Committee on Pediatric Aspects of Physical Fitness, Recreation, and Sports, 1981). However, the Academy states that trampolines should not be part of a physical education program or competitive sports and they should *never* be used in home or recreational settings (Fig. 20-4). The Academy also opposes boxing in any sports program for *any* child or young adult (Committee on Sports Medicine, 1984). The "accumulated destructive effects of repeated blows even when consciousness and posture are not lost are well known and accepted" (Van Allen, 1983).

A variety of injuries can result when an external force is exerted with severe stress on tissue, muscle, and skeletal structures. The body structures attempt to accommodate the force, but when they are unable to do so, injuries occur. Two general types of injury are recognized: (1) *acute overload*, which includes injuries such as dislocations, sprains, and muscle pulls, and (2) *chronic overload (overuse syn-*

drome), which includes stress fractures, tendinitis, bursitis, and fasciculitis. More than 95% of sports injuries involve the soft tissues, not the bony skeleton. About two thirds of these consist of strains and sprains, and most injuries involve the extremities (Committee on Sports Medicine, 1983).

ACUTE INJURIES

Acute overload injuries are those that occur suddenly during an activity and produce immediate symptoms. They can be caused by a blow or overstretching, twisting, or otherwise causing a sudden stress to tissues (Fig. 20-5).

Contusions

Contusions are probably the most common of sports injuries and often considered to be "part of the game." A contusion is damage to the soft tissue, subcutaneous structures, and muscle. The tearing of these tissues and small blood vessels and the inflammatory response lead to hemorrhage, edema, and associated pain when the youngster attempts to move the injured part. The escape of blood into the tissues will be observed as *ecchymosis,* a black and blue discoloration.

The most serious contusions are those involving the quadriceps and are common in strenuous, collision-type sports, usually as a result of getting kicked or "kneed" in

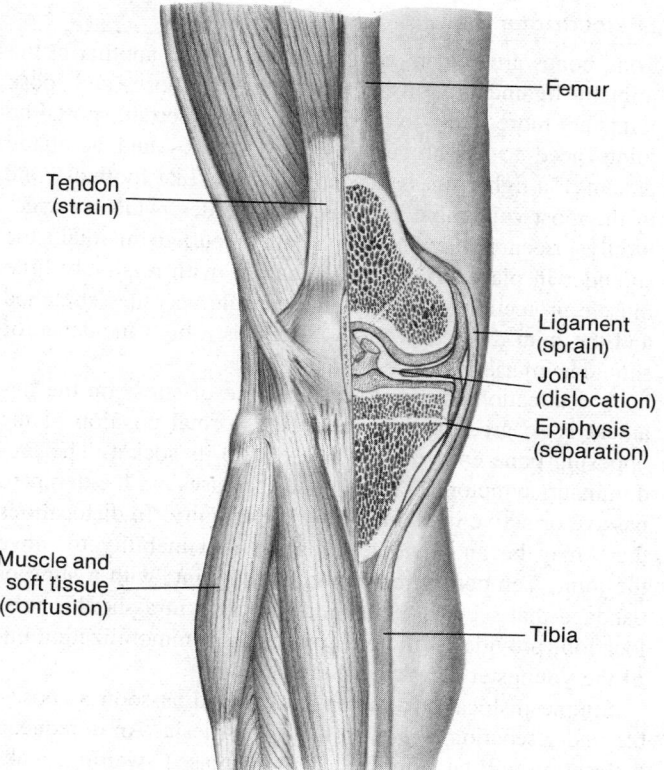

Fig. 20-5. Sites of injuries to bones, joints, and soft tissues.

the thigh. Large contusions cause gross swelling, pain, and disability and usually receive immediate attention from health personnel. The less spectacular smaller injuries may go unnoticed, allowing continued participation. However, they can become disabling after rest because of pain and muscle spasm. The young athlete is frequently instructed to work it out or disregard the pain. Unfortunately, this can result in myositis ossificans, which requires a lengthy recovery.

Immediate treatment consists of cold application as in the treatment of sprains described on p. 847. Return to participation is allowed when the strength and range of motion of the affected extremity are equal to those of the opposite extremity.

Although not always directly related to sports, crush injuries occur in children when they slam their fingers (in doors, folding chairs, or equipment) or hit their fingers (as when hammering a nail). A severe crush injury involves the bone, with swelling and bleeding beneath the nail (subungual) and sometimes laceration of the pulp of the distal phalanx. The subungual hematoma can be released by drilling holes at the proximal end of the nail. The time-honored method of applying a heated paper clip or needle to melt the nail is highly effective and causes few problems. However, any procedure should be performed with aseptic technique. If the bone is fractured, any communication with the skin essentially renders it an open fracture.

Dislocations

Long bones are held in approximation to one another at the joint by ligaments. Joints can be tight or loose, and loose joints are more likely to be dislocated. For certain sports the joints need to be limber (e.g., gymnastics and acrobatic dancing); a tight joint is needed for sports like football. One of the most vulnerable joints is the shoulder, which is structurally insecure, having only a rotator cuff to maintain the shoulder in place. The joint is shallow with relatively little muscle protection; therefore, the capsule becomes stretched and the joint dislocates easily. There is a high incidence of shoulder injuries in male gymnasts.

A dislocation occurs when the force of stress on the ligament is so great as to displace the normal position of the opposing bone ends or the bone end to its socket. The predominant symptom is pain that increases with attempted passive or active movement of the extremity. In dislocations there may be an obvious deformity and inability to move the joint. Temporary restriction of the joint, with a sling or bandage that secures the arm to the chest in a shoulder dislocation, provides sufficient comfort and immobilization until the youngster can receive medical help.

Simple dislocations should be reduced as soon as possible under sedation and often local anesthesia. An unreduced dislocation will be complicated by increased swelling, making reduction difficult and increasing the risk of neurovascular problems. Reduction is accomplished by simple traction and slight flexion followed by immobilization in a splint for 10 to 16 days or up to 3 weeks or more for healing of torn ligaments. See p. 1797 for a discussion of dislocations in small children.

Sprains

A sprain occurs when trauma to a joint is so severe that a ligament is partially or completely torn or stretched by the force created as a joint is twisted or wrenched, often accompanied by damage to associated blood vessels, muscles, tendons, and nerves. As a guideline for management and prognosis, sprains are classified according to degree of injury:

Grade I: mild injury; involves overstretching or microscopic tearing but without hemorrhage or increased instability of the involved joint. Swelling may develop later.

Grade II: moderate injury; involves partial, overt tearing of the ligament with at least some ligamentous continuity remaining; usually immediate pain and swelling with decreased function.

Grade III: severe injury; total loss of ligamentous continuity, that is, disruption of one or more ligaments or the musculotendinous unit. Pain is immediate but subsides because none of the pain fibers are being stretched. Swelling may be minimal because hemorrhage extravasates outside of the area into soft tissues.

The presence of laxity of the joint is the most valid indicator of the severity of a sprain. In a severe injury the athlete complains of the joint "feeling loose" or as if "something is coming apart" and may describe hearing a "snap," "pop," or "tearing." Pain is seldom the principal subjective symptom. There is a rapid onset with swelling, often diffuse, accompanied by immediate disability and appreciable reluctance to use the injured joint.

Strains

A strain is a microscopic tear to the musculotendinous unit and has features in common with sprains. The area is painful to touch and swollen. The severity is evaluated in Grades I, II, and III except that the degree of laxity does not apply. Even with severe Grade III injuries complaints of laxity are rare. Most strains are incurred over time rather than suddenly, and the rapidity of the appearance provides clues regarding severity. In general, the more rapidly the strain occurs, the more severe the injury. When the strain involves the muscular portion, there is more bleeding, often palpable soon after injury and before edema obscures the hematoma.

Therapeutic Management

The first 6 to 12 hours is the most critical period for virtually all soft tissue injuries. Basic principles of managing sprains and other soft tissue injuries are summarized in the acronyms RICE or ICES:

R—rest	I—ice
I—ice	C—compression
C—compression	E—elevation
E—elevation	S—support

Soft tissue injuries should be iced immediately. This is best accomplished with crushed ice wrapped in a towel or encased in a screw-top ice bag or plastic bag (for example, a Ziploc* storage bag). Although the initial application remains in place only 30 minutes, the effects last up to 7 hours.

A wet elastic wrap is applied to provide compression and to keep the ice pack in place. A single layer of the wrap is placed over the injured area to protect the skin under the ice pack, and the remainder of the bandage secures the pack in place. The wet wrap transfers the cold better than a dry wrap (Committee on Sports Medicine, 1983). Some athletic trainers keep wet elastic wraps refrigerated for ready use. There is still controversy regarding the use of heat or ice during the rehabilitative phase of management. Regardless of the method used, it is accompanied by appropriate exercise, depending on the severity of the injury and carried out under the direction of a competent professional experienced in care of sports injuries.

Ice has a rapid cooling effect on tissues that reduces the pain threshold and the magnitude of the stretch reflex by decreasing muscle spindle response, afferent nerve discharge, and the afferent loop response (monosynaptic reflex). Secondary effects are achieved by vasoconstriction, slowing muscle nerve velocity, and increasing muscle viscosity. Also, the decreased temperature slows metabolism, and edema formation is reduced when less histamine-like substances are released. Following 9 to 15 minutes of ice exposure produces a deep-tissue vasodilation without increased metabolism (Hocutt, 1978).

Major sprains or tears to the ligamentous tissue rarely occur in growing children. Ligaments are stronger than bone, and the epiphysis and growth plate are the weakest areas of the bone; therefore the more usual sites of injury are at the growth plate (see Fractures, Chapter 40). Torn ligaments, especially those in the knee, are usually treated by immobilization with a cast for 3 to 4 weeks or strapping of the joint with adhesive or Elastoplast bandage. Passive leg exercises, gradually increased to active ones, are begun as soon as sufficient healing has taken place. Parents and adolescents should be cautioned against using any form of liniment or other heat-producing preparation before examination. If the injury requires casting or splinting, the heat generated in the enclosed space can cause extreme discomfort and may even cause tissue damage.

OVERUSE SYNDROMES

To excel in sports the young athlete is forced to train longer, harder, and earlier in life than previously. The rewards are increased level of fitness, better performances, faster times, and the satisfaction of attaining a personal goal. However, the risk of overuse injury is always present and can be related to several factors: training errors, muscle-tendon imbalance, anatomic malalignment (that is, femoral antever-

sion, excessive lumbar lordosis, or tibial torsion), incorrect footwear or playing surface, an associated disease state, and growth (growth cartilage is less resistant to microtrauma).

The common feature in overuse injuries is the repetitive microtrauma that occurs to a particular anatomic structure. Performing the same movements time and again sometimes causes several types of injury: (1) frictional—rubbing of one structure against another, (2) tractional—repeated pull on a ligament or tendon, or (3) cyclic loading of impact forces (stress fractures). The end result is inflammation of the involved structure with complaints of pain, tenderness, swelling, and disability (Harvey, 1982).

Bursae, tendons, muscles, ligaments, joints, and bones are all subject to overuse. Some of the common overuse syndromes are briefly outlined in Table 20-1. Plantar fasciitis is very common in athletes, and Osgood-Schlatter disease is seen in children who do a lot of jumping.

Stress Fractures

With intensity and duration of training many young athletes suffer stress fractures, especially after a recent increase in training regimens. They occur as a result of repeated muscle contraction and are seen most often in repetitive weight-bearing sports such as running, gymnastics, and basketball. They occur less often in swimmers (upper extremity). The sites in order of frequency are the tibia (50%), metatarsals (18%), fibula (12%), femur (6%), and other (less than 1%) (Orava, 1980).

The most common symptoms of stress fracture are a sharp, persistent, progressive pain or a deep, persistent dull ache located over the bone. Sometimes there is pain on impact (heel strike), but the most important clinical sign is pain over the involved bony surface. Diagnosis is established on the basis of clinical observation. Occasionally a bone scan may be needed.

Therapeutic Management

Development of inflammation is common to all overuse syndromes; therefore the management is directed toward rest or alteration of activities, physical therapies, and medication. Rest is the primary therapy, usually interpreted as reduced activity and use of alternative exercise—*not* bed rest or immobilization with casting. The primary purpose is to alleviate the repetitive stress that initiated the symptoms. It is important to keep the youngster mobile, and training can be continued. Alternative exercise is selected that maintains conditioning without aggravating the injury. For example, pool running (treading water in the deep end of a pool) can use the same movements as running but without the weight-bearing; bicycling, swimming, and rowing are viable alternatives (Harvey, 1982).

Other modalities include cryotherapy and cold whirlpools, and sometimes taping, bracing, splinting, and other orthotics are employed, very specific to the injury. Medications, such as aspirin or nonsteroidal anti-inflammatory drugs, such as tolmetin (the only one recommended for chil-

---

*Dow Chemical Company, Indianapolis, IN 46268.

Table 20-1 Selected overuse injuries

DISORDER	CAUSE	MANIFESTATIONS
Plantar fasciitis	Repetitive stretching of the plantar fascia (calcaneus to metatarsal heads)	Pain in arch or heel
Achilles tendinitis	Repeated forcible traction on short tendon	Pain on palpation; pain with plantar flexion against resistance
Severs disease	Epiphysitis of the calcaneus	Pain over insertion of Achilles tendon into tip of calcaneus
Anterior leg pain ("shin splints")	Irritation of posterior tibial muscle in unconditioned athlete or one not conditioned to a new sport	Pain in leg along anterior or medial edge of midshaft or distal third of tibia
Osgood-Schlatter disease	Traction apophysitis of tibial tubercle	Pain and tenderness; overprominence of involved tubercle
Sinding-Larsen syndrome ("jumper's knee")	A variant of Osgood-Schlatter disease; traction apophysitis on inferior pole of patella	Same as above; pain slightly lower than Osgood-Schlatter
Patellofemoral syndromes	Malalignment of extensors, increased patellar compression, and increased training intensity	Chronic knee pain, especially following forced leg extension from flexion or after running
"Tennis elbow"	Lateral epicondylitis from repetitive strain on elbow	Pain in elbow, aggravated by use
"Little League elbow"	Osteochondritis of the capitellum; tendinitis of flexor origin medial epicondyle from repetitive valgus strain to elbow from throwing	Pain in elbow that increases with activity
"Little League shoulder"	Microfracture of proximal humeral growth plate from repetitive throwing	Pain and characteristic contracture; loss of internal rotation and increased external rotation
"Swimmer's shoulder"	Supraspinatus tendinitis from repetitive shoulder movement	Pain in shoulder that increases with activity

dren), are sometimes prescribed for discomfort. Topical medications are of questionable value.

UNDERWATER SPORTS–RELATED INJURIES

Children who venture into water at least waist deep generally start to play underwater. It is not unusual for children to be able to swim underwater before they are able to swim on the surface. The injuries that are sustained from diving or swimming underwater are serious and deserve brief mention. Near drowning is primarily a respiratory and neurologic problem and is discussed in Chapter 37; the major injury from diving or surfing is damage to the cervical spine (see spinal cord injury, Chapter 40).

Male teenagers are typical victims of shallow-water blackout when they attempt to swim long distances (several lengths of the pool) underwater. Before entering the water the youngster hyperventilates, reducing carbon dioxide to very low levels and thus decreasing the need to breathe. However, this action reduces respiratory stimulation from carbon dioxide accumulation and stretch receptors in the lung. The physical activity of swimming consumes the existing oxygen supply before the Pco_2 level rises sufficiently high to stimulate breathing. Consequently the Po_2 reaches a dangerous level before the respiratory center is stimulated,

resulting in hypoxia and unconsciousness. Unfortunately, hyperventilation does not significantly increase the body's stores of oxygen—mainly stored in arterial hemoglobin and already saturated in normal individuals (Strauss, 1982).

In addition, breath holding with hyperinflated lungs (Valsalva maneuver) causes further decrease in oxygen to the brain. The cerebral hypoxia causes the youngster to lose consciousness before there is the desire to surface for air. Often these youngsters are found at the bottom of a lake or pool. The result is drowning unless the youngster is rescued quickly. Similarly, persons who engage in breath holding while diving in deep water suffer hypoxia as a result of decreasing Po_2 as they ascend from the depths. These are usually older (and experienced) divers.

Other underwater sports injuries include ear squeeze that occurs when middle ear pressures are not equalized during diving, decompression sickness (the bends) and air emboli from too rapid decompression after deep dives, and nitrogen narcosis.

HEALTH CONCERNS ASSOCIATED WITH SPORTS

A number of health concerns that are related to sports activities may affect athletic performance and/or the physical well-being of the participant.

Nutrition

Most athletes are motivated to enhance their performance by any and all means available. They are eager to learn about nutrition, and many become subject to misconceptions, fads, and superstitions regarding certain foods. Physical performance is affected by energy and body composition. The young athlete must maintain a diet that provides sufficient nutrients and energy to meet metabolic needs for optimum functioning. Physical training increases the need for energy as well as for more nutrients that convert food energy into chemical energy for physical performance.

There is no evidence to indicate that food supplements, extra vitamins, or high-protein diets are needed to meet the demands of heavy physical exercise or improve physical performance. However, young athletes need considerably more calories than the recommended daily allowance. When the basic requirements for growth and activity are met by a balanced diet of protein, grains and cereals, fruits and vegetables, and dairy products, the additional calories needed for the extra exertion can be selected as desired. These extra caloric needs can be supplied by eating additional helpings from any of the basic four food groups, but many of the additional calories are provided by complex carbohydrates found in such foods as vegetables, pastas, and bread.

The basic diet will not satisfy the iron requirement of 10% to 15% of female athletes. The largest iron-deficient group are those teenage girls who may become iron depleted after the menarche. Young boys who are experiencing rapid adolescent growth and who are on irregular and inadequate diets also are at risk of iron depletion. These youngsters will need medicinal iron supplements (Smith, 1984).

Energy is derived primarily from glycogen previously stored in muscles and the liver. Energy for prolonged exercise is derived from high-carbohydrate food (such as bread, cereals, pancakes, potatoes, rice, and spaghetti) consumed 24 to 48 hours before the activity, not from a meal eaten just before the activity. The meal before a physical contest should be eaten at least 3 hours before the exertion and consist mainly of carbohydrates. Extra fluids and some added salt are advisable during hot weather; fluids and caloric drinks are allowed during the activity but do not contribute to energy. For more information regarding carbohydrate loading and other techniques for improving athletic performance the readers are directed to excellent texts on sports medicine and sports training.

Control of body weight by restriction of water intake, food restriction, or encouragement of sweat loss is dangerous, and these are highly undesirable means for meeting a minimum weight classification. Young athletes need to learn something about nutrition to dispel the allure of prevalent fads and fallacies about diet and performance (Narins, Belkengren, and Sapala, 1983). The optimum diet for an athlete is one that contains the essential food groups and that is adjusted to the energy requirements of the sport in which the youngster is engaged. Such a diet plan should provide adequate nutrition for top physical efficiency and performance, maintenance of physical fitness and desirable body weight, and optimum function of all organ systems (Lucas, 1981).

Exercise-Related Menstrual Dysfunction

Considerable interest has been generated regarding delayed or secondary amenorrhea associated with the physical stress of ballet dancing and some types of athletics, for example, running and gymnastics. The phenomenon has been attributed to a complex interplay of physical, genetic, hormonal, nutritional, psychologic, and environmental factors that include the stress of competition, decreased protein consumption, and altered lean-to-fat ratio.

Delayed menarche has been reported for girls who engage in strenuous exercise. Except for swimmers, menarche is attained later in athletes than in nonathletes. Gymnasts, figure skaters, and ballet dancers have the latest mean ages of menarche; track athletes have less of a delayed maturity than gymnasts and ballet dancers, who also tend to be smaller, lighter, and leaner than other female athletes. Swimmers, who tend to be larger, have a mean age of menarche that approximates that for nonathletes. Also there appears to be an association between delayed menarche and more advanced competitive levels, that is, athletes at the more advanced levels have a greater delay than those at lower competitive levels (Malina, Meleski, and Shoup, 1982).

It is not clear whether exercise delays menarche or menarcheal delay promotes athletic success. Some observers believe strenuous prepubertal activity delays menarche (Frische and others, 1981; Warren, 1980). It is also postulated that the delayed puberty promotes athletic success, which in turn encourages perseverance (Shangold and Mirkin, 1985). Also, the selection process for various sports may favor certain body types, for example, the smaller, more slender gymnasts (Malina, Meleski, and Shoup, 1982).

Some observers (Frische and McArthur, 1974; Diddle, 1983) attribute delayed menarche and maintenance of regular ovulation to lack of development of body fat with the subsequent effect on feedback mechanisms as the critical factor. These observations established that girls do not begin menses until at least 17% body fat content has been attained. This has been challenged by others who found no level of body fat that can be termed "critical" (Garn, LaVelle, and Pilkington, 1983).

Alterations in established menstrual bleeding patterns are often observed in girls who engage in strenuous exercise. The incidence varies with the type of exercise and the intensity of the exercise program. Circulating gonadotropins are decreased with exercise, but the association between strenuous exercise and menstrual irregularity is still puzzling (Ziporyn, 1984). Increased serum androgen levels have also been reported with intense exercise (Jurkowski and others, 1978). Other factors, including diet and stress, prevent the identification of any typical profile. Not all girls are affected, but the activities that appear to be associated with delayed or altered menstruation are ballet dancing, running, gymnastics, and competitive swimming.

There is consensus regarding a correlation between strenuous exercise and menstruation, although the exact roles played by the various factors have not been defined satisfactorily. No detrimental effects have been detected, and normal patterns are established spontaneously or upon cessation of exercise. A lower incidence of dysmenorrhea has been reported in girls who engage in vigorous exercise (Hale, 1983).

Drug Misuse by Athletes

Young athletes have used various substances in the attempt to augment their athletic performance. These substances, known as *ergogenic aids,* are believed by athletes to increase strength and endurance, delay onset of fatigue, increase the ability to concentrate, and decrease sensitivity to pain. Although use of these substances is prohibited in international Olympic competition, there are no means at present to enforce a prohibition on their use in other sports participation.

The principal drugs misused by athletes are the psychomotor stimulants (for example, amphetamines) and the anabolic steroids. Amphetamines and related drugs, such as methylphenidate (Ritalin) and phenmetrazine (Preludin), are taken to provide a sense of increased alertness and relief of fatigue; however, obscuring fatigue may permit participants to exceed their limits and precipitate a sudden collapse (Dyment, 1982). These drugs can also make the users more aggressive, which can contribute to injuries to themselves and others. Although use of amphetamines is declining, ingestion of caffeine and caffeine-related substances, readily available as cola drinks, tea, and coffee, is increasing (Committee on Sports Medicine, 1983).

Anabolic steroids, such as nandrolone phenpropionate (Durabolin) and methandrostenolone (Dianabol), are a source of concern to health professionals. In the attempt to enhance muscle strength these drugs are administered to athletes by coaches, managers, athletic trainers, and even physicians. The user develops larger-appearing muscles, increased body weight, and body water, but reports on the effectiveness in improving performance have been conflicting (Dyment, 1982). Although the psychologic effect may be beneficial, many valid studies have failed to demonstrate any improvement in performance (Committee on Sports Medicine, 1983).

The dangers of continued use are well known and include hypertension; virilization in females; oligospermia, testicular atrophy, infertility, and gynecomastia in males; and premature closure of the epiphyses, acne, increased blood cholesterol, and hepatocellular carcinoma in both sexes. These health hazards outweigh any potential gain that might be induced, and the American Academy of Pediatrics (1983) and the American College of Sports Medicine both condemn the use of anabolic steroids.

Other drugs that are often misused include nutritional aids, local anesthetic agents, beta blockers (to reduce circulating catecholamines and hence reduce anxiety related to somatic-type stress), and anti-inflammatory drugs, such as dimethylsulfoxide (DSMO) (which is not approved for use and is available only as a veterinary or an industrial preparation) and corticosteroids. The possibility of their use by the adolescent athlete should be considered when performing a health assessment.

Sudden Death

A death associated with sports produces renewed anxiety in both parents and health professionals. The term sudden, or instantaneous, death is applied to death that occurs within minutes of the onset of the cause of death, within an hour or within 24 hours of the episode. Sudden death occurs in three areas: (1) in those sports with a high inherent risk for sport-related sudden death; (2) in children with recognized or unknown underlying medical problems; and (3) in the sport environment (that is, the rules, equipment, practice fields or areas of sports participation, and the ambient temperature of the geographic area), which may be a contributing or causal factor (Luckstead, 1982).

Sports. Sports that create the greatest risk are those involving collision and frequent body contact. Examples of collision sports include football, ice hockey, rugby, and boxing. There is a high potential for serious injury or fatality in sports such as mountain or rock climbing and hang gliding. Sports that involve high velocity objects, such as baseball and ice hockey, may cause death as a result of serious head or chest injuries. Riding vehicles such as mopeds, minibikes, and motorcycles can be considered as sports.

Medical conditions. The most frequent medical causes of sudden death during sports activity are cardiac abnormalities, especially idiopathic hypertrophic subaortic stenosis (hypertrophic cardiomyopathy). Manifestations suggestive of hypertrophic cardiomyopathy include a typical triad of severe chest pain with dizziness, prominent pulses, and a murmur at the left lower sternal border. A history of sudden death of a relative, or relatives, in the second and third decade often offers a clue to recognition.

Well-trained athletes often display evidence of hypertrophic cardiomyopathy, the so-called athlete's heart, but the condition is not pathologic. Congenital heart problems are infrequent causes of sudden death in sports involving children and adolescents. Children with systemic hypertension, some types of cardiac arrhythmias, and some forms of heart block will require restrictions in the type and amount of exercise they can tolerate safely.

Environmental causes. Environmental factors that are potential causes of death include playing conditions, clothing, equipment, rules used by officials governing a sport, and outdoor temperature. Heat stroke and hypothermia are probably the most serious uncontrollable environmental causes of death in athletes.

NURSE'S ROLE IN CHILDREN'S SPORTS

Nurses may become involved in sports activities in the areas of preparation and evaluation for activities, prevention of injury, treatment of injuries, and rehabilitation after injury. Selecting an appropriate sport for both recreation and competition is a joint effort of youngster, parents, and health professionals. Children are introduced to sports as part of family activities, neighborhood games, and school physical education programs, and both parents and children are influenced by media exposure to a variety of sports. Children are highly influenced by the popularity and exposure afforded athletics in the school setting, especially in high school.

The Academy of Pediatrics has established guidelines for programs in elementary school (Committee on Pediatric Aspects of Physical Fitness, Recreation, and Sports, 1981) and for sports for children of all ages (Committee on Sports Medicine, 1983). Nurses who work with children involved in sports activities should be aware of the recommendations regarding children's athletics and understand some of the motivating factors, developmental characteristics of children, and pressures for participation.

The best approach to counseling children and parents regarding sports participation is to encourage activities that are most likely to provide pleasure and physical benefits throughout childhood into adulthood. Exposure to a variety of sports activities is probably better for young children than limiting them to only one sport. Parents should be cautioned against overprogramming children in order that the children have ample time for other activities and associations.

Nurses are sometimes members of a sports medicine team, although the training and rehabilitation are usually managed by certified sports trainers and other specialists in sports medicine. Nurses should be able to provide emergency treatment for any type of injury and know when to refer the injured child for evaluation and care. Sports injuries can occur in free play as well as in organized athletic programs, and a school nurse is often the first person who attends an injured child.

When children sustain athletic injuries, nurses are often responsible for instructing the children and their parents regarding care. Instructions, such as schedule for appointments, application of ice, and any restrictions in activity, should be made clear, preferably accompanied by written directions. The importance of taking medications as prescribed is emphasized, since they may be needed for an extended period of time and compliance may be difficult. For children continuing with activities, drug administration an hour before practice or competition is advantageous.

Prevention of sports injuries is probably the most important aspect of any athletic program. The children should be suited to the activity, the environment and equipment made safe for physical activity, and the children adequately prepared for the sports, especially those requiring strenuous and/or continuous physical exertion. Nurses collaborate with coaches and athletic trainers to ensure that safety measures are carried out. Stretching exercises, warming up and cool-

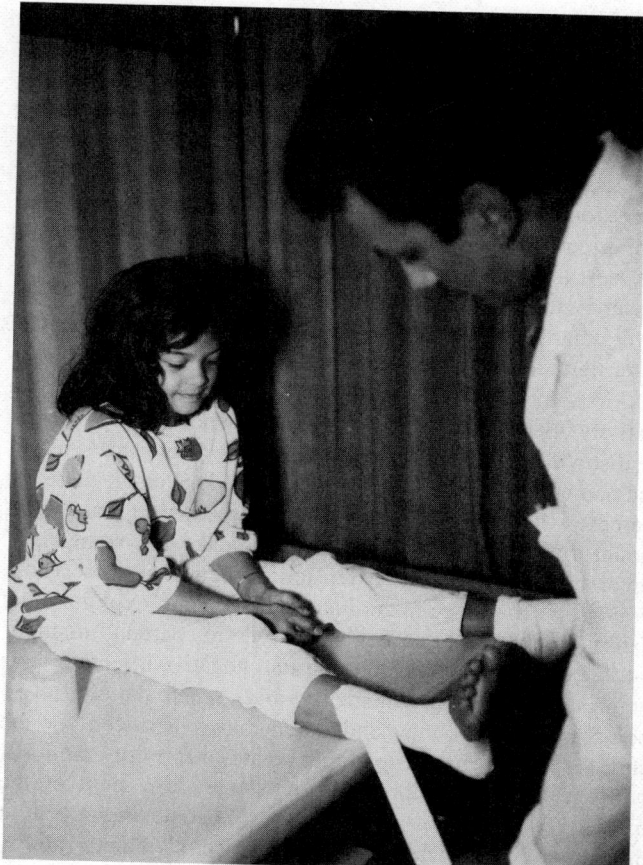

Fig. 20-6. Competent care is essential to prevention of sports injury.

ing down activities, and an appropriate training program are only some of the requisites for safe participation. Protective measures, such as pads, taping, wrapping, or other devices, are employed for areas at risk (Fig. 20-6). Nurses are also on the alert for environmental safety risks.

Parental Pressure

There is a lot of peer and parental pressure to participate in sports, and many children are not enthusiastic. There is much fear of failure related to the pressure to be like friends or parents. When children need medical attention because of repeated injuries, disinterest should be suspected and investigated. It is best to interview the child without the parents so he will feel free to discuss his feelings without undue influence. Alternative sports or other means for gaining self-esteem and regard from parents and peers can be explored and encouraged for children not interested in or suited for athletic competition.

Attrition and exercise aversion are sometimes the aftermath of declining interest in sports after participation during the school years and adolescence. Motivation can be altered or permanently destroyed by failure to appreciate youngsters' needs related to sports activities. Ridicule or derogation during acquisition of motor skills can shatter a youngster's self-esteem, producing anxiety and self-doubt that may result in a lifelong aversion to sports. Every child should have the opportunity to develop a strong sense of personal worth through the process of motor learning and acquisition of skills (Ogilvie, 1982).

Coaches and parents are both guilty of exploiting youngsters for their own purposes. Although the positive aspects are important and inherent in sports activities, nurses should be alert to some parental behaviors and motivations that interfere with a youngster's enjoyment of the activities. However, many parents are notoriously resistant to the idea of altering their behavior.

First, there are parents who are unwilling to allow the activity to remain child-oriented and who often place unrealistic demands on the child. Both the youngster's physical and emotional age must be considered. Second, there are parents who are unable to maintain the appropriate emotional distance from the activity and make the youngsters' involvement in sports an extension of their own egos. These youngsters may recognize that they are being exploited and exhibit extreme forms of rebellion. Third, parents' manipulative behaviors can have a profound negative effect on their youngsters. Guilt-producing verbal manipulation (e.g., pointing out what they and others have sacrificed for the child) is a powerful weapon that creates a form of emotional bondage. Fourth, there are parents who lose sight of the meaning of the sport because they become entrapped in dreams and fantasies that their youngsters' athletic ability can become a passport to status and economic freedom (Ogilvie, 1982).

The pressures that some parents impose on their children negate most of the psychologic values, such as fun, emotional release, and learning to relate effectively with peers. Winning becomes more important than playing. Overemphasis on sports has the potential for interfering with the emotional and social growth of a child, especially when ego integration is tied to recognition and reward through such a narrow range of personal characteristics. Ego vulnerability is great in youngsters whose identity, self-esteem, and feelings of self-worth depend entirely on the psychologic and social rewards of athletic achievement.

Alterations in Growth and Maturation

The absence of sexual maturation at a time when other children are experiencing positive evidence of sexual development and its associated spurt in growth and physical strength is a matter of concern to both parents and affected child. In most instances the slow growth is a simple physiologic or constitutional delay that merely represents one end of the normal genetically influenced variation of pubertal growth. These children will go through normal puberty in their late teens and catch up with their more rapidly developing age-mates. However, this becomes a psychosocial problem for some young people.

Less benign is delayed development caused by endocrine disorders or chromosomal aberrations. In other situations delayed development may be a result of malnutrition or chronic diseases that are serious enough to retard the developmental process, such as malabsorption, chronic asthma, and poorly controlled diabetes mellitus.

ASSESSMENT

Serial measurements of growth are plotted periodically on standard growth charts to determine the pattern of growth and to compare the individual child with the norm for that particular age-group. When assessing children in the extremes of height ranges, it is important to compare their height with the height of their parents and siblings. As a whole, children usually can be categorized into one of the following six groups according to their pattern of maturation:

1. Average children—closely approximate the mean for height and weight at all ages
2. Early-maturing children—tall in childhood but not unusually tall adults
3. Early-maturing children who are also genetically tall—above the mean at all ages
4. Late-maturing children—shorter than average in childhood but not necessarily short adults
5. Late-maturing children who are also genetically short—below the mean at all ages
6. Children who deviate significantly from the normal growth curve—very rapid- and early-maturing children; much later- and slower-maturing children

Diagnostic Evaluation

Clinical diagnosis of delayed development can usually be determined with relative ease on the basis of the following simple criteria.

Family history. Parents and/or other relatives often have a history of a similar type of delayed growth and maturation. Height and weight of siblings at comparable ages and their present measurements are helpful.

Child's history. Prenatal and birth history will reveal whether or not the child's height and weight were appropriate for gestational age, and a pregnancy history might reveal factors that could have influenced a deviation from normal. Concurrent chronic diseases influence growth, and past illnesses such as head injuries and gastrointestinal, renal, or neurologic disorders may provide clues for the examiner.

History of the child's dietary habits, strength, stamina, and susceptibility to infection are investigated as well as attainment of developmental milestones and school progress. Any emotional problems or problems of social adjustment are considered, especially those that may indicate past family instability. It is well known that prolonged emotional upset has a significant influence on growth.

Previous growth pattern. If the growth rate is known, it is often found that it has decreased during the second year of life or just before puberty or that the child has remained relatively small throughout the growth period with a growth curve that is parallel or slightly below the third percentile. If records are not available, information can be obtained regarding when it was first noticed that the child was small compared to other children.

Physical examination. Accurate measurements of height and weight are taken with the child stripped to underclothing. This may also include measurements of body proportions from crown to pubis and pubis to heel to detect any abnormality of body proportion. Signs of sexual development are noted using standard criteria (p. 807). The first evidence of puberty is breast budding in girls and testicular enlargement (testicular volume greater than 2 ml) in boys. If these signs are present, normal sexual development can be expected to follow in 1 to 2 years.

Bone age. Bone age, assessed from wrist x-ray films, is always delayed in these children.

Endocrine studies. Hormonal investigations reveal essentially normal results. Growth hormone (GH) responses, gonadotropin levels, and responses to gonadotropin-releasing factor (GnRF) are usually low for the child's chronologic age but consistent with his bone age. The same is true for the plasma levels of testosterone and estrogen and urinary excretion of 17-ketosteroids. In addition, as these children mature, they have a corresponding change in endocrine response consistent with normal pubertal changes.

SHORT STATURE

Short stature is a nonspecific finding that may be the first manifestation of a serious disorder, or it may be of no consequence medically. It is often the reason an adolescent is brought to the attention of health professionals and is the most common presenting complaint in endocrine clinics. Although it occurs with equal frequency in girls and boys, the problem is more distressful to boys than to girls. Therefore it is boys who more often seek assistance. Since the psychosocial factors are of importance and there are rare situations in which delayed development is caused by a pathogenic condition, it is important to determine the reason for the short stature.

In most instances the cause of short stature is either *familial short stature* or a simple *constitutional growth delay* in which the child appears to be delayed because development is behind that of age-mates. Familial short stature refers to otherwise healthy children who have ancestors with adult height in the lower percentiles, and whose height during childhood is appropriate for genetic background.

Constitutional growth delay refers to individuals (usually boys) with delayed linear growth, in whom commensurate delays in skeletal and sexual maturation suggest that they will reach normal adult height (Ad Hoc Committee on Growth Hormone Usage, The Lawson Wilkins Pediatric Endocrine Society, and Committee on Drugs, 1983). Often there is a history of a similar pattern of growth in one of the parents or other family members of children with constitutional growth delay. The untreated child will proceed through normal changes as expected on the basis of bone age. These changes, although occurring later than in the average child, will appear in normal sequence and manner, and treatment is not usually indicated.

Therapeutic Management

Management consists of continued medical observation, attention to general health and nutrition, and psychologic support. Further assurance can be provided by predicting the youngster's adult height from available tables and other criteria devised from comprehensive studies of child development. Very often the longer a youngster takes to pass through puberty, the better are the prospects for achieving an acceptable adult height, since epiphyseal fusion is more advanced in youngsters who mature earlier.

Most youngsters can be managed with detailed explanation, reassurance, and observation. Unlike growth hormone–deficient children, who do not usually demonstrate

Questions and Controversies

Should children without growth pathology be given growth hormone in an attempt to increase their eventual height?

The approval and availability of a biologically active human growth hormone produced by recombinant-DNA technology has dramatically changed the therapeutic prospects for children with short stature. It has been shown to be effective in facilitating growth in selected cases with no growth hormone failure (Van Vliet and others, 1983; Gertner and others, 1984) (see discussion). It is still not certain precisely which children will benefit from therapy, and the probability of side effects has yet to be thoroughly evaluated.

The Ad Hoc Committee on Growth Hormone Usage, The Lawson Wilkins Pediatric Endocrine Society, and Committee on Drugs (1983) investigated the therapeutic use of growth hormone. Side effects that can occur include formation of antibodies to growth hormone with possible attenuation of growth, hypothyroidism, insulin resistance, hyperinsulinism, and hypertension. Their recommendation is that the only established indication for use of growth hormone is in growth hormone–deficient children. There is still too little experience with the substance to use it indiscriminately.

The multiple questions that arise from the possibilities of accelerating growth will affect health professionals:
1. Should the growth hormone be given to children with familiar short stature in the attempt to gain a height in excess of the expected height?
2. Should it be given to young athletes with normal height in whom additional height might be potentially advantageous (e.g., outstanding basketball players)?
3. Should it be routine treatment for constitutional delay?
4. Will treatment produce a better adjusted adult?
5. Should health professionals be swayed by parental pressures to administer growth hormone?

maladjustment, children with constitutional delay often display characteristic behavioral difficulties (Gordon and others, 1982). Where the growth delay is accompanied by poor self-esteem and incompetence, the psychosocial situation is such that for the youngster (usually a boy) miserable as a result of peer ridicule and indignities, hormonal therapy in addition to psychologic support has proved to be advantageous, and many authorities recommend treatment in these instances.

In a well-known study hormonal therapy was undertaken with caution and consisted of 4 doses of testosterone. A larger number of doses affect epiphyseal closure. The criteria used to identify candidates for treatment are very precise. Treated youngsters were at least 14 years of age, had a height below the fifth percentile, were clearly prepubertal, and displayed significant evidence of poor self-image. The treatment usually resulted in excellent growth, a significant improvement in self-image adjustment, and a dramatic increase in both school-related and extraschool social activity (Rosenfeld, Northcraft, and Hintz, 1982).

Thyroid hormone is of no value unless hypothyroidism is present; and human growth hormone, although capable of increasing height, is expensive, in short supply, and confined to the treatment of growth hormone deficiency (see Chapter 38). With the availability of synthetic growth hormone produced from recombinant DNA technology, the treatment may become commonplace for children of short stature who may require larger amounts of hormone than normally produced or who produce hormone with abnormal structure. The dangers of therapy are a possible diabetogenic effect and overuse in the treatment of short stature. There may be pressures from parents who want their children to be taller than they are genetically constituted. (See Questions and controversies, p. 853.)

Nursing Considerations

Deviation from the normal course of puberty is always of concern to affected adolescents, and to some it assumes monumental proportions. This distress is often so intense that the youngsters hesitate to voice their concerns for fear that their worries and doubts will be confirmed. Nurses, especially school nurses, working with adolescents encounter young people who are delayed in development or who are destined to be shorter in stature than their average age-mates.

Most of the problems of delayed development are those caused by simple constitutional delay of puberty, and in this situation the child can be assured that the normal course of events will eventually take place. This is not always reassuring to such children. They are impatient to grow and are not easily convinced. Even after direct and thorough discussion of growth and the normal variations in rate and timing of maturation, they often doubt that they will grow. It is important to maintain contact with these children, convey to them a concern about their feelings, and let them know that they are accepted as they are.

Those young people who cannot be assured that they will eventually achieve more than a minimum height will need even more acceptance and support. The suffering is especially acute in young boys who may have hoped for success in athletics or those who may have been hurt by thoughtless remarks of their more fortunate associates. They need to know that they have a sympathetic listener who understands their anguish and who can help them develop their potential in areas that do not demand size in order that they will find recognition and acceptance and acquire self-confidence and self-esteem.

One of the difficulties related to a size that is incongruent with chronologic and mental age is the manner in which others, especially adults, relate to the child. People quite naturally respond to children with short stature as though they are younger than their age. Consequently these children often react with babyish or juvenile behavior, thus setting in motion a circular pattern of behavior and response. Conversely, children who are tall or physically advanced for their age are treated as though they are more advanced than their years. They are often considered to be retarded or behaviorally immature when they actually perform according to the normal behavioral expectations for their age.

Listening to distressed adolescents and conveying to them genuine interest and concern are prerequisites to any successful intervention. Counseling and therapy are individualized to meet the needs of each youngster and his problems. Encouraging these children to accentuate the positive aspects of their bodies and personalities with sound health practices and good grooming helps foster a more positive self-image. Helpful devices include a padded brassiere and hairstyling for girls and selection of clothing that adds the illusion of height (or diminishes it in the tall girl). In many areas there are special clothing and footwear stores that cater to persons with atypical sizes and where the youngster can find age-appropriate clothing. Children can also be taught to make their own clothing.

Youngsters with permanent short stature need help to redirect their goals from aspirations that are unattainable to those commensurate with their capabilities. Adjustments may be accompanied by psychophysiologic or behavioral manifestations, and health workers need to be alert for signs and prepare the parents for this possibility with anticipatory guidance.

TALL STATURE

Tallness is rarely a problem to boys, but to the girl who is or is likely to be much taller than her age-mates, it can be a source of acute distress. Although the average height of both boys and girls is steadily increasing, there is still a small group of children who are excessively tall when compared with their contemporaries. In almost all cases the tall girl is expressing an expected genetically determined growth pattern. Many girls like the idea of being tall and manage to cope effectively with any height-related problems that may arise. For others, it can be a source of intense anxiety and a severe social handicap.

When the rate of height change before puberty suggests the probability of excessive adult height, treatment with hormones may be considered. Cyclic administration of estrogens has proved effective in controlling height when therapy is initiated prior to menarche and before the end of the adolescent growth spurt that normally precedes menarche. Estrogen therapy is continued over several years until the epiphyses are fused, as determined by periodic wrist x-ray films. If treatment is stopped before that time, growth will continue. Although estrogen treatment has reduced the height from that estimated on prediction tables in a number of cases, there is still a good deal of controversy regarding its use for this purpose.

Before therapy is instituted, a number of factors must be considered: the prediction of future height based on present height and bone age; determination of whether predicted height is really excessive, that is, greater than 178 cm (70 inches); assessment of the child's and parents' attitudes toward the predicted height; and evaluation of the child's capacity to cope with day-to-day problems associated with such height.

Hormonal therapy has also been shown to be effective in reducing the ultimate height of excessively tall teenage boys. Long-acting testosterone esters administered periodically over 1 year have proved effective in a small sample. The testosterone has the effect of accelerating bone maturation and growth with more rapid epiphyseal closure. As with girls, selection of boys for therapy is made by careful evaluation of physical, psychologic, and social factors.

Nursing Considerations

Nursing intervention with a girl of tall stature has much in common with that for children with short stature. It is primarily directed toward support of the child and the family. Sometimes the concern is primarily that of the parent, especially a tall mother who does not wish to have her daughter experience the same distress as the mother did as a child. The child may not view it as a problem. Therefore the initial goal of care is to determine the source and extent of the perceived problem. Some teenaged girls are overwhelmed by a height of 170 cm (5 feet 7 inches), whereas most youngsters are well adjusted and happy with a height of 178 cm (5 feet 10 inches). Much depends on the social attitudes that affect what is considered to be a desirable or acceptable body image (Bailey, Park, and Cowell, 1981).

If hormone therapy is elected, the parents and the young girl will need to know the anticipated length of treatment, the probability of success, the side effects associated with estrogen administration, such as menorrhagia (progesterone is usually added on the last 7 days of the ovarian cycle to assure sloughing of endometrium), dark pigmentation of areolae, nipples, and labia, and in some cases moderate obesity. Both parents and child will need continued support and encouragement during the extent of therapy.

PRECOCIOUS PUBERTY

Precocious puberty is the manifestation of pubertal development that appears before the expected age of onset. Although puberty is gradually appearing earlier in most societies, manifestations of sexual development before age 10 in boys or age 8½ in girls are considered precocious and should be investigated. Early sexual development can have a number of causes and may result from a disorder of the gonad, the adrenal gland, or the hypothalamic-pituitary gonadal axis. The disorder is nine times more common in girls than in boys (Silver, Gotlin, and Klingensmith, 1984). A familial incidence of male sexual precocity has been observed in some families, but sexual precocity occurs as an isolated event in girls.

True Precocious Puberty

True, or complete, precocious puberty is always isosexual and results from premature activation of the hypothalamic-pituitary-gonadal axis, which produces early maturation and development of the gonads with secretion of sex hormones, development of secondary sex characteristics, and sometimes production of mature sperm or ova. True precocious puberty may be caused by a variety of organic brain lesions, such as tumors, congenital lesions, or postinflammatory disorders, but in most instances no cause can be identified. These cases are termed *functional idiopathic* or *constitutional precocious puberty*. They may occur at any time during childhood and are explained only as an unusually early activation of the maturation process regarded as a normal course of events at a later age. There is early acceleration of linear growth with early epiphyseal fusion and ultimate height less than with later pubertal onset.

Precocious Pseudopuberty

Precocious pseudopuberty, or incomplete puberty (also called pseudosexual precocious puberty), differs from true sexual precocity in that there is no early secretion of gonadotropin. Most cases result from early overproduction of sex hormone, usually caused by a tumor of the ovary or testis, a tumor or hyperplasia of the adrenal gland, or exogenous sources of androgens or estrogens. There is no maturation of the gonads, but there is appearance of secondary sex characteristics. Unlike true sexual precocity, precocious pseudopuberty may be heterosexual. A tumor of the adrenal gland in a girl can cause early and inappropriate female development (e.g., clitoral enlargement and masculinization).

Isolated manifestations that are usually associated with puberty may be seen as variations in normal sexual development. They appear without other signs of pubescence and are probably caused by unusual end organ sensitivity to prepubertal levels of estrogen or androgen. Included are:

premature thelarche Development of breasts in prepubertal females.

premature pubarche (premature adrenarche) Early development of sexual hair.

Therapeutic Management

Treatment of precocious pseudopuberty is directed toward the specific cause when known. Treatment is seldom helpful for idiopathic true precocious puberty. In females, administration of medroxyprogesterone acetate may arrest and reverse the condition either by inhibiting gonadotropin production or by a direct effect on the ovary. Some cases of precocious puberty have responded to the administration of luteinizing hormone–releasing hormone (Pescovitz and others, 1986). Psychologic management of the patient and family is an important aspect of care.

Nursing Considerations

Psychologic support and guidance of the child and family are the most important aspects of management. Although the majority of children do display behavior problems, many girls with true precocious puberty have a high incidence of problem behavior, primarily social difficulties related to age/appearance dysynchrony and moodiness (Sonis and others, 1985).

Parents need a detailed explanation and reassurance of the benign nature of the condition. Dress and activities for the physically precocious child should be appropriate to the chronologic age. Heterosexual interest is not usually advanced beyond the child's chronologic age, and parents need to understand that the child's mental age is congruent with the chronologic age and that the child's normal, overt manifestations of affection are age-appropriate and do not represent sexual advances.

TURNER SYNDROME

Although Turner syndrome is often recognized at birth, it is diagnosed most frequently at puberty because of three outstanding features: short stature, sexual infantilism, and amenorrhea. The incidence of the condition in the population is considered to be from 1:2500 to 1:8000 live female births (Cohen, 1984).

Etiology

Turner syndrome is caused by absence of one of the X chromosomes; as a result the number of chromosomes in these girls is 45—44 pairs of autosomes and one X chromosome (45,X), sometimes referred to as *monosomy X*. The disorder is caused by nondisjunction during germ cell formation and, unlike most nondisjunction phenomena, is related to paternal meiotic error. The reason for the growth retardation is unknown. The child's growth is usually normal until 3 years of age, then slows, gradually drifting away from the normal growth curve. There is no prepubertal growth spurt.

Clinical Manifestations

A tentative diagnosis can be made on the physical appearance in most instances. Only a few persons with this syndrome manifest all of the possible clinical features, which include (Fig. 20-7):

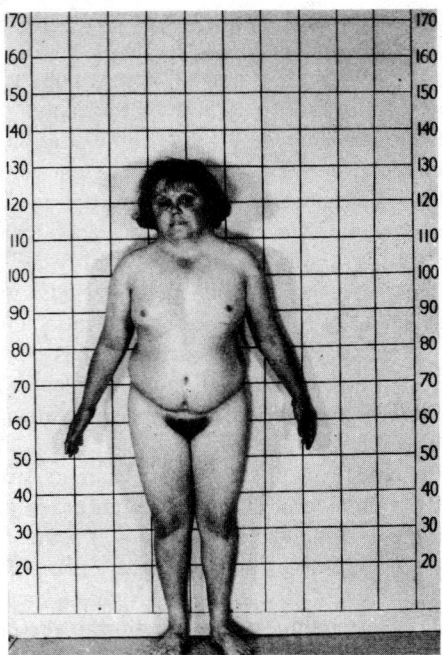

Fig. 20-7. Turner syndrome.
From McKusick, V.A.: J. Chron. Dis. **12**:1-202, 1960.

Significant short stature, which is common to all (many adults are less than 150 cm, or 5 feet, tall) and begins to be apparent at about 4 years, becoming more severe by 8 years of age

Redundant skin folds on the neck (webbed neck) with low posterior hairline (present in 40% to 50% of cases)

Rather "old" facial appearance with micrognathia and low-set and sometimes malformed ears

Shield-shaped chest with widely spaced hypoplastic nipples

Increased carrying angle at the elbow (cubitus valgus)

Cardiac anomalies, principally coarctation of the aorta or aortic valvular stenosis

Moderate degrees of learning difficulty

Abnormal growth patterns; absence of normal growth spurts and sexual development at puberty with primary amenorrhea and sterility; sparse pubic and axillary hair; gonads replaced by fibrous streaks

In the newborn, lymphedema of hands and feet

Diagnostic Evaluation

Diagnosis can be suspected in the newborn period by the presence of lymphedema and characteristic hairline, in childhood by short stature, and at puberty by delayed development. Absence of a Barr body, or negative chromatin, is consistent with the disorder. Definitive diagnosis is confirmed by chromosome analysis.

Therapeutic Management

Therapy is always individualized for these girls and consists primarily of hormone treatment and psychologic counseling for both child and parents. When the diagnosis is made early enough, growth is stimulated with administration of androgen therapy with or without growth hormone at about

10 to 11 years of age. Androgen therapy is followed at about age 14 or 15 by estrogen therapy to promote the development of secondary sex characteristics. When linear growth begins to level off, the dosage is increased and combined with progesterone to effect a normal cyclic pattern. Responses to estrogen therapy vary from girl to girl, but gradual feminization is accomplished to some degree in most individuals, accompanied by a positive effect on the young girl's self-image. Cardiac anomalies, if present, require treatment, and surgical correction of the webbed neck may be undertaken if the defect is disfiguring.

Nursing Considerations

Most of the nursing interventions described for the youngster with short stature apply to the girl with Turner syndrome. The diagnosis should be made as early as possible so that she and her parents can be counseled regarding what to expect. The girl is given some idea of the final height projected in her particular case and the expectations for developing secondary sex characteristics as a result of successful treatment. The girl and parents should understand that the short stature will probably remain despite hormone therapy. It is often reassuring for them to see others who have undergone successful treatment and who are able to adapt to the compromised stature.

It is important that families understand some of the health problems associated with the disorder. The tendency toward obesity may require special attention to diet. The increased tendency for otitis media presents the need for prompt treatment of respiratory infections and regular hearing tests. Other complications commonly associated with Turner syndrome that should be evaluated periodically include hypertension, cardiac anomalies, thyroid disorders, inflammatory bowel disease, and urinary tract anomalies (Cohen, 1984; Conte and Grumbach, 1982).

The fact or decided probability of sterility should be explained to the child and family. This presents a need for special sex education during adolescence, particularly in relation to fertility and alternative routes to parenthood. However, it should be emphasized at the appropriate age that the girl will be able to marry if she wishes and enjoy sexual relationships (Cohen and Durham, 1986).

Several national organizations offer information and support to families with congenital disorders. These include **March of Dimes Birth Defects Foundation,*** **National Easter Seal Society,†** and, in Canada, **Turner Syndrome Society.‡**

KLINEFELTER SYNDROME

Young boys with Klinefelter syndrome are seldom seen for medical evaluation before puberty, at which time varying

*1275 Mamaroneck Ave., White Plains, NY 10605.
†2023 West Ogden Ave., Chicago, IL 60612.
‡Behavioral Science Building, York University, 4700 Keele St., Downsview, Ontario, Canada M3J 1P3.

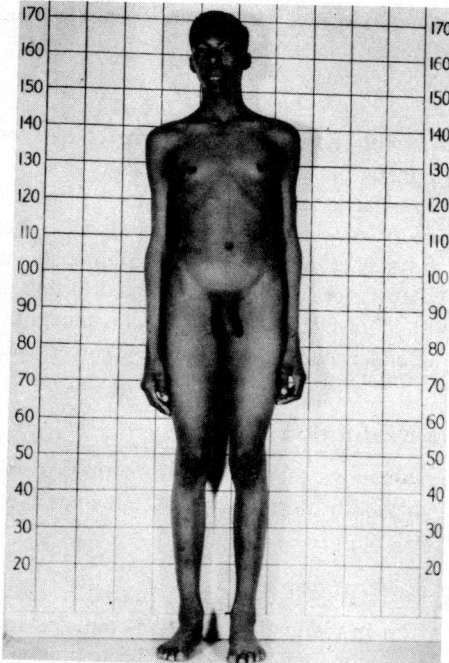

Fig. 20-8. Klinefelter syndrome.
From McKusick, V.A.: J. Chron. Dis. **12:**1-202, 1960.

degrees of failure of adolescent virilization occur. Some males are not detected until they appear for evaluation for infertility. All have absence of sperm in the semen (azoospermia), small testes, and defective development of secondary sex characteristics. The incidence of the disorder is estimated to be approximately 1:500 live male births.

Etiology

The most common of all chromosomal abnormalities, Klinefelter syndrome is caused by the presence of one or more additional X chromosomes, probably as a result of meiotic nondisjunction. The majority of males with this syndrome have a chromosomal complement of 47,XXY, but there are numerous variants in the number of extra sex chromosomes, and the clinical features are essentially the same in all.

Clinical Manifestations

There are no physical characteristics that are helpful in detecting Klinefelter syndrome before the advent of puberty, with the possible exception of mental retardation. Mental impairment of varying degrees is a frequent finding and appears to have a direct relationship to the number of X chromosomes in the cells. The severity of retardation increases with the number of X chromosomes. Characteristic features of the disorder include (Fig. 20-8):

Tall, eunuchoid figure with legs disproportionately long in relation to the trunk
Sparse facial and pubic hair, often with female distribution pattern
Gynecomastia of some degree (seen in half the cases and often the reason for seeking medical advice)

Small, firm, and insensitive testes; small penis in childhood
   (usually normal at adolescence)
Aspermia or oligospermia

Most boys with Klinefelter syndrome have essentially normal intelligence but may have gross motor skill difficulties, developmental language delay, poor verbal skills, and reduced auditory memory. Shyness, passivity, behavioral problems, and school difficulties are often associated with the disorder. However, this may be related to the difference in body build, delayed development, and tendency toward clumsiness (Bender and others, 1983; Walzer and others, 1982).

Diagnostic Evaluation

In 80% of these boys there is a chromatin-positive buccal smear, and the extra chromosome is apparent on chromosomal analysis.

Therapeutic Management

The major effort in medical treatment is directed toward enhancing the masculine characteristics through administration of male hormones, principally testosterone. Cosmetic surgery will eliminate embarrassment for a boy with gynecomastia. As with other pubertal development, psychologic counseling and support are considered along with psychologic problems associated with developmental difficulties.

Nursing Considerations

Special nursing considerations in the care of the youngster with Klinefelter syndrome include counseling or referral for problems associated with peer relationships, techniques for handling difficult social situations, and increasing self-esteem (Cohen and Durham, 1986). The child should be informed at the appropriate time that marriage and sexual relationships are possible, even in the absence of fertility, and alternative reproductive options discussed, such as artificial insemination and adoption.

DELAYED DEVELOPMENT CAUSED BY PATHOLOGIC CONDITIONS

A small group of children suffer delay of growth or onset of adolescence because of disorders that may or may not be amenable to treatment. From a worldwide point of view, the most common cause of short stature and/or delayed development is probably inadequate nutrition; however, the major disorders that produce delayed development are most often caused by chronic diseases, endocrine dysfunction, and primary gonadal dysgenesis, usually Turner or Klinefelter syndromes (see previous section).

Chronic Diseases

Chronic diseases can interfere with growth, but, unless the illness is unduly prolonged, catch-up growth will occur. There are a number of chronic illnesses that fit in this category, and these are discussed where appropriate. Those encountered most frequently are respiratory disorders such as asthma, cystic fibrosis, and recurrent upper respiratory infection; illnesses caused by defective organ or disturbed immune mechanisms; gastrointestinal diseases such as parasitic infestations, cystic fibrosis, and other malabsorption syndromes; cardiac anomalies and blood dyscrasias such as sickle cell anemia; and chronic renal disturbances, especially renal tubular acidosis. It appears that the duration of the illness is more significant than the intensity in its effect on growth, although the precise length of time necessary to affect growth permanently has not been determined.

Skeletal Defects

Skeletal disorders that affect growth in stature are principally those described as dwarfism. Most are caused by a variety of congenital defects and disorders, such as achondroplasia, and some of the inborn errors of metabolism, such as Hurler or Hunter syndrome. Whereas some are readily apparent at or shortly after birth, milder cases may not be recognized until later in life and are diagnosed by x-ray and biochemical examinations.

Endocrine Dysfunction

The major hormones that promote physical growth are thyroid hormone, growth hormone, and sex hormones. Insulin can be said to promote growth by its effect on carbohydrate metabolism, whereas cortisol inhibits growth. Therefore deficiencies of growth-promoting hormones or an excess of cortisol can cause growth retardation in children. Endocrine deficiencies can be the result of abnormal secretory function in the glands responsible for their production, the pituitary hormones that stimulate their secretion, or the releasing factors from the hypothalamus. In some instances growth retardation may be the result of increased production of factors that inhibit hormone secretion. The complex relationships of endocrine function and their disturbances are discussed in Chapter 38; the reader is directed to that segment for further elaboration.

Sex hormone deficiency. Sex hormone deficiency that causes delayed puberty can occur as a result of either pituitary dysfunction or hypogonadism. A hypofunctioning pituitary gland, as briefly discussed in the preceding segment on endocrine dysfunction, can produce a deficiency in either the gonadotropic hormones, which retards maturation of the gonads, or growth hormone, which will diminish total growth during childhood. In addition, there are a large variety of disorders that cause absence or deficiency of sex hormone secretion by their effect on the gonads directly. These may be genital abnormalities that are related to defective gonadal differentiation or those that are associated with functional abnormalities of the already differentiated fetal gonad. The largest group of disorders in which deficient gonadal development is a prominent feature includes the sex chromosomal aberrations. Two of these, Turner and Klinefelter syndromes, are elaborated on pp. 856 and 857.

Cortisol Excess

Cortisol excess as a result of organic factors or of prolonged cortisone therapy also has an adverse effect on growth in children. This effect is produced by direct action on growing cartilage, interference with production of growth hormone, or interference with the response to or production of somatomedin. Because of the growth-suppressing effect of cortisone in excess of minimum requirements, therapy with this drug is limited to short-term administration whenever possible.

PSYCHOSOCIAL DWARFISM

Psychosocial, or deprivation, dwarfism is a term applied to children who are significantly retarded in growth because of environmental circumstances. Children from homes in which they receive little, if any, psychosocial stimulation display markedly delayed skeletal development, and various tests in these children for growth hormone release are consistent with those that indicate a pituitary dysfunction. When these children are removed from the deprived environment, their growth proceeds at a normal or increased rate. This has been repeatedly demonstrated in infants and very young children. Some investigations attribute the growth retardation to malnutrition. Although this may be a factor in infants, it may also be a contributing factor in adolescents with short stature and delayed puberty secondary to psychosocial factors, particularly in the loss of appetite related to the disorder anorexia nervosa.

Although the mechanism is not entirely clear, it is hypothesized that deprivation dwarfism occurs as a response to increased cortisol secretion that results from the prolonged stress of a disturbed environment or unsettled patterns of sleep. Evidence indicates that deprivation dwarfism is also associated with sleep abnormalities. Since growth hormone is secreted in largest amounts during sleep, it follows that anything interfering with normal sleep patterns will interfere with the hormone secretion.

Health Problems of the Male Reproductive System

It is fortunate for the male that most of the parts of the reproductive system are external and therefore visible and palpable. In most instances obvious anomalies have been identified and corrective measures instituted during childhood. A number of the conditions present in the newborn or young child can affect the development of appropriate sexuality during adolescence. Functional disorders such as enuresis may persist, and gynecomastia, a cause of concern in the pubescent male, may become a problem. The most frequent problems related to the reproductive organs are infections, hematuria, voiding dysfunction, penile problems, scrotal conditions, and gynecomastia (Govan and Kessler, 1980).

HEALTH PROBLEMS RELATED TO URINARY FUNCTION

Conditions related to urinary function are frequently those that involve the renal system as a whole and are discussed in Chapter 30. Some conditions are related to trauma; others are associated with sexually transmitted diseases.

Infections

Infections of the male reproductive system are predominantly urethritis of bacterial (primarily *Staphylococcus epidermidis,* and occasionally *Streptococcus faecalis* and enterococci), gonococcal, chlamydial, or candidal etiology. Since the last three organisms are contracted principally through sexual contact, they are discussed later in relation to sexually transmitted diseases. Bacterial infections are seldom asymptomatic, and the young male presents with complaints of burning or stinging on urination, which may or may not be accompanied by urethral discharge. Discharge, if present, can vary according to the organism from a clear mucous fluid to a copious, purulent-appearing discharge. Systemic symptoms are usually absent, although fever is generally a feature of prostate, seminal vesicle, or kidney involvement.

Most urethral infections are the result of sexual contact. Rarely urethritis occurs as a complication of a congenital urethral stricture or valve, foreign body, or trauma. Specific diagnosis is made on identification of the organism by means of smears and cultures of the discharge and/or urine. Treatment is administration of the appropriate antibiotic.

Hematuria

Benign causes of blood in the urine are relatively common in the adolescent, but since hematuria may be a manifestation of a more serious problem, the complaint deserves careful evaluation. The most common cause is acute glomerulonephritis; it may also indicate urinary tract infection, congenital anomalies, drug ingestion (including therapeutic agents such as those used in oncology), and hemorrhagic disorders, including hemophilia, leukemia, thrombocytopenia, and sickle cell disease. Other causes of hematuria include trauma, urinary tract obstruction, tumors, and renal calculi.

Voiding Dysfunction

Voiding dysfunction can vary from a mere increase in frequency to overt incontinence. For most cases of bladder dysfunction a simple explanation can be found. Bladder function can be influenced by a variety of medications (either prescribed or self-administered); it can be of neurologic origin (such as spina bifida, trauma, cerebral palsy, or poliomyelitis); it can be the result of a variety of problems such as enuresis, infection, a foreign body, congenital anomalies; or it can be of a psychosomatic origin.

The diagnosis is made from a careful history, physical examination, and special tests as indicated. Treatment is based on the identified cause.

Nursing Considerations

The adolescent male is extremely self-conscious about his changing body and often refuses a genital examination. Chard (1976) has provided some valuable insights into the problem of assessing the adolescent male. The most successful approach is to assume a matter-of-fact attitude to the examination, explain precisely what will take place, and maintain a continuous commentary about what is being done and the findings at each phase of the examination. Experiencing an erection at an inappropriate moment is one of the greatest fears of the adolescent male. If this occurs during examination of the genitalia, he can be assured that it is a normal physiologic response to touch that is essentially no different from a reflex response in other areas of the body, such as the knee jerk or the pupil response to light.

The adolescent male is approached as someone important as a person, with the nurse interested in his concerns. The health assessment during adolescence is no different from the health assessments that have taken place periodically throughout childhood. The nurse should point out normal changes taking place in other areas of the body, such as developing muscles, and assure the youngster that slower developing changes, such as chest and facial hair, will eventually become apparent.

PENILE PROBLEMS

Common congenital anomalies of the penis are almost always detected and corrected in infancy or early childhood, although some boys who need several operative procedures to repair a hypospadias (the most common congenital deformity of the penis) reach adolescence with a penis that looks different from those of their friends. A few who have received no medical care have uncorrected deformities that can cause serious psychologic problems during this sensitive period of development when being different is intolerable. These young boys need to be identified for surgical repair of the defect.

Since the statement by the Committee on the Fetus and Newborn of the American Academy of Pediatrics (1975) advocated that circumcision not be performed unless there are physiologic or religious reasons for performing the procedure was issued after the birth of the present teenagers, most adolescent males at this time were probably circumcised at birth or during early childhood. Uncircumcised males may encounter some problems during adolescence. Some young men have tight foreskins that cannot be retracted over the enlarging glans; some may not cleanse the area properly even though they know that the foreskin should be retracted and the penis bathed regularly. These boys suffer more frequently from infection.

Trauma to the penis may occur in various ways, including burns and accidental injuries. The frenulum (the fold on the lower surface of the glans that connects it with the prepuce) can be torn after retraction of the foreskin, masturbation, or coitus. It can be terrifying to the young boy but usually heals spontaneously with minimum care. However, any extensive bleeding may require suturing of the tissues.

Other problems include an *adherent penis,* a common condition in which the ventral surface of the penis adheres to the scrotum, producing a severe ventral curvature during erection, thus preventing satisfactory coitus; and *priapism,* a rarer disorder consisting of painful, sustained penile erection without sexual desire. The adherent penis can be surgically corrected; treatment of priapism is directed toward treating conditions with which it is often associated, such as sickle cell disease, leukemia, the use of certain medications, and central nervous system lesions.

A frequent concern of adolescent males is *penile size.* Many boys erroneously assume that the size of the penis is directly related to virility and male prowess; the boy with a small penis is often the object of remarks from more amply endowed age-mates. Rarely, micropenis occurs. This condition may improve somewhat with hormonal treatment but seldom to the extent desired. More often the smaller size is related to late maturation, in which case the youngster can be reassured that the problem will resolve in the normal course of maturation. A concerned young man can also be reassured that the size of the flaccid penis is unrelated to the size of the erect penis and that the length is usually adequate for satisfactory coitus. Repeated follow-up visits are employed for reassurance and to reinforce the fact that the examiner views the adolescent's concern with sincerity.

Nursing Considerations

The nursing care of the adolescent male with specific problems is the same as the general approach and management of all health problems associated with the male reproductive system.

TESTICULAR TUMORS

Tumors of the testes are not a common condition, but when manifested in adolescence they are generally malignant. Testicular cancer constitutes the most common solid tumor in males between ages 15 and 35 (Bosman, 1979). The usual presenting symptom is a heavy, hard, painless mass, palpable on the anterior or lateral aspect of a testis. The tumor may be smooth or nodular and does not transilluminate unless accompanied by a hydrocele. The involved testicle hangs lower and is therefore more susceptible to trauma. Although all scrotal masses are not malignant, any firm swelling of the testis demands immediate evaluation. If a firm swelling is noted, the youth should be subjected to a minimum of preoperative palpation and referred immediately for surgical exploration. There is seldom delay in seeking medical advice if the mass is painful, but in the absence of pain the condition may go unattended for some time.

Treatment for testicular cancer consists of surgical removal of the affected testicle (orchiectomy) and the adjacent lymph nodes, if affected. If metastases are evident in more distant nodes or organs, chemotherapy and radiation therapy are implemented. See also Chapter 23: Impact of life-threatening illness on the child and family.

Nursing Considerations

To supplement routine health assessment, every adolescent male should be taught to perform frequent testicular self-examination (TSE) to familiarize him with his own anatomy and to ensure early detection of any abnormality.* Ideally, self-examination should be performed once a month beginning in early adolescence. Each testicle is examined individually, preferably after a warm bath or shower when scrotal skin is more relaxed, using the thumbs and fingers of both hands and applying a small amount of firm, gentle pressure. The normal testicle is a firm organ with a smooth egg-shaped contour. The epididymis can be palpated as a raised swelling on the superior aspect of the testicle and should not be confused with an abnormality.

VARICOCELE

A varicocele most often appears as a scrotal mass and is characterized by elongation, dilation, and tortuosity of the veins of the spermatic cord superior to the testicle. It is ordinarily small and requires no treatment. Varicoceles are found most often on the left side because of the greater length of the left spermatic vein and its entry into the left renal artery; the right spermatic vein enters the vena cava directly and at a lesser angle, which may be a source of future difficulty. A varicocele can be palpated as a wormlike mass situated above the testicle that decreases in size when the youth is recumbent and becomes distended and tense when he is upright. There may be discomfort during sexual stimulation in some boys. The condition frequently improves spontaneously, and the depressive effect on future fertility is not substantiated; prophylactic repair is contraindicated (Govan and Kessler, 1980).

TESTICULAR TORSION

Torsion of the testicle is a condition in which the tunica vaginalis, which normally encases the testicle, fails to do so and the testis hangs free from its vascular structures. This condition can result in partial or complete venous occlusion with rotation around this vascular axis. In severe torsion the organ can become swollen and painful; the scrotum becomes red, warm, and edematous and appears to be immobile or fixed as a result of spasm of the cremasteric fibers.

Typically the onset is acute and frequently follows intense activity or trauma. Often the patient has a history of a similar pain that was shorter in duration and less intense. An increased incidence of testicular torsion has also been observed in cold weather, presumably caused by contraction of the cremaster muscle (Williamson, 1983). The cold-related torsion is more common in young than in older children because of the more reactive reflex in young children.

Nausea, vomiting, abdominal pain, and a slight fever may accompany the pain. Surgical intervention is mandatory to prevent hemorrhagic necrosis.

Nursing Considerations

Nurses should be alert to the possibility of testicular torsion in children who complain of scrotal pain. Since torsion often results from trauma to the scrotum, school nurses are the persons who are likely to encounter such injuries and refer the youngster for medical evaluation immediately.

OTHER DISORDERS OF THE SCROTUM AND TESTES

Examination of the scrotal contents is part of the routine health assessment (see p. 273). Problems such as cryptorchidism (undescended testes) are usually detected early and corrected in childhood. However, many adolescents have had minimum health care, and the possibility of an imperfectly descended testicle cannot be overlooked in these young men. *Cryptorchid* or *ectopic testes* should be treated as early as possible to reduce the likelihood of malignancy, trauma, or emotional problems resulting from an empty scrotum. A *hydrocele* in the adolescent is most often the result of trauma but rarely may be caused by infection. The fluid generally disappears spontaneously, but aspiration may be required to reduce a large hydrocele or if a hematoma is suspected.

GYNECOMASTIA

Some degree of bilateral or unilateral breast enlargement frequently occurs in young boys during puberty. In most instances it is a transient phenomenon that subsides spontaneously with achievement of male development. Occasionally, however, it is associated with abnormalities such as Klinefelter syndrome or endocrine dysfunction; therefore these possibilities are ruled out by appropriate diagnostic examination. Gynecomastia has also been reported in males receiving oral ketoconazole for fungal infection (Pont and others, 1982) and in a prepubertal child on whom hair cream containing substantial amounts of estrogen was used (Edidin and Levitsky, 1982).

If the condition persists or is extensive enough to cause acute embarrassment or to produce doubts about gender identity in the young boy, plastic surgery is indicated for cosmetic and psychologic considerations. Administration of testosterone has no effect on breast development or regression and may even aggravate the condition.

Nursing Considerations

Treatment usually consists of assurance to the boy and his parents that this is a benign and temporary situation. Since the boy is distressed about his physical integrity and masculinity, he will need reassurance regarding this apparently incongruous development.

---

*To aid in teaching adolescents self-examination an excellent pamphlet, "What you need to know about cancer of the testis," is available from the U.S. Department of Health and Human Services. Material is also available from local branches of the American Cancer Society, Inc. National office: 4 West 35th St., New York, NY 10001.

Health Problems of the Female Reproductive System

Unlike the male, the reproductive organs of the female are located internally; therefore, abnormalities are less apparent and more difficult to detect. Infections are a major source of morbidity, especially those described as sexually transmitted diseases. However, the problems most often brought to the attention of health professionals are those related to menstruation—menstrual delay, irregularities, or discomfort. Any concern is worthy of consideration and understanding from health professionals.

THE GYNECOLOGIC EXAMINATION

One of the most difficult experiences facing the adolescent girl is the gynecologic examination. Whether it is her first experience or not, she is most likely filled with apprehension. Almost all adolescent girls are extremely self-conscious about their bodies and the changes taking place. The girl will need continuing support in the form of anticipatory guidance regarding what she can expect and suggestions of what she can do to help herself relax during the procedure.

The ideal time to begin to prepare the youngster for pelvic examination is during childhood as she is maturing. External genitalia examination is always a part of a routine physical assessment; avoiding the genitals reinforces the attitude that sexuality is wrong and should be avoided. During this time the child and parents are informed that a pelvic examination should be performed during adolescence and is in no way harmful or wrong (Greydanus and McAnarney, 1982).

The timing of the initial pelvic examination is controversial, but examination in early assessment has several advantages. The girl and her parents can be assured that her body is normal, which contributes to a positive body image. It provides an excellent opportunity for health teaching in the areas of hygiene, body functions, and sexuality. The girl should be encouraged to ask questions about her changing body and its implications. For those who object to examination in early adolescence it can be delayed until middle adolescence, although any genitally related problems that arise before that time can be more stressful if the youngster has not experienced the examination before. The pelvic examination should be made as nonstressful as possible.

The teenager is usually given the option of having a parent (usually the mother) present during the pelvic examination. A complete explanation of the examination is offered, including the procedure and draping (which can be optional). The use of models and drawings and a display of equipment to be used facilitate understanding. The youngster is also given the choice of wearing a gown or her own clothing during the procedure (Cavanaugh, 1982).

Usually the stressful experience of being placed in stirrups in the traditional lithotomy position can be avoided.

Most girls favor a semi-sitting position, which has the additional advantage of allowing eye contact during the procedure. The youngster who is relaxed may be examined in the supine position. Girls experiencing their first pelvic examination have been found to be more relaxed when examined by a female. Those having had a previous examination appear to be equally relaxed with a male examiner (Seymore and others, 1986). Sometimes a pillow will help the patient feel more comfortable and less vulnerable. If a female nurse is not the examiner, it is essential for her to remain with the patient during the examination to offer support and guidance. Most examiners provide a mirror that allows the girl to see what is taking place if she so desires, and helps the examiner explain various aspects of anatomy.

Numerous techniques have been described to teach the youngster how to relax, including breathing exercises, imaging, and other stress-reduction strategies (see p. 1071). However, they are not effective with all individuals. When the examination is over the findings are discussed with the youngster (and the parents) and necessary referrals made if indicated. Written teaching materials are useful adjuncts to teaching.

AMENORRHEA/DELAYED MENARCHE

It is not unusual for an adolescent to skip a menstrual period or two when establishing normal menstrual and ovulatory cycles. Delay in initiation of menstruation is ordinarily a temporary problem resulting from late onset of puberty and requires no intervention. This is of little concern unless it creates undue anxiety on the part of the girl and her parents, which can ordinarily be allayed by explanation and reassurance. Careful examination will reveal any congenital defects of the genital tract (a rare cause).

Amenorrhea is considered to be *primary* when menarche is delayed beyond age 17, although some prefer the term *delayed menarche. Secondary* or *postmenarcheal* amenorrhea is prolonged absence of menstruation for 12 months or more between periods in the first 2 years after menarche or when more than three periods have been missed after menses have become established.

Delayed Menarche

Delayed menarche may be the result of absence or malformation of the female genital structures or the inability of normal structures to respond to hormonal stimulation. This can be of hypothalamic, pituitary, ovarian, or uterine origin and can include hypopituitarism, Turner syndrome, tumors, and infections. Pseudoamenorrhea, resulting from imperforate hymen or transverse vaginal septum, is an unusual cause of absent menses in a girl who exhibits all the evidences of estrogen production and sexual maturation and who complains of periodic (usually monthly) lower abdominal pain. The treatment is simple surgical perforation and drainage.

A group of systemic disorders that may affect the functions of the reproductive tract are thyroid hypofunction or hyperfunction, prolonged or severe infections, adrenal hyperplasias, diabetes mellitus, and other chronic diseases. Obesity, malnutrition (including protein, vitamin, or iron deficiencies), or any rapid change in weight either up or down can produce amenorrhea. A common cause of delayed menarche is strenuous physical activity sufficient to reduce body fat content (see p. 849). Management of delayed menarche involves determining and treating the cause or reassurance if the absence of menses is simply delayed normal maturation.

Secondary Amenorrhea

The most common cause of secondary amenorrhea in adolescence is inhibition of the secretion of pituitary hormones. This may be caused by numerous factors including immaturity, pregnancy, extreme physical stress, severe emotional stress, sudden environmental change, hyperthyroidism or hypothyroidism, chronic systemic illness, extreme weight loss or gain, anorexia nervosa (even before marked weight loss), ovarian disturbance, and extrinsic pharmacologic agents (for example, prescribed medications, abused substances, hormones) (Brookman, 1983). Excessive blood levels of carotene also have been implicated. Girls who consumed a diet rich in raw vegetables and no red meat had exceptionally high blood levels of carotene, the one common factor in their amenorrhea (Kemmann and others, 1983). Management of secondary amenorrhea consists of detection and treatment of the cause.

DYSMENORRHEA

A certain amount of discomfort during the first day or two of the menstrual flow is extremely common. Most girls experience cramping, abdominal pain, backache, and leg ache, but in a few the pain is intolerable and incapacitating. The term *primary dysmenorrhea* is applied to these symptoms when there is no pelvic disease to account for cramping discomfort that is severe enough to interfere with normal activity. Primary dysmenorrhea occurs almost always in ovulatory cycles, and commonly appears within 6 to 12 months of the onset of menarche, when ovulatory cycles are usually established. Primary dysmenorrhea is the most common gynecologic complaint, affecting 50% of all female adolescents, and is the leading cause of recurrent school absenteeism among adolescent females in the United States (Klein, 1980; Alvin and Litt, 1982). Therefore the discussion is primarily concerned with this disorder.

Dysmenorrhea beginning more than 2 years after menarche is more suggestive of *secondary dysmenorrhea,* painful menstruation secondary to pelvic pathology. Endometriosis and pelvic inflammatory disease (PID) are the most frequent causes of secondary dysmenorrhea in adolescents. These two health problems are discussed on pp. 864 and 865.

Etiology

No specific etiology of primary dysmenorrhea is known; however, some contributory factors are recognized. The first factor present in all instances of primary dysmenorrhea is the occurrence of prior ovulation. Although it is not invariable, the symptoms do not occur during the first few postmenarchal months or months of irregular anovulatory menses. Estrogen production alone does not appear to be related to uterine discomfort, and progesterone is associated with diminished uterine contractility.

There is a relationship between uterine contractility and the secretion of prostaglandins. Prostaglandins of the F classes cause uterine muscles to contract. The secretion of prostaglandins increases at about the twenty-fifth to the twenty-eighth day of the menstrual cycle and follows the beginning decrease in progesterone secretion. Local discomfort may be related to vascular changes in the endometrial bed during menstruation caused by alternating vasoconstriction and vasodilation of endometrial vessels that induce local ischemia, edema, necrosis, and slough. Nerve terminals also become sensitive to prostaglandins by lowering the threshold of these nerve terminals to the action of chemical and physical stimuli. In some girls the discomfort may be a result of low pain tolerance.

The second factor is psychologic—the reaction of the young girl to this normal female function or an emotional reaction to slight pain. It is not uncommon for girls to outgrow the severity of the symptoms once they have overcome their resentment toward menstruation or resolved the conflict between an unconscious wish to remain a little girl and a conscious drive to gain maturity. There is also a correlation between the incidence of dysmenorrhea in mothers and daughters, possibly related to anxiety transmitted from mother to daughter. These psychic factors, tension, and anxiety can accentuate the local symptoms and produce the associated autonomic nervous system symptoms such as nausea, vomiting, pallor, diaphoresis, and fainting.

Clinical Manifestations

Typical complaints of the girl with dysmenorrhea are lower abdominal cramping, pains or discomfort, and nausea (often with vomiting), diarrhea, and fatigue. Sometimes syncope and collapse occur. The pain usually begins some hours before the appearance of visible vaginal bleeding, is most severe on the first day of menstruation, and may last from a few hours to a day but seldom exceeds 2 to 3 days. The symptoms and degree of discomfort vary considerably from one individual to another and from one period to another in the same youngster. The pain may be only a mild fleeting discomfort or so severe as to be incapacitating, requiring absence from school. After adolescence the menstrual discomfort decreases with age (Alvin and Litt, 1982).

Mittelschmerz, a symptom observed in some girls, is a midcycle lower quadrant pain that sometimes occurs in association with ovulation and is believed to be caused by pelvic irritation from discharged ovarian follicular contents. The discomfort is unilateral and on alternate sides each month, often accompanied by mild bleeding or changes in vaginal secretions. The discomfort may last from several hours to 3 to 4 days.

Therapeutic Management

A thorough gynecologic examination is carried out to exclude any pelvic abnormalities, and a careful history is taken regarding the type and duration of pain, its relationship to menstrual flow, and any associated symptoms. These questions not only provide information to the examiner but also serve to provide the girl with evidence that her problem is being taken seriously. An explanation of the physiology of menstruation helps to give reassurance.

The treatment of choice for adolescents is the administration of nonsteroidal anti-inflammatory drugs, the drugs that block the formation of prostaglandins (called antiprostaglandins, prostaglandin inhibitors, or prostaglandin synthetase inhibitors). Antiprostaglandins are taken for only 2 to 3 days of the menstrual cycle. Prophylactic aspirin has proved effective when begun a few days before the onset of the menses—approximately 11 days after ovulation. The relief appears to be the result of prostaglandin-inhibitory (rather than analgesic) effect.

Drugs that are taken at the onset of the dysmenorrheic symptoms are ibuprofen (Motrin), naproxen (Naprosyn), naproxen sodium (Anaprox), or the fenamates—mefenamic acid (Ponstel) or flufenamic acid (Arlef). The fenamates have the additional benefit of antagonizing the action of already formed prostaglandins. Indomethacin, although effective in alleviating menstrual discomfort or pain, has significant dose-related side effects and is seldom prescribed.

Sometimes cyclic estrogen therapy to prevent ovulation provides dramatic and predictable relief from pain. Oral contraceptives are effective at relieving the discomfort in approximately 90% of cases but are usually reserved for patients who also want contraception control (Dawood, 1983). See Contraception for a discussion of oral contraceptives in adolescence.

Nursing Considerations

The nurse is most frequently the person to whom a young girl turns for advice regarding menstrual problems or problems related to vaginal discharge. Usually all the youngster needs is reassurance about this normal function, but this also provides an opportunity for the nurse to listen to what the adolescent is saying and to engage in health teaching concerning menstrual physiology and hygiene and the importance of a well-balanced diet, exercise, and general health maintenance. It is a time to dispel any myths the girl may have in relation to menstruation and her femininity. When assessment indicates a potential problem and need for evaluation, the girl is referred to a physician, health service, or clinic.

Many of the prostaglandin inhibitors are available without prescription. Whatever drug the girl chooses to use, she needs to be told how the drug produces its effect, how to take the drug for maximum effect, and to try a different drug if one is not effective or if unpleasant side effects are noted. Side effects that have been observed are gastrointestinal symptoms (indigestion, heartburn, nausea, vomiting,

abdominal pain, diarrhea and melena), central nervous system manifestations (headache, dizziness, vertigo, visual or hearing disturbances, irritability, depression, drowsiness, or sleepiness), or other manifestations including allergic reactions, skin rash, edema, and bronchospasm. If no satisfactory relief is achieved, the girl is referred for further evaluation. It is especially important if the girl is using oral contraceptive drugs.

Simple exercises similar to those recommended for relief of prenatal discomfort, such as pelvic rocking, assuming the knee-chest position, and breathing exercises, may also be beneficial. The girl is encouraged to practice good hygiene and participate in regular activities.

PREMENSTRUAL TENSION SYNDROME

Premenstrual tension syndrome (PMS) is a loosely defined congestive dysmenorrhea (sometimes called pelvic congestion syndrome) that begins approximately 7 to 10 days before and ends at the onset of menses. The manifestations most frequently cited are headache, backache, increased fatigue, weight gain, irritability, crying spells, depression, bloating, and breast congestion before menstrual flow.

The etiology is unclear, but water and sodium retention as a result of progesterone production after ovulation appear to be factors. Characteristically these symptoms are present several days before the menstrual period and are relieved at the onset of the menstrual flow. The symptoms do not seem to occur before ovulatory cycles begin and are not ordinarily a problem in adolescence but may occur in some older adolescents.

Therapy is controversial, although relief is sometimes achieved by salt restriction or addition of naturally diuretic foods. Sometimes a mild diuretic during the week preceding the onset of menstrual flow is prescribed.

Nursing Considerations

Nursing care is primarily supportive. Adequate rest, good nutrition, and regular exercise are frequently beneficial in lessening unpleasant symptoms.

ENDOMETRIOSIS

Endometriosis is much more common in adolescents than has previously been thought. This painful disorder is caused by the presence of endometrial tissue refluxed from the fallopian tubes during menstruation or developing from embryonic rests that is seeded anywhere in the pelvis. This ectopic tissue forms multiple small cysts on the ovaries, uterine surface, pelvic ligaments, or peritoneum that swell during the menstrual cycle, irritating nerve endings or creating adhesions between pelvic structures. The resulting pain is localized in the lower abdomen, back, groin, thigh, and/or deep pelvis and can be cyclic or acyclic. It is aggravated by coitus but usually relieved by rest.

Laparoscopic examination confirms the diagnosis. Treatment consists of cyclic hormone administration for 3 to 6 months. However, the disorder tends to become a chronic, recurring condition. Continuing management is usually referred to a gynecologist and surgical intervention may be required, although this is deferred whenever possible until childbearing is completed.

PELVIC INFLAMMATORY DISEASE

Pelvic inflammatory disease (PID) is the term applied to salpingitis, salpingo-oophoritis, and/or endometritis. The onset commonly occurs during or just after menses with intense cramping and pelvic pain. Other symptoms may include lower abdominal pain, vaginal discharge, abnormal bleeding, fever, dysuria, and sometimes malaise, weakness, fainting, dizziness, nausea, and vomiting.

The cause in adolescents is usually gonococcal and/or chlamydial infections (see Sexually Transmitted Disease), but other organisms have been implicated. It is estimated that a sexually active 15-year-old girl has a 1 in 8 chance of acquiring acute PID, compared with a 1 in 80 risk in a 24-year-old woman (Westrom, 1980). Other etiologies that must be ruled out include appendicitis, ectopic pregnancy, ovarian cyst, urinary tract infection, and septic abortion. An accurate diagnosis is essential for adequate management.

DYSFUNCTIONAL UTERINE BLEEDING

Irregularities in the timing, length, or amount of menstrual flow are common conditions in adolescent girls and are caused primarily by either imbalance in the secretion of hormones that control menstrual function or variability in responsiveness of the target organs in adolescence. Anovulatory menstruation is characteristic of the early menstrual periods after menarche and is self-limited for the majority of teenage girls. Occasionally chronic diseases and thyroid dysfunction are causative factors, and abnormal bleeding is associated with systemic diseases that cause bleeding from a variety of mucosal surfaces, such as purpura, scurvy, and leukemia.

In persistent cases hormonal therapy, in the form of oral, cyclic, high-dose estrogen-progesterone combinations available as contraceptive agents, has proved beneficial. The girl needs to know that at the completion of the recommended regimen there will probably be a heavy flow with cramping for 3 to 4 days. If she is not given this information, the youngster may believe that her condition is worse and assume that the treatment was ineffective. This "withdrawal bleeding" requires no additional treatment, but most physicians prescribe a lower-dose cyclic-type combination to begin the fifth day of menstrual bleeding. This medication is continued for 3 weeks and followed a week later by menstruation. The regimen is continued for several months, after which the bleeding irregularities seldom recur.

Dilatation and curettage may be necessary to control hemorrhage in severe cases or if more conservative manage-

ment is not effective. Supplemental iron is sometimes needed to correct anemia if bleeding has been excessive.

Nursing Considerations

Ordinarily only reassurance and attention to general health status are needed, with emphasis on a well-balanced diet, adequate rest, and moderate exercise. Anticipatory supportive care includes preparation for surgical procedures (e.g., dilatation and curettage), if these are a possibility.

VAGINITIS AND VULVITIS (VULVOVAGINITIS)

A small quantity of vaginal mucus is normal and in adolescent girls usually increases at the time of ovulation and before the onset of menstruation. It is characteristically clear and, except in rare instances when it appears in large amounts, causes no discomfort. However, some teenagers mistakenly believe it to be a sign of vaginal infection. After an examination, the girl can generally be reassured. Since increased secretions may be associated with sexual excitement, this association with lovemaking should be discussed with the girl.

Leukorrhea is the term used to describe a glutinous, gray-white discharge, which can be caused by physical, chemical, or infectious agents. Physical causes include foreign bodies (especially in prepubertal girls), a forgotten tampon, an intrauterine device, or even tight jeans. It can also be caused by irritation from pinworms, bubble bath, feminine hygiene products, or improper wiping after defecation. The resulting discharge is purulent, blood tinged, or brown, with an offensive odor. Removal of the foreign material and the use of an acidifying vaginal treatment are all that is usually needed.

Medications that the girl is taking may alter the vaginal environment sufficiently to produce an increased secretion of mucus. The girl receiving tetracycline for severe acne is susceptible to secondary candidiasis, which is often more troublesome than the acne. Contraceptive pills, with their high estrogen content, also increase the quantity of the vaginal discharge. Large quantities of cervical mucus cause the normal acidity of the vagina to become alkaline, which can lead to a change in the vaginal flora. Use of an acidifying agent or a change in the type of contraceptive will usually eliminate the problem.

Many of the infectious causes of vaginitis are sexually transmitted; these are discussed in relation to the specific organisms involved (see Sexually transmitted diseases later in this chapter). However, many cases can and do occur in teenagers who have not experienced coitus. Also, sexual assault is always a possibility (see p. 875). Therapeutic management is directed toward the cause of the inflammation and/or discharge.

Nursing Considerations

Health teaching is important in the prevention and management of vaginitis. Girls should be taught at an early age the

Questions and Controversies

Do the media contribute to the increase in sexual activity among teenagers?

There are data to indicate that television serves as an important source of information about sex for teenagers (Palumbo and Licamele, 1983). Television movies that show sexually suggestive behaviors have increased seven-fold in a 5-year period (Sprafkin and Silverman, 1981). Many overly dramatize the sexual aspect of adolescence, including sexual affairs, rape, teenage prostitution, and pornography. Many "sexploitive" movies made for theaters are directed toward the teenage moviegoer (Strasburger, 1985).

What influence will the increase in the number of homes with videocassette players and the availability of sexually suggestive movies have on teenagers? Can teenagers' access to X-rated movies from adult sources be controlled?

proper hygiene after toileting, that is, wiping from front to back. A careful history can often elicit other causes such as use of irritating substances, foreign bodies, or sexual activity that may be divulged to a sensitive and sympathetic examiner. The youngster will need explanations of how the etiologic agent produced the irritation and the principles behind medical management. The discussion might also elicit questions and concerns the adolescent may have regarding other aspects of her developing body and sexuality.

EXPOSURE TO DIETHYLSTILBESTROL

Intrauterine exposure to diethylstilbestrol (DES) has been associated with the development of clear-cell adenocarcinoma of the genital tract in girls during adolescence. The disease is rare in girls under 14 years of age, but the incidence increases, reaches a peak at age 19, and drops rapidly thereafter. Although the risk is remote (0.14 : 1000 to 1.4 : 1000) (Herbst and others, 1977), all daughters exposed to DES during their mothers' pregnancy should have annual screening examinations beginning no later than menarche or age 14. The screening procedure should include a thorough pelvic examination, including a Papanicolaou (Pap) smear. Any girl should be referred for evaluation if she has abnormal bleeding or discharge at any age or if the parents are concerned (Klein, 1980; Robboy and others, 1984).

Nursing Considerations

Anxiety in both mother and daughter is a common reaction to these findings (although anxiety in the mother does not necessarily cause anxiety in the daughter). Nurses can help by informing families about the need for early and periodic screening examinations and by exploring their feelings regarding the situation, especially the mother's feelings of guilt. Reassurance can be offered concerning the low incidence of problems and the mother's decision to take DES during pregnancy.

Some genital tract deformities resulting from the mother's use of DES have also been described in both males and females, although reports implicating DES exposure in males are conflicting. The most extensive survey conducted to date indicates that there is no increased risk of genitourinary abnormalities, infertility, or testicular cancer (Leary and others, 1984). However, testicular self-examination is still indicated. If a health history reveals that the youngster has been exposed to DES during the mother's pregnancy she or he is referred to a health service or clinic for further evaluation. Fortunately, the problem of DES exposure is time-limited. DES has not been prescribed during pregnancy since 1971; therefore persons born since that date should not be at risk.

Health Problems Related to Sexuality

The biologic maturation that forms the foundation of adolescent development and the transition to adulthood is accompanied by conflicting feelings, attitudes, and social practices related to the developing sexuality. Adolescents have expressed various reasons for wanting to be sexually active: to promote self-esteem, to care about someone else and to have someone care about them, experimentation, reaction to peer pressure, to feel grown up, to touch and be touched by another, to feel good, and for retaliation (Tauer, 1983).

A number of environmental influences may be operating. Sexual enticements by the mass media to enhance physical attractiveness conflict with traditional religious and societal expectations for chastity (see Questions and controversies, above). Easy access to cars, unsupervised after-school activities, removal of other safeguards, and decline of social and religious controls have left youth defenseless against the environmental forces to which they are exposed. The importance of having "popular" daughters frequently causes parents to push young girls into situations they are not mature enough to handle. Biologic and sociologic patterns are proceeding in opposite directions. Young people are maturing earlier and marrying later whereas in earlier times they matured later but married earlier.

Some of the problems engendered by the maturation of sexual capacity, experimentation, acting-out, the need to conform, impulsivity, and the search for a sexual identity are teenage pregnancies and sexually transmitted disease.

ADOLESCENT PREGNANCY

Each year one in 10 adolescent girls in the United States becomes pregnant—approximately 1 million females under the age of 20 years. About 554,000 of these pregnancies result in a birth; more than 400,000 are terminated by abortion (Vernon, Green, and Frothingham, 1983; McAnarney,

1983; Zuckerman and others, 1984). Today most teenage mothers choose to keep their babies, consequently there are 1.3 million infants living with teenage mothers, about half of whom are married (Teenage pregnancy, 1981). Although teenage pregnancy is no longer considered to be biologically disadvantageous to the conceptus, it is still regarded as socially, educationally, psychologically, and economically disadvantageous to the mother.

Medical Aspects

With better facilities available for care, the mortality for teenage pregnancies is decreasing, but the morbidity still remains high. Teenage girls and their unborn infants are at greater risk for complications of both pregnancy and delivery. The most frequent complications are premature labor and infants of low birth weight, high neonatal mortality, preeclampsia, iron-deficiency anemia, fetopelvic disproportion, and prolonged labor. It now appears that the major obstetric difficulties are related to the smaller maternal size rather than the younger age or developmental immaturity (Garn and Petzold, 1983).

A greater weight gain during pregnancy has been noted in younger than in older pregnant women, but it is suggested this is caused by greater fluid retention and/or increased fluid volume (Garn and others, 1984). Although the teenager has special needs, the obstetric risk should be no greater than for any pregnant patient. When quality prenatal care is available early in the pregnancy, the progress and outcome of teenage pregnancies compare favorably with the obstetric performance of older women (Zuckerman and others, 1984).

Developmental. Previously it was believed that pregnancy interfered with normal development when a fetus competed with the maternal needs for nutrients during the rapid growth of early adolescence. Since pregnancy can take place only after the girl has achieved an advanced state of growth and sexual maturity, interference with growth is less of a concern than the dietary habits and the increased incidence of cigarette smoking, alcohol and drug use, and sexually transmitted diseases in this age group.

It does not necessarily follow that early biologic development is accompanied by early emotional and psychologic development. The physically mature young girl is still a teenager who must cope with the developmental tasks of adolescence. When the tasks of motherhood or impending motherhood are superimposed on adolescent needs, the girl is ill prepared to deal appropriately with either. Findings of studies indicate that infants born to adolescent parents are more likely to be at risk for sudden infant death syndrome, infections, and physical injury (Taylor, Wadsworth, and Butler, 1983; Zuckerman and others, 1984).

Complications of pregnancy. The most serious complication of teenage pregnancy is preeclampsia. Girls less than 16 years of age have a five times greater chance of developing preeclampsia than older girls and young women,

and since there is greater likelihood of repeat pregnancy at an earlier age, the threat is not eliminated with the termination of one pregnancy. Younger women are statistically destined to have more than the average number of additional pregnancies, and these earlier and repeated episodes of eclampsia are detrimental to the cardiovascular-renal system. Consequently each subsequent pregnancy bears the risk of increased severity of preeclampsia, and the resulting renal damage can produce chronic renal disease in the young woman by about age 30.

A number of authorities have cited a relatively high incidence of iron-deficiency anemia among pregnant teenage girls (cited in Mahan and Rees, 1984), and the incidence increases sharply when there are repeated pregnancies during the adolescent years. Anemia is not an unusual finding in nonpregnant adolescent girls, but during pregnancy the deficit is increased because of the normal hemodilution associated with pregnancy and the growth demands of the fetus.

There appears to be little difference in the incidence of placental accidents and antepartum and postpartum hemorrhage in teenagers compared to older women, although the findings vary with the observers. Lacerations of the genital tract are more frequent in smaller patients.

Structural. Labor may be prolonged in younger teenagers; this is directly related to fetopelvic incompatibility, and is a reflection of teenagers' smaller stature and incomplete growth process. This is particularly true regarding girls 12 to 16 years of age, and the incidence of prolonged labor is highest in girls less than age 14. Girls 12 and 13 years old have the highest rate of cesarean sections, primarily necessary because of cephalopelvic disproportion. However, older adolescents, 15 to 21 years of age, often have labors that are shorter than average, especially those girls who have previously delivered a baby. The critical point between pelvic disproportion and adequacy appears to occur around 15 years of age in the average adolescent.

Nutritional. Caloric requirements during adolescence closely parallel the growth curve, and the need for protein, calcium, and iron is increased concomitantly. Young adolescents tolerate caloric restriction poorly, and the anabolic need for calories during pregnancy places an added burden on their bodies. The nutritional status at the time of pregnancy is a reflection of lifetime nutritional practices. Unfortunately, because of an attempt to attain fashionably slim figures, denial of the pregnancy, and zealous restriction of diet to control pregnancy weight gain, many teenagers have been placed at risk.

Since there is marked variation in the dietary needs of individual teenagers, no hard and fast rule can be laid down to describe the adequate diet for all pregnant girls. The diet must provide sufficient nutrients to meet growth needs of both the prospective mother and the unborn child without the threat of obesity and other evidences of malnutrition. The best guide for determining nutritional needs is the Rec-

Table 20-2 Calculating calorie requirements for pregnant adolescents*

1. Allow calories for maximal daily growth needs:	123 calories
2. Add RDA† of calories for pregnancy:	300 calories
3. Add average RDA† of calories for age and growth percentile for nonpregnant female:	2100 calories
	2523 total daily calories
4. *Underweight.* Add 500 additional calories per day, 16% of which should be protein (20 g):	3023 total daily calories
5. *Overweight.* Use lower range of "normal" suggested values or 38 calories/kg or 17 calories/lb pregnancy weight.	

From Frank, D., and others: Nutrition in adolescent pregnancy, J. Calif. Perinatal Assoc. **3**(1):21, 1981.
*These calculations are based on the maximum calorie allowance for growth. The best indication of whether a pregnant female is getting sufficient calories is to monitor her growth with a prenatal growth grid. If inadequate or excess weight gain occurs, consultation with a nutritionist is recommended.
†Recommended daily dietary allowance.

ommended Daily Allowances of the Food and Nutrition Board for adolescents of the appropriate age and the added needs for pregnancy. However, these do not take into consideration deviations and deficiencies.

Adolescent girls often adopt unusual dietary patterns that can seriously compromise the health of themselves and their infants. Adolescents are often unresponsive to suggestions about food choices. Experience also indicates that many teenagers do not understand the basic food groups nor the phrasing used to describe nutrients (e.g., grams of protein per day and servings). Table 20-2 provides a formula for calculating caloric needs of the teenage girl, and Table 20-3 outlines sample menus for the average, underweight, and overweight teenager.

Infants. There is a higher incidence of prematurity and low birth weight in infants born to teenagers (Zuckerman and others, 1984). It is difficult to determine if this is a result of the developmental stage of the mother or a reflection of multiple factors associated with teenage pregnancies, including first pregnancy, poor nutrition, lower socioeconomic status, concomitant disease and deleterious habits, and deficiency or lack of prenatal care. Several factors that demonstrate a high degree of association with prematurity, such as first birth, preeclampsia, immaturity, illegitimacy, and the young age of the mother, can create a cumulative effect that places the pregnant teenager in a high-risk situation.

Psychologic and Emotional Aspects

Becoming pregnant is not something that merely happens to a girl. Although she may not be aware of it, she has arrived at the pregnant state through her own actions—conscious or unconscious. She is usually not promiscuous, that is, engaging in sexual intercourse with a variety of partners. Often the pregnancy is planned; however, an unwanted or ill-advised pregnancy can be disruptive and, in the adolescent, catastrophic.

The motivations for and meanings of pregnancy during the teen years are multiple. The pregnant teenager may be a girl who has been submitted to at home and uses the same treatment on herself that her parents have given her. She acts on her impulses with little control over her desires. It is difficult for her to say "no." She may be a girl from a home where the parents are critically demanding, distrustful, and punitive, who chooses pregnancy as an expression of hostility toward the parents. She may be a girl from a home in which something has prevented her from receiving the care and interest that would enable her to think well of herself as a person. When parents are absent, too busy, or preoccupied with their own problems, the girl feels (and often is) neglected. Consequently she turns to another, frequently a boy in similar circumstances, for comfort and love.

Motivation for pregnancy may also reflect maladaptive attempts to solve psychologic conflicts peculiar to the stage of the girl's development. The early adolescent girl has little or distorted information about sexuality, conception, and contraception. Her motivation appears to reflect a complex relationship with her own mother, in which she wishes to break away from her mother and at the same time become dependent on her. Another motivation seems to be a testing of her new and mysterious body functions. She tends to disavow any responsibility for her pregnancy and blames it on a little-known boy or on her mother for failing to provide adequate sex education. This is the type of girl who often denies her pregnancy.

The girl in middle adolescence appears to have sufficient understanding of her sexuality to prevent pregnancy but does nothing to protect herself. She, too, invariably places the blame for her predicament on someone else. At this time sexual activity and pregnancy may reflect a resurgence of the oedipal feelings, in which she indulges in competitive fantasy with her mother and becomes pregnant through a wish to have a baby for her father. It may be a way to express independence of her parents and to break away from them in a less rebellious manner while she is still dependent

Table 20-3 Sample menus

	Day 1		Day 2
Breakfast	Egg and ham on English muffin (fast food)		1 cup cornflakes with 1 cup milk
	1 cup milk		2 T raisins
	1 glass orange juice (6 oz)		1 glass orange juice (6 oz)
Snack	1 pkg peanut butter crackers		1 pkg nuts
	1 can apple juice (6 oz)		1 carton chocolate milk (8 oz)
Lunch	Cheeseburger on bun with lettuce and tomato		"Sub"—1 slice each ham, salami, and cheese with lettuce, tomato, onion, green pepper, 1 T dressing
	1 carton chocolate milk (8 oz)		1 can apple juice (6 oz)
	1 slice watermelon		
Snack	Ice cream cone		1 cup buttered popcorn
Dinner	Baked chicken leg and thigh		2 cups spaghetti and meatballs
	½ cup rice		1 slice Italian bread
	½ cup string beans		Tossed salad—lettuce, tomato, onion
	1 cup milk		1 T dressing
	½ cup fruit cocktail		1 tsp margarine
Snack	1 slice pizza		Milkshake, vanilla

Kcal	Protein (g)	Fat (g)	Cholesterol (g)	Kcal	Protein (g)	Fat (g)	Cholesterol (g)
2604	119	132	286	2857	115	147	248
Underweight—replace cheeseburger with extra-large hamburger deluxe; add 1 cup orange juice to evening snack.				*Underweight*—add 1 carton chocolate milk to afternoon snack, extra cheese or cold cuts to lunch, 2 T dressing for salad.			
3149	133	155	334	3353	137	172	278
Overweight—replace ice cream cone with 1 can apple juice (6 oz).				*Overweight*—replace milkshake with 1 cup skim milk			
2354	111	114	270	2400	112	131	196

From Frank, D., and others: Nutrition in adolescent pregnancy, J. Calif. Perinatal Assoc. **3**(1):21-22, 1981.

on them. She is very conscious of her pregnant state and often takes a romantic view of maternity. This is also the type of girl who identifies with an older, married sister or another young mother and becomes pregnant to emulate these models. Pregnancy can also provide a youngster with positive evidence of maturity.

Girls in late adolescence seem to have a good understanding of conception and contraception and are aware that the pregnancy is their responsibility—the result of a conscious or unconscious slip, such as forgetting to take "the pill." They are rarely surprised at finding themselves pregnant and may even admit that the conception was manipulated in an attempt to force a reluctant boyfriend into a more permanent commitment to them. The late adolescent, unlike the early or middle adolescent, views pregnancy as a happy event under the right circumstances, and the motivation to obtain love and commitment from the boyfriend contrasts sharply with the attitude of the younger girl, to whom the boy is irrelevant and whose pregnancy generally ends their relationship. The older girl shows the beginnings of a genuine wish to love and care for a child.

A teenage pregnancy frequently compels the young girl to cope with several developmental tasks at once—adolescence, pregnancy, marriage, and motherhood. The need for dependency during pregnancy conflicts with the adolescent need for independence. Instead of being an independent person breaking away from her family, she is forced to become more dependent on them for physical, emotional, and financial support. The father of her child, usually a teenager himself and faced with many of the same conflicts, is seldom able to provide the support she needs.

Social and Economic Aspects

The teenage girl who finds herself pregnant and unmarried will frequently become the victim of a forced early marriage that in most cases fails. Statistically teen marriages are notoriously unstable. The highest divorce rate occurs in couples who are married between ages 15 and 19 and is three to four times higher than that among those married at a later age. Teenagers find themselves still dependent on parents for support or, unskilled and inexperienced, in an unfavorable position to earn enough to adequately support a family. A high percentage of young people, especially unmarried mothers, are forced to go on welfare. In addition, the late teen years are considered to be the most fertile; therefore without appropriate intervention, these young mothers tend to fall into a pattern of repeated pregnancies and bearing more children at risk.

Teenage pregnancy is one of the leading causes of school dropout in young female students. Previously the stigma attached to teenage out-of-wedlock pregnancies was such that the girls were not allowed to remain in school. They were considered to be bad influences and publicly condemned for their misconduct. Such punitive behavior was not successful in reducing the number of pregnancies; however, it may have contributed to damaging numerous young lives.

Another significant aspect of school dropout and accelerated maturity is the girl's alienation and isolation from her peers during a stage of development when identity formation is so closely allied with peer identification. She is deprived of the interrelationship with the adolescent social system that is so essential to the development of a sense of identity. The girl believes that she no longer ''belongs'' to the peer group and does not qualify for membership in the older peer group normally associated with marriage and motherhood. On the other hand, the pregnancy may provide the youngster with an entrance into a peer group.

Today most communities have some arrangement for continuation of the girl's education by allowing her to remain in regular classes or providing a curriculum to meet her special needs either within the school system or through programs associated with other community agencies. Most community programs designed for the assistance of pregnant teenagers involve the cooperative efforts of several organizations. The major service components of the programs provide for early and consistent prenatal care, continuing education on a classroom basis, and individual or group counseling.

Mother-Infant Relationship

Not only are infants of teenage mothers at risk medically, but they are also at risk in other aspects of their existence. Although many adolescent mothers want their babies and are prepared to care for them in a mature manner, many others have unrealistic expectations for the child. The young mother often sees the infant as a plaything or a love object for herself. Children of adolescent mothers experience more developmental problems than children of adult mothers. There are conflicting reports of suboptimum cognitive development in children of teenage mothers, but reports indicate an increased risk of child abuse in these children (Elster, McAnarney, and Lamb, 1983). Many are raised by grandparents, a situation that can be fraught with problems and confused identities for the child.

Mother-infant interaction has been observed by numerous investigators. It has been found that infants of teenage mothers display a slight but consistent developmental advantage during their first year of life, but this is reversed in later years (Camp and others, 1984). Adolescent mothers tend to interact with their infants with relatively more physical than verbal exchanges when compared with adult mothers (Sandler, Vietze, and O'Connor, 1981), and nonverbal interaction is most commonly employed by the younger teenage mothers (Epstein, 1980; Ragozin, 1982). Teenage mothers are also more authoritarian in their relationships with their children (Camp and others, 1984).

Researchers have also investigated the various factors that influence the mother-infant relationship. Maternal stresses, including changes in circumstances, influence her ability to cope and her sensitivity to the needs of the infant. The timing of pregnancy is out of phase with the usual course of life events, and role transition and other situational crises of pregnancy all affect the adolescent, who does not have the maturity or the social support to cope adequately (Elster, McAnarney, and Lamb, 1983). Vocational and educational disadvantages of both teenage mothers and fathers further impinge on coping abilities.

There is also a positive correlation between the total amount of social support and the frequency of appropriate maternal behavior (Colletta and Gregg, 1981). The most important source of support is the mother's family of origin, which serves a variety of functions including cognitive guidance, social reinforcement, tangible assistance, social stimulation, and emotional support (Hirsch, 1980). There is more material support and assistance with child care available to the youngster who lives at home.

The cognitive development of the adolescent influences the development of attitudes and realistic expectations regarding childrearing. To cope effectively and solve situational dilemmas, pregnant teenagers must be able to use the problem-solving approach to assess and evaluate consequences of social interactions. The concrete thought and self-centeredness of early adolescence can influence mothers' attentiveness to and evaluation of their infants' needs (Lamb and Easterbrooks, 1981). Adolescent mothers lack knowledge of infant behavior and development, and this directly affects their perception, interpretation, and responsiveness to infant cues. The greater the mothers' knowledge, the more likely they are to interpret the infants' cues correctly and to implement appropriate responses (Elster, McAnarney, and Lamb, 1983).

The characteristics of the infants also influence parental behavior. Teenage parents view their children as more temperamentally difficult than do adult parents, no matter what the infants' temperament (Green and others, 1981). Since temperamentally difficult infants have an adverse effect on sensitive responsiveness of parents, a parent-infant interaction that is not mutually satisfying can alter the parents' feelings of effectiveness and self-worth. This can alter their sensitivity and relationships with the infant. An increased incidence of child abuse has been found in adolescent parents (Leventhal, 1981).

Adolescent Fathers

In the past the role of the father of a child born to an unwed teenage mother was almost completely ignored by health professionals. Contrary to prevalent attitudes, the boy is often concerned about the girl he impregnates and wants to act in a responsible way in supporting the girl and sharing the burden of decisions regarding the new life. With help the couple can explore all the alternatives available regarding the future of the child, including marriage, adoption, or either the mother or father assuming responsibility to care for and rear the child (Redmond, 1985). Most teenage fathers are willing to accept their obligations and demonstrate strong paternal feelings for the newborn child. They also need to be made aware of their legal rights in relation to the child.

Health Care During Pregnancy

The girl who does not choose to marry is faced with a sequence of problems. She must first decide whether to terminate or continue the pregnancy—a difficult decision for a mature woman but even more so for an immature teenager. Liberalized abortion laws have provided a means for terminating an unwanted pregnancy, and a significant number of girls choose this alternative when it is readily accessible to them and the pregnancy is not too far advanced. However, the procedure is not without risk, both physically and psychologically, and those who select this route will require abortion counseling from supportive, nonjudgmental professionals. The girl will have feelings about the therapy, and termination of the pregnancy does not always solve the underlying problem.

The girl who elects to maintain the pregnancy is confronted with the decision of whether to keep the infant and attempt to provide a home, either alone or in some type of family arrangement; to relinquish the child and pursue her educational and career goals; or to provide for the child and pursue her personal goals. The girl who chooses to place her child for adoption, often a difficult and painful decision, will require guidance in selecting a suitable agency to provide this service and support during the trauma of separation from the infant. The girl who decides to keep her child is often faced with loneliness, the burden of responsibility, a new role, and the task of building a new life. She will need assistance and support in providing care for herself and the child.

Medical management of the pregnancy or its alternative, abortion, does not vary significantly for teenage mothers from that of more mature women, with the exception of the special nutritional needs of young teenagers. For routine medical and nursing management throughout the maternity cycle, the reader is referred to an obstetric nursing textbook (see Jensen and Bobak, 1985). However, pregnant teenagers *do* require a broader range of health and auxiliary services for care. This is best accomplished by a team approach toward quality care for the teenager that includes the parents, the school, the father of the child, and, where feasible, social services and sometimes legal counsel in addition to medical and nursing care.

Nursing Considerations

It is evident from the preceding discussion that nurses play a central role in meeting the needs of pregnant teenagers. It is frequently the nurse to whom the young girl turns for help

and guidance in her dilemma and on whom she relies for support and reassurance.

The first goal in nursing care of the pregnant teenager is to obtain medical care for her if she has not already done so. Typically girls in this age-group are reluctant to seek medical help, in part because of anxiety but more often because of a tendency to deny the pregnancy (especially in younger girls) or in an attempt to conceal their condition as long as possible to avoid being dropped from school (older girls). The importance of early prenatal care is well known for the welfare of both mother and infant when the girl chooses to continue the pregnancy and to facilitate a safe abortion when she elects this option. For guidelines, teaching, and general support measures during pregnancy, the reader is directed to the excellent textbooks available on nursing care throughout the maternity cycle.

Basic to the implementation of any program of care is communication and the establishment of a trusting relationship. Initially the adolescent girl frequently appears apathetic and displays little interest in discussing her pregnancy. She may be abrupt, impatient, defensive, hostile, or indifferent. It is important for the nurse to make every effort to put the youngster at ease and avoid undue pressure until a rapport can be developed so that the girl is comfortable in sharing her feelings and concerns. Conveying a nonjudgmental and genuine caring acceptance of the girl and her goals will assist the nurse to gain her confidence and trust, although this may take a good deal of time and several visits to accomplish. The girl may have encountered rejection and open criticism from authority figures and peers depending on the social and cultural attitudes of the school, the community, and her own family structure.

Communication takes time and patience. Asking open-ended questions and listening for cues will help identify physical, emotional, social, and cultural influences that might affect the adolescent's progress through the maternity cycle. For example, various cultural groups have different attitudes toward unsanctioned pregnancies, and it is important to determine other sources of support, such as the family. Factors that might affect her physical status, such as smoking, drug use, and nutritional state and habits, need to be explored and confronted. Each teenager presents a unique situation in relation to background, life-style, support structure, and coping mechanisms.

The young girl needs to know what is happening to her, what is expected of her, and how she can help in developing a plan of care. Adolescents have their own ideas of the type of help they need and support that would be beneficial. They should be consulted and provided with the opportunity to share their ideas and to feel that they make an important contribution to planning their care.

The girl will need help to improve her altered self-image, a crucial factor in adolescence. Giving her as much individual attention as possible, being a sympathetic listener, providing the opportunity for her to know, support, and be supported by other girls in the same situation, and helping her

Table 20-4 Advantages and disadvantages of contraceptive methods in the adolescent

METHOD	ADVANTAGES	DISADVANTAGES
Abstinence	100% effective if carried out Medically ideal contraceptive	Peer pressure to conform Relatively high failure rate from noncompliance
Withdrawal Withdrawal of penis before ejaculation	Reduced risk of pregnancy but high failure rate Popular method with teenagers	Some seminal fluid often released before ejaculation Ejaculate at vaginal orifice may enter vagina
Rhythm Refrain from intercourse during fertile period (time of ovulation)	High failure rate Only method approved by Roman Catholic Church (for family planning)	Requires enormous motivation by the adolescent and partner Requires a regular, predictable menstrual cycle (unusual in early and middle adolescence)

Barrier methods
  Condom
    Penal covering to trap sperm
	Popular with teenagers
	Simple to use
	Available without prescription
	Provides some protection from sexually transmitted disease
	No side effects
	Girl can carry with her for unexpected sexual encounter
		Requires a highly motivated, responsible adolescent male
		Requires premeditated intent for sexual union
		High failure rate
		Requires consistent use

Diaphragm
    Cervical covering to prevent sperm from reaching egg
    For maximum effectiveness, must be used in conjunction with spermicide
	Virgins can be fitted
	May be inserted 4 to 6 hours before intercourse
	Low failure rate when used correctly
	Few contraindications
		High failure rate in adolescents because of inconvenience of use
		Requires consistent use
		Requires fitting and instruction by medical personnel
		If inserted early, should be checked for placement before coitus
		Requires premeditated intent for sexual union
		Requires body awareness for insertion

Sponge
    Cervical covering
    Releases a spermicide
	As effective as the diaphragm
	Can be obtained without a prescription
		Similar to diaphragm

Cervical cap	Can remain in place up to 4 weeks	Not approved for general use Relatively high failure rate
Chemicals—spermicidal foam, jelly, cream, and so on Substance injected into vagina to kill sperm	Available without prescription Inexpensive Easy to use	High failure rate unless combined with mechanical barrier Possible for sperm to be ejaculated directly into uterine os, bypassing spermicide in vagina Must be used shortly before coitus, therefore requires interruption of sexual experience Repeated sexual union requires repeated application Requires premeditated intent for sexual union

Oral contraceptives
    Estrogen and progesterone-like compounds
    Inhibit ovulation by blocking release of gonadotropins from anterior pituitary gland
	Theoretically 100% effective
	Exceedingly safe for adolescents
	Method of choice for most youngsters
	Administered by mouth
	Becomes a ritual not associated with sexual activity
		Higher failure rate in adolescents than in older women
		Need to follow precise instructions; require continued motivation
		Should not be given to immediate postmenarchal females because of critical period in physiologic maturation of hormone system
		Requires prescription
		Price substantial for teenager

Table 20-4 Advantages and disadvantages of contraceptive methods in the adolescent—cont'd

METHOD	ADVANTAGES	DISADVANTAGES
Intrauterine devices (IUDs) Plastic or metal devices worn inside the uterine cavity Local foreign body effect prevents implantation	Effective for teenagers who are at risk for complications from oral contraceptives or who are mentally retarded Eliminates need for motivation or compliance	Increased risk of infection Less readily accepted by nulliparous uterus Side effects include cramps, pelvic discomfort, and excessive bleeding for one to three menstrual cycles Limited supply available
Sterilization	100% effective	Almost universally irreversible

to experience success at every opportunity will facilitate progress toward achieving this goal. Individual or group discussions of clothes, hairstyles, and makeup and involvement in creative and self-improvement activities help to enhance her self-concept.

The nurse also involves the family whenever possible. The parents of the girl and the father of the child need to express feelings and attitudes about the situation. Often they must deal with their own feelings before they are able to provide support and help in problem solving for the pregnant girl. The girl may or may not wish to have these persons involved in her decisions and care. The nurse must attempt to determine the teenager's true feelings regarding these relationships.

Education regarding child care begins during pregnancy, and preparations should be made for continued education and assistance after the birth. The information for which teenage mothers consistently express a need is: (1) medical needs, that is, how to care for an ill child, (2) daily physical care, and (3) protection from injury (Howard and Sater, 1985). Education should also include information on child development, diet, and stress management.

The pregnant adolescent, although still ostensibly under parental control, has legal authority over the conduct of her pregnancy and the disposition of the child. Adolescents who are clearly no longer under parental control, for example, those who are living alone, are married, are economically self-sufficient, or otherwise demonstrate the capacity to give informed consent are considered ''emancipated'' or ''mature'' minors and as such are responsible for their actions in seeking and accepting medical care.

CONTRACEPTION

Family planning services in general have developed and expanded during recent years, and with the increase in sexual activity among the teenage population there is also an increased awareness of the need for contraceptive services as a part of the health care of adolescents. Although all teenagers need sex education, not all of them are candidates for contraception. Among the large adolescent population there

are those youngsters whose voluntary sexual restraint eliminates the need for control measures, and those who are married and wish to have a child. Since contraceptive advice and management of premarital and married teenagers differ little from fertility control offered to older women, little need be added regarding this group of teenagers.

The group that represents the greatest difficulty is that of the unmarried, dependent, sexually active girl, whether she has been pregnant or not. There is considerable controversy about providing medical services to minors without parental consent. The predominant feeling among health professionals is that parental notification is important but that the ''parents' rights'' view is not necessarily sensitive to the health needs and basic rights of youth. There is no evidence to substantiate the belief that providing contraceptive guidance contributes to sexual irresponsibility and promiscuity. Actually a request for contraceptive information indicates a responsible effort on the part of the teenager to avoid an undesirable pregnancy.

Contraceptive Methods

A contraceptive method, to be safe and effective, must be suited to the individual. The choice is based on the youngster's preference and the physician's judgment. Although a girl may prefer to use oral contraceptives, if her menstrual pattern suggests that she is not ovulating normally, she will be guided to another method. The girl must also be motivated to use whatever method is recommended or prescribed. No matter what method is selected, the provision of a birth control device is only part of a comprehensive sex education program. The advantages and disadvantages of various contraceptive methods recommended for use in adolescents are outlined in Table 20-4.

Simple methods. Sometimes, despite the effectiveness of prescription methods, teenagers persist in using less effective methods because of the necessity for medical screening and supervision inherent in the use of superior devices. Commonplace methods such as withdrawal, douches, and reliance on what are hoped to be ''safe'' periods are often reported in teenage obstetric histories. Factual knowledge about more effective methods such as the condom and

Questions and Controversies

Should adolescents under 18 years of age be permitted to obtain contraceptive services, abortions, and treatment for sexually transmitted diseases without the consent of their parents?

With the increase in sexual activity among adolescents, more of them are in need of health care related to conditions associated with sexuality. Many are reluctant to seek medical care because they are often unable to do so without parental knowledge and permission. Some facilities provide health care to these youngsters without the consent of the parents; however, others deny treatment for fear of legal recriminations. Some minors are able to consent for care legally, that is, those who are married, teenage mothers, and/or self-supporting.

The new regulations governing family planning services under Title X of the Public Health Service Act require that any health care providers receiving government funding notify parents when daughters 17 years of age and under receive prescription contraceptives or contraceptive devices. There are both support for and opposition to this regulation.

Many believe that parents have the right to know what is happening to their children who are under 18 years of age. If parents do not know the medications their daughters are receiving, they are unable to observe for side effects or other associated problems. Nor will they know what counseling their youngsters might have received relative to the medications or devices.

Others charge that minors will not attend the clinics for needed services for fear that parents will be notified. Hence this regulation has come to be known as the "squeal rule." Many health professionals insist that young persons have a right to privacy and ownership of their bodies. One of the major reasons youngsters do not seek medical care for sex-related problems is the fear that their parents will find out.

Would notification of parents penalize those teenagers who are mature and responsible enough to seek contraceptive advice? Will the rule exacerbate the already high incidence of teenage pregnancy and sexually transmitted disease?

chemicals and clarifying some of the myths regarding safe times in the menstrual cycle help to reduce the incidence of unwanted pregnancy. Although they may have some small use for infrequent or short-term exposure to pregnancy, the simple methods are generally unpopular with teenagers. Their use requires considerable consistency and care in following directions and inhibits the spontaneity of the activity.

Prescription methods. Birth control methods that require a medical prescription are considered by many teenagers to be too premeditated; as a result they are less popular among teenagers. However, prescription methods are now being used by greater numbers as attitudes are changing in a more open and permissive atmosphere. Oral contraceptives appear to be the preferred method and are usually prescribed unless there are contraindications.

Use of Contraception

Although teenagers frequently seek contraceptive advice and do not wish for a pregnancy, they are inconsistent users of contraception. Studies indicate that a large number had used no contraceptive at the preceding act of intercourse and that only a small number of sexually active youngsters use contraception with regularity. Compliance is positively correlated with postmenarchal age, frequency of intercourse, autonomy in making and paying for a clinic appointment for the purpose of contraception, and acceptance of a method at the time of the initial clinic visit (Litt, Cuskey, and Rudd, 1980). There are several reasons why teenagers are not making better use of contraception.

Lack of information. Sometimes health professionals have a tendency to confuse a teenager's sophistication with knowledge. Although youngsters are acutely aware of their sexuality, their understanding of reproductive anatomy and physiology is incomplete. If they are using contraception, they often do so with little or no instruction and with only vague understanding. Misinformation is commonplace. Lacking a fundamental understanding of fertility, they often believe that they are too young or have sex too infrequently to become pregnant. A majority of girls mistakenly believe that maximum fertility begins with menses and that the safe period occurs midway between menstrual periods.

Anxiety regarding contraception. Teenagers often express the fear of arguments or threats if they seek assistance via health services. Some are concerned that parents will be notified (see Questions and controversies). Many have exaggerated ideas about the hazards of oral contraceptives or intrauterine devices.

Conflict about sexual activity. Many teenagers feel ambivalent regarding their sexual activity and avoid many contraceptives because their use seems too premeditated and implies that sex is planned rather than a spontaneous activity. Most of these girls believe that sex is all right if one is "swept away" (after all, what can one do about it?) but that planning to do something to prevent pregnancy is wrong.

Desire for pregnancy. There are a few teenagers who deliberately expose themselves to the risk of a pregnancy as a conscious or unconscious act of hostility, response to entrapment, or expression of self-assertion. Even though the youngster has an effective contraceptive, she may fail to use it, use it improperly (conveniently forgetting to take a pill), or use a method not suited to her needs. The girl may know how a contraceptive works but fail to put her knowledge to use.

Nursing Considerations

Much of contraceptive education and service is assumed by nurses as part of sex education programs, family planning services, or postpartum health services. The introduction of contraceptive methods should ideally be associated with ongoing sex education. When they are included in this education process, the sexually active school-age adolescent will consider contraceptives as a natural and logical part of sex life. It is important that youngsters learn about sexuality, conception, and contraception from someone who can provide them with accurate information in a straightforward, nonjudgmental manner.

Most youngsters select a family planning clinic when seeking contraceptive advice. Many are reluctant to consult a private physician (especially one they know well) because they fear a lecture on morality or a refusal of their request (Kreutner, 1981). They may fear that a family physician will tell their parents.

Girls need instruction in correct use of their contraceptive. An effective way to test the teenager's understanding of her particular device is to have her explain to the nurse how the device works. Peer counseling has proved to be successful in gaining compliance especially in youngsters who engage in more frequent sexual activity, have sex with one partner, and are worried that they might become pregnant (Jay and others, 1984).

An essential part of contraceptive services to teenagers is follow-up. The recipient is expected to return frequently for a checkup on the effectiveness of the method and her general health and welfare. Prescriptions are usually dispensed for 1 or sometimes 2 months only so that the girl must return at regular intervals to maintain her contraceptive. Intrauterine devices are checked after the first menstrual flow and periodically to ascertain that they are maintained in proper placement and to evaluate any persistent side effects such as excess flow and cramps.

Nurses are continually on the alert for clues that indicate physical, mental, or emotional problems. Discussions about contraception may provide some insight into disturbed interpersonal relationships and other problems related to the health and well-being of the sexually active adolescent. Participation in regularly scheduled "rap sessions" has proved to be a most important means for exchange between nurses and both male and female adolescents.

An organization that provides education and services for adolescents, including both individual and group counseling, is **Planned Parenthood Federation of America.*** It has branches in most cities in the United States.

RAPE

The adolescent girl is particularly vulnerable to sexual assault, and it is estimated that more than 50% of rape victims are between 10 and 19 years of age. In each instance the victim is potentially subject to serious physical or emotional harm or both. Males may also be assaulted (usually homosexually) and experience the same range of symptoms observed in girl victims (Brookman, 1983).

Legal definitions of rape vary from state to state but in-

*810 Seventh Ave., New York, NY 10019.

clude the following categories: *completed rape*, *attempted rape*, and *statutory rape*. Most of the current definitions of rape are expanded to include all forms of sexual victimization, including anal and oral as well as genital penetration. For example, it may include intrusion of any object or body part into the genital or anal area of another person's body. Statutory rape may be charged when the victim is unable to give consent legally by virtue of age (age varies from state to state, but is usually less than 16 years of age), mental deficiency, psychosis, or an altered state of consciousness caused by sleep, drugs (including alcohol), or illness. Fitting the penis between the labia without disruption of the hymen or evidence of ejaculation is also considered sufficient penetration to constitute rape.

Assailants

Three relationships are identified for adolescent assault: stranger, nonstranger, and incest. Although all can have serious and long-lasting effects, they are presumed to be different in a number of important ways: in the nature of the dominant, psychologic, and cognitive behavior they provoke; in the issues they raise for service providers and other potential helpers; and in the techniques that may be helpful for treating existing and new cases (Burgess, 1985).

Stranger rapist. It is believed that stranger rapes probably account for 50% of all rapes reported to police (Rabkin, 1979). Victims are frequently selected at random because they are apparently helpless and are usually in a vulnerable situation, such as the teenage runaway, the unsuspecting hitchhiker, or the youngster walking alone in an unprotected neighborhood.

Nonstranger rapist. A nonstranger may be a date, someone who lives near the adolescent (such as a neighbor), someone who has contact with the victim through recreational activities or sports, or someone in an official association with the teenager, such as a teacher. Some assailants wait for an opportunity when the victim is defenseless, such as the teenager at home alone with an uncle or cousin or the baby-sitter being driven home.

The assailant may be another teenager known through a social activity. Research in recent years has investigated the relationship of rape-supportive behavior and sex-role learning, dating patterns, and adherence to rape myths (Burt, 1980; Koss and Oros, 1982). The nature of sex-role learning in most cultures associates females with softness, nonassertiveness, and dependence on men; socializes young women to be alluring yet sexually unavailable; and assigns women the role of pace-setter in sexual situations. Males are conditioned to be strong, powerful, and aggressive— highly valued measures of masculinity—and to be aggressors in sexual situations (Burgess, 1985).

Findings of studies also indicate that not only are teenagers at risk for rape by peers but they often face multiple assailants or "gang rapes." These variations on teenage rape include: multiple assailants and a single victim, multiple assailants and multiple victims, multiple assailants and multiple serial victims, and peer rape in tandem (for example, offenders who group together specifically to rape) (Burgess and Holmstrom, 1975).

Incest. The most commonly reported incestuous relationships are between daughter and a male in a caretaking role, for example, a father or a stepfather. Significantly, a consistent observation is the unusually high incidence of serious illness or disability in mothers of sexually abused daughters, which places greater responsibility for care of the daughter in the hands of the father (Herman, 1985). The victim's participation is gained through the application of authority, subtle pressure, persuasion, or misrepresentation of moral standards (Burgess and Holmstrom, 1975). For a further discussion of incest see Chapter 16.

Clinical Manifestations

Adolescents who have been raped arrive at the emergency room or physician's office under a variety of circumstances. They are usually brought in by parents, friends, or police, but some girls may seek medical help on their own. They may display a variety of behaviors, such as hysterical crying or giggling, agitation, feelings of degradation, anger and rage, helplessness, nervousness, and rapid mood swings. Adolescents may alternately appear calm and controlled, masking inner turmoil; they may be angry, confused, and filled with self-blame (Committee on Adolescence, 1983).

The rape victim may present with evidence of physical force, including roughness, nonbrutal beating (slapping), brutal beating (slugging, kicking, beating repeatedly with fists), and choking or gagging. The predominant reaction of the victim is fear—of the rape and of injury. Thus the victim is faced with the dilemma of submission or resistance. Resistance increases the victim's chances of escape but also increases the likelihood of violence against him or her.

Therapeutic Management

It is advisable to obtain parental consent for examination, but the examination may be performed without consent if the adolescent is mature and the parents are unavailable. A female nurse should be present during the history and examination of female victims. Whether a parent should be present during the examination is determined on an individual basis. The parent's presence is usually encouraged but only *if the parent is supportive*. Often the presence of a parent or a police officer inhibits the youngster's ability to describe the incident.

Since rape is a legal matter to be determined by the courts, medical examination merely provides evidence of penetration, ejaculation, and, when possible, use of force. The last is difficult to determine, since many young women are left unmarked when forced to comply at the point of a gun or other weapon.

Initial contact. The circumstances of the initial medical evaluation may be frightening and stressful. The initial contact with the rape victim must be supportive, and the fundamental goal (as in any health problem) is to do no further harm. The interrogating and associated activities have the potential to add to the trauma of the sexual assault. First of all the victim needs to know that she is (1) all right and (2) not being blamed for the situation. The first approach is not one of repeated interrogation, but an attempt to reduce the youngster's stress.

History. Although it is important to obtain a clear account of the circumstances of an alleged rape, it is equally essential to minimize any further psychologic trauma that might occur if the adolescent is forced to relive a very painful experience. The youngster will in all likelihood have been questioned by family (or whoever brought the victim for care) and the police (if the rape was reported). If the youngster is too upset, the detailed history may be delayed. The youngster should not be further victimized by insensitive care and unnecessary trauma (Committee on Adolescence, 1983).

The history should be as complete as possible and must be taken and presented in the patient's own words, including any account of force or threats. Some youngsters are able to provide detailed descriptions of the event; others are afraid, stammer, cry, and have difficulty in selecting words or are unable to speak at all. The interview can be more effective if a common vocabulary is established so that both the youngster and the interviewer understand the terms used to describe anatomic features.

Information includes date, time, location, and an accurate description of all types of sexual contact. All related activities are included. For example, evidence can be altered if the victim has bathed, urinated, defecated, douched, or changed clothing; therefore, these activities should be recorded. Use of a condom by the alleged assailant can alter evidence. For adequate care, other important data include date of last menstrual period, date of last intercourse (where applicable), use of contraception, and any possibility of a preexisting pregnancy or sexually transmitted disease. Behavior and emotional state should also be recorded, since responses range from outward calm and controlled behavior and affect to excessive agitation or hysteria. Some girls are inappropriately giddy or nonchalant.

Examination. The physical examination is carried out as soon as possible, since physical evidence deteriorates rapidly. The youngster is always told in advance in understandable terms exactly what to expect in the way of tests and procedures, and the explanation is accompanied by strong emotional support. The victim is examined thoroughly, including nongenital areas for evidence of injury that might substantiate the use of force. Sometimes the stress of the incident makes the girl unaware of physical trauma or even serious injury. The degree and type of injury vary greatly in victims of rape. A few are murdered, many suffer physical injury, and practically all are disturbed emotionally. Photographs are taken of bruises, lacerations, or scratches for evidence, and rips or tears in clothing and the presence of dirt or grass stains are noted and recorded. Perineal or rectal lacerations suggest rape.

Specimens are obtained from the vaginal cul-de-sac, and a hang-drop preparation is examined immediately to assess sperm motility. A cervical smear is prepared and sent to the laboratory. Vaginal secretions are also tested for acid phosphatase, since this enzyme is not normally present in the female genital tract but is found in high concentrations in semen. This is especially important if the assailant has had a vasectomy or is infertile. It is the most accurate test up to 14 hours after the alleged assault; the Pap smear is the most reliable test for documentation of sexual intercourse from 14 to 26 hours after the event.

A baseline serology is drawn, and a gonococcal culture is obtained to prove that the victim did not have any preexisting infection. The girl is reexamined at appropriate intervals (4 to 6 weeks for syphilis; 2 to 3 days for gonorrhea) to determine if the girl acquired disease from the assailant.

Treatment. Any injuries sustained by the victim that require surgical treatment are repaired. Lacerations of the vagina are not uncommon. Most physicians prescribe, and many of the victims and/or their parents prefer the girl to receive, prophylactic administration of penicillin at the time of initial examination. Pregnancy prophylaxis, usually diethylstilbestrol, is offered to the victim who is not using oral contraceptives, pregnant, or menstruating. Follow-up care is needed to observe the youngster for possible development of pelvic inflammatory disease or other sexually transmitted disease.

Rape Trauma Syndrome

Sexual abuse of children, including rape, is being given increasing attention and concern by health professionals, in both the physical aspects and the psychologic reactions to the trauma (see Sexual abuse, p. 689). Burgess, Holmstrom and McCausland (1976), through their observations, have identified what they describe as the *rape trauma syndrome.* The rape trauma syndrome involves two phases: (1) the acute phase of disorganization of life-style and (2) a long-term process of reorganization. These phases encompass behavioral, somatic, and psychologic reactions to the stressful event.

Acute phase of disorganization. During the acute phase victims exhibit either an expressed style or a controlled style of demonstrating emotional reactions. Those with the expressed style are able to express their feelings of fear, anger, and/or anxiety. Those with the controlled style hide or mask their feelings and display a calm, subdued affect. Since a common emotional response to sexual assault is terror, the psychologic mechanisms evoked in an attempt to cope with the stress are equally powerful. Often the emotional shock creates an exaggerated sense of unreality and dissociation; to an untrained observer the victim may appear

indifferent. The controlled victim is equally as upset as the victim who expresses her feelings.

Other acute reactions include physical reactions such as body soreness, disturbances in sleep patterns, and alterations in eating patterns. In addition to fear responses, the victims demonstrate other emotional responses, including anger, self-blame, guilt, shame, and/or feelings of degradation. Feelings of embarrassment are prominent in adolescents. Mood swings, enhanced mood lability, and increased irritability with others are often observed. Almost all victims spend a good deal of time thinking about how the assault might have been prevented. Many concerns of youngsters focus on how the event will affect them at school.

Long-term reorganization process. Changes in lifestyle are often observed during the reorganization phase. Victims may continue previous activities such as attending school but achieve only a minimum level of functioning. A teenager may attend school but be apprehensive that other students know about the incident and are talking about her. When an adolescent girl has been raped by a male student or gang of boys from the school, she is afraid to return to school and may beg to move to a different neighborhood. It is not unusual for the attacker to telephone and taunt the victim or for the girl to receive anonymous obscene calls. Most children experience nightmares, phobias about being left alone, and panic reactions on seeing the assailant, the scene of the crime, or a symbolic reminder of the assault. Sexual fears are prominent and difficult for the victim to discuss.

Feelings of helplessness and powerlessness are experienced as the victim feels that events are totally beyond her control. Many demonstrate a marked degree of self-blame because of society's impression that women provoke sexual attacks. Victims are concerned about the potential effects that the assault will have on their relationships with others, particularly regarding the extent to which persons close to them will blame them for the assault. There are concerns about whom to tell about the event and how to go about telling them. Sexual assault produces varied and profound long-term effects on the victims.

Nursing Considerations

Many of the approaches that have been described for the sexually abused child (p. 692) are applicable to the adolescent. Sexual assault is a devastating experience with long-lasting effects. The primary goal of nursing care is not to inflict further stress on the youngster who is often angry, confused, frightened, embarrassed, and filled with self-blame. Young rape victims fear pregnancy, bodily injury, and the reactions of their parents. Some believe that their bodies are permanently damaged and may even fear death as a consequence of the experience. On the other hand, health professionals are more likely to be angry at the rapist, concerned about sexually transmitted disease, and worried about the youngster's future sexual relations (Mann, 1981).

The nurse must do everything possible to reduce the stress of the interrogation and examination. Application of stress-reduction techniques during the process can help the adolescent manage the immediate experience. Although most health professionals and law enforcement officers are sensitive to the needs of the youngster and attempt to make the process as nonstressful as possible, the nurse should be alert to cues that indicate the victim is being overstressed.

Follow-up care of the rape victim is essential and extends over a long period of time. Consequently, referral to a public health agency, school nurse, and/or mental health agency should be made as soon as possible. Victims who live in areas in which there is an established rape crisis center are fortunate. In areas where they do not exist, nurses can work with communities to establish such a service.

Aside from the universal need for emotional support, there are no firm guidelines for meeting the needs of rape victims. Their needs vary widely and depend on the nature of the incident, when it took place, the physical and emotional injuries sustained by the victim, the actions being considered as a result, the resources available for informal support, and the anticipated reactions of persons in the informal support network (Burgess, 1985). However, the nurse who knows the nature of the rape trauma syndrome and some of the reactions that might be expected is in a better position to assess and meet the needs of the adolescent sexual assault victim.

Family support. In addition to the needs of the adolescent rape victim, the nurse is also sensitive to the needs and reactions of the youngster's parents. Some will be angry and blame the adolescent; others will be guilt ridden. Many reactions can be expected at the time of the incident, ranging from despair to extreme agitation. Frequently the parents require as much support and reassurance as the victim. Agitated, angry, or incapacitated parents are unable to provide support for their youngster. Meeting their needs can facilitate their ability to support the teenager during the crisis.

Prevention. With the increasing incidence of rape many professionals are looking to additional means for preventing rape at all ages. Many schools and organizations arrange for classes on how to avoid an attack and how to behave in the event of an attempted rape. Rape trauma centers and most law enforcement agencies provide this service to schools, organizations, or groups of concerned citizens. Every effort should be made to protect children and adolescents from injury and to teach them how to avoid situations that may promote an attack and how to behave in a threatening situation.

Sexually Transmitted Diseases

Sexually transmitted diseases (STDs) are among the most prevalent and dangerous of the communicable diseases and are now epidemic in the United States, with a disproportion-

ate number occurring in adolescents and young adults. Of the reportable diseases, gonorrhea (GC) ranks first in numbers of cases, with an alarming increase in the adolescent age-group (Frau and Alexander, 1985). Although they constitute only about 20% of the total population in the United States, adolescents experience one of the highest rates for sexually transmitted diseases. Even with the large number of cases that are reported, this is considered to be a conservative estimate of the true incidence because of underreporting of cases and failure to diagnose all cases as they occur. Sexually active adolescents are particularly at risk because they are often late in seeking medical attention. It is important that when a patient is diagnosed with one of the STDs the history and examination should encompass others who may be infected.

Gonorrhea is still considered the most serious STD and is epidemic in adolescents and young adults. The incidence of *Chlamydia trachomatis* is rapidly approaching that of gonorrhea in this age-group, and it is the major cause of nongonorrheal urethritis (NGU). Genital herpes is a source of interest and concern, but although syphilis and some other traditional sexually transmitted diseases occur in adolescents, they are relatively rare.

GONORRHEA

Gonorrhea, also known by such common names as the whites, clap, the drips, and the dose, is a disease that occurs primarily in larger metropolitan areas where the rate of infection is higher than in more rural areas. There are three times as many males affected as females, and it is more prevalent in nonwhite than in white populations.

Gonorrhea is a disease that appears to be everywhere, and an attack confers no immunity to subsequent reinfections. In fact, subsequent infections are often caused by the same untreated partner, and a potentially vicious cycle is created until the infected partner is identified and treated. Gonorrhea is almost always sexually contracted, except when it appears as conjunctivitis. Other manifestations such as pharyngitis and proctitis reflect variant modes of sexual contact.

Pathophysiology

The causative organism is *Neisseria gonorrhoeae,* a grampositive diplococcus. The organisms, commonly known as gonococci, have been divided into four types; types 1 and 2 are pathogenic, and types 3 and 4 are considered nonpathogenic. The difference in pathogenicity appears to be the presence of hairlike projections on types 1 and 2 that cause them to adhere to the mucosa, where they remain attached for 36 to 48 hours, the incubation period of the organism. The organisms have very specific survival requirements. They prefer a moist, alkaline environment (pH 7.2 to 7.6) and a temperature of 35° to 36° C (95° to 96.8° F). They quickly die on drying, exposure to the weakest acids, and an increase of 3° C in temperature. The gonococci survive

Table 20-5 Comparison between gonorrhea and chlamydial infection

CHARACTERISTICS	GONORRHEA	CHLAMYDIAL INFECTION
Incubation period	2-6 days; can be as long as 10-16 days in rare cases	8-21 days
Major site of infection	Urethritis (males) Cervicitis (females)	Urethritis (males) Cervicitis (females)
Local complications	Epididymitis, bartholinitis, salpingitis, prostatitis Conjunctivitis Pharyngitis Proctitis common in homosexual individuals	Epididymitis, bartholinitis, salpingitis Conjunctivitis (trachoma) Pharyngitis Proctitis not yet documented
Systemic complications	Well established; septicemia with resulting arthritis, dermatitis, endocarditis; meningitis; perihepatitis and peritonitis also reported	Possible: arthritis, perihepatitis, peritonitis, endocarditis reported
Carrier state	Recognized, especially in women; can last for months; primary reservoir is the cervix, male urethra a minor one	Recognized, especially in women; can last for months; primary reservoir is the cervix, male urethra a minor one
Effects of maternal infection on newborn	Less well established Ophthalmia neonatorum	Well known: inclusion conjunctivitis and pneumonia
Treatment	Penicillin drug of choice; ampicillin, amoxicillin, streptomycin, tetracycline, spectinomycin Probenecid used in conjunction with antibiotics Shorter period of therapy Treatment of sexual contacts	Tetracycline is drug of choice; erythromycin, sulfonamides, streptomycin, trimethoprim-sulfamethoxazole Regimen of 14 days Treatment of sexual contacts

only on the columnar and transitional epithelium; stratified epithelium is resistant to the onslaught. The organisms spread along the mucosa from the point of entry. They penetrate between the epithelial cells and, when they die, liberate an irritant that produces the inflammatory response characterized by localized capillary dilation, edema, and leukocytosis. This process accounts for the purulent discharge and erosive balanitis and cervicitis observed in affected persons.

Clinical Manifestations

Symptoms can appear as early as 1 day or as late as 2 weeks after sexual contact. Gonococcal infection can occur in many diverse ways with four basic presentations: asymptomatic, uncomplicated symptomatic, complicated symptomatic, and disseminated disease. The infection can involve a number of organs and a wide range of manifestations (see Table 20-5). The pelvic inflammatory disease (PID) in females simulates the inflammatory process caused by other bacterial infections, and differential diagnosis is made for more definitive medical treatment. Since a large percentage of affected persons are asymptomatic, gonorrhea should be considered in the evaluation of all sexually active adolescents. Lack of clinical symptoms is especially characteristic of the rectal and pharyngeal infections.

There is a difference in the way the disease affects children. Whereas uncomplicated urogenital infection in post-

pubescent girls involves the cervix, in prepubescent girls it is seen as vulvovaginitis. Early complaints of vulvovaginitis include dysuria and perineal or vulvar discomfort, often associated with perianal soreness that is increased during defecation. Examination reveals edematous vaginal mucosa, and a greenish yellow discharge may be present; the perianal area often appears inflamed and edematous with some discharge from anal crypts.

Diagnostic Evaluation

The diagnosis is established on identification of the organism from direct smear or culture techniques. In males the diagnosis is relatively easy. Since gram-negative diplococci are not normally present in the male genitourinary tract, their intracellular presence in smears is diagnostic. A false-negative result may be seen in the very early course of the disease, in old, untreated cases, and in persons who have taken penicillin or a wide-spectrum antibiotic within a few hours of the examination.

The diagnosis is more difficult in females, which has been a significant obstacle in effective control programs. Although cervical and urethral smears are fairly reliable in the acute phase of the disease, with less acute or asymptomatic cases there is a high yield of both false-positive and false-negative results. Specimens of pus from the urethra or cervix (not the vagina) should be cultured immediately on special media (Thayer-Martin VCN or Transglow) designed for discriminating these organisms. Because of their adverse effects on organisms, surgical jelly or any fatty substance (including some types of swabs) should not be used in securing the specimen. Presence of menses is not a contraindication; the menstrual secretions provide an optimum environment for growth of the organism.

Therapeutic Management

Effective treatment of both males and females with uncomplicated gonorrhea is administration of penicillin (preferably) or other antibiotic therapy. Resistant strains are treated with spectinomycin or cefoxitin.

Most desirable is an effective single-dose approach in order to prevent problems of follow-up and patient cooperation. Adequate penicillin therapy achieves a 95% success rate in acute genital gonorrhea, but follow-up is essential, since an acute infection may convert to the asymptomatic carrier state and the incidence of reinfection is high. Relief of symptoms cannot be equated with cure. It is important that all affected youngsters have a serologic test for syphilis, and all their sexual contacts should be traced and treated.

Complicated and disseminated infections may require longer antibiotic therapy, and complications are treated appropriately. In all cases of gonorrhea the long-term genitourinary problems in the male and possible occlusion of the fallopian tubes or tuboovarian abscesses in the female from untreated or repeated infections can lead to severe debilitation in later life or even death. Therefore case finding and early treatment are imperative.

Prevention

A genuine prophylaxis against gonorrheal infections is not yet available. There is a protective vaccine in the process of development, but when it becomes available, the decision must be made concerning who should be vaccinated and when they should be vaccinated. Until such time as such protection is in common use, preventive efforts must be directed toward finding and treating affected persons, locating and examining contacts of affected persons, educating young people regarding the facts of the disease and its spread, and encouraging the use of barriers in sexually active young people.

CHLAMYDIAL INFECTION

Recent evidence indicates that chlamydial infection is a major type of sexually transmitted disease in adolescents and young adults and is as important as gonorrhea in its incidence, transmission, range of infection sites, and carrier state. Like gonorrhea, the causative organism is responsible for a variety of disorders, including cervicitis, salpingitis, epididymitis, urethritis, peritonitis, conjunctivitis, pneumonia, and otitis media. However, the main infections are urethritis in males and cervicitis in females.

Pathophysiology

The disease is caused by *Chlamydia trachomatis,* an organism previously thought to be a virus but now known to be bacteria. Like viruses, chlamydiae are intracellular parasites during part of their life cycle. The organisms consist of alternating forms—the extracellular, or elementary, body, and the intracellular, or initial, body. The elementary body attaches to the host cell, where it induces active phagocytosis and is ingested in a vesicle that serves as a setting for the next stage of the cycle.

Unlike other phagocytosed organisms, *C. trachomatis* is able to circumvent host cell defenses and become a part of the cell. Within the host cell, the elementary body reorganizes into the larger initial body, which uses the cell's synthetic functions and energy sources for its own metabolic needs. It divides to produce microcolonies of chlamydiae. After 18 to 24 hours the initial bodies again reorganize into elementary bodies and exit from the disrupted host cell to infect new host cells. The entire process takes about 40 hours, and the result is a slow, steady accumulation of intracellular inclusions that are diagnostic of the infection.

Clinical Manifestations

The signs and symptoms of infection by *C. trachomatis* are similar to those of gonorrhea, which include meatal erythema and tenderness, urethral discharge, dysuria, or urethral itching in males and mucopurulent cervical exudate, usually associated with erythema, edema, congestion, and increased friability of the cervix in females. The symptoms may be mild enough to be ignored or entirely absent (see Table 20-5).

Diagnostic Evaluation

The diagnosis is confirmed by isolation of the organism in a tissue cell culture or serologic evidence of infection. Because the staining techniques are insensitive, smears are not useful in the specific diagnosis of the disease. The complement fixation test is useful in the diagnosis of lymphogranuloma venereum caused by *C. trachomatis,* and the microimmunofluorescent test is often used for other chlamydial infections. Abnormal Pap smears have been associated with antichlamydial antibodies in cervical secretions.

Therapeutic Management

The treatment of choice is oral tetracycline hydrochloride, 1 to 2 g daily for at least 14 days. Also effective are doxycycline (100 mg twice daily) or erythromycin stearate (1 g daily) administered over 1 to 3 weeks. Penicillin and its derivatives are *not* effective against the organism, which probably explains the persistence of infection in those affected persons who are treated for gonorrhea. It is suggested that all patients with gonorrhea receive a course of tetracycline therapy because of the high rate of mixed gonococcal and chlamydial infections. Treatment of sexual partners is also an important part of therapy.

HERPES GENITALIS

Organism: Herpes virus hominis—type II

Incubation period: Virus dormant 3 days or longer

Clinical manifestations: Small, usually painful vesicles on genital area, buttocks, and thighs; itching usually initial symptom; when vesicles break, shallow, circular, extremely painful lesions remain. Other symptoms include fever, malaise, and inguinal lymphadenopathy; may be asymptomatic. Initial infection lasts 2 to 4 weeks; recurrences of infection and symptoms common.

Diagnostic evaluation: Pap smear reveals multinucleated giant cells and nuclear inclusion bodies. Tissue culture necessary for definitive diagnosis.

Therapeutic management: No specific therapy found to be uniformly effective. Acyclovir (Zovirax) as topical ointment has shown a decrease in healing time and in some cases a decrease in viral shedding and pain. The drug is available in intravenous and, recently, oral preparations. Symptomatic relief is sometimes offered by viscous lidocaine applications to painful ulcerations.

Comments: Pregnancy should be prevented in sexually active girls; infection can be transmitted to infant during birth.

TRICHOMONIASIS

Organism: *Trichomonas vaginalis*

Incubation period: Unknown

Clinical manifestations: Pruritus and edema of external genitalia; foul-smelling, greenish vaginal discharge; sometimes postcoital bleeding. May be asymptomatic, especially males.

Diagnostic evaluation: Vaginal secretions examined microscopically via wet mount; Pap smears may show organism; culture of organism made.

Therapeutic management: Oral administration of metronidazole.

Comments: May be contracted by self-infection from toilet bowls, bathtubs, or swimming pools; however, lack of agreement about this. Patient should not consume alcohol while taking medication and for at least 48 hours after last dose.

CANDIDIASIS (MONILIASIS)

Organism: *Candida albicans*

Incubation period: Unknown

Clinical manifestations: Edema and erythema of vulva and thick, white, cheesy vaginal discharge. May be satellite lesions on groin, thighs, and buttocks. May be asymptomatic. Cutaneous lesions on penis.

Diagnostic evaluation: Microscopic examination of vaginal wall scrapings and vaginal discharge.

Therapeutic management: Nystatin vaginal suppositories twice daily for 7 to 14 days; miconazole vaginal cream for 1 week.

Comments: Possibility of predisposing factors such as oral contraceptives, which alter vaginal environment, or antibiotics. Increased risk of neonatal thrush.

SYPHILIS

Organism: *Treponema pallidum,* a fragile spirochete found naturally only in tissues of infected humans

Incubation period: 10 to 90 days

Clinical manifestations: Primary stage characterized by a chancre—a hard, painless, red, sharply defined lesion with an indurated base, raised border, eroded surface, and scanty yellow serous discharge; hard chancre appears at the point of inoculation, usually the penis, vulva, or cervix; extragenital chancres may occur on other areas of body.

Secondary stage characterized by systemic influenza-like symptoms and lymphadenopathy; generalized rash frequently but not invariably develops 1 to 3 months (average, 3 weeks) after spontaneous healing of primary lesion.

Diagnostic evaluation: Positive identification of treponema organism made by examination of exudate from primary or secondary lesions under darkfield microscope.

Serologic tests (mainly screening tests) used for identification of the organism:

1. Nontreponemal or nonspecific reagin antigen tests—Kahn, Kolmer, VDRL (Venereal Disease Research Laboratories) tests, all of which are laboratory tests; Rapid Plasma Reagin (RPR) and plasmacrit (PCT) tests, which are newer tests that do not require laboratory equipment and can be performed in clinic or physician's office.

2. Treponemal or specific antibody tests—*Treponema pallidum* immobilization (TPI) and the fluorescent treponemal antibody absorption (FTA-ABS) tests.

Therapeutic management: Penicillin in doses sufficient to maintain an adequate blood level for a minimum of 10 to 14 days. Alternate drugs for allergic individuals are tetracycline and erythromycin.

Comments: Viability of the organism outside the body is short—rapidly killed by oxygen, soap, common bacterial agents, and drying. About 95% is transmitted sexually; affected person is most infectious during first year of disease, after which communicability diminishes.

NURSING CONSIDERATIONS

Nursing responsibilities encompass all aspects of sexually transmissible disease education, prevention, and treatment. The sex education of young people should include information about these diseases, such as their symptoms and treatment, and dispelling the myths associated with their mode of transmission. These diseases (except possibly trichomoniasis) are not contracted from toilet seats, drinking glasses, and bath towels. Herpes simplex virus has been shown to remain viable on some surfaces and materials that have been in contact with infected lesions; however, the risk is extremely low (Larson and Bryson, 1985; Nerurkar and others, 1983). Most persons in the vulnerable teenage population are uninformed or misinformed about these diseases. Helping to promote the inclusion of venereal disease information in school sex education programs is an important function of the nurse.

No matter what their area of practice, nurses are in a position to disseminate information, identify probable cases, and refer these cases for treatment. In the hospital, school, clinic, or private practice nurses who recognize the signs and symptoms of disease can call these to the attention of the attending physician. This includes not only nurses working in pediatric practice but those in prenatal and obstetric services as well. A characteristic rash or lesion on a pregnant woman may be evidence of disease and a threat to the unborn child. It is nurses who are most successful in persuading pregnant women to receive early and regular prenatal care. The earlier the mother is treated, the less the hazard to the unborn child, especially in the case of syphilis, which does not affect the fetus during the first 4 months of gestation. Gonorrheal and herpes infections are most dangerous to the child during delivery and in the postpartum period.

Nurses, too, should not overlook the need for care in handling infected infants and children to prevent cross-contaminating others or contracting the disease themselves. Gloves should be worn when handling secretions and areas most likely to contain the organisms, and any breaks in the skin should receive special protective covering.

The increasing incidence of STDs in young people is influenced to a great extent by the larger numbers of teenagers who engage in sexual activity more casually, at younger ages, and with more partners. In addition, the changing pattern of contraceptive use is a contributing factor to more promiscuous sexual activity and the concomitant rise in gonorrhea and chlamydial infection. The newer contraceptive methods, oral contraceptives and intrauterine devices, appear to provide no protection against STDs, and barrier devices, such as the condom, that offer some protection are not well accepted by teenagers. Unfortunately, many girls who take oral contraceptive pills mistakenly believe that they are also effective in preventing STDs. To decrease the likelihood of infection, sexually active youngsters should be encouraged to use a mechanical barrier (condom) and/or some substance that alters the environment. Vaginal sprays, lubricants, or douches that lower the vaginal pH are fairly effective, for example, a vinegar douche *soon* after intercourse.

Essential measures for control of the disease are treating the disease, reporting it *promptly,* and tracing and treating contacts (including homosexual contacts). Very often teenagers who suspect they have an STD will seek a trusted nurse for help rather than their parents. It is probably best to try to persuade the youngsters to tell their parents, but, if they are reluctant, the alternative is to refer them to some source where they can receive medical help. The obstacle of the youngster's fear of parental wrath or shame has been overcome in most areas by permitting physicians to treat affected minors without requiring the consent of the parent. Although not all states permit private physicians to treat minors, most public health departments are prepared to accept them for treatment without parental consent, since they are legally allowed to treat persons of all ages for communicable diseases.

In many areas medical clinics and practitioners specializing in members of this age-group have gained the trust of the adolescent, who may readily seek their services in such an emergency. However, there is a dirty connotation to STDs, which must be overcome before many teenagers will cooperate. Most teenagers have intercourse with someone they are fond of, and they do not like to think of the partner in this light. Also, even when youngsters trust the health workers, they may hesitate to be seen entering a clinic that specializes in treatment of STDs.

When dealing with adolescents, nurses need highly developed interviewing skills to elicit a history of sexual contacts. The belief that these diseases are "dirty" and that "nice" people from "nice" families do not contract the diseases, and the fear of parental displeasure and of "squealing" on friends, can be deterrents to getting needed information. To gain youngsters' cooperation the nurse conveys acceptance, helps them feel at ease, and assures them that the information they give will be used to help those persons whom they name as contacts. They can be reassured that their identity and the identities of the persons they name as contacts will be kept confidential. The purpose is not to embarrass or punish but to trace and treat affected persons. This is the most effective means presently available for controlling these diseases.

CONCEPT SUMMARIES

- Typical adolescent health-seeking behaviors center on skin problems, obesity, headaches, abdominal discomfort, menstrual symptoms, and anxieties about physical development and sexual change.

- Acne is prevalent in the teen years; medication and hygiene are the treatments of choice.

- Smoking is a widespread problem among teenagers; reasons for smoking include social pressure, mass media influence, and a need to develop a self-concept.

- Participation in sports predisposes adolescents to acute injuries, such as contusions, dislocations, sprains, and strains, and overuse syndromes, such as stress fractures.

- Health concerns associated with sports are related menstrual dysfunction, drug misuse, and sudden death.

- Alterations in growth and maturation may be manifest in short stature; tall stature; precocious puberty; Turner syndrome; Klinefelter syndrome; pathologic conditions such as chronic disease, skeletal defects, endocrine dysfunction, and cortisol excess; and psychosocial dwarfism.

- Assessment of growth consists of taking a family history, determining previous growth patterns, conducting a physical examination, determining bone age, and conducting endocrine studies.

- The most frequent problems related to the male reproductive system are infections, hematuria, voiding dysfunction, scrotal conditions, and gynecomastia.

- The most frequent problems of the female reproductive system involve menstruation—delays, irregularities, and discomfort—and infections.

- Adolescent pregnancy has profound social, educational, psychologic and economic ramifications; physiologically the pregnancy necessitates special attention to nutrition and psychologic and emotional support for the mother and father.

- Contraception is often not used because of lack of information, anxiety regarding use, conflict over sexual activity, and desire for pregnancy.

- Rape is a serious problem among adolescent females; common forms are rape by stranger, rape by nonstranger, and incest.

- Sexually transmitted diseases frequently found among adolescents are gonorrhea, chlamydial infection, herpes genitalis, trichomoniasis, and candidiasis.

REFERENCES

Ad Hoc Committee on Growth Hormone Usage, The Lawson Wilkins Pediatric Endocrine Society, and Committee on Drugs: Growth hormone in the treatment of children with short stature, Pediatrics **72**:891-894, 1983.

Alpert, G., and Fleisher, G.R.: Complications of infection with Epstein-Barr virus during childhood: a study of children admitted to the hospital, Pediatr. Infect. Dis. **3**:304-307, 1984.

Alvin, P.E., and Litt, I.F.: Current status of the etiology and management of dysmenorrhea in adolescence, Pediatrics **70**:516-525, 1982.

Bailey, J.D., Park, E., and Cowell, C.: Estrogen treatment of girls with constitutional tall stature, Pediatr. Clin. North Am. **28**:501-512, 1981.

Bender, B. and others: Speech and language development in 41 children with sex chromosome anomalies, Pediatrics **71**:262-267, 1983.

Benke, P.J.: The isotretinoin teratogen syndrome, JAMA **251**:3267-3269, 1984.

Biglan, A., and others: A situational analysis of adolescent smoking, J. Behav. Med. **1**:109-114, 1984.

Bosman, S.A.: Testicular tumors in prepubertal children, Urology **13**:581-588, 1979.

Bragg, C., and Hughes, G.H.: Understanding and managing patients who smoke, Fam. Comm. Health **7**:12-21, 1984.

Brookman, R.R.: Adolescent sexuality and related health problems. In Hoffmann, A.D., editor: Adolescent medicine, Menlo Park, CA, 1983, Addison-Wesley Publishing Co.

Burgess, A.W.: The sexual victimization of adolescents, Washington, D.C., 1985, U.S. Government Printing Office, DHHS Publication No. (ADM) 858-1382.

Burgess, A.W., and Holmstrom, L.L.: Sexual trauma of children and adolescents: pressure, sex, and secrecy, Nurs. Clin. North Am. **10**:551-563, 1975.

Burt, M.R.: Cultural myths and supports for rape, J. Pers. Soc. Psychol. **38**:2-220, 1980.

Camp, B.W., and others: Infants of adolescent mothers, Am. J. Dis. Child. **138**:243-246, 1984.

Cavanaugh, R.M.: Pelvic examination of adolescent girls, Am. Fam. Physician **26**:105-108, 1982.

Chassin, L., and others: Self-images and cigarette smoking in adolescence, Pers. Soc. Psychol. Bull. **7**:670-676, 1981.

Cohen, F.L.: Clinical genetics in nursing practice, Philadelphia, 1984, J.B. Lippincott Co.

Cohen, F.L., and Durham, J.D.: Children with sex chromosome variations: implications for pediatric nursing practice, J. Pediatr. Nurs. **1**:12-23, 1986.

Colletta, N.D., and Gregg, C.H.: Adolescent mothers' vulnerability to stress, J. Nerv. Ment. Dis. **169**:50-54, 1981.

Committee on Accident and Poison Prevention: Trampolines, Evanston, IL, 1977, American Academy of Pediatrics.

Committee on Accident and Poison Prevention, and Committee on Pediatric Aspects of Physical Fitness, Recreation, and Sports: Trampolines II, Pediatrics **67**:438-439, 1981.

Committee on Adolescence: Rape and the adolescent, Pediatrics **72**:738-739, 1983.

Committee on Drugs: New therapy for severe cystic acne, Pediatrics **72**:258-259, 1983.

Committee on Environmental Hazards: Smokeless tobacco—a carcinogenic hazard, Pediatrics **76**:1009-1011, 1985.

Committee on Fetus and Newborn: Report of the Ad Hoc Task Force on Circumcision, Pediatrics **56**:610-611, 1975.

Committee on Pediatric Aspects of Physical Fitness, Recreation, and Sports, Pediatrics **67**:927-928, 1981.

Committee on Sports Medicine: Participation in boxing among children and young adults, Pediatrics **74**:311-312, 1984.

Committee on Sports Medicine: Sports medicine: health care for young athletes, Evanston, IL, 1983, American Academy of Pediatrics.

Conte, F.A., and Grumbach, M.M.: Therapeutic issues in Turner's syndrome, West. J. Med. **137**:61-62, 1982.

Dawood, M.Y.: Dysmenorrhea, Clin. Obstet. Gynecol. **26**:719-727, 1983.

Dessendorfer, E.A., Amsterdam, E.A., and Odland, T.M.: Adolescent smoking and its effect on aerobic exercise tolerance, Phys. Sports Med. **11**:109-119, 1983.

Diddle, A.W.: Athletic activity and menstruation, South. Med. J. **76**:619-624, 1983.

Dyment, P.G.: Drug misuse by adolescent athletes, Pediatr. Clin. North Am. **29**:1363-1368, 1983.

Eckert, P.: Beyond the statistics of adolescent smoking, Am. J. Public Health **73**:439-441, 1983.

Edidin, D.V., and Levitsky, L.L.: Prepubertal gynecomastia associated with estrogen-containing hair cream, Am. J. Dis. Child. **136**:587-588, 1982.

Elster, A.B., McAnarney, E.R., and Lamb, M.E.: Parental behavior of adolescent mothers, Pediatrics **71**:494-503, 1983.

Epstein, A.S.: Assessing the child development information needed by adolescent parents with very young children, Final Report, Washington, D.C., 1980, U.S. Department of Health, Education and Welfare.

Evans, R.I., and others: Social modeling films to deter smoking in adolescents: results of a three year field investigation, J. Appl. Psychol. **66**:399,415, 1981.

Flay, B.R., and others: Cigarette smoking: why young people do it and ways of preventing it. In McGrath, P.J., and Firestone, P.: Pediatric and adolescent behavioral medicine: issues in treatment, New York, 1983, Springer Publishing Co.

Frau, L.M., and Alexander, E.R.: Public health implications of sexually transmitted diseases in pediatric practice, Pediatr. Infect. Dis. **4**:453-467, 1985.

Frische, R.E., and McArthur, J.W.: Menstrual cycles: fatness as a determinant of minimum weight for height necessary for their maintenance and onset, Science **186**:949-951, 1974.

Frische, R.E, and others: Delayed menarche and amenorrhea of college athletes in relation to age of onset of training, JAMA **246**:1559-1562, 1981.

Garn, S.M., LaVelle, M., and Pilkington, J.J.: Comparisons of fatness in premenarcheal and postmenarcheal girls of the same age, J. Pediatr. **103**:328-331, 1983.

Garn, S.M., and Petzold, A.S.: Characteristics of the mother and child in teenage pregnancy, Am. J. Dis. Child. **137**:365-368, 1983.

Garn, S.M., and others: Are pregnant teenagers still in rapid growth? Am. J. Dis. Child. **138:**32-34, 1984.

Gertner, J.M., and others: Prospective clinical trial of human growth hormone in short children without growth hormone deficiency, J. Pediatr. **104:**172-176, 1984.

Giarretto, H.: The treatment of father-daughter incest: a psychosocial approach, Child. Today 5(4):2-5, 34-45, 1976.

Gordon, M., and others: Psychosocial aspects of constitutional short stature: social competence, behavior problems, self-esteem, and family functioning, J. Pediatr. **101:**477-480, 1982.

Govan, D.E., and Kessler, R.: Urologic problems in the adolescent male, Pediatr. Clin. North Am. **27:**109-124, 1980.

Green, J.W., and others: Child rearing attitudes, observed behavior, and perception of infant temperament in adolescent versus older mothers, Pediatr. Res. **15:**442, 1981.

Greer, R.O., Jr.: Smokeless tobacco: an unheralded adolescent peril, N.Y. State J. Med. **83:**1370-1371, 1983.

Greydanus, D.E., and McAnarney, E.R.: Menstruation and its disorders in adolescence, Curr. Probl. Pediatr. **12**(10):6-61, 1982.

Guggenheim, J., and others: Changing trends of tobacco use in a teenage population in Western Pennsylvania, Am. J. Publ. Health **76:**196-197, 1986.

Hale, R.W.: Exercise, sports, and menstrual dysfunction, Clin. Obstet. Gynecol. **26:**728-735, 1983.

Harrison, G.N., and others: Peripheral airway function in healthy young cigarette smokers, Lung **156:**205-215, 1979.

Harvey, J.S.: Overuse syndromes in young athletes, Pediatr. Clin. North Am. **29:**1369-1381, 1982.

Herbst, A.L., and others: Age-incidence and risk of diethylstilbestrol-related clear cell adenocarcinoma of the vagina and cervix, Am. J. Obstet. Gynecol. **128:**43-52, 1977.

Herman, J.: Father-daughter incest. In Burgess, A.W., editor: Handbook on rape research, New York, 1985, Garland.

Hirsch, B.J.: Natural support systems and coping with major life changes, Am. J. Community Psychol. **8:**159-172, 1980.

Hocutt, J.E.: Cryotherapy, Am. Fam. Physician **23:**141-144, 1978.

Howard, J.S., and Sater, J.: Adolescent mothers: self-perceived health education needs, JOGN Nurs. **14:**399-404, 1985.

Jarvik, M.E.: Biological influences on cigarette smoking. In U.S. Public Health Service: Smoking and health: a report of the surgeon general, Washington D.C., 1979, U.S. Department of Health, Education and Welfare.

Jay, M.S., and others: Effect of peer counselors on adolescent compliance in use of oral contraceptives, Pediatrics **73:**126-131, 1984.

Jurkowski, J.E., and others: Ovarian hormonal responses to exercise, J. Appl. Physiol. **44:**109-114, 1978.

Kemmann, E., and others: Amenorrhea associated with carotenemia, JAMA **249:**926-929, 1983.

Klein, J.R.: Update: adolescent gynecology, Pediatr. Clin. North Am. **27:**141-152, 1980.

Koss, M.P., and Oros, C.J.: Sexual experience survey: a research instrument investigating sexual aggression and victimization, J. Consult. Clin. Psychol. **50:**455-457, 1982.

Kreutner, A.K.: Adolescent contraception, Pediatr. Clin. North Am. **28:**455-473, 1981.

Lamb, M.E., and Easterbrooks, A.: Individual differences in parental sensitivity: origins, components, and consequences. In Lamb, M.E., and Sherrod, L.R., editors: Infant social cognition: empirical and theoretical considerations, Hillsdale, NJ, 1981, Erlbaum.

Larson, T., and Bryson, Y.J.: Fomites and herpes simplex virus [letter], J. Infect. Dis. **151:**746-747, 1985.

Leary, F.J., and others: Males exposed in utero to diethylstilbestrol, JAMA **252:**2984-2989, 1984.

Leventhal, H., and Cleary, P.D.: The smoking problem: a review of the research and theory in behavioral risk modification, J. Personality Soc. Psychol. **88:**370-405, 1981.

Leventhal, J.M.: Risk factors for child abuse: methodologic standards in case-control studies, Pediatrics **68:**684-690, 1981.

Litt, I.F., Cuskey, W.R., and Rudd, S.: Identifying adolescents at risk for noncompliance with contraceptive therapy, J. Pediatr. **96:**742-745, 1980.

Luckstead, E.F.: Sudden death in sports, Pediatr. Clin. North Am. **29:**1355-1362, 1982.

Mahan, L.K., and Rees, J.M.: Nutrition in adolescence, St. Louis, 1984, Times Mirror/Mosby College Publishing.

Malina, R.M., Meleski, B.W., and Shoup, R.F.: Anthropometric, body composition, and maturity characteristics of selected school-age athletes, Pediatr. Clin. North Am. **29:**1305-1323, 1982.

Mann, E.M.: Interviews reveal multifaceted reactions, Am. Fam. Physician **23:**219-222, 1981.

Marty, P.J., and others: Patterns of smokeless tobacco use in a population of high school students, Am. J. Publ. Health **76:**190-192, 1986.

McAlister, A.L., Krosnick, J.A., and Milburn, M.A.: Causes of adolescent cigaret smoking: tests of a structural equation model, Soc. Psychol. Q. **47:**24-36, 1984.

Melski, J.W., and Arndt, K.A.: Topical therapy for acne, N. Engl. J. Med. **302:**503-506, 1980.

Narins, D.M., Belkengren, R.P., and Sapala, S.: Nutrition and the growing athlete, Pediatr. Nurs. **9:**163-168, 1983.

Nerurkar, L., and others: Survival of herpes simplex virus in water specimens collected from hot tubs in spa facilities and on plastic surfaces, JAMA **250:**3081-3083, 1983.

Ogilvie, B.C.: The orthopedist's role in children's sports, Orthop. Clin. North Am. **14:**361-372, 1983.

Orava, S.: Stress fractures, Br. J. Sports Med. **14:**40-44, 1980.

Palumbo, F.M., and Licamele, W.L.: The adolescent and the media. In Shearin, R.B., and Wientzen, R.L., editors: Clinical adolescent medicine—morbidity and mortality, Boston, 1983, G.K. Hall Medical Publishers.

Pescovitz, O.H., and others: The NIH experience with precocious puberty: diagnostic subgroups and response to short-term luteinizing hormone releasing hormone analogue therapy, J. Pediatr. **108:**47-54, 1986.

Pont, A., and others: Ketoconazole blocks testosterone synthesis, Arch. Int. Med. **142:**2137-2140, 1982.

Rabkin, J.G.: The epidemiology of forcible rape, Am. J. Orthopsychiatry **49:**634-547, 1979.

Ragozin, A.S., and others: Effects of maternal age on parenting role, Dev. Psychol. **18:**627-634, 1982.

Redmond, M.A.: Attitudes of adolescent males toward adolescent pregnancy and fatherhood, Fam. Rel. **34:**337-342, 1985.

Robboy, S.J., and others: Increased incidence of cervical and vaginal dysplasia in 3,980 diethylstilbestrol-exposed young women, JAMA **252:**2979-2983, 1984.

Rosenfeld, R.G., Northcraft, G.B., and Hintz, R.L.: A prospective, randomized study of testosterone treatment of constitutional delay of growth and development in male adolescents, Pediatrics **69:**681-687, 1982.

Sandler, H.M., Vietze, P.M., and O'Conner, S.: Obstetric and neonatal outcomes following intervention with pregnant teenagers. In Scott, K.G., Field, T., and Robertson, E., editors: Teenage parents and their offspring, New York, 1981, Grune & Stratton.

Seymore, C., and others: Influence of position during examination, and sex of examiner on patient anxiety during pelvic examination, J. Pediatr. **108:**312-317, 1986.

Shalita, A.R.: Disorders of sebaceous glands and sweat glands. In Gellis, S.S., and Kagan, B.M.: Current pediatric therapy 12, Philadelphia, 1986, W.B. Saunders Co.

Shangold, M.M., and Mirkin, G.: The adolescent athlete. In Lavery, J.P., and Sanfilippo, J.S., editors: Pediatric and adolescent obstetrics and gynecology, New York, 1985, Springer-Verlag New York, Inc.

Silver, H.K., Gotlin, R.W., and Klingensmith, G.J., editors: Endocrine disorders. In Kempe, C.H., Silver, H.K., and O'Brien, D.: Current pediatric diagnosis and treatment, ed. 8, Los Altos, CA, 1984, Lange Medical Publications.

Smith, N.J.: Nutrition in children's sports. In Micheli, L.J., editor: Pediatric and adolescent sports medicine, Boston, 1984, Little, Brown & Co.

Sonis, W.A., and others: Behavior problems and social competence in girls with true precocious puberty, J. Pediatr. **106**:156-160, 1985.

Sprafkin, J.N., and Silverman, L.T.: Uptake: physically intimate and sexual behavior on prime-time television, J. Commun. **31**:34-40, 1981.

Staff Report on the Cigarette Advertising Investigation: Federal Trade Commission, 1981.

Strasburger, V.C.: Sex, drugs, rock 'n' roll: are solutions possible—a commentary, Pediatrics **76**:704-712, 1985.

Strauss, R.H.: Medical concerns in underwater sports, Pediatr. Clin. North Am. **29**:1431-1440, 1982.

Sumaya, C.V., and Ench, Y.: Epstein-Barr virus infectious mononucleosis in children. II. Heterophil antibody and viral-specific responses, Pediatrics **75**:1011-1019, 1985.

Swinyer, L.J., Swinyer, T.A., and Britt, M.R.: Topical agents alone in acne: a blind assessment study, JAMA **243**:1640-1643, 1980.

Tauer, K.M.: Promoting effective decision-making in sexually active adolescents, Nurs. Clin. North Am. **18**:275-292, 1983.

Taylor, B., Wadsworth, J., and Butler, N.R.: Teenage mothering, admission to hospital, and accidents during the first 5 years, Arch. Dis. Child. **58**:6-11, 1983.

Teenage pregnancy: the problem that hasn't gone away, New York, 1981, Alan Guttmacher Institute.

Tunnessen, W.W.: Acne: an approach to therapy for the pediatrician, Curr. Probl. Pediatr. **14**(5):1-35, 1984.

U.S. Department of Health and Human Services: The health consequences of smoking for women: report of the surgeon general, Washington, D.C., 1980, U.S. Government Printing Office.

U.S. Public Health Service: Smoking and health: A report of the surgeon general, Washington, D.C., 1979, Department of Health and Human Services.

U.S. Public Health Service: The health consequences of smoking: the changing cigarette; a report of the surgeon general, Washington, D.C., 1981, U.S. Department of Health and Human Services.

Van Allen, M.W.: The deadly degrading sport (editorial), JAMA **249**:249-250, 1983.

Van Vliet, G., and others: Growth hormone treatment for short stature, N. Engl. J. Med. **309**:1016-1018, 1983.

Vernon, M.E.L., Green, J.A., and Frothingham, F.E.: Teenage pregnancy: a prospective study of self-esteem and other sociodemographic factors, Pediatrics **72**:632-635, 1983.

Walzer, S., and others: Preliminary observations on language and learning in XXY boys, Birth Defects Original Article Series **18**(18):185-192, 1982.

Warren, M.P.: The effects of exercise on pubertal progression and reproductive function in girls, J. Clin. Endocrinol. Metab. **51**:1150-1155, 1980.

Westrom, L.: Incidence, prevalence, and trends of acute pelvic inflammatory disease and its consequences in industrialized countries, Am. J. Obstet. Gynecol. **138**:880-892, 1980.

Williamson, R.: Cold weather and testicular torsion, Br. Med. J. **286**:1436, 1983.

Wong-McCarthy, W.J., and Gritz, E.R.: Preventing regular teenage cigarette smoking, Pediatr. Ann. **11**:683-689, 1982.

Yonkosky, D.M., and Pochi, P.E.: Acne vulgaris in childhood, pathogenesis and management, Dermatol. Clin. **4**:127-136, 1986.

Ziporyn, T.: Latest clue to exercise-induced amenorrhea, JAMA **252**:1259-1263, 1984.

Zuckerman, B.S, and others: Adolescent pregnancy: biobehavioral determinants of outcome, J. Pediatr. **105**:857-863, 1984.

BIBLIOGRAPHY
General

Clarke, B.A.: Improving adolescent parenting through participant modeling and self-evaluation, Nurs. Clin. North Am. **18**:303-311, 1983.

Eldridge, T.M.: Adolescent health care: the legal and ethical implications, Pediatr. Nurs. **5**(3):51-52, 1979.

Hoffman, A.D., editor: Adolescent medicine, Menlo Park, CA, 1983, Addison-Wesley Publishing Co.

Howe, J.: Nursing care of adolescents, New York, 1980, McGraw-Hill Book Co.

Kempe, C.H., Silver, H.K., and O'Brien, D.: Current pediatric diagnosis and treatment, ed. 8, Los Altos, CA, 1984, Lange Medical Publications.

Krugman, S., and others: Infectious diseases of children, ed. 8, St. Louis, 1985, The C.V. Mosby Co.

Litt, I.F., editor: Symposium on adolescent medicine, Pediatr. Clin. North Am. **27**(1): entire issue, 1980.

Mercer, R.T.: Perspectives on adolescent health care, Philadelphia, 1979, J.B. Lippincott Co.

Acne

Acne products: do fewer teens mean lower sales? Amer. Druggist **192**:117-118, 146, 1985.

De la Cruz, E., and others: Multiple congenital malformations associated with maternal isotretinoin therapy, Pediatrics **74**:428-430, 1984.

Fischer, R.G.: Acne vulgaris: a common disease, Pediatr. Nurs. **4**(2):9-14, 1978.

Lucky, A.W.: Endocrine aspects of acne, Pediatr. Clin. North Am. **30**:495-499,1983.

Matsuoka, L.Y.: Acne, J. Pediatr. **103**:849-854, 1983.

Melski, J.W., and Arndt, K.A.: Topical therapy for acne, N. Engl. J. Med. **302**:503, 1980.

Rasmussen, J.E., and Smith, S.B.: Patient concepts and misconceptions about acne, Arch. Dermatol. **119**:570-573, 1983.

Stone, A.C.: Facing up to acne, Pediatr. Nurs. **8**:229-234, 1982.

Swinyer, L.J.: Topical agents alone in acne, JAMA **243**:640-643, 1980.

Infectious Mononucleosis

McSherry, J.A.: Diagnosing infectious mononucleosis, Am. Fam. Physician **32**:129-132, 1985.

Shurin, S.B.: Infectious mononucleosis, Pediatr. Clin. North Am. **26**:315-326, 1979.

Sumaya, C.V., and Ench, Y.: Epstein-Barr virus infectious mononucleosis in children. I. Clinical and general laboratory findings, Pediatrics **75**:1003-1010, 1985.

Smoking

Coe, R.M., and others: Patterns of change in adolescent smoking behavior and results of a one year follow-up of a smoking prevention program, J. Sch. Health **52**:348-353, 1982.

Demuth, P.J.: Clove cigarettes: a hazardous fad, Am. J. Nurs. **85**:950-951, 1985.

Masironi, R., and Roy, L.: Smoking and youth: a special report, World Smoking and Health **8**(1):27-31, 1983.

McCaul, K.D., and others: Predicting adolescent smoking, J. Sch. Health **52**:342-346, 1982.

Murray, M., Kiryluk, S., and Swan, A.V.: School characteristics and adolescent smoking: results from the MRC/Derbyshire smoking study 1974-8 and from a follow-up in 1981, J. Epidemiol. Comm. Health **38**:167-172, 1984.

Young, T.L., and Rogers, K.D.: School performance characteristics preceding onset of smoking in high school students, Am. J. Dis. Child. **140**:257-259, 1985.

Disorders Related to Sports

Barnes, L.: Cryotherapy—putting injury on ice, Phys. Sportsmed. **7:**130-136, 1979.

Carey, R.J., and Shute, R.E.: Sports trauma management and the high school nurse, J. Sch. Health **52:**156-158, 1982.

Committee on Drugs and Committee on Sports Medicine: Dimethyl sulfoxide (DMSO), Pediatrics **71:**76, 1983.

Frisch, R.E., Wyshak, G., and Vincent, L.: Delayed menarche and amenorrhea in ballet dancers, N. Engl. J. Med. **303:**17-19, 1980.

Garrett, W.E., Jr.: Strains and sprains in athletes, Postgrad. Med. **73**(3):200-209, 1983.

Goldberg, B.: Pediatric sports medicine. In Scott, W.N., Nisonson, B., and Nicholas, J.A., editors: Principles of sports medicine, Baltimore, 1984, Williams & Wilkins.

Kris-Etherton, P.M.: Nutrition, exercise and athletic performance, Food Nutr. **57**(3):13-15, 1985.

Latinis, B.: Frequent sports injuries of children: etiology, treatment, and prevention, Issues Compr. Pediatr. Nurs. **6:**167-178, 1983.

Macvicar, M.G., Harlan, J.D., and Ouellette, M.: What do we know about the effects of sports training on the menstrual cycle? J. Matern. Child Nurs. **7:**55-58, 1982.

Micheli, L.J.: Overuse injuries in children's sports: the growth factor, Orthop. Clin. North Am. **14:**337-360, 1983.

Smith, N.J.: Medical issues in sports medicine, Pediatr. Rev. **2:**229-237, 1981.

Stover, C.N.: Physical conditioning of the immature athlete, Orthop. Clin. North Am. **13:**525-540, 1982.

Sullivan, J.A.: Recurring pain in the pediatric athlete, Pediatr. Clin. North Am. **31:**1097-1112, 1984.

Thomas, K.A.: Screening the child for sports participation, Issues Compr. Pediatr. Nurs. **6:**179-194, 1983.

Thorne, B.P.: A nurse helps prevent sports injuries, J. Matern. Child Nurs. **7:**236-239, 1982.

Altered Growth and Maturation

Blombäck, M., Hall, K., and Ritzén, E.M.: Estrogen treatment of tall girls: risk of thrombosis? Pediatrics **72:**416-419, 1983.

Cohen, F.L., and Durham, J.D.: Update your knowledge of Klinefelter syndrome, J. Psychosoc. Nurs. **23:**19-25, 1985.

Cohen, F.L., and Durham, J.D.: Sex chromosome variations in school-aged children, J. Sch. Health **55:**99-102, 1985.

Davis, J., and Sobel, E.H.: Validity of stature prediction near maturity, J. Pediatr. **95:**992-993, 1979.

Galatzer, A., and others: Intellectual function of girls with precocious puberty, Pediatrics **74:**246-249, 1984.

Grew, R.S., and others: Facilitating patient understanding in the treatment of growth delay, Clin. Pediatr. **22:**685-690, 1983.

Gross, R.T., and Duke, P.M.: The effects of early versus late physical maturation on adolescent behavior, Pediatr. Clin. North Am. **27:**71-78, 1980.

Holmes, C.S., Hayford, J.T., and Thompson, R.G.: Personality and behavior differences in groups of boys with short stature, Child Health Care **11:**61-64, 1982.

Reindollar, R.H., and McDonough, P.G.: Etiology and evaluation of delayed sexual development, Pediatr. Clin. North Am. **28:**267-286, 1981.

Richards, G.E., Marshall, R.N., and Kreuser, I.L.: Effect of stature on school performance, J. Pediatr. **106:**841-842, 1985.

Solomon, S.B.: Children with short stature, J. Pediatr. Nurs. **1:**80-89, 1986.

Stern, N., and Zaiken, H.: Assessing the child with short stature, Pediatr. Nurs. **11:**106-110, 1985.

Tho, P.T., and McDonough, P.G.: Gonadal dysgenesis and its variants, Pediatr. Clin. North Am. **28:**309-329, 1981.

Underwood, L.E.: Growth hormone treatment for short children, J. Pediatr. **104:**237-239, 1984.

Health Problems of the Male Reproductive System

Frank-Stromborg, M.: Nursing's contribution to case finding and early detection of cancer. In Marino, L.B., editor: Cancer nursing, St. Louis, 1981, The C.V. Mosby Co.

Goldbloom, R.B.: Self-examination by adolescents, Pediatrics **76:**126-128, 1985.

Goldenring, J.M., and Purtell, E.: Knowledge of testicular cancer risk and need for self-examination in college students: a call for equal time for men in teaching of early cancer detection techniques, Pediatrics **74:**1093-1096, 1984.

Mitchell, J.R.: Male adolescents' concern about a physical examination conducted by a female, Nurs. Res. **29:**165-169, 1980.

Williams, A.W.: Screening for testicular cancer, Pediatr. Nurs. **7**(5):38-40, 1981.

Health Problems of the Female Reproductive System

Altchek, A.: Vulvovaginitis, vulvar skin disease, and pelvic inflammatory disease, Pediatr. Clin. North Am. **28:**397-432, 1981.

Brown, M.A., and Zimmer, P.A.: Personal and family impact of premenstrual symptoms, JOGN Nurs. **15:**31-38, 1986.

Comerci, G.D.: Symptoms associated with menstruation, Pediatr. Clin. North Am. **29:**177-200, 1981.

Cowell, C.A.: The gynecologic examination of infants, children, and young adolescents, Pediatr. Clin. North Am. **28:**247-266, 1981.

Coyne, C.M., Woods, N.F., and Mitchell, E.S.: Premenstrual tension syndrome, JOGN Nurs. **14:**446-454, 1985.

Emans, S.E.E., and Goldstein, D.P.: The gynecologic examination of the prepubertal child with vulvovaginitis: use of the knee-chest position, Pediatrics **65:**758-761, 1980.

Emans, S.J., Grace, E., and Goldstein, D.P.: Oligomenorrhea in adolescent girls, J. Pediatr. **97:**815-819, 1980.

Frank, E.P.: What are nurses doing to help PMS patients? Am. J. Nurs. **86:**137-140, 1986.

Gantt, P.A., and McDonough, P.G.: Adolescent dysmenorrhea, Pediatr. Clin. North Am. **28:**389-395, 1981.

Gever, L.N.: From arthritis pain to dysmenorrhea, a new indication for prostaglandin inhibitors, Nursing 80 **10:**81, 1980.

Klein, J.R., and others: The effect of aspirin on dysmenorrhea in adolescents, J. Pediatr. **98:**987-990, 1981.

Lavery, J.P., and Sanfilippo, J.S., editors: Pediatric and adolescent obstetrics and gynecology, New York, 1985, Springer-Verlag New York, Inc.

Meyer, M.R.: Adolescent gynecology: problems and ponderings, Pediatr. Nurs. **4**(4):43-47, 1978.

Paradise, J., and Willis, E.D.: Probability of vaginal foreign body in girls with genital complaints, Am. J. Dis. Child. **139:**472-476, 1985.

Peach, E.H.: Counseling sexually active very young adolescent girls, Am. J. Maternal Child Nurs. **5:**191-195, 1980.

Primrose, R.B.: Taking the tension out of pelvic exams, Am. J. Nurs. **84:**72-74, 1984.

Rx drugs switched to OTC, FDA Drug Bull. **13**(3):29-30, 1984.

Sasso, S.C.: Prostaglandin inhibitors for primary dysmenorrhea, J. Matern. Child Nurs. **9:**177, 1984.

Adolescent Pregnancy

Abbott, M.I.: Parenting group for teen-agers fails, Pediatr. Nurs. **6**(5):54-65, 1980.

Abrams, B.: Helping pregnant teenagers eat right, Nursing 81 **11**(3):46-47, 1981.

Admire, G., and Byers, L.: Counseling the pregnant teenager, Nursing 81 **11**(4):62-63, 1981.

Burke, P.J.: A community health model for pregnant teens, J. Matern. Child Nurs. **8:**340-344, 1983.

Cusson, R.M.: Attitudes toward breast-feeding among female high-school students, Pediatr. Nurs. **11:**189-191, 1985.

Daniels, M.B., and Manning, D.: A clinic for pregnant teens, Am. J. Nurs. **83:**68-71, 1983.

Dibble, J.C.: ABC for teens: parent education after the baby comes, Pediatr. Nurs. **7**(4):21-23, 1981.

Donlen, J., and Lynch, P.: Teenage mother: high-risk baby, Nursing 81 **11**(5):51-56, 1981.

Elster, A.B., and Panzarine, S.: Teenage fathers, Clin. Pediatr. **22:**700-703, 1983.

Jensen, M.D., and Bobak, I.M.: Maternity and gynecologic care: the nurse and the family, ed. 3, St. Louis, 1985, The C.V. Mosby Co.

Levine, L., Coll, C.T.G., and Oh, W.: Determinants of mother-infant interaction in adolescent mothers, Pediatrics **75:**23-29, 1985.

Marino, D.D., and King, J.C.: Nutritional concerns during adolescence, Pediatr. Clin. North Am. **27:**125-140, 1980.

McAnarney, E.R., and others: Adolescent mothers and their infants, Pediatrics **73:**358-362, 1984.

Mecklenburg, M.E., and Thompson, P.G.: The adolescent family life program as a prevention measure, Publ. Health Rep. **98:**21-29, 1983.

Mercer, R.: Assessing and counseling teenage mothers during the perinatal period, Nurs. Clin. North Am. **18:**293-301, 1983.

Mercer, R.T.: Teenage motherhood: the first year, JOGN Nurs. **9:**16-27, 1980.

Montagu, A.: The adolescent's unreadiness for pregnancy and motherhood, Pediatr. Ann. **10:**507-511, 1981.

Moore, D.S., Erickson, P.I., and Wurgel, M.: Adolescent pregnancy and parenting: the role of the nurse, Topics Clin. Nurs. **6**(3):72-78, 1984.

Morgan, B.S., and Barden, M.E.: Unwed and pregnant: nurses' attitudes toward unmarried mothers, J. Matern. Child Nurs. **10:**114-117, 1985.

Nakashima, I.I., and Camp, B.W.: Fathers of infants born to adolescent mothers: a study of paternal characteristics, Am. J. Dis. Child. **138:**452-454, 1984.

Poole, C.J., and Hoffmann, M.: Mothers of adolescent mothers: how do they cope? Pediatr. Nurs. **7**(1):28-31, 1981.

Rothenbert, P.B., and Varga, L.E.: The relationship between age of mother and child health and development, Am. J. Publ. Health **71:**810-817, 1981.

Sewall, K.S.: Peer-group reality therapy for the pregnant adolescent, J. Matern. Child Nurs. **8:**67-69, 1983.

Smith, D.L.: Meeting the psychoscoial needs of teen-age mothers and fathers, Nurs. Clin. North Am. **19:**369-379, 1984.

Vukelich, C., and Kliman, D.S.: Mature and teenage mothers' infant growth expectations and use of child development information sources, Fam. Rel. **34:**189-196, 1985.

Zelnick, M., and Kantner, J.: Sexual activity, contraception use, and pregnancy among metropolitan-area teenagers, Fam. Plan. Perspect. **12:**230-237, 1980.

Zuckerman, B., and others: Neonatal outcome: is adolescent pregnancy a risk factor? Pediatrics **71:**489-493, 1983.

Contraception

Babington, M.A.: Adolescent use of oral contraceptives, Pediatr. Nurs. **10:**111-114, 1984.

Gara, E.: Nursing protocol to improve the effectiveness of the contraceptive diaphragm, Am. J. Maternal Child Nurs. **6:**41-45, 1981.

Greydanus, D.E.: Should the media advertise contraceptives? Am. J. Dis. Child. **135:**687-688, 1981.

Hewson, P.M.: Research on adolescent male attitudes about contraceptives, Pediatr. Nurs. **12:**114-116, 1986.

Huxall, L.K.: Update on IUDs, Am. J. Maternal Child Nurs. **5:**186-190, 1980.

Kulig, J.W.: Adolescent contraception: an update, Pediatrics **76:**675-680, 1985.

Taylor, D.: Contraceptive counseling and care. In Mercer, R.T.: Perspectives on adolescent health care, Philadelphia, 1979, J.B. Lippincott Co.

Turetsky, R.A., and Strasburger, V.C.: Adolescent contraception, Clin. Pediatr. **22:**337-341, 1983.

White, J.E.: Initiating contraceptive use: how do young women decide? Pediatr. Nurs. **10:**347-352, 1984.

Rape

Burgess, A.W., and Brodsky, S.L.: Applying flight education principles to rape prevention, Fam. Comm. Health **4**(2):45-51, 1981.

Foley, T.S., and Davies, M.A.: Rape: nursing care of victims, St. Louis, 1983, The C.V. Mosby Co.

Platt, C.R., Hicks, D.J., and Mori, D.M.: Medical care for the rape victim. In Reinhardt, A.M., and Quinn, M.D., editors: Family-centered community nursing, vol. 2, St. Louis, 1981, The C.V. Mosby Co.

Resisting rape without getting killed, Am. J. Nurs. **85:**947-948, 1985.

Warner, C.G.: Comforting and caring for the rape victim using crisis intervention wisely, Nursing Skillbooks, 1979, Nursing 79 Books.

Woodling, B.A., and Kossoris, P.D.: Sexual misuse: rape, molestation, and incest, Pediatr. Clin. North Am. **28:**481-499, 1981.

Sexually Transmitted Diseases

Bell, T.A.: Major sexually transmitted diseases of children and adolescents, Pediatr. Inf. Dis. **2**(2):153-161, 1983.

Bryson, Y.J.: The use of acyclovir in children, Pediatr. Inf. Dis. **3**(4):345-348, 1984.

Bump, R.C., Sachs, L.A., and Buesching, W.J.: Sexually transmissible infectious agents in sexually active and virginal asymptomatic adolescent girls, Pediatrics **77:**488-494, 1986.

Campbell, C.E., and Herten, R.J.: VD to STD: redefining venereal disease, Am. J. Nurs. **81:**1629, 1635, 1981.

Chacko, M.R., and Lovchik, J.C.: Chlamydia trachomatis infection in sexually active adolescents: prevalence and risk factors, Pediatrics **73:**836-840, 1984.

Fraser, J.J., Rettig, P.J., and Kaplan, D.W.: Prevalence of cervical *Chlamydia trachomatis* and *Neisseria gonorrhoeae* in female adolescents, Pediatrics **71:**333-336, 1983.

Greydanus, D.E., and McAnarney, E.R.: *Chlamydia trachomatis:* an important sexually transmitted disease in adolescents and young adults, J. Fam. Pract. **10:**611-615, 1980.

Hammerschlag, M.R.: Chlamydial infections, Pediatr. Rev. **3:**77-84, 1981.

Jaffe, L.R., and Morgentau, J.E.: Syphilis and homosexuality in adolescents, J. Pediatr. **95:**1062-1063, 1979.

Kaplan, K.M., and others: Social relevance of genital herpes simplex in children, Am. J. Dis. Child. **138:**872-874, 1984.

Kathchadourian, H.: Adolescent sexuality, Pediatr. Clin. North Am. **27:**17-28, 1980.

Seidel, J., Zonana, J., and Totten, E.: Condylomata acuminata as a sign of sexual abuse in children, J. Pediatr. **95:**553-554, 1979.

Chapter 21

Behavioral Health Problems of Adolescence

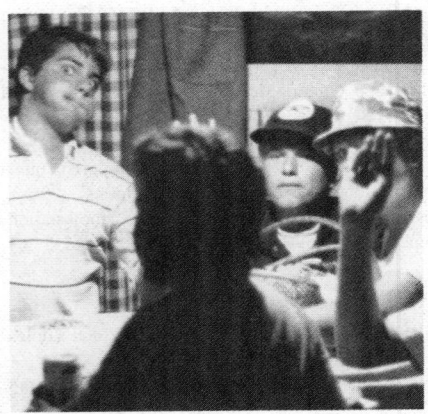

Adolescence is a time of transition, maturational crisis, and adjustment. The peer group becomes increasingly larger and the period of adolescence has become prolonged and intense. The transition to adulthood is characterized by change, growth, and stress. Ineffective and unsuccessful accomplishment of the developmental tasks of adolescence produces a sense of diffuse discomfort within some adolescents, who may use faulty problem solving in their search for relief from the discomfort and stress of this transitional period of life.

Eating Disorders

Eating disorders are among the most frequently encountered health problems of adolescence. Overeating often begins in infancy and continues throughout childhood; deliberate undereating usually does not become apparent until later childhood or adolescence. Either overeating or undereating can have a detrimental effect on health and well-being, and, if extreme, can be a threat to life.

ADIPOSE TISSUE

There is wide variation in the degree of fatness or thinness between individuals at all ages because of a multitude of factors. Fat is contained in connective tissue cells that are usually referred to as adipose tissue; this tissue has a distinct lifetime pattern of development and distribution. Fat is characteristically found in subcutaneous tissues (except those of the eyelids, external ear, nose, scrotum, and backs of hands and feet, which contain very little), in the omentum, and in close relation to some viscera, such as the heart and kidneys. Although it contributes substantially to body weight, whether fat ''grows'' like other tissues is uncertain. The deposits of fat throughout the body function primarily as a means for storing energy. Therefore it is a labile tissue markedly affected by the nutrition of the individual.

Normal fat distribution during childhood follows a definite pattern. Fat first appears in the subcutaneous tissues of the fetus at approximately the sixth month of prenatal life. There is a rapid accumulation from the seventh month through the first 6 postnatal months, and the amount of subcutaneous fat present in the newborn correlates with the weight of the infant. However, at the end of the first year the infant who was lean at birth has approximately the same length and muscle mass as infants who were fatter initially. The significance of subcutaneous fat related to both the specialized ''brown fat'' and gestational age is discussed in relation to problems of prematurity and temperature regulation in the newborn.

After 6 months of age the rate of fat accumulation declines rapidly and then decreases steadily in both sexes until 6 to 8 years of age. All children begin to slim down soon after the first birthday, but the decrease is somewhat less in girls than in boys; thus at any age girls are slightly fatter than boys. From the ages of 6 to 8 years fat again begins to accumulate slowly. It is during this period that obesity may begin in some children. Many children also put on excess fat just before the adolescent growth spurt.

Up to the time of the onset of puberty there is very little difference in fat accumulation and distribution in boys and girls. During the adolescent growth spurt the amount of fat in boys decreases sharply (especially in the limbs) and is not regained until early adulthood. Their increase in body weight and mass is primarily the result of accelerated bone and muscle growth. In many boys a preadolescent period of fat growth, often a source of social concern to both the child and his parents, precedes the general changes of adolescence. In girls the fat accumulation continues but assumes a typical distribution pattern that produces the feminine curves of the mature female.

The amount and distribution of fat are also correlated with a genetically controlled body build that appears to be unrelated to caloric intake. In addition, culturally determined diets, amount of exercise, emotions, and numerous other factors that influence caloric consumption are reflected in increased fat deposits. It is now believed that the number of fat cells is established at an early age and that overfeeding during this time may have a significant influence on obesity at a later age.

OBESITY

There is probably no problem related to adolescence that is so obvious to others, is so difficult to treat, and has such long-term effects on psychologic and physical health status as obesity. It is the most common nutritional disturbance of children and one of the most challenging contemporary health problems at all ages. The incidence of obesity has been conservatively estimated to be 10% to 12% of prepubertal children and anywhere from 10% or 15% to 30% of adolescents. Approximately 80% of obese children perpetuate their obesity into adulthood; 50% of grossly obese adults were obese as children (Lloyd, Wolff, and Whelan, 1981). Since adult obesity is associated with increased mortality and morbidity from a variety of complications, both physical and psychologic, the presence of adolescent obesity is a serious condition that deserves the interest and attention of health professionals.

The definition of obesity has always led to some confusion and, at best, is very imprecise. Because there is such variability in height and weight among normal healthy children, it is often difficult to determine the presence or extent of obesity from comparing a set of numbers with a standardized table of weights and heights. This is especially true in adolescence, when there is normally a period of rapid weight gain and linear growth together with varying rates of muscular development. The greatest amount of confusion is related to the distinction between the terms *overweight* and *obesity*. *Obesity* is an increase in body weight resulting from an excessive accumulation of fat or simply the state of being too fat. *Overweight* refers to the state of weighing more than average for height and body build, which may or may not include an increased amount of fat. It is possible for two children to have the same height and weight and for one to be obese whereas the other is not. This is particularly evident during early adolescence when there are considerable differences in the rates of muscular development. Obesity is easily recognized, although it is difficult to assess its severity, especially in children who are overweight to a lesser degree.

Etiology/Pathophysiology

Obesity results from a caloric intake that consistently exceeds caloric requirements and expenditure. The causes of this disequilibrium are complex and may involve a variety of interrelated influences, including metabolic, hypothalamic, hereditary, social, cultural, and psychologic factors. Birth weight offers no clue in detection and prediction of childhood obesity; obese children do not have higher birth weights than nonobese children. However, there is a high correlation of childhood adiposity with both parental adiposity and children's daytime activity levels (Berkowitz and others, 1985). A brief description of some of the major theories regarding childhood obesity is presented here.

Genetic factors. Heredity has been demonstrated to be an important factor in the development of obesity in some cases. The incidence of obese children born to obese parents is significantly higher than those born to parents of normal weight: 3% to 7% of children born to parents of normal weight are obese, 40% of obese children have one parent who is obese, and 80% of obese children have two obese parents. Comparison of natural and adopted children shows a positive correlation for weight between children and their natural parents (Strunkard and others, 1986; Van Itallie, 1986). In addition, studies of identical and fraternal twins reveal an extremely high correlation between identical twins but not fraternal twins—even identical twins who were reared in different environments (Weil, 1977).

General body build seems to have some effect on obesity. Children who are inclined toward a rounded body build with soft body contours and larger amounts of subcutaneous fat are somewhat predisposed to the accumulation of fat. Some humans may inherit a metabolic defect that interferes with the breakdown of fat once it has been stored in adipose tissue, which makes maintaining an ideal weight more difficult than it is for others.

It is almost impossible to distinguish between hereditary and environmental factors, since both may be operative in any situation, especially when other family members are also obese. Family eating patterns, ethnic diet, and psychologic factors play an important role; to many persons, fat is still considered to be an indication of good health. The tendency to obesity is manifest whenever environmental conditions are favorable, such as an abundance of food and reduced or minimal physical activity (from such causes as excessive television viewing and the availability of automobiles).

Diseases. In less than 5% of cases childhood obesity can be attributed to an underlying disease. These include hypothyroidism, adrenal hypercorticoidism, hyperinsulinism, and dysfunction of or damage to the central nervous system as a result of a tumor, injury, infection, or vascular accident. Obesity is a frequent complication of muscular dystrophy and paraplegia as a result of meningomyelocele.

Five recognized congenital syndromes have obesity as a feature (Laurence-Moon-Biedl, Prader-Willi, Vasquez, and Alstrom syndromes and pseudohypoparathyroidism). The most common of these is Prader-Willi syndrome, a disorder characterized by hypogonadism, slow intellectual development, short stature, and dysmorphic facial features including a narrowed bifrontal diameter, almond-shaped eyes, and triangular-shaped mouth. These children are very hypotonic and will go to great lengths to obtain food.

Metabolic and endocrine factors. The complex interrelationships between hunger, satiety, the central nervous system, and the metabolism of carbohydrates, fats, and protein continue to be investigated in relation to their role in obesity. Theories advanced in an attempt to explain individual variability in energy requirements include increased metabolic efficiency in the obese person that facilitates fat storage, enhanced adipose tissue triglyceride synthesis, and retarded adipocyte lipolysis facilitating fat retention (Merritt, 1982).

A recent theory postulates that obese persons have less heat-producing brown fat than normal persons and that their brown fat works less efficiently. The heat production (thermogenesis) is not linked with working activities or basal metabolism. The hypothesis indicates that the body's heat production influences food intake, and this may explain why some individuals are able to overeat and remain slim (Elliott, 1980; James and Trayhurn, 1981).

It has also been observed that on the whole obese children tend to be taller than average with somewhat larger lean body mass. There is some evidence to indicate that growth is accelerated by overnutrition much the same as it is retarded by undernutrition. Consequently children who are obese in infancy seem to attain relatively greater height than those with later-onset obesity.

It is suggested that obesity may even originate in the prenatal period. Maternal malnutrition during the first trimester, when cells are differentiating and increasing in number, affects the development of the hypothalamus. Disruption of normal development can alter the center that regulates appetite and lead to a lifetime of overeating (Overfield, 1980).

Caloric equilibrium. It is consistently observed that obese children are less active than lean children, but it is uncertain whether the inactivity creates the obesity or if the obesity is responsible for the inactivity. However, it appears that in childhood overeating is the dominant feature, whereas in adult life reduced physical activity with normal intake is more likely to be the rule.

Although the intake of obese persons who are inactive is lower than that of leaner persons, obese persons eat more at a given sitting and eat more rapidly than nonobese persons. It appears characteristic that obese persons not only exhibit an overwhelming appetite but often overeat when they are not hungry or have no appetite. They apparently respond to other cues as well as to the hunger stimulus. It has also been shown that feeding habits and frequency of food ingestion may produce alterations in enzyme activities in both adipose cells and muscle cells. Comparison of individuals who consume similar amounts of calories ingested either as one meal (gorging) or intermittently over a period of time (nibbling) shows an increase of body fat in the "gorgers." It appears that lipogenesis is accelerated following "gorging" patterns of food intake when compared with "nibbling" patterns (Leveille and Romsos, 1974). Obese adolescents are characteristically night eaters and often skip meals, particularly breakfast.

Adipose cell theory. According to this concept obesity may be hyperplastic, hypertrophic, or a mixture of the two. *Hyperplastic,* or hypercellular, obesity occurs when the number of cells in adipose tissue is increased, producing lifelong and intractable obesity (Hirsch, 1976). Hyperplastic obesity is associated with earlier onset. *Hypertrophic* obesity is associated with an increase in cell size and therefore is more likely to be responsive to treatment. There is agreement that fat individuals have larger adipose cells than nonfat counterparts of the same age and sex, and some appear to have more cells. The degree of obesity can be correlated with fat cell number but not with fat cell size. Fat cell size is reduced during weight loss, but fat cell number remains constant (Roche, 1981). The severest degree of obesity will be associated with high adipose cellularity.

It has also been hypothesized that there are sensitive periods when adipose tissue is more liable to undergo hyperplasia with a permanent increase in cell number. These recurrent periods of sensitivity are identified as late in fetal life, the first year, early puberty in girls, and after 17 years of age. It is still speculative whether or not such "sensitive" periods are also "vulnerable" periods with increased predisposition to later obesity (Kirtland and Gurr, 1979).

In both obese and nonobese children fat cell number increases with size until about 2 years of age. In nonobese children adipose cell size remains constant between the ages of 2 and 10, then increases to reach adult level during adolescence (Knittle and others, 1979). In contrast, there is a progressive increase in fat cell number throughout childhood in obese children. Obese children have larger cells that stay the same size once they reach a maximum, and their fat cells appear to increase in number during childhood. It also appears that massive weight gain at any time may trigger an increase in adipose cell number once their age-related maximum size has been reached (Taitz, 1983).

Set point theory. The set point theory states that individuals have a programmed level, or set point, for body weight that remains relatively stable during adulthood. Weight usually returns to this stable level following short periods of weight gain or loss. A hypothalamic feedback mechanism operates to alter intake and output of energy to maintain a specific body mass, which varies among individuals. With increased caloric intake the metabolic rate increases to burn the excess; when intake is reduced, metabolism decreases to conserve energy. Consequently, the body must work harder and restrict calories further in an effort to overcome this mechanism when weight reduction is desired, which may account for some of the plateaus experienced in weight loss programs.

Sociocultural factors. Patterns of eating are culturally and socially based in most instances, and in some the food preferences of the culture contribute to the development of obesity. Many cultures consider plump children to be a sign of health, and some look on obesity as evidence of well-being and foster weight gain as a desirable feature. In others obesity is a status symbol or an indication of affluence. It is not uncommon for obese children to be a product of families in which eating patterns of large meals are emphasized or in which children are admonished for leaving any food on their plates. Parents often have an exaggerated concept of the amount of food children should eat and expect them to eat more than they need.

It has also been observed that in the developed countries such as the United States and those in Western Europe there is a marked difference in the prevalence of obesity between upper- and lower-class children and that these differences are frequently apparent before 6 years of age. Lower socioeconomic groups have a greater prevalence of obesity, especially in girls, and this obese state is established earlier and increases at a more rapid rate.

Psychologic factors. Psychologic factors may provide a basis for eating patterns in childhood. In infancy the child first experiences relief from discomfort through feeding and learns to associate eating with feelings of well-being, security, and the comforting presence of the mothering person. Soon eating is deeply associated with the feeling of being loved. To the infant, to be fed is to be loved; satiety is security. In addition, the pleasurable oral sensation of sucking provides an additional connection between emotions and early eating behavior. Many parents use food, such as candy and other "treats," as a positive reinforcer for desired behavior or as a way to compensate for their own feelings of guilt, especially if the child was unwanted or overvalued because of loss of a previous child. This practice soon acquires symbolic significance to the extent that the child continues to use food as a reward, a comfort, and a means by which to deal with feelings of depression or hostility.

In some children overweight may be the normal state and may simply represent the upper end of the normal distribution curve. These children are most comfortable when they are well filled out, and they may or may not have emotional problems. Others may begin overeating and reducing activity in response to a traumatic or upsetting event in their lives, such as the death of a parent or sibling, separation from parents, or social or scholastic failure, or as a response to illness or surgery.

Obesity may be one manifestation of a disturbed way of life. Typically families of obese children are markedly socially introverted and rely on family members for socialization. Television viewing is the primary source of entertainment. Frequently the family is composed of a domineering, ambitious mother and a passive, docile father. Marital disharmony is common. There are usually only one or two children in the family. The obese child assumes the role of active participant with dependent, submissive, and generally immature behavior. The child follows the family's social pattern of isolation and tends to react to frustration with withdrawal or hostility. On school entrance the child is totally unprepared for experiences outside the shelter of the family group. Consequently the child turns to food for solace, which has become a manner of coping with traumatic experiences, failure, and disappointment. Once obesity has developed, the family patterns of personal and social interaction tend to perpetuate it.

Obesity in Adolescence

Obesity in adolescence may appear simultaneously with the onset of adolescence, or it may have existed before puberty. Although there may be differences in the psychophysiologic dynamics in its development, the effect of the obese condition on the teenager is the same. A great deal has been hypothesized about the psychogenic factors in obesity; however, the psychologic *effects* of being obese are undoubtedly underestimated. Obesity is a serious handicap to the social life of a child and, to an even greater extent, to the life of a teenager. The common emotional sequelae of obesity in adolescence are defective body image, low self-esteem, social isolation, and feelings of rejection and depression.

Adolescent-onset obesity appears to be closely related to the children's inability to master the developmental tasks of adolescence; as a result they regress to the self-satisfying tactic of overeating to compensate. Unfortunately this mechanism only creates an additional obstacle to achieving the desired goal. The obesity, however, serves to ward off the pressures engendered by the internal changes of puberty and the outside world. The obesity becomes the safeguard. As long as they remain fat, children do not have to deal with this repressed emotional material. They may come to view the obesity as a handicap responsible for all their disappointments. Consequently, they avoid making the adaptations necessary to growth and maturation. Eating is their means of coping with the normal drives of adolescence and more closely binds them to the family, especially the mother, who provides the food. Thus they become increasingly dependent on food as a means of gratification. This impedes the normal processes of separation and individuation, since they tend to shy away from their peers and become more closely bound to the family.

Vulnerable personality. Obesity is most often a symptom in passive-dependent, compliant youngsters who are readily controlled by guilt and shame. They are easily influenced by outside forces, such as parents, peers, and school, that they consider to be more powerful than themselves. When faced with an internal or external stress, these youngsters react with helplessness, ambivalence, and a tendency to seek support from someone they see as stronger than themselves, either adult or peer.

There are many psychologic implications in the development and perpetuation of obesity. It may represent aggression directed at the self, an attempt (in younger children) to grow bigger in order to physically deal with a hated person, or a means to bring shame and embarrassment to another (often the mother). Many overweight adolescents use obesity as a means of revenge. However, they easily become a scapegoat for the frustrations and anger of parents and others as a source of embarrassment and shame. A common problem is the ambivalence of mothers who like to see their daughters eat but at the same time desire them to have slender figures.

Self-concept and obesity. Obese adolescents score higher on depression-measurement tests than thinner teenagers and significantly lower on body-image tests, indicating a less positive or a more impaired body concept. Unlike many disorders, the youngster's obesity is a matter of general knowledge, continually on display for others to see. Some of the personality characteristics reflecting the psychologic effects of obesity have been likened to those experienced by ethnic and racial minorities who have been subjected to intense discrimination. These include passivity, obsessive concern with the self-image, expectation of rejection, and progressive withdrawal. This sets into motion a cyclic pattern wherein the youngsters expect rejection, feel awkward and out of place in the social situation, isolate themselves from social contacts, and then experience actual rejection. The decreased opportunity for activity outside the home provides increased exposure to food that leads to an increase in the obesity.

Obese adolescents, particularly obese girls, consider obesity undesirable and intensely dislike their figures and physical characteristics. They are concerned about their obesity, are extremely self-deprecating, and judge other people in terms of degree of adiposity. They express contempt for fat persons and admiration for thin ones. They consider their bodies to be grotesque and are certain that others, too, are contemptuous of them. Stylish, age-appropriate clothing is difficult to find and, when available, is restricted to special shops or departments with labels that further emphasize the negative aspects of appearance. Sexual attractiveness is severely impaired or nonexistent; obese youngsters rarely date.

There are three major factors that contribute to the development of a disturbed body image:

1. Age of onset of the obesity. Body-image disturbances are primarily found in persons who were obese as children and adolescents or as adolescents alone.
2. Presence of emotional disturbances or neuroses. A stable personality and a secure childhood appear to prevent body-image distortion, whereas emotional disturbances caused by the effects of a disturbed family will invite the development of a distorted body image.
3. A negative evaluation of the obesity by others. The child internalizes the attitudes conveyed by significant others.

It appears that there is a critical period for development of a distorted body image that is characteristic of persons who were obese during adolescence. Those who become obese as adults rarely demonstrate this disturbance. During adolescence and when the youngster is establishing a sense of identity, derogatory views by peers and parents are incorporated into enduring views of the self. Fig. 21-1 shows interrelated factors that contribute to adolescent obesity.

Complications of Childhood Obesity

The most prevalent complication of childhood obesity is its persistence into adulthood, with remarkable resistance to

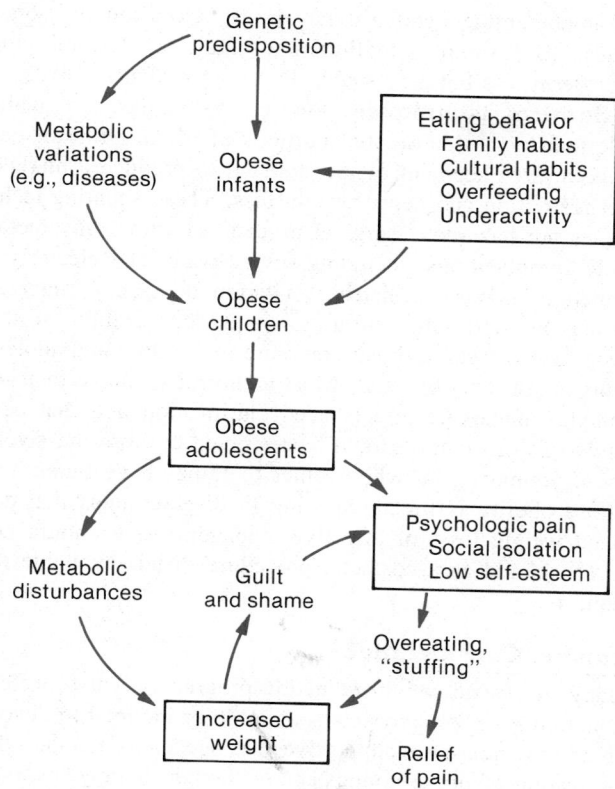

Fig. 21-1. Complex relationships in adolescent obesity.

habits, appetite and hunger patterns, and physical activities. A careful history is taken regarding the development of the obesity, and a physical examination is carried out to help differentiate simple obesity from increased fat resulting from organic causes. Psychologic assessment, accomplished via interviews with the child and standardized personality tests, provides insight into personality and emotional problems that contribute to obesity and that might interfere with therapy. Appropriate diagnostic tests rule out suspected metabolic and endocrine disorders.

It is useful to have an estimation of the degree of fatness in order to have some idea of the component of body weight that can be modified. Several tests, both scientific and unscientific, can be employed to assess obesity. The most widely used means for determining obesity is measurement of skin-fold thickness with special skin-fold calipers. This device, calibrated in millimeters, allows the operator to control the pressure on the skin fold and provides a more precise measurement of its thickness. The Committee on Nutritional Anthropometry of the National Research Council recommends use of the triceps and subscapular areas for skin-fold measurements (see p. 230).

More sophisticated techniques include the *densimetric* method of determining body fat from measures of body density (fat has a low specific gravity); *hydrometry*, which estimates body fat from measurement of total body water; and *radiopotassium*, which evaluates the extent of fat from whole-body potassium content (fat cells contain almost no potassium).

Therapeutic Management

Because of the self-perpetuating nature of obesity, efforts to treat the condition have been universally disappointing. A high proportion of obese children become obese adults. Because most of the nonsurgical approaches to weight reduction and maintenance suffer from a lack of lasting success, a more effective and sustained approach is a preventive one—early recognition and establishment of control measures before the child arrives at an obese state. However, varying degrees of success have been achieved in some highly motivated individuals through weight-reduction techniques, including diet, exercise, behavior modification, and psychologic support.

Diet. Diet modification is essential to any weight-reduction program. The ideal diet regimen for children and adolescents should meet the criteria listed in the box. For extremely obese youngsters calories are markedly restricted, and diet management is under the close supervision of health workers with specialized skills and experience.

Formal calorie-limited diets are more difficult to maintain than more flexible methods. Although short-term weight loss is accomplished, the long-term maintenance is usually unsuccessful. In mildly obese youngsters with good motivation, correction of undesirable food habits and establishment of sensible eating and exercise behavior are sometimes effective. The dietary management requires nutrition reorientation and education.

treatment. With few exceptions, clearly identifiable hazards are rarely present in childhood, but the dangers of obesity increase with its duration. The adult with long-standing obesity is subject to the development of associated medical complications that include hypertension, diabetes, and cardiovascular disease.

The most serious physical effect of severe obesity encountered in childhood is the pickwickian syndrome, named after the Charles Dickens character "Fat Boy Joe," who was continually falling asleep. Although the mechanism is unknown, narcolepsy associated with this obese state is thought to be caused by carbon dioxide narcosis from a decreased ventilatory capacity. There is an increased incidence of certain orthopedic problems in obese children, especially Legg-Perthes disease and genu valgum (knockknee). Probably the most destructive complications are the psychosocial problems that affect obese youngsters as a result of teasing, ridicule, and rejection by peers and family.

Diagnostic Evaluation

The presence of obesity is obvious from appearance alone, and a gross determination can be made by a rough comparison of height and weight with standard growth charts. Children who are 20% over normal for their height and weight should be further evaluated including a height and weight history of the child, parents, and siblings as well as eating

Children below 5 years of age will lose weight on 600 to 800 kcal/day without interference with growth or development of ketosis. A diet containing 800 to 1200 kcal/day is usually suggested for children over 5 years of age (Taitz, 1983). The rate of weight loss varies with the level of physical activity and depends on how large the gap is between intake and normal maintenance requirements. It requires an accumulated deficit of 3500 kcal to lose 1 pound of fat (Merritt and others, 1980). The average caloric maintenance requirements for children over 5 years of age are listed in Table 21-1.

Exercise. Some type of regular exercise is incorporated in a weight-reduction program. In the absence of exercise, both fat and lean body mass are generally lost and weight regained is primarily fat (Fox and Mathews, 1981). For the self-conscious, reluctant youngster it is often more effective to begin the program at the time when some loss has been achieved from dieting and the loss has begun to level off somewhat. The youngster is less likely to feel unwilling to engage in the activity. Parents should be reassured that tapering off in the rate of loss is related not to diet failure but to altered metabolism that must be balanced by increasing activity (Taitz, 1983). Significant decreases in percentage of overweight have been observed in children who exercise in conjunction with diet when compared with those on diet alone (Epstein and others, 1985). Activities should be those that stress self-improvement rather than competition. Teenagers need continued psychologic support and encouragement to prevent the beginning of the destructive cycle of passivity, withdrawal, and rejection.

Behavior modification. Behavior modification approaches to diet loss are based on the observation that obese individuals have abnormal eating practices that can be altered. The attention is focused not on food but on the social and behavioral aspects surrounding food consumption. The technique has been used primarily with older children and adolescents.

Drugs. Prescribing anorexic drugs to children and adolescents is not favored by most practitioners. There is little if any convincing evidence that they are more effective than diet and exercise in maintaining long-term weight loss. Probably more important is a concern regarding habituation to amphetamines and similar drugs. Occasionally some drugs, for example, fenfluramine, may be desirable for short-term loss but are usually discouraged (Taitz, 1983).

Surgical techniques. Surgical techniques are available that bypass substantial portions of the intestine or occlude a large segment of the stomach to produce a marked diet restriction and hence weight loss. These shunting techniques are hazardous surgical procedures with many metabolic complications, including severe water and electrolyte depletion, persistent diarrhea, vitamin deficiency, internal herniation, and fatty infiltration and degeneration of the liver. Use of such a drastic measure in children and adolescents is still controversial. Most authorities believe that the complex metabolic effects need clarification and that certainly this procedure should be restricted to those massively obese youngsters in whom other therapies have failed and whose obesity is life threatening in disease states that demand weight loss for effective management. It should not be considered as a cosmetic procedure that is available on request.

Nursing Considerations

Many successful weight-reduction programs involve professional nurses. Few physicians are able or inclined to devote time to the long-term supportive care needed to maintain the motivation of obese youngsters. Although therapy involves a team approach that includes the physician, dietitian, family, and the children themselves, nurses play a dominant role in any regulated and promising program of weight reduction. Interested nurse practitioners are able to evaluate, treat, and follow overweight adolescents. They also assume an important position in recognizing potential weight problems and assisting parents and their children in programs of prevention.

There are several factors related to the adolescent that health professionals must keep in mind when planning treatment for youngsters in this age-group. First, weight gain and anabolism are normal and necessary to healthy development during adolescent years, and any weight-reduction

Table 21-1 Average calorie requirements for maintenance from age 5 years

AGE	BOYS	GIRLS
5	1350	1300
6	1400	1370
7	1600	1450
8	1650	1500
9	1750	1600
10	1800	1700
11	1900	1800
15	2400	2100
18	2500	2200

Data from Merritt, R.J., and others: Consequences of modified fasting in obese pediatric and adolescent patients. I. Protein-sparing modified fast, J. Pediatr. **96:**13-19, 1980.

program must protect the teenager from prolonged catabolism that may permanently impair growth. Second, energy-absorbing developmental tasks of adolescence are stressful enough in themselves that the psychologic stress of food deprivation may be more than an adolescent can handle.

Motivation to lose weight is the key to success. The reasons behind the desire to lose weight need to be explored with the youngsters, but success is rarely achieved unless they are motivated to lose weight and take personal responsibility for dietary habits and exercise programs. Teenagers who are forced by parents to seek help are seldom sufficiently motivated, become rebellious of parental nagging, and are unwilling to control dietary intake. A rigid approach or one based on parental enforcement of the regimen is usually doomed from the start. The strained relationships between parents and teenager are intensified by parental coercion, and because adolescents get food outside the home, adults simply cannot control their food intake. The result is an angry, sullen, and rebellious youngster who gains rather than loses weight.

Nutrition counseling. Planning caloric restriction for the adolescent during the rapid growth period requires a careful design. Adolescents are unusually sensitive to caloric restriction, both physically and psychologically. It is extremely difficult to achieve the ideal reduction in body fat without concurrent loss in lean body mass. Sharp restriction in calories may result in relatively large losses of lean body mass and is not recommended for children or adolescents.

Sometimes the most realistic approach, especially during growth, is simply to prevent an increase in body fat. Children who are still growing will, by restricting calories, eventually grow into the weight. This can be accomplished by adjusting three aspects of eating: (1) reduce the *quantity* eaten by purchasing, preparing, and serving smaller portions, (2) alter the *quality* consumed by substituting low-calorie foods for high-calorie foods (especially for snacks), and (3) alter the *situations* by severing associations between eating and other stimuli, such as eating while watching television (Copeland and Baucom-Copeland, 1981).

The most successful diets are those that use ordinary foods in controlled portions rather than diets that require the avoidance of any specific food. The youngster and parents are taught how to incorporate favorite foods into the diet and how to select substitutes that are also satisfying. The dieting youngster should eat what the rest of the family eats, but less of it. When parents buy and prepare smaller amounts, tempting second helpings and leftovers are eliminated. For older children exchange diets are useful. There are a multitude of restricted calorie diets available from a number of sources, such as the **American Dietetic Association,** and the caloric values for a wide variety of commercial foods are available to facilitate meal planning.

For the teenager snacking is an integral part of the daily routine, which makes dieting especially difficult for the obese adolescent. Consequently the youngster who is serious about dieting should be helped in elimination or judicious selection of snack foods. For example, getting rid of high-calorie junk foods and placing snack foods out of sight help divert attention away from eating. When snacking, several of a particular item are usually eaten; therefore substituting several items with lower caloric value for one item higher in calories is more satisfying. Foods containing complex carbohydrates are more satisfying than those containing simple sugars. The caloric values for common fast foods and snack items are listed in Table 21-2.

No adolescent should be encouraged to initiate a reduction diet without a health assessment, evaluation, and counseling. It is also important to emphasize the undesirable nature of the fad diets and crash programs that continually appear in various publications. Although some success has been achieved with low-carbohydrate, high-fat diets, their unpalatability and dietary boredom contribute to a high failure rate. Exotic diets have not been successful, and their unbalanced nature makes them potentially dangerous for growing children or adolescents. To be successful from all aspects, a dietary program should be nutritionally sound with sufficient satiety value, produce the desired weight loss, and be accompanied by nutrition education and continued support.

Behavior modification. Altering eating behavior has been found essential to weight reduction, especially in maintaining long-term weight control. This approach emphasizes identification and elimination of inappropriate eating habits. Although the long-term effects of this method are still in need of evaluation, it appears to hold promise for the treatment of obesity in adolescents. The behavior modification programs are based on various concepts, primarily those that incorporate the following (Taitz, 1983):

A description of the behavior to be controlled, such as eating habits

Attempts to modify and control stimuli governing eating

Development of eating techniques designed to control speed of eating

Positive reinforcement for these modifications by a suitable reward system

Some of the techniques used in this approach are listed in the box, p. 897.

Group involvement. Some persons on weight-reduction programs find that the support and mutual reinforcement provided by a group of persons with a similar problem help them adjust to the changes needed for successful accomplishment of their goals, including weight loss. Commercial groups or diet workshops composed primarily of adults may be helpful to a few, but for teenagers a group composed of other adolescents is more acceptable and usually more successful. Types of teenage groups include summer camps designed for obese youngsters and conducted by health professionals, school groups organized and led by a school nurse, and groups associated with special clinics.

*430 N. Michigan Ave., Chicago, IL 60611.

Table 21-2 Caloric values for selected fast food

FOOD	CALORIC VALUE	FOOD	CALORIC VALUE
Burger King		**Cookies and cakes—cont'd**	
Cheeseburger	350	Hostess Twinkie, 1	147
Hamburger	290	Oreo, each	50
Whopper, regular	630	Chocolate chip	50-80
w/cheese	740	Brownie	200
Double beef, plain	850	Fig Newton, 1	60
w/cheese	950	Doughnut, regular, 1 oz	113
French fries, regular	210	old fashioned, 1 oz	151
Onion rings, regular	70	powdered, 1 oz	117
Chocolate shake	365	**Crackers**	
McDonald's		Cheese balls & curls, 1 oz	160
Big Mac	563	Corn chips, 1 oz	150-160
Hamburger	255	Graham crackers, 1 piece	30
Cheeseburger	307	Pretzels, 1 oz	110-116
Chicken McNuggets, (6 pieces)	332	Rye Krisp, 1 triple	25
Quarter Pounder	424	Saltine, 1 piece	12-18
w/cheese	524	Tortilla chips, 1 oz	130-140
Egg McMuffin	327	Trisket, 1 piece	20
French fries, regular	220	Wheat Thins, 1 piece	9
Filet-O-Fish	432	**Candy**	
Milk shake, vanilla	352	Heath, 2½ oz	334
chocolate	383	Hershey's, 1.2 oz bar	187
Wendy's		Nestle's, 1.1 oz bar	159
Hamburger, single	470	Hershey's Kisses, 1 piece	27
w/cheese	580	Krackle bar, .35 oz	52
Hamburger, double	670	Life Savers, 1 piece	10
w/cheese	800	Milk Duds, ¾ oz box	89
Hamburger, triple	850	1¼ oz box	148
w/cheese	1040	M & Ms, peanut, 1½ oz	219
French fries	330	plain, 1½ oz	202
Frostie	390	Mr. Goodbar, 1½ oz	233
Long John Silver's		Snickers, 1.8 oz	247
Fish w/batter, 2 pieces	366	Crackerjacks, ¾ oz	90
3 pieces	549	**Chewing gum**	
Fish sandwich	337	Any brand, 1 stick	10
French fries	288	Dentyne, 1 stick	4
Cole slaw	138	Chiclets, Beechies, 1 piece	6
Hushpuppies (3)	153	**Miscellaneous snacks**	
Taco Bell		Potato chips, 1 oz	150-160
Beef Burrito	466	Pringles, 1 oz	172
Burrito Supreme	457	Yogurt, plain, 8 oz	150-160
Beefy Tostada	291	fruit, 8 oz	230-262
Dairy Queen		Popcorn, plain, 1 cup	54
Brazier Chili Dog	330	**Nuts**	
Super Brazier Dog	518	Almonds, 1 oz	170-178
w/cheese	593	Peanuts, dry roasted, 1 oz	160-173
Super Brazier Chili Dog	555	oil roasted, 1 oz	179
Brazier fries, small	200	Pecans, 1 oz	190-220
Pizza Hut		Pistachios, 1 oz	174
Thin 'n Crispy (¼ medium)		Pumpkin seeds, unshelled, 1 oz	116
Standard cheese	340	Sunflower seeds, shelled, 1 oz	164
Superstyle cheese	410	unshelled, 1 oz	86
Standard pepperoni	370	**Dessert snacks**	
Superstyle pepperoni	430	Popsicle, 1 twin pop	70
Thick 'n Chewy (¼ medium)		Turnover	310-340
Standard cheese	390	Pop Tart	200-220
Superstyle cheese	450	**Baskin-Robbins**	
Standard pepperoni	450	Ice cream, 1 scoop	
Superstyle pepperoni	490	vanilla	147
Supreme	480	French vanilla	181
Super Supreme	590	chocolate	165
Fruit		chocolate fudge	178
Apple w/skin, 2½ in. diameter	66	Sherbet, 1 scoop	99-139
Banana, medium	100	**Beverages**	
Peach w/skin, 2 in. diameter	38	Chocolate milk, 8 oz	213
Cookies and cakes		Skim milk, 8 oz	88
Hostess, 1 cupcake		Whole milk, 8 oz	159
orange	151	Coca Cola, 8 oz	96
chocolate	166	Sprite, 8 oz	95

TREATMENT GUIDELINES FOR MANAGEMENT OF OBESE CHILDREN

Behavioral techniques
Identify eating patterns and behaviors
   Identify food stimuli
      Feelings of hunger
      Television commercials
      Smell or sight of food
   Assess eating environment
      Where food is eaten
      With whom food is eaten, or eaten alone
      Feelings at time of food consumption
      Activity in which engaged while eating
Control food stimuli
   Separate eating from other activities
   Minimize food cues
   Get rid of "junk" food
   Prepare and serve only amount to be eaten
   Put snacks out of sight
   Avoid purchase of problem foods
   Serve food from stove or other place out of reach of the
      established eating place
Change eating patterns
   Eat at a specific place reserved just for eating
   Eat orderly meals at regular hours
   Use smaller plates to make amounts of food appear
      larger
   Slow rate of eating
   Leave a small amount of food on plate
   Eliminate eating during television viewing
   Substitute raw vegetables for "junk" food snacks
Use methods other than eating to deal with emotional
   stress, boredom, fatigue
   Engage in hobby activity, take a walk, straighten up
      room
   Become involved in activities away from food

Increase physical activity
   Have programmed activity such as running, swim-
      ming, cycling
   Engage in routine activity (walking, climbing stairs)
Provide reinforcement for accomplishments
   Focus on short-term goals
   Employ a point system
   Provide tangible rewards such as a movie, concert,
      new record, new item of clothing
   Think positively

Role of the family
Become knowledgeable regarding youngster's therapeutic
   regimen
   Use appropriate reinforcement
   Alter food and eating environment
   Maintain proper attitudes regarding program
Engage in nutrition education
Assist in monitoring eating behavior, food intake, physi-
   cal activity, weight change
Eliminate food as a reward
Encourage youngster with positive statements only

School weight loss program
Employ a buddy system
Use peers as sponsors and positive reinforcers
Employ frequent weigh-ins conducted by involved adult
   nurse, teacher, physical education instructor
Provide reinforcement for weight change
   Social—praise
   Tangible—contract that earns simple rewards
Graph positive weight changes and display where others
   in the program can see it
Provide nutrition education

The group not only is concerned with weight loss but also emphasizes the development of a positive self-image. Nutrition education and diet planning are essential elements of the group function, but equally important are discussions centered around better grooming and improvement of social skills. Improvement is measured by positive changes in all aspects of endeavor. Group support and reinforcement are basic to success.

Family involvement. There is a definite connection between family environment and interaction and obesity (Huse and others, 1982a, 1982b). Involving the family facilitates weight loss, but the nature and extent of the involvement are related to the age of the child. With adolescents parents need education in the purposes of the therapeutic measures and their role in management. The family is given nutrition education and counseled regarding the reinforcement plan, altering the food environment, and maintaining proper attitudes. They assist in monitoring the child's eating behavior, food intake, physical activity, and weight changes (Brownell and Strunkard, 1980). More success has been achieved when counselors meet with adolescents and their parents separately (Brownell, Kelman, and Strunkard, 1983). Younger children and parents meet together, and parents are counseled alone when the children are very young.

Prognosis. Lifelong eating habits and psychologic problems make weight reduction extremely difficult and the failure rate very high. Some predictions can be made on the basis of experience. Weight reduction is more successful in obese adolescents who are older, who have lean parents who are married, who have a good academic performance, who have no affective disorder, and who have had no recent stressful life event (such as parents' divorce or a death).

Huse and others (1982, a) determined that obese youngsters fit into various attitudinal stages indicating stages of problem solving. These stages of problem solving and their relation to weight control are outlined as follows:

Stage 0: Denial. Youngsters have not identified weight control as a personal problem and consider the obesity a result of causes outside themselves. They describe present and future goals that are incompatible with their present weight (e.g., becoming a model). The objective of counseling at this stage is to help the youngsters realize their responsibility in weight control.

Stage I: Awareness. Youngsters recognize that they have a weight-control problem; they feel guilty, helpless, and responsible and are able to identify inappropriate habits or behaviors causing the problem. The objective of counseling is to direct these energies into close self-examination of current energy-balance behaviors.

Stage II: Alterable causes. Youngsters recognize that weight control is a personal problem. They can identify inappropriate habits and behaviors but have not considered alternatives. The objective of counseling is to help the youngsters begin to formulate alternative plans of action.

Stage III: Mechanisms. Youngsters understand the relationship of diet, activity, and weight control. They can identify factors in their lives that are responsible for weight gain and could be modified but have not made the behavioral changes needed for weight control. The objective of counseling is to help the youngsters select the most reasonable mechanisms of change in regard to the obesity-producing factors identified in stage II and to make only those changes that seem reasonable to them.

Stage IV: Implementation. Youngsters have initiated habit and behavioral changes to control the weight problem. They are able to identify persons or situations that affect their ability to manage weight control. They are able to work through the problem-solving stages and handle new threats. The objective of counseling is to encourage the youngsters to exercise the plan whenever it is feasible and to remind them that successful adoption will probably create new difficulties for which they must be alert.

Prevention. Unfortunately weight-loss programs do not enjoy the successes of therapeutic interventions for most other disorders. The failure rate is dismally high. Consequently, the best approach is to identify the infant and child at risk and attempt to prevent obesity. Gradual accumulation of adipose tissue during childhood establishes a pattern of eating that is virtually irreversible by the time a child reaches adolescence (Taitz, 1983). Children who are at risk of obesity, or those considered likely to become fat, are worthy of attempts at prevention. Risk factors in the development of obesity include familial obesity, extreme size at birth, severe disabilities leading to immobility (e.g., meningomyelocele), and syndromes associated with obesity (e.g., Prader-Willi syndrome). Cultural and social factors, including the perception of fat as a sign of good health, are deterrents to prevention.

ANOREXIA NERVOSA

Anorexia nervosa (AN) is the term applied to a long-recognized disorder characterized by severe weight loss in the absence of obvious physical cause. The term *anorexia nervosa* inaccurately describes the disorder in which individuals do not lack hunger but deny its existence. Emaciation occurs as a result of self-inflicted starvation. Anorexia nervosa occurs predominantly in middle-class, well-educated white females between 12 and 25 years of age (McSherry, 1984), and the incidence appears to be increasing significantly. Anorexia nervosa is uncommon in males.

Etiology/Pathophysiology

The onset of anorexia nervosa generally takes place at or near menarche, but it may begin in preadolescence or in adulthood. Young women who have this disorder are most

often from the upper or middle classes, are described as "good children," are academically high achievers, are conforming, are conscientious, and have a high energy level, even with marked emaciation. There is a distinct psychologic component, and the diagnosis is based primarily on psychologic and behavioral criteria. Nevertheless, the physical manifestations of anorexia nervosa lend support to possible organic factors in the etiology. A strong extrinsic motive has, for some reason, suppressed the vital function of eating.

Psychologic aspects. Dominating the psychologic aspects of anorexia nervosa are a relentless pursuit of thinness and a fear of fatness, which are usually preceded by a period of a year or two of mood disturbances and behavior changes. The weight loss is usually triggered by a typical adolescent crisis, such as the onset of menstruation or traumatic interpersonal incidents, that precipitates serious dieting and continues out of control. Frequently there is an exaggerated misinterpretation of the normal fat deposition characteristic of the early adolescent period, or someone may comment that the adolescent girl is putting on weight. The weight loss may be a response to teasing, some change in her life (such as changing schools or going to college), or an incident that requires an independent decision that she is unprepared to make (such as a career choice).

The current emphasis on slimness is a significant factor contributing to the increasing incidence in this disorder among young women. The standard for beauty is one exemplified by the models chosen for advertising clothing. Bigness is considered the ideal for men and smallness is desired for women, and feminine success has long been based on appearance (Garner and others, 1980). Consequently, the pressure to diet and be slim continues relentlessly. Youngsters entering the growth phase of puberty when biological fat accumulation is the normal course of development are particularly vulnerable. However, this standard is not universal. Women in countries where hunger and famine are facts of life do not consider extreme thinness a sign of beauty.

The syndrome of anorexia nervosa consists of three major areas of disordered psychologic functioning (Bruch, 1978):

1. **Disturbed body image and body concept of delusional proportions.** The young girl identifies with her emaciation, defending the skeleton-like appearance as normal, actively maintains it, and denies that it is abnormal. She indicates that it is rewarding to achieve and maintain this emaciated state. She is increasingly fearful of weight gain and interprets the concern of others as attempts to make her fat.

2. **Inaccurate and confused perception and interpretation of inner stimuli.** Inaccurate hunger awareness is pronounced. The adolescent does not recognize signs of nutritional need in herself and is unable to assess the amounts of food taken. She may feel "full" after only a few bites and derives pleasure from the refusal of food. A preoccu-

pation and tremendous involvement with food and related activities are associated with this eating behavior; the girl frequently assumes all meal planning and preparation for others. Girls with anorexia nervosa often increase their activity to help counteract the possibility of weight gain. This hyperactivity may continue until emaciation is far advanced.

3. **Paralyzing sense of ineffectiveness that pervades all aspects of daily life.** Contrary to the defiant and rebellious attitude displayed by anorectic children, they are overwhelmed by a deep sense of ineffectiveness. They are convinced that they only function in response to demands and wishes of others rather than doing as they want or choose to do. They have always been compliant children, but careful analysis reveals this to be mechanical obedience and overconformity that is not recognized as a reflection of a serious problem—a self-doubt regarding their ability to stand up for themselves or even the right for self-assertion.

Some current evidence suggests that anorexia nervosa is a symptom of family psychopathology that is not usually apparent until the child has improved. These girls are usually strongly dependent on their parents, and frequently an ambivalent mother-daughter relationship is present. There is often a history of family strife with the anorexia nervosa being a symptom of the family problems. Two characteristics are common in families with anorectic children: (1) parental conflict with possibility of divorce—to avoid interpersonal conflicts, the family focuses on the symptoms of the anorexia, thereby stabilizing a dysfunctional family (Richardson, 1980); and (2) a sibling who is rebellious and more outgoing and who gets considerable attention as a result of this behavior.

The anorectic youngsters usually feel out of control in all aspects of their lives and choose control of food intake to express their autonomy. Any interventions are viewed as an attempt to remove this control.

Organic etiology. Evidence of organic etiology has been accumulated that may implicate abnormalities of hypothalamic-pituitary and end-organ function in individuals with anorexia nervosa. This is based on the observation that secondary amenorrhea is a common finding and that appetite and satiety are hypothalamic functions. Associated symptoms manifest in anorexia nervosa that relate to hypothalamic dysfunction include abnormalities of thermoregulation, water conservation, and secretion of catecholamines.

Clinical Manifestations

The most obvious manifestation of this disorder is the severe and profound weight loss induced by self-imposed starvation. The youngster identifies with this skeleton-like appearance and does not regard it as abnormal or ugly. She attempts to hide the extreme thinness by wearing bulky sweaters and baggy pants. Anorectic girls also tend to overestimate the size of others (Bruch, 1978). The patient absolutely refuses to eat and has a repertoire of excuses for not eating. Surprisingly, the individual displays a marked preoccupation with food—preparing meals for others, talking about food, and hoarding food. The youngster becomes

obsessed with fasting and engages in frequent strenuous exercise, self-induced vomiting, and/or taking laxatives in an attempt to speed up the weight-loss process.

These youngsters tend to withdraw from peer relationships and engage in self-imposed social isolation. They are continually striving for perfection, which may be demonstrated in other compulsive behaviors such as stinginess. They are usually overachievers and their schoolwork is very important to them.

In the wake of the severe weight loss these young girls exhibit physical signs of altered metabolic activity. They develop secondary amenorrhea, bradycardia, lowered body temperature, decreased blood pressure, and cold intolerance. They have dry skin and brittle nails and develop lanugo hair. The changes are usually reversible with adequate weight gain and improved nutritional status (see also Table 21-1).

Diagnostic Evaluation

Diagnosis is made on the basis of clinical manifestations and conformity to the criteria established by the American Psychiatric Association (1980) (see box).

Therapeutic Management

The treatment and management of anorexia nervosa involve three major thrusts: reinstitution of normal nutrition or reversal of the severe state of malnutrition, resolution of the disturbed patterns of family interaction, and individual psychotherapy to correct deficits and distortions in psychologic functioning. Because of the psychogenic nature of the disorder, treatment is difficult and lengthy.

Nutrition. The initial goal is to treat the life-threatening malnutrition with strict adherence to dietary requirements, which sometimes necessitates intravenous and/or tube feedings, although such methods are usually reserved for severe situations. This is combined with resolution of the family interaction and psychotherapy to improve the underlying psychologic misconceptions about the weight loss. Weight

---

DIAGNOSTIC CRITERIA FOR ANOREXIA NERVOSA

A. Intense fear of becoming obese, which does not diminish as weight loss progresses.
B. Disturbance of body image, e.g., claiming to "feel fat" even when emaciated.
C. Weight loss of at least 25% of original body weight or, if under 18 years of age, weight loss from original body weight plus projected weight gain expected from growth charts combined to equal 25%.
D. Refusal to maintain body weight over a minimum normal weight for age and height.
E. No known physical illness that would account for the weight loss.

From Diagnostic and statistical manual of mental disorders, ed. 3 (DSM-III), Washington, DC, 1980, American Psychiatric Association.

gain alone cannot be considered a cure for the disease and is an unreliable sign of progress. Relapses are frequent as the young girl reverts to previous eating patterns when removed from the therapeutic environment.

Rapid weight gain should be avoided. It can be medically unsafe and it overwhelms the patient, who feels out of control immediately. Many of the deaths associated with anorexia nervosa occur during rehabilitation as a result of cardiovascular overload. A safe and reasonable target weight is calculated by the physician and dietitian—usually 18% fat. Initially the child resists the target weight as "too heavy," but without a target weight she feels out of control and believes people want her to gain weight indefinitely. Establishing a "maintenance weight range" of 1 kg over or under the target weight also helps the youngster feel in control, and teaches how weight is maintained through good dietary habits (e.g., uncontrollable weight gain is not inevitable when an individual consumes a normal diet).

Behavior therapy. The behavior modification approach to therapy has both supporters and detractors. Providing privileges or activities for weight gain or positive eating behaviors has had some success, although this approach alone ignores the youngster's individuality and does not address the conflict precipitating the disorder (Pipes, 1985). A clearly defined behavior modification plan is communicated to the child and maintained through a unified team approach by all persons involved in care.

The team responsible for the management of youngsters with anorexia nervosa arranges a carefully structured environment. A number of aspects are essential. First, there must be consistency. The team decides on an approach and adheres to it. The plan is structured with reality-testing regarding caloric intake and body-image perception as an essential component. The team members provide a unified front to avoid any possibility of manipulation or inconsistency. Second, all members of the team must be involved. The responsibility of the program cannot be left to one person. The role and boundaries of each member are clearly spelled out and understood. Third, it is best to have continuity of team members. If possible it is helpful to have the same staff persons all the time.

Fourth, communication among team members is essential, including clear communication with the patient regarding what is expected from her. Sometimes the limit setting needed may seem unreasonable, and if the youngster does not know the rationale for the limits, she may sabotage the entire program. It is also important to communicate with the family. Fifth, the plan must provide for support of patient, family, and staff. The patient needs positive feedback for accomplishments made in normalizing eating habits and behaviors. Meetings are held to discuss and process feelings and concerns. This includes group meetings of team members, minimeetings of immediate caregivers and the patient, and structured rounds.

All of those involved in therapy must keep in mind the adolescent's distorted sense of body image and self-awareness and her feelings of self-doubt, ineffectiveness, and

Table 21-3 A behavior modification plan for achieving weight gain in anorexia nervosa

WEIGHT (lbs)*	PRIVILEGE LOST OR GAINED
70	Hospitalize
	In room; full bed rest
	No telephone, television, radio, phonograph, and so on
	No books, school work, or craft materials
	No visitors
−3	Tube feeding
+¼	Bathroom privileges
+½	May have books, school work, craft materials
+1	May have radio
+1½	May have television
+2	May have brief visit with parents
+2½	May have telephone
+3	May go out of room
+3½	May have friends visit
+5	May go home
−5	Rehospitalize with all restrictions
−8	Reinstitute tube feedings

From Hofmann, A.D., editor: Adolescent medicine; Menlo Park, CA, 1983, Addison-Wesley Publishing Co., p. 324.
*Privileges should be accorded at ¼ lb gains in the beginning. Later they may be set at ½ lb intervals. This listing is only an example of one behavior modification approach.

helplessness that prompt such bizarre behavior in order to feel in control. The underlying principle in most behavior modification programs is to make conditions extremely uncomfortable and to grant privileges only as a reward for weight gain (Table 21-3). Patients who view the program as coercive and become depressed by this approach seldom maintain weight gain outside the hospital environment.

A *behavioral contract,* an agreement that the patient makes with the others involved to change a maladaptive behavior, has proved to be effective in some cases. The written contract, constructed by the therapeutic team, is approved and signed by the patient. Unless the patient agrees to its terms, the contract can become the source of a power struggle. However, it can be an effective tool by placing the responsibility on the patient for weight gain or other behavior change (Carino and Chmelko, 1983).

Other therapies. Another approach that has sometimes proved effective as an adjunct to therapy is deconditioning by producing a mild euphoria that is incompatible with maintaining an anxiety about eating. There is a decided relationship between anorexia nervosa and depression. Decreasing the patient's consciousness of and vigilance about eating makes her less anxious and more amenable to other suggestions. This includes the administration of antidepressant or antianxiety agents. However, these drugs must be carefully monitored because of their cardiovascular side effects.

Some observations indicate that there may be a link between zinc and some aspects of anorexia nervosa. It is unclear whether the reduced serum zinc levels in these patients are secondary to the inadequate dietary intake or whether a premorbid zinc deficiency precipitates the eating behavior (Bryce-Smith and Simpson, 1984).

Family therapy. Family therapy seems to be effective when begun soon after the onset of illness, but it is less successful when the condition has existed for some time. Therapy is directed toward disengagement and redirection of malfunctioning processes in the family, but this usually requires individual psychotherapy for family members.

Psychotherapy. Psychotherapy for the affected youngster is essential. The patient herself needs to be an active participant in the treatment process and to become aware of the impulses, feelings, and needs originating within herself. It is essential that the patient "rely on her own thinking, become more realistic in her self-appraisal, capable of living as a self-directed, competent individual who can enjoy what life has to offer and no longer needs to manipulate the body and its functions in this bizarre way" (Bruch, 1978).

Children whose illness can be clearly related to a dysfunctional family situation respond to therapy best when separated from the family. Many of those whose therapy plan is implemented in the hospital need a continued behavior modification program after discharge in order to maintain the desired weight. Psychotherapy is aimed at helping the child resolve the adolescent identity crisis, particularly as it relates to a distorted body image.

Prognosis

The complete recovery rate for anorexia nervosa is less than ideal. Only 15% of anorectic individuals attain full recovery; 50% improve substantially although they may relapse during times of stress. The fatality rate for this disorder is approximately 10%, and about 25% to 30% of anorectic persons remain chronically ill (Paige, 1983). Although the changes are often reversible, long-term effects of severe malnutrition may be evident. For many anorexia nervosa will be a lifelong problem.

Evidence indicates that patients restored to normal weight still demonstrate a very low self-esteem, are highly sensitive to social interactions, and remain "obsessoid" (Pillay and Crisp, 1977). There is a strong underlying suicidal tendency and, although the patient may not be aware of it, the efforts to starve themselves may be a manifestation. This should be explored in psychotherapy.

Nursing Considerations

Nurses need to adopt and maintain a kind, supporting, yet firm manner in managing the care of an anorectic child without creating a passive-dependent attitude in the child. The child requires the sustained support and reassurance as she copes with ambivalent feelings related to her own body concept and the desire to see herself as cooperative, reliable, and worthy of the kindness she receives. Encouraging the child with education and activities that strengthen her self-esteem facilitates her resocialization process and social acceptance among her peers.

The goals of nursing care described by Carino and Chmelko (1983) are directed toward assisting patients to:

1. Normalize their eating behaviors
2. Develop realistic perceptions (attitudes) about their body and food
3. Develop adaptive coping mechanisms to deal with their perceptual distortions
4. Obtain a beginning identification and understanding of their underlying issues and conflicts
5. Develop adaptive interactions and relationships with family and other support systems
6. Identify strengths in order to enhance self-worth and self-esteem
7. Use a comfortable, nonthreatening environment (milieu) in which to practice new behaviors and explore sensitive or painful issues

---

Nursing Care Summary: The Adolescent with Anorexia Nervosa

NURSING GOALS	NURSING INTERVENTIONS	EXPECTED PATIENT/FAMILY OUTCOMES
N-MP **Nutrition, alteration in: less than body requirements** **Etiology: self-starvation**		
Restore nutritional status	Implement high-calorie diet as prescribed Explain nutritional plan to child and family Select with dietitian and patient a balanced diet with the prescribed incremental increase in calories Help patient prepare a dietary diary	Child evidences weight gain
Enforce behavior modification plan (if implemented)	Make certain all members of the health team understand the therapeutic plan Make certain that the patient and family understand the conditions of the plan	Expectations are met consistently (specify)

Continued.

NURSING GOALS	NURSING INTERVENTIONS	EXPECTED PATIENT/FAMILY OUTCOMES
Enforce behavior modification plan (if implemented)—cont'd	Involve patient in plans Ensure consistent application of plan by involved health professionals Consult with patient regarding progress Avoid coercive techniques Avoid extensive discussion of food	
Reduce energy expenditure	Monitor physical activity Supervise selection and performance of activity Be alert to evidence of secretive exercising	Child engages in quiet and specified activities

N.D. SP-SCP Self-concept, disturbance in: body image
Etiology: altered perception of self

Provide patient with appropriate feeling of control	Channel need for control and feeling of effectiveness in appropriate directions (rather than control of weight) Obtain psychiatric referral as indicated Encourage patient to monitor own care as appropriate	Child expresses self in acceptable ways
Support patient	Maintain open communications with patient Convey an attitude of caring and protection to patient Avoid conveying an attitude of intrusion Encourage participation in own care	Child expresses feelings and concerns Child becomes actively involved in own care and management
Alter distorted self-image	Support psychiatric plan of care	Child displays evidence of developing a positive self-image

N.D. CSTP Coping, ineffective family: disabling
Etiology: ambivalent family relationships

Resolve disturbed pattern of family interaction	Observe family interaction Explore feelings and attitudes of family members Support psychotherapeutic measures for redirecting malfunctioning family processes Help arrange for referral to individuals and groups that further therapeutic goals	Family patterns of interaction are outlined and evaluated
Prepare for home care	Make certain both patient and family understand therapeutic plan Arrange for follow-up care Refer to special agencies for additional information and support	Family demonstrates an understanding of the etiology of the disorder and conforms to therapeutic program

N.D. CSTP Coping, ineffective individual
Etiology: unrealistic perceptions

Recognize anorexia nervosa	Observe for signs of
	  Malnutrition
	  Behaviors associated with the disorder
	  Evidence of hormonal changes, especially those associated with pubertal changes
	Obtain complete history
	Explore patient's body image perception
		Child with signs of anorexia nervosa is recognized early and receives initial evaluation

Prevent relapse	Maintain consistency in therapeutic approach selected Maintain vigilance to detect signs of sabotaging the therapeutic plan, such as self-induced vomiting, hoarding food, disposing of food, placing weighted material in clothing for weigh-in Provide positive reinforcement for progress Be alert for signs of depression Support psychotherapeutic measures Help arrange for follow-up care	Child and family conform to therapeutic program (specify behaviors)
Monitor progress	Obtain baseline information Observe and record emotional status Observe and record interactions with family and peers	

It is also important for nurses to be aware of some of the physical side effects of anorexia nervosa. Anorectic patients often limit their fluid intake, which can lead to urinary tract problems. Ketones and proteins are frequently detected in the urine as a result of fat and protein breakdown. Vital sign instability can be severe, including orthostatic hypotension; the heartbeat becomes irregular and the pulse rate decreases markedly. The bradycardia and hypothermia can result in cardiac arrest.

Nurses, patients, and families can find assistance and information from organizations that provide services for young persons suffering from this disorder. The **National Anorectic Aid Society, Inc.*** provides information and support services for both patient and families. The **National Association of Anorexia Nervosa and Associated Disorders, Inc. (ANAD)†** provides counseling, referral, and self-help programs for young people with anorexia nervosa. **The American Anorexia/Bulimia Association, Inc.‡** also provides information, referrals, counseling, programs, and activities aimed at combating eating disorders.

Prevention

There are no easy ways to prevent anorexia. However, public and professional awareness of signs and symptoms can help identify patients early so that treatment can be implemented in order to prevent or reduce the long-term adverse consequences. Some of the early signs of anorexia are outlined in the box. Education about the disorder may help prevent some cases.

BULIMIA

Bulimia (from the Greek meaning "ox hunger") is the term applied to an eating disorder, similar to anorexia nervosa, that is characterized by binge eating. The binge behavior consists of secretive, frenzied consumption of large amounts of high-calorie (or "forbidden") foods during a brief period of time (usually less than 2 hours). The binge is counteracted by a variety of weight-control methods (purging), including self-induced vomiting, diuretic and laxative abuse, and rigorous exercise. These binge/purge cycles are followed by self-deprecating thoughts, depressed mood, and an awareness that the eating pattern is abnormal.

Clinical Manifestations

Bulimia is observed more frequently in older adolescent girls and young women; male bulimics are uncommon. Dynamically bulimics have many issues in common with other eating disorders—control being a major issue. Many begin with only occasional binges and purges "just for fun," enjoying the control over their weight while eating amounts of food that would normally produce obesity. As the disease progresses, frequency of binges increases, the amount of

*550 S. Cleveland Ave., Suite F, Westerville, OH 43081.
†Box 271, Highland Park, IL 60035.
‡Cedar Lane, Teaneck, NJ 07666.

WARNING SIGNS OF ANOREXIA NERVOSA

The youngster:
Consumes an inappropriate diet (excessively strict) or may refuse to eat altogether.
Develops peculiar eating habits such as toying with food, food "rituals," preparing and forcing food on family members without eating any herself.
Engages in excessive exercise, such as compulsive jogging, running up and down stairs, rigorous calisthenics to burn off calories—often to the point of exhaustion.
Withdraws from social interaction—starts to spend all her time in her room studying, exercising, or otherwise occupied.
Menstrual periods cease after sudden or excessive weight loss—sometimes almost as soon as dieting begins.
Takes laxatives, diuretics, or enemas to speed intestinal transit time to lose added weight and empty intestines to flatten abdomen.
Vomits deliberately—may go to bathroom after a meal and turn on faucets to avoid being heard.
Denies hunger even after eating practically nothing for days or even weeks.
Develops a distorted body image—states she "feels fat" as she becomes increasingly thinner.
Loses weight—growing girls fail to achieve the 75th percentile on normal growth curves.

---

food consumed increases, and the bulimic gradually loses control over the binge/purge cycle. The binge/purge cycle provides relief from feelings of guilt resulting from the enormous amounts of costly food consumed. The family becomes angry and the bulimic individual becomes frightened, frustrated, and increasingly guilt ridden, which only increases the symptoms in a self-destructive cycle.

Frequency of binging can be anywhere from once per week to seven or eight times per day. Because bulimic persons usually binge on high-calorie foods, especially sweets, ice cream, and pastries, insulin production is stimulated to cope with the added carbohydrate. When the food is vomited, the unused insulin stimulates hunger and the desire to eat. A daily caloric intake of 20,000 to 30,000 calories per day is not unusual. The disorder is almost never seen in lower socioeconomic groups because of the difficulty in obtaining volumes of food.

Characteristically bulimic persons are those who have been unsuccessful dieters, have low impulse control, and may have been self-conscious about overweight in childhood. They may consciously or unconsciously suppress their feelings and have a strong desire to fit into the group.

Bulimic individuals appear to fall into two categories: (1) those who consume vast quantities of food followed by purging but who, if unable to purge, still consume large amounts and (2) those who restrict their caloric intake, especially when unable to purge. Some bulimic women are of normal or (more often) slightly above normal weight; others become as underweight as anorectic individuals. This latter type with a tendency to restrict intake is also called *buli-*

COMPARISON OF ANOREXIA NERVOSA AND BULIMIA

Anorexia nervosa	Bulimia
Turns away from food to cope	Turns to food to cope
Introverted	Extroverted
Avoids intimacy	Seeks intimacy
Negates feminine role	Aspires to feminine role
Maintains rigid control	Loses control
Body distortions	Infrequent body distortions
Denies illness	Recognizes illness
Significant weight loss	Within 5 to 15 lb of normal body weight

marexia. (See the accompanying box for a comparison of anorexia nervosa and bulimia.)

Complications. Bulimic women suffer from several medical complications as a result of the frequent vomiting. Loss of fluids and electrolytes can occur very rapidly as in any other disorder characterized by gastrointestinal losses. Potassium depletion causes diminished reflexes, fatigue, and if severe possible cardiac arrhythmias. Potassium losses are more likely to occur with diuretic abuse. Laxative abuse can interfere with absorption of fat, protein, and calcium as well as produce abdominal complaints, such as cramping, and sluggish bowel function.

Vomiting produces a number of serious complications. Irritation from stomach acid causes erosion of tooth enamel and an increase in dental caries. Chronic esophagitis, chronic sore throat, difficulty swallowing, inflammation, and parotitis are frequent findings. Vomiting may be so severe that the patient suffers esophageal tears, hiatal hernia, and spontaneous bleeding in the eye. Anemia is common.

Diagnostic Evaluation

The diagnosis may be first suspected from the presence of complications. Final diagnosis is made on the basis of criteria established by the American Psychiatric Association (1980) (see box). Distinctive hand lesions have also been observed in bulimic persons. The backs of the hands are often scarred and cut from repeated abrasion of the skin against the maxillary incisors during self-induced vomiting (Williams, Friedman, and Steiner, 1986).

Therapeutic Management

Therapy is similar to the management of anorexia nervosa. Hospitalization may be required, especially for complications, which are treated symptomatically. Intravenous fluids and potassium replacement are the essential elements of care, and cardiac monitoring is indicated.

Two approaches to behavior therapy may be employed. The first advocates eliminating binge/purge opportunity by

wanted behaviors. This approach allows the patient more control as opposed to staff control. (See therapeutic management of anorexia nervosa, p. 899.)

Nursing Considerations

Nursing care is similar to care of the patient with anorexia nervosa. Acute care also involves careful monitoring of fluid and electrolyte alterations and observation for signs of cardiac complications.

FEAR OF FAT SYNDROME

A new phenomenon has been identified that affects preteens and teenagers—the fear of becoming fat (Pugliese and others, 1983). In their enthusiasm to avoid becoming overweight these youngsters restrict their caloric intake to the degree that they stop growing normally and pubertal changes do not take place. The disorder is distinct from anorexia nervosa in which the patients have a distorted body image. Youngsters who are afraid of obesity worry that overweight will make them physically unattractive, jeopardize their health, and shorten their life spans.

The desire for thinness in these youngsters is often triggered by the normal gain in weight and fat accumulation of adolescent growth and development. The dissatisfaction with their appearance often causes young people to resort to fad diets and severely reduce their intake far below the recommended daily allowances for nutrients. The media emphasis on thinness and the nationwide emphasis on preven-

DIAGNOSTIC CRITERIA FOR BULIMIA

A. Recurrent episodes of binge eating (rapid consumption of a large amount of food in a discrete period of time, usually less than 2 hours).
B. At least three of the following:
    1. Consumption of high-caloric, easily ingested food during a binge
    2. Inconspicuous eating during a binge
    3. Termination of such eating episodes by abdominal pain, sleep, social interruption, or self-induced vomiting
    4. Repeated attempts to lose weight by severely restrictive diets, self-induced vomiting, or use of cathartics or diuretics
    5. Frequent weight fluctuations greater than 10 lb because of alternating binges and fasts
C. Awareness that the eating pattern is abnormal and fear of not being able to stop eating voluntarily.
D. Depressed mood and self-deprecating thoughts following eating binges.
E. The bulimic episodes are not due to anorexia nervosa or any known physical disorder.

From Diagnostic and statistical manual of mental disorders, ed. 3 (DSM-III), Washington, DC, 1980, American Psychiatric Association.

tion of obesity may be detrimental to this vulnerable age-group.

Nurses who encounter youngsters who impose unwarranted dieting upon themselves need to focus on education regarding normal changes and the hazards of dieting, which are more serious than the risks associated with unwanted weight gain. Although most authorities suggest a weight maintenance program for overweight children during the growth years, there are those who recommend that no child or adolescent in the growth-spurt be encouraged or counseled to lose weight (Mallick, 1982).

Destructive Behaviors

The turmoil and stress associated with the pubertal changes of adolescence, limited problem-solving capacity, and the struggle for independence experienced by many adolescents make them vulnerable to superimposed stresses. Some youngsters who are unable to cope with these complex problems and feelings indulge in behaviors that are life threatening or harmful.

SUICIDE

The problem of suicide is worldwide and increasing in many countries. A striking feature is the rise among persons in the younger age-groups. Between 1950 and 1981 the suicide rate tripled in young people between the ages of 15 and 24 (Raley, 1985). It is the third leading cause of death during the teenage years, surpassed only by injury and homicide (Friedman and others, 1984; Keidel, 1983).

Suicide is defined as the deliberate act of self-injury with the intent that the injury should kill. Most authorities distinguish between a suicidal gesture and an attempt, and both must be acknowledged. A *gesture* is made without any real attempt to cause either serious injury or death but rather to send out a signal that something is wrong. An *attempt*, unlike a gesture, is intended to cause injury or death. Teenagers sometimes make a number of gestures to draw attention to the fact that they are unable to cope. If the signals are not detected and responded to promptly, they may escalate in seriousness until they become serious attempts or completed acts. Another category, an *impulsive act*, describes a rage response designed to punish or manipulate a loved person perceived as withdrawing that love (Hofmann, 1983).

Incidence

The true incidence of suicide in children and adolescents is not known because of general underreporting. Frequently deaths by suicide are reported as accidental because of pressures exerted by family and society to avoid the cultural and religious stigma associated with self-destruction. There also appears to be some degree of certainty that the high accident rate in persons in this age-group may reflect suicides masked by accidental death or homicide.

There are some differences in suicides in relation to ethnic and racial factors. There is a lower incidence of suicide in Asians and Jews, and although older blacks have a lower incidence, the suicide rate for black teenagers is rapidly approaching that for whites (Maris, 1985). Girls make suicidal gestures or attempts four to eight times more often than boys and account for 90% of suicide attempts, whereas boys account for 70% of successful suicides (Raley, 1985). Gestures are made at home when someone else is nearby, usually in the evening or afternoon. More attempts occur in late winter (Garfinkel and others, 1982). Depression is the most frequent diagnosis and occurs in 35% to 79% of all those who attempt suicide (Friedman and others, 1984).

Etiology

The reasons youngsters attempt suicide are numerous and varied. Some contributing factors include the changing times, especially within families. There is an increase in two-career families, and more separation and divorce, which make youngsters feel more vulnerable and decrease feelings of stability. The youth of today are faced with an increasingly competitive society that encourages them to have high expectations for themselves and fosters a fear of failure that makes them feel highly pressured.

Developmental factors. Adolescence has always been characterized by turmoil, heightened emotionality, and wide variations in mood. Youngsters display moods that range from the depths of depression to the heights of elation. It is sometimes difficult to determine whether a youngster is exhibiting a normal mood swing or is at risk for true depression and suicide. No period in life is fraught with such major changes, and teenagers have limited ability to understand these changes. With limited capacities for problem solving and with fewer and less sophisticated resources for resolving difficulties, they may resort to methods of handling problems that were acquired at an earlier age. It often appears to adults that adolescents ''overreact'' to situations. Actually they experience emotions and react to events more intensely than adults.

Some teenagers have difficulty coping well with critical events, especially a situation that is forced upon them, such as death of a friend, parent, or sibling. Studies have found that suicidal children experienced increasing and significantly greater amounts of stress as they matured, including a number of specific chaotic and disruptive family events that resulted in losses and separations from important people (Cohen-Sandler, Berman, and King, 1982). Most adolescents can function quite well, but when health professionals see those who do not, further investigation is indicated.

A surprising number of children 5 to 9 years of age commit or attempt to commit suicide. This behavior is often wrongly assumed to be accidental. Children in this age-group are unable to think in abstract terms and therefore do not comprehend the permanence and irreversibility of death. Immature adolescents with poor ego development tend to react impulsively to situations much as they did at a younger age. Turning aggression inward in stressful situations, they seek to avoid discomfort, join a lost object, or gain love.

Family factors. Suicidal youngsters almost invariably come from a disturbed family situation, such as economic stresses, family disintegration, medical problems, or psychiatric illness. Broken homes, divorce, separation, abandonment, alcoholism, and death are highly significant factors and are frequently noted in the histories of suicidal youth. In instances in which the family is intact, the disorganization is manifest by marital discord, lack of or disturbed communication, abnormal patterns of interaction, physical aggression, and general lack of unity and solidarity within the family system. Often there is a history of a suicide by another family member.

Parents are often inadequate and unable to cope. There is usually a lack or loss of communication links with parents. Sometimes there is hostility, indifference, or overt rejection by one or both parents. There may be extreme parental control. Younger children who are treated badly at home react with rebellious behavior and may commit suicide for fear of punishment. Parents may set impossibly high expectations for the youngster, or there may be parental indifference with very low expectations. There is often a lack of parental supportive response to the children's problems. Parents have a low understanding of the child and have not noticed the behavior changes displayed by the suicidal youngster. If families seek help immediately after a suicide attempt, there is less possibility of a repeat attempt. If they are negative and apathetic, there is a greater risk of another, more lethal attempt.

Psychoses. When evaluating youngsters for therapy it is important to rule out those with affective disorders, especially borderline and character disorders. Many of these youngsters exhibit self-destructive behavior, such as scratching at their wrists, that is not likely to succeed as a lethal method. It is manipulative behavior and a bid for attention; although these youngsters may talk about suicide dramatically, they rarely want to kill themselves. Most manipulative behaviors are managed by ignoring the behavior, but these youngsters may inadvertently do severe damage as their manipulative behavior increases. There are also those who are psychotic and who may be hearing voices that tell them to kill themselves.

Suicidal Methods

The outcome of suicidal behavior is influenced to some extent by the method used. Violent methods of destruction used by adults, such as jumping from heights or in front of trains, are less frequently employed by younger persons. Overdose of drugs is the method of choice for most adolescents who attempt suicide, and these are usually medications prescribed for parents, such as barbiturates and antidepressants, those intended for household use (such as aspirin), or solvents. Youngsters do not have the sophistication to know the lethality of most drugs. They tend to use drugs that are available.

Ingesting pills and wrist lacerations are the favored methods of females; males tend to use more lethal methods such as knives, guns, automobiles, and jumping from heights (Hofmann, 1983). Younger children (under 13½ years) are more likely to resort to hanging (Garfinkel and others, 1982).

Sometimes an adolescent will threaten suicide in order to manipulate the environment. Unfortunately, with no self-destructive intent, a youngster may make a half-hearted attempt that leads to death or permanent injury. A "partial" or chronic suicide is illustrated by the adolescent with a chronic illness, such as a diabetic youngster who refuses to comply with the prescribed medical regimen, the accident-prone adolescent, and the drug-abusing youngster. Risk factors for suicide are outlined in the box.

Motivation

Suicidal gestures are not uncommon among adolescents, and most are impulsive acts committed to force parents or other significant persons in their lives to pay attention to their need for help. The attempt usually is the culmination of a behavioral pattern. These youngsters often have a history of attention-getting behaviors that range from minor acts to increasingly dramatic ones. With the ultimate act of attempted suicide the teenagers finally make themselves heard. They seldom actually plan a suicidal act because they really want to die; they want to be free from stress created by an intolerable situation. The attempt is made when there is someone around or when they know someone is coming home. These youngsters need someone to act in a controlling manner.

Suicidal ideation is not uncommon in adolescents. It represents numerous fantasies, such as a relief of suffering, a means to gain comfort and sympathy, or a revenge toward those who have hurt them. The youngsters have the erroneous perception that the act of suicide will evoke remorse and pity and that they will be able to return and witness the grief. They expect people to care and be concerned. A frequent motive for suicide in children and younger adolescents is the desire to punish others who will be grieved by their death. Angry children who are unable to directly punish those who have injured or insulted them will take revenge on those who love them through self-destruction ("They'll be sorry when they find me dead"; "They'll be sorry they were mean to me"). This motive is more common in girls and more likely to persist longer. This, of course, is faulty judgment on the part of those attempting suicide.

Occasionally there are adolescents who are so severely depressed that suicide appears to them to be the only means of release from their despair. These youngsters rarely give evidence of their intent, concealing their suicidal thoughts for fear of outside intervention. Sometimes this self-destructive behavior is a desire to punish themselves for guilt-filled actions, such as masturbation or, more often, thoughts. Peer pressure, too, has convinced many young persons that there

RISK FACTORS FOR YOUTH SUICIDE

Past history
History of child abuse or neglect
Death of a parent when child was young (age 3 to 5 years)
Alcohol or substance abuse
Physical/body image problems (delayed puberty, chronic illness, disability)
Thinking disorder (wishes to join a deceased person; hears voices telling to kill self)
Chronic depression; rejects help
Previous suicide attempts
Past psychiatric hospitalization

Family factors
Previous suicide attempts by family member(s)
Family history of suicide (parent or relative)
Depression
Difficult home situation—long, bitter, parent-child conflict
Hostile parents
Overt rejection by one or both parents; may be thrown out of home
Divorce or separation of parents
Recent or impending move
Exposure to unrealistically high expectations from parents
Parental indifference with very low expectations

Mood/affect
Marked persistent depression
Feelings of hopelessness, helplessness, isolation
Deteriorating school work
Remains distant, sad, remote
Flat affect—has "frozen" facial expression
Persistently looks or sounds sad and unhappy
Describes self as worthless
Feelings of self-hatred or excessive guilt
Feelings of humiliation, often brought on by inadequate performance at school
Sudden cheerfulness following deep depression
Wish to be punished

Behavior
Changes in physical appearance—a child previously neat and well groomed will stop bathing and begin to look slovenly

Loss of function due to illness or trauma
Loss of energy—loss of interest, listlessness, exhaustion without obvious cause
Sleep disturbances—difficulty going to sleep or sleeping excessively, takes voluntary naps during afternoon or evening
Increased irritability, argumentativeness, or stubbornness
Physical complaints—recurrent stomachaches, headaches
Repeated visits to doctor's office or emergency room for treatment of injuries
Antisocial behavior—engages in drinking, uses drugs, fights, commits acts of vandalism, runs away from home, becomes sexually promiscuous
*Preoccupation with death—focuses on morbid thoughts; speaks repeatedly about people getting killed
May begin referring to own death

School and interpersonal relationships
Resists or refuses to go to school
May become truant, cut classes, does not complete assignments
Social withdrawal from friends, activities, interests that were previously enjoyed
*Wants to give away cherished possessions
Lacks an effective social support system

Precipitating factors
Environmental change (friend moved away, relocated to new community or school)
Failure to achieve specific goals in school, job, personal life
Fight with close friend
Breakup of important relationship
Discovery of pregnancy plus family crisis and/or rejection by boyfriend
Death of close friend, relative, or pet

Coping skills
Loses reality boundaries
Withdraws and isolates self
No use of support systems
Sees self as totally helpless, a victim of fate

*Absolute red flags.

is something wrong with them if they feel lonely or depressed; therefore they direct these feelings inward to avoid the risk of rejection.

Adolescents often respond to feelings of anger, failure, or loss with overt flight reactions. Some of these adaptive techniques are rebellion, withdrawal into the self with silence, physical withdrawal, such as running away from home, or, the most drastic of all, suicide. Social isolation is seen in many suicidal adolescents, but it appears to be the most significant factor in distinguishing those who will kill themselves from those who will not. It is more characteristic of those who complete suicides than of those who make attempts or threats.

Although suicide is often linked to a specific event, such as a family fight, an important school examination, death of a teen idol, or the breakup of a youthful romance, that produced an impulsive response in the child, careful analysis will usually reveal an ongoing depressive process that has been expressed periodically and behaviorally. Teachers often report changes in the behavior of children who previously had not been behavior problems. They may become easily irritated, demonstrate a low frustration point, or exhibit clowning and active, restless behavior. Older children may begin using drugs and alcohol.

A cluster phenomenon, known as "contagion," has also been observed. Sometimes referred to as a teenage "epidemic," this situation occurs when one suicide appears to trigger several other suicides in a group such as a school or community (Raley, 1985). Suicide of a public figure sometimes serves as a role model and prompts a number of suicides. This has also been termed the *Werther effect,* named for the fictional character who, in love with a girl who belonged to another, penned a farewell love note and shot himself (Phillips, 1985). In the story the act generated considerable sympathy and pity from acquaintances, including the ladylove.

It has often been a general tendency to dismiss a suicide attempt as an impulsive act resulting from a temporary crisis or depression. If this drastic move fails to draw attention to their problems or makes them worse, adolescents may conclude that taking their lives is their only means to solve these escalating, unsolvable, and unbearable problems.

Depression

Depression is a symptom common to all human beings. It is a normal part of life, and even adolescents who are healthy and happy experience alternating periods of depression and elation as a part of the growth process. Depression is part of the breaking-away process. When adolescents break away from their parents, they need something or someone to belong to; belonging to a peer group is a way of coping. However, this and other coping mechanisms are often stretched to the utmost, and adolescents' heightened vulnerability to added stresses sometimes precipitates maladaptive behavior. The ego is under pressure to adapt to the physical changes and instinctual drives of puberty, whereas at the same time the expectations of family and the environment for mature, independent, and responsible behavior must be met. Although some suicides occur in conjunction with a psychotic process, most frequently they are a part of the general picture of depression. When depression appears as a predominant mood, persists for a long time, or is so disabling that the adolescent is unable to fulfill the normal tasks of this period of life, then the condition is serious and warrants special attention and intervention.

Depression is recognized by both subjective symptoms and objective signs that reflect adolescents' grief. Depressed persons describe feelings of sadness, despair, helplessness, hopelessness, boredom, loss of interest, and isolation. They may also feel self-reproach, self-deprecation, and guilt. These subjective symptoms are evidenced by changes in behaviors and attitude.

Therapeutic Management

Suicidal threats should be taken very seriously. Most youngsters quickly respond to intervention. It offers them the opportunity to talk things out. Often the problems are very specific ones that environmental manipulation can solve, such as a change of school or classroom or conferences with parents. Sometimes simply forming an attachment to a sympathetic, caring adult figure (therapist, nurse, or counselor) is sufficient. It can be highly significant in helping children get through a crisis in the face of fear of rejection or anger from the family and feelings of guilt. They need to be made aware that suicide is a permanent solution to a temporary problem and that, given time, the problem will pass if they simply wait it out.

Children need to know that someone cares and must be provided with swift and efficient crisis intervention. Most larger communities have 24-hour service in the form of ''hot lines''—telephone communication that is within reach of troubled youngsters or their families where they can make ready contact with someone to listen to them. The function of the hot line is to help them through the immediate crisis. Through skillful questioning, but without imposing solutions on the callers, the listener helps callers arrive at a course of action that will contribute to a solution for their problem.

Children should be given no false reassurance, but it is essential to make it clear to them that their lives are considered of great importance and that they will be protected from doing themselves harm. Hospitalization, even if brief, is usually recommended. The youngsters need to be removed from the acute situation that troubles them and given the structure and security they need during the crisis period. They need someone to act in a controlling manner to alleviate the desire to die and encourage the wish to live. Hospitalization provides the surveillance that is impossible to accomplish in the home and reinforces the seriousness of a gesture or attempt. It is especially valuable if the youngsters can be placed in a unit where other adolescents can offer warmth, support, and understanding.

Although an acute depressive reaction can be managed without difficulty by ordinary practitioners, the youngster who has made a serious attempt or has made a plan for suicide should receive competent psychiatric care. Antidepressant medication is not usually recommended for acute depression but may be indicated for the youngster who is (1) chronically depressed and suicidal and (2) in an acute crisis situation, that is, when the child is admitted to the hospital for 2 to 3 weeks and is still very agitated and/or depressed. The medications take too long to achieve an antidepressant effect to be used for short-term therapy, and the potential for misuse is always a consideration.

Nursing Considerations

Care of the suicidal adolescent includes early recognition, management, and prevention. Probably the most important aspect of management is the recognition of prodromal signs that indicate that a youngster is troubled and might attempt suicide. Health professionals need to be alert to the signs of adolescent depression, and any youngster who exhibits such behavior, subtle or overt, should be referred for thorough psychologic assessment. Depression can be manifest in two different ways: youngsters who feel depressed may talk about suicide and feelings of worthlessness or they may build themselves a solid defense against such intolerable feelings of depression with behavioral or psychosomatic disturbances.

Too often suicidal threats or minor attempts are confused with bids for attention. No threat of suicide should be ignored or challenged in any way. It is a symptom that must be taken seriously. It is also a mistake to be lulled into a false sense of security when the adolecent's depression is apparently relieved. The improvement in attitude may very well mean that the youngster has made the decision to carry out the threat.

Peers or other confidants are excellent sources of information and valuable observers. They may not be able to diagnose depression, but they can sense when a friend has undergone a marked personality change. It is important to emphasize that the peer who detects any clues should not remain quiet about the observations. Friendship does not imply collusion. A peer who believes that a friend may be suicidal should alert someone who is in a position to help— a parent, teacher, guidance counselor, or other person.

As soon as the youngster who attempts suicide is out of danger from medical problems resulting from the attempt, the data-gathering process should begin. It should include information from several sources to help evaluate the extent to which the child is suffering, direction for therapy, and the probability of a repeated attempt. At least 10% to 15% of those who attempt suicide ultimately *do* commit suicide, and at least 25% of those who commit suicide have made previous attempts (The adolescent in despair, 1985).

The youngster should be questioned directly about the depression or suicidal behavior—it should never be dismissed. Clues to a youngster's feelings may be elicited by questions, such as, "You look so sad. What is troubling you?" or "Sometimes people feel life is no longer worth living. Have you had such thoughts?" Sometimes the youngster is relieved to know others have had similar thoughts. The important objective is to get the teenager to talk about thoughts and feelings. "Where do you see yourself 5 years from now?" may offer clues to future plans. "It's too bad you thought about dying. Have you made any plans?" "What did (do) you think would (will) happen to you as a result of taking the medications (or other means)?" and "When something is not going well is there someone you can go to?" are questions that provide clues regarding the seriousness of the intent.

Some guidelines have been suggested to help evaluate the seriousness of a gesture or an attempt to commit suicide, which include the following areas for exploration (Garfinkel and Golombek, 1974):

1. **Social set.** Determine what steps were taken to prevent rescue, if another person was present in the room or the house during the attempt, and if others were aware of the attempt either before or immediately after.
2. **Intent.** If a suicide note or letter was written, determine how detailed the suicidal plans were. Such communication often expresses the true depth of the youngster's despair.
3. **Method.** Examine the means selected and the child's understanding of the method, for example, the kind, number, and action of the pills taken.
4. **History.** Determine if the attempt was an isolated event and, if not, the number and nature of previous attempts or gestures. A family history of suicide is significant.
5. **Stress.** Determine the nature of the precipitating event, the alternative courses of action available to the child, and previous methods of coping with stress.

6. **Mental status.** Assess the present mental status of the child and compare it with preattempt status as described by others.
7. **Support.** Evaluate the type of support that could be expected from the child's family, friends, peers, teachers, and others.

Not only is it important to treat the suicidal adolescent, but since the suicide attempt is frequently an outgrowth of family distress, it is essential to deal with the family as well. Ideally the most effective approach would be recognition of susceptible youngsters during the early stages of intrafamily distress so that family counseling can be instigated. This emphasizes again the importance of parent-child relationships and the role of the nurse in assessing family interactions and recognizing disturbed relationships. Prevention efforts must be directed toward improving childrearing practices through support and education of parents and changing societal conditions that generate defeat, despair, and maladaptive behavior.

Follow-up care is of utmost importance. Although confidentiality is the usual approach with adolescent counseling, in the case of self-destructive behaviors this cannot be honored. The suicidal behavior is reported to the family and other professionals, and youngsters are informed that this will be done. They are told that the health professional cannot let the youngster do this! Such action conveys an important message to an attempter—that the professionals understand and that they care.

Some schools have instituted suicide prevention programs. Most are designed for high school age youth, but many are attempting to reach the younger ages, including elementary school children. Schools with programs in operation offer services such as drop-in counseling services and a peer counseling telephone line. Information can be obtained from the **American Association of Suicidology.***

SUBSTANCE ABUSE

The use of substances, primarily drugs, by children and adolescents to produce an altered state of consciousness is widespread and is believed to reflect the variety of changes taking place in their lives and the stresses engendered by these changes. The discomfort associated with the growth and changes of this prolonged and intense transitional process encourages the adolescent to search for relief, escape, or self-exploration. To relieve this discomfort, young people often turn to the exhilarating, mind-easing, euphorigenic qualities of drugs.

Most drugs to which young people turn induce changes in perception, a feeling of well-being, and a sense of closeness. To most, they provide a feeling of happiness. With the exception of some stimulant drugs used for practical purposes, such as working better, studying, or increasing cognitive effectiveness, the drugs used are simply pleasure-promoting chemicals used in the hope for altered conscious-

*2459 S. Ash, Denver, CO 80222, 303-692-0985.

ness or the attainment of a different level of functioning. Most of these drugs have some hallucinogenic properties. Far more frequent is the use of alcohol or marijuana as recreational drugs without significant disruption of behavior or performance (Committee on Adolescence, 1983). Since teenagers and parents do not always consider these to be a health issue, the problem may not be called to the attention of health professionals.

Definitions

The greatest area of misinformation and confusion is related to the terms applied to drug use. In order to clarify this discussion, the following terms are defined*:

drug abuse The regular use of drugs for other than accepted medical purposes and to the extent that it results in physical or psychologic harm to the user and/or is used in a way that is detrimental to society.

drug misuse The overzealous use of drugs or the exercise of bad judgment in their use.

narcotic addiction Behavioral pattern of overwhelming involvement with obtaining and using a narcotic for its psychic effects rather than for medical reasons, thereby eliciting social disapproval.

drug tolerance The clinical need to increase the dosage of a drug in order to attain the same desired effect, caused by an increased capacity to metabolize and eliminate the drug or the ability of the individual's tissues to adapt to the drug.

physical dependence An adaptive physiologic state that occurs when a drug is taken in increasing amounts and that is manifest by the development of physiologic symptoms when the drug is withdrawn.

The most important differences among these terms are the distinction between voluntary and involuntary behavior and between culturally defined and physiologically identified events. Drug abuse, misuse, and addiction are culturally defined and are voluntary behaviors. Drug tolerance and physical dependence are involuntary behaviors based on physiologic changes. Consequently, an individual can be addicted to a narcotic with or without being physically dependent, whereas a person may be physically dependent on a narcotic without being addicted, such as patients who are experiencing pain.

The broad term *drug abuse,* which is often applied to all forms of drug misuse, can be a confusing term and does not necessarily define the problem related to drug use. Many of the substances are controlled by law and accompanied by severe penalties for their illegal use; others are sanctioned from a legal, social, and medical standpoint. Problems concerning drug use can therefore be defined as legal, social, medical, and individual.

Legal. Drug use can become a legal problem when the drug being taken is strictly controlled by law and is accompanied by severe penalties for its use or possession. Some youngsters in pursuit of peer approval merely carry a supply of such drugs in order to impress their peers and

achieve acceptance by the group, although they have no intention of actually taking the drug. This is primarily a legal problem.

Social. When the use of a substance by the adolescent leads to disruptive or bizarre behavior that alienates the user from the rest of society, this results in a social problem. The deviant behavior may lead to rejection by family, school, employer, and even the peer group. Such behavior also increases the risk of confrontation with legal authorities and a forced change in life-style.

Medical. When the current or continued use of a substance may adversely affect the physical or mental health of the youngster, it becomes a medical problem. This includes life-threatening situations, such as an overdose or withdrawal in which medical intervention is mandatory, or the demonstration of aberrant behavior patterns that represent acute mental stress, such as panic, toxic psychosis, or acute brain syndrome.

Individual. An individual problem is one that focuses on the person. It requires continued assessment and intervention related to the role that drug use plays in the individual's life and the factors that contribute to his need for the drug.

Patterns of Drug Use

Many factors influence the extent to which drugs are used by teenagers. The type of drug used, mode of administration, duration of use, frequency of use, and single or multiple drug use must be considered in determining the severity of the individual drug problem. Most drug use begins with experimentation. The individual may try a drug only once, it may be used occasionally, or it may become an integral part of a drug-centered life-style. Identification of the pattern of drug use in an individual facilitates the formulation of an approach to the problem. Patterns have been observed based on dose and frequency of use.

There are two broad categories of adolescents who use drugs: the *experimenters* and the *compulsive users*. There is a wide range of use between these groups that represents two ends of a continuum in terms of degree of use. With the exception of a "bad trip" or accidental overdose, the experimenters present few medical problems, although they probably represent the bulk of adolescent drug users. Some of these youngsters with a predisposition to heavy drug use proceed to compulsive use after a time, but by and large they are in the minority.

Between the experimenters and compulsive users is a broad range of *recreational* users of drugs, principally drugs such as marijuana and alcohol. For many, the goal is merely relaxation, and these fit more closely with the experimenting, intermittent users. For others the goal is intoxication, and these are more nearly like the compulsive users. The groups of greatest concern to health workers are those whose patterns of use involve high doses with the danger of overdose and those compulsive users with the threat of dependence, withdrawal syndromes, and altered life-style.

---

*Taken extensively from McCaffery, M.: Nursing management of the patient with pain, ed. 2, Philadelphia, 1979, J.B. Lippincott Co.

Motivation

There are several common motives for drug use. Adolescents try drugs out of curiosity, for kicks. Drugs produce for some persons a dreamy state of altered consciousness and a feeling of power, excitement, heightened acuity, or confidence. Others seek visual hallucinatory experiences and sexual sensation. Many youngsters use drugs not only for the perceptual and sensory experiences but also for the social aspects.

Teenagers are highly influenced by fads and fashions within their society, and they are, developmentally, sensation-hungry risk takers. It is characteristic that they are eager to test their mental and physical capabilities to the utmost. Adolescents are also trying to find a means to cope with their disenchantment with the adult world and its social and technologic concerns and with their powerlessness to change it. They seek escape from reality and want to achieve a sense of closeness and intimacy with other people, to escape from distress or decision making, and to feel a sense of insight into the mysteries of God, death, and rebirth.

During early and middle teenage years, drug use seems to fall into rather distinct groups in relation to motivation.

Social group. These youngsters are members of the same social group who indulge in occasional use as a social act of sharing. They pass around a bottle so that each youngster can take a drink or a marijuana cigarette so that each member can have a puff. The pleasant act of sharing reinforces membership in the group, sets them apart from adults, and provides them with an atmosphere of doing something against the rules—something that is fun to get away with. With most youth drug use is a passing fancy and after a few times is dispensed with and forgotten.

Escapist group. The majority of youth who experiment with drugs are seeking escape from feelings of anger and depression when they are unable to communicate effectively with their parents concerning their problems or to cope with their emotions. Getting drunk or ''freaking out'' seems to work for them. Unfortunately this flight not only leaves the problems unsolved but also interferes with the satisfactory resolution of the problems. Consequently the retreat into use of drugs tends to be repeated.

Punitive group. This smaller group of adolescents seem determined to punish the world for making them angry, depressed, or frustrated. Although they use, sell, and/or push drugs, they do so in the hope that they will be discovered and arrested so that their families will suffer the anguish that the youngsters themselves feel.

Self-destructive group. A few youth are openly self-destructive individuals who internalize their anger to the extent that death seems to provide the only relief from their anger. These youngsters often give evidence of suicidal thoughts or demonstrate suicidal behavior.

Types of Drugs Abused

Any drug can be abused, and most are potentially harmful to adolescents still going through formative life experiences.

Although rarely considered as drugs by society, the chemically active substances most frequently abused are the xanthines and theobromines contained in chocolate and in common beverages such as tea, coffee, and colas. Common analgesics such as aspirin, Darvon Compound, and Fiorinal; ethyl alcohol; and nicotine are others that, although recognized as drugs, are sanctioned by society. Any of these can produce mild to moderate euphoric and/or stimulant effects and can lead to physical and psychic dependence.

A great many factors determine personal preferences for gratification. Many drugs are not harmful for all teenagers, and some, used intermittently, will probably not produce ill effects or result in dependence. Reactions vary according to the drug used and its purity, the expectations of the user, and the context in which the drug is used. These factors determine to a great extent whether the experience is viewed as pleasant or unpleasant. The type of drugs used varies according to geographic location, socioeconomic status, urban as opposed to suburban areas, and various times. A drug that is popular with one ''generation'' of adolescents may not be attractive to another, and changing trends are influenced by the adolescent's constant search for new and different experiences.

The trends in substance abuse have changed markedly in recent years. During the late 1960s the abuse of psychoactive drugs became widespread among teenagers. Large numbers of adolescents used and abused opiates, amphetamines, barbiturates, hallucinogens, and inhalants during the 1970s (Hein, Cohen, and Litt, 1979). The present concern is the use of alcohol, tobacco, cocaine, marijuana, and other intoxicants. Use of alcohol and marijuana has increased dramatically. More than 90% of high school seniors have had some experience with alcohol, and more than half have used marijuana (National Institute on Drug Abuse, 1980).

Drugs with mind-altering capacity that are available on the black market and that are of medical and legal concern are the hallucinogenic, narcotic, hypnotic, and stimulant drugs. In addition, health professionals are concerned about use of alcohol and various volatile substances, such as antifreeze, plastic model airplane cement, organic solvents, and typewriter correction fluid (the most recent craze) that are inhaled to achieve altered sensation in the user. Drugs available on the street are often mixed with other compounds and fillers so that the purity of the drug, its strength, and the nature of additives are highly variable. Many of the hazards associated with drug use are related to driving a car or operating equipment that may be harmful when carelessly used while under the influence of the drug. Some of the more commonly abused substances and their general manifestations are outlined in Table 21-4.

Alcohol. Acute or chronic abuse of ethanol, a socially accepted depressant, is responsible for many acts of violence, suicide, and accidental injury and death. Ethanol reduces inhibitions against aggressive and sexual acting out. Abrupt withdrawal is accompanied by severe physical and psychologic symptoms, and long-term use leads to slow tissue destruction, especially of the brain and liver cells.

Table 21-4 Major drugs abused by adolescents

CHEMICAL AGENT/ROUTE	PHYSICAL SIGNS	BEHAVIOR	COMPLICATIONS
Opiates Heroin, morphine, methadone—injected subcutaneously or intravenously (IV), intranasal (sniffing), oral	Constricted pupils, respiratory depression, cyanosis Needle marks	Initial euphoria, tranquilization, lethargy, coma	Overdose: coma, respiratory arrest, death Injection site infection, hepatitis, abscesses, septicemia, tetanus, pulmonary complications Withdrawal: muscle cramps, stomach cramps, diarrhea, runny nose and eyes, restlessness, convulsions, death Dental caries
Depressants Barbiturates—secobarbital, amobarbital, pentobarbital, amobarbital/secobarbital—oral, IV	Slurred speech, ataxia, slowed reflexes, constricted pupils (barbiturates); dilated pupils (glutethimide)	Short attemtion span, impaired judgment, combativeness, violence	Overdose: respiratory depression, coma, death Injection site infection, hepatitis, septicemia Withdrawal: hyperreflexia, irritability, convulsions, death
Nonbarbiturates—methaqualone (Quaalude), ethchlorvynol (Placidyl)—oral	Incoordination, tremors, ataxia, confusion, slurred speech, hyperreflexia, diplopia, general muscle weakness	Hyperexcitability; euphoria of methaqualone similar to opiate experience	Overdose: delirium and coma, convulsions, hepatic damage, respiratory arrest, death Withdrawal: similar to barbiturates and alcohol
Alcohol (ethanol)—oral	Incoordination	Impaired judgment and perception, loss of inhibitions, emotional lability, quarrelsomeness, aggressiveness, hostility Lethargy	Hazards related to impaired judgment, e.g., automobile accidents, fights Nutritional deficiencies Gastritis Overdose: coma, death, especially when used in combination with barbiturates Withdrawal: anxiety, tremors, hallucinations, hyperreflexia, convulsions, death
Minor tranquilizers Chlordiazepoxide (Librium), diazepam (Valium), meprobamate—oral	Nonspecific	Decreased anxiety and tension Occasional disinhibition	Similar to barbiturates but with reduced intensity
Organic solvents Hydrocarbons and fluorocarbons—glue, cleaning fluid, lighter fluid, aerosol sprays, nail polish, gasoline—sniffed	Nonspecific	Euphoria, dysphoria, confusion, impaired perception and coordination Loss of consciousness	Secondary trauma, asphyxia from plastic bags used to inhale fumes Lead poisoning Possible irreversible damage to central nervous system, kidneys, liver, and bone marrow
Stimulants Amphetamines—amphetamine sulfate, dextroamphetamine, methamphetamine—oral, subcutaneous, IV	Hypertension, weight loss, dilated pupils Sweating (when injected)	Psychologic and motor stimulation Hyperactivity, false bravado, euphoria, increased alertness, insomnia, anorexia, irritability, personality change	Injection site infection Paranoia, severe depression with suicidal tendency when drug stopped
Cocaine—intranasal, IV, smoke	Hypertension, tachycardia, hyperreflexia	Restlessness, hyperactivity, intense euphoria	Nausea and vomiting, inflammation or perforation of nasal septum

Table 21-4 Major drugs abused by adolescents—cont'd

CHEMICAL AGENT/ROUTE	PHYSICAL SIGNS	BEHAVIOR	COMPLICATIONS
Hallucinogens			
Cannabis—marijuana, hashish—smoke, oral	Occasionally tachycardia, delayed response time, poor coordination	Simple euphoria, mild intoxication, heightened sensory awareness, drowsiness	Occasionally depressive or anxiety reactions
LSD, PCP, DMT, STP, THC, mescaline—oral	Dilated pupils, reddened eyes, occasionally hypertension, hyperthermia, piloerection	Euphoria, heightened sensory awareness, increased appetite, hallucinations, confusion, paranoia	Primarily psychiatric: may intensify latent psychotic tendencies, panic, suicide possible, flashbacks

Teenage drinking is not a new phenomenon, but because of its social acceptance, peer pressure, and easy accessibility, alcohol appears to have become the drug of choice. It is the most widely accepted drug, can be purchased legally by adults, is relatively inexpensive, is often used as part of a meal (wine, beer), and is approved by adults throughout the world when used in moderation. Youngsters may be afraid of hard drugs, but they feel comfortable with alcohol. Most have been exposed to alcohol all their lives.

The pattern of frequent, heavy drinking often begins in the eighth grade, increases with age, and peaks between the ages of 18 and 22 years (O'Malley, Bachman, and Johnston, 1984). Some surveys indicate that 11% of eighth graders reported consuming the equivalent of 5.6 oz of absolute alcohol per week, and twelfth grade students admitted to averaging two six-packs of beer per week, often consumed at one or two parties (reported by Schwartz and others, 1986). The majority of youngsters in one study reported high self-esteem, good health, and few psychologic problems, and 63% reported having drunk alcohol at some time. The proportion of youngsters stating that they never drank alcohol becomes progressively smaller with age (Schwartz and others, 1986).

The most noticeable effects of alcohol are on the central nervous system; these include changes in emotional and autonomic functions, such as judgment, memory, learning ability, and other intellectual capacities (Fields, 1979). Marked mood changes are characteristic of adolescent drinkers, who are described as hard to live with, unable to make up their minds, and acting like split personalities. They can be identified by the way in which they use alcohol. Adolescent alcoholics enjoy the effect of the alcohol and look forward to becoming intoxicated. They drink rapidly to obtain a "high" emotional state, often drink alone, cannot predictably control their use of alcohol, and protect their supply, afraid that they will be caught without anything to drink (Fields, 1979).

Teenage alcoholics rely on alcohol as a defense against depression, anxiety, fear, and anger. They become increasingly tolerant to the drug, and there is an increased use of

sedatives with the alcohol. Some alcoholics have difficulty remembering things done while intoxicated and often intend to swear off the drug or cut down on its use. Not all of these characteristics are observed in the alcoholic, but if several of the signs are evident, the youngster should be considered at risk and detoxification therapy should be initiated to ensure safe and complete withdrawal from the drug.

Hydrocarbons and fluorocarbons. Glue "sniffing" and the inhalation of plastic cement and other volatile substances (e.g., gasoline, gold and silver spray paint) that youngsters breathe directly or place in paper or plastic bags from which they rebreathe the fumes produce an immediate euphoria followed by a pleasant drowsiness. The substances are extremely hazardous to the individual, causing rapid loss of consciousness and respiratory arrest. Many persons taking these drugs do not have time to remove the bag from their heads and quickly become asphyxiated.

A current concern is the widespread abuse of fumes from typewriter correction fluid. Because it is such an easily accessible and common substance, youngsters are unaware that the substance is harmful. The pattern of abuse usually begins in preteen years, peaks at about age 15, and then tapers off in favor of other substance abuse (Greer, 1984). The abuse of hydrocarbon is gaining in popularity in the school-age population and is especially prevalent among economically disadvantaged youth groups (King, Smialek, and Troutman, 1985).

Mind-altering drugs. Hallucinogens, also known as psychedelic, psychotomimetic, psychotropic, or illusionogenic drugs, consist of a wide variety of agents that produce vivid hallucinations and euphoria. These substances induce a dreamlike state in which the user experiences a whirl of images and strong emotion accompanied by a feeling of boundless union with the environment, not uncommonly associated with feelings of self-disintegration. These drugs do not produce physical dependence, since they can be abruptly withdrawn without ill effect. However, acute and long-term effects are variable. In some individuals the dissociative behavior may be unduly protracted.

Drugs included in this category are cannabis (marijuana,

hashish), mescaline (peyote), psilocybin, lysergic acid diethylamide (LSD), phencyclidine (PCP), 2,5-dimethoxy-4-methylamphetamine (DOM or "STP," which stands for "serenity, tranquility, peace"), and tetrahydrocannabinol (THC), the active ingredient of cannabis. Street drugs sold as mescaline, psilocybin, or tetrahydrocannabinol rarely contain the stated drug. They more often contain LSD or a combination of two or more chemical agents.

The desirable effects of marijuana depend on the concentration of the substance in the smoke. The youngster's behavior during a "high" may be impulsive and mood unpredictable. The user may become endlessly fascinated by some small trivial item, such as a leaf or wrinkles of the hand. Time seems to pass more slowly, and marijuana-intoxicated drivers may fail momentarily to respond normally to visual cues because of preoccupation with inner thoughts. Unlike alcohol intoxication, a marijuana "high" can be easily overcome so that the user seems normal in appearance, speech, and affect. During the coming-down phase the youngster gradually displays mental and physical torpidity and irritability, is easily provoked to anger, and becomes drowsy. There is a very strong desire for high-calorie sweets, but there is no "hangover." Flashback phenomena have been reported from marijuana but are uncommon (Schwartz, 1984).

Narcotics. Narcotic drugs include opiates such as heroin, morphine, hydromorphone (Dilaudid), and hydrocodone (Dicodid). Codeine, although closely related to these drugs, is less addictive. Chemically different and somewhat less addictive are meperidine (Demerol) and methadone (Dolophine). The direct effect of narcotic substances is to alleviate pain and suffering. They produce a state of euphoria by removing painful feelings and creating a pleasurable experience of specific quality and a sense of success. These feelings are accompanied by clouding of consciousness and a dreamlike state.

Although they produce psychologic and physical dependence, heroin and related narcotics do not cause detectable tissue damage and do not impair coordination and judgment when taken in average doses. However, following dependence and withdrawal, physiologic functions may remain altered for quite some time. The onset of regular use of the most risky drugs usually does not take place until somewhere between 16 and 18 years of age.

Perhaps more important are the indirect consequences related to the illegal status of narcotic use and the problems associated with securing the drug—time-consuming searches and methods used to meet the high cost. Health problems result from self-neglect of physical needs (nutrition, cleanliness, dental care), overdose, contamination, and infection, including acquired immune deficiency syndrome (AIDS). Withdrawal from opiates is extremely unpleasant unless controlled with supervised substitution of methadone.

Central nervous system depressants. A variety of hypnotic drugs that produce physical dependence and withdrawal symptoms on abrupt discontinuance may be used by adolescents. They create a feeling of relaxation and sleepiness, and they impair general functioning. Barbiturates combined with alcohol produce a profound depressant effect.

Central nervous system stimulants. Amphetamines (Benzedrine), methamphetamine (Methedrine), dextroamphetamine (Dexedrine), and cocaine do not produce strong physical dependence and can be withdrawn without much danger. However, psychologic dependence is strong, and acute intoxication can lead to violent aggressive behavior or psychotic episodes manifest by paranoia, uncontrollable agitation, and restlessness. Physical deterioration may occur from loss of appetite and sleep during the time the drug is being taken, and severe suicidal depression is often experienced while "coming down" off the drug. Combined with barbiturates ("goofballs"), the stimulant effect is canceled out by the depressants. However, the euphoric effects of both are synergistic, cumulative, and particularly addictive. Cocaine is the most potent antifatigue agent known and, although it is not a narcotic, is legally categorized as such.

Terminology. Drug users have developed a specialized vocabulary for the substances and behaviors associated with their use (see the boxes on p. 915 and p. 916). The terminology varies in different localities, and new descriptive terms arise spontaneously wherever drugs are part of the environment.

Therapeutic Management

Adolescents experiencing toxic drug effects or withdrawal symptoms are frequently seen in emergency rooms. Experienced emergency room personnel are familiar with the management of acute drug toxicosis; the signs, symptoms, and behavioral characteristics of a variety of substances; and differences and similarities among them. When the drug is questionable or unknown, knowledge of these factors facilitates handling of the youngster and implementation of a treatment regimen.

The treatment for drug toxicity or withdrawal varies according to the drug and the method used. Every effort should be made to determine the type and amount of drug taken, the time it was taken, the mode of administration, and factors related to the onset of presenting symptoms.

It is helpful to know the patient's pattern of use. For example, if two types of drugs are involved, they may require different treatments. Gastric lavage may be employed when the drug has been ingested recently and the cough reflex is intact, but it would be of little value when the drug has been administered by the intravenous ("mainlined") or intranasal ("sniffed") route. Since the actual content of most street drugs is highly questionable, other pharmaceutical agents are administered with caution, except perhaps the narcotic antagonists in cases of suspected opiate overdose. It is necessary to assess for possible trauma sustained while the patient was under the influence of the drug.

Rehabilitation from hard drug use may require withdrawing the youngster from the environment as well as from the chemical agent. Programs must be suited to the individual and may involve foster home placement or residential treat-

GLOSSARY OF DRUG JARGON

Amphetamines

Bams
Beans
Benn
Bennies
Black beauties
Black cadillacs
Black dex
Bombido
  (injectable)
Browns
Cartwheels
Chalk
Co-pilots
Cranks
Cross
Crystal
Dexies

Dice
Doe
Drives
Eyeopeners
Fives (5 mg)
Footballs
Goofballs
Green hearts
Greenies
Greens
Heart(s)
Horse hearts
Jolly babies
Leapers
Lid rollers
Lightning
Meth

Orange hearts
Peaches
Pep pills
Rippers
Roses
Speed
Splash
Thrusters
Truck drivers
Wake-up
White crosses
White dexies
Whites
Yellow bams
Zeeters
Zip

Barbiturates (general)

Barbs
Courage pills
Downers
Golf balls
Goofers

Idiot pills
Nimbie
Nimbles
Peanuts
Sleepers

Barbiturates (specific)

Blue birds (amobarbital)
Blue devils (amobarbital)
Blue heaven (amobarbital)
Canary (pentobarbital)
Christmas trees (mixtures)
Downers (amobarbital)
F-40s (secobarbital)
F-66s (amobarbital sodium
  and secobarbital sodium)
  (gorilla pills)
Mexican yellows (pentobar-
  bital)
Nemmies (pentobarbital)

Phennies
Pink ladies (secobarbital)
Pinks (secobarbital)
Rainbow (secobarbital;
  amobarbital)
Red birds (secobarbital)
Red devils (secobarbital)
Reds (secobarbital)
Seggy, seccy (secobarbital)
Tooies (tuinal)
Yellow jackets (pentobarbital)
Yellows (pentobarbital)

Cocaine

Bernies flake
C
Candy
Cecil
Charlie
Coca-cola
Coke
Cokomo (Kokomo)
Crack
Dust
Flake
Gift of the Sun God
Gold dust
Happy trails
Incentive
Lady snow

Leaf (the)
Movie star drug
Nose
Nose candy
Pimp
Pimp's drug
Rich man's drug
Rock
Schoolboy
Snow
Society high
Star spangled powder
Stardust
White horse
White stuff

Heroin

Big Harry
Blanco
Boy
Caballo
Chiva
Deuce (a $2 packet)
Doojee

Dust
H
Harry; hairy
Horse
Joy powder
Scag
Scat

Smack
Stuff
Sugar
Ticata
White lady
White stuff

Morphine

Dreamer
Dust
Emma (Miss)
Emsel
Hard stuff
Hocus

M
Monkey
Morf
Morpho
Unkie
White stuff

Marijuana

Acapulco gold
  (potent)
Bush
Butter
Flower
Grass
Griffo
Hemp
Hooch
Hooter
Indian hay
J

Jive
Joint
Kif
Mary Jane
Mohasky
Mooters
Mu
Mutah
Panama red
Pot
Reefer (cigarette)
Rockets

Smoke
Splimi
Stick (cigarette)
Straw
Superjoint
Texas tea
Tie stick (mixed
  with opium
  and tied to
  a popsicle stick)
Weed

LSD (lysergic acid diethylamide)

Acid
Blotter acid
  (on paper)
Blue microdot

Cube (the)
D (big)
Heavenly blue
Purple haze

Royal blue
Sugar
Wedding bells
Windowpane

PCP (phencyclidine)

Angel dust
Busy bee
DOA
Elephant
Goon

Hog (also chlora
  (hydrate)
Horse tranquilizer
Magic mist
Peace pills

Rocket fuel
Sherman's
White horizon
Wobble

Other hallucinogens

DMT (dimethyltryptamine):
  businessman's special
DMZ (Benactyzine)
DOM (4-methyl-2, 5-dimeth-
  oxyamphetamine), STP
Hashish: black hash; black
  Russian (potent)

STP (dimethoxymethyl-
  amphetamine), DOM
  (syndicate acid, tran-
  quility)
THC (tetrahydrocanna-
  binol): hallucinogen in
  marijuana and hashish

Mixed substances

Chicago green (marijuana/
  opium)
Double trouble (amobarbital/
  secobarbital)
Fours (acetaminophen with
  60 mg codeine)
Fuel (marijuana/insecticide)
Hog (phencyclidine/vegetable
  material [veterinary drug])

In-betweens (barbiturates/
  amphetamines)
Mickey Finn (chloral hy-
  drate/alcohol)
Speedball (heroin/cocaine;
  Percodan/methedrine)
Star spangled powder
  (heroin/cocaine)

Miscellaneous

Alcohol: mountain dew, alley
  juice (methyl alcohol),
  moonshine (ethyl alcohol),
  sauce, hootch, booze, juice
Amyl nitrite: aimes, snappers
Chloral hydrate: joy juice
Ethchlorvynol (Placidyl):
  dyls, plastic red, K-H, K-N
Meperidine hydrochloride: Diane
Mescaline: chief, mesc, mescalito,
  mescal beans
Methadone: dolls, dollies,
  fizzies (tablets)

Methaqualone (Quaalude):
  714, ludes, sopors,
  westcoast, lemons
Opium for smoking: black
  stuff
Paregoric: licorice, bitter
Peyote: button, cactus, Hikori,
  Kikuli, Huatari, Wokouri,
  seni, tops
Tobacco: coffin, deck (pack),
  fag

TERMINOLOGY ASSOCIATED WITH DRUG USE

Street name	Definition
Ab	Abscess that forms at site of injection
Bag	A small quantity of either heroin or cocaine packaged in cellophane envelopes
Bang	Exhilaration experienced after drug administration
Belongs	On the habit
Bhang	Marijuana, smoking pipe
Binge	An extended period of continued consumption of alcohol
Blanks	Poor quality merchandise
Blow Charlie or snow	To sniff cocaine
Blow horse	To sniff heroin
Blow weed	To smoke marijuana
Bogart	Not to pass the "joint" to a neighbor
Brody	A fit or spasm by an addict to elicit sympathy
Bull jive	Marijuana heavily cut with tea, catnip, or other impurities
Bummer	A bad trip or experience
Burned	Received fake narcotics
Burned out	Sclerotic blood vessel from too many injections; addict who (tired of abuse "hassle") tries to stop drug abuse
Busted	To be caught, usually arrested, by local authorities or to be caught by parents
Cadet	New addict
Candyman	Dealer or pusher of addicting drugs
Cashing a script	Getting a forged or bogus prescription order placed
Catch up	Withdrawal process
Chippin'; chipper	Subcutaneous administration of small dose of heroin; "weekend user" (uses less than daily)
Cleared up	To have withdrawn from drugs
Coasting	Under drug influence
Cold turkey	Withdrawal process
Come down; crash	Dissipation of drug effects
Connect	Make a purchase
Cook it up	To prepare a drug for injection
Cooker	The apparatus used to heat and dissolve a drug before injection (spoons or bottle top)
Cop	To obtain a small quantity of a drug
Crap	Heroin of weak potency
Cut	To adulterate with agents such as quinine, milk sugar
Daytop Lodge	Drug abuse treatment center directed by ex-addicts
Dealer	One who sells drugs
Doper	Regular drug abuser
Dream stick	Opium pipe
Dropped	Consumed an abuse drug
DTs	Delirium tremens (acute alcohol withdrawal syndrome)
Duds	Bags of heroin containing no narcotic agent
Dummy	Drug purchase without purported content
Dynamite	High-grade narcotics; heroin, cocaine
Fix	To inject drugs; satiate addictive needs
Flake out	To pass out from drug use
Flash	Rapid, intense, euphoric reaction
Flashback	Recurrence of some feature of a previous LSD experience
Freak	An addict who enjoys playing with the needle
Freak out	To be intensely affected by something
Garbage	Poor quality merchandise
Garbage head	Individual who takes any kind of drug
Gear	Drugs in general
Gee head	Paregoric user
Get it together	To become mentally organized
Get off	To initially experience the effects of a drug
Glad rag	Cloth or handkerchief that is saturated with a material to be inhaled (e.g., for use in glue-sniffing)
Grasshopper	A marijuana user
Greezy addict	Drug abuser who will take any drug, any time
Habit	Dependence on drugs
Head	User of drugs
Heavy grass high	Strong, stuporous reaction to marijuana
High	Stimulant trip
Hit	Make a purchase; take a drag
Hitting up	Injecting drugs
Holding	Drugs are in user's possession
Hooked	Addicted to drugs
Hop head	Person who smokes opium; addict
Hot shot	Poisons concealed in injectable narcotics for the purpose of homicide

TERMINOLOGY ASSOCIATED WITH DRUG USE—cont'd

Street name	Definition
Hype	A needle addict
Ice cream habit	Small, irregular drug use
In action	To seek narcotics
In flight	To be very high from drugs, especially methamphetamine hydrochloride (Methedrine)
Jabber	A needle addict
Jammed up	An overdose
Joint	Syringe and needle; one stick of marijuana; or an opium smoker's den
Joy popping	Narcotic injections under the skin
Juice freak	One who prefers alcohol
Junk	Narcotics
Junkie	Heroin abuser
Kick	Euphoria
Lay	An opium den
Layout	Equipment for injecting drugs; opium smoker's equipment
Lemon	Bad or fake dope
Luding out	Stupor produced from alcohol and methaqualone
Lumber	Marijuana stems that are found in an ounce of marijuana
Mainliner	One who injects directly into the vein
Mother	Drug peddler
Mud	Stramonium preparation mixed with carbonated beverage
Muggles	Crude marijuana before it is rolled into a cigarette
Narcs	Federal narcotics agents
Nickel bag	A $5 bag of a drug
OD	Overdose; death
Odyssey House	Drug abuse treatment center
On	Using drugs
On the nod	Drowsiness from narcotics
Outfit	Narcotic injection equipment
Papers	Papers generally used to role a marijuana cigarette; popular brands include Zig-Zag, Wheatstraw, Papel del Trigo, Bambu, Job, Roach, Tops
Phoenix House	Drug abuse treatment center
Quill	Matchbook cover for sniffing cocaine
Reader	Prescription order
Reader with tail	Forged prescription order
Roach	Butt of marijuana cigarette
Roll	To make a marijuana cigarette
Run	Period of stimulant abuse
Rush	Rapid, intense, euphoric reaction
Safe	Feeling of protection an addict experiences during trip
Score	To establish a connection with a dealer
Script	Prescription order
Script writer	Sympathetic physician; one who forges prescriptions
Sharps	Needles
Shoot up	To inject drugs
Shooting gallery	Place where addicts inject drugs
Sickie	College student using drugs
Skin pop	Intradermal or subcutaneous injection
Snarf	Nasal inhalation of cocaine
Snort	Inhalation through nose
Space; spaced out	Altered consciousness
Speed freak	Amphetamine abuser
Spike	Needle for injection
Spoon	A gram of cocaine
Stash	Collective term for accumulation of marijuana paraphernalia
Stepped-on	Process of diluting abuse drugs
Stoned	Under influence of narcotics
Straight	Describes one who avoids use of drugs
Strung out	In need of a fix, sedative, trip; hangover
Synanon	Drug abuse treatment center, directed by ex-addicts
Tab	General term to describe drug of solid dosage
Toke	Inhalation of smoke
Tracks; turkey trots	Marks and scars from use of a hypodermic needle
Travel agent	LSD seller
Trips; trippin'	A high mediated by LSD
Wasted	Under influence of drugs
Water pipe	Device for bubbling smoke through water for cooler inhalation
Wired	Intoxicated state due to marijuana
Yen sleep	Somnolent stage during drug withdrawal

ment setting, although many are handled in an ambulatory setting. Programs often include group sessions with other troubled youth.

Nursing Considerations

Nurses in almost every setting are increasingly likely to have contact with youthful drug abusers or to be in position to serve as educator and patient advocate. They are often in a position to serve as listener, confidant, and counselor to troubled youngsters. Nurses are essential members of health teams whose efforts are directed toward short-term and long-term therapy for drug abusers.

Often observation or description of the behavior is more valuable than a report by patients or their friends as to the chemical agent taken. For example, aggressive behavior and disorientation are often seen in barbiturate, alcohol, stimulant, or hallucinogen intoxication but not in opiate intoxication. Overdose from either barbiturates or opiates can result in respiratory failure and coma. Pinpoint pupils are seen only in opiate toxicity. Nurses must be alert for life-threatening consequences of drug toxicity; therefore equipment and personnel should be available or the patient should be transferred to facilities that are prepared to provide supportive measures for physiologic depression and psychogenic phenomena.

Stimulation should be kept to a minimum for agitated, frightened youngsters. Treatment or tests that are not required immediately are best postponed. These youngsters primarily need psychologic support in a nonthreatening environment and close contact with a sympathetic person who can stay with them and help them maintain contact with reality.

Obstetric and nursery personnel sometimes encounter the problem of drug dependence and withdrawal in newborn infants or in a compulsive drug-using mother. Affected infants are at risk and require special surveillance for complications of withdrawal; therefore the nursing staff should be aware of the drug dependence in those mothers who come to the hospital for delivery (see p. 418).

Long-term management. A major factor in the treatment and rehabilitation of young drug users is careful assessment, in the nonacute stage, to determine the function that the drug plays in these youngsters' lives. Adolescents need help to identify the problem that motivated them to resort to drugs and to recognize their own role in self-destructive, inappropriate drug-abuse behavior before they can embark on a rehabilitation program.

The motivated phase of treatment is directed toward exploring the factors that influence drug use and establishing in the youngster a feeling of self-worth and a commitment to self-help. It requires a trust relationship between the youngster and the health team and involves a thorough physical examination and assessment of physical, psychologic, educational, and vocational status. A realistic appraisal of the adolescent's potential and efforts aimed at short-term goal satisfaction with building self-esteem lay the groundwork for a successful rehabilitation program.

Rehabilitation begins when a youngster has decided that, with the help of concerned and supportive adults, he can and is willing to change. Rehabilitation implies not only environmental manipulation and involvement therapy but also commitment on the part of the patient to substitute dependency on people for dependency on drugs and to explore alternative mechanisms for problem solving and coping with stress. Persons working with troubled youth must be prepared for recidivism, or the tendency to relapse, and maintain a plan for reentry into the treatment process.

Organizations that have achieved success in helping others cope with problems of drug abuse are excellent sources for both youngsters and their families. The **Tough Love*** philosophy first employed by Alcoholics Anonymous and Al-Anon is based on the conviction that parents have the right and the responsibility to be the policymakers in the family, set limits on the behavior of their children, and take control of the household from out-of-control teenagers. The premise is that allowing teenagers to experience the negative consequences of their behavior will bring them closer to accepting help and/or changing their behavior (Newton, 1985). Parents no longer take responsibility for the youngsters' behavior and suffer the negative consequences. Adolescents are offered the choice of (1) getting treatment for mental health or drug problem or (2) finding another place to live. It is difficult for parents, and some older youngsters do leave home, but most return when they have rethought their decision after experiencing the real world.

Other groups that provide support and counseling for families experiencing crises with their children include **Parents Anonymous†** and **Parental Stress, Inc.,‡** both of which maintain crisis counseling on a 24-hour basis.

Prevention. Drug abuse in adolescence is both an individual and a community problem, and nurses play an important role in education and legislation as well as in individual observation, assessment, and therapy. In this drug-oriented society patterns of drug use may be established, through parental models and the influence of the media, as an effective means to make the user ''feel better.'' Impressionable youth need to be educated regarding appropriate use of chemicals. More important, those associated with adolescents should listen to what they are saying, determine

---

*Community Service Foundation, P.O. Box 70, Sellersville, PA 18960.
†22330 Hawthorne Blvd., #208, Torrance, CA 90505, 800-352-0386 (California) and 800-421-0353 (elsewhere).
‡617-742-7535 (Massachusetts) and 800-632-8188 (elsewhere). Other sources of information include: National Clearinghouse for Alcohol Information, P.O. Box 2345, Rockville, MD 20852; National Clearinghouse for Drug Abuse Information, P.O. Box 416, Kensington, MD 20795; National Federation of Parents for Drug-Free Youth, 800-554-KIDS or 301-585-5437 (Maryland); National Institute on Drug Abuse Prevention Branch, 800-638-2045 or 301-443-2450 (Maryland); National Cocaine Hotline, 800-COC-AINE.

what is bothering them, and try to help them meet these needs before they resort to drugs.

Some approaches to prevention involve teaching specific skills, including values clarification (e.g., how to use refusal techniques), how to develop alternatives, and problem-solving skills. Peer pressure is a powerful tool and can be used effectively in prevention. A group that has had some success in reducing injury from drunk driving is **Students Against Drunk Driving (SADD),*** an organization designed to help eliminate drunk driving in teenagers. Some of the techniques used by the group include peer counseling, parental guidelines for teenage parties, and community awareness. Also, a model parent-teenager contract regarding drinking and driving is available from the organization. Nurses can encourage the formation of the chapter of SADD in the high schools in their communities.

---

*110 Pleasant St., Corbin Plaza, Marborum, MA 01752.

- Bulimics fall into two categories: those who consume vast quantities of food followed by purging but who, if unable to purge, still consume large amounts; and those who restrict their caloric intake, especially when unable to purge.

- Suicide, the deliberate act of self-injury with the intent to kill, may occur in adolescents because of difficulties in coping with stress, disturbed family environment, and psychoses.

- Substance abuse is a severe problem in adolescence and includes experimentors and compulsive users.

- Classifications of teens who abuse substances are social group, escapist group, punitive group, and self-destructive group.

- Common types of drugs abused include alcohol, hydrocarbons and fluorocarbons, mind-altering drugs, narcotics, central nervous system depressants, and central nervous system stimulants.

CONCEPT SUMMARIES

- The change, growth, and stress accompanying the transition to adulthood may predispose adolescents to faulty problem solving.

- The major eating disorders of adolescence are obesity, anorexia nervosa, and bulimia.

- Obesity may be caused by one of many factors; major categories are disease, metabolic and endocrine, caloric disequilibrium, adipose cell theory, set point theory, sociocultural factors, and psychologic factors.

- Age of onset of obesity, presence of emotional disturbances or neuroses, and negative evaluation of obesity by others may all contribute to the development of a disturbed body image in the adolescent.

- Diet, exercise, and behavior modification are the hallmarks of treatment for obesity.

- The nurse's involvement in obesity control includes nutritional counseling, behavior modification, group programs, and family counseling.

- Anorexia nervosa, a disorder characterized by severe weight loss in the absence of obvious physical cause, consists of three areas of disordered psychologic functioning: disturbed body image and body concept of delusional proportions, inaccurate and confused perception and interpretation of inner stimuli, and paralyzing sense of ineffectiveness that pervades all aspects of daily life.

- Therapeutic management of anorexia involves reinstitution of normal nutrition, resolution of the disturbed patterns of family interaction, and individual psychotherapy to correct deficits and distortions in psychologic functioning.

REFERENCES

The adolescent in despair, Emerg. Med. 17(9): 51-66, 1985.

American Psychiatric Association: Diagnostic and statistical manual of mental disorders, ed. 3 (DSM-III), Washington, DC, 1980, American Psychiatric Association.

Berkowitz, R.I., and others: Physical activity and adiposity: a longitudinal study from birth to childhood, J. Pediatr. 105:734-738, 1985.

Brownell, K.D., Kelman, J.H., and Strunkard, A.J.: Treatment of obese children with and without their mothers: changes in weight and blood pressure, Pediatrics 71:515-523, 1983.

Brownell, K.D., and Strunkard, A.J.: Behavioral treatment for obese children and adolescents. In Strunkard, A.J., editor: Obesity, Philadelphia, 1980, W.B. Saunders Co.

Bruch, H.: Anorexia nervosa, Nutr. Today 13(5):14-18, 1978.

Bryce-Smith, D., and Simpson, R.I.D.: Case of anorexia nervosa responding to zinc sulfate (letter), Lancet 2:350, 1984.

Carino, C.M., and Chmelko, P.: Disorders of eating in adolescence: anorexia nervosa and bulimia, Nurs. Clin. North Am. 18:343-352, 1983.

Cohen-Sandler, R., Berman, A.L., and King, R.A.: Life stress and symptomatology: determinants of suicidal behavior in children, J. Am. Acad. Child Psychiatry 21:178, 1982.

Committee on Adolescence: The role of the pediatrician in substance abuse counseling, Pediatrics 72:251-252, 1983.

Copeland, E.T., and Baucom-Copeland, S.: Childhood obesity: a family systems view, Am. Fam. Physician 24(8):153-155, 1981.

Elliott, J.: Blame it all on brown fat now, JAMA 243:1983-1985, 1980.

Epstein, L.H., and others: Effect of diet and controlled exercise on weight loss in obese children, J. Pediatr. 107:358-361, 1985.

Fields, B.L.: Adolescent alcoholism: treatment and rehabilitation, Fam. Comm. Health 2(1):61-90, 1979.

Fox, E.L., and Mathews, D.K.: The physiological basis of physical education and athletics, Philadelphia, 1981, W.B. Saunders Co.

Friedman, R.C., and others: Family history of illness in the seriously suicidal adolescent: a life-cycle approach, Am. J. Orthopsychiatry 54:390-397, 1984.

Garfinkel, B.D., and Golombek, H.: Suicide and depression in childhood and adolescence, Can. Med. Assoc. J. 110:1278-1281, 1974.

Garfinkel, B.D., and others: Suicide attempts in children and adolescents, Am. J. Psychiatry 129:1257-1261, 1982.

Garner, D.M., and others: Cultural expectations of thinness in women, Psychol. Rep. 47:483-491, 1980.

Greer, J.E.: Adolescent abuse of typewriter correction fluid, South. Med. J. **77**:297-298, 1984.

Hein, K., Cohen, M.I., and Litt, I.F.: Illicit drug use among urban adolescents: a decade in retrospect, Am. J. Dis. Child. **133**:38-42, 1979.

Hirsch, J.: The adipose-cell hypothesis, N. Engl. J. Med. **295**:389-390, 1976.

Hofmann, A.D., editor: Adolescent medicine, Menlo Park, CA, 1983, Addison-Wesley Publishing Co.

Huse, D.M., and others: The challenge of obesity in childhood. I. Incidence, prevalence, and staging, Mayo Clin. Proc. **57**:279-284, 1982a.

Huse, D.M., and others: The challenge of obesity in childhood. II. Treatment guidelines by stage, Mayo Clin. Proc. **57**:285-288, 1982b.

James, W.P.T., and Trayhurn, P.: Thermogenesis and obesity, Br. Med. J. **37**:43-48, 1981.

Keidel, G.C.: Adolescent suicide, Nurs. Clin. North Am. **18**:323-332, 1983.

King, G.S., Smialek, J.E., and Troutman, W.G.: Sudden death in adolescents resulting from the inhalation of typewriter correction fluid, JAMA **253**:1604-1606, 1985.

Kirtland, J., and Gurr, M.I.: Adipose cellularity: a review. 2. The relationship between cellularity and obesity, Int. J. Obesity **3**:15-55, 1979.

Knittle, J.L., and others: The growth of adipose tissue in children and adolescents, J. Clin. Invest. **63**:239-246, 1979.

Leveille, G.A., and Romsos, D.R.: Meal eating and obesity, Nutr. Today **9**(6):4-9, 1974.

Lloyd, J.K., Wolff, O.H., and Whelan, W.S.: Childhood obesity, Br. Med. J. **2**:145-149, 1981.

Mallick, M.J.: Health hazards of obesity and weight control in children: a review of the literature, Am. J. Public Health **73**:73-78, 1982.

Maris, R.: The adolescent suicide problem, Suicide Life Threat. Behav. **15**:91-109, 1985.

McSherry, J.A.: The diagnostic challenge of anorexia nervosa, Am. Fam. Physician **29**:141-145, 1984.

Merritt, R.J., and others: Consequences of modified fasting in obese pediatric and adolescent patients. 1. Protein-sparing modified fast, J. Pediatr. **96**:13-19, 1980.

National Institute on Drug Abuse: National survey of drug abuse: 1979, Rockville, MD, 1980, U.S. Department of Health and Human Services.

Newton, B.: Tough Love: help for parents with troubled teenagers—reorganizing the hierarchy in disorganized families, Pediatrics **76**:691-694, 1985.

O'Malley, P.M., Bachman, J.G., and Johnston, L.D.: Period, age, and cohort effects on substance abuse among American youth, 1976-1982, Am. J. Public Health **74**:882-888, 1984.

Overfield, T.: Obesity: prevention is easier than cure, Nurse Pract. **5**:25, Sept./Oct. 1980.

Paige, D.M., editor: Manual of clinical nutrition, St. Louis, 1983, The C.V. Mosby Co./Nutrition Publications, Inc.

Phillips, D.P.: The Werther effect, Sciences **25**(4):33-39, 1985.

Pillay, M., and Crisp, A.H.: Some psychological characteristics of patients with anorexia nervosa whose weight has been newly restored, Br. J. Med. Psychol. **50**:375-380, 1977.

Pipes, P.L.: Nutrition in infancy and childhood, ed. 3, St. Louis, 1985, The C.V. Mosby Co.

Pugliese, M.T., and others: Fear of obesity: a cause of short stature and delayed puberty, N. Engl. J. Med. **309**:513-518, 1983.

Raley, G.: Youth suicide: the federal response, Soc. Legis. Bull. **29**:65-68, 1985.

Richardson, T.F.: Anorexia nervosa: an overview, Am. J. Nurs. **80**:1470-1471, 1980.

Roche, A.F.: The adipocyte number hypothesis, Child. Dev. **52**:31-34, 1981.

Schwartz, R.H.: Marijuana: a crude drug with a spectrum of underappreciated toxicity, Pediatrics **73**:455-458, 1984.

Schwartz, R.H., and others: Drinking patterns and social consequences: a study of middle-class adolescents in two private pediatric practices, Pediatrics **77**:139-143, 1986.

Strunkard, A.J., and others: An adoption study of human obesity, N. Engl. J. Med. **314**:193-198, 1986.

Taitz, L.S.: The obese child, Boston, 1983, Blackwell Scientific Publications.

Van Itallie, T.B.: Bad news and good news about obesity, N. Engl. J. Med. **314**:239-240, 1986.

Weil, W.B., Jr.: Current controversies in childhood obesity, J. Pediatr. **91**:175-187, 1979.

Williams, J.F., Friedman, I.M., and Steiner, H.: Hand lesions characteristic of bulimia, Am. J. Dis. Child. **140**:28-29, 1986.

BIBLIOGRAPHY
Obesity

Botvin, G.T., and others: Reducing adolescent obesity through a school health program, J. Pediatr. **95**:1060-1062, 1979.

Brownell, K.D., and others: School-based behavior modification, nutrition education and physical education program for obese children, Am. J. Clin. Nutr. **35**:277-281, 1982.

Cecere, M.C.: PIP (Positive Image Program): a group approach for obese adolescents, Nurs. Clin. North Am. **18**:249-256, 1983.

Clark, M.K.: The risks of repeated dieting, Child. Nurse **2**:1, 3-4, 1984.

Dietz, W.H., Jr.: Childhood obesity: susceptibility, cause, and management, J. Pediatr. **103**:676-686, 1983.

Dietz, W.H., Jr., and Gortmaker, S.L.: Factors within the physical environment associated with childhood obesity, Am. J. Clin. Nutr. **39**:619-624, 1984.

Dietz, W.H., Jr., and Gortmaker, S.L.: Do we fatten our children at the television set? Obesity and television viewing in children and adolescents, Pediatrics **75**:807-812, 1985.

Dietz, W.H., Jr., and Hartung, R.: Changes in height velocity of obese preadolescents during weight reduction, Am. J. Dis. Child. **139**:705-707, 1985.

Epstein, L.H., Wing, R.R., and Valoski, A.: Childhood obesity, Pediatr. Clin. North Am. **32**:363-379, 1985.

Epstein, L.H., and others: Effects of weight loss on fitness in obese children, Am. J. Dis. Child. **137**:654-657, 1983.

Hagenbuch, V.E.G.: Obesity and the school-age child, Nurs. Clin. North Am. **17**:207-216, 1982.

Hataway, H., Raines, J.L., and Weinsier, R.L.: Nutrition: its ever-increasing role, Fam. Comm. Health **7**:22-37, 1984.

Hoerr, S.M.: An overlooked factor in adolescent obesity, Food Nutr. News **57**:17-19, 1985.

Hoover, M.L.: The self-image of overweight adolescent females: a review of the literature, Am. J. Maternal Child Nurs. **13**:125-137, 1984.

Jessor, R.: Problem behavior and developmental transition in adolescence, J. Sch. Health **52**:295-300, 1982.

Jonides, L.: Childhood obesity: a treatment approach for private practices, Pediatr. Nurs. **8**:320-322, 1982.

Jung, E., and others: Skinfold measurements in children, Clin. Pediatr. **23**:25-28, 1984.

Kahn, A.N.: Group education for the overweight, Am. J. Nurs. **78**:254, 1978.

Knittle, J.L., and others: Childhood obesity. In Suskind, R.M., editor: Textbook of pediatric nutrition, New York, 1981, Raven Press.

Mendelson, B.K., and White, D.R.: Development of self-body-esteem in overweight youngsters, Dev. Psychol. **21**:90-96, 1985.

Meyer, E.E., and Neumann, C.G.: Management of the obese adolescent, Pediatr. Clin. North Am. **24**:123-132, 1977.

Mogan, J.: Prevention of childhood obesity, Issues Compr. Pediatr. Nurs. **9**:33-38, 1986.

Mowrey, B.D.: Family oriented approach to childhood obesity, Pediatr. Nurs. **6**(2):40-44, 1980.

Orenstein, D.M., and others: The obesity hypoventilation syndrome in children with the Prader-Willi syndrome: a possible role for familial decreased response to carbon dioxide, J. Pediatr. **97**:765-767, 1980.

Potts, N.: The secret pattern of binge/purge, Am. J. Nurs. **84**:32-35, 1984.

Rowe, N.R.: Childhood obesity: growth charts vs. calipers, Pediatr. Nurs. **6**(2):24-27, 1980.

Silber, T., Randolph, J., and Robbins, S.: Long-term morbidity and mortality in morbidly obese adolescents after jejunoileal bypass, J. Pediatr. **108**:318-322, 1986.

Simonson, M.: An overview: advances in research and treatment of obesity, Food Nutr. News **53**:1-4, 1982.

White, J.H.: An overview of obesity: its significance to nursing, Nurs. Clin. North Am. **17**:191-198, 1982.

Anorexia Nervosa/Bulimia

Block, P.J.: Working with anorexic and bulimic adolescents, Food Nutr. News **56**:33-34, 1984.

Bruch, H.: The golden care: the enigma of anorexia nervosa, Cambridge, MA, 1978, Harvard University Press.

Casper, R.C., Offer, D., and Ostrov, E.: The self-image of adolescents with acute anorexia nervosa, J. Pediatr. **98**:656-661, 1981.

Ciseaux, A.: Anorexia nervosa: a view from the mirror, Am. J. Nurs. **80**:1468-1470, 1980.

Claggett, M.S.: Anorexia nervosa: a behavioral approach, Am. J. Nurs. **80**:1471-1472, 1980.

Dexter, J.M.: Anorexia nervosa, Nurs. Times **76**:325-327, 1980.

Doyen, L.: Primary anorexia nervosa: a review and critique of selected papers, J. Psychosoc. Nurs. Ment. Health Serv. **20**(6):12-18, 1982.

Fisher, T.A., and Suskind, R.M.: Nutritional considerations in the development and treatment of anorexia nervosa. In Suskind, R.M., editor: Textbook of pediatric nutrition, New York, 1981, Raven Press.

Garner, D.M., and Garfinkel, P.E.: Handbook of psychotherapy for anorexia nervosa, New York, 1985, Guilford Press.

Garner, D.M., Garfinkel, P.E., and Bemis, K.M.: A multidimensional psychotherapy for anorexia nervosa, Int. J. Eating Disorders **1**:3-46, 1982.

Goodwin, R.A., and Mickalide, A.D.: Parent-to-parent support in anorexia nervosa and bulimia, Child. Health Care **14**:32-37, 1985.

Harding, S.E.: Anorexia nervosa, Pediatr. Nurs. **11**:275-277, 1985.

Inbody, D.R., and Ellis, J.J.: Group therapy with anorexic and bulimic patients: implications for therapeutic intervention, Am. J. Psychother. **39**:411-420, 1985.

Kramer, J.P.: A protocol for outpatient treatment of the adolescent with anorexia nervosa, J. Curr. Adolescent Med. **2**:47-51, 1980.

McNab, W.L.: Anorexia and the adolescent, J. Sch. Health **53**:427-430, 1983.

Misik, I.M.: When the anorectic patient challenges you, Nursing 81 **11**(12):46-49, 1981.

Needleman, H.L.: Why do patients with anorexia nervosa like to cook? Speculations on reward behavior and hypothalamic catecholamines. In Suskind, R.M., editor: Textbook of pediatric nutrition, New York, 1981, Raven Press.

Nussbaum, M., and others: Cerebral atrophy in anorexia nervosa, J. Pediatr. **96**:867-869, 1980.

Potts, N.: The secret pattern of binge/purge, Am. J. Nurs. **84**:32-35, 1984.

Rees, J.M.: Eating disorders. In Mahan, L.K., and Rees, J.M.: Nutrition in adolescence, St. Louis, 1984, The C.V. Mosby Co.

Richardson, T.F.: Anorexia nervosa: an overview, Am. J. Nurs. **80**:1470-1471, 1980.

Sanger, E., and Cassino, T.: Eating disorders—avoiding the power struggle, Am. J. Nurs. **84**:31-35, 1984.

Swift, W.J.: The long-term outcome of early onset anorexia nervosa: a critical review, J. Am. Acad. Child Psychiatry **21**:38-46, 1982.

Unwarranted dieting retards growth and delays puberty, Nutr. Rev. **42**:14-15, 1983.

Yader, J.: Family issues in the pathogenesis of anorexia nervosa, Psychosom. Med. **44**:43-60, 1982.

Suicide

Beardslee, W.R.: Familial influences in childhood depression, Pediatr. Ann. **13**:32-36, 1984.

Carlson, G.A., and Cantwell, D.P.: Suicide behavior and depression in children and adolescents, J. Am. Acad. Child Psychiatry **21**:361-366, 1982.

Carmack, B.J.: Suspect a suicide? RN **46**(44):43-45, 90, 1983.

Committee on Adolescence: Teenage suicide, Pediatrics **66**:144-146, 1980.

Earls, F.: The epidemiology of depression in children and adolescents, Pediatr. Ann. **13**:23-31, 1984.

Eisenberg, L.: Adolescent suicide: on taking arms against a sea of troubles, Pediatrics **66**:315-320, 1980.

Faust, J., Forehand, R., and Baum, C.G.: An examination of the association between social relationships and depression in early adolescence, J. Appl. Dev. Psychol. **6**:291-297, 1985.

Fazen, L.E., Lovejoy, F.H., and Crone, R.K.: Acute poisoning in a children's hospital: a 2-year experience, Pediatrics **77**:144-151, 1986.

Hafen, B.Q., and Peterson, B.: Preventing adolescent suicide. In Hafen, B.Q., and Peterson, B., editors: The crisis intervention handbook, Englewood Cliffs, NJ, 1982, Prentice-Hall, Inc.

Hart, N.A., and Prophit, P., Sr.: Adolescent suicide, Pediatr. Nurs. **5**(6):22-28, 1979.

Hatton, C.L., and Valente, S.M.: Suicide: assessment and intervention, ed. 2, New York, 1984, Appleton-Century-Crofts.

Husain, S.A., and Vandiver, T.: Suicide in children and adolescents, Jamaica, NY, 1984, SP Medical & Scientific Books.

Litt, I.F., Cuskey, W.R., and Rudd, S.: Emergency room evaluation of the adolescent who attempts suicide: compliance with follow-up, J. Adolesc. Health Care **4**:106-109, 1983.

Mitchell, K.: Suicide: a preventable tragedy, Pediatr. Nurs. **11**:165, 1985.

Nursing Grand Rounds: Nursing care of a suicidal adolescent, Nursing 80 **10**(4):56-59, 1980.

Prophit, P., Sr.: The enigma of adolescent suicide. In Mercer, R.T., editor: Perspectives on adolescent health care, Philadelphia, 1979, J.B. Lippincott Co.

Rabin, P.L., and Swenson, B.R.: Teen-age suicide attempts and parental divorce (letter), N. Engl. J. Med. **304**:1048, 1981.

Tishler, C.: Adolescent suicide attempts following elective abortion, Pediatrics **68**:670-671, 1981.

Tishler, C.L.: Adolescent suicide: prevention, practice, and treatment, Feelings Med. Significance **23**:23-26, 1981; **24**:1-4, 1982.

Tishler, C.L.: Depression in children and adolescents: identification and intervention, Public Health Curr. **24**:1-3, 1984.

Tishler, C.L.: Intentional self-destructive behavior in children under age ten, Clin. Pediatr. **19**:451-453, 1980.

Twiname, B.G.: No-suicide contract for nurses, J. Psychiatr. Nurs. Ment. Health Serv. **19**:11-12, 1981.

Valente, S.: Suicide in school aged children: theory and assessment, Pediatr. Nurs. **9**:25-29, 1983.

Valente, S.: The suicidal teenager, Nursing 85 **15**:47-49, 1985.

Wright, L.S.: High school polydrug users and abusers, Adolescence **20**:853-861, 1985.

Substance Abuse

Bachman, J.G., Johnston, L.D., and O'Malley, P.M.: Smoking, drinking, and drug use among American high school students: correlates and trends, 1975-1979, Am. J. Public Health **71**:59-69, 1981.

Burton, J.: Intoxication by centrally acting substances, Crit. Care Update **10**:34-35, 1983.

Coulehan, J.L., and others: Gasoline sniffing and lead toxicity in Navajo adolescents, Pediatrics **71**:113-117, 1983.

Coupey, S.M., and Schonberg, K.: Evaluation and management of drug problems in adolescents, Pediatr. Ann. **11**:653-658, 1982.

Cuddy, P.G.,: Management of acute opioid intoxication, Crit. Care Q. **4**(4):65-74, 1982.

DuPont, R.L.: Teenage drug use: opportunities for the pediatrician, J. Pediatr. **102**:1003-1007, 1983.

Gold, M.S., and others: Opiate withdrawal using clonidine: a safe, effective, and rapid nonopiate treatment, JAMA **243:**343-346, 1980.

Hahn, A.B., Oestreich, S.J.K., and Barkin, R.L.: Mosby's pharmacology in nursing, ed. 16, St. Louis, 1986, The C.V. Mosby Co.

Isralowitz, R., and Singer, M., editors: Adolescent substance abuse: a guide to prevention and treatment, New York, 1983, The Haworth Press.

Kulberg, A.: Substance abuse: clinical identification and management, Pediatr. Clin. North Am. **33:**325-361, 1986.

Lukwikowski, K.L.K.: PPA: an innocent over-the-counter drug? Pediatr. Nurs. **10:**387-390, 1984.

Macdonald, D.I.: Drugs, drinking, and adolescence, Am. J. Dis. Child. **138:**117-125, 1984.

Meyers, F.H.: Drug use among adolescents. In Mercer, R.T., editor: Perspectives on adolescent health care, Philadelphia, 1979, J.B. Lippincott Co.

Pallikkathayil, L., and Tweed, S.: Substance abuse: alcohol and drugs during adolescence, Nurs. Clin. North Am. **18:**313-321, 1983.

Palmer-Erbs, V.K., and DeForge, V.M.: Interventions with the adolescent drug user and the family, Issues Compr. Pediatr. Nurs. **3**(5):15-24, 1979.

Pointer, J.: Typewriter correction fluid inhalation: a new substance of abuse, J. Toxicol. Clin. Toxicol. **19:**493-499, 1982.

Rehrig, M.: Cocaine look-alikes, Crit. Care Update **10:**47-49, 1983.

Rice, M.A., and Kibbee, P.E.: Review: identifying the adolescent substance abuser, Am. J. Maternal Child Nurs. **8:**139-142, 1983.

Roush, G.C., Thompson, W.D., and Berberian, R.M.: Psychoactive medicinal and nonmedicinal drug use among high school students, Pediatrics **66:**709, 1980.

Sanders, J.M.: Adolescents and substance abuse, Pediatrics **76:**630-632, 1985.

Tennant, F.S., Jr., and LaCour, J.: Children at risk for addiction and alcoholism: identification and intervention, Pediatr. Nurs. **6**(1):26-27, 1980.

Wetli, C.V., and Wright, R.K.: Death caused by recreational cocaine use, JAMA **241:**2519-2522, 1979.

Woolf, D.S., Vourakis, C., and Bennett, G.: Guidelines for management of acute phencyclidine intoxication, Crit. Care Update **7**(6):17-24, 1980.

Unit Eight

The Child and Family with Special Needs

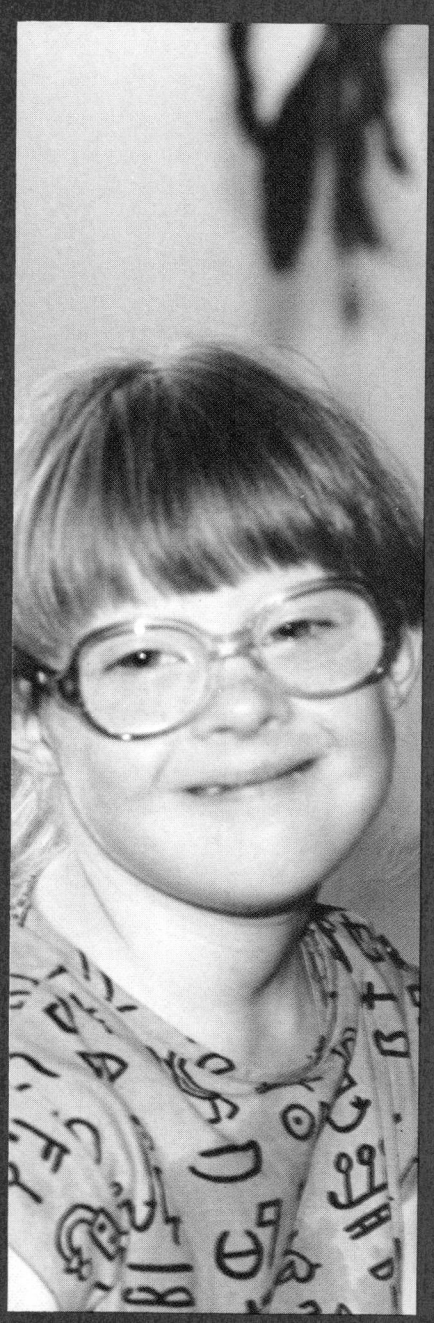

Units Three through Seven have focused on the growth and development of the well child. Most of the health problems discussed for each age-group were those that temporarily incapacitated the child. Unit Eight is concerned with the child who has special needs imposed by a permanent or chronic physical and/or developmental disability. These children need to master the same developmental achievements as children as well, in accordance with their potential abilities and despite the limitations of their condition. Families of these children are faced with exceptional challenges for which there is little guidance or few role models. As a result, the entire family unit is highly vulnerable to psychologic and sometimes physical problems that arise from unsuccessful attempts to deal with the child's special needs.

Chapter 22, *Impact of Chronic Illness or Disability on the Child and Family,* is an overview of the child's and family's reactions to the disorder and nursing interventions that assist each member in adjusting to the condition and developing to his fullest despite the disability. This chapter serves as a basis for understanding the stresses and needs of families when the child is chronically ill, physically disabled, mentally retarded, or sensory impaired. Chapter 23, *Impact of Life-Threatening Illness on the Child and Family,* focuses on the special needs of families when the diagnosis is potentially fatal. Chapter 24, *The Child with Cognitive Impairment,* is primarily concerned with the child who is mentally retarded and the nursing interventions required to help the child develop optimally. Chapter 25, *The Child with Sensory or Communication Impairment,* deals with the child who has a sensory loss or a communication disorder. Emphasis is placed on the effect of the impairment on development, detection of the disorder, and nursing interventions that promote rehabilitation.

Chapter 22

Impact of Chronic Illness or Disability on the Child and Family

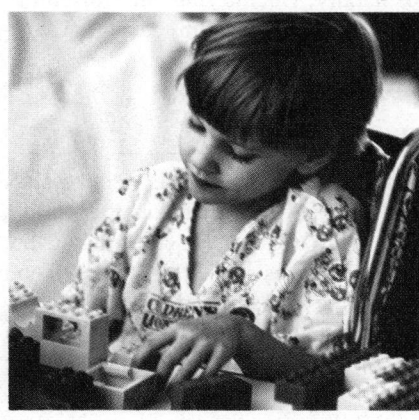

In a complex society there are innumerable abilities necessary for functioning. Loss of any physical or cognitive power immediately poses an obstacle to a person's ability to meet societal expectations. With advances in early diagnosis and treatment of many chronic illnesses and with improved technology for people with physical impairments, there is a growing number of children who need care. Because nurses are intimately involved in care for every type of health deviation, it is inevitable that they will be responsible for some phase of care with families who have children with special needs imposed by a physical or mental limitation. This chapter is primarily concerned with families' responses to the disorder, the effects of chronic illness or disability on the child and family unit, and nursing interventions that promote the optimum adjustment of each family member and acceptance of the child as a unique individual with special attributes as well as needs.

Perspectives in the Care of Children with Special Needs

Children with special needs comprise an increasingly important group of children who require both routine and specialized health care. The following discussion is an overview of the incidence of chronic illness and disability in children and the current trends in caring for these children.

SCOPE OF THE PROBLEM

Despite the interest and concern for children with special needs, exact definitions and incidence rates of chronic illness and disability do not exist. For the purposes of this chapter, the following definitions are used:

chronic illness A condition that interferes with daily functioning for more than 3 months in a year, causes hospitalization of more than 1 month in a year, or (at time of diagnosis) is likely to do either of these (Hobbs and Perrin, 1985).
disability Broadly, refers to a loss of function (Reynolds, 1984).
developmental disability Any severe, chronic disability attributable to a mental or physical impairment or a combination of both that is manifested before age 22 years, is likely to continue indefinitely, and will result in substantial limitation of function (as cited in American Academy of Pediatrics, 1979).

Individuals with chronic illnesses or disabilities are not necessarily handicapped. A *handicap* refers to environmental barriers preventing or making it difficult for full participation or integration, such as curbs or steps for a person in a wheelchair (Rush and League of Human Dignity, 1983).

Statistics regarding chronic illness and disability are at best only estimates of the true incidence of the problem and vary depending on the definitions used, the methods of study, and the population investigated (Gortmaker and Sappenfield, 1984). Overall rates of children with any chronic disorder range from 10% to 15%; approximately 1% to 2% of the total population (1 to 2 million children) have a severe chronic illness (Hobbs and Perrin, 1985). Two thirds of all cases of chronic illness are attributable to asthma and congenital heart defects; however, in terms of mortality, congenital heart defects, spina bifida, and leukemia are the most lethal. While there has been little change in the survival patterns for asthma, cleft lip/palate, and muscular dystrophy in recent years, there have been improvements in other diseases, such as diabetes mellitus, congenital heart disease, cancer, cystic fibrosis, hemophilia, sickle cell disease, and chronic renal failure (Harkey, 1983).

Broadly expanding chronic conditions to include speech, learning, emotional, sensory, and cognitive disorders yields an estimated 40% of children from kindergarten through sixth grade who have a significant long-term condition (Reynolds, 1984). Considering that the average American family has between three and four members, the number of individuals intimately affected by these children is staggering.

The numbers alone suggest that comprehensive nursing approaches are needed to meet the immense problems of children, youth, and families. Clearly nurses have a more crucial role than ever before in early screening, case finding, assessment, and diagnostic studies, as well as supportive interventions that minimize the disruptive effects of the condition on the family. Another major responsibility is preventing disabling disorders by eliminating their known causes. Nurses are responsible for ensuring immunization programs, identifying infants and mothers who may be at risk prenatally or postnatally, identifying the disability early, and implementing innovative health education programs.

CHANGING TRENDS IN CARE

Several changes have occurred in providing services to children with special needs. One is the focus on the child's *developmental* age rather than chronologic age. Using the developmental approach emphasizes the child's abilities and strengths rather than disabilities. In the past health professionals have viewed persons with a disability within a pathologic framework, probing for weaknesses and negative features. While much attention has been given to the technologic aspects of the child's care and health needs, less attention has been paid to the child's individuality, personality, or strengths, the family's needs, and the overall concerns of those who interact with these children. Under the developmental model attention is directed to the child's functional development, changes, and adaptation to the environment. Basic principles underlying rehabilitation efforts using the developmental model are listed in the box. Nurses often are in vital positions to redirect attention from the pathologic to the developmental model to meet the unique needs of the child and family.

Another principle that is increasingly employed is that of *normalization,* which refers to establishing a normal pattern of living (see also p. 945). By applying the principles of normalization, the environment for the child is "normalized" and "humanized." Concurrent with the trend toward normalization has been the earlier discharge of children from acute or chronic care facilities to the family and community. *Home care* represents the return to a system and set of priorities in which family values are as important to the care of a child with a chronic health problem as they are in the care of the well child. Home care seeks to achieve goals that are consistent with the developmental model (Stein, 1985):

1. Normalize the life of a child with special needs, including those with technologically complex care, in a family and community context and setting.

BASIC PRINCIPLES UNDERLYING REHABILITATION

1. The child and family are the primary rehabilitators; professional health team members only assist the family in the process of rehabilitation.
2. The focus of rehabilitation is to treat the *effect* of the condition on the child, not merely the disorder.
3. The goal is to promote optimum development, independence, and emotional adjustment within all family members.
4. The child's developmental age, not chronologic age, is the basis for beginning rehabilitation efforts.
5. Health professionals' role is in preventing the disorder, the treatment regimen, and those working with the child (specifically health team members) from interfering with the development of the child and disrupting the family unit.

2. Minimize the disruptive impact of the child's condition on the family.
3. Foster the child's maximum growth and development.

Throughout the text home care is discussed as appropriate for specific conditions, and the process of transition from hospital to home is elaborated in Chapter 26.

Paralleling normalization and home care, there also has been a trend toward *mainstreaming,* or integrating children with special needs into regular classrooms. Just as the home is the natural environment for children, so school must also be included as an essential component of the children's overall physical, intellectual, and social development. Children who attend school have the advantages of learning and socializing with a wide group of peers. There is an increased focus on individualization as the academic needs of these children are planned along with those of the rest of the students. A variety of supplemental programs have been designed in the school system to accommodate special needs, thus providing these children with an equal educational opportunity. This change has largely been a result of the passage of Public Law 94-142, the Education for All Handicapped Children Act of 1975 (Palfrey, 1980).

Family of the Child with Special Needs

The family of the child with special needs is faced with the crisis of losing a perfect child and the task of adjusting to and accepting the child and his condition. Nurses who understand the responses to the diagnosis and the usual effects the diagnosis have on each family member are able to emotionally support the family, anticipate and prevent potential problems, and foster growth despite the disorder. In addition to the following discussion, the response of parents to a newborn with a physical defect is discussed in Chapter 11 and the family's response to loss, specifically a child with a life-threatening disorder, is presented in Chapter 23.

REACTIONS OF FAMILIES TO A CHRONIC ILLNESS OR DISABILITY

When the diagnosis of a disability or chronic illness is made, the family progresses through a fairly predictable sequence of stages, regardless of the actual nature of the condition. Numerous investigators have studied families' responses and have postulated a number of "stages"; however, no one set of phases is universally accepted (Blacher, 1984). The following discussion focuses on stages that are common to most families, with the exception of the freezing-out stage. Not all families experience this process, and each family member varies widely in the time needed to progress through any of the stages.

Shock and Denial

The initial stage is a period of intense emotion and is characterized by shock, disbelief, and sometimes denial, especially if the disorder is not obvious, such as in chronic illness. Denial as a defense mechanism is a necessary cushion to prevent disintegration and is a normal response to grieving any type of loss. Probably all family members experience various degrees of adaptive denial as they learn of the impact that the diagnosis has on their lives. Denial becomes maladaptive when it prevents recognition of treatment or rehabilitative goals necessary for the child's optimum survival or development. For example, protracted denial may be seen in the response of a family to mental retardation; as long as the family can maintain a fiction of normality and handle the deviance within the present familial roles and values, there may exist no recognition of the diagnosis. Instead the problem is explained as slow maturation or an easily remedied disorder. The denial may be enforced by the child's social development, which belies the degree of motor and speech retardation. Not infrequently this ability to rationalize delayed development is successful until the child enters school, when his differences are compared to other children and become blatantly evident. At this point the family may begin to recognize the diagnosis as a crisis and react with shock and disbelief.

Shock and denial can last from days to months, sometimes even longer. Examples of denial that may be exhibited at the time of diagnosis include: (1) physician shopping, (2) attributing the symptoms of the actual illness to a minor condition, (3) refusal to believe the diagnostic tests, (4) delay in agreeing to treatment, (5) acting very happy and optimistic despite the revealed diagnosis, (6) refusing to tell or talk to anyone about the condition, (7) insisting that no one is telling the truth regardless of others' attempts to do so, (8) denying the reason for admission, and (9) asking no questions about the diagnosis, treatment, or prognosis. Each of these mechanisms allows individuals to distance themselves from the onslaught of a tremendous emotional impact and to collect and mobilize their energies toward goal-directed, problem-solving behaviors.

Partial denial, such as seeking additional professional

consultations or occasionally acting as if nothing were wrong, is used by most people throughout the dying process. Without such a temporary protective mechanism, few people could survive the constant emotional drain of anticipating their own death or the death of a family member. Particularly with parents, anticipating the death of the child is the same as losing part of one's personal hope for achievement, prestige, and accomplishment. There is no comfort or justice in the loss of youth because death occurs before self-fulfillment.

Denial is probably the least understood and most poorly dealt with reaction. Nurses and physicians typically label denial as "maladaptive" and actively attempt to strip it away by repeated and sometimes blunt explanations of prognosis. Mulhern, Crisco, and Camitta (1981) found that physicians had lower prognostic views than parents concerning the child's diagnosis and that neither group displayed an understanding of the disagreement. In fact, the physicians studied were largely unaware of parental hopefulness or denial, suggesting that poor communication existed between the groups.

Waller and associates (1979) present four poignant cases in which the medical and nursing staff could not accept the parents' denial of their child's hopeless prognosis and the hostile, unsupportive relationships that ensued. Of significance, however, was the finding that good relationships existed between the parents and social workers because the social workers were aware that each parent had *varying degrees* of denial and knew that the chance of recovery was small.

In children, the importance of denial has repeatedly been demonstrated as a factor in their positive coping with the diagnosis. O'Malley and others (1979) found that children who used denial to cope with illness were able to deal with anxiety and have a productive attitude about life. Similarly a study by Zeltzer and others (1980) of the coping styles of ill adolescents found that denial allowed even seriously ill adolescents to function adaptively and with hope.

Probably the crucial word here is "hope." Denial allows an individual to maintain hope in the face of overwhelming odds. Like hope, denial may be an adaptive mechanism for dealing with loss that persists until a family or patient is ready or needs other responses. Relatives of critically ill patients also identify hope as a universal need (Molter, 1979).

Adjustment

Adjustment gradually follows shock and is usually characterized by an open admission that the condition exists. This stage is one of "chronic sorrow" and only partial acceptance (Young, 1977) and is manifest by several responses, probably the most universal of which are *guilt* and *self-accusation*. Guilt arises from a human need to find rational causes for events. The concept of cause and effect implies an ability to change future events. It is often greatest when the cause of the disorder is directly traceable to the parent, such as in genetic diseases or from accidental injury. How-

ever, it occurs even without any scientific or realistic basis for parental responsibility. Frequently the guilt stems from a fallacious assumption that the disability is a result of personal failing or wrongdoing, such as drinking, smoking, not eating correctly, having sex or an affair, exercising, or not doing something correctly during pregnancy or the birth (Childs, 1985). Guilt may be related to thoughts of wishing the child dead, especially when the demands of care seem overwhelming and unrelenting. Guilt may also be associated with religious beliefs. Some parents are convinced that they are being punished for some previous misdeed. Others may see the disorder as a sacrifice sent by God to test their religious strength and faith. It is always advisable to pursue the meaning of each person's religious background to identify hidden sources of guilt and punishment, as well as potential support. The ability to master resentful and self-accusatory feelings of having "caused" the child's disorder is a crucial factor in determining the parents' acceptance of their child (Mattsson, 1972).

Children, too, may interpret their serious illness as retribution for past misbehavior. The nurse should be particularly sensitive to the child who passively accepts all painful procedures. This child may believe that such acts are inflicted as punishment that he deserves. It is always vital to assure children that what happens to them during diagnosis or treatment is to make them well.

Other common reactions are bitterness or anger. Anger directed inward may be evident as self-reproaching or punitive behavior, such as neglecting one's health and verbally degrading oneself. Anger directed outward may be manifest in open arguments or withdrawal from communication and may be evident in the person's relationship with any number of individuals, such as the spouse, the child, and siblings. Passive anger toward the ill child may be evident in decreased visiting, refusal to believe how sick he is, or inability to comfort him. One of the most common targets for parental anger is members of the staff. Parents may complain about the nursing care, the insufficient time physicians spend with them, or the lack of skill of those who draw blood or start intravenous infusions.

Children are apt to respond with anger as well, and this includes the sick or disabled child as well as the well siblings. Affected children are aware of the loss engendered by the illness or disability and may react angrily to the restrictions imposed or the feelings of being different. Siblings also feel anger and resentment toward the ill child and parents for the loss of routine and parental attention. It is difficult for older children and almost impossible for younger children to comprehend the plight of the affected child. Their perception is of a brother or sister who has the undivided attention of their parents, is showered with cards and gifts, and is the focus of everyone's concern.

Children of various ages manifest anger differently. Young children may demonstrate their uncooperativeness by yelling, screaming, and physically fighting off the adversary. Older children may verbally express anger through

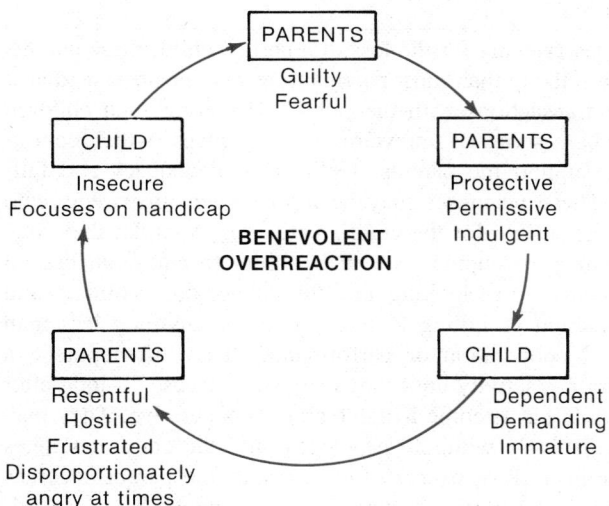

Fig. 22-1. Common cyclical response between parents and child. From Boone, D.R., and Hartman, B.H.: Clin. Pediatr. **11**(5):268-271, 1972.

abusive language. Passive anger, expressed in statements such as, "I don't know" or "I don't care," usually evokes aggressive anger in others. Such passive anger may be misinterpreted as sullen, obnoxious, or hostile reactions. As a result, these statements are effective in keeping people at a distance, when the hidden message really is, "I need to talk. Please help me understand what is happening."

A number of other reactions among family members are typical and include:

1. **Lowered self-esteem,** in which parents perceive a defect in their child as a defect in themselves; their life goals may be abruptly and dramatically altered, and they lose the fantasy of immortality through their child
2. **Shame,** in which parents anticipate social rejection, pity, or ridicule and related loss of social prestige and may experience social withdrawal
3. **Ambivalence,** in which the simultaneous experience of love and hatred normally experienced by parents toward their children is likely to be greatly intensified
4. **Depression,** in which parents experience chronic feelings of sorrow as a reaction to having an affected child; for example, to some parents mental retardation symbolizes the child's death and therefore precipitates a grief reaction
5. **Self-sacrifice,** in which parents become acutely sensitive to implied criticism of their child and may react with resentment and belligerence, or they may deny the existence of the problem and seek professional opinions to substantiate their own belief that "there is really nothing wrong with him"

During the period of adjustment, there are four types of parental reactions to the child that influence the child's eventual response to the disorder (see p. 937) (McDermott and Akina, 1972):

1. **Overprotection,** in which the parents fear letting the child achieve any new skill, avoid all discipline, and cater to every desire to prevent frustration

2. **Rejection,** in which the parents detach themselves emotionally from the child but usually provide adequate physical care or constantly nag and scold the child
3. **Denial,** in which parents act is if the disorder does not exist or attempt to have the child overcompensate for it
4. **Gradual acceptance,** in which parents place necessary and realistic restrictions on the child, encourage self-care activities, and promote reasonable physical and social abilities

The most common initial response, especially among mothers, is *benevolent overreaction* (Boone and Hartman, 1972). It is usually a consequence of unresolved guilt or fear, such as ambivalent feelings or not wanting the child during pregnancy, feeling responsible for the disorder, believing that the child would die at the time of birth or diagnosis, or reactivated feelings about a previous death of a loved one. It results in a vicious cycle of overprotective, permissive parent and dependent, demanding child (Fig. 22-1). It prevents the child from developing self-control, independence, initiative, and self-esteem. It is a reaction that responds to early intervention and prevention but is resistant to change once firmly established. Overprotection is so common a parental reaction that it behooves the nurse to assess for its presence and to begin counseling as soon as possible (see box).

Reintegration and Acceptance

For many families the last stage is characterized by realistic expectations for the child and reintegration of family life with the illness or disability in proper perspective. Since a large portion of the adjustment phase is one of grief for a loss, total resolution is not possible until the child dies or leaves home as an independent adult. Therefore one can re-

---

CHARACTERISTICS OF PARENTAL OVERPROTECTION

1. Sacrifices self and rest of family for the child
2. Continually helps child, even when child is capable
3. Is inconsistent with regard to discipline or employs no discipline; frequently different rules apply to the other siblings
4. Is dictatorial and arbitrary, making decisions without considering child's wishes, such as keeping child from attending school
5. Hovers and offers suggestions; calls attention to every activity, overdoing praise
6. Protects child from every possible discomfort
7. Restricts play, often because of fear that the child will injure himself
8. Denies the child opportunities for growing up and assuming responsibility, such as learning to give his own medications or perform treatments
9. Does not understand the child's capabilities and sets goals too high or too low
10. Monopolizes the child's time, such as sleeping with the child, permitting few friends, or refusing participation in social or educational activities

gard adjustment to chronic sorrow as "increased comfortableness" with everyday living.

This adjustment phase also involves social reintegration in which the family broadens its activities to include relationships outside of the home, with the child as an acceptable and participating member of the group. This last criterion often differentiates the reaction of gradual acceptance during the adjustment period from total acceptance.

One of the most important aspects of acceptance for health professionals to understand is that it is not an "all-or-none" phenomenon. Rather, it is interspersed with periods of intensified sorrow for the loss. Grieving is most likely seen at each period of the child's development. The following developmental crisis points following diagnosis have been identified for families with a mentally retarded child, and somemay also be relevant for families with children having other disorders (Wikler and others, 1981):

1. Time for walking and talking
2. Siblings surpassing child
3. Entry into school
4. Management problems such as discipline
5. Onset of puberty
6. Twenty-first birthday
7. Question of guardianship and placement

Consequently even families who have achieved a high level of adjustment and acceptance are at predictable times in need of professional support.

Freezing-Out Phase

If strategies of coping cannot be employed to minimize the stress and disorganization of maintaining the child within the home to tolerable levels, the affected child may be permanently placed outside the home in a residential setting, usually institutionalization. Evolution of this phase is directly related to the degree of physical and mental disability.

This phase is not necessarily one of maladjustment. Placement may be the only option that will preserve the integrity of the family. Aging parents may be forced to accept this alternative from progressive inability to meet the demands of a severely disabled offspring. Relinquishing the role of primary caregiver is followed by an initial sense of loss, relief, guilt, and ambivalence, a pattern of reactions not unlike that seen following the death of a terminally ill child (see p. 966).

IMPACT OF CHILD'S CHRONIC ILLNESS OR DISABILITY ON FAMILY MEMBERS

Each family who has a child with special needs is affected by the experience. The effects on the parents and their responses are so critical that they directly influence the other members' reactions. In addition, the extended family is affected and their response, as well as the community's acceptance of the child, can further assist or hinder the family's coping with the stresses imposed by caring for a chronically ill or disabled child.

Parents

Besides grieving for the loss of a perfect child, these parents are less likely than most parents to receive positive feedback from transactions with their child. Parenting such children may be a series of unrewarding experiences, which continually support the parents' feelings of inadequacy and failure. These responses may be most evident in parents who are responsible for the child's care. For example, they may become preoccupied with their ability to carry out certain procedures, overlooking the child's personal comfort and satisfaction or failing to praise him for anything less than perfect cooperation or performance. They often pursue a frustrating activity until they achieve "success"—long after the child has become irritable and uncooperative. They may unrealistically withhold privileges until the child completes a certain task or exercise. As a result, the parent becomes caught in a pattern of interaction that is mutually unrewarding and minimally productive. For these parents it may be beneficial to reduce the quantity of time spent with the child to increase the quality of the relationship.

Parents may have excessive demands placed on their time, energy, and financial resources. Depending on the roles assumed by each spouse, the wife often receives the brunt of the time and energy demands and the husband the financial responsibilities. However, with changing sex roles these responsibilities may be shared or shifted more heavily to one member. For example, the working mother may feel the need to continue employment to help defray the expenses, but this also incurs the added burden of additional child/home responsibilities.

The result can eventually be marital conflicts as one partner views his or her share as unequal (see Questions and controversies). In addition, the partner who is not included in the caregiving activities may feel neglected, since all the attention is directed toward the child, and resentful that he or she is not sufficiently informed to be competent in the care. Without active participation in the care of the child, the parent has little appreciation of the time and energy involved in performing those activities. When the less competent partner does attempt to participate, the other parent frequently criticizes the less skillful efforts. As a result, communication breaks down and neither is able to support the other. Unfortunately, the problems are seldom recognized until they are well established rather than early, when intervention can be most effective.

Communication tends to be centered on the affected child, with mothers typically assuming the role of interpreter between the child and other family members. This, combined with mothers' heavy investment in the caregiving role, leads to a very close relationship between the child and parent, usually the mother. However, problems frequently arise as the mother interferes with the child's functioning at maximum potential (Cleveland, 1980). Levels of stress appear to be related to the ease with which mothers can relate to their child and the demands their children make on them. Feelings of restriction and social isolation add further stress (Byrne and Cummingham, 1985), thus compounding the

Questions and Controversies

What are the effects on the marriage of having a child who is chronically ill or disabled?

Numerous reports in the literature support the finding that having a child with special needs places additional stress on the marriage. Reviews of current research document that increased marital discord is common among the partners and that other negative effects include feelings of low self-esteem, helplessness, and unmet dependency needs among the spouses. However, the few controlled studies show that the divorce rate is no higher than that for the general population (Kalnins, 1983; Sabbeth and Leventhal, 1984). The stressors often cited as having an impact on the marriage are: (1) the home care program with the burden of care assumed by primarily one parent, (2) the financial burden, (3) the fear of the child dying, (4) pressure from relatives, (5) the hereditary nature of the disease (if applicable), and (6) fear of pregnancy. Other causes of tension often center on the inconveniences associated with care, such as long waiting for appointments, lack of parking near care facilities, or lack of overnight accommodations (Kalnins, 1983). Certainly these last stressors are within health professionals' domain to minimize, if not eliminate.

Whether having a chronically ill or disabled child brings parents closer together is unclear. Some families report that following the diagnosis there was an immediate upsurge in feelings of closeness but long term the presence of the child neither weakened nor strengthened the marriage (Cleveland, 1980); others contend that the illness brought them closer together (Koocher and O'Malley, 1981). In those families who do divorce it is often not possible to separate the effect of the child's condition from other causes that may have led to marital dissolution.

negative aspects of an overly close and exclusive relationship with the affected child.

Compared to mothers, fathers generally have fewer opportunities to do something directly helpful for the child, such as taking the child to the physician, the drugstore, the physical therapist, the special school, or other special health services. Organizations for parents of children with special needs tend to offer fewer services to fathers. Fathers are less adequately provided for than are mothers by supportive mental health services. As a result, they have fewer opportunities available to them to mourn the loss of the perfect child and to deal with lowered self-esteem associated with fathering a chronically ill or disabled child. Their needs to adjust to the loss of a perfect male child may be even greater than the mother's when the expectations of immortality through a son can no longer be realized.

The main concerns of fathers of chronically ill children often involve the child's future and the unpredictable nature of the illness (McKeever, 1981). Although fathers speak of intense feelings at the time of diagnosis, many believe it is their responsibility to support the wife during the crisis. Many fathers believe their marital relationship has been affected by the child's illness, a major change being less time to enjoy leisure activities together. A significant finding for health professionals is paternal use of denial in coping with the diagnosis and fathers' hesitancy to associate with support groups.

Siblings

Siblings are deeply affected by the affected child's membership in the family. Younger siblings in particular may be affected because they are uprooted and displaced more than older children. For example, if the child with cognitive impairment is first-born, he becomes the "youngest" by virtue of his developmental age. Conversely, the second-born becomes the oldest, often shouldering adultlike responsibilities and achieving parental expectations that would have been reserved for the eldest.

Siblings are likely to show symptoms of irritability, social withdrawal, and fear for their own health. Healthy siblings may have a wide variety of physical complaints, such as headache, abdominal pain, or symptoms mimicking those of the sick or disabled child, as a reflection of their anxiety and fear. Their reactions to the child often do not parallel the severity of the condition. For example, siblings of children with obvious but less serious physical problems may have more adjustment difficulties than siblings of children with less visible but more life-threatening illnesses (Lavigne and Ryan, 1979). However, other findings indicate that the degree of the child's disability has no significant effect on the siblings' adjustment (Breslau, Weitzman, and Messenger, 1981).

Most parents can identify specific behaviors in the well children that have a negative effect on the family, such as jealousy, increased competition and fighting among siblings, anger, hostility, social withdrawal, attention-seeking behavior, and a decline in school performance. However, positive behaviors are also cited, such as increased nurturing, cooperation, sensitivity, compassion, and mastery of new skills. A common pattern among the siblings is periods of good adjustment alternating with times of poorer adjustment (Taylor, 1980). As siblings reach adulthood, they may develop increased altruism, tolerance, and an orientation to humanitarian interests (Siemon, 1984).

Siblings reveal feelings of isolation, deprivation, inferiority, and inadequate knowledge about the child's condition. Their lives are most affected in terms of the parent-child relationship, the medical care and treatment, and play and socialization. For example, the greatest effect of the ill child on the well siblings is a feeling of isolation and of being outside the parent(s)/sick child dyad. This is often increased by social restriction in peer relationships because of additional responsibilities in the home. Many siblings report receiving rewards in terms of "bribes" to overlook shortcomings in their parent-child relationship, but few receive any reward in the form of praise, personal attention, or tangible items. They often feel left out and uninvolved in the child's care, especially when the child is treated away from home. In particular they report feeling ignored by health care members. One study found that only one sibling out of 25 had received information directly from a health care professional (Taylor, 1980). Such findings emphasize that although positive, maturing attitudes can form in these siblings, the responsibility of health professionals is to involve the entire family unit in the adjustment process.

Extended Family Members and Society

Two other groups of people may experience the effects of the chronically ill or disabled child: (1) the significant non-nuclear family members or friends and (2) society as a whole. Although extended family relationships are often helpful to parents in rearing a child with special needs, they may also be sources of stress (Byrne and Cunningham, 1985). Grandparents may have far more difficulty in accepting the diagnosis than the parents themselves do, and parents may have concerns about the best way in which to respond to the grandparents' anger over the diagnosis or criticism regarding parental care. For example, grandparents or other well-meaning relatives may attempt to reassure the parents that the child "will grow out of" his slowness at a time when parents are struggling to accept reality.

Although society's views of individuals with chronic illness or disability are changing toward a more accepting, nonjudgmental, and open attitude, parents, siblings, and the affected child frequently are victims of prejudice, ostracism, or criticism. A great deal of this stems from public ignorance and fear, and this remains a crucial area for intervention by health professionals.

FACTORS AFFECTING THE FAMILY'S ADJUSTMENT

The diagnosis of a child with a serious health problem or disability is a major situational crisis that tremendously affects the entire family system. One nursing goal is to assess which families are at greater or lesser risk for succumbing to the effects of the crisis. Three variables—available support system, perception of the event, and coping mechanisms—influence the resolution of a crisis. Although researchers suggest that approximately 85% of families cope well, the needs of families at risk are great (Schulman, 1983). If they receive emotional support and guidance early, there is an increased likelihood that they will also cope successfully.

Available Support System

The significant others who are available to individuals for emotional strength during periods of crisis comprise their support system. Support systems may be available through a variety of relationships and may consist of one significant other, such as a marital partner, or a group of significant others, such as the extended family or members of the health team. Although a support system exists, it may not be effective unless the individual is able to use the system through mutual channels of communication.

Status of the marital relationship. The marital relationship is a prime source of potential support and overall is considered the best predictor of coping behavior (Friedrich, 1979). When the spouses can openly discuss their feelings, there tend to be much less guilt, anger, blame, and indecision. Each crisis during the long period of chronic illness is successfully resolved, lessening the accumulation and overlapping of multiple stresses.

Unlike the emotionally healthy family, there are other family styles that have less available support. For example, the single-parent family is frequently devoid of immediate support. The single or sole parent bears all the responsibility for decision-making that ordinarily would be shared by two people. In the moderately adjusted family there are no major difficulties between the marital partners until a crisis occurs. Without open communication and mutual sharing of ideas, the spouses react to the crisis with opposing opinions, blame, bitterness, and anger.

In the poorly adjusted family the marital relationship is precarious under the least stressful circumstances. The spouses have few common interests, do not share responsibilities, and communicate ineffectively. During a crisis they react by blaming each other, emphasizing past misdeeds, and searching for reasons to instill guilt in the other partner. Unable to cope constructively with the crisis, they may seek destructive coping mechanisms, such as excessive drinking, drug abuse, promiscuous behavior or physical aggression, or marital dissolution.

Alternate support systems. Support systems may be available with significant others outside the marital relationship. For example, the single-parent family may have the support of extended family, such as that of the parent's own parents. Occasionally parents may be able to communicate with each other but are unable to talk with the child. This is particularly evident with very young children, who communicate least through verbalization, and with adolescents, who may be unwilling to discuss with or listen to adults. In this case the child is left without an available support system.

Ability to communicate. Besides the availability of significant others, family members must have the ability to use the support system. Almost all methods of psychologic intervention, such as support through active listening, counseling, crisis intervention, or psychotherapy, require verbal communication between two individuals. The ability to verbalize about feelings such as anger, fear, guilt, or anxiety helps individuals cope with the particular emotion. Verbalization allows for validation of feelings and thoughts. For example, one mother secretly believed that she had caused her son's illness because before the diagnosis she had had recurrent dreams of his dying. Through discussions about this fear and the unrealistic impact of dreams on future events, the mother was able to resolve her guilt.

Not all individuals are able to communicate verbally. Some rely on religious faith and silent prayers for support. Others, such as children, communicate best through nonverbal methods, such as play, drawing, or writing. Some individuals may not be able to communicate with anyone because of their interpersonal withdrawal and social isolation. These individuals are most at risk because, even if a support system is available, they may be unable to share their problems with others.

Perception of the Illness/Disability

The meaning and significance of the child's condition are influenced by the individual's perception of the diagnosis. In particular the association of guilt may complicate one's ability to realistically view the death and ultimately resolve the grief. Guilt implies a degree of control over one's actions. The more guilt an individual has, the more control that person perceives in the prevention or alteration of the diagnosis. Assessment of specific perceptions concerning the illness or disability aids in evaluating the individual's ability to cope with various aspects of the crisis and identifies possible areas for intervention.

Previous knowledge. Although family members may be shocked to learn that their child has a serious illness or disability, they usually have some knowledge about the disorder from previous associations. It is important to explore the extent of that information, since there is a great tendency to compare the recently disclosed facts with the other knowledge.

Influence of religion. Religious beliefs and spirituality have various meanings for different people. For some, religion comprises the foundation of their support system—all of life revolves around their relationship with God. Healing and faith are synonymous, and any criticism of the family's spirituality can weaken their trust in the medical care. For others, it may intensify feelings of guilt, shame, bitterness, or punishment. For example, some individuals may interpret the illness as a punishment from God. They may exclaim, "What have I done to deserve this?" or "God, why are you punishing me in this way?" It is important to take such statements seriously and to explore reasons why the person believes that this is a punishment.

Imagined cause. Although the cause of many disorders is unknown, parents and children usually supply their own answers. Sometimes this is associated with religious beliefs, but it may also be influenced by previous events. For example, children may interpret the reason for the illness as a punishment for not obeying others. Parents may be convinced that the disease was inherited. Sometimes there is a strong belief in curses, occult witchcraft, or devils as perpetrators of the disorder. Once the fantasied cause is revealed, the person can be helped to deal with the irrationalities of that thinking and, hopefully, will be relieved of feelings of guilt, blame, or anger.

Effects on the family. How the child's illness or disability affects the family reveals how its members perceive the event. For example, the following statements could be representative of a particular reaction:

1. **Denial:** "Everything is the same as it always was."
2. **Inability to express feelings:** "We have more *things* to do."
3. **Anger, blame, or bitterness:** "We never should have had children."
4. **Resentment and hostility:** "My sister gets everything because she is sick."
5. **Acceptance and ability to express feelings:** "The perspective of time has changed because we realize how precious and limited it is."

ASSESSMENT OF COPING BEHAVIORS

Approach behaviors
Asks for information regarding diagnosis and child's present condition
Seeks help and support from others
Anticipates future problems; actively seeks guidance and answers
Endows the illness or disability with meaning
Shares burden of disorder with others
Plans realistically for the future
Acknowledges and accepts child's awareness of diagnosis and prognosis
Expresses feelings, such as sorrow, depression, and anger, and realizes reason for the emotional reaction
Realistically perceives the child's condition; adjusts to changes
Recognizes own growth through passage of time, such as earlier denial and nonacceptance of diagnosis
Verbalizes possible loss of child

Avoidance behaviors
Fails to recognize the seriousness of the child's condition despite physical evidence
Refuses to agree to treatment
Intellectualizes about the illness, but in areas unrelated to the child's condition
Is angry and hostile to members of the staff, regardless of their attitude or behavior
Avoids staff, family members, or child
Entertains unrealistic future plans for child, with little emphasis on the present
Is unable to adjust to or accept a change in progression of disease
Continually looks for new cures with no perspective toward possible benefit
Refuses to acknowledge child's understanding of disease and prognosis
Uses magical thinking and fantasy, may seek "occult" help
Places complete faith in religion to point of relinquishing own responsibility
Withdraws from outside world; refuses help
Punishes self because of guilt and blame
Makes no change in life-style to meet needs of other family members
Resorts to excessive use of alcohol or drugs to avoid problems
Verbalizes suicidal intents
Is unable to discuss possible loss of the child or previous experiences with death

---

Coping Mechanisms

Coping mechanisms are those behaviors aimed at reducing the tension caused by a crisis. *Approach behaviors* are those coping mechanisms that result in movement toward adjustment and resolution of the crisis. *Avoidance behaviors* result in movement away from adjustment or maladaptation to the crisis. Several approach and avoidance behaviors used in coping with a chronic illness or disability are listed in the box. None of the indices can be used singly to assess the possible success or failure in resolving the crisis. Each behavior must be viewed in the context of all the variables affecting the family. For example, the observation of several avoidance behaviors in an emotionally healthy family may denote significantly less risk to the successful resolution of the crisis than an equal number of avoidance behaviors in a poorly adjusted family or in an individual who has few available supports.

Two long-term coping strategies of familial adaptation to chronic and severe childhood illness have been significantly associated with a high level of family functioning (Venters, 1981). The first is the parents' ability to endow the illness with meaning within an existing spiritual or medical/scientific philosophy of life. There is an optimistic belief that all things work out for the good and a focus on the positive qualities of the situation. Statements such as ''God has chosen our family to care for this special child'' are reflective of the religious philosophy.

The second is an ability to share the burdens of the illness with individuals both inside and outside the family constellation. Intrafamilial relationships encourage togetherness of the family members and maintain a mutual acknowledgment that all members are important contributors to the family unit. Extrafamilial supports help preserve meaningful external contacts and provide needed help to the family.

Reactions to previous crises. Exploring the way in which a family dealt with a previous crisis identifies their possible reactions to the present stressful event. The type of family structure frequently offers valuable clues to the general approach the family may use to solve the crisis.

In the authoritarian family one or both parents decide what is best for all its members. As a result, the type of coping behavior demonstrated is usually chosen by a specific individual, regardless of others' needs. In the laissez-faire family new coping mechanisms may be explored, but family members offer little direction, approval, or validation of the effectiveness of the behavior. In the authoritative or democratic family there are flexibility and respect for each other's opinions, although the adults exercise direction and guidance for decision making. This type of family usually demonstrates the most ability in exploring new coping mechanisms that are aimed at successful resolution of the crisis for the ultimate benefit of the entire family.

Concurrent stresses within the family. The ability to deal with the already overwhelming stresses of a potentially terminal illness is challenged when additional stresses are present. These may be related to marital difficulties, financial pressures, or social isolation. Even the more minor stresses such as arranging care for the other siblings, managing the home, and traveling to distant treatment centers can jeopardize the family's ability to cope successfully.

The Child with Special Needs

Children with special needs are in many ways no different from any other children—they have the same requirement for love, security, and self-esteem. But in addition to dealing with all the normal developmental tasks of childhood, they must also cope with the challenges imposed by their illness or disability. While the family's responses are critical to the child's adjustment, other factors, such as the child's age, are important in planning individualized care.

IMPACT OF CHRONIC ILLNESS OR DISABILITY ON THE CHILD

The child's reaction to chronic illness or disability depends to a great extent on his developmental level, available coping mechanisms, and the reactions of significant others to him and to a lesser extent on the condition itself. Knowledge of these variables is essential in providing the kind of support needed by these children to cope with a sometimes overwhelming situation.

Developmental Aspects

The impact of a chronic illness or disability is influenced by the age of onset. Chronic illness affects children of all ages, but the developmental aspects of each age-group dictate particular stresses and risks for the child. An understanding of these factors facilitates planning care to support the child and minimize the risks.

Infancy. During infancy the child is engaged in the task of developing trust, which necessitates a reciprocal satisfying relationship between child and parent. When illness or disability occurs, this relationship is potentially affected. For example, a visible defect can retard parent bonding as the parent mourns the loss of the perfect child. In addition, prolonged illness may impose separations that prevent the child and parent from normal attachment and deprives the infant of the nurturing relationship.

The illness itself affects the infant, especially since sensorimotor experiences are critical at this age. Illness and/or disability often impairs the child's motor abilities, confining the child to a crib and lessening contact with the environment. Certainly the messages transmitted to infants about their body are influenced by the amount of pain and discomfort they experience. This lack of pleasurable sensations can lead to an irritable and unhappy child. Consequently, parents may interpret the behaviors as evidence that they are inadequate in meeting the child's physical and emotional needs, which further affects the parent-child relationship and the acquisition of trust.

To compensate for some of these feelings, parents, especially the mother, may become overly involved with the infant and promote increased dependency. This is significant during infancy when one of the tasks is separation and individuation from the parent. Such a response hinders the child's future self-development and often leads to the pattern of marked dependency, fearfulness, and passivity. One of the critical aspects of this pattern is that it is amenable to change if intervention is begun *early*.

Toddler. The toddler is in the stage of autonomy; the need for mastery of locomotor and language skills is paramount. As the child learns to walk and talk he progresses toward becoming a separate person, both physically and psychologically. However, illness or disability can hinder mobility and deprive the child of mastery. In addition the parents' overprotection can magnify the problem by setting limits on the child's exploration and experimentation for fear of hurting or exerting himself. Even the most basic self-help skills, such as feeding and dressing, may be done for the child. Age-appropriate tasks such as toilet training may be delayed. With such limited opportunities for testing mastery the child soon fears to venture on his own and develops little confidence in his ability. Over time the child may feel defeated and become apathetic, passive, and clinging (Perrin and Gerrity, 1984).

Illness can impose separations that are detrimental to the toddler. Like the infant, separation is the most anxiety-producing event for toddlers. A chronic illness or disability can necessitate repeated hospitalizations and painful procedures. If the need to preserve the parent-child relationship is not appreciated, the child may become depressed and eventually detach from the parent. Children seem to have a tremendous capacity to withstand stress provided their attachment to the parent is preserved.

Preschooler. The preschooler is in the stage of initiative; numerous tasks are achieved during this age that can be severely hampered by chronic illness and disability. Impairment can limit the preschooler's learning about the environment, especially in terms of social development. Rather than being encouraged to play with peers and participate in nursery school activities, the chronically ill preschooler may be confined to the home with socialization limited to the secure and tolerant family. He may be allowed immature behavior because age-appropriate standards and discipline are not enforced. Consequently, when paired with children his own age or placed in school, he is deficient in knowing how to act and can easily be criticized by peers who view him as a "baby." In fact, his illness or disability may provoke much less criticism than his inappropriate behavior. Faced with such reactions from others in contrast to the security of the home, the child may gradually choose a life of social isolation and loneliness, especially during the school-age years.

One of the major tasks of this period is establishing sexual identity, and one of the principal methods is through imitation of sex-related activities. However, the sick child may have fewer opportunities to engage in such activity and may view the parent predominantly in the caregiving role, since this may be the focus of their relationship. In some families it is expected that the mother assume the care of the child while the father provide the financial base by working outside the home. This can limit the child's identification with the male role.

In addition to sexual identity, the child's image of his body is forming. The child's knowledge of his body is limited to what he sees, feels, and uses. If the child is chronically ill, his awareness of his body is focused on its causing him pain and anxiety. For example, the young child may lose control over certain bodily functions, such as newly acquired bowel and bladder function, and feel embarrassed

and inferior. The disabled child may have difficulty forming a mental image of impaired body parts, such as paralyzed extremities. This poorly developed sense of body integrity makes children especially fearful of intrusive or mutilating experiences, which can be frequent during prolonged illness.

One of the more critical influences of chronic illness or disability on the preschooler is the feeling of guilt that he "caused" the condition by a real or imagined misdeed (Gratz and Piliavin, 1984). This is probably less of a factor if the child is born with the disorder than if it occurs during the preschool years. Such guilt can greatly affect the child's developing but fragile self-esteem. Unlike the child with a temporary physical impairment who has additional opportunities for achieving mastery and thus overcome feelings of guilt and inferiority, the child with a chronic illness or disability experiences continual insults. Unless situations are structured for him to succeed, life can become a series of failures—of never being strong enough or good enough to compete with peers.

School-age child. The child of school age is striving to achieve a sense of accomplishment while overcoming a sense of inferiority. Successful mastery of this task depends on the child's ability to cooperate and to compete with others. Consequently, physical impairments can greatly affect the ability to achieve and compete. For example, physical disability may hinder participation in sports and repeated absences from school caused by illness can place the child at an academic disadvantage. To repeat a grade can saddle the child with feelings of shame, inadequacy, and inferiority. However, the decision to remain in the same grade can also enhance feelings of success because the work requirements may be easier and new classmates provide a second chance for forming friendships.

During this age there is a transition from relationships with family members to strong identification with peers. Peers increasingly influence school-age children's view of themselves and their self-esteem. Anything that labels the child as "different" can affect his sense of belonging to the group. Many children cope with their "differentness" by retreating from socialization. As they draw farther from the group their sense of belonging diminishes and intense loneliness and isolation dominate. However, if they are helped to deal with their feelings of not being "normal and perfect" and to recognize their unique abilities, these children can cope very well. It is to be expected that all children are unable to master every task and that they will feel some degree of inferiority. If this is stressed to children with physical impairment, the burden to achieve is lessened.

As school-age children identify more with the peer group and authority figures outside the home, there is a concurrent striving for independence from the family. However, the ill child may be forced into an extended period of dependency either from the disorder or from parental overprotectiveness. Attempts to demonstrate independence may be manifest as resentment toward the parents, refusal to comply with treatment, or risk-taking behavior, such as cheating on the special diet. If parents can understand that these behaviors represent a normal phase of development, they may be more tolerant and able to find appropriate outlets for independence (e.g., increasing child's responsibility for home care).

Adolescence. The impact of illness or disability can be most detrimental during adolescence. Before this age, the child's self-image, self-esteem, and basic adjustment to life were primarily dependent on his relationship with the parents. A young child with impaired health reared in a home with loving parents who are sensitive to his needs generally copes well with the disorder. However, adolescence is different—even with all the benefits of parental love, the adolescent is striving for an independence away from his parents and in many ways must deal with the impact of impairment alone.

The major task of the adolescent is to establish an identity of his own. Pubertal changes must be integrated into the self-image while the teenager is gaining control and mastery over his increased physical capabilities and sexuality. During early adolescence this takes place primarily within the peer group. Illness or injury at this time interferes with the teenager's sense of mastery and control over his changing body. He is different at a stage of development when being different is unacceptable to the peer group, who may view a disability in one member as a threat to the established uniformity by which all are measured. At no time of life is an individual so vulnerable to the emotional stress of biologic impairment (Hofmann, 1980). Appearance, skills, and abilities are highly valued by peers; a teenager who is limited in any of these qualities is subject to rejection by this important group. This is especially marked when a physical disability interferes with sexual attractiveness.

Chronically ill teenagers are faced with the task of incorporating their disability into the changing self-concept. The youngster who develops the illness or acquires the disability during the crucial adolescent years has more difficulty accomplishing this task than does the teenager who has been affected since childhood. It appears that the earlier the onset of a limiting condition, the better the individual is able to adapt to it. The youngster with a newly acquired disorder will have the additional task of grieving for his lost "perfection" while adjusting to the changes taking place as a natural course of events. He often feels rejected because of his appearance or his inability to engage in activities expected of a healthy adolescent (Coupey and Cohen, 1980). The threat is greatest during middle adolescence, when the teenager has less available energy to cope with illness, since his emotional resources are being used to meet the normal demands of this developmental phase.

The severity, type, and visibility of the illness also influence the adjustment process and appear to be sex related. Boys seem to be more concerned about diseases or therapies that interfere with their ability to function independently and to achieve vocational and academic goals. Consequently, they may tolerate wearing a visible device or having a somewhat altered appearance as long as their physical and academic goals are not affected; for them confinement and restricted independence are less tolerable. Girls are more upset by conditions that they perceive to interfere with their ability to attract important others and maintain relationships. Thus they are more likely to tolerate restriction of movement and confinement provided they continue to look attractive; however, disorders or treatments that affect their appearance are devastating (Coupey and Cohen, 1984).

Adolescence is a time for achieving independence from the family and planning for future goals and responsibilities. Adolescents with long-term chronic illness tend to be less future directed and less independent than well peers (Orr and others, 1984). Enforced dependency from physical impairment can exacerbate the parent-child conflicts surrounding independence. Lack of understanding from both parties can result in bitter feelings and intrafamilial turmoil. The tendency toward rebellion may be directed at the disorder and reflected in decreased compliance with treatment, denying the disorder to preserve a sense of normalcy with peers, and risk-taking behavior that can place the teenager in jeopardy, such as driving a car despite a disorder that increases the chance of an injury. Such behaviors can further strain an already tense parent-child relationship.

Coping Mechanisms

Children's innate and learned coping mechanisms are very important in their ability to deal with their disorder. A number of individual factors influence the ability to cope with stress and include (Rutter, 1983):

sex Males are more vulnerable than females.
age Children between ages 6 months and 4 years are considered at greatest risk.
temperament The "difficult child," who is less likely to adapt, is considered more vulnerable than the "easy child."
genetic factors Inborn traits influence the overall ability to adapt.
intelligence Children with above average intelligence tend to have fewer psychiatric problems than children with lower intelligence.

In addition to these variables, the social support afforded these children is critically important. Therefore the better the family copes, the better the child is able to deal with the stressors imposed by the illness or disability.

Because it is often easier to recognize the child who copes poorly with the illness or disability, it is helpful to describe those behaviors typical of the well-adjusted child. The well-adapted child slowly learns to accept his physical limitations but finds achievement in a variety of compensatory motor and intellectual pursuits. He functions well at home, at school, and with peers. He has an understanding of his disorder that allows him to accept his limitations, assume responsibility for care, and assist in treatment and rehabilitation regimens.

He expresses appropriate emotions, such as sadness, anxiety, and anger at times of exacerbations but confidence and guarded optimism during periods of clinical stability (Fig.

22-2). He is able to identify with other similarly affected individuals, promoting positive self-images and displaying pride and self-confidence in his ability to master a productive, successful life despite the disability.

Responses to Parental Behavior

The parents' behavior toward the child, especially in terms of childrearing, is one of the most important influencing factors in the child's adjustment. For example, children whose parents are overprotective tend to have marked dependency, especially on the mother, fearfulness, inactivity, and lack of outside interests. Children who are raised by oversolicitous and guilt-ridden parents are often overly independent, defiant, and high-risk takers. Children who are reared by parents who emphasize their deficits and tend to "hide" or isolate them appear as shy and lonely individuals who harbor resentful and hostile attitudes toward normal persons (Mattsson, 1972). In contrast children who are reared by parents who establish reasonable limits tend to develop independence that is appropriate for their age and achievement commensurate with their limitations. They often display pride and confidence in their ability to cope successfully with the challenges imposed by their disorder.

A common consequence of parental behaviors is progressive control of family functioning by the affected child. Perhaps the most critical factor is the control the child has over the emotional reactions of family members. Many of these children have the ability to cause emotional suffering in their parents and siblings and to ease that suffering by selectively activating parental or sibling feelings of guilt (Cleveland, 1980). Consequently, those families with unresolved guilt are most vulnerable to this type of manipulation.

Despite their ability to control members of the family, these children also may feel responsible for much of the stress created by their condition, such as marital discord, financial problems, additional responsibilities on other members, interruption of previous life-style, and interference with future goals. They may also feel insecure in terms of their true worth to the family. For example, it is not unusual for the child to wonder if the concern and attention focused on him are the result of his condition. He may question his real worth as a person, especially if his disability has received more emphasis than his abilities.

Type of Illness or Disability

The type of illness or disability also influences the child's emotional response. Interestingly, children with *more severe* disorders often cope better than those with milder conditions (Pless, 1984). Considering children's cognitive ability and their delay in achieving abstract thinking until adolescence, it is likely that an obvious condition is easier to accept because its limitations are concrete. For example, the child who is blind or crippled is constantly reminded of his inability to run. However, the child with hemophilia not only lives by rules he does not understand but also only vaguely and occasionally senses his illness, such as when he runs and accidentally initiates a bleeding episode. Therefore

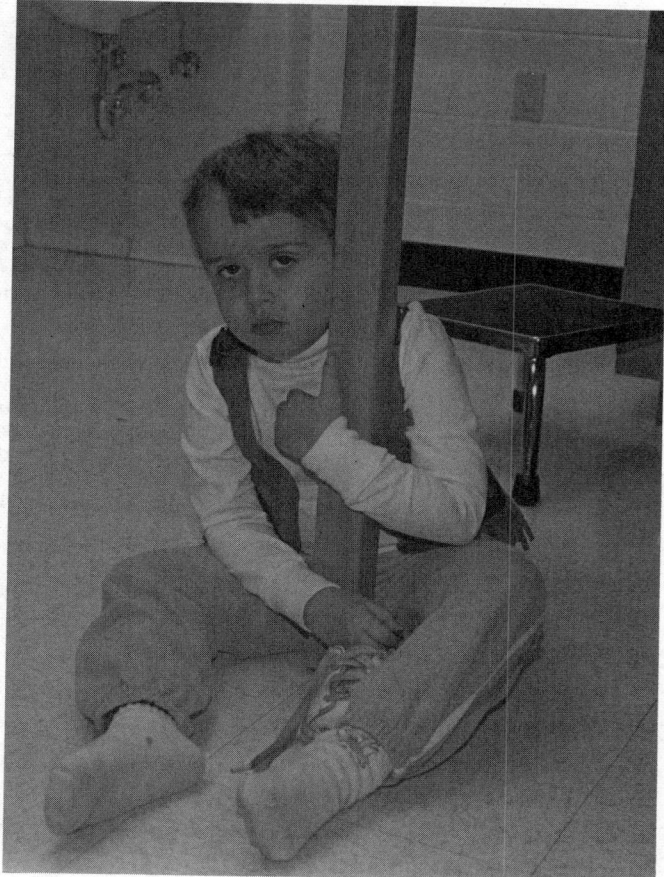

Fig. 22-2. Periods of sadness and anger are appropriate in the child's adjustment to a chronic illness or disability, especially during exacerbations of the disorder.
Photography by Katherine Patterson, University of Kansas Medical Center, Kansas City, KS.

some chronic illnesses pose special threats to the child.

The onset of a crippling condition may generate a state of confusion for the child, who may have trouble differentiating between his actual body functions and his image of his body. He may also experience problems in identifying himself and that extension of himself in the form of wheelchairs, braces, crutches, or other mechanical or prosthetic devices and may have tremendous difficulty in accepting functional aids.

For example, one 8-year-old child who was partially paralyzed from the waist down drew a picture of herself without legs. When asked if she had forgotten anything, the child responded, "No, that's me." When asked if she should draw legs with braces on, she again replied, "No, the braces are not part of me. You said to draw a picture of me." From the drawing and her comments it was obvious that she had dissociated nonfunctional parts of her body from having any meaning in terms of body image. It helped explain why the child refused to wear her braces for ambulation, preferring to be wheeled everywhere by others. Gradually through therapeutic play sessions the child was able to talk about her paralysis and consequently took a

Table 22-1   Assessment of factors affecting family adjustment

FACTORS AFFECTING ADJUSTMENT	ASSESSMENT QUESTIONS
Available support system Status of marital relationship Alternate support systems Ability to communicate	1. Whom do you talk to when you have something on your mind? (If answer is not the spouse, ask for the reason.) 2. When something is worrying you, what do you do? 3. What helps you most when you are upset? 4. Does talking seem to help when you feel upset?
Perception of the Illness/ Disability Previous knowledge of disorder Influence of religion Imagined cause of disorder Effects of illness or disability on family	5. Have you ever heard the word (name of diagnosis) before? Tell me about it (if answer is yes). 6. Has your religion or faith been of help to you? Tell me how (if answer is yes). 7. I know the doctors said there is no known cause of this disorder, but what do you think *really* caused it? 8. How has your child's illness or disability affected you and your family?
Coping Mechanisms Reactions to previous crises Concurrent stresses	9. Tell me one time you've had another crisis (problem, bad time) in your family. How did you solve that problem? 10. What other problems are you facing now? (Be specific—ask about financial, marital, and sibling concerns).

more active role in learning to walk with the orthopedic appliances.

Nursing Care of the Family and Child with Special Needs

The major nursing goal is to help the family remain intact and functioning at maximum levels throughout the child's life. This involves not merely supporting the child and his parents during the critical period of the newborn phase when the infant is being diagnosed or when the parents encounter problems in the child of preschool or school age. It involves using the *mutual participation model* to facilitate better communication and alleviate feelings of parental inadequacy and child inferiority.

This model invites the parents' early input, encourages them to be more accountable and responsible for the child's care, and does not reinforce the dangerous attitude that the professional will "fix" the child and give him back to the parents. It also reinforces the fact that it is not so much the condition itself that affects the child's progress and developmental outcomes but the family's ability to cope successfully with the child's problems. Thus long-term, comprehensive, systematic, family-centered approaches must be applied.

ASSESS THE FAMILY'S STRENGTHS AND LEVEL OF ADJUSTMENT

Since the nurse may meet a family during any phase of the adjustment process, it is essential to assess the family members' individual strengths, coping mechanisms, and reac-

tions to the disorder. Ideally assessment should begin as soon as the family learns the diagnosis. Sample questions designed to elicit information for evaluating the family's adjustment are listed in Table 22-1.

Several instruments can be used to assess the family's overall functioning and support system (see Chapter 6), and specific tools have been developed for the family with a chronically ill or disabled child. The Chronicity Impact and Coping Instrument: Parent Questionnaire (CICI:PQ)* consists of six sections: (1) the child with the condition, (2) parent completing the questionnaire, (3) spouse, (4) other children, (5) hospitalization, and (6) other. Within the sections information concerning stressors and coping strategies is obtained (Hymovich, 1983). A number of other instruments developed by nurses can be used to assess various aspects of the family's needs and resources (Brandt, 1984; Fife, Huhman, and Keck, 1986).

Regardless of the approach, assessment must be a continuous process because approach behaviors during one phase of the illness do not ensure reciprocal coping mechanisms in subsequent phases. Since support systems may change and perception of events may be altered at any point during the illness, nurses must continually evaluate the effectiveness of their interventions.

After assessing the family's strengths or weaknesses in coping with the crisis, nurses can intervene in any or all of the following. If a support system is lacking, they can substitute as a significant person and can locate potential sources of support, such as other parents, extended family

---

*The CICI:PQ and guidelines for scoring may be obtained for a fee of $3.00 from Dr. Debra Hymovich, 929 Longview Road, Gulph Mills, PA 19406.

members, specific service agencies, religious clergy, or community members. If parents are having difficulty in relating to their children, nurses can intervene by serving as interpreters, role models, or temporary supports for the child. When perception of the illness interferes with successful resolution of the crisis, nurses can clarify misconceptions, encourage family members to discuss their feelings, help other professionals to understand the family's reactions, and refer to other specialists for additional assistance in dealing with specific problems.

Families can be helped to explore new coping mechanisms or alter old ones to successfully meet the present crisis. Since a period of crisis is a time for exceptional growth and change, families can be guided toward seeking or avoiding original coping behaviors that may affect their overall functioning as well as adjustment to the crisis.

The nurse also assesses the parents' reaction to the child, using as a guideline the four categories of responses—overprotection, rejection, denial, and acceptance. Questions that may be helpful in revealing childrearing practices and attitudes toward the child include:

"How is this child different from his siblings?"
"Do you find yourself being a little more cautious with this child than your other children?"
"How has your life-style changed since you learned of the diagnosis?"
"When you think of your child's future, what thoughts do you have?"
"Describe your child's personality."

The parents' and child's understanding of the condition is another significant assessment area. Parental knowledge is particularly important since most children seek information from the parents (Nolan and others, 1986). One method of eliciting information is to ask the person how he would explain the child's condition to a stranger. This approach frequently eliminates the use of medical jargon that the family has learned to conveniently cover up their true feelings. For example, if a parent explains that mental retardation means an IQ (intelligence quotient) of 75, the nurse can respond that the stranger is unfamiliar with such numbers and needs to know what it means to have an IQ of 75.

While inquiring about the parents' level of understanding, the nurse also focuses on the child's and siblings' knowledge of the condition. It is not unusual for parents who appear well adjusted and knowledgeable to state that they have never told the children the truth. Although this is less of a problem when the condition is visible, it may occur when the disability can be cloaked in terms such as "a little behind" or "slow learner." Conflict arises when the child or siblings learn of the diagnosis from nonparental sources. Although this issue is similar to the "to tell or not to tell dilemma" when a child has a terminal illness (see p. 961), it has greater ramifications here because the disability may be lifelong, may require assistance from siblings later in life, and influences the entire family's social reintegration as a final phase to acceptance.

There are special challenges in assessing children's feelings about having a disability. Chapter 6 focuses on several approaches to encourage a child to discuss feelings about his diagnosis and future, provided they are appropriate for his developmental age. For example, using drawing and play as a method of communication is usually more appropriate in the developmentally disabled child, who may lack verbal skills.

Traditionally the mother and child have been active participants and receivers of professional care, whereas fathers and siblings have been excluded. However, to achieve the goal of optimum development for the family unit, each member must be included. This involves scheduling office and/or home visits at times when other family members can be present. Although occasionally this necessitates appointments during evenings or weekends, it can also be done late in the afternoon or early morning. Fathers often will change their work schedule to meet with a health professional once an invitation is extended.

The task of including other family members in a visit is approached positively. If they have not been included previously, they may interpret such an invitation as a portent of more bad news or an indication of their own difficulties. One way of welcoming others to join in a visit is to state that after hearing so often about the other siblings and the father the nurse wishes to meet them. This informal, casual approach is nonthreatening and implies only friendly connotations.

Ideally a thorough assessment includes observing the child and family in a variety of settings, including the home and school. Tools that can be used to systematically assess the home environment are the Home Observation for Management of the Environment (HOME) and the Home Screening Questionnaire (see Chapter 6). Both are designed for children up to 3 years of age. However, for developmentally disabled children the tools are applicable for a wider chronologic age range, since they can be used based on the child's developmental or functional age.

The second most important environment for a child is school. Teachers exert a tremendous influence on the child's developmental progress, feelings of self-esteem, learning capacity, and formation of social relationships. Whenever feasible the nurse should visit the school to observe directly the child's behavior and interaction among teachers and classmates. The box on p. 940 presents a summary of objectives for home and school visits.

PROVIDE SUPPORT AT TIME OF DIAGNOSIS

The impact of the crisis usually occurs at the time of diagnosis, which may be at the time of birth, following a long period of physical and/or psychologic testing, or immediately after a tragic injury. It is a critical time for parents. Although they may not hear or remember all that is said to them, they frequently sense a certain attitude of acceptance, rejection, hope, or despair that may influence their ability to absorb the shock and to begin adapting to the family's altered future (Halpern, 1984).

ASSESSMENT OF CHILD'S HOME AND SCHOOL ENVIRONMENT

1. Observe the child's home and classroom behaviors, such as the ability to sit, follow directions, and comply with requests; determine appropriate responses to questions; and determine the child's independence in functioning.
2. Gather data on reported behavioral problems such as "hyperactivity," "noncompliance," or "stubbornness."
3. Observe the child's interactions with siblings and peers.
4. Observe the child's behaviors in structured and non-structured activities.
5. Observe the parents' and teacher's appropriate and nonappropriate interactions with the child.
6. Observe the parents' and teacher's teaching strategies with the child. (Are school strategies consistent with home teaching?)
7. Observe the child's relationships with adults.
8. Determine the parents' and teacher's concerns and expectations of the child.
9. Administer standardized screening tools with the parent or teacher.
10. Observe the child's behavior before, during, and following a medication regimen.
11. Observe the child's eating patterns at home and at school.
12. Collaborate with the parents and teacher in future planning for the child.
13. Determine the effectiveness of programs of care for the child.
14. Coordinate parents, teachers, and others' plans for the child.

Although it is usually the physician's responsibility to inform the family of the diagnosis, nurses are increasingly responsible for acting as a collaborator with the physician, giving follow-up information, and coordinating services with other agencies. Regardless of the exact role nurses assume, they must have guidelines to follow during the informing interview to provide the family with support during this critical time.

Parents are encouraged to be together when they are informed of their child's condition, thus avoiding the problem of one parent having to interpret complex findings and deal with the initial emotional reaction of the other (Fig. 22-3). It also provides an opportunity to observe the interaction between the parents as they are confronted with the tragedy of discovering a serious problem in their child. Expressions on their faces, the times they look down, their ability to maintain eye contact with the nurse, their behaviors that show they are avoiding what the nurse is saying, such as turning their heads, looking around, or looking away, or any other activity that shows that they are indeed dealing with a very difficult subject is observed.

The atmosphere of the informing session should be one in which parents feel free to express their own emotions. If their feelings can be expressed and acknowledged, the parents can be helped to deal openly with them and their need for further counseling can be determined. Their emotional needs are acknowledged by showing acceptance of such expressions as crying, sadness, anger, and disappointment. Emotional support is offered by having tissues available if a family member cries and demonstrating through facial and bodily language that indeed this is a difficult and painful period. Although touching is a powerful expression of empathy, it must be used wisely. For example, it can prematurely terminate free expression of feelings, especially when combined with statements such as "Everything will be all right."

Parents should receive the kind of information they desire. Most parents report wanting a clear, simple explanation of the diagnosis, a prediction of possible futures for the child, advice on what to do next, an opportunity to ask questions, a warm and sympathetic listener, and, most important, time (Halpern, 1984). The nurse should make certain that the parents understand the information with such questions as, "Do you see what I mean?" or "Is this clear to you?" The nurse should then check further and have the parents repeat what they have just been told and to interpret it in their own way, to see if they understood the information. At this point clarification is made if necessary.

For example, if the diagnosis is one of developmental disability, the nurse can intersperse the information with, "Do you agree with these observations?" "Have you made similar observations of your own?" "Is this the kind of behavior you have seen at home or at school?" "Are these the observations that you were hoping we would make about your child?" "Has this been your experience?" "Is this information making sense to you?" and "Do you have any questions?" Waiting for a response, even though it may appear that a long silence is occurring, is important, since the parents should be allowed to think about and comment on what they have just heard. Technical terms are used with constant clarification. If the parents are unaware of the term, they are given written literature or at least a written summary of the diagnosis.

If parents appear overwhelmed, asking questions such as,

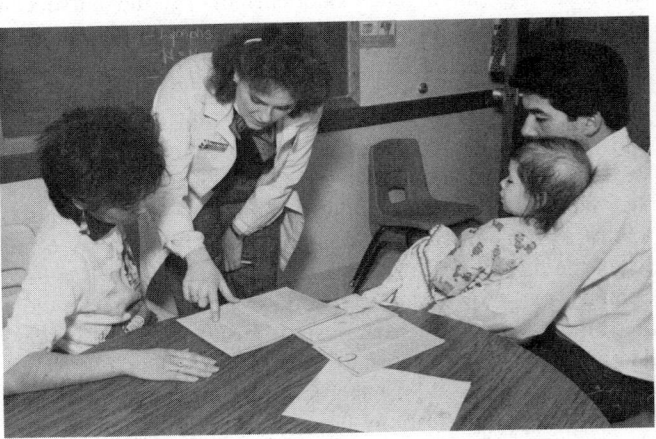

Fig. 22-3. Parents should be together when information about their child is given, especially during the informing conference.
Courtesy University of Kansas Medical Center, Kansas City, KS.

"I can see that this is very difficult for you, am I right?" or "This seems to be pretty overwhelming to you, am I right?" can confirm the observations. It may be appropriate to terminate the conference and continue it at another time with a statement such as, "I know that the diagnosis is serious and a great deal to accept at one time. We can talk again at another time unless there are questions you would like to ask now."

Last, the informing conference should not end with presentation of devastating news. Instead the strengths of the child, his appealing behaviors, his potential for development, and available rehabilitation efforts or treatment are stressed. Parents are encouraged to view life with their child as very similar to life with other children. Their experiences should be thought of as a series of problem-solving processes that they are capable of handling, particularly with available professional feedback. The parents are assured that the nurse will be available to answer questions and to provide further assistance as it is needed in the future.

The preceding discussion relates primarily to the initial informing interview. However, because of the need for long-term follow-up, it is only one in a series of continuing discussions. Although it is not possible to detail every issue that should be discussed with parents throughout the course of the rehabilitation process, the following points are emphasized (Gorham and others, 1975):

1. Be certain that parents clearly understand that imformation regarding treatment or prognosis can change; if a diagnostic label, such as *developmental disability,* has to be used, it is merely a way of communicating about a child; it really tells very little about the child's *current* and *future* capabilities.

2. Remember that parents must understand their child's abilities and assets, not only his negative traits, deficits, disabilities, and dysfunction. Assist the parents in learning to observe even the slightest changes in their child and in being honest with him. Parents need to know that one of their most important contributions to the child's life will be the manner in which they show respect for his appropriate behaviors and help him "feel good about himself." Parents should teach the child as early as possible that his disability cannot be blamed on anyone and is not his fault.

3. Tell parents that some people may dwell on the negatives of their child; this is to be expected. Help them to discover how to reverse this trend by thinking and acting in positive ways so that others can learn from them. Parents need to present their child in positive ways rather than emphasizing his negative traits.

4. Teach parents that they are important and vital contributors to the decision making that is done for their child's welfare and well-being. They should insist that no decisions be made about their child without their input and final approval. Their legal right to all services should be stressed.

5. Encourage parents to become as well informed as possible about their child, his programs, progress, and the ways in which others are treating him. Parents need to learn to interact effectively with other people who help their child and to present their own ideas with tact and confidence.

6. Be supportive of parents as they establish growth-producing and appropriate relationships with various professionals who will work with them on a longitudinal basis.

7. Stress the value of parents keeping their own records, including names, addresses, phone numbers, dates of visits, persons present during visits, and as much as they can remember of what was said.

8. Before giving advice about a problem, remember to ask about what the parent was told by another professional.

9. Encourage parents to speak up and ask professionals when they do not understand what is being said to them. Urge parents to gain confidence in talking openly and honestly with professionals, stating exactly what they want.

10. Guide the parents to appropriate sources of literature and remind them that some literature is out of date and presents only partial descriptions or answers.

11. Help parents get into the habit of seeking out and talking with other parents, to help them evaluate the advantages and disadvantages of all available programs. Encourage them to visit each facility and to ask the nurse to go with them to help them be objective whenever possible.

12. Encourage parents not to discount what their own child is saying to them, just because he is a child, because only the child can tell the parents how he perceives what is happening to him.

13. Remind parents that they are their child's best example of people working together in a mutually supportive, honest, and cooperative manner. Give parents credit for all the strengths they have shown and all the successful interactions they have had. Caution them not to dwell on their weaknesses and fears, but not to discount them either. Convey to parents that they are the primary and best resource for their child and that they should treat themselves with respect because of their many strengths and their powers.

The preceding discussion presented general guidelines; however, some situations require consideration of special problems, which are briefly discussed below.

Cognitive Impairment

Unless cognitive impairment is associated with other physical problems, it is often easy for parents to miss clues to its presence or to make defensive excuses regarding diagnosis. Since the impact of a diagnosis is associated with the reactions of shock and denial, it is important to help parents develop self-awareness of the condition. The best approach lies not so much in careful preparation of how to tell but in planning situations that help them become aware of the problem. This may deliberately involve a prolonged period of evaluation to help the parents gain an appreciation of the child's strengths and weaknesses.

The nurse can encourage parents to discuss their observations of the child without offering diagnostic opinions. For example, the parents may be asked how this child's development compares with that of other siblings or peers, how he is doing in school, if the parents have any concerns about his progress, or what they have been told by others.

By focusing on what the child can do and appropriate interventions to help him progress, such as infant stimulation programs, the nurse can involve parents in their child's care while helping them gain an awareness of his disability.

Physical Disability

If loss of a motor or sensory ability occurs during childhood, there is usually little difficulty in revealing the diagnosis because it is readily apparent. The challenge lies in helping the child and parents over the period of shock and grief toward the phase of acceptance and reintegration. One of the most helpful interventions is to institute early rehabilitation, such as using a prosthetic limb, learning to read braille, learning to read lips, and so on. However, physical rehabilitation usually precedes psychologic adjustment. Therefore persons working with crippled children or those with or sensory impairments must bear in mind that even though the child is proficient in compensatory skills, he may still be grieving for his loss and in great need of emotional support.

A special dilemma exists when the cause of the disability is accidental, since parental and child guilt can be overwhelming. It is imperative at the time of diagnosis to avoid implying that the parents or child was responsible for the injury. However, at the same time the nurse should allow the parents and child the opportunity to discuss feelings of blame. The third-person technique (see p. 195) can be used to encourage parents to express their feelings by stating, "Sometimes it is so difficult for a parent to anticipate hidden dangers in a child's life," or "Parents often feel responsible for things that happen to their child even if there was no way they could have prevented it."

Statements directed at eliciting the child's feelings are, "Sometimes when tragic things happen, people often wonder what they did to deserve them," or "When people tell others not to do things, it is easy to forget their warnings because they may not realize the actual dangers, but then when something happens, they wish they had listened." The nurse can either wait for a response with silence or encourage a reply with a statement such as, "Did you ever feel that way?"

Chronic Illness

Realization of the true impact of a diagnosis of chronic illness may take months or years. Conflict over parents' vs the child's concerns may result in serious problems. For example, whereas parents worry about preventing bleeding episodes and joint deformity, the child with hemophilia may only focus on the activity restriction. Unless each member is able to gain an appreciation of the other's concerns, it is likely that no one's needs will be met.

A special dilemma arises when the illness is inherited, since parents may blame themselves and/or the child may blame the parents. This aspect should be discussed with parents at the time of diagnosis to lessen guilt and accusatory feelings on any person's part. The child should be allowed to express his feelings. Using the third-person technique

helps open discussion in this area. For example, the nurse may comment, "Sometimes when a person has an illness that was passed on by the parents, that person feels angry or bitter toward them."

Multiple Disabilities

The child with multiple disabilities may present special challenges because the child or parent may require additional time for the shock phase. The child or parent may only be able to attend to one diagnosis before hearing significant information regarding the other disorder. When an obvious and a more hidden disability coexist, such as cerebral palsy and mental retardation, the nurse must be careful to acknowledge parents' understanding and acceptance of both diagnoses. Not infrequently the parents intellectualize that any retarded development is the result of the physical impairment and resist in accepting the intellectual deficit.

The nurse must also appreciate the devastating consequences of two disabilities to a child, especially if they interfere with expressive-receptive abilities. The overwhelming example is the blind-deaf child (see Chapter 25). Although both these defects may be present at birth, they may also have different onsets, such as partial deafness at birth with progressive loss of vision. In this situation the child's experiences with the outside world are severely limited.

ACCEPT THE FAMILY'S EMOTIONAL REACTIONS

One of the most supportive interventions is to accept the family's emotional reactions to the diagnosis in as nonjudgmental a manner as possible. Although all families respond differently and in varying degrees of intensity, three responses are so common and often so poorly handled that they deserve special consideration.

Denial

Nurses' response to denial is a critical component of the individual's continuing need for this defense mechanism. The most effective method of support is active listening. Silence neither reinforces nor rejects denial (or any other emotional reaction) but implies a willingness and acceptance of the person's need for this behavior. However, silence alone can be misinterpreted. For example, if the person demonstrates denial, such as by saying, "I am sure the doctors made a mistake," and the nurse responds silently and leaves, the person may infer disapproval, agreement, avoidance, or rejection from this behavior.

To be effective, silence and listening must be accompanied by physical and mental concentration and use of body language to communicate interest and concern. Direct eye contact, touch, physical geographic closeness, and body posture, such as sitting and leaning slightly forward, demonstrate silent but effective communication. Sometimes accepting people where they are, from their own perspective, is likely to give them the acknowledgment necessary to become more aware of their motives and to consider change (Beisser, 1979).

Guilt

Since guilt is such a common response and can cause family members tremendous anxiety, they should be told directly that there is no known cause of the disorder when appropriate and that they are not to be blamed. Using the third-person technique (p. 195) is valuable in eliciting thoughts of guilt. For example, with children an appropriate statement may be, "When people get sick they often wonder if they did anything to make themselves sick." This allows children an opportunity to explore any feelings of responsibility they harbor.

If family members are expressing feelings of guilt, it is important to allow them to talk about their feelings rather than quickly trying to dispel them with long "scientific" explanations. An effective method in lessening guilt is to *encourage the irrationality of thought.* For example, one mother stated that her son probably developed cancer by sitting too close to the television, which she could have prevented by being more strict. By following her reasoning and talking about how *many* children sit close to the television and how *few* of them ever have cancer, the nurse was able to help the mother realize that this activity was not a cause.

Anger

Anger is one of the more difficult reactions to accept and deal with therapeutically. The responses to anger may be reciprocal anger, fear, acceptance, and/or encouragement. The first two reactions close off communication and express disapproval and rejection of the person. They most commonly occur when the listener views the anger as a personal assault. The last two responses allow the individual to ventilate his feelings in an atmosphere of nonjudgmental acceptance. Two basic rules for dealing with the angry person are to avoid losing one's temper and to encourage the person to talk. The following steps encourage expression of emotions, such as anger (Epstein, 1975):

1. Describe the behavior: "You seem angry at everyone."
2. Give evidence of understanding: "Being angry is only natural."
3. Give evidence of caring: "It must be difficult to endure so many painful procedures."
4. Help focus on feelings: "Maybe you wonder why this happened to your child."

One essential element to the successful implementation of this process is to wait for the person to respond to a statement before proceeding to the next step. Since the objective of each statement is for the person to speak freely, the responses should avoid "yes" or "no" type of answers. For example, the behavior can be described as above or the nurse can ask directly, "Are you angry?" The latter question, however, may hinder further expressive communication and places the burden of subsequent conversation on the nurse, who should be the listener.

HELP THE FAMILY COPE

In order for the family to meet the stresses of optimally adjusting to the child's condition, each member must be individually supported so that the family system is strong. Although the family unit can indefinitely support a member who is in need of assistance, its greatest strength lies in every member supporting each other. The nurse should bear in mind that the "member in need" is not necessarily the affected child but may be a parent or sibling who is dealing with stresses that require intervention.

Parents

The nurse can provide support by being attentive to the family's responses to the child. Mothers and fathers need to experience success, joy, and pride in their child to give him the support he needs from them. The child, too, requires support for his interactions, adjustments, and efforts. He must be reinforced for attempts to get to know his care providers and to communicate his needs to them.

Since mothers and fathers of children with special needs have few role models to imitate, they need support to help them adjust. Above all, the nurse should ensure that the parents and siblings learn to perceive the child as a child first with unique and individual needs. The nurse needs to convey a humanistic, accepting approach of the child so that the parents can observe this acceptance. The way the nurse interacts with, approaches, touches, or holds the child makes this obvious. Any signs of rejection of the child, though subtle in nature, are readily interpreted by parents. This attitude of liking, concern for, and acceptance of the child should begin in early infancy and continue throughout the child's life.

Parents are asked for suggestions on care planning, implementation, and evaluation, using the mutual participation model. The nurse can play a valuable role in ensuring that the child learns about his disorder and in fostering communication between child and parents so that the child shares his concerns with them. The parents are helped to realize the child's level of maturity and understanding. The nurse needs to determine if the parents agree on what and when to tell the child about his condition. The parents must stress to the child the hopeful aspects of his condition as well as the problems. Careful consideration should be given to avoid overwhelming him and to support him as he reacts to information about himself.

Communication among all family members is encouraged. Parent group sessions are helpful in assisting parents to verbalize thoughts and feelings to each other but often do not take into account siblings' or the child's viewpoint. Therefore the nurse may need to set up a family session, such as during a home or clinic visit. Although the ideal situation is to have all the members present at once, this is often not possible within the confines of traditional nursing practice. However, inviting members to participate at various visits is an appropriate alternative.

Parents are encouraged to discuss their feelings toward the child, the impact of this event on their marriage, and associated stresses, such as financial burdens. For most families, regardless of their income or insurance coverage, financial concerns exist. The costs of caring for a child with special needs can be overwhelming. For example, the average yearly cost of care for many chronic illnesses is over $10,000, with additional "hidden" costs in out-of-pocket expenses that may be as much as 25% of the family income (Perrin and Ireys, 1984). In addition, the family wage-earner may have to sacrifice job opportunities to remain close to a medical facility or to avoid losing insurance benefits.

Every effort is made to include the father in visits, such as to the nursery, clinic, special school, and stimulation programs. His relationship with the child is observed, noting verbal interactions, tendency to assist the child, ability to give praise or set limits, and sensitivity to the child's needs. He is included in the assessment process with specific emphasis on having him describe the child's strengths and difficulties. It is not unusual to find two parents who have opposing views of the child's abilities, especially in the area of developmental disabilities (Fig. 22-4).

Fathers are encouraged to express their expectations for the child now and in the future. Because fathers tend to repress their feelings and feel less competent, the nurse acknowledges their difficulties and strengths, such as parenting skills and problem- solving abilities. Fathers are also encouraged to be involved with the child's care; maximizing their involvement while minimizing the mother's participation is effective in strengthening family relationships and preventing overdependency between the child and mother (Cleveland, 1980).

Numerous volunteer and community resources are available that provide assistance, rehabilitation, equipment, and funding for a variety of health problems.* National and local disease-oriented organizations may provide needed assistance and support to families that qualify. Many of these are discussed elsewhere in the text under the diagnosis. State and federal departments of health, mental health, social service, and labor may be able to help locate appropriate regional resources. For example, state **Crippled Children's Services** provide financial assistance for children with many disabling conditions. Nurses should become acquainted with those in their communities and with vocational programs for special groups.

Although community resources may exist, it is often very difficult for parents to locate suitable services and coordination among several agencies may be lacking. Fragmented care or "patchwork care" is one of the chief complaints

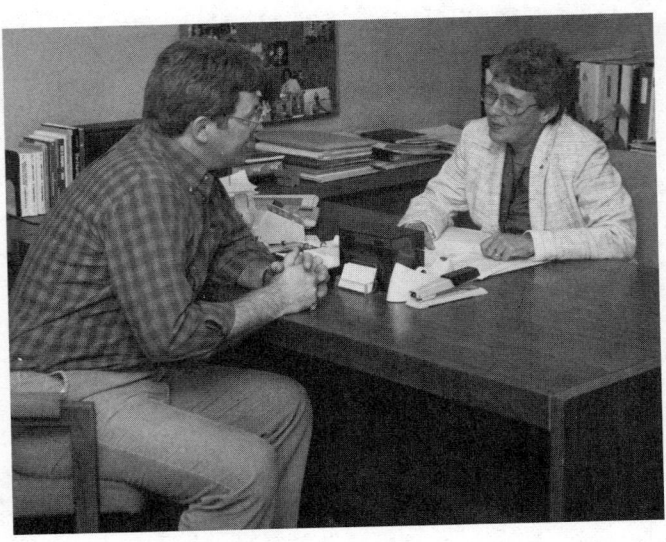

Fig. 22-4. Fathers need to be included in all aspects of the child's care, particularly conferences with health team members. Photography by John Roy, Saint Francis Hospital, Tulsa, OK.

from families, with specific problems of delayed referral and negative experiences with agency personnel cited as other concerns (Strauss and Munton, 1985). Consequently, community networking for improved services is essential (Johnson and Steele, 1983). Although this topic is beyond the scope of the present discussion, nurses can become key figures in coordinating services. Several excellent resources are available* and many projects are currently addressing this significant issue (Bock and others, 1983; Case and Matthews, 1983; Pierce and Freedman, 1983; Stein, 1983;).

Parents' organizations are especially helpful because they provide information and mutual support among the members.† The nurse who is aware of similarly affected families can be instrumental in organizing a self-help parent group.‡ Sometimes all the effort this entails is identifying one or two parents as leaders, sharing with them the names, telephone numbers, and addresses of other families, and guiding them in how to initiate a first meeting. A needs assessment questionnaire is useful for seeking parental opinions for planning meeting topics (Johnson, 1982). Although nurses may not

---

*Guidelines for developing community networks: support for families of children with chronic illness or handicapping conditions, Association for the Care of Children's Health, 3615 Wisconsin Ave. NW, Washington, DC 20016; Workbook series for providing services to children with handicaps and their families, Georgetown University Child Development Center, 3800 Reservoir Road NW, Washington, DC 20007.
†Information about self-help groups, as well as books and pamphlets, is available from The National Self-Help Clearinghouse, Dept. N85, CUNY Graduate Center, 33 W. 42nd St., Room 1227, New York, NY 10036; Self-Help Clearinghouse, CAMAC, Inc., 3737 Van Horne, Montreal, Quebec, Canada H3S 1R9; Directory of Parent Mutual Support Groups is available for a fee of $5.00 from Pediatric Projects, Inc., P.O. Box 1880, Santa Monica, CA 90406.
‡The following resource is recommended: Organizing and maintaining support groups for parents of children with chronic illness and handicapping conditions by Minna Newman Nathanson, available from the Association for the Care of Children's Health, 3615 Wisconsin Ave. NW, Washington, DC 20016.

---

*General sources of information are Clearinghouse on the Handicapped, Office of Special Education and Rehabilitative Services, Room 3132, Switzer Building, C St. SW, Washington, DC 20202, (202) 732-1250; National Information Center for Handicapped Children and Youth, P.O. Box 1492, Washington, DC 20013, (703) 522-3332. A comprehensive list of books and pamphlets for parents and teachers of disabled children is available from The National Easter Seal Society, 2023 W. Ogden Ave, Chicago, IL 60612, (312) 243-8400. Other sources of information are listed in Appendix E.

participate in the actual meeting, they should be available to the parents as resource persons or as intermediaries to locate professional guidance when necessary. It is just as important to recognize personal limitations as abilities in working with a group.

The Child

Through ongoing contacts with the child, the nurse (1) observes the child's responses to his disorder, ability to function, and adaptive behaviors within the environment and with significant others, (2) explores the child's own understanding of the nature of his illness or condition, and (3) supports him while he learns to cope with his feelings. He is encouraged to express his concerns rather than allowing others to express them for him, since open discussions may reduce anxiety.

Parents sometimes convey concern because the child cannot express the anxieties *he feels*. If the child cannot or will not talk, the child may have to play out his feelings. He can be provided with toys to allow him to express threatening or stressful emotions. The nurse may find that the child responds best to drawing pictures or telling stories (see Chapter 6). Puppets can also be used to help him express himself. By demonstrating to parents how useful these techniques are, the nurse also helps them learn new ways of communicating with him. For youngsters with extremely serious handicaps and/or persistent maladjustment, psychiatric evaluation and management may be needed.

One of the most important interventions is alleviating the child's feeling of being different and normalizing his life as much as possible. The principles in the box are fundamental in implementing the normalizing process (Krulik, 1980). Whenever possible the nurse should assess the child's daily routine for indications of lack of normalizing practices. For example, the child who remains in a bedroom all day is in need of a restructured daily routine to provide activities in different parts of the house, such as eating in the kitchen with the family. Such children may also be deprived of social, recreational, and academic activities that can be recognized by applying normalization practices.

Children who are concerned that their condition detracts from their physical attractiveness need attention focused on the normal aspects of appearance and capabilities. Health professionals must help strengthen and consolidate the self-image by emphasizing the normal, while at the same time allowing children to express anger, isolation, fear of rejection, feelings of sadness, and loneliness (Coupey and Cohen, 1980). They need positive reinforcement for compliance and any evidence of improvement. Anything that might improve attractiveness and contribute to a positive self-image is employed, such as makeup for a teenager with a scar; clothing that disguises a prosthesis; a hairstyle or wig to cover a deformity or lost hair.

Siblings

As pointed out, the presence of a child with special needs in a family may result in parents paying less attention to the

---

PRINCIPLES OF NORMALIZATION

1. **Preparation.** Prepare the child in advance for changes that may occur from the illness or disability; for example, the child is told in advance of the possible side effects of drug therapy.
2. **Participation.** Include the child in as many decisions as possible, especially those relating to his care regimen; for example, the child is responsible for taking his medications or scheduling his home treatments.
3. **Sharing.** Allow both family members and the child's peers to be a part of the care regimen whenever possible; for example, the child is given his medication when the other siblings receive their vitamins; mother cooks the same menu for the whole family; and if the child is invited to another's home, the mother advises the family of the child's dietary restrictions.
4. **Control.** Identify areas where the child can be in control so that feelings of uncertainty, passivity, and helplessness are decreased; for example, the child identifies activities that are appropriate to his energy level and chooses to rest when he is fatigued.

---

other children or expecting older siblings to take on greater responsibility for the care of the child. The siblings may respond by developing negative attitudes toward the child or by expressing anger in different forms. The nurse can help by using "anticipatory guidance," questioning the parents about what they believe is the best way to have siblings respond to the child and about whether they have any concerns about the way in which they are assigning responsibility to older siblings. This questioning should take place before serious negative effects occur.

Siblings may also experience embarrassment associated with the stigma of a disorder such as mental retardation. Parents are then faced with the difficulty of responding to this embarrassment in an understanding and appropriate manner without punishing the siblings for feeling the way they do. Parents should talk with the siblings about how they view their affected sibling. For example, siblings of a retarded child may express fears about their ability to bear normal children. Adolescents in particular may not be able to discuss these vital issues with their parents and may prefer to consult with the nurse. Many siblings benefit from sharing their concerns with other young people who are experiencing a similar situation.*

Many parents express concern about when and how to inform the other children in the family about the birth or the presence of a child who is handicapped. The answer depends on each child's level of sophistication and understanding. However, it is usually best to inform the siblings before a neighbor or other nonfamily member does so. Nurses can show by their behavior that they see the parents as being capable in their own unique style of imparting in-

---

*For information on the Sibling Information Network, write Department of Educational Psychology, Box U-64, School of Education, The University of Connecticut, Storrs, CT 06268.

formation about the condition. However, they should make it clear that if the parents postpone informing the siblings they assume the risk of hindering the siblings' ability to develop a realistic understanding of the problem. Uninformed siblings may fantasize or develop apprehensions that are out of proportion to the child's actual condition. Furthermore, if parents choose to be silent or deceptive about the issue, they are setting a negative precedent for the siblings to follow, rather than encouraging the siblings to cope with the experience in a healthy and nurturing way.

The nurse must be sensitive to the reactions of siblings and whenever possible intervene to promote more positive adjustments. For example, siblings often mention that they are expected to take on additional responsibilities to help the parents care for the child. It is not unusual for them to express a positive reaction to assuming the extra duties but a negative response to feeling unappreciated for doing so. Such feelings can often be minimized by encouraging the siblings to discuss this with the parents and by suggesting to parents ways of showing gratitude, such as an increase in allowance, special privileges, and most significantly verbal praise.

Extended Family Members and Society

The nurse must also be sensitive to family's cues regarding sources of stress from extended members, such as grandparents. For example, the nurse may encourage the parents to invite the grandparents to be present during one of the child's visits to a clinic, during the diagnostic workup, or to a parent conference or to provide appropriate literature.* Including grandparents in a discussion in which they can share their concerns may help them deal with their feelings, thus reducing stress on the entire family. Grandparents' feelings of blame and anger as well as any "cure fantasies" they harbor can be brought out in the open and discussed if necessary. Grandparents can be helped to understand the effects of their behavior on the family with an appropriate statement, such as, "Your daughter is currently experiencing a great deal of pain and anguish. We realize that this is difficult for you as well as your daughter; however, you can be of tremendous help by being supportive toward her."

Considerable stress can also arise from nonfamilial sources, such as friends, neighbors, or strangers. Inability to cope with comments about the disorder or curious stares by others may foster the tendency to isolate and protect the child within the home. The family needs guidance in preparing for these inevitable experiences. One approach is encouraging parents to dress the child as much as possible like other children. Good grooming is very important in minimizing differences in appearance. Through role playing parents can practice responses to comments such as, "Is your child retarded?" or "Has he always been crippled?" Through parent groups family members can share experi-

ences and learn from each other how they successfully deal with probing questions or unkind remarks. Such interventions must include the siblings and the affected child, who also must face and deal with these events. Nurses can be instrumental in teaching young children about disabilities to familiarize them with the special needs and abilities of these individuals. For example, school nurses can simulate experiences such as having only one leg by using role playing, can use books or films, or can invite community guests with physical limitations to visit the class (Hedahl, 1981). Special dolls can be used to help children become comfortable and familiar with a variety of disabilities.*

FOSTER REALITY ADJUSTMENT

Fostering a reality adjustment primarily involves education of the parents regarding the disorder, developmental needs of the child, and realistic goal setting. Ideally education should be aimed at preventing problems, rather than at relearning to change existing dilemmas. Like the interventions previously discussed, this goal requires an ongoing process that is part of assessment and emotional support of the family.

Supply Information

Educating the family about the disorder is actually an extension of revealing the diagnosis, especially those points listed on p. 940. Education involves not only supplying technical information but also discussing how the condition will affect the child. For example, it is of little benefit to discuss mental retardation in terms of numbers. Rather parents need to understand what the child can do in terms of self-help, academic learning, and independence. Similarly the child who has lost a limb needs more than an explanation of the prosthetic leg. He must know the limitations it places on his activity as well as the opportunities available to him.

Parents also need guidance in how the condition may interfere with or alter activities of daily living, such as eating, dressing, sleeping, and toileting. One area frequently affected is nutrition. Common problems are undernutrition as a result of food being inappropriately restricted, loss of appetite, or motor deficits that interfere with feeding and overnutrition usually caused by a caloric intake in excess of energy expenditure or boredom and lack of stimulation in other areas. Although the child requires the same basic nutrients as other children, the daily requirements may differ. Special nutritional considerations are discussed as appropriate throughout the text.

Unfortunately few reliable standards exist regarding nutritional requirements for children with special needs. To ensure optimum nutrition, the child's diet is recorded for a 7-day period to determine if deficiencies exist. The nurse

---

*A newsletter, *Especially Grandparents*, for and about grandparents of children with special needs, is available from the King County Advocates for Retarded Citizens, 2230 Eighth Ave., Seattle, WA 98121.

*Hal's Pals for Challenged Kids are available from Mattel, Inc., 5959 Triumph St., City of Commerce, CA 90040, (800)-824-4000.

collaborates with the nutritionist to select a diet that best meets the child's nutritional needs.

Parents also need to be aware of the importance of communicating the child's condition in the event of a medical emergency. Young children are unable to give information about their disorder, and although older children may be reliable sources, after an accident they may be physically unable to speak. Therefore all children with any type of chronic condition that may affect medical care should wear some type of identification, such as a Medic Alert bracelet,* which lists the medical condition and a collect phone number for emergency medical records and other personal information, or a MediScope,† a cylinder-shaped pendant that contains a microfilm medical record and a magnifying lens. Other types of identification usually employ plastic laminated cards, which are less convenient for young children.‡

Children need information about their condition, the therapeutic plan, and how the disease or the therapy might affect their particular situation. Children nearing puberty also need to understand the maturation process and how their disability may alter this event. For example, the youngster with Crohn disease should understand that this disorder is associated with growth failure and delayed puberty; the child with diabetes needs to know that hormonal changes and increased growth needs will alter food and insulin requirements at this time; and the sexually active girl with sickle cell anemia or systemic lupus erythematosus needs to be aware of the hazards of pregnancy. The information should not be given all at once but timed appropriately to meet the changing needs of the youngsters, and it should be described and repeated as often as the situation demands.

The subject of sexuality related to the effects of the disorder is a prominent concern of adolescents, but they rarely initiate a discussion of this sensitive topic. Any probable interference in sexual function because of the disability should be discussed openly and candidly with the teenager. Adults often underestimate the degree to which adolescents engage in unrealistic fantasies regarding sexual activities and related matters. The health professional must be alert to cues that signal when the teenager is ready for more detailed and prognostic information about his condition relative to sexuality and reproduction (Hofmann, 1980).

Throughout the long process of caring for a child with special needs family members become expert in management of their child's care. Unfortunately, this expertise is often not recognized by health professionals who tend to be directive, rather than collaborative, in their approach to the family. This is particularly common during periods of hospitalization, when parents are placed in a "double-bind"— at home they are expected to care for their child yet in the hospital they are ignored as participants in care, especially

treatment regimes (Robinson, 1985). A supportive atmosphere must include coordination of care with family members, respect for their knowledge, and willingness to include their suggestions and recommendations in the treatment plan.

Promote Normal Development

Aside from knowledge of the condition and its effect on the child's abilities, the family must be guided toward fostering appropriate development in their child. Although each stage may take longer to achieve, parents are guided to helping the child fully realize his potential in preparation for the next phase of development.

Early childhood. During infancy the child is achieving basic *trust* through a satisfying, intimate, consistent relationship with his parents. However, the affected child's early existence may be stressful, chaotic, and unsatisfying. Consequently he may need more parental support and expressions of affection to achieve trust. Likewise the parents require assistance in ways of meeting the infant's needs, such as how to hold a rigid or flaccid infant, how to feed a child with tongue thrust or episodes of dyspnea, and how to stimulate a child who seems incapable of achieving any skills. If hospitalizations are frequent or prolonged every effort is made to preserve the parent-child relationship (see also Chapter 26).

During early childhood the goal is to achieve separation from mother, autonomy, and initiative. However, the natural parental response to having a sick child is overprotection. Parents need help in realizing the importance of brief separations from the child, including others in the child's care, and providing social experiences outside the home whenever possible. Respite care, which provides temporary relief for family members, is essential in allowing caregivers time away from the daily burdens* (Warren and Cohen, 1985).

Young children also need the opportunity to develop independence. Frequently the child is able to learn self-help skills, such as holding the bottle, finger-feeding, and removing simple articles of clothing, but the parent continues to perform the act. Therefore the nurse must guide parents to the usual milestones expected from the child. Initially this requires developmental assessment of functional age, such as using the Denver Developmental Screening Test (Appendix B).

Periodically the child's developmental progress is evaluated. Since each child develops at his own rate, there are no rigid guidelines for expecting when particular skills will be achieved. However, lack of progress in any one area is investigated. For example, sometimes a delay in self-feeding is not caused by lack of motor skill but by the parents' im-

---

*P.O. Box 1009, Turlock, CA 95381.

†MicroDesign Systems, P.O. Box 188, Arverne, NY 11692.

‡National Safety Council Medical Information Card, National Health & Safety Awareness Center, Dept. FP, 333 North Michigan Ave., Chicago, IL 60601.

*Information on guidelines to develop a respite care program is available in *Keeping families together: providing respite and other short-term care for people with disabilities,* Alaska Governor's Council for the Handicapped and Gifted, 600 University Ave., University Plaza West, Suite C, Fairbanks, AK 99701.

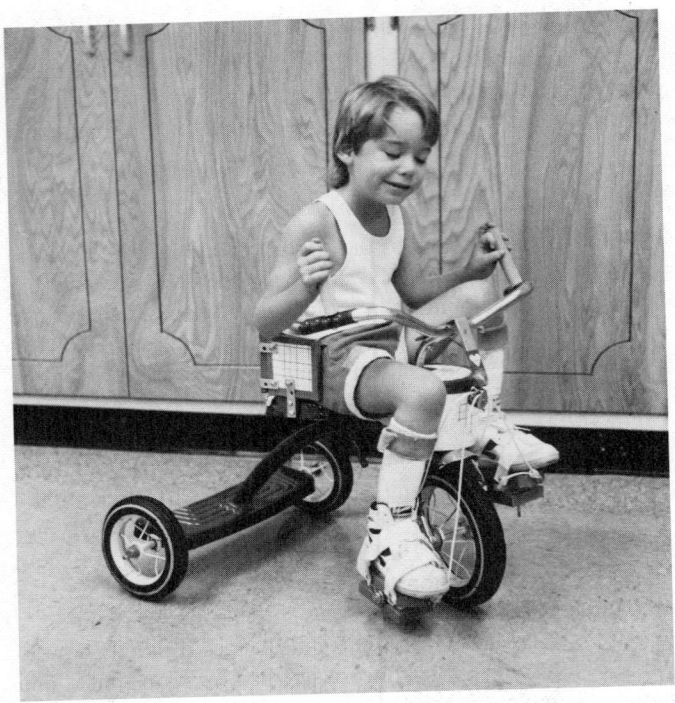

Fig. 22-5. A modified tricycle with block peddles, Velcro straps for support, and modified seat and handle bars can help a child with disabilities gain mobility.
Photography by John Roy, Saint Francis Hospital, on location at Children's Medical Center, Tulsa, OK.

symbolic expression in which words and thoughts replace actions as a way of problem-solving.

When the young child has a disability that interferes with motor development, there is the potential hazard of shifting to development of compensatory intellectual pursuits before the child is ready. If this occurs, achievement of autonomy and initiative may be severely compromised, setting the stage for emotional problems. Therefore intervention must be based on providing activities that allow maximum motor development. For example, if a child has paraplegia, it is not sufficient to strengthen the upper extremities to compensate for the lower ones. Rather the activity must take into account the child's need for social interaction, sense of control over his body, feeling of competence and achievement, and an outlet for aggression. Suitable activities may include ball throwing, swimming and water activities such as races, bubble blowing, and splashing, building blocks, or pounding with a hammer (Bernard and others, 1981).*

With slight modifications, disabled children may be able to ride a tricycle by using Velcro straps to secure the hands and/or feet (Fig. 22-5). Wheelchair races are always a popular activity. Programs such as the Special Olympics† offer children an opportunity to compete with their peers and to achieve athletic skill. Summer camps‡ also provide children with unique opportunities to associate with similarly affected peers and develop a wide variety of skills, including increased independence in activities of daily living and special needs associated with their condition, such as administering medication. With innovation many adaptations can be implemented in children's environment to increase their mobility and independence.§ Technologic advances are mushrooming, especially in the application of computers, and parents should be directed to the latest developments that may help their child (Desch, 1986).

Another critical component for normal child development is discipline. Unfortunately this is one of the earliest child-rearing practices eliminated when parents react with "over-benevolence." Not only does lack of discipline destroy the child's security because he has no boundaries on which to test out his behavior, it also fails to teach the child socially acceptable behavior and creates resentment and hostility among the siblings if different standards are applied to each

patience in waiting for the skill to develop. Cleaning up the spilled food may seem like one more unnecessary task unless the importance of using a cup or spoon is stressed. All that may be necessary to encourage parent participation are suggestions to avoid large accidents, such as pouring only a small amount of juice in a cup or having the child feed himself mashed potatoes (a sticky food) rather than gelatin (a slippery food).

Not all disabled children are capable of achieving normal developmental milestones. For example, the child with mental impairment may never achieve cognitive skills above a preschool level. The child who is deaf may achieve only rudimentary verbal language. In these situations adjustments must be made to compensate for the lack of or severely delayed achievement in one area. However, such adjustments must be based on an understanding of normal development. Since motor limitations are present in a majority of conditions, this disability is used as an example to illustrate psychologic implications in making developmental changes.

During early childhood the basic innate drive for movement is dominant. During toddlerhood there is rapid development of motor skills, which eventually becomes the basis for learning and coping with the complex world. Psychologically this period is critical for developing a desire for independence. Language development, bowel control, locomotion, and fine-motor control all converge to produce a feeling of competency. Gradually during the early school years this basic motor urge shifts to a more goal-directed,

---

*Information on a toy library system for children with sensory deficits, motor disabilities, and developmental delay is available from the National Lekotek Center, 2100 Ridge Ave., Evanston, IL 60204.
†1350 New York Ave., NW, Suite 500, Washington, DC 20005-4709. Several pamphlets are available from the National Easter Seal Society, 2023 W. Ogden Ave, Chicago, IL 60612, and the American Alliance for Health, Physical Education, Recreation and Dance (AAHPERD), 1900 Association Dr., Reston, VA 22091, on sports and recreation for children with disabilities.
‡A directory of camps for children with a variety of chronic illnesses or general physical disabilities is available for a fee of $8.95 from American Camping Association, Publications Service, 100 Bradford Woods, Martinsville, IN 46151.
§An excellent publication is *The more we do together: adapting the environment for children with disabilities*, Monograph No. 31, available for a fee of $5.00 from World Rehabilitation Fund, Inc., 400 East 34th St., New York, NY 10016.

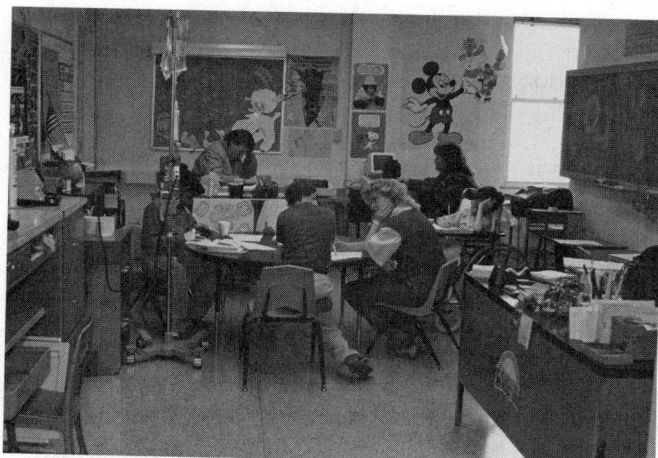

Fig. 22-6. Children with special needs should continue their schooling as soon as their condition permits.
Photography by Katherine Patterson, University of Kansas Medical Center, Kansas City, KS.

child. The nurse's responsibility is to help parents learn successful methods of controlling behaviors before they become problems (see Chapter 14).

School age. For school-age children, the major tasks are entry into school and achieving a sense of industry. While the importance of school in the life of all children is generally acknowledged, studies indicate that school absences are significantly higher among children with chronic illness, especially if psychosocial problems, such as behavior or family difficulties, coexist, than among their healthy peers (Weitzman, Walker, and Gortmaker, 1986). Some children, especially those with potentially terminal illnesses, may not return to school, despite a long period of remission. The more school absences the child experiences, the more difficult it is to return and "school phobia" may result. Psychosocial factors that contribute to the risk of school phobia include depression, change in appearance, fear of separation (child and parents), and resistance on the part of school personnel (Klopovich and others, 1981). To prevent school phobia the child should resume school as quickly as possible following diagnosis (Lansky, 1985).

Preparation for entry to resumption of school is best accomplished through a team approach with the parents, child, school teacher, school nurse, and primary nurse in the hospital. Ideally this planning should begin well before hospital discharge, provided the child is well enough to resume usual activities. A structured plan should be developed, with attention to those aspects of care that must be continued during school hours, such as administration of medication or other treatments (see p. 730). Parents' feelings regarding school resumption also need to be considered. Parents, especially mothers, may have difficulty relinquishing the intensive parenting role, particularly if many of their other social attachments have weakened. A successful approach is to plan school attendance concurrently with the parents' recommencement of prediagnosis activities.

Children also need preparation before entering or resuming school. Having a tutor in the hospital or home as soon as children are physically able helps them realize that school will continue and gives them time to consider this prospect (Fig. 22-6). They need to investigate possible answers to the many questions others will ask. One method of anticipatory preparation is to role play, with the child as the "returned pupil" and the nurse as "other schoolmates." The nurse asks questions about the reason for the child's absence, the name of the disease, and so on. The child is thus provided with a safe opportunity to explore possible answers and to experience some of the possible reactions of others. If the child returns to school with some obvious physical change, such as hair loss, amputation, or visible scar, the nurse might also ask questions about these alterations to prompt preparatory responses from the child.

Plans for entry or return to school must be based on the individual child's ability to resume usual activity. Initially the child may find it easier to attend half-day sessions or to participate in a limited number of activities. It is preferable to plan the school program with as much participation and leadership from the child as possible. For example, during the planning stage of a preadolescent's return to school, a mother had talked to the physical education teacher concerning her daughter's need for limited activity. However, a problem occurred when a substitute teacher taught the class. Since no one had informed her of the child's condition, she expected the child to participate as fully as the others. The child tried to comply but physically was unable. Instead of explaining the situation to the teacher, she became depressed and withdrawn. Because she had not been included in the planning discussions, she assumed this confusion was her mother's fault. However, none of this was disclosed until the child described the events to the nurse. During the next session with the teacher, she and her mother explained the physical limitations imposed by the illness. All agreed that if there were any further changes in teachers, it would be the child's responsibility to clarify the situation.

Once the child returns, regular assessments of his progress are essential to assure a satisfactory adjustment. For example, some children appear to be doing well by investing all of their energies in academic endeavors to the detriment of social and/or physical activities. In essence the scholastic achievement may represent a retreat from other areas of school life that are equally important.

Classroom peers also need preparation, and a joint plan between the school teacher, nurse, and child is best. At a minimum the classmates should be given a description of the child's condition, prepared for any visible changes in the child, and allowed an opportunity to ask questions. The child should have the option of attending this session. As the child's condition changes, particularly if the illness is potentially fatal, school personnel, including the students, need periodic appraisal of the child's status and preparation for what to expect (see also p. 972).*

---

*Several publications are available to help prepare school personnel, health professionals, and families for the child's return to school and are listed at the end of this chapter.

Children with special needs are encouraged to maintain or reestablish relationships with peers and to participate according to their capabilities in any age-appropriate activities. Alternative activities may be substituted for those that are impossible or that place a strain on their condition. It is important for these children to have the opportunity to interact with healthy peers as well as to engage in activities with groups or clubs composed of similarly affected age-mates. Such organizations as ostomy clubs, diabetic clubs, and cerebral palsy groups share information and provide support related to the special problems the members face.

Peer interaction is especially important in relation to cognitive development, social development, and maturation. Cognitive development is facilitated by interaction—by exploration of personal, social, and ethical values with peers, parents, and teachers. Youngsters whose isolation hampers their ability to interact with peers miss this opportunity to expand their thinking (Coupey and Cohn, 1980). Too many of these children withdraw to the passive companionship of television.

Adolescence. Adolescence can be a particularly difficult period for the teenager and family. All the needs discussed before apply to this age-group as well; however, fostering independence and autonomy is particularly important at this time. This can be accomplished by encouraging the teenager to assume responsibility for making and keeping appointments (ideally alone), by encouraging self-management of the disease, and by helping him make decisions regarding his life whenever possible. Age-appropriate pursuits are encouraged, such as driving a car, making plans for college, or securing a job. Planning for the future is a prominent concern.

Establish Realistic Future Goals

One of the most difficult adjustments is setting realistic future goals for the child and for those involved in his continued care. Sometimes the impact of this decision does not surface until the child finishes school or the parents near retirement, when a crisis can arise because all the family roles and relationships that maintained stability are now disrupted.

Planning for the future should be a gradual process. All along the parents should cultivate realistic vocations for the child. For example, if the child has a physical handicap, he is directed to intellectual, artistic, or musical pursuits. If the child is developmentally disabled, he is taught a skill that can be performed in a special workshop. In this way the child's development proceeds in the direction of self-support through gainful employment.

With prolonged survival for many chronic illnesses, surviving young people must deal with new decisions and problems, such as marriage, employment, and insurance coverage (see Questions and controversies). With appropriate guidance many of these individuals are capable of gainful employment* and may choose to marry and raise a fam-

---

*Information about employment is available from The President's Committee on Employment of the Handicapped, Washington, DC 20210.

Questions and Controversies

What ethical issues are young people and families facing as a result of improved survival from chronic illness?

Chronically ill adolescents are faced with a number of serious ethical dilemmas as they enter adulthood. For example, should they share the truth of their condition with dating partners, prospective spouses, or potential employers? Should they seek a job with good health insurance rather than pursue a career with less employee benefits? Should they have the right to refuse further treatment, especially when the prospects for cure or even palliation are minimal? Whose wishes should be upheld when a conflict exists between the parents and young person?

Such questions have no clear-cut answers. Rather, adolescents should be encouraged to weigh decisions, investigate alternatives, and choose their own solution (Silber, 1984). For example, in a study of disabled adolescents concerning their decision to have surgery, assessment of the teenager's view of surgery as "routine" or "nonroutine," the adolescent's and parents' goals, the alternatives to surgical intervention, how much power the teenager had in making the decision, and the young person's feelings regarding the decision-making process were important factors in arriving at an answer (Deatrick, 1984).

Consent and confidentiality are frequent dilemmas in providing care to any minor adolescent and are often made more complex by the teenager's health problem. For example, do these adolescents have the right to request health care without parents' knowledge or permission? If they are engaging in potentially hazardous activities, such as the teenager with cystic fibrosis who begins to smoke or the young man with hemophilia who engages in contact sports, should parents be informed? Two principles may be used in resolving such ethical questions: the principle of *autonomy*, which states that a person should have a say in any action that will affect him, and the principle of *benevolence*, which states that whenever something beneficial can be done, it should be done. Obviously, autonomy and benevolence support the adolescent's right to health care. However, in the best interests of the teenager, parents may need to be informed of activities that jeopardize one's life (Silber, 1984).

---

ily. For those whose conditions are genetic, there is the need for counseling regarding future offspring. Prospective spouses often benefit from an opportunity to discuss their feelings regarding marriage to an individual with continued health needs and possibly a limited life span. Health insurance coverage is a critical issue because some private carriers may no longer insure a young person who leaves home or may be unwilling to reinsure the person who is independent. Life insurance is another dilemma, especially when children have serious defects, such as congenital heart anomalies (Truesdell, Skorton, and Lauer, 1986). These issues are only beginning to receive attention but will become increasingly prominent as the number of survivors increases.

Unfortunately vocational pursuits and independence are not realistic goals for all persons. Persons with multiple or severe disabilities may require lifelong care and assistance. In these situations parents must look to the time when they will no longer be able to care for their child. Residential placement may be very difficult unless the family mutually participates in the decision-making and planning process. Institutionalization should not be viewed as abandonment. Not infrequently it is the only way to preserve the family unit. The nurse should help the family investigate suitable placements, discuss their feelings regarding this decision, and explore measures to maintain meaningful communication with the member who has a disability.

CONCEPT SUMMARIES

- Trends in the treatment of children with chronic illness have focused on developmental age, the child's strengths and uniqueness, family, relationships, establishment of normalization, early discharge, home care, and mainstreaming.

- Families' reactions to disability or chronic illness are manifested in the following stages: shock and denial, adjustment, reintegration and acceptance, and freezing out.

- In response to the child with chronic illness or disability, parents may be affected by feelings of inadequacy and failure; excessive demands on time, energy, and financial resources; and strain on spouse communication.

- Effects of chronic illness on siblings include changes in role status, irritability and physical complaints, jealousy, competition, anger, hostility, attention-seeking behavior, social withdrawal, and decline in school performance.

- Major factors affecting the family's adjustment to a child's chronic illness are the availability of a support system, their perception of the event, and their coping mechanisms.

- The coping mechanisms parents use in dealing with the child with chronic illness are approach behaviors—movement toward adjustment and resolution of crisis—and avoidance behaviors—maladaptation or movement away from adjustment.

- The child's reaction to illness or disability depends on developmental level, coping mechanisms, others' reactions, and the illness itself.

- Mutual participation in care by child and parent facilitates better communication and alleviates feelings of parental inadequacy and child inferiority.

- Assessment of the family's coping mechanisms and reactions entails understanding the family's functioning and observing the child in home and school.

- To help parents cope with their child's chronic illness, nurses must offer attentiveness, humanistic support, solicitation of suggestions for care, facilitation of communication, verbalization of feelings, and referral to volunteer and community agencies.

- Supporting the child involves encouraging self-expression, alleviating feelings of being different, and strengthening self-image.

- Fostering reality adjustment entails supplying information about the disorder, promoting normal development, and establishing realistic future goals.

REFERENCES

American Academy of Pediatrics: Official statement to the Committee on Children with Handicaps, The Developmental Disability Council, U.S. Department of Health, Education and Welfare, April 1979.

Beisser, A.: Denial and affirmation in illness and health, Am. J. Psychiatry 136(8):1026-1030, 1979.

Bernard, B., and others: Exercise for children with physical disabilities, Issues Compr. Pediatr. Nurs. 5:99-107, 1981.

Blacher, J.: Sequential stages of parental adjustment to the birth of a child with handicaps: fact or artifact? Ment. Retard. 22(2):55-68, 1984.

Bock, R.H., and others: There's no place like home, Children's Health Care 12(2):93-96, 1983.

Boone, D.R., and Hartman, B.H.: The benevolent over-reaction, Clin. Pediatr. 11(5):268-271, 1972.

Brandt, P.A.: Clinical assessment of the social support of families with handicapped children, Issues Compr. Pediatr. Nurs. 7:187-201, 1984.

Breslau, N., Weitzman, M., and Messenger, K.: Psychologic functioning of siblings of disabled children, Pediatrics 67(3):344-353, 1981.

Byrne, E.A., and Cunningham, C.C.: The effects of mentally handicapped children on families—a conceptual review, J. Child. Psychol. Psychiatry 26(6):847-864, 1985.

Case, J., and Matthews, S.: CHIP: the chronic health impaired program of the Baltimore City Public School System, Child. Health Care 12(2):97-99, 1983.

Childs, R.: Maternal psychological conflicts associated with the birth of a retarded child, Am. J. Maternal Child Nurs. 14(3):175-182, 1985.

Cleveland, M.: Family adaptation to traumatic spinal cord injury: response to crisis, Family Relations 29:558-565, 1980.

Coupey, S., and Cohen, M.: A developmental approach to the chronically ill adolescent, Feelings Med. Signif. 22(2): 7-10, 1980.

Coupey, S., and Cohen, M.: Special considerations for the health care of adolescents with chronic illnesses, Pediatr. Clin. North Am. 31(1):211-219, 1984.

Deatrick, J.A.: It's their decision now: perspectives of chronically disabled adolescents concerning surgery, Issues Compr. Pediatr. Nurs. 7:17-31, 1984.

Desch, L.W.: High technology for handicapped children: a pediatrician's viewpoint, Pediatrics 77(1):71-87, 1986.

Epstein, C.: Nursing the dying patient, Reston, VA, 1975, Reston Publishing Co.

Fife, B.L., Huhman, M., and Keck, J.: Development of a clinical assessment scale: evaluation of the psychosocial impact of childhood illness on the family, Issues Compr. Pediatr. Nurs. 9(1):11-31, 1986.

Friedrich, W.: Predictors of the coping behavior of mothers of handicapped children, J. Consult. Clin. Psychol. 47:1140-1141, 1979.

Gorham, K.A., and others: Effects on parents. In Hobbs, N., editor: Issues in the classification of children, San Francisco, 1975, Jossey-Bass, Inc., Publishers.

Gortmaker, S.L., and Sappenfield, W.: Chronic childhood disorders: prevalence and impact, Pediatr. Clin. North Am. 31(1):3-18, 1984.

Gratz, R.R., and Piliavin, J.A.: What makes kids sick: children's beliefs about the causative factors of illness, Child. Health Care 12(4):156-162, 1984.

Halpern, R.: Physician-parent communication in the diagnosis of child handicap: a brief review, Child. Health Care 12(4):170-173, 1984.

Harkey, J.: The epidemiology of selected chronic childhood health conditions, Child. Health Care 12(2):62-71, 1983.

Hedahl, K.J.: Helping children establish positive attitudes towards disabled persons, Pediatr. Nurs. 7(6):11-15, 1981.

Hobbs, N., and Perrin, J.M., editors: Issues in the care of children with chronic illness, San Francisco, 1985, Jossey-Bass Inc.

Hofmann, A.D.: Managing handicapped adolescents with impaired body image, Feelings Med. Signif. 22(4):13-18, 1980.

Hymovich, D.P.: The chronicity impact and coping instrument: parent questionnaire, Nurs. Res. 32(5):275-281, 1983.

Johnson, B.H., and Steele, B.B.: Community networking for improved services to children with chronic illnesses and their families, Child. Health Care 12(2):100-102, 1983.

Johnson, M.P.: Support groups for parents of chronically ill children, Pediatr. Nurs. **8**(3):160-163, 1982.

Kalnins, I.: Cross-illness comparisons of separation and divorce among parents having a child with a life-threatening illness, Child. Health Care **12**(2):72-77, 1983.

Klopovich, P., and others: School phobia, J. Kans. Med. Soc. **82**(3):125-127, 1981.

Koocher, G.P., and O'Malley, J.E.: The Damocles syndrome, New York, 1981, McGraw-Hill Book Co.

Krulik, T.: Successful "normalizing" tactics of parents of chronically ill children, J. Adv. Nurs. **5**(6):573-578, 1980.

Lansky, S.B.: Management of stressful periods in childhood cancer, Pediatr. Clin. North Am. **32**(3):62-63, 1985.

Lavigne, J.V., and Ryan, M.: Psychologic adjustment of siblings of children with chronic illness, Pediatrics **63**(4):616-627, 1979.

Mattsson, A.: Long-term physical illness in childhood: a challenge to psychosocial adaptation, Pediatrics **50**(5):801-811, 1972.

McDermott, J.F., and Akina, E.: Understanding and improving the personality development of children with physical handicaps, Clin. Pediatr. **11**(3):130-134, 1972.

McKeever, P.T.: Fathering the chronically ill child, Am. J. Maternal Child Nurs. **6**(2):124-128, 1981.

Molter, N.C.: Needs of relatives of critically ill patients: a descriptive study, Heart Lung **8**(2):332-339, 1979.

Mulhern, R.K., Crisco, J.J., and Camitta, B.M.: Patterns of communication among pediatric patients with leukemia, parents, and physicians: prognostic disagreements and misunderstandings, J. Pediatr. **99**(3):480-483, 1981.

Nolan, T., and others: Knowledge of cystic fibrosis in patients and their parents, Pediatrics **77**(2):229-235, 1986.

O'Malley, J.E., and others: Psychiatric sequelae of surviving childhood cancer, Am. J. Orthopsychiatry **49**(4):608-616, 1979.

Orr, D.P., and others: Psychosocial implications of chronic illness in adolescence, J. Pediatr. **104**(1):152-157, 1984.

Palfrey, J.S.: Commentary: P.L. 94-142: the Education for All Handicapped Children Act, J. Pediatr. **97**(3):417-419, 1980.

Perrin, E.C., and Gerrity, P.S.: Development of children with a chronic illness, Pediatr. Clin. North Am. **31**(1):19-31, 1984.

Perrin, J.M., and Ireys, H.T.: The organization of services for chronically ill children and their families, Pediatr. Clin. North Am. **31**(1):235-257, 1984.

Pierce, P.M., and Freedman, S.A.: The REACH project: an innovative health delivery model for medically dependent children, Child. Health Care **12**(2):86-89, 1983.

Pless, I.B.: Clinical assessment: physical and psychological functioning, Pediatr. Clin. North Am. **31**(1):33-45, 1984.

Reynolds, M.C.: The educational needs of disabled children and youths. In Blum, R., editor: Chronic illness and disabilities in childhood and adolescence, New York, 1984, Grune & Stratton, Inc.

Robinson, C.: Double bind: a dilemma for parents of chronically ill children, Pediatr. Nurs. **11**(2):112-115, 1985.

Rush, W.L., and The League of Human Dignity: Write with dignity: reporting on people with disabilities, Lincoln, NB, 1983, Hitchcock Center.

Rutter, M.: Stress, coping, and development: some issues and some questions. In Garmezy, N., and Rutter, M., editors: Stress, coping, and development in children, New York, 1983, McGraw-Hill Book Co.

Sabbeth, B.F., and Leventhal, J.M.: Marital adjustment to chronic childhood illness: a critique of the literature, Pediatrics **73**(6):762-768, 1984.

Schulman, J.: Coping with major disease: child, family, pediatrician, J. Pediatr. **102**(6):988-991, 1983.

Siemon, M.: Siblings of the chronically ill or disabled child: meeting their needs, Nurs. Clin. North Am. **19**(2):295-307, 1984.

Silber, T.J.: Ethical considerations in the care of the chronically ill adolescent. In Blum, R., editor: Chronic illness and disabilities in childhood and adolescence, New York, 1984, Grune & Stratton, Inc.

Stein, R.: A home care program for children with chronic illness, Child. Health Care **12**(2):90-92, 1983.

Stein, R.E.K.: Home care: a challenging opportunity, Child. Health Care **14**(2):90-95, 1985.

Strauss, S.S., and Munton, M.: Common concerns of parents with disabled children, Pediatr. Nurs. **11**(5):371-375, 1985.

Taylor, S.C.: The effects of chronic childhood illnesses upon well siblings, Am. J. Maternal Child Nurs. **9**(2):109-116, 1980.

Truesdell, S.C., Skorton, D.J., and Lauer, R.M.: Life insurance for children with cardiovascular disease, Pediatrics **77**(5):687-691, 1986.

Venters, M.: Familial coping with chronic and severe childhood illness: the case of cystic fibrosis, Soc. Sci. Med. **15A**:289-297, 1981.

Waller, D.A., and others: Coping with poor prognosis in the pediatric intensive care unit, Am. J. Dis. Child. **133**:1121-1125, Nov. 1979.

Warren, R., and Cohen, S.: Respite care, Rehab. Lit. **46**(3-4):66-71, 1985.

Weitzman, M., Walker, D.K., and Gortmaker, S.: Chronic illness, psychosocial problems, and school absences, Clin. Pediatr. **25**(3):137-141, 1986.

Wikler, L., and others: Chronic sorrow revisited: parent vs. professional depiction of the adjustment of parents of mentally retarded children, Am. J. Orthopsychiatry **51**(1):63-70, 1981.

Young, R.K.: Chronic sorrow: parents' response to the birth of a child with a defect, Am. J. Maternal Child Nurs. **2**(1):38-42, 1977.

Zelter, L., and others: Psychologic effects of illness in adolescence. II. Impact of illness in adolescents—crucial issues and coping styles, J. Pediatr. **97**(1):132-138, 1980.

BIBLIOGRAPHY

Ahmann, E.: An annotated bibliography on respite care for children and families, Child. Health Care **14**(3):183-186, 1986.

American Academy of Pediatrics, Ad Hoc Task Forces on Home Care of Chronically Ill Infants and Children: Guidelines for home care of infants, children and adolescents with chronic disease, Pediatrics **74**(3):434-436, 1984.

Anastasiow, N.J.: Early childhood education for the handicapped in the 1980's: recommendations, Except. Child. **47**(4):276-282, 1981.

Anderson, J.M.: The social construction of illness experience: families with a chronically-ill child, J. Adv. Pediatr. **6**(6):427-434, 1981.

Bakke, K.: Ethical dilemmas: institutionalizing a severely disabled child, Pediatr. Nurs. **7**(6):27-29, 1981.

Baskin, C.H., and others: Helping teachers help children with cancer: a workshop for school personnel, Child. Health Care **12**(2):78-83, 1983.

Beck, J.: The school nurse and the child with cancer. In Spinetta, J., and Deasy-Spinetta, editors: Living with childhood cancer, St. Louis, 1981, The C.V. Mosby Co.

Becker, R.D.C.: Illness and hospitalization in adolescence: a developmental perspective, Paediatrician **9**:242-260, 1980.

Berger, L.R., and Samet, K.P.: Home visits: extending the boundaries of comprehensive pediatric care, Am. J. Dis. Child. **135**:812-814, 1981.

Bernardo, M.L.: Premarital counseling and the couple with disabilities: a review and recommendations, Rehab. Lit. **42**(7-8):213-217, 1981.

Bernardo, M.L.: A conceptual model of children's cognitive adaptation to physical disability, J. Adv. Nurs. **7**:595-601, 1982.

Black, F.W., Gasparrini, B., and Nelson, R.: Parental assessment of temperament in handicapped children, J. Personality Assessment **45**(2):155-158, 1981.

Blum, R.: Chronic illness and disabilities in childhood and adolescence, New York, 1984, Grune & Stratton.

Boren, H.A., and Meell, H.: Adolescent amputee ski rehabilitation program, J. Assoc. Pediatr. Oncol. Nurses **2**(1):16-23, 1985.

Brewster, A.B.: Chronically ill hospitalized children's concepts of their illness, Pediatrics 69(3):355-362, 1982.

Buzinski, P.: Groups for brothers and sisters of developmentally disabled children: one component of a family-centered approach, Issues Compr. Pediatr. Nurs. 4(5-6):45-50, 1980.

Cairns, N., and others: School attendance of children with cancer, J. School Health 52:152-155, 1982.

Cohen, S.: Support families through respite care, Rehab. Lit. 43(1-2):7-11, 1982.

Craft, M.: Help for the family's neglected "other" child, Am. J. Maternal Child Nurs. 4(5):297-300, 1979.

Crummette, B.: Assessing the impact of illness upon an adolescent and family, Am. J. Maternal Child Nurs. 12(3):155-167, 1983.

Darling, R.B., and Darling, J.: Children who are different: meeting the challenges of birth defects in society, St. Louis, 1982, The C.V. Mosby.

Dasson, M.E.: A chance to be normal again, Cancer Nurs. 5(6):453-459, 1982.

Del Campo, E., and Josephson, D.: Accommodating the severely retarded child in our schools, Am. J. Maternal Child Nurs. 3(1):34-37, 1978.

Doernberg, N.L.: Some negative effects on family integration of health and educational services for young handicapped children, Rehab. Lit. 39(4):107-110, 1978.

Drotar, D.: Psychological perspectives in chronic childhood illness, J. Pediatr. Psychol. 6(3):211-228, 1981.

Drotar, D.: Psychosocial functioning of children with cystic fibrosis, Pediatrics 67(3):338-343, 1981.

Fostel, C.: Chronic illness and handicapping conditions: coping patterns of the child and the family. In Brandt, P., and others, editors: Current practice in pediatric nursing, vol. II, St. Louis, 1978, The C.V. Mosby Co.

Fowler, M.G., Johnson, M.P., and Atkinson, S.S.: School achievement and absence in children with chronic health conditions, J. Pediatr. 106(4):683-687, 1985.

Frauman, A.C., and Sypert, N.S.: Sexuality in adolescents with chronic illness, Am. J. Maternal Child Nurs. 4(6):371-375, 1979.

Ganz, R.H.: Chronic illness? Help the family cope, Patient Care 15:23-53, June 1981.

Ganz, R.H.: Child chronically ill? Follow the family, Patient Care 15:199-231, Aug. 1981.

Gearheart, B., and Weishahn, M.: The handicapped child in the regular classroom, ed. 2, St. Louis, 1980, The C.V. Mosby Co.

Geist, R.A.: Onset of chronic illness in children and adolescents: psychotherapeutic and consultative intervention, Am. J. Orthopsychiatry 49(1):4-23, 1979.

Goldberg, R.T.: Toward an understanding of the rehabilitation of the disabled adolescent, Rehab. Lit. 42(3-4):66-74, 1981.

Goldfarb, L.A., and others: Meeting the challenge of disability or chronic illness—a family guide, Baltimore, 1985, Brookes Publishing Co.

Goodell, A.: Peer education in schools for children with cancer, Issues Compr. Pediatr. Nurs. 7:101-106, 1984.

Grant, W.W.: What parents of a chronically ill or dysfunctioning child always want to know but may be afraid to ask, Clin. Pediatr. 17(12):915-917, 1978.

Hall, D.M.B.: The child with a handicap, Boston, 1984, Blackwell Scientific Publications.

Halpern, P.: Respite care and family functioning in families with retarded children, Health Soc. Work 10(2):138-150, 1985.

Harding, R.K., Heller, J.R., and Kesler, R.W.: The chronically ill child in the primary care setting, Primary Care 6(2):311-324, 1979.

Hendahl, K.J.: Helping children establish positive attitudes towards disabled persons, Pediatr. Nurs. 7(6):11-15, 1981.

Henning, J., and Fritz, G.K.: School reentry in childhood cancer, Psychosomatics 24(3):261-269, 1983.

Holaday, B.: Parenting the chronically ill child. In Brandt, P., and others, editors: Current practice in pediatric nursing, vol. II, St. Louis, 1978, The C.V. Mosby Co.

Hughes, J.H., and Hurth, J.L.: Handicapped children and mainstreaming: a mental health perspective; review of model school programs and practices, Pub. No. (ADM) 84-1361, Rockville, MD, 1984, U.S. Department of Health and Human Services Public Health Service, Alcohol, Drug Abuse, and Mental Health Administration.

Hughes, M.C.: Chronically ill children in groups: recurrent issues and adaptations, Am. J. Orthopsychiatry 52(4):704-711, 1982.

Hussey, C.: Surviving a handicap in everday life: how to help, Am. J. Maternal Child Nurs. 4(1):46-50, 1979.

Hymovich, D.P.: Assessing the impact of chronic childhood illness on the family and parent coping, Image 13:71-73, Oct. 1981.

Isaacs, J., and McElroy, M.R.: Psychosocial aspects of chronic illness in children, J. School Health 50:318-321, 1980.

Iscoe, L., and Bordelon, K.: Pilot parents: peer support for parents of handicapped children, Child. Health Care 14(2):103, 1985.

Jelneck, L.J.: The special needs of the adolescent with chronic illness, Am. J. Maternal Child Nurs. 2(1):57-61, 1977.

Kellerman, J., and others: Psychological effects of illness in adolescence. I. Anxiety, self-esteem, and perception of control, J. Pediatr. 97:126-131, 1980.

Kinrade, L.C.: Preventive group intervention with siblings of oncology patients, Child. Health Care 14(2):110, 1985.

Knowles, R.D.: Handling anger: responding vs. reacting, Am. J. Nurs. 81(12):2196, 1981.

Knox, J.E., and Hayes, V.E.: Hospitalization of a chronically ill child: a stressful time for parents, Issues Compr. Pediatr. Nurs. 6:217-226, 1983.

Kodadek, S.: Family-centered care of the chronically ill child, AORN J. 30(4):635-638, 1979.

Kornblatt, E.S., and Heinrich, J.: Needs and coping abilities in families of children with developmental disabilites, Ment. Retard. 23(1):13-19, 1985.

Lansky, S.B., and others: School phobia in children with malignant neoplasms, Am. J. Dis. Child. 129:42-46, 1975.

Lansky, S.B., and others: Childhood cancer: parental discord and divorce, Pediatrics 62(2):184-188, 1978.

Lepler, M.: Having a handicapped child, Am. J. Maternal Child Nurs. 3(1):32-33, 1978.

Levenson, P.M., and Singer, B.: Using computers to help children cope with chronic illness, Child. Health Care 14(2):76, 1985.

Leventhal, J.M.: Psychosocial assessment of children with chronic physical disease, Pediatr. Clin. North Am. 31(1):71-86, 1984.

Lloyd, J.K.: Dietary problems associated with the care of the chronically sick children, J. Hum. Nutr. 33(2):135-139, 1979.

McLane, J.B.: Lekotek: a unique play library for families with handicapped children, Child. Health Care 14(3):178-182, 1986.

Mink, I.R., Nihira, K., and Meyers, C.E.: Taxonomy of family life styles: I. Homes with TMR children, Am. J. Ment. Defic. 87(5):484-497, 1983.

Morrow, G.R., Hoagland, A.C., and Morse, I.P.: Sources of support perceived by parents of children with cancer: implications for counselling, Patient Counselling Health Ed. 4(1):36-40, 1982.

Nathan, S.W., and Goetz, P.: Psychosocial aspects of chronic illness: group interactions in diabetic girls, Child. Health Care 13(1):24-30, 1984.

Neill, K.: Behavioral aspects of chronic physical disease, Nurs. Clin. North Am. 14(3):443-457, 1979.

Nelms, B.C.: Stress during childhood: long-lasting effects? Pediatr. Nurs. 11(2):95-98, 1985.

Oppenheimer, J.R., and Rucker, R.W.: The effect of parental relationships on the management of cystic fibrosis and guidelines for social work intervention, Soc. Work Health Care 5(4):409-419, 1980.

Oremland, E.: Communicating over chronic illness: dilemmas of affected school-aged children, Child. Health Care 14(4):218-223, 1986.

Patton, A.C., Ventura, J.N., and Savedra, M.: Stress and coping responses of adolescents with cystic fibrosis, Child. Health Care 14(3):153-156, 1986.

Pi, E.H.: Congenitally handicapped children and their families: short- and long-term intervention, Pediatr. Basics 31:10-14, 1981.

Pidgeon, V.: Children's concepts of illness: implications for health teaching, Issues Compr. Pediatr. Nurs. 14(1):23-35, 1985.

Pierce, P.M., and Giovinco, G.: Reach: self-care for the chronically ill child, Pediatr. Nurs. 9(1):37-40, 1983.

Pilon, B.H., and Smith, K.A.: A parent group for the Hispanic parents of children with severe cerebral palsy, Child. Health Care 14(2):96-102, 1985.

Pipes, P.L., and Pritkin, R.: Nutrition and feeding of children with developmental delays and related problems. In Pipes, P.L., editor: Nutrition in infancy and childhood, ed. 3, St. Louis, 1985, The C.V. Mosby Co.

Pollard, A., and others: School and the child with cancer: a program to assist school personnel, J. Assoc. Pediatr. Oncol. Nurses 2(3):7-10, 1985.

Redman-Bentley, D.: Parent expectations for professionals providing services to their handicapped children, Phys. Occupational Ther. Pediatr. 2(1):13-27, 1982.

Rose, M.H.: The concepts of coping and vulnerability as applied to children with chronic conditions, Issues Compr. Pediatr. Nurs. 7:177-186, 1984.

Sabbeth, B.: Understanding the impact of chronic childhood illness on families, Pediatr. Clin. North Am. 31(1):47-57, 1984.

Sachs, M.B.: Helping the child with cancer go back to school, J. School Health 50(6):328-331, 1980.

Sahin, S.: The physically disabled child. In Johnson, S., editor: Nursing assessment and strategies for the family at risk, ed. 2, Philadelphia, 1986, J.B. Lippincott Co.

Sargeant, A.: The sick child and the family, J. Pediatr. 102(6):982-987, 1983.

Sargent, J.: The sick child: family complications, Dev. Behav. Pediatr. 4(1):50-56, 1983.

Satterwhite, B.B.: Impact of chronic illness on child and family: an overview based on five surveys with implications for management, Int. J. Rehab. Res. 1(1):7-17, 1978.

Scanlon, M.K.: A chronically ill child's progression through the separation-individuation process, Am. J. Maternal Child Nurs. 14(2):91-102, 1985.

Scheiner, A., and Abroms, F., editors: The practical management of the developmentally disabled child, St. Louis, 1980, The C.V. Mosby Co.

Schonberg, S.K., and Cohen, M.I.: Health needs of the adolescent, Paediatrician 8(Suppl. 1):131-140, 1979.

Seidle, A.H., and Altshuler, A.: Interventions for adolescents who are chronically ill, Child. Today 8(6):16-19, 1979.

Shelly, J.A.: Spiritual care ... planting seeds of hope, Crit. Care Update 9(12):7-15, 1982.

Shields, J.M., Abrams, P., and Siegel, S.: An alternative health care setting for children with cancer: a residential summer camp, Child. Health Care 13(3):135-138, 1985.

Shopper, M.: Chronic illness: long-term management of the child and the family, Child Care Newsletter 4(1):7-11, 1985.

Silberman, M.A., Fochtman, D., and Baum, E.S.: One step at a time: summer camping for children with cancer, J. Assoc. Pediatr. Oncology Nurses 2(1):24-30, 1985.

Silverman, M.: Beyond the mainstream: the special needs of the chronic child patient, Am. J. Orthopsychiatry 49(1):62-68, 1979.

Slonim, M.B.: Depression in the chronically ill or handicapped, Am. J. Maternal Child Nurs. 6(4):266-273, 1981.

Sperling, E.: Psychological issues in chronic illness and handicap. In Gellert, E., editor: Psychosocial aspects of pediatric care, New York, 1978, Grune & Stratton, Inc.

Stearns, S.E.: Understanding the psychological adjustment of physically handicapped children in the classroom, Child. Today 10(1):12-15, Feb. 1981.

Stein, R.E.K.: Growing up with a physical difference, Child. Health Care 12(2):53-61, 1983.

Stein, R.E.K., and Jessop, D.J.: General issues in the care of children with chronic physical conditions, Pediatr. Clin. North Am. 31(1):189-198, 1984.

Stein, R.E.K., and Riessman, C.K.: The development of an impact-on-family scale: preliminary findings, Med. Care 18(4):465-472, 1980.

Steinhausen, H.C.: Chronically ill and handicapped children and adolescents: personality studies in relation to disease, J. Abnormal Child Psychol. 9(2):291-297, 1981.

Stutzman, H.: Explaining leukemia to classmates, J. Assoc. Pediatr. Oncology Nurses 2(1):15, 1985.

Tamlyn, D., and Arklie, M.M.: A theoretical framework for standard care plans: a nursing approach for working with chronically ill children and their families, Issues Compr. Pediatr. Nurs. 9(1):39-45, 1986.

Thomas, R.B.: Nursing assessment of childhood chronic conditions, Issues Compr. Pediatr. Nurs. 7:165-176, 1984.

Wacht, M.: The mentally disabled child. In Johnson, S., editor: Nursing assessment and strategies for the family at risk, ed. 2, Philadelphia, 1986, J.B. Lippincott Co.

Walker, D.K.: Care of chronically ill children in schools, Pediatr. Clin. North Am. 31(1):221-233, 1984.

Weale, J., and Bradshaw, J.: Prevalence and characteristics of disabled children: findings from the 1974 general household survey, J. Epidemiol. Comm. Health 34(2):111-118, 1980.

Weitzman, M.: School and peer relations, Pediatr. Clin. North Am. 31(1):59-69, 1984.

West, M.: The mother, the developmentally disabled child and the nurse, Top. Clin. Nurs. 6:19-29, 1984.

Zamerowski, S.T.: Helping families to cope with handicapped children, Top. Clin. Nurs. 4:41-56, July 1982.

Zelle, R.S.: The developmentally disabled child and the family. In Hymovich, D.P., and Barnard, M.U.: Family health care, New York, 1979, McGraw-Hill Book Co.

Publications for School Attendance

Klopovich, P., and others: Cancer in the classroom: how do you cope? Kansas City, KS, Mid-America Cancer Center and University of Kansas Medical Center.

Morrow, G.: Helping chronically ill children in school, New York, 1985; Parker Publishing Co., Inc.

School nurses working with handicapped children: a statement of the American Nurses' Association Divisions on Nursing Practice, the American School Health Association, and The National Association of School Nurses, ANA Publication No. PN-60, Kansas City, MO, 1980, American Nurses' Association.

Students with cancer: a resource for the educator, U.S. Department of Health and Human Services, National Institutes of Health, NIH Pub. No. 84-2086, Washington, D.C., 1984. (Order from Office of Cancer Communications, National Cancer Institute, Building 31, Room 10A18, Bethesda, MD 20205).

Suggestions for teachers and school counselors, Oak Brook, IL, 1983, The Compassionate Friends.

When your child is ready to return to school, Chicago, 1982, Association for Brain Tumor Research.

Chapter 23

Impact of Life-Threatening Illness on the Child and Family

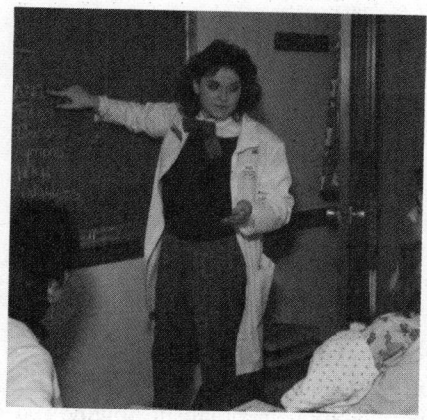

Although most childhood illnesses respond favorably to treatment, some do not. However, with advances in treatment many invariably fatal illnesses are now amenable to a prolonged period of remission and possibly cure. Despite this, families constantly live under the threat of potential loss of their child. As a result, health professionals are faced with the challenge of providing the best care possible to meet the family's psychologic and emotional needs both during the course of the illness and at the time of death.

There is probably no more difficult death to face than that of a child, because the end of life is premature and parents are robbed the fulfillment and joy of seeing their child grow. It is the purpose of this chapter to establish some theoretic and practical guidelines for helping families cope with the loss of a child. An overview of children's concept of death, the grieving process before and after death, each family member's reaction to a life-threatening illness, and nursing interventions to assist the family through each phase of the illness are presented. In providing care during this difficult time, there are no absolute, definitive answers, only the personal willingness to become involved, to feel the child's and family's suffering, and to find one's own answers through individual experiences and dedicated learning.

Children and Death

Most children have relatively little experience with death. However, for some the tragedy of death becomes an indelible memory, and the reactions of others to their loss greatly influence how this event affects their lives. The following discussion is concerned with the development of the death concept in children and awareness of fatally ill children of their own death.

CHILDREN'S UNDERSTANDING OF AND REACTIONS TO DYING AND DEATH

The concept of death is acquired through the sequential development of cognitive abilities, and follows closely Piaget's stages. Although throughout childhood death is greatly influenced by the child's personal experiences with it and the explanations and attitudes offered by others, the abstract adult meaning of death as irreversible, inevitable, and universal is not understood by most children until preadolescence. Unless nurses understand how children perceive death, their fears associated with death in each age-group, and the personal meanings of death and bereavement during various stages of development, they cannot effectively counsel parents and children through the multiple crises associated with expected or unexpected death.

Knowledge about preschool and older children's concept of death is primarily based on the work of Maria Nagy (1948), who asked several hundred Hungarian children ranging in age from 3 to 10 years to draw pictures and write down (if they were old enough) everything they could think of about death. From analyzing their responses, she concluded that there were three main stages of death interpretation. Although more recent studies have corroborated most of her findings, they have not found evidence of the personification seen in school-age children, but support for a concrete connotation of death, with naturalistic explanations about why people die, such as from old age or a gunshot wound (Table 23-1) (Wass, 1985). These findings may reflect differences in the religious and cultural orientation of the children studied by Nagy and those studied by current investigators.

Infants and Toddlers

Exactly how preverbal children view death is a mystery because there is no way of reliably assessing their views of death. It is quite likely, on the basis of their cognitive abilities, that they have no concept of death. Toddlers' egocentricity and vague separation of fact and fantasy make it impossible for them to comprehend absence of life. Although they may repeat what initially sounds like a correct definition of death, such as, "Grandpa is dead; he went to heaven," they may later refer to Grandpa as if he still exists. They can only think about events in terms of their own frame of reference—living.

Table 23-1 Children's concept of death	
COGNITIVE STAGE	**CONCEPT**
Sensorimotor (infancy, toddler)	No concept of death but reacts to loss
Preoperational thought (early childhood)	Death is temporary and reversible Death is seen as a departure or separation
Concrete operations (school age)	Death is irreversible but not necessarily inevitable Death may be personified and viewed as destructive Explanations for death are naturalistic and physiologic
Formal operations (later school age, adolescence)	Death is irreversible, universal, and inevitable Death is still seen as personal but distant event Explanations for death are physiologic and theologic

Reactions to dying. Immobilization, regression to less independent levels of behavior, separation, intrusive or painful procedures, and alteration in ritualistic routine represent the greatest threats to children in this age-group. However, they may perceive the seriousness of their illness from the parents' reactions of anxiety, sadness, depression, or anger. Although the children are unaware of the reason for such emotions, they are disturbed and upset by their parents' behavior. Helping parents deal with their feelings allows them more emotional reserve to meet the needs of their children. Encouraging them to stay in the hospital as much as possible and to participate in the child's care promotes the parents' and child's adjustment to a serious, potentially fatal illness.

Reactions to death. To the amazement and dismay of adults, toddlers may persist in wanting to visit the dead person, request that all that person's possessions and living quarters remain unchanged, and talk about the deceased as if nothing has happened. Dealing honestly and openly with such reactions is preferable to admonishing the child or trying to prove to him what dead means. For example, the parent can restate that the person cannot visit because he is dead and in a special place (cemetery, heaven, or other explanation) and can offer to bring the child to visit the burial plot if possible.

Ritualism is extremely important to toddlers, so any change in the home following the death can produce anxiety. There is no harm in allowing the ritualism, such as setting an extra place at the table for the deceased person, because, for the child, imagining the person to be present is almost as real as life. What is important is to stress that, although the place is set at the table, the dead person will return only in thoughts and memories. As the child grows older, forms new attachments, and develops stronger ego defenses, he will be increasingly able and willing to let go of this fantasy person.

Preschool Children

Several characteristics of preschoolers' cognitive and psychologic development affect their conception of death. Because of their sense of precausality, they are unable to differentiate physical cause from logical or psychologic motivation. In addition, their egocentricity implies a tremendous sense of self-power and omnipotence. Therefore they believe that their thought is sufficient to cause events. The consequence of such magical thinking is the burden of guilt, shame, and punishment.

Concept of death. Children between ages 3 and 5 have usually heard the word "death" and have some connotation of its meaning. They see death as a departure, possibly as a kind of sleep. They may recognize the fact of physical death but do not separate it from living abilities. The dead person in the coffin still breathes, eats, sleeps, and so on. Death is temporary and gradual; life and death can change places with one another. Because of their immature concept of time, there is no real understanding of the universality and inevitability of death. Words such as "forever" and "everyone" have meaning only in the child's egocentric thinking. Waiting until Christmas may be "forever," and anybody the child denotes is "everyone."

Preschoolers' psychosexual development heavily influences their understanding of death. They strongly identify with the parent of the opposite sex and wish to replace the same-sex parent. Casual expressions such as a daughter's desire to marry her father are evidence of this attachment to the opposite-sex parent. Usually this Oedipus or Electra complex is resolved by eventually identifying with the same-sex parent in terms of role functions. However, if the same-sex parent should die during this time, preschoolers feel responsible for the death because of their wishes to rid themselves of the competition. If the opposite-sex parent dies, they may be troubled because the desired object is taken from them.

Reactions to dying. If preschoolers become seriously ill during this time, they conceive of the illness as a punishment for their thoughts or actions. The usual diagnostic and treatment procedures, combined with enforced hospitalization, only confirm their belief that they are being punished. If the parents do not stay with them during hospitalization or prevent the traumatic procedures, they are convinced that the parents are retaliating for the child's previous misdeeds or bad thoughts.

The same principles of magical thinking and omnipotence affect preschoolers when a sibling becomes critically ill or dies. One of the most significant types of death is sudden infant death syndrome (SIDS). Because it occurs unexpectedly to a healthy infant, who may have been rejected and unwanted by a jealous sibling, preschoolers find no evidence to support a physical cause of death. Indeed the parents are frequently unaware of the reason for the fatality and

may question any possible cause. If preschoolers are in any way accused or suspected of having harmed the infant, they may feel extremely guilty and responsible for the tragedy. On observing their parents' acute grief, they may interpret the anger or depression as a rejection of them.

When a sibling becomes ill, the well siblings experience the loss of routine and parental attention. It is natural for them to resent such disruptions and to blame the changes on the ill child. However, preschoolers have less ability to understand the reasons for the parents' prolonged absence from the home than older children. Even though parents may explain how ill the sibling is, what the hospital is like, and why they must be there, preschoolers only see the special attention and the material rewards that the ill sister or brother receives. Because they are also unable to differentiate causes for separation of the parents and ill child, they fear that the parents may never return. If they should learn that the ill child may not get well or come home, they interpret this to mean that the parents will also never return. Their greatest fear concerning death is separation from parents.

Reactions to death. In relation to death, preschoolers may engage in activities that seem strange or abnormal to adults. For example, if a pet dies, preschoolers usually request a "funeral" or some ceremony to symbolize their loss. Perceptive parents realize that the function of such rites of passage is as important to the preschooler for the loss of a pet as to an adult for the loss of a significant person. After the "funeral" and "burial," preschoolers may dig up the remains. Many parents are confused by this behavior and label it morbid. However, children have no concept of the irreversible nature of death and must continually reassure themselves that the animal has not returned or gone somewhere else. If left alone to satisfy their curiosity, they will see that the dead animal is still in the ground.

Because young children accept the literal meaning of words, it is important for others to examine the implications of possible explanations for death. Those with a religious affiliation may equate death with an afterlife and explain that dead animals or people go to heaven. The act of digging up the dead pet may be a result of trying to ascertain whether the animal did go to heaven. Parents who are aware of the reason for this behavior can explain that the "soul" goes to heaven but the body remains in the earth. If parents dismiss this activity without some clarification, the child may interpret the religious message as a lie.

Another common euphemism for death is "gone to sleep." Again preschoolers attach the literal meaning of sleep to death and may fear going to sleep for fear of dying or never waking up. One 5-year-old child who had been told that her aunt died because she was very tired refused to engage in any strenuous activity and took naps frequently. Her parents became concerned about her sudden lassitude and finally asked her why she was always tired. The child exclaimed that she *was not* tired; she took naps to avoid fatigue because she did not want to die like her aunt. When the parents explained that her aunt was tired from old age and sickness, not from playing too much or sleeping too little, the child immediately resumed her usual behaviors.

Because of their fewer defense mechanisms for dealing with loss, young children may react to a less significant loss with more outward grief than to the loss of a very significant person. This can be extremely disconcerting to parents who view their child's undisturbed behavior as evidence of his lack of interest or response to the tragedy. However, the reverse is most likely true. The loss is so deep, painful, and threatening that the child must deny it for the present in order to survive its overwhelming impact. Behavioral reactions such as giggling, joking, attracting attention, or regressing to earlier developmental skills indicate the child's need to distance himself from the tremendous loss. Understanding the function of such behaviors and supporting the child through the reactions until such time as he feels enough self-control to grieve will help him gradually resolve the loss.

School-Age Children

Although school-age children have a better understanding of causality, less egocentricity, and advanced perception of time, they still associate misdeeds or bad thoughts with causing death and feel intense guilt and responsibility for the event. However, because of their higher cognitive abilities, they respond well to logical explanations and comprehend the figurative meaning of words more than children in younger age-groups. Although they are less likely to interpret explanations in a purely literal sense, they are still prone to self-referenced definitions. It is important for adults to clarify the meanings of statements and to repeatedly ask them what they think.

Concept of death. Much of what pertains to the preschool period regarding the understanding of death also relates to school-age children, particularly those near 6 or 7 years of age. However, these children have a deeper understanding of death in the concrete sense. According to Nagy, they attempt to ascribe a more comprehensible meaning to the event by personifying death as a devil, God, ghost, or "bogeyman." According to others, they have naturalistic-physiologic explanations of why death occurs and what happens to the dead body. Factual explanations, such as "When you die, your body decays in the ground," are consistent with their concrete thinking.

By age 9 or 10 years most children have an adult concept of death. They realize that it is inevitable, universal, and irreversible. Their attitudes toward death are greatly influenced by the reactions and attitudes of others, particularly their parents.

Reactions to dying. School-age children's increased ability to comprehend and reason poses additional risks for them. They may fear the reason for the illness, communicability of the disease to themselves or others, consequences of the disease on their functioning and relationships with others, and the process of dying and death itself. They tend to fear the expectation of the event more than its realization. Their fear of the unknown is greater than the known; like

preschoolers, their fantasy explanations for the unexpected or unknown are usually much more frightening and extreme than the actual situation. For this reason anticipatory preparation is very necessary and effective. These children respond well to explanations of the disease, names of drugs, and so on. Inasmuch as the developmental task of this age is industry, helping children maintain control over their bodies by understanding what is happening to them and participating in what is done to them allows these youngsters to achieve independence, self-worth, and self-esteem and to avoid a sense of inferiority.

Because dying is loss of control over every aspect of living, the realization of impending death or failing to recover is a tremendous threat to their sense of security and ego strength. These children are likely to exhibit their fear more through verbal uncooperativeness than actual physical aggression. Health professionals may erroneously interpret this behavior as rude, impolite, insolent, or stubborn. In reality the words are conveying the same meaning as physical attempts to run away or to fight others off. This verbal "flight or fight" reaction to stress is a plea for some control and power. Encouraging children to talk about their feelings and providing outlets for aggression through play are means of dealing with this type of uncooperativeness.

Reactions to death. School-age children are very interested in postdeath services, such as wakes, funerals, and burials. They may be inquisitive about what happens to the body—who dresses it, how the body feels, or what happens in an autopsy. Adults sometimes find these questions distressing, particularly when they concern the death of a significant person. However, such inquiries are children's way of assimilating all the facts about death into a concrete, logical framework. Avoiding such questions or fabricating euphemistic stories only confuses and frustrates children's attempts at understanding what may happen *to them* if they should die.

Adolescents

By the time most children reach adolescence they have a mature understanding of death, and as abstract thinking develops there is more questioning of death and related topics, such as the religious meaning of afterlife. However, their other developmental needs, especially identity, make this an exceptionally difficult time for these young people to cope with the loss of a loved one or their own impending death.

Concept of death. Although adolescents have a mature understanding of death, they are still very much influenced by "remnants" of magical thinking and are subject to the feelings of guilt and shame. Adolescents are exploring many new areas of interpersonal relationships, and are likely to see deviations from accepted behavior as reasons for their illness. It is important to clarify that thoughts and activities, especially sexual experimentation, do not cause diseases, such as cancer.

Reactions to dying. Adolescents by far have the most difficulty in coping with death. Although they have reached the level of adult comprehension of the concept of death, they are least likely to accept cessation of life, particularly if it is their own. Developmentally the rejection of death is understandable because the adolescents' tasks are to establish an identity by finding out who they are, what their purpose is, and where they belong. Any suggestion of being different or nonbeing is a tremendous threat to the answers to such questions. Adolescents' concern is for the present much more than the past or future.

Adolescents strive for group acceptance and independence from parental constraints. As a result, they rely on peer rules and beliefs for personal direction and reject opposing parental demands. However, when they are faced with the crisis of serious illness, they may consider themselves alienated from peer associations and unable to communicate with their parents for emotional support. Therefore they may be virtually alone in their struggle for survival.

Healthy adolescents must deal with several maturational crises, such as acceptance of bodily changes and socialization of intensifying sexual impulses. Any threat to either task increases the vulnerability of adolescents to the stress of coping with such crises. The ravages of a terminal illness and the deleterious effects of chemotherapy may be greater concerns than the prospect of dying. Adolescents' orientation to the present compels them to worry about physical changes even more than the prognosis for future recovery.

Sometimes parents fail to understand the emotional impact on the adolescent of side effects from chemotherapy, such as hair loss, weight gain, fatigue, or skin eruptions. They wonder why the adolescent cannot accept the temporary altered body image for the possible benefit of the treatment. Intellectually adolescents can understand the necessity of treatment, but emotionally they have great difficulty in overcoming the feelings of being different, unable to equal others, and physically compromised because of the illness.

Nurses are in a most advantageous position in working with terminally ill adolescents; in the hospital setting they spend the greatest amount of time with them. They can structure the hospital admission to allow for maximum self-control and independence, while allowing the adolescent the opportunity to learn to know the nurse. Answering adolescents' questions honestly, treating them as mature individuals, and respecting their needs for privacy, solitude, and personal expressions of emotions such as anger, sadness, or fear convey to adolescents the adult's true concern for their physical and emotional welfare. Nurses can help parents to communicate with their adolescent children by acting as a role models, avoiding alliances with either parent or child, and allowing parents the opportunity to ventilate their feelings of frustration, incompetence, or failure in an atmosphere of acceptance and nonjudgment.

Reactions to death. The adolescent's reactions to death straddle the transition from childhood to adulthood. Although some teenagers are able to cope with death by expressing appropriate emotions, talking about the loss, and resolving the grief, others may appear undisturbed by the event, extremely angry, or unusually silent and withdrawn. Because of their idealistic view of the world, they may

criticize funeral rites as barbaric, money making, and unnecessary. Their fear of the unknown and inability to deal with these thoughts may prevent them from attending funeral services. They are sometimes horrified and angry over adults' concerns for practical matters such as immediate financial arrangements. Statements such as, ''Daddy isn't even buried yet and you (mother) are worrying about his money,'' can cause great conflict and misunderstanding between child and parent. Helping adults understand why teenagers have such thoughts can avert an unnecessary and painful strain among family members.

Nursing Considerations

Nurses in almost any area of pediatrics have an opportunity to help children develop positive attitudes toward death. First, they can counsel parents regarding children's age-specific understanding of death and appropriate ways to handle behaviors, such as digging up the dead pet.

Second, nurses can encourage parents to take advantage of ''small deaths'' to help children become familiar and more comfortable with loss. The death of a pet, flowers, or a television character may present such an opportunity. Certainly such events should not be covered up, such as replacing a pet with a new one so the child thinks it is the same animal. Many children's books are available that present death in a sensitive and nonthreatening manner and when read to children offer opportunities for dialogue (Fig. 23-1) (see also discussion on p. 196; sources of books are listed at the end of the chapter).

Third, nurses may take part in organized programs on death education, especially in the schools, or serve as resources for planning such programs (Wass and others, 1980). Through formal curriculum devoted to this topic youngsters are introduced to the many facets of death as a part of life. Such programs can also ease the reentry of children with life-threatening disorders back to school.

Finally, nurses can serve as resources to parents and others involved with children in answering questions about

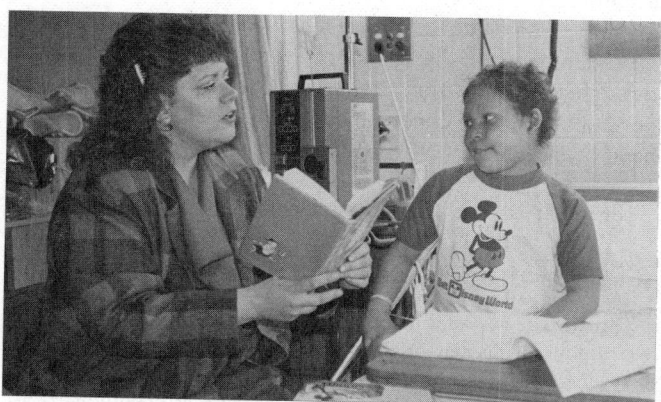

Fig. 23-1. Children can be helped to cope with loss through books with death themes.
Photography by Katherine Patterson, University of Kansas, College of Health Sciences and Hospital, Kansas City, KS.

children and death. For example, many parents are concerned with how to handle "small deaths" constructively or whether young or school-age children should attend funeral or burial services of loved ones (see p. 969). Routine inquiry into such topics should be part of well-child care because it can promote healthy attitudes and prepare chldren to cope with loss when it occurs.

AWARENESS OF DYING IN CHILDREN WITH LIFE-THREATENING ILLNESS

One of the initial reactions of parents (and many health professionals) to the discovery of a life-threatening illness is to protect the child from the impact of the diagnosis. This may result in the "to tell or not to tell" dilemma. One of the choices is not informing the child about his illness and fabricating a plausible story to explain the treatments without implying the seriousness of the actual condition. The other choice is including the child in what is happening by explaining simply and honestly the disease process, the treatments, and the chances of recovery. Although the options seem well defined and absolute, in reality the decision is influenced by the child's level of understanding, the parents' ability to communicate with the child, and the support systems available to both.

Observations of Potentially Fatally Ill Children

The question of whether children realize how ill they are frequently arises in discussions with parents and seems to be an important influencing factor in the final parental decision of whether to tell children about their disease. Several authors have studied the behaviors of terminally ill children and conclude that there is some level of comprehension, even when children are protected from the truth (Waechter, 1985). Anxiety may not be attributable to fear of death but may be demonstrated in relationship to separation, pain, intrusive procedures, bodily change or mutilation, loneliness, immobilization, and punishment. Children as young as 2 or 3 years of age perceive their parents' emotions and react accordingly.

Studies of children' experiences with life-threatening illness demonstrate that children learn about their situation through the acquisition of information, at which time they develop different conceptions of themselves. Five states have been defined (Bluebond-Langner, 1978):

Stage I: Disease is a serious illness. New identity of "sick" child.

Stage II: Discovery of the relationship of medication and recovery. Learns the taboos of disease and death.

Stage III: Marked understanding of the purposes and implications of special procedures. Sense of well-being begins to fade and perceives self as different from other children.

Stage IV: Illness is viewed as a permanent condition. Sense of always being sick and never getting better.

Stage V: Realization that there is only a finite number of medications. Awareness (directly or indirectly) of their fatal prognosis.

Experience is considered the critical factor in the passage through these various stages. The experience of having a disease allows children to assimilate information by relating what they see and hear to what they feel and think. Experience also explains why age and intellectual ability are not related to the speed or completeness with which children pass through the various stages of awareness. Some 3- and 4-year-olds of average intelligence know more about their prognosis than very intelligent 9-year-olds who are still in their first remission, have had fewer clinical experiences, and are aware only that they have a serious illness (Greenham and Lohmann, 1982).

Time lapse between stages tends to be the same for all children regardless of age. Passage from the first stage to the second stage occurs rapidly on relapse. Passage through the second, third, and fourth stages takes somewhat longer, but passage to the fifth stage may take place as soon as the child learns of the death of another, and all knowledge from previous stages is quickly synthesized into a new self-awareness.

Possibly the most significant evidence regarding knowledge of the diagnosis comes from the children themselves. When a large group of survivors of childhood cancer were asked whether they thought children should be told their diagnosis, 70% felt that the child has the right to know, with an additional 20% adding that the child should be emotionally ready. Most felt that some sort of psychosocial support should be available throughout treatment, a finding that has important implications for health providers (O'Malley, 1979).

Symbolic Language

One of the difficulties in attempting to answer the question of whether children are aware of their potentially fatal prognosis is that children frequently speak in symbolic or nonverbal language. Even when asked direct questions and given the opportunity to discuss their thoughts, children may answer in a way that must be interpreted and understood by others in view of the child's age and cognitive abilities, as illustrated in the following example:

One family who had tried to convey openness and honesty to their 9-year-old son was uncertain of his present level of understanding. After several years of remission he had relapsed and chemotherapy was no longer effective. His parents told him that the physician planned to try new drugs but that the leukemic cells had returned and had not responded to the usual treatment. He seemed to accept this information very casually. However, one day as he and his mother returned home from an outpatient visit, he began asking about funerals. He had never attended any wakes or burial ceremonies, but he wanted detailed information regarding disposal of the body. His main concern was, "Who dresses the person—does a man dress a man and a woman dress a woman?" The mother answered as honestly as she could but was disturbed by this question because he exhibited many needs for privacy and usually refused to allow female nurses to dress or bathe him. During her next session with the nurse counselor, she related this conversation and wondered if her son was inquiring about his death. The nurse felt certain that the questions were not random curiosity but were an indication of his awareness of the seriousness of the relapse.

Children may also symbolically communicate their thoughts through writing, telling stories, dreams, drawing, and play. These techniques employ both expressive nonverbal and verbal communication and are discussed in Chapter 6.

The "To Tell or Not To Tell" Dilemma

The initial reaction of parents following discovery of the potentially terminal diagnosis is shock and disbelief. Probably one way of further shielding themselves from the overwhelming reality of the situation is to deny its existence to the child and siblings. Another reason for their inability to deal with the question of preparing the child may be their total concern with the present crisis and lack of emotional reserve to cope with one more stress. As a result, most parents seem to fabricate an alternate excuse as the reason for the child's hospitalization. Frequently health professionals support such improvised explanations because of their own unresolved fears and insecurity in dealing with the truth. With no direction or help in deciding whether to protect the child or openly discuss with him the facts of his illness, many parents persist in fostering this conspiracy.

The decision not to tell. Initially the decision not to tell the child the truth has its superficial advantages. For one, it avoids the entire issue of how to explain the illness. It also solves the problem of the child asking parents or staff any difficult, probing questions. After induction therapy most children attain remission and are physically well and ready to resume prehospital activities. For parents it seems easier to return to normalcy with the diagnosis hidden.

However, the disadvantages of this decision are soon readily apparent. Following the course of remission therapy, there are future courses of treatment and evaluatory procedures, such as lumbar punctures, bone marrow aspirations, and blood tests. There is always the threat of relapse or recurrence of the illness, as well as intermittent problems with infection, hemorrhage, drug toxicity, and so on. What plausible explanation is available for these future problems? The answer is more lies, more excuses, and more flimsy explanations.

Effects on terminally ill children. Children are perceptively aware of conspiracies. They can detect the poorly hidden tears, the look of hopelessness after a conference with the physician, the vague telephone conversations that end abruptly if the child is present, or the whispers in the hallway and the overuse of big words. Children realize from the reactions of others that something is very wrong. But they also know that no one wants to talk about it with them, so they tacitly agree to the "don't tell him game" and protect others by not asking questions. However, such a conspiracy denies these children any opportunity to discuss their fears, questions, or thoughts. They are deprived of the truth and forced to supply their own answers or interpretations to events, which frequently are more extreme, frightening, and bizarre than the truth. Often they learn the truth by accidentally overhearing someone discuss their illness or by listening to the unkind remarks of another child. Such an unfortunate event results in anger and mistrust toward parents.

For example, in a family where the adolescent son had metastatic cancer, the father refused to allow anyone to talk openly to the boy. Although the mother felt strongly that her son knew and needed to discuss his feelings with someone, she also respected the established code of behavior in the Mexican culture of abiding by the patriarch's commands. Members of the medical and nursing staff agreed to the conspiracy, which was facilitated by the adolescent's passive, outwardly accepting behavior. However, one night he had a severe central nervous system reaction to an antiemetic medication. He became extremely upset and panic stricken. The nurse understood that he misinterpreted the reaction as a terminal stage of his disease and spoke softly to him, explaining that the symptoms were caused by a drug, not the illness. He immediately relaxed. The look of relief in his eyes was the clearest message to everyone present that he had feared dying. Although the nurse later tried to discuss with him his behavioral reactions during this episode, he again refused to talk about his illness. As the nurse began to leave, he asked her to stay with him until he fell asleep. She held his hand and reassured him that he was not alone. They communicated in this way for the next several nights until he died.

Effects on siblings. The "to tell or not to tell" dilemma also involves the siblings and the support system that may be available to the family. During the initial hospitalization admission, many parents elect to room-in or stay with their child as much as possible. This is understandable and probably necessary to help them work through their initial grief reactions of denial, disbelief, or anger. If there are other children in the family, they are usually cared for temporarily by a relative or friend. Unless parents give them a reasonable explanation for their continued absence from the home, the siblings will regard the sick child as responsible for the disruption and inconvenience.

To the well children, the brother or sister in the hospital receives the undivided attention of one or both parents and is showered with gifts, cards, and visitors. Consequently the "neglected and forgotten" siblings feel resentful, angry, and jealous of such special treatment. Even when parents do attempt to convey a realistic picture of the hospitalized child's ordeal, few children are able to cast aside their negative feelings for genuine reactions of sympathy and concern. Being truthful with the siblings, including them in family discussions, and encouraging them to visit during the hospital stay help them realize the seriousness of the situation while allowing them the opportunity to be a contributing (not neglected) part of the family.

Many subsequent behavioral problems in well siblings, such as aggressiveness, regression, acting out, and separation anxiety, can be prevented or resolved by including these children in the discussion, decision making, and care of the ill child. Preparing them for expected changes in the child, such as hair loss, physical deterioration, and loss of function, also helps them cope with questions or remarks from other children or adults and facilitates their adjustment to such alterations.

Effects on parents. The conspiracy of hiding or camouflaging the truth also places additional burdens on parents in their social milieu because it robs them of potential support from relatives or friends. It is true that not telling anyone about the child's diagnosis preserves the protective fortress constructed for the ill child and siblings and avoids sometimes distressing questions from others. However, a successful conspiracy is rarely, if ever, possible, and as a result the established code of silence alienates the family from others who are aware of the situation and might wish to help. The more families isolate and close themselves off from their world, the less likely they are to regain emotional strength to help them successfully resolve this crisis. This is particularly significant after the death, when parents wish to reenter their social environment and find their previous relationships and interests affected by their absence.

"Cruel" truth vs "gentle" truth. One of the strongest arguments for protecting the child from knowledge of the disease is that truth dispels hope, unnecessarily increases anxiety, and destroys the will to survive. Many people cite examples of individuals who stopped fighting and died shortly after learning of their terminal illness. Although there is some justification to this because some people do will themselves to die, there is a difference between "cruel" truth and "gentle" truth. To tell someone that he has an incurable illness and that he is going to die can dispel hope and possibly life. On the other hand, to tell someone the name of his illness, its effect on body functioning, and the reason for the treatment instills hope, allows for support from others, and serves as a foundation for explaining and understanding future crises.

Even when parents agree that their child should be told the truth, they encounter difficulty in using such words as "cancer," "leukemia," and "tumor." They believe that such highly emotional words will upset the child by implying hopelessness, disability, or death. However, often these terms have little meaning for children other than the connotations conveyed by others. The emotional impact of the word "cancer" is a learned response. If a cure were suddenly found for all malignancies, the fear, anxiety, and hopelessness presently associated with such diseases would diminish.

Once children know the name of the disease, the treatments, the required laboratory tests, and expected outcomes from each, they are able to deal with what is happening to them by seeking support and understanding from others. The following examples compare the different responses from children who were protected from the truth and those who were exposed to it.

Example A:

Eight-year-old Ann was recently diagnosed as having leukemia. Her parents explained to her that "something was wrong with her blood," which they called anemia. After the initial hospitalization Ann went into remission and returned to school. After 2 days at school a classmate exclaimed, "You have leukemia. You are going to die." Ann was so upset by this that she told the teacher she was sick and consequently was sent home. The following day Ann refused to return to school and was very depressed. She offered no explanation to her parents except that she was not feeling well. Her parents allowed her to remain at home for several weeks, which greatly intensified the child's fear of returning to school. It was not until the family sought professional help that the child was able to disclose the reason for her fear and to understand the actual illness and related facts.

Example B:

Nine-year-old Tom also was recently diagnosed as having leukemia, but his parents decided to be honest and open with their son. They explained what effect the disease has on the blood, the reason for the treatments, and the chances for recovery. They agreed to tell their son that there was no cure for leukemia, that it was a serious illness, but that there were drugs that could kill the leukemia cells indefinitely, possibly forever. They emphasized that at one time such drugs were not available and people died shortly after the diagnosis was made. During the course of the induction therapy Tom went into remission and returned to school. During his first day back at school a classmate said to him, "I heard you had leukemia. I thought you were dead." Tom calmly responded, "I did have leukemia. I don't anymore. Do I look dead?" The other boy shrugged his shoulders and replied, "Come on, let's play." Tom immediately agreed.

Explaining Death to Children

Many adults attempt to shield children from any tragedy, especially death. They argue that children are too young, too fragile, or too vulnerable to cope with grief, sadness, unhappiness, or disappointment. What such individuals fail to understand is that life never shields anyone from eventual tragedy and that allowing children to feel emotions, particularly for less significant or important losses, prepares them for more traumatic events later, as shown by the following example.

A mother of a 5-year-old child decided to spare her son the grief of learning that his cat had been killed by a car. She planned to replace the animal with a substitute before the child returned home that day. However, in the interim she discussed her intended plans with a nurse friend, who emphasized the importance of telling the child the truth because he would realize that the new animal was a replacement and resent its immediate presence. The mother agreed but asked the nurse to be there when she told her son about the accident. The nurse provided the support the parent needed and attended the "burial services" for the animal.

A year later the child's father also died in an accident. The mother used the example of the cat's death to explain this event to her son. She later told her nurse friend that had she shielded her child from the animal's death by substituting a replacement, she did not know how she could have explained the husband's sudden death.

Children need to feel, to express their emotions, and to learn appropriate outlets for anger, sadness, anxiety, or resentment. If others protect them from unhappy truths, children may respond to future stresses with few resources for how to handle their emotions. For example, inappropriate behavior, regression, problems with learning or relating to others, passivity, denial, dependence on drugs, development of psychosomatic symptoms, and withdrawal are a few of the alternative responses children may use to deal with stress.

Exactly how and what to tell children about events such as serious illness, dying, and death is a very individual matter. There is as much danger in telling children too much as there is in telling them too little. However, there are guidelines that can help in determining how to present facts in a way that fosters trust, enhances meaningful communication, and offers emotional support to the child and parents.

Developmental age. A primary concern in any relationship with children is their age, because the level of comprehension is a function of children's cognitive development. As discussed earlier in this chapter, children at various ages have different understandings and fears of death. The younger child fears separation, which can be imposed by any number of circumstances, only one of which is death or illness. The older child fears the results of illness, particularly pain or bodily injury, as well as death itself. Anyone working with children must be aware of such developmental variations, and sensitive to their verbal, nonverbal, and symbolic language.

Previous knowledge. Besides age, another essential principle is first to find out what the child is thinking. Before any explanations (true or false) are offered to children, they have invented their own. Answers to such questions as "What do you think is wrong with you?" or "What have you heard others say?" provide information on which to structure further explanations. Very often a child will respond with an answer of such detailed, accurate information that the only element lacking is the name of the disease. Other answers may reveal possible areas of misconception, which can then be clarified or refocused.

Sometimes parents and other adults hear the child's words but fail to comprehend their meaning. They erroneously assume that because the child recites all the facts he also understands their implications or has dealt with all his fears. This may not be so; intellectualizing about one's condition can be a powerful defense mechanism. For example, an adolescent who was undergoing serious open-heart surgery knew precisely every detail of the operation, preoperative and postoperative care, involved risks, and so on. The medical and nursing staff considered her exceptionally well prepared. However, everyone had failed to ask her about how she felt. When the clinical nurse specialist asked her this before her surgery, the child answered, "I fear that I may die." Once this was verbalized, the child, her parents, and the nurse focused on her fears instead of on the facts of her illness.

Honesty. The last principle in explaining events such as death to children is honesty. Although the truth is usually the most difficult answer to give, in the long run it lessens many of the conflicts or problems that arise from lies, half-truths, or conspiracies. The truth provides answers for future questions. It also fosters trust. Children adeptly perceive the maxim: Do as I say, not as I do. It is very difficult to encourage children to be honest, to confide in others, and to openly discuss their fears if parents refuse to do the same.

Honesty is certainly not the easiest solution; the truth may prompt children to ask other distressing questions. The question many parents and health professionals dread the most is, "Am I going to die?," because what honest answer also implies hope? One possible response is to use the principle of first ascertaining why they are asking questions *now*. Are they asking about dying today? In the future? From the disease? From the treatments? During the relapse? Or from the infection?

If given the opportunity, children will tell others how much they want to know. Asking questions such as, "If the disease came back, would you want to know?" "Do you want others to tell you everything, even if the news isn't good?" or "If someone were not getting better [or more directly, "were dying"], do you think they would want to know?" helps children set the limits for how much truth they can accept and cope with. Children need time to proceed through the stages of denial, shock, and anger before they can assimilate and hopefully accept the inevitable fact of mortality.

The way in which children ask questions also indicates the answer they are seeking. Few children seem to ask such direct questions as, "Am I going to die?" Instead they may ask, "Have the bad cells gone away?" or "Will this medicine make me better?" They tend to avoid final questions, such as, "What happens *if* the bad cells don't go away?" or "What happens *if* there are no more medicines?" In this way they always leave the opportunity for hope.

Grief Process in Expected and Unexpected Death

In response to any loss there is a grief reaction. *Acute grief* develops within hours to days and is characterized by somatic syptoms and intense subjective distress. *Grief work* or *mourning* refers to the lengthy process that begins with acute grief and extends into a period of reorganization of psychologic life, with attachment to new people and interests.

Numerous investigators have contributed greatly to the

present understanding of grief and bereavement, and those whose work is considered classic are presented below. In expected death the child and family must be involved in the plan for intervention both before and after the death. In unexpected death the survivors face the tremendous task of integrating the loss into their lives, with no opportunity for anticipatory grief. In either situation nurses can facilitate the grief process by being aware of expected psychologic and somatic reactions and supporting the grievers through each stage of mourning.

KÜBLER-ROSS: STAGES OF DYING

Although most research on grief has focused on the reactions following a loss, Elisabeth Kübler-Ross (1969) has identified five stages that people experience in terms of expected death. These stages represent a set of *ever-changing behaviors* that surface as the need for them arises within the individual's attempts to cope with expected loss. They are not sequential stages that dying persons progress through. Kübler-Ross maintains that the helping person's role in all stages of dying is to support the person where he or she is, not to maneuver from one stage to another. If support is truly therapeutic, the strength gained from this active intervention will help the person proceed independently to another stage.

The stages of dying can be conceptualized as behavioral reactions of anticipatory grief. One important point to remember when discussing each stage is that it pertains to the dying person and to those experiencing this person's expected death. With children, the "patient" is the ill child, the parents, the siblings, and other significant members of the family.

Denial

In the first stage, denial, the person responds with shock and disbelief. The "No, not me" reaction occurs regardless of whether the person is explicitly told the diagnosis. The duration of the denial depends on the coping mechanisms used by the person in previous crises, the support systems available to the person to help him give up the denial, and the reactions of others, especially physicians and nurses, to the resistance that is demonstrated. Unfortunately the need of others to deny the reality of the situation may be so great that it supports and fosters the patient's own denial and retards progression toward other stages.

Anger

The second stage in the dying process is anger. Although it usually follows denial, it may occur and recur at any time during the dying process. When the denial fails and the reality of the situation penetrates consciousness, the person's reaction is, "Why me?" The anger, rage, hostility, envy, or resentment may be directed at oneself or at others, notably members of the medical and nursing staff. However, unlike denial, anger is not socially approved or condoned. As a result, the person is often harshly judged for his angry refusal to accept mortality and may be further isolated in his struggle for life and death.

To think about why the dying person or the parents of a dying child become enraged and resentful is only to begin to imagine the tremendous consequences of loss. Everything in life that the person dreamed of, hoped for, and expected to achieve is now only painful memories. He is angry toward those who are physically strong, who can make the dreams reality, and who live without pain or suffering. He is not angry at these people but at the things they represent, which for the dying person are no longer possible.

Bargaining

The next stage, and one that is often difficult to identify, is bargaining. It is the dying person's attempt to postpone the inevitable. The bargaining for additional time may be with God, with oneself, or with the most significant other person. One way of exploring a person's silent bargaining is to ask, "If you could do one more thing, what would it be?" Frequently the answer will reveal a hidden desire.

Bargaining also occurs in children. The dying child may wish for additional time for himself, or the child who is facing the loss of a parent may hope for a delay of that person's death. One must listen very carefully to children to understand their symbolic language. One child, who had recently been told that his leukemia had relapsed, casually said to his mother, "Do you know what I wished for on my last birthday? Another birthday."

Depression

Without the denial to protect the person from realizing the seriousness of his condition, the anger to displace the emotional anxiety, and the bargaining to postpone the inevitable, the person eventually experiences depression. Generally there are two types of depression: for past losses and for anticipated or impending losses.

In a chronic terminal illness there are many reasons for the first kind of depression, such as loss of hair from therapy, loss of a body part or function, restricted physical ability, and change in life-style. The second kind of depression signals the person's preparation for the impending loss of all love objects. It is difficult for the dying person because he realizes the enormity of his loss. Unlike the survivors who are saying good-bye to one person, the dying person is saying good-bye to everyone and everything he loved.

Dealing with each loss in a constructive, positive manner can greatly relieve the first type of depression. For example, purchasing an attractive wig, emphasizing the person's ability rather than disability, and manipulating the individual's life-style to accommodate his physical changes help him deal with the depression of each crisis.

During the next period of preparatory grief or depression there is little need for verbal reassurances. Attempts to "lighten the mood" or "cheer up the person" not only are ineffective but may also burden the griever with additional expectations to appear happy in order to meet the needs of those around him. It is a time of listening and of being physically present with the dying person. Toward the terminal stage the person may request the company of only one or two significant people. Children usually desire the presence of their parents more than anyone else.

Acceptance

The final stage of dying is acceptance. The person is no longer angry or depressed. If bargaining occurs, it is usually for a peaceful, painless death rather than for prolongation of life. It is not a happy time but one of inner peace and resolution that death is a certainty. The person may signal his acceptance by being uninterested in present or future events and preoccupied with past events, preferring few visitors, and wanting quiet and solitude.

Such behavior may be very upsetting to others close to him, including health team members who have not reached the same level of acceptance. One critical objective is to recognize the behaviors of acceptance in the patient and help others understand its relevance. Often the medical plan for continued treatment does not allow the patient the opportunity to accept the inevitable end. Nurses can be instrumental in planning care with all members of the health team with the goal of the patient's and family's wishes as the priority. This may involve the willingness to terminate extraordinary or lifesaving measures when death is imminent.

SYMPTOMATOLOGY OF NORMAL GRIEF

Sensations of somatic distress
Feeling of tightness in the throat
Choking, with shortness of breath
Marked tendency to sighing
Empty feeling in abdomen
Lack of muscular power
Intense subjective distress described as tension or mental pain

Preoccupation with image of the deceased
Hears, sees, or imagines that the dead person is present
Slight sense of unreality
Feeling of emotional distance from others
May believe that he or she is approaching insanity

Feelings of guilt
Searches for evidence of failure in preventing the death
Accuses self of negligence or exaggerates minor omissions

Feelings of hostility
Loss of warmth toward others
Tendency to irritability and anger
Wish not to be bothered by friends or relatives

Loss of usual pattern of conduct
Restlessness, inability to sit still, aimless moving about
Continual searching for something to do or what he or she thinks should be done
Lack of capacity to initiate and maintain organized patterns of activity

Modified from Lindemann, E.: Symptomatology and management of acute grief, Am. J. Psychiatry **101**:141-143, 1944. Copyright 1944 American Psychiatric Association.

SYMPTOMATOLOGY OF MORBID GRIEF

Delay in or postponement of grief
None of the expected psychosomatic reactions of grief for the loss of the significant person immediately after death
May see grief for an unresolved earlier loss
Grief reaction may begin as "anniversary reaction"
Acute grief may be postponed because of other immediate tasks, such as sustaining morale of others

Distorted reactions
Overactivity without a sense of loss
Acquisition of symptoms belonging to the last illness of the deceased
Acquisition of a recognized psychosomatic illness, such as ulcers, asthma, or rheumatoid arthritis
Conspicuous alteration in relationship to friends and relatives, usually social isolation
Furious hostility against specific persons
Repression of hostility, resulting in altered affect and conduct, similar to schizophrenic symptoms
Lasting loss of patterns of social interaction, especially lack of decision and initiative
Altered behavior that is detrimental to own social and economic existence, such as unjustified generosity
Agitated depression, with danger signs of suicide

Modified from Lindemann, E.: Symptomatology and management of acute grief, Am. J. Psychiatry **101**:141-148, 1944. Copyright 1944 American Psychiatric Association.

LINDEMANN: SYMPTOMATOLOGY OF GRIEF

Lindemann (1944) analyzed and described the reactions of survivors following the loss of significant others and found that acute grief has the following characteristics:

1. It is a definite syndrome with psychologic and somatic symptoms (see box).
2. The syndrome may appear immediately after a crisis, be delayed, be exaggerated, or be apparently absent.
3. In place of the normal syndrome there may appear distorted reactions that represent one special aspect of the syndrome (see box).
4. Through intervention, distorted reactions can be transformed into normal grief work with successful resolution.

The importance of such work is that health professionals such as nurses can use this theoretic framework to support those individuals who demonstrate adaptive behaviors (approach toward resolution of the crisis) and to intervene in those who exhibit maladaptive behaviors (avoidance or movement away from resolution of the crisis).

One example of emotional support toward the bereaved is to emphasize that reactions such as hearing the dead person's voice, feeling distant from others who want to help, or seeking reassurance that they did everything possible for the lost person are normal, necessary, and expected responses. They in no way signify insanity or approaching mental breakdown. On the contrary such behaviors signify that the survivor is working through the acute grief and will probably satisfactorily resolve the loss and resume or restructure a meaningful role in his social environment.

PARKES: MOURNING

Whereas Lindemann's work focused on the symptoms of acute grief, several other researchers have attempted to analyze the behaviors and responses of the bereaved during the long and difficult process of mourning. Although there are numerous commonalities among the stages proposed by these authorities, the work of C. Murray Parkes with widows and widowers is considered classic (Glick, Weiss, and Parkes, 1974); according to Parkes' findings, the grief process consists of at least four phases, which do not necessarily proceed in sequence and may recur at any time. Contrary to the common belief that mourning is completed in a year, data from clinical studies indicate that resolution of grief may take years and that there may be an *intensification* of grief during the third year (Rando, 1983).

Shock and Disbelief

Shock, numbness, and disbelief are seen during the immediate phase of grief. As one parent described, "We were as prepared for our son's death as anyone could be, but it was a shock when in a moment his life was finished. I just can't get over the rapidity with which life ends." This temporary numbness protects the survivors from the overwhelming pain associated with grief. Often decisions are made automatically and only certain details are remembered.

Expression of Grief

When the numbness fades there begins a period of intense grief characterized by a yearning and loneliness for the deceased. During this stage many of the signs of acute grief are evident, and physical complaints such as inability to sleep and appetite changes are common. There is a tendency to review the events of the deceased's life and to evaluate the relationship with the loved one. At this time feelings of guilt and anger are common.

Disorganization and Despair

During this stage the pain of the loss is replaced primarily by emptiness, apathy, and deep depression. There is a feeling that life has no meaning and that the pain will never end. This is particularly relevant for parents. For example, mothers often comment that they feel they have suffered a double loss—loss of their child and loss of the mothering role (Wong, 1980). Feelings of estrangement from other loved ones are common, and social isolation may foster the depression.

Reorganization

Reorganization refers to recovery from the loss. It is a very gradual process in which the survivors again find meaning in living, readjust to life without the deceased, develop new or renewed relationships, and learn to live with the memory of the deceased with much less pain. It never means that the loved one is forgotten and the pain is gone. There always remains a deep ache that is never totally replaced with happiness and one that returns more intensely, for example, on holidays or anniversaries.

EXPECTED VS UNEXPECTED CHILDHOOD DEATH

Remarkably little research has been conducted comparing grief responses in survivors when the child's death was expected or unexpected. When death is expected there is time for anticipatory grieving, and it has been suggested that this may favorably affect the grief process. However, a comparison of emotional and physical symptoms of parents whose child died after a chronic illness or an accident found no difference between the two groups (Miles, 1985). However, parents of children who died suddenly did experience more guilt, a prolonged period of numbness and shock, intense loneliness and emptiness, anxious fear that someone else would die, and intense anger at those responsible for the injury (Miles and Perry, 1985).

Although the grief process may be relatively unaltered by the timing of the child's death, there are differences for the families. As noted above, the period of shock is shorter when death is expected, a fact that is frequently very difficult for others to understand who are experiencing the child's death as an unexpected event. For example, one mother who had cared for her child at home before his death remarked at the wake services that she wondered if she should be more upset. The visitors cried and were unable to offer any solace to the parents, who frequently reacted to this behavior by stating, "We will be all right. Our son is now in peace." After the funeral services the parents needed to discuss these feelings in order to validate that their more calm acceptance of their son's death was a positive reaction.

In long-term, potentially fatal illnesses the grief for anticipated loss becomes chronic. The parents mourn the loss of their child long before he dies. Unlike parents who experience a sudden loss, these family members are unable to resolve their grief until the child is considered cured or dead. Each time they see the pain the child must endure or anticipate the sudden loss of hope during a relapse, they are reminded of their child's uncertain future.

However, the prolonged period of chronic grief provides families with the precious opportunity to complete all "unfinished business," such as helping the child and siblings understand and cope with a fatal prognosis. Many families reflect on their changed perspective of time after learning of the diagnosis, particularly their heightened awareness of the value and worth of each day. As one father stated, "I used to plan ahead for a better job, more money, and more prestige. But now I find myself wanting to stay home to be with my family. I never before realized how important time really is. Now I only wish we had more of it."

In sudden, unexpected death the family is deprived of any of the advantages of anticipatory grief. There is no opportunity to prepare oneself or others for the death, only the cruel reality that nothing remains of their child except memories. Because of this lack of time to prepare, many families feel great guilt and remorse for not having done something additional or different with the child. For example, they may berate themselves for not having prevented the accident or for depriving the child of some desired material object or privilege.

SPECIAL DECISIONS AT THE TIME OF DYING AND DEATH

Rarely are people prepared to cope with the numerous decisions that must be made when a loved one is dying or dies. When the death is expected there is the opportunity to make plans in advance, such as where the child should spend his last days or what type of funeral arrangements are desired. When death is unexpected the shock is sufficient to render the survivors incapable of making even simple decisions. Those in attendance at the death and those caring for the dying child can be instrumental in initiating discussions that may facilitate the grief process. The following is a brief review of selected instances when nurses can help parents make decisions related to the expected or unexpected death.

Hospice or Hospital Care

When the child is dying, parents should be given the choice of hospice* or hospital care for the terminal stage of illness. Hospital care refers to the traditional practices of caring for dying patients; hospice is a concept, not necessarily a facility. Hospice is holistic care for the patient and family that is intended to maximize the present quality of life whenever there is no reasonable expectation of cure (Corr and Corr, 1985). The three basic ways of providing hospice care are in a hospice, in a facility that employs the hospice concept, or in the child's home. If the home is chosen, the goal is to enable the child and family to enjoy the best possible quality of life until the time of death. The child may or may not die in the home. Reasons for final admission to a hospital vary but may be related to the parent's or sibling's wish to have the child die outside the home, exhaustion on the part of the caregivers, physical problems, such as sudden, acute pain or respiratory distress, and insufficient nursing services in the home (Martinson and others, 1986).

Hospice care is based on a number of important concepts that significantly set it apart from hospital care. First, the family are the principal caregivers, supported by a team of professional and volunteer staff. Second, the priority of care is comfort that considers the child's physical, psychologic, social, and spiritual needs. Third, the needs of family are considered as important as those of the patient. Fourth, hospice is concerned with the family's postdeath adjustment, and care may continue for a year or more.

With children, home care has been the more common environment for implementing the hospice concept, and benefits the family in a variety of ways. Children who are dying are allowed the opportunity to remain with those they love and with whom they feel secure. Many children who were thought to be in imminent danger of death have gone home and lived much longer than anyone would have predicted. Siblings feel more involved in the care and have more positive perceptions of the death (see Questions and

controversies, p. 969). Parental adaptation has been more favorable, as shown by their perceptions of how the experience at home affected their marriage, social reorientation, religious beliefs, and views on the meaning of life and death. They also feel significantly less guilt after the child's death than families whose child died in the hospital (Lauer and others, 1983). There is also the economic advantage of home care (Martinson and others, 1978), although private insurance may not cover all outpatient and related services.

Nurses working in hospice settings and with children dying at home are critical members of the health team. They often provide psychologic support for the family and are responsible for comfort measures, such as pain control (see p. 976 and 1070). They need to be available to the family and cognizant of times when the family may need relief from home care. If the child is at home, all families should have the option of admitting their child to the hospital if they feel they are unable to deal with the death. The child who dies at home must be pronounced dead, and hospice programs have provisions so this may proceed smoothly or the police may be notified with an explanation of the circumstances to prevent unnecessary concern for abuse. Providing the police with the number of the responsible physician is usually all that is necessary to confirm the cause of death. Some parents may wish to keep the body at home for the funeral service. Although state laws vary, usually the wake can be held at home, but if the body is not embalmed, it should not remain for any length of time (usually no longer than 24 to 48 hours). Unless the family can also dispose of the body or has special wishes (e.g., tissue donation or autopsy), arrangements need to be made for mortuary services.

Right to Die

One of the benefits of hospice has been the recognition of patients' right to die as they wish, with emphasis on the *quality* of life. Unfortunately, this is not always the focus of care, especially in the traditional hospital setting. Many families are not given the option of terminating treatment when cure is unlikely, and staff may be reluctant to make decisions about "no code" orders (withholding cardiopulmonary resuscitation in response to cardiac arrest). Some of these situations, such as the dying child's right to refuse additional treatment, often pose difficult ethical questions (See Questions and controversies, p. 968).

As the group of health professionals who are most involved with families, nurses are in a excellent position to ensure that families are given the options available to them at the time of death. The nurse's first responsibility is to explore the family's wishes. This is best done in concert with the physician, but at times may need to be initiated by the nurse. Statements such as, "Tell me about your thoughts for the kind of care you want your child to receive when he is dying" or "Have you considered the kinds of interventions you would like us to use when your child is near death?" can begin discussion of this sensitive but critical aspect of terminal care. If parents choose "no code,"

---

*Information on hospice services for children is available from Children's Hospice International, 501 Slater's Lane, Alexandria, VA 22314.

A list of hospice resources in the United States is in *Dying at Home with Hospice*, by Deborah Chase, St. Louis, 1986, The C.V. Mosby Co.

Questions and Controversies

Does the dying child have the right to refuse further treatment?

Traditionally, minor children (age of minority varies with state law) have not had the legal right to give informed consent for treatment or to refuse treatment. However, there is a growing concern for children in the end stage of fatal disease to have a voice in their care during the terminal phase. One of the major issues is the age at which children have the cognitive ability to understand the implications of their decision (Foley, 1985; Leiken and Connell, 1983; Stanfill and Strong, 1985). According to children's development of the death concept, a mature understanding of death does not occur until about 9 years of age. However, centers that have developed protocols for allowing informed choice by children document that youngsters as young as 6 years of age understand the implications of their disease as incurable and death as irreversible (Nitschke and others, 1982). These findings are consistent with those of Bluebond-Langner, who found that fatally ill children progress through a series of stages that shape their understanding of their disease and death (see p. 960).

Other issues raised by opponents include the concern for dispelling hope in the child once death is pronounced imminent, parents' guilt if they later question the decision, and possible conflict between the child's and parents' wishes (Shumway, Grossman, and Sarles, 1983; Stanfill and Strong, 1985). Although there is insufficient research to answer these concerns, it seems unlikely that they will occur if the family is allowed to choose therapeutic alternatives in an atmosphere of professional support and with sufficient information. In addition, staff need to assess each child's capacity to understand the implications of refusing treatment with documentation of the child's words and actions that support their conclusions (Foley, 1985).

they are assured that this does not mean "no care" and that everything possible will be done to make the child comfortable. Once a decision is made, it must be communicated to all members of the health team, including a *written* medical order for the use or withholding of lifesaving measures. An order of "slow" or "delay" code is not legal (Saunders and Valente, 1986).

Visualization of the Body

Although most institutions recognize the need for parents to hold and spend time with the dead child, a dilemma may arise when the body is mutilated. Although the memory of the child's disfigurement can be extremely upsetting and generate concern for how much the child suffered, not seeing the body leaves the parents with imagined ideas of how their child looked, which can be worse than the reality and can delay the acceptance of the death (Miles and Perry, 1985). However, family members need preparation for this upsetting experience. They should be told what to expect and why certain parts of the body are covered or bandaged (Schultz, 1983). It is desirable to place the body in a private

room, without medical apparatus, and as presentable as the situation allows (Schulman and Rehm, 1983). Some people appreciate the presence of a nurse in the room with them; others desire privacy. Regardless of how badly the body is harmed, parents may want to hold the child. Such options are offered and respected. Family members should be given as much time as they need to say good-bye.

Tissue Donation

A topic that is rarely considered when a child dies is tissue donation. However, for some families this may be a meaningful act—one that benefits another human being despite the loss of their child. Unfortunately, initiating a discussion about tissue donation is often very stressful for staff, and there may be confusion regarding whose responsibility this is. In centers where transplants are performed a full-time transplant coordinator is usually available to inform the family about organ donation and to take care of details.* If such services are not available the staff needs to discuss which members should discuss this topic with the family. Ideally this should be the person who knows the family best, when the death is expected, or who has the opportunity to spend time with the family, when the death is unexpected. Often nurses are in an optimum position to suggest tissue donation. The request should be made in a private and quiet area of the hospital and should be simple and direct, with questions such as "Are you a donor family?" or "Have you ever considered organ donation?" (Weber, 1985). Some states have "required request" statutes that mandate that the hospital make a request for tissue donation from the family of the deceased.

Nurses need to be aware of common questions about organ donation to help families make an informed decision. Healthy children who die unexpectedly are excellent candidates for organ donation, although their age is a determinant of organ suitability. For example, very young donors present technical difficulties in organ removal (Williams, 1985). Children with cancer, chronic disease, or infection, or who have suffered prolonged cardiac arrest may not be suitable candidates, although this is individually determined. The nurse should inquire if organ donation was discussed with the child or if the child ever expressed such a wish. Any number of body tissues or organs can be donated (skin, eyes, bone, kidney, heart, liver), and their removal does not mutilate or desecrate the body or cause any suffering. The family may have an open casket and there is no delay in the funeral. There is no cost to the donor family, but organ donation does not eliminate funeral or cremation responsibilities. Most religions permit organ donation so long as the recipient benefits from the transplant, although Orthodox Judaism forbids it (Carbary, 1985; Gersham, 1985).

---

*Information about organ donation is available from The Living Bank, P.O. Box 6725, Houston, TX 77265, telephone number 1-713-528-2971 (in Texas) or 1-800-528-2971.

Siblings' Attendance at Burial Services

One of the most frequent concerns of parents is whether young or school-age children should attend funeral or burial services (see Questions and controversies). Sharing moments of deep significance with parents helps children understand the experience and deal with their own feelings of shock, sorrow, and grief. However, children need preparation for postdeath services. They should be told what to expect, particularly how the deceased person will look if the coffin is open. Ideally the parent should explain the details to the child, but if the parent's grief prevents this communication, a significant family member or friend should substitute.

It is often helpful to bring the child to the funeral service before many visitors arrive. The child is allowed his private time to say good-bye but is spared some of the unpredictable emotional reactions of others, which can be very distressing to him. Allowing the child to stay as long as he

Questions and Controversies

Should children attend the funeral or burial services of a loved one?

This question generates much controversy among the general public and professionals. Many lay people feel it is too frightening for children to be exposed to the dead and that it is better for them to remember the loved person as he or she was when alive. There is a general attitude of protecting children from unhappy or distressing events. However, among health professionals involved with children there is a fairly general consensus that children should attend such services (Salladay and Royal, 1981; Schultz, 1980), and some authors suggest that no child is too young merely by virtue of age (Foley, 1986). Others recommend that the parents make the decision regarding attendance until children are 6 or 7 years of age, at which time children should choose (Zelauskas, 1981). Children like adults, have "unfinished business," and visiting the dead person may represent an opportunity to complete those affairs. For example, the child may wish to say good-bye (verbally or written) or to leave a memento. Kübler-Ross (1983) tells of a 7-year-old child who chose a puzzle that her brother received shortly before he lost sight from a brain tumor. She matter of factly explained that he could finish it "when he arrives in heaven."

Unfortunately, little research has focused on the difference in adjustment between children who do or do not attend postdeath services. However, one study provides substantial evidence of the benefit of involving children in the experience of their dying sibling. Lauer and others (1985) compared children's perceptions of their sibling's death at home versus in the hospital. The home care group (ages 5 to 23 years) reported they were prepared for the impending death, received consistent information and support from their parents, were involved in most activities, found the funeral experience comforting, and viewed their own involvement as the most important aspect of the experience. The non–home care group (ages 2 to 26 years) had opposite perceptions. Thus it appears that *increased involvement* with the death, not isolation and "protection," benefits children.

wishes but respecting his need to leave provide maximum control for the child over his ability to grieve comfortably.

The Family of the Child with Life-Threatening Illness

In many respects families who are experiencing life-threatening illness in their child respond to the diagnosis in much the same manner as families whose child has a chronic illness or disability. Because of the advances in medical treatment, many fatal illnesses, such as leukemia, are now chronic disorders. However, there remain several differences between families adjusting to a disease such as cancer vs a chronic condition such as diabetes or cystic fibrosis. Many children with cancer may live only a short time after diagnosis, whereas those with diabetes may have a normal life span. With cancer there is the hope of a cure, unlike cystic fibrosis, in which an untimely death usually occurs. Many chronic diseases impose daily reminders of the illness, such as insulin administration or respiratory therapy, whereas treatment for cancer is limited to specific schedules with periods of no therapy and return of health. Because of hope for a cure supported by periods of absence of disease, families of children with cancer may have more difficulty accepting a potential death (Kerner, Harvey, and Lewiston, 1979).

REACTIONS OF THE FAMILY TO A LIFE-THREATENING ILLNESS

All families whose child has some type of physical or cognitive disability experience reactions to the loss of the "perfect" child that are similar despite the diagnosis. The reader is urged to review these concepts in Chapter 22. The following discussion focuses on five phases in which there are significant differences in reactions to chronic disease vs life-threatening illness.

Phase I—Revelation and Dawning Reality: Diagnosis and Treatment

When parents first learn of the diagnosis of cancer, their immediate reactions are similar to those of other parents whose child has a chronic illness, except that the initial impact can be much more pessimistic and overwhelming because of the generally negative connotation regarding the disease.

Almost immediately after the diagnosis is confirmed, induction therapy aimed at total remission of the disease begins. During this period families commonly react with anger, depression, ambivalence, and bargaining. Much of the psychic energy is directed at waiting for the confirmation of a remission. If that does not occur, all the initial reactions may be repeated again, with increased anticipatory grieving.

Shock and disbelief. Many parents relate that after they heard the diagnosis they were deaf to everything else told to them. As one mother described, "All I heard the doctor say was the word leukemia. I didn't hear anything else. All I could think of was that leukemia was fatal. I was certain my child was going to die. My husband heard the doctor say it was curable, but I didn't. I won't believe that until I see it. Even if my child is 50 years old, I will worry about it coming back." The pessimistic response of this mother is typical of many parents who are afraid to believe that their child will recover despite favorable odds. If parents are not helped to understand the improved prognosis of these diseases, they may react by psychologically burying the child.

Guilt. Guilt is probably a universal reaction to the discovery of a catastrophic illness. Parents review every detail of the child's prodromal symptoms, searching for some clue that they missed or overlooked. There is also questioning, either voiced or silent, regarding the genetic influence on the disease. Many parents are greatly concerned about their role in transmitting the condition and the chances of it occurring in other siblings, particularly subsequent children. For example, one father was extremely interested in recent research on the investigation of chromosomal defects in children with leukemia. During this discussion he made no reference to the implication of heredity, but later he asked about the danger of having another offspring develop the disease. These clues led the nurse to question why he thought his child had leukemia. The father admitted his concern over whether he or his wife may have transmitted some genetic defect to their son.

Anger. Anger is closely associated with guilt, and may be directed at oneself or others, such as the parent, the spouse, the child, or members of the staff. One particularly difficult situation is when parents express anger at health professionals for not diagnosing the condition sooner. Because the association of early discovery to more favorable prognosis for cancer is well known, parents understandably wonder if their child's illness was diagnosed as early as possible. In retrospect parents frequently recall signs or symptoms that they now regard as early clues to the disease. Nurses need to be aware of the implications of their responses to parents during such discussions. For example, agreeing that the physician missed an early diagnosis may actually increase the parents' guilt and decrease their trust in the present treatment program. Conversely, defending the physician's medical judgment may weaken the parents' trust in the nurse. Listening to the parents' views and refraining from choosing sides helps them ventilate their anger while maintaining confidence in their child's care.

Children also may feel angry, particularly because of all the traumatic procedures done to them. Once they begin to feel better, they frequently express their anger through uncooperativeness. Parents receive the brunt of much of the child's anger and often find coping with it extremely difficult. A common reaction is to ignore it and try to pacify the child by giving in to his requests whenever possible. Overprotectiveness and permissiveness are typical reactions during remission, and helping parents deal with the child's anger constructively during the hospitalization also prevents some of the potential future problems.

Siblings are not exempt from feelings such as anger. Because of the suddenness and seriousness of the diagnosis, they are forced to cope with a disrupted family life and are often given inadequate explanations for the changes. Their responses are similar to those discussed in Chapter 22, except that if the child dies the surviving siblings may feel very guilty over their feelings of resentment toward the deceased brother or sister.

Anticipatory grieving. Almost immediately after learning of the diagnosis, most parents begin grieving for the loss of a perfect, healthy child. Much of this acute grief remains until there are signs of physical improvement in the child. During the initial days parents may have great difficulty in making decisions concerning what to tell the ill child and how to prepare the siblings. Unfortunately, despite their decreased ability to solve problems, they are forced to make a great many decisions. Nurses can be very helpful in supplying direction in areas in which alternatives are possible. For example, one family decided to move to a new location as soon as they heard that their child had cancer. This sudden uprooting would have been extremely disruptive to the entire family and would have introduced multiple new crises into the already critical stress situation. The nurse was able to intervene by listening to the parents' reasons for wanting to relocate and then discussing with them some of the disadvantages of doing so at the present time. It was stressed that if they still felt inclined to move, they could more effectively plan a change after the child's discharge. The parents realized the tremendous implications of such a decision and decided to wait. After the hospitalization the mother remarked to the nurse, "When I heard the diagnosis, I was in such a state of mental upset that I could have done anything foolish. I am so glad we didn't make any decisions at that time."

Depression and ambivalence. The shock of discovering the diagnosis is followed by depression, which usually lasts until there is physical evidence of improvement. Inasmuch as in many cases the chemical or surgical intervention results in further deterioration of the child's physical status, many parents are ambivalent in their decision to agree to treatment. Although this is rarely voiced, parents may imply their ambivalence in such statements as, "Will the medicine always make him so sick?" "Is surgery really necessary?" "Wouldn't one drug do just as well as so many?" or "Is radiation just an extra measure in case the drugs don't work?" Supplying an automatic answer is less effective than encouraging parents to discuss their thoughts about the treatments. Many parents verbalize that when they consented to the interventions they were not aware of the significance of the side effects, regardless of how well they were informed.

Bargaining. During the initial phase of induction therapy, most of the concern is focused on the child's recovery from the actual disease. Once physical improvement is evident, attention centers on the prospect of a remission. Parents constantly look for signs of a remission, which to them may be indicated by increased appetite, less irritable behavior, more energy, better color, and so on. However, the clinical confirmation of a remission usually takes several weeks or more. During this waiting period parents bargain for a postponement of any pessimistic reports. Parents frequently make comments such as, "If we can make it through this, I think everything will be all right." The significance of the child's attaining a remission cannot be overestimated. For many, it represents a second chance.

Reactions to altered body image. One side effect of chemotherapy or cranial irradiation that has particular psychologic significance for children in different age groups and for parents is hair loss.

Young children. For young children baldness has little significance. Preschoolers may attach superficial concern to the hair loss, particularly if it affects their sex role image. For example, one 4-year-old girl was disturbed about her baldness because she thought she looked like a boy. Once her parents emphasized her femaleness in dress, she was unconcerned about the temporary change.

Parents of young children may have a difficult adjustment. However, they may be unwilling to admit their concern and lack of acceptance. For example, the mother of a 3-year-old boy refused to openly discuss the hair loss in front of her son. She had decided to hide the change from him until new hair grew in. She had formulated a fantastic conspiracy to maintain the secret. For example, she planned to remove all mirrors in the house, to isolate him from children, to keep his head always covered with hats, and to buy a soft brush and groom the hair as if it were still present. She explained that this was necessary because he was very vain. When asked what she would do if he discovered the baldness, she calmly said, "I'll just tell him what happened." It was not possible for her to see the pitfalls of such a scheme until she verbalized her personal feelings about the hair loss.

School-age children. The reactions of school-age children depend on their preparation for the loss and the type of parental adjustment. Much of their anxiety relates to the anticipation of the loss rather than the actual baldness. Telling children about the change before it occurs, stressing that it is temporary, and suggesting ways of camouflaging it, such as with a wig, hat, or scarf, fosters better adjustment to the altered body image.

Adolescents. Adolescents have the most difficulty in accepting and adjusting to hair loss because it occurs at a time when peer acceptance and group conformity are essential. They need the opportunity to express their anger and fears of rejection without being judged or reproached. Sometimes parents try to reason with their adolescent child that the hair loss is a small sacrifice for a possible future recovery. Although true, it does little to comfort the adolescent in his present struggle.

Involving adolescents in selecting a wig *before* the hair falls out provides them with a feeling of participation and allows them to secure a wig that is most similar to their own

hair. For example, a 13-year-old girl whose wig was styled exactly like her hair commented, "I think I like my wig even better than my own hair." Before she began to lose her hair she wore the wig to school to see if anyone could detect the difference. Because no one could, she felt very comfortable about wearing it when it was necessary.

Nursing considerations. The time of diagnosis is a critical period for the development of therapeutic relationships. Ideally, a consistent nurse should be present with family members when the diagnosis is given. The same guidelines as discussed in Chapter 22 apply; parents want information that they consider critical—information related to the diagnosis and prognosis, disease process, need for additional diagnostic tests, immediate therapeutic plan, and availability of the physician (Greenberg, 1984).

In many instances the child's care is so complex that numerous specialists are involved. Consequently the nurse becomes the only consistent person for the family. For example, in the case of a child with Wilms' tumor, a pediatrician, urologist, surgeon, radiologist, and hematologist/oncologist participate in the medical/surgical care of the child. Even under the best of circumstances, parents can receive opposing messages from health team members and can become confused about who can answer their questions. The nurse is in an advantageous position to interpret those messages and to direct the parents to the most appropriate source of information.

In many instances care in the hospital is limited to a few days for diagnosis and initiation of treatment. However, in some cases an extended admission may be necessary. Many parents elect to stay with their child and to participate as much as possible in the care. Because the possibility of death in a child is a highly emotional experience, nurses may unknowingly usurp parents' roles or relinquish nursing responsibilities. They need to be aware of their approach toward parents in order to support them in the way most comfortable for the parents. Planning the child's care *with* family members is a most effective way of communicating genuine concern and avoiding either hazard.

During the remission phase, parents, ill children, and siblings need reassurance that their reactions are normal and expected. The interventions discussed in Chapter 22 apply. Because of the shock usually experienced when a catastrophic illness is diagnosed, the needs of well family members, particularly siblings, may be neglected. Siblings can be helped to understand the reason for the abrupt change in family life by keeping them informed of the child's condition and by continuing as much contact as possible with the hospitalized child (and absent parents if necessary) through visiting, telephone contact, letter writing, cards, or photographs.

Parents and children need thorough, detailed, and repeated explanations of the plan of therapy. They need reassurance that a change in the child's condition is most likely a result of chemotherapy, not the disease. Decreasing the chance for the unexpected lessens the opportunities for increased anxiety. For example, forewarning the family about the side effects of therapy, such as alopecia, weight gain, constipation, stomatitis, and nausea and vomiting, and the necessary laboratory procedures prepares them for these expected events and increases their sense of security and control.

Phase II—Reprieve: Remission and Maintenance Therapy

Once the child is in remission, there is a long period of hope for an eventual recovery and fear of a possible relapse. Parents commonly react to these feelings by overprotecting the child, encouraging dependency, and liberalizing discipline. All of these reactions support the child's sick role and hinder optimum physical and emotional development. Family members may attempt to escape or avoid the problems of this period through social isolation.

Overprotectiveness. Although many children return home in relatively stable and much improved physical health, parents frequently treat them as invalids. One of the most common manifestations of overprotectiveness is parents' inability to set appropriate limits. It is understandable that under the stress of potential loss parents might respond by overindulging the child, giving in to his every desire and wish. Although this is probably part of the grieving process during the initial phase of the illness, persistence of this reaction culminates in special problems during the often long period of remission (see discussion of "benevolent overreaction," p. 929).

For ill children, overprotection and "special" treatment increase their fears of serious illness and failure to recover. In addition, if they are given everything during periods of wellness, they will become very frustrated, unhappy, and demanding children during the terminal phase, when it will be impossible to meet all their requests.

Dependency. Closely associated with the overprotectiveness is increased dependency between parents and child. This is often evident in parents' unwillingness to send their child to school. If not helped toward reintegration of usual activities, they may use the hair loss or frequent visits for treatment as excuses for keeping the child home. The same needs and interventions regarding school that are discussed in Chapter 22 apply. However, the school personnel may have special concerns.* A common, often unvoiced fear of school personnel is that the child will have some dramatic episode, such as massive hemorrhage, while in the classroom, and die (Klopovich and others, 1981). During the discussion of the disease the nurse should include the usual course of the illness and its specific implications, for example, the child's increased susceptibility to common childhood diseases or unexpected epidemics such as chickenpox. In this case the school nurse should report the instance of prevalent illness to the parent.

Several issues should also be approached with the school teacher and nurse, particularly other parents' questions

about the disease, such as the chance of communicability, preparation of the class for expected physical changes, and possible future absences. During the terminal phase the parents should also discuss the likelihood of the child's death and the need for discussing this with the other students. Teachers of siblings who attend the same school should also be included in the discussions. For example, the siblings may be demonstrating in school their difficulties in adjusting to the child's illness. Such behavior may erroneously be interpreted as learning disabilities, behavioral or emotional problems, or delinquency, for example. Unless the teachers are aware of the extenuating circumstances, these children can be saddled with negative labels for the rest of their academic life.

Social isolation. The critical nature of the crisis frequently closes off communication with those people not integrally involved in the child's care. Consequently, when the child returns home the parents may find it easier to keep their secret behind closed doors. Although the community is usually aware of the child's illness, many individuals will avoid the family. If parents are helped to understand the reactions of others and are guided to answer questions, they will be less likely to need protective isolation.

Although friends and relatives may be a significant support system for the family, frequently they are not. For example, unsolicited advice or casual remarks can burden the family with increased guilt. One mother who had returned home with her child after a lengthy hospital stay had gained weight. The neighbors expressed surprise at "how good the mother looked." During the next hospital admission the mother deliberately limited her caloric intake. She commented to the nurse "I can't gain weight this time. They will never understand how difficult this is if I look healthy." It took many discussions before the nurse was able to help the mother realize that what others thought was less important than her physical well-being.

Hope and fear. Throughout the transition period from diagnosis to recovery or death, there is a constant mixing of hope and fear. Accompanying the hope for a cure is the ever-present fear of return of the disease. Any intervening physical crisis, such as infection, drug toxicity, or depressed bone marrow, causes marked parental concern and anxiety. There is a constant need for reevaluation of the child's progress, reassurance that the disease is in remission, and reconfirmation that some children do recover.

If the child is hospitalized during a remission for almost any reason, the parents may respond with what appears to be exaggerated fear and concern. However, health professionals need to understand that any complication magnifies the seriousness of the underlying illness. Nurses should encourage families to express their feelings while emphasizing signs of improvement in the child's condition.

Many parents find that the best times are the most difficult, because in the light of hope lurk the shadows of fear. As one parent explained, "I never can enjoy the good times too much because the fear of leukemia recurring is always there. If I have too much hope and allow my spirits to get

---

*See suggested readings on p. 954 for information concerning students with serious illness.

too high, I am afraid that if something goes wrong I will have too far to fall. I worry that if that happened I would never be able to pick myself up again. So I protect myself by maintaining a cautious level of optimism.''

Anxiety. In addition to the concerns discussed in the preceding paragraphs are many other anxiety-provoking stresses. The financial strain of a chronic illness is a constant worry. Job security is always a necessary consideration, because unemployment may jeopardize insurance coverage. There are also costs besides the actual medical care, such as transportation to the hospital, meals away from home, baby-sitting for other siblings, or temporary housing for distant medical care.* The nurse can provide assistance by referring the family to available organizations, such as the **Leukemia Society of America†** or the **American Cancer Society,‡** who may be able to provide financial help.

Nutrition is also a continuing concern. Many drugs cause severe nausea and vomiting, thereby decreasing the child's appetite. The illness usually results in marked weight loss. Mealtime can become a battleground for family members. The nurse can prevent some of the problems by forewarning parents of the expected change in appetite and by suggesting ways of encouraging children to eat without causing a power struggle (see p. 1115). For example, during the course of steroid therapy, appetite improves dramatically. Parents should be told that the increased hunger is a result of medication, not a change in the child's behavior or attitude. During periods of chemotherapy when the appetite is decreased, providing small, frequent meals of favorite foods often encourages some cooperation. Growth may also be slowed during the treatment phase from the various drugs and use of radiation. If parents are aware of some of these expected changes, they may be more accepting of the child's fluctuating appetite.

Nursing considerations. Often remission and ''going home'' from the cancer center coincide, and a number of problems can be anticipated and often prevented by a thorough discussion at this time: maintenance of normal family patterns, school attendance, and relationships among family and friends (Lansky, 1985). Because of the usual reaction by parents to overprotect the child, they should be advised to continue appropriate discipline of the child and siblings by resuming pre-illness rules and limits. The importance of resuming school and other daily activities as soon as possible is stressed, and other family members, particularly mothers, may benefit from resuming their previous functions, including employment. Parents are encouraged to schedule appointments for visits at times that least interfere with the child's daily routine, such as late on Friday, which leaves the weekend for recuperation from any unpleasant side effects (Fig. 23-2).

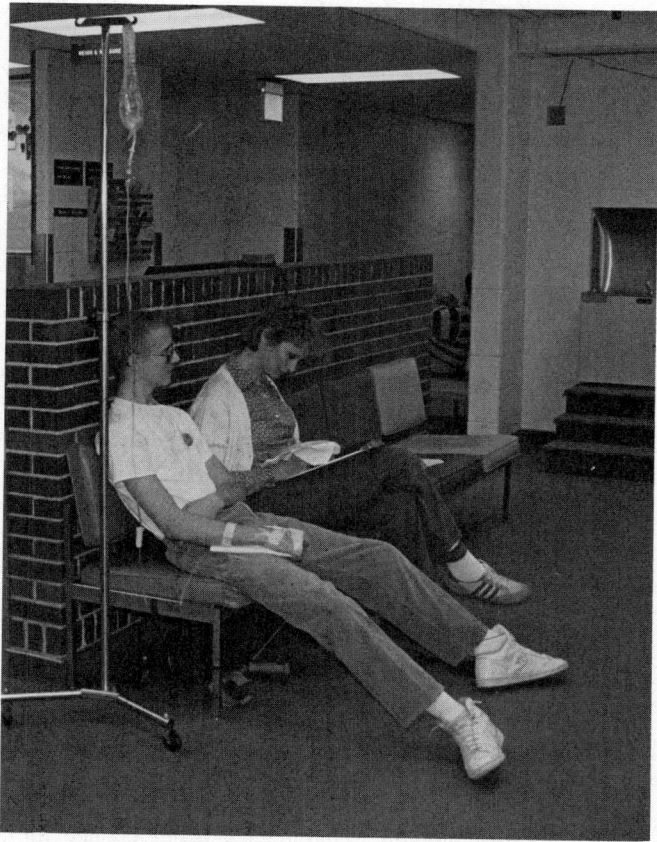

Fig. 23-2. Treatment often involves long periods of outpatient visits that should be scheduled at times that least interfere with the youngster's daily routine.
Photography by Katherine Patterson, University of Kansas, College of Health Sciences and Hospital, Kansas City, KS.

Another concern related to treatment is noncompliance. Among adolescents the rate of treatment refusal may exceed 20%, and is particularly common in nonwhite families in which one parent is not present in the home (Cohen and others, 1985). Poor drug compliance can affect induction and remission therapy and ultimately the prognosis (Smith and others, 1981). Therefore nurses must be aware of the potential for this problem and vigilantly assess adherence to the treatment protocol (see discussion of Compliance, p. 1110).

To avoid unnecessary social isolation the parents need to be prepared for common responses of friends and relatives, such as staying away from the family, fearing the child's illness, especially concern for contagion, and giving unsolicited advice. Families should take the initiative in informing others about the child's condition and asking directly that they remain in contact with each other. Being the first to express, ''I know it's hard to know what to say and do in a situation like this,'' can put others at ease. A more difficult situation is the offering of unsolicited advice regarding treatment, particularly information about ''new'' but unproved methods. Parents need to take a firm but tactful approach; they can comment that they will inquire about the method with their health professional but that they feel

*Ronald McDonald Houses provide inexpensive homelike accommodations for families when distance to the hospital is a major factor. They are located in several large cities and application for lodging is usually made through the social service department of the medical center.
†800 Second Ave., New York, NY 10017.
‡777 Third Ave., New York, NY 10017.

assured that they are receiving the best care available. Many families benefit from associating with other similarly affected families. There is a special camaraderie between these parents that seems to sustain them through the long ordeal. Sources of information about self-help groups are discussed on p. 944.

Because many children are treated in tertiary centers located at a distance from their home, there may not be one primary nurse who can act as liaison and coordinator among the nurses in the hospital, school, clinic, physician's office, and community. Often this results in a lack of preventive intervention. Nurses who are in a particularly advantageous position to become a primary link with the family are nurse practitioners and community nurses, and a nurse network should be established before discharge to ensure continuity of care.

Phase III—Recovery: Cessation of Therapy and Possible Cure

The maintenance period may be followed by cessation of therapy in the hope of a permanent recovery. Although this is a very happy time, it is mixed with feelings of grief, ambivalence, and concern for the future.

Denial and ambivalence. At the time the decision is made to terminate therapy, many parents deny that treatment is no longer warranted. They may express ambivalence with such questions as, "Are you sure that a longer period of drugs wouldn't guarantee a better chance for a cure?" There is great difficulty in giving up the security of the rituals of medication, radiation therapy, and frequent examinations. Occasionally health professionals erroneously label the ambivalence or denial as a psychologic need for the child's sick role.

In general this reaction is characteristic of the grieving for the loss of security afforded by medical intervention and adjustment to the hazards of "waiting it out" again. Parents need almost as much support during this phase as they did when they were told of the diagnosis.

Overprotectiveness. Parents also relate a resurgence of the need to overprotect and isolate their child from any potential physical harm. As one mother stated, "I became fanatical about examining my child for signs of recurring illness when the drugs were stopped. If he had a runny nose or sore throat, I immediately took him to the doctor, requesting a blood count. I was so sure those leukemic cells had returned." She later compared this reaction to the ways in which she treated the child after his first remission. She added, "You would think that after 3 years of living with drugs, side effects, blood tests, and doctors, I would be thrilled to give it all up, but here I am, almost as shaky and nervous as if I had just found out he had the disease."

Concern for the future. When cure is a realistic possibility, parents' concern for the *quantity* of life shifts to the *quality* of life. This is a legitimate concern, because chemotherapy and radiation are not without their immediate and long-term complications (see p. 1573). With increasing numbers of children surviving, it is likely that much more will be known about future consequences. The need for continued medical supervision of these children cannot be overemphasized.

For families who did not have the benefit of anticipatory guidance, the prospect of a cure may represent a rethinking of their childrearing practices. For example, these parents may have indulged the child and tolerated negative or regressive behaviors because of the thought of death. Now that the child's future is much more positive, there may be recognition that changes must occur to reestablish normal behavior. Such families benefit from professional guidance to gradually change behavioral patterns.

Nursing considerations. Probably the most important component of care is acceptance of the parents' need to regress to earlier forms of coping, such as denial or overprotection. Parents need to feel comfortable in calling the nurse or clinic about any concern or problem. They also should be encouraged to verbalize their feelings and thoughts of cessation of therapy. It may be helpful for the nurse to acquaint them with another family who has progressed through this transition period.

Nurses working with these families must be aware of the long-term consequences of treatment and be vigilant of signs indicating problems, such as retarded growth or evidence of a second malignancy. Psychosocial problems may surface, and young people are particularly concerned about fertility and sexuality. Adolescents frequently equate the information about impaired fertility with impaired sexual performance, and even when such concerns are not voiced, they need clarification that sexual performance is not physiologically affected.

Phase IV—Recurrence: Relapse and Death

The most dreaded news other than the initial diagnosis is confirmation of a relapse. For many children the first relapse is followed by another remission, but subsequently by future relapses, with the final one followed by death. The family's reactions during the terminal stage are influenced by their previous acceptance or denial of the child's illness. It is a period of intense anticipatory grieving, characterized by the relapse reactions of depression, loss of hope, and possibly acceptance. As the child's condition worsens, there is intensification of numerous fears.

Heightened anticipatory grieving. Once the remission has ended, there is exacerbation of all the previous stages of grieving. Denial may be present to varying degrees, from minimal disbelief on discovery of the relapse to complete refusal to accept the diagnosis. However, most families tend to practice partial denial. For example, one parent explained that although the leukemic cells were present in the spinal fluid, the physician was not certain "if this is a relapse or a 'slight failure' of the drugs to kill these cells." Children also seem to defend themselves against the complications of a relapse. For example, one adolescent emphasized that Hodgkin disease had not returned. The physician had just found a node that was "missed" during radiation therapy.

During a relapse any of the stages of dying may be exaggerated. Children in particular may become very angry or depressed, especially if they have not been told the truth or if the truth has been distorted to imply that the treatment is a cure. For example, children who may have been very accepting and cooperative during the initial hospitalization may respond to subsequent hospital admissions with hostility and rage. Parents and staff members frequently do not comprehend the reason for the altered behavioral reaction, and instead of trying to understand and deal with it, scold or admonish the child. However, for the child this hospitalization may be more difficult and frightening than the initial one, because the severity and uncertainty of the disease have become a reality.

Loss of hope and depression. One of the most difficult realizations for parents is the knowledge that with each relapse the chances for eventual recovery diminish. The reality of possible death looms before them, particularly during the reinduction phase when a recurrent remission may or may not be feasible. Once another remission is attained, reason for hope is again present.

However, many parents relate that after termination of the primary remission they never again feel as hopeful or optimistic. Some also discuss their silent preparation and grieving for the child's eventual death. Nurses need to be sensitive to such thoughts and aware of the possible beneficial aspect of this reaction, because repeated relapses are associated with poorer prognoses.

The usual reaction to loss of hope is depression. This may be the type of depression for past losses, but most often is anticipatory grieving for impending losses. Nurses need to carefully assess the reason for the depression and realistically plan intervention. For example, if another remission is likely, the nurse should plan to help the parents work through their depression. If this is not done, the parents may psychologically bury the child and end his living prematurely. However, if this relapse is actually the commencement of the terminal stage, the nurse should plan to support the parents in their depression, because it is a necessary precursor of acceptance.

Fear of death. The most prevalent fear is of death itself. Parents frequently ask about death through questions such as, "What will he die from?" "How will we know he is dying?" and "What will happen when he dies?" It is important to listen sensitively to such questions because the real concern may be hidden behind the question. For example, when parents ask, "What will he die from?" they may not be so concerned with the medical cause of death, such as hemorrhage or infection, but may really be asking, "What is hemorrhage like?" Most people have a fantasy idea of how death will occur that is much more horrifying than the actual event. For example, parents will relate that their idea of hemorrhage is uncontrollable gushing of blood from every orifice. In reality it is usually internal bleeding with oozing of blood from the nose. When nurses are aware of the imagined events, they can clarify the misconceptions and supply the correct information.

Fear of pain. The fear of uncontrollable pain is almost universal. Whatever bargaining occurs during the dying stage is for a peaceful, quiet, and quick death. Often parents will relate that the child has pain even when it appears that he is comfortable. It is important for nurses to understand that pain is much more than physical. Watching one's child die is a pain that must certainly be immeasurable and that subjectively shadows one's perception of surrounding events.

Fear of loss of control. A fear that is shared by the dying and the survivors is losing emotional and physical control as death approaches. Some parents attempt to cope with this fear by requesting that their child be heavily sedated during the terminal stage. However, the loss of control imposed by medication may make the child very distraught. Inasmuch as nurses usually regulate the administration of drugs, it is important for them to carefully assess the needs of both the child and the parents. Supporting parents at the time of impending death by being physically present, making the child as comfortable as possible, and talking to the awake child helps parents feel in control without the need for sedating the child.

Fear of isolation and loneliness. Parents fear that their child will die when they are not with him. Dying children often request that their parents stay with them (Fig. 23-3), and this request should always be respected. Although everyone dies alone, no one need die in lonely isolation.

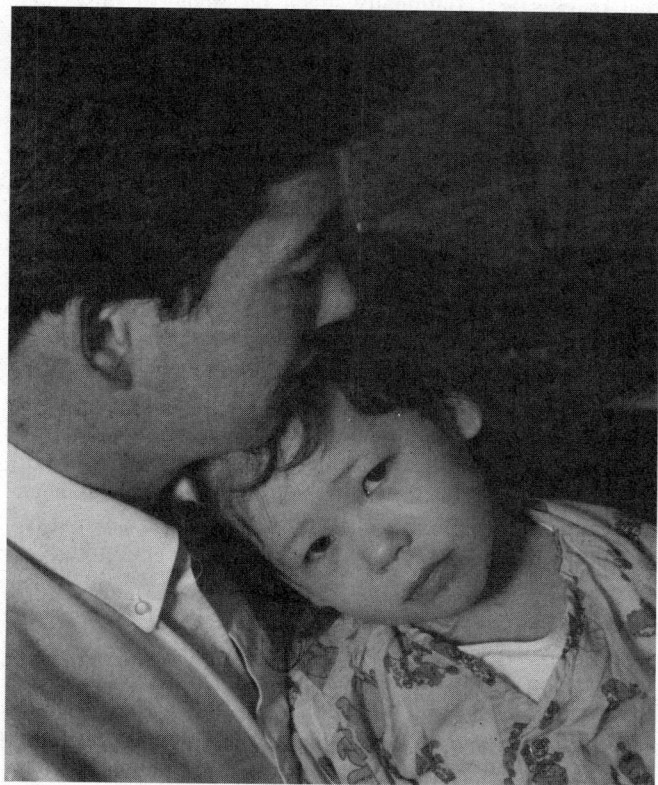

Fig. 23-3. For the dying child there is no greater comfort than the security and closeness of a parent.
Photography by Katherine Patterson, University of Kansas, College of Health Sciences and Hospital, Kansas City, KS.

Nursing considerations. Relapse is a difficult phase for nurses because it often initiates a loss of hope and their own grieving process. One of the dangers during the phase of relapse is that nurses may transfer their feelings of pessimism or optimism to the parents. It is extremely important to assess one's own personal response to the relapse and to plan the intervention according to the person's needs. This seems to be particularly critical during the final relapse. Nurses can help parents and children formulate realistic short-term goals and establish reasonable priorities of care. It is also the time to discuss with parents their wishes and expectations for the terminal phase. For some families the alternative of hospice or home care is a very significant and fulfilling means of sharing their child's last days (see p. 967).

During the terminal stage the fears of parents and children form the foundation for nursing care. These fears may be particularly worrisome for those parents who have chosen home care because they must assume primary responsibility for the child. The nurse's role includes preparing them to deal with each fear and providing assistance through home visits, telephone counseling, and the alternative of hospital admission at any time. As death approaches, nurses should recognize the physical signs (Table 23-2) and summon the parents to the child's bedside. If death approaches sooner than expected, families should be prepared. Sometimes health professionals' need to deny death is so strong that parents are continually given messages of false hope that prevent them from preparing themselves for the worst news. Although others may think such false hope is helpful, in reality it may be extremely painful for family members to live in uncertainty.

The goal in caring for dying children is comfort, and no intervention is more important than control of pain. Ideally pain should be managed all during the terminal phase on a *preventive schedule,* with adjustments made as needed to maintain maximum comfort. This often requires increasing doses of narcotics beyond those normally recommended, decreasing the duration between doses, and changing routes of administration to comply with the child's needs and wishes. Whenever possible the oral route is preferred, but when no longer possible, continuous intravenous infusion or rectal administration may provide the greatest benefit. Any nonpharmacologic measures that may augment pain relief and relaxation are employed, such as cutaneous stimulation (for example, rocking, stroking the skin) or diversion (for example, reading to the child or playing music). (See also p. 1068 for an extensive discussion of pain assessment and management.)

Both the family and the child may have heightened spiritual needs at the time of death. Spiritual support includes respect for the diverse beliefs of families, willingness to discuss matters of spirituality with them, and provision for the rituals and sacraments of organized religion (Conrad, 1985). Many families desire a priest, minister, or rabbi, and the nurse can summon the clergy to be with the family. In those cases in which it may not be possible to reach a clergyman, the nurse may have to provide the spiritual needs by praying with the family, reading from the Bible, or listening to the review of their life.

Phase V—The Beginning: Postdeath

The crisis of loss does not end with the child's death. In many ways it only begins. Families can prepare themselves for the expected loss, but when it occurs there is a period of acute grief, followed by an extended phase of mourning (see p. 966). It is important for families to understand that mourning takes a long time. Whereas acute grief may last only weeks or months, resolving their loss can be measured in years. Holidays and anniversaries can be particularly difficult, and people who previously had been supportive may now expect the family to have "adjusted." Consequently, prolonged mourning is often silent and lonely.

Nursing considerations. Part of the difficulty in helping the bereaved family is lack of opportunity for follow-up in the traditional nursing structure. Consequently many of these families never receive the support and guidance that could help them resolve the loss. Fortunately, hospice programs recognize this need and provide regular follow-up after the death. In addition, self-help groups are present in many communities, such as **The Compassionate Friends,*** an international organization for bereaved parents and siblings, and specialty groups, such as **Parents of Murdered Children.†** When such groups are not available nurses can be instrumental in facilitating parent groups. Lindamood and others (1979) describe the formation, conduct, and follow-up of bereaved groups, which can serve as a prototype for initiating such a program.

Follow-up can help the family understand the process of mourning, particularly its duration and pain, and can provide assistance in making decisions that involve the loss. One especially difficult dilemma faced by many parents is the decision to have additional children. The advisability of having another child soon after the death is controversial. If the grief is unresolved there is the danger of the subsequent offspring becoming a "replacement child" (Poznanski, 1972). However, this view is not shared by all professionals or by bereaved families who have successfully conceived another offspring (Glassman-Feibusch, 1983; Weiss, 1984). Consequently the nurse's role cannot be one of giving answers but of assessing readiness for another pregnancy through knowledge of the parents' progress through grief and their motivations in conceiving.

At times family members may need assistance in their grieving. Mothers, in particular, often feel a great sense of loneliness and emptiness, and part of their resolving the grief is finding a substitute role that is fulfilling and rewarding. Nurses can be instrumental in this process by (1) preparing the mother for anticipating the *normal* feelings of

---

*P.O. Box 3696, Oak Brook, IL 60522-3696.
†100 E. 8th St., Rm. B41, Cincinnati, OH 45202.

Table 23-2 Physical signs of approaching death

SIGNS	INTERVENTIONS
Loss of sensation and movement in the lower extremities, progressing toward the upper body Sensation of heat, although body feels cool	Keep bedsheets untucked Keep child uncovered if sheets are bothersome Apply loose, cool clothing Keep fresh air circulating in room (open window, use small fan) Change child's position only as tolerated Give cool sponge baths Preserve physical closeness with family members (e.g., parent may want to rock child in chair or lie next to child in bed)

Loss of senses
    Tactile sensation decreases
    Sensitive to light
    Hearing is last sense to fail
	Limit care to essentials
	    May need to forego usual hygienic measures such as bath or clothing change but provide comfort measures (e.g., mouth care, wiping forehead, gentle back rub)
	Avoid bright, direct light, but do not keep room too dim
	Sit at head of bed where child can easily see face
	Talk to child in clear, distinct voice, not whispers
	Avoid conversation about the child in his presence

Confusion, loss of consciousness, slurred speech	Talk to child even though may not appear awake Play favorite music; may soothe child Offer calm reassurance and orient child to surroundings when awake Phrase questions for yes or no answers
Muscle weakness	Use pillows or other supports to prop child in comfortable position Carry (if possible) to other areas for diversion if desired
Loss of bowel and bladder control	Place absorbent pads under hips Help child to toilet if he desires
Decreased appetite/thirst Difficulty swallowing	Offer any foods child desires Avoid excessive encouragement to eat or drink Avoid foods with strong odors Serve foods that require the least energy to eat (soups, shakes) Feed slowly Provide mouth care before and after eating; lubricate lips with petrolatum

Change in respiratory pattern
    Cheyne-Stoke respirations (waxing and waning of depth of breathing with regular periods of apnea)
    "Death rattle" (noisy chest sounds from accumulation of pulmonary and pharyngeal secretions)
	Administer anticholinergic drugs (atropine or scopolamine) to reduce secretions (lessens "death rattle," which can be distressing to family)
	Position with head slightly elevated or in well-supported sitting position if tolerated

Weak, slow pulse; decreased blood pressure	No intervention other than reassurance of family Do not disturb child with repeated measurements of vital signs

emptiness, loneliness, and sometimes even failure, (2) helping her reevaluate her role as parent and spouse, stressing that giving up the lost child must occur before she can reestablish emotional relationships, (3) encouraging her to explore fulfilling activities that utilize her special interests, talents, and qualifications, and (4) supporting her as her role changes, particularly assisting with communication between affected family members (Wong, 1980).

Nurses should also be aware of behaviors that indicate siblings' difficulty with resolving their grief, such as persistent blame and guilt, patterns of overactivity with aggressive and destructive outbursts, compulsive caregiving, persistent

anxieties (such as fear of another family death or of their own), excessive clinging to the parent, difficulty with forming new relationships, problems at school, or delinquency (such as stealing) (Krupnick, 1984). In these situations professional assistance may be required and the nurse can provide appropriate referral.

Communication with the bereaved family is essential, but often there is a feeling of not knowing what to say and of helplessness in offering words of comfort. Regrettably, reports from bereaved families indicate that the majority (80%) consider the information or counseling from professionals to be inadequate and even harmful (Segal, Fletcher, and Meekison, 1986). Harmful comments included:

> At stillbirth: "It's horrible; don't look"; "Stop crying."
> During hospital stay: "You need to be strong for your wife"; "You shouldn't be so upset. You should have expected it."
> After unexpected death: "Why did it take you so long to go to Emergency?"

Harmful behaviors included:

> Leaving the parents alone after the child's death
> Prescribing tranquilizers in the first 24 hours after the death
> Not providing explanations when treating the child

In analyzing the type of "helping" statements frequently made in responding to the bereaved, researchers found that 80% were considered nonhelpful (low facilitative). Of the "helpful" statements (high facilitative), those that conveyed feelings were considered most supportive (Davidowitz and Myrick, 1984). The analysis of low and high facilitative statements can provide health professionals with guidelines for effective communication with bereaved families* (see box) (see also Facilitative responding, p. 195).

The Nurse and the Fatally Ill Child

It would not be complete to discuss the nurse's role in caring for the family and dying child without exploring the effects of this stressful, yet extremely rewarding, area of nursing practice on the caregiver. Recognition of the poten-

*Excellent guidelines are also given in the publication, *Suggestions for Doctors and Nurses*, from The Compassionate Friends.

tial stresses is essential in coping successfully with the emotional demands imposed by sharing the family's loss and grief.

NURSES' REACTIONS TO CARING FOR FATALLY ILL CHILDREN

Nurses experience reactions to a fatal illness that are very similar to the responses of family members. Some of these help nurses provide care by protecting them from the emotional impact of the event. Others interfere with the establishment of a therapeutic relationship with family members. Analysis and understanding of these reactions are as important in providing effective care to the dying child as is the recognition of specific responses in the family.

Denial

When children are admitted to a pediatric unit with a suspected diagnosis of a serious illness, the initial response from nurses is shock and denial. However, their behavioral reaction may be withdrawal from the child and family. They choose the "cure" philosophy over the "care" philosophy as a method of distancing themselves from the implications of emotional involvement. Because of their own dependency on denial, nurses may support denial in parents. There are several methods of conveying this message, such as emphasizing only the optimistic "survival statistics," negating the seriousness of the illness, focusing on "cheering up" the family, and engaging in casual conversation to avoid meaningful dialogue. Although this increases nurses' comfort in caring for the dying child, it does little to provide

---

HELPFUL AND NONHELPFUL RESPONSES TO BEREAVED FAMILIES

High facilitative responses
(caring, understanding, warm, respectful, accepting)

Questions are either open or closed and sometimes have advice implied in them. Behind every question is an assumption ("Can I be of any help?" or "Have you decided who the pallbearers will be?"). Questions that help the person to explore ideas and feelings are usually seen as facilitative.

Clarifying and summarizing attempts to seek an understanding of what a person has said or to identify the most salient ideas that seem to be emerging from the conversation ("If I'm following you, you don't want to talk with anyone right now." "Correct me if I'm wrong, but you intend to make all arrangements.").

Feeling-focused conveys that feelings are understood. Requires the use of a feeling word in the statement ("You're uncertain about what to do next." "You're feeling confused, and angry, too." "You're still struggling and feeling the pain."). Communicates the most understanding, acceptance, and respect.

Low facilitative responses
(judgmental, nonaccepting, unconcerned, impersonal)

Advice or evaluation suggests or tells people what they might or ought to do ("You shouldn't question God's will," "You've got to get out more," "Stop feeling sorry for yourself.").

Interpreting or analyzing attempts to connect events, explain behaviors and causative factors ("It was God's will," "It's better now because she is at peace," "You're acting that way because you choose to suffer.").

Reassurance and support are intended to be encouraging but more often than not they also communicate that people need not feel the way they do ("You know, death comes to all of us; it's just a part of life," "At least you still have your father," "Time is a great healer, and you'll be stronger later," "I know how you feel.").

From Davidowitz, M., and Myrick, R.D.: Responding to the bereaved: an analysis of "helping" statements, Death Educ. **8:**1-10, 1984.

family members with an opportunity to progress beyond denial and begin anticipatory grieving.

Some denial is as important for nurses as it is for the child or parents; it protects nurses from the overwhelming reality of death. It would be extremely difficult to participate in the medical treatment plan without some expectation of a cure. Denial is also necessary to prevent feelings of failure. The nursing and medical goal is curing illness and saving lives, not allowing patients to die. However, denial loses its beneficial functions when nurses refuse to admit failure and adhere to the "curing" regimen, regardless of its effectiveness or value.

Anger and Depression

Some nurses may be angry for having been assigned to the "leukemia case," because the very exposure to potential failure in a fatal illness is extremely threatening. Others may feel angry for having to subject the child to painful procedures or for being unable to relieve his physical and emotional suffering. Instead of anger, some nurses may feel depression for any of these reasons.

However, without an understanding of the reason for the emotion, nurses may project the anger onto others, particularly family members. They may be unable to tolerate the child's uncooperative behavior or the parents' continual requests for information. Anger fuels more anger, and parents react with hostility and think the members of the nursing staff are rejecting them. A vicious cycle of resentment, mistrust, and frustration results.

Depression also has adverse effects on a therapeutic relationship, because nurses may withdraw from the child and parents as a method of controlling their sadness. Unaware of the reason for the avoidance, family members interpret it as evidence of inadequate care. This reaction also fosters a nonsupportive cycle of avoidance, withdrawal, resentment, and frustration. However, the messages are usually more covert than when the nurses' reaction is anger, and may prevent a climax that could result in a solution to the problem.

Guilt

Nurses who feel unable to deal with fatal illness in a child often experience guilt. Nurses who become angry or depressed when caring for a dying child often reveal that they are very uncomfortable with this response but are unable to choose a more direct, constructive approach. They express guilt for having been intolerant of the child's or parents' behavior and, even more important, realize the missed opportunity to provide these individuals with professional support and guidance.

Nursing staff may experience guilt even when they can deal effectively with the family. There is often a feeling that the family's needs are never completely met. Such nurses tend to set expectations that are beyond anyone's ability to meet, such as the expectation that they are supposed to save lives, not let people die.

The one important difference between a dying child and an ill child is that there may be no second chance to meet the needs of the dying child. This finality is difficult to comprehend but can be a catalyst toward better understanding of one's own responses to dying. For example, when guilt makes one uncomfortable enough to seek alternate behavior patterns, there is an opportunity for change to occur, provided the individual is given some assistance and support.

Ambivalence

One of the most universal reactions of nurses is ambivalence in their feelings toward a dying child. There is the fluctuating adherence to hope for a cure and fear of a relapse. Sometimes the motivations for either are more for personal needs. For example, they may hope that the child recovers so that he does not return to the hospital. Or they may wish for a remission so that his discharge is assured. Such thoughts are certainly understandable in light of the emotional toll of nursing a dying child.

Ambivalence may be demonstrated in a particular type of bargaining. Rather than bargaining for extra time, nurses may hope that their colleagues are assigned the patient or that a death may occur on a shift other than their own. Bargaining for a temporary absence from the dying child is a healthy response, because it denotes nurses' awareness of their own emotional limits. Nurses who are unable to recognize their personal emotional limits are in danger of seeking from the professional relationship their own needs for gratification, achievements, and fulfillment. This results in the loss of an objective evaluation of therapeutic interventions and the increased potential for subjective overinvolvement with the family.

Coping with Stress

One of the hazards of caring for dying children is the risk of *burnout,* a state of physical, emotional, and mental exhaustion (Pines, 1981). It occurs as a result of prolonged involvement with individuals in situations that are emotionally demanding. Nurses working in intensive care units are particularly prone to this occupational hazard, but staff nurses also can experience it when dealing with groups of children such as those who may die. To cope effectively and therapeutically with children who are dying, while avoiding burnout, requires deliberate and concerted effort on the part of the nurse to cope constructively with the stress generated in this role.

Self-awareness and consciousness raising. The initial step in effectively caring for a dying child is making a deliberate choice to become involved. Many nurses react negatively to the word "involvement" because they believe that professionals must remain uninvolved in order to maintain objectivity. Involvement does not displace objectivity. On the contrary, allowing oneself to feel with the other person expands one's ability to comprehend the meaning and depth of that emotion. Maslach (1979) suggests that the achievement of *detached concern,* in which the health care practitioner provides sensitive, understanding care by being sufficiently detached to make objective, rational decisions, is the ideal.

Involvement does have the potential risk of clouding objectivity, but awareness of one's reactions and investments in the care of a dying child helps prevent such possible hazards. Developing awareness requires the willingness to investigate one's motivations for choosing to work in such an area and an understanding of the stresses inherent in the role, to review one's resolution of past losses, and to contemplate one's own fears of death. Often nurses realize that their cold, impersonal reaction to dying patients stems from previous unresolved conflicts or losses. Once they are able to talk about such experiences, they are usually able to gain insight into their behavior and begin to form alternate methods of reacting.

Knowledge and practice. Intervening therapeutically with terminally ill children and their families requires more than self-awareness. It also necessitates basing nursing practice on sound theoretic formulations and empiric observations that serve as a general, concise analysis of the typical reactions of families. Although every individual is different and responds to events or crises in a way that is influenced by all his or her previous life's experiences, there must be some beginning point for understanding the more typical responses of individuals and for making some decision as to their importance in the eventual resolution of the crisis. In this way nurses can plan care that meets the needs of each family member in terms of prevention as well as intervention of problems.

Nurses also must explore ethical issues surrounding the definition of death, the use of extraordinary, lifesaving measures vs passive or active euthanasia, and patients' rights to know and choose their own destiny. Once they have soundly formulated principles by which to practice, they need opportunities for decision making. When a team approach is used, nurses can be valuable members of the group, provided their own values are clarified and they have critically assessed the family's responses.

Support systems. Support systems are essential to continued functioning in a high-stress environment. They allow for regeneration of energies by sharing feelings and concerns with others. Social supports may be personal family members such as parents or spouses, extended relatives, and friends. Professional supports include colleagues, consultants, teachers, and supervisors. Peers may be sources of technical and practical advice and can provide a frame of reference and feedback for the nurse to gauge her own work (Cherniss as cited in McElroy, 1982). Professional persons may be of their own field or from related disciplines.

Other strategies. Any number of other strategies may be used to reduce stress. These include maintaining good general health practices, especially regular exercise, and diversionary activities that are of personal interest beyond the workplace (Vanchon and Pakes, 1985). Distancing techniques are also effective, such as leaving work at work, informing other staff not to contact them on their days off,

periodically assuming less demanding assignments, and taking time off when needed. For caregivers who find the demands of this kind of nursing too emotionally draining, the ultimate distancing strategy is resignation (Munley, 1985).

A final technique is to focus on the positive aspects of the caregiving role. Despite the difficult times in caring for these children and families there are many rewarding experiences that must be remembered. Dedicated efforts reap numerous rewards, and these must not be forgotten or minimized. Reflection on positive feedback from appreciative families can revitalize self-esteem and job satisfaction. Attending the funeral services can be a supportive act both for the family and the nurse and in no way detracts from the professionalism of care. For the family it conveys a sense of worth and caring by the nurse. For the nurse it provides a sense of "closure" with the family and assists in the resolution of personal grief (Irvine, 1985).

CONCEPT SUMMARIES

- To counsel families and children regarding death, nurses need to understand children's perceptions of death, their fears in each age-group, and personal meanings of death and bereavement during developmental stages.

- Toddlers' egocentricity and separation of fact from fantasy make death incomprehensible; they may still refer to a dead person as if he exists.

- Because of their sense of precausality and self-power, preschoolers may believe that their thoughts actually cause another person's death.

- With their reasoning power and fear of the unknown, school-age children may feel intense guilt and responsibility about someone's death.

- Adolescents have difficulty accepting death because of their preoccupation with developing a sense of identity.

- Nurses may offer the following assistance in assessment and education about death: counseling parents about children's age-specific understanding of death, encouraging parents to help children become familiar and comfortable with loss, taking part in organized death education in schools, and serving as a resource to answer children's questions.

- What children are told about their serious illness is based on several general principles regarding developmental age, previous knowledge, and honesty.

- Kubler-Ross' stages of dying are denial, anger, bargaining, depression, and acceptance.

- According to Lindemann, acute grief is a syndrome with psychologic and somatic symptomatology that may appear after a crisis or be delayed, exaggerated, or apparently absent. Distorted reactions may represent one aspect of the syndrome and can be transformed into normal grief work.

- Parke's grief process consists of four phases that do not necessarily proceed in sequence and may recur at any time: shock and disbelief, expression of grief, disorganization and despair, and reorganization.

- Special decisions at the time of dying and death may involve hospital or hospice care, the child's right to die, visualization of the body, tissue donation, and sibling's attendance at the funeral.

- There are five phases of family reactions to a life-threatening illness: Phase I—shock and disbelief, guilt, anger, anticipatory grieving, depression and ambivalence, bargaining; Phase II—overprotectiveness, dependency, social isolation, hope, fear, and anxiety; Phase III—denial and ambivalence, overprotectiveness, and concern for the future; Phase IV—heightened anticipatory grieving, loss of hope and despair, fear of death, fear of loss of control, and fear of isolation and loneliness; Phase V—acute grief, and extended phase of mourning.

- In coping with stress related to the dying patient, the nurse follows similar patterns: self-awareness, consciousness-raising, knowledge and practice, and need for support system.

REFERENCES

Bluebond-Langner, M.: The private worlds of dying children, Princeton, NJ, 1978, Princeton University Press.

Carbary, L.J.: Easing the family's pain: organ donation, Nurs. Life 5(1):26-28, 1985.

Cohen, D., and others: Psychosocial and family characteristics of adolescents who refuse cancer treatment, J. Assoc. Pediatr. Oncol. Nurs. 3(4):29-30, 1985.

Conrad, N.L.: Spiritual support for the dying, Nurs. Clin. North Am. 20(2):415-426, 1985.

Corr, C.A., and Corr, D.M.: Pediatric hospice care, Pediatrics 76(5):774-780, 1985.

Davidowitz, M., and Myrick, R.: Responding to the bereaved: an analysis of "helping" statements, Death Ed. 8:1-10, 1984.

Foley, G.V.: Facilitating death discussions with children, Pediatrics: Nursing Update, lesson 19, Princeton, NJ, 1986, Continuing Professional Educational Corp.

Foley, G.: Conflicts in practice: the argument for, J. Assoc. Pediatr. Oncol. Nurs. 2(3):22-24, 1985.

Gershan, J.A.: Judaic ethical beliefs and customs regarding death and dying, Crit. Care Nurse 5(1):32-34, 1985.

Glassman-Feibusch, B.: Extremely uncaring [Letter], Am. J. Maternal Child Nurs. 8(6):442, 1983.

Glick, I., Weiss, R., and Parkes, C.: The first year of bereavement, New York, 1974, John Wiley & Sons.

Greenberg, L.W., and others: Giving information for a life-threatening diagnosis, Am. J. Dis. Child. 138(7):649-653, 1984.

Greenham, D.E., and Lohmann, R.A.: Children facing death: recurring patterns of adaptations, Health Social Work 7:89-94, 1982.

Irvine, P.: The attending at the funeral, N. Engl. J. Med. 312(26):1704-1705, 1985.

Kane, B.: Children's concepts of death, J. Gen. Psychiatry 134:141-153, 1979.

Kerner, J., Harvey, B., and Lewiston, N.: The impact of grief: a retrospective study of family function following loss of a child with cystic fibrosis, J. Chron. Dis. 32:221-225, 1979.

Klopovich, P., and others: School phobia, J. Kans. Med. Soc. 82(3):125-127, 1981.

Krupnick, J.: Bereavement during childhood and adolescence. In Osterweis, M., Solomon, F., and Green, M., editors: Bereavement: reactions, consequences, and care, Washington, DC, 1984, National Academy Press.

Kübler-Ross, E.: On death and dying, New York, 1969, Macmillan, Inc.

Kübler-Ross, E.: On children and death, New York, 1983, Macmillan Publishing Co.

Lansky, S.B.: Management of stressful periods in childhood cancer, Pediatr. Clin. North Am. 32(3):625-632, 1985.

Lauer, M.E., and others: Children's perceptions of their sibling's death at home or hospital: the precursors of differential adjustment, Cancer Nurs. 8(1):21-27, 1985.

Lauer, M.E., and others: A comparison study of parental adaptation following a child's death at home or in the hospital, Pediatrics 71(1):107-112, 1983.

Leikin, S.L., and Connell, K.: Therapeutic choices by children with cancer [Letter], J. Pediatr. 103(1):167, 1983.

Lindamood, M.M., and others: Groups for bereaved parents—how they can help, J. Fam. Pract. 9(6):1027-1033, 1979.

Lindemann, E.: Symptomatology and management of acute grief, Am. J. Psychiatry 101:141-148, Sept. 1944.

Martinson, I.M., and others: Home care for children dying of cancer, Pediatrics 62(1):106-113, 1978.

Martinson, I.M., and others: Home care for children dying of cancer, Res. Nurs. Health 9(1):11-16, 1986.

Maslach, C.: The burn-out syndrome and patient care. In Garfield, C., editor: Stress and survival: the emotional realities of life-threatening illness, St. Louis, 1979, The C.V. Mosby Co.

McElroy, A.M.: Burnout—a review of the literature with application to cancer nursing, Cancer Nurs. 5(3):211-217, 1982.

Miles, M.S.: Emotional symptoms and physical health in bereaved parents, Nurs. Res. 34(2):76-81, 1985.

Miles, M.S., and Perry, K.: Parental responses to sudden accidental death of a child, Crit. Care Q. 8(1):73-84, 1985.

Munley, S.A.: Sources of hospice staff stress and how to cope with it, Nurs. Clin. North Am. 20(2):343-355, 1985.

Nagy, M.: The child's view of death, J. Genet. Psychol. 73:3-27, 1948.

Nitschke, R., and others: Therapeutic choices made by patients with end-stage cancer, J. Pediatr. 101(3):471-476, 1982.

O'Malley, J., and others: Psychiatric sequelae of surviving childhood cancer, Am. J. Orthopsychiatry 49(4):608-616, 1979.

Osterweis, M., Solomon, F., and Green, M., editors: Bereavement: reactions, consequences, and care, Washington, DC, 1984, National Academy Press.

Pines, A.: Burnout: a current problem in pediatrics, Curr. Probl. Pediatr. 11(7):2-32, 1981.

Poznanski, E.: The "replacement child"—a sign of unresolved parental grief, J. Pediatr. 81(6):1190-1193, 1972.

Rando, T.: An investigation of grief and adaptation in parents whose children have died from cancer, J. Pediatr. Psychiatry 8(1):3-20, 1983.

Salladay, S.A., and Royal, M.E.: Children and death: guidelines for grief work, Child Psychiatry Hum. Dev. 11(4):203-212, 1981.

Saunders, J.M., and Valente, S.M.: No code: the question that won't go away, Nursing 86 16(3):60-64, 1986.

Schulman, J.L., and Rehm, J.L.: Assisting the bereaved, J. Pediatr. 102(6):992-998, 1983.

Schultz, C.: Grief at sudden death ... you can help, Crit. Care Update 10(2):9-15, 1983.

Schultz, C.: Grieving children, J. Emerg. Nurs. 6:30-36, 1980.

Segal, S., Fletcher, M., and Meekison, W.: Survey of bereaved parents, Can. Med. Assoc. J. 134(1):38-42, 1986.

Shumway, C.N., Grossman, L.S., and Sarles, R.M.: Therapeutic choices by children with cancer [Letter], J. Pediatr. 103(1):168, 1983.

Smith, S., and others: Poor drug compliance in an adolescent with leukemia, Am. J. Pediatr. Hematol. Oncol. 3(3):297-300, 1981.

Stanfill, P., and Strong, C.: Conflicts in practice: the argument against, J. Assoc. Pediatr. Oncol. Nurs. 2(3):25-26, 1985.

Vachon, M.L.S., and Pakes, E.: Staff stress in the care of the critically ill and dying child, Issues Compr. Pediatr. Nurs. 8(1-6):151-182, 1985.

Waechter, E.: Dying children: patterns of coping, Issues Compr. Pediatr. Nurs. 8(1-6):51-68, 1985.

Wass, H.: Concepts of death: a developmental perspective, Issues Compr. Pediatr. Nurs. **8**(1-6):3-24, 1985.

Wass, H., and others: Death education: an annotated resource guide, Washington, DC, 1980, Hemisphere Publishing Corp.

Weber, P.: The human connection: the role of the nurse in organ donation, J. Neurosurg. Nurs. **17**(2):119-122, 1985.

Weiss, R.: Reactions to particular types of bereavement. In Osterweis, M., Soloman, F., and Green, M., editors: Bereavement: reactions, consequences, and care, Washington, DC, 1984, National Academy Press.

Williams, L.: Organ procurement: what nurses need to know, Crit. Care Q. **8**(1):27-30, 1985.

Wong, D.: Bereavement: the empty-mother syndrome, Am. J. Maternal Child Nurs. **5**(6):385-389, 1980.

Zelauskas, B.: Siblings: the forgotten grievers, Issues Compr. Pediatr. Nurs. **5**:45-52, 1981.

BIBLIOGRAPHY

Adams, D.W.: Helping the dying child: practical approaches for nonphysicians, Issues Compr. Pediatr. Nurs. **8**(1-6):95-112, 1985.

Adler, R.: It doesn't end with death: grieving and genetic counseling, Clin. Pediatr. **18**(12):767-768, 1979.

Amado, A., Cronk, B.A., and Mileo, R.: Cost of terminal care: home hospice vs hospital, Nurs. Outlook **27**:522-526, Aug. 1979.

Amenta, M.O.: Hospice in the United States: multiple and varied programs, Nurs. Clin. North Am. **20**(2):269-280, 1985.

Balk, D.: Effects of sibling death on teenagers, J. School Health **53**(1):14-18, 1983.

Baskin, C.H., and others: Helping teachers help children with cancer: a workshop for school personnel, Child. Health Care **12**(2):78-83, 1983.

Benoliel, J.Q.: Nursing research on death, dying, and terminal illness: development, present state, and prospects. In Werley, H.H., and Fitzpatrick, J.J., editors: Annual review of nursing research, vol. 1, New York, 1983, Springer Publishing Co.

Betz, C.L.: Helping children to cope with the death of a sibling, Child Care Newsletter **3**(2):3-5, 1984.

Blotcky, A.D., and Cohen, D.G.: Psychological assessment of the adolescent with cancer, J. Assoc. Pediatr. Oncol. Nurs. **2**(1):8-14, 1985.

Brent, D.A.: A death in the family: the pediatrician's role, Pediatrics **72**(5):645-651, 1983.

Brunnquell, D., and Hall, M.D.: Issues in the psychological care of pediatric oncology patients, Am. J. Orthopsychiatry **52**(1):32-44, 1982.

Cairns, M., and others: Adaptation of siblings to childhood malignancy, J. Pediatr. **95**(3):484-487, 1979.

Carlson, P., and others: Helping parents cope: a model home-care program for the dying child, Issues Compr. Pediatr. Nurs. **8**(1-6):113-128, 1985.

Chase, D.: Dying at home with hospice, St. Louis, 1986, The C.V. Mosby Co.

Chee, C.M.: A child's right to die, Am. J. Maternal Child Nurs. **7**(2):81-88, 1982.

Coleman, F.W., and Coleman, W.S.: Helping siblings and other peers cope with dying, Issues Compr. Pediatr. Nurs. **8**(1-6):129-150, 1985.

Coolidge, C.B.: The dying of Robin: a mother's reflections, J. Pediatr. Psychol. **2**(2):79-81, 1977.

Corr, C.A., and Corr, D.M., editors: Hospice approaches to pediatric care, New York, 1985, Springer Publishing Co.

Counseling the parents whose child is dying due to an accident, Patient Care **16**:168, 1982.

Davidhizar, R.M., and Monhaut, N.: Guidelines for giving bad news by phone, Nursing 85 **15**(4):58-60, 1985.

Davis, A.J.: Breaking the news...to inform relatives of a family member's death, Am. J. Nurs. **83**(10):1457-1478, 1983.

Detwiler, D.A.: The positive function of denial, J. Pediatr. **99**(3):401-402, 1981.

DeVaul, R.A., Zisook, S., and Faschingbauer, T.R.: Clinical aspects of grief and bereavement, Primary Care **6**(2):391-402, 1979.

Dunlop, R.S.: Helping the bereaved, Bowie, Md., 1978, Charles Press.

Edwardson, S.R.: The choice between hospital and home care for terminally ill children, Nurs. Res. **32**(1):29-34, 1983.

Everson, S.: Sibling counseling, Am. J. Nurs. **77**(4):644-646, 1977.

Fanslow, C.A.: Therapeutic touch: a healing modality throughout life, Topics Clin. Nurs. **5**(2):72-79, 1983.

Fischhoff, J., and O'Brien, M.O.: After the child dies, J. Pediatr. **88**(1):140-146, 1976.

Fortunato, R.P., and Komp, D.M.: Death at home for children with acute lymphoblastic leukemia, Va. Med. Monogr. **106**:124-126, Feb. 1979.

Fulton, J., and others: The cadaver donor and the gift of life. In Simmons, R.G., editor: Gift of life: the social and psychological impact of organ transplantation, New York, 1977, John Wiley & Sons, Inc.

Furman, E.: A child's parent dies, New Haven, CT, 1975, Yale University Press.

Garfield, C., editor: Stress and survival: the emotional realities of life-threatening illness, St. Louis, 1979, The C.V. Mosby Co.

Goodell, A.S.: Responses of nurses to the stresses of caring for pediatric oncology patients, Issues Compr. Pediatr. Nurs. **4**(1):1-6, 1980.

Granstrom, S.L.: Spiritual nursing care for oncology patients, Topics Clin. Nurs. **7**(1):39-45, 1985.

Green, M., and Solnit, A.J.: Reactions to the threatened loss of a child: a vulnerable child syndrome. Pediatric management of the dying child. Part III. In Schwartz, J.L., and Schwartz, L.H., editors: Vulnerable infants: a psychosocial dilemma, New York, 1977, McGraw-Hill Book Co.

Greene, P.: The child with leukemia in the classroom, Am. J. Nurs. **75**(1):86-87, 1975.

Gyulay, J.E.: Dealing with the family of a dying child. In Scipien, G.M., and Barnard, M.U., editors: Issues in comprehensive pediatric nursing, New York, 1976, McGraw-Hill Book Co.

Gyulay, J.E.: The dying child, New York, 1978, McGraw-Hill Book Co.

Gyulay, J.E.: The forgotten grievers, Am. J. Nurs. **75**(9):1476-1479, 1975.

Gyulay, J.E., and Miles, M.S.: The family with a terminally ill child. In Hymovitch, D., and Barnard, M., editors: Family health care, New York, 1979, McGraw-Hill Book Co.

Hall, M., Hardin, K., and Conatser, C.: The challenges of psychological care. In Fochtman, D., and Foley, G.V., editors: Nursing care of the child with cancer, Boston, 1982, Little Brown & Co.

Henretta, C.B., and Van Brunt, P.F.: Sudden pediatric death: meeting the needs of family and staff, Nurse Educ. **7**(6):13-16, 1982.

Hogan, N.: Commitment to survival. Part I, Compassionate Friends Newsletter **6**(3):1-6, 1983.

Holland, J.: Understanding the cancer patient, CA **30**(2):103-112, 1980.

Horsley, J.E.: Pulling the plug isn't easy—explaining it is even harder, RN **43**(12):69-74, 1980.

Iles, J.P.: Children with cancer: healthy siblings' perceptions during the illness experience, Cancer Nurs. **2**(5):371-377, 1979.

Johnson, S.: Giving emotional support to families after a patient dies, Nurs. Life **3**(1):34-39, 1983.

Johnson-Soderberg, S.: The development of a child's concept of death, Oncol. Nurs. Forum **8**(1):23-26, 1981.

Johnson-Soderberg, S.: Grief themes, Adv. Nurs. Sci. **3**(4):15-26, 1981.

Kastenbaum, R.J.: Intimations of mortality: in childhood's hour. In Kastenbaum, R.J.: Death, society, and human experience, ed. 2, St. Louis, 1981, The C.V. Mosby Co.

Kinrade, L.C.: Preventive group intervention with siblings of oncology patients, Child. Health Care **14**(2):110, 1985.

Koocher, G.P.: Psychosocial care of the child cured of cancer, Pediatr. Nurs. **11**(2):91-93, 1985.

Krell, R., and Rabkin, L.: The effects of sibling death on the surviving child: a family perspective, Family Process **18**:471-477, 1979.

Krouse, H.J., and Krouse, J.H.: Cancer as crisis: the critical elements of adjustment, Nurs. Res. **31**(2):96-101, 1982.

Krulik, T.: Helping parents of children with cancer during the midstage of illness, Cancer Nurs. **5**(6):441-445, 1982.

Kübler-Ross, E.: Living with death and dying, New York, 1981, Macmillan, Inc.

Kübler-Ross, E., and Warshaw, M.: To live until we say goodbye, Englewood Cliffs, NJ, 1978, Prentice-Hall, Inc.

Kübler-Ross, E.: Death: the final stage of growth, Englewood Cliffs, NJ, 1975, Prentice-Hall, Inc.

Kupst, M.J., and Schulman, J.L.: The CPI subscales as predictors of parental coping with childhood leukemia, J. Clin. Psychol. 37(2):386-388, 1981.

Labson, L.H.: Pediatric oncology. II. Referring children to cancer centers, Patient Care 16:67-94, 1982.

Lansky, S.B., Vats, T., and Cairns, N.U.: Refusal of treatment: a new dilemma for oncologists, Am. J. Pediatr. Hematol. Oncol. 1(3):277-282, 1979.

Lansky, S., and others: Childhood cancer: parental discord and divorce, Pediatrics 62(2):184-188, 1978.

Lascari, A.D.: The dying child and the family, J. Fam. Pract. 6(6):1279-1286, 1978.

Lauer, M.E., and Camitta, B.M.: Home care for dying children: a nursing model, J. Pediatr. 97(6):1032-1035, 1980.

Malecki, M.: Working with families who donate organs and tissues, Child. Today 14(4):26-29, 1985.

Martinson, I.M.: Home care for the dying child: professional and family perspectives, New York, 1976, Appleton-Century-Crofts.

Martinson, I.M.: Parents help each other, Am. J. Nurs. 76 (7):1120-1122, 1976.

Martinson, I.M.: Symposium on child psychiatric nursing: caring for the dying child, Nurs. Clin. North Am. 14:467-474, Sept. 1979.

Martocchio, B.C.: Grief and bereavement: healing through hurt, Nurs. Clin. North Am. 20(2):327-342, 1985.

Martocchio, B.C., and Dufault, K., editors: Symposia on hospice and compassionate care and the dying experience, Nurs. Clin. North Am. 20(2):267-466, 1985.

McEvoy, M., Duchon, D., and Schaefer, D.S.: Therapeutic play group for patients and siblings in a pediatric oncology ambulatory care unit, Topics Clin. Nurs. 7(1):10-18, 1985.

McNeil, J.N.: Death education in the home: parents talk with their children, Issues Compr. Pediatr. Nurs. 8(1-6):293-313, 1985.

Miles, M.S.: Helping adults mourn the death of a child, Issues Compr. Pediatr. Nurs. 8(1-6):219-241, 1985.

Miles, M.S., and Perry, K.: Parental responses to sudden accidental death of a child, Crit. Care Q. 8(1):73, 1985.

Miller, E.L., and Anderson, E.J.: Cancer education for school personnel, J. School Health 49:383-386, Sept. 1979.

Miller, J.F.: Hope doesn't necessarily spring eternal—sometimes it has to be carefully mined and channeled, Am. J. Nurs. 85(1):23-25, 1985.

Moldow, D.G., and Martinson, I.M.: From research to reality—home care for the dying child, Am. J. Maternal Child Nurs. 5(3):159-166, 1980.

Moseley, J.R.: Alterations in comfort, Nurs. Clin. North Am. 20(2):427-438, 1985.

Parkes, C., and Weiss, R.: Recovery from bereavement, New York, 1983, Basic Books, Inc.

Pflaum, M.: Understanding the final messages of the dying, Nursing 86 16(6):26-29, 1986.

Pitel, A.U., and others: Parent consultants in pediatric oncology, Child. Health Care 14(1):46, 1985.

Plank, E.N., and Plank, R.: Children and death. In Solnit, A.J., editor: The psychoanalytic study of the child, New Haven, CT, 1978, Yale University Press.

Rabin, P.L., and Pate, J.K.: Acute grief, South. Med. J. 74(12):1468-1470, 1981.

Rosenthal, P.A.: Short-term family therapy and pathological grief resolution with children and adolescents, Fam. Process 19(2):151-159, 1980.

Ross, J.W.: Childhood cancer: the parents, the patients, the professionals, Issues Compr. Pediatr. Nurs. 4(1):7-16, 1980.

Ross-Alaolmolki, K.: Supportive care for families of dying children, Nurs. Clin. North Am. 20(2):457-466, 1985.

Sahler, O.J., editor: The child and death, St. Louis, 1978, The C.V. Mosby Co.

Schaal, P., and Slemenda, M.B.: Nursing response to transplants, AORN J. 39(1):42-45, 1984.

Schowalter, J.E., Ferholt, J.B., and Mann, N.M.: The adolescent patient's decision to die, Pediatrics 51(1):97-103, 1973.

Schulman, J.L.: Coping with major disease: child, family, pediatrician, J. Pediatr. 102(6):988-991, 1983.

Schulman, J.L.: Coping with tragedy: successfully facing the problem of a seriously ill child, Chicago, 1976, Follett Publishing Co.

Shelton, R.L.: The patient's need of faith at death, Topics Clin. Nurs. 3:55-59, 1981.

Shubin, S.: Burnout: the professional hazard you face in nursing, Nursing 78 7:22-27, July 1978.

Shuler, S.: Death during childhood; reactions in parents and children. In Brandt, P., and others: Current practice in pediatric nursing, vol. 2, St. Louis, 1978, The C.V. Mosby Co.

Siegel, R.K.: Accounting for "afterlife" experiences, Psychol. Today 15(1):65-75, 1981.

Simpson, H.H., II: Understanding the law: organ donation, Nurs. Life 5(1):24-25, 1985.

Smitherman, C.: Dealing with the patient's denial, Nursing 81 11(12):70-71, 1981.

Spinetta, J.J., and Deasy-Spinetta, P., editors: Living with childhood cancer, St. Louis, 1981, The C.V. Mosby Co.

Stickney, S.K., and Gardner, E.R.: Companions in suffering, Am. J. Nurs. 84(12):1491-1493, 1984.

Stowers, S.J.: Nurses cry, too, Nurs. Management 14(4):63-64, 1983.

Sutherland, A.M.: Psychological impact of cancer and its therapy, CA 31(3):159-171, 1981.

van Eys, J., editor: The truly cured child: the new challenge in pediatric cancer care, Baltimore, 1977, University Park Press.

Waechter, E., and others: Concomitants of death imagery in stories told by chronically ill children undergoing intrusive procedures: a comparison of four diagnostic groups, J. Pediatr. Nurs. 1(1):2-11, 1986.

Walker, K.L.: Easing the pain of bereaved parents, Nursing 86 16(4):49-50, 1986.

Wass, H., and Corr, L., editors: Special issue on childhood and death, Issues Compr. Pediatr. Nurs. 8(1-6):3-383, 1985.

Weber, J.A., and Fournier, D.G.: Family support and a child's adjustment to death, Fam. Relat. 34(1):43-49, 1985.

Werner, P.T.: Family medicine and hospice program: a natural alliance, J. Fam. Pract. 12(2):367-368, 1981.

Williams, H.A., Frederick, P.R., and Rothenberg, M.B.: The child is dying: who helps the family? Am. J. Maternal Child Nurs. 6(4):261, 1981.

Williams, L.: Organ procurement: what nurses need to know, Crit. Care Q. 8(1):27-30, 1985.

Wong, D.: The terminally ill child. In Johnson, S., editor: Nursing assessment and strategies for the family at risk, ed. 2, Philadelphia, 1986, J.B. Lippincott Co.

Yoak, M., Chesney, B.K., and Schwartz, N.H.: Active roles in self-help groups for parents of children with cancer, Child. Health Care 14(1):38-45, 1985.

RESOURCES FOR CHILDREN'S BOOKS ON DEATH

Aradine, C.: Books for children about death, Pediatrics 57(3):372-378, 1976.

Bernstein, J.: Literature for young people: non-fiction books about death, Death Ed. 3:111-119, 1979.

Delisle, R., and McNamee, A.: Children's perceptions of death: a look as the appropriateness of selected picture books, Death Educ. 5:1-13, 1981.

Fassler, J.: Helping children cope: mastering stress through books and stories, New York, 1978, The Free Press.

McBride, M.: Children's literature on death and dying, Pediatr. Nurs. 5(3):31-33, 1979.

Mills, G.: Books to help children understand death, Am. J. Nurs. 79(2):291-295, 1979.

Wass, H.: Books for children, Issues Compr. Pediatr. Nurs. **8**(1-6):373-376, 1985.

Wass, H., and Corr, C., editors: Helping children cope with death: guidelines and resources, ed. 2, Washington, DC, 1984, Hemisphere Publishing Corp.

FAMILY-ORIENTED PUBLICATIONS ON LIFE-THREATENING DISORDERS AND DEATH*

Adams, D., and Deveau, E.: Coping with childhood cancer: where do we go from here? Reston, VA, 1984, Reston Publishing Co.

Baker, L.: You and leukemia: a day at a time, Philadelphia, 1978, W.B. Saunders Co.

**Diet and nutrition: a resource for parents of children with cancer, U.S. Department of Health and Human Services, Public Health Service, National Institutes of Health, NIH Publ. No. 81- 2038, Washington, DC, 1981.

Donnelly, K.: Recovering from the loss of a child, New York, 1982, Macmillan Publishing Co., Inc.

**Eating hints: recipes and tips for better nutrition during cancer treatment, U.S. Department of Health and Human Services, Public Health Service, National Institutes of Health, NIH Publ. No. 84-2079, Washington, DC, 1984.

Fox, S.: Good grief: helping groups of children when a friend dies, Boston, 1985, The New England Association for the Education of Young Children.

Frantz, T.: When your child has a life-threatening illness, Washington, DC, 1983, Association for the Care of Children's Health.

Grollman, E.: Talking about death: dialogue between parent and child, Boston, 1976, Beacon Press.

**Help yourself: tips for teenagers with cancer, Bethesda, MD, 1983, National Cancer Institute.

**Hospital days—treatment ways: hematology-oncology coloring book, U.S. Department of Health and Human Services, Public Health Service, National Institutes of Health, NIH Publ. No. 82-2085, Washington, DC, 1982.

LaTour, K.: For those who live: helping children cope with the death of a brother or sister, 1983 (available from the author, P.O. Box 141182, Dallas, TX 75214).

Manning, D.: Don't take my grief away from me, Hereford, TX, 1979, InSight Books, Inc.

Miles, M.: The grief of parents, Oak Brook, IL, 1978, The Compassionate Friends, Inc.

Parent/child handbook, Buffalo, N.Y., 1983, Association for Research of Childhood Cancer.

Pochedly, C.: Cancer in children: reasons for hope, Port Washington, NY, 1979, Ashley Books, Inc.

Roach, N.: The last day of April, New York, 1974, American Cancer Society.

Schiff, H.: The bereaved parent, New York, 1977, Crown Publishers.

Schweers, E., and others: Parents' handbook on leukemia, New York, 1977, American Cancer Society.

Sherman, M.: The leukemic child, U.S. Department of Health, Education and Welfare, National Institutes of Health, NIH Publ. No. 78-863, Washington, DC, U.S. Government Printing Office.

Spinetta, J., and others: Emotional aspects of childhood leukemia; a handbook for parents, New York, 1982, Leukemia Society of America.

**Taking time: support for people with cancer and the people who care about them, U.S. Department of Health and Human Services, Public Health Service, National Institutes of Health, NIH Publ. No. 85-2059, Washington, DC, 1985.

Temes, R.: Living with an empty chair, New York, 1980, Irvington Publishers, Inc.

What happened to you happened to me, New York, 1984, American Cancer Society.

**When someone in your family has cancer, U.S. Department of Health and Human Services, National Institutes of Health, NIH Publ. No. 86-2685, Washington, DC, 1986.

When your brother or sister has cancer, New York, 1984, American Cancer Society.

Wolf, A.: Helping your child to understand death, New York, 1973, Child Study Press.

Young people with cancer: a handbook for parents, U.S. Department of Health and Human Services, National Institutes of Health, NIH Publ. No. 82-2378, Washington, DC, 1982, U.S. Government Printing Office.

ADDITIONAL SOURCES OF INFORMATION

**Coping with cancer: an annotated bibliography of public, patient, and professional information and education materials, NIH Publ. No. 80-2129, Bethesda, MD, 1980, Cancer Information Clearinghouse, Office of Cancer Communications.

**Coping with cancer: a resource for the health professional, NIH Publ. No. 80-2080, Bethesda, MD, 1980, Cancer Information Clearinghouse, Office of Cancer Communications.

Cancer Information Service, a toll-free telephone system for information; dial 1-800-4-CANCER and request number of nearest center.

---

*Other sources of publications are The Compassionate Friends, P.O. Box 3696, Oak Brook, IL 60522-3696; Centering Corporation, P.O. Box 3367, Omaha, NE 68103-0367; Pediatric Projects, P.O Box 1880, Santa Monica, CA 90406.

**Available from Office of Cancer Communications, National Cancer Institute, Bldg. 31, Rm. 10A18, Bethesda, MD 20205.

Chapter 24

The Child with Cognitive Impairment

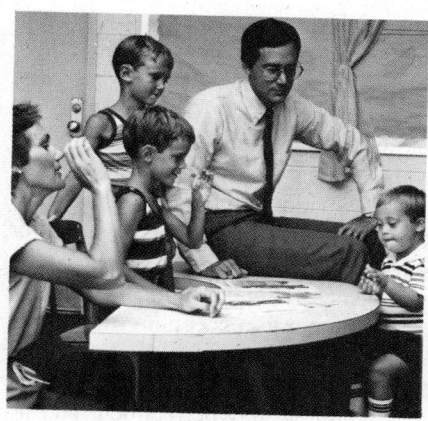

Mental retardation is the most common developmental disability in the United States, affecting some 3% of the population. In recent years, major changes have occurred in the philosophy of care toward people with cognitive impairment. Children with mental retardation are no longer automatically admitted into institutional settings but often remain at home. Therefore parents need role models and adequate preparation to effectively teach the child to function at optimum level within the environment. Nurses are in a strategic position to assume a vital role in assisting these parents with observation, problem solving, and decision making. With expanded roles in nursing, it is not unlikely that nurses will assume additional responsibility for the care of these children in schools, sheltered workshops, residential settings, and ambulatory care centers, as well as in hospitals.

This chapter is concerned with the complex problem of mental retardation—specifically its definition and causes—and strategies that parents can use to successfully rear these children. In addition, two syndromes associated with cognitive impairment are discussed, Down syndrome and fragile X syndrome, a recently recognized disorder. While the needs and concerns of the family are a primary focus throughout the chapter, the reader is encouraged to review Chapter 22, which details the family's adjustment to disabilities in general.

Perspectives in the Care of Children with Cognitive Impairment

Mental retardation is a complex disorder, whose very definition has generated considerable controversy throughout the ages. It is caused by numerous factors, many of which leave families with guilt because of the hereditary component. For families, living with a child with cognitive impairment is more than a challenge of childrearing, particularly if other physical disabilities exist. There are educational dilemmas, the need for other special services, decisions regarding future care, and coping with a society that often denigrates those who are retarded. Nurses can lend support and guidance to help the family cope with the special challenges and concerns associated with the diagnosis of mental retardation.

DEFINITION

The most commonly accepted definition of mental retardation by the American Association on Mental Deficiency (AAMD) refers to it as "significantly subaverage general intellectual functioning existing concurrently with deficits in adaptive behavior and manifested during the developmental period" (Grossman, 1983). Several aspects of this statement are important and require further clarification to understand the implications of the definition. *General intellectual functioning* refers to the results of various individually administered general intelligence tests. *Significantly subaverage intellectual functioning* is defined as an intelligence quotient (IQ) of approximately 70 or below. *Adaptive behavior* is the effectiveness or degree with which individuals meet the standards of personal independence and social responsibility expected for age and cultural group. It is a critical component of the definition, since it implies that intelligence alone is not the criterion for mental retardation. For example, individuals with IQ scores near 70 may not be classified as retarded based on their ability to adapt to the environment. *Developmental period* comprises the period between conception and the 18th birthday. Consequently, if cognitive impairment occurs after this time, such as from injury or disease, the person is not considered retarded.

EARLY BEHAVIORAL SIGNS SUGGESTIVE OF COGNITIVE IMPAIRMENT

Nonresponsiveness to contact
Poor eye contact during feeding
Diminished spontaneous activity
Decreased alertness to voice or movement
Irritability
Slow feeding

From Crocker, A., and Nelson, R.: Mental retardation. In Levine, M., and others: Developmental-behavioral pediatrics, Philadelphia, 1983, W.B. Saunders Co., p. 760.

DIAGNOSIS AND CLASSIFICATION

The diagnosis of cognitive impairment is usually made after a period of suspicion by professionals and/or the family that the child's developmental progress is delayed. In some cases it is made at birth because of recognition of distinct syndromes, such as Down syndrome. At the other extreme, it is made after the child begins school, when problems such as speech delays arouse concern when compared to peer achievement. In all cases a high index of suspicion for developmental delay and behavioral signs (see box, below) is necessary for early diagnosis, and the importance of routine developmental screening with such instruments as the Denver Developmental Screening Test (DDST) (see p. 283) cannot be overemphasized. Delays are commonly seen in gross and fine motor and speech development, although the latter is most predictive. It is suggested that children who show a delay in language on the DDST should be referred for a complete developmental evaluation, not only for speech assessment (Kaminer and Jedrysek, 1982). While gross motor skills such as walking may be delayed, a number of children with even severe retardation may walk at or near the usual age. Hence, age of walking is not necessarily a good predictor of intelligence (Hreidarsson, Shapiro, and Capute, 1983). Other common misconceptions that delay early diagnosis include physical stereotyping ("all retarded children are dumb looking") and that children are too young to be tested. In fact, cute children may be retarded, and no child is too young to be evaluated (Coplan, 1982).

The diagnosis and classification of mental retardation are based on standard intelligence tests. Several tests may be employed depending on the child's age. Two of the most commonly used tests are the Stanford-Binet Test and Wechsler Intelligence Scale for Children (WISC). These tests should be administered only under favorable conditions and individually (never as a group test) by specially trained clinicians, such as psychometrists or child development specialists. Tests available for assessing adaptive behaviors include the Vineland Social Maturity Scale and the AAMD Adaptive Behavior Scale. Informal appraisal of adaptive behavior may be made by those fully acquainted with the child (e.g., teachers, parents, or other care providers). Frequently these observations are what lead parents to seek evaluation of the child's development (Grossman, 1983).

The severity of retardation is based on the IQ scores, which represent mild, moderate, severe, and profound levels of deficit. The classification shown in Table 24-1 is based on the AAMD system, which differs slightly from other classification systems, such as the American Psychiatric Association (DSM-III), in that the cutoff points are flexible to account for different scoring and measurement of error in various tests. In addition, under this system, clinicians are encouraged to use professional judgment in determining adaptive deficit. The revised AAMD system includes a significant change from its previous classification in that *borderline retarded* is eliminated to reflect current thinking in the field and to be consistent with other classification systems (Grossman, 1983).

Table 24-1 Classification of mental retardation

LEVEL (IQ)*	PRESCHOOL (BIRTH-5 YEARS)—MATURATION AND DEVELOPMENT	SCHOOL AGE (6-21 YEARS)—TRAINING AND EDUCATION	ADULT (21 YEARS AND OLDER)—SOCIAL AND VOCATIONAL ADEQUACY
Mild—50-55 to approximately 70	Often not noticed as retarded by casual observer but is slower to walk, feed self, and talk than most children; follows same sequence in development as normal children	Can acquire practical skills and useful reading and arithmetic to a third- to sixth-grade level with special education; can be guided toward social conformity; achieves mental age of 8 to 12 years	Can usually achieve social and vocational skills adequate to self-maintenance; may need occasional guidance and support when under unusual social or economic stress; can adjust to marriage but not childrearing
Moderate—35-40 to 50-55	Noticeable delays in motor development, especially in speech; responds to training in various self-help activities	Can learn simple communication, elementary health and safety habits, and simple manual skills; does not progress in functional reading or arithmetic; achieves mental age of 3 to 7 years	Can perform simple tasks under sheltered condition; participates in simple recreation; travels alone in familiar places; usually incapable of self-maintenance
Severe—20-25 to 35-40	Marked delay in motor development; little or no communication skills; may respond to training in elementary self-help, for example, self-feeding	Usually walks, barring specific disability; has some understanding of speech and some response; can profit from systematic habit training; achieves mental age of toddler	Can conform to daily routines and repetitive activities; needs continuing direction and supervision in protective environment
Profound—below 20-25	Gross retardation; minimal capacity for functioning in sensorimotor areas; needs total care	Obvious delays in all areas of development; shows basic emotional responses; may respond to skillful training in use of legs, hands, and jaws; needs close supervision; achieves mental age of young infant	May walk; needs complete custodial care; has primitive speech; usually benefits from regular physical activity

*Based on classification from American Association on Mental Deficiency.

A more useful approach for clinical application is classification based on educational potential or symptom severity. For educational purposes the terms *educable mentally retarded (EMR)* or *trainable mentally retarded (TMR)* may be used. EMR corresponds to the mildly retarded group and TMR primarily to children with moderate levels of cognitive impairment (Goldman, Stein, and Guerry, 1983). Mild mental retardation is about six times more common than moderate or severe retardation (Coplan, 1982). While nurses should be familiar with the approximate range of IQ for classifying severity, they should refrain from using numbers as the criterion for assessing or evaluating the child's abilities, since numbers are of little value in counseling parents or training these children.

CAUSES

The causes of severe mental retardation are primarily genetic, biochemical, viral, and developmental. In mild retardation, familial, social, and environmental causes predominate. Associated factors include maternal life-styles, such as poor nutrition, cigarette smoking, and chemical abuse, all of which increase the risk of prematurity and intrauterine growth retardation and are preventable (Task Force on Joint Assessment, 1985). Among individuals with severe retardation, chromosome disorders account for 20% to 25% and the majority are Down syndrome. Another quarter of cases are caused by identifiable disorders or syndromes, and about 10% to 20% are associated with severe cerebral palsy, microcephaly, or infantile spasms (Hall, 1984).

Although several etiologic classifications exist, the following is an inclusive list of the prenatal, perinatal, and postnatal causes of mental retardation (Grossman, 1983):

Infection and intoxication, including any agent associated with abnormalities or malformations, such as rubella, syphilis, toxoplasmosis, maternal drug consumption, including alcohol, exposure to industrial chemicals, increased blood levels of lead, Rh incompatibility resulting in kernicterus, or maternal disorders, such as eclampsia

Trauma or physical agent, namely, injury to brain suffered during prenatal, perinatal, or postnatal period, including physical injury, lack of oxygen, or exposure to radiation

Metabolism or nutrition, including imbalances in fat, carbohydrates, and amino acids, inadequate nutrition, and metabolic or endocrine disorders, such as phenylketonuria or congenital hypothyroidism

Gross postnatal brain disease, including diseases characterized by skin eruptions, lesions, and tumors, such as neurofibromatosis and tuberous sclerosis

Unknown prenatal influence, including cerebral, spinal, and craniofacial malformations, such as microcephaly, hydrocephaly, meningomyelocele, and craniostenosis

Chromosomal abnormalities, including chromosomal aberrations resulting from radiation, viruses, chemicals, parental age, and genetic mutations, such as Down and fragile X syndromes

Other conditions originating in the perinatal period, including prematurity, low birth weight, and postmaturity

Psychiatric disorders that have their onset during the child's developmental period up to age 18 years, such as autism

Environmental influences, including evidence of a deprived environment associated with a history of mental retardation among parents and siblings

PREVENTION

Currently there is much concern with prevention of mental retardation. The major intervention is improved support for the small premature infant and other high-risk newborns (Crocker, 1982). Other *primary prevention strategies*—those designed to preclude the occurrence of the condition that causes retardation—include rubella immunization; genetic counseling, especially in terms of Down or fragile X syndrome; education regarding the dangers of ingesting alcohol during pregnancy and lead during childhood; adequate prenatal nutrition; and reduction of nonintentional and intentional (abuse) cerebral injuries.

Secondary prevention activities—those designed to identify the condition early and institute treatment to avert cerebral damage—include prenatal diagnosis or carrier detection of disorders, such as Down syndrome or Tay-Sachs disease, and newborn screening for treatable inborn errors of metabolism, such as congenital hypothyroidism, phenylketonuria, and galactosemia.

Tertiary prevention strategies—those concerned with treatment to minimize long-term consequences—include early identification of conditions and appropriate therapies and rehabilitation services. These include medical treatment of coexisting problems, such as hearing impairment in Down syndrome, and programs for infant stimulation, parent training, preschool education, and counseling services to preserve the integration of the family unit.

Nursing Interventions with Cognitively Impaired Children

The goal of caring for children with mental retardation is to promote their optimum development as individuals within a family and community. Since the general guidelines for coping with and adjusting to the child with special needs are discussed extensively in Chapter 22, the following discussion focuses on principles involved in educating these children, specific interventions to teach self-care skills, guidelines for promoting optimum development, helping families adjust to future care, and caring for these children during hospitalization.

EDUCATING CHILDREN WITH COGNITIVE IMPAIRMENT

In order to learn how to teach children with subaverage intelligence, it is necessary to investigate their learning abilities and deficits. These children have a marked deficit in their ability to discriminate between two or more stimuli because of difficulty in paying attention to relevant cues. Unfortunately, the ability to discriminate between symbols is essential in learning the alphabet for reading or numbers for arithmetic. However, these children can learn to discriminate if the cues are presented in an exaggerated concrete form and all extraneous stimuli are eliminated. For example, the use of colors to exaggerate visual cues or music for auditory cues can help the child learn. The latter is particularly effective for teaching speech by singing the same word rather than only saying it.

These children's deficit in discrimination also implies that concrete ideas are learned much more effectively than abstract concepts. Therefore demonstration is preferable to verbal explanation, and learning should be directed toward mastering a skill rather than understanding scientific principles underlying the procedure.

Another deficit is in short-term memory. Whereas children with average intelligence can remember several words, numbers, or directions at one time, children with cognitive impairment are unable to do so. Thus they need simple one-step directions. They respond to learning how to remember, such as by "clustering" pairs or triads together. This approach is helpful when trying to teach them their telephone number. Rather than having them memorize the entire seven-digit number, the teacher breaks it into pairs. After memorizing the pairs, the child puts them together.

Teaching through a step-by-step process requires the teacher to break down each task into its necessary components. For example, if the child is learning to tie a shoe, the teacher must practice the skill, divide it into steps (task analysis), and teach each step completely before proceeding to the next activity.

One critical area of learning that has had a tremendous impact on education for cognitively impaired individuals is motivation. Programs based on the motivation principles of behavior modification, employing positive reinforcement for specific tasks or behaviors, have demonstrated marked improvement in children's ability to learn. Two techniques are especially important with this group of learners: *fading,* which involves physically taking the child through each sequence of the desired activity and gradually fading out physical assistance to the child so that the child becomes more independent; and *shaping,* which requires waiting for the child to give a response that approximates the desired behavior, then reinforcing the child by social approval, such as touching or talking to him. Such principles can easily be implemented in the home in teaching self-help skills. Main-

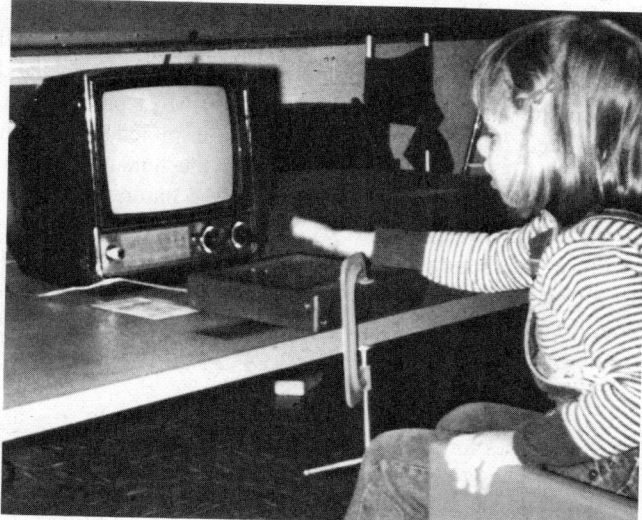

Fig. 24-1. A single push panel allows a child with cognitive impairment to turn a television on and off.

taining feelings of success in accomplishing specified goals also promotes a feeling of self-esteem in the child.

Advances in technology have greatly aided in providing active stimulation,* especially in children who are severely retarded and may have physical disabilities that limit their range of capabilities. For example, with the use of specially designed switches children are given control of some event in the environment, such as turning on the television (Fig. 24-1). The television becomes reinforcement for activating the switch. Repetitive use of these switches provides an early, simplistic association with a technical device that may progress to increasingly complex aids.

Early Intervention Programs

Early intervention or stimulation programs have been widely promoted for children who are at environmental risk, primarily from sociocultural deprivation, and those with developmental disabilities. Since the latter category comprises an extensively diverse group of children with mental retardation, cerebral palsy, language and learning disabilities, sensory disorders, autism, and other conditions, the types of programs vary widely in philosophy and interventions. Because of this the issue of benefit from such programs is often confusing and conflicting (see Questions and controversies).

However, there is considerable evidence that early intervention programs are valuable for cognitively impaired children. Most of the programs are based on one of three models (Marfo and Kysela, 1985):

Parent training/infant curriculum model, which uses a didactic approach in which parents are taught behavioral strategies for teaching their children specific skills and competencies

---

*Information on active stimulation is available from Educational Technology Center, Inc., Box 64, Foster, RI 02825.

Questions and Controversies

How beneficial are early intervention programs (EIP) for children with developmental disabilities?

The effectiveness of early intervention programs is a question of major concern, since it represents a great financial burden for public and private organizations and a considerable time investment for families. Programs should be able to improve functioning or at least minimize regression and help the family cope emotionally with the child's abnormal development. According to Russman (1983), many infant stimulation programs have been judged to be ineffective because their goals are unrealistic. One example is the Doman-Delacata or sensorimotor patterning program, whose basic premise is that a variety of sensory and motor experiences can facilitate "neurological organization" (Storm, 1983). While the program's claims are extraordinary, research has yielded little or no evidence of its effectiveness, which has prompted organizations such as the American Academy of Pediatrics (1982) to issue cautionary statements concerning the treatment.

However, such rigid curricula as that of the Doman-Delacata program are not characteristic of most EIP. On the contrary, most programs are diverse in both their interventions and targeted population, making scientific evaluations and comparisons difficult. One comprehensive review, which concerned itself with an analysis of the factors that complicate study design, concluded that 81% of the studies that incorporated statistical procedures demonstrated effectiveness of EIP and 93% demonstrated effectiveness based on subjective, clinical conclusions (Simeonsson, Cooper, and Scheiner, 1982). The authors propose that the *higher* percentages may reflect more accurately the effectiveness of the programs, since changes in the children's abilities may have been too small to be measured or may have occurred in areas that were not measured, such as feeding. Other authors concur and stress that effectiveness of early intervention programs should not be determined by narrow measures of outcome, such as IQ scores, but should be based on assessment of positive changes in variables related to parental attitudes and coping skills, parent-child and overall family interaction, parental instructional competence, and family's use of support services (Marfo and Kysela, 1985).

Parent/therapy model, which seeks to promote competent parenting through counseling and guidance techniques by focusing on resolving feelings related to the child's impairment

Parent-infant interaction model, which focuses on the quality of the parent/child relationship and considers a mutually satisfying interaction as the prime requisite for the infant's optimum development

Nurses working with these families either through an early stimulation program or individually can incorporate aspects of these models into their intervention plan. They also need to be aware of the types of programs in their community in order to direct families to those whose philosophy is best suited to the family's needs. Early intervention programs are provided by a number of organizations. Under Public Law 94-142, the Education for All Handicapped Children Act, local departments of education are required to

Table 24-2 Self-help skills in children with Down syndrome

SKILL	AVERAGE (MONTHS)	RANGE (MONTHS)
Eating		
Finger feeding	12	8 to 28
Using spoon and fork	20	12 to 40
Toilet training		
Bladder	48	20 to 95
Bowel	42	28 to 90
Dressing		
Undressing	40	29 to 72
Putting clothes on	58	38 to 98

Modified from Pueschel, S.M.: The child with Down syndrome. In Levine, M.D., and others, editors: Developmental-behavioral pediatrics, Philadelphia, 1983, W.B. Saunders Co., p. 359.

provide education programs for children from 3 years of age, and many communities have initiated education programs starting at birth. Other programs may be provided under state **Crippled Children's Program** or by private organizations such as **The National Easter Seal Society*** and **National Association of Retarded Citizens.†** Medical school pediatric departments also may provide direct services or consultation for referrals to existing programs (Russman, 1983). Parents should inquire about these programs by contacting the appropriate agencies as soon as possible. The child's education should not begin at 5 or 6 years of age.

PROMOTING INDEPENDENT SELF-HELP SKILLS

When a child with cognitive impairment is born, parents need assistance in promoting normal developmental skills that are almost automatically learned by other children. There is no way to predict when a retarded child should be able to master self-help skills, and studies demonstrate that there is wide variability in the ages at which children accomplish these functions (Table 24-2). For the nurse to be successful in meeting this goal, the parents must be supported, included as the primary rehabilitators with the child, and provided with detailed written descriptions of the stimulation program. The following discussion is concerned with activities of daily living; promoting gross motor development is discussed on p. 1005. Parents also need to be aware that numerous devices are commercially available that can aid in achievement of independence.‡

*2023 W. Ogden Ave., Chicago, IL 60612.
†2709 Avenue E East, P.O. Box 6109, Arlington, TX 76011. Information on early intervention programs in each state is available from the National Down Syndrome Society, 141 Fifth Ave., New York, NY 10010.
‡A resource for a wide variety of equipment, including self-help devices, is available from J.A. Preston, Catalog: Materials for exceptional children, 60 Page Rd., Clifton, NJ 07012.

Feeding

Self-feeding is recognized as the first major self-help skill that children learn. It involves the integration of fine and gross motor skills and visual perception. Most parents take for granted that they will be successful in teaching their children to feed themselves. Therefore the nurse must also be especially sensitive to the needs of the parent as well as of the child when assistance is offered.

Before beginning a self-feeding program the nurse should do a task analysis, breaking the process of feeding into its smallest component parts. For example, the tasks in self-feeding with a spoon include:

1. Orients to the food by looking at it
2. Looks at the spoon
3. Reaches for it
4. Touches it
5. Grasps it
6. Lifts it
7. Delivers the spoon to the bowl
8. Lowers it into the food
9. Scoops food onto the spoon
10. Lifts it
11. Delivers the spoon to the mouth
12. Opens the mouth
13. Inserts the spoon into the mouth
14. Moves the tongue and mouth to receive the food
15. Closes the lips
16. Swallows the food
17. Returns the spoon to the bowl

It is important to observe the child in an eating situation to determine whether he has mastered any of these small steps that make up the entire task of self-feeding. If so, the nurse should comment about them positively to the parent.

In addition to a task analysis, a number of other factors are assessed, such as the shape of the child's mouth and his control of mouth, lips, and tongue movements (whether the tongue moves forward and backward or from side to side, whether there are rotary movements). The presence of teeth determines the textures and consistencies of food that may be offered to the child. The child's developmental readiness for self-feeding, such as his ability to maintain head and trunk support and to sit without support, his eye-hand coordination, the firmness of his grasp, and his ability to reach for an object, hold it, and release it, are examined. If the child has any physical impairments that interfere with holding or grasping the utensil, specially designed utensils can be substituted (Fig. 24-2) or homemade modifications can be used, such as building the handle up with a sponge or piece of wood or bending it to accommodate arm movement.

The nurse determines whether the child has any dietary deficiencies, as revealed by a 7-day dietary history kept by the parent, whether there have been any changes in the child's eating habits, or if he is on a metabolic diet. Assessment is made of neurologic factors, such as if the child has seizures, is taking medications to control seizures, chokes often, or has difficulty in swallowing or a history of such difficulties.

Further data are obtained from the parent by asking spe-

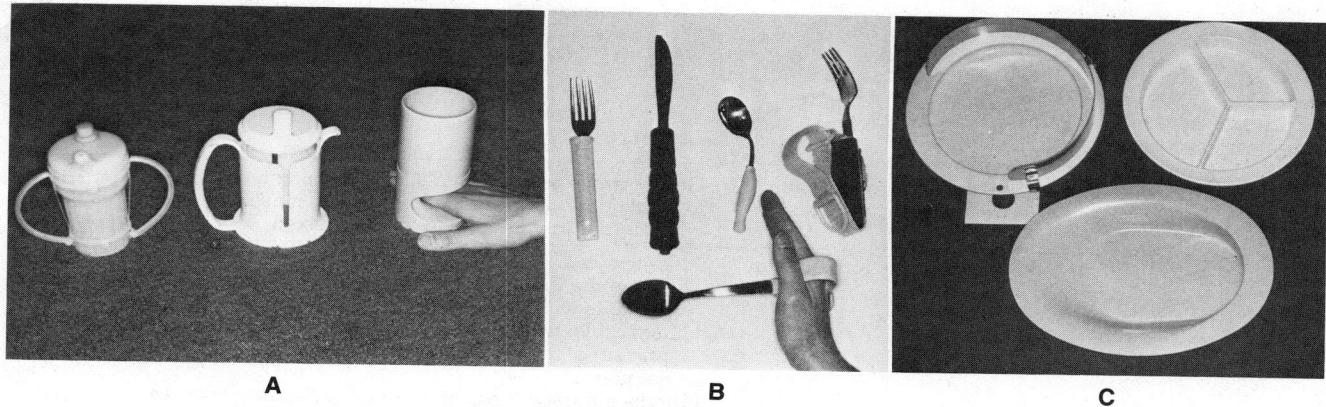

Fig. 24-2. Self-help aids for feeding: **A** *(from left to right)*, modified drinking cup, glass with holder and lid, pedestal cup; **B** *(from left to right)*, soft built-up handle utensil, weighted knife, child's bent spoon, Quad-Quip utensil holder (holds most household utensils), *(at bottom)*, vertical palm self-handle utensil; **C** *(from left to right, top)*, plastic plate with suction feet and optional metal food guard, partitioned scoop dish, *(at bottom)*, scoop dish.

cifically about the family's approach to feeding. For example, who feeds the child regularly? Is the child fed when he is hungry or according to a prescribed schedule? What are the child's appetite patterns? Does the parent know when the child is full? What foods does the child like? How long does feeding take? A short feeding time, such as 10 or 20 minutes, might indicate that the child is being deprived of sensory experiences or appropriate interactions; a long time might indicate frustration and fatigue on the parent's part. Is the feeding environment described as quiet and nondistracting? What is the best time to begin teaching this new task? If the family is going on vacation, if someone is visiting, or if there has been a major stress in the family, this may not be the ideal time to begin a teaching program. The nurse also determines whether the parent is really asking for help by the questions asked, the comments made, and the records kept.

Various principles of learning are discussed before beginning a feeding program. It is crucial not only to continuously reinforce desirable behavior but also to consistently ignore undesirable behavior. Ignoring the child is particularly difficult for many parents, because they may equate ignoring their child with being a "bad parent." Therefore the nurse must be especially supportive as the parent attempts negative reinforcement. The parent should realize that repetition plays an important part in the child's learning. As the child gains mastery, the parent is encouraged to decrease the social or physical reinforcement the child has been offered. The parent should understand that if the feeding program does not move forward successfully, both parent and nurse will reevaluate the last sequence the child mastered to see if they are expecting too much too soon.

Preparation for the feeding activity is also discussed, such as proper placement of the child at the table and protection of the area against spills. The principle of normalization (p. 945) is employed to make feeding a family activity. For example, the child is fed in the kitchen, at the table, or in a highchair in a sitting position, and with other family members whenever possible. Food should be served in attractive receptacles; offered in separate servings, not pureed or mixed together; served at the appropriate temperature, not routinely lukewarm; and of sufficient variety and texture from each of the basic four food groups.

Once the feeding program is begun, the nurse is in an important position to give parents supportive feedback. The parents' observational skills, their ability to share observations, keep records of the child's progress, and establish a goal that is appropriate and realistic for both the child and the parents are praised. By acknowledging these aspects, the nurse promotes mastery of a task that is extremely important to the child who is mentally retarded. Table 24-3 lists activities to help the child learn self-feeding.

Toileting

Independent toileting is another major self-help skill that can be taught using behavior modification principles. It should be started after self-feeding, since this is the normal sequence of development. Plans for a toileting program begin by assessing the child's physical and psychologic readiness (see Table 24-4 and Table 14-4). Because of physical or developmental limitations, certain signs may not be possible. For example, children who cannot walk can be trained once they are able to sit with good balance, and children with poor speech may need to rely on gesturing to signal their toileting needs.

Parents are interviewed regarding their readiness to pursue a toilet-training program that is characterized by a positive, consistent, individualized, nonpunitive, nonpressured style of teaching. It is important to explore the parents' willingness to participate, the time they have to invest in the program, the advantages they see, the inconveniences that toilet training may cause them, the reason they wish to start, and whether this is the best time for both the parents and the child to begin.

Table 24-3 Infant stimulation program for self-feeding

NORMAL AGE OF ACHIEVEMENT (MONTHS)	BEHAVIOR	ACTIVITY
Birth	Has sucking, rooting, and swallowing reflexes	Gently stroke around child's lips and mouth to stimulate puckering in order to strengthen lip muscles if sucking is weak Maintain in midline and slightly flexed
1	Is able to take food from a spoon	Press spoon on the tongue to stimulate jaw closure; press gently above the thyroid cartilage to stimulate swallowing; after spoon is withdrawn, close the mouth by pushing up on the mandible; wipe excess food from the lips in one stroke to prevent disrupting the normal closing and swallowing sequence Introduce pureed foods of different tastes and textures
4-5	Can approximate cup to lips	Offer small amounts of formula from a cup Place hands on lower jaw to provide better lip closure
5-6	Can use fingers to bring food to mouth	Give child dry toast, zwieback, pretzel, or cracker Dip fingers into food and bring hand to his lips Place food in his hand and gradually make him reach for it if child is not used to voluntarily grasping objects
6-7	Is able to chew solids	Introduce soft foods that require some chewing (cooked carrots, baked meats, baked potato, cheese, and so on) Place a small piece of food on the back molar area to stimulate chewing
8-9	Holds a spoon and plays with it during feeding	Give child a small spoon at feeding time Reinforce any attempts at self-feeding (putting spoon in mouth, in food, and so on) Improvise appropriate utensil if child has difficulty in holding spoon
9	Holds own bottle Finger feeds	Place the bottle in child's hands and bring it to his mouth; gradually release your hand Fill it only partway with milk or use a small (4-ounce) bottle Purchase a special nipple with a straw attached that draws milk from the bottom of the bottle if child is unable to tilt the bottle Give firmly cooked food cut into small pieces
12	Drinks from a cup with much spilling	Give child a cup, beginning with the same procedure as for a bottle
15	Drinks from a cup with less spilling	Use a wide, unbreakable cup with two handles Introduce a straw if child is unable to lift a cup; to initiate sucking liquid up the straw, fill the straw with juice, cover the top end with your finger, place the bottom end in child's mouth, and gradually release your finger to let the fluid in when child makes sucking movements Wean child gradually from one bottle at a time, eliminating the nighttime one last
18	Uses a spoon with much spilling	Give child a spoon, a bowl, and "sticky" food (applesauce or mashed potatoes) Guide his hand toward the bowl and then into his mouth if child is unwilling to feed himself; gradually fade out the assistance Anchor the bowl to the table if child has poor motor coordination
24	Holds cup in one hand Uses spoon with little spilling	Give a small-diameter cup that is easily grasped with one hand; add small amount of liquid
36	Begins to use fork; holds it in fist	Give a small-handled and short-pronged fork Guide the hand to pierce the food if child is reluctant
48	Eats with fork held with fingers	Continue encouraging use of fork
72-84	Uses knife	Encourage "spreading" with knife, followed by cutting tender foods Introduce knife and fork cutting

Table 24-4 Child stimulation program for self-toileting

NORMAL AGE OF ACHIEVEMENT (YEARS)	BEHAVIOR	ACTIVITY

1-2½	Is able to
	  Sit unsupported
	  Walk and stand alone
	  Walk alone
	    backward/forward
	  Balance well
	  Climb onto a chair
	  Retain urine for at least 2
	    hours
		Assess physical behaviors that indicate readiness for training; begin after most signs are evident
		Begin bowel training before bladder training
		Record approximate schedule of evacuation
		Place on potty-chair at regular intervals (upon awakening, after meals, before bedtime)
		Stay with child while he is on potty-chair (usually 5-20 minutes)
		Keep potty-chair in bathroom
		Use training pants rather than diapers; whenever possible, leave diapers off child so he can experience feeling of voiding without clothing

	Recognizes urge to let go and hold on Is able to communicate this sensation to parent Has desire to please parent by voluntarily controlling elimination	Assess psychologic readiness for toileting Point out when diapers are wet or dry Use consistent words or gestures to indicate need for elimination Praise for success Avoid punishment or excessive pressure
3 (may be as long as 5 years)	Stays dry during night Seats self on toilet	Take to toilet just before bedtime Do not offer excessive fluids before bedtime When child is trained, gradually reduce use of potty-chair for regular toilet If needed, keep small stool by toilet for climbing onto seat (sitting with legs facing tank reduces feeling of "falling in")
3-3½	Voids standing up (male) Washes/dries hands with supervision	Use imitation of watching father (or other male) Provide small stool for easy access to toilet May need to direct stream initially Turn on faucets for child; provide small stool Make hygiene routine part of toileting
3½-4	Attempts to wipe self but is unsuccessful Undresses/dresses self Flushes toilet Completely cares for self at toilet, including wiping and handwashing	Offer toilet paper Teach correct procedure from front to back Use clothing that is easy to manage (elastic waist pants, dress) Remind to flush toilet after elimination Encourage independence

Any past attempts at toilet training the child are reviewed: When and why did the parents start training? What methods did they use? Did they experience feelings of frustration, indifference, or discomfort? How long did they attempt training, and what were their reasons for discontinuing training efforts? Looking back, how did they view the experience for themselves and the child? Were their efforts consistent? What did they do most consistently? Do they think it is important to try again? If the parents admit to using punishment in any form, including spanking, scolding, withholding privileges, using suppositories, withholding fluid, getting the child up in middle of the night, or making the child wash his soiled sheets or clothes, the nurse appeals to them to discontinue these unnecessary, ineffective methods.

As part of the procedure for determining the readiness of both parents and child to become involved in a successful toilet-training program, parents are asked to keep detailed records for 7 days. They should be cautioned to discontinue record keeping if the child becomes ill or if fluid intake is changed. Record keeping includes the following events:

1. The child ate or drank, no matter how little he consumed.
2. The child's behavior was suddenly distinctly different, for example, when the child was noticeably more quiet or louder, started fussing or tugging at his clothes, pointed toward the bathroom, cried, or squirmed.
3. Parents gave the child positive attention related to toileting behaviors only, in the form of praise, concrete rewards, affection, or approval.
4. Parents gave attention in the form of scolding, threatening, or spanking if the child had wet or soiled his underclothes or did not tell them before eliminating.
5. The child indicated his need to go to the toilet by either gestures or words.

6. The child was noted to have dry underclothes.

7. The child was noted to have wet underclothes.

It is crucial to refrain from beginning any toilet-training program until such records are completed, because they show how parents are responding to the child's behaviors and at what times the child is most likely to eliminate. After the records are completed to the parents' express satisfaction, the nurse should acknowledge their efforts to keep accurate records, their diligence in making observations, and their ability to follow through.

The goal of any toilet-training program is to help the child achieve small goals and experience comfort and success and to help the parents simultaneously experience feelings of adequacy, minimal tension, and success. Parents should understand that they will be capitalizing on the times the child is most likely to eliminate and that they should respond immediately to any cues indicating his need to eliminate. They must be cautioned to ignore accidents.

A task analysis of toileting includes the following steps, which parents must systematically reinforce in positive, natural, spontaneous ways:

1. Sitting on the toilet or potty-chair and playing there without fussing, crying, or attempting to get off
2. Eliminating into the toilet on a regular basis when sitting on it
3. Waiting to eliminate before being placed on the toilet
4. Indicating the need to eliminate before going into the bathroom
5. Asking to go to the toilet or just going to it
6. Remaining dry for longer periods of time
7. Climbing onto the toilet independently
8. Helping undress himself before getting onto the toilet
9. Independently undressing himself before getting onto the toilet
10. Wiping independently
11. Flushing the toilet
12. Dressing
13. Washing his hands with soap in a correct manner
14. Drying his hands with a towel

A positive and relaxed attitude toward toilet training is important and differs little from the approach used with other children (see Chapter 14). Ideally the child should sit on the potty-chair for voiding when he first gets up in the morning, just after breakfast, at midmorning, after snacks, after lunch, at midafternoon, before and after dinner, and again before bedtime. The child cannot be expected to have a regular pattern of elimination unless he is fed at approximately the same times each day. Parents should also remember to help the child only when he needs it. Although this may take longer, it is the best way for a child to learn complete independence. Table 24-4 lists activities to help the child learn independent toileting.

Dressing

Dressing skills develop without special training in most children, usually as a consequence of autonomy and imitation.

For children who are retarded, special training is necessary to promote this skill. Factors that interfere with spontaneous learning include immature motor skills, lack of motivation, physical impairments, or lack of opportunity. The last variable should always be considered when assessing delayed development of independent dressing.

The level of independence in dressing varies according to the degree of retardation. Children with mild and moderate retardation and no accompanying physical limitations can become independent in all dressing skills, except for more complex tasks such as color coordination. Those who are severely retarded can achieve most dressing skills, except the ability to fasten complicated closures such as buttons or ties. Profoundly retarded children are usually able to assist in undressing and dressing but achieve no independent skills.

Before a self-dressing program is instituted, the child's physical readiness is assessed by doing a task analysis of the following gross and fine motor skills:

1. Stands alone
2. Balances in a chair or on the floor without support
3. Leans free from the chair when seated
4. Raises one knee up toward the chest when seated
5. Places either hand on the opposite shoulder
6. Places one or both hands on top of head
7. Has apposition with one or both hands
8. Grasps and holds slim objects with one or both hands
9. Picks up a 2.5 cm (1-inch) button using thumb and forefinger
10. Pushes with one or both hands with all fingers grasped around an object
11. Pulls with one or both hands with all fingers grasped around an object

The child is considered mentally ready for dressing training if he can sit quietly for 3 to 5 minutes while working on a task, can watch what he is doing while working on a task, can follow physical gestures or cues, can follow verbal commands, and can relate clothing to the appropriate body part, such as socks with feet. As with other self-help skills, the child may not be able to master every task but should be evaluated for evidence of willingness to participate at his level of readiness. The use of teaching devices such as dolls with mock closures and reinforcement for success in managing the fasteners has been shown to increase the child's manipulative skills, which may be transferred to ready-to-wear clothing (Lamb, 1977).

After the assessment of the child's readiness, a detailed record is kept of what the child can do in dressing, what is being taught, and how well the child is progressing with the new skill. The program for self-dressing follows the same sequence as normal development: (1) dressing is done for the child but with demonstration of the procedure, (2) the child undresses and then dresses with assistance, (3) the child undresses completely without supervision, (4) the child dresses with little assistance but with supervision, and (5) the child assumes all responsibility for dressing. Table

Table 24-5 Infant stimulation program for self-dressing

NORMAL AGE OF ACHIEVEMENT (MONTHS)	BEHAVIOR	ACTIVITY
15	Cooperates by extending arm or leg	Give child verbal direction ("Put your hands over your head") and assist child in procedure; gradually give only verbal command
18	Takes off mittens, hat, or socks	Demonstrate taking off article of clothing; then give only verbal command Use loose-fitting socks
	Unzips	Place child's finger on zipper head; pull it down with him; gradually reduce assistance until he can do it on verbal command
	Tries to put on shoes	Begin with having child extend foot, put open shoe or slipper in child's hand, and demonstrate getting it over toes; show him how to push foot into shoe and hit the sole with his hand to make sure heel is inside; demonstrate "stepping into" shoes Use oversized shoes at first
21	Undresses	Demonstrate step-by-step procedure, for example, pants: pull down pants to child's ankles, have him pull them off, then pull down to knees, then hips, and last, have child pull them from waist For shirt: unbutton shirt, pull off shoulders and one arm, have child pull off other arm, then pull off shoulders only and have child do both arms
24	Removes shoes	Loosen shoes completely; demonstrate taking them off by pushing from heel; take them off partway, have child do rest; gradually have child do it himself Demonstrate untying shoe by placing two beads or bells at the ends of the laces, grasping each, and pulling the bow out; have child first pull one string with parent until gradually he can do both unaided
	Helps in dressing	Use same technique as for learning to cooperate with undressing (15 months) and self-undressing (21 months) Use simple articles of clothing Concentrate on putting the clothes on first and fastening them later Sew tabs or colorful appliques on shirts and pants to indicate front or back Practice buttoning with large buttons; use front-fastening clothes

24-5 suggests activities for promoting independent dressing. Since most children do not master fastening back closures or tying shoelaces until age 6 or older, it is unrealistic to expect such skills until after this age in children with cognitive impairment.

Choice of clothing is an important aspect of the training program. Clothes should be clean, up-to-date, and well fitted. They should be easy to put on and take off, easy to fasten, comfortable and nonrestricting, capable of disguising a physical disability, and easy to maintain. Minimizing the abnormal appearance of a ''retarded'' child is a major goal in promoting acceptance from others and self-esteem in the child. The following is suggested clothing for use in a training program: undershirts with large neck openings; brassieres that have elastic straps and front fasteners; half-slips; underpants with elastic waists; boxer shorts for boys; slip-on polo shirts with large armholes and wide neck openings (not tight turtleneck sweaters); front-buttoning shirts or dresses; pants with elastic waistbands or large side hook fasteners; wool or cotton ankle socks (not tight nylon knee socks); panty hose with sewn-in panty for girls, and slip-on shoes. If the child cannot manage buttons, hooks, or straps, Velcro fasteners are good substitutes, although they tend to come loose if stressed.*

Grooming

Self-grooming is usually learned along with other independent skills, such as washing hands during toilet training. The same principles are followed in teaching grooming procedures as have already been discussed: assess the child's readiness and present level of competency, proceed with skills in the normal sequence of development, analyze the task into its component parts, and set up an individualized teaching program. As with self-dressing, a major factor in learning independent grooming is the opportunity to practice the skills. Table 24-6 suggests activities for promoting self-grooming. Complete independence for bathing and hair

---

*A helpful book is Hotte, E.: Self-help clothing, available from The National Easter Seal Society, 2023 W. Ogden Ave., Chicago, IL 60612; numerous other resources are listed in the article by Lamb (1977).

Table 24-6 Infant stimulation program for self-grooming

NORMAL AGE OF ACHIEVEMENT (MONTHS)	BEHAVIOR	ACTIVITY
14	Brushes teeth mainly with help	Establish a routine (after each meal and before bedtime) Demonstrate toothbrushing to child on yourself Use small toothbrush with minute amount of pleasant-tasting toothpaste (preferably containing fluoride) Use a mirror for child to observe procedure Place toothbrush in child's hand and assist in brushing Teach child how to rinse toothbrush and mouth
18	Helps with bath	Explain to child what you are doing ("I am washing my face") Give child washcloth and soap, guide his hand to imitate your action; gradually reduce assistance
24	Washes hands with help	Demonstrate procedure Place child by sink with a stool so he can easily reach bowl Regulate water, give him soap, help him rub soap on hands, rinse, and dry; gradually reduce assistance
	Helps with washing hair	Place child's hands in hair while lathering scalp; show him the bubbles on his hands and use a mirror for him to observe shampooing; as he learns to rub scalp, gradually reduce assistance During rinse, give him towel to hold over his eyes Give him a large-toothed comb for his hair; guide his hand in learning to comb his hair
30-36	Brushes teeth alone (but with parents' assistance and supervision)	Demonstrate placing paste on toothbrush Encourage child to brush his own teeth using "any direction" method Reinforce any previously learned skills Remind child to brush according to set routine Begin visits to the dentist (if not begun sooner)
36	Washes hands alone	Place all utensils within easy reach Regulate water for child (safety measure against burning) Teach child to turn off faucets Reinforce all previously learned skills When child has sense of responsibility concerning danger (hot), teach him how to regulate water and check the temperature each time

washing are learned during the school years and therefore are late skills for these children.

Special mention must be made of dental hygiene. An odor-free mouth and a white set of teeth are essential in promoting a positive image. In addition, healthy teeth are necessary for proper mastication and speech. Diseased teeth and gums increase drooling and prevent proper preparation of food for subsequent digestion. Missing teeth interfere with proper tongue positioning for clear speech.

Most causes of dental problems in these children are a result of neglected dental hygiene and excessive quantities of carbohydrates, including the use of candy to reward behavior. Most dental problems are preventable with the same dental hygiene practices discussed in Chapter 14.

If the child has physical impairments that limit his ability to brush, special devices may be necessary, such as a larger handle or a curved toothbrush, to reach all surfaces of the teeth. Electric toothbrushes may be a worthwhile investment for some children. The use of dental disclosing tablets is an excellent aid in visually showing the child (and parent) the thoroughness (or lack) of cleaning. Any devices that help

motivate the child to brush should be used. For example, the parent can place a special "tooth calendar" on the wall and mark each date with stars to represent the number of brushings per day. At the end of a specified number of stars the child can receive a special reward.

The child should be routinely taken to a dentist. To accustom him to this experience, he should go for visits with other members of the family *before* the dentist examines his teeth. It is important to prepare the child for such visits, since it is much more difficult to change an unsatisfactory experience than to prevent one. Once the child is traumatized by the experience, parents may be less inclined to take the child back for fear of temper tantrums or other resisting behavior. The nurse can assist families by locating dentists who are familiar with treating these children and discussing with parents preparatory procedures for the visit.

PROMOTING OPTIMUM DEVELOPMENT

Optimum development involves more than achieving independence. It requires appropriate guidance for establishing acceptable social behavior and personal feelings of self-esteem, worth, and security. These attributes are not simply learned through a stimulation program. Rather they must arise from the genuine love and caring that exists among family members. However, families need guidance in providing an environment that fosters optimum development. Often it is the nurse who can provide continuing assistance in these areas of childrearing.

Play

The child who is retarded has the same need for play as any other child. However, because of his slower development, parents may be less aware of the need to continue appropriate stimulation. They may also feel inadequate in playing with the child, since the usual reciprocal satisfaction between child and parent may be slower in developing. Therefore the nurse guides parents toward selection of suitable toys and interactive activities. Since play has been discussed for children in each age-group in earlier chapters, only the exceptions for these children are discussed.

The type of play is based on the child's developmental age, although the need for sensorimotor play may be prolonged for several years. Parents should use every opportunity to expose the child to as many different sounds, sights, and sensations as possible. Appropriate play includes musical mobiles, stuffed toys, water play, floating toys, rocking chair or horse, swing, bells, and rattles. The child should be taken on outings, such as trips to the grocery store or shopping center; other people should be encouraged to visit in the home; and the child should be related to directly, such as cuddling, holding, rocking, talking to him in the *en face* position, and giving him "rides" on the parents' shoulders.

Toys are selected for their recreational and educational value. For example, a large inflatable beach ball is a good water toy, encourages interactive play, and can be used to learn motor skills, such as balance, rocking, kicking, and throwing. A doll with removable clothes and different types of closures can help the child learn dressing skills. Musical toys that mimic animal sounds or respond with social phrases are excellent ways of encouraging speech. Toys should be simple in design so that the child can learn to manipulate them without help. For children with severe cognitive and physical impairment, electronic switches can be used to allow them to operate toys (Fig. 24-3).

Safety is a major consideration in selection of toys. Toys that may be appropriate developmentally may present dangers to a child who is strong enough to break them. Even if more advanced toys are suitable for the child's developmental skills, the parent must keep in mind the child's level of responsibility in using them properly. For example, the child may be physically able to use a bow and arrow but may lack the judgment in using it to shoot only at a target.

Supervision during play and other activities is stressed, since these children are slow to learn inherent dangers. Parents may need to place reminders around the house to prevent injuries, such as signs to keep the yard gate locked.

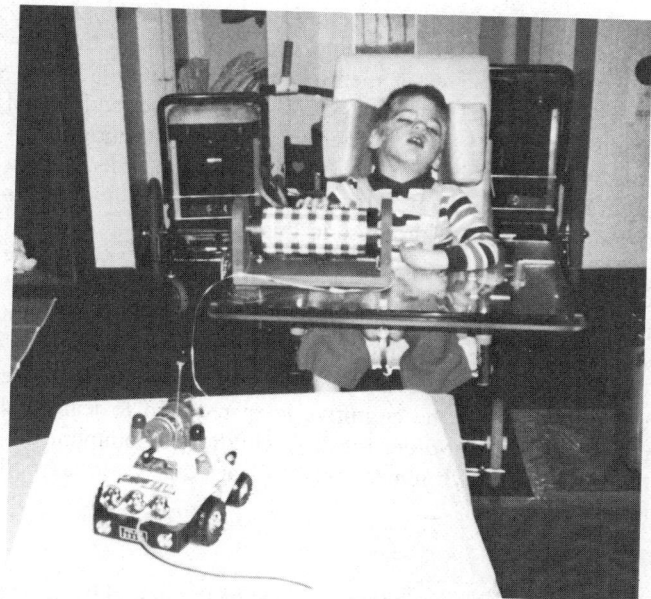

Fig. 24-3. A barrel switch allows a child with cognitive impairment to play with a battery-operated truck.

These children often lack the motivation to institute appropriate play activities on their own. As a result of boredom, they may resort to self-stimulatory behavior such as rocking, head hitting, twirling, masturbating, or finger sucking. Such behaviors are destructive in that they limit developmental progress and impede social acceptance. If such behaviors exist, appropriate play activities, especially as a method of distraction from self-stimulation, are discussed with the parents. Behavior techniques, such as ignoring the child when he engages in such behavior and attending to him when he is behaving acceptably, should also be used.

Communication

Verbal skills are often delayed more than other physical skills and are frequently the first clues of cognitive deficits. Since suggestions for promoting speech development are discussed in Chapter 25, only brief comments are included here.

Speech requires hearing and interpretation (receptive skills) and facial muscle coordination (expressive skills). Both may be impaired in these children. For example, in children with Down syndrome the large protruding tongue often interferes with speech. These children may need tongue exercises to correct the tongue thrust or gentle reminders to keep the lips closed. Deficits in discrimination impede learning of different sounds. Often it helps to associate the sound with other stimuli, such as singing, which attracts the child's attention so that he attends to the cue longer. Parents also must remember that since learning is slower, their teaching must continue longer. The nurse encourages them not to give up or believe that speech is hopeless.

Shaping techniques are useful in fostering meaningful vocalization. Every time the child vocalizes a sound that represents either a letter of the alphabet or an intelligible syllable, the parent reinforces him with praise and social approval. Parents are instructed to record all meaningful vocalizations the child has learned in the past in order to continue reinforcing them. A written record also helps parents monitor evidence of progress in this area.

For some of these children, especially those with severe cognitive and physical impairments, speech acquisition is not possible and nonverbal methods of communication should be employed, such as sign language. Several nonverbal systems are available, but the clinician must be knowledgeable of the cognitive level required to learn and use the method. In order for these children to communicate, others in their environment need to learn the system as well (see also p. 1041).

Discipline

As was discussed in Chapter 22, one of the first childrearing practices eliminated when the parents have a disabled child is discipline. This not only can result in serious behavior problems, but also interferes with the child's developing a sense of security and self-control. It may also foster resentment from siblings who are forced to abide by a double standard.

Discipline must begin early. For children with cognitive impairment, limit-setting measures must be simple, consistent, and appropriate for their mental age. Control measures are based on teaching a specific behavior—not on having the child understand the reasons behind it. Stressing moral lessons is of little value to a child who cannot learn from self-criticism. Behavior modification, especially reinforcement of desired actions, and time out are appropriate forms of behavior control (see Chapter 14).

Socialization

Acquiring social skills is a complex task, as is learning self-care procedures. Active rehearsal with role playing and practice sessions and positive reinforcement for desired behavior have been the most successful approaches (Davies and Rogers, 1985). Parents should be encouraged early to teach their child socially acceptable behavior—waving good-bye, saying hello and thank you, responding to his name, greeting visitors but not being overly affectionate, and sitting modestly. The teaching of socially acceptable sexual behavior is especially important to minimize sexual exploitation (Williams, 1983). Parents also need to expose the child to strangers so he can practice manners, since there is not automatic transfer of learning from one situation to another.

Before preschool age the parents should contact the nearest day-training center or special school. Not only do these centers provide appropriate education and training, they also offer an opportunity for social experiences among the children. As the child grows older, he should have peer experiences similar to those of other children, including group outings, sports, and organized activity, such as Boy Scouts, Girl Scouts, or Special Olympics.* He should be encouraged to form a close relationship with a best friend. Often parents neglect this aspect of the child's life, believing that once he leaves school he should be sheltered in the home. On the contrary, he needs to feel companionship and belonging by being able to invite friends home, talk to them on the telephone, and plan and participate in special events. Siblings can be an important source of companionship, especially if they include the child in their activities or guide in selecting activities the child can manage. If the siblings have an accepting attitude, their friends are likely to accept the child as well.

Adolescents who are retarded also need social outlets for heterosexual experiences. Unfortunately, few schools or communities provide for this recreational need. The nurse can be instrumental in indirectly initiating such activities by encouraging parents to discuss these unmet social needs with educational staff. Clubs, sports, hobby projects, and dances can be organized for the teenagers to provide experience that teaches acceptable social behavior.

Sexuality

Adolescence may be a particularly difficult time for parents, especially in terms of the child's sexual behavior and needs, future plans to marry, and ability to be independent. Frequently little anticipatory guidance has been offered parents to prepare the child for physical and sexual maturation, and the degree of the adolescent's interest in sex has been underestimated. Studies have found that as many as half of the mildly retarded youngsters (a proportion comparable to the general adolescent population), a third of the moderately retarded, and 9% of the severely retarded have had sexual intercourse, and less than one half of the total group used contraception. In addition, these young people have increased rates of sexual abuse or rape, with one third of the mildly retarded and one fourth of the moderately retarded adolescents having been victims (Chamberlain and others, 1984).

Nurses can help in this area by providing parents with information about sex education that is geared to the child's developmental level. For example, the adolescent female needs a *simple* explanation of menstruation and instructions on personal hygiene during the menstrual cycle.†

These adolescents need also practical sexual information regarding anatomy, physical development, and conception. Because of their easy persuasion and lack of judgment, they need a well-defined, concrete code of conduct. The subtleties of social sexual behavior are less beneficial than specific instructions for handling certain situations. For example, a girl should be firmly told never to go alone anywhere with

---

*1350 New York Ave., N.W., Washington, DC 20005-4709.

†Sources of information on sexuality and conception are the National Association for Retarded Citizens, 2501 Avenue J, Arlington, TX 76011; Planned Parenthood Federation of America, 810 Seventh Ave., New York, NY 10019; Coalition on Sexuality and Disability Inc., 853 Broadway, Suite 611, New York, NY 10003.

any man she does not know well. A boy should be warned of intimate advances from other males. To protect him or her from abusive sexual activities, parents must closely observe their teenager's activities and associates.

The question of contraceptive protection for female retarded adolescents is often a parental concern. Of the available methods, medroxyprogesterone, the intrauterine device (IUD), or birth control pills are most commonly used (Chamberlain and others, 1984). However, each has its disadvantages. Medroxyprogesterone (Depo-Provera) requires intramuscular injections every 3 months. Heavy breakthrough bleeding, especially in the first few months, is common, although cessation of menstruation often results, which is a benefit. The IUD requires regular checking of the string's placement and can cause menorrhagia; also, its availability is limited. Birth control pills must be used regularly and may have undesirable side effects. Sterilization is a special dilemma because of moral and ethical questions as well as psychologic effects on the adolescent (see Questions and controversies). Parents seem to be most interested in sterilization of daughters who are more severely retarded and for elimination of menses to avoid the problems of hygiene (Passer and others, 1984).

Parents of these adolescents are often very concerned about the advisability of marriage between two individuals with significant cognitive impairment. There is no conclusive answer; each situation must be judged individually. In many instances marriage would help the couple achieve a mutually satisfying and supportive relationship, meaningful companionship, and a more normal social sexual adjustment. However, parenthood is usually not desirable because of the complexity of childrearing and the problem of perpetuating mental deficiency. The nurse should discuss this topic with parents and with the prospective couple, stressing suitable living accommodations and contraceptive methods to prevent pregnancy.

HELPING FAMILIES ADJUST TO FUTURE CARE

Not all families are able to cope with home care of these children, especially those who are severely or profoundly retarded and/or multiply disabled. Parents may not be able to continue with care responsibilities once they reach retirement or old age. Unfortunately, some parents view institutionalization as the only alternative to coping with problems of retarded adolescents. For families the decision regarding residential placement is a difficult one. The nurse's role is to assist parents in exploring the reasons for desiring placement, especially of adolescents, investigating alternatives to home care before they become necessary, and establishing ways in which to maintain contact and communication with the retarded member of the family.

A number of alternatives exist regarding out of home care, but the availability of these facilities varies widely depending on the community's resources, and in most instances a well-organized, comprehensive system of services is rare in the United States (Cohen, 1982). Basically, care

Questions and Controversies

What are the issues surrounding the question of sterilization of individuals who are mentally retarded?

While parents may ordinarily consent to any necessary medical or surgical treatment for their minor children, consent for sterilization is an exception (Williams, 1983). Currently the decision regarding sterilization of minors and incompetent adults, in particular those who are mentally retarded, is a moral and legal one. State laws vary; some allow no sterilization, and others permit review of sterilization requests. Basically, two opposing viewpoints dominate the controversy: those who feel that the *right to procreate* is fundamental and those who maintain that the *right not to procreate* is equally important. Proponents of the latter view consider laws preventing sterilization to be in violation of human rights (Passer and others, 1984).

In allowing the young person who is mentally retarded to make an informed consent, a basic issue is the individual's level of competency. Assessing competency is a complex process. Silva (1984) presents a detailed review of elements and tests of competency and proposes that the main elements of decision-making competency are (1) internalization of a set of goals and values; (2) ability to comprehend and communicate information; and (3) ability to reason and make choices. Tests of competency must be employed on an individual basis, and nurses may be instrumental in presenting information in a simple and concrete manner that increases the person's understanding and level of competence. Nurses must also be knowledgeable of state laws in their area of practice to ensure the rights of the child and family.

options range from the least to the most restrictive types of environments—foster homes, group foster homes, community residences, and institutions, such as intermediate care facilities, nursing homes, or state boarding homes. Some communities have special vocational and/or day programs, which allow the individual an opportunity for some measure of gainful employment and the family temporary respite from care (see also p. 947 on respite care).

Nurses working with a family may wish to visit each facility to evaluate its suitability for the child or may guide parents on how to assess the facility's adequacy. Guidelines for assessing out of home care facilities are presented in the box p. 1000. Ideally, after a family places the child in a facility, nurses should follow up their adjustment to the change to help them resolve any feelings of loss, self-doubt, or guilt.

CARING FOR HOSPITALIZED CHILDREN WITH COGNITIVE IMPAIRMENT

Caring for children with mental retardation during hospitalization is a special challenge to nurses. Frequently nurses are unfamiliar with these children and cope with the nurses' feelings of insecurity and fear by ignoring or isolating the child. Not only is this approach nonsupportive, it may also be destructive for the child's sense of self-esteem and optimum development and may impair the parents' ability to

GUIDELINES FOR ASSESSING OUT OF HOME CARE FACILITIES

1. Clarify the facility's philosophy of care.
2. Assess the environment for adequacy of inanimate and animate stimuli for the residents.
3. Determine the appropriateness of amounts of stimuli in the environment.
4. Observe care provider–to–resident ratios.
5. Observe care personnel interacting with residents in a variety of teaching and learning experiences.
6. Determine the appropriateness of the setting for the person being considered for placement.
7. Observe the quality of physical care administered.
8. See if the residents are attended to regularly and consistently, instead of when inappropriate behaviors occur.
9. Determine if activities are age appropriate for the residents.
10. Determine the existence of structured and nonstructured activities.
11. Determine if individual plans of care are available and implemented.
12. Determine the functional levels of those who reside in settings, for example, are they ambulatory and is speech encouraged?
13. Determine if speech, physical, and occupational therapies are available.
14. Determine if each person is perceived as unique and distinct and if care is given to residents according to their needs.
15. Determine if and to what degree official standards of care are met.
16. Meet with parents of those who reside in special settings to hear their comments, both positive and negative.

cope with the stress of the experience. In order to prevent use of this nontherapeutic approach, nurses can use the mutual participation model in planning the child's care. Parents are encouraged to room with their child but should not be made to feel as if the responsibility is totally theirs.

Assessment of the child's abilities, special needs, and the family's or other caregiver's successful management techniques is essential. Ideally, a hospital staff should make a prehospital visit to the home or care facility. This not only provides information about the child's usual environment, but also minimizes the unfamiliarity of the hospital setting, since one staff person will be recognized on admission (Wasch, 1981). When the child is admitted, a detailed history (see Chapter 26) is taken, especially in terms of all self-help activity. During the interview the child's developmental age is assessed. While it is not unreasonable to ask about IQ level, such questioning must be done sensitively. Also, the information often tells little about the child's actual abilities.

Questions about the child's abilities are approached positively. For example, rather than asking, "Is he toilet trained yet?" the nurse may state, "Tell me about his toileting habits." The assessment should also focus on any special devices the child uses, effective measures of limit setting, unusual or favorite routines, and any behaviors that may require intervention. For example, if the parent states that the child engages in self-stimulatory activities, the events that precipitate them and techniques the parents use to manage them are assessed. Once the child's functional level is known, he is encouraged to be as independent as possible, even though he is in a hospital setting.

The nurse ensures that the child has toys and other activities to entertain him and that he is included in group activities on the ward. He should be placed in a room with other children of approximately the same developmental age, preferably in an area with two beds in order to prevent overstimulation. The nurse discusses the child's abilities with the other parents the child's abilities and introduces the parents and children to each other. By the nurse's example of treating the child with dignity and respect, others who may be fearful of what they do not understand are encouraged to be accepting.

Procedures are explained to the child using methods of communication that are at his cognitive level. Generally explanations should be simple, short, and concrete, emphasizing what the child will *physically* experience. Demonstration either through actual practice or with visual aids is preferable to verbal explanation. The nurse repeats instructions often and evaluates the child's understanding by asking questions—"What did I say it will feel like?" "What will the doctor look like?" "Show me how you must lie," or "Where will the dressing be?" Parents are included in preprocedural teaching for their learning and to help the nurse learn effective methods of communicating with the child.

During hospitalization the nurse should also focus on growth-promoting experiences for the child. For example, hospitalization may be an excellent opportunity to emphasize to parents abilities the child does have but has not had the opportunity to practice, such as self-dressing. It may also be an opportunity for social experiences with peers, group play, or new educational/recreational activities. For example, one child who had had the habit of screaming and kicking demonstrated a definite decrease in these behaviors after he learned to pound pegs and use a punching bag. Through social services the parents may become aware of specialized programs for the child. Nutritional counseling is available if the child is overweight or has evidence of specific deficiencies, such as iron deficiency. Hospitalization may also offer parents a respite from everyday care responsibilities and an opportunity to discuss their feelings with a concerned professional.

Syndromes Associated with Cognitive Impairment

Numerous chromosomal syndromes are associated with varying degrees of cognitive impairment. Two of them, Down syndrome and fragile X syndrome, are particularly important because of their relative frequency in the general population. The following discussion is concerned with specific aspects of each syndrome. The reader is encouraged to apply the concepts discussed earlier in this chapter and those in Chapter 22 regarding the family's response to the diagnosis and nursing interventions to promote adjustment and acceptance of the child.

DOWN SYNDROME

Down syndrome, also known by the unacceptable name *mongolism*, owing to the particular facial characteristics that resemble those of the Mongol race, is the most common chromosomal abnormality of a generalized syndrome, occurring in 1:800 to 1000 live births. It occurs in slightly more whites than blacks, although the incidence is unchanged in various socioeconomic classes (Pueschel, 1983).

Etiology

The cause of Down syndrome is not known. A number of theories, including genetic predisposition to nondisjunction, radiation prior to conception, and infection, have been proposed, but none of the hypotheses has been substantiated. Recent reports in cytogenetic and epidemiologic studies support the concept of multiple causality.

Although the etiology is unclear, the cytogenetics of the disorder are well established. Approximately 92% to 95% of all cases of Down syndrome are attributable to an extra chromosome 21 (group G), hence the name *trisomy 21*. Although children with trisomy 21 are born to parents of all ages, there is a statistically greater risk in older women, particularly those over 35 years (Table 24-7). However, the majority (53% to 80%) of infants with Down syndrome are born to women under age 35. This trend toward younger families with Down offspring may be caused by the availability of amniocentesis to older women, desire for smaller families, or some unidentified environmental or constitutional factor. Recent evidence is demonstrating that paternal

age is also a factor and may account for 20% to 30% of cases resulting from trisomy 21 in Down syndrome. The risk appears significant only in males 55 years and over (Cohen, 1984).

About 4% to 6% of the cases may be caused by *translocation* of chromosomes 15 and 21 or 22. This type of genetic aberration is usually hereditary and is not associated with advanced parental age. From 1% to 3% of affected persons demonstrate *mosaicism,* which refers to cells with both normal and abnormal chromosomes. The degree of physical and cognitive impairment is related to the percentage of cells with the abnormal chromosome makeup. (For a discussion of the genetics involved in Down syndrome, see Chapter 5.)

Except for mosaicism, the mechanism by which the syndrome occurs has little effect on the characteristics displayed by the affected child and the management of the disorder. However, it is significant for purposes of genetic counseling. Whereas nondisjunction is usually a sporadic event associated with a low risk of recurrence (0.5% to 1%), a translocation is more often hereditary with a recurrence risk that depends on the type of translocation and the sex of the parent (Smith, 1982). In Down syndrome caused by translocation, testing of the parents is necessary to identify the carrier and offer genetic counseling.

Clinical Manifestations

Down syndrome can usually be diagnosed by the clinical manifestations alone, although no one physical feature is diagnostic (see box on p. 1002 and Fig. 24-4) and there is considerable variation in phenotypic expression. In addition, some infants may have characteristics of Down syndrome, such as epicanthal folds, narrow palate, short, broad hands, and a simian crease, but be cytologically normal. Therefore a chromosomal analysis should be done to confirm the genetic abnormality. The following are other outstanding features of the syndrome:

Intelligence Varies from severely retarded to low normal intelligence, but is generally within the mild to moderate range and may be related to parental intelligence (Sharav, Collins, and Shlomo, 1985). Initial development may appear near normal although slow development, especially in speech, is characteristic and highly variable (see Table 24-8). While some reports suggest a relative decline in IQ scores over time, this needs further investigation with the present emphasis on early stimulation

Social development May be 2 to 3 years beyond the mental age, especially during early childhood. Temperamental characteristics show the same range as those found in normal peers, although there is some documentation of a trend toward the early child pattern (Gunn and Berry, 1985).

Congenital anomalies About 30% to 40% have congenital heart disease, especially septal defects. Other structural defects include renal agenesis, duodenal atresia, Hirschsprung disease, and tracheoesophageal fistula. Skeletal defects include patella dislocation, hip subluxation, and instability of the first and second cervical vertebrae (atlantoaxial instability).

Table 24-7 Relationship of Down syndrome to maternal age

MOTHER'S AGE	INCIDENCE OF DOWN SYNDROME
Under 30	Less than 1 in 1000
30	1 in 900
35	1 in 400
36	1 in 300
37	1 in 230
38	1 in 180
39	1 in 140
40	1 in 110
42	1 in 70
44	1 in 40
46	1 in 25
48	1 in 16

Data from Cohen, F.: Clinical genetics in nursing practice, Philadelphia, 1984, J.B. Lippincott Co.; and de la Cruz, F.F., and Muller, J.Z.: Facts about Down syndrome, Child. Today **12**(6):2-7, 1983.

OBSERVABLE PHYSICAL CHARACTERISTICS (STIGMATA) ASSOCIATED WITH DOWN SYNDROME

Head
Brachycephalic
Skull rounded and small
Flat occiput
Sparse hair (variable)
*Separated sagittal suture

Face
Flat profile

Eyes
Inner epicanthal folds
*Oblique palpebral fissures (upward, outward slant)
Speckling of iris (Brushfield's spots)
Short, sparse eyelashes
Blepharitis

Nose
*Small
*Depressed nasal bridge (saddle nose)

Ears
Small
Short pinna (vertical ear length)
Overlapping upper helices
Sometimes low set

Mouth
Small osseous orbit
Protruding tongue, may be fissured at lip and furrowed on the surface
Hypoplastic mandible
Downward curve (especially noted when crying)
*High-arched palate

Teeth
Delayed eruption
Alignment abnormalities common

Neck
Short and broad
*Skin excess and laxity, lateral aspects

Abdomen
Protruding
Muscles lax and flabby
    Diastasis recti
    Umbilical hernia

Genitalia
Small penis
Cryptorchidism
Bulbous vulva

Hands
Broad, short
Stubby fingers
Incurved little finger (clinodactyly)
Transverse palmar crease (simian line)
Characteristic dermal ridge patterns
    Distally located axial triradius
    Increased ulnar loops on fingers

Feet
Broad, stubby
*Wide space between big and second toes
*Plantar crease between big and second toes

Musculoskeleton
Hypotonic
*Hyperextensible and lax joints
*Muscle weakness

Skin
Dry, cracked, and frequent fissuring
Cutis marmorata (mottling)

*Most common findings (Pueschel, 1983).

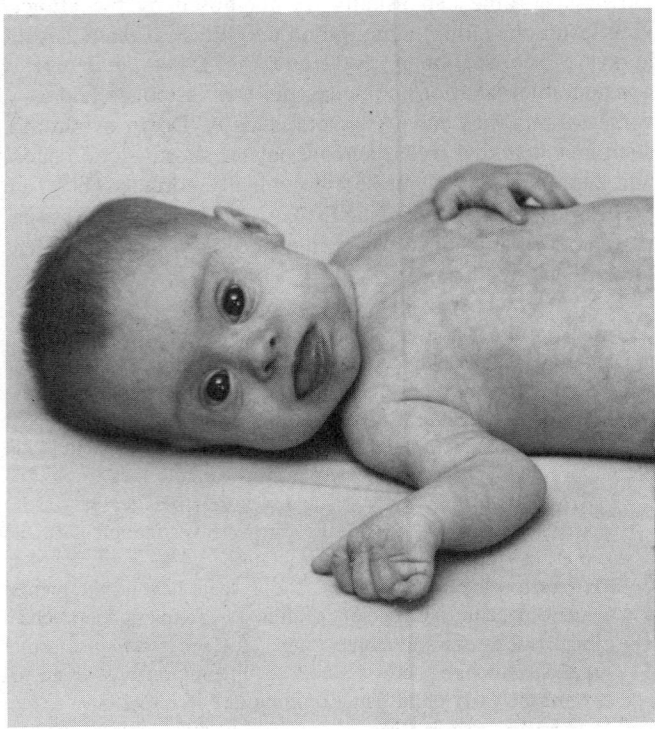

Fig. 24-4. Down syndrome in infant. Note small square head with mongoloid slant to the eyes, flat nasal bridge, protruding tongue, mottled skin, and hypotonia.
Photography by John Roy, Saint Francis Hospital, on location at Children's Medical Center, Tulsa, OK.

Sensory problems Visual problems include strabismus, myopia, nystagmus, cataracts, and conjunctivitis. Conductive hearing loss occurs in a large percentage (up to 80%), probably secondary to otitis media and impacted cerumen in the small ear canals, and is mainly in the mild to moderate range; significantly, binaural loss may be present in over 60% of these children (Balkany and others, 1979).

Other physical disorders Respiratory infections are very prevalent; when combined with cardiac anomalies, they are the chief cause of death, particularly during the first year. The incidence of leukemia is about 14 times more frequent than expected in the general population (Robison and others, 1984) and is thought to be related to immunologic defects. Thyroid dysfunction, including hypothyroidism and hyperthyroidism, is common; the incidence of persistent primary congenital hypothyroidism has been reported as 28 times more frequent than in the general population (Fort and others, 1984).

Growth and sexual development Growth in both height and weight is reduced, and the build is usually stocky because the legs and arms are short in relation to the trunk. Obesity is common and may be related to thyroid dysfunction and/or physical inactivity. Sexual development may be delayed, incomplete, or both. Male genitalia may be underdeveloped, as well as secondary sex characteristics such as facial hair. The breast development of females is mild to moderate. Menstruation usually occurs at the average age, and postpubertal women can be fertile; a small number have had offspring, the majority of whom were born with some type of abnormality. Men with Down syndrome are infertile. Premature aging is common in both sexes, and there are the same types of degenerative changes as in Alzheimer disease, although the relationship between Alzheimer disease and Down syndrome is not well understood (de la Cruz and Muller, 1983).

Therapeutic Management

Although there is no cure for Down syndrome, a number of controversial therapies are advocated, such as megadoses of vitamins and minerals (orthomolecular therapy), use of sicca cells (injection of lyophilized material prepared from embryonic animal organs), surgery to correct the physical stigmata, and administration of drugs, such as thyroid hormone, dimethyl sulfoxide (DMSO), and 5-hydroxytryptophan (Golden, 1984; Pueschel, 1985). Controlled studies have failed to document the effectiveness of any of these treatments, especially the popular orthomolecular therapy (Bennett and others, 1983; Smith and others, 1984).

Children with Down syndrome may require surgery to correct serious congenital anomalies and benefit from regular medical care. Evaluation of sight and hearing is essential, and treatment of otitis media is required to prevent auditory loss, which can influence cognitive function (Libb and others, 1985). Periodic testing of thyroid function is recommended, especially if growth is severely delayed. Children participating in sports that may involve stress on the head and neck, such as gymnastics, diving, butterfly stroke in swimming, high jump, and soccer, should be evaluated for atlantoaxial instability (American Academy of Pediatrics, 1984). Symptoms of the disorder, such as neck pain, weakness, and torticollis, require prompt attention.

Nursing Considerations

Caring for the child with Down syndrome involves several short- and long-term goals. Support for parents from health professionals, especially nurses, is increasingly important with the present trend to rear these children at home. This discussion focuses on supporting parents at the time of diagnosis and preventing physical problems in the child. Long-term psychologic interventions for the child and family are discussed in Chapter 22, and decisions for the future have been explored earlier in this chapter.

Informing parents of diagnosis. Because of the characteristic facies and other stigmata, the infant with Down syndrome is usually diagnosed at birth. However, parents are not always informed of the diagnosis at this time. This presents special difficulties for those caring for the postpartal mother, since she or the father may notice differences in the child and question others about their concern. Therefore the nurse needs some guidelines to help in assessing when, how, and what parents should be told. A general discussion of the informing process is presented on p. 940; therefore only selected aspects are discussed here.

Generally parents wish to know the diagnosis as soon as possible. This approach prevents such dilemmas as telling others that the child has Down syndrome after indicating that he was fine and experiencing unconfirmed doubt over

the child's development. Most parents prefer that both of them be present during the informing interview, because it is a problem that both of them will have to face; they can emotionally support each other, and it eliminates the difficult task of revealing the diagnosis to the other partner. They appreciate receiving reading material about the syndrome* and being referred to others for help or advice, such as parent groups or professional counseling.

The parents' responses to the child may greatly influence decisions regarding future care. Whereas some families willingly plan to take the child home, others consider foster care or adoption. The nurse must carefully answer questions regarding developmental potential, since the responses may influence the parents' decision. It is obvious from ranges such as those in Tables 24-2 and 24-8 that these children's potential for developmental achievement varies greatly. Therefore it would be inaccurate and unfair to predict the child's intellectual capacity at birth.

It is also not possible to predict whether a child will present few problems for childrearing. Although most children with Down syndrome adjust extremely well to the home environment and thrive with appropriate stimulation, those with severe impairments may present difficulties for the family. It is important to stress that a decision regarding placement will affect all of their lives and need not be made at the time of diagnosis. The nurse should emphasize every available source of assistance, such as parent groups, professional guidance, and literature, to help the family learn to live with the child and deal with childrearing problems.

Assisting parents in preventing physical problems. Many of the physical characteristics of Down syndrome present nursing problems. The hypotonicity of muscles and hyperextensibility of joints complicate positioning. The limp, flaccid extremities resemble the posture of a rag doll; as a result, holding the infant is difficult and cumbersome. Sometimes parents perceive this lack of molding to their bodies as evidence of inadequate parenting. The extended body position promotes heat loss because more surface area is exposed to the environment. Parents are encouraged to swaddle or wrap the infant tightly in a blanket before picking him up to provide security and warmth. The nurse also discusses with parents their feelings concerning attachment to the child, emphasizing that the child's lack of

---

*Several publications are available. One that is written very positively in terms of home care and includes a list of other references is Pitt, D.: Your Down syndrome child, available from the National Association for Retarded Citizens, 2709 Avenue E East, P.O. Box 6109, Arlington, TX 76011. Other sources of information are American Association on Mental Deficiency, 5105 Wisconsin Ave., N.W., Washington, DC 20016 (1-800-424-3688); National Down Syndrome Society, 141 Fifth Ave., New York, NY 10010 (1-800-221-4602); Down's Syndrome Congress, 1640 W. Roosevelt Rd., Chicago, IL 60608; Parents of Down's Syndrome Children, 11507 Yates St., Silver Spring, MD 20902; National Association for Down's Syndrome, P.O. Box 63, Oak Park, IL 60301; Association for Children with Down's Syndrome, Inc., 2616 Martin Ave., Bellmore, NY 11710; Caring, P.O. Box 400, Milton, WA 98354.

Table 24-8 Developmental milestones in children with Down syndrome

	AVERAGE (MONTHS)	RANGE (MONTHS)
Smiling	2	1.5 to 4
Rolling over	8	4 to 22
Sitting alone	10	6 to 28
Crawling	12	7 to 21
Creeping	15	9 to 27
Standing	20	11 to 42
Walking	24	12 to 65
Talking, words	16	9 to 31
Talking, sentences	28	18 to 96

From Pueschel, S.M.: The child with Down syndrome. In Levin, M.D., and others, editors: Developmental-behavioral pediatrics, Philadelphia, 1983, W.B. Saunders Co., p. 358.

clinging or molding is a physical characteristic, not a sign of detachment or rejection.

Decreased muscle tone compromises respiratory expansion. In addition, the underdeveloped nasal bone causes a chronic problem of inadequate drainage of mucus. The constant stuffy nose forces the child to breathe by mouth, which dries the oropharyngeal membranes, increasing the susceptibility to upper respiratory infections. Measures to lessen these problems include clearing the nose with a bulb-type syringe, rinsing the mouth with water after feedings, using a cool-mist vaporizer to keep the mucous membranes moist and the secretions liquefied, changing the child's position frequently, and performing postural drainage and percussion if necessary. If antibiotics are ordered, the importance of completing the full course of therapy for successful eradication of the infection and prevention of growth of resistant organisms is stressed.

The large, protruding tongue also interferes with feeding, especially of solid foods. Parents need to know that the tongue thrust does not indicate refusal to feed but is a physiologic response. Parents are advised to use a small but long, straight-handled spoon to push the food toward the back and side of the mouth. If food is thrust out, it should be refed. At times the family may require the assistance of a specially trained speech pathologist to guide them in dealing with feeding problems.

Dietary intake needs supervision. Decreased muscle tone affects gastric motility, predisposing the child to constipation. Dietary measures such as increased residue and fluid promote evacuation. The child's eating habits may need careful scrutiny to prevent obesity. Height and weight measurements should be obtained on a serial basis, especially during infancy, since excessive weight gain can impede motor development. The child should receive calories in accordance with his height and weight, not his chronologic age.

During infancy the child's skin is pliable and soft. However, it gradually becomes rough and dry and is prone to cracking and infection. Skin care involves the use of minimum soap and application of lubricants. Lip balm is applied to the lips, especially when the child is outdoors, to prevent excessive chapping.

Promoting children's developmental progress. The hypotonicity also affects muscular development. Supporting skills such as rolling over, sitting up, standing, or pulling oneself to a sitting or standing position may be delayed. Since it has been found that the child's developmental potential seems greatest during infancy, it is imperative that parents be involved in an infant stimulation program. If a formally organized program is not available, the nurse can individualize one by assessing the infant's present abilities and selecting appropriate activities that he should be learning. Table 24-9 lists several exercises to help a child learn gross motor skills. Suggestions for teaching independent self-help behaviors are discussed earlier in this chapter and are summarized in Tables 24-3 to 24-6.

After a stimulation program is planned, the parents are given detailed written instructions regarding each exercise and how often it should be performed. A return demonstration of each activity is requested to ensure the parents' understanding. The importance of verbally repeating the instructions to the child to enhance his comprehensive and, later, speech development, gradually reducing assistance as the child gains strength and coordination, and praising the child for success and cooperation are emphasized. At regular intervals the child's developmental progress is assessed to ensure compliance with the program. Screening tools such as the Denver Developmental Screening Test are not sufficiently detailed to evaluate indices of progress such as increased strength, balance, coordination, or muscle tone. Therefore the nurse must keep detailed written records of the child's motor abilities in order to distinguish subtle changes in functioning.

With the present trend toward home care, the parents should be encouraged to investigate special day-care programs for the child as soon as possible, since frequently there are long waiting lists. They should also investigate the public school system for special educational classes, including infant stimulation programs and preschools. In essence the same childrearing goals established for normal children are pursued for these children, with attention to preventing the problems of overprotection and including family members, especially the father and siblings, in the caring role.

Prevention. Prevention of the birth of a child with Down syndrome is possible through amniocentesis, since chromosomal analysis of fetal cells can detect the presence of trisomy or translocation. However, analysis will not identify sporadic cases in young women when there is no indication for amniocentesis. The nurse has a role in genetic counseling of women who are of advanced maternal age or who have a family history of the disorder to discuss the possibility of amniocentesis. If the fetus is affected, the nurse must allow the parents to express their feelings concerning elective abortion and support their decision either to terminate or proceed with the pregnancy.

Table 24-9 Infant stimulation program for gross motor development

NORMAL AGE OF ACHIEVEMENT (MONTHS)	BEHAVIOR	ACTIVITY*
Birth	Assumes flexed position, kicks, has dance reflex	Exercise limbs several times each day Place child in flexed position; encourage movement such as kicking Hold child upright with feet touching a flat surface to stimulate dance reflex
3-4	Holds head erect	Hold child prone; encourage him to raise head Place child supine and pull up by arms; encourage him to raise head forward Place child in sitting position, hold head erect, gradually release support on sides of head for him to learn muscle control If child holds head erect, tilt him to one side to learn balance Support child in sitting position with head erect; if head falls forward, attract child's attention to encourage him to look up
4-5	Rolls over—prone to supine	Place child prone but slightly lying on one side; place hand on hip and push down as you are pulling up on the ipsilateral arm; encourage child to push with arm underneath him; gradually encourage child to use free arm to push himself over completely
5-6	Rolls over—supine to prone	Place child supine, cross one leg over the other, and gently push him to one side; reduce assistance as he learns to roll by himself Roll him over and over
8	Sits up unsupported	Place child in sitting position but supported several times each day Support child in sitting position; gently tilt him to one side to learn balance Place child in sitting position with his back against a wall; kneel in front of him and encourage him to lean away from the wall to learn balance Sit child on floor with knees in an Indian position; place his hands on floor so he can balance himself Use same Indian position, kneel down in front of him, and gently push him to one side so that he practices righting himself Sit child on large beach ball with his feet flat on the floor; sway him from side to side to regain balance
9-10	Goes from sitting to standing position	Sit child on a low stool or chair with feet firmly placed on floor; place a towel around his chest and gently pull him up to standing position; help him sit down again; gradually reduce assistance Place child in crib or playpen and in sitting position; encourage him to get up to reach an object
10	Crawls	Place child on abdomen; encourage him to come forward by moving an object away from him (Fig. 24-5) Place child over a large, rolled towel that is high enough to allow him to rest his hands on the floor; encourage him to bear weight on his hands; straighten his arms to increase weight bearing Use same position but with small towel so that elbows and lower arms rest on floor; encourage him to lift up or come forward slightly; press down on his shoulders to stimulate his effort at maintaining this position When bearing weight on hands, place rolled towel or beach ball under his chest to stimulate getting on all fours; gently support him around the waist and pull him up; release assistance as he bears more weight Lay child across beach ball; roll him forward, backward, and to each side to stimulate balance in either direction Play wheelbarrow; hold him at his hips and let him walk forward on his hands; as he bears more weight, hold him by his feet and let him go forward Encourage "walking like a bear" (last step before walking); stand him upright, support him at the hips, and have him lean forward or gently push him over to bear weight on his hands; encourage him to walk in this position and to straighten up
	Stands with support	If child resists standing, place him upright with his back against the wall, grasp his knees, and manually straighten the legs; as he controls his legs, reduce the amount of assistance While child is in crib or playpen, place him in standing position and holding onto railing

Adapted from Gregory, P.: Pediatr. Nurs. 1(4):23-29, 1975.
*With each activity the parent continues the actual behavior with a verbal command and praises the child for each increment in motor development, as well as for cooperation and/or signs of enjoyment.

Continued.

Table 24-9 Infant stimulation program for gross motor development—cont'd

NORMAL AGE OF ACHIEVEMENT (MONTHS)	BEHAVIOR	ACTIVITY*
10—cont'd	Stands with support	While child is in standing position, have him hold your hands; encourage him to bear weight and "jump" up and down
10-12	Stands alone for short periods	With child in standing position, release support for a moment to encourage standing alone
12-14	Walks with support	Hold both his hands in front of you and guide him in walking; gradually hold only one hand Encourage him to cruise around furniture and push a chair or carriage
14	Walks alone	Place child in standing position in front of you; reach out to child but do not actually support him; encourage him to walk forward Hold by one hand; release your grasp while he is walking

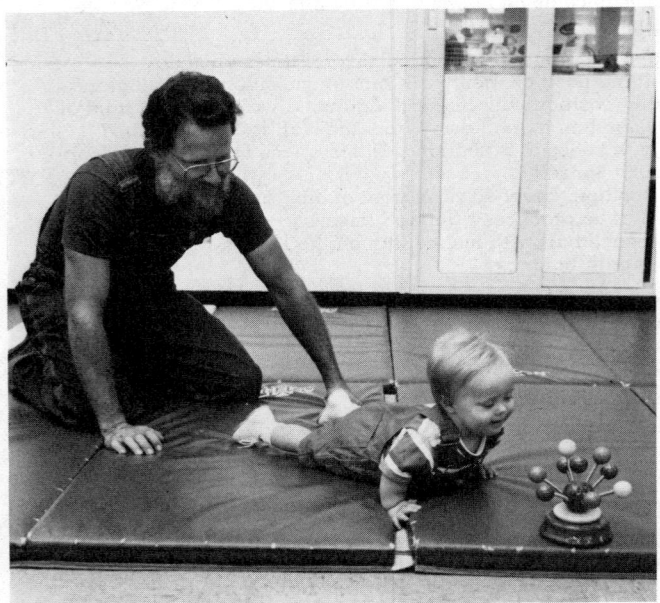

Fig. 24-5. Placing an attractive object out of child's reach encourages crawling movements.
Photography by John Roy, Saint Francis Hospital, on location at Children's Medical Center, Tulsa, OK.

FRAGILE X SYNDROME

One of the most significant cytogenetic advances related to developmental disorders in recent years has been the identification of the fragile X chromosome. The fragile X is a marker found on the X chromosome when the chromosome is placed in a special culture medium that is deficient in folic acid. Although the marker has been found on other chromosomes, the fragile site on the X chromosome is the only one known to be associated with clinical abnormality (Gerald and Meryash, 1983). The fragile X syndrome af-

fects approximately 30% to 50% of families with X-linked mental retardation, making it the second most common specific cause of mental retardation after Down syndrome (Cohen, 1984). Identification of this marker allows for genetic counseling in families of an affected individual that was not possible previously (Carpenter, Leichtman, and Say, 1982).

Clinical Manifestations

In some males with the fragile X chromosome there is a recognizable clinical phenotype and associated developmental characteristics (see box, below). A number of other behavioral manifestations have been found in some males, including autistic tendencies (Fryns, 1984). However, none of these features is specific to individuals with the fragile X site, and there are reports of individuals who have the fragile X site without any of the distinguishing features. Also, females may be affected, and the clinical manifestations are extremely varied. Both affected sexes are fertile and therefore capable of transmitting the fragile X disorder.

CHARACTERISTICS ASSOCIATED WITH FRAGILE X SYNDROME

Short stature
Normal to increased head size
"Long face" with prominent jaw
Large nose with broad nasal bridge
Large or prominent ears
Large testicles (macroorchidism or macrotestes)
Mild to severe mental retardation
Speech or language abnormality
Hyperactivity
Visual-motor incoordination

Nursing Care Summary: The Child with Down Syndrome

NURSING GOALS	NURSING INTERVENTIONS	EXPECTED PATIENT/FAMILY OUTCOMES

HP-HMP   Infection, potential for
Risk factors: hypotonia, increased susceptibility to infection

Prevent respiratory infection	Teach the parents postural drainage and percussion Stress importance of changing child's position frequently, especially sitting posture Encourage use of cool-mist vaporizer Teach suctioning of nares Stress importance of good mouth care (follow feedings with clear water)	Child exhibits no evidence of infection or respiratory distress

HP-HMP   Injury, potential for abnormal development
Risk factors: parental age

Prevent Down syndrome	Discuss with high-risk women risks of giving birth to child with Down syndrome Encourage all pregnant women at risk (over age 35, family history of Down syndrome, or previous birth of child with Down syndrome) to consider amniocentesis during twelfth to sixteenth week of pregnancy to rule out Down syndrome in fetus Discuss option of elective abortion with women who are carrying an affected fetus Discuss with parents of adolescent children with Down syndrome the possibility of conception in a female and the need for contraceptive methods	Pregnant women at risk seek evaluation for Down syndrome Families demonstrate an understanding of options available to them Families of an affected female child seek contraceptive advice

N-MP   Skin integrity, impairment of: potential
Risk factors: hypotonia, increased susceptibility to infection

Prevent skin breakdown	Keep skin well lubricated with topical creams or lotions Use soap sparingly Apply lip balm when the child is outdoors	Skin remains clean and intact with no evidence of inflammation

A-EP   Self-care deficit: feeding, bathing/hygiene, dressing/grooming, toileting (specify level)
Etiology: mental retardation

Facilitate self-care*	Enroll child in stimulation program Reinforce self-care activities	Child participates in self-care to his maximum capabilities
Minimize feeding difficulties in infancy	Suction nares before each feeding, if needed Schedule small, frequent feedings; allow child to rest during feedings Feed solid food by pushing it to back and side of mouth; use long, straight-handled infant spoon Point out to family that tongue thrust does not indicate refusal of food Calculate caloric needs to meet energy requirements; base intake on height and weight, not chronologic age Monitor height and weight at regular intervals Provide sufficient fiber and fluids to prevent constipation	Infant consumes an adequate amount of food for age and size (specify) Family reports satisfactory feeding Infant gains weight in accordance with standard weight tables

*Applicable to any child with mental retardation.

Continued.

Nursing Care Summary: The Child with Down Syndrome—cont'd

	NURSING GOALS	NURSING INTERVENTIONS	EXPECTED PATIENT/FAMILY OUTCOMES
N.D. CPP	**Sensory-perceptual alteration: visual, auditory, kinesthetic, gustatory, tactile, olfactory** **Etiology: mental retardation**		
	Promote optimum development	Involve child and family in an early infant stimulation program	Child and family are actively involved in infant stimulation program
		Assess child's developmental progress at regular intervals; keep detailed records to distinguish subtle changes in functioning	Family applies concepts and continues activities in home care of child
		Help family set realistic goals for child	Child performs activities of daily living at his optimum capacity
		Encourage learning of self-care skills as soon as child achieves readiness	Family investigates educational programs
		Encourage family to investigate special day-care programs and educational classes as soon as possible	Appropriate limit setting, recreation, and social opportunities are provided
		Emphasize that child has same needs as other children	Adolescent issues are explored and implemented as appropriate
		Play	
		Discipline	
		Social interaction	
		Prior to adolescence, counsel child and parents regarding physical maturation, sexual behavior, marriage, and family	
		Encourage optimum vocational training	
N.D. RRP	**Family process, alteration in** **Etiology: birth of a child with mental deficiency**		
	Support family at time of diagnosis*	Inform family as soon as possible after birth	Family expresses feelings and concerns regarding the birth of a mentally retarded child and its implications
		Have both parents present at informing conference	Family members make realistic decisions based on their needs and capabilities
		Give family written information about syndrome	Family members demonstrate acceptance of child
		Discuss with family members benefits of home care vs foster care or adoption; allow them opportunities to investigate all residential alternatives before making a decision	
		Encourage family to meet other families with Down children	
		Refrain from giving definitive answers about the degree of retardation; stress the potential learning abilities of retarded children, especially with early stimulation	
		Demonstrate acceptance of infant through own behavior	
		Emphasize normal characteristics of child	
		Encourage family members to express their feelings and concerns	
	Help family prepare for future care of child	As child grows older, discuss with parents alternatives to home care, especially as parents near retirement or old age	Family identifies realistic goals for future care of child
		Help family investigate residential settings other than institutionalization	Family avails themselves of supportive services
		Encourage family to include retarded member in planning and to continue meaningful relationships with him after placement	
		Refer to agencies that provide support and assistance	

*Applicable to any child with mental retardation.

Nursing Considerations

Since cognitive impairment is a fairly consistent finding in individuals with fragile X syndrome, the care afforded to these families is the same as for any child with mental retardation. Because the disorder is hereditary, genetic counseling is necessary to inform parents of the risks of transmission; a woman who carries a fragile X chromosome has a 25% recurrence risk for transmission to her offspring, regardless of their sex (Cohen, 1984). In addition, any male or female with unexplained or nonspecific mental impairment should be referred for chromosomal analysis and appropriate genetic counseling (see also p. 172) (Brady, 1984).

- For the hospitalized child, nurses must be aware of the child's abilities and needs, provide a familiar setting and support families.

- Down syndrome, a chromosomal abnormality, is characterized by retarded intelligence, slowed social development, congenital anomalies, sensory problems, and diminished growth and sexual development.

- Fragile X syndrome is a recently recognized clinical entity characterized by mental retardation and phenotypic findings in some affected males: It is considered the second leading cause of mental retardation after Down syndrome.

CONCEPT SUMMARIES

- Mental retardation is the most common developmental disability in the United States, affecting about 3% of the population.

- According to the American Association of Mental Deficiencies, mental retardation is a "significantly subaverage general intellectual functioning existing concurrently with deficits in adaptive behavior and manifested during the developmental period."

- Diagnosis of cognitive impairment is based on standard intelligence tests and no child is too young to be assessed.

- Causes of severe mental retardation are primarily genetic, biochemical, viral, and developmental. Mild retardation is associated primarily with familial, social, and environmental causes, whereas severe retardation is more likely associated with specific syndromes.

- Primary prevention efforts focus on support for the premature neonate and other high-risk newborns, rubella immunization, genetic counseling, education regarding alcohol, adequate prenatal nutrition, and reduction of nonintentional and intentional cerebral injuries.

- Secondary prevention activities include prenatal diagnosis or carrier detection.

- Tertiary prevention is aimed at minimizing long-term consequences through medical treatment.

- Education of children with cognitive impairment emphasizes sensory and verbal discrimination, improvement of short-term memory, motivation, and technologic support.

- Intervention programs are based on one of three models: parent training/infant curriculum model, parent/therapy model, and parent-infant interaction model.

- Promotion of independent self-help skills is aimed at feeding, toileting, dressing, and grooming.

- Promoting optimum development may be achieved through family guidance regarding play, communication, discipline, socialization, and sexuality.

REFERENCES

American Academy of Pediatrics: The Doman-Delacato treatment of neurologically handicapped children, Pediatrics **70**(5):810-812, 1982.

American Academy of Pediatrics, Committee on Sports Medicine: Atlantoaxial instability in Down syndrome, Pediatrics **74**(1):152-154, 1984.

Balkany, T.J., and others: Hearing loss in Down's syndrome: a treatable handicap more common than generally recognized, Clin. Pediatr. **18**(2):116-118, 1979.

Bennett, F.C., and others: Vitamin and mineral supplementation in Down's syndrome, Pediatrics **72**(5):707-713, 1983.

Brady, M.A.: Fragile-X syndrome: an overview, Pediatr. Nurs. **10**(3):210-211, 1984.

Carpenter, N.J., Leichtman, L.G., and Say, B.: Fragile X-linked mental retardation, Am. J. Dis. Child. **136**:392-398, 1982.

Chamberlain, A., and others: Issues in fertility control for mentally retarded female adolescents: I. sexual activity, sexual abuse, and contraception, Pediatrics **73**(4):445-450, 1984.

Cohen, F.: Clinical genetics in nursing practice, Philadelphia, 1984, J.B. Lippincott Co.

Cohen, H.J.: Trends in service delivery and treatment of the mentally retarded, Pediatr. Ann. **11**(5):458-469, 1982.

Coplan, J.: Three pitfalls in the early diagnosis of mental retardation, Clin. Pediatr. **21**(5):308-310, 1982.

Crocker, A.C.: Current strategies in prevention of mental retardation, Pediatr. Ann. **11**(5):450-457, 1982.

Davies, R.R., and Rogers, E.S.: Social skills training with persons who are mentally retarded, Ment. Retard. **23**(4):186-196, 1985.

de la Cruz, F.F., and Muller, J.Z.: Facts about Down syndrome, Child. Today **12**(6):2-7, 1983.

Fort, P., and others: Abnormalities of thyroid function in infants with Down syndrome, J. Pediatr. **104**(4):545-549, 1984.

Fryns, J.: Fragile X syndrome: a study of 83 families, Clin. Genet. **26**(6):497-528, 1984.

Gerald, P.S., and Meryash, D.L.: Chromosomal disorders other than Down syndrome. In Levine, M.D., and others, editors: Developmental-behavioral pediatrics, Philadelphia, 1983, W.B. Saunders Co.

Golden, G.S.: Controversies in the therapies for children with Down syndrome, Pediatr. Rev. **6**(4):116-120, 1984.

Goldman, J., Stein, C.L., and Guerry, S.: Psychological methods of child assessment, New York, 1983, Brunner/Mazel.

Grossman, H.J., editor: Manual on terminology and classification in mental retardation, American Association on Mental Deficiency, Baltimore, 1983, Garamond Pridemark Press.

Gunn, P., and Perry, P.: The temperament of Down's syndrome toddlers and their siblings, J. Child Psychol. Psychiatry 26(6):973-979, 1985.

Hall, D.M.B.: The child with a handicap, Boston, 1984, Blackwell Scientific Publications.

Hreidarsson, S.J., Shapiro, B.K., and Capute, A.J.: Age of walking in the cognitively impaired, Clin. Pediatr. 22(4):248-250, 1983.

Kaminer, R., and Jedrysek, E.: Early identification of developmental disabilities, Pediatr. Ann. 11(5):427-437, 1982.

Lamb, J.M.: Clothing for handicapped children: recent developments, Rehabil. Lit. 38(9):278-284, 1977.

Libb, J.W., and others: Hearing disorder and cognitive function of individuals with Down syndrome, Am. J. Ment. Defic. 90(3):353-356, 1985.

Marfo, K., and Kysela, G.M.: Early intervention with mentally handicapped children: a critical appraisal of applied research, J. Pediatr. Psychol. 10(3):305-324, 1985.

Passer, A., and others: Issues in fertility control for mentally retarded female adolescents: II. parental attitudes toward sterilization, Pediatrics 73(4):451-454, 1984.

Pueschel, S.M.: The child with Down syndrome. In Levine, M.D., and others, editors: Developmental-behavioral pediatrics, Philadelphia, 1983, W.B. Saunders Co.

Pueschel, S.M.: Down syndrome: defining problems and exposing useless 'therapy,' Consultant 25(11):77-84, 1985.

Robison, L.L., and others: Down syndrome and acute leukemia in children: a 10-year retrospective survey from Children's Cancer Study Group, J. Pediatr. 105(2):235-242, 1984.

Russman, B.S.: Early intervention for the biologically handicapped infant and young child: is it of value?, Pediatr. Rev. 5(2):51-55, 1983.

Sharav, T., Collins, R., and Shlomo, L.: Effect of maternal education on prognosis of development in children with Down syndrome, Pediatrics 76(3):387-391, 1985.

Silva, M.C.: Assessing competency for informed consent with mentally retarded minors, Pediatr. Nurs. 10(4): 261-265, 306, 1984.

Simeonsson, R.J., Cooper, D.H., and Scheiner, A.P.: A review and analysis of the effectiveness of early intervention programs, Pediatrics 69(5):635-641, 1982.

Smith, D.W.: Recognizable patterns of human malformation: genetic, embryologic and clinical aspects, ed. 3, Philadelphia, 1982, W.B. Saunders Co.

Smith, G.F., and others: Use of megadoses of vitamins with minerals in Down syndrome, J. Pediatr. 105(2):228-234, 1984.

Storm, G.: Alternative therapies. In Levine, M.D., and others, editors: Developmental-behavioral pediatrics, Philadelphia, 1983, W.B. Saunders Co.

Task Force on Joint Assessment of Prenatal and Perinatal Factors Associated with Brain Disorders: National Institutes of Health report on causes of mental retardation and cerebral palsy, Pediatrics 76(3):457-458, 1985.

Williams, J.K.: Reproductive decisions: adolescents with Down syndrome, Pediatr. Nurs. 9(1):43-44 +, 1983.

Wasch, S.W.: Hospitalization of profoundly and severely mentally retarded children, Child. Health Care 9(4):126-131, 1981.

BIBLIOGRAPHY
Mental Retardation

Bernardo, M.L.: Premarital counseling and the couple with disabilities: a review and recommendations, Rehabil. Lit. 42(7-8):213-216, 1981.

Blackwell, M.W., and Roy, S.A.: Surgical "routines" for profoundly retarded patients, Am. J. Nurs. 78(3):402-404, 1978.

Blum, R.W.: Sexual health needs of physically and intellectually impaired adolescents. In Blum, R., editor: Chronic illness and disabilities in childhood and adolescence, New York, 1984, Grune & Stratton, Inc.

Bowness, S., and Zadik, T.D.: Implementing the nursing process at a unit for mentally handicapped children, Nurs. Times 77(16):695-696, 1981.

Bromley, D.: What the parents want ... holiday relief for parents with a mentally handicapped child, Health Soc. Serv. J. 90:191-193, Feb. 1981.

Browder, J.A.: The pediatrician's orientation to infant stimulation programs, Pediatrics 67(1):42-44, 1981.

Cohen, H.J.: Mental retardation: introduction, Pediatr. Ann. 11(5):424-425, 1982.

Colwell, S.O.: The adolescent with developmental disorders. In Blum, R., editor: Chronic illness and disabilities in childhood and adolescence, New York, 1984, Grune & Stratton, Inc.

Crocker, A.C., and Nelson, R.P.: Mental retardation. In Levine, M.D., and others, editors: Developmental-behavioral pediatrics, Philadelphia, 1983, W.B. Saunders Co.

Denhoff, E.: Current status of infant stimulation or enrichment programs for children with developmental disabilities, Pediatrics 67(1):32-36, 1981.

Diamond, D.L.: Medical care of the mentally retarded, Pediatr. Ann. 11(5):445-449, 1982.

Doernberg, N.L.: Issues in communication between pediatricians and parents of young mentally retarded children, Pediatr. Ann. 11(5):438-444, 1982.

Eddington, C., and Lee, T.: Sensory-motor stimulation for slow-to-develop children: a home-centered program for parents, Am. J. Nurs. 75(1):59-62, 1975.

Erickson, M.L.: Care approaches to the child with mental retardation in a hospital setting, Clin. Pediatr. 17(7):539-547, 1978.

Ferry, P.C.: On growing new neurons: are early intervention programs effective? Pediatrics 67(1):38-41, 1981.

Godfrey, A.: Sensory-motor stimulation for slow-to-develop children, Am. J. Nurs. 75(1):56-59, 1975.

Gregory, D.: Family assessment and intervention plan, Pediatr. Nurs. 1(4):23-29, 1975.

Johnson, D.M., and Johnson, W.R.: Sexuality and the mentally retarded adolescent, Pediatr. Ann. 11(10):847-853, 1982.

Koch, R., Martin, G.E., and Sarason, S.B.: Mental retardation: making the tentative diagnosis, Patient Care 12:183-207, Oct. 1978.

Koch, R., Martin, G.E., and Sarason, S.B.: Mental retardation: planning referral and breaking the news, Patient Care 12:210-215, Oct. 1978.

Krajicek, M.J., and Tearney, A.I., editors: Detection of developmental problems in children, Baltimore, 1977, University Park Press.

Lamb, J.M.: Clothing for handicapped children: recent developments, Rehabil. Lit. 38(9):278-284, 1977.

Lepler, M.: Having a handicapped child, Am. J. Maternal Child Nurs. 3(1):32-33, 1978.

Mahoney, G., Finger, I., and Powell, A.: Relationship of maternal behavioral style to the development of organically impaired mentally retarded infants, Am. J. Ment. Defic. 90(3):296-302, 1985.

Myers, P.A., and Warkany, S.F.: Working with parents of children with profound developmental retardation: a group approach, Clin. Pediatr. 16(4):367-370, 1977.

Opitz, J.M.: Mental retardation: biologic aspects of concern to pediatricians, Pediatr. Rev. 2(2):41-50, 1980.

Pipes, P.L., and Pritkin, R.: Nutrition and feeding of children with developmental delays and related problems. In Pipes, P.L., editor: Nutrition in infancy and childhood, ed. 3, St. Louis, 1985, The C.V. Mosby Co.

Roberts, M.J., and Canfield, M.: Behavior modification with a mentally retarded child, Am. J. Nurs. 80(4):679, 1980.

Roberts, S.E., Coffin, G., and Dunn, M.J.: Feeding techniques for the physically impaired child, Pediatr. Basics 21:4-7, 1978.

Smith, M.A.H., and others: Feeding management of a child with a handicap: a guide for professionals, Memphis, TN, 1982, University of Tennessee.

Tudor, M.: Nursing intervention with developmentally disabled children, Am. J. Maternal Child Nurs. 3(1):25-31, 1978.

Ulvund, S.E.: Predictive validity of assessments of early cognitive competence in light of some current issues in developmental psychology, Hum. Dev. 27(2):76-83, 1984.

Wasch, S.W.: Hospitalization of profoundly and severely mentally retarded children, Child Health Care 9:126-131, 1981.

Williams, R.: A community nursing service for mentally handicapped children, Nurs. Times 76:2011-2012, Nov. 1980.

Wilson, B.: Toilet training the mentally handicapped child, Dev. Med. Child Neurol. 22(2):225-229, 1980.

Down Syndrome

Balkany, T.J., and others: Hearing loss in Down's syndrome, Clin. Pediatr. 18(2):116-118, 1979.

Borgaonkar, D.S.: Dermatoglyphic studies and their usefulness in clinical diagnosis by the method of predictive discrimination, Birth Defects: Original Article Series 15(6):621-625, 1979.

Bovicelli, L., and others: Reproduction in Down's syndrome, Obstet. Gynecol. 59(6):(suppl.):135-175, 1982.

Bricker, D., Carlson, L., and Schwarz, R.: A discussion of early intervention for infants with Down's syndrome, Pediatrics 67(1):45-46, 1981.

Brinkworth, R.: Helping the child with Down's syndrome, Midwife Health Visitor & Community Nurse 19:93-96, 1983.

Chatterjee, M.S.: Paternal age and Down's syndrome, Contemp. OB/GYN 21(5):171-174, 1983.

Cranston, J.A.: A Down's baby, Nurs. Times 75(42):1792-1794, 1979.

Fishler, K., Koch, R., and Donnell, G.N.: Comparison of mental development in individuals with mosaic and trisomy 21 Down's syndrome, Pediatrics 58(5):744-748, 1976.

Kerr, R., and Blais, C.: Motor skill acquisition by individuals with Down syndrome, Am. J. Ment. Defic. 90(3):313-318, 1985.

Kihlstrom, A.: A very special boy, Child. Today 12(6):8-11, 1983.

Koch, R.: Down's syndrome: pediatric care, Feelings Med. Signif. 22(1):1-6, 1980.

Long, A.: Down's syndrome, Nurs. Times 76:814-819, May 1980.

Lydic, J.S.: Annotated bibliography: motor development in children with Down syndrome, Phys. Occup. Therapy Pediatr. 2(4):53-74, 1982.

Pipes, P.L., and Holm, V.A.: Feeding children with Down's syndrome, J. Am. Diet. Assoc. 77:277-282, Sept. 1980.

Rex, A.P., and Preus, M.: A diagnostic index for Down syndrome, J. Pediatr. 100(6):903-906, 1982.

Shepperdson, B.: Changes in the characteristics of families with Down's syndrome children, J. Epidemiol. Community Health 39(4):320-324, 1985.

Spencer, K., and Carpenter, P.: Screening for Down syndrome using serum alpha-fetoprotein: a retrospective study indicating caution, Br. Med. J. 290(6486):1940-1943, 1985.

Uchida, I.A., and Freeman, V.C.P.: Trisomy 21 Down syndrome: II. structural chromosome rearrangements in the parents, Hum. Genet. 72(2):118-122, 1986.

Veach, S.A.: Down's syndrome: helping the special parents of a special infant, Nursing 83 13(9):42-43, 1983.

Williams, J.K.: Down syndrome update, Children/s Nurse 3(5):1-4, 1985.

Fragile X Syndrome

Adearce, M., and Kearns, A.: The fragile X syndrome: the patients and their chromosomes, J. Med. Genet. 21:84-91, 1984.

Carmi, R., and others: Fragile X syndrome ascertained by the presence of macro-orchidism in a 5-month-old infant, Pediatrics 74(5):883-886, 1984.

Finelli, P., and others: Neurological findings in patients with the fragile-X syndrome, J. Neurol. Neurosurg. Psychiatry 48(2):150-153, 1985.

Goldfine, P.E., and others: Association of fragile X syndrome with autism, Am. J. Psychiatry 142(1):108-110, 1985.

Hagerman, R., Kemper, M., and Hudson, M.: Learning disabilities and attentional problems in boys with the fragile X syndrome, Am. J. Dis. Child. 139(7):674-678, 1985.

Hogge, W.A., and others: Prenatal diagnosis of fragile "X" syndrome, Obstet. Gynecol. 63(3):suppl.:19S-21S, 1984.

Chapter 25

The Child with Sensory or Communication Impairment

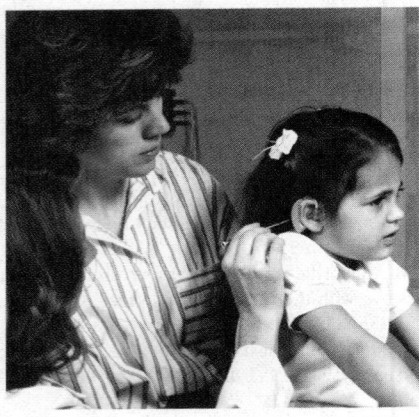

Sensory impairments pose special threats to a child's developmental potential. Deprived of visual or auditory cues, the child must rely more heavily on other sensory experiences to learn about and relate to the environment. The child with a communication disorder may function well during early childhood but be unable to achieve in an academic setting. Without assistance and rehabilitation, these children are vulnerable to the lifelong disadvantages of being an individual with a disability.

Parents are the major rehabilitators of the child. However, they need guidance and support from specially trained professionals to help the child learn. The nurse is often in a strategic position to prevent and identify sensory or communication disorders, support the family in adjusting to the disorder, and assist them in learning methods of overcoming or compensating for the impairment. This chapter is primarily concerned with prevention, identification, and rehabilitation; psychosocial interventions to assist the family in coping with the impairment are discussed in Chapter 22, and the reader is encouraged to review those concepts.

Hearing Impairment

Hearing impairment is one of the most common disabilities in the United States. The exact prevalence of hearing loss is not known, especially in young children with unilateral impairment. National data indicate that about 11 of 1000 children 6 to 17 years of age have a hearing impairment (Gortmaker and Sappenfield, 1984). With improved neonatal detection methods, the incidence of moderate to profound hearing loss in high-risk infants is 2.5% to 5.0% (American Academy of Pediatrics, 1982). About 30% of hearing-impaired children have associated disabilities, such as visual problems or cognitive deficits (Hall, 1984).

DEFINITION AND CLASSIFICATION

A number of definitions exist regarding categories of hearing impairment, including such terms as deaf and dumb, mute, or deaf-mute. However, these terms are unacceptable; hearing-impaired persons are not dumb and, if mute, have no physical speech defect other than that caused by the inability to hear. Acceptable definitions that focus on the child's educational and psychologic potential are (Davis and Silverman, 1978):

hearing impairment A generic term indicating disability that may range in severity from mild to profound and includes the subsets of deaf and hard-of-hearing

deaf Refers to a person whose hearing disability precludes successful processing of linguistic information through audition, with or without a hearing aid

hard-of-hearing Refers to a person who, generally with the use of a hearing aid, has residual hearing sufficient to enable successful processing of linguistic information through audition

Hearing defects may also be classified according to etiology, pathology, or symptom severity. Each is important in terms of treatment, possible prevention, and rehabilitation.

Etiology

The precise cause is not known in about 30% of hearing-impaired children; however, many of these children demonstrate histories of conditions in which the risk of deafness is greatly increased (see the box on p. 1014). Significant causes of hearing impairment from disease are congenital cytomegalovirus and bacterial meningitis; at one time congenital rubella was a leading cause, but mass immunization has reduced the incidence of this infection. Among high-risk newborns factors associated with hearing loss are respirator care, hyperbilirubinemia, and hyponatremia (Bergman and others, 1985).

Of special concern are environmental noise levels. Although exact criteria for damaging noise levels in infants and children are not firmly established, in adults the maximum sound intensity that does not produce sensorineural hearing loss is approximately 80 dB. Depending on duration of exposure to sounds louder than 80 dB, hearing loss may result (Davis and Silverman, 1978). Children are exposed to a wide variety of high-intensity sounds, one of the most common of which is loud rock music. The greatest danger seems to be at dances, concerts, or discotheques, where the noise levels reach between 120 and 140 dB and persist for 3 or more hours. In addition, high-risk neonates who are surviving formerly fatal prenatal or perinatal conditions may be susceptible to hearing loss from continuous humming noises or high noise levels associated with incubators, oxygen hoods, or intensive care units. Continuous exposure to excessive noise levels in the premature infant may represent an even greater risk when combined with the use of potentially ototoxic antibiotics (Bess, Finlayson, and Chapman, 1979).

Pathology

Disorders of hearing can also be classified according to location of the defect within the structures of the ear or the neural pathways. The specific pathologic condition interfering with transmission of sound determines the type of treatment.

Conductive hearing loss. Conductive or middle-ear hearing loss results from interference of transmission of sound to the middle ear. It is the most common of all types of hearing loss and may involve the external auditory canal, tympanic membrane, middle-ear chamber, ossicles (incus, stapes, malleus), or eustachian tube. It may be the result of anatomic anomalies, such as atresia of the external canal, or mesenchymal changes, most frequently as a result of recurrent serous otitis media. A common and temporary cause in children is a blocked external canal from a foreign body or impacted cerumen. Conductive hearing impairment mainly involves interference with loudness of sound. Although air conduction is impaired, bone conduction is intact. Many conductive defects are amenable to medical or surgical treatment, and hearing is improved with the use of a hearing aid to amplify sound.

Sensorineural hearing loss. Sensorineural hearing loss, also called perceptive or nerve deafness, involves damage to the inner ear structures and/or the auditory nerve. In almost half the cases the cause of sensorineural loss is unknown. The most common causes are congenital defects of inner ear structures or consequences of acquired conditions, such as infection, hyperbilirubinemia, administration of ototoxic drugs, or exposure to excessive noise.

Sensorineural hearing loss results in distortion of sound and problems in discrimination. The hearing loss is often selective for various frequencies, especially those in the high range. Loss of discrimination of high frequencies makes perception of consonants such as "s," "z," "ch," or "th" impossible; loss in the middle range eliminates hearing vowels, semivowels, and most consonants. Although the child hears some of everything going on around him, the sounds are distorted, resulting in discrimination and comprehension being severely affected. Medical/surgi-

CONDITIONS ASSOCIATED WITH HEARING LOSS

Familial/genetic factors
Skeletal defects (Treacher Collins and Klippel-Feil syndromes)
Retinitis pigmentosa
Cerebral palsy
Mental retardation
Visual handicaps
Pigment abnormalities (Waardenburg syndrome, albinism)
*Anatomic malformations involving head or neck
Chromosomal abnormalities, such as D and E trisomies
Connective tissue disorders (osteogenesis imperfecta, Hurler syndrome)
*Family history of childhood hearing impairment

Prenatal/intrauterine factors
Diabetes mellitus, alcoholism
Drugs, such as quinine, salicylates, and certain ototoxic antibiotics
Maternal anoxia
Preeclampsia/eclampsia

Perinatal factors
*Birth weight less than 1500 g
Prolonged or difficult birth
*Hyperbilirubinemia at level exceeding indications for exchange transfusion
*Severe asphyxia
*Congenital perinatal infection (cytomegalovirus, rubella, herpes, syphilis, toxoplasmosis)
*Bacterial meningitis

Postnatal factors
Ear infection (chronic otitis media)
Acute infection (mumps, rubella, measles, encephalitis, meningitis)
Respiratory conditions (hypertrophied adenoids, allergy)
Ototoxic drugs, including topical applications to ear (kanamycin, streptomycin, gentamicin, neomycin, vancomycin, viomycin)
Trauma (burns, frostbite, lacerations, perforations, bone fracture)
Exposure to excessive noise (urban living, loud rock music, model airplanes, snowmobiles, sport shooting, motorcycle and sport racing, heavy machinery)

*Indicates the need for hearing assessment by 6 months of age based on recommendation from the American Academy of Pediatrics (1982).

---

cal intervention is rarely of any benefit. Since the defect is not one of intensity of sound, hearing aids are of little value in improving discrimination, since they merely amplify distorted sounds.

Mixed conductive-sensorineural hearing loss. Mixed conductive-sensorineural hearing loss results from interference with transmission of sound in the middle ear and along neural pathways. It frequently results from recurrent serous otitis media, which causes damage to middle- and inner-ear structures. The conductive loss is more amenable to treatment and improvement with a hearing aid than the sensorineural component.

Central auditory imperception. Central auditory imperception includes all hearing losses that do not demonstrate defects in the conductive or sensorineural structures. They are usually divided into organic or functional losses. In the *organic type* of central auditory imperception, the defect involves the reception of auditory stimuli along the central pathways and the expression of the message into meaningful communication. Terms used to describe such receptive-expressive disorders include:

aphasia Inability to express ideas in any form, either written or verbally
agnosia Inability to interpret sound correctly
dysacusis Difficulty in processing details or discrimination among sounds

In each of these conditions the difficulty is in processing, patterning, and interpreting the information within the brain, not in hearing the sound. Perception of sound eventually

Table 25-1 Intensity of sounds expressed in decibels

DECIBELS (dB)	REPRESENTATIVE SOUND
0	Softest sound normal ear can hear
10	Heartbeat, rustling of leaves
20	Whisper at 1.8 m (5 feet)
30-45	Normal conversation
60	Noise in average restaurant
70-80	Street noises
80	Loud radio in home
90-100	Train
120	Thunder, rock music
140	Jet airplane during departure
>140	Pain threshold

becomes so confusing and distressing that it results in complete inhibition of response to all auditory stimuli. Consequently the child acts as if he were deaf.

In the *functional type* of central auditory imperception, there is no organic lesion to support a central auditory loss. Examples of functional hearing loss are conversion hysteria (an unconscious withdrawal from hearing to block remembrance of a traumatic event), infantile autism, and childhood schizophrenia. Another common type is psychogenic selective hearing loss, in which the child who is continually bombarded with auditory stimuli tunes out extraneous sounds. This is in contrast to selective sensorineural loss, in

Table 25-2 Classification of hearing loss based on symptom severity

CLASS	EFFECTIVE ON SPEECH	EDUCATIONAL RECOMMENDATIONS
Slight (hard of hearing)—30 dB or better	Difficulty in hearing faint or distant speech Likely to "get along" in school and to have normal speech	Should be given benefit of favorable seating in regular classrooms May be assisted by special instruction in lipreading
Mild to moderate (hard of hearing)—30-55 dB	Usually understand conversational speech at a distance of 3 to 5 feet without great difficulty May have some defects in articulation of their own speech May have difficulty in hearing adequately in school if talker's voice is faint or if his face is not visible to them	Should wear hearing aids and be given training in their use Should be taught lipreading and be given benefit of speech correction and conservation of speech Should have advantage of favorable seating in classrooms
Marked (hard of hearing)—55-70 dB	Understand conversational speech only if it is loud Have considerable difficulty in group and classroom discussions Language and especially vocabularies may be limited Abnormalities of articulation and voice production are obvious	Hearing aids and auditory training, special training in speech, and special language work are all essential May be able to continue in regular classes; may derive more benefit from special classes
Severe (deaf)—70-90 dB	May hear sound of loud voice about 1 foot from ear May identify some environmental noises and may distinguish vowels but have difficulty with consonants Must be taught both speech and language	Should be taught by means of educational procedures for deaf child, with special emphasis on speech, auditory training, and on language
Extreme (deaf)—90 dB or worse	Are deaf, even though they may hear some very loud sounds Speech and language must be developed through careful and extensive training	Require special educational procedures

Modified from Davis, H., and Silverman, S.R.: Hearing and deafness, ed. 4, New York, 1978, Holt, Rinehart & Winston, p. 436.

which the child has normal hearing for some frequencies and a substantial loss for others.

Symptom Severity

For clinical purposes hearing impairment is described according to the degree or severity of loss. Hearing is expressed in decibels (dB), a unit of loudness (Table 25-1), and is measured at the three frequencies of 500, 1000, and 2000 cycles per second, the critical listening speech range. The term *hearing-threshold level* refers to the measurement of an individual's hearing threshold by means of an audiometer. Hearing impairment can be classified according to hearing-threshold level and the degree of symptom severity as it affects speech (Table 25-2). These classifications offer only general guidelines regarding the effect of the impairment on any individual child, since children differ greatly in their ability to use residual hearing.

Most deaf children have some perception of loud sounds but no usable hearing. Their primary mode of communication is visual (lipreading or sign language). Children who are hard of hearing use auditory cues in conjunction with visual cues to communicate. Educational recommendations based on the severity of hearing are also presented in Table 25-2.

EFFECTS OF HEARING IMPAIRMENT ON DEVELOPMENT

Loss of hearing affects speech, language, and social development. The severity of the impairment depends not only on the extent of the defect but also on the age of occurrence, interval until diagnosis, and adequacy of rehabilitation. To understand the tremendous effect loss of hearing has on a young child, it is necessary to explore the role of hearing in normal childhood development.

The full-term infant is born with auditory sensitivity to all ranges of sound frequencies heard by human beings. From birth, and possibly before, sound acquaints the infant with events in the physical world. Significantly the sound of the parent's voice becomes an important component of parental-infant bonding. Long before he understands the words, the infant learns the emotional intonations of what is said. Likewise, his vocal response, such as small throaty sounds or squeals, gives reciprocal satisfaction and meaning to the parents.

The infant learns from sounds in the environment what is expected of him. For example, when he cries and hears footsteps or his parents' voice, he associates them with anticipated meeting of his needs. He learns that quiet sounds, such as singing when he falls asleep, are soothing. He judges the emotional behavior of others by the way in which they inflect their voices in anger, praise, disapproval, sadness, or joy. From these cues he learns to relate in a complementary manner.

Sounds associated with objects give them additional meaning. For example, a ride in the car is much more stimulating when one hears the myriad of sounds than if one hears only silence or distorted, confusing noise. Much of the child's initial knowledge about objects is related to the sound they make, such as animal sounds or the sound of a clock. Infants with hearing loss compensate for the deficient auditory input with increased visual alertness by as early as 3 months of age (Beratis and others, 1979).

The infant learns speech from the pleasure derived from hearing his own voice, the reinforcement each vocalization evokes, and the usefulness of substituting words for gestures in expressing desires. By the end of the first year he listens to and discriminately behaves according to auditory cues. A primary example is the ability to stop an activity in response to the word "no." Although this may appear to be an insignificant act, it marks the beginning of deliberate socially acceptable behavior, ability to accept frustration, and recognition of a less egocentric existence.

Audition also has a motor component. Although less obvious than the effect of vision on motor development, hearing encourages the child to move rhythmically and later to run, jump, or rock in time with music and use facial muscles for singing. Sounds, such as banging for the resultant noise, striking piano keys for the different notes, or splashing water for the slapping sound, often encourage motor activity. Audition also alerts the child to potential danger, such as a car coming down the street, and to the need for various responses, such as answering the door and coming home when called.

The effect of hearing on academic learning is profound. Most learning is done through auditory cues, primarily verbal language. Even if visual aids are used, the child must understand verbal directions concerning their use and meaning. If the child has some hearing and has learned compensatory visual skills, he may function well in a one-to-one relationship. However, he may have difficulty in school because of his placement distant to the teacher, the teacher's continuous movement while talking (walking back and forth, turning to a blackboard, looking down to a book), group discussions, and extraneous noise.

Socialization depends greatly on communication. Although the infant relies heavily on nonauditory cues, such as vision and tactile sensations, for social interaction, language becomes increasingly important to social development during early childhood. Verbal symbols gradually replace gestures and by school age are a prerequisite for social relationships. The hearing-impaired child is at a great disadvantage. He is often unable to proceed past parallel play within a group because of his inability to follow directions during cooperative play. Even if he has speech, in a group setting his hearing deficit may not allow him to interpret enough of the conversation to join in. Because of his inabil-

ity to quickly grasp the meaning of a discussion, he is often called "slow," "square," or "dumb" by his peers. As a result he learns to stay on the periphery or to avoid social interaction altogether. His self-concept becomes severely damaged, which may result in permanent emotional problems.

While most research has concentrated on effects of binaural hearing loss on children's development, recent studies demonstrate that children with monaural or unilateral hearing loss are also at risk for communication and educational problems. These children are likely to fail a grade in school, to require assistance from school personnel, and to have poorer auditory skills. It is suggested that these children have considerable difficulty in understanding speech in environments with competing sounds, such as a noisy classroom, and that preferential seating may not be sufficient to overcome this handicap (Bess and Tharpe, 1984).

NURSING INTERVENTIONS WITH THE HEARING-IMPAIRED CHILD

Nursing intervention with hearing-impaired children is a specialized area of practice, requiring additional training in hearing assessment and rehabilitation. However, general nursing goals that focus on prevention, detection, and rehabilitation of the child with a hearing impairment are every nurse's responsibility. In addition, nurses may have to care for a hospitalized hearing-impaired child and must know how to meet the child's and the family's special needs.

Prevention

The primary nursing role is prevention of hearing loss. Since the most common cause of impaired hearing is chronic otitis media, it is essential that appropriate measures be instituted to treat existing infections and prevent recurrences (see Chapter 32). Children with histories of ear or respiratory infections or any other condition known to increase the risk of hearing impairment should receive periodic auditory testing.

Routine immunization eliminates the possibility of acquired sensorineural loss from rubella, mumps, and measles (encephalitis). Drugs to treat infections should be used cautiously, with avoidance of ototoxic agents. If ototoxic drugs are used, changes in the child's hearing need to be evaluated for prompt recognition and discontinuation of therapy. Groups at special risk for receiving ototoxic antibiotics are premature or sick neonates and children with chronic illnesses, such as cystic fibrosis, immune-deficiency diseases, and conditions requiring immunosuppressant therapy, such as leukemia or nephrosis.

Pregnant women are counseled regarding the necessity of early prenatal care, including genetic counseling for known familial disorders; avoidance of all ototoxic drugs, especially during the first trimester; tests to rule out syphilis, rubella, or blood incompatibility; medical management of maternal diabetes; control of alcoholism; and adequate dietary intake.

Exposure to excessive noise pollution is a well-established cause of sensorineural hearing loss. The nurse should routinely assess the possibility of environmental noise pollution and advise children and parents of the potential danger. Signals suggesting exposure to excessive noise are ringing or buzzing in the ears and/or perceiving sounds as muffled or dull after leaving the source of the noise. When individuals engage in activities associated with high-intensity noise, such as flying model airplanes, target shooting, or snowmobiling, they wear ear protection such as earmuffs or earplugs (not ordinary dry cotton). However, any protection is better than none. Even common household equipment can be hazardous, such as lawn mowers, power vacuum cleaners, and cordless telephones (Orchik and others, 1985).

Detection

Aside from prevention, the most important nursing responsibility is detection. Discovery of a hearing impairment within the first months of life is essential to prevent social, physical, and psychologic damage to the child. Detection involves (1) screening all children for auditory function, (2) observing for behaviors that indicate a hearing loss, and (3) isolating those children who by virtue of their history are at risk. The American Academy of Pediatrics (1982) recommends that the hearing of any infant manifesting the asterisked items in the box material on p. 1014 be screened by 3 months and no later than 6 months of age. Tests for assessing hearing are discussed in Chapter 7. The following discussion is primarily concerned with behavioral indications of hearing loss.

Infancy. At birth the nurse can observe the neonate's response to auditory stimuli as evidenced by the startle reflex, head turning, eye blinking, and cessation of body movement. The Brazelton Neonatal Behavioral Assessment Scale evaluates the infant's orientation response to the sound of a voice. Scoring is based on the following (Brazelton, 1973):

1. No reaction
2. Respiratory change or blink only
3. General quieting as well as blink and respiratory changes
4. Stills, brightens, no attempt to locate source
5. Shifting of eyes to sound, as well as stills and brightens
6. Alerting and shifting of eyes and head turned to source
7. Alerting, head turned to stimulus, and searching with eyes
8. Alerting prolonged, head and eyes turned to stimulus repeatedly
9. Turning and alerting to stimulus presented on both sides on every presentation of stimulus

The infant may vary in the intensity of the response, depending on the state of alertness. However, a consistent score of "no reaction," especially with absence of the startle reflex, should lead to suspicion of hearing loss.

During infancy children demonstrate developmental changes in response to localizing a source of sound (see Chapter 12). Failure to orient to a sound and to attempt to localize it by age 6 months is an important clue to auditory

loss. Other danger signals suggesting hearing problems in the developing infant are summarized in the box on p. 1018, especially those under "Orientation response."

Childhood. The profoundly deaf child is much more likely to be diagnosed during infancy than the less severely affected one. If the defect is not detected during early childhood, the likelihood is that it will surface at entry to school, when the child has difficulty in learning. Unfortunately some of these children are erroneously placed in special classes for the learning disabled or the mentally retarded.

Signs suggestive of hearing impairment in children are outlined in the box on p. 1018. Of primary significance is the nurse's willingness to *listen* to parents' reports of suspicion regarding hearing loss. The value of a thorough history cannot be overemphasized (see the box on p. 1019). In particular, assessment includes speech development, response to hearing, past history of ear infections, and behavioral patterns.

Of primary importance is the effect of hearing impairment on speech development. Children with hearing impairment often have a monotone, flat type of speech. A child with a mild conductive hearing loss may speak fairly clearly but in a loud voice. A child with a sensorineural or selective hearing loss usually has difficulty in articulation. Depending on the degree of loss, sounds of certain frequencies may not be audible. For example, inability to hear higher frequencies renders the child unable to perceive or to imitate some consonants, especially sounds such as "s," "z," "ch," and "th." Therefore to the child who is unable to discriminate all sounds, the word "spoon" acoustically sounds like "poon." Consequently the child's speech will be a reflection of the distortion of sound.

A child with a central auditory hearing loss presents a special dilemma for diagnosis. During early infancy there is little or no evidence that the child has a hearing impairment because he responds normally to sounds. It is often impossible to ascertain that the child cannot interpret what is heard until 18 months of age or older, at which time associated behavioral characteristics become apparent (Knobloch and Pasamanick, 1974). At this age the child behaves as if he is deaf because he inhibits all response to sounds that are confusing and have little meaning for him.

Communication deficits are important clues to a central auditory hearing loss. The child with a mild loss learns language and can easily give stereotyped responses, such as his name, sex, address, or age. In other words, he can answer questions for which he has learned a patterned response. He can also make appropriate spontaneous remarks or comments. However, when asked a question, such as "What's this?" (pointing to a shoe), he is unable to answer. He may continually repeat the question or answer it incorrectly. Parents frequently become irritated with the monotonous repetition or interpret a wrong response as evidence of stupidity.

He may also experience an inordinate amount of difficulty in learning the correct use of pronouns, especially "you" and "I." Although he may learn usable language, he is unable to manipulate it to express wants, answer ques-

SIGNS SUGGESTIVE OF HEARING IMPAIRMENT IN INFANTS AND YOUNG CHILDREN

Orientation response
Lack of startle or blink reflex to a loud sound
Persistence of Moro reflex beyond 4 months of age (associated with mental retardation)
Failure to be awakened by loud environmental noises during early infancy
Failure to localize a source of sound by 6 months of age
General indifference to sound
Lack of response to spoken word; failure to follow verbal directions
Response to loud noises as opposed to voice

Vocalizations and sound production
Monotone quality, unintelligible speech, lessened laughter
Normal quality in central auditory loss
Lessened experimental sound play and squealing
Normal use of jargon during early infancy in central auditory loss, with persistent use later on
Absence of babble or inflections in voice by age 7 months
Failure to develop intelligible speech by age 24 months
Vocal play, head banging, or foot stamping for vibratory sensation
Yelling or screeching to express pleasure, annoyance, or need
Asking to have statements repeated or answering them incorrectly

Visual attention
Augmented visual alertness and attentiveness
Responding more to facial expression than verbal explanation
Being alert to gestures and movement
Use of gestures rather than verbalization to express desires, especially after age 15 months
Marked imitativeness in play

Social rapport and adaptations
Less interest and involvement in vocal nursery games
Intense preoccupation with things rather than persons
Avoidance of social interaction; often puzzled and unhappy in such situations, prefers to play alone
Inquiring, sometimes confused facial expression
Suspicious alertness, sometimes interpreted as paranoia, alternating with cooperation
Marked reactivity to praise, attention, and physical affection

Emotional behavior
Use of tantrums to call attention to self or his needs
Frequently stubborn because of lack of comprehension
Irritable at not making himself understood
Shy, timid, and withdrawn
Often appears "dreamy," "in a world of his own," or markedly inattentive

Modified from Knobloch, H., and Pasamanick, B., editors: Gesell and Amatruda's developmental diagnosis, New York, 1974, Harper & Row, Publishers.

tions, or engage in social conversation of any complexity. His speech is not as monotonous as that of a child with conductive or sensorineural loss, but it may be so limited that it seems inarticulate. Loud sounds (about 90 dB) are irritating and even painful to the child; as a result he may inhibit such sounds as a banging door or a dropped plate but attend to sounds such as rustling paper or a verbal comment. Obviously such behaviors can lead one to seriously question the existence of a hearing deficit unless there is a high index of suspicion for each type of loss. The best rule to follow is that if the child *acts* as though he were deaf to the human voice, he should be treated as though he has a hearing impairment (Knobloch and Pasamanick, 1974).

The nurse may need to specifically question parents about the child's response to hearing. Some children become so adept at learning visual cues that even a severe loss may go undetected. In particular the nurse inquires about response to vibratory sound, such as music, and to the human voice. Profoundly deaf children enjoy music and may be skillful dancers, not because they hear the sound, but because they sense the rhythm of the vibrations. Such behavior may be mistaken as evidence of hearing. Other clues to vibratory stimulus may be persistent banging activity, such as hammering pegs, playing musical instruments, placing hands against a radio to feel vibrations, or sudden attentiveness to loud noises, such as a door slamming.

Past history of ear disorders may lead to suspicion regarding conductive hearing loss. In addition to inquiry about

ear or throat infection, respiratory allergies, colds, and tonsillitis, the nurse asks about treatment for each disorder and associated complications, such as a "draining" ear or sudden relief of pain (perforation of the membrane). Otoscopic examination may reveal areas of tympanic scarring, perforation, or obstruction, such as from a foreign body or packed cerumen.

Since the deaf child's primary mode of learning is based on visual cues, the nurse also assesses him for visual problems, such as refractive errors, strabismus, and color blindness. The incidence of eye defects is approximately twice as common in hearing-impaired children as in normal children. Although the precise nature of the association between visual and auditory deficiencies is unclear, it follows the frequent biologic adage that one physical defect is often accompanied by others. Correction of visual impairment when possible is essential to reduce additional handicaps to learning. If color blindness is present, teaching aids may need revision to eliminate influence of color in learning situations.

Rehabilitation

Once the diagnosis of hearing impairment is made, parents need extensive support to adjust to the shock of learning about their child's disability. This may be the first time they learn that the child's poor speech development and behavior problems are the result of a hearing deficit, not because of difficulty with his tongue, refusal to talk, or disobedience. Parents may need time to deal with guilt feelings over previous attempts to teach the child to talk or past punishment for the child's misbehavior.

Parents also need an opportunity to realize the extent of the hearing loss. Sometimes parents benefit from a demonstration of what it is like to be deaf or hard of hearing. For example, showing them a moving film without sound helps them appreciate the profound effect of living in a world devoid of hearing and the great difficulty in comprehending the spoken word. If the child has a selective hearing loss, the parents can better understand the distortion of sound and difficulty with discrimination if they are placed in a sound-proof room and allowed to hear only the frequencies the child hears. Central auditory imperception is similar to hearing a foreign language with no understanding of the meaning of the words.

The parents gradually need to adjust to the idea that the child's major obstacle will be the development and use of language. The parents may benefit from being told that with appropriate teaching the child can learn receptive language skills. This step will precede his attempts to use expressive language, because he needs to know and understand what is being communicated to him before he can be expected to communicate expressively to others.

After the parents have been able to assimilate the magnitude of the burden of their child's loss, they may benefit from encouragement and support to set realistic goals for themselves and for their child. A hearing-impaired child's education cannot wait until he is 6 years old. It must begin as early as possible and be continued in the home, where the parents play a significant role in teaching and reinforcing language skills.

Parents need to know how impaired hearing affects a child's normal development. For example, the infant with a hearing loss, especially in the moderate or greater range, is unaware of parental verbal cues. Consequently he is less likely to demonstrate the same degree of reciprocity in relating to his parents as a hearing child. However, he does attend to significant others by looking at them, nestling in their arms during holding, or quieting when his needs are met. These behaviors are stressed to help parents establish meaningful contact with the infant. Although the child is unable to hear, parents are encouraged to talk to him as they would a normal child, supplement his stimulation needs with visual and tactile cues, and relate to him in the *en face* position to help him learn facial expressions.

The initial role in rehabilitation is to help the family accept the defect and participate in an auditory training program.* The nurse encourages the parents to learn role modeling by attending the auditory clinic. It is important that the father and siblings be included in the educational process so that they learn to communicate with the child.

Educational training depends on the severity of hearing

---

*A list of approved programs is available from the Alexander Bell Association for the Deaf, 3417 Volta Place NW, Washington, DC 20007. Home training correspondence programs are sponsored by the John T. Tracy Clinic, 806 West Adams Blvd., Los Angeles, CA 90007. Other sources of information are the National Association of the Deaf, 814 Thayer Ave., Silver Spring, MD 20910; National Association for Hearing and Speech Action, 10801 Rockville Pike, Rockville, MD 20852; National Information Center on Deafness, Gallaudet College, 800 Florida Ave. NE, Washington, DC 20002; SHHH (Self Help for Hard of Hearing People, Inc.), 7800 Wisconsin Ave., Bethesda, MD 20814; National Easter Seal Society, 2023 W. Ogden Ave., Chicago, IL 60612.

ASSESSMENT OF CHILD FOR IMPAIRED HEARING

Family history
Genetic disorders associated with hearing impairment
Family members, especially siblings, with hearing disorders

Prenatal history
Miscarriages
Illnesses during pregnancy (rubella, syphilis, diabetes)
Drugs taken
Exposure to childhood diseases
Eclampsia

Delivery
Duration of labor, type of delivery
Fetal distress
Presentation (especially breech)
Drugs used
Blood incompatibility

Birth history
Apgar score
Weight
Associated anomalies
Cyanosis, oxygen therapy
Jaundice, transfusions

Past health history
Immunizations
Serious illness (e.g., bacterial meningitis)
Convulsions
High unexplained fevers
Ototoxic drugs
No history (adopted child)
Colds, ear infections, allergies
Treatment of ear problems
Visual difficulties

Hearing
Parental concerns regarding hearing loss (what cues, at what age)
Response to name calling, loud noises, sounds of different frequencies (crinkling paper, whisper, bell, rattle)
Results of previous audiometric testing

Speech development
Age of babbling, first meaningful words, phrases
Intelligibility of speech
Present vocabulary

Motor development
Age of sitting, standing, walking
Level of independence in self-care, feeding, toileting, grooming

Adaptive behavior
Play activities
Socialization with other children
Behaviors: temper tantrums, stubbornness, self-vexation, vibratory stimulus
Educational achievement
Recent behavioral/personality changes

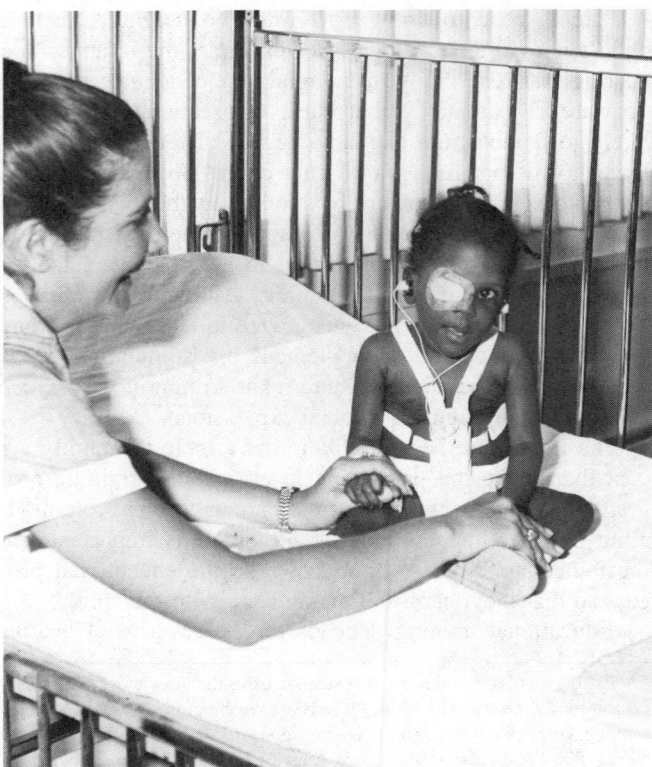

Fig. 25-1. On-the-body hearing aids are convenient for young children, such as this child with bilateral hearing loss. Note the eye patching for strabismus.

Photography by John Roy, Saint Francis Hospital, on location at Children's Medical Center, Tulsa, OK.

loss (see Table 25-2). However, considerable controversy exists about the education of these children. Some educators favor a purely oral approach, arguing that the children must eventually live in a world of hearing people. Others favor the use of nonverbal communication, such as sign language or finger spelling (Hall, 1984). The general trend is toward maximizing children's communication skills with all available means, although verbal skill training is considered the most important method of communication.

Hearing aids. Hearing aids are designed to amplify sound and are of greatest value in conductive hearing losses, although all ambient noise is also amplified, often making conversational speech difficult to hear. Hearing aids are of less benefit in a sensorineural or central auditory loss and constitute only a minor part of rehabilitation, since they amplify distorted sound and are unable to conduct sounds as nerves do. Hearing aids are usually advocated even in profoundly deaf individuals who have some residual hearing to maximize this ability.

The types of hearing aids are:

In the ear: Aid fits directly in the ear canal, supported by the ear shell.

Behind the ear: Aid is housed in a small, curved case that fits behind the ear; microphone, amplifier, and receiver are housed in the case and connected to the ear mold by plastic tubing.

On the body or pocket: Microphone, amplifier, and power supply are enclosed in a case worn in a pocket or attached to clothing; external receiver is attached directly to ear mold and is powered through a flexible wire from the amplifier (Fig. 25-1).

Eyeglass model: Aid is similar to behind-the-ear models except that it is built into the eyeglass frame; convenient for binaural (two-ear) hearing aids.

Basically the hearing aid system consists of a tiny *microphone*, which picks up sound waves and converts them into electrical signals; an *amplifier*, which increases the strength of the electrical signals; a *receiver* or loudspeaker, which

Table 25-3	Care of hearing aids
PART	**INSTRUCTIONS FOR CARE**
Hearing aid casing	Store it away from high heat or excessive cold
	Keep it dry; remove during hair washing, showering, or swimming
	Avoid dropping or bumping it
	Remove it when using any aerosal spray, a hair dryer, or during X-ray study
	Turn switch to off *before* removing aid to prevent accidental drain on batteries
Ear mold	Keep it clean, detach it from receiver, and wash in soap and water; dry thoroughly
	If opening becomes clogged with wax, clean it gently with a pipe cleaner
	Do not use alcohol or other cleaning solutions
Batteries	Store extra batteries in a cool, dry place
	If stored in refrigerator, allow them to warm to room temperature before using
	If carried in a pocketbook, wrap them in plastic to avoid accidental contact with a metal object
	Remove batteries from aid when it is not worn
	Keep battery contacts clean (remove residue with a pencil eraser)
	Insert batteries correctly (proper negative and positive charges to contacts)
	Check periodically with a battery tester
Tubing and cord	Avoid twisting cord or bending tubing
	Replace worn-out tubing or too short cord (on-the-body model)
Microphone	Check microphone openings; if clogged, wipe off particles with a *dry* cloth
	Do not use damp cloth or pipe cleaner to open holes; consult hearing aid dealer for advice

GUIDELINES FOR FACILITATING LIPREADING

Attract child's attention before speaking; use light touch to signal speaker's presence

Stand close to child

Face child directly or move to a 45-degree angle

Stand still; do not walk back and forth or turn away to point or look elsewhere

Establish eye contact and show interest

Speak at eye level and with good lighting on speaker's face

Be certain nothing interferes with speech patterns, such as chewing food or gum

Speak clearly and with a slow and even rate

Use facial expression to assist in conveying messages

Keep sentences short

Do not repeat if child does not understand the words; rephrase message

converts the amplified signals back into sound waves and directs them into the ear via a specially fitted *ear mold;* and a *battery* source, which provides electrical current for operating the device.

Hearing aids are expensive and require care to maintain optimum functioning. The nurse should be familiar with basic care and handling of the device, especially when the child is hospitalized (Table 25-3).* One of the most common problems with the device is *acoustic feedback,* an annoying whistling sound usually caused by improper fit of the ear mold. If this occurs, it may be remedied by reinserting it, making certain that no hair is caught between the ear mold and canal, cleaning the ear mold or ear, or lowering the volume of the aid. Sometimes the whistling may be at a frequency that the child cannot hear but that is annoying to others. In this case, the child is told of the noise and asked to readjust the aid.

As the child grows older, he may be self-conscious about the device. Every effort should be made to make the aid inconspicuous, such as an appropriate hairstyle to cover behind-the-ear or in-the-ear models, attractive frames for glasses, and placement of the on-the-body type where it is not seen, such as under a blouse or sweater. The child is given responsibility for the care of his device as soon as he is able, since fostering independence is a primary goal of rehabilitation.

Lipreading. Even though the child may become an expert at lipreading, only about 40% of the spoken word is understood, and less if the speaker has an accent, mustache, or beard. Exaggerating pronunciation or speaking in an altered rhythm (too slow or too fast) further lessens comprehension. Parents can help the child understand the spoken word by using the suggestions in the box. The child learns to supplement the spoken word with sensitivity to visual cues, primarily body language and facial expression (for example, tightening the lips, muscle tension, and eye contact).

Sign language and finger spelling. Sign language, such as the American Sign Language (ASL) or British Sign Language (BSL), is a visual-gestural language that uses hand signals that roughly correspond to specific words and concepts in the English language. Finger spelling is a manual alphabet that relies on specific hand shapes that represent letters of the English alphabet. Words are spelled out using the manual alphabet. Both are useful nonverbal communication tools, except that finger spelling is slower than signing and both methods are meaningful only when the listener understands the symbols. Family members are encouraged to learn signing or finger spelling because using or watching hands requires much less concentration than lipreading or talking. Also these symbol methods enable some deaf children to learn more and to learn faster. When others who need to communicate with the child do not know these methods, an interpreter is extremely helpful.*

Speech therapy. The most formidable task in the education of a deaf child is learning to speak. Speech is learned through a multisensory approach, using visual, tactile, kinesthetic, and auditory stimulation. Since the usual mechanism for learning language is not available to the deaf child—namely, through imitation and reinforcement—systematic formal education is required. Parents are encouraged to participate fully in the learning process. For example, language that serves a useful purpose is taught. Teaching is related to significant and meaningful experiences. The home environment fosters an atmosphere in which language is used and books are read. While spontaneous language is encouraged, poor articulation, rhythm, and voice quality are corrected.

Additional aids. Everyday activities present problems to the older child. For example, he may not be able to hear the telephone, doorbell, or alarm clock. Several commercial devices† are available to help the deaf person adjust to these dilemmas. Flashing lights can be attached to a telephone or doorbell to signal its ringing. Trained hearing ear dogs can provide great assistance to deaf individuals because they alert the person to sounds, such as someone approaching, a moving car, a signal to wake up, and a child's cry. Special teletypewriters (TYY) or telecommunications devices for the deaf (TDD) help deaf people communicate with each other over the telephone; the typed message is conveyed via the telephone lines and displayed on a small screen.

Any audiovisual medium presents dilemmas to the child because while he can see the picture, he cannot hear the message. However, *closed captioning* is one solution. Through a special decoding device the audio portion of a

---

* Information about hearing aids is available from the National Hearing Aid Society, 20361 Middlebelt Rd., Livonia, MI 48152; 1-800-521-5247 (in Michigan, 1-313-478-2610).

*Information about qualified interpreters for hearing-impaired people is available from the Registry of Interpreters for the Deaf (RID), 814 Thayer Ave., Silver Spring, MD 20910.

†Information about signaling devices is available from the Alexander Graham Bell Association for the Deaf.

television program is translated into captions (subtitles) that appear on the screen.*

As the deaf child learns to compensate for his lack of hearing, he becomes extremely perceptive of visual and vibratory changes. He often knows when another person wishes to talk to him because the person will walk close by him but not pass. He learns to be alert to other people approaching him by seeing their shadows or feeling the vibrations of their footsteps. He is acutely aware of facial expressions and may comprehend the unspoken word more quickly than the spoken word.

Socialization. Since socialization is extremely important to the child's development, the nurse discusses with the family methods of fostering social contact. If the child attends a special school for the deaf, he is able to socialize with peers in that setting. Many programs specifically focus on the ability to relate to peers in a group situation by providing classroom and recreational activities. Classmates become a potential source of close friendships because they communicate more easily among themselves. Parents are encouraged to promote these relationships when possible.

The child with a hearing impairment may need special help in school or social activities. For those children wearing hearing aids, ambient noise should be kept to a minimum. Structural enhancements such as carpeted floor, mounted (not freestanding) blackboards, and quiet heating and air circulation equipment are very helpful. Since many of these children are able to attend regular classes, the teacher may need assistance in adapting methods of teaching for the child's benefit. The school nurse is often in an optimum position to emphasize methods of facilitated communication, such as lipreading (see box). Since group projects and audiovisual teaching aids may hinder the deaf child's learning, these educational methods should be carefully evaluated.

When the child is in a group setting, it is helpful for the other members to sit in a semicircle in front of him so that he can see their faces. Since one of the difficulties in following a group discussion is that the deaf child is unaware of who speaks next, it helps to have someone point out each speaker. This can inconspicuously be accomplished by giving each speaker a number or using his name and marking this down as that person talks. If one person writes down the main topic of the discussion, the child is able to follow lipreading more closely. Such suggestions can increase the child's ability to participate in sports, clubs such as Boy Scouts or Girl Scouts, and group projects.

CARING FOR THE HOSPITALIZED DEAF CHILD

The needs of the hospitalized deaf child are the same as those of any other child, but his disability presents special challenges to the nurse. For example, verbal explanations as the primary method of preparation for admission or proce-

dures must be supplemented with tactile and visual aids, such as books or actual demonstration and practice. The child's understanding of the explanation needs to be constantly reassessed. If the child's verbal skills are poorly developed, he can answer questions through drawing, writing, or gesturing. For example, if the nurse is attempting to clarify where a spinal tap is done, the child is asked to point to where the doctor will insert the needle. Since deaf children often need more time to grasp the full meaning of an explanation, the nurse is careful not to judge the slowness as a sign of retardation and to allow ample time for understanding.

When communicating with the child, the same principles are used as are outlined for facilitating lipreading. Ideally, nurses without foreign accents should be assigned to the child. The child's hearing aid is checked to ensure that it is working properly. If it is necessary to awaken the child at night, nurses should gently shake him to signal their presence or turn on the hearing aid before arousing the child and always makes sure that the child can see them before any procedures, even routine ones such as changing a diaper or regulating an infusion, are performed. It is important to remember that the child may not be aware of another's presence until alerted through visual or tactile cues.

Ideally parents are encouraged to room with the child. However, it must be conveyed to them that this is not to serve as a convenience to the nurse but as a benefit to the child. Although the parents' aid can be enlisted in familiarizing the child with the hospital and explaining procedures, the nurse also talks directly to him, encouraging expression of his feelings about the experience. If there is difficulty in understanding the child's speech, an effort is made to become familiar with his pronunciation of words. Parents often can be helpful by explaining the child's usual speech habits.

The nurse honestly admits if the child cannot be understood and encourages him to write his statements. However, at no time is it implied that the child's speech is imperfect. Rather the nurse lets him know that it will take some time to become familiar with his words and that in the meantime he can help by using gestures or written messages. Expressing an interest in learning sign language, especially useful words, such as "yes," "no," "water," and "toilet," not only improves communication efforts but greatly strengthens the nurse-child-parent relationship. Nonvocal communication devices are also available that employ pictures or words that the child can point to (see p. 1041). Such boards can also be improvised by drawing pictures or writing the words of common needs, such as food, water, toilet, and parent, on cardboard.

The nurse has a special role as child advocate with the deaf and is in a strategic position to alert other health team members and other patients to the child's special needs regarding communication. For example, the nurse should accompany other health team members on visits to the child's room to ensure that they speak to the child and that the child understands what was said. Not infrequently caregivers for-

---

*Additional information is available from the National Captioning Institute, Inc., 5203 Leesburg Pike, Falls Church, VA 22041.

Nursing Care Summary: The Hearing-Impaired Child

NURSING GOALS	NURSING INTERVENTIONS	EXPECTED PATIENT/FAMILY OUTCOMES

HP-HMP   **Injury: potential for tissue damage**
        Risk factors: developmental (maternal infection), chemical (drugs), biologic (genetic),
            environmental

NURSING GOALS	NURSING INTERVENTIONS	EXPECTED PATIENT/FAMILY OUTCOMES
Detect hearing impairment Infancy	Assess neonate's response to a loud noise; observe for signs associated with congenital deafness Assess orientation responses at each well-baby visit (see p. 1018)	*Child's hearing impairment is detected early and appropriate management strategies are implemented
Childhood	Listen carefully to family's concerns regarding hearing loss Take a thorough history regarding factors that support an auditory impairment Evaluate speech development carefully Observe for behaviors that may suggest a hearing impairment (p. 1018) Administer hearing tests and refer for audiometry	Family expresses fears and concerns *Family's concerns are recognized Child is referred for testing
Prevent hearing loss Infancy	Encourage immunization at appropriate age Prevent ear infection; detect early	Infant does not develop hearing loss Children are properly immunized
Childhood	Assess hearing ability of children who are receiving ototoxic antibiotics Promote compliance with treatment regimens for otitis media Discuss with parents measures to prevent otitis media Evaluate auditory ability of children prone to chronic ear or respiratory problems Assess sources of excessive noise in child's environment; institute appropriate measures to decrease sound levels (turn music lower, use ear protection)	Child does not develop hearing loss Child is not exposed to excess noise levels

CPP   **Sensory-perceptual alteration: auditory**
      Etiology: hearing impairment

NURSING GOALS	NURSING INTERVENTIONS	EXPECTED PATIENT/FAMILY OUTCOMES
Promote communication process	Encourage family to attend rehabilitation program in order to continue learning in home; encourage them to learn sign language, finger spelling Teach language that serves a useful purpose Encourage use of language and books in home Encourage spontaneous language but correct speech impairments	Family continues communication practices in home environment Family provides stimulation to child
Facilitate lipreading	Test child for visual problems that may interfere with learning to lipread or use sign language Teach family and others involved with child (e.g., teacher) behaviors that facilitate lipreading (see box, p. 1021)	Child communicates with others in manner taught (specify) Persons communicating with child use good communication techniques
Maximize residual hearing	Help family investigate reliable hearing aid dealers Discuss types of hearing aids and their proper care Teach child how to regulate hearing aid for maximum benefit Help child focus on all sounds in environment and talk to him about them For older child, discuss methods of camouflaging aid to make it less conspicuous	Child acquires and uses hearing aid
Provide opportunities for play/socialization	Guide family in selection of toys that maximize visual and tactile senses, as well as residual hearing Encourage child to participate in group activities Help him follow group discussion by pointing out speaker and arranging group in semicircle Help child develop friendships among hearing and deaf peers Help child achieve a sense of security in his ability to compete with peers	Child engages in activities appropriate to developmental level

*Nursing outcome.

Continued.

Nursing Care Summary: The Hearing-Impaired Child—cont'd

NURSING GOALS	NURSING INTERVENTIONS	EXPECTED PATIENT/FAMILY OUTCOMES
Encourage education within a regular classroom	Discuss with teacher ways of communicating effectively with child (such as through facilitating lipreading) Promote socialization with classmates	Child attends school regularly
Promote independence and development	Help family transfer normal childrearing practices to this child Emphasize importance of attaining independence in self-care Provide child with devices that foster independence (hearing ear dog, special signaling aids for telephone or door bell) Discuss importance of discipline and limit-setting	Child performs activities of daily living appropriate to level of development

N_{of}D

RRP	Family process, alteration in	
	Etiology: situational crisis (diagnosis of deafness in a child)	

Assist family in adjusting to child's loss of hearing	Anticipate usual grief reaction to loss Help family deal with any guilt feelings regarding previous responses to child when true nature of problem was unknown Help family realize extent of child's disability and its tremendous influence on speech and language development Discuss advantages and limitations of amplifying devices with different types of hearing loss Encourage formal rehabilitation as soon as possible	Family expresses feelings and concerns regarding child's loss of hearing Family demonstrates an understanding of implications of hearing loss Family becomes involved in programs
Provide emotional support	Be available to family for assistance Encourage family members to discuss their feelings regarding disability Stress child's abilities rather than disability Become familiar with techniques used for communication if following family on a long-term basis Refer family to appropriate community agencies for medical, psychiatric, educational, vocational, or financial assistance* Involve parents in local parent groups for hearing impaired children	Family expresses feelings and concerns about disability and its ramifications Family members avail themselves of available resources
Promote parent-child attachment	Help family identify clues other than verbal ones that signify infant's communication with them Encourage family to stimulate child with visual and tactile cues Stress importance of continuing to talk to child even though he may not hear their voices Encourage parents to discuss their feelings regarding attachment process	Parents and child demonstrate a positive relationship

get that the child has the abilities to perceive and learn despite a hearing loss and consequently communicate only with the parents. As a result, the child's needs and feelings remain unrecognized and unmet.

Since deaf children often have difficulty in forming social relationships with other children, the child is introduced to his roommates and encouraged to engage in play activities. The hospital setting can provide growth-promoting opportunities for social relationships. With the assistance of a child life specialist, the child can learn new recreational activities, experiment with group games, and engage in ther-

apeutic play. The use of puppets, dollhouses, role playing with dress-up clothes, building with a hammer and nails, finger painting, needle play, and water play can help the deaf child express feelings that previously were suppressed.

Vision Impairment

Visual impairments are a common problem during childhood; prevalence rates for some degree of visual impairment even with corrective glasses is approximately 20 to 35 per

1000 children. Of this group 0.5 to 1.0 per 1000 are considered legally blind (Gortmaker and Sappenfield, 1984). Nearly 50% of blind children under 5 years of age have no useful vision, and for the remainder the visual acuity is unknown (Vision problems in the United States, 1980). The nurse's role is clearly one of detection, referral, and in some instances rehabilitation.

DEFINITION AND CLASSIFICATION

Vision impairment is a general term to refer to visual loss that cannot be corrected with regular prescriptive lenses. However, a more useful system for classifying visual impairments is based on the type of activity in which the child can be expected to engage, which may include the following categories (Helveston and Ellis, 1984):

school vision Visual acuity between 20/70 and 20/200 (also known as partially sighted). The child should be able to obtain an education in the usual public school system with the use of normal-sized print. Near vision is almost always better than distance vision.

legal blindness Visual acuity of 20/200 or less and/or a visual field of 20 degrees or less in the better eye. This is useful only as a legal definition, not as a medical diagnosis. It allows special considerations with regard to taxes, entrance into special schools, eligibility for aid, and other benefits.

travel vision Visual acuity of 20/400. This vision allows the child to travel in unfamiliar surroundings provided he is otherwise healthy. The use of print may be possible but difficult. Learning braille may be required.

light perception This is primarily important for the child's sense of well-being and may be an aid in mobility, but it is not useful for other educational purposes.

ETIOLOGY AND TYPES OF VISUAL PROBLEMS

The etiology of visual impairment can be classified according to a number of divisions. In addition diseases such as cataracts, optic atrophy, or glaucoma may cause any number of visual defects.

familial factors Including genetic diseases associated with visual defects, such as Tay-Sachs disease, albinism, galactosemia, or retinoblastoma.

prenatal/intrauterine factors Especially maternal infections, such as rubella, syphilis, herpes simplex, or toxoplasmosis.

perinatal factors Including prematurity, maternal infection (ophthalmia neonatorum), and oxygen toxicity (retrolental fibroplasia).

postnatal factors Primarily trauma, infections (mumps, measles, rubella, poliomyelitis, and chicken pox), and disorders such as juvenile rheumatoid arthritis, leukemia, and myasthenia gravis.

The following discussion focuses on the most common types of visual disorders in children regardless of the spe-

cific etiology. Clinical manifestations are listed on p. 1032. In many instances, such as with refractive errors, the cause of the defect is unknown.

Refractive Errors

Refractive errors, which refer to those variations within the eye that prevent perfect focusing of light rays on the retina, are the most common causes of visual impairment. Refractive errors may result in myopia, hyperopia, astigmatism, or anisometropia. The following is a brief discussion of how refractive disorders can occur.

The term *refraction* means bending and refers to the bending of light rays as they pass through the lens of the eye. Normally light rays enter the lens and fall directly on the retina (emmetropia), usually at the fovea centralis (center of the macula), the region of greatest visual acuity. However, in refractive disorders the light rays fall either in front of the retina (myopia) or beyond it (hyperopia) (Fig. 25-2).

Three reflexes—accommodation, convergence, and pupillary constriction—are necessary to bring the image into clear focus. The *accommodation reflex* focuses the image sharply on the retina. It causes an increase in the curvature of the lens, constriction of the pupils, and convergence of two eyes. The reflex depends on contraction of the ciliary muscle to change the lens to a more convex shape, thus increasing refractive power. As an object is brought to close range, the pupils constrict (pupillary contraction), and as the object is moved farther away, the pupils dilate (pupillary relaxation).

The *convergence reflex* permits the object seen through each eye to focus on corresponding areas on the retina (binocularity). Convergence refers to the movement of the eyeballs inward as an object is brought closer to the face. The nearer the object, the greater the degree of convergence.

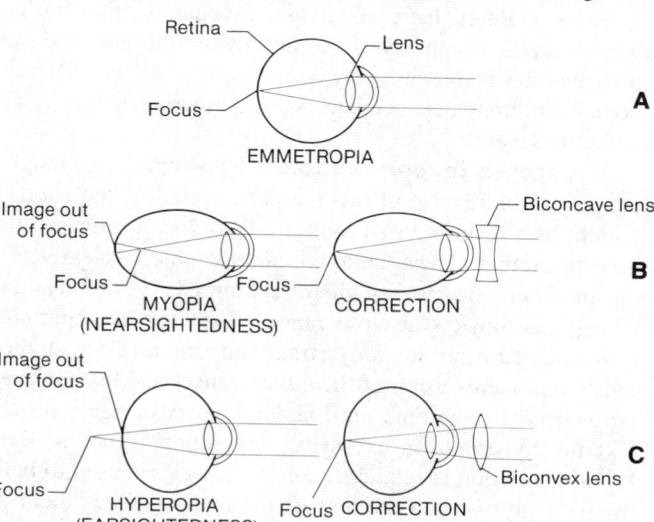

Fig. 25-2. Comparison of normal vision and refractive errors. **A,** Emmetropia (normal vision). **B,** Myopia (nearsightedness). **C,** Hyperopia (farsightedness).

When the eyes do not converge, two images are produced (diplopia).

For an object to be seen there must exist adequate illumination. The amount of light entering the retina is controlled by the *pupillary reflex*. In bright light the pupils constrict; in dim light the pupils dilate. If a bright light is shown into one eye, both eyes constrict (consensual light reflex). Changes in pupillary size are a function of the iris and are controlled by the smooth muscles that surround this pigmented structure.

Refractive errors are evaluated by testing visual acuity (see Chapter 7). They are best assessed by eliminating the accommodative powers of the eye with the use of a cycloplegic drug, such as atropine, that paralyzes the ciliary muscles.

Myopia. Myopia, or nearsightedness, refers to the ability to see objects clearly at close range but not at a distance. In most instances it results from an eyeball that is too long, resulting in the focal point falling in front of the retina. The eye possesses no ability to accommodate itself to this condition. Only when objects are brought close to the eye so that the image falls on the retina is vision clear. The child often squints in an attempt to correct the defect.

Correction involves the use of biconcave lenses, which cause the parallel rays to diverge, thus permitting the lens of the myopic eye to focus the two rays on the retina (see Fig. 25-2, *B*). Since myopia tends to increase in severity until late adolescence when refraction stabilizes, frequent changes of prescription lenses are required to achieve improved vision. While glasses help children see more clearly, there is no evidence to support the concern that minor uncorrected myopia adversely affects children's learning. In fact, children with myopia tend to have higher intelligence scores than emmetropic peers (Stewart-Brown, Haslum, and Butler, 1985).

Some children have congenital myopia. Unlike the acquired type, vision tends to improve with age and approaches normal acuity by adolescence. However, very young children may need to wear corrective lenses if the defect is severe.

Hyperopia (hypermetropia). Hyperopia, or farsightedness, is the reverse of myopia. The eyeball is too short in length; as a result rays of light are theoretically focused behind the retina. These children can see objects clearly at a distance and, because of their accommodative ability, can usually see objects at close range. However, the continual muscular effort produces eyestrain and may result in strabismus from overexertion of the ciliary muscles. Most children are normally hyperopic until about 7 years of age, and unless the hyperopia is excessive, correction is not needed. When correction is required, convex lenses are used to bend the light rays so that the lens of the eye can focus them on the retina (Fig. 25-2, *C*).

Astigmatism. The refractive surfaces of the eye are rarely perfectly spheric. Normally the imperfection is so slight that it does not interfere with refraction or vision. In astigmatism there are unequal curvatures in the cornea or lens so that light rays are bent in different directions, producing a blurred image. Although the eye attempts to accommodate for the distortion, it is unsuccessful, causing eyestrain.

Correction involves the use of specially ground lenses that compensate for errors in refraction. A special chart is used for astigmatism to isolate the exact location of deviation in curvatures along the meridians. Astigmatism may occur with or without other refractive disorders and tends to change with age, necessitating regular eye examinations.

Anisometropia. Anisometropia refers to a difference of refractive strength in each eye. It is a significant problem in early childhood primarily because of the development of amblyopia in the weaker eye (see discussion following). Anisometropia is treated with corrective lenses, preferably contact lenses, to improve vision in each eye so they work as a unit. The lenses must be worn at all times, especially in children less than 9 years of age because of the risk of amblyopia (Kovalesky, 1985).

Amblyopia

Amblyopia or "lazy eye" is a reduced visual acuity in one eye despite appropriate optical correction, and it can occur in the absence of any pathologic defect, (e.g., cataract, scarred cornea, or retrolental fibroplasia) in the affected eye. It affects about 2% of the population, including some 250,00 children under age 4 years in the United States (Kovalesky, 1985). A potential cause of blindness, it is almost always correctable provided treatment is begun early.

Amblyopia results when one eye does not receive sufficient visual stimulation during the critical period of development of the visual cortex. Normally the two eyes work as a unit (binocular vision). Images of an object are focused on the retina of each eye and passed to the brain so that the images are seen as one (fusion). When fusion is disrupted, each retina receives different images, resulting in diplopia (double vision). The brain accommodates for the visual confusion by suppressing the less intense image (formed by those light rays that fall adjacent to but not directly on the macula, the area of sharpest vision). If the defect is not corrected, the visual cortex does not respond to visual stimulation, resulting in loss of vision in the weaker eye (Greenwald, 1983).

Amblyopia can be caused by a number of ocular disorders and may be classified according to the following:

strabismic amblyopia: from prolonged fixation by the dominant eye and suppression of the images in the deviating eye

anisometropic or refractive amblyopia: from different refractive errors in the eyes

deprivation amblyopia: from congenital ocular defects, such as cataracts, that prevent vision on the affected eye

occlusion amblyopia: from prolonged patching of an eye, such as therapeutic patching after an injury, in very young children

The optimum time for correction of amblyopia is during early childhood. The treatment consists of patching the good eye so that the child will be forced to use the weaker eye. If refractive errors are present, corrective lenses are worn. It is more difficult to encourage school-age children to wear the occlusive patch because the poor visual acuity of the uncovered weaker eye interferes with schoolwork and the patch sets them apart from their peers.

Strabismus

Strabismus, which literally means "squinting," refers to malalignment of the eyes. When the eyes are malaligned, the visual axes are not parallel, causing the eyes to see two separate images (diplopia). Because the brain suppresses the images from the weaker or deviating eye, amblyopia can result in children under 9 years of age. Since 80% of all children with strabismus develop the malalignment before 4 years of age, early diagnosis to prevent vision loss is essential.

Terms used to describe strabismus and screening tests for malalignment are discussed in Chapter 7. There are several classifications of strabismus. One is based on the presence or absence of muscle paralysis. In *paralytic* strabismus a deviation of the eye is caused by paralysis of an extraocular muscle (six eye muscles that are innervated by the third, fourth, and sixth cranial nerves). However, more commonly malalignment is *nonparalytic*—there is usually no defect in the action of the individual extraocular muscles or in a specific nerve. Causes of nonparalytic deviations include cataracts, retinoblastoma, high refractive errors, or anisometropia.

The most common type of strabismus is esotropia, an inward deviation of the eye (Fig. 25-3). If the esotropia is evident by 6 to 12 months of age it is considered *infantile* or *early-onset esotropia*. Since young infants normally have malaligned eyes for the first few weeks of life, it is still not clear if this represents congenital strabismus (Nelson, 1983).

Another very common form of inward deviation is *accommodative esotropia,* which occurs between 6 months and 7 years, but most often at about 2½ years. In the accommodative type there is usually a large hyperopic refractive error that requires excessive accommodation to bring the image into clear focus. The child attempts to produce clearer vision by squinting, which forces convergence through increased muscle strength. If this condition is not corrected early, secondary mechanical changes in the muscles can occur that complicate treatment.

Exotropia, outward deviation of the eye or "wall eye," occurs much less frequently in children. Intermittent exotropia is the most common form and usually occurs between infancy and age 4 years. It is most likely to be evident when the child is sick, tired, exposed to bright light, or fixating on distant objects. Since the eyes are aligned most of the time, visual acuity is usually not affected.

Treatment depends on the type of strabismus but may involve surgery of affected muscles, prescription lenses to correct refractive errors, occlusion therapy, and sometimes

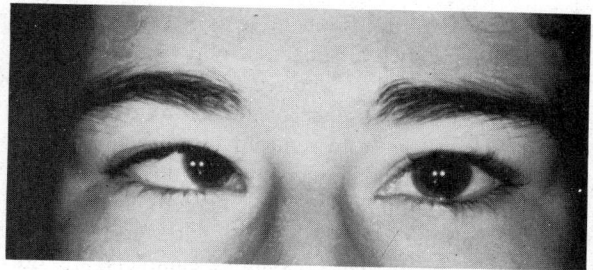

Fig. 25-3. Strabismus. Note obvious malalignment of eyes. Light reflections are centered in left cornea and to side of right cornea. From Havener, W.H., and others: Nursing care in eye, ear, nose, and throat disorders, ed. 3, St. Louis, 1976, The C.V. Mosby Co.

administration of anticholinesterase agents to reduce the accommodative effort. Occlusion therapy is a common procedure and involves patching the stronger eye to increase the visual stimulation to the weaker eye to prevent amblyopia. A careful schedule of patching must be followed to avoid occlusion amblyopia. Some practitioners prescribe 1 week of patching for every year of the child's age, followed by an examination to assess visual acuity in the occluded eye. Other authorities recommend alternative patching and uncovering each day to provide periodic stimulation to the covered eye (Kovalesky, 1985).

The goal in treating strabismus is preservation of vision, binocularity, and improvement in cosmetic appearance. However, all of these goals may not be achieved. Vision loss is always a concern and some children may require low-vision aids to compensate for the impairment. Fortunately lack of binocularity is not a serious handicap for most children. However, it does result in failure to develop stereopsis or depth perception, the ability to locate an object in spatial relationship to another object. The individual has difficulty in judging distances, such as when driving a car or reaching for a close object, and when using binocular instruments, such as a microscope or field glasses. Certain vocations, such as aviation, may not be available for these people and appropriate counseling should begin early.

Cosmetic effects can be difficult for older children. Peers may taunt them with remarks such as "cross-eyed." Other children often have difficulty in looking directly at them because the wandering eye is distracting. This may force the speaker to look away, making the person with strabismus feel insecure. If this occurs, the best advice is to look directly at the focusing or straight eye and avoid contact with the deviated eye, since the person then receives a clear, direct image.

Cataracts

A cataract is an opacity of the crystalline lens. The lens is normally transparent to allow light rays to enter the eye and refract them for a clear image on the retina; a cataract interferes with both of these functions. Cataracts may be congenital, such as those caused by maternal rubella during the first trimester, or acquired, most commonly as a result of penetrating injuries or, less frequently, as a secondary complication to diseases such as galactosemia.

Cataracts are usually identified as a visible white clouding of the lens, from absence of the red reflex on examination of the retina, or from reduced visual acuity in the affected eye. Congenital cataracts are the most common cause of blindness in children and must be removed as early as possible (within the first few weeks of life) to preserve useful vision. If monocular congenital cataracts are not removed early, permanent blindness from amblyopia results. Since the lens has been removed, some type of replacement lens must be used to correct the refractive power. In children prescription glasses or removable contact lenses, such as the extended-wear soft type, are preferred over implantable lenses. Initially the optical correction may provide for sharp vision at only one distance. As the child grows older, a bifocal system is required to correct for both far and near vision (Calhoun, 1983).

Glaucoma

Glaucoma refers to a condition in which intraocular pressure is increased, causing pressure on the optic nerve and eventually atrophy and blindness. Intraocular pressure is the result of pressure exerted by aqueous humor in the anterior cavity of the eye (space posterior to cornea and anterior to lens). Aqueous humor is believed to be produced by the ciliary body and normally passes from the anterior chamber through the pupil, into the canal of Schlemm, and finally into the anterior ciliary veins.

Congenital glaucoma results from defective development of the structures of the eye in the region of the anterior chamber angle (outflow tracts for aqueous humor). Consequently there is obstruction to the flow of fluid, resulting in increased intraocular pressure. Because of the distensibility of the infant's eye, the increased pressure pushes the anterior structures forward, causing thinning of the ocular layers until rupture of the globe may occur.

Surgical treatment (goniotomy) is required to open the outflow tracts (canal of Schlemm) sufficiently to facilitate the flow of aqueous humor. Occasionally more than one operation is necessary to produce an anterior chamber angle that is wide enough.

Acquired glaucoma is rare in children (as opposed to adults, in whom it is the second most common cause of blindness in the United States). It is usually the result of some superimposed obstacle to the flow of aqueous humor. The most common causes are retrolental fibroplasia and retinoblastoma, which result in a narrowing of the anterior angle from forward displacement of the fibrous tissue or tumor, respectively, and trauma or inflammation that results in the formation of synechiae (adhesions) and scarring in the angle. Treatment is aimed at eliminating the cause and is frequently surgical.

Trauma

Trauma is a common cause of vision impairment in children. Injuries to the eyeball and adnexa (supporting or ac-cessory structures such as eyelids, conjunctiva, and lacrimal glands) can be classified as penetrating or nonpenetrating. *Penetrating wounds* damage tissue in the outer coat of the eye, cornea, and sclera and may perforate through the entire thickness of the structures. Penetrating wounds are most often the result of sharp instruments, such as knives or scissors; propulsive objects, such as firecrackers, guns, bows and arrows, slingshots, or twist-off bottle caps; and a powerful contusion by a blunt object, which may occur during a fight, with racquet sports, or from a serious car injury. *Nonpenetrating injuries* damage the outermost surface of the eye and may be the result of foreign objects in the eyes, lacerations, a blow from a blunt object such as a fist, and thermal or chemical burns. Although most instances of eye trauma are unintentional, the possibility of child abuse should be considered, especially when marked facial trauma, bilateral corneal abrasions, unexplained hyphemas, and cigarette burns are present (Frey, 1983).

Visual impairment is not uncommon after serious eye injuries and can be caused by a number of possible posttraumatic events, including:

1. Corneal ulceration and scarring
2. Herniation of the intraorbital contents through a fracture of the orbital floor (blow-out fracture)
3. Complications from a hyphema (hemorrhage into the anterior chamber), such as secondary bleeding, blood staining of the cornea, glaucoma, or sympathetic ophthalmia (autoimmune disease of the uveal tract occurring in the uninjured eye)
4. Damage to the lens and cataract formation
5. Symblepharon (adhesions between the bulbar and palpebral conjunctiva) usually from scarring caused by burns
6. Rupture of the choroid, resulting in scar formation of the retina
7. Damage to the ciliary body
8. Infections of any structures of the eye, including panophthalmitis (see Table 25-4)
9. Retinal detachment from retraction of scar tissue formed along the path of a penetrating wound
10. Therapeutic enucleation

Treatment is aimed at preventing further ocular damage and is primarily the responsibility of the ophthalmologist. It involves adequate examination of the injured eye (with the child sedated or anesthetized in severe injuries), appropriate immediate intervention such as removal of the foreign body or suturing of the laceration, and prevention of complications, such as administration of antibiotics or steroids and complete bed rest to allow the eye to heal and blood to reabsorb. Prognosis varies according to the type of injury. It is usually guarded in all cases of penetrating wounds because of the high risk of serious complications, especially retinal detachment, panophthalmitis, and sympathetic ophthalmia.

Infections

Infections of the adnexa and the structures of the eyeball or globe are not uncommon in children. The most common eye disease is conjunctivitis. Table 25-4 lists the various types of ocular infections. Treatment is usually ophthalmic antibiotics. Severe infections may require systemic antibiotic therapy. Steroids are used cautiously because they exacerbate viral infections such as herpes simplex, increasing the risk of damage to the involved structures.

EFFECTS OF VISUAL IMPAIRMENT ON DEVELOPMENT

Vision is the most sophisticated and objective of all the senses. It is intimately involved with motor development; through sight the child learns spatial relationships, form, size, position, and distance. Without sight the child's mental constructs regarding these visual-motor perceptions are confined to the sense of touch and are limited to the periphery of his reach. Although the child hears, this sense cannot compensate fully for vision. They can, however, offer information about the environment, such as associating the concepts of "near" or "far" with respective sounds.

To comprehend the impact of visual impairment on a child, it is helpful to review the role of sight in childhood development. At birth the newborn is able to distinguish forms at close range. The importance of the first hour of life (sensitive period) to parent-infant bonding has been partly attributed to the neonate's visual alertness. He is able to maintain eye contact with his parents, which evokes a powerful reciprocal response from them. Throughout the attachment process visual responsiveness is extremely influential in assisting parent and child in learning about each other, identifying the parent as a significant caregiver, and perceiving emotional responses and physical needs in the child.

Visual stimulation is intense with the presentation of color, motion, size, and shape. Many blind or partially seeing children develop self-stimulatory habits called *blindisms,* such as eye rubbing, body rocking, finger flicking before the eyes, sniffing and smelling, arm twirling, or repetitive vocal tics, which are thought to serve as substitutes for sensorimotor stimulation. The infant gradually separates himself from his surroundings by learning that blankets, garments, toys, furniture, and other objects are not a part of his body. His body image depends heavily on the visual cues he receives, as well as on tactile sensations.

Visual-motor perception is believed to be a dependent ability. Retinal images supply the data that guide motor function for prehension, manipulation, and locomotion. For example, an infant learns to voluntarily grasp an object by seeing it first and reaching out to prehend it. If he does not see the object, he will have no self-stimulus to reach for it. The stimulus must be provided through another sense, usually touch or sound. For example, the object is taken away and the infant's hand is guided to search for it through touch or toys that make sounds are placed within the child's reach to encourage exploring (Fraiberg, 1977).

When the infant learns to crawl, he is guided in his locomotion through sight. Likewise, as he becomes more mobile he uses his depth perception to learn how to go up and

Table 25-4 Types of ocular infections	
INFECTION (STRUCTURES)	**COMMON CAUSES**
Orbital cellulitis (orbit)	Paranasal sinusitis, meningitis Penetrating injury
Blepharitis (lids)	Bacteria (hordeolum [stye], chalazion, pyodermas) Virus (herpes zoster, herpes simplex)
Conjunctivitis (often called pinkeye) (conjunctiva)	Bacteria (ophthalmia neonatorum) Virus
Keratitis (cornea)	Bacterial (congenital syphilis) Virus (herpes simplex, chicken pox)
Uveitis, panuveitis (uvea [choroid, iris, and ciliary body])	Bacteria (tuberculosis, congenital syphilis) Virus (herpes simplex, herpes zoster, cytomegalic inclusion disease)
Cyclitis (ciliary body) Iritis (iris) Choroiditis (choroid) Choroidoretinitis (choroid and retina)	Fungus Parasita Protozoa (toxoplasmosis) Rheumatoid arthritis Trauma
Endophthalmitis (uvea, retina, and vitreous body)	Bacteria
Panophthalmitis (endothalmitis with involvement of sclera)	Fungi Parasite Penetrating wound Intraocular surgery

down steps and climb off or onto furniture. For the blind child these visual perceptions are learned through experimentation. For example, blind infants will substitute hitching (using legs to propel themselves while in a sitting position) for crawling on all fours so that they may feel for obstacles with their hands rather than their heads.

During the preschool years imitation is a primary form of learning. The child learns appropriate roles by watching and imitating the activities of significant others. Much of social behavior is learned by observing how others relate to one another. It is extremely difficult for a blind child to play cooperatively with peers because he cannot see what they are doing. Although he can hear and follow verbal commands, he may not be able to participate because of limitations in his motor ability. For example, a blind child who is able to walk well may refrain from running for fear of accidental collision with obstacles.

Academic learning depends heavily on visual intactness. The sighted child learns the meaning of words, letters, and numbers by associating the sound with the visual image of the object or symbol. The blind child hears only the word but has no concept of the object other than through touch.

Table 24-5 Anticipatory guidance for prevention of eye injuries

Infants and Toddlers
Avoid any toys with long pointed handles, such as a pinwheel on a stick
Keep pointed instruments and tools out of reach (e.g., scissors, knives, screwdrivers, rulers, pencils, sticks)
Do not allow child to *walk* or *run* with any pointed object in his hand (e.g., spoon, lollipop, toothbrush)
Keep child away from play of older children and adults that involves projectile activities (throwing a ball, golf, target shooting, swings)
Stress importance of fire safety and poison protection in preventing thermal/chemical burns to eye
Shield child's eyes when in direct sunlight

Preschoolers
Supervise use of sharp or pointed objects, especially scissors
Teach proper use of pointed objects, such as toy guns or scissors, namely, to always point them *away* from their face or from anyone else at close range
Teach child to walk carefully (never run) while carrying any sharp or pointed object
Keep child away from projectile activities
Begin teaching respect for firearms

School-age Children and Adolescents
Teach proper use and respect for potentially dangerous equipment such as power tools (flying objects from them), firearms, firecrackers where legally permitted, and racquet sports
Stress use of eye protection when riding motorcycles or using equipment such as power saws or chemistry sets
Teach to open soda bottles with screw cap pointing away from face
Encourage safe use of curling iron
Advise them of danger of excessive sunlight (ultraviolet burns)
Warn to never look directly at the sun even with sunglasses
Monitor duration of wear of contact lens to prevent corneal scratching and possible scarring

He is deprived of the richness of learning provided by pictorial books, photographs, movies, and television. However, despite limitations blind or partially sighted children are able to learn with sighted children, provided they have no additional disabilities.

NURSING INTERVENTIONS WITH THE VISUALLY IMPAIRED CHILD

Nursing interventions with visually impaired children are often a specialized area, requiring additional training in vision assessment and rehabilitation. However, general nursing goals focusing on prevention, detection, and rehabilitation are every nurse's responsibility. In addition, nurses may have to care for a visually impaired child who is hospitalized and must know how to best meet the child's and family's special needs.

Prevention

The primary nursing objective is to prevent visual impairment.* This involves many of the same interventions discussed under hearing impairments, namely (1) prenatal screening for pregnant women at risk, such as those with rubella or syphilis infection and family histories of genetic disorders associated with visual loss; (2) adequate prenatal and perinatal care to prevent prematurity and iatrogenic damage from excessive administration of oxygen; (3) periodic screening of all children, especially newborns through preschoolers, for congenital blindness and visual impairments caused by refractive errors and strabismus; (4) adequate immunization of all children; and (5) safety counseling regarding the common causes of ocular trauma (Table 25-5).

Following detection of eye problems, the nurse has a responsibility to prevent further ocular damage by ensuring that corrective treatment is employed. For the child with strabismus, this often necessitates occlusive patching of the stronger eye. Compliance with the procedure is greatest during the early preschool years and increasingly difficult after school entry. If an older child requires occlusive patching, the nurse discusses the importance of the patch in preserving eyesight, allows the child an opportunity to discuss his feelings regarding the obvious dressing, and attempts to overcome difficulties imposed by the patch, such as unkind remarks from peers.

For the child with refractive errors, the nurse helps the child adjust to wearing glasses. Young children who persist in removing glasses benefit from temporal pieces that wrap around the ears or an elastic strap attached to the frames and around the back of the head to hold them on securely. Once a child appreciates the value of clear vision, he is more likely to wear the corrective lenses.

Older children may refuse to wear glasses for cosmetic reasons. Although this can be a traumatic experience for some children, with support and encouragement, combined with the benefit of improved vision, most children agree to wear them when necessary. Parents may need help to understand the psychologic implications of altered body image, especially in the adolescent. The nurse discusses the importance of including the child in the selection of frames, since they become a significant article of wearing apparel. Frames need not be changed each time further correction is needed. Therefore it is sometimes a worthwhile investment to purchase more expensive, attractive frames, which may induce the child to wear them. Of course, such decisions must be made in light of the child's age and physical activity and the family's financial resources. All corrective lenses should be made from safety glass, which is shatterproof.

Depending on the reason for corrective lenses, some children may be required to wear them continuously whereas others may need them only for close work or distance seeing. If they are to be worn continuously, the nurse dis-

*A resource is the National Society to Prevent Blindness, 79 Madison Ave., New York, NY 10016.

cusses with the physician the feasibility of short periods of disuse for special occasions, such as parties or swimming. Children are usually much more cooperative when they know that there is flexibility in the wearing schedule that permits them to appear at their best with peers.

Glasses should not interfere with any activity. Special protective guards are available to wear during contact sports to prevent accidental injury. Often corrective lenses improve visual acuity so dramatically that children are able to compete more effectively in sports. This in itself is a tremendous inducement to continue wearing glasses.

Contact lenses are desirable alternatives for glasses. Two basic types are available. *Hard lenses* are made of rigid plastic, can be worn for limited periods of time (usually 12 hours, but less than 24 hours), and require gradual wearing time to accustom the eyes to their use. They offer the sharpest vision and are easy to care for. *Soft lenses* are composed mostly of water, are very flexible, are immediately comfortable to use, and, for some types, allow for extended wear up to a month. They are less durable than the hard contact lens and require more care.

Contact lenses have several advantages over conventional spectacles, such as greater visual acuity, total corrected field of vision, and optimum cosmetic benefit. Unfortunately they are quite costly, require more maintenance than glasses, and involve considerable practice in learning techniques for insertion and removal. If they are prescribed, the nurse can be very helpful in teaching parents or older children how to care for the lenses. Nurses should be aware of basic techniques for care and removal, especially during situations when they may be responsible for such procedures (Table 25-6). Contact lenses also have attendant hazards, and proper care and use are necessary to prevent problems such as infection or corneal abrasion. For example, prolonged wearing of hard contact lenses, especially during sleep, damages the cornea because it deprives the corneal layers of their oxygen supply, which is received via exchange of gases in the atmosphere and tears. Normally, when the eyes are closed, the metabolic rate of the cornea decreases so that the oxygen supply via the circulation is sufficient. However, when lenses are worn, the metabolic rate remains high and oxygen in the blood is inadequate to maintain tissue metabolism.

Since treatment of several eye disorders (infection, strabismus, and glaucoma) may require instillation of ophthalmic medication, parents are taught the correct procedure (see Chapter 27). Applying pressure over the lacrimal punctum helps decrease the unpleasant side effects of cholinergic or anticholinesterase agents, such as decreased blood pressure, sweating, salivation, flushing, diarrhea, abdominal cramps, and enuresis.

Since trauma is the leading cause of blindness, the nurse has the major responsibility of preventing further eye injury until the physician orders specific treatment. The major principles in emergency care for eye injuries are presented in the box. Because everyone with an eye injury fears blindness, it is essential to reassure the victim and family that everything possible is being done. It is best to avoid giving false reassurance, however, since the prognosis, especially in penetrating injuries, is usually guarded. Most injuries should be examined by an ophthalmologist and visual acuity checked, even in minor problems. To check for corneal abrasions, the examiner touches a fluorescein strip gently to the conjunctiva; any area where the epithelium has been removed will stain a bright lime green.

Many injuries such as corneal abrasions require patching for optimum healing and minimum discomfort. In penetrating injuries regular eyepatches are not used because they

Table 25-6 Removal and care of contact lenses

REMOVAL	CARE
Hard Contact Lenses	
Manual technique—wash hands; place thumb or finger of one hand on upper lid directly at margin and thumb or finger of other hand on lower lid; separate lids; slowly push lower lid upward until lens is trapped between lids; lower lid ejects lens by breaking suction	Store in sterile saline solution or distilled water
	May be rinsed in sterile saline solution and stored dry to prevent bacterial contamination of soaking solution
Suction method—use same procedure to separate lids, but use a suction cup to lift off lens	Label each lens container as right or left during storage
NOTE: If lens has wandered from center (positioned on sclera, usually under top lid), manipulate lens back onto cornea by gently pushing on lid; if lens does not move freely, instill sterile saline solution	Can be worn again after cleaning and moistening with special wetting solution or sterile saline solution
	Remove before surgery or instilling eye medication
Soft Contact Lenses	
Wash hands; separate lids as for hard lenses; have child look up, slide lens toward bottom lid onto sclera; pinch lens between fingers of hand used to lower bottom lid	Store in sterile distilled saline solution (never dry)
If lens adheres to cornea, moisten with saline solution, then remove	Label each lens container as right or left
Do not use suction cup	Before lenses are worn again, they are sterilized in a special appliance or chemically cleaned
	Do not use tap water in caring for lenses (causes chemical deposits on surface)
	Remove before surgery or instilling eye medication

can exert pressure against the injury. Only curved and perforated metal or plastic shields (Fox shields) are used; the opposite eye is covered as well because when one eye moves both eyes move and the injury is likely to be exacerbated (Melamed, 1982). In very young children patching must be used cautiously to avoid occlusion amblyopia. For those children whose eyes are patched, the same types of suggestions for home care are offered as those discussed for the hospitalized child with temporary loss of vision.

Preservation of sight is such an essential goal that the following preventive health teachings concerning care of the eyes, regardless of the presence or absence of deviations, are emphasized:

1. Avoid excessive eyestrain; when doing close work, periodically look into the distance to relax the muscles of accommodation.
2. Use proper lighting; light should not be glaring or cast shadows on reading material (light source should come from behind the left shoulder in a right-handed individual and vice versa); watch television with a light in a dark room to decrease contrast.
3. Get sufficient amounts of rest.

4. Have the eyes checked regularly by a licensed optometrist or ophthalmologist.

Detection

Equally important as prevention is early detection of eye problems. As has already been pointed out, detection and treatment of many ocular defects, such as strabismus, often prevent any permanent visual impairment. Every child from birth onward should receive periodic visual screening. Chapter 7 includes tests for visual acuity in children in various age-groups. Table 25-7 summarizes the usual signs and symptoms associated with ocular disorders.

Infancy. At birth most infants demonstrate specific orientation responses to visual stimuli, such as a bright or shiny object held in their line of vision. According to the Brazelton Neonatal Behavioral Assessment Scale, the infant may exhibit the following responses (scores) (Brazelton, 1973):

1. Does not focus on or follow stimulus
2. Stills with stimulus and brightens
3. Stills, focuses on stimulus when presented, little spontaneous interest, no following

Table 25-7 Detection of visual impairment

CAUSE	BEHAVIORAL MANIFESTATIONS	SIGNS/SYMPTOMS
Congenital blindness	Does not follow a moving light; no orientation response to visual stimuli Does not initiate eye-to-eye contact with caregiver	Constant nystagmus Fixed pupils Marked strabismus Slow lateral movements
Refractive errors	Rubs eyes excessively Tilts head or thrusts head forward Has difficulty in reading or other close work Holds books close to eyes Writes or colors with head close to table Clumsy; walks into objects Blinks more than usual or is irritable when doing close work Is unable to see objects clearly Does poorly in school, especially in subjects that require demonstration, such as arithmetic	Dizziness Headache Nausea following close work
Strabismus	Squints eyelids together or frowns Has difficulty in focusing from one distance to another Inaccurate judgment in picking up objects Unable to see print or moving objects clearly Closes one eye to see Tilts head to one side If combined with refractive errors, may see any of above	Diplopia Photophobia Dizziness Headache Cross-eye
Glaucoma	Mostly seen in acquired types—loses peripheral vision; may bump into objects that are not directly in front of him; sees halos around objects; may complain of mild pain or discomfort (severe pain, nausea, vomiting if sudden rise in pressure)	Redness Excessive tearing (epiphora) Photophobia Spasmodic winking (blepharospasm) Corneal haziness Enlargement of eyeball (buphthalmos)
Cataract	Gradually less able to see objects clearly May lose peripheral vision	Nystagmus (with complete blindness) Gray opacities of lens Strabismus Absence of red reflex

4. Stills, focuses on stimulus, follows for 30-degree arc, jerky movements
5. Focuses and follows with eyes horizontally for at least 30-degree arc, smooth movement, loses stimulus but finds it again
6. Follows for 30-degree arc with eyes and head, eye movements are smooth
7. Follows with eyes and head at least 60 degrees horizontally, maybe briefly vertically, partly continuous movement, loses stimulus occasionally, head turns to follow
8. Follows with eyes and head 60 degrees horizontally and 30 degrees vertically
9. Focuses on stimulus and follows with smooth, continuous head movement horizontally, vertically, and in a circle; follows for 120-degree arc

Any infant with a response of 1 or with the signs listed in Table 25-7 for congenital blindness is referred for further evaluation.

Of special importance in detecting visual impairment during infancy are the parents' concerns regarding visual responsiveness in their child. Their concerns must be taken seriously, such as lack of eye-to-eye contact from the infant. During infancy the child should be tested for strabismus. Lack of binocularity after 4 months of age is considered abnormal and must be treated to prevent amblyopia.

Childhood. Since the most common visual impairment during childhood is refractive errors, testing for visual acuity is essential. The school nurse usually assumes major responsibility for vision testing in school-age children and adolescents. Besides refractive errors, the nurse should be aware of signs and symptoms that indicate other ocular problems. If a referral is made to the family requesting further eye testing, the nurse is responsible for follow-up concerning the recommendation. Often parents do not willingly neglect their child's care out of disinterest but rather because of contributing factors, such as financial difficulty. The school nurse can be instrumental in seeking financial assistance for the family, such as through health centers that provide care on a sliding-fee basis.

It is also important for the nurse to stress that children continue to need periodic eye examinations. One pair of glasses frequently affords only temporary visual correction. Myopia commonly continues to worsen throughout childhood, necessitating stronger corrective lenses. Conversely, a hyperopic child may outgrow the need for glasses by 7 or 8 years of age.

Rehabilitation

When the child is blind or partially sighted, rehabilitation is a continuous process that relates to every area of the child's life. Nursing goals include (1) helping the family and child adjust to the impairment, (2) promoting parent-child attachment, (3) fostering optimum development and independence, (4) providing for play/socialization, and (5) being aware of educational facilities.

Adjusting to the impairment. The shock of learning that their child is blind or partially sighted is an immense

---

Emergency Treatment: *Eye Injuries*

Foreign object
  Examine eye for presence of a foreign body (evert upper lid to examine upper eye)
  Remove a freely movable object with pointed corner of gauze pad lightly moistened with water
  Do not irrigate eye or attempt to remove a penetrating object
  Caution child against rubbing eye

Chemical burns
  Irrigate eye copiously with tap water for 20 minutes
  Evert upper lid to flush thoroughly
  Hold child's head and eye under tap of running lukewarm water
  Allow child to rest with eyes closed
  Keep room darkened

Ultraviolet burns
  If skin is burned, patch both eyes (make sure lids are completely closed); secure dressing with Kling bandages wrapped around head rather than tape
  Allow child to rest with eyes closed

Hematoma ("black eye")
  Use a flashlight to check for gross hyphema (visible fluid meniscus across iris; more easily seen in light-colored than in brown eyes)
  Apply ice for first 24 hours to reduce swelling if no hyphema is present

Penetrating injuries
  Never remove an object that has penetrated eye
  Follow strict aseptic technique in examining eye
  Observe for:
    Aqueous or vitreous leaks (fluid leaking from point of penetration)
    Hyphema
    Shape and equality of pupils, reaction to light
    Prolapsed iris (not perfectly circular)
  Apply a Fox shield if available (not a regular eye patch)
  Maintain bed rest with child in 30-degree Fowler position
  Apply patch over unaffected eye to prevent bilateral movement
  Caution child against rubbing eye

---

crisis for parents. Of all types of disabilities, many people fear loss of sight the most. Certainly it is one of the senses that is involved in almost every activity of daily living. Parents need support during the initial phase of learning about the diagnosis. They need help to understand that their grief reaction to the loss is normal and that adjustment requires considerable time and emotional working through. The nurse also helps parents gain a realistic understanding of their child's abilities. Although it is impossible to predict the future for the blind child, it is reasonably safe to assume that a blind child without other severe handicaps can live a productive, independent life provided he is afforded the opportunity to learn and develop. For example, blind adults can marry and raise sighted children with remarkably few difficulties (Collis and Bryant, 1981).

Parents should know from the beginning that rearing a blind child is a difficult task for which there are few role models and even fewer ready-made solutions. The nurse discusses with them that the usual reaction is to overprotect the child in an attempt to make the environment as safe as possible for him. However, the destructive effects of the ''benevolent overreaction'' (see Chapter 22), especially to a child who needs encouragement and structured stimulation to learn about his world and venture forth where he cannot see, are emphasized. The family is encouraged to investigate appropriate stimulation and educational programs for the child as soon as possible. Sources of information include state **Commissions for the Blind,** local schools for the blind, the **American Foundation for the Blind,*** **National Federation of the Blind,**† **National Association for Parents of the Visually Impaired, Inc.,**‡ **National Association for the Visually Handicapped,**§ and **American Council of the Blind.**‖

When blindness is not congenital but acquired, the newly blind child needs a great deal of support to help him adjust to the impairment. He is usually frightened and confused by the sudden or progressive loss of sight and benefits from an environment that provides security and familiarity. This is especially important for the nurse to remember when the child is hospitalized. The child needs careful orientation to his immediate surroundings, elimination of as many extraneous stimuli, such as strange noises, as possible, and provision of safety measures to prevent accidents and encourage ambulation. (Interventions for meeting these needs are discussed on p. 1036.) He is encouraged to continue as many independent behaviors as possible and taught methods to help him compensate for the loss of vision, such as localization of objects through sound or touch, organization of personal belongings to facilitate identification of clothes, and grooming aids, and learning braille.

Parent-child attachment. A crucial time in the life of the blind infant is when he and his parents are getting acquainted with each other. Pleasurable patterns of interaction between the infant and his parents may be lacking if there is not enough reciprocity. For example, if the parent gazes fondly at the infant's face and seeks eye contact but the infant fails to respond because he cannot see the parent, a troubled cycle of responses may occur. The nurse can help parents learn to look for cues that indicate the infant's responding to them, such as if his eyelids blink, whether his activity level accelerates or slows, if respiratory patterns change, such as if he breathes faster or slower when they come near, and whether the infant makes throaty sounds when they speak to him. The Brazelton Neonatal Behavioral

Assessment Scale is an excellent tool for acquainting parents with their infant's unique abilities (Als, 1985).

Parents also need advocates for their blind child. The nurse demonstrates by personal example acceptance of the child as a unique and special person. The child's positive aspects, such as physical appearance, cooperative behavior, and developmental progress, are emphasized. The parents are supported in any of their attempts to foster the child's development. Through this approach the nurse indirectly encourages attachment by influencing and strengthening the parents' acceptance of their child.

Development and independence. Motor development is almost as dependent on sight as verbal communication is on hearing. Mobility and locomotion skills are typically delayed in blind children; the majority may not walk independently until 20 months of age (Davidson, 1983). Consequently, from earliest infancy parents are encouraged to expose the infant to as many visual-motor experiences as possible, such as sitting supported in an infant seat or swing and given opportunities for holding up his head, sitting unsupported, reaching for objects, and crawling. Ideally the child should be enrolled in an educational stimulation program for blind infants to develop age-appropriate motor skills. (Many of the activities suggested in Table 24-9 for motor stimulation are applicable for a home program, with modification of those exercises that depend on sight.) It is stressed to parents that the blind child who receives formal instruction in movement can learn and master balance, coordination, and mobility within his environment.

The blind child also must learn to become independent in navigational skills. Orientation and mobility training should begin early. The two main techniques for independent travel are the *tapping* method (use of a cane to survey the environment for direction and avoidance of obstacles) and *guides,* such as a human sighted guide or a dog guide. Newer devices use sensors that convert visual images to tactile impressions on the person's back or directly to the central nervous system by means of optic nerve electrode implants (Davidson, 1983). Partially sighted children may benefit from ocular aids, such as a monocular telescope.

Blind children often lack experiences that help develop fine motor coordination. For example, young sighted children pick up pieces of paper and fine objects from a table or floor surface because they see them. The child who cannot see small objects misses the opportunities for such practice and may have poor fine motor coordinated skills. The nurse suggests to parents that they provide the child with a variety of experiences that include touching small toys and other objects. He should also be introduced to a variety of textures such as silk, satin, coarse burlap, soft cotton, wooly-fuzzy materials, sand, slippery objects, water, hard surfaces, soft toys, and cold and warm temperatures. Such experiences will increase his sensitivity as well as enable him to master braille reading and writing skills more readily.

Despite visual impairment the child can become indepen-

---

*15 W. 16th St., New York, NY 10011.
†1800 Johnson St., Baltimore, MD 21230.
‡ P.O. Box 180806, Austin, TX 78718.
§305 East 24th St., New York, NY 10010.
‖ 1211 Connecticut Ave. NW, Washington, DC 20036.

dent in all aspects of self-care. (See Chapter 24 for a discussion of helping slow-to-develop children learn self-care.) He may need help in dressing, such as special arrangement of clothing for style coordination and various tags (available in braille) or identifying marks to distinguish colors and prints. He should be encouraged to take pride in his appearance, with attention to good grooming and dress, since these assets greatly increase his social acceptance.

The child learns self-feeding as a sighted child would. Some helpful suggestions may be appropriate, such as giving the child a deep bowl and a lightweight spoon so that he is able to scoop food more easily and can determine the quantity by the increased weight of the utensil or securing the dish to the table to make locating it easier, but most children learn easily without these aids. As with all children, eating is messy in the beginning and is particularly so for the blind child, but practice is essential to learning a skill. During the preschool years the child is encouraged to develop table manners. Parents need to realize that without the assistance of imitation they must verbally explain the importance of manners and gently remind the child to practice them.

Toilet training should proceed according to the usual physical and psychologic signs of readiness. Since the child cannot see the toilet or imitate other's toilet habits, he must be verbally instructed regarding its purpose. Using the step-by-step approach outlined in Chapter 24 is often helpful for the blind child to learn independent toileting.

Play/socialization. The blind child does not automatically learn to play. Because he cannot imitate others or actively explore his environment as sighted children do, he is much more dependent on others to stimulate him and to teach him how to play.

Parents need help in selecting appropriate play material. Toys should encourage fine and gross motor development and stimulate the senses of hearing, touch, and smell. (See Tables 12-2 and 14-2 for toys appropriate during early childhood.) Toys with educational value are especially useful, such as dolls with various clothing closures.* Parents need to know that the blind child requires more time and help in learning how to use toys but that this does not indicate slowness or inability to learn. It represents the loss of one sense in the learning process and the compensatory effort required from the other senses.

The blind child has the same needs for socialization as sighted children. Since he has little difficulty in learning verbal skills, he is able to communicate with age-mates and participate in suitable activities. Contact with peers often enables blind children to participate much more easily in activities that require running, jumping, and falling. Parents should take an active part in the socialization process, especially during the phase of parallel play when the blind child may be totally unaware of what the other children are doing, unless someone tells him about the activity. Parents should encourage group activities that are appropriate for the young blind child, such as ring-around-the-rosy, singing nursery rhymes, and playing tag. The nurse discusses with parents opportunities for socialization outside of the home, especially regular nursery schools. The trend is to include these children with sighted children to help them adjust to the outside world for eventual independence.

Blindisms are thought to indicate inadequate compensatory stimulation for the child. Since such habits retard socially acceptable behavior, they should be discouraged. Behavior modification is successful in eliminating these habits and should be employed.

Education. The early education of the blind child must avoid unnecessary confusion. There should be fixed orientation to familiar environments. Each room in the house should be arranged to allow the child maximum mobility and safety. If the child has partial vision, special identifying markers can be used to emphasize certain locations, such as a bright light in the bathroom or a ticking clock near the stairway. When the child is in unfamiliar surroundings, parents should orient him to the room. Some of the "pet peeves" of blind people are leaving doors open, especially on overhead cabinets; moving furniture, such as chairs, or not putting it back; leaving wires stretched across travel areas; and using objects and not putting them away in the same place.

Since strange sounds have no meaning without visual orientation, these are explained whenever necessary. Sighted people often selectively inhibit extraneous sounds because of the more compelling visual cues. However, the blind child is acutely aware of auditory stimuli and can be easily confused or frightened by them unless he is aware of their source. This is similar to deaf children's preoccupation with visual cues, such as facial expressions, which can be upsetting to them if they are not sure of their meaning.

The main obstacle to learning is the child's total dependence on nonvisual cues. Although the child can learn via verbal lecturing, he is unable to read the written word or to write without special education. Therefore he must rely on braille, a system that uses raised symbols in the form of a 6-dot cell to represent letters and numbers. The child can then read the braille with his fingers and can "write" a message using a braille writer. A more portable system for written communication is the use of a slate and stylus (Fig. 25-4) or a microcassette tape recorder. A recorder is especially helpful for notetaking from classroom lecturing. Records and tapes are significant sources of reading material other than braille books, which are large and slow to read. Another device that scans the printed word and converts it into a raised shape identical to the scanned material is the Optacon* (optical to tactile converter). The device is portable but

---

*An excellent resource for fun and learning is *Preschool learning activities for the visually impaired child: a guide for parents* from the National Association for Parents of the Visually Impaired, Inc. For other resources; see p. 948.

*Manufactured by Telesensory Systems, Inc., 455 North Bernardo, P.O. Box 7455, Mountain View, CA 94039-7455.

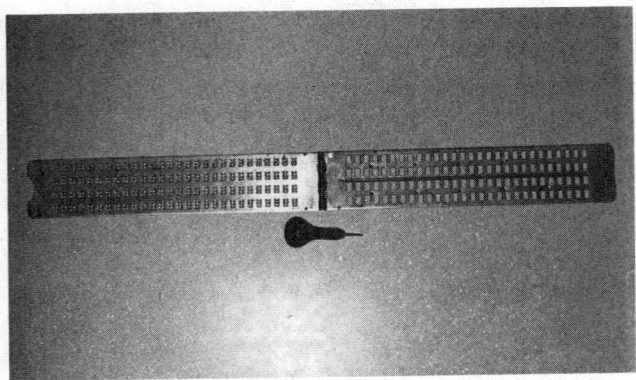

Fig. 25-4. Braille slate and stylus. Hinged slate consists of a series of open rectangles on one side and standard braille cells on the other. Paper is clamped or sandwiched between these two metal bars and appropriate dots are punched with stylus.

expensive (about $1000) and requires training and considerable skill; since it senses only one character at a time, reading is quite slow.

A number of resources are available for braille books, books with enlarged type, or tapes. The **Library of Congress*** has initiated a Talking Books Program that is available at many local libraries. Other sources are the **American Printing House of the Blind, Inc.,†** the **American Foundation for the Blind,** and the **National Association for the Visually Handicapped.** The **Recording for the Blind, Inc.‡** also provides texts and tapes of books, which are very helpful for secondary and college blind students.

Learning to use a regular typewriter is another form of writing, but it has the disadvantage that the blind person is unable to check the accuracy of the typing. Recent developments with computers have eliminated this drawback. A home computer with a voice synthesizer can be adapted to speak each letter or word that has been typed.§

The partially sighted child benefits from specialized visual aids, which produce a magnified retinal image. The basic devices are accommodation, such as bringing the object closer, special plus lenses, hand-held and stand magnifiers, telescopes, video projection systems, and large print. Special equipment is available to enlarge print, such as closed-circuit television and computer programs, such as Viewscan, which displays the materials in enlarged format.‖ Children with low vision often prefer to do close work without their glasses and compensate by bringing the object very near to their eyes. This should be allowed. The exception is the child with vision in only one eye, who should always

wear glasses for protection (Tongue, 1980). To facilitate any useful vision the lighting must be adequate.

CARING FOR THE HOSPITALIZED CHILD WITH TEMPORARY LOSS OF VISION

Children may be hospitalized for ocular surgery that requires temporary patching, such as strabismus or some types of cataract removal, or because of trauma and temporary loss of vision resulting from the injury or treatment. The nursing care objectives in either situation are to (1) reassure the child and family throughout every phase of treatment, (2) orient the child to his surroundings, (3) provide a safe environment, and (4) encourage independence. Whenever possible the same nurse should care for the child to ensure consistency in the approach. These same principles also apply to a blind child who requires hospitalization.

When a sighted child temporarily loses his vision, almost every aspect of his environment becomes bewildering and frightening. He is forced to rely on nonvisual senses for help in adjusting to the blindness without the benefit of any special training. Nurses have a major role in minimizing the effects of temporary loss of vision by talking to the child about everything they are doing, emphasizing aspects of procedures that are felt or heard, approaching the child by always identifying themselves as soon as they enter the room, and explaining unfamiliar sounds that may be frightening to the child. Parents are encouraged to room in and participate in the care. Familiar objects, such as a teddy bear or doll, should be brought from home to help lessen the strangeness of the hospital. As soon as the child is able to be out of bed, he is oriented to his immediate surroundings. If the child is able to see on admission, this opportunity is taken to point out significant aspects of his room and he is encouraged to practice ambulating with his eyes closed to accustom him to this experience.

The room is arranged with safety in mind. For example, a stool or chair is placed next to the bed to help the child climb in and out of bed. The furniture is always placed in the same position to prevent accidental collisions. Cleaning personnel are reminded of the necessity of putting the room back in order. When the child is in bed (even if not asleep), side rails must be up. If the child has difficulty navigating on his own, a rope can be attached from the bed to the point of destination, such as the bathroom. Attention to details such as well-fitting slippers or robes that do not hang on the floor is important in preventing tripping.

The child is encouraged to be independent in self-care activities, especially if the visual loss may be prolonged or potentially permanent. For example, during bathing the nurse sets up all the equipment and encourages the child to participate. At mealtime the nurse explains where each food item is on the tray, opens any special containers, prepares cereal or toast, but encourages the child to feed himself. Favorite finger foods, such as sandwiches, hamburgers, hot dogs, or pizza, may be good selections. The child is praised

---

*Division for the Blind and Visually Handicapped, 1291 Taylor St. NW, Washington, DC 20542.

†1839 Frankfort Ave., Louisville, KY 40206-0085.

‡20 Roszel Rd., Princeton, NJ 08540.

§Additional information is available from Raised Dot Computing, 310 S. 7th Street, Louisberg, PA 17837.

‖ Sources of information on low vision aids are the American Foundation for the Blind and the National Association for the Visually Handicapped.

Nursing Care Summary: The Visually Impaired Child

NURSING GOALS	NURSING INTERVENTIONS	EXPECTED PATIENT/FAMILY OUTCOMES
HP-HMP	**Injury, potential for tissue damage** **Risk factors: environmental hazards**	
Detect eye problems Infancy	At birth assess neonate's response to a bright, shiny object; observe for signs associated with congenital blindness Check for strabismus (lack of binocularity); refer to ophthalmologist for evaluation if malalignment persists past 2 to 3 months of age	*Evidence of visual problems is detected early and appropriate action initiated
Childhood	Test for visual acuity as soon as child is cooperative (sometimes by age 2 years) Advise parents of Home Eye Test for Preschoolers, which is available from National Society for the Prevention of Blindness Observe for signs or behaviors that indicate eye problems (see Table 25-7); include questions regarding behavioral indications of vision impairment in health histories Assume responsibility as school nurse for follow-up care of children who require corrective lenses or other types of treatments, such as patching Stress to parents importance of continued periodic eye examinations, since child's eyesight may change significantly in a short period of time	
Prevent defects of vision	Provide prophylactic eye care at birth Administer oxygen cautiously to premature infant Periodically screen all children from birth through adolescence for visual impairment Participate in immunization programs for children Teach safety regarding common causes of eye injuries Stress importance of good eye care—use of proper lighting, avoidance of excessive close work, proper rest and nutrition, and yearly eye examinations	*Screening and immunization programs are conducted and education programs implemented Healthy child does not acquire visual defect
Infections	Teach family correct procedure for instilling ophthalmic preparations (always in conjunctival cul-de-sac) Ensure proper dosage by holding dropper vertically, slowly closing lids, and having child rotate eyeball for even distribution Wipe excess medication for inner canthus outward to prevent contamination of contralateral eye Emphasize regular administration of drug for entire term of therapy to completely eradicate infection	Family complies with instructions and performs procedures correctly (specify)
Trauma	Prevent further injury by instituting appropriate emergency care (see box, p. 1033) Obtain history of incident; avoid any implication of guilt Reassure parent and child; avoid giving false reassurance; appraise them of each step of treatment, especially if therapy interferes with vision (patching eyes)	Child does not develop complications
Prevent complications of eye defects	Encourage compliance with corrective therapies	Child and family comply with therapy and perform procedures correctly
Strabismus	Discuss with school-age child necessity of patch in preserving vision; allow him to verbalize feelings regarding altered facial appearance Stress importance of wearing corrective lenses, if prescribed Teach parents correct procedures for instilling anticholinesterase drugs, if ordered	

*Nursing outcome.

Continued.

Nursing Care Summary: The Visually Impaired Child—cont'd

NURSING GOALS	NURSING INTERVENTIONS	EXPECTED PATIENT/FAMILY OUTCOMES
Refractive errors	For secure fit of glasses, use ones with rounded temporal pieces or attach elastic strap to handles and around back of head Include older child in selection of frames Encourage parents to compare value of more expensive attractive frames and inducement for wearing them against cost If glasses are recommended for continuous wearing, discuss possibility of temporary removal for special occasions Encourage use of protective shields during contact sports Stress improvement in visual acuity as reason for wearing glasses Discuss feasibility of contact lenses with selected families Know procedures for care, insertion, and removal of lens; teach to parents and older children	Child wears corrective lenses and cares for equipment correctly

CPP   Sensory-perceptual alteration: visual
       Etiology: specify

Provide opportunities for play/socialization	Talk to child about environment Guide family to selection of play material that encourages motor development and stimulates senses of hearing and touch Discuss with family how play for blind children differs from that of sighted children Encourage family to initiate play activities and teach child how to use toys Assess adequacy of environmental stimulation if blindisms are present Use behavior modification to discourage blindisms Discuss importance of consistent limit-setting in helping child learn acceptable behavior and tolerate frustration	Parents engage in appropriate activities with blind child and have realistic expectations for child Blindisms are minimized or eliminated
Promote development and independence	Provide visual-motor activities for infant (e.g., sitting in chair or swing, holding head up, standing, crawling, grasping for objects) Provide an environment that fosters familiarity and security; arrange furniture to allow safe ambulation; place identifying markets to denote steps or other dangerous areas Enroll child in special programs for the blind as soon as possible to learn independent skills, braille reading and writing, and navigational skills (cane method, sighted guide, guide dog) Encourage participation in active play Discuss need for experimenting with active play in safe environment and with other children	Infant or child engages in appropriate activities for level of development (specify) Child demonstrates an attitude of security in his environment

RRP   Family process, alteration in
       Etiology: situational crisis (birth of a blind child; diagnosis of blindness of a child)

Assist family in adjusting to child's loss of sight	Anticipate usual grief reactions to loss Stress to family (and older child) that such feelings are normal and that grief takes time to resolve Help family gain a realistic concept of child's impairment and abilities Encourage formal rehabilitation as soon as realistically feasible Assist family in orienting newly blind child to environment and in making immediate surroundings safe to encourage ambulation Listen to family's concerns of child's visual loss	Parents express their feelings and concerns regarding loss of sight Parents demonstrate an understanding of the child's impairment and its implications

Nursing Care Summary: The Visually Impaired Child—cont'd

NURSING GOALS	NURSING INTERVENTIONS	EXPECTED PATIENT/FAMILY OUTCOMES
Provide emotional support	Be available to family for assistance Encourage child, parents, and siblings to discuss their feelings regarding disability Stress child's abilities rather than disability Refer families to appropriate community agencies for medical, psychiatric, vocational, or financial assistance	Parents express their feelings and concerns regarding child and his special needs Child expresses his feelings and concerns
Promote parent-child attachment	Help parents identify clues other than eye contact from infant that signify communication with them Encourage parents to discuss their feelings regarding lack of visual contact or smiling from child Stress that lack of such responses is not an indication of child's rejection or dislike of parents Demonstrate by own example acceptance of child Emphasize positive abilities or attributes Encourage parents in their attempts to promote child's development	Parents and child exhibit a positive relationship

for efforts at being cooperative and independent, and any improvements he makes in self-care, no matter how small, are stressed.

Appropriate recreational activities are provided. If a child life specialist is available, such planning is done jointly. Since the child with temporary blindness has a wide variety of play experiences to draw on, he is encouraged to select activities. For example, if he liked to read, he may enjoy being read to. If he preferred manual activity, he may appreciate playing with clay or building blocks or feeling different textures and naming them. If he needs an outlet for aggression, activities such as pounding or banging on a drum can be helpful. Simple board and card games can be played if the child has a "seeing partner" or if the opponent helps him with the game. He should have familiar toys from home to play with, since they are more easily manipulated than new ones. If parents wish to bring him presents, they should be things that stimulate hearing and touch, such as a radio, music box, or stuffed animal.

Occasionally children who are blind come to the hospital for procedures to restore their vision. Although this is an extremely happy time, it also requires intervention to help the child adjust to sight. The child needs an opportunity to take in all that he sees. He should not be bombarded with visual stimuli. He may need to concentrate on people's faces or his own to accustom himself to this experience. He often has the need to talk about what he sees and to compare the visual image with his mental one. The child may also go through a period of depression as he begins to realize all that he had lost. This depression must be respected and supported. The nurse or parents should refrain from statements,

such as, "How can you be so sad when you can see again?" Instead it is important that the child be encouraged to discuss how it feels to see, especially in terms of seeing himself.

The child also needs time in adjusting to his ability to engage in activities that were impossible before. For example, he may prefer to use braille to read, rather than learning a new "visual approach" because of his familiarity with the touch system. Eventually, as he learns to recognize letters and numbers, he will integrate these new skills into reading and writing. However, parents and teachers must be careful not to push the child before he is ready. This applies to social relationships and physical activities as well as learning situations.

The Deaf-Blind Child

The most traumatic sensory impairment is loss of sight and hearing. One of the chief causes of deaf blindness was congenital rubella syndrome, but immunization has decreased its incidence. Other causes are usually the result of one congenital sensory impairment combined with an acquired impairment, such as congenital blindness and acquired deafness from meningitis. In most instances those children who have multisensory impairments have some residual hearing and vision to supplement the senses of touch, smell, and taste.

Obviously, auditory and visual impairments have profound effects on the child's development. They interfere with the normal sequence of physical, intellectual, and psychosocial growth. Although the child often achieves the usual motor milestones, they are delayed. Children only learn communication with specialized training. Finger spelling is one desirable method often taught to these children. The letters are spelled into the hand of the deaf-blind person, and the deaf-blind person spells out his ideas to the person with whom he is talking. Children with residual hearing can learn to speak. Whenever possible, speech is encouraged, since it allows communication with individuals not familiar with the preceding list of approaches.

Programs for these children vary. The John T. Tracy Clinic offers a home correspondence course for parents, and the **American Foundation for the Blind**, the **Perkins School for the Blind,*** and **The Foundation for the Junior Blind**† provide special services; the last two organizations have residential educational programs.

NURSING INTERVENTIONS WITH THE DEAF-BLIND CHILD

Caring for children with multisensory impairments is an area in which few nurses have much experience. Obviously, it is an overwhelming adjustment for families, and the educational needs of the child cannot be met in most public school programs. Most of the interventions that were discussed for the hearing or visually impaired child are applicable to the care of these children, such as activities to facilitate learning self-care and increased stimulation for motor development. The following discusses some of the special problems encountered by these families and constructive interventions.

One of the major concerns of families with deaf-blind children is helping them establish communication. The nurse is in a vital position to help parents with this goal. Since the infant cannot coo, laugh, or make eye movements, he is limited in the cues he can send and receive. Therefore initiating and maintaining communication is the responsibility of the caregiver. The nurse discusses with parents behaviors that signal the infant's recognition of them, such as quieting behavior, blinking, and change in respiration. The parents are encouraged to find ways of increasing stimulation for the child, especially cues that help the child identify each parent. For example, each person involved with the child should choose something that he or she, and only he or she, does, such as a kiss on the forehead or a stroke on the cheek. In this way the infant learns to discriminate among people in his environment.

The infant should be held close to the adult with his hands placed on the face while the person talks or changes facial expression. Eventually this technique becomes structured to associate a certain facial vibration with a word. However, such associations take time, patience, and effort on the part of both the child and the parents.

*175 N. Beason St., Watertown, MA 02172-9982.
†5300 Angeles Vista Blvd., Los Angeles, CA 90043.

As many sensory experiences as possible are provided, such as placing the child in different positions during the day in relation to light and providing variation in stimuli so that he will be motivated to move toward, reach, touch, and explore his own environment. Changing position also encourages muscle development and movement patterns. Sounds should be brought near and made interesting to the child. For example, he can participate in hearing by placing his hand on a radio or on a person's throat. Consistent tactile cues should be associated with a change of position and activities so that the movement is experienced as a positive nonthreatening experience. The nurse should encourage family members to urge the child to participate in games that require repositioning and body action, such as peekaboo and pat-a-cake.

The nurse encourages parents to provide secure, safe experiences while the child is learning to walk and gaining confidence. Once ambulatory, the child needs help in exploring the environment on a gradual *planned* basis. The environment should not be haphazard, for the child may become fearful and avoid growth-producing experiences. After the child succeeds in becoming well oriented to his environment and can overcome any abnormal movement patterns, he is ready for a plan of locomotion. Sighted guide, trailing (movement directed by touching objects, such as the wall), and cane walking are three methods. An individually planned mobility program should be based on the child's age, needs, and functional status and shared with the child's therapist, teachers, parents, and siblings.

The future prospects for deaf-blind children are at best unpredictable. Not infrequently congenital blindness and/or deafness is accompanied by other physical or neurologic handicaps, which further lessen the child's learning potential. The most favorable prognosis is often for children who have acquired deaf blindness and have few, if any, associated disabilities. Their learning capacity is greatly potentiated by their developmental progress before the sensory impairments. Although total independence, including gainful vocational training, is the goal, some deaf-blind children are unable to develop to this level. They may require lifelong parental or residential care. The nurse working with such families helps them deal with future goals for the child, including possible alternatives to home care during the parents' advancing years. In this respect much of the nurse's role is similar to that discussed in Chapter 24 for the child with cognitive impairment.

Communication Impairment

One of the most outstanding differences between human beings and lower animals is the human ability to communicate by using verbal language. The profound effect of hearing loss on speech development, discussed on p. 1015, laid a foundation for understanding how inability to communicate hinders every aspect of a child's life. However, hearing impairment is only one of several reasons for communication disorders. Often the child has language and speech but is still unable to communicate effectively. This discussion focuses on types of communication disorders, guidelines for detecting children who require referral, and techniques to promote language/speech development and prevent problems.

DEFINITION AND CLASSIFICATION

Communication impairment is a broad term that refers to the inability to (1) receive and/or process a symbol system, (2) represent concepts or symbol systems, and/or (3) transmit and use symbol systems (Definitions, 1982). Although communication disorders are concerned with verbal symbols of the spoken word, other symbol systems include nonverbal methods, such as gestures, sign language, and braille. With severe communication impairment, these methods may be needed to substitute for the spoken word.

Because of the complexity of communication a number of classification systems are available and there is no universal agreement on one system. Basically, a communication impairment may occur in language, speech, or hearing or any combination of these. The problems encountered when hearing is affected are discussed earlier in this chapter. *Language* primarily refers to the symbol system that is used to convey thoughts or feelings to others. The two major types are *receptive* language, or comprehension of the spoken word, and *expressive* language, or formulation of verbal symbols. *Speech* is the oral production of language, including articulation of sounds, rhythm, and tone.

Language Impairment

Language disorders are the more prevalent type of communication impairment and may be characterized by an inability to:

1. Assign meaning to words (vocabulary)
2. Organize words into sentences
3. Alter word forms to indicate tense, possession, and plurality
4. Produce speech sounds comprising the words of language

The last difficulty is a form of an articulation disorder and is considered below. Some authorities differentiate articulation disorders of language vs speech, but this distinction is less important than recognition that an articulation problem exists. Examples of language disorders are failure to develop vocabulary at the expected age, a reduced vocabulary for age, poor sentence structure, such as "Me see dog," or omitting words from the sentence, such as "Me fun." Such short or "telegraphic" phrases are normal during the first 2 years but should be replaced by more complete statements during the preschool years.

Speech Impairment

Speech impairments include differences from normal in articulation, voice production, and fluency. *Articulation* errors refer to those sounds that a child makes incorrectly or in-

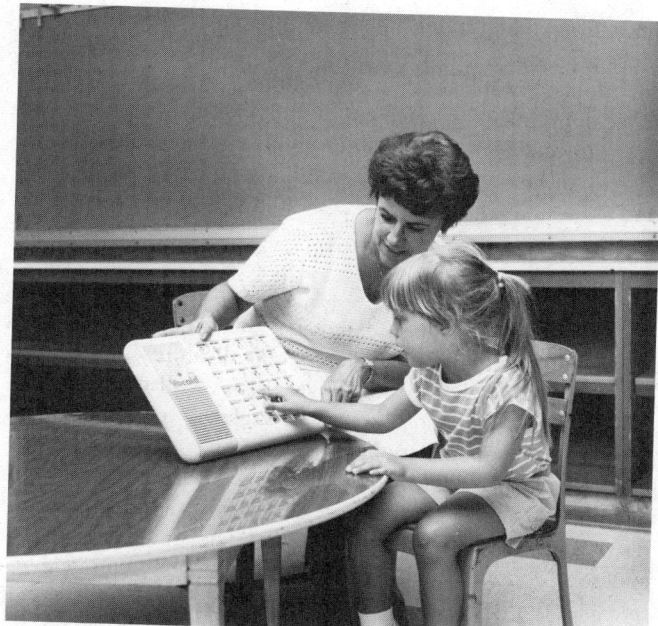

Fig. 25-5. The Vocaid is a communication board with a voice synthesizer. The child pushes the picture he wants and that word or phrase is spoken. Manufactured by Texas Instruments, Dallas, TX.

Photography by John Roy, Saint Francis Hospital, on location at Children's Medical Center, Tulsa, OK.

appropriately. For example, the child tends to distort or substitute a few consonants or blends, especially those that are learned last—"s," "l," "r," and "th"—or child omits many consonants, usually at the end of words, and substitutes the letters "t," "d," "k," or "y" for them.

Voice disorders are defined as differences in terms of pitch, loudness, and quality. *Dysfluency,* or rhythm disorders, usually consist of repetitions of sounds, words, or phrases. One of the most common and serious dysfluencies is stuttering.

Nonspeech Communication

Another category that is receiving increased attention is concerned with those individuals who have severe disabilities, such as cerebral palsy, mental retardation, or multiple physical or cognitive impairments, that prevent acquisition of meaningful verbal speech. Many of these people comprehend language but are unable to speak. Consequently, they benefit from communication methods that employ nonverbal symbols. Besides the use of hand or body gestures, numerous other communication systems exist. For example, *Blissymbols* is a highly stylized system of graphic symbols that represent words, ideas, and concepts (Murray, 1984). Although Blissymbols require education for their use, no reading skill is needed. These symbols or other self-explanatory graphics are usually arranged on a board and the person points to the symbol(s) to convey a message; more sophisticated devices employ voice synthesizers that "speak" the symbol's meaning (Fig. 25-5). For children with physical limitations that prevent fine hand movements, numerous devices are available that facilitate isolating a symbol (Fig. 25-6). Noncommunication systems are allowing severely disabled individuals a much more meaningful life; many children are able to learn more and faster because of the advances in augmentative communication (Lloyd and Karlan, 1984).

CAUSES

Delayed development of language and speech is the most common symptom of developmental disability in children and affects anywhere from 5% to 10% of all children (Coplan, 1985). The most common cause of communication impairment is mental retardation, followed by hearing impairment. Other causes include (1) central nervous system dysfunction, such as attention deficit disorders or learning disabilities; (2) severe emotional disturbance, such as autism and schizophrenia; and (3) organic problems, such as cerebral palsy, cleft palate, vocal cord injury, and paralysis or foreshortening of the soft palate or uvula. In some instances, such as in stuttering, the cause is unknown or speculative. Although the exact influence of environmental factors is controversial, the current thinking deemphasizes the importance of laziness, birth order, or bilingualism on delayed language development (Coplan, 1985).

NURSING INTERVENTIONS WITH THE COMMUNICATION-IMPAIRED CHILD

Nursing goals focus primarily on detection of communication disorders and prevention of primary problems or devel-

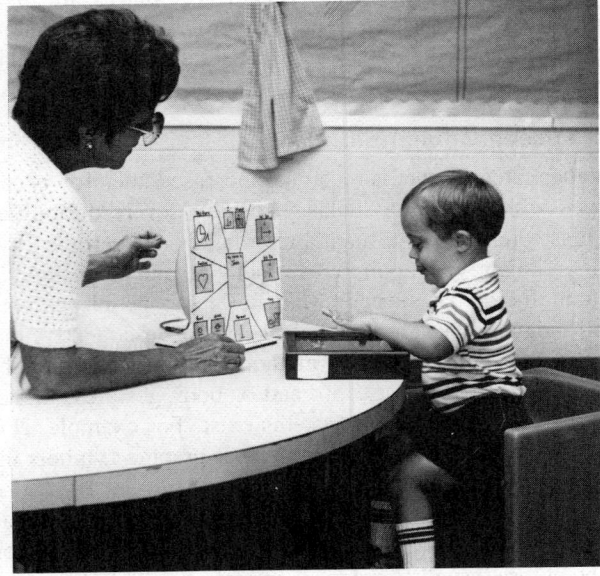

Fig. 25-6. Blissymbols can help a young child communicate nonverbally. This device uses a light behind each symbol; the light is rotated around the board by pressing the push panel.
Photography by John Roy, Saint Francis Hospital, on location at Children's Medical Center, Tulsa, OK.

opment of further difficulties, especially through parent education. Since nurses are frequently involved in preventive health maintenance of well preschool children and care of ill or hospitalized youngsters, they are in an optimum position to assess children for adequate communication development, detect deviations, and begin counseling.

Prevention

The primary intervention for communication disorders is prevention. Much of prevention directly relates to factors that predispose to causes of language/speech impairment, namely, mental retardation and hearing loss. Infants at risk for either condition (see pp. 787 and 1014) should be referred for audiologic evaluation before 6 months of age so that audiologic and speech therapy can be initiated immediately, when required.

Prevention also involves early recognition of children at risk for language delays and involves timely intervention to promote adequate language development. Nurses are often able to provide education for families that foster the child's communication skills. Specific interventions are discussed under Education (p. 1045).

One area that is particularly important in terms of preventing communication impairment through appropriate parental guidance is stuttering. This hesitancy or dysfluency in speech pattern is a *normal* characteristic of language development during the preschool years. It occurs because the child's advancing mental ability and level of comprehension exceed his vocabulary acquisition. The child knows what he wants to say but hesitates or repeats words or sounds as he tries to find the vocabulary to express himself. Eventually his language skills parallel the other abilities and speech becomes fluent.

However, when parents or other significant persons place undue emphasis or stress on this pattern of dysfluency, an abnormal speech pattern may result. Chances for reversal of stuttering are good until about 7 years of age. Therefore prevention must begin early. The nurse discusses with parents the normal dysfluencies in children's speech. When stuttering does occur, parents are advised to use the suggestions listed in the accompanying box in order to prevent inadvertently reinforcing this pattern. If excessive concern on the part of the parent or frustration and struggling behavior from the child are noted, the child is referred for language and speech evaluation. The critical point to remember is that the dysfluency must be arrested before the child develops an awareness or anticipation of the difficulty and begins to mistrust his speech skills.

Detection

Communication disorders can occur at any age but are most commonly found during childhood. The preschool period is considered critical to language development and therefore is a prime age for detection and intervention. Failure to detect communication disorders during early childhood affects the development of social relationships and emotional interactions, increases difficulty in developing academic skills, and

SUGGESTIONS FOR PARENTS REGARDING STUTTERING IN CHILDREN

To be encouraged

Viewing hesitancy and dysfluency as a normal part of speech development

Giving child plenty of time and the impression that you are not rushed or in a hurry

Looking directly at child while he is talking; being patient and never ridiculing or criticizing

Speaking clearly and articulating well but not stressing that all sounds must be perfected too early

Identifying situations when stuttering increases and avoiding them or ignoring the hesitancy

Capitalizing on periods of fluent speech with positive reinforcement such as singing songs or repeating nursery rhymes

To be avoided

The natural tendency to "help" child by supplying word when he is having a block

Telling him to stop and start over, to think before he speaks, or to take it easy and go slowly

Showing great concern, embarrassment, or disapproval for hesitancy

Anything that emphasizes stuttering and calls child's attention to his speech skills

Promising reward for proper speech

lessens the chances for successful correction of deficit skills.

The first step toward detection of abnormalities is knowledge of normal language and speech development. Awareness of when children achieve such milestones enables nurses to distinguish when specific communication characteristics are expected and when they are considered deviations (Table 25-8). Nurses must also be aware of clues that indicate language and speech impairment (Table 25-9), as well as those of hearing or cognitive deficit (see p. 1018 and p. 986).

Three methods are available for assessing speech and language development:

1. Direct observation of the child's verbal skills
2. Questioning of the parents
3. Testing

Direct observation necessitates spontaneous language interaction between the child and the nurse. Suggestions for initiating conversation include showing the child an object and asking him to describe it (asking him to name it often results in one-word responses that are too limited for evaluation of speech, although appropriate for evaluation of language) or posing questions, such as, "If you could have three wishes, what would you want?" The word-imitative procedure may also be used by having the child repeat sen-

Table 25-8 Normal language and speech development during early childhood

AGE (YEARS)	NORMAL LANGUAGE DEVELOPMENT	NORMAL SPEECH DEVELOPMENT	INTELLIGIBILITY
1	Says two to three words with meaning Imitates sounds of animals	Omits most final and some initial consonants Substitutes consonants "m," "w," "p," "b," "k," "g," "n," "t," "d," and "h" for more difficult sounds Height of unintelligible jargon at age 18 months	Usually no more than 25% intelligible to unfamiliar listener
2	Uses two- to three-word phrases Has vocabulary of about 300 words Use "I," "me," and "you"	Uses above consonants with vowels, but inconsistently and with much substitution Omission of final consonants Articulation lags behind vocabulary	At age 2, 65% intelligible in context
3	Says four- to five-word sentences Has vocabulary of about 900 words Uses "who," "what," and "where" in asking questions Uses plurals, pronouns, and prepositions	Masters "b," "t," "d," "k," and "g"; sounds "r" and "l" may still be unclear, omits or substitutes "w" Repetitions and hesitations common	At age 3, 70%-80% intelligible
4-5	Has vocabulary of 1500 to 2100 words Able to use most grammatic forms correctly, such as past tense of verb with "yesterday" Uses complete sentences with nouns, verbs, prepositions, adjectives, adverbs, and conjunctions	Masters "f" and "v"; may still distort "r," "l," "s," "z," "sh," "ch," "y," and "th" Little or no omission of initial or last consonant	Speech is totally intelligible, although some sounds are still imperfect
5-6	Has vocabulary of 3000 words, comprehends "if," "because," and "why"	Masters "r," "l," and "th"; may still distort "s," "z," "sh," "ch," and "j" (usually mastered by age 7½-8 years)	

Table 25-9 Cues for detecting communication impairment

DISORDER	CHARACTERISTICS
Language Disability	
Assigning meaning to words	First words not uttered before second birthday
	Vocabulary size reduced for age or fails to show steady increase
	Difficulty in describing characteristics of objects, although may be able to name them
	Infrequent use of modifier words (adjectives or adverbs)
	Excessive use of jargon past 18 months
Organizing words into sentences	First sentences not uttered before third birthday
	Short and incomplete sentences
	Tendency to omit words (articles, prepositions)
	Misuse of the "be," "do," and "can" verb forms
	Difficulty understanding and producing questions
	Plateaus at an early developmental level; uses easy speech patterns
Altering word forms	Omission of endings for plurals and tenses
	Inappropriate use of plurals and tense endings
	Inaccurate use of possession words
Speech Impairment	
Dysfluency (stuttering)	Noticeable repetition of sounds, words, or phrases after age 4 years
	Obvious frustration when attempts to communicate
	Demonstration of struggling behavior while talking (head jerks, eye blinks, retrials, or circumlocution)
	Embarrassment about own speech
Articulation deficiency	Intelligibility of conversational speech absent by age 3 years
	Omission of consonants at beginning of words by age 3 and at end of words by age 4
	Persisting articulation faults after age 7
	Omission of a sound where one should occur
	Distortion of a sound
	Substitution of an incorrect sound for a correct one
Voice disorders	Deviations in pitch (too high or too low, especially for age and sex); monotone
	Deviations in loudness
	Deviations in quality (hypernasality or hyponasality)

ASSESSMENT OF COMMUNICATION IMPAIRMENT

Key questions for language disorders
1. How old was your child when he began to speak his first words?
2. How old was your child when he began to put words into sentences?
3. Does your child have difficulty in learning new vocabulary words?
4. Does your child omit words from sentences (i.e., do his sentences sound telegraphic?) or use short or incomplete sentences?
5. Does your child have trouble with grammar such as the verbs "is," "am," "are," "was," and "were"?
6. Can your child follow two to three directions given at once?
7. Do you have to repeat directions or questions?
8. Does your child respond appropriately to questions?
9. Does your child ask questions beginning with "who," "what," "where," and "why"?
10. Does it seem that your child has made little or no progress in speech and language in the last 6 to 12 months?

Key questions for speech impairment
1. Does your child ever stammer or repeat sounds or words?
2. Does your child seem anxious or frustrated when trying to express an idea?
3. Have you noticed behavior in your child such as blinking his eyes, jerking his head, or attempting to rephrase his thought with different words when he stammers?
4. What do you do when any of these occur?
5. Does your child omit sounds from his words?
6. Does it seem like your child uses "t," "d," "k," or "g" in place of most other consonants when he speaks?
7. Does your child omit sounds from his words or substitute the correct consonant with another one (such as "rabbit" with "wabbit")?
8. Do you have any difficulty in understanding his speech?
9. Has anyone else ever remarked about having difficulty in understanding him?
10. Has there been any recent change in the sound of his voice?

tences or words. This approach is valid because children are not able to reproduce statements using correct grammatical forms that they have not previously learned to use. Whenever possible, the child's conversation should be tape-recorded for serial documentation of his progressive language/speech development and further evaluation by or consultation with a language or speech therapist.

Indirect assessment relies on parental information obtained through a history. Key questions that reflect problems in language or speech are listed in the box. Information obtained from the history is critically important and parental comments such as "He doesn't say much" or "Her use of words is so much slower than her older brother's was" must be taken seriously. However, caution must also be exercised in evaluating parental comments. Parents may be unaware of the child's difficulties because of lack of comparison with normal language development or they may not realize the degree of unintelligible speech because of familiarity with the child's approximation of words. Conversely, parents may have unrealistic expectations regarding verbal development and may exaggerate the degree of dysfluency, misarticulation, or word usage. Consequently, screening tests are a very important component of objective measurement of speech development.

Denver Articulation Screening Examination. The Denver Articulation Screening Examination (DASE) (see Appendix B) employs the word-imitative procedure and is one of the most frequently used tests. The child repeats 22 words but pronounces 30 different sound elements. The raw score, or the number of correctly pronounced sounds, is then compared to the percentile rank for children in that age-group. The examiner must be careful to evaluate the specific sound rather than the quality of the entire word. For beginning examiners it is helpful to validate the final score by comparing the results with a different examiner, ideally a speech therapist. The child is also scored on intelligibility, by selection of one of four possible categories: (1) easy to understand, (2) understandable half of the time, (3) not understandable, or (4) cannot evaluate. The Denver Articulation Screening Examination is a reliable, effective screening tool because it requires only 10 minutes for the examiner to perform and is designed to discriminate between significant speech delay and normal variations in the acquisition of speech sounds. It also detects common abnormal physical conditions such as hyponasality, hypernasality, tongue thrust, and lateral lisp.

Other tests. A number of other tests are available to either screen or test children for impaired language development. For example, the *Denver Developmental Screening Test,* the most widely used general developmental screening tool used with young children, includes a section on language ability, and delays in that area provide an early indication for those children who require further evaluation. The *Early Language Milestone Scale* (ELM Scale) provides a rapid assessment of auditory expressive, auditory receptive, and visual language skills from birth to 36 months (Coplan and others, 1982). For children 2 ½ to 18 years the *Peabody Picture Vocabulary Test-Revised* is a useful screening instrument for word comprehension (Dunn and Dunn, 1981).

Referral. Following assessment and detection of language or speech problems, the nurse must make a decision regarding appropriate referral. The all too frequent advice of "let's wait and see what happens" or "he will grow out of it" is often to the detriment of the child's future development. Since children normally vary greatly in their development of verbal skills, the nurse needs some guidelines for determining which child's development is abnormal. Table 25-10 lists general recommendations for referring children for specialized audiologic and language evaluations. Information regarding available services for language, speech, and hearing can be obtained from the **American Speech-**Language-Hearing Association* and the **Council for Exceptional Children**† (see also p. 1021 for organizations devoted to hearing impairment).

Education

When a child is delayed in his language development, it becomes very important to try and structure what the parents do so that when they are with their child he has the opportunity to learn. The underlying principle is not to bombard the child with words so that he will learn more language but to plan what will be said to him, how he will be observed, what responses will be expected of him, and how he will be reinforced. The following discussion offers guidelines that can help parents foster their child's attainment of language skills.‡

---

*10801 Rockville Pike, Rockville, MD 20852.
†Division for Children with Communication Disorders, 1920 Association Dr., Reston, VA 22091.
‡Material in this section taken extensively from Kriegsman, 1977.

Table 25-10 Guidelines for referral regarding communication impairment

AGE	ASSESSMENT FINDINGS
2 years	Failure to speak any meaningful words spontaneously
	Consistent use of gestures rather than vocalizations
	Difficulty in following verbal directions
	Failure to respond consistently to sound
3 years	Speech is largely unintelligible
	Failure to use sentences of three or more words
	Frequent omission of initial consonants
	Use of vowels rather than consonants
4 years	Frequent omission of final consonants
5 years	Stutters, stammers, or has any other type of dysfluency
	Sentence structure noticeably impaired
	Substitutes easily produced sounds for more difficult ones
	Omits word endings (plurals, tenses of verbs, and so on)
School age	Poor voice quality (monotonous, loud, or barely audible)
	Vocal pitch inappropriate for age
	Any distortions, omissions, or substitutions of sounds after age 7 years
	Connected speech characterized by use of unusual confusions or reversals
General	Any child with signs suggestive of a hearing impairment (see p. 1018)
	Any child who is embarrassed or disturbed by his speech
	Parents who are excessively concerned or who pressure the child to speak at a level above that appropriate for his age

Comprehensive interaction. No matter what the child's age or level of development, it is important for the parents to try to respond to him by talking to him, praising him, or taking time to listen when he does the following: (1) comes to the parents and tries to tell them something, (2) attempts to follow through with a question the parents have asked or a direction they have given, (3) brings the parents toys or books, (4) tries to imitate what the parents are saying or doing, and (5) seems to enjoy playing near the parents.

Comprehension. It is important to remember that children usually understand many more words than they can say. In addition, a child usually has to understand a word before he can produce it. Many language-delayed children are somewhat more delayed in comprehension of specific words, questions, and directions than in other areas of development. Therefore it is important to concentrate on teaching the meaning of new words to the child, giving him verbal information, and providing listening activities for him as well as helping him produce speech. The nurse can suggest that parents select a small group of words to use each time they are involved in different activities with the child. For example, each time the parent opens a door or a box the parent should say "Open." After doing this many times, the parent only says "Open" and waits to see if the child starts carrying through with the motion. The parent praises the child after he has attempted to respond to a word.

Production of words. When one studies the first words that children use and how they begin to put words together, it is interesting to note that what is actually happening is that children are telling parents how they see the world around them and what is happening to them at the time. Although initially some children do learn the names of common items or people in their environment, such as "mama," "doggie," and "bottle," most of the first meaningful words that they will use indicate egocentric desires, such as "more," "mine," "no," and "I do."

In choosing vocabulary, parents should consider the following: the usefulness of the word to the child, such as the word "more," which can denote more food, another ride in the car, or the desire to be read another story; ease of pronunciation, especially use of vowels and the consonants "b," "d," "m," "k," "t," "p," or "d"; and words whose meaning the child comprehends. Parents can also encourage vocabulary by having the child say a word before some request is fulfilled. For example, each time he wants more cookies, the parent should expect him to try to say part of the word "more."

Children normally learn monosyllabic words, such as "ma ma," and "bye." When learning to pronounce polysyllabic words, they frequently only pronounce the initial sound, such as "ba" for "bottle." Any approximation of words that the child uses should be repeated back to him with a clearer model. At the same time parents should praise him for his attempts to pronounce the word.

Talking and responding to the child. It will help the child if the parents plan ahead in regard to the specific things they will say and how they will respond to him. The child needs the parents to point things out to him. For example, as the child is attending to or is involved in a particular activity, the parents should try to describe what the child is doing. If he is looking at what the parents are doing, the parents should describe what they are doing. *They should reduce the length of what they are saying to approximately one level above the level at which the child is talking.* If he is just beginning to use single-word approximations, they should describe his activities in one or two words. For example, as he points to the "duck," they should say "Duck" or "Quack-quack." If the child is using single words, the parents could add two- or three-word models, such as, "Duck swimming" or "Duck in water."

Sometimes parents ask many questions of the child who has a language delay. The usual reaction from the child is silence. If there is a high frequency of questions, the parents should try to reduce this by making statements about what the child is doing rather than asking questions about it. For example, instead of saying, "What's this?" they should say, "Look, here's a cow." To help the child answer questions, parents should present the question while the child is listening, wait for him to try to answer, praise him if he does so, and, if he has difficulty, give him the answer. For example, if the parent states, "What does the cow say?" and the child has no response, the parent replies, "The cow says moo-moo."

Teaching grammatical forms. Children will begin to use adultlike forms of words only after they are using two-word combinations for an extended period. Parents should remember that when they are using single words and beginning to combine these single words into two-word relationships, the child is talking about ideas and how the world appears to him. For example, when the child says, "Ducky water," he is telling the parent that he sees the duck and the duck is in the water. At that point of development, if he used the word "is" it would not add any meaning for him, because it is the underlying idea that is important rather than the grammatical rules.

When the child is ready, he will begin to apply the "rules of grammar," usually by imitating what he hears around him. He will understand that when "s" is added to the word "dog," it means more than one dog. Children, however, benefit from having the specific word endings emphasized and exaggerated.

Reinforcement. Whenever possible, parents want to respond to the child with what he is trying to say. As mentioned previously, it helps to give him a hug, praise him directly, or comment on what he is saying. However, in order to know what he is trying to say, it is essential that the parents watch and listen to him as carefully as possible. Parents should try to develop a habit of looking at what the child is doing when he is talking. Some attempts on his part to talk will be rather obvious, for example, if he struggles to get out of the parent's arms and says, "Dou," it will be easy for the parent to understand his meaning and imitate him by saying, "Down, good boy, you said down," as he is put down. However, if he points to a dog and says, "Oo," the parent needs to try to think about what he is referring to. Perhaps he is saying to himself that this is a four-legged animal and that all four-legged animals go "moo" like a cow.

It is not always easy to understand what a child is trying to say. Sometimes parents choose the wrong word to stress, and the child becomes frustrated in his attempts to make himself understood. However, success in guessing at the correct meaning of the child's word approximation is greatly reinforcing to him because it symbolizes the usefulness and efficiency of language. The nurse needs to bear this fact in mind, especially when the child is hospitalized and dependent on others to understand him. In these instances it is beneficial to have the parent write a list of the child's vocalizations and related meanings, particularly those that refer to his needs regarding toileting, dressing, bathing, eating, sleep, and play.

CONCEPT SUMMARIES

- Hearing defects may be categorized according to etiology, pathology, or symptom severity; treatment, prevention, and rehabilitation are based on these factors.

- Hearing disorders may be classified according to the location of the defect: conductive, sensorineural, mixed conductive-sensorineural, auditory imperception.

- Some of the effects of hearing loss on growth and development are impaired knowledge of objects, emotional behavior, poor motor development, impaired academic learning, and decreased socialization.

- Prevention of hearing loss is the nurse's major responsibility. Efforts include treatment of infection, auditory testing, immunization, pregnancy and genetic counseling, and reduction of noise pollution.

- Rehabilitation for hearing loss involves parent education and support, hearing aids, lipreading, sign language, speech therapy, and promotion of socialization.

- Visual impairments are often classified, for convenience, by activity: school vision, legal blindness, travel vision, and light perception.

- Visual impairment may result from familial factors, prenatal/intrauterine factors, perinatal factors, and postnatal factors.

- Common visual impairments in childhood are refractive errors, amblyopia, strabismus, cataracts, glaucoma, trauma, and infections.

- Effects of visual impairment on development include impaired motor function, lack of stimulation, and diminished academic learning.

- Prevention of visual impairment focuses on prenatal screening, prenatal and perinatal care, periodic screening of all children, immunization, and safety counseling.

- Nursing goals in visual rehabilitation are helping the family and child adjust to the child's visual impairment, promoting parent-child attachment, fostering optimum development and independence, providing for play and socialization, and being aware of educational facilities.

- For the child undergoing ocular surgery, nursing care is aimed at reassuring the child and family throughout treatment, orienting the child to his surroundings, providing a safe environment, and encouraging independence.

- Nursing interventions for the deaf-blind child are helping the family adjust to the child's impairment, choosing appropriate educational channels, facilitating self-care, promoting communication, and assisting with ambulation.

- Communication impairment broadly refers to the inability to receive and/or process a symbol system, to represent concepts or symbol systems, and to transmit and use symbol systems.

- Three types of communication disorders are language, speech, and non-speech.

- Causes of impaired communication include mental retardation, hearing impairment, CNS dysfunction, severe emotional disturbances, and organic problems.

- Assessing speech and language development is accomplished by direct observation of verbal skills, questioning of parents, and testing.

REFERENCES

Als, H.: Reciprocity and autonomy: parenting a blind infant, Zero to Three **V**(5):8-10, 1985.

American Academy of Pediatrics, Joint Committee on Infant Hearing: Position Statement 1982, Pediatrics **70**(3):496-497, 1982.

Beratis, S., and others: Developmental aspects of an infant with transient moderate to severe hearing impairment, Pediatrics **63**(1):153-155, 1979.

Bergman, I., and others: Cause of hearing loss in the high-risk premature infant, J. Pediatr. **106**(1):95-100, 1985.

Bess, F., Finlayson, B., and Chapman, J.J.: Further observations on noise levels in infant incubators, Pediatrics **63** (1):100-106, 1979.

Bess, F.H., and Tharpe, A.M.: Unilateral hearing impairment in children, Pediatrics **74**(2):206-216, 1984.

Brazelton, T.B.: Neonatal behavioral assessment scale, Philadelphia, 1973, J.B. Lippincott Co.; London, 1973, William Heinemann, Ltd.

Calhoun, J.H.: Cataracts in children, Pediatr. Clin. North Am. **30**(6):1061-1069, 1983.

Collis, G.M., and Bryant, C.A.: Interactions between blind parents and their young children, Child Care Health Dev. **7**(1):41-50, 1981.

Coplan, J.: Evaluation of the child with delayed speech or language, Pediatr. Ann. **14**(3):202-208, 1985.

Coplan, J., and others: Validation of an early language milestone scale in a high-risk population, Pediatrics **70** (5):677-683, 1982.

Davidson, P.W.: Visual impairment and blindness. In Levine, M.D., and others, editors: Developmental-behavioral pediatrics, Philadelphia, 1983, W.B. Saunders Co.

Davis, H., and Silverman, S.R.: Hearing and deafness, ed. 4, New York, 1978, Holt, Rinehart & Winston, Inc.

Definitions: Communicative disorders and variations, Am. Speech Lang. Hear. Assoc. J. **24**:949-950, 1982.

Dunn, L., and Dunn, L.: The Peabody picture vocabulary test-revised, Circle Pines, MN, 1981, American Guidance Service.

Fraiberg, S.: Insights from the blind: comparative studies of blind and sighted infants, New York, 1977, Basic Books, Inc.

Frey, T.: Pediatric eye trauma, Pediatr. Ann. **12**(7):487-497, 1983.

Gortmaker, S.L., and Sappenfield, W.: Chronic childhood disorders: prevalence and impact, Pediatr. Clin. North Am. **31**(1):3-18, 1984.

Greenwald, M.J.: Visual development in infancy and childhood, Pediatr. Clin. North Am. **30**(6):977-993, 1983.

Hall, D.M.B.: The child with a handicap, Boston, 1984, Blackwell Scientific Publications.

Helveston, E., and Ellis, F.: Pediatric ophthalmology practice, ed. 2, St. Louis, 1984, The C.V. Mosby Co.

Knobloch, H., and Pasamanick, B., editors: Gesell and Amatruda's developmental diagnosis, New York, 1974, Harper & Row, Publishers.

Kovalesky, A.: Nurses' guide to children's eyes, New York, 1985, Grune & Stratton, Inc.

Kriegsman, E.: A guide for the language delayed child, unpublished manuscript, University of Washington, 1977.

Lloyd, L.L., and Karlan, G.R.: Non-speech communication symbols and systems: where have we been and where are we going? J. Ment. Defic. Res. **28**:3-20, 1984.

Melamed, M.A.: A generalist's guide to eye emergencies, Emerg. Med. **14**(7):25-47, 1982.

Murray, F.: Language for the handicapped, Point of View **21**(3):8-9, 1984.

Nelson, L.B.: Diagnosis and management of strabismus and amblyopia, Pediatr. Clin. North Am. **30**(6):1003-1014, 1983.

Orchik, D.J., and others: Intensity and frequency of sound levels from cordless telephones, Clin. Pediatr. **24**(12):688-690, 1985.

Stewart-Brown, S., Haslum, M., and Butler, N.: Educational attainment of 10-year-old children with treated and untreated visual defects, Dev. Med. Child. Neurol. **27**:504-513, 1985.

Tongue, A.: Medical management of the child with subnormal vision, Pediatr. Ann. **9**(11):33-45, 1980.

Visions problems in the United States, New York, 1980, National Society to Prevent Blindness.

BIBLIOGRAPHY
Hearing Impairment

Anagnostakis, D., and others: Hearing loss in low-birth-weight infants, Am. J. Dis. Child. **136**(7):602-604, 1982.

Bergstrom, L.: Causes of severe hearing loss in early childhood, Pediatr. Ann. **9**(1):23-30, 1980.

Bess, F.H.: Childhood deafness: causation, assessment and management, New York, 1977, Grune & Stratton, Inc.

Boffman, J.H., and Boffman, R.T.: Early detection of hearing impairment, Issues Compr. Pediatr. Nurs. **5**(1):11-20, 1981.

Brooks, D.N.: Otitis media and child development: design factors in the identification and assessment of hearing loss, Ann. Otol. Rhinol. Laryngol. **88**(suppl. 60, no. 5, part 2):29-47, Sept./Oct. 1979.

Campbell, S.L.: Some sound advice from managing a hearing-impaired patient, Nursing 84 **14**(12):46, 1984.

Downs, M.P.: Hearing development during infancy. In Children are different: behavioral development monograph series, No. 6, Columbus, OH, 1983, Ross Laboratories.

Hanawalt, A., and Troutman, K.: If your patient has a hearing aid, Am. J. Nurs. **84**(7):900-901, 1984.

Holder, L.: Hearing aids: handle with care, Nursing 82 **12** (4):64-67, 1982.

Holm, C.: Deafness: common misunderstandings, Am. J. Nurs. **78**(11):1910-1912, 1978.

Kaplan, S.L., and others: Onset of hearing loss in children with bacterial meningitis, Pediatrics **73**(5):575-578, 1984.

Matkin, N.D.: Early recognition and referral of hearing-impaired children, Pediatr. Rev. **6**(5):151-156, 1984.

McFarland, W.H., and Simmons, F.B.: The importance of early intervention with severe childhood deafness, Pediatr. Ann. **9**(1):13-19, 1980.

McRae, M.J.: Bonding in a sea of silence, Am. J. Maternal Child Nurs. **4**(1):29-34, 1979.

Morgan, R.H.: Breaking through the sound barrier, Nursing 83 **13**(2):112-113, 1983.

Northern, J., and Downs, M.: Hearing in children, ed. 4, Baltimore, 1984, The Williams & Wilkins Co.

Poland, R., and others: Methods for detecting hearing impairment in infancy, Pediatr. Ann. **9**(1):31-44, 1980.

Rapin, I.: Conductive hearing loss: effects on children's language and scholastic skills, Ann. Otol. Rhinol. Laryngol. **88**(suppl. 60, no. 5, part 2):3-12, 1979.

Robinson, T.: Early identification of vision and hearing problems. In Pediatrics: nursing update, vol. 1, no. 12, Princeton, NJ, 1986, Continuing Professional Education Center, Inc.

Rubin, M.: Meeting the needs of hearing-impaired infants, Pediatr. Ann. **9**(1):46-50, 1980.

Sataloff, R.: Pediatric hearing loss, Pediatr. Nurs. **6**(5):16-18, 1980.

Smith, M.P., and Cloonan, P.A.: Meeting the special needs of the hearing-impaired child, Issues Compr. Pediatr. Nurs. **3**(6):21-34, 1979.

Vienny, H., and others: Early diagnosis and evolution of deafness in childhood bacterial meningitis: a study using brainstem auditory evoked potentials, Pediatrics **73**(5):579-586, 1984.

Williamson, W.D., and others: Symptomatic congenital cytomegalovirus: disorders of language, learning, and hearing, Am. J. Dis. Child. **136**(10):902-905, 1982.

Wright, J.: Deaf but not mute, Am. J. Nurs. **76**(5): 795-799, 1976.

Vision Impairment

Bateman, J.B.: Genetics in pediatric ophthalmology, Pediatr. Clin. North Am. **30**(6):1015-1031, 1983.

Beauchamp, G.: Causes of visual impairment in children, Pediatr. Ann. **9**(11):16-22, 1980.

Bischoff, R.W.: Early childhood development of the visually handicapped, Issues Compr. Pediatr. Nurs. **3**(6):35-49, 1979.

Blinding missiles: soft drink twist-off bottle caps, Sightsaving **53**(1):2-7, 1984.

Borders, C.R.: Strabismus/amblyopia: when to refer, Patient Care **18**(17):21-52, 1984.

Bumbalo, J., and Seidel, M.: Identifying and serving a multiple handicapped population, Nurs. Clin. North Am. **10**(2):341-352, 1975.

Carden, R.G.: The ins and outs of contact lenses, RN **48** (2):48-50, 1985.

Chew, E., and Morin, J.D.: Glaucoma in children, Pediatr. Clin. North Am. **30**(6):1043-1060, 1983.

Curson, A.: The blind nursery school child, Psychoanal. Study Child. **34**:51-83, 1979.

Fenwick, A., and others: Traumatic blindness: a flexible approach for helping a blind adolescent, Nursing 79 **9**(1):36-41, 1979.

Herget, M.: For visually impaired diabetics, Am. J. Nurs. **83**(11):1557-1560, 1983.

Jan, J.E., and others: Eye-pressing by visually impaired children, Dev. Med. Child. Neurol. **25**(6):755-762, 1983.

Mannis, M.J., Miller, R., and Krachmer, J.H.: Contact thermal burns on the cornea from electric curling irons, Am. J. Ophthalmol. **98**:336-339, 1984.

McNeer, K.W.: Pediatric ophthalmology, Pediatr. Nurs. **5**(6):47-49, 1979.

Melamed, M.: Complications of contact lenses, Emerg. Med. **14**(4):218-224, 1982.

Nelson, L.B.: The visually handicapped child, Pediatr. Rev. **6**(6):173-182, 1984.

Nelson, L.B., and others: Developmental aspects in the assessment of visual function in young children, Pediatrics **73**(3):375-381, 1984.

O'Brien, R.: Education of the child with impaired vision, Pediatr. Ann. **9**(11):47-58, 1980.

Oglesby, R.: Eye trauma in children, Pediatr. Ann. **6**:5-22, 1977.

Osguthorpe, N.C.: If your patient has contact lenses, Am. J. Nurs. **84**(10):1255-1256, 1984.

Pugh, R.: Effects of visual impairment on children: development in sight, Nurs. Mirror **150**(21):30-32, 1980.

Questions and answers about strabismus, Patient Care **18** (17):184, 1984.

Randall, K.: Contact lenses for infants after congenital cataract surgery, Sightsaving **53**(1):8-13, 1984.

Scheiner, A.P., and Moomaw, M.: Care of the visually handicapped child, Pediatr. Rev. **4**(3):74-81, 1982.

Severtsen, B.M.: Sensory impairment: its effect on the family. In Hymovich, D.P., and Barnard, M.U., editors: Family health care, New York, 1979, McGraw-Hill Book Co.

Steffe, D.R., Suty, K.A., and Delcalzo, P.V.: More than a touch: communicating with a blind and deaf patient, Nursing 85 **15**(8):36-39, 1985.

Tumulty, G., and Resler, M.M.: Eye trauma, Am. J. Nurs. **84**(6):740-744, 1984.

Wassenberg, C.: Common visual disorders in children, Nurs. Clin. North Am. **16**(3):479-485, 1981.

Communication Disorders

Aram, D.M., and Nation, J.E.: Child language disorders, St. Louis, 1982, The C.V. Mosby Co.

Biro, P., and Thompson, M.: Screening young children for communication disorders, Am. J. Maternal Child Nurs. **9** (6):410-413, 1984.

Blager, F.B.: Speech and language development during infancy. In Children are different: behavioral development monograph series, No. 5, Columbus, OH, 1983, Ross Laboratories.

Bloom, L.A., and Rood, S.R.: Voice disorders in children: structure and evaluation, Pediatr. Clin. North Am. **28**(4): 957-963, 1981.

Brown, M.S.: Testing of a young child for articulation skills, Clin. Pediatr. **15**(7):639-644, 1976.

Casper, J.: Disorders of speech and voice, Pediatr. Ann. **14**(3):220-229, 1985.

Cohen, C.: Augmentative communication: a perspective for pediatricians, Pediatr. Ann. **14**(3):232-240, 1985.

Fuller, C.W.: Speech and hearing problems. In Green, M., and Haggerty, R.J., editors: Ambulatory pediatrics, III, Philadelphia, 1984, W.B. Saunders Co.

Goldberg, R.: Identifying speech and language delays in children, Pediatr. Nurs. **15**(4):252-259, 1984.

Graham, J.M., Jr., Bashir, A.S., and Stark, R.E.: Communicative disorders. In Levine, M.D., and others, editors: Developmental-behavioral pediatrics, Philadelphia, 1983, W.B. Saunders Co.

Haber, J.S., and Norris, M.: The Texas Preschool Screening Inventory: a simple screening device for language and learning disorders, Child. Health Care **12**(1):11-18, 1983.

Hixson, P.H.: Recognizing delayed language development in children with hidden hearing impairment, Pediatr. Ann. **9**(1):55-60, 1980.

Langner, B.: Communication between children, Issues Compr. Pediatr. Nurs. **4**(4):1-15, 1980.

Reilly, A.P., editor: The communication game: perspectives on the development of speech, language and nonverbal communication skills, New Brunswick, NJ, 1980, Johnson & Johnson Baby Products Co.

Resnick, T.J., Allen, D.A., and Rapin, I.: Disorders of language development diagnosis and intervention, Pediatr. Rev. **6** (3):85-92, 1984.

Rommel, J.: Referral of children with speech problems, Pediatr. Nurs. **2**(2):28-32, 1976.

Weiss, C.E., and Lillywhite, H.S.: A handbook for prevention and early intervention: communicative disorders, St. Louis, 1976, The C.V. Mosby Co.

Unit Nine

Impact of Hospitalization on the Child and Family

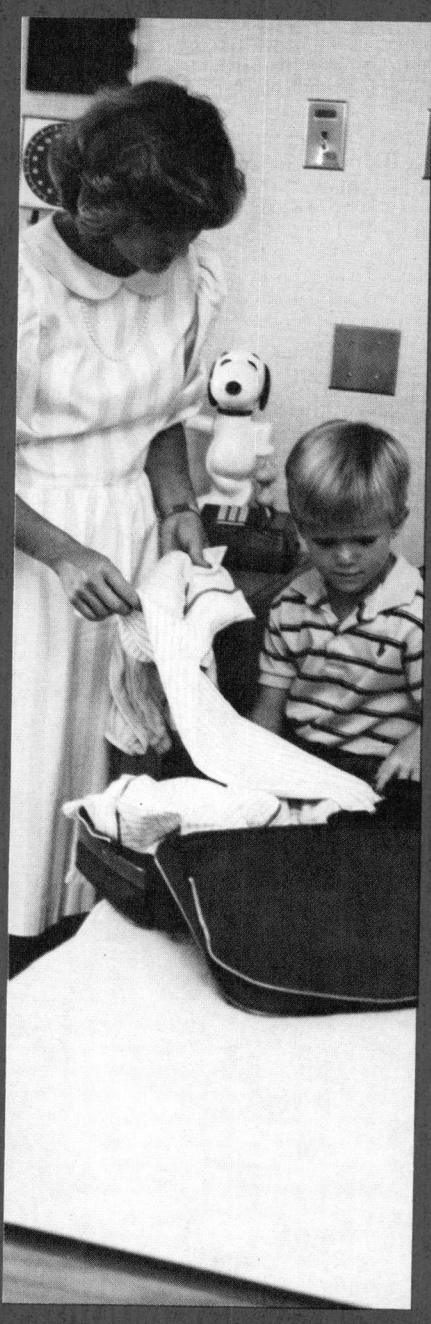

When illness requires hospitalization, it creates a crisis for the child and family. Depending on his age, the child must deal with separation from familiar caregivers and environment, exposure to painful experiences, loss of independence, and disruption of nearly every aspect of his usual life-style. Often the reason for the hospitalization is of much less concern to the child than the consequences of confinement. Emergency and intensive care admissions pose an even greater threat because of the lack of time to prepare the child and the seriousness of the child's condition. In addition, treatments are often painful and frightening.

Chapter 26, *Reaction of Child and Family to Illness and Hospitalization,* is concerned with the child's age-related reactions to illness and hospitalization and with interventions that lessen the psychologic trauma of the experience, particularly parent participation and preparation for admission to the hospital. The effects of the child's hospitalization on the family are discussed and care is extended to these important individuals as well. The needs of the child and family during special hospital admissions are explored. The chapter concludes with a discussion of discharge planning and home care.

Chapter 27, *Pediatric Variations of Nursing Interventions,* deals with pediatric variations of nursing procedures and psychologic and physical preparation of the child for various procedures. It is not designed to present a detailed description of how to perform specific procedures but rather how to safely implement them with children.

Chapter 26

Reaction of Child and Family to Illness and Hospitalization

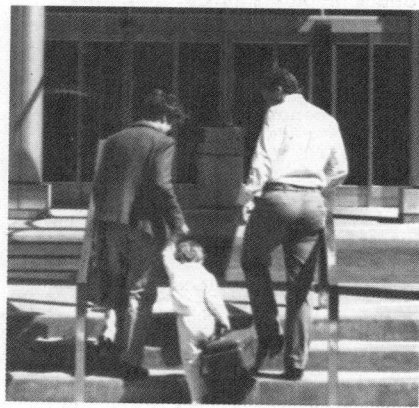

Stressors and Reactions Related to Developmental Stage
Separation anxiety
Early childhood
Later childhood
Loss of control
Toddlers
Preschoolers
School-age children
Adolescents
Bodily injury and pain
Infants
Toddlers
Preschoolers
School-age children
Adolescents
Subsequent effects of hospitalization

Stressors and Reactions of the Family of the Hospitalized Child
Parental reactions
Coping mechanisms
Sibling reactions

Nursing Care of the Hospitalized Child and the Family
Preventing or minimizing separation

Parent participation and "rooming-in"
Strategies to minimize the effects of separation
Minimizing loss of control
Physical restriction
Altered routines
Enforced dependency
Magical thinking
Altered family and social roles
Minimizing bodily injury and pain
Pain assessment
Pain management
Use of play to minimize stress
Diversional activities
Expressive activities
Maximizing potential benefits of hospitalization
Fostering parent-child relationships
Providing educational opportunities
Promoting self-mastery
Providing socialization
Supporting family members
Providing information

Preparation for the Hospital Experience
Guidelines in preparing for hospitalization
Group size and timing of preparation
Setting of the tour
Preparatory materials
Opportunity for discussion
Prehospital counseling by parents
Hospital admission
Nursing admission history
Physical assessment
Placing the child

Nursing care during special hospital admissions
Day hospital
Adolescent unit
Isolation
Emergency admission
Intensive care unit
Discharge planning and home care
Assessment
Planning
Transitional care
Evaluation and continuing support

For children and their families, illness and hospitalization constitute a stressful experience. It is often the first crisis children must deal with and children, especially during the early years, are particularly vulnerable to the crises of illness and hospitalization because (1) stress represents a change from the usual state of health and environmental routine, and (2) children have a limited number of coping mechanisms to resolve the stressful events. Children's reactions to these crises are influenced by their developmental age; previous experience with illness, separation, or hospitalization; available support system; their innate and acquired coping skills; and the seriousness of the diagnosis. This chapter focuses on the various aspects of illness and hospitalization in children to help assist nurses in providing the quality of care that promotes optimum resolution of the crisis and positive growth from the experience for the entire family unit.

Table 26-1   Children's reactions to stress

AGE	DEVELOPMENTAL ACHIEVEMENT AND MAJOR FEARS	BEHAVIOR REACTIONS

Infant	A sense of trust
	Separation
		Early infancy: Global reactions; primarily to change in routine and handling
		Later infancy: Displays separation anxiety:
		    Protest—cries, screams, searches for parent with eyes; clings to parent; avoids and rejects contact with strangers
		    Despair—inactive, withdrawn, depressed, disinterested in environment
		    Detachment—resignation; superficial "adjustment," that is, appears interested in surroundings, happy, friendly

	Pain	Total body reaction (rigidity followed by thrashing) Localized reaction of affected part, cry, facial grimace
Toddler	A sense of autonomy Separatiion	Protest—verbal cries for parent; verbal attack on others; physical fighting, that is, kicks, bites, hits, pinches; tries to escape to find parent, clings to parent and physically tries to force parent to stay Despair—passive, depressed, disinterested in environment, uncommunicative; loss of newly learned skills Detachment—similar to infants; less regressive behaviors
	Loss of control—physical restriction, loss of routine and rituals, dependency Bodily injury and pain	Regression Negativism Temper tantrums Resistance Physical aggression Verbal uncooperativeness
Preschool	A sense of initiative	Protest—less direct and aggressive than toddler, may displace feelings on others
	Separation	Despair—similar to toddler Detachment—similar to toddler
	Loss of control—sense of own power Bodily injury and pain—intrusive procedures, mutilation, castration	Aggression—physical and verbal Regression—dependency; withdrawal; feelings of fear, anxiety, guilt, shame; physiologic responses; immature behavior
School-age	A sense of industry Separation (parents as well as peers)	Usually do not see stage behavior of protest, despair, or detachment Any of following may indicate separation as well as other fears—loneliness, boredom, isolation, withdrawal, depression, displaced anger, hostility, frustration, excessive sleeping or TV watching
	Loss of control—enforced dependency, altered family roles Bodily injury and pain—fear of illness itself, disability, and death; intrusive procedures, especially in genital area	Seeks information Passively accepts pain Groans or whines Holds rigidly still Tries to act brave Communicates about pain May try to postpone an event
Adolescent	A sense of identity Loss of control—loss of identity, enforced dependency Bodily injury and pain—mutilation, sexual changes	Rejection Uncooperativeness Withdrawal Self-assertion Self-control Cooperativeness Fear, anxiety Overconfidence May capitalize on gains from pain
	Separation (especially peer group)	Depression Loneliness Withdrawal Boredom

Stressors and Reactions Related to Developmental Stage

Children's understanding of, reaction to, and method of coping with illness or hospitalization are influenced by the significance of individual *stressors* (those events that produce stress) during each developmental phase. Although the major stressors of separation, loss of control, and bodily injury and their behavioral reactions are discussed in the following section, a review of the previous chapters on normal growth and development will facilitate a more thorough understanding of children's physical, psychosocial, and cognitive abilities and limitations. In addition, Chapters 22 and 23 present an in-depth discussion of children's and family members' reactions to a disability and chronic or life-threatening illness. Table 26-1 summarizes the principal behavioral responses to each stressor during the developmental periods of childhood; appropriate nursing interventions for each are discussed beginning on p. 1063 and are summarized in the Nursing Care Summary on p. 1075.

SEPARATION ANXIETY

The major stress from middle infancy throughout the preschool years, especially for children ages 15 to 30 months, is separation anxiety (also called *anaclitic depression*). The classic work that led to understanding the importance of preventing separation during the early years was done by John Bowlby, John Robertson, and René Spitz on emotional deprivation (see p. 506). Based on these researchers' findings, three distinct phases have been described in the crisis of separation and represent mourning for the loss of the parent. During the phase of *protest,* the child cries loudly, screams for his parent, refuses the attention of anyone else, and is inconsolable in his grief (Fig. 26-1). The child may continue this behavior for a few hours to several days. Some children may protest continuously, ceasing only from physical exhaustion. If a stranger approaches the child, he will initially protest even louder.

During the phase of *despair,* the crying stops. The child is much less active, is disinterested in play or food, and withdraws from others. The child looks sad, lonely, isolated, and apathetic (Fig. 26-2). The major behavior characteristic is depression, a result of increasing hopelessness, grief, and mourning.

The third stage is *detachment,* which is sometimes also called *denial.* Superficially it appears that the child has finally adjusted to the loss. He becomes more interested in his surroundings, plays with others, and seems to form new relationships. However, this behavior is the result of resignation and is not a sign of contentment. He detaches from the parent in an effort to escape the emotional pain of desiring the parent's presence. The child copes by forming shal-

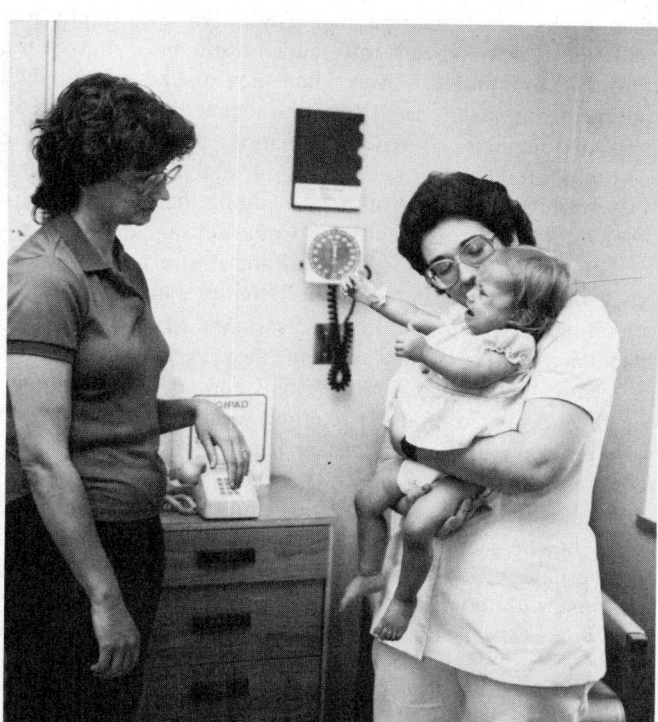

Fig. 26-1. In the stage of protest the child cries loudly and is unconsolable in his grief for the parent.
Photography by John Roy, Saint Francis Hospital, Tulsa, OK.

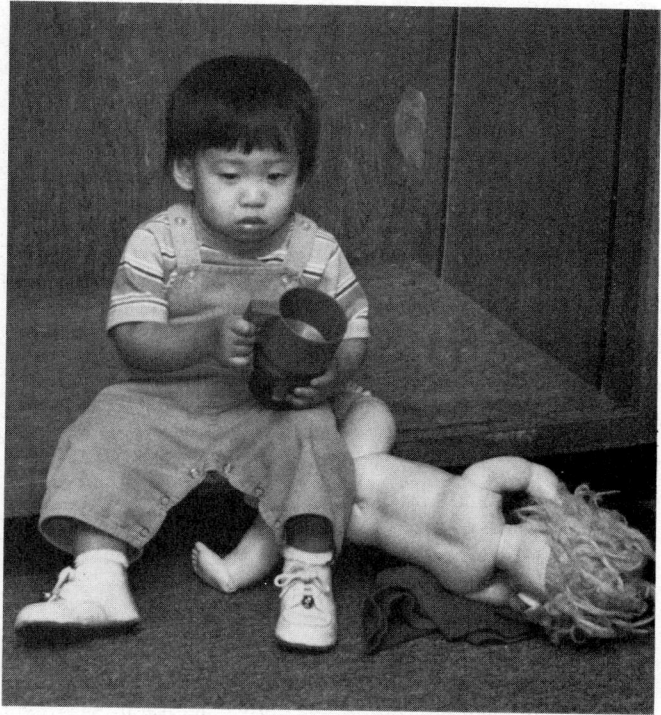

Fig. 26-2. During the stage of despair the child is sad, lonely, and disinterested in play or food.
Photography by John Roy, Saint Francis Hospital, Tulsa, OK.

low relationships with others, becoming increasingly self-centered, and attaching primary importance to material objects. This is the most serious stage in that reversal of the potential adverse effects is less likely to occur once detachment is established. However, in most situations the temporary separations imposed by hospitalization do not cause such prolonged parental absences that the child enters into detachment. In addition there is considerable evidence to suggest that, even with stresses such as separation, children are remarkably adaptable and permanent ill effects are rare (see Questions and controversies, p. 507).

While progression to the stage of detachment is uncommon, the initial stages are frequently observed even with very brief separations from either parent. Without an understanding of the meaning of each stage of behavior, health team members may erroneously label the behaviors as positive or negative. In the stage of protest, they may view the loud crying as "bad" behavior. Since the protesting increases if a stranger approaches, they may interpret the reaction as evidence of their need to stay away. During the quiet, withdrawn phase of despair, they regard the child as finally "settling in" to his new surroundings and the detachment behaviors as proof of a "good adjustment." The faster a child reaches this stage, the more likely he will be regarded as the "ideal patient."

Since children seem to react "negatively" to visits by their parents, uninformed observers feel justified in restricting parental visiting privileges. For example, during the protest stage, children outwardly do not appear happy to see their parents. Instead, they may cry louder than before their visit. If they are depressed, they may reject their parents or begin to protest once more. Often they cling to their parents in an effort to assure their continued presence. Consequently, such behavior reactions may be regarded as "disturbing" the child's adjustment to his surroundings. If the separation has progressed to the phase of detachment, children will respond no differently to their parents than to any other strange or familiar person.

Such reactions are equally distressing to parents, who are unaware of their meaning. If parents are regarded as intruders, parents will view their absence as "beneficial" to the child's adjustment and recovery. They may respond to the child's behavior by staying for short periods of time, decreasing the frequency of visits, or lying to the child when it is time to leave. Consequently a *destructive* cycle of misunderstanding and unmet needs results.

Early Childhood

Separation anxiety is most evident during the ages of 6 to 30 months and is the greatest stress imposed by hospitalization. If separation is avoided, young children have a tremendous capacity to withstand any other stress. During this time the typical reactions described above are seen. However, children in the toddler stage demonstrate more goal-directed behaviors. For example, they may verbally plea for their parents to stay and physically attempt to secure or find them. They may demonstrate displeasure on their return or

departure by having temper tantrums; refusing to comply to the usual routines of mealtime, bedtime, or toileting; or regressing to more primitive levels of development.

Since preschoolers are much more secure interpersonally than toddlers, they can tolerate brief periods of separation from their parents and are more inclined to develop substitute trust in other significant adults. However, the stress of illness usually renders them less able to cope with separation; as a result they manifest many of the stage behaviors of separation anxiety. In general the protest behaviors are more subtle and passive than those seen in younger children. Preschoolers may demonstrate separation anxiety through refusing to eat, difficulty in sleeping, crying quietly for their parents, continually asking when they will visit, or withdrawing from others. They may express anger indirectly by breaking their toys, hitting other children, or refusing to cooperate during usual self-care activities. Nurses need to be sensitive to these less obvious signs of separation anxiety in order to intervene appropriately.

Later Childhood

Although school-age children are better able to cope with separation in general, the stress imposed by illness or hospitalization may increase their need for parental security and guidance. This is particularly true for young school-age children who have only recently left the safety of the home and are struggling with the crisis of school adjustment. Middle and late school-age children may react more to the separation from their usual activities and social attachments than to absence of their parents. Their high level of physical and mental activity frequently finds no suitable outlets in the hospital environment. Even when they dislike school, they admit to missing its routine and associated activities. Feelings of loneliness, boredom, isolation, and depression are common. It is important to recognize that such reactions may occur more as a result of separation than from concern over the illness, treatment, or hospital setting.

School-age children may need and desire parental guidance or support from other adult figures but be unable or unwilling to ask for it. Because the goal of attaining independence is so important to them, they are reluctant to seek help directly for fear that they will appear weak, childish, or dependent. Cultural expectations to "act like a man" or to "be brave and strong" bear heavily on these children, especially males, who tend to react to stress with stoicism, withdrawal, or passive acceptance. Often the need to express hostile, angry, or other negative feelings finds outlets in alternate ways, such as irritability and aggression toward parents, withdrawal from hospital personnel, inability to relate to peers, rejection of siblings, or subsequent behavioral problems in school.

For adolescents separation from home and parents may be a welcomed and appreciated event. However, loss of peer-group contact may be a severe emotional threat because of loss of group status, inability to exert group control or leadership, and loss of group acceptance. Deviations within peer groups are poorly tolerated, and, although members may express concern for the adolescent's illness or need for hospitalization, they continue their group activities, quickly filling the gap of the absent member. During the temporary separation from their usual group, ill adolescents may benefit from group associations with other hospitalized age-mates.

LOSS OF CONTROL

One of the factors influencing the amount of stress imposed by hospitalization is the amount of control (often referred to as locus of control) a person perceives as having. Lack of control increases the perception of threat and can affect children's coping skills (LaMontagne, 1984). Obviously in the hospital numerous situations exist that decrease the amount of control a child feels. Although the usual sensory stimulations are lacking, the additional hospital stimuli of sight, sound, and smell may be bombarding and overwhelming. Without an insight into the type of environment conducive to children's optimum growth, the hospital experience can at best temporarily slow development and at worst permanently retard it. Because the needs of children vary greatly depending on their age, the major areas of loss of control in terms of physical restriction, altered routine or rituals, and dependency are discussed for each age-group.

Toddlers

Toddlers are striving for autonomy and this goal is evident in most of their behaviors—motor skills, play, interpersonal relationships, activities of daily living, and communication. When their egocentric pleasures meet with obstacles, toddlers react with negativism, especially temper tantrums. Any restriction or limitation of movement, such as the simple act of lying toddlers on their back, can cause forceful resistance and noncompliance.

Loss of control also results from altered routines and rituals. Toddlers rely on the consistency and familiarity of daily rituals to provide a measure of stability and control in their complex world of growing and developing. The experience of hospitalization or illness severely limits their sense of expectation and predictability, since practically every detail of the hospital environment differs from that of the home.

Toddlers' main areas for rituals include eating, sleeping, bathing, toileting, and play. When the routines are disrupted, difficulties can occur in any or all of these areas. The principal reaction to such change is regression. For example, when mealtime and food choices differ from those at home, toddlers often refuse to eat, demand a bottle, or request others to feed them. Although regression to earlier forms of behavior may seem to increase toddlers' security and comfort, in reality it is very threatening for them to relinquish their most recently acquired achievements.

Enforced dependency is a chief characteristic of the sick role and accounts for the numerous instances of toddler negativism. For example, rigid schedules, altered caregiving

activities, unfamiliar surroundings, separation from parents, and medical procedures usurp toddlers' control over their world. Although most toddlers initially react negatively and aggressively to such dependency, prolonged loss of autonomy may result in passive withdrawal from interpersonal relationships and regression in all areas of development. Therefore the effects of the sick role are most severe in instances of chronic, long-term illnesses or in those families in which the sick role is fostered despite the child's improved state of health.

Preschoolers

Preschoolers also suffer from loss of control caused by physical restriction, altered routines, and enforced dependency. However, their specific cognitive abilities, which make them feel omnipotent and all-powerful, also make them feel out of control. This loss of control in the context of their sense of self-power is a critical influencing factor in their perception of and reaction to separation, pain, illness, and hospitalization.

Preschoolers' egocentric and magical thinking limits their ability to understand events because they view all experiences from their own self-referenced (egocentric) perspective. Without adequate preparation for unfamiliar settings or experiences, preschoolers' fantasy explanation for such events are usually more exaggerated, bizarre, and frightening than the actual facts. One typical fantasy to explain the reason for illness or hospitalization is that it represents punishment for real or imagined misdeeds. The response to such thinking is usually feelings of shame, guilt, and fear.

Preschoolers' cognitive ability is also concrete. Explanations are understood only in terms of real events. Purely verbal instructions are often inadequate for them because of their inability to abstract and synthesize beyond what their senses tell them. When combined with their egocentric and magical powers, they can interpret any message according to their particular past experiences. Even with the best preparation for a procedure, they may misconstrue the details.

Transductive reasoning implies that preschoolers deduct from the particular to the particular, rather than from the specific to general or vice versa. For example, if preschoolers' concept of nurses is that they inflict pain, preschoolers will think that every nurse (or every one wearing a similar uniform) will also inflict pain.

School-Age Children

Because of their striving for independence and productivity, school-age children are particularly vulnerable to events that may lessen their feeling of control and power. In particular, altered family roles; physical disability; fears of death, abandonment, or permanent injury; loss of peer acceptance; lack of productivity; and inability to cope with stress according to perceived cultural expectation may result in loss of control.

Because of the nature of the patient role, many routine hospital activities usurp individual power and identity. For these children, dependent activities such as enforced bed rest, use of a bedpan, inability to choose a menu, lack of privacy, help with a bed bath, or transport by use of a wheelchair or stretcher can be a direct threat to their security. Although all of these usual hospital procedures seem routine and inconsequential, to children who want to "act grown-up," these activities allow no freedom of choice. However, when children are allowed to exert a measure of control, regardless of how limited it may be, they generally respond very well to any procedure. For example, some of the most cooperative, satisfied, and contented patients are those school-age children who help make their beds, choose their schedule of activities, assist in procedures, and help the nurses care for the younger children. An increased sense of control is usually an outcome of a feeling of usefulness and productivity.

In addition to the hospital environment, illness may also cause a feeling of loss of control. One of the most significant problems of children in this age-group centers on boredom. When physical or enforced limitations curtail their usual abilities to care for themselves or to engage in favorite activities, school-age children generally respond with depression, hostility, or frustration. Keeping a normally active child on bed rest is no small challenge. However, emphasizing areas of control and capitalizing on quiet activities, particularly hobbies such as building models or collecting specific objects, promote their adjustment to physical restriction. Nursing judgment regarding selection of a roommate is one of the most important contributing factors to their overall adjustment to illness and hospitalization.

Adolescents

Adolescents' struggle for independence, self-assertion, and liberation centers on the quest for personal identity. Anything that interferes with this poses a threat to their sense of identity and results in a loss of control. Illness, which limits their physical abilities, and hospitalization, which separates them from usual support systems, constitute major situational crises.

The patient role fosters dependency and depersonalization. Adolescents may react to dependency with rejection, uncooperativeness, or withdrawal. They may respond to depersonalization with self-assertion, anger, or frustration. Regardless of which response they manifest, hospital personnel generally tend to regard them as difficult, unmanageable patients. Parents may not be a source of help because these behaviors serve to further isolate them from understanding the adolescent. Although peers may visit, they may not be able to offer the kind of support and guidance needed. Sick adolescents often voluntarily isolate themselves from agemates until they feel they can compete on an equal basis and meet group expectations. As a result, ill adolescents are left with virtually no support systems.

Loss of control also occurs for many of the reasons discussed under school-age children. However, adolescents are more sensitive to potential instances of loss of control and dependency than younger children. For example, both groups seek information about their physical status and rely heavily on anticipatory preparation to decrease fear and anxiety. However, adolescents react not only to the kinds of information supplied them but also to the means by which it is conveyed. They may feel very threatened by others who relate facts in a derogatory manner. Adolescents want to know that others can relate to them on their own level. This necessitates a careful assessment of their intellectual abilities, previous knowledge, and present needs. It may also require a willingness on the part of the nurse to learn the language of the adolescent.

BODILY INJURY AND PAIN

Fears of bodily injury and pain are prevalent among children and recent research documents that young children, including newborns, react to painful stimuli. In caring for children, nurses must have appreciation of the concerns related to bodily harm and the reactions of children to pain at different developmental periods.

Infants

Of the research exploring children's development of illness concepts and how their understanding of illness relates to fears of bodily injury, no findings are available for preverbal children. Consequently, the following discussion is limited to infants' reactions to pain.

Neonates' general reaction to painful stimuli is body movement associated with brief, loud crying and facial expressions of pain. For example, newborns react to a heelstick by immediate withdrawal of both the affected and unaffected leg, movement of other extremities, facial grimacing (Franck, 1986), and crying for an average of 3 minutes (Owens and Todt, 1984). Physiological indications of pain include palm sweating (Harpin and Rutter, 1982), increased heart rate, and decreased oxygenation (Williamson and Williamson, 1983). Unfortunately, these changes may be less apparent in premature infants; for example, during heelstick procedures they may not demonstrate decreased oxygenation but may be more responsive physiologically to procedures such as suctioning and position changes (Norris, Campbell, and Brenkert, 1982). In caring for both well and sick newborns, many health professionals fail to appreciate the response of infants to painful stimuli and subject newborns to painful procedures without local anesthetic (see Questions and Controversies on circumcision, p. 323). Presently there is no way of knowing what future psychologic effect exposure to multiple, continuous painful procedures, which are so common in neonatal intensive care units, may have.

Infants' response to pain after the neonatal period is quite similar to earlier reactions, although there is marked variability in measures of distress, especially initial cry and heart rate, which may decrease in some infants (Dale, 1986). The most consistent indicator of distress is a facial expression of discomfort. Body movements consist initially of rigidity of the extremities followed by thrashing (Johnston and Strada, 1986). The individual differences may be the result of temperamental characteristics and further study is needed to explore the role that temperament plays in children's response to pain. Some infants may cry loudly following the procedure, whereas others are easily calmed by a gentle hug. It is important to recognize and respect such early signs of individuality and to realize that children who react less intensely may still be experiencing significant discomfort (Chess and Thomas, 1985).

Infants less than 6 months of age seem to have no memory of previous painful experiences and react to a potentially stressful situation with less apprehension and fear than older children. However, after this time, children's response to pain is influenced by their recall of prior painful experiences and the emotional contagion of parents during the procedure (Watson, 1976). Older infants react intensely with physical resistance and uncooperativeness. They may refuse to lie still, attempt to push the person away, or try to escape with whatever motor activity they have achieved. Distraction does little to lessen their immediate reaction to pain, and anticipatory preparation, such as showing them the equipment, tends to increase their fear and resistance. The most supportive intervention is to perform the procedure as quickly as possible and maintain parent-child contact.

Toddlers

Toddlers' concept of body image, particularly the definition of body boundaries, is very poorly developed. Intrusive experiences, such as examining the ears or mouth or taking a rectal temperature, are very anxiety producing. Toddlers may react to such painless procedures as intensely as they do to painful ones.

Toddlers' reactions to pain are similar to those seen during infancy, except that the number of variables influencing the individual response is highly complex and varied. Memory, physical restraint, parent separation, emotional reactions of others, and lack of preparation partially determine the intensity of the behavioral response. In general children in this age-group continue to react with intense emotional upset and physical resistance to any actual or perceived painful experience. Behaviors indicating pain include grimacing, clenching their teeth/lips, opening their eyes wide, rocking, rubbing, and aggressiveness, such as biting, kicking, hitting, or running away. Unlike adults who usually decrease their activity when in pain, young children typically become restless and overly active; frequently this response is not recognized as a consequence of pain.

By the end of this age period toddlers usually are able to communicate about their pain. Although they have not developed the ability to describe the type or intensity of the pain, they usually are able to localize it by pointing to a specific area.

Preschoolers

Concepts of illness begin during the preschool period and are influenced by the cognitive abilities of the preoperational stage. Preschoolers differentiate poorly between themselves and the external world. Their thinking is focused on externally perceived events, and causality is based on the prox-

imity of two events. Consequently, a child defines illness when he is told he is sick or is given external evidence of illness, such as, "You are sick because you have a fever." The cause of illness is seen as a concrete action he does or fails to do, such as, "Catching a cold because you go out into cold weather" (Perrin and Gerrity, 1981) and consequently implies a degree of responsibility and self-blame. Another explanation may be based on contagion, that the proximity of two objects or persons causes the illness—for example—"A person gets a cold when someone else with a cold gets near him" (Bibace and Walsh, 1980).

The psychosexual conflicts of children in this age-group make them very vulnerable to threats of bodily injury. Intrusive procedures, whether painful or painless, are threatening to preschoolers, whose concept of body integrity is still poorly developed. It is not uncommon for preschoolers to react to an injection with as much concern for withdrawal of the needle as for the actual pain. They fear that the intrusion or puncture will not reclose and that their "insides" will leak out.

Concerns of mutilation are paramount during this age period. Loss of any body part is threatening, but preschool boys' fears of castration complicate their understanding of surgical or medical procedures associated with the genital area, such as circumcision, repair of hypospadias or epispadias, cystoscopy, or catheterization. Their limited comprehension of body functioning also increases their difficulty in understanding how or why body parts are "fixed." For example, telling preschoolers that their tonsils are to be removed may be interpreted as "taking out their voice," or having the penis "fixed" may be understood as cutting it off. Words such as "dye," "cut off," "take out," or "draw" (e.g., "draw some blood") are understood literally and can lead to confusion and fear.

For example, a 5-year-old child who had undergone circumcision for phimosis became acutely anxious after surgery and refused to void. After numerous attempts to encourage urinating, the nurse asked the child what he thought had been done during the operation. He stated that his mother had told him that some skin would be removed and the end of the penis stitched together. After surgery he was convinced that the opening had been stitched closed. The nurse then pointed out that the stitches were not near the opening but were below the tip where the skin had been removed. After much reassurance that the opening was still functional, the child voided with no difficulty.

Reactions to pain change during this age period. By the end of the fourth year, many preschoolers exhibit an increasing degree of self-control while experiencing pain. Cultural expectations may be evident, such as the stereotyped sex role of "brave men don't cry," that is often seen in young boys who attempt to be courageous and who, if they fail, feel guilty and ashamed.

Preschoolers' primary reactions to the stress of pain and fear are aggression, verbal expression, and dependency (Smith, 1976). *Aggression* in preschoolers is more specific and goal directed than in younger children and is geared toward fight or flight. Instead of total body resistance, preschoolers may push the person away, try to secure the equipment, or attempt to lock themselves in a safe place. Much more thought is evident in their plan of attack or escape.

Verbal expression in particular demonstrates their advanced development in response to stress. They may verbally abuse the attacker by stating, ''Get out of here'' or ''I hate you.'' They may also use a more cunning approach of trying to persuade the person to give up the intended activity. A common plea is, ''Please don't give me a shot; I'll be good.'' Some statements are not only attempts to avoid the event but also evidence of children's perceptions about the experience.

Dependency very often represents regression to more stable and comforting modes of behavior. Anxiety related to uncertainty, fear, pain, or separation may be expressed through behaviors such as clinging to a parent, refusing to play with other children, reverting to nonverbal means of communication, wanting to be held, or refusing to be left alone. A common expression denoting the need for dependency is, ''Help me.'' It is important to recognize such requests as the need for support from others during a time of stress. Admonishing children to act grown-up or encouraging them to do things by stating, ''I know you can do it yourself,'' deprives them of the support they are requesting and increases their own feelings of guilt and shame.

School-Age Children

Fears of the physical nature of the illness surface at this time. There may be less concern with actual pain than there is for disability, uncertain recovery, or possible death. Girls tend to express more and stronger fears than boys and previous hospitalizations may have no effect on the frequency or intensity of these fears (Aho and Erickson, 1985). Because of their developing cognitive abilities, school-age children are aware of the significance of different illnesses, the indispensability of certain body parts, potential hazards in treatments, lifelong consequences of permanent injury or loss of function, and the meaning of death. A paramount concern of hospitalized school-age children is their fear of not being well again (May and Sparks, 1983). They generally take a very active interest in their health or illness. Even those children who rarely ask questions usually reveal detailed knowledge of their condition by attentively listening to all that is said around them. They request factual information and quickly perceive lies or half-truths. Seeking information tends to be one way of their maintaining a sense of control despite the stress and uncertainty of illness.

The school-age child defines illness by a set of multiple concrete symptoms, such as signs of a cold, and views the cause as primarily germs or bacteria. The germs have a powerful, almost magical quality, so that in the child's mind, illness can be prevented by avoiding people with the germs (Perrin and Gerrity, 1981). There is also the idea of contamination that is similar to the younger age group; for example, the illness occurs because of physical contact or

because the child engaged in a harmful action and became contaminated (Bibace and Walsh). Consequently, feelings of self-blame and guilt may be asociated with the reason for becoming ill (Wood, 1983).

School-age children begin to show concern for the potential beneficial and hazardous effects of procedures. Besides wanting to know if a procedure will hurt, they want to know what it is for, how it will make them better, and what injury or harm could result. For example, these children fear the actual procedure of anesthesia. Unlike preschoolers who fear the mask and the strange surroundings, school-age children fear what may happen while they are asleep, whether they will wake up, and if they may die. Preadolescents also worry about the operation itself, particularly one that will result in visible changes in body image.

Intrusive procedures of a nonsexual nature, such as routine physical examination of the ears, nose, mouth, and throat, are generally well tolerated. However, concerns for privacy become evident and increasingly significant. Although school-age children may be cooperative during examination of, or procedures that are performed on, the genital area, it is usually very stressful for them, especially for preadolescents who are beginning pubertal changes. Nurses who respect children's need for privacy can provide them with much assurance and support.

By the age of 9 or 10, most school-age children show less fright or overt resistance to pain than younger children. They generally have learned passive methods of dealing with discomfort, such as holding rigidly still, clenching their fists or teeth, or trying to act brave by the ''grin-and-bear-it'' routine. If they do display signs of overt resistance, such as biting, kicking, pulling away, trying to escape, crying, or plea bargaining, they may deny such reactions later, especially to their peers for fear of embarrassment.

School-age children verbally communicate about their pain in respect to its location, intensity, and description. Unlike younger children who have difficulty choosing words to describe pain, children 9 years and older use a wide variety of words and phrases, such as throbbing, piercing, bad, terrible, awful, or ''like a torture treatment'' (Savedra and others, 1982). They may also describe pain in psychologic terms, such as ''pain is being afraid, nervous, or getting scolded.'' Boys report being brave more often than girls, who admit being afraid (Schultz, 1971).

School-age children also use words as a means of controlling their reactions to pain. For example, these children may ask the nurse to talk to them during a procedure. Some prefer to participate in a procedure, whereas others choose to distance themselves by not looking at what is happening. Most appreciate an explanation of the procedure and seem less fearful when they know what to expect. Others try to gain control by attempting to postpone the event. A typical request is, ''Give me the shot when I am finished with this.'' Although the ability to make decisions does increase their sense of control, unlimited procrastination results in heightened anxiety. When choices are allowed, such as selection of the injection site, it is best to structure the number of possible sites and to limit the number of "procrastination" techniques.

Similar to their more passive acceptance of pain is their nondirective request for support or help. School-age children will rarely initiate a conversation about their feelings or request someone to stay with them during a lonely or stressful period. In fact, their visible composure, calmness, and acceptance often belie their inner longing for support. It is especially important to be aware of nonverbal clues, such as a serious facial expression, a halfhearted reply of "I am fine," silence, lack of activity, or social isolation, as signs of the need for help. Usually when someone identifies the unspoken messages and offers support, they readily accept it.

Adolescents

Although the development of body image begins at birth, its relevance is paramount during adolescence. Injury, pain, disability, and death are viewed primarily in terms of how each affects the adolescent's view of himself in the present. Any change that differentiates the adolescent from his peers is regarded as a major tragedy. For example, diseases such as diabetes mellitus often present a more difficult adjustment period for children in this age-group than for younger children because of the necessary changes in the adolescent's life-style. Conversely, serious, even life-threatening illnesses that entail no visible body changes or physical restrictions may have less immediate significance for the adolescent. Therefore the nature of bodily injury may be more important in terms of adolescents' perception of the illness than its actual degree of severity.

Adolescents' rapidly changing body image during pubertal development often makes them feel insecure about their bodies. Illness, medical or surgical intervention, and hospitalization increase their existing concerns for normalcy. They may respond to such events by asking numerous questions, withdrawing, rejecting others, or questioning the adequacy of care. Frequently their fear for loss of control and body image change is demonstrated as overconfidence, conceit, or a "know-it-all" attitude.

Because of sexual changes, adolescents are very concerned about privacy. Lack of respect for this need can cause greater stress than physical pain. In addition, adolescents look for signs that indicate that they are developing normally and according to acceptable standards. When illness occurs, they fear that growth may be retarded, leaving them behind their peers. Although they may not voice this concern, they may demonstrate it by carefully observing others' reactions to them during physical examinations or procedures.

Adolescents react to pain with much self-control. Physical resistance and aggression are unusual at this age, unless the adolescents are totally unprepared for a procedure. Like older school-age children they are very concerned with remaining composed and feel embarrassed and ashamed of losing control. They are able to describe their pain experience and to use any of the pain assessment tools developed for adults. However, they may be reluctant to disclose their pain unless the nurse is willing to listen closely and observe physical indications, such as limited movement, excessive quiet, or irritability.

SUBSEQUENT EFFECTS OF HOSPITALIZATION

Children not only react to the stresses of illness and hospitalization during admission but many demonstrate temporary behavioral changes following discharge, especially children under 4 years of age. These effects are a direct result of (1) separation from significant people, (2) a lack of opportunity to form new attachments, and (3) a strange environment (Rutter, 1979).

For example, young children may show some initial aloofness toward the parents, which may be seen as a hesitancy in getting too close right away for fear of being abandoned again. This phase may last from a few minutes (most common) to a few days. This is frequently followed by the reverse—a tendency to cling to the parents, demand their attention, and vigorously oppose any separation, such as staying at nursery school or with a baby-sitter (Patterson, 1979).

Other negative behaviors include new fears, nightmares, insomnia, withdrawal and shyness, hyperactivity, temper tantrums, attachment to blanket or toy, tics or other nervous mannerisms, food finickiness, resistance in going to bed, and regression in self-toileting. Older children may express posthospitalization behaviors such as anger, jealousy, and emotional coldness, followed by intense, demanding dependence on the mother (Freiberg, 1972). Younger children tend to exhibit more of these behaviors for longer periods, usually an average of 3 weeks.

A significant finding from studies done on hospitalization and development of subsequent long-term emotional disturbance relates to the *length* and *number* of hospital admissions. Douglas (1975) and Quinton and Rutter (1976) found that single hospital admissions lasting a *week or less* were not associated with any form of later emotional or behavioral disturbance, regardless of the child's age at the time of hospitalization. However, *repeated* hospital admissions and a single hospitalization of *4 weeks or more* were significantly associated with later disturbances. Children from disadvantaged homes were more at risk for developing emotional problems than children from nondisadvantaged homes. The investigators conclude that children from disadvantaged homes are already insecure and troubled and therefore are more vulnerable to the stresses imposed by hospitalization. However, a more recent review of the relationship between duration of hospital stay in preschool years and behavior at age 6 years does not completely support these findings. Shannon, Fergusson, and Dimond (1984) found no significant association between duration of hospitalization and children's behavior problems when family and social factors were controlled for. The authors propose that the changes in pediatric hospital care currently, as compared to the stricter practices in the 1940s and 1950s, may account for the differences in subsequent behavior of children who are hospitalized during their preschool years.

Until further studies document that hospitalization is a relatively benign experience for most children, the implications from the research by Douglas (1975) as well as Quinton and Rutter (1976) are clear:

1. Avoid unnecessary hospital admissions for all children, especially if diagnosis or treatment can be done on an outpatient basis.
2. Whenever possible, limit hospital stays to less than 1 week.
3. When children from unhappy, deprived, or disrupted homes are admitted, be especially alert to meeting their needs concerning separation, a strange environment, and loss of control or insecurity.

Stressors and Reactions of the Family of the Hospitalized Child

The crisis of childhood illness and hospitalization affects every member of the nuclear family and to varying degrees members of the extended family. The stressors and reactions of families have been discussed in detail in Chapter 22 in relation to chronic illness and in Chapter 23 in relation to life-threatening illness. In many respects they differ little regardless of the diagnosis except for their intensity and persistence, which are proportional to the degree of severity of the illness. Consequently, when a child is admitted to an intensive care facility, the family members' reactions and needs are typically greater than when a child is admitted with a less serious condition to the regular pediatric unit. The following discussion briefly reviews the common reactions of the family; specific reactions during intensive care admissions are discussed on p. 1092.

PARENTAL REACTIONS

Parents' reactions to illness in their child depend on a variety of influencing factors. While it is not possible to predict which factors are most likely to influence their response, a number of variables have been identified, which include:

1. The seriousness of the threat to their child
2. Previous experience with illness or hospitalization
3. Medical procedures involved in diagnosis and treatment
4. Available support systems
5. Personal ego strengths
6. Previous coping abilities
7. Additional stresses on the family system
8. Cultural and religious beliefs
9. Communication patterns among family members.

Almost universally, parents respond to illness and hospitalization in their child with remarkably consistent reactions. Initially parents may react with *disbelief,* especially if the illness is sudden and serious. Following the realization of illness, parents react with *anger, guilt,* or both. There is a tendency to search for self-blame regarding why the child

became ill or to project anger at others for some wrongdoing. Even in the mildest of illnesses, parents question their adequacy as caregivers and review any actions or omissions that could have prevented or caused the illness. When hospitalization is indicated, parental guilt is intensified because they feel helpless in alleviating the child's physical and emotional pain.

Fear, anxiety, and *frustration* are common feelings expressed by parents. Fear and anxiety may be related to the seriousness of the illness and the type of medical procedures involved. Often a great deal of anxiety is related to the trauma and pain inflicted on the child because of the various procedures. Feelings of frustration are often related to lack of information about procedures and treatments, unfamiliarity with hospital rules and regulations, a sense of unwelcomeness from the staff, or fear of asking questions (Freiberg, 1972). It is obvious that much frustration can be alleviated in a pediatric unit in which parents participate in their child's care and are regarded as the most significant contributors to the child's total health.

Parents eventually may react with some degree of *depression.* The depression usually occurs when the acute crisis is over, such as following hospital discharge or complete recovery. Mothers often comment on their feeling of physical and mental exhaustion after all the other family members have adapted to the crisis. Other reasons for anxiety and depression are related to concerns for the child's future well-being, including negative effects produced by the hospitalization and any subsequent financial burden incurred from the hospitalization.

Coping Mechanisms

Coping mechanisms are psychologic processes that temporarily protect individuals from anxiety by providing a measure of security or relief from stress. These defenses are normal and healthy; they may become pathologic when they prevent the person from successfully resolving the crisis situation. The more common defense mechanisms used by parents are denial, intellectualization, regression, projection, displacement, and introjection.

Denial is the avoidance of stressful realities by ignoring or refusing to recognize them. Parents may express denial in any number of ways, such as by asking few questions, focusing primarily on the positive aspects of the child's condition, refusing to accept negative reports of the child's progress, or acting calm in an otherwise stressful situation. However, these behaviors *rarely* signify absolute denial of reality but rather help the family distance themselves temporarily from an overwhelming emotional burden.

Intellectualization is the use of knowledge to control the intense emotional impact of the illness's meaning. Parents intellectualize when they attempt to find out all the information available on their child's illness but fail to face the issues of that disorder. Medical and nursing personnel are frequently caught in this trap because they feel more comfortable in supplying the facts than in helping the family deal with more critical physical or emotional problems.

Regression, or the return to a less stressful level of functioning, is evident in parents as well as children although the behaviors may be more subtle. Fears, "temper tantrums" or sudden outbursts of anger, and demanding behavior toward others such as the spouse or hospital staff are characteristic patterns of regressive behavior.

Projection is resolving conflicts by placing the responsibility outside oneself. For example, parents may project their blame and anger onto the child, other spouse, or hospital staff. Consequently, they accept little or no responsibility for the illness. In this way the parent's own self-esteem can be maintained. Projection can be destructive when it alienates the parent from all potential sources of support.

Displacement is the transference of emotion or concern from one object or event to another, less-threatening one. For example, parents may transfer their fear of the child's recovery into concern for a specific symptom, such as pain from surgery. A common displacement of anger is toward the well siblings. Parents who have tried to be patient and tolerant of the ill child's negative behavior may literally explode with anger at the slightest provocation from other siblings. Siblings interpret such reactions as parental rejection.

Introjection, in which parents turn all their blame, anger, and guilt inward, expecting punishment for their misdeeds, is the opposite of projection. The ultimate result of introjection is self-punishment by suicide. Less severe and more common examples of self-blame are verbally downgrading one's parenting abilities, searching for evidence of responsibility in causing the illness, and neglecting personal physical health.

SIBLING REACTIONS

Siblings' reactions to a sister's or brother's illness or hospitalization are discussed in Chapters 22 and 23 and differ little when a child becomes temporarily ill. Their main reactions are anger, resentment, jealousy, and guilt. A number of factors have been identified that influence the effects of the child's hospitalization on siblings and although they are similar to those seen when a child has a chronic illness, the following are related specifically to the hospital experience and were found to *increase* the effects on the siblings (Craft, Wyatt, and Sandell, 1985):

1. Fear of contracting the illness
2. Younger age
3. Close relationship to sick sibling
4. Out-of-home residence during period of hospitalization
5. Minimal explanation of the sick child's illness
6. Perceived changes in parenting, such as increased parental anger

Parents are often unaware of the number of effects that siblings experience during the sick child's hospitalization nor the benefit of simple interventions to minimize such effects, such as explicit explanations about the illness and provisions for the siblings to remain at home. Although sibling visitation is advocated and is probably advantageous, effects on siblings who do visit the sick child are still evident. The effects may be different, however—those who do not visit may experience more difficulty concentrating in school, feelings of being less healthy, and nail biting, while those who visit are more likely to become angry (Craft and Wyatt, 1986). Nevertheless, more research is needed to document the effects of sibling visitation (see also Questions and controversies, pp. 331 and 389).

Nursing Care of the Hospitalized Child and the Family

Children and their families require competent and sensitive care to minimize the potential negative effects of hospitalization and also to promote positive benefits from the experience. Interventions should focus on (1) eliminating or minimizing the stressors of separation, loss of control, and bodily injury and pain for children and (2) providing specific supportive strategies for family members, such as fostering family relationships and providing information.

PREVENTING OR MINIMIZING SEPARATION

The primary nursing goal is to prevent separation, particularly in children under 5 years of age. However, this is not always possible and in this case measures to minimize the effects of separation must be implemented. The importance of a primary nurse for the child cannot be overemphasized. There is no substitute for the consistency provided by primary nursing and its advantages for the child and family.

Parent Participation and "Rooming-In"

Prevention of separation requires rooming-in facilities in pediatric hospital settings. Although some health facilities provide special accommodations for parents, the concept of "rooming-in" can be instituted anywhere. The first requirement is the staff's positive attitude toward parents. When hospital staff genuinely appreciate the importance of continued parent-child attachment, they foster an environment that encourages parents to stay. When parents are included in the care planning and made to feel as if they are a contributing factor to the child's recovery, they are more inclined to remain with their child and have more emotional reserves to support themselves and the child through the crisis.

Since the mother tends to be the usual family caregiver, she spends more time in the hospital than the father. However, not all mothers feel equally comfortable in assuming responsibility for their child's care. Some may be under such great emotional stress that they need a temporary reprieve from total participation in caregiving activities. Others may feel insecure in participating in specialized areas of care, such as bathing the child after surgery. Individual assessment of each parent's preferred involvement is necessary in order to prevent the effects of separation while supporting parents in their needs as well (Stull and Deatrick, 1986). Both under and overinvolvement of parents' in the child's care can be detrimental; therefore every effort is extended to help parents identify moderate amounts of visiting and participation (O'Donnell as cited in Thompson, 1985).

With life-styles and sexual roles changing, it is conceivable that some fathers may assume all or some of the usual mothering roles in the household. In this case it may be the father-child relationship that requires preservation. Fathers need to be included in the plan of care and respected for their parental role. For some fathers the child's hospitalization may represent an opportunity to alter their usual caregiving role and increase their involvement (Knafl and Dixon, 1984). It is equally important to support the mother's role as family provider or parttime housekeeper in order to meet the needs of each parent. In single-parent families, the caregiver may not be a parent but an extended family member, such as a grandparent or aunt.

One of the potential problems with continuous parent visiting is neglect of the parent's need for sleep, nutrition, and relaxation. Often the sleeping accommodations are limited to a chair and sleep is disrupted by nursing procedures. After a few days parents can become exhausted but feel obligated to stay. Encouraging them to leave for brief periods, arranging for sleeping quarters on the unit but outside the child's room, and planning a schedule of alternating visiting with the other parent or with a family member can minimize the stresses for the parent.

All too often nurses respond to parent participation by abandoning their patient responsibilities. Nurses need to restructure their roles to complement and augment the caregiving functions of parents. Even in units structured to provide care by parents, parents frequently feel anxiety in their caregiving responsibilities; those more involved in direct care may feel increased anxiety over those less involved in direct care. Therefore 24-hour responsibility may be too much for some parents (Monahan and Schkade, 1985). Assistance and relief by nursing personnel should always be available to these families.

Strategies to Minimize the Effects of Separation

When separation cannot be prevented, numerous strategies can be employed to minimize the effects of temporary separation on children. Ideally a primary nurse is assigned to meet the child's needs. Becoming a surrogate parent requires a thorough, detailed nursing history that specifically identifies the child's established daily routine. Usual daily activities such as food preparation and method of feeding help establish a complementary schedule of caregiving practices. It also helps the parent feel as if he or she is participating in the child's care but through another person. A nursing admission history for children is outlined in the boxed material on p. 1088.

The nurse caring for the child must have an appreciation of the child's separation behaviors. As discussed earlier, the phases of protest and despair are normal. The child is allowed to cry. Even if he rejects strangers, the nurse provides support through physical presence in the room. Saying to the child, "I know you are unhappy because you miss your mommy and daddy. It's all right to cry. I will sit here for awhile so you are not alone," reinforces for the child the nurse's awareness of his feelings without abandoning him. If behaviors of detachment are evident, the child's contact with his parents is maintained by frequently talking about them, encouraging him to remember them, and stressing the significance of their visits, telephone calls, or letters.

Separation may be equally as difficult for parents, especially when they do not understand the behaviors of separation anxiety. To avoid the immediate protest, parents may sneak out or lie to the child about leaving. As a result, the child does not learn that absence is associated with a guaranteed return but that absence means loss of parents. Helping parents recognize that separation behaviors are normal and expected can decrease their anxiety and may ease their fears about leaving the child without telling him. Explaining to parents how the child reacts after they leave may also be helpful. Many parents imagine that the child cries for hours after they leave, whereas in reality he may cry for a few minutes but settle down when comforted by someone else.

Toddlers and preschoolers have a very limited concept of time. The young child's question "Will my mommy come yesterday?" symbolizes a lack of understanding for usual measurements of time, such as days, hours, and weeks. Time is measured in associations, such as, "Eating dinner when daddy comes home." Therefore, when helping parents with their fears of separation, nurses need to suggest ways of explaining leaving and returning. For example, if parents must leave to go to work or to make meals for the other family members, they should tell the hospitalized child the reason for leaving. They also need to convey the expected time of return in terms of anticipated events. For example, if the parents return in the morning, they can tell the child that they will see him "After the sun comes up" or "When a favorite program is on television."

The young child's ability to tolerate parental absence is very limited. Therefore parental visits should be frequent. For example, it is better for parents to visit three times a day for short periods than once a day for an extended time. This may necessitate that each parent visit at different times to lessen the length of separation. When parents cannot visit, "on-call lists" of other significant others who can come to the hospital is helpful (Eland, 1985a).

If parents leave after the child is asleep, they still need to communicate their absence. The parents of a five-year-old boy solved this problem by devising a sign; on one side they drew a picture of a telephone and on the other they drew a hamburger. Before they left, they turned the sign to the apppropriate side to tell the child when he awoke that they were out using the telephone or eating.

For older children who know how to tell time, it is helpful to give them a clock or watch. However, these children have the same needs for honesty from their parents regarding visiting schedules. Because peer groups are also important, adolescents often appreciate planning visiting hours with their parents to provide them with some private time for friends.

Familiar surroundings also increase the child's adjustment to separation. If parents cannot room-in, they should leave favorite home articles with the child, such as a blanket, toy, bottle, feeding utensil, or article of clothing. Since young children associate such inanimate objects with significant people, they gain comfort and reassurance from such possessions. They make the association that if the parent left this, the parent will surely return. Placing an identification band on the toy lessens the chances of its being misplaced and provides a symbol that the toy is experiencing the same needs as the child. Other momentos of home include photographs and tape recordings of family members' reading a story, singing a song, saying prayers before bedtime, relating events at home, or taking a "talking walk" through the home. The tapes can be played at lonely times, such as on awakening or before sleeping (McCain, 1982). Some units allow pets to visit, which can be a special event for a child and can have therapeutic benefits (Davis, 1985).

Older children also appreciate familiar articles from home, particularly photographs, a radio, a favorite toy or game, and the usual pajamas. Often the importance of treasured objects for school-age children is overlooked or criticized. However, it is reported that about half of school-age children have a special object to which they formed an attachment in early childhood and that this is a normal and healthy phenomenon (Sherman and others, 1981). Therefore such treasured or transitional objects can help even older children feel more comfortable in a strange environment.

Helping children maintain their usual nonhome contacts by continuing school lessons during the period of illness and confinement, visiting with friends either directly or through letter writing or telephone calls, and participating in extracurricular projects whenever possible also minimizes the effects of separation imposed by hospitalization.

For extended hospitalizations youngsters enjoy personalizing the hospital room to make it "home" by decorating the walls with posters and cards, rearranging the furniture (when possible), and displaying a collection or hobby. Growing plants can also be a constructive activity as it gives the child something to care for (Fig. 26-3). Hardy and fast-growing plants are best, such as beans, sunflowers, and marigolds. A terrarium is useful for a child in an oxygen tent since it can be used to explain the oxygen cycle. When considering plants, the nurse needs to be aware that certain circumstances may preclude this activity, such as children with specific allergies or those who are susceptible to infections (Gough, 1986).

MINIMIZING LOSS OF CONTROL

Feelings of loss of control result from separation, physical restriction, changed routines, enforced dependency, magical thinking, and altered roles within the family or peer group. Although some of these, such as separation from parents,

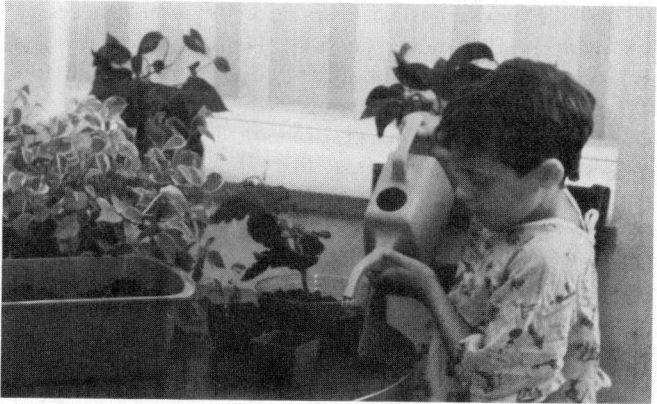

Fig. 26-3. For extended hospitalizations school-age children enjoy having projects to occupy their time, such as caring for plants.
Photography by John Roy, Saint Francis Hospital, Tulsa, OK.

cannot be prevented, most of them can be minimized through individualized planning of nursing care.

Physical Restriction

Younger children react most strenuously to any type of physical restriction or immobilization. Although some restraint, such as immobilizing an extremity for maintenance of an intravenous line, is frequently necessary, most physical restriction can be prevented if the nurse gains the child's cooperation.

For young children, particularly infants and toddlers, preserving parent-child contact is the best means of decreasing the need for or stress of restraint. For example, almost the entire physical examination can be done in a parent's lap, with the parent hugging the child for procedures such as otoscopy. For painful procedures the parents' preferences for assisting, observing, or waiting outside the room are assessed (see also Questions and controversies, p. 1107). Parents may not wish to participate in restraining the child either because of their own fear or because they do not want the child to associate them with the event. In this case the parents can be readily available to console the child immediately following the procedure. Older children may or may not wish their parents' presence, particularly if privacy is a concern.

Most children feel more in control when they know what to expect because the element of fear is reduced. Anticipatory preparation and information-giving is a significant method of lessening stress and often results in little need for physical restraint (see p. 1104 on preparing for procedures).

Environmental factors also influence the need for physical restraint. Keeping children in cribs or playpens may not represent immobilization in a concrete sense, but it certainly limits sensory stimulation. Increasing mobility by transporting children in carriages, wheelchairs, carts, wagons, or on stretchers or beds provides them with mechanical freedom. The choice of a transporting conveyance is discussed on p. 1120.

In some cases physical restraint or isolation is necessary for recovery. Whenever possible, restraints should be removed to allow the child some period of supervised freedom, such as during the bath or when parents visit. In those instances when restraints or isolation cannot be discontinued, such as in severe burns, the environment can be manipulated to increase sensory freedom. For example, moving the bed toward the door or window; opening window shades; providing musical, visual, or tactile toys; and increasing interpersonal contact can substitute mental mobility for the limitations of physical movement.

Altered Routines

Altered daily schedules and loss of rituals are particularly stressful for toddlers and early preschoolers and may increase the stress of separation. As discussed previously, the nursing admission history provides a baseline for planning care around the child's usual home activities.

Children's response to loss of routine and ritualism is often demonstrated in problems with activities such as feeding, sleeping, dressing, bathing, toileting, and social interaction. Although some regression is to be expected in all of these areas, sensitivity to the special needs of children can minimize the negative effects. For example, loss of appetite and marked food preferences are common in ill or hospitalized children. In addition, the food selections on hospital menus may differ greatly from preferred cultural or ethnic food preparation. Encouraging the child to eat while avoiding a battle is often a challenge, yet it is an essential nursing responsibility. Suggestions for feeding hospitalized children are discussed on p. 1115.

Although regression is expected and normal, nurses also have the responsibility of fostering children's optimum growth and development. There are instances during which hospitalization becomes a significant opportunity for learning and advancing. For example, extended hospitalization for long-term chronic illness or situations of failure to thrive, abuse, or neglect represent instances in which regression must be seen as an adjustment period, to be followed by plans for promoting appropriate developmental skills.

One of the aspects of altered routines that is frequently neglected is the change in the child's daily activities. A nonhospitalized child's day, especially during the school years, is structured with specific times for eating, dressing, going to school, playing, and sleeping. However, this time structure vanishes when the child is hospitalized. Although the nurses have a set schedule, the child is frequently unaware of it; new schedules are imposed that may be rigid or flexible. For example, some units have uniform nap and bedtimes for all children while others allow children to stay up very late. Many children obtain significantly less sleep in the hospital than at home; the primary causes are delay in sleep onset and early termination of sleep because of hospital routines (Hagemann, 1981a, 1981b). Not only are hours of sleep disrupted, but waking hours are spent in passive activities. For example, few institutions impose any regulation on the amount of time the child spends watching

ERIC'S DAILY SCHEDULE :

7:00 AM	– Breakfast, Watch TV, Brush Teeth, Wash up	3:00 PM	– Tutor (M,W,F) Study Time (T,Th)
9:00	– Tub Room, Dressing Change	4:00	– Physical Therapy
10:00	– Rest, TV, Snack	5:00	– Dinner
11:00	– Physical Therapy	6:30	– Dressing Change
12:00 PM	– Lunch	7:00 to 9:00	– TV, Reading, Snack, Friends Visit
1:00	– Playroom, Quiet Play, Rest, Friends Visit	9:00	– Brush Teeth, Wash up
		9:15	– Bedtime

Fig. 26-4. Time structuring is an effective strategy for normalizing the hospital environment and increasing the child's sense of control.

television. Studies show that children spend an average of 8 hours a day watching television in the hospital, an amount that is considerably longer than that spent at home (McCain and Bies, 1983).

One technique that can minimize the disruption in the child's routine is *time structuring* (Volz, 1981). This approach is most suitable for the noncritically ill school-age and adolescent child who has mastered the concept of time. It involves scheduling the child's day to include all those activities that are important to the nurse and child, such as treatment procedures, school work, exercise, television, playroom, and hobbies. Together, the nurse, parent, and child then plan a daily schedule with time and activity written down (Fig. 26-4). This is left in the child's room and a clock or watch is available for the child's use. Whenever possible, a calendar is also constructed with special events marked, such as favorite television programs, visits by friends or relatives, events in the playroom, and holidays or birthdays. If specific changes in treatment are expected ("beginning physical therapy in 2 days"), these are added.

Enforced Dependency

The dependent role of the hospitalized patient imposes tremendous feelings of loss on older children. Principal interventions should focus on respect for individuality and the opportunity for decision-making. Although these sound simple, their efficacy lies with nurses who are flexible, tolerant, and personally secure. The last is particularly important because when decision making is geared toward the patient, nurses can feel threatened by a sense of lessened control.

Promoting children's control involves maintaining independence and the concept of *self care* can be most beneficial. Self-care refers to the practice of activities that individuals personally initiate and perform on their own behalf in maintaining life, health, and well-being (Orem, 1985). While self-care is limited by the child's age and physical condition, most children beyond infancy can perform some activities with little or no help. Whenever possible, these activities are encouraged in the hospital. Other approaches include jointly planning care; time structuring; wearing street clothes; making choices in food selections, bedtime, and so on; continuing school activities; and rooming with an appropriate age-mate. For example, although school-age children may enjoy the responsibility of caring for a toddler or preschooler in their room, adolescents generally prefer quarters separate from the pediatric unit (see p. 1091).

Magical Thinking

Loss of control can occur from feelings of too little influence on one's destiny as well as from a sense of overwhelming control or power over fate. Although the cognitive abilities of preschoolers predispose them most significantly to magical thinking and self-power, all children are vulnerable to misinterpreting causes for stresses such as illness and hospitalization. As already pointed out, the principal reason for either crisis is believed to be punishment, which results in feelings of guilt, shame, self-reproach, and depression.

Maintaining a feeling of realistic control involves removing the magic from egocentric, magical thinking. This is best accomplished through age-appropriate preparation for hospitalization and related procedures, which is discussed on p. 1085 and in Chapter 27. It also involves repeatedly clarifying that illness occurs because of germs, accidents, inborn problems, or unknown causes.

Altered Family and Social Roles

In addition to the effects of separation on family roles, loss of parenting, sibling, and offspring roles may affect each family member differently. One of the most common reactions of parents is specialized and intensified attention toward the sick child. The other siblings usually regard this as unfair and interpret the parents' attitude toward them as rejection. Although such responses are usually unconscious and unintended, they place unique burdens on ill children. For example, the ill child may feel obligated to play the sick role in order to meet parents' expectations. This is especially frequent in children who have had limited physical ability and regain normal health status, such as following corrective heart surgery. Parents as well may be unable to perceive the child's recovery and therefore need to continue the pattern of overprotection and indulgent attention.

Ill children may also feel jealousy and resentment from other siblings. Because of their singular position in the family, they may be denied the companionship of their brothers and sisters. Rivalry between siblings tends to be greatest in the sibling who is nearest the ill child's age. Without an understanding of the interpersonal dynamics between siblings, parents are likely to blame the well children for antisocial behavior.

Illness may also result in children's loss of status within either their family or social group. For example, illness in the oldest child may temporarily terminate special privileges as "big" brother or sister. The hospitalized adolescent loses rank within the peer group. The effects of such losses have already been discussed.

MINIMIZING BODILY INJURY AND PAIN

Beyond early infancy all children fear bodily injury either from mutilation, bodily intrusion, body image change, disability, or death. In general, preparation of children for painful procedures decreases their fears. Manipulating procedural techniques for children in each age-group also minimizes fear of bodily injury. For example, since toddlers and young preschoolers are traumatized by insertion of a rectal thermometer, axillary temperatures or electronic temperature probes can effectively be substituted. Whenever procedures are performed on young children, the most supportive intervention is to do them as quickly as possible and maintain parent-child contact.

Children also need permission to express pain. Telling these children that the procedure may be uncomfortable but that it is all right to say "ouch," scream, or cry allows them to express their feelings in an atmosphere of support and acceptance.

Because of young children's poorly defined body boundaries, the use of bandages may be particularly helpful. For example, telling them that the bleeding will stop after the needle is removed does little to relieve their fears, whereas applying a small Band-Aid usually provides much reassurance. The size of bandages is also significant to children in this age-group. The larger the bandage, the more importance is attached to the wound. Using successively smaller surgical dressings is one way of their measuring healing and improvement. Prematurely removing a dressing may cause them considerable concern for their well-being.

In children who fear mutilation of body parts, repeatedly stressing the reason for a procedure and evaluating their understanding is essential in order to minimize fear. For example, explaining cast removal to preschoolers may seem simple enough, but the child's comprehension of the details may vary considerably from the explanation. Asking them to draw a picture of what they think will happen presents substantial evidence of the perceived events.

Children may fear bodily injury from a great variety of sources. X-ray machines, use of strange equipment for examination, unfamiliar rooms, or awkward positions can be perceived as potentially hazardous. In addition, thoughts and actions can be imagined sources of bodily damage. For older children masturbation or sex play may be perceived as powerful weapons of potential destruction. Therefore it is important to investigate imagined reasons, particularly of a sexual nature, for illness. Since children may fear revealing such thoughts, using projective techniques such as drawing or doll play may demonstrate previously undisclosed misconceptions.

Older children fear bodily injury of both internal and external origins. For example, school-age children are aware of the significance of the heart and may fear the actual operation as much as the pain, the stitches, and the possible scar. Adolescents may express concern for the actual procedure but be much more anxious over the resulting scar. An appreciation of each child's special concerns helps nurses focus on critical areas during preparation for proce-

Questions and Controversies

Are hospitalized children adequately medicated for pain?

Several studies have examined the pattern of pain medication for children as compared to adults and have found remarkably consistent findings—that children are grossly undermedicated for pain. Eland and Anderson (1977) investigated the incidence of administration of analgesics to 25 hospitalized children for postoperative pain. Twelve of the children received a total of 24 doses of analgesics; the remaining 13 children were never given any medication for pain relief. In contrast, 18 adults with identical diagnoses received 372 narcotic analgesic doses and 299 nonnarcotic analgesic doses for a total of 671 doses. One of the saddest findings was that more than twice as many children had pain medication ordered as received it. This lack of response to the need for pain medication directly relates to the nurses who failed to administer the analgesic.

Another study investigating analgesic prescriptions given to children and adults after open heart surgery found that all of the adults received medication for a total of 564 doses but only three fourths of the children were given medication for a total of 237 doses during the first 3 postoperative days. This difference was even greater on the fifth postoperative day when 83% of the adults continued to receive analgesics (a total of 136 doses) but only 12% of the children were medicated (a total of 10 doses) (Beyer and others, 1983). Another study on postoperative pain found that 75% of the children reported pain on the day of surgery and if orders for narcotic or nonnarcotic analgesics were written, the nonnarcotic was given exclusively. In addition, the doses ordered were usually too small and/or too infrequent to be maximally effective. The majority of orders were written "PRN," which was often interpreted by nursing staff as "as little as possible" (Mather and Mackie, 1983). Younger children are less likely to have narcotics offered and "PRN" orders may place these children at a further disadvantage because of their inability to communicate their discomfort (Schechter, Allen, and Hanson, 1986).

dures or giving explanations of the disease processes.

Children can grasp information only if it is presented on or close to their cognitive development. This necessitates an awareness of the words used to describe events or processes. The example of a 7-year-old who interpreted the doctor's statement of "there's edema in your belly" as "there's a demon in your belly" is proof of the necessity of choosing words carefully and reevaluating the child's understanding of the intended message (Perrin and Gerrity, 1981).

When a child is upset about his illness, his perception can be changed by (1) providing a somewhat different and less negative account of the disease or (2) by offering an explanation that is characteristic of the next stage of cognitive development (Bibace and Walsh, 1980). An example of the first strategy is reassuring a preschool child who fears that after a tonsillectomy, another sore throat means a second operation. Explaining that once tonsils are "fixed" they do not need fixing again can help relieve the fear. An example of the latter strategy is to explain that germs made the tonsils sick and even though germs can cause another sore throat, they cannot cause the tonsils to ever be sick again. This higher level explanation is based on the school age child's concept of germs as a cause of disease.

Pain Assessment

Pain assessment is a critical component of the nursing process. Several basic assumptions regarding pain perception and expression are important (Smith, 1976):

1. Pain is subjective, personal, and not directly communicable.
2. Pain is integrally interwoven with emotions such as fear, anxiety, anger, loneliness, or depression, and the emotion itself may increase the perception and expression of pain.
3. The expression of pain varies with age.
4. Nonverbal communication, specifically a change in behavior, precedes verbal communication of pain.

The first assumption has significant nursing implications because pain is a personal phenomenon that *cannot* be experienced by any other individual. Therefore defining what pain is in terms of another's perceptions is inappropriate and inaccurate. McCaffery (1979) offers an operational definition that is useful in clinical practice: *pain is whatever the experiencing person says it is, existing whenever he says it does*. This definition implies a very important attitude toward the patient—*that he is believed*. It is meant to encompass both verbal and nonverbal expressions of pain.

Unfortunately this definition is rarely applied in pediatrics (see Questions and controversies). Physicians and nurses tend to underestimate the existence of pain in children and to be conservative in their administration of analgesics. This practice may be attributed in part to the following *myths* (Eland, 1985a):

1. Children tolerate pain better than adults
2. Children cannot tell where it hurts
3. Children always tell the truth about pain
4. Active children are not in pain
5. Narcotics are dangerous drugs for children and cause addiction

Clinical practice and research have disproved such beliefs. Children's tolerance for pain actually increases with age (Haslam, 1969). Children beyond infancy can accurately point to the painful area or mark the site on a drawing. To avoid an injection, children may not admit having pain, or because of constant pain they may not realize how much they are suffering. Overactivity is frequently a behavioral response to hurting. And lastly, narcotics are no more dangerous for children than adults when given correctly; addiction is extremely rare (Porter and Jick, 1980).

Recognition of the existence and evaluation of the severity of pain is facilitated by an understanding of the developmental response to pain of children in each age-group, as well as the influence of factors such as cultural or ethnic background. While studies of cultural components of pain demonstrate some differences in children's descriptions of pain and comfort measures, the differences are slight and should not be overemphasized (Abu-Saad, 1984). Assessment of pain involves three primary areas: observation, questioning, and measurement tools.

Observe the child. A valuable tool in assessing pain is observing behavioral changes and physiologic responses. *Behavioral changes* are common indicators of pain in children, particularly in preverbal youngsters and those with mental retardation or sensory/communication deficits. Such changes include irritability, lethargy, loss of appetite, unusual quietness, disturbed sleep patterns, voluntary resting, increased restless movement or rigid posturing, flat affect, or anger. Specific reactions often indicate discomfort in localized body regions—such as rolling the head from side to side or pulling the ears for an earache, lying on the side with legs flexed on the abdomen for abdominal pain, or favoring a body part during usual activity. However, behavioral manifestations of pain vary widely and some children with more severe pain may show fewer facial and body movements than those with less pain (Hester, 1979).

The child's response to medication is another valuable indicator of pain. For example, in preverbal children who communicate a wide variety of emotions through behavior, obvious change in behavior following administration of an analgesic is evidence of existing pain. This knowledge can help in determining the cause of behaviors suggestive of pain, such as crying or restlessness. If after administering one dose of an analgesic the child's behavior changes, it is likely that the cause was pain, which requires further relief.

Physiologic responses indicating pain include flushing of the skin, increase in sweating, blood pressure, pulse and respiration, restlessness, and dilation of the pupils. However, these signs are very variable—for example, heart rate may actually decrease (Dale, 1986)—and they may be produced by emotions, such as fear, anger, or anxiety. They are seen primarily in acute pain from stimulation of the sympathetic nervous system. If pain persists, the body begins to adapt and there is a decrease or stabilization of these responses. Consequently, if nurses rely primarily on observing these physiologic indications before believing that pain exists, many instances of pain will go unrecognized.

Question the child and parent. Children can be excellent sources of information about pain and a pain history can be invaluable in providing basic information about the child's understanding and previous response to pain (Table 26-2). Although verbal indications are much less common in children than in adults, children can describe pain if asked the right questions. Children, even those up to preadolescence, do not necessarily understand the meaning of terms like "pain" and "discomfort" and have very limited use of descriptive words, such as "burning," "cramping," "severe," or "excruciating." Children may globally describe pain as, "I hurt," or "I don't feel good." Using a variety of words that may be associated with pain, such as "bad," "funny," "hot," "pushing," or "banging," may help them describe the sensation. Asking children to point to where it hurts or having them mark or color the area on a drawing, such as those on p. 1108, is also helpful and children as young as 4 years of age are able to accurately locate their pain on the drawing (Eland and Anderson, 1977).

Parents know their child and are sensitive to changes in behavior. However, there is no documentation of exactly how astute parents are in recognizing pain in their children. Some parents may never have seen their child in severe pain. However, others are aware that certain behaviors signal pain because the child has acted similiarly during previous painful events. To better assess the pain, the nurse can interview the parents about their knowledge of their child's previous pain experiences (Table 26-2). Ideally this questioning should occur before the child is in pain, such as on admission to the hospital.

Children will often reveal how they feel to parents because they are safe and trusted persons. It is not unusual for

Table 26-2 Pain experience inventory

QUESTIONS FOR PARENTS	QUESTIONS FOR CHILD
Describe any pain your child has had before.	Tell me what pain is.
How does your child usually react to pain?	Tell me about the hurt you have had before.
Does your child tell you or others when he/she is hurting?	What do you do when you hurt?
How do you know when your child is in pain?	Do you tell others when you hurt?
What do you do for your child when he/she is hurting?	What do you want others to do for you when you hurt?
What does your child do for him/herself when he/she is hurting?	What don't you want others to do for you when you hurt?
Which of these actions work best to decrease or take away your child's pain?	What helps the most to take away your hurt?
Is there anything special that you would like me to know about your child and pain? (If yes, have parent[s] describe.)	Is there anything special that you want me to know about you when you hurt? (If yes, have child describe.)

From Hester, N., and Barcus, C.: Assessment and management of pain in children. In Pediatrics: Nursing update 1(14):3, Princeton, NJ 1986, Continuing Professional Education Center, Inc.

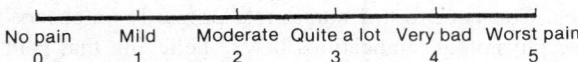

Fig. 26-5. Simple descriptive pain scale.

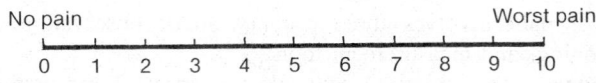

Fig. 26-6. Numeric pain scale.

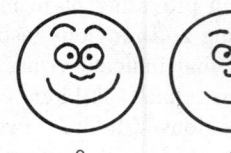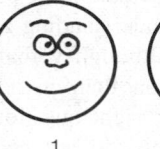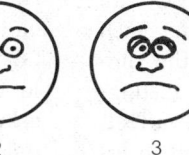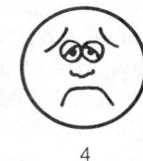

Fig. 26-7. Faces pain scale.

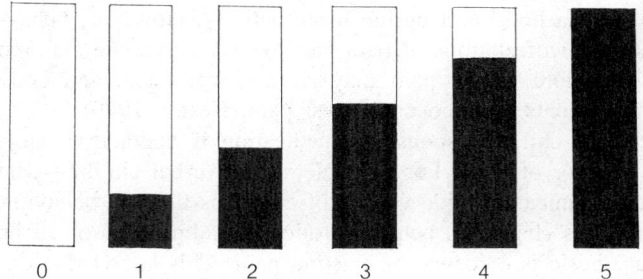

Fig. 26-8. Glasses pain scale.

a child who has been quiet to start crying when the parent visits and complain that he hurts. Nurses sometimes erroneously judge this behavior as seeking attention, when it represents the child's true feelings. The best intervention is to talk with the parent and child and to *believe* that the child hurts.

Use a pain rating scale. Numerous investigators have developed measurement tools or scales that use numeric values (usually from 0 to 5 or 10) to provide a quantitative measure of pain. However, most of the tools are designed for use with adults, although some tools have been developed specifically for children. Very little research has been conducted on the reliability and validity of these tools for children. Tools that are available and may be appropriate for different aged youngsters include the following.

The *simple descriptive scale* uses descriptive words to denote varying intensities of pain. The child chooses the one word that most nearly describes the pain (Fig. 26-5).

The *numeric scale* uses a straight line with the end points identified as "no pain" and "worst pain" and divisions along the line marked in units from 0 to 10. The child chooses the number that best describes the intensity of pain (Fig. 26-6).

The *faces scale* uses a series of faces; the first picture is a very happy smiling face and the last is a sad, tearful face. The pictures in between show varying degrees of happy or sad. The child chooses which face depicts the degree of pain during the procedure (Fig. 26-7).

The *glasses scale* is a drawing of six cylinders or "glasses," five of which are filled with increasing amounts of "pain." The first cylinder is empty and represents "no pain." The completely filled cylinder is the "worst or most pain." The glasses in between have from very little to a whole lot of pain. The child chooses the glass that has the amount of pain that best describes how he is feeling (Fig. 26-8).

The *chips scale* uses four white plastic chips. These chips are compared to pieces of hurt: one chip is a "little hurt" and four chips are the "most hurt." The child chooses the number of chips he feels equals his pain (Hester, 1979).

In the *color scale* the child is given eight crayons or markers (black, brown, purple, blue, green, red, orange, and yellow) and asked to choose a color that is like the "worst or most hurt," then another color that is like a "little less pain," another color for even less pain, and then a color for "no hurt." Another appoach is to ask the child to list painful events he has experienced, rank them from most to least painful, and assign a color to each. When four colors are ranked, a numeric value of 0 to 3 is assigned to the colors. The child then chooses the color that is most nearly like the pain he currently is experiencing (Eland, 1985b).

Pain Management

The reason for assessing pain is to relieve it. Certainly, comfort must be regarded as a basic need of all children, yet nurses and physicians are often reluctant to order analgesics for children. Effective pain management requires that health professionals be willing to try a number of interventions. Basically, methods to relieve pain can be grouped into two categories: nonpharmacologic and pharmacologic. Whenever possible, both of these should be used; however, nonpharmacologic measures should not be viewed as substitutes for analgesics.

Nonpharmacologic management. A number of nonpharmacologic techniques exist for lessening the perception of pain. These include (1) distraction, (2) relaxation, (3) guided imagery, (4) thought-stopping, (5) cutaneous stimulation, and (6) behavioral contracting (see box, p. 1071). These techniques can lessen the perception of pain,

SUGGESTIONS FOR NONPHARMACOLOGIC PAIN MANAGEMENT IN CHILDREN

General strategies

Prepare child in advance of potentially painful procedures but avoid "planting" idea of pain. For example, instead of saying "This is going to (or may) hurt," say "Sometimes this feels like pushing, sticking, or pinching and sometimes it doesn't bother people. You tell me what it feels like to you." This allows for variation in sensory perception, avoids suggesting pain, and gives the child control in describing reactions.

Avoid evaluative statements or descriptions, such as "This is a terrible procedure" or "It really will hurt a lot."

Stay with the child during a painful procedure; parents are often a neglected source of support for the child and can be involved in distracting him.

Use the power of positive suggestion by saying "I am giving you a medicine that *will* take the hurt away."

Reinforce the effect of the analgesic by telling the child he will begin to feel better in x amount of time (according to drug use); use a clock or timer to measure onset of relief with child; reinforce the cause and effect of pain—analgesic, so the child becomes conditioned to *expecting* relief.

Avoid saying "I am going to give you a shot for pain," since this is another pain in addition to the existing pain; if the child refuses an injection, explain that the little hurt from the needle will take away the bigger hurt for a long time.

Give child control whenever possible (e.g., choosing which leg for an injection, taking bandages off, holding the tape or other equipment).

Educate the child about the pain, especially when explanation may decrease anxiety (e.g., that the pain the child is experiencing is expected after surgery and does not indicate that something is wrong; reassure children that they are not responsible for the pain).

For long-term pain control give the child a doll that becomes "his patient" and allow him to do everything to the doll that is done to him; pain control can be emphasized through the doll by stating, "Dolly feels better after her medicine."

Specific strategies

Distraction

Involve parent and child in identifying strong distractors.

Involve child in play; use radio, tape recorder, record player; have him sing or use rhythmic breathing.

Have him concentrate on yelling or saying "ouch" by focusing on "yelling loud or soft as you feel it hurt; that way I know what's happening."

Relaxation

With infant or young child:

Hold in comfortable, well-supported position, such as vertically against chest and shoulder.

Rock in wide, rhythmic arc in rocking chair or sway back and forth, rather than bouncing child.

Repeat one or two words softly, such as "Mommy's here."

With slightly older child:

Ask to take deep breath and "go limp as a rag doll" while exhaling slowly, then ask child to yawn (demonstrate if needed).

Help child assume comfortable position (e.g., pillow under neck and knees).

Begin progressive relaxation: starting with the toes, systematically instruct child to let each body part "go limp" or "feel heavy;" if child has difficulty with relaxing, instruct him to tense or tighten each body part then relax it.

Guided imagery

Have child identify some highly pleasurable experience.

Have child describe the details of the event, write down the script, or record it.

Encourage the child to concentrate only on the pleasurable event during the painful time and/or enhance the image by recalling specific details, such as reading the script or playing the record.

Combine with relaxation.

Thought-stopping

Identify positive facts about painful event, such as "it does not last long."

Identify reassuring information, such as, "If I think about something else, it does not hurt as much."

Condense positive and reassuring facts into a set of brief statements and have child memorize them.

Have child repeat the memorized statements whenever he thinks about or experiences the painful event.

Cutaneous stimulation

Includes simple rhythmic rubbing; use of pressure; electric vibrator; massage with hand lotion, powder, or menthol cream; application of heat or cold, such as ice cube on site before giving injection or application of ice to site opposite the painful area (e.g., if right knee hurts, place ice on left knee).

Is most effective if rhythmic or constant and moderate in intensity.

Behavioral contracting

May be used informally with children as young as 4 or 5; use stars or tokens as rewards. For example, if child is uncooperative and procrastinates during a procedure, give him a limited amount of time (measured by a visible timer) to complete the procedure and if he is unable to comply, proceed as needed; if procedure is accomplished within the set time, reinforce cooperation with reward. With older children a written contract may be used (see p. 1113).

---

and, when used with analgesics, can enhance their effectiveness.

Pharmacologic management. Numerous nonnarcotic and narcotic analgesics exist; however, it is not the purpose of this discussion to describe individual drugs but to present general guidelines in selecting and administering analgesics. Two basic principles govern successful pharmacologic pain control:

1. Schedule the medication for *prevention* of pain
2. Titrate the dosage for maximum comfort

If pain is continuous, which often occurs postoperatively, the goal is relief of pain with maximum mental functioning. Administration of medications as needed (PRN) is not conducive to meeting this goal. Rather, scheduled medication times that are individualized for each child are necessary.

Date	Time[1]	Drug administered	Reason for drug administration[2]	Pain rating[3]	Respirations	Signature

[1]Record time of administering drug and assess analgesic effect 30 minutes later and then hourly.
[2]State reason in behavioral terms.
[3]Use pain rating scale.

Fig. 26-9. Pain assessment record.

The nurse plans such a schedule by anticipating that pain will be continuous, such as after certain procedures, or by recording for at least one 24-hour period the times of day when the child needs pain medication. Based on these findings, a *preventive* schedule of drug administration is plotted. For example, if the child complains of pain at 4- to 6-hour intervals, pain medication is given before the times the child would be expected to ask for it.

Dosage is increased or decreased as necessary to provide maximum relief. For example, if a prescribed dose fails to relieve pain, the dosage is increased until analgesia is achieved. Conversely, if the dosage causes excessive sleepiness, it is decreased gradually until the dose provides analgesia with minimal sedation. Successful manipulation of pain medication requires use of a pain flow chart that lists the time the medication was administered, the medication given, and an assessment or rating of pain at the time the drug is given and every hour thereafter until the next dose of analgesic (Fig. 26-9). This documentation provides evidence of the drug's effectiveness and facilitates collaboration with the physician regarding changes in medication orders.

Whenever possible, the oral form of the safest drug is used. For example, the effective use of oral nonnarcotic analgesics may eliminate the need for injectable narcotics. When pain is more severe, a very effective approach is the combination of a narcotic with a nonnarcotic analgesic. The rationale for combining the two is that pain is attacked at different physiologic levels—the central nervous system (narcotics) and the peripheral nervous system (nonnarcotics). By adding a nonnarcotic, analgesia may be significantly increased without increasing the narcotic dose.

When combining narcotics and nonnarcotics, it is important to take maximum advantage of the nonnarcotic. For example, Tylenol with codeine is available in several preparations, each with a constant dosage of Tylenol and varying amounts of codeine. If inadequate pain relief is achieved, it is preferable to add additional plain Tylenol before doubling the Tylenol with codeine dosage.

Morphine (0.1 to 0.2 mg/kg of body weight) is the narcotic of choice for severe pain; it is superior to Demerol, which has a very short duration of 2 to 4 hours. It is available for parenteral, oral, or rectal administration. The oral form and to a lesser extent the suppository form (Numorphan) are especially useful with children because they provide maximum pain relief without the trauma of an injec-

---

GUIDELINES FOR CONVERTING FROM IV OR IM TO PO ANALGESICS

Convert half the IV or IM dose to a PO dose, using equianalgesic charts.
For example: 10 mg MS, IV

$$\frac{1}{2} \text{ of } 10 \text{ mg} = 5 \text{ mg MS, IV}$$
$$= 30 \text{ mg MS, PO (1:6 parenteral to oral ratio)}$$

Administer half the IV dose and the PO dose.
For example: 5 mg MS, IV
              +30 mg MS, PO

Continue this schedule to ensure that the patient is comfortable.

Gradually decrease the PO dose while maintaining ½ IV dose if sedation is occurring.
For example: 5 mg MS, IV
              +25 mg MS, PO

When IV and PO dose cause analgesia without unwanted sedation, discontinue IV dose and double the PO dose.
For example: 50 mg MS, PO

---

tion. When large doses of morphine are required for intractable pain, continuous morphine infusion is effective.

When parenteral narcotics are required, every effort is made to switch to the oral route as soon as possible. However, conversion from parenteral to oral medication *must* be based on the equianalgesic doses for the drug and is usually best accomplished by gradually decreasing the parenteral dose and increasing the oral dose (see box). For example, if the child is receiving 5 mg of morphine by injection, he needs to receive 30 mg orally to achieve the same amount of analgesia. Table 26-3 lists common narcotics and their equianalgesic doses.

USE OF PLAY TO MINIMIZE STRESS

Play is one of the most important aspects of a child's life and one of the most effective tools for managing stress. Since illness and hospitalization constitute crises in the life of a child and these situations are often fraught with overwhelming stresses, to play out their fears and anxieties affords a means by which children can cope with these stresses.

Play is the "work" of children. It is essential to their mental, emotional, and social well-being, and, like their developmental needs, the need for play does not stop when

Table 26-3 Pediatric and equianelgesic dosages of selected narcotics

DRUG	DOSAGE (IM)*	EQUIANALGESIA IM (MG)	EQUIANALGESIA PO (MG)
Codeine	Newborn—not established Infants and children—0.5 mg per kg q 4 to 6 hours	130	200
Meperidine (Demerol)	1.1 to 1.6 mg per kg q 2 to 4 hours	75	300
Methadone	Children under 6 yrs—0.1 to .7 mg/24 hours Children over 6 yrs—2.5 mg/24 hours†	10	20
Morphine	0.1 to 0.2 mg per kg q 4 to 6 hours Rectal suppositories—dose not established but 5 mg suppository approximately equal in analgesia to 5 mg morphine IM	10	60‡

*IV dose is half IM does, given very slowly.

†In clinical practice a higher dose than that recommended has been found necessary to achieve analgesia. The dose ranged from 2.5 to 40 mg q 4 to 12 hours with a "typical dose" being 5 to 10 mg q 6 to 8 hours. (Martinson, I., and others: Nursing care in childhood cancer: methadone, AJN, **82**(3):432-435, 1982.)

‡For relief of chronic pain, the parenteral-oral ratio may decrease to 1:2 or 1:3, although this is controversial (Kaiko, A.: Controversy in the management of chronic cancer pain: therapeutic equivalents of IM and PO morphine, J. Pain Sympt. Manag. **1**:42-45, 1986.)

NOTE: Research has not proven that the above recommended doses are effective in relieving pain. Rather, clinical experience has shown that these doses are safe for most children.

Children metabolize narcotics faster than adults. Therefore doses need to be given more frequently for optimum pain control. Long-acting drugs such as methadone are preferable in treating prolonged pain.

children are ill or when they enter the hospital. On the contrary, play in the hospital serves many functions:

1. Provides diversion and brings about relaxation.
2. Helps the child feel more secure in a strange environment.
3. Helps to lessen stress of separation and the feelings of homesickness.
4. Provides a means for release of tension and expression of feelings.
5. Encourages interaction and development of positive attitudes toward others.
6. Provides an expressive outlet for creative ideas and interests.
7. Provides a means for accomplishing therapeutic goals (see box, p. 1111).

Probably of all hospital facilities no room does more to alleviate the stressors of hospitalization than the playroom. In this room children temporarily distance themselves from the fears of separation, loss of control, and bodily injury. They can work through their feelings in a nonthreatening, comfortable atmosphere and in the manner that is most natural for them. They also know that the boundaries of this room are safe from intrusive or painful procedures, strange faces, and probing questions. The playroom becomes a sanctuary of peace and safety in an otherwise frightening environment.

Children in various age-groups require different types of play facilities. Infants and toddlers need maximum safety, whereas school-age children and adolescents benefit most from group recreation. Providing space for special needs of children in each age-group can be difficult in overcrowded institutions, but innovative solutions can assure practical answers. Playroom schedules can accommodate children in one age-group at one session and another group at a later

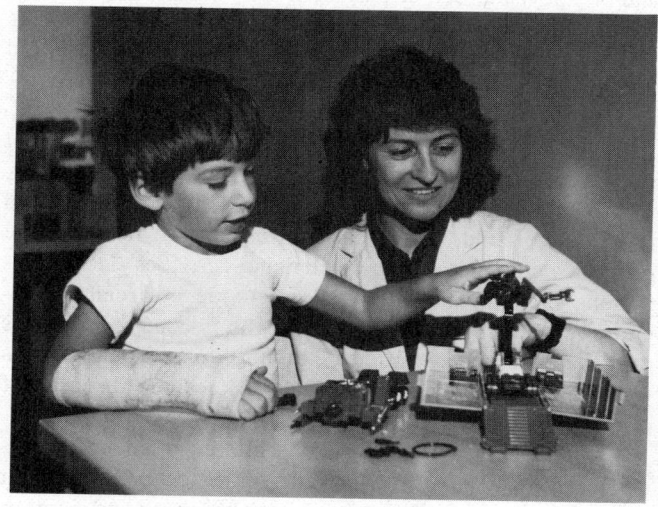

Fig. 26-10. Play materials for hospitalized children need to be appropriate for their age, interests, and limitations.
Photography by John Roy, Saint Francis Hospital, Tulsa, OK.

time; for example, adolescents can use the facility in the evening when younger children are asleep. Older children can also congregate in one patient's room and listen to music, play games, or just talk about their experiences. If the location of the recreational session is rotated each evening, older children can look forward to arranging or setting up for the activities.

Diversional Activities

Almost any form of play can be used for diversion and recreation, but the activity should be selected on the basis of the child's age, interests, and limitations (Fig. 26-10). Children do not necessarily need special direction for using play materials. All they require is the raw materials with which to work and adult approval and supervision to help keep their natural enthusiasm or expression of feelings from getting out of control. Small children enjoy a variety of small, colorful toys that they can play with in bed or in their room or more elaborate play equipment, such as playhouses, sandboxes, rhythm instruments, and large boxes and blocks, that may be a part of the hospital playroom.

Games that can be played alone or with another child or an adult are popular with older children, as are puzzles; reading material; quiet individual activities such as sewing, stringing beads, and weaving; and Tinker-Toys, Lego blocks, and other building materials. Assembling models is an excellent pasttime, but it is a good idea to make certain that all pieces and necessary materials are included in the package. It is disappointing to the child to be ready to begin a project only to find that an essential item, such as glue, is missing from the set.

Well-selected books are of infinite value to the child. Children never tire of stories. To have someone read aloud provides endless hours of pleasure and is of special value to the child who has limited energy to expend in play. A radio and/or television set, a part of most hospital room equipment, is a useful tool for entertaining a child, but parents and nurses should monitor program selection and it should not be used as a substitute for social interaction or therapeutic play.

When supervising play for ill or convalescent children, it is best to select activities that are simpler than would normally be chosen according to the specific developmental level of the child. These children usually do not have the energy to cope with more challenging activities. Other limitations also influence the type of activities. Special consideration must be given to the child who is confined in terms of movement, has a restricted extremity, or is isolated. Toys for isolated children must be capable of being disposed of or disinfected after use.

Toys. Parents of hospitalized children often ask nurses about the types of toys that would be best to bring for their child. Most want to bring new ones to cheer and comfort the child and assuage their own guilt feelings regarding the child's need for hospitalization. It is wise to assure the parents that, although it is natural to want to provide these things for their child, it is often better to wait awhile to bring new things, especially in the case of younger children. Small children need the comfort and reassurance of familiar things, such as the stuffed animal the child hugs for comfort and takes with him to bed at night. These are a link with home and the world outside the hospital.

Large numbers of toys often confuse and frustrate a small child. A few small, well-chosen toys are usually preferred to one large expensive one. Children who are hospitalized for an extended time benefit from changes. Rather than a confusing accumulation of toys, older toys should be replaced periodically as interest wanes. A helpful suggestion is to have parents provide the child with a shoe box, a child's small suitcase, or knapsack to attach to the bed for an easy storage receptacle to prevent small items from becoming lost in the sheets or under the bed. Children love putting things in and taking things out of a larger container. Many simple items, such as a small magnifying glass, a magnet, grooming aids, a small mirror, crayons and coloring books, colorful paper with scissors and paste, a magic slate, small dolls or toy soldiers, small cars, and beads to string, afford endless hours of amusement. It is the responsibility of the nurse to assess the safety of the toys brought to the child.

A highly successful diversion for a child who is hospitalized for a length of time and whose parents are unable to visit frequently is for them to bring a box with seven small, inexpensive, and brightly wrapped items with a different day of the week printed on the outside. The child will eagerly anticipate the time for opening each one. When the parents know when their next visit will be, they can provide the number of packages that corresponds to the days between visits. In this way the child knows that the diminishing packages also represent the anticipated visit from the parent.

Expressive Activities

Play provides one of the best opportunities for encouraging emotional expression, including the safe release of anger and hostility. Nondirective play that allows children freedom for expression can be tremendously therapeutic. Therapeutic play, however, should not be confused with the psychologic technique of play therapy. *Play therapy* is reserved for use by trained and qualified therapists who use the technique as an interpretative method with emotionally disturbed children. *Therapeutic play,* on the other hand, is a very effective nondirective modality for helping children deal with their concerns and fears, whereas at the same time it often helps the nurse to gain insights into their needs and feelings (Clatworthy, 1981).

Tension release can be facilitated through almost any activity and, with younger ambulatory children, large-muscle activity such as use of tricycles and wagons is especially beneficial. A great deal of aggression can be safely directed into pounding and throwing games and activities. Bean bags are often thrown at a target or open receptable with surprising vigor and hostility. A pounding board is employed with enthusiasm by young children; clay and Play-Doh are marvelous media for use at any age. It is not uncommon to see an angry child of 9 or 10 years of age attacking a mound of clay with the same intensity that is observed in his 3- or 4-year-old counterpart.

Creative expression. Drawing and painting are excellent media for expression. The child needs only to be supplied with the raw materials, such as crayons and paper; plots of bright poster color, large brushes, and an ample supply of newsprint supported on easels; or materials for finger painting. Children usually require little direction for

Nursing Care Summary: The Hospitalized Child

NURSING GOALS	NURSING INTERVENTIONS	EXPECTED PATIENT/FAMILY OUTCOMES
A-EP	**Diversional activity, deficit** **Etiology: hospitalization, effects of illness**	
Provide opportunity for play	Allow ample time for play Make play materials available to the child Encourage play activities and diversions appropriate to the child's age, condition, and capabilities Use play as a teaching strategy and an anxiety-reducing technique Provide diversional activities or consult with child-life specialist Encourage interaction with other children Choose a roommate compatible in age, sex, and physical abilities Monitor time spent watching television versus interactive or creative activities	Child engages in age-appropriate diversional activities (specify)
CPP	**Comfort, alteration in: pain** **Etiology: discomfort/pain related to illness or therapies**	

Modify procedures to minimize discomfort	Avoid intrusive procedures
	   Take axillary temperatures
	   Administer medications orally or through an existing intravenous route
	 Use restraints only when necessary
	 Allow child to sit rather than lie down, if feasible, during procedures
	 Maintain child's contact with parent
	 Keep strange and potentially frightening equipment out of view
	 Use correct technique (for intramuscular injections, see p. 1138)
		Child displays evidence of only minimal discomfort

Increase control during procedures	Warn child before implementing a procedure
	   Wake a sleeping child
	 Offer choices only when they exist
	 Avoid undue delay during a procedure
	 Apply a small bandage after injections in young children
	 Allow expression of feelings, such as crying, saying "ouch"
	 Praise for cooperation
	   Give small reward, such as star, sticker, badge
	 See also guidelines for preparing children for procedures, (p. 1104)
		Child expresses discomfort but maintains some degree of control

Assess pain	See suggestions (p. 1068)	
Manage pain	Implement both nonpharmacologic and pharmacologic techniques (p. 1070)	Same as above
SP-SCP	**Anxiety** **Etiology: separation from support system; unfamiliar environment**	

Prevent or minimize separation	Provide consistency of nursing personnel as much as possible; assign a primary nurse
	 Arrange workload and schedule to allow personal contact with the child
	 Encourage parents to room-in whenever possible
	 Provide an atmosphere of warmth and acceptance for both child and parents
	 Encourage parents and others to cuddle, fondle, and otherwise demonstrate affection for the child
	 Recognize the child's separation behaviors as normal
	   Allow the child to cry
	   Provide support through physical presence
		Child has consistent caregivers
		
		 Parents visit as much as possible
		
		 Parents cooperate in care (specify)

Continued.
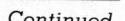

Nursing Care Summary: The Hospitalized Child—cont'd

NURSING GOALS	NURSING INTERVENTIONS	EXPECTED PATIENT/FAMILY OUTCOMES

Prevent or minimize separation—cont'd	Maintain the child's contact with his parents and siblings
	  Talk about his parents frequently
	  Encourage the child to talk about and remember parents
	  Stress the significance of the parents' visits, telephone calls, or letters
		Child discusses his family, including pets

	Help the parents understand the behaviors of separation anxiety and suggest ways of supporting the child
	  Explain to the child when they leave and when they will return
	  Tell the hospitalized child the reason for leaving
	  Convey the expected time of return in terms of anticipated events. For example, if the parents return in the morning, they can tell the child that they will see him, "After the sun comes up," or, "When (a favorite program) is on television"
		Parents demonstrate an understnading of separation behaviors

	Use a clock or calendar for an older child Visit for short but frequent times rather than one long time; encourage parents and relatives to take turns visiting Allow siblings to visit Leave favorite home articles, such as a blanket, toy, bottle, feeding utensil, or article of clothing, with the child Respect treasured objects of older children, such as a stuffed animal	Siblings visit as much as possible Family provides the child with familiar and/or cherished articles from home

	Encourage family to provide photographs of family members and tape recordings of the parents' voices, such as reading a story, singing a song, saying prayers before bedtime, or relating events at home
	  Play tape recordings at lonely times, such as before sleep
	  Encourage child to talk about family members
	Suggest that the family leave small gifts for the child to open each day; if parents know when their next visit will be, have them leave the number of packages that correspond to the days between visits	

	Assign "foster grandparent" or consistent volunteer to the child if available	Assigned person spends time with the child (specify amount of time)
Establish a trusting relationship with the child	Be positive in approach to the child Be honest with the child Convey to the child behaviors expected of him Be consistent in expectations and in relationships with the child Treat the child fairly and help him to feel that he is being treated fairly	Child develops rapport with primary nurse
	Encourage parents to maintain a truthful relationship with the child	Child maintains trust of family.
Allow expression of feelings	Accept expression of feelings Provide an atmosphere that encourages free expression of feelings Provide opportunities for the child to verbalize, "play out," or otherwise express feelings without fear of punishment	Child verbalizes or plays out feelings or concerns

Help the child to feel he is cared for as a person	Maintain the child's identity
	  Address the child by name or usual nickname
	  Avoid assigning a nickname to the child or converting a given name to its counterpart in another language, such as Joe instead of José
		Child interacts with staff
		*Staff demonstrate respect for the child

*Nursing outcome

Nursing Care Summary: The Hospitalized Child—cont'd

NURSING GOALS	NURSING INTERVENTIONS	EXPECTED PATIENT/FAMILY OUTCOMES
	Avoid communicating any signals of rejection, distaste, or other negative feelings to the child Criticize or communicate disapproval of unacceptable *behavior* not disapproval of the *child* Communicate (verbally and nonverbally) to the child that he is a valued person	
Allow for regression during periods of illness	Recognize that regressive behavior is a feature of illness Accept regressive behavior and help the child with his dependency Assist the child in reconquering the negative counterpart of the psychosocial stage to which he has regressed, for example, overcome mistrust; facilitate development of trust	*Staff and parents exhibit an attitude of acceptance of regressive behaviors
Reduce or alleviate fear of the unknown	Help parents to prepare the child for elective hospitalization Explain routines, items, procedures, and events in a language appropriate to the child's developmental level; use simple language Reassure the child and repeat reassurance as necessary Absolve the child from any guilt he might feel regarding his hospitalization Allow the parent(s) to participate in the child's care Allow the child to handle items that he may perceive as strange and/or threatening	Child exhibits understanding of information presented (specify information and means of demonstration)

SP-SCP   Powerlessness
Etiology: health care environment

Modify the hospital environment to resemble home	Determine from parents or other caregiver the child's customary routine and manner of handling (see nursing admission history, p. 1088) Maintain routine similar to the one the child is accustomed to at home Minimize hospital-like environment as much as possible, allow the child to sit at a table to eat meals, wear own pajamas, and so on Use terms familiar to the child, such as those for body functions	Child's routines and environment are similar to those at home (specify)
Provide opportunities for acceptable control	Allow child choices whenever possible, such as food selection, clothing, options for time of basic care (bath, play, bedtime), selection of television channels Use time structuring with older child, a jointly planned and written schedule of daily activities Permit freedom on the unit within defined and enforced limitations Limit use of restraints Encourage self-care according to child's abilities Assign tasks to older child, especially if extended hospitalization—such as making bed, supervising younger children, distributing menus, collating charts Respect need for privacy	Child participates in planning care (specify) Child moves about the unit but respects limits Child participates in care activities (specify activities) Child assumes responsibility for tasks (specify)

*Nursing outcome.

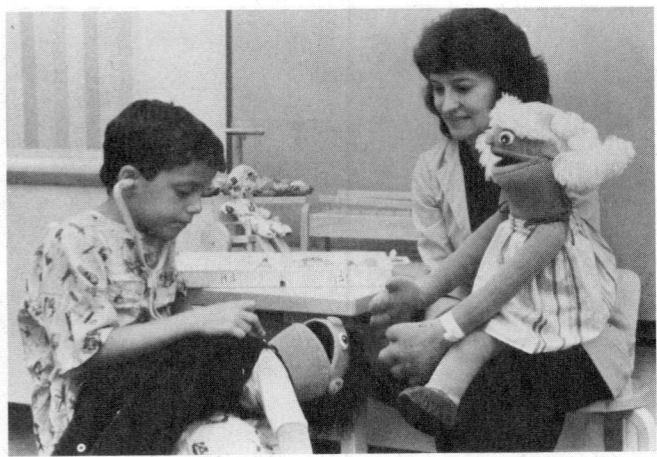

Fig. 26-11. Playing with miniature hospital equipment and puppets allows children to safely explore feelings and concerns. Photography by John Roy, Saint Francis Hospital, Tulsa, OK.

self-expression; however, older children may be given some direction in what to paint or draw. For example, they may be asked to draw the hospital room, draw what they like about the hospital, or draw what they do not like about the hospital. Groups of children can enjoy this creative activity either working individually or, with older children, collaborating on a group project such as a mural painted on a long piece of paper. For children confined to bed, an old sheet (acquired from the laundry) spread over the bed and a large gown that extends down over the bedclothes to cover their own gown provide protection for clean linen.

Holidays provide stimulus and direction for unlimited creative projects. The children can participate in decorating the pediatric unit, and making pictures and decorations for their rooms gives the children a sense of pride and accomplishment. This is especially beneficial for immobilized and isolated children. Making gifts for someone at home helps to maintain interpersonal ties.

Dramatic play. Dramatic play is a well-recognized technique for emotional release, allowing children to reenact frightening or puzzling hospital experiences. Through use of puppets, replicas of hospital equipment, or some actual hospital equipment, children can play out the situations that are a part of their hospital experience. Dramatic play enables children to learn about procedures and events that will concern them and to assume the roles of the adults in the hospital environment.

Puppets are universally effective for communicating with children. Most children view them as peers and readily communicate with them. Children will relate to the puppet feelings that they hesitate to express to adults. Puppets can share children's own experiences and help them to find solutions to their problems. Puppets dressed to represent figures in the child's environment—for example, a physician, nurse, child patient, therapist, and members of the child's own family—are especially useful (Fig. 26-11). Small, ap-

propriately attired dolls are equally effective in encouraging the child to play out situations, although puppets are usually best for direct conversation.

In planning any play activities for the hospitalized child, the nurse must not lose sight of the fact that the reason for the child's hospitalization always takes precedence over other considerations, including the need for play. Play must be scheduled around medical needs and any limitations imposed by the child's condition. For example, it is not uncommon for small children to eat paste and other creative media; therefore, a child who is allergic to wheat should not be given finger paint made from wallpaper paste or play dough made with flour. A child on a restricted salt intake should not play with modeling dough, since salt is one of its major constituents. Treatment schedules and the rules and policies of the institution must be considered, also. At home the play program should be planned around the therapy regimen. However, play can be satisfactorily incorporated into the child's care if the nurse and others involved allow some flexibility and use creativity in planning for play.

MAXIMIZING POTENTIAL BENEFITS OF HOSPITALIZATION

While hospitalization generally represents a stressful time for children and families, it also presents an opportunity for facilitating positive change within the child and among family members. Therefore nursing interventions must also focus on maximizing the potential benefits of the experience.

Fostering Parent-Child Relationships

The crisis of illness and/or hospitalization can mobilize parents into more acute awareness of the needs of their children. For example, one school-age child who was diagnosed with a serious physical condition commented to the nurse that he ''enjoyed'' the hospital because it was the first time that he had seen so much of his parents. He expressed concern over discharge because he anticipated the loss of the intensified love and attention. The nurse was able to discuss these feelings with the parents and to increase their awareness of their child's need for them.

Hospitalization provides opportunities for parents to learn more about their children's growth and development. When parents are helped to understand children's usual reactions to stress, such as regression or aggression, they are not only better able to support the child through the hospital experience but also may extend their insights into child-rearing practices following discharge.

Difficulties in parent-child relationships that may result in feeding problems, negative behavior, and enuresis may decrease during hospitalization. The temporary cessation of such problems sometimes alerts parents to the role they may be playing in propagating the negative behavior. With assistance from health professionals, parents can restructure ways of relating to their children to foster more positive behavior.

Hospitalization may also represent a temporary reprieve or refuge from a disturbed home. Typically abused or neglected children's dramatic physical and social improvement during hospitalization is proof of the growth potential of this experience. Hospitalized children temporarily are able to seek support, reassurance, and security from new relationships, particularly with nurses, hospitalized peers, and others.

Providing Educational Opportunities

Illness and hospitalization represent excellent opportunities for children and other family members to learn more about their bodies, each other, and the health professions. For example, during a hospital admission for a diabetic crisis, the child may learn about his disease, the parents may learn about the child's needs for independence, normalcy, and appropriate limits, and each of them may find a new support system in the hospital staff.

During extended hospitalization, special tutoring can help a child advance his studies and concentrate on subjects that were difficult. The child's relationship with a tutor can foster a more positive attitude toward school and learning.

Illness or hospitalization can also help older children in choosing a vocational career. Frequently children have impressions of physicians or nurses that are disproportionately glorified or horrified. However, actual experience with different health professionals can influence their decision for or against a health career.

For example, an adolescent who was hospitalized for an orthopedic problem related to the nurse that she had no idea of what she would like to do following graduation. She was steadily dating a young man who had asked her to marry him. She admitted that she liked, but did not love, him. However, she saw marriage and child-bearing as a substitute role for a career. She also confided that she was sexually active with him but did not fear a pregnancy, since that would "make up her mind" about marriage. The nurse recognized the adolescent's superficial motives for marriage and focused her discussions on possible careers. The girl stated that she had always wanted to become a nurse but that she did not like "hurting people." She had never seen nurses "supporting" people by talking with them. As a result of her several-week hospital stay and her trusting relationship with her nurse, she made definite plans with her school guidance counselor to begin nursing education, began birth control measures, and continued to see her boyfriend, but with marriage as a possible long-range goal.

Promoting Self-Mastery

The experience of facing a crisis such as illness or hospitalization, coping successfully with it, and maturing as a result of it constitutes an opportunity for self-mastery. Younger children have the chance to test out fantasy vs reality fears. They realize that they were not abandoned, mutilated, castrated, or punished. In fact, they were loved, cared for, and treated with respect for their individual concerns. It is not unusual to hear children who have undergone hospitalization or surgery tell others of how "it was nothing" or proudly display their scars or bandages. For older children hospitalization may represent an opportunity for decision-making, independence, and self-reliance. They are proud of having survived the experience and may feel a genuine self-respect for their achievements. Nurses can facilitate such feelings of self-mastery by emphasizing aspects of personal competence in the child and avoiding paying attention to uncooperative or negative behavior.

Providing Socialization

Hospitalization may offer children a special opportunity for social acceptance. Lonely, asocial, sometimes delinquent children find a sympathetic environment in the hospital. Children who are physically deformed or in some other way "different" from their age-mates may find an accepting social peer group. Although this does not always spontaneously occur, nurses can structure the environment to foster a supportive child group. For example, judicious selection of a roommate can help a child gain a new friend and learn more about himself. Forming relationships with significant members of the health care team, such as the physician, nurse, child life specialist, or minister, can greatly enhance the child's adjustment in many areas of life.

Parents may also encounter a new social group in other parents who have similar problems. The waiting room or hallway "self-help" groups are inherent to every institution. Nurses can capitalize on this informal gathering by encouraging parents to collectively discuss their concerns and feelings. They can also refer parents to organized parent groups or can use the help and support of recovered hospitalized patients.

SUPPORTING FAMILY MEMBERS

The term *family-centered care* defines the focus of pediatric care because nursing of children cannot be optimally performed unless each family member is designated the "patient" or "client." Support involves the willingness to stay and listen to parents' verbal and nonverbal messages. Sometimes the support is not given directly by the nurse. For example, the nurse may offer to stay with the child to allow the parents time alone or may discuss with other family members the parents' need for extra relief. Often extended relatives and friends want to help but do not know how. Suggesting ways such as baby-sitting, preparing meals, tending the garden or home, doing laundry, or transporting the siblings to school lessens the responsibilities that burden parents.

Support may also be provided through the clergy. Parents

GUIDELINES FOR HELPING FAMILIES ELICIT INFORMATION

Find out what the family wants to know.
Teach them to avoid general questions, such as "Why is my child sick?"
Help them prepare specific questions, such as "What is causing my child's pain?" or "What does this drug do?"
Encourage the use of short and open-ended questions.
Have the family write down the questions, preferably in a diary or journal that is kept in an accessible area, such as a pocket, to have available when needed.
Encourage the family to speak up when they do not understand an answer and to have it explained in clearer or easier language.
Have the family repeat the information to be certain they understand it and to record unfamiliar terms.

Modified from Norris, L.: Coaching the question, Nursing 86 **16**(5):100, 1986.

with deep religious beliefs may appreciate the counsel of a clergy member, but because of their stress they may not have sufficient energy to initiate the contact. Nurses can be supportive by arranging for clergy to visit and by respecting and upholding parents' religious beliefs.

Support involves an acceptance of cultural, socioeconomic, and ethnic values. For example, health and illness are defined differently by various ethnic groups. For some, disorders that have few outward manifestations of illness, such as diabetes, hypertension, or cardiac problems, are not viewed as a sickness. Consequently, following a prescribed treatment may be seen as unnecessary. Nurses who appreciate the influences of culture are more likely to intervene therapeutically (see also Chapter 2 for an extensive discussion of cultural and religious influences on health care).

Parents need help in accepting their own feelings toward the ill child. If given the opportunity, parents often disclose their feelings of loss of control, anger, and guilt. They often resist admitting to such feelings because they expect others to disapprove of behavior that is less than perfect. Unfortunately health personnel, including nurses, sometimes do exercise little tolerance for deviation from the expected norm. This only increases the psychologic impact of a child's illness on family members. Helping parents identify the specific reason for such feelings and emphasizing that each is a normal, expected, and healthy response to stress provides them with an opportunity to lessen their emotional burden.

Providing Information

One of the most important nursing interventions is to provide information regarding (1) knowledge of the disease, its treatment, and prognosis; (2) awareness of the child's emotional, as well as physical, reaction to illness and hospitalization; and (3) anticipation of the probable emotional reactions of family members to the crisis.

For many families the child's illness is the first contact they have with hospital personnel and uncertainty about hospital rules often adds to feelings of confusion and anxiety. Therefore the family needs clear explanations about what to expect and what is expected of them. Nurses can also help family members become more adept at seeking information about their child's condition by asking questions that elicit meaningful information (see box).

In giving information, nurses need to be alert to information overload. Signs in adults or children that signal increasing anxiety or decreasing attention from too much information are (Ritchie, 1979):

1. Long periods of silence
2. Wide eyes and fixed facial expression
3. Constant fidgeting or attempting to move away
4. Playing with toys unrelated to the topic of discussion
5. Changing the subject and sudden disruptions, such as asking to go to the bathroom
6. Looking around
7. Yawning

Parents also need to be aware of the effects of illness on the family and strategies that prevent negative changes. Specifically, parents should keep the family well informed and communicating as much as possible. They should treat all the children as equally and as normally as before the illness occurred. Discipline, which initially may be lessened for the ill child, should be continued to provide a measure of security and predictability. When ill children know that their parents expect certain standards of conduct from them, they feel certain that they will recover. Conversely, when all limits are removed, they fear that something catastrophic will happen.

Helping parents understand and accept the meaning of posthospitalization behaviors in the sick child is necessary for them to tolerate and support such behaviors. Consequently, they should be forewarned of the usual continuance of such reactions following discharge. Parents who do not expect such reactions may misinterpret them as evidence of the child's "being spoiled" and demand perfect behavior at a time when the child is still reacting to the stress of illness and hospitalization. If the behaviors, especially the demand for attention, are dealt with in a supportive manner, most children are able to relinquish them and assume precrisis levels of functioning.

Nurses should also forewarn parents of the reactions of siblings to the ill child—particularly anger, jealousy, and resentment. Older siblings may deny such reactions because they provoke feelings of guilt. However, everyone needs outlets for emotions, and the repressed feelings may surface as problems in school, with age-mates, as psychosomatic illnesses, or in delinquent behavior.

Probably one of the most neglected areas involves giving information to siblings. Frequently age becomes the only factor that leads to an awareness of this problem, because older children may begin to ask questions or request expla-

Nursing Care Summary: The Family of the Hospitalized Child

NURSING GOALS	NURSING INTERVENTIONS	EXPECTED PATIENT/FAMILY OUTCOMES
SP-SCP **Anxiety**		
Etiology: situational crisis, threat to role functioning, change in environment		
Help family adjust to the hospital	Introduce family to significant staff members Describe hospital routine that affects the child Acclimate family to the new and strange surroundings 　Physical layout of unit including playroom, unit kitchen, toilet, telephone, where they can stay, etc. Direct family to areas they may need to use outside the unit, (e.g., dining room, chapel) Provide an atmosphere that promotes questioning, expression of doubts and feelings Be available to family Be alert to signs of tension in family members Provide for privacy	Family demonstrates familiarity with hospital environment Family members ask questions
Make family feel important as members of the health team	Employ a polite approach and demeanor Greet family by name when they arrive on the unit Encourage frequent visiting Include family in planning patient care Encourage family to select and assume specific roles in the child's care Offer encouragement for their efforts Ask family to share with the staff what they know about the child's care and needs Convey an attitude of collegiality with family—not competition	Family becomes involved in planning and carrying out care for the child
Reduce apprehension	Allow for expression of feelings about the child's hospitalization Provide needed information Prepare family for what to expect (e.g., procedures, behaviors, happenings) Explore family's concerns and feelings of irritation, guilt, anger, disappointment, inadequacy Explore family's fears and anxieties regarding the child's status and expectations of results of procedures or therapy Introduce parents to other families who have a child in the hospital—especially a child who is similarly affected Provide something legitimate for them to focus on (e.g., a small task such as assuring a specified amount of fluid, collecting a specimen)	Family members verbalize feelings and concerns Family demonstrates an understanding of procedures and behaviors (specify manner of demonstration and learning) Family interacts with other families Family complies with directions (specify)
Prepare family for special procedures (x-ray, diagnostic tests, surgery)	Assess family's understanding of the procedure and its purpose Provide needed information, clarify misconceptions Explain special preparation needed (e.g., NPO, shaving, preprocedure medication or equipment) Describe 　Where the child will be during the procedure 　Whether the family can be with the child 　Where the family can wait 　Approximate length of time procedure requires Reassure family that they will be notified regarding progress of the procedure	Family demonstrates an understanding of procedures and tests (specify)
Support the family during child's absence	Provide a comfortable place for the family to wait Suggest activities to help reduce anxiety (e.g., go to the coffee shop or dining room, take a short walk [specify activity]) Be available to family Make contact with family at frequent intervals to relay information, provide comforts, etc.	Family takes advantage of suggestions (specify)

Continued.

Nursing Care Summary: The Family of the Hospitalized Child—cont'd

NURSING GOALS	NURSING INTERVENTIONS	EXPECTED PATIENT/FAMILY OUTCOMES

Help family adjust to the child's appearance and behavior following procedure(s) or in special care unit	Remain calm
	Describe the environment, if appropriate (e.g., ICU)
	Apply principles of learning to explanations
	    Begin with small amounts of information
	    Begin with very general information
	    Allow ample time for family to absorb information and to ask questions
	Explain how the child will look and the reasons for his appearance and equipment
	Explain what the child is experiencing
	Prepare the child and his environment to lessen the impact of first impression
	    Tidy the bed
	    Personalize the bed and bedside with a toy or other item(s)
	    Provide chairs for the family
	    Be prepared for possible adverse reaction (e.g., fainting)
	Convey an attitude of caring *about* as well as *for* the child
	Accompany the family to the child's bedside
		Family comes to child's bedside without evidence of distress

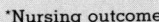

SP-SCP   Fear
Etiology: knowledge deficit, environmental stimuli

Alleviate fears	Help family distinguish between realistic and unfounded fears
	Help eliminate unfounded fears
	Discuss with family their fears regarding
	    Child's signs and symptoms
	    Child's anxiety
	    Dire consequences of disease or therapy
	    Deterioration of child's condition
	    Tests and procedures
	    Death
	Answer questions
		Family members verbalize fears and explore nature and ramifications of these fears

SP-SCP   Powerlessness
Etiology: health care environment

Provide a sense of control	Encourage family visiting at times convenient for them (there will be cultural variations in the amount and type of visiting)
	Allow expression of concerns regarding the child's care and progress
	Explore the family's feelings regarding prescribed therapies
	Permit the family as much control as possible in the child's management
	    Encourage participation in the child's care
	    Include family in setting goals for care
	    Involve family in scheduling and other aspects of care
	    Explain what family can do for the child and how to handle him or her to maintain therapy, e.g., how to pick up the child with an IV
	    Employ family's suggestions regarding the child's care whenever possible
		Family schedules visiting times
		Family readily discusses feelings and concerns
		
		Family contributes to care and management of the child
		
		*Families suggestions are incorporated into plan of care

*Nursing outcome.

Nursing Care Summary: The Family of the Hospitalized Child—cont'd

NURSING GOALS	NURSING INTERVENTIONS	EXPECTED PATIENT/FAMILY OUTCOMES

RRP   **Family process, alteration in**
Etiology: situational crisis (threat to role functioning, hospitalization of a child)

NURSING GOALS	NURSING INTERVENTIONS	EXPECTED PATIENT/FAMILY OUTCOMES
Help family understand the child's illness	Recognize family concern and need for information and support Assess family's understanding of the diagnosis and the plan of care Reinforce and clarify physician's explanation of the child's condition, suggested procedures and therapies, and the prognosis Use every opportunity to increase the family's understanding of the disease and its therapies Repeat information as often as necessary Interpret technical information Help family interpret the infant's or child's behaviors and responses Do not appear rushed—if time is inappropriate, set a date for discussion as soon as feasible Keep appointment meticulously	Family demonstrates an understanding of the disease and its therapies (specify knowledge)
Help alleviate guilt feelings	Provide accurate and specific information regarding the causes of the illness Clarify misconceptions and false assumptions	Family verbalizes their understanding of the cause of the illness (specify)
Support family	Respect parental rights Convey an attitude of respectful caring of both the child and the family Support and emphasize the strengths and abilities of the family Provide feedback and praise for compliance Refer to other professionals for additional interpersonal and concrete support (e.g., social service clergy)	Family exhibits behaviors that indicate a feeling of self-respect
Help family cope with the child's behavior	Determine family's understanding of the normal childhood responses to stress of illness and hospitalization Explain child's regression, magical thinking, egocentricity, separation anxiety, etc. Explain behavioral reactions generally expected of the child (specify according to age and developmental level) Explain what the child is (family are) permitted to do in coping with the child's behavior Reinforce family's endeavors	Family members demonstrate an understanding of the child's unfamiliar behaviors (specify manner of demonstration—verbalization, physical attitude, behaviors with child)
Help family to assist the child to cope with his or her hospitalization	Help parents determine the best way to prepare the child for hospitalization, procedures, etc. Provide family with precise information about what will take place so that they know what the child is likely to experience Encourage the family to trust the child's capacity to cope Impress upon the family the need for honesty in relating to the child Encourage the family to use play as a coping strategy Suggest appropriate items to bring to the child (e.g., pajamas, favorite toys) See also The hospitalized child, p. 1075	Family members help in planning strategies Family members are honest with the child and staff Family uses play as a tool for relating with the child
Promote and foster positive family relationships	Recognize that the family members know the child best and are "cued in" to his or her needs Allow unlimited visiting times Encourage the family to bring other significant family members to visit (e.g., siblings, grandparents, and [where permitted] pets) Encourage family to provide the child with significant, but manageable, items from home	Child and family exhibit behaviors that indicate positive coping Family members visit child at appropriate times and in appropriate numbers Child demonstrates an attitude of security with familiar persons and things

Continued.

Nursing Care Summary: The Family of the Hospitalized Child—cont'd

NURSING GOALS	NURSING INTERVENTIONS	EXPECTED PATIENT/FAMILY OUTCOMES
Promote family health	Stress the importance of maintaining health during the child's illness and hospitalization	Family shows no evidence of illness
	Encourage adequate rest	
	Provide sleeping facilities where possible	
	Encourage members to alternate visiting with the child to allow some time at home	Family members appear well-rested
	Explore means for respite care of dependent family members	
	Convey to the family the assurance that the child will receive optimal care in their absence	
	Provide relief for family members from direct care of child as needed	
	Promote adequate nutrition	
	Provide meals for parents if possible	
	Direct family to nutritious resources for meals	
	Encourage regular mealtimes away from unit	
Promote a smooth transition from hospital to home	Assess the learning needs of the family	Child and family demonstrate the ability to provide needed care in the home
	Outline and carry out a teaching plan	
	Determine services needed and make necessary referrals	
	Include family in planning and problem-solving	
	Maintain open communication between the family and health care providers	
Prepare for discharge	Assess the family's knowledge	Family demonstrates the procedures needed to provide care to the child in the home (specify learning and method of demonstration)
	Teach family the skills needed to carry out the therapeutic program (specify)	
	Allow ample time for preparation	
	Teach necessary techniques and observations	
	Help family by demonstration	
	Distribute appropriate Home Care Instructions or other educational materials or both	
	Encourage questions and expression of feelings and concerns	
	Allow sufficient time for family to perform procedures under supervision	
	Inform parents of	
	Signs of progress to observe for	
	Any unfavorable signs to be alert for	
	Problems that can be anticipated (e.g., care of equipment or devices)	
	Behaviors that indicate special needs (e.g., pain medication, imminent seizures)	
	A course of action to follow (e.g., seizure care, CPR)	
	Make certain family knows how to contact appropriate persons if or when needed	Family is aware of how to seek help
	Prepare family for possible post-hospital behaviors of the child	
	Ensure family's comprehension of the child's needs before discharge	
Maintain continuity of care	Inform family of community resources available	Family seeks appropriate assistance
	Refer to agencies as appropriate (specify)	
	Help identify support group(s) for family	
	Be available to family by telephone or other means	
	Schedule follow-up appointments as needed	Family keeps appointments

nations. However, even in this situation the information may be seriously inadequate. Children in every age-group deserve some explanation of the child's illness or hospitalization. Although the exact wording may differ, the answer should focus on the following concerns: (1) "Will I get sick and have to go to the hospital?" (2) "Did I cause the illness?" (for actual or imagined reasons), and (3) "Will my parents abandon me if my brother or sister doesn't recover?" If parents or nurses address the explanations to these three questions, the siblings' own fears of illness, guilt, and abandonment are minimized.

Nursing approaches with siblings can be direct or indirect. Direct services might include (1) incorporating siblings into hospital admission programs; (2) liberalizing visiting regulations; (3) extending parent participation programs to include sibling involvement, such as through family dining or group play sessions; and (4) developing programs designed specifically for siblings, such as group sessions to discuss their concerns or posthospital discharge visits to evaluate the siblings' adjustment.

Indirect services, which are amenable to any existing nursing role, involve helping parents understand, cope with, and support the siblings' reactions to the experience. Measures, such as being certain the siblings understand what is happening and provisions for them to remain at home rather than with a neighbor or relative, can help minimize some of the negative effects* (Knafl and Dixon, 1983; Craft, Wyatt, and Sandell, 1985).

Preparation for the Hospital Experience

The rationale for preparing children for the hospital experience and related procedures is based on the principle that fear of the unknown (fantasy) exceeds fear of the known. Therefore decreasing the elements of the unknown results in less fear. When children do not have paralyzing fear to cope with, they are then able to direct their energies toward dealing with the other unavoidable stresses of hospitalization and to benefit optimally from the growth potential of the experience.

For children past infancy and early toddlerhood, in-hospital and/or home preparation for hospitalization reduces children's stress (Wolfer and Visintainer, 1979). Even when children are too young to benefit from direct preparation, parents need prehospital counseling to lessen their fears and, thereby, increase their ability to psychologically support the child. Prehospital counseling has two major goals:

1. To make the hospital less strange and frightening to parents and children

2. To establish a positive atmosphere and trusting relationship with hospital staff and family members.

GUIDELINES IN PREPARING FOR HOSPITALIZATION

While preparation for hospitalization is a common practice, there is no universal standard or program that is advocated in both general and children's hospitals. Some hospital admission programs focus on group preparation before actual admission, whereas others prepare each child either before or on the day of admission. There is also a trend to prepare well children for future hospitalizations although the benefits and disadvantages are controversial (Azarnoff, 1985). The primary audience of most hospital preparation programs is children who are experiencing an initial hospitalization. However, readmission is also stressful—children's fear and fantasies may not subside with repeated hospital stays but may intensify (Johnston and Salazar, 1979). These children need preparation as well although the type of program needs to be individualized and may differ from the following guidelines for planning prehospital tours for groups or individual families who have not yet experienced hospital admission.

Ideally preparatory procedures should be:

1. Planned by the hospital staff before any child's admission to the hospital
2. Appropriately designed for each child's developmental age
3. Sufficiently individualized to account for different children's previous experience with hospitalization, present reason for admission, and available support system

Group Size and Timing of Preparation

Group size should be small (about 10 children to a group) to provide individualized attention and facilitate discussion (Huth, 1983). If tours are arranged for each child, the parents should be included and possibly the well siblings, although the actual benefit to these children has not been researched.

Prehospital admission programs should be scheduled for the time of day when hospital staff is most available and the majority of treatment procedures are completed. They should take place before actual admission occurs. However, there is no firm consensus on the timing of the event. Some authorities recommend preparing children 4 to 7 years of age about 1 week in advance so they can assimilate the information and ask questions. For older children, the time may be longer. However, for young children, who may begin to fantasize about what they observed, 1 or 2 days before admission is sufficient time for anticipatory preparation (Petrillo and Sanger, 1980). Other research has found that children ages 5 to 12 years prefer to know about impending hospitalization from several weeks to a few minutes before the event, suggesting that the optimum approach is one that is individualized for each child (Ross and Ross, 1984). The

---

*A helpful book about siblings' needs is *Becky's Story: A Book to Share* by Donna Baznik available for purchase from the Association for the Care of Children's Health, 3615 Wisconsin Ave., N.W., Washington, DC 20016.

length of the session should be suited to the children's attention span—the younger the child, the shorter the program.

Setting of the Tour

The setting of the tour should avoid any frightening aspects of the hospital environment and should typically include an inpatient room, the playroom (a highlight of the tour), the parents' waiting room, the nurses' station, and other special areas, such as the group dining room. Other areas that may be visited are the x-ray department and laboratory area, the slumber or induction room, and the recovery room. Different hospitals may tailor this tour to include special rooms, such as the "OR playroom," where children and parents first go before any induction is administered. Children who are undergoing serious surgery requiring special postoperative care may be taken to visit the intensive care unit. Children scheduled for special tests, such as cardiac catheterization or cystoscopy, are sometimes shown these areas. Young children may respond better to shorter tours that concentrate on the areas of most concern, such as the pediatric unit, playroom, and recovery room. In any case, throughout the tour, the nurse (or other guide) must be alert to signs of concern or fear in the children. Strange noises, sights, sounds, and smells that are routine to hospital personnel can be frightening to children.

Preparatory Materials

The most suitable type of presentation for children includes a wide variety of preparatory materials, including films, lecture, demonstration, and play. The following discussion explores some of the typical methods that may be used in preparing children for elective surgery. A puppet show may reenact the basic steps of hospitalization—admission procedures; preparation for surgery, the operating room, and the recovery room; and postsurgical treatment. The main focus of each scene is the use of concrete actions and models to familiarize the family members with what will actually occur. The puppets talk about children's common fears—pain, anesthesia, and parent separation. Although the sophistication of the materials varies, the basic characters should include a puppet family (mother, father, child) and hospital staff (physician, nurse) that are racially representative of the patient and hospital population. For example, both black and white dolls are required in many urban areas. Hospital equipment includes mask, cap, gloves, gown, intravenous bottle, stand, tubing, syringes, thermometer, blood pressure machine, stethoscope, scale, oxygen mask, suture removal set, bandages, bed, and sheets. If children are routinely admitted for diagnostic evaluations, miniature replicas of machinery, such as x-ray equipment, or the use of slides as visual aids may be used. The use of scaled-down models is especially beneficial for young children who may be frightened by the actual proportions of some equipment. However, it is the intent of what is conveyed that greatly surpasses the sophistication of the materials used.

Opportunity for Discussion

Any type of preparatory program needs to provide ample opportunity for discussion both before and after the tour. During the tour family members are encouraged to ask questions and to familiarize themselves with the environment by sitting on a bed, using the electric bed controls, riding in a wheelchair, or handling the equipment in the special rooms. Ideally the tour should also be an opportunity for meeting the child's primary nurse. Although this is not always possible because of staffing schedules, the nursing staff should be introduced to the children by name. Introducing them to one specific nurse, such as the head nurse or clinical specialist, helps them feel more comfortable in knowing who is available for questions or concerns during the hospital stay.

Following the tour there should be a question-and-answer period, monitored by a nurse. Sometimes the group is reticent about asking questions. In this case the nurse can stimulate discussion by posing a question to the audience or inviting the children to see and touch the puppets and equipment. Allowing children to play with the equipment and draw pictures about what they observed are excellent methods of evaluating the learning process and clarifying any misconceptions.

The tour may conclude with serving refreshments, which

OUTLINE OF ADMISSION PROCEDURES

Preadmission

Assign a room based on developmental age, seriousness of diagnosis, communicability of illness, and projected length of stay

Prepare roommate(s) for the arrival of a new patient; when children are too young to benefit from this consideration, prepare parents

Prepare room for child and family, with admission forms and equipment nearby to eliminate need to leave child

Admission

Introduce primary nurse to child and family

Orient child and family to inpatient facilities, especially to assigned room and unit; emphasize positive areas of pediatric unit

  Room: explain call light, bed controls, television, etc.; direct to bathroom, telephone, etc.

  Unit: Direct to playroom, desk, dining area, or other areas

Introduce family to roommate and his parents

Apply identification band to child's wrist, ankle, or both (if not done)

Explain hospital regulations and schedules (e.g., visiting hours, mealtimes, bedtime, limitations [give written information if available])

Perform nursing history

Take vital signs, blood pressure, height, and weight

Obtain specimens as needed and order needed laboratory work

Support child and assist physician with physical examination (for purposes of nursing assessment)

helps people relax, gather their thoughts, and ask a last-minute question. By informally visiting each table, the nurse has an excellent opportunity to discuss individual concerns. At this time the parents can also be invited to call the pediatric unit for any reason before admission, since questions may arise during this interval.

Prehospital Counseling by Parents

In many situations the preparation of children for the hospital experience is left up to parents. Parents may abdicate this responsibility for a variety of reasons. For example, they sometimes think the child is too young to understand or is better off not knowing beforehand; often they are unable to prepare the child because of their own lack of knowledge and understanding.

Professionals can help parents prepare their children by adequately informing them of the specific details of hospitalization and related procedures, through both direct discussion and written material. Responsibility for such guidance often rests with office and clinic nurses. They can discuss with parents appropriate timing of the preparation and preparation methods, such as picture books about going to the hospital (see resources, p. 1100). Nurses working with these parents should also assess their level of anxiety regarding the impending hospitalization to prevent emotional contagion to the child (Vardaro, 1978).

HOSPITAL ADMISSION

The preparation that children require on the day of admission depends on the kind of prehospital counseling they have received. If they have been prepared in a formalized program, they will usually know what to expect in terms of initial medical procedures, inpatient facilities, and nursing staff. However, prehospital counseling does not preclude the need for support during procedures such as drawing blood, x-ray tests, or physical examination. For example, undressing young children before they feel comfortable in their new surroundings can be very upsetting. Causing needless anxiety and fear during admission may adversely affect the nurse's establishment of trust with these children. Therefore nursing assistance during the admission procedure is vital, regardless of how well prepared any child is for the experience of hospitalization. In addition, spending this time with the child gives the nurse an opportunity to evaluate understanding of subsequent procedures, such as surgery (Fig. 26-12). The usual admission procedures for children are outlined on p. 1088.

Nursing Admission History

The nursing admission history refers to a systematic collection of data about the child and family that allows the nurse to plan individualized care. The nursing admission history presented in the box is organized according to the Functional Health Patterns outlined by Gordon (1985) (see p.

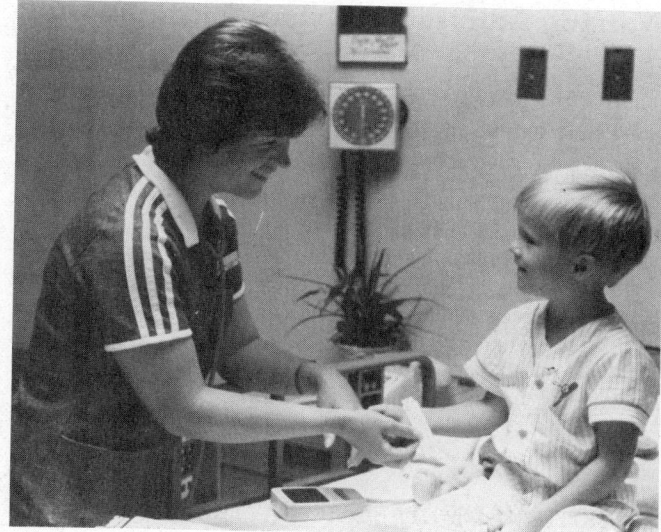

Fig. 26-12. The initial admission procedures allow the nurse an opportunity to begin knowing the child and assessing his understanding of the hospital experience.
Photography by John Roy, Saint Francis Hospital, Tulsa, OK.

21), which facilitates the formulation of nursing diagnoses. One of the main purposes of the history is to assess the child's usual health habits at home to promote a more normal environment in the hospital. Therefore questions related to activities of daily living are a major part of the assessment. The questions found under the health-perception—health-management pattern are directed toward evaluation of the child's preparation for hospitalization and are key factors in determining if additional preparation is needed.

As with any history form, the questions are only guidelines; for maximum communication nurses should ask these questions as a part of conversation, not as a direct questionnaire. Answers to questions, such as, "What does your child know about this hospitalization?" that are broad and nonspecific, need to be followed by more directive questions, such as, "Tell me what you told him." Children may respond to questions regarding their knowledge of hospitalization with statements such as, "I don't know why I am here." Although this may be correct, frequently they have been given some explanation concerning the reason for hospitalization. Such an answer may mean that the explanation was inadequate, their anxiety blocked the recall, or they are testing out the explanation by prompting the nurse to supply additional information.

Once the data is collected it must be applied to the nursing process and communicated to other staff. It makes little sense to assess a child's home routine if none of this knowledge is integrated into the plan of care. Most nursing units have provisions for care plans in which specific information about the child's habits and needs are recorded.

Nursing Admission History According to Functional Health Patterns*

HEALTH-PERCEPTION–HEALTH-MANAGEMENT PATTERN

1. Why has your child been admitted?
2. How has your child's general health been?
3. What does your child know about this hospitalization?
   a. Ask the child why he came to the hospital.
   b. If answer is "For an operation or for tests," ask the child to tell you about what will happen before, during, and after the operation or tests.
4. Has your child ever been in the hospital before?
   a. How was that hospital experience?

   b. What things were important to you and your child during that hospitalization? How can we be most helpful now?
5. What medications does your child take at home?
   a. Why are they given?
   b. When are they given?
   c. How are they given (if a liquid, with a spoon; if a tablet, swallowed with water, or other)?
   d. Does he have any trouble taking medication? If so, what helps?
   e. Does he have any allergies to medications?

NUTRITIONAL-METABOLIC PATTERN

1. What are the family's usual mealtimes?
2. Do family members eat together or at separate times?
3. What are you child's favorite foods, beverages, and snacks?
   a. Average amounts consumed or usual size portions
   b. Special cultural practices, such as family eats only ethnic food
4. What goods and beverages does your child dislike?
5. What are his feeding habits (bottle, cup, spoon, eats by self, needs assistance, any special devices)?
6. How does he like his food served (warmed, cold, one itme at a time)?

7. How would you describe his usual appetite (hearty eater, picky eater)?
   a. Has being sick affected your child's appetite?
8. Are there any known or suspected food allergies; is your child on a special diet?
9. Are there any feeding problems (excessive fussiness, spitting up, colic); any dental or gum problems that affect feeding?
10. What do you do for these problems?

ELIMINATION PATTERN

1. What are your child's toilet habits (diaper, toilet trained—day only or day and night, use of word to communicate urination or defecation, potty chair, regular toilet, other routines)?
2. What is his usual pattern of elimination (bowel movements)?

3. Do you have any concerns about elimination (bed-wetting, constipation, diarrhea)?
4. What do you do for these problems?
5. Have you ever noticed that your child sweats a lot?

SLEEP-REST PATTERN

1. What is your child's usual hour of sleep and awakening?
2. What is his schedule for naps; length of naps?
3. Is there a special routine before sleeping (bottle, drink of water, bedtime story, nightlight, favorite blanket or toy, prayers)?
4. Is there a special routine during sleep time, such as waking to go to the bathroom?
5. What type of bed does he sleep in?
6. Does he have his own room or share a room; if he shares a room, with whom?

7. What are the home sleeping arrangements (alone or with others, such as sibling, parent, or other person)?
8. What is his favorite sleeping position?
9. Are there any sleeping problems (falling asleep, waking during night, nightmares, sleep walking)?
10. Are there any problems awakening and getting ready in the morning?
11. What do you do for these problems?

*The focus of the admission history is the child's psychosocial environment. For an assessment of physical aspects, see Chapter 7. Most of the questions are worded in terms of parental responses. Depending on the child's age, they should be addressed directly to the child when appropriate.

ACTIVITY-EXERCISE PATTERN

1. What is your child's schedule during the day (nursery school, daycare center, regular school, extracurricular activities)?
2. What are his favorite activities or toys (both active and quiet interests)?
3. What is his usual television viewing schedule at home?
   a. What are his favorite programs?
   b. Are there any TV restrictions?
4. Does your child have any illness or disabilities that limit his activity? If so, how?
5. What are his usual habits and schedule for bathing (bath in tub or shower, sponge bath, shampoo)?
6. What are his dental habits (brushing, flossing, fluoride supplements or rinses, favorite toothpaste); schedule of daily dental care?
7. Does your child need help with dressing or grooming, such as hair combing?
8. Are there any problems with the above (dislike of or refusal to bathe, shampoo hair, or brush teeth)?
9. What do you do for these problems?
10. Are these special devices that your child requires help in managing (eyeglasses, contact lenses, hearing aid, orthodontic appliances, artificial elimination appliances, orthpedic devices)?

NOTE: Use following code to assess functional self-care level for feeding, bathing/hygiene, dressing/grooming, toileting:

O: Full self-care
I: Requires use of equipment or device
II: Requires assistance or supervision from another person
III: Requires assistance or supervision from another person and equipment or device
IV: Is dependent and does not participate

COGNITIVE-PERCEPTUAL PATTERN

1. Does your child have any hearing difficulty?
   a. Does he use a hearing aid?
   b. Have "tubes" been placed in your child's ears?
2. Does your child have any vision problems?
   a. Does he wear glasses or lenses?
3. Does your child have any learning difficulties?
   a. What is his grade in school?
4. For information on pain, see Table 26-00.

SELF-PERCEPTION–SELF-CONCEPT PATTERN

1. How would you describe your child (e.g., takes time to adjust, settles in easily, shy, friendly, quiet, talkative, serious, playful, stubborn, easy going)?
2. What kinds of things make your child angry, annoyed, anxious or sad? What helps?
3. How does your child act when he is annoyed or upset?
4. What have been your child's experiences with and reactions to temporary separation from you (parent)?
5. Does your child have any fears (places, objects, animals, people, situations)? How do you handle them?
6. Do you think your child's illness has changed the way he thinks about himself (e.g., more shy, embarrassed about appearance, less competitive with friends, stays at home more)?

ROLE-RELATIONSHIP PATTERN

1. Does your child have a nickname he wishes to be called?
2. What are the names of other family members or others who live in the home (relatives, friends, pets)?
3. Who usually takes care of your child during the day/night (especially if other than parent, such as babysitter, relative)?
4. What are the parents' occupations and work schedule?
5. Are there any special family considerations (adoption, foster child, stepparent, divorce, single parent)?
6. Have any major changes in the family occurred lately (death, divorce, separation, birth of a sibling, loss of a job, financial strain, mother beginning a career, other)? Explain child's reaction.
7. Who are your child's play companions or social group (peers, younger or older children, adults, prefers to be alone)?
8. Do things generally go well for your child in school or with friends?
9. Does your child have "security" objects at home (pacifier, thumb, bottle, blanket, stuffed animal or dqll)? Did you bring any of these to the hospital?
10. How do you handle discipline problems at home? Are these methods always effective?
11. Does your child have any speech or hearing problems? If so, what are your suggestions for communicating with him?
12. Will your child's hospitalization affect family's financial support or care of other family members, such as other children?
13. What concerns do you have about your child's illness and hospitalization?
14. Who will be staying with your child while he is in the hospital?
15. How can we contact you or another close family member outside of the hospital?

SEXUALITY-REPRODUCTIVE PATTERN

(Answer questions that apply to your child's age-group.)

1. Has your child begun puberty (developing physical sexual characteristics, menstruation)? Have you or your child had any concerns?
2. Does your daughter know how to do breast self-examination?
3. Does your son know how to do testicular self-examination?
4. How have you approached topics of sexuality with your child? Do you feel you might need some help with some topics?
5. Has your child's illness affected the way he or she feels about being a male or female? If so, how?
6. Do you have any concerns with behaviors in your child, such as masturbation, asking many questions or talking about sex, not respecting others privacy or wanting too much privacy?

7. Initiate a conversation about adolescent's sexual concerns with open-ended to more direct questions and using the terms ''friends'' or ''partners'' rather than ''girlfriend'' or ''boyfriend:''
   a. Tell me about your social life.
   b. Who are your closest friends? (If one friend is identified, could ask more about that relationship, such as how much time they spend together, how serious they are about each other, if the relationship is going the way the teenager hoped it would)
   c. Might ask about dating and sexual issues, such as the teenager's views on sex education, ''going steady,'' ''living together,'' or premarital sex.
   d. Which friends would you like to have visit in the hospital?

COPING-STRESS TOLERANCE PATTERN

(Answer questions that apply to your child's age-group.)

1. If your child is tired or upset, what does he do?
   a. If he is upset, does he have a special person or object he wants? If so, explain.
2. If your child has temper tantrums, what causes them and how do you handle them?
3. Who does your child talk to when something is worrying him?

4. How does your child usually handle problems or disappointments?
5. Have there been any big changes or problems in your family recently? How did you handle them?
6. Has your child ever had a problem with drugs or alcohol or tried suicide?
7. Do you think your child is ''accident prone?'' If so, explain.

VALUE-BELIEF PATTERN

1. What is your religion?
2. How is religion or faith important in your child's life?

3. What religious practices would you have continued in the hospital, such as prayers before meals/bedtime; visit by minister, priest, or rabbi, prayer group?

Physical Assessment

Although physical examinations by physicians are a required part of the admission procedure, nurses should also use the valuable information gained from physical assessments in their planning of care (Chapter 7). Subjecting children to two separate examinations is unnecessary if the nurse and physician cooperate during the procedure. For example, when the nurse is present to psychologically support the child, the opportunity can also be used to observe the child's body for any bruises, rash, signs of neglect, deformities, or physical limitations.

The nurse should also listen to the heart and lungs to assess overall physical status. For example, it is impossible to evaluate improvement in respiratory function in a child admitted with pulmonary disease unless there is baseline data with which to compare subsequent findings. Collaboration also prevents the often frustrating and needless waste of the family's time in repeating histories and examinations, especially when the child has a chronic condition that necessitates numerous hospitalizations.

Placing the Child

Room assignments are usually made before the child is admitted to the pediatric unit. The minimum considerations for room assignment are age, sex, and nature of the illness. Ideally, however, room selection should be based on a variety of developmental and psychobiologic needs. Determining compatible roommates, both for the children and for rooming-in parents, greatly influences the growth potential from the hospital experience.

Although there are no absolute rules to govern room selection, in general placing children of the same age-group and with similar types of illness in the same room is both psychologically and medically advantageous. However, there are many exceptions. For example, a school-age child may thrive on the responsibility of caring for a younger child. A child in traction may be very therapeutic for another child confined to bed because of a serious illness. A child who is very independent despite physical disabilities may help another child with similar or different limitations and his parents achieve deeper insight and acceptance of the disorder.

NURSING CARE DURING SPECIAL HOSPITAL ADMISSIONS

In addition to admission to a general pediatric unit children may be admitted to special facitilies, such as a day hospital, an adolescent unit, an isolation room, or an intensive care unit. Some admissions are unexpected and frequently constitute medical emergencies. Such situations require special preparation of the child and family and nursing care interventions based on an awareness of the child's needs and the unique stressors associated with these hospital facilities.

Day Hospital

The concept of a day hospital is to provide needed medical services for the child while eliminating the necessity of overnight admission. Among the benefits of a day hospital are (1) minimization of the stressors of hospitalization, especially separation from the family, (2) reduced chance of infection, and (3) economic saving. Typically admission to the day hospital is for operative or diagnostic procedures such as insertion of tympanostomy tubes, hernia repair, cystoscopy, or bronchoscopy (Koop, 1981).

Because of the limited contact with the child, nursing admission procedures are extremely important. Ideally, each child and family should receive preadmission counseling, including a tour of the facility and a review of the expected day's procedures. However, when it is not possible, surgery should be scheduled to allow some time for children to get acquainted with their surroundings and nurses to assess, plan, and complement appropriate teaching.

Adolescent Unit

In recent years there has been increased awareness of children's needs based on developmental considerations. To meet the unique needs of adolescents, special units have been developed that provide privacy, increased socialization, and appropriate activities for these young people. Typically these units are set apart from the general pediatric facility so that the teenagers do not share space with younger children, who are often perceived as a threat to their maturity. Such units also provide more flexible routines and activities, such as more group activity, wearing of street clothes, provisions to temporarily leave the adolescent unit, and access to the paraphenalia that is so critical to teenagers—telephones, record and tape players, video recorders, and televisions. Because adolescents' food habits are rarely limited to the three traditional meals a day, a ready supply of snacks should be available. However, the most important benefit of these units is increased socialization with peers; in addition, the staff are usually individuals who enjoy working with this age group and are well suited to establishing the trust that is so essential for communication.

Despite the advantages of adolescent units all young people require preparation for the experience. They need orientation to the unit, introduction to staff and other patients, and an atmosphere of warmth and welcome. Just as teenagers form "cliques" in the course of normal social relationships, this same tendency occurs in the hospital and staff must be aware of exclusivesness of group membership, especially when new patients are admitted. Scheduled and supervised group meetings are effective in preventing feelings of "nonbelonging" and in facilitating introductions and new friendships. They also provide an excellent opportunity for discussions about typical teenager concerns, such as sexuality, drugs, drinking, and parental relations, and special concerns of ill adolescents, such as peer rejection for being different (Pazola and Gerberg, 1985).

Isolation

Admission to an isolation room increases all the stressors typically associated with hospitalization. There is further separation from familiar persons, additional loss of control, and added environmental changes such as sensory deprivation and the strange appearance of visitors. These stressors are compounded by children's limited understanding of isolation. Preschool children have difficulty understanding the rationale for isolation as they are unable to comprehend the cause-and-effect relationship between germs and illness. They are likely to view isolation as punishment. Older children understand the causality better but still require factual information to decrease fantasizing or misinterpretation (Broeder, 1985).

When a child is placed in isolation, preparation is essential for the child to feel in control. With young children the best approach is a simple explanation, such as, "You need to be in this room to help you get better. This is a special place to make all the germs go away. The germs made you sick and you could not help that." If the child is in protective isolation, one can emphasize that other people's germs can make him sick and this is a special place that keeps the germs from coming in. With older children and parents the explanation can be based more on the cause-and-effect relationship, including how germs enter another's body, such as "by breathing them in." Family members are more likely to practice good hand washing, toileting hygiene, and so on if they are aware of their value.

All children, but especially younger ones, need preparation in terms of what they will see, hear, or feel in isolation. Therefore they are shown the mask, gloves, and gown and are encouraged to "dress up" in them. Playing with the strange apparel lessens the fear of seeing "ghostlike" people walk into the room. Before entering the room, nurses and other health personnel should introduce themselves and let the child see their face before donning a mask. In this way the child associates them with significant experiences and gains a sense of familiarity in an otherwise strange and lonely environment.

When the child's condition improves, appropriate play activities are provided to minimize boredom. Rather than dwelling on the negative aspects of isolation, the child can be encouraged to view this experience as challenging and positive. For example, the nurse can help the child look at isolation as a method of keeping others out and letting only special people in. Children often think of intriguing signs for their doors, such as "Enter at your own risk" or "Many have entered but few have left." These posterlike signs also encourage people "on the outside" to enter and talk with the child about the ominous greetings.

Emergency Admission

One of the most traumatic hospital experiences for the child and parents is an emergency admission. The sudden onset of an illness or the occurrence of an injury leaves little time for preparation and explanation. Sometimes the emergency admission is compounded by admission to an intensive care unit or the need for immediate surgery. However, even in those instances requiring outpatient treatment, the child is exposed to a strange, frightening environment and to people who often inflict pain. Therefore every medical emergency requires psychologic intervention to reduce the fear and anxiety frequently associated with the experience.

There is a wide discrepancy between what constitutes a medically defined emergency and a client-defined emergency. Studies show that acute life-threatening emergencies account for less than 1% of all emergency visits and that acute non-life-threatening emergencies account for approximately 6%. In pediatric populations the majority of visits are for respiratory infections, with skin conditions, gastrointestinal disorders, and trauma such as poisoning accounting for the remainder of the cases. The most common reason parents give for bringing the child to the emergency room is concern for the illness worsening. However, physicians generally do not consider the progressive symptoms as necessitating emergency care (McFarlane, 1976). Therefore it is obvious that "emergency" is a term perceived differently by various people. One of nursing's primary goals is to assess the parents' perception of the events and their reason for considering it serious or life threatening.

Lengthy preparatory admission procedures are often inappropriate for emergency situations. In such instances nurses must focus their nursing interventions on the essential components of admission counseling, which include the following:

1. Appropriate introduction to the family
2. Use of child's name, not terms such as "honey" or "dear"
3. Determination of child's age and some judgment made about developmental age (if the child is of school age, asking about his grade level will offer some evidence for concurrent intellectual ability)
4. Information about child's general state of health, any problems that may interfere with medical treatment, such as sensitivity to medication, and previous experience with hospital facilities
5. Information about the chief complaint from both the parent and the child

Unless an emergency is life threatening, children need to participate in their care to maintain a sense of control. Because emergency rooms are frequently hectic, there is a tendency to rush through procedures in order to save time. However, the extra few minutes needed to allow children to participate may save many more minutes of useless resistance and uncooperativeness during subsequent procedures. Other supportive measures include assuring privacy, accepting various emotional responses to fear or pain, preserving parent-child contact, explaining all events before or as they occur, and personally remaining calm.

There are occasions when, because of the child's physical condition, little or no preparatory counseling for emergency hospitalization can be done. In such situations the implementation of postvention, or counseling subsequent to the event, has therapeutic value. The process of postvention involves evaluating children's thoughts regarding admission and related procedures. It is similar to precounseling techniques; however, instead of supplying information, the nurse listens to the explanations offered by the child. Projective techniques such as drawing, doll play, or storytelling are especially effective. The nurse then bases additional information on what has already been revealed, as in the following example.

A child who was admitted to the hospital for an emergency appendectomy described the usual admission and preoperative procedures correctly but had no understanding of why they were done. His most prominent recollection focused on all the "shots" he had received (blood tests, intravenous fluid, sedation). When the nurse asked him why he had received so many (he had stated "millions of shots"), he responded *too* appropriately, "To make me better." Because the nurse sensed that he had been programmed or taught to view injections in this way, he was asked, "Why wouldn't one shot have been enough?" He thought for a moment, then replied, "I guess because I didn't tell my mommy about my stomachache soon enough." Based on this statement, which supports self-blame, guilt, and punishment, the nurse described the entire admission and preoperative procedure, stressing the reason for each shot. The child was also asked to confirm the details and to count the number of injections to lessen the enormity of "millions" of shots.

Intensive Care Unit

Admission to an intensive care unit (ICU) can be a particularly traumatic event for both the child and the parents. The nature and severity of the illness and the circumstances surrounding the admission are major factors, especially for parents. Parents experience significantly more stress when the admission is unexpected than expected (Eberly and others, 1985). In addition, the physical environment of the ICU can be awesome, frightening, and intimidating. Lights are on constantly, making a normal day-night orientation impossible, and sleep deprivation is common. There are strange, loud, and monotonous noises. Unfamiliar people speak *about* the child but rarely to him, creating a feeling of depersonalization, and there is little chance for privacy. Despite the constant turmoil there is social isolation from usual patterns of relations, especially in terms of the parent-child relationship. The atmosphere is often charged with a sense of urgency, over which the child has little control and no means of escape. In addition to all of these external factors, the child is often in pain, immobilized, and subjected to numerous frightening and traumatic procedures (Lybarger, 1979; Kleck, 1984; Baker, 1984).

While the effects of such a setting on adult patients have been well documented, relatively little research has been done on pediatric patients. Most observations of the emotional reactions of children to the pediatric ICU have been described as remarkably mild and no more severe than those of other children to routine pediatric hospitalization. On admission, children tend to be solemn, serious, egocentric, and preoccupied with their physical condition. Their major concern is themselves. They scarcely notice the machines or environment not directly involved with them and attend to those things they can feel (May, 1972). Verbalizations by wake and alert children are uncommon, their affect tends to be neutral or negative, and passivity toward the environment predominates (Cataldo and others, 1979). Only when children are much improved is there more concern with the ICU environment and other patients. However, this increased concern is more common in older children than younger ones, who tend to remain egocentric (May, 1972).

Prolonged admission to the ICU is associated with more severe adjustment problems following discharge. Children who spend 1 to 2 days in the ICU often recover quickly when transferred. Children who stay longer than 3 to 4 days may have an extended period of adjustment characterized by irritability, fearfulness, anorexia, and increased need for sleep (Lybarger 1979).

Parents are also under considerable stress. The major parental stressors that have been identified for both fathers and mothers are (Miles and others, 1984):

Child's behavior and emotion, which includes demanding, crying, whining, and unresponsive behavior

Concern regarding their parental role, which includes inability to visit at will; inability to ease fear, help the child, and hold him; and separation from the crying child

The emotional needs of the family are paramount when a child is admitted to an intensive care unit. While the same interventions that were discussed earlier for the stressors of separation, loss of control, and bodily injury and pain apply here, frequently they are not implemented or adjustments need to be made to accommodate the needs of the family despite the often hectic and stressful atmosphere.

When an ICU admission is expected, such as for postoperative care after cardiac surgery, the child and parents should be prepared for the event. Some units advocate a tour, while others use picture books of the unit to familiarize the family with the environment and usual equipment (see resources, p. 1100). Dolls can be used to demonstrate the types of tubes that the child may have. Special care or effects of the tubes are discussed, such as the need to move despite the presence of chest tubes and inability to talk with an endotracheal tube. As much reassurance as possible should accompany the introduction of stressful information. For example, children should be reassured that they can talk when the tube is removed and that in the meantime they can use a communication board to convey their needs.

When parents first visit the child in the ICU, they need preparation for how the child will look and what he is experiencing if awake. Ideally the nurse should accompany the family to the bedside to provide emotional support and answer any questions. If siblings visit they need the same preparation as parents. Whether they should visit soon after the child is admitted and usually critically ill or after the child's condition is stabilized is controversial. Early visiting minimizes the opportunity for siblings to fantasize about the experience and imagine fears that are probably greater than the actual situation (Shonkwiler, 1985). However, visiting early may be frightening, especially when the child is in pain or unresponsive and attached to numerous tubes and machinery. The length of time for sibling visitation should be planned ahead and monitored during the visit to prevent the well child from becoming overwhelmed.

Children admitted to the ICU need their parents' comfort and security and parents are encouraged to stay with their child. If visiting hours are limited, there should be flexibility in the schedule to accommodate parental needs. Family members should be given a written schedule of the times permitted and assured that they can call the unit at any time. With liberalization of visiting hours, many parents feel that they must stay and nurses need to be sensitive to their needs, suggesting periodic respites from the tense, stressful ICU environment.

Since altered parental roles is a major stress for parents, nurses need to implement interventions to minimize this concern, such as (1) educating and preparing parents for the expected role changes, (2) identifying ways in which parents can continue to fulfill parenting functions, such as helping with the bath or feeding and touching and talking to the child, and (3) determining new roles, such as helping with procedures (Miles and others, 1984; Rennick, 1986). Information sharing can increase parents' sense of control and responsibility, but facts must be conveyed simply, repeated often, and monitored to prevent overwhelming family members. Since medical jargon abounds in a complex environment such as the ICU, unfamiliar terms need to be clarified and simpler terms such as *tube, TV screen,* and *sample* can be substituted for *catheter, monitor,* and *specimen* (Johnson, 1986).

There is the same tendency in the ICU to perform procedures quickly and without attention to the child's preparational needs as in emergency admissions. Therefore nurses need to remember the special concerns of children in each age-group about bodily injury. Explaining each procedure, altering it whenever possible to decrease the child's fears, and supporting the child are essential. Giving children an object that symbolizes their courage, such as a "hero badge" or an "ICU diploma," helps them face their fears and anxiety. It is a positive memento of an otherwise stressful experience. Because of the numerous procedures performed on the child and the nature of the illness, pain management needs to receive a high priority.

Of particular importance in decreasing fear is ensuring that discussions that do not directly include the family are held where the child and family cannot overhear them. Casual conversation in the nursing station or in the halls can often be overheard and taken out of context. When discussions are held at the bedside, it is very easy to forget the patient and make remarks that are misunderstood. Usually a quiet reminder of how frightened the child can become from listening to these discussions is sufficient. If bedside conferences are necessary, the nurse interprets them for family members in language they can comprehend or if appropriate, asks the family to leave the area during report.

Extensive monitoring makes a usual day-night cycle difficult in an ICU. However, some schedule should be established that maintains a similarity to daily events in the child's life. These include organizing care during normal waking hours, keeping regular bedtime schedules, including quiet times when televisions and radios are lowered or turned off, closing and opening drapes as appropriate, dimming lights, placing a curtain around the bed for privacy and decreased stimulation, and having clocks or calendars in easy view for older children. In particular staff members must be cognizant of the need for quiet and refrain from loud talking or laughing. Equipment noise should be kept to a minimum by turning alarms as low as safely possible, performing treatments requiring equipment at one time, turning off bedside equipment that is not in use, such as suction and oxygen, and avoid loud, abrupt noises, such as clattering bedpans or toilet flushing (Synder-Halpern, 1985). Such measures can reduce the sensory overload and the sleep deprivation commonly associated with ICU admissions.

Despite the stresses normally associated with ICU admission, a special security develops from being carefully monitored and receiving individualized care. Therefore planning for transition to the regular unit is essential and should include (1) assignment of a primary nurse on the regular unit who visits before the transfer, (2) continued visits by the ICU staff to assess the child's and parents' adjustment and to act as a temporary liaison with the nursing staff, (3) explanation of the differences between the two units and the rationale for the change to less intense monitoring of the child's physical condition, and (4) selection of an appropriate room, such as one that is close to the nursing station, and a compatible roommate.

DISCHARGE PLANNING AND HOME CARE

Most hospitalizations necessitate some type of discharge planning. Often this involves education of the family for continued care and follow-up in the home. Depending on the diagnosis, this may be relatively simple or considerably complex. With the current concern for cost containment and recognition of children's emotional needs, home care for children with technologically complex care, such as youngsters on ventilators, has become increasingly common. Preparing the family for home care demands a high degree of competence in planning and implementing discharge instruction. Although this is usually a team effort, nurses are often key individuals in initiating the process and collaborating with others in the planning and implementing stages. While it is not possible to present all the details needed for effective discharge planning and home care, a brief overview of the more critical aspects is presented. More specific details are discussed throughout the text for conditions such as home apnea monitoring, tracheostomy care, or hyperalimentation, and numerous sources of information exist in the literature (Steele and Harrison, 1986).

Assessment

Discharge planning for home care must begin with an assessment of the family's desire and capability in assuming care responsibilities. Ideally, at least two individuals should be committed to learning the skills needed for home care. A thorough assessment of the family and home environment should be done to ensure that the family's emotional and physical resources are sufficient to manage the tasks of home care (for a discussion of family and home assessment strategies, see Chapter 6). In addition to adequate family resources, an investigation of community services, including respite care, is needed to ensure that appropriate support agencies are available, such as emergency facilities, home health agencies, and equipment vendors. To coordinate the immense task of assessment and plan implementation, a case coordinator should be appointed early in the discharge program (Stein, 1985).

Planning

Ideally, preparation for hospital discharge and home care begins during the admission assessment with the establishment of short- and long-term goals. These goals are concerned with the child's physical needs as well as the psychologic needs of the youngster and family. In terms of home care for children with complex care, discharge planning is concerned with those skills that parents or children are expected to continue at home. In planning appropriate teaching, nurses need to assess (1) the actual and perceived complexity of the skill, (2) the parents' or child's ability to learn the skill, and (3) the parents' or child's previous or present experience with such procedures (See also p. 1113 for guidelines for effective teaching).

The teaching plan should incorporate levels of learning,

such as observing, participating with assistance, and finally acting without help or guidance. The skill should be divided into discrete steps and each step taught to the family member until it is learned. Return demonstration of the skill should be requested before new skills are introduced. A record of teaching and performance provides an efficient checklist for evaluation. All families should receive detailed *written* instructions about home care before they leave the hospital with telephone numbers for assistance.*

Transitional Care

Once the family is competent in performing the skill, they should be given responsibility for the care. Whenever possible, the family should have a transition or trial period to assume care with minimal supervision. This may be arranged on the unit, during a home pass, or in a facility, such as a motel, near to the hospital. Some programs incorporate a hospital trial into their discharge criteria, necessitating that the family successfully manage this phase before discharge to home (Steele and Harrison, 1986). Such transitions provide a safe practice period for the family with assistance readily available when needed and are especially valuable when the family lives at a distance to the treating center.

Evaluation and Continuing Support

Evaluation is a critical part of any discharge plan and assumes even more importance in home care of children with complex needs. Factors to consider in home care programs are need for subsequent hospitalization, child's developmental and physical progress, effects of home care on the family, actual vs expected use of resources by the family and home care team, financial costs and savings, and improved survival (American Academy of Pediatrics, 1984).

In most instances parents need only simple instructions and understanding of follow-up care. However, the often overwhelming care assumed by some families necessitates continued professional support after discharge. Appropriate referrals and resources may include visiting nurse or home health agencies, private nurse services, the school system, physical therapist, mental health counselor, social worker, or any number of community agencies, including special organizations, such as SKIP.† Sharing the important issues surrounding the child's and family's needs is essential. Referral summaries should be concise, specific, and factual. When numerous support services are involved, periodic collaboration among the professionals involved and the family is an excellent strategy to ensure efficient usage and comprehensive delivery of services.

---

* Home care instructions for a wide variety of technical skills are available in Wong, D., and Whaley, L.: Clinical handbook of pediatric nursing, ed. 2, St. Louis, 1986, The C.V. Mosby Co.

†SKIP (Sick Kids need Involved People) serves as an educational, support, and resource agency that provides assistance to families who have chosen home care for their hospitalized child. National headquarters is at 216 Newport Drive, Severna Park, MD 21146.

CONCEPT SUMMARIES

- Children are particularly vulnerable to the stresses of illness and hospitalization because stress represents a change from the usual state of health and routine and because they possess limited coping mechanisms.

- The three phases of separation anxiety are protest, despair, and detachment.

- Feelings of loss of control are caused by unfamiliar environmental stimuli, physical restriction, altered routine, and dependency.

- Fear of bodily pain may be manifested in the following ways: infants—expressions, body movements; toddlers—intense emotional upset, physical resistance; preschoolers—aggression, verbal expression, dependency; school-age children—precise verbalization of pain, passive requests for support or help, procrastination technique; adolescents—self-control, irritability, limited movement.

- Because of their separation from significant people, hospitalized children may lack the opportunity to form new attachments in the strange environment and exhibit negative behaviors after discharge.

- Family reactions are influenced by the seriousness of illness, experience with illness or hospitalization, diagnostic or therapeutic procedures, available support systems, personal ego strengths, coping abilities, additional stresses, cultural and religious beliefs, and family communication patterns.

- Common parental coping mechanisms include intellectualization, denial, regression, projection, displacement, and introjection.

- Fear of contracting illness, their younger age, a close relationship with the ill sibling, substitute child care, minimum explanation of the illness, and perceived changes in parenting all increase the deleterious effects of a brother's or sister's illness/hospitalization on siblings.

- Nursing care of the hospitalized child and family is aimed at preventing or minimizing separation, decreasing loss of control, minimizing bodily injury and pain, using play to lessen stress, maximizing potential benefits of hospitalization, and supporting family members.

- Pain assessment includes observing the child, questioning the child and parents, and using pain rating scales. Pain management should incorporate both pharmacologic and nonpharmacologic methods.

- Diversional or expressive play is an effective tool in minimizing stress.

- The nurse can maximize potential benefits of hospitalization by fostering parent-child relations, providing educational opportunities, promoting self-mastery, and encouraging socialization.

- Supporting family members involves listening to parents' verbal and nonverbal messages, providing clergy support, accepting cultural, socioeconomic, and ethnic values, and giving information to families and siblings.

- The major goals of prehospital counseling are to make the hospital less strange and frightening to parents and children and to establish a positive atmosphere and trusting relationships with hospital staff and family members.

- In preparing families for hospitalization, the nurse should consider small group size and timing of event, setting tour, inclusion of preparatory materials, time for discussion, and prehospital counseling for parents.

REFERENCES

Abu-Saad, H.: Cultural group indicators of pain in children, Maternal Child Nurs. J. **13**(3):187-196, 1984.

Aho, A.C., and Erickson, M.T.: Effects of grade, gender, and hospitalization on children's medical fears, Dev. Behav. Pediatr. **6**(3):146-153, 1985.

American Academy of Pediatrics, Ad Hoc Task Forces on Home Care of Chronically Ill Infants and Children: Guidelines for home care of infants, children, and adolescents with chronic disease, Pediatrics **74**(3):434-436, 1984.

Azarnoff, P.: Preparing well children for possible hospitalization, Pediatr. Nurs. **11**(1):53-56, 1985.

Baker, C.F.: Sensory overload and noise in the ICU: sources of environmental stress, Crit. Care Q. **6**(4):66-80, 1984.

Beyer, J., and others: Patterns of postoperative analgesic use with adults and children following cardiac surgery, Pain **17**:71-81, 1983.

Bibace, R., and Walsh, M.E.: Development of children's concepts of illness, Pediatrics **66**(6):912-918, 1980.

Broeder, J.L.: School-age children's perceptions of isolation after hospital discharge, Maternal Child Nurs. J. **14**(3): 153-174, 1985.

Cataldo, M.F., and others: Behavioral assessment for pediatric intensive care units, J. Appl. Behav. Anal. **12**:83-97, 1979.

Chess, S., and Thomas, A.: Temperamental differences: a critical concept in child health care, Pediatr. Nurs. **11**(3):167-171, 1985.

Clatworthy, S.: Therapeutic play: effects on hospitalized children, Child. Health Care **9**(4):108-113, 1981.

Craft, M.J., and Wyatt, N.: Effect of visitation upon siblings of hospitalized children, Maternal Child Nurs. J. **15**(1):47-59, 1986.

Craft, M.J., Wyatt, N., and Sandell, B.: Behavior and feeling changes in siblings of hospitalized children, Clin. Pediatr. **24**(7):374-378, 1985.

Dale, J.C.: A multidimensional study of infants' responses to painful stimuli, Pediatr. Nurs. **12**(1):27-31, 1986.

Davis, J.H.: Children and pets: a therapeutic connection, Pediatr. Nurs. **11**(5):377-379, 1985.

Douglas, J.W.B.: Early hospital admissions and later disturbances of behaviour and learning, Dev. Med. Child Neurol. **17**(4):456-480, 1975.

Eberly, T.W., and others: Parental stress after the unexpected admission of a child to the intensive care unit, Crit. Care Q. **8**(1):57-65, 1985.

Eland, J.M.: The child who is hurting, Semin. Oncol. Nurs. **1**(2):116-122, 1985a.

Eland, J.M.: Pediatrics. In Pain, Springhouse, PA, 1985b, Springhouse Corporation.

Eland, J.M., and Anderson, J.E.: The experience of pain in children. In Jacox, A., editor: Pain: a source book for nurses and other health professionals, Boston, 1977, Little, Brown and Co.

Franck, L.S.: A new method to quantitatively describe pain behavior in infants, Nurs. Res. **35**(1):28-31, 1986.

Freiberg, K.H.: How parents react when their child is hospitalized, Am. J. Nurs. **72**(7):1270-1272, 1972.

Gordon, M.: Manual of nursing diagnosis, New York, 1985, McGraw-Hill Book Co.

Gough, W.C.: A growing interest, Am. J. Nurs. **86**(2):165-166, 1986.

Hagemann, V.: Night sleep of children in a hospital. Part 1. Sleep duration, Maternal Child Nurs. J. **10**:1-13, 1981a.

Hagemann, V.: Night sleep of children in a hospital, Part 2. Sleep disruption, Maternal Child Nurs. J. **10**:127-142, 1981b.

Harpin, V.A., and Rutter, N.: Development of emotional sweating in the newborn infant, Arch. Dis. Child. **57**:691-695, 1982.

Haslam, D.R.: Age and the perception of pain, Psychonom. Sci. **15**:86, 1969.

Hester, N.: The preoperational child's reaction to immunization, Nurs. Res. **28**(4):250-255, 1979.

Huth, M.M.: Guidelines for conducting hospital tours with early school-age children, Pediatr. Nurs. **9**(6):414-415, 1983.

Johnson, S.H.: Ten ways to help the family of a critically ill patient, Nursing 86 **16**(1):50-53, 1986.

Johnston, C.C., and Strada, M.E.: Acute pain response in infants: a multidimensional description, Pain **24**(3):373-382, 1986.

Johnston, M., and Salazar, M.: Preadmission program for rehospitalized children, Am. J. Nurs. **79**(8):1421-1422, 1979.

Kleck, H.G.: ICU syndrome: onset, manifestations, treatment, stressors, and prevention, Crit. Care Q. **6**(4):21-28, 1984.

Knafl, K.A., and Dixon, D.M.: The role of siblings during pediatric hospitalization, Issues Compr. Pediatr. Nurs. **6**: 13-22, 1983.

Knafl, K.A., and Dixon, D.M.: The participation of fathers in their children's hospitalization, Iss. Compr. Pediatr. Nurs. **7**(4-5):269-281, 1984.

Koop, C.E.: Pediatric surgery: the most important advances of the last ten years, Pediatr. Consult. **2**(1):1-8, 1981.

LaMontagne, L.L.: Children's locus of control beliefs as predictors of preoperative coping behavior, Nurs. Res. **33** (2):76-79, 1984.

Lybarger, P.M.: The intensive care environment: its effect on the child and parents, Issues Compr. Pediatr. Nurs. **3**(6):50-57, 1979.

Mather, L., and Mackie, J.: The incidence of postoperative pain in children, Pain **15**:271-282, 1983.

May, B.K., and Sparks, M.: School-age children: are their needs recognized and met in the hospital setting?, Child. Health Care **11**(3):118-121, 1983.

May, J.G.: A psychiatric study of a pediatric intensive therapy unit, Clin. Pediatr. **2**(2):76-82, 1972.

McCaffery, M.: Nursing management of the patient with pain, ed. 2, Philadelphia, 1979, J.B. Lippincott Co.

McCain, G.C.: Parent-created tape recordings for hospitalized children, Child. Health Care **10**(3):104-105, 1982.

McCain, G.C., and Bies, D.C.: Television viewing and the hospitalized child, Pediatr. Nurs. **9**(1):33-35, 1983.

McFarlane, J.M.: Pediatric care in the emergency room, Pediatr. Nurs. **2**(2):22-25, 1976.

Miles, M.S., and others: Maternal and paternal stress reactions when a child is hospitalized in a pediatric care unit, Issues Compr. Pediatr. Nurs. **7**:333-342, 1984.

Monahan, G.H., and Schkade, J.K.: Comparing care by parent and traditional nursing units, Pediatr. Nurs. **11**:463-648, 1985.

Norris, S., Campbell, L.A., and Brenkert, S.: Nursing procedures and alterations in transcutaneous oxygen tension in premature infants, Nurs. Res. **31**(6):330-336, 1982.

Orem, D.: Nursing: concepts of practice, ed. 3, New York, 1985, McGraw-Hill Inc.

Owens, M.E., and Todt, E.H.: Pain in infancy: neonatal reaction to a heel lance, Pain **20**(1):77-86, 1984.

Patterson, P.: Chospitology, Dimen. Health Serv. **56**(5):12-15, 1979.

Pazola, K.J., and Gerberg, A.K.: Teen group: a forum for the hospitalized adolescent, Am. J. Maternal Child Nurs. **10**(4):265-269, 1985.

Perrin, E.C., and Gerrity, P.S.: There's a demon in your belly: children's understanding of illness, Pediatrics **67**(6):841-849, 1981.

Petrillo, M., and Sanger, S.: Emotional care of hospitalized children, ed. 2, Philadelphia, 1980, J.B. Lippincott Co.

Porter, J., and Jick, H.: Addiction rare in patients treated with narcotics, NEJM **302**(2):123, 1980.

Quinton, D., and Rutter, M: Early hospital admissions and later disturbances of behaviour: an attempted replication of Douglas' findings, Dev. Med. Child Neurol. **18**(4):447-459, 1976.

Rennick, J.: Reestablishing the parental role in a pediatric intensive care unit, J. Pediatr. Nurs. **1**(1):40-44, 1986.

Ritchie, J.A.: Preparation of toddlers and preschool children for hospital procedures, Can. Nurse **75**(11):30-32, 1979.

Ross, D.M., and Ross, S.A.: Childhood pain: the school-age child's viewpoint, Pain **20**(2):179-191, 1984.

Rutter, M.: Separation experiences: a new look at an old topic, J. Pediatr. **95**(1):147-154, 1979.

Savedra, M., and others: How do children describe pain? a tentative assessment, Pain **14**:95-104, 1982.

Schechter, N.L., Allen, D.A., and Hanson, K.: Status of pediatric pain control: a comparison of hospital analgesic usage in children and adults, Pediatrics **77**(1):11-15, 1986.

Schultz, N.V.: How children perceive pain, Nurs. Outlook **19**(10):670-673, 1971.

Shannon, F.T., Fergusson, D.M., and Dimond, M.E.: Early hospital admissions and subsequent behavior problems in 6-year-olds, Arch. Dis. Child. **59**:815-819, 1984.

Sherman, M., and others: Treasured objects in school-aged children, Pediatrics **68**(3):379-386, 1981.

Shonkwiler, M.A.: Sibling visits in the pediatric intensive care unit, Crit. Care Q. **8**(1):67-72, 1985.

Smith, M.E.: The preschooler and pain. In Brandt, P.A., Chinn, P.L., and Smith, M.E.: Current practice in pediatric nursing, St. Louis, 1976, The C.V. Mosby Co.

Snyder-Halpern, R.: The effect of critical care unit noise on patient sleep cycles, Crit. Care Q. **7**(4):41-50, 1985.

Steele, N., and Harrison, B.: Technology-assisted children: assessing discharge preparation, J. Pediatr. Nurs. **1**(3):150-158, 1986.

Stein, R.: Home care: a challenging opportunity, Child. Health Care **14**(2):90-95, 1985.

Stull, M.K., and Deatrick, J.A.: Measuring parental participation; Part I, Issues Compr. Pediatr. Nurs. **9** (3):157-165, 1986.

Thompson, R.H.: Psychosocial research on pediatric hospitalization and health care: a review of the literature, Springfield, IL, 1985, Charles C Thomas, Publisher.

Vardaro, J.A.: Preadmission anxiety and mother-child relationships, Maternal Child Nurs. J.: **7**(2):8-15, 1978.

Volz, D.D.: Time structuring for hospitalized school-aged children, Iss. Compr. Pediatr. Nurs. **5**:205-210, 1981.

Watson, J.: Research and literature on children's responses to injections: some general nursing implications, Pediatr. Nurs. **2**(1):7-8, 1976.

Williamson, P.S., and Williamson, M.L.: Physiologic stress reduction by a local anesthetic during newborn circumcision, Pediatrics **71**(1):36-40, 1983.

Wolfer, J., and Visintainer, M.: Prehospital psychological preparation for tonsillectomy patients: effects on child's and parents' adjustment, Pediatrics **64**:646-655, 1979.

Wood, S.P.: School-aged children's perceptions of the causes of illness, Pediatr. Nurs. **9**(2):101-104, 1983.

BIBLIOGRAPHY
Hospitalization: The Child and Family

Algren, C.L.: Role perception of mothers who have hospitalized children, Child. Health Care **14**(1):6-9, 1985.

American Academy of Pediatrics Committee on Hospital Care: Hospital care of children and youth, Elk Grove Village, IL, 1986, The Academy.

American Academy of Pediatrics, Committee on Hospital Care and Pediatric Section of the Society of Critical Care Medicine: Guidelines for pediatric intensive care units, Pediatrics **72** (3):364-371, 1983.

Becker, R.D.C.: Illness and hospitalization in adolescence: a developmental perspective, Paediatrician **9**(3-4):242-260, 1980.

Betz, C.L., and Poster, E.C.: Incorporating play into the care of the hospitalized child, Issues Compr. Pediatr. Nurs. **7**: 343-355, 1984.

Birchfield, M.E.: Nursing care for hospitalized children based on different stages of illness, Am. J. Maternal Child Nurs. **6**(1):46-52, 1981.

Brown, C.C., and Gottfried, A.W., editors: Play interactions: the role of toys and parental involvement in children's development, 1985, Johnson & Johnson Baby Products Co.

Calkin, J.: Are hospitalized toddlers adapting to the experience as well as we think? Am. J. Maternal Child Nurs. **4**(1):18-23, 1979.

Cave, N.: What a little care can do, Can. Nurse **75**(11):38-40, 1979.

Chinn, P.L.: Activities of daily living for the hospitalized child. In Brandt, P., Chinn, P.L., and Smith, M.E., editors: Current practice in pediatric nursing, vol. II, St. Louis, 1978, The C.V. Mosby Co.

Clark, D.: Parents' meeting in a pediatric unit: helping parents cope with their child's hospitalization, J. Assoc. Care Child. Hosp. **8**(2):32-35, 1979.

Clements, D.B.: Reminiscence: a tool for aiding families under stress, Am. J. Maternal Child Nurs. **11**(2):114-117, 1986.

Coucouvanis, J.A., and Solomons, H.C.: Handling complicated visitation problems of hospitalized children, Am. J. Maternal Child Nurs. **8**(2):131, 1983.

Crummette, B.D., Mills, H.H., and Beale, A.V.: One latency-age child's coping with hospitalization, Maternal Child Nurs. J. **13**(3):167-175, 1984.

Denehy, J.: What do school-age children know about their bodies? Pediatr. Nurs. **10**(4):290-292, 1984.

Denholm, C.J.: Hospitalization and the adolescent patient: a review and some critical questions, Child. Health Care **13**(3):109-116, 1985.

Dorn, L.D.: Children's concepts of illness: clinical applications, Pediatr. Nurs. **10**(5):325-327, 1984.

Droske, S.C.: Children's behavioral changes following hospitalization—have we prepared the parents? J. Assoc. Care Child. Hosp. **7**(2):3-7, 1978.

Everson, S.: Sibling counseling, Am. J. Nurs. **77**(4):644-646, 1977.

Facteau, L.M.: Self-care concepts and the care of the hospitalized child, Nurs. Clin. North Am. **15**(1):145-155, 1980.

Fadden, T.C., and Seiser, G.K.: Nursing diagnosis: a matter of form, Am. J. Nurs. **84**(4):470-472, 1984.

Fassler, D., and Wallace, N.: Children's fear of needles, Clin. Pediatr. **21**(1):59-60, 1982.

Fletcher, B.: Psychological upset in posthospitalized children: a review of the literature, Maternal Child Nurs. J. **10** (3):185-195, 1981.

Ferraro, A.R., and Longo, D.C.: Nursing care of the family with a chronically ill, hospitalized child: an alternative approach, Image: The Journal of Nursing Scholarship **XVII**(3):77-81, 1985.

Fore, C.V., and Holmes, S.S.: A care-by-parent unit revisited, Am. J. Maternal Child Nurs. **8**(6):408-410, 1983.

Fosson, A., and deQuan, M.M.: Reassuring and talking with hospitalized children, Child. Health Care **13**(1):37-44, 1984.

Galligan, A.C.: Using Roy's concept of adaptation to care for young children, Am. J. Maternal Child Nurs. **4**(1):24-28, 1979.

Garot, P.A.: Therapeutic play: work of both child and nurse, J. Pediatr. Nurs. **1**(2):111-116, 1986.

Gohsman, B.: The hospitalized child and the need for mastery, Issues Compr. Pediatr. Nurs. **5**:67-76, 1981.

Gohsman, B., and Yunck, M.: Dealing with the threats of hospitalization, Pediatr. Nurs. **5**(5):32-35, 1979.

Goslin, E.R.: Hospitalization as life crisis for the preschool child: a critical review, J. Commun. Health **3**(4):321-346, 1978.

Gratz, R.R., and Piliavin, J.A.: What makes kids sick: children's beliefs about the causative factors of illness, Child. Health Care **12**(4):156-162, 1984.

Green, C.S.: Larry thought puppet-play "childish," but it helped him face his fears, Nursing 75 **5**(3):30-33, 1975.

Guerin, L.S.: Hospitalization as a positive experience for poverty children, Clin. Pediatr. **16**(6):509-513, 1977.

Guttentag-Waldner, D.N.: Daytime television viewing by hospitalized children, Pediatrics **68**(5):672-676, 1981.

Hill, C.: The mother on the pediatric ward: insider or outlawed, Pediatr. Nurs. **4**(5):26-29, 1978.

Hong, S.D., and Kim, S.P.: Self-concept and body-image of children during physical illness, Psychosomatics **22**(2):128-135, 1981.

Jerrett, M.D., and Ross, M.M.: Learning to nurse: the family as the unit of care, J. Adv. Nurs. **7**:461-468, 1982.

Johnston, M.: Toward a culture of caring: children, their environment, and change, Am. J. Maternal Child Nurs. **4**(4):210-214, 1979.

Jolly, J.D.: Through a child's eyes—the problems of communicating with sick children, Nursing **1**:1012-1014, 1981.

Kerr, N.J.: The effect of hospitalization on the developmental tasks of childhood, Nurs. Forum **18**(2):109-131, 1979.

King, J., and Ziegler, S.: The effects of hospitalization on children's behavior: a review of the literature, Child. Health Care **10**(1):20-28, 1981.

Knafl, K.A., and Dixon, D.M.: The role of siblings during pediatric hospitalization, Issues Compr. Pediatr. Nurs. **6**:13-22, 1983.

Koss, T., and Teter, M.: Welcoming a family when a child is hospitalized, Am. J. Maternal Child Nurs. **5**(1):51-54, 1980.

Lamb, J.M., and Rodgers, D.R.: Assisting the hostile, hospitalized child, Am. J. Maternal Child Nurs. **8**(5): 336-339, 1983.

LaMontagne, L.L.: Three coping strategies used by school-age children, Pediatr. Nurs. **10**(1):25-28, 1984.

Maheady, D.C.: Cultural assessment of children, Am. J. Maternal Child Nurs. **11**(2):129, 1986.

Maheady, D.C.: Health concepts of preschool children, Pediatr. Nurs. **12**(3):195-197, 1986.

Marchant, R.: Caring for hospitalized inner-city children, Pediatr. Nurs. **11**(2):129-131, 1985.

McLellan, C.L.: Hero badges mean more than courage, Pediatr. Nurs. **2**(3):7, 1976.

Meer, P.A.: Using play therapy in outpatient settings, Am. J. Maternal Child Nurs. **10**(6):378-380, 1985.

Meng, A.: Parents' and children's reactions towards impending hospitalization for surgery, Maternal Child Nurs. J. **9**:89-98, 1980.

Millstein, S.G., Adler, N.E., and Irwin, C.D., Jr.: Conceptions of illness in young adolescents, Pediatrics **68**(6):834-839, 1981.

Mishel, M.H.: Parents' perception of uncertainty concerning their hospitalized child, Nurs. Res. **32**(6):324-330, 1983.

Nelson, M.: Identifying the emotional needs of the hospitalized child, Am. J. Maternal Child Nurs. **6**(3):181-183, 1981.

Norberta, S.: Caring for children with the help of puppets, Am. J. Maternal Child Nurs. **1**(1):22-26, 1976.

Norris, L.: Coaching the question, Nursing 86 **16**(5):100, 1986.

Pidgeon, V.: Functions of preschool children's questions in coping with hospitalization, Res. Nurs. Health **4**:229-235, 1981.

Pidgeon, V.: Children's concepts of illness: implications for health teaching, Maternal Child Nurs. J. **14**(1):23-35, 1985.

Plank, E.N.: Working with children in hospitals, Chicago, 1971, The Press of Case Western Reserve University.

Poster, E.C.: Stress immunization: techniques to help children cope with hospitalization, Maternal Child Nurs. J. **12**:(2):119-134, 1983.

Poster, E.C., and Betz, C.L.: Allaying the anxiety of hospitalized children using stress immunization techniques, Issues Compr. Pediatr. Nurs. **67**:227-233, 1983.

Riffee, D.M.: Self-esteem changes in hospitalized school-age children, Nurs. Res. **30**(2):94-97, 1981.

Robinson, C.A.: When hospitalizataion becomes an ''everyday thing'', Issues Compr. Pediatr. Nurs. **7**:363-370, 1984.

Rumfelt, J.J.M.: How five-year old children perceive the role of the nurse, Maternal Child Nurs. J. **9**:13-27, 1980.

Smitherman, C.: Parents of hospitalized children have needs, too, Am. J. Nurs **79**(8):1423-1424, 1979.

Sweeney, L., and others: Hospitalization enhances creativity, J. Assoc. Care Child. Hosp. **7**(3):14-16, 1979.

Tesler, M., and Savedra, M.: Coping with hospitalization: a study of school-age children, Pediatr. Nurs. **7**(2):35-40, 1981.

Verzemnieks, I.L.: Developmental stimulation for infants and toddlers, Am. J. Nurs. **84**(6):749-752, 1984.

White, J.E.: Special nursing needs of hospitalized children with learning disabilities, Am. J. Maternal Child Nurs. **8**:209-212, 1983.

Zweig, C.D.: Reducing stress when a child is admitted to the hospital, Am. J. Maternal Child Nurs. **11**(1):24-26, 1986.

Pain Assessment and Management

Abu-Saad, H., and Holzemer, W.L.: Measuring children's self-assessment of pain, Issues Compr. Pediatr. Nurs. **5**:337-349, 1981.

Ahmann, E.: The child at home with chronic pain, Am. J. Maternal Child Nurs. **9**(4):264-266, 1984.

Beyer, J.E., and Byers, M.L.: Knowledge of pediatric pain: the state of the art, Child. Health Care **13**(4):150-159, 1985.

Beyer, J.E., and Knapp, T.R.: Methodologic issues in the measurement of children's pain, Child. Health Care **14**(4):233-241, 1986.

Chapman, C.R., and others: Pain measurement: an overview, Pain **22**:1-31, 1985.

D'Apolito, K.: The neonate's response to pain, Am. J. Maternal Child Nurs. **9**(4):256-257, 1984.

Hawley, D.D.: Postoperative pain in children: misconceptions, descriptions, and interventions, Pediatr. Nurs. **10**(1):20-23, 1984.

Hester, N., and Barcus, C.: Assessment and management of pain in children. In Pediatrics: Nursing update, **1**(14):3, Princeton, N.J., 1986, Continuing Professional Education Center, Inc.

Jeans, M.E.: The measurement of pain in children. In Melzack, R., editor: Pain measurement and assessment, New York, 1983, Raven Press.

Jerrett, M.D.: Children and their pain experience, Child. Health Care **14**(2):83-89, 1985.

Kaiko, R.: IM/PO morphine controversy, J. Pain Symptom Manag. **1**(1):42-45, 1986.

Korberly, B.H.: Pharmacologic treatment of children's pain, Pediatr. Nurs. **11**(4):292-294, 1985.

Koster, M.K.: Self-care: health behavior for the school-age child, Top. Clin. Nurs. **5**(1):29-40, 1983.

Lutz, W.J.: Helping hospitalized children and their parents cope with painful procedures, J. Pediatr. Nurs. **1**(1):24-32, 1986.

Lynn, M.R.: Pain in the pediatric patient: a review of research, J. Pediatr Nurs. **I**(3):198-201, 1986.

McCaffery, M.: Pain relief for the child: problem areas and selected nonpharmacological methods, Pediatr. Nurs. **3**(4):11-16, 1977.

McGuire, L., and Dizard, S.: Managing pain in the young patient, Nursing 82 **12**(8):52-57, 1982.

Owens, M.E.: Assessment of infant pain in clinical settings, J. Pain Symptom Manag. **1**(1):29-31, 1986.

Owens, M.E.: Pain in infancy: conceptual and methodological issues, Pain **20**(3):213-230, 1984.

Pilowsky, I., and others: Childhood hospitalization and chronic intractable pain in adults: a controlled retrospective study, Int. J. Psychiatry Med. **12**(1):75-84, 1982.

Ross, D.M., and Ross, S.A.: Stress reduction procedures for the school-age hospitalized leukemic child, Pediatr. Nurs. **10** (6):393-395, 1984.

Ross, D.M.: Thought-stopping: a coping strategy for impending feared events, Issues Compr. Pediatr. Nurs. **7**(2-3):83-89, 1984.

Scott, J.G., and Rigney-Radford, K.: Factors affecting the management of pain, Am. J. Maternal Child Nurs. **9**(4):253-255, 1984.

Sheredy, C.: Factors to consider when assessing responses to pain, Am. J. Maternal Child Nurs. **9**(4):250-252, 1984.

Smith, D.: Using humor to help children with pain, Child. Health Care **14**(3):187-188, 1986.

Tan, S.: Cognitive and cognitive-behavioral methods for pain control: a selective review, Pain **12**:201-228, 1982.

Wofford, L.G.: Pain in children with cancer: an assessment, J. Assoc. Pediatr. Oncol. Nurs. **2**(2):34-37, 1985.

Wright, Z.: From IV to PO: titrating your patient's pain medication, Nursing 81 **11**:39-43, 1981.

Zollo, M.: Management of pain in critically ill children, Am. J. Maternal Child Nurs. **9**(4):258-261, 1984.

Hospital Preparation and Special Admissions

Alcock, D., and others: Evnironment and waiting behaviors in emergency waiting areas, Child. Health Care **13**(4):174-180, 1985.

Azarnoff, P.: Preparing children for hospitalization. In Preparing children and families for health care encounters, Washington, DC, 1980, Association for the Care of Children's Health.

Azarnoff, P.: Preparation of young healthy children for possible hospitalization, Monograph No. 1, Santa Monica, CA, 1983, Pediatrics Projects, Inc.

Azarnoff, P., and Woody, P.D.: Preparation of children for hospitalization in acute care hospitals in the United States, Pediatrics **68**(3):361-368, 1981.

Beglinger, J.E.: Coping tasks in critical care, Dimens. Crit. Care Nurs. **2**(2):80-89, 1983.

Bellack, J.P., and Fore, C.V.: The young children in the critical care unit, Crit. Care Update **8**(5):26-38, 1981.

Bozett, F.W., and Gibbons, R.: The nursing management of families in the critical care setting, Crit. Care Update **10**(2):22-27, 1983.

Broome, M.E.: Working with the family of a critically ill child, Heart Lung **14**(4):368-372, 1985.

Canright, P., and Campbell, M.J.: Nursing care of the child and his family in the emergency department, Pediatr. Nurs. **3**(4):43-45, 1977.

Carty, R.: Observed behaviors of preschoolers to intensive care, Pediatr. Nurs. **6**(4):21-25, 1980.

Colainni, J.A.: Parents care in intensive care, Pediatr. Nurs. **1**(2):16-19, 1975.

deChesnay, M.: Promoting healthy family functioning in acute care units, J. Pediatr. Nurs. **1**(2):96-101, 1986.

Epsersen, S., and Hardy, C.D.: Pediatric care plan for adult ICU nurses, Crit. Care Nurse **5**(2):14-18, 1985.

Etzler, C.A.: Parents' reaction to pediatric critical care settings: a review of the literature, Issues Compr. Pediatr. Nurs. **7**:319-331, 1984.

Ferguson, B.: Preparing young children for hospitalization: a comparison of two methods, Pediatrics **64**(5):656-664, 1979.

Ferguson, C.K.: Childhood coping: adaptive behavior during intensive care hospitalization, Crit. Care Q. **6**(4):81-93, 1984.

Goldbloom, R.B., and Macleod, M.U.: Impact of preadmission evaluations on elective hospitalization of children, Pediatrics **73**(5):656-660, 1984.

Green, M.: Parent care in the intensive care unit, Am. J. Dis. Child. **133**:1119-1120, 1979.

Hansen, M., Young, D.A., and Carden, F.E.: Psychological evaluation and support in the pediatric intensive care unit, Pediatr. Ann. **15**(1):60-69, 1986.

Hazinski, M.F.: Nursing care of the critically ill child: a seven-point check, Pediatr. Nurs. **11**(6):453-461, 1985.

Hedenkamp, E.A.: Humanizing the intensive care unit for children, Crit. Care Q. **3**(1):63-73, 1980.

Hedenkamp, E.A.: Preparing parents for a visit to the intensive care unit. In Preparing children and families for health care encounters, Washington, DC, 1980, Association for the Care of Children's Health.

King, S.L., and Gregor, F.M.: Stress and coping in families of the critically ill, Crit. Care Nurse **5**(4):48-51, 1985.

Lewandowski, L.: Psychosocial aspects of pediatric critical care. In Hazinski, M.F., editor: Nursing care of the critically ill child, St. Louis, 1984, The C.V. Mosby Co.

Making the right moves in discharge planning, Am. J. Nurs. **79b**(8):1439-1454, 1979.

McGarvey, M: Preschool hospital tours, Child. Health Care **11**(3):122-124, 1983.

McGuire, M., Shepherd, R., and Greco, A.: Hospitalized children in confinement, Pediatr. Nurs. **4**(6):31-35, 1978.

Miles, M.S.: Impact of the intensive care unit on parents, Issues Compr. Pediatr. Nurs. **3**(7):72-90, 1979.

Miles, M.S., and Carter, M.C.: Sources of parental stress in pediatric intensive care units, Child. Health Care **11**(2):65-69, 1982.

Miles, M.S., and Carter, M.C.: Assessing parental stress in intensive care units, Am. J. Maternal Child Nurs. **8** (5):354-359, 1983.

Miles, M.S., and Carter, M.C.: Coping strategies used by parents during their child's hospitalization in an intensive care unit, Child. Health Care **14**(1):14-21, 1985.

O'Mears, K., and others: Preadmission programs: development, implementation, and evaluation, Child. Health Care **11**(4):137-141, 1983.

Pearson, J.E.R., and others: Pediatric intensive care unit patients: effects of play intervention on behavior, Crit. Care Med. **8**(2):64-67, 1980.

Play and preparation: an annotated bibliography, Washington, DC, 1984, Association for the Care of Children's Health.

Pomarico, C., Marsh, K., and Doubrava, P.: Hospital orientation for children, AORN J. **29**(5):864-875, 1979.

Soupios, M., Gallagher, J., and Orlowski, J.P.: Nursing aspects of pediatric intensive care in a general hospital, Pediatr. Clin. North Am. **27**(3):621-632, 1980.

Stevens, K.R.: Humanistic nursing care for critically ill children, Nurs. Clin. North Am. **16**(4):611-622, 1981.

Stevens, K.R.: Psychosocial care. In Vestal, K.W., editor: Pediatric critical care nursing, New York, 1981, John Wiley & Sons, Inc.

Thompson, R.: Recent research on preparation: an annotated bibliography, In Preparing children and families for health care encounters, Washington, D.C., 1980, Association for the Care of Children's Health.

Vestel, K.W., and Richardson, K.: The nature of pediatric critical care nursing: perspectives of patient, family, and staff, Nurs. Clin. North Am. **16**(4):605-610, 1981.

Zweig, I.K.: A new way to get acquainted with the hospital—pediatric open house for well children, Am. J. Maternal Child Nurs. **1**(4):217-219, 1976.

Discharge Planning and Home Care

Bock, R., and others: There's no place like home, Child. Health Care **12**(2):93-96, 1983.

Goldberg, A.I., and others: Home care for life-supported persons: an approach to program development, J. Pediatr. **104**(5):785-795, 1984.

Goldfarb, L., and others: Meeting the challenge of disability or chronic illness—a family guide, Baltimore, 1986, Paul H. Brookes Publishing Co.

Jones, M.: Home care for the chronically ill or disabled child: a manual and sourcebook for parents and professionals, New York, 1985, Harper & Row, Publishers, Inc.

Kasprisin, C.: Home care instructions. In Wong, D., and Whaley, L.: Clinical handbook of pediatric nursing, ed. 2, St. Louis, 1986, The C.V. Mosby Co.

Kruger, S.F., and Rawlins, P.: Pediatric dismissal protocol to aid the transition from hospital care to home care, Image **16**:120, 1984.

McCorkle, R., and others: What nurses need to know about home care, Oncol. Nurs. Forum **11**(6):63-69, 1984.

McHatton, M.: A theory for timely teaching. Am. J. Nurs. **85**(7):798-800, 1985.

Miller, A.: When is the time ripe for teaching? Am. J. Nurs. **85**(7):801-804, 1985.

Morris, E.M., and Fonseca, J.D.: Home care today: an interview with E. Griffith, Am. J. Nurs. **84**(3), 340-342, 1984.

Sanborn, C.W., and Blount, M.: Standard plans for care and discharge, Am. J. Nurs. **84**(11):1394-1396, 1984.

Steele, B.: Home care for children: an annotated bibliography, Washington, DC, 1984, Association for the Care of Children's Health.

Stein, R.: A home care program for children with chronic illness, Child. Health Care **12**(2):90-92, 1983.

SELECTED BOOKS FOR CHILDREN ABOUT HOSPITALIZATION

Chase, F., and Coleman, L.: A visit to the hospital, New York, 1974, Grosset & Dunlap.

Clark B.: Pop-up going to the hospital, New York, 1970, Random House, Inc.

Collier, J.: Danny goes to the hospital, 1970, W.W. Norton & Co., Inc.

Howe, J.: The hospital book, New York, 1981, Crown Publishers Inc.

Rey, M., and Rey, H.: Curious George goes to the hospital, New York, 1966, Houghton Mifflin Co.

Sobol, H.: Jeff's hospital book, New York, 1975, Henry Z. Walck, Inc.
(NOTE: deals with corrective eye surgery for crossed eyes)

Stein, S.: A hospital story, New York, 1974, Walker & Co.

Weber, A.: Elizabeth gets well, New York, 1970, Thomas Y. Crowell Co.

RESOURCES FOR FAMILIES ABOUT HOSPITALIZATION

The following publications are available from the Association for the Care of Children's Health (ACCH), 3615 Wisconsin Avenue, N.W., Washington, DC 20016:

Caring for your child in the emergency room
Caring for your hospitalized baby
A child goes to the hospital
For teenagers: your stay in the hospital
Going to the hospital
Preparing your child for the hospital: a checklist
Preparing your child for repeated or extended hospitalizations
Selected books for children and teenagers about hospitalizaiton, illness, and handicapping conditions
When you visit the ICU
Your hospital: meeting the special needs of children

Talk's About the Hospital, series written by Fred Rogers is available from Family Communications, Inc., 4802 Fifth Avenue, Pittsburgh, PA 15213.

Bibliographies for children about health and illness are available from Pediatric Projects, Inc., P.O. Box 1880, Santa Monica, CA 90406.

An annotated list of books on various aspects of illness and hospitalization is in Fassler, J.: Helping children cope: mastering stress through books and stories, New York, 1978, The Free Press.

Chapter 27

Pediatric Variations of Nursing Interventions

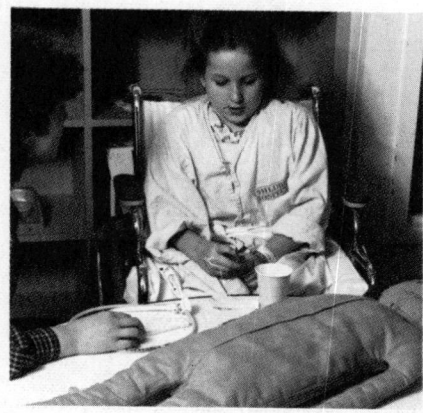

Informed Consent
Requirements for obtaining informed consent
Eligibility for giving informed consent
Informed consent of parents or legal guardian
Informed consent of persons other than parents or legal guardian
Oral informed consent
Informed consent of mature and emancipated minors
Treatment without parental consent
Parental negligence

Preparation for Procedures
Psychologic preparation
Establish trust and provide support
Provide an explanation
Performance of procedure
Expect success
Involve the child
Provide distraction
Allow expression of feelings

Postprocedural support
Encourage expression of feelings
Praise child
Use of play in procedures

Compliance
Assessment
Factors that influence compliance
Measurement of compliance
Compliance strategies
Organizational strategies
Educational strategies
Behavioral strategies

General Hygiene and Care
Bathing
Oral hygiene
Hair care
Feeding the sick child
Control of fever
Physiology of fever
Therapeutic management
Health teaching

Safety
Environmental factors
Limit-setting
Transporting infants and children
Restraints
Jacket restraint
Mummy restraint
Arm and leg restraints
Elbow restraint
Positioning for procedures
Jugular venipuncture
Femoral venipuncture
Extremity venipuncture
Lumbar puncture
Bone marrow aspiration/ biopsy
Other procedures

Collection of Specimens
Urine specimens
Clean-catch specimens
Twenty-four-hour collection
Special techniques
Stool specimens
Blood specimens
Sputum specimens

Administration of Medication
Determination of drug dosage
Body surface area
Preparation for safe administration
Checking dosage
Identification
Parents
Child
Oral administration
Preparation
Administration
Intramuscular administration
Selecting syringe and needle
Determining site
Administration
Intravenous administration
Rectal administration
Optic, otic, and nasal administration
Family teaching and home care

Gastric Feeding Techniques
Gavage feeding
Preparation
Procedure
Gastrostomy feeding
Family teaching and home care

Procedures Related to Elimination
Enema
Ostomies
Family teaching and home care

Procedures Related to Surgery
Psychologic preparation
Preoperative care
Perioperative care
Postoperative care

Children are not simply small adults. They differ from their older counterparts in the areas of biologic, cognitive, and emotional function and response. Consequently many of the standard techniques employed in nursing practice must be altered to meet the special needs of children at various developmental stages. The chapter presents an overview of psychologic preparation of children for procedures, strategies to enhance compliance, application of principles of growth and development in planning, implementing, and evaluating nursing procedures, and selected aspects of skills that require modification in caring for infants and children.

Informed Consent

Informed consent refers to the legal and ethical requirement that the patient clearly, fully, and completely understand the medical treatment to be performed and all the risks, consequences, or results that may or may not occur from the medical treatment. The patient must also be informed of alternative treatments that could be offered, including their benefits and risks. For an informed consent to be valid, three conditions must be met (Hogue, 1986):

1. The person must be capable of giving consent; he must be over the age of majority and must be considered competent—that is, possess the mental capacity to make choices and understand their consequences.
2. The person must receive the information needed to make an intelligent decision.
3. The person must act voluntarily when exercising freedom of choice without force, fraud, deceit, duress, or other forms of constraint or coercion.

Because of the numerous variations of the laws within different regions of the United States, the following discussion of informed consent is presented in general terms and is not to be interpreted as legal advice. Although informing patients of the risks, benefits, and alternatives of a procedure is the physician's responsibility, nurses frequently are responsible for securing the person's signature on the consent form (Cushing, 1984). In caring for children special dilemmas may arise regarding who may sign the consent for treatment when parental consent is not available. The age of majority is especially important when caring for adolescents, and competence is a key issue in decisions involving minors who are retarded (see Questions and controversies, p. 1103). Consequently, nurses need to be familiar with the issues involved in this highly significant and complex subject and must keep current on legal aspects of practice within their community.

REQUIREMENTS FOR OBTAINING INFORMED CONSENT

Written informed consent of the parent or legal guardian is usually required for medical or surgical treatment, including many diagnostic procedures. One blanket consent is not sufficient. Separate informed permissions must be obtained for each surgical or diagnostic procedure, including:

1. Major surgery
2. Minor surgery, for example, cutdown, biopsy, dental extraction, suturing a laceration (especially one that may have a cosmetic effect), removal of a cyst, and closed reduction of a fracture
3. Diagnostic tests with an element of risk, for example, bronchoscopy, needle biopsy, angiography, electroencephalogram, lumbar puncture, cardiac catheterization, ventriculography, and bone marrow aspiration
4. Medical treatments with an element of risk, for example, blood transfusion, thoracentesis or paracentesis, radiation therapy, and shock therapies

In addition, there are certain situations, such as the following, that are not directly related to medical treatment but that require parental consent:

1. Taking photographs for medical, educational, or other public use
2. Removal of the child from the hospital against the advice of the physician
3. Postmortem examinations except in unexplained deaths, such as sudden infant death, violent death, or suspected suicide
4. Examination of medical records by unauthorized persons, such as attorneys or insurance representatives (family members have legal right to medical records)

The need for informed consent is also an issue in research involving children. While parents of minor children must give written informed consent, the researcher must also obtain *assent* from children with a mental age of 7 years or older. Informed assent, which refers to the child's express permission to participate in the research after the purposes and procedures have been explained, is not a legal requirement but an ethical one to protect the rights of children. There is considerable controversy over the use of children as research subjects (see Questions and controversies), and any nurse involved in such research must be aware of the ethical issues and follow ethical guidelines in initiating pediatric research (Rae and Fournier, 1986).

ELIGIBILITY FOR GIVING INFORMED CONSENT

In most situations the parent or legal guardian gives informed consent. However, problems may arise when parents are not available to give informed consent, the child is a borderline or emancipated minor, or the parents neglect or refuse care for their minor children.

Informed Consent of Parents or Legal Guardian

Parents have been considered to have full responsibility for the care and rearing of their minor children, including legal control over them. Therefore as long as a child remains classified as a minor, the parent or the person designated as

Questions and Controversies

What are the ethical arguments regarding use of children as research subjects?

Although the ethics involved in the use of children in experimental research are complex, basically the ethical arguments center on two opposing views: (1) that research on children should never be done, as it is impossible to obtain the children's informed consent (Ramsey, 1978), and (2) that certain forms of research on children without their consent is acceptable if the benefits are high and the risks minimal (Fried, 1978). Obviously, the two issues in each argument are informed consent and risk vs benefit. The requirement for obtaining assent in children over 7 years of age is aimed at providing a vehicle for consent to protect children's rights. However, the question of consent still remains in relation to children with a mental age below 7 years and presented dilemmas in research studies on infants and young children and those with cognitive deficit.

The second issue relates to the risk vs benefit factor. Rae and Fournier (1986) define three types of risk in research: (1) *no risk*, such as retrospective studies using medical records that involve no interaction with children, (2) *minimal risk*, in which the probability and magnitude of physical or psychologic harm is no greater than encountered in daily life or normal medical care, and (3) *more than minimal risk*, in which children are subjected to experimental procedures apart from the necessary care or treatment. These authors conclude that the benefit must greatly exceed the risk in any research involving more than minimal risk and might be justified in such situations in which the results offer hope of curing a life-threatening condition but that in psychosocial research such degrees of benefit can rarely be substantiated.

Currently these ethical issues remain unresolved. Most institutions have an Institutional Review Board (IRB) whose function is to review proposals, educate investigators, and identify potential problems in human-subjects research (Shaffer and Pfeiffer, 1986). Because specific IRB procedures vary according to institutional policy, nurses need to be familiar with the IRB guidelines in their institution and be prepared to document issues such as consent and risk vs benefit in seeking research approval.

legal guardian for the child is required to give informed consent before medical treatment is implemented or any procedure is performed on the child.

Informed Consent of Persons Other than Parents or Legal Guardian

In the absence of the parents or legal guardian, a person in charge of the child is usually allowed to give informed consent for treatment. Depending on state law, this person, *in loco parentis,* may be a relative or other person who is caring for the child while the parents are away.

Temporary caregivers, such as school officials, camp counselors, neighbors, babysitters, foster parents, and court-appointed welfare workers, need written permission from parents for treatment in the event of an emergency (Selbst, 1985). Special forms are available in many hospitals to authorize emergency care to minors. At the least these individuals should know the location of the parents and the child's home address to contact the persons able to give consent.

Oral Informed Consent

When the parent is not immediately available to sign a consent form, oral informed consent may be obtained. This may be a telephone consent or an oral consent from a parent who is for some reason unable to sign, such as because of an injury following an accident. When verbal informed consent is being secured, it is wise to have a witness, such as another nurse, on a telephone extension. Both nurses can record that informed consent was given and the name, address, and relationship of the person giving consent, together with their signatures indicating that they witnessed the consent. As in any other situation, the nurse must be aware of state laws governing oral informed consent.

Informed Consent of Mature and Emancipated Minors

One of the areas in which modifications have been made in the usual view of parental obligation is in regard to borderline minors, that is, youngsters who are legally minors but who are considered to possess the maturity to give consent for their own medical care. Most states have enacted legislation that permits young people to give consent for their medical and surgical treatment.

An *emancipated minor* is one who is legally underage but is recognized as having the legal capacity of an adult under circumstances prescribed by state law. Minors may become emancipated by the following (Selbst, 1985):

Pregnancy
Marriage
High school graduation
Living independently
Military service

The majority of states provide a specific statutory age (usually 15 or 16 years) at which a minor may consent to medical or surgical treatment without parental consent. In this case the child is known as a *mature minor* even though he is not considered emancipated (Leiken, 1983). Examples of medical conditions that can be treated without parental consent include (Selbst, 1985):

Sexually transmitted disease
Contraceptive services
Pregnancy
Drug or alcohol abuse
Emergency care

Consent regarding abortion is more complex. Although state laws vary, the Supreme Court has held that parents have no veto over a daughter's decision for an abortion.

State laws differ in their interpretation of when a child attains the age of majority. Even within the same state a child may be considered an adult in certain situations, for instance, in being responsible for necessities of life (food, clothing, and shelter) but may not be considered an adult in other situations. Many states now consider a child, male or female, an adult upon the eighteenth birthday. However, this may vary; some states may even differentiate between the sexes on attainment of majority. Because the age of majority and definitions of emancipation vary within jurisdictions, nurses need to be aware of the way in which the law functions in their state regarding medical care to children (Selbst, 1985).

Treatment Without Parental Consent

An exception to the general rule that parental consent is obtained before medical treatment of minor children occurs in situations in which children need prompt medical or surgical treatment and a parent is not readily available to give consent. Many states recognize this exception and permit treatment if the life or health of such a minor is in jeopardy or if delayed treatment would create a risk to the health of the minor. When surgical intervention is indicated in such situations, the procedure is usually begun only after consultation with another physician.

Parental Negligence

The state is able to intervene in situations that jeopardize the health and welfare of children. Children may need protection from their parents in cases in which parents neglect or impose excessive or improper punishment on a child. In most communities there are procedures by which custody of the child can be transferred to a governmental or a private agency when parental neglect can be proved. In many cases the state interferes with the parental rights in the interest and protection of minor children.

Preparation for Procedures

Children, regardless of their age, require preparation for procedures. With appropriate preparation the fear and discomfort are minimized and the child is helped to feel success and mastery from a potentially traumatic experience. However, nurses must be aware that a child's responses are strongly influenced by developmental characteristics such as physical and cognitive abilities; environmental factors, including past experiences with hospitalization, procedures, and health personnel; and his perception of the present situation. The child's general temperament and behavior patterns should be assessed, as well as his condition and the degree of regression he has experienced as a result of his illness. All of these areas are considered in planning an approach best suited to the child as an individual.

PSYCHOLOGIC PREPARATION

The principles governing preparation for hospital procedures, such as diagnostic tests, medical treatments, surgery, and other therapeutic interventions, are similar and include the following:

1. Determine the details of the exact procedure to be performed
2. Review the parents' and child's present level of understanding
3. Plan the actual teaching based on the child's developmental age and existing level of knowledge
4. Incorporate parents in the teaching if they desire and especially if they plan to participate in the care
5. While preparing the child, allow for ample discussion to prevent information overload and ensure adequate feedback

The exact timing of the preparation for a procedure varies with the child's age and type of procedure. There are no exact guidelines to govern timing, but in general, the younger the child, the closer the explanation should be to the actual procedure to prevent undue fantasizing and worrying. With complex procedures more time may be needed for assimilation of information, especially with older children. For example, the explanation for an injection can immediately precede the procedure for all ages, but preparation for surgery may begin the day before for young children and a few days before for older children, although older children's preferences should be elicited (see p. 1085).

In addition to these general principles, certain guidelines apply to the actual preparation process and are discussed here. Specific suggestions for each age-group based on developmental characteristics are included in Table 27-1.

Establish Trust and Provide Support

The nurse who has spent time with and who has established a positive relationship with a child will usually find it easy to gain his cooperation. If the relationship is based on trust, the child will associate the nurse with caregiving activities that give him comfort and pleasure most of the time and not as someone who brings discomfort and stress. If the nurse does not know the child, it is best if she is introduced by another staff person whom the child trusts. The first visit with the child should avoid any painful procedure and ideally should focus on the child first, then on the explanation of the procedure. When talking with the child, the nurse uses the same guidelines for communicating with children that are discussed in Chapter 6.

Children need support during procedures, and for young children the greatest source of support is the parents. However, controversy exists regarding the role parents should assume during the procedure, especially if discomfort is involved (see Questions and controversies), and nurses need to consider the issues in deciding whether parental presence is beneficial. The parents' preferences for assisting, observing, or waiting outside the room should be assessed. Parents who wish to stay need preparation for what will occur and how they can help. Simple instructions such as clarifying where parents can stay in the room and positioning them where they have eye contact with the child provide support and lessen anxiety. Parents who do not wish to be present or participate are supported in their decision and encouraged to remain close by so that they can be available to console the child immediately following the procedure.

Table 27-1 Guidelines for preparing children for procedures

DEVELOPMENTAL CHARACTERISTICS	RESPONSIBILITIES
Infancy: developing trust	
Attachment to parent	Involve parent in procedure if desired Keep parent in infant's line of vision If parent is unable to be with infant, place familiar object with infant, such as stuffed toy
Stranger anxiety	Have usual caregivers perform or assist with procedure Make advances slowly and in nonthreatening manner Limit number of strangers from entering room during procedure
Sensorimotor phase of learning	During procedure use sensory soothing measures (e.g., stroking skin, talking softly, giving pacifier) Use analgesics (e.g., local anesthetic, sedation) to control discomfort Cuddle and hug child after procedure; encourage parent to comfort child
Increased muscle control	Expect older infants to resist Restrain adequately Keep harmful objects out of reach
Memory for past experiences	Realize that older infants associate objects or persons with prior painful experiences Keep in mind that older infants will cry and resist at sight of objects or persons that inflict pain Keep frightening objects out of view Perform painful procedures in a separate room, not in crib
Imitation of gestures	Model desired behavior (e.g., opening mouth)
Toddler: developing autonomy	Use same approaches as above in addition to following:
Egocentric	Explain procedure in relation to what child will see, hear, taste, smell, and feel Emphasize those aspects of procedure that require cooperation, such as lying still Tell child he can cry, yell, or use other means to verbally express discomfort
Negative behavior	Expect treatments to be resisted; child may try to run away Use firm, direct approach Ignore temper tantrums Use distraction techniques Restrain adequately
Limited language skills	Communicate using behaviors Use few and simple terms that are familiar to child Give one direction at a time, such as "Lie down" and then "Hold my hand" Use small replicas of equipment; allow child to handle equipment Use play; demonstrate on doll but avoid child's favorite doll as he may think doll is really "feeling" procedure Prepare parents separately to avoid child's misinterpreting words
Limited concept of time	Prepare child shortly or immediately before procedure Keep teaching sessions short (about 5 to 10 minutes) Have preparations completed before involving child in procedure Have extra equipment nearby (e.g., alcohol swabs, new needle, or Band-Aids) to avoid delays Tell child when procedure is completed
Striving for independence	Allow choices whenever possible but realize that child may still be resistant and negative Allow child to participate in care and to help whenever possible (e.g., drink medicine from a cup, hold a dressing)
Preschooler: developing initiative	
Preoperational thought; egocentric	Explain procedure in simple terms and in relation to how it affects child (as with toddler, stress sensory aspects) Demonstrate use of equipment Allow child to play with miniature or actual equipment Encourage "playing out" experience on a doll both before and after procedure to clarify misconceptions Use neutral words to describe the procedure (see box, p. 1108)
Increased language skills	Use verbal explanation but avoid overestimating child's comprehension of words Encourage child to verbalize ideas and feelings

Continued.

Table 27-1 Guidelines for preparing children for procedures—cont'd

DEVELOPMENTAL CHARACTERISTICS	RESPONSIBILITIES
Concept of time and frustration tolerance still limited	Implement same approaches as for toddler but may plan longer teaching session (10 to 15 minutes); may divide information into more than one session
Illness and hospitalization often viewed as punishment	Clarify why all procedures are performed, such as "This medicine will make you feel better" Ask child his thoughts regarding why a procedure is performed State directly that procedures are never a form of punishment
Fears of bodily harm, intrusion, and castration	Point out on drawing, doll, or child where procedure is performed Emphasize that no other body part will be involved Use nonintrusive procedures whenever possible (e.g., axillary temperatures, oral medication) Apply a Band-Aid over puncture site Realize that procedures involving genitals provoke anxiety Allow child to wear underpants with gown Explain unfamiliar situations, especially noises or lights
Striving for initiative	Involve child in care whenever possible (e.g., hold equipment, remove dressing) Give choices whenever possible but avoid excessive delays Praise child for helping and cooperating; never shame child for lack of cooperation

School-age: developing industry

Increased language skills; interest in acquiring knowledge	Explain procedures using correct scientific/medical terminology Explain reason for procedure using simple diagrams of anatomy and physiology Explain functioning and mechanism of equipment in concrete terms Allow child to manipulate equipment; use doll or another person as model to practice using equipment whenever possible (doll play may be considered "childish" by older school-age child) Allow time before and after procedure for questions and discussion
Improved concept of time	Plan for longer teaching sessions (about 20 minutes) Prepare in advance of procedure
Increased self-control	Gain child's cooperation Tell child what is expected Suggest ways of maintaining control (e.g., deep breathing, relaxation, counting)
Striving for industry	Allow responsibility for simple tasks, such as collecting specimens Include in decision making, such as time of day to perform procedure, preferred site Encourage active participation, such as removing dressings, handling equipment, opening packages
Developing relationships with peers	May prepare two or more children for same procedure or encourage one to help prepare another peer Provide privacy from peers during procedure to maintain self-esteem

Adolescents: developing identity

Increasingly capable of abstract thought and reasoning	Supplement explanations with reasons why procedure is necessary or beneficial Explain long-term consequences of procedures Realize that adolescent may fear death, disability, or other potential risks Encourage questioning regarding fears, options, and alternatives
Conscious of appearance	Provide privacy Discuss how procedure may affect appearance, such as scar, and what can be done to minimize it Emphasize any physical benefits of procedure
Concerned more with present than future	Realize that immediate effects of procedure are more significant than future benefits
Striving for independence	Involve in decison making and planning, for example, choice of time, place, individuals present during procedure (such as parents), clothing to wear Impose as few restrictions as possible Suggest methods of maintaining control Accept regression to more childish methods of coping Realize that adolescent may have difficulty in accepting new authority figures and may resist complying with procedures
Developing peer relationships and group identity	Same as for school-age child but assumes even greater significance

Questions and Controversies

Should parents be allowed to stay with their children during stressful procedures?

Health professionals have basically adopted two opposing philosophies in relation to parental presence during procedures. One view purports that parents should not be present since the child may view the parent's presence and/or participation as complicity and then blame the parent for allowing such indignities to be inflicted on him. Since children normally associate parents with a comforting, "make it better" role, these professionals believe that parents should be a source of comfort and security to the child, which is best served by reuniting the child and parents after the procedure. The opposite view holds that not allowing the parents to be present inflicts the additional stress of separation on the child and deprives him of his parent's support. There is no consensus on whether parents who are present with the child should participate in the procedure, such as assisting in restraint.

While relatively little research has focused on this important issue, most of the available research finds that parental presence is supportive. Vernon, Foley, and Schulman (1967) compared preschoolers' responses to stress during admission and anesthesia induction with the parent present or absent. They found no differences in the preschoolers' behavior during admission procedures but considerably more distress in children whose parent was not present during induction, especially at the final phase after the mask was placed on the face. A more recent study found similar results when parents were permitted to stay with unpremedicated children during induction anesthesia in an outpatient setting (Hannallah and Rosales, 1983).

Shaw and Routh (1982) assessed the effect of parental presence on young children during an injection and found that the children separated from the parent cried less and for a shorter duration. They concluded that the increased negative behavior in the children when the parent was present was not an indication of greater upset but evidence of the children's greater expression of emotion in a supportive atmosphere. Another study on parental presence during dental treatment, which did not find a statistically significant difference between children's stress levels and parental presence or absence, did find that children whose parents were with them were more relaxed (Venham, Bengston, Cipes, 1978). While some health professionals maintain that parents are disruptive during a procedure, Savedra (1981) found that most parents choose to participate, are not disruptive of the procedure, and are able to support their children even when they find the experience difficult and stressful.

Provide an Explanation

Children need an explanation for anything that involves them directly. Before performing a procedure, the nurse explains to the child what is to be done and what is expected of him. The explanation should be short, simple, and appropriate to the child's level of comprehension. Long explanations are not necessary and may only increase anxiety in a small child. This is especially true regarding painful procedures. When explaining the procedure to parents with the child present, the nurse uses language appropriate to the child because unfamiliar words can be misunderstood. If the parents need additional preparation, this is done in an area away from the child. Teaching sessions are planned at times most conducive to the child's learning, for example, after a rest period, and for the usual span of attention.

Special equipment is not necessary for preparing a child, but for young children who cannot yet think in concepts, using objects to supplement verbal explanation is important. Allowing children to handle actual items that will be used in their care, such as a stethoscope, sphygmomanometer, or oxygen mask, helps them to develop familiarity with these items and to reduce the threat often associated with their use. Miniature versions of hospital items such as gurneys and x-ray and intravenous equipment can be used to explain what the children can expect and permit them to safely experience the situations that are unfamiliar and potentially frightening. Written and illustrated materials are also valuable aids to preparation.*

Although the precise words used to describe a procedure will vary for children in each age-group and for each specific event, several important considerations apply to any situation:

1. Use concrete, not abstract, terms and visual aids to describe the procedure. For example, use a simple line drawing of a boy or girl (Fig. 27-1) and mark the body part that will be involved in the procedure.
2. Emphasize that no other body part will be involved.
3. Use words appropriate to the child's level of understanding (a rule of thumb for number of words is the age in years plus 1).
4. Avoid words/phrases with dual meanings (see box, p. 1108).
5. Clarify all unfamiliar words, such as "anesthesia is a *special* sleep."
6. Allow the child to practice those procedures that will require his cooperation, such as turning, coughing, deep breathing, using a blow bottle or mask, or breathing on an intermittent positive pressure (IPPB) machine.
7. Emphasize the sensory aspects of the procedure—what the child will feel, see, smell, and touch and what he can do during the procedure, such as lie still, count out loud, squeeze a hand, or hug a doll.
8. If the body part is associated with a specific function, stress the change or noninvolvement of that ability, for example, following tonsillectomy, the child can still speak.
9. Introduce anxiety-laden information last, such as the preoperative injection.
10. Be honest with the child about the unpleasant aspects of a procedure but avoid creating undue concern. When discussing that a procedure may be uncomfortable, state that it feels different to different people and the child can tell you how it felt.

*Sources of preparatory materials are the *You're Gonna Do What?* series of diagnosis and treatment procedures available from Arkansas Children's Hospital Companies, 1916 Maryland Ave., Little Rock, AR 72202; *Talks About the Hospital Series* by Fred Rogers and available from Family Communications, Inc., 4802 Fifth Ave., Pittsburgh, PA 15213; and *Child Care Series—Patient Education for Children* available from the Centering Corp., P.O. Box 3367, Omaha, NE 68103-0367.

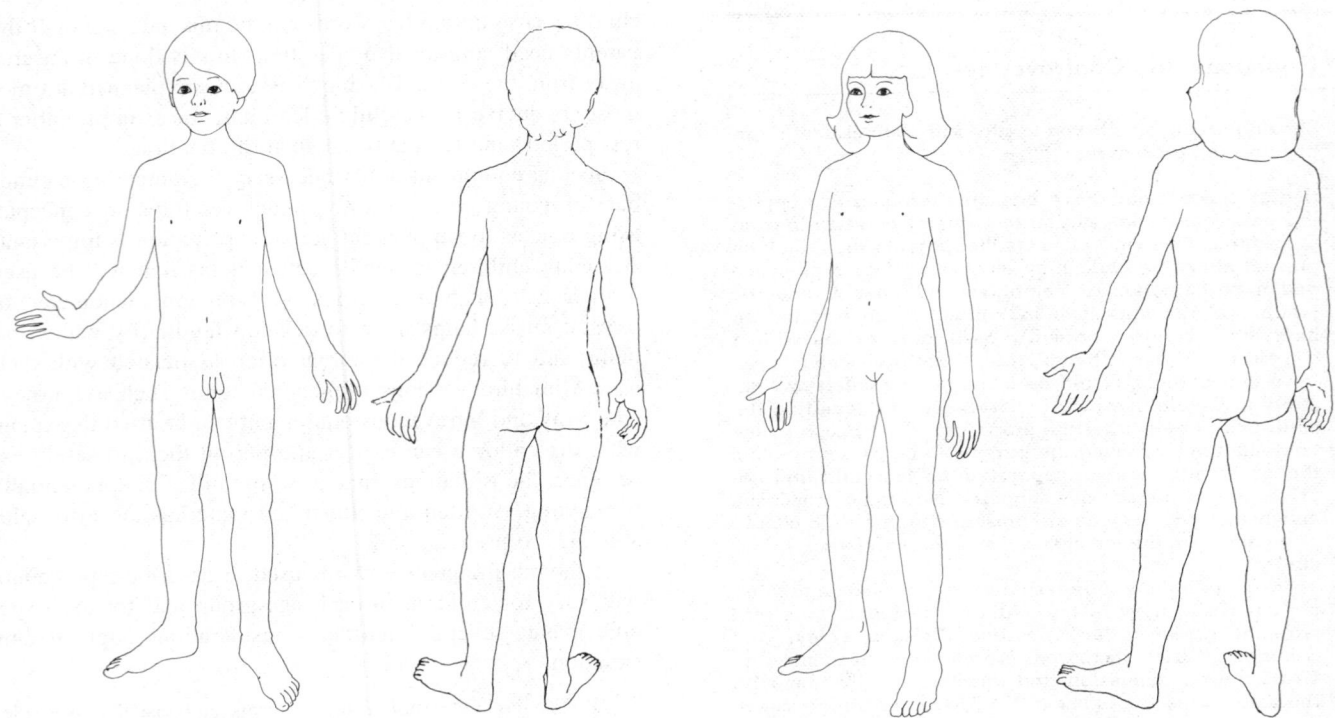

Fig. 27-1. Examples of line drawings to be used in preparing child for procedures.

GUIDELINES FOR SELECTING NONTHREATENING WORDS OR PHRASES

Words/phrases to avoid	Suggested substitutions
Shot	Medicine under the skin
Organ, tissue	Special place in body
Test	See how _____ is working
Incision	Special opening
Edema	Puffiness
Stretcher	Rolling bed
Stool	Child's usual term
Dye	Special medicine
Pain	Hurt, discomfort, "owie"
Deaden	Numb, make sleepy
Cut, fix	Make better
Take (as in "take your temperature")	See how warm you are
Put to sleep	Special sleep

11. Emphasize the end of the procedure and any pleasurable events afterward, such as going home or seeing the parent. Stress the positive benefits of the procedure, for example, "After your tonsils are made better, you won't have as many sore throats."

PERFORMANCE OF PROCEDURE

Supportive care continues during the procedure and can be a major factor in a child's ability to cooperate and achieve mastery. Ideally the same nurse who explains the procedure should perform it or assist. Before beginning, all equipment is assembled and the room is readied to prevent unnecessary delays and interruptions that only serve to increase the child's anxiety. If at all possible, procedures should be performed in a special treatment room rather than the child's bedroom. Procedures should never be performed in "safe" areas, such as the playroom. If the procedure is lengthy, conversation that could be misinterpreted by the child is avoided. As the procedure is nearing completion the nurse should inform the child that it is almost over.

Expect Success

Nurses who approach children with confidence and who convey the impression that they expect to be successful are less likely to encounter difficulty. It is best to approach a child as though he is expected to cooperate. Children sense anxiety in another and will respond to a perceived threat by striking out or with active resistance. Although it is not possible to eliminate such behavior in every child, a firm approach with a positive attitude on the part of the nurse tends to convey a feeling of security to most children.

Involve the Child

As in any other aspect of care, involving children helps to gain their cooperation. Permitting them to make choices gives them some measure of control. However, a choice is given only in situations in which one is available. To ask a child, "Do you want to take your medicine now?" or "I'm going to give you a shot now, okay?" leads him to believe that there is an option and provides him with the opportunity to legitimately refuse or delay the medication. This places the nurse in an awkward, if not impossible, position. It is much better to state firmly, "It's time to drink your medicine now." Children usually like to make choices, but the choice must be one that they do indeed have, for example, "It's time for your medicine. Do you want to drink it plain or with a little water?"

Many children respond to tactics that appeal to their maturity or courage. This also gives them a sense of participation and achievement. For example, preschool children will be proud that they can hold the dressing during the procedure or remove the tape. The same is true for the school-age child who cooperates with minimal resistance.

Provide Distraction

When a child is occupied with some activity that interests him, he is less likely to focus on the procedure. For example, when an injection is given, it is helpful to give the child something to do or something on which to focus his attention. For example, asking the child to point the toes inward and wiggle them not only helps relax the gluteal muscles but provides a diversion. Other strategies for diverting attention are to have the child tightly squeeze the hands of a parent or an assistant, count aloud, sing a familiar song such as a nursery rhyme, or verbally express his discomfort. Other interventions that may lessen the discomfort are relaxation, imagery, and cutaneous stimulation (see box, p. 1071).

Allow Expression of Feelings

The child should be allowed to express feelings of anger, anxiety, fear, frustration, or any other emotion. It is natural for children to strike out in frustration or to try to avoid stress-provoking situations. The child needs to know that it is alright to cry. Whatever the response, it is important that the nurse accept the behavior for what it is. Telling a child with limited verbal skills, such as a toddler, to stop kicking, biting, or otherwise expressing his frustration conveys to him that he is not being understood. Behavior is his primary means of communication and coping and should be permitted unless it inflicts harm on the child or those caring for him.

POSTPROCEDURAL SUPPORT

After the procedure the child continues to need reassurance that he performed well and is accepted and loved. If the parents did not participate, the child is united with them as soon as possible so that they can comfort him.

Encourage Expression of Feelings

Some planned activity after the procedure is helpful in encouraging expression of feelings in a constructive way. Infants and young children are given the opportunity for gross

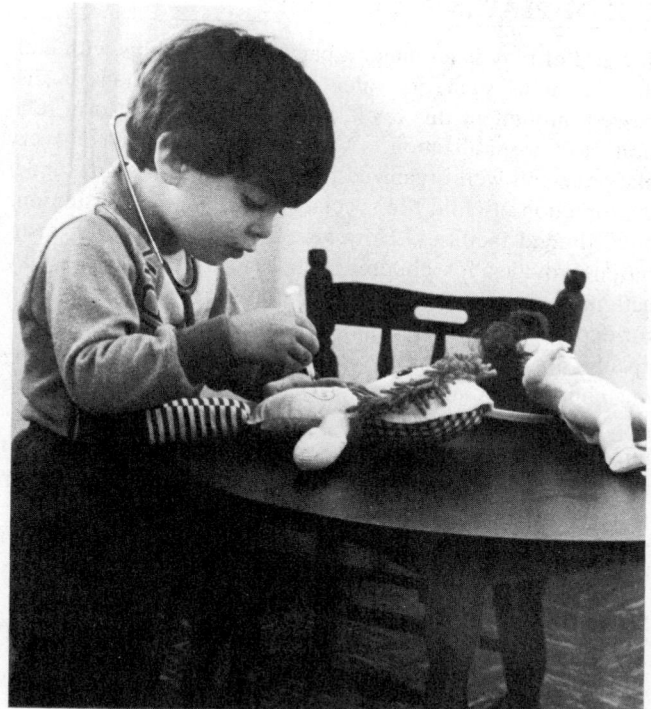

Fig. 27-2. Needle play provides child with opportunity to play out fears and concerns.

motor movement. Even older children are able to vent their anger and frustration in acceptable pounding or throwing activities. Play-Doh is a remarkably versatile medium for pounding and shaping. Dramatic play provides an outlet for anger and places the child in a position of control, in contrast to his position of helplessness in the real situation. One of the most effective interventions is therapeutic play, which includes activities such as permitting the child to give a "shot" to a doll or stuffed toy to reduce the stress of injections (Fig. 27-2).

Praise Child

The child needs to hear from others that they know that he did the best he could in the situation—no matter how he behaved. It is important for the child to know that his worth is not being judged on the basis of his behavior in a stressful situation. Reward systems, such as earning stars or tokens or saving the empty medicine cup as evidence of achievement, are often helpful. Children who require distasteful medications or injections over a period of time can look with pride on a series of stars or stickers on a calendar, especially if an accumulated number represents a special privilege or reward.

Returning to the child a short while after the procedure helps the nurse to strengthen a supportive relationship. Relating with the child in a relaxed and nonstressful period allows him to see the nurse not only as someone associated with stressful situations but as someone with whom to share pleasurable experiences as well.

USE OF PLAY IN PROCEDURES

The use of play is an integral part of relationships with children, and, as such, its value in specific situations is discussed throughout this book, such as in Chapter 26 in relation to hospitalization. Many institutions have very elaborate and well-organized play areas and programs under the direction of child life specialists, while other institutions have limited facilities. However, no matter what the institution provides for children, nurses can still include play activities as part of nursing care. Play can be used to teach, for expression of feelings, or as a method to achieve a therapeutic goal. Consequently, it should be included in preparing children for and encouraging their cooperation during procedures. Play sessions after procedures can be structured, such as directed toward needle play, or general, with a wide variety of equipment available for children to play with. Even "routine" procedures such as temperature taking and oral administration of medication may be of concern to children (Ellerton, Caty, and Ritchie, 1985). The box presents suggestions for incorporating play into nursing procedures and activities for the hospitalized child that facilitate learning and adjustment to a new situation.

Compliance

One of the most significant problems in terms of procedures that must be repeated in the hospital and/or continued at home is related to compliance. Compliance refers to the extent to which the patient's behavior in terms of taking medication, following diets, or executing other life-style changes coincides with the prescribed regimen (Blum, 1984). Estimates on patient noncompliance vary but conservatively up to 50% of patients do not follow instructions in taking medicines (Moree, 1985). Reviews of compliance rates in children with chronic diseases estimate that the rate of noncompliance may be as high as 88% (Rapoff and Christophersen, 1982). Since nurses are frequently responsible for teaching families about treatment protocols, they must have knowledge of factors that influence compliance, methods to measure compliance, and strategies to enhance adherence to prescribed treatment.

ASSESSMENT

In developing strategies to improve compliance the nurse must first assess the level of compliance in the patient. Since many children are too young to assume partial or total responsibility for their care, parents are usually the primary caregivers in terms of home management. Consequently the nurse needs to assess their ability to carry out instructions. The first approach to assessment is knowledge of those factors that influence compliance and the second is to apply methods to more objectively assess the child's and parents' levels of compliance.

Factors that Influence Compliance

Research concerned with compliance has identified several factors that influence compliance, and these are summarized in the box. The first area relates to factors about the patient. Contrary to what might be expected, there are no typical characteristics of noncompliers and even education is not correlated with compliance (Haynes, 1982; McCord, 1986). There is some evidence that higher levels of self-esteem and increased autonomy favorably affect adolescent compliance (Litt, Cuskey, and Rosenberg, 1982). However, family factors are important and characteristics that are associated with good compliance include family support, good communication, and expectations for successful completion of therapeutic regimen.

Factors relating to the care setting are very important in determining compliance and provide useful guidelines in planning strategies to improve compliance. Basically any aspect of the health care setting that increases the family's satisfaction with the physical setting and the relationship with the practitioner positively influences adherence to the treatment regimen. In addition the type of care required to manage the disorder is important. The more complex, expensive, inconvenient, longer, and disruptive the treatment protocol, the less likely the family is to comply. Obviously, during long-term conditions that involve multiple treatments and considerable rearrangement of life-style, compliance is most severely affected.

Measurement of Compliance

While it is helpful to know those factors that influence compliance, especially in assessing the likelihood of compliance in a family, assessment must include more direct measurement techniques. A number of methods exist, each with their advantages and disadvantages. The most successful approach includes a combination of at least two of the following methods (Haynes, 1982; Westfall, 1986):

clinical judgment The nurse judges family compliance. This is a very poor method that is subject to bias and inaccuracy unless the nurse carefully evaluates the criteria used in evaluation.

self-reporting The family is asked about their ability to carry out the prescribed treatments. While a simple method, most people overestimate their compliance by about 20%, even when they admit to lapses in treatment.

direct observation The nurse directly observes the patient or family perform the treatment. Although this approach is very effective in identifying errors related to the correct procedure, it is difficult to employ outside the health care setting and the family's awareness of being observed frequently affects their performance.

monitoring appointments The family's attendance at scheduled appointments is recorded. Keeping appointments indicates general levels of compliance but only indirectly indicates compliance with the prescribed care.

monitoring therapeutic response The child's response in terms of benefit from treatment is monitored, preferably re-

PLAY ACTIVITIES FOR SPECIFIC PROCEDURES

Fluid intake

Make freezer pops using child's favorite juice

Cut Jell-O into fun shapes

Make game of taking sip when turning page of book or in games like "Simon Says"

Use small medicine cups; decorate the cups

Color water with food coloring or Kool Aid

Have tea party; pour at small table

Let child fill a syringe and squirt it into his mouth or use it to fill small decorated cups

Cut straws in half and place in small container (much easier for child to suck liquid)

Decorate straw—cut out small design with two holes and pass straw through; place small sticker on straw

Use a "crazy" straw

Make a "progress poster"; give rewards for drinking a predetermined quantity

Deep breathing

Blow bubbles with bubble blower

Blow bubbles with straw (no soap)

Blow on pinwheel, feathers, whistle, harmonica, balloons, toy horns

Practice band instruments

Draw face on rubber glove to expand when blown up

Have blowing contest using balloons, boats, cotton balls, feathers, marbles, Ping-Pong balls, pieces of paper

Blow such objects on a table top without falling over a goal line, over water, through an obstacle course, up in the air, against an opponent, or up and down a string

Suck paper or cloth from one container to another using a straw

Use blow bottles with colored water to transfer water from one side to the other

Dramatize stories, as "I'll huff and puff and blow your house down" from the Three Little Pigs

Do straw blowing painting

Take a deep breath and "blow out the candles" on a birthday cake

Range of motion and use of extremities

Throw bean bags at fixed or movable target, wadded paper into wastebasket

Touch or kick balloons held or hung in different positions (if child is in traction, hand balloon from trapeze)

Play "tickle toes"; wiggle them on request

Play Twister game or "Simon Says"

Play pretend and guess games, such as imitate a bird, butterfly, horse

Have tricycle or wheelchair races in safe area

Play kick or throw ball with soft foam ball in safe area

Position bed so that child must turn to view television or doorway

Climb wall like "spider"

Pretend to teach "aerobic" dancing or exercises; encourage parents to participate

Encourage swimming, if feasible

Play video games or pinball (fine motor movement)

Play "hide and seek" game—hide toy somewhere in bed (or room, if ambulatory) and have child find using specified hand or foot

Provide clay to mold with fingers

Paint or draw on large sheets of paper placed on floor or wall

Encourage combing own hair; play "beauty shop" with "customer" in different positions

Soaks

Play with small toys or objects (cups, syringes, soap dishes) in water

Wash dolls or toys

Bubbles may be added to bath water if permissible; move bubbles to create shapes or "monsters"

Pick up marbles, pennies from bottom of bath container

Make designs with coins on bottom of container

Pretend to make a boat or submarine by keeping it immersed

Have "Instant Products"* for child (a capsule filled with a design that when immersed in warm water dissolves and foam rubber animals or other surprises appear)

Read to child during soaks, sing with child, or play game, such as cards, checkers, or other board game (if both hands are immersed, move the board pieces for the child)

Sitz bath—give child something to listen to (music, stories) or look at (Viewmaster, book, etc.)

Injections

Let child handle syringe, vial, alcohol swab and give a "shot" to doll or stuffed animal

Use syringes to decorate cookies with frosting, squirt paint, or target shoot into a container

Draw a "magic circle" or area before injection

Allow child to have a "collection" of syringes (without needles); make "wild" creative objects with syringes

If multiple injections or venipunctures, make a "progress poster;" give rewards for predetermined number of injections

Ambulation

Give child something to push

    Toddler—push-pull toy

    School age—wagon or decorated IV

    Teenage—a baby in a stroller or wheelchair

Have a parade—make hats, drums, etc.

Extending environment (patients in traction, etc.)

Make bed into a pirate ship or airplane with decorations

Put up mirrors so patient can see around room

Move patient's bed frequently, especially to playroom, hallway, or outside

*Instant Products, Inc., P.O. Box 33068, Louisville, KY 40232.

corded on a graph or chart. Unfortunately, few treatments yield directly measurable results, such as decreased blood pressure or weight loss, making this a less satisfactory method for most types of therapies.

pill counts The nurse counts the number of pills remaining in the original container and compares the amount missing to the number of days the medication should have been taken. Although this is a simple method, families may forget to bring the container or deliberately alter the number of pills to avoid detection. This method is also poorly suited to liquid medication, which is so commonly prescribed in pediatrics.

chemical assay For certain drugs, such as digoxin and phenytoin, measurement of plasma drug levels provides information on the amount of drug recently ingested. However, this method is expensive, indicates only short-term compliance, and requires precise timing of the assay for accurate results.

COMPLIANCE STRATEGIES

Strategies to improve compliance are concerned with those interventions that encourage families to follow the prescribed treatment regimen. Ideally such strategies should be implemented before or concurrent with the initiation of therapy to avoid compliance problems. A number of strategies have been identified as effective but, like measurement methods, no one approach is always successful and the best results occur when at least two strategies are employed. The following is an overview of compliance strategies.

Organizational Strategies

Organizational strategies refer to those interventions that are concerned with the care setting and the therapeutic plan and include manipulating the factors listed in the box below that are known to positively affect compliance (Young, 1986). Depending on the individual situation, this may involve increasing the frequency of appointments, designating a primary practitioner, reducing the cost of medication by purchasing generic brands, reducing the disruption of the treatment on the family's life-style, and the use of "cues" to minimize forgetting. Numerous devices are available commercially or can be improvised for cueing, such as pill dispensers; watches with alarms; charts to record completed

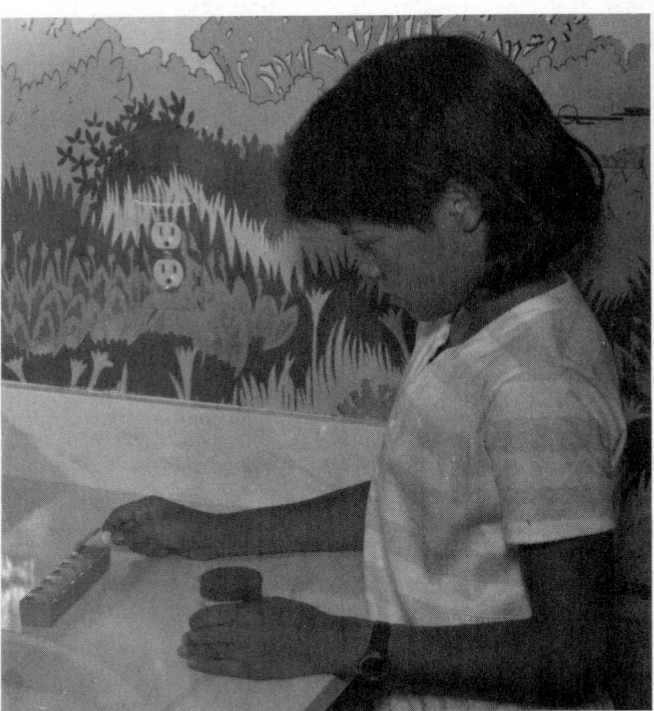

Fig. 27-3. Pill dispensers can help children assume responsibility for their care at home, serve as reminders that medication needs to be taken, and facilitate checking compliance.

therapy; reminders, such as messages on the refrigerator or morning coffee pot; and treatment schedules that incorporate the treatment plan into the daily routine, such as physical therapy after the evening bath (Fig. 27-3).

Educational Strategies

Educational strategies are concerned with instructing the family about the treatment plan. Although education is an important component in enhancing compliance and patients who are more knowledgeable about their condition are more likely to comply, education alone does not ensure compliant behavior. Also, for education to be effective it must incorporate teaching principles known to enhance understanding and retention of material (see box). Written materials are essential, especially in any regimen requiring multiple or complex treatments, and need to be readable by the average individual, which appears to be at the fourth grade level (50% of health care clients have difficulty or are unable to read at a fifth grade level) (Streiff, 1986).

Behavioral Strategies

Behavioral strategies encompass those interventions designed to directly modify behavior. Several strategies exist that are effective in encouraging the desired behavior and are very useful with children. Ideally positive reinforcement should be employed to strengthen the behavior and may consist of earning stars or tokens, which gains the child a special privilege or gift. A more formal method is the use

---

FACTORS THAT POSITIVELY INFLUENCE COMPLIANCE

Individual/family factors
High self-esteem
Positive body image
High degree of autonomy (increased locus of control)
Supportive and well-adjusted family
Effective family communication
Family expectation for successful completion of therapy

Care setting factors
Perceived satisfaction with care
Positive interactions with practitioners
Continuity of care
Individualized care
Minimum waiting time for appointments
Convenient care setting

Treatment factors
Simple
Minimum disruption in usual life-style
Short duration
Inexpensive
Visible benefits
Tolerable side effects

GUIDELINES FOR EFFECTIVE TEACHING

Establish rapport; reduce anxiety and fear

Assess what family knows and expects to learn, especially if they have concerns, and address their concerns before beginning teaching

Assess family's learning style; ask if they are the type of people who like to have everything explained in detail or if they prefer knowing only the major facts

Use a variety of teaching materials (lecture, demonstration, video or slide presentation, written material)

Speak family's language, avoid jargon, and clarify all terms

Be specific when giving information; divide information into small steps

Keep information short, simple, and concrete

Introduce most important information first

Use "verbal" headings to organize information, such as "There are two things you need to learn: how to give the medicine and what side effects to look for. First, how to give. . . . Second, what side effects . . ."

Stress how important instructions are and expected benefits; explain detrimental effects of inadequate treatment but avoid fear tactics

Evaluate teaching by eliciting feedback to ensure that family understands information

Repeat information as needed

Reward family for learning through verbal praise

of contracting (see below). However, at times disciplinary techniques, such as time out for young children (see p. 608) or withholding privileges for older children, may be needed to reduce noncompliance (Rapoff, 1986).

Contracting. Contracting is a process in which the exact elements of desired behavior are explicitly outlined in the form of a written contract (Steckel, 1982). Based on behavior modification it is a very effective method of shaping behavior, especially with older children who are involved in the process of defining the rules of the agreement. Ideally it should involve tangible rewards but it may include negative consequences, such as demerits or "checks" for failing to comply. In deciding whether to use positive or negative reinforcers, the nurse should question parents about their opinion regarding powerful motivators for the child. Often the contract includes a commitment from the parent, such as agreeing to stop nagging about taking medication.

An effective contract includes the following components:

1. The goal or desired behavior is realistic and seems possible.
2. The behavior is measurable, for example, agreeing to take the drug before leaving for school without reminding.
3. The contract is written and signed by all those involved in any of the agreements.
4. The contract is dated and, if appropriate, a date is specified when a goal should be reached, such as number of pounds of weight loss in 2 weeks.
5. The identified rewards or consequences are reinforcing.
6. The goal can be evaluated, such as using counting the number of pills or using a scale for weight measurement.

Once the contract is implemented it should be evaluated at the end of the time specified in the agreement and revisions

made, such as extending the time or terminating the contract. If the contract has not been successful, every effort should be made to ascertain if the goals were realistic, the time period was sufficient for accomplishing the goal, and the rewards or consequences were motivating.

General Hygiene and Care

Hygienic care is continued throughout the child's hospital stay and is essentially no different from that provided to persons of any age. The primary differences are those related to the size of the patient. Grooming aids and attractive attire are important adjuncts to hygienic care. Children are delighted with anything that makes them feel more attractive.

Certain caregiving activities present special challenges, especially feeding the sick child. In addition children often have high fevers that require attention. Any of these activities presents excellent opportunities for family health teaching.

BATHING

Unless contraindicated, most infants and children can be bathed in a tub at the bedside, on the bed, or in a standard bathtub located on the unit, which is often conveniently adapted for pediatric use. For infants and young children confined to bed the towel method can be used. Two towels are immersed in a dilute soap solution and wrung damp. With the child lying supine on a dry towel, one damp towel is placed on top of the child and used to gently clean the body. This towel is discarded, then the child is dried and turned prone. The procedure is repeated using the second damp towel.

Infants and small children are *never* left unattended in a bathtub, and infants who are unable to sit alone are securely held with one hand during the bath. The infant's head is supported securely with one hand or the farther arm is firmly grasped in the nurse's hand while the head rests comfortably on the wrist. This provides secure control of the infant while the other hand is free to wash the infant's body (Fig. 27-4). Infants or children who are able to sit without assistance need only close supervision and a pad placed in the bottom of the tub to prevent slipping and loss of balance, which could result in a bumped head or submersion of the face.

Older children may enjoy a shower if it is available. School-age children may be reluctant to bathe, and many are not accustomed to a daily bath. However, most children who feel well require little encouragement to participate in their daily care. Nurses will need to use judgment regarding the amount of supervision the child requires. Some can be trusted to assume this responsibility unaided, whereas others will need someone in constant attendance. Retarded children, those with physical limitations such as severe anemia

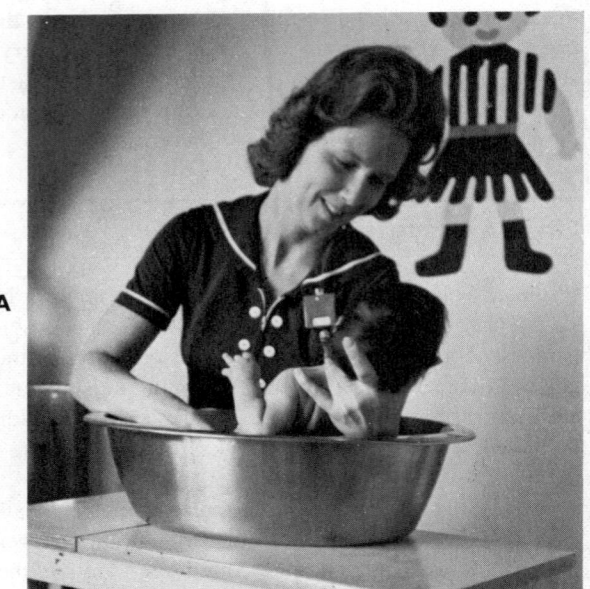
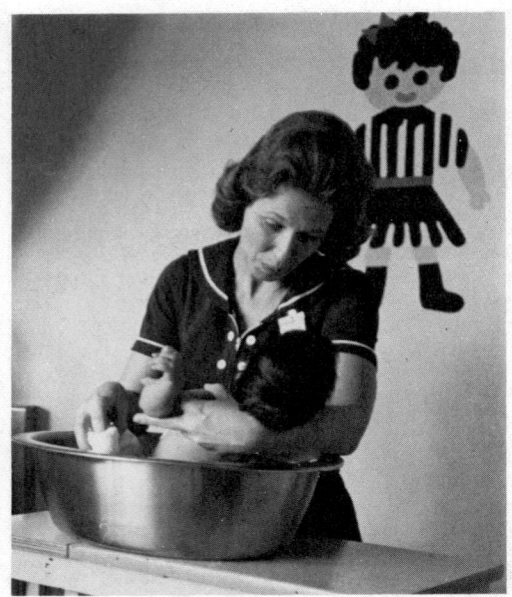

Fig. 27-4. Proper method for holding infant for tub bath. **A,** Supporting neck; **B,** neck supported on wrist.

or leg deformities, and suicidal or psychotic children (who may commit bodily harm) require close supervision.

Areas that require special attention during bed baths and for children performing their own care are the ears, between skin folds, the neck, the back, and the genital area. The genital area should be carefully cleansed and dried with particular care to skin folds, and in uncircumcised boys the foreskin should be gently retracted and the exposed surfaces cleansed and then the foreskin replaced. Older children have the tendency to avoid these areas; therefore they may need a gentle reminder.

Children who are ill or debilitated will need more extensive assistance with bathing and other aspects of hygienic care, but they should be encouraged to perform as much as they are capable without overtaxing their energies. Increasing involvement can be expected with improved strength and endurance. Children who are limited in the capacity for self-help and who have no other contraindications benefit a great deal from tub baths. They can be transported to the tub and, with the aid of lifting devices and/or an appropriate number of persons to assist, gain the advantages of a tub bath.

ORAL HYGIENE

Mouth care is an integral part of daily hygiene and should be continued in the hospital. Infants and debilitated children will require the nurse to perform mouth care. Although small children can manage a toothbrush and should be encouraged to use it, most will need assistance to perform a satisfactory job. Older children, although capable of brushing without assistance, sometimes need to be reminded that this is a part of their hygienic care. Most hospitals have equipment available for those children who do not have

toothbrush or toothpaste of their own. (See p. 613 for specific oral hygiene techniques and p. 1582 for mouth care of children with mucosal ulcers.)

HAIR CARE

Brushing and combing hair are a part of the daily care for all persons in the hospital, including infants and children. If the child does not have a brush or comb, many hospitals provide one as part of the usual admission kit. If not, the parents should be asked to bring hair care equipment for the child's use. Both boys and girls should be helped to comb or brush their hair, or it should be done for them, at least once daily. There is no special hairstyle that is prescribed for hospitalized children. The hair should be styled for comfort and in a manner pleasing to the child and parents. A satisfactory style for girls with longer hair is the French braid, which is created by starting with three equal portions of hair from the top of one side of the scalp; as the hair is braided, segments of hair are added at successive intervals until all the hair has been incorporated into one neat, head-hugging braid on each side of the head. The ends are firmly anchored with a malleable holder or barrette. The hair should not be cut without parental permission, although shaving hair to provide access to a scalp vein for intravenous needle insertion is frequently carried out without permission.

If children are hospitalized for more than a few days, the hair may need shampooing. With infants, the hair may be washed during the daily bath or less frequently. For most children washing the hair and scalp once or twice weekly is sufficient, unless there is an indication to wash it more frequently, such as following a high fever and profuse sweating. Some hospitals have shampoo basins, but almost any child can be conveniently transported by a gurney to an accessible sink or washbasin for shampooing. Those who are unable to be transported can receive a shampoo in their beds with adequate protection and/or specially adapted equipment or positioning. A convenient method involves positioning the child near the edge of the bed, placing towels under the shoulders, and draping a large plastic garbage bag at the edge of the bed with one open side under the shoulders and the other side opened away from the head so that the hair is inside the opening. Water can be transported in a basin or placed in an empty enema bag that is hung from an intravenous pole. The clamp on the bag's tubing is used to adjust the flow of water (Bourgault, 1985).

Teenagers, with their normally increased oily sebaceous secretions, are particularly in need of frequent hair care and usually require more frequent shampoos. Commercial "dry shampoo" products also may prove useful on a short-term basis.

Black children require special hair care, and this need is frequently neglected or inadequately managed. For the black child with kinky hair, most standard combs are inadequate and may cause hair breakage and discomfort to the child. If a special comb with widely spaced teeth is not available on the unit, the parent can be reminded to bring a comb, if possible, for the child's use. This type of hair also requires a special hair dressing or pomade, which usually has a coconut oil base. The preparation is rubbed on the hands and then transferred to the hair to make it more pliable and manageable. The child's parents should be consulted regarding the preparation they wish to be used on their child's hair and asked if they can provide some for use during the child's hospitalization. Petroleum jelly should *not* be used.

FEEDING THE SICK CHILD

Loss of appetite is a symptom common to most childhood illnesses and is frequently the initial evidence of illness, preceding fever and other overt signs of infection. In most cases the child can be permitted to determine his own need for food. Since an acute illness is usually short, the nutritional state is seldom compromised. In fact, urging foods on the sick child may precipitate nausea and vomiting and in some cases even cause an aversion to the feeding situation that can extend into the convalescent period and beyond.

Refusing to eat may also be one way children can exert power and control in an otherwise helpless situation. For young children, loss of appetite may be related to the depression of separation from their parents and their natural tendency toward negativism. Parents' concern with eating can intensify the problem. Forcing a child to eat only meets with rebellion and reinforces the behavior as a control mechanism. Parents are encouraged to relax any pressure during the period of acute illness. Although it is best to encourage high-quality nutritious foods, the child may desire foods and liquids that contain mostly calories. Some well-tolerated foods include gelatin, clear soups, carbonated drinks, popsicles, dry toast, crackers, and hard candy. Even

though these substances are not nutritious, they can provide necessary fluid and calories.

Dehydration is always a hazard when children are febrile or anorexic, especially when this is accompanied by vomiting or diarrhea. An adequate fluid intake should be encouraged by offering small amounts of favored fluids at frequent intervals and by salty foods if allowed. High-calorie liquids such as colas, fruit juices, water flavored and sweetened with corn syrup, or similar drinks help prevent catabolism and dehydration. Fluids should not be forced, and the child should not be wakened from his rest to take fluids. Forcing fluids may create the same difficulties as urging unwanted food. Gentle persuasion with preferred beverages will usually meet with success. Using play techniques can also be very effective.

In general, hotdogs, hamburgers, peanut butter and jelly sandwiches, spaghetti, and pizza are favorite foods of most children. Although alone they may not typify well-balanced diets, they can be adjusted to include sufficient amounts from the basic four food groups. It is better to work with preferred food choices than with selections that children rarely eat. A number of creative approaches to food preparation can increase the child's interest in eating (see box on p. 1116).

An understanding of children's feeding habits can also increase food consumption. For example, if children are given all of their food at one time, they will generally eat the dessert first. Likewise, if they are presented with large portions, they often push the food away because the amount overwhelms them. If young children are not supervised during mealtime, they tend to play with the food rather than eat it. Therefore nurses should present food in the usual order, such as soup first, followed by small portions of meat, potatoes, and vegetables, and ending with dessert. The principles of conservation discussed in Chapter 15 can also be used to increase food consumption.

Once the child is feeling better, his appetite usually begins to improve. It is best to take advantage of any hungry period by serving high-quality foods and snacks. If the child still refuses to eat, nutritious fluids, such as prepared breakfast drinks, should be encouraged. Parents can be very helpful by bringing in these food items from home. This is especially important if the family's cultural eating habits differ from the hospital's food services.

Frequently, children are placed on special diets, such as clear liquids after surgery or during episodes of diarrhea. When children are on these diets, assessment of their intake and readiness to advance to more complex foods is essential. Guidelines for evaluating diet intolerance include (Farrell and McKiernan, 1977):

1. Evidence of vomiting or diarrhea
2. Evidence of a decrease in appetite
3. Signs of abdominal cramping, distention, or bowel sounds
4. Signs of dehydration or weight loss

Regardless of the type of diet, charting of the amount consumed is an important nursing responsibility. Descriptions

SUGGESTIONS FOR FEEDING THE SICK CHILD

Take a dietary history (see p. 212) and use information to make eating time as much like home as possible.

Encourage parents or other family members to feed child or to be present at mealtimes.

Have children eat at tables in groups; bring nonambulatory children to eating area in wheelchairs, beds, strollers, gurneys, or wagons.

Use familiar eating utensils, such as a favorite plate, cup, or bottle for small children.

Make mealtimes pleasant; avoid any procedures immediately before or after eating; make sure child is rested and pain-free.

Have a nurse present at mealtimes to offer assistance, prevent disruptions, and praise children for their eating.

Serve small, frequent meals rather than three large meals or serve three meals and nutritious between-meal snacks.

Bring in foods from home, especially if food preparation is markedly different from hospital; consider cultural differences.

Provide finger foods for young children.

Involve children in food selection and preparation whenever possible.

Serve small portions, and serve each course separately, such as soup first, followed by meat, potatoes, and vegetables, and ending with dessert; with young children camouflage size of food by cutting meat thicker so less appears on plate or by folding a cheese slice in half; offer second helpings; ensure a variety of foods, textures, and colors.

Provide food selections that are favorites of most children, such as peanut butter/jelly sandwiches, hot dogs, hamburgers, macaroni and cheese, pizza, spaghetti, tacos, fried chicken, and corn on the cob.

Avoid foods that are highly seasoned, have strong odors, are served hot, or are all mixed together, unless typical of cultural practices.

Provide fluid selections that are favorites of most children, such as fruit punch, cola, ginger ale, sweetened tea, ice pops, sherbet, ice cream, milk and milk shakes, eggnog, pudding, gelatin, clear broth, or creamed soups.

Offer nutritious snacks, such as frozen yogurt or pudding, ice cream, oatmeal or peanut butter cookies, hot cocoa, cheese slices or "kisses," pieces of raw vegetable or fruit, and dried fruit or cereal.

Make food attractive and different, for example:

Serve a "picnic lunch" in a paper bag.

Pack food in a Chinese-food container; decorate container.

Put a "face" or a "flower" on a hamburger or sandwich with pieces of vegetable.

Use a cookie-cutter to shape a sandwich.

Serve pudding, yogurt, or juice frozen as a popsicle.

Make slurpies or snowcones by pouring flavored syrup on crushed ice.

Add vegetable coloring to water or milk.

Serve fluids through brightly colored or unusually shaped straws.

Make "bowtie" sandwiches by cutting them in triangles and placing two points together.

Slice sandwiches into "fingers."

Grate mounds of cheese.

Cut apples horizontally to make circles.

Put a banana on a hotdog bun and spread with peanut butter.

Break uncooked spaghetti into toothpick lengths and skewer cheese, cold meat, vegetables or fruit chunks.

Praise child for what he does eat.

Do *not* punish children for not eating by removing their dessert or putting them to bed.

---

need to be detailed and accurate, such as "4 ounces of orange juice, one pancake, no bacon, and 8 ounces of milk." Comments such as "ate well" or "ate poorly" are inadequate. If parents are involved in the child's care, they are encouraged to keep a list of everything eaten. Using a premeasured cup for fluids ensures a more accurate estimate of intake. A comparison of the intake at each meal can isolate food deficiencies, such as insufficient intake of meat or vegetables. Behaviors associated with mealtime also identify possible factors influencing appetite. For example, the observation that "Child eats well when with other children but plays with food if left alone in room" helps the nurse plan mealtime activities that stimulate the appetite.

CONTROL OF FEVER

Fever, one of the most common symptoms of illness in children, is also one of the most frequently misunderstood manifestations of disease and a great source of concern to parents. To facilitate an understanding of fever, the following terms are defined (McCarthy, 1985):

set point The temperature around which body temperature is regulated

fever An elevation in set point such that body temperature is regulated at a higher level

hyperthermia A situation in which body temperature exceeds the set point, which usually results from the body creating more heat than it can eliminate, such as in heat stroke, aspirin toxicity, or hyperthyroidism

Although definitions of temperature elevation to describe fever vary, the following are generally accepted:

fever Rectal temperature above 38° C (100.4° F); oral temperature above 37.8° C (100° F); axillary temperature above 37.2° C (99° F)

high fever Temperature above 40.4° C (105° F)

harmful fever Temperature at or above 41.7° C (107° F)

Physiology of Fever

Body temperature is regulated by a thermostat-like mechanism in the hypothalamus. This mechanism receives input from centrally and peripherally located receptors. When temperature changes occur, these receptors relay the information to the thermostat, which either increases or decreases heat production to maintain a constant set point temperature. However, during an infection, pyrogenic substances cause an increase in the body's normal set point, a process that is mediated by prostaglandins. Consequently the hypothalamus increases heat production until the core temperature reaches the new set point.

Most fevers in children are of viral origin, are of relatively brief duration, and have limited consequences (Lovejoy, 1978). In addition, there is mounting evidence that fever plays a role in enhancing the development of both specific and nonspecific immunity and aiding recovery and survival from infection (McCarthy, 1985). Contrary to popular belief the rise in temperature does not indicate the severity of infection, which casts doubt on the value of using fever as a diagnostic or prognostic indicator (Musher and others, 1979).

Therapeutic Management

Treatment of fever is based on an understanding of the body's control mechanisms and the attendant consequences of therapy. The principal rationale for treating fever is the relief of discomfort, and there is no general level of temperature that requires treatment. Relief measures include pharmacologic and/or environmental intervention. In treating fever the most effective intervention is the use of antipyretics to lower the set point. Cooling procedures such as sponging or tepid baths have been shown to be ineffective in treating fever either when used alone or in combination with antipyretics and inflict considerable discomfort on the child (Newman, 1985). Conversely, antipyretics are of no value in hyperthermia because the set point is already normal, but cooling measures are beneficial and are discussed below for application in these situations. The use of antipyretics and/

Table 27-3 Dosage recommendations for acetaminophen (Tylenol)*

AGE	WEIGHT (POUNDS)	DOSE (MG)	FORM†
Under 3 months	6-11	40	½ dropper
4-11 months	12-17	80	1 dropper or ½ tsp elixir
12-23 months	18-23	120	1½ dropper or ¾ tsp elixir or 1½ chewable tablet
2-3 years	24-35	160	2 droppersful or 1 tsp elixir or 2 chewable tablets
4-5 years	36-47	240	3 droppersful or 1½ tsp elixir or 3 chewable tablets
6-8 years	48-59	320	4 droppersful or 2 tsp elixir or 4 chewable tablets or 2 swallowable tablets
9-10 years	60-71	400	5 droppersful or 2½ tsp elixir or 5 chewable tablets or 2½ swallowable tablets
11 years	72-95	480	3 tsp elixir or 6 chewable tablets or 3 swallowable tablets
12-14 years	96+	640	4 swallowable tablets

*Doses should be administered four or five times daily, but not to exceed five doses in 24 hours.
†1 dropper = 80 mg/0.8 ml; elixir = 160 mg/5 ml; chewable tablet = 80 mg each; junior strength swallowable tablets = 160 mg each.

or cooling measures in febrile seizures is controversial. The use of antipyretics has not been shown to reduce the incidence of febrile seizures and there is no documentation that seizures cause permanent damage, such as intellectual deficits (Consensus statement, 1980; Ellenberg, Hirtz, and Nelson, 1986).

Pharmacologic management. Aspirin and acetaminophen are the preferred drugs for management of fever, although aspirin should not be given to children possibly infected with influenza virus or chicken pox because of the risk of Reye syndrome (Hurwitz and others, 1985). Acetaminophen is preferred for infants or young children because it is available in liquid form. Over the counter ibuprofen (Nuprin, Advil) also is an effective antipyretic but is not recommended for children under 12 years of age. Antipyretic drugs appear to exert their action by inhibiting prostaglandin synthesis, thereby lowering the set point.

The recommended dosages of aspirin and acetaminophen are given in Tables 27-2 and 27-3. Aspirin should not be given more often than every 4 hours, since there is risk of toxic effects from accumulation. Acetaminophen should also be given every 4 hours, but chronic overdose in young

Table 27-2 Recommended dosage of aspirin (1¼-grain tablets) for children by age and weight*

AGE (YEARS)	WEIGHT (POUNDS)	DOSAGE (TABLETS)
Under 2	Below 27	As directed by physician
2-3	27-35	2
4-5	36-45	3
6-8	46-64	4
9-10	66-76	5
11	77-83	6
12+	84+	8

Modified from Done, A., and others: J. Pediatr. **95**(4):617-629, 1979.
*If child's weight falls outside the range for his age, give dosage according to weight, not age. Aspirin may be given every 4 hours, but not to exceed five times a day unless prescribed by a physician.
NOTE: Children should not be given aspirin for chicken pox or flu symptoms because of the association between aspirin and Reye syndrome (see also p. 1655).

children probably does not occur (Rumack, 1986). Since body temperature normally decreases at night, three to four doses in 24 hours are usually sufficient to control most fevers. The temperature is usually retaken 30 minutes after the antipyretic is given to assess its effect but should not be repeatedly measured; the child's level of discomfort is the best indication for continued treatment.

Sometimes full doses of aspirin and acetaminophen are given alternately for high fevers, such as aspirin at 2, 6, and 10 PM and acetaminophen at 4 and 8 PM and 12 AM. However, there are no controlled studies to document the efficacy of this treatment and it is is a potentially dangerous home practice because of the risk of chronic salicylate toxicity if aspirin is mistakenly administered at 2-hour intervals. This practice also conveys to parents that fever is a grave condition, thus adding to parental fear (Schmitt, 1984). Another approach is to give full doses of both drugs *concurrently,* which increases the effect on the fever and prolongs temperature reduction time to 6 rather than 4 hours. This approach may be effective in conditions of high and persistent fevers (Temple, 1983).

The usual method of administration is oral in either tablet or liquid preparations. Older children are able to swallow the tablet; younger ones chew the flavored variety or can be given the tablet crushed and mixed in syrup or jelly. The tablet must be well crushed in order to avoid chunks that might be aspirated into the larynx or trachea. Sometimes the rectal route, using aspirin or acetaminophen suppositories, is easier, especially for infants or children with sore, swollen throats. However, unless the suppository contains the exact dose, the oral route should be encouraged. Some children respond well to aspirin incorporated into a chewing gum (Aspergum), although the dosage must be calculated carefully since each piece contains 228 mg, an amount that differs from the usual dosages prescribed for children.

Environmental management. Environmental measures to reduce fever are used if tolerated by the child and if they do not induce shivering. Shivering is the body's way of maintaining the set point by producing heat. Environmental measures such as minimal clothing, exposing the skin to the air, reducing room temperature, increasing air circulation, and cool moist compresses to the skin, such as the forehead, are most effective if employed approximately 1 hour *after* an antipyretic is given so that the hypothalamic set point is lowered.

Environmental measures are the primary therapy to reduce body temperature from hyperthermia. Cool applications to the skin help to reduce the core temperature. Cooled blood from the skin surface is conducted to inner organs and tissues, and warm blood is circulated to the surface where it is cooled and recirculated. The surface blood vessels dilate as the body attempts to dissipate heat to the environment and facilitate this cooling process.

Cool applications can be given in a tub or in the bed or crib. Tepid tub baths are fast, simple, and effective for reducing an elevated temperature in a child. When using the tub, it is usually best to start with warm water and gradually add cool water until the desired water temperature of 37° C (98.6° F) is reached. In this way the child becomes more easily accustomed to the lower water temperature. The child is placed directly into the tub of tepid water for 20 to 30 minutes while water is gently squeezed from a washcloth over his back and chest or gently sprayed over his body from a sprayer. The bath is even more effective if the child can tolerate lying down in the water with his head supported on the nurse's arm or a padded support. This is more easily accomplished with a small infant or an older child. Small children dislike lying down and often resist any efforts to force them into the horizontal position. For conscious children a floating toy or other distraction can be employed during the bath. The child is never left alone in the tub.

The cooling bath can also be given in the bed or crib. The child is completely undressed and placed on an absorbent blanket or towel spread over the bed. He is covered with a large towel or lightweight, absorbent cotton blanket. A cool washcloth or ice pack is placed on the child's forehead and changed as it warms. One area of the body is exposed at a time and sponged with a washcloth soaked in tepid water. The sponge bath is continued for approximately 30 minutes.

A safe, easy, and effective alternate method of temperature reduction is the towel method. The child is undressed and placed on an absorbent towel or blanket, and a cool cloth or ice bag is applied to the forehead. Each extremity is wrapped in a towel moistened in tepid water, one is placed under the back, and another covers the neck and torso. Special care is taken to make certain that opposing body surfaces, such as the groin and lateral torso between the arms and chest, are covered. The towels are changed as they warm. This is continued for approximately 30 minutes.

After the tub or sponge bath, the child is dried and dressed in lightweight pajamas, nightgown, or diaper and placed in a dry bed. The temperature is retaken 30 minutes after the tub bath or sponge bath. The child is dried by gently rubbing the skin surface with a towel to stimulate circulation. The bath or sponge should not be continued or restarted until the skin surface is warm or if the child feels chilled. Chilling causes vasoconstriction, which defeats the purpose of the cool applications. In this condition little blood is carried to the skin surface but remains primarily in the viscera to become heated.

HEALTH TEACHING

Nurses have a unique opportunity for teaching the family about health care practices while the child is hospitalized. Although most children have learned self-care and hygiene in the home or at school, many have not. For some young children this is their first introduction to the use of a toothbrush. A great deal of health teaching can be accomplished even when the child is hospitalized for only a short time. The daily bath, hand washing before meals and after bowel and bladder evacuation, and conscientious dental hygiene are taught by example during routine care. Clean hair, nails, and clothing as well as good grooming are emphasized as essential to a pleasing appearance. Positive reinforcement of good hygiene practices helps to create a positive body image, promote the development of self-esteem, and prevent health problems, for example, teaching girls to wipe the genital area from front to back after toileting.

While sick children's appetite may be poor and not characteristic of their home eating habits, the hospital stay provides numerous opportunities for nurses to assess the family's knowledge of good nutrition and to implement teaching as needed to improve nutritional intake. Creative games can be employed that not only teach but provide diversion as well (Dininny, 1977; Mandelbaum, 1983).

Parental education about fever is essential since many parents are unaware of what constitutes a fever, have unrealistic fears about the dangers of fever, and are apt to overmedicate the febrile child (Kramer, Naimark, and Leduc, 1985; Schmitt, 1980). They need guidelines for when to seek professional care (see box) and instruction in safe and effective measures to reduce fever. They should know how to take the child's temperature and read the thermometer accurately.* If the use of aspirin or acetaminophen is indicated, the parents may need instruction in administering the drug.* It is important to emphasize accuracy in both the amount of drug given and the time intervals at which the drug is administered in order to avoid cumulative effects. Since many forms of acetaminophen are available, the nurse must be certain of the type being used in the home when discussing dosage. For example, the specially coated swallowable tablets for older children contain *twice* the amount of drug in the chewable tablets.

Safety

Since small children are separated from their usual environment and do not possess the capacity for abstract thinking and reasoning, it is the responsibility of everyone who comes in contact with them to maintain protective measures throughout their hospital stay. Nurses need a good understanding of the age level at which each child is operating and plan for safety accordingly.

Name bands, a part of hospital safety practices, are particularly important for children in the pediatric age-group. Infants and unconscious patients are unable to tell or respond to their names. Toddlers may answer to any name or to a nickname only. It is not uncommon for older children to exchange places, give an erroneous name, or choose not to respond to their own names as a form of a joke, unaware of the hazards of such practices.

*Home care instructions on Measuring your child's temperature and giving medications to children are available in Wong, D., and Whaley, L.: Clinical handbook of pediatric nursing, ed. 2, St. Louis, 1986, The C.V. Mosby Co.

GUIDELINES FOR PARENTS OF CHILD WITH FEVER

Call immediately if:
  Child is <2 months of age
  Fever is >40.5°C (105°F)
  Child is crying inconsolably
  Child is difficult to awaken
  Child is confused or delirious
  Child has had a seizure
  Child has a stiff neck
  Child has purple spots on the skin
  Breathing is difficult and child does not feel better after nose is cleared
  Child is acting very sick
  Child has an underlying risk factor for serious infection (e.g., sickle cell disease)
Call during office hours if:
  Child is 2-4 months old (unless fever is due to a DPT shot)
  Fever is between 40° and 40.5°C (104° and 105°F), especially if child is <2 years old
  Burning or pain occurs with urination
  Fever has been present for >72 hours
  Fever has been present for >24 hours without an obvious cause or location of infection
  Fever went away for >24 hours and then returned
  Child has a history of febrile seizures
  Parents have other questions

Modified from Schmitt, B.D.: Fever in childhood, Pediatrics **74**(5)(suppl.):934, 1984.

ENVIRONMENTAL FACTORS

All the environmental safety measures in operation for the protection of adults apply to children as well, such as good illumination, floors clear of fluid or other objects that might contribute to falls, and nonskid surfaces in showers and tubs; electrical equipment that is maintained in good working order, is used only by personnel familiar with its use, and is not in contact with moisture or near tubs where it could prove to be a shock hazard; beds of ambulatory patients locked in place and at a height that allows easy access to the floor; proper care and disposal of small breakable items such as thermometers and bottles; and a well-organized fire plan known to all staff members. Medical asepsis and isolation techniques differ very little from those in any other hospital unit and should be strictly adhered to by personnel, since infants and small children are highly susceptible to cross-infection.

All windows should be securely screened and elevators and stairways made safe. Ideally electrical outlets should be provided with covers to prevent burns in small children whose exploratory activities may extend to inserting objects into the small openings. Bath water is carefully checked before placing the child in it, and children must never be left alone in a bathtub. Infants are helpless in water, and small children (and some older ones) may turn on the hot water faucet and be severely burned.

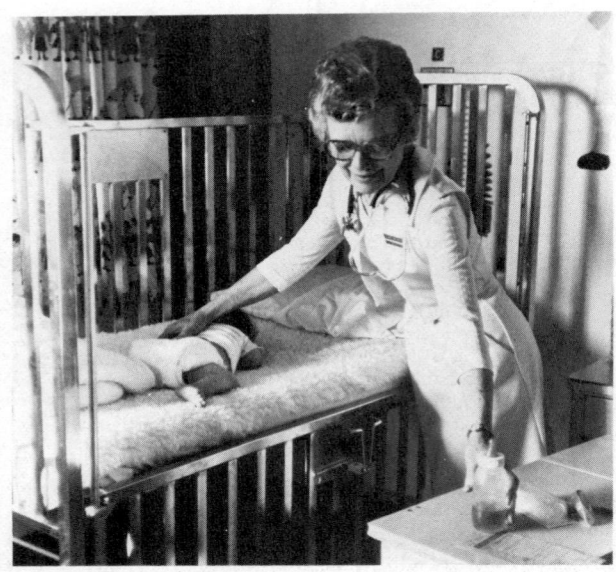

Fig. 27-5. Nurse maintains hand contact when back is turned.

Furniture is safest when scaled to the child's proportions, sturdy, and well balanced to prevent its being easily tipped over. Infants and small children must be securely strapped into infant seats, feeding chairs, and strollers. Infants and small, agitated, or mentally retarded children should not be left unattended on treatment tables, on scales, or in treatment areas. Even tiny premature infants are capable of surprising mobility; therefore portholes in Isolettes must be securely fastened when not in use.

Crib sides should be kept up and fastened securely unless an adult is at the bedside. It is safer to leave crib sides up, even when the crib is unoccupied, to remove the temptation to climb in. Anyone attending an infant or small child in a crib with the sides down should never turn away without maintaining hand contact with the child; that is, one hand should be kept on the child's back or abdomen to protect him from rolling, crawling, or jumping from the open crib (Fig. 27-5). The crib bars should be spaced close enough together to prevent a child's head from being caught between them. A child who is apt to or has demonstrated the inclination to climb over the sides of the crib is safest when placed in a specially constructed crib with a cover or one that has a safety net placed over the top. If the net is used, it must be tied to the frame in such a manner that there is ready access to the child in case of emergency. Nets are never tied to the movable crib sides, and the knots should be tied in a manner that permits quick release. Cribs should not be placed within reach of heating units, appliances, dangling cords, or other objects that can be grabbed by curious hands, and toys should not be tied to or across crib rails once children are old enough to reach them.

LIMIT-SETTING

Setting limits is essential to a child's safety. Children must understand where they are permitted to go and what they are permitted to do in the hospital. These limitations should be made clear to them, consistently enforced, and repeated as frequently as necessary to make certain that they are understood. The nurse is responsible for where children are at all times. Children can easily wander off unnoticed. Normally active older children often become restless when their activity is restricted and may resort to pillow fights, water fights, and other rough play that might endanger the safety of the involved children or of bystanders (other children, staff, visitors). Children in the hospital require surveillance, and appropriate tension-reducing activities can be planned and supervised by nurses and/or by the play therapist. A useful discipline technique is the use of time-out (see p. 608).

TRANSPORTING INFANTS AND CHILDREN

In the course of a hospital stay, infants and children usually need to be transported within the unit and to areas outside the pediatric unit. It is ordinarily safe to carry infants and small children for short distances within the unit, but for more extended trips the child should be securely transported in a suitable conveyance.

Small infants can be held or carried in the horizontal position with the back supported and the thigh grasped firmly by the carrying arm (Fig. 27-6, A). In the football hold the infant is carried on the nurse's arm with the head supported by the hand and the body held securely between the nurse's body and elbow (Fig. 27-6, B). Both of these holds leave the nurse's other arm free for activity. The infant can be held in the upright position with the buttocks on the nurse's forearm and the front of the body resting against the nurse's chest. The infant's head and shoulders are supported by the nurse's other arm to allow for any sudden movement by the infant (Fig. 27-6, C). Older infants are able to hold their heads erect but are still subject to sudden movements.

Infants can be transported to other areas, such as the x-ray department, in their bassinet or crib. Baby carriages are sometimes used for infants who are not likely to stand up. Strollers and wheeled feeding chairs or tables are also convenient transporters in some situations, such as trips to the playroom, nurse's station, or sun porch.

The method of transporting children is determined by their age, condition, and destination. Most older children are safe in wheelchairs or in gurneys. Younger children can be transported in their crib, on a gurney, in a wagon with raised sides, or in a wheelchair with a safety belt. Gurneys should be equipped with high sides and a safety belt, both of which are kept in place during transport.

RESTRAINTS

Frequently some method of restraint is needed for a child's safety or comfort, to facilitate examination, or to carry out diagnostic and therapeutic procedures. Restraint can be accomplished with the hand or with physical devices. Restraining the child with the hand provides an element of hu-

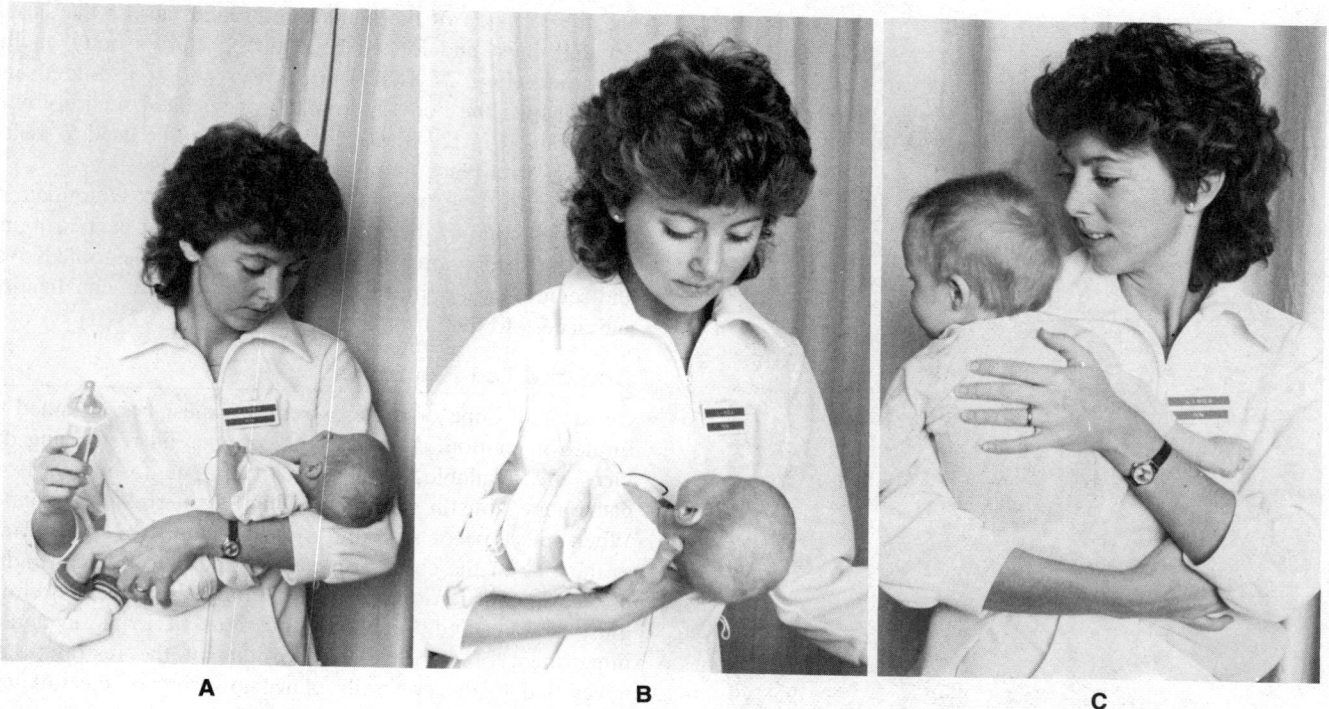

Fig. 27-6. Transporting infants. **A,** Infant's thigh firmly grasped in nurse's hand; **B,** football hold; **C,** back supported.

man contact that is lacking in restraint by mechanical means. For example, a large infant or small child can be effectively restrained by having him sit astride the lap facing an assistant. The assistant hugs him close against the body to provide both comfort and restraint while the nurse safely carries out the necessary procedures.

Mechanical restraints are never used as a punishment or as a substitute for observation. When a child must be restrained, he and his parents need a simple explanation, and if the restraint is applied for an extended time, the explanation must be repeated often to gain his cooperation and to help him understand that it is not a punishment. Restraining devices are not without risk and must be checked frequently to make certain that they are accomplishing the purpose for which they are intended, that they are applied correctly, and that they do not impair circulation.

Parents need to know the purpose of restraints, how to remove and reapply them, and the signs of complications from their use. Parents are sometimes upset when their child must be restrained and need to understand how they can help to ensure the maximum benefit and minimize the stress related to their use. Children, too, should be prepared for both the procedure or the circumstance for which the restraint is required.

Removing restraints whenever possible (at least every 2 hours) is an essential part of nursing care of children who are restrained for treatments or other purposes. Alternate methods may be devised to replace the need for passive restraints. Holding the child for periods is a pleasant alternative, as is restraining him in a highchair where he can ob-

serve the activities around him. If feasible, distraction techniques such as play and reading to the child should be employed to gain the child's cooperation without resorting to restraints. Parental participation is always encouraged in these efforts.

Jacket Restraint

A jacket restraint is sometimes used as an alternative to the crib net to prevent the child from climbing out of the crib or to keep the child safe in various kinds of chairs. The jacket is put on the child with the ties in back so that the child is unable to manipulate them, and the long tapes, secured to the understructure of the crib, keep the child inside the crib (Fig. 27-7). The jacket restraint is also useful as a means to maintain the child in a desired horizontal position. A Posey belt scaled to fit the child is an alternative device.

Mummy Restraint

When an infant or small child requires short-term restraint for examination or treatment that involves the head and neck—such as venipuncture, throat examination, and gavage feeding—the mummy device effectively controls the child's movements. A blanket or sheet is opened on the bed or crib with one corner folded to the center. The infant is placed on the blanket with shoulders at the fold and feet toward the opposite corner (Fig. 27-8, *A*). With the infant's right arm straight down against the body, the right side of the blanket is pulled firmly across the infant's right shoulder and chest and secured beneath the left side of the body (Fig. 27-8, *B*). The left arm is placed straight against his side,

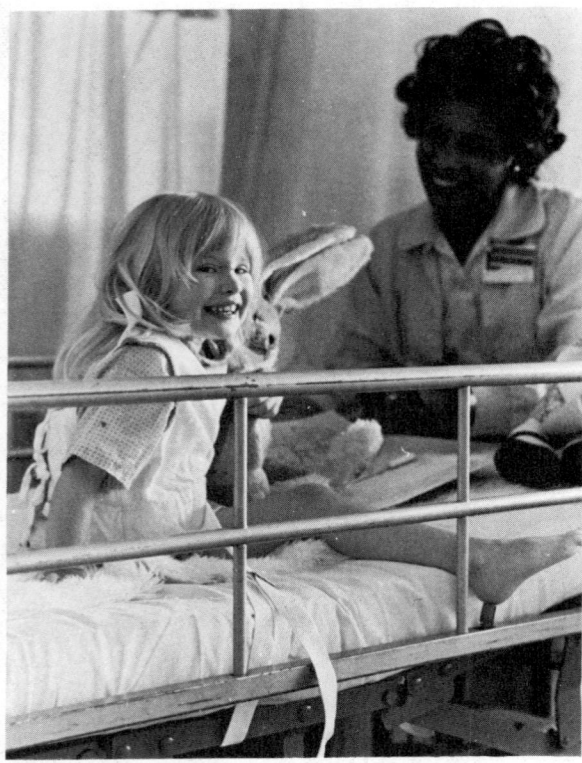

Fig. 27-7. Jacket restraint.

and the left side of the blanket is brought across the shoulder and chest and locked beneath the child's body on the right side (Fig. 27-8, *C*). The lower corner is folded and brought over the body and tucked or fastened securely with safety pins (Fig. 27-8, *D*). Safety pins can be used to fasten the blanket in place at any step in the process.

To modify the mummy restraint for chest examination, the folded edge of the blanket is brought over each arm and under the back, after which the loose edge is folded over and secured at a point below the chest to allow visualization and access to the chest.

Arm and Leg Restraints

Occasionally one or more extremities must be restrained or limited in motion. A number of commercial restraining devices are available, or a restraint can be fashioned from gauze tape, muslin strips, or a length of narrow stockinette. When this type of restraint is used, it must be appropriate to the size of the child, it must be padded to prevent undue pressure, constriction, or tissue injury, and the extremity must be observed frequently for signs of irritation and/or impairment of circulation. The ends of the restraints are never tied to the crib rails, since lowering of the rail will disturb the extremity, frequently with a jerk that may hurt or injure the child.

The *clove hitch* restraint is fashioned from a length of

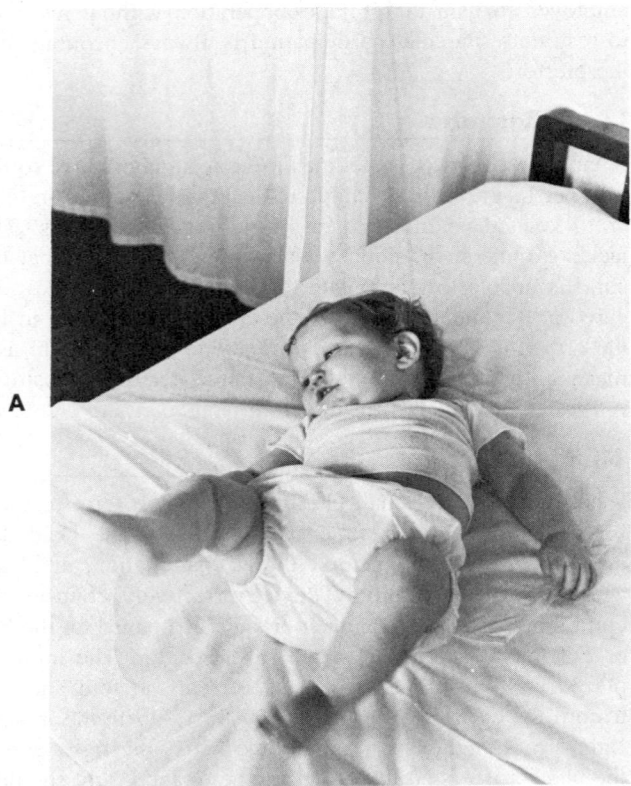

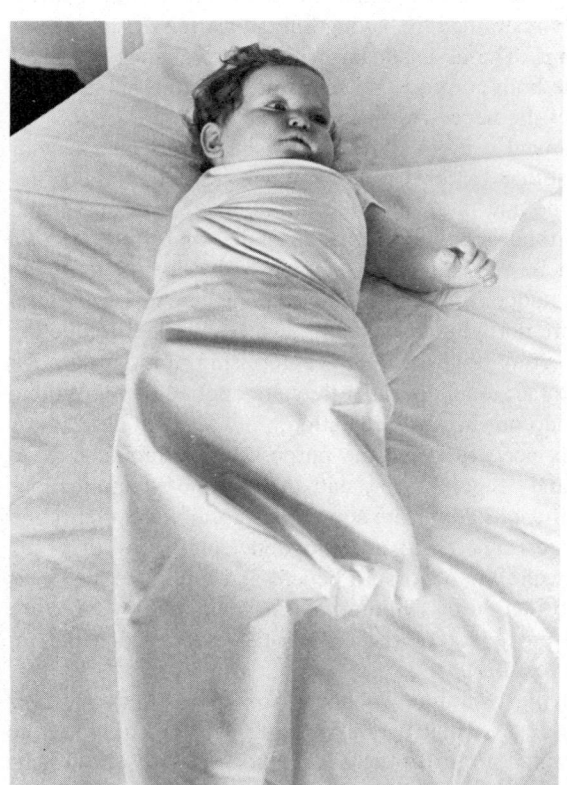

Fig. 27-8. Application of mummy restraint. **A,** Infant placed on folded corner of blanket; **B,** one corner of blanket brought across body and secured beneath body;

gauze or muslin tape. When properly applied, the restraint should provide a snug fit with minimum danger of pulling too tightly. Fig. 27-9 illustrates the method of tying and applying a clove hitch restraint.

Elbow Restraint

Sometimes it is important to prevent the child from reaching his head or face, for example, after lip surgery, when a scalp vein infusion is in place, or to prevent scratching in skin disorders. For this purpose, elbow restraints fashioned from a variety of materials function very well. The most common form of elbow restraint consists of a piece of muslin long enough to reach comfortably from just below the axilla to the wrist with a number of vertical pockets into which tongue depressors are inserted (Fig. 27-10). The restraint is wrapped around the arm and secured with tapes or pins. It may be necessary to pin the top of the restraint to undershirt sleeve to prevent the restraint from slipping.

Similar restraints can be made from padded large-diameter towel rollers or appropriately sized plastic containers from which the tops and bottoms have been removed. Both types need to be padded and to have some means to prevent the restraint from slipping from the extremity. Adjustable restraints can be fashioned from tongue blades placed vertically against strips of adhesive and then covered with adhesive; the restraint is then applied and secured with tape.

POSITIONING FOR PROCEDURES

Infants and small children are unable to cooperate for many procedures; therefore the nurse is responsible for minimizing their movement and discomfort with proper positioning. Older children usually need only minimum, if any, restraint. Careful explanation and preparation beforehand and support and simple guidance during the procedure are usually sufficient.

Jugular Venipuncture

The large, superficial external jugular vein is frequently used to obtain blood specimens from infants and young children. For easy access to the vein, the child is first placed in a mummy restraint in which the top edge of the restraint is low enough to permit access to the vein. The child is placed so that his head and shoulders extend over the edge of a table or a small pillow with his neck extended and his head turned sharply to the side (Fig. 27-11). One alternate method for restraining arms and legs is with the nurse holding the child's arms and legs at the same time that the child's head is restrained and positioned. It is important for the nurse holding the infant to maintain control of the infant's head without interfering with the operator's approach to the vein. The infant's crying during the procedure increases intravenous pressure, which facilitates visualization of the vein. Following venipuncture, digital pressure is ap-

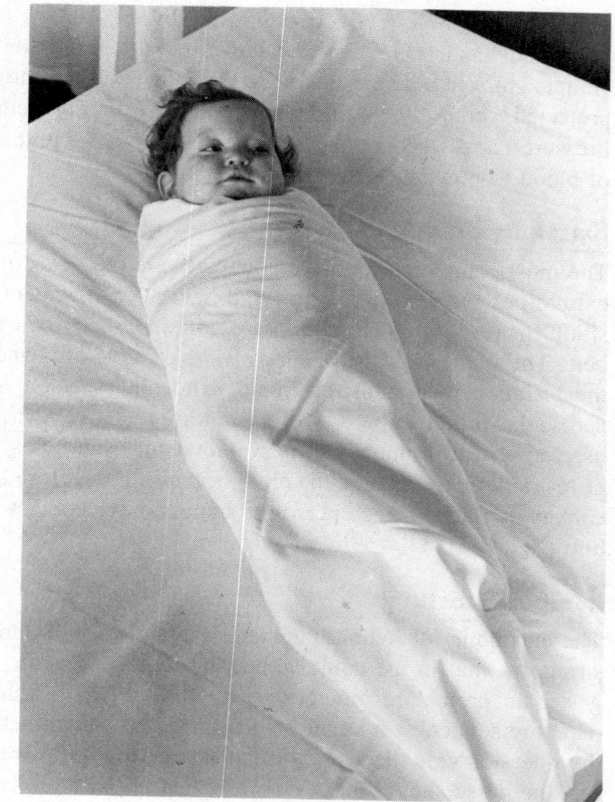
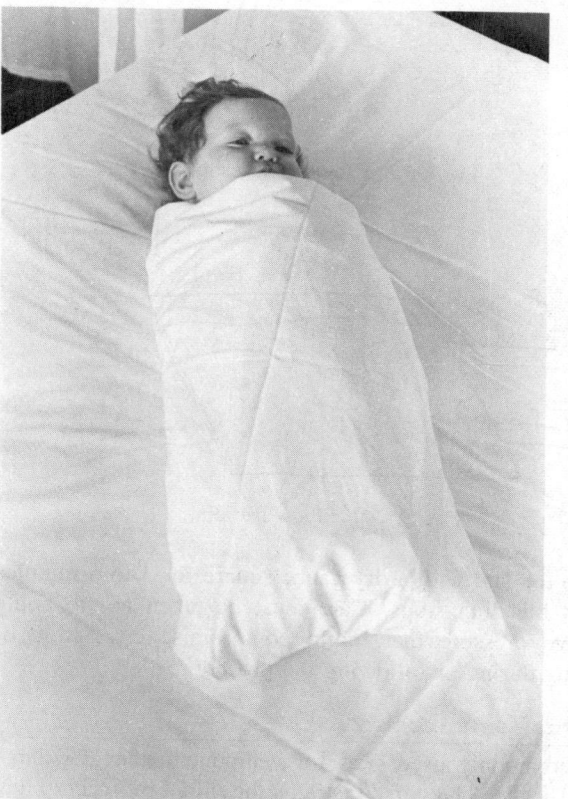

Fig. 27-8, cont'd. C, second corner brought across body and secured; **D,** lower corner folded and tucked or pinned in place.

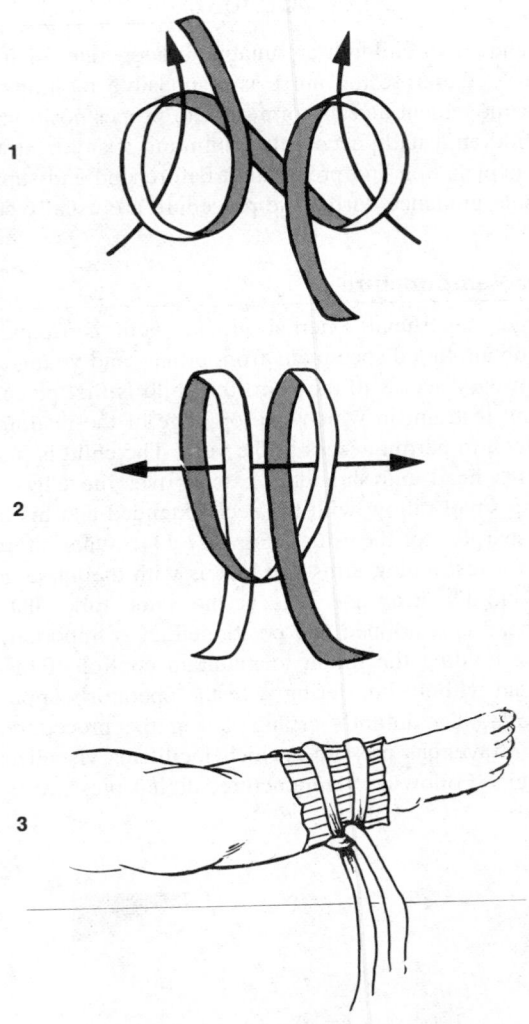

Fig. 27-9. Clove hitch restraint.

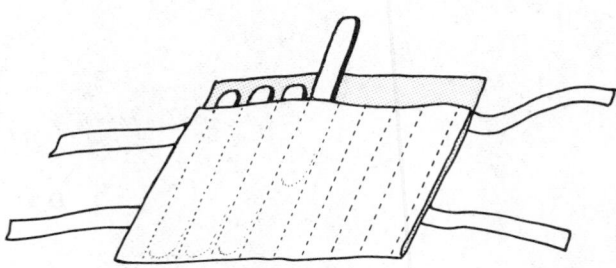

Fig. 27-10. Elbow restraint.

plied to the site with a dry gauze square for 3 to 5 minutes or until bleeding stops. Care must be taken not to apply excessive pressure that might compromise circulation or breathing during or following the procedure.

Femoral Venipuncture

Other commonly used sites for venipuncture are the large femoral veins. The nurse restrains the infant by placing him supine with his legs in a frog position to provide extensive exposure of the groin area. Both the arms and the legs of

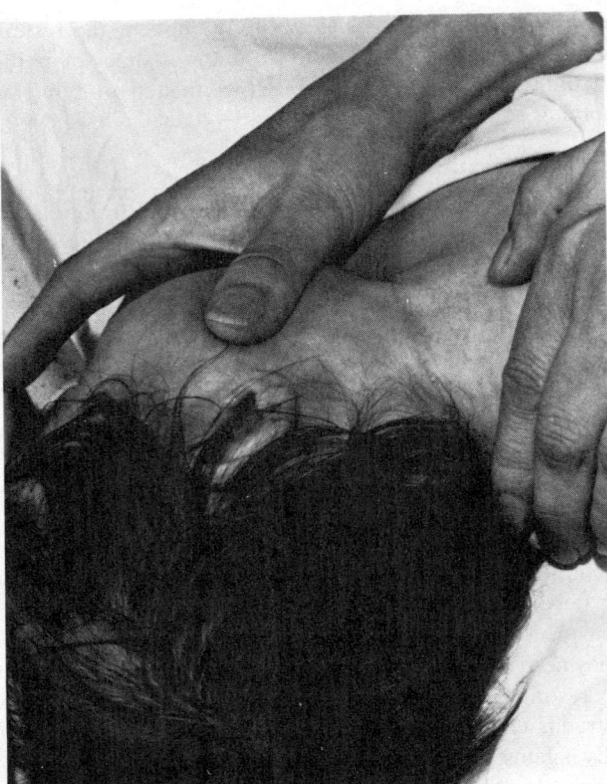

Fig. 27-11. Restraining child for jugular vein puncture.

the infant can be effectively controlled by the nurse's forearms and hands (Fig. 27-12). Only the side used for the venipuncture should be uncovered, so that the operator is protected should the child urinate during the procedure. Pressure should be applied to the site after the withdrawal of blood to prevent oozing from the site.

Extremity Venipuncture

The most common sites of venipuncture are the veins of the extremities, especially the arm and hand. A convenient position for restraint is having one person on either side of the bed. The child's outstretched arm is partially stabilized by the technician drawing the blood. The other person leans across the child's upper body, preventing its movement, and uses an arm to immobilize the venipuncture site. This type of restraint also comforts the child because of the close body contact and allows each person to maintain eye contact with him (Fig. 27-13).

Lumbar Puncture

The technique for lumbar puncture in infants and children is similar to that in the adult, although modifications are suggested in premature infants (see p. 409). Pediatric lumbar puncture sets contain smaller spinal needles, but sometimes the operator will specify a particular size or type of needle that the nurse should make certain is placed on the tray.

Children are usually controlled best in the side-lying position, with the head flexed and the knees drawn up toward

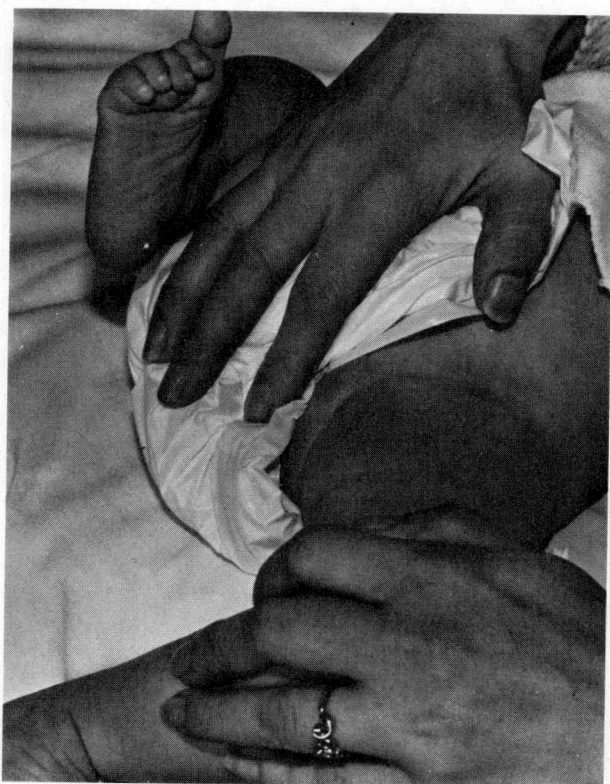

Fig. 27-12. Restraining infant for femoral vein puncture.

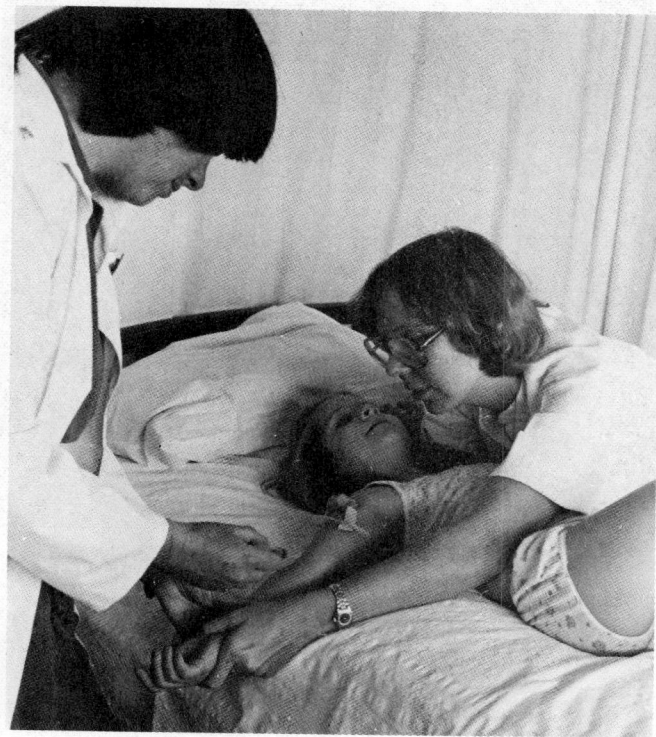

Fig. 27-13. Restraining child for extremity vein puncture.

the chest. Even cooperative children need to be restrained to prevent possible trauma from unexpected, involuntary movement. They can be reassured that, although they are trusted, the restraint will serve as a reminder to maintain the desired position. It also provides a measure of support and reassurance to them.

The child is placed on the side with the back close to the edge of the examining table on the side from which the operator is working. The nurse maintains the child's spine in a flexed position by holding the child with one arm behind his neck and the other behind his thighs. The position can be effectively stabilized if the nurse's hands are clasped in front of the child's abdomen (Fig. 27-14, *A*). The flexed position enlarges the spaces between the lumbar vertebral spines, which facilitates access to the spinal fluid space. It is helpful to wrap the legs before positioning to decrease leg movement.

An alternate position used with small infants and some older children is the sitting position. The child is placed with the buttocks at the edge of the table and with the neck flexed so that the chin rests on the chest. The infant's arms and legs are immobilized by the nurse's hands (Fig. 27-14, *B*). Since this position may interfere with chest expansion and diaphragm excursion, the child is observed for difficulty in breathing. In addition, the soft, pliable trachea of the infant is subject to collapse.

Another position that employs close and comforting contact for the child involves holding the child upright against

the nurse's (or parent's) chest with the child's legs wrapped around the adult's waist. The adult's arms are used to hug and restrain the child. For ease of the examiner, the adult should be standing. A small pillow is placed between the child's abdomen and the adult to help arch the child's back. If the pillow proves unsuccessful, a third person can place an arm in this space to achieve the desired position (Brown, 1984).

Specimens and spinal fluid pressure are obtained, measured, and sent for analysis in the same manner as for the adult patient. It is advisable for the child to lie quietly for an hour following the procedure to decrease the likelihood of headache, and he is offered fluids to drink. Vital signs are taken as ordered, and the child is observed for any changes in level of consciousness, motor activity, or other neurologic signs.

Bone Marrow Aspiration/Biopsy

Position for a bone marrow aspiration or biopsy depends on the location of the chosen site. In children the posterior or anterior iliac crest is most frequently used, although in infants the tibia may be selected because of easy access to the site and restraint of the child. The sternum, which is the most frequent site in adults, is generally avoided in children because the bone is more fragile and adjacent to vital organs.

If the posterior iliac crest is used, the child is positioned prone. Sometimes a small pillow or folded blanket is placed

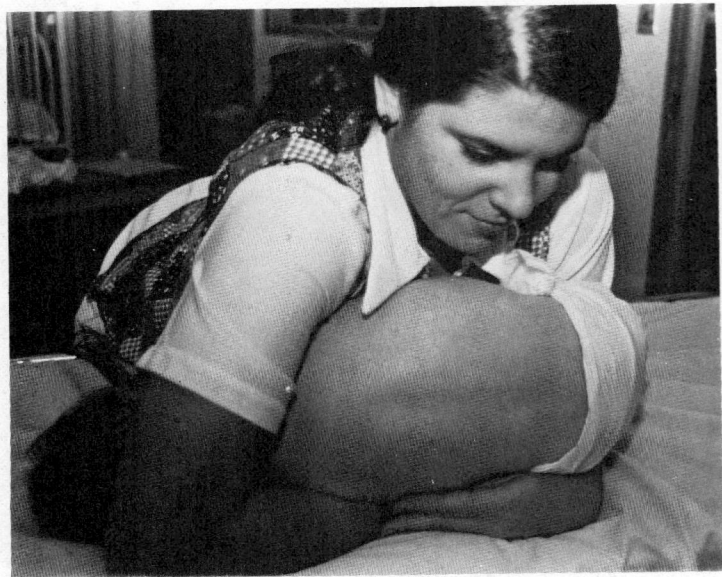

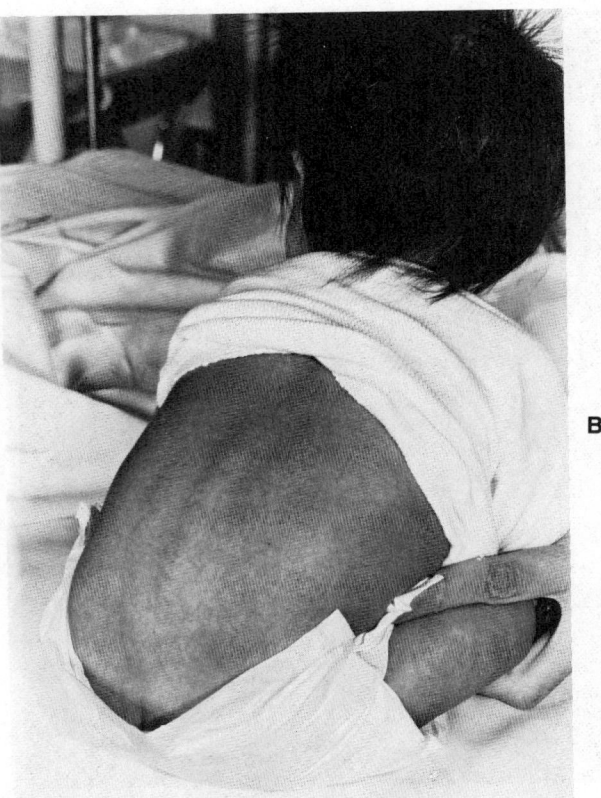

Fig. 27-14. Position for lumbar puncture. **A,** Lying on side. **B,** Sitting.

under the hips to facilitate obtaining the bone marrow specimen. Since few children can be trusted to remain still, restraint is needed and is best applied with two people—one person to immobilize the upper body and a second person to immobilize the lower extremities. If the other sites are used, the child is placed supine and restraint is applied in a similar manner with modifications made for access to the tibia or sternum.

Other Procedures

For subdural puncture through a fontanel or burr hole, the infant is wrapped in a mummy restraint and placed in the supine position with the head accessible to the examiner. To control the head the nurse uses a firm hold on each side of it. Procedures for immobilizing the head for examining the ears, nose, or throat are discussed in Chapter 7.

Collection of Specimens

Many of the specimens needed for diagnostic examination of children are collected in much the same way as they are for adults, and older children are able to cooperate if given proper instruction regarding what is expected from them. Infants and small children, however, are unable to follow directions or control body functions sufficiently to help in collecting some specimens.

URINE SPECIMENS

Children admitted to the hospital or seen in a clinic or office may require a urine specimen as a routine diagnostic procedure. Older children and adolescents will readily use the bedpan or urinal or can be trusted to follow directions for collection in the bathroom. However, they may have special needs. School-age children are cooperative but curious. They are concerned about the reasons behind things and are likely to ask questions regarding the disposition of their specimen and what one expects to discover from it. Self-conscious adolescents may be reluctant to carry a specimen bottle through a hallway or waiting room and appreciate a paper bag or other means for disguising the container. The presence of menses is sometimes an embarrassment to teenage girls; therefore it is a good idea to ask them if it might be that particular time of the month and make adjustments as necessary. The specimen can be delayed or a notation made on the laboratory slip to explain the presence of red blood cells.

Preschoolers and toddlers are less cooperative primarily because they are usually unable to void on request. It is often best to offer them water or other liquids that they enjoy and wait about 30 minutes until they are ready to void voluntarily or set a timer to alert the child that he needs to void shortly. The child will better understand what is expected if the nurse uses his terms for the function, such as "pee-pee" or "tinkle." Some will have difficulty voiding

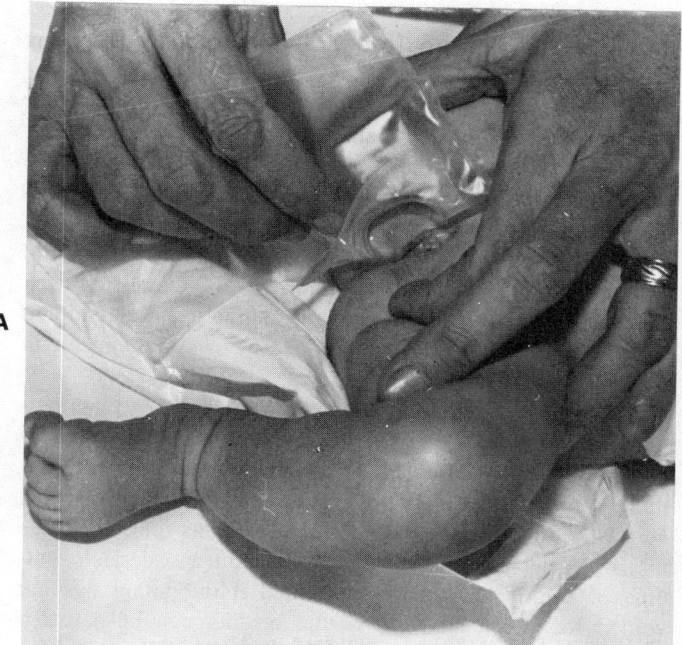
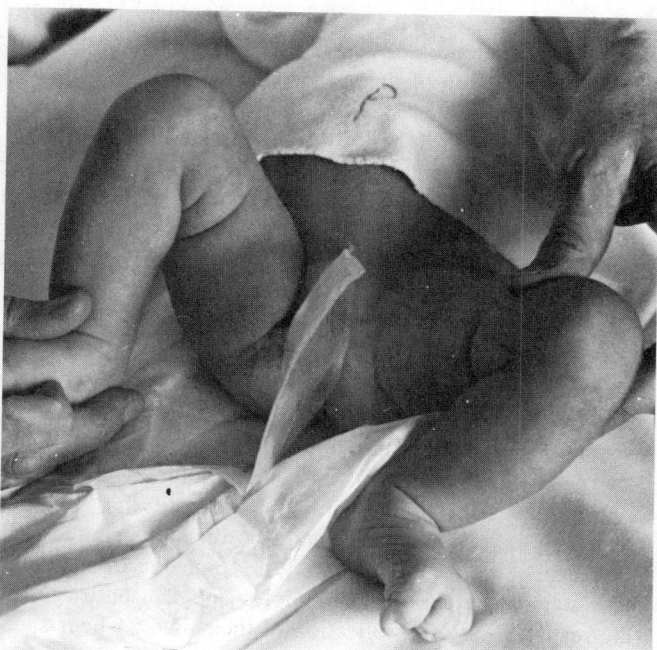

A

B

Fig. 27-15. Application of urine collection bag. **A,** For female infants adhesive portion is applied to exposed and dried perineum first. **B,** Bag adheres firmly around perineal area to prevent urine leakage.

in an unfamiliar receptacle. Potty-chairs or a bedpan placed on the toilet will ordinarily prove satisfactory. Toddlers who have recently acquired bladder control may be especially reluctant, since they undoubtedly have been admonished for "going" in places other than those approved by parents. A useful approach is to enlist the help of parents; they are likely to be successful, and this helps them to feel a part of the child's care.

For infants and toddlers who are not toilet trained, special urine collection devices are used. These devices are clear plastic single-use bags with self-adhering material around the opening at the point of attachment. To prepare the infant, the genitalia, perineum, and surrounding skin are washed and dried thoroughly, since the adhesive will not stick to a moist, powdered, or oily skin surface. The collection bag is easiest to apply if attached first to the perineum, progressing to the symphysis (Fig. 27-15). With little girls the perineum is stretched taut during application to that area to ensure a leak-proof fit. With small boys the penis and scrotum are placed inside the bag. The adhesive portion of the bag must be firmly applied to the skin all around the genital area to avoid possible leakage. The diaper is carefully replaced. Cutting a small slit in the diaper and pulling the bag through allows room for urine to collect and facilitates checking on the contents. The bag is checked frequently and removed as soon as the specimen is available, since the moist bag may become loosened on an active child. For some types of urine testing, such as checking specific gravity, urine can be aspirated directly from the diaper (Strohbach and Kratina, 1982). If diapers with absorbent

gelling material that trap urine are used, a small gauze dressing placed inside the diaper can be used to collect urine.

At times parents may be requested to bring a urine sample to a health care facility for examination, especially when infants are unable to void during an outpatient visit. In this instance parents need instruction on applying the collection device and storage of the specimen.* Ideally the specimen should be brought to the designated place as soon as possible; if there is a delay, the sample should be refrigerated and the lapsed time reported to the examiner (see p. 1128).

Clean-Catch Specimens

Although older children can be instructed in the proper technique, the nurse performs the cleansing procedure on infants and young children. The perineum is cleansed with a soap- or an antiseptic-soaked sterile pad, wiping from front to back only once with each pad. This is repeated at least two times. The area is then wiped with sterile water to prevent accidental contamination of the urine with a solution that may destroy the pathogens, although minute amounts of antiseptic such as iodine do not alter bacterial counts.

To collect the urine, the nurse holds the infant over a sterile container or applies a sterile plastic collecting bag. The infant can be encouraged to void by applying pressure over the suprapubic area or by stroking the paraspinal mus-

---

*Home care instructions on obtaining a urine sample are available in Wong, D., and Whaley, L.: Clinical handbook of pediatric nursing, ed. 2, St. Louis, 1986, The C.V. Mosby Co.

cles to elicit a Perez reflex. This reflex, which usually disappears by 4 to 6 months of age, results in crying, extension of the back, flexion of the arms and legs, and urination.

When voiding has occurred, the bag is removed immediately. Urine that has been allowed to remain at room temperature is unacceptable as a sample for culture because the number of bacteria doubles every 20 to 30 minutes. If the urine is not tested within 30 minutes, the specimen is refrigerated. If the child has not voided within 45 minutes, the bag must be removed and the cleansing procedure repeated.

Twenty-Four-Hour Collection

Collection of urine voided over a 24-hour period creates some special problems in infants and children. Collection bags and sometimes restraining methods are required to collect specimens from infants and small children. Older children require special instruction about notifying someone when they need to void or have a bowel movement so that urine can be collected separately and not discarded. Some older school-age children and adolescents can be trusted to take responsibility for collection of their own 24-hour specimens. They can keep output records and transfer each voiding to the 24-hour collection container if this is permitted.

As in any 24-hour urine collection, the collection period always starts and ends with an empty bladder. At the time the collection begins the child is instructed to void and the specimen is discarded. All urine voided in the subsequent 24 hours is saved in a refrigerated container. Twenty-four hours from the time the precollection specimen was discarded, the child is again instructed to void, the specimen is added to the container, and the entire collection is taken to the laboratory for examination.

Infants and small children who are bagged for 24-hour urine collection will require a special collection bag; frequent removal and replacement of adhesive collection devices can produce skin irritation. A thin coating of tincture of benzoin applied to the skin helps to protect it and aids adhesion. Plastic collection bags with collection tubes attached are ideal when the container must be left in place for a time. These can be connected to a collecting device or emptied periodically by aspiration with a syringe. When such devices are not available, a regular bag with a feeding tube inserted through a puncture hole at the top of the bag serves as a satisfactory substitute. However, care must be taken to empty the bag as soon as the infant urinates to prevent leakage and loss of contents.

Special Techniques

Catheterization or *suprapubic aspiration* is employed when a specimen is urgently needed or when the child is unable to void or otherwise provide an adequate specimen. Catheterization is most often used when urethral obstruction or anuria caused by renal failure is believed to be the cause of the child's failure to void. Suprapubic aspiration is useful in clarifying the diagnosis of suspected urinary tract infection in acutely ill infants.

Catheterizing a child requires aseptic technique, good light, and gentle, thorough cleansing of the vulva or glans penis. Most children, including female infants, accommodate a size 8 or 10 French catheter, but in male infants or when the larger catheters cannot be passed, a smaller, soft plastic feeding tube may be needed. Most children are frightened of this procedure, and few small children are entirely cooperative; therefore even when the procedure is adequately explained, an assistant is needed to help restrain and reassure the child. Special care must be exercised when catheterizing young males to avoid trauma to the ductal and glandular openings into the urethra, which might result in sterility.

Suprapubic aspiration, which is performed by a practitioner skilled in the procedure, involves aspirating bladder contents by inserting a 20- or 21-gauge needle in the midline approximately 1 cm above the symphysis and directed vertically downward. The skin is prepared as for any needle insertion, but the bladder should contain an adequate volume of urine. This can be assumed if the infant has not voided for at least 1 hour or the bladder can be palpated above the symphysis. This technique is especially useful for obtaining clean specimens from young infants. The bladder is an abdominal organ at this time and is easily accessible.

STOOL SPECIMENS

Stool specimens are frequently collected in children to identify parasites and other organisms that cause diarrhea, to assess gastrointestinal function, and to check for occult (hidden) blood. Ideally stool should be collected without contamination with urine, but in children wearing diapers this is difficult unless a urine bag is applied. Children who are toilet trained should urinate first, flush the toilet, then defecate in the toilet or in a bedpan (preferably one that is placed on the toilet to avoid embarrassment). An ample amount of stool is collected using a tongue blade and placed in the appropriate container that is covered and labeled. If several specimens are needed, the containers are marked with the date and time and kept in a specimen refrigerator. Special care is exercised in handling the specimen because of the risk of contamination.

BLOOD SPECIMENS

Most blood specimens are obtained by the laboratory staff, physicians, or specially trained nurses, such as those in intensive care units where specimens are frequently needed. However, all nurses are often responsible for making certain that specimens, such as serial examinations and fasting specimens, are collected on time and that the proper equipment is available, such as correct collection tubes and ice for blood gas samples.

Venous blood samples can be obtained by venipuncture or by aspiration from an intravenous infusion site. When using an intravenous infusion site for specimen collection, it is important to consider the type of fluid being infused. For example, a specimen collected for glucose determination would be inaccurate if removed from a catheter through which glucose-containing solution is being administered.

No matter how or by whom the specimen is collected, nurses should be aware that children, even some older ones, fear the loss of their blood. This is particularly true for children whose condition requires frequent blood specimens. Ignorant about the process of hemopoiesis, they mistakenly believe that blood removed from their bodies is a threat to their lives. Explaining to them that their blood is continually being produced by their bodies provides them with a measure of reassurance regarding this aspect of the stress-provoking procedure. When the blood is drawn, a simple comment, such as, "Just look how red it is. You're really making a lot of nice red blood," confirms this information and affords them an opportunity to express their concern. A Band-Aid gives them added assurance that the vital fluids will not leak out through the puncture site.

Capillary blood samples are taken from children by finger or earlobe stick methods, just as in the adult patient. The best method for taking peripheral blood samples from infants is by a heel stick. Before the blood sample is taken, the heel is warmed with warm, moist compresses for 5 to 10 minutes in order to dilate the vessels in the area. The area is cleansed with alcohol, and with the infant's foot firmly restrained with the free hand, the heel is punctured with a Bard-Parker no. 11 or Redi-Lance blade.

The most serious complication of infant heel puncture is necrotizing osteochondritis from lancet penetration of the underlying calcaneus bone. To avoid this, the puncture should be no deeper than 2.4 mm and should be made at the outer aspect of the heel. The boundaries of the calcaneus can be marked by an imaginary line extending posteriorly from a point between the fourth and fifth toes and running parallel to the lateral aspect of the heel and another line extending posteriorly from the middle of the great toe and running parallel to the medial aspect of the heel (Fig. 27-16) (Blumenfeld, Turi, and Blanc, 1979). In addition, repeated trauma to the walking surface of the heel can cause fibrosis and scarring that may interfere with locomotion. Frequent heel punctures have been associated with development of plantar warts at a later age.

The needed specimens are quickly collected and pressure applied to the puncture site with a dry gauze square until bleeding stops. The site is then covered with a Band-Aid. Applying warm compresses to ecchymotic areas increases circulation, helps remove extravasated blood, and decreases pain.

SPUTUM SPECIMENS

Older children and adolescents are able to cough as directed and supply sputum specimens when given proper directions. It must be made clear to them that a coughed specimen, not what is cleared from the throat, is needed. It is helpful to

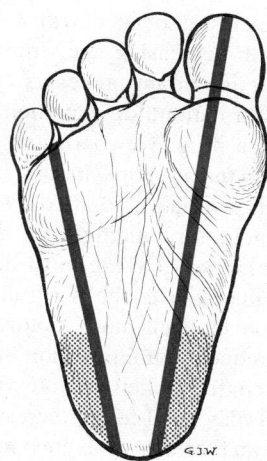

Fig. 27-16. Puncture site *(red stippled area)* on sole of infant's foot.

demonstrate a deep cough so that communication is clear. Infants and small children are unable to follow directions to cough and will swallow any sputum produced when they do; therefore gastric washings (lavage) may be used to collect a specimen. Sometimes it is possible to get a satisfactory specimen by using a suction device such as a mucous trap if the catheter is inserted into the trachea and the cough reflex elicited. A catheter that is inserted into the back of the throat is not sufficient. For children with a tracheostomy, a specimen is easily aspirated from the trachea or major bronchi by attaching a collecting device to the suction apparatus.

Administration of Medication

The administration of medications to children presents a number of problems that are not encountered when giving medication to adult patients. Children vary widely in age, weight, surface area, and the ability to absorb, metabolize, and excrete medications. Nurses must be particularly alert when computing and administering drugs to infants and children.

DETERMINATION OF DRUG DOSAGE

It is the physician's responsibility to prescribe drugs in the correct dosage to achieve the desired effect without endangering the health of the child. However, nurses must have an understanding of the safe dosage of medications they administer to children as well as the expected action, possible side effects, and signs of toxicity. Unlike adult medications, there are no standardized dosage ranges for children in the pediatric age-groups, and, with a few exceptions, drugs are prepared and packaged in average adult-dosage strengths.

Factors related to growth and maturation significantly alter the capacity of an individual to metabolize and excrete drugs, and deficiencies associated with immaturity become more important with decreasing age. Immaturity or defects in any or all of the important processes of absorption, distribution, biotransformation, or excretion can significantly alter the effects of a drug. Newborn and premature infants with immature enzyme systems in the liver (where most drugs are broken down and detoxified), lower plasma concentrations of protein for binding with drugs, and immaturely functioning kidneys (where most drugs are excreted) are particularly vulnerable to the harmful effects of drugs. Many drugs are metabolized more rapidly by the liver, necessitating more frequent administration. This is particularly important in pain control, when the interval between administering analgesics may need to be decreased.

Other factors that create problems in drug dosages in children include the difficulty in evaluating drug response. For example, how is a toxic manifestation such as ringing in the ears assessed in a preverbal child? In disease states, particularly in children, water losses and water requirements are both increased, whereas the fluid intake decreases. Since water is required to excrete the drug, dehydration poses the danger of toxic accumulation. For example, aspirin, which is commonly prescribed for fever, is excreted in the kidney, and its excretion is decreased with diminished urine pH and renal blood flow, both of which are associated with fever.

Various formulas involving age, weight, and body surface area (BSA) as the basis for calculations have been devised to determine children's drug dosage from a standard adult dose. Since the administration of medication is a nursing responsibility, nurses need not only a knowledge of drug action and patient responses but some resources for estimating safe dosages for children. The method most often used to determine children's dosage is based on surface area.

Body Surface Area

The most reliable method for determining children's dosage is to calculate the proportional amount of body surface area to body weight. The ratio of body surface area to weight varies inversely to length; therefore the infant who is shorter and weighs less than an older child or adult has relatively more surface area than would be expected from his weight.

The usual determination of surface area requires the use of the West nomogram (Fig. 27-17). Body surface area is estimated from height and weight of the child, and then this information is applied to a formula for dosage, such as either of the following formulas, which require different types of information:

$$\frac{\text{Body surface area of child}}{\text{Body surface area of adult}} \times \text{Adult dose} = \begin{array}{l}\text{Estimated}\\\text{child's dose}\end{array}$$

$$\text{Surface area of child (m}^2) \times \text{Dose/m}^2 = \begin{array}{l}\text{Estimated}\\\text{child's dose}\end{array}$$

PREPARATION FOR SAFE ADMINISTRATION

Unit dose packaging, which is gaining wide usage in hospital pharmacies, frequently does not extend to pediatric medications. Therefore the ability to calculate fractional doses from larger dosages is absolutely essential. In addition, measuring doses, identifying patients, and gaining cooperation create problems not usually encountered in giving medications to adults.

Checking Dosage

Administering the correct dosage of a drug is a shared responsibility between the physician who orders the drug and the nurse who carries out that order. Children react with unexpected severity to some drugs, and ill children are especially sensitive to drugs. Therefore checking the dose if there is any doubt about its accuracy is a valuable habit to acquire. When a dose is ordered that is outside the usual range or if there is some question regarding the preparation or the route of administration, the nurse should always check with the physician before proceeding with the administration, since the nurse is legally liable for any drug administered.

Administering some medications requires added safeguards. Even when it has been determined that the dosage is correct for a particular child, there are many drugs that are potentially hazardous or lethal. Most hospital units or other facilities where medications are given to children have regulations requiring that specified drugs be double-checked by another nurse before they are given to the child. Among those drugs that require such safeguards are digoxin, heparin, and insulin. Others that are frequently included are epinephrine, narcotics, and sedatives. Even if this precaution is not mandatory, nurses would be wise to take such precautions for their own sense of security.

Identification

Before the administration of any medication, the child must be correctly identified, since children are not totally reliable in giving correct names on request. An infant is unable to give his name, a toddler or preschooler may admit to any name, and a school-age child may deny his identity in an attempt to avoid the medication. Children sometimes exchange beds for a while. Parents may be present to identify their child, but the only safe method for identifying children is to check their hospital identification bands with the medication card.

Parents

Parents can be useful sources of information regarding the child and his capabilities. Nearly all parents have given some kind of medication to their child and can describe the approaches that they have found to be successful. They can also provide information regarding the child's reaction to similar experiences if the child has been hospitalized before or if he has been given medication in a physician's office or clinic. In some cases it is less traumatic for the child if a parent gives the medication, provided the nurse prepares the medication and supervises its administration and the practice is consistent with hospital or ward policy. Children being given daily medications at home are accustomed to the par-

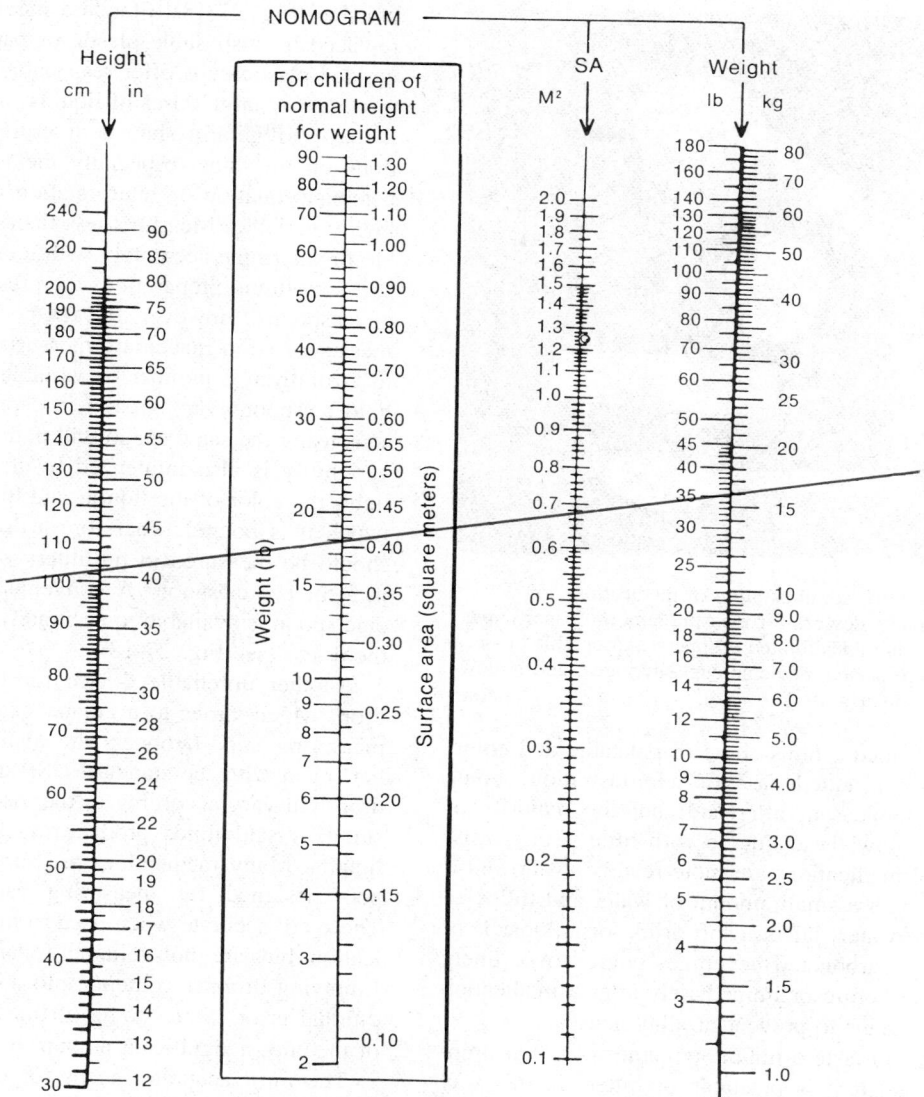

Fig. 27-17. West nomogram (for estimation of surface areas). Surface area is indicated where a straight line connecting height and weight intersects surface area (SA) column, or if patient is roughly of normal proportion, from weight alone (enclosed area). Red line shows SA determination ($0.78M^2$) for child 115 cm tall who weighs 19 kg.

Nomogram modified from data of E. Boyd by C.D. West; from Behrman, R.E., and Vaughan, V.C., editors: Nelson textbook of pediatrics, ed. 12, Philadelphia, 1983, W.B. Saunders Co.

ent functioning in this capacity and are less apt to fuss than they would if the medication were administered by a stranger. Individual decisions need to be made regarding parental presence and participation, such as in helping with restraint, during injections (see Questions and controversies, p. 1107).

Child

Every child requires psychologic preparation for parenteral administration of medication and supportive care during the procedure (see p. 1108). Even if children have received several injections, they rarely become accustomed to the discomfort and have as much right to understanding and patience from those involved in giving the injection as any

other child. Safe administration of any drug requires meticulous attention to the safeguards discussed here.

ORAL ADMINISTRATION

The oral route is preferred for administering medications to children whenever possible. Because of the ease of administration of oral medications, most are dissolved or suspended in liquid preparations. Although some children are able to swallow or chew solid medications at an early age, solid preparations are not recommended for young children. There is danger of aspiration in any oral preparation, but solid forms (pills, tablets, capsules) are especially hazardous if their administration causes marked resistance or crying.

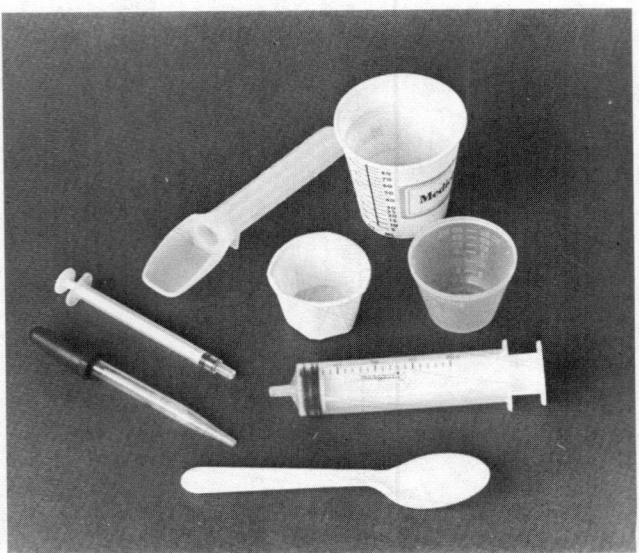

Fig. 27-18. Devices for administration of medications to children. Unacceptable devices for measurement are paper cups, household spoons, and uncalibrated droppers. Acceptable devices for measurement are plastic medicine cups, syringes, and hollow-handled medicine spoons.

Most pediatric medications come in palatable and colorful preparations for added ease of administration. Some have a slightly unpleasant aftertaste, but the majority of children will swallow these liquids with little if any resistance. Many oral medications are more readily swallowed if they are diluted with a small amount of water and followed by a "chaser" of water, juice, a soft drink, or a Popsicle or frozen juice bar. Carbonated beverages poured over finely crushed ice given before or immediately after a medication are an excellent means to prevent or allay nausea.

The nurse should taste a minute amount of an oral preparation to ascertain if it is palatable or bitter. In this way legitimate complaints of dislike from the child can be accepted and the taste camouflaged whenever possible. Most pediatric units have preparations available for this purpose. Sweet-tasting substances that are suitable include honey (except in infants because of the risk of botulism), flavored syrups, jam, and fruit purees. Syrups are ideal for mixing with medicines that do not dissolve in water and for powdered drugs or pulverized tablets. When drugs are mixed, only a small amount of liquid or food is used, since the child may refuse to take the entire amount and thus receive only a partial dose of the medication. When selecting a substance to mix with a medication, *essential food items,* such as milk, cereal, and orange juice, are avoided. If they are used, children may become adversely conditioned against them and refuse these foods in their diet.

Preparation

Selecting a vehicle to measure and administer a medication requires careful consideration. The devices available to measure medicines are not always sufficiently accurate for measuring the small amounts needed in pediatric nursing

practice (Fig. 27-18). Standard medicine glasses have been replaced by disposable plastic or paper cups. Although the molded plastic cups offer reasonable accuracy in measuring moderate or large doses of liquids, the paper cups are likely to have irregularly shaped or crumpled bottoms. Calibrations on the cups (especially the teaspoon mark) and the personal equation or interpretation of a given measure are highly variable. Measures less than a teaspoon are impossible to determine accurately with a cup.

Many liquid preparations are prescribed in measurements of teaspoons. However, the teaspoon (and other household measures) is an inaccurate measuring device and is subject to error from a number of variables. For example, household teaspoons vary greatly in capacity, and different persons using the same spoon will pour different amounts. This variability is also influenced by the adequacy of available light, the color of the liquid, and the size of the bottle from which it is poured. Therefore a drug ordered in teaspoons should be measured in milliliters—the established standard is 5 ml per teaspoon. A convenient hollow-handled medicine spoon is available to accurately measure and administer the drug* (see Fig. 27-18).

Another unreliable device for measuring liquids is the drop, which varies to a greater extent than the teaspoon or measuring cup. Droppers are available in numerous sizes but, even with the standard USP dropper, the volume of a drop will vary according to the viscosity of the liquid measured. Viscid fluids produce much larger drops than thin liquids. Many medications are supplied with caps or droppers designed for measuring each specific preparation. These are accurate when used to measure that specific medication but are not reliable for measuring other liquids. Emptying dropper contents into a medicine cup invites additional error. Since some of the liquid clings to the sides of the cup, a significant amount of the drug can be lost.

The most accurate means for measuring small amounts of medication is the plastic disposable (never glass) syringe, especially the tuberculin syringe for volumes less than 1 ml. Not only does the syringe provide a reliable measure, but it also serves as a convenient means for transporting and administering the medication. The medication can be placed directly into the child's mouth from the syringe. For added safety, a short length of flexible tubing can be placed on the tip of the syringe to prevent injury to the mouth, although the tubing must be completely emptied of medication.

Small children and some older children as well have difficulty in swallowing tablets or pills. Since a number of drugs are not available in pediatric preparations, the tablet will need to be crushed before it can be given to these children. To minimize loss of the drug, the tablet can be crushed between two spoons or placed either in a medicine cup or between two small paper soufflé cups and crushed in a mortar and then mixed with syrup or juice for the child to swallow. The nurse must make certain that the bits of pul-

---

*Manufactured by Apex Medical Corp., P.O. Box 20171, Bloomington, MN 55420.

verized medication that tend to cling to the sides of the medicine cup or spoon are not lost.

Not all drugs can be crushed, for example, medication with an enteric or protective coating or formulated for slow release. For some children it may be possible to encourage swallowing the tablet or capsule by using a special glass designed with a shelf that holds the drug (manufactured by Apex Medical Corp.). The child drinks normally and the tablet is carried to the back of the throat. For children who must take solid oral medication for an extended period training sessions using progressively larger candy to teach the child to swallow can be beneficial (Funk, Mullins, and Olson, 1984).

Since pediatric doses often require dividing adult preparations of medication, the nurse may be faced with the dilemma of accurate dosage. With tablets, only those that are scored can be halved or quartered accurately. If the medication is soluble, the tablet or contents of a capsule can be mixed in a small premeasured amount of liquid and the appropriate portion given. If half a dose is required, the tablet is dissolved in 5 ml of water and 2.5 ml is given.

Administration

While administering liquids to infants is relatively easy, care must be observed to prevent aspiration. With the infant held in a semireclining position, the medication is placed in his mouth from a spoon, plastic cup, plastic dropper, or plastic syringe (without needle). The dropper or syringe is best placed along the side of the infant's tongue and administered slowly to avoid causing him to choke. Medicine cups can be used effectively for older infants who are able to drink from a cup. Because of the natural outward tongue thrust in infancy, medications may need to be retrieved from lips or chin and refed. Allowing the infant to suck the medication that has been placed in any empty nipple* or inserting the syringe or dropper into the side of the mouth, parallel to the nipple, while the infant nurses are other convenient methods for giving liquid medications to infants. Medication is not added to the infant's formula feeding.

The small child who refuses to cooperate or resists consistently despite explanation and encouragement may require mild physical coercion. If so, it is carried out quickly and carefully. Every effort is made to determine why the child resists, and the reasons for this alternative are explained to the child in such a way that he will know that it is being carried out for his well-being and is not a form of punishment. There is always a risk in using even mild forceful techniques. A crying child can aspirate a medication, particularly when he is lying on his back. If the nurse holds the child in the lap with the child's right arm behind the nurse, the left hand firmly grasped by the nurse's left hand, and the head securely restrained between the nurse's arm and body, the medication can be slowly poured into the mouth (Fig. 27-19).

INTRAMUSCULAR ADMINISTRATION

Injections constitute some of the most traumatic health-related experiences for children. No one likes an injection, especially young children, who may associate the procedure with other meanings such as fear of body mutilation and punishment. At times it can be no less stressful to the nurse who must inflict the distress. Consequently, injections are given only when the drug cannot be given by any other route.

Selecting Syringe and Needle

The volume of medication prescribed for small children and the small amount of tissue for injection require that a syringe be selected that can measure very small amounts of solution. For volumes less than 1 ml the tuberculin syringe, calibrated in one-hundredth increments, is appropriate. Very minute doses may require the use of a 0.5 ml, low-dose syringe. These syringes with specially constructed needles minimize the possibility of inadvertently administering incorrect amounts of a drug because of dead space, which allows fluid to remain in the syringe and needle after the plunger is pushed completely forward. A minimum of 0.2 ml of solution remains in a standard needle hub; therefore when very small amounts of two drugs are combined in the

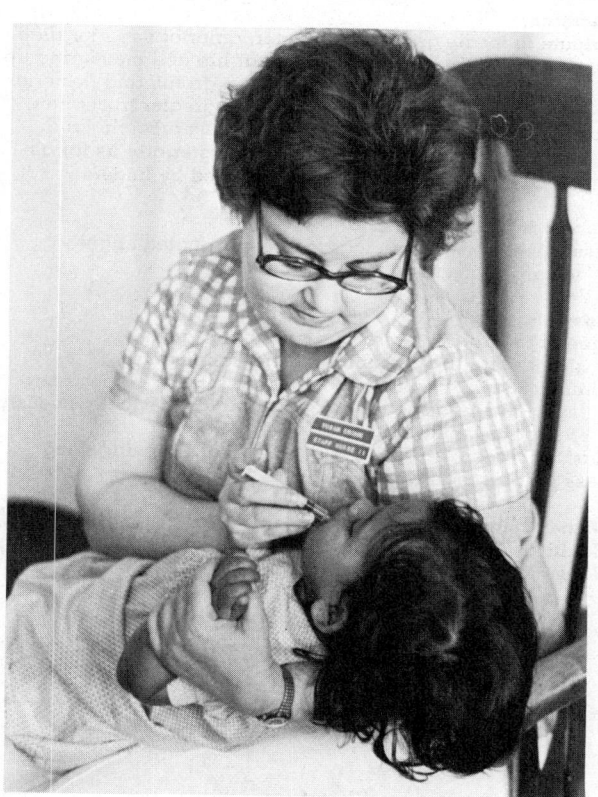

Fig. 27-19. Nurse partially restrains child for easy and comfortable administration of oral medication.

*A commercial nipple (NUK Medi-Nurser) is designed with a reservoir to hold the liquid and is available from Reliance Products Corp., 108 Mason St., P.O. Box 1220, Woonsocket, RI 02895.

Table 27-4 Intramuscular injection sites in children

SITE	DISCUSSION

Vastus lateralis

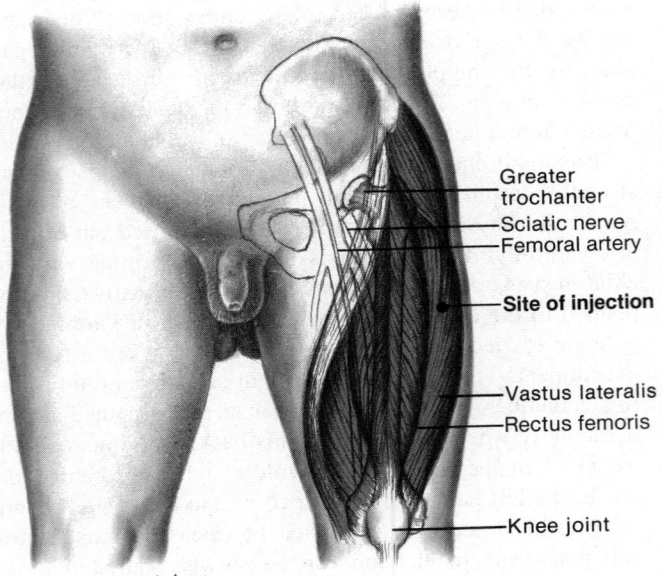

Greater trochanter
Sciatic nerve
Femoral artery

Site of injection

Vastus lateralis
Rectus femoris

Knee joint

G.J.Wassilchenko

Location
Palpate to find greater trochanter and knee joints; divide vertical distance between these two landmarks into quadrants; inject into middle of upper quadrant.

Needle insertion
Insert needle at 45-degree angle toward knee in infants and in young children or needle perpendicular to thigh or slightly angled toward anterior thigh.

Advantages
Large, well-developed muscle that can tolerate larger quantities of fluid
No important nerves or blood vessels in this location
Easily accessible if child is supine, side-lying, or sitting
A tourniquet can be applied above injection site to delay drug hypersensitivity reaction if necessary

Disadvantages
Thrombosis of femoral artery from injection in midthigh area
Sciatic nerve damage from long needle injected posteriorly and medially into small extremity

---

Ventrogluteal

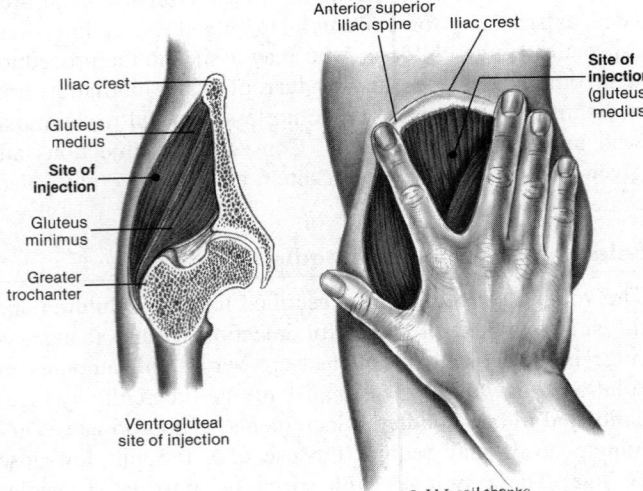

Iliac crest
Gluteus medius
Site of injection
Gluteus minimus
Greater trochanter

Ventrogluteal site of injection

Anterior superior iliac spine   Iliac crest

Site of injection (gluteus medius)

G.J.Wassilchenko

Location
Palpate to locate greater trochanter, anterior superior *iliac* tubercle (found by flexing thigh at hip and measuring up to 1 to 2 cm above crease formed in groin), and posterior iliac crest; place palm of hand over greater trochanter, index finger over anterior superior ilac tubercle, and middle finger along crest of ilium posteriorly as far as possible; inject into center of V formed by fingers.

Needle insertion
Insert needle perpendicular to site but angled slightly toward iliac crest.

Advantages
Free of important nerves and vascular structures
Easily identified by prominent bony landmarks
Thinner layer of subcutaneous tissue than in dorsogluteal site, thus less change of depositing drug subcutaneously rather than intramuscularly
Easily accessible if child is supine, prone, or side-lying
Less painful than vastus lateralis

Disadvantages
Health professionals' unfamiliarity with site
Not suitable for use of a tourniquet

Table 27-4 Intramuscular injection sites in children—cont'd.

SITE	DISCUSSION

Dorsogluteal

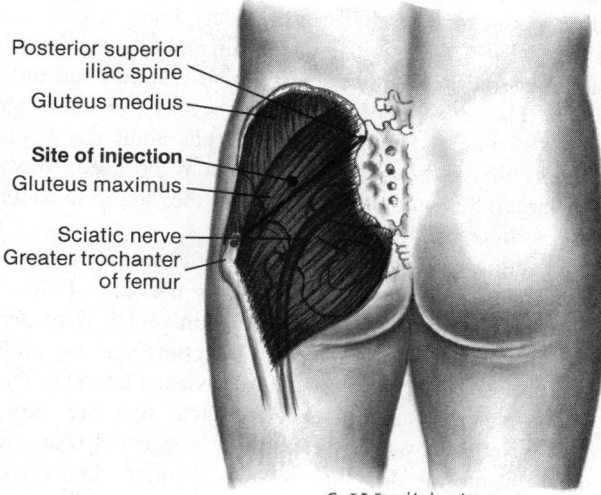

Posterior superior iliac spine
Gluteus medius
Site of injection
Gluteus maximus
Sciatic nerve
Greater trochanter of femur

G.J.Wassilchenko

Location

Locate greater trochanter and posterior superior iliac spine; draw imaginary line between these two points and inject lateral and superior to line into gluteus muscle.

Needle insertion

Insert needle perpendicular to surface on which child is lying when prone.

Advantages

In older child large muscle mass; well-developed muscle can tolerate greater volume of fluid
Child does not see needle and syringe
Easily accessible if child is prone or side-lying

Disadvantages

Contraindicated in children who have not been walking for at least 1 year
Danger of injury to sciatic nerve
Thick, subcutaneous fat, predisposing to deposition of drug subcutaneously rather than intramuscularly
Not suitable for use of a tourniquet
Inaccessible if child is supine
Exposure of site may cause embarrassment in older child

Deltoid

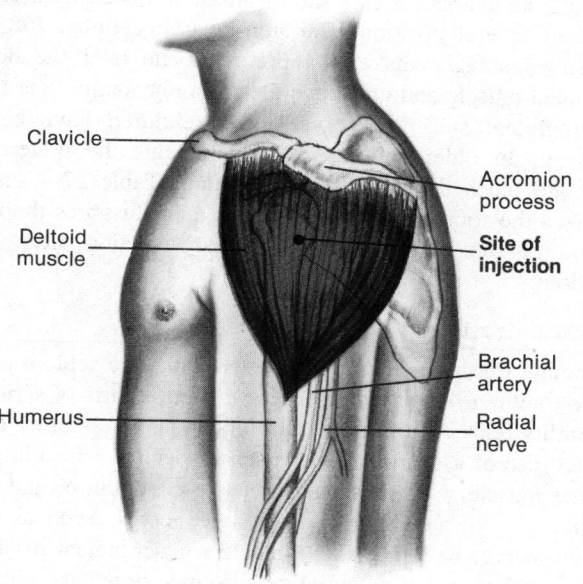

Clavicle
Acromion process
Deltoid muscle
Site of injection
Brachial artery
Humerus
Radial nerve

G.J.Wassilchenko

Location

Locate acromion process; inject only into upper third of muscle that begins about 2 finger-breadths below acromion.

Needle insertion

Insert needle perpendicular to site but angled slightly toward shoulder.

Advantages

Faster absorption rates than gluteal sites
Tourniquet can be applied above injection site
Easily accessible with minimum removal of clothing

Disadvantages

Small muscle mass; only limited amounts of drug can be injected
Small margins of safety with possible damage to radial nerve
Pain with repeated injections

Continued.

syringe, such as atropine and meperidine or mixtures of insulin, the ratio of the two drugs can be altered significantly (Wong, 1982).

Dead space is also a significant factor to consider when injecting medication, since flushing the syringe with an air bubble or parenteral fluid adds an additional amount of medication to the prescribed dose. This can be hazardous when very small amounts of a drug are given. For example, a tuberculin syringe filled to the 0.05 ml mark can deliver *more than twice* the calculated dose of medication when it is flushed with parenteral fluid from an intravenous line. This has resulted in overadministration of digoxin, a drug with a narrow margin of safety between therapeutic and toxic dose (Berman and others, 1978).

Consequently flushing is not advisable, especially when less than 1 ml of medication is given. Syringes are calibrated to deliver a prescribed drug dose and the amount of medication left in the hub and needle is not part of the syringe barrel calibrations. However, the air-bubble technique (drawing up about 0.2 ml of air into the syringe after withdrawing the medication) may be beneficial with certain drugs, such as iron dextran and diphtheria and tetanus toxoid, to avoid tracking the drug through the tissue (Chaplin, Shull, and Welk, 1985). Other techniques to minimize tracking include changing the needle after withdrawing the fluid from the vial and using the Z track method.

The needle length must be sufficient to penetrate the subcutaneous tissue and deposit the medication well in the body of the muscle. One method of estimating this distance is grasping the vastus lateralis or deltoid muscle and measuring half the distance between the thumb and index finger. This is the approximate needle length required to penetrate that muscle. With the ventrogluteal or dorsogluteal site, only the subcutaneous tissue is grasped and half this distance is the *minimum* needle length needed to reach the muscle. Additional length is required to penetrate the muscle (Lenz, 1983). In both instances needle length must also allow for a small portion of the needle to be exposed at the skin surface as a precaution if the needle should break off from the hub. The most satisfactory needles for intramuscular injections to children are the 25- to 27-gauge needles with a length of ½ to 1 inch. Regular intramuscular needles are too large, in both length and gauge, for pediatric use except for very large, obese children.

Determining Site

Factors that are considered when selecting a site for an intramuscular injection on an infant or child include:

1. The amount and character of the medication to be injected
2. The amount and general condition of the muscle mass
3. The frequency or number of injections to be given during the course of treatment
4. The type of medication being given

5. Factors that may impede access to or cause contamination of the site
6. The ability of the child to assume the required position safely

Ordinarily older children and adolescents pose few problems in selecting a suitable site for intramuscular injections, but infants with their small and underdeveloped muscles have fewer available sites. It is sometimes difficult to assess the amount of fluid that can be safely injected into a single site. Usually 1 ml is the maximum volume that should be administered in a single site to small children and older infants. The muscles of small infants may not tolerate more than 0.5 ml. As the child approaches adult size, volumes approaching those given to adults may be used. However, the larger the amount of solution, the larger must be the muscle into which it is injected.

Injections must be placed in muscles large enough to accommodate the medication, yet major nerves and blood vessels must be avoided. There is no universal agreement regarding the best intramuscular injection site for children. The preferred site for infants is the vastus lateralis. General recommendations for using the gluteal sites are after children have been walking (length of suggested time varies), since the muscle develops with locomotion. Unfortunately, this recommendation is often applied to the ventrogluteal muscle site as well as the dorsogluteal site. However, there are significant differences between these two sites that warrant recognition. The ventrogluteal site is relatively free of major nerves and blood vessels, is a relatively large muscle with less subcutaneous tissue than the dorsal site, has well-defined landmarks for safe site location, and is easily accessible in several positions (Intramuscular injections, 1985). These advantages make it a preferred site over the dorsogluteal muscle and challenge the recommendation that the ventrogluteal site not be used until children have been walking. In older children and adolescents the preferred sites are much the same as in the adult. Table 27-4 summarizes the four major injection sites and illustrates the location of the preferred intramuscular injection sites for children.

Administration

Although injections that are executed with care seldom produce trauma to the child, there have been reports of serious disability related to intramuscular injections in children. Repeated use of a single site has been associated with fibrosis of the muscle with subsequent muscle contracture, and injections in the neighborhood of large nerves, such as the sciatic nerve, have been responsible for permanent disability, especially when potentially neurotoxic drugs are administered. There are several reports of tissue damage from penicillin; one of the difficulties in administering the opaque preparations, such as Bicillin, is that aspirated blood cannot be detected at the bottom of the syringe, thus increasing the risk of injecting into a blood vessel. When such drugs are injected, great care must be used in locating the correct site. When aspirating, the nurse should look for blood at the *top* of the syringe near the plunger since blood may be drawn up through the column of penicillin (Stoller and Losey, 1985).

A reported potential hazard with medication in glass ampules is the presence of glass particles in the ampule after the container is broken. When the medication is withdrawn into the syringe, the glass particles are also withdrawn and are subsequently injected into the patient. As a precaution, medication from glass ampules should only be drawn up through a needle with a filter or injected intravenously through a site in the tubing that is distal to an intravenous filter (Shaw and Lyall, 1985). Another precaution that does not relate to patient but to nursing safety is proper disposal of the needle to prevent contamination with organisms such as hepatitis. To prevent needle-stick injuries, used needles should not be recapped, broken, or bent by hand and should be placed in specially designed puncture-resistant containers (Garner and Simmons, 1983). Other safety precautions for administering chemotherapeutic drugs are discussed on p. 1575.

Most children are unpredictable and few are totally cooperative when receiving an injection. Even children who appear to be relaxed and constrained can lose control under the stress of the procedure. It is advisable to have someone available to help restrain the child if needed. Since children often jerk or pull away unexpectedly, it is a good idea to carry an extra needle to exchange for a contaminated one so that there is a minimum of delay. The child, even a small one, is told that he is getting an injection, and then the procedure is carried out as quickly and skillfully as possible to avoid prolonging the stressful experience. Delay caused by lengthy explanations, attempts to hide the syringe from sight, or efforts to soothe the child will only serve to increase his anxiety. It must be kept in mind that intrusive procedures such as injections are especially anxiety provoking in preschool children and that small children usually associate any assault to the ''behind'' area with punishment.

Small infants offer little resistance to injections. Although they squirm and may be difficult to hold in position, they can usually be restrained without assistance. The muscle mass of the thigh to be injected is firmly grasped in one hand to stabilize the limb and compress the muscle mass for injection with the other hand. The body of a larger infant can be securely restrained between the nurse's arm and body (Fig. 27-20).

If medication is given around the clock, the nurse must be careful to wake the child before giving the injection. Although it may seem easier to surprise the sleeping child and get it over with as quickly as possible, performing the procedure in this way can cause the child to fear going back to sleep. If he is awakened first, the child will know that nothing will be done to him unless he is forewarned. The box on p. 1138 summarizes administration techniques that maximize safety and minimize the discomfort often associated with injections.

INTRAVENOUS ADMINISTRATION

The intravenous route for administering medications has gained widespread use in pediatric therapy. For some important drugs it is the only effective route of administration. This method is used for giving drugs to children who have poor absorption as a result of diarrhea, dehydration, or peripheral vascular collapse; children who need a high serum concentration of a drug; and those with resistant infections that require parenteral medication over an extended time.

Insertion sites and observation of the intravenous infusion are discussed in Chapter 28. However, there are a number of factors that need to be considered in relation to intravenous medication. When a drug is administered intravenously, the effect is almost instantaneous and further control is limited. Most drugs for intravenous administration require a specified minimum dilution and/or rate of flow, and many

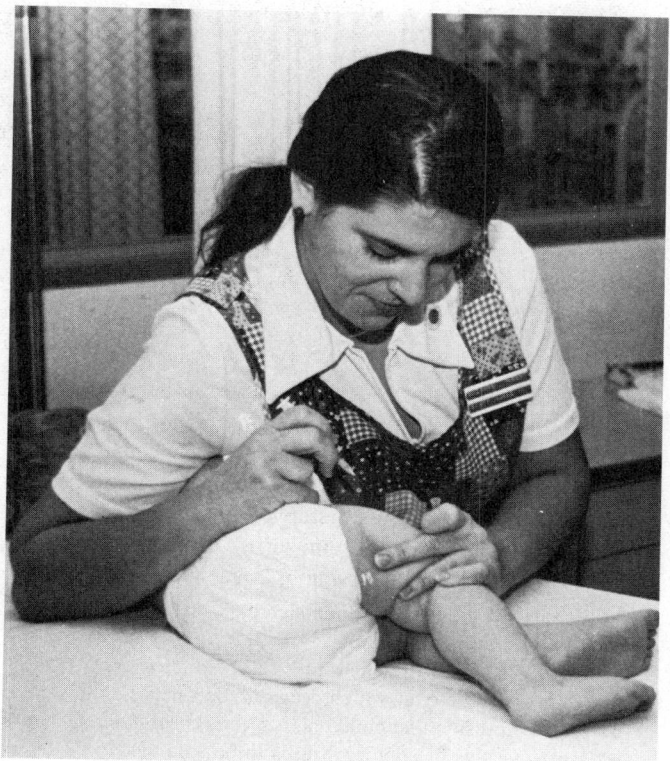

Fig. 27-20. Restraining small child for intramuscular injection. Note how nurse isolates and stabilizes muscle.

GUIDELINES FOR INTRAMUSCULAR ADMINISTRATION OF MEDICATION

1. Use universal precautions for safety in administering medications.
2. Prepare medication.
   a. Select needle and syringe appropriate to following:
      (1) Amount of fluid to be administered
      (2) Viscosity of fluid to be administered
      (3) Amount of tissue to be penetrated
   b. Maximum volume to be administered in a single site is 1 ml for older infants and small children.
3. Determine the site of injection (Table 27-8); make certain muscle is large enough to accommodate volume and type of medication.
   a. Older children—select site as with adult patient; allow child some choice of site, if feasible.
   b. Following are acceptable sites for infants and small or debilitated children:
      (1) Vastus lateralis muscle
      (2) Ventrogluteal muscle
   c. Dorsogluteal muscle is insufficiently developed to be a safe site for infants and small children.
4. Administer medication.
   a. Provide for sufficient help in restraining child; children are often uncooperative, and their behavior is usually unpredictable.
   b. Explain briefly what is to be done and, if appropriate, what child can do to help.
   c. Expose injection area for unobstructed view of landmarks.
   d. Select a site where the skin is free of irritation and danger of infection; palpate for and avoid sensitive or hardened areas.
   e. Place child in a lying or sitting position; child is not allowed to stand because:
      (1) Landmarks are more difficult to assess.
      (2) Restraint is more difficult.
      (3) Child may faint and fall.
   f. Use a new sharp needle with smallest diameter that permits free flow of the medication.
   g. Grasp muscle firmly between thumb and fingers to isolate and stabilize muscle for deposition of drug in its deepest part; in obese children spread skin with thumb and index finger to displace subcutaneous tissue and grasp muscle deeply on each side.
   h. Allow skin preparation to dry completely before skin is penetrated.
   i. Have medication at room temperature.
   j. Decrease perception of pain:
      (1) Distract child with conversation.
      (2) Give child something on which to concentrate, such as squeezing a hand or bed rail, pinching his own nose, humming, counting, or yelling "ouch."
      (3) Place a cold compress or wrapped ice cube on site about a minute before injection or apply cold to contralateral site.
      (4) Say to child, "If you feel this, tell me to take it out please."
   k. Insert needle quickly.
   l. Aspirate for blood.
      (1) If blood is found, remove syringe from site, change needle, and reinsert into new location.
      (2) If no blood is found, inject into a relaxed muscle:
         (a) Dorsogluteal—place child on abdomen with his legs and toes rotated inward.
         (b) Ventrogluteal—place child on side with upper leg flexed and placed in front of lower leg.
   m. Avoid tracking any medication through superficial tissues:
      (1) Replace needle after withdrawing medication or wipe medication from needle with sterile gauze.
      (2) If withdrawing medication from an ampule, use a needle equipped with a filter that removes glass particles and use a second needle for injection.
      (3) Use the Z-track and/or air bubble technique as indicated.
      (4) Avoid any depression of the plunger during insertion of needle.
   n. Aspirate to be sure the needle is not in a blood vessel; if it is, begin again with a new needle and syringe.
   o. Inject medication slowly (over a period of 20 seconds.)
   p. Remove needle quickly; hold gauze sponge firmly against skin near needle when removing it to avoid needle's pulling on tissue.
   q. Apply firm pressure to site after injection; massage site to hasten absorption unless contraindicated, as with irritating drugs and heparin.
   r. Place a small Band-Aid on puncture site; with young children decorate Band-Aid by drawing a smiling face or other symbol of acceptance.
   s. Hold and cuddle young child and encourage parents to comfort him; praise older child.
   t. Allow expression of feelings.
5. Record time of injection, drug, dose, and injection site.

---

are highly irritating or toxic to tissues outside the vascular system. In addition to the precautions and nursing observations related to intravenous therapy, factors that are considered when preparing and administering drugs to infants and children by way of the intravenous route include:

1. Amount of drug to be administered
2. Minimum dilution of drug
3. Type of solution in which drug can be diluted
4. Length of time over which drug can be safely administered
5. Rate of infusion that child and his vessels can tolerate safely
6. Time that this or another drug is to be administered
7. Compatibility of all drugs that child is receiving intravenously

Before any intravenous infusion the site of insertion is checked for patency. Medications are never administered by way of blood products.

When a drug with poor stability, such as ampicillin, is being administered, it should be kept in mind that the Volutrol (or similar container, such as Burette, Pediatrol, and Metriset) must be emptied of the drug-containing solution and that the tubing from the Volutrol to the insertion site contains the drug as well. The child does not receive the full dose of the drug until the 10 ml or more of solution within the tubing has also been infused. This is a significant consideration when drugs are given in small amounts of fluid. For example, if a drug is added to 10 ml of fluid in the Volutrol, it does not reach the bloodstream until all of the fluid in the tubing is absorbed.

As a general rule, all antibiotics administered via Volutrol should infuse within 1 hour. The nurse calculates the infusion to allow for the drug to be administered in the proper amount of time, including in the calculation the 10 ml of fluid that occupies the tubing (if extension tubing is added, the fluid occupying that space must also be considered). For example, if ampicillin is added to 10 ml of solution and the pediatric Soluset is regulated at 10 drops/minute, by the end of 1 hour the 10 ml of the medication will remain in the tubing. To ensure that the antibiotic is infused within the 1-hour limit, the microdropper must be set at 20 drops/minute (to infuse the 10 ml in the tubing and the 10 ml in the Volutrol) and then reset to its former rate.

Only one antibiotic should be administered at a time. If the intravenous solution contains other medications such as some electrolytes or vitamins, an antibiotic is not added because the other drugs may inactivate it. In this situation another bottle of intravenous solution is hung and attached via a stopcock to the main infusion line. This "piggyback" setup allows antibiotics to be infused without mixing with the other solution.

Another method of intravenous infusion is the *retrograde technique,* in which the medication is injected directly into the intravenous tubing at the site of the Y connection. However, the drug is injected *back* toward the Soluset while the tubing is pinched between the Y connection and the venipuncture site. After the drug is injected, the tubing is no longer pinched and the intravenous infusion is allowed to flow. This allows for slower administration of the drug and greater dilution in the fluid than if it were placed in the open tubing toward the vein. It is advantageous in administering medication when fluid intake is limited, such as in neonates with congestive heart failure.

Several other methods of long-term venous access are available and include the heparin lock device, Hickman or Broviac atrial catheters, and implantable infusion ports. These devices are discussed in Chapter 28. Instilling medication through the injection cap is easily accomplished with the heparin device or atrial catheter. With the implanted device the port must be palpated for placement and stabilized, the overlying skin cleansed, and only special Huber needles used to pierce the port's diaphragm. To avoid repeated skin punctures a special infusion set with a 90-degree prebent Huber needle and extension tubing with Luer connection can be used. With this attached the injection procedure is the same as for the heparin device or atrial catheters. To prevent infection meticulous aseptic technique must be used anytime the devices are entered, including instillation of heparin to prevent clotting. Because these methods of venous access are preferred for long-term administration of medication, families are usually required to learn the skills necessary for their care at home.*

RECTAL ADMINISTRATION

The rectal route for administration is less reliable but sometimes used when the oral route is difficult or contraindi-

---

*Home care instructions on caring for heparin lock and caring for a Hickman/Broviac catheter are available in Wong, D., and Whaley, L.: Clinical handbook of pediatric nursing, ed. 2, St. Louis, 1986, The C.V. Mosby Co.

cated. Some of the drugs available in suppository form are aspirin, sedatives, analgesics (morphine), and antiemetics. The difficulty in using the rectal route is that, unless the rectal ampulla is empty at the time of insertion, the absorption of the drug may be delayed, diminished, or prevented by the presence of feces. Sometimes the drug is later evacuated, securely surrounded by stool. However, the rectal route is used most frequently in children who are unable to take anything by mouth and are unlikely to have large amounts of stool. It is also used when oral preparations are unsuitable to control vomiting.

The wrapping on the suppository is removed. Using a glove or finger cot, the suppository is quickly but gently inserted into the rectum, making certain that it is placed beyond both of the rectal sphincters. The buttocks are then held or taped together firmly to relieve pressure on the anal sphincter until the urge to expel the suppository has passed—5 to 10 minutes. Sometimes the amount of drug ordered is less than the dosage available. The irregular shape of most suppositories makes the process of dividing them into a desired dose difficult if not dangerous. If it must be halved, it should be cut lengthwise. However, there is no guarantee that the drug is evenly dispersed throughout the petrolatum base.

If medication is administered via a retention enema, the same procedure is used. Drugs given by enema are diluted in the smallest amount of solution possible to minimize the likelihood of being evacuated.

OPTIC, OTIC, AND NASAL ADMINISTRATION

There are few differences in administering eye, ear, and nose medication to children and to adults. The major difficulty is in gaining their cooperation or employing restraining techniques. The infant or young child's head is immobilized in the same manner as described in Fig. 7-34. Older children need only explanation and direction. For greater comfort medications stored in the refrigerator should be warmed to room temperature before instillation. For example, cold solutions striking the tympanic membrane may produce pain or vertigo.

To instill eye medication the child is placed supine or sitting with the head extended and the child is asked to look up. One hand is used to pull the lower lid downward; the hand that holds the dropper rests on the head so that it may move synchronously with the child's head, thus reducing the possibility of trauma to a struggling child or dropping medication on the face (Fig. 27-21). As the lower lid is pulled down, a small conjunctival sac is formed; the solution or ointment is applied to this area, never directly on the eyeball. Another effective technique is to pull the lower lid down and out to form a cup effect, into which the medication is dropped.

The lids are gently closed to prevent expression of the medication, and the child is asked to look in all directions to enhance even distribution of the preparation. Excess medication is wiped from the inner canthus outward to prevent

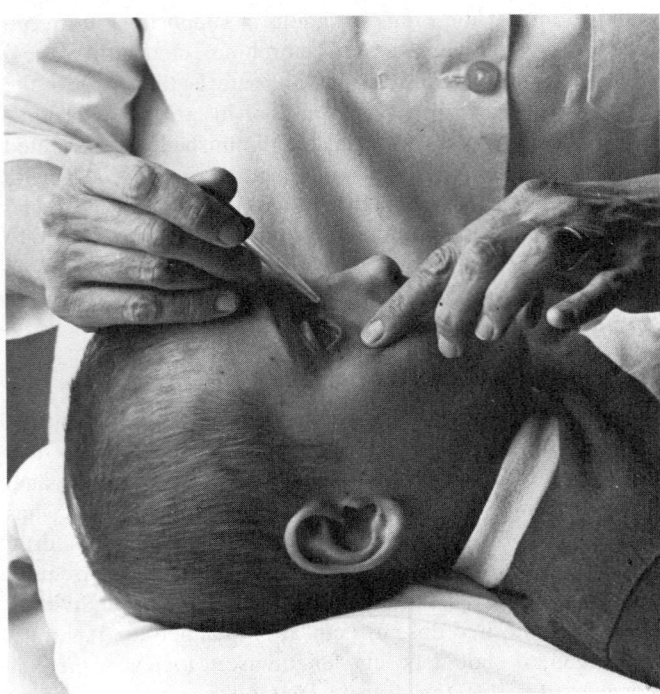

Fig. 27-21. Administering eye drops.

contamination to the contralateral eye. Applying finger pressure to the lacrimal punctum at the inner aspect of the lid for 1 minute prevents drainage of medication to the nasopharynx and eliminates the unpleasant "tasting" of the drug.

Instilling eye drops in infants can be most difficult since infants often clench the lids tightly closed. One approach is to place the drops in the nasal corner where the lids meet. The medication pools in this area and when the child opens the lids the medication flows onto the conjunctiva. For young children playing a game can be helpful, such as instructing the child to keep the eyes closed until the count of 3, then to open them, at which time the drops are quickly instilled. Ointment can be applied when the child is sleeping by gently pulling down the lower lid and placing the ointment in the lower conjunctival sac.

Ear drops are instilled with the child restrained in the supine position and the head turned to the appropriate side. For children younger than 3 years of age, the external auditory canal is straightened by gently pulling the pinna downward and straight back. The pinna is pulled upward and back in children older than 3 years of age (see Fig. 7-29). After instillation, the child should remain lying on the unaffected side for a few minutes. Gentle massage of the area immediately anterior to the ear facilitates the entry of drops into the ear canal. The use of cotton pledgets prevents medication from flowing out of the external canal. However, they should be loose enough to allow any discharge to exit from the ear.

Nose drops are instilled in the same manner as in the adult patient. Unpleasant sensations associated with medi-

cated nose drops are minimized when care is taken to position the child with the head extended well over the edge of the bed or a pillow (Fig. 27-25). Depending on the size of the infant, he can be positioned in the football hold (p. 1121), in the nurse's arm with the head extended and stabilized between the nurse's body and elbow and the arms and hands immobilized with the nurse's hands, or with the head extended over the edge of the bed or a pillow. Strangling sensations are caused by medication trickling into the throat rather than up into the nasal passages. Following instillation of the drops, the child should remain in position for 1 minute to allow the drops to come in contact with the nasal surfaces.

FAMILY TEACHING AND HOME CARE

It is usually the nurse who assumes the responsibility for preparing families to administer medications at home. The family should have an understanding of why the child is receiving the medication and the effects that might be expected, as well as the amount, frequency, and length of time the drug is to be administered. Instruction should be carried out in an unhurried, relaxed manner, preferably in an area away from busy ward or office routine following the same guidelines for teaching as outlined on p. 1113.

The caregiver is carefully instructed regarding the correct dosage, and it is the nurse's responsibility to prepare parents for the specifics of the task. Some persons have difficulty in understanding or interpreting terminology from the pharmacy, and just because they nod or otherwise indicate an understanding, it cannot be assumed that the message is clear. It is important to ascertain their interpretation of a

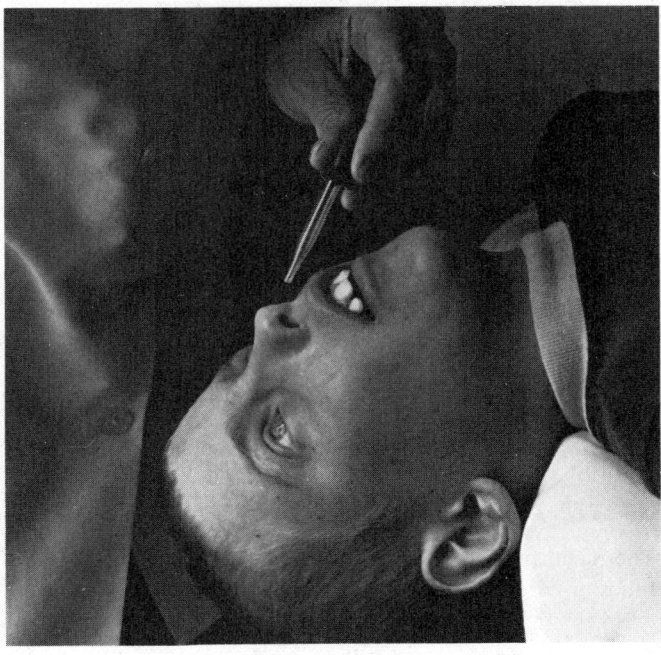

Fig. 27-22. Proper position for instilling nose drops.

teaspoon, for example, and to be certain they have acceptable devices for measuring the drug. If the drug is packaged with a dropper, syringe, or plastic cup, the nurse should show the point on the device that indicates the prescribed dose and demonstrate how the dose is drawn up into a dropper or syringe and measured and the bubbles eliminated. If the nurse has any doubts about the parent's ability to administer the correct dose, the parent should give a return demonstration. This is especially important when the drug has potentially serious consequences from incorrect dosage, such as insulin or digoxin, or when more complex administration is required, such as parenteral injections. When teaching a parent to give an injection, adequate time for instruction and practice must be allotted.

The time that the drug is to be administered is clarified with the parent. For instance, when a drug is prescribed in association with meals, the number of meals that the family is accustomed to eat influences the amount of drug the child receives. Do they have meals twice a day or five times a day? When a drug is to be given several times during the day, together the nurse and parents can work out a schedule that accommodates the family routine. This is particularly significant if the drug must be given at equal intervals throughout a 24-hour period. For example, telling them that the child needs 1 teaspoon of medicine four times a day is subject to misinterpretation, since parents may routinely schedule the doses at incorrect times. Instead, a preplanned schedule based on 6-hour intervals should be set up with the number of days required for therapeutic dosage listed. Written instruction should accompany all drug prescriptions.*

Gastric Feeding Techniques

Children who are unable to take nourishment by mouth because of conditions such as anomalies of the throat, esophagus, or bowel, impaired swallowing capacity, severe debilitation, respiratory distress, or unconsciousness are frequently fed by way of a tube inserted orally or nasally to the stomach (gastric gavage) or duodenum/jejunum (enteral gavage) or by a tube inserted directly into the stomach (gastrostomy) or jejunum (jejunostomy). Such feedings may be intermittent or by continuous drip. Because enteral feedings are used less often than gastric feedings, the following discussion is limited to gastric gavage and gastrostomy.

GAVAGE FEEDING

Infants and children can be fed simply and safely by a tube passed into the stomach through either the nares or the mouth. The tube can be left in place or inserted and removed with each feeding. In older children it is usually less

*Home care instructions on giving medications to children are available in Wong, D., and Whaley, L.: Clinical handbook of pediatric nursing, ed. 2, St. Louis, 1986, The C.V. Mosby Co.

traumatic to tape the tube securely in place between feedings. When this alternative is used, the tube should be removed and replaced with a new tube according to hospital policy, specific orders, and the type of tube used. Meticulous hand washing should be practiced during the procedure to prevent bacterial contamination of the feeding, especially during continuous drip feedings.

Preparation

The equipment needed for gavage feeding includes:

A suitable tube selected according to the size of the child and the viscosity of the solution being fed; for infants a 15-inch French catheter or feeding tube size 5 to 6 is appropriate. In larger children a longer catheter with a larger diameter, usually size 8 French, is needed.

A receptacle for the fluid; for small amounts a 10 to 30 ml syringe barrel or Asepto syringe is satisfactory; for larger amounts a 50 ml syringe with a catheter tip is more convenient.

A syringe to aspirate stomach contents and/or to inject air after the tube has been placed.

Water or water-soluble lubricant to lubricate the tube; sterile water is used for infants.

Paper or nonallergenic tape to mark the tube and to attach the tube to the infant's or child's cheek.

A stethoscope to determine the correct placement in the stomach.

The solution for feeding.

A number of types of feeding tubes are available, including those made of silicone rubber, polyurethane, polyethylene, or polyvinylchloride. The last two types lose their flexibility and need to be replaced frequently, usually every 3 to 4 days. The polyurethane and silicone rubber tubes remain flexible so that they can remain in place longer and afford more patient comfort. They are smaller in diameter than the less flexible tubes (they are often referred to as *small bore tubes,* although the diameter inside the polyurethane tube is wider than the silicone tube with equivalent outside diameters). While the increased softness and flexibility of the tubes are advantages, they also cause disadvantages, such as difficult insertion (may require a stylet—a metal guide wire), collapse of tube during aspiration of gastric contents to test for correct placement, dislodgement during forceful coughing, and unsuitability for thick feedings (Moore and Green, 1985).

Procedure

Infants will be easier to control if they are first wrapped in a mummy restraint (p. 1121). Even tiny infants with random movements can grasp and remove the tube. Premature infants do not ordinarily require restraint, but, if they do, a small towel folded across the chest and secured beneath the shoulders is usually sufficient. Care must be taken so that breathing is not compromised.

Gavage feeding is usually carried out with the infant or child lying on the back or toward the right side and the head and chest elevated slightly. A folded blanket under the head

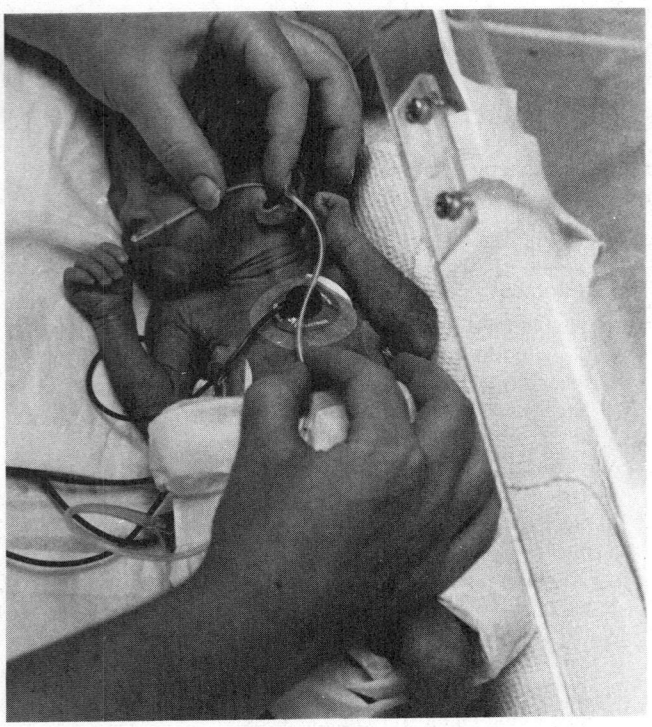

Fig. 27-23. Measuring tube for gavage feeding from tip of nose to earlobe and to tip of sternum.

and shoulders is satisfactory for infants, and a pillow is useful for small children. The head of the bed is raised for larger children. The feeding tube can be passed through either the nose or the mouth. Since most young infants are obligatory nose breathers, insertion through the mouth causes less distress and helps to stimulate sucking. A tube passed through one of the nares in older infants and children is satisfactory once the tube is in place. An indwelling tube is almost always placed through the nose; the tube is alternated between nares with each insertion to minimize irritation, chance of infection, and possible breakdown of mucous membranes from pressure that occurs over a period of time.

The procedure for gavage feeding is carried out as follows:

1. Measure the tube for correct length of insertion and mark the point with a small piece of tape. Correct length can be determined by one of two methods: (a) measuring from the bridge of the nose to the umbilicus or (b) measuring from the tip of the nose to the earlobe (or vice versa) and then to the tip of the xiphoid process (ensiform cartilage) of the sternum (Fig. 27-23). However, the tube may need to be advanced a few centimeters farther for correct placement as verified by aspiration of stomach contents in step 3 (Ziemer and Carroll, 1978).

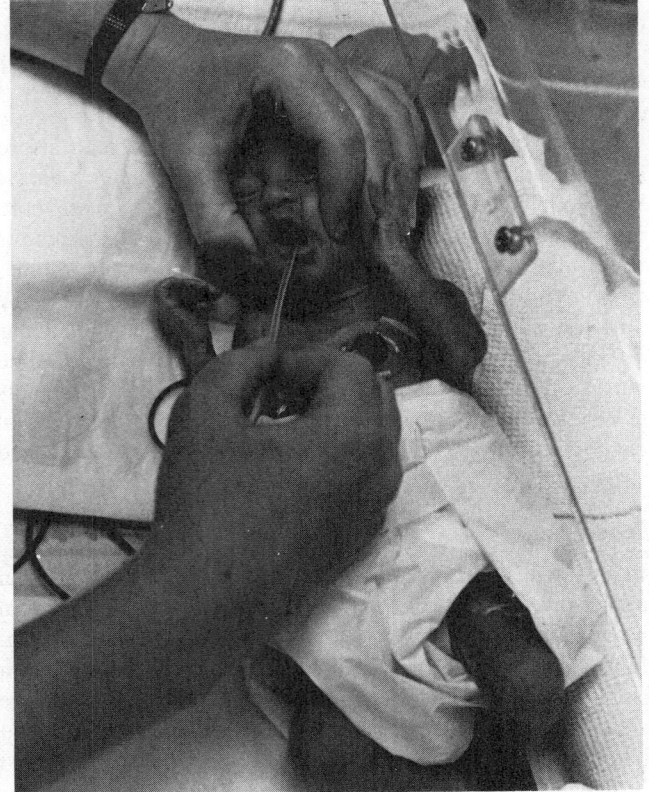

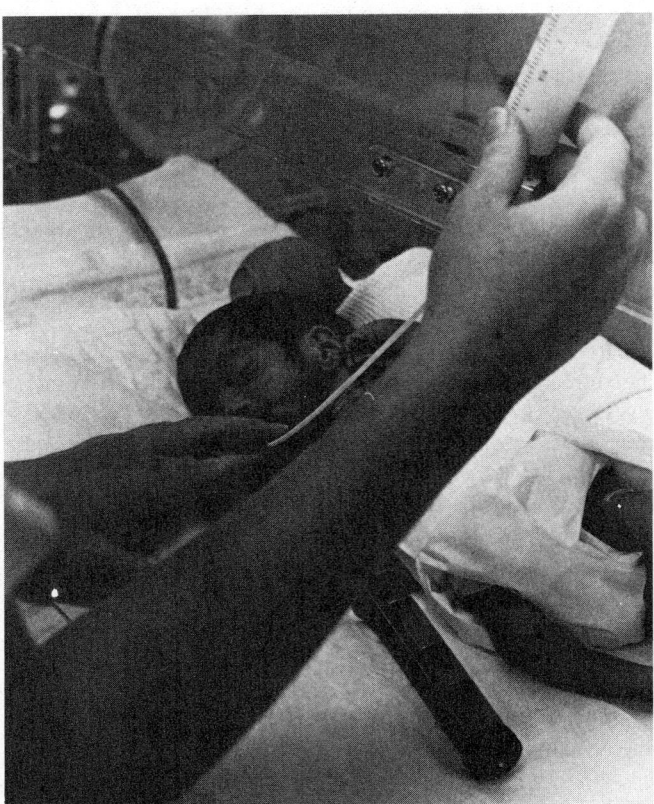

Fig. 27-24. Gavage feeding. **A,** Inserting tube. **B,** Allowing formula to flow into tube by gravity.

2. Insert the tube that has been lubricated with sterile water or water-soluble lubricant through either the mouth or one of the nares to the predetermined mark. Since the esophagus is situated behind the trachea, the tube is more easily inserted when the child's head is hyperflexed. This reduces the chance of the tube entering the trachea. When using the nose, the tube is slipped along the base of the nose and directed straight back toward the occiput; when entering through the mouth, the tube is directed toward the back of the throat (Fig. 27-24, *A*). The tube is passed quickly and, if the child is able to swallow on command, synchronized with swallowing.

3. Check the position of the tube by using one or both of the following:

  a. The syringe is attached to the feeding tube and gentle negative pressure is applied. Aspiration of stomach contents indicates proper placement. The amount and character of any fluid aspirated are noted and the fluid returned to the stomach. Absence of fluid is not necessarily evidence of improper placement. The stomach may be empty or the tube may not be in contact with stomach contents.

  b. With the syringe, inject a small amount of air into the tube while simultaneously listening with a stethoscope over the stomach area. Sounds of gurgling or growling will be heard if the tube is properly situated in the stomach. The air is then withdrawn. The amount of air injected is determined by the size of the child: 0.5 to 1 ml in premature or very small infants to 5 ml in larger children.

4. Stabilize the tube by holding or taping it in place to maintain correct placement. When taped, the tube is secured to the cheek, not to the forehead because of possible damage to the nostril.

5. Feed the formula, which has been warmed to room temperature. Formula is poured into the barrel of the syringe attached to the feeding tube (Fig. 27-24, *B*). To start the flow a gentle push with the plunger may be required, but the plunger should then be removed and the fluid allowed to flow into the stomach by gravity. The rate of flow should not exceed 5 ml every 5 to 10 minutes in premature and very small infants and 10 ml/minute in older infants and children to prevent nausea and regurgitation. The rate is determined by the diameter of the tubing and the height of the reservoir containing the feeding and is regulated by adjusting the height of the syringe. A usual feeding may take from 15 to 30 minutes to complete.

6. Flush the tube with sterile water (1 or 2 ml for small tubes to 5 ml or more for large ones) to clear it of formula. Indwelling catheters are capped or clamped to prevent loss of feeding and entry of air into the stomach.

7. If the tube is to be removed, first pinch it firmly to prevent escape of fluid as the tube is withdrawn. Withdraw the tube quickly.

8. Position the child on the right side or abdomen for at least 1 hour in the same manner as following any infant feeding to minimize the possibility of regurgitation and aspiration. If the child's condition permits, he can be bubbled after the feeding.

9. Record the feeding, including the type and amount of residual, the type and amount of formula, and the manner in which it was tolerated. For most infant feedings any amount of residual fluid aspirated from the stomach is refed to prevent electrolyte imbalance and the amount subtracted from the prescribed amount of feeding. For example, if the infant is to receive 30 ml and 10 ml is aspirated from the stomach before the feeding, the 10 ml of aspirated stomach contents is refed plus 20 ml of feeding.

10. Provide emotional care. Give the infant a pacifier during feeding time and hold or cuddle him if his condition permits. If the child is bedfast, spend time talking or reading with him during feeding. Encourage parents to participate in the care.

Nonnutritive sucking has been shown to have several advantages, such as increased weight gain and decreased crying (Anderson, 1986). However, only pacifiers with a safe design must be used to prevent the possibility of aspiration. Using improvised pacifiers made from bottle nipples is not a safe practice (see p. 534).

GASTROSTOMY FEEDING

Feeding by way of gastrostomy tube is a variation of tube feeding that is often used for children in whom passage of a tube through the mouth, pharynx, esophagus, and cardiac sphincter of the stomach is contraindicated or impossible or to avoid the constant irritation of a nasogastric tube in children who require tube feeding over an extended period. Placement of a gastrostomy tube may be performed under general anesthesia or percutaneously using an endoscope under local anesthesia (Benkov and others, 1986). The tube is inserted through the abdominal wall into the stomach about midway along the greater curvature and secured by a purse-string suture. The stomach is anchored to the peritoneum at the operative site. The tube used can be a Foley, wing-tip, or mushroom catheter. Immediately after surgery the catheter is left open and attached to gravity drainage for 24 hours or more. Postoperative care of the wound site is directed toward prevention of infection and irritation. The area is cleansed and covered with a sterile dressing daily or as often as needed to keep the area dry. After healing takes place meticulous care is needed to keep the area surrounding the tube clean and dry to prevent excoriation and infection. Daily applications of antibiotic ointment or other preparations may be prescribed to aid in healing and prevention of irritation. Care is exercised to prevent excessive pull on the catheter that might cause widening of the opening and subsequent leakage of highly irritating gastric juices. Sliding the tube through a sterile disposable nipple whose tip is cut off and whose base is then taped to the abdomen keeps the tube from rotating and causing erosion and enlargement of the skin opening (Perez and others, 1984).

Positioning and feeding of water, formula, or pureed foods are carried out in the same manner and rate as gavage feeding. However, residual may not be aspirated and is measured as the amount of feeding left in the tube and syringe. After feedings the infant or child is positioned on the

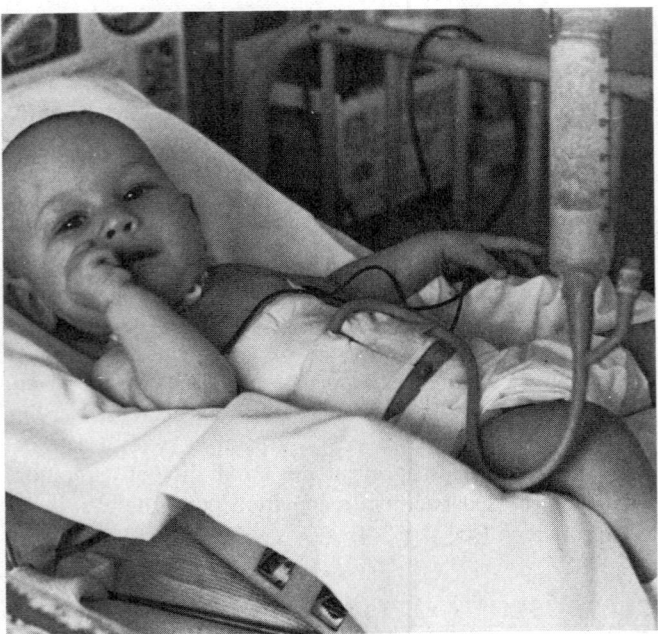

Fig. 27-25. Gastrostomy feeding. Syringe barrel suspended to allow thick formula to enter stomach by gravity. Note child sucking on thumb for oral gratification.

right side or in Fowler position, and the tube may be left open and suspended or clamped between feedings, depending on the child's condition (Fig. 27-25). A clamped tube allows more mobility but is only appropriate if the child can tolerate intermittent feedings without vomiting or prolonged backup of feeding into the tube. Sometimes a Y tube is used to allow for simultaneous decompression during feeding. If a Foley catheter is used as the gastrostomy tube, very slight tension is applied and the tube securely taped to maintain the balloon at the gastrostomy opening and prevent its progression toward the pyloric sphincter where it may occlude the stomach outlet. As a precaution the length of the tube should be measured postoperatively and then remeasured each shift to be sure it has not slipped. When the gastrostomy tube is no longer needed, it is removed; the skin opening ordinarily closes spontaneously by contracture.

FAMILY TEACHING AND HOME CARE

When gastric tube feedings are needed for an extended period, the child may be discharged home before the tube is removed. The family will require appropriate instruction and preparation for performing the skill. The same principles discussed earlier in this chapter for compliance, especially in terms of education (see p. 1112), and in Chapter 26 for discharge planning and home care are applied.*

---

*Home care instructions for gavage and gastrostomy feeding are available in Wong, D., and Whaley, L.: Clinical handbook of pediatric nursing, ed. 2, St. Louis, 1986, The C.V. Mosby Co.

Procedures Related to Elimination

Children seldom have problems with elimination, but in cases of severe constipation or when an empty rectum is needed before surgery or diagnostic procedures, an enema may be administered to stimulate rectal emptying. A number of conditions in the newborn and childhood period also require formation of an ostomy for purposes of elimination.

ENEMA

The procedure for giving an enema to an infant or child does not differ essentially from that for an adult with the exception of the type and amount of fluid administered and the distance for inserting the tube into the rectum (see box). An isotonic solution is used in children; if prepared saline is not available, it can be made by adding 1 tsp table salt to 500 ml (1 pint) tap water. Plain water is not used in children because, being hypotonic, it can cause rapid fluid shift and fluid overload.

The Fleet enema is not advised for children because of the harsh action of its ingredients (sodium biphosphate and sodium phosphate). Commercial enemas can be dangerous to patients with megacolon and to dehydrated or azotemic children. The osmotic effect of the Fleet enema may produce diarrhea, which can lead to metabolic acidosis. Other potential complications are extreme hyperphosphatemia, hypernatremia, and hypocalcemia, which may lead to neuromuscular irritability and coma (Uy, 1981).

Since infants and small children are unable to retain the solution after it is administered, the buttocks must be held together for a short time to retain the fluid. The enema is administered and expelled while the child is lying with the buttocks over the bedpan and his head and back supported with pillows. Older children are ordinarily able to hold the solution if they understand what to do and if they are not expected to hold it for too long a period. It is well to have the bedpan handy or, for the ambulatory child, to make certain that the bathroom is readily available before beginning the procedure. An enema is an intrusive procedure and thus threatening to the preschool child; therefore a careful explanation is especially important to ease possible distress.

GUIDELINES FOR ADMINISTRATION OF ENEMAS TO CHILDREN

Age	Amount (ml)	Insertion distance (cm/inches)
Infant	120-240	2.5 (1 inch)
2-4 years	240-360	5.0 (2 inches)
4-10 years	360-480	7.5 (3 inches)
11 years	480-720	10.0 (4 inches)

OSTOMIES

Children may require stomas for various health problems. The most frequent causes are necrotizing enterocolitis and imperforate anus in the infant, less often Hirschsprung disease. In the older child the most frequent causes are inflammatory bowel disease, especially Crohn disease and ureterostomies for distal ureter or bladder defects.

Care and management of ostomies in the older child differ little from the care of ostomies in the adult patient. The major emphasis in pediatric care is the preparation of the child for the procedure and teaching care of the ostomy to the child and his family. The basic principles of preparation are the same as for any procedure (p. 1104). Simple, straightforward language is most effective together with the use of illustrations and a replica model; for example, drawing a picture of a child with a stoma on the abdomen and explaining it as "another opening where bowel movements [or any other term the child uses] will come out." At another time the nurse can draw a bag over the opening to demonstrate how the contents are collected. Using a doll to demonstrate the process is an excellent teaching strategy and special books are available.*

Because the stoma is edematous after surgery, an appliance is usually not fitted for several days. Once an appliance is in place, drainage is directly measured from the collecting bag. In order to accurately measure colostomy drainage before a collecting appliance is in place, the nurse weighs the dry dressing and reweighs it when wet. The difference in weight is calculated as fluid because 1 g equals 1 ml. If formed stool is passed, it is not weighed and calculated as part of fluid loss.

Ostomies performed on infants create special problems. The fragile nature of the skin increases the risk of breakdown, and the small surface area of the abdomen is ill suited to the standard appliances. Regardless of the type of stoma (ileostomy or colostomy), initially most infants are left with a gauze dressing over the stoma that is secured to the opening by Kerlix or similar expansible wrap. The dressing may or may not be saturated with petroleum jelly or other protective material. The skin is cleansed well after each bowel movement; a nonporous substance, (e.g., zinc oxide ointment, aluminum paste, or karaya products) is applied.

A variety of inexpensive techniques have been devised to absorb drainage around the stoma. Squares of tissue paper, facial tissue, or gauze with openings cut to fit the stoma are gently pressed against the layer of protective substance on the area around the stoma. They can be kept in place with a diaper or Montgomery straps and are replaced after each bowel movement. As a rule, if a sigmoid colostomy is to be performed on an infant, a colostomy appliance is usually not used because the stools are formed and less likely to irritate the skin. Usually only diapers and a nonporous ointment such as zinc oxide around the stoma are used.

When the stoma is healed and the infant has grown to a size that permits their use, appropriate infant-sized stoma bags are introduced. Until then, sometimes the small urine collection bags prove to be sufficient, although they require frequent changes. When either stoma bags or urine collection bags are used, the skin is prepared with tincture of benzoin and karaya powder, paste, or gum to prevent breakdown and to facilitate adherence.

FAMILY TEACHING AND HOME CARE

Since these children are almost always discharged with a functioning colostomy, preparation of the family should begin as early as possible in the hospital. The family is instructed in the application of the device (if used), care of the skin, and instructions regarding appropriate action in case skin problems develop. Early evidence of breakdown should be brought to the attention of the physician, the nurse, or the stoma specialist (see p. 1421). The same principles discussed earlier in this chapter for compliance, especially in terms of education (see p. 1112), and in Chapter 26 for discharge planning and home care are applied.*

Procedures Related to Surgery

Some of the most traumatic procedures for children involve surgery. Both the psychologic and physical aspects of care are significant in the child's adjustment and recovery. Although procedures related to surgery differ according to the type of surgery, the following is an overview of general nursing interventions.

PSYCHOLOGIC PREPARATION

In general, psychologic preparation is similar to that discussed earlier in the chapter for any procedure and employs many of the same techniques used in preparing a child for hospitalization, such as films, books, play, and tours (see Chapter 26). However, there are some important differences. Even though children are asleep for the actual surgical intervention, they are subjected to numerous preoperative and postoperative procedures, which require a series of preparatory sessions to prevent overstressing the child with too much information. Six stress points before and after surgery have been identified as being significant in terms of causing anxiety (Visintainer and Wolfer, 1975):

1. Admission
2. The blood test
3. The afternoon of the day before surgery
4. Injection of preoperative medication
5. Before and during transport to the operating room
6. Return from the recovery room

Psychologic intervention consisting of systematic preparation, rehearsal of the forthcoming events, and supportive care at each of these points has been shown to be more effective than a single session preparation (which is a common method of preoperative preparation) or consistent supportive care without systematic preparation and rehearsal. Play is always an effective strategy in preparing children, and increased familiarity with medical procedures decreases anxiety (Siaw, Stephens, and Holmes, 1986).

Another stress often imposed on the child undergoing surgery is that more than one nurse is often responsible for different aspects of care. Although the same supportive nurse should remain with the child through as many of the procedures as possible, the child may have other nurses, especially if he returns to a special care unit postoperatively. However, joint planning of care between the various nursing staffs, such as in pediatrics and the recovery room, can overcome some of the disadvantages of unfamiliar nurses caring for the child. Many hospitals have surgical tours for children and parents to familiarize them with the strange environment and to introduce them to other individuals who will be involved in their care.

Special fears are often associated with surgery that are not present with other procedures. One special fear is of anesthesia. Children under 5 years of age primarily worry about what will happen when they wake up, such as where they will be and who will be with them. Showing youngsters the recovery room whenever possible, telling them where their parents will visit them after surgery, and encouraging the parents to be with the children as soon as possible after surgery decreases these fears. School-age children fear the anesthesia itself. Seeing the mask and learning how the "gas" or "medicine" works help minimize their concerns. Children about age 9 years and older fear the anesthesia, the operation itself, and possible death. They may ask, "Will I wake up?" or "What happens if I don't wake up?" Adolescents share these concerns with a special anxiety for change in body image. They fear the loss of control while under anesthesia, both in terms of their behavior and for their body integrity. Reassuring them that only what is supposed to be done will be performed is essential.

Because anesthesia is a type of sleep, children often supply their own definitions to this concept. Children worry about whether they will awaken during the procedure and how the doctor knows when to awaken them. Stressing that anesthesia is a "special sleep," caused by the mask and gas or medicine that is controlled by a special person, called the anesthesiologist, is important in minimizing children's fear-provoking fantasies.

PREOPERATIVE CARE

Besides psychologic preparation, children usually require various types of physical care before surgery, such as those listed in the nursing care summary. Infants require special attention to fluid needs. They should not be without oral fluids for an extended period and should receive carbohy-

drate in an oral mixture until 3 hours preoperatively to avoid glycogen depletion and dehydration.

Although most of the preoperative care procedures are routine, nurses should keep in mind that they can be anxiety provoking for children and parents. For example, for young children having to wear a loose-fitting hospital gown without the security of underpants or pajama bottoms can be traumatic. The most upsetting event for children is generally the preoperative injection. Unfortunately little research has been done on the value of this practice, but there is evidence to suggest that the injection does little to relieve anxiety even in adult patients (Catchpole, 1984). Some hospitals administer oral drug combinations, such as promethazine, atropine, and meperidine, to achieve sedation without the trauma of an injection. Whenever possible, such practices should be implemented and formal research initiated to document the effectiveness of such practices.

PERIOPERATIVE CARE

Perioperative care refers to care given immediately before, during, and after surgery and has received little attention in the pediatric literature. Like the preoperative injection, the practice of separating the child and parent before the child enters the surgical unit has been accepted as standard policy. However, there is no theoretical basis for the practice since the effects of separation on children are well known and research indicates that parents are able to support their child and that the child has less anxiety when parents remain until induction of anesthesia in underway (Hannallah and Rosales, 1983).

Other practices that can minimize anxiety in the operative suite are (1) disguising the unpleasant odor of anesthetic gases by applying a pleasant smelling substance on the mask; (2) using a transparent plastic mask rather than an opaque black mask and *gradually* bringing it toward the face; if the child still resists, a stream of gas can be directed toward the child's face from the bare tube until the child becomes drowsy and no longer objects; (3) allowing the child to sit up rather than lie down for anesthesia induction; (4) leaving a favorite possession with the child during surgery and recovery; and (5) having the child recover in his own room in the company of his parents rather than in the recovery unit whenever possible, such as in relatively simple operative procedures (tonsillectomies, insertion of ear tubes, or strabismus) (Jones, 1985).

POSTOPERATIVE CARE

After surgical procedures, various physical interventions and observations are required to prevent or minimize possible untoward effects (see nursing care summary). Although most of these interventions are prescribed by physicians, it is the nurse's responsibility to exercise judgment in their implementation. For example, vital signs are taken as frequently as necessary until they are stable. Simply recording temperature, pulse, respiration, and blood pressure without

Nursing Care Summary: The Child Undergoing Surgery

Preoperative Care

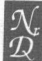

NURSING GOALS	NURSING INTERVENTIONS	EXPECTED PATIENT/FAMILY OUTCOMES
HP-HMP	**Injury: potential for**	
	Etiology: surgical procedure	

Ensure legal authorization	Check chart for signed informed consent form
	Obtain informed consent
	  Contact physician to determine if parents have
	    been informed of procedure (informed consent
	    is physician's responsibility)
	Obtain and/or witness signature if not obtained
	  earlier
		*Appropriate permissions are
		  obtained

Provide hygienic
preparation
	Bathe child
	Cleanse site according to prescribed method, if
	  ordered
	Remove any makeup and/or nail polish (to observe
	  for cyanosis)
	Remove jewelry and/or prosthetic devices (e.g.,
	  mouth retainers)
	Check for loose teeth
	  Inform anesthesiologist if detected
		Child is cleansed and prepared
		  appropriately (specify)

Provide physical
preparation
	Attire child appropriately (e.g., special operating
	  room gown)
	  Allow child to wear underwear or pajama
	    bottoms, if possible
	  Label personal articles and clothing
		Child is prepared appropriately
		  (specify)

	Maintain child NPO (nothing by mouth) usually 12
	  hours before surgery (prevents aspiration from
	  vomiting during anesthesia [gag reflex is
	  depressed]; last feeding indicated by physician)
	Be sure child is well hydrated before NPO begins,
	  especially infants
	Take and record vital signs
	  Report any deviations from admission readings,
	    especially elevated temperature, which may
	    indicate infection
		Child is NPO for designated time
		  preoperatively

	Have child void before preoperative medication is
	  administered to prevent bladder distention or
	  incontinence during anesthesia
	  Record time of last voiding if unable to void
		Child voids

Prevent complications	Be certain allergies are clearly indicated on chart
	Check laboratory values for any sign of systemic
	  abnormality, such as infection (increased white
	  blood cells), anemia (decreased hemoglobin
	  and/or hematocrit), or bleeding tendencies
	  (reduced platelets or prolonged bleeding or
	  clotting time)
		*Pertinent information about child is
		  visible

	Be certain physical preparation is completed	*Child is physically prepared
SP-SCP	**Anxiety**	
	Etiology: separation from support system; unfamiliar environment	

Increase child's sense of
security
	Institute preoperative teaching
	Orient child to strange surroundings
	Explain where parents will be while child is in
	  operating room
	Place child in quiet room with minimal distraction
		Child demonstrates minimum
		  insecurity or anxiety

	Do not leave child unattended
	Explain what is happening, unless child is asleep
	Encourage parents to accompany child as far as
	  possible, preferably through induction of
	  anesthesia
	Allow for significant objects to accompany child
	  (e.g., a favorite toy)
		Child is not left alone

*Nursing outcome.

Continued.

Nursing Care Summary: The Child Undergoing Surgery—cont'd

Preoperative Care

NURSING GOALS	NURSING INTERVENTIONS	EXPECTED PATIENT/FAMILY OUTCOMES
HP-HMP	**Injury: potential for**	
	Etiology: surgical procedure, anesthesia	
Admit to room	Place child in bed (unless transported in own bed or crib) Hang IV and connect any needed equipment (e.g., suction apparatus, traction)	

Acquire baseline information	Take vital signs, including BP
	Inspect operative area
	  Check dressing if present
	  Outline any bleeding area on dressing or cast with pen
	  Reinforce, but do not remove, loose dressing
	  Observe areas below surgical site for blood that may have drained toward bed
	  Assess for bleeding and other symptoms in areas not covered with a dressing, such as throat following tonsillectomy, external auditory meatus after ear procedures
	Observe skin color, activity, level of consciousness, etc.
	Perform specific assessments based on type of surgery, e.g., circulation in extremities, movement of part(s), specific appliance (e.g., tension apparatus)
	Notify physician of any irregularities
		*Child's baseline status is determined
		Vital signs are within expected limits for age (see inside front cover); skin is pink and dry
		Child responds appropriately (for age) when stimulated; is not unduly agitated
		Operative area is clean and intact

Achieve optimum relaxation and sedation before child arrives in operating room	Place child in quiet room with minimal distraction Encourage parents to stay with child as long as permitted Permit parent to hold child until he falls asleep, if desired	Child falls asleep or lies quietly
Ensure safety	Ascertain that identification band is securely fastened Check identification band with surgical personnel Fasten side rails of bed or crib Use restraints during transport by use of stretcher (or other conveyance) Do not leave child unattended Explain what is happening, unless child is asleep	Child is safe from immediate harm Child is not left alone
Prepare room and bedside area to receive child on return from surgery	Collect needed equipment for assessment and recording (e.g., record sheets, IV pole, restraints, thermometer, BP apparatus, etc.) Turn down covers or prepare surgical bed as appropriate	Child is transferred to bed with minimum stress
Monitor physiologic status	Take vital signs as ordered; blood pressure cuff kept in place, deflated in order to lessen amount of disturbance to child Take and record more frequently if any value fluctuates Report any deviations from normal	*Alterations in status are determined early and appropriate interventions initiated

Prevent complications	Encourage to turn, cough, and deep breathe
	  Splint operative site with hand or pillow if possible before coughing
	Maintain child NPO until fully awake
	  Start with small sips of water and advance as tolerated
	  Avoid brown- or red-colored fluids (to distinguish old and fresh blood from oral fluids) in oral or abdominal surgery
	For gastrointestinal procedures listen for bowel sounds before and after beginning fluids
	Encourage to void when awake
	  Offer bedpan
	  Boys may be allowed to stand at bedside
	Notify physician if unable to void
		Lungs remain clear
		Child takes and retains fluid when allowed (specify)
		Child is free of complications

*Nursing outcome.

Nursing Care Summary: The Child Undergoing Surgery—cont'd

Preoperative Care

NURSING GOALS	NURSING INTERVENTIONS	EXPECTED PATIENT/FAMILY OUTCOMES
CPP Comfort, alteration in: pain		
Etiology: surgical incision		
Relieve discomfort	Assess need for pain medication (see p. 1068) Implement appropriate nonpharmacologic pain reduction techniques (see p. 1071) Encourage parental visiting as soon as child is awake	Child exhibits minimum evidence of pain (specify)
RRP Family process, alteration in		
Etiology: child who is undergoing a surgical procedure		
Keep family informed	Explain preparation procedures Direct family to appropriate waiting area Be available to family	Family complies with directives (specify)

Nursing Interventions Related to Medical Management

PREOPERATIVE CARE
Prevent complications
  Consult with physician for appropriate change in schedule or route of administration of any medication child ordinarily receives
Achieve relaxation
  Administer preoperative sedation (preferably oral), as ordered
Provide information needed
  Make certain the following procedures have been performed and evidence is in chart:
    Urinalysis
    Blood work such as blood count, bleeding and clotting times, and type and cross-match, if ordered
    Roentgenograms
    Electrocardiogram
    Note by anesthesiologist

POSTOPERATIVE CARE
Determine specifics of care
  Review surgeon's orders after completing initial assessment
  Perform stat (immediate) activities
Provide nutrition
  Begin and advance diet as prescribed
Prevent complications
  Dangle and ambulate as soon as feasible according to physician's orders
Relieve discomfort
  Administer analgesics prescribed
  Administer antiemetics as ordered
  Monitor effectiveness of analgesics
Provide for hydration
  Monitor intravenous infusion at prescribed rate
    Attach pediatric intravenous apparatus if not done in operating room
    Begin oral intake as ordered
Provide for nutrition
  Feed diet as ordered
  Advance as appropriate

*Nursing outcome.

comparing the present readings to previous ones is a useless technical function. Each vital sign is evaluated in terms of side effects from anesthesia and signs of impending shock. Pain is assessed and the child given analgesics as needed to provide comfort and facilitate his cooperation in postoperative procedures, such as ambulating, coughing, and deep breathing. Routinely scheduled analgesics, rather than p.r.n. orders, afford more satisfactory pain control.

During the recovery period some time should be spent with the child to assess his perception of surgery. Play, drawing, and story telling are excellent methods of discovering the child's thoughts. With such information the nurse can support or correct his perceptions and assist the child in achieving mastery for having endured a stressful procedure.

CONCEPT SUMMARIES

- Informed consent is valid when the person is capable of giving consent (is over the age of majority and is competent), the person is supplied with information needed to make an intelligent decision, and the person acts voluntarily when exercising freedom of choice.

- Informed consent is needed for major surgery, minor surgery, and diagnostic tests and medical treatments with an element of risk.

- The major principles in psychologic preparation of the child for surgery are to establish trust, provide support, and give an explanation in easy-to-understand terms.

- In the performance of a procedure the nurse should expect success, involve the child when possible in the procedure, provide distraction, and allow for expression of feelings.

- In giving postprocedural support, the nurse should encourage the child to express his feelings and praise him for completion of the procedure.

- Assessment of compliance entails measuring factors that affect compliance (through clinical judgment, self-reporting, and direct observation), monitoring therapeutic response, taking pill counts, and performing chemical assay.

- Compliance strategies may be classified as organizational, educational, and behavioral.

- Knowledge of the sick child's eating habits and favorite foods can help in maintaining adequate nutrition.

- Control of fever may be accomplished by pharmacologic means (administration of antipyretics) and environmental means (minimum clothing, increased air circulation, or cool compresses).

- Ensuring safety in the hospital setting is a major concern and can be achieved through environmental measures, limit-setting, and safe transportation.

- Common types of physical restraints for children are jacket, mummy, arm and leg, and elbow.

- Factors that affect drug dosage determination are growth and maturation, difficulty in evaluating drug response, and body surface area.

- Family teaching regarding medication administration includes telling parents why the child is receiving the drug, its possible effects, and the amount, frequency, and length of time the drug is to be administered.

- The major forms of gastric feeding for children are gavage feeding and gastrostomy feeding.

- In the care of children with ostomies, nurses play an important role in family support and instruction in care of the stoma site.

- Six stressful times before and after surgery that produce anxiety in children are the day of admission, blood tests, the afternoon of the day before surgery, injection of preoperative medication, transportation to the operating room, and return from the recovery room.

REFERENCES

Anderson, G.C.: Pacifiers: the positive side, Am. J. Maternal Child Nurs. 11(2):122-124, 1986.

Benkov, K., and others: Percutaneous endoscopic gastrostomies in children, Pediatrics 77(2):248-249, 1986.

Berman, W., and others: Inadvertent overadministration of digoxin to low-birth weight infants, J. Pediatr. 92(6):1024-1025, 1978.

Blum, R.W.: Compliance with therapeutic regimens among children and youths. In Blum, R., editor: Chronic illness and disabilities in childhood and adolescence, New York, 1984, Grune & Stratton, Inc.

Blumenfeld, T.A., Turi, G.K., and Blanc, W.A.: Recommended site and depth of newborn heel skin punctures based on anatomical measurements and histopathology, Lancet 1(8110):230-233, 1979.

Bourgault, A.: A hair piece, Nursing 85 15(9):80, 1985.

Brown, S.R.: An anxiety reduction technique during lumbar punctures in infants and toddlers, J. Assoc. Pediatr. Oncology Nurs. 1(3):24-25, 1984.

Catchpole, M.: Does preop medication promote stress? Am. J. Nurs. 84(10):1202, 1984.

Chaplin, G., Shull, H., and Welk, P.C., III: How safe is the air-bubble technique for I.M. injections? Nursing 85 15 (9):59, 1985.

Consensus statement: Febrile seizures: long-term management of children with fever-associated seizures, Pediatrics 66(6):1009-1012, 1980.

Cushing, M.: Informed consent: an MD responsibility? Am. J. Nurs. 84(4):437-440, 1984.

Dininny, J.B.: Food rummy, the game of nutrition, Am. J. Maternal Child Nurs. 2(2):90-91, 1977.

Ellenberg, J., Hirtz, D., and Nelson, K.: Do seizures in children cause intellectual deterioration? N. Engl. J. Med. 314(17):1085-1088, 1986.

Ellerton, M.L., Caty, S., and Ritchie, J.A.: Helping young children master intrusive procedures through play, Child. Health Care 13(4):167-173, 1985.

Farrell, Sr. E., and McKiernan, B.: A positive approach to nutrition for hospitalized children, Am. J. Maternal Child Nurs. 2(2):113-117, 1977.

Fried, C.: Children as subjects for medical experimentation. In van Eys, J., editor: Research on children: medical imperatives, ethical quandries, and legal constraints, Baltimore, 1978, University Park Press.

Funk, M.J., Mullins, L.L., and Olson, R.A.: Teaching children to swallow pills: a case study, Child. Health Care 13(1):20-23, 1984.

Garner, J.S., and Simmons, B.P.: Guideline for isolation precautions in hospitals, Infect. Control 4(4)(suppl.): 245-325, 1983.

Hannallah, R., and Rosales, J.: Experience with parents' presence during anaesthesia induction in children, Can. Anaesth. Soc. J. 30(3):287-290, 1983.

Haynes, R.B.: Strategies for enhancing patient compliance, Drug Ther. 12(1):33-40, 1982.

Hogue, E.: What you should know about informed consent, Nursing 86 16(6):46-48, 1986.

Hurwitz, E.S., and others: Public health service study on Reye's syndrome and medications, N. Engl. J. Med. 313(14):849-857, 1985.

Intramuscular injections: a guide to sites and techniques, Philadelphia, 1985, Wyeth Laboratories.

Jones, S.T.: Reducing children's psychological stress in the operating suite, Ophthalmic Plast. Reconstr. Surg. 1:199-203, 1985.

Kramer, M.S., Naimark, L., and Leduc, D.G.: Parental fever phobia and its correlates, Pediatrics 75(6):1110-1113, 1985.

Leikin, S.L.: Minors' assent or dissent to medical treatment, J. Pediatr. 102(2):169-176, 1983.

Lenz, C.L.: Make your needle selection right to the point, Nursing 83 13(2):50-51, 1983.

Litt, I.F., Cuskey, W.R., and Rosenberg, A.: Role of self-esteem and autonomy in determining medication compliance among adolescents with juvenile rheumatoid arthritis, Pediatrics 69(1):15-17, 1982.

Lovejoy, F.H., Jr.: Aspirin and acetaminophen: a comparative view of their antipyretic and analgesic activity, Pediatrics 62(suppl.):904-909, 1978.

Mandelbaum, J.: The food square: helping people of different cultures understand balanced diets, Pediatr. Nurs. 9(1): 20-21, 1983.

McCarthy, D.O.: The adaptive value of fever during infection, Diet. Curr. 12(3):13-18, 1985.

McCord, M.A.: Compliance: self care or compromise? Top. Clin. Nurs. 7(4):1-8, 1986.

Moore, M.C., and Greene, H.L.: Tube feeding of infants and children, Pediatr. Clin. North Am. 32(2):401-417, 1985.

Moree, N.A.: Nurses speak out on patients and drug regimens, Am. J. Nurs. 85(1):51-54, 1985.

Musher, D.M., and others: Fever patterns: their lack of clinical significance, Arch. Intern. Med. 139:1225-1228, 1979.

Newman, J.: Evaluation of sponging to reduce body temperature in febrile children, Can. Med. Assoc. J. 132:641-642, 1985.

Perez, R.C., and others: Care of the child with a gastrostomy tube: common and practical concerns, Issues Compr. Pediatr. Nurs. 7(2-3):107-119, 1984.

Rae, W.A., and Fournier, C.J.: Ethical issues in pediatric research: preserving psychosocial care in scientific inquiry, Child. Health Care 14(4):242-248, 1986.

Ramsey, P.: Ethical dimensions of research on children. In van Eys, J., editor: Research on children: medical imperatives, ethical quandries, and legal constraints, Baltimore, 1978, University Park Press.

Rapoff, M.A.: Helping parents to help their children comply with treatment regimens for chronic diseases, Issues Compr. Pediatr. Nurs. 9(3):147-156, 1986.

Rapoff, M.A., and Christophersen, E.R.: Improving compliance in pediatric practice, Pediatr. Clin. North Am. 29(2):339-357, 1982.

Rumack, B.H.: Acetaminophen overdose in children and adolescents, Pediatr. Clin. North Am. 33(3):691-701, 1986.

Savedra, M.: Parental responses to a painful procedure performed on their child. In Azarnoff, P., and Hardgrove, C., editors: The family in child health care, New York, 1981, John Wiley & Sons.

Schmitt, B.D.: Fever phobia: misconceptions of parents about fevers, Am. J. Dis. Child. 134(2):176-181, 1980.

Schmitt, B.D.: Fever in childhood, Pediatrics 74(5) (suppl):929-936, 1984.

Selbst, S.M.: Treating minors without their parents, Pediatr. Emerg. Care 1:168-173, 1985.

Shaffer, M.K., and Pfeiffer, I.L.: Nursing research and patients' rights, Am. J. Nurs. 86(1):23-24, 1986.

Shaw, N., and Lyall, E.: Hazards of glass ampoules, Br. Med. J. 291(6506):1390, 1985.

Shaw, E.G., and Routh, D.K.: Effect of mother presence on children's reaction to aversive procedures, J. Pediatr. Psychol. 7(1):33-42, 1982.

Siaw, S.N., Stephens, L.R., and Holmes, S.S.: Knowledge about medical instruments and reported anxiety in pediatric surgery patients, Child. Health Care 14(3):134-141, 1986.

Steckel, S.: Patient contracting, New York, 1982, Appleton-Century-Crofts.

Stoller, K.P., and Losey, R.: Inadvertent intra-arterial injection of penicillin: an unseen danger, Pediatrics 75(4):785-786, 1985.

Streiff, L.D.: Can clients understand our instructions, Image: J. Nurs. Scholarship 18(2):48-52, 1986.

Strohbach, M.E., and Kratina, S.H.: Diaper versus bag specimens: a comparison of urine specific gravity values, Am. J. Maternal Child Nurs. 7:198-201, 1982.

Temple, A.R.: Review of comparative antipyretic activity in children, Am. J. Med. 75(5A):38-46, 1983.

Uy, C.: Complications of sodium phosphate enemas, Pediatr. Rev. 2(8):238, 1981.

Venham, L.L., Bengston, D., and Cipes, M.: Parent's presence and the child's response to dental stress, J. Dentistry Child. 45(3):213-217, 1978.

Vernon, D.T.A., Foley, J.M., and Schulman, J.L.: Effect of mother-child separation and birth order on young children's responses to two potentially stressful experiences, J. Personality Social Psychol. 5(2):162-174, 1967.

Visintainer, M.A., and Wolfer, J.A.: Psychological preparation for surgical pediatric patients: the effect of children's and parents' stress responses and adjustment, Pediatrics 56(2):187-202, 1975.

Westfall, U.E.: Methods for assessing compliance, Top. Clin. Nurs. 7(4):23-30, 1986.

Wong, D.L.: Significance of dead space in syringes, Am. J. Nurs. 82 (8):1237, 1982.

Young, M.S.: Strategies for improving compliance, Top. Clin. Nurs. 7(4):31-38, 1986.

Ziemer, M., and Carroll, J.S.: Infant gavage feeding, Am. J. Nurs. 78:1543-1544, 1978.

BIBLIOGRAPHY
Informed Consent

Bernzweig, E.P.: Don't cut corners on informed consent, RN 47(12):15, 1984.

Creighton, H.: Law every nurse should know, ed. 5, Philadelphia, 1985, W.B. Saunders Co.

Dunn, L.J.: Legal aspects of communication with and about the pediatric patient, Issues Compr. Pediatr. Nurs. 4:13-18, 1980.

Frost, N.: Parental control over children, J. Pediatr. 103(4):571-572, 1983.

Gargaro, W.J.: Informed consent. Part I. A good thing for patients: a better thing for doctors and nurses, Cancer Nurs. 1(1):81-82, 1978.

Gargaro, W.J.: Informed consent. Part II. How much to tell the patient, Cancer Nurs. 1(2):167-168, 1978.

Gargaro, W.J.: Informed consent. Part III. The nurse's right to inform, Cancer Nurs. 1(3):249-250, 1978.

Holder, A.R.: Parents, courts, and refusal of treatment, J. Pediatr. 103(4):515-520, 1983.

Lovett, J., and Wald, M.S.: Physician attitudes toward confidential care for adolescents, J. Pediatr. 106(3): 517-521, 1985.

Moore, D.S., and Bauer, C.S.: Effect of prepodyne as a perineal cleansing agent for clean catch specimens, Nurs. Res. 25(4):259-261, 1976.

Ormond, E.A.R., and Caulfield, C.: A practical guide to giving oral medications to young children, Am. J. Maternal Child Nurs. 1:320-325, 1976.

Plotkin, R.: When rights collide: parents, children, and consent to treatment, J. Pediatr. Psychol. 6(2):121-130, 1981.

Silva, M.C.: Assessing competency for informed consent with mentally retarded minors, Pediatr. Nurs. 10(4):261-265, 306, 1984.

Preparing for Hospital Procedures and Surgery/ Use of Play

American Academy of Pediatrics, Committee on Infectious Diseases, Committee on Drugs, and Section on Surgery: Antimicrobial prophylaxis in pediatric surgical patients, Pediatrics 74(3):437-439, 1984.

Beckemeyer, P., and Bahr, J.E.: Helping toddlers and preschoolers cope while suturing their minor lacerations, Am. J. Maternal Child Nurs. 5(5):326-330, 1980.

Broome, M.E.: The relationship between children's fears and behavior during a painful event, Child. Health Care 14(3):142-145, 1986.

Burton, F., and Salminen, C.A.: Controlling postoperative infection, Nursing 84 14(9):43-46, 1984.

Crawford, C., Finke, L., and Henning, M.A.: Nursing management of the postoperative pediatric patient, Issues Compr. Pediatr. Nurs. 6:157-165, 1983.

Demarest, D.S., Hooke, J.F., and Erickson, M.T.: Preoperative intervention for the reduction of anxiety in pediatric surgery patients, Child. Health Care 12(4):179-183, 1984.

Droske, S.C., and Francis, S.A.: Pediatric diagnostic procedures: with guidelines for preparing children for clinical tests, New York, 1981, John Wiley & Sons, Inc.

Fernald, C.D., and Corry, J.J.: Empathic versus directive preparation of children for needles, Child. Health Care 10(2):44-47, 1981.

Gelfant, B.B.: Minimizing the stress of surgery through patient and family orientation and education, Point of View 23(1):9, 1986.

Griffith, N.L.: A review of the literature: the patient and the perioperative period, Point of View 22(1):14-15, 1985.

Hansen, B.D., and Evans, M.L.: Preparing a child for procedures, Am. J. Maternal Child Nurs. 6(6):392-397, 1981.

Hunsberger, M., Love, B., and Byrne, C.: A review of current approaches used to help children and parents cope with health care procedures, Am. J. Maternal Child Nurs. 13(3):145-165, 1984.

Johnson, J.E.: Coping with elective surgery. In Werley, H.H., and Fitzpatrick, J.J., editors: Annual review of nursing research, vol. 2, New York, 1984, Springer Publishing Co.

Johnson, J.E., Kerchhoff, K.T., and Endress, M.P.: Easing children's fright during health care procedures, Am. J. Maternal Child Nurs. 1(4):206-210, 1976.

Jones, S.T.: Unnecessary psychological complications in children after ocular surgery, J. Pediatr. Ophthalmol. Strabismus 22(6):218-219, 1985.

Kline, J.: Recovery room care for the child in pain, Am. J. Maternal Child Nurs. 9(4):261-264, 1984.

Knudsen, K.: Play therapy: preparing the young child for surgery, Nurs. Clin. North Am. 10:679-686, 1975.

Luciano, K., and Shumsky, C.J.: Pediatric procedures, Nursing 75 5(1):49-52, 1975.

McHatton, M.: A theory for timely teaching, Am. J. Nurs. 85(7):798-800, 1985.

Miller, A.: When is the time ripe for teaching? Am. J. Nurs. 85(7):801-804, 1985.

Norberta, Sr. M.: Caring for children with the help of puppets, Am. J. Maternal Child Nurs. 1(1):22-25, 1976.

Petrillo, M., and Sanger, S.: Emotional care of hospitalized children, ed. 2, Philadelphia, 1980, J.B. Lippincott Co.

Play and preparation: an annotated bibliography, Washington, DC, 1984, Association for the Care of Children's Health.

Pontious, S.L.: Practical Piaget: helping children understand, Am. J. Nurs. 82(2):114-117, 1982.

Ritchie, J.A.: Preparation of toddlers and preschool children for hospital procedures, Can. Nurse 75(11):30-32, 1979.

Robinson, S.J.: A nurse's role in preparing children for surgery, AORN J. 30(4):619-621, 1979.

Schulz, J.B., and others: The effects of a preoperational puppet show on anxiety levels of hospitalized children, Child. Health Care 9(4):118-121, 1981.

Schwartz, B.H., Albino, J.E., and Tedesco, L.A.: Effects of psychological preparation on children hospitalized for dental operations, J. Pediatr. 102(4):634-638, 1983.

Thompson, R.H.: Recent research on preparation: an annotated bibliography. In Preparing children and families for health care encounters, Washington, DC, 1980, Association for the Care of Children's Health.

Waidley, E.K.: Show and tell: preparing children for invasive procedures, Am. J. Nurs. 85(7):811-812, 1985.

Compliance

Baer, C.L.: Compliance: the challenge for the future, Top. Clin. Nurs. 7(4):77-85, 1986.

Burckhardt, C.S.: Ethical issues in compliance, Top. Clin. Nurs. 7(4):9-16, 1986.

Clark, S.R.: Compliance and health behaviors, Top. Clin. Nurs. 7(4):39-46, 1986.

Connaway, N.: My patient won't follow the medical plan treatment. what should I do to protect myself—legally? . . . home health care, Home Healthcare Nurse 3(4):6-8, 1985.

Davidson, S.B.: Using compliance research in clinical practice, Top. Clin. Nurs. 7(4):65-76, 1986.

Kaufman, D.H.: An interview guide for helping children make health-care decisions, Pediatr. Nurs. 11(5):365-367, 1985.

Klopovich, P.M., and others: Adherence to chemotherapy regimens among children with cancer, Top. Clin. Nurs. 7(1):19-25, 1985.

Korsch, B.M.: Compliance. In Green, M., and Haggerty, R.J., editors: Ambulatory pediatrics, ed. 3, Philadelphia, 1984, W.B. Saunders Co.

Korsch, B.M.: What do patients and parents want to know? what do they need to know? Pediatrics 74(5)(suppl.):917-920, 1984.

Lucas, C.M.: Compliance and illness responses, Top. Clin. Nurs. 7(4):47-56, 1986.

McLean, J.C., and others: Improving patient compliance in pediatric outpatient surgery . . . nurse practitioner telephones the parents one to two days before the appointment, AORN J. 40(5):676-680, 1984.

Morse, D.L., and others: Waning effectiveness of mailed reminders on reducing broken appointments, Pediatrics 68 (6):846-849, 1981.

O'Connell, K.A., and Marvin, N.G.: Improving adherence to medication regimens, J. Kans. Med. Soc. 80(3):130-134, 1979.

Padrick, K.P.: Compliance: myths and motivators, Top. Clin. Nurs. 7(4):17-22, 1986.

Sallis, J.F.: Improving adherence to pediatric therapeutic regimens, Pediatr. Nurs. 11(2):118-120, 1985.

Sloan, M.R., and Schommer, B.T.: Want to get your patient involved in his care? use a contract, Nursing 82 12(12): 48-49, 1982.

Williams, R.L., and others: Educational strategies to improve compliance with an antibiotic regimen, Am. J. Dis. Child. 140(3):216-220, 1986.

Yoos, L.: Factors influencing maternal compliance to antibiotic regimens, Pediatr. Nurs. 10(2):141-147, 1984.

General Care and Hygiene

Bishop, B.: How to cool a feverish child, Pediatr. Nurs. 4(1):19-20, 1978.

Brown, B.S., and Younger, J.B.: Facts about fever, Child. Nurse 2(3):1-3, 1984.

Burson, J.Z., and Brannigan, C.N.: The use of play in the nutritional support of hospitalized children, Issues Compr. Pediatr. Nurs. 7(4-5):283-289, 1984.

Casey, R., and others: Fever therapy: an educational intervention for parents, Pediatrics 73(5):600-605, 1984.

Done, A., and others: Aspirin dosage for infants and children, J. Pediatr. 95(4):617-629, 1979.

Gladtke, E.: Use of antipyretic analgesics in the pediatric patient, Am. J. Med. 75(5A):121-126, 1983.

Grier, M.E.: Hair care for the black patient, Am. J. Nurs. 76:1781, 1976.

Handbook of nonprescription drugs, ed. 7, Washington, DC, 1982, American Pharmaceutical Association, The National Professional Society of Pharmacists.

How to take your child's temperature, Patient Care 14: 141-148, Sept. 1980.

Kauffman, R.E.: Fever. In Shirkey, H.E., editor: Pediatric therapy, ed. 6, St. Louis, 1980, The C.V. Mosby Co.

McCarthy P.L., and others: History and observation variables in assessing febrile children, Pediatrics 65(6):1090-1095, 1980.

Mancini, R.E., and Yaffe, S.J.: The feverish child—aspirin or acetaminophen? Drug Ther. 10(5):103-114, 1980.

Reynolds, J.: How to take a temperature, Pediatr. Nurs. 4(6):67-68, 1978.

Snell, B., and McClellan, C.: Whetting hospitalized preschooler's appetites, Am. J. Nurs. 76:413-415, 1976.

Stern, R.C.: Pathophysiologic basis for symptomatic treatment of fever, Pediatrics 59:92-97, 1977.

Wong, D.: Dosage of aspirin (letter to the editor), J. Pediatr. 95(5):956-957, 1980.

Younger, J.B., and Brown, B.S.: Fever management: rational or ritual? Pediatr. Nurs. 11(1):26-28, 1985.

Safety/Collection of Specimens

Chavigny, K.H., and Moore-Nunnally, D.S.: A comparison of methods for collecting clean-catch urine specimens in a clinic population of obstetric patients, Am. J. Obstet. Gynecol. 122(1):34-42, 1975.

Hargiss, C.O., and Larson, E.: How to collect specimens and evaluate results, Am. J. Nurs. 81(12):2166-2174, 1981.

Mason, G.: Bottle type restraints, Am. J. Nurs. 76:1258, 1976.

Misik, I.: About using restraints—with restraint, Nursing 81 11(8):50-55, 1981.

Perry, A.G., and Potter, P.A.: Clinical nursing skills and techniques: basic, intermediate, and advanced, St. Louis, 1986, The C.V. Mosby Co.

Utley, R.M.: A collector's item, Nursing 85 15(1):94, 1985.

Administration of Medications

Bavin, R.: Obtaining therapeutic antibiotic blood levels in children, J. Pediatr. Nurs. **1**(3):164-169, 1986.

Bergeson, P.A., Singer, S.A., and Kaplan, A.M.: Intramuscular injections in children, Pediatrics **70**(6):944-948, 1982.

Birdsall, C., and Uretsky, S.: How do I administer medication by NG? Am. J. Nurs. **84**(10):1259-1260, 1984.

Eland, J.M.: Minimizing pain associated with prekindergarten intramuscular injections, Comp. Pediatr. Nurs. **5**:361-372, 1981.

Evans, M.L., and Hansen, B.D.: Administering injections to different-aged children, Am. J. Maternal Child Nurs. **6**(3):194-199, 1981.

Feingold, A., and Walther, P.: Volume of syringe-needle dead space, Am. J. Hosp. Pharm. **33**:758-759, 1976.

Feldstein, A.: Detect phlebitis and infiltration, Nursing 86 **16**(1):44-47, 1986.

Frank, T., and Fischer, R.G.: What are some of the most common reasons for medication errors? Pediatr. Nurs. **10**(4): 294, 1984.

Geolot, D., and McKinney, N.: Administering parenteral drugs, Am. J. Nurs. **75**(5):788-789, 1975.

Grabinski, P.Y.: I.M. injections—deltoid or gluteal site? PRN Forum **2**(3):1-2, 1983.

Hicks, A.: Give it a shot, Nursing 84 **14**(12):70, 1984.

Howry, L.B., Bindler, R.M., and Tso, Y.: Pediatric medications, Philadelphia, 1981, J.B. Lippincott Co.

Hughes, W.T., and Buescher, E.S.: Injections. In Hughes, W.T., and Buescher, E.S., editors: Pediatric procedures, ed. 2, Philadelphia, 1980, W.B. Saunders Co.

Hussar, D.A.: Your role in patient compliance, Nursing 79 **9**(11):48-53, 1979.

Jerrett, M.D.: Taking the ouch out of injections, Can. Nurse **79**(1):24-27, 1983.

Lang, S., Zawacki, A., and Johnson, J.: Reducing discomfort from IM injections, Am. J. Nurs. **76**(5):800-801, 1976.

McCloskey, J.R., Stanley, M.K., and Chung, M.K.: Quadriceps contracture as a result of multiple intramuscular injection, Am. J. Dis. Child. **131**:416-417, 1977.

McConnell, E.A.: The subtle art of really good injections, RN **45**(2):24-34, 1982.

Mitchell, J.F., and Liadis, M.: Oral solid dosage forms that should not be crushed prior to administration, Hosp. Pharmacy **17**:148-156, 1982.

Nahata, M.C.: Methods of intravenous drug infusion in pediatric patients, Am. J. Intraven. Ther. Clin. Nutr. **11**(5):6-7, 1984.

Newton, D.W., and Newton, M.: Route, site, and technique: three key decisions in giving parenteral medication, Nursing 79 **9**(7):18-25, 1979.

No more teaspoons, Nurs. Life **4**(2):13, 1984.

Perez, S.: Reducing injection pain, Am. J. Nurs. **84**(5):645, 1984.

Rettig, F.M., and Southby, J.R.: Using different body positions to reduce discomfort from dorsogluteal injection, Nurs. Res. **31**(4):219-221, 1982.

Rimar, J.M.: Guidelines for the intravenous administration of medications used in pediatrics, Am. J. Maternal Child Nurs. **7**(3):184-197, 1982.

Sbravati, E.C., and Fischer, R.G.: What medication do parents need to get up and give their child at night? Pediatr. Nurs. **8**(2):126, l982.

Shainfeld, F.J.: Errors in insulin doses due to the design of insulin syringes, Pediatrics **56**(2):302-303, 1975.

Shaw, B.: Crushing tablets, Nursing 83 **13**(2):6, 1983.

Shepherd, M.J., and Swearington, P.L.: Z-track injections, Am. J. Nurs. **84**(6):746-747, 1984.

Thomas, N.P.: Preparing cancer patients to administer medication, Patient Counselling Health Ed. **3**(4):137-143, 1982.

Tso, Y.: Drug dosing for pediatric patients, Nurse Pract. **2**:35-37, Sept./Oct. 1977.

Walson, P.D.: Giving medicine to children, Pediatr. Consult. **2**(4):1-7, 1984.

Weeks, H.F.: Administering medication to children, Am. J. Maternal Child Nurs. **5**(1):63, 1980.

Wertsching, J.H.: Reconstituting parenteral antibiotics for children, Am. J. Maternal Child Nurs. **7**(2):128-133, 1982.

Wezel-Bolen, G.: Technological advances in the care of children with chronic illness, Pediatrics: Nursing Update Series **1**(11), Princeton, NJ, 1986, Continuing Professional Education Center, Inc.

Yaffe, S.J.: Prescribing drugs in infants and children—the unique problems, Drug Ther. **12**(4):178-193, 1982.

Yaffe, S.J.: Overview of drug usage in infants and children: developmental background, Fam. Commun. Health **6**(3):31-40, 1983.

Yetka, P.: When your child must take antibiotics for ten days, Pediatr. Nurs. **4**(6):65, 1978.

Zeanah, P.D., and Bross, R.A.: Emergency drug guidelines: a pediatric reference, Pediatr. Nurs. **11**(3):194-202, 1985.

Zenk, K.E.: The intravenous administration of antibiotics to infants and children, Am. J. Intraven. Ther. **6**:28-34, 1979.

Gastric Feeding Techniques/Procedures Related to Elimination

Bayer, L.M., Scholl, D.E., and Ford, E.G.: Tube feeding at home, Am. J. Nurs. **83**(9):1321-1325, 1983.

Bishop, W.S., and Head, J.J.: Care of the infant with a stoma, Am. J. Maternal Child Nurs. **1**:315-319, 1976.

Bjeletich, J., and Hickman, R.O.: The Hickman indwelling catheter, Am. J. Nurs. **80**(1):62-65, 1980.

Broadwell, D.C., and Jackson, B.S., editors: Principles of ostomy care, St. Louis, 1982, The C.V. Mosby Co.

Cooney, D.E., and Grosfeld, J.L.: Care of the child with a colostomy, Pediatrics **59**(3):469-472, 1977.

Forman, J., Baluarte, H.J., and Gruskin, A.B.: Hypokalemia after hypertonic phosphate enemas, J. Pediatr. **94**(1):149-151, 1979.

Guiness, R.: How to use the new small-bore feeding tubes, Nursing 86 **16**(4):51-56, 1986.

Jensen, T.G.: Home enteral nutrition, Diet. Curr. **9**(4):17-20, 1982.

Konstantinides, N.N., and Shronts, E.: Tube feeding: managing the basics, Am. J. Nurs. **83**(9):1312-1320, 1983.

Metheny, N.M.: 20 ways to prevent tube-feeding complications, Nursing 85 **15**(1):47-50, 1985.

Paarlberg, J., and Balint, J.P.: Gastrostomy tubes: practical guidelines for home care, Pediatr. Nurs. **11**(2):99-102, 1985.

Padilla, G.V.: Psychological aspects of tube feeding, Diet. Curr. **8**(5):21-24, 1981.

Paludetto, R., and others: Transcutaneous oxygen tension during nonnutritive sucking in preterm infants, Pediatrics **74**(4):539-542, 1984.

Patterson, R., and Andrassy, R.J.: Needle-catheter jejunostomy, Am. J. Nurs. **83**(9):1325-1326, 1983.

Perry, S., Johnson, S., and Trump, D.: Gastrostomy and the neonate, Am. J. Nurs. **83**(7):1030-1033, 1983.

Pollack, P.F., and others: 100 patient years' experience with the Broviac silastic catheter for central venous nutrition, J. Parenteral Enteral Nutr. **5**(1):32-36, 1981.

Price, S.: The phenomena of imperforate anus in newborns, J. Enterostom. Ther. **7**(6):16-17, 1980.

Rowbotham, J.L.: Managing colostomies, **31**(6):336-345, 1981.

Schreiner, R.L., and others: Environmental contamination of continuous drip feedings, Pediatrics **63**(2):232-237, 1979.

Smith, D.B.: The ostomy: how is it managed? Am. J. Nurs. **85**(11):1246-1249, 1985.

Sotos, J.F., and others: Hypocalcemic coma following two pediatric phosphate enemas, Pediatrics **60**:305, 1977.

van Someren, V., and others: An investigation into the benefits of resiting nasoenteric feeding tubes, Pediatrics **74**(3): 379-383, 1984.

Ward, J.: Evaluation of enteral feeding pumps for pediatric use, J. Pediatr. Nurs. **1**(2):133-136, 1986.

Wink, D.M.: The physical and emotional care of infants with gastrostomy tubes, Comp. Pediatr. Nurs. **6**:195-203, 1983.

Unit Ten

The Child with Disturbance of Fluid and Electrolytes

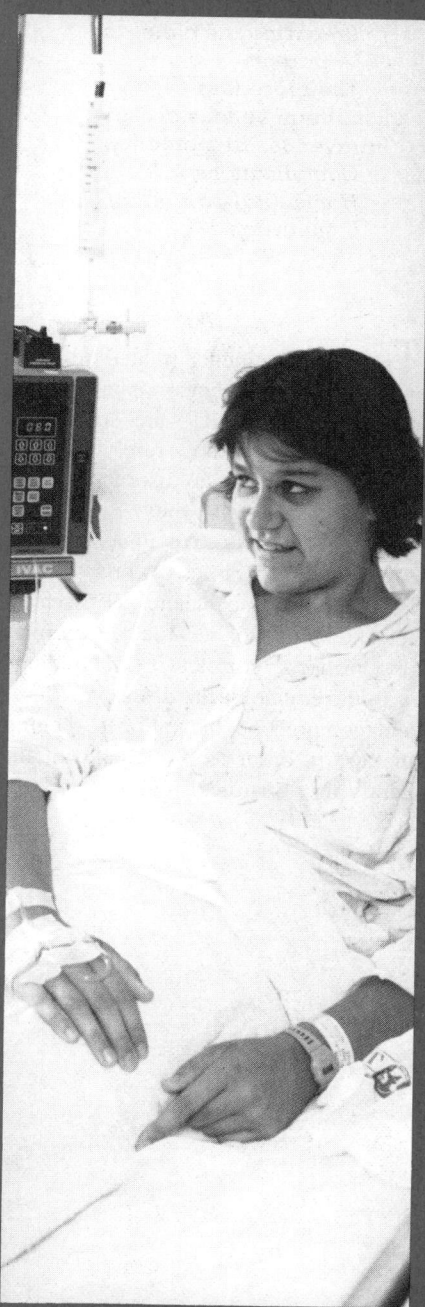

Some of the most common problems associated with the care of infants and children are related to the assessment and maintenance of fluid balance. The physiologic characteristics of young children render them more susceptible to fluid imbalances, and almost any early childhood illness is complicated by fluid disturbances. These differences are particularly noted in the infant, whose proportion of total body water is considerably greater than that of the adult or older child. In addition, the usual childhood responses to illness, such as fever and loss of appetite, further contribute to water depletion and dehydration.

It is essential that nurses who work with children have an understanding of the basic principles underlying the pathologic processes that produce fluid and electrolyte disturbances, the rationale behind fluid therapy, and the role of the nurse in maintaining or restoring fluid balance. Chapter 28, *Balance and Imbalance of Body Fluids*, provides a brief review of the basic concepts of fluid and electrolyte balance and imbalance and the nurse's role in fluid administration. Chapter 29, *Conditions that Produce Fluid and Electrolyte Imbalance*, discusses some of the major causes of fluid disturbance, and Chapter 30, *The Child with Renal Dysfunction*, deals with the more specific fluid problems of renal dysfunction.

Chapter 28

Balance and Imbalance of Body Fluids

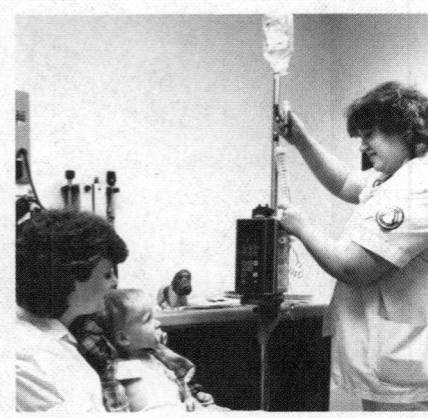

The basic elements related to fluid and electrolyte balance—body water, electrolytes, and pH—are so closely interrelated that they rarely can be separated in clinical disorders; however, for simplicity they will be reviewed separately. An understanding of the basic principles of fluid dynamics and acid-base balance is essential for the nurse to be able to interpret observations, correlate these findings with the course of the disease process, and comprehend the rationale behind therapy in order to participate intelligently in a treatment regimen.

Distribution of Body Fluids

Water is the major constituent of body tissues, and the total body water (TBW) in an individual ranges from 45% to 75% of total body weight. Its importance to body function is related not only to its abundance but also to the fact that it is the medium in which body solutes are dissolved and all metabolic reactions take place. Since these metabolic processes are affected by even small alterations in fluid composition, precise regulation of the volume and composition of the fluid is essential. In healthy individuals body water remains singularly constant, but marked alterations in either its volume or distribution that occur in many disease states can produce severely damaging physiologic consequences.

WATER BALANCE

Under normal conditions the amount of water ingested closely approximates the amount of urine excreted in a 24-hour period, and the water in food and from oxidation balances that lost in feces and through evaporation. In this way equilibrium is maintained.

Mechanisms of Fluid Movement

Water is retained in the body in a relatively constant amount and, with few exceptions, is freely exchangeable between all body fluid compartments. However, water volume is continually subject to change, and its distribution and maintenance are largely determined by:

1. **Solutes** dissolved in the body water—especially sodium and colloids
2. **Physical forces** that act at the site of the partitioning membranes—hydrostatic pressure, osmotic pressure (especially serum proteins), diffusion (including facilitated diffusion), active transport, and vesicular transport
3. **Internal control mechanisms**—thirst, antidiuretic hormone (ADH) release, aldosterone secretion, and the renin-angiotensin system
4. **Boundary organs** through which external exchanges take place—gastrointestinal tract, respiratory tract, kidneys, and skin. Table 28-1 shows electrolyte concentrations of various body fluids.

Table 28-1 Electrolyte concentration of body fluids (mEq/l)

SOURCE	Na$^+$	K$^+$	CL$^-$
Stomach	20-80	5-20	100-150
Ileostomy	45-135	3-15	20-115
Diarrhea	10-90	10-80	10-110
Sweat	10-30	3-10	10-35
Burn	140-145	4-5	110

Table 28-2 Maintenance requirements

WEIGHT (kg)	SURFACE AREA (m^2)	WATER (ml/kg)	Cal/kg	Na$^+$/kg (mEq)	K$^+$/kg (mEq)
3	0.20	100	40-50	3-4	3-4
5	0.27	90	50-70	3-4	2-3
10	0.45	75	40-60	2-3	2-3
15	0.64	65	40-50	2-3	2-3
30	1.10	55	35-45	2-3	1-2
50	1.50	45	25-40	1-2	1-2
70	1.75	40	15-20	1-2	1-2

From Barness, L.A.: Fluid and electrolyte therapy. In Gillis, S.S. and Kagan, B.M., editors, Current pediatric therapy 12, Philadelphia, 1986, W.B. Saunders Co., p. 762.
Requirements/m^2; Water 1500 ml Na$^+$ 60 mEq, K$^+$ 45 mEq.

Maintaining water balance. Maintenance water requirement is the volume of water needed to replace insensible water loss (through the skin and respiratory tract) and losses through urine and stool formation. In afebrile patients at rest the maintenance water requirement is approximately 100 ml for each kcal expended (Barness, 1986). Calculations are based on any of the following parameters: metabolic rate, surface area, or weight (Table 28-2).

Maintenance fluids contain both water and electrolytes and are used for conditions in which a child is in a normal state of hydration, for example, preoperative preparation. Children with fluid losses or other alterations require adjustment of these basic needs to accommodate abnormal losses of both water and electrolytes as a result of a disease state.

Changes in Fluid Volume Related to Growth

The percentage of total body water varies among individuals and in adults and older children is related primarily to the amount of body fat. Consequently females, who have significantly more body fat than males, and obese persons have less water content in relation to weight.

The embryo is composed primarily of water with little tissue substance. As the organism grows and develops, there is a progressive decrease in total body water, with the fastest rate of decline taking place during fetal life. The changes in water content and distribution that occur with age reflect the changes that take place in the relative amounts of bone, muscle, and fat comprising the body. The percentage of total body water falls from 90% in the 1-month-old embryo to 75% or 80% of total body weight at birth. In a child 3 years of age total body water comprises 63% of body weight and decreases slowly until age 12, when it reaches approximately 58%. At maturity the percentage of total body water is somewhat higher in the male than in the female and is probably a result of the differences in body composition, particularly fat and muscle content (Fig. 28-1).

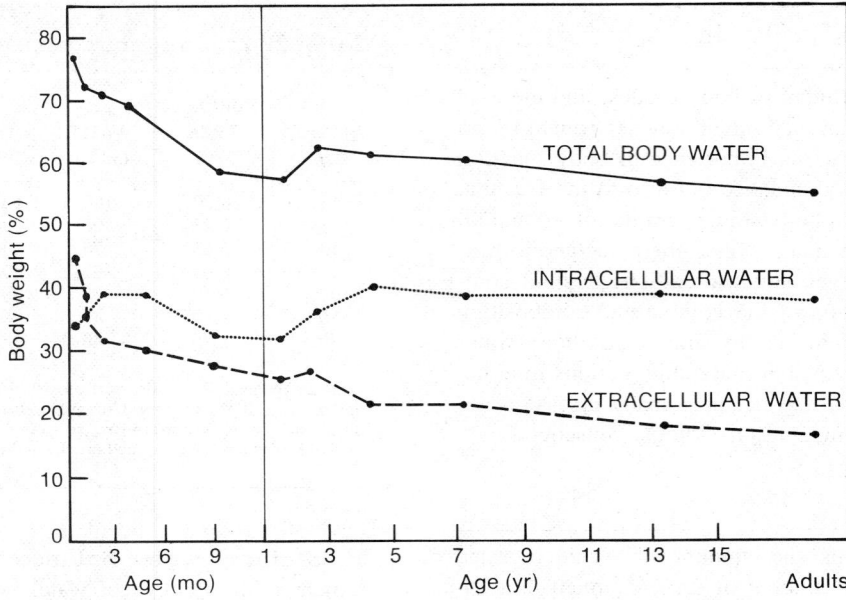

Fig. 28-1. Changes in total body water, extracellular water, and intracellular water in percentages of body weight.
After Friis-Hansen, B.: Pediatrics **28**:169, 1961.

Another important aspect of growth change as it corresponds to water distribution is related to the intracellular and extracellular fluid compartments. In the fetus and prematurely born infant, the largest proportion of body water is contained in the extracellular compartment. As growth and development proceed, the proportion within this fluid compartment decreases as the intracellular fluid and cell solids increase.

Water Balance in Infants

Because of several characteristics, infants and young children have a greater need for water and are more vulnerable to alterations in fluid and electrolyte balance. Newborns have an appreciably larger water content than children and adults. This is partially because the newborn has less fat and a greater proportion of body mass, especially the larger percentage of mass composed of the visceral organs. Compared to older children and adults, infants have a greater fluid intake and output relative to size; water and electrolyte disturbances occur more frequently and more rapidly; and they adjust less promptly to these alterations. The extracellular fluid compartment comprises over half of the total body water at birth and contains a greater relative content of extracellular sodium and chloride. Most of this neonatal "excess" extracellular fluid is lost in the first 10 days of life through insensible perspiration, which can amount up to 10% of the infant's birth weight.

Until about 2 years of age, the infant maintains a larger relative amount of extracellular fluid than the adult, and this fluid volume, together with other anatomic and physiologic differences, contributes to greater and more rapid water loss during this age period. Infants are subject to rapid and profound water depletion in dehydration states as a result of intake restriction or excessive losses from disease. Similarly, overhydration from excessive intake, especially in intravenous fluid administration, is more serious in infants.

During the first year there is a sharp decrease in total body water when expressed as a percentage of body weight. The percentage of extracellular fluid also decreases from approximately 45% to 27%. The gradual alteration in water distribution that accompanies growth and maturation is a result of several changes that occur from infancy to childhood. Muscle growth associated with expanding size of individual cells increases the actual and relative intracellular fluid volume and decreases the relative volume of extracellular fluid. In addition to muscle growth, other organs also increase in size; for example, the size of nerve cells grows with a corresponding decrease in extracellular fluid volume, and the fraction of total body water contained in the skin diminishes during growth. Furthermore, the daily volume of secretions into the gastrointestinal tract is relatively much higher in infants than in children. The net result of these changes is a decrease in the proportion of extracellular fluid as the infant grows older.

Surface area. The infant's relatively greater surface area to body mass allows larger quantities of fluid to be lost in insensible perspiration through the skin. It is estimated that the body surface area of the premature neonate is proportionately five times as great, and that of the newborn is two to three times as great, as that of the older child or adult. The gastrointestinal tract, sometimes considered to be an extension of the body surface area, is also relatively larger in infancy and is a source of proportionately greater fluid loss, especially from diarrhea. The large surface area is an important factor in metabolism and heat production, which also influence fluid loss.

Table 28-3 Ranges of daily water requirements of infants and children at different ages under normal conditions

AGE	AVERAGE BODY WEIGHT (kg)	TOTAL WATER REQUIREMENTS PER 24 HOURS (ml)	WATER REQUIREMENTS PER KG PER 24 HOURS (ml)
3 days	3.0	250-300	80-100
10 days	3.2	400-500	125-150
3 months	5.4	750-850	140-160
6 months	7.3	950-1100	130-135
9 months	8.6	1100-1250	125-145
1 year	9.5	1150-1300	120-135
2 years	11.8	1350-1500	115-125
4 years	16.2	1600-1800	100-110
6 years	20.0	1800-2000	90-100
10 years	28.7	2000-25000	70-85
14 years	45.0	2200-2700	50-60
18 years	54.0	2200-2700	40-50

From Behrman, R.E. and Vaughan, V.C., III, editors: Nelson's textbook of pediatrics ed. 12, Philadelphia, 1983, W.B. Saunders Co., p. 138.

Metabolic rate. The rate of metabolism in infancy is significantly higher than in adulthood because of the larger surface area in relation to the mass of active tissue. Consequently there is a greater production of metabolic wastes that must be excreted by the kidneys. Any condition that increases metabolism causes a rise in heat production, with its concomitant insensible fluid loss and growing need for water for excretion.

Kidney function. The kidneys of the infant are functionally immature at birth and are therefore inefficient in excreting waste products of metabolism. Of particular importance for fluid balance is the inability of the infant's kidneys to concentrate or dilute urine, to conserve or excrete sodium, and to acidify urine. Therefore the infant is less able to handle large quantities of solute-free water than the older child and is more apt to become dehydrated when given concentrated formulas.

Fluid requirements. As a result of these characteristics, infants ingest and excrete a greater amount of fluid per kilogram of body weight than older children. Since electrolytes are excreted with water and the infant has limited ability for conservation, maintenance requirements include both water and electrolytes. The daily exchange of extracellular fluid in the infant is much greater than that in older children, which leaves little fluid volume reserve in dehydration states. Water requirements for infants and children at various ages are listed in Table 28-3.

Disturbances of Fluid and Electrolyte Balance

Disturbances of fluids and their solute concentration are closely interrelated. Alterations in fluid volume affect the electrolyte component, and changes in electrolyte concentration influence fluid movement. Intracellular water and elec-

trolytes depend on diffusion and transport to and from the extracellular fluid compartment; thus any imbalance in the intracellular fluid is reflected by an imbalance in the extracellular fluid. Disturbances in the extracellular fluid involve either an excess or a deficit of fluid and/or electrolytes; of these, fluid loss occurs more frequently.

Depletion of extracellular fluid, usually caused by gastroenteritis, is one of the most common problems encountered in infants and children. Until modern techniques for fluid replacement were perfected, it was one of the chief causes of infant mortality. Fluid and electrolyte problems related to specific diseases and their management are discussed throughout the book where appropriate. The major fluid and electrolyte disturbances, their usual causes, and clinical manifestations are outlined in Table 28-4, and the most common disturbances—dehydration and edema—will be elaborated further. Problems of fluid and electrolyte disturbance always involve both water and electrolytes; therefore replacement always includes administration of both, calculated on the basis of ongoing processes and laboratory serum electrolyte values.

In disturbance problems that involve alterations in the amount and composition of body fluid compartments, the following five areas are considered when planning medical management:

1. Volume of the body fluids, that is, the water content of the patient
2. Osmolality of the body fluids, a factor that has an effect on the distribution of body water among the various compartments
3. Hydrogen ion status, that is, whether or not there has been a disturbance in the pH of body fluids or a disturbance in the homeostatic mechanisms that maintain the pH
4. Electrolyte deficits from cells as well as extracellular water
5. Disturbances in the equilibrium between the mineral skeleton and body fluids

TABLE 28-4 Disturbances of fluid and electrolyte balance

PRIMARY DISTURBANCE	MECHANISMS	CLINICAL SITUATIONS	CLINICAL MANIFESTATIONS	LABORATORY FINDINGS

Water depletion	Complete sudden cessation of water intake
	 Prolonged diminished intake
	 Failure to absorb or reabsorb water
	 Loss from gastrointestinal tract
	 Excessive renal excretion
	  Extrarenal causes
		Neglect of intake by self or caregiver—confused, psychotic, unconscious, or helpless (infant, handicapped)
		 Diarrhea or other intestinal disorders, such as obstruction
		 Vomiting, diarrhea, fistula, nasogastric suction
		 Disturbed body fluid chemistry
		  Inappropriate antidiuretic hormone secretion (head injury, diabetes insipidus)
		  Glycosuria of diabetes mellitus
			General symptoms:
			  Thirst
			  Variable temperature—can be increased (infection) or decreased (shock states)
			  Dry skin and mucous membranes
			  Poor skin turgor
			  Longitudinal wrinkles in tongue
			  Weight loss
			  Fatigue
				High specific gravity of urine (except in inappropriate antidiuretic hormone secretion)
				 Increased blood urea nitrogen
				 Serum sodium concentration variable
				 Potassium levels normal or increased
				 Increased hematocrit

	Renal causes Iatrogenic	Renal disease Overzealous use of diuretics Improper postoperative fluid replacement	Oliguria Depressed fontanel (infant) Irritability and lethargy Sunken eyeballs	

	Loss through skin or lungs
	  Excessive perspiration or vaporization
	
	 Impaired integrity of skin
		Febrile states
		 Hyperventilation
		 Increase in ambient temperature, such as by use of an overheated warmer
		 Heat prostration
		 Transudate from injuries such as burns, wounds
		 Hemorrhage
			Severe symptoms—
			  Signs of shock
			  Soft eyeballs
			  Rapid pulse and respirations
			  Low blood pressure
			 Symptoms depend to some extent on proportion of electrolytes lost with water	

Interstitial fluid-to-plasma shift	Recovery from plasma-to-interstitial fluid shift (remobilization of edema fluid) Volume replacement after hypovolemia	Recovery from burns Hemorrhage Administration of excessive amounts of blood, plasma, blood expanders, or hypertonic solutions	Signs of hypervolemia—bounding pulse, peripheral vein engorgement, moist rales in lungs, weakness, pallor, hyperpnea	Decreased red blood cell count, packed cell volume, hemoglobin concentration (hemodilution)

Table 28-4 Disturbances of fluid and electrolyte balance—cont'd

PRIMARY DISTURBANCE	MECHANISMS	CLINICAL SITUATIONS	CLINICAL MANIFESTATIONS	LABORATORY FINDINGS
Water excess	Water intake in excess of output	Excessive oral intake Overloading with hypotonic solutions Plain water enemas	Edema: Generalized Pulmonary (moist rales) Intracutaneous, particularly noted in loose areolar tissue of eyelids and scrotum	Low specific gravity of urine Dilution of electrolytes Decreased hematocrit Variable urine volume Hemodilution
	Failure to excrete water in presence of normal intake	Kidney disease Congestive heart failure Malnutrition	Elevated venous pressure Bradycardia Weight gain Lethargy Increased spinal fluid pressure Cerebral manifestations such as convulsions, coma	
Plasma-to-interstitial fluid shift	Portal hypertension Decreased oncotic pressure with increased capillary permeability: Cutaneous	Chronic liver disease Malnutrition Starvation edema	Ascites Peripheral edema Signs of hypovolemia—pallor, tachycardia, low blood pressure, weak pulse, cold extremities, disorientation	Elevated hematocrit, red blood cell count, packed cell volume
	Renal Vasodilatation Decreased venous return	Burns Massive crushing injury Nephrotic syndrome Shock		
Sodium depletion (hyponatremia)	Inadequate sodium intake Loss through perspiration	Prolonged low-sodium diet Fever Excess sweating Cystic fibrosis	Associated with water loss: Same as with water loss— dehydration, weakness, dizziness, nausea, abdominal cramps, apprehension Mild—apathy, weakness, nausea, soft pulse Moderate— decreased blood pressure	N = 140 mEq/liter; Sodium concentration may be high, low, or normal Specific gravity depends on water deficit or excess
	Loss through nonintact skin Loss through gastrointestinal tract Excessive renal excretion May be associated with water deficit or excess	Burns and wounds Vomiting, diarrhea, nasogastric suction, fistulas Adrenal insufficiency Renal disease Diabetic acidosis		
Sodium excess (hypernatremia)	Increased intake without increase in output Decreased output (renal disease)	High salt intake— nasogastric or intravenous Renal disease	Intense thirst Dry, sticky mucous membranes Flushed skin Temperature may be increased Hoarseness Oliguria Nausea and vomiting Firm tissue turgor Irritability and possible progression to disorientation, convulsions	Serum sodium concentration increased or normal High plasma volume Alkalosis

Continued.

Table 28-4 Disturbances of fluid and electrolyte balance—cont'd

PRIMARY DISTURBANCE	MECHANISMS	CLINICAL SITUATIONS	CLINICAL MANIFESTATIONS	LABORATORY FINDINGS
Potassium depletion (hypokalemia)	Inadequate intake of potassium	Starvation Clinical conditions associated with poor food intake Intravenous fluid without added potassium	Muscle weakness, stiffness, paralysis, hyporeflexia Hypotension Cardiac arrhythmias, gallop rhythm	N = 4.1-5.6 mEq/liter Decreased serum potassium concentration Abnormal ECG—flat T waves, prolonged ST segment
	Loss from gastrointestinal tract	Diarrhea, vomiting, fistulas, nasogastric suction Diuresis	Tachycardia or bradycardia Ileus	
	Excessive renal excretion	Administration of diuretics Administration of cortiocosteroids Diuretic phase of nephrotic syndrome Healing stage of burns Potassium-losing nephritis Hyperglycemic diuresis Familial periodic paralysis	Apathy, drowsiness Irritability Fatigue	
	Movement from extracellular to intracellular fluid	Intravenous administration of insulin in ketoacidosis Alkalosis		
Potassium excess (hyperkalemia)	Inadequate excretion	Renal disease Renal shutdown Adrenal insufficiency (Addison disease) Associated with metabolic acidosis	Muscle weakness, flaccid paralysis Twitching Hyperreflexia Bradycardia Ventricular fibrillation and cardiac arrest	High serum potassium concentration Variable urine volume Flat P wave on ECG
	Increased intake	Too rapid administration of intravenous potassium chloride Transfusion with old donor blood	Oliguria Apnea—respiratory arrest	
	Movement from intracellular to extracellular fluid	Severe dehydration Crushing injuries Burns Hemolysis from sudden massive water intake		
	Hemoconcentration	Dehydration		
Chloride depletion (hypochloremia)	Inadequate intake	Starvation Inadequate replacement of losses	Symptoms associated with alkalosis—lethargy, muscle hypertonicity	N = 100 mEq/liter High carbon dioxide combining power
	Excessive excretion	Vomiting Pyloric obstruction Nasogastric suction	Depressed respirations Metabolic alkalosis	Low plasma chloride concentration
Chloride excess (hyperchloremia)	Excessive ingestion	Treatment with ammonium chloride	Tachypnea Weakness	Low carbon dioxide combining power
	Decreased output	Renal disease	Symptoms associated with acidosis	High plasma chloride concentration

Table 28-4 Disturbances of fluid and electrolyte balance—cont'd

PRIMARY DISTURBANCE	MECHANISMS	CLINICAL SITUATIONS	CLINICAL MANIFESTATIONS	LABORATORY FINDINGS
Calcium depletion (hypocalcemia)	Inadequate intake	Inadequate dietary calcium	Neuromuscular irritability	N = 4-5 mEq/liter
		Vitamin D deficiency	Tingling of nose, ears, fingertips, toes	Decreased serum calcium concentration
	Malabsorption from gastrointestinal tract	Rapid transit through gastointestinal tract		
	Excessive losses of calcium	Advanced renal insufficiency	Tetany	
	Decreased bone resorption	Hypoparathyroidism	Laryngospasm	
	Unavailable for use as ionized calcium	Alkalosis	Generalized convulsions	
		Trapped in diseased tissues	May be changes in clotting	
		Cow's milk formula—tetany of the newborn	Positive Chvostek sign	
		Exchange transfusion with titrated blood	Cardiac arrest	
Calcium excess (hypercalcemia)	Converted from nonionized to ionized form	Acidosis	Few problems	Increased calcium concentration in urine—may cause formation of kidney stones
		Prolonged immobilization	Constipation	
		Conditions associated with increased bone catabolism	Anorexia	
			Dryness of mouth	
			Muscle hypotonicity	
	Inadequate elimination	Kidney disease		
	Increased absorption of calcium from gastrointestinal tract	Hypervitaminosis D		
	Increased resorption of calcium by kidney	Hyperparathyroidism		

The following discussion is concerned with the general concepts of two common fluid volume disturbances, dehydration and edema, that are a feature of a variety of conditions. Specific disorders are discussed in Chapters 29 and 30, and elsewhere in the book when appropriate.

DEHYDRATION

Dehydration is a common body fluid disturbance encountered in the nursing of infants and children; it occurs whenever the total output of fluid exceeds the total intake, regardless of the underlying cause. Although dehydration can result from lack of oral intake (especially in elevated environmental temperatures), more often it is a result of abnormal losses, such as those that occur in vomiting or diarrhea, when oral intake only partially compensates for the abnormal losses. Other significant causes of dehydration are diabetic ketoacidosis and extensive burns.

Types of Dehydration

Sodium is the primary osmotic force that controls fluid movement between the major fluid compartments; therefore describing dehydration according to plasma sodium concen-

trations (i.e., isonatremic, hyponatremic, or hypernatremic) would be more descriptive. However, other osmotic forces may play the dominant role in dehydration, such as glucose in diabetic dehydration and protein in nephrotic syndrome. Consequently dehydration is conventionally classified as (1) isotonic, (2) hypotonic, and (3) hypertonic.

Isotonic dehydration. Isotonic (isosmotic or isonatremic) dehydration occurs in conditions in which electrolyte and water deficits are present in approximately balanced proportion. The observable fluid losses are not necessarily isotonic, but losses from other avenues make adjustments so that the sum of all losses, or the net loss, is isotonic. Since there is no osmotic force present to cause a redistribution of water between the intracellular and extracellular fluid, the major loss is sustained from the extracellular compartments. This significantly reduces the plasma volume and hence the circulating blood volume with its effect on skin, muscle, and kidneys. Shock is the greatest threat to life in isotonic dehydration, and the child with isotonic dehydration displays symptoms characteristic of hypovolemic shock. Plasma sodium remains within normal limits, between 130 and 150 mEq per liter.

Hypotonic dehydration. Hypotonic (hyposmotic or

Table 28-5 Physical signs of dehydration

	ISOTONIC (LOSS OF WATER AND SALT)	HYPOTONIC (LOSS OF SALT IN EXCESS OF WATER)	HYPERTONIC (LOSS OF WATER IN EXCESS OF SALT)
Skin			
Color	Gray	Gray	Gray
Temperature	Cold	Cold	Cold or hot
Turgor	Poor	Very poor	Fair
Feel	Dry	Clammy	Thickened
Mucous membranes	Dry	Slightly moist	Parched
Tearing and salivation	Absent	Absent	Absent
Eyeball	Sunken and soft	Sunken and soft	Sunken
Fontanel	Sunken	Sunken	Sunken
Body temperature	Subnormal or elevated	Abnormal	Subnormal or elevated
Pulse	Rapid	Very rapid	Moderately rapid
Respirations	Rapid	Rapid	Rapid
Behavior	Irritable to lethargic	Lethargic to comatose; convulsions	Marked lethargy with extreme hyperirritability on stimulation

hyponatremic) dehydration occurs when the electrolyte deficit exceeds the water deficit. Since intracellular fluid is more concentrated than extracellular fluid in hypotonic dehydration, water transfers from the extracellular to the intracellular fluid to establish osmotic equilibrium. This movement further increases the extracellular fluid volume loss, and shock is a frequent result. Because there is a greater proportional loss of extracellular fluid in hypotonic dehydration, the physical signs tend to be more severe with smaller fluid losses than isotonic or hypertonic dehydration. Plasma sodium concentration is less than 130 mEq per liter.

Hypertonic dehydration. Hypertonic (hyperosmotic or hypernatremic) dehydration results from water loss in excess of electrolyte loss and is usually caused by a proportionately larger loss of water and/or a larger intake of electrolytes. This sometimes occurs in infants with diarrhea who are given fluids by mouth that contain large amounts of solute or in children receiving high protein nasogastric tube feedings that place an excessive solute load on the kidneys. In hypertonic dehydration, fluid shifts from the lesser concentration of the intracellular fluid to the extracellular fluid. Plasma sodium concentration is greater than 150 mEq per liter.

Since the extracellular fluid volume is proportionately larger, hypertonic dehydration has a large degree of water loss for the same intensity of physical signs. Shock is less apparent in hypertonic dehydration. However, neurologic disturbances, such as seizures, are more likely to occur. Cerebral changes are serious and may result in permanent damage. Table 28-5 outlines the general physical signs of dehydration.

Degree of Dehydration

The magnitude of fluid loss is best ascertained by a comparison of pre-illness weight and current weight, because any

weight loss is substantially equivalent to the amount of water lost. If pre-illness weight is unknown, the degree of dehydration is estimated by assessing the intensity of clinical signs. In infants, who are most vulnerable to rapid and extensive fluid losses, isotonic dehydration is usually described as 5% (mild), 10% (moderate), and 15% (severe). Older children and adolescents, with proportionally less total body water, display smaller proportional losses; therefore the estimates of 3%, 6%, and 9% values more nearly describe mild, moderate, and severe dehydration in these age-groups.

At each of these levels certain manifestations, in addition to weight, provide clues to the extent of dehydration. The first of these appear when about 5% of the weight has been lost; the child is nearly moribund when water loss approaches 15%. Initial and ongoing losses can be determined from body weight loss with a high degree of reliability. Compensatory mechanisms attempt to maintain fluid volume by adjusting to these losses. Interstitial fluid moves into the vascular compartment to maintain the blood volume in response to hemoconcentration and hypovolemia, and vasoconstriction of peripheral arterioles helps maintain pumping pressure. When fluid losses exceed the body's ability to sustain blood volume and blood pressure, circulation is seriously compromised and the blood pressure falls. This results in tissue hypoxia with accumulation of lactic acid, pyruvate, and other acid metabolites, which contributes to the development of metabolic acidosis.

Renal compensation is impaired by reduced blood flow through the kidneys, and little urine is formed. Increased serum osmolality stimulates the secretion of antidiuretic hormone to conserve fluid and initiates the renin-angiotensin mechanisms in the kidney, causing further vasoconstriction. Aldosterone is released to promote sodium retention and conserve water in the kidneys. If dehydration increases in

---

Table 28-6 Intensity of clinical signs associated with varying degrees of isotonic dehydration in infants

| | DEGREE OF DEHYDRATION | | |
	MILD	MODERATE	SEVERE
Body weight	Up to 5%	5%-9%	10%-15%
Skin color	Pale	Gray	Mottled
Skin turgor	Decreased	Poor	Very poor
Mucous membranes	Dry	Very dry	Parched
Urine output	Decreased	Oliguria	Marked oliguria and azotemia
Blood pressure	Normal	Normal or lowered	Lowered
Pulse	Normal or increased	Increased	Rapid and thready

---

severity, urine formation is markedly diminished and metabolites and hydrogen ions that are normally excreted by this route are retained.

Shock is a common manifestation of severe depletion of extracellular fluid volume accompanied by tachycardia and low blood pressure. Peripheral circulation is poor as a result of reduced blood volume; therefore the skin is cool and mottled, with poor capillary filling after blanching. Impaired kidney circulation often leads to oliguria and azotemia. Skin and mucous membranes are dry, skin turgor is poor, and in infants the anterior fontanel is depressed. A mild degree of dehydration, however, is associated with barely discernible physical signs and absence of shock (Table 28-6).

Therapeutic Management

Medical management is directed at correcting the fluid imbalance and treating the underlying cause. To initiate a therapeutic plan, there are several factors that must be determined: the degree of dehydration based on physical assessment; the type of dehydration based on the pathophysiology of the specific illness responsible for the dehydrated state, specific physical signs other than general signs, and initial plasma sodium concentrations; and associated electrolyte (especially serum potassium) and acid-base imbalances. Initial and regular ongoing evaluations are carried out to assess the patient's progress toward equilibrium and the effectiveness of therapy. Assessment is based on two major types of information:

1. Clinical observation—accurate body weight measurements, circulatory status, urinary output, and the presence and intensity of signs of dehydration
2. Chemical analysis—blood plasma electrolyte (sodium, potassium, and chloride ion) concentrations, blood urea nitrogen (BUN), acid-base status, hemoglobin, and plasma protein concentrations; urine specific gravity; pH; and the presence or absence of sugar and ketone bodies.

When the child is alert, awake, and not in shock, dehydration can be corrected with oral fluid administration. Most dehydration is mild and can be managed at home by this method. Several commercial rehydration fluids are available for home use. Rehydration management consists of 50 ml per kg body weight within 4 hours for mild dehydration and 100 ml per kg over 6 hours for moderate dehydration (Barness, 1986; Robson, 1983). Amounts and rates are increased if rehydration is incomplete or if excess losses continue. Full diet is usually withheld until the child is well hydrated and the basic problem is under control.

Parenteral fluid therapy is instituted whenever the child is unable to ingest sufficient amounts of fluid and electrolytes to (1) meet ongoing daily physiologic losses, (2) replace previous deficits, and (3) replace ongoing abnormal losses. Patients who usually require intravenous fluids are those with severe dehydration, those with uncontrollable vomiting, those who are unable to drink for any reason (such as extreme fatigue or coma), and those with severe gastric distention (Barness, 1986).

Since dehydration constitutes the greatest threat to life, the first priority is the restoration of circulation by rapid expansion of the extracellular fluid volume in order to treat shock or prevent its occurrence. Intravenous administration of fluid is begun immediately, even though the exact nature of the dehydration and the serum electrolyte values are not known. The solution selected is based on what is known regarding the probable type and cause of the dehydration—usually a saline solution. Sodium bicarbonate may be added, since acidosis is usually associated with severe dehydration, but potassium is not administered until kidney function is restored, unless the child is known to be hypokalemic (as in diabetic ketoacidosis). As the circulation improves, the glomerular filtration pressure increases to improve renal function, which is essential to electrolyte readjustments.

The goal of the next phase is the restoration of extracellular fluid volume. With improved circulation, water and electrolyte deficits can be evaluated and acid-base status corrected either directly through the administration of fluids or indirectly through improved renal function. Next, potassium lost in intracellular fluid must be replaced slowly by way of the extracellular fluid. Finally, the body fat and protein stores are replaced through diet. If the child is unable to eat or if feeding aggravates the condition (such as diarrhea), intravenous alimentation is provided to prevent serious malnourishment.

While the initial phase of fluid replacement is rapid in both isotonic and hypotonic dehydration, it is contraindicated in hypertonic dehydration because of the risk of water intoxication, especially in the brain cells. There is an apparent physiologic difference in the manner and length of time for diffusion of sodium into and out of brain cells. There is a significant time lag for sodium to reach a steady state in these cells, whereas water diffuses almost instantaneously. Consequently rapid administration of fluid will cause equally rapid diffusion of water into the dehydrated brain cells, causing marked cerebral edema. Since extracellular fluid volume is maintained relatively well in hypertonic as opposed to the other types of dehydration, shock is not a usual manifestation.

WATER INTOXICATION

Water intoxication, or water overload, is observed less often than dehydration. However, it is important that nurses and others who care for children are aware that this can occur and be alert to the possibility in certain situations. Patients who ingest excessive amounts of fluid develop a concurrent decrease in serum sodium and central nervous system symptoms. There is a large urine output and, because water moves into the brain more rapidly than sodium moves out, the child also exhibits irritability, somnolence, headache, vomiting, diarrhea, and generalized seizures. The affected child usually appears well hydrated but may be edematous or even dehydrated.

Fluid intoxication can occur during acute intravenous water overloading, too rapid dialysis, tap water enemas, or with too rapid reduction of glucose levels in diabetic ketoacidosis. Patients with central nervous system infections occasionally retain excessive amounts of water. Administration of inappropriate hypotonic solutions (such as 5% dextrose in water) may cause a rapid reduction in sodium and result in symptoms of water overload.

Infants are especially vulnerable to fluid overload. Their thirst mechanism is not well developed; therefore they are unable to "turn off" fluid intake appropriately. A decreased glomerular filtration rate does not allow for repeated excretion of a water load, and antidiuretic hormone levels may not be maximally reduced. Consequently infants are unable to excrete a water overload effectively.

Administration of inappropriately prepared formula is one of the more common causes of water intoxication, often related to feeding mismanagement (Schulman, 1980; Partridge and others, 1981). Families who cannot afford to buy enough expensive formula may dilute the formula to increase the volume or even substitute water for the formula. A family may run out of formula and dilute the remaining amount to make it last until they are able to purchase replacement formula. In addition, water is sometimes used for pacification. Water intoxication has also been observed in an infant who received overly vigorous hydration during a febrile illness (Etzioni, Benderly, and Levi, 1979).

A number of clinicians have observed water intoxication in infants following swimming lessons (Goldberg and others, 1982; Kropp and Schwartz, 1982; Bennett, Wagner, and Fields, 1983). Although they hold their breath, infants apparently swallow a large amount of water during repeated submersion. Therefore anticipatory guidance to parents should include a discussion of swimming instruction and advice to stop a lesson if the child is observed to swallow unusual amounts of water or exhibit any symptoms of hyponatremia.

EDEMA

Edema is the presence of excess fluid in the interstitial spaces as a result of some defect in the normal circulation of body fluids that causes increased pressure in the interstitial spaces. Fluid removal from the interstitial spaces depends on the following:

1. Venous hydrostatic pressure
2. Colloidal osmotic pressure of both the intravascular and interstitial spaces
3. Intact semipermeable capillary wall
4. Tissue tension
5. Lymphatic flow

Mechanisms of Edema Formation

A defect in any of the homeostatic mechanisms maintaining fluid balance can cause accumulation of interstitial fluid. Disequilibrium results from anything that (1) alters the retention of sodium, such as renal disease or hormonal influences; (2) affects the formation or destruction of plasma proteins, such as starvation or liver disease; and (3) alters membrane permeability, such as nephrotic syndrome or trauma.

Edema may be localized to a small or large area, such as that occurring in urticaria, infection, and pulmonary congestion, or it can be generalized, as in the the nephrotic syndrome and starvation. A severe, generalized accumulation of great amounts of fluid in all body tissues is termed *anasarca*.

Increased venous pressure. The colloidal osmotic pressure of the plasma proteins draws fluid back into the vascular system as long as this force is greater than the venous hydrostatic pressure. However, when the venous pressure is increased, fluid tends to be retained in the interstitial spaces. This occurs when an individual remains in the same position for a long time, such as swollen ankles and feet after standing or sitting for long periods. Constrictive dressings or restraints applied too tightly to extremities will obstruct venous return, increase venous and capillary pressure, and cause edema. The most graphic pathologic illustrations are pulmonary edema caused by pulmonary circulation overload in cardiac defects with a left-to-right shunt and ascites caused by portal hypertension. Edema from any cause is increased in dependent areas because of this added factor of increased venous hydrostatic pressure and the gravitational effects in these areas.

Capillary permeability. Damage to capillary walls or alteration in their permeability will permit exudation of plasma protein into the interstitial space. Most often this occurs as local edema, such as manifested in inflammatory and hypersensitivity reactions. Capillary damage from burns allows extensive exudation of protein-rich fluid into the interstitial spaces to compound edema formation.

Diminished plasma proteins. A fall in plasma protein levels hampers the osmotic pull back into the vessels. Consequently fluid remains in the interstitial spaces. Although other factors play a role, such as hydrostatic pressure of both the arterial vascular system and the tissues and sodium ion concentration, significantly low protein levels (below 4.5 mg per dl) are associated with edema. Examples of this are the massive albumin losses of the nephrotic syndrome, diminished serum protein from insufficient dietary protein, and (sometimes) hemodilution of plasma proteins from intravenous fluid administration in chronic dehydration.

Lymphatic obstruction. Obstruction of lymph flow creates edema high in protein content. This is uncommon in childhood but can result from trauma to the lymphatic glands or removal of lymph nodes.

Tissue tension. Tissue hydrostatic pressure is ordinarily of little consequence. However, it plays a significant role in determining distribution of edema fluid in certain pathologic conditions. Loose tissues allow a greater amount of fluid accumulation than tissues that are tightly bound by dense fibrous bands in which tissue pressure rapidly increases to limit further extravasation of fluid. Edema appears earlier and more readily in loose structures such as those in the periorbital and genital tissues. The areolar structure of lung tissue is probably a contributing factor in pulmonary edema as well as in increased hydrostatic pressure in the pulmonary vessels.

Other factors in edema formation. Any factor that causes sodium retention by the kidneys will produce or augment edema formation. This includes stimulation of the renin-angiotensin-aldosterone mechanisms for sodium reabsorption created by the diminished plasma volume in edema, which resulted from primary causes. The salt-retaining property of steroids is responsible for the edema associated with their administration.

A particularly threatening form of edema is cerebral edema caused by trauma, infection, or other etiologic factors, including vascular overload or injudicious intravenous administration of hypotonic solutions. The problems and assessment of cerebral edema are always nursing considerations in fluid administration.

Therapeutic Management

The primary goal in the management of edema is treatment of the basic disease process, which will be discussed in relation to the specific disorders. However, an essential aspect in the management of any fluid overload is early recognition, in which nurses play a vital role.

Disturbances of Acid-Base Balance

The ability of the body to regulate the acid-base status is one of its most crucial physiologic functions. Many disease states, such as diarrhea, vomiting, or febrile conditions, are complicated by disturbances in the acid-base balance, which are often more hazardous to the child's survival than the primary disease process. Sometimes simply providing adequate hydration, replacing electrolytes, and correcting acid-base disturbances are all that is needed to sustain an infant or child until the primary disorder has run its course.

ACID-BASE IMBALANCE

A disturbance of acid-base equilibrium in the direction of acidosis or alkalosis may come about in a variety of ways. However, very simply stated, *acidosis (acidemia)* results from either accumulation of acid or loss of base, and *alkalosis (alkalemia)* results from either accumulation of base or loss of acid.

Hydrogen Ion Concentration

The pH represents the concentration of hydrogen ions in solution and only indicates whether the imbalance is acidosis or alkalosis. It does not reflect the nature of the imbalance, that is, whether it is of metabolic or respiratory origin. Body metabolism affects primarily the base bicarbonate; therefore alterations in the concentration of base bicarbonate are termed *metabolic* disturbances of acid-base balance, and since the amount of carbon dioxide exhaled through the lungs affects the carbonic acid concentration, changes in the carbonic acid concentration are referred to as *respiratory* disturbances. Consequently the simple disturbances (those with a single primary cause) are categorized as metabolic acidosis or alkalosis and respiratory acidosis or alkalosis.

It is also significant that the major signs and symptoms of hydrogen ion imbalances, acidosis and alkalosis, reflect central nervous system involvement. Depression of the central nervous system, manifested by lethargy, diminished mental capacity, delirium, stupor, and coma, is observed in acidosis of either metabolic or respiratory origin. On the other hand, alkalosis produces clinical manifestations of nervous system stimulation and excitement, including overexcitability, nervousness, tingling sensations, and tetany that may progress to convulsions. Persons with epilepsy are particularly susceptible to seizures, which can be precipitated by hyperventilation.

The extent and severity of signs and symptoms depend on the length of time the imbalance has existed and the magnitude or degree of the deviation from normal. A rapid, severe imbalance will seriously compromise the compensatory mechanisms to the point where it is incompatible with life, whereas the body will be able to compensate adequately for a mild, gradual distortion and produce few if any observable signs or symptoms.

Compensatory Mechanisms

When the fundamental acid-base ratio is altered for any reason, the body attempts to correct the deviation. In a simple disturbance there is a single *primary* factor that affects one component of the acid-base pair and is usually accompanied by a *compensatory* or *secondary* change in the component that is not primarily affected. For example, increased formation of metabolic acid rapidly reduces the base bicarbonate in the formation of carbonic acid. The respiratory mechanism immediately attempts to compensate for the imbalance by eliminating the carbonic acid through exhaled carbon dioxide and water. The imbalance is corrected when the kidneys excrete hydrogen and ammonium ions in exchange for reabsorbed sodium bicarbonate.

When the secondary changes (the hyperventilation and urine acidification in the preceding example) succeed in preventing a distortion of the acid-base ratio and the pH is restored to normal, the disturbance is described as *compensated*. A *partially compensated* state is one in which the serum pH is not within normal limits but in which there is no discernible compensatory effect. The *uncompensated* state exists when there is no compensatory effect and the pH remains uncorrected. The imbalance is said to be *corrected* when physiologic mechanisms fully correct the primary abnormality.

Laboratory Measurements

Several laboratory tests are employed to assess the nature and extent of acid-base disturbances. The importance of these data is readily apparent when a clinical observation such as hyperventilation can represent either the primary factor in respiratory alkalosis or a secondary or compensatory factor in metabolic acidosis. The laboratory tests of value in the assessment of acid-base status are outlined in Table 28-7. To determine the acid-base status, three variables—the respiratory component (Pco_2), the metabolic component (base bicarbonate, or carbon dioxide), and the serum pH—must be determined. Measurement of any two will allow computation of the third. A summary of relationships between these and other variables is outlined in Table 28-8.

Associated Disturbances in Acid-Base Imbalance

Physiologic functions of the body take place optimally when the pH is maintained within a normal range. The disequilibrium created by moderately altered pH can produce disordered function of physiologic and enzyme systems, but great divergences are incompatible with life. In addition, electrolyte shifts that take place in response to changes in pH alter the electrolyte concentration in the fluid compartments to disturb the normal concentrations. For example, cell membrane permeability is affected by changes in pH. A lowered pH allows potassium to move from the intracellular fluid to the extracellular fluid. Serum potassium levels increase with acidosis and decrease with alkalosis.

Serum potassium. One of the disturbances that complicates both fluid losses and acid-base imbalance is an alteration in potassium levels. During dehydration, fluid moves out of the intracellular fluid compartment into the extracellular fluid compartment in an attempt to balance the fluid losses. In the process, potassium also moves out, creating a total body potassium depletion. Since renal function is drastically reduced in dehydration, normal excretion of potassium does not take place. This causes elevated serum levels that can produce all the signs and symptoms of hyperkalemia. During rapid rehydration therapy for gastroin-

---

Table 28-7 Laboratory tests employed in assessment of acid-base status

ABBREVIATION	TEST	NORMAL VALUES*	DESCRIPTION
pH	Partial pressure of hydrogen	Birth: 7.11-7.36 1 day: 7.29-7.45 Child: 7.35-7.45	Expression of hydrogen ion concentration
Pco_2	Partial pressure of carbon dioxide or carbon dioxide tension	Newborn: 27-40 Infant: 27-41 Girls: 32-45 Boys: 35-48	Measure of carbon dioxide tension; reflects carbonic acid concentration of plasma
HCO_3 (serum) arterial	Carbon dioxide content or carbon dioxide combining power	Infant: 21-28 mEq/liter	Concentration of base bicarbonate
BE	Base excess (whole blood)	Newborn: -2 to -10 Infant: -1 to -7 Child: $+2$ to -4 Thereafter: $+3$ to -3	Used to express extent of deviation from normal buffer base concentration; indicates quantity of blood buffers remaining after hydrogen ion is buffered

*Data from Behrman, R.E., and Vaughan, V.C., III, editors: Nelson textbook of pediatrics, ed. 12, Philadelphia, 1983, W.B. Saunders Co.

Table 28-8 Summary of simple acid-base disturbances (partially compensated)			
DISTURBANCE	PLASMA pH	PLASMA Pco_2	PLASMA HCO_3
Respiratory acidosis	↓	↑	↑
Respiratory alkalosis	↑	↓	↓
Metabolic acidosis	↓	↓	↓
Metabolic alkalosis	↑	↑	N or ↑

testinal losses and diabetic ketoacidosis, the extracellular fluid potassium moves back into the intracellular fluid compartment, thereby posing the risk of hypokalemia unless there is an anticipated replacement. However, potassium is not replaced until the intravascular fluid is sufficient to restore adequate renal function.

Serum calcium. Disturbed extracellular fluid calcium levels may occur in various types of dehydration. Usually the disturbance is in the form of reduced serum calcium levels, especially where there is a concomitant potassium loss; therefore therapy includes adequate replacement of potassium losses. However, tetany may result from an acute calcium imbalance associated with metabolic alkalosis. Long-term calcium imbalance results from the effects of chronic acidosis are related to bone resorption from renal disturbances.

Oxygen combination. The capacity of oxygen to combine with hemoglobin is also affected by changes in pH. The affinity of hemoglobin for oxygen decreases with a decrease in pH so that, in a state of acidosis, less oxygen will be picked up by the hemoglobin as blood travels through the lungs. However, oxygen is more easily released to the tissues when the pH is lowered. The opposite effects operate during an increase in pH.

Blood flow. Blood flow in various areas is altered by changes in pH. Pulmonary circulation constricts in acidosis, whereas decreased pH (acidosis) causes vasodilation in systemic vessels.

RESPIRATORY ACIDOSIS

Respiratory acidosis results from diminished or inadequate pulmonary ventilation that causes an elevated plasma Pco_2 with an increased concentration of dissolved carbon dioxide, which leads to elevated carbonic acid and hydrogen ion concentration. Conditions that produce respiratory acidosis can originate at three levels in the respiratory system and result in inadequate gas exchange. These are:

1. Factors that depress the respiratory center, such as head injury, depressant or narcotizing drugs, and infections of the central nervous system

2. Factors that affect the lung proper, such as obstructive pulmonary disease, pneumonia, cystic fibrosis, acute pulmonary edema, atelectasis, and occlusion of respiratory passages

3. Factors that interfere with the bellows action of the chest wall, including trauma to the chest wall, skeletal diseases or deformities, and diseases of the thoracic muscles or their innervation (e.g., muscular dystrophy or muscular atrophy)

Compensation is mediated through the kidneys, which are stimulated to conserve and thus increase the plasma bicarbonate concentration and to excrete hydrogen ions. Laboratory findings in respiratory acidosis include elevated plasma bicarbonate concentration (over 29 mEq per liter in older children, over 28 mEq per liter in young children), and elevated Pco_2 (above 38 mm Hg, arterial).

The treatment of respiratory acidosis is aimed at correcting the primary defect, improving gas exchange at the alveolar level to provide more efficient removal of carbon dioxide, and administration of buffers such as bicarbonate to reduce hydrogen ion concentration during critical periods.

RESPIRATORY ALKALOSIS

Conversely, respiratory alkalosis is caused by a primary increase in the rate and depth of pulmonary ventilation, resulting in unusually large amounts of carbon dioxide being exhaled or "blown off." This reduces the plasma Pco_2, carbonic acid, and hydrogen ion concentration and leaves an excess of base bicarbonate. Conditions that cause stimulation of the respiratory center to produce hyperventilation include:

1. Primary central nervous system stimulation resulting from emotions, including hysteria, fear, or apprehension; central nervous system infection (encephalitis); and certain drug reactions, such as early salicylate intoxication (a primary respiratory stimulant)

2. Reflex central nervous system stimulation from peripheral chemoreceptors as a result of hypoxia, which provides the stimulus for hyperventilation at high altitudes, fever or high environmental temperatures, and cardiac conditions

3. Reflex central nervous system stimulation from intrathoracic stretch receptors, which is believed to be the cause of hyperventilation in localized pulmonary disease

A frequent cause of hyperventilation in children is voluntary hyperventilation before underwater swimming. It is also a consideration in the care of persons having assisted ventilation. Incorrectly set mechanical ventilators can cause respiratory rates and tidal volumes in excess of physiologic needs.

Compensation of respiratory alkalosis takes place in the kidneys and consists of excretion of bicarbonate in association with sodium and potassium ions to conserve hydrogen ions. Laboratory findings include elevated plasma pH (over 7.43), depressed plasma bicarbonate concentration (less than 23 mEq per liter in older children, less than 20 mEq per liter in young children), and lowered P_{CO_2} (less than 35 mm Hg).

Treatment of respiratory alkalosis consists of correction of the primary defect and prevention of lost anions and the associated potassium deficit. Carbon dioxide administered by mask slows respirations and provides rapid relief.

METABOLIC ACIDOSIS

Metabolic acidosis is a lowered plasma pH caused by any process that reduces the base bicarbonate concentration. Metabolic acidosis can be produced by the gain of nonvolatile acids or the loss of base bicarbonate. Strong acid is gained by several specific mechanisms, primarily the following:

1. Gain of exogenous acid (e.g., ammonium chloride) by ingestion or infusion
2. Incomplete oxidation of fatty acids, which occurs in conditions such as diabetic ketoacidosis, starvation (including patients receiving nothing by mouth for therapeutic purposes), and salicylate poisoning
3. Incomplete oxidation of carbohydrate which produces large amounts of lactic acid as a result of primary lactic acidosis (rare) or secondary to tissue hypoxia from excessive exercise, serious trauma, and severe infection
4. Inability of the renal system to excrete the normal, ongoing volume of inorganic acid metabolites, which results from the azotemic acidosis of advanced renal failure

Base bicarbonate is lost from the extracellular fluid by the following two general routes:

1. Losses from the gastrointestinal tract—secretions distal to the pyloric sphincter contain large amounts of bicarbonate, which may be lost during conditions that produce diarrhea or vomiting, including fistula drainage and suction
2. Losses as a result of inappropriate bicarbonate excretion in the kidneys because of renal tubular acidosis

Compensation of metabolic acidosis is achieved through the respiratory system. Strong acids are immediately buffered to generate the weaker carbonic acid, which the respiratory system attempts to eliminate through increased alveolar ventilation. In this respiratory effort the breathing is deep and rapid—the Kussmaul or air-hunger type of respirations. Bicarbonate conservation and excretion by the kidneys is a slower mechanism. Laboratory findings of uncompensated metabolic acidosis include lowered plasma pH (below 7.33), diminished plasma bicarbonate concentration (below 23 mEq per liter in older children, below 20 mEq per liter in young children), and carbon dioxide combining power that is lowered and approximately equivalent to the plasma bicarbonate in concentration.

Treatment is directed at correcting the basic defect and replacing the excessive losses of bicarbonate with sodium or potassium bicarbonate or sodium lactate.

METABOLIC ALKALOSIS

Metabolic alkalosis is an elevated plasma pH that occurs when there is a reduction in hydrogen ion concentration and an excess of base bicarbonate. This can be caused by a gain in base or a loss of acid, which is almost the same as base gain. Loss of acid can result from the following:

1. In children the most common cause of hydrogen ion depletion is loss of hydrochloric acid (HCl) incident to hypertrophic pyloric stenosis. The infant produces large amounts of hydrochloric acid, which is vomited with repeated feedings.
2. Less often, hydrogen ions are lost through the kidneys in diuretic therapy, potassium depletion, or administration of adrenocortical hormones.

A gain in base is usually iatrogenic and relatively uncommon in children but can result from the following:

1. Gain of exogenous bicarbonate from ingestion or infusion
2. Oxidation of salts or organic acid from infusion or ingestion of lactate, citrate, or acetate

Compensation in metabolic alkalosis theoretically should be respiratory; however, such compensation is irregular and unpredictable. In addition, renal correction is complicated by losses of sodium, potassium, and chloride ions, which are lost through vomiting in pyloric stenosis. The kidneys will attempt to conserve the sodium and potassium ion concentration at the expense of hydrogen ion concentration and acid-base balance. Laboratory findings include elevated urine pH (often above 7; may be lowered if associated with potassium ion depletion), elevated plasma pH (above 7.43), elevated plasma bicarbonate concentration (above 29 mEq per liter in older children, above 28 mEq per liter in young children), and, if in conjunction with chloride deficit, reduced chloride ion concentration (below 98 mEq per liter).

Treatment of metabolic alkalosis is aimed at preventing further losses of acid and replacement of lost electrolytes.

Nursing Responsibilities in Fluid and Electrolyte Disturbances

Nursing observation and intervention are essential to the detection and therapeutic management of disturbances in fluid and electrolyte balance. There are a wide variety of circumstances in which imbalances may be precipitated, and the balance is so precarious, especially in infants, that changes can take place in a very short time. Therefore an important nursing responsibility is perceptive observation for any signs of imbalance, particularly in those situations and conditions in which imbalance is likely to occur. Conditions in which changes can develop with surprising rapidity in young children include diarrhea; vomiting; sweating; fever; disorders such as diabetes, renal disease, and cardiac anomalies; administration of certain drugs, such as diuretics and steroids;

and trauma, such as major surgery, burns, and other extensive injury.

Nurses need to be comfortable with equipment used to deliver fluids to infants and children and be familiar with the knowledge and techniques for assessment. An understanding of normal serum levels provides additional data on which to base assessments and interventions and to validate observations. Data that are helpful in assessment related to fluid and electrolyte balance are the medical diagnosis, the treatment that the child is receiving (especially medications and fluid therapies), laboratory reports, history, and records of intake and output. An important nursing role in child care is teaching parents to recognize early signs of dehydration.

ASSESSMENT

The assessment of suspected or potential fluid and electrolyte disturbance begins with the observation of general appearance. Ill children usually have drawn, flaccid expressions, and their eyes lack luster. Loss of appetite is one of the first behaviors observed in the majority of childhood illnesses, and the infant's or child's activity level is diminished. The cry of an ill infant is less vigorous, often whining, and higher pitched than usual. The child is irritable, seeks the comfort and attention of the parent, and displays purposeless movements and inappropriate responses to people and familiar things.

As the child's illness becomes more severe, the irritability progresses to lethargy and even unconsciousness. Much of this information can be elicited from the parent, along with a history of excessive fluid losses, diminished output, and other clues to body fluid disturbance, for example, the number and consistency of stools the child has passed in the past 24 hours, the number of times the child voided, and the type and amount of food and fluid ingested or vomited. Parents frequently omit this information from their discussion with the health professional. They tell how much has been taken but not how much was excreted.

Other observations, as outlined in Table 28-9, are used to arrive at a meaningful assessment. Vital signs are assessed as often as every 15 to 30 minutes, and weight is recorded frequently during the initial phase of therapy. It is important to use the same scale each time the child is weighed and to predetermine the weight of any equipment

Table 28-9 Significance of observations and probable problem

OBSERVATION	SIGNIFICANT VARIATION	PROBABLE IMBALANCE	COMMENTS
Temperature	Elevated	Early water depletion Sodium excess	Elevated temperature will increase rate of water loss
	Lowered	Fluid volume deficit	Caused by reduced energy output Shock is outcome of severe fluid deficit
Pulse	Rapid, weak, thready, easily obliterated	Circulatory collapse may result from fluid deficit, hemorrhage, plasma-to-interstitial fluid shift	Pulse rate should include assessment of volume and quality as well as rate
	Bounding, easily obliterated	Impending circulatory collapse Sodium deficit	Pulse may be influenced by activity or emotions
	Bounding, not easily obliterated	Fluid volume excess Interstitial fluid-to-plasma shift	
	Weak, irregular, rapid	Severe potassium deficit	
	Weak, irregular, slowing	Severe potassium excess	
	Increased	Sodium excess Magnesium deficit	
	Decreased	Magnesium excess	
Respiration	Slow, shallow	Respiratory alkalosis	Rapid respirations increase water loss
	Rapid, deep	Metabolic acidosis	Not a reliable sign of respiratory alkalosis in infants
	Dyspnea	Fluid volume excess either general or pulmonary	
	Moist rales	Fluid volume excess Pulmonary edema	
	Shallow	Potassium excess or deficit	
	Stridor	Severe calcium deficit	
Blood pressure	Increased	Fluid volume excess Sodium deficit	Blood pressure not a reliable sign in young children
	Decreased	Diminished vascular volume (loss or plasma-to-interstitial fluid shift) Severe potassium excess or deficit	Elasticity of blood vessels may keep blood pressure stable

Continued.

Table 28-9 Significance of observations and probable problem—cont'd

OBSERVATION		SIGNIFICANT VARIATION	PROBABLE IMBALANCE	COMMENTS
Skin				
	Color	Pallor	Protein deficit Fluid deficit Fluid compartment shifts Sodium excess	
		Flushed		
	Temperature	Cold extremities	Severe fluid volume deficit, even with fever Severe sodium depletion	Caused by decreased peripheral blood flow
	Feel	Dry	Fluid depletion Sodium excess	
		Clammy, cold	Sodium deficit Plasma-to-interstitial fluid shift Hypotonic dehydration	
		Poor capillary filling	Fluid volume deficit	
	Turgor	Poor to very poor	Fluid depletion	Pinch of skin from abdomen or inner thigh is lifted and remains raised for several seconds
	Pitting edema	Slight to severe	Fluid volume excess Plasma-to-interstitial fluid shift	Obese infants may appear normal
Mucous membranes		Dry Longitudinal wrinkles on tongue	Fluid volume depletion	
		Sticky; rough, red, dry tongue	Sodium excess Hypertonic dehydration	
Salivation and tearing		Absent	Fluid volume deficit	
Fontanel		Sunken	Fluid volume deficit	
Eyeballs		Sunken Soft	Fluid volume deficit	
Sensory alterations		Tingling in fingers and toes	Calcium deficit Alkalosis	Sensory alterations unreliable in infants and young children who are unable to communicate symptoms
		Abdominal cramps	Sodium deficit Potassium excess	
		Muscle cramps	Calcium deficit Potassium deficit	
		Lightheadedness Nausea	Respiratory alkalosis Calcium excess Potassium excess Potassium deficit	
		Thirst	Fluid deficit Sodium excess Calcium excess	May be difficult to assess in infants May be masked by nausea Any condition that reduces intravascular volume will stimulate thirst receptors
Neurologic signs		Hypotonia	Potassium deficit Calcium excess	
		Flaccid paralysis	Severe potassium deficit Severe potassium excess	
		Weakness	Metabolic acidosis	
		Hypertonia 　Positive Chvostek sign 　Tremors, cramps, 　　tetany	Calcium deficit Alkalosis with diminished calcium 　ionization Calcium deficit	Children may suffer calcium deficit easily, since growing bones do not readily relinquish calcium to circulation
		Twitching	Magnesium deficit	

Table 28-9 Significance of observations and probable problem—cont'd

OBSERVATION	SIGNIFICANT VARIATION	PROBABLE IMBALANCE	COMMENTS
Behavior	Lethargy	Fluid volume deficit	Behavioral changes among the first indications of dehydration as reported by parents
	Irritability	Fluid volume deficit	
	Comatose condition	Hypotonic fluid deficit Profound acidosis or alkalosis	
	Lethargy with hyperirritability on stimulation	Hypertonic fluid deficit	
	Extreme restlessness	Potassium excess	

Weight	Loss
	    Up to 5%
	    5% to 9%
	    10% or higher
		Fluid deficit
		    Mild
		    Moderate
		    Severe
		Protein or calorie deficiency	

	Gain	Edema—general or pulmonary Ascites	

Urine	Increased (polyuria)	Interstitial fluid-to-plasma shift
		Increased renal solute load
			Normal range*
			  Newborn: 2.0-12.5 ml/hr
			  Neonatal period: 11-18 ml/hr
			  Infant: 14.5-22.9 ml/hr
			  Child: 20-40 ml/hr
			  Adolescent: 20-62 ml/hr
			    (varies with intake and other factors)

	Diminished	Mild fluid deficit	
	Oliguria	Moderate to severe fluid deficit Plasma-to-interstitial fluid shift Sodium deficit Potassium excess Severe sodium excess Renal insufficiency	
	Specific gravity Low (1.010 or less)	Adequate hydration Fluid excess Renal disease Sodium deficit	Used to monitor hydration status in infants Fixed low reading occurs in renal disease
	High (1.030 or more)	Fluid deficit Sodium excess Glycosuria Proteinuria	
	pH Acid	Acidosis—metabolic or respiratory Alkalosis accompanied by severe potassium deficit	
	Alkaline	Alkalosis—metabolic or respiratory Hyperaldosteronism Acidosis accompanied by chronic renal infection and renal tubular dysfunction Diuretic therapy with carbonic anhydrase inhibitors	

*Data from Behrman, R.E., and Vaughan, V.C., III, editors: Nelson textbook of pediatrics, ed. 12, Philadelphia, 1983, W.B. Saunders Co.

or device that must remain attached during the weighing process, including armboards and sandbags. Routine weights should be taken at the same time each day.

Intake and Output (I & O) Measurement

One of the most important roles of the nurse in fluid and electrolyte disturbance is related to intake and output. Accurate measurements are essential to the assessment of fluid balance. Measurements—include both gastrointestinal and parenteral intake and output from urine, stools, vomitus, fistulas, nasogastric suction, sweat, and drainage from wounds. Although the physician usually indicates when intake and output are to be recorded, it is a nursing responsibility to keep an accurate intake and output record on patients in the following situations:

Receiving intravenous therapy
After major surgery

Severe thermal burns or injuries
Renal disease or damage
Congestive heart failure
Dehydration
Diabetes mellitus
Oliguria
Diuretic therapy
Corticosteroid therapy

Infants or small children who are unable to use a bedpan or those who have bowel movements with every voiding will require the application of a collecting device (p. 1127). Collecting bags may not be suitable for all infants, for example, preterm and other infants whose fragile skin does not tolerate self-adhesive appliances. If collecting bags are not used, wet diapers or pads are carefully weighed to ascertain the amount of fluid lost. This includes liquid stool, vomitus, and other losses. The volume of fluid in milliliters is equivalent to the weight of the fluid measured in grams. The specific gravity as a measure of osmolality is determined with a urinometer or a refractometer and assists in assessing the degree of hydration.

There are disadvantages to the weighed diaper method of fluid measurement. It is impossible to differentiate one type of loss from another because of admixture; the total excreted may not be collected on the diaper (especially in male infants), and the frequency is unknown unless the infant is observed voiding. When accurate urine evaluation is needed, the urine must be caught before it soaks into the diaper. Also, evaporative losses render measurements inaccurate unless the diaper is weighed and measured for specific gravity at least every 30 minutes when critical values are needed. There is a significant error in measurements delayed more than 60 minutes (Williams and Kanarek, 1982). Evaporative losses are greater in infants under radiant warmers or being treated with phototherapy.

At home parents are advised to observe the number of times and how much the child voids. Infants younger than 1 year of age normally void every 1 to 2 hours; toddlers urinate approximately every 3 hours. As children get older, they void less frequently. The parents are instructed to notify the nurse or clinician if the child appears to be voiding an insufficient amount or persistently losing fluid through vomiting or diarrhea.

ORAL FLUID INTAKE

Under ordinary circumstances an adequate oral intake is no problem in children who are able to respond to thirst cues. Hydration becomes a nursing problem when infants or children are unable to respond to the thirst mechanism and when fatigue or discomfort makes them reluctant to swallow. Children with elevated temperatures, those with continued gastrointestinal losses, and those with labile diabetes are especially prone to dehydration. Occasionally dehydration, caused by inadequate intake has been observed in breast-fed infants (Rowland and others, 1982).

Table 28-10 Sodium, potassium, and caloric content of commonly administered oral fluids

FLUID	Na+ (mEq/liter)	K+ (mEq/liter)	CALORIES (Kcal/liter)
Water	0	0	0
Sugar water (5%)	0	0	200
Lytren	25	25	280
Pedialyte	30	20	280
Coca-Cola	*	*	435
Pepsi Cola	*	*	480
Ginger ale	*	*	380
7-Up	*	*	420
Orange juice	2	48.5	410
Apple juice	1.8	26.7	517
Gatorade	0.23	2.5	167

*Varies according to mineral content of water used for bottling.

A number of common fluids found in hospitals and in the home are acceptable for the management of dehydration, including diluted fruit juice, liquid or solid gelatin, sweetened tea, Popsicles, and decarbonated cola or ginger ale. A carbonated drink is easily decarbonated (or made "flat") by pouring some in a glass with a spoon in it and allowing the liquid to stand at room temperature for a short time. When teaching parents about fluid management, it is always wise to determine whether or not they understand the concept of clear liquids. Any liquid through which newsprint can be read is considered to be clear. It is important to emphasize that milk is not a liquid, since it forms curds when it comes in contact with stomach renin.

If an electrolyte formula is prescribed, it is advisable to have the parents demonstrate their ability to prepare it, because a mistake or misunderstanding of measurements, for example, substitution of a tablespoon for the teaspoon measure, using heaping rather than level measurements, or adding other ingredients, such as milk, can significantly alter the electrolyte concentration. Parents are cautioned about including broth as fluid intake. When prepared as directed on the labels, most commercial broths contain unusually high sodium concentrations. Parents should consult with a dietician or the physician for proper dilution of these fluids before offering them to a child who is suffering from large fluid losses. The calorie content and electrolyte composition of some common fluids are listed in Table 28-10.

Getting a reluctant child to drink fluids can be a nursing problem and is not uncommon in the care of infants and children. Older children will often respond to the challenge of meeting a specific goal for fluid intake (or deprivation) and can be active participants in planning an intake schedule. Contracts and rewards are effective strategies. However, young children require more creative tactics. A number of suggestions for encouraging children to drink fluids are discussed on p. 1115.

NASOGASTRIC ALIMENTATION

Special problems are encountered with infants and children who must be fed through a nasogastric or gastrostomy tube and those who require nasogastric suction. Nasogastric suction removes important electrolytes and fluid from the stomach and intestine, which must be replaced by the parenteral route. If replacement is omitted or inadequate, imbalance is likely to occur; therefore an accurate record of the amount and type of fluid entering and leaving the tube is crucial. When the tube requires irrigation to maintain patency, an electrolyte solution, usually saline, is used to prevent further depletion of electrolytes, since plain water irrigation stimulates electrolyte secretion and removal.

Tube-fed children are vulnerable to imbalances, principally in relation to solute load, with the ever-present threat of fluid deficit. This is especially true when tube feedings contain a large concentration of protein and the water intake is limited. An osmotic diuresis associated with the solute load can cause water to be drawn from tissues to supply a deceptively adequate urine output. Eventually hypernatremic dehydration and accumulation of nitrogenous waste products will occur. It is the nurse's responsibility to ensure an adequate water intake because most of these children, such as infants and unconscious, confused, or mentally retarded children, are unable to perceive or respond to the stimulus of thirst. These children are unable to communicate the need for fluid. They must rely on the nurse's competency to assess the adequacy of hydration, to recognize signs of fluid deficit or hyperelectrolytemia, and to take appropriate action.

Infants or children who are unable to take fluid by mouth will require special mouth care. Oral hygiene, a part of routine hygienic care, is especially important when fluids are restricted or withheld. The mouth can be cleaned and kept moist by swabbing with moistened gauze or Toothettes. Water sprayed into the mouth from a perfume atomizer is refreshing and relieves a dry mouth. A thin layer of white petrolatum helps to keep lips soft and prevents cracking and caking. To meet the need to suck, infants should be provided with a pacifier, preferably an acceptable commercial variety. Aspiration of a nipple used to construct a pacifier has been reported (Millunchick and McArtor, 1986).

Complications

To prevent imbalances resulting from the inadvertent substitution of salt for sugar in infant or nasogastric formulas, great care should be exerted in their preparation. Children, especially infants, can be quickly subject to life-threatening hypernatremic dehydration from this rare but conceivable accident. It is important to stress to parents and others responsible for mixing formula feedings the harm that excessive sodium intake can cause and the simple modes of prevention. The hazard is not limited to infants. A teenager who had recently undergone surgery for an esophageal stricture and was receiving nasogastric tube feedings was given formula in which salt had been substituted for sugar during preparation. He developed a fever, physical signs of dehydration, and extreme lethargy before the cause was detected by serum electrolyte examination. Laboratory electrolyte values were hematocrit, 44%; sodium, 187 mEq/liter; chloride, 169 mEq/liter; carbon dioxide, 18 mEq/liter; and potassium, 3.4 mEq/liter. Intravenous fluid therapy produced a gradual reduction of sodium and chloride to normal levels over 48 hours, cleared his sensorium, and relieved other signs of dehydration. In this instance it was the nurse who persistently pointed out the significant observations that resulted in the correct diagnosis.

Aspiration. The danger of aspiration is reduced in children with nasogastric tubes in place. However, the child may dislodge the tube with random or purposeful movements and pose the risk of aspirating fluids that remain in the tube or from reflux of stomach contents following feedings. Aspiration is usually manifested by coughing, choking, gurgling sounds with respiration, and signs of respiratory distress including restlessness, diaphoresis, and pallor or cyanosis.

It is best to call for assistance, especially if suction equipment is not readily available. The tube is removed immediately; no effort should be made to replace the tube. The child is placed on the left side with the head of the bed lowered. The left bronchus is less vertical than the right, and therefore the left side position makes it less likely that any remaining solution will move further into the respiratory tree. The mouth and pharynx are suctioned followed by administration of oxygen. Deep tracheal suctioning may be indicated, and a manual resuscitation bag should be at hand in case the child stops breathing. The physician is notified, and preparations are made for possible diagnostic tests including radiographs and blood gases. Vital signs are monitored frequently and observed for signs of respiratory distress. The child may need to be transferred to the intensive care unit.

PARENTERAL FLUID THERAPY

Since most hospitalized infants and children with serious disturbance of fluid and electrolyte balance are maintained with intravenous fluids, monitoring intravenous fluid replacement is a major nursing responsibility. Most of the general principles of intravenous therapy apply to infants and children, but with a number of important variations.

Preparation

Before an intravenous infusion is started, several preparatory activities must take place. All needed equipment is gathered so that the operator can proceed without interruption. More importantly, the child and the family must be prepared for this universally stressful procedure.

Solution. The composition of intravenous solution is selected on the basis of tonicity (osmolality) and electrolyte content. A solution that is *isotonic* has the same osmolality, or tonicity, as body fluids such as plasma. A *hypertonic*

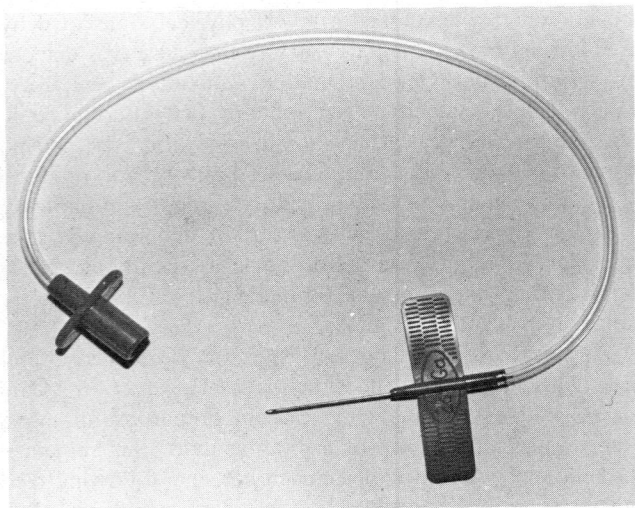

Fig. 28-2. Scalp vein needle.

solution is one that has a greater concentration of solutes than plasma; a *hypotonic* solution has a lower concentration. Examples of isotonic solutions are 0.9% saline solution and 5% dextrose in water; 10% glucose in water is a hypertonic solution; plain water and 0.2% sodium are hypotonic solutions. Although it is larger, one molecule of glucose has only half the osmolality of one molecule of sodium chloride because the sodium chloride ionizes in solution into two particles, the sodium and the chloride ions. Thus one molecule of sodium chloride exerts twice the osmotic pressure of one molecule of glucose.

Because infants and young children are subject to rapid fluid shifts, any intravenous solution given to them contains at least 0.2% sodium chloride to prevent brain edema, a disorder to which they are susceptible if given plain water. Glucose is rapidly metabolized; therefore the osmolality of 5% glucose is further diminished.

Equipment. For most intravenous infusions in children, a scalp-vein (butterfly) needle, size 21 or 23, is used with flexible winged tabs that are easily secured to the skin (Fig. 28-2). For long-term therapy a 22- or 24-gauge over-the-needle catheter is preferred, and in situations in which fluids are urgently needed and there is difficulty in entering a vein, a polyethylene tube inserted by the surgical cutdown procedure may be necessary. The vein of choice for this alternative is the internal saphenous vein located just anterior to the medial malleolus of the tibia.

Other equipment needed includes alcohol or povodine-iodine swabs to clean the site, a tourniquet, an appropriate-sized padded armboard (when an extremity is used), sandbags, rolled towels or small blankets for maintaining position of head or extremity, tape (or dressing and bacteriostatic ointment if hospital dictates), and a device to protect the IV site after insertion. The prescribed solution, tubing, filter, and infusion pump are prepared in advance, ready to connect to the needle after insertion.

Infusion pumps. There are several modifications in equipment used for intravenous infusion for children. A gravity drainage apparatus used for children is much the same as that for adults except that it is designed to deliver a reduced drop size (60 drops per ml) and contains a calibrated volume control chamber (such as a Buretrol or Soluset) that regulates the amount of fluid that can be infused. A microdropper greatly facilitates calculation of flow rate because a prescribed number of milliliters per hour equals the number of drops per minute. For example, if the solution is to infuse at a rate of 30 ml per hour, the infusion is regulated to deliver 30 drops per minute.

A variety of types of pumps are available, but all have a limited capacity, refillable from the bottle above, to minimize the possibility of overloading the circulation (Fig. 28-3). When using this device, it is important that the tubing between the bottle and the chamber is firmly clamped to prevent additional fluid from dripping into the chamber. When pumps with collapsible chambers and rigid cylinders with an automatic shutoff valve are employed, the infusion stops automatically when the chamber is empty. It is an important nursing responsibility to calculate the amount to be

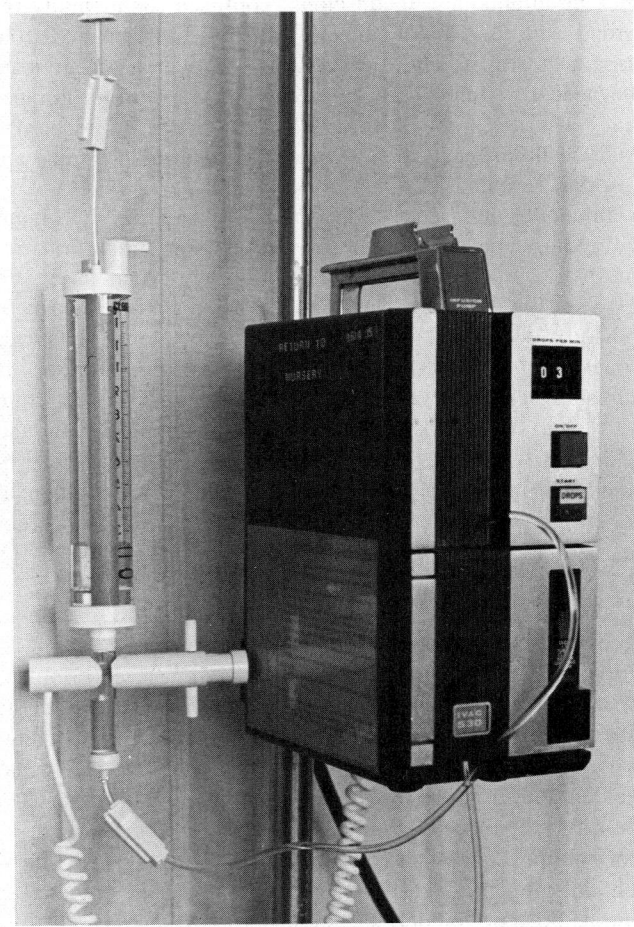

Fig. 28-3. Gravity drainage apparatus attached to an infusion pump for administration of intravenous fluids.
IVAC Corp.

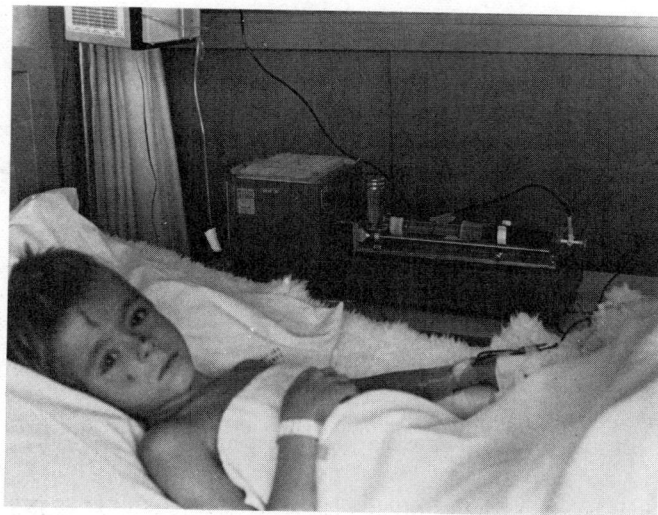

Fig. 28-4. Syringe (Harvard) pump for infusion of a very small amount of fluid over a specified period of time.

infused in a given length of time, set the infusion rate, and monitor the apparatus frequently to make certain that the desired rate is maintained and the infusion does not stop.

To facilitate a more precise flow rate, a number of continuous infusion pumps are now available and are used almost exclusively for pediatric intravenous fluid administration. Most of these devices pump a given amount of fluid by peristaltic action on the tubing, governed by a flow rate setting, and regulated by a drop sensor that activates an alarm when no drops are formed. Some of the newer devices have a volume control built into the major mechanism. For administering a very small amount of fluid over a specific time, precision-controlled syringe pumps may be preferable (Fig. 28-4). These devices, although convenient and efficient, are not without attendant risks. Overreliance on the accuracy of the machine can cause either too much or too little fluid to be infused; therefore its use does not obviate careful periodic assessment by the nurse. Excess pressure can build up if the machine is set at a rate faster than the vein is able to accommodate (or continues to pump when the needle is out of the lumen). This is especially true in very small infants and when circumstances necessitate the use of a capillary. No matter what device is used, a thorough understanding of the apparatus is essential for safe fluid administration.

Preparing the Child and Parents

Children of any age are anxious and fearful of injections, and unless the intravenous infusion is implemented as an emergency procedure, there will be time to prepare the child (see p. 1104 for Preparation for procedures). Many children have never undergone the procedure, and those who have will retain memories of the experience. It is useful to ask each child what he thinks about the procedure and why it is needed for him specifically. Children's perceptions of the anticipated experience furnish information on misconceptions that need to be clarified and help the nurse prepare children for what they can expect. In addition, children's observations provide some insight into how to cope with a child's reactions during the insertion procedure and throughout the course of the intravenous therapy (Guhlow and Kolb, 1979).

Play, always an excellent stress-reducing technique, can be employed during the preparation process. Allowing children to handle the equipment and to "start" an intravenous infusion on a toy animal or doll helps familiarize them with the frightening aspects of the procedure. In some instances it may be helpful to introduce a child to another child who is coping well in the same situation (Piercy, 1981).

It is best to arrange for a quiet, private setting for the child during the insertion. The assurance of privacy relieves the child of some anxieties concerning loss of control in front of others. It also avoids subjecting other children to the potentially stress-provoking scene. The child should be provided with some distracting activity, such as those described for injections, and perhaps be allowed to "help" by holding supplies such as a gauze square, helping to clean the site with alcohol, and assisting in taping the site after the procedure.

Children will usually cooperate better and feel more in command if they are allowed to sit up during the process, although this may not be possible even with some older, normally cooperative children. It is a mistake to assume that children will not lose control even after they promise to cooperate. It is wise to have ample assistance available in the event a child cannot control his anxieties. The child need not be restrained until necessary, but the assisting nurse should be prepared to grasp the child gently but firmly during the insertion. Explaining to children what is being done during each step of the procedure and how they can participate helps to obtain their cooperation and reduce their stress.

Parents should be told about the procedure, including the reason for the procedure, how long the needle must remain in place, and what they can expect during and after the insertion. Sometimes the parents are encouraged to participate by providing support and comfort to the child during the procedure; at other times they are advised to remain outside but ready to comfort the child after the insertion. Many parents find it too distressful and become upset because they are unable to comfort and protect the child from pain. If the parents remain with the child during venipuncture, they should not be responsible for restraining the child. They can be reassured that children usually handle the situation well, and they should be told exactly what to expect in order to avoid communicating their own anxiety to the child (Piercy, 1981).

The Procedure

The site selected for intravenous infusion depends on accessibility and convenience. In older children any accessible vein may be used. Whenever possible, it is best to avoid the child's favored hand in order to reduce the disability related

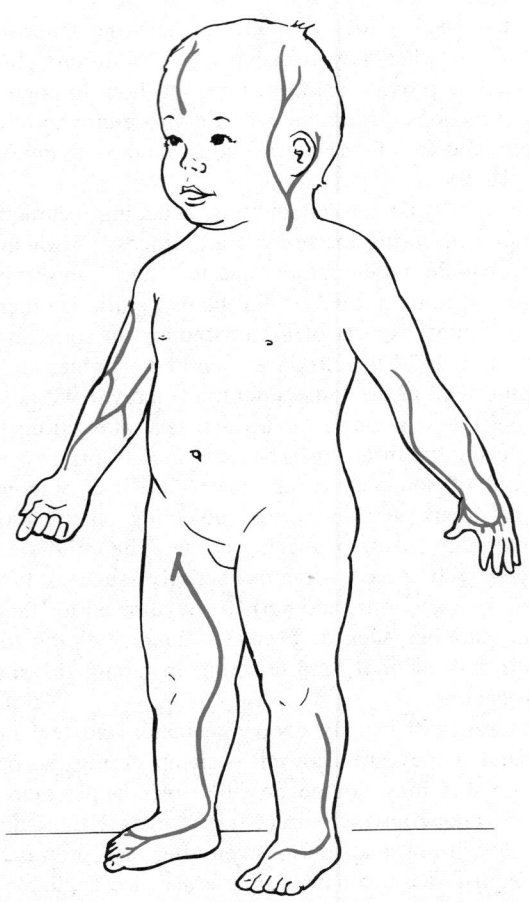

Fig. 28-5. Superficial veins used most often for intravenous infusion in infants and very young children.
From Kempe, C.H., Silver, H.K., and O'Brien, D.: Current pediatric diagnosis and treatment, ed. 9, Los Altos, Calif., 1986, Lange Medical Publications.

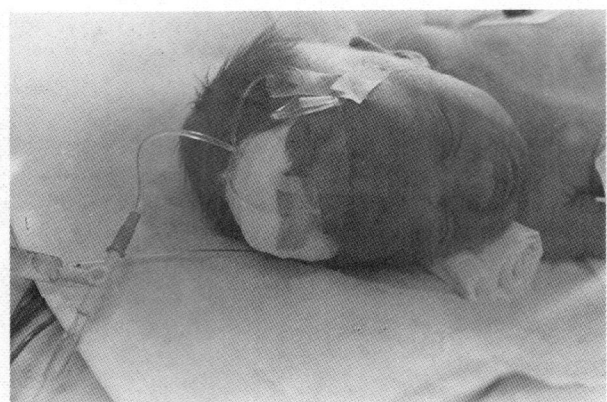

Fig. 28-6. Scalp vein infusion.

to the procedure. A site is chosen that restricts the child's movements as little as possible—a site over a joint in an extremity is avoided. An older child can help to select the site and thereby maintain some measure of control. In small infants a scalp vein or a superficial vein of the wrist, hand, foot, or arm is usually convenient and most easily stabilized (Fig. 28-5).

Most children have 1 or 2 possible intravenous sites on each arm and foot and 4 to 8 sites on the scalp. Since superficial veins of the scalp have no valves, they can be infused in either direction and are frequently used for intravenous therapy in infants less than 9 months of age. The temporal and forehead areas are suitable and do not interfere with side-to-side head movements. Scalp veins have little subcutaneous tissue to obscure visualization of the vein, and there are no joints to interfere with movement. However, the use of a scalp vein site requires shaving the area around the site to better visualize the vein and provide a smooth surface on which to tape the tubing (Fig. 28-6). Shaving off a portion of the infant's hair is very upsetting to parents; therefore they should *always* be told what to expect and reassured that the hair will grow in again rapidly (save the

hair because parents often wish to keep it). As little as possible is removed directly over the insertion site. A rubber band slipped onto the head from brow to occiput will usually suffice as a tourniquet.

The extremity or head should be restrained for easier venipuncture and to minimize trauma resulting from the child's inadvertent movement. Extremities are secured to the armboard when those sites are used, and head movements are restrained for scalp venipuncture. (See also p. 1120 for additional restraining methods.) For a scalp site it is helpful to visualize the way in which the needle will be secured following insertion (Arthur, 1984).

Locating a vein may be difficult because the veins are smaller and children have a significant amount of subcutaneous fat. When veins are not readily visible, applying a warm compress to the site or, when using an extremity, holding the limb in a dependent position below body level will help fill the veins for better visualization. Gentle tapping sometimes causes the veins to stand out. A flashlight held against the skin below the intended site sometimes assists in locating vessels. If these measures do not help, a tourniquet applied with light pressure medially to the site may be needed. Although the tourniquet makes the veins more visible and provides a more rapid blood return, the added venous pressure may cause fragile veins to "blow" when punctured, producing a hematoma.

The needle must be placed in the direction of the blood flow, which creates no problem when an extremity is used. Scalp veins are more difficult to assess. In general, the venous blood flows from the top of the head toward the neck. To test the direction before insertion, the forefinger is placed on the vein at the site chosen for venipuncture. While the finger gently presses the vein, a second finger is used to "strip" the vein in the direction of the top of the head. The pressure from the second finger is released. If the vein fills distal to the compressing finger, the direction of flow is toward the stationary finger (Arthur, 1984).

To maintain the integrity of the intravenous site, adequate restraint will be required for the child. An attempt is made to place the extremity in a natural anatomic position

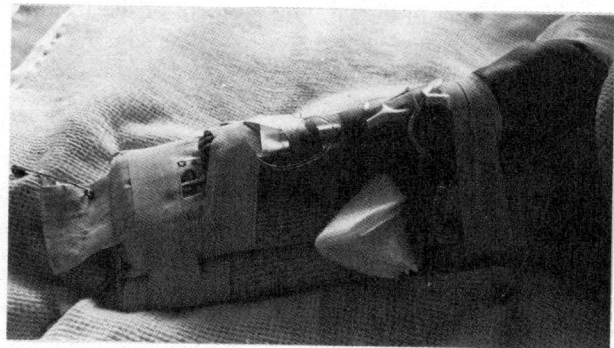

Fig. 28-7. Extremity immobilized with board and firmly secured to bedding with pins.

with the use of gauze pads or rolls as needed. A sandbag or a small board, well padded with plastic foam and a cloth or stockinette cover, provides a suitable means for immobilization (Fig. 28-7). Some form of resilient padding is required to prevent areas of pressure necrosis over bony prominences such as the ankle or pressure on the peroneal nerve on the lateral aspect of the knee. The head can be immobilized with covered sandbags. To prevent trauma to the skin from removal of tape, gauze can be placed between the skin and the adhesive.

Following insertion, the needle is firmly secured at the puncture site with nonallergenic tape and protected from becoming dislodged by immobilization of the extremity. The insertion site and about 1 inch of skin beyond the site are left uncovered for early detection of infiltration. Clear plastic dressings are ideal because they allow ready visualization of the insertion site. Some finger or toe areas are left unoccluded by dressings or tape to allow for assessment of circulation. The thumb is never immobilized because of the danger of contractures with limited movement later on. A plastic or wax paper cup that is cut in half (with the rigid edges covered with tape) and applied directly over the needle site will further protect the infusion. Some needle containers make excellent protective covers. A colorful and interesting sticker can be applied to the armboard or protective device to add a positive note to the procedure.

Older children who are alert and cooperative can usually be trusted to protect the intravenous site. Infants, small children, and uncooperative children require varying degrees of immobilization, and sometimes complete restriction of movement may be needed to prevent removal of the intravenous infusion. The board is secured to the bed, and extremities that might be used to dislodge the needle are restrained. This includes feet as well as hands, since most infants will attempt to brush away the offending attachment by rubbing it against another extremity or body part.

Immobilization is intolerable to the naturally active child, and every effort should be extended to relieve the stress of immobilization (see Chapter 40). Frequent removal of the restraints provides the child with the opportunity to move the extremities. Whenever possible, the infant or child

Questions and Controversies

Should a nurse irrigate an intravenous catheter that is not running and may be clotted?

A great deal of controversy has been generated by the question of whether or not an intravenous catheter can be safely irrigated to reestablish flow. The problem is rarely addressed in textbooks, and no controlled scientific studies have been conducted to confirm or refute the practice. Although most hospital policies discourage this alternative, the practice is widespread and supports the justification for irrigating. No confirmed pulmonary embolism from irrigating a peripheral or central intravenous catheter has been reported (Feldstein, 1985).

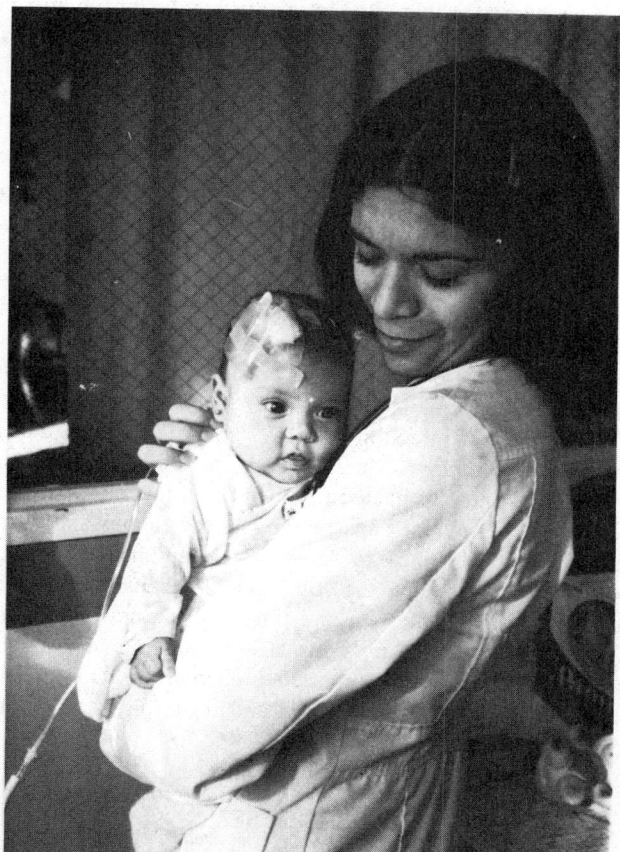

Fig. 28-8. Intravenous infusion does not prevent infant from being picked up and cuddled.

should be held and cuddled to help meet his emotional needs during this trying time (Fig. 28-8). Range of motion exercises are employed on infants and children who are too ill or unable to move their extremities, but others should be encouraged to move their arms and legs in response to a natural stimulus. Most infants or small children will instinctively move their extremities when released. If not, a toy or other stimulus can provide incentive.

The same precautions regarding maintenance of asepsis, prevention of infection, and observation for infiltration are carried out with patients of any age. However, infiltration is more difficult to detect in infants and small children than it is in adults. The increased amount of subcutaneous fat and the amount of tape used to secure the needle often obscure the signs of early infiltration. When the fluid appears to be infusing too slowly or ceases, the usual assessment for obstruction within the apparatus, that is, kinks, screw clamps, shutoff valve, and positioning interference (e.g., a bent elbow), often locates the difficulty. When these actions fail to detect the problem, it may be necessary to carefully remove some of the tape and other material that obscures a clear view of the venipuncture site. Dependent areas, such as the palm and undersides of the extremity or the occiput and behind the ears, are examined.

Whenever possible, the intravenous infusion should be placed in an extremity to which the identification band (or bracelet) is not attached. Serious circulatory impairment can result from infiltrated solution distal to the band, which acts as a tourniquet preventing adequate venous return. To check for return blood flow through the needle, the bottle is lowered below the level of the infusion site. If the tubing is connected to an infusion pump, it must be removed from the pump before lowering.

An intravenous infusion is not always a deterrent to mobility. When the child is feeling well and the insertion site is well secured, the child can be held or be walked, but precautions must be observed to preserve the integrity of the intravenous system.

Prevention of infection is a major nursing function during intravenous therapy. The infusion site is protected from trauma and entry of bacteria. When an intravenous infusion continues for several days or longer, the tubing and bottle are changed every 24 to 48 hours depending on hospital policy. To ensure that the equipment is changed regularly, it is labeled with the date and time that the new bottle and tubing are attached. Any signs of inflammation such as redness or pain should be reported immediately. This usually requires removal of the infusion and restarting it at another site.

LONG-TERM VENOUS ACCESS

Even greater mobility is possible with the use of the heparin lock system. The heparin lock is used as an alternative for a keep-open infusion when extended access to a vein is required without the need for fluid. It is most frequently employed for intermittent infusion of medication into a preestablished venous route. A short, flexible catheter or scalp vein needle is used for the heparin lock device, and a site is selected where there will be minimum movement, such as the forearm. The needle is inserted and secured in the same manner as any intravenous infusion device, but the needle hub is occluded with a stopper.

The type of device used may vary among medical establishments, and the care and use of the heparin lock are carried out according to the specific protocol of the institution or unit. However, the general concept is the same. The needle remains in place and is flushed with heparin following infusion of the medication. The heparin solution prevents blood from clotting in the needle between infusions. Children may be discharged with a heparin lock in place in order that they can continue receiving medications without hospitalization. Heparin locks are usually reserved for children who require medications on a short-term basis. Those who require long-term chemotherapy are best managed with a central venous catheter.

The children and parents are taught the procedure before discharge from the hospital, including preparation and injection of the prescribed medication, the heparin flush, and dressing changes. A protective device may be recommended for some active children to prevent their accidentally dislodging the needle. An eye bubble shield taped over the needle provides excellent protection. Many children take responsibility for preparing and administering medications (Fig. 28-9). The procedure is explained and demonstrated. Both verbal and written step-by-step instructions are provided for the learners as well as ample opportunities for questions and practice (see Home care instructions on caring for a heparin lock*).

Other alternatives for long-term venous access include the indwelling central venous catheters (Broviac or Hickman catheters) and implantable infusion ports (Infuse-A-Port, MediPort, Port-A-Cath). With the patient under local or general anesthesia, the central venous catheter is placed with meticulous aseptic technique. The jugular or subclavian vein is entered through a small cutdown site and threaded to the right atrium, confirmed by fluoroscopic dye injection, and then sutured in place. To stabilize the catheter, the remainder is tunneled beneath the skin to exit through a small incision at a convenient location on the anterior aspect of the chest (Fig. 28-10). The cutdown site is surgically closed, the catheter is sutured to the skin at the exit site, and a sterile dressing applied. An alternative method eliminates the second site by simply introducing the catheter into the central venous location through a single cutdown or percutaneous puncture site into the vein of choice, usually the subclavian vein.

The smaller Broviac catheter is used most often in children. No matter which catheter is used, the child and family are taught the care and management of the device with provision for practice under supervision (Fig. 28-11). It can be frightening to the child and parents to know that the catheter tip is situated in the heart. They need reassurance that they will do no harm to the apparatus. It is often useful to introduce the family to other children and families who are using central venous catheters successfully. They are able to share concerns and helpful tips regarding care and management. This sharing is especially valuable for teenage patients. Because teenagers usually have a positive attitude toward the

---

*Wong, D.L., and Whaley, L.F.: Clinical handbook of pediatric nursing, ed. 2, St. Louis, 1986, The C.V. Mosby Co.

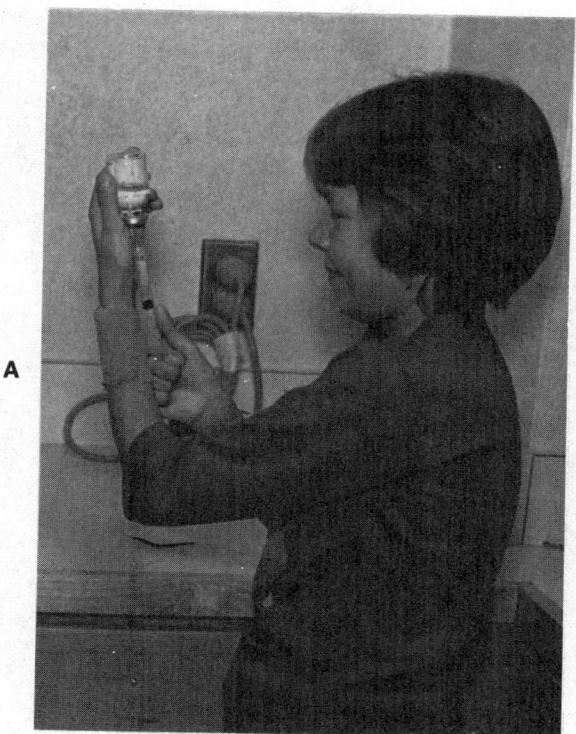

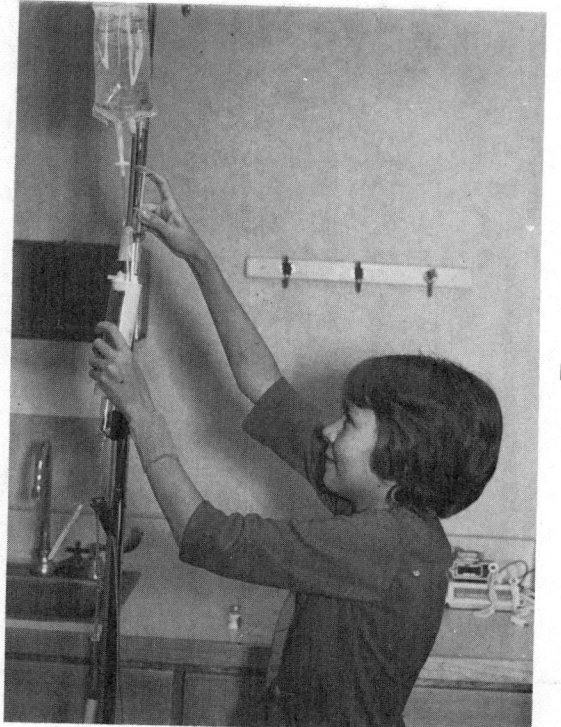

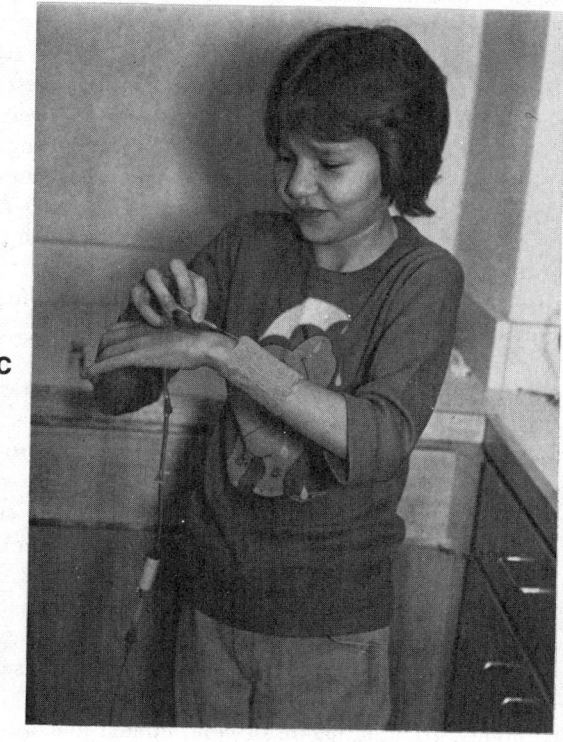

Fig. 28-9. Child preparing and injecting medication by way of heparin lock. **A,** Withdrawing medication. **B,** Injecting medication into Soluset. **C,** Injecting intravenous line into heparin lock.

catheter, it is beneficial for them to share their experiences with adolescents who face the prospect of catheter placement (Bergman, 1985).

Parents of children who engage in outside activities, go to school, or are otherwise under the supervision of another adult should inform the teacher, coach, and baby-sitter about the presence of the central venous catheter. Grandpar-

ents and other family members who care for the child are taught the care and management of the catheter by the nurse or the parents.

Procedures and published standards for catheter care vary widely among organizations, and there is no evidence that one method is superior to another. For example, some advocate covering the healed catheter site with a dressing; others do not. All companies that manufacture central venous catheters have patient and professional teaching kits. (See also Home care instructions on caring for a Hickman/Broviac Catheter*.)

The Broviac catheter is not a deterrent to most activities, including showers or even swimming. However, the physician should be consulted before either of these is attempted. The site is covered with a plastic dressing before entering the water, and a fresh dressing is applied immediately after getting out of the shower or pool.

Infection and a clotted catheter are possible complications of central venous catheters, but neither is an emergency. Uncapping can be prevented by taping the cap securely to the catheter and the clamped line to the dressing. Leaks can be prevented by using a smooth-edged clamp dur-

---

*Wong, D.L., and Whaley, L.F.: Clinical handbook of pediatric nursing, ed. 2, St. Louis, 1986, The C.V. Mosby Co.

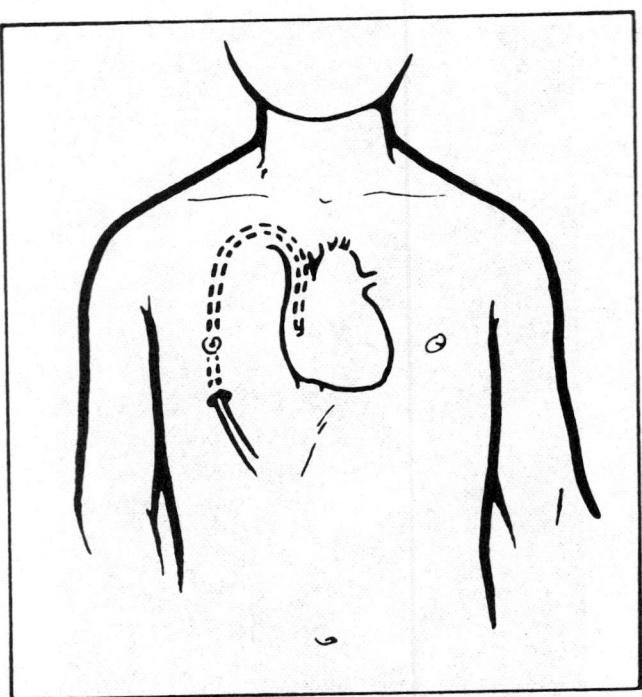

Fig. 28-10. Central venous catheter insertion site.

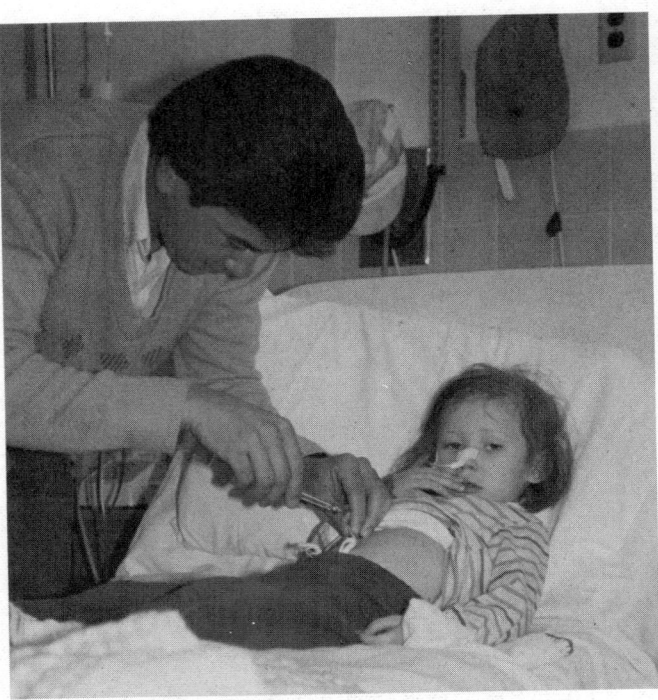

Fig. 28-11. A parent flushing a central venous catheter.
Photography by Katherine L. Patterson, University of Kansas Medical Center, Kansas City, KS.

ing dressing changes. Parents should be cautioned to keep scissors away from the child to prevent accidental cutting of the catheter. If the catheter leaks, they are instructed to tape it above the leak and then clamp the catheter at the taped site. The child should be taken to the physician as soon as possible to prevent infection or clotting following a catheter leak, although this is no longer considered an emergency (Vogel and McSkimming, 1983).

Adolescents may benefit from the implantable ports, which consist of a small circular "port-of-entry" that is placed under the skin (while the patient is under local anesthesia) over a bony prominence to provide a stable surface—usually under the distal third of the clavicle. A tunnel is created from the port to the point where the catheter enters a central vein leading to the right atrium. Medication or other solution is injected with a special needle through the skin into the port. The device can remain situated indefinitely. Adolescents who are highly concerned about body image and may be troubled by the highly visible Broviac catheter often prefer this method of venous access. One disadvantage of an infusion port is that it requires repeated skin punctures, which may make it less acceptable to children.

INTRAVENOUS ALIMENTATION

Another advance in intravenous therapy is total parenteral nutrition (TPN), also known as intravenous alimentation, which provides for the total nutritional needs of infants or children whose lives are threatened because feeding by way of the gastrointestinal tract is impossible, inadequate, or hazardous. Common conditions for which total parenteral

nutrition is used therapeutically include chronic intestinal obstruction from peritoneal sepsis or adhesions, bowel fistulas, inadequate intestinal length, chronic nonremitting severe diarrhea, extensive body burns, abdominal tumors treated by surgery, irradiation, and chemotherapy. It may also be initiated prophylactically in situations in which prolonged starvation is expected.

Hyperalimentation therapy involves intravenous infusion of highly concentrated solutions of protein, glucose, and other nutrients. The hyperalimentation solution is infused either through conventional tubing with a Millipore filter attached to remove particulate matter or microorganisms that may have contaminated the solution or through a Broviac catheter if long-term therapy is anticipated. The highly concentrated solutions require infusion into a vessel with sufficient volume and turbulence to allow for rapid dilution. The wide-diameter vessels selected are the superior vena cava and innominate or intrathoracic subclavian veins approached by way of the external or internal jugular veins. In some situations the inferior vena cava from a femoral vein serves as an alternative route.

The highly irritating nature of concentrated glucose precludes the use of the small peripheral veins in most instances. However, dilute glucose-protein hydrolysates that are appropriate for infusing into peripheral veins are being used with increasing frequency. When peripheral veins are used, intralipids become the major calorie source. Since this fat solution cannot be mixed with the glucose solutions, it requires administration through a separate bottle and tubing that enters the circuit near the venous entry site through a Y type of injection adapter. There is controversy regarding whether this secondary route should be used for intravenous administration of medication, open central venous pressure monitoring, and blood withdrawal. Most authorities believe that the risk of infection is great enough to warrant an additional intravenous infusion site for purposes other than total parenteral nutrition; however, this is a source of dispute.

Complications

Complications from total parenteral nutrition are numerous, and a major nursing responsibility is to prevent these when possible and to be alert to signs of their development. Complications either are related to the infusate (metabolic complications) or result from the presence of the indwelling catheter. Metabolic complications are associated with the infant's or child's tolerance for the various components of the hyperalimentation solution. Excessive intake of any of the components will create an imbalance, for example, hyperglycemia, azotemia, acid-base disorders, hyperosmotic dehydration and coma, fluid overload, and a variety of electrolyte imbalances. With the increased use of long-term therapy, vitamin and mineral deficiencies are being observed (Rombeau and Caldwell, 1986).

Liver disease is the most important gastrointestinal complication in pediatric populations. The cause is obscure, but liver disease appears to be more prevalent in preterm infants who have minimum enteral feedings and who were begun on TPN at an early age (Ament, 1986). Affected children develop cholestasis, hepatocellular necrosis, and, in advanced disease, cirrhosis or hepatic failure. Manifestations include hepatomegaly, jaundice, and elevated serum transaminase, bilirubin, and alkaline phosphatase levels, which become evident approximately 2 weeks after initiation of TPN. Cholelithiasis is an uncommon but possible occurrence in pediatric patients. Therefore children on TPN should be assessed periodically for signs and symptoms of cholelithiasis and/or cholecystitis (Roslyn and others, 1983).

Catheter-related complications include those involving catheter placement, such as pneumothorax, hemothorax, perforation, and catheter dislodgement. The major complication associated with the catheter is infection: infection at catheter entrance site, catheter "seeding" sepsis, venous thrombosis with infection and embolization, and endocarditis.

Meticulous monitoring of patients on total parenteral nutrition is needed to avoid complications. General physical assessment and special observations of vital signs, daily weights, intake and output measurements, and monitoring acid-base status, as well as checking results of laboratory tests, facilitate early detection of infection or fluid and electrolyte imbalance. Additional amounts of potassium and sodium chloride are often required in total parenteral nutrition; therefore observation for signs of potassium or sodium deficit or excess is part of nursing care. This is rarely a problem except in children with reduced renal function or metabolic defects. Vitamin and mineral deficits are a possible complication of TPN unless appropriate mineral replacements are added to the hyperalimentation solution. Signs of possible deficits include rashes from zinc deficiency and bone changes from rickets.

Another problem may occur during the first few days as the child adapts to the high-glucose load of the hyperalimentation solution. The addition of insulin to the solution may be required to assist the body's adjustment to the hyperglycemia. Nursing responsibilities include Dextrostix or other spot tests for the presence of glucose and thus the effectiveness of the insulin therapy. To prevent hypoglycemia at the time the hyperalimentation is disconnected, the rate of the infusion and the amount of insulin are decreased gradually. The high concentration of glucose may produce an osmotic diuresis with the risk of hypertonic dehydration.

The total parenteral nutrition solutions must be prepared under rigid aseptic conditions best accomplished in the pharmacy by specially trained technicians. The solution and tubing are changed and the infusion site redressed by specially trained nurses every 24 hours, using meticulous aseptic precautions. In many institutions this may be a nursing responsibility. The infusion site is carefully exposed and examined for kinks, catheter displacement, loose sutures, and signs of inflammation, such as redness, edema, or observable sediment in the line (an indication of possible infection). The area around the infusion site is first defatted with acetone, followed by application of povidone-iodine (Betadine) solution and covered with a sterile occlusive dressing. An antibiotic ointment (such as bacitracin) is often applied to the infusion site.

The tubing is changed with rapid transfer of insertion ends to reduce the likelihood of microorganism entry and to prevent air embolism. To reduce the risk of air entry during the tubing change, the child is instructed to perform the Valsalva maneuver, that is, to increase the intrathoracic pressure by attempting to forcibly exhale with the glottis closed. If the nurse demonstrates the procedure, the child should have no difficulty imitating it. It can also be described as similar to the breath-holding that accompanies a bowel movement. An infant is stimulated to cry and the change timed to coincide with the breath-holding phase of the cry. If an air bubble is detected in the tubing, it should be removed by milking the bubble back toward the bottle or removed by aspirating the bubble with an empty, sterile syringe inserted into the special rubber diaphragm on the tubing. The tubing should not be disconnected. A hemostat with padded prongs is used to clamp off the central venous lines during the change. Air can easily be drawn into the open end of the line with negative pressure during the inspiratory phase of respiration.

The infusion is maintained at a uniform rate by means of a constant infusion pump to ensure proper concentrations of glucose and amino acids. This requires accurate calculation of the rate required to deliver a measured amount in a given length of time. Since alterations in flow rate are relatively common, the drip should be checked frequently to ensure an even, continuous infusion. If for some reason the infusion rate slows, the rate should not be increased to compensate for the uninfused amount.

Because many children are treated with hyperalimentation regimens for long periods of time, it is especially important to be attuned to developmental needs. Allen and Harper (1983) found significant developmental delays in infants receiving long-term (greater than 3 months) TPN, especially in the areas of gross motor and language skills. An infant stimulation program is initiated as early as feasible to prevent developmental delays (see Infant stimulation, p. 385). The program is maintained throughout the hospital stay and extended into the home, where home hyperalimentation is implemented. In most instances children achieve a satisfactory developmental level by 2 years of age (Cannon and others, 1980; Ralston and others, 1984).

Home Total Parenteral Nutrition

Some children require total parenteral nutrition over an extended period, often weeks or months. A promising therapeutic approach to the problem is the recent implementation of home total parenteral nutrition (HTPN) for selected children as an alternative to long-term hospitalization. The child must be one who is unable to maintain adequate enteral alimentation, has no medical problems requiring hospitalization, has a parent who is able to manage the home care (or is an older child who can participate in his own care), and has the potential to benefit from the treatment (Bothe and others, 1979).

Before a home care program can be implemented, a thorough assessment is made of the family and the home situation. The parents must be capable of performing the technical aspects of the procedure and be able to adapt to the changes inherent in the home program. Family support systems and practical considerations are investigated including availability of a pharmacy to prepare the hyperalimentation solution, a physician to handle day-to-day emergency needs, and a cooperating insurance company or agency (because of the exorbitant cost of maintaining long-term parenteral feeding). In most areas home health care agencies are able to assume the major management of TPN for families.

A plan of care for the child and family is developed and instituted based on the needs of the particular child and the family situation. The parent (or parents) and child are tutored by a specially trained nurse, and they learn to carry out the procedure under his or her supervision; detailed, step-by-step instructions are written out. Before discharge the parent (or parents) is prepared for taking over the child's total care. Either a room is provided at the hospital or the parent and child are housed at a nearby motel for 3 to 4 days. The parent assumes full responsibility for the child's total care, with help readily available if needed.

The emotional and economic benefits of this approach are readily apparent. The familiar environment and the atmosphere of normality are enormously therapeutic, and the stress of separation is avoided. With support from health professionals, a home care program can be the ideal alternative to hospitalization for a capable, motivated family of a child who requires total parenteral nutrition.

CONCEPT SUMMARIES

- Water distribution and maintenance are determined by solutes, physical forces, internal control mechanisms, and boundary organs through which external exchanges occur.

- Infants are subject to fluid depletion because of their relatively greater surface area, their high rate of metabolism, and their immature kidney function.

- Management of fluid volume disturbances focuses on the following areas: volume of body fluids, osmolality, hydrogen ion status, electrolyte deficits, and disturbances in mineral skeleton and body fluid equilibrium.

- Fluid disturbances experienced by children are dehydration, water intoxication, and edema.

- Dehydration may be classified as isotonic, hypotonic, and hypertonic.

- Parenteral fluid therapy is initiated to meet ongoing, daily physiologic losses, restore previous deficits, and replace ongoing abnormal losses.

- Fluid gains or losses from the interstitial spaces depends on the following factors: venous hydrostatic pressure, colloidal osmotic pressure, semipermeable capillary wall, tissue tension, and lymphatic flow.

- Edema formation is caused by increased venous pressure, capillary permeability, diminished plasma proteins, lymphatic obstruction, or decreased tissue tension.

- Disturbances in acid-base balance are respiratory acidosis, respiratory alkalosis, metabolic acidosis, and metabolic alkalosis.

- Respiratory acidosis may result from factors that depress the respiratory center, factors that affect the lung, and factors that interfere with the bellows action of the chest wall.

- Respiratory alkalosis results primarily from CNS stimulation.

- Metabolic acidosis is a lowered plasm pH caused by any process that reduces base bicarbonate concentration or increases metabolic acid formation.

- Metabolic alkalosis is elevated plasma pH that occurs when there is a reduction of hydrogen ion concentration or an excess of base bicarbonate.

- Nursing assessment of fluid and electrolyte disturbances entails observation of general appearance, vital signs, and intake and output measurement.

- Long-term venous access is accomplished by heparin lock or indwelling central venous catheters.

- Intravenous alimentation provides total nutritional needs when feeding via the gastrointestinal tract is impossible, inadequate, or hazardous.

- Before initiating home total parenteral nutrition, the following factors are assessed: parents' ability to perform the procedure, existence of family support systems, availability of nearby pharmacies, and insurance coverage.

REFERENCES

Allen, S.S., and Harper, K.L.: Developmental delays in infants on long-term TPN, Nutr. Support Serv. **3**:42-43, 1983.

Ament, M.E.: Home parenteral nutrition in infants and children. In Rombeau, J.L., and Caldwell, M.D., editors: Parenteral nutrition, Philadelphia, 1986, W.B. Saunders Co.

Arthur, G.M.: When your littlest patients need IVs, RN **47**(4):30-35, 1984.

Barness, L.A.: Fluid and electrolyte therapy. In Gellis, S.S., and Kagan, B.M., editors: Current pediatric therapy 12, Philadelphia, 1986, W.B. Saunders Co.

Bennett, H.J., Wagner, T., and Fields, A.: Acute hyponatremia and seizures in an infant after a swimming lesson, Pediatrics **72**:125-127, 1983.

Bergman, T.: Verbal responses of adolescents to right atrial catheters, J. Assoc. Pediatr. Oncol. Nurses **3**:31-36, 1985.

Bothe, A., and others: Home hyperalimentation, Compr. Ther. **5**(12):54-61, 1979.

Cannon, R.A., and others: Home parenteral nutrition in infants, J. Pediatr. **96**:1098-1104, 1980.

Etzioni, A., Benderly, L.A., and Levi, Y.: Water intoxication by the oral route in an infant, Arch. Dis. Child. **54**:551-553, 1979.

Feldstein, A.G.: Consultation: irrigating question, Nursing 85 **15**(8):22, 1985.

Goldberg, G.N., and others: Infantile water intoxication after a swimming lesson, Pediatrics **70**:599-600, 1982.

Guhlow, L., and Kolb, J.: Pediatric I.V.s, RN **42**:40-51, 1979.

Kropp, R.M., and Schwartz, J.F.: Water intoxication from swimming, J. Pediatr. **101**:947-948, 1982.

Millunchick, E.W., and McArtor, R.D.: Fatal aspiration of a makeshift pacifier, Pediatrics **77**:369-370, 1986.

Partridge, J.C., and others: Water intoxication secondary to feeding mismanagement, Am. J. Dis. Child. **135**:38-41, 1981.

Piercy, S.: Children on long-term I.V. therapy, Nursing 81 **11**(9):66-69, 1981.

Ralston, C.W., and others: Somatic growth and developmental functioning in children receiving prolonged home total parenteral nutrition, J. Pediatr. **105**:842-846, 1984.

Robson, A.M.: Parenteral fluid therapy. In Behrman, R.E., and Vaughan, V.C.,III, editors: Textbook of pediatrics, ed. 12, Philadelphia, 1983, W.B. Saunders Co.

Roslyn, J.J., and others: Increased risk of gallstones in children receiving total parenteral nutrition, Pediatrics **71**:784-789, 1983.

Rowland, T.W., and others: Malnutrition and hypernatremic dehydration in breast-fed infants, JAMA **247**:1016-1017, 1982.

Schulman, J.: Infantile water intoxication at home, Pediatrics **66**:119-122, 1980.

Vogel, T.C., and McSkimming, S.A.: Teaching parents to give indwelling C.V. catheter care, Nursing 83 **13**(1):55-56, 1983.

Williams, P.R., and Kanarek, K.S.: Urine evaporative loss and effects on specific gravity and osmolality, J. Pediatr. **100**:626-628, 1982.

BIBLIOGRAPHY

General

Aberman, A.: The ins and outs of fluids and electrolytes, Emerg. Med. **14**:121-127, 1982.

Aperia, A., and others: Salt and water homeostasis during oral rehydration therapy, J. Pediatr. **103**:364-369, 1983.

Burton, J.: Compensation of acid-base disturbances, Crit. Care Update **9**(11):15-16, 1982.

Carroll, P.F.: Aspirated feeding solution, Nursing 86 **16**(1):33, 1986.

Done, A.K.: The toxic emergency, Emerg. Med. **8**:68-84, 1981.

Felver, L.: Understanding the electrolyte maze, Am. J. Nurs. **80**:1591-1595, 1980.

Finberg, L.: Treatment of dehydration in infancy, Pediatr. Rev.**3**:113-120, 1981.

Finberg, L., Kravath, R.E., and Fleischman, A.R.: Water and electrolytes in pediatrics, Philadelphia, 1982, W.B. Saunders Co.

Folk-Lighty, M.: Solving the puzzles of patients' fluid imbalances, Nursing 84 **14**(2):34-41, 1984.

Forlaw, L.: The critically ill patient: nutritional implications, Nurs. Clin. North Am. **18**:111-117, 1983.

Glass, L.B., and Jenkins, C.A.: The ups and downs of serum pH, Nursing 83 **13**(9):34-41, 1983.

Guyton, A.C.: Textbook of medical physiology, ed. 6, Philadelphia, 1981, W.B. Saunders Co.

Hochman, H.I., Grodin, M.A., and Crone, R.K.: Dehydration, diabetic ketoacidosis, and shock in the pediatric patient, Pediatr. Clin. North Am. **26**:803-826, 1979.

Hurley, J.K.: Acid-base balance: normal regulation and clinical application, Curr. Probl. Pediatr. **9**(9):5, 1979.

Lander, J.D.: Nursing care of children with fluid and electrolyte disorders, Issues Compr. Pediatr. Nurs. **2**(2):41-52, 1980.

Menzel, L.K.: Clinical problems of fluid balance, Nurs. Clin. North Am. **15**:549-558, 1980.

Menzel, L.K.: Clinical problems of electrolyte balance, Nurs. Clin. North Am. **15**:559-576, 1980.

Perkins, C., and Bralley, H.K.: Metabolic alkalosis, Nursing 83 **13**(1):57, 1983.

Perkins, R.M., and Levin, D.L.: Common fluid and electrolyte problems in the pediatric intensive care unit, Pediatr. Clin. North Am. **27**:567-586, 1980.

Quinlin, M.: Edema: what really causes it, how to control it, RN **47**(4):54-57, 1984.

Strom, J.A.: When diuretics affect electrolytes, Patient Care **16**:62-95, 1982.

Urrows, S.T.: Physiology of body fluids, Nurs. Clin. North Am. **15**:537-547, 1980.

Wink, D.M.: Fluid-induced hyponatremia in infancy: a preventable problem, Am. J. Nurs. **83**:765-767, 1983.

Wright, T.R., and Murray, M.: Potassium problems: Which patient's in danger? RN **45**(6):57-61, 1982.

Parenteral Therapy

Bosque, E., and Weaver, L.: Continuous versus intermittent heparin infusion of umbilical artery catheters in the newborn infant, J. Pediatr. **108**:141-143, 1986.

Cozad, J.: Indwelling central venous catheters, Point of View, **22**(3):14-16, 1985.

Ellerhorst-Ryan, J.M.: Troubleshooting the venous access system, Am. J. Nurs. **85**:795, 1985.

Fay, M.J.: The special challenges of pediatric IVs, Dimens. Crit. Care Nurs. **2**:23-29, 1983.

Feldstein, A.: Detect phlebitis and infiltration before they harm your patient, Nursing 86 **16**(1):44-47, 1986.

Fischer, A.Q., and Strasburger, J.: Footdrop in the neonate secondary to use of footboards, J. Pediatr. **101**:1003-1004, 1982.

Goodman, M.S., and Wickham, R.: Venous access devices: an overview, Oncol. Nurs. Forum **11**(5):16-23, 1984.

Gould, T., and Roberts, R.J.: Therapeutic problems arising from the use of the intravenous route for drug administration, J. Pediatr. **95**:465-471, 1979.

Gruber, D.: Helping the child accept I.V. therapy, Am. J. I.V. Ther. **4**:50-55, 1977.

Hodder, S.L., and Stern, R.C.: Safety of long duration intravenous heparin-lock needles for administration of antibiotics to cystic fibrosis patients, J. Pediatr. **99**:312-314, 1981.

Koszuta, L.E.: Choosing the right infusion control device for your patient, Nursing 84 **14**(3):55-57, 1984.

Levitt, D.Z.: Use of the heparin lock on an outpatient basis, Cancer Nurs. **4:**115-119, 1981.

McGrath, B.J.: Fluids, electrolytes, and replacement therapy in pediatric nursing, Am. J. Maternal Child Nurs. **5:**58-62, 1980.

Nelson, R., and Miller, H.: Keeping air out of I.V. lines, Nursing 86 **16**(3):57-59, 1986.

Peck, N.: Perfecting your I.V. therapy techniques, part I, Nursing 85 **15**(5):38-43, 1985.

Peck, N.: Perfecting your I.V. therapy techniques, part II, Nursing 85 **15**(6):48-51, 1985.

Peck, N.: Perfecting your I.V. therapy techniques, part III, Nursing 85 **15**(7):32-35, 1985.

Poichuk, N., and Fraser, C.: I.V. therapy for children, Dimens. Health Serv. **57**(8):32, 1980.

Roderick, B.: How to manage CVP lines, RN **48**(8):22-25, 1985.

Rombeau, J.L., and Caldwell, M.D.: Parenteral nutrition, Philadelphia, 1986, W.B. Saunders Co.

Tanner, S.: Toward impeccable IV technique: IV bolus leaves no room for error, RN **44**(10):54-55, 1981.

Wittig, P., and Semmler-Bertanzi, D.J.: Pumps and controllers—a nurse's assessment guide, Am. J. Nurs. **83:**1022-1025, 1983.

Intravenous Alimentation

Atkins, J.M., and Oakley, C.W.: A nurse's guide to TPN, RN **49**(6):20-24, 1986.

Birdsall, C.: When is TPN safe? Am. J. Nurs. **85:**73, 1985.

Carr, P.: When the patient needs TPN at home, RN **49**(6):25-27, 1986.

Colley, R., and Wilson, J.: Meeting patients' nutritional needs with hyperalimentation: how to begin hyperalimentation therapy, Nursing 79 **9**(5):76-83, 1979.

Colley, R., and Wilson, J.: Meeting patients' nutritional needs with hyperalimentation: managing the patient on hyperalimentation, Nursing 79 **9**(6):57-61, 1979.

Colley, R., and Wilson, J.: Meeting patients' nutritional needs with hyperalimentation: providing hyperalimentation for infants and children, Nursing 79 **9**(7):50-53, 1979.

Committee on Nutrition: Commentary on parenteral nutrition, Pediatrics **71:**547-552, 1983.

Dahlstrom, K.A., and others: Nutritional status in children receiving home parenteral nutrition, J. Pediatr. **107:**219-224, 1985.

Davis, J., Jedlicka, L., and Johnson, F.: Sure-fire asepsis for your TPN patients, RN **44**(12):39-41, 1982.

Doran, E.: Care of the Hickman catheter in children, Nurs. Clin. North Am. **18:**79-81, 1983.

Forlaw, L.: Parenteral nutrition in the critically ill child, Crit. Care Q. **3:**1-20, 1981.

Fox, B., and Stegall, B.: TPN: take precautions now, Nursing 85 **15**(5):48-49, 1985.

Geertsma, M.A., and others: Feeding resistance after parenteral hyperalimentation, Am. J. Dis. Child. **139:**255-256, 1985.

Heird, W.C., and Greene, H.L.: Panel report on nutritional support of pediatric patients, Am. J. Clin. Nutr. **34:**1223-1228, 1981.

Hoelzer, D.J., and L'Hommedieu, C.S.: Central venous catheter complications (letter), Pediatrics **71:**865, 1983.

Koop, C.E.: The most important advances of the last ten years, Pediatr. Consult. **2**(1):1-3, 1981.

Levy, J.S., Winters, R.W., and Heird, W.C.: Total parenteral nutrition in pediatric patients, Pediatr. Rev. **2**(4):99-104, 1980.

Munro-Black, J.: The ABCs of total parenteral nutrition, Nursing 84 **14**(2):50-56, 1984.

Should you infuse anything else through a TPN line? RN **44**(10):32-33,1981.

Vileisis, R.A., Inwood, R.J., and Hunt, C.E.: Prospective controlled study of parenteral nutrition—associated cholestatic jaundice: effect of protein intake, J. Pediatr. **96:**893-897, 1980.

Wesley, J.: Home parenteral nutrition: indications, principles and cost-effectiveness, Compr. Ther. **9:**29-36, 1983.

Wilhelm, L.: Helping your patient "settle in" with TPN, Nursing 85 **15**(4):60-64, 1985.

Wilkes, G., Vannicola, P., and Starck, P.: Long-term venous access, Am. J. Nurs. **85:**793-796, 1985.

Wilson, J., and Colley, R.: Meeting patients' nutritional needs with hyperalimentation: teaching patients to administer hyperalimentation infusions at home, Nursing 79 **9**(8):56-63, 1979.

Wilson, J., and Colley, R.: Meeting patients' nutritional needs with hyperalimentation: administering peripheral and enteral feedings, Nursing 79 **9**(9):62-69, 1979.

Zlotkin, S.H., Stallings, V.A., and Pencharz, P.B.: Total parenteral nutrition in children, Pediatr. Clin. North Am. **32:**381-400, 1985.

Home Intravenous Alimentation

Cannon, R.A., and others: Home parenteral nutrition in infants, J. Pediatr. **96:**1098-1104, 1980.

Goldberger, J.H., and others: A home program of long-term total parenteral nutrition in children, J. Pediatr. **94:**325-328, 1979.

Parfitt, D.M., and Thompson, V.D.: Pediatric home hyperalimentation: educating the family, Am. J. Maternal Child Nurs. **5:**196-202, 1980.

Chapter 29

Conditions that Produce Fluid and Electrolyte Imbalance

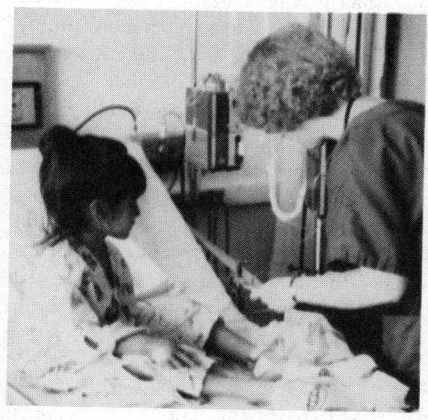

Fluid and electrolyte disturbances are common in the pediatric age-group. Acute attacks of vomiting and diarrhea are so common in this group that they can almost be regarded as part of the normal way of life. However, the nature of the anatomic and physiologic structure of the infant and small child renders them particularly vulnerable to imbalances when pathologic changes affect the fluid compartments. The most serious disturbances are those involving the gastrointestinal tract, the cardiovascular system, and losses resulting from massive burn injury.

Gastrointestinal Disorders

The numerous secretions of the gastrointestinal tract are produced in large amounts, but under ordinary conditions most of the fluid is reabsorbed in the lower bowel. With the exception of saliva, which is hypotonic, the total solute concentration in most of the gastrointestinal secretions is similar to that of interstitial fluid, but there are marked differences among the secretions in electrolyte composition. Therefore the consequences of fluid lost from the gastrointestinal tract depend a great deal on the composition of the fluid that is lost. Fluid losses from the gastrointestinal tract in vomiting, diarrhea, or other routes (fistula, nasogastric tube) not only produce rapid and profound depletion of extracellular volume but can cause marked distortion of the electrolyte composition as well. Most illnesses create some disturbance in body fluids or electrolytes, and in many children these disturbances are more threatening than the primary disorder. Replacement requires careful attention to both volume and solute composition.

DIARRHEA

Diarrhea is an increase in the number of stools or a decrease in their consistency. It is a symptom with diverse origins and results from disorders involving digestive, absorptive, and secretory functions. However, a precise definition and identification of what constitutes diarrhea pose a problem in terms of number or consistency of stools, because there are wide variations in colonic function between individuals. For example, normally one infant may have one firm stool every second or third day, whereas another normally passes from five to eight small, soft stools daily. Therefore more important are (1) a noticeable or sudden increase in number of stools, (2) a reduction in their consistency with an increase in fluid content, and (3) a tendency for the stools to be greenish in color.

Diarrhea is one of the symptoms encountered most frequently in infants and children and was at one time a chief cause of death in infancy. With improved public health measures, the incidence has been dramatically reduced during the past century, and although it still remains a major health problem in many areas of the world, a greater understanding of the pathophysiology of diarrhea and more effective management of the disorder have also reduced the death rate from the consequences of diarrhea. Severe cases, however, continue to present serious problems, especially with more widespread adoption of bottle-feeding throughout the world.

Diarrhea may be acute or chronic, inflammatory or noninflammatory, and the physiologic consequences vary considerably in relation to its severity, duration, associated symptoms, the age of the child, and the child's nutritional status before the onset of diarrhea. Diarrhea related to inflammatory processes is usually described as *gastroenteritis*, and the terms are often used interchangeably.

Etiology/Pathophysiology

Diarrhea can be attributed to a large number of specific causes, mechanisms, and predisposing factors that include:

1. **Age.** As a rule, the younger the child the more susceptible he is to diarrhea and the more severe the diarrhea is likely to be. Diarrhea occurs more frequently in infancy, is a lesser threat in early childhood, and usually constitutes only a minor problem in older children.
2. **Impaired health.** Children who are malnourished or debilitated from disease are more susceptible to diarrhea, and it tends to be more severe in these children.
3. **Climate.** In areas in which sanitation and refrigeration are a problem, saprophytic organisms (organisms that grow more readily in the warmer weather) are more apt to proliferate. Most organisms that cause diarrhea are more prevalent in warmer weather. In addition, the dehydration that accompanies diarrhea is aggravated by hot weather.
4. **Environment.** Diarrhea occurs with greater frequency in circumstances in which living conditions are inadequate. Crowding, substandard sanitation, poor facilities for preparation and refrigeration of food, and generally inadequate health care and education all tend to increase the likelihood for spread of pathogens. The frequency of diarrhea in infancy is closely related to the ingestion of contaminated milk. Significantly, there is a lower incidence of diarrhea in breast-fed infants even where formula preparation is satisfactory.

Specific etiologic mechanisms. There are several major mechanisms that produce diarrhea in infants or children who are susceptible or exposed to a causative agent. In some cases more than one mechanism may be operative. There are numerous agents that are responsible for causing diarrhea by way of these mechanisms. Some agents create their effect by direct invasion of the intestinal tract, whereas others exert their effect through parenteral means, that is, not by way of the intestinal tract. The following mechanisms are known to produce diarrhea (Silverman and Roy, 1983):

1. **Osmotic factors.** Water is passively absorbed as a function of solute transport and normally accompanies solute movement in isotonic proportions across the intestinal mucosa in response to osmotic gradients. The presence of unabsorbed solutes creates an osmotic gradient, causing movement of sodium and water in the intestinal lumen (for example, ingestion of nonabsorbable solutes and malabsorption of water-soluble nutrients).
2. **Diminished absorption or increased secretion of water and electrolytes.** Diminished absorption of solutes will also cause decreased absorption of water and electrolytes (for example, mucosal disease). Increased secretion can be either passive secretion secondary to inflammation or active secretion secondary to stimulation of mucosal cells (for example, toxin-producing bacteria).
3. **Reduction in anatomic or functional surface area.** There is reduced absorptive surface to absorb all ingested substances in the anatomically short bowel.
4. **Altered motility.** Both hypermotility and hypomotility reduce the amount of substance absorbed by the intestinal mucosa.

Specific causes. A variety of factors can produce diarrhea in the infant or child either as the initial symptom or an associated symptom. Often a specific etiologic diagnosis is lacking. *Acute* diarrhea, sudden change in frequency and consistency of stools, is often caused by an inflammatory process of infectious origin but may also be the result of toxic reaction to ingestion of poisons, dietary indiscretions, or associated with infection outside the alimentary tract (see box below). Most are self-limited and will ultimately subside without specific treatment if consequent dehydration does not create a serious complication. *Chronic* diarrhea, passage of loose stools with increased frequency of more than 2 weeks duration, is likely to be associated with disorders of malabsorption, anatomic defects, abnormal bowel motility, hypersensitivity (allergic) reaction, or an long-term inflammatory response (see box, p. 1190).

Diarrheal disturbances can involve the stomach and intestine *(gastroenteritis)*, the small intestine *(enteritis)*, the colon *(colitis)*, or the colon and intestine *(enterocolitis)*. *Dysentery* is a term that describes intestinal inflammation, especially of the colon, that is accompanied by cramping abdominal pain, tenesmus, and watery stools containing blood and mucus. Enteropathologic organisms are frequent causes of diarrhea in infancy and childhood and are further discussed in relation to gastroenteritis p. 1195.

Antibiotic therapy is a common cause of diarrhea in children. Antibiotics such as ampicillin, neomycin, and tetracyclines cause a decrease in glucose absorption and disaccharidase activity. They should be discontinued and a lactose-free diet implemented if diarrhea occurs. Antibiotics can also cause diarrhea by allowing an overgrowth of a bacterium responsible for pseudomembranous colitis.

Dietary indiscretions and sensitivities are observed at any age. However, the most common causes, especially in infancy, are high osmolar formulas and food sensitivities, discussed in Chapter 13. Children can have an innate sensitivity to certain foods, but more often the sensitivity develops from repeated exposure to specific antigenic substances. Another dietary cause of diarrhea that has been reported is ingestion of dietetic candies made with sorbitol, a hexahydric sugar alcohol that acts as an osmotic laxative.

Chronic nonspecific diarrhea. Chronic nonspecific diarrhea (CNSD) (sometimes called irritable bowel syndrome) is the most common cause of prolonged diarrhea in young children and appears to be caused by decreased transit time in the alimentary tract. Characteristically there is diarrhea for at least 3 weeks, normal growth, and no evidence of enteric pathogens. Ingestion of apple juice has been implicated in a number of young children (Hyams and Leichtner, 1985). Excessive intake of fluid appears to have been associated with the development of CNSD in some children. The incidence has increased significantly since the implementation of oral rehydration therapy, and affected children developed normal stool patterns following fluid restriction (Greene and Ghishan, 1983).

It has also been observed that persistent diarrhea is an important side effect of exogenous prostaglandins administered to pregnant women to initiate labor. Prostaglandins have also been implicated as a cause of diarrhea associated with some tumors. Increased circulating prostaglandin levels have been found in some children with CNSD. These children respond well to administration of prostaglandin synthetase inhibitors such as aspirin or indomethacin (Dodge and others, 1981).

CAUSES OF ACUTE DIARRHEA

Dietary
Overfeeding
Introduction of new foods
Unripe fruit
Reinstituting milk too soon after diarrheal episode
Osmotic diarrhea from excess sugar or fat in formula

Toxic
Ingestion of
   Heavy metals (arsenic, lead, mercury)
   Organic phosphates
   Ferrous sulfate
   Antibiotics

Enteropathologic
Bacteria: *Escherichia coli, Shigella, Salmonella, Yersinia enterocolitica, Campylobacter, Staphylococcus aureus, Clostridium perfringens, Vibro cholerae, Vibro parahaemolyticus,* tuberculosis
Viruses: Adenoviruses, rotavirus, parvovirus-like organisms
Infestations*: Amebiasis, giardiasis, ascariasis, coccidiosis

Parenteral infection
Communicable diseases
Upper respiratory tract infections
Urinary tract infections
Otitis media

Inflammatory bowel disease
Necrotizing enterocolitis of the newborn

Emotional
Episodes of nervous excitement
Periods of emotional tension
Fatigue
Psychogenic "irritable colon syndrome" in hyperactive children

*See Chapter 16.

CAUSES OF CHRONIC DIARRHEA*

Anatomic or mechanical
Small bowel syndrome
Hirschsprung disease
Partial small bowel obstruction (stenosis)
Malrotation
Fistula
Intestinal lymphangiectasis
Chronic idiopathic intestinal pseudo-obstruction

Biochemical causes
Celiac disease
Specific carbohydrate or fat malabsorption syndromes caused by enzyme deficiencies such as lactase deficiency, bile-salt deficiency

Endocrinopathies
Hyperthyroidism
Congenital adrenal hyperplasia
Addison disease

Hepatic and pancreatic disorders
Cystic fibrosis
Cirrhosis
Hepatitis
Chronic pancreatitis
Pancreatic exocrine deficiency
Pancreatic hypoplasia
Nonspecific enterocolitis of infancy

Neoplastic disorders
Lymphoma
Neuroblastoma
Polyposis
Adenocarcinoma
Pancreatic islet cell tumor
Ganglioneuroma
Medullary thyroid carcinoma

Immune deficiencies
Acquired hypoglobulinemia
Wiskott-Aldrich syndrome
Agammaglobulinemia
Severe combined immune deficiency disease
Thymic hypoplasia
Selective IgA deficiency
Acquired immune deficiency syndrome

Food allergy
Milk colitis
Allergic gastroenteropathy

Inflammatory bowel disease
Ulcerative colitis
Regional enteritis (Crohn disease)
Nonspecific enterocolitis of infancy
Pseudomembranous enterocolitis

Malnutrition
Protein malnutrition (kwashiorkor)
Protein-calorie malnutrition (marasmus)

*See Chapter 34 for discussion of chronic gastrointestinal disorders.

Clinical Manifestations

The most serious and immediate physiologic disturbances associated with severe diarrheal disease are (1) dehydration, (2) acid-base derangements with acidosis, and (3) shock that occurs when dehydration progresses to the point that circulatory status is seriously disturbed.

Dehydration, which can be isotonic (isonatremic; 70% of cases), hypotonic (hyponatremic; 15%), or hypertonic (hypernatremic; 5%), is the result of:

Voluminous losses of fluid and electrolytes in frequent watery stools
Losses when there is frequent vomiting
Reduced fluid intake resulting from nausea or anorexia
Increased insensible losses from fever, hyperpnea, and sometimes, high environmental temperature
Continued (although diminished) obligatory renal losses

All of these losses contribute to the rapid deterioration in diarrheal disease in infancy, and although the fluid deficit cannot be stated precisely, it can be estimated from changes in body weight and objective clinical signs (see p. 1164). The metabolic acidosis of severe diarrhea is the result of several factors:

Losses of bicarbonate, sodium, and potassium in diarrheal stools

Impaired renal function
Accumulation of lactic acid from tissue hypoxia
Ketosis from fat metabolism when glycogen stores are depleted in untreated diarrheal dehydration or inadequate carbohydrate intake

In association with both fluid losses and acidosis, there are alterations in body potassium. Potassium is continually lost in stools, cellular potassium leaves the cells in exchange for sodium and hydrogen ions entering the cells, and potassium is lost from cells damaged by hypoxia. Thus the cellular potassium is seriously depleted. However, because renal excretion is impaired as a result of the circulatory adjustments, the serum levels of potassium are normal or even elevated. When circulatory volume and renal function are restored, potassium redistribution and excretion may produce a potassium deficit unless adequate amounts are restored at this time.

Diagnostic Evaluation

The history provides valuable information regarding exposure to infectious agents, personal contact, travel, or probable contact with contaminated foods. Allergic and dietary history may indicate food allergies. Crowding and close person-to-person contact, as in institutions, make epidemics with any enteric pathogen more likely.

The age of the child provides clues to the cause of diarrheal disturbances. For example, with the exception of nursery epidemics, infectious enteritis is uncommon during the first days of life. *Escherichia coli* is the usual agent after the first week of life, with a peak incidence from 1 to 3 months of age in bottle-fed infants; it is uncommon after 1 year of age. In breast-fed infants the time sequence is later. Shigellosis is most common from ages 2 to 4 years, but the most severe form is more apt to occur in children older than 5 years. Although *Salmonella* infection is encountered in children in any age group, it appears to be most prevalent in children younger than 2 years, as are the viral diarrheas. Rotavirus occurs most commonly in infants.

It is characteristic that multiple cases in a household are usually shigellosis, whereas a single case is more typical of enteropathogenic *E. coli*. Likewise, milk allergy or intolerance of other formula constituents is suspected in early infancy. In later infancy new foods added to the diet are frequent offenders. Parenteral infections are very common causes of diarrhea in infancy.

Most acute, inflammatory diarrheas are infectious, and the type of stools and symptoms associated with diarrhea provide clues to the organism. For example, fever is not a symptom of *E. coli* disease until late, whereas it is a common early feature even in mild cases of shigellosis. Abdominal cramps are common in shigellosis. Explosive onset of diarrhea accompanied by or preceded by vomiting suggests food poisoning. Although vomiting may occur in all infectious diarrheas, it is not a major feature. Children with a cluster of three historical commonalities—abrupt onset, more than four stools per day, and absence of vomiting before onset of diarrhea—have been found to have a high incidence of positive stool cultures for bacterial diarrhea (DeWitt, Humphrey, and McCarthy, 1985).

Laboratory examination. Peripheral blood leukocyte count is of little value in differentiating organisms, but the presence of many band forms in the differential white blood count is characteristic of shigellosis but not of most other infectious diarrheas.

Examination of the stool for leukocytes often differentiates between some bacteria. No leukocytes appear in normal stools or in diarrheal disease of viral or enterotoxin-producing bacteria, but many leukocytes or clumps of pus cells are seen in infections caused by enteroinvasive organisms. The stool specimen is obtained from evacuated stool and should include mucus or tissue shreds, if present. The specimen is also examined for the presence of red blood cells. Rectal swabs for culture are indicated whenever a bacterial agent is suspected.

Stool examination with indicator paper for pH and a Clinitest tablet will detect the acid stool containing sugar that is characteristic of disaccharide intolerance. Bulky stools containing fat suggest malabsorption diarrhea.

The breath hydrogen test for carbohydrate malabsorption (lactose, sucrose) provides a simple, rapid, and noninvasive method to detect a variety of gastrointestinal disorders. The end products of many metabolic processes, carbon dioxide and hydrogen, are normally absorbed, transported by the bloodstream, and eliminated by the lungs. In children with carbohydrate malabsorption the breath hydrogen excretion rate is two to eight times greater than normal after ingestion of the specific testing carbohydrate. The test has also been perfected to detect bacterial overgrowth (Davidson, Robb, and Kirubakaran, 1984).

Serum electrolyte values are obtained in the young infant who is hospitalized with diarrhea because of the likelihood of complicating dehydration and associated electrolyte imbalances, particularly in relation to sodium and potassium alterations. Dehydrated infants will have an elevated hematocrit as a result of volume loss, and elevated blood urea nitrogen will be found in the presence of reduced renal circulation.

Therapeutic Management

Mild or moderate diarrhea is usually managed by simple measures and seldom requires hospitalization. Mild diarrhea is described as a few loose stools each day without other evidence of illness, that terminates in a few days. With moderate diarrhea the child is sicker, may have a fever, vomits, appears fretful and irritable, and passes several loose or watery stools daily. Although the child may not gain weight or may even show a slight loss, signs of dehydration are usually absent.

The extent to which the child should be examined and observed by a nurse or a physician depends a great deal on the intelligence and cooperation of the caregiver in following instructions and assessing the progress of treatment. When the competency of the caregiver is questionable in regard to estimating the child's condition, the child should be seen daily by a health worker. If the diarrhea persists, if the child loses weight, if there is blood in the stools, or if associated signs develop, such as deep breathing, listlessness, or reduced urinary output that may signal complications, the child should be seen by the physician. When the moderate diarrhea becomes worse or does not respond to simple measures, hospitalization is indicated. This provides the opportunity for closer observation and examination and for a brief course of parenteral fluid therapy, which usually results in rapid improvement.

Rehydration. In mild cases of noninflammatory diarrhea fruit juices and caffeine-free soft drinks are adequate for fluid replacement (see p. 1193). Orally administered rehydration solutions (ORS) are currently the therapy of choice in treatment of diarrhea of any cause and in a wide range of age groups except in severe dehydration or other complicating circumstances.

The ORS recommended by the Diarrheal Disease Control Program of the World Health Organization is used successfully throughout the world, but seldom in the United States. The Committee on Nutrition of the American Academy of Pediatrics (1985) states that it is appropriate for rapid rehydration but is not suitable for maintaining fluid balance in infants with ongoing losses. The large amount of sodium in the solution contributes to the risk of hyperelectrolytemia.

Table 29-1 Composition of oral rehydration solutions

FORMULA	Na⁺ (mEq/L)	K⁺ (mEq/L)	Cl⁻ (mEq/L)	BASE (mEq/L)	CARBOHYDRATE (g/L)
Lytren (Mead-Johnson)	50	25	45	30 (citrate)	20 (dextrose, corn syrup, solids)
Pedialyte	45	20	35	30 (citrate)	25 (dextrose)
Pedialyte RS	75	20	65	30 (citrate)	25 (dextrose)
Infalyte powder (Pennwalt)	50	20	40	30 (bicarbonate)	20 (glucose)
WHO (World Health Organization)	90	20	80	30 (bicarbonate)	18 (dextrose)

In addition, it is typically prepared in powder form, which must be mixed with water for administration; thus the chance of inaccurate measurement increases the likelihood of error in preparation. In the United States commercially prepared formulas are available (Table 29-1) and used almost exclusively for oral rehydration.

The usual approach is to administer ORS, 50 ml/kg body weight, within 4 hours for mild dehydration, and 100 ml/kg over 6 hours for moderate dehydration. The amounts and rates are increased if the patient does not appear fully hydrated or continues to have diarrhea. The amounts are decreased if the patient appears to be fully hydrated earlier than expected or signs of overhydration develop, for example, periorbital edema. Infants can be allowed to continue breast-feeding as desired after treatment has been started; other infants are offered plain water (Robson, 1983).

When oral rehydration is complete, maintenance therapy is begun. Most mild to moderate diarrhea can be managed at home under careful health supervision. The recommended maintenance schedule is ORS 100 ml/kg/24 hours until diarrhea ceases, with continuation of breast-feeding or supplemental water intake (Robson, 1983; Barness, 1986). The volume of ORS ingested should equal the volume of stool losses. ORS 10 to 15 ml/kg/hr is an appropriate amount when stool volume cannot be measured. Some authorities advocate ad libitum intake of ORS with in addition one bottle of plain or flavored water for every two bottles of ORS (Bass and Walker, 1986).

The issue of continued or delayed feedings has not been resolved. Some advocate continuing the child's regular diet; others advise removing all milk for 24 to 36 hours. Lactose-free formulas are often substituted (Brown and MacLean, 1984), but research has indicated that infants recover from mild disease regardless of the carbohydrate ingested (Groothuis, Berman, and Chapman, 1986). Breast milk is generally well tolerated by infants. Investigators have found that introduction of a soy-based, lactose-free formula (usually diluted 50%) after the initial 4 hours of rehydration re-

duced stool output and duration of diarrhea in most infants (Santosham and others, 1985).

Hypernatremic diarrheal dehydration is usually managed by *slow* oral rehydration (over 12 hours) to avoid cerebral edema with accompanying seizures (Pizarro, Posada, and Levine, 1984). In many children a secondary lactase deficiency may cause a temporary intolerance to milk and exacerbation of diarrhea; therefore, reintroduction of lactose is attempted progressively. Milk is usually withheld until at least a week after the disappearance of symptoms, and the feeding consists of some type of hydrolyzed lactose-free formula.

Medications. Antimicrobial therapy is instituted in some types of diarrhea. It significantly shortens the course of shigellosis and appears to be beneficial in *E. coli* infections but does not affect the course of *Salmonella* disease. It is always indicated in bacteremia, and parenteral infections are treated with appropriate drugs.

Antidiarrheal medications such as opiates (paregoric), which inhibit peristaltic action, are seldom employed in treatment of diarrhea in the pediatric age-group. They have little or no effect on the course of infantile diarrhea and are more likely to cause toxicity. Diphenoxylate hydrochloride with atropine sulfate (Lomotil) is sometimes prescribed for older children, but is contraindicated in infants and children younger than 2 years of age because of its narrow margin of safety.

Adsorbents, such as kaolin and pectin, alter consistency and cosmetic appearance of stools and decrease the frequency of evacuation but do not reduce the amount of fluid loss and may actually mask significant fluid losses. Although of questionable value, they are sometimes prescribed to provide parents with a sense that something is being done for the child. Antidiarrheal agents are not administered to infants, but may be of limited value in older children.

Severe diarrhea. Severe diarrhea is largely a problem of infants and very young children, and regardless of the cause, successful management relies primarily on appropriate treatment of physiologic disturbances and is only secondarily concerned with specific treatment of the etiologic agent. Severe diarrhea warrants hospitalization, comprehensive evaluation, and parenteral fluid therapy. Intravenous fluid therapy is directed toward rapid replacement of (1) the fluid deficit, (2) ongoing normal losses, and (3) ongoing abnormal losses. The magnitude of the deficit is determined from loss of body weight and ongoing losses by calculating the energy requirements of the child. The energy requirements include not only predicted caloric expenditure for age and size but other factors that increase the use of energy, such as elevated temperature (metabolism increases by about 12% for each 1° C) and hyperventilation. Additional replacement covers abnormal losses as determined by output measurement, weight, and electrolyte determinations.

Once the severe effects of dehydration are under control, specific diagnostic and therapeutic measures are instigated to detect and treat the cause of the diarrhea. This includes mild sedation, antimicrobial therapy when indicated, and treatment of secondary effects of the illness or its therapy. For example, secondary bacterial growth may be countered with a short course of nonabsorbable antibiotics or oral administration of lactobacilli to recolonize the normal flora of the gastrointestinal tract.

Typically the frequency and volume of stools will subside within 48 hours in fasted patients receiving intravenous fluids. If the child is alert and no intervening complications, such as persistent vomiting or distention, arise, an ORS is generally initiated. The caloric intake is increased gradually until the usual dietary intake is reestablished, usually within 7 to 8 days.

Nursing Considerations

The observation of children who receive treatment at home is often the responsibility of a nurse. Management involves assessment, therapy, and education. The status of the child must be evaluated to determine the extent of disease—the nature and frequency of stools, associated signs such as tenesmus, cramping, vomiting, or fever, and assessment of the state of hydration. When the diarrhea consists of a few loose stools each day without evidence of illness, it is managed with continued observation and diet management.

The parent is allowed to give fluids to the child. The duration of time before initial feedings and the amount and type of fluids suggested depend on the philosophy of the physician. Fluids are usually tolerated best at room temperature, and the parent should be cautioned against giving other than those prescribed by the physician. The ORS is usually well tolerated by infants, but older children find them unpalatable. Some type of flavoring may improve the taste, but many flavorings contain glucose; therefore caution should be observed in their selection. The fluids recommended for dehydration (p. 1174) are well-tolerated by children.

Soft foods are gradually added when liquids are well tolerated, as evidenced by no vomiting and an increased consistency and decrease in number of stools. Appropriate soft foods include gelatin desserts, soups (not creamed), bananas, applesauce, strained carrots, crackers (including pretzels), rice, and toast with jelly.

Part of the home assessment includes taking a history to help elicit probable etiologic agents, such as introduction of a new food, travel to an area of high susceptibility, contact with foods that might be contaminated, and contact with pets that are known to be sources of enteric infections. Unrefrigerated milk and egg products provide excellent media for growth of *Staphylococcus,* and fowl, both wild and domestic, is a well-known source of *Salmonella.* Animals of all varieties can be infected by other animals and birds. Recent evidence has implicated pet chickens, mammals, such as dogs, cats, and mice, and reptiles, especially turtles, as sources of infection in children. Home assessment should include detection of such sources of contamination as well as observation of general cleanliness and sanitation in preparation and storage of food.

Infants. Infants take ORS readily, and there is seldom difficulty in encouraging an adequate intake. Vomiting may occur during the first 2 hours of ORS administration but is not an indication to discontinue the feedings. Vomiting can be reduced by giving the solution slowly, in small amounts, and at more frequent intervals. Sustained vomiting should be reported; intravenous therapy may be required.

Following rehydration infants are often given soy formula for a short time or milk is added to the diet cautiously. Foods are then reintroduced, and the customary diet is gradually resumed as described in therapeutic management. Progress is assessed frequently, with weights when possible and observation of other signs of adequate hydration.

Severe diarrhea. The infant or child admitted to the hospital with diarrhea is always isolated from other children, and appropriate precautions are implemented to prevent possible spread to other children and personnel. Each hospital has a policy regarding isolation and enteric precautions.

The child is weighed on admission and frequently during the emergency phase of rapid hydration. Accurate intake and output measurement is imperative, and a urine collection bag is placed to determine the volume of output, to measure specific gravity, and ascertain that renal blood flow is sufficient to permit administration of potassium. Unless urine is separated from stool, this essential information cannot be obtained.

Children who are sufficiently ill to require hospitalization are almost always given parenteral fluid therapy with nothing by mouth for 12 to 48 hours. Monitoring the intravenous infusion is a primary nursing function, with careful attention to ascertain that the correct fluid and electrolyte concentration is infused, the flow rate is adjusted to deliver the desired volume over a given period, and the intravenous site is maintained. Restraint of some type is needed with infants and small children, whose purposeful or random movements might disturb the needle placement (pp. 1178). Frequent assessment of the intravenous site for infiltration and of the restrained limbs for circulation and pressure areas is neces-

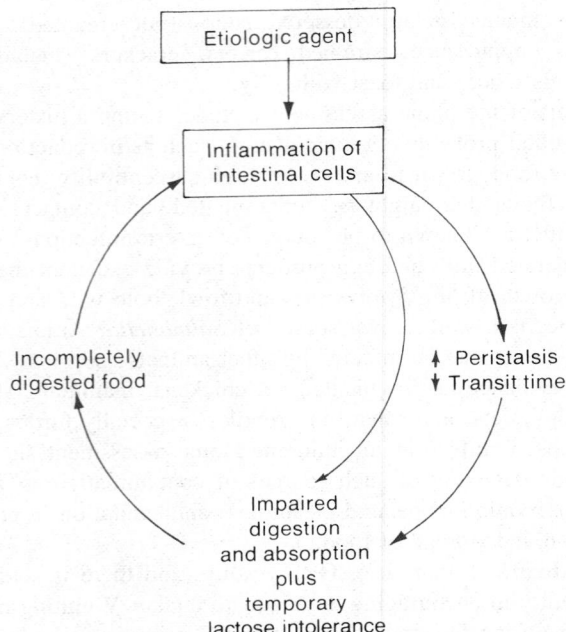

Fig. 29-1. Vicious pathologic cycle in diarrhea with temporary lactose intolerance.

sary. Restraints should be released as frequently as possible to allow the child to move the extremities. Children are sufficiently active that range of motion exercises are seldom necessary when they are unconstrained and not in severe pain.

The nurse is responsible for examination of stools and the collection of specimens for laboratory examination. Care is exerted in obtaining and transporting stools to prevent possible spread of infection. Specimens are manipulated and transported to the laboratory in appropriate media and containers and in accordance with hospital policy. Tests for pH, blood, and sugar can be done without removing the stool from the diaper. A clean tongue depressor can be used to obtain specimens for laboratory examination when a larger volume is needed or as an applicator for transfer to a culture medium.

Because diarrheal stools are highly irritating to the skin, extra care is needed to protect the skin of the diaper region from becoming excoriated. Exposing the reddened areas to heat and light is an effective method to facilitate healing. An excellent way to provide dry heat to the area is by means of a goose-necked lamp, but the lamp must be placed at a sufficient distance that the child is unable to reach any part of it. The heat source should be no closer than 18 inches (45 cm). The child will require close observation during treatment, and the duration of any application should not exceed 20 minutes. Active children will require restraint to maintain proper exposure, prevent any possibility of injury, and minimize possible spread of any feces that may be expelled. Contamination is especially likely in children with explosive bowel movements. Holding an infant or small

child in the lap, protected with blankets or diapers, during the heat application serves as an excellent means for observing and restraining the child as well as providing tactile stimulation.

Oral feedings are begun according to the philosophy of the attending practitioner, and resumption of feedings is usually begun with a diluted soy formula (such as Isomil or ProSobee), which is gradually strengthened as tolerated until the full-strength formula is taken without exacerbation of the diarrhea. Milk and lactose-containing formulas are usually withheld for at least a week in children with severe diarrhea. Hydrolyzed protein formulas with nonlactose sugar (such as Nutramigen or Pregestimil) are substituted until the gastrointestinal tract is again able to tolerate milk and milk products.

INTRACTABLE DIARRHEA OF INFANCY

Intractable diarrhea of infancy is a syndrome defined as diarrhea occurring in the first 3 months of life that persists for longer than 2 weeks with no recognized pathogens and is refractory to treatment. It is classified as either primary, which is identified as nonspecific enterocolitis, or secondary, associated with disease entities such as allergy, bowel anomalies, or a variety of congenital diseases. The age of onset ranges from 4 days to 3 months.

The primary form, although the triggering factor is not well defined, may be secondary to such trivial causes as an infection or feeding difficulties, but in most cases no predisposing cause can be identified. The immediate concerns are dehydration and electrolyte imbalances, but these children universally suffer from malnutrition and its consequences. Because the diarrhea occurs during a period of high caloric need, affected infants can quickly become severely ill.

The diarrhea rapidly becomes self-perpetuating through a combination of secondary consequences: malnutrition deprives the infant of the elements protein, vitamins, calcium, and magnesium needed for mucosal regeneration; the villi of the small intestine atrophy; the bowel wall becomes inflamed and irritated by undigested foodstuffs or microorganisms; and secondary digestive and absorptive disorders develop as a result of malnutrition, various patterns of motility, and overgrowth of bacteria caused by the infant's debilitated state (Fig. 29-1).

Therapeutic Management

The selection of a rehydration method is based on the infant's clinical status as well as biochemical findings. Mildly affected infants who are not malnourished may do well with an orally administered rehydration solution followed by an elemental diet as described for severe diarrhea. Moderately or severely ill infants require hospitalization. The initial concern in the first 24 to 48 hours is correction of acidosis, dehydration, and electrolyte disturbances, with nothing by mouth, to place the bowel at rest.

In relatively mild cases an elemental diet is initiated, and gradually increased in concentration and volume over several days. Daily weight, stool volume and stool-reducing substances, and pH are followed as a guide to therapy. Infants who have difficulty adjusting to oral feedings require peripheral alimentation with dextrose and amino acids to supplement enteral feedings. Intralipid may be given slowly to provide additional calories. The orally administered formula is usually increased in concentration while the infant is receiving peripheral alimentation. When full-strength formula is tolerated, the volume is gradually increased and the intravenously administered fluids decreased accordingly (Bass and Walker, 1986).

Infants who are moderately ill and are unable to tolerate the initial enteral feedings may be able to tolerate continuous nasogastric feedings at 0.5 ml/kg/hr, and the volume and concentration gradually increased and parenteral feeding decreased. If the infant is unable to tolerate full-volume feedings, the concentration may be increased to provide adequate caloric intake.

Severely ill infants who are unable to tolerate continuous enteral feedings are usually provided with peripheral alimentation with lipids. If sufficient caloric intake is not achieved by this route, a central venous catheter is required. Central alimentation may be needed for several weeks before the infant is able to tolerate enteral feedings. When an elemental diet is established and weight gain is satisfactory, the infant is discharged with careful follow-up care and observation. Parents are usually instructed to avoid feeding the infant milk protein and lactose for at least 6 months (Bass and Walker, 1986).

Nursing Considerations

Nursing care of the infant with intractable diarrhea is the same as for any infant receiving graduated oral feedings, intravenous therapy, and intravenous alimentation. Because the recovery in severe disease is frequently a lengthy process, the family will need considerable support and encouragement during both the period of hospitalization and home management. An important aspect of care that is common to all infants and children who require lengthly hospitalization and treatment is meeting growth and development needs. It is a nursing responsibility to ensure that adequate and appropriate stimulation activities are planned and implemented for the infant.

ACUTE INFECTIOUS GASTROENTERITIS

When diarrhea is presumed or established to be caused by a microorganism the terms "infectious gastroenteritis" or "bacterial gastroenteritis" are applied. In the pediatric age group infectious gastroenteritis is second only to upper respiratory tract infections as a cause of illness (Silverman and Roy, 1983). Although they are ordinarily benign and self-limited, they are a major pediatric problem and account for a significant number of hospital admissions.

Epidemiology

A variety of organisms are responsible for gastrointestinal tract disorders in infants and children. The disorders are transmitted by individuals or animals or by way of foods, and most of the illnesses show seasonal variations. Some are more prevalent at one age group than at another.

Sources and transmission. Most organisms that cause diarrhea are spread by the fecal-oral route. Some are transmitted by direct person-to-person contact, especially where sizable groups are in direct contact such as in day care centers. These include *Shigella*, *Giardia*, and sometimes *Campylobacter* and *Cryptosporidium*. A number of organisms are transmitted through contaminated food or water, for example, *Salmonella* and *Escherichia coli*. Raw milk and poultry have been sources of *Salmonella* and *Campylobacter jejuni*, and the Norwalk-like viruses are associated with consumption of drinking water, swimming water, and food. Family pets can be reservoirs of enteric pathogens (e.g., *Yersinia enterocolitica*, *C. jejuni*, and *Salmonella*).

Seasonal variability. Viral gastroenteritis is seen more frequently in winter months, whereas bacterial disorders are more prevalent during the summer and fall. There are some exceptions, however. For example, *Y. enterocolitica* infections are more common in winter months (Silverman and Roy, 1983).

Age. Although acute gastroenteritis affects all age groups, certain patterns are discernible. There is a greater frequency of diarrheal disease in younger children. *E. coli* is a prominent pathogen in the newborn. Rotaviruses are the most common cause of winter diarrhea in children younger than 2 years of age. *Giardia* and *Shigella* are common pathogens in toddlers 13 to 24 months old, and *Yersinia* and *Campylobacter* are also more likely to be associated with diarrhea in this age-group. The relative chance of a given illness being associated with *C. jejuni* is greater in older children, and the Norwalk-like viruses are a frequent cause of epidemics in school-age children (Guerrant, Lohr, and Williams, 1986).

Adolescents who are sexually active are subject to enteric pathogens that are transmitted by sexual contact (e.g., *Shigella*, *C. jejuni*, *Giardia*, *Entamoeba histolytica*) as well as the traditional sexually transmitted organisms that present with diarrhea or proctitis (e.g., *Neisseria gonorrhoeae*, syphilis, *Chlamydia*, and herpes simplex).

Other situations. Traveler's diarrhea is a common problem for some persons traveling to other countries. It is most often caused by enterotoxigenic *E. coli*. Other persons at risk are children with immune system disorders.

Daycare centers are a prime source of infection in younger children, especially in centers that care for children in diapers (see the discussion of infections in daycare centers in Chapter 16). The most common cause of diarrhea in daycare centers is *Giardia lamblia*. Other etiologic organisms include rotaviruses, *Shigella*, and *Campylobacter*. Outbreaks with *Clostridium difficile* and *Cryptosporidium* have been reported. *Salmonella* is a less common cause. The incidence is greatest in children younger than 3 years of age. Not only do toddlers explore their environment with their mouths, but many are not toilet trained and engage in direct contact with other children and caregivers.

Etiology/Pathophysiology

There are many organisms that can cause diarrheal disturbances in children, especially in infants. These can be enteric pathogens primarily, such as the *Shigella* and *Salmonella* groups of bacteria, or other organisms that have the potential to produce diarrhea under favorable circumstances, such as *Staphylococcus aureus*. Most infectious organisms are transmitted through contaminated feedings or by infected "carriers," including animal reservoirs such as dogs, cats, hamsters, birds, and turtles.

Bacterial invasion of the gastrointestinal tract produces diarrhea and related symptoms by interaction with intestinal mucosa in the following ways (Silverman and Roy, 1983):

1. **Enterotoxin production.** The organisms do not invade the mucosal epithelium. They produce their effect by multiplication in the gastrointestinal tract, followed by adhesion to the mucosa, where they release an exotoxin that binds to the small bowel villi. Interaction of this toxin and mucosa stimulates profuse secretion of water and electrolytes. Examples include *Shigella*, *E. coli*, and *Vibrio cholerae*.
2. **Invasion and destruction of epithelial cells.** The organisms directly invade and destroy the cells of the intestinal epithelium. The infection proceeds from the upper to the lower intestines, producing bloody mucoid stools. They also produce a powerful endotoxin that promotes loss of fluids and electrolytes into the intestine. Within the epithelium the organisms multiply and cause superficial ulcerations of the mucosa. Examples include *Shigella* and *E. coli*.
3. **Penetration and systemic invasion.** There is stimulation and excretion of intestinal fluids. Local inflammation is produced as organisms invade the thin layer of connective tissue (lamina propria) lying immediately beneath the epithelium of the mucous membrane in the distal small bowel and colon. The mucosa becomes hyperemic and edematous. From this point the organism has access to the systemic circulation, in which it can produce foci of infection elsewhere in the body. An example is *Salmonella*.
4. **Adherence without destruction of mucosa and without enterotoxin production** (unconfirmed). Enteropathic organisms (*E. coli*) penetrate the covering (glycocalyx) of some cells and adhere to the enterocyte surface. They disrupt the microvilli and have a blunting effect on the villi, interfering with villi functioning.

Organisms that are considered "normal flora" in most situations are enteropathic under certain conditions and in susceptible children, particularly newborn and young infants. These include certain strains of *E. coli* and *Staphylococcus aureus*. Some strains of *E. coli* produce diarrhea by invasion of the intestinal mucosa, and others by elaboration of enterotoxins. *S. aureus* can cause diarrhea by (1) food poisoning from contamination (especially milk or egg products) with exotoxin production, (2) enteritis as a result of prolonged broad-spectrum antibiotic therapy that destroys and eliminates enteric organisms that normally control staphylococcal invasion, (3) enteritis as a complication of staphylococcal infection elsewhere (skin or lungs), and (4) primary staphylococcal infection in newborn infants who have not yet established competing enteric flora.

The leading cause of noninflammatory bacterial disease in children worldwide is enterotoxigenic *E. coli*, which also remains the primary organism causing diarrhea in travelers. However, it is relatively uncommon in the United States. Enteropathologic *E. coli* is an important cause of diarrhea in the tropics, and *Cryptosporidium* is being recognized with increased frequency in tropical areas. Major causes of diarrhea in the United States are those that produce inflammatory diarrhea, including *C. jejuni*, *Shigella*, *Salmonella*, *Yersinia enterocolitica*, and *C. difficile*.

The enteropathic organisms are briefly outlined in Table 29-2. Other agents such as *Pseudomonas*, *Klebsiella*, and *Proteus* may cause diarrhea but do not ordinarily have a tendency to do so. Amebic dysentery seldom occurs in infants.

Clinical Manifestations

Infectious diarrheas have some features in common, such as vomiting, and there is frequently abdominal discomfort. Bacterial infections and some viral infections are accompanied by fever. The severity is variable among the various forms (see Table 29-2).

Diagnostic Evaluation

Laboratory confirmation of the specific organism confirms the diagnosis and serves as a guideline for appropriate medical therapy.

Therapeutic Management

The primary concern in infectious gastroenteritis, as in all conditions in which fluid is lost in large amounts, is dehydration and the attendant deterioration. Fluid replacement and monitoring of electrolyte status with replacement are the same as for any diarrheal disorder. When the organism is identified appropriate antibiotics are prescribed for those diarrheas for which specific therapy has been found to be effective.

Preliminary tests of a preventive vaccine for rotavirus infection (Vesikari and others, 1984) have been developed. When its effectiveness is established, infants and children at risk can be protected against this common cause of diarrhea in the pediatric age-group.

Nursing Considerations

Basic nursing care for the infant or child with infectious gastroenteritis is the same as for any diarrheal disease. However, appropriate isolation precautions are carried out to prevent the spread of the infection to others. The degree of isolation varies with the type of organism, from strict precautions to appropriate stool management.

Table 29-2 Enteropathologic causes of infectious gastroenteritis

ORGANISM	PATHOLOGY	CHARACTERISTICS	COMMENTS

Viral agents
Rotavirus
  Incubation period: 2-3
  days
	Remains unexplained
	Severely distorted mucosal
	  architecture with
	  atropic mucosa and
	  severe inflammatory
	  changes
		Abrupt onset
		Fever (38° C or above)
		  lasting approximately
		  48 hours
		Associated upper
		  respiratory tract
		  infection
		Diarrhea may persist for
		  more than a week
			Incidence higher in cool
			  weather (80% in winter)
			Affects all age groups; 6 to
			  24-month-old infants
			  more vulnerable
			Usually mild and self-
			  limited

Norwalk-like organisms
 	
  Incubation period: 1-2
  days
	Mechanism of affect
	  unknown
	Blunting of villi and
	  inflammatory changes
	  in lamina propria
	Reduced enzymes
		Fever
		Loss of appetite
		Nausea/vomiting
		Abdominal pain
		Diarrhea
		Malaise
			Source of infection:
			  drinking water,
			  recreation water, food
			  (including shellfish)
			Affects all ages
			Benign; seldom lasts more
			  than 3 days
			Self-limited

Bacterial agents
Pathogenic
  Escherichia coli
  Incubation period: highly
  variable
	Enterotoxin production
	  (small bowel)
	Reduces absorption and
	  increases secretion of
	  fluids and electrolytes
		Onset gradual or abrupt
		Variable clinical
		  manifestations
		Most—green, watery
		  diarrhea with mucus;
		  becomes explosive
		Vomiting may be present
		  from onset
		Abdominal distention
		Diarrhea
		Fever; appears toxic
			Incidence higher in
			  summer
			Usually interpersonal
			  transmission but may
			  transmit via inanimate
			  objects
			A cause of nursery
			  epidemics
			With symptomatic
			  treatment only, may
			  continue for weeks
			Full breast-feeding has a
			  protective effect
			Symptoms generally
			  subside in 3-7 days
			Relapse rate approxi-
			  mately 20%

Salmonella groups
  (nontyphoidae)—
  gram-negative,
  nonencapsulated,
  nonsporulating
  Incubation period:
    6-72 hours for
    intraluminal
    7-21 days for
    extraluminal
	Penetration of lamina
	  propria (small bowel
	  and colon)
	Local inflammation—no
	  extensive destruction
	Stimulation of intestinal
	  fluid excretion
	Systemic invasion of other
	  sites
		Rapid onset
		Variable symptoms—mild
		  to severe
		Nausea, vomiting, and
		  colicky abdominal pain
		  followed by diarrhea,
		  occasionally with blood
		  and mucus
		Chills not uncommon
		Hyperactive peristalsis
		  and mild abdominal
		  tenderness
		Symptoms usually subside
		  within 5 days
		May have fever,
		  headache, and cerebral
		  manifestations, for
		  example, drowsiness,
		  confusion,
		  meningismus, or
		  seizures
		Infants may be afebrile
		  and nontoxic
		May result in life-
		  threatening septicemia
		  and meningitis
			Two thirds of patients are
			  younger than 20 years
			  of age; highest
			  incidence in children
			  younger than age 9
			  years, especially
			  infants
			Highest incidence occurs
			  July through October,
			  lowest from January
			  through April
			Transmission primarily via
			  contaminated food and
			  drink—most from
			  animal sources,
			  including fowl,
			  mammals, reptiles,
			  and insects
			Most common sources are
			  poultry and eggs
			In children—pets, e.g.,
			  dogs, cats, hamsters,
			  and especially pet
			  turtles
			Communicable as long as
			  organisms are excreted

Continued.

Table 29-2 Enteropathologic causes of infectious gastroenteritis—cont'd

ORGANISM	PATHOLOGY	CHARACTERISTICS	COMMENTS
Vibrio cholerae (cholera) groups Incubation period: usually 1-3 days; range from few hours to 5 days	Enterotoxin causes increased secretion of chloride and possibly bicarbonate Intestinal mucosa congested with enlarged lymph follicles Intact mucosal surface	Sudden onset of profuse, watery diarrhea without cramping, tenesmus, or anal irritation, although children may complain of cramping Stools are intermittent at first, then almost continuous Stools are whitish, almost clear, with flecks of mucus—"rice water stools"	Rare in infants younger than 1 year old Mortality high in both treated and untreated infants and small children Transmitted via contaminated food and water Endemic in Bengal Attack confers immunity
Food poisoning *Staphylococcus* Incubation period: 4-6 hours	Produce heat-stable enterotoxin	Nausea, vomiting Severe abdominal cramps Profuse diarrhea Shock may occur in severe cases May be a mild fever	Transferred via contaminated food—inadequately cooked or refrigerated, e.g., custards, mayonnaise, cream-filled or -topped desserts Self-limited; improvement apparent within 24 hours Excellent prognosis
Clostridium perfringens Incubation period: 8-24 hours	Produces heat-resistant and heat-sensitive toxins	Moderate to severe crampy, midepigastric pain	Self-limited illness Transmission by commercial food products—most often meat and poultry
Botulism *Clostridium botulinum* Incubation period: 12 hr–3 days	Highly potent neurotoxin	Nausea, vomiting Diarrhea CNS symptoms with curarelike effect (see p. 000) Dry mouth, dysphagia	Transmitted by contaminated food products Variable severity—mild symptoms to rapidly fatal within a few hours Antitoxin administration
S. typhi	Rapid invasion of bloodstream from minor sites of inflammation Marked inflammation and necrosis of intestinal mucosa and lymphatics	Variable in infants Older children—irregular fever, headache, malaise, lethargy Diarrhea occurs in 50% at early stage Cough is common In a few days, fever rises and is consistent; fatigue, cough, abdominal pain, anorexia, and weight loss develop; diarrhea begins	Decreased incidence in last decade Acute symptoms may persist for a week or more
Shigella groups—gram-negative, nonmotile, anaerobic bacilli Incubation period: 1-7 days	Enterotoxin Stimulates loss of fluids and electrolytes Invasion of epithelium with superficial mucosal ulcerations *S. dysenteriae* forms exotoxin	Onset variable but usually abrupt Fever and cramping abdominal pain initially Fever—may reach 40.5° C Convulsions in about 10%—usually associated with fever Patient appears sick Headache, nuchal rigidity, delirium	Approximately 60% of cases in children younger than age 9 years with more than one third between ages 1 and 4 years Peak incidence late summer Transmitted directly or indirectly from infected persons Communicable for 1-4 weeks

Table 29-2   Enteropathologic causes of infectious gastroenteritis—cont'd

ORGANISM	PATHOLOGY	CHARACTERISTICS	COMMENTS
Shigella groups— cont'd		Watery diarrhea with mucus and pus starts about 12-48 hours after onset Stools preceded by abdominal cramps; tenesmus and straining follow Symptoms usually subside in 5-10 days	Self-limited disease Treat with antibiotics Severe dehydration and collapse can affect all patients Acute symptoms may persist for a week or more
Yersinia enterocolitica Incubation period: 7-10 days		Diarrhea—may be bloody Fever (>38.7° C) Abdominal pain (RLQ) Vomiting, diarrhea	Seen more frequently in winter Majority in first 3 years of life Transmitted by food and pets Can resemble appendicitis May be relapsing and last for months
Campylobacter jejuni Incubation period: 2-11 days	Precise mechanism unclear Jejunum and ileum involvement Extensive ulceration with hemorrhagic ileitis Broadening and flattening of mucosa	Fever Abdominal pain—often severe, cramping, periumbilical Watery, profuse, foul-smelling diarrhea Vomiting	Person-to-person transmission May be transmitted by pets (e.g., cat, dog, hamster) Food (especially chicken) and water-borne transmission Relapse possible Most patients recover spontaneously Antibiotics advocated to speed recovery Peak incidence in summer
Clostridium difficile Incubation period: variable	Enterotoxin Irritates and degenerates colonic membranes	Tenesmus, cramping Diarrhea—frank blood and pus in stools	Most cases in adults Seen with increasing frequency in children May be a cause of chronic diarrhea Newborn may be asymptomatic carrier

It may be necessary to obtain stool specimens from the child and other family members who are affected or suspected to be carriers of infectious organisms. The parents are provided with specimen containers and instructed in collection and disposition of stool samples.

Recent reports suggest that traveler's diarrhea can be prevented by prophylactic administration of trimethoprim/sulfamethoxazole (Bactrim, Septra) (Freeman and others, 1983), doxycycline (Vibramycin, Vibra-Tabs) (Dupont and others, 1983), or subsalicylate bismuth suspension (Pepto-Bismol) (Dupont and others, 1980; Graham and others, 1983). Although the medications appear to be safe for adults, parents should be cautioned against giving any of the drugs to children. The drugs may be inappropriate or untested for use in children. For example, the large doses of Pepto-Bismol recommended for adults may contain toxic amounts of salicylates when given to children, and the bismuth may cause neurologic deficits.

Until vaccines or other prophylactic measures are proved safe for children, the best prevention is to allow children to drink only bottled water and carbonated beverages (from the container through a straw supply brought from home). Tap water, ice, unpasteurized dairy products, raw vegetables, and unpeeled fruits should be avoided. Meats and seafoods may be risky as well.

VOMITING

Vomiting, a very common symptom in childhood, is usually of little concern. Often it is of a minor and temporary nature, but when vomiting is persistent and prolonged, the consequences to the infant or child can be rapid and serious.

Nursing Care Summary: The Child with Gastroenteritis (Acute Diarrhea)

	NURSING GOALS	NURSING INTERVENTIONS	EXPECTED PATIENT/FAMILY OUTCOMES
N.D	**HP-HMP Infection: potential for** **Risk factors: presence of infectious organisms**		

	Prevent spread of infection	Isolate affected child from contact with others
		Implement protective techniques as dictated by
		  hospital policy, including
		    Disposal of excreta and laundry
		    Appropriate handling of specimens
		Maintain careful hand washing
		Apply diaper snugly to reduce likelihood of fecal
		  spread
		Instruct others (parents, members of staff) in
		  protective procedures
		Teach affected children protective methods to
		  prevent spread of infection, for example,
		  remaining in restricted area, hand washing,
		  handling genital area, care after using bedpan or
		  toilet, and so on
		Endeavor to keep infants and small children from
		  placing hand and objects in contaminated areas
		Assess home situation and implement protective
		  measures as feasible in individual circumstances
			Infection does not spread to others

N.D	**HP-HMP Injury, potential for (trauma)** **Risk factors: therapies, dehydration**		

	Prevent complications from
	  restraining devices
		Remove restraints from extremities as often as
		  possible
		Change position at least every 2 hours
		Frequently observe circulation, position, and
		  pressure points
			Extremities remain free of
			  construction and pressure

	Observe for signs of
	  complications
		Assess frequently
		  Vital signs—temperature, pulse, respiration, and
		    blood pressure
		  Skin characteristics
		  Sensory response
		  Neurologic signs
		  Behavior
			Vital signs remain within normal
			  limits for age (see inside front
			  cover for normal variations)

N.D	**N-MP Fluid volume deficit: actual (2)** **Etiology: excessive losses**		
	Rehydration	Offer appropriate fluids as tolerated	Child exhibits signs of adequate hydration (specify)

	Assess progress of
	  hydration
		Maintain accurate record of intake
		Weigh child daily or as ordered
		Assess all parameters, for example, vital signs,
		  skin characteristics
		Apply urine collection device when indicated
		Measure urine volume and specific gravity	

	Prevent interference with
	  therapeutic regimen
		Apply appropriate restraining methods where
		  indicated
			*Therapy(ies) are maintained

N.D	**N-MP Nutrition, alteration in: less than body requirements** **Risk factors: nothing by mouth, diarrheal losses**		

	Reestablish diet
	  appropriate for age
		Gradually reintroduce foods as indicated (specify)
		Observe response to feedings
		Describe feeding behavior
			Child takes prescribed nourishment
			*Observations are recorded
			  accurately

N.D	**N-MP Oral membranes, alteration in** **Etiology: dehydration, nothing by mouth**		

	Relieve dryness	Administer special mouth care while fluids by mouth
		  are restricted
			Mucous membranes remain moist
			  and clean

*Nursing outcome.

Nursing Care Summary: The Child with Gastroenteritis (Acute Diarrhea)—cont'd

	NURSING GOALS	NURSING INTERVENTIONS	EXPECTED PATIENT/FAMILY OUTCOMES
N-MP	**Skin integrity, impairment of: potential** **Risk factors: frequent loose stools**		
	Prevent skin breakdown	Change diaper and wash and dry area thoroughly after each soiling; disposable diapers absorb poorly, cloth diapers are preferred; may need to apply thick cotton panties to keep stool contained in diaper Cleanse buttocks and genital area well Apply protective lotion or ointment Expose reddened area to heat and air where feasible (risk of contamination great in explosive diarrhea)	Skin exhibits no evidence of discoloration or irritation
EP	**Bowel elimination, alteration in: diarrhea** **Etiology: inflammation, irritation**		
	Assess status of diarrhea	Record urine output Record fecal output—number, volume, characteristics Observe and record presence of associated signs—tenesmus, cramping, vomiting	*Extent of intestinal losses is determined
SP-SCP	**Anxiety** **Etiology: separation from parents, strange environment, distressing procedures**		
	Provide comfort measures	Provide pacifier for infants who are receiving nothing by mouth Bubble child periodically to help expel swallowed air Hold infant or child when this does not interfere with therapy Touch, talk, and otherwise comfort child who cannot be held Provide sensory stimulation and diversion appropriate to child's level of development Encourage family members to visit and allow them to comfort and care for child to the extent possible	Child engages in nonnutritive sucking Child exhibits no signs of distress
RRP	**Family process, alteration in** **Etiology: situational crisis (child's illness and/or hospitalization)—cont'd**		

	Support family	Reassure family, especially mother
		Explain therapeutic measures that may be distressing to family
		  Nothing by mouth
		  Parenteral fluids
		  Restraints necessary
		  Shaving of infant's head for intravenous therapy
		  Isolation from other children
		  Need for precautions that family must observe
		Help family provide comfort and support for child
		See also The family of the hospitalized child, p. 1081.
			Family displays an understanding of the child's condition and therapies and becomes actively involved in physical and emotional care

	Educate family	Instruct in diet planning (see general plan for dietary management, which follows) Help caregiver plan diet to meet needs of affected child in relation to family diet plan Instruct in preparation and storage of food, based on assessment of individual family needs and facilities Instruct in care and disposal of waste materials Teach and emphasize importance of good hygiene and sanitation	Family demonstrates and understands child's care and management

*Nursing outcome.

Continued.

Nursing Care Summary: The Child with Gastroenteritis (Acute Diarrhea)—cont'd

NURSING GOALS	NURSING INTERVENTIONS	EXPECTED PATIENT/FAMILY OUTCOMES
Arrange for follow-up care	Emphasize importance of posthospitalization health assessment Refer to community health agency for care and instruction when indicated	Family complies with instructions

Nursing Interventions Related to Medical Management

Rehydrate child
 Administer fluids as ordered
  Intravenous
   Administer correct fluid
   Maintain desired drip rate
   Add appropriate electrolytes as prescribed
   Maintain integrity of infusion site
  Oral
   Feed electrolyte-containing solutions as prescribed
Eradicate infectious agent
 Administer antimicrobial medications as prescribed
 Administer other medications as prescribed

Assess progress of diarrhea
 Collect specimens as needed
 Make appropriate diagnostic tests and record
  Stools—pH, blood, sugar, frequency
  Urine—pH, specific gravity, frequency
Detect source of infection
 Examine other members of household and refer for treatment where indicated
 Collect stool specimens from household members where indicated

An associated hazard, especially in very young and debilitated infants and children, is the risk of aspiration, with the possibility of asphyxiation, atelectasis, or pneumonia.

The amount and character of the vomiting are important observations, and nurses should be able to distinguish between and describe the various forms this behavior takes. *Vomiting* is the forcible ejection of stomach contents and is usually accompanied by nausea. In *projectile vomiting* vomitus is forcefully ejected as far as 2 to 4 feet (0.6 to 1.2 m) from the child. Projectile vomiting is not associated with nausea. Spitting up and regurgitation, characteristic of infants, are described in Chapter 9.

Vomiting in childhood can be caused by numerous intrinsic and extrinsic factors, but is usually caused by readily detected infections or psychologic causes. Vomiting and diarrhea are common manifestations of a variety of infectious disorders, responses to an allergen or ingestion of drugs or other toxic substances, and symptoms associated with appendicitis or gastrointestinal tract obstruction. Recurrent, prolonged, or persistent vomiting is also associated with encephalographic variations and results from increased intracranial pressure caused by space-occupying lesions.

Many children are prone to motion sickness when riding in an automobile or airplane or even when swinging in a swing. Some children, especially overly dependent children, maladjusted children, or children who react to environmental stress (e.g., a high-anxiety home environment), with somatic symptoms, respond to tension or stress with stomach upset and vomiting.

Occasionally children will vomit as an oral defense mechanism, such as when children resist feedings they do not want. They may think eating is an obligation they are powerless to resist. Other children resort to contentious vomiting when they become angry with someone they know loves and cares for them. For example, struggles over independence in 2-year-old children can trigger intense emotions. A child who vomits during a conflict with parents soon realizes that this inadvertent occurrence causes concern in the parents, who view kicking and screaming as behavior but vomiting as illness. Consequently, the reflexive vomiting may become conditioned and reinforced by the parents' response to it (Fleisher, 1986).

The *cyclic vomiting syndrome* usually begins between 2 and 9 years of age with episodes that tend to be stereotypic and self-limited. Typically they begin at night or on rising and last 12 to 48 hours, although some children may have symptoms for as little as a few hours, and others for as long as 10 days. Attacks occur regularly in most patients and may occur weekly or months apart. In the majority of cases specific events trigger an attack, such as vacations or other nonnoxious excitement, noxious emotional experiences, and colds or flu. There is no cure, but in most children the disorder remits during adolescence (Fleisher, 1986).

Older children may practice vomiting as an act of malingering, deceiving parents or others in order to gain something or to be relieved of some obligation. This manipulative behavior stops as soon as it ceases to work. Bulimia, practiced by some adolescents, is described in Chapter 21.

Pathophysiology

Vomiting, one of the most primitive protective functions with which animals are endowed, is controlled through the vomiting center located in the reticular core of the medulla. The vomiting center receives stimuli from three sources:

1. Higher cortical centers—either deep-seated or superficial psychologic disturbances. Stimuli include those associated with unpleasant sights, repugnant odors, and fright.
2. A chemosensitive trigger zone located on the floor of the fourth ventricle posterior to the medullary surface, which transmits impulses to the center. Stimuli include chemical stimulation by drugs such as apomorphine, morphine, ipecac, and some digitalis derivatives, and toxins such as metabolic substances that result from uremia, infections, or radiation; cerebral hypoxia from decreased cerebral blood supply; the direct effect of increased intracranial pressure; and disturbances of the semicircular canals of the inner ear.
3. Reflex excitement from vagal and sympathetic afferent nerves resulting from disturbed gastrointestinal and other viscera. Stimuli include irritation, inflammation, or mechanical disturbance at any level of the gastrointestinal tract, such as distention or obstruction; irritation of other viscera, such as the heart, renal pelvis, and bladder; and pain of many sources.

Vomiting involves a complex reflex that is associated with widespread autonomic discharge that causes salivation, pallor, sweating, and tachycardia. Motor reaction, transmitted to the upper gastrointestinal tract, causes the vomiting act. The stomach antrum and duodenum contract; the remainder of the stomach, the esophagus, and its sphincters relax; the glottis closes to occlude the pulmonary airway; and the soft palate closes the nasopharynx. Then the diaphragm and abdominal muscles contract sharply, raising the intraabdominal pressure, which compresses the abdominal contents and propels them into the esophagus and out through the mouth. Actual vomiting is usually preceded by severe cycles of reflux into the esophagus.

Assessment

Vomiting is the first symptom of a variety of common infections as well as a manifestation of more serious conditions. It is a relatively frequent symptom during the neonatal period, usually caused by simple regurgitation from overfeeding or insufficient bubbling, and has little clinical significance. However, it can indicate the presence of gastrointestinal tract disorders or increased intracranial pressure. The following nursing observations can provide valuable information for evaluating the nature and importance of vomiting.

Character of vomitus. Vomitus that contains unchanged food and no gastric juice is esophageal. A relaxed cardiac sphincter or rumination (habitual regurgitation) will produce frequent small amounts of vomitus emitted with little force. The presence of sour milk curds with no green or brown color indicates vomitus from the stomach and excludes an esophageal cause. Uncurdled milk may also be vomited during or shortly after feedings. Vomitus containing greenish material indicating the presence of bile pigment is most likely to occur when an obstruction is situated below the ampulla of Vater; bile in the vomitus almost always excludes pyloric stenosis. Vomitus with a fecal odor suggests a lower intestinal obstruction or peritonitis.

Blood in the vomitus may appear as bright red, bloody streaks or brown coffee grounds emesis and may be insignificant or of major importance. Hematemesis is sometimes observed in the immediate neonatal period in infants who have swallowed maternal blood during delivery or occasionally from a cracked nipple. Other causes of hematemesis in early infancy include hemorrhagic disease of the newborn or other defects of coagulation and early esophageal erosion associated with regurgitation of gastric juice in diaphragmatic hernia. Trauma from nasogastric tubes or tracheal catheters may cause bleeding followed by vomiting of swallowed blood.

In older children hematemesis may be caused by swallowed blood from epistaxis or after nose or throat surgery. Rupture of esophageal varices and peptic ulcer can cause profuse hematemesis. Coagulation defects or vascular damage may cause bloody vomiting in many diseases.

Frequency and persistence. Frequent or persistent vomiting indicates that the causative factor is still operating. The primary danger is loss of fluids and electrolytes, which increases with the frequency and duration of vomiting. In early infancy the most frequent causes are pylorospasm, pyloric stenosis, adrenocortical insufficiency, and urinary tract infections. Recurrent vomiting suggests gastrointestinal allergy, an epileptic equivalent ("abdominal epilepsy"), a childhood form of migraine, or inconsistent intestinal obstruction, as might occur with malrotation of the colon. It is frequently associated with the onset of a febrile illness or a period of increased emotional tension.

Amount. The amount of the emesis should be measured and recorded because it often furnishes information regarding the amount of fluid lost in relation to intake. This provides a clue to the extent of dehydration. Overfeeding or too rapid feeding may cause the child to vomit part of the feeding.

Force of vomiting. Repeated regurgitation is most often related to rumination or gastroesophageal reflux. Forceful vomiting during or after a meal is usually caused by overdistention with milk and air. Repeated forceful vomiting of a projectile nature is one of the cardinal signs of pyloric stenosis in early infancy and can be a result of a brain tumor at any age. When combined with abdominal distention, it suggests intestinal obstruction.

Relationship to feeding. Emesis in infants may be related to the nature of their formula. Highly diluted formula may cause hungry infants to consume so much that they vomit from overdistention. High-fat or acidified formulas may cause others to vomit. Food that is contaminated by bacteria or food that is inappropriate for the child, such as unripe fruits or rich, highly seasoned foods, may cause a child to vomit.

Vomiting soon after eating may be the result of food allergy or a symptom of an acute, febrile illness. More often it is caused by gastric distention associated with improper feeding techniques. Overdistention by milk and air initiates vomiting, which is caused by such feeding practices as failure to bubble the infant during and immediately after feedings, feeding formula through nipples with holes so small that the infant takes in air while sucking for milk, improper positioning of the bottle so that air instead of milk enters the nipple, feeding too rapidly, swallowing air from prolonged sucking on an empty breast, and underfeeding, which leads to hunger and causes the infant to swallow air while sucking on fingers or fists. Unwarmed formula may cause a few infants to vomit, and hurried eating at any age may precipitate vomiting, particularly when the child is excited or overly tired.

History. Sometimes the cause of vomiting is readily apparent from the history. Vomiting associated with diarrhea is usually caused by gastroenteritis; vomiting that occurs suddenly in a previously healthy child suggests the early stages of an infection. When several children or members of a family who have eaten together vomit, food poisoning is the most likely possibility. Vomiting accompanied by fever and abdominal pain and tenderness is a common symptom of appendicitis or other conditions of the abdomen requiring surgical repair. Vomiting is not an uncommon reaction to toxins and to drugs taken as prescribed or ingested accidentally.

Diagnostic Evaluation

When vomiting is persistent and cannot be attributed to an obvious and temporary condition, a more comprehensive evaluation is warranted. It may be the only symptom the child has; however, more often it is only one clinical feature of any one of a variety of disorders. The importance of vomiting in relation to the associated disease is also variable. It may be a minor manifestation of a serious illness or the dominant clinical feature. Vomiting that is not associated with feeding may be an indication of a space-occupying lesion.

Diagnostic tests. Physical examination and routine tests of blood and urine are performed, but special laboratory tests are seldom employed. Radiographic studies can detect anomalies of the alimentary tract. If vomiting has persisted to the degree that dehydration and electrolyte imbalance are present, the weight and serum electrolyte, blood urea nitrogen, and carbon dioxide content of the blood are determined to assess the state of hydration and to serve as the basis for therapy.

Therapeutic Management

Management is directed toward detection and treatment of the cause of the vomiting and prevention of complications of the vomiting. Vomiting that results in fluid loss of considerable degree may require parenteral fluid therapy. Fluids are administered in the same manner and in a similar electrolyte composition to those administered in diarrhea. This includes both parenteral and oral fluids.

Although most children respond well to these measures, centrally acting antiemetic drugs may be prescribed when the cause of the vomiting is known and the vomiting is pre-

dictable and of limited duration. Several antiemetics are safe for children: antihistamines, such as dimenhydrinate (Dramamine) and cyclizine (Marezine), which exert their effect on neural labyrinth pathways; dopamine antagonists, for example, promethazine (Phenergan), chlorpromazine (Thorazine), and metoclopramide (Reglan), which depress the chemoreceptor trigger zone and the vomiting center; and miscellaneous drugs including diphenidol (Vontrol), which acts on the aural vestibular apparatus, and trimethobenzamide (Tigan), which acts on the chemoreceptor trigger zone.

Nursing Considerations

The major emphasis of nursing care of the vomiting infant or child is on observation and reporting of vomiting behavior and associated symptoms and the implementation of measures to reduce the vomiting. Accurate assessment of the type of vomiting, the appearance of the vomitus, and the child's behavior associated with the vomiting greatly aids in establishing a diagnosis of disorders that have vomiting as a clinical manifestation.

Nursing interventions will be determined by the cause of the vomiting. When the vomiting is identified as a manifestation of improper feeding methods, establishing proper techniques through teaching and example will usually correct the situation. If the vomiting is assessed as a probable manifestation of a gastrointestinal obstruction, food is usually withheld or special feeding techniques are implemented. In situations in which vomiting is related to concurrent infection, dietary indiscretion, or emotional factors, efforts are directed toward maintaining hydration or preventing dehydration by offering small amounts of palatable fluids such as ice chips, ginger ale, or diluted fruit juices, much the same as the oral intake described for dehydration (p. 1174).

The thirst mechanism is the most sensitive guide to fluid needs, and ad libitum administration of a glucose-electrolyte solution to an alert child will restore water and electrolytes satisfactorily. It is important to include carbohydrate to spare body protein and to avoid ketosis resulting from exhaustion of glycogen reserves. Once vomiting has abated, more liberal amounts can be offered, followed by simple foods such as gelatin, crackers, clear broth, and buttered toast in small amounts, when the child desires, followed by gradual resumption of the regular diet. Some physicians believe that small, frequent feedings actually induce further losses through activation of the gastrocolic reflex, and prescribe large volumes initially at less frequent intervals. Care must be exercised in the use of electrolytes to avoid the possibility of hyperelectrolytemia.

HYPERTROPHIC PYLORIC STENOSIS

Obstruction at the pyloric sphincter by hypertrophy of the circular muscle of the pylorus is one of the most common surgical disorders of early infancy. This functional anomaly is seen soon after birth with vomiting that becomes progres-

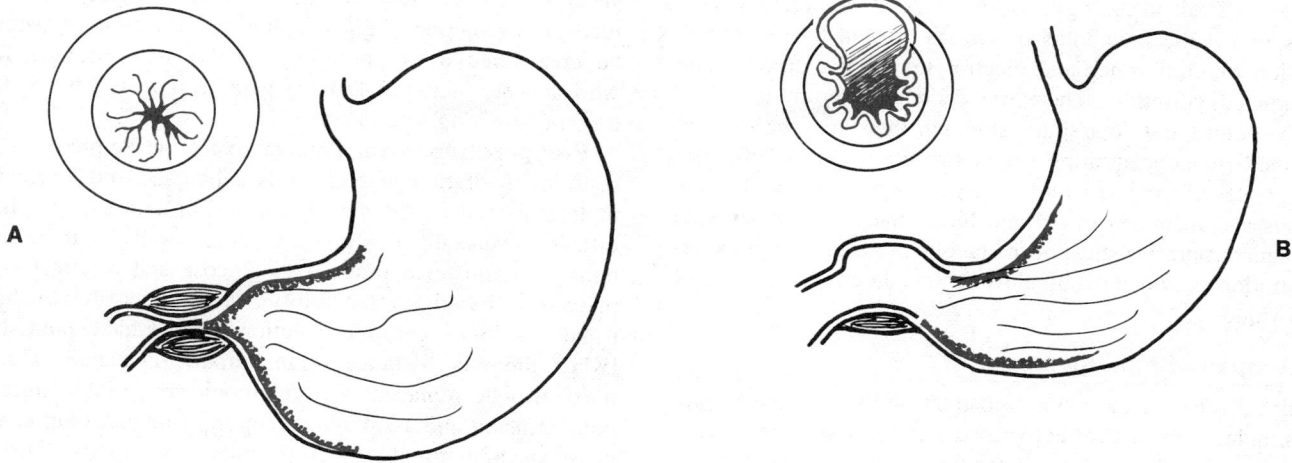

Fig. 29-2. Hypertrophic pyloric stenosis. **A,** Enlarged muscular tumor nearly obliterates pyloric channel. **B,** Longitudinal surgical division of muscle down to submucosa establishes adequate passageway.

sively more severe and projectile. It is five times more common in male than in female infants, affecting approximately five of 1000 males and only one of 1000 females (Cohen, 1984). It is seen less frequently in black and Oriental than in white infants. It is more likely to affect a full-term than a premature infant.

The cause of the increased size of the pyloric musculature is unknown. A higher incidence in first-degree relatives and in monozygotic as opposed to dizygotic twins implicates heredity in the etiology, although the nature of the hereditary factors is only speculative.

Pathophysiology

The circular muscle of the pylorus is grossly enlarged as a result of both hypertrophy and hyperplasia. This produces severe narrowing of the pyloric canal between the stomach and the duodenum. Consequently the lumen at this point is partially obstructed. Over a period of time inflammation and edema further reduce the size of the opening until the partial obstruction may progress to complete obstruction. The muscle is thickened to as much as twice its usual size—2 to 3 cm (¾ to 1¼ inches) long—and is almost cartilaginous in consistency. The distal portion ends abruptly and is externally distinct and easily palpated, but the proximal end merges into the gastric antrum. The stomach is usually dilated (Fig. 29-2, *A*).

Clinical Manifestations

The age of onset and pattern of vomiting are variable. Typically infants with pyloric hypertrophy are well during the first weeks of life. Initially there is only regurgitation or occasional nonprojectile vomiting that begins about the second to the fourth week after birth, although in a few infants symptoms begin at birth. Others do well for the first few weeks and then suddenly develop projectile vomiting that rapidly leads to dehydration. The projectile vomiting usually develops within a week and may lead to complete obstruc-

tion by 4 to 6 weeks. The vomitus may be ejected 2 to 4 feet (0.6 to 1.2 m) from the child in a side-lying position, and 1 foot (0.3 m) or more when the infant is lying on the back. Vomiting occurs most often shortly after a feeding, although it may occur as long as several hours later. In some instances the vomiting may follow each feeding; in others it appears intermittently. The infant is hungry and an avid nurser who eagerly accepts a second feeding after a vomiting episode. The vomitus is nonbilious, containing only gastric contents, but may be blood tinged. The infant does not appear to be in pain other than the discomfort of chronic hunger.

The infant fails to gain weight or may lose weight, the stools diminish in number and size from the reduced intake, and evidence of dehydration becomes increasingly obvious. There is decreased elasticity of the skin, loss of subcutaneous tissue, and sunken eyeballs. The upper abdomen is distended, and diagnosis can be established on the basis of (1) a readily palpable olive-shaped tumor in the epigastrium just to the right of the umbilicus and (2) visible gastric peristaltic waves that move from left to right across the epigastrium. The pyloric tumor is most easily felt when the abdominal muscles are relaxed during a feeding or immediately after vomiting. Positive identification of these physical signs is sufficient evidence to establish a diagnosis (usually corroborated by a second physician).

Difficulty in diagnosis is related to children with feeding difficulties associated with disturbed mother-child relationships or hyperkinetic infants, who are exceptionally reactive to external stimuli and vomit more frequently than usual in the early weeks of life.

Diagnostic Evaluation

If diagnosis is inconclusive from the history and physical signs, ultrasound or upper gastrointestinal radiographic studies will reveal delayed gastric emptying and an elongated, threadlike pyloric channel. A palpable "olive" mass can usually be felt in the right upper quadrant. Laboratory findings reflect the metabolic alterations created by severe depletion of both water and electrolytes from extensive and prolonged vomiting. There are decreased serum levels of both sodium and potassium, although these may be masked by the hemoconcentration from extracellular fluid depletion. Of greater diagnostic value are a decrease in serum chloride levels and increases in pH and bicarbonate (carbon dioxide content) characteristics of metabolic alkalosis. Hemoconcentration is evidenced by elevated hematocrit and hemoglobin values.

Therapeutic Management

Surgical relief of the pyloric obstruction by pyloromyotomy is simple, safe, and effective and is, with very few exceptions, the standard treatment for this disorder. Nonoperative management is possible but seldom employed today because the treatment is lengthy and the results uncertain.

Inasmuch as the surgery is not an emergency procedure, the initial efforts are directed toward rehydration of the infant, replenishment of body potassium stores, and correction of alkalosis with parenteral fluid and electrolyte administration. In well-hydrated infants with no evidence of electrolyte imbalance, surgery is performed without delay. Replacement fluid therapy usually delays surgery for 24 to 48 hours. Some surgeons prefer the stomach to be empty during surgery to diminish postoperative vomiting from gastric irritation. For these infants, gastric lavage with isotonic saline solution is part of preoperative preparation. The lavage tube is often left in place during the surgical procedure to keep the stomach empty of fluid, air, or barium from radiographic procedures.

The surgical procedure is performed through a right upper quadrant muscle-splitting incision and consists of a longitudinal incision through the circular muscle fibers of the pylorus down to but not including the submucosa (Fredet-Ramstedt operation) (Fig. 29-2, *B*). The procedure has a very high success rate when infants receive careful preoperative preparation to correct fluid and electrolyte imbalances.

Feedings are usually begun 4 to 6 hours postoperatively, beginning with small, frequent feedings of glucose in water or electrolyte solution. If clear fluids are retained, about 24 hours after surgery formula is started in the same stepwise increments, gradually increasing the amount and the interval between feedings until a full feeding schedule is reinstated, which usually takes about 48 hours. The infant is ready to be discharged from the hospital by about the fourth postoperative day. The prognosis is excellent, and the mortality is low.

Nursing Considerations

Nursing care of the infant with hypertrophic pyloric stenosis involves primarily observation for physical signs and behaviors that help establish the diagnosis, careful regulation of fluid therapy, and reestablishment of normal feeding behaviors. Nurses are in a position to recognize signs of the disorder in infants and to refer them for medical evaluation. Hypertrophic pyloric stenosis should be considered as a possibility in the very young infant who appears alert but fails to gain weight and has a history of vomiting after meals.

Preoperative care. Preoperatively the emphasis is on restoring hydration and electrolyte balance and beginning replacement of depleted body fat and protein stores. These infants are usually not given feedings orally, but intravenously administered fluids with glucose and electrolyte replacement based on laboratory serum electrolyte values, usually sodium chloride solution with added potassium (when there is adequate urine output). Depleted calcium must also be replaced. Careful monitoring of the intravenous infusion and assiduous attention to intake, output, and urine specific gravity measurements are important to the success of fluid replacement. Accurate description of any vomiting, as well as the number and character of stools, is recorded.

If the infant is fed either thickened or unthickened feedings, special techniques are needed to minimize the likelihood of vomiting. Feedings are given slowly with the infant held in a semi-upright position. Because these infants tend to suck their fingers and hands, they swallow a considerable amount of air; therefore, bubbling before and frequently during feedings will lessen gastric distention. After a feeding the infant is turned slightly on the right side in high-Fowler position in an infant seat or propped in the crib to facilitate gastric emptying. Minimal handling, especially after a feeding, helps prevent vomiting. If vomiting occurs, the type, amount, character, and its relationship to the feeding are observed and recorded. Refeeding of formula is usually ordered in an amount equivalent to the volume lost.

Observations include assessment of vital signs, particularly those that might indicate fluid or electrolyte imbalances. These infants are especially prone to metabolic alkalosis from loss of hydrogen ions and to potassium, sodium, and chloride depletion, all of which are contained in gastric secretions (see Table 28-4 for signs of deficits). The skin and mucous membranes are assessed for alterations in hydration status, and daily weight measurement provides added clues to water gain or loss.

When stomach decompression and gastric lavage are part of preoperative management, it is the responsibility of the nurse to ensure that the tube is patent and functioning properly and to measure and record the type and amount of drainage. The infant is usually positioned flat or with the head slightly elevated. The infant who is receiving intravenous fluids or has a nasogastric tube for continuous drainage must be adequately restrained to prevent the needle or tube from becoming dislodged.

General hygienic care, with particular attention to skin and mouth in dehydrated infants, is an important part of care. Protection from infection is also important, because infants with impaired nutritional status are even more susceptible than normal newborn infants. As with any child in the hospital, parents are encouraged to visit and become involved in the child's care. Vomiting of a projectile nature is frightening to parents, and they often believe that they may have done something wrong. Most parents need support and reassurance that the condition is caused by a structural problem and is in no way a reflection of their parenting skills and capacities.

Postoperative care. Postoperative vomiting is not uncommon, and most infants, even with successful surgery, exhibit some vomiting during the first 24 to 48 hours. Intravenous fluids are administered until the infant is taking and retaining adequate amounts by mouth. Therefore much of the same care that was instituted before surgery is continued postoperatively, that is, observation of physical signs, monitoring of intravenous fluids, and careful observation and recording of intake and output. In addition, the infant is observed for responses to the stress of surgery. The nasogastric tube may be maintained after surgery for a variable length of time. Feedings are usually instituted rela-

tively soon, beginning with clear liquids containing glucose and electrolytes. They are offered slowly and at frequent intervals as ordered by the physician. If the infant has been breast-fed, breast milk, expressed by the mother, is given by bottle when the infant is able to tolerate feedings, and breast-feeding is resumed as soon as feasible. Observation and recording of feedings and the infant's responses to feedings and feeding techniques are a vital part of postoperative care. Positioning with the head elevated is usually continued postoperatively. Care of the operative site consists of observation for any drainage or signs of inflammation, and care of the incision as directed by the surgeon.

Sensory stimulation is incorporated into the infant's care, and parental involvement is encouraged and promoted, and parents require support and reassurance. Illness and surgery in an infant is a frightening event for families, especially following a frustrating preoperative experience. Parents are involved in the infants care as soon as possible after surgery and encouraged to provide comfort and stimulation appropriate to the needs of the infant.

Nursing Care Summary: The Child with Pyloric Stenosis

NURSING GOALS	NURSING INTERVENTIONS	EXPECTED PATIENT/FAMILY OUTCOMES
HP-HMP **Injury: potential for (trauma)** **Risk factors: operative repair**		
Avoid overdistention	Offer small, frequent feedings	Abdomen does not become overdistended Sutures remain intact
N-MP **Fluid volume deficit, potential** **Risk factors: vomiting**		
Provide fluids	Offer fluids as tolerated	Child exhibits no evidence of dehydration
Assess adequacy of intake	Weigh daily Assess status of skin and mucous membranes Measure carefully 　Intake—oral and/or parenteral 　Output—vomitus, nasogastric tube drainage, 　　stools, and urine 　Urine specific gravity	
N-MP **Nutrition, alteration in: potential for less than body requirements** **Risk factors: vomiting**		
Prevent vomiting	Give small, frequent feedings; feed slowly Bubble before and frequently during feedings Position in high Fowler position and slightly on right 　side after feeding Handle minimumly and gently after feeding	Child does not vomit
SP-SCP **Anxiety** **Etiology: separation from accustomed routine and environment**		
Provide comfort	Provide pacifier to meet oral needs Provide sensory stimulation Encourage parents' visitation and involvement in care Whenever possible, arrange to hold or have others 　hold infant	Infant's nonnutritive sucking needs are met; appears alert Family is involved in care

Continued.

Nursing Care Summary: The Child with Pyloric Stenosis—cont'd

NURSING GOALS	NURSING INTERVENTIONS	EXPECTED PATIENT/FAMILY OUTCOMES
RRP	**Family process, alteration in** **Etiology: situational crisis (illness and hospitalization of infant)**	
Support family	Keep family informed regarding infant's progress Assure mother or other caregiver that the problem is organic and is in no way a reflection of inadequate mothering skills Allow to express concerns and anxieties	Family discusses infant's condition and care realistically

Teach family	Instruct family in feeding and positioning techniques
	Instruct in care of incision
	Instruct regarding signs of
	  Expected behavior
	  Behaviors and signs that should be reported
		Family demonstrates ability to administer optimum care to the infant

Provide follow-up care	Instruct parents regarding posthospitalization evaluation Refer to public health agency if needed See also The family of the hospitalized child, p. 1081	Parents comply with instructions

Nursing Interventions Related to Medical Management

Help establish diagnosis
Recognize signs of pyloric stenosis and refer for medical evaluation
Obtain specimens and assist with diagnostic tests and procedures
Observe and record
  Physical signs of upper gastrointestinal obstruction, hyperperistalsis
  Amount, type, and character of vomiting
  Amount, type, and character of stools
Observe oral behaviors, including eating, hand sucking, and so on
Provide nutrition
  Administer feedings as ordered
Promote gastric decompression
  Give nothing by mouth

Carry out lavage as ordered
Maintain patency of nasogastric tube
Measure and record amount and type of drainage
Prevent removal of intravenous or nasogastric tube
  Apply and maintain adequate restraining devices
Recognize signs of complications
  Observe, report, and record any signs of upper gastrointestinal fluid loss
    Alkalosis
    Hypokalemia
    Hypocalcemia
    Dehydration
    Altered neurologic signs
    Shock
Postoperatively, check incision site

Shock States

A number of conditions constitute medical and nursing emergencies. Severe shock is one of these conditions. Nurses should be prepared for this possibility and intervene early and appropriately when patients display signs that indicate circulatory impairment.

SHOCK

Shock, or circulatory failure, is a clinical syndrome characterized by prostration and tissue perfusion that is inadequate to meet the metabolic demands of the body, resulting in depressed vital cell function. Although the causes are different, the physiologic consequences are the same: hypotension, tissue hypoxia, and metabolic acidosis.

Stages of Shock

Because of the progressive nature of shock, it can be divided into three stages or phases: *compensated, uncompensated,* and *irreversible*.

Compensated shock. When vital organ function is maintained by intrinsic compensatory mechanisms, it is said to be compensated. In this early stage blood flow is usually normal or increased but is generally uneven or maldistributed in the microcirculation. It is difficult to differentiate between the normal and compensated shock states by nonspecific measures such as vital signs and cardiac output (Perkin and Levine, 1982a).

Uncompensated shock. As shock progresses to an uncompensated state the efficiency of the cardiovascular system gradually diminishes, until perfusion in the microcirculation becomes marginal despite compensatory adjust-

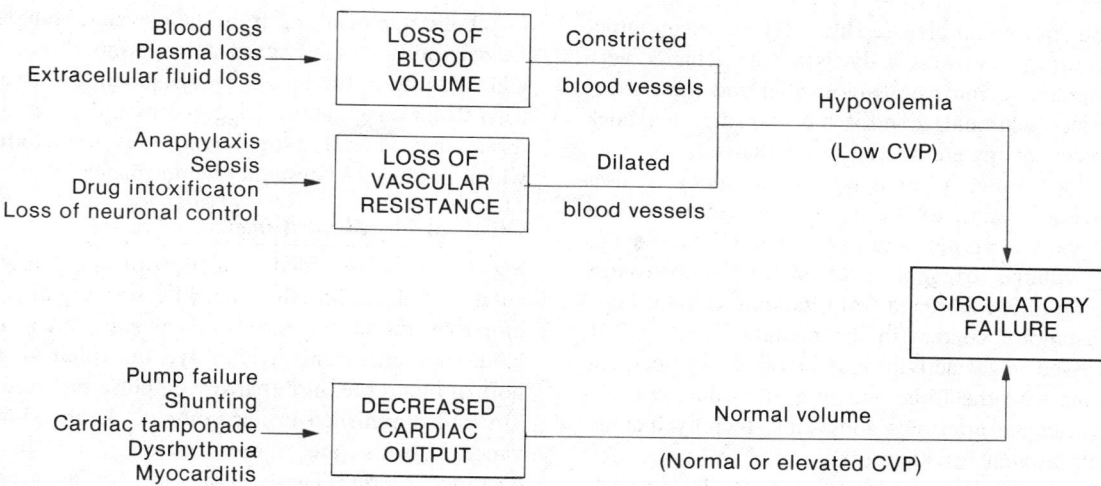

Fig. 29-3. Causes of circulatory failure in children.
Redrawn from Crone, R.K.: Pediatr. Clin. North Am. **27:**525-538, 1980.

ments. Eventually circulatory impairment becomes self-sustaining, and compensatory mechanisms may actually contribute to progression and perpetuation of the shock state (Perkin and Levin, 1982a). The outcomes of circulatory failure that progress beyond the limits of compensation are tissue hypoxia, metabolic acidosis, and eventual dysfunction of all organ systems.

Irreversible shock. Irreversible or terminal shock implies damage to vital organs such as the heart or brain of such magnitude that the entire organism will be disrupted regardless of therapeutic intervention. Death occurs even if cardiovascular measurements return to normal levels with therapy (Perkin and Levin, 1982a).

Types of Shock

Circulatory failure in children is the result of hypovolemia, altered peripheral vascular resistance, or pump failure (Fig. 29-3).

Hypovolemic shock. The most common type of circulatory failure in children is hypovolemia, or *hypovolemic shock,* which follows a reduction in the circulating blood volume. There is a reduction in the size of the child's vascular compartment, accompanied by falling blood pressure, poor capillary filling, and low central venous pressure. The reduction in the circulating blood volume is related to blood, plasma, or extracellular fluid losses beyond the child's physical ability to compensate (Crone, 1980). The most frequent causes of acute hypovolemia in children are:

Blood loss *(hemorrhagic shock)*—caused by trauma, gastrointestinal bleeding, intracranial hemorrhage
Plasma loss—caused by increased capillary permeability associated with sepsis and acidosis, hypoproteinemia, burns, peritonitis
Extracellular fluid loss—caused by vomiting, diarrhea, glycosuric diuresis, sunstroke

Distributive shock. Reduction in peripheral vascular resistance leads to profound inadequacies in tissue perfusion. There is an associated increase in venous capacity and pooling, which produces an acute reduction in return blood flow to the heart and a consequent diminished cardiac output. Reduction in peripheral vascular resistance is observed in the following types of shock:

Anaphylaxis *(anaphylactic shock)*—caused by an extreme allergy or hypersensitivity to a foreign substance (see p. 1213)
Sepsis *(septic shock, bacteremic shock, endotoxic shock)*—caused by overwhelming sepsis and circulating bacterial toxins
Loss of neuronal control *(neurogenic shock)*—caused by interruption of neuronal transmission such as observed in spinal cord injury. (Myocardial depression and peripheral dilation can also result from exposure to anesthesia or ingestion of barbiturates, tranquilizers, narcotics, antihypertensive agents, or ganglionic blocking agents.)

Cardiogenic shock. *Cardiogenic shock* resulting from decreased cardiac output is not common in children, but it can be caused by the following:

Congenital heart disease—in infancy, usually caused by outflow obstruction or systemic-to-pulmonary shunting
Inflow or outflow obstruction—associated with cardiac tamponade, tension pneumothorax, or pericardial effusion
Primary pump failure—associated with myocarditis, myocardial trauma, biochemical derangements
Dysrhythmias—such as paroxysmal atrial tachycardia, atrioventricular block, and ventricular arrhythmias; secondary to myocarditis or biochemical abnormalities (occasionally)

Pathophysiology

In the healthy child the circulation is able to transport oxygen and metabolic substrates to meet the essential needs of body tissues, which demand varying amounts of nutrients in relation to one another and relative to alterations in conditions such as exercise and disease states. The cardiac output and distribution to the various body tissues can change very rapidly in response to intrinsic (myocardial and intravascular) or extrinsic (neuronal) control mechanisms. In shock states these mechanisms are altered or challenged.

Reduced blood flow, as in hypovolemic shock, causes diminished venous return to the heart, low central venous pressure, low cardiac output, and hypotension. The reduced intravascular volume triggers a chain of compensatory mechanisms. Fluid is mobilized from the extracellular compartment. Vasomotor centers in the medulla are signaled, causing depressed vagal activity and increased sympathetic activity that increase the force and rate of cardiac contraction and constrict the arterioles and veins, thereby increasing peripheral vascular resistance.

Simultaneously the lowered blood volume also leads to the release of large amounts of catecholamines, antidiuretic hormone, adrenocorticosteroids, and aldosterone in an effort to conserve body fluids. The catecholamines augment the vasomotor activity to produce vasoconstriction and reduce blood flow to the skin, kidneys, muscles, and splanchnic viscera in order to shunt the available blood to the brain and heart. Consequently the skin feels cold and clammy, there is poor capillary filling, and glomerular filtration and urine output are significantly reduced.

Impaired perfusion to peripheral tissues also produces metabolic alterations. Oxygen depletion causes the cells to revert to anaerobic glycolytic metabolism, forming pyruvic acid, which is then converted to lactic acid, thus producing lactic acidosis. The acidosis places an extra burden on the lungs as they attempt to compensate for the metabolic acidosis by increased rate. Impaired cellular uptake and metabolism of glucose create hyperglycemia. When plasma fluid is lost, hemoconcentration and diminished blood flow increase the viscosity of the blood and further impair perfusion.

Prolonged vasoconstriction results in fatigue and atony of the resisting peripheral arterioles and, augmented by the release of vasodilator substances such as histamine, leads to vessel dilation. Venules, less sensitive to vasodilator substances, remain constricted for a time, causing massive pooling in the capillary and venular beds and transudation of plasma fluid into the tissues to further deplete blood volume. In all types of shock these circulatory alterations take place, but in neurogenic, septic, and anaphylactic shock there are some variations.

In neurogenic shock control mechanisms that maintain vascular tone are interrupted, causing reduced vascular resistance and peripheral pooling of blood; with this increased vascular capacity, there is loss of effective circulating blood volume. Septic shock produces a hyperdynamic state in which there is often an elevated plasma volume and reduced peripheral resistance that leads to widespread vasodilation. In many cases there is a high cardiac output caused by the vasodilation in infected tissues and elsewhere plus a high

metabolic rate resulting from the elevated body temperature. Degenerating tissues cause aggregation of red blood cells and sludging of the blood. Development of disseminated intravascular coagulation, triggered by either the degenerating tissue or bacterial toxins, consumes the clotting factors, which produces widespread hemorrhages.

Clinical Manifestations

Shock can be regarded as a form of compensation for circulatory failure. Initially, the child's ability to compensate is effective; therefore, early clinical signs are subtle and include apprehension, irritability, unexplained tachycardia, normal blood pressure, narrowing pulse pressure, thirst, pallor, and diminished urinary output. As the shock state advances, signs are more obvious and indicate early decompensation. These signs are confusion and somnolence, tachypnea, moderate metabolic acidosis, oliguria, and cool, pale extremities with decreased skin turgor and poor capillary filling. Thready, weak pulse, hypotension, periodic breathing or apnea, anuria, and stupor or coma are signs of impending cardiopulmonary arrest. Additional signs or modifications of these more universal signs may be present depending on the type and cause of the shock.

Complications of shock create further hazards. Central nervous system hypoperfusion may eventually lead to cerebral edema, cortical infarction, or intraventricular hemorrhage. Renal hypoperfusion causes renal ischemia with possible tubular or glomerular necrosis and renal vein thrombosis. Reduced blood flow to the lungs can interfere with surfactant secretion and result in "shock lung," which is characterized by sudden pulmonary congestion and atelectasis with formation of a hyaline membrane. Gastrointestinal tract bleeding and perforation are always a possibility following splanchnic ischemia and necrosis of intestinal mucosa. Metabolic complications of shock may include hypoglycemia, hypocalcemia, and other electrolyte disturbances.

Hypovolemic shock. Cardiac and peripheral compensatory adjustments may sufficiently restore cardiac output, systemic arterial blood pressure, and organ perfusion to normal or near normal. However, changes in blood flow to various organs and regions are altered. There is a decrease in central venous blood pressure and in stroke volume as well as other signs of early shock. Systemic arterial blood pressure is frequently normal. With continued blood loss compensatory mechanisms fail to maintain perfusion and signs of decompensation appear. There is pronounced systemic vasoconstriction and hypoxia of visceral and cutaneous circulations causing hypotension, acidosis, lethargy or coma, and oliguria or anuria.

Septic shock. The mechanisms producing septic (bacteremic) shock are not clear, but appear to be the result of many interrelated factors. There is uneven flow and inadequate tissue oxygenation, which result in progressive decompensation of the capillary circulation and the cells it

MANIFESTATIONS OF SEPTIC SHOCK

Hyperdynamic stage (warm shock, pink shock)	Normodynamic stage (cool shock)	Hypodynamic stage (cold shock)
Objective observations		
Tachycardia	Tachycardia	Tachycardia
Tachypnea	Hyperventilation	Respiratory distress
Chills and fever	Normal temperature	Profound hypothermia
Skin flushed, warm	Skin cool	Skin cold, clammy
Warm extremities	Cool extremities	Cold, pale extremities
Bounding pulses	Normal pulses	Weak, thready pulses
Normal or elevated systemic blood pressure	Normal blood or slightly elevated systemic blood pressure	Severe hypotension
Wide pulse pressure	Normal to slightly narrow pulse pressure	Narrow pulse pressure
Normal urine output or polyuria	Oliguria	Severe oliguria or anuria
Mental confusion	Depressed sensorium	Lethargy or coma

supports. Three stages have been identified in septic shock (Lamb, 1982; Perkin and Levin, 1982a) (see box):

1. **Hyperdynamic,** warm, or hyperdynamic-compensated shock—Early signs reflect vascular tone abnormalities and hyperdynamic compensatory responses. The patient has the best chance for survival from this stage.
2. **Normodynamic,** cool, or hyperdynamic-uncompensated shock—the signs progress with advancing disease through decompensatory manifestations deteriorating to manifestations of the cardiogenic phase. This stage lasts for only a few hours, and the signs of circulatory collapse are indistinguishable from late shock of any cause.
3. **Hypodynamic,** cold, or cardiogenic shock—Cardiovascular function progressively deteriorates even with aggressive therapy. This is the most dangerous stage of shock.

In early septic shock there are chills, fever, and vasodilation with increased cardiac output that results in warm, flushed skin—*hyperdynamic* or "hot shock." A later and ominous development is disseminated intravascular coagulation, which is evidenced by petechiae or purpura fulminans, a severe form of subcutaneous hemorrhage. Disseminated intravascular coagulation is the major hematologic complication of septic shock.

Diagnostic Evaluation

The cause of shock can be discerned from the history and the physical examination. The extent of the shock is determined by measurement of vital signs, including central venous pressure and capillary filling. Laboratory tests that assist in assessment are blood gas measurements, pH, and sometimes various liver function tests such as serum glutamic oxaloacetic transaminase (SGOT), bilirubin, and total serum protein (TSP). Coagulation status (prothrombin time [PT], partial thromboplastin time [PTT], platelet count, fibrinogen, fibrin) is evaluated when there is evidence of bleeding, such as oozing from a venipuncture site, bleeding from any orifice, or petechiae. Cultures of blood and other sites are indicated when there is a high suspicion of sepsis.

Renal function tests are performed when impaired renal function is evident.

Therapeutic Management

Treatment of shock consists of three major thrusts: (1) ventilation, (2) fluid administration, and (3) improvement of the pumping action of the heart. The first priority is to establish an airway and administer oxygen. Once the airway is ensured, circulatory stabilization is the major concern. Placement of an intravenous catheter for rapid volume replacement is the most important action for reestablishment of circulation. Where individuals are familiar with and skilled in the technique, percutaneous cannulation of the internal jugular or subclavian veins is preferred. An alternative is rapid surgical cutdown cannulation of the saphenous vein. The vein is anatomically accessible, can accommodate the volumes of fluid needed, and is situated where it does not interfere with any resuscitation procedures that might be necessary. It is the only practical route in profound circulatory collapse or in obese infants.

Cardiovascular support. In the majority of cases rapid restoration of blood volume is all that is needed for resuscitation of the child in shock. The nature of the fluid depends primarily on the availability of the appropriate fluid and the kind of fluid loss incurred. It may be a crystalloid solution such as lactated Ringer's solution, a colloid in the form of fresh-frozen plasma, or blood. Successful resuscitation will be reflected by an increase in blood pressure and a reduction in heart rate. An increased cardiac output will result in improved capillary circulation and skin color. For these children effective monitoring includes accurate measurements and recording of vital signs and objective observations. Urinary output measurement is an important indicator of adequacy of circulation.

For the critically ill child with shock and multisystem dysfunction more aggressive monitoring is needed. Central venous measurements of right atrial pressure or pulmonary wedge pressure help guide fluid therapy. In children with persistent shock a Swan-Ganz catheter should be placed for more accurate monitoring. Determination of arterial blood gases, hematocrit, serum electrolytes, glucose, and calcium concentrations provides additional information concerning composition of circulating blood. Correction of acidosis, hypoxemia, and any metabolic derangements is mandatory.

Temporary pharmacologic support may be required to enhance myocardial contractility, to reverse metabolic or respiratory acidosis, and to maintain arterial pressure. The principal agents used to improve cardiac output and circulation are the sympathetic amines administered by constant infusion pump. Those given most often to pediatric patients are the sympathomimetic amines dopamine (Intropin) and dobutamine (Dobutrex). Dopamine is the preferred drug because it also improves renal perfusion. The more potent isoproterenol (Isuprel) may be used as a second-line agent. Digitalis may be given to augment myocardial contractility in a failing heart, thereby increasing cardiac output.

Other drugs with vasopressor action may be used in specific situations, including phenylephrine and methoxamine. Vasodilators that are sometimes employed include nitroprusside (Nipride) and hydralazine (Apresoline). Nitroprusside is both a venous and an arteriolar vasodilator with immediate action, but it can be toxic to central nervous system tissues and therefore is reserved for short-term treatment. Apresoline, a relatively pure arteriolar dilator, is difficult to titrate but may be used for more extended treatment.

Metabolic acidosis is usually corrected with adequate tissue perfusion and improved renal function. This is accomplished with adequate ventilatory support, including oxygen, and restoration of blood volume and peripheral circulation. The administration of sodium bicarbonate may be associated with complications; therefore it is used only to partially correct the pH to levels that do not pose a threat to life (Perkin and Levin, 1982b).

Calcium chloride may be administered to improve cardiac function and to offset the reduced ionized calcium associated with large amounts of albumin, whole blood, or fresh-frozen plasma. Diuretics, such as furosemide (Lasix), cause a reduction in the ventricular filling pressures without changing cardiac output or heart rate and promote sodium and water excretion by the kidney in cases where pulmonary congestion is a problem.

Ventilatory support. The lung is the organ most sensitive to shock. The decreased or redistribution of blood flow to respiratory muscles plus the increased work of breathing can rapidly lead to respiratory failure. Critically ill patients are unable to maintain an adequate airway. To place the lung at rest and improve ventilation, tracheal intubation is initiated early with positive-pressure ventilation and supplemental oxygen. Blood gasses and pH are monitored frequently.

Increased extravascular lung water caused by edema—both hydrostatic and permeable—contributes to the development of respiratory complications. Hydrostatic edema occurs from elevation of pulmonary microvascular pressure as

a result of left ventricular dysfunction; permeable edema occurs when damage to alveolar cell and pulmonary capillary epithelium causes fluid to leak into the interstitial space resulting in the so-called adult respiratory distress syndrome or shock lung (see p. 1373). Therapy is directed toward maintaining normal arterial blood gas measurements, normal acid-base balance, and circulation. Efforts are made to remove fluid and prevent its accumulation by increasing oncotic pressure and decreasing microvascular hydrostatic pressure. Elevated oncotic pressure is promoted by diuresis with furosemide or mannitol, colloid administration, or both (Perkin and Levin, 1982b).

Other therapies. Appropriate antibiotics are administered to patients in septic shock. Peritoneal dialysis may be necessary if hyperkalemia, acidosis, hypervolemia, or altered mental status occurs. Gastrointestinal problems, such as paralytic ileus and stress ulceration, are managed appropriately. Nutritional support is provided by both enteral and parenteral routes. Prevention of infection is a primary concern because host resistance is depressed in patients in shock. Other complicating disorders, for example, disseminated intravascular coagulation, are treated appropriately.

Corticosteroids are controversial in the treatment of shock. When used they are given in massive doses on a short-term basis. They may be administered for anaphylactic shock, but time is required for their effects to develop. Extracorporeal oxygenation is used occasionally as a last resort where this therapy is available.

Nursing Considerations

The child in shock requires intensive observation and care. When shock is a likely complication, the child should be observed carefully for any early signs such as irritability, unexplained increase in heart rate, thirst, pallor, or diminished urinary output. Appearance of any of these signs requires further evaluation and initiation of therapy.

The initial action in care of the child in shock is assuring adequate tissue oxygenation. The nurse should be prepared to administer oxygen by the appropriate route and to assist with any intubation and ventilatory procedures indicated. Other procedures and activities that require immediate attention are establishing an intravenous line, weighing the child, obtaining baseline vital signs, placing an indwelling catheter, obtaining blood gas and other measurements, and administering medications as indicated.

The child is best positioned flat with legs elevated. Hypotensive patients show no benefit from the traditional Trendelenburg position. Head-down positioning tends to increase intracranial pressure, decrease diaphagmatic excursion and lung volume, and decrease venous return to the heart because of the altered thoracic pressure. Elevating the lower extremities decreases pooling in the extremities, thereby returning blood supply to the heart.

The nurse's responsibilities are to monitor the intravenous infusion, intake and output, vital signs (including central venous pressure), and general systems assessments on a routine basis. Intravenous medications are titrated according to patient responses, and vital signs are taken every 15 minutes during the critical periods and thereafter as needed. Urine output is measured hourly, and blood gases, hematocrit, pH, and electrolytes are monitored frequently to assess the status of the child and the efficacy of therapy. Apnea and cardiac monitors are attached and used continuously. In the initial stages of acute shock the care of the child often requires the attendance of more than one nurse in order to manage all the necessary activities that must be carried out simultaneously.

Throughout the intense activity the parents must not be overlooked. Someone should contact them at frequent intervals to inform them about what is being done and if there is any progress. Ideally, someone should remain with the parents to serve as liaison between them and the intensive care team. However, this is not always feasible in such a critical situation. As soon as possible they should be allowed to see the child. A clergyman may be called to help provide comfort and support.

ANAPHYLAXIS

Anaphylaxis is the acute clinical syndrome resulting from the interaction of an allergen and a patient who is hypersensitive (Zimmerman, 1985). Severe reactions are immediate in onset, are often life threatening, and frequently involve multiple systems, primarily the cardiovascular, respiratory, gastrointestinal, and integumentary. Exposure to the antigen can be by ingestion, inhalation, or injection. The most common allergens are listed in the box.

Prevention of a reaction is the primary goal of anaphylaxis. Preventing exposure is more easily accomplished in children known to be at risk, including those with (1) a history of previous allergic reaction to specific antigen, (2) a history of atopy, (3) a history of severe reactions in immediate family members, and (4) a reaction to a skin test, although skin tests are not available for all allergens.

Pathophysiology

An anaphylactic reaction occurs as a result of interaction between an allergen and preexisting specific immunoglobulin E (IgE). When the antigen enters the circulatory system, a generalized reaction rapidly takes place. Vasoactive amines (principally histamine or histamine-like substance) are released and cause vasodilation, bronchoconstriction, and increased capillary permeability. Consequently there is increased venous capacity and pooling, reduced arterial pressure, and rapid loss of fluid into interstitial spaces, causing a marked decrease in venous return to the heart.

Clinical Manifestations

The onset of clinical symptoms usually occurs within seconds or minutes of exposure to the antigen, and the rapidity of the reaction is directly related to its intensity—the sooner the onset, the more severe the reaction. Typically the

---

COMMON ALLERGENS ASSOCIATED WITH ANAPHYLAXIS

Drugs
Antibiotics (penicillin, cephalosporins, tetracyline, aminoglycosides, streptomycin, amphotericin B)
Analgesics (aspirin, indomethacin, codeine, phenylbutazone)
Local anesthetics (lidocaine, procaine, bupivacaine, tetracaine)
Chemotherapeutic agents (adriamycin, bleomycin, cisplatin, cyclophosphamide, L-asparaginase, melphalan)
Diagnostic contrast media (sulfobromophthalein sodium [BSP] dye, dehydrocholic acid [Decholin], iodinated contrast media, iopanoic acid [Telepaque])

Foods
Eggs
Seafood (fish, shellfish)
Milk and milk products
Chocolate
Nuts and seeds
Berries
Legumes (soybeans, beans, lentils, peanuts)
Wheat
Citrus fruits

Venoms
Hymenoptera (bee, yellow jacket, hornet, wasp, fire ant)
Snake
Jellyfish
Spider

Biologics
Allergen extracts
Antisera (snake, tetanus, diphtheria)
Enzymes
Hormones
Immune globulin (gammaglobulin, cryoprecipitate, blood, plasma)

---

reaction is preceded by one or more prodromal signs and symptoms including vague complaints of uneasiness or impending doom, restlessness, irritability, severe anxiety, headache, dizziness, paresthesia, and disorientation. The patient may lose consciousness. Cutaneous signs are the most common initial sign, and the child may complain of feeling warm. Angioedema is most noticeable in the eyelids, lips, tongue, hands, feet, and genitalia.

Any or all of several reactions may affect one or more organ systems, as follows:

Cardiovascular—Tachycardia, dysrhythmia, hypotension, relative hypovolemia
Respiratory—Rhinitis (sneezing, nasal itching, rhinorrhea), laryngeal edema (stridor), bronchospasm (cough, wheezing)
Gastrointestinal—Nausea and vomiting, abdominal pain, diarrhea
Skin—Diffuse flushing, urticaria, angioedema (periorbital, perioral)
Central nervous system—Seizures, loss of consciousness

Cutaneous manifestations are often followed by bronchiolar constriction. Bronchiolar constriction causes a narrowing of the airway, dilated pulmonary circulation produces pulmonary edema and hemorrhages, and there is often life-threatening laryngeal edema. Shock occurs as a result of mediator-induced vasodilation and sudden inadequacy of the circulation. The hypovolemia is further enhanced by increased capillary permeability and loss of intravascular fluid into the interstitial space. Laryngeal edema with its acute upper airway obstruction and related hypovolemic shock carry a more ominous prognosis.

Therapeutic Management

Successful outcome of anaphylactic reactions depends on rapid recognition and institution of treatment. The goals of treatment are to provide ventilation, restore adequate circulation, and prevent further exposure by identifying and removing the cause when possible.

A mild reaction with no evidence of respiratory distress or cardiovascular compromise can be managed with antihistamines, such as diphenhydramine (Benadryl) and epinephrine. Moderate or severe distress presents a potentially life-threatening emergency and requires immediate intervention. Severely unresponsive patients are transferred to hospital intensive care units when possible.

As in any shock state, the airway is the first concern. The most important drug is aqueous epinephrine 1:1000 (0.1 to 0.5 ml [0.01 mg/kg]) administered subcutaneously for mild reactions and intramuscularly for moderate reactions. The dose may be repeated three times at 15- to 20-minute intervals. When cardiovascular collapse is present or imminent, the drug may be diluted in 10 ml saline solution and administered slowly over several minutes by the intravenous route (Bailit, 1986). If the site of the antigen injection is known (e.g., drug, sting), the site is isolated by application of a tourniquet proximal to the site and this epinephrine injected directly to the area (Morriss, 1984).

Other drugs that may be used but are not universally applied are aminophylline and diphenhydramine (Benadryl). Vasopressors may be required for severe shock from any cause. Corticosteroids are controversial, but some authorities advocate their use for control of persistent or recurrent symptoms. The time required for them to achieve their effect diminishes their value for emergency therapy.

The child is positioned and monitored the same as any shock patient. If this is the initial anaphylactic reaction it is especially important to identify the allergen and implement measures to prevent any future reaction. A MedicAlert bracelet, tag, or other identification should be carried by the patient at all times. Desensitization may be recommended in certain cases.

Nursing Considerations

The major nursing responsibility in anaphylaxis is anticipating which children are likely to develop a reaction, recognizing the early signs, and intervening appropriately. When an anaphylactic reaction is suspected, both immediate intervention and preparation for medical therapy are nursing responsibilities. Help will be needed and the physician noti-

fied, but the nurse must not leave the patient. Ventilation is ensured by placing the child in a head-elevated position, unless contraindicated by hypotension, to facilitate breathing and administer oxygen. If the child is not breathing, cardiopulmonary resuscitation is initiated.

If the cause can be determined, measures are implemented to slow the spread of the offending substance. For example, a tourniquet is applied above the point of entry (e.g., sting or injection) or intravenous medication or dye infusion is discontinued. If an intravenous infusion line is not in place, one is established immediately and the flow rate monitored carefully. Vital signs are monitored every 15 minutes, and urine output measured at regular intervals. Medications are administered as prescribed, with regular assessment to monitor effectiveness and to detect signs of side effects of medication and fluid overload.

To prevent an anaphylactic reaction parents are always asked about possible allergic responses to foods, medications, and environmental conditions. These are displayed prominently on the patient's chart. The specific allergen and the type and severity of the reaction are noted. Parents are excellent historians, especially when the child has displayed a pronounced reaction to a substance. Drugs, including related drugs (e.g., penicillin and nafcillin), that have produced a reaction previously are *never* given to a patient.

The child and the parents need as much reassurance as can be provided without giving false hope. They are kept informed of the child's progress, the reasons for the therapies, and what they can reasonably expect. It is a frightening experience and one which the family will remember and will make every effort to prevent recurring. The idea of medical information in a convenient and visible form, such as the Medic-Alert items, is reinforced. For the child who is allergic to insect venom, the family is instructed to purchase an emergency kit to be kept with the child at all times (e.g., Ana-Kit,* EpiPen Auto-Injector, or EpiPen Jr. Auto-Injector†). Both the family and the child, if the child is old enough and is likely to be away from the family (e.g., at school), are taught how to use the equipment (see also p. 1133).

TOXIC SHOCK SYNDROME

Toxic shock syndrome (TSS) is a relatively rare disease that occurs predominantly (but not exclusively) in previously healthy young women during their menstrual periods. Studies have shown a striking relationship between the disease and the use of tampons (Centers for Disease Control, 1980), although other foci have been identified, including contraceptive sponges (Faich and others, 1986; Dart and Levitt, 1985), nasal packing (Hull and others, 1983; Barbour, Shlaes, and Guertin, 1984), and burns and osteotomy (Buchdahl and others, 1985). Some cases reported in chil-

---

*Hollister-Stier Laboratories.
† Center Labs.

dren were unrelated to any identifiable foci (Wiesenthal and Todd, 1984; Surh and Read, 1984).

Pathophysiology

Evidence from several sources suggests that TSS occurs secondary to infection with phage group-1 *Staphylococcus aureus*. The organism is believed to produce an epidermal toxin, but the precise mode of transmission is not known. The disease has been observed primarily in women who use tampons during a menstrual period. The tampons may carry the organism from the fingers or the vulva into the vagina during insertion, the tampon might traumatize the vaginal wall and provide a focus of infection, or the tampon itself may provide a favorable environment for growth of the organism or elaboration of its toxin. The superabsorbent tampons appear to be more likely to contribute to development of the disease. Persistent use throughout the menstrual cycle also alters the vaginal mucosa by absorbing protective secretions and subjects it to greater mechanical trauma and microulcerations.

Clinical Manifestations

The sudden development of high fever, vomiting and diarrhea, profound hypotension, shock, oliguria, and an erythematous macular rash with subsequent desquamation are characteristic manifestations of toxic shock syndrome. Other manifestations might include headache, blurred vision, purulent conjunctivitis, abdominal guarding, and purulent vaginal discharge. Inasmuch as various signs and symptoms are associated with the disease and affected individuals seldom exhibit all of them, the Centers for Disease Control has published a case definition of toxic shock syndrome (see box).

Complications of the shock state are respiratory distress, cardiac dysfunction, hematologic changes (particularly disseminated intravascular coagulation), and abnormal liver function. Impaired perfusion to extremities may become severe, with eventual necrosis and loss of extremities.

Diagnostic Evaluation

Diagnosis is established on the basis of the criteria of the Centers for Disease Control's toxic case definition. A history of tampon use contributes to the diagnosis. Additional laboratory tests include cultures from blood, vagina, cervix, and discharge from any suspected source of infection. Other laboratory tests are those that facilitate the management of shock.

Therapeutic Management

The management of toxic shock syndrome is the same as management of shock of any cause. Because the disease is highly varied in intensity, therapy is directed toward supportive care in mild cases to hospitalization and intensive care in severe cases. Appropriate parenteral antibiotics are usually administered after cultures are obtained. Penicillinase-resistant penicillin or cephalosporins are the drugs of choice. The drugs do not appear to alter the course of the disease but seem to be effective in preventing recurrences.

CASE DEFINITION OF TOXIC SHOCK SYNDROME

1. Fever (temperature at or above 38.9° C, or 102° F)
2. Rash (diffuse macular erythroderma)
3. Desquamation 1 to 2 weeks after onset of illness, particularly of the palms and soles
4. Hypotension (systolic blood pressure at or below 90 mm HG for adults or below the fifth percentile for age for children younger than 16 years of age, or orthostatic syncope)
5. Involvement of three or more of the following organ systems:
   a. Gastrointestinal (vomiting or diarrhea at onset of illness)
   b. Muscular (severe myalgia or creatine phosphokinase level above 2 times the upper limits of normal)
   c. Mucous membrane (vagina, oropharyngeal, or conjunctival hyperemia)
   d. Renal (blood urea nitrogen or creatinine levels above 2 times the upper limits of normal or above 5 white blood cells per high-power field—in the absence of a urinary tract infection)
   e. Hepatic (total bilirubin, SGOT [serum glutamic oxaloacetic transaminase], or SGPT [serum glutamic pyruvic transaminase] above 2 times the upper limits of normal)
   f. Hematologic (platelets below 100,000/mm³)
   g. Central nervous system (disorientation or alterations in consciousness without focal neurologic signs when fever and hypotension are absent)
6. Negative results on the following tests, if obtained:
   a. Blood, throat, or cerebrospinal fluid cultures
   b. Serologic tests for Rocky Mountain spotted fever, leptospirosis, or measles

From Centers for Disease Control: Morbid. Mortal. Weekly Rep. **29**:442, 1980.

Preventing complications of impaired circulation demands constant observation and immediate therapeutic intervention for hypotension, pulmonary dysfunction, acidosis, hematologic changes, and renal impairment.

Nursing Considerations

Nursing care and observation of the acutely ill patient are the same as those described for shock of any cause. Because the disease is relatively rare, the major efforts of nursing are directed toward prevention. The association between the disease and the use of tampons provides some direction for education. Avoiding the use of tampons offers the most certain preventive measure, although this approach is probably unacceptable to most adolescent girls. Most young women prefer the freedom, comfort, and inconspicuousness that tampons afford, and are unlikely to comply with this advice.

Adolescent girls who use tampons can be advised to modify their use. For example, tampons may be used intermittently during the menstrual cycle, alternating with sanitary napkins—perhaps using the napkins during the night and tampons during the day. It is probably advisable to encourage young girls not to use superabsorbent tampons and not to leave any tampon in the body for more than 12 hours. Instruction in general hygienic measures, such as hand washing before insertion of the tampon, is an important part of patient teaching.

It is also advisable to teach patients how to recognize the early symptoms of toxic shock syndrome. They should understand that they should remove the tampon and consult their physician if they develop a sudden high fever, vomiting and diarrhea, muscle pain, dizziness, fainting or near fainting when standing up, or rash (that resembles a sunburn). Excellent posters and handout materials for use as teaching aids are available from the **Food and Drug Administration.***

Burns

Minor thermal injuries are experienced by everyone in day-to-day living and are relatively commonplace in nursing practice. Extensive burns, on the other hand, are relatively uncommon; however, they account for some of the most difficult nursing problems encountered in the pediatric age-group. Serious burn injury accounts for a very large number of children who must undergo prolonged, painful, and restrictive hospitalization, many of whom emerge from the experience with scars to both body and personality that profoundly affect their social and emotional development. It is tragic, too, that the great majority (75%) of burn injuries are preventable.

OVERVIEW

Although severe burns are manifest primarily in damage to the skin, they produce a complex illness that requires the utmost in nursing skill and care. Every organ system becomes involved, and sometimes the treatment even creates additional problems. Nursing care of patients with extensive burns involves an understanding of a variety of specialized areas, including surgical principles and techniques, respiratory physiology, fluid and electrolyte physiology, nutrition, bacteriology, growth and development, occupational therapy, physical therapy, and principles of psychiatric nursing.

Epidemiology

More than two million persons each year in the United States sustain significant burns. At least half of these injuries occur in the pediatric age group (Dyer, 1980) and account for approximately 3000 deaths from burn injury in persons younger than 15 years of age (Harmel, Vane, and King, 1986). The second most important cause of death from *trauma* in childhood, burns are outranked only by motor vehicle casualties. Figures contributed from major burn centers that specialize in the care of children reveal that the largest percentage of burns in the pediatric age group occurs in children younger than 5 years of age. Until age 9 years there is no sex differences in the incidence of burns, but after age 9 years boys outnumber girls 3:1 (Herrin and Crawford, 1977).

*FDA, HFE-88 (or HFW-40 for multiple copies), Rockville, MD 20857.

Table 29-3 describes the types of burn that are most often associated with children at different developmental levels.

House fires cause three fourths of all fire deaths, especially of young children and elderly persons. Cigarettes used by adults are the leading cause of ignition of fatal house fires—from 30% to 45% of deaths. Approximately 2% of residential fire deaths are attributed to children playing with matches or other ignition sources (Baker, O'Neill, and Karpf, 1984).

Age. Children younger than age 5 years sustain 70% of burn injuries, and the incidence is often related to the quality and quantity of adult supervision. Very young children have limited perception of danger, less control of elements in their environment, and limited ability to react promptly and properly to a fire or burn situation (McLoughlin and Crawford, 1985). Burns in children in this age-group occur more often in large than in small families. The most hazardous periods are the early morning hours when parents are still in bed and the interval between the time school is out and the evening meal. Many children die or are seriously injured in burning buildings, especially when left unattended. A significant number of burns occur in garages and basements in which there is an open gas heating unit or pilot light.

Whereas young children receive more scalds, older children are likely to be burned severely by flaming clothing from open flames, heaters, and explosions—very often in an unsupervised play situation in which combustible materials, such as gasoline and matches or cigarette lighters, are present. Fascination with fire seems to be a normal trait, and natural curiosity will lead young children who have access to matches or cigarette lighters to experiment with them (McLoughlin and Crawford, 1985). Match play generally occurs in the bedroom, where the child goes to be alone. Somewhat older children (especially boys) playing with matches or gasoline tend to be with friends, out of sight of adults (Libber and Slayton, 1984).

Electric burns of the mouth from chewing on an electric cord are more typical of children in the crawling or toddler stage of development. Younger children are more likely to be burned by poking metal objects into electric outlets, whereas burns from tension wires occur in older children.

Seasonal incidence. Burns also have a seasonal incidence. Inasmuch as furnaces and other heating devices are used most extensively during cold weather, burns from heaters, wood stoves, and house fires are more frequent in the winter months. Flash burns from explosive ignition of outdoor barbecues with volatile liquids increase in summer months. Burns caused by clothing catching fire from campfires occur in summer, and from burning leaves in autumn. Some types of burns occur on specific dates, for example, sunburns on Memorial Day weekend and blast and burn injuries from Independence Day firecrackers (McLoughlin and Crawford, 1985). In all seasons young girls sustain burn injuries to the chest and arms when loose, frilly clothes (especially nightwear) are ignited by an open fire, gas ranges or heaters, and candelabra. Fortunately these burns have de-

Table 29-3 Burn hazards of children

AGE-GROUP	TYPE OF BURN	HAZARD	TIME/PLACE
Toddler (6-24 months)	Scalds	Playing underfoot in kitchen, overturning cups, pulling electric cords off coffeepots or frying pans; bath water too hot; parental neglect/abuse	Daytime/home
	Electric burns	Chewing extension cords	
Young children (2-6 years)	Flame burns	Playing with matches, climbing on stove, warming with heating source	Early morning/kitchen, bedroom, and so on
6- to 14-year-old children	Scalds	Water too hot	
Boys	Flame burns	Playing/working with gasoline, campfires, barbecues, chemistry sets, firecrackers, rockets, matches, and so on	After school, holidays/outdoors, indoors
	Electric burns	Climbing around high-tension wires	
Girls	Flame burns	Reaching over stove, candles, making candles, "innocent bystander" (observing others play with fire or gasoline)	Morning, evening/kitchen; after school/yard
All children	Flame burns	House fires; gas tank explosion during automobile accident	Usually night, anytime

Courtesy Northern California Burn Council, San Francisco, and Elizabeth McLoughlin, Director of Burn Injury Project, Shriners Burns Institute, Boston, Mass.

creased significantly since regulation of inflammable clothing has been established.

Psychologic factors. Psychologic factors are often related to burn injury in children. For example, burns inflicted as punishment are a common form of child abuse, and it is the unwanted or least desirable child who is the last to be rescued from a burning building. Approximately 30% of pediatric burns are the result of child abuse; therefore, when abuse is suspected, it is important to look for associated injuries. The frequency of burn injury, as well as other accidental injuries, is increased in families in which there is emotional disturbance, such as marital discord, a disturbed parent, or a disturbed or retarded child. Setting fires by small boys and burns of either boys or girls can often be interpreted as a signal of distress related to loss of a parent to whom the child had a strong attachment. In many children difficult behavior for varying periods of time precedes the burn injury. Not only do these psychologic and behavioral problems contribute to the injury, but they also influence the child's hospitalization and convalescence (Herrin and Crawford, 1977).

Etiology

Burns can be caused by thermal, chemical, electric, or radioactive agents. Most burn injuries are caused by thermal agents, principally flame, direct contact (stove, heater), and hot water (scalding water, steam), and to a lesser extent by friction and frostbite. Chemical burns can be caused by either acids or alkalis, and radiation burns by either x-rays or ultraviolet radiation. The extent of tissue destruction is determined by the intensity of the heat source, the duration of contact or exposure, and the speed with which the heat energy is dissipated by the burned surface. For example, a brief exposure to high-intensity heat, such as a flame, or a longer exposure to low-intensity heat, such as hot water, can produce similar burns. Burns caused by boiling oil or liquid fat tend to cause deep partial-thickness burns. Prolonged exposure to the sun or to a heated object, such as a sidewalk, is also capable of producing significant burns.

Full-thickness destruction frequently occurs when clothing is ignited. Cotton and nylon clothing burns most easily, whereas clothing made from wool or other animal fibers burns less readily. Synthetic fabrics melt and stick to the skin surface. Contact burns from heated metal or liquids (e.g., tar) at extreme temperatures, prolonged immersion in hot water, chemical burns without rinsing with water, and electric burns all can cause severe burn trauma. Chemical agents continue to cauterize the tissues until the injurious agent is chemically united with tissue elements, neutralized, or removed by washing with running water.

Electric burns are especially deceptive, because they are characterized by more extensive thrombosis that is not evident until 24 to 36 hours after injury. Electricity is converted to thermal energy as it encounters resistance. Inasmuch as body tissues vary in the degree of resistance they offer, the type of tissue through which an electric current passes plays a role in the extent of the burn injury. Bone offers the greatest amount of resistance. Other tissues in descending order of resistance are fat, tendon, skin, muscle, blood, and nerves. Although blood offers less resistance than most tissues, it is an extremely good conductor of electric current. All other things being equal, the greater the skin resistance, the more severe the local burn; the less the skin resistance, the greater the systemic effects. The extensive destruction of an electric burn has been described as resembling a crush injury.

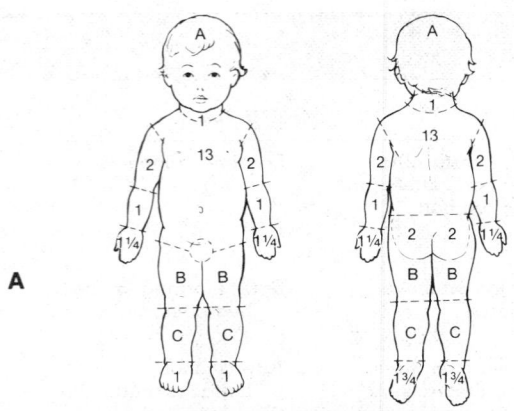

RELATIVE PERCENTAGES OF AREAS AFFECTED BY GROWTH

AREA	BIRTH	AGE 1 YR	AGE 5 YR
A = ½ of head	9½	8½	6½
B = ½ of one thigh	2¾	3¼	4
C = ½ of one leg	2½	2½	2¾

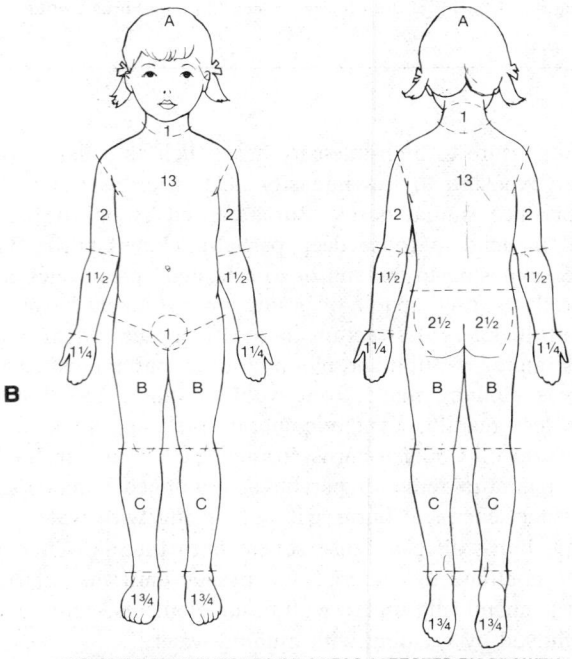

RELATIVE PERCENTAGES OF AREAS AFFECTED BY GROWTH

AREA	AGE 10 YR	AGE 15 YR	ADULT
A = ½ of head	5½	4½	3½
B = ½ of one thigh	4½	4½	4¾
C = ½ of one leg	3	3¼	3½

Fig. 29-4. Estimation of distribution of burns in children. **A,** Children from birth to age 5 years. **B,** Older children.

BURN WOUND CHARACTERISTICS

The physiologic responses, therapy, prognosis, and disposition of the injured child are all directly related to the *amount of tissue destroyed;* therefore the severity of the burn injury is assessed on the basis of percentage of body

surface burned, depth of the burn, and location of the burn(s).

Also important in determining the seriousness of the injury are age of the child, etiologic agent, extent of respiratory tract involvement, general health of the child, and presence of any associated injury or condition.

Extent of Injury

The extent of a burn is usually expressed as a percentage of total body surface area, which is most accurately estimated by using specially designed age-related charts (Fig. 29-4). Because of the body proportions, especially the head and lower extremities, the standard "rule of nines" charts used for adults are not applicable to small children.

Depth of Injury

A thermal injury is a three-dimensional wound and therefore is also assessed in relation to depth of injury. Traditionally the terms *first-, second-,* and *third-degree* have been used to describe the depth of tissue injury. However, with the current emphasis on burn healing, these are gradually being replaced by more descriptive terms based on the extent of destruction to the epithelializing elements of the skin. Partial-thickness burns heal in time; full-thickness burns require skin grafting for closure. Partial-thickness injury is further categorized by many as superficial or deep dermal burns, depending on how rapidly they heal. Because both terminologies are used, often interchangeably, both are presented in describing the characteristics of burn wounds (Fig. 29-5.)

Superficial (first-degree) burns are usually of minor significance. There is frequently a latent period followed by erythema. Tissue damage is minimal, protective functions remain intact, and systemic effects are rare. Pain is the predominant symptom.

Partial-thickness (second-degree) burns are deeper and involve not only the epithelium but also a minimal to substantial portion of the corium. The severity of the injury and the rate of healing are directly related to the amount of un-

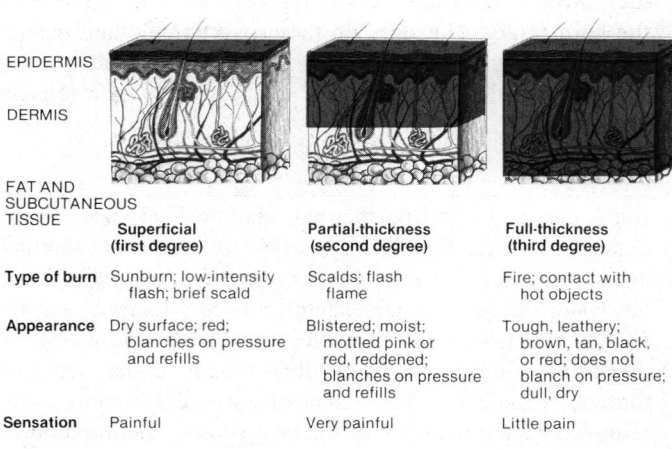

	Superficial (first degree)	Partial-thickness (second degree)	Full-thickness (third degree)
Type of burn	Sunburn; low-intensity flash; brief scald	Scalds; flash flame	Fire; contact with hot objects
Appearance	Dry surface; red; blanches on pressure and refills	Blistered; moist; mottled pink or red, reddened; blanches on pressure and refills	Tough, leathery; brown, tan, black, or red; does not blanch on pressure; dull, dry
Sensation	Painful	Very painful	Little pain

Fig. 29-5. Classification of burn depth.

damaged corium from which new tissue can regenerate. Superficial burns are often classified with first-degree burns and heal uneventfully. Deep dermal burns, although classified as second-degree or partial-thickness burns, in many respects resemble third-degree burns. There is hyperemia in areas with less heat, and leakage of protein in areas with the most heat. Systemic effects are similar to those that occur with deeper burns. Whereas first-degree and superficial partial-thickness burns are painful, deep dermal burns are often anesthetic for the first 1 or 2 days after injury.

Full-thickness (third-degree) burns are serious injuries in which all layers of the skin are destroyed, may involve underlying tissues as well, and are usually combined with extensive partial-thickness damage. Presence of visible thrombosed veins in the burn wound is pathognomonic of a full-thickness burn. Systemic effects can be life threatening and involve every organ system in the body. Although a notable characteristic of third-degree burns is lack of sensation at the wound surface, this is misleading. Superficial nerve endings are destroyed in the full-thickness areas, but nerve endings are hypersensitive on wound edges (described by Kibbee, 1984). In addition, deep somatic pain is present in the full-thickness area as a result of inflammation and ischemia (LaMotte and Thalhammer, 1982).

Sometimes additional categories are used to further describe full-thickness burns. Fourth-degree burns involve fat and are difficult to prepare for grafting. Burns involving muscle may be designated as fifth-degree burns. Because of the myoglobin released from muscle destruction, burns involving muscle may lead to kidney damage. Burns that destroy bone are sixth-degree burns, are usually hard and dry, and lead to amputation of the affected part (Jacoby, 1984).

Severity of Injury

Burns are also appraised on the basis of their severity. This is useful in determining the disposition of the patient for treatment. Burned patients can usually be distinguished as (1) those with a critical burn who require the services and equipment of a special burn facility, (2) those with moderate burns who may be treated in any hospital unit, and (3) those with minor burns who are able to be treated on an outpatient basis. Although each burn unit and specialist in the field of burn management has criteria for admission to special units, there are many factors that influence the effects of the injury, the probability of recovery, and response to therapy.

Initial assessment to estimate the extent of skin destruction is made on the basis of observation and simple diagnostic techniques. The extent of surface involvement is readily calculated, and the surface appearance of the wound provides clues to whether the injury involves the full thickness of the skin or only a portion of the skin layers. The extent to which the wound is capable of regeneration depends on the areas destroyed. Epithelial regeneration can take place from residual basilar cells and from the epithelial lining of sweat glands and hair follicles.

Blisters do not occur in full-thickness burns, but with superficial burns in general, the deeper the burn, the more common is blister formation. Blisters increase in size in the hours immediately after the burn occurs, and usually the larger the blister, the deeper the burn. Touching injured surfaces gives more additional information. Testing for capillary filling by blanching and refilling indicates whether circulation in the area is intact. Because the sensory end organs are concentrated in the deep dermal areas, presence of sensation indicates tissue viability; absence of sensation suggests full skin thickness destruction. This is easily determined by pricking the skin with a sterile needle.

The burn source can help to estimate and classify the extent of the injury. Hot liquids may result in partial-thickness injury, whereas full-thickness injury is associated with flame burns. This can vary with the age of the child, however. Because infants' skin is so thin, it is readily destroyed by thermal agents. This makes estimation of depth difficult in children in this age-group, especially in scalds. Electric burns appear to be less serious than they actually are, because they often involve deep structures. The electric current will follow nerves and blood vessels, and it may cause thrombosis with subsequent severe tissue destruction. Children with facial burns, those with burns acquired in an enclosed area, or those in whom inhalation injury is suspected for other reasons are at risk for developing airway obstruction or severe hypoxia during the hours after inhalation.

In calculating the risk related to thermal injuries, children younger than 2 years have a significantly higher mortality than older children with burns of similar size. They are subject to rapid fluid shifts, which places them in jeopardy in the early hours, and their immune competence is not well developed; thus sepsis is a frequent complication. Burn classification according to severity is outlined in the box.

BURN SEVERITY CRITERIA

Minor burns
Partial-thickness burns of less than 15% of body surface
Full-thickness burns of less than 2% of body surface

Moderate burns
Partial-thickness burns of 15% to 25% of body surface
Full-thickness burns of less than 10% of body area, except in small children and when the burns involve critical areas, such as the face, hands, feet, or genitalia

Major or critical burns
Burns complicated by respiratory tract injury
Partial-thickness burns of 25% total area or greater
Burns of face, hands, feet, or genitalia, even if they appear to be partial thickness
Full-thickness burns of 10% of body surface or greater
Any child younger than 2 years of age, unless the burn is very small and very superficial
Electric burns that penetrate
Deep chemical burns
Respiratory tract damage
Burns complicated by fractures or soft tissue injury
Burns complicated by concurrent illness, such as obesity, diabetes, epilepsy, and cardiac and renal diseases

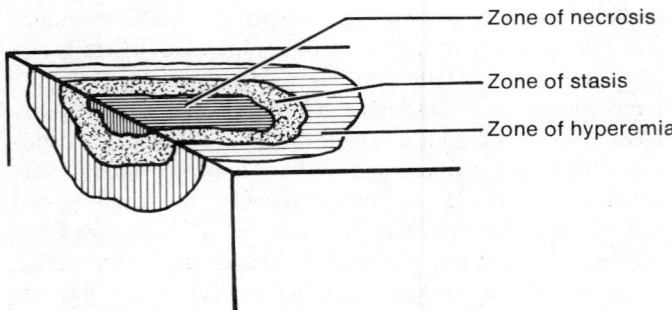

Fig. 29-6. Zones of injury in burn.
After Zawacki, B.: Ann. Surg. **180**:98-102, 1974.

Local Responses

Local changes at the site of the burn injury begin to occur at approximately 45° C (113° F); tissues die at 65° C (149° F) and higher because of coagulation necrosis. The tissue coagulates, desiccates, or becomes carbonized, depending on the extent of exposure to the source of heat. At the same time, changes in the intercellular cement that binds the epidermis to the dermis cause the epidermis to detach and either peel away or form a blister between the two layers. In infants and young children the skin is so thin and contains such shallow dermal appendages that full-thickness loss occurs easily on exposure to heat. There are also fewer skin appendages in prepubescent children than in adolescents.

The burn wound consists basically of three distinct layers (Fig. 29-6) (Zawacki, 1974):

1. **Zone of coagulation.** In this zone, beneath the obviously destroyed tissue, capillary flow has ceased and tissue destruction is irreversible. The tissue is dead.
2. **Zone of stasis.** Beneath and surrounding the zone of coagulation there is a zone with markedly reduced capillary flow. The tissue is severely damaged from heat but is not coagulated. The tissue in this zone can be saved with prevention of further injury and adequate perfusion.
3. **Zone of hyperemia.** An area metabolically active and displaying the usual response to tissue injury.

It is the two outer zones in which significant changes take place and that are involved in the pathophysiology of the burn wound and the systemic responses to the initial burn injury.

Edema formation. Increased capillary permeability in these two outer zones is caused by thermal injury to the vessels. At the same time vasodilation causes an increase in hydrostatic pressure within the capillaries. The increased hydrostatic pressure plus the increased capillary permeability cause loss of water, protein, and electrolytes from the intravascular compartment into the interstitial spaces. This shift is further enhanced by a diminishing intravascular oncotic pressure, as protein and sodium are lost to the interstitial spaces. Although the edema involves both burned and nonburned areas, at the site of injury the accumulation of edema fluid beneath and around the burn can reach tremendous proportions until the extravasation of fluid is limited by tissue tension.

In addition, there are also changes in the permeability of tissue cells in and around the burned area that allow an abnormal exchange of electrolytes between the cells and the interstitial fluid; that is, sodium enters the cells in exchange for potassium, causing further depletion of intravascular sodium.

Fluid loss. Without the protective skin, fluid loss at the air-wound interface can be extremely high. These losses reach a maximum about the fourth day after the burn occurs but continue to pose problems until the denuded surfaces are debrided and grafted.

Circulatory stasis. Significant circulatory alterations take place in the zone of stasis located around the coagulated dead tissue. When red blood cells are heated, they become spherical in shape. These heat-damaged cells, together with hemoconcentration from fluid loss, depressed cardiac output, and tissue edema, reduce the blood flow in the burn area, causing capillary stasis. Thrombi develop that further impede circulation, producing tissue ischemia and eventual necrosis. This may also prolong the edema phase. Further hyperviscosity and impaired blood flow are attributed to the release of substances from damaged cells, such as thromboplastin and clot-activating factors, that cause the production of microthrombi, platelet adhesiveness and aggregation, and increased pain and swelling.

In partial-thickness burns circulation around the burn area ceases immediately after injury but is rapidly restored within 24 to 48 hours. In full-thickness burns, however, the vascular supply is completely occluded, and no appreciable circulation is reestablished until granulation takes place at the interface between burned and unburned tissue.

Burn wound. In first-degree destruction of the vascular epithelium, tissue damage is minimal. Protein loss is insignificant and edema barely perceptible. The burning sensation and pain resolve in 48 to 72 hours, and in 5 to 10 days the damaged epithelium peels off in small scales or sheets, leaving no scar.

In second-degree, partial-thickness burns there is considerable edema and more severe capillary damage. In 3 to 5 days a crust of dried exudate and injured tissue covers the wound to form a protective seal while healing takes place from underneath. With reasonable care superficial burns heal spontaneously and uneventfully through the generative capacity of the stratum germinativum and epithelial cells of appendageal linings. The crust separates in 10 to 14 days with minimal or no scarring.

Deep dermal burns heal more slowly by regeneration from the epithelial lining of skin appendages, sweat glands, and hair follicles. A thin epithelial covering develops in 25 to 35 days, but this type of burn may require several months to heal. Scarring is common, and trauma or infection can easily convert a partial-thickness burn to a full-thickness injury, especially in young children with their normally thinner skin. Fluid loss and metabolic effects may be considerable.

In third-degree, full-thickness burns there is cell destruction by coagulation necrosis. The dead tissue and exudate convert to a thick leathery eschar in 48 to 72 hours, which liquefies and begins to separate in 12 to 21 days as a result of autolysis, leukemic digestion, and disintegration of collagen fibers. New granulation tissue will form on the wound bed, which, if not grafted, will heal by slow proliferation from the edges with severe scarring. In full-thickness burns there is severe edema with fluid and electrolyte shifts and extensive metabolic changes.

Systemic Responses

Along with and subsequent to the pathophysiologic response at the site of thermal injury, a number of systemic responses occur.

Circulation. The immediate postburn period is marked by dramatic alterations in circulation, known as *burn shock*. There is a precipitous drop in cardiac output (about 50% of normal resting values) that precedes any changes in circulating blood or plasma volume. With the large fluid losses through denuded skin, vasodilation, and edema formation, the blood volume decreases rapidly and cardiac output is reduced even further, usually leveling off at 20% of normal resting values. Cardiac output returns to normal spontaneously in 24 to 36 hours, although the plasma volume lags far behind.

The initial decrease in cardiac output is attributed to a circulating myocardial depressant factor, associated with severe burn injury, that affects the contractility of heart muscle directly. The blood volume deficit, although slower in onset, can be profound and appears to be directly proportional to the extent and depth of the burn.

Capillary permeability with leakage of fluid takes place in noninjured areas including bowels, brain, and other organs, as well as in the outer zones of the burn wound. The edema fluid accumulates rapidly in the first 18 hours after injury to reach a maximum in about 48 hours. Capillary permeability returns to normal and the fluid is reabsorbed, chiefly by way of the lymphatics. Reabsorption usually proceeds at the rate of fluid accumulation, although it may persist longer. Redistribution of fluid is often complex and unpredictable. After a time the lymphatics become incompetent, and inapparent lymph accumulation may take place in compartments within the trunk or extremities.

In most children the cardiovascular system is able to withstand the demands placed on it, although shock is a prominent feature of large thermal injuries, and many children are prone to congestive heart failure and pulmonary edema. In addition, peripheral circulation in the infant is less efficient and more labile, which complicates burn response and therapy in children in this age-group.

Anemia. Loss of circulating red cell mass is significantly reduced and is associated predominantly with deep burns. The anemia characteristic of thermal injury is attributed to several factors—red blood cells are destroyed by heat; circulating red blood cells are lost in the zone of stasis;

red blood cells are damaged by heat; hemolysis from circulating plasma and from *Pseudomonas* invasion occurs; there is direct bleeding from the wound; bone marrow is depressed as a result of sepsis; and (later) loss from bleeding during repeated debridement of the wound surface occurs.

Renal. The loss of fluid from the intravascular compartment causes renal vasoconstriction that in turn leads to reduced renal plasma flow and depressed glomerular filtration. When adequate fluids are provided, the glomerular filtration rate returns to normal, and by the third or fourth day of fluid therapy, urine output increases as edema fluid is mobilized and eliminated. In the first few days oliguria is more commonly the result of inadequate fluid replacement than of acute renal failure. If the patient does not respond to treatment or if there is inadequate fluid resuscitation, acute renal failure may develop with permanent kidney damage. Children with a history of a prior kidney disorder are at increased risk.

Blood urea nitrogen and creatinine levels are elevated from tissue breakdown and oliguria. Hematuria may also be evident from hemolysis of red blood cells, and oliguria may develop as a consequence of the increased pigment load the kidneys must handle, especially myoglobin from extensive electric burn destruction, which blocks the kidney tubules. Renal failure is uncommon in burns involving less than 20% of the body surface. It occurs more frequently following flame burns sustained indoors than after scalds.

Metabolism. The metabolic rate in burned patients is greatly accelerated, and the nitrogen losses are far in excess of those seen in other types of injuries. The magnitude of energy requirements of a burned child frequently exceeds the requirements of a normal active child, and when the burned area is extensive, may approach twice the normal requirements.

The response to the stress of injury places high demands on the body. The stress-invoked glycogen breakdown depletes the energy stores in 12 to 24 hours, after which the body resorts to glyconeogenesis for high energy needs. Blood glucose levels are elevated and, inasmuch as insulin resistance is evident, remain elevated for some time. Protein breakdown is rapid, as reflected in blood urea nitrogen and urine urea nitrogen levels. Each gram of urinary urea nitrogen represents a loss of 30 g of lean body mass.

Many of the metabolic consequences of extensive burn injuries are attributed to the amount of energy needed for the energy-consuming process of evaporation of water from the damaged skin surface. The infant or young child is especially vulnerable because of the large surface area relative to metabolically active tissue. Burning destroys a lipid layer and converts skin that is normally virtually impermeable to water to a freely water-permeable state that transmits water vapor at least four times as rapidly as normal skin. In partial-thickness burns this loss is greatest the day of injury; in full-thickness areas it rises slowly at first and then rapidly increases to reach a peak about the fourth day after the burn occurs. Evaporative losses are maintained until partial-thickness burns are healed and full-thickness injuries are grafted. Thus body stores of energy are rapidly depleted unless sufficient replacement is provided or losses are reduced.

Neuroendocrine system. As occurs in response to any stress, the hypothalamic-hypophyseal mechanism restores equilibrium by secreting tropic hormones, which stimulate various target organs of the neuroendocrine system. Adrenal activity is stimulated maximally. The medulla responds by secreting increased amounts of the catecholamines epinephrine and norepinephrine, which appear to have a sustained elevation. Adrenocortical hormones are elevated and reach a peak immediately after injury but remain high for some time. Aldosterone secretion is elevated and sustained at a high level throughout hospitalization, and there is release of antidiuretic hormone. Despite this increased adrenal activity, adrenal insufficiency is a rare complication.

Acidosis. Most burned patients exhibit some degree of metabolic acidosis. Reduced blood volume and cardiac output result in diminished tissue perfusion with resultant tissue hypoxia, which causes a shift to anaerobic metabolism with formation of metabolic acids. However, this is usually sufficiently compensated by increased ventilation as a result of pulmonary irritation or an independent respiratory alkalosis. Renal compensatory mechanisms are impaired by the decreased blood flow.

Growth changes. Changes in the growth pattern are frequently observed, particularly in older children who have burns covering large areas of their body. As in any severely burned individual, nail and hair growth essentially ceases during the catabolic phase of burn response. It is believed that bone growth is also affected; weight loss is marked. During convalescence following full recovery, there is a catch-up spurt in bone growth and weight recovery. In prepubertal children who suffer thermal injury, there is frequently a rapid acceleration of pubertal changes, with development of secondary sex characteristics, which may occur 2 to 3 years before usual. It is believed that these changes are probably caused by a prolonged and heavy production of growth hormone.

Complications

Thermally injured children are subject to a number of serious complications, both from the wound and from systemic alterations resulting from the wound. The immediate threat to life is asphyxia resulting from irritation and edema of the lungs and respiratory passages. In the first 48 to 72 hours the greatest hazard is unremitting shock, followed by possible renal shutdown and potassium excess during the first week. During healing, infection—both local and generalized sepsis—is the primary complication. Mortality associated with thermal injury in children decreases with the age of the child and increases with the extent of the burn. In children older than age 3 years the fatality rate is similar to that in adults, but below this age resistance to the burn or its complications is considerably lessened. Although the cause for

this is unknown, it may be a function of physiologic immaturity.

Pulmonary. Pulmonary problems persist as the major cause of fatality in patients with thermal burns or a result of injury to or complications in the respiratory tract. A full range of respiratory insufficiency can occur, including inhalation injury, aspiration in unconscious patients, bacterial pneumonia, pulmonary edema, pulmonary embolus, and posttraumatic pulmonary insufficiency.

Inhalation injury may be caused by heat injury to the tissues of the airway or inhalation of carbon monoxide or other noxious gases. Although direct thermal injury to the upper airway may occur, heat damage below the vocal cords is rare. Above the glottis the damage is thermal (laryngeal edema); below the glottis damage is chemical. The inspired heated air is cooled in the upper airway before reaching the trachea, and reflex closure of the cords and laryngeal spasm prevent full inhalation. Evidence of direct thermal injury to the upper airway includes burns of the face, lips, and nasal hairs and signs of pharyngeal swelling or necrosis. Acute edema formation may lead to airway obstruction and asphyxiation. Symptoms may not develop for as long as 24 hours. Wheezing, prolonged expiratory phase, wet rales, and sooty secretions are signs of respiratory tract involvement. In such situations tracheal intubation or tracheostomy with gentle suction to clear the bronchial tree is indicated.

Inhalation of carbon monoxide is suspected when the injury occurs in a closed space (see p. 1373 for a discussion of carbon monoxide inhalation). Inhalation of other byproducts of combustion, that is, smoke and toxic chemicals, can produce varying degrees of lung damage, depending on the type of burning material. Burning wood smoke is extremely irritating, and smoke from burning plastic material, especially polyvinyl chloride, is the most irritating. Poisonous gases such as chlorine, sulfuric acid, or cyanide can be lethal if absorbed into the bloodstream. Respiratory injury is manifest as severe mucosal edema followed by sloughing of the mucosa and replacement by a mucopurulent membrane. This purulent material together with edema seriously compromises respiration. Acute bronchitis and bronchopneumonia commonly develop within a few days of injury.

The most common etiologic factor in respiratory failure in the pediatric age-group is bacterial pneumonia, which may be secondary to airway injury or contamination from a tracheostomy or acquired through hematogenous spread of bacteria, usually from the burn wound. However, the largest percentage (65%) is caused by airborne infection, which occurs early in the postburn period and is associated with poor mentation, abdominal distention, and immobilization. The hematogenous variety occurs later from either the septic burn wound or other foci, such as phlebitis at an old cutdown site.

Less common pulmonary complications are pulmonary emboli and pulmonary edema resulting from fluid overload during early fluid replacement. Sometimes deep burns of the chest may cause restriction of chest movement secondary to the effect of the binding, inelastic eschar formation. This is relieved by longitudinal incision of the eschar to prevent fatal hypoxia. Posttraumatic pulmonary insufficiency, which is difficult to distinguish from bacterial pneumonia, is sometimes a consequence of severe burns and is associated with sepsis and intravascular coagulation. It is the result of pulmonary capillary damage and leaking of fluid and protein into interstitial spaces of the lung, which cause loss of compliance and interference with oxygenation.

Wound sepsis. Sepsis is the most critical problem in burn treatment and is an ever-present threat after the shock phase. Initially burns are relatively pathogen free, unless the wound is contaminated with potentially infectious material (e.g., as dirt and polluted water). However, dead tissue and exudate provide a fertile field for bacterial growth. Early colonization of the wound surface by a preponderance of gram-positive organisms (primarily staphylococci) changes, on about the third postburn day, to predominantly gram-negative organisms, particularly *Pseudomonas aeruginosa* organisms. By the fifth postburn day the bacterial invasion is well underway beneath the wound surface.

Characteristics of the burn wound contribute to the proliferation of pathogenic organisms. The vascular supply to full-thickness burns is occluded immediately, and there is no appreciable blood supply to the area for approximately 3 weeks after the injury. In partial-thickness burns the circulation to the burn area stops immediately, but returns in about 24 to 48 hours, unless infection supervenes. Thrombosis from bacterial invasion will impair circulation sufficiently to convert the partial-thickness injury to full-thickness destruction. These large amounts of nonviable tissue provide an excellent medium for the growth of microorganisms.

Occlusion of the local blood supply is believed to impair the delivery of both humoral and cellular defense mechanisms to the burn area. Initially there is a decrease in inflammatory and phagocytic cells to the area, but the number of phagocytes gradually increases until they are present in abundance by the third postburn week, when good granulation tissue is forming. Granulating tissue, with its rich blood supply, affords increasing resistance to infection. Inasmuch as organisms are normally a part of skin flora, cultures that reveal an organism concentration of 10^5/g of tissue have been arbitrarily set as the level at which burn wound invasion occurs.

Normally there is a cyclic variation in the ability of phagocytes to kill ingested bacteria, and it appears that burn injury accentuates this process markedly. Burn wound sepsis occurs only during the periods when this phagocytic killing power is depressed. Although the amount of complement (the system of plasma enzymes that mediate the antigen-antibody response) is also depressed, it is still present in sufficient quantities. This has led to development of a specific antibody against *P. aeruginosa*, the primary organism involved in burn wound sepsis. The success of this approach is presently being evaluated.

Disorientation in the patient is one of the first signs of overwhelming sepsis. A spiking fever and usually paralytic ileus develop and progressively increase in severity over 2 to 3 days, after which the temperature falls to below normal. At this time the wound deteriorates, the white blood cell count is depressed, and septic shock becomes manifest.

Gastrointestinal. Recurrent or intermittent bleeding resulting from Curling, or stress, ulceration is a major non-infectious complication of burns. Routine antacid administration has reduced the incidence of this complication in recent years, but these superficial erosive lesions still occur in a number of burn injuries. The cause is obscure, and although gastric ulcers are more common in the total burn population, duodenal ulcers occur twice as frequently in children as in adults. Whereas gastric ulcers are observed in persons in all age-groups during the first postburn month, the peak occurrence of duodenal lesions is in the first week in adults but not until the third or fourth week in children. Children with significant (greater than 50% total body surface area) burn injury may be given cimetidine intravenously.

Children with burns covering more than 20% of body surface usually develop a partial paralytic ileus that lasts for 2 to 3 days in the early postburn period. Gastric decompression and parenteral nutrition are needed until bowel motility is reestablished and oral feedings are started.

Central nervous system. In children a frequent complication of both large and small burn injuries is central nervous system dysfunction. The manifestations range from hallucinations, personality change, and delirium to seizures and coma. Postburn seizures seem to be unique to children. In most cases the cause of this burn encephalopathy can be attributed to hypoxemia, electrolyte imbalance (hyponatremia), hypovolemia, septicemia, and drug administration. When the cause is determined, appropriate treatment can be initiated. Although the cause is unknown in one third of cases, full neurologic recovery is usual, even with prolonged and serious manifestations.

Hypertension. Approximately one third of children with severe thermal injuries develop arterial hypertension. The cause is unclear but may be related to the increased secretion of catecholamines or high plasma renin levels. Hypercalcemia caused by immobilization is occasionally a factor. It may appear at any time during the burn course and may persist for a few days or several months. Control is achieved by administration of diuretic and antihypertensive drugs. Mild hypertension is managed with administration of morphine sulphate or furosemide (Lasix); hydralazine may be required for more refractory problems (Harmel, Vane, and King, 1986).

THERAPEUTIC MANAGEMENT

The treatment of burns is commonly divided into phases because of the nature of the pathologic processes. The phases are described and titled differently by various authorities.

However, for the purpose of this discussion, the emergency care is discussed first, followed by the medical management for minor and major burns. No phases are delineated.

Emergency Care

The aims of immediate treatment of thermal injury are to stop the burning process, begin emergency procedures, cover the burn, transport the child to medical aid, and provide reassurance.

Stop burning process. In flame burns the chief aim in rescue is to smother the fire, not to fan it. Children tend to panic and run, which only serves to fan the flames and make assistance more difficult. The victim should not run and should not remain standing. The injured child should be placed in a horizontal position and rolled in a blanket, rug, or similar article, being careful not to cover the head and face because of the danger of the child's inhaling the toxic fumes. If no such article is available, the child should be made to lie down and roll over slowly. If the victim remains in a vertical position, the hair may be ignited or it may cause him to inhale flames, heat, or smoke.

Spontaneous cooling of burns by slow immersion in cool water or any nonflammable liquid helps to relieve the pain, inhibit edema formation, and slow the process of heat damage, especially in the zone of stasis. Ice water or ice packs are contraindicated because the resulting vasoconstriction interferes with capillary perfusion and carries the risk of further damage from cold burn. Unless there is nothing else available, no dirt or sand should be thrown on the burn. In chemical burns it is particularly important to wash the burn with copious amounts of cool running water. The exception to this rule is when the chemical irritant is a powder. The addition of water will spread the caustic agent.

Burned clothing is removed to prevent further damage from smoldering fabric or hot beads of melted synthetic material. This also provides better access to the wound and precludes more painful removal later on.

Emergency procedures. As soon as the flames are extinguished the condition of the victim is assessed. Airway, breathing, and circulation are the priority concerns. Cardiopulmonary or cerebral emergencies are always a possibility following a severe injury. Cardiopulmonary resuscitation is begun if indicated from the assessment. Cardiopulmonary complications may result from hypovolemic (or electric) shock and seizures may be caused by lack of oxygen to the brain, inhalation of noxious fumes, or aggravation of a preexisting tendency to convulsions by stress of the injury.

Cover burn. The burn wound should be covered with a clean cloth to prevent contamination and to alleviate pain by avoiding air contact. The child with extensive burns is covered to prevent hypothermia and help ease pain from contact with the air. No attempt should be made to treat the burn. Application of topical ointments, oils, or other home remedies is avoided.

Transport child to medical aid. The child with an extensive burn should not be given anything by mouth because of the risk of aspiration and water intoxication. The child is transported to the nearest place where medical aid is available. If this cannot be accomplished within a relatively short time and if facilities for intravenous fluid therapy and oxygen administration are available, they should be instigated to prevent burn shock. A report of the initial assessment is given to the person assuming charge of the child's care.

Provide reassurance. Providing reassurance and psychologic support to both the parents and the child helps immeasurably during postinjury crisis. Reducing anxiety helps to conserve energy needed to cope with the physiologic and emotional stress of a traumatic injury.

Management of Minor Burns

Treatment of burns classified as minor usually can be managed adequately on an outpatient basis when it is determined that the parents can be relied on to carry out instructions for care and observation. Children with burns of the hands and most children with burns of the feet are admitted to the hospital so that they can receive careful local wound care and proper splinting to prevent deformity. In addition, burns of the face should be observed for airway obstruction.

The wound is cleansed and debrided (all foreign material and devitalized tissue removed) with a tepid or cool, dilute, nonirritating soap solution and rinsed with sterile saline solution. Coolness reduces pain and probably reduces edema that can interfere with capillary flow in the zone of stasis. Blisters may or may not be debrided. Whereas removal of the dead skin makes a cleaner wound and reduces the chance of infection in the blister fluid, it is more painful and the intact blister skin provides a biologic dressing.

Most physicians favor covering the wound with a dry dressing or fine-mesh gauze lightly lubricated with water-soluble antiseptic or antimicrobial cream and then wrapping it with bulky dry gauze dressings. This helps to keep the wound clean and to protect it from trauma. Some physicians prefer that an occlusive dressing be left in place for 7 to 10 days if the dressing remains clean and the child afebrile. The parents are instructed to cleanse the wound with mild soap and tepid water, change the dressings once or twice daily, and return to the office or clinic as directed for wound observation.

If there is a high probability of infection or other complications or if there is doubt about their ability to carry out the directions, the parents may be directed to return daily for dressing change and inspection or a nurse may be assigned to make a home visit for that purpose. Frequent removal of dressings is an effective mode of debridement. Soaking the dressing in tepid water before removal will help loosen the dressings and debris and reduce the discomfort. Burns about the face are usually treated by exposure; a protective crust will form in 24 to 36 hours if the atmosphere is cool and dry.

A tetanus history is obtained on admission. When there is no history of immunization, human tetanus antitoxin should be administered. Administration of antibiotics for minor burns is controversial. If medication is needed for discomfort, acetaminophen is usually adequate to control pain of superficial burns.

Most mild burns heal with little difficulty, but if the wound margin becomes erythematous, gross purulence is noted, or the child develops evidence of systemic reaction, such as fever or tachycardia, hospitalization is indicated. A mild analgesic such as acetaminophen is usually sufficient to relieve any discomfort, and the antipyretic effect of the drug helps alleviate the sensation of heat.

Management of Major Burns

When a child with serious burns is admitted to the hospital for treatment, a variety of assessments are made and therapies initiated. Of these, the priority concerns are to (1) establish and maintain an adequate airway, (2) establish a lifeline for fluid resuscitation, and (3) care for the burn wound. Although the order of implementation may vary from institution to institution and from patient to patient, a number of procedures and activities generally are initiated on admission. Some are carried out simultaneously.

Ascertain the adequacy of the airway and provide oxygen, intubation, and ventilatory assistance as indicated

Provide intravenous sedation only if necessary

Remove clothes and examine for trauma to head, skeleton, or nervous system

Insert an intravenous line to deliver fluids at a rapid rate, and in patients with extensive injury to accommodate a central venous pressure line

Weigh the child

Insert an indwelling Foley catheter to obtain specimens and measure hourly output

Empty stomach through nasogastric tube

Obtain blood sample for baseline laboratory studies

Examine the burn wound and evaluate the extent and depth of injury

Carry out an escharotomy (incision through the eschar) for constricting circumferential eschar of chest or extremities

Cover flame or contact burns and apply topical medication and gauze dressings

Calculate fluid requirements and establish appropriate regimen

Administer appropriate protection against tetanus

Initiate low-dose penicillin prophylaxis

Obtain history regarding the injury and other pertinent data

Other needs and therapies, including nutritional support, splinting to prevent contractures, treatment of anemia and hypoproteinemia, and the rehabilitative aspects of burn management, are initiated as appropriate throughout the course of treatment.

Establishment of adequate airway. The first priority of care is airway maintenance. Thermal injuries to the face, nares, or upper torso, history of fire in an enclosed area, or examination of the oral and nasal membranes that reveals edema of these membranes, hyperemia, burns of mucous membranes, or evidence of trauma to upper respiratory passages all suggest inhalation of noxious agents or presence of respiratory burn. Oxygen is administered and blood gases, including carbon monoxide, are quickly determined. If the child exhibits air hunger or otherwise appears

---

Emergency Treatment: Burns

Minor burns
  Stop burning process:
    Apply cool water to burn or hold burned area under cool running water
  Do not disturb any blisters that form
  Do not apply anything to wound
  Leave small burns exposed to air
  Apply dry, nonstick dressing if risk of damage or contamination
  Observe for signs of infection
Major burns
  Stop burning process:
    Flame burns—smother fire
    Place victim in horizontal position
    Roll victim in blanket or similar object—avoid covering head
    Immerse in cool water or any nonflammable liquid
  Remove burned clothing
  Assess for adequate airway and breathing
    If not breathing, begin mouth-to-mouth resuscitation
  Cover wound with clean cloth
  Transport to medical aid

---

in critical condition, an endotracheal tube is inserted to maintain the airway. The usual practice is to place a tube if there is any question regarding the possibility of respiratory problems. Pharyngeal edema may make delayed intubation difficult, and the child will become restless from hypoxia.

Tracheostomy is rarely employed, because it has been associated with serious complications and significant mortality in childhood burn injuries, such as a high incidence of infection, tracheobronchitis, delayed hemorrhage, and cannula obstruction from secretions and granulations. Inasmuch as early edema subsides within 24 to 48 hours and many have been managed successfully for longer periods without significant damage, nasotracheal intubation is the safer and preferred approach. It allows for the delivery of humidified air with oxygen, the easy removal of secretions from respiratory passages, and the use of a pressure ventilator if needed.

Frequently placing the child in a Croupette or under an oxygen hood with a high flow of oxygen and maximum humidity is sufficient to reduce reflex bronchospasm produced by trauma to the bronchial mucosa. To combat continued respiratory distress, frequently a large dose of an antiinflammatory corticosteroid compound is given rapidly by the intravenous route to augment the already elevated blood level of circulating steroids. This therapy still remains somewhat controversial, however.

Fluid replacement therapy. The objectives of fluid therapy are to (1) compensate for water and sodium lost to traumatized areas and interstitial spaces, (2) replenish sodium deficits, (3) restore plasma volume, (4) obtain adequate perfusion, (5) correct acidosis, and (6) improve renal function.

Fluid and electrolyte therapy for children in the first 24 hours after a burn is still controversial. This controversy is centered primarily around whether colloid solution, usually albumin, dextran, Plasmanate, or plasma, should be part of the resuscitation phase of fluid therapy. Those who favor crystalloid solutions believe that during this time the altered capillary membrane is unable to provide a structural barrier and that, therefore, colloid solutions are of questionable value in restoring the plasma oncotic pressure. Instead, the colloid crosses the membrane and becomes trapped in the interstitial spaces as capillary permeability is restored during the next 24 hours, augmenting the extravascular fluid retention. This has serious implications for fluid accumulation in the lungs and brain.

The composition of the fluid selected varies with the philosophy of the individual physician or the burn unit and may consist of isotonic saline solution, a near-isotonic solution (such as Ringer's lactate), or even a hypertonic saline solution. Needs are determined by several parameters, such as vital signs, including blood pressure, urine volume and character, pulse, adequacy of capillary filling, and state of sensorium. In complicated cases arterial, central venous, and pulmonary artery pressures are monitored. These criteria, based on individual needs, are more effective for fluid resuscitation. Periodic monitoring of potassium, chloride, carbon dioxide, blood urea nitrogen, and osmolality help determine the adequacy of fluid therapy and evidence of acidosis (Herndon and others, 1985).

After diuresis, in 48 to 72 hours when capillary permeability is restored, fluid requirements decrease to a constant that remains so long as the burn wound is open. Sometimes colloid solutions such as albumin or plasma are used in maintaining plasma volume. During this phase interstitial fluid is returning rapidly to the vascular compartment, and increasing intake to match urine output may cause circulatory overload. Oral fluids are usually withheld in the early resuscitative phase but may be administered in 24 to 48 hours. Fluid balance may continue to be a problem throughout the course of treatment, especially during the periods in which there may be considerable evaporative loss from the wound.

Nutrition. The high metabolic requirements and catabolism in severe burns make nutritional needs of paramount importance and often difficult to provide. Hypermetabolism, increased glucose flow, and severe protein and fat wasting are characteristic of the response to major trauma and infection. Children with multiple trauma and who are respiratory dependent can have metabolic requirements 30% to 75% above normal. The metabolic rate of those with burns greater than 40% total body surface is 100% greater than normal (Herndon and others, 1985) and may reach 200% of normal resting energy expenditure (Harmel, Vane, and King, 1986).

The diet must provide sufficient protein to avoid protein breakdown, and extra calories to utilize the proteins, sustain the adaptive hypermetabolism, and spare protein breakdown. Normal protein requirements may be three times the standard adult intake, and increase proportionately as a result of trauma and stress. The child's proportionately less body fat and substantially smaller muscle mass predispose to the rapid development of protein-calorie malnutrition (Harmel, Vane, and King, 1986). Extra calories should be derived from carbohydrates, because fat, although higher in total calories, will not spare protein. The normal energy stores of glycogen are depleted; therefore exogenous glucose must be provided early. Intravenous 5% glucose can supply minimal requirements, but these are inadequate to meet added needs.

Most burn patients are able to eat, and the child is given oral feedings as soon as possible. A liquid diet is instituted, and gradually advanced to a regular diet. Because burned children have poor appetites and the caloric requirements may be as much as two to three times their usual requirements for size and age, the diet is high in calories and protein, supplemented with high doses of vitamins B and C and iron. An adequate anabolic state is reached when the blood urea nitrogen level begins to fall.

Nasogastric feedings may be needed to supplement oral intake, and intravenous hyperalimentation has been used to provide a large amount of concentrated glucose and amino acids, especially in infants. The anorexia, delayed gastric emptying, and osmotic diarrhea secondary to high-solute tube feedings lead to this mode of nutrition despite difficulties encountered in placement of the catheter and the increased risk of sepsis.

Medication. Controversy also exists regarding the use of antibiotics during the first few days after injury. Some authorities believe that low doses of penicillin should be given prophylactically to all children with serious burns because of (1) their susceptibility to rapidly spreading cellulitis as a result of γ-hemolytic streptococci, and (2) lowered immunoglobulin levels. Others prefer to treat the streptococci only when they become a problem. Fevers are evaluated and antibiotics administered if no immediate source of the elevation can be identified. Broad-spectrum antibiotics are avoided to prevent the possibility of a superimposed infection. In addition, impaired circulation in the wound area prevents their access to the site.

Some form of sedation and analgesia is required in the care of burned children. During the first 12 to 24 hours sedation is kept at a minimum to allow for observation of sensorium to assess brain perfusion and to evaluate cerebral status when head trauma is established or suspected. Also, there is increased risk of respiratory distress in some patients. Suitable narcotics such as morphine sulfate are administered intravenously and titrated as needed. The unstable circulatory status precludes the use of intramuscular injections. Beyond 24 hours the amount and type of sedation are determined by the individual patient and the philosophy of the burn unit. General anesthesia is required for extensive debridement, but during dressing changes and tubbing a number of methods are available.

Morphine sulfate is the drug of choice for severe burn injuries. Morphine has been found to have a rapid and extensive distribution in burn patients, although it is eliminated more rapidly (Perry and Intrisi, 1983). Consequently, more frequent administration is needed for burn pain management. Meperidine hydrochloride (Demerol) and acetaminophen with codeine are also effective for less severe injury. Meperidine varies widely in peak action and often produces paradoxical agitation and nausea; it should be used less frequently for burn pain. For a more extensive discussion of pain see Chapter 26.

To facilitate growth and proliferation of epithelial cells, administration of vitamin A is begun early in the postburn period. Zinc sulfate is also administered by some physicians, because zinc stores are depleted during catabolism and it appears to facilitate wound healing and epithelialization.

Management of Burn Wound

After the initial period of shock and restoration of fluid balance, the primary concern is the burn wound. The objective of management for epidermal and superficial (first- and second-degree) burns is to prevent infection by providing an environment as aseptic as possible. Occlusive dressings help to reduce pain by minimizing exposure to air. The exposure method allows the wound to dry and is used primarily for mild to moderate face wounds. All methods employ topical

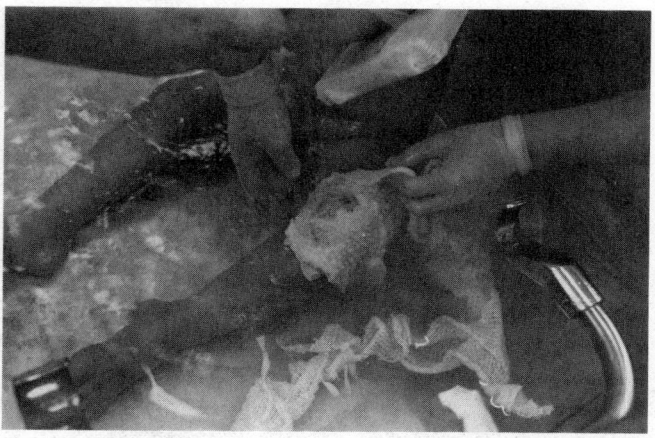

Fig. 29-8. Removal of dressings during tubbing.
Photography by Sharon Bornstein, San Jose, CA.

antibacterial applications, or daily hydrotherapy or tubbing, or both, to remove loose tissue and debris and to allow inspection of the wound. The objectives for management of full-thickness wounds are prevention of invasive infection, removal of dead tissue, protection from mechanical trauma, and closure of the wound.

Debridement. The use of hydrotherapy has reduced the need for surgical debridement under general anesthetic. Debridement is painful and requires some type of analgesic before the procedure (Fig. 29-7). Soaking in the Hubbard tank for 20 to 30 minutes once or twice daily facilitates the loosening and removal of sloughing tissue, eschar, exudate, and topical medications. The mesh gauze serves to entrap exudative slough and is readily removed during the tubbing procedure (Fig. 29-8). Any loose tissue or eschar is carefully trimmed away before redressing (Fig. 29-9). Morphine is the current drug of choice in most units. Ketamine hydrochloride in subanesthetic doses has proved highly effective in children, and nitrous oxide inhalation is employed in a number of burn units. The child will require instruction in how to breathe the gas at the appropriate time and coaching during its use.

Methods. There are several methods for covering the burn wound. All meet the objective of preparation for permanent wound coverage. Four methods are employed in the management of burn wounds:

Exposure—the wounds are left open to the air; crust forms on partial-thickness wounds, eschar forms on full-thickness wounds

Open—a topical antimicrobial ointment is applied directly to the wound surface, but the wound is left uncovered

Modified—ointment is applied directly to wound or impregnated into thin gauze and applied to the wound; a stretched gauze or net covering secures the area (Fig. 29-10)

Occlusive—ointment-impregnated gauze or ointment covered with a gauze layer is placed on the burn wound; multiple layers of bulky gauze are placed over the primary layer and secured with stretched gauze or net

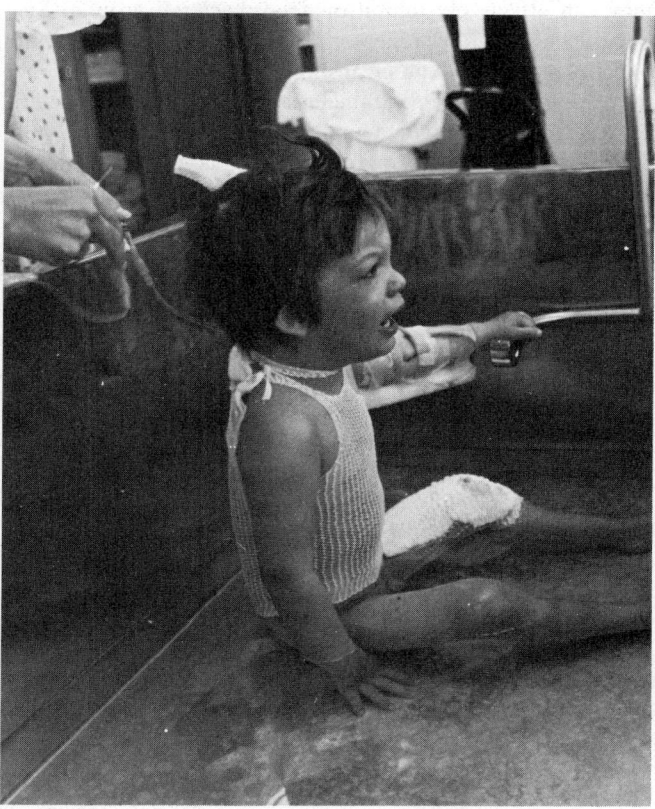

Fig. 29-7. An analgesic is administered before removal of dressings and debridement. In this instance analgesic is injected directly into intravenous line at time of tubbing.
Photography by Sharon Bornstein, San Jose, CA.

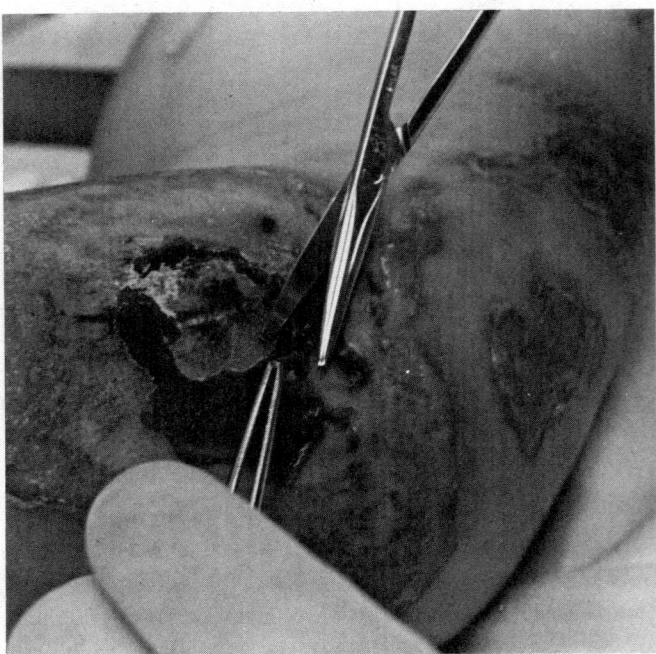

Fig. 29-9. Dead skin and debris are carefully trimmed away before dressing is applied.
Photography by Sharon Bornstein, San Jose, CA.

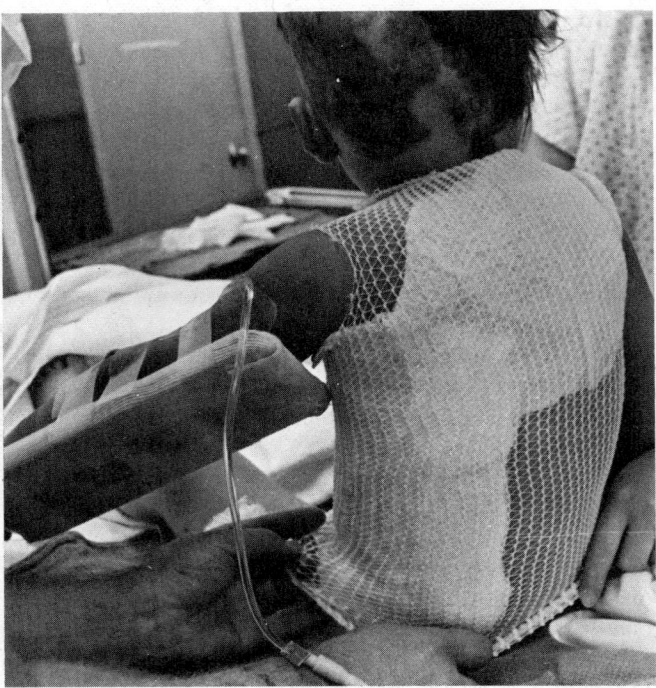

Fig. 29-10. Burn wound covered with gauze dressings and secured with tabular elastic netting.
Photography by Sharon Bornstein, San Jose, CA.

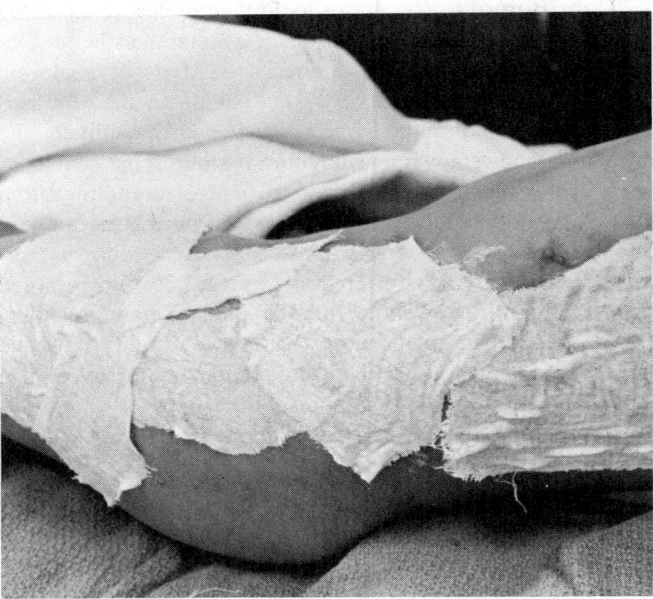

Fig. 29-11. Gauze impregnated with ointment applied to burn wound.
Photography by Sharon Bornstein, San Jose, CA.

Topical antimicrobial agents. Before the development of effective topical agents for reducing the incidence of invasive organisms, wound sepsis was the major cause of mortality from burn injury. Systemic administration cannot reach the area because of thrombosed vessels. Topical agents do not eliminate organisms from the burn wound, but they can effectively inhibit or delay bacterial growth. Successful burn therapy relies on both topical antibacterial applications and thorough cleansing and debridement to reduce the amounts of necrotic material on which the bacteria grow. To be effective, a topical application must be nontoxic, capable of diffusing through eschar, harmless to viable tissue, nonallergenic, not conducive to causing an increase in resistant strains, inexpensive, and easy to apply (Artz, Moncrief, and Breitt, 1979) (Fig. 29-11).

A number of topical agents are employed, but those used most frequently are 0.5% silver nitrate solution, 10% mafenide acetate (Sulfamylon), and 1% silver sulfadiazine (Silvadene). All three are effective bacteriostatic agents, but each has advantages and disadvantages. Less frequently used are 0.1% gentamicin sulfate (Garamycin) and povidone-iodine (Betadine) ointment. Furacin-saturated gauze dressings have been used by some burn units, but renal impairment has been observed in some patients, caused by the polyethylene glycol base in which it is prepared (Food and Drug Administration, 1982). The significant aspects of each are summarized in Table 29-4.

Biologic skin coverings. Biologic dressings are used during the acute phase of therapy to cover wound surfaces, protect wound from bacterial invasion, limit fluid and protein loss, reduce pain, and increase rate of epithelialization (Herndon and others, 1985). These temporary grafts are:

allografts (homografts) Skin obtained from genetically different members of the same species, living or dead—usually cadavers—that are free from disease.

Table 29-4 Comparison of common topical preparations

AGENT	DRESSINGS	ADVANTAGES	DISADVANTAGES
Silver nitrate, 0.5% (AgNO₃)	Exposure, modified or occlusive Impedes joint movement Dressings changed twice daily	Greatly reduces evaporative losses, thus lower metabolic rate and lower weight loss Effective in controlling *Pseudomonas* Does not interfere with wound healing Nonallergenic Inexpensive Effective against major burn flora, including *Pseudomonas* and *Staphylococcus*	Cannot allow dressings to become dry; requires frequent wetting (at least every 2 hours) Difficult to use Ineffective on established burn wound infections Does not penetrate eschar; therefore, should be applied before bacterial growth established Hypotonicity pulls electrolytes from wound, causing depletion of sodium, chloride, potassium, and magnesium that necessitates continuous monitoring and replacement Little effect on *Klebsiella* and *Aerobacter* groups
Mafenide acetate (Sulfamylon), 10%	Usually exposure Occasionally with dressings Reapplied twice daily	Diffuses rapidly into burn wound and underlying tissues Rapidly excreted Easily applied Penetrates through eschar and deeply into burn wound; therefore, effective in deep flame, electric, and older wounds Effective against many gram-positive and gram-negative organisms, including *Pseudomonas* and *Clostridium*	Mild acidosis caused by inhibition of carbonic anhydrase in kidney Hypersensitivity reaction in many children Causes discomfort during application Inhibits wound healing
Silver sulfadiazine (Silvadene), 1% (AgSD)	Occlusive Motion of joints maintained Applied once or twice daily	Nontoxic Combines advantages of silver nitrate and mafenide acetate Painless Easy to apply Absorbs slowly Bactericidal for up to 48 hours Effective against gram-positive and gram-negative bacteria and *Candida albicans*	Does not penetrate eschar as well as mafenide acetate or gentamicin sulfate May cause neutropenia
Gentamicin sulfate (Garamycin), 0.1%	Exposure, modified or occlusive	No pain associated with use Relatively nontoxic Penetrates burn wound quickly Especially effective against *Klebsiella* and *Enterobacter*	40% of pseudomonal organisms have become resistant Occasionally nephrotoxicity and ototoxicity
Povidone-iodine (Betadine) ointment	Exposure, modified or occlusive Impedes joint movement	Apparently nontoxic Effective against broad spectrum of organisms	Elevation of protein-bound iodine (PBL) Use associated with considerable pain Causes eschar to "tan" and become very stiff, making debridement and evaluation of burn wound difficult May cause acidosis

xenografts (heterografts) Skin obtained from members of a different species. At present most grafts are derived primarily from pig skin, either fresh or frozen.

The type of graft particularly suitable and used most frequently for temporary covering in children is the porcine xenograft (Fig. 29-12). The split-thickness pig skin is available commercially and is an effective covering agent after eschar separation. Changed regularly, it reduces evaporative loss, protects the wound bed, and is believed to protect the wound from infection and trauma. The grafts usually adhere within a few hours, and dressings are not needed. They are particularly effective in children with second-degree scald burns of hands and face, because they allow relatively pain-free movement, which reduces contracture and has the

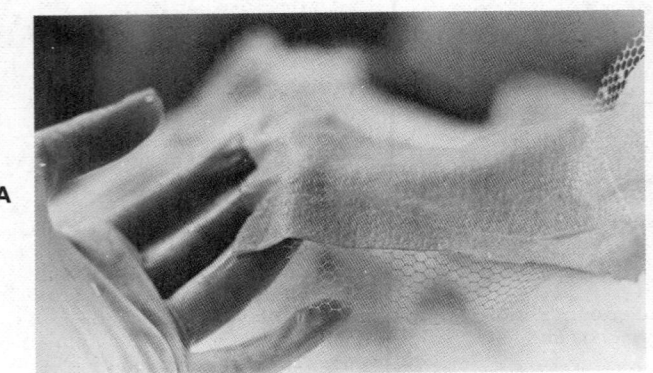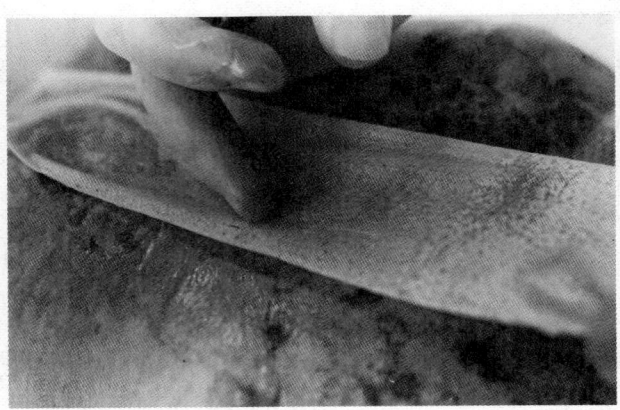

Fig. 29-12. Porcine dressing. **A,** Removed from net backing. **B,** Applied to wound.
Photography by Sharon Bornstein, San Jose, CA.

added benefit of improved appetite and morale. Pig skin dressings are replaced daily or at least every 3 to 4 days; as a result acceptance of the graft is minimal. When they are left in place for longer periods, antibody development causes increasingly rapid rejection.

Other allografts that are used are from human cadavers, when available. Rejection of these grafts occurs in about 14 days. Skin allografts from closely histocompatible living related donors, used in conjunction with immunosuppression therapy, maintain wound coverage continuously over a longer period of time. Short-term coverage can be accomplished with human amnion (obtained by stripping the amniotic membrane from the placenta).

Synthetic skin coverings. A number of satisfactory biologic dressings and skin subtitutes are available for burn wound management. Ideally the dressing should provide many of the properties of human skin—adherent, elastic, durable, and hemostatic—and be inexpensive and available.

Synthetic skin substitutes are available in several forms. Examples include dressings consisting of a layer of polyurethane foam laminated to outer sheets of microporous polypropylene film, a silicone polymer membrane, a semisynthetic membrane composed of Silastic nylon and collagen (Biobrane), and a mixture of polymer powder and polyethylene glycol liquid that forms a flexible, adherent, transparent, water-soluble dressing (Hydron). Synthetic adhesive, vapor-permeable polyurethane film dressings (Op-Site, Clingfilm, Via-film, and Tegaderm) are also available and especially valuable for fresh, small partial-thickness wounds treated on an outpatient basis. All synthetic dressings are reputed to hasten the healing of some partial-thickness burns and donor sites and to reduce wound discomfort.

Combined biologic and synthetic skin substitutes have been developed for covering burns and skin graft sites. This is the collagen wound dressing, and contains a porous collagen fibrillous "dermal" layer combined with an impermeable "epidermal" layer of Silastic. The synthetic skin is gradually replaced with normal vascularized connective tissue elements as it is slowly biodegraded. This new tissue is then ready to support a standard split-thickness skin graft that is placed as the Silastic is removed (Burke and others, 1981).

Permanent skin covering. Permanent skin grafting is part of the rehabilitative stage to restore cosmetic appearance and to achieve maximum functional capacity. Permanent grafting of full-thickness burns is usually accomplished with a split-thickness skin graft, which can be obtained from only two sources:

autografts Tissues obtained from undamaged areas of the patient's own body
isografts Histocompatible tissue obtained from genetically identical individuals, that is, the patient's identical twin

A permanent skin graft consists of the epidermis and part of the dermis being removed from an undamaged area by a special instrument, the dermatome, which is designed to excise split-thickness skin. The priority areas for coverage are the face, neck, and areas around joints, especially the hands. With extensive burns it is often difficult to find enough viable skin to cover the wounds; therefore, available donor sites are used to the best advantage by special techniques. The various methods of applying split-thickness grafts are:

full-cover graft—A sheet of skin, removed from the donor site, is placed intact over the recipient site. It may be sutured or maintained in place by pressure dressings.
postage-stamp graft—A sheet of skin from the donor site is cut into postage-stamp pieces and placed on the recipient bed. Spaces between grafts allow for drainage. These may be covered with a dressing or, when possible, left exposed for inspection and for rolling serum from beneath the graft to aid contact between surfaces. These are not removed from the site as readily as large sheet grafts.
mesh, lace, or slit graft—A sheet of skin, removed from the donor site, is run through a special instrument to make multiple slits so that, when stretched, the skin expands to cover from one and one half to nine times (usually three

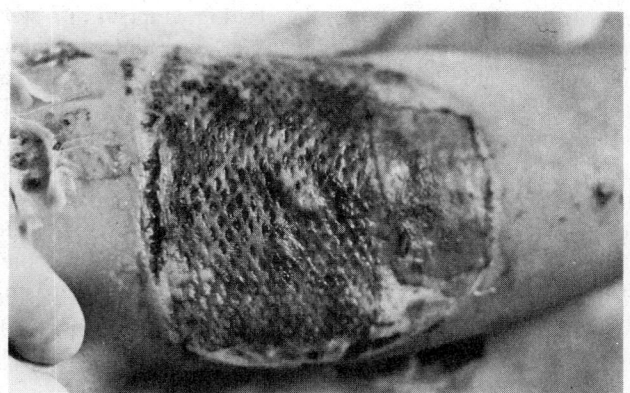

Fig. 29-13. Mesh graft.
Photography by Sharon Bornstein, San Jose, CA.

times) the area of a full-cover graft. This type of graft requires suturing to maintain tension. The openings allow drainage of serum and bacteria, thus allowing earlier closure of the burn. The graft may be exposed or covered with an occlusive dressing for about 48 hours. Mesh grafts are an effective method of covering large areas with a small amount of donor skin (Fig. 29-13).

Full-sheet grafts are used in areas in which a cosmetic effect is desired. Patch and mesh grafts result in a less desirable appearance. Requirements for a successful "take," regardless of graft type, are:

Sufficient nourishment until new blood supply grows in from the base of the recipient bed

Primary tissue contact, that is, actual contact between cut surface of the graft and the recipient bed

Avoidance of bleeding; the possibility of even the slightest bleeding must be controlled with light pressure

Prevention of infection, especially in full-cover grafts; postage-stamp grafts will often "take" in contaminated areas

Until blood supply is established, the grafted skin is nourished by osmotic interchange with the recipient bed. Wound healing takes place as the recipient area throws out fibrin that attaches the graft to the new bed. The fibrin is infiltrated by leukocytes and fibroblasts, and the capillary buds of the granulation tissue spread through the fibrin. Within 3 days there is vascularization of the graft; after 2 weeks the graft is attached to the base by connective tissue.

The donor site is dressed with either a xenograft or fine-mesh gauze and left exposed until the dressing falls off in about 10 to 14 days. Dressings are not changed on donor sites to prevent tearing the new, delicate epithelium.

When burns are extensive and donor sites for split-thickness grafts are inadequate for coverage, it is possible to culture epidermal cells from a small skin biopsy and produce coherent epithelial sheets that can be grafted to generate a permanent epidermal surface (Green, Kelrinde, and Thomas, 1979). Some children have been successfully treated with this autologous cultured epithelium method (Gallico and others, 1984; O'Conner and others, 1981).

Primary excision. Excision and immediate grafting of small full-thickness and deep partial-thickness burns hastens recovery in selected cases (Gray and others, 1982). In some areas this is replacing standard topical therapy. Primary excision should take place as early as possible after restoration of physical balance.

NURSING CONSIDERATIONS

Nursing care is the most important aspect of burn therapy. Because the care of severely burned children encompasses such a broad range of skills and foci, it is divided into segments that correspond with the major phases of burn treatment: the *acute phase* (also referred to as the resuscitative, emergent, or metabolic phase), which involves the first 24 to 48 hours; the *management phase,* which extends from the time a child has been adequately resuscitated until the major rehabilitative aspects of care are initiated; and the *rehabilitative phase,* which begins with permanent grafting. This phase continues until all full-thickness injuries are covered and reconstructive procedures and corrective measures have been accomplished. This often extends over a period of months or years. Because pain is a major initial nursing consideration, it is discussed before these three phases.

Burn Pain

The severe pain of the wound and the therapies, the anxiety generated by these experiences, and the conscious and unconscious interpretations of traumatic events contribute to the psychologic reactions frequently observed in burned children. Much of the difficulty encountered in managing burned children is related to these factors. Soon after hospitalization many burned children become irritable, depressed, hostile, and aggressive toward the members of the health team. When pain is not a factor, as in the case of burns to a paralyzed area, this behavior has not been observed. In their helplessness, children often resort to angry outbursts against anything and anybody.

The burn pain is overwhelming, engulfing, and irrepressible. Consequently the pain causes anxiety and a feeling of profound helplessness in a child and can produce reactions of confusion, fear, and panic. Compounding the pain is a child's interpretation of it and of the procedures; this is closely related to the developmental level of a child. Many burned children believe their pain is punishment for past misdeeds and therefore deserved. There are often feelings of anger, guilt, and depression, and, as in all illness, regressive behavior. When children appear to accept their pain and show little or no aggressive behavior, psychologic consultation is usually in order.

It is always difficult to deal with children in pain, and to inflict pain on helpless children is contrary to the empathetic nature of nursing. Adequate management of pain is essential to reduce discomfort of the burn and the necessary therapeutic procedures. Management of pain consists of (1) choosing the correct analgesic (narcotics are often needed for severe pain), (2) adequate dosage, and (3) appropriate timing. For example, to relieve pain adequately, the *onset* of action of the drug must be considered in order that the peak effect occurs when the treatment is performed. An analgesic administered shortly before the procedure will exert its effect *after* the procedure is completed.

Management of pain follows the principles described in Chapter 26.

Acute Phase

The primary emphasis during the initial phases of burn care is prevention of burn shock. Checking vital signs, monitoring the intravenous infusion line, and measuring urinary output are ongoing nursing activities in the hours immediately after injury. The intravenous infusion is started immediately by intracatheter or cutdown and is regulated according to urine output and specific gravity, laboratory data, and objective signs of adequate hydration. Urine volume, measured at least every hour, should be (Jacoby, 1984):

> 20 to 30 ml/hour in a child older than 2 years of age
> 10 to 20 ml/hour in a child younger than 2 years of age

Children are observed for all parameters outlined in the Nursing Care Summary. They require constant observation and assessment with special attention to signs of complications. Respiratory, cardiac, and renal complications may appear early in the postburn period.

Care of the burn wound is secondary to the more critical problems of circulatory or respiratory failure. When a special burn facility is available, the child is wrapped in a sterile sheet and covered with a blanket to keep him warm during transfer, and the burn wound is attended to after arrival at the unit. If no burn unit is available, the wound is cleansed and dressed in the emergency department. Many units take photographs of the burn wound initially and periodically as a record of wound progress and for legal purposes, if needed—especially in cases of suspected child abuse. Evaluation of the wound is more accurately accomplished during or after cleansing. Ideally the cleansing should take place in a hydrotherapy tub. Water is maintained at body temperature (about 37.2° C or 99° F) and is disinfected with chlorine (pool chlorine or Clorox).

The burn wound is treated according to the protocol of the specific burn facility. Extensive wounds may require the use of special beds such as CircOlectric beds, flotation beds, and alternating pressure mattresses, and many other devices, depending on the extent and location of the wound. When inhalation injury is suspected, the nurse observes the child for evidence of pulmonary involvement. Activities include listening for inspiratory wheezing, observing for carbon particles in the sputum, being alert for "smoky" smell on the breath, and detecting increasing hoarseness.

Throughout the acute phase of care the child's emotional needs must not be overlooked. The child is frightened, uncomfortable, and often confused. He is isolated from familiar persons and surroundings, and the often overwhelming physical needs at this time are the primary focus of staff and parents. The child needs to be reassured that he is all right and that he will get better.

Nursing Care Summary: The Child with Burns

ACUTE PHASE OF BURN CARE		
NURSING GOALS	NURSING INTERVENTIONS	EXPECTED PATIENT/FAMILY OUTCOMES
HP-HMP	**Injury: potential for tissue damage**	
	Risk factors: presence of infective agents, smoke inhalation, metabolic derangements	
Implement care	Have respiratory resuscitation equipment ready	Skin is visible for evaluation
	Remove all clothing, jewelry, and so on	Essential information is obtained from family
	Evaluate level of consciousness	
	Summon medical assistance if not present	Family consents to treatment
	Ascertain religious affiliation	
	Get parental consent for treatment or notify parents if not present	
	Begin "critical care" record keeping according to unit policy	
Obtain baseline information	Take vital signs	Child's physiologic status is determined
	Weigh child	
	Help evaluate extent and depth of burn wound	
	Help assess condition	
Obtain history of burn injury	Ascertain information concerning burn	*Extent of injury is determined
	Time of occurrence (needed for assessment of fluid shifts)	

*Nursing outcome.

Nursing Care Summary: The Child with Burns—cont'd

ACUTE PHASE OF BURN CARE

NURSING GOALS	NURSING INTERVENTIONS	EXPECTED PATIENT/FAMILY OUTCOMES
	Nature of burning agent	
	Duration of contact with agent (to help assess depth)	
	If occurred in enclosed area (clue to possible respiratory involvement)	
	Pain—severe, mild (can affect blood pressure)	
	Any medications given	
	Preburn weight	
	Preexisting illnesses	
	Any known allergies	
Prevent eye damage	Check eyes; irrigate with saline solution and apply protective ointment if indicated	Eyes remain moist and unirritated
Prevent respiratory failure	Observe for signs of respiratory distress	Respirations remain within acceptable limits (see inside front cover for normal variations)
	Check for constricting eschar of chest	
	Observe nasopharynx for edema or redness	
Prevent fluid overload	Monitor vital signs frequently	Child remains adequately hydrated and exhibits no evidence of fluid overload
	Observe for signs of impending overhydration	
	Be alert for altered behavior or sensorium	
Prevent circulatory impairment	Check circulation in extremities or other areas peripheral to burns—color, capillary filling, pulses, sensation	Circulatory impairment is detected early, and appropriate interventions are initiated
	Check for constricting eschar	
Assess cardiac function	Monitor vital signs	*Deviations from normal are detected
Assess renal function	Measure intake and output accurately	Output is at or greater than minimum acceptable output (specify)
	Check hourly for amount, color (dark brown indicates blood or products of hemoglobin breakdown)	
Prevent heat loss	Maintain warm, humid environment	Child does not complain of chilliness
	Monitor temperature at least every 2 hours; in severe burns keep continuous record with direct-reading probe	Temperature remains within acceptable limits less than 38° C (100.4° F)
	Adjust ambient temperature according to child's temperature	
	Use direct-probe thermometer when feasible	
	Avoid drafts	

N-MP   Skin integrity, impairment of: actual
Etiology: burns

Treat burn wound	Assess depth and extent of wound	*Extent of wound is determined
	Shave hair from wound and area immediately surrounding burn	Wound area is clean
	Thoroughly cleanse wound and surrounding skin; debride of devitalized tissues	
Control bacterial growth on wound	Implement and maintain protective isolation precautions	Possible sources of infection are eliminated
	Maintain careful handwashing by members of staff and visitors	
	Wear clean or sterilized gown, cap, mask, and sterile gloves when handling wound area	
	Avoid injury to crust and eschar	
	Avoid patient contact with persons who have upper respiratory tract or skin infection	
	Cover wound and/or patient according to protocol of unit	
	Administer mouth care	

*Nursing outcome.

Continued.

Nursing Care Summary: The Child with Burns—cont'd

ACUTE PHASE OF BURN CARE

NURSING GOALS	NURSING INTERVENTIONS	EXPECTED PATIENT/FAMILY OUTCOMES
N-MP	**Fluid volume deficit, actual (2)** Etiology: active loss through body surface	
Monitor hydration	Monitor vital signs (including central venous pressure, if employed) Monitor urinary output, specific gravity, and pH (sometimes protein) every ½ to 1 hour	There is no evidence of dehydration
Prevent further losses	Cover denuded areas Maintain high-humidity atmosphere	Burned area shows no evidence of fluid loss
CPP	**Comfort, alteration in: pain** Etiology: trauma to skin	
Relieve pain	Assess need for pain medication Position for comfort Employ appropriate nonpharmacologic pain-reduction techniques	Child exhibits evidence of tolerable discomfort
Prevent pain	Avoid touching or moving painful areas Reduce irritation, for example, avoid drafts, movement	Same as above
RRP	**Family process, alteration in** Etiology: situational crisis (child with a serious injury)	
Support child psychologically	Reassure child and family Allow family to visit child Facilitate family-child interaction Do not allow isolation technique to unduly separate parent and child Allow child to express anger and distress Answer questions as honestly as possible	Family interacts with child appropriately Child expresses feelings and emotions
Support family	Reinforce factual information Answer questions regarding therapy Allow for expression of feelings Help alleviate feelings of guilt Instruct in techniques required for visiting child Isolation procedures Help to devise means for providing tactile contact with child Help family deal with anxiety regarding child's pain See also The child in the hospital, p. 1075; Family of the hospitalized child, p. 1081	Family expresses feelings and concerns Family makes appropriate contacts with child, employing correct procedure

Nursing Interventions Related to Medical Management

Implement care
  Give analgesia if ordered
  Insert Foley catheter
  Insert nasogastric tube
  Request laboratory studies as ordered—hematocrit, sodium, chloride, potassium, carbon dioxide, blood urea nitrogen, creatinine, and serum protein levels
Prevent shock
  Help establish intravenous line
  Administer fluids as ordered
  Monitor intravenous infusion closely
  Obtain needed specimens for examination or perform needed studies

Prevent complications
  Abdominal distention
    Insert nasogastric tube and attach to low Gomco suction
    Administer nothing by mouth
  Tetanus
    Administer tetanus prophylaxis (see p. 529)
  Infection
    Administer penicillin prophylaxis, if ordered
    Obtain cultures of wound, nose, throat, and stool as ordered
  Acute respiratory distress
    Administer humidified oxygen
    Obtain blood for blood gas determination, if indi-

Nursing Interventions Related to Medical Management—cont'd

Treat burn wound
  Apply topical medication as ordered
  Dress or leave exposed as ordered
  Perform or request laboratory studies
Relieve pain
  Administer analgesics as indicated
  Monitor effectiveness of analgesics (p. 1071)

  cated
    Have respiratory resuscitation equipment available
    Have tracheostomy tray available
    Obtain chest x-ray film
  Cardiac failure
    Order electrocardiogram, if indicated
    Give digitalis as ordered
  Seizures
    Monitor serum electrolytes and blood gases

Management Phase

After the patient's condition is stabilized, the long management phase begins. The major goals for this period are (1) care of the wound to facilitate healing and prepare for permanent closure, (2) prevention and minimization of infection, both local and generalized, (3) provision of adequate nutrition and reduction of metabolic losses, and (4) meeting the emotional and developmental needs of the child.

One of the most difficult aspects of burn care, especially in children, is the impact it has on nurses. The appearance and smell of the burn and the necessary discomfort that must be inflicted on the child as a part of the therapy are often beyond the nurse's ability to cope and remain therapeutic. Throughout the entire process of burn management, nurses must deal with their own feelings and anxieties regarding their therapeutic role in burn care.

Children should begin early to do as much for themselves as possible and to be active participants in their care. It takes a great deal of warm firmness and fortitude on the part of the nurse to force these children to do this. Moving hurts. Many children are able to move and help themselves. Others need considerable help and encouragement. If children are unable to move, they should be told firmly but gently that it must be done, that the nurses will help them, and that it will be done as quickly as possible. They should be told how they can help to make it easier.

It is difficult to handle children with extensive burns. It is almost impossible to move and turn them without touching a burned area. Fortunately the discomfort lasts only for the short time they are being handled; once repositioned it hurts no longer. Children may cry, but they usually stop once the procedure is over. Some children cry in anticipation of the move and may continue to cry afterward, but even small children learn that the hurt stops when the moving is over. Special frames and beds can be used to facilitate the process and to keep children positioned in an attitude that prevents contracture deformity. Fowler position is comfortable but may produce hip and knee contractures that take months to correct.

Children should be encouraged to participate in as many aspects of their care as possible. With illness, children always regress to the developmental level that allows them to deal with the stress. However, there are limits to how long they should be permitted to remain at a lower level of functioning. To lie passively while others tend to their needs is not "normal" and may be detrimental. As their condition permits, children can be expected to do things that they were capable of doing for themselves before they were burned, such as oral hygiene, face washing, feeding themselves, and playing. Allowing children to make choices and to help make decisions about the time of their care and recreational activities makes them feel a part of the team and provides them a small measure of control. They will probably require assistance; however, as children see themselves contributing to their care, they gain confidence and self-esteem. Fears and anxieties diminish with accomplishment and self-confidence.

Activities are selected and encouraged according to each child's level of development and interest, but, as with any ill child, the activity should be somewhat simpler and less challenging than would be expected in a state of health. Otherwise the child's already taxed energies may be further depleted and self-esteem threatened. Quiet games and activities such as reading, coloring, drawing, games, and puzzles are always appropriate. Television is a satisfactory diversion but should not replace active participation and should not substitute for contacts with others. Play that encourages the expression of feelings of guilt, frustration, and anger is especially therapeutic. During the acute, resuscitative phase, children are frequently isolated, but should be moved to where they have contact with others, especially other children, as soon as their physical condition allows. School-age children should continue with schoolwork.

Children need to be bolstered in other ways. They like to look and smell nice, and the unattractive burns, dressings, and assorted paraphernalia do little to foster a positive self-image. They know how they appear to others, and small things such as careful hair combing and a bright ribbon, colorful nightgown or pajamas (when possible), slippers, or any decoration (a flower, pin, necklace, badge) will help make them feel that they look better and are worthwhile to others.

All hospitalized children, especially those who must undergo painful procedures, must be allowed to express their anger and frustration appropriately through verbalization or play. They need to know that their injury and the treatments are not punishment for specific or general, real or imagined transgressions and to know that nurses understand their fears, anger, and discomfort. They also need body contact. This is often difficult to arrange for the child with massive injury. The discomfort associated with moving, the bulky, messy dressings or the bare open wound are deterrents and frequently provide justification for the nurse to avoid such action because of fear or repulsion. Even older children enjoy sitting on the nurse's or parent's lap and being cuddled and hugged. This can be a comfort in times of stress or used as a reward, but most of all it should be kept in mind that it is a natural part of childhood.

Care of burn wound. The nurse has the major responsibility for cleansing, debriding, and applying topical medication and dressings to the burn wound. Because dressing removal is a painful procedure, children should receive adequate analgesia about 30 minutes before the scheduled tubbing. Both nurses and children must recognize it for exactly what it is—a dreadful but absolutely necessary procedure. Because it is painful, children should know that it is all right to cry when the treatment hurts, but only *when it hurts*. Because it is easy for children to give way to emotional excesses they cannot control, they need the firm control and guidance of a caring adult. This includes both actual and anticipated hurt. Children need help to gain and maintain control of their emotions. They benefit from knowing why things are being done to them, how these things will help them get better, and how they can contribute.

Recent research has demonstrated that children are more cooperative and demonstrate less anxiety and depression when they are allowed to be active participants in their care (Kavanagh and Freeman, 1984). Predictability and controllability are promoted during dressing changes. Predictability is increased by providing cues (nurses wearing specific clothing for dressing changes), focusing the patient on the procedure, and providing children with information about physical sensations they are likely to experience (e.g., pulling, stinging, pressure) before they experience them. Controllability is enhanced by providing the children with as many choices as possible during the burn care and encouraging active participation. These strategies are unlike the traditional approaches of distraction and passivity. "Learned helplessness" is most intense when the outcomes are unpleasant and when the situation is perceived to be unchangeable (Murphy, 1982).

New procedures or changes in routine need to be explained. When possible, there should be consistency in members of the staff who care for the children and the routine for procedures and activities. Providing some order in their world reduces the anxieties related to apprehension about the unknown. Children feel comfortable with the known, the routine.

Outer dressings (if any) are removed before a child is placed in the tub, but adherent dressings are more easily removed after soaking in the water. It is helpful to involve children in the process. Whereas children will cry and protest vigorously when others remove the dressings, they will remove adherent gauze with a minimum of fuss. In this way they maintain some control of the situation. Loose or easily detached tissue is also removed during hydrotherapy, and children are encouraged to move about as much as possible to exercise muscles and reduce contracture formation. They need encouragement and every little bit of healing pointed out as evidence that they are getting better. Merely saying that they are better is insufficient as they gaze at unsightly wounds. Providing something constructive for a child to do during dressing application, such as holding a package of dressings or a roll of Kerlix or simply holding someone's hand, helps to focus on something other than the procedure. In dressing the wound, it is important that all areas be clean, that medication be amply applied, and that no two burned surfaces touch, such as fingers or toes.

Ointments are applied directly to the burn wound surface with sterile tongue blades or the sterile gloved hand. The layer of cream or ointment should be applied thick enough so that the wound cannot be seen. It can be left uncovered or covered with a layer of fine-mesh gauze and secured with stretch gauze or elastic tubular netting. For areas that are small or difficult to cover, strips of fine-mesh gauze are impregnated with the medication and then applied to the wound.

There are some psychologic implications that may influence a child's reaction to the tubbing and application of medication. Children who acquired the burn from hot water are particularly fearful, especially if the injury was inflicted as a punishment (battered child). Application of the medication can be a painful experience also, when mafenide (Sulfamylon) cream is the agent employed. Both the nurse and the children must understand that there is a painful sensation often described as "burning" that may have special significance for burned children. These children must be reassured that the medication is not inflicting further injury.

When occlusive dressings are applied, elastic bandages are worn over dressings to prevent epithelial breakdown, to stimulate circulation, and to make mobility easier. This is especially important when the children are ambulatory.

There are other aspects of burn care of which nurses should be aware. Many children are placed in protective isolation, which severely limits their contact with others. Complete coverings on all who enter their presence, including most of the face, serve to further isolate these children. Children who are accustomed to having someone nearby continuously, as in the intensive care burn unit, may become anxious and uneasy when transferred to a transitional unit or a regular unit where staff members are available only intermittently or when summoned.

Nutrition. After the initial phase of care, children are usually allowed oral feedings (unless paralytic ileus persists). If they will not eat, tube feeding is necessary, but every effort should be made to encourage oral intake. Serving regular meals even though a child may take only a small amount helps to maintain the habit of eating by mouth. For older children, forming a contract with them that regulates the need for supplemental tube feeding based on the amount of oral food consumed often encourages them to eat solids in order to avoid tube feedings.

Because children frequently lack appetite and their caloric needs and protein needs are markedly increased, a great deal of encouragement, help, and patience is required on the part of the nursing staff. Consultation with the parents and the dietitian is arranged to determine the best way to provide needed nutrients in foods the child will be more likely to eat. Children who are old enough to participate should be included in the planning. Nourishing snacks are provided between regularly scheduled mealtimes, and if children eat better at times other than scheduled mealtimes, that is when they should be fed. Most important, meals should not be scheduled immediately after a dressing change. Most children are too physically exhausted and too emotionally upset to eat at this time.

Many children eat better when they can feed themselves and when they can eat in an atmosphere more nearly like what they are accustomed to at home. Even if they are unable to feed themselves (for example, if their arms are bandaged), they do better if they can sit up or at least see the tray of food so that they can instruct the person feeding them how they prefer their food and what they want to be fed next. When their condition allows, children enjoy sitting at a table for their meals. Parents are encouraged to bring a child's favorite dish from home.

Prevention of complications. Attempts should be made to decrease the excess metabolic expenditures of burned children. This means avoiding overheating and underheating. The hypermetabolic response is temperature sensitive but not temperature dependent. Environmental temperatures greater than skin temperature cause the metabolic rate of patients with burns in excess of 40% to increase twice the normal rate. Therefore the environmental temperature in the child's room should be maintained between 28° and 33° C (82.4° to 91.4° F) to minimize metabolic expenditure and maximize comfort (Herndon and others, 1985).

Hypothermia is also a threat, and a means must be provided to prevent heat loss, such as expeditious dressing changes to avoid prolonged exposure and intermittent hypothermia that result in "cold stress." An overhead warming unit may be provided to maintain body heat. Although evaporative heat loss is unchanged, the warmer air reduces the conductive, convective, and radiant heat losses from the denuded areas. Heat is often provided by means of a heat cradle over the child, but, if employed, the heat source should be situated well away from the child's body. Other methods include electric heaters, which should be situated 4 to 5 feet (1.2 to 1.5 m) away to avoid overheating, and maintaining room temperature sufficiently elevated to reduce evaporative loss. This can be extremely uncomfortable for persons attending the child, however.

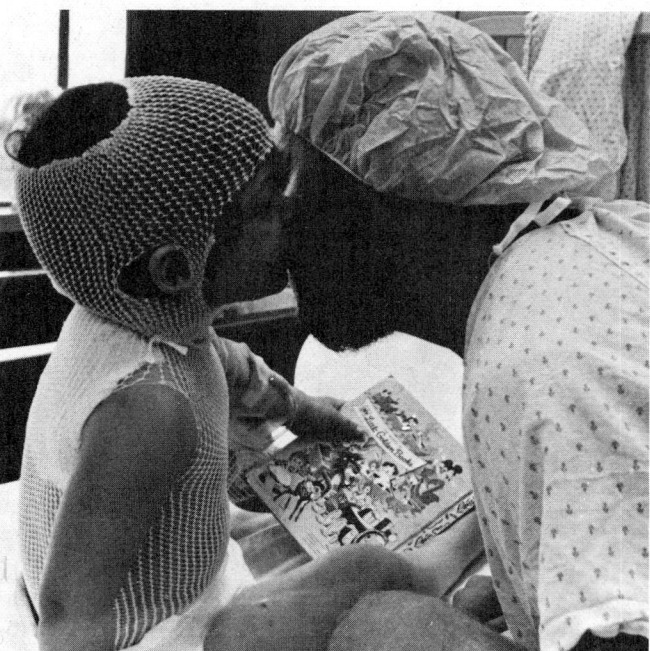

Fig. 29-14. Visitors wear cover gowns and hair coverings while child is in a protected environment.
Photography by Sharon Bornstein, San Jose, CA.

The chief danger in this phase of burn care is infection—wound infection, generalized sepsis, and bacterial pneumonia. All burn patients are treated in a protected environment. Staff and visitors change into "scrub" clothing when entering the burn unit (Fig. 29-14). Children on open units are placed in protective isolation. It is important to make accurate ongoing assessments of all parameters that provide clues for diagnosis. For example, wound cultures are done at least three times weekly, and a blood culture is indicated in any child with a rectal temperature of 39.5° C (103° F) or higher.

Antacids are usually administered prophylactically to prevent or minimize the effect of Curling ulcer, but nurses must be alert for any signs of bleeding.

Continued observations are made to detect any indication of other complications associated with burns and their management. Rashes are not uncommon in children and may be of viral origin or a reaction to medications. They should be evaluated. The nurse must be alert to the possibility of any of the complications described previously—hypertension, renal disorders, and convulsion disorders.

Because children are reluctant to move because doing so causes pain or discomfort, stiffness and joint contracture develop easily. In an effort to prevent this complication, they are encouraged to move whenever feasible and active physiotherapy is included as an essential aspect of burn care. When children are resting or sleeping, contracture is prevented by proper splinting. Children's natural tendency is to be active, and they will usually move spontaneously unless the pain is severe.

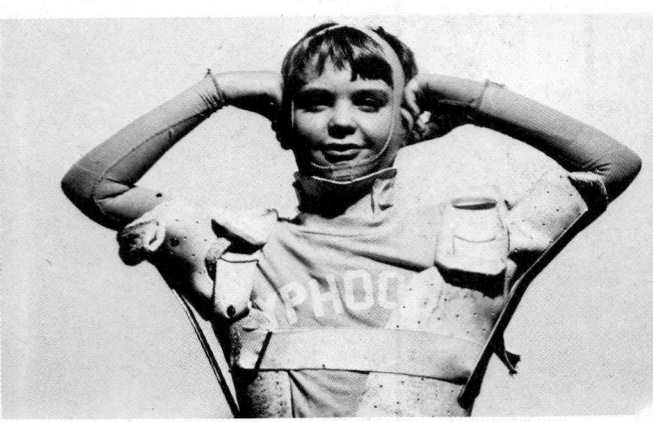

Fig. 29-15. Child in elasticized (Jobst) garment and "airplane" splints.

Rehabilitative Phase

The rehabilitative phase of burn care begins when permanent closure of the wound is implemented. The primary focus of this phase is to obtain functional use of burned areas and cosmetic results as nearly normal as possible. Efforts in the care of children with skin grafts are directed toward facilitating a "take." Trauma, infection, and bleeding must be avoided for a successful transplantation to occur. When the grafted area is left exposed, children must be immobilized to prevent the graft from becoming dislodged. Flat surfaces usually pose few problems, but grafts over irregular or mobile areas may require special techniques such as splints or skeletal traction. Small children usually need to be restrained, and sedation is sometimes needed for very restless or uncooperative children for the first 2 or 3 days after surgery.

The exposed method allows for easier inspection of the grafts, and collection of fluid under the graft can be removed by gently rolling the fluid out with a sterile applicator. This should be attempted with collections of fluid 1.25 cm (½ inch) or less from the edge of the graft. For those farther toward the middle, a tiny slit is made in the graft tissue through which the fluid can be rolled. The less disturbance to any fibrous attachments, the better.

Some plastic surgeons prefer to use occlusive pressure dressings over the grafted tissue or secured with sutures attached to normal surrounding skin and tied over the grafted skin to hold it in place. Wet dressings are occasionally applied over lace grafts and kept moist with antimicrobial agents, silver nitrate, or normal saline solution. Moist dressings are covered with dry absorbent gauze. Plastic wraps are contraindicated because they cause buildup of heat and moisture that may cause maceration of the graft.

Wound contraction and scar tissue formation are normal parts of wound healing. Scar tissue is metabolically active tissue that continually rearranges itself; as a result disabling contractures, deformity, and disfigurement are ever-present possibilities. Physical therapy, splints, and other methods are employed to minimize these long-term effects. Pressure splints and elastic bandages or elasticized (Jobst) garments help reduce scar hypertrophy and are sometimes worn for months after hospitalization (Fig. 29-15). Parents should be advised that these garments are expensive and need to be replaced frequently. It is also advisable to have two garments if the child wears it 24 hours a day, to allow for laundering and care.

Scar tissue has some properties that are significant, particularly for growing children. Scar tissue does not grow as normal tissues, which may create difficulties, especially in areas such as hands. Additional surgery is sometimes needed to maintain function in contracted areas. Because scar tissue has no sweat glands, children with extensive scarring may have difficulty during hot weather or when they develop a fever. Parents need to be informed of this characteristic so that they can be prepared to find alternative cooling methods when indicated.

Severely burned children must return to the hospital periodically for additional skin grafts and scar revisions, especially to release contractures over joint spaces and for cosmetic considerations. Achievement of optimum results frequently requires years. In the meantime, burn scars are unsightly, and although improvements can be made, hope should not be extended to the parents and child for cosmetic and functional repair.

The psychologic pain and sequelae of severe burn trauma are as intense as the physical trauma. Each burned child has a tremendous amount of pain, often continuous for varying periods, and is separated from his family for extended periods. During the painful ordeal of hospitalization, children develop coping mechanisms for dealing with the acute and ever-present pain. Self-induced hypnosis is not uncommon. In addition, a continual barrage of painful therapeutic and diagnostic procedures is inflicted by others. This pain, however, is usually psychologically repressed, as the child attempts to forget these painful incidents.

Life becomes a struggle for the child after burn trauma. He is puzzled, confused, and bombarded by a new way of life in a frightening world of strange people, things, and language. He wonders why this has happened to *him*—what he has done that he should be punished so. Past experiences cannot serve him in this crisis. He does not understand the "ugliness" and disfigurement he sees as his body. He wonders, "Am I going to die?"

Preparation for facing friends and classmates may be more than he is able to cope with; some severely burned children are ashamed to show their bodies in the hospital. In addition, pressure garments and other therapeutic measures greatly intensify the child's feeling of being different. It is not difficult to imagine how the child dreads facing a world of stares or imagined stares. Undressing at school can be a painful experience. It is not surprising that many children withdraw from contacts with others, even at a very early age. In time, as understanding and acceptance increase, they may feel more comfortable with themselves, and the emotional scars may fade somewhat.

The impact of such severe injury taxes the capabilities of

children at all ages, but the young child, who suffers acutely from separation anxiety, and the adolescent, who is developing an identity, are probably most affected psychologically. The toddler cannot begin to comprehend why the parents whom he loves and who have protected him from hurt can leave him in such a dreadful place and allow others to inflict such painful indignities on him. The adolescent, in the process of achieving independence from the family and seeking to find out who he is in the world, finds himself in a dependent position with a damaged body. Being different from others at a time when conformity and being like his peers are so important is difficult to accept. These children need understanding adults to help them deal with the struggles concerning resentment and other feelings generated by such a catastrophe. A psychiatric nurse is often an integral member of the burn team and is invaluable to the total management of the child and his family.

Family Support

Members of the family as well as the child feel the impact of severe burn injury. They are concerned about the child's survival, recovery, and future appearance. Because they, too, have overwhelming anxieties, fears, frustrations, and feelings of guilt, their needs must be met in order that they, in turn, can provide the support and encouragement so desperately needed by the child. It is the family, particularly the parents, who are the most significant persons in the child's life.

As in any emergency situation, all attention is focused on the child, and the parents are forced to abandon their child to others. Often they do not know what is happening, how the child is doing, or if he is even alive. They feel powerless and ineffectual. Nurses can alleviate parents' anxiety simply by acknowledging that they appreciate their concern, explain what is being done, explain why the child is crying, and offer whatever physical comfort is available.

Most parents feel overwhelming guilt about the child's illness. Whether justified or not, they feel responsible for the accident or injury—as if in some way they should have been able to prevent it. These feelings sometimes impede the child's rehabilitation. Parents may indulge the child and give in to his every whim. Some are unable to look at or touch the child as they see him grow edematous, lethargic, and covered with unsightly eschar. Parents need to be told what to expect in the child, concerning both appearance and behavior. The burn wound will look worse before it looks better, and the child may exhibit unpredictable behavior when the parents are present. Ill children often cry when the parents are around, almost certainly when they prepare to leave; at other times they may reject the parents.

Nurses are in the most opportune position to assist parents to cope with the stresses of the child's illness and their own feelings of guilt and helplessness. The parents need to be informed of the child's progress and helped in their efforts to cope with their feelings while providing support to the child. The nurse is the person who can help them understand that it is not selfish to look after themselves and their own needs in order that they can better meet the needs of the child. For parents whose response to the illness is too severe or whose response to stress is manifest in destructive behavior, professional help may be needed.

Prevention of Burn Injury

Nurses have an obligation to be active in educating parents, children, and others in prevention of burn injuries. Children can be taught the hazards of flame and what to do in case of fire. They should be taught respect for matches, lighters, and other items, such as firecrackers and torches, that might cause fires or catch clothing afire. Any heating unit, flame heater, or fire is a potentially lethal device, and children must learn to maintain a safe distance from the heat source. They can learn to be ''fire marshals'' and inspect their homes and neighborhood for fire hazards.

Children can also be taught how to behave in case of fire. Every family should practice fire drills and designate specific responsibilities for the child in getting himself to safety from any location. Special decals are available that can be placed in windows to help firemen identify children's rooms in burning buildings. Older children should know how to report a fire and the location of the nearest fire alarm box. All children should be taught to crawl to safety. Children have a tendency to crawl under beds or into cupboards, where they are difficult to locate. They should also be taught how to behave if their clothing becomes ignited. For example, a child who calmly walked to the kitchen where her mother was working and reported that her nightgown was afire received much less severe burns than a child in a similar situation who ran around in a panic.

Parent education should be aimed at prevention and emergency care for burns. Parents can be taught common-sense safety precautions. Many persons are not aware that simple acts that can prevent tragedy. Small or helpless children should not be left alone in the kitchen or bathroom. The child can turn on a gas range, especially where the knobs are situated at the front of the stove, run hot water, and pull hot items onto himself. It is also characteristic of small children in a bathtub of hot water to remain still or even to squat down rather than to climb out. Crawling infants or toddlers should be kept away from electric cords on which they might chew. Parents should recognize that children's thin skin is sensitive to direct sunlight and limit the time the child is exposed to the sun. Preventive measures regarding burns are discussed in Chapters 12 and 14. A handy resource for parents, the Fire Safety Book,* outlines activities for presenting safety messages appropriate for preschoolers.

Instruction in emergency first-aid measures should be part of parent education. Most lay persons still treat burns with application of butter or petroleum jelly. They need to be aware that current treatment is cooling the area with cool water. It is important that they have some criteria for deter-

---

*Available for $2.00 from The Children's Television Workshop, Community Education Service Division, Dept. FS, One Lincoln Plaza, New York, NY 10023

mining when the injury can be treated with a simple dressing and when to seek medical aid.

Public education through community groups, the communication media, and offices, clinics, and homes is part of nurses' responsibility in preventive care. Information regarding safety devices for the home, such as sprinkling systems, smoke detectors, and fire extinguishers, can be disseminated to a large audience. Nurses can be effective campaigners for safety legislation, such as fireproofing children's clothing and for improvement of substandard hous-ing. As health professionals, their voices can and should be heard. Additional information on burn care and prevention can be obtained from the **Institute for Fire and Burn Education,** * the **American Burn Association,** † and the **National Safety Council.** ‡

*1377 K Street, N.W., Suite 667, Washington, DC 20005.
†New York-Cornell Medical Center, 525 E. 68th St., Rm. F758, New York, NY 10021.
‡444 North Michigan Ave., Chicago, IL 60611.

Nursing Care Summary: The Child with Burns

MANAGEMENT AND REHABILITATIVE PHASES OF BURN CARE

NURSING GOALS	NURSING INTERVENTIONS	EXPECTED PATIENT/FAMILY OUTCOMES
HP-HMP Injury: potential for hypothermia, bleeding, and CNS complications **Risk factors: presence of infective organisms, depleted body defenses**		
Prevent evaporative heat loss	Maintain critical environmental temperature at wound and air interface Prevent drafts	Child's temperature remains within acceptable limits (28-30° C)
HP-HMP Infection, potential for **Risk factors: denuded skin, presence of pathogenic organisms**		
Recognize signs of complications	Assess for abdominal discomfort Check for recurrent or intermittent bleeding from GI tract Observe for seizures, alterations in sensorium, behavioral changes	*Deviations from baseline findings are detected early and appropriate interventions initiated
Recognize signs of infection	Take vital signs (temperature, pulse, respirations, blood pressure) as ordered Record intake and output Observe for signs of septicemia Observe for signs of pneumonia Check blood pressure regularly Observe amount, color, specific gravity, and reaction of urine daily or as ordered Carefully cleanse and observe for signs of infection	
N-MP Nutrition, alteration in: less than body requirements **Etiology: increased catabolism, loss of appetite**		
Maintain adequate nutrition and prevent nitrogen loss	Provide high-calorie, high-protein meals and snacks	Child maintains a positive nitrogen balance—no weight loss
Stimulate appetite	Encourage oral feeding Provide foods child likes Allow self-help Provide meals when child is most likely to eat well Provide attractive meals and surroundings Provide companionship at meals Employ "contract" with older children	Child consumes a sufficient amount of nutrients (specify) Child interacts with other children

Nursing Care Summary: The Child with Burns—cont'd

MANAGEMENT AND REHABILITATIVE PHASES OF BURN CARE

NURSING GOALS	NURSING INTERVENTIONS	EXPECTED PATIENT/FAMILY OUTCOMES
N-MP **Skin integrity, impairment of: actual** **Etiology: thermal injury**		
Facilitate wound healing	Keep child from scratching and picking at wound Provide distraction Older child: explain reasons Young child: apply restraining devices as needed Maintain care in handling wound to avoid damaging epithelializing and granulating tissues Offer high-calorie, high-protein meals and snacks Prevent infection	Wound heals without evidence of damage or inflammation
Control bacterial growth on wound	Maintain clean environment Maintain careful handwashing Wear sterile gown, mask, and gloves when handling burn wound Carefully cleanse wound and remove devitalized tissue and eschar Administer good oral hygiene Avoid injury to crusts and eschar Avoid contact with infected persons Assess wound for signs of invasive infection, including redness, purulent drainage, unpleasant odor	Wound displays minimum or no evidence of infection
Protect graft area	Position for minimum disturbance of graft site Restrain if necessary	Skin graft remains intact
N-MP **Skin integrity, impairment of: potential** **Risk factors: immobility**		
Prevent pressure necrosis	Turn frequently Stimulate circulation	Skin has no evidence of pressure or irritation
EP **Bowel elimination, alteration in: constipation** **Etiology: less than adequate intake, immobility**		
Stimulate elimination	Record bowel movements Administer enema or remove impacted feces as needed Encourage foods that stimulate bowel function Encourage ample fluid intake	Child has regular bowel movements
A-EP **Mobility, impaired physical (specify level)** **Etiology: pain, impaired joint movement**		
Promote optimum functioning (physical)	Carry out range of motion exercises Encourage mobility if child is unable to move extremities Ambulate as soon as feasible Splint involved joints at night and rest periods Encourage and promote self-help activities	Joints remain flexible with maximum functional capacity

*Nursing outcome.

Continued.

Nursing Care Summary: The Child with Burns—cont'd

MANAGEMENT AND REHABILITATIVE PHASES OF BURN CARE

NURSING GOALS	NURSING INTERVENTIONS	EXPECTED PATIENT/FAMILY OUTCOMES
Minimize scar formation	Position in functional attitude for minimum deformity and optimum function Apply splints as ordered and designed Wrap healing tissue with elastic bandage or dress in elastic garments as ordered Carry out physical therapy	Wound heals with minimum scar formation; joints remain flexible and functional

𝒩𝒟 | **A-EP** Self-care deficit: feeding, bathing/hygiene, dressing/grooming, toileting (specify level)
Etiology: variable disability, immobility

Promote self-care	Assist with self-care activities as needed Encourage self-care according to capabilities	Child assists with care as able

𝒩𝒟 | **CPP** Comfort, alteration in: pain
Etiology: burn wound, donor graft site

Relieve pain	Assess need for pain medication (see p. 1068) Implement appropriate nonpharmacologic pain reduction techniques	Child exhibits only minimum evidence of pain

𝒩𝒟 | **SP-SCP** Self-concept, disturbance in: body image
Etiology: perception of appearance and mobility

Meet emotional needs	Convey positive attitude toward child Encourage parents to visit Encourage as much independence as condition allows Arrange for continued schooling Promote peer contact where possible	Child accepts efforts of family and caregivers Child engages in activities with others according to age and capabilities

Help build self-esteem and a positive self-image	Explore feelings concerning physical appearance
	Discuss feelings about returning to home and family, school, and friends
	Provide reinforcement of positive aspects of appearance and capabilities
	Point out evidence of healing
	Discuss aids that camouflage disfigurement
	   Wigs
	   Clothing, for example, turtleneck sweaters
	   Makeup
	Provide recreational and diversional activities
	Promote constructive thinking in child
		Child discusses feelings and concerns regarding appearance and perceived reactions of others
		Child verbalizes positive suggestions for adjusting to appearance

Prepare child for discharge	Begin early in hospitalization to discuss "going home" Accept regressive behavior where appropriate Help child develop independence and self-help capabilities	Child verbalizes and otherwise demonstrates interest in going home Child engages in self-help activities

𝒩𝒟 | **RRP** Family process, alteration in
Etiology: situational crisis (child with a severe injury)

Prepare family for discharge	Teach wound care to caregiver Discuss diet, rest, and activity Explore attitudes toward child's reentry into the family Explore family's concept regarding child's capabilities and the possible restrictions and freedom they will allow	Family demonstrates an understanding of the needs of the child and the impact his condition will have on them Family sets realistic goals for selves, child, and others

Nursing Care Summary: The Child with Burns—cont'd

MANAGEMENT AND REHABILITATIVE PHASES OF BURN CARE

NURSING GOALS	NURSING INTERVENTIONS	EXPECTED PATIENT/FAMILY OUTCOMES
	Help family set realistic goals for themselves, child, and other family members	
	Help family acquire needed equipment and supplies	
Participate in follow-up care	Coordinate team management of child and family	Family maintains contact with health providers
	Arrange for return visits	
	Assess needs of family	
	Arrange for referral to agencies based on need assessment	
	Collaborate with school nurse to help with child's reintegration into school and the world of peers	Child attends school regularly and interacts with age-mates
	Visit school to prepare teacher and peers, if possible	
	See also The child in the hopital, p. 1075; Family of the hospitalized child, p.1087	

Nursing Interventions Related to Medical Management

Facilitate wound healing
Administer supplementary vitamins and minerals—vitamins A, B, and C and zinc sulfate
Apply prescribed topical antimicrobial preparation and dressings (if ordered) to wound
Obtain wound cultures three times per week to ascertain any increase in wound flora
Relieve pain
Administer analgesics as needed
Monitor effectiveness of analgesics using a pain assessment record

Prevent constipation
Administer stool softeners as needed
Prevent and/or treat complications
Obtain blood culture of child with temperature of 39.5° C (103° F) or over
Administer antacids as ordered
Determine hematocrit
Send urine specimens for laboratory examination periodically

CONCEPT SUMMARIES

- Acute gastrointestinal disorders of childhood that cause fluid depletion are diarrhea, acute infectious gastroenteritis, and vomiting.

- Mechanisms known to produce diarrhea are osmotic factors, diminished absorption or increased secretion of water and electrolytes, reduction in anatomic or functional surface area, and altered bowel motility.

- Acute infectious gastroenteritis is caused by enterotoxin production, invasion and destruction of epithelial cells, penetration and system invasion, or adherence without destruction of mucosa and without enterotoxin production.

- Vomiting may result from infectious disorders, responses to an allergen or ingestion of drugs or other toxic substances, symptoms associated with appendicitis or gastrointestinal obstruction, motion sickness, environmental stress, and oral-defense mechanisms.

- Nurses should observe character, frequency, amount, and force of vomitus.

- Hypertrophic pyloric stenosis is relieved by pyloromyotomy. Nursing care is aimed at feeding regulation and sensory stimulation.

- Shock is divided into three stages: compensated, uncompensated, and irreversible.

  Types of shock are hypovolemic, including hemorrhagic, plasma loss, and extracellular fluid loss; distributive, including anaphylactic, septic, and neurogenic; and cardiogenic, resulting from congenital heart disease, inflow or outflow obstruction, primary pulmonary failure, and dysrhythmias.

  Persons at risk for of anaphylaxis may be identified by a history of previous allergic reaction, history of atopy, history of severe reactions in family, and positive skin test to the allergen.

- Nursing management of the patient with toxic shock syndrome focuses on prevention and education.

- Burns are caused by thermal, chemical, electric, or radioactive agents.

- Burns are assessed on the basis of percentage of body surface burned, depth, location, age, etiologic agent, respiratory involvement, general health, and presence of associated injury or condition.

- Emergency measures for severe burns include stopping the burning process covering the burn, transporting the child to medical aid, and providing reassurance to child and family.

- Management of minor burns is facilitating wound healing, relieving discomfort, and preventing complications.

- Management of major burns is facilitating wound healing, relieving discomfort, replacing destroyed skin, preventing and/or treating complications, and providing rehabilitation.

REFERENCES

Artz, C.P., Moncrief, J.A., and Breitt, B.A.: Burns—a team approach, Philadelphia, 1979, W.B. Saunders Co.

Bailit, I.W.: Anaphylaxis. In Gellis, S.S., and Kagan, B.M., editors: Current pediatric therapy 12, Philadelphia, 1986, W.B. Saunders Co.

Baker, S.P., O'Neill, B., and Karpf, R.: The injury fact book, Lexington, 1984, Lexington Books.

Barbour, S.D., Shlaes, D.M., and Guertin, S.R.: Toxic-shock syndrome associated with nasal packing: analogy to tampon-associated illness, Pediatrics 73:163-165, 1984.

Barness, L.A.: Fluid and electrolyte therapy. In Gellis, S.S., and Kagan, B.M., editors: Current pediatric therapy 12, Philadelphia, 1986, W.B. Saunders Co.

Bass, D.M., and Walker, W.A.: Acute and chronic nonspecific diarrhea syndromes. In Gellis, S.S., and Kagan, B.M., editors: Current pediatric therapy 12, Philadelphia, 1986, W.B. Saunders Co.

Brown, K.H., and MacLean, W.C., Jr.: Nutritional management of acute diarrhea: an appraisal of the alternatives, Pediatrics 73:119-125, 1984.

Buchdahl, R., and others: Toxic shock syndrome, Arch. Dis. Child. 60:563-567, 1985.

Burke, J.F., and others: Successful use of a physiologically acceptable artificial skin in the treatment of extensive burn injury, Ann. Surg. 194:413-428, 1981.

Centers for Disease Control: Follow-up on toxic-shock syndrome, Morbid. Mortal. Weekly Rep. 29:441-445, 1980.

Cohen, F.L.: Clinical genetics in nursing practice, Philadelphia, 1984, J.B. Lippincott Co.

Committee on Nutrition: Use of oral fluid therapy and posttreatment feeding following enteritis in children in a developed country, Pediatrics 75:358-361, 1985.

Crone, R.K.: Acute circulatory failure in children, Pediatr. Clin. North Am. 27:525-538, 1980.

Dart, R., and Levitt, A.: Toxic shock syndrome associated with the use of the vaginal contraceptive sponge, JAMA 253:1877, 1985.

Davidson, G.P., Robb, T.A., and Kirubakaran, C.P.: Bacterial contamination of the small intestine as an important cause of chronic diarrhea and abdominal pain: diagnosis by breath hydrogen test, Pediatrics 74:229-235, 1984.

DeWitt, T.G., Humphrey, K.F., and McCarthy, P.: Clinical predictors of acute bacterial diarrhea in young children, Pediatrics 76:551-556, 1985.

Dodge, J.A., and others: Toddler diarrhea and prostaglandins, Arch. Dis. Child. 56:705-707, 1981.

Dupont, H., and others: Prevention of traveler's diarrhea (emporiatic enteritis): prophylactic administration of subsalicylate bismuth, JAMA 243:237-241, 1980.

Dupont, H., and others: Prevention of traveler's diarrhea with trimethoprim-sulfamethoxazole and trimethoprim alone, Gastroenterology 84:75-80, 1983.

Dyer, C.: Burn care in the emergent period, J. Emerg. Nurs. 6:9-16, 1980.

Edelman, R., and Levine, M.M.: Acute diarrheal infections in infants. II. Bacterial and viral causes, Hosp. Pract. 15:97-101, 1980.

Faich, G., and others: Toxic shock syndrome in the vaginal contraceptive sponge, JAMA 255:216-218, 1986.

Fleisher, D.R.: Nausea and vomiting. In Gellis, S.S., and Kagan, B.M., editors: Current pediatric therapy 12, Philadelphia, 1986, W.B. Saunders Co.

Food and Drug Administration: Topical PEG in burn ointments, FDA Drug Bull. 12(3):25-26, 1982.

Freeman, L., and others: Brief prophylaxis with doxycycline for the prevention of traveler's diarrhea, Gastroenterology 84:276-280, 1983.

Gallico, G.G., and others: Permanent coverage of large burn wounds with autologous-cultured human epithelium, N. Engl. J. Med. 311:448-451, 1984.

Graham, D.Y., and others: Double-bind comparison of bismuth subsalicylate and placebo in the prevention and treatment of enterotoxigenic *Escherichia coli*–induced diarrhea in volunteers, Gastroenterology 85:1017-1022, 1983.

Gray, D.T., and others: Early surgical excision versus conventional therapy in patients with 20 to 40 percent burns, Am. J. Surg. 144:76-80, 1982.

Green, H., Kelrinde, O., and Thomas, J.: Growth of cultured epidermal cells into multiple epithelia suitable for grafting, Proc. Natl. Acad. Sci. U.S.A. 76:5665-5668, 1979.

Greene, H.L., and Ghishan, F.K.: Excessive fluid intake as a cause of chronic diarrhea in young children, J. Pediatr. 102:836-840, 1983.

Groothuis, J.R., Berman, S., and Chapman, J.: Effect of carbohydrate ingested on outcome in infants with mild gastroenteritis, J. Pediatr. 108:903-906, 1986.

Guerrant, R.L., Lohr, J.A., and Williams, E.K.: Acute infectious diarrhea. I. Epidemiology, etiology and pathogenesis, Pediatr. Infect. Dis. 5:353-359, 1986.

Harmel, R.P., Vane, D.W., and King, D.R.: Burn care in children: special considerations, Clin. Plastic Surg. 13:95-105, 1986.

Herndon, D.N., and others: Treatment of burns in children, Pediatr. Clin. North Am. 32:1311-1332, 1985.

Herrin, J.T., and Crawford, J.D.: The seriously burned child. In Smith, C.A., editor: The critically ill child, ed. 2, Philadelphia, 1977, W.B. Saunders Co.

Hull, H.F., and others: Toxic shock syndrome related to nasal packing, Arch. Otolaryngol. 109:624-626, 1983.

Hyams, J.S., and Leichtner, A.M.: Apple juice: an unappreciated cause of chronic diarrhea, Am. J. Dis. Child. 139:503-505, 1985.

Jacoby, F.: Care of the massive burn wound, Crit. Care Q. 7(3):44-53, 1984.

Kavanagh, C.K., and Freeman, R.: Burn care and the pediatric patient: a preliminary report, PRN Forum, 3(2):1-3, 1984.

Kibbee, E.: Burn pain management, Crit. Care Q. 7(3): 54-62, 1984.

Lamb, L.S.: Think you know septic shock? Nursing 82 12(1):34-43, 1982.

LaMotte, R., and Thalhammer, J.: Peripheral neural mechanisms of cutaneous hyperalgesia following mild injury by heat, Neuroscience 2:765-781, 1982.

Libber, S.M, and Slayton, D.J.: Childhood burns reconsidered: the child, the family, and the burn injury, J. Trauma 24:245-252, 1984.

McLoughlin, E., and Crawford, J.D.: Burns, Pediatr. Clin. North Am. 32:61-75, 1985.

Morriss, F.C.: Anaphylaxis. In Levin, D.L., Morriss, F.C., and Moore, G.C., editors: A practical guide to pediatric intensive care, ed. 2, St. Louis, 1984, The C.V. Mosby Co.

Murphy, S.A.: Learned helplessness: from concept to comprehension, Perspect. Psychiatr. Care **20**(2):27-32, 1982.

O'Conner, N.E., and others: Grafting of burns with cultured epithelium prepared from autologous epidermal cells, Lancet **1**:75-78, 1982.

Perkin, R.M., and Levin, D.L.: Shock in the pediatric patient. Part I, J. Pediatr. **101**:163-169, 1982a.

Perkin, R.M., and Levin, D.L.: Shock in the pediatric patient. Part II. Therapy, J. Pediatr. **101**:319-323, 1982b.

Perry, S., and Intrisi, C.: Analgesia and morphine disposition in burn patients, J. Burn Care Rehab. **4**:276-279, 1983.

Pizarro, D., Posada, G., and Levine, M.M.: Hypernatremic diarrheal dehydration treated with ''slow'' (12-hour) oral rehydration therapy: a preliminary report, J. Pediatr. **104**:316-319, 1984.

Reed, M.: Vaccine against traveller's diarrhea nearing readiness for clinical trials, JAMA **247**:24, 1982.

Robson, A.M.: Parenteral fluid therapy. In Behrman, R.E., and Vaughan, V.C., III, editors: Textbook of pediatrics, ed. 12, Philadelphia, 1983, W.B. Saunders Co.

Santosham, M., and others: Role of soy-based, lactose-free formula during treatment of acute diarrhea, Pediatrics **76**:292-298, 1985.

Silverman, A., and Roy, C.C.: Pediatric clinical gastroenterology, ed 3, St. Louis, 1983, The C.V. Mosby Co.

Surh, L., and Read, S.E.: Staphylococcal tracheitis and toxic shock syndrome in a young child, J. Pediatr. **105**:585-587, 1984.

Vesikari, T., and others: Protection of infants against rotavirus diarrhoea by RIT 4237 attenuated bovine rotovirus strain bacteria, Lancet **1**:977-981, 1984.

Wiesenthal, A.M., and Todd, J.K.: Toxic shock syndrome in children aged 10 years or less, Pediatrics **74**:112-117, 1984.

Zawacki, B.: Reversal of capillary stasis and prevention of necrosis in burns, Ann. Surg. **180**:93-102, 1974.

Zimmerman, S.S.: Anaphylaxis. In Zimmerman, S.S., and Gildea, J.H.: Critical care pediatrics, Philadelphia, 1985, W.B. Saunders Co.

BIBLIOGRAPHY

General

Barkin, R.M., and Rosen, P., editors: Emergency pediatrics, St. Louis, 1984, The C.V. Mosby Co.

Behrman, R.E., and Vaughan, V.C.,III, editors: Textbook of pediatrics, ed. 12, Philadelphia, 1983, W.B. Saunders Co.

Book, L.S.: Vomiting and diarrhea, Pediatrics **74**:(suppl.)950-954, 1984.

Dickerman, J.D, and Lucey, J.F.: The critically ill child: diagnosis and medical management, ed. 3, Philadelphia, 1985, W.B. Saunders Co.

Gellis, S.S., and Kagan, B.M., editors: Current pediatric therapy 12, Philadelphia, 1986, W.B. Saunders Co.

Guyton, A.C.: Textbook of medical physiology, ed. 6, Philadelphia, 1981, W.B. Saunders Co.

Kempe, C.H., Silver, H.K., and O'Brien, D.: Current pediatric diagnosis and treatment, ed. 9, Los Altos, Calif., 1986, Lange Medical Publications.

Khamapirad, T., and Athey, P.A.: Ultrasound diagnosis of hypertrophic pyloric stenosis, J. Pediatr. **102**:23-26, 1983.

Krugman, S., and others: Infectious diseases of children, ed. 8, St. Louis, 1985, The C.V. Mosby Co.

Levin, D.L., Morriss, F.C., and Moore, G.C., editors: A practical guide to pediatric intensive care, ed. 2, St. Louis, 1984, The C.V. Mosby Co.

Oakes, A.R., editor: Critical care nursing of children and adolescents, Philadelphia, 1981, W.B. Saunders Co.

Smith, J.B., editor: Pediatric critical care, New York, 1983, John Wiley & Sons.

Vestal, K.W., editor: Pediatric critical care nursing, New York, 1981, John Wiley & Sons.

Zimmerman, S.S., and Gildea, J.H.: Critical care pediatrics, Philadelphia, 1985, W.B. Saunders Co.

Diarrhea

Boyne, L.J., Kerzner, B., and McClung, H.J.: Chronic nonspecific diarrhea: the value of a preliminary observation period to assess diet therapy, Pediatrics **76**:557-561, 1985.

Copeland, L.: Chronic diarrhea in infancy, Am. J. Nurs. **77**:461-463, 1977.

Davidson, M., and Silverberg, M.: Acute and chronic diarrhea. In Shirkey, H.C., editor: Pediatric therapy, ed. 6, St. Louis, 1980, The C.V. Mosby Co.

DeBenham, J.J., and others: Initial assessment and management of chronic diarrhea in toddlers, Pediatr. Nurs. **11**:(4)281-285, 1985.

Fitzgerald, J.F.: Management of the infant with persistent diarrhea, Pediatr. Infect. Dis. **4**:6-9, 1985.

Fitzgerald, J.F., and Clark, J.H.: Chronic diarrhea, Pediatr. Clin. North Am. **29**:221-231, 1982.

Hamilton, J.R.: Treatment of acute diarrhea, Pediatr. Clin. North Am. **32**:419-427, 1985.

Hughes, J.G.: Synopsis of pediatrics, ed. 5, St. Louis, 1979, The C.V. Mosby Co.

Jonas, A., and others: Disturbed fat absorption following infectious gastroenteritis in children, J. Pediatr. **95**:366-372, 1979.

Lifschitz, C.H., and others: Carbohydrate malabsorption in infants with diarrhea studied with the breath hydrogen test, J. Pediatrics **102**:371-375, 1983.

Linshaw, M.A., and others: Hypochloremic alkalosis in infants associated with soy protein formula, J. Pediatr. **96**:635-640, 1980.

Lo, C.W., and Walker, W.A.: Chronic protracted diarrhea of infancy: a nutritional disease, Pediatrics **72**:786-800, 1983.

Morgan, S.R., and Parks, B.: What is the role of oral electrolyte solution in diarrheal dehydration in children? Pediatr. Nurs. **11**(3):215, 227, 1985.

Pickering, L.K.: Antimicrobial therapy of gastrointestinal infections, Pediatr. Clin. North Am. **30**:373-388, 1983.

Pickering, L.K., and others: Diarrhea caused by *Shigella*, rotavirus, and *Giardia* in day-care centers: prospective study, J. Pediatr. **99**:51-56, 1981.

Pizarro, D., and others: Oral rehydration in hypernatremic and hyponatremic diarrheal dehydration: treatment with oral glucose/electrolyte solution, Am. J. Dis. Child. **137**:730-734, 1983.

Santosham, M., and others: Oral rehydration therapy for acute diarrhea in ambulatory children in the United States: a double-blind comparison of four different solutions, Pediatrics **76**:159-166, 1985.

Sharifi, J., and Ghavami, F.: Oral rehydration therapy of severe diarrheal dehydration, Clin. Pediatr. **23**:87-90, 1984.

Wehrle, P.F., and Top, F.H., editors: Communicable and infectious diseases, ed. 9, St. Louis, 1981, The C.V. Mosby Co.

Infectious Gastroenteritis

Bartlett, A.V., and others: Diarrheal illness among infants and toddlers in day care centers. I. Epidemiology and pathogens, J. Pediatr. **107**:495-502, 1985.

Bartlett, A.V., and others: Diarrheal illness among infants and toddlers in day care centers. II. Comparison with day care homes and households, J. Pediatr. **107**:503-509, 1985.

Donta, S.T., and Myers, M.G.: *Clostridium difficile* toxin in asymptomatic neonates, J. Pediatr. **100**:431-434, 1982.

Goodman, R.A., and others: Infectious diseases and child day care, Pediatrics **74**:134-139, 1984.

Hamm, P., and Jemison-Smith, P.: *Salmonella*, Crit. Care Update **9**:41-44, 1982.

Hyams, J.S., and others: *Salmonella* bacteremia in the first year of life, J. Pediatr. **96**:57-59, 1980.

Hyams, J.S., Krause, P.J., and Gleason, P.A.: Lactose malabsorption following rotavirus infection in young children, J. Pediatr. **99:**916-918, 1981.

Keswick, B.H., and others: Prevalence of rotavirus in children in day care centers, J. Pediatr. **103:**85-86, 1983.

Kim, K., DuPont, H.L., and Pickering, L.K.: Outbreaks of diarrhea associated with *Clostridium difficile* and its toxin in day-care centers: evidence of person-to-person spread, J. Pediatr. **102:**376-382, 1983.

Pickering, L.K., and Woodward, W.E.: Diarrhea in day care centers, Pediatr. Infect. Dis. **1:**47-52, 1982.

Radetsky, M.: Laboratory evaluation of acute diarrhea, Pediatr. Infect. Dis. **5:**230-238, 1986.

Raucher, H.S., and others: Treatment of *Salmonella* gastroenteritis in infants: the significance of bacteremia, Clin. Pediatr. **22:**601-604, 1983.

Riesenberg, D.E.: How to protect day-care center children from infectious disease? JAMA **255:**1245-1251, 1986.

Steinhoff, M.C.: Rotavirus: the first five years, J. Pediatr. **96:**611-622, 1980.

Thompson, C.M., Jr., and others: *Clostridium difficile* in a pediatric population, Am. J. Dis. Child. **137:**271-274, 1983.

Zedd, A.J., and others: Nosocomial *Clostridium difficile* reservoir in a neonatal intensive care unit, Pediatr. Infect. Dis. **3:**429-432, 1984.

Hypertrophic Pyloric Stenosis

Martin, L.W.: Pediatric surgery—general. In Shirkey, H.C., editor: Pediatric therapy, ed. 6, St. Louis, 1980, The C.V. Mosby Co.

Silverberg, M., and Davidson, M.: Vomiting. In Shirkey, H.C., editor: Pediatric therapy, ed. 7, St. Louis, 1980, The C.V. Mosby Co.

Shock

Barrows, J.J.: Shock demands drugs—but which one's best for your patient? Nursing 82 **12**(2):34-41, 1982.

Cohen, M.R.: Action stat! Drug-induced anaphylaxis, Nursing 85 **15**(2):43, 1985.

Corse, K.M., and Lambert, L.E.: Multisystem disorders: shock and trauma. In Smith, J.B., editor: Pediatric critical care, New York, 1983, John Wiley & Sons.

Ellner, J.J.: Septic shock, Pediatr. Clin. North Am. **30:**365-371, 1983.

Hackleman, N.: The unwritten rules that saved Katie, RN **47**(1):52-53, 1984.

Hochman, H.I., Grodin, M.A., and Crone, R.K.: Dehydration, diabetic acidosis, and shock in the pediatric patient, Pediatr. Clin. North Am. **26:**803-826, 1979.

Holt, M., McKenny, S., and Pribyl, C.: Shock—detecting it soon enough to save your patient: seven fast refreshers. Part I, Nurs. Life **4**(6):33-40, 1984.

Holt, M., McKenny, S., and Pribyl, C.: Shock—detecting it soon enough to save your patient: nine more fast refreshers. Part II, Nurs. Life **5**(1):33-40, 1985.

Kaplan, S.L., and Vargo, T.A.: Endotoxin shock in children. In Dickerman, J.D., and Lucey, J.F., editors: The critically ill child: diagnosis and medical management, ed. 3, Philadelphia, 1985, W.B. Saunders Co.

Keely, B.R.: Septic shock, Crit. Care Q. **7**(4):59-67, 1985.

Lamb, L.S.: You think you know septic shock, Nursing 82 **12**(1):34-43, 1982.

McConnell, E.A.: Septic shock: recognizing it can be the hardest part of dealing with it, Nurs. Life **3**(5):33-40, 1983.

Morse, T.S.: Shock in infants and children. In Pierog, J.E., and Pierog, L.J., editors: Pediatric critical illness and injury, Rockville, MD, 1984, Aspen Systems Corporation.

Perry, A.G., and Potter, P.A., editors: Shock: comprehensive nursing management, St. Louis, 1983, The C.V. Mosby Co.

Purcell, J.A.: Shock drugs: standardized guidelines, Am. J. Nurs. **82:**965-974, 1982.

Randall, B.J.: Reacting to anaphylaxis, Nursing 85 **16**(3):34-40, 1986.

Rice, V.: Shock management. Part I. Fluid volume replacement, Crit. Care Nurse **4**(6):69-82, 1984.

Rice, V.: Shock management. Part II. Pharmacologic, intervention, Crit. Care Nurse **5**(1):42-46, 48-49, 51-57, 1985.

Yabek, S.M.: Management of septic shock, Pediatr. Rev. **2:**83-87, 1980.

Toxic Shock Syndrome

Brown, B.S.: Tampons, teen-agers, and toxic shock (editorial), Pediatr. Nurs. **7**(3):7, 1981.

Brown, L.K.: Toxic shock syndrome, Am. J. Maternal Child Nurs. **6:**57-60, 1981.

Stein, A.P., and Baughman, D.C.: Nursing implications of toxic shock syndrome, Crit. Care Update **8**(6):17-19, 1981.

Todd, J., and others: Toxic shock syndrome associated with phage-group-1 staphylococci, Lancet **2:**1116-1118, 1978.

Toxic shock syndrome: an update, Crit. Care Update **8**(2):33-35, 1981.

Toxic shock syndrome: an update on symptoms and treatment, Nursing 85 **15**(9):74, 1985.

Weinberg, H.D.: Toxic shock in the teenage patient, Am. J. Dis. Child. **135:**244-245, 1981.

Whettam, J.: Update on toxic shock: how to spot it and treat it, RN **47**(2):55-56, 58, 60, 1984.

Wroblewski, S.S.: Toxic shock syndrome, Am. J. Nurs. **81:**82-85, 1981.

Burns

Acres, C., and Kraft, E.R.: Skin transplantation, Am. J. Nurs. **81:**1466-1467, 1981.

Arneson, S.W., and Triplett, J.L.: How children cope with disfiguring changes in their appearance. In Fore, C., and Poster, E.C., editors: Meeting psychosocial needs of children and families in health care, Washington, DC, 1985, Association for the Care of Children's Health.

Berger, L.R., and Kalishman, S.: Floor furnace burns to children, Pediatrics **71:**97-99, 1983.

Bingham, H.: Electrical burns, Clin. Plastic Surg. **13:**75-85, 1986.

Brown, A.S., and Barot, L.R.: Biologic dressings and skin substitutes, Clin. Plastic Surg. **13:**69-74, 1986.

Cameron, C.O., Juszczak, L., and Wallace, N.: Using creative arts to help children cope with altered body image, Child. Health Care **12:**108-112, 1984.

Charnock, E.L., and Meehan, J.J.: Postburn respiratory injuries in children, Pediatr. Clin. North Am. **27:**661-676, 1980.

Clark, A.M.: Thermal injuries: the care of the whole child, J. Trauma **20:**823-829, 1980.

Conrad, F.L.: Tips for treating corrosive burns, Nursing 83 **13**(2):55-57, 1983.

Dittemore, I.L.: Behavioral responses in the early recovery of a severely burned 4-year-old child, Am. J. Maternal Child Nurs. **12**(1):21-34, 1983.

Finlayson, L.: Emergent care of the burn patient, Crit. Care Update **7**(10):18-23, 1980.

Fonger, L.: Emergency! First aid for burns, Nursing 82 **12**(9):70-77, 1982.

Gaston, S.F., and Schumann, L.L.: Burn wound management, Crit. Care Update **7**(10):5-17, 1980.

Gordon, E.F., Gordon, R.C., and Passal, D.B.: Zinc metabolism: basic, clinical, and behavioral aspects, J. Pediatr. **99:**341-349, 1981.

Grossman, E.R.: Floor furnace burns (letter), Pediatrics **73:**568-569, 1984.

Harris, J.R., Kobayashi, J.M., and Frost, F.: Injuries from fireworks, JAMA **249:**2460, 1983.

Hemenway, B.: Major thermal injury: initial assessment and treatment, Emerg. Nurs. **1**(20):1-8, 1981.

Hight, D.W., Bakalar, H.R., and Lloyd, J.R.: Inflicted burns in children, JAMA **242:**517-520, 1979.

Hobel, M.: Plasma expanders, Crit. Care Update **8**(3):14-20, 1981.

Hurt, R.A.: More than skin deep: guidelines on caring for the burn patient, Nursing 85 **15**(6):52-57, 1985.

Katcher, M.L.: Scald burns from hot tap water, JAMA **246:**1219-1222, 1981.

Kavanagh, C.: Psychological intervention with the severly burned child: report of an experimental comparison of two approaches and their effects on psychological sequelae, J. Am. Acad. Child Psychiatry **22:**145-156, 1983.

Kenner, C., and Manning, S.: Emergency care of the burn patient, Crit. Care Update **7**(10):24-33, 1980.

Knudson-Cooper, M.S.: Adjustment to visible stigma: the case of the severly burned, Soc. Sci. Med. **15B:**31-44, 1981.

Langley, J.: Description and classification of childhood burns, Burns **10:**231, 1984.

Lushbaugh, M.A.: Critical care of the child with burns, Nurs. Clin. North Am. **16:**635-646, 1981.

Luterman, A., Adams, M., and Curreri, P.W.: Nutritional management of the burn patient, Crit. Care Q. **7**(3):34-43, 1984.

Marvin, J.A.: Planning home care for burn patients, Nursing 83 **13**(8):65-67, 1983.

Marvin, J.A., and Einfeldt, L.E.: Infection control for the burn patient, Nurs. Clin. North Am. **15:**833-842, 1980.

McHugh, M.L., Dimitroff, K., and Davis, N.D.: Family support group in a burn unit, Am. J. Nurs. **79:**2148-2150, 1979.

McLoughlin, E., and others: Project burn prevention: outcome and implications, Am. J. Public Health **72:**241-247, 1982.

Miller, R.E., and others: Pediatric counseling and subsequent use of smoke detectors, Am. J. Public Health **72:**329-393, 1982.

Moylan, J.A.: Outpatient treatment of burns, Postgrad. Med. **73**(3):2135-242, 1983.

Puczynski, M., Rademaker, D., and Gatson, R.L.: Burn injury related to the improper use of a microwave oven, Pediatrics **72:**714-715, 1983.

Rausch, T.: Minor thermal injury: initial assessment and treatment, Emerg. Nurs. **1**(19):1-8, 1980.

Robertson, K.E., Cross, P.J., and Terry, J.C.: Burn care: the crucial first days, Am. J. Nurs. **85:**30-50, 1985.

Solomon, J.R.: Care and needs in a children's burn unit, Prog. Pediatr. Surg. **14:**19-32, 1981.

Stoddard, F.J.: Coping with pain: a developmental approach to treatment of burned children, Am. J. Psychiatry **139:**736-740, 1982.

Surveyer, J.A.: Smoke inhalation injuries, Heart Lung **9:**825-830, 1980.

Surveyer, J.A., and Halpern, J.: Age-related burn injuries and their prevention, Pediatr. Nurs. **7**(5):29-34, 1981.

Thomas, K.A., Hassanein, R.S., and Christophersen, E.R.: Evaluation of group well-child care for improving burn prevention practices in the home, Pediatrics **74:**879-882, 1984.

Thompson, J.C., and Ashwal, S.: Electrical injuries in children, Am. J. Dis. Child. **137:**231-235, 1983.

Tobiasen, J., Hiebert, J.M., and Edlich, R.F.: The abbreviated burn severity index, Ann. Emerg. Med. **11:**260-262, 1982.

Wagner, M.M., editor: Care of the burn-injured patient, Littleton, MA, 1981, PSG Publications Co., Inc.

Wingate, E.: Emergent burn care: a time for life-saving measures, Crit. Care Update **10**(8):49-53, 1983.

Wooldridge, M., and Surveyer, J.A.: Skin grafting for full-thickness burn injury, Am. J. Nurs. **80:**2000-2004, 1980.

Yanofsky, N.N., and Morain, W.D.: Upper extremity burns from woodstoves, Pediatrics **73:**722-726, 1984.

Chapter 30

The Child with Renal Dysfunction

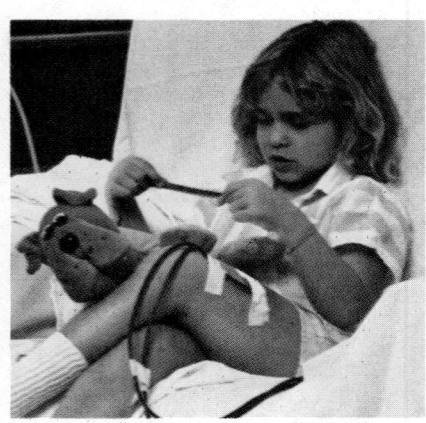

Diseases involving the kidneys are relatively common in childhood and are caused by a variety of etiologic factors. To better understand the way in which the pathologic processes produce an effect, the basic kidney structure and function are briefly reviewed and the most frequently used tests of renal function are outlined to help the reader understand the relationship of these studies to renal physiology and pathology. Discussion of the more common disorders of renal function is followed by discussion of the critical therapies of dialysis and renal transplant.

Renal Structure and Function

The primary responsibility of the kidney is to maintain the composition and volume of the body fluids in equilibrium. To maintain this constant internal environment, the kidney must respond appropriately to alterations in the internal environment caused by variations in dietary intake and extrarenal losses of water and solutes. This is accomplished by the formation of an ultrafiltration of plasma, with subsequent reabsorption of most of the water and electrolytes by the renal tubules and the secretion of certain other substances into the tubular urine. *Reabsorption* is the transport of a substance from the tubular lumen to the blood in surrounding vessels. *Secretion* is transport in the opposite direction, that is, from the blood to the lumen. These processes can be active or passive. *Excretion* is the elimination of a substance from the body, in this case urine.

A secondary function of the kidney is the production of certain humoral substances. One such substance is an enzyme, *erythropoietic stimulating factor (ESF, or erythrogenin),* which acts on a plasma globulin to form erythropoietin, which in turn stimulates erythropoiesis in the bone marrow. Its production is increased in the presence of hypoxia and androgens. Few red blood cells are formed in the absence of erythropoietin, which accounts in some measure for the anemia associated with advanced renal disease. Another enzyme, *renin,* is also secreted by the kidney in response to reduced blood volume, decreased blood pressure, or increased secretion of catecholamines. Renin stimulates the production of the angiotensins, which produce arteriolar constriction and an elevation in blood pressure and stimulate the production of aldosterone by the adrenal cortex.

RENAL PHYSIOLOGY

The structural and functional unit of the kidney is the nephron, which is composed of a complex system of tubules, arterioles, venules, and capillaries. The nephron itself consists of *the Bowman capsule,* enclosing the capillary tuft of the *glomerulus,* which is joined successively to the *proximal convoluted tubule, the Henle loop,* the *distal convoluted tubule,* and the *straight,* or *collecting duct.* Collecting tubules join larger ducts, and all the larger collecting ducts of one renal pyramid join to form a single duct that opens into a *minor calyx.* A number of calyces empty into one of several *major calyces* that converge into the *renal pelvis.* The renal pelvis narrows after it leaves the kidney and forms what then becomes a *ureter,* through which urine drains into the *urinary bladder.*

The blood supply to the kidneys constitutes about one fifth of the total cardiac output; therefore profuse bleeding can accompany renal trauma. Because interstitial tissue is sparse, individual nephrons with their blood vessel component are closely packed together. Each nephron is supplied by a sizable *afferent arteriole,* which separates into capillary loops that comprise the glomerular tuft. Blood leaves by a smaller *efferent arteriole.* From there the efferent arterioles branch into a *peritubular capillary* network and hairpin loops called the *vasa recta,* which parallel the Henle loops and the collecting ducts. The total surface area of the renal capillaries is approximately equal to the total surface of the tubules.

In the Bowman capsule the *glomerular capsule* is composed of two cellular layers that separate the blood from the glomerular filtrate—the capillary endothelium and a layer of tubular epithelial lining cells. Situated between these layers is the basal lamina, or basement membrane. The permeability of this glomerular membrane is a result of its structure; the capillary endothelium is fenestrated with pores or *fenestrae,* and the outer surface of the glomerular epithelium consists of fingerlike projections *(pseudopodia,* or *podocytes),* which cover the entire surface to form slits called *slit pores.* The basement membrane has no visible openings but behaves as if it contains pores or channels. Consequently the glomerular filtrate, which has essentially the same composition as plasma except for the large protein molecules and cellular elements, passes through these three layers and does so at a very rapid rate. The structure of these layers becomes altered in kidney disease.

Glomerular Filtration

Filtration through the glomerular capillaries is governed by the same mechanisms as filtration across other capillaries in the body, that is, the size of the capillary bed, the permeability of the capillaries, and the hydrostatic and osmotic pressure gradients across the capillaries. The filtration capacity of the glomerulus is the product of three pressure forces—the glomerular hydrostatic pressure, the colloidal osmotic (oncotic) pressure (COP), and the intracapsular pressure—and permeability of the glomerular capillaries.

Blood enters the nephron at a substantial pressure. This hydrostatic pressure forces plasma fluid and solutes through the capillary membrane into the collecting apparatus of the unit. As this filtrate travels through the renal tubules, water and solutes are selectively reabsorbed back into the vascular compartment. That which is not reabsorbed is excreted as urine. Filtration takes place as long as hydrostatic pressure within the glomerular capillaries exceeds the opposing colloidal osmotic pressure (COP) of the plasma proteins. If the pressure becomes equal through decreased hydrostatic pressure or decreased colloidal osmotic pressure, no further filtration takes place. In a state of dehydration, more water is reabsorbed; when water intake is increased, more is excreted as urine. In conditions that produce osmotic diuresis (i.e., when large solutes, such as glucose, are filtered through the capillaries in such excessive amounts that they cannot be reabsorbed), the osmotic attraction of the solute causes less water to be reabsorbed, resulting in water being excreted in the urine with the solute.

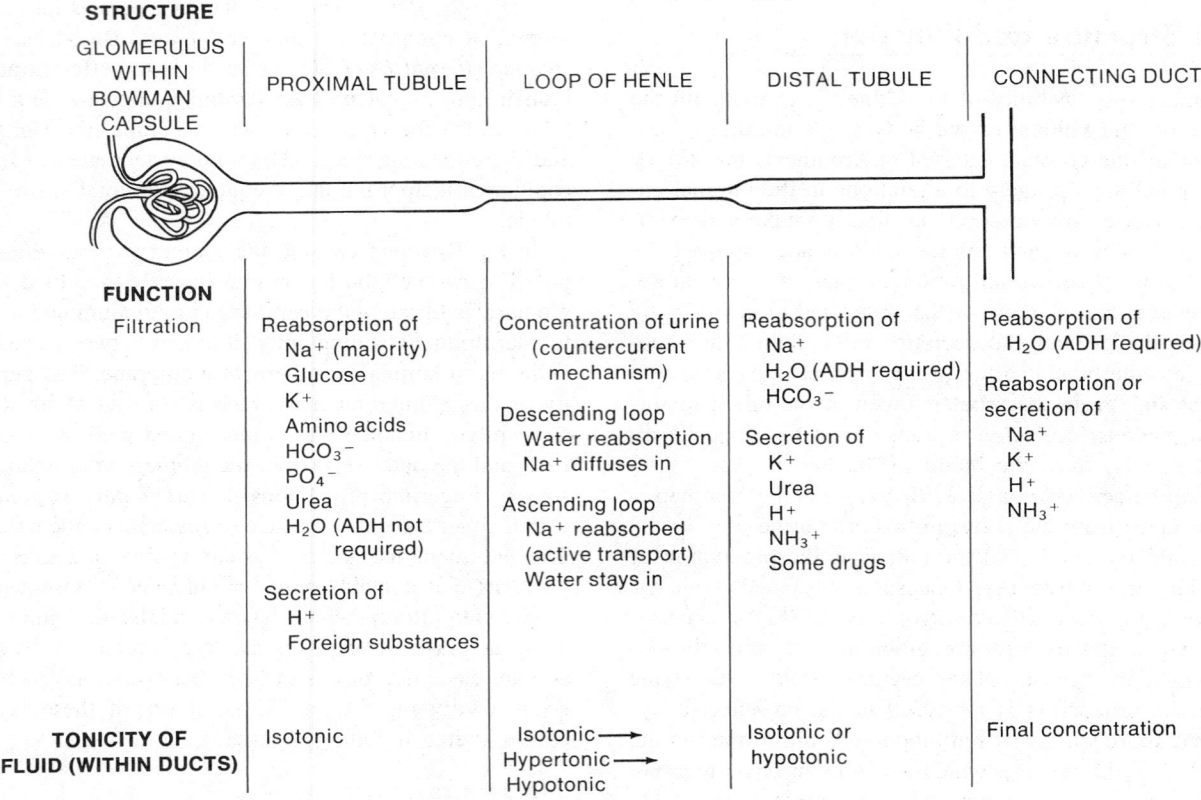

Fig. 30-1. Major functions of nephron components.

Tubular Function

The function of the renal tubules is to modify the glomerular filtrate. Tubular cells may add more of a substance to the filtrate (tubular secretion), remove some or all of a substance from the filtrate (tubular reabsorption), or both. The reabsorption is selective and discriminating for substances essential to body processes and equilibrium, whereas nonessential substances are eliminated as waste. The substances are secreted or reabsorbed in the tubules by osmosis, passive diffusion down a chemical or electric gradient, or actively transported against these gradients. These processes operate throughout the length of the tubules, but there are variations in the types, amounts, and mechanisms by which substances are secreted or reabsorbed in the different tubular segments, caused in large part by the cellular characteristics of each segment (Fig. 30-1).

Active transport mechanisms move vital substances both inward and outward from the tubular filtrate. For example, essential items such as glucose, amino acids, and sodium ions are reabsorbed in the proximal tubule and returned directly to the blood. Active transport mechanisms, as elsewhere, have a limited capacity, or threshold, for moving the solute. When the maximum of the transport mechanism is reached, no more of the substance is reabsorbed and the remainder is excreted in the urine. For example, when blood glucose concentrations exceed their transport capacity, the surplus remains in the filtrate to be excreted in the urine

(glycosuria). When two substances share a common transport mechanism, the first substance may be blocked by the addition of a second substance (selective inhibition). The effect of many therapeutic agents, for example, diuretics, depends on this process.

Electrolytes are moved by both active transport and diffusion, and the transport of some, particularly sodium, has important effects on other substances. For example, sodium is actively transported from all parts of the nephron. The movement of sodium ions produces both an electric and an osmotic gradient, which causes chloride ions and water to diffuse from the tubules in an effort to establish equilibrium. This is the obligatory water reabsorption in the kidneys. There is a limit to the concentration gradient against which sodium can be transported out; therefore when larger than normal amounts of sodium ions remain in the tubules, water is obliged to remain with the sodium.

Under normal conditions the kidneys are able to adjust the urine and solute excretion in response to the requirements for body water and electrolyte balance. They are able to excrete or conserve both water and most electrolytes in addition to excreting end products of protein metabolism, principally urea. The volume of urine excreted by the kidneys in a given period of time depends on the water balance (including intravascular filtration pressure), the quantity of solutes presented to the kidneys, and the capacity of the kidneys to dilute or concentrate the filtrate.

Renal Development and Function in Early Infancy

Development of the kidney begins within the first weeks of embryonic life but is not completed until about the end of the first year after birth. The nephrons increase in number throughout gestation and reach their full complement by birth. However, they are immature and less efficient than at later ages. Many of the tubular sections are not fully formed, and the glomeruli enlarge considerably after birth.

Glomerular filtration and absorption are relatively low and do not reach adult values until the child is between 1 and 2 years of age. This appears to be related to a barrier imposed by more cuboidal-shaped glomerular epithelial cells and higher afferent arteriole resistance. Consequently, the newborn is unable to dispose of excess water and solute rapidly or efficiently.

There is large variation in the tubular length between nephrons, although glomerular size is less variable. The juxtaglomerular nephrons show more advanced development than cortical nephrons. The loop of Henle, the site of the urine-concentrating mechanism, is short in the newborn, which is reducing the ability to reabsorb sodium and water and produces a very dilute urine, although adequate amounts of antidiuretic hormone are secreted by the newborn pituitary gland. The length gradually increases until the concentrating ability reaches adult levels about the third month of life. Urea synthesis and excretion are slower during this time, and the newborn retains large quantities of nitrogen and essential electrolytes in order to meet needs for growth in the first weeks of life. Consequently the excretory burden is minimized. The lower concentration of urea, the principal end product of nitrogen metabolism, reduces concentrating capacity, since it also contributes to the concentration mechanism.

Other characteristics of the newborn's kidneys create differences in renal function from that of older children and adults. Because of some as yet undetermined cause, newborn infants are unable to excrete a water load at rates similar to older persons. Hydrogen ion excretion is reduced, acid secretion is lower for the first year of life, and plasma bicarbonate levels are low. As a result of these inadequacies of the kidney and less efficient blood buffers, the newborn is more liable to develop severe acidosis. Sodium excretion is reduced in the immediate newborn period, and the kidneys are less able to adapt to deficiencies and excesses of sodium. For example, an isotonic saline infusion may produce edema because the ability to eliminate excess sodium is impaired. Conversely, inadequate reabsorption of sodium from tubules may compound sodium losses in disorders such as vomiting or diarrhea. In addition, infants have a diminished capacity to reabsorb glucose and, during the first few days, to produce ammonium ions.

Because of the small, conical pelvis, the urinary bladder is an abdominal organ in infancy, but, as the pelvis expands with growth, the bladder settles into it to become a pelvic organ. The kidney functions during fetal life and produces urine that contributes to the amniotic fluid volume. The 24-hour urine volume is low at birth, rapidly increases in the neonatal period, and steadily increases with normal growth (see Appendix B).

ASSESSMENT OF RENAL INTEGRITY

Assessment of kidney and urinary tract integrity and the diagnosis of renal or urinary tract disease are based on several evaluative tools. Physical examination, history, and observation of symptoms are the initial procedures. In suspected urinary tract disorders, further assessment by laboratory, radiologic, and other evaluative methods is carried out.

Clinical Manifestations

As in most disorders of childhood, the incidence and type of kidney or urinary tract dysfunction change with the age and maturation of the child. In addition, the presenting complaints and the significance of these complaints varies with

---

SIGNS AND SYMPTOMS OF URINARY TRACT INFECTIONS AT DIFFERENT AGES

Neonatal period (birth to 1 month)
Poor feeding
Vomiting
Failure to gain weight
Rapid respiration (acidosis)
Frequent urination
Screaming on urination
Poor urinary stream
Jaundice
Convulsions
Dehydration
Other anomalies or stigmata
Enlarged kidneys or bladder

Infancy (1 to 24 months)
Poor feeding
Vomiting
Failure to gain weight
Excessive thirst
Frequent urination
Straining or screaming on urination
Foul-smelling urine
Pallor
Fever
Persistent diaper rash
Convulsions (with or without fever)
Dehydration
Enlarged kidney or bladder

Childhood (2 to 14 years)
Poor appetite
Vomiting
Growth failure
Excessive thirst
Enuresis, incontinence, frequent urination
Painful urination
Swelling of face
Convulsions
Pallor
Fatigue
Blood in urine
Abdominal or back pain
Edema
Hypertension
Tetany

maturation. For example, a complaint of enuresis has greater significance at age 8 years than at age 4. In the newborn, urinary tract disorders are associated with a number of obvious malformations of other body systems, including the curious and unexplained but frequent association between malformed or low-set ears and urinary tract anomalies. Important signs and symptoms that suggest possible renal or urinary tract disease in children at different ages are outlined in the box on p. 1251.

Many of the clinical manifestations are common to a variety of childhood disorders, but their presence is an indication to obtain further information from past history, family history, and laboratory studies as part of a complete physical examination. Suspected renal disease can be further evaluated by means of radiographic studies and renal biopsy.

Laboratory Tests

Both urine and blood studies contribute vital information for detection of renal problems. The single most important test is probably the routine urinalysis. Specific urine and blood tests provide additional information. Since nurses are usually the persons who collect the specimens for examination and who often perform many of the screening tests, they should be familiar with the test, its function, and factors that can alter or distort the results of the test (see Chapter 27 for collection of urine specimens).

Glomerular filtration rate is a measure of the amount of plasma from which a given substance is totally cleared in 1 minute. Clearance is calculated from the ratio of substance excreted to the concentration of that substance in the plasma. A number of substances can be used, but the most useful clinical estimation of glomerular filtration is the clearance of creatinine, an end-product of protein metabolism in muscle and a substance that is freely filtered by the glomerulus and secreted by renal tubular cells. The production and secretion of creatinine remain relatively constant from day to day, and its appearance in the urine is determined by the serum level. When the collection is complete and accurately timed, the results are fairly reliable and compare favorably with clearance of other substances, such as inulin, that require special equipment to evaluate and long immobilization of the child. Any significant degree of renal disease can diminish the glomerular filtration rate, but diseases of the glomerulus and renal vascular disease have the most immediate effect. The nurse's responsibility in this test is collection of urine, usually a 12- or 24-hour specimen.

The major blood and urine tests are outlined in Tables 30-1 and 30-2. Special tests and nursing responsibilities are briefly described in Table 30-3.

Table 30-1 Urine tests of renal function

TEST	NORMAL RANGE	DEVIATIONS	SIGNIFICANCE OF DEVIATIONS
Physical tests			
Volume	Age related	Polyuria	Osmotic factors (urinary glucose level in diabetes mellitus)
		Oliguria	Retention caused by obstructive disease
			Inadequate bladder emptying caused by neurogenic bladder or obstructive disorder
Specific gravity	With normal fluid intake: 1.016-1.022 Newborn: 1:001-1.020 Others: 1.001-1.030	High	Dehydration
			Presence of protein or glucose
			Presence of radiopaque contrast medium after radiologic examinations
		Low	Excessive fluid intake
			Distal tubular dysfunction
			Insufficient antidiuretic hormone
			Diuresis
		Fixed at 1.010	Chronic glomerular disease
Osmolality	Newborn: 50-600 mOsm/liter Thereafter: 50-1400 mOsm/liter	High or low	Same as for specific gravity
			More sensitive index than specific gravity
Appearance	Clear pale yellow to deep gold	Cloudy	Contains sediment
		Cloudy reddish pink to reddish brown	Blood from trauma or disease
			Myoglobin following severe muscle destruction
		Light	Dilute
		Dark	Concentrated

Table 30-1   Urine tests of renal function—cont'd

TEST	NORMAL RANGE	DEVIATIONS	SIGNIFICANCE OF DEVIATIONS
Chemical tests			
pH	Newborn: 5-7 Thereafter: 4.8-7.8 Average: 6	Weak acid or neutral	If associated with metabolic acidosis, suggests tubular acidosis If associated with metabolic alkalosis, suggests potassium deficiency Urinary infection
		Alkaline	Metabolic alkalosis
Protein level	Absent	Present	Abnormal glomerular permeability, for example, glomerular disease, changes in blood pressure Most kidney disease Orthostatic in some individuals
Glucose level	Absent	Present	Diabetes mellitus Infusion of glucose-containing fluids Impaired tubular reabsorption
Ketone levels	Absent	Present	Conditions of acute metabolic demand (stress)
Microscopic tests			
White blood cell count	Less than 1 or 2	More than 5 polymorphonuclear leukocytes/field	Urinary tract inflammatory process
		Lymphocytes	Allograft rejection Malignancy
Red blood cell count	Less than 1 or 2	4-6/field in centrifuged specimen	Trauma Stones Infection Neoplasms
Presence of bacteria	Absent to a few	More than 100,000 organisms/ml in centrifuged specimen	Urinary tract infection
Presence of casts	Occasional	Protein casts	Pronounced renal malfunction Tubular or glomerular disorders
		White blood cell casts	Pyelonephritis
		Red blood cell casts	Glomerulonephritis
		Epithelial casts	Glomerulonephritis
		Hyaline casts	Usually temporary; must be correlated with other findings

Table 30-2   Blood tests of renal function

TEST	NORMAL RANGE (mg/dl)	DEVIATIONS	SIGNIFICANCE OF DEVIATIONS
Blood urea nitrogen (BUN)	Newborn: 4-18 Infant, child: 5-18	Elevated	Renal disease—acute or chronic (the higher the BUN, the more severe the disease) Increased protein catabolism Dehydration Hemorrhage High protein intake Corticosteroid therapy
Uric acid	Child: 2.0-5.5	Increased	Severe renal disease
Creatinine	Infant: 0.2-0.4 Child: 0.3-0.7 Adolescent: 0.5-1.0	Increased	Severe, long-standing renal impairment

Table 30-3 Radiologic and other tests of renal function

TEST	PROCEDURE	PURPOSE	COMMENTS AND NURSING RESPONSIBILITIES
Radiologic tests			
Intravenous pyelography (IVP) (intravenous urogram; excretory urogram)	Intravenous injection of a contrast medium Medium secreted and concentrated by tubules X-ray films made 5, 10, and 15 minutes after injectiion	Defines urinary tract Provides information about integrity of kidneys, ureters, and bladder Retroperitoneal masses visualized when they shift position of ureters	Preparation for test: Infants less than 2 years of age—no solid food, omit one bottle on morning of examination, studies should be done early to avoid withholding of fluids Children aged 2-14 years—administer cathartic evening before examination, nothing is given orally after midnight, enema (Fleet or soapsuds) is given morning of examination
Time-sequence IVP	Modification of those for IVP Films made every 5 minutes after injection of contrast medium	More accurately distinguishes differences between kidneys Differences in times of excretion indicate unilateral disease	Support during procedure Normal kidneys show dye before abnormal ones
Retrograde pyelography	Contrast medium injected through catheter inserted into kidney pelvis via urethra, bladder, and ureter	Visualizes pelvic calyces, ureters, and bladder	Rarely necessary during childhood
Renal angiography	Contrast medium injected directly into renal artery via catheter placed in femoral artery (or umbilical artery in newborn) and advanced to renal artery	Visualizes renal vascular system, especially for renal arterial stenosis	Give cathartic if ordered Give preoperative medication if ordered Observe for reaction to contrast medium
Radioisotope renography and renal scanning	Radioisotopes injected intravenously and recorded with special camera and computer analysis	Records appearance and disappearance of radioactivity in each kidney Gives detailed picture of excretory performance Helps define intrarenal masses	Give sedation as ordered Insert or assist insertion of intravenous infusion Monitor intravenous infusion
Voiding cystourethrography	Contrast medium injected into bladder through urethral catheter until bladder is full; films taken before, during, and after voiding	Visualizes bladder outline and urethra, reveals reflux of urine into ureters, and shows complications of bladder emptying	
Scout film (KUB)	Flat plate roentgenogram of abdomen and pelvis	Detects and establishes renal outlines, presence of calculi, or opaque foreign bodies in bladder	Prepare as for routine x-ray film
Miscellaneous tests			
Cystoscopy	Direct visualization of bladder and lower urinary tract through small scope inserted via urethra	Investigation of bladder and lower tract lesions; visualizes urethral openings, bladder wall, trigone, and urethra	Give nothing orally after midnight Carry out preoperative preparations

Table 30-3 Radiologic and other tests of renal function—cont'd

TEST	PROCEDURE	PURPOSE	COMMENTS AND NURSING RESPONSIBILITIES
Renal biopsy	Removal of kidney tissue by open or percutaneous technique for study by light, electron, or immunofluorescent microscopy	Yields histologic and microscopic information about glomeruli and tubules; helps to distinguish between types of nephrotic syndromes Distinguishes other renal disorders	Give nothing orally 4-6 hours before test Premedicate as ordered Prepare setup for procedure Assist with procedure Take vital signs Apply pressure to area with pressure dressing and, if feasible, a sandbag Bed rest for 24 hours Observe for abdominal pain, tenderness Monitor input and output; surgical incision may be required in infants
Nephrosonography	Transmission of ultrasonic sound waves through kidney areas to outline kidney mass	Distinguishes between cystic and solid masses and renal and nonrenal masses, localizes kidneys, and delineates nonfunctional kidney	Administer sedation if needed
Tomography	Narrow beam x-rays and computer analysis provide precise reconstruction of area	Visualizes vertical or horizontal cross section of kidney Especially valuable to distinguish tumors and cysts	Noninvasive Similar to preparation for pyelography
Urine culture and sensitivity	Collection of sterile specimen	Determines presence of pathogens and the drugs to which they are sensitive	Does not require specific parental permission Send specimen to laboratory immediately after collection Catherization, clean-catch, or suprapubic specimen

Inflammatory Disorders of the Genitourinary Tract

Kidneys react to tissue injury in the same manner as all other body tissues. Acute inflammation evokes a pattern of exudation, white blood cell accumulation, and tissue damage; chronic long-standing inflammation results in scarring and permanent destruction of tissue elements. This discussion focuses on inflammations of the renal system, including bacterial infections and those nonsuppurative disorders, collectively described as *nephritis*.

URINARY TRACT INFECTION

Urinary tract infection (UTI) is the term used to describe a clinical condition that may involve the urethra, bladder (lower urinary tract), and/or the ureters, renal pelvis, calyces, and renal parenchyma (upper urinary tract). Because it is often impossible to localize the infection, the broad designation UTI is applied to the presence of significant numbers of microorganisms anywhere within the urinary tract (except the distal one third of the urethra, which is usually colonized with bacteria) (Underwood, 1980).

Classification

Infection of the urinary tract may be present with or without clinical symptoms. As a result, the site of infection is often difficult to pinpoint with any degree of accuracy. Various terms used to describe urinary tract disorders include the following:

bacteriuria Growth of bacteria in uncontaminated urine (greater than 100,000 colonies/ml)

asymptomatic bacteriuria Significant bacteriuria with no clinical evidence of active infection

symptomatic bacteriuria Significant bacteriuria accompanied by physical symptoms

recurrent UTI Repeated symptomatic episodes, usually caused by entry of new organisms from the perineal-fecal flora (sometimes termed *reinfection*)

relapse of UTI Relapse is persistence of the same organism despite appropriate antibiotic therapy
urethritis Inflammation of the urethra
cystitis Inflammation of the bladder
ureteritis Inflammation of the ureters
pyelonephritis Inflammation of the kidney and upper tract (may be acute or chronic)

Incidence

The prevalence of UTI in childhood is second only to infections of the respiratory tract and is a significant cause of hospitalization and morbidity in children (Sidor and Resnick, 1983). Although its exact incidence is not known, it is estimated that 1.5% to 2% of children age 1 to 5 years will develop symptomatic UTI (Siegel and others, 1980). In children 5 to 10 years of age the incidence is about 1% to 2% (Kunin, 1979). The peak incidence of UTI not caused by structural anomalies occurs between 2 and 6 years of age. Except for the neonatal period, females have a 10 to 30 times greater risk for developing UTI than males. It has been estimated that approximately 5% of school-age females will develop bacteriuria by 18 years of age.

UTI in newborns differs in some respects from infections occurring in older children. In this group males outnumber females. At all ages asymptomatic bacteriuria is more common than symptomatic disease and recurrence is not uncommon, especially in girls. An increased incidence of UTI is observed in adolescents, especially those with evidence of sexual activity (Weir and Lampe, 1984).

Etiology

A variety of organisms can be responsible for UTI. *Escherichia coli* (80% of cases) and other gram-negative enteric organisms are most frequently implicated; all are common to the anal, perineal, and perianal region. Other organisms associated with UTI include *Proteus, Pseudomonas, Klebsiella, Staphylococcus aureus, Haemophilus,* and coagulase-negative *Staphylococcus* (Ogra and Faden, 1985).

Some children appear to be more susceptible to UTI. There is some evidence that suggests a genetic predisposition to UTI, for example, an association between blood group B antigen in blood groups B and AB (persons lacking anti-B isohemagglutinin) (Lomberg and others, 1983; Kinane and others, 1982). In addition there are a number of factors that contribute to the development of UTI. These include anatomic, physical, and chemical conditions or properties of the host urinary tract.

Anatomic and physical factors. The structure of the lower urinary tract is believed to account for the increased incidence of bacteriuria in females. The short urethra, which measures about 2 cm (¾ inch) in young females and 4 cm (1½ inches) in mature women, provides a ready pathway for invasion of organisms. In addition, the closure of the urethra at the end of micturition may return contaminated bacteria to the bladder.

The longer male urethra (as long as 20 cm [8 inches] in an adult) and the antibacterial properties of prostatic secretions inhibit the entry and growth of pathogens. Recently there have been reports of an increased incidence of UTI in infants who are not circumcised compared to infants who are circumcised (Roberts, 1986). Of the UTIs in male infants less than 8 months of age, 95% occurred in the uncircumcised (Wiswell, Smith, and Bass, 1985). The incidence of renal scarring is greatest in patients whose first infection occurs during infancy.

The single most important host factor influencing the occurrence of UTI is urinary stasis. Ordinarily urine is sterile, but at 37° C (98.6° F) it provides an excellent culture medium. Under normal conditions the act of completely and repeatedly emptying the bladder flushes away any organisms before they have an opportunity to multiply and invade surrounding tissue. However, urine that remains in the bladder allows bacteria from the urethra to rapidly become established in the rich medium.

Incomplete bladder emptying (stasis) may result from reflux (see p. 1259 for a discussion of reflux), anatomic abnormalities (especially those involving the ureters), dysfunction of the voiding mechanism, or extrinsic ureteral or bladder compression. Pressure of overdistention within the bladder may increase the risk of infection by decreasing host resistance, probably as a result of lessened blood flow to the mucosa. This frequently occurs in neurogenic bladder or as a consequence of voluntarily holding back urine despite the urge to void.

Extrinsic factors that may be responsible for *functional* bladder neck obstruction are chronic and intermittent constipation and pregnancy. In both conditions, the full rectum or uterus displaces the bladder and posterior urethra in the fixed and limited space of the bony pelvis, causing obstruction, incomplete micturition, and urinary stasis. Treating constipation along with antibiotic therapy for UTI reduces the recurrence of infection, whereas failure to relieve the fecal retention in spite of adequate treatment of the UTI may result in recurrence. Hormones of pregnancy also cause decreased bladder and ureteral tone, hydroureter, and increased residual bladder urine.

Other extrinsic factors that can contribute to UTI include catheters, especially short-term indwelling catheters, and administration of antimicrobial agents. Antimicrobials alter the host's normal perineal flora, allowing easier colonization with uropathogens. Tight clothing or diapers, poor hygiene, and local inflammation, such as from vaginitis, masturbation, or pinworm infestation, may also increase the risk of ascending infection. The essential oils in bubble baths and shampoos have been found to irritate the urethra of both boys and girls, causing painful and frequent urination (Rogers, 1985). Consequently, bubble baths are discouraged. There is no evidence that plain tub baths increase the risk of UTI, but infections have been related to the use of hot tub or whirlpool baths (Salmen, 1983). Sexual intercourse produces transient bacteriuria in females and is associated with an increased risk of UTI.

Altered urine and bladder chemistry. Several chemical characteristics of the urine and bladder mucosa help maintain urinary sterility. An increased fluid intake promotes flushing of the normal bladder and lowers the concentration of organisms in the infected bladder. Water diuresis also seems to enhance the antibacterial properties of the renal medulla. One effect of water diuresis is increased blood flow to the medulla (where it is normally low), thereby increasing the availability of white cells at the site of inflammation.

Most pathogens favor an alkaline medium. Normally urine is slightly acidic, but it can be made more acidic by diet (apple or cranberry juices, large amounts of ascorbic acid, animal protein) or acid-forming drugs. When the urine pH is about 5, bacterial multiplication is hampered, although the acidification rarely eliminates the bacteriuria. However, it may enhance the therapeutic effectiveness of drugs and of the natural defense mechanisms, as well as help relieve some of the symptoms. Infection by some organisms, such as *Proteus,* increases the pH by decomposing urea to ammonia, thereby increasing the favorable conditions for the continued growth of the organism.

The bladder mucosa seems to have bactericidal effectiveness by destroying the bacteria in the very thin layer of urine left on the walls after complete voiding. Since close contact of the bacteria with the mucosa is essential for lysis to occur, any residual urine prevents the mechanism from functioning.

Pathophysiology

Inflammatory changes are usually confined to the bladder (cystitis) in uncomplicated infection. However, recurrent infection of the bladder may produce changes that distort the normal anatomic relationships of the ureter as it traverses the bladder wall causing incompetence of the vesicoureteral valve. This may permit reflux of urine during voiding, which can allow access of organisms to the upper urinary tract.

Infection of the upper collecting system (pyelitis) and kidney (pyelonephritis), although much less common than cystitis, is usually acquired through an ascending infection from the lower tract. Infection of the renal parenchyma may also be introduced hematogenously, especially in infants in whom this is the more common route. Infection causes acute and chronic inflammatory changes in the pelvis and medulla with resulting scarring and loss of renal tissue, usually symmetric. Recurrent or chronic episodes cause an increase in fibrotic tissue and kidney contraction. In acute pyelonephritis the kidney is swollen and edematous with diffuse infiltration of polymorphonuclear cells. The scarring in relation to reflux appears to occur mainly in children under 5 years of age (Kroovand and Perlmutter, 1983).

Clinical Manifestations

The clinical manifestations of UTIs depend on the age of the child. In newborn infants and children less than 2 years of age the signs are characteristically nonspecific. They more nearly resemble gastrointestinal tract disorders: failure to thrive, feeding problems, vomiting, diarrhea, abdominal distention, and jaundice. Newborns may have fever or hypothermia and/or sepsis. Other evidence that may be observed includes frequent or infrequent voiding, constant squirming and irritability, strong-smelling urine, and abnormal stream. A persistent diaper rash may also be a helpful clue.

The classic symptoms of UTI are often observed in children over 2 years of age. These include enuresis or daytime incontinence in the child who has been toilet trained, fever, strong- or foul-smelling urine, increased frequency of urination, dysuria, or urgency. They may also complain of abdominal pain or costovertebral angle tenderness (flank pain). Some will present with hematuria; preschoolers may vomit. There is a high frequency of obstructive uropathy in young infants and boys that is characterized by dribbling of urine, straining with urination, or a decrease in the force and size of the urinary stream. High fever and chills accompanied by flank pain, severe abdominal pain, and leukocytosis suggests pyelonephritis. However, flank pain and tenderness may be the only indication of pyelonephritis on physical examination.

Manifestations in adolescents are more specific. Symptoms of lower tract infections include frequency and painful urination of a small amount of turbulent urine that may be grossly bloody. Fever is usually absent. Upper tract infection is characterized by fever, chills, flank pain, and lower tract symptoms, which may appear 1 or 2 days after the upper tract symptoms.

A large proportion (40%) of UTIs in children are asymptomatic or atypical in clinical presentation, and many complaints may be unrelated to the urinary tract (Hellerstein and others, 1984). Many are treated as respiratory or gastrointestinal infections. It is important that these children be identified so that treatment can be initiated. Significant scarring can take place, especially in infants and very young children.

Diagnostic Evaluation

Urine characteristic of possible infection appears cloudy, hazy, or thick with noticeable strands of mucus and pus; it also smells fishy and unpleasant even when fresh. Presumptive UTI diagnosis can be made on the basis of microscopic examination of the urine, which often reveals pyuria (5 to 8 white blood cells/ml of uncentrifuged urine), and the presence of at least one bacterium in a Gram stain. However, a normal urinalysis may also be present in conditions of asymptomatic bacteriuria.

Diagnosis of UTI is confirmed by detection of bacteriuria in urine culture, but urine collection is often difficult, especially in infants and very small children (see Collection of specimens, p. 1126). Several factors may alter a urine specimen. Contamination of a specimen by organisms from sources other than the urine is the most frequent cause of false-positive results. Bag urine specimens are frequently contaminated by perineal and perianal flora and are usually considered inadequate for a definitive diagnosis. More accurate estimates are obtained from clean-catch midstream specimens but these may be contaminated. Unless the specimen is a first morning sample, a recent high fluid intake may indicate an falsely low organism count. Therefore children should not be encouraged to drink large volumes of water in an attempt to obtain a specimen quickly.

Urine obtained by (1) suprapubic aspiration or (2) from catheterization is normally sterile. Catheterized specimens are usually excellent as long as the first few milliliters are excluded from collection. Suprapubic aspiration is equally reliable and is frequently used for collecting specimens in infants. Care of a urine specimen obtained for culture is an important nursing aspect related to diagnosis. The specimen should be taken to the laboratory for culture immediately.

Recently developed tests to detect bacteriuria are being used with increased frequency in screening for UTI. The plastic dipstick, Chemstrip, and the agar-coated slide tests are quick and inexpensive alternatives to microscopic examination and, in some instances, are replacing routine culture.

Localization of the infection site may involve more specific tests, including ureteral catheterization and bladder washout procedures. Other tests, such as ultrasonography, voiding cystourethrogram (VCUG), intravenous pyelogram (IVP), and cystoscopy, are often performed after the infection subsides to identify anatomic abnormalities contributing to the development of infection and existing kidney changes from recurrent infection.

Therapeutic Management

The objectives of treatment of children with UTI are (1) to eliminate the infection, (2) to detect and correct functional or anatomic abnormalities, (3) to prevent recurrences, and (4) to preserve renal function (Krugman and others, 1985). Antibiotic therapy should be initiated based on identification of the pathogen, the child's history of antibiotic use, and the location of the infection. A variety of antimicrobial drugs are available for treating UTI, but all of them can occasionally be ineffective because of resistance of organisms. Antibacterial compounds used in the management of UTI include (1) systemic penicillins and sulfonamides, which are used for a short, intensive course of therapy; and (2) antiseptic preparations, which are often continued over longer periods to maintain urinary sterility, especially in children with long-term susceptibility to infection, such as those with neurogenic bladder.

The optimum length of therapy for UTI in children is not well established. Conventional therapy for uncomplicated infection, a single oral antibiotic (e.g., ampicillin, a sulfonamide, or nitrofurantoin) that the patient has not taken recently, can be administered for 10 to 14 days. Three-day administration of nitrofurantoin has been proven effective (Lohr and others, 1981; Khan, Kumar, and Evans, 1981) and single-dose therapy with amoxicillin is reported to be equally effective (Shapiro and Wald, 1981; Avner and others, 1983; Fine and Jacobson, 1985). The short-term therapy is not universally accepted nor is it effective against upper tract infections. It is usually restricted to children be-

yond the newborn period with their first UTI. In all cases follow-up laboratory evaluation is needed.

Children with suspected pyelonephritis and fever are admitted to the hospital and given appropriate antibiotics intravenously for a minimum of 48 hours. Blood and urine cultures are obtained on admission and following therapy. The cultures are usually repeated at monthly intervals for 3 months and at 3-month intervals for 6 months (Smith, 1986).

Newborn infants with documented UTI, UTI in boys of any age, and females 2 to 3 years of age with a second or subsequent UTI infection warrant sonographic or radiographic evaluation (Hellerstein and others, 1984). If anatomic defects such as primary reflux or bladder neck obstruction are present, surgical correction of these abnormalities may be necessary to prevent recurrent infection.

Follow-up study is an important component of medical management, since the relapse rate is high and recurrent infection tends to occur 1 to 2 months after termination of treatment. Even with recurrent infections, renal damage is rare if no anatomic abnormalities complicate the condition. The aim of therapy and careful follow-up in such cases is to prevent morbidity rather than reduce the chance of renal failure. However, the hazard of progressive renal injury is greatest when infection occurs in young children (especially under 2 years of age) and is associated with congenital renal malformations and reflux. Therefore early diagnosis of children at risk is particularly important during infancy and toddlerhood.

Nursing Considerations

Objectives of nursing care include identification of children with UTI and education of parents and child regarding prevention and treatment of infection. Aside from the influence of renal abnormalities, females between the ages of 2 and 6 years are in general a high-risk group. Since they are not a captive population, mass screening is difficult. However, the annual health examinations should include a routine urinalysis. In addition, nurses should instruct parents to observe regularly for clues suggesting UTI. Unfortunately the signs of UTI are not as evident as those of upper respiratory infection. Therefore many cases go undetected because no one thought to investigate this very common problem.

Since infants and young children are unable to express their feelings and sensations verbally, it is difficult to detect discomfort they may be experiencing from dysuria. A careful history regarding voiding habits and episodes of unexplained irritability may assist in detecting less obvious cases of UTI. Consequently parents should be cautioned to observe for specific clues of UTI in suspected cases, such as checking the diaper every ½ hour, which increases the opportunity for observing the stream for such findings as straining or fretting before voiding begins, signs of discomfort before and during urinating, starting and stopping the stream intermittently, and frequent dripping of small amounts of urine.

When infection is suspected, collecting an appropriate specimen is essential. It is the nurse's responsibility to take every precaution to obtain acceptable clean-voided specimens in order to avoid the use of other collecting procedures except where absolutely indicated.

Frequently other tests are performed to detect anatomic defects. Children are prepared for these tests as appropriate for their age. Except for intravenous pyelography (IVP), voiding cystography and cystoscopy are usually performed under general anesthesia. However, children who are old enough to understand still need an explanation of the procedure, its purpose, and what they will experience (see Preparing for procedures, p. 1104). Sometimes a simple description of the urinary system is helpful. Especially for preschool children, the nurse must clarify that the urinary tract is separate from any sexual function and that the test is for a problem that they did not cause. It is not uncommon for children to associate blame for perceived wrongdoing (e.g., masturbation) or unacceptable thoughts with the reason for the illness or the tests. For young children under 3 to 4 years of age, the procedure can be explained on a doll. For those who are older, a simple drawing of the bladder, urethra, ureters, and kidneys makes the explanation more understandable.

Children may be treated as outpatients to avoid overnight separation from home for such procedures. In such cases nurses must be careful not to overlook the need for adequate preparation, since if surgery is subsequently indicated, the child will be able to undergo the impending operation with facts and understanding from these procedures, which will help to decrease his fear and anxiety of more extensive medical-surgical intervention.

Since antibacterial drugs are indicated in UTI, the nurse advises parents of proper dosage and stresses the importance of administering the drug as prescribed. When antiseptics such as nitrofurantoin are used for prolonged therapy to maintain urine sterility, parents need an explanation of their continued necessity when no signs of infection are present.* For all children an adequate or increased fluid intake is encouraged.

Prevention. Prevention is the most important goal in both primary and recurrent infection, and most preventive measures are simple to very simple, ordinary hygienic habits that should be a routine part of daily care. Parents are taught to cleanse their infant's genital areas from front to back to avoid contaminating the urethral area with fecal organisms. Female children are taught to wipe from front to back after voiding or defecating. Clothing that is tight in the perineal area may contribute to spread of bacteria and absorbent cotton briefs are preferred to those made from synthetic fibers.

Any signs of intestinal parasites (e.g., scratching between the legs and around anal area) should be investigated

and treated appropriately. The child is taught to avoid "holding" urine and is encouraged to void before beginning an activity where toilet facilities are less accessible (e.g., an automobile trip). Sexually active adolescent females are advised to urinate as soon as possible after intercourse to flush out bacteria introduced during sex play.

Children with disabilities involving the bladder are frequently on a prophylactic regimen, such as acidifying agents and prescribed fluid intake. The importance of compliance should be reinforced in parents and responsible children.

VESICOURETERAL REFLUX

Vesicoureteral reflux (VUR) refers to the retrograde flow of bladder urine into the ureters. Reflux increases the chance for and perpetuates infection, since with each void urine is swept up the ureters and then allowed to empty after voiding. Therefore the residual urine from the ureters remains in the bladder until the next void (Fig. 30-2). The International Classification System describes the degree of reflux from the bladder into upper genitourinary tract structures (see box on p. 1260).

Primary reflux results from the congenitally abnormal insertion of the ureters into the bladder and predisposes to development of infection. *A familial incidence of VUR is sometimes observed. Secondary reflux* occurs as a result of infection. Normally the ureters enter the bladder wall in such a manner that the accumulating urine compresses the submucosal segment of the ureter, preventing reflux. However, the edema caused by bladder infection renders this mechanism at the ureterovesicular junction incompetent. In addition, in infants and young children the shortness of the submucosal portion of the ureter decreases the effectiveness of this antireflux mechanism. Other causes of secondary reflux are neurogenic bladder from either chronic obstruction or neural dysfunction or as an iatrogenic result from progressive dilation of the ureters following surgical urinary diversion.

Reflux with infection can lead to kidney damage, since refluxed urine ascending into the collecting tubules of the nephrons allows the microorganisms to gain access to the renal parenchyma, initiating renal scarring. Forty-six percent of infants younger than 23 months and as many as 9% of children 24 to 60 months of age with UTI exhibit vesicoureteral reflux (Siegel and others, 1980). Also, most renal scars associated with reflux are present at the time of diagnosis; few develop after 5 years of age. However, between 30% and 60% of children with VUR have evidence of renal scarring and scarring is almost always found in association with reflux (Ehrlich, 1982). Therefore VUR is an important cause of renal damage and careful examination for its presence is indicated. Careful routine follow-up is a critical part of management of children with urinary tract infection (UTI), and children with reflux, documented by voiding cystoureterography, are assessed repeatedly during ensuing years (Hellerstein, 1984).

---

*See Home care instructions for giving medications to children. In Wong, D.L., and Whaley, L.F.: Clinical handbook of pediatric nursing, ed 2. St. Louis, 1986, The C.V. Mosby Co.

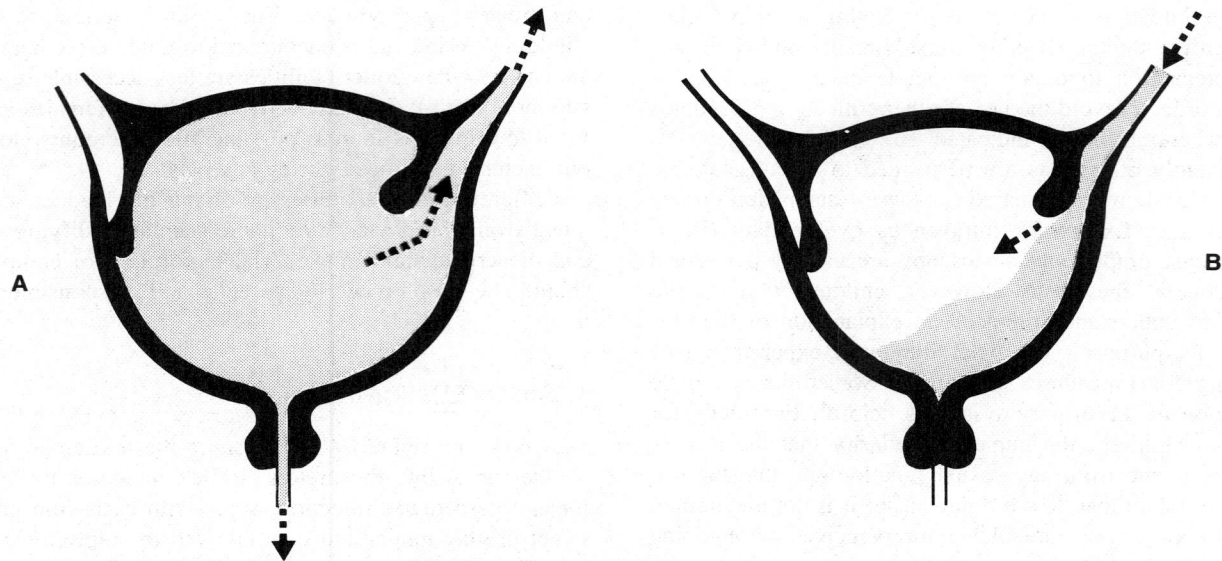

Fig. 30-2. Mechanisms of vesicoureteral reflux. **A,** During voiding, urine refluxes into ureter. **B,** After voiding, residual urine from ureter remains in bladder.

Therapeutic Management

Conservative, nonoperative therapy is effective in controlling infection in most cases of VUR. There is a high incidence of spontaneous resolution over time—approximately 20% to 30% for each 2-year period throughout childhood (Ehrlich, 1982). An 80% probability of remission may occur in Grades I and II reflux when managed medically (Hensle and Burbige, 1986). Therapy consists of continuous low-dose antibacterial therapy with frequent urine cultures, which can usually be done at home by the dip slide or Chemstrip methods. This long-term therapy requires medical supervision and reliable, cooperative parents. Surgical correction of reflux may be required for Grades IV and V reflux. Grade III is managed conservatively unless complications interfere.

The major indications for surgical intervention include significant anatomic abnormality at the ureterovesical junction, recurrent UTI, high grades of VUR, noncompliance with medical therapy, intolerance to antibiotics, and VUR after puberty in females (Hensle and Burbige, 1986). Antireflux surgery consists of reimplantation of the ureters. Postsurgical antibiotic therapy is continued until a voiding cystourethrogram demonstrates no further VUR. Postoperative excretory urograms are performed before discharge, at 3 months, at 1 year, and 3 years after surgery to assess renal growth. Accelerated renal growth is observed in some children after surgery.

Nursing Considerations

The primary nursing goal for children in medical therapy is encouraging compliance. The importance of maintaining the medical regimen should be emphasized to parents and older

---

VESICOURETERAL REFLUX GRADING SYSTEM

Grade I: VUR into the lower ureter only
Grade II: Ureteral and pelvic filling without calyceal dilation
Grade III: Ureteral and pelvic filling with mild calyceal blunting
Grade IV: Marked distention of pelvis, calyces, and ureter
Grade V: Massive VUR associated with severe hydronephrosis

---

children. The medications prescribed are usually well tolerated by children but parents may need help in encouraging children to take the medication. The methods described in Chapter 27 provide some guidelines for administration and encouraging compliance. The importance of hygiene and a frequent voiding schedule is also discussed.

NEPHROTIC SYNDROME

Nephrotic syndrome is the most common presentation of glomerular injury in children. It is defined as massive proteinuria, hypoalbuminemia, hyperlipemia, and edema, but the disorder is a clinical manifestation of a large number of distinct glomerular disorders in which increased glomerular permeability to plasma protein results in massive urinary protein loss. Following a description of the three major forms of nephrotic syndrome, the remainder of the discussion is devoted to minimal change disease.

Types of Nephrotic Syndrome

Nephrotic syndrome can be classified as *primary,* when the syndrome is restricted to glomerular injury, or *secondary*, when it develops as part of a systemic illness. Although it may have several different histologic variations, the most descriptive term for the primary disease is *minimal change nephrotic syndrome*. A congenital form is also recognized.

Minimal change nephrotic syndrome (MCNS). Approximately 80% of cases of nephrotic syndrome in children occur in the absence of recognizable systemic disease or preexisting renal disease and are categorized as idiopathic. MCNS can present at any age but is predominantly a disease of the preschool child. In 74% of children, the onset of the disease occurs between the ages of 2 and 7 years (McEnery and Strife, 1982). The disease is rare in children younger than 6 months of age, uncommon in infants younger than 1 year of age, and unusual after the age of 8. The incidence of the disease in North America is approximately 2:100,000 children per year and males outnumber females 2:1 (Drummond, 1983). In adolescence the ratio is 1:1.

The cause of minimal change nephrotic syndrome (also known as idiopathic nephrosis, "minimal lesion" nephrosis, childhood nephrosis, lipoid nephrosis, or uncomplicated nephrosis) remains obscure. Often a nonspecific illness, usually a viral upper respiratory infection, precedes the manifestations by 4 to 8 days but is considered to be a precipitating factor rather than a cause. Familial or genetic factors are found in a few cases and HLA antigen B12 is said to be more common in these children than in the general population (Drummond, 1983).

Secondary nephrotic syndrome. Nephrotic syndrome may occur after or in association with glomerular damage of known or presumed etiology. Prominent among causes of glomerular damage is acute or chronic glomerulonephritis. Less commonly, secondary nephrotic syndrome occurs during the course of collagen diseases (such as disseminated lupus erythematosus and anaphylactoid purpura) or as the result of toxicity to drugs (such as trimethadione and heavy metals), stings, or venom. Diverse, rare causes are sickle cell disease, malaria, cyanotic heart disease, diabetes mellitus, amyloidosis, tuberculosis, infected ventriculojugular shunts, renal vein thrombosis, or malignancies.

Congenital nephrotic syndrome. The hereditary form of nephrotic syndrome is caused by a recessive gene on an autosome. Infants who have nephrotic syndrome are small for gestational age, and proteinuria and edema are manifest early. The disease does not respond to the usual therapy, and death in the first year or two of life is the rule. Renal transplant in the newborn periods has been attempted with a few successes.

Pathophysiology

The pathogenesis of this disorder is not understood. There may be a metabolic, biochemical, or physicochemical disturbance in the basement membrane of the glomeruli that leads to increased permeability to protein, but the causes and mechanisms are only speculative.

The glomerular membrane, which is normally impermeable to albumin and other large proteins, becomes permeable to proteins, especially albumin, which leak through the membrane and are lost in urine (hyperalbuminuria). This reduces the serum albumin level (hypoalbuminemia), which decreases the colloidal osmotic pressure in the capillaries. As a result, the hydrostatic pressure exceeds the pull of the colloidal osmotic pressure and fluid accumulates in the interstitial spaces and body cavities, particularly the abdominal cavity (ascites). The shift of fluid from the plasma to the interstitial spaces reduces the vascular fluid volume (hypovolemia), which in turn stimulates the renin-angiotensin system and the secretion of antidiuretic hormone and aldosterone. Tubular reabsorption of sodium and water are increased in an attempt to increase intravascular volume. The elevation of serum cholesterol, phospholipids, and triglycerides is unexplained. The sequence of events in nephrotic syndrome is diagrammed in Fig. 30-3.

Clinical Manifestations

A previously well child begins to gain weight, which progresses insidiously over a period of days or weeks. Puffiness of the face, especially around the eyes, is apparent on arising in the morning but subsides during the day, when swelling of the abdomen and lower extremities is more prominent. The generalized edema develops so slowly that parents may consider it to be a sign of healthy growth. Although an acute infection may precipitate severe generalized edema (*anasarca*), the usual course is one of progressive weight gain until either rapid or gradual increase in edema prompts the family to seek medical evaluation. Usually present are abdominal swelling from ascites, respiratory difficulty from pleural effusion, and labial or scrotal swelling (Fig. 30-4). Edema of the intestinal mucosa may cause diarrhea, loss of appetite, and poor intestinal absorption. The volume of urine is decreased, and it appears darkly opalescent and frothy. Neurologic examinations are negative, and the sensorium is clear.

Extreme skin pallor is often present, and the child has a tendency toward skin breakdown during periods of edema. The child is irritable and may be easily fatigued or lethargic but does not appear seriously ill. Malnutrition from poor appetite and loss of protein is not uncommon, although it is frequently obscured by edema. However, changes in the quality of the hair give evidence of the malnourished state. The blood pressure is usually normal or slightly decreased. The child is more susceptible to infection, especially cellulitis, pneumonia, peritonitis, or septicemia.

In children who have minimal change nephrotic syndrome, there may be an absence of significant or persistent hypertension, gross or persistent hematuria, significant or persistent azotemia (presence of increased nitrogenous products in the blood), as well as depression of serum $\beta 1_c$ globulin.

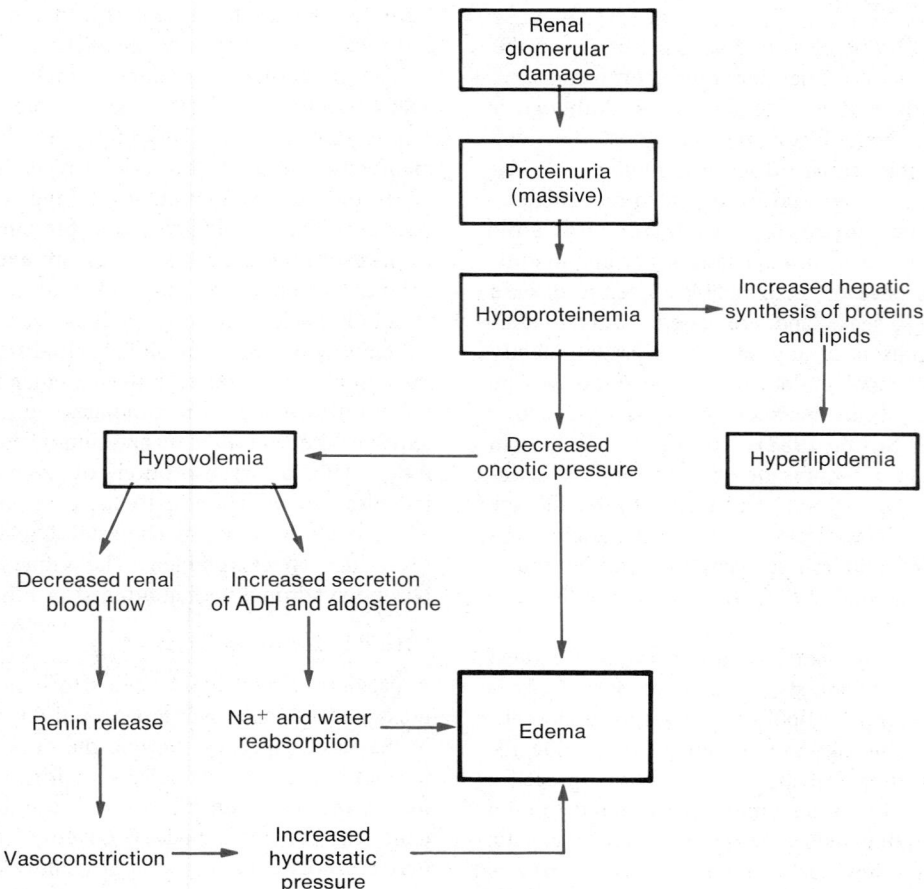

Fig. 30-3. Sequence of events in nephrotic syndrome.

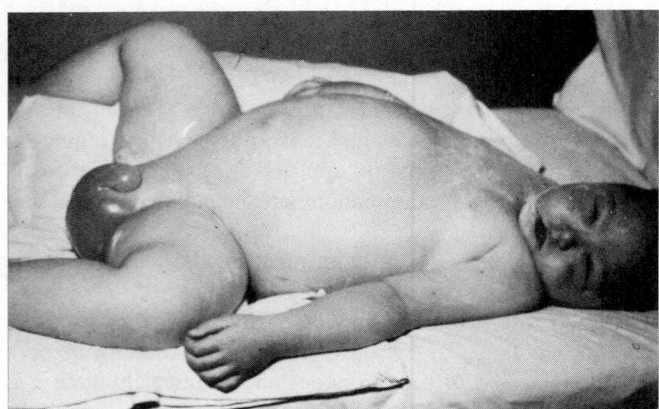

Fig. 30-4. Two-year-old child with nephrosis.

From Shirkey, H.C., editor: Pediatric therapy, ed. 6, St. Louis, 1980, The C.V. Mosby Co.

Diagnostic Evaluation

The diagnosis is made on the basis of remarkably consistent history, typical clinical manifestations, and proteinemia. Massive proteinuria is reflected in urine excretion of protein that frequently reaches levels in excess of 2 g/m²/day of body surface with relatively greater clearance of low molec-

ular weight proteins. Hyaline casts from high protein and sluggish flow and oval fat bodies, as well as a few red blood cells, can be found in the urine of most affected children although there is seldom gross hematuria. Specific gravity is high and proportionate to the amount of protein concentration. If hypovolemia is not significant and the child is well hydrated, the glomerular filtration rate is usually normal.

Total serum protein concentrations are reduced, with the albumin fractions significantly reduced (less than 2 g/dl) and elevation of α_2 globulins and plasma lipids. Serum cholesterol may be as high as 450 to 1500 mg/dl. Hemoglobin and hematocrit are usually normal or even elevated as a result of hemoconcentration. Serum sodium concentration is usually low, about 130 to 135 mEq/L.

Renal biopsy and the appearance of renal tissue under the light and electron microscope provide information regarding the glomerular status and type of nephrotic syndrome, response to drugs, and probable course of the disease. Under the microscope the foot processes of the basement membrane appear fused. The major focuses in differential diagnosis are to establish the edema as renal in origin and to distinguish minimum change nephrotic syndrome from other glomerulopathies with nephrotic syndrome as a manifestation.

Therapeutic Management

The medical management consists of both general and specific measures. The primary objective is to reduce the excretion of urinary protein and maintain a protein-free urine. Additional objectives include prevention or treatment of acute infection, control of edema, establishment of good nutrition, and readjustment of any disturbed metabolic processes. Children with severe symptoms or whose disease is newly recognized are hospitalized for assessment and observation for evidence of infection and response to therapy.

General measures. General treatment is principally supportive. During the edema phase the child is often placed on bed rest, but activity is not restricted during remission. Children can be remarkably active with no evidence that restriction affects the ultimate outcome. Acute and intercurrent infections are treated with appropriate antibiotics, and efforts are made to eliminate possible infection.

Diet. The child who is in remission is allowed a regular diet; however, during periods of massive edema, salt is restricted in the form of no added salt at the table and excluding foods with very high salt content. This is usually tolerated by the child for a time, but it should be adjusted to the child's appetite and must not interfere with nutrient intake. Although edema cannot be removed by a low-sodium diet, its rate of increase may be reduced. Water is seldom restricted. A diet generous in protein is logical but there is no evidence that it is beneficial or alters the outcome of the disease (Kim and Grupe, 1986). The presence of azotemia and renal failure is a contraindication for high-protein intake.

Corticosteroid therapy. The response of most affected children to corticosteroids has established these drugs as prime therapeutic agents in management of nephrotic syndrome. Corticosteroid therapy is begun as soon as the diagnosis has been determined and administered orally in a dosage of 2 mg/kg of body weight or 60 mg/m^2/day in evenly divided doses. Prednisone, the safest and least expensive drug, is the steroid of choice. The drug is continued until the urine is free from protein and remains normal for 10 days to 2 weeks (Drummond, 1983).

The course of the disease is fairly predictable. There is little change during the first few days of therapy. In most patients diuresis occurs, urine protein excretion disappears within 7 to 21 days, and other clinical manifestations stabilize or return to normal. Almost 95% of patients between 1 and 10 years of age with no hypertension, hematuria, or renal insufficiency and whose laboratory measurements of C3 complement and a renal clearance of IgG less than 10% of the renal clearance of transferrin will have complete resolution of proteinuria with therapy (Kim and Grupe, 1986). In 90% of cases protein excretion returns to normal within 4 weeks with an average response time of 10 days (Drummond, 1983).

If the child has not responded to therapy in 28 days of daily administration, the likelihood of subsequent response diminishes rapidly. When the child is free of proteinuria and

edema, the daily dose is usually increased one and one half to two times and the medication is given as a single dose every 48 hours for a time. It is then gradually tapered to discontinuation over a variable period, from several days to weeks or months, depending on the philosophy of the physician. When the larger single dose is given intermittently, it is less likely to depress the pituitary-adrenal function and fewer side effects are produced during prolonged therapy. If a tendency to relapse is demonstrated, the number of relapses can be reduced by an interrupted schedule of prednisone therapy that continues for 6 months to 1 year, as measured from the initial daily dose.

Children with nephrotic syndrome are often described according to their response to corticosteroid therapy: (1) 20% to 40% of children are "steroid-sensitive" and have little tendency to recurrence after a single course of therapy; (2) 60% to 80% are "steroid-dependent" and respond well to steroid therapy, but their course is dominated by intermittent exacerbations and remissions over several years before they clear completely and lose the tendency to active disease (relapses are defined as three or more relapses within a year); and (3) less than 5% are "steroid-resistant," or are resistant to steroids at some stage and eventually go on to chronic renal failure. There is some evidence that relapse may be related to prolonged postprednisone adrenocortical suppression (Leisti and Koskimies, 1983). It has been suggested that long remissions can be maintained in some patients by long-term administration of low doses of hydrocortisone, which supplements impaired adrenal corticosteroid production (Schoeneman, 1983).

Children who require frequent courses of steroid therapy are highly susceptible to complications of steroids, such as growth retardation, hypertension, gastrointestinal bleeding, Cushing syndrome, bone demineralization, infections, and diabetes mellitus. Children who do not respond to steroid therapy, those who have frequent relapses, and those in whom the side effects threaten their growth and general health are considered for a course of immunosuppressant drug therapy.

Immunosuppressant therapy. It is often possible to reduce the relapse rate and induce long-term remission with administration of an oral alkylating agent, usually cyclophosphamide (Cytoxan), alternating with prednisone. Both drugs are administered for up to 2 months, after which cyclophosphamide is discontinued abruptly and the prednisone is decreased by decrements. Chlorambucil has also proven effective when given with corticosteroids. The two drugs share many characteristics and response to both appears to depend on dose, duration of therapy, age, and the duration of the disease.

There are significant side effects of cyclophosphamide that must be considered and discussed with parents of children for whom this drug is contemplated. Leukopenia and alopecia, although uncommon in the recommended dosage, must be anticipated, and evidence suggests that cyclophosphamide may cause azoospermia with sterility in males treated for more than 2 to 3 months and variable effects on gonadal function in females.

Diuretics. One characteristic of the edema of nephrotic syndrome is its usual lack of responsiveness to diuretic agents. However, in cases in which edema interferes with respiration or there is hypotension, hyponatremia, or evidence of skin breakdown, loop diuretics are sometimes useful, usually spironolactone in combination with hydrochlorothiazide. Furosemide may be given but its potent diuretic effect may induce hypovolemic shock from massive diuresis. In addition, plasma expanders such as salt-poor human albumin may be administered to severely edematous children requiring prompt control; however, they must be administered frequently, since the glomeruli are readily permeable to albumin in the acute stage.

Antimicrobials. The increased susceptibility to infection during the edematous phase of the disease and the lowered resistance associated with corticosteroid therapy are a constant hazard of nephrotic syndrome. Therefore a broad-spectrum antimicrobial agent is often administered in an effort to reduce the risk of infection until the initial phase of treatment is completed and the child is receiving reduced dosages of corticosteroids.

Prognosis. The prognosis for ultimate recovery in most cases is good. It is a self-limiting disease and in children who respond to steroid therapy, the tendency to relapse decreases with time. With early detection and prompt implementation of therapy to eradicate proteinuria, progressive basement membrane damage is minimized so that when the tendency to exacerbations is past, renal function is usually normal or near normal. It is estimated that approximately 80% of nephrotic children have this favorable prognosis, although half the children have relapses even after 5 years and 20% after 10 years (Kim and Grupe, 1986).

Nursing Considerations

Children hospitalized with nephrotic syndrome are placed on bed rest during the edema phase of the disease. They seldom offer resistance, since they are usually lethargic and easily fatigued and their cumbersome edematous bulk is not conducive to movement. Most are content to lie in the prone position. These children must be encouraged and helped to turn regularly to prevent tissue breakdown. Areas that are particularly edematous, such as the scrotum, abdomen, and legs, may require support, and skin surfaces should be cleaned and separated with clothing, cotton, or antiseptic powder to prevent intertrigo.

Infection is a constant source of danger to edematous children and those in corticosteroid therapy. These children are particularly vulnerable to upper respiratory infection; therefore, they must be kept warm and dry, turned frequently, and protected from contact with infected roommates, visitors, and personnel. Vital signs are monitored to detect any early signs of an infective process.

Continuous monitoring of fluid retention or excretion is an important nursing function. Strictly accurate records of intake and output are essential but may be difficult in very young children. Application of collection bags is highly irritating to edematous, sensitive skin, already subject to breakdown. Application of diapers or weighing wet pads may be necessary, or sometimes estimating the size of the wet area may be allowed. If so, it is wise to pour a measured amount of water on a similar pad as a comparison. Other methods of monitoring progress include urine examination for specific gravity and albumin, daily weight, and measurement of abdominal girth. Assessment of edema such as increased or decreased swelling around eyes and dependent areas, degree of pitting (if noted), and color and texture of skin are part of nursing care.

The loss of appetite that accompanies active nephrosis creates a perplexing problem for nurses. During this time the combined efforts of nurse, dietitian, parents, and the child himself are needed to formulate a nutritionally adequate and attractive diet. Salt is usually restricted, but not eliminated, during the edema phase. A generous protein intake is highly desirable to minimize negative nitrogen balance but is poorly accepted by most children. Fluid restriction is limited to short-term use during massive edema. Every effort should be made to serve attractive meals with a minimum of fuss, but it usually requires a considerable amount of ingenuity and enticement to get the child to eat. Games, rewards, and special treats often help, but each child is unique, and it may require considerable trial and error to arrive at a successful strategy. Also, the same strategy may not work consistently (see Feeding the sick child, p. 1115).

As the edema subsides, children are allowed increased activity. Although they are easily fatigued, they are usually able to adjust activities according to their individual tolerance but may require guidance in selection of play activities. Suitable recreational and diversional activities are an important part of their care. Once edema fluid has been lost, children are allowed to resume their usual activities with discretion. Irritability and mood swings accompanying the inactivity, disease process, and steroid therapy are not unusual manifestations in these children, which create an additional challenge to the nurse and the family.

Family Support and Home Care

Many children are treated at home during exacerbations. Parents are taught to detect signs of relapse and to bring the child for treatment at the earliest indications. Unless the edema and proteinuria are severe or the parents, for some reason, are unable to care for the ill child, home care is preferred. Parents are instructed in testing urine for albumin, administration of medications, and general care. Salt is restricted to no additional salt during relapse, but a regular diet is suitable for the child in remission. Parents are instructed regarding avoiding contact with infected playmates, but the child is permitted to attend school. It is important for parents of children in corticosteroid therapy to be aware of the common side effects of steroid therapy,

Nursing Care Summary: The Child with Nephrotic Syndrome

	NURSING GOALS	NURSING INTERVENTIONS	EXPECTED PATIENT/FAMILY OUTCOME
N/D	**HP-HMP** Infection: potential for Risk factors: lowered body defenses		
	Prevent and control acute infection	Protect child from contact with infected persons Observe medical asepsis Keep child dry and warm Monitor vital signs for early signs of infectious processes Collect specimens, such as urine for culture, blood	Child displays no evidence of infection
N/D	**N-MP** Fluid volume, alteration in: deficit (intravascular) Etiology: protein and fluid loss, edema		
	Detect evidence of intravascular fluid loss	Monitor vital signs to detect physical signs Assess pulse quality and rate Take blood pressure Report deviations	Child displays no evidence of hypovolemic shock *Deviations from baseline findings are detected and appropriate interventions are initiated (specify parameters) (see inside front cover for normal variations in vital signs)
N/D	**N-MP** Fluid volume, alteration in: excess (total body) Etiology: impaired renal excretion of water		

	Detect evidence of fluid retention	Assess intake relative to output
		  Measure and record intake and output accurately
		  Weigh daily (or more often if needed)
		Assess changes in edema
		  Measure abdominal girth at umbilicus
		  Test urine for specific gravity, albumin
		  Collect specimens for laboratory examination
			*Child's intake and output are recorded and evaluated
			Child exhibits no evidence of increased edema (specify parameters)

	Prevent fluid retention	Limit fluids as indicated	Child displays no evidence of increased fluid accumulation (specify parameters)
N/D	**N-MP** Nutrition, alteration in: less than body requirements Etiology: loss of appetite		
	Provide good nutrition Stimulate appetite	Offer high-protein, high-carbohydrate diet (restrict sodium during edema) Enlist aid of child, parents, and dietitian in formulation of diet Provide cheerful, clean, relaxed atmosphere during meals Serve small quantities initially to stimulate appetite; encourage seconds Provide special and preferred foods Serve foods in an attractive manner (see p. 1115 for feeding the sick child)	Child consumes an adequate diet (specify amounts)
N/D	**N-MP** Skin integrity, impairment of: potential Risk factors: edema, lowered body defenses		
	Prevent skin breakdown	Provide meticulous skin care Cleanse and powder opposing skin surfaces several times per day Separate opposing skin surfaces with soft cotton Support edematous organs, such as scrotum Cleanse edematous eyelids with warm saline wipes Change position frequently; maintain good body alignment	Child displays no evidence of redness or irritation

*Nursing outcome.

Continued.

Nursing Care Summary: The Child with Nephrotic Syndrome—cont'd

NURSING GOALS	NURSING INTERVENTIONS	EXPECTED PATIENT/FAMILY OUTCOME
A-EP Activity intolerance **Etiology: bed rest, fatigue**		
Conserve energy	Maintain bed rest initially Balance rest and activity when ambulatory Plan and provide quiet activities Instruct child to rest when he begins to feel tired	Child engages in activities appropriate to his capabilities
SP-SCP Self-concept, disturbance in: body image **Etiology: change in appearance**		
Establish good mental hygiene	Encourage activity within limits of tolerance Encourage socialization with persons without active infection Provide positive feedback Explore areas of interest and encourage their pursuit	Child discusses his feelings and concerns Child engages in activities appropriate to his interests and capabilities
RRP Family process, alteration in **Etiology: situational crisis (child with a serious illness)**		
Support family	Listen to family Assist family with problem solving Provide education when indicated Provide positive feedback Refer to parent groups See also The child in the hospital, p. 1075; Family of the hospitalized child, p. 1081	Family members discuss their feelings and anxieties

Prepare for home care	Instruct family
	   Testing urine for albumin daily
	   Administration of medications
	   Initial signs of relapse
	   Side effects of drugs
	   Prevention of infection
	 Impress on family importance of following prescribed regimen
		Family conveys an understanding of the instructions; repeats instructions; demonstrates procedures

Continue follow-up care	Maintain contact with family Refer to appropriate persons or agencies for assistance	Family complies with instructions

Nursing Interventions Related to Medical Management

Assist with diagnosis
  Collect specimens as needed
  Assist with diagnostic procedures
Control edema
  Provide salt-restricted diet
  Administer steroids and diuretics, if ordered

Administer salt-poor albumin intravenous infusion if
  ordered
Limit intake, if ordered
Ensure adequate nutrition
  Administer supplementary vitamins and iron as or-
  dered

such as rounding of the face, increased appetite, abdominal distention, and hirsutism, and to distinguish some of these from the edema formation of the disease. They should be reassured that the symptoms will disappear gradually after discontinuation of the drug. The child should receive close medical and/or nursing observation to detect unusual but more serious side effects.

The prolonged course of the relapsing form of nephrotic syndrome is taxing to both the child and the family. The up-and-down course of remissions and exacerbations with periodic disruption of family life by hospitalization places a severe strain on the child and the family, both psychologically and financially. Parents and children over 5 or 6 years of age need reassurance regarding this characteristic of the course of the disease so that they will not become discouraged with the frequent relapses. At the same time it is im-

Table 30-4   Childhood glomerulonephritis: some clinical forms and characteristics

TYPE	ETIOLOGY	MICROSCOPIC CHANGES	MAJOR CLINICAL MANIFESTATIONS
Acute poststreptococcal	Antecedent group A hemolytic streptococcal infection	Diffuse, proliferative neutrophil exudation	Edema Hypertension Hematuria Proteinuria
Rapidly progressive	Unknown	Diffuse Glomerular necrosis Epithelial crescents in more than 80% of glomeruli	Oliguria and/or anuria Azotemia Acute nephrotic syndrome or progressive renal failure
Proliferative	Unknown; occasional streptococcal infection	Diffuse, proliferative Hypercellularity	Variable manifestations
Membranoproliferative	Unknown; sometimes with lipodystrophy	Diffuse Glomerular enlargement Basement membrane thickening Histologically, three clinical groups: types I, II, and III	Nephrotic syndrome Occasional hypertension
Focal segmented	Unknown	Focal or segmented glomerulosclerosis Hypercellularity	Nephrotic syndrome Hematuria
Focal segmented proliferative	Unknown	Focal, proliferative	Hematuria
Childhood nephrosis; minimal change nephrotic syndrome	Unknown	Foot process fusion	Nephrotic syndrome

portant to impress on them the importance of long-term care to gain their cooperation. A satisfactory response is more likely when relapses are detected and therapy is instituted early, and remissions are prolonged when instructions are carried out faithfully. For example, one child had an exacerbation when his mother reduced the dosage of his drug because it was so expensive.

Social isolation is a concomitant problem for these children. Isolation is related to frequent hospitalization or confinement during relapse, the risk of infection that may precipitate an exacerbation, lack of energy, and the child's reluctance to face friends at home or school because of the changes in his appearance resulting from the disease or the medication. Both parents and child need someone to listen to their complaints, to assist them to cope with both short-term and long-term problems associated with the disease, and to find solutions to their problems. Continuous support of the child and family is one of the major nursing considerations.

ACUTE GLOMERULONEPHRITIS

Acute glomerulonephritis (AGN) as a classification includes a number of distinct entities (Table 30-4). It may be a primary event or a manifestation of a systemic disorder (Table 30-5), and the disease can range from minimal to severe. The common features include oliguria, edema, hypertension and circulatory congestion, hematuria, and proteinuria. Most are postinfectious and have been associated with pneu-

mococcal, streptococcal, and viral infections. All postinfectious diseases are presumed to result from immune complex formation and glomerular deposition, and the clinical presentations may be indistinguishable.

Acute poststreptococcal glomerulonephritis (APSGN) is the most common of the noninfectious renal diseases in childhood and the one for which a cause can be established in the majority of cases. APSGN can occur at any age but affects primarily early school-age children with a peak age of onset of 6 to 7 years. It is uncommon in children younger than 2 years of age, and males outnumber females 2:1 (Jordan and Lemire, 1982).

Etiology

It is now generally accepted that APSGN is an immune-complex disease, that is, a reaction that occurs as a by-product of an antecedent streptococcal infection with certain strains of the group A β-hemolytic *Streptococcus*. Most streptococcal infections do not cause APSGN. The development of the disease follows a limited number of subtypes, principally types 4, 12, and 49, and the clinical pattern of the disease is the same whether the disease is associated with type 12 or type 49 pharyngitis, which produces the skin disease, impetigo. There is a latent period of 10 to 14 days between the streptococcal infection and the onset of clinical manifestations. The peak incidence of disease corresponds to the incidence of streptococcal infections. Disease secondary to streptococcal pharyngitis is more common in the winter or spring, but, when associated with pyoderma

Table 30-5 Renal involvement associated with a systemic disease process

DISEASE	MECHANISM	RENAL MANIFESTATION	COMMENTS
Systemic lupus erythematosus (SLE)	Deposition of autoantibody-antigen complexes in kidney	Variable degrees of hematuria and proteinuria More severe—nephrotic syndrome, hypertension, renal insufficiency	Responsive to corticosteroid and antimetabolite therapy Renal failure most common cause of death from SLE Rare before adolescence but may occur in school-age children
Anaphylactoid (Henoch-Schönlein) purpura	Unknown	Hematuria (gross or microscopic) Less common—edema, hypertension Nephrotic syndrome with oliguria and hypertension indicates severe involvement Rarely—acute renal failure	Incidence from 20% to 70% of cases Renal involvement most serious manifestation of the disease More common in children over age 6 years Responsive to corticosteroid therapy Management similar to that for persistent glomerulonephritis
Sickle cell disease	Infarction of renal vessels by sickled cells (especially medullary) Results in decreased circulation in vasa recta and impaired sodium and chloride ion reabsorption in collecting ducts	Hematuria Nephrotic syndrome Defective urine collection Progressive glomerulonephritis	Irreversible with increasing age Severe urinary tract infections with bacteremia not uncommon
Polyarteritis nodosa	Fibroid necrosis of arterial walls Large vessels—patchy renal infarction Microscopic vessels—necrotizing glomerulitis	Proteinuria Hematuria Severe hypertension	Kidney involvement of secondary importance in infancy Variable course Long-term prognosis guarded
Bacterial endocarditis	Focal or diffuse, immune-complex deposition related to chronic bacteremia Some embolization of glomeruli by bacteria and fibrin from endocardial vegetations	Proteinuria Hematuria	Seen in about 50% of cases Renal involvement seldom of major significance
Prolonged bacteremia (infected atrioventricular shunts)	Immune-complex deposition with exudation and cellular proliferation	Variable degrees of persistent nephrotic syndrome	Vigorous antibiotic therapy and/or removal of infected shunt required

(principally impetigo), it may be more prevalent in later summer or early fall, especially in warmer climates. Multiple cases tend to occur in families. Second attacks are rare.

Pathophysiology

The mechanism by which the reaction takes place is still speculative. The most popular proposal to explain the pathologic process is that the streptococcal infection is followed by the release of a membranelike material from the specific organism into the circulation. Because it is antigenic, antibody is formed, and, after the appropriate period of time, an immune-complex reaction occurs. These immune complexes become trapped in the glomerular capillary loop, much the same as experimental serum sickness.

The kidney itself appears normal or moderately enlarged, but microscopic examination reveals a diffuse proliferative and exudative process. Glomerular capillary loops are almost obliterated by swelling, and infiltration with polymorphonuclear leukocytes adds to the appearance of increased cellularity. Consequently, the glomeruli appear dense and bloodless. Further examination reveals discrete nodules or "humps" on the basement membrane, which are identified

COMPARISON OF POSTSTREPTOCOCCAL GLOMERULONEPHRITIS AND NEPHROTIC SYNDROME

Manifestations	Acute poststreptococcal glomerulonephritis	Minimal change nephrotic syndrome
Streptococcal antibody titers	Present	Absent
Blood pressure	Elevated	Normal or decreased
Edema	Primarily periorbital and peripheral	Generalized severe
Circulatory congestion	Common	Absent
Proteinuria	Moderate	Massive
Hematuria	Gross or microscopic	Microscopic or none
Casts	Present	Present
Azotemia	Present	Absent
Serum potassium levels	Increased	Normal
Serum protein levels	Minimum reduction	Markedly decreased
Serum lipid levels	Normal	Elevated
Fatigue	Present	Present
Age at onset (years)	5-7	2-3

as deposits of immune complexes. These deposits are not evident after about 6 weeks.

Endothelial cell proliferation and edema occlude the capillary lumen of affected glomeruli, and the afferent arteriole is probably constricted by vasospasm, both of which significantly reduce the glomerular filtration rate. This occurs without a proportional decrease in renal blood flow and results in a reduced capacity to form filtrate from the glomerular plasma flow. Vascular and tubular changes are mild and nonspecific; tubular function is less severely impaired.

The decreased filtration of plasma results in an excessive accumulation of water and an avid retention of sodium. These cause expanded plasma and interstitial fluid volumes that lead to circulatory congestion and edema. It is unclear whether the decreased glomerular filtration rate, increased capillary permeability, or vascular spasm is responsible for these various manifestations. The cause of the hypertension associated with acute glomerulonephritis is also unexplained. Plasma renin activity is low during the acute phase, but the hypervolemia may be a factor.

Clinical Manifestations

Typically, affected children are in good health until they experience the antecedent infection. In some instances there is no history of an infection, or it is only described as a mild cold. The onset of nephritis appears after an average latent period of about 10 days. Since the child appears well during this time, the association is not recognized by parents.

Initial signs of nephrotic reaction include puffiness of the face, especially around the eyes (periorbital edema), anorexia, and passage of dark-colored urine. The edema is more prominent in the face in the morning but spreads during the day to involve the extremities and abdomen. The edema is only moderate and may not be appreciated by someone unfamiliar with the child's normal appearance.

The urine is cloudy, smoky brown, or what parents describe as resembling tea or cola, and severely reduced in volume.

The child is pale, irritable, and lethargic. He appears unwell but seldom expresses specific complaints. Older children may complain of headaches, abdominal discomfort, and dysuria. Vomiting is not uncommon. On examination there is usually a mild to moderate elevation in blood pressure (diastolic, 80 to 120 mm Hg; systolic, 120 to 180 mm Hg). Occasionally a child will have an atypical mode of onset with severe symptoms such as convulsions (secondary to cerebral ischemia and/or hypertension), pulmonary and circulatory congestion, minimal urine findings, or hematuria in the absence of hypertension and edema. For a comparison between APSGN and MCNS see the box above.

Clinical course. The acute edematous phase of glomerulonephritis usually persists from 4 to 10 days but may persist for 2 or 3 weeks, during which time the child remains listless, anorexic, and apathetic. The weight fluctuates, the urine remains thick and smoky brown in color, and the blood pressure may suddenly reach dangerously high levels at any time during this phase.

The first sign of improvement is a small increase in urine output with a corresponding decrease in body weight, followed in 1 or 2 days by copious diuresis. With diuresis the child begins to feel better, the appetite improves, and the blood pressure decreases to normal with the reduction of edema. Gross hematuria diminishes, in part because of dilution of the red blood cells in the more dilute urine, but microscopic hematuria may persist for weeks or months. The blood urea nitrogen level decreases during diuresis, but it, along with a slight to moderate proteinuria, may persist for several weeks.

Almost all children correctly diagnosed as having APSGN recover completely, and specific immunity is conferred so that subsequent recurrences are uncommon. Deaths from complications still occur but are, fortunately, rare. A few of these children may develop chronic disease, but many of these cases are believed to be probably different glomerular diseases misdiagnosed as poststreptococcal disease.

Complications. The major complications that may develop during the acute phase of glomerulonephritis are hypertensive encephalopathy, acute cardiac decompensation, and acute renal failure. Normally cerebral blood flow responds to acute arterial hypertension by vasoconstriction. However, acute and severe hypertension may cause this protective autoregulation of cerebral blood flow to fail, leading to hyperperfusion of the brain and cerebral edema. The premonitory signs of encephalopathy are headache, dizziness, abdominal discomfort, and vomiting. If the condition progresses there may be transient loss of vision and/or hemiparesis, disorientation, and generalized convulsions of the grand mal type.

Cardiac decompensation during the acute edematous phase of nephritis is caused by hypervolemia and not by cardiac failure. Signs of circulatory congestion are evident, however. The heart is enlarged, and increased pulmonary vascular markings are evident on roentgenographic examination. Increased pulmonary capillary permeability is also believed to be an important factor in the development of pulmonary edema.

Acute renal failure with persistent oliguria or anuria is an uncommon complication but one that requires an appropriate treatment regimen.

Diagnostic Evaluation

Urinalysis during the acute phase characteristically shows hematuria, proteinuria, and increased specific gravity. The specific gravity is moderately elevated and seldom exceeds 1.020. Proteinuria generally parallels the hematuria, and the content usually shows 3+ or 4+ but is not the massive proteinuria seen in nephrotic syndrome. Gross discoloration of urine reflects its red blood cell and hemoglobin content. Microscopic examination of the sediment shows many red blood cells, leukocytes, epithelial cells, and casts, primarily composed of epithelial and red blood cells. Bacteria are not seen, and urine cultures are negative.

Blood examination reveals normal electrolytes (sodium, potassium, and chloride ions) and carbon dioxide levels, unless the disease has progressed to renal failure. Azotemia resulting from impaired glomerular filtration is reflected in elevated blood urea nitrogen and creatinine levels in at least 50% of cases. When proteinuria is heavy, there may be changes associated with nephrotic syndrome, that is, transient hypoproteinemia and hyperlipidemia.

Cultures of the pharynx are positive for streptococci in only a few cases, and the numbers are not significantly greater than the normal carrier incidence in many communities. Positive cultures help to establish a diagnosis. Cultures should be obtained from other household members, and persons positive for group A streptococci should receive a course of antistreptococcal therapy.

Some serologic tests may help in diagnosis. Antibody responses to the extracellular products of the streptococcus provide indirect evidence of previous streptococcal infection. These include antistreptolysin-O (ASO), antistreptokinase (ASKase), antihyaluronidase (AHase), antideoxyribonuclease-B (ADNase-B), and antinicotyladenine dinucleotidase (ANADase). The ASO titer is the most familiar and readily available test for streptococcal antibodies. ASO appears in the serum about 10 days after the initial infection and persists for 4 to 6 weeks; however there is no correlation between the degree of elevation and its duration and the severity or prognosis of the glomerulonephritis. It is a useful diagnostic tool when nephritis follows a pharyngeal infection but is of less value after pyoderma. An ASO titer of 250 Todd units or higher is of diagnostic significance, as is a rising titer in two samples taken a week apart. More consistent and reliable antibody tests following streptococcal skin infections are elevated AHase and ADNase-B titers.

Nonspecific acute-phase reactants that reflect acute inflammatory processes, such as the erythrocyte sedimentation rate (ESR), C-reactive protein (CRP), and serum mucoprotein tests are elevated during the early stages of acute disease and then gradually return to normal as healing takes place. The ESR is sometimes used as a guide to the progress of the nephritis.

Since glomerulonephritis is an immune-complex disease, there is reduced total serum complement activity in the early stages of acute disease. The simpler measurements of the C3 complement component (β_1 globulin) is used as an index of total complement activity. The test is most useful in children with no edema or minimal urine findings.

Other studies that are employed include a chest x-ray examination, which shows characteristic generalized cardiac enlargement, pulmonary congestion, and pleural effusion during the edematous phase of acute disease. Electrocardiography reveals elevation or depression of the ST segment, prolonged QRS and ST segments, lengthening of the P-R interval, and flattened or inverted T waves. Renal biopsy for diagnostic purposes is seldom required but may be useful in the diagnosis of atypical cases.

Correlations between laboratory and morphologic findings indicate a significant relationship between creatinine clearance and severity of glomerular damage. Greater damage is reflected in a reduced creatinine clearance and is also associated with a higher blood urea nitrogen level. An increased excretion of cellular protein is associated with increasing glomerular capillary obliteration. There appears to be no correlation between the extent of glomerular damage and ASO titer, oliguria, or blood pressure.

Therapeutic Management

There is no specific treatment for acute glomerulonephritis, and recovery is spontaneous and uneventful in most cases. Management consists of general supportive measures and early recognition and treatment of complications. Children who have normal blood pressure and a satisfactory urine output can generally be treated at home. Those with substantial edema, hypertension, gross hematuria, and/or significant oliguria should be hospitalized because of the unpredictability of complications. Short hospitalization is the rule in uncomplicated cases; prolonged hospitalization is required only for children with severely impaired renal function.

General measures. Bed rest is recommended during the acute phase, but ambulation does not seem to have an adverse effect on the course of the disease once the gross hematuria, edema, hypertension, and azotemia have abated. Since they are generally listless and experience fatigue and malaise, most children voluntarily restrict their activities during the most active phase of the disease. After diuresis has occurred, ambulation is allowed for those children without hypertension and gross urine abnormalities. Occasionally a rebound phenomenon, characterized by a transient increase in blood urea nitrogen level, hematuria, and/or proteinuria, may appear after ambulation but does not require resumption of bed rest.

Fluid balance. Regular measurement of vital signs, body weight, and intake and output is essential in order to monitor the progress of the disease and to detect complications that may appear at any time during the course of the disease. A record of daily weight is the most useful means to assess fluid balance and should be kept for children treated at home as well as for those who are hospitalized. Water restriction is seldom necessary unless the output is significantly reduced (less than 2 to 3 dl/24 hours). In these children the water allowed is equivalent to the calculated insensible loss plus the volume of urine excreted. Children on restricted fluids, especially those who are severely edematous or those who have lost weight, should be observed for signs of dehydration.

Diuretics are usually of limited value, since very little sodium reaches the distal tubules as a result of the reduced filtration rate. However, diuretic therapy, usually hydrochlorothiazide, is helpful if significant edema and fluid overload are present, and furosemide has been used with some success in severe cases. Digitalis may be employed sometimes, although there is question regarding its effectiveness in acute nephritis. Rarely children with acute glomerulonephritis develop acute renal failure with oliguria that significantly alters the fluid and electrolyte balance. These children require careful management that may include peritoneal dialysis or hemodialysis.

Loss of glomerular filtration may produce electrolyte imbalances in children with severe forms of PSGN, especially hyperkalemia, acidosis, hypocalcemia, and hyperphosphatemia. Management of these electrolyte disturbances is described under acute renal failure.

Hypertension. Acute hypertension must be anticipated and identified early. Blood pressure measurements are taken every 4 to 6 hours. Significant but not severe hypertension is controlled with hydralazine (Apresoline), usually in conjunction with reserpine or furosemide (Lasix). Oral hydrochlorothiazide is used to control mild hypertension. Seizure activity associated with hypertensive encephalopathy requires anticonvulsant therapy as well as antihypertensive agents (see Renal failure, p. 1282 for management of severe hypertension).

Nutrition. Dietary restrictions depend on the stage and severity of the disease, especially the extent of edema. Regular diet is permitted in uncomplicated cases, but the intake of sodium is usually limited (no salt is added to foods). Moderate sodium restriction is usually instituted for children with hypertension or edema. Severe sodium restriction is not well tolerated by children and may interfere with caloric intake in those children with poor appetites. Foods with substantial amounts of potassium are generally restricted during the period of oliguria. Protein restriction is reserved only for children with severe azotemia resulting from prolonged oliguria. The loss of appetite associated with the disease usually limits the protein intake sufficiently. During the acute stage calories may be restricted to carbohydrates and fats.

Antibiotics. Antibiotic therapy is indicated only for those children with evidence of persistent streptococcal infections. The antibiotics do not alter the course of the disease but are often recommended to prevent transmission of nephritogenic streptococci to other family members (Fish and Fouser, 1986). Authorities are divided in their use of prophylactic antimicrobials for other family members.

Nursing Considerations

Nursing care of the child with glomerulonephritis involves careful assessment of the disease status, with regular monitoring of vital signs (including frequent measurement of blood pressure), fluid balance, and behavior. Vital signs provide clues to the severity of the disease and early signs of complications. They are carefully measured and any abnormalities reported and recorded. The volume and character of urine are noted, and the child is weighed daily. Assessment of the child's appearance for signs of cerebral complications is an important nursing function, since the severity of the acute phase is variable and unpredictable. The child with edema, hypertension, and gross hematuria may be subject to complications, and anticipatory preparations such as seizure precautions and intravenous equipment are included in the nursing care plan.

For most children a regular diet is allowed, but it should contain no added salt. Foods high in sodium and salted treats are eliminated, and parents and friends should be advised not to bring items such as potato chips or pretzels. However, the total amount of salt ingested is usually less than prescribed because of poor appetite. Fluid restriction, if prescribed, is more difficult, and the amount permitted should be evenly divided throughout the waking hours and served in small cups to give the illusion of larger servings. Meal preparation and service require special attention, since the child has a poor appetite and is indifferent to meals during the acute phase. Again, collaboration with parents and the dietitian and special consideration for food preferences facilitate meal planning.

During the acute phase children are generally quite content to lie in bed, but activities should be those that require little expenditure of energy. As they begin to feel better and their symptoms subside, activities should be planned to allow for frequent rest periods and avoidance of fatigue.

Children with mild edema and no hypertension as well as convalescent children being treated at home need follow-up care. Parents are instructed regarding general measures, including activity, diet, and prevention of infection. The children are permitted to be ambulatory but should not attend school or participate in outside games and sports until the risk of complications has passed. Strenuous activity is usually restricted until there is no microscopic evidence of proteinuria or hematuria, which may persist for months. No diet restrictions are imposed, but many parents continue to limit salt intake, "just in case."

Health supervision is continued with weekly, followed by monthly, visits for evaluation and urinalysis. Parent education and support in preparation for discharge and home care include education in home management and the need for follow-up care and health supervision.

CHRONIC OR PROGRESSIVE GLOMERULONEPHRITIS

The majority of cases of renal glomerular disease are acute glomerulonephritis, minimal change nephrotic syndrome, and glomerulonephritis associated with systemic diseases. These pose relatively few problems of diagnosis, and their natural course is fairly predictable. A few cases present a prolonged course and a poor ultimate prognosis. They are a rather heterogeneous group, defined by correlating the clinical manifestations, pathologic conditions, and natural course of the individual diseases.

Persistent glomerulonephritis is used to describe those cases of glomerulonephritis that have no specific histologic picture but that fail to show the rapid recovery expected in acute nephritis. *Chronic glomerulonephritis (CGN)* describes advanced glomerular disease, which includes a variety of different disease processes. *Rapidly progressive glomerulonephritis* is used to describe an acute illness with severe, acute onset resembling acute poststreptococcal glomerulonephritis but that causes rapidly progressive deterioration of renal function in 6 to 12 months.

Pathophysiology

In most cases of CGN immunologic mechanisms can be implicated either through direct attack on the kidney or secondary to the accumulation of immune complexes in the glomerular filter or fibrin deposition from previously damaged glomeruli. Either can contribute to further glomerular damage and can initiate chronic changes in the glomerular structure. In many cases there is no history of an attack of acute glomerular disease. In other cases it may represent one of a succession of exacerbations of a preexisting disease. CGN that is not associated with other diseases may go undetected for years and be relatively asymptomatic until kidney destruction produces marked reduction in renal function. Consequently, the disease is more common in adolescents than in younger children. Renal insufficiency with all its manifestations occurs as the ultimate event.

Clinical Manifestations

The varied clinical manifestations and laboratory findings generally reflect deteriorating renal function. Nephrotic syndrome, with its usual manifestations, frequently develops. Hypertension, edema, proteinuria, cardiac failure, dyspnea, osteodystrophy, and anemia are common manifestations of progressive disease.

Diagnostic Evaluation

Laboratory findings may include proteinuria, with casts and red and white blood cells. Failing renal function is evidenced by elevated blood urea nitrogen, creatinine, and uric acid levels. Electrolyte alterations include metabolic acidosis, decreased sodium from the chronic salt-losing state, elevated potassium, elevated phosphorus, and decreased calcium levels. As the disease progresses, urine specific gravity eventually stabilizes at an isotonic state (about 1.012) as a result of the inability of the kidney to reabsorb solutes or respond to antidiuretic hormone. The renal insufficiency may extend from 5 to 15 years and even longer, or rapid deterioration may cause death in 1 to 2 years.

Therapeutic Management

Early in the course of the disease, treatment is appropriate to the underlying disease and is largely symptomatic in most cases. Efforts are directed toward providing optimal conditions for the child's physical, psychologic, and social development. As few restrictions as feasible are imposed, and the child is allowed to live as normal a life as possible for as long as possible. Drug treatment offers little lasting benefit, although diuretic therapy may be helpful occasionally for edema or hypertension. Marked hypertension is controlled with antihypertensive agents, and anemia may require periodic transfusion with fresh packed cells. Salt is only moderately restricted. Ultimately dialysis and transplantation may restore relatively good health; however, these are usually not available alternatives until renal failure is far advanced. (See Chronic renal failure, p. 1284, for more detailed management of specific problems.) Children with rapidly progressive glomerulonephritis are usually referred to a center specializing in renal disease.

Nursing Considerations

The problems of chronic glomerular nephritis and those encountered in chronic renal insufficiency from any cause are discussed in association with chronic renal failure.

Renal Tubular Disorders

Disorders of renal tubular function include a variety of conditions in which there are one or more abnormalities in specific mechanisms of tubular transport or reabsorption, whereas initially glomerular function is normal or comparatively less impaired. Eventually there may be more widespread kidney destruction with renal failure. In some cases the dysfunction has little, if any, effect on renal function. These disorders may be permanent or transient and may originate as primary defects or arise as a secondary effect of metabolic disease or exogenous toxins. Renal tubular disorders may be congenital (usually displaying characteristic patterns of genetic transmission), appear without evidence of hereditary transmission, or be acquired as a result of known or unknown causes.

Unlike the classic manifestations of glomerular diseases, edema and hypertension are absent and the blood urea nitrogen level and routine urinalysis are usually normal. Proteinuria may be demonstrated but only by elaborate tests. Manifestations of tubular disorders are primarily metabolic disturbances or deficiencies, such as failure to thrive, metabolic bone disease, or persistent acidosis. The variety of these disorders is extensive and the incidence rare.

TUBULAR FUNCTION

The function of the proximal tubules is the reabsorption of substances from the glomerular filtrate, including sodium, potassium, chloride, bicarbonate, glucose, phosphate, and amino acids. A number of disorders feature impairment of reabsorption of one or more filtrate constituents and most involve defects in the transport mechanisms for these substances. Impaired tubular reabsorption of any specific substance will cause that substance to appear in the urine, usually with reduced levels in the blood.

The primary functions of the distal renal tubules are acidification of urine, potassium secretion, and the selective and differential reabsorption of sodium, chloride, and water, which determines the final urinary concentration. Since the contribution of the distal tubule to urine composition depends in part on the volume and composition of the filtrate from the proximal tubule, the net contribution of the distal tubule is related to proximal tubular function and glomerular filtration.

RENAL TUBULAR ACIDOSIS

Renal tubular acidosis (RTA) is a syndrome of sustained metabolic acidosis in which there is impaired reabsorption of bicarbonate and/or excretion of net hydrogen ion, but where glomerular function is normal or comparatively less impaired. On the basis of underlying pathophysiology, renal tubular acidosis is divided into *proximal renal tubular acidosis,* which results from a defect in absorption of bicarbon-

ate, and *distal renal tubular acidosis,* which results from an inability to establish an adequate gradient of pH between blood and tubular fluid.

Proximal Tubular Acidosis (Type II)

Proximal tubular, or bicarbonate wasting, acidosis is caused by impaired bicarbonate reabsorption in the proximal tubule. It may occur as an isolated defect (primary); however, more often it appears in association with other proximal tubular disorders (secondary). As a result of a depressed renal threshold, bicarbonate reabsorption in the proximal tubule is incomplete, causing the plasma concentration of bicarbonate to stabilize at a lower level than normal. This results in a hyperchloremic metabolic acidosis. There is no impairment of distal tubular integrity or, in most cases, of the distal acidifying mechanism. A more complex abnormality in the proximal tubules is the *Fanconi syndrome* in which transport mechanisms are damaged by the accumulation of toxic metabolites or the tubular epithelium is damaged by heavy metals such as lead or arsenic.

The cause of the primary disorder is unknown, but it appears to be almost entirely restricted to male infants. The major clinical manifestation and presenting symptom is growth failure. Tachypnea from hyperchloremic metabolic acidosis is also evident. Dehydration, vomiting, episodic fever, nephrolithiasis secondary to hypercalciuria, muscle weakness or paralysis as a result of hypokalemia, and episodes of severe, life-threatening acidemia (sometimes triggered by a concurrent infection) may be seen also.

Complications are rare. The disorder appears to be transient and resolves spontaneously in time.

Distal Tubular Acidosis (Type I)

Distal tubular acidosis is caused by the inability of the kidney to establish a normal pH gradient between tubular cells and tubular contents. Its most characteristic feature is the inability to produce a urinary pH below 6.0 despite the presence of severe metabolic acidosis.

Distal renal tubular acidosis may occur as a primary, isolated defect or in association with other diseases or disorders. Most secondary causes are rare. The primary disorder is usually considered to be a hereditary defect with a variable degree of expression and a greater penetrance in females. After the age of 2 years the child usually has growth failure, although there is often a history of vomiting, polyuria, dehydration, anorexia, and failure to thrive. Evidence of bone demineralization (see hypophosphatemic rickets) may be present along with, occasionally, the formation of urinary calculi (urolithiasis) in older children.

The inability to secrete hydrogen ion causes an accumulation of the ion in the body, which soon depletes the available hydrogen buffer, producing a sustained acidosis. Acidosis retards normal somatic growth, and demineralization of bone occurs as bone salts are mobilized to buffer the excessive hydrogen ions. Increased serum levels of both calcium and phosphorus contribute to the development of stones within the renal system. Both sodium and potassium are secreted in larger amounts. Serum potassium levels are depleted as the distal tubules excrete large amounts of potassium ions in an attempt to conserve sodium, since hydrogen ions are unable to participate in the exchange. Hyponatremia stimulates increased aldosterone secretion, which further aggravates the hypokalemia. With the depletion of bicarbonate ions, more chloride is reabsorbed in the proximal tubule to create a hyperchloremia.

The primary disorder is usually permanent, but with early diagnosis and therapy secondary effects on growth and stone formation can be avoided. When it occurs as a secondary complication and renal damage is prevented, the prognosis is good.

Therapeutic Management

Treatment of both proximal and distal disorders consists of administration of sufficient bicarbonate or citrate to balance metabolically produced hydrogen ions and maintain the plasma bicarbonate level within normal range and to correct associated electrolyte disorders, especially hypokalemia. Proximal disorders require large volumes of bicarbonate to compensate for urinary losses; in distal disorders the alkali required to maintain a normal plasma concentration is low. Most authorities favor a mixture of sodium and potassium bicarbonate (or citrate) in order to prevent deficiencies of either cation. The citrate solutions (Bicitra, Polycitra, or Shohl solution) are usually more easily tolerated than bicarbonate solutions. Shohl is very effective but has the disadvantage of requiring preparation by a pharmacist.

Nursing Considerations

Nursing goals include recognizing the possibility of RTA in children who fail to thrive or display other symptoms suggestive of the disorders and referring these children for medical evaluation. Helping parents understand the importance of compliance in administration of medications on a long-term basis is a primary goal of nursing management (see p. 1110). Children who must continue the medication indefinitely are taught the importance of taking the medications as soon as they are old enough to assume responsibility for their own care.

NEPHROGENIC DIABETES INSIPIDUS

Nephrogenic diabetes insipidus (NDI) is the major disorder associated with a defect in the ability to concentrate urine. In this disorder the distal tubules and collecting ducts are insensitive to the action of antidiuretic hormone or its exogenous counterpart, vasopressin. The nature of the defect is unknown but it occurs primarily in males, which supports X-linked recessive inheritance. The disease is more variable in female carriers of the defective gene who may exhibit only a mild defect in urine-concentrating ability. Sometimes nephrogenic diabetes insipidus can result from chronic obstructive renal disorders, sickle cell disease, renal tuberculosis, and other renal disorders.

Clinical Manifestations

The disease is manifest in the newborn period by vomiting, unexplained fever, failure to thrive, and severe recurrent dehydration with hypernatremia. The passage of copious amounts of dilute urine, which produces severe dehydration and hypoelectrolytemia, is a serious threat to life during this period and may be responsible for the high incidence of mental and motor retardation found in affected persons. Growth retardation is probably related to diminished food intake and poor general health because of uncontrolled polydipsia. Diagnosis is suspected on the basis of patient and family history and confirmed by a urine osmolality value consistently below that of plasma. Lack of response to vasopressin administration rules out other causes.

Therapeutic Management

Therapy involves provision of adequate volumes of water to compensate for urinary losses. As a result of an insatiable thirst, most of the child's time is spent drinking and voiding, with little time for activity and stimulation. These children may go to great lengths to satisfy their thirst. A low-sodium/low-solute diet and the use of chlorothiazide or ethacrynic acid diuretics to increase the reabsorption of sodium and water in the proximal tubule help to reduce the amount of tubular fluid delivered to the distal tubules and diminish the volume of water excreted. Urine output has been reported to be reduced when prostaglandin inhibitors such as tolmetin sodium, indomethacin, ibuprofen, and aspirin are administered in conjunction with chlorothiazide (Chevalier and Rogol, 1982; Garin and Richard, 1983; Libber, Harrison, and Spector, 1986). Supplemental potassium may be required to prevent hypokalemia as a result of thiazide therapy. If the disease is recognized early and treatment instituted and maintained, normal growth can be expected and a normal life span anticipated.

Nursing Considerations

Nursing goals for children and families with NDI are to recognize signs of the disorder early and assist them in coping with the long-term inconvenience of the continual thirst and elimination problems. Families need to be taught to administer medications and help with diet planning for those on sodium restriction and who need supplemental potassium. The problem of ensuring adequate hydration is lifelong and families need to adapt to away-from-home fluid needs and to avoid activities that contribute to dehydration when fluids may not be available. Genetic counseling is recommended.

Miscellaneous Renal Disorders

Renal damage occurs as a major or minor complication in many systemic diseases and with varying degrees of severity. In some cases the renal complications may be the principal cause of death or one of several complications with fatal consequences. In other cases it may be only a source of discomfort but no direct threat to life. Sometimes renal complications provide a clue to diagnosis of the underlying disease; at other times renal involvement confuses the diagnosis. Some of the disorders in which renal dysfunction is acquired as a manifestation of a systemic disease have been outlined previously.

There are a wide variety of hereditary disorders of renal function, some of which have been mentioned. It is estimated that 15% of renal diseases are genetically determined. These may be glomerular function disorders, tubular defects, metabolic disorders that may lead to renal damage, disorders involving more than one system, or structural abnormalities and tumors. In addition, there are a number of miscellaneous renal conditions for which a cause is unknown.

OBSTRUCTIVE UROPATHY

Structural or functional abnormalities of the urinary system that obstruct the normal flow of urine can produce renal disorders. When there is interference with urine flow, the collecting system above the obstruction causes *hydronephrosis* (the collection of urine in the renal pelvis to the point of cyst formation from the distention) with eventual pressure destruction to renal parenchyma, although the dilating ureters form a reservoir that reduces the effect on the kidneys for a long time.

Obstruction may be congenital or acquired, unilateral or bilateral, complete or incomplete, and the manifestations acute or chronic. The obstruction can occur at any level of the upper or lower urinary tract (Fig. 30-5). Partial obstruction may not be symptomatic unless there is a water or solute diuresis. Boys are affected more commonly than girls and malformations should be suspected when patients have some other congenital defects (e.g., prune belly syndrome, chromosome anomalies, hypospadias, anorectal malformations, and aural defects).

Pathophysiology

The pathologic changes depend on the location and nature of the defect, the site of obstruction, the duration of the obstruction, and complications such as infection or urinary calculi. With hydronephrosis, glomerular filtration ceases when intrapelvic pressure equals the filtration pressure in glomerular capillaries. However, a pressure gradient usually is established because of some flow beyond the obstruction as a result of periodic relaxation of ureteral wall musculature. There is also an exchange of solutes and water between the pooled urine in the renal pelvis and fluid in the adjoining tissues and fluid compartments (such as interstitial fluid in the pelvic wall and inner kidney medulla), resulting from an intrarenal vascular adjustment caused by a corresponding increase in peritubular capillary pressure.

Damage to distal nephrons in chronic uropathy alters the ability to concentrate urine, which contributes to increased urine flow. Metabolic acidosis occurs from decreased excretion of acid secondary to impaired ability of the distal neph-

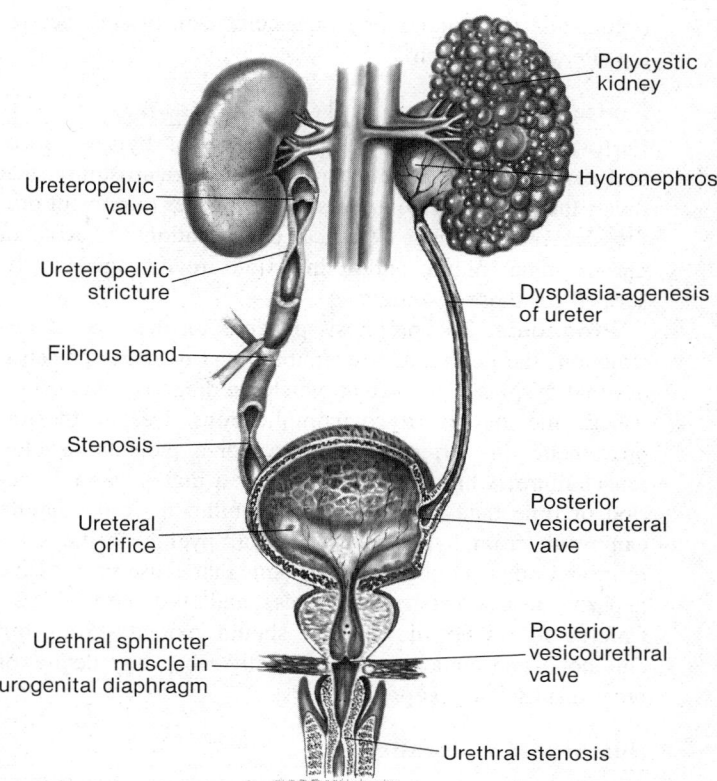

Fig. 30-5. Major sites of urinary tract obstruction.

ron to secrete hydrogen ions. Partial obstruction results in progressive loss of renal function as a result of irreversible damage to the nephrons. Pooled urine serves as a medium for bacterial growth; therefore, urinary tract infections further increase the extent of renal damage.

Clinical Manifestations

The clinical manifestations depend on whether the obstruction is acute or chronic, partial or complete, and the extent of complications (e.g., infection). There may be pain or strangury (slow and painful urination, drop by drop) and hematuria (if caused by calculi). The type and location of pain are related to the area of obstruction (e.g., abdominal, flank, suprapubic, or radiating to the testicle or inguinal region).

Chronic obstruction may cause polyuria and polydipsia as a result of inability to concentrate urine, anemia caused by renal damage that impairs the secretion of erythropoietin, failure to thrive, unexplained febrile episodes caused by urinary infection, frequent voiding, weak or forceful urinary stream, and daytime and nocturnal enuresis. A full bladder and/or enlarged kidney may be evident on examination of the abdomen (Kaplan, 1983).

Diagnostic Evaluation

Laboratory examination reveals findings of acute or chronic renal failure. A voiding cystoureterogram may demonstrate the presence of posterior ureteral valves or vesicoureteral reflux, and ultrasonography may help identify and localize the site of obstruction.

Therapeutic Management

Early diagnosis and surgical correction or bypass procedures, such as ileal conduit or cutaneous ureterostomy, that divert the flow of urine are essential in order to prevent progressive renal damage. Medical complications of acute or chronic renal failure and/or infection are managed as described for those disorders.

Prognosis. The prognosis depends on the type of obstruction, the degree of irreversible renal damage, presence of renal dysplasia, the age at which the diagnosis was established, and the severity of complications. Despite the improvements in corrective surgery, some patients develop renal failure, which may evolve over a highly variable period of time that can extend into adulthood. Renal failure can result from hypoplasia-dysplasia, pyelonephritic scarring, and other proposed mechanisms that cause progressive nephron loss (Warshaw, Hymes, and Woodard, 1982). Careful follow-up of children should extend throughout childhood and adolescence, especially when any degree of renal insufficiency is present.

Nursing Considerations

Nursing goals in urinary tract obstruction include helping to identify cases, assisting with diagnostic procedures, and caring for children with complications (described elsewhere). Preparing parents and children for procedures is a major nursing responsibility, especially preparation for urinary diversion procedures (see Preparation for procedures, p. 1104).

Parents and children need emotional support and counseling during the lengthy management of these disorders. Parents are the primary target during infancy and very early childhood when most reparative surgery is performed. They will need assistance in managing the apparatus that accompanies many temporary and permanent repair procedures. Many children are discharged with ureteral drainage systems in place that must be protected from damage, and the danger of infection is a constant concern. Parents are taught to care for the equipment and recognize the signs of possible obstruction or infection within the system (see discharge planning and home care in Chapter 26, p. 1094).

Children with external diversional systems will need psychologic support and guidance, especially as they reach adolescence and body image concerns assume more prominence. Those with progressive renal deterioration may face the prospect of dialysis and/or transplantation and the emotional aspects that accompany these procedures.

HEMOLYTIC-UREMIC SYNDROME

Hemolytic-uremic syndrome (HUS) is an uncommon acute renal disease that is characterized by a triad of manifestations: acute renal failure, hemolytic anemia, and thrombocytopenia. HUS occurs primarily in infants and small chil-

dren between the ages of 6 months and 3 years. It has been recognized predominantly in whites and, although it occurs worldwide, is more prevalent in South Africa, Argentina, and the West coasts of North and South America. There have also been reports of increased incidence in families (Fong, de Chadarevian, and Kaplan, 1982). Although uncommon, HUS represents one of the most frequent causes of acute renal failure in children.

Etiology

In the majority of cases no causative agents have been identified, although recent theories implicate genetic factors, prostacyclin deficiency, neuraminidase and agglutination, endotoxins (especially *Shigella* endotoxin), antithrombin-III deficiency, deficiency of antioxidants, and reduced platelet aggregation. The appearance of the disease has been associated with *Rickettsia,* viruses (especially Coxsackie, ECHO, and adenovirus), pneumococci, *Shigella,* and *Salmonella* and may represent an unusual response to these infections. The disease usually follows an acute gastrointestinal or upper respiratory infection and tends to occur in scattered outbreaks in small geographic areas. HUS is clinically and pathologically similar to thrombocytopenic purpura, except for the hypertension that is associated with HUS. Some have speculated that thrombocytopenic purpura may be the adult version of the hemolytic-uremic syndrome of infancy and early childhood.

Pathophysiology

The primary site of injury appears to be the endothelial lining of the small glomerular arterioles, although other organs and tissues may be involved (e.g., the liver, brain, heart, pancreatic islet cells, and muscles). The endothelium becomes swollen and occluded with deposition of platelets and fibrin clots (intravascular coagulation). Red blood cells are damaged as they move through the partially occluded blood vessels. These fragmented red blood cells are removed by the spleen, causing acute hemolytic anemia. Fibrinolytic action on the precipitated fibrin causes these fibrin-split products to appear in the serum and urine. The platelet aggregation within damaged blood vessels or the damage and removal of platelets produce the characteristic thrombocytopenia.

Clinical Manifestations

The disease is preceded by a prodromal period during which there is an episode of diarrhea and vomiting. Less often the illness is an upper respiratory infection and occasionally varicella, measles, or urinary tract infection.

The hemolytic process persists for several days to 2 weeks. During this time the child is anorectic, irritable, and lethargic. There is marked and rapid onset of pallor, accompanied by hemorrhagic manifestations such as bruising, purpura, or rectal bleeding. Severely affected patients are anuric and are frequently hypertensive. Convulsions and stupor suggest central nervous system involvement, and there may be signs of acute heart failure. Mild cases demonstrate anemia, thrombocytopenia, and azotemia; urine output may be reduced or increased.

Diagnostic Evaluation

The triad of anemia, thrombocytopenia, and renal failure is sufficient for diagnosis. Renal involvement is evidenced by proteinuria, hematuria, and presence of urinary casts; blood urea nitrogen and serum creatinine levels are elevated. A high reticulocyte count confirms the hemolytic nature of the anemia.

Therapeutic Management

In general, treatment is directed toward control of the complications and hematologic manifestations of renal failure. The initial supportive measures for most children are those used in managing renal failure—fluid replacement (calculated with great care), treatment of hypertension, and correction of acidosis and electrolyte disorders. The most consistently effective treatment is early and repeated peritoneal dialysis, which is instituted in any child who has been anuric for 24 hours or who demonstrates oliguria with hypertension and seizures. Blood transfusions with fresh, washed packed cells are administered for severe anemia but are used with caution to prevent circulatory overload from added volume.

There is no substantial evidence that heparin, corticosteroids, or fibrinolytic agents are beneficial, and in some instances they may aggravate the condition. With prompt treatment the recovery rate is about 95%, but residual renal impairment ranges from 10% to 50% in various areas. Death is usually caused by residual renal impairment or central nervous system injury.

Nursing Considerations

Nursing care is the same as that provided in acute renal failure and, for children with continued impairment, includes management of chronic disease.

BENIGN RECURRENT HEMATURIA

Benign recurrent hematuria is characterized by recurrent episodes of gross hematuria in the absence of systemic disease. The etiology is unknown, but the episodes of hematuria are frequently precipitated by viral respiratory infections, other mild febrile illnesses, or strenuous exercise.

The disorder may be confused with other forms of renal disease; therefore, renal biopsy is indicated to confirm the diagnosis and rule out more serious renal disease. There is no loss of renal function, and treatment is seldom indicated.

FAMILIAL GLOMERULOPATHY (ALPORT SYNDROME)

The syndrome of chronic hereditary nephritis consists of hematuria, nerve deafness, ocular disorders, and chronic renal failure. The disease appears to be inherited as an autosomal-dominant trait, which suggests a possible X-linked dominant trait, although rare male-to-male transmission occurs. It is uncommon but not rare and accounts for a significant percentage of persistent glomerular disease in childhood.

The clinical manifestations are indistinguishable from mild acute nephritis. Initial symptoms include hematuria, proteinuria, malaise, and mild edema. The symptoms are often associated with an acute respiratory infection. The average age of onset is 6 years but the condition may be noted in infancy. It begins slowly and progresses until uncontrollable renal failure develops in adolescence or early adulthood. There is a positive family history. Most untreated boys develop severe symptoms, whereas affected girls generally have a milder disease and a normal life expectancy.

Treatment is symptomatic and supportive, and every effort should be made to restrict the activities of affected children as little as possible. Dialysis and renal transplantation are ultimate therapeutic measures for renal involvement. Hearing loss and ocular disorders should receive appropriate attention, and families should be counseled regarding the genetic implications of the disease.

UNEXPLAINED PROTEINURIA

Often apparently healthy children with no suggestion of renal disease will demonstrate proteinuria on routine urinalysis. The percentage of children with unexplained proteinuria ranges from 1% at 6 years of age to 11% at puberty, reaching a maximum prevalence at age 13 in girls and age 16 in boys.

Unexplained proteinuria can be categorized as (1) *transient (inconstant),* (2) *persistent,* or (3) *orthostatic,* or *postural.* Transient proteinuria is a common finding with no known cause, but it sometimes increases with febrile illness, exercise, cold, or emotions.

Persistent proteinuria usually signifies renal disease but may occur consistently in children with no impairment of renal function. Orthostatic proteinuria is seen in 3% to 5% of adolescents and young adults, and although proteinuria is evident in the recumbent as well as the erect position, it is readily detected by qualitative tests. Reactions of 2 + or 3 + are frequently encountered. The cause is unknown, but minor glomerular changes occur in many instances. The condition is benign and generally resolves over a period of time.

In cases of unexplained proteinuria, it is important to confirm or exclude renal disease with appropriate diagnostic tests. Repeated examination for proteinuria; an orthostatic test; and, if proteinuria is persistent, more definitive tests, including 24-hour protein excretion, intravenous pyelogram, and urine culture, are indicated.

RENAL TRAUMA

Serious injuries of the genitourinary tract are not uncommon in the pediatric age-group, the peak incidence occurring between the ages of 10 and 20 years. The kidneys are among the organs most often injured in children, despite their relatively protected location. However, the kidneys in children are more mobile than they are in the adult and the outer borders are less well protected. They are separated from the skin surface by only 2 to 3 cm (¾ to 1¼ inches) in young children. Most injuries are of the nonpenetrating or "blunt" type, usually involving falls, athletic injuries, and motor vehicle accidents. Penetrating trauma (e.g., gunshot or stab wound) occurs much less frequently in children. In many children preexisting renal abnormalities, particularly congenital anomalies associated with mild to moderate hydronephrosis, are found that were unrecognized before the accident.

Renal injury can be suspected in children who complain of flank pain, and frequently there are abrasions or contusions on the overlying skin. Hematuria is consistently present, but the amount of blood in the urine is not a reliable indicator of the seriousness of the injury. Many relatively insignificant injuries are associated with grossly bloody urine, whereas some of the most severe injuries are found in children with only microscopic hematuria.

Renal injuries are classified according to the extent of injury (Hoover, 1984):

Type I A relatively mild renal contusion where the capsule, parenchyma, and collecting system are usually intact but subcapsular bleeding frequently occurs into the parenchyma and appears in the urine. Renal contusion is an important cause of gross hematuria in active children.

Type II Laceration of the kidney, injury to a major renal vessel, or injury to the collecting system with intracapsular extravasation of urine.

Type III Multiple renal lacertions or injury to the main renal artery.

Renal rupture involves the actual splitting open of the kidney capsule, causing extravasation of blood or a mixture of blood and urine into the surrounding retroperitoneal space. Renal vascular injury, although unusual, requires immediate recognition and surgical intervention. Since the volume per minute blood flow through the kidney is greater (25% of cardiac output) than to any other abdominal organ, injury to the kidney may result in a rapid loss of blood (Hoover, 1984).

In active children there may or may not be history of unusual trauma. Abdominal or flank pain and tenderness are caused by bleeding around the kidney and may or may not be associated with fever. Clots passing down the ureter may cause pain similar to that of renal colic, and dysuria is common. Patients with more severe injuries may complain of nausea or abdominal pain. There may be a palpable abdominal mass caused by loss of blood and/or urine loss into the retroperitoneum. The fibrous capsule enclosing the kidney prevents expansion of a hematoma; therefore exsanguination and shock are seldom observed even in severe renal trauma.

Diagnosis is made on the basis of intravenous pyelography, angiography, and/or retrograde pyelography. Unsuspected hydronephrosis often is first detected as a result of traumatic injury.

Therapeutic Management

Severe injury requires close observation in the hospital intensive care unit as well as blood replacement if there is severe internal or external bleeding. In most cases bleeding subsides spontaneously. Surgical exploration is indicated in multiple injuries, extravasation of blood around the kidneys, or disruption of the major vessels or the collecting system. Children with less severe injury, such as contusions only, are placed on bed rest. They should remain on bed rest for 3 days after cessation of gross bleeding, since the substance released from injured renal tissue (urinary urokinase) has strongly fibrinolytic properties that may precipitate serious bleeding.

Nursing Considerations

Nursing management is directed toward recognizing and assisting in the diagnosis of renal injury. Care of both child and family is primarily supportive. All the concepts related to emergency hospitalization and care are implemented (see Chapter 26). Postsurgical care, if indicated, is the same as for any other surgical patient.

Renal Failure

Renal failure is the inability of the kidneys to excrete waste material, concentrate urine, and conserve electrolytes. The disorder can be acute or chronic and affects most of the systems in the body. Two terms that are often used in relation to renal failure need some clarification: *azotemia* is the accumulation of nitrogenous waste within the blood; *uremia* is a more advanced condition in which retention of nitrogenous products produces toxic symptoms. Azotemia is not life threatening, whereas uremia is a serious condition that often involves other body systems.

ACUTE RENAL FAILURE

Acute renal failure (ARF) is said to exist when the kidneys suddenly are unable to regulate the volume and composition of urine appropriately in response to food and fluid intake and the needs of the organism. The principal feature is oligoanuria* associated with azotemia, acidosis, and diverse electrolyte disturbances. ARF is not common in childhood, but the outcome depends on the cause, associated findings, and prompt recognition and treatment.

Etiology

ARF can develop as a result of a large number of related or unrelated clinical conditions—poor renal perfusion, acute renal injury, or the final expression of chronic, irreversible renal disease. The most common cause in children is transient renal failure resulting from dehydration or other causes of poor perfusion that respond to restoration of fluid vol-

---

*The definition of oligoanuria varies extensively, from 1.8 to 4 dl/m²/24 hours, in the literature.

ume. Causes of ARF are usually classified as to *prerenal*, *intrinsic renal*, and *postrenal* causes (see the boxed material below). This implies that only renal causes are characterized by damage to the renal parenchyma while prerenal and postrenal causes can be more easily remedied. However, severe or long-standing prerenal or postrenal etiologies can produce severe secondary renal damage.

Prerenal causes. Prerenal causes of ARF are most common in children and are always related to reduction of renal perfusion in an anatomically and physiologically normal kidney and collecting system. Dehydration secondary to diarrheal disease or persistent vomiting is the most frequent cause of prerenal failure in infants and children. Surgical shock and trauma (including burns) are also common causes. Hypovolemia and decreased renal perfusion cause a decreased glomerular filtration rate and stimulate the secretion of renin, aldosterone, and antidiuretic hormone, which further diminish urine flow. Extended and severe hypoperfusion can produce cortical or tubular necrosis; however, where medical care is available, this is seldom allowed to occur. Azotemia that accompanies this type of renal failure generally is rapidly reversible with prompt attention to expansion of the extracellular fluid volume. Prerenal failure is often difficult to distinguish from tubular or cortical necrosis.

Intrinsic renal causes. Intrinsic renal causes of ARF comprise the largest group that requires extended management. These include diseases and nephrotoxic agents that damage the glomeruli, tubules, or renal vasculature. Glomerular disease is the most common cause of glomerular damage, whereas tubular destruction is more often caused by ischemia or nephrotoxins. Vascular damage is an uncommon cause of renal failure in childhood. The type and extent of damage determine the degree and duration of renal insufficiency, and it is difficult to predict in any given case whether or not acute necrosis will develop.

Postrenal causes. ARF resulting from obstructive uropathy is uncommon in children except during the first year of life. However, renal function can be restored by relief of the obstruction. The degree of recovery is dependent on the duration of the renal failure. When the obstruction persists for more than 3 weeks, complete recovery is unlikely.

Pathophysiology

ARF is usually reversible, but the deviations of physiologic function can be extreme and mortality in the pediatric age-group is still high. There is severe reduction in glomerular filtration rate, an elevated blood urea nitrogen level, and decreased tubular reabsorption of sodium from the proximal tubule. Consequently, there is increased concentration of sodium in the distal tubule, which causes stimulation of the

---

ETIOLOGY OF ACUTE RENAL FAILURE IN INFANTS AND CHILDREN

Prerenal (decreased perfusion)
Hypovolemia
  Hemorrhage (within or outside kidney)
  Gastrointestinal losses (vomiting, diarrhea, nasogastric tubes)
  Sequestered or isolated accumulation (local injury, trauma, disease)
  Burns
  Hypoproteinemia (nephrotic syndrome)
  Diabetic acidosis
Circulatory insufficiency
  Congestive heart failure
  Cardiac defects
  Shock
  Acute anemia (hemolytic crises, including sickle cell crisis and blood incompatibility)
Peripheral vasodilation
  Sepsis
  Drug-induced (antihypertensives, anesthesia)
Increased vascular resistance
  Anesthesia
  Surgery
Renal arterial occlusion
  Renal vein thrombosis or embolus
  Narrowing of arteries (congenital stricture)
  External compression (tumor)
Intrinsic

Renal
Diseases of kidney
  Glomerulopathies
  Pyelonephritis
  Cortical or medullary necrosis
  Diseases associated with systemic disease
  Hemolytic-uremic syndrome
  Tumors
  Intravascular coagulation
Tubular destruction
  Nephrotoxins (drugs, chemicals, dyes)
  Intravascular hemolysis (hemoglobinuria)
  Crush injury (myoglobinuria)
  Transfusion reaction
Vascular
  Thrombosis
  Polyarteritis or systemic vasculitis
  Acute and/or chronic rejection
Hypoxic ischemia
  Near drowning
  Shock
  Septicemia (especially if associated with calculi or obstruction)
  Structural anomalies (renal dysplasia, polycystic kidneys)

Postrenal
Upper tract obstruction
  Stones
  Tumors
  Uric acid or sulfonamide crystals
  Ureterocele
  Structural anomalies (stricture, bladder neck obstruction, posterior ureteral valves, pelviureteric junction obstruction)

renin mechanism. The local action of angiotensin causes vasoconstriction of the afferent arteriole, which further reduces glomerular filtration and prevents urinary losses of sodium. There is a significant reduction in renal blood flow.

The pathologic conditions that produce acute renal failure caused by glomerulonephritis, hemolytic-uremic syndrome, and other renal disorders have been discussed in relation to those disease processes. The necrotic processes within the nephron can be cortical, tubular, or both.

Cortical necrosis. Complete cortical necrosis usually results from severe ischemia, infection, or intravascular coagulation and represents a severe irreversible cause of acute renal failure. In the pediatric age-group this occurs as a fatal event most frequently during the neonatal period as a result of hypoxia and shock. When cortical destruction is incomplete, some recovery of renal function may occur. Intravascular coagulation is believed to play a significant role as an intermediate factor in the development of ARF, especially in cases related to sepsis.

Tubular necrosis. Damage to the renal tubules can be broadly classified as (1) secondary to renal ischemia and (2) associated with the ingestion or inhalation of substances toxic to the kidneys. Renal tubules are particularly vulnerable to a wide variety of toxic agents that produce vasoconstriction and to focal patches of ischemia that cause a uniform necrosis of the tubular epithelium down to, but not including, the basement membrane. A lesion produced by sustained reduction in renal blood flow involves the basement membrane as well, which may become fragmented and ruptured to the extent that the continuity of tubular structure is disrupted. The lesions may affect any segment of the tubules, appearing at irregular intervals along with normal segments throughout the kidney.

Healing of tubular lesions is accomplished by reepithelialization in the areas with intact basement membrane. In those areas in which the basement membrane has been disrupted, such healing is unable to take place and connective tissue grows through the ruptured membrane, thus preventing reestablishment of tubular integrity. Individual cells within the nephron are capable of regeneration, but the entire nephron is not capable of this.

Clinical course. The clinical course of the child with ARF is variable and depends on the cause. In reversible ARF there is a period of severe oliguria, or the low-output phase, followed by an abrupt onset of diuresis, or a high-output phase, followed by a gradual return to, or toward, normal urine volumes. The length of the oliguric phase in older children and adolescents is 10 to 14 days, although it is highly variable at all ages. It tends to be shorter (3 to 5 days) in infants, children, and milder cases. The onset of the diuretic phase appears unexpectedly and over several days proceeds in stepwise fashion from very low to above normal urine volumes. During the oliguric phase manifestations of uremia are present but may also be accompanied by other clinical disorders that make assessment difficult, such as infection, anoxia, and shock.

Clinical Manifestations

In many instances of ARF the infant or child is already critically ill with the precipitating disorder and the explanation for development of oliguria is readily apparent. Often the underlying illness overshadows the renal failure and frequently assumes the priority of care—for example, the patient who is in shock from endotoxemia, the infant who is severely dehydrated from gastroenteritis, or a child who is subject to seizures as a result of hypertensive encephalopathy associated with acute glomerulonephritis.

The prime manifestation of ARF is oliguria, generally a urine output less than 50 ml/24 hours. Anuria is uncommon except in obstructive disorders. Other symptoms related to ARF include edema, drowsiness, circulatory congestion, and cardiac arrhythmia from hyperkalemia. Seizures may be caused by hyponatremia or hypocalcemia and tachypnea from metabolic acidosis. With continued oliguria, biochemical abnormalities can develop rapidly and circulatory and central nervous system manifestations appear.

Diagnostic Evaluation

When a previously well child develops ARF without obvious cause, a careful history is taken to reveal symptoms that may be related to glomerulonephritis, to obstructive uropathy, or regarding exposure to nephrotoxic chemicals, such as ingestion of heavy metals or inhalation of carbon tetrachloride or other organic solvents or drugs, such as methicillin, sulfonamides, neomycin, polymyxin, and kanamycin. Laboratory data reflect the kidney dysfunction—hyperkalemia, hyponatremia, metabolic acidosis, hypocalcemia, anemia, or azotemia (Table 30-6).

Therapeutic Management

The most effective management of ARF is prevention. The development of ARF is a known risk in certain situations. This should be anticipated, recognized, and adequate therapy implemented—for example, fluid therapy for children with hypovolemia in such conditions as dehydration, burns, and hemorrhage. Nephrotoxic drugs should be used with caution or avoided in children with renal disease, and all personnel should be knowledgeable about precautions related to their administration. For example, a generous fluid intake is needed for children receiving antimetabolite drugs and after radiotherapy.

The treatment of ARF is directed toward (1) treatment of the underlying cause, (2) management of the complications of renal failure, and (3) provision of supportive therapy within the constraints imposed by the renal failure. Treatment of poor perfusion resulting from dehydration consists of volume restoration, as was described previously in the treatment of dehydration. If oliguria persists after restoration of fluid volume or the renal failure is caused by intrinsic renal damage, the physiologic and biochemical abnormalities that have resulted from kidney dysfunction must be corrected or controlled. Central venous pressure monitoring is usually implemented.

Table 30-6 Laboratory findings associated with acute renal failure

CLINICAL PROBLEM	MECHANISM	CLINICAL CONSIDERATIONS
Azotemia		
Elevated BUN levels	Ongoing protein catabolism Significantly decreased excretion	Lower rate of production in neonates and persons with depleted protein stores Increased in situations involving large amounts of necrotic tissue or extravasated blood
Elevated plasma creatinine levels	Continued production Significantly decreased excretion	Production less affected by other factors More sensitive measure of intensity of azotemia Low in neonate because of small muscle mass relative to size
Metabolic acidosis	Continued endogenous acid production Significantly decreased excretion Depletion of extracellular and intracellular fluid buffers	Compensatory hyperventilation Opisthotonos Major threat to life
Hyponatremia	Dilution of extracellular fluid Decreased excretion of water	May develop cerebral signs
Hyperkalemia	Ongoing protein catabolism Decreased excretion compounded by metabolic acidosis	Most important electrolyte to be considered in acute renal failure May contribute to cardiac arrhythmia With ECG changes, major threat to life May be lost from gastrointestinal tract
Hypocalcemia	Associated with metabolic acidosis and hyperphosphatemia	During alkali therapy, may cause tetany

Initially a Foley catheter is inserted to rule out urine retention, to collect available urine for analysis, and to monitor results of diuretic administration. The catheter may or may not be removed. Many authorities who believe that it serves little purpose during the oliguric phase and predisposes to bladder infection prefer collection bags for measuring urine output. Others maintain a catheter for hourly urine measurements.

Oliguria. When there is persistent oliguria in the presence of adequate hydration and no lower tract obstruction, mannitol, furosemide, or both are administered rapidly as a test to provoke a flow of urine. When glomerular function is intact, the administration of these substances will behave as nonreabsorbable solute in the tubular fluid to evoke an osmotic diuresis. The presence of mannitol in tubular fluid and the obligatory water that follows it also serve to dilute the concentration of any nephrotoxin that may be present in the tubules below toxic levels. The furosemide blocks reabsorption of tubular filtrate. If urine flow is generated to the extent of 6 to 10 ml/kg of body weight in 1 to 3 hours, the initial dosage is reduced and continued, if needed, to sustain the flow. If no urine is produced within 2 hours after the single dose, the drugs are not repeated and an oliguric regimen is instituted to control water balance and other abnormalities.

Fluid and calories. The amount of exogenous water provided should not exceed the amount needed to maintain zero water balance. It is calculated on the basis of estimated endogenous water formation and losses from sensible (primarily gastrointestinal) and insensible sources. No allotment is calculated for urine as long as oliguria persists.

The child with ARF has a tendency to develop water intoxication and hyponatremia, which make it difficult to provide calories in sufficient amounts to meet the needs of the child and reduce the tissue catabolism, metabolic acidosis, hyperkalemia, and uremia. If the child is able to tolerate oral foods, concentrated food sources high in carbohydrate and fat but low in protein, potassium, and sodium may be provided. However, many children have functional disturbances of the gastrointestinal tract, such as nausea and vomiting; therefore the intravenous route is generally preferred and usually consists of highly concentrated carbohydrate solutions in small volumes of water administered by the central venous route.

Control of water balance in these patients requires careful monitoring of feedback information, such as accurate intake and output, body weight, and electrolyte measurements. In general during the oliguric phase no sodium, chloride, or potassium is given unless there are other large ongoing losses. Regular measurement of plasma electrolyte, pH, blood urea nitrogen, and creatinine levels is required to assess the adequacy of fluid therapy and to anticipate complications that require specific treatment.

Hyperkalemia. Elevated serum potassium is the most immediate threat to the life of the child with ARF. Potassium ions are not being excreted, whereas at the same time release of potassium from cells is accelerated by acidosis, stress, and tissue breakdown in cases associated with internal bleeding or trauma. Since cardiac arrhythmia and cardiac arrest may result, electrocardiograms as well as serum potassium ion levels are monitored regularly. Hyperkalemia can be minimized and sometimes avoided by eliminating potassium from all food and fluid, by reducing tissue catabolism, and by correcting acidosis. Serum potassium concentrations in excess of 7 mEq/L or the presence of ECG abnormalities, such as prolonged QRS complex, depressed ST segment, high peaked T waves, bradycardia, or heart block, constitute an emergency situation.

Several measures are available to reduce the serum potassium concentration, and the priority of implementation is usually based on the rapidity with which the measures are effective. Temporary measures that produce a rapid but transient effect are:

1. Calcium gluconate, 0.5 ml/kg, administered intravenously over 2 to 4 minutes, with continuous ECG monitoring, exerts a protective effect on cardiac conduction.
2. Sodium bicarbonate, 2 to 3 mEq/kg, administered intravenously over 30 to 60 minutes, elevates the serum pH to cause a transient shift of extracellular fluid potassium into the intracellular fluid. However, there is risk of hypocalcemia, tetany, and fluid overload.
3. Glucose, 50%, and insulin, 1 U/kg, administered intravenously, accelerate glycogen synthesis, causing glucose and potassium to move into the cells. Insulin facilitates the entry of glucose into cells.

These effects produce only transient protection by redistributing existing potassium stores; they do not remove potassium from the body. However, they provide relief while more definitive but slower-acting measures are being implemented. Potassium can be removed by:

1. Administration of an ion-exchange resin such as polystyrene sodium sulfonate (Kayexalate), 1 g/kg, administered orally or rectally, to bind potassium and remove it from the body. This requires time to be effective, and a sodium ion is exchanged for each potassium ion. This increased sodium concentration adds to the body fluids, which may potentially contribute to fluid overload, hypertension, and cardiac failure.
2. Dialysis (discussed on p. 1289). Hemodialysis is efficient but requires specialized facilities. Peritoneal dialysis is simpler and can be carried out in almost any hospital setting. Indications for dialysis in ARF are continued oliguria associated with any of the following:
Severe, persistent acidosis
Inability to reduce serum potassium levels to a safe range with other methods
Clinical uremic syndrome, consisting of nausea and vomiting, drowsiness, and progression to coma
Circulatory overload, hypertension, and evidence of cardiac failure

A popular philosophy is to institute dialysis after 24 to 48 hours of oliguria, regardless of other symptoms. Supporters of this approach believe that early and frequent dialysis is associated with reduced morbidity and mortality and that it permits improved nutrition with relaxed diet restrictions. The combination of dialysis and nutrition tends to reduce the complications of ARF.

Hypertension. Hypertension is a frequent and serious complication of ARF, and, to detect it early, blood pressure determinations are taken every 4 to 6 hours. The most common cause of hypertension in ARF is overexpansion of the extracellular fluid and plasma volume together with activation of the renin-angiotensin system. The goal of therapy is to prevent hypertensive encephalopathy and avoid overtaxing the cardiovascular system.

When there is a threat of encephalopathy, diazoxide is administered intravenously as rapidly as possible, sometimes in conjunction with furosemide, and repeated in 20 minutes if there is no response. Sodium nitroprusside may be given but requires close monitoring. For less urgent situations, hydralazine and reserpine are administered together intramuscularly and repeated in 2 to 3 hours if needed. Other drugs that may be given singly or in combination are oral methyldopa (Aldomet), hydrochlorothiazide, hydralazine, propranalol, and furosemide (Lasix). Another drug, labetalol, with both β and α blocking activity is attracting increased interest for management of severe hypertension (Drummond, 1983).

Other complications. Other complications that may occur with ARF are anemia, convulsions and coma, cardiac failure, and pulmonary edema. *Anemia* is frequently associated with ARF, but transfusion is not recommended unless the hemoglobin level drops below 6 g/dl. Transfusions, if used, consist of fresh, packed red blood cells given slowly to reduce the likelihood of increasing blood volume, hypertension, and hyperkalemia.

Seizures occur rather often when renal failure progresses to uremia and are also related to hypertension, hyponatremia, and hypocalcemia. Treatment is directed to the specific cause when known. More obscure etiologies are managed with anticonvulsant drugs.

Cardiac failure with pulmonary edema is almost always associated with hypervolemia. Treatment is directed toward reduction of fluid volume, with water and sodium restriction and administration of diuretics. Digitalis is ineffective and can be hazardous.

Diuretic, or high-output, phase. When the output begins to increase, either spontaneously or in response to diuretic therapy, the intake of fluid, potassium, and sodium must be monitored and adequate replacement provided to prevent depletion and its consequences. In some cases the high-output phase is mild and lasts only a few days; in others enormous amounts of electrolyte-rich urine are passed.

Prognosis. The prognosis of ARF depends largely on the nature and severity of the causative factor or precipitating event and the promptness and competence of management. The mortality rate is less than 20%. The outcome is least favorable in children with rapidly progressive nephritis and cortical necrosis. Children in whom ARF is a result of hemolytic-uremic syndrome or acute glomerulitis may recover completely, but residual renal impairment or hypertension is more often the rule. Complete recovery is usually expected in children whose renal failure is a result of dehydration, nephrotoxins, or ischemia. ARF following cardiac surgery is less favorable. It is often impossible to assess the extent of recovery for several months.

Nursing Considerations

Nursing care of the infant or child with ARF involves care of the underlying cause plus careful observation and management of the renal status. The major goal is reestablishment of renal function, with emphasis on providing an adequate caloric intake to minimize reduction of protein stores, prevention of complications, and monitoring of fluid balance, laboratory data, and physical manifestations. The probability of dialysis must be considered and the necessary equipment made available in anticipation of such an eventuality. Because the child requires intensive observation and often specialized equipment, he is usually admitted to an intensive care unit in which needed equipment and personnel trained in its use are available.

Meticulous attention to the fluid intake and output is mandatory, including all the physical measurements discussed previously in relation to problems of fluid balance. Monitoring of fluid balance is a continuous process, and nursing measures, such as maintaining an optimum thermal environment, reducing any elevation of body temperature, and reducing restlessness and anxiety, are employed to decrease the rate of tissue catabolism. Although these children are usually quite ill and voluntarily diminish their activity, infants may become restless and irritable and children are often anxious and frightened. There are frequent painful and stress-producing treatments and tests that must be performed. The presence of a supportive, empathetic nurse can provide comfort and stability in a threatening and unnatural environment.

The nurse must be continually alert for changes in behavior that indicate the onset of complications. Infection from reduced resistance, anemia, and general morbidity is a constant threat. Fluid overload and electrolyte disturbances can precipitate cardiovascular complications such as hypertension and cardiac failure. Fluid and electrolyte imbalances, acidosis, and accumulation of nitrogenous waste products can produce neurologic involvement manifested by coma, convulsions, or alterations in sensorium.

Parental support and reassurance are among the major nursing responsibilities. The seriousness and emergency nature of ARF are stressful to parents, and most parents feel some degree of guilt regarding the child's condition, especially when the illness is the result of ingestion of a toxic substance, dehydration, or genetic disease. They need reassurance and a sympathetic listener. They also need to be kept informed of the child's progress and provided explanations regarding the therapeutic regimen. The equipment and the child's behavior are sometimes frightening and anxiety provoking. Nurses can do much to help them comprehend and deal with the stresses of the situation.

Nursing Care Summary: The Child with Acute Renal Failure

NURSING GOALS	NURSING INTERVENTIONS	EXPECTED PATIENT/FAMILY OUTCOMES
HP-HMP **Potential for infection** **Risk factors: diminished body defenses, fluid overload**		
Prevent infection	Observe medical asepsis Avoid contact with infected persons Keep skin clean and dry Change position at least every 2 hours	Child exhibits no evidence of infection
N-MP **Fluid volume, alteration in: excess/fluid volume deficit, actual** **Etiology: failure of or compromised regulator mechanisms**		
Maintain fluid balance	Monitor fluid balance Weigh child daily or as needed Measure intake and output accurately Measure urine specific gravity Observe for signs of dehydration or fluid overload Monitor vital signs Blood pressure Heart rate Respiratory status Central venous pressure, if indicated Regulate fluid intake and output	Child exhibits no evidence of fluid imbalance Child's physiologic signs are recorded *Evidence of deviations from normal findings are detected early and appropriate interventions implemented (see inside front cover for normal variations) Child's intake is appropriate (specify type and amount)

*Nursing outcome.

Continued.

Nursing Care Summary: The Child with Acute Renal Failure—cont'd

NURSING GOALS	NURSING INTERVENTIONS	EXPECTED PATIENT/FAMILY OUTCOMES
N-MP Nutrition, alteration in: less than body requirements **Etiology: altered diet, loss of appetite**		
Provide nutritious meals within dietary limitations	Become well acquainted with protein, potassium, and sodium content of common foods and beverages	Child exhibits no harmful accumulation of electrolytes and nitrogenous waste
Stimulate appetite	Make mealtime a pleasant experience Offer preferred foods whenever possible Arrange food and setting attractively	Child consumes a sufficient amount of nutrients
SP-SCP Fear **Etiology: hospitalization**		
Support child	Remain with child Provide as much comfort as possible within limitations imposed by treatment regimen Provide means for child to express feelings	Child is not left alone Child expresses his feelings and concerns
RRP Family process, alteration in **Etiology: hospitalization of child**		
Support family	Allow family to visit child Explain or reinforce explanations of treatments Keep family informed of child's progress Allow family to express feelings and concerns Provide reassurance where possible Refer to agencies for social service and financial aid See also The child in the hospital, p. 1075; Family of the hospitalized child, p. 1081	Family demonstrates an understanding of information presented (specify information and method of demonstration) Family expresses their feelings and concerns

Nursing Interventions Related to Medical Management

Help establish cause of failure and extent of renal function
  Assist with diagnostic procedures
  Collect specimens for laboratory examinations
  Perform tests as ordered
  Observe, record, and report clinical manifestations
Distinguish between urine retention and diminished urine formation
  Insert Foley catheter
  Send urine obtained (if any) for laboratory analysis
Prevent dehydration
  Replace fluid losses as ordered (such as gastrointestinal and perspiration)
Remove excess fluid and elevated levels of electrolyte and nitrogenous waste
  Assist with periotoneal dialysis
    Gather necessary equipment
    Warm dialysate solution

  Assist with catheter insertion
  Carry out procedure as ordered
  Observe response to treatment
  Monitor vital signs frequently
  Collect specimens as ordered
  Transport to hemodialysis unit as ordered
  Administer diuretics if ordered
Provide nutrition
  Provide low-protein, low-sodium, and low-potassium diet
  Administer hyperalimentation formula as ordered
Prevent infection
  Administer aseptic care of intravenous, hyperalimentation, or dialysis sites
  Administer antibiotics if ordered
Reduce blood pressure
  Administer antihypertensives if ordered

CHRONIC RENAL FAILURE

The kidneys are able to maintain the chemical composition of fluids within normal limits until more than 50% of functional renal capacity is destroyed by disease or injury. Chronic renal failure (CRF) or insufficiency begins when the diseased kidneys can no longer maintain normal chemi- cal structure of body fluids under normal conditions. Progressive deterioration over months or years produces a variety of clinical and biochemical disturbances that eventually culminate in the clinical syndrome known as *uremia*. When the kidneys can no longer function, even with medical intervention, and the patient must resort to dialysis for clearing wastes, the term *end-stage renal disease (ESRD)* is applied. The pattern of renal dysfunction is remarkably uniform no matter what disease process initiates the advanced disease.

Etiology

A variety of diseases and disorders can result in CRF. The most frequent causes of CRF before age 5 years are congenital renal and urinary tract malformations (particularly renal hypoplasia and dysplasia) and vesicoureteral reflux. Glomerular and hereditary renal disease predominate in children 5 to 15 years of age. Glomerular diseases that most frequently lead to CRF are chronic pyelonephritis, chronic glomerulonephritis, and glomerulonephropathy associated with systemic diseases such as anaphylactoid purpura and lupus erythematosus. Hereditary nephritis, congenital nephrotic syndrome, Alport syndrome, polycystic kidney, and several other hereditary disorders result in renal failure in childhood. Renal vascular disorders such as hemolytic-uremic syndrome, vascular thrombosis, or cortical necrosis are less frequent causes.

Pathophysiology

Early in the course of progressive nephron destruction, the child remains asymptomatic with only minimal biochemical abnormalities. Unless its presence is detected in the process of routine assessment, signs and symptoms that indicate advanced renal damage frequently emerge only late in the course of the disease. Midway in the disease process, as increasing numbers of nephrons are totally destroyed and most others are damaged in varying degree, the few that remain intact are hypertrophied but functional. These few normal nephrons are able to make sufficient adjustments to stresses to maintain reasonable degrees of fluid and electrolyte balance. Definitive biochemical examination at this time will reveal restricted tolerance to excesses or restrictions. As the disease progresses to the terminal stage, because of severe reduction in the number of functioning nephrons, the kidneys are no longer able to maintain fluid and electrolyte balance and the features of the uremic syndrome appear.

The pathophysiology of specific biochemical abnormalities is briefly summarized in the following sections.

Retention of waste products. Moderate decrease in renal function is not associated with a rise in fasting blood urea nitrogen concentration. With progressive nephron destruction and diminished function, the serum level of these end products of protein metabolism is increasingly. However, the blood urea nitrogen level is affected by protein intake, whereas the creatinine concentration is not; therefore creatinine is a more reliable index of renal failure.

Water and sodium retention. The damaged kidneys are able to maintain sodium and water balance under normal circumstances, although the few remaining functional nephrons are required to increase their rate of filtration and reabsorption in proportion to their numbers. The limitations of this capacity become apparent under stress. The nature of abnormalities in adjustment depends on the underlying renal disease: infants and small children with kidney dysplasia or urinary obstructive disease tend to excrete large volumes of dilute urine low in sodium content, children with glomerular disease tend to retain both sodium and water as a result of a greater reduction in glomerular filtration than of tubular reabsorption, and children with defective sodium reabsorption from tubular disease tend to lose sodium with a corresponding osmotic water loss. Consequently, sodium excesses may cause edema and hypertension, whereas sodium deprivation can result in hypovolemia and circulatory failure. Only in end-stage renal disease is markedly reduced glomerular filtration inadequate to handle normal amounts of sodium and water. Retention of these substances then leads to edema and vascular congestion.

Hyperkalemia. Dangerous hyperkalemia is an infrequent occurrence in CRF until the terminal stages. However, the kidneys are unable to adjust readily to increased ingestion of potassium, and they require a longer period of time to rid the body of this excess.

Acidosis. A sustained metabolic acidosis is characteristic of CRF; it results from the inability of the damaged kidney to excrete a normal load of metabolic acids generated by normal metabolic processes. There is reduced capacity of the distal tubules to produce ammonia and impaired reabsorption of bicarbonate. Although there is continual hydrogen ion retention and bicarbonate loss, the plasma pH is maintained at a level compatible with life by other buffering mechanisms, particularly the bone salt.

Calcium and phosphorus disturbances. One of the distressing features of CRF is its effect on calcium and phosphorus homeostasis. Profound and complex disturbances in the metabolism of these substances result in significant bone demineralization and impaired growth. This appears to be related to several factors:

1. In a state of acidosis there is dissolution of the alkaline salts of bone, which serve as buffers, and the release of phosphorus and calcium into the bloodstream.
2. Reduced glomerular filtration and excretion of inorganic phosphate lead to an elevation of plasma phosphate with a concomitant decrease in serum calcium.
3. Decreased serum calcium concentration stimulates the secretion of parathyroid hormone (PTH), which results in resorption of calcium from bones. Under normal circumstances parathyroid hormone inhibits the tubular reabsorption of phosphates.
4. Diseased kidneys are unable to complete the synthesis of vitamin D to its most active form, 1,25-dihydroxycholecalciferol, which is necessary for the absorption of calcium from the gastrointestinal tract and deposition of calcium in bone. This acquired resistance to vitamin D decreases calcium absorption, permits retention of phosphorus, and contributes to secondary hyperparathyroidism.

In CRF the result of these complex disturbances in calcium, phosphorus, and bone metabolism produces growth arrest or retardation, bone pain, and deformities known as *renal osteodystrophy,* sometimes called *renal rickets,* since the disorganization of bone growth and demineralization is similar to that caused by vitamin D end resistant rickets.

Anemia. A consistent feature of chronic renal insufficiency is anemia that appears to result from:

1. Shortened life span of red blood cells caused by some extracorpuscular factor associated with the uremic state
2. Impaired red blood cell production resulting from decreased production of erythropoietin
3. Increased tendency to bleed, associated with a prolonged bleeding time probably related to impaired platelet function
4. Superimposed nutritional anemia

Growth disturbance. One of the most striking effects of CRF in childhood is retarded growth, and one which can have profound psychologic and social consequences for the developing child. The cause is poorly understood but may be related to:

1. Renal osteodystrophy
2. Poor nutrition associated with dietary restrictions (especially protein) and loss of appetite
3. Biochemical abnormalities associated with renal failure, such as sustained acidosis, hyperkalemia, chronic hyposmolarity secondary to hyposthenuria (secretion of urine with low specific gravity), and phosphorus depletion

Sexual maturation may be delayed or may not occur in children with CRF, and secondary amenorrhea frequently develops in girls past puberty. CRF can also cause sexual dysfunction by creating imbalances in gonadal hormone levels. Decreased testosterone levels impair spermatogenesis in males; decreased estrogen, luteinizing hormone, and progesterone in females cause anovulation and menstrual irregularities (usually amenorrhea) in females. Autonomic neuropathy and anemia are also factors that can alter sexual function.

Other disturbances. Children with CRF seem to be more than usually susceptible to infection, especially pneumonia, urinary tract infection, and septicemia, although the reason for this is not entirely clear. Hyperventilation, a manifestation of the respiratory compensatory mechanism for metabolic acidosis, and pulmonary edema may contribute to upper respiratory infection. These children become extraordinarily sensitive to changes in vascular volume that may cause, in addition to pulmonary overload, cerebral symptoms and circulatory manifestations such as hypertension and cardiac failure.

Numerous neurologic manifestations appear with advanced renal failure, although no specific toxin or biochemical defect has been identified. However, disturbances in enzyme function, disturbances in water and electrolyte balance, altered calcium ion concentration, hypertension, and accumulation of various "uremic toxins" have been implicated.

Clinical Manifestations

The first evidence of difficulty is usually loss of normal energy and increased fatigue on exertion. For example, the child may prefer quiet, passive activities rather than participation in more active games and outdoor play. The child is usually somewhat pale, but it is often so inconspicuous that the change may not be evident to parents or others. Sometimes the blood pressure is elevated.

As the disease progresses, other manifestations may appear. The child eats less well (especially breakfast), shows less interest in normal activities, such as schoolwork or play, and has an increased urinary output and a compensatory intake of fluid. For example, a previously dry child may wet the bed at night. Pallor becomes more evident as the skin develops a characteristic sallow, muddy appearance as the result of anemia and deposition of urochrome pigment in the skin. The child may complain of headache, muscle cramps, and nausea. Other signs and symptoms include weight loss, facial puffiness, malaise, bone or joint pain, growth retardation, dryness or itching of the skin, bruised skin, and sometimes sensory or motor loss. Amenorrhea is common in adolescent girls.

Therapy is generally instigated before the appearance of the *uremic syndrome,* although there are occasions in which the symptoms may be observed. Manifestations of untreated uremia reflect the progressive nature of the homeostatic disturbances and general toxicity. Gastrointestinal symptoms include loss of appetite, nausea, and vomiting. Bleeding tendencies are apparent in bruises, bloody diarrheal stools, stomatitis, and bleeding from lips and mouth. There is intractable itching, probably related to hyperparathyroidism, and deposits of urea crystals appear on the skin as "uremic frost." There may be an unpleasant "uremic" odor to the breath. Respirations become deeper as a result of metabolic acidosis, and circulatory overload is manifest by hypertension, congestive heart failure, and pulmonary edema. Neurologic involvement is reflected by progressive confusion, dulling of sensorium, and, ultimately, coma. Other signs may include tremors, muscular twitching, and seizures.

Diagnostic Evaluation

The diagnosis of CRF is usually suspected on the basis of any of a number of manifestations, history of prior renal disease, and/or biochemical findings. The onset is usually gradual and the initial signs and symptoms vague and nonspecific. Laboratory and other diagnostic tools and tests are of value in assessing the extent of renal damage, biochemical disturbances, and related physical dysfunction. Often they can help establish the nature of the underlying disease and differentiate between other disease processes and the pathologic consequences of renal dysfunction.

Therapeutic Management

In irreversible renal failure the goals of medical management are to promote effective renal function, to maintain body fluid and electrolyte balance within acceptable limits, to treat systemic complications, and to promote as active and normal a life as possible for the child for as long as possible. This becomes increasingly difficult as the disease progresses toward its inevitable end. Even therapeutic measures designed to relieve one manifestation may prove detrimental to another. For example, antihypertensive agents may further impair renal function, and sodium bicarbonate given to correct acidosis may precipitate tetany.

Activity. The child is allowed unrestricted activity and to set his own limits regarding rest and extent of exertion. He is encouraged to attend school as long as he is able. When the effort is too great, home tutoring is arranged.

Diet. Regulation of diet is the most effective means, short of dialysis, for reducing the quantity of materials that require renal excretion. The goal of the diet in renal failure is to provide sufficient calories and protein for growth while limiting the excretory demands made on the kidney, to minimize metabolic bone disease (osteodystrophy), and to minimize fluid and electrolyte disturbances. Dietary phosphorus, principally the intake of cow's milk, is restricted. This reduces the excretory load on the kidneys, the phosphorus content in the diet, and one of the principal sources of metabolic acids.

Limited protein in the diet should include foods high in essential amino acids; those foods with protein of lesser value can be omitted. Bottle-fed infants are placed on a low-protein, low-electrolyte formula with additional caloric supplements. When given with meals, substances that bind phosphorus in the intestines prevent its absorption and allow a more liberal intake of phosphorus-containing protein. Sodium and water are not usually limited, unless there is evidence of edema or hypertension.

Potassium is not restricted as long as creatinine clearance remains at acceptable limits (greater than or equal to 30 to 35 ml/min). Restrictions are instituted for patients with oliguria or anuria, however. Restrictions of any or all these minerals may be imposed in later stages or at any time in which factors cause abnormal serum concentrations.

Because of modified dietary intake, altered metabolism, and poor appetite, some dietary supplementation is usually needed. Because fat-soluble vitamins can accumulate in patients with CRF, vitamins A, E, and K are not supplemented beyond normal dietary intake. Vitamin D is prescribed and water-soluble vitamin supplementation may be required if diet is inadequate. Other dietary needs are discussed in relation to osteodystrophy and anemia.

Osteodystrophy. Measures directed at prevention or correction of the calcium/phosphorus imbalance are reduction of dietary phosphorus, administration of a phosphorus-binding agent, provision of supplemental calcium, control of acidosis, and administration of vitamin D.

Dietary phosphorus is controlled by the reduction of protein and milk. Phosphorus levels can be further reduced by the oral administration of aluminum hydroxide gel (Amphojel) or tablets that combine with the phosphorus to decrease gastrointestinal absorption and thus the serum levels of phosphate. However, aluminum phosphate binders have been shown to cause aluminum loading when used on a continuous basis in children; therefore, these substances are used only for very short periods to treat hyperphosphatemia (Sedman, 1986a; Griswold and others, 1983). These chil-

dren should be monitored for aluminum accumulation and evidence of aluminum intoxication, such as altered sensorium, inability to talk, atoxia, or seizures. Serum calcium levels are increased with supplementary calcium preparations, calcium gluconate, calcium carbonate, or calcium lactate.

When serum phosphate levels are within a normal range, appropriate vitamin D therapy is instituted. The drugs that are administered to increase the absorption of calcium through the gastrointestinal tract dihydrotachysterol (Hytakerol) or 1,25-dihydroxyvitamin D_3 (Rocaltrol). The serum calcium level is monitored weekly during periods when the drugs are being changed or regulated.

Osseous deformities that result from renal osteodystrophy, especially those related to ambulation, are troublesome and require correction as soon as feasible. It has been found that noticeable deformities develop in one third of patients with osteodystrophy despite medical therapy (Hsu and others, 1982). Deformities are particularly frequent and severe in children whose renal failure develops in infancy. However, until the osteodystrophy is healed and under control, the deformities will recur.

Acidosis. In addition to reducing the formation of metabolic acids by decreasing the dietary intake of protein, acidosis is alleviated by alkalizing agents such as sodium bicarbonate or a combination of sodium and potassium citrate (Bicitra, Polycitra, or Shohl solution*). Correction of acidosis is best attempted after calcium levels are elevated, since rapid correction may precipitate tetany in a hypocalcemic child.

Anemia. Because the anemia associated with renal failure is related to decreased production of erythropoietin, it usually cannot be successfully managed with hematinic agents. However, sufficient sources of folic acid and iron should be provided in the diet, although this is difficult when protein sources are restricted. Inadequate intake and iron losses that may occur are managed by supplemental iron, usually ferrous sulfate. Providing adequate sources of ascorbic acid at the same time that iron-rich food or supplementation is given enhances the absorption.

Blood transfusions carry the risk of aggravating or precipitating cardiovascular disturbances and also tend to inhibit erythropoiesis. If needed for symptomatic anemia, packed red blood cells are given slowly over several hours.

Hypertension. Hypertension of advanced renal disease may be managed initially by cautious use of a low-sodium diet, fluid restriction, and perhaps diuretics such as furosemide. Strict restriction of sodium intake may be necessary in oliguric patients. Severe hypertension requires the use of a combination of beta blocker and a vasodilator (propranolol and hydralazine). Other drugs that may be used include reserpine, methyldopa, minoxidil, prazocin, captopril, or labetalol singly or in combinations.

Growth retardation. One major consequence of CRF

---

*Each milliliter of Shohl solution contains 1 mEq of citrate ion, which metabolizes to yield 1 mEq of bicarbonate. Citric acid exerts no effect on acid-base balance but enhances the palatability of the mixture.

is growth retardation, especially in the preadolescent. These children grow poorly both before and after initiation of hemodialysis. Depletion of body protein is characteristic of children with CRF, in addition to a number of metabolic abnormalities. Some success has been reported in the use of the anabolic steroid, oxandrolone, which was selected because of its powerful anabolic but weak androgenic properties. The boys on whom this drug has been used demonstrated accelerated growth velocity, which suggests that this therapy may be of value in reducing the incidence or overcoming the effects of growth retardation connected with CRF (Jones and others, 1980).

Miscellaneous complications. Intercurrent infections are treated with appropriate antimicrobials at the first sign of infection. Most of these drugs are excreted through the kidneys; therefore, the dosage is usually reduced in proportion to the decrease in renal function and the interval between doses extended in these children to avoid possible toxic effects from accumulation. Any drug eliminated through the kidneys is administered with caution. Serum levels of ototoxic and/or nephrotoxic drugs (e.g., gentamicin or kanamycin) are assessed regularly to assure a safe nontoxic level.

Dental defects are common in children with chronic kidney disease and the earlier the onset of the disease the more severe are the dental manifestations. These include hypoplasia, hypomineralization, tooth discoloration, alteration in size and shape of teeth, malocclusion (secondary to deficient skeletal growth), ulcerative stomatitis, occasional oral hematomas, and an increase in calcific deposits around the teeth (Cooley and Sobel, 1982). Regular dental care is especially important in these children. Other nondental complications are treated symptomatically, for example, chlorpromazine (Thorazine) or prochlorperazine (Compazine) are given for nausea, anticonvulsants for seizures, and diphenhydramine (Benadryl) for pruritus.

Once evidence of ESRD appears in a child, the disease runs its relentless course and terminates in death in a few weeks, unless waste products and toxins are removed from body fluids by dialysis and/or kidney transplantation. Since these techniques have been adapted for infants and small children, the outlook for children with ESRD has improved remarkably. These alternatives are implemented in most cases of renal failure once palliative management is no longer effective.

Nursing Considerations

The child with CRF is a prime example of an individual whose life is maintained by drugs and artificial means, and the multiple stresses placed on these children and their families are often overwhelming. The unrelenting course of the disease process is one of progressive deterioration. There is no means to prevent the irreversible progress of renal insufficiency, nor is there any known cure. As the affected child progresses from renal insufficiency to uremia and then to hemodialysis and transplantation with a need for intensity of therapy, the need for supportive nursing care is also inten-

sified. Team effort is more important than ever and involves coordination of personnel from medicine, nursing, social services, dietetics, and psychologic or psychiatric specialties.

Progressive disease places a number of stresses on the child and his family. There is continuing need for repeated examinations that often entail painful procedures, side effects, and frequent hospitalizations. Diet therapy becomes progressively more restricted and intense, and parents may need help in learning to select appropriate foods, reading labels carefully for sodium and potassium content, and modifying meals to accommodate the special needs of the child. The child is required to take a variety of medications. Compliance is difficult when long-term therapies are involved. Ever present in all aspects of the treatment regimen is the agonizing realization that without treatment death is the inevitable outcome.

End-stage renal disease (ESRD) presents the same nonspecific stresses on child and family as any other chronic (Chapter 22) or life-threatening illness (Chapter 23). The reactions and adaptation of the child and family depend on the age and developmental stage of the child, the cultural and socioeconomic background of the family, the quality of the interpersonal relationships of family members, and the communication patterns within the family. In general the problems observed and emotional responses to the stress of the illness are influenced less by the nature of the illness than by the characteristics of the family relationships and the personalities of its members.

One of the first and most noticeable changes is the alteration in physical appearance—fluctuations in weight, pallor, and failure to grow. Children must adjust to the fact that they will always be different from their peers in some ways. They will be shorter, often more tired, and unable to participate in all the activities that are attractive to young people. Children who have had diversion procedures, dialysis shunts, and other surgeries or who urinate into a bag must learn to adjust to these differences. Children must educate their friends to accept them as they are, or affected children must learn to bear the teasing if they are unable to adjust. Such difficulties can lead to behavior problems in these children.

School is often difficult for these children. Frequent absences for illnesses, evaluations, or treatments disrupt the educational process and socialization. Teachers and school systems are not always sympathetic to the rights and needs of a chronically ill child—e.g., the right to equal education and the need for flexibility and special help at times, which places an additional burden on the parents. Sometimes a teacher will pass a failing child because of pity (Dracopoulos and Weatherly, 1983).

In some families illness and stressful experiences act as a unifying force; in others stress aggravates preexisting problems and contributes to family disharmony. The relentless nature of the disease and its therapies not only place physical and emotional stresses on the family but are also a chronic drain on the family finances. Insurance rarely covers the full cost of the multiple hospitalizations and outpatient expenses. Hidden costs abound, such as transportation to special treatment centers, meals, and sometimes lodging away from home. Some temporary assistance may be provided by private foundations, churches, and community groups, and nurses should become familiar with those in the area of their practice that can be of financial and educational service to these families. For example, the **National Kidney Foundation*** and numerous other agencies provide services and information for families, including pamphlets and descriptive literature. Particularly useful are easily understandable booklets for children with renal disease.

Some specific stresses related to end-stage renal disease and its treatment are predictable. When it first becomes apparent that kidney failure is inevitable, both parents and child experience great depression and anxiety. Acceptance is particularly difficult if renal failure progresses rapidly after diagnosis. Denial and disbelief are usually pronounced, especially among parents. Once the kidney failure is established and symptoms become progressively more distressing, the initiation of hemodialysis is usually perceived as a positive experience, and, after the initial concerns of implementing the treatment, the child begins to feel better and parental anxiety is relieved for a time.

DIALYSIS

Dialysis is the process of separating colloids and crystalline substances in solution by the difference in their rate of diffusion through a semipermeable membrane. This movement across the membrane is accomplished by three processes:

1. **Osmosis,** the passive movement of water from a solution of lower concentration to a solution of higher concentration of particles
2. **Diffusion,** the random movement of particles from an area of greater concentration to an area of lower concentration
3. **Ultrafiltration,** the movement of fluid, under pressure, through filtering material with minute pores

Two methods of dialysis are currently available for clinical management of renal failure:

1. **Peritoneal dialysis,** wherein the abdominal cavity acts as a semipermeable membrane through which water and solutes of small molecular size move by osmosis and diffusion according to their respective concentrations on either side of the membrane
2. **Hemodialysis,** in which blood is circulated outside the body through artificial cellophane membranes that permit a similar passage of water and solutes

As a rule, hemodialysis is reserved for children who are in ESRD since it requires creation of a vascular access and special equipment. Peritoneal dialysis is preferred for children in acute renal failure, because it is usually a temporary therapy, is generally an emergency procedure, and therefore

*National Kidney Foundation, 116 East 27th St., New York, NY 10016.

is more readily available, requires less expertise, and does not require specialized facilities.

Peritoneal Dialysis

Peritoneal dialysis is used in children to treat a number of acute disorders, as well as acute and chronic renal failure. Examples include such acute conditions as severe metabolic acidosis, accidental poisoning, intractable heart failure, hypernatremia, hyperkalemia, and hepatic coma.

The absolute indications for dialysis are life-threatening electrolyte abnormalities and severe volume overload. Although each child is assessed on an individual basis, indications for instituting dialysis in chronic renal failure are biochemical abnormalities such as blood urea nitrogen level greater than 100 mg/dl, serum bicarbonate concentration less than 12 mEq/L, serum potassium concentration greater than 6 mEq/l, and severe hypocalcemia (less than 7 mg/dl) and hyperphosphatemia (greater than 15 mg/dl) (Sedman, 1986b).

Other indications may be a falling hematocrit less than 20 mg/dl requiring transfusion in the face of the attendant hazards of hypertension and hyperkalemia, evidence of deteriorating central nervous system function, or congestive heart failure that is unresponsive to other therapy. Growth failure, severe osteodystrophy, insufficient caloric intake, and inability to carry out normal activities are sometimes criteria for dialysis. The only contraindication for use of peritoneal dialysis is intraabdominal bleeding from a coagulation disorder.

Procedure. After urethral catheterization of the child's bladder and administration of an analgesic and local anesthetic, the abdomen is surgically prepared and a trocar and catheter are inserted through the anterior abdominal wall. The trocar is removed and the catheter maneuvered into the desired position. Any abdominal fluid is aspirated, after which commercially prepared dialysis solution is allowed to flow by gravity into the abdominal cavity where it remains while equilibration between plasma and the dialysis fluid takes place. The amount of fluid instilled is approximately 30 to 50 ml/kg for each instillation. The fluid then flows out by gravity drainage, and fresh dialysate is again instilled.

Each pass generally takes about 30 minutes: 5 minutes for the fluid to flow into the peritoneal cavity, 20 minutes for equilibration, and 5 to 10 minutes for removal (Sedman, 1986b). The procedure is usually continued for 48 hours, although a shorter time may suffice if it is being used to reduce hyperkalemia. After a period of 48 hours, the risk of peritoneal infection increases considerably. The catheter is removed and a sterile dressing applied. The procedure is repeated as needed until renal function is restored, poisons are reduced, or, in prolonged need, treatment is converted to hemodialysis.

The length of the dialysis period requires the child to remain relatively quiet for long periods, and the attendant risk of peritonitis makes peritoneal dialysis relatively unsuited to the long-term dialysis for chronic renal failure. Accidental perforation of bowel or bladder during trocar insertion is an added hazard.

Hemodialysis

Hemodialysis is better suited to long-term therapy, although when facilities are available, it is sometimes used for prolonged episodes of acute renal failure to allow better dietary intake and to minimize symptoms. Dialysis is absolutely essential in children with bilateral neoplastic disease or bilateral nephrectomies performed for intractable hypertension. Many children are being successfully managed on hemodialysis either as a maintenance procedure while awaiting kidney transplant or as a means in itself.

Hemodialysis requires the use of special dialysis equipment—the hemodialyzer, or so-called artificial kidney. Hemodialyzers are available in three forms—coil, parallel flow (plate), and hollow fiber—but not all are suited to pediatric patients. Hollow fiber dialyzers are preferable for children because the blood compartment of the dialyzer is relatively small and rigid (Novello, 1986a). Pediatric dialysis can be safely carried out when the fluid volume required to fill both hemodialyzer and blood tubing does not exceed 10% of the child's calculated blood volume.

Hemodialysis also requires blood access by three types of means: shunts, fistulas, and temporary access. For children weighing less than 15 kg or who are less than 5 years of age, the Thomas femoral shunt is preferred. The goal with any shunt is to implant a cannula that fits comfortably without damage to the vessel lining. Special pediatric cannulas have been developed that allow an access route even in infants.

Children weighing over 15 kg who must undergo long-term dialysis are usually provided with an atriovenous fistula. The preferred site for cannula placement is the radial artery and a forearm vein. Sometimes alternate vessels are used including the tibial artery and the long saphenous vein, especially for home dialysis. An alternative to the external Teflon shunt is the creation of a subcutaneous (internal) arteriovenous fistula by anastomosing a segment of a saphenous vein autograft or a bovine arterial xenograft to the brachial artery and brachiocephalic vein, which produces dilation and thickening of the superficial vessels of the forearm to provide easy access for repeated venipuncture. There appear to be fewer complications and less restriction of activity with this approach; however, it requires needle insertion at each dialysis. For temporary vascular access, percutaneous catheters are inserted in the femoral, subclavian, or internal jugular veins, even in very small children.

Various hemodialysis schedules are employed, but most centers recommend dialysis three times a week for 4 to 6 hours, depending on the size of the child. For a complete description of the highly specialized process of hemodialysis, the reader is directed to the numerous references available on this topic.

Dietary limitations are necessary in chronic dialysis to avoid biochemical complications and to facilitate adequate dialysis. Fluid and sodium are restricted to prevent fluid overload with its associated symptoms of hypertension, cerebral manifestations, and congestive heart failure. Potassium is restricted to prevent complications related to hyperkalemia; phosphorus restriction helps to prevent parathyroid hyperactivity and its attendant risk of abnormal calcification in soft tissues. Limited protein intake reduces high levels of blood urea nitrogen. Fluid is usually limited to 5 dl/m^2/day plus an amount equal to daily urine output.

Response to Dialysis

Most children show rapid clinical improvement with the implementation of dialysis, although it is directly related to the duration of uremia before dialysis and the extent to which dietary regulations are followed. Growth rate and skeletal maturation usually improve, but recovery of normal growth is uncommon. In many cases sexual development, although delayed, has progressed to completion.

Seizures during or after hemodialysis are not uncommon. The cause is uncertain, but they probably result from cerebral edema caused by alterations in osmolality in the brain when the blood urea nitrogen level is lowered rapidly. Hyponatremia may be a factor as well. Seizures are most likely to occur at the time dialysis is first initiated, when large changes in serum osmolality may occur.

Home Dialysis

With appropriate implantation or cannulization and proper training and education of both the child and parents, either peritoneal dialysis or hemodialysis can be performed at home. Time spent in transportation is eliminated, the environment is more pleasant and secure, and the child is able to assume a more active role in the treatment program. Home dialysis is especially advantageous for children waiting for a transplant who live a great distance from the dialysis center or for children who have had one or more kidney transplant failures.

Home hemodialysis units are available to some children, and the preparation and management are similar to those required for hemodialysis in the hospital. The patient is equipped with a dialysis unit that is used with the vascular access established for outpatient dialysis.

The development of satisfactory methods for *continuous ambulatory peritoneal dialysis (CAPD)* and its alternative *continuous cycling peritoneal dialysis (CCPD)* has provided additional means for managing end-stage renal disease at home. In both methods commercially available sterile dialysate solution is instilled into the peritoneal cavity through a surgically implanted indwelling catheter sutured in place. The warmed solution is allowed to enter the peritoneal cavity by gravity and remains a variable length of time according to the procedure used.

In CAPD the dialysate is instilled, the line clamped off, and the empty solution bag rolled up and worn attached to the abdomen or thigh or even placed in a pocket. The solution is allowed to remain in the peritoneum for 4 to 6 hours.

The bag is then unrolled and placed on the floor, the line is unclamped, and the fluid is drained into the bag by gravity. Another heated bag is hung and the process is repeated so that there is fluid in the abdomen continuously. The procedure is performed 3 times during the day and once at night. For an active child CAPD has proved to be a satisfactory alternative to hemodialysis that can be continued for an indefinite time.

CCPD is a modification of CAPD and intermittent peritoneal dialysis. The dialysis exchange is performed only at night using an automatic dialysis machine, which controls the timed cycles of inflow and outflow of dialysate. The catheter is opened only at night rather than four times per day, although an additional exchange may be prescribed during the day. The nighttime dialysis allows the child more freedom during the day and relieves parents from having to perform muliple exchanges (Alliapoulos and others, 1984).

The care and management of the procedure are the responsibility of the parents of young children. School nurses can perform the procedure for younger school-age children. Older children and adolescents are able carry out the procedure themselves, thus providing them with some control and less dependency. This is especially important for adolescents.

Complications. CAPD and CCPD are presently considered to be the methods of choice for most children who require dialysis because they are easier to initiate and maintain than hemodialysis. Peritonitis is the major complication of home peritoneal dialysis but no differences in the incidence of infection have been found between the two methods (Warady and others, 1984; Alliapoulos and others, 1984). The patients are treated with antibiotics and some may require catheter replacement. Although the risk of infection is continuously present, most practitioners believe that it is not great enough to discourage the use of these methods (Fine and others, 1983).

However, other complications have been noted in patients on home peritoneal dialysis. Tunnel infections are evidenced by swelling, warmth, and tenderness along the subcutaneous catheter tract; however, they can be managed with administration of antibiotics. Peritoneal leaks and ventral hernias caused by the sustained hydraulic pressure that develops within the peritoneum have also been found in a significant number of children. Most of these patients respond to reduction in dialysate volume.

Nursing Considerations

Initiating a hemodialysis regimen is a traumatic and anxiety-provoking experience for most children. It involves surgery for implantation of the shunt or fistula, and the initial experience with the hemodialysis machine and its implication are frightening to most children. They need reassurance about the nature of the preparations for dialysis and conduct of the treatment. They are anxious concerning repeated venipunctures (with implanted shunts and for blood chemistries) and the sight of their blood leaving their body and entering the machine. Once the initial fear of the machine has been resolved, younger children adjust fairly well to maintenance hemodialysis.

Adolescents, with their increased need for independence and their urge for rebellion, usually adapt less well. They resent the control and enforced dependence imposed by the rigorous and unrelenting therapy program. They resent being dependent on a machine, parents, and professional staff. Depression, hostility, or both are common in adolescents undergoing hemodialysis. The adverse consequences of the disease include the need for diet restrictions, limitations to physical activity (resulting from lack of energy, frequent illnesses, and specific restrictions related to the shunt, such as no swimming with an external shunt), and simply the sense of being different from other children. Withdrawal from peers and social isolation are the rule, and noncompliance with the therapeutic regimen is not uncommon in the adolescent.

Body changes related to the disease process, such as growth retardation, skin color, and lack of sexual maturation, are stress provoking. Dietary restrictions are particularly burdensome for both children and parents. Children feel deprived when unable to eat foods previously enjoyed and unrestricted for other family members. Consequently, failure to cooperate is not uncommon. Diet restrictions are interpreted as punishment and, since they may not be able to fully understand the purpose of the restrictions, some will sneak forbidden food items at every opportunity. Allowing children, especially adolescents, maximum participation in and responsibility for their own treatment program is helpful. The extent of compliance and adjustment depends on the personalities of the involved persons, the quality of their relationships, and their coping mechanisms.

After weeks or months of hemodialysis, parents and child feel anxiety associated with the prognosis and continued pressures of the treatment. The relentless need for treatment interferes with family plans. Transportation to and from the dialysis unit and the time spent on the machine restrict the time available for outside activities, including school. Shunt and fistula problems are not uncommon and present a common source of aggravation. Shunts and fistulas are prone to infection and are easily subject to clogging, which may necessitate further surgery. The occurrence of seizures during dialysis is highly stressful to both child and family. Eventually most severely affected children face nephrectomy, which predictably causes depression in both child and family. Most families have maintained some hope throughout dialysis, but imminent nephrectomy necessitates final acceptance of the diagnosis.

The availability of home dialysis has offered a greater degree of freedom for persons undergoing long-term dialysis. The need for a residence convenient to a dialysis unit and the necessity for frequent trips to the unit are eliminated except for monthly evaluations. The nurse is responsible for teaching the family. Education focuses on (1) the disease, its implications, and the therapeutic plan; (2) the possible psychologic effects of the disease and the treatment; and (3) the technical aspects of the procedure.

The family must learn how to take vital signs before and after the dialysis and how to interpret the significance of blood pressure and temperature variations. They need to know how to vary the composition of the dialysate to compensate for variations in the vital signs and to maintain an accurate record of all aspects of the treatment. Parents of children on hemodialysis must know how to operate the equipment, connect the unit to the vascular access, protect the shunt, change the dressing, and assess the status of the child. They must palpate an internal shunt for evidence of patency and auscultate it for a bruit sound. Rarely an external shunt may become detached at the site of entry, and the family should know how to clamp and reconnect the tubing using aseptic technique before excess bleeding can take place.

Parents of the young child using CAPD are taught how to exchange bags and manage the procedure at home. Even newborn infants are able to benefit from peritoneal dialysis. Older children can be taught to take responsibility for their own treatments as much as possible. The family is encouraged to ask questions throughout the preparation time, including those that clarify anatomy and physiology, mechanical functioning, and side effects of the disease and the treatment. The peritoneal dialysis schedule is outlined to meet the individual needs of the patient and the family. Most schedules are arranged for uninterrupted sleep at night and to coordinate the dialysis with school and other activities. The diet, medication, and activity are discussed, and feelings about the entire therapeutic program are explored with the child and the family.

Infection is the greatest hazard of both hemodialysis and peritoneal dialysis; therefore the family is instructed to contact the appropriate persons at the earliest evidence of shunt infection or peritonitis. In most instances of peritonitis the infection can be controlled with administration of antibiotics. Unfortunately there is a high incidence of peritonitis; episodes occur approximately 6 months to a year apart (Sedman, 1986b). Repeated infections may necessitate replacement of the catheter or its removal and abandonment of the peritoneum as an access route. An infected or occluded shunt usually requires changing the access site, which involves another surgical procedure for its replacement.

The importance of emotional as well as material support cannot be overemphasized. The National Kidney Foundation, mentioned previously, provides a number of services and information for families of children with renal disease. A relatively new organization, the **National Association of Patients on Hemodialysis and Transplantation (NAPHT),** * has been organized to promote the interest of and welfare of kidney patients. It provides education and support for patients and public education regarding all areas of kidney disease.

*150 Nassau St., New York, NY 10038.

TRANSPLANTATION

Renal transplantation is now an acceptable and effective means of therapy in the pediatric age-group. While peritoneal dialysis and hemodialysis are life-preserving and are able to be carried out in the home in a large number of cases, neither method is compatible with a normal life-style. Transplantation, on the other hand, offers the opportunity for a relatively normal life and does not impair physical growth. It is presently regarded as the preferred form of treatment for many children with chronic renal failure.

Kidneys for transplant are available from two sources: a living related donor (LRD), usually a parent or sibling, and cadaver donor (CD), wherein the family of a dead or brain-dead patient consent to donation of a healthy kidney. The criteria for selection of kidney recipients are quite liberal, but uniform criteria have not been established among the various centers that specialize in the procedure. In general there is no limit to age. In some cases, a person's mental status (e.g., mental retardation, emotional instability, or noncompliant behavior) may be reason to defer transplantation until the recipient's psychoemotional status improves and it is reasonable to assume that the posttransplant regimen will be carried out (Novello, 1986b).

Possible recipients with preexisting malignancy (e.g., Wilms tumor) are at risk and there may be reason for delay. Generalized infection must be eradicated before attempted transplantation, and the recipient should have adequate bladder capacity, although this is not considered to be a contraindication. Children with abnormal bladders may be subject to more posttransplant urologic complications and infection than they would otherwise be. Nevertheless, many children with systemic disease and tumors have had successful transplants. On the other hand, there is a high incidence of recurrent disease in the donor kidney in children who receive a transplant for rapidly progressive glomerulonephritis with irreversible renal failure.

Procedure

The kidney graft is placed in the extraperitoneal space, usually the anterior iliac fossa, and the renal artery is anastomosed to the internal iliac or hypogastric artery, the renal vein is anastomosed to the hypogastric vein, and the ureter is implanted into the bladder or anastomosed to the recipient's ureter. Small children receiving a large donor kidney may require placement within the abdomen with vessel anastomoses to the aorta and inferior vena cava. Unless there is medical contraindication, the recipient's failed kidneys are left in place. Severe hypertension, neoplasm, and immunologic glomerulonephritis with antibody formation against the recipient's kidney tissue are the usual causes for nephrectomy.

The primary goal in transplantation is the long-term survival of the grafted tissue. The means by which this is attempted is (1) securing tissues that are antigenically similar to that of the recipient and (2) suppressing the recipient's immune mechanism.

Questions and Controversies

Who should be denied renal transplantation?

The criteria for selection of renal transplant recipients sometimes creates dilemmas for professionals. In most cases the decision is simply a matter for the transplant team and the family to resolve for the benefit of the child involved. However, in some situations, especially in view of the scarcity of donor kidneys and the expense of the procedure, the solution is less clear. The matter creates more questions than answers.

For example, should a child with a severe mental or physical disability take priority over one without these disabilities? Should financial responsibility be a consideration? Some youngsters with renal transplants have discontinued taking their medications thereby either causing damage to their kidney or losing the graft (Korsch, 1981). Should these youngsters receive a second transplant? Should very young children whose families have proven too unreliable in complying with a therapeutic regimen be given a transplant when the success of the graft depends on following a prescribed therapeutic plan? Are very young, unwed adolescent mothers likely to be less compliant in following the prescribed medical regimen? Can persons on limited incomes manage to acquire the costly medications? If not, should the government subsidize payment?

What solutions to these dilemmas are available and how are decisions justified? Who should make the decisions?

Selection of Donor Tissue

The source of a donor kidney is either a live person or a cadaver soon after death. The closer the genetic relationship between the donor and recipient, the better the possibility of long-term survival. The only truly compatible tissue match is that between identical twin siblings. The next best possible match is a sibling, then a parent, and finally an uncle or aunt. Use of siblings is impossible, however, until the possible donor is of age to give consent for removal of a kidney. Unrelated donors are least likely to be compatible. Careful studies are carried out to determine the donor whose kidney is least likely to be rejected by the recipient.

Suppression of the Immune Response

After the best possible tissue match is obtained for a transplant, the survival time can be significantly lengthened by suppressing the immune response of the recipient. The immunosuppressant therapy of choice in kidney transplantation is corticosteroids (prednisone) in conjunction with cyclosporine or azathioprine. Other therapies include antilymphoblast globulin, administered intravenously for 14 days posttransplant.

The administration of these drugs is not without hazard. The major problem encountered with nonspecific immunosuppression is that it not only suppresses the immune response to the grafted tissue but also suppresses the body's capacity to respond to other antigenic stimuli. Consequently, the child is vulnerable to overwhelming infections.

Prednisone is a powerful immunosuppressant and anti-inflammatory agent that acts to stabilize cell walls, reduce migration of white blood cells into the inflamed area, and inhibit deposition of fibrin and collagen. It also depresses T-cells, B-cells, and phagocytes. A number of complications that are directly attributable to corticosteroid therapy are cause for concern for children in steroid therapy. Interference with calcium absorption retards linear growth, and in some centers alternate-day administration is being used in an effort to improve growth rates. Other corticosteroid-induced side effects may include the characteristic fat redistribution of Cushing syndrome (see Fig. 38-3), cataracts, fluid and sodium retention, and gastric ulcer.

Cyclosporine is a powerful immunosuppressant that acts to decrease production of T-cells. Side effects of this drug are arterial hypertension, which may appear within 3 weeks of transplant; hirsutism; and nephrotoxicity, a major concern in renal transplantation. A response to these side effects is to reduce the drug dosage until the child exhibits some sign of rejection and then to increase it to an ideal level needed to maintain the transplanted kidney. After the initial intravenous therapy immediately posttransplant, the drug is administered orally. It has a rather unpleasant taste; however, this can be satisfactorily disguised by the addition of chocolate milk at a level of at least 10 times the amount of the drug.

Azathioprine is a powerful immunosuppressant that interferes with cellular protein synthesis. The problem related to the toxic effect of azathioprine is mainly hepatic dysfunction, which is usually managed by reduced dosage. (See Chapter 36 for a discussion of immunosuppressant therapy and related nursing care.)

Rejection

Rejection of a transplanted kidney is the most frequent cause of transplant failure. Rejection can be one of three types—hyperacute, acute, or chronic. Hyperacute rejection is irreversible, develops immediately or within a few hours after revascularization, and is related to circulating antibodies preformed in the recipient against the donor tissue antigens. These are seen in second transplants or in persons sensitized from blood transfusions.

Acute rejection usually occurs between the first few days and 6 months after transplantation but may occur as late as 1 or 2 years later. Rejection is evidenced by both biochemical and clinical abnormalities. The most frequent finding is fever, which is usually accompanied by swelling and tenderness over the graft, hypertension, and diminished urine output. A severe reaction may cause oliguria. Increases in serum blood urea nitrogen and creatinine levels are laboratory evidence of decreased transplant function. Most acute rejection episodes respond to intravenous administration of methylprednisolone sodium succinate (Solu-Medrol).

Chronic rejection is characterized by slow, gradual deterioration of renal function that typically begins 6 months or more after transplantation. Evidence of rejection may be heralded by proteinuria and/or hematuria, and the rejection may have symptomatology indistinguishable from the original kidney disease. No present therapy can halt the progressive process, which inevitably leads to loss of the implanted kidney.

Prognosis

The 2-year survival rate of transplants varies from 65% to 95% for relative donors and 42% to 80% for cadaver grafts. Complications that have been reported are hypertension, steroid-induced diabetes, cataracts, bone demineralization, and aseptic necrosis (Lum, Wassner, and Martin, 1985). Although growth retardation is a problem, it appears to be less in recipients receiving their transplants under age 10. In very small children who are almost always severely growth retarded, good graft function generally ensures some catchup growth and consistently near-normal rates of growth thereafter (Sheldon and others, 1985).

Nursing Considerations

The possibility of renal transplantation often comes as a hope for relief from the rigors of hemodialysis and the hated diet restrictions. Except for children with preexisting personality problems or residual physical disabilities, most children and families respond well to kidney transplant and the majority return to normal life within a year after surgery. The dynamics related to accepting and donating kidneys are fraught with emotional overtones, caused in part by the issues related to the child's receiving an organ from another person.

A variety of serious emotional and psychologic conflicts may arise as a consequence of donor selection, including ambivalence of donors faced with surgery and relinquishing a kidney, feelings of guilt if one should prove to be unacceptable as a donor, and the emotional impact of having a live-relative donated kidney rejected by the recipient. This is especially guilt-producing when a parent is the donor.

The child recipient responds in various ways to kidney transplant. The concept of having a foreign body, especially a cadaver kidney, inside their own body is sometimes disturbing to children. They often speculate about the age, sex, personality, and physical characteristics of the donor. They may fear that the kidney will wear out if it came from an older person. Some children are distressed to find that their donor kidney came from a person of the opposite sex. Corticosteroid therapy, necessary in kidney transplants, creates undesirable side effects—for example, growth failure, obesity, characteristics of Cushing syndrome, acne, and hirsutism—that are frequently a source of emotional and social problems for older children.

The most frequent reason for noncompliance in childhood renal transplant recipients is dislike of undesirable side effects. The cosmetic implications of the side effects can be overwhelming, especially to adolescent girls. Deliberate discontinuation of the drugs is most commonly observed in teenage girls. Noncompliance is also seen frequently in children from poorly communicating families who are not very

supportive (see Chapter 27). These children have the lowest results on personality tests.

Working with children and their families during the various stages of renal failure, dialysis, and transplantation is a difficult and challenging experience. Nurses must become familiar with the family; assess family strengths, weaknesses, and coping mechanisms; and be prepared to provide intensive support and guidance during the prolonged experience. The child and family need help in accepting what is happening to them, learning anticipatory guidance regarding predictable stresses, and dealing constructively with the physical, emotional, and financial burdens that are an ongoing part of this prolonged disability.

CONCEPT SUMMARIES

- The main function of the kidney is to maintain the composition and volume of body fluids in equilibrium.
- Common inflammatory disorders of the genitourinary tract include urinary tract infection, nephrotic syndrome, and acute glomerulonephritis.
- UTIs constitute the second largest group of infections, next to respiratory tract disease.
- Management of UTIs is directed at eliminating infection, detecting and correcting functional or anatomic abnormalities, preventing recurrences, and preserving renal function.
- Vesicoureteral reflux is the retrograde flow of bladder urine into the ureters.
- Nephrotic syndrome is characterized by increased glomerular permeability to protein.
- Management of nephrotic syndrome is aimed at reducing excretion or protein, reducing or preventing fluid retention by tissues, and preventing infection and other complications, dietary control, corticosteroid therapy,, immunosuppressant therapy, use of diuretics, and use of antimicrobials.
- Common features of acute glomerulonephritis are oliguria, edema, hypertension, circulatory congestion, hematuria, and proteinuria.
- Therapeutic management of acute glomerulonephritis is maintenance of fluid balance, treatment of hypertension, and antibiotic therapy.
- Primary functions of the distal renal tubules are acidification of urine, potassium secretion, and selective and differential reabsorption of sodium, chloride, and water.
- The most common renal tubular disorders are renal tubular acidosis and nephrogenic diabetes insipidus.
- Obstructive uropathy is the result of structural or functional abnormalities of the urinary system that obstruct the normal flow of urine.
- Management of hemolytic-uremic syndrome is aimed at control of complications and hematologic manifestations of renal failure.
- In acute renal failure, management is directed at determining treatment of underlying cause, management of complications of renal failure, and supportive therapy.

- Abnormalities in chronic renal failure are waste product retention, water and sodium retention, hyperkalemia, acidosis, calcium and phosphorus disturbance, anemia, and growth disturbances.

- When the child will need home dialysis, the nurse educates the family on the disease, its implications, the therapeutic plan, possible psychologic effects of the disease, and the treatment and technical aspects of the procedure.

- The major concerns in renal transplantation are tissue matching and prevention of rejection; psychologic concerns involve self-image as related to possible body changes as a result of the effects of corticosteroid therapy.

REFERENCES

Alliapoulos, J.C., and others: Comparison of continuous cycling peritoneal dialysis with continuous ambulatory peritoneal dialysis in children, J. Pediatr. **105:**721-725, 1984.

Avner, E.D., and others: Single-dose amoxicillin therapy of uncomplicated pediatric urinary tract infections, J. Pediatr. **102:**623-627, 1983.

Chevalier, R.L., and Rogol, A.D.: Tolmetin sodium in the management of nephrogenic diabetes insipidus, J. Pediatr. **101:**787-789, 1982.

Cooley, R.O., and Sobel, R.S.: Dental treatment considerations for the medically compromised child, Pediatr. Clin. North Am. **29:**613-629, 1982.

Dracopoulos, D.T., and Weatherly, J.B.: Chronic renal failure: the effects on the entire family, Issues Compr. Pediatr. Nurs. **6:**141-146, 1983.

Drummond, K.N.: Developmental abnormalities. In Behrman, R.E., and Vaughan, V.C., III, editors: Textbook of pediatrics, ed. 12, Philadelphia, 1983, W.B. Saunders Co.

Ehrlich, R.M.: Vesicoureteral reflux: a surgeon's perspective, Pediatr. Clin. North Am. **29:**827-834, 1982.

Fine, J.S., and Jacobson, M.S.: Single-dose versus conventional therapy of urinary tract infections in female adolescents, Pediatrics **75:**916-920, 1985.

Fine, R.N., and others: Peritonitis in children undergoing continuous ambulatory peritoneal dialysis, Pediatrics **71:**806-809, 1983.

Fish, A.J., and Fouser, L.S.: Glomerulonephritis. In Gellis, S.S., and Kagan, B.M., editors: Current pediatric therapy 12, Philadelphia, 1986, W.B. Saunders Co.

Fong, J.S.C., de Chadarevian, J., and Kaplan, B.S.: Hemolytic-uremic syndrome, Pediatr. Clin. North Am. **29:**835-856, 1982.

Garin, E.H., and Richard, G.A.: Prostaglandin inhibitors in treatment of nephrogenic diabetes insipidus, J. Pediatr. **104:**174, 1983.

Griswold, W.R., and others: Accumulation of aluminum in a nondialyzed uremic child receiving aluminum hydroxide, Pediatrics **71:**56-58, 1983.

Hellerstein, S., and others: Consensus: roentgenographic evaluation of children with urinary tract infection, Pediatr. Infect. Dis. **3:**291-293, 1984.

Hensle, T.W., and Burbige, K.A.: Vesicoureteral reflux. In Gellis, S.S., and Kagan, B.M., editors: Current pediatric therapy 12, Philadelphia, 1986, W.B. Saunders Co.

Hoover, D.L.: Genitourinary trauma. In Pierog, J.E., and Pierog, L.J., editors: Pediatric critical illness and injury, Rockville, MD, 1984, Aspen Systems Corp.

Hsu, A.C., and others: Renal osteodystrophy in children with chronic renal failure: an unexpectedly common and incapacitating complication, Pediatrics **70:**742-750, 1982.

Jones, R.W.A., and others: The effects of anabolic steroids on growth, body composition, and metabolism in boys with chronic renal failure on regular hemodialysis, J. Pediatr. **97:**559-566, 1980.

Jordan, S.C., and Lemire, J.M.: Acute glomerulonephritis, Pediatr. Clin. North Am. **29:**857-873, 1982.

Kaplan, B.: General considerations of obstructive lesions of the urinary tract. In Behrman, R.E., and Vaughan, V.C., III, editors: Textbook of pediatrics, ed. 12, Philadelphia, 1983, W.B. Saunders Co.

Khan, A.J., Kumar, K., and Evans, H.E.: Three-day antimicrobial therapy of urinary tract infection, J. Pediatr. **99:**992-994, 1981.

Kim, M.S., and Grupe, W.E.: The nephrotic syndrome. In Gellis, S.S., and Kagan, B.M., editors: Current pediatric therapy 12, Philadelphia, 1986, W.B. Saunders Co.

Kinane, D.F., and others: ABO blood group, secretor state and susceptibility to recurrent urinary tract infection in women, Br. Med. J. **285:**7-9, 1982.

Korsch, B.: The impact of end-stage renal disease. In Azarnoff, P., and Hardgrove, C., editors: The family in child health care, New York, 1981, John Wiley & Sons.

Kroovand, R.L., and Perlmutter, A.D.: The genitourinary system. In Behrman, R.E., and Vaughan, V.C., III, editors: Textbook of pediatrics, ed. 12, Philadelphia, 1983, W.B. Saunders Co.

Krugman, S., and others: Infectious diseases of children, ed. 8, St. Louis, 1985, The C.V. Mosby Co.

Kunin, C.: Diagnosis, prevention, and management of urinary tract infection, ed. 3, Philadelphia, 1979, Lea & Febiger.

Leisti, S., and Koskimies, O.: Risk of relapse in steroid-sensitive nephrotic syndrome: effect of stage of post-prednisone adrenocortical suppression, J. Pediatr. **103:**553-557, 1983.

Libber, S., Harrison, H., and Spector, D.: Treatment of nephrogenic diabetes insipidus with prostaglandin synthesis inhibitors, J. Pediatr. **108:**305-311, 1986.

Lohr, A.A., and others: Three-day therapy of lower urinary tract infection with nitrofurantoin macrocrystacs: a randomized clinical trial, J. Pediatr. **99:**990-995, 1981.

Lomberg, H., and others: Correlation of P blood group, vesicoureteral reflux, and bacterial attachment in patients with recurrent pyelonephritis, N. Engl. J. Med. **308:**1189-1192, 1983.

Lum, C.T., Wassner, S.J., and Martin, D.E.: Current thinking in transplantation in infants and children, Pediatr. Clin. North Am. **32:**1203-1232, 1985.

McEnery, P.T., and Strife, C.F.: Nephrotic syndrome in childhood, Pediatr. Clin. North Am. **89:**875-894, 1982.

Novello, A.C.: Hemodialysis. In Gellis, S.S., and Kagan, B.M., editors: Current pediatric therapy 12, Philadelphia, 1986a, W.B. Saunders Co.

Novello, A.C.: Renal transplantation. In Gellis, S.S., and Kagan, B.M., editors: Current pediatric therapy 12, Philadelphia, 1986b, W.B. Saunders Co.

Ogra, P.L., and Faden, H.S.: Urinary tract infections in childhood: an update, J. Pediatr. **106:**1023-1028, 1985.

Roberts, J.A.: Does circumcision prevent urinary tract infection, J. Urol. **135:**991-992, 1986.

Rogers, W.B.: Shampoo urethritis, Am. J. Dis. Child. **139:**748-749, 1985.

Salmen, P., and others: Whirlpool-associated *Pseudomonas aeruginosa* urinary tract infection, JAMA **250:**2025-2026, 1983.

Schoeneman, M.J.: Minimal change nephrotic syndrome: treatment with low dose of hydrocortisone, J. Pediatr. **102:**791-793, 1983.

Sedman, A.B.: Chronic renal failure. In Gellis, S.S., and Kagan, B.M., editors: Current pediatric therapy 12, Philadelphia, 1986a, W.B. Saunders Co.

Sedman, A.B.: Peritoneal dialysis. In Gellis, S.S., and Kagan, B.M., editors: Current pediatric therapy 12, Philadelphia, 1986b, W.B. Saunders Co.

Shapiro, E.D., and Wald, E.R.: Single dose amoxicillin treatment of urinary tract infection, J. Pediatr. **99:**989-992, 1981.

Sheldon, C.A., and others: Improving survival in the very young renal transplant recipient, J. Pediatr. Surg. **6:**622-626, 1985.

Sidor, T.A., and Resnick, M.I.: Urinary tract infection in children, Pediatr. Clin. North Am. **30:**323-332, 1983.

Siegel, S.R., and others: Urinary infection in infants and preschool children, Am. J. Dis. Child. **134:**369-372, 1980.

Smith, F.G.: Urinary tract infections. In Gellis, S.S., and Kagan, B.M., editors: Current pediatric therapy 12, Philadelphia, 1986, W.B. Saunders Co.

Underwood, M.A.: Urinary tract infections, Crit. Care Q. **3**(3):63-70, 1980.

Warady, B.A., and others: Peritonitis with continuous ambulatory peritoneal dialysis and continuous cycling peritoneal dialysis, J. Pediatr. 726-730, 1984.

Warshaw, B.L., Hymes, L.C., and Woodard, J.R.: Long-term outcome of patients with obstructive uropathy, Pediatr. Clin. North Am. **29**:815-826, 1982.

Weir, M.R., and Lampe, R.M.: Urinary tract infections in children, Am. Fam. Physician **29**:147-153, 1984.

Wiswell, T.E., Smith, F.R., and Bass, J.W.: Decreased incidence of urinary tract infections in circumcised male infants, Pediatrics **75**:901-903, 1985.

BIBLIOGRAPHY

General

Anderson, G.F., and Smey, P.: Current concepts in the management of common urologic problems in infants and children, Pediatr. Clin. North Am. **32**:1133-1149, 1985.

Brundage, D.J.: Nursing management of renal problems, ed. 2, St. Louis, 1980, The C.V. Mosby Co.

Droske, S.C., and Francis, S.A.: Pediatric diagnostic procedures, New York, 1981, John Wiley & Sons.

Grupe, W.E.: Nutritional considerations in the prognosis and treatment of children with renal disease. In Suskind, R.M., editor: Textbook of pediatric nutrition, New York, 1981, Raven Press.

Guyton, A.C.: Textbook of medical physiology, ed. 6, Philadelphia, 1980, W.B. Saunders Co.

Hetrick, A., Frauman, A.C., and Gilman, C.M.: Nutrition in renal disease: when the patient is a child, Am. J. Nurs. **79**:2152-2154, 1979.

International Reflux Study Committee: Medical versus surgical treatment of primary vesicoureteral reflux, Pediatrics **67**:392-400, 1981.

Kallen, R.J.: What's causing the hematuria? Contemp. Pediatr. **8**:55-71, June 1986.

Kaplan, M.R.: Hematuria in childhood, Pediatr. Rev. **5**:99-105, 1983.

Mathews, K.P., and Calvallo, T.: Immune aspects of renal disease, JAMA **248**:2701-2703, 1982.

Murphy, L.M., and Cole, M.J.: Renal disease: nutritional implications, Nurs. Clin. North Am. **18**:57-70, 1983.

Nace, G.: Preventing adverse drug reactions in patients with renal failure, J. Nephr. Nurs. **2**:30-32, 1985.

Oestreich, S.J.K.: Rational nursing care in chronic renal disease, Am. J. Nurs. **79**:1096-1099, 1979.

Orr, M.L.: Drugs and renal disease, Am. J. Nurs. **81**:969-971, 1981.

Stark, J.L.: BUN/creatinine: your keys to kidney function, Nursing 80 **10**(5):33-38, 1980.

Tichy, A.M.: Renal failure, Crit. Care Update **7**(3):5-18, 1980.

Vehaskari, V.M., and Rapola, J.: Isolated proteinuria: analysis of school-age population, J. Pediatr. **101**:661-668, 1982.

Vernier, R.L.: Commentary, J. Pediatr. **100**:235-236, 1982.

Urinary Tract Infection

Bergstein, J.M.: Hematuria, proteinuria, and urinary tract infections, Pediatr. Clin. North Am. **20**:55-66, 1982.

Brogna, L., and Lakaszawski, M.L.: The continent urostomy, Am. J. Nurs. **86**:160-163, 1986.

Hellerstein, S.: Recurrent urinary tract infections in children, Pediatr. Infect. Dis. **1**:271-281, 1982.

Hellerstein, S., and others: Localization of the site of urinary tract infections with the bladder washout test, J. Pediatr. **98**:201-206, 1981.

Kaplan, G.W.: Recurring urinary infections: current dilemmas, observations, reflections, Pediatr. Consult. **1**:1-8, 1980.

LaFave, J.B., and others: Office screening for asymptomatic urinary tract infections, Clin. Pediatr. **18**:53-59, 1979.

Luke, R.J.: Reflux nephropathy—not "chronic pyelonephritis," Kidney **14**:46, 1981.

McCracken, G.H., and others: Evaluation of short-term antibiotic therapy in children with uncomplicated urinary tract infections, Pediatrics **67**:796-801, 1981.

Roberts, K.B., and others: Urinary tract infection in infants with unexplained fever: a collaborative study, J. Pediatr. **103**:864-867, 1983.

Selden, R.V., and others: Managing urinary-tract infections in children, Pediatr. Ann. **10**:12-24, 1981.

Stann, J.H.: Urinary tract infections in children, Pediatr. Nurs. **5**:49-52, 1979.

Thomas, C.K.: Childhood urinary tract infection, Pediatr. Nurs. **8**:114-119, 1982.

Wientzen, R.L., and others: Localization and therapy of urinary tract infections of childhood, Pediatrics **63**:467-474, 1979.

Winberg, J., and others: Clinical pyelonephritis and focal renal scarring, Pediatr. Clin. North Am. **29**:801-814, 1982.

Nephrotic Syndrome

Callis, L., and others: Chlorambucil treatment in minimal lesion nephrotic syndrome: a reappraisal of its gonadal toxicity, J. Pediatr. **97**:653-656, 1980.

Cornfield, D.: Nephrosis in childhood, Hosp. Med. **14**:98-99, 1978.

Early identification of frequent relapsers among children with minimal change nephrotic syndrome, J. Pediatr. **101**:514-518, 1982.

MacDonald, N.E., and others: Role of respiratory viruses in exacerbations of primary nephrotic syndrome, J. Pediatr. **108**:378-382, 1986.

Mahan, J.D., and others: Congenital nephrotic syndrome: evolution of medical management and results of renal transplantation, J. Pediatr. **105**:549-553, 1984.

Report of International Study of Kidney Disease in Children: The primary nephrotic syndrome in children. Identification of patients with minimal change nephrotic syndrome from initial response to prednisone, J. Pediatr. **98**:561-564, 1981.

Glomerulonephritis

Earle, D.P.: Poststreptococcal acute glomerulonephritis, Hosp. Pract. **20**(7):48E-48J, 48O-P, 48U, 48Z, 48AA-BB, 1985.

Kleinknecht, C., and others: Membranous glomerulonephritis and hepatitis B surface antigen in childhood, J. Pediatr. **95**:946-952, 1979.

Renal Tubular Disorders

Chan, J.C.M.: Renal tubular acidosis, J. Pediatr. **102**:327-340, 1983.

Donckerwolcke, R.A.: Diagnosis and treatment of renal tubular disorders in children, Pediatr. Clin. North Am. **29**:895-906, 1982.

Rodriguez-Soriano, J., and others: Natural history of primary distal renal tubular acidosis treated since infancy, J. Pediatr. **101**:669-676, 1982.

Hemolytic-Uremic Syndrome

Friedman, A., and Chesney, R.W.: Hemolytic-uremic syndrome. In Novello, A.C., editor: Current pediatric therapy, ed. 12, Philadelphia, 1986, W.B. Saunders Co.

Gomperts, E.C., and Lieberman, E.: Hemolytic-uremic syndrome, J. Pediatr. **97**:419-420, 1980.

O'Regan, S., and others: Aspirin and dipyridamole therapy in the hemolytic-uremic syndrome, J. Pediatr. **97**:473-476, 1980.

Acute Renal Failure (ARF)

Anand, S.K.: Acute renal failure in the neonate, Pediatr. Clin. North Am. **29**:791-800, 1982.

Engle, W.D.: Evaluation of renal function and acute renal failure in the neonate, Pediatr. Clin. North Am. **33**:129-151, 1986.

Kon, V., and Ichikawa, I.: Research seminar: physiology of acute renal failure, J. Pediatr. **105**:351-357, 1984.

Stark, J.L.: How to succeed against acute renal failure, Nursing 82 **12**(12):26-33, 1982.

Tichy, A.M.: Renal failure, Crit. Care Update **9**:7-21, 1982.

Chronic Renal Failure

Broyer, M.: Growth in children with renal insufficiency, Pediatr. Clin. North Am. **29:**991-1003, 1982.

Fennell, R.S., and others: Effects of kidney transplantation on cognitive performance in a pediatric population, Pediatrics **74:**273-278, 1984.

Fennell, R.S., and others: Growth in children with various therapies for end-stage renal disease, Am. J. Dis. Child. **138:**28-31, 1984.

Frauman, A.C., and Lansing, L.: The child with chronic renal failure. I. Change and challenge, Issues Compr. Nurs. **6:**127-133, 1983.

Frauman, A.C., and Lansing, L.: The child with chronic renal failure. II. Developmental habilitation, Issues Compr. Nurs. **6:**135-139, 1983.

Geary, D.F., and others: Encephalopathy in children with chronic renal failure, J. Pediatr. **96:**41-44, 1980.

Hodson, E.M., and others: Growth retardation and renal osteodystrophy in children with chronic renal failure, J. Pediatr. **103:**735-740, 1983.

Klein, K.L., and Maxwell, M.H.: Renal osteodystrophy, Orthop. Clin. North Am. **15:**687-695, 1984.

Langman, C.B., and others: 25-hydroxyvitamin D$_3$ (calcifediol) therapy of juvenile renal osteodystrophy: beneficial effect on linear growth velocity, J. Pediatr.**100:**815-820, 1982.

Lewis, S.M.: Pathophysiology of chronic renal failure, Nurs. Clin. North Am. **16:**501-513, 1981.

Lopes, G.S.: A dietary approach to chronic renal failure, Issues Compr. Pediatr. Nurs. **6:**23-62, 1983.

McGraw, M.E., and Haka-Ikse, K.: Neurologic-developmental sequelae of chronic renal failure in infancy, J. Pediatr. **106:**579-583, 1985.

Norman, M.E., and others: Early diagnosis of juvenile renal osteodystrophy, J. Pediatr. **97:**226-232, 1980.

Rodriguez, D.J., and Hunter, V.M.: Nutritional intervention in the treatment of chronic renal failure, Nurs. Clin. North Am. **16:**573-585, 1981.

Stark, J.L., and Hunt, V.: Helping your patient with chronic renal failure, Nursing 83 **13**(9):56-63, 1983.

Topor, M.: Chronic renal disease in children, Nurs. Clin. North Am. **16:**587-597, 1981.

Tyndall, M.G.: Chronic renal failure: past and future trends, Nurs. Clin. North Am. **16:**489-499, 1981.

Warshaw, B.L., and others: Progression to end-stage renal disease in children, J. Pediatr. **100:**183-187, 1982.

Wassner, S.J.: The role of nutrition in the care of children with renal insufficiency, Pediatr. Clin. North Am. **29:**973-990, 1982.

Dialysis

Binkley, L.S.: Keeping up with peritoneal dialysis, Am. J. Nurs. **84:**729-733, 1984.

Brem, A.S., and Toscano, A.M.: Continuous-cycling peritoneal dialysis for children: an alternative to hemodialysis treatment, Pediatrics **74:**254-258, 1984.

Ceccarelli, C.M.: Hemodialytic therapy for the patient with chronic renal failure, Nurs. Clin. North Am. **16:**531-550, 1981.

Chambers, J.K.: Assessing the dialysis patient at home, Am. J. Nurs. **81:**750-754, 1981.

Davis, V., and Lavandero, R.: Caring for the catheter carefully ... before, during, and after peritoneal dialysis, Nursing 80 **10**(12):67-71, 1980.

Denniston, D.J., and Burns, K.T.: Home peritoneal dialysis, Am. J. Nurs. **80:**2022-2026, 1980.

Duffy, M.M.: Peritoneal dialysis, Crit. Care Update **10**(8):7-22, 1983.

Fear of floating to a renal unit, Nursing 82 **12**(12):42-43, 1982.

Fine, R.N.: Peritoneal dialysis update, J. Pediatr. **100:**1-7, 1982.

Fleming, L.M., and Kane, J.: Step-by-step guide to safe peritoneal dialysis, RN **47**(2):44-47, 1984.

Gross, S.: Teaching young patients—and their families—about home peritoneal dialysis, Nursing 80 **10**(10):72-73, 1980.

Hewitt, I.K., and others: Renal osteodystrophy in children undergoing continuous ambulatory peritoneal dialysis, J. Pediatr. **103:**729-734, 1983.

Irwin, B.C.: Hemodialysis means vascular access ... and the right kind of nursing care, Nursing 79 **9**(10):49-53, 1979.

Reed, S.B.: Giving more than dialysis, Nursing 82 **12**(4):58-63, 1982.

Salusky, I.B., and others: Continuous ambulatory peritoneal dialysis in children, Pediatr. Clin. North Am. **29:**1005-1012, 1982.

Salusky, I.B., and others: Role of aluminum hydroxide in raising serum aluminum levels in children undergoing continuous ambulatory peritoneal dialysis, J. Pediatr. **105:**717-720, 1984.

Sorrels, P.A.J.: Peritoneal dialysis: a rediscovery, Nurs. Clin. North Am. **16:**515-529, 1981.

Spinnozi, N.S.: Teaching nutritional management to children on chronic hemodialysis, J. Am. Diet. Assoc. **75:**157-159, 1979.

Stefanidis, C.J., Hewitt, I.K., and Balfe, J.W.: Growth in children receiving continuous ambulatory peritoneal dialysis, J. Pediatr. **102:**681-685, 1983.

Tank, E.S., and Hatch, D.A.: Hernias complicating chronic ambulatory peritoneal dialysis in children, J. Pediatr. Surg. **21:**41-42, 1986.

Walker, L.: Adolescent dialysands in group therapy, Soc. Casework **66:**21-19, 1985.

Zappacosta, A.R., and Perras, S.T.: Continuous ambulatory peritoneal dialysis, Philadelphia, 1984, J.B. Lippincott Co.

Transplantation

Cianci, J., Lamb, J., and Ryan, R.K.: Renal transplantation, Am. J. Nurs. **81:**354-355, 1981.

Conley, S.B., and others: Use of cyclosporine in pediatric renal transplant recipients, J. Pediatr. **106:**45-49, 1985.

Enthusiastic cyclosporine consensus, Am. J. Nurs. **85:**861-862, 1985.

Fine, R.N., and others: Long-term results of transplantation in children, Pediatrics **61:**641-649, 1978.

Golden, D., and others: Understanding the magic of cyclosporine, RN **48**(6):53-54, 1985.

Gradus, D., and Ettenger, R.B.: Renal transplantation in children, Pediatr. Clin. North Am. **29:**1013-1038, 1982.

Irwin, B.C.: The renal transplant patient, Crit. Care Update **8**(9):30-41, 1981.

Kobrzycki, P.: Renal transplant complications, Am. J. Nurs. **77:**641-643, 1977.

Miller, L.C., and others: Transplantation of the adult kidney into the very small child: long-term outcome, J. Pediatr. **100:**675-680, 1982.

Moel, D.I., and Butt, K.M.H.: Renal transplantation in children less than 2 years of age, J. Pediatr. **99:**535-539, 1981.

Rasbury, W.C., Fennell, R.S., III, and Morris, M.K.: Cognitive functioning of children with end-stage renal disease before and after successful transplantation, J. Pediatr. **102:**589-592, 1983.

Rimar, J.M.: Cyclosporine for organ transplantation, J. Maternal Child Nurs. **10:**237, 1985.

Unit Eleven

The Child with Problems Related to Transfer of Oxygen and Nutrients

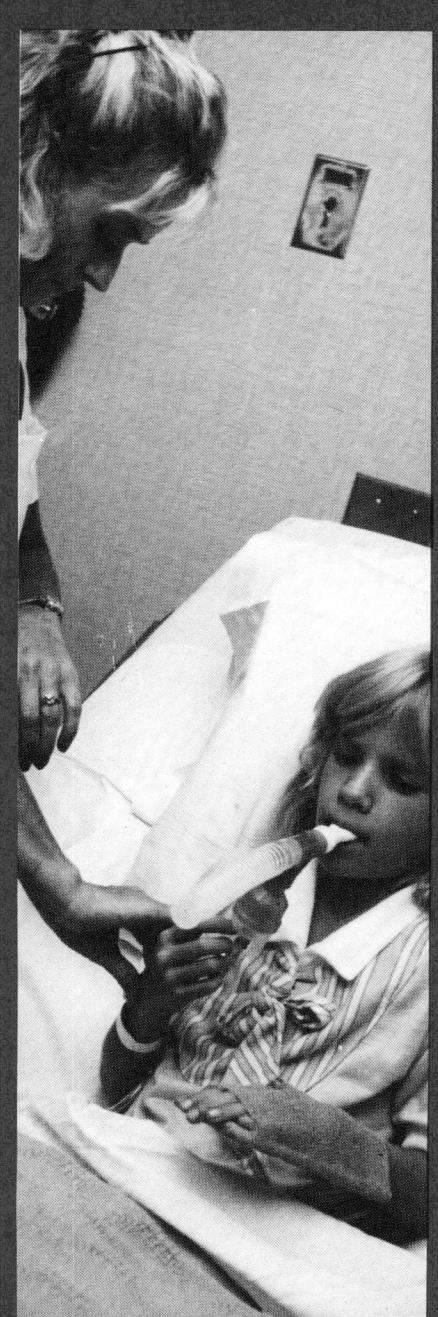

The survival of an individual depends on a continuous supply of energy for maintaining the function of all the cells in the body. This energy is obtained through oxygen and nutrients incorporated by the body and converted to energy by the process of oxygenation-reduction. Any circumstance or condition that requires an increase in energy requires a concomitant increase in the materials that the body converts into energy.

The need for oxygen is acute. Without this vital substance, the body is unable to survive more than a few minutes without permanent damage to vital structures or death. Therefore oxygen must be supplied constantly. Nutrients and water, on the other hand, can be stored within the body for use at times of increased need or diminished supply.

Alterations in the ability to supply oxygen or nutrients are some of the most common health problems of childhood. Interference with respiratory and gastrointestinal function is encountered at all ages, but very young children are especially vulnerable to dysfunctions in these systems. Respiratory and gastrointestinal disorders are encountered more frequently and the effects are more serious in children in the younger age-groups. Chapter 31, *The Child with Disturbance of Oxygen and Carbon Dioxide Exchange*, and Chapter 32, *The Child with Respiratory Dysfunction*, describe the more common conditions that impair the exchange of oxygen and carbon dioxide. Chapter 33, *The Child with a Gastrointestinal Disorder*, is concerned with factors that interfere with digestion or absorption of body nutrients. There are other situations in which there are disturbances in the availability of oxygen and nutrients for energy, for example, diabetes mellitus and disorders of fluid and electrolyte balance, but these are more appropriately discussed elsewhere.

Chapter 31

The Child with Disturbance of Oxygen and Carbon Dioxide Exchange

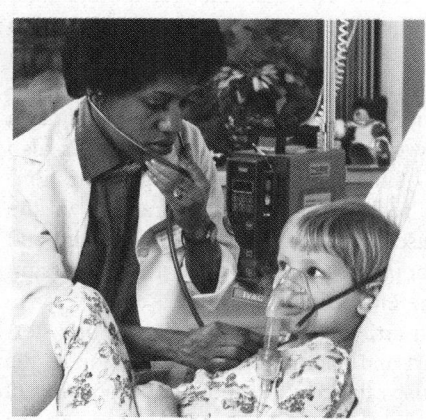

Disorders involving the respiratory tract, many of which can be life-threatening, are very common in infancy and childhood. A number of factors influence the development of respiratory disease in infancy and childhood. To enhance understanding of the way in which pathologic processes produce an effect, the basic anatomy and physiology of the respiratory tract are reviewed. The physiologic responses are no different in the child than in the adult; for example, gas exchange, oxygen and carbon dioxide tension, and the activity of chemoreceptors are very much the same in children and in adults. Anatomically, however, there are a number of differences that influence the way in which children, and particularly infants, respond to respiratory disturbances.

Respiratory Tract Structure and Function

The respiratory tract consists of a complex of structures that function under neural and hormonal control. The primary responsibility of these structures is to distribute air and exchange gases so that cells are supplied with oxygen for body metabolism and the volatile product of the metabolism (carbon dioxide) is removed. The organs of the respiratory system—nose, pharynx, larynx, trachea, bronchi, and lungs—provide the means whereby gases enter the body; the circulatory system distributes gases to and from the millions of cells throughout the body. All the structures of the respiratory system, except the minute air sacs (alveoli) of the lung tissue, function in air distribution. It is within the alveoli that the gas exchange takes place.

STRUCTURE

The thoracic cavity, which is encased in the bony framework provided by the ribs, vertebrae, and sternum, consists of three major partitions: the three-lobed lung on the right, the two-lobed lung on the left, and the space between them—the mediastinum—which contains the esophagus, trachea, large blood vessels, and heart. The entire thoracic cavity is lined by the smooth parietal pleura, which adheres to the ribs and superior surface of the diaphragm. Each lung is encased in a separate visceral pleural sac that, when inflated, lies against the parietal pleura. Normally the two pleural membranes are separated by only enough fluid to lubricate the surface for painless movement during filling and emptying of the lungs. In disease states this space may contain air (*pneumothorax*) or fluid (*pleural effusion*), more specifically serum (*hydrothorax,*), blood (*hemothorax*), or pus (*pyothorax*, also known as *empyema*.) Inflammation of the pleura causes the painful friction of pleurisy during respiratory movements.

General Aspects

The chest has a relatively round configuration at birth but changes gradually to one that is more or less flattened in the

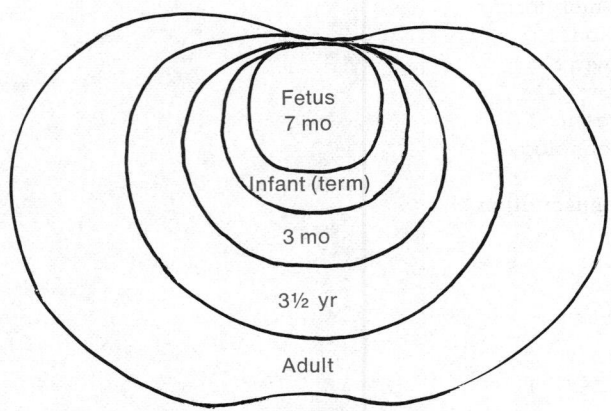

Fig. 31-1. Changes in chest shape with age.

anteroposterior diameter in adulthood (Fig. 31-1). In certain lung diseases chronic overinflation causes changes in these measurements. For example, in severe obstructive lung disease (such as asthma and cystic fibrosis) the anteroposterior measurement approaches the transverse measurement to produce the so-called barrel chest. Periodic measurements provide clues to the course of lung disease or the efficacy of therapy.

The elliptic shape of the ribs and the angle at which they are attached to the spine allow the thorax to change size during respiration. Contraction of the intercostal muscles lifts the ribs from a downward angle to a more horizontal angle, which increases both the anteroposterior and the lateral dimensions of the chest. This also changes the diameter of the bronchi. The diameter increases during inspiration and decreases during expiration, an important factor when the bronchi are narrowed as a result of obstruction or inflammation. Contraction and relaxation of the diaphragm cause the chest cavity to lengthen and shorten, which also increases the volume of the chest cavity during inspiration. Normal expiration is passive, although contraction of the internal intercostal muscles pulls the rib cage downward and contraction of the abdominal muscles forces the diaphragm upward to decrease the chest size actively.

The ribs of an adult articulate with the vertebrae and sternum from a downward and lateral angle. Contraction of the intercostal muscles raises the ribs to a horizontal position in a "bucket-handle" type of respiratory motion, causing the chest cavity to enlarge. In the newborn infant the ribs articulate with the spine at a horizontal rather than a downward slope and, if raised further, decrease the diameter of the chest (Fig. 31-2). Therefore the infant relies almost entirely on diaphragmatic-abdominal breathing. During inspiration the diaphragm is forced downward, increasing the available space for lung expansion. The intercostal muscles serve primarily as stabilizing forces.

Also facilitating respiration are (1) the elastic properties of lung tissue, which allow the lungs to expand with increasing volume (compliance) and to collapse away from the pleural wall with decreased volume (elastic recoil), and (2) the presence of a lipoprotein (surfactant) layer at the air-fluid interface, which allows even alveolar expansion and prevents alveolar collapse.

Compliance also changes with age. It is very high in the newborn, facilitated in part by a more pliant rib cage. This increased compliance in the newborn causes the rib cage to be easily distorted with increased negative pressure in the pleural cavity or when factors inhibit the stabilizing action of the intercostal muscles. This can be observed in the infant with lung disease. Inspiration causes an inward movement of the rib cage as the abdomen moves outward, because the greater negative pleural pressure required to move the lungs pulls in the soft, compliant, and easily distorted rib cage. Factors that interfere with compliance and recoil increase the work of respiration, for example, a deficiency of surfactant in respiratory distress syndrome or reduced compliance from fibrotic changes as a result of chronic lung

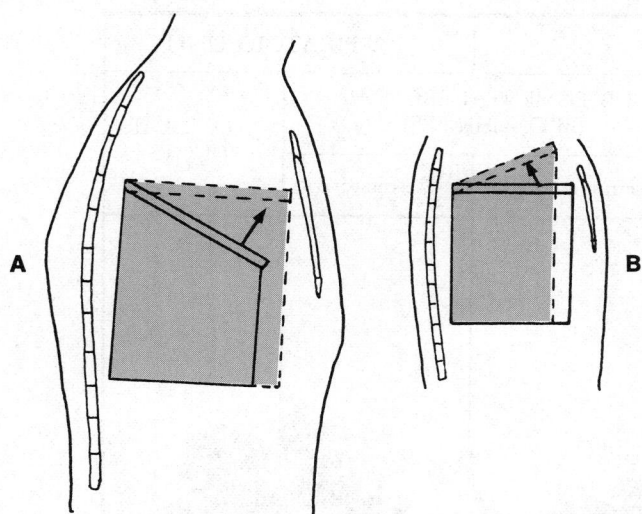

Fig. 31-2. Mechanisms of respiratory excursion. **A,** Downward and lateral position of rib in adult and expansion of lung capacity on thoracic inspiration. **B,** More horizontal position of rib in infant and decreased expansion of lung capacity of thoracic inspiration.

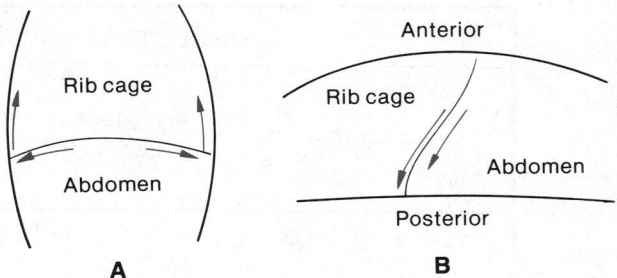

Fig. 31-3. Relationship of diaphragm and abdominal contents in **A,** upright, and **B,** supine positions.

disorders such as cystic fibrosis and chronic asthma.

There are also variations in lung volume relative to posture. In the upright position the evenly distributed weight of the abdominal contents contributes to uniform application of negative intrathoracic pressure. However, in the supine position the abdominal contents apply weight caudally to create a nonuniform distribution of positive pressure to the diaphragm. Consequently, lung volume is increased in the upright position and decreased in the supine position. In addition, the mechanical attachment of the diaphragm to the rib cage is such that contraction will elevate the rib cage in the upright position but in the supine position tends to pull the rib cage in (Muller and Bryan, 1979) (Fig. 31-3).

In the newborn the diaphragm is attached higher in front and consequently is longer. Therefore this already stretched diaphragm is unable to contract as far or as forcefully as that of the older infant or child. Also, young infants are less able to withstand diaphragmatic fatigue because of fewer energy-producing components. Abdominal distention from gas or fluid can impede diaphragmatic excursion significantly.

Airways. The rigid nasal structures, which are lined with ciliated mucous membranes, serve as passageways for air, warming and moistening air and filtering it of impurities. In infancy the nasal passages are narrow, and infants are primarily nose-breathers, which substantially increases airway resistance. Any factor that decreases the size of the passages and further increases airway resistance, such as nasal mucosal swelling and mucous accumulation, hampers the breathing and feeding of infants.

The upper airway is common to both the respiratory and the alimentary tracts, and many of the muscles in this area participate in several complex acts. However, the sequence of airway muscle activation is different in breathing and swallowing. The upper airway dilates during inspiration and constricts during exhalation. During certain activities these dimensions are modified; for example, inspiration is short during crying, coughing, and sneezing, but with crying the larynx and pharynx dilate. The net result of swallowing is closure of the upper airway with interruption of airflow. Consequently, the timing and magnitude of muscle activation have important implications for airway dimension and patency.

The pharynx is also a passageway for the entry and exit of air, but in addition it plays a role in phonation by helping produce vowel sounds. The pharynx contains the palatine and lingual tonsils, which play an important role in infection control.

The larynx, situated at the upper end of the trachea, is constructed of a rigid circular framework of cartilage and contains the epiglottis and the glottis (vocal cords). These structures prevent solids or liquids from entering the airway during swallowing, and the vibrations of the vocal cords produce voice sounds. In infancy the glottis is located more cephalad than in later childhood and the laryngeal reflexes are very active. The epiglottis is longer and projects further posteriorly. The narrowest portion of the larynx is at the level of the cricoid cartilage. In the infant and young child the ciliated columnar epithelium below the vocal cords is loosely bound with areolar tissue and is therefore more susceptible to edema formation. Swelling of the glottis and epiglottis produces hoarseness and often life-threatening obstruction of this narrow portion of the airway (croup).

The trachea, which is composed of smooth muscle supported by C-shaped rings of cartilage, ensures an open airway to the bronchi and lungs. The trachea divides into two primary bronchi, the right one situated slightly more vertical than the left, which causes aspirated objects to lodge more frequently in the right bronchus. Each bronchus enters the lung on its respective side, where it divides into secondary bronchi that continue to branch and divide into progressively smaller bronchioles. The entire bronchial tree is lined with mucous membrane and is composed of spiral smooth muscle supported by rings of cartilage. As the bronchioles become smaller, the cartilaginous rings become increasingly irregular and then disappear completely in the smallest bronchioles, the walls of which consist of only a single layer of cells (Fig. 31-4).

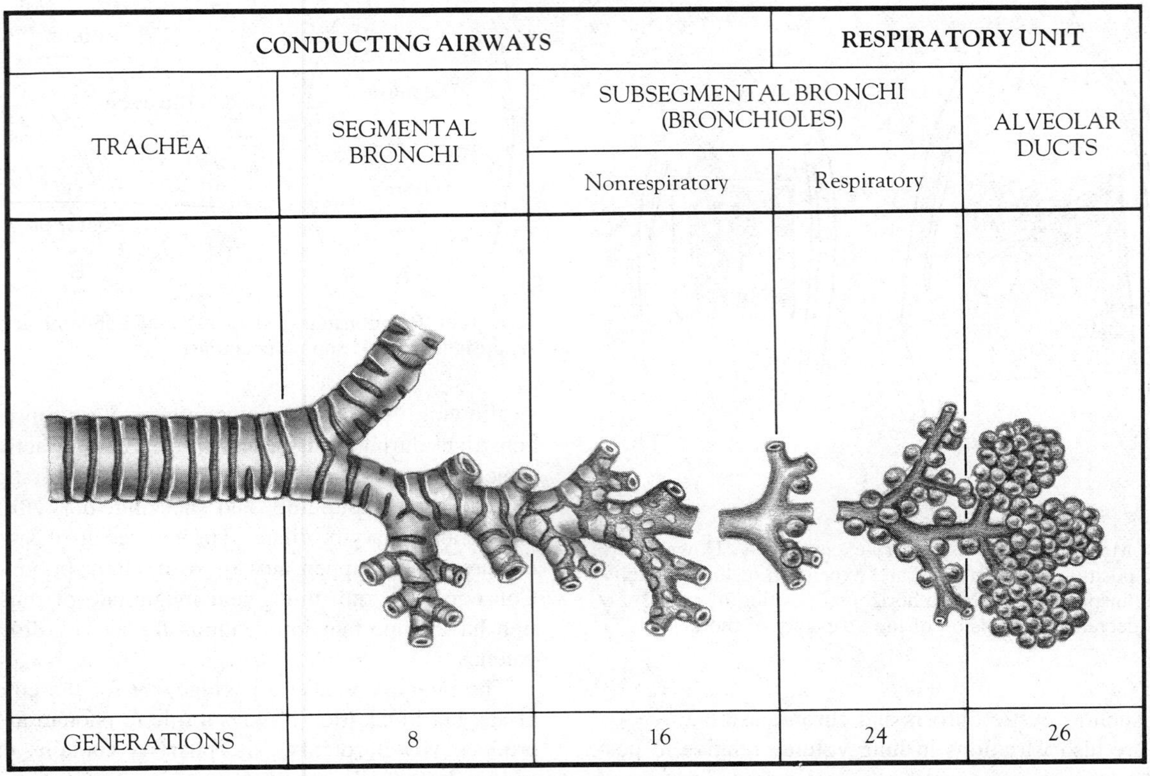

CONDUCTING AIRWAYS				RESPIRATORY UNIT
TRACHEA	SEGMENTAL BRONCHI	SUBSEGMENTAL BRONCHI (BRONCHIOLES)		ALVEOLAR DUCTS
		Nonrespiratory	Respiratory	
GENERATIONS	8	16	24	26

Fig. 31-4. Structures of the lower airway.

From Thompson, J.M., and others: Clinical nursing, St. Louis, 1986, The C.V. Mosby Co., p. 116.

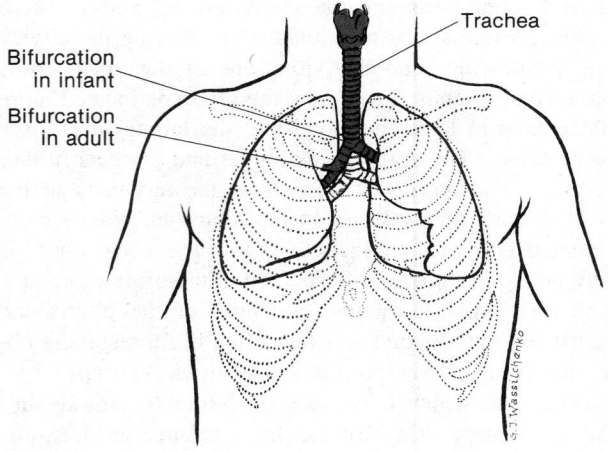

Fig. 31-5. Difference in level of bifurcation of trachea in infant and adult.

All the structures are subject to obstruction from edema or foreign objects, but there are differences in the degree of obstruction from constriction of smooth muscle. The diameter of the relatively rigid upper airway is less subject to constriction than the lower airways, which contain very little cartilaginous support. The highly reactive bronchiolar smooth muscle of the lower airways can cause life-threatening obstruction during bronchoconstriction. The airway cartilage in young infants is very soft and compressible; therefore the intrathoracic airways are highly reactive to stimuli, for example, vagal stimulation.

The airways of the newborn have very little smooth muscle, but in children 4 to 5 months of age they contain sufficient muscle to cause narrowing in response to irritating stimuli. Smooth muscle development and reactivity are comparable to those in the adult by 1 year of age. Growth of the respiratory system follows the general growth curve during the early weeks of life, but the airways grow faster than the thoracic and cervical portions of the vertebral column. Consequently, the larynx and trachea descend in relation to the upper spine. For example, the bifurcation of the trachea that lies opposite the third thoracic vertebra in the infant descends to a position opposite the fourth in adulthood (Fig. 31-5). Likewise, the cricoid cartilage descends from a position opposite the fourth cervical vertebra in the infant to opposite the sixth cervical vertebra in the adult. These anatomic changes produce differences in the angle of access to the trachea at various ages and must be considered when the infant or child is to be positioned for purposes of resuscitation and airway clearance.

The function of the tracheobronchial tree is to distribute air to the alveoli of the lung. A variety of diseases and conditions, such as mucosal swelling, muscular contraction, and mechanical obstruction by mucus or a foreign body, can cause localized or generalized airway occlusion.

Respiratory units. The two cone-shaped structures, the lungs, consist of the bronchi, bronchioles, and innumerable small air sacs, or alveoli. It is through these thin-walled structures that gas exchange takes place between the inspired air and the bloodstream. The amount of gas exchanged depends on many factors, for example, the amount and composition of air inhaled, thickness of the alveolar wall, adequacy of circulation to the alveoli, and substances within the alveoli that either prevent their inflation (the surface-active substance surfactant) or prevent gas exchange, such as fluids.

With age, changes take place in the air passages that increase respiratory surface area. The major changes are in the number and size of alveoli and in the increased branching of terminal bronchioles. Whereas the number of conducting airways is complete early in fetal life, the air sacs are shallow and wide-necked but have few septa at birth. This promotes patency but limits surface area for gas exchange. The alveoli are large with thick septa that have little elastic recoil (not unlike the emphysemic lung). During the first year bronchioles continue to branch, and the earlier globular alveoli in the terminal units rapidly increase in number as they partition and divide existing alveoli to form smaller lobular units separated by thinner septa, thus enlarging the area available for gas exchange.

The number of alveoli continues to increase steadily, but it is unclear when septal division ceases and an increase in size begins. It appears to occur sometime during middle childhood, although there is evidence to indicate that an increase in number of alveoli for each terminal airway takes place at puberty. At age 12 there are approximately nine times as many as were present at birth. In later stages of growth the structures lengthen and enlarge. In addition, collateral pathways of ventilation develop, including pores through alveolar walls and possibly pathways between bronchioles.

All of these factors have significance for respiratory disorders in young children; infants and young children have less alveolar surface area for gas exchange, the narrow branching peripheral airways become easily obstructed, and lack of collateral pathways inhibits ventilation beyond obstructed units. Consequently, young children are more readily subject to obstruction and atelectasis, especially as a result of repeated infection.

A variety of pathologic conditions can affect lung growth. A postural defect such as kyphoscoliosis causes a reduction in the number of alveoli, and acute infections of the respiratory tract can permanently alter lung development, resulting in decreased numbers of small airways. Replication of alveoli is inhibited so that the remaining alveoli are large but decreased in number. Lung growth can also be enhanced by changes in levels of hormones. Glucocorticosteroids promote lung maturation, and prenatal administration of corticosteroids has reduced the incidence of neonatal respiratory distress syndrome. Thyroxine and prolactin also enhance lung development, and lack of thyroid hormone results in immature lungs. Biochemical substances that enhance lung growth are theophylline, estrogen, isoxsuprine, epidermal growth factor, and heroin ingested during pregnancy. Lung growth is inhibited by phenobarbital or excess insulin (Inselman and Mellins, 1981).

Ventilation

Respiratory movements are first evident at approximately 20 weeks' gestation, and throughout fetal life there is an exchange of amniotic fluid in the alveoli. In the neonate the respiratory rate is rapid to meet the needs of a high metabolism. During growth the rate steadily decreases until it levels off at maturity (see inside front cover). The volume of air inhaled increases with the growth of the lungs and is closely related to body size. In addition, there is a qualitative difference in expired air at different ages. The amount of oxygen in the expired air gradually decreases and the amount of carbon dioxide increases during growth.

Ventilation takes place as air moves in and out of the lungs as the result of changes in pressure gradients created by changes in the size of the thoracic cavity. Contraction of the diaphragm and external intercostal muscles increases the size of the thorax and decreases the intrathoracic pressure. As a result, air moves from the atmosphere, which has a higher pressure, into the lungs, which have a lower pressure. The principles of artificial ventilation are based on this concept. Artificial respiratory devices increase the pressure entering the air passages (positive-pressure breathing devices), lower the pressure around the body (negative-pressure ventilator), or increase the negative pressure within the thoracic cavity (rocking bed). The shorter abdominal length of infants makes this last method ineffectual for them.

The alveoli are surrounded by pulmonary capillaries, and in most areas of the lung the membranes that separate these structures are exceedingly thin. The gas exchange takes place by simple diffusion in the alveoli; gas in other parts of the respiratory tract is unavailable for exchange with capillary blood.

The diameter of the airways and thus the air flow are determined by the balance of forces that tend to widen or narrow the airways. One of these is neural regulation of bronchial smooth muscles mediated through autonomic nerves. Sympathetic impulses relax the airways; parasympathetic impulses constrict them. Reflex constriction occurs in response to irritating inhalants such as dust, smoke, or sulfur dioxide; arterial hypoxemia and hypercapnia; cold air; and some drugs, such as acetylcholine and histamine. Other factors that alter airway size are peribronchial pressure, which tends to narrow the airways, and intraluminal pressure, which tends to keep airways open. For example, forced expiration causes increased peribronchial pressure and hence narrowing of the airways; positive-pressure breathing apparatus increases intraluminal pressure, keeping airways open.

Gas exchange. The exchange of gases in the lungs takes place between the alveolar air and the capillary blood. The amount of alveolar ventilation must be adequate to keep the Po_2 and Pco_2 at values that promote the escape of carbon dioxide from pulmonary capillaries and uptake of oxygen from the alveoli. Each gas moves in both directions through the alveolar-capillary membrane by diffusion in accordance with the pressure gradient for each gas. The pressure gradients of the gases between alveolar air and pulmonary blood cause outward diffusion of carbon dioxide from lung capillary blood and inward diffusion of oxygen from alveolar air. This exchange lowers the PCO_2 and raises the PO_2, converting the blood from its venous to its arterial saturation. In health, arterial PO_2 is approximately 95 to 100 mm Hg and arterial PCO_2 is 40 mm Hg.

Since carbon dioxide diffuses 21 times faster than oxygen, there is no impairment of diffusion for carbon dioxide from the blood to the alveoli. The amount of oxygen that diffuses into the blood depends on several factors:

1. The pressure gradient between alveolar air and capillary blood—when the oxygen content of alveolar air is increased with administration of oxygen, more oxygen enters the blood; when concentration of inspired alveolar PO_2 is reduced by large amounts of air trapped in the alveoli (as in asthma), the amount that enters the blood is decreased.
2. The total functional surface area of the alveolar-capillary membrane—when the surface area is decreased in conditions such as emphysema or pneumonia, the amount that can cross the membrane is also reduced.
3. The minute volume (the amount of air inhaled with each breath times the number of respirations per minute)—conditions that reduce the respiratory rate, such as depressant drugs, or reduce the capacity, such as paralysis, will significantly alter the amount of oxygen.
4. Alveolar ventilation, or the amount of air that reaches the alveoli—obstruction of air flow in the bronchi prevents air from reaching the respiratory unit.

Oxygen transport. Once oxygen has diffused from the alveolus to the pulmonary capillary, it is transported throughout the body in two ways. A small amount (PO_2) is transported as a solute dissolved in the plasma and the water of the red blood cells. A larger portion (40 to 70 times as much) is carried by the hemoglobin as oxyhemoglobin. Since each gram of hemoglobin can combine with 1.34 ml of oxygen, the transport capacity is largely determined by the amount of hemoglobin present. For example, children with severe anemia tend to be fatigued, be somewhat cyanotic, and breathe more rapidly. In addition, increasing the amount of oxygen delivered to the alveoli can increase the amount carried by the blood only in relation to the amount of hemoglobin present. For example, at a PO_2 of 100 mm Hg, hemoglobin is 97.5% saturated.

The oxygen, in order to combine with hemoglobin molecules, must diffuse from the plasma into the red blood cells. The degree to which oxygen combines with hemoglobin is affected by several factors. An increasing PO_2 and a decreasing PCO_2 both accelerate the hemoglobin association with oxygen to form oxyhemoglobin, and a decreasing PO_2 and an increasing PCO_2 accelerate the dissociation from oxyhemoglobin. A decrease in pH or an increase in temperature also increases the dissociation of oxygen from oxyhemoglobin. Therefore the percent saturation of PO_2 is less under conditions of acidosis or hyperpyrexia.

Carbon dioxide is carried in the blood in a number of ways. A small amount (PCO_2) is transported dissolved in the plasma and the water of red blood cells; a large amount, more than half, hydrates to form carbonic acid, which dissociates and is carried as bicarbonate and hydrogen ions; and the remainder combines with certain plasma proteins and hemoglobin. The association of carbon dioxide with hemoglobin is accelerated by an increasing PCO_2 and a decreasing PO_2 and is decreased by the opposite conditions. The diffusion of carbon dioxide into the alveoli is very rapid; thus the equilibrium between the PCO_2 of the pulmonary capillaries and the alveoli is achieved promptly.

Transport between blood and tissue cells is accomplished down a diffusion gradient just as it is between the blood and the alveoli.

Regulation of respiration. The mechanisms that control respiration can be divided into the following two large categories: (1) a neural system that maintains a coordinated, rhythmic respiratory cycle and regulates the depth of respiration and (2) a chemical (neurohumoral) system that regulates alveolar ventilation and maintains normal blood gas tensions.

Neural control in the respiratory center is sited in three areas: (1) a *pneumotaxic center,* which modulates respiratory frequency and depth; (2) an *apneustic center,* which produces inspiratory spasm and is modulated by pneumotaxic and medullary centers and by vagal afferent impulses; and (3) *medullary respiratory centers,* both inspiratory and expiratory, which regulate rhythmicity of respirations.

Impulses from other areas also affect the respiratory centers. *Proprioceptive vagal* impulses in the lung parenchyma are sensitive to stretching. When lungs become stretched, impulses are transmitted by the vagus nerve to the respiratory center, which inhibits further inflation and prevents overdistention—the *Hering-Breuer reflex.* The cerebral cortex also helps to control respirations by voluntary inhibition or acceleration of rate and depth of respirations. Reflex apnea can result from sudden painful stimulation, sudden cold stimulation, and stimulation to the larynx or pharynx (the choking reflex, which serves to prevent aspiration).

Chemical, or neurohumoral, control is mediated by specialized structures that respond to changes in pH, PCO_2, and PO_2—central chemoreceptors, probably located in the medulla, and peripheral chemoreceptors located in the great vessels. Peripheral chemoreceptors of greatest physiologic importance are the carotid bodies located at the division of the common carotid artery into its external and internal branches and the aortic bodies that lie between the ascending aorta and the pulmonary artery. Carbon dioxide and hydrogen ions control respiration by acting directly on the respiratory center; the peripheral chemoreceptors respond to changes in oxygen tension. Thus an increase in ventilation can result from either (1) stimulation of the respiratory center by an increased PCO_2 or hydrogen ion concentration or (2) a decreased PO_2 that stimulates the carotid and aortic bodies, which in turn transmit signals to the brain to excite the respiratory center.

The lungs also have an important role in acid-base balance. Less rapid than the chemical buffers, the respiratory mechanism begins to act within 1 to 3 minutes to make adjustments in pH by eliminating or retaining carbon dioxide. When the levels of carbon dioxide are altered sufficiently, the respiratory centers in the brain respond by either increasing or decreasing the rate and depth of respirations. For example, when the pH of the blood drops, as from increased exercise, there is a compensatory increase in respirations to rid the body of carbon dioxide derived from carbonic acid formed from buffered acid metabolites. Carbon dioxide buildup from breath holding will produce the same response, again increasing the carbonic acid and reducing the serum pH. The lungs therefore are the compensatory organs in metabolic disturbances and relatively prompt in their response.

Defenses of Respiratory Tract

The respiratory tract has several anatomic and biochemical characteristics that provide natural defenses against the multitude of both biologic and inanimate agents that can damage respiratory tissues. Intact defenses help to repel and resist the impact of deleterious agents; factors that reduce the integrity of these mechanisms increase the vulnerability of these tissues to invasion and disease.

lymphoid tissues Faucial, lingual, and pharyngeal tonsils (adenoids) and other pharyngeal lymphoid tissues, which form a protective circle around the entrance to the respiratory tract, help to localize and contain invading organisms where they can be destroyed by the body's humoral defense mechanisms.

viscid secretions The epithelium of the respiratory tract secretes a sticky mucus to which airborne organisms adhere.

ciliary action The mucus secreted by the columnar epithelium of the respiratory tract is kept flowing, carrying microorganisms and other hostile agents away from the lungs to be coughed or swallowed.

epiglottis The epiglottis and the epiglottis reflex protect the respiratory tract from invading material, including infectious exudate from the upper tract, and prevent such material from being aspirated into the lower tract.

cough The expulsive force of the cough reflex propels foreign material out of the lower tract.

tracheobronchial dynamics The tracheobronchial tree elongates and dilates on inspiration and shortens and narrows on expiration.

position changes Changes in body position encourage drainage of tracheobronchial passages.

lymphatics Lymphatics draining the terminal bronchi and bronchioles remove invading organisms to be filtered and destroyed in the regional lymph nodes.

humoral defenses Organisms and other foreign material are removed and/or destroyed by the action of phagocytes, enzymes, and immune globulins, especially immunoglobulin A (IgA).

Effective as these natural barriers are, they are frequently breached. For example, there are children who have conditions that predispose to infection resulting from interference with the efficiency of these mechanisms, such as chronic asthma, cystic fibrosis, and the various immune-deficiency disorders. Frequent intense exposure to organisms that accompanies conditions of crowding or continual exposure to irritating substances in the air results in breakdown of healthy defenses. Concurrent illness, malnutrition, or fatigue reduces the efficiency of natural defenses.

Diagnostic and Therapeutic Procedures

A variety of procedures relating to respiratory function are available to assist in diagnosis and provide therapy. Some can be performed by most health professionals; others require specialized skills and/or equipment. Only the more common ones are presented here.

DIAGNOSTIC PROCEDURES

Various procedures are available for assessing respiratory function and diagnosing respiratory disease. For nurses caring for the child with respiratory disorders, understanding how the tests are carried out helps them to devise the best strategies for preparing children for the tests, gaining their cooperation, and supporting them during the procedure. Moreover, this knowledge provides nurses with information on which to base nursing interventions, such as positioning, use of supplemental oxygen, and assistance with coughing or deep breathing.

Physical Examination

A great deal can be determined about the child's respiratory status from simple observations of physical signs and behavior. However, to make a useful assessment, the nurse needs to know what to look for, and what is observed must have meaning (see physical assessment of the chest, p. 258). To assess deviations from the usual, the observer must know the normal type and rate of respiration in relation to the size and age of the child (see inside front cover), which is best observed when the child is sleeping or quietly awake.

Much can be determined from the configuration of the chest and the pattern of respiratory movement, including rate, regularity, symmetry of movements, amplitude (deep or shallow), effort expended in respiration, and use of accessory muscles of respiration. Increased respiratory rate is observed with anxiety, with elevated temperature, with severe anemia, as the result of metabolic acidosis, and sometimes associated with respiratory alkalosis caused by psychoneurosis, salicylate ingestion, and some central nervous system disturbances. The progress of disorders that contribute to low compliance, such as the pneumonias, pulmonary edema, and pleural effusion, can be followed and evaluated by observing changes in respiratory rate.

Alterations in the depth of respirations—too deep *(hyperpnea)* or too shallow *(hypopnea)*—are recognized as abnormal only in the extremes. Hyperpnea is noted with fever, severe anemia, respiratory alkalosis associated with psy-

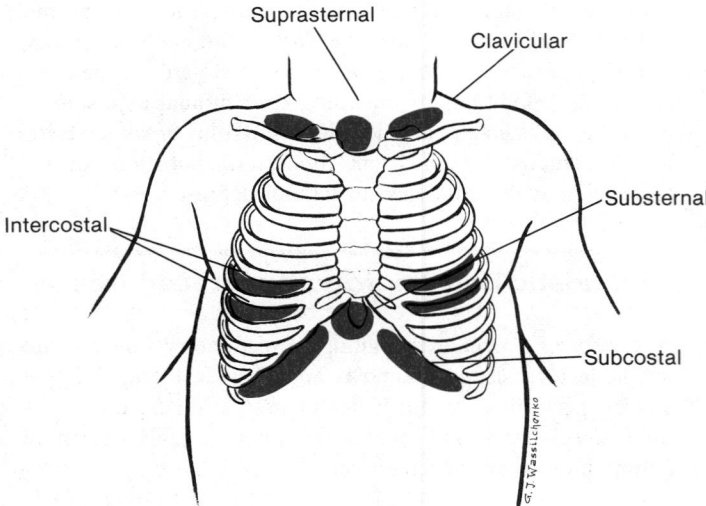

Fig. 31-6. Location of retractions.

chosis, salicylate ingestion, central nervous system disturbances, and respiratory acidosis that accompanies disorders such as diabetes mellitus or diarrhea. Hypoventilation is less easily detected and occurs with metabolic alkalosis in conditions such as pyloric stenosis and respiratory acidosis that accompanies diaphragmatic paralysis or central nervous system depression.

Retractions, or a sinking in of soft tissues relative to the cartilaginous and bony thorax, may be noted in some pulmonary disorders. Although slight intercostal retractions are normal, in disease states (particularly in severe airway obstruction) retraction becomes extreme. Subcostal retraction, observed anteriorly at the lower costal margins, indicates a flattened diaphragm, as it not only lowers the floor of the thorax but also pulls on the rib cage in response to a greater than normal decrease in intrathoracic pressure. In severe obstruction, retractions extend to the supraclavicular areas and the jugular notch. Palpation and percussion provide information regarding areas of pain and tissue density, and auscultation is essential to determine the patency of airways. (See Fig. 31-6 for location of retractions.)

The type of sound heard helps to identify specific areas of obstruction to airflow. For example, *wheezing* usually indicates small bronchiolar narrowing, *rhonchi* are more characteristic of obstruction to large airways, and *rales* are related to secretions in the respiratory unit. However, in infants wheezing often originates in the larger airways because of their smaller diameter.

Associated observations contribute to assessment. For example, *head bobbing* in a sleeping or exhausted infant is a sign of dyspnea. The head, supported on the mother's arm only at the suboccipital area, will bob forward with each inspiration. This is caused by neck flexion resulting from contraction of the scalene and sternocleidomastoid muscles. Noisy breathing such as ''snoring'' is frequently associated with hypertrophied adenoidal tissue, choanal obstruction,

polyps, or a foreign body in the nasal passages. *Stridor,* a harsh inspiratory sound, is usually caused by laryngeal or tracheal obstruction. Audible wheezes are heard in children with bronchial asthma and foreign bodies in the trachea or bronchi. *Grunting* is frequently a sign of chest pain, suggesting acute pneumonia or pleural involvement. It is also observed in pulmonary edema and is a characteristic of respiratory distress syndrome. It serves to increase end-expiratory pressure and thus prolong the period of oxygen and carbon dioxide exchange across the alveolocapillary membrane.

Color changes of the skin, specifically the distribution, degree, and duration of *cyanosis,* are noted. Except for the peripheral bluish discoloration resulting from circulatory stasis in the newborn, cyanosis is significant and usually indicates cardiopulmonary disease. The most common causes of cyanosis in children are (Waring, 1983):

1. Acute or chronic alveolar hypoventilation, as seen in airway obstruction, weakness of the respiratory muscles, or a depressed respiratory center
2. Uneven distribution of gas and blood throughout the lungs, as might occur in bronchopneumonia
3. Anatomic right-to-left shunts of blood that occur in some forms of congenital heart disease or congenital arteriovenous aneurysms of the lung
4. Disturbances of alveolocapillary diffusion, a rare cause of cyanosis as a result of interstitial pneumonia or pulmonary fibrosis

Chest pain may be a complaint of older children and may have a variety of causes, both pulmonary and nonpulmonary. It may be caused by disease of any of the chest structures—esophagus, pericardium, diaphragm, pleura, or chest wall. Parietal pleural pain is usually localized over the affected area and is aggravated by respiratory movements. It is not uncommon for the pain of diaphragmatic pleural irritation to be referred to the base of the neck posteriorly and anteriorly or to the abdomen. Most pleural pain is related to respiration; therefore respiratory movements are shallow and rapid.

Clubbing, or proliferation of tissue about the terminal phalanges, accompanies a variety of conditions, frequently those associated with chronic hypoxia, primarily cardiac defects and chronic pulmonary disease. The degree of clubbing reflects the severity of the hypoxia, and serial measurements provide clues to the progress of the disease. For example, increased clubbing correlates with worsening of the condition and indicates a poor prognosis in cystic fibrosis. On the other hand, diminished clubbing often occurs with intensive pulmonary therapy. The degree of clubbing is determined by the extent to which the nail base is lifted on the dorsal surface of the phalanx by the tissue proliferation. The greater the angle formed above the finger at the skin-nail junction, the more pronounced the clubbing, especially when there is a decided curvature to the nail (Fig. 31-7).

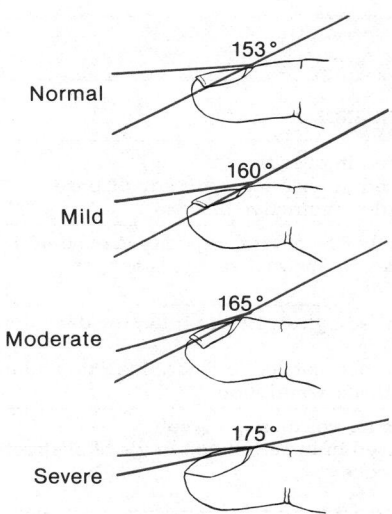

Fig. 31-7. Stages of clubbing. Degree of angle formed above finger at skin-nail junction indicates extent of clubbing. Angle greater than 160 degrees and decided curvature of nail are good criteria for presence of clubbing.

Modified from Waring, W.W.: The history and physical examination. In Kendig, E.L., Jr., and Chernick, V., editors: Disorders of the respiratory tract in children, ed. 4, Philadelphia, 1983, W.B. Saunders Co.

Cough. Cough is often associated with respiratory disease. A cough can be initiated voluntarily, although it is usually a result of a complex reflex consisting of three components: afferent nerve fibers, the cough center, and efferent nerve fibers. Much of the respiratory epithelium contains afferent receptors that are sensitive to mechanical or chemical stimuli. These receptors are concentrated in the areas of the larynx, carina, and the bifurcations of the large and medium-sized bronchi. When a stimulus is applied to these areas, impulses are transmitted via the vagus nerve to the cough center in the brain stem. Efferent impulses travel via the vagus, phrenic, and spinal motor nerves to the larynx, intercostal muscles, diaphragm, abdominal muscles, and pelvic floor. An inspiratory gasp and closure of the glottis are followed by contraction of muscles in the chest wall, diaphragm, abdomen, and pelvic floor. The resulting compression and increase in pleural, alveolar, and subglottic pressure cause a sudden opening of the glottis and immediate release of trapped air at extremely rapid expiratory flow rates, forcing undesirable material from the respiratory tract.

Inflammation or infection almost anywhere in the upper or lower respiratory tract may produce coughing. Some types of cough are characteristic of specific diseases. For example, severe cough is associated with measles and cystic fibrosis, and the paroxysmal cough accompanied by an inspiratory ''whoop'' is pathognomonic of pertussis. A brassy cough is part of the symptomatology of croup and foreign body aspiration, and a nervous cough is not uncommon in older children and adolescents. Because there are no cough receptors in the alveoli, a cough may be absent in a child with lobar pneumonia in the early stages of the disease.

Cough is assessed according to a number of significant features, including (Chow and others, 1984):

Onset and duration
Type—dry, hacking, moist, barking, brassy, paroxysmal (a sudden attack, outburst, or intensification of symptoms)
Progress—better, worse, unchanged, persistent
Pattern—daytime, nighttime, both, different intensity with time or activity
Associated symptoms—sore throat, dyspnea, pain and its location
Secretions—sputum presence, consistency, color, frequency, evidence of swallowing sputum, postnasal drip

Pulmonary Function Tests

Pulmonary function tests are used less frequently in children than in adults, since most tests require the understanding and active participation of the child. For those children who are able to cooperate, the tests provide valuable information that assists in the diagnosis and management of many types of pulmonary disease. Most children over 5 can be taught to perform the simpler tests when personnel involved are trained in the use of the equipment and know how to relate to children. Children need to know what is expected of them and to have time to practice the expected maneuver in a pleasant laboratory environment free from distractions. The most useful tests and applications are shown in Table 31-1.

Radiology and Other Diagnostic Procedures

X-radiography is used frequently in diagnostic evaluation of children. Although there is no definitive information on the effects of low-dose radiation, measures are carried out to protect vulnerable areas from possible damage. When possible, technicians and others try to prevent unnecessary exposure of the child (and personnel), and the more radiosensitive areas should be protected. Careful protection of the immature gonads of the infant or child is essential. Other sensitive areas are the thyroid gland, ocular lens, and bone marrow.

Although nurses have limited control over the length, frequency, and correct application of the x-ray beam, they can make certain that the infant or child receives proper protection from possible hazards. Lead shields, correctly placed and consistently applied to areas not needed for diagnostic purposes, are essential. Play and modification of methodology can be used effectively to reduce the trauma sometimes associated with the procedure and to gain the cooperation of the child. Special radiologic examinations used in respiratory diagnosis are outlined in Table 31-2.

Several diagnostic procedures are employed to assist in diagnosis of lung disorders (Table 31-3). Most require specialized equipment and skills. All require some type of preparation of the child.

Blood Gas Determination

Blood gas measurements are sensitive indicators of change in respiratory status in acutely ill patients. They provide val-

Table 31-1 Pulmonary function tests used in children

TEST	DEFINITION	SIGNIFICANCE
Vital capacity	Maximum amount of air that can be expelled from the lungs after maximum inspiration	Reduced in obesity Reduced in obstructive airway disease Normal in restrictive disease
Forced expiratory volume in 1 (FEV_1) or 3 (FEV_3) seconds	Amount of air that can be forced from the lungs after maximum inspiration in 1 and 3 seconds	Normally 80% of vital capacity is exhaled in 1 second Reduced in obstructive disease
Tidal volume (TV or V_T)	Amount of air inhaled and exhaled during any respiratory cycle	Multiplied by respiratory rate provides minute volume Information needed to determine rate and depth of artificial ventilation
Functional residual volume (FRV); functional residual capacity (FRC)	Volume of air remaining in the lungs after passive expiration	Allows for aeration of alveoli Increased in hyperinflated lungs of obstructive lung disease

Table 31-2 Radiologic examinations

TEST	DESCRIPTION	PURPOSE	COMMENT
Radiography	Pictures obtained by passing x-rays through body and recording them on sensitized film	Produces images of internal structures of chest, including air-filled lungs, airways, vascular markings, heart, and great vessels	Requires cooperation of child
Fluoroscopy	Electronically intensified image to allow its projection on a viewing screen	Used primarily to study diaphragmatic excursion and respiratory motion of the lungs Examination of barium-filled esophagus to outline mediastinal abnormalities	Requires cooperation of child
Bronchography	Contrast medium is instilled directly into bronchial tree through opaque catheter inserted via orotracheal tube	Most valuable to demonstrate and inspect bronchiectasis Detects distal bronchial obstruction Detects malformations	Carried out under general anesthesia Used less frequently than other examinations
Esophagoscopy	Esophagus is outlined when barium solution or colloid is swallowed	Esophageal displacement defines mediastinal masses Detects swallowing disorders and malformations, e.g., tracheoesophageal fistula	Valuable adjunct for diagnosis Usually performed under fluoroscope
Angiography	Injection of dye to produce image of pulmonary vasculature	Investigation of pulmonary vascular anomalies and pulmonary hypertension	Seldom used in child
Tomography	Sequence of x-rays, each representing a cross section or "cut" through the lung tissue at a different depth	Useful in identifying the presence of calcium or a cavity within a lesion, hilar adenopathy, mediastinal masses, or abnormalities	Usually reserved for children old enough to be able to suspend respiration voluntarily

Table 31-2   Radiologic examinations—cont'd

TEST	DESCRIPTION	PURPOSE	COMMENT
Radioisotope scanning	Intravenous injection of albumin labeled with radioisotopes or inhalation of radioactive aerosols or xenon gas followed by radiation scanning	Delineates defects in pulmonary arterial perfusion and diseased areas of lung Detects location of aspirated foreign body	Requires cooperation of child
Ultrasonography	Transmission of sound waves through chest	Identifies opacification	Limited use in diagnosis of respiratory disorders

Table 31-3   Diagnostic procedures used in respiratory disorders

PROCEDURE	DESCRIPTION	PURPOSE
Tracheal aspiration	Sputum obtained by direct aspiration from trachea	Obtains secretions for examination culture
Bronchoscopy	Direct observation of tracheobronchial tree via bronchoscope	Localizes abnormalities in major airways Provides access to (1) remove aspirated foreign bodies from major airways, (2) remove obstructive mucous plugs, and (3) perform bronchial lavage
Lung puncture	Needle aspiration of lung fluid via syringe and needle through intercostal space	Obtains lung aspirate for histologic study or culture
Lung biopsy	Removal of lung tissue via open thoracotomy or closed needle procedures	Diagnosis of protracted pulmonary disease unexplained by other means
Brush biopsy	Material for biopsy obtained with a nylon brush on the end of a wire passed through a tube placed via the nose, pharynx, trachea, and airways (via fluoroscope) to the involved lung segment	Obtains material for culture and histologic examination
Diagnostic pneumoperitoneum	Injection of air into peritoneal cavity sharply outlines the diaphragm on radiography	Indicates position of diaphragm Differentiates eventration of diaphragm from extralobular sequestration
Percutaneous transtracheal aspiration	Needle and catheter aspiration of tracheal secretions through thyroid cartilage	Obtains secretions for laboratory examination and culture
Arterial puncture	Arterial blood obtained from temporal (neonates), brachial, radial, and femoral arteries	Obtains blood for gas analysis (Po_2, Pco_2)

uable information regarding lung function, lung adequacy, and tissue perfusion. They are invaluable for monitoring conditions involving hypoxemia, carbon dioxide retention, or both. For the nurse who cares for the acutely ill respiratory patient, this information provides cues for decision making regarding therapeutic interventions, such as adjusting the respirator, increasing chest physical therapy, administration of oxygen, or positioning the child for maximum ventilation.

Blood gas measurements include the Po_2 and Pco_2 in as-sociation with the pH. Often the oxygen saturation and base excess values are also included. The P represents the partial pressure of the gas being measured, and the figures following indicate the pressure in millimeters of mercury. The pH indicates the hydrogen ion concentration (see acid-base balance, p. 1167). Arterial blood samples are expressed as Pao_2 or $Paco_2$. Venous blood does not indicate the true values and is not used for blood gas determination.

For continuous monitoring of blood gases, noninvasive measurements are used whenever possible. Electronic

NORMAL ARTERIAL BLOOD GAS AND pH MEASUREMENTS AT SEA LEVEL (21% OXYGEN)*

pH: Normal range = 7.35-7.45

Acidosis	Mild:	7.300-7.350
	Mod.:	7.250-7.300
	Severe:	<7.250
Alkalosis	Mild:	7.450-7.500
	Mod.:	7.500-7.550
	Severe:	>7.550

P_{CO_2}: Normal range = 35 − 45 mm Hg

Hypercapnia	Mild:	45-50
	Mod.:	50-60
	Severe:	>60
Hypocapnia	Mild:	30-45
	Mod.:	25-30
	Severe:	<25

P_{O_2}: Normal range = 83 − 108 mm Hg

Hypoxemia	Mild:	55-85
	Mod.:	40-55
	Severe:	<40

Bicarbonate: Normal values = 21 − 28 mEq/liter

Depression	Mild:	19-22
	Mod.:	17-19
	Severe:	< 17
Elevation	Mild:	28-31
	Mod.:	31-35
	Severe:	>35

Base excess: Normal values = −3 to +3

Depression	Mild:	−3 to −7
	Mod.:	−7 thru −10
	Severe:	< −10
Elevation	Mild:	+4 to +8
	Mod.:	+8 thru +12
	Severe:	> +12

*Ranges are for children and infants beyond the newborn period. See Appendix D for newborn and premature values.

equipment has proved valuable in the treatment of both inpatients and ambulatory patients. The most frequently used noninvasive device is the tcPo$_2$ monitor, which measures Po$_2$ and Pco$_2$. The device provides a reasonably accurate reflection of Pao$_2$ in critically ill children. However, when critical assessment of the degree of hypoxemia is needed, the device is no substitute for arterial measurements (Yip and others, 1983). Patients need adequate peripheral circulation and sometimes the response time varies, frequent calibration is needed, and change of site is required to prevent skin damage. For these reasons others favor the oximeter, which measures O$_2$, because of its rapid response (Fanconi and others, 1985).

There is some controversy regarding the collection of ''arterialized'' capillary blood for blood gas measurements; however, many believe it to be a safe, convenient, and relatively accurate method. The blood samples are obtained by taking a deep heel stick after dilation of the vascular bed by warming (see Fig. 27-16). The first drop of blood is discarded, and subsequent blood is collected directly into heparinized capillary tubes held in a horizontal position. The filled tube is sealed on one end with wax or clay, a small piece of iron wire is placed inside, and the other end is sealed. The blood is thoroughly mixed by passing a magnet back and forth along the length of the tube, then the tube is placed in a basin of cracked ice and delivered to the laboratory as soon as possible.

Samples are obtained through an indwelling catheter or by way of arteriopuncture. The artery most frequently used is the radial artery, since there are no nearby veins. The temporal and umbilical arteries can be used effectively in the newborn. Other arteries that may be used are the femoral or brachial arteries. The normal values are much the same for all ages and depend on the concentration of the gases in the ambient air the child is breathing. The normal values for ambient oxygen concentration are lower at high altitudes than at sea level, and the arterial Po$_2$ should rise in proportion to the oxygen concentration being inhaled. Therefore when one is assessing the significance of blood gas values, the data should include the percentage of oxygen administered (if any), the child's body temperature, since as little as 1° F can alter the blood gas values 5% to 8%, and the presence of anxiety, which causes many children to hyperventilate and blow off extra carbon dioxide.

Unclotted blood is required; therefore a syringe rinsed with heparinized solution is used to draw blood samples, and no air bubbles should enter the syringe to alter the blood gas concentration. The amount collected depends on the size of the child. Ideally 2.5 ml of blood is drawn for blood gas analysis, but depending on the laboratory facilities as little as 0.1 ml may be sufficient in small infants. See the boxed material for normal arterial blood gas and pH measurements in patients breathing room air at sea level.

The significance of blood gas determinations is related primarily to the relationships among these three determinations: pH, Po$_2$, and Pco$_2$. Much of this is discussed in relation to acid-base imbalance in Chapter 28. Any change in a blood gas value must be compared to the other values and to previous readings as well as to the child's clinical appearance and behavior, his medical history, and associated physiologic factors. It is essential to understand the relationship between pH and Pco$_2$ readings.

The nurse has several responsibilities in monitoring blood gases. The first is to determine when a blood gas sample should be taken. Sometimes a specified schedule is ordered; at other times the sample is to be drawn as indicated by clinical observations. In this situation the nurse must understand the factors influencing blood gas levels and be able to recognize the need for a blood gas examination. Factors that influence blood gas levels include the amount and method of oxygen administration, the position of the child, and the nature of the respiratory disorder.

Signs that indicate the need for blood gas examination

include a change in color, depth, or rate of respirations, behavior, or sensorium, and sometimes other vital signs. The nurse may or may not be able to obtain the blood sample by arteriopuncture, depending on the policies of the institution. Nurses are usually able to withdraw the sample from an arterial catheter, and they should become skilled in the techniques of drawing blood and flushing the line. No matter who obtains the sample, the nurse is responsible for its speedy transport to the technician for analysis.

The results of the gas analysis provide the nurse with information on which to base further nursing action. Nurses must be able to understand the significance of the report and to implement nursing activities, for example, adjusting the concentration of oxygen the patient is receiving, changing the position, administering suction, administering prescribed drugs, or notifying the attending physician, according to the interpretation of the gas analysis.

THERAPEUTIC PROCEDURES

Procedures to improve ventilation are employed with increasing frequency in the prevention and management of pulmonary dysfunction. Most of these involve the nurse in the hospital or the home situation.

Inhalation therapy is an all-inclusive term that encompasses a variety of therapies that involve changing the composition, volume, or pressure of inspired gases. This includes primarily increasing the oxygen concentration of inspired gas *(oxygen therapy)*, increasing the water vapor content of inspired gas *(humidification)*, addition of airborne particles with beneficial properties *(aerosol therapy)*, and various means for controlling or assisting respiration *(artificial ventilation*, or *intermittent positive pressure breathing)*.

Although the major responsibility for providing therapies is assumed by the respiratory therapist, in most institutions nurses take a prominent role in observation and ongoing management. Nonmechanical means for improving ventilation are often the responsibility of nurses, including chest physiotherapy and breathing exercises.

Oxygen Therapy

The indication for administration of oxygen is *hypoxemia* as evidenced by reduced arterial oxygen tension and cyanosis. Cyanosis is a late sign but remains the single best criterion for supplemental oxygen. Dyspnea, on the other hand, is not necessarily relieved by oxygen. Oxygen is administered by mask, hood, nasal cannula, face tent, intermittent positive-pressure breathing apparatus, or oxygen tent. The mode of delivery is selected on the basis of the concentration needed in the inspired air and the ability of the child to cooperate in its use. The concentration of oxygen delivered should be regulated according to the needs of the individual child. For most conditions an ambient oxygen concentration of 40% to 50% is satisfactory and should be analyzed periodically for percent concentration. There are hazards related to its use; therefore oxygen should not be continued after

the indication for its use (such as cyanosis) is no longer present. Since oxygen is dry, it is always humidified in some manner.

Oxygen therapy is primarily carried out in the hospital, although increasing numbers of children are receiving oxygen in the home. Oxygen delivered to the infant Isolette is satisfactory when lower levels are adequate to prevent cyanosis, but the highest concentration (almost 100%) is supplied by way of a plastic hood (Fig. 31-8). The gas should not be allowed to blow directly into the infant's face. Cold fluid or air applied to the face stimulates receptors that trigger the diving reflex, which causes bradycardia and shunting of blood from peripheral to central circulation. The oxygen hood should not rub against the infant's neck, chin, or shoulder. Older cooperative children can use a nasal cannula or prongs, which can supply a concentration of about 50%. A nasal catheter or a mask is not well tolerated by children.

For most children beyond early infancy the oxygen tent, or canopy, is the most satisfactory means for administration of oxygen (Fig. 31-9). A tent does not require any device to come into direct contact with the face, but the concentration of oxygen within the tent is difficult to control and to maintain above about 40%. The comfort to the child makes it the method of choice except in cases of marked respiratory distress. A major difficulty with the use of the tent is keeping the tent closed so that oxygen concentration is maintained.

To reduce oxygen loss, nursing care should be planned carefully so that the tent is opened as little as possible. Since oxygen is heavier than air, loss will be greater at the bottom of the tent; therefore the tent should be tucked in snugly without open edges. The bottom of the tent should be examined more often when the child is restless and fussy and liable to pull the covers loose. Some tents are even open at the top. Because of the rapid diffusing qualities of carbon dioxide, the levels of the gas do not build up within these enclosures. After the tent has been opened for an extended

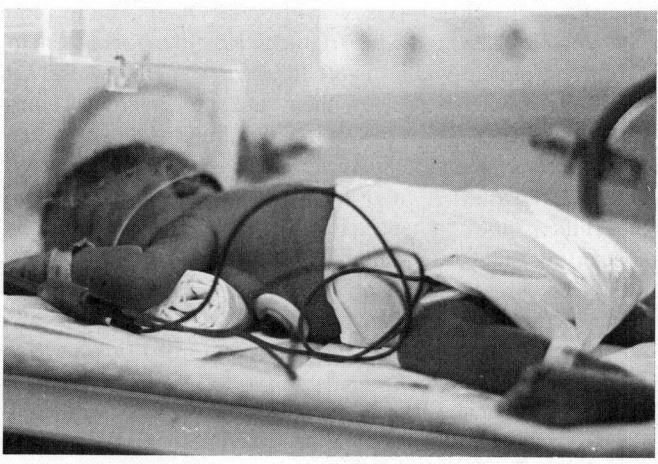

Fig. 31-8. Oxygen administered to infant by plastic hood.

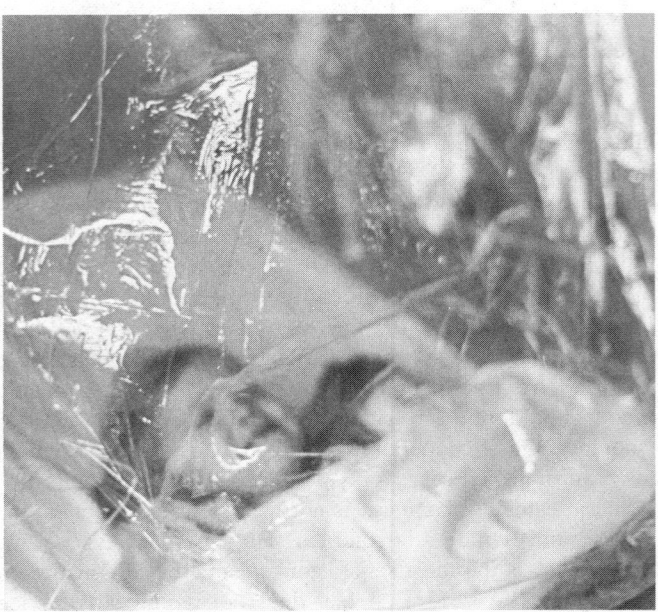

Fig. 31-9. The tent provides a comfortable method for oxygen administration but may be frightening to a small child, even when shared by a familiar "friend."

period, it is flushed with oxygen by increasing the flowmeter for a few minutes to raise the oxygen and mist concentration within the tent quickly. The flowmeter is then reset to the prescribed number of liters per minute.

The enclosed tent becomes very warm; therefore some type of refrigeration unit is provided. The temperature inside the tent must be checked periodically to be certain that it is maintained at the desired level. It is important to make certain that the child is kept warm and dry. Mist is usually prescribed in conjunction with oxygen therapy, and the moisture condenses on the tent walls. The child's bedding and clothing are examined periodically and changed as needed to prevent chilling.

The reactions of children to the oxygen tent vary. Some, especially older children, feel comfortable in the tent and like the cozy, close privacy it affords. Others, more often younger children, may be frightened by the forced enclosure. The plastic walls distort their view of the world and constitute a barrier between them and their source of comfort, the parents. Their distress can be minimized if they are able to see someone nearby and are reassured that they will not be left alone. A favorite toy or object can accompany the child inside the tent. However, all toys should be inspected for safety and suitability. The high oxygen environment makes any source of sparks (such as metal toys and some mechanical toys) a potential fire hazard. Other familiar items can be placed at the foot of the bed or otherwise in view.

In most instances the child can be removed from the oxygen tent for activities such as feeding and bathing, whereas in other cases the child is placed in the tent only during periods of rest. Still others may require oxygen continuously and can be removed from the tent or Isolette only if an oxygen source is held close to the child's face. Any change in color, increased respiratory effort, or restlessness is an indication to return the child to the oxygen tent.

The oxygen content within the device is analyzed periodically (always at a point near the child's head) to determine the rate of flow needed to maintain the desired concentration. The equipment is changed and/or cleaned at regular intervals (at least once weekly) to prevent bacterial growth when the child requires oxygen over an extended period.

Oxygen toxicity. Oxygen is essential to life and a valuable therapeutic aid. However, prolonged exposure to high oxygen tensions can be damaging to lung tissue. Although the exact pathogenesis of the pulmonary changes is unclear, there is evidence to indicate damage to lung capillaries, which causes diffuse microhemorrhagic changes, diminished mucous flow, inactivation of surfactant, and altered ciliary function. The total effect appears to be the direct result of "lung burn" and is therefore a result of the alveolar oxygen ($P_{A}O_2$) and not the arterial oxygen tension (PaO_2). The result of these changes is a gradual impairment of alveolar ventilation.

Atelectasis may occur as the result of the "washing out" of nitrogen from the alveoli by the high concentrations of oxygen. This is more likely to occur in persons with low tidal volume and retention of mucus or other secretions (Wade, 1982).

Oxygen-induced carbon dioxide narcosis is a physiologic hazard of oxygen therapy that may occur in persons with chronic pulmonary disease. It is seldom encountered in children except those with cystic fibrosis. These children have chronic alveolar hypoventilation with a concomitant chronic carbon dioxide retention and hypoxemia. In these patients the respiratory center has adapted to the continuously higher P_{CO_2} levels, and therefore hypoxia becomes the more powerful stimulus to respiration. When the P_{O_2} is elevated during oxygen administration, the hypoxic drive is removed, causing progressive hypoventilation and increased P_{CO_2} levels, and the child rapidly becomes unconscious. Carbon dioxide narcosis can also be induced by the administration of sedation in these patients.

Other toxic effects of oxygen that are suspected include changes in the renal tubules, sympathoadrenal medullary stimulation precipitating neurogenic seizures, and an increased rate of destruction of red blood cells.

Aerosol Therapy

The inhalation and subsequent deposition of airborne water particles within the airway are the function of aerosol therapy. This may be merely saline to help moisten the airway and help liquefy secretions, or the particles may contain mucolytic, bronchodilating, decongestant, or antimicrobial agents. The particles can vary in size, depending on the mode of delivery, and may be administered intermittently and briefly or continuously and for a prolonged period. In all forms of aerosol therapy the nebulized substance is distributed according to the gas flow. Large droplets are usually deposited in larger airways, and any unventilated areas receive none of the aerosol. The smaller the droplets formed, the more widely they are distributed.

For continuous aerosol therapy a misting device is attached to or incorporated into the mist tent. Distilled water is used most commonly, although propylene glycol in aqueous solution is often employed, especially in jet-type nebulizers. For intermittent administration of small quantities of an agent with specific pharmacologic action, a small nebulizer can be used powered by a small electric motor or in association with a positive-pressure breathing apparatus.

Aerosol therapy is widely used in treatment of both upper and lower respiratory tract disease, including croup, bronchitis, pneumonia, asthma, cystic fibrosis, and conditions in which there is weakness of the muscles of respiration. In some instances aerosol therapy is employed prophylactically (e.g., cystic fibrosis) to prevent complicating pulmonary problems. There is a decided relationship between aerosol therapy and bronchial drainage. Drainage is much more effective immediately after aerosol therapy.

Aerosol therapy is usually performed under the guidance of a respiratory therapist, although nurses may assume this responsibility in the home or in association with the therapist. Nebulizers attached to mist tents are monitored to be certain that the fluid is maintained within the desired level and that the nebulization takes place. When mist cannot be observed, the apparatus is checked for interruption of patency or other malfunction. Children using nebulization by mask or other device are taught how to use the aerosol effectively and are supervised in its operation. Nurses need to know how the apparatus works and to recognize when it is functioning properly. Because of the danger of bacterial growth, equipment is thoroughly cleaned daily. For use of hand nebulization see p. 1387.

Bronchial (Postural) Drainage

Bronchial drainage is indicated whenever excessive fluid or mucus in the bronchi is not being removed by normal ciliary activity and cough. The techniques of segmental drainage, percussion, and vibration assist the normal cleansing mechanisms of the lung. Positioning the child to take maximum advantage of gravity further facilitates removal of secretions. The effect is sometimes dramatic in children with chronic lung disease characterized by thick mucous secretions, such as asthma and cystic fibrosis.

Postural drainage is carried out three to four times daily and is more effective when it follows other respiratory therapy, such as bronchodilator and/or nebulization medication. Bronchial drainage is generally performed before meals (or 1 to 1½ hours after meals) to minimize the chance of vomiting and is repeated at bedtime. The length and duration of treatment depend on the child's condition and tolerance level—usually 20 to 30 minutes. There are positions to facilitate drainage from all major lung segments (Fig. 31-10), but all positions are not employed at each session. Children will usually cooperate for four to six positions, but more than six tend to exceed their limits of tolerance. Older children can be expected to tolerate longer periods.

In the hospital an older child can be positioned over an elevated knee rest. Small children and infants can be positioned with pillows or on the therapist's lap and legs (Fig. 31-13). Special modifications of the techniques are required in children whose conditions contraindicate the standard positioning, such as head injuries, some types of surgical incisions or burns, and casts or traction. At home small children can be positioned on a padded ironing board. Children who require postural drainage over months or years may benefit from specially constructed tables padded and adjusted to their individual needs. The position used and the frequency and duration of treatment are individualized.

Chest Physical Therapy

Chest physical therapy maneuvers are effective in helping to remove secretions when combined with postural drainage. Viscid secretions may not drain from the bronchi by gravity alone. Methods used to facilitate drainage include deep breathing, reinforced cough, thoracic "squeezing," percussion, and vibration. These techniques are frequently taught to parents who will continue to carry out the physical therapy at home.*

"Squeezing." A squeeze is sometimes a useful maneuver while the child is in the drainage position. He is directed to take a deep breath and then to exhale through the mouth rapidly and as completely as possible. The depth of the expiratory effort is increased by brief, firm pressure from the therapist's hands compressing the sides of the chest. This decreases the volume of the tracheobronchial tree and facilitates the expression of secretions. The inspiration after the activity often stimulates a deep, productive cough (reinforced by the operator).

Percussion. Percussion—clapping or cupping—is performed intermittently during postural drainage. The operator's hands are held in the cupped position and vigorously and repeatedly strike the chest wall under which the specific lung segment to be drained is situated. The simile used to illustrate this concept is that of a freshly opened catsup bottle. Even when the bottle is inverted, the catsup will not flow until it is loosened and ejected by repeated blows to the bottom of the bottle.

Performed properly, percussion is painless. The operator's hand should not strike the bare skin. A light cotton undershirt or gown is an appropriate covering to protect the skin from possible irritation. The hand does not slap but conforms to the contour of the chest wall, the entire circumference of the cupped hand touching the chest wall at the same instant. When correctly applied, the clapping emits a loud, hollow sound. Care is exerted to clap over the *rib cage only*. For an infant whose chest is too small for conventional hand percussion, a small face mask is substituted for the operator's hand (see Fig. 10-15).

---

*See home care instructions on performing postural drainage in Wong, D.L., and Whaley, L.F.: Clinical handbook of pediatric nursing, ed. 2, St. Louis, 1986, The C.V. Mosby Co.

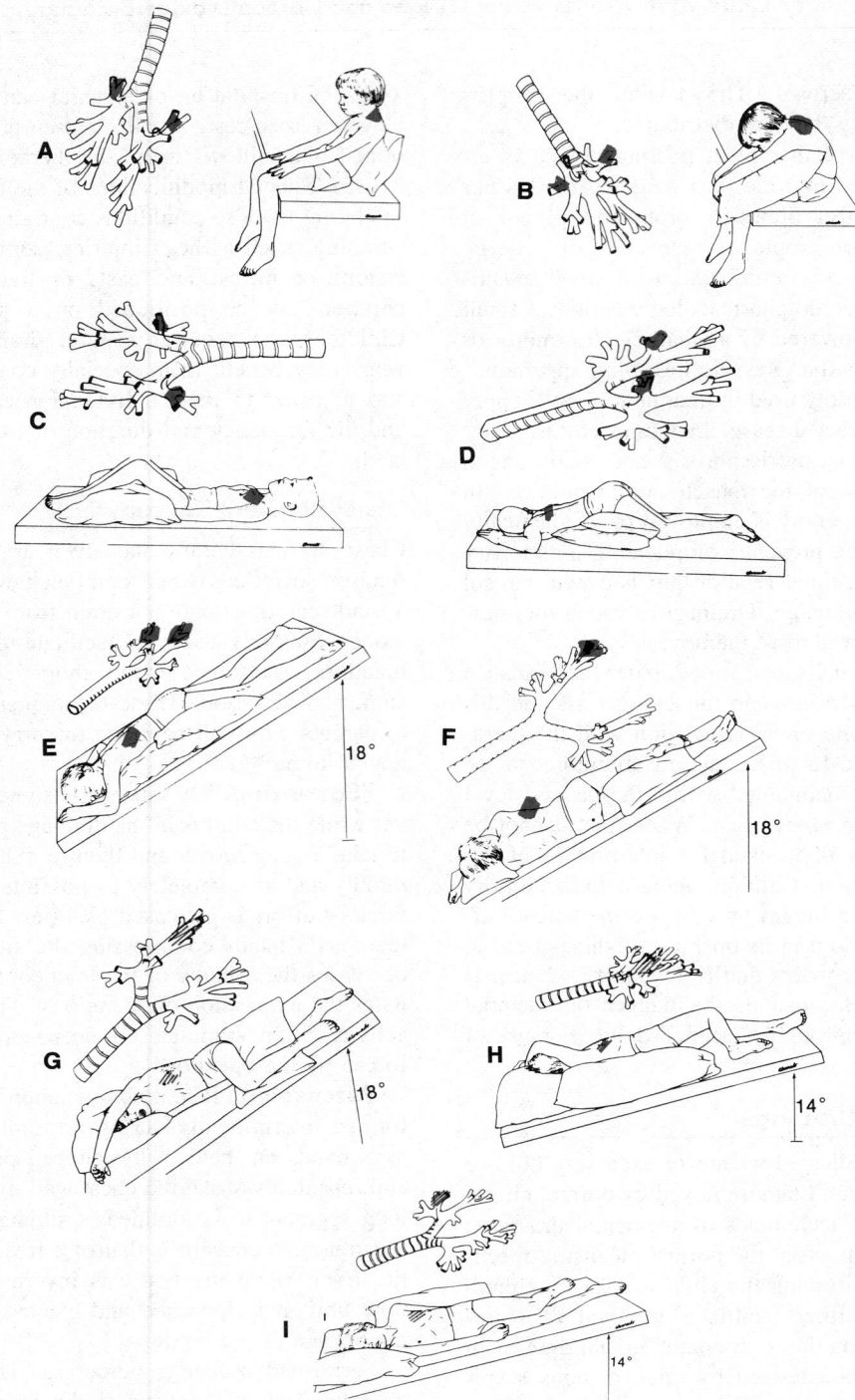

Fig. 31-10. Bronchial drainage positions for all major segments of child. For each position, model of tracheobronchial tree is projected beside child in order to show segmental bronchus *(striped)* being drained and pathway *(arrow)* of secretions out of bronchus. Drainage platform is horizontal unless otherwise noted. Striped area on child's chest indicates area to be cupped or vibrated by therapist. **A,** Apical segment of right upper lobe and apical subsegment of apical-posterior segment of left upper lobe. **B,** Posterior segment of right upper lobe and posterior subsegment of apical-posterior segment of left upper lobe. **C,** Anterior segments of both upper lobes; child should be rotated slightly away from side being drained. **D,** Superior segments of both lower lobes. **E,** Posterior basal segments of both lower lobes. **F,** Lateral basal segments of right lower lobe; left lateral basal segment would be drained by mirror image of this position (right side down). **G,** Anterior basal segment of left lower lobe; right anterior basal segment would be drained by mirror image of this position (left side down). **H,** Medial and lateral segments of right middle lobe. **I,** Lingular segments (superior and inferior) of left upper lobe (homologue of right middle lobe).

From Kendig, E.L., Jr., editor: Disorders of the respiratory tract of children, ed. 4, Philadelphia, 1983, W.B. Saunders Co.

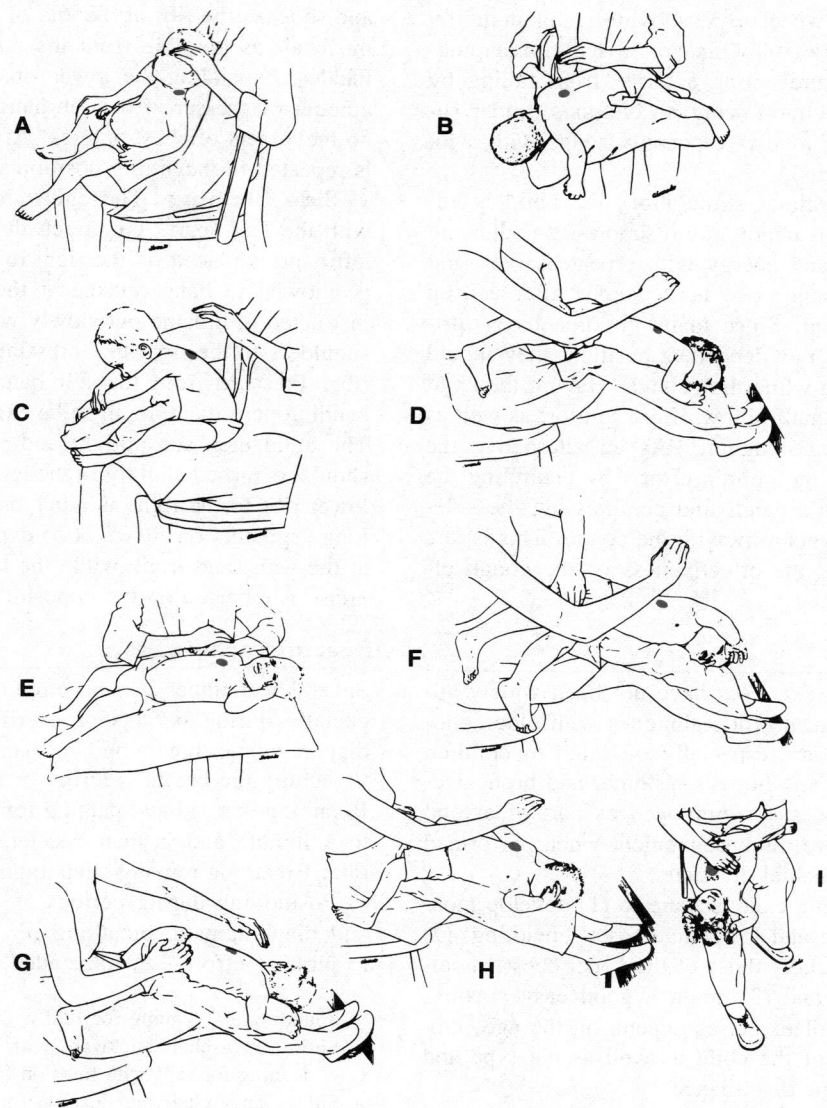

Fig. 31-11. Bronchial drainage positions for major segments of all lobes in infant. Procedure is most easily carried out in therapist's lap. Therapist's hand on chest indicates area to be cupped or vibrated. **A,** Apical segment of left upper lobe. **B,** Posterior segment of left upper lobe. **C,** Anterior segment of left upper lobe. **D,** Superior segment of right lower lobe. **E,** Posterior basal segment of right lower lobe. **F,** Lateral basal segment of right lower lobe. **G,** Anterior basal segment of right lower lobe. **H,** Medial and lateral segments of right middle lobe. **I,** Lingular segments (superior and inferior) of left upper lobe.
Modified from Infant segmental bronchial drainage. Reprinted with permission of Cystic Fibrosis Foundation, Rockville, MD.

Vibration. Vibration, a more difficult procedure, is performed only during the exhalation phase of breathing. The child is instructed to take a deep breath and exhale slowly through pursed lips. The operator places one hand on top of the other over the target lung segment and, as the child exhales, transmits a rapid vibratory impulse through the chest wall by a tensing contraction of the forearm flexor and extensor muscles. After full expiration, pressure is released. In infants whose respirations are too rapid, the handle of an electric toothbrush (suitably padded) serves as an excellent mechanical vibrator.

Deep breathing. When the child is relaxed in the desired position for drainage, he is directed to take several deep breaths, using diaphragmatic breathing. The use of deep breathing enlarges the tracheobronchial tree, enabling air to circulate around and through secretions that are not affected by usual tidal volumes. Expirations after these deep breaths often carry secretions and may stimulate a cough. Other methods that can be employed to stimulate deep breathing are blow bottles of various types, incentive spirometers, and incorporation of play that extends the expiratory time and increases expiratory pressure, for example, play items such as pinwheel toys, moving small items by blowing through a straw, blowing cotton balls or a ping-pong ball on a table, preventing a tissue from falling by blowing it against a wall, blowing up balloons (under supervision), and singing loudly (especially songs with a lot of words between breaths).

Cough. With or without stimulation, the child is encouraged to cough. He is taught not to suppress a cough and not to waste strength and energy with repeated weak and ineffective coughs. One or two hard coughs after a deep breath are more efficient. Since many children have difficulty in coughing when in a dependent position, they should be encouraged to sit up while they cough. Having the child hug a stuffed toy or a small pillow offers comfort as well as physical support during coughing. As an alternative the therapist can reinforce the child's efforts by encircling the chest with the therapist's hands and compressing the sides of the lower chest in synchrony with the cough. This is less fatiguing and increases the effectiveness of the cough efforts.

Breathing Exercises

Breathing and postural exercises have not been widely applied to children but are useful techniques with older, motivated children. They are especially of value to children with kyphoscoliosis, cystic fibrosis, asthma, and bronchiectasis. Breathing exercises are employed as part of a total therapy program and are more convenient when performed in association with bronchial drainage.

The goals of breathing exercises are to (1) develop more effective diaphragmatic and lower intercostal breathing, (2) relax all muscles, especially those of the upper chest, shoulder girdle, and neck, and (3) attain a good easy posture. The number and type of exercises depend on the age, motivation, and strength of the child as well as the type and extent of the physiologic disturbance.

A variety of exercises are employed, but any individual child is unable to tolerate all of them; therefore they are either selected to meet the needs of the specific child or alternated in their use. The most important exercises are diaphragmatic breathing and side bending, concentrating on both abdominal expansion and lateral expansion.

Diaphragmatic breathing. This exercise is performed lying down on the floor or mat after a short rest in the supine position, which stretches the pectoral, chest, and upper back muscles in preparation for the exercise. For abdominal expansion the child lies on the back with knees flexed, with one hand placed on the upper chest and one on the abdomen. He breathes out *slowly* while compressing the lower rib cage and upper abdomen and then inhales, relaxing and expanding the upper abdomen. There should be no movement in chest or neck. The exercise is also carried out in the sitting position with the back supported.

To concentrate on lateral expansion, the child lies on the back with knees flexed and palms of hands on the sides of the lower rib cage. The child is instructed to breathe out *slowly* while compressing the lower ribs and upper abdomen

and squeeze the ribs at the end of expiration to get rid of as much air as possible from the base of the lungs. He then inhales, expanding the lower ribs outward against a small amount of pressure from the hands. Again there should be no movement of chest or neck. After back lying the exercise is repeated in the sitting position with the back supported.

Side bending. The child sits comfortably in a chair with the feet apart. To stretch the rib cage on the left, the left hand is placed on the right lower ribs and the right arm is allowed to hang relaxed at the right side. The child is instructed to breathe out slowly while bending the head and shoulders to the right and pressing the left hand against the ribs. Pressure from the left hand together with the torso bending permits more air to be expelled from the right lung. The child then sits upright and inhales with the head and shoulders turned slightly to the left, thus expanding the right lower ribs to the right as much as possible. This allows the lung segments on the right to expand. Bending takes place at the waist and trunk while the hips remain level. The exercise is repeated on the opposite side.

Special Techniques

Several techniques can be employed to aid relaxation, especially during periods of exertion or stress. Accelerated diaphragmatic breathing, or panting, is often useful for "catching the breath" during or after episodes of dyspnea. Breathing is rapid and panting for approximately 30 seconds to 1 minute and is then decelerated slowly to the normal rate. Breathing remains diaphragmatic.

Positioning during periods of stress promotes relaxation and diaphragmatic breathing for easier and more efficient respiratory effort. Recommended positions include:

Squatting and leaning forward with elbows on knees
Sitting on a chair backward with forearms on chair back and leaning forward with head on forearms
Sitting on a chair and leaning forward with elbows on knees and forearms relaxed
Leaning forward against a wall or railing
Lying on side with top shoulder and side leaning over pillows placed as follows—one between knees, one under head and upper trunk, and one between arms and under head

When engaged in an activity such as climbing stairs, the child should be taught to regulate breathing with the activity. For example, when climbing stairs, the child inhales while taking two steps and exhales while taking six steps. The expiratory phase should be extended as long as possible; however, the expiration should be three times the length of the inspiration.

Respiratory Dysfunction

Disorders of respiratory structure and function that may result in ventilatory failure are a significant cause of childhood illness. They may have a variety of causes, both pulmonary and nonpulmonary, and the pulmonary dysfunction can result in disturbances in other organs and systems. The primary function of the lungs is to provide sufficient oxygen for metabolic needs and to remove the carbon dioxide produced. Inadequacy of the oxygen-supplying role results in *hypoxemia* and tissue *hypoxia;* inadequate carbon dioxide removal causes *hypercapnia.* Often both gases may be insufficiently exchanged.

RESPIRATORY FAILURE

In general, the term *respiratory insufficiency* is applied to two conditions: (1) children with increased work of breathing while preserving gas exchange function near normal—ventilatory insufficiency, and (2) children who are unable to maintain normal blood gas tensions and develop hypoxemia and acidosis secondary to carbon dioxide retention.

Respiratory failure is defined as the inability of the respiratory apparatus to maintain adequate oxygenation of the blood, with or without carbon dioxide retention.

Respiratory arrest is the cessation of respiration.

Apnea is absence of airflow (breathing). Apnea can be (1) central, in which respiratory efforts are absent, (2) obstructive, in which respiratory efforts are present, and (3) mixed, in which both central and obstructive components are present.

Effective pulmonary gas exchange requires clear airways, normal lungs and chest wall, and adequate pulmonary circulation. This functional pulmonary unit plus normal respiratory control mechanisms ensures adequate total alveolar ventilation and perfusion, which are reflected in oxygen and carbon dioxide tensions in arterial blood leaving the lung. Anything that affects these functions or their relationships can compromise respiration.

Respiratory dysfunction may have an abrupt or an insidious onset. Respiratory failure therefore can occur as an emergency situation or may be preceded by gradual and progressive deterioration of respiratory function. Physical examination does not reveal the presence of either hypoxemia or hypercapnia. Most clinical manifestations are nonspecific and are affected by variations among individuals and differences in severity and duration of inadequate gas exchange.

The diagnosis of respiratory failure is determined by the combined application of three sources of information (Wade, 1982):

1. Presence or history of a condition that might predispose to respiratory failure
2. Observation of respiratory failure
3. Measurement of arterial blood gases and pH

Conditions that Predispose to Respiratory Failure

Respiratory disorders are more conveniently classified according to three dominant functional abnormalities, although all three types may be present in the disease. The three primary types of functional disorders and examples of each are:

1. *Obstructive lung disease,* in which there is increased resistance to airflow in either the upper or the lower respiratory tract (Table 31-4).
2. *Restrictive lung disease,* in which there is impaired lung expansion resulting from loss of lung volume, decreased distensibility, or chest wall disturbance (Table 31-5).
3. *Primary inefficient gas transfer,* in which there is insufficient alveolar ventilation for carbon dioxide removal or impaired oxygenation of pulmonary capillary blood as a result of dysfunction of the respiratory control mechanism or a diffusion defect (Table 31-6).

Table 31-4 Causes of obstructive respiratory disease

SITE OF DISTURBANCE	SPECIFIC DISEASE CONDITIONS	
	NEWBORN AND EARLY INFANCY	LATE INFANCY AND CHILDHOOD
Upper airway		
Anomalies	Choanal atresia, Pierre-Robin syndrome, flabby epiglottis, laryngeal web, tracheal stenosis, vocal cord paralysis, tracheomalacia, vascular ring	Tracheal stenosis, vocal cord paralysis, vascular ring, laryngotracheomalacia
Aspiration	Meconium, mucus, vomitus	Foreign body, vomitus
Infection	Pneumonia, pertussis	Laryngotracheitis, diphtheria, epiglottitis, peritonsillar or retropharyngeal abscess
Tumors	Hemangioma, cystic hygroma, teratoma	Papilloma, hemangioma, lymphangioma, teratoma, hypertrophy of tonsils and adenoids
Allergic or reflex	Laryngospasm from local irritation (intubation) or tetany	Laryngospasm from local irritation (aspiration, intubation, drowning) or tetany, allergy, smoke inhalation

From Pagtakhan, R.D., and Chernick, V.: Intensive care for respiratory disorders. In Kendig, E.L., and Chernick, V., editors: Disorders of the respiratory tract in children, ed. 4, Philadelphia, 1983, W.B. Saunders Co.

Continued.

Table 31-4 Causes of obstructive respiratory disease—cont'd

SITE OF DISTURBANCE	SPECIFIC DISEASE CONDITIONS	
	NEWBORN AND EARLY INFANCY	LATE INFANCY AND CHILDHOOD
Lower airway		
Anomalies	Bronchostenosis, bronchomalacia, lobar emphysema, aberrant vessels	Bronchostenosis, lobar emphysema, aberrant vessels
Aspiration	Amniotic contents, tracheoesophageal fistula, pharyngeal incoordination, gastroesophageal reflux	Foreign body, vomitus, pharyngeal incoordination (Riley-Day syndrome), drowning, gastroesophageal reflux
Infection	Pneumonia, pertussis	Bronchiolitis, pneumonia, tuberculosis (endobronchial, hilar adenopathy), cystic fibrosis, bronchiectasis
Tumors		Bronchogenic cyst, teratoma
Allergic or reflex		Asthma, bronchospasm secondary to inhalation of noxious gases

Table 31-5 Causes of restrictive respiratory disease

SITE OF DISTURBANCE	SPECIFIC DISEASE CONDITIONS	
	NEWBORN AND EARLY INFANCY	LATE INFANCY AND CHILDHOOD
Parenchymal		
Anomalies	Agenesis, hypoplasia, lobar emphysema, congenital cyst, pulmonary sequestration	Hypoplasia, congenital cyst, pulmonary sequestration
Atelectasis	Hyaline membrane disease	Thick secretions, foreign body
Infection	Pneumonia	Pneumonia, cystic fibrosis, bronchiectasis, pneumatocele
Alveolar rupture	Pneumothorax (spontaneous or iatrogenic), intestinal emphysema	Pneumothorax (trauma, asthma)
Others	Pulmonary hemorrhage, pulmonary edema, Wilson-Mikity syndrome, sudden infant death syndrome	Pulmonary edema, lobectomy, chemical pneumonitis, pleural effusion, near-drowning
Chest wall		
Muscular	Diaphragmatic hernia, eventration, edema	Amyotonia congenita, poliomyelitis, diaphragmatic hernia, eventration, myasthenia gravis, muscular dystrophy, botulism
Skeletal malformations	Hemivertebrae, absence of ribs, thoracic dystrophy	Kyphoscoliosis, hemivertebrae, absence of ribs
Others	Abdominal distention	Obesity, flail chest

From Pagtakhan, R.D., and Chernick, V.: Intensive care for respiratory disorders. In Kendig, E.L., and Chernick, V., editors: Disorders of the respiratory tract in children, ed 4, Philadelphia, 1983, W.B. Saunders Co.

Recognition of Respiratory Failure

Respiratory failure that occurs as the result of acute obstruction of a major airway or cardiac arrest is sudden and readily apparent. Gradual and more covert development of signs and symptoms is less easily recognized. Insufficient alveolar ventilation from any cause ultimately leads to hypoxemia and hypercapnia. However, there are situations in which severe respiratory distress may be present without significant carbon dioxide retention, and hypoxemia may occur without clinically detectable cyanosis. Therefore evaluation of respiratory adequacy is based on both clinical assessment and laboratory studies. Nursing observation and judgment are vital to successful management of respiratory failure. Nurses must be able to assess a situation and initiate appropriate action within moments.

Unless respiratory arrest occurs suddenly, signs of hypoxemia and hypercapnia are usually subtle in their development and become more obvious as respiratory failure pro-

Table 31-6 Causes of primary inefficient gas transfer

SITE OF DISTURBANCE	SPECIFIC DISEASE CONDITIONS
Pulmonary diffusion defect	
Increased diffusion path between alveoli and capillaries	Pulmonary edema, pulmonary fibrosis, collagen disorders, *Pneumocystis carinii* infection, sarcoidosis
Decreased alveolocapillary surface area	Pulmonary embolism, sarcoidosis, pulmonary hypertension, mitral stenosis, fibrosing alveolitis
Inadequate erythrocytes and hemoglobin	Anemia, hemorrhage
Respiratory center depression	
Increased cerebrospinal fluid pressure	Cerebral trauma (birth injuries), intracranial tumors, central nervous system infection (meningitis, encephalitis, sepsis)
Excessive central nervous system depressant drugs	Maternal oversedation, overdosage with barbiturates, morphine, or diazepam
Excessive chemical changes in arterial blood	Severe asphyxia (hypercapnia, hypoxemia)
Toxic	Tetanus

From Pagtakhan, R.D., and Chernick, V.: Intensive care for respiratory disorders. In Kendig, E.L., and Chernick, V., editors: Disorders of the respiratory tract in children, ed. 4, Philadelphia, 1983, W.B. Saunders Co.

gresses. The unknowing observer may attribute early signs such as mood changes and restlessness to other causes, and some signs can be altered by other factors, for example, anemia. Hemoglobin is needed to show some cyanosis; therefore it may not be observed in the child with a hemoglobin less than 6 g/dl. Cyanosis is usually apparent at a Po_2 of 40 to 50 mm Hg. The signs of respiratory failure are outlined in the box on p. 1322.

In clinical situations in which impaired ventilation can be anticipated or clinical manifestations indicate impending hypoxemia, serial measurements of blood gases should be obtained and monitored in order to detect impending respiratory failure and implement therapy before respiratory acidosis becomes extreme.

MANAGEMENT AND RELATED NURSING CONSIDERATIONS

The interventions used in the management of respiratory failure are often dramatic, requiring special skills, and are frequently emergency procedures. If respiratory arrest occurs, the primary objectives are to recognize the situation and initiate resuscitative measures within moments. When the situation is not an arrest, the suspicion of respiratory failure is confirmed by diagnosis and the type defined by arterial blood gas analysis. When severity is established, an attempt is made to determine the underlying cause by thorough evaluation.

Treatment of respiratory dysfunction involves both specific and nonspecific therapy. Specific therapies are directed toward reversal of the causative factors. However, sometimes nonspecific measures are needed to maintain oxygenation and enhance CO_2 removal until specific methods take effect. The major reasons for implementing nonspecific

treatments are: (1) unknown etiology, (2) lack of specific treatment for a known cause, (3) lack of time for a specific treatment to take effect, and (4) need for specialized personnel or equipment for specific treatment.

The principles of management are: (1) maintain oxygenation, (2) maintain ventilation, (3) apply specific and nonspecific therapy, and (4) anticipate complications. Monitoring the patient's condition is critical, and some of the techniques employed to maintain oxygenation and assist ventilation include artificial ventilation, artificial airway, and cardiopulmonary resuscitation.

Observation and Monitoring

The child is monitored to evaluate the cause of the failure, help determine a course of action, and assess the patient's response to treatment. If close continuous monitoring is required, the child is transferred to an intensive care unit and appropriate treatment modalities are applied according to the specific functional disturbance and the underlying etiology.

The child's cardiac and respiratory status are monitored by observation and by electronic means. However, no monitoring equipment can replace conscientious nursing observations, including:

1. Visual inspection of skin color to estimate the level of arterial oxygen saturation
2. Observation of respiratory effort or distress—nasal flaring, grunting, gasping, retraction
3. Observation of diaphragmatic movement, lung expansion, and use of accessory muscles—depth, symmetry, inspiration/expiration ratio
4. Auscultation of the thorax to assess
   a. Breath sounds—presence, intensity, quality, symmetry

b. Abnormal sounds—stridor, wheezes, rales, rhonchi, rubs, crepitation, increase or decrease in sounds

c. Tube placement and the need for endotracheal suction when the child is intubated

Hourly temperature assessments are needed, and assessments should be performed more often if the child, usually an infant, requires a thermally controlled environment. Optimum temperature is maintained, since fever increases the need for oxygen and increases respiratory efforts. Blood gases are usually monitored continuously via electronic devices or regular measurements by laboratory analysis as described previously.

Artificial Ventilation

There are a variety of methods for controlling or assisting ventilation. Temporary assistance can be provided by a hand-operated self-inflating ventilation bag with mask and a nonreturnable valve to prevent rebreathing (Ambu bag). With the mask placed on the nose and mouth (an open airway is established by correct positioning with the chin forward and the neck extended to the ''sniffing'' position), the bag is rhythmically compressed, forcing the gas from the bag into the patient's lungs.

For more prolonged assistance, mechanical ventilation is employed to replace the bellows function of the diaphragm and thoracic wall muscles. The lungs are inflated by the application of either positive or negative pressure. The positive-pressure machine inflates the lung by increasing airway pressure above atmospheric pressure, and a negative-pressure ventilator creates a subatmospheric pressure around the chest wall, whereas airway pressure remains atmospheric. Application of positive pressure by mechanical means usually improves the distribution of gas within the lung and often reinflates partially collapsed lung segments. The overall effect is the improvement of gas exchange.

Types of ventilators. Ventilators, or respirators, are characterized by the way in which gas is generated (constant pressure or constant flow) and by the way in which the gas is cycled to change from the respiratory to the expiratory phase of respiration. They are classified as *pressure cycled, volume cycled,* and *time cycled.* The pressure-cycled ventilator produces a preset pressure and ceases to deliver gas once this pressure is reached. With this type, changes in compliance allow changes in volume of gas delivered. Volume-cycled ventilators deliver a fixed volume of gas and are more effective in maintaining alveolar ventilation when compliance is severely diminished, as in asthma or pulmonary edema. Time-cycled ventilators terminate inspiration and expiration by a preset cycle duration and gas flow rate. Most negative-pressure ventilators are time cycled.

Pressure ventilators can be regulated to either assist or substitute for the patient's respiratory effort. When used to assist ventilation, the ventilator transmits the prescribed volume of gas in response to the patient's own respiratory effort. In controlled ventilation the machine automatically controls both the rate and the depth of ventilation at fixed settings (see Table 10-4). Ventilators are attached to the patient by mask, endotracheal tube, or tracheostomy.

Care of the patient. The regulation and maintenance of mechanical ventilators are the responsibility of respiratory therapists. However, nurses should understand the function of the ventilator in use and be able to detect signs of malfunction and deviations from the desired settings. The nurse also promotes the effectiveness of ventilation by suctioning, positioning, and providing support and reassurance to the child receiving mechanical respiration. See Chapter 10 for assisted and controlled respiration in the neonate.

Weaning the patient from a ventilator involves gradual physical and psychologic withdrawal from dependence on the mechanical device. The child is ready for weaning when there is (1) no evidence of the primary disease, (2) intact central nervous system function (especially a gag reflex), (3) adequate muscular strength and nutritional status, (4) Pco_2 less than 50 mm Hg in children with an acute disease, and (5) Po_2 greater than 100 mm Hg in 50% oxygen. The child should be able to generate a tidal volume of 5 cc per kg (Crowley and Morrow, 1980). The child should be free of infection and have stable hemodynamics and a hematocrit of at least 30%.

The child who is to be weaned from the respirator is deprived of oral intake for approximately 6 hours before scheduled extubation (this is shorter in infants) and at least 4 hours after. If edema persists the time may be longer. Sedation or other respiratory depressants are contraindicated so that the child can be observed for respiratory activity, and the child is placed on a cardiac and apnea monitor if one is not already attached. Resuscitation and reintubation

---

SIGNS OF RESPIRATORY FAILURE

Cardinal signs
Restlessness
Tachypnea
Tachycardia
Diaphoresis

Early but less obvious signs
Mood changes, such as euphoria or depression
Headache
Altered depth and pattern of respirations
Hypertension
Exertional dyspnea
Anorexia
Increased cardiac output and renal output
Central nervous system symptoms (decreased efficiency, impaired judgment, anxiety, confusion, restlessness, and irritability)
Flaring nares
Chest wall retractions
Expiratory grunt
Wheezing and/or prolonged expiration

Signs of more severe hypoxia
Hypotension or	Dyspnea
hypertension	Depressed respirations
Dimness of vision	Bradycardia
Somnolence	Cyanosis, peripheral
Stupor	or central
Coma	

equipment is available at the bedside. Vigorous chest physiotherapy and suctioning are ordinarily performed just before tube removal, and cool mist is begun immediately after extubation. The child is monitored for clinical signs of a reaction to the removal, and blood gas measurements are observed. The most common reactions are airway edema, fatigue, and atelectasis. Airway edema often responds to racemic epinephrine.

Endotracheal Airways

An artificial airway is usually used in association with artificial ventilation and in children with upper airway obstruction. Endotracheal (ET) intubation can be accomplished by the nasal (nasotracheal), oral (orotracheal), or direct tracheal (tracheostomy) routes. Oral intubation is usually the method of choice for emergency situations, but for prolonged intubation a nasotracheal tube is more often used. Although it is more difficult to place technically, nasotracheal intubation is preferred to orotracheal intubation because it facilitates oral hygiene and provides more stable fixation, which reduces the complication of tracheal erosion and the danger of accidental extubation.

ET tubes may be cuffed to provide an airtight seal or uncuffed. Most children do not require a cuffed tube, because they have sufficient tracheal compliance and pressure from cuffed tubes predisposes to subglottic stenosis. Cuffed tubes are used when high inflation pressures are needed. They are inflated to the minimum volume, and the pressure cuff must be deflated hourly for 2 to 5 minutes to minimize the possibility of pressure necrosis. However, pressure cuffs are rarely used in children younger than 10 years of age. Air or gas delivered directly to the trachea must be humidified as in tracheostomy.

Although newborn infants have been successfully maintained on nasotracheal tubes for longer periods, in older children who require intubation beyond a week, tracheostomy is usually performed. The decision to change from ET tube to tracheostomy is made on an individual basis. The tracheostomy allows for speaking and eating and also facilitates clearing of secretions. Some authorities consider 24 hours the maximum time for ET intubation if edema of the airway is present. Suctioning is carried out with the same care as suctioning a tracheostomy.

Complications. Complications are a risk of intubation. Some occur immediately; others are not apparent until after extubation. Those related to immediate intubation include trauma to mouth and teeth and reflex-mediated changes in vital signs. The most common sequela of intubation is sore throat, which is benign and disappears within 48 to 72 hours without therapy, although a humidified atmosphere is beneficial. Other complications include traumatic laryngitis, infection, glottic edema, and mucosal lesions of the larynx secondary to entrapment of mucosa between the two rigid structures, the tube and the nonexpansible cartilage. The most severe sequela of intubation is laryngeal stenosis secondary to fibrosis (approximately 8%) (Morriss, 1984).

Tracheostomy

Tracheostomy can be a lifesaving procedure. It is performed as an emergency or an elective procedure and may be combined with mechanical ventilation. The number of children who have tracheostomies performed is increasing because of the sophistication of the practice and the availability of intensive care units and specialized nursing care for infants and children. The usual indications for tracheostomy are (Waring, 1983):

1. Mechanical obstruction of the upper airway, for example, croup, foreign body, and laryngeal paralysis
2. Disease of the central nervous system, for example, head injury, craniotomy, and drug depression
3. Neuromuscular disease, for example, poliomyelitis, tetanus, myasthenia gravis, amyotonia congenita, and Guillain-Barré syndrome
4. Secretional obstruction, such as debility with weak cough, severe thoracic or chest pain (from incision or injury)
5. Conditions with disturbances of gas diffusion or distribution, such as blunt chest injuries, smoke inhalation, and widespread pneumonia
6. Prophylaxis for radical neck or head surgery—an unusual need in children

Infants and children with tracheostomies require skilled and intensive nursing care. The diameter of the pediatric trachea is very small and can become occluded easily and quickly, leaving the infant or child who is unable to signal for help at risk of respiratory and cardiac arrest. Children with tracheostomies are usually placed in hospital units where constant surveillance is available, preferably in an intensive care setting.

Plastic and Silastic have largely replaced silver as the preferred material for tracheostomy tubes, especially for pediatric use. These materials can be constructed with a more acute angle, and since they soften at room temperature are better able to conform to the contours of the airway. The flexibility of the material resists kinking, and the smooth surface reduces crust formation; therefore most tubes are constructed without an inner cannula. The tube is held in place by an appropriate length of sturdy cloth tape around the child's neck. Umbilical cord tape is ideal (Fig. 31-12).

A simple method for securing a tracheostomy tube consists of looping a sufficient length of tape through one or both openings in the sides of the tube. If both sides are secured, the ends of the tapes are tied at the back of the neck (Fig. 31-13, A). If one side is secured in the middle of the tape, one end is passed through the remaining opening and tied securely at the side (Fig. 31-13, B). A better fit can be achieved if the child's head is flexed, rather than extended, while the tape is fixed. If the cord is too loose, the tube may be coughed out. The ties should fit snugly enough so that one finger can be inserted with difficulty between the tape and the child's neck (Fig. 31-14). To reduce the possibility that the tracheostomy tube may come out, the new ties are attached before the old ties are removed. The obturator is kept in a sterile package taped to the head of the bed.

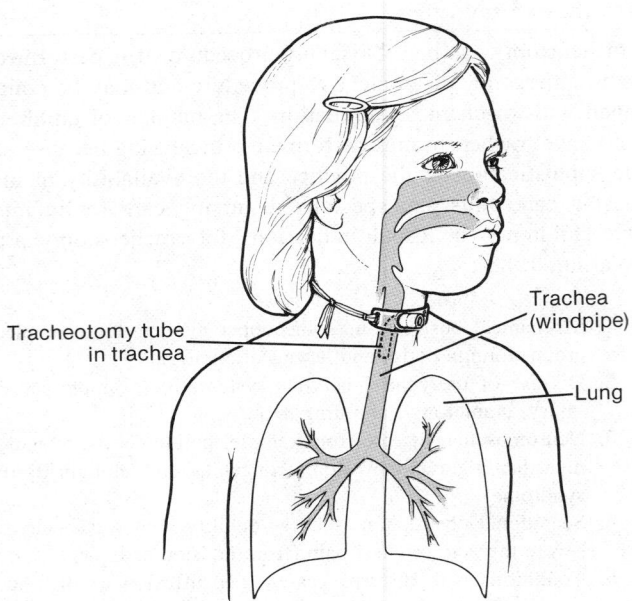

Fig. 31-12. Tracheostomy tube in trachea and securely tied with tape.

Since the normal warming, wetting, and filtering functions of the upper airway are inoperative, air entering the tracheostomy opening is humidified by attaching a special tracheostomy mask or "collar" to deliver humidified gas directly to the tracheostomy opening, or by direct attachment to a mechanical ventilator (Fig. 31-15). The humid gas helps to loosen mucus and reduce the chances of crust formation and a mucous plug. Moisture from the humidified gas tends to accumulate on the inner surface of the flexible plastic tubing and must be eliminated periodically to prevent occlusion of the tube and/or accidental aspiration. The tubing is disconnected at the collar or tracheostomy tube and drained into a container. It is not allowed to flow back into the humidifying receptacle.

The tracheostomy requires daily care the same as any other surgical skin opening. Children usually return from surgery with two long sutures, one attached to each side of the tracheostomy opening and both taped to the child's chest. These help identify the opening to aid in replacing a tube in the event the tube becomes dislodged. The dressing around the stoma is changed three times daily (after the initial change by the surgeon) until healed, then twice daily if a dressing is needed. Special dressings slit to the center fit neatly around the tube and cover the opening. An alternative dressing can be constructed from gauze dressings folded and placed one on each side of the tube and taped together. Regular gauze dressings are not cut to fit because of the risk of aspirating gauze fibers. Careful aseptic technique is used throughout care of the tracheostomy.

Suctioning. The airway must remain patent and requires frequent suctioning during the first few hours after tracheostomy to remove mucous plugs and excess secretions. Tracheal suction catheters are available in a variety of sizes. The catheter selected should have a diameter one-half

the diameter of the tracheostomy tube. If the catheter is too large it can obliterate the airway. The catheter is constructed with a side port so that the catheter can be introduced without suction and removed while simultaneously intermittent suction is applied by obliterating the port with the thumb (Fig. 31-16). A small amount of sterile isotonic saline injected into the tube helps to loosen the secretions and crusts for easier aspiration. The amount of saline used (0.5 to 2 ml) depends on the size of the child. The amount of suction applied should not exceed 40 mm Hg, and the pressure of the suction machine is checked daily. These precautions reduce the likelihood of mucosal damage.

Each pass of the suction catheter should take no longer than 5 seconds in an infant and 10 to 15 seconds for an older child, especially when respiratory status is compromised. Counting 1-one thousand, 2-one thousand, etc., while suctioning is a simple means for monitoring the time. Without a safeguard the airway may be obstructed for too long a period of time.

Suctioning is carried out at frequent intervals to prevent buildup of crusts and as often as needed for signs of mucus in the airway, such as bubbling, noisy breathing, or coughing. The cough, although noisy, is ineffectual, because the glottis, which normally closes and releases suddenly to effect a cough, is bypassed by the tracheostomy. The child is allowed to rest for 30 to 60 seconds after each aspiration to allow oxygen tension to return to normal, then the process is repeated until the trachea is clear.

Aseptic technique is essential during care of the tracheostomy. Secondary infection is a major concern, since the air entering the lower airway bypasses the natural defenses of the upper airway. If the suction tubes are not the type that comes equipped with a plastic sleeve, a sterile glove is worn during the aspiration procedure. A fresh tube and

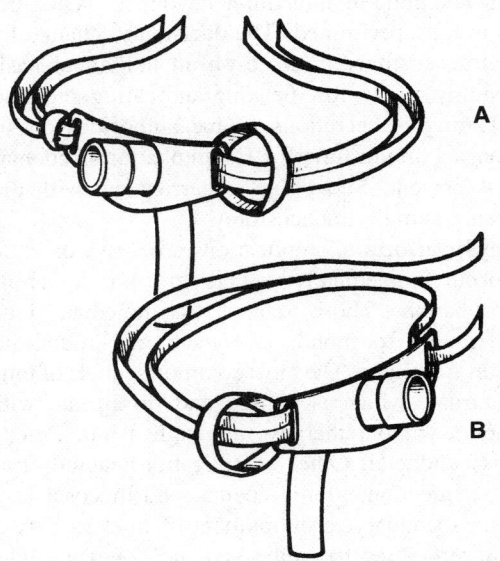

Fig. 31-13. Pediatric tracheostomy tube. **A,** Tape secured at both sides to be tied in back. **B,** Tape secured on one side and looped through other side to be tied at side.

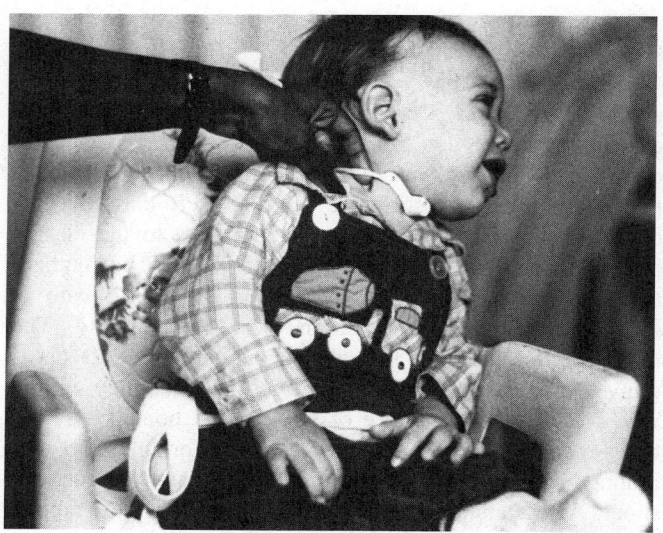

Fig. 31-14. Securing tracheostomy tube. A snug fit, but finger can be inserted beneath ties.

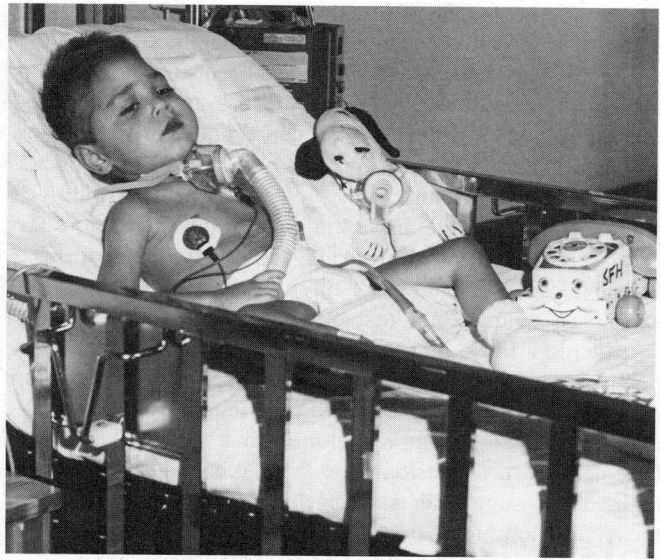

Fig. 31-15. Child with a tracheostomy and a mist collar.
Photography by John Roy, Saint Francis Hospital, Tulsa, OK.

glove are used each time. Both types of suction tubes are discarded after suction. Sterile saline solution used to moisten and clean the tube should be discarded after each use. A container of saline for multiple use is discouraged; it serves as a reservoir for organisms from secretions aspirated through the tube.

Routine care. A duplicate tracheostomy tube (with obturator) and equipment needed for its insertion are kept at the bedside in the event that the tube becomes dislodged and needs to be replaced. For a "fresh" tracheostomy a tube one size smaller is also placed at the bedside in the event the duplicate cannot be replaced. If the tube accidentally becomes dislodged, the attending nurse should maintain the patency of the incision by spreading the edges with a sterile clamp until the tube can be replaced. The child's head is *gently* extended with a towel roll or small pillow under the shoulders to help keep the stoma open. In an emergency when the child is in distress and unable to move air, a large size (number 10 to 14) French catheter can be inserted about 4 inches and cut off a few inches from above the stoma to provide an airway until a tracheostomy tube can be replaced. Children with tracheostomies that must remain in place for months or years require a weekly tube change.

A child with a tracheostomy requires continuous nursing attendance. Vital signs are monitored regularly, and the patency of the tube is maintained. An infant or small child must be placed on a cardiac/apnea monitor continuously while not under *direct* nursing observation. A child with a new tracheostomy requires chest auscultation every hour initially, then every 2 hours to assess the tube for patency. Once every 24 hours is usually sufficient for the established tracheostomy. The child is observed closely for any signs of distress or complications, including infection, atelectasis, cannula occlusion, tracheal bleeding, expulsion of the tube, tracheal ulceration and granulation, tracheal stenosis, air swallowing, and delayed healing of the stoma. Nursing ob-

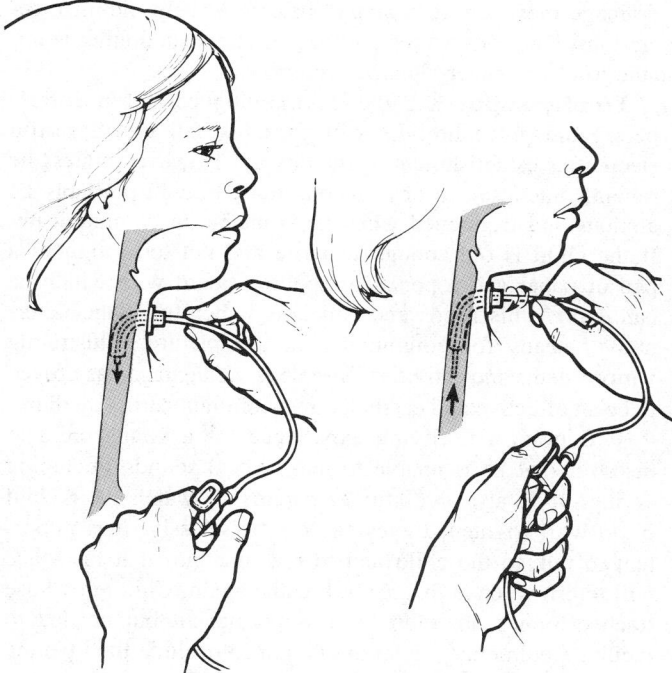

Fig. 31-16. Tracheostomy suctioning. **A,** Insertion, port open. **B,** Withdrawal, port occluded.

servation is vital to the child who is unable to signal for help. Signs of impending difficulty include restlessness, dyspnea, pallor or cyanosis, changes in pulse or blood pressure, overt bleeding from the trachea or around the incision site, retractions, and noisy respirations.

The tracheostomy tube is removed as soon as it is no longer needed. Diseases of short duration, such as croup, usually allow early removal, but some conditions, such as tracheomalacia, tracheal stenosis, or paralysis, may require the tube to remain in place indefinitely. Opinions differ regarding the best means for removing a tube, especially after it has been in place for an appreciable length of time. More commonly the diameter of the tube is reduced daily by inserting tubes of decreasing size. When a tube several sizes smaller than the original is tolerated without difficulty, the tube is plugged. If the child has no problems after 24 hours, the plugged tube is removed. Plugging the tube would occlude too much of the airway in small infants; therefore the tube is removed and the opening covered with a dressing the next day. Any air leaks through the wound nearly always cease within 72 hours.

Attention must be given to ensure that children with tracheostomies are well hydrated to keep secretions loose enough for removal by cough or suction. Also, these children frequently use more calories than normal; therefore they need to have nutritionally sound diets and may require high-calorie supplements. The children are weighed daily; those with long-term tracheostomies are weighed and measured for height regularly. Because they have more difficulty generating sufficient pressure on expiration to remove secretions effectively, chest physiotherapy and postural drainage may be a regular part of care to help mobilize secretions. These measures are used anytime suctioning is unable to clear deeper-situated secretions.

Family support. If the child is fatigued and in distress before the procedure, he will probably fall into a restful sleep after establishment of the airway. However, unless he remains unconscious or semiconscious, he will probably be anxious and frightened when he is unable to communicate. If the child is old enough to write and not too fatigued, a pad of paper and a pencil or spelling board with which he can express his needs and concerns is helpful. Other alternative means for communication are pictures illustrating various items and activities. Simple sign language has proved to be an effective and easily learned communication medium.

It is often a terrifying experience for a young child to discover that he is unable to make vocal sounds, including crying. It is also stressful to parents to watch their child plead with frightened eyes and cry noiselessly. It is important to talk to the child and to reassure him that his voice will return when he is able to breathe again. Children whose tracheostomies are more or less permanent but needed to facilitate pulmonary toilet are taught to occlude the opening with a clean finger so that they can use the vocal cords to communicate.

Parents have numerous concerns relative to the procedure. If time allows before the procedure, the reasons for the decision to perform the tracheostomy, the expected results, and the approximate length of time it will remain in place should be discussed with them. Parental concern is centered around the (often) life-threatening implications generated by the need for the procedure and the possible long-term effects on the child, both physiologic and psychologic. They are concerned about the visible wound and the scar that will remain. Parents who must face the possibility of caring for the child with a tracheostomy at home have additional worries regarding their ability to assume this responsibility.

Some children may be discharged from the hospital with tracheostomy tubes. Before discharge the parents will need careful instruction and practice in the care and management of the tracheostomy,* including cardiopulmonary resuscitation (CPR). Some institutions provide CPR classes especially for families; others refer the families to the classes offered by the **American Red Cross.**† During hospitalization the parents should be involved in the child's care as soon as possible in anticipation of this eventuality. The more comfortable they are with all the aspects of tracheostomy care, the more confident and less anxious they will be when faced with total care of the child at home. It sometimes requires weeks before they feel comfortable with suctioning, cleaning, and changing the tube. Instructions should be detailed and explicit. To facilitate their adjustment, supplies identical to the ones they are accustomed to should be available to the parents. Parents often become anxious when they encounter even small differences from the familiar. In the event of substitution, they need to be reassured that the unfamiliar equipment is safe to use on their child.

A nurse from the public health department or other service should be available to the family and should periodically assess the family's ability to carry out the activities needed in care of the child. The parents may find it helpful to talk to other parents of children with tracheostomies. They also need to know whom to call and where they can get help and support in times of uncertainty or in an emergency.

Parents should be encouraged to provide as normal a life as possible for their child and other family members. The child who is physically able (e.g., a child with a tracheostomy without respiratory disability such as recurrent laryngeal polyps) can usually be allowed to engage in most activities that are appropriate for his age. He may even play outdoors with a scarf or other protection to cover the tracheostomy stoma. Both child and parents must be cautioned regarding play near any collection of water, such as a swimming pool or stream, and informed about safety precautions in the bathtub. The child should not be exposed to noxious fumes (e.g., paint, varnish, hair spray) and baby powder. Young children who may spill food near the stoma should wear a fabric bib (without plastic lining) or other device to prevent dribbled food or crumbs from being aspirated.

Pharmacologic Agents

Several drugs may be used in the treatment of respiratory failure, and an intravenous route for administration is started

---

*See home care instructions on caring for the child with a tracheostomy in Wong, D.L., and Whaley, L.F.: Clinical handbook of pediatric nursing, ed. 2, St. Louis, 1986, The C.V. Mosby Co.

†Make referral to classes available through the local chapter of the American Red Cross. Most units keep a list of dates and times of classes in their areas.

after the initial establishment of an airway (unless it was already in existence before the respiratory failure). To correct metabolic acidosis, sodium bicarbonate is usually the drug of choice, although tromethamine (THAM) has been employed successfully in some instances. Cardiac stimulants are given in cardiac arrest or severe bradycardia, vasopressors for hypotension, atropine for excessive vagal tone (especially bradycardia), and calcium gluconate or chloride to correct electromechanical dissociation. Bronchodilators are essential in cases of status asthmaticus.

Narcotic antagonists are administered in cases of depression caused by drugs, most often in the newborn after placental transfer during labor and delivery or the adolescent victim of narcotic overdose. Nurses should anticipate the need for drugs during respiratory failure, maintain an adequate emergency supply, and be familiar with their administration and the nursing responsibilities related to their use.

HOME CARE OF THE TECHNOLOGY-ASSISTED CHILD

Advanced technology and medical knowledge have improved the survival of children with a number of respiratory problems formerly considered fatal. Children have been sent home on low or intermittent oxygen therapy for quite some time. But the ventilator-dependent child is now able to be managed at home with proper equipment and dedicated family. This has created a new category of disabled children—one created by technology.

Nurses are the persons who prepare families for care of their child at home and the persons who serve as liaison between the family and other members of the health team. Discharge planning begins in the hospital when it is determined that the child can be managed at home and the family is willing to provide the needed care. It is essential that all elements of the proposed management be examined in order to orchestrate the best possible care for the child. An assessment of the caregiving ability of the family and their perception of the child is mandatory. For example, do they view the child as "ill"? What does "quality of life" mean to the family? The family should be able to provide optimum, holistic care with minimum intervention from health professionals.

The length and intensity of preparation vary by family, as does the content of the program. At least two persons must be educated in the care of the child. The mother is ordinarily the primary caregiver, and the participation of fathers may vary among families. These caregivers should be identified early and a means provided for assuring their continued involvement in the training sessions. A signed contract may be employed specifying the time and commitment of the primary caregiver and the backup person or persons (Steele and Harrison, 1986).

Clear objectives should be established describing the goals and outcomes of a successful program. Details should not be overlooked. The family is encouraged to become in-

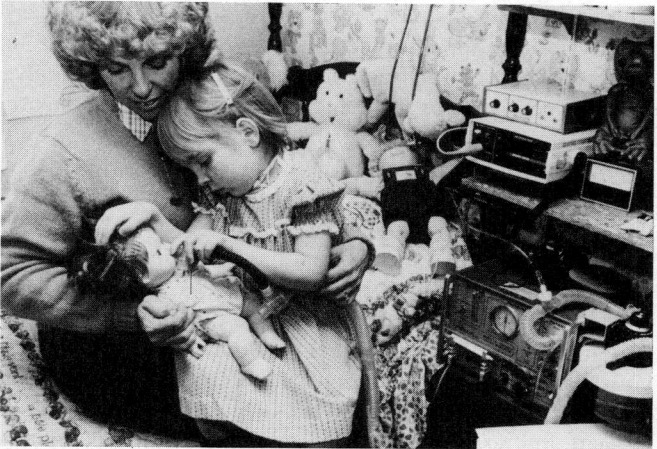

Fig. 31-17. Child with tracheostomy being managed at home.
Courtesy Karen Shannon, Saverna Park, MD.

volved with the care of the child as soon as they demonstrate a willingness to do so. They should begin with relatively simple care and activities. Bringing the child his own clothes and toys from home is a good beginning (most families do this before home care is recognized as an option). Bathing and feeding are activities that are pleasant and nonthreatening to families. Complex procedures, such as changing a tracheostomy tube, that are frightening tasks are usually left until the family is comfortable with other aspects of care (Calvi, 1985).

As the family become increasingly comfortable with the care of the child, short excursions out of the care setting offer the family some control over the child and expose the child to the normal aspects of daily living. Gradually the family assumes more and more responsibility for care in the hospital setting until the child is allowed short periods at home. Discussions with the family regarding emergencies and the proper actions to take help reduce anxiety. Practice sessions are essential. Eventually families become knowledgeable about their child's condition and therapies and adept at managing routine care and emergency situations (Fig. 31-17).

Several practical decisions must be made. For example, what is needed in the home for safe care? Will needed equipment be purchased or rented? The family needs to find the best buy when purchasing equipment and supplies. How is the equipment packaged? It is especially important to find vendors who provide service—at all hours. Backup equipment, such as mouth suction apparatus that can be used when a mechanical suction machine malfunctions and as an alternative when the child is away from the machine for a short period (e.g., in another room or in the yard), should be at hand.

The nurse makes at least one visit to the home to assess the situation and participate with the family in making decisions they can live with when they have complete care of the child. The problem of round-the-clock care is discussed with some decisions made regarding respite for the primary caregiver. The child should be as portable as possible to allow for more normal activity for both child and family. Families need to recognize that isolation may be an unanticipated stress. Visitors are either not allowed or kept to a highly selective minimum. The changes in the life of the family will be endless with many surprises and disappointments.

The child must be merged and integrated into the family. Other siblings should not be neglected because of the needs of the disabled child, and the care of the child should not be left to only one of the parents. Both should become involved in his care, and the presence of both should be encouraged at follow-up conferences. Most parents are eager to share the responsibilities but need the continued support and reassurance of the nurse and other health care providers.

As the child grows and develops, many of the problems of rearing a child are altered (see Care of the chronically ill or disabled child, Chapter 22). Providing education is probably one of the most difficult problems facing the family. Traveling creates unanticipated barriers, and community issues may be a prime source of difficulty. The multiple problems that might be encountered by the child and family with a respiratory disability are beyond the scope of this discussion. A beginning list of references dealing with both general and specific aspects of home care is provided in the bibliography. Organizations such as the **American Lung Association***, those providing services for disabled children in general (see list of resources in Appendix E) and those devoted to special health problems (see the specific disease) offer education and support to families. Of particular interest are organizations such as **SKIP (Sick Kids Need Involved People, Inc.),†** an organization that provides information, planning, education, and referral services for families of children on home care. Numerous other organizations are designed to meet the special needs of these families‡.

CARDIOPULMONARY RESUSCITATION

Complete apnea signals the need for rapid and vigorous action to prevent cardiac arrest. In such situations nurses must be prepared to initiate action immediately. Neurologically intact survival has been only in those children who receive immediate resuscitation and respond promptly (Torphy, Minter, and Thompson, 1984). In the hospital, emergency equipment should be readily available in areas in which respiratory arrest might take place, and the status of this resuscitation equipment should be checked at least once daily. Regardless of the cause of the arrest, some very basic procedures are carried out, modified somewhat according to the size of the child. The following actions are based on the Standards and Guidelines for cardiopulmonary resuscitation (CPR) and emergency cardiac care (ECC) published by the American Medical Association (1986).

Outside the hospital situation, the first action in an emergency is to assess quickly the extent of any injury and determine whether the child is unconscious. A child who is struggling to breathe but conscious should be transported immediately to an advanced life support (ALS) facility, allowing the child to maintain whatever position affords the most comfort. An unconscious child is managed with care to prevent additional trauma if the child has sustained a head or spinal cord injury. The circumstances in which the child is found offer some clues to a possible injury. For example, a child who has been thrown from a bicycle or fallen from a tree is more likely to sustain trauma than a child who is discovered in bed. The child should be turned as a unit with firm support to the head and neck to prevent rolling, twisting, or tilting backward or forward.

Resuscitation

For effective CPR the victim is placed on the back on a firm flat surface, employing appropriate precautions (see Emergency Treatment: Child with Cardiopulmonary Arrest for outline of procedure).

With loss of consciousness the tongue, which is attached to the lower jaw, relaxes and falls back, obstructing the airway. To open the airway, the head is positioned with either head tilt/chin lift (Fig. 31-18, *A*) or jaw thrust (Fig. 31-18, *B*). After restoration of a patent airway by removal of foreign material and secretions (if indicated) and if the child is not breathing, continuation of the airway is maintained and rescue breathing is initiated. To ventilate the lungs in the infant and small child, the mouth of the operator is placed in such a way that both the mouth and the nostrils are included (Fig. 31-18, *C*). Older children are ventilated through the mouth while the nostrils are firmly pinched for airtight contact (Fig. 31-18, *D*).

The volume of air in an infant's lungs is small and the air passages are considerably smaller with resistance to flow potentially higher than in adults. However, since the differences are relative and vary according to the size of the child, the correct volume of air and force of the rescue breaths cannot be stated with certainty. If air enters freely and the chest rises, the airway is assumed to be clear. Breaths should be given slowly; the necessary volume can be provided without causing abdominal distention. Gastric distention, which interferes with diaphragmatic excursion, frequently occurs when breaths are delivered too rapidly.

After an initial two breaths, a peripheral pulse is palpated to ascertain the presence of a heartbeat. The carotid is the most central and accessible artery (Fig. 31-18, *E*). The very short and often fat neck of the infant renders the carotid pulse (ordinarily used in the adult) difficult to palpate. Therefore it is preferable to use the brachial pulse, located on the inner side of the upper arm midway between the el-

---

*1740 Broadway, New York, NY 10019.

†216 Newport Drive, Severna Park, MD 21146.

‡Ventilator Dependent Children/Home Care Program, Children's Hospital of Philadelphia, 34th and Civic Center Blvd., Philadelphia, PA 19104; Life Care, 5505 Central Ave., Boulder, CO 80301; Rancho Los Amigos Hospital, 7601 E. Imperial Hwy., Downey, CA 90242; Home Care Associates, Ltd., 299 Chandler, Elmhurst, IL 60126

Emergency Treatment: *Child with Cardiopulmonary Arrest*

Assessment

1. Determine responsiveness or respiratory difficulty.
2. Call for help.
3. If alone with child: perform CPR for 1 min. before calling for help.
4. If second rescuer present: one rescuer continue CPR; second rescuer call emergency medical system (EMS), giving the following information:
   —Location of emergency
   —Telephone number from which call is being made
   —Circumstances of emergency
   —Condition of victim
   —Nature of aid being given
   —Any other information requested (caller should hang up last)

Resuscitation

1. Position victim on back on firm, flat surface, taking precautions if evidence of head and/or neck injury.
2. Check mouth and remove foreign material, e.g., vomitus or foreign body.
3. Open airway.
   No neck injury: tilt head gently back to "sniffing" or neutral position. Lift chin from airway.
   Suspected neck injury: lift jaw by placing two or three fingers at its angle and lifting upward.
4. Check for evidence of breathing.
   a. Look at chest for movement.
   b. Listen for exhaled air.
   c. Feel for exhaled air flow.
5. Breathe for victim.
   a. Take a breath.
   b. Open mouth wide and place over mouth and nose of child. For larger child place mouth over child's mouth and occlude nostrils with rescuer's cheek or pinch nares tightly with fingers.
   c. Force breaths into victim's mouth, using just enough air pressure to cause child's chest to rise.
   d. Give two slow breaths (1.0 to 1.5 seconds per breath), pausing to inhale between breaths.
6. Check pulse of a large central artery.
   Children—carotid artery
   Infants—brachial artery

Resuscitation—cont'd

7. Continue as follows:
   If pulse present: initiate rescue breathing and continue until spontaneous breathing resumes.
   Infant—every 3 seconds, or 20 times per minute.
   Child—every 4 seconds, or 15 times per minute.
   If pulse not present: initiate chest compressions and coordinate with breathing.

NOTE: If second rescuer present, breathing and compressions are shared.

Chest Compressions:

Infants:
1. Place index finger of hand farthest from infant's head just under imaginary line drawn between nipples.
2. Move index finger to a position one fingerbreadth below this intersection (compression area).
3. Using two or three fingers, compress sternum to depth of ½ to 1 inch (1.3 to 2.5 cm).
4. Release pressure without moving fingers from position.
5. Repeat at rate of at least 100 times per minute.

Children:
1. Using hand farthest from child's head, locate notch on child's chest where rib cage meets sternum.
2. With middle finger on notch, place index finger next to middle finger.
3. Place heel of other hand next to index finger with long axis of heel of hand parallel to sternum.
4. Compress chest with one hand to depth of 1 to 1½ inches (2.5 to 3.8 cm).
5. Compress at rate of 80 to 100 times per minute.

Coordinate compressions and breathing

1. Pause at end of every fifth compression to allow for a ventilation.
2. Maintain 5:1 ratio for one or two rescuers.
3. Reassess after 10 cycles of compression and ventilation and every few minutes thereafter.

NOTE: Adult standards are applied to children over 8 years of age.

---

bow and shoulder (Fig. 31-18, *F*). Absence of carotid or temporal pulse is considered sufficient indication to begin external cardiac massage.

Chest Compression

External chest compression consists of serial, rhythmic compressions of the chest to maintain circulation to vital organs until the child achieves spontaneous vital signs or ALS can be provided. Chest compressions are always accompanied by simultaneous ventilation of the lungs. For optimum compressions it is essential that the child's spine is supported during compression of the sternum, and sternal pressure must be forceful but not traumatic. In an infant the hard surface can be the palm of the hand not performing compressions. The child is positioned for optimum airway opening. Head tilt is provided by the weight of the head and

a slight uplift of the shoulders. It is best to prevent overextension of the head of small babies, since some authorities argue that this tends to close the flexible trachea.

The placement of the fingers for compression in infants is now determined to be lower than previously thought, that is, at a point on the lower rather than the middle sternum (Orlowski, 1984). The site is one fingerbreadth below the intersection of the sternum and an imaginary line drawn between the nipples (Fig. 31-18, *G*) (see Emergency treatment). Compressions on the child age 1 to 8 years of age are applied to the lower sternum two fingerbreadths above the sternal notch (Fig. 31-18, *H*) (see also Emergency treatment). Sternal compression to infants is applied with two or three fingers on the sternum exerting a sharp downward thrust; on children pressure is applied with the heel of one

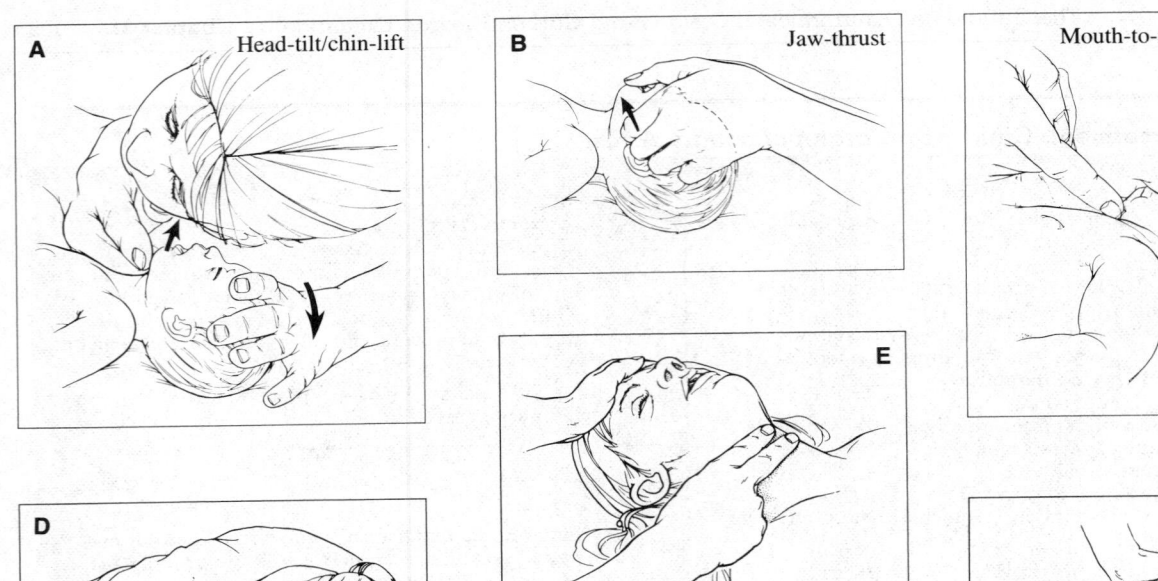

A Head-tilt/chin-lift

B Jaw-thrust

C Mouth-to-mouth and nose seal

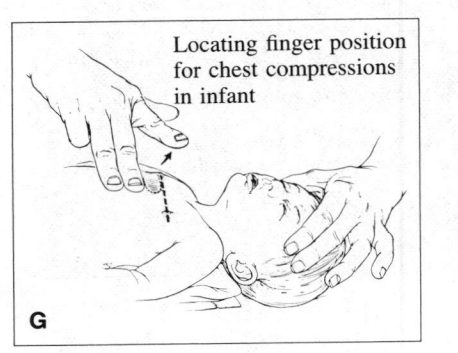

D Mouth-to-mouth seal

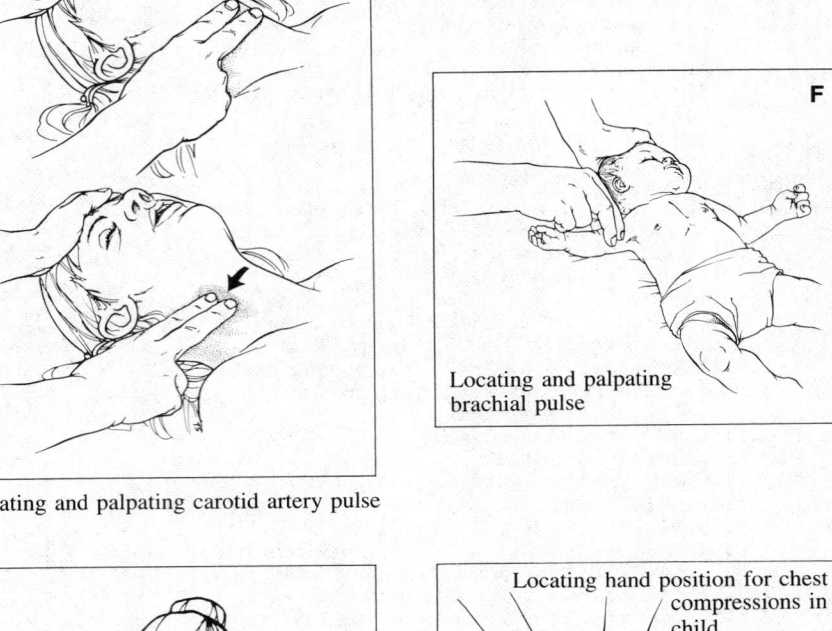

E

Locating and palpating carotid artery pulse

F

Locating and palpating brachial pulse

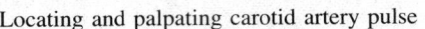

G Locating finger position for chest compressions in infant

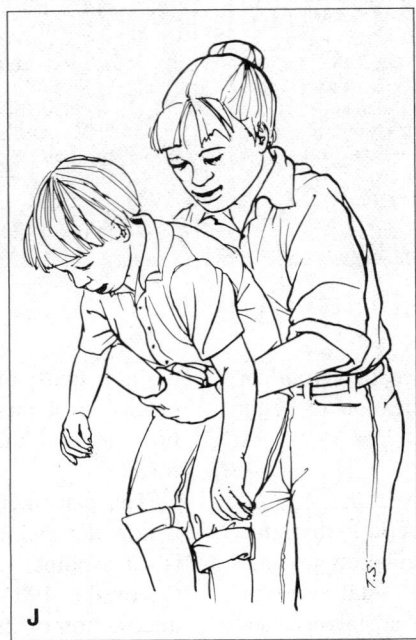

J Heimlich maneuver with child standing

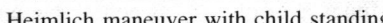

H Locating hand position for chest compressions in child

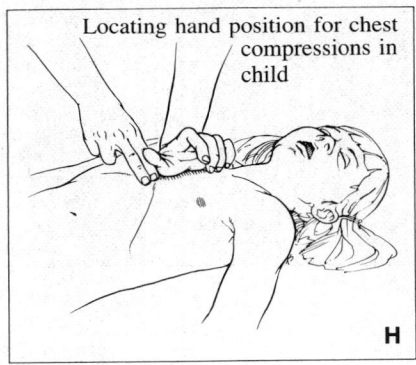

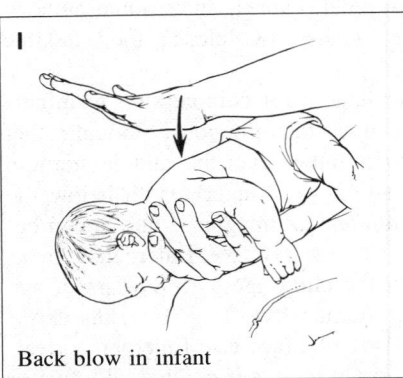

I Back blow in infant

K Heimlich maneuver with child lying

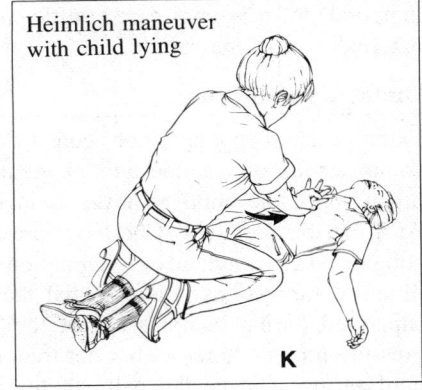

Fig. 31-18. Procedures for cardiopulmonary resuscitation *(A-H)* and airway obstruction *(I-J)*.
From Standards for Cardiopulmonary Resuscitation (CPR) and Emergency Cardiac Care
(ECC): Part IV. Pediatric basic life support, JAMA **225** (21):2954-2960, 1986.

hand. The depth of compression is also adapted to the size of the child (see Emergency treatment). The location, rate, and depth for children over 8 years are the same as for adults (Standards for CPR and ECC, 1986). There previously was concern regarding the possibility of rib fractures during CPR; this has been found to be a rare occurrence (Feldman and Brewer, 1984).

Ventilation and compression are continued by the mouth-to-mouth method or artificial ventilator, at a ratio of one breath for five compressions until there are signs of recovery, as evidenced by palpable peripheral pulses, return of pupils to normal size, and the disappearance of mottling and cyanosis.

AIRWAY OBSTRUCTION

Attempts at clearing the airway should be considered for (1) children in whom aspiration is witnessed or strongly suspected and (2) unconscious, nonbreathing children whose airways remain obstructed despite the usual maneuvers to open them (Standards, 1986). When a child is obviously choking, the initial step is to open his mouth and attempt to visualize and remove the object. *No blind finger sweeps should be used.* If this fails, the next step is to apply mechanical force in an attempt to dislodge the object.

There is strong controversy concerning the optimum method for relieving foreign-body obstruction in children. The methods currently offered are a combination of *back blows* and *chest thrusts* and the *Heimlich maneuver*. Because of the risk of injury to abdominal organs, abdominal thrusts should not be used for infants of 1 year of age or less.

Infants

A choking infant is placed face down over the rescuer's arm with his head lower than his trunk and his head supported (Fig. 31-18, *I*). Additional support can be achieved if the rescuer supports his arm firmly against his thigh (Committee on Accidents and Poison Prevention, 1986). Four quick, sharp, back blows are delivered between the infant's shoulder blades with the heel of the rescuer's hand. Less force is required than would be applied to an adult. After delivery of the back blows, the rescuer's free hand is placed flat on the infant's back so that the infant is "sandwiched" between the two hands, making certain the neck and chin are well supported. While the rescuer maintains support with the infant's head lower than the trunk, the infant is turned and placed supine on the rescuer's thigh, where four chest thrusts are applied in rapid succession in the same manner as external chest compressions described for CPR (see Emergency treatment).

Children

The Heimlich maneuver, a series of subdiaphragmatic abdominal thrusts, is recommended for children. The maneuver creates an artificial cough that forces air, and with it the

Emergency Treatment: Airway Obstruction

Infant
1. Check inside of infant's mouth for foreign object.
2. If foreign body observed, insert middle finger inside child's mouth on side farthest from rescuer, taking great care not to push object farther into throat.
3. Position child prone over forearm of rescuer with head down and infant's jaw firmly supported in rescuer's hand.
4. Rest supporting arm on thigh.
5. Deliver four back blows forcefully between infant's shoulder blades with heel of free hand.
6. Place free hand on infant's back so infant is sandwiched between both hands: one supporting neck, jaw, and chest, the other supporting back.
7. Turn infant and place supine head down, with head and neck supported, and apply four chest thrusts to same location as chest compressions but at a slower rate.

ALTERNATIVE POSITION: Place infant face down on rescuer's lap, head lower than trunk, and head firmly supported. Apply back blows, turn infant, and apply chest thrusts as above.

Child
Heimlich maneuver with victim standing or sitting
1. Stand behind victim.
2. Wrap arms around victim's waist with one hand made into fist.
3. Place fist on victim's abdomen in midline slightly above navel and well below tip of sternum with thumb side of fist resting against victim's abdomen.
4. Grasp fist with other hand and press into victim's abdomen with a quick upward thrust.
5. Repeat if needed. Each thrust should be a separate and distinct movement.

Heimlich maneuver with victim lying (conscious or unconscious)
1. Position child face up on back.
2. Kneel at child's feet (child on floor) or stand at child's feet (child on table).
3. Place heel of *one hand* on child's abdomen in midline slightly above navel and well below rib cage.
4. Place other hand on top of first hand and press into victim's abdomen with a quick upward thrust.
5. Repeat thrusts if needed (6 to 10 in rapid succession).

NOTE: The astride position is not recommended for children.

foreign body, out of the airway. The procedure is carried out with the child in a standing, sitting, or lying position (Figs. 31-18, *J* and Fig. 31-18, *K*). Upward thrusts are delivered to the upper abdomen with the fisted hand at a point just below the rib cage (see Emergency treatment). To prevent damage to the internal organs, the rescuer's hands should not touch the xiphoid process of the sternum or the lower margins of the ribs. Six to 10 thrusts are repeated in rapid succession until the foreign body is expelled.

It is neither necessary nor desirable to squeeze or compress the arms during the procedure. It is not a punch or a bear hug. The child may vomit after relief of the obstruction and should be positioned to prevent aspiration. After breathing is restored, the child should receive medical attention so he can be assessed for complications.

The success of the technique is primarily a result of the fact that obstruction takes place at the end of a maximum respiration. The victim is most likely to choke on food during inspiration; therefore the tidal volume plus expiratory reserve volume is present in the lungs. When pressure is exerted on the diaphragm by the maneuver, the food bolus is ejected with considerable force by this trapped air.

CONCEPT SUMMARIES

- The major functions of the respiratory tract are to distribute air and exchange gases in order to supply cells with oxygen and to remove carbon dioxide.

- Gas exchange depends on the amount and composition of air inhaled, the thickness of the alveolar wall, the adequacy of circulation to the alveoli, and substances within the alveoli that prevent their inflation or gas exchange.

- Artificial respiratory devices increase the pressure entering the air passages, lower the pressure around the body, or increase the negative pressure within the thoracic cavity.

- The amount of oxygen that diffuses into the blood depends on a pressure gradient between alveolar air and capillary blood, the total functional surface area of the alveolar-capillary membrane, the minute volume, and alveolar ventilation.

- Defense mechanisms of the respiratory tract include lymphoid tissues, viscid secretions, ciliary action, epiglottis, cough reflex, tracheobronchial dynamics, body position changes, lymphatics, and humoral defenses.

- Assessment of respiratory function involves a detailed physical examination, pulmonary function tests, radiography, and blood gas determination.

- Improvement of ventilatory functions may be accomplished with measures such as oxygen therapy, humidification, aerosol therapy, artificial ventilation, and intermittent positive pressure breathing.

- Oxygen is administered by mask, hood, nasal cannula, face tent, IPPB apparatus, or oxygen tent.

- Techniques for improving ventilatory capacity include postural drainage, chest physical therapy, and breathing exercises.

- The term *respiratory insufficiency* applies to two conditions: increased breathing efforts with near-normal gas exchange and carbon dioxide retention with hypoxemia and acidosis.

- Three types of functional respiratory disorders are obstructive lung disease, restrictive lung disease, and primary inefficient gas transfer.

- Management of respiratory failure is to provide oxygenation, maintain ventilation, apply appropriate therapy, and anticipate complications.

- Ventilators are classified by the way gas is generated: pressure cycled, volume cycled, and time cycled.

- Indications for tracheostomy in children include upper airway obstruction, CNS dysfunction, neuromuscular disease, secretional obstruction, and disturbances of gas diffusion or distribution.

- Two essential principles of cardiopulmonary resuscitation are to support the patient's spine and apply forceful but not traumatic sternal pressure.

- Airway clearance measures are reserved for children for whom aspiration is witnessed or strongly suspected and for unconscious, nonbreathing children whose airways are obstructed despite usual maneuvers to open them.

REFERENCES

Calvi, A.: Care of the child requiring long-term mechanical ventilation, Pediatr. Nurs. Update 1(6):1-8, 1985.

Chow, M.P., and others: Handbook of pediatric primary care, New York, 1979, John Wiley & Sons, Inc.

Committee on Accidents and Poison Prevention, American Academy of Pediatrics: Revised first aid for the choking child, Pediatrics 78:177-178, 1986.

Crowley, C.M., and Morrow, A.I.: A comprehensive approach to the child in respiratory failure, Crit. Care Q. 3(6):27-43, 1980.

Fanconi, S., and others: Pulse oximetry in pediatric intensive care: comparison with measured saturations and transcutaneous oxygen tension, J. Pediatr. 107:362-366, 1985.

Fedlman, K.W., and Brewer, D.K.: Child abuse, cardiopulmonary resuscitation and rib fractures, Pediatrics 73:339-342, 1984.

Inselman, L.S., and Mellins, R.B.: Growth and development of the lung, J. Pediatr. 98:1-15, 1981.

Morriss, F.C.: Postintubation sequelae. In Levin, D.L., Morriss, F.C., and Moore, G.C., editors: A practical guide to pediatric intensive care, ed. 2, St. Louis, 1984, The C.V. Mosby Co.

Muller, N.L., and Bryan, A.C.: Chest wall mechanics and respiratory muscles in infants, Pediatr. Clin. North Am. 26:503-516, 1979.

Orlowski, J.P.: Optimal position for external cardiac massage in infants and children, Crit. Care Med. 12:224-229, 1984.

Standards for Cardiopulmonary Resuscitation (CPR) and Emergency Cardiac Care (ECC): Part IV. Pediatric basic life support, JAMA 255(21):2954-2960, 1986.

Steele, N.F., and Harrison, B.: Technology-assisted children: assessing discharge preparation, J. Pediatr. Nurs. 1(3):150-158, 1986.

Torphy, D.E., Minter, M.G., and Thompson, B.M.: Cardiorespiratory arrest and resuscitation in children, Am. J. Dis. Child. 138:1099-1102, 1984.

Wade, J.F.: Respiratory nursing care: physiology and technique, ed. 3, St. Louis, 1982, The C.V. Mosby Co.

Waring, W.W.: Diagnostic and therapeutic procedures. In Kendig, E.L., and Chernick, V., editors: Disorders of the respiratory tract in children, ed. 4, Philadelphia, 1983, W.B. Saunders Co.

Yip, W.C.L., and others: Reliability of transcutaneous oxygen monitoring of critically ill children in a general pediatric unit, Clin. Pediatr. **22**:431-434, 1983.

BIBLIOGRAPHY
General

Eigen, H.: The clinical evaluation of chronic cough, Pediatr. Clin. North Am. **29**:67-78, 1982.

Gregory, G.A.: Respiratory care of the child, Crit. Care Med. **8**(10):582-587, 1980.

Kendig, E.L., and Chernick, V., editors: Disorders of the respiratory tract in children, ed. 4, Philadelphia, 1983, W.B. Saunders Co.

Mathew, O.P.: Maintenance of upper airway patency, J. Pediatr. **106**:863-869, 1985.

Neilsen, L.: Pulmonary oxygen toxicity and other hazards of oxygen therapy, Am. J. Nurs. **80**:2213-2215, 1980.

Pagtakhan, R.D., and Chernick, V.: Respiratory failure in the pediatric patient, Pediatr. Rev. **3**(8):247-256, 1982.

Signor, G., and Del Bueno, D.J.: A sinfully easy way to interpret ABGs, RN **45**(9):45-49, 1982.

Standards for Cardiopulmonary Resuscitation (CPR) and Emergency Cardiac Care (ECC): Part V. Pediatric advanced life support, JAMA **255**(21):2961-2968, 1986.

Diagnostic Procedures

Cameron, T.J.: Fiberoptic bronchoscopy, Am. J. Nurs. **81**:1462-1464, 1981.

Cardin, S.: Acid-base balance in the patient with respiratory disease, Nurs. Clin. North Am. **15**:593-601, 1980.

D'Agostino, J.S.: Set your mind at ease on oxygen toxicity, Nursing 83 **13**(7):55-56, 1983.

Gammon, S.S.: Respiratory acidosis, Nursing 82 **12**(8):65, 1982.

Nielsen, L.: Interpreting arterial blood gases, Am. J. Nurs. **80**:2197-2201, 1980.

Rokosky, J.S.: Assessment of the individual with altered respiratory function, Nurs. Clin. North Am. **16**:195-209, 1981.

Wimsatt, R.: Unlocking the mysteries behind the chest wall, Nursing 85 **15**(11):58-64, 1985.

Therapeutic Procedures

Alderson, S.H., and Warren, R.H.: Pediatric aerosol therapy guidelines, Clin. Pediatr. **23**:553-557, 1984.

Colombo, J.L., Hopkins, R.L., and Waring, W.W.: Steam vaporizer injuries, Pediatrics **67**:661-663, 1981.

Finer, N.N.: Newer trends in continuous monitoring of critically ill infants and children, Pediatr. Clin. North Am. **27**:553-566, 1980.

McFadden, R.: Decreasing respiratory compromise during infant suctioning, Am. J. Nurs. **81**:2158-2161, 1981.

Weaver, T.E.: New life for lungs through incentive spirometers, Nursing 81 **11**(2):54-58, 1981.

Artificial Ventilation

Belitz, J.: Minimizing the psychological complications of patients who require mechanical ventilation, Crit. Care Nurse **3**(3):42-46, 1983.

Craven, D.E., and others: Contamination of mechanical ventilators with tubing changes every 24 or 48 hours, N. Engl. J. Med. **306**:1505-1509, 1982.

Hess, D.: Bedside monitoring of the patient on a ventilator, Crit. Care Q. **6**(2):23-31, 1983.

Janowsky, M.J.: Accidental disconnections from breathing systems, Am. J. Nurs. **84**:241-244, 1984.

Jonson, B., and others: Continuous positive airway pressure: modes of action in relation to clinical applications, Pediatr. Clin. North Am. **27**:687-699, 1980.

Landis, K., and Smith, S.: The mechanically ventilated patient: a comprehensive nursing care plan, Crit. Care Q. **6**(2):43-52, 1983.

Vincent, J.E.: Medical problems in the patient on a ventilator, Crit. Care Q. **6**(2):33-41, 1983.

Endotracheal Airways

Browning, D.H., and Graves, S.A.: Incidence of aspiration with endotracheal tubes in children, J. Pediatr. **102**:582-584, 1983.

Corbo, B.H.: Endotracheal intubation: adolescent ICU experiences, Crit. Care Q. **8**(1):35-46, 1985.

Finer, N.N., and others: Limitations of self-inflating resuscitators, Pediatrics **77**:417-420, 1986.

Fuchs, P.L.: Streamlining your suctioning techniques, Part I. Nasotracheal suctioning, Nursing 84 **14**(5):55-61, 1984.

Fuchs, P.L.: Streamlining your suctioning techniques, Part II. Endotracheal suctioning, Nursing 84 **14**(6):46-51, 1984.

Nieves, J.: Avoiding spontaneous extubation of nasotracheal or oral tracheal tubes, Pediatr. Nurs. **12**:215-218, 1986.

Riegel, B., and Forshee, T.: A review and critique of the literature on preoxygenation for endotracheal suctioning, Heart Lung **14**:507-518, 1985.

Scott, P.H., and others: Predictability and consequences of spontaneous extubation in a pediatric ICU, Crit. Care Med. **13**:228-232, 1985.

Smith, A.E.: Endotracheal suctioning: "Are we harming our patients?," Crit. Care Update **10**(1):29-31, 1983.

Spitzer, A., and Fox, W.W.: Post extubation atelectasis: the role of oral versus nasal endotracheal tubes, J. Pediatr. **100**:806-809, 1982.

Tracheostomy

Benchot, R.J.: Tracheostomy care in infants and young children, Point View **18**(4):8-9, 1981.

Feaster, S.C., West, C., and Ferketich, S.: Hyperinflation, hyperventilation, and hyperoxygenation before tracheal suctioning in children requiring long-term respiratory care, Heart Lung **14**:379-384, 1985.

Fuchs, P.L.: Providing tracheostomy care, Nursing 83 **13**(4):139-143, 1983.

Geron, G.R., and Tucker, G.F.: Infant tracheostomy, Ann. Otol. Rhinol. Laryngol. **91**:413-416, 1982.

Harris, R., and Hyman, R.: Clean vs. sterile tracheostomy care and level of pulmonary infection, Nurs. Res. **33**:80-85, 1984.

Oermann, M.H., and others: Patient sensations following a tracheostomy: a discussion, Crit. Care Q. **6**(2):53-58, 1983.

Wetmore, R., Handler, S., and Potsic, W.: Pediatric tracheostomy experience during the past decade, Ann. Otol. Rhinol. Laryngol. **91**:628-632, 1982.

Home Care

Antibiotic therapy at home, Am. J. Nurs. **84**:348-350, 1984.

Aradine, C.E.: Home care for young children with long-term tracheostomies, Am. J. Maternal Child Nurs. **5**:121-125, 1980.

Aradine, C.: Young children with long-term tracheostomies: health and development, West. J. Nurs. Res. **5**:115-124, 1983.

Bendell, D., and others: Behavioral treatment of CPR anxiety: a case study, Child. Health Care **13**:77-81, 1984.

Burr, H.B., and others: Home care for children on respirators, N. Engl. J. Med. **309**:1319-1323, 1983.

Cagan, J., and Meier, P.: Evaluation of a discharge planning tool for use with families of high-risk infants, JOGN Nurs. **12**:275-281, 1983.

Czarniecki, L.: Caring for a young child with a tracheostomy, Caring **4**(5):30-32, 1985.

Fanconi, S.: Outcome of home mechanical ventilation (letter), J. Pediatr. **108**:791, 1986.

Foster, S., and Hoskins, D.: Home care of the child with a tracheotomy tube, Pediatr. Clin. North Am. **28**:855-857, 1981.

Frates, R.C., and others: Outcome of home mechanical ventilation in children, J. Pediatr. **106**:850-856, 1985.

Giovannoni, R.: Chronic ventilator care: from hospital to home, Rx Home Care **7**(1):51-52, 54, 56-57, 1985.

Goldberg, A.I., and others: Home care for life-supported persons: an approach to program development, J. Pediatr. **104**:785-795, 1984.

Groeneveld, M.: Sending infants home on low-flow oxygen, JOGN Nurs. **15**:237-241, 1986.

Hazinski, M.F.: Pediatric home tracheostomy care: a parent's guide, Pediatr. Nurs. **12**:41-48, 69, 1986.

Home care today, Am. J. Nurs. **84**:340-342, 1984.

Kahn, L.: Ventilator dependent children heading home, Hospitals **58**(5):54-55, 1984.

Kennedy, A.H., Johnson, W.G., and Sturdevant, E.W.: An educational program for families of children with tracheostomies, Am. J. Maternal Child Nurs. **7**:42-49, 1982.

Kopacz, M.A., and Moriarty-Wright, R.: Multidisciplinary approach for the patient on a home ventilator, Heart Lung **13**:255-262, 1984.

Kruger, S., and Rawlins, P.: Pediatric dismissal protocol to aid the transition from hospital to home care, Image **16**:120-125, 1984.

Make, B., and others: Rehabilitation of ventilator-dependent subjects with lung diseases, Chest **86**:358-365, 1984.

McCrory, L.: Pediatric home tracheostomy care alternatives (letter), Pediatr. Nurs. **12**:223, 1986.

Mizuki, J.A.: There's no place like home, Am. J. Nurs. **84**:646-648, 1984.

Nelson, D.: Nurse managed rehabilitation, Nurs. Management **15**(3):30-39, 1984.

Rathlev, M.C., and McNamara, M.A.: Teaching families to give trach care at home, Nursing 82 **12**(6):70-71, 1982.

Rehm, R.S.: Teaching cardiopulmonary resuscitation to parents, Am. J. Maternal Child Nurs. **8**:411-414, 1983.

Special teams in home care, Am. J. Nurs. **84**:342-345, 1984.

Splaingard, M.L., and others: Home positive pressure ventilation—twenty years experience, Chest **84**:376-382, 1983.

Talabere, L.: The child with a tracheostomy: a holistic approach to home care, Topics Clin. Nurs. **2**:27-44, 1980.

Wasserman, A.L.: A prospective study of the impact of home monitoring on the family, Pediatrics **74**:323-329, 1984.

Wills, J.: Concerns and needs of mothers providing home care for children with tracheostomies, Maternal Child Nurs. J. **12**:89-107, 1983.

Cardiopulmonary Resuscitation

Brill, J.E.: Cardiopulmonary resuscitation, Pediatr. Ann. **15**:24-29, 1986.

Kulberg, A.: CPR in the very young, Emerg. Med. **13**:154-176, 1981.

Longo, A.: Teaching parents CPR, Pediatr. Nurs. **9**:445-447, 1983.

Phillips, G.W.L., and Zideman, D.A.: Relation of infant heart to sternum: its significance in cardiopulmonary resuscitation, Lancet **1**:1024-1025, 1986.

Rehm, R.S.: Teaching cardiopulmonary resuscitation to parents, J. Maternal Child Nurs. **8**:411-414, 1983.

Rogers, M.C.: New developments in cardiopulmonary resuscitation, Pediatrics **71**:655-658, 1983.

Scientific Board, California Medical Association: Transmission of disease via mouth-to-mouth resuscitation, West. J. Med. **143**:468, 1985.

Airway Obstruction

Day, R.L.: Differing opinions on the emergency treatment of choking, Pediatrics **71**:976-977, 1983.

Day, R.L., and Dubois, A.B.: Treatment of choking, Pediatrics **71**:300-306, 1983.

Eigen, H.: Treatment of choking (letter), Pediatrics **71**:300-301, 1983.

Hoffman, J.R.: Treatment of the choking child (letter), Pediatrics **71**:468-469, 1983.

Mofenson, H.C., and Greensher, J.: Management of the choking child, Pediatr. Clin. North Am. **32**:183-192, 1985.

Montgomery, W.H.: Back blows and choking (letter), Pediatrics **71**:982-983, 1983.

Thompson, S.W.: How to use the Heimlich maneuver on choking infants and children, Pediatr. Nurs. **9**:13-16, 1983.

Torrey, S.B.: The choking child—a life-threatening emergency: evaluation of current recommendations, Clin. Pediatr. **22**:751-754, 1983.

Chapter 32

The Child with Respiratory Dysfunction

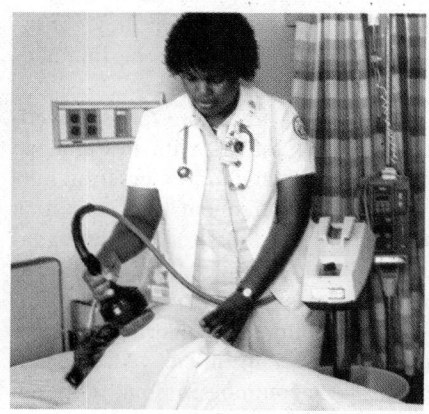

Some of the most common problems in the pediatric age-group are related to disturbed respiratory function, and respiratory failure is the chief cause of morbidity in the newborn period. Respiratory illness can be caused by disease, trauma, or physical anomalies or can be seen as a manifestation of a disturbance in another organ or system, such as neurologic disorders involving the respiratory center or innervation to the respiratory musculature. Most communicable diseases have respiratory symptoms.

The type and pattern of respiratory disturbances also vary tremendously according to the age of the child. There are differences in susceptibility to infections and in response to various organisms and conditions at various ages. Moreover, manifestations of illness vary according to the age of the child and may involve different organ systems. For example, diarrhea is often the manifestation of a viral infection in infancy that produces a pharyngoconjunctivitis in the older child. This chapter is primarily concerned with infectious, allergic, and mechanical disturbances.

Respiratory Infection

Acute infection of the respiratory tract is the most common cause of illness in infancy and childhood. Young children ordinarily have four or five such infections each year that manifest a wide range of severity from trivial to severe or even fatal illness. The type of illness and the physical response are also related to a variety of factors, including the type of infectious agent, the age of the child, and the integrity of the child's defense mechanisms. Despite the effectiveness of the natural defense mechanisms in the respiratory tract, circumstances alter their ability to repel invading organisms.

GENERAL ASPECTS OF RESPIRATORY INFECTIONS

Infections of the respiratory tract are described in a number of different ways according to the general areas of involvement in the more common infections. The upper respiratory tract, or upper airway, consists primarily of the nose and pharynx. The lower respiratory tract consists of the bronchi and bronchioles, which constitute the reactive portion of the airway because of their smooth muscle content and ability to constrict, and the primary respiratory unit, the lungs. It is the structurally stable or nonreactive portion of the airway, including the epiglottis, larynx, and trachea, that is a point of disagreement among authorities. Some consider these structures to be part of the lower respiratory tract while others categorize them as upper tract structures. For the purpose of this discussion the trachea is considered with lower tract disorders, and infections of the epiglottis and larynx are categorized as croup syndromes.

Etiology and Characteristics

The etiology and course of respiratory tract infections are influenced by a number of factors. They are seldom localized to a single anatomic structure or area but tend to spread to a variable extent as a result of the continuous nature of the mucous membrane lining the respiratory tract. Consequently infections of the respiratory tract generally involve several areas rather than a single structure, although the effect on one may predominate in any given illness.

Numerous factors, including the nature of the agent, the age of the child, and the resistance offered by natural defenses, influence the incidence and severity of respiratory infections.

Infectious agents. The respiratory tract is subject to a wide variety of infective organisms, but the largest percentage of infections are caused by viruses, particularly in the upper respiratory passages. The organism *Chlamydia trachomatis* is considered in the diagnosis more often in afebrile pneumonitis with onset in the first months of life. Other organisms that may be involved in primary or secondary invasion are group A β-hemolytic streptococci, *Staphyloccus aureus, Haemophilus influenzae,* and pneumococci. Of special significance is the β-hemolytic Streptococcus because of the relationship between respiratory infection with this organism and the incidence of subsequent nephritis or rheumatic fever. *C. trachomatis* respiratory infection may be acquired by the newborn during descent through the birth canal.

Size and frequency of dose. The larger the dose of an infectious agent, the greater the likelihood of a significant infection. Pathogenic bacteria are natural inhabitants of the oropharynx, as evidenced by positive throat cultures from healthy persons. These organisms increase in number when the local defenses are lowered by damage to the mucous membranes from viral infections or when they are affected by concurrent respiratory, debilitating, or immunologic disorders.

Age. The pattern of respiratory infection varies considerably with the age of the child. Infants with few outside contacts acquire fewer infections than children entering nursery school or grade school with frequent exposure to a wider circle of contacts. The susceptibility to specific organisms varies with age as well; for example, there is a lower incidence of infection in infants exposed to group A beta-hemolytic streptococci than in children in older age-groups. The incidence of influenza is lower in infants. Also, pneumococcal lobar pneumonia is uncommon in small children and pneumonia caused by *Mycoplasma* infection is uncommon during the first 3 to 4 years of life.

In infants beyond the newborn period lack of specific antibodies against common viral pathogens causes an increased incidence of respiratory tract infections. This incidence peaks at 1 year of age. Some of the viral agents produce a mild illness in older children but cause severe lower respiratory tract illness and croup in infants. The amount of lymphoid tissue increases throughout middle childhood, and repeated exposure to organisms confers increasing immunity as the child grows older; thus older children have a greater resistance to most organisms. Whooping cough is a relatively harmless tracheobronchitis in childhood but a serious disease in infancy.

Risk of aspiration is increased during the first year, partially related to the feeding and postfeeding positions. During feeding the infant is in a recumbent position that facilitates entry of fluids into the airway that can cause upper lobe changes. In children beyond infancy most aspiration occurs when they are in the upright position.

Size. In the young child the diameter of the respiratory tract is smaller than in older children and is therefore subject to considerable narrowing from edematous mucous membranes and increased production of secretions. In addition, the distance between structures within the tract is shorter anatomically in the young child; therefore organisms move more rapidly down the respiratory tract for more extensive involvement. Also, the relatively short and open eustachian tube in infants and young children allows pathogens easy access to the middle ear.

Resistance. The ability to resist invading organisms depends on several factors. Deficiencies of the immune system place the child at risk for any infectious process. The general conditions that appear to decrease resistance to infection are malnutrition, anemia, fatigue, and chilling of the body. Conditions affecting the respiratory tract that weaken its defenses and predispose to infection include allergies such as allergic rhinitis and asthma, cardiac anomalies that have the tendency to pulmonary congestion, and cystic fibrosis of the pancreas.

Seasonal variations. The most common respiratory tract pathogens appear in epidemics during the winter and spring months, but *Mycoplasma* infections occur more often in autumn and early winter. To differentiate from asthma symptoms, asthma pollen-related symptoms appear more often in spring, summer, and early fall, whereas symptoms caused by house dust and molds are more likely to occur when children are confined to the house during cold winter months. Infection-related asthma (e.g., asthmatic bronchitis) occurs more frequently during cold weather.

Clinical Manifestations

Infants and young children react more severely to acute respiratory tract infection than older children, and they appear to be much more ill than their local manifestations would indicate. This is especially true for children between 6 months and 3 years of age. Young children display a number of generalized signs and symptoms as well as local manifestations that differ from those seen in older children and adults. An infant or child may display any or all of the following signs and symptoms.

Fever. A characteristic of illness in newborn infants is the presence of sepsis without an elevation of temperature. Even severe infections in newborns can occur without fever. The temperature may even be subnormal. However, the infant tends to develop fever more readily with advancing age. This capacity is greatest at ages 6 months to 3 years. Even with mild infections the temperature may reach 39.5° to 40.5° C (103° to 105° F). Children may have a fever before any other sign of infection is evident; therefore any child with a fever should be observed for development of symptoms.

Although an elevated temperature usually makes children listless and irritable, they may become somewhat euphoric and more active than normal, temporarily. Some children talk with unaccustomed rapidity when they have a fever, and parents learn to recognize this as a sign of illness. The tendency to develop high temperatures with infection seems to occur in certain families.

Febrile convulsions. In some small children a sudden temperature rise to 40° C (104° F) or higher will precipitate febrile convulsions of a tonic-clonic character (see p. 1670). A more gradual temperature rise will not elicit a seizure.

Approximately one third of these children have a family history of febrile convulsions that appear to be unrelated to epilepsy in most cases. Febrile convulsions are uncommon after 3 or 4 years of age.

Meningismus. Meningeal signs without infection of the meninges may be present in small children who have an abrupt onset of fever. The signs of fever, which may include headache, pain and stiffness in the back and neck, and presence of Kernig and Brudzinski signs, subside as the temperature drops. Cerebrospinal fluid is normal but its pressure may be slightly elevated.

Anorexia. Loss of appetite is a symptom common to most childhood illnesses, and it almost invariably accompanies acute infections in small children. It is frequently the initial evidence of illness, preceding fever and other overt signs of infection. When a child who usually has a good appetite develops a distaste for food, he should be observed for impending infection. The loss of appetite persists to a greater or lesser degree throughout the febrile stage of illness and often into convalescence. Return of appetite is a well-recognized sign that the peak of illness has passed.

Vomiting. Small children vomit readily with illness, and vomiting occurs so frequently at the onset of infection that its appearance for no obvious reason is a clue to the advent of infection. It often precedes other signs, such as fever, by several hours. Although usually short lived, vomiting may persist during the illness to become the dominant feature, with the associated risk of dehydration and electrolyte imbalance.

Diarrhea. Mild transient diarrhea often accompanies respiratory infections in small children, particularly viral infections. However, the diarrhea may be severe, creating a greater problem than the respiratory aspects of the illness.

Abdominal pain. Abdominal pain, sometimes indistinguishable from the pain of appendicitis, is a common complaint in small children with acute respiratory infections. Mesenteric lymphadenitis that accompanies throat infection may be a cause of acute symptoms. Muscle spasms from vomiting may be a factor or a manifestation in a nervous, tense child.

Nasal blockage. The small nasal passages of the infant are easily blocked by mucosal swelling and exudation. Infants have difficulty breathing through their mouth; therefore this occlusion can interfere with respiration and feeding. The infant becomes restless, feeding is difficult, and fluid intake is compromised. It also contributes to the development of complications such as otitis media and sinusitis.

Nasal discharge. A nasal discharge frequently accompanies respiratory infections. The discharge may be thin and watery (rhinorrhea) or thick and purulent, depending on the type and/or stage of the infection. The child often rubs his nose in an attempt to relieve the associated itching, and the discharge may irritate the upper lip and the skin surrounding the nose.

Cough. A cough is a common feature of respiratory disease. It is one method by which the respiratory tract is cleared of secretions. The cough may be evident only during the acute phase of an illness or persist several months following a disease such as viral bronchiolitis. A cough may be an ever-present reminder of a chronic lung disease, such as cystic fibrosis, chronic atelectasis, or bronchiectasis.

Respiratory sounds. Many sounds are associated with respiratory disease. Cough, hoarseness, stridor, and wheezing are readily audible, and auscultation reveals such chest sounds as rhonchi, rales, hyperresonance, and absence of sound. (For a detailed description of breath sounds and their assessment see p. 263.)

Presence or absence of sore throat. Young children who are able to describe symptoms often do not complain of sore throat, even when the throat is highly inflamed. It may be that the elastic nature of the tissues in young children causes less pressure on sensitive nerve endings. However, older children frequently complain of sore throat.

Complications. There is a higher incidence of complications with acute respiratory infection in young children, probably because of decreased resistance to infection and because of local circumstances such as a greater degree of nasal and paranasal blockage, large adenoid tissue, and shorter distance between structures (shorter and straighter eustachian tube). Complications that are common include otitis media, cervical adenitis, retropharyngeal abscess, and downward extension of infection to lower respiratory structures. Septicemia and meningitis also occur more frequently after respiratory infections in children.

Therapeutic Management

Effective antimicrobial therapy is available for the eradication of most microorganisms (except viruses) responsible for upper respiratory infections in children. The penicillins are the drugs of choice for bacterial pneumonia because of maximum bacterial activity plus absence of toxicity (sensitization is a problem in some children). They come in forms that can be given orally or parenterally and are prescribed according to their pattern of absorption. At present there are no specific therapies for viral infections or their symptoms.

Other management consists of providing symptomatic relief of symptoms and preventing dehydration and other complications (see Nursing considerations). Medical management for specific infections is considered in relation to those disorders.

Nursing Considerations

Since the majority of children with upper respiratory tract infections are treated at home, most of the nursing care is directed toward education and guidance of parents in caring for their child and serving as resources for problem solving. If the physician has given the parents written instructions, these can be explained and reinforced as appropriate. If written instructions have not been furnished, the nurse should provide the parents with written guidelines and, in some cases, outlines of procedures to be carried out.

Rest. Any child who has an acute febrile illness should be placed on bed rest. This is usually not difficult while the temperature is elevated but may be difficult when the child feels fairly well, particularly in young children. When parents take the advice seriously and consistently keep the child in bed, most children learn to cooperate during illness. Often the child is more apt to comply if he is allowed to lie quietly on the couch where he can watch television or participate in an alternate quiet activity. If he is unreasoning and expends an inordinate amount of energy in protest, playing quietly on the floor serves the purpose of rest better than crying excessively in bed. A number of entertainment devices can be employed to keep the child quiet, based on the child's individual interests.

Every endeavor should be made to remove the child from contact with other children. Ideally the ill child should be isolated in a separate bedroom at the first sign of illness. This is seldom a problem with an only child but is often difficult when living arrangements are crowded and there are several children in the family. If the child has no bedroom of his own, sometimes another child can sleep on a couch or cot or with relatives or friends. Well children can be taught to stay away from the ill child if the living conditions allow for segregation and the rule is rigidly enforced.

Nutrition. Loss of appetite is characteristic of acute infections in children, and in most cases the child can be permitted to determine his own need for food. Many children show no decrease in appetite, and others respond well to certain foods such as gelatin, soup, and puddings (see also Feeding the sick child, p. 1115). Since the illness is relatively short, the nutritional state is seldom compromised. In fact, urging foods on the anorexic child may precipitate nausea and vomiting and in some cases even cause an aversion to the feeding situation that can extend into the convalescent period and beyond. Sometimes reducing the milk intake of formula-fed infants is helpful during the initial phase of an acute respiratory infection.

Dehydration is always a hazard when children are febrile or anorexic, especially when vomiting or diarrhea is also present. An adequate fluid intake should be encouraged by offering small amounts of favored fluids at frequent intervals. High-calorie liquids such as colas, fruit juices, water flavored and sweetened with corn syrup, or similar drinks help prevent catabolism and dehydration. Fluids should not be forced, and the child should not be wakened from his rest to take fluids. Forcing fluids may create the same difficulties as urging unwanted food. Gentle persuasion with preferred beverages will usually meet with success. The parent should be advised to observe the frequency of voiding and notify the nurse or physician if the child does not seem to be voiding sufficiently.

Control of fever. If the child has a significantly elevated temperature, controlling the fever becomes a major nursing task. The parent should know how to take the child's temperature and read the thermometer accurately. Most parents are able to do this, but nurses cannot make this assumption. Those who cannot will require instruction in use of the thermometer.

If the physician has prescribed aspirin or acetaminophen for the child, the parents may need help in administering the drug. Most parents can read the label and calculate the desired dosage, but some have difficulty and will require careful instruction or precise direction. It is important to emphasize accuracy in both the amount of drug given and the time intervals at which the drug is administered in order to avoid accumulation effects. Cool liquids are encouraged to help reduce the temperature and to minimize the chances of dehydration. (See p. 1116 for management of fever and administration of antipyretic drugs.)

Local measures. Older children are usually able to manage nasal secretions with little difficulty. They should be taught to use a tissue when they cough or sneeze and to dispose of the tissues properly. The parents are instructed concerning the correct administration of nose drops and throat irrigations, if ordered. For very young infants, who normally breathe through their noses, an infant nasal aspirator or a rubber ear syringe is helpful in removing nasal secretions before feeding. This, followed by instillation of saline nose drops, may be all that is necessary to clear nasal passages and promote feeding. Saline nose drops can be prepared at home by dissolving 1 teaspoon of salt in 1 pint of warm water.

For older infants and children who can better tolerate decongestants, vasoconstrictive nose drops may be administered 15 to 20 minutes before feeding and at bedtime. Two drops are instilled, and since this shrinks only the anterior mucous membranes, 2 more drops are instilled 5 to 10 minutes later. Phenylephrine (Neo-Synephrine) 0.25% is the usual choice of decongestant nose drops, although others such as ephedrine 1% may be prescribed. Older cooperative children often prefer nasal sprays. They are taught to compress the plastic container at the moment of inspiration to gain relief. Spray bottles and bottles of nose drops should be used for one child only and only for one illness, since they become easily contaminated with bacteria.

Hot or cold applications sometimes provide relief to older children with painful cervical adenitis. An ice bag or heating pad applied to the neck may decrease the discomfort, but safety precautions must be observed in order to prevent burns. The ice bag or heating device must be covered, and the heating pad should not be set at the high ranges.

Warm or cool mist has been a common therapeutic measure for symptomatic relief of respiratory discomfort. The moisture soothes inflamed membranes and seems to be especially beneficial when there is hoarseness or any laryngeal involvement. Mist tents and hoods are frequently employed in the hospital for liquefying secretions and relieving discomfort. However, moisturizing air by use of vaporizors in the home is not advised and should be discouraged because of the hazards related to their use and the little evidence to support their efficacy (Colombo, Hopkins, and Waring, 1981). Alternate suggestions are available, such as humidification systems. Shallow pans with wide surface areas for evaporation increase humidity but should be placed where they do not pose a safety hazard. A large, wet beach towel hung with one end in shallow water in the bathtub will increase humidity if the bathroom door remains open.

A time-honored method of producing steam is the shower. Running the shower of hot water into the empty bathtub or open shower stall with the bathroom door closed produces a quick source of steam. Keeping a child in this environment for 10 to 15 minutes offers the same advantages as the croup tent without the fear and restraint often associated with the confines of a tent. A small child can be held on the lap of a parent or other adult. Older children can sit in the bathroom under the supervision of an adult.

Medication. In addition to antipyretics and nose drops, the child may require antibiotic therapy. It is usually the nurse who instructs the parents regarding continuing medication begun in the hospital or initiating medications at home, especially antibiotics. Parents of children who are sent home with oral antibiotics need to understand the importance of regular administration and to continue the drug for the prescribed length of time, regardless of whether the child appears to be ill or not.

Parents are also cautioned against giving the child any medications that are not prescribed. Adverse effects have been noted in children who have received some preparation intended for adults, for example, some long-acting nose drops (Neo-Synephrine II) and dextromethorphan cough squares (mistaken for candy). They are also cautioned regarding giving the child unprescribed antibiotics left over from a previous illness. Self-medication with unprescribed antibiotics is a significant problem (Cunningham and others, 1983). It should be emphasized that some drugs interact with others to produce serious side effects, and such a likelihood is increased when medications are administered to a child without consultation with the physician. The nurse is in an excellent position to provide drug information to families. It has been found that when patients have questions concerning medications they are more likely to ask a nurse than a physician (Morris and others, 1984). (See Chapter 27 for administration of medications and teaching parents.)

Nursing Care Summary: The Child with Acute Respiratory Infection

NURSING GOALS	NURSING INTERVENTIONS	EXPECTED PATIENT/FAMILY OUTCOMES

HP-HMP Infection, potential for
Risk factors: presence of infective organisms

NURSING GOALS	NURSING INTERVENTIONS	EXPECTED PATIENT/FAMILY OUTCOMES

Prevent spread of infection	Isolate child from other family members as much as possible
	   Provide separate bedroom if possible
	   Avoid close contact between well persons and ill child
	   Discourage parents and others from lying down with ill child
	Keep others from using child's eating and drinking utensils
	Use separate washcloth and towel for ill child
	Teach child proper behavior when coughing or sneezing and proper disposal of tissues
	Teach all family members good handwashing technique and encourage frequent use
		Others remain free from infection

HP-HMP Injury, potential for (airway obstruction)
Risk factors: inflammatory process (croup, epiglottitis)

NURSING GOALS	NURSING INTERVENTIONS	EXPECTED PATIENT/FAMILY OUTCOMES

Assess respiratory status and detect impending airway obstruction	Monitor respirations for rate, depth, pattern, presence of retractions, and flaring nares
	Auscultate lungs
	   Evaluation of breath sounds
	   Detection of presence of rales or rhonchi
	Observe color of skin and mucous membranes for pallor and cyanosis
	Observe for presence of hoarseness, stridor, and cough
	Monitor heart rate and regularity
	Observe behavior
	   Restlessness
	   Irritability
	   Apprehension
	Report and record significant observations
		*Deviations from normal (for the specific child) are detected early (see inside front cover for normal variations)
		
		*Any deviations from normal (for the individual child) are detected (specify parameters)

Prevent respiratory arrest	Avoid throat examination (epiglottitis) Have emergency equipment available	

N-MP Body temperature, alteration in: potential
Risk factors: inflammatory process

NURSING GOALS	NURSING INTERVENTIONS	EXPECTED PATIENT/FAMILY OUTCOMES
Control fever	Implement measures to decrease temperature Provide cool environment Monitor temperature to detect status of temperature Place in lightweight clothing and bed linen Encourage cool liquids	Body temperature remains within the acceptable limits—between 37.8° – 38.0°C (100° = 100.4°F)

N-MP Swallowing, impaired
Etiology: edema of nasopharynx and pharynx, discomfort

NURSING GOALS	NURSING INTERVENTIONS	EXPECTED PATIENT/FAMILY OUTCOMES
Facilitate swallowing	Offer cool fluids	Child swallows fluids

N-MP Fluid volume deficit, potential
Risk factors: difficulty swallowing due to inflammatory process, increased metabolic rate, insensible fluid losses

NURSING GOALS	NURSING INTERVENTIONS	EXPECTED PATIENT/FAMILY OUTCOMES
Prevent dehydration	Observe for signs of dehydration Monitor intake, output, urine specific gravity, and daily weight Encourage fluids when tolerated	Child remains well hydrated and exhibits no evidence of dehydration Child drinks adequate amounts of fluid (specify)

*Nursing outcome.

NURSING GOALS	NURSING INTERVENTIONS	EXPECTED PATIENT/FAMILY OUTCOMES

N-MP   Nutrition, alteration in: less than body requirements
Etiology: difficulty swallowing, loss of appetite

| Provide nutrition | Encourage high-calorie fluids when tolerated, then progress to diet as tolerated | Child ingests adequate amounts of nourishment (specify amounts) |

A-EP   Breathing pattern, ineffective
Etiology: infective process

Monitor respiratory status	Observe respiratory rate and pattern
	Auscultate to determine type and location
	    Breath sounds
	    Presence of rales, rhonchi, wheezing
	    Areas of consolidation
	    Effectiveness of chest therapy
	Assess skin color, presence or absence of retractions, nasal flaring
		*Deviations from normal (for the individual child) are detected early (see inside front cover for normal variations)
		Color remains pink; no visible retractions

Detect complications early	Carry out periodic assessment of respiratory status
	Change position every 2 hours
	Observe for signs of
	    Chest pain
	    Abdominal pain
	    Dyspnea
	    Pallor or cyanosis
		Respirations unlabored
		Child exhibits no evidence of discomfort
		Color remains pink

Prevent aspiration of secretions	Administer nothing by mouth during acute stage of dyspnea Position to promote drainage of secretions from airway Prevent aspiration of secretions	Airways remain clear
Maintain patent airway Ease respiratory efforts	Suction secretions as needed Promote rest Maintain patent airway Provide high-humidity atmosphere Position for comfort and maximum lung expansion Reduce anxiety Organize activities to allow for minimum expenditure of energy	Airway remains clear Child rests and sleeps quietly Respirations unlabored Respirations remain within normal limits (see inside front cover for normal variations)
Reduce anxiety and apprehension	Provide constant attendance during acute phase of illness Encourage presence of parents Provide comfort and cuddling when possible Remove restraining devices when and as often as possible Provide quiet diversion appropriate to child's age and condition	Child exhibits no signs of distress Parents remain with child and provide comfort Child engages in quiet activities appropriate for age, interest, and condition

A-EP   Activity intolerance, potential for
Risk factors: imbalance between oxygen supply and demand

| Conserve energy | Promote rest
Organize nursing care to disturb as little as possible
Remove or minimize sources of anxiety
Avoid stimulating excessive coughing | Child rests quietly |

SP-SCP   Fear
Etiology: hospitalization, difficulty breathing

| Reduce child's apprehension | Remain in constant attendance
Hold and cuddle child whenever possible—preferably by parent or other familiar person
Provide security devices such as familiar toy, blanket
Encourage parental attendance and, when possible, involvement in child's care | Child responds positively to comforting measures |

*Nursing outcome.

Nursing Care Summary: The Child with Acute Respiratory Infection—cont'd

NURSING GOALS	NURSING INTERVENTIONS	EXPECTED PATIENT/FAMILY OUTCOMES
Keep child calm	Do nothing to make child more anxious than he already is Maintain relaxed manner Establish rapport with child and parents Instill confidence in both parents and child Try to avoid intrusive procedures	Child exhibits no signs of apprehension Parents relate readily with personnel and calmly with child

RRP   Family process, alteration in
Etiology: situational crisis (hospitalization of child)

Reduce parental anxiety	Recognize parental concern and need for information and support Explain therapy and child's behavior Provide support as needed Encourage to become involved in child's care	Parents ask appropriate questions, discuss child's condition and care calmly, and become involved positively in child's care
Prepare parents for child's discharge	Teach parents needed skills for home care, e.g., administration of medications Refer to appropriate health agency as indicated	Family demonstrate evidence of understanding instructions for care

Nursing Interventions Related to Medical Management

Ease respiratory efforts
Place in mist tent or Croupette with cool vapor
Provide oxygen as prescribed
Give nothing by mouth to prevent aspiration of fluids (severe tachypnea)
Be prepared to assist with tracheostomy (croup)
Have tracheostomy equipment at beside
Obtain parental permission for procedure
Remove excess secretions
Carry out percussion, vibrations, and drainage and/or suctioning
Control fever
Administer antipyretics as indicated (acetaminophen)
Promote rest
Administer sedatives as indicated if ordered for restlessness and pain

Ease discomfort
Administer analgesic medication
Prevent dehydration
Administer fluids as prescribed
Monitor intravenous infusion during acute phase
Provide nutrition
Administer intravenous glucose during acute phase (if prescribed)
Determine causative organisms
Collect specimens as needed
Assist with diagnostic procedures
Radiographs
Thoracentesis
Venipuncture
Eradicate causative organisms
Administer antimicrobial medications if prescribed
Support body's natural defenses

Upper Respiratory Tract Infections

Upper respiratory infections (URI) include infectious processes involving any or all of the structures in the upper respiratory tract. Most are caused by viruses and are self-limited. The average North American preschooler or young school-age child has five or six minor respiratory infections per year (Goldbloom, 1986). However, secondary infection or extension of URIs can cause serious or long-lasting effects, especially in infants and very young children. A primary site for extension is the middle ear.

ACUTE NASOPHARYNGITIS

Acute nasopharyngitis (the equivalent of the "common cold" in adults) is caused by any of a number of different viruses, usually rhinoviruses, respiratory syncytial virus, adenovirus, influenza virus, or parainfluenza virus.

Clinical Manifestations

Symptoms of nasopharyngitis are more severe in infants and children than in adults. Fever is common, especially in young children, although very young infants may be afebrile. Older children have low-grade fevers. The fever appears early and suddenly in children 3 months to 3 years of age in association with irritability, restlessness, and sneezing. Nasal discharge begins in a few hours. Other symptoms (e.g., vomiting and diarrhea) may be evident in some children.

The initial symptoms in older children are dryness and irritation of nasal passages and sometimes the pharynx, followed in a few hours by sneezing, chilly sensations, muscular aches, an irritating nasal discharge, and sometimes cough. Nasal inflammation may lead to obstruction, and continual wiping away of secretions causes skin irritation to nares.

The disease is self-limited and usually resolves within 4 to 10 days without complications. The most common complication is otitis media, especially in infants, and this should be suspected if fever recurs. It may occur early or after the initial phase of nasopharyngitis is past. Pneumonia is a less frequent complication and found more often in infants.

Therapeutic Management

Children with nasopharyngitis are managed at home. There is no specific treatment, and effective vaccines are not yet available. These children are managed symptomatically with antipyretics and decongestants. The decongestants that exert their effect by vasoconstriction are usually less effective when taken orally than when applied topically as nose drops. Since these drugs affect *all* vascular beds they should be given with caution to children with diabetes. The decongestants prescribed most frequently are pseudoephedrine (Sudafed), phenylephrine (Neo-Synephrine), and phenylpropylmethylamine (Vonedrine).

If the child is coughing but has a profuse nasal discharge, potent antitussives are avoided since depressing the cough reflex may greatly increase the risk of aspiration of the secretions (Boat and others, 1983). A dry, hacking cough serves no useful purpose and antitussives that act on the central nervous system to depress the cough reflex may be helpful. Dextromethorphan is the safest antitussive. Some preparations contain up to 22% alcohol; they should not be administered to young children continuously and they must be stored out of reach of the child.

Antihistamines, although effective in treatment of allergic rhinitis, are largely ineffective for treating nasopharyngitis. The drugs have a weak atropine-like side effect that tends to dry secretions. However, they can cause drowsiness and, paradoxically, have a stimulatory effect in children. There is no support for the usefulness of expectorants, and antibiotics are usually contraindicated because they can sensitize a child who may need the drugs in a severe illness. Administration of vitamin C has not been shown to have significant therapeutic or prophylactic value (Goldbloom, 1986).

Recent reports indicate some success with the intranasal administration of interferon (from human white blood cells) or alpha-2-interferon (from recombinant DNA) in preventing nasopharyngitis caused by rhinovirus and coronavirus infections (Hayden and others, 1985). Virucidal-treated paper tissues have been reported and are presumed to reduce the spread of infection from person to person (Dick and others, 1986; Hayden and others, 1985). However, since children are the major source of spread, the logistics regarding effective use are apparent and positive results questionable.

Nasopharyngitis is so widespread in the general popula-

tion that it is impossible to prevent. In addition, children are more susceptible to colds because they have not yet developed resistance to many types of viruses. Very young infants are subject to relatively serious complications; therefore some attempt should be made to protect them from exposure. Rest in bed is recommended until the child is free of fever for at least 1 day.

Nursing Considerations

Parents are assisted in managing the infant or child as described for general care. Most of the distress of nasopharyngitis is related to the nasal obstruction, especially in small infants. Placing the child in a prone position (unless respirations are compromised), suctioning, and vaporization may help provide relief. Saline nose drops and gentle suction with an ear syringe, particularly before feeding, are sometimes useful. Parents are instructed to notify a health professional if any signs of complications appear or if the child does not improve within 2 or 3 days.

Because nasopharyngitis is spread from secretions the best means for prevention is avoiding contact with affected persons. This is difficult in places where large numbers of people are confined in a small area for a long time, like classrooms. Family members with a cold should try to "keep it to themselves" by carefully disposing of tissues, not sharing towels, glasses, or eating utensils, covering the mouth and nose with tissues when coughing or sneezing, and washing the hands thoroughly after noseblowing or sneezing. The most frequent carriers of infection are the human hands, which deposit viruses on doorknobs, faucets, and other everyday objects. Therefore children should be taught to wash their hands thoroughly before putting them near nose, mouth, or eyes.

ACUTE PHARYNGITIS

Acute pharyngitis (sore throat) may be part of a generalized upper respiratory infection or the dominant feature of the illness. The term refers to all acute infections of the pharynx, including the tonsils and pharyngotonsillitis. However, this discussion is restricted to pharyngitis; tonsillitis is discussed in the next segment. The usual organisms responsible for pharyngitis are the viruses. Although others may proliferate during acute viral infections, sore throat of bacterial origin is caused by group A beta-hemolytic streptococci.

Clinical Manifestations

The signs and symptoms of pharyngitis vary depending on whether or not the causative organism is viral or bacterial, although sufficient overlapping occurs that differentiation on the basis of symptoms is often difficult (see box, p. 1344).

Viral pharyngitis. In general, viral infections have a relatively gradual onset, produce a shorter and milder illness with less intense inflammation, and cause few complications. The sore throat may be present initially or appear a day or two after the onset of other symptoms to reach a peak by the second or third day. Hoarseness, cough, and rhinitis

---

COMPARISON OF SIGNS AND SYMPTOMS OF VIRAL vs BACTERIAL PHARYNGITIS (TONSILLITIS)

Viral pharyngitis
Gradual onset
Low-grade fever

Headache, rhinitis, cough, and hoarseness occur after 1 to 2 days of fever

Slight erythema of pharynx and slight or moderate enlargement of tonsils

Firm, tender cervical lymph nodes may be present
Child is moderately ill for 1 to 5 days

Bacterial (streptococcal) pharyngitis
More abrupt onset
Fever increased to 40° C (104° F)

Conjunctivitis, rhinitis, cough, or hoarseness uncommon
Headache, severe sore throat, and abdominal pain more common

White exudate on posterior pharynx and tonsils; erythema and enlargement of tonsils

Localized firm, tender cervical lymph nodes common
Child is acutely ill for as long as 2 weeks

---

are common. The pharyngeal inflammation may be relatively slight but occasionally is severe. Cervical lymph nodes are usually enlarged slightly, and laryngeal involvement is common. The illness can last from 24 hours to over 5 days, but complications are rare.

Streptococcal pharyngitis. The onset of a bacterial infection is more rapid. Children over 2 years of age may complain of headache and abdominal pain associated with a high fever (40° C or 104° F), although fever may not be noted for 12 hours or more. The child may vomit. Sore throat appears in a few hours accompanied by tonsillar enlargement, exudation, and a variable amount of pharyngeal erythema. Pain can be relatively mild to severe enough to make swallowing difficult. Anterior cervical lymphadenopathy usually occurs early and the nodes are often tender. Fever may continue for 1 to 4 days. Severe illness may last up to 2 weeks.

Therapeutic Management

Although 80% to 90% of all cases of acute pharyngitis are viral, a throat culture should be done to rule out group A β-hemolytic *Streptococcus* (GABHS) infection, and (in some cases) *Corynebacterium diphtheriae*. Because some children normally harbor streptococci in their throats, a positive culture is not always conclusive of active disease.

Rapid identification of GABHS is possible with diagnostic test kits that can be used in the office or clinic setting. However, some authorities question their sensitivity as a substitute for culture.

If streptococcal sore throat infection is present, oral penicillin G is prescribed in a dosage sufficient to control the acute local manifestations and to maintain an adequate level for at least 10 days to eliminate any organisms that might remain to initiate rheumatic fever symptoms. Penicillin does not appear to prevent the development of acute glomerulonephritis in susceptible children; however, it may prevent the spread of nephrogenic strain of GABHS to others in the family (Gerber and Markowitz, 1985). Penicillin usually produces a prompt response within 24 hours.

The disease is short and self-limiting, and there is some question whether or not antibiotic therapy is always warranted (Denny, 1983; Nelson, 1984), especially with the dramatic decline in rheumatic fever. It has been observed that a combination of penicillin and rifampin is more effective in eradicating GABHS than penicillin alone and is recommended for carriers and persons resistant to penicillin (Chaudhary and others, 1985; Tanz and others, 1985). Erythromycin is the alternative medication most often used for children who are sensitive to penicillin.

Nursing Considerations

The nurse is often the person who performs a throat smear for culture and instructs the parents regarding administration of penicillin and analgesics as prescribed. Special emphasis is placed on completing the course of penicillin (see Compliance, p. 1110). Most children prefer to remain in bed during the acute phase of the illness. Cold or warm compresses to the neck may provide relief. In children old enough to cooperate, warm saline gargles offer some relief of throat discomfort. Pain may interfere with oral intake but the child should not be forced to eat. Cool liquids or ice chips are usually more acceptable than solids and are encouraged.

Children with streptococcal infection are noninfectious to others within a few hours after initiation of penicillin therapy, but those with viral disease remain infectious for several days (Behrman, 1983). The streptococcus is not virulent when dried but is acquired from close droplet transmission; therefore fomites are not usually a hazard. Household pets have been implicated as reservoirs for persistent streptococcal sore throats (Copperman, 1982).

INFLUENZA

Influenza, or "flu," is one of the most common disorders and one that has been overused in diagnosis of relatively nondescript respiratory infections. Influenza is caused by three of the orthomyxoviruses, which are antigenically distinct: types A and B, which cause epidemic disease, and type C, which is unimportant epidemiologically. Type A also has three distinct hemagglutinin subtypes (H1, H2, and H3) and two neuraminidases (N1 and N2), and specific antibodies to these various antigens determine immunity. The viruses may undergo significant changes from time to time. Major changes that occur at intervals of years (usually 5 to 10) are called *antigenic shift;* minor variations within the same subtypes, *antigenic drift,* occur almost annually. Consequently, antigenic drift that takes place over several years can alter the virus sufficiently to result in susceptibility of an individual to a type for which he was previously immunized or infected.

The disease is spread from one individual to another by direct contact (large-droplet infection) or by articles recently contaminated by nasopharyngeal secretions. There is no predilection for a specific age-group, but attack rates are highest in young children who have not had previous contact with a strain. It is frequently most severe in infants. During epidemics, infection among school-age children is believed to be a major source of transmission in a community. Influenza is more common during the winter months.

The disease has a 1- to 3-day incubation period, and affected persons are most infectious for 24 hours before and after onset of symptoms. The virus has a peculiar affinity for epithelial cells of the respiratory tract mucosa, where it destroys ciliated epithelium with metaplastic hyperplasia of the tracheal and bronchial epithelium with associated edema. The alveoli may also become distended with a hyaline-like material. The viruses can be isolated from nasopharyngeal secretions early after onset of the infection, and serologic tests identify the type by complement fixation or the subgroups by hemagglutination inhibition.

Clinical Manifestations

The manifestations of influenza may be subclinical, mild, moderate, or severe. In most cases of overt illness, the throat and nasal mucosa are dry, there is a dry cough, and there is a tendency toward hoarseness. There is a sudden onset of fever, accompanied by flushed face, photophobia, myalgia, hyperesthesia, and sometimes prostration. Subglottal croup is common, especially in infants. The symptoms last for 4 to 5 days. Complications include severe viral pneumonia (often hemorrhagic), encephalitis, and secondary bacterial infections, such as otitis media, sinusitis, or pneumonia may develop. Reye syndrome can be a serious complication of influenza A or B at any age but occurs most often in school-age children. Therefore children with influenza should not receive aspirin.

Therapeutic Management

Uncomplicated influenza in children usually requires only symptomatic treatment—acetaminophen for fever, dextromethorphan for cough (if needed), and sufficient fluids to maintain hydration. Amantadine hydrochloride (Symmetrel) has been effective in reducing symptoms associated with type A disease if administered within 24 to 48 hours after onset. It is ineffective against type B or C influenza or other

viral diseases. It should not be given to children under 1 year of age but is recommended for unvaccinated high-risk children, as is late immunization. Ribavirin (Virazole), an antiviral agent, has been used successfully in the treatment of acute influenza when administered as an aerosol.

Prevention. Immunization against influenza is available and recommended for children with chronic or acute conditions that make them susceptible to serious complications of the disease. This includes (1) cardiac disease, (2) chronic bronchopulmonary disease (e.g., asthma, cystic fibrosis) or other instances in which the pulmonary system is compromised, (3) chronic metabolic disease (diabetes mellitus), (4) renal dysfunction, (5) anemia, (6) immunosuppression, and (7) chronic neurologic disorders, especially those that involve ventilation. Children being treated with long-term aspirin therapy (e.g., Kawasaki disease, rheumatoid disorders) should be immunized. For information on immunization see Chapter 12.

Nursing Considerations

Nursing care is the same as for any child with an upper respiratory infection, including helping the family implement measures to relieve symptoms.

TONSILLITIS

The tonsils are masses of lymphoid tissue located in the pharyngeal cavity. Their function is to filter and protect the respiratory and alimentary tracts from invasion by pathogenic organisms. They also may have a role in antibody formation. Although the size of tonsils varies, children generally have much larger tonsils than adolescents or adults. This difference is thought to be a protective mechanism at a time when young children are especially susceptible to upper respiratory infection.

Pathophysiology

Several pairs of tonsils are part of a mass of lymphoid tissue encircling the nasal and oral pharynx, known as Waldeyer tonsillar ring (Fig. 32-1). The *palatine,* or *faucial,* tonsils are located on either side of the oropharynx, behind and below the pillars of the fauces (opening from the mouth). A free surface of the palatine tonsils is usually visible during oral examination. The palatine tonsils are those removed during tonsillectomy. The *pharyngeal* tonsils, also known as the *adenoids,* are located above the palatine tonsils on the posterior wall of the nasopharynx. Their proximity to the nares and eustachian tubes causes difficulties in instances of inflammation. The *lingual* tonsils are located at the base of the tongue and only rarely are removed. The *tubal* tonsils, found near the posterior nasopharyngeal opening of the eustachian tubes, are not part of Waldeyer tonsillar ring.

Etiology

Tonsillitis usually occurs in association with pharyngitis. Because of the abundant lymphoid tissue and the frequency of upper respiratory infections, tonsillitis is a very common

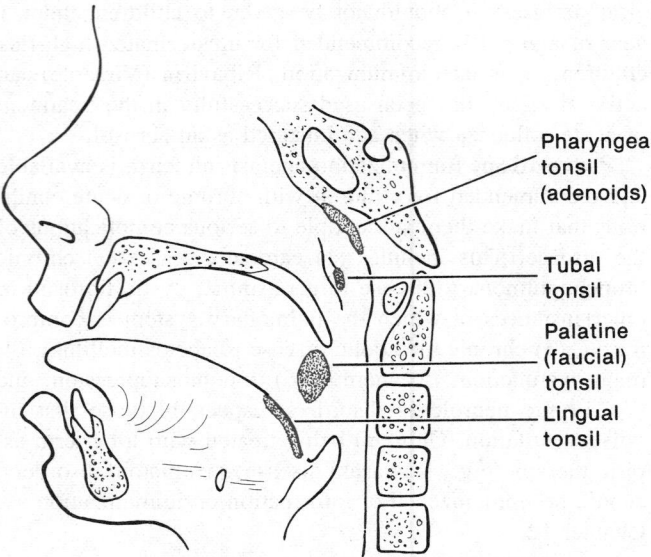

Fig. 32-1. Location of various tonsillar masses.

Pharyngeal tonsil (adenoids)

Tubal tonsil

Palatine (faucial) tonsil

Lingual tonsil

cause of morbidity in young children. The causative agent may be viral or bacterial.

Clinical Manifestations

The manifestations of tonsillitis are chiefly caused by inflammation. As the palatine tonsils enlarge from edema, they may meet in the midline (kissing tonsils), obstructing the passage of air or food. The child has difficulty in swallowing and breathing. Enlargement of the adenoids blocks the space behind the posterior nares, making it difficult or impossible for air to pass from the nose to the throat. As a result, the child breathes through the mouth.

If mouth breathing is continuous, the mucous membranes of the oropharynx become dry and irritated. There may be an offensive mouth odor and impaired senses of taste and smell. Because air cannot be trapped for proper speech sounds, the voice has a nasal and muffled quality. A persistent, harassing cough is also common. Because of the proximity of the adenoids to the eustachian tubes, this passageway is frequently blocked by swollen adenoids, interfering with normal drainage and frequently resulting in otitis media and/or difficulty hearing.

Therapeutic Management

The diagnosis is established from visual examination of the throat. The majority of children with tonsillitis respond to medical treatment. However, a significant number undergo surgical intervention, although the exact criteria for this common procedure are controversial.

Medical. Since the illness is self-limiting, treatment of viral pharyngitis is symptomatic. Throat cultures that are positive for group A beta-hemolytic streptococci warrant antibiotic treatment. A 10-day schedule of oral drug therapy, such as penicillin, is necessary to totally eradicate the bacilli. If the child is not seriously ill and follow-up care is reasonably certain, antibiotic therapy may be delayed for a few days to allow antibody formation against the streptococcus to occur.

Surgical. Surgical treatment of chronic tonsillitis is a very controversial subject. Tonsillectomy is the most frequently performed pediatric surgical procedure, but many authorities believe that the majority of these surgeries are unwarranted and unnecessary. Others, who have seen children improve measurably after tonsillectomy and adenoidectomy, continue to recommend it for selected patients (Paradise and others, 1984). For a small number of severely affected children surgery is clearly indicated, for a larger number it is not indicated, and a considerable number fall between these two extremes. It is these children over whom most of the controversy occurs.

Tonsillectomy (removal of the palatine tonsils) is indicated for massive hypertrophy that results is difficulty eating or extreme discomfort breathing. Absolute indications are malignancy and obstruction of the airway that result in cor pulmonale. *Adenoidectomy* (removal of the adenoids) is recommended for children with recurrent otitis media, especially when associated with hearing loss and in those children where hypertrophied adenoids obstruct nasal breathing. Their removal may be warranted in the child under 3 years of age and should be performed without a tonsillectomy. Follow-up after adenoidectomy should include assessment of hearing, smell, and taste for expected improvement. Contraindications to either tonsillectomy or adenoidectomy are (1) cleft palate, since both tonsils help minimize escape of air during speech, (2) acute infections at the time of surgery, since the locally inflamed tissues increase the risk of bleeding, and (3) uncontrolled systemic diseases or blood dyscrasias.

Generally removal of the tonsils should occur after 3 or 4 years of age because of the problem of excessive blood loss in small children and the possibility of regrowth or hypertrophy of lymphoid tissue. Tubal and lingual tonsils often enlarge to compensate for lost lymphoid tissue, resulting in continued pharyngeal and eustachian tube obstruction.

Nursing Considerations

Nursing care of the child with tonsillitis mainly involves providing comfort. A soft to liquid diet is generally preferred. A cool-mist vaporizer helps keep the mucous membranes moist during periods of mouth breathing. Warm salt-water gargles, throat lozenges, and analgesic/antipyretic drugs such as acetaminophen (Tylenol) are useful to promote comfort.

If antibiotics are prescribed, parents need counseling regarding their correct administration (see p. 1140) and the need for completing the treatment period. If injections are given, they must be administered deep into a large muscle mass, such as the vastus lateralis or gluteus muscle in older children. Parents need to be aware of the residual tenderness, which may cause the child to limp for a day or two. Local applications of heat are helpful in relieving some of the discomfort.

If surgery is needed, the child requires the same psychologic preparation and physical care as for any other operation (see Chapters 26 and 27). The following focuses on specific nursing care for tonsillectomy and adenoidectomy.

Preoperative care. A complete history is taken with special notation of any bleeding tendencies, since the operative site is highly vascular. Bleeding and clotting times are included in the usual blood work. During physical assessment the presence of any loose teeth is noted.

Postoperative care. Postoperative nursing objectives include (1) comfort measures to relieve the pain, (2) proper positioning to avoid aspiration, and (3) observation of signs of hemorrhage. The throat is very sore after surgery. An ice collar may provide relief, but many children find it bothersome and prefer not to have it. Analgesics are usually ordered but may need to be given rectally or intramuscularly to avoid the oral route. If children are very irritable, mild sedation is helpful to lessen crying, which irritates the operative site, increasing the chance of bleeding.

Food and fluid are restricted until the child is fully alert and there are no signs of hemorrhage. Cool water, crushed ice, Popsicles, or dilute fruit juice is given first, although fluids with a red or brown color are avoided to distinguish fresh or old blood in emesis from the ingested liquid. Citrus juice is usually poorly tolerated because of the discomfort it causes. Milk, ice cream, or pudding is not offered until clear fluids are retained, because milk products coat the mouth and throat, causing the child to clear the throat more often, which may initiate bleeding. Soft foods, particularly gelatin, cooked fruits, sherbet, soup, and mashed potatoes, are started on the first or second postoperative day or as the child tolerates feeding. Eating promotes healing because it increases the blood supply to the tissues.

Until the child is fully awake, he is placed on his abdomen or side to facilitate drainage of secretions, and needed suctioning is performed carefully to avoid trauma to the oropharynx. When alert the child may prefer sitting up, although he should remain in bed for the remainder of the day. Some secretions are common, particularly dried blood from surgery. Dark brown blood is usually present in the emesis, as well as in the nose and between the teeth. If parents do not expect this, they may be frightened at a time when they need to be calm and reassuring for the child.

Postoperative hemorrhage is unusual but can occur. The most obvious early sign is the child's continuous swallowing of the trickling blood. Therefore the nurse observes the throat directly for evidence of bleeding, using a good source of light and, if necessary, carefully inserting a tongue depressor. While the child is sleeping, the frequency of swallowing is noted. Other signs of hemorrhage are increased pulse (above 120 beats/minute), pallor, frequent clearing of the throat, and vomiting of bright red blood. Restlessness, an indication of hemorrhage, may be difficult to differentiate from general discomfort after surgery. Decreasing blood pressure is a later sign and signals impending shock.

If continuous bleeding is suspected, the physician is notified immediately, since a child can lose a considerable amount of blood before overt signs of blood loss are observed. Surgery may be required to ligate a bleeding vessel. Airway obstruction may occur as a result of edema or accumulated secretions and is indicated by progressive cyanosis. Suction equipment should be available after tonsillectomy.

Discharge instructions include (1) avoiding foods that are irritating or highly seasoned, (2) avoiding the use of gargles or vigorous toothbrushing, (3) discouraging the child from coughing or clearing his throat or putting objects in his mouth, and (4) using mild analgesics or an ice collar for pain. Hemorrhage may occur 5 to 10 days after surgery, as a result of tissue sloughing from the healing process. Any sign of bleeding warrants immediate medical attention. Objectionable mouth odor and slight ear pain with a low-grade fever are common occurrences for a few days postoperatively. However, persistent severe earache, fever, or cough necessitates medical evaluation. Most children are ready to resume normal activity within 1 to 2 weeks after the operation.

Nursing Care Summary: The Child with a Tonsillectomy

NURSING GOALS	NURSING INTERVENTIONS	EXPECTED PATIENT/FAMILY OUTCOMES
PREOPERATIVE CARE		
SP-SCP **Fear** **Etiology: separation from support system in a potentially threatening situation (hospitalization)**		
Prepare for hospitalization and surgery	See preparation for hospitalization and surgery, p. 1104 Additional preparation includes: Explain to child that he will have a sore throat when he awakens but will be able to talk Explain what he can expect when he returns to his room, especially positioning in bed and expectoration of blood and mucus	Child repeats information with reasonable degree of accuracy (specify information)

Continued.

Nursing Care Summary: The Child with a Tonsillectomy—cont'd

NURSING GOALS	NURSING INTERVENTIONS	EXPECTED PATIENT/FAMILY OUTCOMES
POSTOPERATIVE CARE		

N̲R̲ **HP-HMP   Injury: potential for (hemorrhage)**
Risk factors: raw, denuded surfaces of tonsil sockets

NURSING GOALS	NURSING INTERVENTIONS	EXPECTED PATIENT/FAMILY OUTCOMES

Detect extent of bleeding	Take pulse and respiration frequently
	Assess skin color
	Be alert for signs of covert bleeding: restlessness, frequent swallowing, frequent clearing of throat, nausea and vomiting
	Inspect throat for signs of oozing
	    Insert tongue depressor carefully
	    Use good light source
	Inspect any vomitus for evidence of fresh bleeding (blood-tinged mucus expected; may be small amounts of old blood)
		Vital signs remain within normal limits (specify) (see inside front cover for normal variations)
		Child demonstrates no evidence of
		Restlessness
		    More than usual frequency of swallowing
		    Frequent clearing of throat
		    Nausea and vomiting

Prevent bleeding	Discourage child from coughing frequently or clearing his throat Avoid use of gargles or hard objects (such as toothbrush) in mouth	Child does not aggravate the operative site No evidence of bleeding

N̲R̲ **N-MP   Fluid volume deficit: potential**
Risk factors: NPO prior to surgery, reluctance to swallow

NURSING GOALS	NURSING INTERVENTIONS	EXPECTED PATIENT/FAMILY OUTCOMES

Promote adequate hydration	Monitor intravenous infusion (if any)
	Offer fluids as tolerated after child has fully reacted from anesthetic and there is no evidence of bleeding
	    Ice chips
	    Cool water
	    Bland juices
	    Jell-O
	Avoid fluids with red or brown color that may be confused with bleeding
	Avoid fluids containing acids
	Assess state of hydration
		Child consumes an adequate amount of fluid (specific amounts according to age)
		Child consumes appropriate fluids
		Child appears well hydrated
		    Skin turgor
		    Mucous membranes
		    Color

N̲R̲ **N-MP   Swallowing, impaired**
Etiology: discomfort from surgical site

NURSING GOALS	NURSING INTERVENTIONS	EXPECTED PATIENT/FAMILY OUTCOMES

Provide nonirritating nourishment	Offer diet as tolerated
	    Cool liquid diet for 12-24 hours
	    Soft diet thereafter
	    Advance to regular diet as recommended
	Avoid substances that irritate denuded areas
	    Acid juices
	    Rough foods
	    Highly seasoned foods
		Child consumes an adequate amount of appropriate foods

N̲R̲ **A-EP   Airway clearance, ineffective**
Etiology: discomfort when swallowing

NURSING GOALS	NURSING INTERVENTIONS	EXPECTED PATIENT/FAMILY OUTCOMES
Facilitate drainage	Position on side or stomach while sleeping Discourage swallowing mucous secretions	Breathing remains unlabored Child disposes of mucus appropriately

N̲R̲ **C-PP   Knowledge deficit**
Etiology: unfamiliarity with situation

NURSING GOALS	NURSING INTERVENTIONS	EXPECTED PATIENT/FAMILY OUTCOMES

Instruct family regarding home care	Provide specific information
	    Avoid foods that are irritating or highly seasoned
	    Encourage cool liquid or semi-soft foods
		Family demonstrates an understanding of instructions (specify manner of demonstration and specific information)

Nursing Care Summary: The Child with a Tonsillectomy—cont'd

NURSING GOALS	NURSING INTERVENTIONS	EXPECTED PATIENT/FAMILY OUTCOMES
Instruct family regarding home care—cont'd	Avoid the use of gargles or vigorous toothbrushing Discourage child from coughing or clearing throat Use mild analgesics or an ice collar for pain Notify designated health professional if there is any sign of bleeding (most likely 5-10 days following surgery)	

SP-SCP   **Fear**
Etiology: unfamiliar surroundings; discomfort

Reduce anxiety	Explain source of discomfort Remain with child and/or allow significant persons to be with child Anticipate needs Keep child and bed free from any blood-tinged excretions Reassure child regarding any blood-tinged drainage Keep emesis basin within easy reach Make certain child has call light or other signal device within reach	Child rests quietly and readily attends to verbal and nonverbal communication Child communicates needs and wants in a calm manner

RRP   **Family process, alteration in**
Etiology: situational crisis (hospitalization of child)

Reassure parents	Explain what to expect
	    Appearance of child following surgery
	    Expectoration of blood-tinged mucus
	    Temporary alteration in voice
	    General morbidity
	Answer questions
	Explore fears and anxieties regarding child's status and expectations
	Explain what child is permitted to do
		Family members are able to express their concerns calmly, react to child's postoperative appearance in a positive manner, and respond to child's needs without hesitation

Nursing Interventions Related to Medical Management

Prepare for surgery
    Order bleeding and clotting times
    Collect urine specimen
    Administer preoperative medication as prescribed

Relieve discomfort
    Assess need for pain medication
    Administer analgesics as prescribed
Prepare for discharge
    Provide written instructions

OTITIS MEDIA

Otitis media (OM) is one of the most prevalent diseases of early childhood. It has been determined that approximately 70% of children have had at least one episode and 33% have had three or more episodes by 3 years of age. The incidence is highest in children age 6 months to 2 years, then it gradually decreases with age, except for a small increase at age 5 and 6 years, the time of school entry. OM is uncommon in children over 7 years of age. Boys are affected more frequently than girls in children less than school age; later the sexes are affected equally. The incidence of acute OM is highest in the winter months. Children living in households with many members (especially smokers) are more likely to have OM than those living with fewer persons, and children with siblings or parents who had a history of chronic OM have a higher incidence than those who do not (McFadden and others, 1985; Teele, Klein, and Rosner, 1980).

OM has been defined in a variety of ways. The acute disease has been known as "suppurative," "purulent," or "bacterial" OM and OM with effusion as "serous," "secretory," "nonsuppurative," and "glue ear." The standard terminology that has been established to describe OM is as follows (Senturia and others, 1980):

otitis media An inflammation of the middle ear without reference to etiology or pathogenesis

acute otitis media (AOM) A rapid and short onset of signs and symptoms lasting approximately 3 weeks

otitis media with effusion (OME) An inflammation of the middle ear in which a collection of fluid is present in the middle ear space

subacute otitis media Middle ear effusion lasting from 3 weeks to 3 months

chronic otitis media with effusion Middle ear effusion that persists beyond 3 months

Etiology

AOM is most frequently caused by *Streptococcus pneumoniae, Haemophilus influenzae,* and *Staphylococcus aureus.* The etiology of the noninfectious type is unknown, although it is a frequent result of blocked eustachian tubes from the edema of allergic rhinitis or hypertrophic adenoids. Chronic OM is frequently an extension of an acute episode.

A relationship has been observed between the incidence of OM and the feeding methods in early infancy. Breast-fed infants have a lower incidence of OM compared to formula-fed infants (Cunningham, 1984; Paradise and Elster, 1984). Breast-feeding may protect infants against respiratory viruses and allergy and limits the exposure of the eustachian tube and middle ear mucosa to microbial pathogens and foreign proteins (Saarinen, 1982). Also, reflux of milk up the eustachian tubes is less likely in breast-fed infants because of the semivertical positioning during breast-feeding compared to bottle-feeding. The admonition is to "prop the baby, not the bottle."

Pathophysiology

Otitis media is primarily the result of dysfunctioning eustachian tubes. The eustachian tubes are part of a contiguous system composed of the nares, nasopharynx, eustachian tube, middle ear, and mastoid antrum and air cells (see Fig. 7-30). Eustachian tubes have three important functions relative to the middle ear: (1) protection of the middle ear from nasopharygeal secretions, (2) drainage of secretions produced in the middle ear into the nasopharynx, (3) and ventilation of the middle ear to equalize air pressure with atmospheric pressure in the external ear canal.

Mechanical or functional obstruction of the eustachian tube causes accumulation of secretions in the middle ear. Intrinsic obstruction can be caused by infection or allergy; extrinsic obstruction is usually the result of adenoids or nasopharyngeal tumors. Persistent collapse of the tube during swallowing can cause functional obstruction associated with decreased stiffness or an inefficient opening mechanism. Eustachian tube obstruction results in negative middle ear pressure and, if persistent, produces a transudative middle ear effusion. Drainage is inhibited by sustained negative pressure and impaired ciliary transport within the tube. When the passage is not totally obstructed, contamination of the middle ear can take place by reflux, aspiration, or insufflation during crying, sneezing, nose blowing, and swallowing when the nose is obstructed.

Several factors predispose infants and young children to development of otitis media:

1. The eustachian tubes are short, wide, and straight and lie in a relatively horizontal plane (Fig. 32-2).
2. The cartilage lining is undeveloped, making the tubes more distensible and therefore more likely to open inappropriately.
3. The normally abundant pharyngeal lymphoid tissue readily obstructs the eustachian tube openings in the nasopharynx.
4. Immature humoral defense mechanisms increase the risk of infection.
5. The usual lying-down position of infants favors the pooling of fluid, such as formula, in the pharyngeal cavity.

Complications. The consequences of prolonged middle ear disorders can be either functional or structural. The principal functional consequence is *hearing loss,* although loss in the majority of cases is conductive in nature and mild in severity. The causes of hearing loss are negative middle ear pressure, the presence of effusion in the middle ear, or structural damage to the tympanic membrane. However, the most feared consequence of hearing loss is its adverse effect on development of speech, language, and cognition. It has been observed that children who had spent prolonged periods of time with middle ear effusion performed less well on speech and language tests that those who had few if any middle ear diseases. The association is most strong when the effusion occurred during the first 6 to 12 months of life (Teele and others, 1984).

Structural complications or sequelae involve primarily the tympanic membrane. *Tympanic membrane retraction* or *retraction pocket* occurs when continued negative middle ear pressure draws the tympanic membrane inward, and in areas of low tensile strength or atrophic segments of the drum head, retraction pockets appear. This retraction may result in impaired sound transmission, perforation of the thinned-out areas, or infection in the pockets and, later, cholesteatoma.

Tympanosclerosis (eardrum scarring) is the deposition of hyaline material into the fibrous layer of tympanic membrane. It is commonly seen in children with inflammatory middle ear disease or those with repeated tympanoplasty tube placement. Eardrum *perforation* is a common complication in AOM and often accompanies chronic disease. Persistent perforation is a complication of tympanostomy tube placement. Surgery is required to close some perforations.

Adhesive otitis media (glue ear) is a thickening of the mucous membrane by proliferation of fibrous tissue that can cause fixation of the ossicles with a resultant hearing loss.

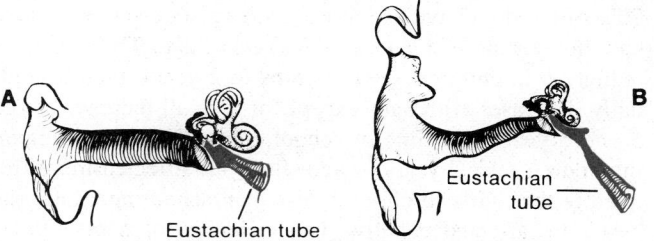

Fig. 32-2. Comparison of anatomic position of eustachian tube in **A,** child, and **B,** adult.

Chronic suppurative otitis media, an inflammation of the middle ear and mastoid, is evidenced by perforation and discharge (otorrhea). *Labyrinthitis,* infection of the inner ear, and *mastoiditis,* infection of the mastoid sinus, are rare occurrences since the advent of antibiotic therapy. *Meningitis* and other suppurative intracranial complications are possible complications of extension of infection from the middle ear or mastoid. However, these complications are uncommon when adequate antibiotic therapy is implemented. *Facial paralysis* may occur during the course of AOM.

Cholesteatoma is one of the least common but most potentially dangerous sequelae of OME. A cholesteatoma is formed when the keratinizing stratified squamous epithelial cell lining desquamates to form scales that accumulate within the middle ear space. As it enlarges, the cholesteatoma erodes all the structures it encounters, especially bone, destroying the ossicles and gaining entry to the inner ear and meninges. Clinical signs are a foul-smelling, grayish yellow discharge, sometimes pain, and permanent progressive hearing loss. Treatment is surgical excision of the entire cholesteatoma.

Clinical Manifestations

As purulent fluid accumulates in the small space of the middle ear chamber, pain results from the pressure on surrounding structures. Infants become irritable and indicate their discomfort by holding or pulling at their ears and rolling their head from side to side. Young children will usually verbally complain of the pain. A temperature as high as 40° C (104° F) is common, and postauricular and cervical lymph glands may be enlarged. Rhinorrhea, vomiting, and diarrhea as well as signs of concurrent respiratory or pharyngeal infection may also be present. Loss of appetite is common, and sucking or chewing tends to aggravate the pain. As the exudate accumulates and pressure increases, the tympanic membrane may rupture spontaneously. As a result, there is immediate relief of pain, a gradual decrease in temperature, and the presence of purulent discharge in the external auditory canal.

Severe pain or fever is usually absent in OME, and the child may not appear ill. Instead there is a feeling of "fullness" in the ear, a popping sensation during swallowing, and a feeling of "motion" in the ear if air is present above the level of fluid. Since chronic serous otitis media is the most frequent cause of conductive hearing loss in young children, audiometry may reveal deficient hearing.

Diagnostic Evaluation

In AOM otoscopy reveals an intact membrane that appears bright red and bulging, with no visible landmarks or light reflex. The usual landmarks of the bony prominence from the long and the short process of the malleus are obscured by the outwardly bulging membrane. In the OME otoscopic findings may include a slightly injected, dull gray membrane, obscured landmarks, and a visible fluid level or meniscus behind the eardrum if air is present above the fluid.

Pressure to the tympanic membrane is applied by means of a bulb attached to the head of the otoscope. Normally the tympanic membrane moves inward with positive pressure and outward with negative pressure to the external auditory canal. When positive then negative pressure is applied, the normal membrane moves rapidly inward and outward. Presence of fluid or high negative pressure within the middle ear diminishes tympanic membrane mobility.

Tympanometry is a simple, reliable, and easily performed procedure that measures the compliance of the tympanic membrane and middle ear pressure. Pneumatic otoscopy also provides an assessment of mobility of the tympanic membrane. Diminished movement of the tympanic membrane is a reliable and significant indication of middle ear effusion. The technique is difficult to perform in children less than 7 months of age. For additional information on these procedures, see p. 255.

Acoustic reflectometry measures the level of sound transmitted and reflected from the middle to a microphone located in a probe tip placed against the ear canal opening and directed toward the tympanic membrane. The information provides a measure of canal length and presence of effusion. The greater the cancellation of transmitted sound by reflected sound, the greater the probability of middle ear effusion (Lampe and others, 1985).

Diagnosis is usually based on clinical manifestations, but if purulent discharge is present, it should be cultured and a specific antibiotic chosen for that organism.

Therapeutic Management: Acute Otitis Media

Some children with AOM will improve without antibiotic therapy, but many have persistent acute signs and some may develop complications. The antimicrobial of choice for initial treatment is amoxicillin or ampicillin. A variety of other antibiotics may be prescribed individually or in combination. With appropriate therapy most children improve within 48 to 72 hours. If not, the child is reexamined and medication altered if indicated by laboratory tests.

The usual length of therapy is 10 to 14 days. However, compliance with the recommended schedule is a serious problem. Other measures include the use of analgesic/antipyretic drugs such as acetaminophen (Tylenol) to reduce the pain and/or fever. Oral decongestants, such as pseudoephedrine hydrochloride, may relieve nasal congestion and antihistamines may provide relief from known or suspected nasal allergy. The efficacy of these drugs in treatment of OM is questioned, but they may provide relief from symptoms of associated upper respiratory infection or allergy. Although they may promote comfort, ear drops are not recommended because they obscure a clear view of the tympanic membrane. Myringotomy (incision of the eardrum) may be required to relieve the symptoms in some children, especially those with acute suppuration who are in severe pain.

Children with AOM should be seen following antibiotic therapy to evaluate the effectiveness of the treatment and to identify potential complications, such as effusion or hearing impairment. Hearing loss may not be noticed by parents but should be determined by audiometric testing. (Screening tests for hearing are discussed in Chapter 7.)

Recurrent otitis media. Children who have recurrent episodes of AOM may require preventive therapy during periods of greatest susceptibility—either immunoprophylaxis with pneumococcal vaccine or chemoprophylaxis with a modified course of an antibiotic agent, usually a combination of amoxicillin and sulfisoxazole. Antibacterial prophylaxis has reduced ear infection in children at high risk but can cause toxicity and resistance. The pneumococcal vaccine can reduce the incidence by 50% but currently is not recommended for infants or children under 2 years of age (Klein, 1986).

Children on antibiotic prophylaxis are evaluated once a month to detect any evidence of effusion. Any acute infection during prophylaxis is treated with an alternate antibiotic regimen. If acute episodes are frequent and close together, additional treatment similar to that for OME may be indicated. This includes myringotomy with insertion of typanostomy tubes to improve middle ear ventilation. The efficacy of these therapies as prophylaxis has not been established.

Therapeutic Management: Otitis Media with Effusion

Many children have fluid that persists in the middle ear for weeks or months, and most have some impairment of hearing. The major goal of therapy is to establish and maintain an aerated middle ear that is free of fluid with a normal mucosa and to achieve normal hearing. The medical management of OME is uncertain and controversial. The widespread use of decongestants and antihistamines to shrink the mucous membranes and increase eustachian tube function is of unproved benefit. Occasionally attempts at middle ear inflation by the Valsalva maneuver are successful. Because of the spontaneous improvement in a large percentage of children, one simple method is observation, especially if the child speaks well and has only unilateral involvement (Rapkin, 1980).

Surgical management. When medical intervention is unsuccessful in achieving the goals of therapy, surgical intervention may be required. Myringotomy and needle aspiration have been tried with variable degrees of success. Some children benefit from adenoidectomy alone or in combination with tonsillectomy. More often the surgical treatment involves tympanostomy or insertion of ventilating tubes. Mechanical drainage promotes better healing of the membrane and prevents scar formation and loss of elasticity. Tympanostomy tubes (pressure-equalizer [PE] tubes, grommets, or dottles) facilitate continued drainage of fluid and allow ventilation of the middle ear. The objective is to allow the eustachian tube a period of recovery while the tubes perform its functions.

Tympanostomy tubes are usually inserted while the child is under general anesthesia in an outpatient surgical department. The tubes remain in the ear an average of 6 months before being spontaneously rejected. Although an extremely common practice in the United States, the insertion of PE tubes is not without complications and therefore controversial (Paradise and Rogers, 1986). Some argue that there are no solid data to support the efficacy of the procedure and that the risk of eardrum complications is greater with tubes (Stickler, 1984). Others cite the loss of hearing and risk of delayed speech and language development as sufficient justification for use of tubes (Teele and others, 1984). Additional disadvantages relative to the surgery include the psychologic trauma of surgery, anesthetic risks, and secondary infection (Paradise, 1981).

Tubes also tend to plug and often require reinsertion. The complications of repeated or long-term tube placement are tympanosclerosis, localized or diffuse atrophy of the membrane, persistent perforation, or, in rare instances, cholesteatoma.

Nursing Considerations

Nursing objectives for the child with OM include relief of pain, facilitation of drainage when possible, and prevention of complications or recurrence. Analgesics are often very helpful to reduce the severe earache. Although acetaminophen (Tylenol) is usually recommended for children, aspirin may be more effective in alleviating the pain. High fever, particularly in infants, should be reduced with antipyretic drugs and/or cool sponges to avoid febrile convulsions. The application of heat with a heating pad on low setting may reduce the discomfort. Local heat should be placed over the ear with the child lying on the affected side. This position also facilitates drainage of the exudate if the eardrum has ruptured or if myringotomy was performed. An ice bag placed over the affected ear may also be beneficial since it reduces edema and pressure. If the child is cooperative, either procedure can be tried to determine which offers maximum relief.

If the ear is draining, the external canal may be cleansed with sterile cotton swabs or pledgets soaked in hydrogen peroxide. If ear wicks or lightly rolled sterile gauze packs are placed in the ear after surgical treatment, they should be loose enough to allow accumulated drainage to flow out of the ear; otherwise the infection may be transferred to the mastoid process. Parents should be told to keep these wicks dry during shampoos or baths. Occasionally drainage is so profuse that the auricle and skin surrounding the ear become excoriated from exudate. This is prevented by frequent cleansing and application of petrolatum or zinc oxide to the area.

Parents require some anticipatory guidance regarding temporary hearing loss that accompanies OM. For example, they may need to speak louder, at closer proximity, and while facing the child. They are reminded that the child is not ignoring them but is unaware that he is being spoken to. Persistent difficulty hearing beyond the acute stage should be evaluated.

Preventing recurrence requires adequate parent education regarding antibiotic therapy. Antibiotics are frequently regarded as ''miracle'' drugs or as the ''one-dose'' cure for everything. Since the symptoms of pain and fever usually subside within 24 to 48 hours, the rapid outward signs of recovery support such thinking. Nurses must emphasize that, although the child looks well in a couple of days, the infection is not completely eradicated until all of the prescribed medication is taken. At the risk of alarming parents, it is important to stress the potential complications of otitis media, especially hearing loss, which can be prevented with adequate treatment and follow-up care (see Administration of medications and Compliance in Chapter 27).

A concern presented by the use of tympanostomy tubes is the possibility of water entering the middle ear. Several studies indicate that small amounts of water pose little hazard and that even swimming without earplugs or occlusive bathing caps carries no higher risk for an increased incidence of OM (Lounsbury, 1985; Strome, 1983). However, diving, jumping, and submerging may be forbidden by some physicians. It is recommended that bath and shampoo water be kept out of the ear, if possible, since soap reduces the surface tension of water, facilitating entry through the tube. Lake water as well as bath water is contaminated; therefore wearing ear plugs, although not watertight, prevents total flooding of the external canal and provides sufficient protection. Parents should be aware of the appearance of a grommet (usually a tiny, white, plastic, spool-shaped tube) so that they can observe if it falls out. They are reassured that this is normal and requires no immediate intervention.

Parents sometimes ask about preventing ear discomfort in their infants during ascent or descent of an airplane. During ascent, air in the middle ear expands but decompression takes place through a normal eustachian tube. If the tissues are congested with an upper respiratory infection, the passage of air may be blocked. A nasal mucosa–shrinking spray or oral decongestant before the trip may be helpful. During descent, the air within the middle ear decreases as atmospheric pressure increases. Swallowing is the simplest and most effective method for inflating the middle ear on descent; therefore feeding or offering a pacifier to infants during descent is beneficial.

Reducing the chances of otitis media is possible with some simple measures, such as sitting or holding an infant upright for feedings. Forceful nose blowing during an upper respiratory infection is discouraged. Any evidence of hearing impairment should be investigated. Early detection of possible middle ear effusion is a primary nursing goal in prevention of complications. Infants and preschool children should be screened for effusion and all schoolchildren tested for middle ear effusion, especially those with learning disabilities. Frequent audiologic evaluations, medical consultation, and education of parents and children are advised when middle ear effusion is detected.

OTITIS EXTERNA

Infections of the external ear may result from normal ear flora (*Staphylococcus epidermidis* and *Corynebacterium*,

---

Nursing Care Summary: The Child with Acute Otitis Media

NURSING GOALS	NURSING INTERVENTIONS	EXPECTED PATIENT/FAMILY OUTCOMES
HP-HMP **Hyperthermia** **Etiology: infectious process**		
Reduce body temperature	Remove bed clothes, extra clothing Reduce environmental temperature	Child's temperature remains less than 38.0° C (100.4° F)
N-MP **Skin integrity, impairment of: potential** **Etiology: ear drainage**		
Prevent skin breakdown	Keep skin around ear and pinna clean and dry Protect skin with protective coating of zinc oxide or petrolatum (if permitted) If used, change ear wicks when soiled	Skin remains smooth, intact, and exhibits no evidence of irritation
CPP **Comfort, alteration in: pain** **Etiology: inflammatory process**		
Promote comfort	Assess need for pain medication (p. 1068) Position for comfort according to needs of individual child Apply external heat (with heating pad on low setting) or cool compresses Avoid chewing by offering liquid or soft foods	Child sleeps and rests quietly and exhibits no signs of discomfort Restlessness Irritability Crying
Facilitate drainage	Position with affected ear in dependent position; have child lie on affected side	Child lies on affected side

Continued.

Nursing Care Summary: The Child with Acute Otitis Media—cont'd

NURSING GOALS	NURSING INTERVENTIONS	EXPECTED PATIENT/FAMILY OUTCOMES
CPP Knowledge deficit **Etiology: unfamiliarity with situation**		
Educate parents	Stress importance of follow-up care Stress importance of regular hearing tests to assess early signs of impairment Teach parents to recognize signs of hearing impairment in the infant or child (pp. 1018-1019) Avoid excessive water in ear if polyethylene tubes or myringotomy was part of therapy	Parents comply with instructions (specify)
Prevent recurrence or complications	Emphasize importance of following instructions, especially regarding administration of antibiotics Maintain regularity of administration Complete course of therapy	Family members comply with instructions (specify)

	Employ simple preventive practices such as
	  Sit or hold child upright for feedings
	  Promote aeration of middle ear
	    Encourage gentle nose blowing
	    Employ modified Valsalva maneuver, i.e., pinch nose, close lips, and force air up eustachian tube (except during upper respiratory infections)
	    Use blowing games
	    Chew gum (older child)
	  Eliminate tobacco smoke and known allergens from child's environment
	  Avoid injury to ear or eardrum
		Child has no more episodes of infection

SPECIFY Growth and development, altered **Etiology: impaired hearing**		
Identify developmental deficit(s)	Perform developmental tests (see Chapter 7) Perform hearing tests (see Chapter 25)	Child demonstrates responses appropriate for age Child exhibits hearing within normal range
Restore hearing and prevent further hearing loss	Refer for medical examination	Child receives medical care Child exhibits hearing within normal range
Overcome developmental deficit	Facilitate development Encourage in activities appropriate for age Provide stimulating activities appropriate for age	Child exhibits behaviors appropriate for age
RRP Family process, alteration in **Etiology: situational crisis (hospitalization of child)**		
Provide emotional support	See Family of the hospitalized child, p. 1081 Refer to community agencies as appropriate	Family demonstrates appropriate coping (specify)

Nursing Interventions Related to Medical Management

Recognize overt and covert signs and symptoms
  Assess for evidence of discomfort
  Inspect external auditory canal
    Observe for drainage in external auditory canal
  Inspect tympanic membrane for redness, bulging, and/or puncture
  Assess for hearing impairment
  Be alert to sudden relief of pain (rupture of eardrum)
Eliminate infective agent
  Administer antibiotics as prescribed
Reduce inflammation
  Administer decongestants as prescribed

Promote comfort
  Administer analgesics as needed and prescribed
  Administer at regular intervals for maximum comfort
Reduce fever
  Administer antipyretic drugs as needed
Reduce middle ear pressure
  Assist with myringotomy
  Prepare patient for insertion of PE tubes
Facilitate drainage
  Maintain wick
    Insert loosely
    Change as needed

primarily) that assume pathogenic characteristics under conditions of excessive wetness or dryness. Ordinarily the external ear canal is protected by a waxy, water-repellent coating composed of highly viscid secretions of the sebaceous glands and the watery, pigmented secretions of apocrine glands in combination with exfoliated surface cells. Inflammation occurs when this environment is altered by swimming, bathing, or increased environmental humidity *(swimmer's ear);* by infection, dermatoses, or insufficient cerumen; or by trauma from a foreign body or a finger.

Secondary invasion of foreign pathogens also occurs. In addition to the resident flora the offending agents can be *Pseudomonas aeruginosa* (most commonly), *Enterobacter aerogenes, Proteus mirabilis, Klebsiella pneumoniae,* streptococci, and fungi such as *Candida* and *Aspergillus.* The ear canal becomes irritated and maceration takes place.

The predominant symptom of external ear infection is ear pain accentuated by manipulation of the pinna, especially pressure on the tragus. The pain may appear to be out of proportion to the degree of inflammation. Conductive hearing loss may be present as a result of the edema, secretions, and accumulation of debris within the canal. Edema, erythema, and a greenish purulent discharge may accompany acute disease. The external canal may be so tender and swollen that visualization is difficult. There may be fever.

Treatment involves removal of the debris with gentle suction and wisps of cotton on metal cotton carriers. Otic preparations containing neomycin with either colistin or polymyxin and corticosteroids are instilled in the canal. A gauze wick is usually inserted to facilitate the medication reaching the site of inflammation. The wick is removed after swelling and pain have subsided, but the drops are continued for at least 3 days following relief of pain. Pain is managed with analgesics.

The best management for external ear inflammation is prevention. Nurses can teach patients to place alcohol in the ear canal routinely after swimming (the most common cause of external otitis) or bathing. A combination of white vinegar and rubbing alcohol (50/50) is highly effective in preventing recurrence.

Croup Syndromes

Croup is a general term applied to a symptom complex characterized by hoarseness, a resonant cough described as "barking" or "brassy" (croupy), varying degrees of inspiratory stridor, and varying degrees of respiratory distress resulting from swelling or obstruction in the region of the larynx. Acute infections of the larynx are of greater importance in infants and small children than they are in older children, in part because of the increased incidence in children in this age-group and the smaller diameter of the airway, which renders it subject to significantly greater narrowing with the same degree of inflammation (Fig. 32-3).

Acute respiratory infections of the nonreactive airway involve all areas to some extent and are seldom restricted to one area. Croup syndromes affect to varying degrees the

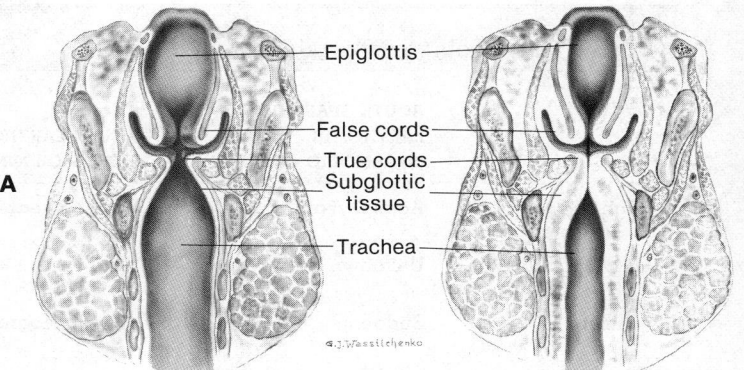

Fig. 32-3. A, Normal larynx; **B,** obstruction and narrowing resulting from edema of croup.

larynx, trachea, and bronchi. However, the laryngeal involvement often dominates the clinical picture because of the severe effects on the voice and breathing. Croup is usually described according to the primary anatomic area affected, that is, epiglottitis, laryngitis, laryngotracheitis, laryngotracheobronchitis, and spasmodic laryngitis (spasmodic croup). In general, laryngotracheobronchitis tends to occur in very young children, whereas epiglottitis is more characteristic of older children. Table 32-1 compares and contrasts the major types of croup.

Croup appears more often in males, commonly between the ages of 3 months and 3 years and is more prevalent in the winter months; laryngitis tends to recur in the same child. The principal etiologic agents in croup are viruses, except those cases associated with diphtheria, pertussis, and epiglottitis. The viral croup is more common in children in the younger age-group, 3 months to 5 years of age, whereas croup caused by *H. influenzae* and *C. diphtheriae* is more often seen in children ages 3 to 7 years. A positive family history for croup is a common finding (Stern, 1983).

In most children the disease is relatively mild, with cough, stridor, and mild retractions and gradual improvement to recovery in 3 to 7 days. However, complications of viral croup occur in a number of children, the most common of which are extensions of the infection to other areas of the respiratory tract to cause otitis media, bronchiolitis, and pneumonia. The most serious complication, and the one responsible for most deaths from croup, is laryngeal obstruction. Complications of nasotracheal intubation or tracheostomy are other hazards related to these disorders.

ACUTE LARYNGITIS

Mild laryngitis is characterized by hoarseness and a barking cough that is usually worse at night. There can be a wide range of manifestations from few symptoms to severe obstructive laryngitis. There may be a low-grade fever, loss of appetite, and malaise but there is little or no difficulty breathing. A more severe type, *acute infectious laryngitis,*

Table 32-1 Comparison of croup syndromes

	ACUTE SPASMODIC LARYNGITIS (SPASMODIC CROUP)	ACUTE LARYNGO-TRACHEOBRONCHITIS	ACUTE TRACHEITIS	ACUTE EPIGLOTTITIS (SUPRAGLOTTITIS)
Age-group affected	Ages 2-years	Under 3 years	1 month-6 years	2-6 years
Etiologic agent	Unknown	Viral	Bacterial, usually *aureus*	Bacterial, usually *H. influenzae*
Onset	Sudden	Slowly progressive	Moderately progressive	Rapidly progressive
Major symptoms	URI Croupy cough Stridor Hoarseness Dyspnea Restlessness Symptoms waken child	URI Stridor Brassy cough Hoarseness Restlessness Irritability Low-grade fever Nontoxic	URI Croupy cough Stridor Purulent secretions High fever No response to LTB therapy	Dysphagia Stridor aggravated when supine Drooling High fever Toxic Rapid pulse and respirations

begins in the same manner as the mild disease but progresses rapidly to the stage of obstruction. Breathing becomes rapid and labored, with inspiratory stridor, retractions, and restlessness.

Physical examination reveals evidence of inflammation. The main area of obstruction is below the vocal cords. The mucosa is deep red and velvety. If the disorder is limited to the larynx, the lungs are clear to auscultation except for inspiratory stridor and generally diminished aeration.

Therapeutic Management and Nursing Considerations

Afebrile children with mild laryngitis and a croupy cough are usually managed at home with symptomatic treatment. Rest in bed and humidified air during sleep may be helpful. Severe cases often require hospitalization (see Acute laryngotracheobronchitis).

ACUTE LARYNGOTRACHEOBRONCHITIS

Acute laryngotracheobronchitis (LTB) is the most common form of croup. The disease is usually preceded by an upper respiratory infection for several days. The infection rapidly proceeds to laryngitis, then descends rapidly to the trachea and sometimes the bronchi (see box). Fever and prostration increase. There is respiratory distress with inspiratory dyspnea, substernal and suprasternal retractions, and expiratory difficulty with prolonged expirations. The child is irritable and restless and may be pale or cyanotic. Auscultation reveals scattered rales of various types, rhonchi, expiratory wheeze, and localized areas of diminished to absent breath sounds bilaterally.

As distress increases, the child becomes increasingly restless and anxious. He dozes, wakens startled, and makes visible efforts to draw in air. Tracheostomy is usually performed at this stage of distress. If not, the inspiratory stridor

---

PROGRESSION OF SYMPTOMS IN LARYNGOTRACHEOBRONCHITIS

Stage I
Fear
Hoarseness
Croupy cough
Inspiratory stridor when disturbed

Stage II
Continuous respiratory stridor
Lower rib retraction
Retraction of soft tissue of neck
Use of accessory muscles of respiration
Labored respiration

Stage III
Signs of anoxia and carbon dioxide retention
Restlessness
Anxiety
Pallor
Sweating
Rapid respiration

Stage IV
Intermittent cyanosis
Permanent cyanosis
Cessation of breathing

As described by Forbes from Krugman, S., and others: Infectious diseases of children, St. Louis, 1985, The C.V. Mosby Co., p. 275.

---

and retractions progress until he becomes markedly pale or ashen, his skin is cold and clammy, and all his attention and effort are focused on fighting for air. He becomes increasingly agitated, thrashes about, and tries to climb the sides of the Croupette in his efforts to breathe. His status is critical. An artificial airway is mandatory for survival. The child may or may not be cyanotic; cyanosis is often a late sign.

Therapeutic Management

The major objective in medical management of infectious laryngotracheitis or laryngotracheobronchitis is maintaining an airway and providing for adequate respiratory exchange. Although many children with croup and significantly elevated temperatures (above 39° C [102.2° F]) can be managed at home, hospitalization is often advised. Those for whom hospitalization is indicated are children with:

Presence or suspicion of epiglottitis, progressive stridor, and respiratory distress (especially during the daytime)

Presence of hypoxia, restlessness, cyanosis, pallor, and/or depressed sensorium

A high temperature and toxic appearance

Facilities and equipment for tracheostomy or intubation, as well as reliable observation, are readily available in the hospital setting. If the hospital does not provide close, skilled observation, the child may be safer at home where the parents can maintain vigilance. The admission examination of the child with LTB should be as noninvasive as possible to disturb the child as little as possible. It is easy to underestimate the child's distress. The major part of the history and physical examination can be accomplished from a distance.

Children with LTB, whether treated at home or in the hospital, require close observation for signs of respiratory obstruction. They are placed in high humidity, preferably in a mist tent or Croupette with cool mist vapor. Since a rapidly rising heart rate is an early signal of hypoxia and impending airway obstruction, regular monitoring of cardiac rate is instituted, preferably using a cardiac monitor. Oxygen therapy is also indicated to alleviate hypoxia and reduce apprehension.

Fluid by the intravenous route is indicated to lessen physical exertion and to reduce the likelihood of vomiting with the attendant risk of aspiration. Infants with rapid respirations may aspirate feedings.

Severe cases of airway obstruction often require insertion of an artificial airway. The trend is to employ nasotracheal intubation rather than perform a tracheostomy. However, nasotracheal tube placement for longer than 24 hours frequently results in subglottic stenosis, which necessitates a tracheostomy for a long and indefinite time following the procedure, with periodic mechanical dilation. The stenosis is caused by fibrosis of the cricoid area, as denuded epithelium from the pressure of the tube is replaced with fibrotic tissue. Consequently, if lengthy intubation is anticipated, a tracheostomy may be the preferred technique. Indications for tracheostomy are increased patient fatigue, cyanosis, increased obstruction, and decreased response to epinephrine.

Medications. Since LTB is viral in origin, antibiotics are administered only in specific cases of bacterial disease. Use of corticosteroids for reduction of inflammation is controversial. Advocates acknowledge that the antiinflammatory effect is not an immediate one, but administration when the infection is progressing toward obstruction may stabilize the disease and avoid intubation or tracheostomy. Steroids appear to decrease the severity and duration of the disease (Mobley and Mansmann, 1986).

Racemic epinephrine by nebulizer lessens or abolishes moderately severe symptoms. Where facilities are available the drug is sometimes administered by intermittent positive-pressure breathing (IPPB) with face mask, although this is difficult with an anxious, struggling child and may serve to increase the work of breathing and hypoxia.

Nursing Considerations

The most important nursing function in the care of children with croup is vigilant observation for signs of respiratory embarrassment and relief of laryngeal obstruction. The child is placed in a cool high-humidity environment with oxygen, usually administered by way of a mist tent or Croupette and with skilled nursing personnel in attendance to observe for any indications of respiratory distress. Vital signs are monitored frequently, and the child's appearance and behavior are observed to detect early signs of impending airway obstruction, such as increased pulse and respiratory rate; substernal, suprasternal, and intercostal retractions; flaring nares; and increased restlessness.

Equipment for performing a tracheostomy or endotracheal intubation should be at hand in case an artificial airway must be supplied immediately; it remains until respiratory difficulty has subsided completely. Any child with laryngeal stridor requires constant surveillance. Laryngeal stridor is a shrill, harsh respiratory sound, often described as a "crowing" sound, that is particularly marked during inspiration.

Fortunately only a small percentage of children with croup require a tracheostomy. Immediately after the procedure the child becomes more relaxed as a result of the relief from laryngeal obstruction, breathing becomes regular, and he usually falls asleep from exhaustion. Later he may become frightened to discover that he is unable to speak or to cry. One of the greatest fears is that he will be unable to call someone to his side. He will need continued emotional support as well as physical vigilance required in tracheostomy care (see p. 1323). The tracheostomy is usually left in place only as long as needed to relieve respiratory distress.

To conserve energy, the child is given every opportunity to rest. Fluids are administered intravenously during the acute phase of illness, and other measures are implemented to promote rest and to reduce anxiety. An infant or small child finds that being enclosed within the mist tent, coughing, laryngeal spasms, and restraint for intravenous therapy are additional sources of distress. He needs the security of the parent's or the nurse's presence. When his condition allows, a small child can be removed for short periods for comfort and reassurance, especially to reduce apprehension during coughing spells.

The rapid progression of croup, the alarming sound of the cough and stridor, and the child's apprehensive behavior and ill appearance combine to create a very frightening experience for the parents. They need reassurance regarding the child's progress and an explanation of treatments. They may feel guilty for not having suspected the seriousness of the condition sooner, especially if an artificial airway is needed. The nurse can provide them with an opportunity to express their feelings, thus minimizing any blame or guilt. Fortunately, as the crisis subsides and the child responds to therapy, his breathing becomes easier and recovery is generally prompt. Home care after discharge includes continued humidity, adequate hydration, and nourishment. Parents are encouraged to ask questions about home care and preparation for discharge. Referral to a public health agency for follow-up care may be advisable.

ACUTE SPASMODIC LARYNGITIS

Acute spasmodic laryngitis (spasmodic croup) is distinct from laryngitis and laryngotracheobronchitis and characterized by paroxysmal attacks of laryngeal obstruction that occur chiefly at night. Signs of inflammation are absent or mild and there is frequently a history of previous attacks that last for 2 to 5 days followed by uneventful recovery. It usually affects children aged 1 to 3 years. Some children appear to be predisposed to the condition; allergy and psychogenic factors are implicated in some cases.

The child goes to bed well or with some very mild respiratory symptoms but awakes suddenly with characteristic barking, metallic cough, hoarseness, noisy inspirations, and restlessness. He appears anxious, frightened, and prostrated. Dyspnea is aggravated by excitement, but there is no fever, the attack subsides in a few hours, and the child appears well the following day.

Therapeutic Management and Nursing Considerations

Children with spasmodic croup are managed at home. Cool mist is recommended for the child's room, but if symptoms return, warm mist provided by steam from hot running water in a closed bathroom, if a shower is available, may be advised. This quick and easy treatment usually provides almost immediate relief of acute laryngeal spasm and respiratory distress. The parents are cautioned to avoid overheating the child, however. Sometimes the spasm is relieved by sudden exposure to cold air (as when the child is taken out into the night air to see the physician). Parents are usually advised to have the child sleep in humidified air until the cough has subsided so that subsequent episodes may be prevented. Children with moderately severe symptoms may be hospitalized for observation and therapy with cool mist and racemic epinephrine as for LTB.

ACUTE EPIGLOTTITIS

Acute epiglottitis, or acute supraglottitis, is a serious obstructive inflammatory process that occurs principally in children between 2 and 6 years of age (mean age, 3.1 years) and requires immediate attention. The obstruction is supraglottic as opposed to the subglottic obstruction of laryngitis.

The responsible organism is usually *H. influenzae;* croup and epiglottitis do not occur together.

Clinical Manifestations

The onset of epiglottitis is abrupt and rapidly progressive to severe respiratory distress. The child usually goes to bed asymptomatic to awaken later complaining of sore throat and pain on swallowing. The child has a fever, appears toxic out of proportion to the clinical findings, and presents a classic picture; the child generally insists on sitting upright, leaning forward, with chin thrust out, mouth open, and tongue protruding (tripod position). Drooling of saliva is common because of the difficulty or pain on swallowing and excessive secretions.

The child is irritable and markedly restless, and has an anxious, apprehensive, and frightened expression. He has a thick, muffled voice and a ''froglike'' croaking sound on inspiration. The child is not hoarse. Suprasternal and substernal retractions may be visible. The child seldom struggles to breathe, and slow quiet breathing provides better air exchange. The sallow color of mild hypoxia may progress to frank cyanosis. The throat is red and inflamed, and a distinctive large, cherry-red, edematous epiglottis is visible on careful throat inspection.

Therapeutic Management

The course of epiglottitis may be fulminant with respiratory obstruction appearing suddenly. Progressive obstruction leads to hypoxia, hypercapnia, and acidosis followed by decreased muscular tone, reduced level of consciousness, and, when obstruction becomes more or less complete, a rather sudden death. A presumptive diagnosis of epiglottitis constitutes an emergency.

The child suspected of epiglottitis should be examined where facilities are available for coping with this type of emergency. The child is best transported while sitting in a parent's lap to reduce distress. Examination of the throat with a tongue depressor is contraindicated until properly experienced personnel and equipment are at hand to proceed with immediate intubation or tracheostomy in the event that the examination precipitates further or complete obstruction.

If a lateral neck film is indicated, the same experienced personnel should accompany the child to the radiology department. However, most practitioners prefer that the child not be transported but remain on the parent's lap in the examination area during portable radiology.

Endotracheal intubation or tracheostomy is usually considered for *H. influenzae* epiglottitis with severe respiratory distress. It is recommended that the intubation or tracheostomy and any invasive procedure, such as starting an intravenous infusion, be performed in the operating room. Whether the child has an artificial airway or not he requires intensive observation by experienced personnel. The epiglottal swelling usually decreases after 24 hours and is near normal by the third day. Intubated children are generally extubated at this time.

Children with suspected bacterial epiglottitis are given

ampicillin and/or amoxicillin and chloramphenicol intravenously followed by oral administration to complete a 7- to 10-day course. The use of corticosteroids for reducing edema is controversial but may be of benefit during the early hours of treatment. Most intubated children will have had a course of corticosteroids for 24 hours before extubation.

Nursing Considerations

Nurses who suspect epiglottitis do not attempt to visualize the epiglottis directly with a tongue depressor and refer the child to a physician immediately. Epiglottitis is a serious and frightening disease for child, family, and health professionals. It is important to act quickly but calmly and provide support without unduly increasing anxiety. The child is allowed to remain in the position that provides the most comfort and security, and parents are reassured that everything possible is being done to obtain relief for their child.

Acute care of the child is that described for the child with acute respiratory distress and artificial airways in Chapter 31. Continuous monitoring of respiratory status including blood gases is part of the nursing observations, and the intravenous infusion is maintained as described in Chapter 28.

Prevention. The Committee on Infectious Diseases of the American Academy of Pediatrics (1985) and the Immunization Practices Advisory Committee (1985) recommend that all children over 24 months of age receive the *Haemophilus* type B polysaccharide vaccine. As administration of the vaccine becomes a routine part of the regular immunization schedule, a decline in the incidence of epiglottitis can be anticipated. (See also Immunization in Chapter 12.)

BACTERIAL TRACHEITIS

Bacterial tracheitis, an infection of the mucosa of the upper trachea, is a distinct entity with features of both croup and epiglottitis. The disease is seen in children ages 1 month to 6 years and may be a serious cause of airway obstruction—severe enough to cause respiratory arrest. It is believed to be a complication of LTB, and although *Staphylococcus aureus* is the most frequent organism responsible, group A β-hemolytic streptococci and *H. influenzae* have also been implicated.

Many of the manifestations of bacterial tracheitis are similar to LTB but are unresponsive to LTB therapy. There is a history of previous upper respiratory infection with croupy cough, stridor unaffected by position, toxicity, and high fever. A prominent manifestation is the production of thick, purulent tracheal secretions. Respiratory difficulties are secondary to these copious secretions.

Therapeutic Management and Nursing Considerations

Bacterial tracheitis requires vigorous management. Humidified oxygen, antipyretics, and antibiotics are prescribed. Most children require endotracheal intubation and frequent tracheal suctioning to prevent airway obstruction. The emphasis in this disorder is early recognition in order to prevent catastrophic airway obstruction.

Infections of the Lower Airways

The reactive portion of the lower respiratory tract includes the bronchi and bronchioles in children. Cartilaginous support of the large airway is not fully developed until adolescence. Consequently the smooth muscle in these structures represents a major factor in the constriction of the airway, particularly in the bronchioles, that portion that extends from the bronchi to the alveoli.

The infectious disorders involving the reactive portion of the airway are diverse in nature and etiology. Inflammation of the bronchi (bronchitis) as an isolated clinical entity is uncommon in childhood, if it exists at all. Bronchial inflammation is usually seen as tracheobronchitis or laryngotracheobronchitis. Infection of the bronchioles (bronchiolitis, or capillary bronchitis) is an entirely different illness that is more closely related to interstitial pneumonia. Asthmatic bronchitis is often confused with bronchiolitis and represents a peculiar response to a variety of upper respiratory tract infections. Table 32-2 compares some of the major features of bronchial and bronchiolar infections. Most of the following discussion is focused on bronchiolitis.

ASTHMATIC BRONCHITIS

Asthmatic bronchitis is an exaggerated response of the bronchi to upper respiratory infection with spasm and exudation similar to that seen in children with asthma. It is a disease of early infancy and early childhood. The affected children are seldom ill, but wheezing, productive cough, and signs of moderate emphysema are apparent. There is usually a history of attacks associated with upper respiratory infections.

Therapeutic Management and Nursing Considerations

Asthmatic bronchitis is effectively treated with high-humidity atmosphere and administration of sympathomimetic bronchodilators and expectorants. Immediate relief of dyspnea and wheezing is obtained by subcutaneous administration of epinephrine, and the effect is maintained with oral administration of an ephedrine preparation (pseudoephedrine [Sudafed], triprolidine [Actifed]). The stimulant effect of these drugs is offset or counterbalanced by small doses of phenobarbital. An expectorant may help liquefy and remove bronchial secretions. Since the majority of attacks are triggered by viral infections, antimicrobials are rarely indicated.

BRONCHITIS

Bronchitis, although an isolated condition and unusual in childhood, may be associated with either upper or lower res-

Table 32-2 Comparison of acute infections of the airways

	ASTHMATIC BRONCHITIS	BRONCHITIS	BRONCHIOLITIS
Description	Exaggerated response of bronchi to infection Spasm and exudation similar to asthma in older children	Usually occurs in association with URI Seldom an isolated entity	A more common infectious disease of lower airways Maximum obstructive impact at bronchiolar level
Age-group affected	Late infancy and early childhood	Affects children in first 4 years of life	Usually children 2-12 months; rare after age 2 Peak incidence approximately age 6 months
Etiologic agents	Most commonly viruses but may be any of a variety of URI pathogens	Usually viral (same as croup) Other agents, (e.g., bacteria, fungi, allergic disorders, airborne irritants) can trigger symptoms	Viruses, predominantly respiratory syncytial viruses; also adenoviruses, parainfluenza viruses, and *Mycoplasma pneumoniae*
Onset	Sudden onset at night	Abrupt onset	Gradual onset of respiratory symptoms
Predominant characteristics	Wheezing, productive cough, moderate signs of emphysema	Persistent dry, hacking cough (worse at night) becoming productive in 2-3 days	Dyspnea, paroxysmal cough, tachypnea with retractions and flaring nares, emphysema, may be wheezing

piratory tract conditions and affects children in the first 4 years of life. Noxious chemicals in urban air pollution and households with smokers are becoming important in triggering symptoms. Viral agents are the primary cause of the disease, which is characterized by a dry, hacking, and nonproductive cough that is worse at night and becomes productive in 2 to 3 days.

Bronchitis is a mild self-limiting disease that requires only symptomatic treatment directed primarily toward cough control. Although fluids are usually sufficient, cough suppressants may be needed if the cough interferes with sleep or causes vomiting. High humidity or mist helps liquefy secretions and provides symptomatic relief, and percussion and postural drainage promote the mobilization of secretions.

BRONCHIOLITIS

Bronchiolitis is represented by severe infectious and mechanical changes in the bronchioles. The causative agent in 50% to 75% of diagnosed cases is the respiratory syncytial virus (RSV). Other organisms that have been implicated are adenoviruses, parainfluenza viruses, and, in older children, *Mycoplasma pneumoniae*.

Pathophysiology

Bronchiole mucosa is swollen, and lumina are filled with mucus and exudate, the walls of the bronchi and bronchioles are infiltrated with inflammatory cells, and peribronchiolar

interstitial pneumonitis is usually present. The variable degrees of obstruction produced in small air passages by these changes lead to hyperinflation, obstructive emphysema resulting from partial obstruction, and patchy areas of atelectasis. Dilation of bronchial passages on inspiration allows sufficient space for intake of air, but narrowing of the passages on expiration prevents air from leaving the lungs. Thus air is trapped distal to the obstruction and causes progressive overinflation (*emphysema*).

Clinical Manifestations

Bronchiolitis begins as a simple upper respiratory infection with serous nasal discharge that may be accompanied by fever. The child gradually develops increasing respiratory distress, paroxysmal cough, and irritability. The chest appears barrel shaped from overinflation, and respiratory excursions are usually shallow and rapid with flaring nares and suprasternal and subcostal retractions. This in turn causes increased alveolar oxygen tension (PA_{O_2}). Severe disease may be followed by a rise in arterial carbon dioxide tension (hypercapnia), leading to respiratory acidosis. Hypoxemia may persist for 4 to 6 weeks after the peak of the illness. Auscultation reveals fine rales, diminished breath sounds, hyperresonance, scattered consolidation, and a prolonged expiratory phase. There may be wheezing.

The disease lasts about 7 to 10 days, and the prognosis is generally good. The disorder is most often confused with infantile asthma and asthmatic bronchitis. Diagnosis of asthma is favored in repeat attacks, where there is a family history of asthma, and if the child responds favorably to administration of epinephrine, which is frequently used to differentiate between viral bronchiolitis and asthmatic conditions.

Therapeutic Management

Bronchiolitis is treated with an atmosphere of high humidity, an adequate fluid intake, and rest. Hospitalization is usually recommended, and the child is placed in a mist tent or Croupette to help loosen tenacious secretions and minimize fluid loss from the lungs. Mist therapy is generally combined with oxygen in concentrations sufficient to alleviate dyspnea and hypoxia, after which mist alone is continued for mild dyspnea. Fluids by mouth may be contraindicated because of tachypnea, weakness, and fatigue; therefore intravenous fluids are preferred until the crisis of the disease has passed.

Most authorities use the conservative approach regarding medications. Antibiotics are not routinely employed, bronchodilators are ineffectual since bronchospasm is not part of the disorder, although in selected cases of severe illness aminophylline may be useful. Corticosteroids have not been proved to be of universal value, cough suppressants and expectorants have not been found to be useful, and sedatives are contraindicated. Digitalization is indicated in the presence of cardiac decompensation from cor pulmonale (heart failure secondary to pulmonary disease).

Arterial blood gas analysis and pH determination to detect impending respiratory failure are carried out. Acute respiratory failure and threatened asphyxia require endotracheal intubation and positive-pressure ventilation, often accompanied by administration of a skeletal muscle relaxant such as curare, which is given so that the ventilation can be slowed and the expiratory phase extended. This serves to more effectively empty the hyperexpanded lungs.

Nursing Considerations

Care of the child with a lower respiratory tract infection is similar whether the infection is primarily one of the airways or the lung parenchyma (see Nursing care of the child with acute respiratory tract infection, p. 1340). The child is placed in a bed away from others, frequently in a small, segregated area used only for children who have respiratory infections. Ideally, a cohort system of nurses should be assigned to these children with responsibility for no other children.

Because RSV has been found to be readily transmitted by close contact with hospital personnel (Hall and Douglas, 1981), precautions against cross-infection are especially important. The virus is readily transmitted to personnel, families, and other children by both direct contact (especially cuddling) and fomites, particularly hard smooth surfaces. Therefore infection control should stress handwashing of all persons caring for affected children and wearing cover gowns while in the room. Wearing masks and gowns appears to have limited if any value (Murphy and others, 1981).

Pneumonia

Pneumonia, inflammation of the pulmonary parenchyma, is common in childhood but occurs more frequently in infancy and early childhood. Pneumonias can be classified according to morphology, etiologic agent, and clinical forms. Clinically pneumonia may occur either as a primary disease or as a complication of some other illness. Morphologically pneumonias are recognized as:

1. *Lobar pneumonia,* in which all or a large segment of one or more pulmonary lobes is involved. When both lungs are affected, it is known as bilateral or "double" pneumonia.
2. *Bronchopneumonia,* which begins in the terminal bronchioles that become clogged with mucopurulent exudate to form consolidated patches in nearby lobules; also called lobular pneumonia.
3. *Interstitial pneumonia,* in which the inflammatory process is more or less confined within the alveolar walls (interstitium) and the peribronchial and interlobular tissues.

Other terms that describe pneumonias are hemorrhagic, fibrinous, and necrotizing. *Pneumonitis* is a localized acute inflammation of the lung without the toxemia associated with lobar pneumonia.

The most useful classification of pneumonia is based on the etiologic agent. In general pneumonia is caused by four etiologic processes: viruses, bacteria, mycoplasmas, and aspiration of foreign substances. Less often pneumonia may be caused by histomycosis, coccidioidomycosis, and other fungi. The clinical manifestations of pneumonia vary greatly depending on the etiologic agent, the age of the child, the child's systemic reaction to the infections, the extent of the lesions, and the degree of bronchial and bronchiolar obstruction. The etiologic agent is identified largely from the clinical history, the child's age, the general health history, the physical examination, radiography, and the laboratory examination.

VIRAL PNEUMONIA

Viral pneumonias occur more frequently than bacterial pneumonia and are seen in children in all age-groups. They are often associated with viral upper respiratory infections, and the pathologic changes involve interstitial pneumonitis with inflammation of the mucosa and the walls of bronchi and bronchioles. Of the many viruses that produce pneumonia in children, the respiratory syncytial virus (RSV) accounts for the largest percentage. Others are the influenza virus, parainfluenza virus, psittacosis, rhinovirus, and adenovirus. There are few clinical symptoms to distinguish between the responsible organisms, and differentiations between viruses can be made only by laboratory examination.

Clinical Manifestations

The onset may be acute or insidious, and symptoms are variable, ranging from mild fever, slight cough, and malaise to high fever, severe cough, and prostration. Early in the

Table 32-3 Comparison of the major bacterial pneumonias

	PNEUMOCOCCAL PNEUMONIA	STAPHYLOCOCCAL PNEUMONIA	STREPTOCOCCAL PNEUMONIA
Organism	Pneumococci	S. aureus S. epidermidis	Group A β-hemolytic streptococci Group B streptococcus
Age-group affected	Highest in first 4 years	Greatest incidence in first 2 years of life, usually less than 1 month of age	Not age specific Group B is most common cause of neonatal pneumonia
Time of year	More often in winter and early spring	Most often in winter months	No seasonal variation
Area of pathology	Lobar but may be lobular	Bronchopneumonia	Interstitial pneumonia
Radiology	Areas of consolidation (usually patchy) in one or more lobes	Patchy clouding in one or more lobes Pneumatoceles of various sizes	Disseminated infiltration
Prominent	Usually follows URI Infants: poor feeding followed by abrupt onset of fever Children: chills and fever, pleurisy, pain that may simulate appendicitis	Abrupt onset Rapid progression of symptoms Shock-like state may be present	Occasionally only mild symptoms, sometimes prostration Tachypnea usually mild Chills

course of the illness the cough is likely to be unproductive or productive of small amounts of whitish sputum. There is often evidence of obstructive emphysema as bronchi become plugged by necrotic material from ulceration and necrosis of tracheal and bronchial mucosa. The alveoli are generally free of fluid. Chest signs are noncontributory but may include a few rhonchi or fine crepitant rales. Radiography reveals diffuse or patchy infiltration with a peribronchial distribution.

Therapeutic Management and Nursing Considerations

The prognosis is generally good, although viral infections of the respiratory tract render the affected child more susceptible to secondary bacterial invasion, especially when there is denuded bronchial mucosa. Treatment is usually symptomatic. Although some authorities recommend antimicrobial therapy in hope of reducing or preventing secondary bacterial infection, it is usually reserved for cases in which the presence of such infection is demonstrated by appropriate cultures.

PRIMARY ATYPICAL PNEUMONIA

Approximately 10% to 20% of hospital admissions of children with pneumonia are caused by *Mycoplasma pneumoniae*. It occurs principally in fall and winter months and is more prevalent where there are crowded living conditions.

Clinical Manifestations

The onset may be sudden or insidious and is usually manifest first by general systemic symptoms, including fever,

chills (in older children), headache, malaise, anorexia, and muscle pain (myalgia). These are followed by rhinitis, sore throat, and a dry, hacking cough. The cough, initially nonproductive, becomes productive of seromucoid sputum that later becomes mucopurulent or blood streaked. The duration and degree of fever vary widely and may last from several days to 2 weeks. Dyspnea is uncommon.

Radiographic examination reveals evidence of pneumonia before physical signs are apparent. Fine crepitant rales over various areas of the lung fields are the most prominent sign. The pathologic process consists of interstitial round cell infiltration and edema of alveolar septa and varying distribution of areas of inflammation, necrosis, and ulceration of the mucosal lining of bronchi and bronchioles. Areas of consolidation and emphysema are present.

Therapeutic Management and Nursing Considerations

Most affected persons recover from acute illness in 7 to 10 days with symptomatic treatment, followed by a week of convalescence. Hospitalization is rarely necessary.

BACTERIAL PNEUMONIA

The three major organisms causing pneumonia are pneumococci, streptococci, and staphylococci. Since the availability of antimicrobial agents, the incidence of pneumococcal and streptococcal pneumonia has dropped sharply, although pneumococcal pneumonia is still the most common form encountered in childhood. Staphylococcal pneumonia has not shown a similar decline but remains a serious disease and is seen more frequently in infants than in children.

The major bacterial pneumonias are compared in Table 32-3. *H. influenzae* pneumonia is seen less frequently in children and *Chlamydia trachomatis* pneumonia is principally a disease of the newborn; therefore they will not be discussed here.

Etiology and Epidemiology

The pneumococcus is the most common agent in lobar pneumonia and is transmitted by droplet infection. It occurs most often in late winter and early spring. The attack rate is highest during the first 4 years, then declines with increasing age.

Staphylococcal pneumonia is the most common agent in bronchopneumonia and is usually contracted as a primary infection. Cross-contamination in hospitals is common. The highest incidence is in the first 2 years of life; 30% of cases occur in children less than 3 months of age, 70% before age 1 year (Stern, 1983). The infection occurs most often in winter months.

Streptococcal pneumonia is more often lobular and is less common than other bacterial pneumonias. It usually occurs as a complication of influenza or measles.

Pathophysiology

In children beyond the neonatal period, bacterial pneumonias display distinct clinical patterns that facilitate their differentiation from other causes, and each individual microorganism produces a distinctive clinical picture. In very small infants (younger than 3 to 4 months of age), however, bacterial pneumonias appear as a diffuse process indistinguishable from viral pneumonia. The largest percentage of bacterial pneumonias in childhood is caused by the pneumococcus. Onset is abrupt and is generally preceded by a viral infection that disturbs the natural defense mechanisms of the upper respiratory tract and allows the pathogenic bacteria normally harbored in the upper passages to increase in number.

Pneumococcal pneumonia. Pneumococcal pneumonia is usually lobar but may be lobular. The disease process progresses through four stages:

engorgement—lobe is congested, heavy, and dark with effusion of blood and serum into the alveoli.

red heparinization—lobe is solid, dark red, and airless; alveoli contain fibrin, serum, red blood cells, neutrophils, and pneumococci.

gray heparinization—lobe is larger than normal, firm, and gray, and pleural surface appears dull; fibrin is present in alveoli but there are fewer cellular elements and bacteria.

resolution

Radiography shows areas of consolidation in one or more lobes. This is usually patchy in children but may involve the entire lung.

Staphylococcal pneumonia. Exotoxin produced by the organisms causes necrosis and sloughing of bronchial mucous membranes, resulting in peribronchial abscesses.

The abscesses are localized in older children but more diffuse in infants. Frequently the abscesses erode the bronchial wall and abscess material is discharged into the airway lumen. Air enters the abscess cavity and becomes trapped to form *pneumatoceles* that are pathognomonic of staphylococcal pneumonia. These pneumatoceles, visible on radiography, usually develop during the first 10 days of illness; most disappear within a few weeks. Patchy clouding in one or more lobes is visible on radiographs, and pneumatoceles of varying sizes appear as thin-walled translucencies.

Streptococcal pneumonia. Streptococcal pneumonia is an interstitial infection that spreads via the lymphatics. Although ordinarily lobular, areas of consolidation may coalesce to become lobar. Radiography shows disseminated infiltration.

Clinical Manifestations

The clinical manifestations vary among the bacterial pneumonias depending on the causative agent, the age of the child, the child's systemic reaction to the infection, the presence of any underlying conditions, the extent of the lesions, and the degree of bronchial and bronchiolar obstruction.

Pneumococcal pneumonia. Pneumococcal pneumonia is usually, but not always, preceded by an upper respiratory infection. Vomiting or a seizure may be the first sign in an infant. Infants become fretful and eat poorly, then there is an abrupt onset of fever (39° to 40° C [102° to 105° F]), which may be accompanied by seizures. The infant is restless, apprehensive, or stuporous, and there is often stiff neck, bulging anterior fontanel, or Brudzinski sign. The infant is in respiratory distress with moderate to severe air hunger, flushed cheeks, and circumoral cyanosis. The child appears acutely ill. On auscultation there may be diminished breath sounds and crackling rales, exaggerated breath sounds on the opposite side, and a pleural friction rub.

Older children may complain of headache, abdominal pain, or chest pain and have shaking chills followed by high fever (40° to 40.5° C [104° to 105° F]). They are drowsy with intermittent periods of restlessness. There is rapid pulse, rapid shallow respirations, and hot dry skin. Rales are heard on auscultation. About the second day of illness the child develops a hacking, unproductive cough, expiratory grunt, dilated nares, and circumoral cyanosis. Splinting of the side caused by pleurisy pain is observed, and occasionally a child is delirious. Auscultation reveals dullness, diminished breath sounds, and tactile and vocal fremitus. Consolidation on the second to third day is evidenced by tubular breath sounds and disappearance of rales. As the disease resolves, moist rales are heard and the cough becomes productive with large amounts of blood-tinged mucus.

Staphylococcal pneumonia. The disease usually occurs in infants less than 1 year, often with a history of staphylococcal skin infection. There are abrupt onset of fever, listlessness and lethargy when disturbed, irritability on arousal, loss of appetite, nasal discharge, cough, grunting respirations, and progressively severe dyspnea that may include subcostal and sternal retractions and cyanosis. The child appears to be in a shocklike state. Early in the disease auscultation reveals diminished breath sounds, rales, and rhonchi with effusion or pneumothorax. There are dullness on percussion, respiratory lag on affected side, exaggerated excursion on opposite side, and tubular breathing above the fluid level and on the unaffected side.

Streptococcal pneumonia. The disease may appear without evidence of illness but may follow a streptococcal upper respiratory infection or be a complication of contagious disease. Symptoms are similar to those of pneumococcal pneumonia with sudden onset, fever, chills, signs of respiratory distress, and, at times, extreme prostration. Occasionally there are only mild symptoms. Rales are generally unilateral and exaggerated by deep inspiration.

Diagnostic Evaluation

Radiographic examination reveals the characteristic pictures described earlier. Laboratory examination shows elevated white blood cell counts (may be normal in infants with staphylococcal disease) and positive blood cultures in a number of patients. Children with streptococcal disease have an elevated antistreptolysin-O titer.

Therapeutic Management

Antimicrobial therapy has significantly reduced the morbidity and mortality from bacterial pneumonia. Penicillin G is effective in treatment of pneumococcal and streptococcal pneumonia and is implemented as soon as the diagnosis is suspected. Other antibiotics may be used, however. Because staphylococcal infections are caused by penicillinase-producing (penicillin G–resistant) staphylococci, semisynthetic penicillins are administered. In the hospital medications are given parenterally for rapid action and maximum effect. Sometimes a single daily dose of procaine penicillin G or oral penicillin every 6 to 8 hours for 7 to 10 days may be given for pneumococcal pneumonia.

The majority of older children with pneumococcal pneumonia can be treated at home, especially if the condition is recognized and treatment initiated early. Antibiotic therapy, bed rest, liberal oral intake of fluid, and administration of aspirin for fever constitute the principal therapeutic measures. Hospitalization is indicated when pleural effusion or empyema accompanies the disease and is mandatory for children with staphylococcal pneumonia. Pneumonia in the infant or young child is best treated in the hospital, since the course of illness is more variable and complications are more common in very young patients. In addition, fluids usually are given intravenously, and oxygen administration greatly reduces the restlessness associated with respiratory distress.

The prognosis for pneumococcal infections is generally good with rapid recovery when they are recognized and

treated early. Streptococcal infections vary in duration but usually resolve spontaneously. The course of staphylococcal pneumonia is generally prolonged. The prognosis varies with the length of the illness before treatment, although early recognition and treatment are usually beneficial.

Use of pneumococcal polysaccharide vaccine is recommended for use in selected individuals such as children over age 2 years who are at risk of acquiring pneumococcal infection or are at risk of serious disease. (See Pneumococcal vaccine, p. 530).

Complications. At present the classic features and clinical course of pneumonia are rarely seen because of early and vigorous antibiotic and supportive therapy. However, a large number of children, especially infants, with staphylococcal pneumonia develop empyema, pyopneumothorax, or tension pneumothorax. Pneumococci are the most common cause of acute otitis media and a frequent complication of pneumococcal infection. Pleural effusion is not uncommon in children with lobar (pneumococcal) pneumonia. A diagnostic thoracentesis is performed if fluid is suspected to be in the pleural cavity. Nonpurulent effusions, such as occur in pneumococcal pneumonia, do not require surgical drainage.

Continuous closed chest drainage is instituted when purulent fluid is aspirated, a frequent finding in staphylococcal infections. If a large amount of purulent drainage is obtained, an appropriate antibiotic is instilled into the cavity and the suction is discontinued for approximately 1 hour after the instillation. Closed drainage is continued until drainage fluid is free of pathogens—rarely more than 5 to 7 days. Sometimes repeated pleural taps are sufficient to remove fluid; however, the purulent drainage accumulates so rapidly and is so highly viscous that continuous drainage is preferred. In addition, continuous drainage is less traumatic to the child than repeated thoracentesis.

Thoracentesis. Dyspnea resulting from pressure from fluid accumulation in the pleural cavity requires removal by thoracentesis. Thoracentesis is also performed to obtain fluid for culture or to instill antibiotics directly into the pleural cavity. Equipment and preparation for the procedure are the same as for an adult. Nursing responsibilities include obtaining and setting up equipment, preparing the child physically and psychologically, and assisting the physician with the procedure. If continuous closed chest drainage is anticipated, this equipment should also be available. Thoracentesis is performed with the child in a sitting position, preferably with arms and trunk bent forward over pillows or over an overbed table with a pillow. Infants are positioned in a semirecumbent position on the unaffected side. The child will need to be physically restrained in the desired position by the nurse. The nurse provides explanation, offers emotional support during the procedure, and observes the child for any changes in color, respiration, and pulse and any alterations in behavior (such as coughing) and sensorium.

After the procedure the child is made comfortable, and observations and recording of physical and emotional responses are continued. The amount and description of the fluid obtained and any medication instilled are recorded, and specimens are sent to the laboratory for culture. Continuous closed chest drainage is managed according to the same protocol as for the child with a thoracotomy.

Nursing Considerations

Nursing care of the child with a lower respiratory tract infection is primarily supportive and symptomatic to meet the needs of each child. The child is assigned a bed away from others, frequently in a small, segregated ward used only for children who have respiratory infections. Children with staphylococcal infections are isolated to prevent cross-contamination. Rest and conservation of energy are encouraged by relief of physical and psychologic stresses. The child is disturbed as little as possible. Since rapid improvement is the rule in most types of pneumonia, feedings may be omitted, especially when the respiration is rapid, in order to prevent possible aspiration. To prevent dehydration, fluids are frequently administered intravenously during the acute phase. Oral fluids, if allowed, are given cautiously to avoid aspiration and to decrease the possibility of aggravating a fatiguing cough.

The child is placed in a mist tent with oxygen. Cool mist moistens the airways, helps mobilize secretions, reduces bronchial edema, and provides a cool atmosphere that aids in temperature reduction. The child often requires frequent clothing and linen changes to prevent chilling in the damp atmosphere. He is usually more comfortable in a semierect position but should be allowed to determine his position of comfort. Lying on the affected side (if pneumonia is unilateral) splints the chest on that side and reduces the pleural rubbing that often causes discomfort. Fever is usually controlled by the cool environment and administration of antipyretic drugs as prescribed. Temperature is monitored regularly to detect a rapid rise that might trigger a febrile seizure.

Vital signs and chest sounds are monitored to assess the progress of the disease and to detect early signs of complications. Children with ineffectual cough or those with difficulty handling secretions, especially infants, will require suctioning to maintain a patent airway. A simple bulb syringe is usually sufficient for clearing the nares and nasopharynx of infants, but mechanical suction should be readily available if needed. Older children can usually handle secretions without assistance. Percussion, vibration, and suctioning or drainage are generally prescribed every 4 hours or more often, depending on the child's condition.

The child in the hospital is apprehensive, and many of the treatments and tests are frightening and stress producing. Reducing anxiety and apprehension reduces psychologic distress in the child and, when the child is more relaxed, the respiratory efforts are lessened. Easing respiratory ef-

forts makes the child less apprehensive, and encouraging the presence of the caregiver provides the child with his customary source of comfort and support.

CHLAMYDIAL PNEUMONIA

Chlamydia trachomatis is an intracellular microorganism that has a number of properties similar to gram-negative bacteria. It is currently classified as a specialized bacteria. The organism is responsible for one of the most common sexually transmitted diseases, and newborn infants acquire pulmonary infection from their mothers via ascending infection just before birth or in the process of the birth itself. Chlamydial infection is the cause of up to one third of cases of pneumonia in infants 1 to 6 months of age (Stagno and others, 1981).

Chlamydial pneumonia is a severe, diffuse disease; its onset is in children between 1 and 3 months, and it features a persistent cough, tachypnea, but minimum or absent fever. Radiographs show nonspecific abnormalities. Treatment with erythromycin and sulfa drugs shortens the course of the illness. Nursing care is the same as for any infant with pneumonia.

Other Infections of the Respiratory Tract

Although less common than the previously described illnesses, several infectious disorders are capable of causing significant morbidity, especially in the infant and very young child.

PERTUSSIS (WHOOPING COUGH)

Pertussis, or whooping cough, is an acute respiratory infection caused by *Bordetella pertussis* that occurs chiefly in children younger than 4 years of age who have not been immunized. It is highly contagious and is particularly threatening in young infants, in whom there is a higher morbidity and mortality rate. (See Table 16-1 for signs, symptoms, and management of pertussis.) The incidence is highest in the spring and summer months, and a single attack confers lifetime immunity. Pertussis vaccine is effective but the immunity diminishes with time after the initial infection or immunization. A small number of asymptomatic adults and immunized children have been shown to be carriers of organisms and transmit the infection to susceptible contacts (Mertsola and others, 1983).

TUBERCULOSIS

Tuberculosis (TB, Tbc) is an ancient disease and, although controlled in most developed countries, still remains a health hazard and a leading cause of death throughout many parts of the world. Tuberculosis in children is still a problem. In many areas of the United States the incidence has increased, especially in large cities. This is attributed, in part, to the influx of foreign-born persons and recognition of the disease in the native-born population (Inselman, 1986).

Etiology

Tuberculosis is caused by *Mycobacterium tuberculosis,* an acid-fast bacillus (i.e., the organism is not readily decolorized by acids after staining). The main types of tubercle bacilli that cause disease in man are the human *(M. tuberculosis)* and the bovine *(M. bovis).* Children are susceptible to both varieties, and in parts of the world where tuberculosis in cattle is not controlled or pasteurization of milk is not practiced, the bovine type is a common source of infection in children.

Although the causative agent is the tubercle bacillus, other factors influence the degree to which the organism is able to produce an altered state in the host. Resistance to the bacillus can be modified by several factors:

1. **Heredity.** There is no positive evidence to indicate a hereditary tendency to tuberculosis infection, but there is evidence that resistance to the infection may be genetically transmitted. For example, there is a higher disease rate in the nonwhite population, particularly in the American Indian. However, this may be related to environmental factors, including circumstances that are not hygienic, poor housing conditions, and crowded conditions that result in more frequent contact between infected and noninfected persons.

2. **Sex.** There are no sex differences in the incidence of the disease in early years, but in later childhood and adolescence the morbidity and mortality are higher in girls than in boys.

3. **Age.** The age of the child has a decided influence on resistance to tuberculosis infection. Infants have a diminished resistance to infection, and during puberty and adolescence there is an increased tendency to develop the disease. In infancy this may be ascribed to a delay in development of acquired immunity. Infants also have a diminished capacity to resist extension of the infective process. The heightened tendency to acquire the disease during adolescence may be caused by a new infection superimposed on an old one associated with increased contacts or as a result of indigenous reinfection stimulated by metabolic changes or suboptimal diets during a period of rapid growth. There are also age differences in the type of lesions initiated, which are discussed later.

4. **Stress states.** Temporary circumstances that produce a state of stress, such as injury or illness, undernutrition, and emotional distress or chronic fatigue, may increase susceptibility to infection. Increased secretion of adrenal steroids that occurs during stress suppresses the protective inflammatory response, which permits the infection to spread. Therapeutic administration of corticosteroids causes a similar effect; therefore they are reserved for cases with meningitis and complications such as pleural effusion.

5. **Nutrition.** It is difficult to distinguish between the effects of poor nutrition and socioeconomic factors in resistance to tuberculosis. However, active disease is inversely proportional to the state of nutrition, and excellent nutrition is essential to young children's recovery from the disease.

6. **Intercurrent infection.** Infectious diseases have been implicated in activation of latent tuberculosis, especially measles and pertussis. There are also indications that corticosteroid therapy may precipitate the disease (Krugman and others, 1985).

Pathophysiology

The source of infection in children is in most situations an infected adult or a teenager, usually a member of the household. It can also be a baby-sitter, domestic worker, or a frequent visitor to the household. The tubercle bacillus from a lung lesion is expelled in microdroplets from the respiratory tract during a cough or a sneeze where they disperse into the air; therefore the lung is the most frequent portal of entry in human beings. Less often the organism gains entrance to the body by ingestion. Because droplet transmission accounts for most initial infections, most primary lesions are in the lungs. At the focal site there is first an inflammatory reaction with accumulation of polymorphonuclear leukocytes, then localized acute bronchopneumonia.

There is a proliferation of epithelial cells that surround and encapsulate the multiplying bacilli in an attempt to wall off the invading organisms, thus forming the typical tubercle. During the inflammatory process some of the bacilli leave the focal area and are carried to the regional lymph nodes that drain the anatomic area of the organism; as a result the child develops a fever. Radiographic examinations may be positive if such tests are made, as in cases in which the child is known to have been exposed. The tuberculin test is positive. Outcomes of pulmonary tuberculosis can vary.

Extension of the primary lesion at the original site causes progressive tissue destruction as it spreads within the lung, discharges material from foci to other areas of the lungs (e.g., bronchi or pleura), or produces pneumonia. Erosion of blood vessels by the primary lesion can cause widespread dissemination of the tubercle bacillus to near and distant sites (miliary tuberculosis). Areas that are frequently affected include lymph nodes, meninges, and bone.

Clinical Manifestations

Clinical manifestations of tuberculosis in children are extremely variable. The disease may be asymptomatic or produce a broad range of symptoms, including general responses such as fever, malaise, anorexia, and weight loss or more specific symptoms related to the site of infection (e.g., lungs, bone, brain, kidneys). Lung disease may or may not include cough (which progresses slowly over weeks to months), aching pain and tightness in the chest, and (rarely) hemoptysis.

As increasing amounts of lung tissue become involved, the respiratory rate increases, the lung on the affected side does not expand as well as the other, auscultation reveals diminished breath sounds and rales, and there is dullness to percussion. In children (usually infants) who are unable to contain the spread of infection, the fever persists, the generalized symptoms are manifest, and they develop pallor, anemia, weakness, and weight loss.

Diagnostic Evaluation

Several tests and procedures are employed to establish a diagnosis. In addition, it must be determined whether the lesion is in the active, quiescent, or healed stage. A definitive diagnosis is made by demonstrating the presence of the organisms, but in the absence of this positive evidence diagnosis is based on information derived from physical examination, history, reaction to tuberculin tests, and radiographic examinations.

History. Symptoms generally do not contribute significantly to a diagnosis. History of possible contact with a person known to be infected or subsequently found to be infected is helpful. All contacts of an affected child are examined for the disease.

Tuberculin test. This is the single most important test to determine whether a child has been infected with the tubercle bacillus. A primary infection initiates a hypersensitivity reaction to the protein fraction of the tubercle bacillus. This can be detected 2 to 10 weeks after the infection. (See p. 530 for a discussion of this test.)

Various factors can affect the response to the test and produce false reactions. A negative reaction will usually mean that the child has never been infected with the organism. However, circumstances that may produce a false-negative reaction include:

1. **Intercurrent diseases,** especially viral diseases such as measles, rubella, influenza, mumps, varicella, and probably others, which suppress the tuberculin reaction for about 4 weeks
2. **Viral vaccines,** such as measles, mumps, and rubella, which suppress the reaction for about 4 weeks
3. **Corticosteroids** and other **immunosuppressive agents** that suppress the reaction
4. **Cellular immune deficiency disease**
5. **Severe malnutrition**
6. **Too early testing** before the body develops a sensitivity to the protein fraction of the tubercle bacillus
7. **Use of impotent, outdated testing material,** as a result of a mixture that has been prepared for too long or has been exposed to sunlight
8. **Faulty technique,** such as too deep an injection, no wheal formed, improper measurement of solution, or leaking of solution from a defective or loosely fitting syringe
9. **Overwhelming tuberculosis infections,** such as end-stage and terminal miliary disease, which may cause the allergy to disappear

Bacteriologic examination. The organism can be isolated by several bacteriologic examinations: (1) microscopic examination of properly prepared and stained smears from a lesion, sputum, gastric washings, spinal fluid, draining lymph nodes, and so on; (2) guinea pig inoculations with any of these materials, which produce the disease in the animal; and (3) culture, the most effective method.

Radiographic studies. Radiographic examinations are usually carried out, but numerous chronic intrathoracic diseases may simulate tuberculous lesions; therefore the use of x-ray examinations is chiefly supplementary to other diagnostic methods.

Therapeutic Management

Medical management of tuberculous lesions in children consists of adequate nutrition, chemotherapy, general supportive measures, unnecessary exposure to other infections that further compromise the body's defenses, prevention of reinfection, and sometimes surgical procedures. The child is placed on bed rest to conserve energy, avoid fatigue, and decrease metabolic demands. Bed rest is continued until the child is free of fever, exhibits evidence of returning strength, has no manifestations that limit ambulation, and desires to be up and about. Since metabolic deficits, particularly negative calcium and nitrogen levels, occur easily in infected children, special attention is given to planning an adequate intake of the necessary nutritional elements.

The need for hospitalization varies. If possible, children with recent PPD conversions or active disease are hospitalized to obtain culture material, ascertain tolerance and compliance with medication, investigate household contacts for exposure, identify and initiate treatment for the index case, and remove active sources from the environment before returning the child to the home. It also serves as an excellent opportunity for family education regarding the importance of medication and follow-up care.

Chemotherapy. Chemotherapy is the single most important therapeutic modality available for management of tuberculosis. A variety of chemical agents can be employed, and a regimen involving two or more drugs simultaneously has been found to be effective and is usually the mode of choice. The most commonly used combinations of drugs are isoniazid (INH) and rifampin (RMP). INH with ethambutol (EMB) or another combination of drugs is used if the child is intolerant of the other drug(s). For severe, life-threatening disease the triple combination of INH, RMP, and either EMB or streptomycin (STM) is used. Drugs used to treat tuberculosis are listed in Table 32-4.

The optimum duration of therapy is unknown, but the usual course of treatment is no less than 12 months for an initial treatment or 18 to 24 months for more serious forms of the disease. The most valuable drug, INH, is rapidly conjugated to an inactive form by approximately 25% of the population. In these persons the drug must be tailored to the individual's needs. The only serious side effect of the drug is peripheral neuritis, which seems to be related to a deficiency of pyridoxine. Supplementary administration of pyridoxine is advisable in children in whom dietary meat and milk do not provide sufficient amounts of pyridoxine, such as adolescents, preadolescents, and malnourished children.

Surgical procedures. Surgical procedures may be required to remove the source of infection in tissues that are inaccessible to chemotherapy or that are destroyed by the disease. Orthopedic operations for correction of bone de-

Table 32-4 Drug therapy in pulmonary tuberculosis

DRUGS/DURATION OF TREATMENT	COMMENTS
Isoniazid (INH) 12-18 mo	Most universally used drug About 25% of population rapidly inactivate INH Administer orally, intramuscularly, or intravenously Few neurotoxic symptoms if pyridoxine administered in conjunction with INH
Para-amino-salicylic acid (PAS) 6-18 mo	Give *after* meals Given as sodium (NaPAS), potassium (KPAS), or calcium (CaPAS) salt Can be given orally or intramuscularly Used with decreasing frequency since newer drugs available
Streptomycin (STM) 2-4 mo	Must be given intramuscularly Reserved for serious cases Frequent testing of auditory function
Rifampin (RMP) 12-18 mo	Administer orally Used in conjunction with INH May cause reddish color to urine and other body secretions Used with increasing frequency
Ethambutol (EMB) 12-18 mo	Not recommended for children less than age 5 years because of difficulty in testing visual fields in young children Replacing use of PAS in older persons
Ethionamide (ETA) 12-18 mo	Used in conjunction with INH Used in treatment of bacilli resistant to more usual drugs

formities, bronchoscopy for removal of a tuberculous granulomatous polyp, or resection of a portion of a diseased lung may also be performed.

Prognosis. Most children recover from primary tuberculosis infection and are often unaware of its presence. However, very young children have a higher incidence of disseminated disease. It is a serious disease during the first 2 years of life and during adolescence. Except in cases of tuberculous meningitis, death seldom occurs in treated children. Antibiotic therapy has decreased the death rate and the hematogenous spread from primary lesions.

Prevention. The only certain means to prevent tuberculosis is to avoid contact with the tubercle bacillus. Maintaining an optimum state of health with adequate nutrition and avoidance of fatigue and debilitating infections promotes natural resistance but does not prevent infection. There is no means to induce reliable immunity.

Pasteurization of milk and routine testing and elimination of diseased cattle have helped reduce the incidence of bovine tuberculosis. Infants and children should be given only pasteurized milk from tuberculosis-free cattle.

In general, primary pulmonary tuberculosis in young children is noninfectious for older children or adults (Krugman and others, 1985). The contagiousness of chronic pulmonary tuberculosis in older children and adolescents is comparable to similar disease in adults. Of concern to hospital personnel is that infected family members may spread the disease when visiting a child in the hospital. Therefore the child and all visitors may be restricted to the child's room until the family can be screened for evidence of the disease.

Limited immunity can be produced by administration of the only successful vaccine to date, BCG (bacillus Calmette-Guérin) vaccine containing bovine bacilli with reduced virulence. The freshly prepared vaccine, injected intradermally, produces a definite although incomplete protection against tuberculosis. In most instances positive tuberculin reactions develop after inoculation. The distribution of BCG vaccine is controlled by local or state health departments, but the vaccine is not used extensively, even in areas with a high prevalence of disease. Greater protection is afforded by daily prophylactic administration of INH. The drug is given to children with a high probability of exposure to tuberculosis despite the disadvantage of the need for continuous therapy. The drug has no effect on the child's reaction to tuberculin; therefore the test continues to be useful in detecting acquired infection.

Nursing Considerations

Most children with pulmonary tuberculosis are almost always noninfectious; therefore they seldom need to be isolated. There are few bacilli in the sputum, the amount of sputum produced is quite small, and it is swallowed rather than expectorated. Exceptions are children with draining fistulas from cervical adenitis or other infectious lesions and the rare child with cavitating tuberculosis.

Hospitalization is seldom necessary except for needed diagnostic tests. Only those children with the more serious forms are placed in the hospital for therapy; others are managed satisfactorily at home. Therefore the major nursing care of children with tuberculosis involves nurses in ambulatory settings—outpatient departments, schools, and especially public health agencies.

Asymptomatic children are able to lead an essentially unrestricted life. They can, and should, attend school (or nursery school), but older children are restricted from vigorous activities such as competitive games and contact sports during the active stage of primary tuberculosis. They should be protected from stresses, including parental anxieties, overprotection, and pressures regarding nutritional intake. The regular immunization schedule should be continued. Care should be exerted to maintain an optimum health status with proper diet, adequate rest, and avoidance of infection.

Diagnosis. Nurses assume several important roles in management of the disease, including assisting with radiographic examinations, performing skin tests, and obtaining specimens for laboratory examination. Skin tests, used as screening tools or diagnostic aids, must be carried out correctly for results to be accurate. A wheal 6 to 10 mm in diameter is formed in the skin when the solution is injected. If a wheal is not formed, the procedure is repeated.

Sputum specimens are difficult or impossible to obtain in an infant or young child, since they swallow any mucus coughed from the lower respiratory tract. Therefore the best means for obtaining material for smears or culture is by gastric washing, that is, aspiration of lavaged contents from the fasting stomach. The procedure is carried out and the specimen obtained early in the morning before the customary breakfast time.

Ambulatory care. Nursing supervision of the child at home involves teaching parents and child about the disease and its ramifications. Since children usually acquire the disease from an adult in the home, parents often feel guilty. Historically the disease has been regarded with fear, and numerous misconceptions need to be clarified. Reducing parental anxieties helps them to deal with the illness more constructively and to collaborate more effectively in planning for the child's continued care. The success of therapy depends on the acceptance and cooperation of the family. The nurse can help the family to understand the rationale of diagnostic procedures and therapy and the importance of maintaining the therapeutic plan over the extended period needed for recovery. Promoting optimum general health and preventing intercurrent infections and reinfections with the tubercle bacillus are also of primary importance.

Case finding. Case finding and follow-up of known contacts are important nursing responsibilities. Every case of tuberculosis identified in the community involves nurses in follow-up of known contacts—contacts from which the affected person may have acquired the disease and persons who may have been exposed to the diseased individual. Early diagnosis affords a means for early protection or treatment and prevents further spread of the disease.

Periodic skin testing of all school children and adults could serve to identify positive reactors, particularly in populations in which there is a high incidence of the disease. Annual skin tests are recommended for high-risk children such as American Indian children and children of parents who have immigrated from Asia, Africa, the Middle East, Latin America, and the Caribbean. Annual testing is not recommended for children from areas where there is a low prevalence of the disease. For these children testing is recommended at three stages: (1) at 12 to 15 months, (2) before school entry, and (3) during adolescence (Committee on Infectious Diseases, 1986).

Pulmonary Disturbance Caused by Noninfectious Irritants

Inflammation of lung tissue can occur occasionally as the result of irritation from foreign material. Aspiration of food, oral secretions, or other substances by otherwise normal in-fants or children can set up an inflammatory response or chemical pneumonia. Young children are especially prone to aspiration of foreign substances, and weak and debilitated children are subject to aspiration of food or secretions. Infants may aspirate talcum powder, especially during diaper changes (see p. 534). The major problems associated with aspiration in children are asphyxia or respiratory tract inflammation as the result of inhaling foreign material. Medical and nursing care of a subsequent pneumonitis and/or bronchitis is similar to that for lower respiratory tract inflammation resulting from infectious agents.

FOREIGN BODY ASPIRATION

Small children characteristically explore matter with their mouths and are therefore particularly prone to aspirate foreign bodies into the air passages. Aspiration of a foreign body (FB) can occur at any age but is most commonly seen in children ages 1 to 3 years. The signs and changes produced depend on the degree of obstruction and the nature of the foreign body. For example, dry vegetable matter, such as a seed, nut, or piece of carrot or popcorn, that does not dissolve and that may swell when wet creates a particularly difficult problem. The high fat content of potato chips and peanuts may cause the added risk of lipoid pneumonia. "Fun foods" of any kind are among the worst offenders.

The types of food items are significant. In a study by Harris and others (1984), over 90% of deaths from food-related asphyxiation occurred in children less than 5 years of age and 65% in infants. Offending foods in the order of frequency of aspiration are: hot dog, round candy, peanut or other nut, grape, cookie or biscuit, other meat, carrot, apple, and peanut butter. Round foods are the most frequent offenders. The first four items together contribute more than 40% of all specified food items.

A sharp or irritating object produces irritation and edema. A round, pliable object that does not readily break apart is more likely to occlude an airway than an object with a different shape. Balloons are especially hazardous. A small object may cause little if any pathologic changes, whereas an object of sufficient size to obstruct a passage can produce various changes, including atelectasis, emphysema, inflammation, and abscess.

Pathophysiology

A foreign body may be arrested in any portion of the air passages from the larynx to the bronchi. The site is usually determined by the size, weight, and configuration of the object. For example, heavy objects such as bullets, coins, and nails are more likely to drop into the most dependent portions of the tracheobronchial tree. The object may remain in the same location or change its situation in the airway. It can be coughed from a smaller to a larger airway and reaspirated in a different passage—or it might be ejected forcefully into the mouth and subsequently swallowed.

Signs characteristic of obstruction caused by a foreign body in a bronchi can be explained by the same mechanisms

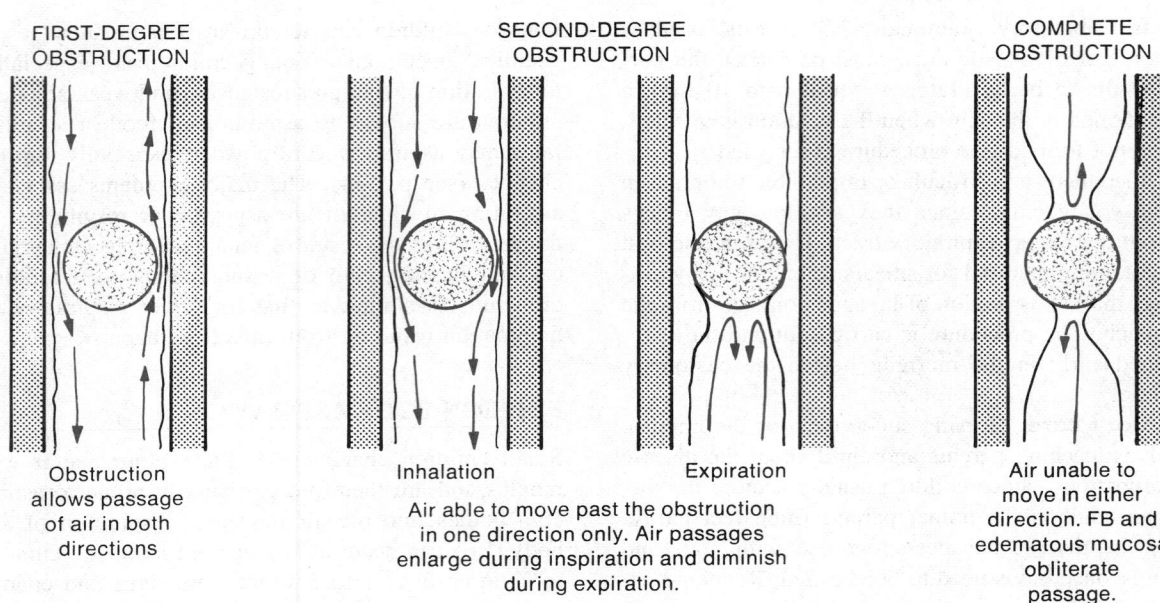

FIRST-DEGREE OBSTRUCTION

Obstruction allows passage of air in both directions

SECOND-DEGREE OBSTRUCTION

Inhalation

Expiration

Air able to move past the obstruction in one direction only. Air passages enlarge during inspiration and diminish during expiration.

COMPLETE OBSTRUCTION

Air unable to move in either direction. FB and edematous mucosa obliterate passage.

Fig. 32-4. Mechanisms of airway obstruction by foreign body *(FB)*.

that control the flow of fluids in pipes (Fig. 32-4). During normal respiration the caliber of bronchi and bronchioles becomes larger during inspiration and smaller during expiration. When a small object partially obstructs a passage, air passes around the obstruction during both inspiration and expiration (bypass valve). In this type of obstruction a wheeze is heard. A somewhat larger obstruction will allow air to enter the distal portion when bronchioles enlarge during inspiration, but when they diminish in caliber during expiration, the lumen becomes occluded and air becomes trapped distal to the obstruction (check valve). This type of obstruction produces obstructive emphysema. When there is complete blockage of the bronchus by a foreign body or by the foreign body and swollen mucosa, air is unable to move in either direction (stop valve), and the air distal to the obstruction is soon absorbed, leaving an area of obstruction atelectasis. The right bronchus, with its shorter length and straighter angle, is the usual site of bronchial obstruction.

Clinical Manifestations

Initially a foreign body in the air passages produces choking, gagging, wheezing, or cough. The child's face may become livid and sometimes he falls unconscious and dies of asphyxiation if the object is not removed. If obstruction is partial, there is often an interval of hours, days, or even weeks without symptoms after the initial period. Secondary symptoms are related to the anatomic area in which the foreign body is lodged and are usually caused by a persistent respiratory infection focused distally to the obstruction. A history of recurrent intractable pneumonia is reason to consider a foreign body in an airway. Often, by the time secondary symptoms appear, the parents have forgotten the initial episode of coughing and gagging.

Manifestations related to anatomic location. A foreign body in the *larynx* produces hoarseness, cough that rapidly becomes croupy with inspiratory stridor, and inability to speak. There may be hemoptysis, dyspnea with wheezing, and cyanosis. Obstruction of the airway from the foreign body alone or in combination with the local inflammatory reaction constitutes an emergency that requires prompt recognition and relief of the obstruction. The foreign body is located and removed by direct laryngoscopy.

A foreign body in the *trachea* may produce cough, hoarseness, dyspnea, and cyanosis, but characteristically there is an asthmatic wheeze, an audible slap, and a palpable thud as air becomes trapped at the subglottic level.

When a foreign body becomes lodged in a *bronchus*, the initial symptoms are similar to those described previously—cough, blood-tinged sputum, and dyspnea. The symptoms are largely determined by the degree of obstruction created by the foreign body and the stage at which the child is seen. A nonobstructive, nonirritating object may cause few symptoms; an obstructive object quickly produces signs of pathologic changes; and a slight obstruction may only be evidenced by a wheeze. A foreign body is always a possibility in acute or chronic pulmonary lesions. Symptoms may include limited expansion (unilateral), decreased vocal fremitus, and diminished breath sounds distal to the obstruction. Percussion may reveal hyperresonance (caused by emphysema) or impaired sounds (resulting from atelectasis).

Diagnostic Evaluation

The diagnosis of a foreign body is usually suspected on the basis of history and physical signs. Radiographic examination reveals opaque foreign bodies but may be of limited use in localizing vegetable matter. Bronchoscopy is usually required for a definitive diagnosis of foreign bodies in the larynx and trachea. Fluoroscopic examination is a valuable aid in detecting and localizing foreign bodies in the bronchi.

On fluoroscopy a check-valve–obstructed lung will remain expanded, the diaphragm will remain low and fixed on the obstructed side, and the heart and mediastinum will shift to the unobstructed side during expiration. In a stop-valve obstruction the heart and mediastinum are drawn to the obstructed side and remain there during both inspiration and expiration. The diaphragm on the obstructed side remains high, whereas that on the unobstructed side moves normally.

Therapeutic Management

Foreign bodies rarely are coughed up spontaneously; therefore they must be removed instrumentally by direct laryngoscopy or bronchoscopy. This should be carried out as soon as possible, since the progressive local inflammatory process triggered by the foreign material hampers removal, a chemical pneumonia soon develops, and vegetable matter begins to macerate within a few days, causing it to be even more difficult to remove.

Some advocate removal with a Foley catheter inserted to a point beyond the object, inflated, and used to draw the object into the bronchoscope or withdrawn simultaneously with the scope. After removal of the foreign body, the child is placed in a high-humidity atmosphere, and any secondary infection is treated with appropriate antibiotics.

Nursing Considerations

All persons working with children should be prepared to deal effectively with aspiration of a foreign body. Choking on food or other material should not be fatal. Two very simple procedures, back blows and the Heimlich maneuver, which can be used by both health professionals and lay persons, can save lives. It is the obligation of nurses to learn the techniques and teach them to parents and other groups. (See p. 1331 for the procedure.)

To aid a child who is choking, nurses need to recognize when he is indeed in distress. Not every child who gags or coughs while eating is truly choking. The child in distress (1) *cannot speak,* (2) *becomes cyanotic,* and (3) *collapses.* These three signs indicate that the child is truly choking and requires immediate and quick action to save his life. He can die within 4 minutes.

Prevention. Small children should not be allowed access to enticing small objects that they might place in their mouth. Prevention based on ages of the child is discussed on pp. 532 and 622.

Nurses, as child advocates, are in a position to teach prevention in a variety of settings. They can educate parents singly or in groups about hazards of aspiration in relation to the developmental level of their children and encourage them to teach their children safety. Parents teach by example; therefore they should be cautioned about behaviors that their children might imitate, for example, holding foreign objects, such as pins, nails, and toothpicks, in their lips or mouth.

FOREIGN BODY IN THE NOSE

Children will sometimes introduce a foreign object into the nose. This includes such items as food, crayons, small toys, pieces of plastic, beans, beads, erasers, wads of paper, and small stones. A foreign body can be suspected when there is evidence of local obstruction with sneezing, mild discomfort, and (rarely) pain. The irritation produces local mucosal swelling and, with items that increase in size as they absorb moisture (hygroscopic), the signs of obstruction and discomfort increase with time. Infection usually follows as evidenced by foul breath and a purulent or bloody discharge from one nostril.

Although the object is usually situated anteriorly, unskilled attempts at removal may move it further posteriorly. Removal is carried out as soon as possible to prevent the risk of aspiration and to prevent local tissue necrosis. Removal can usually be accomplished with topical anesthesia and either forceps or suction. Sometimes phenylephrine added to the topical anesthesia will help shrink swollen membranes (Templer, 1982). Infection and irritation usually disappear promptly following removal.

FOREIGN BODY IN THE EAR

A variety of objects can be inserted in the external ear canal by children. Such foreign bodies are a common occurrence in childhood. First an attempt should be made to remove the object by straightening the ear canal by pulling on the pinna and gently shaking the child's head. A smooth object (such as a bead) can often be removed by applying a cotton-tipped applicator with warmed dental wax or collodion against the object for 1 to 2 minutes, then withdrawing the applicator. The object remains attached to the wax or collodion. Irregularly shaped objects might be removed with bayonet forceps, and steel objects (e.g., a ball bearing) can sometimes be removed with a magnetic probe. A right-angle hook or ear curette can be inserted behind the object and the hook withdrawn, pushing the object ahead of it.

Other options include irrigation by placing the tip of the irrigation tube past the object and directing the flow toward the tympanic membrane to flush the object out of the canal. Irrigating is contraindicated for attempted removal of vegetable matter that may swell on contact with water. In this case 70% alcohol is substituted. Using a suction machine is another alternative. However, if the object is large or wedged in place, the child is referred to an otolaryngologist for removal to avoid the risk of damage to the tympanic membrane or ossicles.

ASPIRATION PNEUMONIA

Aspiration of fluid or food substances is a particular hazard in the child who has difficulty with swallowing or is unable to swallow because of paralysis, weakness, debility, congenital anomalies such as cleft palate or tracheoesophageal fistula, or absent cough reflex (unconscious) or who is force fed, especially while crying or breathing rapidly. The newborn may develop a severe pneumonia from aspirating amniotic fluid and debris during the process of birth. Rarely aspiration causes immediate death from asphyxia; more often the irritated mucous membrane becomes a site for secondary bacterial infection. In addition to fluids, food, vomitus, and nasopharyngeal secretions, other substances that cause pneumonia are hydrocarbons, lipids, or powder.

Hydrocarbon Pneumonia

Children frequently develop pneumonia secondary to the ingestion of various forms of hydrocarbons, such as kerosene, gasoline, solvents, and lighter fluid. Petroleum distillates are generally impure substances and contaminated with heavy metals or other toxic chemicals that can cause systemic as well as local effects. Many, but not all, hydrocarbons are made from petroleum (e.g., turpentine is made from pine oil), and many are found in the home or garage.

Hydrocarbons are usually packaged in attractive containers and many have a pleasant aroma. Therefore they are frequently ingested accidentally by young children. They are not often swallowed with the intent of committing suicide, however (National Clearinghouse for Poison Control Centers, 1980). On the average children will swallow less than 30 ml (often about 3 to 4 ml). They begin coughing severely and swallow no more. Although central nervous system abnormalities, gastrointestinal irritation, myocardiopathy, and renal toxicity can all occur, the most serious complication is pneumonitis.

On the whole distillates that have high volatility, decreased viscosity, and low surface tension are more likely to be aspirated and produce respiratory complications. Lower viscosity enhances penetration into more distal airways; lower surface tension facilitates spread over a larger area of lung surface. Consequently, ingestion of lighter fluid or gasoline frequently causes a pathologic condition whereas petroleum jelly or tar rarely does.

The pathogenesis of the pulmonary involvement is the subject of conflicting interpretations, but the most generally accepted explanation is irritation from aspiration during swallowing, vomiting, or gastric lavage. Reactions include bronchospasm, atelectasis, and emphysema; pathologic changes consist of signs of inflammation (edema, hyperemia, and infiltration of polymorphonuclear cells), vascular thrombosis and hemorrhage, and necrosis of bronchial, bronchiolar, and alveolar tissues. Even in small amounts the hydrocarbon spreads over the surface of tissues. In the lungs it interferes with gas exchange. Coughing and vomiting occur almost immediately after ingestion and probably contribute to aspiration. Central nervous system symptoms may consist of agitation and restlessness, confusion, drowsiness, or coma. The temperature is elevated (37.8° to 40° C [100° to 104° F]).

After swallowing, coughing, and choking the child becomes short of breath; older children complain of dyspnea. There are varying degrees of cyanosis, tachycardia, tachyp-nea, nasal flaring, and retractions. Intercostal retractions, grunting, cough, and fever may appear within 30 minutes or be delayed a few hours. Localized areas of dullness are felt on percussion and moderately intense rhonchi, wheezes, and rales are usually heard. Severe injury causes hemoptysis and pulmonary edema that develop rapidly, more severe cyanosis, and death within 24 hours of aspiration.

Inducing the child to vomit is contraindicated because of the renewed danger of aspiration (see p. 670). Hydrocarbons are readily absorbed by the gastrointestinal tract and excreted by the lungs. Bronchitis or pneumonia usually develops early (within the first 24 hours) but may be delayed. Recovery from pulmonary involvement occurs in most instances despite a severe clinical course. Death, if it occurs, is generally the result of hepatic failure complicated by pulmonary factors. Treatment is the same as for any lower respiratory tract inflammation and consists of high humidity, oxygen, hydration, and treatment of any secondary infection.

Lipoid Pneumonia

Oily substances aspirated into the respiratory passages cause progressive changes to take place in the lung tissues. First, an interstitial proliferative inflammation occurs that may include an exudative pneumonia. The next stage involves a diffuse, chronic, proliferative fibrosis that is often complicated by acute bronchopneumonia. The final stage features multiple localized nodules or tumorlike paraffinomas. There are no characteristic manifestations. Cough is usually present, and dyspnea is seen in severe cases. Secondary bronchopneumonia infections are common. The outcome depends on the extent of pulmonary damage, the general condition of the infant, and discontinuation of the oily inhalation. There is no specific treatment.

Powder

The use of powder has been discouraged for infants; however, although the incidence has decreased, a significant number of infants suffer talcum powder aspiration. Commercial talcum powder is predominantly a mixture of talc (hydrous magnesium silicate) and other silicates. The true incidence of powder inhalation is unknown, but of those with respiratory distress serious enough to be brought to medical attention, the mortality is high (Mofenson and others, 1981). Severe respiratory distress occurs immediately as a result of an inflammatory reaction in small bronchioles initiated by deep inhalation of the extremely light powder (see p. 534 for further discussion of powder inhalation).

Nursing Considerations

Care of the child with aspiration is the same as that described for the child with pneumonia from other causes. However, the major thrust of nursing care is aimed at prevention of aspiration. Proper feeding techniques should be carried out for weak, debilitated, and uncooperative children, and preventive measures are used to prevent aspiration of any material that might enter the nasopharynx.

Oily nose drops and oil-based vitamin preparations are not appropriate for infants and small children. Solvents, lighter fluid, and other hydrocarbon substances should be kept away from older infants and small children who are apt to put anything in their mouths and who may be attracted by their slightly sweet smell.

Infants and debilitated children should be positioned on the abdomen or the right side after feedings to minimize the possibility of aspirating vomitus or regurgitated feeding. Nurses are major forces in education for injury prevention (see Injury prevention in Chapters 12 and 14).

ADULT RESPIRATORY DISTRESS SYNDROME

Adult respiratory distress syndrome (ARDS) is now recognized in children as well as adults and poses a major threat to a child recovering from a primary insult. It is characterized by respiratory distress and hypoxemia that occur within 72 hours of a serious injury or surgery in a person with previously normal lungs (Holbrook and others, 1980). It is a syndrome and not a disease and has been variously described as *shock lung, wet lung, stiff lung, congestive atelectasis,* and *posttraumatic lung,* among others. Shock is the most common event associated with the onset of the syndrome.

Compromised circulation to the lung tissue apparently results in disruption at the alveolar-capillary membrane, causing release of enzymes. Subsequent damage from the enzymes produces swelling, increased capillary permeability, and fluid accumulation within the interstitial spaces. The lungs become stiff, gas diffusion is impaired, and eventually there is bronchiolar mucosal swelling and congestive atelectasis. The net effect is decreased functional residual capacity and increased intrapulmonary right-to-left shunting of pulmonary circulation. Surfactant secretion is reduced, and the atelectasis and fluid-filled alveoli provide an excellent medium for bacterial growth.

The first evidence of the disorder is acute tachypnea beginning several hours to days after injury, followed by dyspnea, tachycardia, anxiety, and restlessness. As it progresses, hypoxemia becomes unresponsive to inspired oxygen reflecting the increased shunting. Auscultatory findings are normal in early stages, but bronchial breath sounds may be heard in the later stage. Diagnosis is made on the basis of clinical manifestations, blood gas analysis, and evaluation of shunting. Chest radiographs, often normal in the early stages, reveal characteristic bilateral diffuse alveolar infiltration, which increases as the disease progresses.

Treatment involves general measures such as prevention of infection, adequate nutrition, comfort measures, and positioning to improve functional residual capacity. Definitive therapy is primarily directed toward improvement of oxygenation. For the child who is ventilating adequately, respiratory assistance with continuous positive airway pressure (CPAP) may be sufficient. Patients may require positive pressure ventilation with positive end-expiratory pressure (PEEP).

Nursing care involves careful monitoring of pulse, heart rate, perfusion, capillary filling, and urine output, as well as assessment of respiratory status. Blood gas analysis is an important evaluation tool. Respiratory distress is a frightening situation for both the child and the parents, and attention to their psychologic needs is a major element in the care of these children.

SMOKE INHALATION INJURY

A number of noxious substances that may be inhaled are toxic to humans. They are primarily products of incomplete combustion and are believed to cause more deaths from fires than flame injuries. The severity of the injury depends on the nature of the substances generated by the material being burned and whether the victim is confined in a closed space.

General Aspects

Possible inhalation injury is suspected when there is a history of flames in a closed space whether burns are present or not. Sooty material around the nose or in the sputum, singed nasal hairs, or mucosal burns of the nose, lips, mouth, or throat are all signs that the affected person demands observation for possible pulmonary injury from inhalants. A hoarse voice and cough are further evidence of airway involvement, and increased inspiratory and expiratory stridor indicates severe damage to the upper passages. Signs of respiratory distress are further indicated by tachypnea, tachycardia, and abnormal breath sounds, including rales, rhonchi, wheezes, and diminished breath sounds. Smoke inhalation causes three different types of injury: heat, local chemical, and systemic.

Heat injury. Heat causes thermal injury to the upper airways, but since air has low specific heat, the injury goes no farther than the upper airway. Reflex closure of the glottis prevents injury to lower airways. Heat may reach the middle airway occasionally but it rarely penetrates to the lungs.

Chemical injury. A wide variety of gases may be generated during the combustion of materials such as clothing, furniture, and floor coverings. Acids, alkalis, and their precursors in smoke can produce chemical burns. These substances can be carried deep into the respiratory tract, including the lower respiratory tract, in the form of insoluble gases. Soluble gases tend to dissolve in the upper respiratory tract.

Synthetic materials are especially toxic, producing gases such as oxides of sulfur and nitrogen, acetaldehyde, formaldehyde, hydrocyanic acid, and chlorine. Heated plastics are the source of extremely toxic vapors, including chlorine and hydrochloric acid from polyvinylchloride and hydrocarbons, aldehydes, ketones, and acids from polyethylene. Irritant gases such as nitrous oxide or carbon dioxide combine with water in the lungs to form corrosive acids; aldehydes cause denaturation of proteins, cellular damage, and edema of pulmonary tissues. Chemical burns to the airways are similar to burns on the skin except they are painless because the tracheobronchial tree is relatively insensitive to pain.

Inhalation of small amounts of noxious irritants produces alveolar and bronchiolar damage that can lead to obstructive bronchiolitis. Severe exposure causes further injury, including alveolar-capillary damage with hemorrhage, necrotizing bronchiolitis, inhibited secretion of surfactant, and formation of hyaline membranes—manifestations of the adult respiratory distress syndrome described in the previous section.

Systemic injury. Gases that are nontoxic to the airways (e.g., carbon monoxide and hydrogen cyanide) can cause injury and death by interfering or inhibiting cellular respiration. Carbon monoxide is an extremely dangerous gas and is responsible for more than half of fatal poisonings in the United States (Burton, 1979). It is a colorless, odorless gas with an affinity for hemoglobin 230 times greater than that of oxygen. Carbon monoxide combines at the same point on the hemoglobin molecule as does oxygen. When it enters the bloodstream, carbon monoxide readily binds reversibly with hemoglobin to form carboxyhemoglobin (COHb). Because it combines more readily and is released less readily, very low levels of tissue oxygen levels must be reached before appreciable amounts of oxygen are released from the hemoglobin. Therefore tissue hypoxia reaches dangerous levels before oxygen is available to meet tissue needs.

Accidental poisoning is most often the result of exposure to fumes of heaters or smoke from structural fires, although poorly ventilated recreational vehicles with improperly operated or maintained gas lamps or stoves and cooking in underventilated areas with charcoal grills or hibachis are also frequent causes. Carbon monoxide is produced by incomplete combustion of carbon or carbonaceous material such as wool or charcoal.

The signs and symptoms of carbon monoxide poisoning are secondary to tissue hypoxia and vary with the level of carboxyhemoglobin. Mild manifestations include headache, visual disturbances, irritability, and nausea, whereas more severe intoxication causes confusion, hallucinations, ataxia, and coma (see box). Carbon monoxide may increase cerebral blood flow, increase cerebral capillary permeability, and increase cerebrospinal fluid pressure, which further contribute to the central nervous system signs observed. The bright, cherry-red lips and skin often described are less often observed; more frequently pallor and cyanosis are seen.

Therapeutic Management

When inhalation injury is suspected, the patient is given humidified 100% oxygen by mask, and blood is drawn to determine baseline arterial blood gases and carboxyhemoglobin levels. Surprisingly arterial oxygen partial pressure may be within normal limits unless there is marked respiratory depression. If carbon monoxide poisoning is confirmed, 100% oxygen is continued until carboxyhemoglobin levels fall to the nontoxic range of about 10%, and artificial ventilation may be implemented in selected cases. Where a hyperbaric oxygen chamber is available, the breakdown of the carbon monoxide–hemoglobin bond is greatly accelerated. Other therapies that may be employed but that remain controversial are the administration of 5% to 7% carbon dioxide to stimulate the respiratory center, transfusion with washed red blood cells to increase the oxygen carried to tissues, and hypothermia to reduce the tissue demand for oxygen and to prevent central nervous system complications.

Respiratory distress may occur early in the course of smoke inhalation as a result of hypoxia, or patients who are breathing well on admission may later develop sudden respiratory distress. Therefore intubation and/or tracheostomy equipment should be available at the bedside. More often distress is related to transient edema of the airways, which can occur at any level in the tracheobronchial tree. Assessment and localization of the obstruction should be accomplished before severe swelling of head, neck, or oropharynx takes place. Intubation is often necessary when (1) severe burns in the area of the nose, mouth, and face increase the likelihood of developing oropharyngeal edema and obstruction, (2) vocal cord edema causes obstruction, (3) the patient has difficulty handling secretions, and (4) progressive respiratory distress requires artificial ventilation. There is a good deal of controversy regarding tracheostomy, but many prefer this procedure when the obstruction is proximal to the larynx and reserve nasotracheal intubation for lower tract involvement.

Use of corticosteroids, although controversial, may be of value in reducing edema, and bronchodilators (usually isoproterenol) are often given intravenously or by nebulizer. A broad-spectrum antibiotic is sometimes administered prophylactically but this too is controversial.

INHALATION INJURY RELATED TO CARBOXYHEMOGLOBIN CONCENTRATION

Signs and symptoms	Percentage of COHb concentration
Usually none (often questioned)	0-5
Tightness across forehead, may or may not be headache, cutaneous blood vessel dilation	5-15
Throbbing headache plus above	15-30
Severe headache, weakness, dizziness, dimmed vision, nausea, vomiting, cardiovascular collapse (especially infants, anemic children, and those with pulmonary disease)	30-40
Same as above but worse, with greater possibility of cardiovascular collapse, syncope, coma, and lactic acidemia	40-50
Syncope, tachycardia, poor cardiac output, seizures, Cheyne-Stokes respirations, death	50-60
Coma, seizures, decreased cardiac output, respiratory depression, death if not treated*	60-80

*Death can occur with lower concentrations in infants and in children with pulmonary disease or anemia.

Nursing Considerations

Nursing care of the child with inhalation injury is the same as that for any child with respiratory distress. Vital signs and other respiratory assessments are performed frequently, and the pulmonary status is carefully observed and maintained. Pulmonary physical therapy is usually part of the therapeutic program, and mechanical ventilation or periodic intermittent positive-pressure breathing with bronchodilators is employed.

In addition to the observation and management of the physical aspects of inhalation injury, the nurse also deals with the psychologic needs of a frightened child and distraught parents. As with any accidental injury, the parents feel overwhelming guilt, even when the injury occurred through no fault of their own. More often, however, the injury could have been prevented, which compounds their guilt feelings. They need a great deal of support and reassurance, as well as information regarding the child's condition, treatment, and progress.

The increased use of wood-burning stoves as a primary or supplementary source of heat has produced additional air-pollutant particles in residential air. Investigators have noted an increase in respiratory illness in infants and children from households heating with wood-burning stoves (Honicky, Osborne, and Akpom, 1985). A family assessment that reveals frequent respiratory infections in children during the cold winter months provides the nurse with a clue to inquire about this possibility.

PASSIVE SMOKING

Many researchers have investigated the effects of environmental pollution on children's health and have determined that the worst pollutant is parental smoking, especially maternal smoking. Children are at particular risk for health problems as a result of passive smoking. It has been found that children in passive smoking situations have an increased number of respiratory illnesses when compared to children of nonsmoking parents and that the number of illnesses is positively correlated with the number of cigarettes smoked (Bonham and Wilson, 1981; Ogston, 1985; Pattishall and others, 1985; Pedreira and others, 1985).

The incidence of respiratory disease related to passive smoking also correlates with the smoking members of the family. Maternal cigarette smoking is associated with increases of 20% to 35% in the rates of respiratory illnesses and respiratory symptoms. Paternal smoking is associated with smaller but still substantial increases (Ware and others, 1984). Other researchers have found that children of smoking parents have reduced performance on pulmonary function tests (Tager and others, 1983; White and Froeb, 1980), and parental smoking may have a deleterious effect on children's growth (Rona and others, 1981).

Nursing Considerations

Passive smoking during childhood may well be the most important precursor of chronic lung disease in the adult.

Nurses and other health professionals need to be aware of this problem and include this information in all health assessments of children, especially those with respiratory illnesses. The American Academy of Pediatrics has renewed its statement on hazards of passive smoking (Committee on Environmental Hazards, 1986). Armed with this knowledge, nurses should play a stronger role in ridding children's environments of tobacco smoke by informing parents, setting an example for children and families, and advocating "no smoking" ordinances in public places.

Long-Term Respiratory Dysfunction

Respiratory disorders that assume a long-term aspect are not uncommon in childhood. They are responsible for significant morbidity and school absenteeism as well as altering the quality of life and physical and social development of children. Bronchial asthma is prominent among these, and cystic fibrosis of the pancreas is the most common inherited disease of children.

ALLERGIC RHINITIS

Allergic rhinitis is the most common of all allergic disorders and, although not life threatening, is a significant cause of morbidity in all age-groups. The manifestations may be episodic or perennial. Seasonal allergic rhinitis, also known as "hay fever" or "summer cold," occurs during certain months of the year and does not develop until the individual has been sensitized by two or more pollen seasons. Although the peak incidence is in the postadolescent teenage group, younger children are affected occasionally.

The development of allergic rhinitis requires two conditions: a familial predisposition to develop allergy and exposure of a sensitized person to the allergen. Inhalants in the form of microscopic airborne particles are the principal allergens, including pollens, mold, animal danders, and environmental dusts. It is thought that water-soluble allergens diffuse into the respiratory epithelium from airborne foreign particles that enter the upper respiratory tract with each inhalation. Following diffusion, immunoglobulin E antibody production is stimulated in the genetically susceptible child and subsequent sensitization of respiratory tissues takes place. Repeated exposure of these sensitized membranes to specific aeroallergens results in antigen-antibody interactions with the release of mast cell mediators, inflammation, and clinical allergic disease (Mathews, 1982).

Clinical Manifestations

Symptoms of allergic rhinitis may include paroxysms of sneezing; itching of the nose, eyes, palate, pharynx, and conjunctiva; nasal stuffiness progressing to partial or total obstruction of airflow; and mucous secretion, frequently accompanied by postnasal drainage. Other symptoms may appear during peak symptom periods, including tearing and soreness of the eyes and gelatinous conjunctival discharge in the morning, irritability, fatigue, depression, and loss of appetite. Symptoms related to an accompanying otitis media with effusion and eustachian tube dysfunction may be present, especially in children.

Therapeutic Management

Therapy is directed toward avoidance of offending allergens, medication, and immunotherapy (hyposensitization or desensitization). Avoidance measures involve removing allergens from the environment and are usually effective for allergy to foods, drugs, and animals, and allergy-proofing the household (see p. 1387).

If a patient is unable to avoid the allergens, symptoms can be controlled with drugs in many cases. Antihistamines are the preferred medications and any of a variety of these drugs are effective. If nasal obstruction is a prominent feature, relief can often be obtained from an α-adrenergic decongestant, such as phenylephrine, phenylpropanolamine, or pseudoephedrine, given singly or in combination with an antihistamine. Topical nasal applications of α-adrenergic vasoconstrictors often provide symptomatic relief but should not be used for any length of time. After 7 to 10 days many persons develop a rebound vasodilation and, occasionally, habituation (Fagin, Friedman, and Fireman, 1981). For cases that cannot be controlled with the previous therapies some suggest the use of topical corticosteroids.

Immunotherapy may be necessary if drug therapy and avoidance of allergens are ineffective in controlling symptoms or if drugs evoke undesirable side effects. Skin tests are performed to determine the offending antigens and desensitization injections are carried out. About 80% to 90% of patients achieve significant clinical improvement, but the duration of immunotherapy injections depends on the patient's overall clinical response (Fagin, Friedman, and Fireman, 1981). If improvement is not obtained after a 2-year trial the child is reevaluated and therapy usually discontinued. With clinical improvement patients are given the opportunity to stop the immunotherapy after approximately 5 years of injections.

Nursing Considerations

The major nursing goal in care of the child with allergic rhinitis is preparation for skin tests and desensitization injections that are the source of greatest stress to children. It is difficult to make them understand how inflicting discomfort regularly over a long period of time is going to make them better. Adolescents can intellectualize the rationale behind the procedures and tolerate the discomfort but still need the support that is provided by sympathetic nursing.

To help allay children's fears of skin tests, they need a careful and thorough explanation of what is to be done, how many shots are involved (usually series of eight on each site, for a total of 30 tests). Very young, anxious patients may benefit from one prick on the arm to demonstrate how it feels. The skin is pricked with a stylet rather than a regular needle and syringe, then a drop of allergen is placed on the pierced skin. A helpful strategy is to have the child

count off the number of pricks with the nurse as a distraction.

BRONCHIAL ASTHMA

Bronchial asthma is a reversible process, often called reactive airway or hyperreactive airway disease, which is characterized by variations in central and/or peripheral airway obstruction over short periods of time, with a decrease in the degree of airway obstruction demonstrated clinically and physiologically as a direct response to bronchodilator drugs (Hen, 1986). It is manifest by labored breathing, bilateral wheezing, prolonged expiration, and an irritative tight cough caused by a reduction in the diameter of the airway. The symptoms can vary from a mild cough to severe respiratory distress with hypoxemia, retention of carbon dioxide, and respiratory acidosis that may result in prostration and even fatal asphyxia.

Asthma is a common disorder and one of the leading causes of chronic illness in childhood, which accounts for substantial school absence. It is believed by many to be the single most important cause of morbidity in childhood. Asthma occurs more than twice as often in boys as in girls during childhood, and parental asthma, early eczema, and wheeze in the first year are significant risk factors. In girls the only significant risk factor is early eczema (Horwood and others, 1985). This has led some to speculate that asthma may be sex influenced, with expression in genetically susceptible males (Fergusson, Horwood, and Shannon, 1983). During adolescence boys and girls are affected equally; in adulthood women slightly outnumber men. Onset is rare in the first year of life but not uncommon in the second, and the majority of childhood cases have their onset before the seventh year. Socioeconomic level appears to have no effect on the incidence, but urban dwellers appear to be more prone to asthma than persons who live in the country.

Etiology

The usual cause of the asthmatic manifestations is an allergic hypersensitivity to foreign substances, usually those carried in the air, such as plant pollens. However, in some instances no allergic process can be detected. It is a complex disorder in which biochemical, immunologic, infectious, endocrine, and psychologic factors are involved to varying degrees in different persons. A prominent feature of asthma is the heightened airway irritability, manifested by hyperreactivity of the trachea and bronchi to irritants (Boushey and others, 1980; Gurwitz, Mindorff, and Levison, 1981).

Asthma is classified variously as *allergic* (reaginic) and *nonallergic* (nonreaginic). Most asthma in children is caused by an allergic reaction in the bronchi, but there may be nonallergic precipitating factors such as bronchial compression from external pressure, a foreign body in the airway, a diffuse endobronchial inflammation, or postexercise bronchial constriction. Asthma is also described as (1) *extrinsic asthma,* caused by allergens or other external factors, (2) *intrinsic asthma,* caused by nonallergic factors such as bacterial infection, cold, or emotional stimuli, and (3) *mixed asthma,* having components of both extrinsic and intrinsic asthmas.

Asthma is further described as:

spasmodic, intermittent, or **mild asthma** Attacks occur intermittently (fewer than six times per year) with long symptom-free intervals.

frequent or **moderately severe asthma** Airway obstruction is found several times per month.

continuous asthma Daily wheezing is present.

exercise-induced asthma An asthma attack is triggered by physical exercise.

intractable or **severe asthma** Symptoms are constant and unrelieved by bronchodilators.

status asthmaticus There is little or no response to bronchodilators, and respiratory metabolism is unbalanced.

The familial association among asthma, allergic rhinitis, and atopic dermatitis suggests a common genetic basis for these disorders. There is frequently a family history of allergy and the tendency appears to come from both sides of the family: the likelihood of asthma is greater if one parent has asthma than if neither does and greater still if both parents are asthmatic (Bierman and Pearlman, 1983). The relationship between asthma and IgE-mediated diseases (especially allergic rhinitis) is established. There is a higher incidence of these diseases in families although the specific form may vary. Usually the child has other manifestations of allergy such as nasal allergy, eczema, or urticaria.

Pathophysiology

There is general agreement that heightened airway reactivity is characteristic of children with asthma. The reasons for this are less clear, and most theories do not explain all types and causes of asthma. Some of the theories attribute the hyperreactivity to (1) an exaggeration of the normal defenses of the respiratory tract, (2) abnormal tissue reactions in the bronchioles, possibly immunologically induced, or (3) an imbalance of normally balanced responses. However, the mechanisms responsible for the obstructive symptoms of asthma are (Fig. 32-5):

1. Edema of the mucous membranes
2. Accumulation of tenacious secretions from mucous glands
3. Spasm of the smooth muscle of the bronchi and bronchioles, which decreases the caliber of the bronchioles

The role that each of these mechanisms plays varies from patient to patient and during the course of the disease. In some patients, smooth muscle contraction is the major factor early in the episode, followed by mucosal edema and increased mucous secretion, which are predominant in contributing to the obstruction. In others the sequence of the responses is reversed.

Precipitating factors. Many of the stimuli that provoke asthmatic episodes may do so by being directly toxic or irritative, such as smoke (especially parental smoking), fumes, odors, or infection, by eliciting the immune response, or by a combination of mechanisms. Other factors that contribute to the responses are rapid changes in environmental temperature (especially cold), physical stress

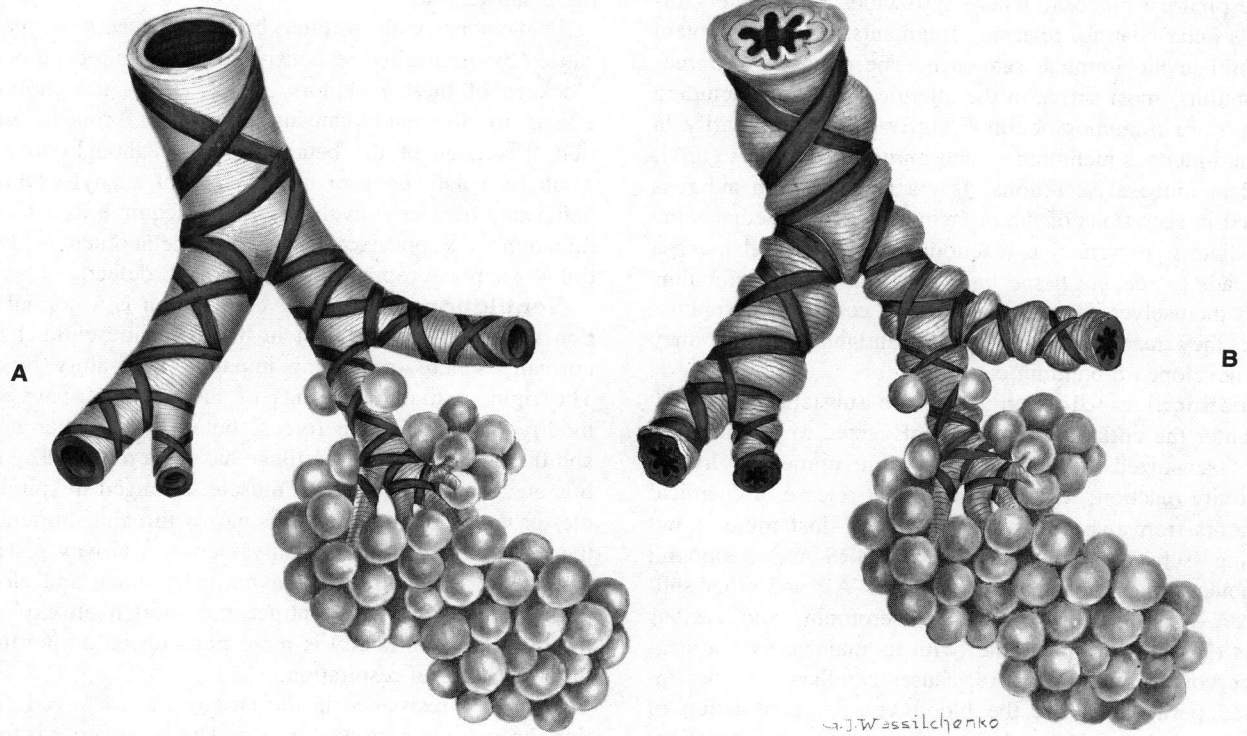

Fig. 32-5. Mechanisms of obstruction in asthma. **A,** Normal bronchus; **B,** asthmatic bronchus.

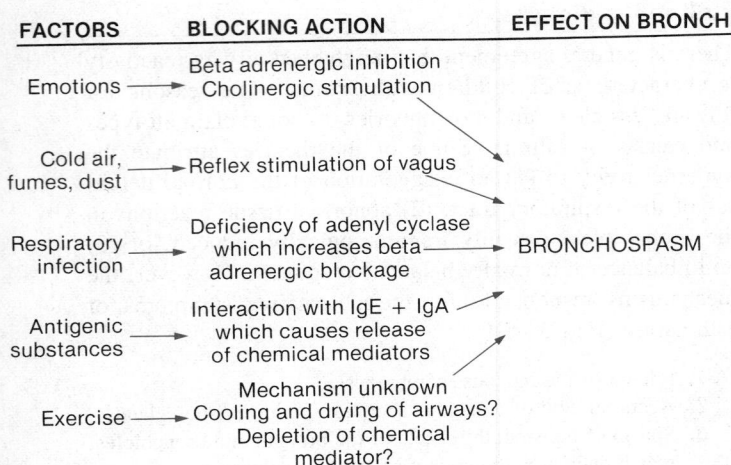

FACTORS	BLOCKING ACTION	EFFECT ON BRONCHI
Emotions	Beta adrenergic inhibition Cholinergic stimulation	
Cold air, fumes, dust	Reflex stimulation of vagus	
Respiratory infection	Deficiency of adenyl cyclase which increases beta adrenergic blockage	BRONCHOSPASM
Antigenic substances	Interaction with IgE + IgA which causes release of chemical mediators	
Exercise	Mechanism unknown Cooling and drying of airways? Depletion of chemical mediator?	

Fig. 32-6. Precipitating factors and mechanism of bronchospasm.

(fatigue, exertion), additive substances (sulfites in dried fruits and produce), medications (aspirin), psychologic stress (tension, fear, anxiety), or infections in the respiratory tract or nearby structures (such as the ears or sinuses) (Fig. 32-6).

Immunologic factors. In the majority of cases of childhood asthma there is a very strong allergic component. A vast number of substances in the environment are capable of inducing an asthmatic response, but the most significant are those that are antigenic, that is, that evoke the immune response. The antigen (or foreign substance) is deposited on the respiratory mucosa, where lysozymes immediately digest its outer coating, releasing fragments of foreign protein that initiate the immune sequence. The antibodies (immunoglobulins) most active in the allergic disorders, including asthma, are immunoglobulin E (IgE), located primarily in skin and mucous membranes, and immunoglobulin A (IgA), found in mucosal secretions. IgA acts on foreign antigens trapped in secretions of the bronchial tree. IgE mediates the immediate hypersensitive reaction in the bronchial mucosa that leads to *specific tissue binding*. Both immunoglobulins attach themselves to surfaces of mast cells and basophils, where they react with the specific antigen to which they have developed a bonding capacity.

Chemical mediators. Antigenic substances, as they encounter the antibodies (IgA or IgE) fixed to the lung tissue of sensitized individuals, trigger an immediate hypersensitivity reaction, with the subsequent release of chemical mediators from mast cells and basophils—histamine, slow-reacting substance of anaphylaxis (SRS-A), eosinophil chemotactic factor of anaphylaxis (ECF-A), and other substances, including prostaglandins, serotonin, and various kinins (Fig. 32-5). Histamine, with its major effect on central nervous system receptors, causes capillary dilation, increased permeability of the blood vessels, contraction of smooth muscle, and stimulation of mucous gland secretion. SRS-A, although its effects are less well defined, produces

contraction of bronchial muscles, with a delayed and more prolonged action than histamine.

Vagal stimulation. Normally the balance of vagal and sympathetic nerve influences maintains the tone of bronchial smooth muscle. Irritant receptors on the bronchial mucosa stimulated by various antigenic (pollens, dust) or nonantigenic (smoke, fumes, cold) stimuli trigger a reflex bronchospasm that narrows the airway. This normal reflex mechanism is designed to protect the alveoli from harmful stimuli in the bronchi; however, in the asthmatic person the bronchial constriction is abnormally severe. Acetylcholine, a neurotransmitter, mediates the vagal response.

β-Adrenergic system. The two basic adrenergic receptors, alpha and beta, are located in the smooth muscle of the bronchi. Normally the physiologic tone of the bronchial airway represents a balance between bronchorelaxation, induced by sympathetic (β-adrenergic) stimulation, and bronchoconstriction, caused by vagal (cholinergic) stimulation and, to some extent, by α-adrenergic stimulation. Beta receptors are located in the glands, smooth muscle, and blood vessels of the bronchi. Stimulation of β-adrenergic receptors activates the enzyme *adenyl cyclase*, which catalyzes the synthesis of another essential intracellular substance, *cyclic adenosine monophosphate (cyclic 3'-5'-AMP, or cyclic AMP)*. Cyclic AMP inhibits the release of mediator substances from mast cells and also activates the mechanism that either prevents contraction or induces relaxation of bronchial smooth muscle. Cyclic AMP is degraded by the enzyme *phosphodiesterase*. The tissue level of cyclic AMP is modulated by these two enzymes, and drug therapy for bronchial asthma is based on the intracellular activities of these substances.

In persons with asthma bronchial reactions may be caused by diminished responsiveness of beta receptors or by blockage of these receptors, which allows the cholinergic effects to dominate, causing unopposed bronchoconstriction. Blockage of the beta receptors is thought to be the result of a deficiency or malfunction of adenyl cyclase. A deficiency of adenyl cyclase may be acquired as a result of infection, the presence of certain metabolites or certain drugs, such as propranolol, or a genetic defect.

Ventilation. Bronchiolar constriction is a normal reaction to foreign stimuli, but in the asthmatic child it is abnormally severe, producing impaired respiratory function. The rigid cartilaginous rings of the upper airways act to modify the constrictive forces, but in the smaller bronchi and the bronchioles the cartilage has been replaced by membranous tissue. The smooth muscle, arranged in spiral bundles around the airway, causes narrowing and shortening of the airway, which significantly increases airway resistance to airflow. Since the bronchi normally dilate and elongate during inspiration and contract and shorten on expiration, the respiratory difficulty is more pronounced during the expiratory phase of respiration.

Increased resistance in the airway causes forced expiration through the narrowed lumen. The volume of air trapped in the lungs increases as airways are functionally closed at a point between the alveoli and the lobar bronchi by the combined mechanisms just described. As the severity of the asthma increases, the airways close at higher residual volume. This gas trapping is the central physiologic feature in the clinical manifestations of asthma, as it forces the individual to breathe at a higher and higher lung volume. This in turn increases the elastic work of breathing and decreases the mechanical efficiency of respiratory muscles. Consequently the person with asthma fights to inspire sufficient air, and there is hyperinflation of alveoli, which increases the diameter of the airways by exerting lateral traction on bronchiolar walls. This helps gas exchange but requires more energy during inspiration to overcome the tension of already stretched elastic lung tissues. This expenditure of effort for breathing causes fatigue, decreased respiratory effectiveness, and increased oxygen consumption and cardiac output at a time when the gas exchange and cardiac output are already compromised. In addition, the inspiration occurring at higher lung volumes reduces the effectiveness of the cough. The child becomes progressively dyspneic, cyanotic, and tachypneic.

Gas exchange. The degree to which impaired respiration interferes with gas exchanges depends to a large measure on the ratio of poorly ventilated and hyperextended alveoli to well-ventilated alveoli. Other factors that reduce the ventilatory efficiency include atelectasis and pneumonia. When the number of poorly ventilated alveoli increases, the degree of arterial hypoxemia also increases; in cases of complete airway obstruction there is a right-to-left pulmonary shunt with total absence of ventilation.

While there are a sufficient number of well-ventilated alveolar-capillary units, perfusion remains adequate and carbon dioxide elimination is not impaired. As the severity of obstruction increases, there is a reduced alveolar ventilation with carbon dioxide retention, hypoxemia, respiratory acidosis, and eventually respiratory failure.

Complications. The most prominent complications associated with asthma are:

Infection resulting from diminished efficiency of defenses and mucous growth media
Atelectasis—partial, recurrent, or chronic
Emphysema caused by chronic hyperinflation
Pneumothorax
Collapsed lung
Status asthmaticus
Cor pulmonale with right-sided heart failure
Misuse of medications (sedatives, aerosols, tranquilizers, theophylline)
Emotional and behavior problems

Clinical Manifestations

Bronchial asthma in children is sometimes confused with acute middle and lower respiratory tract infections, congenital stridor, upper airway edema resulting from multiple causes, a foreign body in the bronchi or trachea, bronchial or tracheal compression, and cystic fibrosis. There is often a history of atopic dermatitis or allergic rhinitis in the child and/or a history of familial allergic disease. The age of the child is often a significant factor, since the onset of most cases occurs between ages 3 and 8 years. In infancy an attack usually follows a respiratory infection. If the child has a history of asthma, the diagnosis is almost assured.

Children with bronchial asthma may show signs and experience symptoms that range from discrete, acute episodes of shortness of breath, wheezing, and cough followed by a quiescent period to a relatively continuous pattern of chronic symptoms that fluctuate in severity. The onset of an attack may develop gradually or appear abruptly and may be preceded by an upper respiratory infection. As a rule, episodes associated with infections are insidious in onset and prolonged; those caused by a specific allergen are acute and short lived if the causative agent is removed.

It has been observed that children may experience a prodromal itching localized at the front of the neck or over the upper part of the back just before an attack (David and others, 1984). An asthmatic episode begins with a hacking, paroxysmal, irritative, and nonproductive cough caused by bronchial edema. Accumulated secretions, acting as a foreign body, stimulate the cough. As the secretions become more profuse, the cough becomes rattling and productive of frothy, clear, gelatinous sputum. Bronchial spasm and mucosal edema reduce the size of the bronchial lumen, which is, as a result, more easily occluded by mucous plugs.

The child appears short of breath, he tries to breathe more deeply, and the expiratory phase becomes prolonged and is accompanied by an audible wheezing. He often appears pale but may have a malar flush and red ears. His lips assume a deep, dark red color that may progress to cyanosis observed in the nail beds and skin, especially around the mouth. The child is restless and apprehensive, and his facial expression is anxious. Sweating may be prominent as the attack progresses. Older children have a tendency to sit upright with shoulders in a hunched-over position, hands on the bed or chair, and arms braced to facilitate the use of accessory muscles of respiration. The child speaks with short, panting, broken phrases. Infants and small children are restless, irritable, and difficult to make comfortable. The severity of the attack can be evaluated on the basis of the child's refusal to lie down and sweating. A nonsweating child who remains upright is moderately ill; one who remains recumbent is the least ill.

The prolonged expiratory phase is less apparent in infants and young children because of a more pliable chest and the normal rapid respiratory rate. Therefore expiratory and inspiratory dyspnea are more difficult to differentiate. Infants may display intercostal and suprasternal retractions.

Examination of the chest reveals hyperresonance on percussion. Breath sounds are coarse and loud, with sonorous rales throughout the lung fields. Expiration is prolonged. Coarse rhonchi, as well as generalized inspiratory and expiratory wheezing that becomes more high pitched as obstruction progresses, can be heard. With minimal obstruction, wheezing may be only slight or even absent, but it can be accentuated by rapid, deep breathing.

With severe spasm or obstruction, breath sounds and rales may become almost audible. Cough is ineffective despite repeated, hacking maneuvers. This represents lack of air movement and may be misinterpreted as improvement by unknowing examiners. Shallow or irregular respirations and a sudden rise in the rate of respiration are ominous signs indicating ventilatory failure and imminent asphyxia.

Children with chronic asthma develop generalized vascularization, mucosal thickening, and hypertrophy of the mucous glands and fibers of the bronchial musculature. With repeated episodes the thoracic cavity becomes fixed in a hyperventilated state (barrel chest) with depressed diaphragm, elevated shoulders, and use of accessory muscles of respiration. The child's face takes on a typical appearance with flattened malar bones, circles beneath the eyes, narrow nose, and prominent upper teeth.

Diagnostic Evaluation

The diagnosis is determined on the basis of clinical manifestations, history, physical examination, and to a lesser extent laboratory tests. Radiographic examinations are used primarily to rule out other diseases and to evaluate coexisting disease. Sputum examination shows large numbers of eosinophils and colorless crystalloid fragments representing degeneration of eosinophils—Charcot-Leyden crystals, a unique feature of asthma.

There may be leukocytosis resulting from stress, dehydration, or infection. Most asthmatic children tend to have above-average hematocrit values and hemoglobin concentration, which are probably related to chronic hypoxemia with dehydration as a contributing factor. The eosinophil count is frequently over 5% and may reach 30% to 40% in longstanding, severe disease. There is no conclusive proof concerning significant alterations in gamma globulin levels.

Measurements of total and specific immunoglobulin E (IgE) levels in serum determine the sensitivity of the patient's leukocytes for antigen-induced histamine release. The paper radioimmunosorbent test (PRIST) or the double antibody radioimmunoassay procedure provides quantitative measures of IgE. Individuals with allergic disorders have higher concentrations of IgE. There are tests that determine IgE levels against specific antigens such as ragweed, grass, house dust, and some other inhalants, and the radioallergosorbent test (RAST) helps identify antigens against various foods.

Skin testing is useful in identifying specific allergens, and those obtained by the puncture technique correlate better than intracutaneous tests with symptoms and measurements of specific IgE antibody. Provocative testing, direct exposure of the mucous membranes to a suspected antigen in increasing concentrations, helps to identify inhaled allergens.

Pulmonary function tests are helpful in diagnosis and follow-up of patients with asthma. Measurements of forced expiratory volume at 1 second (FEV_1), forced vital capacity (FVC), and their ratios (FEV_1/FVC) give some indication of the degree of obstruction and are used both for diagnosis and as guidelines for management. A simple mechanical spirometer is available for use in offices and clinics as well as a pediatric flow meter for measurements in young children at home. The children are taught the necessary maneuver by practice on a party favor.

Challenge tests. Airway hyperreactivity to substances forms the basis of the challenge tests for asthma. Inhalation of an antigen to which the patient has a positive skin test is used to test the relevance of skin tests and the effects of drugs or other therapy on the bronchial response. These are potentially dangerous and are used only when other methods fail to provide the information needed, and they are only performed by specialists with training in their use and with emergency drugs and equipment at hand.

Exercise tolerance tests are useful for providing information on the individual child's ability to exercise and to participate in sports and normal recreational activities. Adolescents and children over 6 years of age are challenged on a treadmill to precipitate a response in children who have a history of exercise-induced bronchospasm. The test is also employed to measure the efficacy of drug control.

A safe and simple test for diagnosis of asthma is the cold air inhalation challenge test. Asthmatic children respond to isocapneic hyperventilation with cold air differently than nonasthmatic children. There is a significant decrease in vital capacity, forced expiratory volume, peak flow rate, and maximum midexpiratory flow rate in asthmatic children, and there has been no respiratory distress following testing (McLaughlin and Dozor, 1983).

Therapeutic Management: General

The overall goal of asthma management is to prevent disability and to minimize physical and psychologic morbidity—to assist the child to live as normal and happy a life as possible (see box). This includes facilitating the child's social adjustments in the family, school, and community and normal participation in recreational activities and sports (Bierman and Pearlman, 1983). To accomplish these goals the efforts are directed toward recognizing acute episodes early and implementing appropriate therapy, identifying and eliminating irritant and allergic factors from the child's environment, educating parents to the long-term nature of the disease and how to manage exacerbations, and helping the child to deal constructively with the disease. Compliance to the prescribed regimen is essential to successful management.

Periodic pulmonary function tests are performed to follow the course of the disease, evaluate the response to therapy, and regulate the duration and form of therapy. Most children learn to perform the necessary maneuvers with reliability after a short period of patient and careful instruction. Younger children (less than 6 years) may require longer practice.

Allergen control. Basic to any therapeutic plan is an evaluation of the child's general health and an assessment

GOALS OF ASTHMA THERAPY

1. Control symptoms to the maximum possible with a minimum number of the safest medications.
2. Participate in normal daily activities and sports without restrictions or with minimum and specific restrictions.
3. Prevent acute episodes that require emergency treatment.
4. Reduce the number and frequency of hospitalizations.
5. Educate the patient and family to understand, accept, and manage asthma within the context of the family's life-style.
6. Relieve airway obstruction and normalize pulmonary function.
7. Improve the long-term prognosis.
8. Achieve normal growth and development.
9. Minimize school absenteeism.

Modified from Hen, J., Jr.: An overview of pediatric asthma, Pediatr. Ann. 15:92-96, 1985.

of the specific allergenic factors and the nonspecific factors that precipitate symptoms. House dust mites and other components of house dust are the agents identified most often in children allergic to inhalants. Other causes are animal dander (especially cats and dogs), fungi, and allergenic pollens. Irritants that can cause bronchoconstriction in asthmatic individuals whether there is also allergy or not are cigarette smoking, especially maternal smoking (the most common source of local air pollution), wood-burning stoves, kerosene heaters, and fireplaces.

Once the specific allergens are identified and confirmed by provocative tests, steps are taken to eliminate or avoid the offending allergens. Often simply removing environmental factors will provide protection from attacks, for example, removal of a dog or cat from the home of a child sensitive to animal dander. Allergenic foods are eliminated from the diet. Nonspecific factors that may trigger an attack, such as extremes of temperature, are sometimes controlled by humidifiers or air conditioners, and the child can be helped to develop a tolerance to temperature fluctuations by gradual or systematic exposure to temperature differences.

Drug therapy. Most children do not require medication continuously. The goal is to control the acute attack; therefore early recognition and treatment at the onset are most important. Rapid relief of the bronchospasm reduces the need for drastic measures and increases the likelihood that relief will be complete. Parents and older asthmatic children are taught to implement therapy at the onset of symptoms or when exposed to symptom-provoking situations.

Rapid-acting bronchodilators are the major therapeutic agents for the relief of bronchospasm. These are the β-adrenergic agonists and the methylxanthines. Each appears to work differently, and they may be synergistic in their actions on the airways. The β-adrenergic agonists provide relief from an acute attack and can be used to prevent exercise-induced asthma. They are available in syrups, tablets,

injectable solutions, metered dose inhalers, and solutions for inhalation therapy. The most effective method of administration is by metered-dose inhaler (metaproterenol, fenoterol, and albuterol). Inhalers are difficult to use with very young children. Children age 3 to 6 years old are best managed with a Spinhaler or other device that does not require coordinating delivery of the drug with inspiration. Table 32-5 outlines the major pharmacologic agents used in the treatment of asthma.

The methylxanthine drugs, principally theophylline, are probably the most effective and versatile asthmatic drugs. They are prepared for intravenous, intramuscular, oral, or rectal administration. The xanthines block the effect of phosphodiesterase to prevent the breakdown and thus prolong the action of adenyl cyclase, the adrenergic activator.

The administration of a corticosteroid preparation may provide significant relief of an attack when symptoms are not controlled by other therapies. The drugs can be given intravenously, orally, or topically by aerosol. The corticosteroids are not actually drugs but act by their hormonal effect; therefore results are delayed for up to 6 hours. The antiinflammatory effect diminishes the inflammatory component of asthma and thereby reduces the airway obstruction. The hormonal effects are less clear. There is also evidence to indicate that they in some way increase beta-adrenergic sensitivity and induce a decreased phosphodiesterase activity in tissues, thus allowing accumulation of cyclic AMP. Corticosteroids are lifesaving in status asthmaticus.

Cromolyn sodium is neither a bronchodilator nor an antiinflammatory agent but acts superficially to inhibit the release of chemical mediators, especially histamine, in the human lung. The action is essentially prophylactic and is of no value when the drug is administered after the allergic reaction. Its chief value is to prevent an attack, and it is especially useful in preventing exercise-induced bronchospasm.

Antihistamines are sometimes useful by decreasing postnasal drip–induced cough that may lead to bronchospasm, but they are not a routine part of medical management. In the case of infection the appropriate antibiotic is administered. Expectorants, long used in asthma therapy, have not been shown to be effective.

Exercise. Vigorous physical activity is frequently followed by an asthmatic attack; therefore children with asthma are often excluded from exercise by parents, teachers, and physicians as well as the children themselves because they are reluctant to provoke an attack. This can seriously hamper peer interaction. It has been found that moderate exercise or even strenuous exercise is advantageous for children with asthma. In fact some investigators have found significant improvement in work tolerance and cardiopulmonary fitness (Nickerson and others, 1983; Orenstein and others, 1985).

The Committee on Children with Disabilities and the Committee on Sports Medicine of the American Academy

Table 32-5 Pharmaceutic agents used in the treatment of asthma

DRUG	ADMINISTRATION	ACTION	NURSING CONSIDERATIONS
Beta adrenergics Terbutaline (Bricanyl, Brethine)	Oral Subcutaneous (IV available)	High potency Primarily β_2 effects Provides prolonged effects up to 6 hours	Minimum side effects Not recommended for children less than 12 yr of age Subcutaneous: repeat dose in 30 min if no response; not to exceed total of 0.5 mg/4 hr
Albuterol (Proventil)	Oral Inhalation	High potency Primarily β_2 stimulation	No side effects Not recommended for children less than 12 yr of age Better results from nebulized administration; not to exceed 12 inhalations/day
Metaproterenol (Metaprel, Alupent)	Oral Inhalation	Moderate potency Acts on both alpha and beta receptors	Lacks potency for acute attacks Avoid excess heat; refrigerate unit dose vial; store inhalant at room temperature
Isoetherine (Bronkosol-2, Dey-Lute)	Aerosol administration per IPPB	Mild potency Acts on alpha and beta receptors	Pediatric dosage not standardized
Epinephrine (adrenalin)	0.01 mg/kg/dose (max. 0.5 ml) of 1:100 aqueous IM Subcutaneous Aerosol	High potency Rapid action; short duration α, β_1 and β_2 effects	Repeat in 20 min if no relief; repeat 2-4 times Destroyed by light; store only in dark glass vials Brown color indicates deterioration Observe child for sympathetic nervous system stimulation (tachycardia, increased blood pressure)
Sus-Phrine	0.05-0.3 ml of 1:200 solution Subcutaneous	High potency Released slowly over 4-8 hr α, β_1, and β_2 effects	Observations same as for epinephrine Contains 50% epinephrine and 80% crystalline epinephrine to prolong action
Isoproterenol (Isuprel, Aerolone)	Aerosol per IPPB or aerosolized IV Sublingual	Rapid relief of symptoms Primarily β_2 stimulation Increases velocity of mucous transport in trachea	Potentiates side effects of epinephrine; should not be given within 1 hr after epinephrine or Sus-Phrine Dosage individualized Freon-propelled aerosol units not recommended for children
Ephedrine	PO Subcutaneous IM	Moderately high potency Less potent than epinephrine; more prolonged action Acts on α, β_1, and β_2 receptors	Watch for side effects of beta stimulation Often combined with phenobarbital
Methylxanthines Theophylline (Bronkodyl, Elixophyllin)	Oral IV Rectal suppository	Blocks phosphodiesterase to prevent breakdown of and prolong action of adenyl cyclase (adrenergic activator) Inhibits release of histamine and other mediators Improves diaphragm contractility	Wide individual variation in rate of metabolism Children metabolize drug faster than adults Available as short- or long-acting preparations Serum levels must be monitored Oral preparations should be given with food Observe for signs of toxicity: fever, restlessness, nausea, vomiting, hypotension, and abdominal discomfort
Aminophylline (Phyllocontin)	Oral IV Rectal suppository	Same as theophylline Contains 78% anhydrous theophylline and 12% ethylenediamine	Same as above

Table 32-5 Pharmaceutic agents used in the treatment of asthma—cont'd

DRUG	ADMINISTRATION	ACTION	NURSING CONSIDERATIONS
Corticosteroids			
Hydrocortisone (Solu-Cortef) Methylprednisolone (Solu-Medrol)	IV	All: Potentiate an increase in cyclic AMP that promotes bronchodilation; inhibits cyclic GMP, which induces smooth muscle contraction	Given for shortest time and smallest dose possible to achieve desirable effect Life-saving in status asthmaticus Undesirable effects on systemic growth
Prednisone	Oral	Shorter acting	Protect child from infection
Triamcinolone (Aristocort, Kenocort) Betamethasone Dexamethasone (Decadron)	Oral	Longer acting	
Beclomethasone dipropionate (Vanceril, Aldicin, Becotide, Viarex)	Inhalation	Deactivated first time through liver	Fewer steroid side effects Not recommended for children less than 6 yr of age
Prophylactic agent Cromolyn sodium (Aarane, Intol)	Inhalation	Acts primarily through local effect on respiratory tract mucosa Prevents release of histamine and leukotrienes from mast cells	Taken to prevent asthmatic attack

of Pediatrics (1984) agree that physical activities are useful to asthmatic children and that the majority can participate in activities at school and in sports with minimum difficulty, provided the asthma is under control. Participation is encouraged but should be evaluated on an individual basis in terms of tolerance for duration and intensity of effort. Appropriate prophylactic treatment with β-adrenergic agents administered by aerosol or orally before exercise will usually permit full participation in strenuous exertion. Restrictions are invoked only when the condition of the child makes it necessary.

Asthma camps have become popular in recent years as a means of encouraging physical activity in a more homogeneous, controlled, and less competitive environment. Not all persons subscribe to this practice. There are those who support the positive benefits, which are primarily that the denominator of asthma is removed as a factor. Everyone at the camp has asthma; therefore no child is different from the others. On the other hand, many believe that such segregation from family and peers serves only to reinforce the sick role.

Physical therapy. Physical therapy is one of the standard adjuncts to treatment of chronic, or frequent, asthma. This includes chest physical therapy, breathing exercises, physical training, and inhalation therapy. These therapies help to produce physical and mental relaxation, improve posture, strengthen respiratory musculature, and develop more efficient patterns of breathing. Postural drainage, which includes percussion, vibration, deep breathing, and assisted coughing, helps to clear mucus from the bronchial tree (see p. 1315). For the motivated child, breathing exercises and controlled breathing are of value in preventing overinflation and in improving the strength of respiratory muscles and the efficiency of the cough. Stretch exercises sometimes help to increase the flexibility of the ribs. Sit-ups and leg exercises strengthen abdominal muscles and aid expiration.

Hyposensitization. The role of hyposensitization in childhood asthma has not been clarified. In many cases the child demonstrates multiple sensitivities, which makes such therapy impractical. Moreover, the injections can be uncomfortable. When the allergen can be defined and is one that cannot be avoided or controlled satisfactorily by drugs, specific hyposensitization is seriously considered. Immune therapy is not recommended for allergens that can be eliminated effectively, for example, food sensitivities, drugs, and animal dander. Inhalant allergens such as house dust, pollens, and molds are most often the allergens considered for immune therapy.

Injection therapy is usually limited to clinically significant allergens. The initial dose of the offending allergen(s), based on the size of the skin reaction, is injected subcutaneously. The amount is increased at weekly intervals until a maximum tolerance is reached, after which a maintenance dose is given at 4-week intervals. This may be extended to 5- or 6-week intervals during the off-season for seasonal allergens. Successful treatment is continued for a minimum of 3 years and then stopped. If no symptoms appear, the acquired immunity is said to be retained; if symptoms recur, the treatment is reinstituted.

Prognosis. The outlook for children with asthma varies widely. An impressive number of children lose their symptoms at puberty, but there is no factor that can predict which children will "outgrow" their asthma. Some develop other forms of allergy in adulthood. It has been postulated that, just as the skin manifestations of infancy (eczema) shift to the bronchi in childhood, there may be another shift in the susceptible tissues (shock organ) at adulthood—most frequently to the nose.

The prognosis for control of symptoms or disappearance of symptoms will differ from children who have rare and infrequent attacks to those who are constantly wheezing or some who are subject to status asthmaticus. In general, the more severe and numerous the symptoms, the longer they have been present, and the prognosis for improvement is poorer when there is a family history of allergy. Many who outgrow them are subject to exercise-induced asthma as adults, and the associated disorders such as growth impairment, chest deformity, and airway obstruction are maintained throughout life.

Therapeutic Management: Specific

Children are subject to asthmatic attacks at varying intervals, and the severity can also vary from wheezing to life-threatening status asthmaticus. The modes of management vary according to the frequency and severity of the disease.

Intermittent (mild) asthma. Children with intermittent asthma need rapid relief of symptoms and drugs are prescribed for attacks only. Some find the most rapidly effective drug for these children is aerosol albuterol or fenoterol, which provides sustained bronchodilation and long-lasting inhibition of exercise-induced asthma (Sly, 1986). Others may prescribe different drugs, but all are intended for fast relief.

Because the bronchoconstriction is likely to persist for several days following relief of symptoms, the children are prescribed a bronchodilator for 4 to 5 days after resolution of coughing and wheezing. The most frequently prescribed drug is theophylline (usually a sustained-release preparation), which is available in tablets (Theo-Dur tablets) for children who can swallow tablets and sustained-release beads from a capsule (e.g., Theo-Dur Sprinkle, Slo-Bid Gyrocaps, or Somophylline-CRT) that are sprinkled on applesauce. Metaproterenol and terbutaline are alternative drugs. Infants and toddlers require liquid preparations of theophylline or metaproterenol.

Frequent asthma. Children with attacks several times each month require continual drug therapy when allergens are difficult to avoid. Sustained-release theophylline is prescribed with β-adrenergic oral or aerosol medication (e.g., terbutaline or metaproterenol) for attacks that occur despite

continual treatment. Sometimes cromolyn sodium is preferred over theophylline because of its paucity of side effects. When these drugs afford inadequate control, corticosteroids may be needed.

Exercise-induced asthma. If asthma on exercise is ineffectively controlled by nasal breathing or other measures, such as a cold weather mask or a muffler or scarf wrapped around the nose and mouth, medication before anticipated exercise may be needed. Pretreatment with a bronchodilator provides relief through the exercise period. Inhaled albuterol or fenoterol can inhibit an attack for 4 to 6 hours; cromolyn sodium is most effective during the first hour after inhalation but some effect remains for 4 hours. Sustained-release theophylline is probably most convenient for the youngster who may be exercising unpredictably at any time in the day, but optimum effectiveness can be achieved only if the drug is administered on a continual basis or a very large dose given to maintain the needed serum levels. Sometimes combinations of an inhaled β agonist with cromolyn or theophylline are more effective (Sly, 1986).

Bronchodilation for 1 to 2 minutes occurs in some children following strenuous exercise, whereas 5 to 6 minutes of sustained but moderate exercise causes airway obstruction. These children better tolerate activities that require only intermittent, brief intervals of exercise (e.g., baseball, sprinting, gymnastics, or skiing) rather than activities that involve endurance exercise (e.g., soccer, basketball, distance running). Swimming, even long-distance swimming, is well tolerated by children with asthma. This is partly because they are breathing air fully saturated with moisture, but it may also be a result of the type of breathing required. Exhaling under water prolongs each expiration and increases the end-expiratory pressure within the respiratory tree (essentially pursed-lip breathing).

Severe asthma. Children who continue to have incapacitating dyspnea, cough, and obstructed airways regardless of treatment prescribed for moderate asthma may require long-term corticosteroid therapy. Detracting from their use are dangers of steroid dependency and undesirable side effects, including cushingoid changes, increased susceptibility to infection, and growth suppression. When oral steroids are used over a long period, they are gradually reduced to the smallest possible maintenance dose and replaced with aerosol steroids because the hypothalamic-pituitary-adrenal axis can take up to a year to recover normal responsiveness. The drug is then discontinued as soon as possible.

Status asthmaticus. Children who continue to display respiratory distress despite vigorous therapeutic measures, especially injections of epinephrine, are considered to be in status asthmaticus. The condition may develop gradually or rapidly, often coincident with complicating conditions such as pneumonia that can influence the duration and treatment of the attack. These children are acutely ill and require hospitalization, preferably where intensive care is available. They need continuous nursing attendance with frequent monitoring and observation.

The drug most frequently prescribed in emergency rooms for acute, severe asthma in the United States is aqueous epinephrine 1:1000 followed by epinephrine 1:200 (Sus-Phrine) when there has been a satisfactory response (terbutaline is equally effective). An inhaled β agonist is often as effective as injections of epinephrine but requires longer observation. Nebulization better delivers the drug to the lower airways than a metered-dose inhaler during severe airway obstruction. Failure to respond to these drugs establishes the diagnosis of status asthmaticus.

Persistent hypoventilation leads to accumulation of carbon dioxide, with a decrease in arterial pH and respiratory acidosis. As a result, compensatory buffering mechanisms become overtaxed and the pH may drop to dangerous levels. Vomiting and dehydration cause further reduction of arterial pH by promoting retention of metabolic acids. Therapy of status asthmaticus is directed toward correction of dehydration and acidosis, improvement of ventilation, and treatment of any concurrent infection.

The child is given intravenous fluids and nothing by mouth except liquids if his condition permits. The intravenous infusion provides a means for hydration, liquefying secretions, and administering medications. The correction of dehydration, acidosis, hypoxia, and electrolyte derangements is guided by frequent determination of arterial pH, PO_2, PCO_2, and serum electrolytes. Acidosis is corrected by administration of sodium bicarbonate in sufficient amounts to maintain pH at acceptable levels.

A loading dose of aminophylline (5 mg/kg) is infused intravenously over 20 minutes, followed by constant infusion of 0.5 to 1.1 mg/kg/hr to maintain serum concentrations of 10 to 20 µg/ml (ideally 14 to 18 µg/ml if tolerated). Metaproterenol or terbutaline is administered every 2 hours by inhalation after nebulization. (These drugs are not recommended for children less than 12 years of age.) Isoproterenol may be given intravenously to children less than 14 years of age; there is increased frequency of cardiac arrhythmias in adolescents. Adrenal corticosteroids, either hydrocortisone 4 mg/kg or methylprednisolone 1 mg/kg, are administered intravenously every 4 hours. Sedatives, tranquilizers, morphine, and antihistamines are contraindicated (Sly, 1986). However, mild sedatives, usually chloral hydrate or a tranquilizing agent, may be given with caution to children whose agitation is not caused by hypoxia.

Humidified oxygen is administered by tent, face mask, or cannula to maintain an arterial PO_2 greater than 65 torr but less than 100 torr to avoid the danger of oxygen narcosis. Since oxygen is a stimulus for respiration, high levels may significantly depress respirations. Controlled ventilation with endotracheal intubation may be needed when the condition progresses to respiratory failure. When assisted ventilation is used, volume respirators are usually more satisfactory than pressure-cycled respirators for children. Volume-type respirators ensure proper alveolar ventilation without overinflation and prevent high pressure caused by sudden obstruction.

Antibiotics are frequently advisable in therapy, since infection may be masked or may not always be evident and is always a threatening complication. As the attack subsides, fluids and medication are given orally and postural drainage and breathing exercises help remove secretions. Administration of steroids is withdrawn as rapidly as possible.

Psychologic Aspects

Emotional factors are known to be associated with childhood asthma; however, it is not known whether emotional disturbance is present before the onset of asthma and is a probable etiologic factor in its development or whether it occurs as a result of the asthma. Although no decisive evidence is available regarding the relative importance of all etiologic factors, the consensus accepts a multicausal etiology for childhood asthma in which hereditary, allergic, infectious, and psychologic factors assume importance independently or, more often, in combination.

Studies of children with behavioral problems indicate that family interactions play an important role in the child's adjustment to the disease. There is a high correlation between the level of disturbed family relationships and the child's psychosocial adjustments. The severity and course of illness do not appear to be related to the level of family adjustment, however.

Both short- and long-term adaptation of the asthmatic child to the disease depends to a great extent on the family's acceptance of the disorder. The task of living day to day with an asthmatic child involves the family continually. There are periodic crises and the ever-present threat of a crisis, requiring parental vigilance, sleepless nights, frequent emergency trips to the hospital, and often overwhelming medical expenses. Throughout these stresses the parents are expected and encouraged to promote as normal a life as possible for the asthmatic child without neglecting the needs of the siblings.

Parental responses to the asthmatic child with emotional disturbances range from rejection to overprotection. A significant number are overprotective, babying the child even during symptom-free periods. Frequently, believing that physical activity precipitates the attacks, the parents attempt to limit the physical activities of their child—in some cases to the point of confining the child to the home. The child appears fearful, is usually physically inactive, and lacks self-confidence. The child has few friends, and the parental protective behavior further alienates him from his peers. On reaching adolescence the overprotected child may rebel against the control to become defiant and overactive, often accompanied by a careless attitude toward the management of his illness that places him at risk for serious respiratory events.

Although encountered less frequently, the child of negligent parents feels insecure and will often associate the nonaccepting behavior of the parents with provoking or worsening an attack of asthma. This may or may not be the case. However, the nonaccepting parental attitudes have usually been present before the onset of the child's asthma.

Not uncommonly parents of asthmatic children accuse

the child of manipulating his environment by deliberately precipitating an attack to gain his own ends—to gain a special consideration or to avoid a responsibility. This accusation is difficult to verify; however, there are some children who actually claim to have the power of controlling their symptoms and use this as a threat. There is some question that this behavior may represent an effort on the part of these children to master their anxiety regarding attacks by proclaiming to be in control of the onset and course of the asthmatic attacks, particularly when others fail to prevent them.

Where family relationships are determined to produce an adverse effect on the asthmatic child, psychiatric help is recommended; where disturbances are marked, foster placement or respite care in institutions providing residential care for asthmatic children is advised. A number of these facilities are available throughout the United States. A significant finding is that asthmatic symptoms are relieved when the child is removed from the parents, such as when the child is hospitalized or is away from home for other reasons. It is in these rapidly remitting children with asthma, in contrast to the steroid-dependent children, that psychologic factors assume greater significance than allergic or infectious factors in triggering symptoms. For example, an attack can be precipitated by major emotions such as anger, anxiety and worry, sadness and depression, and either pleasurable or nonpleasurable excitement. When a child repeatedly improves during separation from family members, it is strongly suspected that emotional and family interactional factors are contributing to the course of the disease.

Nursing Considerations

Nursing care of children with asthma involves both acute and long-term care and includes therapies and observations described in previous discussions of respiratory disturbances.

Acute asthma. Children who are admitted to the hospital with acute asthma are ill, anxious, and uncomfortable. In most instances the child is admitted as an emergency with status asthmaticus and is in acute distress. An intravenous infusion is begun immediately, and medication, usually corticosteroids and aminophylline, is administered to relieve bronchospasm. The child is monitored closely and continuously during aminophylline administration for relief of respiratory distress and signs of side effects or toxicity. The pulse, respiration, and blood pressure are taken and recorded every 5 minutes during rapid infusion and every 15 minutes for at least an hour after the drug has been absorbed.

It is especially important that the child receive sufficient fluid either orally or intravenously to replace losses through diaphoresis and hyperventilation. Liquids are best tolerated if they are warm or room temperature. Cold liquids can trigger reflex bronchospasm and should be avoided (Seaman-Bates, 1980). Nourishment is provided in small frequent feedings to avoid abdominal distention that might interfere with diaphragm excursion.

The child usually prefers the high-Fowler position, although he may be more comfortable sitting upright or leaning slightly forward. When possible, the nurse communicates with him in such a way that he need only reply in a few words to avoid fatigue. Shortness of breath makes talking difficult. Since oxygen is indicated, he is placed in a mist tent for relief of dyspnea and cyanosis, but an older child may prefer a nasal cannula. Oxygen is not administered indiscriminately but regulated according to the blood gas analysis and objective observation of color, respiratory effort, and sensorium. Associated treatments such as intermittent positive-pressure breathing or postural drainage, and tests, such as blood gases or pulmonary function tests, are often performed by specialized personnel, or they may be the nurse's responsibility.

The child with status asthmaticus is apprehensive and anxious. Moreover, he is usually tired from his respiratory efforts and loss of sleep. The calm, efficient presence of a nurse helps to reassure him that he is safe and will be cared for during this stressful period. It is important to ensure the child that he will not be left alone and that his parents are allowed to be near and available when he needs them.

Parents need reassurance too. They want to be informed of their child's condition and the therapies being employed. They are upset, apprehensive regarding the child's condition, and feeling guilty. Often they feel that they may have in some way contributed to the child's condition or could have prevented the attack. They may even feel, consciously or unconsciously, anger toward the child for continuing to display symptoms despite their efforts to prevent or control the attack. Reassurance regarding their efforts expended on the child's behalf and their parenting capabilities can help alleviate their stress. All efforts to reduce the parental apprehension will, in turn, help reduce the child's distress. Anxiety is easily communicated to the child from parents and members of the staff.

Long-term support. Nurses who are involved with asthmatic children in the home, clinic, or physician's office play an important role in helping the children and their families learn to live with the condition. The disease can be tolerated if it does not interfere with family life, physical activity, or school attendance or if it does not require hospitalization.

Nurses are involved in the initial assessment and workup to determine the cause and extent of the asthma. They assist with diagnostic tests, pulmonary function tests, and general health assessment. Parents need to know the nature of the disease and, when the allergens are determined, how they can avoid and/or relieve asthmatic attacks. The nurse assists the parent in planning and carrying out an elimination diet to detect foods that may precipitate symptoms. When the allergen or allergens are identified, nurses can provide valuable assistance to the parents in modifying the environment to reduce contact with the offending allergen(s) (see box on p. 1387).

The parents are cautioned to avoid exposing the child to excessive cold, wind, or other extremes of weather and to smoke, sprays, or other irritants. Although foods are an unusual cause of asthma, foods known to provoke symptoms should be eliminated from the diet. The foods most likely

"ALLERGY PROOFING" THE HOME

Reduce house dust
Child's bedroom should be for sleeping, not playing
Dust room daily and clean thoroughly weekly; child should not be in house during housecleaning activities
Floors should be bare and damp mopped daily
Remove from room unnecessary furniture, rugs, stuffed animals, upholstered furniture, etc.
Walls should be covered with washable paint or wallpaper
Hot-air heating vents should be covered to prevent circulation of dust (e.g., when heat is turned on after summer accumulation of dust); substitute electric heater (properly protected) if possible
Bedcovers, curtains, and scatter rugs should be made of smooth cotton or synthetic fabric and laundered frequently
Closets should be free of stored articles, especially woolens
If possible, install air purification unit; small unit can be placed in child's bedroom

Reduce pollen and other allergens
Bedding should be free of allergens:
 Use foam rubber or dacron pillows, synthetic blankets
 Wool or feather items should be encased in nonallergenic coverings
Use foam mattress or cover mattress and box springs with nonallergenic covers
Windows and doors should remain closed during pollen season
Pets, furry or feathered, should be excluded from home
Use only furniture upholstered in foam rubber

Reduce exposure to molds and mildew
Avoid cellars as play area
Clean showers and tile areas; spray with antimold agent (e.g., Lysol)
Keep vaporizers, air conditioners (including automobile) clean and free of mold
Keep plants and aquariums out of child's room

become distressing. A simple, inexpensive peak flow meter is available for use in the home to help parents assess the extent of the child's symptoms.* Many children are administered theophylline or other medication, and parents should understand the importance of taking the drugs as prescribed.

Older children who use a nebulizer or aerosol device to deliver adrenergic drugs need to be taught how to use the device. The metered-dose inhaler (MDI) is the device most frequently prescribed (Fig. 32-7). It combines portability with a rapid and reliable dose for patients managed at home. To achieve the greatest effect, the child is instructed to (Levison, Reilly, and Worsley, 1985):

1. Shake the inhaler
2. Remove the cap
3. Tilt the head back
4. Perform a slow, deep expiration
5. Place the inhaler in the mouth, with lips sealed
6. In the middle of a slow deep inspiration, activate the canister
7. After a full inspiration, hold the breath for at least 5 seconds

It is important to breath slowly and deeply for better distribution to narrowed airways. Rapid inspiration causes the drugs to move through unobstructed bronchioles to patent airways where they are less needed. After reaching full lung capacity, the child should count to five slowly before exhaling so that the drugs can be deposited in the obstructed airway. The child waits a prescribed length of time, then repeats the process. There is controversy regarding the amount of time to wait between puffs; the recommendations range from 3 to 10 minutes.

Young children and those who are otherwise unable to

*HealthScan Products Inc., 882 Pompton Ave., Cedar Grove, NJ 07009.

to be allergenic are eggs, peanuts and peanut butter, milk, and chocolate. Parents should be advised to read labels on prepared foods and snacks to determine the presence of allergens. For example, a tremendous number of foods contain sodium caseinate or dried milk products.

Since approximately 2% to 6% of asthmatic children are sensitive to aspirin, nurses caution the parents to use other analgesic/antipyretic drugs for discomfort or fever. Acetaminophen appears to be a safe drug for these children and is recommended as the analgesic of choice (Fischer and others, 1983). Those children with aspirin-induced asthma may also be sensitive to nonsteroidal antiinflammatory drugs and tartrazine (yellow dye number 5, a common food coloring) (Tan and Collins-Williams, 1982). Other drugs that should be avoided by asthmatic children are antihistamines (dry airway secretions, making expectoration difficult), cough suppressants (impair clearance of secretions), and sedatives (depress respirations and aggravate hypoventilation).

The parents and the older child need to learn how to use the medications prescribed to relieve bronchospasm. They are taught to recognize early signs and symptoms of an impending attack so that it can be controlled before symptoms

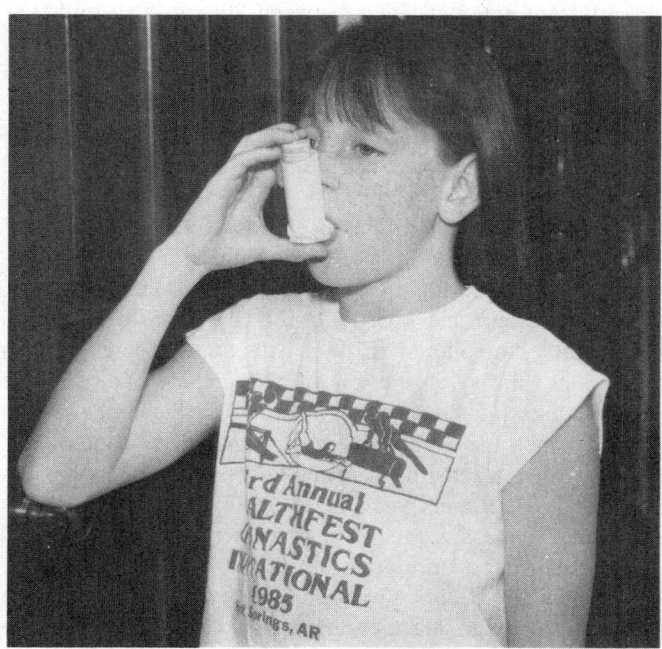

Fig. 32-7. Child using metered-dose inhaler.

manipulate the device or coordinate breathing with activation of the MDI inhaler are able to use special chambers called add-on devices, spacers, or extension tubes. These permit an operator to deliver the medication from the MDI into the spacer from which the child inhales. Some simple alteratives to the spacer have been suggested, including a modified freezer bag and a styrofoam cup with a hole made in the bottom for the MDI (Henry, Milner, and Davies, 1983). Compressor-nebulizers are now available for use with younger children.

The child and parents also need to be cautioned about the adverse effects of the drugs and the dangers of overuse. They should know that it is important to use the drugs when needed but not indiscriminately or as a substitute for avoiding the symptom-provoking allergen. Persons can become refractive to the prescribed medication. When a drug is no longer effective, this may be because of altered drug metabolism, a large causative load, or an emotional overlay. If a drug is given long enough, the body frequently develops a resistance to it. Parents and child are taught to report any changing reaction to a drug or if the drug appears to be losing its effectiveness, as evidenced by more frequent need for the drug.

Incidents of drug abuse have been reported in which children used their aerosols to experience the hallucinations the drug produced in excessive dosages. Nonasthmatic children have used the aerosols in much the same manner as glue sniffing in order to get "high" or to relieve tension and anxiety (Brennan, 1983; Thompson and others, 1983).

Parents of children who are taking prescribed theophylline should also be advised regarding side effects (which appear when serum levels exceed 40 μg/ml) and some of the substances and factors that alter the effects of the drug. Minor toxic symptoms, such as nausea, headache, and irritability, are noted at levels between 20 and 40 μg/ml; seizures have been reported for very high toxicity (Richards and others, 1985). Symptoms of depression have also been noted in susceptible children. These include sleep disturbance, headaches, abdominal pain, restlessness, hyperactivity, irritability, negativity, and unhappiness (Brumback and others, 1984).

Theophylline toxicity has been observed in patients taking their accustomed dosage of the drug after influenza immunization or during a flu epidemic (Fischer and others, 1982; Goldstein and others, 1982). Therefore they should be carefully monitored in these situations. There are also variations in the absorption of slow-release theophylline preparations related to food intake. The bioavailability is greater when the drug is taken in a fasting state than when taken with a standardized meal (Pederson and Møoller-Peterson, 1984; Rogers and others, 1985). Parents should be cautioned about the possibility of toxic reactions if the child alters the usual pattern of medication and meals.

The child should be protected from a respiratory infection that can trigger an attack or aggravate the asthmatic state, especially in young children. Their airways are mechanically smaller and more reactive; therefore edema from infection causes wheezing and other signs of respiratory obstruction. Also, the equipment used for the child, such as nebulizers, must be kept absolutely clean to decrease the chances of contamination with bacteria and fungi. Oral candidiasis is a major complication of aerosolized steroids; therefore children with severe asthma who are taking steroids by this route are taught to rinse the mouth thoroughly with water following each treatment to minimize the risk of infection.

Breathing exercises and controlled breathing are taught and encouraged for the motivated youngster, and the nurse can help him select activities suitable to his capacity. Anything that promotes proper diaphragmatic breathing, side expansion, and generally improved mobility of the chest wall is encouraged. If the child requires segmental drainage and percussion, someone in the family must assume responsibility for carrying out the procedure. It is the responsibility of the physical therapist or the nurse to teach the parent the proper technique (see Chapter 31 for description of physical therapy techniques).

Children with emotional overtones associated with their asthma create additional problems. In these children an attack can be triggered by emotional experiences mediated through several central nervous system pathways to precipitate asthmatic symptoms. Even some respiratory behaviors (such as crying, laughing, coughing, and hyperventilation) that accompany strong emotions may trigger a mechanical or reflex narrowing of the airway.

The interactions of members of the family need careful assessment to identify maladaptive behaviors and precipitating factors. A team approach is usually employed especially when family interaction may be a contributing factor in the child's illness. Sometimes all the members of the family need reassurance, education, and referral to persons or agencies that can help meet their needs with continued support and encouragement. Parent groups can be very effective in providing support to parents in dealing with their frustrations.

Sometimes it is necessary to remove the child from the family for short-term respite care and provide the family with crisis therapy. In severe cases long-term respite care is the only satisfactory solution. The children live in a residential treatment center in which the needs of the child are met by professionals. The child is removed from the interactional stress of the home environment and educated regarding the nature of his illness and how he can live with it.

The nurse working with asthmatic children can provide them with support in a number of ways. Many asthmatic children voice frustration about the ways their attacks interfere with their goal achievements and social lives. They need education concerning their disease and to realize that is it not as bad as they might think. Children, their families, and their peers need to know what to do to prevent an attack and what to do during an attack. These children need much reassurance from the health team and reinforcement of their coping mechanisms. Last of all, they need "grit"—the courage to help them live and cope with their condition 1 day at a time.

Self-management. Self-care is hallmark of effective asthma management, and self-management programs are important in helping the child and family to learn as much as possible about the factors that precipitate an asthma attack and the most effective means of bringing the disease under control. Self-managment programs have three main objectives (Lewiston, 1986):

1. To remove the stigma of self-fault for the condition
2. To integrate the reality of asthma into the life-style of the individual's choice
3. To learn management skills to avoid or minimize conditions that cause asthma attacks

Most self-management programs have four principles that are conveyed to the child and family regarding the disease and its management. First, asthma is a very common disease and to have asthma is annoying but not disgraceful. Even though emotions have been implicated in asthma, psychologic aspects are primarily a response rather than a cause. Emotions and stress can be major triggers but the disease, not the individual, is responsible for the symptoms. Absolution of the individual from the responsibility for the etiology makes the concept of a therapeutic plan more sensible and acceptable.

Second, persons with asthma are able to live full and active lives. Learning about others who have accomplished their goals (e.g., Theodore Roosevelt) and meeting children of the same age who are dealing effectively with their disease, including engaging in age-related activities, such as sports, provide positive examples of what is possible.

Third, it is much easier to prevent than to treat an asthmatic attack. The importance of compliance to a therapeutic program and learning the activities or factors that trigger an attack are emphasized. The sustained-release medications and appropriate drug administration before exercise or with a respiratory infection have made it possible for asthmatic children to avoid an attack.

Fourth, individuals do not become addicted to asthma medication but they do prefer to breathe more freely whenever possible. Emphasis is on management rather than cure. The cost/benefit of each medication is explained and attempts are a made to assess the "wheezogenic" potential by tapering the medication periodically to demonstrate that the management process is a dynamic one in which the child and the parent are active participants (Lewiston, 1986).

Several approaches are used to facilitate self-management. Self-contained programs and brochures for patient education are available through the national office of the **Asthma and Allergy Foundation of America (AAFA).*** the **American Lung Association**† also has brochures about asthma available through the local offices. One that is highly recommended is "Superstuff," a workbook for elementary and junior high school children that includes self-management techniques using a variety of educational aids. A more structured individual management product is the

workbook, "Teaching Myself About Asthma," for children 7 to 12 years.* Both have been tested and found effective for teaching (Green, Goldstein, and Parker, 1983).

Self-management instruction in group settings (e.g., camps for asthmatic children) is a very popular means for education and training. Three such packaged programs are available that have proved to be successful. Many are funded by organizations with support from local health professionals, institutions, and interested families. One, ACT (Asthma Care Training), a five-session program with the theme "You're in the driver's seat," using driving and traffic analogies, is available without charge through the Asthma and Allergy Foundation of America. Another program, which can be purchased for a nominal fee,† is "Camp Wheeze," designed for integration with recreational activities in a daycamp format. WOW (Winning Over Wheezing) is a cassette-workbook developed for group instruction distributed without charge from William H. Rorer, Inc.‡. Other programs are also available, such as Camp Broncho Junction, which offers a short-term practical program for holistic management of asthmatic children.§

Asthma education and awareness are an important aspect of asthma management. Although the principles of self-management are very general and the programs designed for general use, each child and family have their own special needs that require individualized care and attention.

CYSTIC FIBROSIS

Cystic fibrosis of the pancreas is the most common inherited disease of children. Cystic fibrosis is a generalized dysfunction of the exocrine (mucous-producing) glands and is one of the most serious chronic diseases that affect white children. It accounts for a large percentage of lung disease in children; however, the disease affects multiple organ systems in varying degrees of severity, which presents some problems with early recognition.

In the past the mortality has been high in young children with the disease, but with early diagnosis and treatment the mortality has decreased significantly. Consequently more persons with the disease reach the reproductive age.

Etiology

Cystic fibrosis is believed by most authorities to be inherited as an autosomal-recessive trait; therefore the affected child inherits the defective genes from both parents with an overall incidence of 1:4. However, there are some who suggest that the disease may be a symptom complex caused by more than one gene. The incidence of the disease is estimated at approximately 1:1600 births in predominantly white popu-

---

lations and with an equal sex distribution (Shwachman, 1983). Although the disease is found in all racial and socioeconomic groups, it is almost nonexistent in the mongoloid races and is far less prevalent in blacks, occurring primarily in areas in which there is apt to be mixed ancestry.

Pathophysiology

Although it has now been determined that the gene responsible for cystic fibrosis is located on chromosome 7 (Newmark, 1985), the basic biochemical defect in cystic fibrosis is unknown. It is assumed, however, that it is probably caused by alteration in a protein, perhaps an enzyme. The defect gives rise to several apparently unrelated clinical features—increased viscosity of mucous gland secretions, a striking elevation of sweat electrolytes, an increase in several organic and enzymatic constituents of saliva, and abnormalities in autonomic nervous system function.

There is some evidence for overactivity of the autonomic nervous system, which stimulates the cholinergic glands. This is plausible since this system innervates all exocrine glands, but findings are not conclusive. Altered cell membrane permeability may be a factor. Abnormalities of the non-mucous-producing glands are primarily evidenced in the saliva and sweat. There is an increase in sodium and chloride in both saliva and sweat in children with cystic fi-

brosis, which forms the basis for one of the most reliable diagnostic procedures, the sweat chloride test.

The sweat electrolyte abnormality is present from birth throughout life and is unrelated to the severity of the disease or the extent to which other organs are involved. The sodium and chloride content of sweat in children with cystic fibrosis is two to five times greater than that of the controls and occurs in 98% to 99% of affected children. It has been recently demonstrated that a decrease in cellular permeability to chloride may explain the observation of electrolyte alterations in cystic fibrosis and might be the basic generalized biochemical abnormality in this disorder (Quinton and Bijman, 1983).

The primary factor, and the one that is responsible for the multiple clinical manifestations of the disease, is mechanical obstruction caused by the increased viscosity of mucous gland secretions (Fig. 32-8). Instead of forming a thin, freely flowing secretion, the mucous glands produce a thick, inspissated mucoprotein that accumulates and dilates them. Small passages in organs such as the pancreas and bronchioles become obstructed as secretions precipitate or coagulate to form concretions in glands and ducts.

In the pancreas the thick secretions block the ducts, leading to cystic dilations of the acini (small lobes of the gland), which then undergo degeneration and progressive diffuse fi-

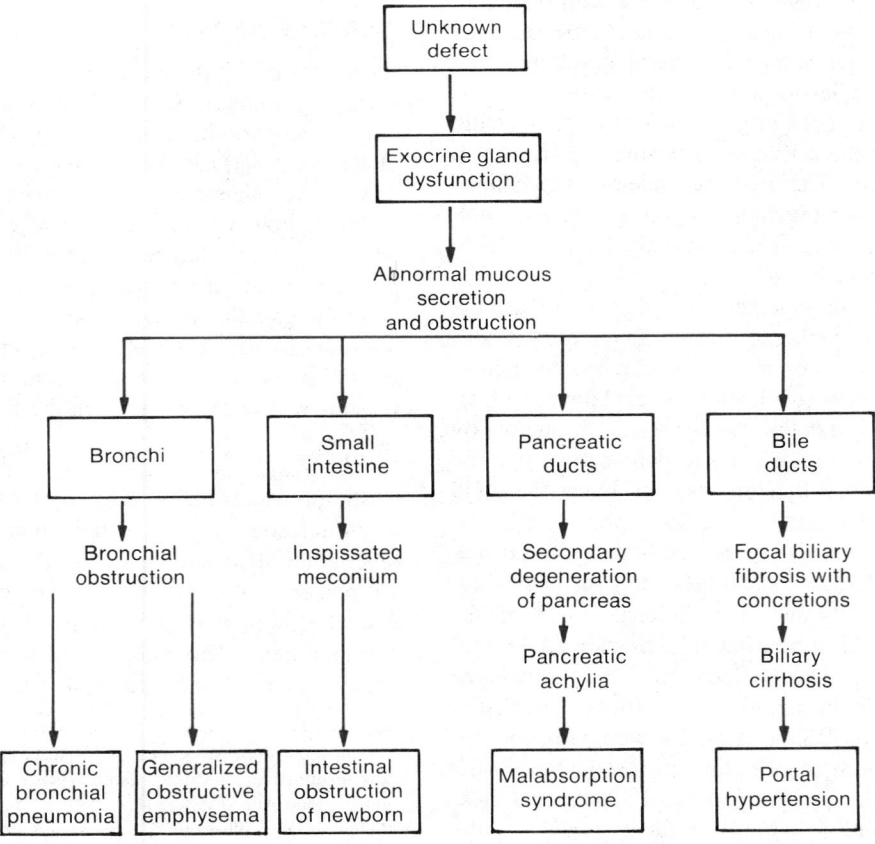

Fig. 32-8. Various effects of exocrine gland dysfunction in cystic fibrosis.

brosis. Grossly the pancreas is smaller, thinner, and firmer than normal. Because essential pancreatic enzymes (trypsin, amylase, and lipase) are unable to reach the duodenum, digestion and absorption of nutrients—particularly fats, proteins, and, to a lesser degree, carbohydrates—are markedly impaired. The disturbed absorption is reflected in excessive stool fat (steatorrhea) and protein (azotorrhea). The islands of Langerhans remain unaffected but may decrease in number as pancreatic fibrosis progresses. However, the incidence of diabetes mellitus is greater in these children than in the general population.

In the liver focal biliary obstruction and fibrosis are common and become more extensive with time, eventually giving rise to a distinctive type of multilobular biliary cirrhosis. A few children develop extensive liver involvement, resulting in portal hypertension, splenomegaly with hypersplenism, ascites, and/or esophageal varices with gastrointestinal hemorrhage. Jaundice is sometimes observed in newborn infants with cystic fibrosis. The gallbladder is small and contains a firm, gelatinous material that also fills the cystic duct. Findings similar to those in the pancreas are found in the salivary glands and contribute to a dry mouth and susceptibility to infection as a result of interference with salivation.

Pulmonary complications are present in almost all children with cystic fibrosis and constitute the most serious threat to life. Bronchial and bronchiolar obstruction by the abnormally thick, tenacious mucus causes patchy atelectasis with both lobar and generalized hyperinflation. Because of the increased viscosity of the mucus, there is greater resistance to ciliary action, a slower mucous flow rate, and reduced expectoration, which also contributes to the mucous obstruction. This retained mucus serves as an excellent medium for any bacterial growth. Reduced oxygen–carbon dioxide exchange causes variable degrees of hypoxia, hypercapnia, and acidosis. In severe, progressive lung involvement, compression of pulmonary blood vessels and progressive lung dysfunction frequently lead to pulmonary hypertension, cor pulmonale, respiratory failure, and death.

The disease is sometimes expressed in other ways, for example, hypoelectrolytemia caused by massive losses through the sweat, especially in high environmental temperatures or febrile episodes. Infants with cystic fibrosis who fail to thrive frequently demonstrate hypoalbuminemia resulting from diminished absorption of protein, which in severe cases causes generalized edema.

The variability in clinical expression of the disease has lead to the conclusion that there are different clinical expressions of cystic fibrosis. Some children have normal fat absorption, milder clinical symptoms, and less lung involvement than other children (Gaskin and others, 1982).

Clinical Manifestations

Because the disease is variable in severity and extent of manifestations and can simulate a number of clinical entities, the diagnosis is not readily apparent in most cases, especially when there is no familial evidence of disease. Some children display symptoms at birth, whereas symptoms in others are not apparent until several years have passed. Some show only mild forms of the disease with only limited impairment of digestion and respiratory problems, whereas others have severe malabsorption and life-threatening pulmonary complications. Although most affected children display both pulmonary and gastrointestinal symptoms, a few children have only enzyme deficiency without pulmonary disease; a few have only pulmonary disease without pancreatic insufficiency.

Gastrointestinal tract. The earliest manifestation of cystic fibrosis is *meconium ileus* in the newborn. The lumen of the small intestine is blocked with thick puttylike, tenacious, mucilaginous meconium, usually at or near the ileocecal valve, which gives rise to signs of intestinal obstruction, including abdominal distention, vomiting, failure to pass stools, and rapid development of dehydration with associated electrolyte imbalance. After the newborn period intestinal obstruction is often referred to as "meconium ileus equivalent."

As the disease progresses, obstruction of pancreatic ducts and the absence of enzymes (trypsin, amylase, lipase) in the duodenum prevent conversion of ingested food into compounds that can be absorbed by the intestinal mucosa. Consequently the nondigested food is excreted, chiefly unabsorbed fats and proteins, which increases the bulk of feces two or three times the normal amount. The bulky nature of the stools may go unnoticed at first, but usually by 6 months of age the child passes large, loose stools with normal frequency or a chronic diarrhea of unformed stools. As solid foods are added to the diet, the excessively large stools become frothy and extremely foul smelling.

Because so little is absorbed from the intestine, the child compensates with a voracious appetite (with advanced disease the appetite diminishes markedly); however, since he is unable to compensate for the fecal wastage, he loses weight with marked wasting of tissues and failure to grow. The abdomen is distended and the extremities are thin, and the sallow skin droops from wasted buttocks. The impaired ability to absorb fats results in a deficiency of the fat-soluble vitamins A, D, E, and K (which causes easy bruising), and anemia is a common complication. These gastrointestinal symptoms are similar to those seen in children with celiac disease, and failure to thrive is a frequent initial diagnosis in young children with cystic fibrosis. When the child is ill with an infection, especially *Pseudomonas,* the appetite usually decreases with subsequent weight loss. Sometimes hospitalization is necessary.

The most common gastrointestinal complication associated with cystic fibrosis in untreated children is *prolapse of the rectum,* which occurs most often in infancy and childhood. Affected children of all ages are subject to peptic ulcers, pancreatic insufficiency, and intestinal obstruction from inspissated or impacted feces. Abdominal cramps may be excessive, and foul flatus is a common complaint. Malnutrition is another commonly associated problem.

Respiratory tract. Pulmonary problems are present in almost all children with cystic fibrosis, but the time of appearance is variable. The majority show evidence before 1 year of age; others may not develop symptoms for weeks, months, or years. Initial manifestations are often wheezing respirations and a dry, nonproductive cough. Eventually diffuse bronchial and bronchiolar obstruction leads to irregular aeration with progressive pulmonary disturbance and secondary infection. Dyspnea increases, the cough often becomes paroxysmal, and the mucoid impactions within the small air passages cause a generalized obstructive emphysema and patchy areas of atelectasis.

Progressive pulmonary involvement with hyperaeration of functioning alveoli produces the overinflated, barrel-shaped chest in which the anteroposterior diameter approaches the lateral diameter. When ventilation is significantly impaired, there are cyanosis and clubbing of fingers and toes. The child suffers repeated episodes of bronchitis and bronchopneumonia, primarily caused by *Staphylococcus aureus* and/or *P. aeruginosa*, and is subject to chronic sinusitis and nasal polyps. Respiratory symptoms mimic diseases such as pneumonia, bronchitis, asthma, whooping cough, tuberculosis, and bronchiectasis.

There is a high percentage of children with cystic fibrosis who have sinusitis, and nasal polyps are relatively common in these children. The incidence of ear, nose, and throat surgeries is higher in this group of children when compared to the general population.

Genital tract. Females with cystic fibrosis have increased viscosity and dehydration of cervical mucus. They may be able to reproduce, although the mucus acts as a plug and blocks the entry of sperm, which is thought to be the mechanism responsible for the decreased fertility in females. There is also an increased incidence of cervical polyps in affected females. With few exceptions males are sterile, which may be caused by blockage of the vas deferens with abnormal secretions or by failure of normal development of the wolffian duct structures (vas deferens, epididymis, and seminal vesicles) resulting in aspermia.

Diagnostic Evaluation

An initial evaluation is conducted with general appraisal in the areas of general activity, physical findings, nutritional status, and findings on chest radiographs. The diagnosis of cystic fibrosis is established on the basis of (1) a history of the disease in the family, (2) the absence of pancreatic enzymes, (3) an increase in electrolyte concentration of sweat, and (4) chronic pulmonary involvement. All four criteria are not always present but, for a positive diagnosis, the presence of elevated sweat electrolytes plus either pulmonary disease or pancreatic insufficiency should be present.

Family history. A history of one or more previously affected siblings alerts health personnel to the possibility of the disease in a child born to that family. When diagnosis can be established early, treatment can be initiated to reduce the complications in many instances.

Sweat electrolytes. For a definitive test, the quantitative sweat test is employed. The consistent finding of abnormally high sodium and chloride concentrations in the sweat is a unique characteristic of cystic fibrosis. Parents frequently observe that their infants taste "salty" when they kiss them. For diagnostic purposes the quantitative test is performed on sweat obtained by iontophoresis of pilocarpine, in which a small electric current carries the cholinergic drug pilocarpine into a small patch of skin (the forearm in older children, the thigh in infants) to stimulate the sweat glands locally. The sweat is then collected on a filter paper and the chloride content measured in the laboratory.

Application of electrodes and the amount and duration of current are carried out according to the manufacturer's instructions. It is important to make certain that the positive electrode is completely covered with gauze and moistened with pilocarpine and that the entire surface of the 4 square inches electrode makes contact with the skin surface. The small amount of current spread over this area is almost indiscernible, but if contact is poor, the current becomes concentrated in a smaller area and may produce a burn.

Sweat tests are included in the workup of children with recurrent respiratory infections, malabsorption, or failure to thrive. Since sweat glands function inadequately during the first weeks of life, reliable sweat tests are difficult to obtain. Normally the sweat chloride content is less than 40 mEq/L, with a mean of 18 mEq/L; a chloride concentration greater than 60 mEq/L is diagnostic of cystic fibrosis, and levels of 40 to 60 mEq/L are highly suggestive of the disease. The test is repeated if results are questionable or if results are negative in a case in which clinical symptoms are strongly suggestive. A new sweat patch test (SPT) has been devised for use when there is insufficient sweat. Results indicate that the test is reliable (Yeung and others, 1984).

Pancreatic enzymes. Measurements of duodenal enzyme activity may be made to confirm a diagnosis. These enzymes are absent or diminished in children with cystic fibrosis. Usually only trypsin and chymotrypsin are measured. Trypsin is absent in over 80% of patients with the disease.

Fat-absorption tests. Impaired fat absorption in the intestines causes large volumes to be excreted in the stools (steatorrhea). In fat-absorption tests impaired fat absorption is measured in a 5-day stool collection and calculated as a percentage of intake.

Radiography. Evidence of generalized obstructive emphysema is highly suggestive of cystic fibrosis. With advanced disease, patchy atelectasis and a disseminated infiltrative pattern of bronchopneumonia are observed.

Screening. Several neonatal screening tests have been developed but are not yet sufficiently reliable for mass screening. The relatively simple dried blood immunoreactive trypsinogen (IRT) assay has generated the most interest. However, the Ad Hoc Committee Task Force on Neonatal Screening, Cystic Fibrosis Foundation (1983), recommends that until information on a number of issues is obtained "no mass screening for cystic fibrosis be implemented, even if a valid and reliable test is available.'' No test is presently available for detecting heterozygotes.

Therapeutic Management

Early diagnosis before irreversible pulmonary changes take place and individualized treatment have reduced the morbidity and increased the longevity of children with cystic fibrosis. Pulmonary function tests and blood gas determinations detect lung changes before they are evident on chest x-ray examinations, and new drugs and pulmonary hygiene provide better control of complications. Wherever possible, the goals of care are aimed at promoting a normal life for the affected child. This includes maintaining good nutrition, prevention and control of pulmonary infections, and promoting a satisfactory psychologic adjustment to the disease and all of its ramifications.

Diet. The impaired intestinal absorption necessitates a diet significantly higher in calories and protein than is normally required in a child of similar size. Fats are generally allowed as tolerated although, if steatorrhea is not controlled with pancreatic enzymes, fat content may be reduced. High-protein formulas with low-curd tension are recommended during the first weeks of life, followed by low-fat or skim milk and homogenized milk in older children if they can tolerate it. Medium-chain triglycerides (MCTs) are more readily absorbed than longer chain fats and are sometimes given as a dietary supplement. However, they represent an added expense associated with an already financially burdensome disease.

Water-miscible preparations of vitamins A, D, and E are provided daily in twice the usually recommended dosage. Vitamin K is indicated if hypoprothrombinemia is present as a result of accompanying liver involvement or in small infants with achylia to prevent hypoprothrombinemia. The nutritional status of most patients is compromised, especially during the second decade of life. Supplementary iron is prescribed, and frequently diet supplements (such as Carnation Instant Breakfast, Ensure or Ensure Plus, Sustacal, or Sustacal pudding) are given to provide additional protein, vitamins, and calories. Short-term parenteral nutrition may be implemented in some cases. A relationship between improved nutritional status and increased pulmonary muscle strength following parenteral nutritional supplementation of malnourished children has been demonstrated (Mansell and others, 1984). Improved nutrition has also been noted when malnourished children receive nocturnal supplemental feedings via gastrostomy tube (Levy and others, 1985).

Pancreatic enzyme replacement is given in conjunction with meals and snacks and is regulated in order to obtain normal bowel movements, nutrition, and growth. The dosage is determined by the degree of enzyme deficiency, the destruction of the exogenous enzymes by gastric hydrochloric acid, and the food intake. Each enzyme unit will digest only a specific amount of protein, fat, or complex carbohydrate. Simple sugars are absorbed directly. Less enzyme is needed if the child becomes constipated; more is required if the stools remain loose and fatty.

A variety of preparations are available that provide missing enzymes. The most recent and preferred preparation is Pancrease, which consists of enteric-coated microspheres contained in a capsule (Cotazym-S, Pancrease). The enteric coating delays release of the enzyme and its destruction in the acid environment of the stomach. The capsules may be swallowed intact or broken apart and the contents sprinkled on soft food, such as applesauce or pudding. Occasionally an infant or young child may require a preparation that does not require an alkaline environment for release of the enzymes. For these children, some of the older preparations are available, including pancrelipase (Cotazym) and pancreatin (Panteric, Viokase). The average dose is three capsules per meal, with a range of one to six. A slightly smaller amount may be used for smaller meals or snacks (Doershuk and Stern, 1986). Sometimes an antacid (such as Maalox) or cimetidine (Tagamet) is administered with the enzymes to lower the gastric acidity.

Since salt depletion through sweating is a hazard, children are allowed to use salt generously. Most children are able to adjust this to their needs, and older children often exhibit a preference for salty foods. Additional salt should be taken during hot weather or febrile periods.

Pulmonary therapy. Management of pulmonary problems is directed toward prevention and treatment of pulmonary infection by improving aeration, removing mucopurulent secretions, and administering antimicrobial agents. Once infection becomes established in relatively defenseless lungs, it is difficult to eradicate, becoming chronic with recurrent episodes of bronchopneumonia sometimes complicated by atelectasis and bronchiectatic abscesses and stimulating pulmonary fibrosis, which eventually terminates in cor pulmonale.

Physical therapy is implemented to maintain good pulmonary hygiene by way of postural drainage and breathing exercises. Postural drainage through positioning, clapping with the cupped hand over the lung segment to be drained, and vibration over the segment during exhalation has been described (p. 1315) and is carried out to encourage coughing and assist in removal of mucus and exudate. The procedure should be carried out several times daily prophylactically and during infections as often as the child is able to tolerate it without undue fatigue. Chest physiotherapy should not be performed before or immediately after meals. Planning the activity so that it does not coincide with meals is difficult in the hospital situation. However, it is very important and is often overlooked by nursing personnel.

Breathing exercises (p. 1318) are recommended for the majority of children with cystic fibrosis, even those with minimal pulmonary involvement. The exercises are usually performed twice daily, preceded by postural drainage. Exercises to improve posture and mobilize the thorax are added, such as swinging the arms and trunk bending and twisting. Children are encouraged to increase physical activity and participate in sports. The ultimate aim of these exercises and activities is to establish a good habitual breathing pattern.

Moisture-laden air is a major modality in pulmonary therapy of cystic fibrosis. It moistens bronchial secretions to assist in their evacuation. Moist air is provided by intermittent inhalation therapy, usually used in conjunction with postural drainage, and by mist tent therapy. In order to be effective, the particles of moisture must be small enough to penetrate to the smaller bronchi; therefore nebulization must produce particles 0.5 to 5 μg in diameter.

Medications that are used in conjunction with nebulization include antibiotics and bronchodilators such as terbutaline, metaproterenol, and cromolyn sodium. Intermittent therapy is provided by hand-held nebulizers, either the hand-bulb variety or the jet-aerosol or cartridge-type devices that employ Freon propellants, and ultrasonic nebulizers that produce smaller droplets of a more consistent size. The recommended schedule for intermittent, or interrupted, therapy to be carried out at least twice daily (morning and evening), and more often if needed, consists of three steps:

1. Postural drainage for 5 to 10 minutes
2. Nebulization with appropriate solution
3. Postural drainage for 10 to 20 minutes

Nebulization after postural drainage permits deeper penetration of the droplet particles. There is not total agreement regarding the benefits of bronchodilators or mucolytic agents used in the nebulizing solution. Most favor a solution of 10% propylene glycol and 90% distilled water. Propylene glycol stabilizes the mist in droplet form and prevents vaporization of the droplet. Normal saline is sometimes employed on a short-term basis.

Most children do not use oxygen tents, but a small number feel more comfortable in the water-saturated atmosphere. Mist-tent use is confined to use in the hospital for some children during acute episodes of pulmonary disease. Oxygen therapy is usually recommended for children with acute episodes, and since many of these children have chronic carbon dioxide retention, the unsupervised use of oxygen can be harmful. Expectorants and mucolytic agents may be used to relieve bronchial obstruction.

During acute exacerbations of pulmonary disease, intensive antibiotics are employed to control pulmonary infection. Many physicians prefer to use antibiotics only when there is evidence of infection, whereas others prescribe their use as a prophylactic measure. When used therapeutically, it is important that the drugs be given over a long enough period and in sufficient dosage to be effective. Oral antibiotics are best selected on the basis of sputum cultures, but in acute situations a broad-spectrum drug is employed pending results of the culture. Antibiotics used for long-term prophylactic therapy are frequently rotated to reduce the chance of developing resistance to any single drug.

The most frequent organism found in sputum is hemolytic *S. aureus*. After extended use of antibiotics, the predominant organism is *Pseudomonas*, which is resistant to most oral antibiotics. During acute disease the child is frequently hospitalized and the appropriate antibiotic administered parenterally. Sometimes antibiotics are given by nebulization to provide a high concentration of antibiotic in the respiratory passages, where it can attack the microorganisms directly.

Because high doses are frequently used, blood serum levels are monitored closely to prevent toxicity. When the aminoglycosides are used extensively, vigilance is needed to detect early signs of renal toxicity and ototoxicity. Children who receive these drugs over a prolonged period should have frequent audiograms. Also children taking long-term antibiotics need vitamin K.

Exercise. Numerous investigations have reported that exercise training is often effective in improving the ability of a patient to clear accumulated lung secretions and increase the capacity to endure exercise before experiencing dyspnea. Conversely, patients who voluntarily restrict physical activities because of increased respiratory difficulty may have muscle deterioration, increased shortness of breath, and loss of exercise tolerance. Consequently, an exercise program is often included as an integral part of the therapeutic regimen (Edlund and others, 1986; Orenstein, Henke, and Cerney, 1983). Activities that are encouraged are swimming and walking/jogging. The exercise and increased feeling of well-being have the added benefit of improving self-image, self-confidence, and quality of life for the youngster with cystic fibrosis.

Complications. Other complications are treated symptomatically. Meconium ileus usually responds to the administration of diatrizoate methylglucamine (Gastrografin) or acetylcysteine (Mucomist) enemas. Rectal prolapse is reduced by gently pressing against the everted rectum with a gloved, lubricated finger while the child is in the knee-chest position. The buttocks are then strapped together with tape. Nasal polyps, to which children with cystic fibrosis are predisposed, are removed surgically to relieve blockage of nasal passages.

Prognosis. It is the pulmonary involvement that determines the ultimate outcome of the disease. Pancreatic enzyme deficiency is less of a problem if adequate nutrition is ensured. Hemorrhage from liver cirrhosis and massive salt depletion in hot weather are occasional hazards. With early diagnosis and improved therapeutic measures, the life expectancy has improved. Many more children are reaching adulthood; however, the variation in severity of the disease is an important factor in determining the ultimate outcomes. It has been observed that children whose presenting symptoms were gastrointestinal at diagnosis have a good clinical course; those whose initial symptoms at diagnosis were pulmonary frequently demonstrate subsequent clinical deterioration (Katz and others, 1986).

No exact figures are available regarding the life expectancy of a child with cystic fibrosis. Many still die in infancy and early childhood, but increasing numbers are living into the the third and fourth decades and even beyond. More than 50% of the patients now live into adulthood (Barbero, 1982). However, the survival rate appears to favor boys. Almost twice as many boys as girls survive to adulthood, and the sex difference becomes pronounced after age

15. There is a marked relationship between survival and pulmonary function, which is positively correlated with weight (Gurwitz and others, 1979).

Nursing Considerations

Nursing care of infants and children with cystic fibrosis involves both acute and chronic management. These children require regular observation and medical supervision, including ongoing assessment of general health and nutritional and pulmonary status.

The nurse's contact with an affected child usually begins when the child is brought to the hospital or clinic for confirmation of the diagnosis. Perhaps the reason for hospitalization is failure to thrive or recurrent respiratory infections. Later, during recurrent admission to the hospital or during ongoing follow-up in the clinic or at home, the nurse and the child develop a sustained relationship.

Diagnosis. On the initial contact, frequently in the hospital setting, nurses are involved in performing or assisting with diagnostic tests and obtaining primarily sweat for laboratory analysis of chloride content and, less often, stool specimens for trypsin and fat. The child, usually an infant, needs comfort during the procedures; young children need distraction while they are confined during iontophoresis. Even short periods of inactivity seem long to an active child. Children beyond very early childhood need explanation of the strange, and sometimes painful, procedures and the equipment used for tests and treatments.

At first the respiratory equipment, oxygen mask, mouthpiece, and mist tent are frightening, especially to infants and very young children. The mist tent (if prescribed) can be a source of either fear or comfort and security. The child needs patient support and guidance in using the equipment. Accepting uncharacteristic behavior and explaining this normal stress response to parents are important nursing functions.

Parents are anxious and puzzled. Few of them have any understanding of the disease process and the long-term implications it has for their family. They need patient and careful explanations of the disease, how it might affect their family, and what they can do to provide the best possible care for their child.

The shock associated with the diagnosis is overwhelming to parents. They must face the impact of the chronic, life-threatening nature of the disease and the prospect of intensive treatment, for which they must assume a major part of the responsibility and for which they are ill prepared. They often fear that they will be unable to provide the care the child needs. One of the most difficult aspects of the diagnosis is the implications inherent in its etiology, that is, the recognition that each parent contributed the gene responsible for the defect in their child.

Hospital care. When the child is hospitalized for confirmation of the diagnosis or for pulmonary complications, aerosol therapy is instituted or continued. The child may or may not be placed in a mist tent, but nebulization is almost always central to hospital management. Respiratory therapy is usually initiated and supervised by a trained respiratory therapist or physiotherapist. In institutions with large support staffs, they may provide all treatments. Otherwise, it becomes the responsibility of the nurse to perform the prescribed nebulization, postural drainage, percussion, and vibration and to teach supervised breathing exercises.

The child who receives mist therapy requires frequent observation to make certain that the equipment is operating properly and that the reservoir contains the prescribed solution (usually distilled water with a mucolytic agent). The mist should be of sufficient density that the child is barely visible through the moisture. The child requires frequent changes of linen, which becomes wet from the high humidity within the tent or Isolette. Oxygen is cautiously administered to children in respiratory distress but the child requires frequent assessment. The hazard of oxygen narcosis is a constant threat in children with long-standing disease who receive oxygen (see p. 1314). Intensive aerosol therapy may cause large volumes of sputum to be thinned suddenly in the early hours of treatment; therefore the child requires close observation to assist him with expectoration and to prevent deeper aspiration. Expectorant drugs are administered orally, which further facilitates the expectoration of mucus.

The diet is implemented for the newly diagnosed child or continued for the child who is hospitalized for pulmonary disease. Children in the early stages of the disease maintain a good appetite, and some will eat excessively. With infection and increased lung involvement, the appetite diminishes, however. Eventually it becomes a challenge to tempt failing appetites (see Feeding the sick child in Chapter 27). Some younger children may object to the extra fluids that are encouraged to promote thinning of mucous secretions. Food should be considered as therapy for these patients. The caloric intake should be about two to three times that of normal children. Enzymes are supplied for each meal or snack, and adequate salt is provided, especially for febrile children.

Frequent skin care is carried out to prevent irritation and skin breakdown over bony prominences. Particular attention is necessary after use of the bedpan or when the diaper is changed. Careful cleansing helps to reduce irritation and odor from offensive stools.

The child will need support for the many treatments and tests that are a necessary part of the hospital therapy. Intravenous fluids and blood tests are almost always a part of the treatment, and the child soon associates hospitalization with these stress-provoking procedures. These children are usually quite thin with little muscle mass, which requires careful selection of injection sites.

Support to both child and family is a vital part of nursing care. The progressive nature of the disease makes each illness requiring hospitalization a potentially life-threatening event. Skilled nursing care and sympathetic attention to the emotional needs of the child and family help them cope with the stresses associated with repeated respiratory infections and hospitalization.

Home care. After the diagnosis is confirmed and a treatment program determined, parents will need help in finding inhalation equipment available for home use that best meets their needs. They will need opportunities to learn about and practice the use of the equipment as well as some of the problems they may encounter.

They need to learn about the preferred diet of nutritious meals with tolerated fat and ample protein and carbohydrate and the administration of pancreatic enzymes. Children usually adjust well to taking pancreatic enzymes. For infants and young children, they can be mixed with pureed fruit, such as applesauce, and fed with a spoon. The capsules are suitable for older children. It is important to stress to parents that the enzymes, in the amount regulated to the child's needs, are to be administered with all meals or at bedtime. They are cautioned about not restricting salt, especially during hot weather, and ensuring an adequate fluid intake since dehydration aggravates the thick mucous secretions. Oral hygiene is important because of interference with salivation and the increased susceptibility to oral infections.

One of the most important aspects of educating parents for home care is teaching postural drainage and breathing exercises. The success of a therapy program depends on conscientious performance of these treatments regularly as prescribed. The number of times these therapies are performed each day is determined on an individual basis, and often parents readily learn to adjust the number and intensity of the treatments to the child's needs. Whether the nurse or therapist instructs the parents, nurses are frequently the persons who can follow up the care in the home and assist the family with innovative approaches to the therapy. For example, using games and normal childhood activities to provide postural drainage reduces the likelihood that treatment will meet with resistance from the child.

Simple activities that are fun, such as hanging by the knees from a bar or low-hanging trapeze that can be easily built in the backyard (or indoors), turning somersaults, or playing "wheelbarrow" with the child suspended head down and propelling himself on his hands while the adult holds onto his feet, should be encouraged. Most children respond to a challenge, such as, "How long can you stand on your head?" Small children can "stand on their heads" with their heads on the cushion of a large chair with or without the adult holding on to their feet. Parents soon learn to respond to cues from their children and incorporate spontaneous activities into the treatment regimen.

During the end-stage of the disease, home intravenous antibiotics may be prescribed. With the use of the venous access devices the parents and/or the child are taught the technique of direct administration into the intravenous line.* Unfortunately the need for around-the-clock administration may be difficult for some families because it requires waking at least once during the night to give the drug.

The nurse can assist the family to contact resources that provide help to families with affected children. The various Special Child Health Services, many local clinics, private agencies, service clubs, and other community groups often offer equipment and medications either free or at reduced rates. The **Cystic Fibrosis Foundation*** has chapters throughout the United States to provide education† and services to families and professionals.

Psychologic support. One of the most important and difficult aspects in providing care for the family of a child with cystic fibrosis is coping with the emotional needs of the child and family. The diagnosis, treatment, and prognosis are fraught with a multiplicity of problems, frustrations, and feelings. The diagnosis with all its implications evokes feelings of guilt and self-recrimination in the parents. These feelings may be particularly marked if the newly diagnosed child is the second affected child in the family and the parents had been counseled regarding the 1:4 risk of such an event occurring.

The long-range problems are those encountered in the care of a child with a chronic illness (Chapter 22). Both the child and the family must make many adjustments, the success of which depends on their ability to cope and also on the quality and quantity of support they receive from outside sources. Combined efforts of a variety of health professionals offer the most comprehensive services to families. It is often the responsibility of the nurse to organize and coordinate these services, to assess the home situation, and to collect the data needed to evaluate the effectiveness of the services in meeting the family's needs.

For the family the illness means modification of numerous family activities. Meals require planning in order not to place too many restrictions on the affected child or deprive the other members of the family. Limits on mobility restrict family recreational activities, especially when the child's therapy includes respiratory equipment that is not transportable. Postural drainage must be continued wherever the child may be. In addition, members of the family hesitate to take the child too far from familiar and trusted medical care. The illness even determines the family's place of residence and employment, as the child's condition dictates that he should remain near medical care facilities that offer the specialized care he needs.

The persistent need for treatment several times daily also places a strain on the family. Someone must perform the procedures, such as percussion and vibration, even on older children who are able to assume responsibility for their own exercises and respiratory therapy. Children often balk at the treatments, and the parents are placed in the position of insisting on compliance. Sometimes the stress and anxiety related to this continual routine generate feelings of resent-

---

*For home care instructions see Wong, D.L., and Whaley, L.F.: Clinical handbook of pediatric nursing, St. Louis, 1986, The C.V. Mosby Co.

*6000 Executive Blvd., Suite 309, Rockville, MD 20852.
†Two excellent publications are "What everyone should know about cystic fibrosis" and "Cystic fibrosis: a summary of symptoms, diagnosis, and treatment."

ment, which are frequently focused on one aspect of the regimen, such as the diet or equipment. When possible, occasional trusted respite care should be made available to the parent or parents to allow them the opportunity to leave the situation for short periods without undue anxiety regarding the child's welfare.

The affected child also may become resentful about his disease, its relentless routine of therapy, and the necessary curtailment it places on his activities and relationships. The child's activities are interrupted or built around treatment, medications, and diet that imposes hardships (such as carrying medication to school and other places where he may eat away from home), and growth retardation that is associated with most chronic illness may be trying to the child. Any of these aspects of the disease may be the cause of ridicule from other children. However, these children should be encouraged to attend school and join age-appropriate groups, such as scouting, to foster a life that is as normal and productive as possible.

A constant source of anxiety for both parents and child is the ever-present fear of death. The increased survival of these patients has altered the prognosis and expectations. It may be the result of better and earlier diagnosis, especially with patients with mild disease, or improved management. It is now possible to express a hopeful attitude about a newly diagnosed patient. Also, this improved longevity has created some new counseling and supportive needs (see Chapter 22).

The expected life span, although significantly increased during the past years, offers only limited encouragement regarding prognosis for some patients. The future is always uncertain. These families need all the support and skill the nurse can offer to cope with the guarded prognosis (see Chapter 23). During the terminal phase in particular *anticipatory* planning should occur, in which aspects of medical intervention are clearly defined, such as cardiopulmonary resuscitation efforts. When the health care team and parents are prepared for the death, efforts can be focused on making the child as comfortable as possible and on supporting the family.

Nursing Care Summary: The Child with Cystic Fibrosis

NURSING GOALS	NURSING OUTCOMES	EXPECTED PATIENT/FAMILY OUTCOMES
HP-HMP Infection, potential for **Risk factors: impaired body defenses**		
Prevent infection	Restrict contact with persons who have respiratory tract infections, including family, other children, friends, and members of staff	Child displays no evidence of an infective process
Maintain optimum health	Promote good health practices Nutrition Hygiene	Child and family apply good health practices
N-MP Nutrition, alteration in **Etiology: inability to digest nutrients**		
Maintain nutrition	Provide diet high in carbohydrate and protein Discourage use of foods high in fat; provide appropriate fat if recommended by physician Ensure adequate intake of salt	Child consumes a well-balanced diet (specify)
A-EP Activity intolerance **Etiology: imbalance between oxygen supply and demand**		
Conserve energy	Provide or encourage activities appropriate to child's developmental level and physical capacity (specify) Encourage frequent rest periods Enforce regular sleep times	Child engages in activities appropriate to his/her age and physical capabilities (specify)
A-EP Airway clearance, ineffective **Etiology: secretion of thick, tenacious mucus**		
Assist patient to expectorate sputum	Perform postural drainage Teach and/or supervise breathing exercises	Child manages secretions with minimum distress

Continued.

Nursing Care Summary: The Child with Cystic Fibrosis—cont'd

NURSING GOALS	NURSING OUTCOMES	EXPECTED PATIENT/FAMILY OUTCOMES
A-EP Breathing pattern, ineffective **Etiology: tracheobronchial obstruction**		
Improve aeration	Supervise breathing exercises Encourage good posture and active exercises suitable to child's needs, capabilities, and preferences	Child breathes easily and without dyspnea
SRP Sleep pattern disturbance **Etiology: frequent coughing, ineffective breathing**		
Promote rest	Organize activities for maximum sleep time Encourage regular bedtime and nap time Implement measures to ensure sleep, such as quiet, darkened room	Child appears rested when awake
SP-SCP Self-concept, disturbance in: body image, self-esteem, personal identity **Etiology: perception of being "different"**		

Promote self-care	Teach child about disease and treatment
	Encourage child to assist in his own care
	    Food selection
	    Use of pancreatic enzymes
	    Use of equipment
	    How he can cooperate during treatments and tests
		Child demonstrates an understanding of his disease and complies with therapies

Determine extent of disturbance	Encourage verbalization of feelings and perceptions Convey attitude of understanding and acceptance Assist child to identify his assets, strengths, and capabilities	Child verbalizes his feelings and concerns about his disease, its therapies, and implications Child is able to identify his capabilities, etc., realistically
Improve self-concept	Point out positive aspects of his coping, appearance, and other capabilities Assist with improving appearance and grooming Promote successful undertakings	Child demonstrates a positive appearance and attitude
RRP Family process, alteration in **Etiology: situational crisis (child with a chronic illness)**		
Provide material support to child and family	Guide to available resources equipped to deal with their special needs Provide counseling services Collaborate with family and health team in assessing family needs and coping mechanisms	Family members avail themselves of resources within their community and identify strengths and assets
Support family emotionally	Listen to family members—singly or collectively Act on cues that indicate a family member's reaction to child Help family to gain confidence in their ability to cope with child, the disability, and its impact on other family members Encourage unaffected siblings to discuss their feelings regarding possibility of being a carrier of disease Encourage interaction with other families who have a similarly affected child See also The family of the hospitalized child, p. 1081	Family members demonstrate an attitude of confidence in their ability to cope
Promote optimum home care	Assess home situation Help devise individualized regimen based on assessment Teach family home care Help family acquire needed drugs and equipment Arrange for regular follow-up care to reassess effectiveness of home management Assist family in problem solving	Family members comply with prescribed home care

Nursing Care Summary: The Child with Cystic Fibrosis—cont'd

NURSING GOALS	NURSING OUTCOMES	EXPECTED PATIENT/FAMILY OUTCOMES
Increase knowledge of disease and therapies	Prepare child and family for diagnostic tests Provide information regarding the disease Reinforce information given by others Provide accurate information at a rate family can absorb Provide or arrange for genetic counseling regarding inherited aspects of disease when requested	Child and family comply with therapeutic regimen Family demonstrates understanding of the disease and therapies (specify knowledge and method of demonstration)
Provide therapies to child	Teach family (and child) proper performance of therapies Use of equipment Exercises and procedures Diet and administration of pancreatic enzymes Administration of drugs Protection from infection	

RRP   Grieving, anticipatory
Etiology: perceived potential loss of child

Help family face possibility of child's death	Provide consistent contact with family Assign primary nurse Clarify, refocus, and supply information as needed Help family plan care of child, especially at terminal stage (e.g., extent of extraordinary life-saving measures)	Family remains open to counseling and nursing contacts Family and child discuss their fears, concerns, needs, and desires at terminal stage

RRP   Social interaction, impaired
Etiology: hospitalization, confinement to home, fatigue

Promote growth and development	Encourage to maintain usual activities Arrange for continued family contacts during hospitalization Arrange for continued schooling while hospitalized Encourage relationships with peers Promote development of a positive self-image Arrange for spiritual support in accordance with family's beliefs and/or affiliation Be especially alert to family's needs when another sibling (siblings) is affected with disease	Child associates with peers and family Child attends school with reasonable regularity Family receives appropriate religious representative (specify)

Nursing Interventions Related to Medical Management

Assist in diagnoses
  Perform nursing assessment of child
  Take family history and health history
  Encourage medical evaluation for any child who displays suggestive signs of the disease
    Frequent respiratory tract infection
    Large, bulky stools
    Prolapsed rectum
    Failure to gain weight
  Assist with diagnostic procedures
    Collect stool specimens
    Perform sweat test
    Assist with radiographs
Assist child to expectorate sputum
  Provide nebulization with appropriate solution and equipment as prescribed
  Place in mist tent as ordered; make certain compressor or ultrasonic mechanism provides very small droplets in ample supply
  Administer expectorants
  Administer bronchodilators, if ordered

Improve aeration
  Perform postural drainage
  Administer medications that promote breathing (bronchodilators, expectorants)
  Administer oxygen, if indicated and prescribed
  Provide nebulization
Prevent infection
  Administer antibiotics as prescribed
  Manage respiratory tract infections as in pneumonia
Facilitate digestion
  Administer pancreatic enzyme replacement with meals and snacks
Provide optimum nutrition
  Administer water-miscible vitamins, iron, and calorie supplement

CONCEPT SUMMARIES

- Acute infection of the respiratory tract is the most common cause of illness in infancy and childhood.

- The incidence and severity of respiratory tract infections are influenced by the infectious agent involved, the child's age, and the child's natural defenses.

- Symptoms of respiratory tract infections include fever, febrile convulsions, meningismus, anorexia, vomiting, diarrhea, abdominal pain, nasal blockage and discharge, cough, respiratory sounds, presence or absence of sore throat.

- Common respiratory tract infections of childhood include acute nasopharyngitis, acute pharyngitis, influenza, tonsillitis, and otitis media.

- Factors that predispose children to otitis media are the shape and position of eustachian tubes, undeveloped cartilage lining, abundant pharyngeal lymphoid tissue, immature humoral defense mechanisms, and the recumbent position (in infants).

- Croup syndromes include acute laryngitis, acute laryngotracheobronchitis, acute spasmodic laryngitis, and acute epiglottitis.

- The primary nursing function in the care of children with croup is observation for signs of respiratory embarrassment and relief of laryngeal obstruction.

- Common infections of the lower airway include bacterial tracheitis, asthmatic bronchitis, bronchitis, and bronchiolitis.

- Pneumonias are generally classified either by site (lobar, bronchial, or interstitial) or by etiologic agent (viruses, bacteria, mycoplasmas, or associated with foreign bodies).

- In tuberculosis, resistance to the bacillus can be altered by heredity, sex, age, stress states, poor nutrition, and intercurrent infection.

- Signs of choking include inability to speak, cyanosis, and collapse.

- Allergic rhinitis, bronchial asthma, and cystic fibrosis represent long-term respiratory dysfunctions in children.

- Asthma is one of the leading causes of chronic illness in children.

- In asthma, hyperreactivity of airways is thought to be attributed to exaggeration of normal defenses of the respiratory tract, abnormal tissue reactions, or imbalance of normally balanced responses.

- General therapeutic management of asthma includes allergen control, drug therapy, controlled exercise, physical therapy, and hyposensitization.

- Family support for the child with asthma includes teaching about proper positioning, removing allergens from child's environment, reducing exposure to irritants, understanding medications and their overuse, practicing breathing exercises, and self-management.

- Diagnosis of cystic fibrosis is based on family history, absence of pancreatic enzymes, increase in electrolyte concentration of sweat, and chronic pulmonary involvement.

REFERENCES

Ad Hoc Committee on Definition and Classification of Otitis Media with Effusion: Report, Ann. Otol. Rhinol. Laryngol. (Suppl.) 89(Pt. 3):3-4, 1980.

Ad Hoc Committee Task Force on Neonatal Screening, Cystic Fibrosis Foundation: Position paper, Pediatrics 72:741-745, 1983.

Barbero, G.J.: Commentary: the clinical forms of cystic fibrosis, J. Pediatr. 100:914-915, 1982.

Behrman, R.E.: Acute pharyngitis. In Behrman, R.E., and Vaughan, V.C., III: Textbook of pediatrics, ed. 12, Philadelphia, 1983, W.B. Saunders Co.

Bierman, C.W., and Pearlman, D.S.: Asthma. In Kendig, E.L., and Chernick, V., editors: Disorders of the respiratory tract in children, Philadelphia, 1983, W.B. Saunders Co.

Boat, T.F., and others: Acute nasopharyngitis. In Behrman, R.E., and Vaughan, V.C., III, editors: Textbook of pediatrics, ed. 12, Philadelphia, 1983, W.B. Saunders Co.

Bonham, G.S., and Wilson, R.W.: Children's health in families with cigarette smokers, Am. J. Public Health 71:290-293, 1981.

Boushey, H.A., and others: Bronchial hyperreactivity, Am. Rev. Respir. Dis. 121:389-393, 1980.

Brennan, P.O.: Inhaled salbutamol: a new form of drug abuse? Lancet 2:1030, 1983.

Brumback, R.A., and others: Behavioral problems in children taking theophylline, Lancet 1:958, 1984.

Burton, J.: Carbon monoxide poisoning, Crit. Care Update 6(12):33-35, 1979.

Chaudhary, S., and others: Penicillin V and rifampin for the treatment of group A streptococcal pharyngitis: a randomized trial of 10 days penicillin vs 10 days penicillin with rifampin during the final 4 days of therapy, J. Pediatr. 106:481-486, 1985.

Colombo, J.L., Hopkins, R.L., and Waring, W.W.: Steam vaporizer injuries, Pediatrics 67:661-663, 1981.

Committee on Children with Disabilities and Committee on Sports Medicine: The asthmatic child's participation in sports and physical education, Pediatrics 74:155-156, 1984.

Committee of Environmental Hazards: Involuntary smoking—a hazard to children, Pediatrics 77:755-757, 1986.

Committee on Infectious Diseases: *Hemophilus* type b polysaccharide vaccine, Pediatrics 76:322-324, 1985.

Committee on Infectious Diseases: Recommendations for using pneumococcal vaccine in children, Pediatrics 75:1153-1158, 1985.

Committee on Infectious Diseases: Report of the committee on infectious diseases, ed. 12, Elk Grove Village, IL, 1986, American Academy of Pediatrics.

Copperman, S.M.: Household pets as reservoirs of persistent or recurrent streptococcal sore throats in children, N.Y. State J. Med. 82:1685-1687, 1982.

Cunningham, A.S.: Morbidity in breast-fed and artificially fed infants: II, J. Pediatr. 95:685, 1984.

Cunningham, D.G., and others: Unprescribed use of antibiotics in common childhood infections, J. Pediatr. 103:747-749, 1983.

David, T.J., and others: Prodromal itching in childhood asthma, Lancet 2:154-155, 1984.

Denny, F.W.: Effect of treatment on streptococcal pharyngitis: is the issue really settled? Pediatr. Infect. Dis. 4:352-354, 1983.

Dick, E.C., and others: Interruption of transmission of rhinovirus colds among human volunteers using virucidal paper handkerchiefs, J. Infect. Dis. 153:352-356, 1986.

Doershuk, C.G., and Stern, R.C.: Cystic fibrosis. In Gellis, S.S., and Kagan, B.M., editors: Current pediatric therapy 12, Philadelphia, 1986, W.B. Saunders Co.

Edlund, L.D., and others: Effects of swimming program on children with cystic fibrosis, Am. J. Dis. Child. 140:80-83, 1986.

Fagin, J., Friedman, R., and Fireman, P.: Allergic rhinitis, Pediatr. Clin. North Am. 28:797-806, 1981.

Fergusson, D.M., Horwood, L.J., and Shannon, F.T.: Parental asthma, parental eczema and asthma and eczema in early childhood, J. Chron. Dis. 36:517-524, 1983.

Fischer, R., and others: Influence of trivalent influenza vaccine on serum theophylline levels, J. Can. Med. Assoc. 126:1312-1313, 1982.

Fischer, T., and others: Adverse pulmonary responses to aspirin and acetaminophen in chronic childhood asthma, Pediatrics 71:313-318, 1983.

Gaskin, K., and others: Improved respiratory diagnosis in CF patients with normal fat absorption, J. Pediatr. 100:875-878, 1982.

Gerber, M.A., and Markowitz, M.: Management of streptococcal pharyngitis reconsidered, Pediatr. Infect. Dis. 4:518-526, 1985.

Goldbloom, R.B.: Nasopharyngitis. In Gellis, S.S., and Kagan, B.M., editors: Current pediatric therapy 12, Philadelphia, 1986, W.B. Saunders Co.

Goldstein, R., and others: Decreased elimination of theophylline after influenza vaccination, J. Can. Med. Assoc. 126:470, 1982.

Green, L., Goldstein, R., and Parker, S.: Workshop proceedings on self-managment of childhood asthma, J. Allergy Clin. Immunol. 72:519-526, 1983.

Gurwitz, D., and others: Perspectives in cystic fibrosis, Pediatr. Clin. North Am. 26:931-942, 1979.

Gurwitz, G., Mindorff, C., and Levison, H.: Increased incidence of bronchial reactivity in children with a history of bronchiolitis, J. Pediatr. 98:551-555, 1981.

Hall, C.B., and Douglas, R.G., Jr.: Nosocomial respiratory syncytial viral infections: should gowns and masks be used? Am. J. Dis. Child 135:512-515, 1981.

Harris, C.S., and others: Childhood asphyxiation by food: a national analysis and overview, JAMA 251:2231-2235, 1984.

Hayden, G.F., and others: The effect of placebo and virucidal paper handkerchiefs on viral contamination of the hand and transmission of experimental rhinovirus infection, J. Infect. Dis. 152:403-407, 1985.

Hen, J.: An overview of pediatric asthma, Pediatr. Ann. 15:92-94, 96, 1986.

Henry, R., Milner, A., and Davies, J.: Simple drug delivery system for use by young asthmatics, Br. Med. J. 286:2021, 1983.

Holbrook, P.R., and others: Adult respiratory distress syndrome in children, Pediatr. Clin. North Am. 27:677-685, 1980.

Honicky, R.E., Osborne, J.S., III, and Akpom, C.A.: Symptoms of respiratory illness in young children and the use of wood-burning stoves for indoor heating, Pediatrics 75:587-593, 1985.

Horwood, L.J., and others: Social and familial factors in the development of early childhood asthma, Pediatrics 75:859-868, 1985.

Immunization Practices Advisory Committee (ACIP): Polysaccharide vaccine for prevention of Haemophilus influenzae type b disease, MMWR 34:201-205, 1985.

Inselman, L.S.: Tuberculosis. In Gellis, S.S., and Kagan, B.M., editors: Current pediatric therapy 12, Philadelphia, 1986, W.B. Saunders Co.

Katz, J.N., and others: Clinical features as predictors of functional status in children with cystic fibrosis, J. Pediatr. 108:352-358, 1986.

Klein, J.O.: Otitis media. In Gellis, S.S., and Kagan, B.M., editors: Current pediatric therapy 12, Philadelphia, 1986, W.B. Saunders Co.

Krugman, S., and others: Infectious diseases of children, ed. 8, St. Louis, 1985, The C.V. Mosby Co.

Lampe, R.M., and others: Acoustic reflectometry in the detection of middle ear effusion, Pediatrics 76:75-79, 1985.

Levison, H., Reilly, P.A., and Worsley, G.H.: Spacing devices and metered-dose inhalers in childhood asthma, J. Pediatr. 107:662-668, 1985.

Levy, L.D., and others: Effects of long-term nutritional rehabilitation on body composition and clinical status in malnourished children and adolescents with cystic fibrosis, J. Pediatr. 107:225-230, 1985.

Lewiston, N.J.: Asthma self-management programs and education, Pediatr. Ann. 15:127-136, 1986.

Lounsbury, B.F.: Swimming unprotected with long-shafted middle ear ventilation tubes, Laryngoscope 95:340-343, 1985.

Mansell, A.L., and others: Short-term pulmonary effects of total parenteral nutrition in children with cystic fibrosis, J. Pediatr. 104:700-705, 1984.

Mathews, K.P.: Respiratory atopic disease, JAMA 248:2587-2610, 1982.

McFadden, D.M., and others: Age-specific patterns of diagnosis of acute otitis media, Clin. Pediatr. 24:571-575, 1985.

McLaughlin, F.J., and Dozor, A.J.: Cold air inhalation challenge in the diagnosis of asthma in children, Pediatrics 72:503-509, 1983.

Mertsola, J., and others: Intrafamilial spread of pertussis, J. Pediatr. 103:359-363, 1983.

Mobley, S.L., and Mansmann, H.C., Jr.: The croup syndrome. In Gellis, S.S., and Kagan, B.M., editors: Current pediatric therapy 12, Philadelphia, 1986, W.B. Saunders Co.

Mofenson, H.C., and others: Baby powder—a hazard! Pediatrics 68:265-266, 1981.

Morris, L., and others: A survey of patient sources of prescription drug information, Am. J. Public Health 74:1161, 1984.

Murphy, D., and others: The use of gowns and masks to control respiratory illness in pediatric hospital personnel, J. Pediatr. 99:746-750, 1981.

National Clearinghouse for Poison Control Centers Bull. 24(10):1, 1980.

Nelson, J.D.: The effect of penicillin therapy on the symptoms and signs of streptococcal pharyngitis, Pediatr. Infect. Dis. 3:10-13, 1984.

Newmark, P.: Testing for cystic fibrosis, Nature 318:309, 1985.

Nickerson, B., and others: Distance running improves fitness in asthmatic children without pulmonary complications or changes in exercise-induced bronchospasm, Pediatrics 71:147-152, 1983.

Ogston, S.A.: The Tayside infant morbidity and mortality study: effect on health of using gas for cooking, Br. Med. J. 290:957-960, 1985.

O'Neill, J.A., Jr., Holcomb, G.W., Jr., and Neblett, W.W.: Management of tracheobronchial and esophageal foreign bodies in childhood, J. Pediatr. Surg. 18:475-479, 1983.

Orenstein, D.M., Henke, K.G., and Cerney, F.J.: Exercise and cystic fibrosis, Physician Sports Med. 11:57-63, 1983.

Orenstein, D.M., and others: Exercise conditioning in children with asthma, J. Pediatr. 106:556-560, 1985.

Paradise, J.L.: Otitis media during early life: how hazardous to development? A critical review of the evidence, Pediatrics 68:869-873, 1981.

Paradise, J.L., and Elster, B.A.: Evidence that breast milk protects against otitis media with effusion in infants with cleft palate, Pediatr. Res. 18:283A, 1984.

Paradise, J.L., and Rogers, K.D.: On otitis media, child development, and tympanostomy tubes: new answers or old questions? Pediatrics 77:88-92, 1986.

Paradise, J.L., and others: Efficacy of tonsillectomy for recurrent throat infection in severely affected children: results of parallel randomized and nonrandomized clinical trials, N. Engl. J. Med. 310:674-683, 1984.

Pattishall, E.N., and others: Serum cotinine as a measure of tobacco smoke exposure in children, Am. J. Dis. Child. 139:1101-1104, 1985.

Pederson, S., and Møoller-Peterson, J.: Erratic absorption of a slow-release theophylline sprinkle product, Pediatrics 74:534-538, 1984.

Pedreira, F.A., and others: Involuntary smoking and incidence of respiratory illness during the first year of life, Pediatrics 75:594-597, 1985.

Quinton, P.M., and Bijman, J.: Higher bioelectric potentials due to decreased chloride absorption in the sweat glands of patients with cystic fibrosis, N. Engl. J. Med. 308:1185-1189, 1983.

Rapkin, R.H.: Spontaneous improvement of abnormal tympanograms, Pediatr. Rev. 2(5):153, 1980.

Richards, W., and others: Theophylline-associated seizures in children, Ann. Allergy 54:276-279, 1985.

Rogers, R.J., and others: Inconsistent absorption from a sustained-release theophylline preparation during continuous therapy in asthmatic children, J. Pediatr. 106:496-501, 1985.

Rona, R.J., and others: Parental smoking at home and the height of children, Br. Med. J. 283:1363, 1981.

Saarinen, U.M.: Prolonged breast-feeding as prophylaxis for recurrent otitis media, Acta Paediatr. Scand. 71:567, 1982.

Seaman-Bates, N.J.: Emergency management of status asthmaticus, J. Emerg. Nurs. **6**(5):9, 1980.

Senturia, B.H., and others: Report of the ad hoc committee on definition and classification of otitis media and otitis media with effusion, Ann. Otol. Rhinol. Laryngol. (Suppl.)**89**:3-4, 1980.

Shwachman, H.: Cystic fibrosis. In Kendig, E.L., and Chernick, V., editors: Disorders of the respiratory tract in children, ed. 4, Philadelphia, 1983, W.B. Saunders Co.

Sly, R.M.: Asthma. In Gellis, S.S., and Kagan, B.M., editors: Current pediatric therapy 12, Philadelphia, 1986, W.B. Saunders Co.

Stagno, S., and others: Infant pneumonitis associated with cytomegalovirus, chlamydia, pneumocystis, and ureaplasma: a prospective study, Pediatrics **68**:322-329, 1981.

Stern, R.C.: Bacterial pneumonia. In Behrman, R.E., and Vaughan, V.C., III: Textbook of pediatrics, ed. 12, Philadelphia, 1983, W.B. Saunders Co.

Stern, R.C.: Infectious croup. In Behrman, R.E., and Vaughan, V.C., III, editors: Textbook of pediatrics, ed. 12, Philadelphia, 1983, W.B. Saunders Co.

Stickler, G.B.: The attack on the tympanic membrane, Pediatrics **74**:291-292, 1984).

Strome, M.: Must children with tympanostomy tubes avoid swimming? Pediatr. Alert **8**(7):28, 1983.

Tager, I.B., and others: Longitudinal study of the effects of maternal smoking on pulmonary function in children, N. Engl. J. Med. **309**:699-703, 1983.

Tan, Y., and Collins-Williams, C.: Aspirin-induced asthma in children, Ann. Allergy **48**:1-5, 1982.

Tanz, R.R., and others: Penicillin plus rifampin eradicates pharyngeal carriage of group A streptococci, J. Pediatr. **106**:876-880, 1985.

Teele, D.W., and others: Otitis media with effusion during the first three years of life and development of speech and language, Pediatrics **74**:282-287, 1984.

Teele, D.W., Klein, J.O., and Rosner, B.A.: Epidemiology of otitis media in children, Ann. Otol. Rhinol. Laryngol. **682**(Suppl. 89):5-6, 1980.

Templer, J.: Removal of foreign body from the nose, Hosp. Med. :77, 1982.

Thompson, P.J., and others: Addiction to aerosol treatment: the asthmatic alternative to glue sniffing, Br. Med. J. **287**:1515-1516, 1983.

Ware, J.H., and others: Passive smoking, gas cooking, and respiratory health of children living in six cities, Am. Rev. Respir. Dis. **129**:366-374, 1984.

White, J.R., and Froeb, H.F.: Small-airway dysfunction in nonsmokers chronically exposed to tobacco smoke, N. Engl. J. Med. **302**:720-723, 1980.

Yeung, W.H., and others: Evaluation of a paper-patch test for sweat chloride determination, Clin. Pediatr. **23**:603-607, 1984.

BIBLIOGRAPHY
General

Anas, N.G., and Perkin, R.M.: Resuscitation and stabilization of the child with respiratory disease, Pediatr. Ann. **15**:43-57, 1986.

Bass, J.W.: Pertussis: current status of prevention and treatment, Pediatr. Infect. Dis. **4**:614-619, 1985.

Bean, B., and others: Survival of influenza viruses on environmental surfaces, J. Infect. Dis. **146**:47-51, 1982.

Daum, R.S., and Granoff, D.M.: A vaccine against *Haemophilius influenzae* type b, Pediatr. Infect. Dis. **4**:355-357, 1985.

Fulginiti, V.A.: Current topics in immunization, Pediatr. Consult **4**(2):1-8, 1985.

Granoff, D.M., and Cates, K.L.: *Haemophilus influenzae* type b polysaccharide vaccines, J. Pediatr. **107**:330-336, 1985.

Immunization Practices Advisory Committee (ACIP). Prevention and control of influenza, MMWR **33**:253-260, 265-266, 1984.

Jones, M.L.: Home care for the chronically ill or disabled child, New York, 1985, Harper & Row, Publishers.

Mandell, G.L., Douglas, R.G., and Bennett, J.E., editors: Principles and practice of infectious diseases, ed. 2, New York, 1985, John Wiley & Sons.

Mansell, K.A.: New immunization against *H. influenzae* type b, Pediatr. Nurs. **11**:433-435, 1985.

Mendelsohn, J.: Pediatric respiratory emergencies. In Pierog, J.E., and Pierog, L.J., editors: Pediatric critical illness and injury, Rockville, MD, 1984, Aspen Systems Corp.

Miller, D.L., Alderslade, R., and Ross, E.M.: Whooping cough and whooping cough vaccine: the risks and benefits, Epidemiol. Rev. **4**:1-24, 1982.

Moxon, E.R.: *Haemophilus influenzae* vaccine, Pediatrics **77**:258-260, 1986.

Murphy, S., and Florman, A.L.: Lung defenses against infection: a clinical correlation, Pediatrics **72**:1-15, 1983.

Rimar, J.M.: *Haemophilus influenzae* type b polysaccharide vaccine, Am. J. Maternal Child Nurs. **11**:57, 1986.

Simons, F.E.R., and Simons, K.J.: H1 receptor antagonists: clinical pharmacology and use in allergic disease, Pediatr. Clin. North Am. **30**:899-914, 1983.

Smoke inhalation. In Pulmonary crises: hydrocarbon ingestion, smoke inhalation, and near drowning, Consultant **23**(7):33-42, 1983.

Welliver, R.C.: Viral infections and obstructive airway disease in early life, Pediatr. Clin. North Am. **30**:819-828, 1983.

Upper Respiratory Infection

Breese, B.B., and others: Consensus: difficult management problems in children with streptococcal pharyngitis, Pediatr. Infect. Dis. **4**:10-13, 1985.

Castiglia, P.T., and Aquilina, S.: Streptococcal pharyngitis: a persistent challenge, Pediatr. Nurs. **8**:377-381, 1982.

Douglas, R.M., and others: Prophylactic efficacy of intranasal alpha$_2$-interferon against rhinovirus infections in the family setting, N. Engl. J. Med. **314**:65-70, 1986.

Gerber, M.A., Randolph, M.F., and Tilton, R.C.: Enzyme fluorescence procedure for rapid diagnosis of streptococcal pharyngitis, J. Pediatr. **108**:421-423, 1986.

Hammerschlag, M.R.: Infections due to *Chlamydia trachomatis*, Pediatr. Ann. **13**:673-681, 1984.

Hayden, F.G., and others: Prevention of natural colds by contact prophylaxis with intranasal alpha$_2$-interferon, N. Engl. J. Med. **314**:71-75, 1986.

Kim, K.S., and Kaplan, E.L.: Association of penicillin tolerance with failure to eradicate group A streptococci from patients with pharyngitis, J. Pediatr. **107**:681-684, 1985.

Meltzer, E.O., and others: Chronic rhinitis in infants and children: etiologic, diagnostic, and therapeutic considerations, Pediatr. Clin. North Am. **30**:847-871, 1983.

Radetsky, M., and others: Comparative evaluation of kits for rapid diagnosis of group A streptococcal disease, Pediatr. Infect. Dis. **4**:274-281, 1985.

Randolph, M.F., and others: Effect of antibiotic therapy on the clinical course of streptococcal pharyngitis, J. Pediatr. **106**:870-875, 1985.

Roddey, O.F., and others: Comparison of a latex agglutination test and four culture methods for identification of group A streptococci in a pediatric office laboratory, J. Pediatr. **108**:347-351, 1986.

Rubin, B.K.: The evaluation of the child with recurrent chest infections, Pediatr. Infect. Dis. **4**:88-98, 1985.

Walson, P.D.: Coughs and colds, Pediatrics **74**(suppl.):937-940, 1984.

Antibiotic Therapy

Byrd, H.J., and Fischer, R.G.: Cephalosporins: a brief overview of three generations, Pediatr. Nurs. **9**:330-332, 1983.

Cunningham, D.G., and others: Unprescribed use of antibiotics in common childhood infections, J. Pediatr. **103**:747-749, 1983.

Eichenwald, H.F.: Antimicrobial therapy in infants and children: update 1976-1985. Part I, J. Pediatr. **107**:161-168, 1985.

Eichenwald, H.F.: Antimicrobial therapy in infants and children: update 1976-1985. Part II, J. Pediatr. **107**:337-345, 1985.

Langslet, J., and Habel, M.L.: The aminoglycoside antibiotics, Am. J. Nurs. **81**:1144-1146, 1981.

Teele, D.: Pneumonia: antimicrobial therapy for infants and children, Pediatr. Infect. Dis. **4**:330-335, 1985.

Yoos, L.: Factors influencing maternal compliance to antibiotic regimens, Pediatr. Nurs. **10**:141-147, 1984.

Tuberculosis

Abernathy, R.S., and others: Short-course chemotherapy for tuberculosis in children, Pediatrics **72**:801-806, 1983.

Chest x-ray screening statements, FDA Drug Bull. **13**(2):13-14, 1983.

Coleman, D.A.: TB: the disease that's not dead yet, RN **47**(9):49-59, 1984.

Hauser, M., and Baier, H.: Interactions of isoniazid with foods, Drug Intell. Clin. Pharm. **16**:617-618, 1982.

Jacobs, R.F., and Abernathy, R.S.: The treatment of tuberculosis in children, Pediatr. Infect. Dis. **4**:513-517, 1985.

Lorin, M.I., Hsu, K.H.K., and Jacob, S.C.: Treatment of tuberculosis in children, Pediatr. Clin. North Am. **30**:333-348, 1983.

Perez-Stable, E.J., and others: Tuberculin skin test reactivity and conversions in United States–and foreign-born Latino children, Pediatr. Infect. Dis. **4**:476-479, 1985.

Foreign Substances

Anas, N.G., and Perkin, R.M.: Aspiration of a balloon by a 3-month-old infant, JAMA **250**:385-386, 1983.

Anas, N.G., and others: Criteria for hospitalizing children who have ingested products containing hydrocarbons, JAMA **246**:840-843, 1981.

Baker, S.P., and Fisher, R.S.: Childhood asphyxiation by choking or suffocation, JAMA **244**:1343-1346, 1980.

Breslin, E.H., and Lery, M.J.: Prevention and treatment of aspiration pneumonitis secondary to massive gastric aspiration, Crit. Care Q. **6**(2):73-82, 1983.

Ciresi, S.A.: Pulmonary aspiration: a review, AANA J. **50**:266-269, 1982.

Corkery, C.M.: Removal of a child's tonsils and adenoids, Nurs. Times **75**:742-743, May 1979.

Cotton, E., and Yasuda, K.: Foreign body aspiration, Pediatr. Clin. North Am. **31**:937-941, 1984.

Tonsils and Adenoids

Dupont, J.: EENT emergencies, Nursing 79 **9**(11):65-70, 1979.

Gladwin, B.: Adenotonsillectomy: bearing up with Paddington, Nurs. Mirror **150**(6):42-44, 1980.

Kornblut, A.D.: Surgery of the tonsils and adenoids, Ear Nose Throat J. **59**(11):65-75, 1980.

Maurer, J.A.: The care and feeding of a T & A, Point of View **18**(4):10, 1981.

Paradise, J.L.: Tonsillectomy and adenoidectomy, Pediatr. Clin. North Am. **28**:881-892, 1981.

Wolfer, J.A., and Visintainer, M.A.: Prehospital psychological preparation for tonsillectomy patients: effects on children's and parents' adjustment, Pediatrics **64**:646-655, 1979.

Otitis Media

Adams, J.L., Evans, G.A., and Roberts, J.E.: Diagnosing and treating otitis media with effusion, Am. J. Maternal Child Nurs. **9**:22-28, 1984.

Barfoed, C., and Rosborg, J.: Secretory otitis media: long-term observations after treatment with grommets, Arch. Otolaryngol. **106**:553-556, Sept. 1980.

Biles, R.W., and others: Epidemiology of otitis media: a community study, Am. J. Public Health **70**(6):593-598, 1980.

Bluestone, C.D., and others: Workshop on effects of otitis media on the child, Pediatrics **71**:639-652, 1983.

Bluestone, C.D., and others: Consensus: management of the child with a chronic draining ear, Pediatr. Infect. Dis. **4**:607-612, 1985.

Bluestone, C.D., and others: Controversies in screening for middle ear disease and hearing loss in children, Pediatrics **77**:57-70, 1986.

Bresolin, D., and others: Facial characteristics of children who breathe through the mouth, Pediatrics **73**:622-625, 1984.

Castiglia, P.T., Aquilina, S.S., and Kemsley, M.: Focus: nonsuppurative otitis media, Pediatr. Nurs. **9**:427-430, 1983.

Downs, M.P.: Identification of children at risk for middle ear effusion problems, Ann. Otol. Rhinol. Laryngol. **89**(suppl. 68, no. 3, part 2):168-171, 1980.

Glass, R.: The association of middle ear effusion and auditory learning disabilities in children, Rehab. Lit. **42**:81-85, 1981.

Hayden, G.F., and Schwartz, R.H.: Characteristics of earache among children with acute otitis media, Am. J. Dis. Child **139**:721-723, 1985.

Mäkelä, P.H., and Karma, P.: Can otitis media be prevented with pneumococcal vaccine? Prog. Clin. Biol. Res. **47**:95-106, 1980.

Marchant, C.D., and Shurin, P.A.: Therapy of otitis media, Pediatr. Clin. North Am. **30**:281-296, 1983.

Moran, D.M., and others: The use of an antihistamine-decongestant in conjunction with an anti-infective drug in the treatment of acute otitis media, J. Pediatr. **101**:132-136, 1982.

Paradise, J.L.: Otitis media in infants and children, Pediatrics **65**(5):917-943, 1980.

Sataloff, R.T., and Colton, C.M.: Otitis media: a common childhood infection, Am. J. Nurs. **81**(8):1480-1483, 1981.

Smelt, G.J.C., and Yeoh, L.H.: Swimming and grommets, J. Laryngol. Otol. **98**:243-245, 1984.

Study identifies children at risk for otitis media, AORN J. **31**(6):1014-1015, 1980.

Teele, D.W., and others: Epidemiology of otitis media in children, Ann. Otol. Rhinol. Laryngol. **89**(suppl. 68, no. 3, part 2):5-6, 1980.

Teele, D.W., and Teele, J.: Detection of middle ear effusion by acoustic reflectometry, J. Pediatr. **104**:832-836, 1984.

Tos, M.: Pathogenesis and pathology of chronic secretory otitis media, Ann. Otol. Rhinol. Laryngol. **89**(suppl. 68, no. 3, part 2):91-97, 1980.

Croup Syndromes

Bass, J.W., and others: Sudden death due to acute epiglottitis, Pediatr. Infect. Dis. **4**:447-449, 1985.

Davis, H.W., and others: Acute upper airway obstruction: croup and epiglottitis, Pediatr. Clin. North Am. **28**:859-880, 1981.

Denny, F.W., and others: Croup: an 11-year study in a pediatric practice, Pediatrics **71**:871-876, 1983.

Eavey, R.D.: A sound workup for evaluating airway obstruction, Contemp. Pediatr. **3**:78-83, 1986.

Fogel, J.M., and others: Racemic epinephrine in the treatment of croup: nebulization alone versus nebulization with intermittent positive pressure breathing, J. Pediatr. **101**:1028-1031, 1982.

Grossman, T.W.: An orderly approach to diagnosis in children and adults, Consultant **23**(8):63-91, 1983.

Kulberg, A.: Keeping little airways open, Emerg. Med. **13**:173, 177, 180-181, 186, 188-189, 1981.

Pierog, J.E.: Acute supraglottitis (epiglottitis) in children. In Pierog, J.E., and Pierog, L.J., editors: Pediatric critical illness and injury, Rockville, MD, 1984, Aspen Systems Corp.

Sofer, S., Duncan, P., and Chernick, V.: Bacterial tracheitis—an old disease rediscovered, Clin. Pediatr. **22**:407-411, 1983.

Thomas, D.O.: Are you sure it's only croup? RN **47**(12):40-43, 1984.

Pneumonia

Giebink, G.S.: Preventing pneumococcal disease in children: recommendations for using pneumococcal vaccine, Pediatr. Infect. Dis. **4**:343-348, 1985.

Long, S.S.: Treatment of acute pneumonia in infants and children, Pediatr. Clin. North Am. **30:**297-321, 1983.

Noninfectious Irritants

Burton, J.: Carbon monoxide poisoning, Crit. Care Update **10**(2):19-21, 1983.

Desai, M.H.: Inhalation injuries in burn victims, Crit. Care Q. **7**(3):1-7, 1984.

Feyerabend, C., and others: Nicotine concentration in urine and saliva of smokers and non-smokers, Br. Med. J. **284:**1002-1004, 1982.

Friedman, G.D., Petitti, D.B., and Bawol, R.D.: Prevalence and correlates of passive smoking, Am. J. Public Health **73:**401-405, 1983.

Gozal, D., and others: Accidental carbon monoxide poisoning: emphasis on hyperbaric oxygen treatment, Clin. Pediatr. **24:**132-135, 1985.

Greenberg, R.A., and others: Measuring the exposure of infants to tobacco smoke, nicotine and cotinine in urine and saliva, N. Engl. J. Med. **310:**1075-1078, 1984.

Jarvis, M.J., and others: Passive exposure to tobacco smoke: saliva cotinine concentration in a representative population sample of non-smoking school children, Br. Med. J. **291:**927-929, 1985.

Kent, J.M.: How serious is that smoke inhalation? Patient Care **18**(13):172-176, 179-180, 185-186, 1984.

Klein, B.L., and Simon, J.E.: Hydrocarbon poisonings, Pediatr. Clin. North Am. **33:**411-419, 1986.

O'Sullivan, B.P.: Carbon monoxide poisoning in an infant exposed to a kerosene heater, clinical and laboratory observations, J. Pediatr. **103:**249-250, 1983.

Adult Respiratory Distress Syndrome

Fanconi, S., and others: Long-term sequelae in children surviving adult respiratory distress syndrome, J. Pediatr. **106:**218, 1985.

Holbrook, P.R., and others: Adult respiratory distress syndrome in children, Pediatr. Clin. North Am. **27:**677, 1980.

Lyrene, R., and Truog, W.: Adult respiratory distress syndrome in a pediatric intensive care unit: predisposing conditions, clinical course and outcome, Pediatrics **67:**790, 1981.

Pfenninger, J., and others: Adult respiratory distress syndrome in children, J. Pediatr. **101:**352-356, 1982.

Bronchial Asthma

Aubier, M., and others: Aminophylline improves diaphragmatic contractility, N. Engl. J. Med. **305:**249-252, 1981.

Berman, B.A.: Cromolyn: past, present, and future, Pediatr. Clin. North Am. **30:**915-930, 1983.

Blessing-Moore, J., Fritz, G., and Lewiston, N.J.: Self-management programs for childhood asthma, Chest **87:**1-5, 1985.

Chryssanthopoulos, C., and others: Cardiopulmonary responses of asthmatic children to strenuous exercise, Clin. Pediatr. **23:**384-387, 1984.

Conboy, K.: Nursing care plan for the child with status asthmaticus, Crit. Care Nurse **5**(2):8-9, 12, 1985.

Dahms, T.E., Bolin, J.F., and Slavin, R.G.: Passive smoking: effects on bronchial asthma, Chest **80:**530-534, 1981.

DiPalma, J.R.: Beta$_2$ agonists for acute asthma, Am. Fam. Physician **31**(5):184-187, 1985.

Eitches, R.W., and others: Methylprednisone and troleandomycin in treatment of steroid-dependent asthmatic children, Am. J. Dis. Child. **139:**264-268, 1985.

Fireman, P., and others: Teaching self-management skills to asthmatic children and their parents in an ambulatory care setting, Pediatrics **68:**341-348, 1981.

Fischer, T.J., and others: Adverse pulmonary responses to aspirin and acetaminophen in chronic childhood asthma, Pediatrics **71:**313-318, 1983.

Galant, S.P.: Current status of beta-adrenergic agonists in bronchial asthma, Pediatr. Clin. North Am. **30:**931-942, 1983.

Galdès-Sebaldt, M., McLaughlin, F.J., and Levison, H.: Comparison of cold air, ultrasonic mist, and methacholine inhalations as tests of bronchial reactivity in normal and asthmatic children, J. Pediatr. **107:**526-530, 1985.

Goldstein, R.A., editor: Advances in the diagnosis and treatment of asthma, Chest (Suppl.)**87:**1S-113S, 1985.

Gortmaker, S.L., and others: Parental smoking and the risk of childhood asthma, Am. J. Public Health **72:**574-579, 1982.

Haltom, J.R., and Szefler, S.J.: Theophylline absorption in young asthmatic children receiving sustained-release formulations, J. Pediatr. **107:**805-810, 1985.

Hen, J.: Office evaluation and management of pediatric asthma, Pediatr. Ann. **15:**111-124, 1986.

Isles, A., and Levison, H.: Treatment of childhood asthma, J. Respir. Dis. (Suppl.) **3:**60-71, 1982.

Jennings, C.: Controlling the home environment of the allergic child, Am. J. Maternal Child Nurs. **7:**376-381, 1982.

Josephs, S.H.: Immunologic mechanisms in pulmonary disease, Pediatr. Clin. North Am. **31:**919-936, 1984.

Kirilloff, L.H., and Tibbals, S.C.: Drugs for asthma: a complete guide, Am. J. Nurs. **83:**55-61, 1983.

Kjellman, N.-I.M.: Prediction and prevention of atopic allergy, Allergy **37:**463-473, 1982.

Kubly, L.S., and McClellan, M.S.: Effects of self-care instruction on asthmatic children, Issues Compre. Pediatr. Nurs. **7:**121-130, 1984.

Kubo, M., and others: Intraindividual changes in theophylline clearance during constant aminophylline infusion in children with acute asthma, J. Pediatr. **108:**1011-1015, 1986.

Lee, H., and Evans, H.E.: Aerosol bag for administration of bronchodilators to young asthmatic children, Pediatrics **73:**230-232, 1984.

Lewis, C.E., and others: A randomized trial of A.C.T. (asthma care training) for kids, Pediatrics **74:**478-486, 1984.

Mitsuhashi, M., and others: Hyperresponsiveness of cough receptors in patients with bronchial asthma, Pediatrics **75:**855-858, 1985.

Murray, A.B., and Ferguson, A.C.: Dust-free bedrooms in the treatment of asthmatic children with house dust or house dust mite allergy: a controlled trial, Pediatrics **71:**418-422, 1983.

Murray, A.B., and others: Diagnosis of house dust mite allergy in asthmatic children: what constitutes a positive history? J. Allerg. Clin. Immunol. **71:**21-28, 1983.

Neijens, H.J., Duiverman, E.J., and Kerrebijn, K.F.: Bronchial responsiveness in children, Pediatr. Clin. North Am. **30:**829-846, 1983.

Neild, J.E., and Cameron, I.R.: Bronchoconstriction in response to suggestion: its prevention by an inhaled anticholinergic agent, Br. Med. J. **290:**674, 1985.

Nickerson, B.G.: Approach to the wheezing infant, Pediatr. Ann. **15:**99-104, 1986.

Nickerson, B.G., and others: Distance running improves fitness in asthmatic children without pulmonary complications or changes in exercise-induced bronchospasm, Pediatrics **71:**147-152, 1983.

Rachelefsky, G.S.: Asthma self-management programs for children, Child Care Newsletter **3**(2):5-8, 1984.

Rachelefsky, G.S.: The wheezing child, Pediatrics **74**(suppl.):941-947, 1984.

Rachelefsky, G.S., and others: ACT for kids, Chest (suppl.) **87:**98S-100S, 1985.

Rimar, J.M.: Albuterol: a selective beta$_2$ bronchodilator, Am. J. Maternal Child Nurs. **11:**169, 1986.

Rubin, D.H., and others: Educational intervention by computer in childhood asthma: a randomized clinical trial testing the use of a new teaching intervention in childhood asthma, Pediatrics **77:**1-10, 1986.

Schwartz, R.H.: Children with chronic asthma: care by the generalist and the specialist, Pediatr. Clin. North Am. **31:**87-105, 1984.

Sedlacek, K.K.: Asthma in children: facilitating self-care, Pediatr. Nurs. Update **1**(1):1-8, 1985.

Shapiro, G.G.: Corticosteroids in the treatment of allergic disease: principles and practice, Pediatr. Clin. North Am. **30:**955-971, 1983.

Silver, R.B., and Ginsburg, C.M.: Early prediction of the need for hospitalization in children with acute asthma, Clin. Pediatr. **23**:81-84, 1984.

Söderman, P., Sahlberg, D., and Wiholm, B.E.: CNS reactions to nose drops in small children (letter), Lancet **1**:573, 1984.

Stempel, D.A., and Mellon, M.: Management of acute severe asthma, Pediatr. Clin. North Am. **31**:879-890, 1984.

Sulfites in foods and drugs, FDA Drug Bull. **13**(2):11-12, 1983.

Szefler, S.J.: Practical considerations in the safe and effective use of theophylline, Pediatr. Clin. North Am. **30**:943-954, 1983.

Tal, A., and others: Response to cold air hyperventilation in normal and in asthmatic children, J. Pediatr. **104**:516-521, 1984.

Towns, S.J., and Mellis, C.M.: Role of acetyl salicylic acid and sodium metabisulfite in chronic childhood asthma, Pediatrics **73**:631-637, 1984.

Willert, C., and others: Short-term holding room treatment of asthmatic children, J. Pediatr. **106**:707-711, 1985.

Wolf, S.I., and Nicklas, R.A.: Sulfite sensitivity in a seven-year-old child, Ann. Allergy **54**:420-422, 1985.

Zwerdling, R.G.: Status asthmaticus, Pediatr. Ann. **15**:105-109, 1986.

Cystic Fibrosis

Canam, C.: Talking about cystic fibrosis within the family—what parents need to know, Issues Compre. Pediatr. Nurs. **9**:167-178, 1986.

Cowen, L., and others: Psychologic adjustment of the family with a member who has cystic fibrosis, Pediatrics **77**:745-753, 1986.

Desmond, K.J., and others: Immediate and long-term effects of chest physiotherapy in patients with cystic fibrosis, J. Pediatr. **103**:538-542, 1983.

Glendon, M.: Teaching Harry what we'd thought he knew, Nursing 85 **15**(7):44-46, 1985.

Harder, L., and Bowditch, B.: Siblings of children with cystic fibrosis: perceptions of the impact of the disease, Child. Health Care **10**:116-120, 1982.

Hymovich, D.P., and Baker, C.D.: The needs, concerns and coping of parents of children with cystic fibrosis, Fam. Relations **34**:91-97, 1985.

Kruger, S., Shawver, M., and Jones, L.: Reactions of families to the child with cystic fibrosis, Image **12**:67-72, 1980.

Lewis, B.L., and Kaw, K-T.: Family functioning as a mediating variable affecting psychosocial adjustment of children with cystic fibrosis, J. Pediatr. **101**:636-640, 1982.

Marks, M.I.: The pathogenesis and treatment of pulmonary infections in patients with cystic fibrosis, J. Pediatr. **98**:173-179, 1981.

Matthews, L.W., and Drotar, D.: Cystic fibrosis—a challenging long-term chronic disease, Pediatr. Clin. North Am. **31**:133-152, 1984.

Nolan, T., and others: Knowledge of cystic fibrosis in patients and their parents, Pediatrics **77**:229-235, 1986.

Patterson, J.M.: Critical factors affecting family compliance with home treatment for children with cystic fibrosis, Fam. Relations **34**:79-89, 1985.

Patton, A.C., Ventura, J.N., and Savedra, M.: Stress and coping responses of adolescents with cystic fibrosis, Child. Health Care **14**:153-156, 1986.

Pumariega, A.J.: The adolescent with cystic fibrosis: developmental issues, Child. Health Care **11**:78-81, 1982.

Shepard, R., Cooksley, W.G.E., and Cooke, W.D.D.: Improved growth and clinical, nutritional, and respiratory changes in response to nutritional therapy in cystic fibrosis, J. Pediatr. **97**:351-357, 1980.

Shwachman, H., Mahmoodian, A., and Neff, R.K.: The sweat test: sodium and chloride values, J. Pediatr. **98**:576-578, 1981.

Spotting and sustaining patients with CF, Patient Care **16**:16-53, 1982.

Stewart, A.: Care in the hospital: cystic fibrosis. Part 3, Nurs. Times **80**(22):44-45, 1984.

Chapter 33

The Child with a Gastrointestinal Disorder

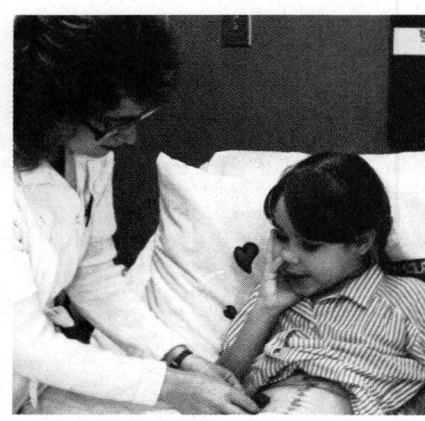

Disorders of the gastrointestinal tract are very common and constitute one of the largest categories of illnesses that occur in infancy and childhood. Structural and obstructive defects interfere with the ingestion and transport of foodstuffs, and inflammatory, malabsorptive, and maldigestive disturbances impair the functional integrity of the gastrointestinal tract. Furthermore, in most of the disorders the primary defect can produce additional complications. For example, obstructive or inflammatory conditions affect digestion and absorption because bowel motility, mucosal functioning, enzymatic activity, and bacterial flora are altered. This chapter is concerned with those conditions that in some way interfere with normal digestion and absorption of nutrients.

Gastrointestinal Structure and Function

Knowledge of the basic structure and physiology of digestion and absorption is foundational to the understanding of gastrointestinal disorders. The following discussion is an overview of the development of the gastrointestinal tract during early childhood and of the basic physiology of digestion and absorption. For a review of the major anatomic structures within the abdominal cavity, the reader is referred to Fig. 7-46.

GASTROINTESTINAL DEVELOPMENT AND FUNCTION IN EARLY CHILDHOOD

The gastrointestinal (GI) system serves several essential functions: (1) processes and absorbs nutrients necessary to maintain metabolic processes and to support growth and development, (2) performs an excretory function for both digestive residue and other waste products that pour into the intestine from the blood or are excreted in the bile, (3) provides detoxification while other routes of elimination (kidneys, liver, skin) are still immature, and (4) participates in maintaining fluid and electrolyte balance in infancy. All actions of the gastrointestinal tract are subject to a variety of outside influences at all ages. They are sensitive to tensions and anxieties, and many diseases and disorders are reflected in altered gastrointestinal function.

The primitive digestive system forms during the fourth week of gestation, but the most rapid and extensive development occurs just before birth. As a result, most biochemical and physiologic functions are established at the time of birth. Before birth the exchange of nutrients and waste is assumed by the placenta; therefore the demands on the alimentary tract are minimum. However, the presence in the intestine of a thick, sticky, greenish black material *(meconium)* composed of cast-off epithelial cells, digestive tract secretions (e.g., mucus and bile), and residue from swallowed amniotic fluid attests to prenatal activity. The passage of this meconium after birth provides evidence of the patency of the tract.

The mechanical functions of digestion are relatively immature at birth. Sucking and swallowing are established prenatally but do not become fully developed until after birth. Swallowing is an automatic reflex action for the first 3 months, and the infant has no voluntary control of swallowing until the striated muscles in the throat establish their cerebral connections. This begins at approximately 6 weeks of age. By 6 months the infant is capable of swallowing, holding food in the mouth, or spitting it out at will. The mechanism of sucking is also a reflexive activity in the newborn, and the muscular action of the tongue has a typical forward thrust. With neural and muscular development, the infant gradually acquires the ability to perform the coordinated muscular action typical of the adult type of swallowing (see p. 497). The chewing function is facilitated by

STOMACH CAPACITY (APPROXIMATE) AT VARIOUS STAGES OF DEVELOPMENT

AGE	CAPACITY (ml)
Newborn	10-20
1 week	30-90
2-3 weeks	75-100
1 month	90-150
3 months	150-200
1 year	210-360
2 years	500
10 years	750-900
16 years	1500
Adult	2000-3000

eruption of the primary teeth. The timing of dietary changes closely parallels these progressive capabilities. First to develop are those that require merely swallowing, then those that need no mastication, and finally those that require biting and chewing.

The stomach, which lies horizontally, is round until the child is approximately 2 years of age. It then gradually elongates until at about 7 years of age it assumes the shape and anatomic position of the adult. This anatomic placement of the stomach in infancy influences positioning practices during and after feeding (p. 325). At birth the capacity of the stomach is only about 10 to 20 ml, but the stomach, a distensible organ, rapidly expands to triple its capacity in 3 weeks and to reach 5 to 10 times its original birth capacity at the age of 1 month (see box, above).

The immaturity of the digestive system in the infant is demonstrated by the rapidity with which swallowed food is propelled through the entire tract. The frequency and character of stools are affected by the rate of peristalsis and the nature of ingested food. For example, the frequent, yellow stools of the neonate gradually assume a more adult regularity and character in the infant. The emptying time of the stomach increases from 2½ to 3 hours in the newborn to 3 to 6 hours in older infants and children. The small stomach capacity with a rapid transit time has implications for determining the amount and frequency of feedings during this period of growth. In addition, peristalsis is more rapid in infancy than at other periods of life, and it is not uncommon for peristaltic waves to reverse and cause spitting up or, if vigorous, vomiting of stomach contents. An immature, relaxed cardiac sphincter in infancy and early childhood contributes to this ease of regurgitation.

During the prenatal period the large intestine grows more rapidly than the small intestine, but after birth this rate is reversed. The length of the intestine in infants is 6 times the body length and is proportionately greater than that of the full-grown individual, which is 4 to 5 times the body length. There are two periods of accelerated growth of the intestine that correlate with nutritional and physiologic changes taking place: (1) between 1 and 3 years of age, during a period of diet transition, and (2) between 10 and 15 years of age, a period that coincides with the adolescent growth spurt.

The secretory cells of the gastrointestinal tract are believed to be functional at birth. However, since most of the digestive enzymes depend on a specific pH relationship that is gradually acquired with age, their efficiency may be impaired. The newborn produces only small amounts of saliva, which contains some of the starch-splitting enzyme ptyalin; therefore its primary purpose at this time is to moisten the mouth and throat. It has little time to act on starches in the rapidly swallowed food. By the end of the second year the salivary glands have increased in size about 5 times to reach their full size and function.

Gastric acidity varies during childhood. The acidity of gastric juice is low during infancy and rises during childhood to level off at approximately 10 years of age. At the time of the adolescent growth spurt there is an increase in free hydrochloric acid. It is particularly marked in males, which probably contributes to the simultaneous increase in consumption of food. Most of the chemical activity is functional within these limitations and to the extent that it is dependent on the development of hormonal and neurologic maturation.

DIGESTION

Digestion refers to the catabolism of foodstuffs from their original complex form to simple, assimilable nutrients. Foodstuffs are composed of six substances: water, vitamins, mineral salts, carbohydrates, proteins, and fats. The processes of digestion are mainly *mechanical* (mixing and propulsion of food along the alimentary tract) and *chemical* (conversion of carbohydrates, proteins, and fats into assimilable forms, namely, simple sugars, amino acids, and fatty acids and glycerol, respectively).

Mechanical digestion begins in the mouth. The chewing movements of the teeth and tongue mix the food with saliva and reduce the size of the particles into what is called a *bolus*. Besides moistening the food sufficiently to aid in swallowing, saliva initiates digestion. The enzyme ptyalin, also called amylase, catalyzes the more complex carbohydrates or starches into simpler forms, such as maltose. Once the bolus is swallowed, the remainder of mechanical digestion is involuntary.

The pharynx and esophagus are primarily concerned with deglutition, or swallowing. As the tongue pushes the food backward into the pharynx, the food is propelled into the esophagus by two mechanisms, which prevent its entry up into the nasal cavity or respiratory tract. First, the soft palate and uvula elevate to block off the nasopharynx. Second, the epiglottis closes over the larynx to prevent food from passing into the airway. As food enters the esophagus, it is propelled forward into the stomach by movements called *peristalsis*. These wavelike movements squeeze the food along the entire length of the alimentary tract. The passage

of stomach contents is controlled by the cardiac sphincter between the esophagus and stomach and by the pyloric sphincter between the stomach and duodenum, the beginning of the small intestine.

As the bolus passes into the stomach, gastric movements churn the particles back and forth, mixing them with gastric juice. Gastric juice contains water, pepsin, hydrochloric acid, rennin, lipase, and mucin. Pepsin (also called protease), hydrochloric acid, and rennin partially digest proteins; lipase initiates the digestion of fats. Mucin serves primarily to buffer the strong acid and forms a protective barrier between the acid and the stomach. The entire alimentary tract is protected from the digestive action of its various secretions by the production of mucus and the rapid replacement of mucosal cells.

The partially digested food, now called *chyme*, passes from the stomach into the small intestine, where churning movements cause it to mix thoroughly with intestinal juices and to come in contact with the mucosal lining for absorption. The intestinal epithelial cells contain large quantities of digestive enzymes, which appear to complete digestion while the substances are being absorbed into the cells. These enzymes include (1) peptidases for splitting peptides into amino acids, (2) sucrase, maltase, isomaltase, and lactase for converting disaccharides into the monosaccharides glucose, galactose, and fructose, and (3) lipase for splitting fats into fatty acids and glycerol.

Secretions from the liver and pancreas complete digestion in the small intestine. Bile, formed in the liver, contains no enzymes but is important for digestion because it (1) lowers the surface tension of fat, forming an emulsion that allows the water-soluble lipase to exert its enzymatic effect on the fat globules, and (2) increases the absorption of the end products of fat digestion by the intestinal wall. The absence of bile causes about half of the ingested fat to appear in the feces, a condition called *steatorrhea,* and impairs the absorption of the fat-soluble vitamins A, D, E, and K.

Pancreatic juice contains three important digestive enzymes: (1) trypsin (also called protease), which converts partially digested proteins, namely proteoses and peptones, and intact proteins into the final end product, amino acids, (2) lipase, which catalyzes the bile-emulsified fats into their final end products, fatty acids and glycerol, and (3) amylase, which hydrolyzes most starches and carbohydrates to the disaccharides maltose, sucrose, and lactose. Each of these three enzymes becomes active only after the inactive forms are secreted into the small intestine. For example, enterokinase is necessary for trypsinogen to be converted into trypsin. If this were not the case, the activated enzymes would digest the pancreas and pancreatic duct.

After the digestion and absorption of the nutritional end product in the small intestine, the remainder of the intestinal contents, namely nondigestible residue and a small amount of undigested fat and protein, pass through the ileocecal valve into the large intestine. Here the contents are prepared for excretion as *feces.* Most of the remaining water and electrolytes is absorbed from the proximal colon. The bacterial flora form vitamin K, vitamin B_{12}, thiamine, riboflavin, and various gases. The odor of feces is primarily the result of the products of bacterial action and depends on the type of colonic flora and ingested food. Defects in digestion or absorption notably alter the odor, as well as the appearance, of feces. The color is caused by the end products of bilirubin, which is converted by bacteria to urobilinogen and then oxidized to urobilin.

As the rectum becomes distended with feces, powerful peristaltic waves are stimulated, which propel the colonic contents toward the anus. At the same time, the internal anal sphincter relaxes, and, if the external sphincter voluntarily or involuntarily relaxes, defecation occurs.

ABSORPTION

The principal absorbing site in the gastrointestinal system is the small intestine. The inner lining of the small intestine contains many folds called *valvulae conniventes,* or *plicae circulares,* and the entire surface of these folds is covered with small, fingerlike projections called *villi.* Millions of *microvilli* make up the luminal surface of the intestinal epithelial cells covering each villus, forming what is called the *brush border* of the villi. These structures or coats have been estimated to increase the surface area of the intestine by 600 to 700 times (Klish and Putnam, 1981). In each villus are *crypts of Lieberkühn,* whose main purpose is to replace the absorptive cells that are constantly being extruded at each villus tip. This process of regeneration is so effective that normally the intestinal epithelium replaces itself every 5 days.

Unlike this type of surface, the stomach and large intestine are devoid of villi. Most of the absorption that takes place there is by *diffusion,* or the movement of substances from an area of higher concentration to one of lower concentration. Absorption in the small intestine may be by simple diffusion or *active transport,* which requires energy to transport a substance across an opposing pressure gradient or against an electric potential. The mechanisms of active transport are not completely understood but are thought to be carried on by the epithelial cells of the intestinal mucosa.

The end products of carbohydrate and protein digestion, the monosaccharides and amino acids, are absorbed into the intestinal capillaries and circulated to the liver by the portal vein, where they are metabolized and either used for energy or stored as the body's reserves. The end products of fat digestion, the fatty acids and glycerol, are absorbed by the epithelial cells of the villi, where they are reconverted to the triglyceride fat molecule, which then moves out of the cells into the lymph capillaries (lacteals) of the villi. The lymphatics carry them to the venous circulation by the thoracic duct to the left subclavian vein, superior vena cava, heart, and general circulation. Some undigested emulsified fats directly enter the circulation by the intestinal capillaries.

All of the vitamins are believed to be absorbed in the small intestine. The fat-soluble vitamins are absorbed along with digested fats in the presence of bile. The water-soluble vitamins, vitamin B complex and C, are quickly absorbed, although absorption of vitamin B_{12} takes place only in the ileum. Water and electrolytes are also absorbed primarily in the small intestine, although some absorption also takes place in the large intestine.

ASSESSMENT OF GASTROINTESTINAL FUNCTION

A number of tests may be employed to assess gastrointestinal function. One of the most common is *fecal examination* to evaluate the absorptive function of the intestine, especially the amount of fecal fat and levels of electrolytes. Stool specimens may also be collected to check for the presence of blood, bacteria, and parasites (see p. 1129 for collection of stool specimens). More complicated procedures may be used to examine other products of the GI tract, such as gastric contents and duodenal secretions.

Radiologic examination of the GI tract involves the introduction of a contrast medium, such as barium, into the upper or lower tract to visualize outlines of structures or pathologic conditions. The oral introduction of barium into the upper GI tract *(upper GI series)* permits radiographic visualization of the esophagus, stomach, and small bowel. Introduction of barium via enema *(lower GI series)* permits radiographic visualization of the colon. Since children may not like to drink the barium and generally dislike enemas, they need preparation for the GI series (see Preparation for procedures in Chapter 27).

Direct visualization of the GI tract is possible through *fiberoptic endoscopy,* which consists of a flexible tube that contains bundles of thin, transparent fibers through which light can be transmitted to different regions of the GI tract. Light is transmitted down some of the fibers; from the illuminated area the light is then reflected back up the remaining fibers to produce an image. The endoscope is equipped with channels through which various instruments can be passed, for example, to take a biopsy or retrieve foreign objects (Tilkian, Conover, and Tilkian, 1983). Another procedure permitting direct visualization of the sigmoid colon and rectum is *sigmoidoscopy,* which may use the traditional rigid scope or the fiberoptic scope. *Fiberoptic colonoscopy* can be used to reach the cecum, and if used by skilled practitioners, it is a safe method with young children (Hassall, Barclay, and Ament, 1984).

Tests to measure GI motility and pressure may be required in those instances when sphincter function or motility of the esophagus or colon must be assessed. Such tests include *esophageal manometry,* to measure the pressure gradients generated by peristalsis as the peristaltic wave progresses from the hypopharynx to the stomach, and *anorectal manometry,* to measure anal sphincter function. These tests and other special procedures are discussed in more detail later in the chapter when specific conditions are presented.

Ingestion of Foreign Substances

Children are prone to ingesting foreign substances as they place their hands and any attractive object or substance into their mouths. Infants and small children in particular explore items with their mouths instinctively. Older children often place items in their mouths and accidentally swallow them. Rarely, a child deliberately swallows unusual objects or substances. Hands come into contact with dirt and contaminated objects that contain ova or larvae of a variety of parasites. The following is an overview of ingestion of foreign objects; discussion of specific substances, such as lead or parasites, is presented in Chapter 16.

PICA

Pica is the Latin word for magpie, a bird of voracious and indiscriminate appetite. The use of the term today refers to the habitual, purposeful, and compulsive ingestion of nonfood substances in the environment. The list of ingested substances is practically endless but most commonly includes clay, dirt, ashes, paint chips, laundry starch, cornstarch, paper, pencils, erasers, crayons, cigarette butts, and matches. Most children have a particular craving for a few items, which is largely determined by the availability of the substance.

It is believed by some that certain forms of pica are manifestations of a deficiency in the diet, especially of minerals. For example, clay-eating has been related to zinc deficiency and eating chalk to calcium deficiency. In most instances pica is relatively harmless, but if the substance ingested contains a harmful ingredient (e.g. lead in paint), the practice becomes a serious matter. If the eating of a specific substance persists, it should probably be evaluated. Certainly if a potentially harmful substance is involved, it should be removed from the environment or the child denied access to it.

FOREIGN BODIES

Children ingest a variety of foreign objects. Most ingested foreign bodies, such as marbles, coins, beads, and small safety pins, pass through the alimentary tract without difficulty once they reach the stomach. Larger items and straight or sharp objects, such as bobby pins, hairpins, pull tabs on beverage cans, needles, tacks, and large safety pins, may become lodged in the esophagus or duodenal loop.

Once an ingested object passes the pylorus, its progress is followed by radiograms, and the stools are examined for its presence. The child is fed his customary diet. If serial radiographs indicate that the object remains stationary, it is removed by an endoscope or in rare cases by laparotomy. Surgical removal is indicated in instances of perforation, bleeding, or obstruction and when large or long objects have not cleared the stomach within 3 to 5 days (Webb, McDaniel, and Jones, 1984).

Foreign bodies that become lodged in the esophagus require immediate attention since they may adhere to the esophageal wall, where they cause erosion of the epithelium. Of particular concern is the increasing incidence of ingestion of "button" batteries commonly found in watches, hearing aids, cameras, and calculators. Some have been found to leak their alkaline electrolytes and other corrosive substances or have been acted upon by stomach and intestinal secretions. While most button battery ingestions are benign, the most difficulty arises from the larger diameter batteries, which become impacted in the esophagus. Recommendations for treating battery ingestions include (1) confirming the location by radiographic examination, (2) removing immediately those lodged in the esophagus, (3) observing those beyond the esophagus on an outpatient basis, (4) repeating radiography after 48 hours if the ingested battery is larger than button size and removing those that still remain in the stomach, and (5) repeating radiography if a small battery has not passed in the stool by 4 to 7 days (Litovitz, 1985).

Nursing Considerations

The primary nursing intervention is prevention of foreign body ingestion through preventive family teaching. All children who are old enough to understand should be told not to put anything in their mouths before asking permission. Infants and young children who cannot follow such advice must have their environment protected for them. Small objects are placed out of their reach or properly discarded. The best suggestion is to get down on the floor and look for and remove objects that are accessible to inquisitive young children.

Once an object is swallowed, parents need guidelines on seeking treatment (see box). When no treatment is instituted, parents should examine the stool for verification that the object has passed safely through the gastrointestinal tract, usually in 3 to 4 days. For children in diapers this is easily accomplished by squeezing the stool between the diaper to locate the object, but in toilet-trained children it requires more effort. A piece of plastic wrap placed across the toilet bowl to collect the stool makes it easier to examine the feces, although a tongue blade or some other disposable object may be needed to break up the stool.

Malabsorption Syndromes

The term *malabsorption syndrome* is applied to a long list of disorders associated with some degree of impaired digestion and/or absorption. Most are classified according to the locations of the supposed anatomic and/or biochemical defect.

GENERAL CLASSIFICATION

Digestive defects mainly include those conditions in which the enzymes necessary for digestion are diminished or absent, such as (1) cystic fibrosis, in which pancreatic enzymes are absent, (2) biliary or liver disease, in which bile production is affected, or (3) lactase deficiency, in which there is congenital or secondary lactose intolerance.

Absorptive defects include those conditions in which the intestinal mucosal transport system is impaired. It may be because of a primary defect, such as in celiac disease, or secondary to inflammatory disease of the bowel that results in impaired absorption because bowel motility is accelerated, such as ulcerative colitis. Obstructive disorders, such as Hirschsprung disease, can also cause secondary malabsorption from enterocolitis, chronic inflammation of the distended small and large bowel.

Anatomic defects, such as short bowel syndrome, affect digestion by decreasing the transit time of substances with the digestive juices and affect absorption by severely compromising the absorptive surface.

Emotional Factors

There are also some disorders that result in malabsorption but for which no specific organic cause can be found. One of the classic examples is nonorganic failure to thrive, in which malnutrition results despite adequately functioning body systems and is reversed by a program of emotional stimulation rather than medical intervention.

CELIAC SYNDROME

Celiac syndrome and *malabsorption syndrome* are terms used to describe a symptom complex associated with several different diseases that have four characteristics in common: (1) steatorrhea (fat, foul, frothy, bulky stools), (2) general malnutrition, (3) abdominal distention, and (4) secondary vitamin deficiencies.

Celiac disease and cystic fibrosis are the two most common malabsorptive disorders in children. Presently celiac disease refers to a specific condition, callled *gluten-sensitive enteropathy.* In adults this same condition is often referred to as nontropical sprue.

CELIAC DISEASE (GLUTEN ENTEROPATHY)

Celiac disease, also referred to as gluten enteropathy (GE), gluten-sensitive enteropathy (GSE), and celiac sprue, is second only to cystic fibrosis as a cause of malabsorption in children. Recent reports indicate that the incidence of celiac disease is declining, from 49:100,000 live births between 1970 and 1974 to 21:100,000 live births between 1975 and 1979 (Simila and others, 1981). Although the exact reason is not known, there is an association between changes in feeding practices—specifically, delayed introduction of solid foods and encouragement of breast-feeding—and the declining incidence of celiac disease (Dossetor, Gibson, and McNeish, 1981; Littlewood and Crollick, 1980). It is seen more frequently in Europe than in America and is rarely reported in Asians or blacks. Although the exact mode of transmission is not known, there is a tendency for the disease to occur in several members of the same family. An

important link between the disease and genetic factors is the finding of a significant increase in the incidence of certain histocompatibility antigens. HLA-B8 is found in 60% to 90% of affected individuals, which is a fourfold increase over that found in the general population (Silverman and Roy, 1983). Celiac disease is also more common in children with insulin-dependent diabetes mellitus, particularly those carrying the HLA-B8 and DR3 antigens (Savilahti and others, 1986).

Pathophysiology

The disease is characterized by an intolerance for gluten, one of the proteins found in wheat, barley, rye, and oats. Gluten consists of two fractions, glutenin and gliadin. It is the gliadin fraction to which susceptible individuals are sensitive. Although the precise mechanism by which gliadin produces cell damage is not known, inability to fully digest gliadin results in accumulation of the amino acid glutamine, which is toxic to the mucosal cells. As a result the newly forming epithelial cells in the crypts of Lieberkühn die before they can migrate to the surface of the villi to replace worn-out cells. This causes the villi to eventually atrophy, thus greatly reducing the absorptive surface of the small intestine and in addition affecting various absorptive processes.

The basic defect is believed to be either an inborn error of metabolism or an immunologic response. The former theory holds that there is an absence of peptidase in intestinal mucosal cells that results in an inability to digest gliadin. The immunologic theory proposes that gliadin acts as an antigen that evokes an injurious response from the mucosal cells. The resulting peptidase deficiency is a consequence of the antigenic response rather than the primary defect.

In the early stages of celiac disease fat absorption is primarily affected, resulting in elimination of large quantities of digested fat (soaps and fatty acids) in the stool. The frothy appearance, foul odor, and excessive quantity of stool are the result of altered bacterial flora on the digested,

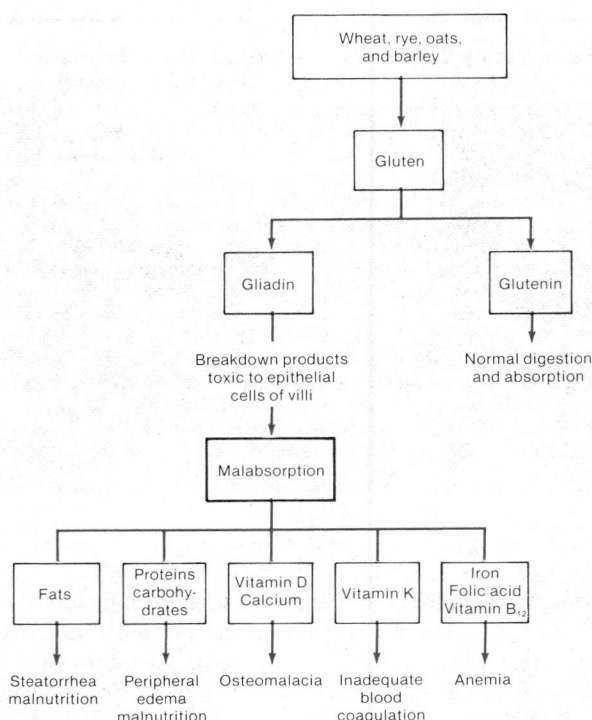

Fig. 33-1. Malabsorptive defect in celiac disease.

Clinical Manifestations

Symptoms of celiac disease do not begin until the child is ingesting grains (the chief source of gluten), usually within 3 to 6 months of the introduction of gluten. The clinical manifestations are usually insidious and chronic. The first evidence of the disease may be failure to regain weight or appetite after a bout of diarrhea. Although steatorrhea is a common symptom, it is absent in 10% to 20% of children. Constipation, vomiting, and abdominal pain may also be initial presenting signs. Behavioral changes, such as irritability, fretfulness, uncooperativeness, or apathy, are common. As the disease progresses, signs of general wasting become evident.

Some children do not manifest symptoms until later in life, usually after the age of 5 years. The symptoms are mainly those of retarded growth and delayed sexual development, with diarrhea less of a problem. The reasons why some individuals have symptoms later in life or remain asymptomatic despite mucosal abnormalities are unknown (Shah and Lebenthal, 1983).

Celiac disease may be characterized by acute, severe episodes of profuse, pale, bulky, rancid, poorly formed stools and vomiting, called *celiac crisis*. Other manifestations are a wasted appearance, especially of extremities and buttocks, dependent edema, and a smooth tongue. Celiac crises may be precipitated by infections, especially of the gastrointestinal tract, prolonged fasting, dietary sources of gluten, or anticholinergic drugs, such as the preanesthetic agents atropine or scopolamine.

Diagnostic Evaluation

Several tests are available for establishing the diagnosis of celiac disease, many of which are based on the expected pathologic findings, such as stool analysis for fecal fat excretion; hematologic studies for hypoproteinemia, anemia, hypoprothrombinemia, serum iron, folic acid, and vitamin B_{12} levels; immunoglobulin levels; roentgenographic studies for bone age; evidence of osteoporosis and osteomalacia; and bowel studies for dilated, flaccid bowel loops and thickening of the mucosal folds. Pancreatic function studies and a sweat test are usually included in the general laboratory evaluation to rule out the possibility of cystic fibrosis. Currently several procedures are under investigation to permit screening of individuals at risk for developing the disease. These tests detect antibodies that may form as a result of the immune response, such as gliaden antibody (circulating antibody to wheat gliadin fractions) or reticulin antibody (an autoantibody that is thought to be directed against reticulin from animal food sources) (Burgin-Wolff and others, 1983; Maki and others, 1984).

However, definitive diagnosis is based on a small bowel biopsy, which demonstrates the atrophic changes in the architecture of the mucosal wall. The peroral jejunal biopsy is performed by passing a polyethylene tube through the mouth along the alimentary tract to the jejunum of the small bowel. The child is given nothing by mouth for 4 to 8 hours before the procedure and is not sedated, because the passage

but unabsorbed, fats and proteins. At this time the disease is sometimes called *idiopathic steatorrhea,* which is a general term to describe fat in the stools resulting from unknown causes. However, as the pathologic processes in the villi continue, the absorption of protein, carbohydrates, calcium, iron, folic acid, and vitamins D, K, and B_{12} is greatly impaired and contributes to the typical clinical picture seen in the child (Fig. 33-1).

If the disease process is not arrested, *growth failure* results from fecal loss of fat, protein, and carbohydrates and the concurrent anorexia. Generally weight is compromised more than height, although bone growth is also arrested. Muscle wasting is especially severe in the extremities and buttocks, which appear thin, flabby, and wrinkled. The abdomen becomes progressively more distended as a result of a weakened musculature, accumulation of intestinal secretions and gas, altered peristaltic activity, and fluid from altered osmotic pressure resulting from protein loss. Rarely, constipation and fecal impaction rather than diarrhea may be present because of decreased peristalsis. Peripheral edema, usually confined to the lower extremities, is also a result of hypoproteinemia.

Anemia is caused by low serum iron and inadequate supplies of vitamin B_{12} and folic acid. *Disturbed blood coagulation* occurs because of inadequate vitamin K and may result in epistaxis, ecchymosis, or intestinal hemorrhage. Low levels of vitamin D impair calcium absorption and result in demineralization of bone *(osteoporosis)* and softening of the bone *(osteomalacia)*. Because bone growth is arrested, actual rickets is not commonly seen.

of the tube is slowed as a result of preanesthetic drugs. Older children need preparation for this test in order to enhance their cooperation. Younger children can be prevented from biting the tube by passing it through a rigid plastic tube held between their teeth. In infants the tube can be threaded through a pacifier. Three biopsies are recommended—one at the time of diagnosis, a second one following a trial gluten-free period to demonstrate repair of the mucosa, and a third following a challenge test of reintroducing gluten into the diet.

Although bleeding after biopsy is rare, prothrombin time, platelet count, and bleeding time should be evaluated before the procedure and vitamin K administered prophylactically. Since hemorrhage and perforation are potential complications, the nurse should observe for signs of shock after the test.

The other essential criterion of diagnosis is dramatic clinical improvement after adherence to a gluten-restricted diet. Within 2 weeks of instituting the diet, most children with celiac disease demonstrate a favorable personality change, followed by weight gain, improved appetite, and disappearance of diarrhea and steatorrhea.

Therapeutic Management

Treatment of chronic celiac disease is primarily dietary management. Since gluten is found mainly in the grains of wheat and rye, but also in smaller quantities in barley and oats, these four foods are eliminated. Corn, rice, and millet are substitute grain foods.

In those children with severe malnutrition, specific deficiencies are treated with supplemental vitamins, iron, and calories. At times peripheral parenteral alimentation with glucose, amino acids, and fatty acids may be required. Because absorption of fat-soluble vitamins is impaired, these are supplied in a water-miscible form.

Since a celiac crisis is a life-threatening event, prompt medical intervention to correct the dehydration and metabolic acidosis is essential. Usually treatment involves use of a nasogastric tube attached to intermittent suction to decrease abdominal distention; intravenous fluids with supplements of potassium, calcium, and magnesium where indicated; albumin infusions to prevent shock if hypoproteinemia is severe; and intravenous steroids to decrease the inflammation of the bowel. The prompt improvement in response to steroids is believed to support the immunologic theory that gluten acts as an antigen to the mucosal cells.

Nursing Considerations

The main nursing consideration is helping the parents and child adhere to diet therapy. This involves considerable time in explaining the disease process to the parents, the specific role of gluten in aggravating the disorder, and those foods that must be restricted. It is especially difficult to maintain a diet indefinitely when the child has no symptoms and temporary transgressions result in no difficulties. Although the chief source of grain is cereal and baked goods, grains are frequently added to processed foods as thickeners or fillers. To compound the difficulty, gluten is added to many foods but obscurely listed on the label as "hydrolyzed vegetable protein." The nurse must advise parents of the necessity of reading all label ingredients carefully to avoid hidden sources of gluten.

Although at first it may appear that eliminating wheat, rye, barley, and oats is a relatively simple matter, it soon becomes obvious that some of children's favorite foods contain these ingredients, including bread, cake, cookies, crackers, doughnuts, pies, spaghetti, pizza, prepared soups, some processed ice cream, many types of chocolate candy, milk preparations such as malts, hot dogs, luncheon meats, meat gravy, some prepared hamburgers, and many soups. Many of these products can be eliminated from the infant's or young child's diet fairly easily, but monitoring the diet of a school-age child or adolescent is a much more difficult situation. Many "favorite" foods, such as hot dogs, pizza, and spaghetti, are chief offenders. Luncheon preparation away from home is particularly difficult, since bread, luncheon meats, and instant soups are not allowed. For families on restricted food budgets, adhering to the diet adds an additional financial burden, since many inexpensive or convenience foods cannot be used. It may be more economical for these families to buy rice or corn flour directly from the milling company. Because the flour is a dietary prescription, the cost is a tax-deductible medical expense (Hartwig, 1983).

In addition to restricting gluten, other dietary alterations may also be necessary. For example, in some children who have more severe mucosal damage, the digestion of disaccharides is impaired, especially in relation to lactose. Therefore these children often need a temporary lactose-free diet, which necessitates eliminating all milk products.

Another deterrent to dietary adherence is the recommendation that the child continue it indefinitely. This is especially difficult for parents and children to understand when there have been no symptoms of the disease for an extended time and occasional dietary indiscretions have not caused untoward effects. However, evidence demonstrates that the majority of individuals who relax their diet will experience a relapse of their disease and possibly exhibit growth retardation, anemia, or osteomalacia. In addition, there is evidence that terminating the diet predisposes affected adults to the risk of developing malignant lymphoma of the small intestine, esophageal cancer, and other gastrointestinal cancers.

When parents and older children are being counseled in regard to the necessity of a lifelong gluten-restricted diet, it is important to stress these long-range complications, as well as to remind parents of the child's physical status before dietary treatment and his dramatic improvement after it was begun. For the child, however, these arguments may not be as convincing because the future is less significant than the present and the past has little meaning. The nurse can be instrumental in allowing the child to express these feelings, while focusing on ways in which the child can still be "normal" like his friends. For example, the usual prepared foods, such as hot dogs and hamburgers, may be restricted, but tacos and other Mexican dishes made with corn tortillas are acceptable. Many children complain that their diet is boring because the parent prepares the same food all the time. One way of dealing with this is encouraging the child to find new recipes using suitable ingredients.* With the present emphasis on natural health foods, the nurse can encourage the child to investigate new foods, such as sesame seeds and rice flour, to enhance their choices, while still being in vogue with peer interests. In some children permanent growth retardation is another emotional crisis.

Since celiac crises can be life-threatening events, the nurse also counsels parents regarding those factors that precipitate a crisis. The need for dietary control has already been discussed. However, the nurse also emphasizes the importance of maintaining good health to prevent infections. Whereas avoiding known sources of infection, such as other children who are ill, is certainly sound advice, the nurse also stresses the dangers of excessive overprotection. Since anticholinergic drugs can precipitate a crisis, the nurse advises the parents to inform any other treating physician of the celiac disorder. For example, orthodontic care requiring preanesthetic sedation can be a greater risk to these children, even when the celiac condition is well controlled.

The importance of consistent long-term follow-up care of parents and children with celiac disease cannot be overemphasized. Each phase of child development brings various types of problems related to dietary management and prevention of crises. The nurse is in an optimum position to provide continuous counseling, support, and encouragement to parents and children regarding adjustment to a lifelong disorders.

SHORT GUT (BOWEL) SYNDROME

The short gut syndrome refers to a condition in which there is a loss of intestine resulting in a diminished ability to normally digest and absorb a regular diet. The major causes in children are (1) congenital, such as small intestine atresias or gastroschisis, (2) volvulus involving a large segment of bowel, and (3) inflammation, such as from necrotizing enterocolitis or Crohn disease.

Both the amount of gut lost and its location, especially the ileum, are important factors in determining the severity of the condition. As much as 50% of the intestine can be lost without affecting the health of the child, unless it includes the distal ileum. A loss of greater than 75% of the small bowel results in malabsorption. However, the remaining intestine and stomach can adapt to the loss provided the child is kept alive through nutritional support. Adaptation

*A source of information for gluten-free recipes is the American Celiac Society, 45 Gifford Ave., Jersey City, NJ 07304; a booklet, *Pointers for Parents: Coping with Celiac Sprue,* is available from Clinical Dietetics Dept., Children's Memorial Hospital, 2300 Children's Plaza, Chicago, IL 60614.

occurs in a compensatory growth of all coats of the bowel wall with increased length and diameter of the remaining gut (Klish and Putnam, 1981).

Therapeutic Management

The goals of treatment are (1) to preserve as much length of bowel surgically as possible and (2) to maintain the child's nutritional status until adaptation of the bowel occurs. Small amounts of dilute formula should be started as soon as possible, since the bowel must be challenged with formula for it to develop enzymes to tolerate feedings. This necessitates a planned schedule of gradually increased concentration of formula; enteral feedings may be prescribed, and severely affected children require total parenteral nutrition to provide sufficient nutrition.

Nursing Considerations

Nursing care is directed toward maintaining the child's nutritional state, and prescribed orders for oral or enteral feedings must be followed exactly. If parenteral alimentation is required, every effort is made to preserve the intravenous line and to prevent complications such as infection. When long-term parenteral nutrition is required, preparing the family for home care of the child is a major nursing responsibility (see pp. 1094 and 1184). Since hospitalization may be prolonged, the child's developmental and emotional needs must be attended to as well.

Obstructive Disorders

Obstruction of the bowel occurs when the passage of intestinal contents is mechanically impeded by a constricted or occluded lumen or when there is interference with normal muscular contraction. Intestinal obstruction from any cause is characterized by similar signs and symptoms, although the progression may vary greatly. For example, in acute conditions, such as intussusception, the clinical manifestations are apparent within a few hours of the onset of the disorder. In other conditions, such as pyloric stenosis (see p. 1204), the signs and symptoms may be more gradual and may be missed during early stages of the disorder.

GENERAL SIGNS OF OBSTRUCTION

Classically, acute mechanical intestinal obstruction is characterized by colicky abdominal pain, nausea and vomiting, abdominal distention, and constipation. *Abdominal distention* is the result of accumulation of gas and fluid above the level of the obstruction. As these secretions continue to accumulate, the gut becomes excessively irritated and stimulates the vomiting center in the medulla to rid itself of the irritants with or without nausea. *Vomiting* is often the earliest sign of a high obstruction and a later sign in lower obstructions. Conversely, *constipation* and *obstipation* are early signs of low obstructions and later signs of higher obstructions. For example, a child with a high obstruction can have normal stools for a couple of days as the bowel evacuates itself distal to the defect.

If the obstruction is below the stomach, reflux from the small intestine causes intestinal secretions to flow back into the stomach, where they are vomited along with stomach contents. As this progresses, large quantities of fluid and electrolytes are lost, causing *dehydration.*

As distention progresses, the abdomen may be rigid and boardlike, with moderate to severe *tenderness. Bowel sounds* gradually diminish and cease. *Respiratory distress* occurs as the diaphragm is pushed up into the pleural cavity. As proteins are lost from the bloodstream into the intestinal lumen, the plasma volume diminishes and *shock* may occur.

INTUSSUSCEPTION

Intussusception is one of the most frequent causes of intestinal obstruction during infancy. Half of the cases occur in children younger than 1 year, more commonly between 3 and 12 months of age, and most of the others occur in children during the second year. Intussusception is three times more common in males than females. Although specific intestinal lesions can be found in a small percentage of the children, generally the cause is not known. The occurrence of intussusception is increased in children with cystic fibrosis and celiac disease.

Pathophysiology

Intussusception is an invagination or telescoping of one portion of the intestine into another. The most common site is the ileocecal valve, in which the ileum invaginates into the cecum and then further into the colon (Fig. 33-2). This type of intussusception is termed *ileocolic.* Other forms include *ileoileal* (one part of the ileum invaginates into another section of the ileum) and *colocolic* (one part of the colon telescopes into another area of the colon). The apex of the invagination is usually at the hepatic or splenic flexure or at some point along the transverse colon.

As a result of the invagination, there is an obstruction to the passage of intestinal contents beyond the defect. In addition, the two walls of the intestine press against each other, causing inflammation, edema, and eventually decreased blood flow. As incarceration continues, necrosis results with hemorrhage, perforation, and peritonitis. If untreated, this condition is incompatible with life.

Clinical Manifestations

Classic presentation of intussusception is a healthy, thriving child, usually between 3 and 12 months of age, who suddenly has an episode of acute abdominal pain. Typical behavior includes screaming and drawing the knees up to the chest. These episodes of severe pain are characterized by intervals in which the child appears normal and comfortable.

During this initial period vomiting usually occurs and the child passes one normal brown stool. However, as the con-

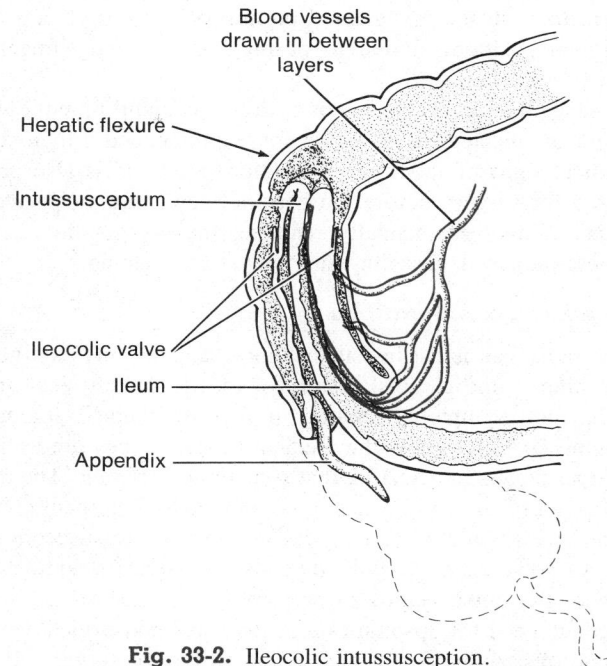

Fig. 33-2. Ileocolic intussusception.

dition worsens, the vomiting increases, the child becomes apathetic, and subsequent stools are red and currant jelly–like from the passage of stool mixed with blood and mucus.

The abdomen becomes tender and distended. A sausage-shaped mass may be felt in the upper right quadrant. In contrast, the lower right quadrant usually feels empty (Dance sign) as the bowel distal to the obstruction is less involved and free of contents. If treatment is not sought, the child becomes acutely ill with fever, prostration, and signs of peritonitis (see p. 1426).

Although the classic signs and symptoms of intussusception are intermittent abdominal pain, vomiting, and currant-jelly stools, a more chronic picture may occur, characterized by diarrhea, constipation, occasional vomiting, and periodic colic. Since this condition is potentially life threatening, the nurse must recognize such signs and closely observe and refer these children for further medical investigation.

Diagnostic Evaluation

Frequently the diagnosis can be made on subjective findings alone. However, definitive diagnosis is based on a barium enema, which clearly demonstrates the obstruction to the flow of barium. A rectal examination reveals mucus, blood, and occasionally a low intussusception itself.

Therapeutic Management

In most cases the initial treatment of choice is nonsurgical hydrostatic reduction by barium enema. Usually correction of the invagination is carried out at the same time as the diagnostic testing. The principle behind this procedure is that the force exerted by the flowing barium will be sufficient to push the invaginated portion of the bowel into its original position, similar to pushing an inverted "finger" out of a glove.

Since this procedure is not always successful (about 75% in uncomplicated cases) and is not recommended if there are clinical signs of shock or perforation, the child is also prepared for surgery before the barium enema. Surgical intervention involves manually reducing the invagination and, where indicated, resecting any nonviable intestine.

Nursing Considerations

The nurse can assist in establishing a diagnosis by carefully listening to the parents' history of the child's physical and behavioral symptoms relating to the complaint. Although parents may not know the medical problem, they are astute diagnosticians in detecting that something is wrong. The description of the child's severe colicky abdominal pain combined with vomiting is a significant clue to intussusception.

As soon as a possible diagnosis of intussusception is made, the nurse begins to prepare the parents for the immediate need for hospitalization, the usual nonsurgical technique of barium enema, and the possibility of surgery. It is important at this time to explain the basic defect of intussusception, which can be easily demonstrated by pushing the end of a finger on a rubber glove back into itself or using the example of a telescoping rod. The principle of reduction by hydrostatic pressure can be simulated by filling the glove with water, which pushes the "finger" into a fully extended position. By using such demonstrations, the parents are aware of why surgery is sometimes necessary. Without this preparation, they may be left with the feeling that the physician "failed" or that their child had "complications."

Since this hospitalization may be the child's first separation from his parents, it is especially important to preserve the parent-child relationship by encouraging rooming-in or extended visiting. It may also be the parents' first experience with hospital care for their child, necessitating their preparation for procedures such as intravenous therapy, frequent vital sign and blood pressure monitoring, dressings, and special orders, such as nothing by mouth. Because of the rapidity of the onset, diagnosis, and treatment, parents may be left with the feeling of stunned numbness. They may ask few questions or they may constantly make inquiries, sometimes the same ones several times. If the nurse realizes the circumstances surrounding this condition, the parents' reactions are more likely to be understood and accepted.

Physical care of the child with intussusception differs little from that for any child undergoing abdominal surgery. Even though nonsurgical intervention may be successful, usual preoperative procedures, such as withholding fluids, routine laboratory testing (complete blood count and urinalysis), signed parental consent, and preanesthetic sedation, are done. For the child with signs of electrolyte imbalance, hemorrhage, or peritonitis, additional medical preparation such as replacement fluids, whole blood or plasma, and na-

sogastric suctioning may be performed. Before surgery the nurse monitors all stools. Passage of a normal brown stool usually indicates that the intussusception has reduced itself. This is immediately reported to the physician, who may choose to alter the diagnostic/therapeutic plan of care.

Postprocedural care includes the usual postoperative observations, such as vital signs, blood pressure, intact sutures and dressing, and the return of bowel sounds. In the case of hydrostatic reduction or autoreduction, the nurse observes for passage of barium and the stool patterns, since recurrences of the intussusception are most likely to occur within the first 36 hours after reduction. For this reason the child is kept in the hospital for 2 to 3 days. Overall recurrence of intussusception after nonsurgical or operative reduction is between 4% and 10% (Silverman and Roy, 1983).

Disorders of Motility

A number of gastrointestinal disorders are caused by disturbance in motility. Some, such as Hirschsprung disease and gastroesophageal reflux, are seen primarily in infancy and cause problems in elimination or feeding. Others, such as constipation, can occur at any age and produce few serious effects, unless the primary disorder can lead to obstruction. The common problems of diarrhea and vomiting are discussed in Chapter 29 because of the importance of the fluid and electrolyte changes they can produce.

CONSTIPATION

Constipation is the regular passage of firm or hard stools or of small, hard masses with associated symptoms such as difficulty in expulsion of the stools, blood-streaked bowel movements, and abdominal discomfort. The frequency of bowel movements is not considered a diagnostic criterion because it varies widely among children. General guidelines for stool frequency suggest a lower limit of six per week in children younger than 3 years and four per week in older children (Corazziari and others, 1985). However, less frequent bowel movements may be normal. Extremely long intervals between defecation is termed *obstipation*. Constipation with fecal soiling is *encopresis*. The following discussion is concerned primarily with causes of constipation in different age-groups and the treatment of simple constipation during childhood. For a discussion of encopresis, see Chapter 18.

Constipation can be a symptom of a number of abdominal disorders, primarily those that cause an obstruction in the lower intestinal tract, such as Hirschsprung disease or imperforate anus. Physical and mental disorders are often associated with defecation problems, for example, neurologic disorders, mental retardation, hypothyroidism, and hypercalcemia. However, the development and course of constipation can be influenced by a number of familial, cultural, and social factors. Psychologic factors play an important role in bowel habits as well as toilet-training techniques, diet, overuse of laxatives, and enemas. The most common cause of constipation in children is environmental change, such as change in feeding habits, using a new toilet, birth of a sibling, and relocation of housing or school (Johns, 1985).

Newborn

Normally the newborn passes a first meconium stool within 24 to 36 hours of birth. Any infant who does not do so should be assessed for evidence of intestinal atresia or stenosis, congenital aganglionic megacolon (50% of cases), hypothyroidism, meconium plugs, or meconium ileus. Meconium plugs are caused by meconium that has reduced water content and are usually evacuated following digital examination, but they may require irrigations of normal saline or the iodinated contrast medium *diatrizoate meglumine (Gastrografin)*.

Meconium ileus, the initial manifestation of cystic fibrosis, is the presence of thick, mucilaginous meconium that clings to the abdominal wall, making it difficult, if not impossible, to pass. Treatment is the same as for a meconium plug. Rarely, surgical intervention may be necessary.

Infancy

Medical causes such as Hirschsprung disease, hypothyroidism, and strictures must be ruled out in chronic cases of constipation. However, the most frequent cause in infancy is dietary mismanagement. It is almost unknown in breast-fed infants, who typically have fewer stools than bottle-fed infants. Constipation may accompany the change from human milk or modified cow's milk formula to whole cow's milk, presumably because of the greater protein-to-carbohydrate ratio of whole cow's milk. Some bottle-fed infants pass hard stools and develop anal fissures. To avoid the pain in defecation these infants voluntarily withhold stool. The infant's behavior during withholding of stools is often misinterpreted by parents as constipation. He grunts and appears to be straining while his face turns red and he draws his legs up on his abdomen.

Simple measures ordinarily correct the problem, such as increasing the amount of fluid or sugar in the formula in the very young infant or adding or increasing the amount of cereal, vegetables, and fruit in the diet of the older infant. If the child has anal fissures, the temporary use of stool softeners or mineral oil is usually sufficient to break the pain cycle on defecation.

Childhood

Children between 1 and 3 years of age are most likely to have constipation (Abrahamian and Lloyd-Still, 1984). Most constipation is due to environmental changes, but if there are associated manifestations, such as vomiting, abdominal distention, or pain, and evidence of growth failure,the condition merits further investigation. Constipation may result from some medications, such as iron preparations, diuretics, antacids, and anticonvulsant agents. Constipation frequently accompanies enuresis, and treatment of

the constipation often results in resolution of the enuresis (O'Regan and others, 1986).

The management of simple constipation is based on a plan to keep the bowel relatively empty of stool and dietary management to prevent further constipation. Although authorities differ on the methods to clean out the bowel, all agree that use of laxatives is not usually recommended because of their tendency to produce dependency. Some regimens employ the use of enemas to initially rid the bowel of stool and additional enemas if voluntary evacuation does not occur within 48 hours. During this time a high-fiber diet is instituted and any foods known to be constipating are eliminated, such as all milk and milk products, apples, apple juice, carrots, bananas, rice, and Jell-O. Supplemental bran may be given also (Olness, 1984). When high-fiber foods are added, additional sources of fluid must be given to the child to prevent the fiber from having a binding effect. Other regimens may include a stool softener such as dioctyl sodium sulfosuccinate (Colace) to keep the stool of a consistency that is more easily evacuated.

Nursing Considerations

Constipation, unfortunately, tends to be self-perpetuating. If the child has difficulty or discomfort when attempting to evacuate his bowels, he has a tendency to retain the bowel contents and thus begins a vicious cycle. Nursing assessment begins with an accurate history of bowel habits, diet, events that may be associated with the onset of constipation, drugs or other substances that the child may be taking, and the consistency, color, frequency, and other characteristics of the stool. If there is no evidence of a pathologic condition that requires further investigation, the major task of the nurse is to educate the parents regarding normal stool patterns and to relieve the cause of the constipation.

Dietary modifications are usually essential in preventing constipation. During infancy simply increasing the carbohydrate (sugar or corn syrup) in an infant formula will often relieve the problem. During childhood the diet should contain increased amounts of fiber and fluid. Parents will benefit from guidance in dietary planning, especially regarding foods that facilitate bowel movements (Table 33-1). If bran is added to the diet, creative ways to disguise the consistency are needed. For example, it can be added to cereal, peanut butter, mashed potatoes, fruit shakes, and baked goods.

Parents also need reassurance concerning the benign nature of the condition. It is important to discuss with them their attitudes and expectations regarding toilet habits and to discourage the use of stool softeners, laxatives, and enemas. If such measures have been prescribed by a physician, parents should understand that these are merely temporary and not to be continued beyond the current need.

HIRSCHSPRUNG DISEASE (CONGENITAL AGANGLIONIC MEGACOLON)

Hirschsprung disease is a congenital anomaly that results in mechanical obstruction from inadequate motility in part of

Table 33-1 High-fiber foods

FOOD GROUP	SELECTIONS
Bread, grains	Whole-grain bread or rolls Whole-grain cereals Bran Pancakes, waffles and muffins with fruit or bran Unrefined (brown) rice
Vegetables	Raw vegetables, especially broccoli, cabbage, carrots, cauliflower, celery, lettuce, and spinach Cooked vegetables, such as those listed above and asparagus, beans, brussels sprouts, corn, potatoes, rhubarb, squash, string beans, turnips
Fruits	Raw fruits, especially those with skins or seeds, other than ripe banana or avocado Raisins, prunes, or other dried fruits
Miscellaneous	Nuts, seeds, legumes, popcorn

the intestine. It accounts for about one fourth of all cases of neonatal obstruction, although it may not be diagnosed until later in infancy or childhood. It is four times more common in males than females, follows a familial pattern in a small number of cases, and is considerably more common in children with Down syndrome. Depending on its presentation, it may be an acute, life-threatening condition or a chronic disorder.

Pathophysiology

The term *congenital (aganglionic) megacolon* describes the disorder. The primary defect is absence of autonomic parasympathetic ganglion cells of the submucosal (Meissner) and myenteric (Auerbach) plexuses in one segment of colon, hence the term *aganglionic,* or absence of ganglia. The defect is probably the result of defective migration of parasympathetic ganglion cell precursors during embryonic development. The functional defect as a result of lack of innervation is absence of propulsive movements (peristalsis), causing accumulation of intestinal contents and distention of the bowel proximal to the defect, hence the term *megacolon,* or large colon. In addition, there is failure of the internal rectal sphincter to relax, which adds to the clinical manifestations because it prevents evacuation of solids, liquids, and gas.

The length of aganglionic bowel varies greatly, from involving only the internal sphincter to the entire colon. The latter condition is rare (about 12% of all cases) and significantly influences prognosis and mortality (about 54%), although newer surgical techniques have dramatically improved the outlook for these children (Jordan, Coran, and Wesley, 1981). The most commonly affected site is the rectosigmoid colon (Fig. 33-3).

Clinical Manifestations

Clinical manifestations vary according to the age when symptoms are recognized and the occurrence of complications, such as enterocolitis. In the newborn the chief signs and symptoms are failure to pass meconium within 24 to 48 hours after birth, reluctance to ingest fluids, bile-stained vomitus, and abdominal distention. If the disorder is allowed to progress, other signs of intestinal obstruction develop, such as respiratory distress and shock.

During infancy the child does not thrive and has constipation, abdominal distention, and episodes of diarrhea and vomiting. The occurrence of explosive, watery diarrhea, fever, and severe prostration is ominous because it often signifies the presence of enterocolitis (inflammation of the small bowel and colon), which greatly increases the risk of fatality. Enterocolitis may also be present without diarrhea and is first evidenced with unexplained fever and poor feeding.

During childhood the symptoms are chronic and include constipation, passage of ribbonlike, foul-smelling stools, abdominal distention, and visible peristalsis. Fecal masses are easily palpable. The child is usually poorly nourished, anemic, and hypoproteinemic from malabsorption of nutrients.

Diagnostic Evaluation

In the neonate diagnosis is suspected on clinical signs of intestinal obstruction and failure to pass meconium. In infants and children the history is an important part of diagnosis and typically details a chronic pattern of constipation. On rectal examination the rectum is empty of feces, the internal sphincter is tight, and there is leakage of liquid, offensive, pale stool and accumulated gas. Radiographic studies using a barium enema often demonstrate the transition zone between the dilated proximal colon (megacolon) and

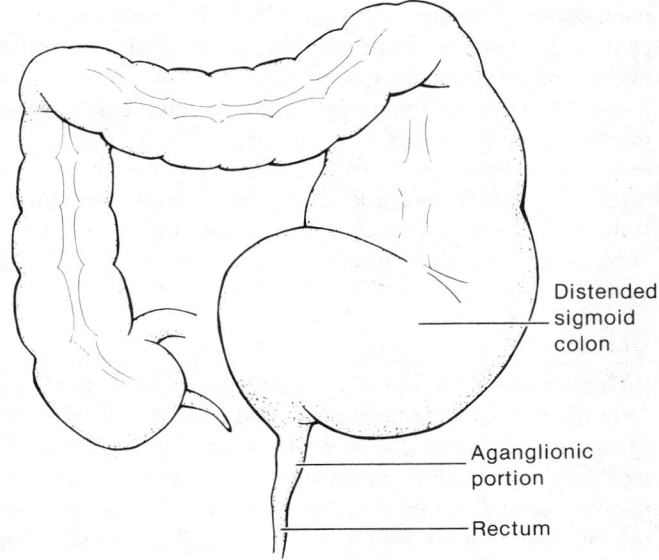

Distended sigmoid colon

Aganglionic portion

Rectum

Fig. 33-3. Hirschsprung disease.

the aganglionic distal segment. However, this typical megacolon and narrow distal segment may not develop until 3 to 4 weeks or even months after birth in some children.

To confirm the diagnosis rectal biopsy is performed either surgically, to obtain a full-thickness biopsy for histologic evidence of aganglionic cells, or by suction biopsy, a newer test that is performed without anesthesia to detect the presence of ganglia in the submucosa and increased amounts of the enzyme acetylcholinesterase in a biopsy specimen. Another noninvasive procedure that may be used is anorectal manometry. In this test a cylinder with three balloons attached to it is inserted partway into the rectum. Two of the balloons are positioned at the internal sphincter and the third at the external sphincter. The test records the reflex response of the sphincters to distention of the balloons. A normal response is relaxation of the internal sphincter followed by contraction of the external sphincter. In Hirschsprung disease the external sphincter contracts normally, but the internal sphincter fails to relax or contract.

Therapeutic Management

Treatment is primarily surgical intervention to remove the aganglionic bowel and ensure continence. In a very small number of children with chronic, but not severe, symptoms of megacolon conservative treatment with occasional enemas may be instituted to establish a regular pattern of defecation. However, these children represent a distinct exception and may be at continued risk for the development of fatal enterocolitis (Martin and Torres, 1985).

Surgical correction usually involves a three-stage approach. In most cases a temporary colostomy is performed in part of the bowel with normal innervation (usually the sigmoid or transverse colon) and at a site that would permit the corrective operation to be performed without closing the colostomy until after the rectal area has healed. The colostomy allows the bowel a period of rest in order to resume its normal caliber and tonicity and provides an opportunity for the child to gain weight before the more extensive repair is undertaken.

Definitive correction is usually performed when the child is 8 months to 1 year of age or has reached approximately 20 pounds (Polley, Coran, and Wesley, 1985). The type of surgical procedure for reanastomosis involves "pulling" the end of the intact bowel down to a point near the rectum. The most common surgical techniques are the Swenson, the Soave (endorectal pull-through), and the Duhamel operations, which usually require both an abdominal and a perineal incision.

The third stage involves closure of the colostomy, which is normally performed within a few (usually 3) months of the definitive repair. The prognosis after complete surgical repair depends on the child's ability to adjust to a normal diet and to learn bowel control and varies depending on the type of surgery. However, most children are able to attain satisfactory defecatory function (Martin and Torres, 1985; Polley, Coran, and Wesley, 1985).

Nursing Considerations

Many of the nursing concerns depend on the child's age and the type of treatment. If the disorder is diagnosed during the neonatal period, the main objectives are helping the parents adjust to a congenital defect in their child, fostering infant-parent bonding, preparing them for the medical/surgical intervention, and assisting them in colostomy care after discharge.

When the disorder is not discovered during this period, the nurse can facilitate establishing a diagnosis by carefully listening to the parents' history, with special emphasis on bowel habits. In Hirschsprung disease several areas must be investigated: (1) onset of constipation, especially if present since birth, (2) character of stools, particularly ribbonlike and foul smelling, and (3) frequency of bowel movements. Other clues in the history and physical examination include poor feeding habits, fussiness and irritability, a distended abdomen, and signs of undernutrition, such as thin extremities, pallor, muscle weakness, and fatigue.

The following discussion is limited to the care of the child undergoing surgical correction. For the rare child who is managed with occasional enemas the nurse needs to teach the parents the correct procedure, as well as inform them of the dangers of using tap water, concentrated salt solutions, soap solutions, or phosphate preparations. Normal saline solution can be purchased without a prescription from a pharmacy or can be prepared at home by adding 1 level measuring teaspoon of noniodized salt to 1 pint of tap water. Since the instructions for preparing the solution and administering the enema require several steps, all the directions should be written down as well as verbally explained.* Suggested amounts of solution according to the child's age are listed on p. 1144.

Preoperative care. Much of the child's preoperative care depends on his age and clinical condition. Physical preoperative preparation entails the same measures that are common to any surgery (see p. 1145). In the newborn, whose bowel is sterile, no additional preparation is necessary. However, in children beyond the newborn period emptying the bowel with repeated saline enemas and decreasing bacterial flora with systemic antibiotics and colonic irrigations using antibiotic solution are usually ordered. A nasogastric tube may be inserted to prevent abdominal distention, and antibiotic solution may be instilled through the tube to further prepare the gastrointestinal tract. All intake and output of irrigant and drainage are noted, particularly a marked discrepancy in retention or loss of fluid. A rectal tube may also be inserted to allow for escape of accumulated fluid and gas. Because of the rectal tube and to prevent damage to the mucosa, only axillary temperatures are taken.

In children with enterocolitis, emergency preoperative care includes frequent monitoring of vital signs and blood

---

*Home care instructions on giving an enema are available in Wong, D., and Whaley, L.: Clinical handbook of pediatric nursing, ed. 2, St. Louis, 1986, The C.V. Mosby Co.

pressure for signs of shock, monitoring fluid replacement with electrolytes, plasma, or other blood derivatives, and observing for symptoms of bowel perforation, such as increasing abdominal distention, vomiting, increased tenderness, irritability, dyspnea, and cyanosis.

Since progressive distention of the abdomen is a serious sign, abdominal circumference is measured at the largest diameter, usually at the level of the umbilicus. The point of measurement is marked with a pen to assure reliability. In order to lessen any stress to the acutely ill child, the tape measure should be left under the child, rather than removed each time. As a rule of thumb, abdominal measurement can be performed at the same time that vital signs are taken. It is best to record the measurement in serial order so that a change will be readily apparent.

The age of the child dictates the type and extent of psychologic preparation. Since a colostomy is usually performed, the child of at least preschool age is told about the procedure in concrete terms. For example, this can be illustrated by drawing a picture of a child with a stoma on the abdomen and explaining it as "another opening where bowel movements [or any other term the child uses] will come out." At another time the nurse can draw a bag over the opening to demonstrate how the contents are collected.

Whenever possible, the stoma can also be illustrated by drawing or cutting a small hole on a plastic doll and applying a bag over it. A urine-collecting bag works very well as an example of a colostomy appliance. Since an abdominal dressing is present immediately after surgery, the child should be made aware of this fact. Dressings or "bandages" are especially important to preschoolers, who see them as a form of preserving body integrity. However, it is important to space explanations to prevent anxiety and confusion from too much information.

Parents also need preparation before surgery. Since a colostomy represents a change in body function and appearance, the nurse should investigate parents' previous knowledge of this procedure. It is not uncommon for parents to have some knowledge about a colostomy. For example, one mother related that a friend's father had a permanent colostomy because of cancer. As soon as the mother heard that her child needed this procedure, she was convinced that the mass in her child's abdomen was a cancerous tumor.

It is best not to assume that parents understand a verbal explanation of a colostomy. Drawing a picture or using the doll is excellent for parents as well as children. During this teaching session, the nurse should briefly mention methods of care since presenting too much information can overwhelm the parents.

It is important to stress to parents and older children that the colostomy for Hirschsprung disease is temporary. The nurse should also keep in mind that although a temporary colostomy is favorable in terms of future health and adjustment, it also necessitates additional surgery, which may be very stressful to parents and children.

Since feeding and associated behavioral problems are frequently associated with a chronic pattern of megacolon, the nurse should inform parents that although the defect can be corrected, it will take some time for the child's physical status and feeding practices to improve. Although this should not be stated in such a way as to minimize the benefit of surgery, it is necessary to avoid implying that surgical correction is a panacea to all previous physical and behavioral complaints.

Postoperative care. Physical postoperative care usually includes (1) nothing by mouth until bowel sounds return and the colostomy and/or anastomosed bowel are ready for feedings, (2) intravenous fluid to maintain hydration and replace lost electrolytes, (3) nasogastric suctioning to prevent abdominal distention, (4) frequent abdominal dressing changes, and (5) perineal dressing changes.

To prevent contamination of the abdominal wound with urine, the diaper should be pinned below the dressing. Sometimes a Foley catheter is used in the immediate postoperative period to divert the flow of urine away from the abdomen. Drainage from the nasogastric tube and the colostomy is measured, since fluid and electrolyte replacement is partially calculated on these losses.

When parents initially visit their child postoperatively, they are frequently unprepared for the numerous tubes and intravenous lines attached to various body parts. Even when all the procedures are explained beforehand, the actual visual shock can be great. The nurse should explain the function of each piece of equipment, stressing safety features that permit the child to be safely moved and handled, such as length of tubing, use of armboards at intravenous sites, and tape to secure the nasogastric tube to the nose. In this way parents are encouraged and assisted in holding and stimulating their child.

The nurse emphasizes the expected changes in the appearance of the stoma, which initially is large, protruding, red, and raw looking. Since the stomal site appears painful, it is also important to stress that bowel mucosa is nonsensitive but that the surrounding abdominal skin must be protected.

Home care. Postoperatively, parents need instruction concerning colostomy care at home* (see p. 1145). During the early postoperative period, including parents and the older child in dressing changes can enhance teaching of colostomy care when an appliance is fitted and promotion of gradual acceptance of the body change. Even a preschooler can be included in the care by handing articles to the parent, rolling up the colostomy bag after emptying, or applying cream to the surrounding skin. Since these children may have had difficulties with bowel training before surgery because of constipation and erratic stool patterns, the period during the temporary colostomy can relieve the pressures previously associated with bowel control. Older children should be involved in colostomy care to the point of total responsibility.

---

*Home care instructions on caring for the child with a colostomy are available in Wong, D., and Whaley, L.: Clinical handbook of pediatric nursing, ed. 2, St. Louis, 1986, The C.V. Mosby Co.

In some institutions an enterostomal therapist is available to provide expert assistance in planning procedures for home care, such as preparation of skin, application of the collecting appliance, care of the appliance, control of odor, and signs of stomal complications, such as ribbonlike stools, excessive diarrhea, bleeding, prolapse, or failure to pass flatus or stool. Whenever possible, this person should be used in preparing for colostomy care.

In those children with delayed correction of Hirschsprung disease, feeding problems may be present, including the discomfort from abdominal distention after eating and the likelihood of parental pressure to eat. Hospitalization provides an excellent assessment period for the nurse to observe parent-child interaction during mealtime. Once specific problems are discovered, the nurse can initiate steps to reverse the pattern. It is important to remember that relearning must take place because the behavior has probably been reinforced for a long time.

Behavior modification techniques tend to be especially effective in changing eating patterns but require a thorough assessment and identification of reinforcement factors. Other helpful suggestions include establishing regular frequent mealtimes with small servings, avoiding an argument or any type of parental pressure at mealtime, and serving as many of the child's favorite foods as possible.

Referral to a public health nurse establishes continuity of care, especially in relation to colostomy care and dietary management. The community nurse can also assist parents and children in anticipating subsequent surgery. Sometimes families require financial assistance and additional psychologic support. Therefore a referral to a social worker or other service agency may be necessary.

Nursing Care Summary: The Child Undergoing Abdominal Surgery

PREOPERATIVE CARE

NURSING GOALS	NURSING INTERVENTIONS	EXPECTED PATIENT/FAMILY OUTCOMES
HP-HMP Injury: potential for **Etiology: surgical procedure**		
Provide physical preparation	For general preparatory interventions, see Nursing care summary, p. 1147	
Observe for complications Shock	Monitor vital signs and blood pressure	
Intestinal obstruction	Observe for decreased or absent bowel sounds, increasing abdominal distention, vomiting, absence of stools, pain	*Complications are recognized and reported
Perforation and peritonitis	Observation for sudden relief from pain followed by increased diffuse abdominal pain, absence of bowel sounds, tachycardia, pallor, high temperature, abdominal splinting, and rapid, shallow respirations	

Prevent and observe for abdominal distention	Give the child nothing by mouth as ordered
	 Maintain patency of nasogastric tube, if present
	    Check functioning of suction machine
	        Irrigate tube if no drainage is obtained but the child vomits around the tube
	    Check proper placement of tube
	    Secure tube by taping to nose or upper lip (not forehead) to maintain proper stomach placement
		Child receives nothing by mouth
		 *Patency of tube is maintained

	Keep the child in semi-Fowler position or as ordered to facilitate drainage of abdominal contents and to promote respiratory expansion	Child remains in proper position
	Measure abdominal circumference at widest point (mark with pen, usually at umbilicus); record measurements on graph or in sequence to detect changes Check often for bowel sounds	*Information regarding bowel circumference and bowel sounds is obtained
Prevent dehydration	Record all output (urinary, stool, vomiting, nasogastric) and input (intravenous, oral if allowed, and nasogastric irrigant); notify physician of marked discrepancies Monitor intravenous infusion, if present Take temperature often; notify physician of elevations	Child remains well hydrated

*Nursing outcome.

Continued.

Nursing Care Summary: The Child Undergoing Abdominal Surgery—cont'd

PREOPERATIVE CARE

NURSING GOALS	NURSING INTERVENTIONS	EXPECTED PATIENT/FAMILY OUTCOMES
SP-SCP **Anxiety**		
Etiology: Separation from support system; unfamiliar environment		
Prepare child and parents for expected surgical procedure and postoperative care	Prepare for postoperative procedures, as indicated, such as nasogastric tube, intravenous fluids, nothing by mouth, dressing changes, and wound drains if necessary	Family is knowledgable of forthcoming events (specify methods of learning and evaluation)
	Explain reason for surgery; if bowel diversion is to be performed, explain basic principle of ostomy and brief outline of bowel care	
	Explain all preoperative procedures, such as blood work, nasogastric tube, bowel preparation, and any other laboratory test	
	In emergency situation, explain most essential components of surgery, such as where child will be before and after surgery, anesthesia, and dressing on abdomen	
	Accept behavioral reactions of parents and child	Family's behavioral reactions are accepted and supported

POSTOPERATIVE CARE

HP-HMP **Infection: potential for**		
Etiology: Surgical wound		
Prevent wound infection	Use proper hand washing techniques, especially if wound drainage is present	No signs of wound infection are evident
	Change dressings (abdominal and/or perineal), if indicated, whenever soiled; carefully dispose of soiled dressings	
	Pin diapers below abdominal dressing to prevent contamination	
	Assess wound for signs of complications, unless ordered not to remove dressing	
	Change dressings as prescribed by surgeon	
	Report any unusual appearance or drainage	
	Carry out special wound care as prescribed: irrigation, drain care, etc.	
Prevent respiratory complications	Assess need for pain medication before respiratory hygiene	Lungs remain clear
	Assist to turn, cough, deep breathe	
	Stimulate infat to cry	
	Assist with use of spirometer or blow bottle	
	Perform percussion and vibration, if indicated	
	Suction secretions if needed	

HP-HMP **Injury: potential for**		
Etiology: Surgical procedure; anesthesia		
Assess general status	Monitor vital signs as ordered	*Alterations in physical status are determined early and interventions initiated
	Check dressings for bleeding or other abnormalities	
	Assess level of consciousness	
	Assess for evidence of discomfort	
	Place in position of comfort in accordance with surgeon's orders	
	Check bowel sounds	
Detect early signs of complications	Observe for signs of	Complications are detected and reported
	Shock	
	Abdominal distention	
	Wound infection	
	Other infections	

*Nursing outcome.

Nursing Care Summary: The Child Undergoing Abdominal Surgery—cont'd

PREOPERATIVE CARE

NURSING GOALS	NURSING INTERVENTIONS	EXPECTED PATIENT/FAMILY OUTCOMES
N-MP **Fluid volume deficit, potential** **Risk factors: NPO prior to and/or after surgery**		
Promote adequate hydration	Monitor intravenous infusion (if any) Offer fluids as soon as ordered or child tolerates	Child exhibits no evidence of dehydration
N-MP **Nutrition, alteration in: less than body requirements** **Risk factors: NPO prior to and/or after surgery, lack of appetite due to discomfort**		
Provide nourishment	Offer diet as tolerated Offer favorite foods Avoid foods that may produce gas	Child consumes an adequate diet (specify)
CPP **Comfort, alteration in: pain** **Etiology: Surgical incision**		
Provide comfort measures	Assess need for pain medication (see p. 1068) Implement appropriate nonpharmacologic pain reduction techniques (see p. 1071) Administer mouth care Lubricate nostril to decrease irritation from nasogastric tube, if present Allow the child position of comfort if not contraindicated (usually side-lying or prone with legs flexed on chest) Perform procedures (e.g., dressing change, deep breathing) after administering analgesics	Child exhibits minimal evidence of pain (specify)
CPP **Knowledge deficit** **Etiology: Unfamiliarity with situation**		
Instruct family regarding home care Wound care	If dressing changes are required at home, teach parents sterile or aseptic procedures; provide written list of necessary equipment and instructions	Family demonstrates an understanding of instructions (specify methods of learning and evaluation)
Administration of medications Special procedures	Instruct parents regarding administration of medications (if ordered) Instruct parents in care and management of special procedures such as ostomy care, irrigations	
RRP **Family process, alteration in** **Etiology: Situational crisis (hospitalization and surgical intervention)**		
Support and reassure parents and child	Explain all procedures Keep informed of progress Encourage expression of feelings If emergency procedure, review child's memory of previous events Refer to public health nurse if necessary Refer to appropriate agency for specific help	Family demonstrates an awareness of child's progress (specify method of evaluation) Appropriate referrals are made

Nursing Interventions Related to Medical Management

PREOPERATIVE
Assist in preparing bowel for surgery (if indicated)
   Administer colonic enemas as ordered, using only saline solution
   Administer antibiotics as ordered, observing for known side effects
   Order and/or assist with special tests such as radiographs

POSTOPERATIVE
Prevent infection
   Administer antibiotics as prescribed
   Advance drains as ordered
Provide comfort
   Administer analgesics as appropriate

GASTROESOPHAGEAL REFLUX

Gastroesophageal reflux (GER, chalasia, cardiochalasia) denotes relaxation or incompetence of the lower esophageal sphincter, causing frequent return of stomach contents into the esophagus. In newborns this is considered a normal phenomenon because of immature neuromuscular control of the gastroesophageal sphincter. However, in a small percentage of infants reflux continues, producing symptoms that warrant investigation. The exact cause is not known, although it is thought to result from delayed maturation of lower esophageal neuromuscular function or impaired local hormonal control mechanisms. GER is also more common in children with cystic fibrosis, although the mechanisms responsible for the increased prevalence are not clear (Scott, O'Loughlin, and Gall, 1985).

Clinical Manifestations

The most common symptoms are vomiting, weight loss, respiratory problems, and bleeding. Vomiting is the most common symptom and in infants is quite forceful. It is frequently so severe that there is a loss of calories sufficient to cause weight loss and failure to thrive.

Reflux of stomach contents to the pharynx predisposes to aspiration and the development of respiratory symptoms, especially pneumonia. Repeated irritation of the esophageal lining with gastric acid can lead to esophagitis and consequently bleeding. Blood loss in turn causes anemia and is seen as hematemesis or melena (blood in stools). Heartburn is also a frequent symptom in older children, who can describe it, but may go unrecognized in infants.

Diagnostic Evaluation

The history is an important part of the diagnostic evaluation, including observation of the child's feeding habits. Several tests are available to evaluate the presence of reflux. The initial test is the barium esophagram. Reflux of barium from the stomach to the esophagus can be seen by fluoroscopy, although it may be missed because of the intermittent nature of the disorder. Other tests include manometry to measure esophageal sphincter pressure; the acid reflux (Tuttle) test, which uses a probe to directly measure the pH of the distal esophagus; and gastroesophageal scintigraphy, which scans the esophagus after a feeding of a radioactive compound to detect reflux or aspiration.

Therapeutic Management

Therapeutic management of GER depends on its severity. In most instances of GER in infants who are thriving, no therapy is needed other than parental reassurance that the child will outgrow the condition. For the symptomatic child modification of feeding with small, frequent feedings of thickened formula and positioning may be helpful to minimize the symptoms of the reflux until the child grows and a normal physiologic barrier to reflux develops. However, there is considerable controversy regarding the type of positioning. Traditionally, the upright position (usually in an infant

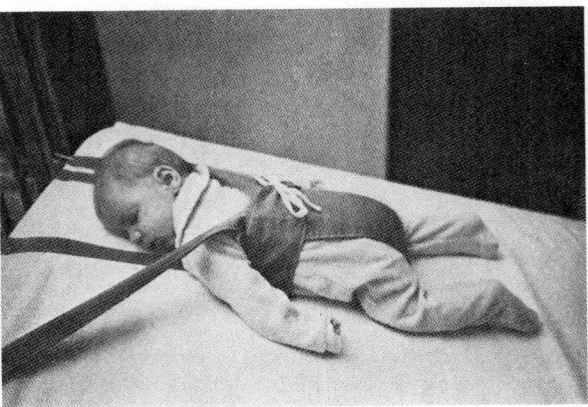

Fig. 33-4. Five-week-old infant positioned in harness.
From Orenstein, S.R., and Whitington, P.F.: Positioning for prevention of infant gastroesophageal reflux, J. Pediatr. **103:**534-537, 1983.

seat) has been recommended, but research in infants less than 6 months of age demonstrated that positioning the child prone with the body inclined at about a 30-degree angle for 24 hours a day was more effective (Orenstein and Whitington, 1983). This position is easily maintained by use of an upper body harness (Fig. 33-4). Length of time to recovery is variable but is usually within a couple of weeks, although recommendations to continue the treatment for considerably longer may be given.

Various drugs that promote gastric emptying and/or relax the pyloric sphincter have been used with some success, including bethanechol (a cholinergic agent), metoclopramide (a dopamine blocker), and domperidone (a benzimidazole derivative with peripheral dopamine antagonist properties). Surgical intervention is selected for those children with severe complications, such as respiratory distress (choking, aspiration, recurrent apnea), esophagitis, or esophageal stricture (Herbst, 1983). A commonly used surgical procedure is the Nissen fundoplication, which creates a valve mechanism by wrapping the greater curvature of the stomach (fundus) around the distal esophagus.

Nursing Considerations

Nursing care is directed at (1) identifying children with symptoms suggestive of gastroesophageal reflux, (2) helping parents with home care of feeding and positioning when indicated, and (3) if appropriate, caring for the child undergoing surgical intervention. For the majority of infants parental reassurance of the benign nature of the condition and its relationship to physiologic maturity is the most important intervention. To help parents cope with the inconvenience of vomiting, simple measures such as using bibs and protective cloths during feeding are beneficial.

Feeding modification may require some rescheduling of the family's routine to accommodate more frequent feeding times. Formula is thickened with cereal and the nipple opening may need to be enlarged for easier sucking. If the mother is breast-feeding her infant, a decision regarding the benefit of feeding modification must be made; she can express the milk or change to commercial formula if thickening is recommended.

For the very young infant positioning can be accomplished by raising the mattress at the head end and using a harness. Once the infant is older and more mobile, positioning becomes increasingly difficult; a special procedure has been described for constructing a bed that comfortably maintains the child's position. It consists of a cradle bed or bassinet that incorporates a wooden base with a wooden spindle under the mattress. The spindle protrudes through a hole cut in the mattress and is padded. The infant is positioned prone with his legs straddling the spindle, and the head end of the bassinet is raised at a 30-degree angle (Boyd, 1981).

If medication is prescribed or surgery performed, the same nursing responsibilities for helping parents administer the drug at home (see p. 1140) and postoperative care (see p. 1146) are instituted. After surgery symptoms are completely controlled in most cases, with these children attaining normal health and growth. Minor problems that may occur following surgery are gas bloat, inability to vomit, slow eating habits, and choking on solids (Harnsberger and others, 1983). Families should be aware of such subsequent changes in order to take appropriate actions, such as increased precaution with foods that can be aspirated and allowing children longer time at the table.

Inflammatory Conditions

Inflammatory conditions involving large or small segments of the gastrointestinal tract are not uncommon in childhood. They may be acute or chronic, and some are more likely to affect one age-group than another. For example, Meckel diverticulum is seen primarily in children under age 2 years, ulcerative colitis occurs most frequently in the prepubescent and adolescent child, and acute appendicitis appears at any age.

ACUTE APPENDICITIS

Appendicitis, inflammation of the vermiform appendix, or blind sac, at the end of the cecum, is the most common reason for abdominal surgery during childhood. It is often an acute condition that, if undiagnosed, rapidly progresses to perforation and peritonitis. It occurs in all age-groups but is rare in children younger than 2 years of age. However, appendicitis is associated with increased complications and mortality in children in this age-group because of the difficulty in establishing an early diagnosis. The condition is more common in those children with a family history of appendicitis (Brender and others, 1985c).

Appendicitis is a significant pediatric problem. While mortality has decreased greatly since the advent of antibiotics, the incidence of appendiceal rupture has still remained high, occurring in about 28% of patients (Berry and Malt, 1984). The most significant factor associated with perforation is delay in treatment, primarily on the part of professionals, not parents. Other contributing factors are young age, lower social class, presence of fecaliths, absence of family history, and advice given by the first health professional the family contacted, especially the advice to observe the child at home (Brender and others, 1985a).

Etiology

The exact cause of appendicitis is poorly understood but it is almost always a result of obstruction of the lumen, usually by a fecalith (a hard fecal concretion). Sometimes a fold of peritoneum causes the appendix to adhere to the cecum, resulting in an obstructive kink. Other causes include lymphoid hyperplasia, fibrous stenosis from an earlier inflammation, and tumors. Although worms are frequently found in the appendix, their role in the pathophysiology is unclear. There is mounting evidence that dietary habits play a role; children with diets high in fiber foods have a lower incidence of appendicitis than those whose fiber intake is low (Barker, Morris, and Nelson, 1986; Brender and others, 1985b). Fiber increases intestinal transit time and increases the bulk and softness of the stool—factors that minimize the chance of obstruction.

Pathophysiology

With acute obstruction the outflow of mucous secretions is blocked and pressure builds within the lumen, resulting in compression of blood vessels. The resulting ischemia is followed by ulceration of the epithelial lining and bacterial invasion. Subsequent necrosis causes perforation or rupture with fecal and bacterial contamination of the peritoneal cavity, resulting in *peritonitis,* inflammation of the lining of the peritoneal cavity—especially in young children who are unable to localize infection and who have a thinner appendiceal wall. The omentum, which is not fully developed, is less efficient in walling off the inflammation, sealing perforated viscera, and confining an intraperitoneal disease process. The proximity of all abdominal and pelvic organs favors the spread of peritonitis to accessory digestive and reproductive organs. Progressive peritoneal inflammation results in functional intestinal obstruction of the small bowel, since intense gastrointestinal reflexes severely inhibit bowel motility. Since the peritoneum represents a major portion of total body surface, the loss of extracellular fluid to the peritoneal cavity leads to electrolyte imbalance and hypovolemic shock.

Clinical Manifestations

The most common signs and symptoms of appendicitis are colicky abdominal pain, tenderness, and fever. Initially the pain is generalized or periumbilical; however, it usually descends to the lower right quadrant. The most intense site of pain may be at McBurney point, which is located midway between the anterior superior iliac crest and the umbilicus. Other important signs are a rigid abdomen, decreased or absent bowel sounds, and rebound tenderness (the sudden pain at the point of tenderness elicited by pressing firmly over a part of the abdomen distal to the area of tenderness). Jumping or riding over bumps in an automobile or gurney aggravates the pain.

Vomiting commonly follows the onset of pain, especially in younger children, and constipation or diarrhea may be present. Anorexia is a constant feature. Low-grade fever is typically seen early in the disease but can rise sharply once peritonitis has begun. Probably the most significant clinical manifestation is a change in the child's behavior. The younger, nonverbal child will assume a rigid, motionless, side-lying posture with the knees flexed on the abdomen. The older child may exhibit all of these behaviors, while complaining of abdominal pain.

Signs of peritonitis in addition to fever include sudden relief from pain after perforation, subsequent increase in pain, which is usually diffuse and accompanied by rigid guarding of the abdomen, progressive abdominal distention, tachycardia, rapid shallow breathing as the child refrains from using abdominal muscles, pallor, chills, irritability, and restlessness.

Diagnostic Evaluation

Diagnosis is based primarily on history and examination. The chief clues that should alert the practitioner to appendicitis are the progression of abdominal pain, location of abdominal tenderness, decreased peristalsis, pain on rectal examination, and absence of any other symptoms or findings suggesting another disorder, such as pneumonia.

Laboratory evaluation includes a white blood cell count, which is usually elevated but is seldom higher than 15,000 to 20,000/mm^3, and roentgenographic studies of the abdomen may reveal possible contributing causes of appendicitis, such as fecaliths or a foreign body.

Diagnosis is not always straightforward. Numerous infectious processes have features in common. Fever, vomiting, abdominal pain, and elevated blood count are associated with inflammatory bowel disease, gastroenteritis, urinary tract infection, pneumonia, and numerous hematologic disorders, for example. Therefore practitioners must have a high degree of suspicion for appendicitis in the differential diagnosis.

Therapeutic Management

Treatment of appendicitis before perforation is surgical removal of the appendix (appendectomy). Recovery is rapid and generally uneventful unless peritonitis has occurred. The following discussion is concerned with the special care of the child with a ruptured appendix.

Ruptured appendix. Management of the child diagnosed with peritonitis caused by a ruptured appendix often begins preoperatively with intravenous administration of fluid and electrolytes, systemic antibiotics, and nasogastric

suction. Postoperative management includes fluid and electrolyte balance maintenance, continued administration of antibiotics, and nasogastric suction for abdominal decompression until intestinal activity returns.

Most surgeons provide for external drainage when abscess formation has occurred, when there is necrotic or severely damaged tissue, or where there are purulent collections within the peritoneum. This is accomplished by sump drainage or a Penrose drain and wound irrigations. The child is maintained in semi-Fowler position to reduce spread of the infection to other parts of the peritoneum, one of the most common of which is the subdiaphragmatic area.

Nursing Considerations

Because successful treatment of appendicitis is based on prompt recognition of the disorder, a primary nursing objective is assisting in establishing a diagnosis. Even though in many instances nurses may not perform the complete history and examination, they are often in a strategic position to make judgments regarding the child's care. For example, nurses in private physicians' offices, ambulatory settings, or emergency units often have the responsibility of counseling parents or triaging patients regarding additional treatment. When the child with an *acute abdomen* (a general term used to describe conditions associated with acute abdominal pain) is admitted to the pediatric unit, staff nurses usually decide where to place the child, how quickly to arrange for laboratory evaluation, and how much observation and assessment of the child are required and by whom. Even outside the strictly professional relationship, parents may ask nurse friends for advice regarding abdominal pain. Without an appreciation of the signs and symptoms suggestive of appendicitis, these nurses may not make decisions that facilitate rapid diagnosis.

Since abdominal pain is the most common childhood complaint, the nurse needs to make some preliminary assessment of the severity of pain (see p. 1068). One of the most reliable estimates is the degree of change in behavior. A child who stays home from school and voluntarily lies down or refuses to play is much more likely to have considerable pain than the child who is absent from school but plays contentedly at home. For those nurses involved in primary ambulatory care, the responsibility of recognizing a possible instance of appendicitis and prompt medical/surgical referral is particularly great. A detailed history and careful abdominal examination cannot be overstressed. Techniques for assessment of the abdomen are discussed in Chapter 7.

Preoperative care. Physical preparation of the child with appendicitis is the same as that for any child with abdominal surgery (see p. 1421). Any skin preparation, such as shaving the abdomen of an adolescent, must be done very gently because of the area's extreme tenderness. In situations in which medical treatment is required to correct problems associated with peritonitis, the nurse must anticipate expected procedures and set up equipment as quickly as possible to prevent any delay in preparing the child for surgery. In any instance when severe abdominal pain is expected, the nurse must be aware of the danger of administering laxatives or enemas or applying heat to the area. Such measures stimulate bowel motility and increase the risk of perforation. Psychologic preparation of the child and parents is similar to that employed in other emergency situations (see p. 1092).

Postoperative care. Postoperative care for the nonperforated appendix is the same as for most abdominal operations. Care of the child with a ruptured appendix and peritonitis involves more complex care. The course of recovery is considerably longer and may require up to 2 weeks of hospitalization, in contrast to about 4 days for an uncomplicated appendectomy.

The child is maintained on intravenous fluids, is allowed nothing by mouth, and remains on low intermittent gastric decompression until there is evidence of intestinal activity. The nurse listens for bowel sounds as part of the routine assessment and observes for other signs of bowel activity such as passage of stool. Management of intravenous therapy is the same as for any child, and parenteral antibiotics are usually infused for 7 to 10 days, after which oral preparations may be continued even longer.

Positioning the child in semi-Fowler position or lying on the right side after surgery for a ruptured appendix facilitates drainage from the peritoneal cavity and prevents the formation of a subdiaphragmatic abscess. A Penrose drain is placed in the wound, and frequent dressing changes with meticulous skin care are essential to prevent excoriation of the surgical area. Sometimes the abdominal wound is irrigated with antibacterial solution.

Nursing Care Summary: The Child with Appendicitis

NURSING GOALS	NURSING INTERVENTIONS	EXPECTED PATIENT/FAMILY OUTCOMES
 **HP-HMP** **Infection: potential for** **Etiology: presence of infective organisms**		
Prevent spread of infection	Position in low Fowler position to localize and prevent upward spread of infection Implement appropriate isolation precautions Careful wound care and disposal of wound dressings	Infection remains confined to lower right quadrant of abdomen
Detect presence of infection	Take vital signs every 2-4 hours Collect or request needed specimens Inspect wound for signs of infection—redness, swelling, heat, pain, purulent drainage	Child exhibits no evidence of infection
HP-HMP **Injury: potential for** **Etiology: inflammation of appendix**		
Prevent aggravation of condition	Maintain complete bed rest Avoid heat to abdomen Apply cold applications (ice pack) to abdomen Caution against administering laxatives	Condition remains stable
Assess status of bowel activity	Gently palpate abdomen to determine degree of distention (if present) Auscultate abdomen for sounds of peristaltic activity Observe and record type and amount of any bowel movement	*Bowel activity is detected
Prevent abdominal distention	Allow nothing by mouth Insert rectal tube if indicated	Child does not exhibit signs of discomfort; abdomen remains soft
Prevent other complications	Turn, cough, deep breathe every 2 hours Ambulate as prescribed Assess for bladder distention Encourage to void	Child does not exhibit signs of complications
N-MP **Fluid volume deficit, potential** **Etiology: loss of appetite, vomiting, NPO**		
Maintain hydration	Offer fluids when tolerated	Child takes sufficient amount of fluid

*Nursing outcome.

Continued.

Nursing Care Summary: The Child with Appendicitis—cont'd

NURSING GOALS	NURSING INTERVENTIONS	EXPECTED PATIENT/FAMILY OUTCOMES
C-PP Comfort, alteration in: pain **Etiology: inflammation of appendix**		
Relieve discomfort	Assess need for pain medication (p. 1068) Position for comfort Semi-Fowler position Side-lying position Implement appropriate nonpharmacologic pain reduction techniques (see p. 1071) Monitor effectiveness of interventions	Child displays a minimum of discomfort preoperatively
Preoperative	Avoid palpating the abdomen unless necessary Apply cold applications to abdomen	
Postoperative	Insert rectal rube, if indicated Encourage to void, if appropriate	Child rests quietly and displays no evidence of discomfort
SP-SCP Fear **Etiology: hospitalization, discomfort**		
Relieve anxiety in child and parents	Maintain calm, reassuring manner Explain procedures and other activities before initiating Answer questions and explain purposes of activities Keep informed of progress	Child rests quietly and calmly Discusses procedures and activities without evidence of anxiety
Provide reassurance	Remain with child as much as possible Explain activities and procedures Give encouragement and positive feedback for cooperation in care See also The child in the hospital, p. 1075	
RRP Family process, alteration in **Etiology: situational crisis (emergency hospitalization of child)**		
Support and reassure child and family	Explain all procedures Prepare child and family for surgery Keep family informed of child's progress Encourage expression of feelings Review child's memory of events, if an emergency procedure Refer to public health nurse if indicated Refer to appropriate agency or persons for specific help (e.g., social service, clergy) See also The family of the hospitalized child, p. 1081	Family discusses child's condition and therapies confortably Family members avail themselves of appropriate assistance

Nursing Interventions Related to Medical Management

Assist with diagnosis
   Obtain history, if appropriate
   Observe for symptoms of appendicitis
   Order or collect necessary specimens
      Collect urine specimens
      Order blood work
Anticipate possible surgery
Administer analgesics cautiously (if ordered) to prevent
   masking of symptoms
Initiate nothing by mouth
Collect and order needed specimens
Relieve discomfort
   Administer analgesics as prescribed
   Record effectiveness of analgesics

RUPTURED APPENDIX
Eradicate organisms
   Administer antibiotics as prescribed
Ensure adequate hydration
   Monitor intravenous infusion
   Provide fluids and foods by mouth as ordered when
      bowel activity evident
Facilitate wound healing
   When child begins oral feedings, provide nutritious
      diet as ordered
   Careful wound care
      Keep wound clean and dry
      Cleanse with prescribed preparation
      Advance Penrose drain as ordered (if present)
      Apply antibacterial solutions and/or ointments as
         ordered

Nursing Interventions Related to Medical Management—cont'd	
NURSING GOALS **NURSING INTERVENTIONS**	**EXPECTED PATIENT/FAMILY OUTCOMES**

Prevent abdominal distention
   Maintain abdominal decompression as ordered
     Assess and ensure patency of nasogastric tube; irrigate with normal saline solution as indicated
     Maintain intermittent suction at appropriate negative pressure
	Maintain adequate nutrition and hydration
	   Monitor IV infusion
	   Provide fluids and food by mouth as ordered when bowel activity is evident
	   Provide progressive diet as tolerated
	Reduce fever
	   Administer antipyretics as indicated

Psychologic care after surgery is also important. Parents and older children need an opportunity to express their feelings regarding the events surrounding the hospitalization. It is especially important for the nurse to encourage the child to relate all the events he remembers concerning admission and treatment in order to clarify misconceptions.

MECKEL DIVERTICULUM

Meckel diverticulum results when the omphalomesenteric or vitelline duct, which connects the midgut to the yolk sac during embryonic development, fails to completely obliterate. Although several different types of malformations can result, such as cysts, fistulas, or fibrotic cords, Meckel diverticulum is the most common and consists of an outpouching of the ileum, most commonly in proximity to the ileocecal valve. It may vary in size from a small appendiceal process to a segment of bowel several inches long and wide. At times it may be connected to the umbilicus by a cord.

It is the most common congenital malformation of the gastrointestinal tract and is present in 1% to 2% of the population. It is more common in males than females, and complications are several times more frequent in males. Often it exists without causing symptoms. Most symptomatic cases are seen in the first 2 years of life.

Pathophysiology

Meckel diverticulum is a sac subject to inflammation (diverticulitis) in the same manner as appendicitis. In over half the cases the diverticulum contains gastric mucosa, which produces hydrochloric acid and pepsin. The acid continually irritates the bowel and erodes the surface, which results in bleeding and, in some instances, may lead to perforation. Mechanical obstruction can occur as a result of volvulus, or twisting of the bowel around the fibrotic Meckel cord. Intussusception can occur if the diverticulum acts as a lead point for invagination.

Clinical Manifestations

Signs and symptoms are based on the specific pathologic process, such as diverticulitis or intestinal obstruction. Rectal bleeding, however, is the chief presenting sign in more than half of the cases. Bright red or dark red rectal bleeding is much more common than black tarry stools and represents acute hemorrhage. Usually there is no evidence of abdominal pain. Severe anemia and shock are consequences of the hemorrhage.

Diagnostic Evaluation

Diagnosis is usually based on the history. Rectosigmoidoscopy and barium enema are usually performed to eliminate other possible diagnoses, such as anal fissure, polyps, and intussusception. Radiologic studies are not helpful in confirming the diagnosis because the diverticulum may be too small to be visualized or may fail to fill with barium. Blood studies are usually part of the general laboratory workup to rule out any bleeding disorder and to evaluate the severity of the anemia.

Therapeutic Management

Treatment is surgical removal of the diverticulum. In instances in which severe hemorrhage increases the surgical risk, medical intervention to correct hypovolemic shock (e.g., blood replacement, intravenous fluids, and oxygen) may be necessary. In diverticulitis antibiotics may be used preoperatively to control infection. If intestinal obstruction has occurred, appropriate preoperative measures are used to reverse electrolyte imbalances and prevent abdominal distention.

Nursing Considerations

Nursing objectives are similar to those listed in the Nursing care summary on p. 1421 regarding abdominal surgery. Since the onset is usually rapid, psychologic support parallels that for other conditions, such as appendicitis. It is important to remember that the occurrence of massive rectal bleeding is most often traumatic to both the child and the parents and may significantly affect their emotional reaction to hospitalization and surgery.

Specific preoperative considerations when rectal bleeding is present include (1) frequent monitoring of vital signs and blood pressure for shock, (2) keeping the child on bed rest, and (3) recording the approximate amount of blood lost in stools. In the absence of rectal hemorrhage, the nurse tests the stools for occult blood.

INFLAMMATORY BOWEL DISEASE

Inflammatory bowel disease (IBD) is a general term used to designate two chronic intestinal disorders—ulcerative colitis

Table 33-2 Comparison of inflammatory bowel diseases—ulcerative colitis and Crohn disease

CHARACTERISTICS	ULCERATIVE COLITIS	CROHN DISEASE
Pathologic changes		
Extent of involvement	Diffuse, mucosal	Focal, transmural (entire wall)
Ulceration	Superficial, extensive	Deep
Distribution of lesions	Contiguous, symmetric	Segmental, asymmetric with "skip" areas
Lymph nodes	Normal	Affected
Primary areas of involvement	Colon, rectum	Ileum, colon, rectum (10%-20%)
Clinical features		
Rectal bleeding	Common	Uncommon
Diarrhea	Often severe	Moderate to absent
Pain	Less frequent	Common
Anorexia	Mild or moderate	Can be severe
Weight loss	Moderate	Severe
Growth retardation	Usually mild	Often marked
Anal and perianal lesions	Rare	Common
Fistulas and strictures	Rare	Common
Surgical resection of affected bowel	Curative	Unsatisfactory because of frequent recurrence
Risk of carcinoma	Related to duration of disease	Occurs less frequently
	Prevented by surgery	Not prevented by surgery

and Crohn disease. The term should not be confused with *irritable bowel syndrome (IBS)*, which refers to a functional disorder generally thought to be brought on by stress that is unaccompanied by any structural defect.

Although these two diseases are grouped under the classification of IBD because they have similar epidemiologic, immunologic, and clinical features, they are two distinct conditions with very significant differences (see Table 33-2 for a comparison of these diseases). The most important reason for differentiating between the two is prognosis. Crohn disease is considered the more serious and disabling disorder, and medical/surgical treatment is much less effective than in ulcerative colitis. Unfortunately, the incidence of Crohn disease is increasing in the population, although the reason for this change is not known.

Etiology

The cause of IBD is unknown, although infectious, nutritional, immunologic, and psychogenic etiologies have been proposed. The current thinking is that IBD is the result of a genetically conditioned susceptibility to one or more environmental influences. Psychologic factors such as stress or personality characteristics do not play a role in the pathogenesis of the disease but may accentuate symptoms and the severity of a relapse (Silverman and Roy, 1983).

Several genetic and environmental factors influence the incidence of IBD: (1) there is a familial tendency in about 5% to 15% of the cases, (2) individuals from higher socio-economic levels and more whites than nonwhites are affected, (3) the incidence is several times greater in Jews living in Europe and North America than in the general population, and (4) there is a higher occurrence of the disease in children living in urban settings than rural areas.

ULCERATIVE COLITIS

Ulcerative colitis is a disease characterized by a chronic inflammatory reaction involving the mucosa and submucosa of the large intestine. It occurs in both sexes and in all age-groups. It is basically a disease of young adults, although close to 15% of the cases begin in children younger than 16 years. The mean age of onset in children is around 11.

Pathophysiology

The inflammatory changes in ulcerative colitis are primarily limited to the mucosa of the colon and rectum. The mucous membranes become hyperemic and edematous with the formation of patchy granulations over the intestinal surface that bleed easily and eventually develop irregular areas of superficial ulcerations. The ulcerated and damaged mucosa is ineffective in reabsorbing nutrients, fluid, and electrolytes. The more extensive the involvement, the more severe is the diarrhea and resulting growth retardation. In long-standing disease the bowel becomes narrowed, smooth, and inflexible, with thin or absent mucosa heavily infiltrated by scar

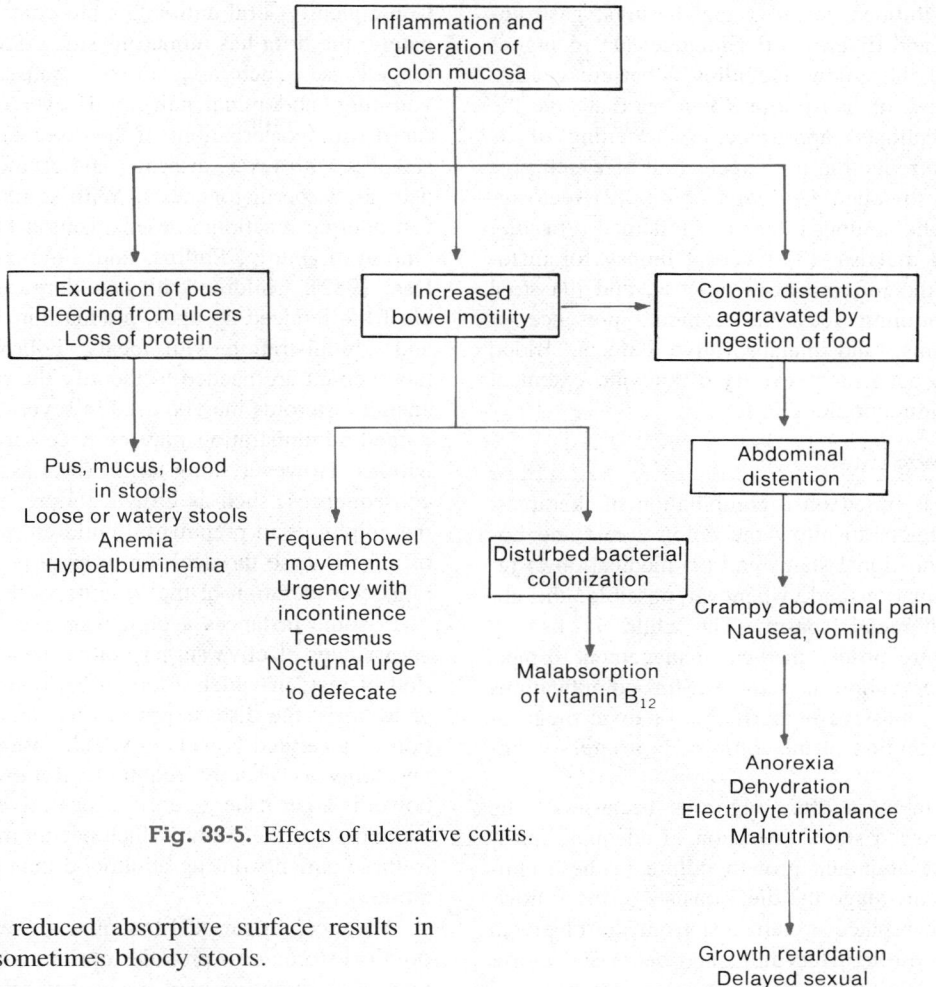

Fig. 33-5. Effects of ulcerative colitis.

tissue. The greatly reduced absorptive surface results in loose, watery, and sometimes bloody stools.

Clinical Manifestations

The most common feature of ulcerative colitis is persistent or recurring diarrhea. In the acute, fulminating disease there is bloody diarrhea preceded by cramping abdominal pain and followed by abdominal distention. Diarrhea may be severe with marked urgency and frequency (20 to 30 stools daily). It is usually associated with fever, weight loss, anorexia, and sometimes nausea and vomiting. Nocturnal diarrhea is common and is associated with more involvement. Pallor and anemia may result from bleeding and reduced dietary intake, and the numerous watery bowel movements often cause depletion of water and electrolytes. Growth retardation and delayed puberty are common findings, especially with more severe disease, although stunted growth may also be seen with few gastrointestinal symptoms (Fig. 33-5). A number of other symptoms unrelated to the gastrointestinal manifestations may be seen, such as low-grade fever peaking in the evening, aphthous stomatitis (ulcerated areas in the mouth), joint pain, and conjunctivitis.

The clinical course varies markedly in terms of severity, response to therapy, and prognosis. In general, the disease follows one of two patterns: acute remitting type or chronic continuous course. Children afflicted with either type are usually healthy before the onset of the disease.

The *acute remitting* type is more common and follows a pattern of remissions and exacerbations. During the period of remission, the child is usually well, with few or no symptoms of the disease. However, periods of exacerbation are severe and acute, although they usually respond well to medical treatment. The disease may terminate in a permanent remission or ultimately follow the course of chronic colitis.

In *chronic continuous colitis* there are no definitive periods of severe disease with intermittent good health. Intestinal symptoms tend to be less severe, but chronic malnutrition and anemia are common. These children often respond poorly to medical therapy and are more likely to suffer from complications, especially carcinoma of the colon.

Diagnostic Evaluation

Diagnosis is usually based on a combination of findings from the history, physical examination, and laboratory testing. Specific diagnostic tests to confirm the diagnosis and rule out other possibilities, such as anal fissures, gastrointestinal infections, and diverticulitis, include: (1) roentgenographic studies of the colon, including a barium enema, which may show loss of haustration (pouches that give the normal colon a scalloped appearance), shortening of its length, and uniform reduction in diameter, all of which give the picture of the so-called *lead-pipe colon,* (2) rectosigmoidoscopy, which demonstrates an inflamed, friable, bleeding, ulcerated mucosa, (3) mucosal biopsy for histologic evidence of the inflammatory process, and (4) stool samples for determining fecal fat content, presence of pathologic organisms, and malabsorptive defects. Blood studies are done to determine severity of anemia, extent of albumin loss, and immunoglobulin levels.

Therapeutic Management

Medical treatment is based on a combination of therapies: (1) dietary management to allow the colon a rest and improve the child's nutritional status and (2) medication to reduce bowel inflammation and, whenever possible, the abdominal pain and rectal spasm. The child is usually hospitalized to ensure proper medical management. Emergency surgical intervention is required for complications such as perforation, massive hemorrhage, or toxic megacolon (fulminating distention of the colon with progressive inflammation).

Dietary management is often vigorous because of the child's poorly nourished state. Provision of adequate nutrition can reverse the attendant growth failure in these children. During the acute stage the diet consists of the following: *high protein* to replace protein lost from the ulcerated bowel, plasma lost through bleeding, and decreased intake resulting from anorexia; *high calories* to restore daily losses in the stool, to combat weight loss, and to promote positive nitrogen balance; *normal to low fat;* and *low fiber* to decrease bowel irritation. Elimination of lactose-containing foods may be needed temporarily. Vitamin and mineral supplements are usually provided to correct the anemia (iron), to promote tissue synthesis (ascorbic acid and vitamin B complex), and to correct deficiencies (zinc, folate, magnesium, vitamin B_{12}) (Motil and Grand, 1985). Supplemental nutrition may be provided through intermittent or continuous drip gastric feedings. Intermittent feedings are preferred because they can be given at night and interfere less with the child's usual activities if they are continued at home. Other therapies that may be warranted include intravenous fluids to correct dehydration and associated electrolyte imbalances and parenteral alimentation when malnutrition is severe and the colitis is further aggravated by oral diet.

Drug therapy primarily involves the use of sulfasalazine. Although the action of the drug is not well established, it appears to be an inhibitor of both the synthesis and the degradation of prostaglandins in the colonic mucosa. The active component is 5-aminosalicylic acid (5-ASA), which acts locally on the mucosa to reduce inflammation (Singleton, 1982). The therapeutic efficacy of the drug depends on colonic bacteria to split the molecule for the release of 5-ASA.

Consequently, oral antibiotics are contraindicated. Unfortunately, the drug has numerous side effects that limit its prolonged use, such as anorexia, nausea, bloody diarrhea, vomiting, abdominal pain, and fever (which may be confused with exacerbations of the disease); anemia; serum-like sickness with fever, arthritis, and erythema multiforme; and decreased spermatogenesis. With some patients who manifest allergic reactions, desensitization has been successfully employed (Purdy, Philips, and Summers, 1984; Taffet and Das, 1982). Children with nonallergic symptoms may benefit from reduced dosages, gradual introduction of the drug, and administration with meals. Follow-up studies of the blood count are needed to identify the possibility of aplastic anemia. Steroids may be used in severe cases, in which prolonged administration may be necessary to prevent exacerbations. However, long-term use is associated with serious consequences, such as growth failure, premature closure of the epiphyses in prepubertal children, and increased chance of infection, so the decision to employ steroids always warrants consideration of the benefits vs the risks.

In some instances a poor response to medical treatment necessitates elective surgery either to allow the bowel a period of rest, in which a temporary colostomy is performed, or to arrest the disease process by removing the entire section of ulcerated bowel, in which case a total colectomy or ileostomy is usually required. Removal of the diseased bowel is a permanent cure for ulcerative colitis and prevents carcinoma of the colon, which occurs much more frequently in these patients during adulthood than in the general population.

Advances in surgical techniques over the incontinent abdominal stoma now provides options for some children. One possible alternative to a permanent colectomy or ileostomy is the *continent (Koch) ileostomy.* In this procedure an intraabdominal pouch or reservoir is constructed from the terminal ileum. The feces are stored in the pouch until the patient drains it with a catheter. A surgically implanted valve prevents leakage of feces. The stoma is less than an inch in diameter, is almost level with the skin, and requires no appliance (Cassell, 1984).

Another option is the *continent colectomy.* After resection of the diseased colon and removal of the rectal mucosa from the muscular wall of the rectum, the ileum is reanastomosed to the anus (ileoanal-endorectal pull through). While this procedure eliminates the need for an intestinal stoma on the abdomen and is likely to ensure continence, it results in frequent loose stools and a sense of fecal urgency. To lessen this problem a fecal reservoir may be constructed immediately proximal to the ileoanal anastomosis and drained with a rectal tube in much the same manner as the Koch procedure. Results with this approach have been satisfactory, although some complications can occur, such as distention of the reservoir and incomplete emptying of feces (Fonkalsrud, 1982). However, both procedures offer young people with ulcerative colitis a more acceptable means of elimination than the traditional stoma and pouch.

Psychotherapy may also prove helpful in reducing

stresses that have resulted from the colitis. A particularly difficult stress for these children to cope with is the consequent growth retardation and delayed sexual maturation because of chronic colitis. Supportive therapy may also be of benefit to those children facing the adjustment of a permanent ileostomy.

Nursing Considerations

Many of the nursing considerations relate directly to the therapeutic management in treating colitis. However, the scope of nursing responsibilities extends beyond the immediate period of hospitalization and involves (1) continued guidance of families in terms of dietary management and drug compliance, (2) adjusting to a disease of remissions and exacerbations or one of chronic ill health, and (3) when indicated, preparing the child and parents for the possibility of diversionary bowel surgery.

Since diet therapy is a very important component of therapy, encouraging the anorexic child to consume sufficient quantities of this diet is of primary importance and is frequently a nursing challenge. An approach that is more likely to meet with success involves including the child in meal planning; encouraging small, frequent meals or snacks rather than three large meals a day; serving meals around medication schedules when diarrhea, mouth pain, and intestinal spasm are controlled; and preparing high-protein, high-calorie foods, such as eggnog, milk shakes, cream soups, puddings, or custard (if lactose is tolerated) (see also Feeding the sick child, p. 1115). Foods that are known to aggravate the condition are avoided as are high-fiber foods (see Table 33-1). Occasionally the occurrence of aphthous stomatitis further complicates adherence to dietary management. Good mouth care before eating and the selection of bland foods help relieve the discomfort of mouth sores.

The importance of continued drug therapy despite remission of symptoms must be stressed to the parents and child. Failure to adhere to the pharmacologic regimen can result in exacerbation of the disease process (see Chapter 27 for a discussion of compliance).

Attending to the emotional components of a chronic disease requires a thorough assessment of those stress factors that are disease related. Frequently the nurse can be instrumental in helping these children adjust to the problems of growth retardation, delayed sexual maturation, dietary restrictions, feelings of being "different" or "sickly," inability to compete with peers, and necessary absence from school during exacerbations of the illness (see Chapter 22).

In the event that a permanent colectomy/ileostomy is required, the nurse can assist the child and family in accepting and adjusting to the change by teaching them how to care for the ileostomy, by emphasizing the positive aspects of surgery, particularly accelerated growth and sexual development, permanent recovery, and eliminated risk of colonic cancer, and by stressing the normalcy of life despite bowel diversion. Introducing the child and parents to other ostomy patients, especially those of the child's age, can be the greatest therapeutic measure in fostering eventual accep-

tance. Whenever possible the newer continent ostomies should be offered as options to the child, although they are not performed in all centers throughout the United States.

Because of the chronic and often life-long nature of the disease, families benefit from many of the services provided by organizations such as the **National Foundation for Ileitis and Colitis, Inc.,*** which has branches in many major communities and provides education regarding the management of inflammatory bowel disease. If diversionary bowel surgery is indicated, the **United Ostomy Association**† is available to assist with information concerning the ileostomy care and provides important psychologic support through its self-help groups.

CROHN DISEASE (REGIONAL ENTERITIS)

Crohn disease is an inflammatory disease of the bowel that is being recognized in both children and adolescents with increasing frequency. It occurs in both sexes and, like ulcerative colitis, is more prevalent in the adolescent and young adult. Since many of the features of Crohn disease are similar to ulcerative colitis, the following discussion is concerned primarily with the differences in the two bowel disorders (see also Table 33-2).

Pathophysiology

Crohn disease may involve any part of the gastrointestinal tract but most commonly affects the terminal ileum. The disease characteristically involves all layers of the bowel wall (transmural). Acute edema and inflammation eventually progress to deep, transverse or longitudinal ulcerations often associated with fissure formation. The thickened bowel wall may lead to obstruction. The asymmetric and patchy distribution of the lesions helps to differentiate Crohn disease from the contiguous and symmetric lesions of ulcerative colitis. Local lymph nodes are enlarged.

Clinical Manifestations

The onset of Crohn disease is usually insidious, with nonspecific symptoms including anorexia, lethargy, fever, and fatigue. Diarrhea and intermittent, cramping pain that often resembles that of acute appendicitis occur. The pain is often triggered by eating. As the disease progresses, however, the abdominal pain becomes a constant aching or soreness. The diarrhea may contain blood, but it is a less frequent finding in children. Weight loss, pallor, anemia, and finger clubbing are not uncommon and may precede the abdominal symptoms.

Diagnostic Evaluation

The diagnosis is established by sigmoidoscopic examination and biopsy. Barium enema and small bowel series demonstrate characteristic bowel changes. The stool is examined for occult blood, white blood cells, fat, and ova and para-

---

*295 Madison Ave., New York, NY 10017.
†2001 W. Beverly Blvd., Los Angeles, CA 90057-2491.

sites to help rule out infectious processes. An elevated erythrocyte sedimentation rate is usually found, and a red cell count and hemoglobin analysis reveal the extent of anemia.

Therapeutic Management

The general principles of care outlined for ulcerative colitis are applied to children with Crohn disease, although the results are often less satisfactory. Management includes primarily nutritional management with a high-protein, high-energy diet with vitamin/mineral supplements, sulfasalazine and/or corticosteroids, antibiotics, and general supportive therapy. Sometimes total parenteral nutrition is needed for short periods to alleviate severe malnutrition, and enteral feedings using elemental formula such as Vivonex may be instituted as an alternative when oral feedings are poorly tolerated. Sedatives and analgesics are administered as indicated according to the individual case. Surgical removal of affected areas is not curative; the disease tends to recur in 20% of the children after 2 years and in 40% after 4 years (Silverman and Roy, 1983). However, surgery may be recommended to reverse the severe effects of growth retardation. In most instances the continent ileostomy or colectomy is contraindicated.

Nursing Considerations

The nursing care for Crohn disease is the same as that discussed for the child with ulcerative colitis. However, the chronic and often unrelenting nature of this condition and the lack of a cure with surgery pose extra stresses on the child and family. If surgery is performed, the family can expect resumption of growth and abatement of the symptoms, but they need a realistic knowledge of the incidence of recurrence. Although the incidence of carcinoma of the bowel is lower than in ulcerative colitis, there is still a substantial risk that requires appropriate screening throughout life for early detection.

PEPTIC ULCER

A *peptic ulcer* is an erosion of the mucosal wall of the stomach, pylorus, or duodenum. A *gastric ulcer* affects the lining of the stomach, whereas a *duodenal ulcer* involves the pylorus or duodenum. Although peptic ulcers are more common in adults, they are also a significant pediatric problem, occurring most frequently between 12 and 18 years. Males are affected more than three times as often as females.

Etiology

Both genetic and environmental factors appear to be important in the etiology of peptic ulcers. There is an increased frequency among relatives and a positive relationship to blood group O. However, emotional stress has been implicated as an important contributing factor toward the development, severity, and prognosis of peptic ulcers.

Secondary ulcers are also known to occur as a complication of a number of acute disorders, such as encephalitis, meningitis, or sepsis, and several chronic conditions, such as burns, rheumatoid arthritis, cirrhosis of the liver, or chronic obstructive lung disease, except cystic fibrosis. They are termed *stress ulcers,* although the exact disease process is not known. Certain drugs, particularly aspirin and corticosteroids, are ulcerogenic.

Pathophysiology

The precise mechanism is not understood, but one of two mechanisms probably reflects the basic defect: (1) an increase in the rate of production of gastric juice or (2) interference with the normal protective mechanisms of the mucosal lining. As a result of either of these two conditions, the gastric mucosa is highly vulnerable to the digestive effects of gastric juice. Prolonged contact with the highly acidic contents of the stomach and duodenum causes an erosion of the mucosal wall, especially in those areas least protected, such as the cardia and lesser curve of the stomach and the area immediately beyond the pylorus. Factors that can result in hypersecretion or decreased protection are outlined in Fig. 33-6.

Clinical Manifestations

Signs and symptoms of peptic ulcers vary according to the age of the child and the location of the ulcer (Table 33-3). The typical pain-food-relief syndrome seen in adults with peptic ulcer is often absent in young children. Suggestive symptoms of peptic ulcer include chronic abdominal pain, especially when the stomach is empty, such as during the night or early morning, recurrent vomiting after meals, chronic anemia with occult blood in the stools, and vague gastrointestinal complaints with a positive family history for peptic ulcer.

Diagnostic Evaluation

Diagnosis is based on the history (pattern of pain), physical examination (pain in the epigastric area), and diagnostic testing such as radiologic studies, barium swallow, and endoscopy. Other tests include blood studies (anemia), stool samples (occult blood), and, occasionally, gastric acid measurements (to isolate hypersecretors).

Therapeutic Management

The major objectives of therapy for children with peptic ulcers are to relieve discomfort, promote healing, and prevent complications and recurrence. The management of ulcers is primarily medical and consists of administration of medications that reduce or neutralize gastric acid secretion and, when possible, measures to eliminate or reduce stresses.

The child is provided with a nutritious diet but advised to avoid foods that are associated with aggravation of symptoms (see discussion under Nursing considerations). Milk and other dairy products at frequent intervals are no longer recommended for treatment of ulcers. Milk contains protein and calcium, both of which stimulate gastric acid production. Milk also distends the stomach, further stimulating acid secretion, and exits from the stomach rapidly, thereby

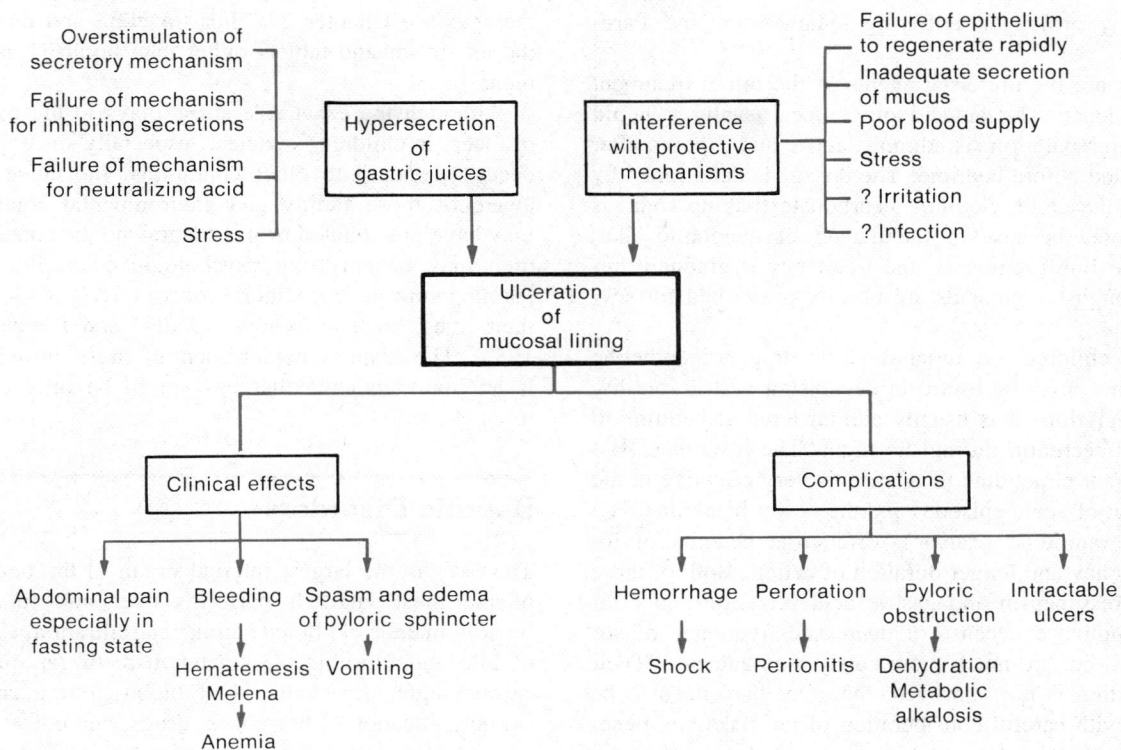

Fig. 33-6. Possible causes and effects of peptic ulcer.

Table 33-3 Clinical manifestations of peptic ulcers

AGE-GROUP	TYPE OF ULCER	MANIFESTATIONS	COMMENTS
Neonates	Usually gastric	Usually perforation Often massive hemorrhage Almost the same as seen in stress ulcers	Usually catastrophic More likely in infants with hypoxia, sepsis, difficult labor/delivery, or nasogastric feeding Prognosis often poor
Infants to 2-year-old children	Gastric or duodenal, primary or secondary	Poor eating, vomiting, crying spells after feeding, abdominal distention, tarry stools, melena Vague discomfort Irritability	Primary ulcers more likely to be gastric with slow onset Usually bleed rather than perforate
2- to 6-year-old children	Gastric or duodenal	No really positive physical findings May have vomiting related to eating, generalized or periumbilical pain, melena, hematemesis Wake at night crying with pain	Diagnosis often made on basis of social history Duodenal ulcers 5:1 over gastric Perforation more likely in secondary ulcers
6- to 9-year-old children	Usually duodenal and primary Often with obstruction	Pain—burning or gnawing sensation in epigastrium related to fasting state, melena, hematemesis, vomiting	Often related to school achievement, change, relationship with peers and/or teachers
Children over 9 years	Usually duodenal	Same as above	More typical of adult type Chances of recurrence greater than 50%

negating any prolonged buffering (Mathewson and Farnham, 1984).

Antacids are the preferred agents in the initial treatment of peptic ulcers. The antacid of choice, usually a liquid magnesium preparation, is administered 1 and 3 hours after each meal and before bedtime. The dosage is determined by the size of the child. Sodium bicarbonate (baking soda) is contraindicated because of the danger of metabolic alkalosis. As healing progresses, the frequency is gradually reduced although the antacids are usually prescribed for several weeks.

In some children the anticholinergic drug propantheline (Pro-Banthine) may be useful in decreasing gastric motility and acid secretion. It is usually administered at bedtime to reduce acid secretion during the night. The histamine (H_2) blocking agent cimetidine (Tagamet) is very effective in the management of acute episodes and the newer histamine (H_2) antagonist, ranitidine (Zantac), offers the benefits of increased potency and longer duration of action. Both of these drugs suppress pepsin and gastric acid secretion and offer greater compliance because of decreased frequency of administration, but are much more costly than antacids. Their use in children is not approved; therefore they need to be prescribed with careful consideration of the risks and benefits. Sucralfate (Carafate), which exerts a local effect by covering the ulcer, may also be used for short-term treatment.

A child with an acute ulcer who has developed complications, such as massive hemorrhage, requires emergency care. A nasogastric tube is inserted to remove the blood, prevent abdominal distention, and provide a means of calculating blood loss. Blood replacement, intravenous fluids, and oxygen are usually necessary. Surgical closure of the perforation or bleeding point may be required to stop the hemorrhage.

Surgical management is rarely used in children, except for patients with complications of intractable pain, perforation, hemorrhage, and obstruction. Vagotomy with pyloroplasty is the preferred technique. Gastric resection is rarely performed.

Nursing Considerations

The main nursing objective is to promote healing of the ulcer through compliance with the dietary and medication regimen. The diet is usually liberal, with avoidance of those foods that enhance gastric secretion, such as tea, coffee, spices, carbonated beverages, and meat extractives (beef broth), and any food that causes the child discomfort. Substances that irritate the gastric wall are also avoided, such as alcohol, smoking, and aspirin. However, these present no problem in children, although use of alcohol and tobacco may be an issue in adolescents with ulcers. If an analgesic/antipyretic is needed during the course of therapy, acetaminophen is substituted for aspirin.

Drug compliance is essential and can be a problem with frequent administration of antacids. Therefore strategies to improve compliance are instituted early in the course of

therapy (see Chapter 27). For traveling and during school the use of antacid tablets rather than liquid is more convenient.

Although the exact role stress plays in the pathogenesis of ulcers in children is unclear, especially since many ulcers occur secondary to other conditions, the nurse should be aware of those family and environmental conditions that may have precipitated or may aggravate the condition. Children may benefit from psychologic counseling and from learning how to cope more constructively with stresses in their lives, such as school, family, and friends (Sibinga, 1983). The adaptive management of stress during childhood is an important area that has yet to be fully explored or researched.

Hepatic Disorders

The liver is the largest internal organ in the body and one of the most vital. It performs over 400 functions that broadly include (1) blood storage and filtration, (2) secretion of bile and bilirubin, (3) metabolism of fat, protein, and carbohydrate and synthesis of blood-clotting components, (4) detoxification of hormones, drugs, and other substances, and (5) storage for glycogen, iron, and vitamins A, D, E, and B_{12}. Inflammatory, obstructive, or degenerative disorders that affect the liver will affect all or some of these functions. The following discussion is concerned with two disorders that affect the liver during childhood—hepatitis and cirrhosis. Biliary atresia, a congenital anomaly, is discussed in Chapter 11.

ACUTE HEPATITIS

Hepatitis, inflammation of the liver, is rapidly emerging as one of the major causes of morbidity and a significant cause of mortality in children. The discussion that follows is primarily concerned with acute hepatitis; yet the chronic form of the disease may involve many of the same mechanisms.

Etiology

Hepatitis of viral origin is caused by at least four types of virus, hepatitis A virus (HAV, formerly referred to as "infectious" hepatitis), hepatitis B virus (HBV, formerly referred to as "serum" hepatitis), hepatitis D (HDV), and non-A, non-B virus (NANBV). HDV is a newly described, unique viral agent in that it replicates only in the presence of HBV. NANBV agents have not been identified; they refer to instances of hepatitis when other viral agents are excluded (Krugman, 1985). NANBV is the most common cause of posttransfusion hepatitis in the United States (Hamm and Jemison-Smith, 1983). The following discussion is concerned with HAV and HBV. Although these viruses produce the same pathologic changes in the liver and similar clinical manifestations, they are distinct in their epidemiologic and immunologic characteristics. Table 33-4 compares the various features of HAV and HBV.

Table 33-4 Comparison of types A and B hepatitis

CHARACTERISTICS	TYPE A	TYPE B
Incubation period	15-40 days, average 25 days	6 weeks to 6 months
Period of communicability	Unknown Virus in blood and feces 2 to 3 weeks before onset of jaundice and for at least 1 week after onset of jaundice	Variable Virus in blood (probably in stool but no direct proof) during late incubation period and acute stage of disease; may persist in carrier state for years
Mode of transmission	Principal route—oral-fecal Less frequent route—parenteral	Principal route—parenteral Less frequent route—oral, venereal (semen, menstrual secretions, saliva) Fetal transfer—from transplacental blood during last trimester, but more commonly at time of delivery
Clinical features		
Onset	Usually rapid, acute	More insidious
Fever	Common and early	Less frequent
Anorexia	Extreme	Mild to moderate
Nausea and vomiting	Common	Less common
Rash	Rare	Common
Arthralgia	Rare	Common
Pruritus	Rare	Sometimes present
Jaundice	Present	Present
Immunity	Present after one attack, but no crossover to type B	Present after one attack, but no crossover to type A
Carrier state	None	Yes
Prophylaxis		
Immune serum globulin (ISG)	Passive immunity Successful, especially during early incubation period and for preexposure prophylaxis	Passive immunity Inconsistent benefits; probably of no use
Hepatitis B immune globulin (HBIG)	No benefit	Postexposure protection possible if given immediately after definite exposure
Hepatitis B vaccine (Heptavax-B)	Not indicated	Provides active immunity Recommended for those persons at high risk of exposure

Hepatitis A. Hepatitis A is a relatively benign, self-limiting, but highly contagious disease that is spread primarily by the fecal-oral route, usually from ingestion of contaminated food or water. This includes eating shellfish caught in contaminated water and from swimming in such water. HAV can affect individuals at any age but is seen primarily in children under 15 years of age, especially those in low socioeconomic groups, where housing conditions are crowded. Recent concern with outbreaks of HAV are in daycare centers that care for children in diapers. An estimated 30% of HAV outbreaks in the United States have started in daycare centers (Marwick and Simmons, 1984). Because most of the infected children may have only mild symptoms or be asymptomatic, the disease is usually spread long before it is recognized.

Hepatitis B. Hepatitis B causes a more insidious and serious form of the disease. HBV is most commonly transmitted by direct (needles) or indirect (cuts, burns, abrasions) parenteral means, although it can be spread to mucous surfaces (intimate contact, contaminated secretions splashed into mouth or eyes during irrigations) and by certain fomites (contaminated equipment, gloves). The virus can be found in almost all body fluids and secretions (except perhaps feces)—saliva, tears, sweat, urine, genital secretions, nasopharyngeal secretions, and possibly breast milk, although these fluids probably are not sources of transmittable HBV. Persons at risk include close family contacts, clients and staff of custodial institutions for retarded children, those requiring frequent blood transfusions and hemodialysis, and health workers—especially those in operating rooms, emergency rooms, dialysis units, intensive care units, laboratories, and dental care units. With the abuse of parenteral drugs, the incidence of HBV is significant in adolescent drug users and their contacts. Most HBV in children is acquired by the nonparenteral route. Newborns are also at risk for neonatal hepatitis, especially if the mother is infected with HBV or was a carrier of HBV during pregnancy. Infection can occur in utero, at birth, or postnatally. Possible routes of maternal-fetal (infant) transmission include (1) leakage of virus across the placenta late in pregnancy or during labor, (2) ingestion of amniotic fluid or maternal blood, and (3) breast-feeding, especially if the mother has cracked nipples (Krugman and others, 1985). The severity of hepatitis in the infant varies from no liver disease to a fulminant or chronic, active type.

Pathophysiology

The pathologic changes occur primarily in the parenchymal cells of the liver and result in variable degrees of swelling, infiltration of liver cells by mononuclear cells, subsequent degeneration, necrosis, and autolysis. Structural changes within the hepatocyte are thought to account for altered liver functions, such as impaired bile excretion, elevated transaminase and alkaline phosphatase levels, and decreased albumin synthesis.

The disorder is usually self-limiting, with complete regeneration of liver cells without scarring occurring within 2 to 3 months. There are, however, forms of hepatitis that do not result in complete return of liver function. These include *fulminant hepatitis,* which is characterized by a severe, acute course with death frequently occurring within 1 to 2 weeks, and *subacute* or *chronic active hepatitis,* characterized by progressive liver destruction and uncertain regeneration with the possibility of scarring.

Clinical Manifestations

The clinical manifestations for both types of viral hepatitis are similar except for a more rapid, acute onset in type A and a slower, more insidious onset in type B. Both types may have flulike symptoms and may never be recognized as actual cases of hepatitis.

However, the classic picture begins with initial symptoms of nausea and vomiting, extreme anorexia, malaise, easy fatigability, and slight to moderate fever. The child may have abdominal pain, especially in the epigastrium or upper right quadrant. He usually acts ill, preferring to rest in bed, and is fretful or irritable. The most significant finding on physical examination is liver tenderness with or without enlargement. This initial anicteric (absence of jaundice) phase usually lasts 5 to 7 days.

Following this period, evidence of jaundice (the icteric phase) is present, beginning with darkening of the urine and the presence of light-colored stools and followed by yellowing of the sclera and skin. Usually as the jaundice worsens, the child begins to feel better, with improved appetite and behavior and the absence of nausea, vomiting, and fever. This opposing course of rising bilirubin and improved clinical signs is regarded as a significant diagnostic and prognostic sign of benign viral hepatitis. The appearance of jaundice with worsening constitutional symptoms is regarded as a poorer prognostic sign, with a majority of these children developing fulminant, subacute, or chronic active hepatitis. Some children never develop jaundice; however, although their course is usually milder, they are still infectious.

The icteric phase commonly lasts less than 4 weeks.

Complete recovery with return of normal liver function and a feeling of well-being with absence of fatigue or malaise may take 1 to 3 months. Generally children recover promptly. However, it is not unusual for the child to experience a short relapse of slight jaundice and clinical symptoms 10 to 12 weeks after the illness. Unless the symptoms persist and continue to worsen, this relapse is considered benign.

Not all affected children exhibit signs of disease. Because the manifestations of hepatitis are the body's response to the viral antigen, individuals who are unable to muster an adequate defense will develop few if any symptoms. However, they will still harbor the virus as carriers. In newborns of mothers with HBV who have been exposed to the virus during prenatal life the virus is not recognized as a foreign protein and therefore these newborns become chronic carriers.

Diagnostic Evaluation

Diagnosis is based on history, physical examination, laboratory evidence of the virus, and liver function tests. Besides the history of the chief complaint and present illness, several other factors are significant in confirming exposure to hepatitis virus, such as (1) contact with a person known to have hepatitis, especially a family member, (2) questionable sanitation practices, such as drinking impure water, (3) eating certain foods, such as clams or oysters (especially from polluted water), (4) recent immunizations or blood transfusions, (5) ingestion of hepatotoxic drugs, such as salicylates, sulfonamides, several antineoplastic agents, and many other medications, and (6) parenteral administration of illicit drugs or sexual contact with a person who uses these drugs. The last event is especially important when hepatitis is suspected in an adolescent and should be coupled with a careful examination for signs of needle marks, especially in the antecubital fossa.

Diagnosis is confirmed by the detection of various antibodies or antigens that are produced in response to the infection. HAV is diagnosed by the presence of hepatitis A antibody (anti-HAV). During the initial infective period anti-HAV of the IgM class is present, but after about 3 to 6 months this antibody declines and anti-HAV of the IgG class increases. Therefore detection of anti-HAV IgM indicates active infection and anti-HAV IgG indicates past infection and immunity (Krugman, 1985).

Several antibodies and antigens are important in the diagnosis of HBV and include:

HBsAg Hepatitis B surface antigen (found on the surface of the antigen)
anti-HBs Antibody to hepatitis B surface antigen
HBcAg Hepatitis B core antigen (found on the core of the antigen)
anti-HBc Antibody to hepatitis B core antigen
HBeAg The e antigen, which is closely associated with HBV infection
anti-HBe Antibody to the e antigen

Tests are available for detection of all the HBV antigens and antibodies except hepatitis B core antigen (HBcAg). The presence of hepatitis B surface antigen (HBsAg) and hepatitis B e antigen (HBeAg) indicates active infection. Clinical improvement is usually associated with a decrease and disappearance of these antigens, followed by the appearance of their antibodies. Hepatitis B core antibody (anti-HBc) of the IgM class is seen early in the disease followed by a rise in anti-HBc of the IgG class. Since the antibodies persist indefinitely, they are used to identify the carrier state (individuals with the HBV who have no clinical disease but are able to transmit the organism). Presence of the antigens or antibodies indicates immunity to HBV, but there is no crossover immunity to HAV.

Therapeutic Management

There is no specific treatment for either type of viral hepatitis. Management is primarily treatment of symptoms. For example, antiemetics may be helpful to reduce the nausea or vomiting. The value of bed rest in promoting overall recovery is controversial. Since the child feels ill and tired in the anicteric phase, he usually chooses to stay in bed. However, once improvement of physical complaints begins, the child prefers to resume normal activity gradually. The best approach is probably to allow the child to regulate his own pace. Hospitalization is rarely necessary, although proper isolation practices at home are imperative.

The child is allowed to choose foods he prefers, especially during the initial stage when anorexia is severe. Generally low-fat foods cause less stomach distention and are better tolerated than foods high in fat content. Carbohydrates should be encouraged to ensure an adequate caloric intake to spare proteins for cell growth. Vitamin K is administered if prothrombin time is prolonged.

Prevention. Isolation or quarantine of the infected child is not necessary as long as measures are employed to prevent spread of the virus. An attack of either virus confers long-lasting immunity to that virus; however, there is no crossover protection to the other virus. Prophylactic use of immune serum globulin (ISG) is effective in preventing hepatitis virus A in situations of preexposure, such as anticipated travel to areas where HAV is prevalent, or in situations of postexposure during the early part of the incubation period and, to a lesser extent, before the onset of the disease. It is of inconsistent benefit in preventing type B virus.

Passive immunity to HBV can be achieved with hyperimmune gamma globulin (hepatitis B immune serum globulin, HBIG), which is very expensive. However, it is used for postexposure prophylaxis in the following situations: (1) newborn infants born to HBsAg-positive mothers, (2) accidental needle stick or mucosal exposure to HBsAg-positive blood, or (3) sexual contact with an HBsAg-positive person. The hepatitis B vaccine (Heptavax), the first to be manufactured from human blood, is highly effective in providing protection against HBV and may be used alone or with

HBIG. It is expensive (about $100 quires three injections (the first two apart followed by a third dose 6 (Krugman, 1985). At present the v for those persons with frequent exp cussion under hepatitis B).

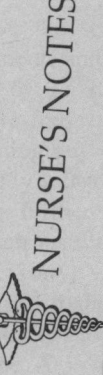

Nursing Considerations

Nursing objectives depend largely hepatitis, the rigidity of medical tre encing the control and transmissi children with benign viral hepatiti at home, the responsibility of exp apies and control measures is freq office nurse. In instances in wl needed for parents to comply with lic health nursing referral may be

The emphasis is on encouragir a realistic schedule of rest anc child's condition. Since hepatiti within a week or so after onset feel well enough to resume school shortly thereafter. The parents are also cautioned about administering any medication to the child without the physician's knowledge, since normal doses of many drugs may become dangerous because of the liver's inability to detoxify and excrete them. Common drugs that are affected by hepatic failure include acetaminophen (Tylenol), ferrous sulfate (oral iron), and propoxyphene hydrochloride (Darvon).

Handwashing is the single most effective measure in prevention and control of hepatitis in any setting (for a discussion of preventive measures in daycare center, see p. 640). Parents and children need an explanation of the usual ways in which hepatitis virus A (oral-fecal route) and hepatitis virus B (parenteral route) are spread; they may benefit from receiving a written list of precautions (see box, p. 1440).

Hospitalized children are not usually isolated in a separate room unless they are fecally unreliable or incontinent or if their toys and other items might become contaminated with feces. They are discouraged from sharing their toys; other precautions for prevention of spread of HAV or HBV are listed in the box on p. 1440. All personnel should wear gowns and gloves when caring for the child directly in addition to following other enteric precautions. Contaminated items (such as a stethoscope) are cleaned with a detergent solution and appropriate disinfectant. Special attention must be given to handling and disposing of all blood products and invasive equipment. The nurse explains to parents and older children the reason for isolation if required and specific precautions to help them adjust to hospitalization and to reinforce practice of control measures before and after discharge.

In those children with type B virus who have a known or suspected history of illicit drug use, the nurse has the additional responsibility of helping them realize the associated dangers of drug abuse, stressing the parenteral mode of

PRECAUTIONS TO PREVENT SPREAD OF HEPATITIS

Precautions for HAV

Wash hands after touching the child or potentially contaminated articles, such as diapers

Discard articles soiled with feces in special container marked for decontamination

Use gowns and gloves when it is anticipated or possible that clothing will be soiled by feces while attending the child

Place child in private room if child is fecally incontinent or if the child's hygiene practices are questionable

Eliminate specific sources of contamination, such as impure water, milk, or food, if these are identified

Clean soiled surfaces with a 1:10 dilution of household bleach

Precautions for HBV

Wash hands after handling blood or blood-soiled articles

Discard articles soiled with blood in special container marked for decontamination

Use gowns and gloves when it is anticipated or possible that clothing will be soiled by blood while attending the child

Place child in private room if profuse bleeding is likely to cause environmental contamination

Handle sharp items (e.g., needles, scalpels) that are contaminated with blood with extraordinary care; do not recap or bend needles; dispose of needles in puncture-resistant containers

Discourage sharing of razors

Clean soiled surfaces with a 1:10 dilution of household bleach

transmission, and encouraging them to seek counseling from a drug program.

CIRRHOSIS

Cirrhosis is a chronic disease in which there is generalized destruction of hepatic cells. It is a result, not a primary cause, of liver dysfunction. It represents the end stage of chronic disease in which there is generalized destruction of hepatic cells. While cirrhosis is not a common cause of morbidity or mortality in children, it is becoming an increasingly significant pediatric health problem. With the alarming escalation in the number of adolescents who are at risk for contracting hepatitis type B from illicit parenteral drug use, it is likely that the occurrence of cirrhosis will also increase. Likewise, improved treatment of genetic diseases, such as cystic fibrosis or sickle cell anemia, will also affect the number of children who are at risk for developing this complication.

Pathophysiology

Cirrhosis is believed to be the result of some type of injury or insult to the liver. The hepatocellular injury (with or without inflammation) activates fibroblasts that respond by synthesizing collagen, thus forming fibrous connective tissue. The balance among fibrogenesis, the mechanisms for fibrous tissue removal, and hepatocyte regeneration appear to determine the degree of permanent hepatic fibrosis.

Once mature fibrous tissue is formed, a vicious cycle ensues. Vascular pathways form within the fibrotic tissues, depriving hepatocytes of their blood supply. The consequent cellular hypoxia, inflammation, and necrosis stimulate further fibroblastic activity. As a result normal hepatic architecture is sufficiently distorted to affect both hepatocellular function and hepatic blood circulation.

The consequences of liver malfunction are evident in the various processes that depend on the products of liver function. For example, diminished formation of blood proteins results in hypoproteinemia and impaired coagulation, inability to conjugate bilirubin produces jaundice, reduced bile causes malabsorption of fats, and depressed detoxification and destruction result in accumulation of toxic substances. Interference with liver circulation causes hypertension in the portal circulation. This together with the decreased protein in the blood leads to fluid accumulation in the abdomen (ascites).

Clinical Manifestations

Clinical manifestations depend on the etiology. In cirrhosis from congenital biliary atresia, jaundice is usually the first sign. In cirrhosis from other causes, the symptoms are usually vague and the onset insidious.

The three major complications of chronic liver disease are (1) bleeding from esophageal varices, (2) ascites, and (3) hepatic encephalopathy (hepatic coma). Not infrequently the first evidence of severe liver decompensation is failure to thrive, ascites, or bleeding esophageal varices.

Diagnostic Evaluation

Diagnosis rests on (1) the history, especially evidence of prior liver disease, such as hepatitis, (2) physical examination, particularly hepatosplenomegaly, and the cutaneous changes from hemodynamic alterations and increasing hormone levels, and (3) laboratory evaluation, especially liver function tests (Table 33-5), such as serum bilirubin level, serum enzyme assays (glutamic oxaloacetic transaminase [SGOT], serum glutamic pyruvic transaminase [SGPT], and lactic dehydrogenase [LDH]), serum protein level, and blood ammonia level. Definitive diagnosis rests on a liver biopsy for evidence of histologic changes.

Therapeutic Management

There is no specific treatment for cirrhosis, except in those cases in which a treatable cause, such as an infection, exists. Therapy is directed primarily toward (1) frequent assessment of liver status with physical examination and liver function tests and (2) management of pathologic changes based on these findings. Liver transplant is becoming a more viable option for some children, although children with progressive disease, such as cystic fibrosis, are unlikely candidates. Most of the liver transplant recipients are children with extrahepatic biliary atresia and biliary hypoplasia and those with metabolic disorders, such as glycogen storage disease (Gartner and others, 1984).

For cirrhosis uncomplicated by ascites or encephalopathy

Table 33–5 Liver function tests

TEST	NORMAL FUNCTION OF LIVER	ABNORMAL FINDING AND SIGNIFICANCE
Blood		
Serum bilirubin level	Conversion of indirect (unconjugated) bilirubin to direct (conjugated) bilirubin for excretion in bile	Increased indirect bilirubin level denotes damage to hepatic cells Increased direct bilirubin level denotes some blockage of bile duct
Thymol turbidity or cephalin flocculation	Globulins produced by liver	Abnormal globulins produced, especially in acute liver disease
Bromsulphalein (BSP) excretion	Filtration and excretion	Removal of this dye is similar to mechanisms used in excreting bilirubin; therefore excess dye in bloodstream can indicate problems in hepatic blood flow, liver cells, or bile ducts
Blood ammonia level	Detoxification of ammonia to urea	Increased level reflects poorly functioning hepatic cells and impaired hepatic blood flow
Prothrombin time	Prothrombin manufactured by liver	Prothrombin time increased but usually only reflected in severe liver disease
Serum protein levels	Albumin manufactured chiefly by liver; globulins manufactured by liver, spleen, lymphatics, and bone marrow	Albumin usually decreased, whereas globulins increased
Alkaline phosphatase level	Enzyme produced by liver and excreted with bile	Increased level reflects *acute* liver cell disease or bile duct obstruction.
Serum glutamic oxaloacetic transaminase (SGOT) level, serum glutamic pyruvic transaminase (SGPT) level, and lactic dehydrogenase (LDH) level	Metabolic enzymes produced by liver	All elevated in *acute* liver destructions as the damaged cells release their enzymes SGOT—found also in heart tissue SGPT—found mostly in liver but a less sensitive indicator than SGOT LDH—found in several organ tissues, therefore not specific for liver disease
Urine		
Urine bilirubin level	Normally bilirubin excreted in bile, broken down to urobilinogen in stool, and therefore not excreted in urine	Present in urine, produces deep yellow to brown color Reflects direct bilirubin level because only this form is water soluble
Urine urobilinogen level	Normally contains only small amounts from filtration of blood	Increased
Stool		
Stool sample	Urobilinogen oxidized to pigment urobilin (stercobilin), which gives stool its characteristic color	If bile is not being produced or if its flow is obstructed, stool will be white or clay-colored from lack of bile pigments

the diet is one that provides sufficient calories and essential nutrients to maintain growth and prevent specific deficiencies. A high-calorie diet with low or moderate fats, moderate high-quality protein, and high carbohydrates is recommended. In addition, supplements of water-soluble preparations of vitamins A, D, E, and K are given. In children with vitamin B_{12} deficiency, injectable supplements are necessary.

The child and his parents are advised against strenuous physical exercise and cautioned regarding the role of trauma, infection, and hepatotoxic drugs as factors that can aggravate his condition.

Complications. The complications of cirrhosis require special treatment:

Hemorrhage from esophageal varices is managed, as in adults, with blood transfusions, fluid and electrolyte replacement, administration of vitamin B complex and vitamin K, and, in life-threatening bleeding, with a Sengstaken-Blakemore balloon tube and oxygen.

Ascites is managed with diuretics and restriction of dietary sodium, limitation of protein, and sometimes intravenous administration of albumin. Fluid restriction may be necessary but drainage by paracentesis is rarely needed unless abdominal pain or respiratory distress is present.

Hepatic encephalopathy is related to the harmful effects of ammonia; therefore much of the management is aimed at reducing ammonia formation. Treatment attempts to (1) reduce dietary protein, (2) inhibit the growth of organisms active in the formation of ammonia by administration of lactulose, (3) reduce the bacterial flora by administration of antibiotics, and (4) correct any other causes that might precipitate coma, such as infections or fluid and electrolyte imbalances.

Nursing Considerations

Nursing objectives in caring for the child with cirrhosis depend on several factors, including the precipitating cause of the cirrhosis, the severity of complications, and the prognosis. Overall the last factor has the greatest impact because the prognosis for life is poor. Since treatment of cirrhosis ideally is treatment of the cause, in many instances a fatal outcome is determined by the inability to surgically correct or reverse the underlying problem. Therefore nursing care of this child is the same as that for any ill child with a life-threatening illness (Chapter 23). Hospitalization is usually required when complications such as ascites, bleeding esophageal varices, or hepatic coma occur.

Prevention, however, is an important nursing responsibility in terms of those diseases that may ultimately lead to cirrhosis. For example, genetic counseling would reduce the number of children afflicted with many genetic-metabolic disorders, such as galactosemia, sickle cell disease, or cystic fibrosis. Proper prenatal care and immunization can lessen the possibility of neonatal hepatitis. Public health education regarding the dangers of hepatitis and in particular the usual modes of transmission of hepatitis B virus may eventually decrease the human reservoir.

CONCEPT SUMMARIES

- The essential functions of the gastrointestinal system are to process and absorb nutrients necessary to maintain metabolic processes and support growth and development, to perform excretory functions, to provide detoxification, and to maintain fluid and electrolyte balance, especially in infancy.

- Digestion is the catabolism of foodstuffs (water, vitamins, mineral salts, carbohydrates, proteins, and fats) from their original complex form to simple, assimilable nutrients.

- The small intestine is the principal absorbing site in the gastrointestinal system.

- Assessment of the gastrointestinal function may be performed through one of the following procedures: fecal examination, radiologic examination, direct visualization (fiberoptic endoscopy or sigmoidoscopy), and esophageal or anorectal manometry.

- Malabsorption syndromes are disorders associated with some degree of impaired digestion and/or absorption. They include digestive defects, absorptive defects, and anatomic defects.

- Celiac disease, the second leading cause of malabsorption in children, is characterized by an intolerance for gluten. It is thought to be either an inborn error of metabolism or an immunologic response.

- The major role of the nurse in the management of celiac disease is helping parents and child adhere to diet therapy and preventing infections.

- General signs of obstruction include colicky abdominal pain, nausea and vomiting, abdominal distention, and constipation.

- Intussusception is one of the most common causes of intestinal obstruction during infancy. Treatment is either nonsurgical hydrostatic reduction by barium enema or surgical reduction.

- Surgical correction in Hirschsprung disease is a three-stage approach: a temporary colostomy, reanastomosis at 8 months to 1 year of age, and closure of the colostomy three months later.

- Nursing care of gastrointestinal reflux is aimed at identifying children with suggestive symptoms, helping parents with home care feeding and positioning, and caring for the child undergoing surgical intervention.

- Although the cause of appendicitis is poorly understood, it is commonly a result of obstruction of the lumen, usually by a fecalith. Common signs and symptoms are colicky abdominal pain, tenderness, and fever.

- Postoperative care of the child with appendicitis is aimed at maintaining IV fluids, proper positioning, and psychologic support.

- Meckel diverticulum, the most common congenital malformation of the GI tract, is characterized by extreme rectal bleeding.

- Inflammatory bowel disease refers to ulcerative colitis and Crohn disease. Persistent and recurring diarrhea is the most common feature of ulcerative colitis, usually associated with fever, weight loss, anorexia, and nausea and vomiting. It follows one of two patterns: acute remitting type or chronic continuous course. It is treated by dietary management and medication.

- Management of Crohn disease includes nutritional management with high protein diet, vitamin/mineral supplements, sufasalazine and/or corticosteroids, antibiotics, and general supportive therapy.

- Peptic ulcers are poorly understood, but one of two mechanisms probably reflects the basic defect: an increase in the rate of production of gastric juice, or interference with the normal protective mechanisms of the mucosal lining.

- Viral hepatitis is caused by at least four types of virus—hepatitis A virus, hepatitis B virus, hepatitis D virus, and non-A, non-B virus.

- Hepatitis A virus is spread by the fecal-oral route, whereas hepatitis B virus is transmitted primarily by the parenteral route. The single most effective measure in prevention and control of hepatitis in any setting is handwashing.

REFERENCES

Abrahamian, F.P., and Lloyd-Still, J.D.: Chronic constipation in childhood: longitudinal study of 186 patients, J. Pediatr. Gastroenterol. Nutr. 3:460-467, 1984.

Barker, D.J.P., Morris, J., and Nelson, M.: Vegetable consumption and acute appendicitis in 59 areas in England and Wales, Br. Med. J. 292(6525):927-930, 1986.

Berry, J., Jr., and Malt, R.A.: Appendicitis near its centenary, Ann. Surg. 200:567-575, 1984.

Boyd, C.W.: A bed for infants with gastroesophageal reflux, Pediatr. Nurs. 7(5):53-55, 1981.

Brender, J.D., and others: Childhood appendicitis: factors associated with perforation, Pediatrics 76(2):301-306, 1985a.

Brender, J.D., and others: Fiber intake and childhood appendicitis, Am. J. Public Health **75**(4):399-400, 1985b.

Brender, J.D., and others: Is childhood appendicitis familial? Am. J. Dis. Child. **139**(4):338-340, 1985c.

Burgin-Wolff, A., and others: A reliable screening test for childhood celiac disease: fluorescent immunosorbent test for gliadin antibodies, J. Pediatr. **102**(5):655-660, 1983.

Cassell, B.L.: The new trend in ileostomy surgery, RN **47** (1):48-51, 1984.

Corazziari, E., and others: Gastrointestinal transit time, frequency of defecation, and anorectal manometry in healthy and constipated children, J. Pediatr. **106**(3):379-382, 1985.

Dossetor, J.F.B., Gibson, A.A.M., and McNeish, A.S.: Childhood coeliac disease is disappearing, Lancet **1**(8215):322-323, 1981.

Fonkalsrud, E.W.: Continence following colectomy for ulcerative colitis, Pediatr. Ann. **11**(11):921-925, 1982.

Gartner, J.C., and others: Orthotopic liver transplantation in children: two-year experience with 47 patients, Pediatrics **74**(1):140-145, 1984.

Hamm, P., and Jemison-Smith, P.: Viral hepatitis, Crit. Care Update **10**(2):37-44, 1983.

Harnsberger, J.K., and others: Long-term follow-up of surgery for gastroesophageal reflux in infants and children, J. Pediatr. **102**(4):505-508, 1983.

Hartwig, M.S.: Sticking to a gluten-free diet, Am. J. Nurs. **83**(9):1308-1310, 1983.

Hassall, E., Barclay, G.N., and Ament, M.E.: Colonoscopy in childhood, Pediatrics **73**(5):594-599, 1984.

Herbst, J.J.: Diagnosis and treatment of gastroesophageal reflux in children, Pediatr. Rev. **5**(3):75-79, 1983.

Johns, C.: Encopresis, Am. J. Nurs. **85**(2):153-156, 1985.

Jordan, F.T., Coran, A.G., and Wesley, J.R.: Modified endorectal procedure for management of long-segment aganglionosis, Ann. Surg. **194**(1):70-75, 1981.

Klish, W.J., and Putnam, T.C.: The short gut, Am. J. Dis. Child. **135**:1056-1061, 1981.

Krugman, S.: Viral hepatitis: 1985 update, Pediatr. Rev. **7**(1):3-11, 1985.

Krugman, S., and others: Infectious diseases of children, ed. 8, St. Louis, 1985, The C.V. Mosby Co.

Litovitz, T.L.: Battery ingestions: product accessibility and clinical course, Pediatrics **75**(3):469-476, 1985.

Littlewood, J.M., and Crollick, A.J.: Childhood coeliac disease is disappearing, Lancet **2**(8208):1359-1360, 1980.

Maki, M., and others: Evaluation of a serum IgA-class reticulin antibody test for the detection of childhood celiac disease, J. Pediatr. **105**(6):901-905, 1984.

Martin, L.W., and Torres, A.M.: Hirschsprung's disease, Surg. Clin. North Am. **65**(5):1171-1180, 1985.

Marwick, C., and Simmons, K.: Changing childhood disease pattern linked with day-care boom, JAMA **251**:1245-1251, 1984.

Mathewson, M., and Farnham, C.: Milk therapy in ulcer disease: yes or no? Home Healthcare Nurse **2**(4):8, 1984.

Motil, K.J., and Grand, R.J.: Nutritional management of inflammatory bowel disease, Pediatr. Clin. North Am. **32** (2):447-469, 1985.

Olness, K.: Constipation and soiling, Pediatr. Basics **38**:4-7, 1984.

O'Regan, S., and others: Constipation: a commonly unrecognized cause of enuresis, Am. J. Dis. Child. **140**(3):260-261, 1986.

Orenstein, S.R., and Whitington, P.F.: Positioning for prevention of infant gastroesophageal reflux, J. Pediatr. **103**(4):534-537, 1983.

Polley, T.Z., Jr., Coran, A.G., and Wesley, J.R.: A ten-year experience with ninety-two cases of Hirschsprung's disease, Ann. Surg. **202**(3):349-354, 1985.

Purdy, B.H., Philips, D.M., and Summers, R.W.: Desensitization for sulfasalazine skin rash, Ann. Intern. Med. **100**(4):512-514, 1984.

Savilahti, E., and others: Celiac disease in insulin-dependent diabetes mellitus, J. Pediatr. **108**(1):690-693, 1986.

Scott, R.B., O'Loughlin, E.V., and Gall, D.G.: Gastroesophageal reflux in patients with cystic fibrosis, J. Pediatr. **106** (2):223-227, 1985.

Shah, P.C., and Lebenthal, E.: Gluten sensitive enteropathy (GSE): a practical approach, Pediatr. Basics **34**:4-8, 1983.

Sibinga, M.S.: The gastrointestinal tract. In Levine, M.D., and others, editors: Developmental-behavioral pediatrics, Philadelphia, 1983, W.B. Saunders Co.

Silverman, A., and Roy, C.C.: Pediatric clinical gastroenterology, ed. 3, St. Louis, 1983, The C.V. Mosby Co.

Simila, S., and others: Childhood coeliac disease, Lancet **1**(8218):494-495, 1981.

Singleton, J.W.: Current therapy of inflammatory bowel diseases, Drug Ther. **12**(2):89-96, 1982.

Taffet, S.L., and Das, K.M.: Desensitization of patients with inflammatory bowel disease to sulfasalazine, Am. J. Med. **73**:520-524, 1982.

Tilkian, S.M., Conover, M.B., and Tilkian, A.G.: Clinical implications of laboratory tests, ed. 3, St. Louis, 1983, The C.V. Mosby Co.

Webb, W.A., McDaniel, L., and Jones, L.: Foreign bodies of the upper gastrointestinal tract: current management, South. Med. J. **77**:1083-1086, 1984.

BIBLIOGRAPHY
Malabsorption Syndromes

Cacciari, E., and others: Can antigliadin antibody detect symptomless celiac disease in children with short stature? Lancet **1**(8444):1469-1471, 1985.

Congdon, P., and others: Small-bowel mucosa in asymptomatic children with celiac disease, Am. J. Dis. Child. **135**:118-121, 1981.

Gantt, L., and Thompson, C.: Short gut syndrome in the infant, Am. J. Nurs. **85**(11):1263-1266, 1985.

Lamb, C.: Simplifying diagnosis of malabsorption, Patient Care **15**(17):128-178, 1981.

Robinson, L.A.: Nontropical sprue (gluten intolerance and vitamins), Pediatr. Nurs. **7**(5):61, 1981.

Weizman, Z., Stringer, D.A., and Durie, P.R.: Radiologic manifestations of malabsorption: a nonspecific finding, Pediatrics **74**(4):530-533, 1984.

Obstructive Disorders/Disorders of Motility

Alterescu, K.B.: The ostomy: what about special procedures? Am. J. Nurs. **85**(12):1363-1367, 1985.

American Academy of Pediatrics, Committee on Infectious Diseases, Committee on Drugs, and Section on Surgery: Antimicrobial prophylaxis in pediatric surgical patients, Pediatrics **74**(3):437-439, 1984.

Andrassy, R.J., Isaacs, H., and Weitzman, J.J.: Rectal suction biopsy for the diagnosis of Hirschsprung's disease, Ann. Surg. **193**(4):419-424, 1981.

Berquist, W.E.: Gastroesophageal reflux in children: a clinical review, Pediatr. Ann. **11**(1):135-142, 1982.

Binder, H.J.: Rational use of laxatives, Drug Ther. **11** (11):83-88, 1981.

Boarini, J.: The ostomy: what can go wrong? Am. J. Nurs. **85**(12):1358-1362, 1985.

Boyd, C.W.: Postural therapy at home for infants with gastroesophageal reflux, Pediatr. Nurs. **8**(6):395-398, 1982.

Cargile, N.D.: Buying time when you face a bowel obstruction, RN **48**(8):40-46, 1985.

Crummette, B.D., Mills, H.H., and Beale, A.V.: One latency-age child's coping with hospitalization, Am. J. Maternal Child Nurs. **13**(3):167-175, 1984.

Doering, K.J., and LaMountain, P.: Flowcharts to facilitate caring for ostomy patients: 2. Immediate postop care, Nursing 84 **14**(10):47-49, 1984.

Doering, K.J., and LaMountain, P.: Flowcharts to facilitate caring for ostomy patients: 4. Discharge outcome assessment, Nursing 84 **14**(12):47-49, 1984.

Grill, B.B., and others: Effects of domperidone therapy on symptoms and upper gastrointestinal motility in infants with gastroesophageal reflux, J. Pediatr. **106**(2):311-316, 1985.

Herbst, J.J.: Gastroesophageal reflux, J. Pediatr. **98**(6):859-870, 1981.

Hoffman, M.J., Kodner, I.J., and Fry, R.D.: Internal intussusception of the rectum: diagnosis and surgical management, Dis. Colon Rectum **27**(7):435-441, 1984.

Kurer, M., Lowson, J., and Pambakian, H.: Techniques for diagnosing suction biopsy of Hirschsprung's disease, Arch. Dis. Child. **61**(1):83-84, 1986.

Lynn, M.R.: Use of infant seats for gastroesophageal reflux, J. Pediatr. Nurs. **1**(2):127-129, 1986.

Okamoto, E., and Ohashi, S.: Simple modification of Duhamel's operation for the treatment of Hirschsprung's disease, Am. J. Surg. **142**:302-304, 1981.

Puri, P., and Guiney, E.J.: Small bowel tumours causing intussusception in childhood, Br. J. Surg. **72**(6):493-494, 1985.

Rosenberg, A.J., and Vela, A.R.: A new simplified technique for pediatric anorectal manometry, Pediatrics **71**(2):240-245, 1983.

Sasso, S.C.: Metoclopramide and chalasia, Am. J. Maternal Child Nurs. **8**(5):361, 1983.

Scallen, C., Puri, P., and Reen, D.: Identification of rectal ganglion cells using monoclonal antibodies, J. Pediatr. Surg. **20**(1):37-40, 1985.

Sugar, E.C.: Hirschsprung's disease, Am. J. Nurs. **81**(11):2065-2067, 1981.

Weissbluth, M.: Gastroesophageal reflux, Clin. Pediatr. **20**(1):7-14, 1981.

Werlin, W.L., and others: Mechanisms of gastroesophageal reflux, J. Pediatr. **97**(2):244-249, 1980.

Inflammatory Conditions

Adkins, R.B., Jr., and others: The management of gastric ulcers: a current review, Ann. Surg. **201**(6):741-750, 1985.

Blumer, J.L., and others: Pharmacokinetic determination of ranitidine pharmacodynamics in pediatric ulcer disease, J. Pediatr. **107**(2):301-306, 1985.

Buchmann, P., and others: The prognosis of ileorectal anastomosis in Crohn's disease, Br. J. Surg. **68**:7-10, 1981.

Catching an early appendicitis early, Emerg. Med. **13**(15):49-52, 1981.

Chong, S.K.F., and others: Endocrine dysfunction in children with Crohn's disease, J. Pediatr. Gastroenterol. Nutr. **3**:529-534, 1984.

Dickson, A.P., and MacKinlay, G.A.: Rectal examination and acute appendicitis, Arch. Dis. Child. **60**(7):666-676, 1985.

Euler, A.R.: Youngsters with ulcers, Emerg. Med. **13**(17):100-101, 1981.

Gryboski, J.D.: Crohn's disease in children, Pediatr. Rev. **2**(8):239-244, 1981.

Hagenah, G.C., Harrigan, J.F., and Campbell, M.: Inflammatory bowel disease in children, Nurs. Clin. North Am. **19**(1):27-39, 1984.

Harrison, M.W., and others: Acute appendicitis in children: factors affecting morbidity, Am. J. Surg. **147**:605-609, 1984.

Kroner, K.: Are you prepared for your ulcerative colitis patient? Nursing 80 **10**(4):43-49, 1980.

Labson, L.H.: Which drug for which peptic ulcer? Patient Care **15**(16):49-90, 1981.

Lessman, M.: Painful chronicle, Am. J. Nurs. **85**(5):551-552, 1985.

Lewicki, L.J., and Leeson, M.J.: The multisystem impact on physiologic processes of inflammatory bowel disease, Nurs. Clin. North Am. **19**(1):71-80, 1984.

Meyers, S., and others: Fecal alpha-1-antitrypsin measurement: an indicator of Crohn's disease activity, Gastroenterology **89**(1):13-18, 1985.

Motil, K.J., Altchuler, S.I., and Grand, R.J.: Mineral balance during nutritional supplementation in adolescents with Crohn disease and growth failure, J. Pediatr. **107**(3):473-479, 1985.

Myers, S.A.: Crohn's disease, Crit. Care Update **7**(1):12-23, 1980.

Nord, K.S., Rossi, T.M., and Lebenthal, E.: Peptic ulcer in children, Am. J. Gastroenterol. **75**(2):153-157, 1981.

Nursing grand rounds: supporting the patient with Crohn's disease, Nursing 83 **13**(11):46-51, 1983.

Postuma, R., and Moroz, S.P.: Pediatric Crohn's disease, J. Pediatr. Surg. **20**(5):478-482, 1985.

Prior, P., and others: Mortality in Crohn's disease, Gastroenterology **80**:307-312, 1981.

Rosenthal, S.R., and others: Growth failure and inflammatory bowel disease: approach to treatment of a complicated adolescent problem, Pediatrics **72**(4):481-490, 1983.

Simmons, M.A.: Using the nursing process in treating inflammatory bowel disease, Nurs. Clin. North Am. **19**(1):11-25, 1984.

Sparacino, L.L.: Psychosocial considerations for the adolescent and young adult with inflammatory bowel disease, Nurs. Clin. North Am. **19**(1):41-49, 1984.

Stotts, N.A., Fitzgerald, K.A., and Williams, K.R.: Care of the patient critically ill with inflammatory bowel disease, Nurs. Clin. North Am. **19**(1):61-70, 1984.

Wilson, C.: The diagnostic work-up for the patient with inflammatory bowel disease, Nurs. Clin. North Am. **19**(1):51-59, 1984.

Hepatic Disorders

Brainerd, E.: Nursing management of chronic infectious diseases in children, Pediatrics Nurs. Update **1**(17):2-7, 1986.

Chin, J.: Prevention of chronic hepatitis B virus infection from mothers to infants in the United States, Pediatrics **71**(2):289-292, 1983.

Fredette, S.L.: When the liver fails, Am. J. Nurs. **84**(1):64-67, 1984.

Genesca, J., Esteban, J.I., and Esteban, R.: Hepatitis B immunoprophylaxis of low-birth-weight infants, Pediatrics **76**(6):1020, 1985.

Guenter, P.: Hepatic disease: nutritional implications, Nurs. Clin. North Am. **18**:71-80, 1983.

Gurevich, I.: Hepatitis in critical care: area of concern, Crit. Care Update **10**(4):14-17, 1983.

Gurevich, I.: Viral hepatitis, Am. J. Nurs. **83**:572-586, 1983.

Keith, J.S.: Hepatic failure: etiologies, manifestations, and management, Crit. Care Nurse **5**(1):60-86, 1985.

Kirkman-Liff, B., and Dandoy, S.: Hepatitis B: what price exposure? Am. J. Nurs. **84**(4):988-990, 1984.

Recommendation of the Immunization Practices Advisory Committee (ACIP): Immune globulins for protection against viral hepatitis, Morbid. Mortal. Weekly Rep. **30**(34):423-435, 1981.

Recommendation of the Immunization Practices Advisory Committee (ACIP): Inactivated hepatitis B virus vaccine, Morbid. Mortal. Weekly Rep. **31**(24):317-328, 1982.

Wimpsett, J.: Trace your patient's liver dysfunction, Nursing 84 **14**(8):56-57, 1984.

Xu, Z., and others: Prevention of perinatal acquisition of hepatitis B virus carriage using vaccine: preliminary report of a randomized, double-blind placebo-controlled and comparative trial, Pediatrics **76**(5):713-718, 1985.

Unit Twelve

The Child with Problems Related to Production and Circulation of Blood

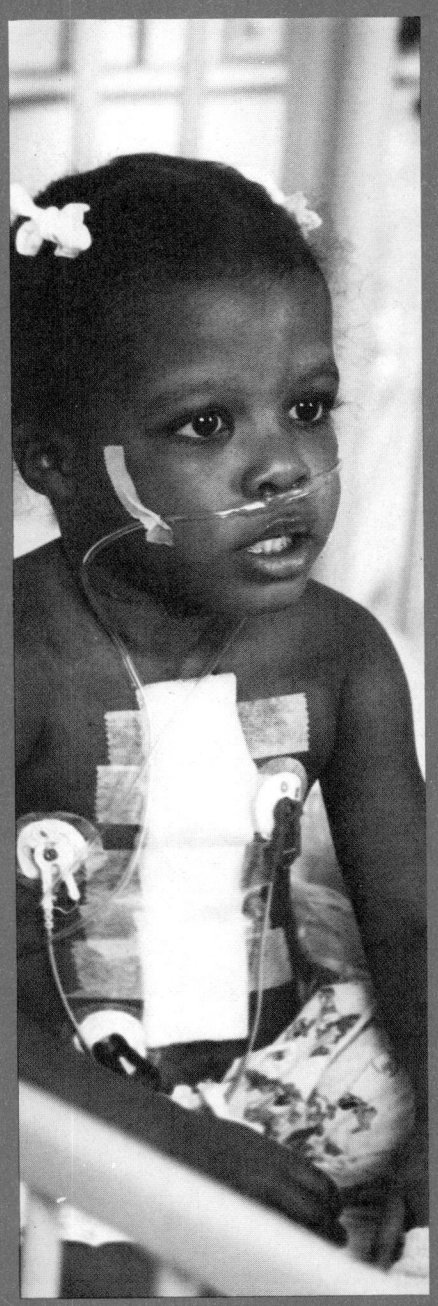

Some of the most common and serious childhood conditions are related to the heart and formed elements of the blood. Many of these disorders, especially those of the blood, are inherited and present at birth, whereas others are acquired. Most of them necessitate medical and/or surgical intervention to prevent complications, some of which can be life threatening. Nursing care at the time of diagnosis, before and during corrective/palliative procedures, and after treatment is essential to promote physical and emotional recovery.

Chapter 34, *The Child with Cardiovascular Dysfunction*, discusses the types of congenital and acquired cardiac disorders and the physical consequences of impaired functioning. It focuses on caring for the child with heart disease, preparation of the family for diagnostic procedures and surgery, and postoperative nursing interventions, including discharge planning to help the child and parents adjust to improved physical status. Chapter 35, *The Child with Hematologic Dysfunction*, deals with several disorders related to the formed elements of the blood. Since many of these conditions are inherited and chronic, nursing interventions stress helping the family adjust to the disorder and cope with and prevent its complications.

Chapter 34

The Child with Cardiovascular Dysfunction

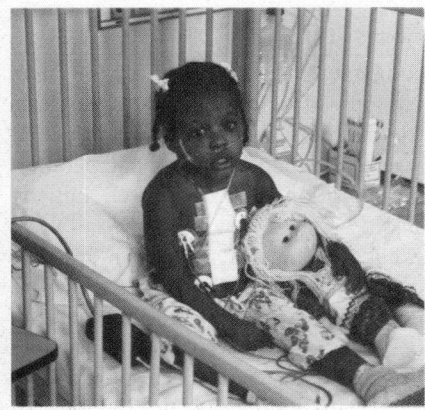

Disorders involving the heart and blood vessels include those that are present at birth and those that are acquired as the result of some disease process that directly or indirectly affects cardiovascular function. Some conditions are asymptomatic and detected only on examination. Many conditions place minimal limitations on a child's activities, while others are serious enough to impose severe restrictions. A few are incompatible with life.

The most common form of cardiac disease in children is congenital heart disease, predominantly structural defects that result from developmental arrest or deviation. Congestive heart failure is a serious consequence of congenital or acquired heart disease, and it is also a complication of other diseases, including chronic lung disease, muscular dystrophy, advanced kidney disease, and a variety of acute disorders and infections that place undue demands on the heart. Other disorders that occur less frequently include rhythm disturbances, rheumatic fever, and Kawasaki disease. Although hypertension is seen primarily in adults, it is of concern in children in terms of preventing the long-term consequences associated with high blood pressure.

Any disorder that affects the heart provokes anxiety in the family. In many instances this anxiety is not unfounded, but in some cases it is greater than called for by the seriousness of the condition. To help the child and family adjust to a heart condition and to be prepared for the medical and/or surgical management require guidance and support from many health professionals, particularly nurses.

Cardiac Structure and Function

Understanding the effects of congenital and acquired heart defects requires knowledge of the normal heart's structure and function, including embryologic development, fetal circulation, and the changes that occur with postnatal growth. In addition to the following general overview, the specific embryologic changes resulting in each major heart defect are discussed later in the chapter.

CARDIAC DEVELOPMENT

The heart is a muscular four-chambered organ whose primary purpose is to pump blood throughout the body. It is located slightly to the left of the sternum in the space between the two pleural cavities, called the *mediastinum.* The main mass of the heart is formed by the muscular tissue, the *myocardium.* Lining the inner surface of the myocardium is the *endocardium,* a thin layer of endothelial tissue. The heart also has its own special covering, a double-walled membrane called the *pericardium.* The outer membrane is the *fibrous pericardium.* The inner membrane, the *serous pericardium,* also consists of two layers, the *parietal* layer, which lines the inside of the fibrous pericardium, and the *visceral* layer *(epicardium),* which lines the heart muscle. Between these two layers is a slight space *(pericardial space),* which is filled with a few drops of serous fluid *(pericardial fluid).* These layers provide for frictionless movement of the heart muscle.

The interior of the heart is divided into four chambers. The two upper chambers are called *atria* and include a right atrium (RA) and a left atrium (LA). The two bottom chambers are *ventricles,* a right ventricle (RV) and a left ventricle (LV). The chambers are separated by walls called the atrial septum and ventricular septum. Located within the heart chambers are four *valves,* whose main function is to prevent the backflow of blood. The valves are attached to the heart muscle by several cordlike structures called *chordae tendineae.* The *tricuspid* valve, so named because it has three flaps or cusps of endocardial tissue projecting into the ventricles, is located between the right atrium and ventricle. The *bicuspid,* or *mitral,* valve has two flaps and is located between the left atrium and ventricle. Together these two valves are often termed *atrioventricular* valves. The *semilunar* valves are located in the pulmonary artery (pulmonic valve) and the aorta (aortic valve). Heart sounds (S_1 and S_2) are thought to be related to the vibrations that result during closing of these valves (see Chapter 7).

Embryologic Development

The heart and other components of the circulatory system (blood, blood vessels, lymph) develop from the mesoderm beginning during the fourth week of gestation and are completed by the eighth week. Cardiac development parallels the embryo's increasing nutritional needs, which initially were supplied by diffusion.

During the first 3 weeks the lateral mesoderm splits to form two layers, the somatic and the splanchnic mesoderm. The somatic mesoderm eventually gives rise to limb muscle, while the splanchnic mesoderm forms two endocardial tubes that fuse to become the *heart tube.* As the tube elongates it begins to coil to the right. This looping occurs by approximately the twenty-eighth day when the heart begins to beat. The mesodermal tissue surrounding the heart tube differentiates into two layers: the *endocardium* and *myoepicardium.* Concentrations of mesenchymal cells enlarge and cause the endocardium to bulge into the lumen of the heart. These internal bulges are called *endocardial cushions* and eventually merge to divide the heart chambers.

The developing heart tube bulges until it finally lies in the pericardial cavity. The tube remains attached to the pericardium at its cephalic and caudal ends but is free at the midsection. During the fifth week the midcardiac tube grows rapidly and assumes a characteristic convoluted shape with identifiable structures. These structures ultimately give rise to the chambers and vessels of the heart and include (1) a *common atrium,* (2) a *common ventricle,* (3) the *bulbus cordis,* which eventually helps form the outflow tracts of the ventricles, (4) the *sinus venosus,* which develops into the inferior and superior vena cava and coronary sinus, and (5) the *truncus arteriosus,* which divides into the pulmonary artery and aorta.

The formation of the internal structures of the heart, particularly the cardiac septa, takes place almost simultaneously. During this partitioning process, congenital defects may result if the formation of various structures is disturbed; the various pathologic changes are discussed later in this chapter for each major defect. The structure of the fetal heart provides for a pattern of circulation that is markedly different from that required during postnatal life. During prenatal life it distributes oxygen and nutrients, supplied via the placenta, to the developing fetus through an efficient

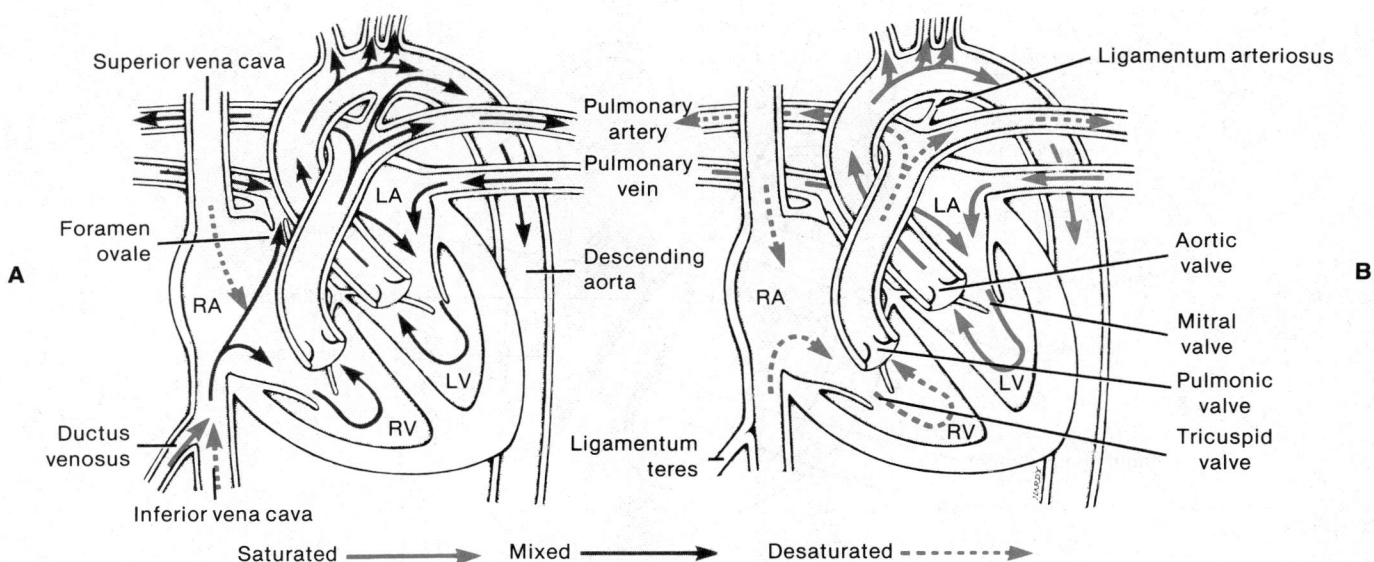

Fig. 34-1. Changes in circulation at birth. **A,** Prenatal circulation. **B,** Postnatal circulation. Arrows indicate direction of blood flow. *RA,* Right atrium. *LA,* Left atrium. *RV,* Right ventricle, *LV,* Left ventricle. Although four pulmonary veins enter the left atrium, for simplicity this diagram shows only two.

system of shunts that partially bypass the nonfunctioning lungs.

Fetal circulation. The normal growth and development of the fetus rely on an active, independent metabolism, but they also require an efficient circulation. During fetal life the lungs are essentially nonfunctional and the liver only partially functional; therefore less blood is needed in these organs than is required after birth. The fetal brain requires the highest oxygen concentration, and the heart must pump a large amount of blood through the placenta. The characteristics of fetal circulation ensure that the most vital organs and tissues receive the maximum concentration of vital materials for growth.

Blood carrying oxygen and nutritive materials from the placenta enters the fetal system through the umbilicus via the large umbilical vein (Fig. 34-1, *A*). The blood then travels upward to the underside of the liver where it separates—part of the blood enters the portal and hepatic circulation of the liver and the remainder travels directly to the inferior vena cava by way of the *ductus venosus.* Because of the higher pressure of blood entering the right atrium from the inferior vena cava, it is directed posteriorly in a straight pathway across the right atrium and through the *foramen ovale* to the left atrium. In this way the better-oxygenated blood enters the left atrium and ventricle to be pumped through the aorta to the head and upper extremities. Blood from the head and upper extremities entering the right atrium from the superior vena cava is directed downward through the tricuspid valve into the right ventricle. From here it is pumped through the pulmonary artery, where the major portion is shunted to the descending aorta via the *ductus arteriosus.* A small amount flows to and from the non-

functioning fetal lungs. Blood is returned to the placenta from the descending aorta through the two umbilical arteries.

Before birth the high pulmonary vascular resistance created by the collapsed fetal lung causes greater pressures in the right side of the heart and the pulmonary arteries. At the same time the free-flowing placental circulation and the ductus arteriosus produce a low systemic vascular resistance in the remainder of the fetal vascular system. With the clamping of the umbilical cord and the expansion of the lungs at birth, the hemodynamics of the fetal vascular system undergo pronounced and abrupt changes. These changes are the direct result of cessation of the placental blood flow and the beginning of lung respiration. The changes occurring at birth are discussed on p. 294 and the circulatory changes in the heart are shown in Fig. 34-1, *B*.

Postnatal Development

In infancy the size of the heart in relation to total body size is larger, and it occupies a larger space within the lung enclosure. It lies at a transverse angle, but with growth and the enlarging lungs it comes to lie lower and more obliquely at maturity (see Fig. 7-42). The ventricle walls are more or less equal in thickness at birth (some believe that the right ventricle may be somewhat larger). With the increased demand of the postnatal peripheral circulation, the left side becomes thicker than the right. During the first years the weight of the heart is doubled; by 5 years, it is increased fourfold, and by 9 years, sixfold (Lowrey, 1986). An increase in heart size accompanies the adolescent growth spurt with a resulting increase in blood pressure and decrease in heart rate. The heart rate at any age shows an inverse relationship to body size (see inside front cover).

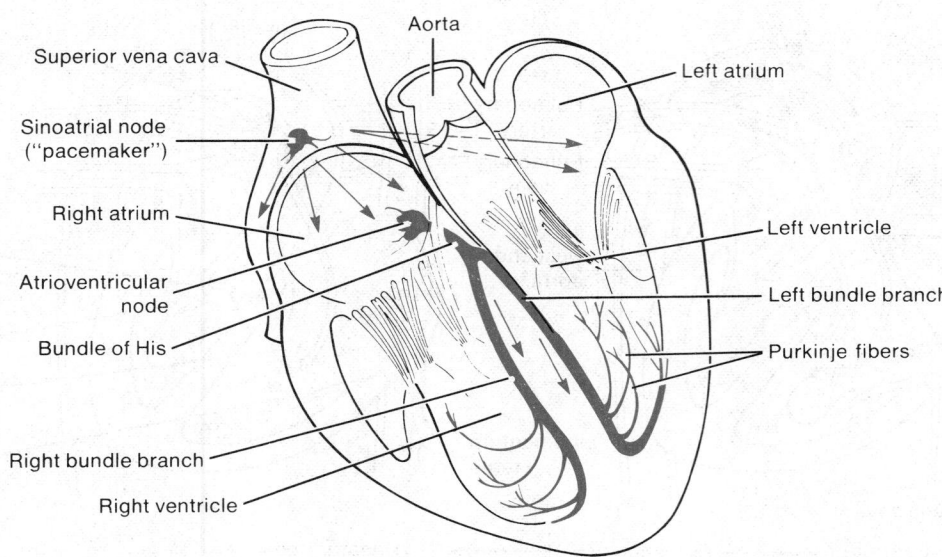

Fig. 34-2. Conduction system of heart.

The arteries and veins elongate to keep pace with expanding body dimensions, and the vessel walls thicken to cope with the increased pressure. The systolic blood pressure after birth is low, reflecting the weaker left ventricle of the neonate. With the developing strength and power of the left side of the heart, the systolic pressure rises rather sharply during the first 6 weeks and continues to rise but at a much slower rate until shortly before puberty, at which point it rises rapidly to adult levels (see inside front cover).

Postnatal circulation. Once the cardiorespiratory system adjusts to the changes necessary to support extrauterine life, the circulation through the heart assumes a pathway that allows for oxygenation of venous blood by the lungs and delivery of saturated blood to the systemic circulation. Blood returning from the body via the superior vena cava (SVC) and inferior vena cava (IVC) is received in the RA. It is then pumped to the RV through the tricuspid valve. The LV pumps the blood through the pulmonic valve into the pulmonary artery where the blood becomes saturated with oxygen in the lungs. The blood is then returned from the lungs via the pulmonary veins into the LA, where it is pumped through the bicuspid valve to the LV, and finally through the aortic valve to the aorta into the systemic circulation (Fig. 34-1, *B*).

Arteries are blood vessels that carry blood away from the heart and serve primarily the function of distributing highly oxygenated blood to the capillaries. Veins are blood vessels that carry poorly oxygenated blood to the heart and function as both collectors and reservoirs. Their function as a reservoir helps maintain normal circulation. For example, if there is increased resistance to blood flow through the right side of the heart (e.g., as the result of severe pulmonary valvular stenosis), right ventricular end-diastolic and right atrial pressures may rise. As a result, central venous pressure rises and hepatomegaly may occur. The function of the

arterioles is mainly to provide resistance to blood flow to maintain blood pressure and circulation.

Although major blood vessels enter and leave the heart, the heart muscle receives its own coronary blood supply. The *right* and *left coronary arteries,* which arise above the aortic valve, supply all of the myocardium. *Coronary veins* collect the blood and return it directly to the right atrium or through a common venous channel called the *coronary sinus,* which drains into the right atrium.

Conduction system. To maintain an orderly and effective pumping action, the heart has a specialized electrical conduction system—electrical impulses generated within the heart initiate the mechanical contraction leading to circulation of blood. Although all myocardial cells are capable of developing an action potential and depolarizing without external stimulation, certain specialized cells exist that make up the heart's normal pacemaker. These structures include (Fig. 34-2) (Anthony and Thibodeau, 1983):

1. The *sinoatrial (SA) node,* located within the right atrial wall near the opening of the superior vena cava
2. The *atrioventricular (AV) node,* also located within the right atrium but near the lower end of the septum
3. The *atrioventricular bundle (bundle of His),* which extends from the atrioventricular node along each side of the interventricular septum and then divides into right and left bundle branches
4. *Purkinje fibers,* which extend from the atrioventricular bundle into the walls of the ventricles

The sinoatrial (SA) node initiates the heart's conduction system and normally is the heart's pacemaker. The impulse spreads from the SA node throughout the atria to cause depolarization. As the atria depolarize, impulses spread to the atrioventricular node to stimulate the ventricles. The atrioventricular node is the major pathway by which the impulses from the atria can be transmitted to the ventricles. The impulses then spread to the atrioventricular bundle and Purkinje fibers to cause simultaneous depolarization of the ventricles.

A *cardiac cycle* is composed of sequential contraction (systole) and relaxation (diastole) of both the atria and the ventricles. First, the atria contract, ejecting blood into the relaxed ventricles. Then, as the atria relax, the ventricles contract to eject blood into the pulmonary artery and aorta. During the period of atrial diastole blood enters the atria from the systemic and pulmonary veins, thus completing one cardiac cycle.

ASSESSMENT OF CARDIAC FUNCTION

Diagnosis of congenital or acquired heart disease is aided by a comprehensive history and physical examination. In addition several specialized diagnostic procedures are available to help confirm the diagnosis. The following discussion is an overview of the major techniques. Specific positive findings are included under the discussion of the heart defect.

History and Physical Assessment

A complete history is essential regardless of the type of heart condition. The major categories to investigate include a history of:

1. Poor weight gain, poor feeding habits, and fatigue during feeding
2. Frequent respiratory infections and difficulties (tachypnea, dyspnea, shortness of breath)
3. Cyanosis with or without clubbing of fingers
4. Evidence of exercise intolerance

In taking a history the nurse should elicit the concerns of the parents. Often they have vague, nonspecific complaints, such as "baby doesn't feed well" or "baby is too quiet," that offer clues to a less obvious cardiac defect. In addition, a history of previous defects in a sibling, maternal rubella infection during pregnancy, the use of medications or chemicals during pregnancy, and a chronic illness in the mother can be important clues to diagnosis. Children with chromosomal abnormalities, such as Turner or Down syndrome, are especially likely to have associated heart defects and the history is essential in evaluating their overall health. A history of a viral infection or toxic exposure is important if myocarditis is suspected, and a history of a previous streptococcal infection is of primary importance in rheumatic fever.

Several aspects of the physical examination may yield evidence of heart disease. (See Chapter 7 for a discussion of how to assess each of the following characteristics.) The most important is auscultation to:

1. Assess heart rate and rhythm, heart sounds, and adventitious sounds, such as friction rubs or murmurs
2. Determine physiologic splitting of the second heart sound
3. Locate sounds, including murmurs
4. Assess approximate anatomic size from the point of maximum impulse
5. Determine blood pressure

Palpation and percussion are used to:

1. Assess the quality and symmetry of all pulses
2. Locate the cardiac, hepatic, and splenic borders for evidence of organ enlargement
3. Determine thrills

Inspection of nutritional status, skin color (especially signs of cyanosis), respiratory rate and rhythm, posturing, chest deformities or asymmetry, distended veins, and abnormal cardiac pulsations may help substantiate evidence of a cardiac defect.

Murmurs. Although most murmurs are benign, they can also be an important sign of cardiac defects. Auscultation of murmurs is discussed on p. 267. The following discussion is an overview of the types of murmurs heard in heart defects.

The most common cause of murmurs is an abnormal shunting of blood between two heart chambers or between vessels. However, murmurs can also be produced by disturbing the flow of fluid through a vessel as a result of (1) increasing the rate of flow, (2) constricting or dilating the lumen, and (3) creating some type of irregularity on the vessel wall, such as an aneurysm, which vibrates as fluid flows past.

Murmurs are classified according to their timing within the cardiac cycle (Fig. 34-3):

systolic Between S_1 and S_2.
diastolic Between S_2 and S_1.
systolic ejection Begin after the S_1, attain a peak during mid-systole, and terminate before the S_2.
pansystolic or **holosystolic** During all of systole.
pandiastolic or **holodiastolic** During all of diastole.
prodiastolic Early diastolic.
presystolic Late diastolic.
continuous Continue through all of systole and all or part of diastole.

Murmurs caused by congenital defects involving the septum or great vessels are usually heard best near the sternal borders or over the base of the heart. Those of valvular origin are typically loudest over the respective auscultating valvular area, in the direction of blood flow. Murmurs that originate on the right side of the heart are subject to change during respiration as a result of intrathoracic pressure that prolongs right ventricular filling. Thus murmurs originating on the right side of the heart increase during inspiration.

Although the determination of the significance of murmurs is generally a medical decision, nurses should be aware of those murmurs that are most likely associated with cardiac defects. Pathologic murmurs generally include those that are diastolic, pansystolic, systolic, continuous, or very loud (Rosenthal, 1984).

TESTS OF CARDIAC FUNCTION

A variety of invasive and noninvasive tests may be employed in the diagnosis of heart disease. The more fre-

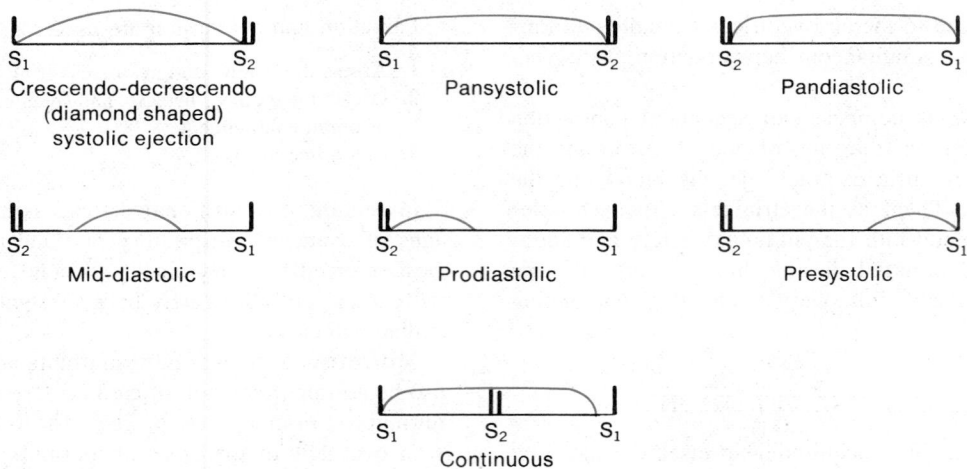

Fig. 34-3. Diagrammatic representation of murmurs.

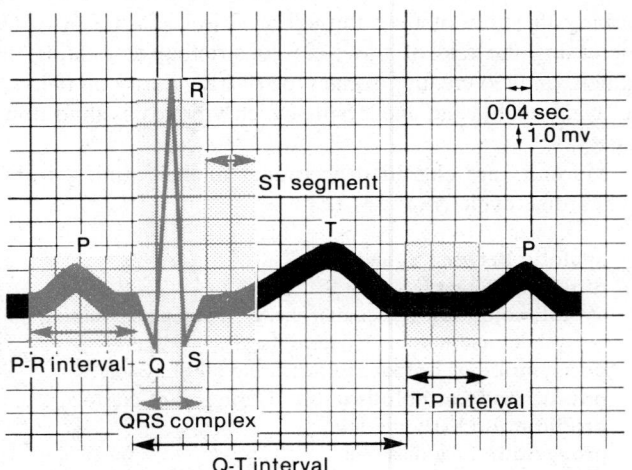

Fig. 34-4. Normal electrocardiogram pattern.

quently conducted tests are described here. Cardiac catheterization, which generates more anxiety than any other test, is discussed in detail.

Laboratory Tests

Alterations in cardiac function are frequently reflected in compensatory increases in erythrocyte count, hemoglobin level, and hematocrit. Physiologic basis for polycythemia in cyanotic heart defects is discussed later in this chapter.

In children with cyanosis, blood gas analysis and laboratory tests for hemostasis are usually performed. In children with cyanotic heart disease, a number of hemostatic abnormalities are common, including thrombocytopenia, thrombocytopathia (decreased platelet function), and low levels of prothrombin and factors V, VII, and IX (Henriksson, Gunilla, and Lundstrom, 1979).

Radiography

Radiographic tests frequently ordered for the child with suspected cardiac problems include a chest x-ray examination

and fluoroscopy, although the latter procedure is being replaced by more sophisticated tests, such as echocardiography. A chest film provides a permanent record of the size and configuration of the heart, its chambers, and the great vessels and the pattern of blood flow, especially in the pulmonary vessels.

Electrocardiography

Electrocardiography (ECG or EKG) summarizes and records graphically the depolarization and repolarization (electrical current) of cardiac tissue. This allows evaluation of the sequence and magnitude of these electrical currents (Fig. 34-4). The following describes the impulses recorded:

P wave Represents sinoatrial node depolarization and the spread of the impulse over the atria.

QRS complex (wave) Is actually composed of three separate waves, the Q wave, the R wave, and the S wave, that are caused by currents generated when the ventricles depolarize before their contraction. Because ventricular depolarization requires septal and right and left ventricular depolarization, the electrical wave depicting these events is more complex than the smooth P wave.

P-R interval Is measured from the beginning of the P wave to the beginning of the QRS complex. It is termed P-R instead of PQ because frequently the Q wave is absent. This interval represents the time that elapses from the beginning of atrial depolarization to the beginning of ventricular depolarization.

T wave Represents repolarization of the ventricles.

Q-T interval Begins with the QRS complex and ends with the completion of the T wave. It represents ventricular depolarization and repolarization. This interval varies with the heart rate. The faster the rate, the shorter the Q-T interval. Therefore in children this interval is normally shorter than in adults.

S-T segment Is normally an isoelectric (flat) line that includes the interval between the S wave and the beginning of the T wave.

An electrocardiogram is taken by placing leads or electrodes on the skin to transmit electric impulses back to a recording machine. The position of the electrodes on the body and the manner in which they are attached to the electrocardiogram machine influence the type of recording. Usually the electrodes are attached to the body with a rubber strap or a type of adhesive (for continuous monitoring). An electrolyte lubricant or electrolyte-soaked gauze is placed between the skin and lead to increase conductivity.

The PQRST complex is plotted on graph paper. Each small block represents 0.04 second horizontally and 1 mv (millivolt) vertically. By counting the number of squares intersected by the complex, the various intervals, such as the P-R or Q-T interval, and the amplitude (height) of each wave can be calculated, although the normal values vary with the child's age. Other information supplied by an electrocardiogram includes heart rate, rhythm, abnormalities of conduction, muscular damage (ischemia), hypertrophy, effects of electrolyte imbalance, influence of various drugs, and pericardial disease. However, the electrocardiogram gives no direct information concerning the mechanical performance of the heart as a pump (Berne and Levy, 1986).

Special uses of the ECG include (1) continuous ambulatory monitoring, which employs a Holter monitor, a transistorized tape recorder that is attached to chest leads, and (2) exercise stress ECG, monitoring of the ECG during controlled exercise, usually on a treadmill. Although all of these tests are painless, they can be traumatic for children. The leads can be frightening, and the child is undressed and must remain still for the standard electrocardiogram. Children old enough to understand benefit from an explanation of what is to occur. Infants and young children may be more cooperative if held in the parent's lap during the procedure.

Echocardiography

After electrocardiography, echocardiography is one of the most frequently used tests for detecting cardiac dysfunction in children. In selected instances it can confirm the diagnosis without resorting to cardiac catheterization. It involves the use of ultrahigh-frequency sound waves to produce an image of the structure of the heart. A transducer placed directly on the chest wall delivers repetitive pulses of ultrasound and processes the returned signals (echoes). Various types of echocardiography may be performed, such as the two-dimensional time and motion image, the single-cross sectional view (M-mode), or the use of pulse or continuous Doppler. Depending on the type of test, the following information can be obtained: integrity of septa; chamber size, position, and contractility; presence, position, size, and functioning of valves; velocity of blood flow; and the relationship and size of the great vessels.

Although the test is noninvasive, painless, and associated with no known side effects, it can be traumatic for children. The child must lie quietly in the standard echocardiographic positions; crying, nursing, or sitting up often leads to diagnostic errors or omissions (Snider, 1984). Therefore infants and young children may need a mild sedative; older children benefit from psychologic preparation for the test.

CARDIAC CATHETERIZATION

The most diagnostic invasive procedure is cardiac catheterization, in which a radiopaque catheter is inserted through a peripheral blood vessel into the heart. It is usually combined with angiography (angiocardiography), in which a radiopaque contrast material is injected through the catheter into the circulation. Cardiac catheterization provides information regarding:

1. Oxygen saturation of blood within the chambers and great vessels
2. Pressure changes within these structures
3. Changes in cardiac output or stroke volume (the amount of blood pumped out of the left ventricle into the aorta with each contraction)
4. Anatomic abnormalities, such as septal defects or obstruction to flow

The two main types of cardiac catheterizations are: (1) *right-sided or venous catheterization,* in which the catheter is introduced from a vein into the right atrium, and (2) *left-sided or arterial catheterization,* in which the catheter is threaded by way of a systemic artery retrograde into the aorta and left ventricle or from a right-sided approach to the left atrium by means of a septal puncture or through an existing abnormal septal opening. In children the most common method is a right-sided catheterization, since septal defects permit entry into the left side of the heart.

The catheter is usually introduced through a percutaneous puncture into the femoral vein (the catheter is threaded over a guidewire that is inserted through a large-bore needle). Rarely, a cutdown procedure is needed to gain access to the vein, but this approach is associated with increased risk of infection, hemorrhage, and obstruction. Once the vessel is entered, the catheter is guided through the heart with the aid of fluoroscopy. As the tubing is advanced, the child may feel pressure at the insertion site and vasospasm (fluttering) of the small vessels. Once the catheter is within the heart, blood samples and pressure readings are taken for analysis. Then the contrast material may be injected and films taken of the dilution and circulation of the material. As the contrast medium is administered, the child may experience warmth, nausea, vomiting, restlessness, or headache.

Nursing Considerations

Although cardiac catheterization has become a routine diagnostic procedure, it is not without risks, especially in neonates and seriously ill infants and children. Therefore good nursing judgment before and after the procedure is essential. Since cardiac catheterization is performed more frequently than cardiac surgery, attention to this necessary but potentially frightening procedure is of utmost importance.

Preprocedural care. Preparing the child and his family for the procedure is the joint responsibility of physician, nurse, and parents. The cardiologist usually explains the procedure to the parents, but nurses can reinforce and clarify the information. Many parents and older children who undergo both cardiac catheterization and cardiac surgery

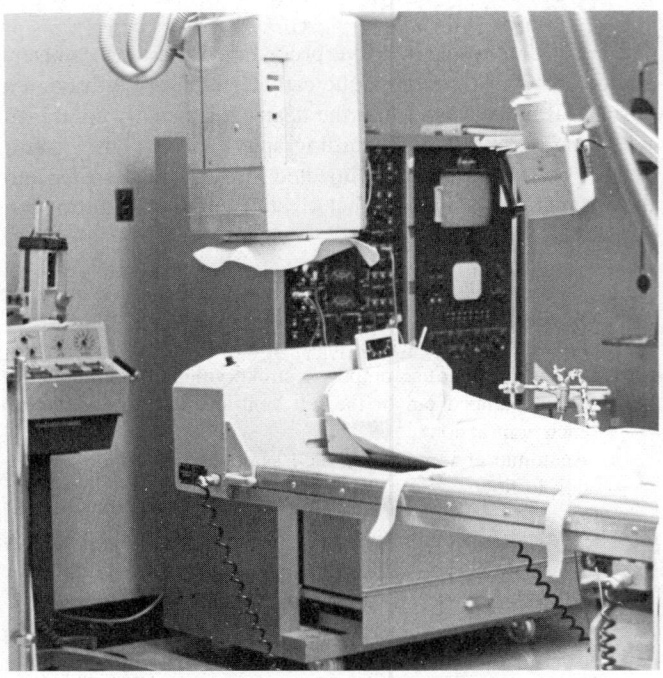

Fig. 34-5. Cardiac catheterization room.

say, in retrospect, that they were more anxious about cardiac catheterization than about the surgery.

Little psychologic preparation can be given to infants and toddlers, who comprise the majority of candidates for cardiac catheterization. The preparation of children of preschool age and above must be individualized to their level of understanding (especially their cognitive skills), their past experiences, and their understanding and perception of the situation. They should be neither underprepared nor overprepared for the experience. Overpreparing the child, especially a preschooler, can *add* to the level of anxiety rather than decrease it.

Preparation for cardiac catheterization requires the same attention to the principles of preparation for procedures described in Chapter 27. As a general guideline, the child is best informed about what he will see, feel, and hear during the procedure; what he will be expected to do to cooperate; and who will be there to help him. He needs to know what preparations will be made before he goes to the cardiac catheterization laboratory. Familiar and strange aspects are explained and, if possible, related to past experiences, such as electrocardiographic leads on the chest. Including parents and enlisting their aid as participants is helpful since parents are often aware of the child's fears and concerns.

For older children, the nurse explains the basic principles of the test, such as where the ''tube'' will go and what the physician will see, or the procedure can be demonstrated on a doll or described by reading to the child a book that explains what will happen. If the nurse is unaware of the child's concept of the heart, it is useful to have the child draw a picture so that the nurse can make certain that the explanation coincides with his level of understanding. Tak-

ing the time to establish an understanding of basic heart anatomy and physiology in preparation for this test is advantageous if heart surgery is anticipated. It is important to describe what the catheterization (''cath'') room looks like, because the x-ray machinery can appear frightening. Some institutions routinely take children on a brief tour of the area before the test. Although this is a controversial practice, it has been shown to help decrease children's anxiety (Naylor, Coates, and Kan, 1984). If this is not permitted, the child can be shown a picture (Fig. 34-5).

Other aspects of the procedure that should be explained (using words the child understands) include, specifically, that (1) the groin (or sometimes the antecubital fossa) is cleansed with a special brown solution, (2) he will receive some medicine (lidocaine) in that area so that the skin will go to sleep, (3) a tube will be placed in a blood vessel and the child may feel a little pushing at times, (4) when a special ''medicine'' (referring to the contrast material) is put into the tubing, the child may feel warm for a few seconds, and (5) as soon as the medicine is put in, the lights will go off and a machine will begin to take pictures. The last point is important to stress because younger children may associate the lights going off with ''causing'' the warm feeling from the contrast agent. As a result, they may become fearful of the dark and the noise from the machines.

Older children may appreciate a more detailed explanation of how the contrast agent aids in the diagnostic procedure, and this point can be elaborated during the test to prevent boredom. An adequate explanation is helpful in ensuring the older child's cooperation during the long procedure, which may last 2 hours or more. Diversions for children (depending on their age) include reading them stories during the test, allowing them to hold a favorite toy, or playing tapes of favorite stories or music (especially using an earphone set) (Caire and Erickson, 1986).

Before the test the child may be sedated with drugs, such as meperidine (Demerol) with or without promethazine (Phenergan) and/or chlorpromazine (Thorazine). Ideally the medication should be administered orally to avoid the added trauma of an injection. General anesthesia is not induced because of the risk of cardiovascular side effects associated with general anesthesia and the occasional need to elicit cooperation from children to assist in advancing the catheter (Agamalian, 1986). The child is allowed nothing by mouth for 4 to 6 hours before the catheterization, although polycythemic infants and children may require intravenous fluids to prevent dehydration and neonates may need dextrose solution up to 2 to 3 hours before the procedure to prevent hypoglycemia. Since young children often wonder why they do not receive breakfast, it is important to explain that this is because of the test and that, after it is over, they can have their breakfast and lunch. Ideally the child should be kept in a room with other children who are receiving nothing by mouth or allowed to spend time in the playroom, since watching others eat may make him irritable. Usually the morning dose of all oral medications is withheld, although this is clarified beforehand with the physician.

Postprocedural care. Essentially the care following cardiac catheterization is the same as general postoperative care. However, since the child is not anesthetized during the procedure, he usually returns directly to his room. Several complications can occur following a cardiac catheterization, including arrhythmias, cardiac perforation, hemorrhage, arterial obstruction, reactions to contrast media, infection, phlebitis, and hypoxia. The most important nursing responsibility is observation of the following for signs indicating these problems:

1. Vital signs, which are taken as frequently as every 15 minutes, with special emphasis on heart rate counted for 1 full minute for evidence of arrhythmias or bradycardia
2. Blood pressure, especially for hypotension, which may indicate hemorrhage from cardiac perforation or bleeding at the site of initial catheterization
3. Pulses, especially below the catheterization site, for equality and symmetry (pulse distal to the site may be weaker for the first few hours after catheterization but should gradually increase in strength)
4. Temperature and color of the affected extremity, since coolness or blanching may indicate arterial obstruction
5. Dressing for evidence of bleeding or hematoma formation in the femoral or antecubital area

Depending on hospital policy the child may be kept in bed with the affected extremity kept straight for 4 to 6 hours after venous catheterization and 6 to 8 hours after arterial catheterization to facilitate healing of the cannulated vessel. If a younger child has difficulty complying, he can be held in the parent's lap with the leg maintained in the correct position. If bleeding occurs, direct continuous pressure is applied 2.5 cm (1 inch) *above* the percutaneous skin site to localize pressure over the vessel puncture (Agamalian, 1986). The child's usual diet can be resumed as soon as tolerated, beginning with sips of water and advancing as his condition allows. The child is encouraged to void to clear the contrast material from the blood. Generally there is only slight discomfort at the percutaneous site. To prevent infection the catheterization area is protected from possible contamination. If the child wears diapers, the dressing can be kept dry by covering it with a piece of plastic film and sealing the edges of the film to the skin with tape. The nurse must be careful, however, to continue to observe the site for any evidence of bleeding.

It is important at this time to evaluate the child's ideas of what occurred during the procedure in order to clarify any misconceptions and allow the child a feeling of triumph and satisfaction in having gone through the experience. Questions such as "Was the test like what you expected?" or "How was it different (or the same) from what you expected?" can encourage the child to discuss his concerns. Play and drawing are especially valuable tools. One 7-year-old child's drawing of his tiny body on a large examining table with a huge x-ray machine hovering over of him clearly demonstrated his feeling of powerlessness and insecurity. However, when the nurse remarked, "Look at how small you are next to that big machine," the child proudly answered, "Yes, but I made it!"

Nursing Care Summary: The Child Undergoing Cardiac Catheterization

NURSING GOALS	NURSING INTERVENTIONS	EXPECTED PATIENT/FAMILY OUTCOMES
HP-HMP **Injury: potential for trauma** **Risk factors: surgical procedure**		
Preprocedural Care		
Prepare child for procedure	See Preoperative preparation, p. 1145	
Take to cardiac catheterization laboratory	Transport infants in bassinets, crib, or Isolette with extra diapers, blanket, and glucose water and/or pacifier Transport older children by gurney Prepare requests to accompany child, such as x-ray, cardiopulmonary, according to routine of hospital Provide pacifier and/or sugar nipple for smaller infants if irritable Provide K-pad or other device for warming small infant Provide extra diapers for infants	Child is transported to the cardiac catheterization laboratory with a minimum of distress to child and family
Postprocedural Care		
Assess physiologic status	Check vital signs until stable (frequency determined by policy) Pulse (apical) Respirations Temperature Blood pressure (if prescribed)	Child's vital signs remain within normal limits for age (see inside front cover for normal variations)

Continued.

Nursing Care Summary: The Child Undergoing Cardiac Catheterization—cont'd

NURSING GOALS	NURSING INTERVENTIONS	EXPECTED PATIENT/FAMILY OUTCOMES
Assess physiologic status—cont'd	Assess general color Assess circulation in involved extremity and compare with opposite extremity 　Pedal pulses 　Color 　Temperature 　Capillary filling time Assess operative site for bleeding and/or swelling Report any compromise in circulation to physician	*Signs of bleeding or inflammation are detected early
Prevent complications	Keep catheterized leg as straight as possible Keep incision and dressing clean and dry Apply pressure if oozing or bleeding noted Carry out routine physical assessments Keep child relatively quiet Avoid undue excitement	Child remains free of complications
Maintain optimum body temperature	Provide warmth if infant or child is chilled from exposure during procedure Avoid either overheating or chilling	Child's temperature remains below 38° C (100.4° F)

N-MP　**Fluid volume deficit, potential**
Risk factors: nothing by mouth prior to procedure

Provide nutrition and hydration	Give sips of water first Advance intake to include other fluids and foods as tolerated, when fully awake	Child tolerates fluids and food as offered

SP-SCP　**Fear**
Etiology: unfamiliar environment, new experience

Provide psychologic preparation 　Explain procedure	Describe what child will experience 　Honestly 　In simple terms 　In terms appropriate to the child's level of development and past experiences Stress familiar and relate unfamiliar to known objects or experiences Avoid overpreparing child with 　Too much information 　Unneeded information 　Information beyond child's ability to comprehend Allow child to experience unfamiliar pieces of equipment in safe environment of play 　Ride a gurney in hallway 　Wear gown and mask 　Play with real hospital equipment and/or miniature replicas or models Allow child to see and hold catheter Describe sensations child will feel, in simple terms, at the appropriate time (not far in advance of experience)	Child displays an attitude of understanding; is able to repeat information in his own words; asks pertinent questions
Provide comfort	Allow child the comfort of a familiar toy or object such as a favorite blanket Offer distractions, such as music or tapes Permit family to be with child as long as possible Be available and accessible to child Answer questions Maintain a calm, reassuring manner See also The child in the hospital, p. 1075	Child is calm and quiet

*Nursing outcome.

Nursing Care Summary: The Child Undergoing Cardiac Catheterization—cont'd

NURSING GOALS	NURSING INTERVENTIONS	EXPECTED PATIENT/FAMILY OUTCOMES
RRP **Family process, alteration in** **Etiology: situational crisis (hospitalization of child)**		

Support and reassure family	Reinforce and clarify information given by physician
	Explain associated diagnostic tests and procedures such as x-ray examinations, ECG
	Explain child's schedule
	  When child will receive premedication
	  Time child will leave for cardiac catheterization laboratory
	  Where parents can wait for child to return
	  Room to which child return
	  Postprocedural care and routines
	Explore family's feelings regarding procedure and its implications
	Include parents in preparation of child
	See also The family of the hospitalized child, p. 1081
		Family demonstrates an understanding of procedure (specify manner of demonstration) and related information (specify)

Prepare for home care	Teach procedures and observations
	  Wound care
	  Bathing instructions
	  Activity
	  Signs for which to observe
	Make certain family knows whom to contact if needed
		Family demonstrates ability to provide postprocedural care (specify understanding and method of evaluation)

Nursing Interventions Related to Medical Management

PREPROCEDURAL CARE
Check that parental consent for procedure has been obtained
Arrange for preoperative diagnostic procedures as ordered: electrocardiogram, complete blood count, chest radiograph, vectorcardiogram, phonocardiogram, echocardiogram
Provide physical preparation
  Ensure nothing by mouth for a stated period of time prior to procedure (usually 4-6 hours depending on age of child)

Cyanotic, polycythemic infants are usually allowed dextrose water 2-3 hours prior to procedure to prevent dehydration and/or hypoglycemia
Take and record vital signs
Administer preoperative medication to older infants and children

POSTPROCEDURAL CARE
Administer withheld digitalis and other medications if ordered

Congenital Heart Disease

The incidence of congenital heart disease (CHD) in children is generally reported to be 8:1000 live births, although recent findings indicate the rate to be lower (4:1000 live births) (Ferencz and others, 1985). About a third of these children have insignificant defects, another third demonstrate significant findings beyond the first year, and a third have serious, even critical manifestations within the first year of life (Nadas, 1984). CHD is the major cause of death in the first year (other than prematurity). Depending on the defect, the sexes are affected differently (Table 34-1). Although there are over 35 well-recognized individual defects, the most common heart anomaly is ventricular septal defect.

Reports on its incidence indicate that the defect is increasing in frequency in the United States. While the reason for this increase is not known, at least a portion of it is probably due to better case finding methods and more complete diagnosis (Newman, 1985).

The etiology of most congenital heart defects is not known in over 90% of the cases. However, several factors are associated with a higher than expected incidence of the disease. These include prenatal factors such as (1) maternal rubella during pregnancy, (2) maternal alcoholism, (3) maternal age over 40 years, and (4) maternal insulin-dependent diabetes. Heart defects are found in a much higher percentage of stillbirths, spontaneous abortions, and low-birth-weight infants, especially those small for age (Noonan,

Table 34-1 Incidence and recurrence risks of selected congenital heart defects and association with other conditions

ANOMALY	MALE TO FEMALE RATIO	RISK OF RECURRENCE IN CHILD HAVING ONE PARENT WITH CHD* (%)	PERCENTAGE OF INCIDENCE OF CHD IN INFANTS†	DISORDERS ASSOCIATED WITH INCREASED INCIDENCE‡
Ventricular septal defect (VSD)	1:1	5.0	28.3	Down syndrome Holt-Oram syndrome Fetal alcohol syndrome
Patent ductus arteriosus (PDA)	1:3	3.5	12.5	Rubella syndrome Down syndrome
Atrial septal defect (ASD)	1:3	3.2	9.7	Noonan syndrome Holt-Oram syndrome Down syndrome Fetal alcohol syndrome
Coarctation of aorta	4:1	2.4	8.8	Turner syndrome Apert syndrome
Transposition of great vessels (TGV)	3:1		8.0	Diabetes or prediabetes in mother
Tetralogy of Fallot	1:1	3.2	7.0	Down syndrome Fetal alcohol syndrome
Pulmonic stenosis	1:1	2.9	6.0	Rubella syndrome Noonan syndrome
Aortic stenosis	4:1	2.1	3.5	Turner syndrome

*Data from Nora, J.J., and Nora, A.H.: Circulation **53**(4):701-702, 1976.
†Data from Campbell, M. In Watson, A., editor: Paediatric cardiology, London, 1968, Lloyd-Luke, Ltd., Chapter 5.
‡Data from Noonan, J.A.: Pediatr. Clin. North Am. **25**(4):797-816, 1978.

1978). Children with CHD are also more likely to have extracardiac defects, such as tracheoesophageal fistula, renal agenesis, and diaphragmatic hernia.

Several genetic factors are also implicated in CHD, although the influence is multifactorial. The risk of recurrence in families with an affected parent is variously reported in the literature but may be as high as 16% (Whittemore, Hobbins, and Engle, 1982), especially if the mother has the defect (Rose and others, 1985). The rising recurrence rates may be the result of more children with previously fatal heart defects surviving to adulthood and having offspring. Certain chromosomal aberrations, such as Down syndrome, are associated with increased risk of cardiac defects. Table 34-1 summarizes the incidence and recurrence risks of major cardiac defects and the increased risk in various disorders.

TYPES OF DEFECTS

Congenital heart defects may be divided into various categories, but two commonly used divisions are based on the alteration in circulation:

acyanotic in which there is no mixing of desaturated (poorly oxygenated venous) blood in the systemic arterial circulation

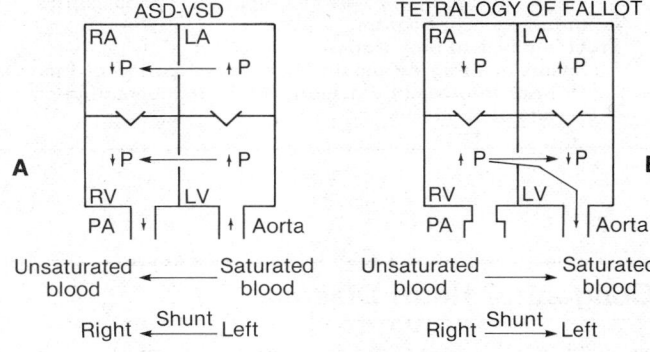

Fig. 34-6. Shunting of blood in congenital heart disease. **A,** Acyanotic defect; **B,** cyanotic defect.

cyanotic in which desaturated blood enters the systemic arterial circulation, regardless of whether cyanosis is clinically evident

Clinical manifestations depend on the severity of the defect and the amount of pulmonary blood flow. In acyanotic defects no associated signs and symptoms may be apparent if the defect is small and the heart is able to compensate for the extra workload.

Altered hemodynamics. To understand the physiol-

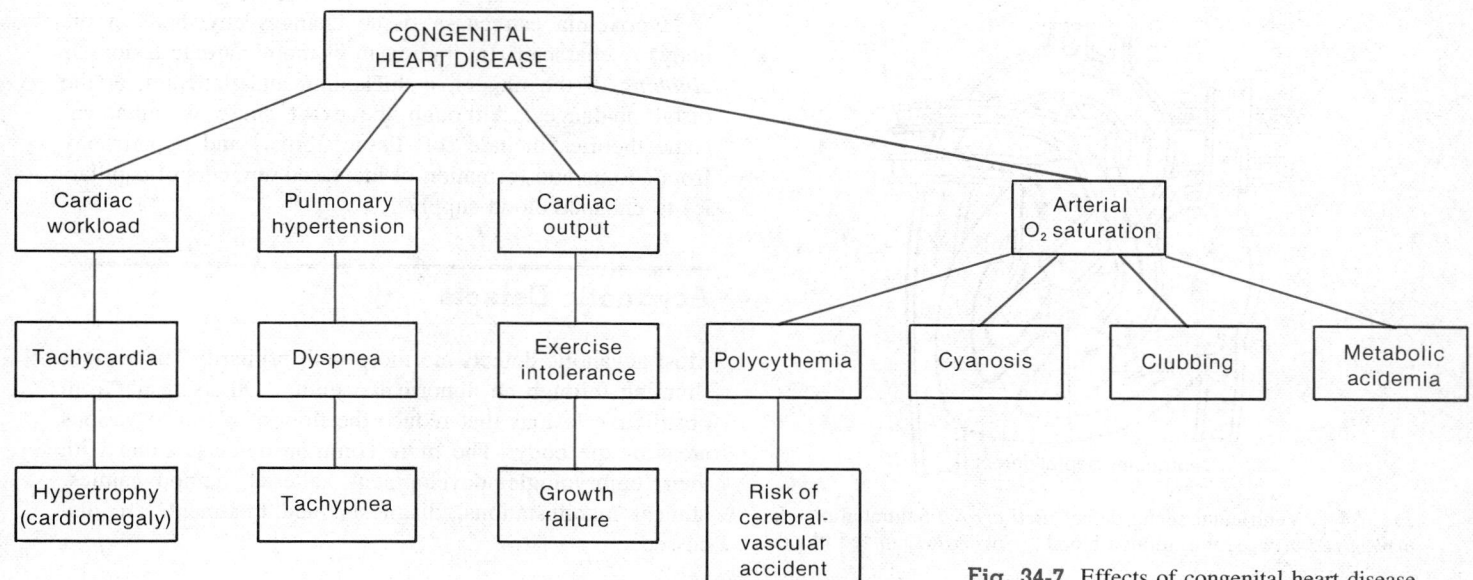

Fig. 34-7. Effects of congenital heart disease.

ogy of heart defects, it is necessary to review the role of pressure gradients, flow, and resistance within the circulation. Blood flows as a result of pressure gradients existing in different parts of the body and because of the pumping action of the heart. Like any fluid, blood flows from an area of high pressure to one of low pressure and toward the path of least resistance. The rate of flow is directly proportional to the pressure gradient (that is, the higher the pressure gradient, the greater the rate of flow) and inversely proportional to the resistance (that is, the higher the resistance, the less the rate of flow). However, increased resistance does not always decrease flow. If the proximal cardiac chamber can increase the driving pressure proportionately, flow can remain unchanged.

Normally the pressure on the right side of the heart is lower than that on the left side, and the resistance in the pulmonary circulation is less than that in the systemic circulation. Likewise, vessels entering or exiting from these chambers have corresponding pressures (for example, lower pressure in the pulmonary artery and higher pressure in the aorta). Therefore if there is an abnormal connection between the heart chambers, such as a septal defect, blood flows from an area of higher pressure (left side) to one of lower pressure (right side). This directional flow of blood is termed a *left-to-right shunt*. If the opening is small, the amount of blood shunted to the atrium or ventricle may be minimal. In this instance no unoxygenated blood flows directly into the left side of the heart, hence the term *acyanotic defect* (Fig. 34-6, *A*).

However, severe acyanotic defects are potentially cyanotic as a result of pulmonary vascular changes. *Eisenmenger complex (syndrome)* refers to the clinical situation in which a left-to-right shunt becomes a right-to-left shunt because of progressive increase in pulmonary vascular resistance. With increasing pulmonary vascular thickening the resistance in the pulmonary circulation can exceed or

equal that in the systemic circulation, causing a reversal of blood flow from the right to the left ventricle (Macartney, 1979).

Cyanotic heart defects may be the result of anomalies that cause a change in pressure so that the blood is shunted from the right to the left side of the heart (hence the term *right-to-left shunt*) because of either increased pulmonary vascular resistance or obstruction to blood flow through the pulmonic valve/artery (Fig. 34-6, *B*). Cyanosis may also occur because of a defect that allows mixing of blood between the pulmonary and systemic circulations, such as truncus arteriosus or transposition of the great vessels.

PHYSICAL CONSEQUENCES

The general effects of heart malformation may be summarized as (1) increased workload in terms of systolic or diastolic overloading of the chambers, (2) pulmonary hypertension (increased vascular resistance), (3) inadequate systemic cardiac output, and (4) in cyanotic defects arterial desaturation from shunting of unoxygenated blood directly into the systemic circulation, which produces hypoxemia and, if severe enough, may result in tissue hypoxia. Also decreased tissue perfusion can produce acidosis and death if cardiac performance is severely compromised. The principal physical consequences of these changes, which may vary in severity, are growth retardation, decreased exercise tolerance, dyspnea, tachypnea, tachycardia, cyanosis, and tissue hypoxia (Fig. 34-7).

Growth retardation is primarily the result of feeding difficulties, which lead to decreased nutrient intake, and increased caloric need related to the tachypnea and tachycardia. Failure to gain weight, even during the neonatal period, is a consistent finding. *Decreased exercise tolerance* is a direct consequence of inadequate nutrient intake and increased metabolic demands. Exercise intolerance is usually

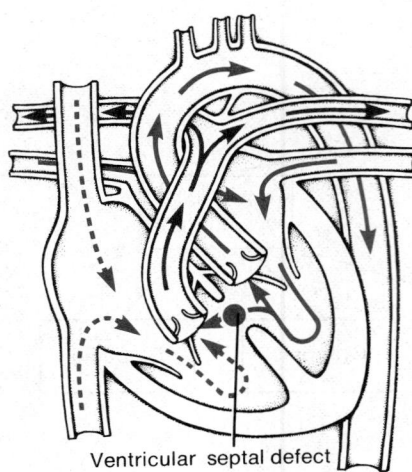

Fig. 34-8. Ventricular septal defect. *Red arrow,* Saturated blood; *broken red arrows,* unsaturated blood; *gray arrows,* mixed blood.

first noted by the parent during feedings when the infant is too fatigued to consume the entire formula.

Dyspnea occurs as a result of decreased lung compliance and the increased work of breathing or it may be a result of arterial oxygen desaturation. It may be associated with *tachypnea* as the lungs try to compensate through an increased respiratory effect. Tachypnea is also a reflex response to hypoxemia, which may be present in cyanotic defects. Respiratory infections in these children have a tendency to be severe.

Cardiac changes include increased cardiac workload to meet the body's oxygen demands, principally through increasing the rate of contractions *(tachycardia).* Increased cardiac effort eventually results in an increased size of the heart muscle *(cardiomegaly).*

A number of consequences can occur as a result of reduced arterial oxygen saturation. *Cyanosis,* the blue color observed in the skin and mucous membranes, results when at least 5 g of desaturated or reduced hemoglobin (hemoglobin not bound to oxygen) is present per 1 dl of blood. In polycythemic patients, cyanosis appears more readily because of the large amount of total hemoglobin present. Cyanosis indicates that hypoxemia (reduced arterial oxygenation saturation) is present but it does not necessarily mean that hypoxia (reduced tissue oxygenation) has occurred. However, if tissue hypoxia does develop as the result of progressive arterial oxygen desaturation, metabolic acidosis and death can occur. (See p. 235 for a discussion of evaluation of skin color.)

Persistent hypoxemia stimulates erythropoiesis, resulting in polycythemia (increased number of red blood cells). When polycythemia is present the viscosity of the blood increases. However, the resultant viscosity and volume of blood lead to further problems: increased risk of complications such as emboli and cerebrovascular accident (stroke), slowed circulation, and an increased workload on the heart, which may lead to congestive heart failure.

Hypoxemia can cause tissue changes anywhere in the body. A characteristic finding in cyanotic cardiac lesions is *clubbing* of the fingers, a thickening and flattening of the distal phalanges. Although the exact cause is unknown, some theories include soft tissue fibrosis and hypertrophy from anoxia and formation of increased numbers of capillaries to enhance blood supply.

Acyanotic Defects

Most acyanotic defects are those with primarily left-to-right shunting through an abnormal opening. Others result from obstructive lesions that reduce the flow of blood to various areas of the body. The more common defects, along with their embryologic development, altered hemodynamics, clinical manifestations, diagnosis, and treatment, are discussed.

VENTRICULAR SEPTAL DEFECT

A ventricular septal defect (VSD) is an abnormal opening between the right and left ventricles (Fig. 34-8). It may vary in size from a small pinhole to absence of the septum, resulting in a common ventricle. It is frequently associated with other defects, such as pulmonary stenosis, transposition of the great vessels, patent ductus arteriosus, atrial defects, and coarctation of the aorta. About 80% of the children with a small VSD will experience spontaneous closure of the defect, usually by age 10 years, as a result of growth and proliferation of the muscular septum, apposition of a cusp of the tricuspid valve against the defect, or formation of a membranous diaphragm across the opening (Alpert and others, 1979).

Embryologic Development

Between the fourth and eighth weeks of gestation, the single ventricular chamber is divided in two by fusion of the membranous portion of the ventricular septum, the endocardial cushions, and the bulbus cordis. Inadequate development of any of these structures results in an abnormal communication between the two ventricles.

Altered Hemodynamics

The hemodynamic consequences of VSD depend on the size of the opening, its location, and the reactivity of the child's pulmonary vascular bed. Because of the higher pressure within the left ventricle and because the systemic arterial circulation offers more resistance than the pulmonary circulation, blood flows through the defect into the pulmonary artery. The increased blood volume is pumped into the lungs, which may eventually result in increased pulmonary vascular resistance. Increased pressure in the right ventricle as a result of left-to-right shunting and pulmonary resistance causes the muscle to hypertrophy. If the right ventricle is unable to accommodate the increased workload, the right atrium may also enlarge as it attempts to overcome the resistance offered by incomplete right ventricular emptying. In severe defects Eisenmenger syndrome may develop (p. 1459).

Clinical Manifestations

One of the most characteristic signs of VSD is a loud, harsh, pansystolic murmur that is generally heard best at the left lower sternal border and radiating throughout the precordium. The intensity of the murmur is not necessarily an indication of the defect's size. In neonates the murmur may be absent because of the normally high pulmonary vascular resistance, which tends to equalize the pressure between the two ventricles. A systolic thrill is associated with loud murmurs.

Severe overloading of the right ventricle and occasionally the right atrium causes hypertrophy and an obvious cardiac enlargement. With increased pulmonary blood flow under high pressure the infant is likely to develop congestive heart failure (p. 1488).

Diagnostic Evaluation

The electrocardiographic and echocardiographic findings of left ventricular hypertrophy and cardiomegaly, and prominent pulmonary markings on chest radiograph usually confirm the diagnosis of VSD. Cardiac catheterization may be done to demonstrate the exact location of the defect and assess pulmonary pressures.

Therapeutic Management

If the defect is small and the child is asymptomatic, the child is usually followed to allow for spontaneous closure of the VSD. These children are candidates for antibiotic prophylaxis to prevent bacterial endocarditis (see p. 1496). When surgery is required, the recommended treatment is total surgical correction using deep hypothermia. During open-heart surgery, the defect is closed with sutures or a knitted cloth patch. If the defect is associated with complex heart disease or if the infant is too ill to tolerate corrective surgery, a banding procedure may be performed to decrease the pulmonary blood flow and prevent pulmonary vascular disease.

Mortality after repair of a VSD depends on the presence or absence of pulmonary vascular disease, the age of the child, and his general condition at the time of surgery. Beyond the age of 2 years, elective closure of an uncomplicated defect carries a mortality of 1% or less in most qualified centers (Moss, 1979), although the mortality in infants is close to 5% (Graham, 1984). The major complications following repair are conduction defects and residual ventricular shunts. Congestive heart failure may be observed postoperatively if it is present preoperatively or if a right ventriculotomy cardiac incision is required for the repair. Conduction disturbances are the result of damage to the ventricular conduction system. A fatal complication may be late-onset heart block. Residual VSDs may result from incomplete closure, subsequent breakdown of sutures, or additional septal defects undetected at the initial repair.

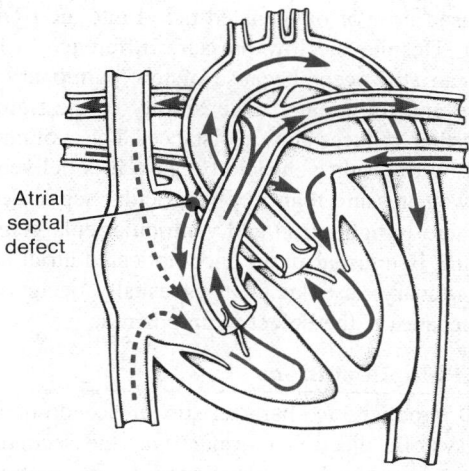

Fig. 34-9. Atrial septal defect. *Red arrows,* Saturated blood; *broken red arrows,* unsaturated blood; *gray arrows,* mixed blood.

ATRIAL SEPTAL DEFECT

An atrial septal defect (ASD) is an abnormal opening between the two atria (Fig. 34-9). The defect may be one of three types: ostium primum, ostium secundum, or sinus venosus defect.

Embryologic Development

From about the fourth to the sixth week of gestation, the common atrium is divided into two chambers. The first septum originates in the dorsal wall of the atrium and grows toward the endocardial cushions. The space between these two structures is called the *ostium primum* (first hole). As the first septum continues to grow, a hole called the ostium secundum (second hole) appears in its center. At about the same time a second septum, *septum secundum,* begins to grow; eventually the two septa form the *foramen ovale.*

Failure in any stage of this development leads to an abnormal opening between the two atria. If the hole is in the center of the septum, it is an *ostium secundum defect.* If the opening is at the lower end of the septum, it is an *ostium primum defect.* Ostium primum defects are generally associated with mitral valve abnormalities, since the valve is derived from the endocardial cushions, and may extend to the upper portion of the ventricles, creating an atrioventricular communication. In this instance the defect is referred to as an *endocardial cushion defect.* If the opening is near the junction of the superior vena cava and the right atrium, it is called a *sinus venosus defect.* Sinus venosus defects may be associated with partial anomalous pulmonary venous return, since the right pulmonary veins may join the right atrium at the level of the defect. Small defects located high on the septum, such as ostium secundum or sinus venosus defects, may result in no apparent clinical symptoms.

Altered Hemodynamics

Because left atrial pressure slightly exceeds right atrial pressure, blood flows from the left to the right atrium, causing an increased flow of oxygenated blood into the right side of the heart. Despite the low pressure difference, a high rate of flow can still occur because of low pulmonary vascular resistance and the greater distensibility of the right atrium, which further reduces flow resistance. This volume is well tolerated by the right ventricle because it is delivered under much lower pressure than in a ventricular septal defect. Although there is right atrial and ventricular enlargement, cardiac failure is unusual in an uncomplicated atrial septal defect. Pulmonary vascular changes usually occur only after several decades if the defect is unrepaired.

Clinical Manifestations

An ASD produces a characteristic crescendo-decrescendo type of systolic ejection murmur over the second to third interspace along the left sternal border. The murmur is not produced by blood flow across the defect as in ventricular septal defect but represents increased blood flow through the normal pulmonic valve.

Although the heart sounds are normal in intensity, there is a wide fixed splitting of the second sound. Normally the splitting between the two components of the second sound occurs because closure of the aortic valve precedes closure of the pulmonic valve during inspiration. The split normally widens because the increased venous return prolongs right ventricular emptying, causing a delay in pulmonic valve closure. When an ASD is present, the fixed overload of the right ventricle further prolongs its ejection time, thus widening the delay in closure of the pulmonic valve.

Diagnostic Evaluation

The most suggestive sign of ASD is its characteristic murmur and fixed splitting of the second sound. Cardiac catheterization definitively demonstrates the abnormal opening in the atrial septum and increased oxygen saturation on the right side of the heart. Radiographic findings include right atrial and ventricular hypertrophy, and pulmonary vascular marking may be present as the result of increased pulmonary blood flow. The electrocardiogram may demonstrate right atrial and right ventricular enlargement.

Therapeutic Management

Surgical closure of ASD is reserved for moderate to large shunts and is similar to the corrective procedures employed in ventricular septal defects. Postoperative complications are unusual, and survival is greater than 99%. The most common complication is atrial arrhythmias, which may require pacemaker implantation. Residual mitral valve insufficiency is common but causes few difficulties (Portman and others, 1985). Recently, closure of an ASD has been reformed during cardiac catheterization with the use of an umbrella-tipped catheter.

ENDOCARDIAL CUSHION DEFECT

Endocardial cushion defect is incomplete fusion of the endocardial cushions. It consists of a low atrial septal defect

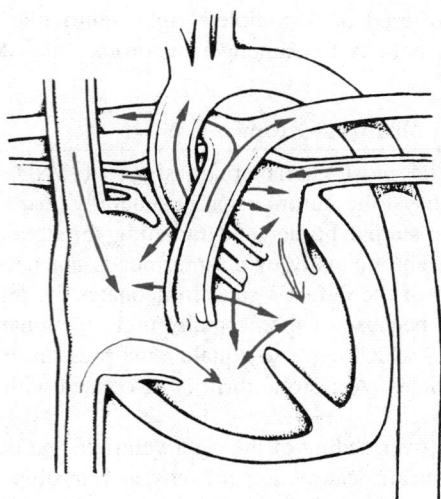

Fig. 34-10. Endocardial cushion defect.

that is continuous with a high ventricular septal defect and clefts of the mitral and tricuspid valves. This creates a large central atrioventricular valve that allows blood to flow between all four chambers of the heart (Fig. 34-10). There are varying degrees of the defect, which is often classified as incomplete, intermediate, and complete. The most severe form (complete atrioventricular canal) consists of a primum ASD and a single, common atrioventricular valve, with or without a VSD.

Embryologic Development

The embryologic development of the endocardial cushions has already been described for both ventricular and atrial septal defects. Inadequate development of the endocardial cushions during the period of fusion results in failure of the septum to fuse, and the defect may be complete or partial absence of the septum and atrioventricular valves. Because of the failure of the septum to form between the atria and ventricles, the conduction system is affected.

Altered Hemodynamics

The alterations in the hemodynamics depend on the severity of the defect and on the child's pulmonary vascular resistance. Immediately after birth, while the newborn's pulmonary vascular resistance is high, there is minimal shunting of blood through the defect. Once this resistance falls, left-to-right shunting occurs and pulmonary blood flow increases. The resultant pulmonary vascular engorgement predisposes to development of congestive heart failure.

Clinical Manifestations

At birth signs and symptoms may be minimal except during crying or on exertion, when cyanosis occurs. If the defect consists of an ostium primum atrial septal defect and mild mitral valve insufficiency, the child is usually asymptomatic. If a complete atrioventricular canal is present, cyanosis will be more severe. Murmurs characteristic of an ASD or VSD may be found.

Diagnostic Evaluation

The electrocardiogram may demonstrate biventricular hypertrophy and a left axis deviation. Echocardiography may reveal separate mitral and tricuspid valves with a primum ASD and continuity between these valves with a complete atrioventricular canal. Cardiac catheterization findings are characteristic of a left-to-right shunt and indicate the presence and location of septal defects.

Therapeutic Management

Surgical intervention involves closure of the ASD and repair of the mitral valve. If the septal defect is large a patch may be required; with a severe mitral valve defect a valve replacement may be needed. Operative mortality depends on the severity of the defect and the age of the child at the time of surgery and varies from 10% to 35% (Feldt and others, 1983). Complications include bleeding, heart block, arrhythmias, and congestive heart failure. These patients are at risk for bacterial endocarditis and require antibiotic prophylaxis.

PATENT DUCTUS ARTERIOSUS

A patent ductus arteriosus (PDA) is present when the normal fetal structure fails to close completely after birth (Fig. 34-11). In fetal life the ductus arteriosus connects the pulmonary artery to the aorta and shunts oxygenated blood directly into the systemic circulation, bypassing the lungs. At birth functional closure of the ductus arteriosus occurs within a few hours as a result of constriction of smooth muscle in its vessel walls from exposure to increased oxygen tension. Complete anatomic closure may take several weeks. However, under certain circumstances the ductus arteriosus remains open.

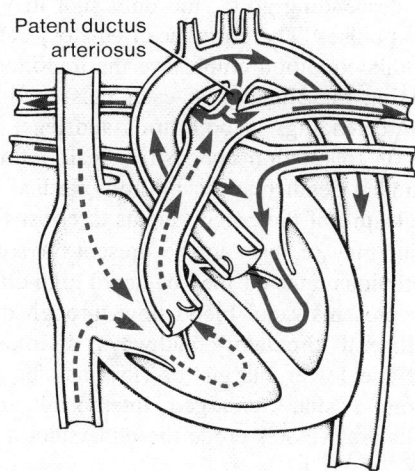

Fig. 34-11. Patent ductus arteriosus. *Red arrows,* Saturated blood; *broken red arrows,* unsaturated blood; *gray arrows,* mixed blood.

Embryologic Development

During the fifth and seventh weeks of gestation the aortic arch system develops and begins as six paired arches growing from the apex of the truncus arteriosus. The sixth paired arch branches toward each lung, forming the proximal portion of the pulmonary artery. On the right side the distal portion of the arch disappears, but on the left side it remains attached to the aorta, forming the ductus arteriosus. In a strict sense, a PDA is not a congenital malformation, since the ductus develops normally.

Altered Hemodynamics

The hemodynamic consequences of PDA depend on the size of the ductus and the pulmonary vascular resistance. A small ductus offers high resistance to flow, limiting the volume of the shunted blood. At birth the resistance in the pulmonary and systemic circulations is almost identical, thus equalizing the resistance within the aorta and pulmonary artery. However, as the pulmonary resistance falls, a gradient is created between the aorta and the pulmonary artery. Blood is then shunted from the aorta to the pulmonary artery.

The additional blood is recirculated through the lungs and returned to the left atrium and left ventricle. The effect of this altered circulation is increased workload on the left side of the heart, increased pulmonary vascular congestion and possibly resistance, and potentially increased right ventricular pressure and hypertrophy.

Clinical Manifestations

The turbulent flow of blood from the aorta through the patent ductus arteriosus to the pulmonary artery results in a characteristic machinery-like murmur, which is heard best at the middle to upper left sternal border. Since there is a continuous flow of blood across the shunt, the murmur is heard during all of systole and most of diastole beyond the neonatal period. It is usually associated with a thrill. Another common feature is a widened pulse pressure.

Enlargement of the left atrium, left ventricle, and possibly right ventricle is a consistent finding. If the left ventricle cannot accommodate the volume overload, the diastolic pressure increases, leading to an increase in left atrial pressure and pulmonary venous engorgement. Consequently signs of congestive heart failure result.

Diagnostic Evaluation

The machinery-type murmur is almost diagnostic of PDA, but it may be absent in neonates or premature infants because of the normally high pulmonary resistance that tends to equalize the pressure between the two vessels. Radiographic examinations usually demonstrate left atrial and ventricular enlargement and evidence of increased pulmonary blood flow. The electrocardiogram is generally normal, although it may demonstrate left ventricular or biventricular enlargement. Cardiac catheterization may not be necessary to confirm the diagnosis because of the characteristic auscultatory and radiographic findings. An echocardiogram is

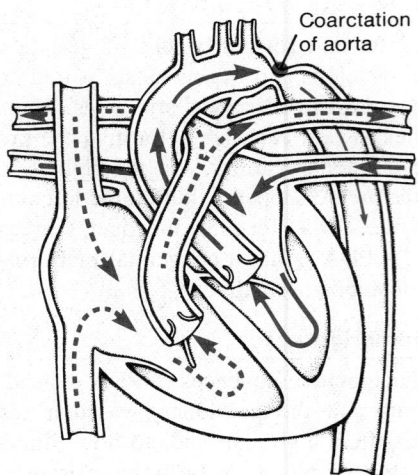

Fig. 34-12. Coarctation of aorta (postductal). *Red arrows,* Saturated blood; *broken red arrows,* unsaturated blood.

useful, since it may demonstrate an increased left atrial to aortic ratio, which is characteristic of a defect producing increased pulmonary blood flow and increased venous return, as is seen in PDA.

Therapeutic Management

Surgical intervention involves surgical division or ligation of the patent vessel. Since the defect is outside the heart, cardiopulmonary bypass is not necessary. However, it is still a major operative procedure, since the thoracic cavity must be entered.

In the asymptomatic infant with a patent ductus arteriosus, the recommended time for repair is at 1 to 2 years of age (Emmanouilides and Baylen, 1981). Because of the low surgical risk (less than 1%) and the possible occurrence of bacterial endocarditis later in life, surgical correction is recommended for all affected children. In critically ill newborns with PDA, pharmacologic closure of the ductus may be attempted with indomethacin, a prostaglandin inhibitor (see also p. 411). If surgical correction is performed on these neonates, operative risk is much higher.

COARCTATION OF AORTA

Coarctation of the aorta (COA) is a narrowing of the aorta (Fig. 34-12). The position of the narrowing is described as follows:

preductal Proximal to the insertion of the ductus arteriosus, commonly between that vessel and the left subclavian artery
postductal Distal to the ductus arteriosus
juxtaductal At the level of the ductus arteriosus

A coexisting bicuspid aortic valve is found in about 50% of patients.

Embryologic Development

The development of coarctation of the aorta is related to the embryologic development of the aortic arch (see discussion of embryologic development for patent ductus arteriosus). The right fourth arch gives rise to the right subclavian artery, and the left fourth arch becomes the definitive aortic arch. For some unknown reason the area of the aorta near the attachment of the ductus arteriosus may develop improperly, resulting in a constricted lumen. Only a localized area or the entire aorta can be affected.

Altered Hemodynamics

The effect of a narrowing within the aorta is increased pressure proximal to the defect and decreased pressure distal to it. In the preductal type the lower half of the body is supplied with blood by the right ventricle through the ductus arteriosus. In the postductal type of coarctation right ventricular outflow cannot maintain blood flow to the descending aorta. Therefore collateral circulation develops during fetal life to maintain flow from the ascending to the descending aorta.

Clinical Manifestations

The cardinal sign of coarctation of the aorta is a marked difference in the blood pressure and pulses of the upper and lower extremities. In those areas of the body that receive blood from vessels proximal to the defect, blood pressure is high and the pulses are bounding. In the postductal type hypertension is present in both upper extremities and head. However, if the constriction is between the insertion of the innominate and left subclavian arteries, the right arm will have bounding radial pulses and high blood pressure, whereas the left arm will have diminished pulses and pressure. Because of hypertension, the child occasionally may experience dizziness, headaches, fainting, and epistaxis.

In those areas of the body distal to the defect, the blood pressure is decreased. The femoral pulses are weak or absent, the lower extremities may be cooler than the upper ones, and muscle cramps may result during increased exercise from tissue anoxia (a condition called claudication). If adequate collateral pathways have developed to maintain blood flow to the descending aorta, the only sign may be diminished femoral pulses. Therefore the circulatory changes associated with this condition emphasize the importance of routinely assessing the equality of each pulse and comparing blood pressure readings in both arms and legs. In the preductal type of coarctation congestive heart failure is common and sudden death may occur from cardiac decompensation and closure of the patent ductus arteriosus in infants.

A murmur may or may not be present. A soft high-frequency continuous murmur may be heard high on the sternal border. It represents rapid blood flow through the coarcted area or collateral circulatory pathways. In older children notching of the lower margin of ribs may be evident on roentgenograms, since enlarged intercostal arteries that serve as collateral vessels erode the underside of the ribs.

Diagnostic Evaluation

Diagnosis is based on the characteristic physical findings including hypertensive upper extremities and hypotensive lower extremities. Radiographic studies may also demonstrate the rib notching and dilation of the aorta proximal to the stricture. The electrocardiogram usually demonstrates left ventricular hypertrophy; biventricular hypertrophy is present if preductal coarctation is present. Echocardiography and/or cardiac catheterization may be done to confirm the diagnosis.

Therapeutic Management

Treatment depends on the type and severity of the defect. Infants with congestive heart failure are usually managed medically until they are able to tolerate surgery. In infants who depend on patency of the ductus arteriosus to provide adequate systemic blood flow, prostaglandins may be used to keep the ductus arteriosus open and perfuse the kidneys and lower part of the body until surgical correction can be safely performed. The timing of the surgery is significant, since repair during infancy is associated with a higher incidence of recoarctation. The recommended age for elective surgical repair in asymptomatic children is 4 to 5 years, but if upper extremity pressures approach 140 to 150 mm Hg, then repair is performed earlier (Graham, 1984). There is a trend toward earlier repair to prevent or reduce the problem of persistent postoperative hypertension (Moss, 1983).

Surgical treatment consists of either resection of the coarcted portion with an end-to-end anastomosis of the aorta or enlargement of the constricted section using a graft of prosthetic material or a portion of the left subclavian artery. Because the defect is outside the heart and pericardium, cardiopulmonary bypass is not required and a thoracotomy incision is used.

Beyond early infancy the operative mortality is less than 1%. Late cardiovascular problems following repair include systemic hypertension, restenosis, mitral valve disease, bicuspid aortic valve, and possible bacterial endocarditis (Moss, 1979). After coarctectomy there may be symptoms of gastrointestinal disturbance, such as abdominal pain, distention, nausea, and vomiting. These are believed to be caused by increased blood pressure in vessels that have previously received blood under lower pressure. Careful attention to control of blood pressure and assessment of bowel sounds, abdominal distention, and tenderness must be implemented.

PULMONIC STENOSIS

Pulmonic stenosis is a narrowing at the entrance to the pulmonary artery (see Fig. 34-13). The valve may be normal but the raphae (divisions between the cusps) are fused so that blood flow through the valve is restricted or the valve may be malformed. Stenosis may also occur from infundibular hypertrophy. Pulmonary atresia is the extreme form of pulmonary stenosis in that there is total fusion of the commissures and no blood flows to the lungs.

Embryologic Development

Between the sixth and ninth weeks of gestation the pulmonic valve develops within the truncus arteriosus as the

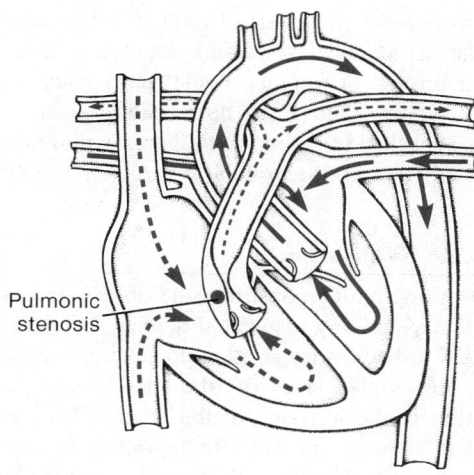

Fig. 34-13. Pulmonic stenosis. *Red arrows,* Saturated blood; *broken red arrows,* unsaturated blood.

result of enlargement of three tubercles within the lumen of the vessel. These enlargements eventually are hollowed out at their attachment to the wall of the pulmonary artery, giving rise to the valve leaflets. At about the same time the infundibulum (muscular narrowing that forms the right ventricular outflow tract) is being formed from the bulbus cordis. Failure of normal development of the three leaflets or the infundibulum results in pulmonic stenosis.

Altered Hemodynamics

When pulmonic stenosis is present, resistance to blood flow causes right ventricular hypertrophy. If right ventricular failure develops, right atrial pressure will increase; this may result in reopening of the foramen ovale, shunting of unoxygenated blood into the left atrium, and systemic cyanosis. If pulmonic stenosis is severe, congestive heart failure occurs, and systemic venous engorgement will be noted. An associated defect such as a patent ductus arteriosus partially compensates for the obstruction by shunting blood from the aorta to the pulmonary artery and into the lungs.

Clinical Manifestations

Symptoms depend on the degree of the stenosis and can range from only the presence of a murmur to cyanosis and congestive heart failure. A systolic ejection murmur is heard best over the second intercostal space at the left sternal border, radiating to the infraclavicular area. It is usually accompanied by a systolic thrill caused by the flow of blood through a narrowed orifice. Because of the prolongation of right ventricular ejection, the pulmonary component of the second heart sound is widely split. With severe stenosis the pulmonary component of the second heart sound becomes less distinct or totally disappears and pulmonic valve insufficiency may be present.

Children with moderate defects generally experience dyspnea and fatigue, especially on exertion, since blood flow to the lungs is insufficient to accommodate demands for increased cardiac output. Occasionally, severe pulmonary stenosis is associated with a small right ventricle and an intact ventricular septum. These infants develop a large right-to-left shunt through a foramen ovale; pulmonary blood flow is greatly reduced and acute heart failure ensues. Without immediate surgical intervention to increase pulmonary blood flow and relieve right ventricular obstruction, death will occur.

Diagnostic Evaluation

An echocardiogram demonstrates the obstruction to the pulmonary artery and any associated defects such as atrial septal defect. Cardiac catheterization documents increased pressure in the right side of the heart, and decreased oxygenation in the left side of the heart will be noted if a right-to-left shunt is present. Radiographic studies show a normal size heart, usually with normal or decreased pulmonary vascular markings and poststenotic dilation of the pulmonary artery. An electrocardiogram may show several changes, including right atrial and ventricular hypertrophy.

Therapeutic Management

Children with mild degrees of stenosis may not require surgical intervention but are followed medically with appropriate antibiotic administration to prevent bacterial endocarditis. Although children with severe stenosis may require surgery, many pulmonic defects are being successfully treated with *balloon angioplasty.* Through a percutaneous puncture (similar to cardiac catheterization) a catheter is inserted across the stenotic pulmonary valve into the pulmonary artery, and a balloon at the end of the catheter is inflated and rapidly passed through the narrowed opening. The procedure is associated with few complications, although transient bradycardia following balloon valvuloplasty can occur. Currently the long-range results of the repair are not known (Rocchini and Kveselis, 1984).

Surgical intervention consists of a pulmonary valvotomy. An incision in the right ventricle may be required to gain access to the stenotic area, so open-heart surgery is generally performed. In critically ill infants, a transventricular (closed) valvulotomy, known as the Brock procedure, may be used. Surgery is recommended whenever the child demonstrates a significant pressure gradient across the pulmonic valve, since continued right ventricular hypertension contributes to the development of right ventricular fibrosis.

The operative risk of elective pulmonary valvotomy is very low (less than 1%), but the risk of surgical intervention in critically ill neonates is higher. Long-term postoperative problems are uncommon, although the child is susceptible to bacterial endocarditis and residual pulmonary stenosis or insufficiency may occur, necessitating eventual valve replacement.

AORTIC STENOSIS

Aortic stenosis is a narrowing or stricture of the aortic outflow tract. *Valvular* stenosis, the most common type, is usu-

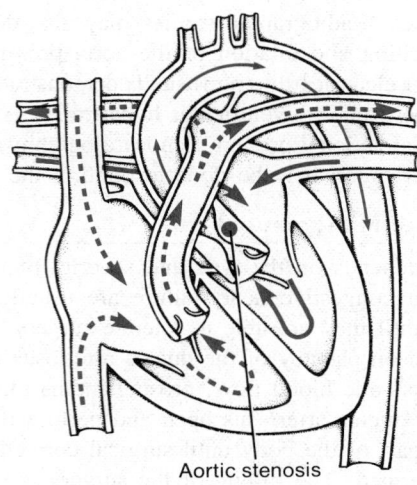

Fig. 34-14. Aortic stenosis. *Red arrows,* Saturated blood; *broken red arrows,* unsaturated blood.

ally caused by malformed cusps resulting in a bicuspid rather than tricuspid valve or fusion of the cusps (Fig. 34-14). *Subvalvular* stenosis is a stricture caused by a fibrous ring below a normal valve. *Supravalvular* stenosis occurs above the valve and is uncommon, but when present it is often seen as a part of a syndrome that includes mental retardation and elfin facies. Embryologic development of the valve is similar to that described for pulmonic stenosis.

Valvular aortic stenosis is a serious defect for the following reasons: (1) the obstruction tends to be progressive, (2) sudden episodes of myocardial ischemia or low cardiac output can result in sudden death, and (3) surgical repair rarely results in a normal valve. This is one of the rare instances in which strenuous physical activity may be curtailed because of the cardiac condition (Moss, 1979).

Altered Hemodynamics

A stricture in the aortic outflow tract causes resistance to ejection of blood from the left ventricle. The extra workload on the left ventricle causes hypertrophy. If left ventricular failure develops, left atrial pressure will increase; this causes increased pressure in the pulmonary veins, resulting in pulmonary vascular congestion (pulmonary edema).

Clinical Manifestations

A serious form of critical aortic stenosis may occur during the neonatal period. Symptoms of left ventricular failure and low cardiac output—respiratory distress, faint peripheral pulses, decreased urine output, and poor feeding—occur during the first 2 weeks of life. Children with less severe stenosis may not show signs of the defect until preadolescence. Clinical manifestations such as fainting, epigastric or anginal pain, exercise intolerance, and dizziness after prolonged standing may occur. Sudden death after exertion has been reported among children with aortic stenosis and is thought to be due to the development of sudden arrhythmias.

A murmur is typically produced by blood flow through the stenotic area. It is heard best at the upper right sternal border at the second interspace (aortic space) and radiates to the suprasternal notch, clavicular area, and neck. Sometimes it is transmitted along the left sternal border to the apex. It is usually associated with a thrill.

The second heart sound is characteristically affected. Because the closure of the aortic valve is delayed, the normal splitting of S_2 is narrowed. With severe stenosis the left ventricular ejection may be so prolonged that the closure of the aortic valve occurs simultaneously with or after that of the pulmonic valve. In the former instance there is no splitting. In the latter event the usual splitting of S_2 narrows with inspiration (the pulmonic component being delayed) and widens with expiration, a phenomenon referred to as paradoxic splitting.

Diagnostic Evaluation

Diagnosis may be made on the basis of the history and physical findings alone. Cardiac catheterization is necessary to determine the location and severity of the stenosis, especially in those children with minimal symptoms who are at risk for sudden arrhythmias. The catheterization is also diagnostic in terms of the surgical approach; if a thin membrane is present, this is easily removed with excellent results.

Radiographic studies may confirm left ventricular enlargement and a dilated aorta in the poststenotic area; increased pulmonary vascular markings and cardiomegaly may be noted if congestive heart failure is present. An electrocardiogram may show left ventricular hypertrophy in mild defects. Depression of the ST segment indicates myocardial ischemia and is a very important finding in determining the need for immediate surgery. Echocardiography may show a thick, poorly contractile left ventricular wall and an abnormal aortic valve.

Therapeutic Management

Surgical intervention for valvular aortic stenosis involves opening the valve orifice (commissurotomy). It may be indicated in children with minimal symptoms who demonstrate myocardial ischemia. Surgical repair of subvalvular aortic stenosis may involve incising a membrane if one exists or cutting the fibromuscular ring. If the obstruction is the result of a narrowing of the left ventricular outflow tract and a small aortic valve annulus, a patch may be required to enlarge the entire left ventricular outflow tract and annulus, an approach known as the *Konno* procedure (Konno and others, 1975). Supravalvular aortic stenosis may also involve incising a membrane if present; however, an extensive area of narrowing requires enlargement with a patch graft. All types of aortic valve stenosis require open-heart surgery and are performed through a median sternotomy.

Overall postoperative mortality varies with the type of valvular repair: it is much higher in infants with critical aortic stenosis than in older children who are treated on an elective basis. Unfortunately there is a high incidence in later life of restenosis following a valvotomy, which requires additional surgery on the valve or prosthetic replacement. If replacement is needed in young children, additional replacements will be required as the child grows. Because of the increased risk of bacterial endocarditis, antibiotic prophylaxis is necessary.

Cyanotic Defects

Cyanotic defects refer to those congenital heart anomalies in which desaturated blood mixes with blood saturated with oxygen in the systemic arterial circulation. Cyanosis is usually caused by right-to-left shunting of blood through an intracardiac communication, mixing of blood in a common chamber, and/or abnormal development of major blood vessels. Advancements in surgical techniques have significantly improved the prognosis for children with these defects.

TETRALOGY OF FALLOT

Tetralogy of Fallot (TOF) is the most common cyanotic heart defect. The anatomic definition includes four defects: (1) ventricular septal defect, (2) pulmonic stenosis, (3) an aorta that overrides the ventricular septal defect, and (4) right ventricular hypertrophy (Fig. 34-15). However, there are various degrees of the condition. For example, in some instances the pulmonary stenosis is so severe that there may be no anatomic connection between the right ventricle and the pulmonary artery. This condition is referred to as pulmonary atresia. The following discussion, however, is concerned with the classic pattern of TOF.

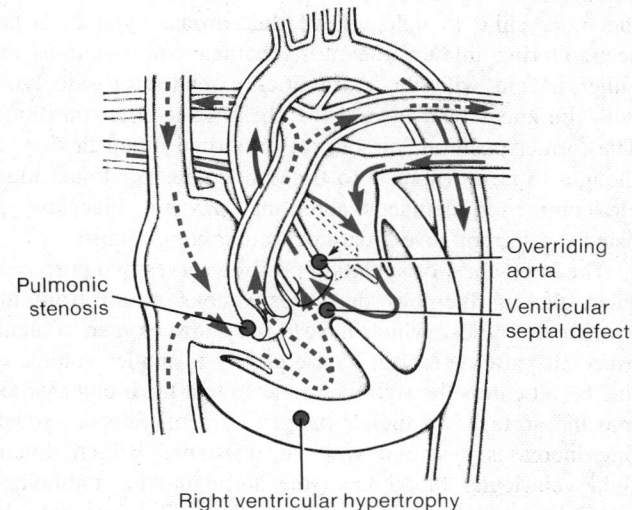

Pulmonic stenosis

Overriding aorta

Ventricular septal defect

Right ventricular hypertrophy

Fig. 34-15. Tetralogy of Fallot. *Red arrows,* Saturated blood; *broken red arrows,* unsaturated blood; *gray arrows,* mixed blood.

Embryologic Development

The development of the defects in tetralogy of Fallot is the result of abnormal embryologic development of the pulmonary infundibulum. This contributes to infundibular narrowing and a ventricular septal defect.

Altered Hemodynamics

Right-to-left shunting of blood through the ventricular septal defect occurs if significant pulmonic stenosis is present, since this causes an increased resistance to pulmonary flow. Consequently, the degree of cyanosis is related to the severity of the stenotic defect. Desaturated blood is then forced through the septal defect almost directly into the aorta. The increased workload on the right ventricle causes hypertrophy. The decreased pulmonary blood flow and right-to-left shunt increase the amount of desaturated blood reaching the systemic arterial circulation. The body attempts to compensate for the chronic hypoxia through polycythemia.

Clinical Manifestations

Newborns usually do not demonstrate cyanosis because of a patent ductus arteriosus that shunts blood to the lungs, bypassing the pulmonic stenosis. However, hypoxic spells become evident when the infant's oxygen requirements exceed the blood supply, usually during crying or after feeding. In addition, acute, severe paroxysmal hypercyanotic episodes may occur, in which the child suddenly becomes deeply cyanotic and hyperpneic and may lose consciousness or develop seizures because of the acute hypoxemia. The infant characteristically assumes a hypotonic extended position. The spells may be very brief or prolonged. Although hypercyanotic episodes can occur in other cyanotic defects, in TOF they are often called "blue" or "tet" spells and are thought to result from pulmonary infundibular spasm, which abruptly occludes all blood flow to the lungs.

In most instances surgical repair is done early and the characteristic squatting posture automatically assumed by the older child to help relieve the chronic hypoxia is not seen. During infancy the most characteristic positions are either flaccid with the extremities extended or side lying with the knees bent toward the chest (knee-chest position). The former position, in contrast to normal infant flexion, is thought to be a response to tissue hypoxia. Continual muscle contraction demands additional oxygen. Flaccidity is usually a sign of severe cardiovascular compromise.

The knee-chest or squatting position serves two purposes. First, flexing the legs decreases venous return from the lower extremities, which have a very low oxygen content, especially after exercise. Consequently a smaller volume of this blood enters the right ventricle so that the blood shunted into the aorta has a higher oxygen content. Second, squatting increases systemic vascular resistance, which diverts right ventricular blood from the aorta into the pulmonary artery, increasing pulmonary blood flow. This increases the amount of oxygenated blood in the left side of the heart and eventually into the systemic circulation (Perloff, 1978).

The child also demonstrates clubbing of the fingers (see

Fig. 31-7) and markedly delayed physical growth and development if the repair is delayed or if the child is severely cyanotic. There is some indication of cognitive impairment, especially perceptual-motor deficits, the longer the surgery is delayed, and these are believed to be sequelae of chronic hypoxemia (Newburger and others, 1984). Typically these children do not develop congestive heart failure because the pulmonary blood flow is decreased.

A pansystolic murmur is usually heard at the middle to lower left sternal border. It is usually associated with a thrill, which may be felt along the lower left sternal border. Typically the pulmonic component of the second heart sound is faint or absent, as a result of decreased flow through the pulmonic valve. As a result, a single second heart sound, caused by closure of the aortic valve, is heard.

Diagnostic Evaluation

A diagnosis is usually made on the history and physical findings alone. However, a cardiac catheterization and/or echocardiogram is performed to evalute the severity of the anatomic defects and cardiac changes. Laboratory tests determine the degree of polycythemia and arterial oxygen saturation.

Radiographic studies reveal a "boot-shaped" or "golf-club–shaped" configuration of heart and great vessels. Right ventricular hypertrophy is noted, and the left ventricle may be small because of the decreased pulmonary venous return. The pulmonary artery is typically small in size. Pulmonary vascularity is normal or decreased.

Hematologic tests are performed to evaluate the severity of polycythemia. The red blood cell count is elevated (above 6 million/mm^3), the hematocrit is high (above 55%) as a result of both the absolute increase in erythrocytes and the increased ratio of red blood cells to plasma, and hemoglobin levels are usually elevated. However, the change in hemoglobin may be falsely high, since the test measures the quantity of hemoglobin per 1 dl of whole blood, which contains excess numbers of red blood cells, not the quantity of hemoglobin within each cell. Because of the body's demand for iron during erythropoiesis, the child may actually be in a state of iron-deficiency anemia despite the usual laboratory findings in polycythemia. The red cell indices, especially the mean corpuscular hemoglobin (MCH), more accurately reflect the true hemoglobin levels. (See Chapter 35 for a discussion of these tests.)

Therapeutic Management

The current trend is to repair the defects in TOF early; the exact timing depends on the child's overall condition and the size of the pulmonary arteries, but elective repair is usually performed between 18 and 36 months. Indications for earlier repair include increasing cyanosis with the hematocrit approaching or exceeding 60% or the systemic oxygen saturation falling below approximately 75%. In children with minimum cyanosis and mild hypercyanotic episodes, propranolol (Inderal) may be administered to relieve infundibular spasm and allow the child an opportunity to grow

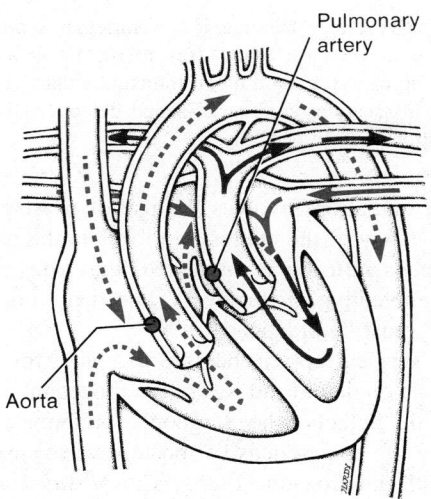

Fig. 34-16. Transposition of the great vessels. *Red arrows,* Saturated blood; *broken red arrows,* unsaturated blood; *gray arrows,* mixed blood.

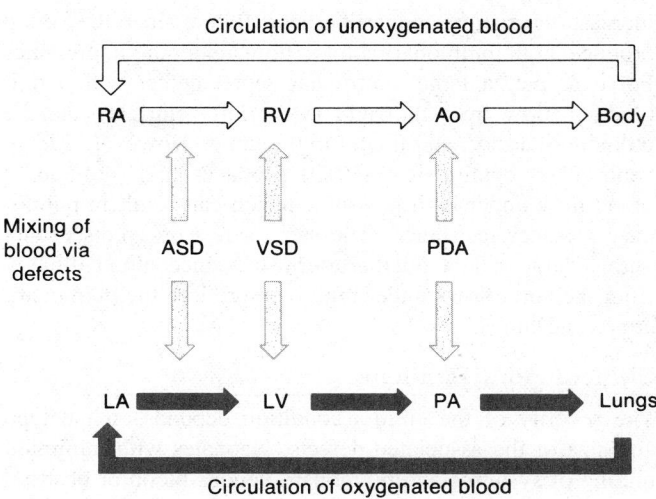

Fig. 34-17. Hemodynamics in transposition of great vessels.

before attempting corrective repair (Graham, 1984). In addition, these children are usually placed on supplemental iron to prevent iron-deficiency anemia, which may precipitate paroxysmal hypercyanotic spells, and they are kept well hydrated to decrease the risk of thrombic emboli. They require antibiotic prophylaxis for bacterial endocarditis. If they are hospitalized and have an intravenous infusion, it is imperative that no air enter the line since systemic venous blood may shunt directly into the aorta and the air may cause a cerebral air embolus (Hazinski, 1984).

Complete repair involves closure of the ventricular septal defect and resection of the infundibular stenosis, possibly with a pericardial patch to enlarge the right ventricular outflow tract. The procedure requires a median sternotomy and the use of cardiopulmonary bypass.

In infants whose pulmonary arteries are not large enough to accommodate the increased blood flow once the ventricular septal defect is closed, a palliative procedure may be done to increase pulmonary blood flow. The construction of a shunt serves the same purpose as the ductus arteriosus—to increase the flow of blood to the lungs by bypassing the pulmonic stenosis. Several palliative procedures have been devised but currently the preferred procedure is the *Blalock-Taussig* or *modified Blalock-Taussig anastomosis,* which creates a communication between the right or left subclavian artery and the ipsilateral pulmonary artery. Because of the higher resistance in the systemic circulation, blood flows from the subclavian artery to the pulmonary artery and to the lungs for oxygenation. The small diameter of the subclavian artery (as opposed to the aorta) automatically restricts the volume of blood flow to the pulmonary artery. This procedure sacrifices the brachial and radial pulse on the affected side, and the hand initially may be slightly cooler and paler until collateral circulation develops.

The operative mortality for total correction of TOF in children beyond the neonatal period is less than 5%. How-

ever, total correction is a misnomer because late complications are common and include residual ventricular septal defects, pulmonary insufficiency, and conduction disturbances. In particular sudden death has been reported in approximately 7% of individuals following TOF repair (Katz and others, 1982).

TRANSPOSITION OF THE GREAT VESSELS

By definition, transposition of the great vessels (TGV) refers to a condition in which the pulmonary artery leaves the left ventricle and the aorta exits from the right ventricle (Fig. 34-16). Obviously this type of circulation is incompatible with extrauterine life because the body receives only desaturated blood and progressive hypoxemia will develop. For survival the parallel circuits must communicate to allow adequate mixing of saturated blood in the pulmonary circulation and desaturated blood in the systemic circulation. This is accomplished through associated defects such as septal defects or a patent ductus arteriosus (Fig. 34-17).

Embryologic Development

From the third to the fourth weeks of gestation the truncus arteriosus is divided into the aorta and pulmonary artery. There is a spiral growth of the truncoconal ridges (ridges from the truncus and the conus or ventricular infundibulum), which eventually results in correct anatomic placement of the great vessels. If a disruption occurs in the spiral growth, the vessels are transposed to the opposite ventricle.

Associated Defects and Hemodynamics

The most common defect associated with TGV is a patent foramen ovale. At birth there is also a patent ductus arteriosus, although in most instances this closes beyond the neonatal period. Another associated anomaly may be a ventricular septal defect. However, presence of these defects can increase the risk of congestive heart failure since they often produce high pulmonary blood flow under high pressure. For example, a large ventricular septal defect will permit blood to flow from the right to the left ventricle, into the pulmonary artery, and finally to the lungs. However, a large ventricular septal defect (VSD) produces high pulmonary blood flow under high pressure, which can result in pulmonary vascular resistance. The same series of events occurs with a large patent ductus arteriosus, since blood directly from the aorta flows under high pressure into the pulmonary artery and lungs.

Clinical Manifestations

The severity of the child's condition depends on the type and size of the associated defects. Neonates with minimum mixing of systemic and pulmonary venous blood or obstruction to pulmonary blood flow are severely cyanotic at birth. Those with large septal defects or a patent ductus arteriosus may be less severely cyanotic but develop symptoms of congestive heart failure during the first weeks of life. In these infants the only signs at birth may be cyanosis after crying or feeding and progressive hyperpnea. However, hypercyanotic episodes can occur and are thought to be the result of an increased oxygen demand that the cardiovascular system cannot meet.

There is no murmur associated with simple TGV and if one is present, it is characteristic of the associated defects. Cardiomegaly from right and left ventricular hypertrophy may be evident a few weeks after birth. Signs of congestive heart failure (see p. 1489) will be present in those infants with a large ventricular septal defect.

Diagnostic Evaluation

Definitive diagnosis is made on the findings of echocardiography. Cardiac catheterization, especially selective angiography of the ventricles, may be used to delineate the exact communication between the systemic and pulmonary circulations and also permits the performance of a balloon atrial septostomy (see below). Radiographic studies may reveal right and left ventricular hypertrophy and increased pulmonary vascularity. An electrocardiogram also demonstrates ventricular enlargement. Laboratory studies are helpful in assessing the degree of cyanosis and acidosis.

Therapeutic Management

Both palliative and corrective surgical procedures can be performed. The objective of the palliative approaches is to prevent pulmonary vascular resistance and congestive heart disease until the child is able to tolerate complete cardiac repair. There are several palliative procedures:

1. Enlargement of an existing atrial septal defect by pulling a balloon through the defect (balloon septostomy) during a cardiac catheterization (Rashkind procedure) (preferred procedure unless corrective repair using Senning approach is planned)
2. Creation of a systemic-pulmonary shunt if pulmonic stenosis is present (Blalock-Tarrearg anastamosis)
3. Pulmonary artery banding if a ventricular septal defect is present to decrease blood flow to the lungs and increase shunting of oxygenated blood intraventricularly to the aorta
4. Surgical creation of an atrial septal defect (Blalock-Hanlon operation) (rarely performed)

Medical palliation involves the use of prostaglandins to maintain patency of the ductus arteriosus in the newborn. If an intravenous infusion is employed, the same precautions regarding preventing air in the IV line that were discussed under TOF must be practiced.

Several surgical approaches are available for correction of TGV. The choice of the reparative procedure depends on the anatomic defects, the surgeon's preference, and the availability of comprehensive postoperative management (Malinowski and Elixson, 1985). The *Mustard* or *Senning* operation involves the creation of an intraatrial baffle to tunnel or divert systemic venous blood to the mitral valve (and the left ventricle and pulmonary artery) and divert pulmonary venous blood to the tricuspid valve (and the right ventricle and aorta). Therefore the operation does not attempt to transplant the transposed arterial vessels but reverses the function of the atria. An advantage of the Senning operation is the use of patient's own atrial septum to create the baffle rather than pericardium or prosthetic material, which is used in the Mustard operation. The use of little or no foreign material allows for growth of the biologic baffle.

Another approach is the *Jatene* operation, which involves switching the great vessels to their correct anatomic placement and reimplanting the coronary arteries. It is a technically difficult procedure because the coronary arteries must be removed from the aorta before the switch is performed and then they must be reimplanted into the aorta at its new location. Reimplantation of the coronary arteries is critical to the infant's survival, and they must be reattached without torsion or kinking to provide the heart with its supply of oxygen.

A fourth surgical option is the *Rastelli* procedure, which is the operative choice in infants with TGV, VSD, and severe pulmonic stenosis. It involves closure of the VSD with a baffle, directing left ventricular blood through the VSD into the aorta. The pulmonic valve is then closed and a conduit is placed from the right ventricle to the pulmonary artery, creating a physiologically normal circulation. Unfortunately, this procedure requires multiple conduit replacements as the child grows.

The optimum time for the repair is controversial, but it is generally recommended that it be done before 1 year of age. Mortality following repair is influenced by the type of surgical procedure, complexity of the lesion, maturity of the infant, and degree of pulmonary vascular changes. Mortality risks may be summarized as follows (Gutgessel, Garson, and McNamara, 1979): a mortality of about 10% in the neonatal period, up to 15% risk of death between balloon septostomy and baffle repair, an operative mortality of about 10% or higher with a ventricular septal defect, and a late postoperative mortality of 8%. There is also significant morbidity associated with repair, although the long-term problems of the various procedures are unknown. For example, there is concern for right ventricular failure and tricuspid valve insufficiency from the constant high systemic pressures created in these structures by the intraatrial baffle procedures. A long-term benefit of anatomic correction may be elimination of this potential problem because the left ventricle becomes the systemic ventricle. Complications associated with the various procedures are summarized in Table 34-2.

TRUNCUS ARTERIOSUS

Truncus arteriosus results from failure of normal septation and division of the common trunk into the pulmonary artery and aorta. As a result, a single vessel arises from both ventricles and may receive blood for the pulmonary, systemic, and coronary circulations. There are four major types of truncus arteriosus:

Type I A single pulmonary trunk arises near the base of the truncus and divides into the left and right pulmonary arteries
Type II The left and right pulmonary arteries arise separately from the posterior aspect of the truncus
Type III The pulmonary arteries arise independently and from the lateral aspect of the truncus (Fig. 34-18)
Type IV No main pulmonary artery exists and the pulmonary arterial circulation is supplied from the systemic arterial circulation through collateral vessels of the bronchial arteries

Embryologic Development

The embryologic development of truncus arteriosus is similar to that described for transposition of the great vessels.

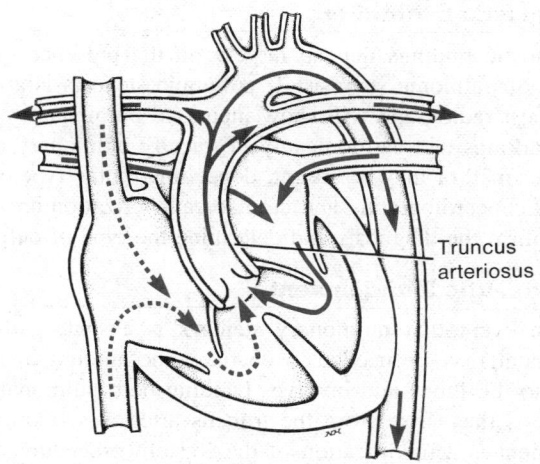

Fig. 34-18. Truncus arteriosus. *Red arrows,* Saturated blood; *broken red arrows,* unsaturated blood; *gray arrows,* mixed blood.

However, in this defect septation of the common trunk fails to occur altogether. In addition, since the septum of the truncus arteriosus normally fuses with the bulbar ridges, which eventually meet with the endocardial cushions and membranous portion of the ventricular septum to divide the ventricles, arrested truncal septation results in a ventricular septal defect.

Altered Hemodynamics

Blood ejected from the left and right ventricles enters the common artery and flows either to the lungs or to the aortic arch and body. Since the pressure in the combined ventricles is high, the blood flow to the lungs may be increased, unless stenosis of the pulmonary arteries is present. Other indications of this defect are a harsh systolic murmur heard at the lower left sternal border and a single second heart sound, caused by the presence of only one semilunar valve.

Clinical Manifestations

Clinical manifestations depend on the source and volume of the infant's pulmonary blood flow and the presence of other intracardiac anomalies. The infant without pulmonary stenosis often demonstrates mild or moderate cyanosis within the first days of life, which worsens upon crying or exertion. However, as pulmonary vascular resistance falls, the lungs receive an increased volume of blood and signs of severe congestive heart failure develop. If pulmonic stenosis is present, the cyanosis is severe, particularly once the patent ductus arteriosus begins to close. However, these infants are less likely to develop congestive heart failure.

A harsh systolic ejection murmur is heard along the left sternal border as a result of the VSD and is usually accompanied by a thrill. Opening of the truncal valve may produce a click immediately after the first heart sound. If pulmonary blood flow is increased, the child may demonstrate bounding pulses and a widened pulse pressure.

Table 34-2 Complications associated with surgical correction of transposition of great vessels

Mustard or Senning
   Arrhythmias (may produce sudden death)
   Superior and/or inferior vena caval obstruction
   Baffle leaks or obstruction
   Tricuspid regurgitation
   Right ventricular failure (late)
   Pulmonary venous obstruction (late)

Jatene
   Coronary artery insufficiency
   Pulmonic outflow obstruction
   Aortic outflow obstruction

Rastelli
   Arrhythmias
   Conduit obstruction
   Risks related to conduit replacement
   Residual ventricular shunts
   Obstruction to left ventricular outflow tract

Data from Malinowski, P., and Elixson, E.: Transposition of the great arteries, Crit. Care Nurs. 5(3):35-48, 1985.

Diagnostic Evaluation

Diagnostic findings depend largely on the presence or absence of pulmonic stenosis. If pulmonic stenosis is absent, the chest radiograph will show increased pulmonary vascular markings and cardiomegaly. Typically pulmonary arteries are small or may be absent, depending on the type of defect. Echocardiography and cardiac catheterization are done to confirm the diagnosis and determine the type of defect.

Therapeutic Management

In the event that pulmonary stenosis is absent, palliative treatment may be needed to decrease the amount of blood flow to the lungs and involves banding both pulmonary arteries as they arise from the truncus arteriosus. Corrective treatment is a modification of the Rastelli procedure; it involves closing the ventricular septal defect so that the truncus arteriosus receives the outflow from the left ventricle, excising the pulmonary arteries from the aorta, and attaching them to the right ventricle by means of a prosthetic valve conduit.

The success of corrective surgery depends on the child's age and the severity of existing pulmonary vascular disease. Elective repair is recommended during infancy or early childhood to prevent severe congestive heart failure, severe growth failure, or increasing pulmonary vascular disease. Postoperative complications include persistent heart failure, arrhythmias, and residual ventricular septal defects. These children require repeated operations to replace the conduit as its size becomes inadequate in relation to the children's growth.

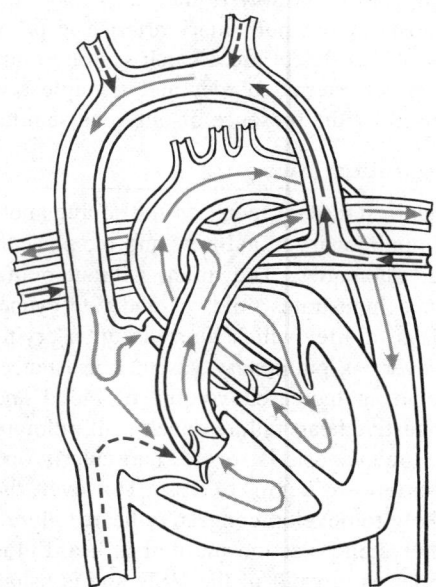

Fig. 34-19. Supracardiac total anomalous pulmonary venous connection. *Red arrows,* Saturated blood; *broken red arrows,* unsaturated blood; *gray arrows,* mixed blood.

TOTAL ANOMALOUS PULMONARY VENOUS CONNECTION

Total anomalous pulmonary venous connection (TAPVC), also called total anomalous pulmonary venous return (TAPVR) or total anomalous pulmonary venous drainage (TAPVD), is a rare defect characterized by the abnormal connection of the pulmonary veins to the systemic venous circuit (right atrium or various veins draining toward the right atrium, such as the superior vena cava or innominate vein) instead of the left atrium. Usually the pulmonary veins come together to form a channel close to the left atrium before their attachment to the right atrium or vein. The abnormal attachment results in desaturated blood being returned to the right atrium and mixed blood shunting from the right to the left through an arterial septal defect (ASD) or a patent foramen ovale. The type of TAPVC is classified according to the pulmonary venous point of attachment as:

Type 1, supracardiac Attachment above the diaphragm, such as to the superior vena cava (most common form) (Fig. 34-19)

Type 2, cardiac Direct attachment to the heart, such as to the right atrium or coronary sinus

Type 3, subdiaphragmatic or **infradiaphragmatic** Attachment below the diaphragm, such as to the inferior vena cava (most severe form)

Type 4, mixed lesions

Embryologic Development

Beginning in the third week of gestation, the pulmonary venous drainage system develops. In the common atrium there is an outpouching known as the common pulmonary vein. It grows to join the splanchnic plexus, which is in communication with the lung buds, the umbilical vitelline veins, and the cardinal veins. Eventually these veins lose their connection with the splanchnic plexus, leaving them to drain into the left atrium through the common pulmonary vein. Gradually the common pulmonary vein is absorbed and the four veins drain directly into the left atrium. Any disruption in this process necessitates the development of another route of communication between the common pulmonary vein and the heart.

Altered Hemodynamics

The right atrium receives all the blood that normally would flow into the left atrium. As a result, the right side of the heart hypertrophies, whereas the left side, especially the left atrium, may remain small. An associated atrial septal defect allows systemic venous blood to shunt from the higher pressured right atrium to the left atrium and into the left side of the heart. As a result the oxygen saturation of the blood in both sides of the heart (and ultimately, in the systemic arterial circulation) is the same. If the pulmonary blood flow is large, pulmonary venous return is also large and the amount of saturated blood is relatively high. However, if there is obstruction to pulmonary venous drainage, pulmonary venous return is impeded, pulmonary venous pressure rises, and pulmonary interstitial edema develops and eventually contributes to congestive heart failure. Subdiaphragmatic and, to a lesser extent, supracardiac types are often associated with obstruction to pulmonary venous drainage.

Clinical Manifestations

Most infants with TAPVC develop cyanosis early in life, although children with the cardiac or supracardiac types may have symptoms similar to those seen in ASD. The degree of cyanosis is inversely related to the amount of pulmonary blood flow—the more pulmonary blood, the less cyanosis. Consequently, the symptoms become worse in the presence of pulmonary obstruction; once obstruction occurs, there is usually rapid deterioration of the infant's physical condition.

Auscultatory findings depend on the hemodynamics. A blowing systolic murmur from tricuspid regurgitation may be heard at the lower left sternal border. A continuous murmur or venous hum may be present from blood flow through the anomalous venous channels. Because the right side of the heart is hyperdynamic, a gallop rhythm is common.

Diagnostic Evaluation

The chest radiograph reveals increased pulmonary vascular markings and right atrial and ventricular enlargement, although both findings will be altered by pulmonary venous obstruction. The electrocardiogram shows right ventricular hypertrophy and the echocardiogram demonstrates the abnormal connections. The cardiac catheterization provides evidence of the changes in oxygen saturation of the blood within various chambers and vessels and angiography identifies the site of the pulmonary venous connection.

Therapeutic Management

Palliation involves the Rashkind balloon septostomy to ensure an unobstructed interatrial communication. The surgical approach varies with the anatomic defect; however, in general the common pulmonary vein is anastomosed to the left atrium, the ASD is closed, and the anomalous pulmonary venous connection is ligated. Any other defects, such as patent ductus arteriosus (PDA), are also repaired.

The success of corrective surgery depends on the location of the defect, absence or presence of pulmonary venous obstruction, and left ventricular function. The current trend is toward corrective repair during early infancy (Turley and others, 1980). Cardiac types are most successfully repaired because of ease in restructuring the channels and less chance of pulmonary vein obstruction. The subdiaphragmatic type has the greatest incidence of morbidity and mortality.

TRICUSPID ATRESIA

Tricuspid atresia is failure of the tricuspid valve to develop; consequently there is no communication between the right atrium and right ventricle (Fig. 34-20). Tricuspid atresia is also associated with right ventricular hypoplasia and de-

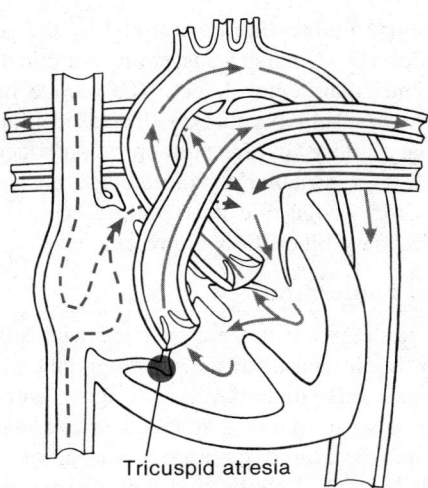

Fig. 34-20. Tricuspid atresia. *Red arrows,* Saturated blood; *broken red arrows,* unsaturated blood; *gray arrows,* mixed blood.

fects, such as septal defects, that allow some shunting of blood to the left side of the heart, then back to the right ventricle or pulmonary artery. About a quarter of these children also have transposition of the great vessels and as many as half have pulmonic stenosis.

Embryologic Development

At about the fifth week of gestation the tricuspid valve is formed by the progressive meeting of the anterior and posterior endocardial cushions, a segment of the interventricular septum, and the ventricular muscle. Any disruption in this process results in a valve deformity, in this case complete absence of valvular tissue. In addition, the decreased blood flow to the right ventricle during fetal life results in right ventricular hypoplasia.

Altered Hemodynamics

At birth the presence of a patent foramen ovale (or other atrial septal opening) permits blood to flow across the septum into the left atrium; as a result complete mixing of saturated and unsaturated blood occurs in the left side of the heart. The patent ductus arteriosus allows blood to flow to the pulmonary artery for oxygenation into the lungs. A ventricular septal defect allows a modest amount of blood to enter the right ventricle and pulmonary artery for oxygenation. Usually pulmonary blood flow is diminished.

Clinical Manifestations

The degree of cyanosis depends on the amount of pulmonary blood flow. Severe cyanosis, dyspnea, anoxic spells, and signs of congestive heart failure are evident early during infancy, especially if blood flow to the lungs is restricted by a closing patent ductus arteriosus. If the child survives later into infancy, systemic consequences of cyanosis and polycythemia may develop.

Auscultatory findings are determined by the presence of associated defects. A harsh pansystolic murmur usually indicates a ventricular septal defect. The second heart sound may be narrowly split because of decreased blood flow to the pulmonary artery, or the pulmonic component may be absent when no ventricular septal defect is present. Pulmonary findings of congestive heart failure occur early if increased pulmonary blood flow is present.

Diagnostic Evaluation

Laboratory findings are those associated with any cyanotic defect (hypoxemia and acidosis). Radiographic studies usually reveal a small, underdeveloped right ventricle, large atria (which give the heart a rounded or apple-shaped appearance), and decreased pulmonary vascularity. Echocardiography is helpful in confirming the presence of tricuspid atresia. An electrocardiogram shows significant right atrial and left atrial and ventricular enlargement. Confirmation of the diagnosis is made by cardiac catheterization, which reveals flow of right atrial blood to the left atrium, inability to enter the right ventricle, and presence of associated defects, such as TGV, VSD, and pulmonic stenosis.

Therapeutic Management

Palliative treatment is the same as for tetralogy of Fallot (pulmonary-to-systemic artery anastomoses) to increase blood flow to the lungs. If the atrial septal defect is small, an atrial septostomy is done during cardiac catheterization. Some children have increased pulmonary blood flow and require pulmonary artery banding to lessen the volume of blood to the lungs.

Total correction is now possible by converting the right atrium into an outlet for the pulmonary artery. This is called the *Fontan procedure* and involves placement of a tubular conduit with or without a valve between the two and closing the atrial septal defect. The Fontan procedure physiologically corrects tricuspid atresia by preventing any mixing of systemic blood in the left atrium and shunting the entire venous blood to the lungs for oxygenation. This operation is most effective in children with normal left ventricular function, pulmonary artery anatomy, and vascular resistance, who are able to delay surgery until approximately 4 or 5 years of age (Graham, 1984). While initial results have been encouraging, long-term survival and morbidity must await future studies.

INOPERABLE CARDIAC DEFECTS

Despite the advances in corrective cardiac surgery there still remain a number of congenital heart anomalies for which no successful corrective procedure exists. The most common inoperable cardiac defect is hypoplastic left heart syndrome, a spectrum of uniformly fatal congenital cardiovascular malformations—underdeveloped left ventricle and aortic and/or mitral valve stenosis or atresia. Experimental palliative procedures are being attempted, but the long-term results are unknown and it is improbable that the heart could sustain normal activity should the child survive.

Heart Transplantation

In an attempt to cure these unfortunate infants, heart transplantation is being attempted. Cardiac xenotransplantation (cross-species transplant) using a baboon heart has been performed when a suitable human heart was not available and may prove to be an important adjunct to care of these infants while an allograft (same-species) donor is located (Bailey and others, 1985). While human heart transplants have been performed in infants, there are serious long-term problems. Aside from the initial concerns of rejection, the heart recipient must receive large doses of immunosuppressant drugs, such as steroids, azathioprine (Imuran), antithymocyte globulin (ATG), and cyclosporine, which can cause serious and complex additional problems. For example, steroids suppress growth, which is a major consequence when the drug is administered to infants. All of the drugs depress the immune system, rendering the infant highly susceptible to life-threatening infections. Aside from the physical problems, heart transplantation and drug maintenance are extremely costly—the average cost of the transplant operation and follow-up during the first year approaches $130,000 (Pennock and others, 1982) and monthly medication bills can amount to $1000. Because of the shortage of suitable heart donors, the same ethical questions are of concern here as in other major organ transplants (see Questions and controversies, p. 1293, on renal transplants).

Nursing Care of the Family and Child with Congenital Heart Disease

When a child is born with a severe cardiac anomaly, the parents are faced with the immense psychologic and physical tasks of adjusting to the birth of a child with special needs. The reactions and nursing interventions required to support the family differ little from those discussed in Chapters 11 and 22. Since corrective surgery is increasingly being performed at an earlier age, the interventions are primarily directed toward the family of an infant who has a serious heart defect that requires home care before definitive repair and toward preparation and care of the child and family when heart surgery is performed.

OBSERVE FOR INDICATIONS OF CHD

Nursing care of the child with a congenital heart defect (CHD) begins once the diagnosis is suspected. However, in some instances symptoms suggestive of a cardiac anomaly are not present at birth or, if manifest, are so subtle as to be missed. Many heart defects are not evident until postnatal circulatory changes occur, such as closure of a patent ductus arteriosus or fall in pulmonary vascular resistance.

Since the onset of symptoms may be gradual, the child may curtail his activity so that the signs of exercise intolerance are less obvious. However, a careful history yields important clues to this change. For example, infants are normally extremely mobile and their energies are directed toward learning gross motor skills. Most infants suck vigorously and fall asleep after finishing a feeding. It is very unusual to hear of a child who prefers to sit rather than crawl or walk or who falls asleep shortly after beginning a feeding. Likewise, a child who needs frequent rests or naps after limited play periods may also be exhibiting exercise intolerance. Such histories should alert the nurse to assess cardiac function.

Other clues, already discussed on p. 1451, are a history of retarded weight gain; poor feeding habits, especially the need to pause during feeding; poor suck; difficulty in coordinating sucking, swallowing, and breathing; frequent respiratory infections; cyanosis; and any unusual posturing, such as squatting. Since parents may not view any of these findings as abnormal, the nurse must specifically ask about them during a physical assessment.

Another indication of heart defects is murmurs. In Chapter 7 the usual distinguishing characteristics between innocent and organic murmurs are discussed. Nurses who perform primary health assessments must be knowledgeable of the differences in order to correctly refer children with heart murmurs of possible organic origin to a cardiologist. There has been controversy over informing parents of innocent murmurs, since some physicians believe that the parent may be unduly worried and transfer that concern to overprotectiveness of the child. However, this problem is most often avoidable by stressing to parents that although a murmur was heard, no heart disease is present, no further cardiac study is needed, and the heart is normal (Folger, 1981).

SUPPORT THE FAMILY

Helping families adjust to the diagnosis involves several principles: (1) allowing the family a period of time to grieve for the loss of a perfect child, (2) assessing the level of the parents' and child's understanding of the heart, (3) helping the family cope with the effects of the defect, and (4) fostering family patterns of interaction that enhance the optimum growth and development of each of its members.

Allow Period of Grief

Once parents learn of the heart defect, they are initially in a period of shock, followed by high anxiety, especially fear of the child's death. This reaction may occur soon after the child's birth or at a later period in life. Whatever its timing, the family needs a period of grief before assimilating the meaning of the defect. Unfortunately the demands for medical treatment may not allow this, necessitating that the parents be informed of the condition in order to give informed consent for diagnostic/therapeutic procedures. The nurse can be instrumental in supporting parents in their loss, assessing their level of understanding, supplying information as needed, and helping other members of the health team to understand the parents' reactions.

Severely distressed newborns usually remain in the hospital. This can seriously affect parent-infant attachment unless parents are encouraged to hold, touch, and look at their child. The symptoms of cyanosis, dyspnea, and extreme fatigue may discourage parents from physical contact with the infant. However, every effort must be made by health personnel to foster attachment, especially when parents may be required to continue the care at home. (See Chapter 10 for suggestions in promoting attachment between parents and their hospitalized newborn.)

A congenital heart defect may constitute a long-term family crisis. Frequently, the continuing unremitting stresses of care—physical exhaustion, financial costs, emotional upset, fear of death, and concern for the child's future—are not fully appreciated by those caring for the family. Even when the child's condition is stabilized or corrected, the family may need to make new adjustments in their life-style. Introducing them to other families with similarly affected children can help them adjust to the daily stresses.* As one mother remarked, "By the time my child was discharged from the nursery, I felt confident in her care. I thought I had my home organized for her arrival. However, I really didn't know what to expect. I only wish that I could have spoken to another mother who had gone through the experience. Every time I saw my child turn blue or gasp for air, I felt inadequate and scared. That only added to the difficulty of coping with all the physical things I had to do." This mother later worked with other parents who had newborns with heart defects.

Assess Level of Understanding

Once parents are ready to hear about the heart condition, it is essential that they be given a clear explanation, based on their level of understanding. Fundamental ignorance of the cardiovascular system may be a major reason for lack of parental understanding, and it is usually helpful to review the basic structure and function of the heart before describing the defect (Kaden and others, 1985). One method of simplistically illustrating heart defects is to depict the heart as a four-room structure (house) that normally has exits and entrances (representing the valves and vessels) (Fig. 34-21). A septal defect can then be illustrated as an abnormal entrance to another room that allows mixing of blood that should remain only in one room. Although this explanation may not suffice for all parents, it does allow for clarification of basic information. It is certainly more explanatory than the usual colloquial expression, "a hole in the heart," for septal defects, since this is frequently misinterpreted to mean that blood leaks out of the heart. Parents appreciate receiving written information about the specific defect.[†]

Another fact to remember is that different health personnel may convey the same information using different diagrams and medical terms. To prevent this from becoming a problem (which often happens when several members of a health team work with a family), the same type of diagram

---

*Some local American Heart Associations have organized parent groups.
[†]A booklet that can be given to parents is "If your child has a congenital heart defect," available from the American Heart Association, 7320 Greenville Ave., Dallas, TX 75231.

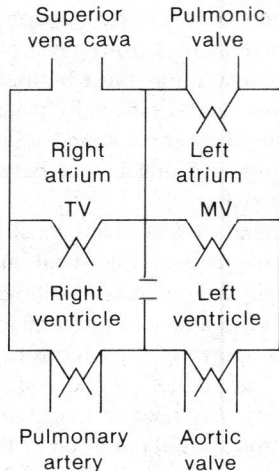

Superior vena cava   Pulmonic valve

Right atrium   Left atrium

TV   MV

Right ventricle   Left ventricle

Pulmonary artery   Aortic valve

Fig. 34-21. Use of four-room structure to explain cardiac defect; in this instance an abnormal opening *(red)* between ventricles.

should be used and the parents should write down any terms that are unclear or ask for clarification. Sometimes it is helpful to provide the family with a glossary of frequently used words for reference. For example, one mother told the nurse that her child had three heart defects—a hole in the heart, an abnormal opening, and a defect between two ventricles. She understood that the surgeon was to repair all of them at the same time and wondered if her child's heart "could stand it." The nurse clarified that all three terms meant the same thing. However, no expression had any meaning until the nurse showed the mother where the abnormal opening was and how it would be repaired.

Parents are primarily interested in two kinds of information—prognosis and surgery (Kupst and others, 1976). They are frequently upset about indefinite answers to either. The family should be assured that the health care team will be honest in keeping them informed of the child's condition and of decisions regarding future procedures and treatments. The nurse needs to be aware of alterations in the plan of therapy in order to convey similar messages to the family.

Children of various ages have different ideas about their heart (Reif, 1972). Children between 4 and 6 have heard about the heart, know its approximate anatomic location in the chest or back, illustrate it as valentine shaped, and characterize it by the sounds tick-tock, thump, and so on. Children 7 to 10 have a clearer concept of the heart, realizing that it is not shaped like a valentine and that it has vital functions, such as, "It makes you live." However, their knowledge of its integrated functions to pump blood through a system of vessels to all parts of the body is still hazy. By the age of 10 or 11 children have a much more involved concept of the heart with knowledge of veins, valves, pumping action, and circulation. They are beginning to appreciate why death occurs when the heart stops.

Information given to the child must be tailored to the child's developmental age and, as the child matures, the level of information upgraded to meet the child's present

cognitive level of understanding. Preschoolers need basic information about what they will experience more than what is actually occurring physiologically. School-age children benefit from a concrete explanation of the defect. Use of the "house model" can be very effective. Preadolescents and adolescents often appreciate a more detailed description of how the defect affects their heart. Children of all ages need to express their feelings concerning the diagnosis.

For example, one 14-year-old girl who had been told that she had an atrial septal defect and was undergoing cardiac catheterization was well informed by her two physician parents. However, no one had asked the adolescent how she felt. Before the procedure, the nurse remarked, "I know you are aware of everything that is going to happen, but what do you think about all of this?" The child replied, "I really wonder if I may die." The nurse allowed her to express her unspoken fears. Later, when the nurse mentioned the conversation to her parents, they too remarked that despite all their knowledge of "low risks, complications, and mortality statistics," they too secretly worried for their child's welfare. This opened communication between the parents and child, allowing the youngster and parents to be optimally prepared for open-heart surgery.

Help Family Cope with Effects of Defect

Parents also need an explanation regarding the symptoms of the disease. Many children have few symptoms but may develop congestive heart failure. Therefore parents should be aware of early signs of worsening physical status, such as sweating, sudden weight gain, decreased exercise tolerance, and increased effort breathing. These symptoms need medical evaluation, but the family is assured the symptoms usually respond quickly to therapeutic intervention. Because of the anxiety typically associated with a heart defect, the nurse should be cautious in giving information that can increase the family's concern.

For those children with cyanotic heart disease, the family needs instruction regarding hypercyanotic spells. Watching a child turn cyanotic and dyspneic is frightening, and parents must be prepared for how to help the child. After a cyanotic/dyspneic episode, the child needs to rest and attain a position of comfort, usually side lying with knees flexed and head and chest elevated. He is kept warm to prevent increased metabolism and vasoconstriction. Most importantly, he should be kept calm. This requires treating the cyanotic spell casually to prevent transfer of parental emotions to the child. Supplemental oxygen may be helpful but is not always available. In selected instances cardiopulmonary resuscitation may be taught to parents or another emergency plan may be implemented (Cloutier and Measel, 1982), although some authorities suggest that all parents should know resuscitative care in case of any childhood emergency.*

---

*Home care instructions on performing cardiopulmonary resuscitation are available in Wong, D., and Whaley, L.: Clinical handbook of pediatric nursing, ed. 2, St. Louis, 1986, The C.V. Mosby Co.

Another area of parental concern is the child's level of physical activity. For children there is no need to restrict activity and the best approach is to treat the child normally and allow self-limited activity. Even in infants, there is little need to prevent crying because it usually ceases when hypoxia increases. Deliberately attempting to prevent crying should be avoided because it can establish a maladaptive parental pattern of relating to the infant. There are exceptions to self-determined activity and they primarily involve strenuous recreational and competitive sports. Although these decisions need to be made on an individual basis, children with aortic stenosis or insufficiency are usually not permitted to engage in strenuous activity (Freed, 1984).

Children with CHD require good nutrition. The infant may need to be fed small amounts of formula every 2 to 3 hours to ensure adequate nutrition. If several nighttime feedings are required, the nurse should discuss with parents the need to share the responsibility and enlist the help of others whenever possible. Often parents do not feel confident leaving the child in anyone else's care because they believe that the child will be upset by a change in routine and that the baby-sitter will be unable to cope with the cyanosis and dyspnea. This often sets up a trap for parents, especially mothers, who become locked into the child's care with no relief. Although the parents' fears are justified, they can be minimized by gradually teaching someone (a reliable relative or neighbor) how to care for the child and by seeking baby-sitters who are more familiar with these children, such as nursing students and retired nurses. It also may be helpful to introduce parents to other families with children who have heart disease so that as a group they can share such responsibilities.

Feeding the cyanotic infant in the knee-chest position has been found to help the infant suck more strongly, ingest more, tire less, establish more predictable feeding times, and consequently gain weight (D'Antonio, 1979). The infant is placed on the parent's lap and is positioned on his side facing away from the parent with the knees flexed on the abdomen. However, this position is awkward and many parents dislike the lack of eye contact with the infant. Other helpful techniques include using a soft "premie" nipple, frequent burping, and pauses for rest.

Since growth retardation is a result of inadequate caloric intake, the nurse assists parents in ways of providing highly nutritious foods. Sometimes protein/calorie/fat supplements are prescribed, such as polycose or MCT oil. Some supplements can be fed separately while others are mixed with milk or formula. Another approach is early feeding of solids with a spoon or concentrating the formula by adding less water. For example, a 24-calorie formula can be prepared by diluting the 13-ounce can of liquid concentrate with 9 ounces of water instead of 13 (Cloutier and Measel, 1982).

Children with severe cardiac defects are often anorexic. Encouraging them to eat can be a tremendous challenge. Because of the parents' concern over eating, children learn early to manipulate parents through eating, such as making unrealistic demands for foods that are not available. The nurse advises parents of this potential problem, since prevention yields greater success than intervention. For example, the child should be given a choice of available high-quality foods. Suggestions for encouraging sick children to eat are discussed on p. 1115.

The family also needs to be knowledgeable regarding the therapeutic management of the disorder, especially in terms of the medications that the child is receiving. Specific drugs, such as digoxin and diuretics, are discussed later in the chapter in relation to congestive heart failure and bacterial endocarditis. Supplemental iron may be prescribed to prevent iron deficiency and ensure maximum hemoglobin levels. Parents are taught the correct procedure for giving drugs* and cautioned to keep them in a safe area to prevent accidental ingestion.

Foster Growth-Promoting Family Relationships

The effect of a child with a serious heart defect on the family is complex. No member, regardless of the degree of positive adjustment, is unaffected. Mothers frequently feel inadequate in their mothering ability because they gave birth to a child with a defect and are unable to keep their child well. For example, they may view the child's failure to feed as evidence of their failure, not as a direct consequence of the disease. Mothers often feel constantly exhausted from the pressures of caring for these children and the other members of the family.

Likewise fathers and siblings may feel neglected and resentful, a reaction that is similar to the feelings of family members toward other chronic conditions (see Chapter 22). These feelings are normal—they are the expected consequences of a chronic illness. However, they can be lessened by encouraging family members to discuss how they feel toward one another, encouraging parents to arrange "time off" from home responsibilities, and fostering normal expectations from all the siblings.

The need to maintain discipline and set consistent limits cannot be overemphasized. Using behavior modification techniques, either in the form of concrete awards, such as a favorite food, or social reinforcement, such as approval, can be effective. However, it is most beneficial if employed *before* the child learns to control the family. Therefore guiding parents toward the need for discipline while the child is in infancy is necessary to prevent problems later on. It also teaches these children how to tolerate frustration and delayed gratification, which so often are lacking because of immediate satisfaction of all their needs.

Another problem that may develop within family relationships is the child's overdependency. This is often the result of parental fear that the child may die and overcompensation through what has been termed the benevolent overreaction (see p. 929). The best approach to dealing with this dilemma is prevention. Parents need guidance to

---

*Home care instructions on giving medications to children are available in Wong, D., and Whaley, L.: Clinical handbook of pediatric nursing, ed. 2, St. Louis, 1986, The C.V. Mosby Co.

Nursing Care Summary: The Child with Congenital Heart Disease

	NURSING GOALS	NURSING INTERVENTIONS	EXPECTED PATIENT/FAMILY OUTCOMES
HP-HMP	**Infection: potential for** **Risk factors: debilitated physical status**		

	Prevent infection	Avoid contact with infected persons
		Provide for adequate rest
		Be alert for signs of complications
		    Congestive heart failure (CHF) (p. 1489)
		    Maintain high index of suspicion regarding digitalis toxicity
		    Increased respiratory effort—tachycardia, retraction, grunting, cough, cyanosis
		    Hypoxemia—cyanosis, restlessness, tachycardia
		    Cerebral thrombosis—compensatory polycythemia (in cyanotic heart disease) is particularly hazardous when child is dehydrated
		    Cardiovascular collapse—pallor, cyanosis, hypotonia
			Infant remains free of infection
			
			*Evidence of complications is detected early and interventions are implemented without delay

HP-HMP	**Injury: potential for (defective development, tendency toward fluid accumulation in lungs)** **Risk factors: prenatal insult to cardiac tissues**		
	Observe for signs or symptoms of congenital heart disease	Be alert for physical and behavioral characteristics that indicate congenital heart disease Report suspected heart murmurs	*Signs of cardiac disease are detected early and appropriate actions implemented

	Recognize signs of complicating factors	Be alert for signs in
		    History—poor weight gain, poor feeding, exercise intolerance, unusual posturing, or frequent respiratory tract infections
		    Physical assessment—color, pulse (apical and peripheral), respiration, blood pressure, and examination and auscultation of chest	

N-MP	**Nutrition, alteration in: less than body requirements** **Etiology: fatigue, reduced circulation to tissues**		

	Maintain nutrition
	    Prevent potassium depletion
	    Improve iron-carrying capacity of blood
		Ensure well-balanced diet
		Help plan a diet with potassium-rich foods to prevent depletion
		Encourage iron-rich foods in the diet
			Infant or child consumes an adequate amount of nutrients (specify amounts)

	Reduce fluid retention	Discourage food with high- or added-salt content	Infant exhibits no evidence of nutritional deficiency
	Facilitate feeding	Administer small, frequent meals Encourage child to eat (see p. 1115)	Child consumes sufficient food (specify)
A-EP	**Activity intolerance** **Etiology: imbalance between oxygen supply and demand**		
	Reduce energy expenditure	Feed infant slowly Allow for frequent rest periods Encourage quiet games and activities Caution family to consult with child's cardiologist before taking child on an airplane or to a higher altitude Schedule nursing activities to allow for maximum rest Help child select activities appropriate to his age, condition, and capabilities Avoid extremes of environmental temperature	Infant rests quietly and breathes easily Child determines and engages in activities commensurate with his capabilities

*Nursing outcome

NURSING GOALS	NURSING INTERVENTIONS	EXPECTED PATIENT/FAMILY OUTCOMES

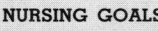

SP-SCP   Self-concept, disturbance in: body image
Etiology: activity intolerance, feeling of differentness

| Improve self-concept | Allow child to express feelings about heart condition
Explore child's feelings regarding his disorder
Clarify misconceptions child may have acquired
Support positive coping mechanisms and extinguish negative ones | Child openly discusses feelings and concerns about his condition |

SP-SCP   Fear
Etiology: serious illness

| Reduce family's fears and anxieties | Explore family's concerns and feelings of irritation, guilt, anger, disappointment, inadequacy
Help family distinguish between realistic fears and eliminate unfounded fears
Discuss with parents their fears regarding
  Child's symptoms, such as pounding heart, cyanotic spells, irritability
  Dealing with child's anxiety about his condition
  Fear of dreadful developments
  Fear of death
  Fear of tests and procedures | Family is able to discuss their fears and concerns |

CPP   Knowledge deficit
Etiology: unfamiliarity with disease and prescribed treatments

Increase family's understanding of child's condition	Assess family's understanding of diagnosis Reinforce and clarify physician's description of child's condition and the prognosis Explore their feelings regarding prescribed therapies Reinforce and clarify physician's explanation of suggested diagnostic procedures and palliative or corrective surgeries	Family demonstrates an understanding of the disease (specify)
Help family cope with symptoms of disease	During dyspneic/cyanotic spell, place child in knee-chest position, with head and chest elevated or over the shoulder Keep child warm; encourage rest and sleep Decrease child's anxiety by remaining calm Encourage family to include others in child's care to prevent their own exhaustion Assist family in determining appropriate physical activity and disciplining methods for child	Family copes with child's symptoms in a positive way Child engages in appropriate activities for age and condition (specify)
Help child understand his defect	Assess level of understanding Use visual aids to describe heart defect Provide written information Keep technical information simple Convey same information as other health team members Stress that prognosis and plans for surgery may change Base explanation of heart on child's developmental level of understanding	Child demonstrates an understanding of his disease and its implications
Prepare for diagnostic tests and surgery	Explain or clarify information presented to family by physician and surgeon Prepare child and parents for procedure Assist with family's decision regarding surgery Explore feelings regarding palliative or corrective surgery	Family demonstrates an understanding of tests, surgery, etc. (specify learning and manner of demonstration) Family expresses feelings and concerns

Continued.

Nursing Care Summary: The Child with Congenital Heart Disease—cont'd

NURSING GOALS	NURSING INTERVENTIONS	EXPECTED PATIENT/FAMILY OUTCOMES
RRP **Family process, alteration in** **Etiology: situational crisis (child with a defect, hospitalization of child)**		
Help family and child adjust to diagnosis	Allow period of grief Accept initial shock and disbelief Repeat information as often as necessary Encourage family to express their concerns Foster parent-child attachment, especially of newborn Introduce parents to other families who have similarly affected child	Family demonstrates an attitude of acceptance and adjustment (specify)
Foster growth-promoting family relationships	Assess family's support systems Reinforce positive coping mechanisms Encourage family members to discuss their feelings about each other Impress upon parents importance of providing as normal a life as possible for affected child	Family demonstrates positive, growth-promoting behaviors
	Help family feel adequate in their parental roles by emphasizing growth and developmental progress of their child Help family foster child's development by stimulating child to age-appropriate goals consistent with his activity tolerance	Child engages in activities appropriate for his age and capabilities
Prepare family for home care of infant or child	Encourage family to participate in care of child Administration of medications Feeding techniques Interventions for conserving energy and those directed toward relief of frightening symptoms Signs that indicate complications Where and whom to contact for help and guidance Anticipate need for further information and support	Family demonstrates the ability and motivation for home care of the infant
	Refer family to local chapter of the American Red Cross for instruction in cardiopulmonary resuscitation	Family members learn cardiopulmonary resuscitation technique
Support family	Be available to family Refer to family support groups such as those provided through local branch of the American Heart Association See also The family of the hospitalized child, p. 1081	Family becomes involved with local support groups
Assist in providing financial support	Investigate state and local agencies that may be able to provide financial assistance, such as state, Special Child Health Services, American Heart Association† Collaborate with social service agency to ensure optimum utilization of community services	Parents avail themselves of assistance
RRP **Social isolation** **Etiology: hospitalization, frequent illness, activity intolerance**		
Promote interpersonal relationships	Encourage relationships with children his own age Arrange for continued family contacts during hospitalization Promote development of a positive self-image	Child engages in age-appropriate activities within the limits of his capabilities

---

Nursing Interventions Related to Medical Management

Assist with diagnosis
  Order or draw blood for CBC
  Perform or assist with electrocardiography
  Order and/or assist with x-ray examinations, echocardiography, angiography, fluoroscopy, ultrasonography
  Prepare child and family for and assist with cardiac catheterization
Prevent anemia
  Administer iron preparations as prescribed

Prevent fluid accumulation
  Administer diuretics as prescribed
  Provide low-sodium diet
Prevent hypokalemia
  Provide high-potassium diet
  Administer supplemental potassium as prescribed
Palliate or correct defects
  Perform needed preoperative procedures and tests

---

recognize the eventual hazards of continuing dependency and protectiveness as the child grows older, and the nurse can assist parents in learning ways to foster optimum development. For example, the parents should stimulate the infant toward feasible goals, such as holding his own bottle, learning to amuse himself for short periods rather than always being held, and picking up finger foods. Unless parents are helped to see what activities the child can do, they may focus on physical limitations and encourage dependency.

The child also needs opportunities for social development. These children do not need to be isolated from known sources of infection or prevented from playing with other children because of concern regarding overexertion. Such practices only add to the dangers of increased dependency in the home environment. Parents need to be encouraged to seek appropriate social activity, especially before kindergarten. One approach is to locate families with a similar problem and form a play group. One parent found that her child's first contact with other children was during hospitalization for diagnostic procedures. As she observed the beginning interaction between the children, she introduced herself to the other parents and on discharge continued a friendship with a family who had a child with neurologic impairment.

PROVIDE PREOPERATIVE CARE

Few surgical procedures demand as much planning for preoperative preparation and postoperative care as heart surgery. The general principles for preparing children for procedures, such as surgery, are discussed in Chapter 27, and the reader is urged to review them. This discussion focuses on those measures specific to the cardiovascular procedure. There are technical differences between closed- and open-heart surgery, since the latter involves the use of cardiopulmonary bypass (extracorporeal circulation). Consequently there are some additions to physical care postoperatively in open-heart surgery. However, in general the term *heart surgery* is used regardless of the actual procedures and the same nursing interventions apply.

The child is usually admitted to the hospital 1 to 2 days before surgery for diagnostic tests. This interval allows time to prepare the child and parents for surgery, although with the present concern on health care costs, less time may be appropriated for admission procedures. With infants the focus of preoperative teaching is directed to the parents. Since a great deal of information is conveyed, it is important to schedule teaching to prevent information overload and to be alert to signs of overload (see p. 1080). There is no well-documented research on how extensive preoperative preparation should be, and the nurse must use considerable judgment in planning the aspects of teaching. Preparation can be divided into three categories: equipment, environment, and procedures. The following discussion assumes that the child and/or parents have an understanding of the defect.

Introduce the Child and Family to the Environment

Ideally, when the child is admitted he should be assigned to one nurse for each shift. In some institutions the nurse who will care for the child postoperatively in the intensive care unit is also assigned to the child at admission to facilitate forming a relationship with the family and to share preoperative teaching, such as introduction to the recovery room and intensive care unit. To increase familiarity all nurses should call the child and parents by name and refer to themselves by name. Wearing an obvious name tag reinforces this point. Postoperatively the family will feel more at ease recognizing familiar names, faces, and voices.

If a visit to the recovery room and/or intensive care unit is planned, it should take place when there is least activity in the area, the parents can accompany the child, and the child is well rested. Usually the day before surgery is ample time to allow the child to ask questions and to prevent undue fantasizing about the experience. If a visit is included in the teaching plan, the nurse can use a book that explains the environment to the child (for a list of resources, see p. 1100).

During the visit to the intensive care unit, the child and parents should experience everything that directly affects the child's care, such as the sounds of electrocardiogram monitors, oxygen tents, and placement of the bed. All positive, nonfrightening aspects of the environment are emphasized, such as the play area, visitors' section, pictures or mobiles in the room, or television. If it is a pediatric intensive care unit, the nurse can introduce the family to other children who may be recovering from surgery. The child should be protected from the frightening sights in the unit, and equipment not in his view postoperatively, such as equipment located behind or below the bed, needs less attention. The child and parents are encouraged to ask questions or to explore further any equipment in the room, but they should not be pushed to assimilate more information than they appear to be tolerating.

Familiarize the Child and Family with Equipment

Some of the equipment, such as the stethoscope, blood pressure apparatus, and thermometer, will already be familiar to the child and parents. However, the nurse emphasizes that procedures involving such equipment will be done more frequently. If continuous monitoring devices are used, such as for temperature, the child is told about the placement of the sensor on the skin. If blood pressure cuffs are to be left on, he should also be aware of this.

Types of equipment that are new to many families are the oxygen mask, oxygen tent, suction, chest tubes, endotracheal tubes, incentive spirometers, nasogastric tube, and intravenous tubing. Each of these is shown to the child and demonstrated either on him or on a doll, if he appears ready. With a younger child the use of miniaturized equipment that is suitable for use with a doll or puppet is often less anxiety producing than the actual samples. If other children in the unit have an intravenous infusion or are in oxygen tents, the older child may benefit from seeing them, but this must be planned carefully to avoid frightening the child.

Several intravenous lines are inserted perioperatively: (1) an ordinary line for infusion of fluids, inserted in a peripheral vein, (2) a venous pressure line, inserted into the right subclavian or jugular vein, and (3) an arterial line for direct measurement of arterial pressure. Younger children need only know the location of each tubing and that both arms may be restrained to prevent dislodging the tubing. Older children may appreciate knowing the reason for each infusion, especially when venous and arterial measurements are taken. Since the lines are inserted during surgery, they are not painful, only uncomfortable because of the restricted movement.

The type and size of dressing the child will have after surgery are discussed and can be shown on a doll. Usually one of two types of incisions is made: a median sternotomy, which splits the sternum, or a lateral thoracotomy, which extends from the midaxillary line to the scapula. In either instance the incision and dressing are extensive. Frequently no sutures are visible because subcuticular, absorbable sutures may be used. If this is done, it should be pointed out to the child and parents, who may fear the incision will open. Sometimes a butterfly incision is used for cosmetic reasons in girls instead of the regular median sternotomy.

The child may be told about chest tubes and their purpose in draining fluid from around the heart and lungs. He can be shown a picture of the equipment used for drainage, or the setup can be assimilated by attaching one end of the tubes to a doll with a chest dressing and the other end to small bottles (such as empty medicine vials). The nurse stresses that the child must move even though the tubes are in place. It can be demonstrated on the doll that the tubing is long enough to permit turning. Since this information may be anxiety producing, it is best left to the end of teaching or eliminated if the child appears too anxious.

An endotracheal (ET) tube is inserted during surgery and may be left in place for ventilatory assistance and tracheobronchial suctioning. However, it may be best to prepare older children for the ET tube only if *prolonged* ventilatory support is planned. The ET tube can be presented as a "breathing tube" or straw that is placed in the nose or mouth (Rushton, 1983). The nurse explains that while the tube is in, the child will feel it in his throat and he will not be able to talk, but nothing is wrong. The child can express his desires by pointing or using a picture communication board. The nurse stresses that the tube will be removed as soon as possible, often during the first postoperative day.

Preoperative physical care differs little, if any, from that for any other surgery and is discussed in Chapter 27. The child should be assured that his parents will be there when he wakes up, and they should be allowed to accompany him as far as possible to the operating suite (see Questions and controversies, p. 1107). After all the equipment and procedures have been explained, it is important to talk about "getting well" and going home. If a doll was used during the preparatory session, the tubes can be removed and the doll can be dressed in regular clothes in anticipation of discharge.

Assess Preoperative Behaviors and Physiologic Status

There are several observations that, when made preoperatively, facilitate care planning postoperatively. Although it is not always possible to implement the same type of care after surgery as before the operation (for example, maintaining the child's usual sleep patterns) every effort should be made to decrease additional sources of stress in the postoperative period.

Vital signs. Vital signs and blood pressure are recorded at rest and with activity to establish a baseline of the child's energy tolerance. Temperature is carefully evaluated, since an elevation may be the first indication of a preoperative infection, which ordinarily is a contraindication to surgery because it increases the risk of postoperative infective endocarditis. Any sudden change in vital signs is reported to the physician immediately. For example, an increase in pulse and respirations during periods of rest may be an early sign of congestive heart failure.

Sleep/awake patterns. Sleep and activity patterns are recorded to allow the child optimum rest during the postoperative period and maximum tolerance to stress. With increasing evidence of the importance of identifying an individual's biorhythms, a sleep and activity record illustrates those periods when the child is most tolerant of activity and most in need of sleep. For example, the body's ability to withstand stress is correlated with the usual diurnal pattern of hydrocortisone secretion. Normally hydrocortisone secretion is highest between 6 and 9 AM and lowest between 9 PM and midnight. By maintaining the usual sleep/awake periods, these levels are maintained so that stressful procedures performed in the morning are best tolerated by the body (Stephenson, 1977).

Elimination. Elimination patterns are observed to avoid constipation postoperatively. The child's toilet habits, including expressions for urinating or defecating, are recorded on the care plan. If the child uses a potty-chair, this is also noted. The child should be allowed every opportunity to continue newly learned skills and maintain bodily control. Children who are toilet trained should not be forced to regress by having diapers placed on them. It is often surprising how quickly children recover from extensive heart surgery and how helpful it is for them to remain independent.

Weight and height. Accurate weight measurement is imperative, since it is the basis for calculation of postoperative medication dosages and evaluation of fluid status. Height is also recorded on admission for accurate determination of body surface area.

Laboratory values. Preoperative laboratory values are also important to note to identify problems before surgery, such as fluid and electrolyte imbalance, low hemoglobin/hematocrit levels in anemia, or high white blood cell counts in infections. In evaluating anemia, it is necessary to compare hemoglobin and hematocrit levels to the total red blood cells because this affects the values.

Fluid intake. Fluid intake should be recorded before surgery to estimate the child's usual fluid consumption and to identify which fluids are preferred. Postoperatively fluids are usually restricted to prevent circulatory overload. By identifying the child's pattern of intake, especially in relation to sleep/awake periods, intake restrictions can be planned to allow fluids when the child usually prefers them.

PROVIDE POSTOPERATIVE CARE

Immediate postoperative care is usually provided by specially trained nurses in intensive care units. Many of the procedures, such as arterial and central venous pressure monitoring and the observations related to vital functions, require advanced educational training (the reader should refer to critical care texts, such as Hazinski [1984] for further information). However, nurses caring for the child before surgery and during the convalescent period need to be familiar with the major principles of care.

Observe Vital Signs and Arterial/Venous Pressures

Vital signs and blood pressure are recorded frequently until stable. Heart rate and respirations are counted for 1 full minute, compared with the electrocardiogram monitor, and recorded with activity. The heart rate is normally increased after surgery. The nurse observes cardiac rhythm and noti-

fies the physician of any changes in regularity.

At least hourly the lungs are auscultated for breath sounds. Diminished or absent sounds most likely indicate an area of atelectasis, which necessitates further medical assessment. Auscultation guides the nurse's selective use of postural drainage and percussion to those pulmonary lobes most in need of it. It also allows a more objective evaluation of effective ventilation.

Temperature changes are usual during the early postoperative period. Hypothermia is expected immediately after surgery from hypothermia procedures, effects of anesthesia, and loss of body heat to the cool environment. During this period the child is kept warm to prevent additional heat loss. Infants may be placed under radiant heat warmers. During the next 24 to 48 hours the body temperature may rise to 37.7° C (100° F) or slightly higher as part of the inflammatory response to tissue trauma. After this period an elevated temperature is most likely a sign of infection and warrants immediate investigation for probable cause.

Intraarterial monitoring of blood pressure is almost always used following open-heart surgery, because residual vasoconstriction after the use of cardiopulmonary bypass makes indirect blood pressure readings less reliable and because intraarterial monitoring permits continuous rather than intermittent observation. A catheter is passed into the radial artery or the dorsalis pedis or posterior tibial artery and the other end is attached to an electronic monitoring system, which provides a continuous recording of the blood pressure on an oscilloscope. Continuous blood pressure readings are compared with those taken indirectly with a sphygmomanometer, since a discrepancy between the two may indicate a change in peripheral vascular resistance, a malfunction in the electronic device, or human error in using the wrong size blood pressure cuff. The nurse also observes for potential complications of intraarterial monitoring, such as arterial thrombosis, infection, air emboli, or blood loss through the catheter. Prevention of each of these hazards is similar to care for any other type of infusion.

The intraarterial line is irrigated frequently or maintained with a low-rate constant infusion of heparinized saline to prevent clotting. The amount of irrigant is recorded as intake fluid. The dressing at the site is changed daily. In some institutions a bactericidal ointment is applied to the puncture site. If the child's condition remains stable, the arterial catheter is removed in 24 to 48 hours.

Central venous pressure (CVP) is often measured after heart surgery. This is a measurement of the pressure of the right side of the heart. Therefore it indicates right atrial filling pressure, right ventricular function, the relationship between blood volume (venous return) and cardiac output, and early signs of right-sided congestive heart failure. The central venous pressure catheter is inserted into the right atrium or threaded through a large vein into the superior vena cava or inferior vena cava and the other end is attached to a monitor.

The central venous pressure continually changes according to blood volume, heart rate, and myocardial function. If the blood volume decreases, such as in shock, the central venous pressure falls. If the efficiency of the left side of the heart decreases, the resistance to right ventricular ejection will ultimately result in an elevated central venous pressure but decreased intraarterial pressure. Congestive heart failure and/or hypervolemia raise the central venous pressure.

The complications of central venous pressure lines are similar to other infusions, with the addition of atrial arrhythmias from irritation of the atrial wall, hemothorax, pneumothorax, or hydrothorax from accidental puncture as the catheter enters the thorax, and fluid overload, since the intravenous line is kept patent by a continuous drip. The nurse observes for signs and symptoms indicative of each of these risks.

Movement of the central venous pressure catheter into the right ventricle can result in life-threatening ventricular arrhythmias and falsely elevated central venous pressure readings. Signs of migration are vigorous fluctuations of the manometer fluid with the heartbeat, which indicates placement in the right ventricle, or consistently elevated central venous pressure readings without further evidence of hypervolemia or congestive heart failure, which indicates entry into the right ventricle. The nurse alerts the physician to these signs. A chest radiograph or echocardiogram is necessary to confirm misplacement. Treatment is to withdraw the catheter until it is again in the right atrium. The catheter should be marked with tape close to the site of insertion to readily detect any further advancement or the length marked before insertion to detect migration.

Maintain Respiratory Status

If respirations are impaired, the child may temporarily be placed on a mechanical ventilator. Otherwise, he is kept in a humidified environment, such as an oxygen tent or oxygen hood, to liquefy secretions. The child is kept warm and dry, since excessive chilling from wet linens causes an increased metabolic need and consequent increased cardiac demand. The child is encouraged to cough, turn, and deep breathe at least hourly. Every measure is employed to enhance ventilation and decrease pain, such as splinting of the operative site and judicious use of analgesics. Although crying increases heart rate, it is beneficial in promoting deep respirations.

Postural drainage is done frequently, usually every 2 to 4 hours. It is helpful to have two nurses work together, one to position the child while the other percusses and vibrates. Since the procedure is uncomfortable, it is important to emphasize to the child the necessity of performing it and to clarify that the percussion, sometimes mistakenly viewed as hitting, is done to loosen secretions in the lungs and is not a form of punishment. The child is usually comforted by his parents, and if they wish to participate, they can be very helpful in positioning him.

Suctioning is performed as needed. Deep suctioning is performed carefully to avoid vagal stimulation (cardiac arrhythmias) and laryngospasm, especially in infants. Suctioning is intermittent and maintained for no more than 5 seconds at a time to prevent depleting the oxygen supply. Supplemental oxygen is administered with a manual resuscitator (Ambu bag) before and after the procedure. Heart rate is monitored after suctioning to detect changes in rhythm or rate, especially bradycardia. The child should always be positioned so that he faces the nurse, allowing for assessment of the child's color and tolerance to the procedure.

Chest tubes are inserted into the pleural and/or mediastinal space during surgery or in the immediate postoperative period to remove secretions and air in order to allow reexpansion of the lung. The chest tube is attached to a water-seal drainage system, usually a disposable type such as Pleurevac. The purpose of the underwater drainage is to prevent air from traveling up the tube into the pleural space, causing a pneumothorax. The nursing considerations are the same as those for adults and include the following essential interventions: (1) do not interrupt water-seal drainage unless the chest tube is clamped, (2) check for tube patency (fluctuation in the water-seal chamber, and (3) maintain sterility.

Drainage is checked hourly for color and quantity. Immediately postoperatively the drainage may be bright red, but afterward it should be serous. The largest volume of drainage occurs in the first 12 to 24 hours and is more copious in extensive heart surgery. Chest tube drainage greater than 3 ml/kg/hour for more than 3 consecutive hours is excessive and may indicate postoperative hemorrhage (Mills and others, 1984). The surgeon is notified immediately as cardiac tamponade can develop rapidly and is life threatening (see p. 1487).

Chest radiographs are taken when the tubes are inserted to check their location and after they are removed to evaluate the inflation of the lungs. Chest tubes are usually removed on the second to third postoperative day. Lung expansion is evidenced by decreased fluctuation in the tube and absence of drainage.

Removal of chest tubes is a painful and frightening experience. Analgesics such as morphine sulfate (0.1 mg/kg) should be given before the procedure. Children are forewarned that they will feel a sharp momentary pain. After e suture is cut, the tubes are quickly pulled out at the end of full inspiration to prevent intake of air into the pleural cavity. A purse-string suture (placed at the time the tubes were inserted) is pulled tight to close the opening and a petrolatum-covered gauze dressing is immediately applied over the wound and securely taped on all four sides to the skin so an airtight seal is formed. The dressing should be checked for signs of drainage, any evidence of infection, or loosening and the lungs auscultated for breath sounds.

Provide Maximum Rest

After heart surgery maximum rest should be provided to decrease the workload of the heart and promote healing. With a great many procedures and observations to be performed, this objective is met through organized nursing care, which is planned according to the child's usual activity/sleep patterns. The simplest way to ensure individualized, efficient, high-quality care is to plan at the beginning of the shift the nursing procedures to be done. For example, each hour is divided into 15-minute intervals and appropriate observations/procedures are scheduled. Periods of rest are identified. The schedule should be shared with parents to allow them to visit at the most advantageous times, such as after a rest period when no special treatments are anticipated.

Provide Comfort

Heart surgery is both a painful and a frightening experience for children, and comfort should be a primary nursing concern. Unfortunately, children are often poorly medicated for pain after surgery (see Questions and controversies, p. 1068), especially young children who are unable to verbally communicate their discomfort. During the initial 24 hours when an intravenous line is in place, narcotic analgesics, such as morphine sulfate, should be given intravenously on a regular schedule (not p.r.n.) for maximum pain control. Once the intravenous line is discontinued, analgesics should be given orally to avoid the additional trauma of an injection. If an intramuscular injection must be given, the child may benefit from an explanation that the ''little hurt'' from the injection will take away the ''bigger hurt'' from the operation. Every effort is made to minimize the discomfort of procedures, such as using a firm pillow or favorite stuffed animal placed against the chest incision during coughing, and performing treatments *after* pain medication is given, preferably at a time that coincides with the peak effect of the drug. Nonpharmacologic measures are employed to lessen the perception of pain (see p. 1071), and parents are encouraged to comfort their child as much as possible.

Monitor Fluids

Intake and output of all fluids must be accurately calculated. Intake is primarily intravenous fluids. However, the nurse must keep a record of fluid used to flush the arterial and central venous pressure lines or to dilute medications. Output includes hourly recordings of urine (usually a Foley catheter is inserted and attached to a closed collecting device), drainage from chest and nasogastric tubes, and blood drawn for analysis. Urine is also analyzed for specific gravity to assess the concentrating ability of the kidneys and to approximately assess the body's degree of hydration. The nurse measures pH to evaluate metabolic acidosis. Kidney failure is a potential risk from a transient period of low cardiac output and is most likely to occur in the presence of preexisting renal disease. The signs of kidney failure are decreased urine output (less than 1 ml/kg/hour) and elevated levels of blood urea nitrogen and serum creatinine (van Breda, 1985).

Fluids are restricted during the immediate postoperative period to prevent hypervolemia, which places additional demands on the myocardium, predisposing to cardiac failure. Two factors influence increased blood volume. In open-heart surgery the cardiopulmonary pump is primed with a large volume of fluid (usually electrolyte solution), which may greatly dilute the patient's blood. During circulation

through the body, some of this priming fluid diffuses into the interstitial spaces but postoperatively diffuses back into the systemic circulation.

In addition, the physiologic changes of open- or closed-heart surgery stimulate the adrenal cortex to secrete aldosterone, which increases renal reabsorption of sodium. This results in water retention but increased excretion of potassium. Concurrently the hypothalamus secretes additional antidiuretic hormone (ADH), which causes the distal and collecting tubules to reabsorb more water. Not only can this process result in hypervolemia, but it also may cause electrolyte imbalances, principally hypokalemia. Decreased potassium affects myocardial function and may increase the risk of arrhythmias. The nurse assesses electrolyte imbalances by observing for signs of hypokalemia and checking all blood electrolyte analysis reports.

Fluid requirements are based on the child's weight and body surface area. The child is weighed daily, and the same scale is used at approximately the same time each day to avoid errors in measurement. The child is usually given nothing by mouth for the first 24 hours. If an endotracheal tube is inserted, oral fluids are usually withheld until the child is extubated. Fluid restriction is usually imposed even when oral fluids are given. Therefore the nurse plans how many milliliters are allowed per 8-hour shift, basing this calculation on the child's preoperative drinking habits. For example, if the child is allowed 10 dl/24 hours, a typical fluid schedule might be 5 dl during the day shift, 3.5 to 4 dl during the evening shift, and 1 to 1.5 dl during the night shift. If additional or less fluid is taken on one shift, an adjustment is made during the next 8-hour period.

Plan for Progressive Activity

Fatigue and weakness are common after heart surgery, as a result of both the surgical trauma to the heart and sleep deprivation during the immediate postoperative period. However, moderate activity is essential to prevent pulmonary and vascular complications. Initially, turning, coughing, and deep breathing are sufficient to promote respiratory expansion. However, passive range of motion exercises, especially to the lower extremities, are instituted to prevent venous stasis. All infusion sites are inspected for evidence of thrombophlebitis and emboli. The areas are passively exercised to promote circulation.

A progressive schedule of ambulation and activity is planned, based on the child's preoperative activity patterns and postoperative cardiovascular and pulmonary function. For some children the ability to regain independence in self-care may be more of a priority than sitting up to read. Therefore the nurse conserves the child's energy for what is most important to him. Toys that were enjoyed before surgery are provided to encourage movement. It is important to plan the activity at times when the child is well rested, is comfortable (usually has had analgesic medication), and is not scheduled for any strenuous procedure or treatment immediately afterward.

Ambulation is initiated early, usually by the second postoperative day, when chest tubes, arterial lines, and assisted ventilatory equipment may be removed. The nurse begins ambulation for this child as for a child who had undergone any other postsurgical procedure, progressing from sitting on the edge of the bed and dangling the legs to standing up and to sitting in a chair. Heart rate and respirations are carefully monitored to assess the degree of cardiac demand imposed by each activity. Tachycardia, dyspnea, progressive fatigue, or arrhythmias indicate the need to limit further energy expenditure. Even if the child is able to ambulate to a chair with a moderate increase in heart rate, the nurse keeps in mind the effort required to return to bed. After ambulation a rest period is scheduled.

Provide Emotional Support

It is not uncommon for children to become depressed after surgery. This is thought to be caused by preoperative anxiety, postoperative psychologic and physiologic stress, and sensory overstimulation. Typically the disposition of the child improves on leaving the intensive care unit. (See care of the child in the intensive care unit, p. 1092.) The nurse should be aware of the possible reasons for such behavioral changes and manipulate the environment to accommodate the child's needs. The following example illustrates this point.

A child in the adult surgical intensive care unit became severely depressed and withdrawn postoperatively. She continually requested that the drapes be kept drawn around her bed. The nurse, realizing the sensory overload from the patient activity around the child, had her transferred to a private room in the unit. Almost immediately the child's mood improved. In 2 days she returned to her own room on the pediatric unit, where she recovered rapidly.

The child may also be angry and uncooperative after surgery as a response to the physical pain and to the loss of control imposed by the surgery and treatments. He needs an opportunity to express his feelings, either verbally or through activity. The nurse can be supportive by reassuring the child that the procedures that require cooperation, such as coughing and deep breathing, are difficult to perform, praising him for any effort he makes to cooperate, and refraining from expecting too much "courage" or "bravery." For example, rather than fostering cooperation with statements such as "Big boys can stand this pain," the nurse reassures the child that "Even the bravest of men cry when they hurt." With this approach the child is allowed to express his feelings with acceptance from the nurse, regardless of his emotional response.

The nurse also accepts any negative remarks from the child, realizing that pain has been inflicted on him. It is not unusual for children to tell nurses that they hate them during a treatment. Rather than becoming defensive or overly apologetic, nurses should reply that they understand why the child feels that way but that the treatment is necessary for his recovery and is *never* performed as a punishment. They can also help parents and other caregivers accept the child's

negativism by explaining that the outburst is a response to the treatment, not to the person.

The nurse can support the parents by being available for information and explaining all the procedures to them. The first few postoperative days are particularly difficult because parents see their child in pain and realize the potential risks from surgery. They often are overwhelmed by the physical environment of the intensive care unit and feel useless because they can do so little for their child. The nurse can minimize such feelings by including parents in caregiving activities if they wish, such as a partial bath, turning, or positioning for postural drainage; providing information about the child's condition; and being sensitive to their emotional and physical needs. The importance of their presence in making the child feel more secure is stressed, even if they cannot physically care for him.

Nurses in the intensive care unit should be aware of statements they make that can be misinterpreted by parents. For example, remarking that the electrocardiogram does not look good can immediately raise parental concern for their child's survival, when actually the nurse may be referring to the machine's functioning. Casual statements or jokes made by nurses and other members of the health team can be viewed as lack of concern for the child. Such misconceptions can be greatly lessened if one nurse assumes responsibility for the child's care and maintains constant communication with the family.

Observe for Complications of Heart Surgery

Several complications can occur after heart surgery, the majority of which are related to open-heart surgery and use of cardiopulmonary bypass. Many of the procedures discussed in the preceding paragraphs are aimed at preventing these problems. Only those that have not already been discussed are included in the following paragraphs. A serious complication, bacterial endocarditis, is discussed on p. 1496.

Hematologic changes. While passing through the heart-lung machine, blood is exposed to substantial trauma by direct contact with oxygen, mechanical action, foreign substances, and massive doses of anticoagulants. The result of this injury is red blood cell hemolysis and potential renal tubular necrosis, clotting abnormalities from decreased thrombin and prothrombin, heparinization of the blood during extracorporeal circulation, decreased platelets, and altered platelet aggregation.

Hemolysis of red blood cells results in blood loss and anemia, which may require packed red blood cell transfusion. The nurse monitors results of complete blood counts in order to identify the severity of the hemolysis. If transfusions are required, the child is closely observed for signs of reaction and fluid overload. The necessity of measuring urine output hourly has already been discussed.

Since blood clotting mechanisms are affected, signs of hemorrhage are watched for, especially frank bleeding from the chest tubes and a fall in arterial/venous pressures. Hemorrhage is more likely to occur in patients who have repair of cyanotic heart defects because of the physiologic thrombocytopenia associated with these defects.

Normally the filter and bubble trap on the machine remove air emboli, tiny clots, fat debris, and organisms from the arterialized (oxygenated) blood before its return to the body. However, impure blood entering the systemic circulation can cause fat emboli, thromboemboli, and infection anywhere in the body, but most importantly in the brain. Hepatitis and acquired immune deficiency disease from multiple donor transfusions during the bypass procedure are also a concern.

Cardiac changes. Cardiac failure may result from increased workload on ventricles that have been hypertrophied before surgery. Consequently, signs of heart failure are watched for, including elevation of the central venous pressure.

Low cardiac output syndrome and decreased peripheral perfusion can occur as a result of hypothermia or from inability of the left ventricle to maintain systemic circulation. The most important signs of adequate peripheral perfusion are good skin color, warm extremities, and strong pulses. Evidence of low cardiac output is similar to signs of shock, namely decreased blood pressure, decreased pulse pressure, cool extremities, metabolic acidosis, and oliguria.

Arrhythmias can result from electrolyte imbalance, especially hypokalemia, and surgical intervention of the septum or myocardium. The heart rate and rhythm are carefully monitored by observing the electrocardiographic pattern and by counting the apical pulse for 1 full minute. Dysrhythmias that impair cardiac performance are bradycardias (heart rate less than 80 beats/minute), tachycardia (ventricular rate greater than 180 to 200 beats/minute), extrasystole, or heart block. Epicardial pacing wires may be inserted during surgery for monitoring of cardiac arrhythmias postoperatively.

Cardiac tamponade is compression of the heart by blood and other effusion (clots) in the pericardial sac, which severely restricts the normal heart movement. A characteristic sign is *paradoxic pulse pressure,* in which the systolic pressure drops during inspiration because accumulated blood compresses the heart, resulting in a drop in cardiac output. Other signs include a rising venous pressure, falling arterial pressure, narrowing pulse pressure, dyspnea, cyanosis, apprehension, and a compensatory posture of sitting and leaning forward. Any evidence of this potentially fatal complication is immediately reported to the physician. Treatment consists of prompt pericardiocentesis to remove the blood. If active hemorrhage and coagulopathy are present, steps are taken to enhance blood clotting.

Pulmonary changes. Areas of atelectasis are common immediately after surgery as a result of deflation of the lung during cardiopulmonary bypass. Two other pulmonary complications are pneumothorax, especially caused by faulty chest tubes, and pulmonary edema, from increased pulmonary blood flow or heart failure. Signs of pneumothorax are persistent decreased breath sounds, sudden dyspnea, tachycardia, rapid, shallow respirations, cyanosis, and sometimes sharp chest pain. Signs of pulmonary edema are rales, wheezing, moist dyspneic respirations, tachycardia, cyanosis, and restlessness.

Neurologic changes. Cerebral edema and brain damage may occur during open-heart surgery. Although the exact cause is unknown, it is thought to be a result of tissue ischemia or emboli. The nurse checks the equality of strength and reflexes in both extremities for evidence of paralysis; assesses the pupil size, equality, and reaction to light and accommodation; and assesses the child's orientation to his environment. Any evidence of cerebral damage is immediately reported to the physician.

Postpericardiotomy syndrome. This syndrome of fever, leukocytosis, pericardial friction rub, and/or pericardial and pleural effusion can occur anytime the pericardium is opened, either in the immediate postoperative period or after surgery, typically around the seventh to twenty-first day. The cause is unknown, although theories of etiology include a viral infection, autoimmune response to myocardial tissue, or a reaction to blood in the pericardium. It is self-limited and is treated with rest, salicylates, and sometimes steroids.

Plan for Discharge and Home Care

Ideally discharge planning begins soon after admission for cardiac surgery and includes an assessment of the parents' adjustment to the child's altered state of health. As mentioned earlier, one of the most common parental reactions is overprotection, and the nurse needs to be aware of instances in which the family may need help in recognizing the child's improved health status. With surgical correction of heart anomalies occurring during infancy, there is less likelihood of this pattern of overdependency being firmly established.

The family needs clear instructions on the child's care at home, such as checking the chest wound for signs of infection and administering any medications prescribed. Almost all congenital heart defects require prophylactic antibiotics after surgery to prevent bacterial endocarditis, and some children may still have signs of congestive heart failure that must be managed medically. Most children do not have any activity restrictions, although this should be clarified with the cardiologist, especially in terms of resumption of strenuous activity. Parents also need guidance regarding when to seek medical care in the event of cardiac complications. Since postpericardiotomy syndrome may occur after discharge, the nurse alerts the parents to signs suggesting this, namely, unexplained fever, any chest pain, difficulty in breathing, or a loss of energy. It is best not to place undue emphasis on this syndrome to avoid creating anxiety over its occurrence.

Although there have been dramatic improvements in surgical correction of heart defects, it is still not possible to totally reverse many of the complex anomalies. For many children repeat operations are required to replace conduits or grafts or manage complications, such as restenosis. Consequently, the long-term prognosis is uncertain and full recovery is not always possible. For these families medical follow-up and continued emotional support are essential. The nurse can often serve as an important primary health professional and as a resource for referrals when needed.

Acquired Cardiovascular Disorders

Acquired cardiovascular disorders, as opposed to congenital heart disease, may occur as a result of a previously existing disease or defect, as a complication of an acute disease, or from unknown causes. The most common condition classified as an acquired cardiovascular disorder is congestive heart failure, usually as a complication of congenital heart disease. Bacterial endocarditis is a major concern either before or after the correction of most congenital heart defects. Rheumatic fever, once a common and serious sequela of streptococcal infection, has decreased dramatically in recent years. However, there is continuing concern regarding hypertension in children and Kawasaki disease, a serious disorder of unknown etiology that seriously can damage the cardiovascular system. Cardiomyopathy, once an invariably fatal disease if medical management was ineffective, is increasingly being treated with heart transplants. Nursing care often plays a critical role in the identification and supportive management of these cardiovascular disorders.

CONGESTIVE HEART FAILURE

Congestive heart failure (CHF) is inability of the heart to pump an adequate amount of blood to the systemic circulation to meet the body's metabolic demands. Causes of heart failure can be classified according to the following changes:

Increased volume, especially with left-to-right shunts that may cause the right ventricle to hypertrophy in order to compensate for the additional blood volume

Increased afterload (resistance against which the ventricles must pump when ejecting blood), primarily resulting from obstructive lesions, such as valvular stenosis or coarctation of the aorta

Decreased contractility, primarily factors that affect the contractility of the myocardium, such as cardiomyopathy or myocardial ischemia from severe anemia or asphyxia, heart block, acidemia, and low levels of potassium, glucose, calcium, or magnesium

High cardiac output demands, in which the body's need for oxygenated blood exceeds the heart's cardiac output (even though the volume may be normal), such as in obstructive lung disease, hyperthyroidism, and severe anemia. *Cor pulmonale* is the term applied to CHF that results from obstructive lung disease, such as cystic fibrosis

In children CHF occurs most frequently secondary to structural abnormalities that result in increased blood volume and pressure. It is a symptom caused by an underlying cardiac defect, not a disease in itself, since it is usually the result of an excessive workload imposed on a normal myocardium. The majority of children who experience CHF are infants, and more than 50% are younger than 1 month of age (Sulayman and Thilenius, 1981).

Pathophysiology

Heart failure may be theoretically divided into two classifications: right-sided or left-sided failure. In *right-sided failure* right ventricular function is suboptimal. Right ventricular end-diastolic pressure rises, causing increased central venous pressure and systemic venous engorgement. Systemic venous hypertension causes hepatomegaly and may cause edema in the extremities. In *left-sided failure* left ventricular dysfunction occurs and left ventricular end-diastolic pressure rises, resulting in increased pressure in the left atrium and pulmonary veins. The lungs become congested with blood, causing elevated pulmonary pressures and pulmonary edema.

Although each type of heart failure produces different signs and symptoms, clinically it is unusual to observe solely right- or left-sided failure in children. Since both sides of the heart depend on adequate function of the other side, failure of one chamber causes a reciprocal change in the opposite chamber.

Compensatory Mechanisms

During the initial stages of CHF compensatory mechanisms occur to increase cardiac function in accordance with metabolic requirements. Since most of the signs and symptoms result from decompensation, it is helpful first to review the compensatory processes that attempt to preserve cardiac function (Fig. 34-22).

Sympathetic stimulation. When the cardiac output begins to fall, the atrial and venous stretch receptors and the aortic and carotid baroreceptors stimulate the sympathetic nervous system, which exerts two major effects. It increases the force and rate of myocardial contraction, resulting in a more efficient pumping action. It also increases venous return by increasing the tone of blood vessels and decreasing peripheral circulation to the limbs, splanchnic bed (viscera), and kidneys. Stimulation of the sympathetic cholinergic fibers in the skin causes increased sweating, which is especially prominent on the scalp during periods of exertion, such as crying or feeding.

Renal system. In response to decreased renal blood flow and reduced renal perfusion, the renin-angiotensin-aldosterone mechanism is activated and results in changes aimed at increasing venous return through increased blood volume. First, there is an increase in aldosterone production in response to increased renin secretion from decreased renal blood flow and sympathetic stimulation. Aldosterone increases the rate of sodium reabsorption by the distal tubules, promoting osmosis of water into the blood. The absorbed sodium increases the osmotic concentration of the extracellular fluid, stimulating release of antidiuretic hormone (ADH) from the hypophysis, which promotes increased water reabsorption by the tubules.

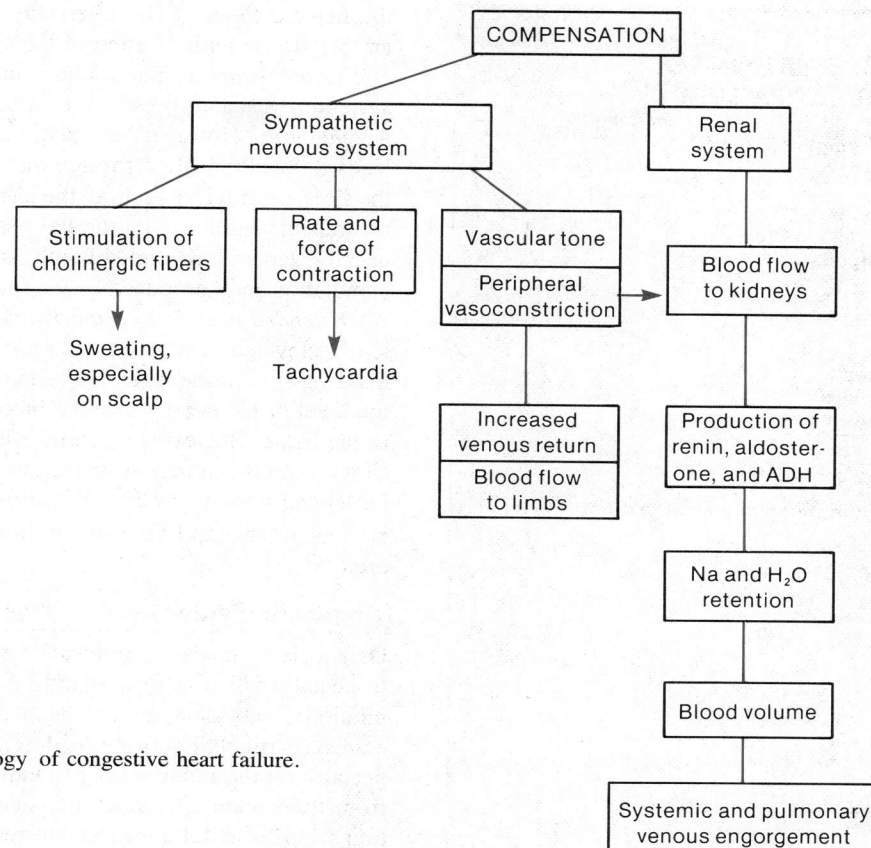

Fig. 34-22. Pathophysiology of congestive heart failure.

Clinical Manifestations

Despite compensatory mechanisms, the heart may be unable to maintain an adequate cardiac output to meet the body's metabolic needs. Decreased blood flow to the kidneys continues to stimulate sodium and water reabsorption, leading to hypervolemia, increased workload on the heart, and congestion in the pulmonary and systemic circulations. Because these hemodynamic changes occur at different times, the signs and symptoms can vary.

Impaired myocardial function. One of the earliest signs of congestive heart failure is *tachycardia* (sleeping heart rate above 160 beats/minute in infants), as a direct result of sympathetic stimulation. It is elevated even during rest but becomes markedly rapid with the slightest exertion.

Increased blood volume causes the ventricles to dilate, stretching the myocardial fibers until they are no longer as contractile. Ventricular dilation results in extra heart sounds, S_3 and/or S_4. The addition of these extra sounds to S_1 and S_2 produces a *gallop rhythm*. Variations in the strength of ventricular contraction result in *pulsus alternans,* regular alternation of one strong pulse and one weak one. It is best detected by palpating the pulse while taking the blood pressure. The increased pressure from the inflated cuff occludes the weak beats, so that only the stronger beats are counted. As a result, the pulse is half the actual rate.

Cardiomegaly results from dilation of the ventricle to ac-

commodate increasing volumes of blood and from hypertrophy, as a result of persistent lengthening and thickening of the myocardial fibers. Decreased cardiac output results in poor peripheral perfusion, which is manifest by cold extremities, weak pulses, low blood pressure, mottled skin, and eventually death.

Pulmonary congestion. As the left ventricle fails, blood volume and pressure increase in the left atrium, pulmonary veins, and lungs. Eventually the pulmonary capillary pressure exceeds the plasma osmotic pressure, forcing fluid into tissues, causing pulmonary edema. Increased pressure also decreases compliance (expansion) of the lungs.

Dyspnea is one of the earliest signs of heart failure and is thought to be caused by a decrease in the distensibility of the lungs. *Costal retractions* occur as the pliable chest wall in the infant is drawn inward when the infant attempts to ventilate the noncompliant lungs. Initially dyspnea may only be evident on exertion, but it may progress to the point that even slight activity results in labored breathing. In infants dyspnea at rest is a prominent sign and may be accompanied by flaring nares.

Tachypnea (respiratory rate above 60 breaths/minute in infants) occurs in response to decreased lung compliance. Inability to feed with resultant weight loss is primarily a result of tachypnea and dyspnea on exertion.

Orthopnea (dyspnea in the recumbent position) is caused

CLINICAL MANIFESTATIONS OF CONGESTIVE HEART FAILURE

General signs and symptoms
Tachycardia
Tachypnea
Sweating (inappropriate)
Weight gain
Decreased urine output
Fatigue
Weakness
Restlessness
Anorexia
Pale, cool extremities
Weak peripheral pulses
Decreased blood pressure
Gallop rhythm
Cardiomegaly

Left-sided heart failure (pulmonary congestion)
Dyspnea
Retractions (infants)
Flaring nares
Exercise intolerance
Orthopnea
Cough, hoarseness
Cyanosis
Wheezing
Grunting

Right-sided heart failure (systemic congestion)
Hepatomegaly
Peripheral edema, especially periorbital
Ascites
Neck vein distention (children)

by increased blood flow to the heart and lungs from the extremities. It is relieved by sitting up, because blood pools in the lower extremities, decreasing venous return. In addition, this position decreases pressure from the abdominal organs on the diaphragm. In infants orthopnea may be evident in their inability to lie supine and their desire to be held upright.

Edema of the bronchial mucosa may produce *cardiac wheezing* from obstruction to airflow. Mucosal swelling and irritation result in a persistent, dry, hacking *cough*. As pulmonary edema increases, the cough may be productive from increased secretions. Pressure on the laryngeal nerve results in *hoarseness*. A late sign of heart failure is *gasping* and *grunting respirations*. An uncommon sign in infants is rales.

Cyanosis may occur without a right-to-left shunt and is the result of impaired respiratory gas exchange. On exertion, such as crying or feeding, the infant may demonstrate mottling of the skin or generalized transient duskiness. Extreme pallor or persistent duskiness is an ominous sign of CHF.

Systemic congestion. Systemic congestion from right-sided failure results in increased pressure and pooling of blood in the venous circulation. *Hepatomegaly* is usually the earliest sign of heart failure and occurs from pooling of blood in the portal circulation and transudation of fluid into

the hepatic tissues. The liver may be tender on palpation, and its size is an indication of the course of heart failure.

Edema forms as the sodium and water retention cause systemic vascular pressure to rise. The earliest sign is *weight gain*. However, as additional fluid accumulates, it leads to swelling of soft tissue that is dependent and favors the flow of gravity, such as the sacrum and scrotum (when recumbent) and loose periorbital tissues. In infants edema is usually generalized and difficult to detect. Gross fluid accumulation may produce *ascites* and *pleural effusions*.

Distended neck and *peripheral veins* result from a consistently elevated central venous pressure. Normally neck and hand veins collapse when the head or hands are raised above the level of the heart, since the blood drains by gravity back to the heart. However, when the venous pressure is high, it slows venous return, causing the veins to remain distended. Distended neck veins are difficult to detect in the short, fat neck of infants and are usually observed only in older children.

Diagnostic Evaluation

Diagnosis is made on clinical symptoms such as dyspnea (especially when at rest), flaring nares, moist grunting respirations, subcostal retractions, tachycardia, activity intolerance (particularly during feeding), excessive sweating (especially on the infant's scalp), and unexplained weight gain from fluid retention. Since the signs of pulmonary congestion from heart failure resemble respiratory infections, it is imperative to differentiate between the two. Signs selectively indicative of CHF are cardiac enlargement, edema, sweating, hepatomegaly, and auscultatory findings such as tachycardia, gallop rhythm, and pulsus alternans.

Therapeutic Management

Treatment of CHF is to remove the cause and allow the heart to compensate for the temporary failure. The goals of treatment are to (1) improve cardiac function, (2) remove accumulated fluid and sodium, (3) decrease cardiac demands, and (4) improve tissue oxygenation (unless shock is present).

Improve cardiac function. Myocardial efficiency is improved using digitalis glycosides. Digitalis has three major actions:

1. Increases the force of contraction (positive inotropic)
2. Decreases the heart rate (negative chronotropic) and slows the conduction of impulses through the atrioventricular node (negative dromotropic)
3. Indirectly enhances diuresis by increased renal perfusion

The beneficial effects are increased cardiac output, decreased heart size, decreased venous pressure, and relief of edema.

In pediatrics digoxin (Lanoxin), rather then digitoxin, is used almost exclusively because of digoxin's rapid onset and decreased risk of toxicity as a result of a short half-life.

Table 34-3 Diuretics used in congestive heart failure (CHF)

DRUG	ACTION	COMMENTS	NURSING CONSIDERATIONS
Furosemide (Lasix)	Blocks reabsorption of sodium and water in proximal renal tubule and interferes with reabsorption of sodium in Henle loop and in most proximal portion of distal tubule	Drug of choice in severe congestive heart failure Causes excretion of chloride and potassium (hypokalemia may precipitate digitalis toxicity)	Begin to record output as soon as drug is given Observe for dehydration caused by profound diuresis Observe for side effects (nausea and vomiting, diarrhea, ototoxicity, hypokalemia, dermatitis, postural hypotension) Encourage foods high in potassium and/or give potassium supplements Monitor chloride and acid-base balance in chronic therapy Observe for signs of digitalis toxicity
Chlorothiazide (Diuril)	Acts directly on distal tubules and possibly proximal tubules to decrease sodium, water, potassium, chloride, and bicarbonate absorption Decreases urinary diluting capacity	Most commonly used drug, inexpensive Causes hypokalemia, acidosis from large doses May be given on alternate days or for 4-5 days and stopped for 2 days to allow for reabsorption of potassium	Observe for side effects (nausea, weakness, dizziness, paresthesia, muscle cramps, skin eruptions, hypokalemia, acidosis) Encourage foods high in potassium and/or give potassium supplements
Hydrochloro-thiazide (Hydro-Diuril)	Same as chlorothiazide	Effect is 10 times more potent than chlorothiazide; therefore dose is decreased by one tenth	Same as chlorothiazide
Spironolactone (Aldactone)	Blocks action of aldosterone, which promotes retention of sodium and excretion of potassium	Has potassium-sparing effect, frequently used with thiazides, furosemide Poorly absorbed from gastrointestinal tract, expensive Beneficial for children who are resistant to other diuretics	Observe for side effects (skin rash, drowsiness, ataxia, hyperkalemia) Do not administer potassium supplements
Hydrochlorothiazide plus spironolactone (Aldactazide)	Same as two components	Combines benefits of both drugs	Same as two components

It is available as an elixir (0.05 mg/ml) for oral administration or in a parenteral preparation (0.1 mg/ml). For infants the dose is often calculated in micrograms (1000 μg = 1 mg). Because digoxin has a very narrow margin of safety, the dosage must be calculated exactly; premature infants are more sensitive to digoxin and require smaller doses because the drug accumulates in the blood faster than in infants and children (Hastreiter and others, 1985). If life-threatening toxicity occurs, a specific antidote, Digibind, is available. However, the product is very expensive and criteria for its use need to be developed (Lewander, 1986).

Treatment is based on a digitalizing dose, given intravenously, orally, or intramuscularly in divided doses over a short time span to bring the child's serum digoxin level into the therapeutic range, and a maintenance dose, usually one eighth of the digitalizing dose, given orally twice a day to maintain blood levels. During digitalization the child is monitored by means of an electrocardiogram to observe for the desired effects (prolonged P-R interval and reduced ventricular rate) and detect side effects, especially arrhythmias. Therapeutic serum digoxin levels range from 1 to 2 ng/ml (Park, 1986).

Remove accumulated fluid and sodium. Treatment consists of diuretics, fluid restriction, and possible sodium restriction. Diuretics are the mainstay of therapy to eliminate excess water and salt to prevent reaccumulation. The most commonly used agents are listed in Table 34-3. Since furosemide and the thiazides cause loss of potassium, potassium supplements and rich dietary sources of the electrolyte are given. A fall in serum potassium enhances the

GUIDELINES FOR ADMINISTERING DIGOXIN

1. Give digoxin at regular intervals, usually every 12 hours, such as 8 AM and 8 PM.
2. Plan the times so that the drug is given *1 hour before* or *2 hours after* feedings.
3. Use a calendar to mark off each dose that is given or post a reminder, such as a sign on the refrigerator.
4. Have the prescription refilled *before* the medication is completely used.
5. Administer the drug carefully by slowly directing it on the side and back of the mouth.
6. Do not mix it with other foods or fluids, since refusal to consume these results in inaccurate intake of the drug.
7. If the child has teeth, give him water after administering the drug; whenever possible, brush the teeth to prevent tooth decay from the sweetened liquid.
8. If a dose is missed and more than 4 hours has elapsed, withhold the dose and give the next dose at the regular time; if less than 4 hours has elapsed, give the missed dose.
9. If the child vomits do not give a second dose.
10. If more than two consecutive doses have been missed, notify the physician.
11. Do not increase or double the dose for missed doses.
12. If the child becomes ill, notify the physician immediately.
13. Keep digoxin in a safe place, preferably a locked cabinet.
14. In case of accidental overdose of digoxin, call the nearest poison control center immediately.

Modified from Jackson, P.L.: Digoxin therapy at home: keeping the child safe, Am. J. Maternal Child Nurs. 4(2):105-109, 1979.

effects of digitalis, increasing the risk of digitalis toxicity. Therefore serum potassium levels must be carefully monitored.

Fluid restriction may be required in the acute states of CHF and must be carefully calculated to avoid dehydrating the child, especially if cyanotic CHD and significant polycythemia are present.

Sodium-restricted diets are used less often in children than in adults to control CHF because of their potential negative effects on the child's appetite and ultimate growth. If salt intake is restricted, the diet usually consists of avoiding additional table salt and highly salted foods, and a low-salt formula (Lonalac) may be used to feed infants.

Decrease cardiac demands. To lessen the workload on the heart, metabolic needs are kept to a minimum by providing a neutral thermal environment to prevent cold stress in infants, treating any existing infections, reducing the effort of breathing (semi-Fowler position), and using medication to sedate an irritable child (usually morphine sulfate, 0.1 mg/kg).

Improve tissue oxygenation. All of the preceding measures serve to increase tissue oxygenation either by improving myocardial function or by lessening tissue oxygen demands. However, supplemental cool humidified oxygen may also be administered to increase the amount of available oxygen during inspiration. An oxygen hood is preferred

with infants to provide increased concentration of the gas. Cool humidification is necessary to counteract the drying effect of oxygen. The amount of cool humidity is carefully regulated to prevent chilling.

Nursing Considerations

The objectives of nursing care are to (1) assist in measures to improve cardiac function, (2) decrease cardiac demands, (3) reduce respiratory distress, (4) maintain nutritional status, (5) assist in measures to promote fluid loss, and (6) provide family support. Although the objectives are the same, the interventions differ depending on the child's age, especially with infants as compared to older children.

Assist in measures to improve cardiac function. The nurse's responsibility in administering digitalis includes observing for signs of toxicity, calculating and administering the correct dosage, and instituting parental teaching regarding drug administration at home. Digitalis is a potentially dangerous drug because the margin of safety of therapeutic, toxic, and lethal doses is very narrow; there is no known antidote. Many toxic responses are extensions of its therapeutic effects. Therefore the nurse must maintain a high index of suspicion when administering digitalis for the following signs of toxicity.

Cardiac toxicity. The principal manifestations of cardiac toxicity are abnormalities in heart rate, rhythm, and conduction. An early sign is bradycardia. Therefore the child's apical pulse is always checked before administering digitalis. As a general rule the drug is not given if the pulse is below 90 to 110 beats/minute in infants and young children or below 70 beats/minute in older children (the cutoff point for adults is 60). However, since the pulse rate varies in children in different age-groups, the physician should specify with the written drug order at what heart rate the drug is withheld. The nurse should also use judgment in evaluating the pulse rate. If it is significantly lower than the previous recording, the dose should be withheld until the physician is notified.

The apical rate is taken because a pulse deficit (radial pulse rate lower than apical) may be present with decreased cardiac output. It is auscultated for 1 full minute to evaluate alterations in rhythm. If the child is monitored by means of an electrocardiogram, a rhythm strip is obtained and attached to the chart for rate and rhythm analysis, such as abnormal lengthening of the P-R interval (more than a 50% increase over predigitalization interval) and signs of ectopic beats, especially premature ventricular contractions (PVCs) (QRS complex is wide and bizarre in shape).

Digitalis toxicity can occur from accidental overdose. To avoid confusion between the two preparations, Lanoxin is usually used to differentiate digoxin from digitoxin. Anyone administering the drug must carefully read the container's label to ensure use of the correct preparation. Since margins of safety between therapeutic and toxic doses are narrow, great care must be taken in properly calculating and measuring the dosage. It is essential that the exact number of milliliters be given. When converting milligrams to micrograms to milliliters, the nurse carefully checks the placement of the decimal point, since an error causes a significant change in dosage. For example, 0.1 mg is 10 times the dosage of 0.01 mg. To ensure safety, the nurse compares the calculations with another staff member before giving the drug.

These same principles are taught to parents in preparation for discharge, although the correct dose in milliliters is usually specified on the container, thus reducing potential errors in calculation. The nurse observes the parent measure the elixir in the dropper and stresses the level mark as the meniscus of the fluid that is observed at eye level. Other instructions for administering digoxin are listed in the boxed material.

Parents are also advised of the signs of toxicity. According to the physician's preference they may be taught to take the pulse before giving the drug. A return demonstration of the procedure from both parents or other principal caregiver is included as part of the teaching plan. Their level of anxiety in counting the pulse is assessed, since overconcern about the heart rate may result in excessive withholding of the drug.

Extracardiac signs and symptoms. The earliest manifestation of toxicity is vomiting, usually with anorexia and nausea, caused by stimulation of the emetic control center in the medulla. Although vomiting should alert the nurse to observe for other evidence of cardiac toxicity, one episode of vomiting does not warrant cessation of the drug because vomiting from other causes is common, especially in infants. When in doubt regarding the cause of the vomiting and if another dose of digoxin should be given, the nurse should seek the physician's advice before administering the next dose of digitalis. Other extracardiac signs of toxicity are neurologic or visual disturbances (box, p. 1493), which are extremely difficult to identify in children and consequently are of little value in assessing toxicity in infants.

Decrease cardiac demands. The infant requires provision of rest and conservation of energy for the task of feeding. Every effort is made to organize nursing activities

to allow for uninterrupted periods of sleep. Whenever possible, parents are encouraged to stay with their infant to provide the holding, rocking, and cuddling that help children sleep more soundly. To minimize disturbing the infant, changing bed linen and complete bathing are done only when necessary. Feeding is planned to accommodate the infant's sleep and wake patterns. He is fed as soon as he appears hungry, such as when sucking on his fists rather than when crying for a bottle, since the stress of crying exhausts his limited energy supply. If he is sleeping, he is fed after he awakens.

Every effort is made to minimize unnecessary stress. With infants this primarily involves preserving the parent-child relationship and meeting their needs to reduce frustration. Older children need an explanation of what is happening to them to decrease anxiety over their deteriorating physical status. For example, if they are monitored by an electrocardiogram or placed in an oxygen tent, the nurse first explains the procedure. Sometimes the sense of urgency associated with admission of a child in severe CHF overshadows the need for psychologic preparation of the child. However, the few minutes it takes to reassure a child that electrocardiographic leads do not hurt or to familiarize him with the world through a plastic tent result in lessening physiologic responses to stress.

Temperature is carefully monitored for hyperthermia (a sign of infection) or hypothermia (loss of heat to ambient air). Fever is reported to the physician, since infection must be promptly treated. If body temperature is low, the child is kept warm with additional blankets or the use of a radiant heater. Maintaining body temperature is very important for the child who is receiving cool, humidified oxygen and for one who tends to be diaphoretic, losing heat via evaporation.

Respiratory infection and skin breakdown from edema accumulation are minimized or prevented if possible. The child is placed on sheepskin, egg crate mattress, or alternating pressure mattress and turned every 2 hours (from side to side while in semi-Fowler position). The skin, especially over the sacrum, is checked for evidence of redness from pressure. The child is placed in a room with noninfectious patients. With an older child, it is advantageous to choose a roommate who is also confined to bed and relatively quiet in order to promote a restful environment. Visitors and hospital personnel with active respiratory infections are isolated from the child. Good hand washing is practiced before and after caring for any hospitalized child. Antibiotics may be given to combat respiratory infection or to prevent bacterial endocarditis. The nurse ensures that the drug is given at equally divided times over a 24-hour schedule to maintain high blood levels of the antibiotic.

Reduce respiratory distress. To reduce the work of breathing the infant or child is positioned in semi- to high-Fowler position in an infant or cardiac seat. Infants and children with cyanotic heart disease often breathe better in the knee-chest position. Infants can be maintained in this position by placing them on their side with the knees bent toward the chest and pillows propped behind the back and

---

SIGNS OF DIGOXIN TOXICITY

Gastrointestinal signs
*Vomiting
Anorexia
Nausea
Diarrhea
Salivation
Abdominal pain

Cardiac signs
*Bradycardia (below 90 to
    110 in infants;
    below 70 in children)
Arrhythmias
Hypotension

Neurologic signs
Fatigue
Muscle weakness
Headache
Drowsiness
Insomnia
Vertigo
Confusion
Delirium

Ocular signs
Yellow-green halos around
    dark objects
Blurred vision
Light flashes

*Most common signs.

buttocks. If they must be transported, the position that maximizes breathing is maintained. Shirts and diapers are pinned loosely to allow maximum chest expansion. Safety restraints, such as those used with the infant seats, are applied low on the abdomen and loosely enough to provide safety and maximum expansion.

Respirations are counted for 1 full minute during a resting state and any evidence of increased respiratory distress is reported to the physician, since this may indicate worsening heart failure. If morphine sulfate is given, the nurse observes for respiratory depression from the drug.

The infant or child is often placed in an oxygen hood or tent with cool humidified oxygen; supplemental oxygen may or may not be helpful in relieving the respiratory distress or cyanosis. If a trial period is ordered to determine its effectiveness, the child's response is evaluated by noting the respiratory rate, ease of respiration, color, and interval of sleep, and blood gas measurements are taken to objectively assess benefit from the procedure.

Maintain nutritional status. The same interventions discussed on p. 1476 (under Help the family cope with effects of defect) apply here. Attention to nutrition is essential and is a nursing challenge because of the fatigue associated with CHF. If the child is hospitalized, parents are encouraged to feed the infant and employ whatever strategies have been successful at home. If such measures are still exhausting to the infant, he may be fed by gavage.

Assist in measures to promote fluid loss. When diuretics are given, the nurse continues to record fluid intake and output and monitors body weight at the same time each day to evaluate benefit from the drug. Since profound diuresis may cause dehydration and electrolyte imbalance (loss of sodium, potassium, chloride, bicarbonate), the nurse observes for signs indicating either complication, as well as signs and symptoms suggesting reactions to the drugs (Table 34-3). Diuretics should be given early in the day to children who are toilet trained to avoid the need to urinate at night. If potassium-losing diuretics are given, the nurse encourages foods high in potassium, such as bananas, oranges, whole grains, legumes, and leafy vegetables. If potassium supplements are given, the elixir may be mixed with fruit juice (red punch or grape juice works well) to disguise the bitter taste and to prevent intestinal irritation from a concentrated solution. The nurse observes for signs of hypokalemia (muscle weakness, hypotension, arrhythmias, tachycardia or bradycardia, irritability, drowsiness) or hyperkalemia (muscle weakness, twitching, bradycardia, ventricular fibrillation, oliguria, apnea) from supplemental overdose and for digitalis toxicity (low potassium enhances effects of digitalis toxicity).

Fluid restriction is rarely necessary in infants because of their difficulty in feeding. However, if fluids are restricted, the nurse plans fluid intake schedules using the same principles discussed under postoperative cardiac care (p. 1485). With toddlers and preschoolers it is psychologically advantageous to give small amounts of liquid in small cups so the

containers appear full. Suitable utensils are decorated medicine cups, paper Dixie cups, doll-sized teacups, or measuring cups. It is also important to avoid leaving extra fluids at the bedside, since older children may help themselves to additional servings. Older children's cooperation is gained by placing them in charge of recording fluid intake.

If salt is limited, the nurse discusses food sources of sodium with the family and discourages their bringing salt-containing treats to the child. At mealtime the child's tray is checked to make sure the appropriate diet is given.

Provide family support. CHF is a serious complication of heart disease. Parents and older children are usually acutely aware of the critical nature of the condition. Since stress places additional demands on cardiac function, the nurse should focus on reducing anxiety through anticipatory preparation, frequent communication with the parent regarding the child's progress, and constant reassurance that everything possible is being done.

The placement of the child in an oxygen tent can severely limit physical contact between the child and the parents and in the neonatal period can interfere with bonding. The nurse can minimize this separation by encouraging parents to participate in care, such as feeding, bathing, positioning, and stimulating the child. As mentioned earlier, active parent participation also optimally meets the infant's physical and emotional needs with minimum exertion. However, parents must feel comfortable and well accepted by the staff. For example, positioning the child may be cumbersome with the interfering electrocardiographic leads, but with practice parents become expert in functioning despite such equipment.

Home care involves many of the same interventions as discussed for postoperative surgery—teaching the family about the medications that need to be administered and alerting them to the signs of worsening CHF that need medical attention, such as increased sweating, decreased urine output (noted in fewer wet diapers or infrequent use of the toilet), and any cardiac dysrhythmia. Compliance is a major issue and every effort is extended to improve the family's adherence to the medication schedule (see p. 1110). Written instructions regarding correct administration of digoxin are essential,* including an explanation regarding signs of toxicity.

If CHF is the end stage of a severe heart defect, the nurse cares for this child as for any terminally ill child, using the principles discussed in Chapter 23.

BACTERIAL (INFECTIVE) ENDOCARDITIS

Bacterial endocarditis (BE) or infective endocarditis (IE), also referred to as subacute bacterial endocarditis (SBE), is an infection of the valves and inner lining of the heart. Although it can occur without underlying heart disease, it most often is a sequela of bacteremia in the child with congenital

---

*Home care instructions on giving medications to children are available in Wong, D., and Whaley, L.: Clinical handbook of pediatric nursing, ed. 2, St. Louis, 1986, The C.V. Mosby Co.

Nursing Care Summary: The Infant with Congestive Heart Failure

NURSING GOALS	NURSING INTERVENTIONS	EXPECTED PATIENT/FAMILY OUTCOMES
HP-HMP Infection, potential for **Risk factors: reduced body defenses, debilitated physical status**		
Prevent infection	Avoid exposure to persons with infections Employ thorough handwashing techniques and meticulous cleansing of any equipment coming in contact with infant	Infant remains free of infection
N-MP Fluid volume, alteration in: excess **Etiology: compromised cardiac function**		
Assess cardiac status Assess fluid gain or loss	Attach cardiac monitor Carry out frequent assessments of vital signs Weigh daily at same time and on same scale Maintain strict intake and output Assess for evidence of increased or decreased edema Provide or restrict fluids as determined by amount of fluid retention	*Deviations from normal findings are recognized early and interventions implemented
N-MP Nutrition, alteration in: less than body requirements **Etiology: fatigue, circulatory impairment**		
Maintain nutrition	Provide feedings appropriate to age and capabilities relative to feeding techniques	Infant consumes an adequate amount with minimum effort (specify amount)
A-EP Activity intolerance **Etiology: imbalance between oxygen supply and demand**		
Reduce cardiac demands and oxygen consumption	Maintain neutral thermal environment for minimum oxidative metabolism Place infant in Isolette with servocontrol or under warmer Maintain in resting state at 10 to 30 degrees Feed small volumes at frequent intervals (every 2-3 hours) using soft nipple with moderately large opening Implement gavage feeding if infant becomes fatigued before taking an adequate amount Use nutritional supplements Time nursing activities to disturb infant as little as possible Implement measures to reduce anxiety Respond promptly to crying or other expressions of distress	Infant rests quietly
A-EP Cardiac output, alteration in: Decreased **Etiology: structural defect**		
Improve ventilation Reduce venous return to heart (cyanotic heart disease)	Place in inclined posture of 10 to 30 degrees; tilt mattress support of Isolette; place older infant in cardiac chair or infant seat Avoid any constricting clothing or restraints around abdomen and chest Place in knee-chest position	Respirations remain within normal limits, color is good, and infant rests quietly (see inside front cover for normal variations in respirations)

*Nursing outcome.

Nursing Care Summary: The Infant with Congestive Heart Failure—cont'd

NURSING GOALS	NURSING INTERVENTIONS	EXPECTED PATIENT/FAMILY OUTCOMES
SP-SCP Anxiety **Etiology: unmet needs, discomfort**		
Reduce anxiety	Employ flexible feeding schedule that reduces fretfulness associated with hunger Handle child gently Hold and comfort infant Employ comfort measures found to be effective in individual cases Encourage family to provide comfort and solace	Infant rests quietly and breathes easily
RRP Family process, alteration in **Etiology: hospitalization of child**		
Support family	Employ active listening techniques Explain and clarify child's behavior and therapies prescribed Keep family informed of child's condition Reassure family that everything is being done for child Encourage parents to remain with child Ask family how they think child is doing; respect their observations and concerns Demonstrate acceptance of family's willingness to participate in child's care If this is terminal stage for child, support family's grief, make child as comfortable as possible, and remain with family	Family displays an attitude of understanding and discusses the infant's condition and prognosis calmly

Nursing Interventions Related to Medical Management

Improve efficiency of heart
  Administer digoxin (Lanoxin) as ordered, using established precautions to prevent toxicity
  Make certain dosage is within safe limits
  Ascertain correct preparation for route
  Check dosage with another nurse
  Count apical pulse for 1 full minute prior to giving drug
    Withhold medication and notify physician if pulse rate is less than 90 to 110 beats per minute (infants) or 70 to 85 (older children), depending on previous pulse readings
  Often an ECG rhythm strip is taken to assess cardiac status prior to administration
  Ensure adequate intake of potassium
  Monitor serum potassium levels (decrease enhances digitalis toxicity)
Reduce respiratory distress
  Administer oxygen via Isolette, Croupette, or hood
Remove accumulated tissue fluid
  Administer diuretics as prescribed
  Observe for side effects of electrolyte depletion, especially potassium

  Administer early in day to avoid need for frequent voiding at night
Prevent complications
  Replace electrolytes as indicated
    Mix potassium supplements with fruit juice to camouflage bitter taste and prevent intestinal irritation
  Administer antibiotics if prescribed
  Take ECG as prescribed and/or indicated by infant's condition
  Perform percussion, vibration, and suction as ordered
Provide adequate systemic oxygen transport
  Administer supplemental iron preparation as prescribed
Relieve distress
  Administer morphine sulfate judiciously, if ordered
  Monitor effectiveness of analgesia (p. 1072)
Prevent increased accumulation of fluids
  Feed low-salt formula
    Lonalac (Mead-Johnson)
    Similac PM 60/40 (Ross)
  Administer diuretics as prescribed

cardiac anomalies, especially tetralogy of Fallot, ventricular septal defect with aortic regurgitation, aortic stenosis, prosthetic valves, and recent cardiac surgery and in children with rheumatic heart disease. The most common causative agent is *Streptococcus viridans;* other causative agents are *Staphylococcus aureus,* gram negative bacteria, and fungi, such as *Candida albicans* (Newburger and Nadas, 1982).

Pathophysiology

The microorganisms usually grow on a section of the endocardium that has been subjected to abnormal blood streaming and turbulence, such as occurs when the flow of blood is restricted by an anatomic narrowing or forced through an abnormal opening. Growth may also begin where the abnormal jet of blood strikes the opposing endocardium, causing a thickening of the lining. Changes in the endocardium predispose it to the growth of invading organisms.

Organisms may enter the bloodstream from any site of localized infection. The most common portals of entry are oral from dental work *(S. viridans);* urinary tract, such as from urinary tract infection after catheterization (gram-negative bacilli); heart, from cardiac surgery, especially if synthetic material is used (valves, patches, or conduits); and the bloodstream from long-term indwelling catheters. The microorganisms grow on the endocardium, forming vegetations (verrucae), deposits of fibrin; and platelet thrombi. The lesion may grow to invade adjacent tissues, such as aortic and mitral valves and myocardium, and may break off and embolize elsewhere, especially in the spleen, kidney, central nervous system, lung, skin, and mucous membranes.

Clinical Manifestations

The onset of symptoms is usually insidious, with unexplained low-grade, intermittent fever. Other common nonspecific symptoms are anorexia, malaise, and weight loss. A new murmur or a change in a previously existing one is frequently found as a result of damage to valves or perforation of the myocardium. Another finding, especially in those with prolonged illness, is splenomegaly. Other signs that result from emboli formation elsewhere in the body include splinter hemorrhages (thin black lines) under the nails, Osler nodes (red, painful intradermal nodes with white centers found on the pads of the phalanges), Janeway spots (painless hemorrhagic areas on the palms and soles), and petechiae on the oral mucous membranes.

Diagnostic Evaluation

Several laboratory findings may indicate infectious endocarditis, such as electrocardiographic changes (prolonged P-R interval), roentgenographic evidence of cardiomegaly, anemia, elevated erythrocyte sedimentation rate, leukocytosis, and microscopic hematuria. Definitive diagnosis can be made after growth of the organism and identification of the causative agent in the blood and visualization of the vegetations on two-dimensional echocardiography. Usually several blood specimens are drawn for culturing to rule out contamination during venipuncture and dilution technique. As soon as an organism is isolated, sensitivity studies are done to determine appropriate antibiotic therapy.

Therapeutic Management

Treatment is administration of high-dose antibiotics (usually penicillin, ampicillin, methicillin, cloxacillin, streptomycin, and/or gentamicin for specific bacteria or amphotericin B and/or flucytosine for fungi) given intravenously for at least 4 to 6 weeks. Blood cultures are taken periodically to evaluate response to antibiotic therapy. In instances when antibiotic therapy is unsuccessful, congestive heart failure develops, or recurrent systemic emboli are present, surgical intervention is warranted and may include replacing damaged valves with prostheses, debriding and draining myocardial abscesses, excising areas of infection, and removing vegetations (Karchmer, 1981).

PROCEDURES FOR WHICH ENDOCARDITIS PROPHYLAXIS IS INDICATED

All dental procedures likely to induce gingival bleeding (not simple adjustment of orthodontic appliances or shedding of deciduous teeth)
Tonsillectomy and/or adenoidectomy
Surgical procedures or biopsy involving respiratory mucosa
Bronchoscopy, especially with a rigid bronchoscope
Incision and drainage of infected tissue
Genitourinary and gastrointestinal procedures such as most invasive diagnostic and therapeutic procedures (cystoscopy, urethral catheterization, colonoscopy, endoscopy with biopsy)

Data from Shulman, S., and others: Prevention of bacterial endocarditis, Circulation **70**(6):1123A-1127A, 1984.

Successful early medical treatment, especially with bacterial endocarditis, occurs in approximately 80% of affected patients (Stinson, 1979). However, cases diagnosed late, those caused by antibiotic-resistant organisms or fungi, or those occurring in infants or patients without preexisting heart disease carry a higher mortality and may necessitate surgical intervention. Death is most often caused by congestive heart failure, myocardial infarction from coronary emboli, or cardiac perforation. Nonfatal complications result from embolism to other organs, especially to the central nervous system (causing hemiplegia, aphasia, meningitis, convulsions), kidney (resulting in hematuria, proteinuria), spleen, and bowel.

Prevention of infective endocarditis in susceptible children is of utmost importance and includes all children with CHD except those with (1) isolated secundum ASD or repair without a patch 6 months or more earlier and (2) PDA repair 6 months or more earlier (Shulman and others, 1984). Prevention involves administration of prophylactic antibiotic therapy both shortly before and for a brief period after procedures known to increase the risk of entry of organisms (see box). Published recommendations provide guidelines for antibiotic prophylaxis, but they are complex and must be individualized for the individual child (Shulman and others, 1984). Drugs of choice are penicillin, ampicillin, erythromycin, and vancomycin. The drugs may be given orally or parenterally depending on the type of procedure to be performed.

Nursing Considerations

Ideally the objective of nursing care is counseling parents of high-risk children concerning the need for prophylactic antibiotic therapy before procedures such as dental work. The family's regular dentist should be advised of existing cardiac problems in the child as an added precaution to ensuring preventive treatment. These children should also maintain the highest level of oral health to reduce the chance of bacteremia from oral infections. Dental education using materials such as videotapes can increase children's knowledge of dental health-care needs and promote good dental habits, including brushing, flossing, low cariogenic diet, fluoride treatment, and regular dental examinations (Uzark, Messiter, and Rosenthal, 1986) (see also discussion on dental care in Chapter 14).

Parents should also have a high index of suspicion regarding potential infections. Without unduly alarming them, the nurse stresses that any unexplained fever, weight loss, and change in behavior (lethargy, malaise, anorexia) must be brought to the attention of the physician. Such symptoms should not be self-diagnosed as a cold or flu. Early treatment is important in preventing further cardiac damage, embolic complications, and growth of resistant organisms.

Treatment of endocarditis requires long-term hospitalization for the duration of parenteral drug therapy. Nursing goals during this period are (1) preparation of the child for intravenous infusion, usually a heparin-lock device and several venipunctures for blood cultures, (2) prevention of boredom and depression, especially from restricted mobility caused by hospitalization and need for partial bed rest (if required), (3) observation for side effects of antibiotics, especially inflammation along venipuncture sites, and (4) observation for complications, including embolism and congestive heart failure. Follow-up after treatment is also important, and the nurse can be instrumental in arranging for convenient appointments.

RHEUMATIC FEVER

Rheumatic fever is an inflammatory disease affecting the heart, joints, central nervous system, and subcutaneous tissue. It derives its name from involvement of joints and the presence of fever in the acute stage. The major sequela to rheumatic fever is heart damage, especially scarring of the mitral valve, then referred to as *rheumatic heart disease*.

The incidence of rheumatic fever is approximately 0.5 per 100,000 children ages 5 to 9 years for both white and black populations and represents a dramatic decline during the past three decades (Gordis, 1984). Although the reason for this epidemiologic change is not known, speculative causes include antibacterial control of streptococcal infection, successful treatment of rheumatic fever, a decrease of recurrences, and a change in the organism itself (DiSciascio and Taranta, 1980).

Etiology

There is strong evidence to support a relationship between upper respiratory infection with group A streptococci and subsequent development of rheumatic fever (usually within 2 to 6 weeks). In almost all the cases of rheumatic fever a previous infection with group A streptococci can be documented by laboratory evidence of rising antibody titers. Prevention or treatment of group A streptococcal infection prevents rheumatic fever.

Clinical Manifestations

The principal manifestions of rheumatic fever are observed in the heart, joints, skin, and central nervous system. In the heart inflammatory hemorrhagic bullous lesions, called *Aschoff bodies,* are formed that cause swelling, fragmentation, and alterations in the connective tissue. Subsequent endocarditis produces vegetations, which when healed become fibrous, scarred areas. The structures of the heart most affected are the mitral and aortic valves. With progressive involvement of the valves, signs of mitral and aortic valve stenosis are evident, especially murmurs. Other signs of carditis are tachycardia that is out of proportion to the degree of fever, especially during rest or sleep, precordial pain from pericarditis, pericardial friction rub, muffled heart sound from pericardial effusion, and an accentuated third sound (prediastolic gallop).

Pathologic changes in the joints are mainly caused by edema, inflammation, and effusion in joint tissue. They are reversible and migratory in nature, favoring large joints, such as the knees, elbows, hips, shoulders, and wrists. The affected joint is swollen, hot, red, and exquisitely painful for 1 to 2 days, after which a different joint is affected. The manifestations usually accompany the acute febrile period, most often the first 1 to 2 weeks.

The skin manifestation is an erythematous macule with a clear center and wavy, well-demarcated border. The transitory, nonpruritic rash is most commonly found on the trunk and proximal extremities. Subcutaneous nodules are small (0.5 to 1 cm), nontender swellings that persist indefinitely after onset of the disease and gradually resolve with no resulting damage. They are rare but may be found in crops over bony prominences, such as feet, hands, elbows, scalp, scapulae, and vertebrae.

Central nervous system involvement is characterized by chorea, which is referred to as St. Vitus dance or Sydenham chorea. Chorea is characterized by sudden, aimless, irregular movements of the extremities, involuntary facial grimaces, speech disturbances, emotional lability, and muscle weakness that can be profound. It is usually exaggerated by anxiety and attempts at deliberate fine motor activity and relieved by rest, especially sleep.

In addition to these major manifestations, other vague signs and symptoms include low-grade fever, usually spiking in the late afternoon, unexplained epistaxis, abdominal pain that may be severe enough to simulate appendicitis, arthralgia without arthritic changes, weakness, fatigue, pallor, anorexia, and weight loss.

Diagnostic Evaluation

Diagnosis is based on a set of guidelines recommended by the American Heart Association known as modifications of the Jones criteria. The criteria include evidence of (1) the major manifestations of the disease, (2) minor manifestations, such as arthralgia or fever, (3) laboratory findings, including increased erythrocyte sedimentation rate or leukocytosis, and (4) supportive findings, such as a positive throat culture for streptococci or an elevated or rising antistreptolysin-O (ASO) titer.

Streptolysin-O (O because it is oxygen labile) is a streptococcal extracellular product that produces lysis of the red blood cell. Antistreptolysin-O titers measure the concentration of antibodies formed in the blood against this product. Normally the titers begin to rise about 7 days after onset of the infection and reach maximum levels in 4 to 6 weeks. Therefore a rising titer demonstrated by at least two antistreptolysin-O tests is the most reliable evidence of recent streptococcal infection. Normal values are between 0 and 120 Todd units. Elevations over 333 Todd units indicate recent streptococcal infection in children.

Therapeutic Management

The goals of medical management are (1) eradication of hemolytic streptococci, (2) prevention of permanent cardiac damage, (3) palliation of the other symptoms, and (4) prevention of recurrences of the disease. Penicillin is the drug of choice, with erythromycin as a substitute in penicillin-sensitive children. Salicylates are used to control the inflammatory process, especially in the joints, and reduce the fever and discomfort. Bed rest is recommended during the acute febrile phase but need not be strict. In patients with carditis physical exercise should be limited, at least until the pulse rate returns to normal (Kashani, 1981).

Prophylactic treatment against recurrence is started after the acute therapy and involves monthly intramuscular injections of benzathine penicillin G (1.2 million U), two daily oral doses of penicillin (200,000 U), or one daily dose of sulfadiazine (1 g). The duration of long-term prophylaxis is uncertain. Because of the risk of bacterial endocarditis in rheumatic heart disease, the same prophylaxis discussed earlier is implemented here. The antibiotic regimens used to prevent recurrences of acute rheumatic fever are inadequate for the prevention of bacterial endocarditis.

Nursing Considerations

The objectives of nursing care are to (1) encourage compliance with drug regimens, (2) facilitate recovery from the illness, (3) provide emotional support, and (4) prevent the disease. Since compliance is a major concern in long-term drug therapy, every effort should be expended to encourage adherence to the therapeutic plan (see p. 1110). When compliance is poor, monthly injections may be substituted for daily oral administration of antibiotics, and children need preparation for this often dreaded procedure.

Interventions during home care are primarily concerned with providing rest and adequate nutrition. Usually once the febrile stage is over, children can resume moderate activity and their appetite improves. If carditis is present, the family must be aware of any activity restrictions and may need help in choosing less strenuous activities for the child.

One of the most disturbing and frustrating manifestations of the disease is chorea. The onset is gradual and may occur weeks to months after the illness, sometimes even occurring in children who have not been diagnosed with rheumatic fever. It may be mistaken for nervousness, clumsiness, behavioral changes, inattentiveness, and learning disability. It is usually a source of great frustration to the child because the movements, incoordination, and weakness severely limit

physical ability. The child needs an opportunity to verbalize his feelings. Of utmost importance is stressing to parents and schoolteachers the involuntary, sudden nature of the movements, that the chorea is transitory, and that all manifestations eventually disappear.

Nurses also have a role in prevention, primarily in screening school-age children for sore throats caused by group A streptococci. This may involve actively participating in throat culture screening programs or in referring children with a possible streptococcal infection to a physician. Because of the decline in rheumatic fever, however, there is controversy regarding the continued benefit of screening, although many practitioners continue to consider throat culture an important control measure for identifying streptococcal infections and instituting treatment.

SYSTEMIC HYPERTENSION

Hypertension is the consistent elevation of the blood pressure beyond values considered the upper limits of normal. The two major categories of hypertension are *essential* (no identifiable cause) and *secondary* (subsequent to an identifiable cause) hypertension. Traditionally, essential hypertension has been considered to be a disease of middle-aged or older persons and is a major health problem. Hypertension is the most common cause of cerebral vascular accident and is a major risk factor in myocardial infarction. However, in recent years there has been increasing interest in this disorder as it occurs in adolescents and children, particularly in terms of prevention of fatal consequences in adulthood.

Routine blood pressure measurements of children have detected hypertension similar to essential hypertension in adults with surprising frequency in asymptomatic children, especially teenagers. A conservative estimate suggests at least 1% to 2% incidence of sustained hypertension in the age-groups under 20 years (Cranwell, 1984), although many authorities believe that the incidence is considerable higher (Rocchini, 1984). The prevalence of the condition in adolescents is difficult to evaluate, since no firm criteria have been established to determine what constitutes hypertension in the pediatric age-groups or which of the three blood pressure levels (supine, sitting, standing) provides the most significant prognostic information. However, evidence is accumulating to indicate that the essential hypertension of adulthood may have its origin in childhood; thus its early detection has significance for prevention and treatment.

Etiology

Most instances of hypertension observed in young children occur secondary to a structural abnormality or an underlying pathologic process, although this is being challenged by screening programs of relatively healthy children. The most common cause of secondary hypertension is renal disease (80%), followed by cardiovascular, endocrine, and some neurologic disorders (Mentser, 1982). Miscellaneous conditions such as lead poisoning and ingestion of excessive amounts of licorice are causes unique to children. As a rule,

CONDITIONS ASSOCIATED WITH SECONDARY HYPERTENSION IN CHILDREN

Renal disorders
Congenital defects
    Polycystic kidney, ectopic kidney, horseshoe kidney, etc.
    Obstructive anomalies
    Hydronephrosis
Renal tumor
    Wilms tumor
    Renovascular
Abnormalities of renal arteries
Renal vein thrombosis
Acquired disorders
    Glomerulonephritis—acute or chronic
    Pyelonephritis
    Nephritis associated with collagen disease

Cardiovascular disease
Coarctation of aorta
Arteriovenous fistulas
Patent ductus arteriosus
Aortic or mitral insufficiency

Metabolic and endocrine diseases
Adrenal tumors
    Adenoma
    Pheochromocytoma
    Neuroblastoma

Cushing syndrome
Adrenogenital syndrome
Hyperthyroidism
Aldosteronism
Hypercalcemia
Diabetes mellitus

Neurologic disorders
Space-occupying lesions of cranium (increased intracranial pressure)
    Tumors, cysts, hematoma
    Cerebral edema
    Encephalitis (including Guillain-Barré and Reye syndromes)

Miscellaneous causes
Drugs (corticosteroids, oral contraceptives, pressor agents, amphetamines)
Burns
Genitourinary surgery
Trauma (e.g., stretching of femoral nerve with leg traction)
Insect bites (e.g., scorpion)
Intravascular overload (blood, fluid)
Hypernatremia
Toxemia of pregnancy
Heavy metal poisoning

---

the younger the child and the more severe the hypertension, the more likely it is to be secondary. The conditions associated with secondary hypertension in children and adolescents are listed in the boxed material.

Essential hypertension is seen more often in adolescents than the secondary forms are (Loggie and others, 1984). The causes of essential hypertension are undetermined, but there is evidence to indicate that both genetic and environmental factors play a role. Hypertension has been shown to be increased in children whose parents are hypertensive. American blacks have a higher incidence of hypertension than whites, and in these persons it develops earlier, is frequently more severe, and results in mortality at an earlier age. In fact, hypertension among American blacks is more prevalent and more fatal than sickle cell disease. In such susceptible persons emotional and mental stresses, excessive salt ingestion (often associated with "soul foods"), smoking, and obesity are significant environmental factors.

Clinical Manifestations

Although clinical manifestations associated with hypertension depend largely on the underlying cause, there are some observations that can provide clues to the examiner that an elevated blood pressure may be a factor. Adolescents and older children with hypertension complain of frequent headaches, dizziness, and/or changes in vision. In infants or young children who cannot communicate symptoms, observation of behavior provides clues, although gross behavioral changes may not be apparent until complications are present. Parents of infants and small children who have been treated for hypertension report that their child had previously been irritable, often indulged in an abnormal degree of head banging or rubbing, and may have wakened screaming in the night (when blood pressure tends to be highest).

Blood pressure levels vary widely within a normal range in children of the same age and in the same child on any given day. In addition, the pressures are subject to false readings because of the stress associated with the examination, use of improper size blood pressure cuffs, incorrect interpretation, or mechanical factors. Most of the confusion regarding hypertension is related to a cutoff point to differentiate normal from abnormal blood pressure in children, especially in borderline cases.

Diagnostic Evaluation

It is clear from the increasing numbers of hypertensive or potentially hypertensive children and adolescents being identified that a blood pressure determination should be a routine part of assessment in children over 3 years of age. The blood pressure of children at *any* age should be measured if they are diagnosed as having or suspected of (1) coarctation of the aorta, (2) unexplained heart failure, (3) unexplained heart murmurs, (4) unexplained seizures or other neurologic signs, (5) an abdominal mass or masses, (6) edema, ascites, and/or evidence of renal failure, (7) hypernatremia, (8) failure to thrive, (9) raised intracranial pressure, (10) tumors of the orbit, or (11) respiratory distress. Black teenagers of both sexes are at greater risk to develop primary hypertension than the teenage population as a whole.

The National Heart, Lung and Blood Institute's Task Force on Blood Pressure Control in Children has determined that elevated blood pressure levels in children or its presence in the parents is the best indicator of hypertension later in life (Blumenthal and others, 1977). The Task Force recommends that blood pressure measurements *sustained* above the 95th percentile, for the patient's age and sex (see inside front cover), on *at least three separate occasions* should be considered abnormal. The pressures are taken in the right upper extremity while the child is seated. Because there has been considerable controversy concerning the validity of these standards, some authorities suggest using the 90th percentile, taking three readings on each visit, and recording the average of the last two measurements (Rocchini, 1984).

To obtain an accurate reading, care should be taken to quiet the child or relax the adolescent while the measurement is recorded to avoid false readings caused by excitement. The chief cause of falsely elevated blood pressure readings is the use of improperly fitting, narrow cuffs. Sphygmomanometer cuffs must be selected according to the individual's build and weight (see p. 233 for selection of blood pressure cuff and method of measurement).

Detection of elevated blood pressure calls for a full diagnostic evaluation to determine the etiology. When there is a strongly positive family history of hypertension, and in the absence of other signs or symptoms, the youngster with borderline readings is not usually submitted to an intensive barrage of diagnostic tests. The blood pressure is monitored for at least 6 to 12 months to rule out possible transient hypertension, after which the tests are more likely limited to renal function tests, intravenous pyelography, and echocardiography. In adolescents with more severe hypertension a full diagnostic evaluation is indicated.

Therapeutic Management

Therapy for secondary hypertension involves diagnosis and treatment of the underlying cause. In those cases amenable to surgical repair, the nature of the condition, the type of surgery, and the age of the child are all essential considerations. For example, vascular repair in a child with renovascular hypertension is usually delayed when possible to allow for sufficient growth of both the child and his blood vessels. Most surgeons prefer that the child be kept on a medical regimen until he weighs at least 18 kg (40 pounds). On the other hand, coarctation of the aorta is frequently repaired at an early age to avoid prolonged preoperative hypertension and its associated sequelae (see p. 1464). Pheochromocytoma, a rare benign tumor that secretes the hypertensive catecholamines (norepinephrine and epinephrine), is usually removed as soon as a diagnosis is confirmed (see p. 1701).

Children or adolescents who have consistently elevated blood pressure readings with no known etiology or those in whom secondary hypertension is not amenable to surgical correction may be treated with a combination of nonpharmacologic and pharmacologic interventions. Since the long-term effects of antihypertensive agents on hormonal cycles regulating growth are not known, drug treatment of asymptomatic children with mild or borderline hypertension is controversial. General measures that carry no risk should be initiated for all children, such as limitation of dietary salt, weight control, increased exercise, and avoidance of stress and smoking (McCrory, 1982).

Since there is a close association between overweight and hypertension, a weight-reduction program is recommended for overweight youngsters. It has also been confirmed that high salt intake increases the risk of hypertension in genetically predisposed persons and aggravates existing hypertension unless salt intake is limited. This is not uniformly seen in children, however, and decreasing salt intake is often poorly tolerated. Regular exercise augments weight reduction and alone has been shown to normalize blood pressure. The exercise regimen should be tailored to the child's interest; recommended activities are swimming, running, or bicycling. The exercise should be sufficiently aerobic to raise the heart rate to approximately 150 beats per minute. The exercise should be continued at that intensity for 45 minutes and performed 4 times per week (Goldring and Hernandez, 1982). Stress reduction strategies may be beneficial and include biofeedback and relaxation. Smoking is discouraged, although it is difficult to encourage a young person to stop smoking. If the adolescent is taking birth control pills, these need to be discontinued.

Indications for hypotensive drug therapy are significant elevation of diastolic pressure (greater than 90 mm Hg in children less than 12 years and greater than 100 mm Hg in children older than 12 years) and/or evidence of target organ involvement (cardiomegaly, headaches, dizziness, seizures, retinopathy, renal involvement) (McCrory, 1982; Rocchini, 1984). The initial drug is usually a diuretic, such as hydrochlorothiazide (see Table 34-3). If this produces an unsatisfactory response, an antihypertensive drug is administered. The drugs of choice are the beta blockers (propranolol) and methyldopa (Table 34-4).

The drug is tailored to meet the needs of individual children and is determined by the hypotensive effect produced and the appearance of any side effects. The aim is to achieve a normotensive state throughout the day without any accompanying side effects. The drug regimen is kept simple, preferably with a single antihypertensive agent in combination with a suitable diuretic. If the teenager is unreliable in taking a drug pharmacologically best suited to his particular form of hypertension several times a day, the physician may prescribe a less optimum drug that can be taken only once a day if it produces an adequate lowering of the pressure. In addition, a drug such as guanethidine that has a tendency to cause postexercise syncope is not advised for the athletic youngster. The choice of agent may need to be changed if it is found to produce depression, as reserpine does, for example.

Nursing Considerations

The nurse is a valuable link in the health care delivery system in relation to hypertension in the pediatric age-group. Active in detection, diagnosis, and therapy in any setting—hospital, school, clinic, private office, public health services, and private practice—nurses are frequently the per-

Table 34-4 Antihypertensive drugs most frequently used in treatment of hypertension

DRUG	MODE OF ACTION	PATIENT TEACHING*
Methyldopa (Aldomet)	Acts on vascular smooth muscle Reduces blood pressure by lowering peripheral vascular resistance; also lowers norepinephrine levels; sodium and water retention may occur if a diuretic is not given with drug	Will require frequent blood studies if on long-term therapy Drug may cause drowsiness and abdominal symptoms such as distention, flatus, diarrhea Notify physician if fever develops
Propranolol (Inderal)	Acts as a beta blocker Blocks response to beta stimulation and depresses renin output	Take drug with meals Monitor pulse and blood pressure (causes bradycardia and hypotension) Drug may cause fatigue, decrease in exercise tolerance, weakness, cold extremities Warn sexually active males of impotence
Reserpine (variety of trade names, including Serpasil, Sandril, Serfin, Reserpoid, Rau-Sed)	Acts on sympathetic nervous system Reduces norepinephrine levels in sympathetic nerves by altering ability of nerve cells to bind norepinephrine, which inhibits stimulation of vascular smooth muscle	Take drug with meals Expect nasal stuffiness; may require drugs for relief Relieve mouth dryness with chewing gum, sour hard candy, ice chips Drug may cause drowsiness; use caution in potentially hazardous situations Notify physician if depression or nightmares develop
Hydralazine (Apresoline)	Acts on vascular smooth muscle Thought to produce its effect by direct action on blood vessels to cause arterial vasodilation	Take drug with meals Drug may cause drowsiness; use caution in potentially hazardous situations Notify physician if sore throat, fever, muscle and joint aches, or skin rash develops
Guanethidine (Ismelin)	Acts on sympathetic nervous system Causes release and subsequent depletion of norepinephrine from adrenergic nerve endings to produce dilation of both arterial and venous vessels; sodium and water retention if not given with a diuretic	May be subject to weight gain, nasal stuffiness, fatigue Warn sexually active males about impotence and failure of ejaculation Warn to avoid strenuous exercise if postexercise syncope is present

*For the use of all drugs youngster should be instructed to:
  Rise slowly from a horizontal position and avoid sudden position changes
  Take drug as prescribed
  Notify physician if unpleasant side effects appear, but do not discontinue drug
  Avoid alcohol and stay on prescribed diet

sons who operate well child care and follow-up units and are usually the primary contact between health services and the child and his family.

A blood pressure measurement should always be a part of the routine assessment of infants and children. In carrying out the procedure, it is most important to make certain that the cuff used is suited to the individual child and that any questionable reading is repeated, using different instruments if necessary. When an elevated pressure is detected, the procedure should be carried out in the standing, sitting, and supine positions and comparison readings made between both upper extremities and between upper and lower extremities to ascertain if they are equal.

Nursing counseling and guidance of the hypertensive teenager pose a number of problems. In the hospital situation diet and medication regimens can be carefully regu-

lated. Home management necessitates motivating older youngsters and their parents to cooperate in carrying out a treatment plan. The major problem in hypertensive children is compliance in relation to maintaining contact with the physician or clinic for follow-up care, taking antihypertensive drugs as prescribed, and allowing home blood pressure to be taken (see discussion of compliance, p. 1110). An important aspect of nursing care is to convince these youngsters that their disorder is probably a lifelong concern and that management must include drug therapy, perhaps some modification in diet and activity, and regular follow-up care.

Home blood pressure measurements greatly facilitate surveillance in youngsters with chronic hypertension. Someone in the hypertensive child's family, such as a parent, sibling, or other responsible person, must be assisted in securing proper equipment and instructed in its use. He or she needs to know about fluctuations in readings that can be expected in relation to the time of day, posture (sitting, lying, standing), activity, and stress. He or she needs to be told at what levels to seek advice. The nurse can help this person set up a system for recording the measurements, usually using a graphic record.

The drug therapy program, including the need for taking the drug, how the drug works and its duration of action, any side effects that may be expected, and what to do if such effects are experienced, must be explained to the youngster and his family. It is important to impress on the youngster the importance of taking the drug continuously as prescribed and that it is effective only during the time it is taken regularly. The child who has no symptoms and feels no ill effects may discontinue taking the medication, having his blood pressure checked, or visiting the office or clinic for checkups. For these youngsters nursing follow-up and guidance are extremely important. Young hypertensive women should avoid oral contraceptives because of their pressor effects, which may have broader implications in relation to compliance to a regimen by the sexually active teenager.

Unfortunately not all children and their families are able to accept the responsibility and the stress of continuous management. In such cases the school nurse may need to assume the responsibility for taking blood pressure measurements regularly or making arrangements for another individual to do so. It is simple to stress the importance of weight control or reduction and suggest restricting salt intake to teenagers, but it is another matter to see that they follow through on these instructions. The family may be reluctant to impose necessary modifications to the usual family diet, and the youngster who enjoys food-related activities with friends is less likely to comply. Both the teenager and the parent will need guidance in the avoidance of high-sodium foods and preparation and selection of palatable, low-salt foods. For example, the child can select unsalted peanuts or popcorn instead of the salted variety and substitute unsalted French fries for potato chips. Exercise prescriptions may be difficult for youngsters to follow unless they are enjoyable. For example, enrolling in an aerobic dance class may be more appealing than the use of a stationary bicycle. The exercise sessions need to be planned and routinely scheduled; outside play time, such as riding a bicycle in the neighborhood, is rarely sufficiently strenuous to produce desired results. If peers and family members can be encouraged to participate in any of the management strategies, the child's compliance is likely to be greater.

Learning needs vary greatly among affected children. Some require a great deal of support, education, and guidance; others need only education and periodic follow-up. Scolding the noncompliant child is useless and may serve only to alienate him from the nurse and continued health care. Exploring with him the reasons for difficulty in following the prescribed regimen will assist both nurse and youngster in problem solving. Continued reinforcement for positive behavior is a major nursing responsibility, and a good nurse-patient relationship is essential to the continued

compliance. The child and family need education and guidance as well as support and reassurance.

CARDIAC DYSRHYTHMIAS

Cardiac dysrhythmias occur less frequently in children than in adults; however, they are not rare. Approximately 1% of newborn infants have disorders of cardiac rhythm and conduction, although the majority outgrow their abnormality by 3 months of age (Southall and others, 1981). In addition, dysrhythmias are a complication of several types of cardiac repair; with the increasing number of children surviving these operations, more are experiencing such complications. Nurses need to have a basic knowledge of the types of dysrhythmias seen in children and their respective treatment.

Classification

Dysrhythmias can be classified according to various criteria, such as effect on heart rate and rhythm (Gillette, 1981):

bradydysrhythmias Abnormally slow rate
tachydysrhythmias Abnormally rapid rate
conduction disturbances Irregular heart rate

Another useful system is to group dysrhythmias according to their site of origin:

dysrhythmias originating in the ventricles (bundle branches and Purkinje fibers) Ventricular tachycardia, bundle branch block
dysrhythmias originating in the atria Paroxysmal atrial tachycardia (PAT)
dysrhythmias originating in the atrioventricular (AV) junction (AV node and bundle of His) AV block, Wolff-Parkinson-White syndrome

Although a number of dysrhythmias are found in children, the more common ones include:

sinoatrial dysrhythmias Influenced by autonomic nervous system, thus they are common in children. Sinus tachycardia may accompany fever, hemorrhage, crying, and infections; sinus arrhythmia, in which rate increases with inspiration and decreases with expiration, is a normal variation.
premature contractions (PC) (atrial [PAC], atrioventricular, or ventricular [PVC]) May be seen in children with a normal heart and are usually benign, disappearing with exercise; may result from specific causes such as digitalis toxicity, acute rheumatic fever, and acid-base disturbances.
tachycardia-bradycardia syndrome (sinus node dysfunction, sick sinus syndrome) Consists of sinus bradycardia, sinus arrest, sinoatrial block, and dysrhythmias. A complication of the Mustard procedure for transposition of the great vessels and atrial septal repair, this syndrome has also been seen in healthy adolescents, especially following strenuous physical exercise in males. It may require a permanent pacemaker and can result in sudden death.
complete AV block May be congenital but not always found at birth; it carries a better prognosis if found later. It is usually acquired as a result of tetralogy of Fallot repair and has a worse prognosis than the congenital type. AV block may require a permanent pacemaker.

Supraventricular tachycardia is a frequently used term that broadly refers to any tachycardia originating above the bundle of His. Currently the term more specifically refers only to paroxysmal atrial tachycardia (PAT) without heart block and AV junctional tachycardia (Alpert, 1980); PAT is one of the most common dysrhythmias in children.

PAT arises from atrial or nodal focus, causing a rapid, regular heart rate in the range of 160 to 300 beats/minute. It occurs most often in infants 1 to 3 months of age, especially males, but can occur at any age, even in utero. It can last from minutes to several hours. Onset is sudden; the arrhythmia frequently terminates abruptly and spontaneously.

The clinical course in infants is more serious than in children; if the dysrhythmia continues, congestive heart failure develops within 24 to 48 hours. Early signs of the dysrhythmia, in addition to the rapid heart rate, are poor response to feeding and extreme irritability.

A number of infants with PAT manifest the Wolff-Parkinson-White syndrome (WPW) on the ECG after establishment of a normal sinus rhythm. In WPW the sinus impulses bypass all or part of the normal AV conduction system through an accessory AV muscle connection. Consequently the ventricular myocardium is preexcited or activated earlier than would be expected if the impulse traveled through the normal AV conduction pathway (Prystowsky, 1982). The majority of infants with WPW improve dramatically during the first year, possibly because of postnatal resorption of the accessory AV connections.

Diagnostic Evaluation

Several advances in the diagnosis of cardiac dysrhythmias have greatly improved the understanding and treatment of these conditions in children. The basic diagnostic procedure is the electrocardiogram (ECG), including 24-hour Holter monitoring (see p. 1453). However, more definitive procedures include both noninvasive and invasive techniques. Transtelephonic electrocardiogram allows for monitoring at any time and anywhere a telephone is available. The transtelephonic ECG system consists of a battery-powered transmitter. One side of the transmitter is placed against the child's chest and the other side is adapted to fit over an ordinary telephone receiver. The ECG is then transmitted over the telephone line to a central ECG receiving facility. This noninvasive and painless procedure allows the family immediate diagnosis of dysrhythmias without a trip to an emergency unit.

An invasive procedure that allows for precise identification of the conduction disturbance and immediate investigation of drugs that are effective in halting the dysrhythmia is electrophysiologic monitoring. Electrode catheters are introduced percutaneously to the right ventricle. The heart is then selectively stimulated to induce dysrhythmias; once a dysrhythmia occurs, different antiarrhythmic drugs are administered intravenously to monitor which pharmacologic agent is most successful in terminating it.

Other procedures employed are transesophageal recording, in which an electrode catheter is passed to the lower esophagus and, when in position at a point proximal to the heart, is used to stimulate and record dysrhythmias, and epicardial pacing, in which wire electrodes are placed in the heart at the time of cardiac surgery to monitor and manage rhythm and conduction disturbances postoperatively.

Therapeutic Management

Treatment of dysrhythmias depends on the cause and severity. Whenever possible the underlying cause is treated. However, in the majority of instances this is not possible, and the use of antidysrhythmic drugs is required; rarely a permanent pacemaker may be needed to take over the conduction function of the heart. Some types of dysrhythmias are life threatening and require immediate intervention. For example, in the infant with PAT the heart rate must be rapidly converted to a normal sinus rhythm to prevent heart failure. The classic treatment consists of intravenous digitalis or cardioversion. Some authorities prefer to use digitalis first and cardioversion only if digitalization is unsuccessful, whereas others recommend cardioversion initially, since it is almost universally successful and is more dangerous if done after digitalization. Intravenous verapamil, a calcium channel blocker, has also been found to be effective (Dick and Campbell, 1984). Digitalis, verapamil, or other antidysrhythmic drugs are usually administered for almost a year and then discontinued, usually with no recurrence of PAT. In Wolff-Parkinson-White syndrome selected children who require long-term drug therapy may be candidates for surgical division of the accessory pathway.

Nursing Considerations

An initial nursing responsibility is recognition of an abnormal heartbeat, either in rate or in rhythm. Assessment of heart rate is discussed in Chapter 7, and normal pulse rates are listed on the inside front cover. Consistently high or low heart rates should be regarded with suspicion and correlated with expected changes with exercise or rest. Although no absolute standard exists for lower limits of normal heart rates, a general rule for resting rates is (Gillette, 1983):

Newborn to 3 months—below 100
3 months to 2 years—below 80
2 to 10 years—below 70
10 years and older— below 55

The infant with PAT often requires hospitalization, especially in the event of congestive heart failure. The child must be observed closely, and any worsening of the condition must be reported immediately. Heart rate is monitored and charted with any sign of activity. The child is given the same care as that discussed under congestive heart failure, including home care instructions to the parents for safe administration of digoxin (see box on p. 1492). If surgery or implantation of a pacemaker is required, the parents and child need an explanation of what to expect.

In some instances the parents and older child may be instructed in various types of reflex stimulation to terminate PAT. These include (Dick and Campbell, 1984):

diving reflex Immersing the face in cold or ice water or placing a cold washcloth on the face

Valsalva maneuver Exhaling against a closed glottis (e.g., blowing on the thumb as if it were a trumpet for 30 to 60 seconds), or deep inspiration, expiration, or coughing

baroreceptor reflex Standing on the head for 2 to 3 minutes

gag reflex Inducing gagging or vomiting by irritating the throat

In those instances when the dysrhythmia may be life threatening, parents should be taught cardiopulmonary resuscitation.

The onset and diagnosis of a cardiac dysrhythmia are frightening experiences for parents and the older child. Sometimes the dysrhythmia rapidly leads to heart failure and an emergency medical crisis. In this situation parents need a great deal of support to express their feelings, understand the diagnosis, and comply with home therapy such as daily drug administration. In working with the family, the nurse must not forget the impact of the diagnosis of a heart problem. As one mother stated, ''The heart is the body''; there is acute awareness of the necessity of the heart as a vital organ. Often an unspoken fear of potential death exists even if the dysrhythmia is benign, and repeated explanations are needed to allay the anxiety. In dealing with parents of an infant diagnosed with a dysrhythmia, the nurse must be sensitive to the care needed by parents facing the birth of a child with a congenital anomaly (see Chapter 11).

MUCOCUTANEOUS LYMPH NODE SYNDROME (KAWASAKI DISEASE)

Mucocutaneous lymph node syndrome (MLNS), or Kawasaki disease (KD), is an acute febrile illness of unknown etiology that occurs primarily in infants and young children. In the United States the peak incidence is at 3 years of age, with a slightly higher incidence in males. In Japan, where it was first described, the peak incidence is at 9 to 12 months of age. There appears to be no regional, seasonal, or socioeconomic prevalence associated with the disease, and no organism or environmental toxins have been definitively implicated. There is some evidence that susceptibility is associated with histocompatibility antigens, however.

Pathophysiology

The principal area of involvement is the cardiovascular system. During the initial stage of the illness there is progressive inflammation of the microvessels and pancarditis. During the second stage there may be progression to macrovessel inflammation and formation of coronary aneurysms (dilations of the vessel wall) and occasionally of peripheral vessel aneurysms in the cervical, axillary, brachial, iliac, and renal arteries. In the third stage much less inflammation occurs, and during the convalescent stage the inflammation ceases. However, there may be scar formation and calcification of the coronary arteries, stenosis, and/or recanalization of the coronary vessel lumen and myocardial fibrosis (Crowley, 1984). If death occurs, it is usually the result of coronary thrombosis or severe scar formation and stenosis of the main coronary artery.

Clinical Manifestations

The disease manifests in three stages. In stage one the child is ill with a prolonged high fever that is unresponsive to antipyretics and antibiotics. Within 3 to 4 days of onset the child develops inflamed mucous membranes of the eye and oropharynx, diffuse and tender indurative swelling and erythema of the extremities, and an erythematous rash. The second or subacute stage begins by 7 to 10 days with a decrease in the fever, followed by characteristic desquamation, especially of the tips of the fingers and toes. The cervical lymph nodes are often enlarged. In addition, the child may display other signs, including diarrhea, photophobia, tympanitis, and arthralgia and arthritis, especially involving the larger joints such as elbows, wrists, knees, and ankles. It is in this stage that the characteristic cardiovascular changes occur and when the diagnosis is typically made. The third or convalescent stage begins when symptoms have ended and lasts until laboratory findings of platelet count and sedimentation rate return to normal, usually 6 to 8 weeks after onset of the disease (Crowley, 1984).

Of major concern is the occurrence of myocardial infarction resulting from thrombotic occlusion in a coronary aneurysm. These usually occur within the first year of the disease but may occur for a considerable period of time beyond the disease process. The main symptoms of acute myocardial infarction in children are shock, unrest, vomiting, abdominal pain, and chest pain, which is seen mostly in older children. About a third of the patients may be asymptomatic and the majority of infarctions occur during sleep or rest (Kato, Ichinose, and Kawasaki, 1986).

Diagnostic Evaluation

Diagnosis is established on the basis of the clinical findings. The child must exhibit five of the following six criteria, including fever:

1. Fever for 5 or more days
2. Bilateral congestion of the ocular conjunctiva without exudation
3. Changes of the mucous membranes of the oral cavity, such as erythema, dryness, and fissuring of the lips, oropharyngeal reddening, or ''strawberry tongue''
4. Changes in the extremities, such as peripheral edema, peripheral erythema, and desquamation of palms and soles—particularly periungual peeling
5. Polymorphous rash, primarily of the trunk
6. Cervical lymphadenopathy

No laboratory tests are of significant value in diagnosis of the disease. Yet baseline cardiologic studies, such as chest radiograph, electrocardiogram, and echocardiogram, should be done to evaluate progressive cardiovascular changes.

Therapeutic Management

There is no definitive treatment for the disease; therefore the management is primarily supportive and aimed at controlling fever, preventing dehydration, and minimizing possible cardiac complications. Large doses of aspirin are administered in the acute stage to control fever and symptoms of inflammation and during the recovery period to prevent platelet aggregation. There is some evidence that administering high doses of salicylates (100 mg/kg/day) (Koren and others, 1985) or reduced amounts of salicylates with intravenous gamma globulin is effective in decreasing risk of coronary disease (Furusho and others, 1984). Monitoring cardiac status for possible complications is essential in follow-up.

Nursing Considerations

The nursing care of children with Kawasaki disease is primarily concerned with assisting in the diagnosis and case finding, supportive treatment as outlined by the physician, and supportive care to the child and family during both the acute and the chronic phases of the illness. Nurses should be aware that children with prolonged fever may be victims of this disorder and should encourage early medical evaluation. Administration of aspirin involves an understanding of the reasons for administration and teaching the family how it can best be given, the importance of compliance, and the early signs of toxicity. During the acute phase comfort measures are important and include relieving eye discomfort by darkening the room, having the child wear dark glasses, providing cool washcloths to cover the eyes, and instilling artificial tears. To minimize skin discomfort, cool baths, soothing lotion, and soft, loose clothing are helpful (Anderson and Thibault, 1981). Mouth care is important to prevent infection and increase comfort during feeding times. Because the child's appetite is poor during the febrile stage, favorite fluids and foods should be offered.

The child requires careful monitoring during the acute phase and conscientious follow-up in the chronic phase. It is during the long-term stage of the disease that the nurse can be especially valuable in monitoring progress and preparing the child for health visits and diagnostic tests that may be ordered to assess cardiac status, such as echocardiography and electrocardiography. Parents need to be aware of signs of complications, such as myocardial infarction, and seek medical assistance immediately. The importance of nutrition, hygiene, and normal activities is emphasized.

CARDIOMYOPATHY

Cardiomyopathy refers to abnormalities of the myocardium. Although the incidence of pediatric cardiomyopathy is only 1% of that of congenital heart disease, it accounts for 4% to 8% of all cardiac deaths in childhood and about half the survivors have chronic cardiac disability (Tripp, 1984).

Cardiomyopathy is classified according to two major types: (1) primary or idiopathic, in which the cause is unknown and the abnormality is not associated with systemic disease, and (2) secondary, in which the disorder is associated with an identifiable underlying cause. In the majority of instances the cardiomyopathy is primary, although some types demonstrate an increased incidence in families. Some of the known causes of secondary cardiomyopathy are anthracycline toxicity (the antineoplastic agents doxorubicin and daunomycin), hemochromatosis (from excessive iron storage), Duchenne muscular dystrophy, Kawasaki disease, collagen diseases, and thyroid dysfunction (French, 1981; Tripp, 1984).

Idiopathic cardiomyopathy is further classified according to its anatomic and functional features and, although the classification systems vary, may include hypertrophic, endocardial fibroelastosis, congestive, restrictive, and obliterative types. *Hypertrophic cardiomyopathy,* also known as *idiopathic hypertrophic subaortic stenosis (IHSS),* is characterized by massive ventricular hypertrophy, left ventricular outflow tract obstruction, various degrees of myocardial fibrosis, and mitral valve dysfunction. It occurs in all age-groups, but especially in the second and third decades and is the most frequent cause of sudden cardiac death in athletes (Luckstead, 1982).

Endocardial fibroelastosis (EFE) usually consists of a dilated hypocontractile heart and is a disease of infants and young children. In approximately 75% of the children EFE occurs in conjunction with congenital lesions such as aortic atresia, patent ductus arteriosus, or coarctation of the aorta, in which case it is termed *secondary EFE* (French, 1981). The cause of primary EFE is unknown but a prenatal viral infection is postulated.

Congestive or *dilated cardiomyopathy* is characterized by massive cardiomegaly as a result of the dilated ventricles; ventricular hypertrophy is mild to moderate. All age-groups are affected, including infants. The least common types are *restrictive* or *obliterative cardiomyopathy.* Poor ventricular compliance is the major abnormality in the restrictive type, and in the obliterative type abnormal tissue invades the ventricular cavity. The classic example of obliterative cardiomyopathy is endomyocardial fibrosis (EMF), a disease primarily of tropical areas, such as Africa and South America.

Therapeutic Management

Treatment is directed toward correcting the underlying cause whenever possible. However, in the majority of affected children this is not possible and treatment is aimed at managing congestive heart failure (see p. 1490) and dysrhythmias (see p. 1504). Since sudden arrhythmias can be fatal, careful monitoring and treatment are essential. Restriction of activity, especially in IHSS, is recommended to reduce the workload on the heart muscle. Propranolol (Inderal) is often prescribed for the child with IHSS because it may reduce the progressive left ventricular outflow tract obstruction. Anticoagulants may be given to reduce the risk of thromboemboli—a complication of the sluggish circulation and restricted activity of the patient with cardiomyopathy. Surgical intervention may be attempted to repair or replace affected valves or to remove part of the enlarged heart muscle.

Heart transplantation. Another option for treatment is heart transplantation in those children with end stage disease and a life expectancy of less than 6 months despite maximum medical management (Tripp, 1984). Although there have been several advancements in cardiac transplantation, especially in terms of less organ rejection with immunosuppressant drugs such as cyclosporine, heart transplantation offers palliation, not a cure. Survival rates for patients at major heart transplant centers in the United States are 50% at 5 years after surgery (Frazier and others, 1985). Most authorities restrict cardiac transplantation to children 12 years of age or older because of the extreme growth suppression associated with immunotherapy, especially steroids. Other problems with transplantation in children are the limited availability of donors, since size compatibility between donor and recipient is an important factor (English, 1983; Levitt and Karp, 1985). There is also the ethical issue of subjecting children to an essentially palliative procedure without the child's full awareness of the risks and limited benefits. These and the other issues previously discussed on p. 1474 are major concerns in use of heart transplantation.

Nursing Considerations

Because of the poor prognosis in the majority of children with cardiomyopathy, nursing care is consistent with that for any child with a life-threatening disorder (see Chapter 23). One of the most difficult adjustments for the child may be the need for restricted activity, especially the normally active youngster with IHSS. The child should be included in decisions regarding activity and allowed to discuss his feelings, particularly if the disease follows a progressively fatal course. Once symptoms of CHF or dysrhythmias develop, the same nursing interventions are implemented as discussed on p. 1491 and p. 1504. If cardiac transplantation is considered, the needs of the child and family are great in terms of psychological preparation and postoperative care. The nurse plays an important role in assessing the family's understanding of the procedure and long-term consequences. Children of school age and older should be fully informed to give their assent to the procedure.

CONCEPT SUMMARIES

- Congenital heart disease is the most common form of cardiac disease in children.

- Major categories to investigate in the cardiac history are poor weight gain, poor feeding habits, and fatigue during feeding, frequent respiratory infections and difficulties, cyanosis with or without clubbing, and evidence of exercise intolerance.

- The most common tests used in assessing cardiac function are radiography, electrocardiography, echocardiography, and cardiac catheterization.

- Cardiac catheterization provides important information about oxygen saturation of blood within the chambers and great vessels, pressure changes, changes in cardiac output or stroke volume, and anatomic abnormalities.

- Several prenatal factors may predispose children to congenital heart disease: maternal rubella during pregnancy, maternal alcoholism, maternal age above 40 years, and maternal insulin-dependent diabetes.

- Congenital heart disease is usually classified as acyanotic or cyanotic.

- Physical consequences of congenital heart disease are growth retardation, decreased exercise tolerance, dyspnea, tachypnea, tachycardia, cardiomegaly, cyanosis, and clubbing.

- Common acyanotic defects in children are ventricular septal disease, atrial septal defect, endocardial cushion defect, patent ductus arteriosus, coarctation of the aorta, pulmonic stenosis, and aortic stenosis.

- Common cyanotic defects in children are tetralogy of Fallot, transposition of the great vessels, truncus arteriosus, total anomalous pulmonary venous connection, and tricuspid atresia.

- Caring for the child with congenital heart disease and the family requires allowing for a period of grief, assessing the family's level of understanding, helping the family cope with the effects of the defect, and fostering growth-promoting family relationships.

- Preoperative care of the child with a congenital defect involves introducing the child and family to the hospital, preparing them for preoperative and postoperative procedures, and assessing physiologic status (vital signs, sleep-wake patterns, elimination, weight and height, laboratory values, and fluid intake) to determine baseline data.

- Providing postoperative care includes observing vital signs and arterial venous pressures, maintaining respiratory status, allowing maximum rest, providing comfort, monitoring fluids, planning for progressive activities, giving emotional support, observing for complications of surgery, and planning for discharge and home care.

- Acquired cardiovascular disorders include congestive heart failure, bacterial endocarditis, rheumatic fever, systemic hypertension, cardiac dysrhythmias, Kawasaki disease, and cardiomyopathy.

- Clinical manifestations of congestive heart failure (CHF) are impaired myocardial function (tachycardia, cardiomegaly), pulmonary congestion (dyspnea, tachypnea, orthopnea, cyanosis), and systemic congestion (hepatomomegalogy, edema, distended veins).

- Nursing measures in the care of a child with CHF are to assist in improving cardiac function, decrease cardiac demands, reduce respiratory distress, maintain nutritional status, promote fluid loss, and provide family support.

- Prevention of bacterial endocarditis in certain children with CHD involves administration of prophylactic antibiotics when specific procedures are performed.

- Education of the child and family with hypertension focuses on drug therapy, diet control, and appropriate exercise.

- Common dysrhythmias in children are sinoatrial dysrythmia, premature contractions, tachycardia-bradycardia syndrome, and complete atrioventricular block.

REFERENCES

Agamalian, B.: Pediatric cardiac catheterization, J. Pediatr. Nurs. **1**(2):73-79, 1986.

Alpert, B., and others: Spontaneous closure of small ventricular septal defects: ten-year follow-up, Pediatrics **63**(2):204-206, 1979.

Alpert, M.A.: Cardiac arrhythmias: a bedside guide to diagnosis and treatment, Chicago, 1980, Year Book Medical Publishers, Inc.

Anderson, D.J., and Thibault, J.: Nursing management of the pediatric patient with Kawasaki's disease, Issues Compr. Pediatr. Nurs. 5(1):1-10, 1981.

Anthony, C., and Thibodeau, G.: Textbook of anatomy and physiology, ed. 11, St. Louis, l983, The C.V. Mosby Co.

Bailey, L., and others: Baboon-to-human cardiac xenotransplantation in a neonate, JAMA 254(23):3321-3329, 1985.

Berne, R.M., and Levy, M.N.: Cardiovascular physiology, ed. 5, St. Louis, 1986, The C.V. Mosby Co.

Blumenthal, S., and others: Report of the task force on blood pressure control in children, Pediatrics 59(5)(suppl.):797-820, 1977.

Caire, J.B., and Erickson, S.: Reducing distress in pediatric patients undergoing cardiac catheterization, Child. Health Care 14(3):146-152, 1986.

Cloutier, J., and Measel, C.P.: Home care for the infant with congenital heart disease, Am. J. Nurs. 82(1):100-103, 1982.

Cranwell, P.D.: Blood pressure teaching and screening programs for school children in grades 5-8, Home Healthcare Nurse 2(3):42-46, 1984.

Crowley, D.C.: Cardiovascular complications of mucocutaneous lymph node syndrome, Pediatr. Clin. North Am. 31(6):1321-1329, 1984.

D'Antonio, I.G.: Cardiac infant's feeding difficulties, West. J. Nurs. Res. 1(1):53-55, 1979.

Dick, M., II, and Campbell, R.M.: Advances in the management of cardiac arrhythmias in children, Pediatr. Clin. North Am. 31(6):1175-1195, 1984.

DiSciascio, G., and Taranta, A.: Rheumatic fever in children, Am. Heart J. 99(5):635-658, 1980.

Emmanouilides, G.C., and Baylen, B.G.: Structural congenital heart disease in the newborn: its differentiation from nonstructural cardiac or pulmonary disease, Paediatrician 10:46-84, 1981.

English, T.A.H.: Is cardiac transplantation suitable for children? Ped. Cardiol. 4:57-58, 1983.

Feldt, R., and others: Atrial septal defects and atrioventricular canal. In Adams, F.H., and Emmanouilides, G.C., editors: Moss' heart disease in infants, children, and adolescents, ed. 3, Baltimore, 1983, The Williams & Wilkins Co.

Ferencz, C., and others: Congenital heart disease: prevalence at livebirth: the Baltimore-Washington Infant Study, Am. J. Epidemiol. 121(1):31-36, 1985.

Folger, G.M.: The murmur in the well appearing child—functional or organic? Pediatr. Basics 29:4-10, 1981.

Frazier, O.H., and others: Cardiac transplantation at the Texas Heart Institute: comparative analysis of two groups of patients (1968-1969 and 1982-1983), Ann. Thoracic Surg. 39(4):303-307, 1985.

Freed, M.D.: Recreational and sports recommendations for the child with heart disease, Pediatr. Clin. North Am. 31(6):1307-1320, 1984.

French, J.W.: Diseases of the myocardium. In Kelley, V.C., editor: Practice of pediatrics, Philadelphia, 1981, Harper & Row.

Furusho, K., and others: High-dose intravenous gammaglobulin for Kawasaki disease, Lancet 2(8411):1055-1058, 1984.

Gillette, P.C.: Cardiac dysrhythmias in infants and children, Cardiovasc. Clin. 11(2):79-95, 1981.

Gillette, P.C.: Dysrhythmias. In Adams, F.H., and Emmanouilides, G.C., editors: Moss' heart disease in infants, children, and adolescents, ed. 3, Baltimore, 1983, The Williams & Wilkins Co.

Goldring, D., and Hernandez, A.: Hypertension in children, Pediatr. Rev. 3(8):235-246, 1982.

Gordis, L.: Changing risk of rheumatic fever. In Management of pharyngitis in an era of declining rheumatic fever, report of the Eighty-Sixth Ross Conference on Pediatric Research, Columbus, OH, 1984, Ross Laboratories.

Graham, T.P., Jr.: When to operate on the child with congenital heart disease, Pediatr. Clin. North Am. 31(6):1275-1291, 1984.

Gutgessel, H.P., Garson, A., and McNamara, D.G.: Prognosis of the newborn with transposition of the great arteries, Am. J. Cardiol. 44:96-100, July 1979.

Hastreiter, A.R., and others: Maintenance digoxin dosage and steady-state plasma concentration in infants and children, J. Pediatr. 107(1):140-146, 1985.

Hazinski, M.F.: Cardiovascular disorders. In Hazinski, M.F., editor: Nursing care of the critically ill child, St. Louis, 1984, The C.V. Mosby Co.

Henriksson, P., Gunilla, V., and Lundstrom, N.: Haemostatic defects in cyanotic congenital heart disease, Br. Heart J. 41:23-27, 1979.

Kaden, G.G., and others: Physician-patient communication: understanding congenital heart disease, Am. J. Dis. Child. 139(10):995-999, 1985.

Karchmer, A.W.: Active infective endocarditis: when to operate, J. Cardiovasc. Med. 6(10):1015-1031, 1981.

Kashani, I.A.: Acute rheumatic fever: a review of pathogenesis, diagnosis, and a modified approach to Jones criteria and management, Paediatrician 10:158-176, 1981.

Kato, H., Ichinose, E., and Kawasaki, T.: Myocardial infarction in Kawasaki disease: clinical analyses in 195 cases, J. Pediatr. 108(6):923-927, 1986.

Katz, N., and others: Late survival and symptoms after repair of tetralogy of Fallot, Circulation 65(2):403-410, 1982.

Konno, S., and others: A new method for prosthetic valve replacement in congenital aortic stenosis associated with hypoplasia of the aortic valve ring, J. Thorac. Cardiovasc. Surg. 70:909-917, 1975.

Koren, G., and others: Probable efficacy of high-dose salicylates in reducing coronary involvement in Kawasaki disease, JAMA 254(6):767-769, 1985.

Kupst, M.J., and others: Improving physician-parent communication, Clin. Pediatr. 15(1):27-30, 1976.

Levitt, J.M., and Karp, R.B.: Heart transplantation, Surg. Clin. North Am. 65(3):613-635, 1985.

Lewander, W.J.: Introduction of a specific antidote for digoxin, Pediatr. Alert 11(17):65-66, 1986.

Loggie, J.M.H., and others: Juvenile hypertension: highlights of a workshop, J. Pediatr. 104(5):657-663, 1984.

Lowrey, G.: Growth and development of children, ed. 8, Chicago, l986, Year Book Medical Publishers, Inc.

Luckstead, E.F.: Sudden death in sports, Pediatr. Clin. North Am. 29(6):1355-1362, 1982.

Macartney, F.J.: Heart and circulation. In Godfrey, S., and Baum, J.D.: Clinical paediatric physiology, London, 1979, Blackwell Scientific Publications.

Malinowski, P., and Elixson, E.M.: Transportation of the great arteries, Crit. Care Nurse 5(3):35-48, 1985.

McCrory, W.W.: Essential hypertension in childhood, Pediatr. Ann. 11(7):585-590, 1982.

Mentser, M.: Diagnosis and treatment of hypertension in children, Pediatr. Clin. North Am. 29(4):933-945, 1982.

Mills, L.J., and others: Cardiothoracic surgery: perioperative principles. In Levin, D.L., Morriss, F.C., and Moore, G.C., editors: A practical guide to pediatric intensive care, ed. 2, St. Louis, 1984, The C.V. Mosby Co.

Moss, A.J.: What every primary physician should know about the postoperative cardiac patient, Pediatrics 63(2):320-330, 1979.

Moss, A.J.: Coarctation of the aorta: current status, J. Pediatr. 102(2):253-255, 1983.

Nadas, A.S.: Update on congenital heart disease, Pediatr. Clin. North Am. 31(1):153-164, 1984.

Naylor, D., Coates, T.J., and Kan, J.: Reducing distress in pediatric cardiac catheterization, Am. J. Dis. Child. 138(8):726-729, 1984.

Newburger, J.W., and Nadas, A.S.: Infective endocarditis, Pediatr. Rev. 3(7):226-230, 1982.

Newburger, J.W., and others: Cognitive function and age at repair of transposition of great arteries in children, N. Engl. J. Med. 310:1495-1499, 1984.

Newman, T.B.: Etiology of ventricular septal defects: an epidemiologic approach, Pediatrics 76(5):741-749, 1985.

Noonan, J.A.: Association of congenital heart disease with syndromes or other defects, Pediatr. Clin. North Am. 25(4):797-816, 1978.

Park, M.: Use of digoxin in infants and children, with specific emphasis on dosage, J. Pediatr. 108(6):871-877, 1986.

Pennock, J., and others: Cardiac transplantation in perspective for the future: survival, complications, rehabilitation, and cost, J. Thorac. Cardiovasc. Surg. 83(2):168-177, 1982.

Perloff, J.K.: The clinical recognition of congenital heart disease, ed. 2, Philadelphia, 1978, W.B. Saunders Co.

Portman, M.A., and others: A 20-year review of ostium primum defect repair in children, Am. Heart J. 110(5):1054-1058, 1985.

Prystowsky, E.N.: Wolff-Parkinson-White syndrome, Drug Ther. 12(2):137-141, 1982.

Reif, K.: A heart makes you live, Am. J. Nurs. 72(6):1085, 1972.

Rocchini, A.P.: Childhood hypertension: etiology, diagnosis, and treatment, Pediatr. Clin. North Am. 31(6):1259-1273, 1984.

Rocchini, A.P., and Kveselis, D.: The use of balloon angioplasty in the pediatric patient, Pediatr. Clin. North Am. 31(6):1293-1305, 1984.

Rose, V., and others: A possible increase in the incidence of congenital heart defects among the offspring of affected parents, J. Am. Coll. Cardiol. 6:376-382, 1985.

Rosenthal, A.: How to distinguish between innocent and pathologic murmurs in childhood, Pediatr. Clin. North Am. 31(6):1229-1240, 1984.

Rushton, C.H.: Preparing children and families for cardiac surgery: nursing interventions, Issues Compr. Pediatr. Nurs. 6:235-248, 1983.

Shulman, S.T., and others: Prevention of bacterial endocarditis: a statement for health professionals by the Committee on Rheumatic Fever and Infective Endocarditis of the Council on Cardiovascular Disease in the Young, Circulation 70(6):1123A-1127A, 1984.

Snider, A.R.: Use and abuse of echocardiogram, Pediatr. Clin. North Am. 31(6):1345-1366, 1984.

Southall, D.P., and others: Frequency and outcome of disorders of cardiac rhythm and conduction in a population of newborn infants, Pediatrics 68(1):58-66, 1981.

Stephenson, C.A.: Stress in critically ill patients, Am. J. Nurs. 77(11):1806-1809, 1977.

Stinson, E.B.: Surgical treatment of infective endocarditis, Prog. Cardiovasc. Dis. 22(3):145-168, 1979.

Sulayman, R.F., and Thilenius, O.G.: Complications of heart disease in children: congestive heart failure, cyanotic spells, and infective endocarditis, Paediatrician 10:99-116, 1981.

Turley, K., and others: Total anomalous pulmonary venous connection in infancy: influence of age and type of lesion, Am. J. Cardiol. 45:92-97, 1980.

Tripp, M.E.: Congestive cardiomyopathy of childhood, Adv. Pediatr. 31:179-206, 1984.

Uzark, K., Messiter, E., and Rosenthal, A.: Promoting dental health care in children with congenital heart disease, Pediatr. Nurs. 12(2):96-99, 152, 1986.

van Breda, A.: Postoperative care of infants and children who require cardiac surgery, Heart Lung 14(3):205-208, 1985.

Whittemore, R., Hobbins, J.C., and Engle, M.A.: Pregnancy and its outcome in women with and without surgical treatment of congenital heart disease, Am. J. Cardiol. 50(3):641-651, 1982.

BIBLIOGRAPHY
Diagnostic Procedures

Armstrong, F., and Finesilver, C.: Cardiac catheterization, Crit. Care Update 10(7):39-46, 1983.

Engle, M.A.: Heart sound and murmurs in diagnosis of heart disease, Pediatr. Ann. 10:18-31, 1981.

Fahey, V.A., and Finkelmeier, B.A.: Iatrogenic arterial injuries, Am. J. Nurs. 84(4):448-451, 1984.

Gersony, W.M., and Bierman, F.Z.: Cardiac catheterization in the pediatric patient, Pediatrics 67(5):738-740, 1981.

Haughey, C.W.: Preparing your patient for echocardiography, Nursing 84 14(5):68-71, 1984.

Hinz, E.: Coping strategies of a two year old girl hospitalized for cardiac catheterization, Am. J. Maternal Child Nurs. 9(1):1-6, 1980.

Laird, W.P.: Echocardiography. In Levin, D.L., Morriss, F.C., and Moore, G.C., editors: A practical guide to pediatric intensive care, ed. 2, St. Louis, 1984, The C.V. Mosby Co.

Liebman, J.: Diagnosis and management of heart murmurs in children, Pediatr. Rev. 3(10):321-332, 1982.

Malinowski, L.M., and Doyle, J.E.: Cardiac catheterization of the neonate, Am. J. Nurs. 85(1):60-62, 1985.

Slota, M.: Pediatric cardiac catheterization: complications and interventions, Crit. Care Nurse 2:22-26, 1982.

Sumner, S.M., and Grau, P.A.: Guidelines for running a 12-lead E.K.G., Nursing 85 15(12):30-33, 1985.

Youssef, M.M.: Self control behaviors of school-age children who are hospitalized for cardiac diagnostic procedures, Am. J. Maternal Child Nurs. 10:219-284, 1981.

Congenital Heart Disease

Adams, F.H., and Emmanouilides, G.C., editors: Moss' heart disease in infants, children, and adolescents, ed. 3, Baltimore, 1983, The Williams & Wilkins Co.

Bove, E.L.: Infradiaphragmatic total anomalous pulmonary venous drainage: surgical treatment and long-term results, Ann. Thorac. Surg. 31:544-550, 1981.

Clark, E.B.: Cardiac embryology: its relevance to congenital heart disease, Am. J. Dis. Child. 140(1):41-44, 1986.

Donahoo, J.S.: Prostaglandin E₁ as an adjunct to emergency cardiac operation in neonates, J. Thorac. Cardiovasc. Surg. 81:227-231, 1981.

Gersony, W.M.: Patent ductus arteriosus in the neonate, Pediatr. Clin. North Am. 33(3):545-560, 1986.

Harlan, J.L., and others: Coarctation of the aorta in infants, J. Thorac. Cardiovasc. Surg. 88:1012-1019, 1984.

Jimenez, M.Q.: Ten common congenital cardiac defects: diagnosis and management, Paediatrician 10:3-45, 1981.

Linde, L.M.: Psychiatric aspects of congenital heart disease, Psychiatric Clin. North Am. 5(2):399-406, 1982.

Marcelletti, C.: Fontan's operation: an expanded horizon, J. Thorac. Cardiovasc. Surg. 80:764-769, 1980.

Nadas, A.S.: Role of general pediatrician in pediatric cardiology, Pediatr. Rev. 3(4):103-107, 1981.

Newfeld, E.A.: Cyanotic congenital heart disease. In Levin, D.L., Morriss, F.C., and Moore, G.C., editors: A practical guide to pediatric intensive care, ed. 2, St. Louis, 1984, The C.V. Mosby Co.

Rowland, T.W.: The pediatrician and congenital heart disease—1979, Pediatrics 64(2):180-186, 1979.

Rubin, J.D., and Ferencz, C.: Subsequent pregnancy in mothers of infants with congenital heart disease, Pediatrics 76(3):371-374, 1985.

Sacksteder, S.: Congenital heart defects—embryology and fetal circulation, Am. J. Nurs. 78:262-264, 1978.

Sacksteder, S., Gildea, J.H., and Dassy, C.: Common congenital cardiac defects, Am. J. Nurs. 78(2):266-272, 1978.

Sasso, S.C.: Prostaglandin E¹ for infants with congenital heart disease, Am. J. Maternal Child Nurs. 8(1):29, 1983.

Stanton, R.E., and others: The Fontan procedure for tricuspid atresia, Circulation 64 (suppl. II):140-146, 1981.

Tucker, W.Y.: Management of symptomatic tetralogy of Fallot in the first year of life, J. Thorac. Cardiovasc. Surg. 78:494-501, 1979.

Werner, B.L.: Cardiovascular crises. In Vestal, K.W.: Pediatric critical care nursing, New York, 1981, John Wiley & Sons.

Nursing Care of the Family and Child

Bindler, R.M.: Home care for a child with a cardiac defect, Issues Compr. Pediatr. Nurs. 3(7):48-60, 1979.

Cohen, S.: Programmed instruction: how to work with chest tubes, Am. J. Nurs. 80(4):685-712, 1980.

Dance, D., and Yates, M.: Nursing assessment and care of children with complications of congenital heart disease, Heart Lung 14(3):209-214, 1985.

Engle, M.A.: Management of the child after cardiac surgery, Pediatr. Ann. 10(4):53-60, 1981.

Erickson, R.: Chest tubes: they're really not that complicated, Nursing 81 11(5):34-42, 1981.

Filipek, J.E.: Post-operative care of the pediatric cardiac patient, Crit. Care Q. 3(1):45-52, 1980.

Furgal, C.L.: Pediatric cardiology: stressors, reactions, and interventions, Issues Compr. Pediatr. Nurs. **5**:21-31, 1981.

Gay, W.A.: Cardiac surgery in infancy, Pediatr. Ann. **10**(4):48-52, 1981.

Gildea, J.H., and others: Congenital heart defects, pre- and postoperative nursing care, Am. J. Nurs. **78**:273-278, 1978.

Gottesfeld, I.B.: The family of the child with congenital heart disease, Am. J. Maternal Child Nurs. **4**:101-104, 1979.

Hazinski, M.F.: Critical care of the pediatric cardiovascular patient, Nurs. Clin. North Am. **16**(4):671-697, 1981.

Kashani, I.A., and Higgins, S.S.: Counseling strategies for families of children with congenital heart disease, Pediatr. Nurs. **12**(1):38-40, 1986.

Kotchabhakdi, P., and Beardslee, C.: School-age children's conceptions of the heart and its function: part I. Review of literature, Am. J. Maternal Child Nurs. **14**(3):139-152, 1985.

Lewandowski, L.A.: Stresses and coping styles of parents of children undergoing open-heart surgery, Crit. Care Q. **3**:75-84, 1980.

Loeffel, M.: Developmental considerations of infants and children with congenital heart disease, Heart Lung **14**(3):214-217, 1985.

Mims, B.C.: You can manage chest tubes confidently, RN **48**(1):39-44, 1985.

Peterson, M.C.: Preparation of the cardiac child and the family for surgery, Issues Compr. Pediatr. Nurs. **3**:61-71, Dec. 1979.

Rogers, T.R., and others: Heart surgery in infants: a preliminary assessment of maternal adaptation, Child. Health Care **13**(2):52-58, 1984.

Shor, V.Z.: Congenital cardiac defects: assessment and case findings, Am. J. Nurs. **78**(2):256-261, 1978.

Shor, V.Z.: Long-term implications of cardiovascular disease, Issues Compr. Pediatr. Nurs. **2**(5):36-50, 1978.

White, R.C.: Action stat: dislodged chest tube, Nursing 85 **15**(12):25, 1985.

Congestive Heart Failure

Barry, W.H., and Smith, T.W.: Digitalis: how does it work? J. Cardiovasc. Med. **7**(2):217-220, 1982.

Cohen, S.: New concepts in understanding congestive heart failure. Part I. How the clinical features arise, Am. J. Nurs. **81**(1):119-142, 1981.

Cohen, S.: New concepts in understanding congestive heart failure. Part II. How the therapeutic approaches work, Am. J. Nurs. **81**(2):357-380, 1981.

Friedman, W.F., and George, B.L.: New concepts and drugs in the treatment of congestive heart failure, Pediatr. Clin. North Am. **31**(6):1197-1227, 1984.

Friedman, W.F., and George, B.L.: Treatment of congestive heart failure by altering loading conditions of the heart, J. Pediatr. **106**(5):697-706, 1985.

Horvath, P.T., and Depew, C.C.: Toward preventing digitalis toxicity, Nurses Drug Alert **IV**(4):25-32, 1980.

Jackson, P.L.: Digoxin therapy at home: keeping the child safe, Am. J. Maternal Child Nurs. **4**(2):105-109, 1979.

Koren, G.: Interaction between digoxin and commonly coadministered drugs in children, Pediatrics **75**(6):1032-1037, 1985.

Levin, D.L.: Congestive heart failure. In Levin, D.L., Morriss, F.C., and Moore, G.C., editors: A practical guide to pediatric intensive care, ed. 2, St. Louis, 1984, The C.V. Mosby Co.

McCauley, K., and Burke, K.G.: Your detailed guide to drugs for C.H.F., Nursing 84 **14**(5):46-50, 1984.

Modrcin, M.A., and Schott, J.: An update of congestive heart failure in infants, Issues Compr. Pediatr. Nurs. **3**(7):6-22, 1979.

Norsen, L.H., and Fox, G.B.: Understanding cardiac output—and the drugs that affect it, Nursing 85 **15**(4):34-41, 1985.

Smith, K.M.: Recognizing cardiac failure in neonates, Am. J. Maternal Child Nurs. **4**(2):98-100, 1979.

Bacterial Endocarditis

Dajani, A.S.: Prevention of bacterial endocarditis, Pediatr. Infect. Dis. **4**(4):349-352, 1985.

Fordham, C., and others: Infective endocarditis: an analysis based on strict case definitions, Ann. Intern. Med. **94**(Part 1):505-518, 1981.

Guntheroth, W.G.: How important are dental procedures as a cause of infective endocarditis? Am. J. Cardiol. **54**:797-801, 1984.

Jenkins, J.: Infective endocarditis: a clinical overview, Crit. Care Update **10**(5):42-47, 1983.

Special statement: prevention of bacterial endocarditis, Pediatrics **75**(3):603-607, 1985.

Van Hare, G.F., and others: Infective endocarditis in infants and children during the past 10 years: a decade of change, Am. Heart J. **107**:1235-1240, 1984.

Rheumatic Fever

Bisno, A.L.: The rise and fall of rheumatic fever, JAMA **254**(4):538-541, 1985.

Diehl, A.M.: Clinical aspects of rheumatic fever: an update, Issues Compr. Pediatr. Nurs. **2**:69-76, April 1980.

Lue, H., and others: Rheumatic fever recurrences: controlled study of 3-week versus 4-week benzathine penicillin prevention programs, J. Pediatr. **108**(2):229-304, 1986.

Markowitz, M.: The decline of rheumatic fever: role of medical intervention, J. Pediatr. **106**(4):545-550, 1985.

Nordin, J.D.: Recurrence of rheumatic fever during prophylaxis with monthly benzathine penicillin G, Pediatrics **73**(4):530-531, 1984.

Wannamaker, L.W.: Changes and changing concepts in the biology of group A streptococci and in the epidemiology of streptococcal infections, Rev. Infect. Dis. **1**(6):967-975, 1979.

Wannamaker, L.W., and Kaplan, E.L.: Acute rheumatic fever. In Adams, F.H., and Emmanouilides, G.C., editors: Moss' heart disease in infants, children, and adolescents, ed. 3, Baltimore, 1983, Williams & Wilkins.

Systemic Hypertension

Alpert, B.S., and others: Blood pressure response to dynamic exercise in healthy children—black vs white, J. Pediatr. **99**:556-560, 1981.

Bailie, M.D., and Mattioli, L.F.: Hypertension: relationships between pathophysiology and therapy, J. Pediatr. **96**:789-797, 1980.

Britton, C.V.: Blood pressure measurement and hypertension in children, Pediatr. Nurs. **7**(4):13-17, 1981.

Buckley, K.M.: Pediatric and adolescent hypertension, Crit. Care Update **6**(2):14-26, 1979.

Fixler, D.E., and Laird, W.P.: Validity of mass blood pressure screening in children, Pediatrics **72**(4):459-463, 1983.

Fixler, D.E., Laird, W.P., and Dana, K.: Usefulness of exercise stress testing for prediction of blood pressure trends, Pediatrics **75**(6):1071-1075, 1985.

Grim, C.M., and Grim, C.E.: The nurse's role in hypertension control, Fam. Commun. Health **4**(1):29-40, 1981.

Grimm, R.H., Jr., and Hunninghake, D.B.: Lipids and hypertension: implications of new guidelines for cholesterol management in the treatment of hypertension, Am. J. Med. **80**(suppl. 2A):56-63, 1986.

Gruskin, A.B.: The adolescent with essential hypertension, Am. J. Kidney Dis. **VI**(2):86-90, 1985.

Hutchins, L.N.: Drug treatment of high blood pressure, Nurs. Clin. North Am. **16**(2):365-376, 1981.

Jorde, L.B., and Williams, R.R.: Innovative blood pressure measurements yield information not reflected by sitting measurements, Hypertension **14**(4):252-257, 1986.

Kaplan, M.R., and Hernandez, L.G.: The pathogenesis and diagnosis of hypertension in children, Pediatr. Ann. **11**(7):592-602, 1982.

Lieberman, E.: Blood pressure and primary hypertension in childhood and adolescence, Curr. Probl. Pediatr. **10**(4):1-35, 1980.

Loggie, J.M.H.: Systemic hypertension. In Adams, F.H., and Emmanouilides, G.C., editors: Moss' heart disease in infants, children, and adolescents, ed. 3, Baltimore, 1983, The Williams & Wilkins Co.

Loggie, J.M.H., New, M.I., and Robson, A.M.: Hypertension in the pediatric patient: a reappraisal, J. Pediatr. **94**:685-699, 1979.

Loustau, A., and Blair, B.J.: A key to compliance: systematic teaching to help hypertensive patients follow through on treatment, Nursing 81 **11**:84-87, 1981.

McCrory, W.W.: Finding an elevated blood pressure—what does it mean? Pediatr. Ann. **11**(7):581-584, 1982.

Moore, L.C., and Pulliam, C.B.: An on-the-spot guide to antihypertensive drugs, Nursing 86 **16**(1):54-57, 1986.

Nauright, L.P., and others: Identifying hypertensive adolescents, Pediatr. Nurs. **5**(2):34-37, 1979.

The 1984 Report of the Joint National Committee on Detection, Evaluation, and Treatment of High Blood Pressure, Arch. Intern. Med. **144**:1045-1057, 1984.

Oberfield, S.E., and others: Long-term treatment of childhood hypertension with captopril, Pediatr. Ann. **11**(7):614-621, 1982.

Olson, R.E.: Mass intervention vs screening and selective intervention for the prevention of coronary heart disease, JAMA **255**(16):2204-2207, 1986.

Plunkett, L.W., and Dustan, H.P.: Mild hypertension: the continuing dilemma of treatment, Fam. Commun. Health **7**(1):38-46, 1984.

Pruitt, A.W.: Pharmacologic approach to the management of childhood hypertension, Pediatr. Clin. North Am. **28**:135-144, 1981.

Reisman, L., and Selden, R.V.: Management of systemic hypertension in children, Pediatr. Ann. **11**(7):604-613, 1982.

Roy, C.C., and Galeano, N.: Childhood antecedents of adult degenerative disease, Pediatr. Clin. North Am. **32**(2):517-533, 1985.

Cardiac Dysrhythmias

Campbell, R.M., and others: Atrial overdrive pacing for conversion of atrial flutter in children, Pediatrics **75**(4):730-736, 1985.

Dunnigan, A., Benson, D.W., Jr., and Benditt, D.G.: Atrial flutter in infancy: diagnosis, clinical features, and treatment, Pediatrics **75**(4):725-729, 1985.

Gillette, P.C., and others: Dysrhythmias. In Adams, F.H., and Emmanouilides, G.C., editors: Moss' heart disease in infants, children, and adolescents, ed. 3, Baltimore, 1983, The Williams & Wilkins Co.

Johnson, D.L.: Pediatric arrhythmias: a nursing approach, Dimen. Crit. Care Nurs. **2**(3):147-157, 1983.

Mahoney, L.T., and others: Pacemaker management for acute onset of heart block in childhood, J. Pediatr. **107**(2):207-211, 1985.

Mantakas, M.E., McCue, C.M., and Miller, W.W.: Natural history of Wolff-Parkinson-White syndrome discovered in infancy, Am. J. Cardiol. **41**:1097-1103, May 1978.

Mason, J.W.: The role of surgery in the treatment of arrhythmias, Hosp. Pract. **16**(12):66-74, 1981.

Mofenson, H.C., Caraccio, T.R., and Schauben, J.: Poisoning by antidysrhythmic drugs, Pediatr. Clin. North Am. **33**(3):723-738, 1986.

Moser, S., and Flaker, G.: Get ready: the new antiarrhythmics are coming, Nursing 85 **15**(9):56-58, 1985.

Pickoff, A.S., and others: Arrhythmias and conduction system disturbances in infants and children—recent advances and contributions of intracardiac electrophysiology, Cardiovasc. Clin. **11**(1):203-219, 1980.

Shakibi, J.G.: Arrhythmias in infants and children, Paediatrician **10**:117-122, 1981.

Yabek, S.M., and others: Symptomatic sinus node dysfunction in children without structural heart disease, Pediatrics **69**(5):590-593, 1982.

Kawasaki Disease

Anderson, T.M., Meyer, R., and Kaplan, S.: Long-term echocardiographic evaluation of cardiac size & function in patients with Kawasaki disease, Am. Heart J. **110**(1)(part 1):107-115, 1985.

Koren, G., and others: Kawasaki disease: review of risk factors for coronary aneurysms, J. Pediatr. **108**(3):388-392, 1986.

L'Orange, C.: Kawasaki disease: a new threat to children, Am. J. Nurs. **83**:558-562, 1983.

Lynch, M.H., and Gray, J.L.: Kawasaki disease, Pediatr. Nurs. **8**:96-101, 1982.

Nakano, H., and others: Clinical characteristics of myocardial infarction following Kawasaki disease: report of 11 cases, J. Pediatr. **108**(2):198-203, 1986.

Turner-Gomes, S., and others: High persistence rate of established coronary artery lesions secondary to Kawasaki disease among a panethnic Canadian population, J. Pediatr. **108**(6):928-932, 1986.

Cardiomyopathy

Gillum, R.F.: Idiopathic cardiomyopathy in the United States, 1970-1982, Am. Heart J. **111**(4):752-755, 1986.

Hanukoglu, A., Fried, D., and Somekh, E.: Inheritance of familial primary endocardial fibroelastosis, Clin. Pediatr. **25**(5):272-275, 1986.

Hazinski, M.F.: Sudden cardiac death in children, Critical Care Quarterly **7**(2):59-70, 1984.

Maron, B.J.: Cardiomyopathies. In Adams, F.H., and Emmanouilides, G.C., editors: Moss' heart disease in infants, children, and adolescents, ed. 3, Baltimore, 1983, Williams & Wilkins.

Rao, P.S.: Chronic afterload reduction in infants and children with primary myocardial disease, J. Pediatr. **108**(4):530-534, 1986.

Vetter, V.L.: Sudden death in infants, children, and adolescents, Cardiovasc. Clin. **15**(3):301-313, 1985.

Heart Transplantation

Allender, J., and others: Stages of psychological adjustment associated with heart transplantation, Heart Transplantation **2**(3):228-233, 1983.

Bolman, R.M., III: Cardiac transplantation: realities in 1985, Ann. Thoracic Surg. **39**(4):301-302, 1985.

Cardin, S., and Clark, S.: A nursing diagnosis approach to the patient awaiting cardiac transplantation, Heart Lung **14**(5):499-504, 1985.

Goldman, M.H., and others: Cyclosporine in cardiac transplantation, Surg. Clin. North Am. **65**(3):637-659, 1985.

Hess, M.L., and others: Status of cardiac transplantation 1981-1982, National Registry Report, J. Am. Coll. Cardiol. **1**(2):721, 1983.

Hunt, S.A.: Complications of heart transplantation, Heart Transplantation **3**(1):70-74, 1983.

Marsden, C.: Ethical issues in a heart transplant program, Heart Lung **14**(5):495-499, 1985.

Mathias, J.M.: Immunosuppression: postoperative management of heart transplant recipients, AORN J. **41**(4):748-753, 1985.

McAleer, M.J., and others: Psychological aspects of heart transplantation, Heart Transplantation **4**(2):232-233, 1985.

O'Brien, V.C.: Psychological and social aspects of heart transplantation, Heart Transplantation **4**(2):229-231, 1985.

Painvin, G.A., and others: Cardiac transplantation: indications, procurement, operation, and management, Heart Lung **14**(5):484-489, 1985.

Penkoske, P.A., and others: The future of heart and heart-lung transplantation in children, Heart Transplantation **3**(3):233-237, 1984.

Wiles, H.B., and others: Repeated endomyocardial biopsy without complication in an infant after heart transplantation, J. Thoracic Cardiovasc. Surg. **91**(4):637-638, 1986.

Chapter 35

The Child with Hematologic Dysfunction

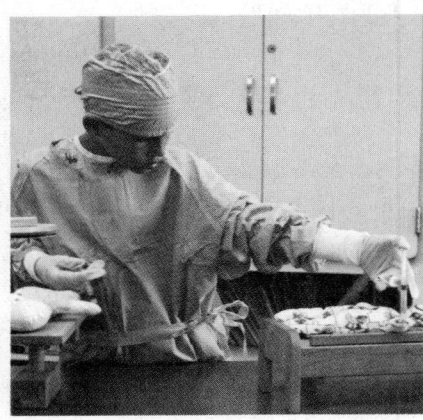

Disorders related to the blood and/or blood-forming organs in childhood encompass a wide range of diseases and pathologic states. Since the blood is a multipurpose fluid involved in the functions of so many tissues and organs, either primary or secondary changes in the blood are reflected in the essential functions of these structures. Hematologic disorders in childhood include the anemias, defects in hemostasis, and the immunologic-deficiency diseases. Related neoplastic disorders—the leukemias and lymphomas—are discussed in Chapter 36.

The Hematologic System and Its Function

The hematologic system, composed of the blood and blood-forming tissues, is responsible for a complex system of homeostatic mechanisms that produces cells with specific functions and provides for oxygenation and distribution of nutrients and other chemicals to the cells, collection of wastes from the cells, and regulation of heat. Any disturbance within this system can result in widespread alteration of function almost anywhere in the body, including rapid death from acute loss of blood. The following is an overview of the formation of the various elements of the blood and a brief discussion of assessment of hematologic function. More detailed information is provided when specific disorders are presented.

ORIGIN OF FORMED ELEMENTS

Blood has two major components: a fluid portion called plasma and a cellular portion known as the formed elements of the blood. The two components are approximately equal in volume. Plasma is about 90% water and 10% solutes. The principal solutes are the proteins albumin, globulin, and fibrinogen. The cellular elements are red blood cells *(erythrocytes)*, white blood cells *(leukocytes)*, and platelets *(thrombocytes)*.

The major blood-forming (hemopoietic) organs of the body are the red bone marrow (myeloid tissue) and lymphatic system, which consists of lymph (fluid), lymphatic vessels, and lymphoid structures—the lymph nodes, spleen, thymus, and tonsils. However, not all structures of the lymphatic system produce blood cells, especially during postnatal life. Another system that is involved in blood cell production is the *reticuloendothelial system*. Although not a discrete anatomic entity, it refers to widely dispersed cells of mesodermal origin that line the vascular and lymph channels. These cells, called *reticular cells* because they form a network, are capable of phagocytosis (ingestion and digestion of foreign substances), formation of immune bodies, and differentiation into other cells, such as hemocytoblasts, myeloblasts, or lymphoblasts.

All of the formed elements of the blood, except to some extent the agranulocytes, are believed to be formed in myeloid tissue during postnatal life. During embryonic development the mesenchyme, spleen, liver, thymus, and yolk sac serve as additional sites of blood cell formation. In certain blood disorders these sites, particularly the spleen, can be stimulated to produce blood cells, and constitute *extramedullary hemopoiesis*. In infants and young children all of the bone contains red marrow (so called because of its color from formation of erythrocytes), but as bone growth ceases near the end of adolescence, only the ribs, sternum, vertebrae, and pelvis continue to produce blood cells. The remainder of the bone marrow becomes yellow from deposition of fat. However, in conditions of increased demand for blood cells, the yellow marrow can revert to red marrow as another hemopoietic source.

Although the progressive development of each blood cell is fairly well delineated, there is considerable controversy regarding the origin of the blood cell. One of the most widely held theories (monophyletic) is that each blood cell originates from a primordial (primitive) cell called a *blast,* or *stem,* cell. This *hemocytoblast* in turn gives rise to the erythroblast, myeloblast, monoblast, lymphoblast, and megakaryoblast (Fig. 35-1).

Erythrocytes

The erythrocyte is formed from the hemocytoblast in the red bone marrow. As illustrated in Fig. 35-1, the *hemocytoblast* forms the proerythroblast. The initial cell of this series has a deep blue (basophilic) staining cytoplasm and therefore is called a *basophilic erythroblast*. The chief change in the erythroblast is accumulation of hemoglobin in the cytoplasm. As the basophilic material decreases and the amount of hemoglobin increases, the cell is called a *polychromatic erythroblast,* which describes its mixture of staining properties. At the same time as the nucleus is decreasing in size, the basophilic material disappears, so that the cell is uniformly stained by eosin dye, hence the name *orthochromatic erythroblast,* or *normoblast*. Finally the normoblast completely loses its nucleus by a process of extrusion as it squeezes through the pores of the membrane into the capillary. As a result of losing its nucleus, the cell caves in on both sides, giving the mature *erythrocyte* its characteristic appearance as a biconcave disc. During each of these stages the different cells continue to undergo mitosis so that increasingly greater numbers of cells are produced.

The *reticulocyte* is the last stage of development before the mature erythrocyte. Reticulocytes are slightly larger than erythrocytes and are used as an indicator of active erythropoiesis. Ordinarily the total proportion of circulating reticulocytes (known as the reticulocyte count) is between 0.5% and 1.5%. A change in the number of reticulocytes is an indicator of increased red blood cell production or hyperfunctioning of the bone marrow. The *reticulocyte* (or ''retic'') *count* is a simple laboratory test frequently used to indirectly analyze hemopoiesis.

Regulation of erythrocyte production. The usual life span of the mature erythrocyte is 120 days. Apparently as red blood cells grow old, their membranes become fragile and eventually rupture. The contents of the cell fragment as they circulate through the blood vessels and are phagocytized by the reticuloendothelial cells in the spleen, liver, and bone marrow. The hemoglobin is broken down into the iron-containing pigment hemosiderin and the bile pigments biliverdin and bilirubin. Most of the iron is reused by the bone marrow for production of new red blood cells or stored in the liver and other tissues for future use. The bile pigments are excreted by the liver in bile.

Normally there is a homeostatic balance between the regulation of red blood cell production and destruction. This

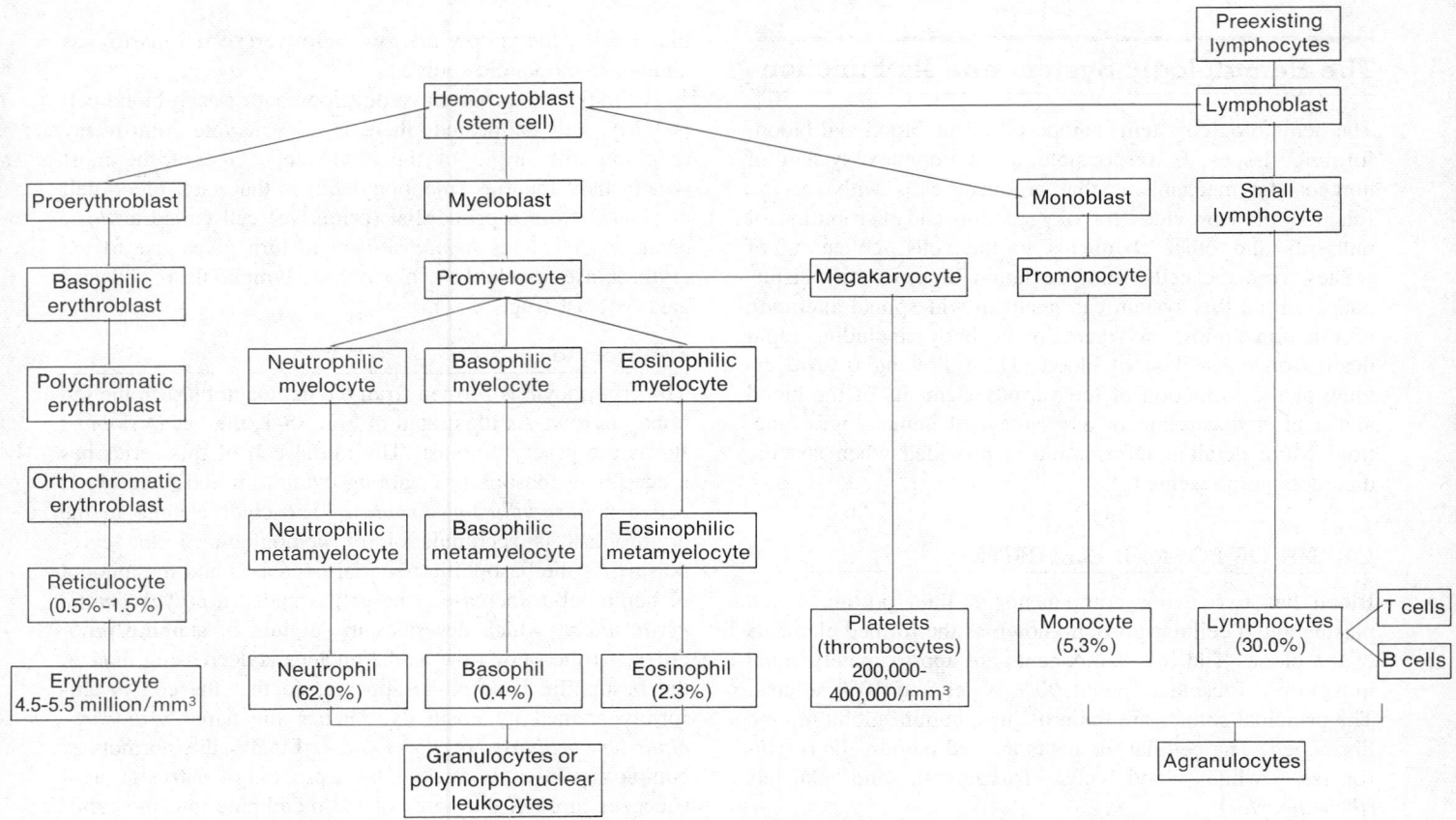

Fig. 35-1. Formation of blood cells. Erythrocyte values are averages for older children. (For blood values at each age, see Appendix D.)

balance ensures adequate tissue oxygenation and a blood viscosity that allows the blood to flow freely through the vessels. The basic regulator of erythrocyte production is believed to be tissue oxygenation. In states of tissue hypoxia, *erythropoietin* (also called *erythropoietic stimulating factor* or *hemopoietin*) is released by the kidneys into the bloodstream. As a result, the bone marrow is stimulated to produce new red blood cells. The major activity seems to be an increase in both the maturation rate and mitosis of all stages of erythrocyte production, but primarily at the stem cell level.

During this rapid increase of red blood cell production, the circulating erythrocytes may not be totally mature. Consequently, the number of reticulocytes may increase dramatically (as high as 30% or more of the total red blood cell count). Even normoblasts may appear in the blood. Failure to observe this rise in erythrocyte and reticulocyte count is an indicator of bone marrow failure.

Once tissue oxygenation is adequate, the production of erythropoietin ceases. Thus tissue oxygen requirements control both the stimulation and termination of erythrocyte production. It is important to note that it is the function of red blood cells to transport oxygen to the tissues in response to their needs, not the circulating numbers of erythrocytes, that is the basic regulatory mechanism. This explains why *polycythemia* (increase in the number of erythrocytes) occurs in conditions of prolonged tissue hypoxia, such as cyanotic

heart defects (see p. 1460). If the circulating numbers of erythrocytes controlled erythropoietin release, this feedback mechanism would control erythrocyte production at a constant level (4.5 to 5.5 million/mm³ of blood) regardless of existing tissue hypoxia.

Functions of erythrocytes. The major function of red blood cells is to transport hemoglobin, which in turn carries oxygen to all cells of the body. However, erythrocytes have other significant functions: (1) they contain quantities of carbonic anhydrase, an enzyme that catalyzes the reaction between carbon dioxide and water, allowing large quantities of carbon dioxide to react with blood for transportation to the lungs, and (2) the hemoglobin, a protein, serves as an effective acid-base buffer, maintaining the blood pH at a constant level.

Leukocytes

The leukocytes refer to a number of cells with similar yet distinct functions. They are divided into two major classifications—granulocytes and agranulocytes—based on the presence or absence, respectively, of granules within the cytoplasm of the cells.

Granulocytes. There are three types of granulocytes: *neutrophils, basophils,* and *eosinophils.* The name of each of these refers to the granule's characteristic staining property during laboratory analysis. Neutrophils stain neutral to the dyes, whereas basophils stain a purple color to the basic methylene blue dye and eosinophils take on a red color to the acidic eosin dye. Because the nuclei of these cells have two or more lobules that are connected by fine chromatin strands, the term *polymorphonuclear* (meaning "many-formed nuclei") *leukocytes,* or simply "polys," is collectively used to refer to the granulocytes.

The granulocytes, like erythrocytes, are produced in the bone marrow. For this reason these cells are sometimes referred to as *myelogenous leukocytes.* It is believed that these cells originate from primitive stem cells, which develop into myeloblasts. As Fig. 35-1 illustrates, the genesis of neutrophils, basophils, and eosinophils is similar to the stages observed during erythrocyte production. The differentiation of myeloblasts into various mature white blood cells is primarily the result of specialization within the cytoplasm and degeneration of the nucleus. Unlike the erythrocyte, however, all of the white blood cells are nucleated.

Bands or *band forms* are slightly immature forms of granulocytes. Increased numbers of bands in the peripheral circulation (referred to as a "shift to the left" on the complete blood count) indicate an accelerated production of granulocytes to meet the body's needs, such as in bacterial infection.

Agranulocytes. The agranulocytes comprise two cell types, the *monocytes* and *lymphocytes.* Characteristically these cells do not develop granules, and the nuclei are not lobulated. They are believed to have their origin in various lymphogenous organs and for this reason are sometimes referred to as *lymphogenous leukocytes.* However, since stem cells and reticular cells are capable of differentiating into monocytes or lymphocytes, the origin of these cells is frequently designated as the *lymphomyeloid complex,* which includes the bone marrow, lymph nodes, spleen, liver, thymus, subepithelial lymphoid tissue (tonsils, vermiform appendix, and intestinal lymphoid tissues), and connective tissues (mesenchymal cells of the reticuloendothelial system).

The monocytes follow the same sequence of development from the stem cell as the granulocytes (see Fig. 35-1). The monocytes, in turn, have the ability to develop into *macrophages,* large cells that are highly effective phagocytes.

Lymphocyte formation *(lymphocytopoiesis)* is believed to take place anywhere in the lymphomyeloid complex. Lymphocytes develop from blast (stem) cells (see Fig. 35-1). The lymphocyte has the potential to develop into other cells. For example, lymphocytes may become T-cells or B-cells (see p. 1549).

Regulation of leukocyte production. The exact life span of the leukocytes is not as clearly defined as that of the erythrocytes, because their existence in the circulation is primarily for transportation to extravascular areas, where they reside in reservoirs or where they are needed to resist infection. Therefore their survival rate has been divided into three phases: (1) the *hemopoietic phase,* extending from the development of the blast cell to the delivery of the mature leukocyte into the circulation, (2) the *intravascular phase,* or the period within the circulation, and (3) the *extravascular phase,* or the time spent in the viscera or tissues.

Granulocytes have a half-life of 6 to 8 hours in the blood and, after entering the tissues, die over 4 to 5 days (Chessells, 1979). Agranulocytes live for an extended period because they remain in inflamed tissue areas longer than the granulocytes. Because monocytes wander back and forth between the blood and tissues and are capable of becoming macrophages, their life span is still unknown.

The regulation of leukocytes is based on the body's need for them. Tissue damage from bacterial or viral agents promotes leukocyte circulation and production. However, *leukocytosis* (increase in leukocytes) results from tissue destruction from almost any factor, such as hemorrhage, neoplastic disease, toxicity, operative procedures, chemical and thermal injury, or tissue ischemia.

The leukocytes probably die as a result of their activity at the site of injury and are phagocytized by other newly formed white blood cells. Effective control of the inflammatory process with subsequent tissue recovery most likely results in a feedback mechanism to the bone marrow and causes lymphogenous organs to cease increased production of white blood cells.

Functions of leukocytes. Although all of the leukocytes play some role in the immune process, each of the white blood cells plays a specific role. Neutrophils and monocytes are effective phagocytes and as a result are primarily involved in inflammatory reactions. *Neutrophilia* (increased numbers of neutrophils) is most evident in an acute inflammation, whereas *monocytosis* (increased number of monocytes) is more evident in chronic conditions. The reason for this is that as the affected area becomes acidic from tissue necrosis, neutrophils, which prefer a neutral environment, become less efficient, and the monocytes, which become macrophages, become more powerful. Since lymphocytes have the ability to become monocytes and then macrophages, these cells also increase during chronic inflammation. The other functions of lymphocytes in terms of the immune process are discussed on p. 1549.

The function of eosinophils is still not completely known. They seem to have parasiticidal properties because they can selectively destroy parasites. They may also function in the immediate type of allergic or anaphylactic hypersensitivity reactions, since *eosinophilia* (increased numbers of eosinophils) is well documented in such conditions. Eosinophils also are thought to release a substance called *profibrinolysin,* which, when activated to form fibrinolysin, digests *fibrin,* thereby helping dissolve a clot.

The function of basophils is also poorly understood, although *basophilia* (increased numbers of basophils) occurs during the healing phase of inflammation and during prolonged inflammation. Since basophils closely resemble mast cells, which liberate heparin (a substance that prevents blood coagulation), it is possible that the basophilia that occurs in these two conditions helps prevent the agglutination process that is peculiar to prolonged inflammation.

Platelets

Platelets are actually small fragments of cells. They are smaller than blood cells, do not possess a cellular structure, and consist of a clear substance containing granules. The origin of platelets is the megakaryocytes, which are part of the myelogenous group of white blood cells (see Fig. 35-1). Platelets are formed when the megakaryocytic membrane invaginates, fuses within the cell to separate the cytoplasm, and then fragments.

Regulation of platelet production. The life span of platelets has been estimated as 8 to 10 days. Apparently the body regulates platelets to maintain a fairly constant level (between 200,000 and 400,000/mm³). Platelet production is probably regulated by a hormone, thrombopoietin, but the source and mode of action of this substance are unknown. Old platelets are most likely removed by the liver and spleen.

Function of platelets. The term *thrombocyte* means "clot" (thrombo) and "cell" (cyte) and accurately describes the main function of platelets. When there is a break in the continuity of a blood vessel, the platelets, which are normally round or oval discs, come in contact with the wet vessel surface and dramatically change their shape to become swollen spheres with long irregular projections called *pseudopodia* (false feet). As a result, the platelets begin to adhere to the wet endothelium and to each other. The initial platelets at the site of injury release substances that attract other thrombocytes to the area. This causes a layering of platelets, which eventually forms a plug. This plug is large enough to partially or totally occlude the opening in the vessel wall but small enough to allow blood flow to continue unimpaired through the vessel.

In small vessel tears, the platelet plug is sufficient to produce hemostasis and additional blood coagulation is not necessary. However, when platelet counts are low, these numerous small ruptures, which occur continually in the body as a result of general functioning, are not repaired. Consequently, small hemorrhagic areas called *petechiae* form under the skin. Their appearance is similar to reddish freckles.

Platelets also influence hemostasis by releasing a substance called *serotonin* at the site of injury. This substance is a vasoconstrictor that produces vascular spasm to decrease the amount of blood flow to the injured area.

ASSESSMENT OF HEMATOLOGIC FUNCTION

Several tests can be performed to assess hematologic function, including additional procedures to identify the cause of the dysfunction. The following discussion is limited to a description of the most common and one of the most valuable tests, the complete blood count (CBC). Other procedures, such as those related to iron, coagulation, and immune status, are discussed throughout the chapter as appropriate.

The CBC consists of the following determinations: red blood cell count (RBC), white blood cell count (WBC), hematocrit (Hct), hemoglobin (Hb or Hgb), differential WBC, RBC indices (mean corpuscular volume [MCV], mean corpuscular hemoglobin [MCH], and mean corpuscular hemoglobin concentration [MCHC]), and peripheral smear. Additional tests may be included, such as the reticulocyte count and platelet count. Each of these is summarized in

Table 35-1. Most of the determinations can be performed on a small quantity of blood (micromethod) and are automatically computed. The nurse should be familiar with the significance of the findings from the CBC and aware of normal values for age, which are listed in Appendix D.

As with any other disorder, the history and physical examination are essential to identification of hematologic dysfunction, and the nurse is often the first person to suspect a problem based on information from these sources. Comments by the parent regarding the child's lack of energy, food diary of poor sources of iron, frequent infections, and bleeding that is difficult to control offer clues to the more common disorders affecting the blood. A careful physical appraisal, especially of the skin, can reveal findings such as pallor, petechiae, or bruising that may indicate minor or serious hematologic conditions. Nurses need to be aware of the clinical manifestations of blood diseases in order to assist in recognizing symptoms and establishing a diagnosis.

Disorders Related to the Red Blood Cell

The most common disorders affecting the blood are those that in some way alter the function or production of red blood cells. In broad terms all of the disorders produce anemia, but the causes of reduction in erythrocyte volume or hemoglobin production vary tremendously. The following presents an overview of anemia in general and specific disorders in children that produce an anemic state.

ANEMIA

Anemia is defined as reduction of red cell volume or hemoglobin concentration to levels below normal. It is not a disease itself but a manifestation of an underlying pathologic process. The anemias are the most common hematologic disorders of infancy and childhood. The following discussion is primarily concerned with an overview of the classification of anemia. Specific anemic conditions such as iron-deficiency anemia, the hemoglobinopathies, and aplastic anemia are then presented in greater detail.

Classification

Anemias can be classified using two basic approaches: (1) etiology or physiology, the causes of erythrocyte and hemoglobin depletion, or (2) morphology, the characteristic changes in red cell size, shape, and color. While the morphologic classification is more useful in terms of laboratory evaluation of the anemia, the etiologic approach is more relevant to nurses because it helps direct the planning of nursing care. In anemia caused by decreased red cell production, the etiology may be dietary deficiency of iron and the principal intervention is replenishing iron stores.

Etiology. The basic causes of anemia are (1) blood loss, (2) increased destruction of red blood cells, or (3) impaired or decreased rate of production. An etiologic classification is based on the various conditions that can result from any of these physiologic changes.

Table 35-1 Tests performed as part of the complete blood count*

TEST	DESCRIPTION	COMMENTS
Red blood cell (RBC) count	Number of RBCs/mm^3 of blood	Indirectly estimates Hb content of blood Reflects function of bone marrow
Hemoglobin (Hb) determination	Amount of Hb/dl of whole blood	Total blood Hb primarily depends on number of circulating RBCs, but also on amount of Hb in each cell
Hematocrit (Hct)	Percentage or volume of packed RBCs to whole blood	Indirectly measures Hb content Is approximately three times Hb content
Red blood cell indices Mean corpuscular volume (MCV)	Average or mean volume (size) of a single RBC $$MCV = \frac{Hct\,(\%) \times 10}{RBC\ count\ (millions/mm^3)}$$	MCV and MCH depend on accurate counts of RBCs, whereas MCHC does not; therefore MCHC is often more reliable All indices depend on *average* cell measurements and do not show individual RBC (anisocytosis) variations MCV values expressed as cubic microns (μm^3) or femtoliters (fl)
Mean corpuscular hemoglobin (MCH)	Average or mean quantity (weight) of Hb of a single RBC $$MCH = \frac{Hb\,(g)/dl \times 10}{RBC\ count\ (millions/mm^3)}$$	MCH values expressed as picograms (pg) or micromicrograms ($\mu\mu$g)
Mean corpuscular hemoglobin concentration (MCHC)	Average concentration of Hb in a single RBC $$MCHC = \frac{Hb\,(g)/dl \times 100}{Hct\,(\%)}$$	MCHC values expressed as % Hb/cell or Hb/dl RBC
Reticulocyte count	% Reticulocytes to RBCs	Index of production of mature RBCs by red bone marrow Decreased count indicates depressed bone marrow function Increased count indicates erythrogenesis in response to some stimulus When reticulocyte count is extremely high, other forms of immature RBCs (normoblasts, even erythroblasts) may be present Indirectly estimates hypochromic anemia
White blood cell (WBC) count	Number of WBC/mm^3 of blood	Total number of WBCs less important than differential count
Differential WBC count	Inspection and quantification of white blood cell types present in peripheral blood	Values are expressed as percentages. To obtain absolute number of any type of WBCs, multiply its respective percentage by total number of WBCs
Neutrophils (polys)		Primary defense in bacterial infection. Capable of phagocytizing and killing bacteria
Bands		Immature neutrophil Increased numbers in bacterial infection Also capable of phagocytosis and killing
Eosinophils		Named for their staining characteristics with eosin dye Increased in allergic disorders, parasitic diseases, certain neoplasms, and other diseases
Basophils		Named for their characteristic basophilic stippling Contain histamine, but their function is unknown
Lymphocytes		Involved in development of antibody and delayed hypersensitivity reactions
Monocytes		Large phagocytic cells that are involved in early stage of inflammatory reaction
Platelet count		Cellular fragments that are necessary for clotting to occur
Stained peripheral blood smear	Visual estimation of amount of Hb in RBCs and overall size, shape, and structure of RBCs	Various staining properties of RBC structures may be evidence of immature forms of erythrocyte Shows variation in size and shape of RBCs—microcytic, macrocytic, poikilocytic (variable sizes)

*See Appendix D for normal values.

Blood loss. Acute or chronic hemorrhage results in loss of plasma and all formed elements of the blood. After acute hemorrhage the body replaces plasma within 1 to 3 days, maintaining blood volume. However, this results in a low concentration of red blood cells, which are gradually replaced within 3 to 4 weeks. During this period there is usually a normocytic (normal size), normochromic (normal color) anemia, provided there are sufficient iron stores for hemoglobin synthesis.

In chronic blood loss the actual number of red blood cells may be normal because of continual replacement. However, insufficient iron is available to form hemoglobin as quickly as it is lost. As a result, erythrocytes are usually small in size (microcytic) and pale in color (hypochromic).

Excessive destruction. Excessive destruction or hemolysis of erythrocytes can occur from a variety of causes. One of the most common is a result of a defect within the red blood cell (intracorpuscular) that shortens the life span of the cell so that production cannot keep pace with destruction. The two examples discussed in this chapter, sickle cell anemia and thalassemia, have decreased erythrocyte life spans because of a hemoglobin defect.

Extracorpuscular factors are those conditions that cause hemolysis in otherwise normal red blood cells. A classic example is blood group incompatibility, such as hemolytic disease of the newborn or consequent to mismatched blood transfusion. Other causes can be toxic drugs, burns, poisonings (such as from lead), infections such as malaria, and splenic sequestration (hypersplenism).

Impaired or decreased production. Production of red blood cells can occur as a result of either bone marrow failure or deficiency of essential nutrients. Bone marrow failure may be caused by (1) replacement of bone marrow by fibrosis or by neoplastic cells, such as in leukemia, (2) depression of marrow activity from irradiation, chemicals, or drugs, or (3) interference with bone marrow activity from other systemic diseases, such as severe infection, chronic renal disease, widespread malignancy (without marrow infiltration), collagen diseases, or hypothyroidism. When depression of the hematologic system is extensive, aplastic anemia develops.

The reason for various systemic disorders affecting erythrocyte production varies according to the condition. For example, in severe chronic infection there is evidence that depression of erythropoiesis is caused by a defect in the conversion of protoporphyrin into hemoglobin. In addition, there is some degree of hemolysis, although the exact mechanism is not known.

The most common childhood anemia is a result of deficient iron supply. Besides iron as an essential component of hemoglobin synthesis, red blood cell production is dependent on amino acids, vitamins B_6, B_{12}, and C, folic acid, copper, and possibly cobalt. Chronic malnutrition causes in anemia as a result of generalized protein, mineral, and vitamin deficiencies.

Pernicious anemia develops when the gastric mucosa fails to secrete sufficient amounts of intrinsic factor, which is essential for absorption of vitamin B_{12}. This type of anemia is common in the elderly as a result of physiologically decreased gastric secretions. Deprived of vitamin B_{12}, the bone marrow produces fewer but larger (macrocytic) red blood cells. The erythrocytes are usually immature and because of their extremely fragile cell membranes are more rapidly destroyed during circulation.

Morphology. The morphologic classification provides an orderly method for ruling out certain diagnoses when establishing a cause for a particular anemia. The major characteristics of the red blood cell that are affected are (1) its size—which may be *normocytic* (normal), *microcytic* (small), or *macrocytic* (large)—and (2) its color—*normochromic* (normal) or *microchromic* (pale), which reflects reduced hemoglobin in the cell. These changes are also reflected in tests that measure the average or mean volume of a single RBC (mean corpuscular volume [MCV]), the mean quantity of hemoglobin in a single RBC (mean corpuscular hemoglobin [MCH]), and the mean concentration of hemoglobin in a single RBC (mean corpuscular hemoglobin concentration [MCHC]) (see Table 35-1). For example, a hypochromic microcytic anemia is characterized by a reduced mean cell volume (MCV) and mean cell hemoglobin (MCH).

Pathophysiology and Clinical Manifestations

The basic physiologic defect caused by anemia is a decrease in the oxygen-carrying capacity of blood and consequently a reduction in the amount of oxygen available to the tissues. When the anemia has developed slowly, the child usually adapts to the declining hemoglobin level, and most children seem to have a remarkable ability to function quite well despite low levels of hemoglobin. Also, compensatory mechanisms such as a shift in the oxyhemoglobin dissociation curve may delay the development of any obvious signs.

When the hemoglobin falls sufficiently to produce clinical manifestations, the signs and symptoms are directly attributable to tissue hypoxia. Muscle weakness and easy fatigability are common. The skin is usually pale and may take on a waxy pallor in severe anemia. Cyanosis is typically not evident, because it is the result of the quantity of deoxygenated hemoglobin in arterial blood. Hemoglobin levels generally must *exceed* 5 g/dl before cyanosis is evident. Anemia is caused by decreased hemoglobin and/or red blood cells, not inadequate oxygen saturation of existing hemoglobin.

Central nervous system manifestations include headache, dizziness, light-headedness, irritability, slowed thought processes, decreased attention span, apathy, and depression. Growth retardation resulting from decreased cellular metabolism and coexisting anorexia is a common finding in chronic severe anemia. It is frequently accompanied by delayed sexual maturation in the older child.

The effects of anemia on the circulatory system can be profound. A reduction in hemoglobin concentration that results in decreased oxygen-carrying capacity of the blood is associated with a compensatory increase in heart rate and cardiac output. Initially this greater cardiac output compensates for the lower oxygen-carrying capacity of the blood, since blood replenished with oxygen returns to the tissues at a faster than normal rate. However, if the body's demand on the pumping action of the heart increases, such as during exercise, infection, or emotional stress, cardiac failure may ensue.

Diagnostic Evaluation

The diagnosis depends largely on the cause of the anemia. In general, anemia may be suspected from findings on the history and physical examination, such as lack of energy, easy fatigability, and pallor, but unless the anemia is severe the first clue to the disorder may be alterations in a complete blood count (CBC), such as decreased RBCs, hemoglobin, and hematocrit levels. Although some authorities define anemia by a hemoglobin below 10 or 11 g/dl, this arbitrary cutoff is inappropriate for children, whose hemoglobin levels normally vary with age (see Appendix D).

Various findings on the CBC are also significant, such as increased reticulocytes, which indicates the body's increased demand for RBCs, such as in severe anemia hemolysis. A peripheral smear may demonstrate significant changes in the shape of RBCs, such as sickled cells. As mentioned previously, tests to measure the amount of hemoglobin in a single cell are helpful in determining the cause of the anemia (Table 35-1). Rarely, a bone marrow aspiration may be necessary to evaluate the body's ability to produce normal cells, such as in leukemia and aplastic anemia. In leukemia the bone marrow is hyperplastic (producing increased numbers of cells), whereas in aplastic anemia the bone marrow is hypoplastic (producing decreased numbers of cells) or aplastic (producing no cells).

Tests for hematologic function do not always reflect the *immediate* changes occurring in the blood. For example, in acute massive hemorrhage the hemoglobin and hematocrit may not be reliable, since the plasma volume may not reequilibrate for several hours. Without the hemodilution caused by the reexpansion of the vascular space, the red blood cell loss may not be apparent in these laboratory tests. Consequently, assessing the quantity of blood loss in a seriously ill child may be difficult. The estimated volume of blood loss must be analyzed in conjunction with the total blood volume of the child to determine the percent of blood loss. Blood specimens obtained from central lines may more accurately reflect the patient's status than specimens obtained from an extremity, because of the vasoconstriction of the peripheral vasculature. Systolic blood pressure can be a sensitive indicator of blood loss. For example, systolic blood pressure less than 65 mm Hg in children under age 4, or 75 mm Hg in children aged 5 to 8, or 85 mm Hg in 9- to 12-year-olds, or 99 mm Hg in adolescents, may signal 30% or greater reduction in blood volume (Oski, 1981).

Therapeutic Management

The objective of medical management is to reverse the anemia by treating the underlying cause. For example, in nutritional anemias the specific deficiency is replaced. In blood loss from acute hemorrhage, red blood cell transfusion may be given. In instances of severe anemia, supportive medical care may include oxygen therapy, restoration of adequate blood volume, intravenous fluids, and bed rest. In addition to these general measures, more specific interventions may be implemented depending upon the cause, and these are discussed in the next sections.

Nursing Considerations

Since anemia is not a disorder but a symptom of some underlying problem, nursing care is related to determining the cause, fostering appropriate supportive and therapeutic treatments, and decreasing tissue oxygen requirements.

Assist in establishing a diagnosis. Although the physical examination yields valuable evidence regarding the severity of the anemia and some indication of its possible etiology, diagnosis primarily rests on hematologic blood studies and a careful history. In interviewing parents the nurse stresses the following areas that include tentative information regarding common causes of childhood anemia: (1) nutrition, especially dietary intake of iron, (2) past history of chronic, recurrent infection, (3) eating habits, particularly pica and ingestion of lead-based paint or other toxic agents, (4) bowel habits and presence of frank blood in stools or black, tarry stools, and (5) familial history of hereditary diseases, such as sickle cell anemia or thalassemia.

The nurse should also be aware of the significance of blood tests. For example, if the blood studies show a microcytic, hypochromic anemia suggestive of iron deficiency but the parent reports an iron-rich diet, the nurse needs to pursue the nutritional history for possible discrepancies.

Prepare child for laboratory tests. Usually a battery of blood tests are ordered, but since they are generally done sequentially rather than at one time, the child is subjected to multiple fingersticks and/or venipunctures. Laboratory technicians frequently are not aware of the trauma that repeated punctures represent to a child. Therefore it is the nurse who has the responsibility of preparing the child for the tests by (1) explaining the significance of each test, particularly why the tests are not done at one time, (2) physically being with the child during the procedure whenever possible, and (3) allowing the child to play with the equipment on a doll and/or participate in the actual procedure, for example, by cleansing the finger with an alcohol swab. Older children may appreciate the opportunity to observe the blood cells under a microscope or in photographs. This is an especially important consideration if a serious blood disorder, such as leukemia, is suspected, since it serves as a foundation for explaining the pathophysiology of the disorder.

Multiple blood samples may present a problem with cumulative blood loss, necessitating blood replacement. This situation occurs most often in infants or young children with severe anemia. To prevent this, blood may be withdrawn through a continuous intravenous line and replaced after the exact amount needed has been tested and discarded. As a precaution, a record should be kept of the volume of blood being withdrawn. Another measure is to use micromethods of testing whenever possible to minimize the amount of blood required for the test. The nurse needs to observe for cumulative effects of blood loss, particularly signs of shock and increased hypoxia, and to explain to parents the necessity of multiple blood samples and the reason for blood replacement. Bone marrow aspiration is not a routine hematologic test but is essential for definitive diagnosis of the leukemias and aplastic anemias.

Decrease tissue oxygen needs. Since the basic pathology in anemia is a decreased oxygen-carrying capacity in the red blood cells, a nursing responsibility is to minimize tissue oxygen needs when anemia is severe enough to affect the child's energy level. In most instances of anemia this is not necessary, but when it is, several important interventions should be implemented. The child's level of tolerance for activities of daily living and play is assessed and adjustments are made to allow as much self-care as possible without undue exertion. During periods of rest the nurse takes vital signs and observes behavior to establish a baseline of nonexertion energy expenditure. During periods of activity the nurse repeats these measurements and observations to compare them with resting values. Signs of exertion include tachycardia, palpitations, tachypnea, dyspnea, shortness of breath, hyperpnea, breathlessness, dizziness, light-headedness, diaphoresis, and change in skin color. The child looks fatigued (sagging, limp posture; slow, strained movements; inability to tolerate additional activity).

Once a baseline of physical tolerance has been established, the nurse anticipates those activities that are physically taxing, such as dressing, feeding, or getting out of bed, and allows for conservation of energy by assisting the child as needed. However, since dependency can be threatening to a child, he is allowed as much control in the environment as possible. For example, a child with severe anemia may be unable to walk to the bathroom but may be able to use a bedside commode or be transported in a wheelchair to the lavatory rather than having to use a bedpan. Scheduling activities throughout the day with planned rest periods in between maximizes the child's energy potential without causing undue exertion.

Diversional activities are planned that promote rest but prevent boredom and withdrawal. Since short attention span, irritability, and restlessness are common in anemia and increase stress demands on the body, appropriate activities are planned, such as listening to music; using a tape recorder; watching television; reading or listening to stories or comics; continuing a favorite hobby, such as stamp collecting, coloring, or drawing; playing board and card games; or being wheeled in a carriage or chair. Choosing the appropriate roommate, such as a child of similar age with a diagnosis that also requires restricted activity, is a major asset in preventing the boredom of imposed bed rest.

If infants or young children are hospitalized, the importance of preventing separation from parents must be consid-

ered. Crying and fretfulness place increased stress demands on the body, which increases oxygen needs. Parents need help in understanding the importance of their presence, even though the child may be less responsive than usual. The nurse also explains the reason for mood changes and the necessity of allowing the child's dependency.

Anemic children are prone to infection because tissue hypoxia causes cellular dysfunction and the disturbed metabolic processes weaken the host's defenses against foreign agents. Infection also worsens the anemia by increasing metabolic needs and in instances of chronic infection also interferes with erythropoiesis and shortens the survival time of red blood cells. All the usual precautions are taken to prevent infection, such as appropriate room selection in a noninfectious area, restricting visitors or hospital personnel with active infection, practicing good handwashing, and maintaining adequate nutrition. The nurse also observes for signs of infection, particularly temperature elevation and leukocytosis. However, an elevated white blood cell count sometimes occurs in anemia without the presence of systemic or local infection.

Implement safety precautions. Children with chronic anemia usually adjust to the low levels of hemoglobin remarkably well. Often it is difficult for others unfamiliar with the child's condition to recognize the actual degree of physical tolerance. The nurse needs to inform all health personnel caring for the child to be alert to signs of overexertion and to anticipate the need for assistance, particularly when getting out of bed or going for a walk. Since young children cannot verbalize their fatigue or weakness, others must rely on observation to prevent accidental injuries. The importance of safety measures such as raised side rails or the use of restraints when the young child is in a high chair or stroller should be emphasized.

Observe for complications. The main complication of anemia is cardiac decompensation, which can result from excessive demands on the heart as a result of increased metabolic needs or of cardiac overload during rapid blood transfusion. Signs and symptoms of heart failure are tachycardia, dyspnea, rales, moist respirations, cough, shortness of breath, and sweating. Obviously, preventing heart failure through minimizing hypoxia and transfusing blood slowly is of first priority. Packed red blood cells are usually administered to prevent circulatory hypervolemia. When blood transfusions are required in severe anemia to increase the hemoglobin level, all the usual precautions for administering blood and observing for signs of transfusion reactions are instituted. (See Table 35-2.)

Oxygen may be administered to provide optimum environmental conditions for hemoglobin saturation. However, oxygen is of limited value because each gram of hemoglobin is able to carry a limited amount of the gas. In addition, prolonged supplemental oxygen can decrease erythropoiesis. Therefore the child is monitored closely for evidence of decreasing benefit from oxygen. One of the first signs of hypoxia is restlessness.

Nursing Care Summary: The Child with Anemia

NURSING GOALS	NURSING INTERVENTIONS	EXPECTED PATIENT/FAMILY OUTCOMES
HP-HMP Infection, potential for **Risk factors: lowered body defenses**		
Prevent and observe for infection	Place child in room with noninfectious children; restrict visitors with active illnesses Advise visitors (and hospital personnel) to practice good handwashing Report any temperature elevation to physician Observe for leukocytosis Maintain adequate nutrition	Child exhibits no signs of infection
A-EP Activity intolerance **Etiology: generalized weakness**		
Minimize physical exertion	Assess child's level of physical tolerance Anticipate and assist child in those activities of daily living that may be beyond his tolerance Provide diversional play activities that promote rest and quiet but prevent boredom and withdrawal Choose appropriate roommate of similar age and interests who requires restricted activity	Child plays and rests quietly and engages in activities appropriate to his capabilities
Minimize emotional stress	Anticipate child's irritability, short attention span, and fretfulness by offering to assist him in activities rather than waiting for him to ask Assess parents' awareness of child's need for dependency to conserve strength Explain to older children and parents reason for behavioral changes caused by anemia Encourage parents to remain with child	Child remains calm and quiet
PRP Family process, alteration in **Etiology: situational crisis (child in the hospital)**		
Support family	Keep family informed regarding child's progress Explain procedures and precautions related to child's care Encourage expression of feelings and concerns See also The child in the hospital, p. 1075; Family of the hospitalized child, p. 1081	Family demonstrates understanding of information given (specify information and manner of demonstration) Family members verbalize fears and concerns
IRON-DEFICIENCY ANEMIA		
N-MP Nutrition, alteration in: less than body requirements **Etiology: reported inadequate iron intake less than RDA**		

Promote adequate intake of iron-rich foods	Take careful diet history to identify deficiencies
	Provide diet counseling to caregiver; emphasize:
	   Food sources of iron, e.g., meat, liver, fish, egg yolks, green leafy vegetables, legumes, nuts, whole grains
	   Milk is undesirable as entire or predominant food in infant's diet
		Diet modifications are implemented

Provide iron supplement	Instruct family regarding correct administration of oral iron preparation
	   Give in divided doses (specify)
	   Give between meals
	   Administer with fruit juice or multivitamin preparation
	   Do not give with milk, antacids, or tea
		Family relates a diet history that verifies that child complies with these suggestions
		Child is given iron supplement as evidenced by green, tarry stools

Prevent discoloration of teeth	Instruct family to administer liquid preparation with dropper, syringe, or straw to prevent contact with teeth	Child takes medication appropriately

Continued.

Nursing Care Summary: The Child with Anemia—cont'd

NURSING GOALS	NURSING INTERVENTIONS	EXPECTED PATIENT/FAMILY OUTCOMES
SP-SCP Fear **Etiology: strange environment**		
Prepare child for laboratory tests	Explain to older children need for repeated venipunctures or fingersticks for blood analysis, particularly why a sequence of tests is required Allow children to play with laboratory equipment and/or participate in test Older children may enjoy looking at blood smears under a microscope or at pictures of blood cells Observe for signs of shock and hypoxia from repeated blood samples Explain to parents reason for replacing withdrawn blood and necessity of performing tests	Child is calm and cooperative

Nursing Interventions Related to Medical Management

Assist in establishing diagnosis
Take careful history regarding common causes of anemia in childhood
Be aware of significance of various blood tests
Improve tissue oxygenation
Administer oxygen as indicated
Monitor for benefit of oxygen but avoid prolonged use

Determine cause of anemia
Assist with diagnostic tests
Iron-deficiency anemia
Replace iron
Administer iron as prescribed

IRON-DEFICIENCY ANEMIA

Anemia caused by an inadequate supply of dietary iron is the most prevalent nutritional disorder in the United States and the most common mineral disturbance. It most frequently occurs in children between 6 and 36 months of age with a peak between 10 to 15 months (Lanzkowsky, 1985). Adolescents are also at risk because of their rapid growth rate combined with poor feeding or eating habits. Premature infants are especially at risk because of their reduced fetal iron supply.

Reports on the prevalence of iron deficiency vary widely and are complicated by the lack of acceptable definitions of anemia. However, using a diagnosis of anemia as hemoglobin level below 10 g/dl, the reported incidence of iron deficiency in children between 6 and 36 months varies from 17% to 44% (Lanzkowsky, 1985). In general, iron-deficiency anemia is more common in black children and in children from inner city areas attending clinics than in children from private practice settings (Lukens, 1984). Although no socioeconomic group is spared, this difference probably reflects the influence of socioeconomic status on adequate nutritional intake. However, this may be changing; recent evidence indicates that supplemental programs, such as Women, Infants, and Children (WIC), are improving the iron intake in infants by altering feeding patterns (increased breastfeeding and use of commercial formula rather than whole cow's milk) (Ryan and Martinez, 1985; Miller, Swaney, and Deinard, 1985).

Etiology

Iron-deficiency anemia can be caused by any number of factors that decrease the supply of iron, impair its absorption, increase the body's need for iron, or affect the synthesis of hemoglobin (see box, p. 1523). Although the clinical manifestations and diagnostic evaluation are quite similar regardless of the cause, the therapeutic and nursing considerations depend on the specific reason for the iron deficiency. The following discussion is limited to iron-deficiency anemia resulting from inadequate dietary supply of iron.

At birth the full-term infant's supply of iron is approximately 300 mg, or 75 mg/kg of body weight. The majority of iron has been transferred from the mother at the rate of 4 mg per day during the last trimester. The bulk of the iron is stored in the circulating hemoglobin of the erythrocytes; the rest is deposited in the liver, spleen, and bone marrow. Maternal iron stores are adequate for the first 5 to 6 months of age in the full-term infant but only for about 2 to 3 months in premature infants or infants of multiple births. When exogenous sources of iron are not supplied to meet the infant's growth demands following depletion of fetal iron stores, iron-deficiency anemia results. Physiologic anemia should not be confused with iron-deficiency anemia resulting from nutritional causes (see p. 496).

Pathophysiology

Iron is required for the production of hemoglobin. One hemoglobin molecule consists of protein (globin) combined

CAUSES OF IRON-DEFICIENCY ANEMIA

1. Inadequate supply of iron
   a. Deficient dietary intake
      (1) Rapid growth rate
      (2) Excessive milk intake, delayed addition of solid foods
      (3) Poor general eating habits
   b. Inadequate iron stores at birth
      (1) Low birth weight, premature, multiple births
      (2) Severe iron deficiency in mother (hemoglobin level below 9 g/dl)
      (3) Fetal blood loss at or before delivery
2. Impaired absorption
   a. Presence of iron inhibitors
      (1) Phytates, phosphates, or oxalates
      (2) Gastric alkalinity
   b. Malabsorptive disorders
   c. Chronic diarrhea
3. Blood loss
   a. Acute or chronic hemorrhage
   b. Parasitic infestation
4. Excessive demands for iron required for growth
   a. Prematurity
   b. Adolescence
   c. Pregnancy
5. Inability to form hemoglobin
   a. Lack of vitamin B_{12} (pernicious anemia)
   b. Folic acid deficiency

with four molecules of a pigmented compound (heme). Each molecule of heme contains one atom of iron. When iron stores are deficient, the production of hemoglobin is reduced. Consequently, the main effect of iron deficiency is decreased hemoglobin and reduced oxygen-carrying capacity of the blood.

Clinical Manifestations

The clinical manifestations are directly attributed to the reduction in the amount of oxygen available to tissues and resemble those seen in any type of anemia. Usually the signs are insidious and obscure and the severity is directly related to the duration of the dietary deficiency.

Although the majority of infants with iron-deficiency anemia are underweight, many are overweight because of excessive milk ingestion (known as *milk baby*). These children become anemic because milk, a poor source of iron, is given almost to the exclusion of solid foods. Although chubby, these infants are pale, usually demonstrate poor muscle development, and are prone to infection. The skin color may be described as porcelain-like.

Although the mechanism is unknown, iron-deficiency anemia enhances the leakage of plasma proteins in infants, causing edema, retarded growth, and decreased serum concentration of the proteins albumin, gamma globulin, and transferrin, a protein that binds iron and transports it through the plasma. Other less common manifestations of iron deficiency include glossitis, angular stomatitis, and koilonychia (concave or ''spoon'' fingernails). The precise relationship of iron-deficiency anemia to behavioral and intel-

lectual functioning is not clear, but increasing evidence suggests that iron deficiency, alone or with anemia, results in impaired cognitive skills that may or may not reverse after correction of the iron-deficient state (Walter, Kovalskys, and Stekel, 1983; Deinard and others, 1986).

Diagnostic Evaluation

Since iron deficiency primarily affects hemoglobin synthesis, laboratory tests that measure or describe hemoglobin, the morphologic changes in the red blood cell, and iron concentration are usually performed. The RBC count may be normal, borderline, or moderately reduced. Typically the almost normal number of erythrocytes is strikingly out of proportion to the hemoglobin concentration, which is below normal for the child's age. No absolute lower limit of hemoglobin is diagnostic of iron-deficiency anemia because the values vary with age; also normal values for black children are 0.5 mg/dl lower than for white children (Dallman and others, 1978). Although the RBC count may be normal, red blood cells are typically small in size. Consequently, this alteration is expressed in a lowered hematocrit level (usually below 33%), since the microcytic red blood cells pack together into a smaller volume, regardless of their actual number. The mean corpuscular volume is decreased, since the size of the RBC is affected. For infants near 1 year of age, a mean corpuscular volume below 70 μm^3 is considered diagnostic, whereas in the preschool and older child an MCV of 75 μm^3 is usually the lower limit of normal.

The reticulocyte count is usually normal or slightly reduced because of decreased stores of iron. However, in severe anemia when tissue hypoxia exerts an erythropoietic response, the reticulocyte count may be elevated to 3% or 4%. The level of erythrocyte protoporphyrin (EP), the immediate precursor of heme, becomes elevated in red blood cells whenever heme synthesis is disturbed. An EP level of 35 $\mu g/dl$ or above can be used as a screening test for anemia (Yip, Schwartz, and Deinard, 1983).

In terms of differential diagnosis, a stool analysis for occult blood (guaiac test) is commonly performed to confirm or rule out the possibility of chronic fecal blood loss, especially from milk intolerance or structural anomalies such as diverticulitis.

Iron studies. In addition to those tests that indirectly indicate the level of iron by the effects of iron deficiency on the red blood cell, several other tests are usually performed that more directly measure the amount of circulating iron. The serum-iron concentration (SIC) measures the amount of circulating iron and normally is about 70 $\mu g/dl$ in infants and slightly higher in older children. Lower limits of serum iron vary not only with age but also time of day; it is highest in the morning, when the test should be performed (Lanzkowsky, 1985).

The total iron-binding capacity (TIBC) measures the amount of transferrin or iron-binding globulin, which is necessary for the transport of iron in the bloodstream. When combined with transferrin, the iron is loosely bound to the globulin molecule so that it can be released easily to tissue

RECOMMENDATIONS FOR INFANT FEEDING TO PREVENT IRON-DEFICIENCY ANEMIA

Begin iron supplementation (preferably iron-fortified commercial formula or in breastfed infants, iron-fortified infant cereal) to provide 1 mg/kg/day of iron by 4 to 6 months of age in full-term infants and by 2 months in preterm infants.

Administer iron (ferrous sulfate) drops at a dose of 2 to 3 mg/kg/day to a maximum of 15 mg/day to breastfed preterm infants after 2 months of age and iron-fortified infant cereal when solid foods are introduced.

Use commercial infant formula or other sterilized milk products, rather than fresh whole cow's milk, as substitutes for breast milk during first 9 to 12 months.

Limit amount of milk or formula feeding to no more than 1 L/day to encourage intake of iron-rich solid foods.

Adapted from Committee on Nutrition: Pediatric nutrition handbook, ed. 2, Elk Grove Village, IL, 1985, American Academy of Pediatrics.

cells anywhere in the body. In iron-deficiency anemia the TIBC is elevated above the normal range of 250 μg/dl. The elevated TIBC represents the body's compensatory mechanisms to absorb more exogenous sources of iron during states of deficiency than normally. The combination of a reduced SIC and an elevated TIBC is of significant diagnostic value because it is not found in any other condition, except hypochromic, microcytic anemia caused by inadequate intake or absorption of iron. The transferrin saturation is calculated by dividing the SIC by the TIBC and multiplying the result by 100 to express the value as a percentage. A transferrin saturation of 10% suggests anemia.

Therapeutic Management

Prevention is the primary goal and is achieved through optimum nutrition and appropriate iron supplementation. In infants the American Academy of Pediatrics has set forth guidelines to prevent iron deficiency (see box above). The recommendations for feeding include iron supplementation primarily through food sources, except for preterm breastfed infants, whose iron needs may exceed those supplied through human milk. In formula-fed infants the most convenient and best sources of supplemental iron are iron-fortified commercial formula and iron-fortified infant cereal. Iron-fortified formula provides a relatively constant and predictable amount of iron and is not associated with an increased incidence of gastrointestinal symptoms, such as colic, diarrhea, or constipation (Oski and Landaw, 1980). Children receiving cow's milk formula should be given heat-treated milk products such as evaporated milk rather than fresh cow's milk to decrease the possibility of iron deficiency from gastrointestinal blood loss occurring from allergy to the milk protein.

Past infancy, prevention is accomplished through sound nutritional practices. Unfortunately, this becomes increasingly difficult to ensure during adolescence, when the growth rate is increased and the food practices of these youngsters are less than ideal. Consequently, daily iron supplementation may be needed, especially in menstruating girls, to prevent the development of iron deficiency.

Iron-deficiency anemia is usually treated with oral iron supplements. Dietary addition of iron-rich foods is usually inadequate to provide sufficient supplemental quantities of iron. Ferrous iron is more readily absorbed than ferric iron, resulting in higher hemoglobin levels. Ingested iron is absorbed largely from the duodenum, and absorption is facilitated by an acid environment. Children absorb an average of 10% to 20% of oral iron supplements, but during periods of iron deficiency they absorb an additional 5% to 10%. Oral iron supplements are prescribed in daily doses of 10 to 15 mg for approximately 4 months to replace body stores. Ideally the daily dose of iron should be given in two or three divided doses between meals. Side effects of oral iron therapy include nausea, gastric irritation, diarrhea or constipation, and anorexia, but they occur infrequently, especially in infants (Reeves and Yip, 1985). If the iron produces vomiting and diarrhea, it should be administered with meals and in gradually increasing doses.

Response to oral iron therapy is reflected in a peak increase in reticulocyte count by the fifth to the tenth day of administration. Following the reticulocyte rise, the hemoglobin and hematocrit levels and red blood cell count increase. The hemoglobin level rises an average of 0.17 to 0.25 g/dl/day; therefore a substantial increase should occur by the end of 1 month.

Parenteral iron therapy may be used if hemoglobin levels fail to raise after 1 month of oral therapy. The most common cause of failure of oral iron therapy is noncompliance. Since parenteral iron can cause a fatal anaphylactic reaction, every attempt should be made to encourage adequate therapy with oral supplements. If iron dextran (Imferon) is ordered, it must be injected deeply into a large muscle mass using the Z-tract method to minimize skin staining and irritation.

Transfusions are indicated for the severest degree of anemia (usually a hemoglobin value of 4 mg/dl or less), in cases of serious infection, cardiac dysfunction, or surgical emergency when anesthesia is required. Packed red cells, not whole blood, should be used to minimize the chance of circulatory overload. Supplemental oxygen is administered when tissue hypoxia is severe.

Nursing Considerations

The main nursing objective is prevention of nutritional anemia through parent education. Nurses need to be aware of recommendations regarding iron supplementation during infancy and appropriate sources of dietary iron. One of the difficulties in terms of infant feeding is encouraging parents to limit the quantity of milk and introduce solid foods when they believe milk is best for the infant and equate the resultant weight gain with a "healthy child." Although milk is an excellent food, it is deficient in iron, vitamin C, zinc, and fluoride. Sources of each of these nutrients and the role they play in preventing deficiencies need to be discussed with the family, especially the person who is responsible for feeding the infant. For example, the mother may have less decision-making power regarding feeding than the grandmother who cares for the child.

It is also stressed that overweight is not synonymous with good health. If the infant has obvious signs of anemia such as pallor, listlessness, frequent infections, and muscular weakness, they are pointed out as evidence of suboptimum health. In some instances it is helpful to chart the hemoglobin or hematocrit values to visually impress on parents the change in iron levels. Often increased blood values correspond to improved physical status and reinforce the benefit of dietary or oral iron supplementation.

Instructing parents regarding proper administration of oral iron supplements is an essential nursing responsibility. Several factors affect the absorption of iron, such as stomach acidity (see p. 555). Ideally iron supplements are administered in two divided doses between meals when the presence of free hydrochloric acid is greatest and are accompanied with a citrus fruit or juice, which helps reduce iron to its most soluble state. An adequate dietary intake of calcium helps bind and remove agents such as phosphates and phytates that react with iron to render it insoluble. In cultures in which tea is drunk as a common beverage, iron should be administered with some other liquid, because the tannins in tea form an insoluble complex with iron from foods other than meat (Merhav and others, 1985).When adequate dosage is reached, the stools usually turn a tarry green color. The nurse advises parents of this normally expected change and inquires about its occurrence on follow-up visits. Absence of the greenish-black stool may be a clue to poor compliance. If compliance is an issue, every effort should be made to institute strategies to improve adherence to the medication regimen, such as administering the drug once a day at the most convenient time (see Compliance, p. 1110).

Oral iron supplements are available in liquid or tablet form. Since liquid preparations may temporarily stain the teeth, the medication should be taken through a straw or given through a syringe or medicine dropper placed toward the back of the mouth. Brushing the teeth after administration of the drug lessens the discoloration. Because iron ingested in excessive quantities is toxic, even fatal, parents should keep no more than a 1-month supply in the home and store it safely away from the reach of children.

Counseling families whose children are anemic is often a difficult and challenging task. Meal planning must be based on their budget, cultural pattern, and food preferences. Often this requires more than a brief discussion with the mother or usual caregiver about foods high in iron (see p. 555). For teaching to be effective, the nurse may need to offer recipes, assist in planning a shopping list, and investigate food prices for economy. Since the physical effects of anemia are insidious, parents may not consider their child ill and consequently may view the medication and diet changes as unnecessary. Stressing what the physical and behavioral improvements will be and what effect the improved diet will have on all family members may encourage parents to adhere to the treatment plan.

SICKLE CELL ANEMIA

Sickle cell anemia is part of a group of diseases called *hemoglobinopathies*. In these diseases the normal adult hemoglobin (hemoglobin A or HbA) is partly or completely replaced by a hemoglobin variant, including fetal hemoglobin (HbF). Sickle cell disease includes all those hereditary disorders, the clinical, hematologic, and pathologic features of which are related to the presence of sickle hemoglobin (HbS).

In the United States the most common forms of sickle cell disease are:

1. Sickle cell trait, the heterozygous form of the disease (HbA and HbS or HbSA)
2. Sickle cell anemia, the homozygous form of the disease (HbSS)
3. Sickle cell–hemoglobin C disease, a variant of sickle cell anemia including both HbS and HbC
4. Sickle cell–hemoglobin E disease, a variant of sickle cell anemia in which glutamic acid has been substituted for lysine in the number 26 position of the beta chain
5. Sickle cell–thalassemia disease, a combination of sickle cell trait and β-thalassemia trait

Sickle cell anemia is found primarily in the black race, although infrequently it affects whites, especially those of Mediterranean descent. The incidence of the disease varies in different geographic locations. Among American blacks, the incidence of sickle cell trait is about 8%. In West Africa the incidence is reported to be as high as 40% among native blacks. The high incidence of sickle cell trait in these individuals is believed by some to be the result of selective protection of trait carriers against malaria caused by *Plasmodium falciparum* (Pearson, 1984).

Of the sickle cell diseases, sickle cell anemia is the most common form in black Americans in the United States, followed by sickle cell–hemoglobin C disease. Another beta chain variant, hemoglobin E, is found primarily in people of Southeast Asian origin. People who carry the trait for hemoglobin E are completely asymptomatic, but those who are homozygous exhibit a disease clinically similar to hemoglobin C disease.

Mode of Transmission

Sickle cell anemia is an autosomal disorder. The expected pattern of transmission from two parents who carry the heterozygous gene HbSA is illustrated on p. 155. In the United States it is estimated that one in 12 black persons carries the trait; therefore the risk of two black parents having a child with the disease is 0.7%. The occurrence of other forms of sickle cell disease is the result of union between two individuals who carry the heterozygous form of variants of sickle cell trait.

Basic Defect

The basic defect responsible for the sickling effect of erythrocytes is in the globin fraction of hemoglobin, which is composed of 574 amino acids. Hemoglobin S differs from hemoglobin A in the substitution of only one amino acid (valine) for another (glutamine) at the sixth position of the β-polypeptide chain. Under conditions of decreased oxygen tension and lowered pH, the relatively insoluble hemoglobin S changes its molecular structure to form long, slender crystals. The rapid growth of these filamentous crystals causes tenting of the cell membrane and the formation of crescent- or sickle-shaped red blood cells. The filamentous forms are associated with much greater viscosity than the normal holly-leaf structure of hemoglobin A.

The tendency to sickle is also related to the concentration of hemoglobin within the cell. Since hypertonicity of the blood plasma increases the intracellular concentration of hemoglobin, dehydration promotes sickling. In most instances the sickling response is reversible under conditions of adequate oxygenation and hydration. During this time the red blood cells are indistinguishable from normal erythrocytes on peripheral examination.

Although the defect is inherited at the time of conception, the sickling phenomenon is usually not apparent until later in infancy because of the presence of fetal hemoglobin (HbF). HbF is composed of two alpha and two gamma polypeptide chains. At 32 weeks' gestation, the production of beta and delta chains begins. These combine with alpha chains to form the major adult hemoglobins, HbA (two alpha and two beta chains) and HbA$_2$ (two alpha and two delta chains). As long as HbF persists, sickling does not occur, because there are no beta chains carrying the defect. The newborn has from 60% to 80% fetal hemoglobin, but this rapidly decreases during the first year, so that sickling becomes apparent after 4 months of age (Vichinsky and Lubin, 1980).

Sickle cell trait. Persons with sickle cell trait have the same basic defect, but only about 34% to 45% of the total hemoglobin is hemoglobin S (Pearson, 1984). The remainder is HbA. Normally these individuals are asymptomatic. However, under conditions of extreme or prolonged deoxygenation, such as strenuous physical exercise, anesthesia, infection, pulmonary disease, anemia, high-altitude environments, underwater swimming, or pregnancy, sickling crises may occur. The higher the percentage of hemoglobin S, the more likely the occurrence of symptomatic responses.

Pathophysiology and Clinical Manifestations

The pathologic changes from sickle cell anemia are primarily the result of (1) increased blood viscosity and (2) increased red blood cell destruction (Fig. 35-2). The entanglement and enmeshing of rigid sickle-shaped cells with one another increases the internal friction of the suspension, thus increasing blood viscosity. The thickened blood slows the circulation, causing capillary stasis, obstruction by elongated and pointed erythrocytes, and thrombosis. Eventually tissue ischemia and necrosis result with pathologic changes in the following sites.

Spleen. Initially the spleen becomes enlarged from congestion and engorgement with sickled cells. Eventually the sinuses are compressed and infarctions result. The functioning cells are gradually replaced with fibrotic tissue, until eventually in severe stages of the disease the spleen is decreased in size and totally replaced by a fibrous mass, resulting in functional asplenia. Without the spleen to filter bacteria and to promote the release of large numbers of phagocytic cells, these individuals are highly susceptible to infection.

Liver. The liver is also altered in form and function. Liver failure and necrosis are the result of severe impairment of hepatic blood flow from anemia and capillary obstruction. The liver is usually enlarged as a result of blood stasis and is occasionally tender. With progressive focal necrosis and subsequent scarring, cirrhosis eventually occurs.

Kidney. Kidney abnormalities are probably the result of the same cycle of congestion of glomerular capillaries and tubular arterioles with sickle cells and hemosiderin, tissue necrosis, and eventual scarring. The principal results of kidney ischemia are hematuria, inability to concentrate urine, enuresis, and occasionally nephrotic syndrome.

Bones. The hyperplasia and congestion of the bone marrow result in osteoporosis, widening of the medullary spaces, and thinning of the cortices. As a result of the weakening of bone, especially in the lumbar and thoracic regions, skeletal deformities, particularly lordosis and kyphosis, may occur. From chronic hypoxia, the bone becomes susceptible to osteomyelitis, frequently from *Salmonella*. Aseptic necrosis of the femoral head from chronic ischemia is an occasional problem.

Vaso-occlusive crises can result in a variety of skeletal problems. One of the more frequent is the *hand-foot syndrome*, which occurs primarily in young children ages 6 months to 2 years. It is caused by infarction of short tubular bones and is characterized by pain and swelling of the soft tissue over the hands and feet. It usually resolves spontaneously within a couple of weeks. Localized swelling over joints with arthralgia can occur from erythrostasis with sickle cells.

Central nervous system. Changes in the central nervous system are primarily vascular from the same cyclic reaction of stasis, thrombosis, and ischemia. Stroke or cerebrovascular accident is a major complication and can result in permanent paralysis or death. Any number of neurologic symptoms can herald a minor cerebral insult, such as headache, aphasia, weakness, convulsions, or visual disturbances. Loss of vision is usually the result of progressive retinopathy and retinal detachment.

Heart. Cardiac problems are mainly attributable to the stress of chronic anemia, which can eventually result in decompensation and failure. Myocardial infarctions may also occur from stasis and thrombosis.

Blood. With the formation of sickled erythrocytes, me-

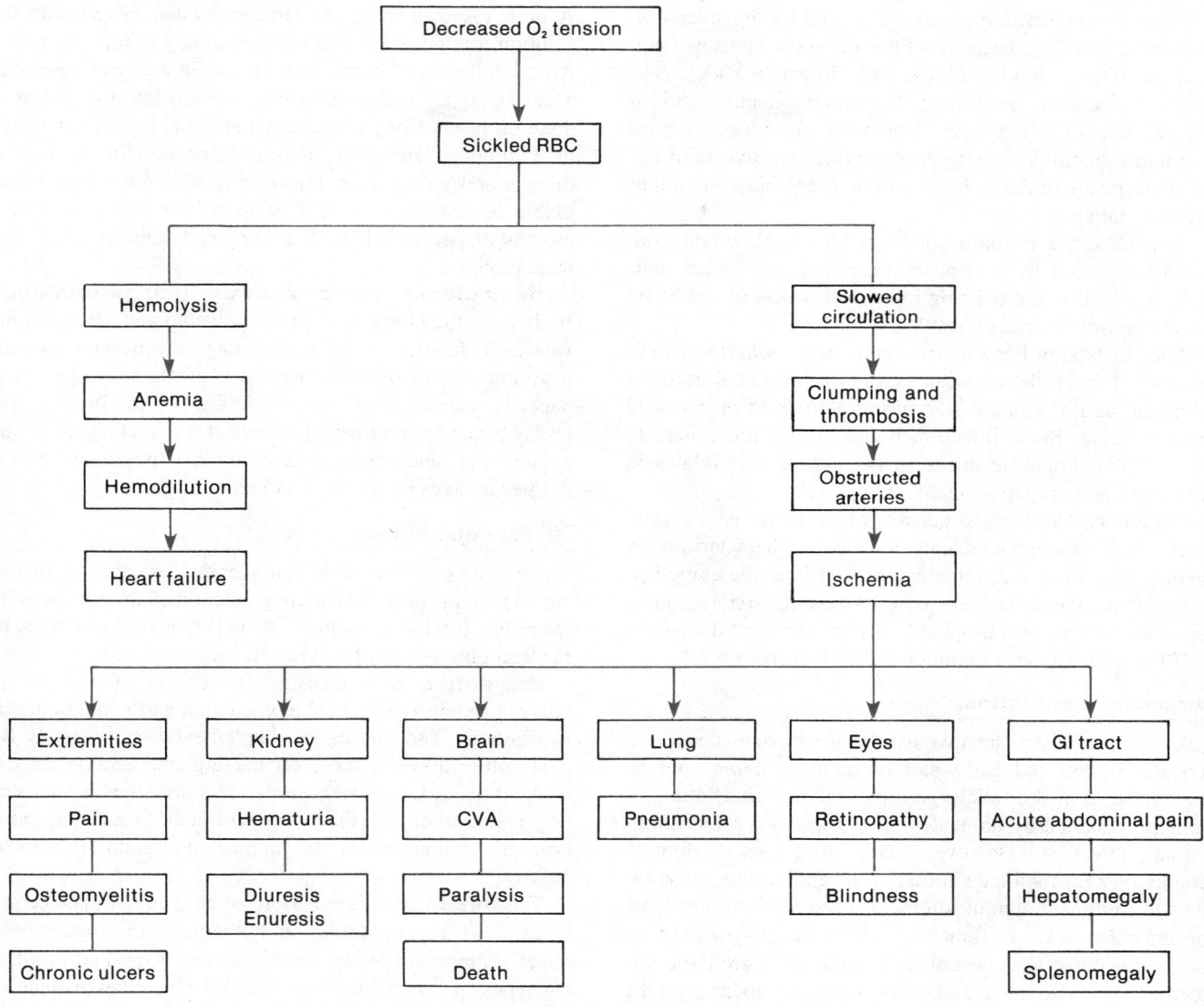

Fig. 35-2. Tissue effects of sickle cell anemia.

chanical fragility is increased, thereby decreasing the red blood cell's life span. Hemolysis occurs both during intravascular circulation and as a result of stagnation of sickled cells in the congested spleen. Although the body attempts to compensate through stimulated erythropoietic activity, as evidenced by a hyperplastic bone marrow, the rate of destruction exceeds the rate of production. A normocytic, normochromic anemia results. With increased hemolysis, hemosiderosis (increased storage of iron) is present in the liver, spleen, bone marrow, kidneys, and lymph nodes (see p. 1534).

Other signs and symptoms. In addition to the effects of sickling on various organ structures, the child with sickle cell anemia may have a variety of complaints, such as weakness; anorexia; joint, back, and abdominal pain; fever; and vomiting. Chronic leg ulcers are common in adolescents and adults and are thought to be the result of thrombosis

and decreased peripheral circulation. Other generalized effects include growth retardation in both height and weight, delayed sexual maturation, decreased fertility, and priapism (constant penile erection). If the child reaches adulthood, sexual development and adult height are usually achieved.

Sickle cell crisis. The clinical manifestations of sickle cell anemia vary markedly in severity and frequency. The most acute symptoms of the disease occur during periods of exacerbation called *crises,* which are usually precipitated by infection. There are four types of episodic crises—vaso-occlusive, splenic sequestration, aplastic, and hyperhemolytic.

Vaso-occlusive crises are the most common and the only painful ones. They are the result of sickled cells obstructing the blood vessels, causing occlusion, ischemia, and potentially necrosis. The major symptoms of this crisis are fever, acute abdominal pain from visceral hypoxia, hand-foot syndrome, and arthralgia, without an exacerbation of anemia.

Splenic sequestration crises are caused by the spleen sequestering (pooling) large quantities of blood, causing a precipitous drop in blood volume and ultimately shock. The crisis may be acute or chronic. The chronic manifestation is termed *functional asplenia*. The acute form occurs most commonly in children between 8 months and 5 years of age and may result in death from profound anemia and cardiovascular collapse.

Aplastic crisis is diminished red blood cell production, usually triggered by a viral or other infection. When it is superimposed on the existing rapid destruction of red blood cells, a profound anemia results.

Another type of bone marrow crisis is *megaloblastic anemia,* which is attributed to an excessive nutritional need for folic acid and/or vitamin B_{12} during periods of pronounced erythropoiesis. Since infection is not always antecedent to aplastic or hypoplastic crises, it is possible that folic acid deficiency is a causative agent.

Hyperhemolytic crisis occurs when there is an even greater rate of red blood cell destruction characterized by anemia, jaundice, and reticulocytosis. It is a rare complication and frequently suggests other coexisting abnormalities, such as glucose-6-phosphate dehydrogenase deficiency (G6PD), which is also common in black persons.

Diagnostic Evaluation

Although sickle cell anemia has been reported during the neonatal period and early part of infancy, it may not be recognized until the toddler and preschool period, during a crisis precipitated by an acute upper respiratory or gastrointestinal infection. However, early diagnosis (before 3 months of age) facilitates initiation of appropriate interventions to minimize complications. Several tests are available for detecting sickle cell anemia. Although most of the routine hematologic tests described in Table 35-1 are done primarily to evaluate the anemia, this discussion focuses on the tests specifically used to detect the homozygous or heterozygous form of the disease.

For screening purposes the Sickledex is commonly used. If the test is positive, hemoglobin electrophoresis is necessary to distinguish between those children with the trait and those with the disease. Screening for sickle cell trait has become a controversial subject, especially among the black community, since there is no method of preventing the disease other than selective birth procedures. This subject is discussed in more detail under Nursing considerations.

Stained blood smear. Examination of the stained smear of blood may reveal a few sickled red blood cells. However, since the erythrocyte assumes its normal discoid shape under adequate oxygenation, no sickled cells may be present even in the homozygous form of the disease. Whenever sickle cells are found, the diagnosis is usually positive for sickle cell anemia, not sickle cell trait.

Sickle-turbidity test (Sickledex). In this test anticoagulated blood is mixed with a special solution. Since hemoglobin S is normally much less soluble than hemoglobin

A or F (as well as other variants), when mixed with this solution it is insoluble and forms a cloudy or turbid mixture. All other forms of hemoglobin result in a clear suspension. This test is a reliable screening method because it can be done on blood from a fingerstick and yields accurate results in 3 minutes. However, it is not specific for the trait or disease and yields false negatives in children whose hemoglobin is less than 10 g/dl or in infants less than 4 to 6 months of age who have not completely converted to adult hemoglobin.

Hemoglobin electrophoresis ("fingerprinting"). In this test the blood is specially prepared and separated into various hemoglobins by high-voltage electrophoresis. The resulting pattern of the separated peptides as it appears on paper is referred to as "fingerprinting" of the protein. This test is accurate, rapid, and specific for detecting the homozygous and heterozygous forms of the disease, as well as the percentages of the various hemoglobins.

Therapeutic Management

There is no cure for sickle cell anemia. The aims of therapy are (1) to prevent the sickling phenomenon, which is responsible for the pathologic sequelae, and (2) to treat the medical emergency of sickle cell crisis.

Prevention of sickling. Prevention of sickling involves promoting adequate oxygenation and maintaining hemodilution. The successful implementation of these two goals often depends more on nursing intervention than on medical therapies. Current research is investigating antisickling agents such as ethacrynic acid analogs and the induction of hyponatremia to induce hydration (Charache, 1986).

Treatment of crises. More often medical management is directed at supportive and symptomatic treatment of crises. Although specific treatments are warranted in different types of crises, the main general objectives include (1) bed rest to minimize energy expenditure and oxygen utilization at the child's discretion, (2) hydration for hemodilution through oral and intravenous therapy, (3) electrolyte replacement, since hypoxia results in metabolic acidosis, which also promotes sickling, (4) analgesics for the severe abdominal and joint pain, (5) blood replacement to treat anemia and to reduce the viscosity of the sickled blood, and (6) antibiotics to treat any existing infection. The administration of pneumococcal, *Haemophilus* type B, and meningococcal vaccines is recommended for those children who are over 2 years of age because of their susceptibility to infection from asplenia (see also p. 529). In addition, it is recommended that they receive prophylaxis with oral penicillin by 4 months of age (Gaston and others, 1986).

Short-term oxygen therapy may be helpful in severe crises, especially in children with cardiac failure. Although oxygen may prevent more sickling, it usually is not effective in reversing sickling, because with the vessels clogged with cells, the oxygen is not able to reach the enmeshed sickled erythrocytes. In addition, prolonged administration

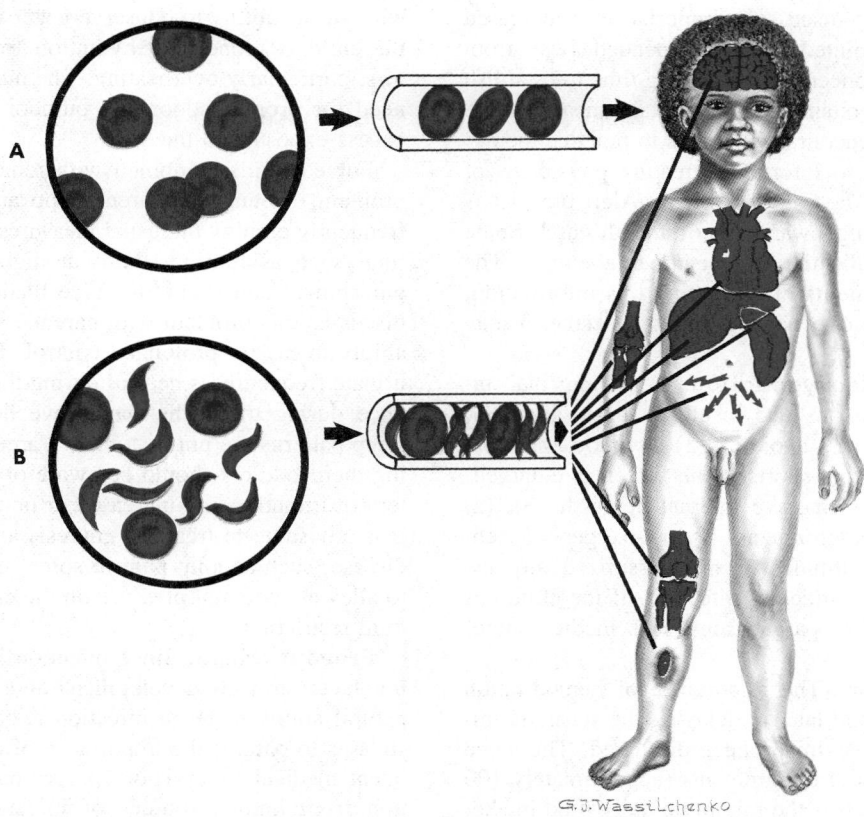

G.J.Wassilchenko

Fig. 35-3. Differences between effects of **A,** normal, and **B,** sickled red blood cells on circulation with selected consequences in child.

of oxygen can depress bone marrow activity, further aggravating the anemia.

The use of blood transfusions is another important component of care. Exchange transfusions have been successful in reducing the number of circulating sickle cells and therefore slowing down the vicious cycle of hypoxia, thrombosis, tissue ischemia, and injury. They are used in aplastic, hyperhemolytic, and sequestration crises, as well as after a stroke to prevent recurrence and further cerebral damage (Reindorf, 1980). Routine transfusions to maintain the hemoglobin above 10 g/dl in children with central nervous system disease can minimize the chances of further neurologic problems. In the event of surgery, preoperative exchange or partial exchange transfusions are given to prevent anoxia and suppress the formation of new sickle cells and postoperatively to replace lost blood. However, multiple transfusions carry the risk of hepatitis, hemosiderosis, and transfusion reactions.

In children with recurrent splenic sequestration, splenectomy may be a life-saving measure. However, because the spleen usually atrophies on its own through progressive fibrotic changes, routine splenectomy is not recommended, especially since any surgical procedure has increased risk for these children. Warranted surgical or autosplenectomy has several advantages, since the spleen is the major site of sickling, sequestration, and destruction of red blood cells.

Priapism, a painful condition, may be treated with aspiration of the corpora cavernosum. This complication is particularly frequent in vaso-occlusive crises.

Nursing Considerations

The primary nursing objectives are to (1) teach the family how to recognize and prevent sickling, (2) manage pain during sickling crises, and (3) help the child and parents adjust to a lifelong, potentially fatal, hereditary disease. Many of the measures that prevent sickling are also appropriate when a crisis occurs. In addition, special cautions are mandatory when the child undergoes surgery of any kind. Nurses may also be involved in sickle cell screening and genetic counseling.

Explain the disease. Since sickle cell anemia is first recognized when the child is a toddler, most of the nurse's counseling is with parents. The nurse explains to parents the basic effect of tissue hypoxia on red blood cells and the effect of sickling on circulation (Fig. 35-3). One simple yet graphic way of illustrating the difference between normal discoid red blood cells and sickle cells is to roll round or oval objects, such as marbles, through a tube to demonstrate normal blood cell circulation and then roll pointed objects such as screws or jacks through the tube. The effect of sickling and clumping of the pointed objects is especially noticeable at a bend or slight narrowing of the tube. This same idea can be expanded to discuss the importance of increased fluid in keeping the pointed objects suspended away from each other to prevent concentration. Taking time to establish a sound basis of understanding why certain measures are beneficial to the child encourages parents to practice them.*

Parents are advised to inform all treating physicians of the child's condition. The use of a Medic Alert bracelet is another way of ensuring awareness of the disease. Some people view such identification as "negative labeling." The nurse can stress the benefits of displaying this information, especially in emergencies when the use of anesthesia may be required.

Prevent tissue deoxygenation. Anything that increases cellular metabolism also results in tissue hypoxia. For the child this includes avoiding (1) strenuous physical activity (especially contact sports if the spleen is enlarged, since rupture will cause massive internal hemorrhage), (2) emotional stress, (3) environments of low-oxygen concentration, such as high altitudes or nonpressurized airplane flights, and (4) known sources of infection. If the child has even a mild infection, the parents must seek medical attention at once.

Promote hydration. The importance of hemodilution in preventing sickling and later in delaying the stasis-thrombosis-ischemia cycle has already been discussed. The nurse calculates the child's fluid requirements (approximately 100 to 125 ml/kg/day), which is the minimum daily fluid intake. The nurse also assesses the child's usual fluid consumption to evaluate its adequacy and makes adjustments based on this knowledge. It is not sufficient to advise parents to "force fluids" or "encourage drinking." They need specific instructions on how many glasses or bottles of fluid are required. Many foods are also a source of fluid, particularly soups, Jell-O, and puddings, and these can be included as liquid sources.

Children can be encouraged to drink by giving them a "special" cup or glass, using a straw, taking advantage of thirsty times, such as on awakening or after playing, serving frequent, small portions, and leaving the cup in easy reach for self-service. Frozen popsicles, crushed ice "slurpies," and flavored ice cubes are sources of fluid commonly accepted by children.

Since the kidneys' ability to concentrate urine is impaired, the child is especially prone to dehydration. Dilute urine or low specific gravity is no longer a valid sign of adequate hydration. Parents are taught to observe for other indications of fluid loss, such as dry mucous membranes, weight loss, and sunken fontanel in infants. In addition,

without the ability to conserve water by concentrating urine, the child is prone to dehydration from environmental factors, particularly overheating. The nurse alerts parents to the need for proper indoor and outdoor clothing and avoiding excess exposure to the sun.

Forced fluids combined with renal diuresis result in the problem of enuresis. Parents who are unaware of this fact frequently employ the usual measures to discourage bedwetting, such as limiting fluids at night, and many revert to punishment and shame to force bladder control. The nurse discusses this problem with parents, stressing the child's inability to master prolonged control. Reminding the child to urinate frequently is helpful during the day, and waking him once during the night may prove beneficial if the child's sleep patterns are not disturbed. Parents who are toilet training their toddlers should be aware of the more frequent pattern of urination and increased difficulty in learning control. It is advisable to treat the enuresis as a complication of the disease, such as joint pain or some other symptom, in order to alleviate parental pressure on the child and to prevent any fluid restriction.

Prevent crises. Since infection is the major predisposing factor toward development of a crisis and the body's natural ability to resist infection is compromised, the nurse stresses to parents the importance of adequate nutrition, frequent medical supervision, proper handwashing, and isolation from known sources of infection. The last measure must be tempered with an awareness of the child's need for living a normal life. Overprotection can be equally as devastating emotionally as an infection is physically. Parents need to be aware of the necessity of seeking prompt medical care at the first sign of any infection.

The family should be taught the signs and symptoms of crises and advised to seek medical attention immediately. There is some evidence that teaching parents spleen palpation for earlier detection of splenic sequestration can reduce mortality from this serious complication (Emond and others, 1985).

Promote supportive therapies during crises. The success of many of the medical therapies relies heavily on nursing implementation. Management of pain is an especially difficult problem and often involves experimenting with various analgesics, including narcotics, and schedules before relief is achieved. Unfortunately, these children tend to be undermedicated, resulting in "clock watching" and demands for additional doses sooner than might be expected. Often this incorrectly raises suspicions of drug addiction, when in fact the problem is one of improper dosage (Reindorf, 1980). In choosing and scheduling analgesics, the goal should be *prevention* of pain.

An effective approach has been the use of parenteral morphine sulfate every 2½ hours for the first 48 hours, followed by a gradual tapering of the narcotic within dosages that continue to provide pain relief. Once the dose has been lowered to half the initial dose, oral narcotics are substituted

---

*A Sickle Cell Home Study Kit For Families is available from the National Association for Sickle Cell Disease, Inc., 4221 Wilshire Blvd., Los Angeles, CA 90010. Additional resources are Howard University, Center for Sickle Cell Disease, 2121 Georgia Ave., N.W., Washington, DC 20059; National Sickle Cell Disease Program, National Heart, Lung, and Blood Institute, 7550 Wisconsin Ave., Room 504, Bethesda, MD 20205.

using equianalgesic dosages and are given every 4 hours and after discharge if needed (Vichinsky, Johnson, and Lubin, 1982). Any pain program should be combined with psychologic support to help the child deal with the depression, anxiety, and fear that accompany the disease. This includes regular visits with the child to discuss his concerns during the hospitalization and positive reinforcement of adaptive coping skills, such as successful methods of dealing with the pain and compliance with treatment prescriptions. (For a general discussion of assessment and management of pain see pp. 1068 and 1071.)

Frequently heat to the affected area is soothing. Cold compresses are not applied to the area, because this enhances sickling and vasoconstriction. Bed rest is usually well tolerated during a crisis, although actual rest depends a great deal on pain alleviation and organized schedules of nursing care. Although the objective of bed rest is to minimize oxygen consumption, some activity, particularly passive range of motion exercises, is beneficial to promote circulation. Usually the best course of action is to let the child dictate his activity tolerance.

If blood transfusions or exchange transfusions are given, the nurse has the responsibility of observing for signs of transfusion reaction (see p. 1537). Since hypervolemia from too rapid transfusion can increase the workload of the heart, the nurse also is alert to signs of cardiac failure.

In splenic sequestration the size of the spleen is gently measured, since increasing splenomegaly is an ominous sign. A decreasing spleen denotes response to therapy. Vital signs and blood pressure are also closely monitored for impending shock. Anemia is typically not a presenting complication in vaso-occlusive crises but is a critical problem in other types of crises. The nurse monitors for evidence of increasing anemia and institutes appropriate nursing intervention.

If oxygen is administered, the child's response in terms of decreased pain and improved physical status is noted. However, since prolonged oxygen can aggravate the anemia, signs of lack of therapeutic benefit, such as restlessness, increased pallor, and continued pain, are reported.

Intake, especially of intravenous fluids, and output are recorded. The child's weight should be taken on admission, since it serves as a baseline for evaluating hydration. Since diuresis can result in electrolyte loss, the nurse also observes for signs of hypokalemia and should be familiar with normal serum electrolyte values to report changes to the physician.

Decrease surgical risks. The main surgical risk is hypoxia from anesthesia. However, emotional stress, the demands of wound healing, and the possibility of infection potentially increase the sickling phenomenon, both in children with the disease and in those with the trait. The primary nursing objectives are aimed at minimizing each of these threats preoperatively and postoperatively by keeping the child well hydrated, preparing the child psychologically, and preventing infection.

Provide screening and genetic counseling. Screening is recommended during the neonatal period, since early diagnosis allows earlier, more prevention-oriented treatment, such as prophylactic antibiotic therapy (Gaston and others, 1986). The advantages of trait identification lie in selective reproduction of offspring not afflicted with hemoglobin SS. Alternate methods of childbearing include artificial insemination, adoption, or abortion of afflicted fetuses. However, these alternatives may be viewed as unacceptable.

To be effective, screening must be combined with genetic counseling and long-term follow-up. The nurse can be instrumental in such programs by conducting parent education sessions, following the family in the home, disseminating correct information about the disease and trait to the community, and rendering support to parents of newly diagnosed children. A primary consideration in genetic counseling is informing parents who both carry the trait of the chances of having a child with the disease (see Chapter 5).

Prenatal diagnosis is possible through amniocentesis or fetoscopy and fetal blood sampling. Analysis of amniotic cells for a DNA fragment associated with the gene responsible for sickled β-globulin chain synthesis can be done at the sixteenth week of gestation (Vichinsky and Lubin, 1980). In the event of an affected fetus, the decision regarding termination of the pregnancy should be left to the couple rather than viewed as an automatic selection of abortion.

Support the family. Parents need the opportunity to discuss their feelings regarding transmitting a potentially fatal, chronic illness to their child. Some parents are able to cope with this fact; some feel great guilt and remorse for giving their child the disease, whereas others regret not knowing that they carried the trait. For many parents the decision regarding subsequent pregnancies is viewed with doubt and ambivalence.

Because of the sometimes poor prognosis for children with sickle cell anemia, many parents express their fear of death. Prognosis varies; approximately 20% to 30% of children under 5 years of age die, mainly from overwhelming infection (sepsis) and sequestration (Pearson, 1984). However, as the child grows older, the crises usually become less severe and less frequent. There is an increasing number of adults who survive with the disease, and as palliative treatment and antisickling techniques advance, prognosis will continue to improve. However, since there is no way to predict which child will follow a favorable course, the nurse should care for the family as she would for any family with a child who has a chronic and life-threatening illness, with particular emphasis on the siblings' reactions, the stress on the marital relationship, and the childrearing attitudes displayed toward the child (see Chapters 22 and 23).

Nursing Care Summary: The Child with Sickle Cell Anemia

NURSING GOALS	NURSING INTERVENTIONS	EXPECTED PATIENT/FAMILY OUTCOMES

HP-HMP Infection, potential for
Risk factors: altered body defenses

Prevent infection	Stress importance of adequate nutrition, protection from known sources of infection, and frequent medical supervision Report any sign of infection to physician immediately Promote compliance with antibiotic administration	Child remains free of infection

HP-HMP Injury: potential for tissue damage
Risk factors: physiologic (abnormal hemoglobin, decreased ambient oxygen,
dehydration)

Promote tissue oxygenation	Explain preventive measures
	    Avoidance of strenuous physical exertion
	    Avoidance of emotional stress
	    Prevention of infection
	    Avoidance of low-oxygen environment
		Child avoids situations that reduce tissue oxygenation

Promote hydration	Calculate recommended daily fluid intake and base child's fluid requirements on this *minimum* amount Give parents written instructions regarding specific quantity of fluid required Encourage child to drink Teach family signs of dehydration Stress importance of avoiding overheating as source of fluid loss	Child drinks adequate amount of fluid and shows no signs of dehydration
Decrease surgical risks	Explain reason for preoperative blood transfusion Keep child well hydrated Decrease fear through appropriate preparation Avoid unnecessary exertion Promote pulmonary hygiene postoperatively Use passive range of motion exercises to promote circulation Observe for signs of infection	Child undergoes surgical procedure without crisis
Observe for complications (crisis)	Monitor for evidence of increasing anemia; use appropriate nursing interventions Measure size of spleen; continually monitor for shock Observe mental status for evidence of cerebrovascular accident	Child exhibits no evidence of crisis

RRP Family process, alteration in
Etiology: situational crisis (child with a physiologic defect)

Increase understanding of disease	Inform family and older children of basic defect and measures that prevent sickling Stress importance of informing significant health personnel of child's condition and benefit of Medic Alert tag Explain signs of developing crisis, especially fever, pallor, and pain Reinforce basics of trait transmission, especially concerning subsequent pregnancies	Parents and child demonstrate understanding of disease, its etiology, and its therapies
Support child and family	Allow family to express feelings regarding transmitting disease to offspring Encourage siblings to discuss their feelings regarding possibility of being a carrier of disease Refer to public health nurse for follow-up in home	Child and family verbalize their fears and concerns regarding implications of disease

Nursing Care Summary: The Child with Sickle Cell Anemia—cont'd

NURSING GOALS	NURSING INTERVENTIONS	EXPECTED PATIENT/FAMILY OUTCOMES
Support child and family —cont'd	Refer to special organization such as National Association for Sickle Cell Disease, Inc. Refer child for medical care through comprehensive sickle cell clinic Discuss prognosis, especially increased chances of survival when sickling is prevented Care for child as one with life-threatening illness Be especially alert to family's needs when two or more members are affected	Family takes advantage of community services (specify)
Prevent psychologic problems	Encourage normal activities and relationships within child's capabilities Implement measures to reduce unpleasant side effects of disease, such as enuresis Explore feelings and attitudes toward disease, its side effects, and its complications	Child participates in activities appropriate for age

SICKLE CELL CRISIS

N-MP   Fluid volume deficit, potential
Risk factors: sickling phenomenon, pain, immobility

Ensure adequate intake	Record intake and output Observe for signs of dehydration; diuresis is not a valid indication Observe for signs of electrolyte imbalance	Child does not exhibit signs of dehydration

A-EP   Tissue perfusion, alteration in: cardiopulmonary
Etiology: interruption of flow, arterial

Increase tissue oxygenation	Promote circulation through passive range of motion exercises	Extremities remain free of pain

A-EP   Activity intolerance
Etiology: generalized weakness

Promote rest	Schedule care-giving activities to allow for optimum rest Enforce bed rest	Child remains quiet and relaxed

C-PR   Comfort, alteration in: pain
Etiology: tissue ischemia

Relieve pain	Assess need for pain medication (p. 1068) Implement appropriate nonpharmacologic pain reduction techniques (p. 1071) Position for comfort Apply warmth to affected area	Child rests quietly; facial expression remains free of stress

Nursing Interventions Related to Medical Management

Assist with diagnosis
  Assist with diagnostic procedure
  Prepare child and family for procedures
Relieve pain
  Administer analgesics as ordered, especially on preventive schedule
  Record effectiveness of analgesics (see p. 1072)
Prevent infection
  Administer antibiotic
  Administer immunization as ordered

Sickle cell crisis
Replace blood
  Administer blood
  Observe for signs of transfusion reactions and cardiac overload
Increase tissue oxygenation
  Administer oxygen
  Monitor for evidence of benefits from oxygen
  Avoid prolonged use
Provide fluids
  Monitor intravenous fluids carefully

β-THALASSEMIA (COOLEY ANEMIA)

The term *thalassemia* comes from the Greek word *thalassa*, meaning "sea," and is applied to a variety of inherited blood disorders characterized by deficiencies in the rate of production of specific globin chains in hemoglobin. The name appropriately refers to those people living near the Mediterranean Sea who have the highest incidence of the disease, namely, Italians, Greeks, and Syrians. There is evidence to suggest that the high incidence of the disorder among these groups is a result of selective advantage of the trait to malaria, as is postulated in sickle cell disease. However, the disorder has a wide geographic distribution, probably as a result of genetic migration through intermarriages or possibly as a result of spontaneous mutation.

The thalassemias are classified according to the hemoglobin chain affected and by the amount of the globin chain that is synthesized; for example, if alpha chains are affected, alpha thalassemia. Each of the abnormal genes that cause thalassemia is seen in particular populations; for example, beta thalassemia, Greeks, Italians, and Syrians; alpha thalassemia, Chinese, Thai, African, and Mediterranean peoples.

Beta thalassemia is the most common form, and it is the entity that will be discussed further. *Silent carriers* are individuals who carry the gene but demonstrate no clinical symptoms. Persons with *thalassemia trait*, the heterozygous form, usually have mild anemia, hypochromic and microcytic cells, and elevated HbA$_2$ and/or HbF. *Thalassemia intermedia* presents with splenomegaly and severe anemia. Skeletal deformities, frequent fractures, and arthritis complicate the clinical course. The homozygous form, *thalassemia major (Cooley anemia)*, results in a severe anemia that is not compatible with life unless transfusion support is given. Ordinarily homozygous alpha thalassemia results in hydrops fetalis, which usually ends in death in utero. However, supportive therapy has resulted in live births and survival through the neonatal period (Beaudry and others, 1986; Bianchi and others, 1986).

Mode of Transmission

Thalassemia is an autosomal-recessive disorder with varying expressivity. Sometimes the trait is found in only one parent of a child with severe thalassemia. In this situation the likelihood is that the other parent carries a gene for some variant of sickle cell anemia or other hemoglobinopathy. The exact mode of transmission between parents who are heterozygous for thalassemia is illustrated on p. 155.

Pathophysiology

Normal postnatal hemoglobin (HbA) is composed of two α- and two β-polypeptide chains. In β-thalassemia there is a partial or complete deficiency in the synthesis of the β-chain of the hemoglobin molecule. Consequently, there is a compensatory increase in the synthesis of α-chains, and γ(gamma)-chain production remains activated, resulting in defective hemoglobin formation. This unbalanced polypeptide unit is very unstable, disintegrates, and damages the red blood cells, causing severe anemia. To compensate for the hemolytic process, an overabundance of red blood cells is formed. The body also attempts to balance the low level of circulating hemoglobin A by producing large concentrations of fetal hemoglobin, which normally does not contain β-chains.

Clinical Manifestations

The clinical effects of thalassemia major are primarily attributable to (1) defective synthesis of hemoglobin A, (2) structurally impaired red blood cells, and (3) shortened life span of the erythrocyte. The major consequences of thalassemia are caused by the pathologic condition, resultant chronic hypoxia, and the supportive treatment of multiple blood supplements (Fig. 35-4). The onset is usually insidious and not recognized until the latter half of infancy. Signs of anemia, unexplained fever, poor feeding, and a markedly enlarged spleen, particularly in a child of Mediterranean extraction, are descriptive.

Anemia. Anemia results from the body's inability to maintain a level of erythropoiesis commensurate with hemolysis. The bone marrow compensates by increasing production of large numbers of immature cells, such as normoblasts and erythroblasts, large cells that are extremely thin and form bizarre shapes, and nonspecific macrocytes called *target cells,* which have abnormal staining properties. As a result of the excessive production of abnormal red blood cells, their life span is severely shortened.

Anemia also is exaggerated by aplastic crises after infection, folic acid deficiencies from demands of bone marrow hyperplasia, splenic sequestration, and progressive hemolysis from repeated blood transfusions. The spleen becomes greatly enlarged as a result of extramedullary hemopoiesis, rapid destruction of the defective erythrocytes, and, rarely, progressive fibrosis from hemochromatosis. Splenomegaly may progress until the organ's very size interferes with the function of other abdominal organs and respiratory expansion.

With progressive anemia, signs of chronic hypoxia, namely, headache, precordial and bone pain, decreased exercise tolerance, listlessness, and anorexia, may develop. Another common symptom in these children is frequent epistaxis, although the exact reason is unknown. Hyperuricemia and gout from rapid cellular catabolism are also seen.

Hemosiderosis and hemochromatosis. *Hemosiderosis* is excess iron storage in various tissues of the body, especially the spleen, liver, lymph glands, heart, and pancreas, but without associated tissue injury. *Hemochromatosis* refers to excess iron storage with resultant cellular damage. Although the exact mechanism for the conversion of iron storage to tissue destruction is not known, chronic hypoxia is believed to be an important contributing factor.

In thalassemia, excess hemosiderin, the iron-containing pigment from the breakdown of hemoglobin, results from decreased hemoglobin synthesis and increased hemolysis of transfused erythrocytes. Decreased production of hemoglobin results in an excess supply of available iron. In addition,

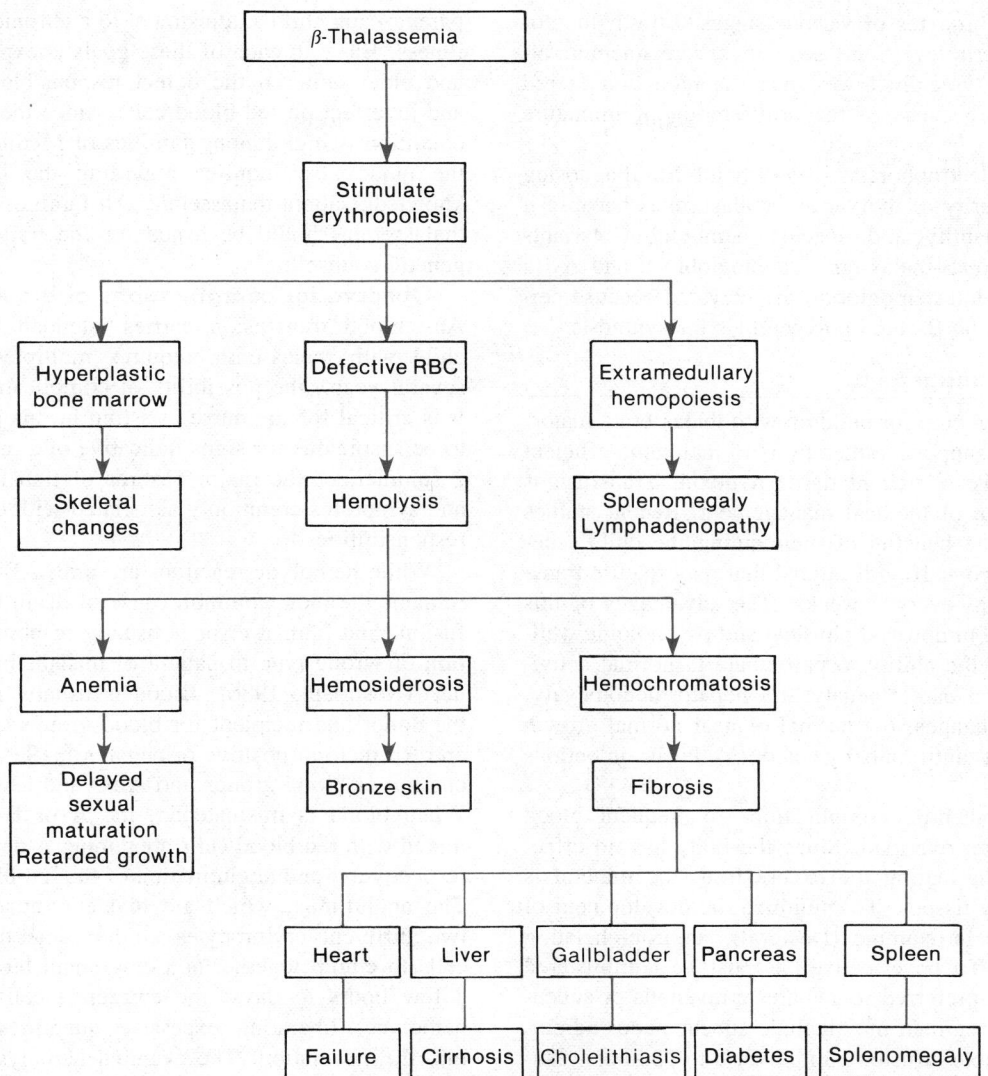

Fig. 35-4. Effects of Cooley anemia.

the body probably responds to the anemia by increasing the rate of gastrointestinal absorption of dietary iron, since ineffective erythropoiesis is a potent controlling factor regarding exogenous iron use. However, the primary source of additional iron is from the hemolysis of supplemental erythrocytes and rapid destruction of defective red blood cells. With the prophylactic use of deferoxamine to minimize excess iron storage, the characteristic changes in body structures from hemochromatosis have been greatly reduced. Before the advent of this aspect of therapy, specific bone changes produced characteristic facies in older children— enlarged head, prominent frontal and parietal bosses, prominent malar (cheekbone) eminences, a flat or depressed bridge of the nose, enlargement of the maxilla, with protrusion of the lip and upper central incisors and eventual malocclusion, and a mongoloid appearance to the eyes.

Growth and sexual maturation. Retarded growth and especially delayed sexual maturation are common find-

ings. There is evidence that both may also be caused by pituitary failure, although the exact reasons for this are unclear, but the impaired growth is probably related to hemochromatosis. It is possible that the endocrine glands are extremely sensitive to iron toxicity and that even small amounts of deposited iron can produce organ dysfunction. Children with severe disease usually achieve normal growth rates until puberty, when height becomes markedly retarded. Secondary sexual characteristics are delayed or absent in as many as 40% of adolescents (Borgna-Pignatti and others, 1985).

Diagnostic Evaluation

The classic picture of Cooley anemia in a child of Mediterranean background provides ample evidence of the disease. Hematologic studies reveal the characteristic changes in the red blood cell, namely microcytosis, hypochromia, anisocytosis, poikilocytosis, target cells, and basophilic stippling of immature erythrocytes of various stages. Low hemoglobin and hematocrit levels are seen in severe anemia, although they are typically lower than the reduction in red blood cell count because of the proliferation of immature erythrocytes.

Hemoglobin electrophoresis is very helpful in diagnosing the type and severity of the various thalassemias because it analyzes the quantity and specific hemoglobin variants found in blood. In β-thalassemia, hemoglobin F and A$_2$ (a type of normal adult hemoglobin) are elevated because neither is dependent on β-chain polypeptides for synthesis.

Therapeutic Management

There is no known cure for children with thalassemia major. The objective of supportive therapy is to maintain sufficient hemoglobin levels to prevent tissue hypoxia. Transfusions are the foundation of medical management. Recent studies have evaluated the benefits of maintaining the child's hemoglobin level above 10 g/dl, a goal that may require transfusions as often as every 3 weeks. The advantages of this therapy include (1) improved physical and psychologic well-being because of the ability to participate in normal activities, (2) decreased cardiomegaly and hepatosplenomegaly, (3) fewer bone changes, (4) normal or near normal growth and development until puberty, and (5) fewer infections (Festa, 1985).

One of the potential complications of frequent blood transfusions is iron overload. Since the body has no effective means of eliminating the excess iron, the mineral is deposited in body tissues. To minimize the development of hemosiderosis, deferoxamine (Desferal), an iron-chelating agent, is given. To be effective, it must be administered parenterally. The preferred routes are intravenous or subcutaneous, and the regimen may include subcutaneous administration via portable infusion pump over 8 to 10 hours (usually during sleep) for 6 days a week and intravenous administration over 8 hours at the time of transfusion (Festa, 1985).

In some children with severe splenomegaly who require repeated transfusions, a splenectomy may be necessary to decrease the disabling effects of abdominal pressure and to increase the life span of supplemental red blood cells. There is evidence that with repeated blood transfusions, a hemolytic factor develops in the spleen that increases the rate of erythrocyte destruction. After a splenectomy children generally require many fewer transfusions, although the basic defect in hemoglobin synthesis remains unaffected. A major postsplenectomy complication is severe and overwhelming infection. Therefore these children are kept on prophylactic antibiotics with close medical supervision for many years and should receive the pneumococcal, meningococcal, and *Haemophilus influenza* vaccines (see also p. 529).

Nursing Considerations

The objectives of nursing care are to (1) observe for complications of multiple blood transfusions, (2) assist the child in coping with the effects of the illness, and (3) foster the parents' and child's adjustment to a chronic, life-threatening illness. Basic to each of these goals is explaining to parents and older children the defect responsible for the disorder and its effect on red blood cells. Since the incidence of this condition is high among families of Mediterranean descent, the nurse also inquires regarding the family's previous knowledge about thalassemia. All families with a child with thalassemia should be tested for the trait and referred for genetic counseling.

Observe for complications of blood transfusions. Any blood transfusion carries attendant risks. Since the child with thalassemia requires multiple transfusions for several years, the possibility of complications is increased. It is critical for the nurse assisting in this procedure always to be suspicious for signs indicative of a reaction. Table 35-2 summarizes the major hazards of transfusions, the signs and symptoms commonly associated with each, and nursing responsibilities.

While hemolytic reactions are rare, ABO incompatibility remains the most common cause of death from blood transfusion, and human error is usually responsible (administration of wrong type to patient or mislabeling of blood product) (Kasprisin, 1986). Blood is usually matched between the donor and recipient for blood groups (A, B, AB, or O) and Rh factors (positive or negative). (See p. 349 for a discussion of blood groups and ABO and Rh incompatibility.) When blood is mismatched, the A or B antiagglutinin is mixed with red blood cells containing A or B agglutinogens, respectively, and agglutination of the red blood cells occurs. The agglutinins, which are bivalent, attach themselves to two different erythrocytes at the same time, causing the cells to clump together and clog small blood vessels. Over a few hours to days, the entrapped cells degenerate and hemolyze, liberating excessive quantities of hemoglobin into the circulation. The eventual hemolysis of large numbers of red blood cells decreases the blood volume, causing circulatory failure and *shock*. Treatment is aimed at replacing lost blood and using plasma volume expanders.

Acute kidney shutdown and eventual *renal failure* are the result of renal vasoconstriction from antigen-antibody complexes derived from the red cell surface. The greatly reduced blood flow causes complete renal failure and death within 7 to 12 days. Treatment involves promoting diuresis with rapid dilute intravenous fluids and diuretics, such as furosemide and mannitol, and alkalinizing body fluids, which render hemoglobin more soluble.

Another consequence of hemolysis is the release of large quantities of phospholipids, which are capable of stimulating disseminated intravascular coagulation (DIC) (p. 1547). As a result, the plasma is depleted of the necessary coagulation factors needed to prevent hemorrhage. Without treatment with heparin to prevent the coagulation and blood components to initiate clotting, death from generalized hemorrhage can occur.

Besides the nursing precautions and responsibilities outlined in Table 35-2, some general guidelines that apply to all transfusions include:

Table 35-2 Nursing care of the child receiving blood transfusions

COMPLICATION	SIGNS/SYMPTOMS	PRECAUTIONS/NURSING RESPONSIBILITIES
Immediate reactions		
Hemolytic reactions—most severe type, but rare Incompatible blood Intradonor incompatibility in multiple transfusions	Chills Shaking Fever Pain at needle site and along venous tract Nausea/vomiting Sensation of tightness in chest Red or black urine Headache Flank pain Progressive signs or shock and/or renal failure	Positively identify donor and recipient blood types and groups before transfusion is begun; verify with one other nurse or physician Transfuse blood slowly for first 15 to 20 minutes and/or initial 1/5 volume of blood; remain with patient In event of signs or symptoms, stop transfusion immediately, maintain patent intravenous line, and notify physician Save donor blood to re-crossmatch with patient's blood Monitor blood pressure for shock Insert urinary catheter and monitor hourly outputs Send sample of patient's blood and urine to laboratory for presence of hemoglobin (indicates intravascular hemolysis) Observe for signs of hemorrhage resulting from disseminated intravascular coagulation (DIC) Support medical therapies to reverse shock
Febrile reactions Leukocyte or platelet antibodies Plasma protein antibodies	Fever Chills	May give acetaminophen for prophylaxis Use of leukocyte-poor red blood cells is less likely to cause reaction Stop transfusion immediately; report to physician for evaluation
Allergic reactions—recipient reacts to allergens in donor's blood	Urticaria Flushing Asthmatic wheezing Laryngeal edema	Give antihistamines for prophylaxis to children with tendency toward allergic reactions Stop transfusions immediately Epinephrine may be used for wheezing or anaphylactic reaction
Circulatory overload Too rapid transfusion (even if small quantity) Excessive quantity of blood transfused (even if slowly)	Precordial pain Dyspnea Rales Cyanosis Dry cough Distended neck veins	Transfuse blood slowly Prevent overload by using packed red blood cells or administering divided amounts of blood Use infusion pump to regulate and maintain flow rate If signs of overload, stop transfusion immediately Place child upright with feet in dependent position to increase venous resistance
Air emboli—may occur when blood is transfused under pressure	Sudden difficulty in breathing Sharp pain in chest Apprehension	When infusing blood under pressure, normalize pressure before container is empty If air is observed in tubing, clamp tubing immediately below air bubble, clear tubing of air by aspirating air with syringe or disconnecting tubing and allowing blood to flow until air has escaped
Hypothermia	Chills Low temperature Irregular heart rate Possible cardiac arrest	Allow blood to warm at room temperature (less than 1 hour) Use an electric warming coil to rapidly warm blood Take temperature if patient complains of chills; if subnormal stop transfusion
Electrolyte disturbances Hyperkalemia (only in massive transfusions or in patients with renal problems)	Nausea, diarrhea Muscular weakness Flaccid paralysis Paresthesia of extremities Bradycardia Apprehension Cardiac arrest	Use washed red blood cells or fresh blood if patient at risk
"Citrate" intoxication (hypocalcemia)	Tingling in fingers Tetany Muscular cramps Carpopedal spasm Hyperactive reflexes Convulsions Laryngeal spasm Respiratory arrest	Infuse blood slowly (citrate reaction less likely to occur) If signs of tetany occur, clamp tubing immediately, maintain patent intravenous line, and notify physician

Continued.

Table 35-2 Nursing care of the child receiving blood transfusions—cont'd

COMPLICATION	SIGNS/SYMPTOMS	PRECAUTIONS/NURSING RESPONSIBILITIES
Delayed reactions		
Transmission of infection	Signs of infection after trans-	Blood is tested for HB$_s$Ag (hepatitis B), syphilis, and in
Hepatitis	fusion, e.g.,	most centers HTLV-III (AIDS); positive units are
AIDS	jaundice from	destroyed. Individuals at risk for carrying certain
Malaria	hepatitis	viruses are deferred from donation
Syphilis	Bacterial or toxin	Report any sign of infection, and if occurring during
Bacteria or viruses	contamination—	transfusion, stop transfusion immediately, send
Other	high fever, se-	sample for culture and sensitivity tests, and notify
	vere headache	physician
	or substernal	
	pain,	
	hypotension,	
	intense flush-	
	ing,	
	vomiting/diarrhea	
Alloimmunization	Increased risk of	Occurs in patients receiving multiple transfusions
(antibody formation)	hemolytic,	Use limited number of donors
	febrile, and	Observe carefully for signs of reactions
	allergic	
	reactions	
Delayed hemolytic reaction	Destruction of red	Observe for posttransfusion anemia and decreasing
	blood cells and	benefit from successive transfusions
	fever 5 to 10	
	days after	
	transfusion	

1. Take vital signs and blood pressure *before* administering blood to establish baseline data for posttransfusion comparison, then every 15 minutes for 1 hour while blood is infusing
2. Check the identification of the recipient with the donor's blood group and type, regardless of the blood product used
3. Administer the first 50 ml of blood or 1/5 volume (whichever is smaller) *slowly* and stay with the child
4. Administer with normal saline on a piggyback setup
5. Administer blood through an appropriate filter to eliminate particles in the blood and prevent the precipitation of formed elements
6. Use blood within 30 minutes of its arrival from the blood bank; if it is not used, return to blood bank—do not store in regular unit refrigerator
7. If a reaction of any type is suspected, stop the transfusion, maintain a patent intravenous line with normal saline and new tubing, notify the physician, and do not restart the blood until the child's condition has been medically evaluated

When the blood is started, the filter chamber is filled to allow the total filter to be used. The drip chamber is partially filled with blood to permit counting of the drops. In adjusting the flow rate, it is important to remember that blood administration sets do not use microdrops (60 drops/ml) but regular drops (usually 10 or 15 drops/ml). Therefore, when administering the first 50 ml of blood, the nurse adjusts the flow rate to 16 drops per minute to infuse this amount in 30 minutes. If no reaction occurs, the flow rate is increased accordingly to infuse the remainder of blood within 2 hours. For example, if a unit of 275 ml of blood is to be given, a flow rate of 19 drops per minute permits the remaining 225 ml to be infused in 2 hours. (These calculations are based on 10 drops/ml.) A unit of blood should be infused within 4 hours. If the infusion will exceed this time, the blood should be divided by the blood bank and the unused portion refrigerated under controlled conditions.

Assist in coping with effects of disorder. Body image alterations, decreased growth, and sexual immaturity are frequently difficult adjustment problems for older children. These children feel different from their peers, and the delayed sexual development with ramifications on sexual function are major issues for the maturing adolescent with an improved life expectancy (see Questions and controversies, p. 950). Adolescents need an opportunity to express their thoughts and feelings about these complex issues. Adolescents can learn grooming aids that make them appear more sexually mature, such as up-to-date clothing, new hairstyles, and well-applied makeup. Children with the characteristic bone changes may benefit from surgery or orthodontic appliances to improve facial structure.

With frequent transfusion therapy there is less restriction imposed on physical activity because of severe anemia, and these children should be encouraged to pursue activities commensurate with their exercise tolerance. However, the frequency of treatment can interfere with a normal life style. To minimize disruptions, the nurse can be instrumental in arranging for blood transfusions and medical supervision at times that interfere least with the child's regular activities, especially school. In addition, children are more likely to cooperate with medical treatments that do not interfere significantly with their routine.

Support the family. As with any chronic, life-threatening illness, the needs of the family must be met for optimum adjustment to the stresses imposed by the disorder. These needs are discussed in Chapter 22. Sources of information for the family are the **Cooley's Anemia Foundation*** and the **AHEPA Cooley's Anemia Foundation.**† Genetic counseling for the parents and fertile offspring is mandatory, and both prenatal diagnosis using amniocentesis at 10 weeks or fetal blood sampling at 20 weeks' gestation (Alter, 1985) and screening for thalassemia trait are available.

Even though the prognosis for children with thalassemia major is improving and will probably continue to improve, a proportion of these children die before adulthood, and for the survivors the life expectancy is significantly reduced. The chief cause of death is heart failure, and once signs of this complication become evident, death may occur within a year. Unfortunately, it is not possible to predict which severely afflicted child will follow a more favorable course. The nurse must care for families of these children in light of this knowledge, be willing to discuss the future prospects with the parents and child as appropriate, and plan realistic goals for the thalassemic child. (See also Chapter 23.)

APLASTIC ANEMIA

Aplastic anemia refers to a condition in which all formed elements of the blood are simultaneously depressed. The peripheral blood smear demonstrates pancytopenia or the triad of profound anemia, leukopenia, and thrombocytopenia. *Hypoplastic anemia* is characterized by a profound depression of erythrocytes but normal or slightly decreased white blood cells and platelets.

A type of hypoplastic anemia is pure red cell anemia, a congenital condition marked by complete or almost complete absence of all cells of the erythroid series with normal production of the other myeloid cells. Its treatment, which consists of transfusions, splenectomy, and administration of corticosteroids, is similar to that of other diseases, such as the thalassemias, that result in profound anemia. Prognosis varies, although long-term survival is possible. The principal causes of death are cardiac failure, hepatitis from transfusion therapy, and sepsis. Hemosiderosis and hemochromatosis (p. 1534) also affect vital tissues necessary for survival.

Acquired hypoplastic anemia can result from several factors, including suppressed erythropoiesis from multiple

transfusion therapy, hemolytic syndromes, such as sickle cell anemia, infections, toxic substances, drugs, and autoimmune or allergic states. The following discussion, however, focuses on aplastic anemia, which carries a much poorer prognosis and follows a more rapidly fatal course.

Etiologic Factors

Aplastic anemia can be primary (congenital) or secondary (acquired). Of the congenital variety, one of the best known disorders of which aplastic anemia is an outstanding feature is *Fanconi syndrome*. Besides pancytopenia, the condition is associated with a large number of congenital anomalies, including microcephaly; dwarfism; mental retardation; anomalies of ears, skeleton, kidneys, and heart; strabismus; ptosis; nystagmus; deafness; and excess deposits of melanin in areas of the skin. The syndrome appears to be inherited as an autosomal-recessive trait with varying penetrance; therefore affected siblings may demonstrate several different combinations of defects. The treatment is the same as for other causes of aplastic anemia. Prognosis is variable but is better than for acquired types.

The most common causes of acquired aplastic anemia are:

1. Irradiation
2. Drugs, such as the chemotherapeutic agents and several antibiotics, one of the most notable being chloramphenicol
3. Industrial and household chemicals, including benzene and its derivatives, which are found in petroleum products, dyes, paint remover, shellac, and lacquers
4. Infections, especially hepatitis or overwhelming infection
5. Infiltration and replacement of myeloid elements, such as in leukemia or the lymphomas
6. Idiopathic, in which no identifiable precipitating cause can be found

Clinical Manifestations and Diagnosis

The clinical manifestations, which include anemia, leukopenia, and decreased platelet count, are usually insidious. The onset is not unlike that seen in leukemia. Definitive confirmation is based on bone marrow aspiration or biopsy, which demonstrates the conversion of red bone marrow to yellow, fatty bone marrow.

Therapeutic Management

The objectives of treatment are based on the recognition that the underlying disease process is failure of the bone marrow to carry out its hematopoietic functions. Therefore therapy is directed at restoring function to the marrow and involves two main approaches: (1) immunosuppressive therapy to remove the presumed immunologic functions that prolong aplasia and/or (2) replacement of the bone marrow through transplantation (Gordon-Smith, 1985). Bone marrow transplantation is the treatment of choice in severe aplastic anemia when a compatible donor exists.

Two agents have been found to be effective in restoring function to the bone marrow. Currently, antilymphocyte

---

*104 E. 22nd St., New York, NY 10017.
†1422 K St., N.W., Washington, DC 20005.

globulin (ALG) or antithymocyte globulin (ATG) is the preferred agent over androgens, which previously constituted the principal treatment for aplastic anemia. The specific globulin is prepared by immunizing suitable animals, usually horses or rabbits, with lymphocytes (ALG) obtained from patients undergoing surgery or with lymphocytes obtained by thymectomy (ATG). The cells are then harvested and commercially prepared. ALG and ATG are similar products; therefore the terms are used interchangeably. The rationale for using ATG is based on the theory that aplastic anemia may be the result of autoimmunity. ATG suppresses T-cell-dependent autoimmune responses but does not cause bone marrow suppression. The optimum schedule for ATG administration is still under investigation. It is usually given intravenously over 12 to 16 hours, after a test dose to check for hypersensitivity. Subsequent doses are given depending upon the reduction in circulating lymphocytes.

Androgens may be used to stimulate erythropoiesis. Although the exact mechanism of erythropoietic action is unclear, testosterone increases production of erythroid elements, converting the fatty, hypocellular bone marrow to one of erythroid hyperplasia. Several testosterone preparations are available. Those most commonly used and their methods of administration are oxymetholone and fluoxymesterone in daily oral doses or nandrolone decanoate and testosterone enanthate in weekly intramuscular doses.

Response to immunosuppressive therapy is gradual. Elevations in hemoglobin and red blood cells may take as long as 3 to 6 months. During this period the child must be protected from infection and hemorrhage and treated for the pancytopenia with transfusions. Unfortunately, the prognosis is poor. In children with severe aplastic anemia treated with ATG about 40% may attain independent bone marrow function; 10% to 20% may subsequently relapse (Gordon-Smith, 1985). Mortality associated with androgens is about 70% for acquired aplastic anemia; almost 50% of these children die within 12 months after diagnosis (Goldstein, 1980).

Because of the relatively poor prognosis in aplastic anemia treated with drug therapy, bone marrow transplantation should be considered *early* in the course of the disease if a compatible donor can be found. Transplantation is more successful when performed before multiple transfusions have sensitized the child to leukocyte and HLA antigens. Children who are eligible for transplantation should be transferred to one of the medical centers that specialize in this procedure. For nontransfused patients, pretransplantation immunosuppressive therapy consists of administration of near lethal doses of cyclophosphamide. Those patients who have received transfusions undergo total body irradiation with immunosuppressives (e.g., cyclophosphamide, ATG, or cyclosporine). Bone marrow transplantation is associated with a 60% to 80% survival rate (Kamani, 1985).

Nursing Considerations

The care of the child with aplastic anemia is similar to that of the child with leukemia, namely, preparing the family for the diagnostic and therapeutic procedures, preventing complications from the severe pancytopenia, and emotionally supporting them in terms of a potentially fatal outcome (Chapters 23 and 36). Since each of these has already been discussed, only the exceptions are presented here. Bone marrow transplantation is discussed on p. 1565.

During administration of ATG, vigilant attention must be directed to the intravenous infusion to prevent extravasation. To prevent sclerosing from extravasation, a central vein should be used. Because of the child's susceptibility to infection, meticulous care of the venous access catheter is essential. Although anaphylactic reactions to ATG are rare, emergency preparations should be planned in advance, with epinephrine readily available. The nurse should observe for other reactions. Immediate reactions to ATG are common and include fever and skin rash. Delayed reactions (serum sickness) may also occur within 7 to 14 days of a course of ATG, and the manifestations are similar to immediate reactions. The symptoms are reversed and in the case of serum sickness may be prevented with corticosteroids.

Testosterone produces several undesirable effects that result in dramatic body image alterations, including deepening of the voice, hirsutism, growth of pubic hair, enlargement of the penis in males, flushing of the skin, and acne. Potentially, testosterone can cause muscular and skeletal maturation, resulting in severely retarded height in a young child. Not only are these changes difficult to accept, they are especially difficult to explain to children not approaching puberty. Parents may feel embarrassed because they are unprepared for the sexual changes. The nurse can help by deemphasizing the sexual nature of the effects and matter-of-factly explaining each. Expressing embarrassment or surprise to the child at observing mature sexual characteristics must be prevented. New members of the staff who may be assigned to care for the child, such as nursing students, need to be prepared for the experience of seeing a "sexually mature 6-year-old male with a slight beard and a deep masculine voice."

Since chemotherapeutic agents may be used, many of the reactions, such as nausea and vomiting, alopecia, and mucosal ulceration, can be encountered. In addition, extensive ecchymotic areas of the oral mucosa from thrombocytopenia require meticulous mouth care to prevent breakdown, bleeding, and infection. Fortunately, these lesions, which look painful, cause little or no discomfort. Local anesthetics are not necessary, but anorexia is still a consequence because of the edematous nature of the lesions. Liquid, bland, and soft diets are usually tolerated best.

Defects in Hemostasis

The body controls excessive bleeding through three processes: (1) vascular spasm, (2) platelet aggregation, and (3) coagulation and clot formation. Defects in platelets and clotting factors are the most common causes of bleeding during childhood. The following discussion focuses on the major conditions that require nursing intervention. The reader is urged to apply these principles to other medical conditions that involve similar nursing considerations.

MECHANISMS INVOLVED IN NORMAL COAGULATION

To understand the role that factor deficiencies play in promoting bleeding tendencies, it is necessary to review the normal coagulation process of the blood. Although the process is complex, clotting takes place in essentially three phases:

1. A substance called *prothrombin activator* is formed in response to an extrinsic or intrinsic mechanism.
2. The prothrombin activator catalyzes the conversion of *prothrombin* into *thrombin*.
3. Thrombin acts as an enzyme to convert *fibrinogen* into the *fibrin* threads that enmesh the red blood cells and plasma to form a clot.

Phase I

Blood clotting is initiated either by an *extrinsic* mechanism, in which an extract called *thromboplastin* is released from the damaged tissues into the blood, or by an *intrinsic* mechanism, in which the blood itself is damaged and the platelets respond by releasing a substance called *platelet factor 3* into the blood. In both instances several factors, collectively termed a prothrombin activator, are present in the plasma and are necessary to initiate clotting. Table 35-3 lists the various clotting factors and their common synonyms; there is no Factor VI. In addition, calcium ions must be available in the plasma for the reactions to take place.

Phase II

After prothrombin activator has been formed, it catalyzes the conversion of prothrombin to thrombin. Prothrombin is a plasma protein formed in the liver that is dependent on vitamin K for its synthesis. The rate of formation of thrombin from prothrombin is directly proportional to the amount of prothrombin activator or blood-clotting factors. Therefore a low level of prothrombin in the blood is potentially an indirect estimate of a factor deficiency, since the prothrombin complex is dependent on factors II, V, VII, and X.

Phase III

Thrombin, a protein enzyme with proteolytic ability, acts on fibrinogen, a plasma protein produced by the liver, to form a molecule called fibrin. The fibrin molecule polymerizes to form long fibrin threads that run in all directions, shorten, and eventually form a clot by entrapping blood cells and plasma in the web. Phase III factors include factors I and XIII.

A few minutes after clot formation, the clot retracts, expressing most of the plasma from itself and pulling the broken ends of the blood vessels closer together. Clot retraction is dependent on an adequate number of platelets, which may provide the energy for the fibrin threads to shorten. Since

Table 35-3 Blood-clotting factors

FACTOR NUMBER	SYNONYMS
I	Fibrinogen
II	Prothrombin
III	Platelet factor 3, thromboplastin
IV	Calcium
V	Labile factor, proaccelerin, Ac globulin
VII	Serum prothrombin conversion accelerator (SPCA), proconvertin, stable factor
VIII	Antihemophilic factor (AHF), antihemophilic globulin (AHG)
IX	Plasma thromboplastin component (PTC), Christmas factor
X	Stuart-Prower factor
XI	Plasma thromboplastin antecedent (PTA)
XII	Hageman factor
XIII	Fibrin stabilizing factor (FSF)

the proteolytic ability of thrombin is capable of initiating more clotting by breaking down prothrombin to form more thrombin in a cyclical reaction, clot formation is controlled by the rate of blood flowing past the injured site to remove excess fibrin. This is also one of the reasons why an injured area is immobilized initially to promote adequate clot formation and why early resumption of too vigorous movement may reinitiate bleeding.

HEMOPHILIA

Hemophilia refers to a group of bleeding disorders in which there is a deficiency of one of the factors necessary for coagulation of the blood. Although the symptomatology is similar despite the missing factor, the identification of specific factor deficiencies has allowed definitive treatment with replacement agents. The two most common forms of the disorder are *classic hemophilia* (hemophilia A or factor VIII deficiency) and *Christmas disease* (hemophilia B or factor IX deficiency). The following discussion is primarily concerned with the classic form, which accounts for about 75% of all cases.

A major feature of hemophilia is that its expression varies markedly in the degree of bleeding severity. Hemophilia is generally classified into three groups according to the severity of factor deficiency as described below; approximately 60% to 70% of children with hemophilia demonstrate the severe form of the disorder:

Clinical severity	Factor VIII activity	Bleeding tendency
Severe	1%	Spontaneous bleeding without trauma
Moderate	1%- 5%	Bleeding with trauma
Mild	5%-50%	Bleeding with severe trauma or surgery

Table 35-4 Laboratory tests for hemostasis*

TEST	DESCRIPTION	COMMENTS
Platelet function		
Bleeding time	Measures time interval for bleeding from small superficial wound to cease	Function depends on platelet aggregation and vasoconstriction; two common methods used: Ivy (incision made on forearm) and Duke (incision made on earlobe)
Tourniquet test	Measures platelet function and capillary fragility; apply pressure to forearm with tourniquet for 5 to 10 minutes	Normal response is absence of petechiae or fewer than 10 Abnormal in platelet and connective tissue disorders
Clot retraction test	Measures degree to which clot shrinks and expresses serum	Depends on platelet function
Blood clotting mechanisms		
Whole blood clotting time	Measures time it takes for clot to form *within* blood	Prolonged clotting time indicates problem in thrombin-to-fibrin phase or in any factor in intrinsic clotting mechanism; difficult test to standardize, therefore often unreliable results
Prothrombin time (PT)	Measures activity of prothrombin, as well as factors necessary for its conversion to thrombin and fibrinogen	Actually does not measure prothrombin levels, but activity; since it bypasses intrinsic-extrinsic mechanism, detects deficiencies of factors V, VII, X, and fibrinogen, as well as prothrombin
Partial thromboplastin time (PTT) test	Similar to PT but measures activity of thromboplastin, which depends on intrinsic clotting factors	Specific for factor deficiencies, except factor VII, which results in a normal PTT but prolonged PT
Thromboplastin generation test (TGT)	Measures blood's ability to generate thromboplastin	Allows for determination of specific factor deficiencies, especially distinguishing between factors VIII and IX
Prothrombin consumption test	Indirectly measures thromboplastin generation and prothrombin response	Normally, as blood clots, prothrombin is converted to thrombin so that serum is depleted of prothrombin; if thromboplastin is decreased (as a result of extrinsic factor deficiencies), not all prothrombin will be converted and removed from serum
Fibrinogen level	Directly measures fibrinogen levels in blood	Not dependent on phase I or II deficiencies

*Normal values are listed in Appendix D.

Modes of Transmission

Hemophilia is transmitted as an X-linked recessive disorder; however, only about 60% of affected children have a positive family history for the disease. As many as one third of the cases of hemophilia may be caused by gene mutation (Karayalcin, 1985). The most frequent pattern of transmission is between an unaffected male and a trait-carrier female (see p. 155). With improved treatment for persons with hemophilia, it is important to consider the results of mating between an affected male and a normal female or a carrier female. For example, the mating of an affected male with a carrier female results in a 1:4 chance of producing either an affected son or daughter, a carrier daughter, or a normal son. This is one of the few ways in which a female inherits the disorder. Other mechanisms responsible for female expression of the disease include a symptomatic carrier of classic hemophilia with a moderate defect of factor VIII and a female with an autosomal dominant transmitted form of factor VIII deficiency, such as von Willebrand disease.

Pathophysiology

In hemophilia A the factor VIII molecule is present but is defective in its clotting function. Factor VIII-related antigen (FVIIIR:Ag) is normal. In hemophilia B there may be a defect or a deficiency of factor IX.

Clinical Manifestations

The effect of hemophilia is prolonged bleeding anywhere from or in the body. With severe factor deficiencies, hemorrhage can occur as a result of minor trauma, such as after circumcision, during loss of deciduous teeth, or as a result of a slight fall or bruise. In children with less severe deficiencies the bleeding tendency may not be noted until onset of walking.

Subcutaneous and intramuscular hemorrhages are common. *Hemarthrosis,* which refers to bleeding into the joint cavities, especially the knees, elbows, and ankles, is the most frequent form of internal bleeding and often results in bone changes and consequently crippling, disabling deformities. Early signs of hemarthrosis are a feeling of stiffness,

Table 35-5 Plasma products used to treat patients with hemophilia

PRODUCT/MAJOR CONTENTS	CLINICAL INDICATIONS	ADVANTAGES	DISADVANTAGES
Fresh frozen plasma (all coagulation factors)	Unknown type of hemophilia Mild hemophilia A or B with history of few prior transfusions von Willebrand disease	Low risk of hepatitis Readily available	Transfusion reactions Volume overload Inconvenient Impossible to raise factor level over 15%-20%
Cryoprecipitate (factor VIII; fibrinogen)	Hemophilia A von Willebrand disease	Moderate hepatitis risk Less expensive than concentrates	Bags contain widely variable amounts of factor VIII Inconvenient to use
Factor VIII concentrate*	Hemophilia A	Convenient Ability to infuse known number of units	Hepatitis Hemolytic anemia (FVIII) Venous thrombosis (FIX) Expensive ($50-$120 per vial)
Factor IX (prothrombin complex) concentrate† (Factor IX; factors II, VII, X; contaminating procoagulants)	Hemophilia B Hemophilia A with inhibitor	Same as F VIII	Same as F VIII

Modified from Buchanan, G.R.: Pediatr. Clin. North Am. **27**(2):309-326, 1980.
*Products currently available in the United States include Profilate (Abbott), Factorate (Armour), Koate (Cutter), Hemofil (Hyland), and Humafac (Parke-Davis).
†Products currently available in the United States include Konyme (Cutter) and Proplex (Hyland).

tingling, or ache in the joint, followed by a decrease in the ability to move the affected joint. Obvious signs and symptoms are warmth, redness, swelling, and severe pain with considerable loss of movement (Sergis-Deavenport, Miller, and Gomperts, 1983). Spontaneous hematuria is not uncommon. Epistaxis may occur but is not as frequent as other kinds of hemorrhage. Petechiae are uncommon in persons with hemophilia because repair of small hemorrhages is dependent on platelet function, not on blood-clotting mechanisms.

Bleeding into the tissue can occur anywhere but is serious if it occurs in the neck, mouth, or thorax, since the airway can become obstructed. Intracranial hemorrhage can have fatal consequences and is one of the major causes of death. Hemorrhage anywhere along the gastrointestinal tract can lead to obstruction, and bleeding into the retroperitoneal cavity is especially hazardous because of the large space for blood to accumulate. Hematomas in the spinal cord can cause paralysis.

Diagnostic Evaluation

The diagnosis is usually made on a history of bleeding episodes, evidence of X-linked inheritance, and laboratory findings. To understand the significance of various tests of hemostasis, it is helpful to recall the usual mechanisms to control bleeding, namely, the function of platelets and of clotting factors. Tests that measure platelet function, such as the bleeding time, tourniquet test, and clot retraction test, are all normal in persons with hemophilia, whereas tests that assess clotting factor function may be abnormal (Table 35-

4). The tests specific for hemophilia are those that depend on specific factors for a reaction to occur, such as the partial thromboplastin time test, thromboplastin generation test, and prothrombin consumption test. Specific determination of factor deficiencies requires assay procedures normally done by specialized laboratories.

Carrier detection is possible in classic hemophilia and is an important consideration in families in which female offspring may have inherited the trait. The test involves an assay and comparison of factor VIII coagulant activity (FVIII-c) and factor VIII-related antigen (FVIII R:Ag), a protein found in the plasma that is antigenically similar to FVIII-c but has no measurable coagulant activity. To increase the accuracy of the test, DDAVP (1-desamino-8-D-arginine vasopressin), a synthetic derivative of vasopressin, may be given intravenously. In unaffected individuals, DDAVP produces an increase in FVIII-c and FVIII R:Ag, but in carriers, the increase in FVIII-c, not FVIII R:Ag, is less pronounced, thus increasing the difference in the ratio between the two factors (Kobrinsky and others, 1984). Prenatal diagnosis includes sex determination through amniocentesis or fetal blood sampling to detect FVIII R:Ag.

Therapeutic Management

The primary therapy for hemophilia is preventing spontaneous bleeding by replacement of the missing factor. The products currently used are summarized in Table 35-5. Vigorous therapy is instituted to prevent chronic crippling effects from joint bleeding. If factor replacement therapy is begun immediately, local measures such as ice applications and splinting are seldom needed and preservation of the joint is good. One of the major concerns with the use of factor replacement is the risk of hepatitis and especially acquired immune deficiency syndrome (AIDS) (see p. 1550). Since the risk of infections is lower with the use of cryoprecipitate or fresh frozen plasma than factor concentrates, these products should be used whenever possible, especially in children under age 4 and newly identified patients never treated with concentrates (Karayalcin, 1985).

A number of other drugs may be included in the therapy plan depending on the source of the hemorrhage. Corticosteroids are administered to reduce inflammation in the joints; nonsteroidal antiinflammatory agents, such as aspirin, indomethacin (Indocin), and phenylbutazone (Butazolidin) should not be used because they inhibit platelet function. Ibuprofen (Motrin, Advil, or Nuprin) has been demonstrated to be safe despite its anti-platelet aggregation effect (Karayalcin, 1985). DDAVP may be helpful in children with mild to moderate hemophilia because of the transient rise in FVIII-c. Local application of epsilon aminocaproic acid (Amicar) prevents clot destruction; however, its use is limited to mouth or trauma surgery.

A regular program of exercise and physical therapy is an important aspect of management. Physical activity, within reasonable limits, strengthens muscles around joints, which helps control bleeding in the area. Pain management with appropriate nonnarcotic and narcotic drugs, such as acetaminophen with or without codeine, is essential to ensure compliance with the physical therapy plan.

Treatment without delay results in more rapid recovery and a decreased likelihood of complications; therefore most children are treated at home. The family is taught the technique of venipuncture and the administration of the replacement factor to children over 3 years of age. The child learns the procedure for self-administration between ages 9 and 12. Home treatment is highly successful, and the rewards, in addition to the immediacy of treatment, are less disruption of family life, fewer school or work days missed, and enhancement of the child's independence and self-esteem.

Nursing Considerations

The objectives for nursing care can be divided into immediate needs and long-term goals. Obviously, the most immediate consideration is control of bleeding episodes. However, the ultimate adjustment and prognosis for the child rely heavily on the family's ability to cope with the disorder, to learn effective methods of control and prevention, and to temper child-rearing practices with judicious protection from injury while fostering independence and development.

Prevent bleeding by decreasing risk of injury. Prevention of bleeding through control of behavior is no easy task. During infancy and toddlerhood the normal acquisition of motor skills creates innumerable opportunities for falls, bruises, and minor wounds. Restraining the child from mastering motor development can herald more serious long-term problems than allowing the behavior. However,

the environment can be made as safe as possible to minimize the incidental injuries, with close supervision maintained during playtime.

For older children the family usually needs assistance in preparing for school. A nurse who knows the family can be instrumental in discussing the situation with the school nurse and in jointly planning an appropriate schedule of activity. Since almost all persons with hemophilia are boys, the physical limitations in regard to active sports are a difficult adjustment, and activity restrictions must be tempered with sensitivity to the child's emotional as well as physical needs. Noncontact sports, especially swimming, are suitable activities and should be encouraged.

To prevent oral bleeding, some readjustment in terms of dental hygiene may be needed to minimize trauma to the gums. For example, the nurse can recommend the use of a water irrigating device, softening the toothbrush in warm water before brushing, or using a sponge-tipped disposable toothbrush available in many drugstores. A regular toothbrush should be soft bristled and small in size. Adolescents also need to be advised of the dangers of shaving with razor blades and encouraged to use an electric shaver.

Since any trauma can lead to a bleeding episode, all persons caring for these children must be aware of their disorder. These children should wear Medic Alert identification, and older children should be encouraged to recognize situations in which disclosing their condition is important, such as dental extraction or injections. Health personnel need to take special precautions to prevent the use of procedures such as intramuscular injections or venipunctures. A peripheral fingerstick is better for blood samples, and the subcutaneous route is substituted for intramuscular injections. Neither aspirin nor any aspirin-containing compound should be used. Acetaminophen (Tylenol) is a suitable aspirin substitute, expecially for use during control of pain at home. Another common drug that should not be used is glyceryl guaiacolate (guaifenesin), an expectorant found in several over-the-counter cough preparations.

Recognize and manage bleeding. The earlier a bleeding episode is recognized, the more effectively it can be treated. Children are often aware of internal bleeding before clinical manifestations are evident, and they must be taken seriously when they report their concerns. In addition to the signs of hemarthrosis that have been discussed, the family also needs to be aware of signs and symptoms indicating internal tissue bleeding, such as headache, slurred speech, and loss of consciousness from bleeding within the brain and black tarry stools, hematemesis, and loss of consciousness from gastrointestinal bleeding, which require immediate medical attention.

Factor replacement therapy should be instituted according to established medical protocol and supportive measures implemented, such as (1) applying pressure to the area for at least 10 to 15 minutes to allow clot formation, (2) immobilizing and elevating the area above the level of the heart to decrease blood flow, and (3) applying cold to promote vasoconstriction. When parents and older children are taught such measures beforehand, they can be prepared to initiate immediate treatment before blood loss is excessive. Plastic bags of ice or Cryogel* cold packs should be kept in the freezer for such emergencies. However, such measures should not take the place of factor replacement.

Prevent crippling effects of joint degeneration. From repeated hemarthrosis, incompletely absorbed blood in the joints, and limitation of motion, bone and muscle changes occur that result in flexion contractures and joint fixation. Obviously, prevention of bleeding is the ideal goal. However, since spontaneous bleeding is not uncommon in persons with severe hemophilia, definitive measures, including replacement therapy and physical therapy, are necessary to limit joint damage.

During bleeding episodes the joint is elevated and immobilized. Passive range of motion exercises are usually instituted after the acute phase. Physical therapy is beneficial to promote maximum function of the joint and unaffected body parts. Success of a physical therapy plan involves control of pain by administering analgesics before therapy and adjusting the dose to provide maximum benefit.

If an exercise program is instituted in the home, a physical therapist or public health nurse may need to supervise compliance with the regimen. Occasionally orthopedic intervention such as casting, application of traction, or aspiration of blood may be necessary to preserve joint function. Diet is also an important consideration, since excessive body weight can increase the strain on affected joints, especially the knees, and predispose to hemarthrosis. Consequently, calories need to be supplied in accordance with energy requirements.

Since many individuals are unaware of the serious effects of joint involvement, the nurse has the responsibility of educating the child and family concerning the long-range consequences of this complication. Surgical joint replacement in instances of total disability offers new hope to some persons with hemophilia.

Prepare for home care. The discovery of factor concentrates has greatly changed the outlook for these children. With scheduled infusions of the missing factor, bleeding can be prevented and the child can live a much more normal, unrestricted life. To foster maximum independence, home-care programs that teach the parent and/or child to administer the drug have been instituted. The same principles discussed in Chapter 26 regarding preparing families for home management apply here. The nurse, skilled in venipuncture techniques, is often the person who teaches the families to administer antihemophilic factor concentrates.

In addition, the nurse must be familiar with the properties of the concentrates (see Table 35-5) and their preparation. For example, to hasten the mixing process of reconstituting dried antihemophilic factor with diluent, the solution may be warmed or the vial gently rotated. Excessive heating or shaking of the container will result in loss of active antihemophilic factor. A filtered intravenous setup is usually supplied with the drug to filter any particles in the solution. If the solution is not thoroughly mixed before administration, the filter will also remove the active factor.

Transfusion reactions and infection with viral hepatitis and AIDS are potential complications from replacement products. The nurse teaches the parents and/or child the signs of transfusion reactions or hepatitis and stresses the necessity of notifying a physician of their occurrence. If the child tests positive for AIDS, the family may need additional support in dealing with this diagnosis and the often unsympathetic responses of the community (see also p. 1552).

Not all children with hemophilia are eligible for or have the opportunity of a home-care program. For these children, repeated hospitalizations may be needed to control the bleeding episodes. Ideally a core of nurses should work with these children to maintain consistency of care during each hospitalization. Besides the physical goals of controlling bleeding and preventing disability, the nursing objectives should include fostering independence and self-care, providing an opportunity for the children to discuss their feelings regarding the disease, and a continuous reevaluation of those factors that may influence a bleeding episode. Every effort is made to discharge the child as soon as possible and continue treatment on an outpatient basis.

Support the family. Not only is hemophilia a chronic, potentially fatal, hereditary condition, it is also one of unpredictable emergencies that impose additional emotional stress on family members. Children with the moderate or mild form may be undiagnosed until an accident occurs or elective medical procedure is performed. Then, coping with the diagnosis may be hindered by the circumstances surrounding its discovery. At other times parents are aware of the severity of the defect from birth and are immediately faced with the birth of a defective child. Whatever the situation, constructive teaching about the disease and measures to control or prevent bleeding must follow a period of parental adjustment to the diagnosis. For the nurse this involves (1) carefully listening to the parents' statements regarding their understanding of the condition, (2) awareness of the parents' feelings, particularly those of the mother concerning transmitting the disorder, and (3) an assessment of those factors that promote or retard coping with a crisis, such as marital stability, previous patterns of coping, and the ability to seek out and use help (see Chapter 22).

Genetic counseling as soon as possible after diagnosis is essential and must include evaluation of parental understanding and counseling about feelings as well as transmission of information. Unlike many other disorders in which both parents carry the trait, the feeling of responsibility for this condition rests on the mother.

The needs of the family are best met through a comprehensive team approach of physicians (pediatrician, hematologist, orthopedist), nurse, social worker, and physical therapist. Parent-group discussions are beneficial in addressing those needs often best met by similarly affected families. For example, with the improved prognosis for these chil-

---

*Manufactured by 3M Co., Medical Products Division, St. Paul, MN.

dren, adolescents with hemophilia are faced with vocational, employment, and financial problems (see Questions and controversies, p. 950). Further, factor replacement therapy and other treatments for the child with severe hemophilia can cost in excess of $10,000 a year. The **National Hemophilia Foundation*** provides numerous services and publications for both health providers and families.

VON WILLEBRAND DISEASE

von Willebrand disease is a hereditary bleeding disorder characterized by a moderate to severe factor VIII deficiency and low levels of factor VIII–related antigen (FVIII R:Ag). In addition, the functional component of the factor VIII molecule that is required for platelet adhesion to vascular subendothelium (known as von Willebrand factor or ristocetin cofactor) is reduced. This results in prolonged bleeding time because the platelets fail to adhere to the walls of the ruptured vessel to form a platelet plug.

The most characteristic clinical feature of von Willebrand disease is an increased tendency to bleeding from mucous membranes. The most common symptom is frequent nosebleeds, followed by gingival bleeding, easy bruising, and menorrhagia in females. Unlike hemophilia, it affects both males and females because its inheritance is autosomal dominant. However, the treatment and final outcome are similar in both disorders. Treatment of bleeding is with cryoprecipitate or fresh frozen plasma.

Nursing Considerations

The nursing goals are similar to those for hemophilia with special considerations related to epistaxis (p. 1548) and menorrhagia. Replacement therapy may be beneficial before the menstrual cycle to lessen the flow. Teaching the adolescent methods to prevent embarrassing accidents during menstruation, such as wearing plastic-lined underpants and using double sanitary pads, helps her adjust to the inconvenience. Interestingly, these females frequently do not experience excessive bleeding at the time of delivery. This is thought to be because of increased levels of factor VIII during pregnancy. Decisions regarding childbearing are difficult because of the dominant pattern of inheritance.

IDIOPATHIC THROMBOCYTOPENIC PURPURA

Idiopathic thrombocytopenic purpura (ITP) is an acquired hemorrhagic disorder that results from excessive destruction of platelets. Although the exact cause is unknown, it is believed to be an autoimmune response to disease-related antigens and is the most commonly occurring thrombocytopenia of childhood.

Clinical Manifestations

ITP occurs in one of two forms: an acute, self-limiting course or a chronic condition interspersed with remissions.

*19 W. 34th St., New York, NY 10011.

The acute form is most commonly seen after upper respiratory infections or the childhood diseases measles, rubella, mumps, and chickenpox. The most common clinical manifestations of either type include (1) easy bruising with petechiae and/or ecchymoses, particularly over bony prominences, (2) bleeding from mucous membranes, such as epistaxis, bleeding gums, and internal hemorrhage with evidence of hematuria, hematemesis, melena, hemarthrosis, and menorrhagia, and (3) hematomas over the lower extremities that may result in chronic leg ulcers.

Diagnostic Evaluation

In ITP the platelet count is reduced to below 20,000 mm³/dl; therefore tests that depend on platelet function are abnormal, such as the tourniquet test, bleeding time, and clot retraction. Although there is no definitive test on which to establish a diagnosis of ITP, several tests are usually performed to rule out other disorders in which thrombocytopenia is a manifestation, such as systemic lupus erythematosus, lymphoma, or leukemia.

Therapeutic Management

Management is primarily supportive, because the course of the disease is self-limited in the majority of cases. Activity is restricted at the onset while the platelet count is low and active bleeding or progression of lesions is occurring. This restriction is most easily accomplished in the hospital. Corticosteroids are employed for children with the highest risk for serious bleeding (platelet count less than 30,000); it is hypothesized that steroids inhibit removal of sensitized platelets by the reticuloendothelial system. The use of intravenous gamma globulin has also been advocated and has demonstrated some effectiveness in increasing platelet production until spontaneous recovery takes place, although the mechanism of action is unknown. Splenectomy is reserved for symptomatic children who do not respond to drug therapy and who have life-threatening hemorrhage. Any child undergoing splenectomy is at risk for overwhelming sepsis and should receive the pneumococcal and meningococcal vaccines and antibiotic therapy of indefinite duration.

Nursing Considerations

Nursing care is largely supportive and directed toward restricting the activity of an otherwise normal child. Children and parents need careful explanations of the rationale behind the therapies employed and support in their efforts to comply. As in any condition with an uncertain outcome, the family needs emotional support, especially during periods of hospitalization.

The nursing considerations of controlling bleeding, preventing bruising, and preventing crippling effects of hemarthrosis are similar to those discussed for hemophilia. The deleterious effects of using aspirin to control joint pain are critical for these children; therefore salicylate substitutes should always be used. The family also needs to be aware of signs and symptoms indicating internal bleeding, which although rare requires immediate medical attention.

HENOCH-SCHÖNLEIN PURPURA

Henoch-Schönlein purpura (HSP) (Schönlein-Henoch vasculitis, allergic purpura, anaphylactoid purpura) is a relatively common acquired disorder in children characterized by a nonthrombocytopenic purpura, arthritis, nephritis, and abdominal pain. The etiology is unknown, but the disease often follows an upper respiratory infection, and allergy or drug sensitivity plays a role in some instances. The disease occurs in children aged 6 months to 16 years but more frequently between ages 2 to 8 years. It is observed more often in white children than in other races and in boys three times more often than in girls.

Pathophysiology

The disease is characterized by inflammation of small blood vessels, and the manifestations observed are influenced by the size and distribution of the affected vessels. A generalized vasculitis of dermal capillaries (and to a lesser extent small arterioles and veins) causing extravasation of red blood cells produces the petechial skin lesions. Inflammation and hemorrhage may also occur in the gastrointestinal tract, synovium, glomeruli, and central nervous system.

Clinical Manifestations

The onset of the disease may be abrupt with simultaneous appearance of several manifestations or gradual with sequential appearance of different manifestations. The primary feature, however, is a symmetrical purpura that involves the buttocks and lower extremities but may extend to include the extensor surfaces of the upper extremities and, less commonly, the upper trunk and face. The rash may be associated with maculopapular lesions and variable elements of urticaria and erythema. There is often marked edema of scalp, eyelids, lips, ears, and dorsal surfaces of hands and feet—especially in infants and younger children.

Arthritic effects are evident in two thirds of affected children and range from asymptomatic swelling around a single joint to painful tender swelling of several joints, most often the knees and ankles. The involvement is periarticular and resolves in a few days without permanent damage or deformity.

Two thirds of the children have gastrointestinal involvement manifested by recurrent colicky midabdominal pain often associated with nausea and vomiting. The stools contain gross or occult blood and mucus.

Renal involvement occurs in up to 50% of affected children and is potentially the most serious long-term complication. Initially the nephritis is manifested as hematuria, casts, and proteinuria. Although the majority of children with renal involvement recover completely, some develop chronic renal disease with eventual renal failure.

Diagnostic Evaluation

Diagnosis is usually established on the basis of clinical manifestations. Laboratory tests are employed to assess gastrointestinal and renal involvement and to determine adequacy of hemostatic function. Although no test is diagnostic, increased levels of immunoglobin A are a frequent finding (Saulsbury, 1986).

Therapeutic Management

Management is primarily supportive with close observation for signs of renal or gastrointestinal manifestations. Edema, rash, malaise, and arthralgia are usually managed with appropriate analgesics, such as acetaminophen, and mild sedation if necessary. Corticosteroids may be prescribed for relief of more severe edema, arthralgia, and colicky abdominal pain but are not warranted in all cases.

The majority of children recover without the need for hospitalization, and in most instances a single acute episode clears spontaneously within a month. Others may have periodic recurrences for as long as 2 to 3 years before permanent remission from symptoms. Rarely death occurs from severe gastrointestinal complications, acute renal failure, or central nervous system involvement.

Nursing Considerations

Nursing care of the child hospitalized with Henoch-Schönlein purpura is primarily supportive with vigilant observation for signs of complications. Vital signs are taken and recorded at regular intervals, specimens obtained for laboratory examination, and medication administered as prescribed. Urine and stools are carefully observed for fresh and occult blood.

If the child suffers from joint pain, positioning, careful movement, and administration of analgesics help reduce discomfort. Nonnarcotic analgesics also relieve the discomfort of fever and malaise. More severe involvement such as gastrointestinal symptoms and nephritis is managed as for any such disorder (see appropriate nursing care).

The child may be concerned about the unsightly appearance of the rash. He and his parents can be reassured that it is only a temporary phenomenon, and he can be encouraged to wear clothing that helps hide the rash, such as long sleeves, pants, and robe. Emphasizing good grooming and attractive apparel helps promote a more positive self-image.

DISSEMINATED INTRAVASCULAR COAGULATION

Disseminated intravascular coagulation (DIC), also known as *consumption coagulopathy,* is not a primary disease but a secondary disorder of coagulation that complicates a number of pathologic processes (such as hypoxia, acidosis, shock, and endothelial damage [burns]) and many severe systemic disease states (such as congenital heart disease, necrotizing enterocolitis, gram-negative bacterial sepsis, rickettsial infections, and some severe viral infections). The disease is characterized by inappropriate systemic activation and acceleration of the normal clotting mechanism.

Pathophysiology

DIC occurs when the first stage of the coagulation process is abnormally stimulated. Although there is no well-defined sequence of events, two distinct phases can be identified.

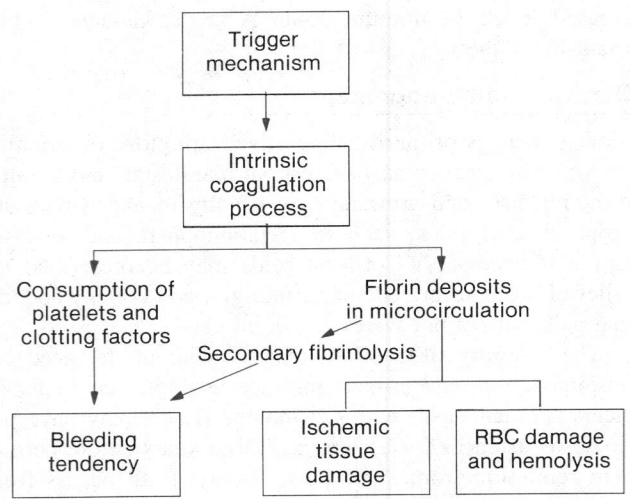

Fig. 35-5. Effects of disseminated intravascular coagulation.

First, when the clotting mechanism is triggered in the circulation, thrombin is generated in greater amounts than can be neutralized by the body. Consequently, there is rapid conversion of fibrinogen to fibrin with aggregation and destruction of platelets. If local and widespread fibrin deposition in blood vessels takes place, obstruction and eventual necrosis of tissues occur. Second, the fibrinolytic mechanism is activated, causing extensive destruction of clotting factors. With a deficiency of clotting factors the child is vulnerable to uncontrollable hemorrhage into vital organs. An additional complication is damage and hemolysis of red blood cells (Fig. 35-5).

Clinical Manifestations

Signs of DIC are those of many other diseases, which often confuses the diagnosis. There is evidence of bleeding—petechiae, purpura, bleeding from openings in the skin (such as a venipuncture site or surgical incision), hypotension, and dysfunction of organs from infarction and ischemia.

Diagnostic Evaluation

DIC is suspected when there is an increased tendency to bleed, as from venipuncture or blood taken from the heel, and bleeding from the umbilicus, trachea, or gastrointestinal tract. Hematologic findings include prolonged prothrombin (PT), partial thromboplastin (PTT), and thrombin times. There is a profoundly depressed platelet count, fragmented red blood cells, and depleted fibrinogen.

Therapeutic Management

Treatment is directed toward control of the underlying or initiating cause, which in most instances stops the coagulation problem spontaneously. Platelets and fresh frozen plasma may be needed to replace lost plasma components, especially in the child whose underlying disease remains uncontrolled. The very ill newborn infant may require exchange transfusion with fresh blood. The administration of heparin to inhibit thrombin formation is most often restricted to severe cases.

Nursing Considerations

The goals of nursing care are to be aware of the possibility of DIC in the severely ill child and to recognize signs that might indicate its presence. The skills needed to monitor intravenous infusion and blood transfusions and to administer heparin are the same as for any child receiving these therapies. Since the child is usually cared for in an intensive care unit, the special needs of the family must be considered (see p. 1092).

EPISTAXIS (NOSEBLEEDING)

Isolated and transient episodes of epistaxis, or nosebleeding, are common in childhood. The nose is a highly vascular structure, and bleeding usually results from direct trauma, including blows to the nose, foreign bodies, and nose picking, or from mucosal inflammation associated with allergic rhinitis and upper respiratory infections or drying of the mucous membranes in environments with low humidity. Ordinarily the bleeding stops spontaneously or with minimal pressure and requires no medical evaluation or therapy.

Recurrent epistaxis and severe bleeding may indicate an underlying disease, particularly vascular abnormalities, leukemia, thrombocytopenia, and clotting factor deficiency diseases such as hemophilia and von Willebrand disease. Sometimes nosebleeds are associated with administration of aspirin, even in normal amounts. Persistent nosebleeding requires medical evaluation.

Nursing Considerations

Nosebleeds are often a frightening experience for the child and parents. A calm, reassuring manner can alleviate anxiety and promote the child's cooperation. Since most of the nosebleeding originates in the anterior part of the nasal septum, bleeding can be controlled by applying pressure to the nose with the thumb and forefinger. (See Emergency box). During this time the child breathes through his mouth.

In the event that hemorrhage continues, the child should be evaluated by a physician, who may pack the nose with epinephrine-soaked gauze. After a nosebleed, petroleum or water-soluble jelly can be inserted into each nostril to prevent crusting of old blood and to lessen the likelihood of the child's picking at his nose and restarting the hemorrhage. Whenever possible, factors believed to increase the likelihood of epistaxis are eliminated, such as discouraging nose picking or altering the household humidity by placing a cool-mist vaporizer in the child's room.

Immunologic-Deficiency Disorders

A number of disorders can cause profound, often life-threatening alterations within the body's immune system. The most serious are those conditions that completely depress immunity, such as severe combined immunodeficiency disease. However, the one disorder that generates the most anxiety, within both the family and the community at large, is acquired immune deficiency syndrome (AIDS).

Immunodeficiency disorders can be classified into five groups according to the site of immune alteration (Cohen, 1984):

stem cell defects, which usually lead to a combined immunodeficiency of both the cell-mediated and humoral components

T-cell defects, which cause defective cellular immunity

B-cell defects, which result in impaired humoral immunity

phagocytic defects, which affect the ability of the white blood cells to control infection

In order to enhance understanding of immunologic-deficiency disorders, the following overview is presented of the body's immune system.

MECHANISMS INVOLVED IN IMMUNITY

In simple terms, the function of the immune system is to recognize "self" from "non-self" and to initiate responses to eliminate the non-self or the foreign substance known as *antigen*. However, the specific processes involved in this function are complex and interrelated, and advances in the understanding of immunologic mechanisms are helping to further elucidate the intricacies of this system.

The immune system includes the *primary lymphoid organs* (thymus, bone marrow, and probably liver) and the *secondary lymphoid organs* (lymph nodes, spleen, and gut-associated lymphoid tissue [GALT]). The functions of the immune system are basically two types: nonspecific and specific (Fig. 35-6). *Nonspecific immune defenses* are activated on exposure to any foreign substance but react similarly regardless of the type of antigen; they are unable to identify the antigen. The principal component of this system is *phagocytosis,* the process of ingesting and digesting foreign substances. Phagocytic cells are composed of neutrophils and monocytes (see p. 1514).

Specific Immune Mechanisms

Specific (adaptive) defenses are those that have the ability to recognize the antigen and respond selectively. The components of adaptive immunity are *humoral immunity* and *cell-mediated immunity*. The cells responsible for these two forms of immunity are the lymphocytes, specifically B-lymphocytes and T-lymphocytes.

Humoral Immunity

Humoral immunity is involved with antibody production and complement. The principal cell involved in antibody production is the B-lymphocyte. In humans the exact site of production of the B-lymphocyte is speculative, although it is probably the bone marrow. In chickens the site is clearly identified as a hind-gut organ known as the bursa of Fabri-

---

Emergency Treatment: Epistaxis

1. Have child sit up and lean forward (not lying down)
2. Apply continuous pressure to nose with thumb and forefinger for at least 10 minutes
3. Insert cotton or wadded tissue into each nostril and apply ice or cold cloth to bridge of nose if bleeding persists
4. Keep child calm and quiet

---

cius, hence the term "B-lymphocyte," or "B-cell." When challenged with an antigen, B-cells divide and differentiate into *plasma cells*. The plasma cells produce and secrete large quantities of antibodies specific to the antigen. Five classes of antibodies of immunoglobulins (Ig) have been identified: G, M, A, D, and E, each serving a specific function.

On initial exposure to an antigen, the B-lymphocyte system begins to produce antibody, predominantly IgM, which appears in 2 to 3 days. This process is referred to as the *primary antibody response*. With subsequent exposure to the antigen, a *secondary antibody response* occurs. Antibody, chiefly IgG, is produced in much greater quantities within 1 to 2 days. An example of the secondary response is consecutive administration of immunizations, often called boosters. Memory B-cells allow the immune system to recognize the same antigen for months or years.

When antibody reacts with antigen, they bind to form an antigen-antibody complex. This binding serves several functions. Antibody aids in the phagocytosis of antigen by sensitizing it in such a manner that it is more readily destroyed by phagocytes, a process known as *opsonization*.

Antibody also activates or fixes complement, the second component of humoral immunity. The complement system is a series of nine major factors (C_1 to C_9) present in serum that results in a cascade of enzymatic actions and death of a viable antigen. It also serves to bridge cellular and humoral immunity. After being activated by antibody, complement produces a chemotactic factor that summons T-lymphocytes and macrophages to the antigen site.

Cell-Mediated Immunity

Cell-mediated immunity is involved in a variety of specific functions mediated by the T-lymphocyte. The T-lymphocyte is so named because it passes through the thymus during the differentiation process, which leads to the mature T-cell. T-lymphocytes do not carry typical immunoglobulins on their surfaces as do the B-cells. However, they are functionally heterogenous in that several subsets have been identified, including cytotoxic T-cells, inducer T-cells, helper T-lymphocytes, and suppressor T-lymphocytes. T-cells may also be classified structurally by their surface antigens. Once mature, T-cells display either the T_4 or the T_8 antigen. The T_4, which comprises 60% to 70% of circulating T-cells, consists

Fig. 35-6. Components of immune system.

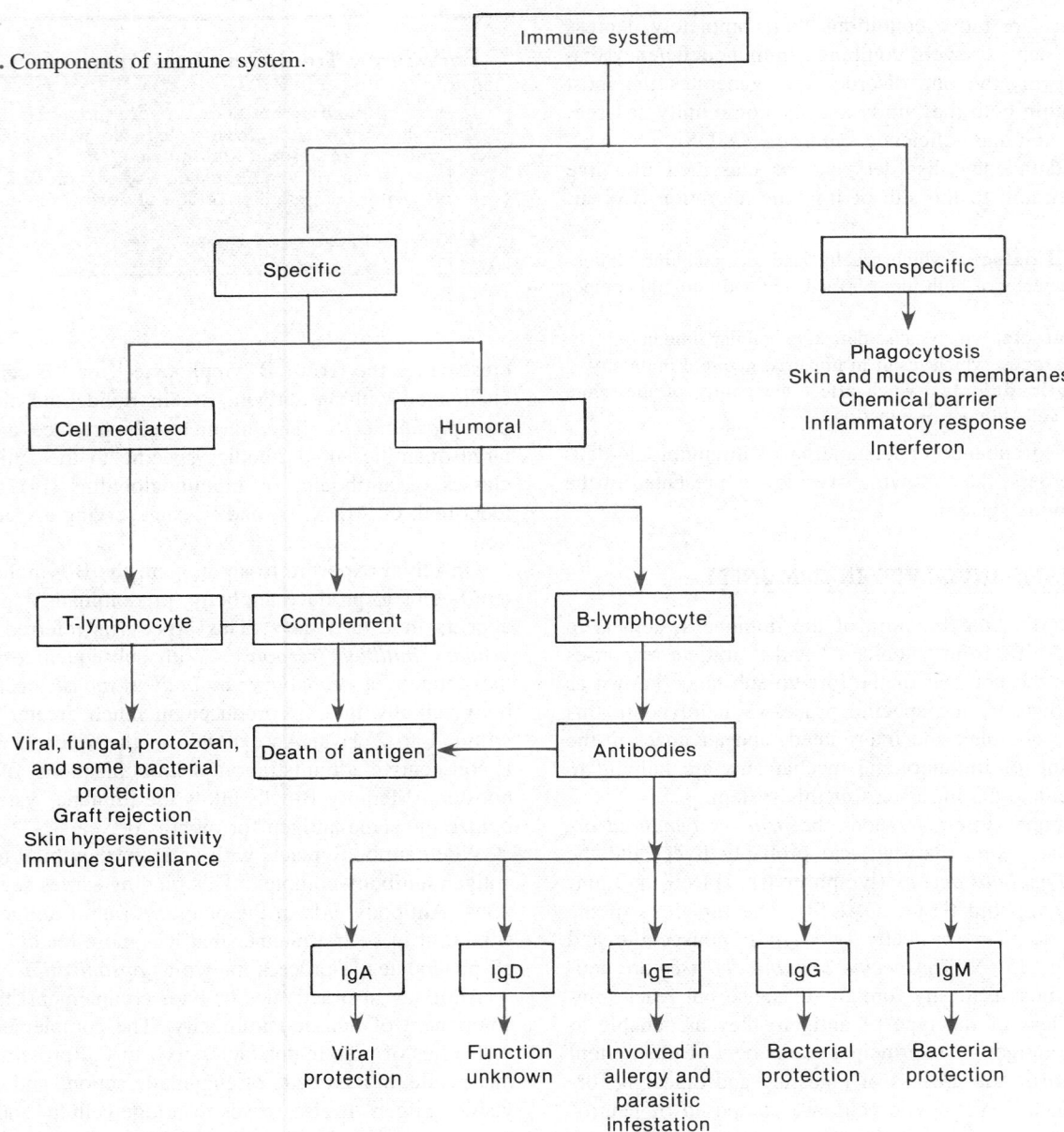

mainly of helper/inducer cells, while the T_8 subset contains cytotoxic/suppressor cells.

Specific functions of T-lymphocytes include: (1) protection against most viral, fungal, and protozoan infections and slow-growing bacterial infections, such as tuberculosis, (2) rejection of histoincompatible grafts, (3) mediation of cutaneous delayed hypersensitivity reactions, such as in tuberculin testing, and (4) probably immune surveillance for malignant cells. In addition, they also have regulatory functions within the immune system. For example, helper T-lymphocytes assist B-lymphocytes and other types of T-cells to mount an optimum immune response.

The cellular immune response is initiated when a T-lymphocyte is sensitized by antigen. In response to this contact the T-cell releases numerous humoral factors called *lymphokines,* which eventually bring about death of the antigen.

For example, *chemotactic factor* promotes the migration of phagocytes and other T-lymphocytes to the antigenic area, *migratory inhibitor factor* prevents their leaving the site, *transfer factor* transforms nonsensitized T-cells into sensitized T-lymphocytes, *blastogenic factor* initiates the rapid mitosis of sensitized T-cells, and *macrophage activation factor* transforms local macrophages to highly phagocytic cells. Another lymphokine is *interferon,* which nonspecifically inhibits viral replication, promotes phagocytosis, and stimulates the killer activity of sensitized lymphocytes.

ACQUIRED IMMUNE DEFICIENCY SYNDROME

Acquired immune deficiency syndrome (AIDS) is a recently recognized disorder that has generated intense medical investigation and even greater public concern and fear. The first published reports of unusual opportunistic infections in previously healthy individuals appeared in 1981; retrospective analysis of data demonstrated the existence of cases since 1978. In 1983 and 1984, a retrovirus (RNA virus) found in AIDS patients was characterized and named. The French researchers named the virus *Lymphadenopathy Associated Virus (LAV)*, and the United States team labeled it *Human T-cell Lymphotrophic Virus Type III (HTLV-III)*. Current evidence suggests that these viruses are one and the same; the term *Human Immunodeficiency Virus (HIV)* is also used to refer to the virus.

Etiology and High-Risk Groups

The HTLV-III virus is believed to cause AIDS. It is suspected that infection with the virus is not solely responsible for the development of AIDS, but that other co-factors determine pathogenicity, such as repeated antigenic stimulation, prematurity, unhygienic living conditions, viral illnesses, and factors that suppress the immune system (Church, Allen, and Stiehm, 1986). The virus has been found in blood and almost all body fluids (semen, saliva, urine, breastmilk, and tears), but to date there is evidence that the virus is transmitted only through direct contact with blood or blood products and intimate sexual contact in which semen and blood mix (primarily anal intercourse). There is no evidence that *casual* contact between affected and unaffected individuals can spread the virus (Kaplan and others, 1985; Centers for Disease Control, 1986).

Initially AIDS was identified in sexually active homosexual males; since then additional high-risk groups have been identified, which include bisexual males, intravenous drug abusers, recipients of multiple transfusions (e.g., hemophiliacs), sexual partners of risk group and members, newborns of high-risk mothers (e.g., intravenous drug use in mother or father, maternal promiscuity, Haitian extraction). The majority of children with AIDS are less than 2 years of age and constitute a small percentage of the AIDS population. Approximately 75% of these cases resulted from perinatal transmission and 15% from blood transfusions (Church, Allen, and Stiehm, 1986). Children with hemophilia are especially at risk because factor concentrates are prepared from pooled plasma that is obtained from up to 20,000 donors, thus exposing these children to tens of thousands of blood donors (Speck, 1983). However, recent advances in the preparation of concentrates and screening for the antibody to the HTLV-III virus in blood products will probably reduce the risk to these children and other children who require frequent blood transfusions.

Of major concern is the rapidly rising incidence of the disorder. In the United States the current doubling time for cases is 11 to 12 months. More than 50% of risk-group members in certain areas of the country have been infected with the virus; it is estimated that between 1 million and 2 million people (mostly adults) have already been exposed to the virus, with perhaps 1,000 new cases a day (Selwyn, 1986). While individuals exposed to the virus may demonstrate a positive antibody test to HTLV-III, it is uncertain

who are carriers of the virus and who will eventually develop the clinical syndrome of AIDS or AIDS-related complex (ARC), the presence of various symptoms, such as lymphadenopathy, fever, or diarrhea.

Pathophysiology

AIDS is characterized by a generalized dysfunction of the immune system. In adult onset AIDS, the primary immunologic abnormality includes decreased T-cells (especially T helper cells of the T_4 subset). In normal individuals there are more helper than suppressor T-cells (T_8 subset), but in AIDS victims there is a reverse helper to suppressor ratio. There is also cutaneous anergy to delayed hypersensitivity antigens. Similar pathologic findings are found in children with AIDS, but they occur later in the disease course.

Abnormal B-cell function is apparent early in pediatric AIDS. Often there are an increased number of B-cells and increased levels of IgG, IgM, and IgA, but deficiencies of IgG subclasses have been identified. Despite the hypergammaglobulinemia, the immunoglobulins are nonfunctional, leaving the body defenseless to many opportunistic infections (Iazzetti, 1986).

Clinical Manifestations

The clinical presentation of pediatric AIDS includes failure to thrive, interstitial pneumonitis, and hepatosplenomegaly (present in greater than 90% of patients). Diffuse lymphadenopathy is found in more than half of the children. Less common findings are protracted diarrhea, thrombocytopenia, low birth weight (less than 2500 g), eczematoid rash, recurrent otitis media, developmental failure, and microcephaly. Kaposi sarcoma, one of the hallmarks of the adult disease, is found in less than 10% of the affected children. Clinical and laboratory signs of AIDS in children with maternal transmission is 2 to 4 months. Earlier clues in these children include a complex of craniofacial features: increased inner and outer canthal distance, mildly oblique eyes, prominent triangular philtrum (vertical groove in middle of upper lip) and patulous (widely spread apart) lips (Krug, 1986).

Diagnostic Evaluation

The Centers for Disease Control (CDC) have defined specific criteria for the diagnosis of AIDS in children. These include any child who has had:

1. A reliably diagnosed disease at least moderately indicative of underlying cellular immunodeficiency
2. No known cause of underlying cellular immunodeficiency or any other cause of reduced resistance reported to be associated with that disease

Because of the number of disorders that may mimic AIDS, such as severe combined immunodeficiency disease and Wiskott-Aldrich syndrome, the diagnosis is often one of ruling out other probable causes, demonstrating the principal immunologic abnormalities in AIDS, and establishing a positive antibody to HTLV-III. A positive HTLV-III antibody test is not sufficient to establish a diagnosis of AIDS, because HTLV-III virus infections result in a spectrum of responses, from asymptomatic seroconversion to complete immunologic incompetence (Church, Allen, and Stiehm, 1986).

Therapeutic Management

Currently, there is no cure for AIDS and the disease is uniformly fatal. Treatment is directed at the prevention and management of the opportunistic infections. The most common infections are chronic candidiasis and interstitial pneumonia, especially *Pneumocystis carinii,* which occurs in greater than 70% of affected children. Combination therapy for *P. carinii* includes trimethoprim/sulfamethoxazole (Bactrim, Septra) and pentamidine. If a skin reaction, fever, or cytopenia occurs secondary to the trimethoprim/sulfamethoxazole, the drug is discontinued.

Gamma globulin administration may be helpful to compensate for the deficiency of B-lymphocytes. Ongoing studies are investigating the benefits of periodic administration of intravenous gamma globulin. Preliminary results suggest that the treated group may have fewer episodes of bacterial infection (Rubinstein and others, 1986).

Nursing Considerations

Nursing considerations are primarily directed at preventing the transmission of the virus, caring for the child with AIDS, and educating the public regarding the *realistic* concerns in terms of communicability of the virus. Recommendations for preventing spread of the virus consist of the same precautions for preventing the transmission of other blood-borne diseases, such as hepatitis B virus (see box, p. 1440). These precautions should be routinely enforced regardless of whether the child is a known carrier.

The nursing care of the child with AIDS is primarily supportive, both physiologically and psychologically. Since the child is immunodeficient, every precaution to prevent infection is implemented (see Nursing care summary p. 1554). The nurse must carefully and frequently monitor for changes in status that may indicate impending sepsis or other complications. Fever is a cardinal sign of infection, especially since other responses to infection are usually absent.

Psychologic support of the family is essential. Unfortunately, the public is very fearful of contracting the disease from AIDS victims, and criticism and ostracism of the child and family are common. In an effort to protect the child and deal with the community's fear, the family may keep the child at home in an atmosphere of overprotection. While certain precautions are justified in limiting exposure to sources of infection, they must be tempered with concern for the child's normal developmental needs. Both the family and the community need education about AIDS virus to dispel many of the myths that have been perpetuated by the uninformed.*

Of major concern for both family and community has been school attendance for children with AIDS. Both the

Centers for Disease Control (1985) and the American Academy of Pediatrics (1986) have published guidelines regarding school attendance, which include the following:

1. Unrestricted school attendance for most school-aged children and adolescents, with the approval of their personal physician, is recommended, including children with AIDS or AIDS-related complex, or who have antibody to the virus
2. Students who do not have control of their bodily secretions, who display behaviors such as biting, or who have open sores that cannot be covered may present a greater risk and should be given a more restricted school environment until more is known about the disease

Nurses need to be knowledgeable of these guidelines and of changes that may occur as additional information about the virus is known. School nurses, in particular, play a vital role in educating the public and in monitoring the needs of the affected child. Confidentiality is a major factor—the number of personnel aware of the child's condition should be kept to a minimum. In addition, school personnel must be aware of sanitary practices to prevent spread of the virus, including proper disposal of items contaminated with blood, for example, sanitary napkins, tissues from caring for a bloody nose, or bandages used in cleaning a wound.

SEVERE COMBINED IMMUNODEFICIENCY DISEASE

Severe combined immunodeficiency disease (SCID) is a defect characterized by absence of both humoral and cell-mediated immunity. The terms *Swiss-type lymphopenic agammaglobulinemia,* an autosomal-recessive form of the disease, and *X-linked lymphopenic agammaglobulinemia* have been used to describe this disorder, which, as the names imply, can follow either mode of inheritance.

Pathophysiology

The exact cause of SCID is unknown. The theories include (1) a defective stem cell that is incapable of differentiating into B- or T-cells, (2) defective organs responsible for the differentiating process, primarily the thymus and lymphoid complex, or (3) an enzymatic defect that suppresses lymphocytic cell function.

The consequence of the immunodeficiency is an overwhelming susceptibility to infection and to the *graft-vs-host reaction,* which can occur when any histoincompatible (unmatched) tissue from an immunocompetent donor is infused into the immunodeficient recipient. Because of its immunodeficiency, the body is unable to reject the foreign incompatible tissue. Therefore the antigenic donor cells attack the host's tissues. The graft-vs-host reaction is a serious complication in the only known treatment for SCID, bone marrow transplantation.

Clinical Manifestations

The most common manifestation is susceptibility to infection early in life, most often by 3 months of age when prenatal acquired immunity is exhausted. Specifically, the disorder in children is characterized by chronic infection,

---

*Information is available from the AIDS hotline: 1-800-447-AIDS (Atlanta area: 1-404-329-1295).

failure to completely recover from an infection, frequent reinfection, and infection with unusual agents. In addition, the history reveals no logical source of infection. Failure to thrive is a consequence of the persistent illnesses.

If the child should receive a foreign tissue, such as blood supplements, signs of graft-vs-host reaction, such as fever, skin rash, alopecia, hepatosplenomegaly, and diarrhea, are expected. Since the reaction requires 7 to 20 days for tissue damage to become evident, the symptoms may be mistaken for an infection. However, the presence of a graft-vs-host reaction increases the child's susceptibility to overwhelming infection and therefore is a grave complication.

Diagnostic Evaluation

Diagnosis is usually based on a history of recurrent, severe infections from early infancy, a familial history of the disorder, and specific laboratory findings, which include lymphopenia, lack of lymphocyte response to antigens, and absence of plasma cells in the bone marrow. Documentation of immunoglobulin deficiency is difficult during infancy because of the normally delayed response of the infant to produce his own immunoglobulins and material transfer of immunoglobulin G.

Therapeutic Management

The only definitive treatment is a histocompatible bone marrow transplant. The most suitable donor is a sibling with a matched HLA bone marrow. Because SCID is inherited, an identical twin, who usually is a perfect donor, is not a candidate, since that offspring would also display the disorder. Since the host's immunologic system is incompetent, graft rejection is not a problem. However, a graft-vs-host reaction is always a possibility, and once it occurs, little can be done to reverse the process.

Other approaches to SCID are providing passive immunity with intravenous immune globulin and maintaining the child in a sterile environment. The latter is effective only if instituted before the existence of any infectious process in the infant, and it represents an extreme effort to prevent life-threatening infections. Other investigational transplant procedures include nonidentical HLA bone marrow grafts and fetal liver or thymus transplants. However, the results are still uncertain, although they provide potential hope for future children born with the disorder.

Nursing Considerations

Nursing care depends on the type of therapy employed. If bone marrow transplantation is attempted, the care is consistent with that needed for bone marrow transplantation for any condition (see p. 1565). To prevent infection, all interventions aimed at protecting the immunocompromised child are implemented (see Nursing care summary, p. 1554). However, even with exacting environmental control, these children are prone to opportunistic infection. Chronic fungal infections of the mouth and nails with *Candida albicans* are frequent problems despite vigorous efforts at prevention or treatment. A hoarse voice may result from repeated esophageal and vocal cord erosions from the fungus. It is important to stress to parents that such conditions are not a result of laxity on their part in preventing them but are the result of the severe immunologic disorder. Parents should be encouraged to immediately notify a physician regarding any evidence of a worsening infection.

Since the prognosis for SCID is very poor if a compatible bone marrow donor is not available, nursing care is directed at supporting the family in caring for a child with a life-threatening illness (Chapter 23). Genetic counseling is essential because of the modes of transmission in either form of the disorder.

WISKOTT-ALDRICH SYNDROME

The Wiskott-Aldrich syndrome is an X-linked recessive disorder characterized by a triad of abnormalities: (1) thrombocytopenia, (2) eczema, and (3) immunodeficiency of selective functions of B- and T-lymphocytes.

Pathophysiology

The exact defect is unknown, although recent evidence suggests a basic hematopoietic cell abnormality specifically related to cell energy metabolism (Shapiro and others, 1978). A variety of pathologic findings are evident. The platelets are abnormally small in size and have a shortened life span, possibly because of a metabolic defect in their synthesis. The primary immunologic defect consists of the inability of phagocytes (macrophages) to process foreign antigens, particularly polysaccharides such as pneumococcus. As a result, immunologically competent cells fail to produce normal immunoglobulin patterns. Early in life the immunoglobulin levels may be normal, but later low levels of IgM are observed. Typically isohemagglutinins (anti-A and anti-B agglutinins in the blood) are decreased or absent.

The thymus and lymph nodes are normal at birth but become progressively dysfunctional with age until a profound cellular immunodeficiency results. Consequently, these children are highly susceptible to infection and malignancy, especially of the lymphoreticular system.

Clinical Manifestations

At birth the major effect of the disorder is bleeding because of the thrombocytopenia. As the child grows older, recurrent infection and eczema become more severe and the bleeding becomes less frequent.

Eczema is typical of the allergic type and readily becomes superinfected. Chronic infection with herpes simplex is a frequent problem and may lead to chronic keratitis with loss of vision. From infection, chronic pulmonary disease, sinusitis, and otitis media result. In those children who survive the bleeding episodes and overwhelming infections, malignancy presents an additional threat to survival.

Diagnostic Evaluation

Diagnosis can usually be made during the neonatal period because of the thrombocytopenia. Specific tests for immunologic function confirm the diagnosis. Carrier detection is also possible (Hill, 1980).

Nursing Care Summary: The Child with Immunosuppression

NURSING GOALS	NURSING INTERVENTIONS	EXPECTED PATIENT/FAMILY OUTCOMES
HP-HMP Infection: potential for **Risk factors: altered body defenses**		
Minimize risk of infection	Place child in private room Advise all visitors and staff to practice handwashing Screen all visitors and staff for signs of infection Use scrupulous aseptic technique for all invasive procedures Teach child and family principles of protective isolation (if ordered) Evaluate child for any potential sites of infection (needle punctures, mucosal ulceration, minor abrasions, dental problems) Provide nutritionally complete diet for age Serve cooked foods; avoid raw, unpeeled vegetables or fruits Teach preventive measures at discharge (handwashing and isolation from crowds) Stress importance of isolating child from any known cases of chickenpox or other childhood diseases; work with school nurse and physician to determine optimum time for school reattendance	Child remains in private room *Staff and visitors comply with infection precautions *Signs of infection are recognized and reported. Note: usual signs of infection may not be present in all immunocompromised children Child consumes diet appropriate for age (specify) Family demonstrates knowledge of instructions (specify methods of learning and evaluate)
A-EP Diversional activity, deficit **Etiology: restricted environment**		
Provide diversion	Provide age-appropriate toys that can be properly cleaned Involve child life specialist or other supportive services in planning diversional activities	Child engages in activities appropriate for age and interests Suitable toys are provided
RRP Grieving, anticipatory **Etiology: perceived potential loss of child**		
Support family	Allow family time and place to openly discuss their fears and concerns Discuss with family their preferences for care if death is imminent Arrange for appropriate spiritual care in accordance with family's beliefs and/or affiliations	Family expresses fear, concerns, and any special desires for terminal child *Appropriate religious representation is contacted (specify)
RRP Alteration, family process, alteration in **Etiology: situational crisis (child with life-threatening illness)**		
Support family	Teach parents about disease process Explain all procedures that will be done to child Encourage discussion and expression of feelings and concerns Schedule time for family to be together, without interruptions from staff	Family demonstrates knowledge of child's disease and treatments (specify methods of learning and evaluation) Family expresses feelings and concerns and spends time with child

*Nursing outcome.

Therapeutic Management

Medical treatment mainly involves (1) counteracting the bleeding tendencies with platelet transfusions, (2) using intravenous immune globulin to provide passive immunity, and (3) administering prophylactic antibiotics to prevent and control infection. Splenectomy may be performed to reverse the thrombocytopenia, but asplenia imposes the additional risk of fulminant infection. These children require the same prophylactic measures as any child with asplenia—appropriate immunizations and continuous antibiotics—and despite their immune deficiency they are able to mount an adequate immunologic response to the inactivated vaccines. When an HLA-matched donor exists, bone marrow transplantation is the treatment of choice.

Nursing Considerations

Because of the grave prognosis for these children, the main nursing consideration is supporting the family in the care of a child with a life-threatening illness (see Chapter 23). Physical care is directed at controlling the problems imposed by the disorder. The measures used to control bleeding are similar to those discussed under hemophilia and epistaxis. Another major goal is related to preventing or controlling infection. Since eczema is a troublesome problem, nursing measures specific to this condition are especially important (see p. 577).

The genetic implications of this X-linked recessive disorder differ little from those of hemophilia. However, because of the multiplicity of defects, the emotional adjustment and physical care required for these children are greater than those of many other conditions. The nurse can be especially supportive by providing short-term goals during periods of hospitalization and by focusing on long-range needs through coordinated efforts with a public health nurse.

CONCEPT SUMMARIES

- Major functions of the hematologic system include production of cells, oxygenation, nutrient distribution to the cells, collection of wastes from the cells, and heat regulation.

- The major blood-forming organs of the body are red bone marrow, lymphatic system, and reticuloendothelial system.

- Anemia is defined as reduction of red cell volume or hemoglobin concentration to levels below normal; disorders are classified either by etiology/physiology or by morphology.

- The nurse's role in treatment of anemia is to assist in establishing a diagnosis, prepare the child for laboratory tests, decrease tissue oxygen needs, implement safety precautions, and observe for complications.

- The main nursing goal in prevention of nutritional anemia is parent education regarding correct feeding practices.

- Four types of sickle cell crisis are: vasoocclusive, splenic sequestration, aplastic, and hyperhemolytic.

- Nursing care of the child with sickle cell disease is aimed at teaching the family how to recognize and prevent sickling, managing pain during splenic crises, and helping the child and parents adjust to lifelong, potentially fatal disease.

- Nursing care of the child with Cooley anemia entails observing for complications of multiple blood transfusions, assisting the child to cope with the effects of illness, and fostering parent-child adjustment to long-term illness.

- Common causes of aplastic anemia include irradiation, drugs, industrial and household chemicals, infections, infiltration and replacement of myeloid elements, and idiopathic conditions.

- The human body controls bleeding through three processes: vascular spasm, platelet aggregation, and coagulation and clot formation.

- Nursing care of the hemophiliac child involves preventing bleeding by decreasing the risk of injury, recognizing and managing bleeding, preventing the crippling effects of joint degeneration, preparing and supporting the child and family for home care.

- Immunodeficiency disorders can be classified into groups according to the site of immune alteration: stem cell defects, T-cell defects, B-cell defects, and phagocytic defects.

- Pediatric clinical manifestations of AIDS include failure to thrive, interstitial pneumonitis, and hepatosplenomegaly.

REFERENCES

Alter, B.P.: Antenatal diagnosis of thalassemia: a review. In Bank, A., Anderson, W.F., and Zaino, E.C., editors: Fifth Cooley's anemia symposium, vol. 445, New York, 1985, Ann. N.Y. Acad. Sci.

American Academy of Pediatrics, Committee on School Health, and Committee on Infectious Diseases: School attendance of children and adolescents with human T lymphotropic virus III/lymphadenopathy-associated virus infection, Pediatrics 77(3):430-432, 1986.

Beaudry, M.A., and others: Survival of a hydropic infant with homozygous α-thalassemia-1, J. Pediatr. 108(5):713-716, 1986.

Bianchi, D.W., and others: Normal long-term survival with α-thalassemia, J. Pediatr. 108(5):716-718, 1986.

Borgna-Pignatti, C., and others: Growth and sexual maturation in thalassemia major, J. Pediatr. 106(1):150-155, 1985.

Centers for Disease Control: Apparent transmission of HTLV-III/LAV from a child to a mother providing health care, Morb. Mort. Weekly Rep. 35(5):76-79, 1986.

Centers for Disease Control: Education and foster care of children infected with human T-lymphotropic virus type III/lymphadenopathy-associated virus, Morb. Mort. Weekly Rep. 34(34):517-521, 1985.

Charache, S.: Advances in the understanding of sickle cell anemia, Hosp. Pract. 21(2):173-190, 1986.

Chessels, J.M.: Blood. In Godfrey, S., and Baum, J.D., editors: Clinical paediatric physiology, London, 1979, Blackwell Scientific Publications.

Church, J.A., Allen, J.R., and Stiehm, E.R.: New scarlet letter(s), pediatric AIDS, Pediatrics 77(3):423-427, 1986.

Cohen, F.: Clinical genetics in nursing practice, Philadelphia, 1984, J.B. Lippincott Co.

Dallman, P.R., and others: Hemoglobin concentration in white, black and Oriental children: is there a need for separate criteria in screening for anemia? Am. J. Clin. Nutr. 31:377, 1978.

Deinard, A.S., and others: Cognitive deficits in iron-deficient and iron-deficient anemic children, J. Pediatr. **108**(1):681-689, 1986.

Emond, A.M., and others: Acute splenic sequestration in homozygous sickle cell disease: natural history and management, J. Pediatr. **107**(2):201-206, 1985.

Festa, R.S.: Modern management of thalassemia, Pediatr. Ann. **14**(9):597-606, 1985.

Gaston, M.H., and others: Prophylaxis with oral penicillin in children with sickle cell anemia, N. Engl. J. Med. **314**(25):1593-1599, 1986.

Goldstein, M.: The aplastic anemias, Hosp. Pract. **15**:85-94, 1980.

Gordon-Smith, E.C.: Treatment of aplastic anemias, Hosp. Pract. **20**(5):69-84, 1985.

Hill, H.R.: Laboratory aspects of immune deficiency in children, Pediatr. Clin. North Am. **27**(4):805-830, 1980.

Iazzetti, L.: Nursing management of the pediatric AIDS patient, Issues Compr. Pediatr. Nurs. **9**(2):119-129, 1986.

Kamani, N.: Marrow transplantation in pediatric hematologic disorders, Pediatr. Ann. **14**(9):661-670, 1985.

Kaplan, J.E., and others: Evidence against transmission of human T-lymphotropic virus/lymphadenopathy-associated virus (HTLV-III/LAV) in families of children with the acquired immunodeficiency syndrome, Pediatr. Infect. Dis. **4**(5):468-471, 1985.

Karayalcin, G.: Current concepts in the management of hemophilia, Pediatr. Ann. **14**(9):640-659, 1985.

Kasprisin, C.A.: Recipient considerations. In Reynolds, A.W., and Steckler, D., editors: Practical aspects of blood administration, Arlington, VA, 1986, American Association of Blood Banks.

Klug, R.: Children with AIDS, Am. J. Nurs. **86**(10):1126-1132, 1986.

Kobrinsky, N.L., and others: Improved hemophilia A carrier detection by 1985.

Lanzkowsky, P.: Problems in diagnosis of iron deficiency anemia, Pediatr. DDAVP stimulation of factor VIII, J. Pediatr. **104**(5):718-724, 1984.

Lanzkowsky, P.: Problems in diagnosis of iron deficiency anemia, Pediatr. Ann. **14**(9):618-636, 1985.

Lukens, J.N.: Iron metabolism and iron deficiency anemia. In Miller, D.R., and others, editors: Blood diseases of infancy and childhood, ed. 5, St. Louis, 1984, The C.V. Mosby Co.

Merhav, H., and others: Tea drinking in infants may cause anemia, Am. J. Clin. Nutr. **41**(6):1210-1213, 1985.

Miller, V., Swaney, S., and Deinard, A.: Impact of the WIC program on the iron status of infants, Pediatrics **75**:100-150, 1985.

Oski, F.A., and Landaw, S.A.: Inhibition of iron absorption from human milk by baby food, Am. J. Dis. Child. **134**:459-460, 1980.

Oski, F.A.: Red cell transfusion and phlebotomy. In Nathan, D.G., and Oski, F.A., editors: Hematology of infancy and childhood, Philadelphia, 1981, W.B. Saunders Co.

Pearson, H.A.: Sickle cell syndromes and other hemoglobinopathies. In Miller, D.R., and others, editors: Blood diseases of infancy and childhood, ed. 5, St. Louis, 1984, The C.V. Mosby Co.

Reeves, J.D., and Yip, R.: Lack of adverse side effects of oral ferrous sulfate therapy in 1-year-old infants, Pediatrics **75**(2):352-355, 1985.

Reindorf, C.A.: Sickle cell anemias: current concepts, Pediatr. Nurs. **6**(2):E-G, 1980.

Rubinstein, A., and others: Periodic intravenous gammaglobulin in children with AIDS or AIDS related complex (ARC), Pediatr. Res. **20**(4):299A, 1986.

Ryan, A.S., and Martinez, G.A.: Iron intake in the United States during the first year of life according to demographic characteristics, Ecology of Food and Nutrition **16**:21-32, 1985.

Saulsbury, F.: IgA rheumatoid factor in Henoch-Schonlein purpura, J. Pediatr. **108**(1):71-76, 1986.

Sergis-Deavenport, E., Miller, R., and Gomperts, E.: Overview of hemophilia, Issues Compr. Pediatr. Nurs. **6**(5-6):317-328, 1983.

Selwyn, P.A.: AIDS: what is now known. II. Epidemiology, Hosp. Pract. **21**(6):127-164, 1986.

Shapiro, R., and others: A metabolic abnormality in platelets from Wiskott-Aldrich syndrome heterozygotes, Lancet **1**:121, 1978.

Speck, W.: Acquired immune deficiency syndrome, J. Pediatr. **103**(1):161-163, 1983.

Vichinsky, E.P., Johnson, R., and Lubin, B.H.: Multidisciplinary approach to pain management in sickle cell disease, Am. J. Pediatr. Hematol./Oncol. **4**(3):328-333, 1982.

Vichinsky, E.P., and Lubin, B.H.: Sickle cell anemia and related hemoglobinopathies, Pediatr. Clin. North Am. **27**(2):429-447, May 1980.

Walter, T., Kovalskys, J., and Stekel, A.: Effect of mild iron deficiency on infant mental development scores, J. Pediatr. **102**(4):519-522, 1983.

Yip, R., Schwartz, S., and Deinard, A.S.: Screening for iron deficiency with the erythrocyte protoporphyrin test, Pediatrics **72**(2):214-219, 1983.

BIBLIOGRAPHY
General

Bank, A., Anderson, W.F., and Zaino, E.C., editors: Fifth Cooley's anemia symposium, vol. 445, New York, 1985, Ann. N.Y. Acad. Sci.

Klopovich, P.M.: An overview of anemia in children, Issues Compr. Pediatr. Nurs. **6**(5-6):277-282, 1983.

McConnell, E.A.: Leukocyte studies: what the counts can tell you, Nursing 86 **16**(3):42-43, 1986.

Miller, D.R.: Anemias: general considerations. In Miller, D.R., and others, editors: Blood diseases of infancy and childhood, ed. 5, St. Louis, 1984, The C.V. Mosby Co.

Patterson, K.L.: The childhood anemias, Pediatrics: Nursing Update **1**(4):2-7, 1985.

Silinsky, J.: Understanding white cell morphology, RN **47**(12):82-84, 1984.

Iron-Deficiency Anemia

Calbreath, D.: Serum iron and iron-building capacity, J. Nurs. Care **12**(9):30, 1979.

Czajka-Narins, D.M.: Iron absorption in the young infant, Pediatr. Basics **32**:11-15, 1982.

Dallman, P.R., Siimes, M.A., and Stekel, A.: Iron deficiency in infancy and childhood, Am. J. Clin. Nutr. **33**:86-118, Jan. 1980.

Deinard, A. and others: Iron deficiency and behavioral deficits, Pediatrics **68**(6):828-833, 1981.

Gever, L.N.: Parenteral iron supplements, Nursing 80 **10**(8):60, 1980.

Oski, F.A.: The nonhematologic manifestations of iron deficiency, Am. J. Dis. Child. **133**(3):315-322, 1979.

Oski, F.A.: Iron deficiency—facts and fallacies, Pediatr. Clin. North Am. **32**(2):493-497, 1985.

Oski, F.A., and Stockman, J.A.: Anemia due to inadequate iron sources or poor iron utilization, Pediatr. Clin. North Am. **27**(2):237-253, 1980.

Reeves, J.D., and others: Iron deficiency in infants: influence of mild antecedent infection, J. Pediatr. **105**(6):874-879, 1984.

Robinson, L.A., Brown, A.L., and Underwood, T.: Iron therapy helps and hazards, Pediatr. Nurs. **4**(6):9-13, 1978.

Stockman, J.A.: Infections and iron, too much of a good thing? Am. J. Dis. Child. **135**(1)18-20, 1981.

Waskerwitz, M.J.: Iron deficiency anemia in children, Issues Compr. Pediatr. Nurs. **6**(5-6):283-294, 1983.

Weeks, H.F.: Iron supplements, Am. J. Maternal Child Nurs. **5**(5):354, 1980.

Sickle Cell Anemia

Anglin, D.L., and others: Effect of penicillin prophylaxis on nasopharyngeal colonization with *Streptococcus pneumoniae* in children with sickle cell anemia, J. Pediatr. **104**(1):18-22, 1984.

Bainbridge, R., and others: Clinical presentation of homozygous sickle cell disease, J. Pediatr. **106**(6):881-890, 1985.

Conyard, S., Krishnamurthy, M., and Dosik, H.: Psychosocial aspects of sickle-cell anemia in adolescents, Health Soc. Work **5**(1):20-26, Feb. 1980.

Flanagan, C.: Home management of sickle cell anemia, Pediatr. Nurs. **6**(2):B-D, 1980.

Gradolf, B.: Sickle cell anemia in children, Issues Compr. Pediatr. Nurs. **6**(5-6):295-306, 1983.

Greene, P.: Teaching aid for children with sickle cell disease, Am. J. Nurs. **77**(12):1953, 1977.

Hathaway, G.: The child with sickle cell anemia: implications and management, Nurse Pract. **9**(10):16-22, 1984.

Johnson, F.L., and others: Bone marrow transplantation in patients with sickle cell anemia, N. Engl. J. Med. **311**:780-783, 1984.

Lamb, C., editor: Managing sickle cell emergencies, Patient Care **19**(1):92-141, 1985.

Pearson, H.A., and others: Developmental pattern of splenic dysfunction in sickle cell disorders, Pediatrics **76**(3):392-397, 1985.

Phebus, C.K., Glonger, M.F., and Maciak, B.J.: Growth patterns by age and sex in children with sickle cell disease, J. Pediatr. **105**(1):28-33, 1984.

Richardson, E.A.W., and Milne, L.S.: Sickle-cell disease and the child-bearing family: an update, Am. J. Maternal Child Nurs. **8**:417-422, 1983.

Smith, J.A.: Management of sickle cell disease: progress during the past 10 years, Am. J. Pediatr. Hematol./Oncol. **5**(4):360-366, 1983.

Weintrub, P.S., and others: Long-term follow-up and booster immunization with polyvalent pneumococcal polysaccharide in patients with sickle cell anemia, J. Pediatr. **105**(2):261-263, 1984.

Thalassemia

Giordano, V.: Psychosocial impacts on a thalassemic patient's life. In Bank, A., Anderson, W.F., and Zaino, E.C., editors: Fifth Cooley's anemia symposium, vol. 445, New York, 1985, Ann. N.Y. Acad. Sci.

Modell, B., and others: Effect of fetal diagnostic testing on birth rate of thalassemia major in Britain, Lancet **2**:1383-1386, 1984.

Ohene-Frempong, K., and Schwartz, E.: Clinical features of thalassemia, Pediatr. Clin. North Am. **27**:403-420, 1980.

Pearson, H.W., and others: Low risk of hepatitis B from blood transfusions in thalassemic patients in Connecticut, J. Pediatr. **108**(2):252-253, 1986.

Piomelli, S., and others: Current strategies in the management of Cooley's anemia. In Bank, A., Anderson, W.F., and Zaino, E.C., editors: Fifth Cooley's anemia symposium, vol. 445, New York, 1985, Ann. N.Y. Acad. Sci.

Sherman, M., and others: Thalassemic children's understanding of illness: a study of cognitive and emotional factors. In Bank, A., Anderson, W.F., and Zaino, E.C., editors: Fifth Cooley's anemia symposium, vol. 445, New York, 1985, Ann. N.Y. Acad. Sci.

Smith, L.G.: Reactions to blood transfusions, Am. J. Nurs. **84**:1096-1101, 1984.

Wolfe, L., Sallan, D., and Nathan, D.G.: Current therapy and new approaches to the treatment of thalassemia major. In Bank, A., Anderson, W.F., and Zaino, E.C., editors: Fifth Cooley's anemia symposium, vol. 445, New York, 1985, Ann. N.Y. Acad. Sci.

Aplastic Anemia

Alter, B.P.: Bone-marrow failure in children, Pediatr. Ann. **8**(7):53-70, 1979.

Griner, P.F.: A survey of the effectiveness of cyclophosphamide in patients with severe aplastic anemia, Am. J. Hematol. **8**:55-60, 1980.

Hunter, R.F., Roth, P.A., and Huang, A.T.: Predictive factors for response to anti-thymocyte globulin in acquired aplastic anemia, Am. J. Med. **79**(1):73-78, 1985.

Heimpel, H., and Heit, W.: Drug-induced aplastic anaemia: clinical aspects, Clin. Haematol. **9**(3):641-662, 1980.

Sanders, J.E., and others: Bone marrow transplantation experience for children with aplastic anemia, Pediatrics **77**(2):179-186, 1986.

Weinblatt, M.E., Higgins, G., and Ortega, J.A.: Aplastic anemia in Down's syndrome, Pediatrics **67**(6):896-897, 1981.

Defects in Hemostasis

Buchanan, G.R., and others: Hepatitis in household contacts of patients with hemophilia who have received multiple transfusions, J. Pediatr. **108**(6):937-939, 1986.

Buchanan, G.R.: Hemophilia, Pediatr. Clin. North Am. **27**(2):309-326, 1980.

Buchanan, G.R., and Moore, G.C.: Disseminated intravascular coagulation. In Levin, D.L., Morriss, F.C., and Moore, G.C., editors: A practical guide to pediatric intensive care, ed. 2, St. Louis, 1984, The C.V. Mosby Co.

Bussel, J.B., and others: Treatment of acute idiopathic thrombocytopenia of childhood with intravenous infusions of gammaglobulin, J. Pediatr. **106**(6):886-890, 1985.

Byrnes, J.J.: Thrombotic thrombocytopenic purpura, Adv. Intern. Med. **26**:131-157, 1980.

Dressler, D.: Understanding and treating hemophilia, Nursing 80 **10**(8):72-73, 1980.

Dubansky, A.S., and Oski, F.A.: Controversies in the management of acute idiopathic thrombocytopenic purpura: a survey of specialists, Pediatrics **77**(1):49-52, 1986.

Gaddy-Cohen, D.: Idiopathic thrombocytopenic purpura in children, Issues Compr. Pediatr. Nurs. **6**(5-6):307-316, 1983.

Gill, J.C., and others: HTLV-III serology in hemophilia: relationship with immunologic abnormalities, J. Pediatr. **108**(4):511-516, 1986.

Karpatkin, M.: Screening tests in hemostasis, Pediatr. Clin. North Am. **27**(4):831-841, 1980.

Kasprisin, D.O., and Kasprisin, C.A.: Introduction to transfusion therapy: a programmed text, New York, 1980, Medical Examination Publishing Co., Inc.

Klosky, L.: Nose picking in children, Pediatr. Nurs. **4**(6):47-48, 1978.

Koch, P.M.: Thrombocytopenia: don't let it make a big problem out of nothing, Nursing 84 **14**(10):55-57, 1984.

Lightsey, A.L., Jr.: Thrombocytopenia in children, Pediatr. Clin. North Am. **27**:293-308, 1980.

McConnell, E.A.: APTT and PT: the tests of time, Nursing 86 **16**(5):47, 1986.

O'Brian, B.S., and Woods, S.: The paradox of DIC, Am. J. Nurs. **78**:1878-1880, 1978.

Persky, M.S.: Stanching a nasal bleed, Emerg. Med. **14**(1):108-115, 1982.

Sergis-Deavenport, E., and Varni, J.W.: Behavioral techniques in teaching hemophilia factor replacement procedures to families, Pediatr. Nurs. **8**(6):416-419, 1982.

Shende, A.: Idiopathic thrombocytopenic purpura in children, Pediatr. Ann. **14**(9):609-616, 1985.

Stuart, M.J., and others: Bleeding time in hemophilia A: potential mechanisms for prolongation, J. Pediatr. **108**(2):215-218, 1986.

Walker, R.W., and Walker, W.: Idiopathic thrombocytopenia: initial illness and long-term follow-up, Arch. Dis. Child. **59**:316-322, 1984.

Immunologic-Deficiency Disorders

Boland, M., and Gaskill, T.B.: Managing AIDS in children, Am. J. Maternal Child Nurs. **9**(6):384-389, 1984.

Brainerd, E.: Nursing management of chronic infectious diseases in children, Pediatrics: Nursing Update **1**(17):2-7, 1986.

Conley, M.E., Park, C.L., and Douglas, S.D.: Childhood common variable immunodeficiency with autoimmune disease, J. Pediatr. **108**(6):915-922, 1986.

Durandy, A., and others: Prenatal diagnosis of severe combined immunodeficiency, J. Pediatr. **101**(6):995-997, 1982.

Fidler, R.: Deciphering diagnostic studies: complement assays, Nursing 83 **13**(6):17-19, 1983.

Groenwald, S.L.: Physiology of the immune system, Heart Lung **9**(4):645-650, 1980.

Henley, W.L.: Mechanisms of autoimmunity, Pediatr. Ann. **11**(3):293-300, 1982.

Jemison-Smith, P., and Hamm, P.: Immune responses, Crit. Care Update **10**(8):45-46, 1983.

Lind, M.: The immunologic assessment: a nursing focus, Heart Lung **9**(4):658-661, 1980.

Lum, L.G.: Splenectomy in the management of the thrombocytopenia of the Wiskott-Aldrich syndrome, N. Engl. J. Med. **30**(16):892-896, 1980.

Meuwissen, H.J., and others: Long-term survival after bone marrow transplantation: a 15-year follow-up report of a patient with Wiskott-Aldrich syndrome, J. Pediatr. **105**(3):365-369, 1984.

Puri, S., and Chandra, R.K.: Nutritional regulation of host resistance and predictive value of immunologic tests in assessment of outcome, Pediatr. Clin. North Am. **32**(2):499-516, 1985.

Stiehm, E.R.: Clinical and laboratory evaluation of the child with suspected immunodeficiency, Pediatr. Rev. **7**(2):53-61, 1985.

Taylor, D.L.: Immune response: physiology, signs, and symptoms, Nursing 84 **14**(5):52-54, 1984.

AIDS

Ammann, A.J., and Shannon, K.: Recognition of acquired immune deficiency syndrome (AIDS) in children, Pediatr. Rev. **7**(4):101-107, 1985.

Bennett, J.A.: AIDS epidemiology update, Am. J. Nurs. **85**(9):968-972, 1985.

Bennett, J.A.: HTLV-III AIDS link, Am. J. Nurs. **85**(10):1086-1089, 1985.

Black, J.L.: AIDS: preschool and school issues, J. Sch. Health **56**(3):93-95, 1986.

Centers for Disease Control: Recommendations for assisting in the prevention of perinatal transmission of human T-lymphotropic virus type III/lymphadenopathy-associated virus and acquired immunodeficiency syndrome, Morb. Mort. Weekly Rep. **34**(48):721-732, 1985.

Centers for Disease Control: Summary: recommendations for preventing transmission of infection with human T-lymphotropic virus type III/lymphadenopathy-associated virus in the workplace, Morb. Mort. Weekly Rep. **34**(45):681-695, 1985.

Centers for Disease Control: Update: acquired immunodeficiency syndrome (AIDS) among patients with hemophilia—United States, Morb. Mort. Weekly Rep. **32**(47):613-615, 1983.

Church, J.A., and Isaacs, H.: Transfusion-associated acquired immune deficiency syndrome in infants, J. Pediatr. **105**(5):731-737, 1984.

Marion, R., and others: Human T-cell lymphotropic virus type III (HTLV-III) embryopathy, Am. J. Dis. Child. **140**(7):638-640, 1986.

Selwyn, P.A.: AIDS: What is now known, I. History and immunovirology, Hosp. Pract. **21**(5):67-82, 1986.

Shannon, K.M., and Ammann, A.J.: Acquired immune deficiency syndrome in childhood, J. Pediatr. **106**(2):332-342, 1985.

Shannon, K., and others: Transfusion-associated cytomegalovirus infection and acquired immune deficiency syndrome in an infant, J. Pediatr. **103**(6):859-863, 1983.

Sullivan, J.L., and others: Hemophiliac immunodeficiency: influence of exposure to factor VIII concentrate, LAV/HTLV-III, and herpes viruses, J. Pediatr. **108**(4):504-510, 1986.

Thompson, S.W., and Gietz, K.R.: Acquired immune deficiency syndrome in infants and children, Pediatr. Nurs. **11**(4):278-280, 1985.

Unit Thirteen

The Child with a Disturbance of Regulatory Mechanisms

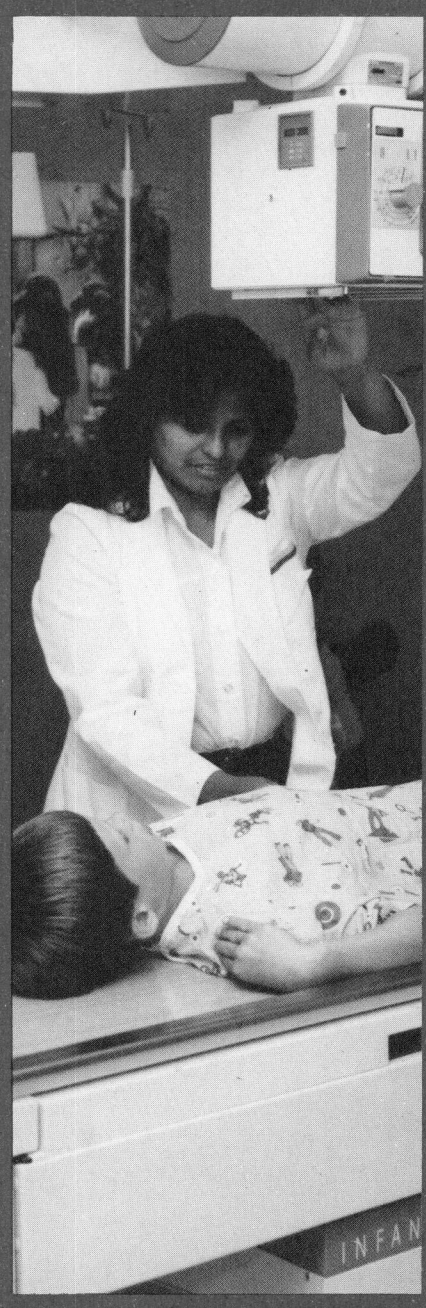

In an organism such as a human being, the maintenance of dynamic equilibrium involves a complex interaction of many systems and subsystems. All the activities within the individual cells, tissues, and organs that comprise these systems depend on the function of other systems, and, like all systems, each component has one or more factors that act on it or affect it. A change in one component can affect all other components.

Regulation enables the organism to maintain the function of cells, tissues, organs, and systems within the parameters described as normal for that system despite changes in the internal or external environment. Communication between the various systems and subsystems is carried by chemical or neural mechanisms. Disturbances in the regulatory processes can create disturbances in one or more of the interrelated components of the system with consequences that affect other systems and the organism as a whole.

The major regulatory mechanisms of the body are the endocrine and neural systems. Dysfunction in the central nervous system is discussed in Chapter 37, *The Child with a Disturbance of Cerebral Function*. Defects in the integrity of the peripheral nervous system are elaborated in Unit Fourteen. It is sometimes difficult to determine if dysfunctions in this interrelated system are caused by impaired function in the target glands that secrete the hormones, the pituitary tropic substances that stimulate the target glands to secrete hormones, or the portions of the midbrain that produce releasing factors that stimulate the pituitary gland. Defects within the complex neuroendocrine regulatory system and the pancreatic hormones are discussed in Chapter 38, *The Child with an Endocrine Dysfunction*. Genetic and other chemical regulatory mechanisms, for example, acid-base equilibrium and oxygen–carbon dioxide disturbances, are discussed in previous segments.

Chapter 36, *The Child with Cancer*, is concerned with disordered cell proliferation. Although the mechanism is unknown, it is believed that altered cell regulation is caused by a genetic abnormality, which is in some way provoked by environmental or other influences into initiating uncontrolled abnormal cell proliferation—the malignant process. It is speculated that some regulatory mechanism is affected, probably the immune response.

Chapter 36

The Child with Cancer

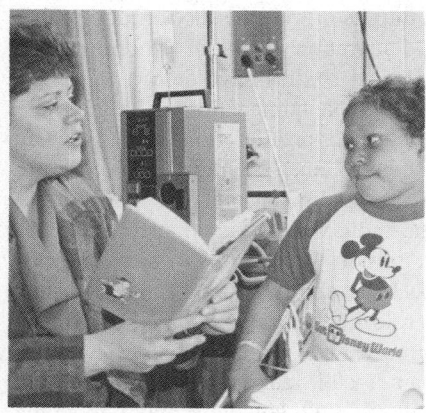

There are few situations in nursing that exceed the challenges of caring for a child with the diagnosis of cancer. Despite the dramatic improvements in survival rates for these children, the needs of the family are tremendous as they cope with a serious physical illness as well as the fear that the child will not be cured. This chapter is concerned primarily with the physical problems associated with several types of childhood cancer. The general psychologic needs of these children and their families are discussed in Chapter 22 in terms of chronic illness and in Chapter 23 for situations when the outcome becomes life-threatening and death is a possibility. Except for specific emotional concerns of the family that are unique to the type of cancer, the interventions thoroughly explored in these earlier chapters are not repeated here. Nurses are encouraged to apply the psychologic principles of care whenever they are involved with these children and their families. The child's future, not just his cancer, must be viewed as the priority. If a cured child is a possible outcome, then a *truly cured child* is an essential outcome—that is, a child who is not just free of disease but who is developmentally commensurate with his age and well adjusted to the experience of having cancer (van Eys, 1977).

The purpose of discussing types of childhood cancer in one chapter is to present a comprehensive model of the nursing care that applies to these diseases. For example, most of the emphasis focuses on the discussion of leukemia, because it is the most frequent form of cancer and because it serves as a prototype for problems and needs encountered in other cancers. In addition, since many of the diagnostic procedures and medical therapies differ little from one type of malignancy to another, discussing them together allows for a detailed exploration without undue repetition.

Cancer in Children

Cancer is the leading cause of death from disease in children ages 3 to 15 years and the second cause of death from all causes, exceeded only by injuries. The incidence of cancer in this age-group is approximately 12.1 per 100,000 white children and 9.3 per 100,000 black children (Pratt, 1985). If the present rates continue, the projected number of new cases will be about 6555, with about 2175 deaths in 1986 (Cancer facts, 1986).

During childhood there are changing incidences for various types of cancer. For children in all pediatric age-groups, leukemia is the most frequent type of cancer, followed by brain tumors and lymphomas (Table 36-1). However, there are some important differences between the two groups. Tumors of the kidney and soft tissue are more common in blacks, whereas tumors of the bone are more common in whites. Males are affected more often by cancer than females (ratio of 1.2:1), although this varies with the type of cancer. The most frequent forms of cancer occur in more males, but tumors of the skin and gonads are found in more females (Pratt, 1985).

Probably the most significant aspect of childhood cancer is the improved prognosis during the last three decades. Mortality among children with cancer has declined from 8.3 per 100,000 in 1950 to 4.1 per 100,000 in 1983 (Cancer facts, 1986). Currently, more than 50% of all children with malignant neoplasms treated at major cancer centers will become long-term survivors. The cancers demonstrating the greatest improvements in survival rates are acute leukemia, lymphomas, Wilms tumor, rhabodomyosarcoma, and osteosarcoma (Sutow, 1984). However, black children with cancer do more poorly than white children.

Although survival is discussed in terms of "cure," the term *biologic cure* is not absolute, as it is not possible to definitively demonstrate complete eradication of all cancer cells and late recurrences of the disease do occur. The definition of cure includes the criteria of (1) cessation of therapy, (2) continuous freedom from clinical and laboratory evidence of cancer, and (3) minimal or no risk of relapse as determined by previous experience with the disease (Pinkel, 1979). The time that must elapse before a child clinically free of cancer is considered cured varies with each type of cancer but typically ranges from 2 to 5 years.

ETIOLOGIC FACTORS

The cause of cancer is not known. While there are numerous hypotheses concerning its origin, the most enduring theory is that some genetic alteration results in the unregulated proliferation of cells. Recent studies have demonstrated the existence of genes activated in human tumors that are capable of causing uncontrolled proliferation of cells when transmitted to normal cells. Genes having the potential to transform normal cells into malignant ones are called *oncogenes*. What causes the induction of cell transformation is speculative, but RNA tumor viruses (also called retroviruses, because they have the ability to translate RNA back to DNA) may play a role in the transfer of DNA from a malignant cell to a normal cell (Krontiris, 1983). The identification of the human T-cell leukemia-lymphoma virus (HTLV) in some forms of adult leukemia and lymphoma and the Epstein-Barr (EB) virus, a type of herpes virus, in Burkitt lymphoma has lent support to this theory (Gallo, 1983). While these viruses have been isolated, there is no firm evidence that childhood cancer is communicable.

Despite the lack of knowledge about the origin of cancer, there is considerable information on risk factors that increase the likelihood of children developing specific types of cancer. The following is a brief overview of some of the etiologic factors implicated in childhood cancer.

Several environmental agents that are carcinogenic (capable of producing cancer) in adults have been described, but only one of these—ionizing radiation—has been implicated in children. Low doses of radiation have been known to cause thyroid cancer and leukemia. There is some evidence that exposing pregnant women to diagnostic radiographic procedures increases the occurrence of leukemia and other forms of cancer among their children (Harvey and others, 1985).

Although drugs, particularly those containing radioisotopes and immunosuppressive agents, can increase the risk of developing childhood cancer, the one drug most notably recognized for its carcinogenic effect is diethylstilbestrol. Large doses of this hormone given to pregnant women to prevent abortion cause adenocarcinoma of the vagina in a significant proportion of the female offspring when they reach adolescence and early adulthood.

Some childhood cancers, in particular retinoblastoma, Wilms tumor, and neuroblastoma, may demonstrate patterns of inheritance that suggest a genetic basis for the disorder. In addition, children with certain types of chromosomal ab-

Table 36-1 Cancer incidence by site for children under 15, SEER Program, 1973-1982

SITE	PERCENT OF TOTAL	RATE PER 1,000,000 CHILDREN
Leukemia	30.1	37.8
Central Nervous System	19.1	24.1
Lymphomas	12.3	15.5
Sympathetic Nervous System	8.1	10.4
Kidney	6.5	8.2
Soft Tissue	6.3	7.9
Bone	4.8	6.1
Retinoblastoma	2.7	3.4
Liver	1.1	1.4
All Others	9.0	11.5
All Sites	100.0	126.3

From the Surveillance Epidemiology and End Results (SEER) study, National Cancer Institute. In Silverberg, E.: Cancer statistics, 1986, CA **36**(1):32-42, 1986.

normalities, especially those syndromes caused by abnormal numbers of chromosomes, have an increased incidence of cancer. For example, in children with Down syndrome the probability of developing leukemia is about 14 times greater than the normal rate for whites (Robison and others, 1984). Other chromosome syndromes associated with a predisposition to cancer are Fanconi syndrome (a deficiency of all cellular elements of the blood), Bloom syndrome (dwarfism and skin changes), ataxia-telangiectasia (progressive cerebellar ataxia and oculocutaneous vascular lesions), and Klinefelter syndrome. In addition, some of the cancers have been associated with nonrandom chromosome changes, such as translocation of chromosomes 4 and 11 and a specific chromosome marker called the Philadelphia (Ph[1]) chromosome in different types of leukemia (Cohen, 1984; Esseltine and others, 1982).

Children with immune deficiencies, such as Wiskott-Aldrich syndrome or acquired immune deficiency syndrome, or children whose immune system has been suppressed, such as following transplant procedures, are at a greater risk for developing various cancers. Of major concern is the increased risk of secondary cancers in some children successfully treated for their primary malignancy.

A familial tendency of clustering of cancer also occurs. For example, there are some families who have a higher than expected incidence of cancer, although no environmental or host factor can explain the event. When cancer has occurred in one child, the risk of cancer in the remaining siblings is three times the expected risk for the general population, but the actual risk is considered low because of the rarity of childhood cancer (Pratt, 1985). However, in leukemias the risk among monozygous twins is extremely high—nearly 100% if the disease is diagnosed in the twin before 1 year of age, about 15% between years 1 to 4, and then four times the average risk after 4 years (Strong, 1984). Clustering of cases of cancer within a geographic location that exceeds the incidence expected by chance also occurs, but it is thought that these are unusual, random events. Unfortunately, such situations can cause considerable concern and even panic in the community.

Prevention

Knowledge of the risk factors that increase the likelihood of cancer holds the promise of prevention. Unfortunately, in children the known carcinogens are limited to radiation and a few drugs given to the mother during pregnancy. Therefore at present there is really no known prevention.

Health professionals do have two roles, however. One is aimed at preventing adult-type cancers by educating parents and children about the hazards of known carcinogens, particularly the effects of cigarette smoking and excessive exposure to sunlight. Lung cancer is the leading cause of death from cancer in adults, and malignant melanoma is the leading cause of death from diseases of the skin. Children at higher risk for skin cancer are those with light-colored eyes, complexion, and hair, those who sunburn easily, and those who live near the equator (Friedman, Rigel, and Kopf,

Table 36-2 Cardinal symptoms of cancer in children

Symptom	Probable malignancy
Fever	Leukemia, lymphoma, neuroblastoma, Wilms tumor
Pain	Leukemia, bone tumors, brain tumors (headache)
Mass	Wilms tumor, neuroblastoma, lymphoma
Purpura	Leukemia, neuroblastoma
Changes in balance, gait, or personality	Brain tumors
Changes in eye	Retinoblastoma

Adapted from Fernbach, D.: The role of the family physician in the care of the child with cancer, CA **35**(5):258-270, 1985.

1985). Not only these children but all children should be protected from overexposure to the sun (see also p. 776). In addition, to prevent other types of cancer males should be taught testicular self-examination; female adolescents should be taught breast self-examination and encouraged to seek periodic health examinations, including a Papanicolaou (Pap) smear.*

Second, health professionals need to be aware of the cardinal symptoms of childhood cancer (Table 36-2). Unfortunately, fever and pain are manifestations of common childhood disorders, and without a high index of suspicion, they may be attributed to minor ailments. The other signs are subtle and easily missed. If parents suspect an abnormality, their concerns must be taken seriously. The greatest weapons against all forms of cancer are early detection and treatment.

PROPERTIES OF MALIGNANT CELLS

Malignant or cancer cells are cells that have the specific properties of anaplasia, invasion, and metastasis. An appreciation of the unique properties of these abnormal cells facilitates an understanding of the pathologic changes that occur in cancer:

Growth rate—usually very rapid, in contrast to other cells of the body (except bone marrow, gastrointestinal mucosa, and hair follicles, which divide slowly)

Anaplasia—loss of orderly differentiation and organization of cells to perform a specific function

Competition—rapidly proliferating, nonfunctional cells compete with normal cells for essential nutrients, until eventually the normal cells die and are replaced by cancer cells

Expansion—abnormal, unrestricted growth of cancer cells produces organ damage by compressing adjacent tissues, until the tissues' normal functions are altered

*Information on self-instructional materials on testicular and breast self-examination is available from the local chapters of the American Cancer Society, Inc., or the national office, 90 Park Ave., New York, NY 10016.

Invasion—malignant cells invade adjacent tissues and eventually the normal cells may be replaced by cancer cells that are incapable of performing the original cells' functions

Metastasis—the ability to spread to distant sites within the body and establish secondary colonies of malignant growth; may occur by natural seeding via the bloodstream or lymph system or iatrogenically, such as during surgery or needle biopsy, when cancer cells are dislodged and implant elsewhere in the body

Neoplasms are any new and abnormal growth and may be benign or malignant. Benign neoplasms do not demonstrate the degree of anaplasia or metastasis that malignant neoplasms do, but they may still be serious, especially when they occur in confined spaces, such as the brain. Malignant neoplasms can arise from any tissue of the body and are classified according to tissue and cell type. The major classifications are:

Embryonal tumor, arising from embryonic tissue, such as the blastomas

Lymphomas of the lymphatic system

Leukemias of the blood-forming organs

Sarcoma, derived from connective and supporting tissue, such as bone, cartilage, nerve, and fat

Carcinoma, derived from epithelial tissue such as skin and lining of the body cavities

Adenocarcinoma, a carcinoma of glandular tissue, such as the breast or prostate

Childhood cancers occur most frequently in rapidly growing tissue, especially the bone marrow. Carcinoma and adenocarcinoma are primarily adult types of cancer and may result from prolonged contact with various carcinogens, such as excessive sunlight on the skin or tobacco products in the lungs.

Metastasis of cancer cells seems to occur more readily in children than adults. For example, the dissemination of cancer cells during surgery, nonsurgical manipulation, or biopsy occurs more frequently in children than is generally expected. However, spontaneous regression of even widely metastasized malignancy occasionally occurs in children. Although the reason is not known, one theory suggests that embryonal tumors undergo maturation to become benign masses.

ASSESSMENT OF MALIGNANCY AND METASTASIS

When a child is suspected of having cancer, extensive diagnostic procedures are carried out to locate the primary (original) site and any evidence of metastasis. In addition to the initial work-up, diagnostic tests are repeated regularly to assess the effectiveness of treatment. Consequently, the child is subjected to numerous noninvasive and invasive procedures, many of which cause considerable pain and anxiety. The following is an overview of the more typical diagnostic procedures employed to assess a malignancy and metastasis and the nursing interventions needed to support the child and family. Specific tests and nursing considerations that are unique to a particular type of cancer are discussed later in the chapter.

History and Physical Examination

The history and physical examination often yield the first clues to the presence of cancer. Vague complaints, such as fatigue, pain in a limb, night sweating, lack of appetite, headache, and general malaise, may be the earliest clues and need to be taken seriously. Most children have a great deal of energy and if sick with a cold or other childhood affliction recover quickly and completely. Any evidence of a lingering disorder is often the first sign of leukemia. Parents are often the first persons to detect physical signs, such as enlarged lymph nodes (lymphoma), a strange glint in the eye (retinoblastoma), or an abdominal mass (Wilms tumor). Any such complaints must be thoroughly followed with a complete examination.

Laboratory Tests

Any number of laboratory tests may be performed, but most commonly a complete blood count and chemistry and urinalysis will be done. Malignancies of the blood-forming organs manifest signs early, and these frequently cause decreased elements of the blood, increased production of immature cells, and/or overproduction of some cells, such as leukocytosis. Since many of the chemotherapeutic agents depress bone marrow function, repeated blood counts are a constant feature of follow-up care.

Blood chemistry yields important information concerning renal and liver function and electrolyte balance. Evaluation of renal and liver function is important not only for detection of cancer or metastasis to these organs, but also for monitoring during treatment because of the extra burden placed on these systems to metabolize and excrete the chemotherapeutic drugs. Consequently, regular blood chemistries and urinalysis are standard procedures through the course of the disease.

A lumbar puncture is a routine test employed in leukemia, brain tumors, and other cancers that may metastasize to the spinal cord and brain. Lumbar punctures are also performed to administer intrathecal drugs, such as methotrexate, when this mode of administration is part of the treatment protocol.

Imaging Techniques

Advances in imaging procedures have greatly aided in the diagnosis of solid tumors and have minimized the need for invasive techniques. Depending on the suspected site of the malignancy, initial preliminary radiologic studies include conventional films of the chest, abdomen, bone, and skull and more specialized tests such as the intravenous pyelogram for kidney involvement. However, these radiographs are generally followed by much more sophisticated imaging procedures, including computerized axial tomography (CAT), ultrasound, nuclear scan, and magnetic resonance imaging (MRI) (see Table 37-4).

Biopsy

As part of the diagnostic evaluation, biopsies are essential to determine the classification and stage of the disease. *Classification* refers to the biologic characteristics of the tumor in relation to the tumor (T) itself, the involvement of regional lymph nodes (N), and the presence of metastasis (M). *Staging* refers to the extent of the disease at the time of diagnosis in regard to TNM (McCalla, 1982). While the classification of the tumor may not change, the stage frequently does and is usually directly related to prognosis (the higher the stage, the poorer the prognosis).

Biopsies may be performed during surgical removal of the tumor, or in the case of lymphomas, surgery may be performed specifically to obtain tissue samples of the spleen and involved lymph nodes. Easily accessed nodes, such as those in the cervical or axillary region, may be removed for biopsy. Whenever there is concern for metastasis to the hematologic system or when the primary site is the blood-forming organs, bone marrow studies are performed.

Access to the bone marrow may be accomplished by the following techniques: (1) *aspiration,* which consists of aspirating marrow through a large- or fine-bore needle; (2) *biopsy,* which consists of aspirating a piece of bone through a special type of needle; and (3) *open,* which is a surgical biopsy of a section of bone. Aspiration is the method of choice, unless the cells are so tightly packed that suction is inadequate to remove a sample. In that case a biopsy is performed.

Nursing Considerations

The diagnostic procedures initially employed to confirm the diagnosis and those that are repeated to monitor treatment are often a source of discomfort and stress to the child and family. Even noninvasive procedures such as radiologic tests are frightening to a young child. Many of these tests require the child to lie absolutely motionless for a prolonged period of time in a confined space with little or no communication with a supportive adult. Consequently, infants and young children are usually sedated, and older children need an explanation of what to expect and reminders during the test of how much longer they must remain still. The same principles for preparing children for procedures that are discussed in Chapter 27 apply here, including the option of having parents stay with the child whenever possible (see Questions and controversies, p. 1107). It is a mistake to assume that children who undergo repeated tests do not need additional preparation or emotional support. Children are more likely to become conditioned to the discomfort and to experience *increasing,* not decreasing, levels of stress (Katz, Kellerman, and Siegel, 1980).

Two procedures, bone marrow studies and lumbar punctures, are so commonly employed in many types of childhood cancer that they deserve special consideration in preparing children. Both tests can be frightening to children, because they are done behind the child's field of vision (unless the sternum or anterior iliac crest is used for the bone marrow test). In some institutions sedation is administered before the test, but since it is often in the form of an injection, it can add to the trauma of the experience. Typically (but not always) the puncture site is anesthetized with a local anesthetic, which may be given by subcutaneous injection or with a pressurized air gun. In a lumbar puncture, when a local anesthetic is given, this is the only discomfort the child feels. However, in a bone marrow test, the insertion of the needle into the bone as it passes through the periosteum and the withdrawal of the marrow also cause pain. In addition, pressure must be exerted to facilitate entry through the bone, which is upsetting to some children.

Although it is an infrequent practice, some institutions are recognizing the extreme stress associated with these invasive procedures and are offering children the option of having general anesthesia on an outpatient basis. Parents are allowed to stay with the child from induction of anesthesia through recovery. Preliminary results indicate that the majority (80%) of children choose to have the procedure performed under general anesthesia and that the technique is safe (Perin and Frase, 1985).

For both procedures, children of preschool age and beyond should be prepared beforehand. If this is not possible, the nurse should explain each step of the procedure as it occurs, stressing what will be done and what it will feel like. If each step is explained beforehand, having the child recall the next step during the procedure can be a distraction mechanism.

Physical care after the procedures is minimal. A small pressure bandage is applied to the bone marrow puncture site, and an adhesive bandage is applied to the lumbar puncture site. No activity restriction is necessary after the bone marrow test, although the site is usually sore and the child may prefer to remain quiet. Recommendations after the lumbar puncture vary, but usually the child is advised to remain flat for 30 minutes or more to minimize the development of a headache. If medication was instilled, the child may be placed in a slight Trendelenburg position to facilitate circulation of the medicated spinal fluid.

MODES OF THERAPY

Several advances in the understanding of cancer and improvements in technical procedures have greatly influenced present modes of therapy, including (1) surgery, (2) chemotherapy, (3) radiotherapy, (4) immunotherapy, and (5) bone marrow transplantation. While there have been significant developments in new modes of treatment, one of the major reasons for more effective treatment regimens has been the use of clinical trials and protocols. Because of the relatively small number of children with cancer, The National Cancer Institute (NCI) set up cooperative groups of pediatric oncologists from different regions of the United States to systematically pool their information regarding treatment and other aspects of cancer care. Based on the evaluation of success from different types of treatment, these experts plan and initiate *comparative clinical trials.* Although clinical trials may involve any aspect of cancer care (prevention, treatment, or long-term effects), they are frequently concerned with evaluating investigational drugs. For example, one group of patients (control group) typically receives the best possible treatment presently known. The experimental group(s) receives the same treatment plus another form of treatment that is believed to be even better. The formalized outline of the clinical study, which among other details includes the treatment plan (administration and evaluation), is called a *protocol* (Pochedly, 1978).

Over the past 30 years the use of clinical trials and protocols has been responsible for major changes in the approaches to cancer treatment. Some of the recent strategies include reduction of toxicity with prolonged and continuous rather than intermittent intravenous infusion; shortening of duration of maintenance therapy; and the use of intensive combination therapy (the administration of as many effective agents as possible in the highest doses possible during the initiation of therapy) (Bleyer, 1985). The following is an overview of the major modes of therapy. In addition, specific aspects of therapy are discussed later in the chapter when applicable to the individual type of cancer.

Surgery

The main goal of surgery, besides its use to obtain biopsies, is to remove all traces of tumor and restore normal body functioning. Surgery is most successful when the tumor is encapsulated and localized (confined to the site of origin). It may only be palliative when the cancer is regional (metastasized to an area adjacent to the original site) or advanced (widespread throughout the body). Obviously, the best prognosis is directly related to early detection of the tumor.

The recent trend is toward more conservative surgical excision. For example, in some types of bone cancer, such as osteosarcoma, patients are successfully treated with resection of the diseased portion of the bone rather than amputation. There is an increasing emphasis on the use of combination drug therapy and radiotherapy after limited surgical intervention.

Chemotherapy

Chemotherapy, the use of drugs with antineoplastic capabilities, may be the primary form of treatment, or it may be used as an adjunct to surgery and/or radiotherapy. Although several agents have been found effective in treating different forms of cancer, the remarkable survival rates have been the result of improved combination-drug regimens. Combining drugs allows for optimum cell-cycle destruction with minimum toxic effects and decreased resistance by the cancer cells to the agent. For example, the combination MOPP (mechlorethamine [Mustargen], vincristine [Oncovin], procarbazine, and prednisone) combines complementary cytotoxic effects with nonsimilar side effects. Mechlorethamine and procarbazine are myelosuppressive, vincristine is neurotoxic, and prednisone produces mild bone marrow depression with beneficial effects of improved appetite and a feeling of well-being.

In addition to more effective combinations of drugs, several advances in the administration of chemotherapy have permitted continuous or intermittent intravenous administration without multiple venipunctures. The use of venous access lines, especially indwelling atrial catheters (Hickman/Broviac catheters) and implantable infusion ports, has greatly facilitated safe and effective drug administration with a minimum of discomfort to the child (see p. 1180). Subcutaneous continuous infusions using syringe pumps have made possible the administration of certain drugs, such as cytosine arabinoside, in higher doses with less toxicity than when the drug is administered intermittently (Holmes, 1985).

Another advance in intrathecal administration is the *Ommaya reservoir,* which eliminates the need for repeated lumbar punctures. In this procedure a silicone rubber tube is surgically inserted into one of the ventricles and connected to a reservoir placed beneath the scalp. To instill medication, the area of scalp covering the reservoir is cleansed with an antiseptic and a small needle is inserted through the skin into the reservoir. The drug is then injected into the reservoir and, by gentle compression of the skin over this site, is pumped into the ventricles. If no complications develop, such as a misplaced reservoir or infection that does not respond to treatment, the device can function for months and in some instances for years (Rahr, 1986). In addition to facilitating the administration of chemotherapy, venous access devices and the Ommaya reservoir can be used to obtain blood or cerebrospinal fluid, respectively, and to administer other drugs, such as antibiotics and analgesics.

Chemotherapeutic agents are classified according to their cytotoxic action. The agents are discussed in the following paragraphs, and the principal drugs used in treatment of childhood cancer are summarized in Table 36-3. An understanding of drugs' actions and side effects is essential to nursing care of children with cancer. Unfortunately, the drugs are not selectively cytotoxic for malignant cells, and other cells with a high rate of proliferation, such as the bone marrow elements, hair, skin, and epithelial cells of the gastrointestinal tract, are also affected. Frequently the problems related to the destruction of these normal cells require more nursing care than the disease itself.

Alkylating agents. Alkylation is the replacement of a hydrogen atom of a molecule by an alkyl group. The irreversible combination of alkyl groups with nucleotide chains, particularly DNA, causes unbalanced growth of unaffected cell constituents so that the cell eventually dies. They are radiomimetic, in that their action is similar to irradiation.

Antimetabolites. These agents resemble essential metabolic elements needed for cell growth but are sufficiently altered in molecular structure to inhibit further synthesis of DNA and/or RNA.

Plant alkaloids. These agents from the periwinkle plant *Vinca rosea* arrest cells in metaphase (a phase of mitosis) by binding to microtubular protein needed for spindle formation. The two agents, vincristine and vinblastine, differ structurally by only one oxygen atom but are markedly different from each other with regard to dose, toxicity, and

Table 36-3 Summary of chemotherapeutic agents used in the treatment of childhood cancers*

AGENT/ADMINISTRATION	SIDE EFFECTS AND TOXICITY	COMMENTS AND SPECIFIC NURSING CONSIDERATIONS
Alkylating agents		
Mechlorethamine (nitrogen mustard, Mustargen) IV. IT†	N/V‡ (½-8 hours later) BMD§ (2-3 weeks later) Alopecia Local phlebitis	Infuse through free-flowing infusion; extravasation causes necrosis and sloughing of skin
Cyclophosphamide (Cytoxan, CTX, Endoxan) PO, IV, IM†	N/V (3-4 hours later) BMD (10-14 days later) Alopecia Hemorrhagic cystitis Severe immunosuppression Stomatitis (rare) Hyperpigmentation Transverse ridging of nails Infertility	BMD has platelet-sparing effect Give dose early in day to allow adequate fluids afterward Force fluids before administering drug and for 2 days after to prevent chemical cystitis; encourage frequent voiding, even during night Warn parents to report signs of burning on urination or hematuria to physician
Chlorambucil (Leukeran) PO	N/V BMD Diarrhea Dermatitis Less commonly may be hepatotoxicity	Usually slow onset; side effects related to high doses
Antimetabolites		
Cytosine arabinoside (Ara-C, Cytosar, Cytarabine, arabinosyl cytosine) IV, IM, SC,† IT	N/V BMD (7-14 days later) Mucosal ulceration Immunosuppression Hepatitis (usually subclinical)	Crosses blood-brain barrier Use with caution in patients with hepatic dysfunction
5-Azacytidine (5-AzaC) IV	N/V BMD Diarrhea	Infuse slowly to decrease severity of N/V
Mercaptopurine (6-MP, Purinethol) PO	N/V Diarrhea Abdominal pain Anorexia Stomatitis BMD (4-6 weeks later) Immunosuppression Dermatitis Less commonly may be hepatic dysfunction	Abdominal pain usually relieved by defecation 6-MP is an analog of xanthine; therefore allopurinol (Zyloprim) delays its metabolism and increases its potency
Methotrexate (MTX, Amethopterin) PO, IV, IM, IT	N/V Diarrhea Mucosal ulceration (2-5 days later) BMD (10 days later) Immunosuppression Dermatitis and sensitivity to sun Photosensitivity Alopecia (uncommon) Toxic effects include Hepatitis (fibrosis) Osteoporosis Nephropathy Pneumonitis (fibrosis)	Potency and toxicity increased by salicylates, sulfonamides, and aminobenzoic acid; avoid use of these substances, such as aspirin Citrovorum factor (folinic acid or leucovorin) decreases cytotoxic action of MTX; used as an antidote for overdose and to enhance normal cell recovery following intense therapy; avoid use of vitamins during drug administration unless prescribed by physician Increased toxicity with IT use—pain at injection site, meningismus (signs of meningitis without actual inflammation), especially fever and headache; potential sequelae— transient or permanent hemiparesis, convulsions, dementia, and death

*A general discussion of side effects common to many drugs is presented on page 1580-1584.
†IV, intravenous; IT, intrathecal; PO, by mouth; IM, intramuscular; SC, subcutaneous.
‡N/V, nausea and vomiting.
§BMD, bone marrow depression
‖Abbreviations stand for chemical compound.

Continued.

Table 36-3 Summary of chemotherapeutic agents used in the treatment of childhood cancers—cont'd

AGENT/ADMINISTRATION	SIDE EFFECTS AND TOXICITY	COMMENTS AND SPECIFIC NURSING CONSIDERATIONS
Methotrexate (MTX, Amethopterin) PO, IV, IM, IT—cont'd	Hemorrhagic enteritis	Meningeal irritation can be minimized by (1) using a preservative-free diluent, (2) allowing it to warm to room temperature, and (3) filtering it through a Millipore filter before administration; use of an Ommaya reservoir also decreases side effects

6-Thioguanine (6-TG, Thioguan) PO	N/V
	BMD
	Stomatitis
	Rarely
	    Dermatitis
	    Photosensitivity
	    Liver dysfunction
		Side effects are unusual

Plant alkaloids Vincristine (Oncovin) IV	BMD (especially anemia) Alopecia Neurotoxicity—paresthesia (numbness), ataxis, weakness, foot drop, hyporeflexia, constipation (adynamic ileus), hoarseness (vocal cord paralysis), abdominal, chest, and jaw pain, mental depression Fever	Extravasation causes cellulitis; administer through free-flowing infusion Individuals with underlying neurologic problems may be more prone to neurotoxicity Institute safety precautions when ambulation is impaired (side rails, wheelchair, assistance when walking) Monitor stool patterns closely; administer stool softener Report signs of neurtoxicity because may necessitate cessation of drug Excreted primarily by liver into biliary system; administer cautiously to anyone with biliary disease
Vinblastine (Velban) IV	N/V BMD (especially neutropenia) Alopecia Neurotoxicity (same as for vincristine but less severe)	Same as for vincristine
Antibiotics Actinomycin-D (Dactinomycin, Osmegen, ACT-D) IV	N/V (2-5 hours later) BMD (especially platelet) Immunosuppression Mucosal ulceration Abdominal cramps Diarrhea Anorexia (may last few weeks) Alopecia Acne Erythema or hyperpigmentation of previously irratiated skin Fever Malaise	Extravasation causes skin necrosis and pain; administer through free-flowing infusion Enhances cytotoxic effects of radiation therapy but increases toxic effects May cause serious desquamation of irradiated tissue

Doxorubicin, adriamycin (Doxyrubicin) IV	N/V
	Stomatitis
	BMD
	Fever, chills
	Local phlebitis
	Alpecia
	High-dose toxicity includes
	    Cardiac abnormalities
	    ECG changes
	    Heart failure
		Use only sterile distilled water as a diluent
		Administer through free-flowing infusion to minimize vascular irritation (extravasation may *not* cause pain)
		Observe for any changes in heart rate or rhythm and signs of failure
		Cumulative dose must not exceed 550 mg/m^2
		Warn parents that drug causes urine to turn red (for up to 12 days after administration); this is normal, not hematuria

Table 36-3 Summary of chemotherapeutic agents used in the treatment of childhood cancers—cont'd

AGENT/ADMINISTRATION	SIDE EFFECTS AND TOXICITY	COMMENTS AND SPECIFIC NURSING CONSIDERATIONS
Antibiotics—cont'd		
Daunorubicin (Daunomycin, Rubidomycin) IV	Similar to adriamycin	Similar to adriamycin
Bleomycin (Blenoxane) IV, IM, SC	Allergic reaction—fever, chills, hypotension, anaphylaxis N/V Stomatitis Cumulative dose effects include Skin—rash, hyperpigmentation, thickening, ulceration, peeling, nail changes, alopecia Lungs—Pneumonitis with infiltrate that can progress to fatal fibrosis	Should have test dose before therapeutic dose administered Have Benadryl and epinephrine at bedside Hypersensitivity occurs with first one to two doses Concentration of drug in skin and lungs accounts for toxic effects
Hormones		
Corticosteroids (prednisone most frequently used; many proprietary names such as Meticorten, Deltasone, Paracort) PO; also IM or IV but rarely used	For short-term use, no acute toxicity Usual side effects are mild: moon face, fluid retention, weight gain, mood changes, increased appetite, gastric irritation, susceptibility to infection	Explain expected effects, especially in terms of body image, increased appetitie, and personality changes Monitor weight gain; evaluate true weight (muscle mass) from water retention May recommend moderate salt restriction Administer with antacid and early in morning (sometimes given every other day to minimize side effects) May need to disguise bitter taste Observe for potential infection sites; usual inflammatory response and fever are absent
	Long-term effects of chronic steroid administration are mood changes, hirsutism, trunk obesity (buffalo hump), thin extremities, muscle wasting and weakness, osteoporosis, poor wound healing, bruising, potassium loss, gastric bleeding, hypertension, diabetes mellitus	All of above; in addition, encourage foods high in potassium (bananas, raisins, prunes, coffee, chocolate) Test stools for occult blood Monitor blood pressure Test urine for sugar and acetone
Enzymes		
L-asparaginase (Elspar) IV, IM	Allergic reactions (including anaphylactic shock) Fever N/V Anorexia Weight loss Toxicity— Liver dysfunction Hyperglycemia Renal failure	Have epinephrine (1:1000) at bedside (usual dose 0.01 mg/kg) Record signs of allergic reaction, such as urticaria, facial edema, hypotension, or abdominal cramps Check weight daily Normally, BUN and ammonia levels rise as a result of drug—not evidence of liver damage Check urine for sugar
Nitrosoureas		
Carmustine (BCNU)‖ IV Lomustine (CCNU) PO	N/V (2-6 hours later) BMD (3-4 weeks later) Burning pain along IV infusion BCNU—flushing and facial burning on infusion	Should be used cautiously if BMD already present Prevent extravasation; contact with skin causes brown spots Oral form—give 4 hours after meals when stomach is empty Crosses blood-brain barrier

Continued.

Table 36-3 Summary of chemotherapeutic agents used in the treatment of childhood cancers—cont'd

AGENT/ADMINISTRATION	SIDE EFFECTS AND TOXICITY	COMMENTS AND SPECIFIC NURSING CONSIDERATIONS
Other agents		

Hydroxyurea (Hydrea) PO	N/V
	Anorexia
	Less commonly
	  Diarrhea
	  BMD
	  Mucosal ulceration
	  Alopecia
	  Dermatitis
		Must be given cautiously in patients with renal dysfunction

Procarbazine (Matulane) PO	Severe N/V
	BMD (3-4 weeks later)
	Lethargy
	Dermatitis
	Myalgia
	Arthralgia
	Less commonly
	  Stomatitis
	  Neuropathy
	  Alopecia
	  Diarrhea
		Central nervous system depressants (phenothiazines, barbiturates) enhance central nervous system symptoms
		Monoamine oxidase (MAO) inhibition sometimes occurs; therefore sympathomimetic drugs and foods such as aged cheese, yogurt, alcohol, and bananas should be avoided

Dacarbazine (DTIC-Dome) IV	N/V (especially after first dose) BMD Flulike syndrome Burning sensation in vein during infusion (not extravasation)	Must be given cautiously in patients with renal dysfunction Decrease IV rate or use warm moist towels on IV site
Cisplatin (Platinol) IV	Renal toxicity (severe) N/V (severe, 1-4 hours later) BMD (mild, 2-3 weeks later) Ototoxicity Neurotoxicity (similar to that for vincristine) Anaphylactic reactions	Renal function must be assessed before giving drug Must maintain hydration before and during therapy (specific gravity of urine is used to assess hydration) Monitor intake and output Administer antiemetic, especially chlorpromazine Advise patient of possible ototoxicity and neurotoxicity; signs to be reported immediately Observe for signs of allergic reactions Have oxygen, suction, and emergency drugs at bedside

antitumor activity. Although both are neurotoxic, vincristine causes more severe side effects than vinblastine.

Antitumor antibiotics. These agents are natural products that interfere with cell division by reacting with DNA in such a way as to prevent further replication of DNA and transcription of RNA.

Hormones. Both adrenal and gonadal hormones have antineoplastic properties. The precise mechanism of action is still unclear. Adrenocorticosteroids are thought to bind with DNA and alter the transcription process. Although there are a number of cortisone preparations, prednisone is most frequently used. Androgens and estrogens are effective against certain cancers usually found in adults, such as prostate and breast cancers. Consequently, they have little applicability in childhood cancer.

Miscellaneous agents. A number of agents are not categorized according to the preceding classifications. The most commonly used ones are described in the following:

L-*asparaginase* is an enzyme isolated from extracts of bacterial cultures of *Escherichia coli* or *Erwinia carotovora*. It hydrolyzes L-asparagine, an amino acid, to L-aspartic acid, which prevents the cell from synthesizing protein needed for DNA and RNA synthesis.

L-asparaginase is unique because it is selectively cytotoxic only for certain cancer cells. L-asparagine is synthesized by normal cells but must be exogenously supplied to certain leukemic and lymphoma cells. Administration of the enzyme L-asparaginase destroys the essential exogenous supply while sparing normal cells of untoward effects.

Hydroxyurea, a cell-cycle dependent agent, inhibits ribonucleotide reduction to deoxyribonucleotide. DNA synthesis is impaired, but protein and RNA synthesis are less affected; therefore the unbalanced growth results in eventual cellular death.

Nitrosoureas, of which a number of compounds are available, act similarly to alkylating agents and are sometimes classified as such because they replace an essential DNA molecule, thus inhibiting DNA, RNA, and protein synthesis. One of their unique properties is the ability to cross the blood-brain barrier.

Procarbazine is a weak monoamine oxidase (MAO) inhibitor. (MAO is an enzyme that destroys the neurohormones epinephrine, norepinephrine, and serotonin. MAO inhibitors act as psychic energizers.) Its exact cytotoxic action is not known, although it inhibits DNA, RNA, and protein synthesis.

Dacarbazine is an analog of aminoimidazole carboxamide. It interferes with purine synthesis and also exhibits alkylating properties in DNA synthesis. It has shown significant antitumor activity when combined with other drugs, especially doxorubicin.

Cisplatin is a heavy-metal derivative containing a central platinum atom bounded by ammonia and chloride groups. It inhibits DNA synthesis by the formation of intrastrand and interstrand crosslinks, similar to alkylating agents.

Radiotherapy

Radiotherapy is frequently used in the treatment of childhood cancer, usually in conjunction with chemotherapy and/or surgery. It can be used for curative purposes and is often employed for palliation to relieve symptoms by shrinking the size of the tumor. Recent advances in radiation therapy have optimized its beneficial effects and minimized many of the undesirable side effects, although high-dose radiation is associated with many serious late effects.

Ionizing radiation is cytotoxic in at least three different ways: (1) damaging the pyrimidine bases cytosine, thymine, and uracil needed for the synthesis of nucleic acids, (2) causing single-strand breaks in the DNA or RNA molecule, or (3) causing double helical–strand breaks in these molecules. The effect of disturbing cellular metabolic and reproductive functions is either sublethal or lethal damage.

Lethal damage refers to the death of the cell. *Sublethal* damage refers to injured cells that may subsequently be repaired. Many of the acute side effects are the result of lethal damage to radiosensitive tissue, particularly proliferating cells such as those of the bone marrow, gastrointestinal tract, and hair follicles. Late effects are usually the result of cell death.

The acute untoward reactions from radiotherapy depend primarily on the area to be irradiated. Total-body irradiation (TBI) is associated with the most severe reactions and is employed to prepare the immune system for bone marrow transplantation. Table 36-4 summarizes the acute effects of radiation therapy and nursing interventions that may be helpful in lessening or preventing them.

Immunotherapy

Another research area in the treatment of certain cancers has been the stimulation of the body's natural immune defenses to combat malignant cells. One of the theories behind the development of immunotherapy is that since cancer cells are constantly developing in the body, there must be a natural immunity that prevents the cells from proliferating to cause

Table 36-4 Early side effects of radiotherapy

SITE/EFFECTS	NURSING INTERVENTIONS
Gastrointestinal tract	
Nausea/vomiting	Give antiemetic on regular schedule
	Measure amount of emesis to prevent dehydration
Anorexia	Encourage fluids and foods best tolerated, usually light, soft diet
	Monitor weight loss
Mucosal ulceration	Use frequent mouthwashes and oral hygiene to prevent mucositis
Diarrhea	Can be controlled with antispasmodics and kaolin pectin preparations
	Observe for signs of dehydration
Potential effects:	
Pancreatitis	May need analgesics to relieve discomfort
Parotitis	
Loss of taste	Combat severe dryness of mouth with oral hygiene and liquid diet
Skin	
Alopecia (within 2 weeks; begins to regrow by 3-6 months)	Introduce idea of wig
	Stress necessity of scalp hygiene and need for head covering in cold weather
Dry or moist desquamation	Do not refer to skin change as a "burn" (implies use of too much radiation)
	Keep skin clean
	Wash daily, using soap sparingly
	Do not remove skin marking for radiation fields
	Avoid exposure to sun
	For dryness, apply lubricant
	For desquamation, consult physician for skin hygiene and care
Head	
Nausea/vomiting	Same as for gastrointestinal tract
Alopecia	Regular dental care, fluoride treatments
Potential effects	
Parotitis	
Loss of taste	
Xerostomia (dry mouth)	
Urinary bladder	
Rarely cystitis	More likely to occur with concomitant use of cyclophosphamide
	Encourage liberal fluid intake and frequent voiding
Bone marrow	
Myelosuppression	Institute bleeding and infection precautions
	Observe for signs of anemia

disease. Also, cancer cells contain antigens that may be capable of eliciting an immune response in the host. If it were possible to introduce these specific antigens into the body, the accelerated immune response would then selectively attack the malignant cells. Based on theories and several documented reports linking cancer to the immune system, such as the increased incidence of cancer in immunosuppressed individuals, immunotherapy has become an increasingly important area of research.

To date there have been many disappointments in the development of specific agents, such as interferon, in acting selectively against tumor cells. Much of the current work in immunotherapy is directed toward the use of *monoclonal antibodies* in diagnosis and treatment of cancers. Through a complex process, special cells are fused to form a hybrid clone or hybridoma that produces antibodies that recognize a single specific antigen, hence the term *monoclonal antibody* ("mono" meaning one and "clone" meaning exact duplicate). These clones are then frozen, maintained in culture, or grown as tumors in mice to produce large quantities of the antibody in ascites fluid (Moldawer and Murray, 1985). While there are many prospective uses for monoclonal antibodies, their current role has been in diagnosing subclasses of leukemia cells to enhance understanding of which types of leukemia respond to different treatments and if the subclass is related to prognosis. Monoclonal antibodies have also been used to deplete allogeneic bone marrows of T-cells to reduce graft-versus-host disease and to selectively eliminate malignant cells from autologous marrow for transplanting back into the patient (Bernstein and others, 1985). Results from these studies have been encouraging, but further work is needed to define the role monoclonal antibodies will have in cancer care.

Bone Marrow Transplantation

Another approach to the treatment of some forms of cancer, in particular the leukemias but also non-Hodgkin lymphoma and neuroblastoma, is bone marrow transplantation. Candidates for transplantation are children with suitable donors and who have malignancies that are unlikely to be cured by other means. Basically, the principle behind bone marrow transplantation is that once the marrow is totally free of malignant cells and the immune system is suppressed to prevent rejection of the transplanted marrow, the donor marrow cells will begin to produce functioning nonmalignant blood cells. In essence, a new blood-forming organ will be accepted by the recipient.

Presently three types of bone marrow transplants may be done:

Allogeneic, which involves the matching of a histocompatible donor, usually a sibling, with the recipient

Autologous, which uses the patient's own marrow that was collected from disease-free tissue and frozen

Syngeneic, which uses marrow from an identical twin

The most common type of bone marrow transplantation is allogeneic. To understand the selection process of a suit-able donor and the potential complications in transplantation, it is necessary to review the human leukocyte antigen (HLA) system complex. The HLA (major histocompatibility) system is a group of antigens that are shared by many tissues in the body. The genes that determine the HLA system are located close together on chromosome number 6 and are inherited as a unit. Some of the major HLA antigens are A, B, C, D, and DR. There is a wide diversity for each of these HLA loci. There are more than 20 different HLA-A antigens that can be inherited and more than 40 different HLA-B antigens.

HLA-A, B, and C genes and HLA-D/DR genes are inherited as a single unit or haplotype. A child inherits one unit from each parent; thus a child and each parent have one identical and one nonidentical haplotype. Since the possible haplotype combinations among siblings follow the laws of Mendelian genetics, there is a one in four chance that two siblings have two identical haplotypes and are perfectly matched at the HLA loci. Since many patients have more than one sibling and certain HLA genotypes are more common among families prone to leukemia, approximately 35% of leukemia patients have a matched sibling (Quinn, 1985).

The importance of HLA matching is to prevent the grave complication known as *graft-versus-host disease (GVHD)*. Since the child's immune system is essentially rendered nonfunctional prior to surgery, there is little difficulty with bone marrow rejection by the recipient. However, the donor's marrow may contain antigens not matched to the recipient's antigens, and these antigens begin attacking body cells. The more closely the HLA systems match, the less likely GVHD is to develop. However, it can occur even with a perfect HLA match, because there are as yet unidentified and thus unmatched histocompatibility antigens (Quinn, 1985).

Although the actual transplant procedure is simple and involves harvesting several bone marrow specimens from the donor (which is done under general anesthesia) and diluting the marrow and administering it intravenously similar to any blood product to the recipient, the preoperative and postoperative care are complex. The first stage is identifying a compatible donor in the case of an allogeneic transplant. The second phase is cytoreduction to produce a totally aleukemic immunosuppressed state, which involves intense chemotherapy (usually administration of high-dose cyclophosphamide) and total-body irradiation.

The third phase is preventing complications. During the preoperative aplastic phase and for the 10- to 20-day period after transplantation before the new marrow begins adequately replacing granulocytes, the child is extremely susceptible to infection. Interstitial or nonbacterial pneumonia is another serious complication with a high mortality rate. However, the most common complication is GVHD, which can affect the skin, gastrointestinal tract, liver, heart, lungs, lymphoid tissue, and marrow. GVHD is characterized by a hardening of the tissues and drying of the mucous membranes. The severity of the manifestations varies, but once vital organs are affected, death can ensue. Treatment involves the use of steroids and/or azathioprine (Imuran). However, these immunosuppressive drugs further increase the risk of infection. All blood products should be irradiated to minimize the introduction of additional antigens (Woods, 1984). Another unfortunate posttransplant possibility is recurrence of the leukemia after engraftment.

Supportive Therapies

Cancer care encompasses more than treatments aimed at eliminating the malignant cells. Because of the delicate balance between killing malignant cells and preserving functional cells, supportive therapy is frequently needed during those times that serious damage occurs to normal body tissues. For example, infection is a constant threat from the immunosuppressant effects of antineoplastic agents. Prophylactic antibiotics, such as trimethoprim/sulfamethoxazole (Bactrim, Septra) and nystatin or amphotericin B, may be given to reduce the incidence of serious infection (Wolff, 1984). Other supportive therapies include replacement of blood elements as needed in anemia, agranulocytopenia, and thrombocytopenia. However, the use of granulocyte transfusions and preventive infusions of platelets is controversial because of the lack of documented effectiveness and the risk of developing antibodies to the foreign antigens, respectively (Strauss, 1984; Feusner, 1984).

Allopurinol, a xanthine-oxidase inhibitor, may be administered to prevent renal damage. Massive cellular damage from cytotoxic therapy releases large amounts of uric acid, which can accumulate and precipitate in the renal tubules, eventually causing tubular obstruction. Allopurinol prevents the metabolic breakdown of xanthine to uric acid. Other supportive measures include alkalinization of the urine and adequate hydration.

Nutritional support has been increasingly recognized as a significant component of cancer treatment. Optimum nutrition is believed to promote the body's tolerance to antineoplastic agents and preserve immunologic responsiveness. Excellent nutrition prior to intensive therapy provides nutrient stores during periods of anorexia, nausea, and vomiting. The most common nutritional problem is children's unwillingness to consume sufficient food to maintain a nutritional balance. Oral supplementation with fortified foods, such as commercial preparations (Ensure), may be helpful, but nonoral routes may be necessary, such as nasogastric tube feedings, gastrostomy, or parenteral alimentation (Lukens, 1984).

A final supportive therapy is the effective use of analgesics, especially when the malignant process is uncontrolled and causes pain. Dosages of narcotics *titrated to the child's needs* should be administered *around the clock* for optimum pain control. Nonpharmacologic strategies should be implemented as needed but should not be regarded as substitutes for pharmacologic management. The reader is encouraged to review the principles of pain assessment and management presented in Chapter 26 in caring for the child with cancer.

Long-Term Sequelae of Treatment

Vigorous treatment of childhood cancers has resulted in dramatically improved survival rates. However, treatment programs combining surgery, irradiation, and chemotherapy are not without their complications. Some may occur immediately, such as loss of a limb from surgical amputation or asplenia from splenectomy in Hodgkin lymphoma. However, current concern is with late effects—adverse changes related to treatment modalities, interactions between modes of treatment, individual characteristics of the child, and the disease process that may appear months to years after lifesaving treatment (Ruccione, 1985). Because of the greater number of children who are cured and surviving into adulthood, increasing documentation of late effects is emerging (Table 36-5). Almost no organ is exempt, and almost every antineoplastic agent and especially irradiation are responsible for some adverse effect. Although many factors influence the development of late effects from radiation, some of the more important ones include the total cumulative dose given, the age of the child (the younger the child, the more radiosensitive the body organs are), and the location of the tumor.

In addition to physical effects, there is also concern for the psychologic sequelae of surviving cancer (see Questions and controversies, p. 1575). Regardless of the level of functioning at the time of cure, having cancer is a stressful experience, and nurses can play an important part in ameliorating many of the frightening and painful aspects of care.

Nursing Considerations

Nurses working with cancer patients have a significant supportive role in helping the family understand the various therapies, preventing or managing expected side effects or toxicities, and observing for late effects of treatment. Education is a constant feature of the nursing role, especially in terms of new treatments, clinical trials,* and home care. Because of the anxiety generated by the diagnosis of cancer, some families may resort to unproven methods of treatment that are frequently referred to as "cancer quackery." These unorthodox approaches are a threat to every cancer family; they may produce unnecessary harm by themselves or, if benign, render injury because other proven modes of therapy are avoided. In many instances this causes financial burden and emotional strife among family members.

Nurses can be instrumental in working against cancer quackery by being aware of factors that increase a family's likelihood of seeking unproven remedies, such as social pressure to "leave no stone unturned" and feelings of depression, helplessness, and hopelessness (Holland, 1982). Communicating effectively with families about the diagnosis and forms of therapy and providing all possible support and reassurance during treatment are also important interventions to counteract the factors that lead to dissatisfaction

---

*A helpful resource is *What are clinical trials all about?*, which is available at no cost from the Office of Cancer Communications, National Cancer Institute, Bldg. 31, Room 10A18, Bethesda, MD 20205.

Table 36-5 Late effects of cancer treatment	
SYSTEMIC EFFECTS	**ASSOCIATED MODE OF TREATMENT**
Central nervous system (CNS)	
Leukoencephalopathy (syndrome ranging from lethargy, dementia, and seizures to quadriplegia and death)	Methotrexate and/or CNS irradiation
Mineralizing microangiopathy (headaches, focal seizures, incoordination and gait abnormalities)	Methotrexate and/or CNS irradiation
Peripheral neuropathy (foot drop)	Vincristine
Cognitive deficitis (IQ, nonlanguage skills)	Intrathecal chemotherapy and/or cranial irradiation (especially before age 5 years)
Cardiovascular	
Cardiomyopathy	Anthracyclines (doxorubicin and daunorubicin) and/or irradiation to heart
	High-dose cyclophosphamide
Pericardial damage	Mediastinal irradiation
Respiratory	
Pneumonitis	Lung irradiation, alkylating agents, possibly bleomycin,
Pulmonary fibrosis	vinblastine, cisplatin
Gastrointestinal	
Chronic enteritis	Abdominal irradiation, methotrexate, cytosine arabinoside
Hepatitis fibrosis	Methotrexate, 6-mercaptopurine
Urinary	
Hemorrhagic cystitis, bladder fibrosis, renal tubular necrosis	Cyclophosphamide, cisplatin, irradiation, especially with radiomimetic chemotherapeutic agents (i.e., doxorubicin and daunorubicin)
Endocrine	
Growth retardation, thyroid dysfunction, gonad dysfunction	Irradiation
Reproductive	
Possible gonadal damage (both sexes)	Cyclophosphamide, chlorambucil, busulphan
Skeletal	
Linear growth retardation	Irradiation, long-term steroids
Spinal deformities, asymmetric growth, pathologic fractures	Irradiation
Immune	
Asplenia (overwhelming infection)	Splenectomy (Hodgkin lymphoma)
Sensory organs	
Cataracts	Cranial irradiation, high-dose steroids
Hearing	Cisplatin
Additional effects	
Dental problems	
Increased caries, periodontal disease, hypoplastic teeth, hypodontia (delayed or absent tooth development)	Irradiation to maxilla and mandible
Second malignancies	Irradiation
Bone and soft tissue tumors	Alkylating agents
Leukemia	Irradiation, procarbazine
Nonlymphocytic leukemia	

with conventional care. Nurses must be fortified with knowledge to substantiate present treatment protocols and to discredit unauthorized methods. The American Cancer Society and local and state medical societies are reliable sources of information concerning research on investigational vs quack methods of cancer therapy.

General needs. Children in particular need psychologic preparation for the various treatment modalities, which often involve surgery, intravenous injections, and lumbar punctures for intrathecal administration. Even noninvasive treatments such as radiotherapy can be frightening to the unprepared child. Instruction regarding home care fre-

Questions and Controversies

What are the long-term psychologic consequences of surviving childhood cancer?

With increasing numbers of children surviving childhood cancer, there is concern for their emotional as well as their physical health. Among the studies that have investigated the psychologic and social adjustment of these young people, the findings have been conflicting. One study found that more than 50% of survivors had mild psychiatric symptomatology, including anxiety, depression, and poor self-esteem (O'Malley and others, 1979). However, those who adjusted well did so regardless of the degree of residual physical impairment, such as loss of a limb (O'Malley and others, 1980). Factors related to fewer adjustment problems included: (1) young age at time of diagnosis, (2) short treatment course with minimum side effects, (3) absence of relapse or recurrence of the disease, and (4) absence of unresolved concerns about the outcome of the disease (Koocher and O'Malley, 1981).

Another study, long-term survivors reported that their illness disrupted school attendance, resulted in academic difficulties, and altered future plans and peer relationships. While most youngsters adapted well, some developed emotional problems, specifically, symptoms related to depression and/or alcoholism (Lansky and others, 1985). Other researchers have found that the majority of children are psychologically healthy with few differences between them and healthy groups of youngsters (Zeltzer and others, 1980). In addition, there have been findings of a high quality of life among survivors, with the majority reaching or surpassing their preillness goals (Holmes and Holmes, 1975). Obviously, additional research is needed in this area with unaffected children serving as controls.

quently involves teaching about medication schedules, observation for side effects or toxicities that require further evaluation, measures to prevent or manage these problems, and care of special devices such as central venous catheters.* Compliance is a very important issue, since poor adherence to drug regimens can result in a relapse. Every effort must be made to ensure that the family understands the importance of adhering to the prescribed treatment schedule and measures to improve compliance (see p. 1110).

General well-child care must also continue. Sometimes the overwhelming needs and demands placed on the family coupled with the singular concern focused on the cancer result in a lack of attention to normal health care needs. In particular, dental care must be stressed. Irradiation to the head and neck can cause a number of late complications (Hazra and Shipman, 1982). Some are irreversible, such as facial asymmetry, but those affecting the teeth and gums (caries, periodontal disease) benefit from excellent oral hygiene, including regular use of systemic and topical fluoride (see Dental health, p. 613). There is also evidence of de-

layed or absent development of the permanent teeth (Welbury and others, 1984). Depending on the child's age, this can be a source of acute psychologic distress, especially during early school-age years when "losing a tooth" is a status symbol. Therefore children need to be aware of this possibility and helped to explain the delay to peers.

Bone marrow transplantation. The needs of the family are enormous when bone marrow transplantation is expected. These children may be hospitalized from 30 to 60 days and are usually in a medical center that specializes in this procedure. Because of the risk of infection, the unit generally employs strict reverse isolation, including laminar air flow to sterilize the air. Consequently, the child is faced with the additional trauma of isolation (see also p. 1091). Numerous procedures are performed, such as insertion of a Broviac catheter, intensive chemotherapy and irradiation, and meticulous personal hygiene. In addition, side effects and complications may occur after the preoperative cytotoxic regimen and include severe mucositis, parotitis, nausea, vomiting, diarrhea, inappropriate secretion of antidiuretic hormone, nephropathy, and heart failure (Wiley and Decuir-Whalley, 1983). Throughout this long ordeal there is the family's concern for successful engraftment and fear of fatal complications. Consequently, nurses involved with the child and family need to provide sensitive care and maintain a supportive attitude during the many crises that may arise. If the procedure is not successful, the care needed by these families is consistent with that required by the family of any child with a life-threatening disorder (see Chapter 23).

Follow-up care. At the other end of the spectrum, care does not end when the child completes therapy. With the increasing awareness of late effects, nurses play an important role in the assessment of the child for problems such as delayed growth, secondary malignancies, and disturbances in any body system. These children require regular follow-up, and the family needs to be aware of the importance of continued medical supervision. Other health care professionals caring for the child, such as school nurses, family physicians, and dentists, should be informed of the child's previous diagnosis of cancer. As children reach adulthood they may benefit from genetic counseling regarding cancers that are likely to be inherited. If the possibility of sterility exists, pretreatment sperm banking may be offered to adolescent boys, which allows additional options regarding family planning in adulthood (Ruccione, 1985).

Precautions in handling neoplastic agents. In addition to the many responsibilities nurses have in regard to the child and family, they must also use safeguards to protect themselves. Handling chemotherapeutics may present risks to the handler and to her offspring, although the exact degree of risk is not known. Several publications are available that describe the safeguards that should be practiced (Stolar, Power, and Veile, 1983; Bergemann, 1983; ASHP, 1985).* Basic guidelines include the following:

---

*Home care instructions on giving medications to children and caring for a Hickman/Broviac catheter are available in Wong, D., and Whaley, L.: Clinical handbook of pediatric nursing, ed. 2, St. Louis, 1986, The C.V. Mosby Co.

---

*Complimentary information is also available from Germfree Laboratories, Inc., 7435 NW 41 St., Miami, FL 33166.

1. Use utmost care and strict aseptic technique in handling chemotherapeutic agents to prevent any physical contact with the substance
2. Prepare drugs in a properly ventilated room or biologic safety cabinet (incorporates protective front panel and vertical laminar air flow to reduce potential for inhalation during preparation)
3. Wear disposable gloves and protective clothing and discard in special container after each use
4. Use a sterile gauze pad when priming IV tubing, connecting and disconnecting tubing, inserting syringes into vials, breaking glass ampules, or any other procedure in which antineoplastic drugs may be inadvertently discharged
5. Dispose of all contaminated needles, syringes, IV tubing, and other contaminated equipment in a leakproof and puncture-resistant container; do not recap or bend needles

Cancers of the Blood and Lymph Systems

Three of the most common cancers in children, leukemia, Hodgkin lymphoma, and non-Hodgkin lymphoma, arise in the blood and lymph systems. Children with all of these cancers have benefited from improved methods of treatment in recent years, and a significant portion of affected children will be long-term survivors.

LEUKEMIAS

Leukemia, cancer of the blood-forming tissues, is the most common form of childhood cancer. The annual incidence in white children under 15 years of age is 4.2 per 100,000 and in black children is 2.4 per 100,000 (Poplack, 1985). It occurs more frequently in males than females after age 1 year, and the peak onset is between 2 and 6 years. It is one of the forms of cancer that have demonstrated dramatic improvements in survival rates. Before the use of antileukemic agents in 1948, a child with acute lymphocytic leukemia (ALL) lived 2 to 3 months. Current 5-year survival rates for children with ALL exceed 60% in major research centers, and the majority of these children may be cured (Poplack, 1985).

Classification

Leukemia is a broad term given to a group of malignant diseases of the bone marrow and lymphatic system. Current research has revealed that it is a complex disease of varying heterogeneity. Consequently, classification has become increasingly complex, sophisticated, and essential, since identification of the subtype of leukemia has therapeutic and prognostic implications. The following is an overview of the major classification systems currently being used.

Morphology. Leukemia is classified according to its predominant cell type and level of maturity, as described by the following:

Lympho—for leukemias involving the lymphoid or lymphatic system

Myelo—for those of myeloid (bone marrow) origin
Blastic and acute—for those involving immature cells
Cytic and chronic—for those involving mature cells

Prior to modern treatment, the classifications of acute or chronic were applied to the cells' level of maturity because they correlated with the course of the disease—the immature form of the disease demonstrated a rapid or acute course of deterioration. Now this distinction is less likely to be seen, and the acute disease refers primarily to the presence of immature blast cells that accumulate and inhibit production of normal functioning cells (Ruccione, 1983). (For a review of the origin and development of blood cells, see p. 1513.)

In children two forms are generally recognized: *acute lymphoid leukemia (ALL)* and *acute nonlymphoid (myelogenous) leukemia (ANLL or AML)*. Synonyms for ALL include lymphatic, lymphocytic, lymphoblastic, and lymphoblastoid leukemia. Usually the terms *stem cell* or *blast cell leukemia* also refer to the lymphoid type of leukemia. Synonyms for the ANLL type include granulocytic, myelocytic, monocytic, myelogenous, monoblastic, and monomyeloblastic. There are also much rarer forms of leukemia that are named for the specific cell involved, such as basophilic or eosinophilic leukemia.

Morphology. Because of the confusion and inconsistency in classifying the leukemias, acute lymphoblastic and acute nonlymphoblastic leukemias are further subdivided according to another system known as the *French-American-British (FAB) system*. In the FAB system the subtypes are determined after a thorough study of the morphology (structure) and cytochemical reactivity of the leukemic cells. Accordingly, ALL is divided into three subtypes: L_1, L_2, and L_3. L_1 morphology is the most common subtype, accounts for 84% of children with ALL, and has the best prognosis. ANLL is classified into six subtypes that comprise 10% to 20% of the leukemias in children. The subtypes of ANLL are not clearly related to prognosis as is the case with ALL.

Biochemical markers. Leukemic cells also demonstrate different reactions when they are exposed to certain chemicals. For example, terminal deoxynucleotidyl transferase is able to provide excellent differentiation between ALL and ANLL. Several other chemicals are available to further differentiate various cell types.

Cell-surface markers. A number of cell-surface antigens have permitted differentiation of ALL into three broad classes: T-lymphocytes (T-cells), B-lymphocytes (B-cells), and "null" cells, those cells that lack T- or B-cell characteristics. Within the null cell category are those that react with an antigen called the common acute lymphoblastic leukemia antigen (CALLA). This further classification of lymphocytic leukemia appears to have prognostic importance in that persons with leukemias of the "null" category (about 85% of ALL), especially those who are CALLA-positive, demonstrate better survival rates. At present, cell-surface markers for ANLL are still rudimentary, although there is current research with monoclonal antibodies that may provide significant information about the non-lymphoid cells.

Staging and Prognostic Factors

There is general agreement among researchers that the most important prognostic factors in determining long-term survival for children with ALL are the initial white blood count (WBC) and the patient's age at diagnosis, followed by the histologic type of the disease and sex, which favors females. These factors have been used to predict the eventual prognosis as defined by the stages in Table 36-6.

No such staging exists with ANLL, and prognostic indicators are less clearly defined. Initial evidence suggests that high myeloblast count and age below 2 years are associated with a poorer prognosis (Grier and Weinstein, 1985).

From the time of establishment of the diagnosis, the nurse has some idea of the expected course the child will follow. However, in some instances, because of the variety of cell types observed and the marked undifferentiation of immature cells, a definitive classification cannot be made or the diagnosis may be changed. The nurse should be aware of the importance of such events in counseling and supporting family members.

Pathologic and Related Manifestations

Leukemia is an unrestricted proliferation of immature white blood cells in the blood-forming tissues of the body. Although not a "tumor" as such, the leukemic cells demonstrate the neoplastic properties of solid cancers. Therefore the resultant pathology and clinical manifestations of the disease are caused by infiltration and replacement of any tissue of the body with nonfunctional leukemic cells. Highly vascular organs of the reticuloendothelial system are most severely affected.

In order to understand the pathophysiology of the leukemic process, it is important to clarify two common misconceptions. First, although leukemia is an overproduction of white blood cells, most often in the acute form the leukocyte count is low. Instead, the peripheral blood smear and, more definitive, the bone marrow examination reveal greatly elevated counts of immature cells or "blasts." Second, these immature cells do not deliberately attack and destroy the normal blood cells or vascular tissues. Cellular destruction is by the process of infiltration and subsequent competition for metabolic elements. The following discussion elaborates on the pathologic process and related clinical manifestations in the most susceptible organs of the body (Fig. 36-1).

Bone marrow dysfunction. In all types of leukemia the proliferating cells depress bone marrow production of the formed elements of the blood by competing for and depriving the normal cells of the essential nutrients for metabolism. The three main consequences are (1) *anemia* from decreased erythrocytes, (2) *infection* from neutropenia, and (3) *bleeding tendencies* from decreased platelet production.

The invasion of the bone marrow with leukemic cells

Table 36-6 Staging system for acute lymphoblastic leukemia

STAGE	PROGNOSIS	CRITERIA
1	Good	2-9 years of age WBC <10,000/mm^3 ≥90% L$_1$ morphology in marrow lymphoblasts Excludes boys with platelet count <100,000/mm^3
2	Intermediate	Ineligibility for other prognostic groups
3	Poor	WBC >50,000/mm^3 or 10,000-50,000/mm^3 <90% L$_1$ morphology in marrow lymphoblasts
4	Poor	Lymphoma-leukemia (bulky extramedullary disease)
5	Poor	Infants <1 year of age

From Bleyer, W.A.: Acute lymphoid leukemia, Pediatr. Ann. 12(**4**):277-292, 1983.

gradually causes a weakening of the bone and a tendency toward fractures. As leukemic cells invade the periosteum, increasing pressure causes severe pain.

The most frequent presenting signs and symptoms of leukemia are a result of infiltration of the bone marrow. These include fever, pallor, fatigue, anorexia, hemorrhage (usually petechiae), and bone and joint pain. In the presence of neutropenia the body's normal bacterial flora can become aggressive pathogens. Any break in the skin is a potential site of infection. Frequently, vague abdominal pain is caused by areas of inflammation from normal flora within the intestinal tract.

Disturbance of involved organs. The organs of the reticuloendothelial system, namely, the spleen, liver, and lymph glands, demonstrate marked infiltration, enlargement, and eventually fibrosis. Hepatosplenomegaly is typically more common than lymphadenopathy. Chemotherapeutic agents seem to account for more liver and spleen damage than does the disease process.

The next most important site of involvement is the central nervous system. Initially, at the time of diagnosis, leukemic cells do not tend to invade this area, probably as a result of the protective blood-brain barrier. However, this normal protective mechanism also prevents the antileukemic drugs, with the exception of a few agents, from entering the brain in sufficient therapeutic doses to be effective. Before prophylactic use of cranial irradiation and intrathecal methotrexate, central nervous system involvement was frequent in children who survived 6 months or more. However, newer modes of therapy have significantly changed the course of the disease, although central nervous system complications still occur, even during bone marrow remission.

The usual effect of leukemic infiltration of the meninges is increased intracranial pressure. The pathogenesis is pre-

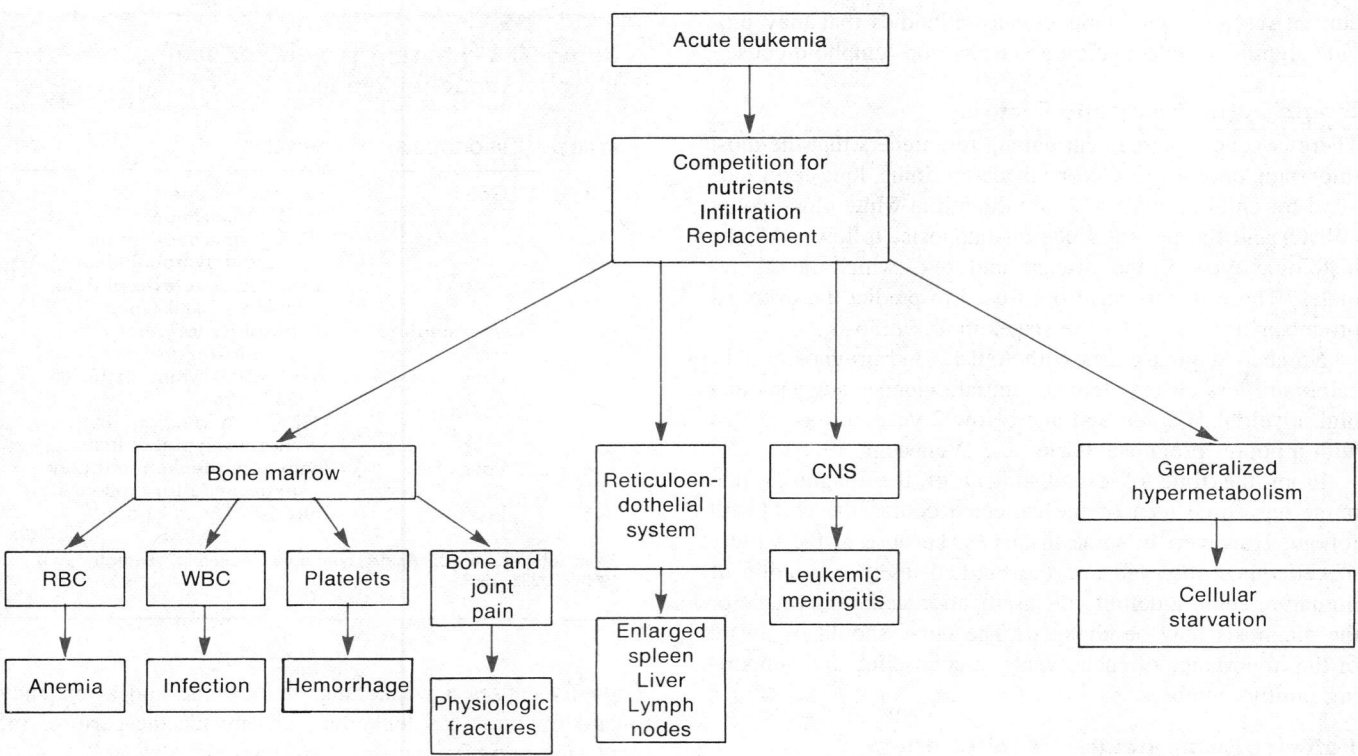

Fig. 36-1. Principal sites of tissue involvement in leukemia.

sumably attributable to invasion of the arachnoid by proliferating cells, which then interfere with the flow of cerebrospinal fluid in the subarachnoid space and at the base of the brain. The increased fluid pressure causes dilation of all four ventricles and consequently the signs and symptoms normally associated with this condition, such as severe headache, vomiting, papilledema, irritability, lethargy, and eventually coma. Irritation of the meninges also causes pain and stiffness in the neck and back.

Additional sites of involvement may be the cranial nerves, most often cranial nerve VII, or the facial nerve, and spinal nerves, particularly of the lumbar-sacral plexus, hypothalamus, and cerebellum. Clinical manifestations for these sites are directly related to the area involved. For example, with lumbar-sacral invasion, there is weakness in the lower extremities, pain radiating down the legs to the feet, and difficulty in voiding. Although such signs may suggest a brain tumor, the absence of localized signs often leads to the discovery of central nervous system involvement in leukemia.

Other long-term sites of involvement include the kidneys, testes, prostate, ovaries, gastrointestinal tract, and lungs. With long-term survivors becoming increasingly common, such extramedullary sites of leukemic invasion, especially the testes, are becoming more important clinically.

Hypermetabolism. The immense metabolic needs of proliferating leukemic cells eventually deprive all body cells

of nutrients necessary for survival. Muscle wasting, weight loss, anorexia, and fatigue are natural consequences. Obviously, in addition to the risk of death from infection and hemorrhage, uncontrolled growth of leukemic cells can terminate in metabolic starvation.

Onset

The precise onset of leukemia is unknown. Its clinical appearance varies markedly from acute to insidious. In most instances the child displays remarkably few symptoms. For example, it is quite typical for leukemia to be diagnosed when a minor infection, such as a cold, fails to completely disappear. The child continues to be pale, listless, irritable, febrile, and anorexic. Parents often suspect some underlying problem when they observe the weight loss, petechiae, bruising without cause, and continued complaints of bone and joint pain.

At other times leukemia is diagnosed after an extended history of signs and symptoms mimicking such conditions as rheumatoid arthritis or mononucleosis. There are also occasions when the diagnosis of leukemia accompanies some totally unrelated event, such as a routine physical examination or accidental injury.

The history not only yields valuable medical information regarding the subsequent course of the illness but also bears heavily on the parents' emotional reaction to the discovery of the diagnosis. In most instances the diagnosis is an unexpected revelation of catastrophic proportion.

Diagnostic Evaluation

Leukemia is usually suspected from the history, physical manifestations, and a peripheral blood smear that contains immature forms of leukocytes, frequently combined with low blood counts. Definitive diagnosis is based on bone marrow aspiration or biopsy. Typically the bone marrow is hypercellular with primarily blast cells. Once the diagnosis is confirmed, a lumbar puncture is performed to determine if there is any central nervous system involvement, although a very small number of children have CNS involvement and most are asymptomatic.

Therapeutic Management

Treatment of leukemia involves the use of chemotherapeutic agents with or without cranial irradiation in three phases: (1) *induction,* which achieves a complete remission or disappearance of leukemic cells; (2) *sanctuary therapy,* which prevents leukemic cells from invading or destroys leukemic cells in those areas of the body normally protected from cytotoxic drug levels; and (3) *maintenance,* which serves to maintain the remission phase. Although the combination of drugs and radiation may vary according to the institution, the prognostic or risk characteristics of the patient, and the type of leukemia being treated, the following general principles for each phase are consistently employed.

Remission induction. Almost immediately after confirmation of the diagnosis, induction therapy is begun and lasts for 4 to 6 weeks. The principal drugs used for induction in ALL are the corticosteroids (especially prednisone), vincristine, and L-asparaginase, with or without doxorubicin (see Table 36-3). Since combination-drug therapy has been more successful in inducing remissions than single-agent schedules, these drugs are used concurrently. Oral steroids are administered daily in divided doses to maintain consistently high blood levels. Vincristine is given by intravenous infusion once a week for a total of four to six doses, and L-asparaginase or doxorubicin is given at various schedules. Some treatment regimens include a period of *consolidation* or *intensification therapy* with one or more of the usual remission drugs. A complete remission is determined by the absence of clinical signs or symptoms of the disease and the presence of less than 5% blast cells in the bone marrow (may be described as an M_1-type bone marrow).

With AML the drug therapies differ from those used for lymphoid leukemia. The principal drugs used for induction therapy in AML are doxorubicin or daunomycin and cytosine arabinoside; various other drugs may be added.

Since many of the drugs also cause myelosuppression of normal blood elements, the period immediately following a remission can be critical; the body is defenseless against invading organisms (especially normal bacterial flora) and highly susceptible to spontaneous hemorrhage. Consequently, supportive therapy during this time is essential.

Sanctuary therapy. Sanctuary therapy refers to treatment directed at those anatomic areas that are protected to some degree from systemic chemotherapy—the central nervous system (protected by the blood-brain barrier) and the testes (lie outside the body). The second phase involves prophylactic treatment of the central nervous system with cranial irradiation and/or intrathecal administration of methotrexate. Because of the concern regarding late effects of cranial irradiation, this mode of therapy is generally reserved for high-risk patients and/or those with CNS disease. Therapy is usually begun during the first 6 to 8 weeks after diagnosis and may consist of daily high-dose radiation treatments for about 2 weeks and weekly or twice weekly doses of methotrexate for a total of five to six injections. Another approach is intrathecal chemotherapy, such as a combination of methotrexate, cytosine arabinoside, and steroids, without irradiation.

A second site that is resistant to chemotherapy and is responsible for leukemic relapse is the testes. A minority of males experience relapse during maintenance therapy or have occult disease after cessation of therapy. Most authorities believe in routine bilateral testicular biopsies at the time of terminating treatment to identify occult disease, followed by aggressive treatment for affected males, including bilateral testicular irradiation, intensive systemic chemotherapy, and central nervous system reinforcement therapy (Askin and others, 1981).

Maintenance. Maintenance, or continuation, therapy is begun after completion of successful induction and sanctuary therapy to preserve the remission and further reduce the number of leukemic cells. It begins when blood values start to approach normal levels. As with induction therapy, combined-drug regimens have been more successful in maintaining remissions and preventing drug resistance. Although a variety of combinations are used, a frequent schedule includes daily doses of oral 6-mercaptopurine and weekly doses of oral methotrexate. Intermittent short-term intensified therapy with prednisone and vincristine may be included. Depending on the type of leukemia and the risk factors of the child, several other drugs may be added to the intensification protocol.

During maintenance therapy, weekly or monthly complete blood counts are taken to evaluate the marrow's response to the drugs. If myelosuppression becomes severe (usually indicated by a white blood cell count below 2000/mm^3) or toxic side effects occur, therapy is temporarily stopped or the dose decreased.

Duration of therapy has been based on clinical experience comparing survival rates for various time intervals and is concerned with preventing deleterious effects of excessive treatment. While the optimum time for discontinuing therapy is not known, current research indicates that girls do not need therapy for longer than 1.5 years. Because of the risk of testicular relapse in boys, some centers favor longer maintenance programs, but in general the additional maintenance therapy appears to delay, not prevent, relapses (Bleyer, 1983). All children after cessation of therapy require regular medical evaluation for surveillance of relapse and long-term sequelae of treatment. Most relapses (16%)

occur during the first year off therapy, about 2% to 3% of the relapses occur during each of the next 3 years, and very few relapses occur after 6 years (Simone and Rivera, 1984).

Reinduction. For many children a fourth phase of therapy becomes necessary when a relapse occurs, as evidenced by the presence of leukemic cells within the bone marrow, which is described as type M_2 or M_3, depending on the percentage of leukemic cells. Usually reinduction for ALL includes the use of prednisone and vincristine with a combination of other drugs not previously used. Sanctuary and maintenance therapy follow as already outlined if a remission is induced. Although remissions may be achieved after more than one relapse, each relapse heralds an increasingly poor prognosis. However, more long-term second and subsequent remissions are occurring, and these may have better outlooks than previously thought (Musgrave, Dickerman, and Land, 1986).

Bone marrow transplantation. Bone marrow transplants have been used successfully in treating some children with ALL and ANLL. In general, bone marrow transplantation is not recommended for children with acute lymphocytic leukemia (ALL) during the first remission because of the excellent results possible with chemotherapy. The group with the best results have been those with ALL who receive the graft during the second remission (Poplack, 1985). Because of the poorer prognosis in children with acute nonlymphocytic leukemia (ANLL), transplantation may be considered during the first remission when a suitable donor is available (Grier and Weinstein, 1985).

Prognosis after transplantation varies with the timing of the procedure and the type of leukemia; reported ranges for long-term survival are between 25% and 50% (Wiley and DeCuir-Whalley, 1983). However, many of the transplanted children faced almost certain death without transplantation, so that even these low figures represent a major advance in eliciting a cure.

Nursing Considerations

Nursing care of the child with leukemia is directly related to the regimen of therapy. Secondary complications that necessitate supportive physical care are caused by myelosuppression, drug toxicity, and leukemic infiltration. Although this discussion is primarily concerned with the physical problems requiring nursing care, it also focuses on the specific emotional needs during diagnosis, treatment, and relapse. General aspects of care have been discussed under Nursing considerations for modes of therapy (p. 1573), and the psychologic interventions during significant phases of therapy are discussed in Chapter 23.

Prepare the family for diagnostic/therapeutic procedures. From the time before diagnosis to cessation of therapy, children must undergo several tests, the most traumatic of which are bone marrow aspiration or biopsy and lumbar punctures. Multiple fingersticks and venipunctures for blood analysis and drug infusion are common occurrences for several years after the diagnosis. Therefore the child needs an explanation of why each procedure is done and what can be expected (see also p. 1565).

Depending on the age of the child, one way of beginning such preparation is to explain the basic elements of the blood.* Using a drawing or letting the child look at a drop of blood under a microscope not only teaches but also encourages trust between the nurse and child. It also allows the nurse to assess the child's level of understanding. An error many health professionals make is to overestimate children's knowledge about their bodies. For example, a bone marrow aspiration makes sense only when it is clarified that the center of a bone is hollow and contains the cells that later become "working" blood cells or leukemic cells.

Prevent complications of myelosuppression. The leukemic process and most of the chemotherapeutic agents cause myelosuppression. The reduced numbers of blood cells result in secondary problems of infection, bleeding tendencies, and anemia. Supportive care involves both medical and nursing management. Because they are so closely linked, they are discussed together rather than separately.

Infection. The most frequent cause of death from leukemia is overwhelming infection secondary to neutropenia (defined as an absolute neutrophil count below 1000/mm^3) (Henschel, 1985). The child is most susceptible to overwhelming infection during three phases of his disease: (1) at the time of diagnosis and relapse when the leukemic process has replaced normal leukocytes, (2) during immunosuppressive therapy, and (3) after prolonged antibiotic therapy that predisposes to the growth of resistant organisms.

The organisms most lethal to these children are (1) viruses, particularly varicella (chickenpox), herpes zoster, herpes simplex, measles, rubella, mumps, and poliomyelitis; (2) *Pneumocystis carinii* (a protozoan); (3) fungi, especially *Candida albicans;* (4) gram-negative bacteria, such as *Pseudomonas aeruginosa, Escherichia coli, Proteus,* and *Klebsiella;* and (5) gram-positive bacteria, especially *Staphylococcus aureus, S. epidermidis,* and group A β-hemolytic streptococcus. As prophylaxis against these various organisms, broad-spectrum antibiotics are usually prescribed. Ensuring compliance with this long-term regimen is an important nursing responsibility.

Because the usual viral infections of childhood are particularly dangerous, immunizations against these diseases (measles, rubella, mumps, and polio) are not given until the child's immune system is capable of responding appropriately to the vaccine (at least 3 months after termination of chemotherapy during remission) (American Academy of Pediatrics, 1986). If immunization is given when the immune system is depressed, the attenuated virus can result in an overwhelming infection. Exceptions are the use of the Salk (inactivated) vaccine for poliomyelitis and the newly developed varicella (chickenpox) vaccine, which has been shown

---

*Appropriate literature is listed on p. 984; especially recommended is Baker, L.: You and leukemia: one day at a time.

to be effective in preventing varicella in high-risk children (Gershon and others, 1984).

The first defense against infection is prevention. When the child is hospitalized, the nurse employs all measures to control transfer of infection. These typically include the use of a private room, restriction of all visitors and health personnel with active infection, and strict handwashing technique with an antiseptic solution. The use of protective (reverse) isolation is controversial; however, research provides evidence that protective isolation does *not* decrease the risk of infection nor improve survival (Nauseef and Maki, 1981). Therefore any decision to implement protective isolation must be seriously evaluated in terms of its doubtful benefit and the psychologic stress it imposes on the child.

The child is evaluated for potential sites of infection, such as from a needle puncture, mucosal ulceration, or minor abrasion or skin tears, such as a hangnail. Although the body is unable to mount an adequate inflammatory response to the infection and the usual clinical signs of infection may be partially expressed or absent, fever will occur. Consequently, any elevation of temperature is considered a sign of infection (Henschel, 1985). To identify the source of infection, blood, stool, urine, and nasopharyngeal cultures and chest x-ray films are taken. Broad-spectrum intravenous antibiotic therapy is begun before the organism is identified and continued for the usual 7- to 10-day period, regardless of whether a specific agent is isolated. If the child does not have an intraarterial line (Broviac/Hickman catheter or implanted infusion port), a heparin lock should be inserted to prevent the inconvenience of multiple venipunctures to maintain a patent intravenous line and limited activity imposed by an immobilized body part.

Prevention of infection continues as a priority after discharge from the hospital. However, rigid social restriction must be tempered with the child's need for resuming normal activity. Ordinarily the child can return to school when the absolute neutrophil count is above 500/mm^3. If the level falls below this value, cautious isolation from crowded areas, such as shopping centers or subways, is advisable. At all times family members are encouraged to practice good handwashing to prevent introducing pathogens into the home.

A very important indication for isolation is an outbreak of childhood disease, especially chickenpox. The child is confined from all known sources of the infection, such as schoolmates, until the epidemic is over. Ideally the school nurse should work with the treating physician to decide the optimum time for school reattendance. If the child has been exposed to the varicella virus, varicella-zoster immune globulin (VZIG) given within 96 hours may favorably alter the course of the disease, or antiviral agents, such as acyclovir, may be given. These antiviral agents are very effective in preventing serious disease if given during the first 3 days of the appearance of symptoms (Shulman, 1985). Without treatment, death from disseminated varicella (about 7%) is usually caused by pneumonia; other serious although non-fatal complications include hepatitis, pancreatitis, meningitis, and bacterial skin infections.

Nutrition is another important component of infection prevention. An adequate protein-calorie intake provides the child with better host defenses against infection and increased tolerance to chemotherapy and irradiation. However, providing optimum nutrition during periods of anorexia and vomiting from chemotherapy is a tremendous challenge. Every effort is made to encourage the child to eat (see suggestions on p. 1116), and if nonoral feedings are instituted, meticulous care in terms of the feeding procedure is implemented to prevent infection.

Hemorrhage. Before the use of transfused platelets, hemorrhage was a leading cause of death in leukemia. Now most bleeding episodes can be prevented or controlled with judicious administration of platelet concentrates or platelet-rich plasma. Severe spontaneous internal hemorrhage usually does not occur until the platelet count is 10,000/mm^3 (Allegretta, Weisman, and Altman, 1985).

Since infection increases the tendency toward hemorrhage, and bleeding sites become more easily infected, special care is taken to avoid performing skin punctures whenever possible. When fingersticks, venipunctures, intramuscular injections, and bone marrow aspirations are performed, aseptic technique must be employed with continued observation for bleeding. Meticulous mouth care is essential, since gingival bleeding with resultant mucositis is a frequent problem. Since the rectal area is prone to ulceration from various drugs, feces and urine are removed immediately and the perianal area washed. To prevent additional trauma, rectal temperatures are not taken. Frequent turning, the use of a flotation or alternating-pressure mattress, and sheepskin under bony prominences prevent development of pressure areas and decubital ulcers.

Platelet transfusions are generally reserved for active bleeding episodes that do not respond to local treatment and that may occur during induction or relapse therapy. Epistaxis and gingival bleeding are the most common. The nurse teaches parents and older children measures to control nose bleeding (see p. 1549). Pressure at the site without disturbing clot formation is the general rule.

Two of the problems with multiple platelet transfusions are the risk of febrile reactions and decreased life span of the platelets. Platelet concentrates normally do not have to be crossmatched for blood group or type. However, because platelets contain specific antigen components similar to blood group factors, children who receive multiple transfusions may become immunized to a platelet group other than their own. Therefore it is advisable to crossmatch platelets with the donor's blood components whenever this is possible.

Transfused platelets generally survive in the body for 1 to 3 days. The peak effect is reached in about 2 hours and decreased by half in 24 hours. Therefore after a transfusion the nurse observes and records the approximate time when hemostasis of bleeding sites occurs. Delayed hemostasis is evidence of platelet destruction. For long-term leukemia patients, multiple transfusion therapy becomes progressively less effective.

During bleeding episodes the parents and child need much emotional support. The sight of oozing blood is very upsetting. Often parents will request a platelet transfusion, unaware of the necessity of trying local measures first. The nurse can be instrumental in allaying anxiety by explaining the reason for delaying a platelet transfusion until absolutely necessary. Since compatible donors decrease the risk of antigen formation in the recipient, the nurse should encourage parents to locate suitable donors for eventual blood use.

Children at home who have low platelet counts (usually below 100,000 mm³) are advised to avoid those activities that might cause injury or bleeding, such as riding bicycles or skateboards, roller skating, and contact sports. These restrictions can be terminated once the platelet count rises, such as after platelet transfusion. In addition, parents must be aware that aspirin and aspirin-containing products are avoided; for mild pain or significantly elevated temperature, acetaminophen is substituted.

Anemia. Initially anemia may be profound from complete replacement of the bone marrow by leukemic cells. During induction therapy, blood transfusions with packed red cells may be necessary to raise hemoglobin to levels approaching 10 g. The usual precautions in caring for the anemic child are instituted (see p. 1520).

Anemia is also a consequence of drug-induced myelosuppression. Although not as severely affected as the white blood cells, erythrocyte production may be delayed. Since children have an amazing capacity to withstand low hemoglobin levels, the best approach is to allow the child to regulate his activity with reasonable adult supervision. It may be necessary for the parents to alert the schoolteacher to the child's physical limitations, particularly in terms of strenuous activity.

Manage problems of irradiation and drug toxicity. Irradiation and chemotherapy present several challenges to providing effective care. The complexity of the treatment protocols alone is often overwhelming to families, who can benefit from receiving a monthly calendar of anticipated treatment dates. In addition, each therapy is associated with a number of predictable side effects (see Tables 36-3 and 36-4). The following is a discussion of these reactions and appropriate interventions.

Nausea and vomiting. The nausea and vomiting that occur shortly after administration of several of the drugs and as a result of cranial radiation can be profound. Although a number of antiemetic agents are available, no product is uniformly successful in controlling the vomiting. For mild to moderate vomiting, antiemetics such as promethazine (Phenergan), chlorpromazine (Thorazine), prochlorperazine (Compazine), or trimethobenzamide (Tigan) may be effective. Metoclopramide (Reglan) is a more effective antiemetic for severe vomiting, especially that induced by cisplatin (the chemotherapeutic agent with the highest emetic potential) (Flaherty, 1985). Unfortunately, the drug causes a number of side effects in children, particularly extrapyramidal reactions, such as muscle tremors or twitching, agi-

tation, grimacing, dysarthria, and oculogyric crisis (fixation of eyes in one position for minutes or hours) (Terrin, McWilliams, and Maurer, 1984). Another drug that has yielded promising results is THC (delta-9-tetrahydrocannabinol), the active component of marijuana. As of this writing the drug is available only from major cancer centers and is not uniformly effective for all patients.

The most beneficial regimen for antiemetic control has been the administration of the antiemetic *before* the chemotherapy begins (30 minutes to 1 hour before) and regular (not PRN) administration every 2, 4, or 6 hours for at least 24 hours after chemotherapy (Yasko, 1985). The goal is to prevent the child from ever experiencing nausea or vomiting, since this can prevent the development of anticipatory symptoms (the conditioned response of developing nausea and vomiting before receiving the drug) (Dolgin and others, 1985). Other nonpharmacologic interventions (similar to those discussed for pain management on p. 1071) can be useful in controlling posttherapy and anticipatory nausea and vomiting (Morrow and Morrell, 1982; Yasko, 1985; Hockenberry and Cotanch, 1985). Giving the antineoplastic drug with a mild sedative at bedtime is also helpful for some children, and there is evidence that nighttime administration of drugs such as methotrexate and 6-mercaptopurine may be more effective cytotoxically than morning administration (Rivard and others, 1985).

Anorexia. Loss of appetite is a direct consequence of the chemotherapy, irradiation, and nausea and vomiting. It is a major problem for parents because it is the one area they feel responsible for, particularly when so many other facets of care are outside their control. There are no universally successful techniques for encouraging a sick child to eat. However, the guidelines on p. 1116 can be helpful during the anorexic period and can prevent additional problems during the remission.

Some children still do not eat despite these approaches. The following theories have been postulated to explain persistent anorexia: (1) a physical cause related to the cancer that is nonspecific; (2) a conditioned aversion to food from nausea and vomiting during treatment; (3) stress in the environment, related to eating and/or to the child's condition; (4) depression; (5) a control mechanism when so much else has been imposed on him; and (6) an opportunity to express anger at his parents and punish them for "allowing" him to become sick. When loss of appetite and weight persist, the nurse should investigate the family situation to determine if any of these variables are contributing to the problem. To prevent conditioned aversion to food, it is best to offer few foods and no favorite foods prior to chemotherapy (Bernstein, Webster, and Bernstein, 1982).

Mucosal ulceration. One of the most distressing side effects of several drugs is gastrointestinal mucosal cell damage, which results in ulcers anywhere along the alimentary tract. Oral ulcers (stomatitis) are red, eroded, painful areas in the mouth and/or pharynx. They may extend along the esophagus and frequently occur in the rectal area. They greatly compound anorexia, because eating is extremely uncomfortable. When oral ulcers develop, the following interventions are helpful: (1) a bland, moist, soft diet, (2) use of a soft sponge toothbrush (Toothettes)* or cotton-tipped applicator, (3) frequent mouthwashes with normal saline, and (4) local anesthetics such as Chloraseptic spray, viscous lidocaine, or nonprescription preparations, such as Orabase. Although local anesthetics are effective in temporarily relieving the pain, many children dislike the taste and numb feeling they produce. Viscous lidocaine is not recommended for young children; if applied to the pharynx, it may depress the gag reflex, increasing the risk of aspiration. Insensitivity to the temperature of food can also cause burns.

Other solutions that help coat the denuded areas and may be effective if accepted by children are Kaopectate (with or without Benadryl) and sucralfate (Carafate). Agents such as lemon glycerin swabs, hydrogen peroxide, and milk of magnesia are avoided because of the drying effects on the mucosa. In addition, lemon may be irritating to eroded tissue and can decay the teeth (Daeffler, 1980). A strategy that may be helpful is massaging the area on the backs of both hands between the thumb and index finger with an ice cube for 5 to 7 minutes until the area becomes numb. This procedure, based on acupuncture, has been successful in decreasing dental pain (Melzack, Guite, and Gonshor, 1980).

Administering mouth care is particularly difficult in infants and toddlers. A satisfactory method of cleaning the gums is to wrap a piece of gauze around a finger, soak it in saline or plain water, and swab the gums, palate, and inner cheek surfaces with the finger. Mouthwashes are best accomplished with plain water or saline, because the child cannot gargle or spit out excess fluid. Mouth care should be done routinely before and after any feeding and as often as every 2 to 4 hours to rid mucosal surfaces of debris, which becomes an excellent medium for bacterial and fungal growth.

Dental hygiene can become a serious problem if the child wears an orthodontic appliance. The accumulated debris on braces is difficult to remove without vigorous brushing, and the appliance itself traumatizes the gums. Sometime braces are removed to allow chemotherapy to continue.

Difficulty in eating is a major problem with stomatitis and may warrant hospitalization if the child refuses fluids. The child will usually choose the foods that are best tolerated. Surprisingly, some children prefer salty foods to more bland ones. Drinking can usually be encouraged if a straw is used to bypass the ulcerated oral mucosa. The nurse should encourage parents to relax any eating pressures, because the anorexia accompanying stomatitis is well justified. In addition, since it is a temporary condition, once the ulcers heal the child can resume good food habits. Ordinarily severe mucosal ulceration indicates a need for decreased chemotherapy until complete healing takes place, usually within a week.

If rectal ulcers develop, meticulous toilet hygiene, warm sitz baths after each bowel movement, and periodic exposure of the ulcerated area to warm heat promote healing, and the use of stool softeners is necessary to prevent further

discomfort. Sometimes a rectal ulcer can be so uncomfortable that the child prefers to spend as much time as possible in the bathtub. Parents should be advised to record bowel movements, since the child may voluntarily avoid defecation to prevent discomfort. Rectal temperatures are not taken because the thermometer may further traumatize the area.

Neuropathy. Vincristine and to a lesser extent vinblastine can cause various neurotoxic effects, one of the more common of which is severe constipation from decreased bowel innervation. The nurse advises parents to record bowel movements and to notify the physician of a change in stool habits. Physical activity and stool softeners are helpful in preventing the problem, but laxatives, such as Peri-Colace, or enemas are often necessary to stimulate evacuation. Dietary changes such as increased fiber are not advised, because the increased bulk tends to increase fecal distention and discomfort without producing the necessary mechanical stimulation (Cimprich, 1985).

Footdrop and weakness and numbing of the extremities may cause difficulty in walking or fine hand movement. The nurse should warn parents of these side effects, which are reversible once the drug is stopped. If the child is on bed rest, a footboard should be used to preserve proper alignment. If weakness occurs while the child is attending school, a temporary alteration of activity may be necessary. The teacher should be apprised of the situation so that unrealistic expectations of the child's abilities are not made.

Another side effect that can be severe is jaw pain. Analgesics may be necessary to relieve the discomfort. Avoiding movement by not talking or chewing is usually self-imposed, although continuous chewing, such as with gum, may actually reduce the pain. Since the pain is temporary, usually lasting for a day or two, the child can be given fluids through a straw.

A neurologic syndrome (postirradiation somnolence) may develop 5 to 8 weeks after central nervous system irradiation and may last for 4 to 15 days. It is characterized by somnolence with or without fever, anorexia, and nausea and vomiting. Parents should be warned of the possibility of such symptoms and encouraged to seek medical evaluation, since somnolence may be an early indicator of long-term neurologic sequelae after cranial irradiation (Ch'ien and others, 1980).

Hemorrhagic cystitis. Sterile hemorrhagic cystitis is a side effect of chemical irritation to the bladder from cyclophosphamide. It can be prevented by (1) a liberal fluid intake (at least one and one-half times the recommended daily fluid requirement (2 liters per meter squared per day), (2) frequent voiding immediately after feeling the urge, including immediately before bed and after arising (some authorities include one nighttime void), and (3) administering the drug early in the day to allow for sufficient intake of oral fluids and frequent voiding. If signs of cystitis such as burning on urination occur, prompt medical evaluation is needed. Hemorrhagic cystitis warrants cessation of the drug and is more frequently a complication of oral cyclophosphamide than of intravenous administration. In the latter instance intravenous fluids are given before, during, and after the drug to ensure adequate hydration, thereby eliminating the need for the child's drinking large amounts of fluid. If oral home administration is prescribed, the family needs *specific* instructions on exactly how much fluid the child must have.

Alopecia. Hair loss is a side effect of several chemotherapeutic drugs and cranial irradiation. Not all children lose their hair during drug therapy; however, retaining hair is the exception rather than the rule. It is better to warn children and parents of this side effect than to allow them to think that it is only a remote possibility. Encouraging a child to choose a wig similar to his own hairstyle and color *before* the hair falls out is helpful in fostering later adjustment to hair loss. The family should know that the hair falls out in clumps, causing patchy baldness. To lessen the trauma of seeing large amounts of hair on bed linen or clothing, the child can wear a disposable surgical cap to collect the shed hair during the period of greatest hair loss or cut the hair short. Families should also be aware that wigs are tax deductible and that hair regrows in 3 to 6 months. The hair frequently is darker, thicker, and curlier than before.

If the child chooses not to wear a wig, attention to some type of head covering is important, especially in cold or sunny climates. Scalp hygiene is also important. The scalp should be washed regularly like any other body part.

Many children demonstrate increased tolerance to hair loss on reinduction therapy. Rather than complete baldness, the child may experience thinning of the hair. If the hair is cut short, kept clean, and blow-dried with an electric hair drier, it usually can look full enough to make a wig unnecessary. This can be a tremendous psychologic boost to the child who is already depressed about learning of a relapse and the need for additional chemotherapy.

Although nothing can prevent alopecia from cranial irradiation, the use of a scalp tourniquet or hypothermia cap may prevent hair loss from drugs. A scalp tourniquet is a wide rubber band that is placed around the head near the hairline during drug infusion and kept in place for several minutes after administration of the drug. The hypothermia cap* is a durable polyurethane cap filled with cryogel for maximum cooling. The use of the tourniquet and cap is controversial; widely disseminated cancers such as leukemia and lymphoma and most solid tumors are contraindications. Exceptions may be made for adolescents who refuse treatment because of alopecia or children with isolated tumors during maintenance therapy.

Moon face. Short-term steroid therapy produces no acute toxicities and often results in two beneficial reactions—increased appetite and a sense of well-being. However, it does produce alterations in body image, which, although not clinically significant, can be extremely distressing to older children. One of these is moon face. The child's face becomes rounded and puffy (see Fig. 38-3).

*Manufactured by Con Med International Inc., Los Angeles, CA.

Unlike hair loss, little can be done to camouflage this obvious change, although careful avoidance of salt and salt-containing foods can help reduce fluid accumulation. It is not unusual for other children to make fun of the child with such remarks as "porky-pig" or "fat face." For the child who experiences such name-calling, it is helpful to reassure him that after cessation of the drug the facial contours will return to normal. If the child resumes activity early in the course of treatment, the change may be less noticeable to peers than after a long absence. Also, the use of loose-fitting clothes, such as warm-up outfits, can help camouflage the change in weight.

In contrast, parents may appreciate the full-rounded appearance because it simulates the look of a well-nourished, healthy child. Because of their own needs, they may be less able to understand the child's misery over his altered body image. The nurse can foster a better understanding between the parents and child if both parties are encouraged to openly discuss their feelings.

Children on steroid therapy do look healthy. The moon face, red cheeks, supraclavicular fat pads, protuberant abdomen, and fluid retention indicate weight gain. However, the actual weight gain resulting from increased muscle mass and subcutaneous tissue may be small. Therefore the nurse should evaluate weight gain carefully during steroid therapy to make certain that some of it is a result of increased dietary intake. This is done by observing the extremities and measuring skinfold thickness and arm circumference.

Mood changes. Shortly after beginning steroid therapy, children may experience a number of mood changes, which range from feelings of well-being and euphoria to depression and irritability. If parents are unaware of these drug-induced changes, they may become unduly concerned. Therefore the nurse should warn them of the reactions and encourage them to discuss the behavioral changes with each other and the child.

Provide continued emotional support. The preceding discussion of nursing care of the child with leukemia is based on typical problems with which the family is confronted during the treatment phases. It is not unusual for a child who discontinues therapy after 2 or 3 years and maintains a permanent remission to experience many of these side effects. Therefore the nurse's role is continually one of support, guidance, clarification, and judgment. Parents need to know how to recognize symptoms that demand medical attention. Although some of the reactions discussed are expected, parents still should report them to their physician. Warning parents of their possible occurrence beforehand also allows parents the opportunity to prepare for them. At the same time it reassures them that these reactions are not caused by a return of leukemic cells.

The nurse must also use judgment in recognizing which side effects are normal reactions and which indicate toxicity. Frequently it is the office or clinic nurse who screens such telephone calls and gives advice when appropriate. Usually nausea and vomiting are not indications for drug cessation. However, severe vomiting may require immediate intervention to prevent dehydration. Signs of infection, mucosal ulceration, hemorrhagic cystitis, peripheral neuropathy, and obstipation require medical evaluation.

Another aspect of continued emotional support involves prognosis. Certainly leukemia can no longer be defined as invariably fatal. However, present statistics must also be correctly interpreted; while more than 95% of children with ALL will achieve an initial remission and as many as 60% of them will live 5 years or longer, it must be remembered that these are *average* estimates and are applicable to those children treated with the latest protocols since diagnosis. For the low-risk child the chances may be better, but for the high-risk child they may be significantly poorer. Of those who do survive after discontinuing therapy, a portion will relapse. Therefore at present only the passage of time is positive confirmation of the child who is ultimately "cured" of the disease.

The nurse must be familiar with these statistics in order to interpret them correctly to parents. At the same time the nurse must realize that a realistic understanding of the chances for survival requires an adjustment period. For example, it is not unusual for parents to interpret the "95% remission" as the probability for a cure. When a relapse occurs, parents may for the first time be able to "hear" the correct facts.

Statistics are numbers. Sometimes they bring hope and at other times despair. Although very important in terms of research, better treatment, and identification of high- or low-risk populations, they present a general picture of what to expect. The nurse who is working with family members must individualize the "numbers" to relate to the people. An understanding of each member's emotional needs, as well as competent care of physical ones, is essential to the positive, growth-promoting support of the family. Comprehensive emotional support for the family through all phases of the illness is discussed in Chapter 23.

Nursing Care Summary: The Child with Cancer

NURSING GOALS	NURSING INTERVENTIONS	EXPECTED PATIENT/FAMILY OUTCOMES
HP-HMP	**Infection: potential for**	
	Risk factors: reduced body defenses (myelosuppression)	
Minimize risk of infection	See Nursing care summary of the child with immunosuppression, p. 1554	
HP-HMP	**Injury: potential for tissue damage, hemorrhage**	
	Risk factors: undiagnosed tumor, fatigue, antimetabolites, intracranial trauma (brain tumor)	
Recognize cancer early	Be alert to signs and symptoms that might indicate cancer (see Table 36-2, 7, and 8) Obtain thorough history Carry out thorough physical assessment, especially regarding affected area, including Functional status Signs of inflammation, anemia Size of mass Regional lymph node involvement Ocular changes Weight loss	*Cancer is detected early and appropriate action implemented
Prevent hemorrhagic cystitis	Observe for signs (burning and pain on urination) Give liberal (3000 ml/m²/day) fluid intake Encourage frequent voiding, including during nighttime	Urine remains clear; voids without discomfort; sufficient output (urinary)
Prevent hemorrhage	Use all measures to prevent infection, especially in ecchymotic areas Use local measures to stop bleeding Restrict strenuous activity that could result in accidental injury Involve child in responsibility for limiting activity when platelet count drops	No evidence of bleeding
POSTOPERATIVE CARE (BRAIN TUMOR)		
Prevent hyperthermia	Place hypothermia blanket on bed prior to child's return to room View any temperature elevation as potential sign of infection	Temperature remains within acceptable limits (specify)

*Nursing outcome.

Continued.

Nursing Care Summary: The Child with Cancer—cont'd

NURSING GOALS	NURSING INTERVENTIONS	EXPECTED PATIENT/FAMILY OUTCOMES
Monitor vital functions	Take vital signs, blood pressure, and ocular signs every 15-30 minutes until stable Auscultate respiratory status, especially for evidence of decreased breath sounds Institute tests for function after child is alert Observe level of consciousness, noting sleep pattern and response to stimuli	*Deviations from baseline findings are detected early
Prevent pneumonia	Institute breathing exercises (incentive spirometer) when child is awake.	Lungs remain clear; respirations within acceptable limits (see inside front cover for normal variations)
Maintain desired position Prevent fluid overload or dehydration	Turn child cautiously to maintain proper position Check gag and swallowing reflexes before offering clear oral fluids Stop oral fluids if vomiting occurs Calculate all fluids very carefully to prevent overload Measure urinary output, especially if hypertonic solutions for brain edema are given	Child remains in desired position Child exhibits no signs of fluid overload or dehydration
Prevent eye damage	Apply ice compresses to eyes for short intervals to relieve edema Keep eyes closed or apply eye dressings May need to instill normal saline eye drops to prevent corneal ulceration if blink reflex is depressed	Eyes remain clear with no evidence of irritation

Provide special postoperative care	Observe dressings for drainage
	    Reinforce with sterile gauze pads but do not remove bandage
	    Circle area of drainage to note further seepage
	    Report evidence of clear fluid (cerebrospinal fluid) immediately
	    Restrain child's hands as necessary to preserve intact dressing
		Dressing remains intact
		*Observations are noted and recorded

N-MP   Nutrition, alteration in: less than body requirements
Etiology: loss of appetite

Stimulate appetite	Encourage parents to relax; stress legitimate nature of loss of appetite Allow child *any* food he tolerates; plan to improve quality of food selections when appetite increases Stress expected increase in appetite from steroids Take advantage of any hungry period; serve small "snacks" Fortify foods with nutritious supplements, such as powdered milk or commercial supplements Allow child to be involved in food preparation and selection Make food appealing Remember usual food practices of children in each age-group, such as food jags in toddlers or normal occurrence of physiologic anorexia Assess family for additional problems (e.g., use of food by child as a control mechanism if appetite does not improve despite improved physical status) See Feeding the sick child, p. 1115	Child consumes adequate amounts of appropriate foods

*Nursing outcome.

Nursing Care Summary: The Child with Cancer—cont'd

NURSING GOALS	NURSING INTERVENTIONS	EXPECTED PATIENT/FAMILY OUTCOMES
N-MP Oral mucous membrane, alteration in **Etiology: administration of antimetabolites, disease process**		

Prevent ulceration	Inspect mouth daily for oral ulcers
	Institute meticulous oral hygiene as soon as a drug is used that causes oral ulcers
	  Use soft-sponge toothbrush, cotton-tipped applicator, or gauze-wrapped finger
	  Administer frequent (at least every 4 hours and after meals) mouthwashes (normal saline)
	Report evidence of ulcers to physician
	Apply local anesthetics to ulcerated areas before meals and as needed
	Serve bland, moist, soft diet
	Encourage fluids; use a straw to help bypass painful areas
		Mucous membranes remain intact

N-MP Skin integrity, impairment of; potential **Risk factors: administration of antimetabolites, radiotherapy, immobility**		
Prevent skin breakdown	Provide meticulous skin care, especially in mouth and perianal regions Change position frequently Encourage adequate calorie-protein intake	Skin remains intact

Reduce undesirable effects of therapy	Suggest and/or implement measures to reduce physical effects of radiotherapy
	  Select loose-fitting clothing over irradiated area to minimize additional irritation
	  Protect area from sunlight and sudden changes in temperature (avoid ice packs, heating pads)
		Child and family comply with suggestions (specify)

EP Bowel elimination, alteration in: constipation **Etiology: medications, pain on defecation**		
Prevent or reduce effects of rectal ulcers	Wash perianal area after each bowel movement Use warm sitz baths or tub baths as frequently as necessary for comfort Expose ulcerated area to warm heat to hasten healing Observe for constipation resulting from child's voluntary refusal to defecate or from chemotherapy Do not take rectal temperatures or use suppositories Record bowel movements; use stool softener to prevent constipation; may need stimulants for evacuation	Rectal mucosa remains clean and intact Ulcerated areas heal without complications
A-EP Activity intolerance, potential **Risk factors: anemia, reduced energy and fatigue**		
Promote rest and reduce fatigue	Allow child to monitor his activity Encourage rest periods throughout day and at least 8 to 10 hours of sleep at night *For severe anemia, see Nursing care summary, p. 1521	Child engages in activities according to his abilities

*Nursing outcome.

Continued.

Nursing Care Summary: The Child with Cancer—cont'd

NURSING GOALS	NURSING INTERVENTIONS	EXPECTED PATIENT/FAMILY OUTCOMES

A-EP   Mobility, impaired physical
Etiology: decreased strength and endurance, pain and discomfort, neuromuscular
impairment, amputation of lower extremity (osteosarcoma)

NURSING GOALS	NURSING INTERVENTIONS	EXPECTED PATIENT/FAMILY OUTCOMES
Reduce effects of peripheral neuropathy	Encourage ambulation when child is able Alter activity to prevent accidents if weakness occurs, including school attendance Use footboard to prevent footdrop Provide fluids and soft foods to lessen chewing movements	Child ambulates without incident
Assist with managing loss of limb	Assist with early ambulation and use of temporary prosthesis Arrange for, carry out, or supervise physical therapy as prescribed Arrange for preparation of permanent prosthesis Teach use of auxiliary appliances such as wheelchair or crutches	Child and family adjust to loss of limb

CPP   Comfort, alteration in: pain
Etiology: physiologic effects, neoplasia

NURSING GOALS	NURSING INTERVENTIONS	EXPECTED PATIENT/FAMILY OUTCOMES
Relieve pain	Assess need for pain management (see p. 1168) During terminal stage, appreciate that pain control is necessary component of physical and emotional care Avoid excessive noise or light Place all commodities within easy reach Use gentle, minimal physical manipulation Avoid pressure (bedclothes, sheets) on painful areas Experiment with using heat or cold on painful areas (use cautiously because of easy skin breakdown) Change position frequently; if difficult for child, coordinate with pain relief from analgesics Avoid pressure on bony prominences or painful sites (water bed, bean bag chair, flotation mattress); ensure good body alignment Evaluate effectiveness of pain relief with degree of alertness vs sedation Implement appropriate nonpharmacologic pain reduction techniques (see p. 1071)	Child rests quietly, exhibits no evidence of discomfort, verbalizes no complaints of discomfort

CPP   Sensory-perceptual alteration: visual, auditory, kinesthetic, gustatory, tactile, olfactory
Etiology: altered sensory reception, transmission, and/or integration related to brain tumor

NURSING GOALS	NURSING INTERVENTIONS	EXPECTED PATIENT/FAMILY OUTCOMES
Observe progress of signs and symptoms	Keep daily records of signs and symptoms to assess child's physical capabilities and to assist family in adjusting to insidious or acute deterioration (see Table 36-7)	*Child's physical signs and behaviors are observed and recorded *Deviations from normal findings are determined early, and appropriate interventions are implemented

SP-SCP   Self-concept, disturbance in: body image
Etiology: loss of hair, moon face, debilitation, loss of limb (osteosarcoma)

NURSING GOALS	NURSING INTERVENTIONS	EXPECTED PATIENT/FAMILY OUTCOMES
Help child and family cope with hair loss	Introduce idea of wig prior to hair loss Administer good scalp hygiene	Child verbalizes concern regarding hair loss

*Nursing outcome.

Nursing Care Summary: The Child with Cancer—cont'd

NURSING GOALS	NURSING INTERVENTIONS	EXPECTED PATIENT/FAMILY OUTCOMES
Help child and family cope with hair loss—cont'd	Provide adequate covering during exposure to sunlight, wind, or cold Suggest keeping thin hair clean, short, and fluffy to camouflage partial baldness Stress that hair begins to regrow in 3-6 months and may be a slightly different color or texture Stress that alopecia during a second treatment with same drug may be much less severe	Child helps determine methods to reduce effects of hair loss and applies these methods
Promote adjustment to altered facial appearance	Encourage rapid reintegration with peers to lessen contrast of changed facial appearance Stress that this reaction is temporary Evaluate weight gain carefully (in weight gain resulting from administration of steroids, extremities remain thin)	Child resumes former activities and relationships within capabilities
Assist child to adjust to disability (amputation)	Encourage visits from friends before discharge to prepare child for reactions and questions Encourage early and consistent interaction with peers Assist child to become adept in use of appliances Assist child to select clothing to camouflage prosthesis	Child resumes former contacts and activities commensurate with limitations
	Encourage good hygiene, grooming, and sex-appropriate items to enhance appearance, such as wig (for hair loss from antimetabolites), makeup, attractive, sex-appropriate clothing	Child appears clean, well-groomed, and attractively dressed

RRP   Grieving, anticipatory
Etiology: perceived potential loss of child, prospect of loss of limb or other bodily function

NURSING GOALS	NURSING INTERVENTIONS	EXPECTED PATIENT/FAMILY OUTCOMES
Help family face possibility of child's death	Provide consistent contact with family Primary nurse Clarify, refocus, and supply information as needed Help family plan care of child, especially at terminal stage (e.g., extent of extraordinary life-saving measures) Arrange for spiritual support in accordance with family's beliefs and/or affiliations	Family remains open to counseling and nursing contacts Family and child discuss their fears, concerns, needs, and desires at terminal stage Appropriate religious representative is contacted (specify)
Prepare child and family for possible amputation or limb salvage procedure	Employ straightforward honesty Avoid disguising diagnosis with terms such as "infection" Emphasize lack of alternatives Answer questions regarding information presented by surgeon and clarify any misconceptions Avoid overwhelming child or parents with too much information Be available and willing to listen and to talk to child and parents about their concerns Allow for and encourage expression of feelings	Family and child express feelings regarding potential loss Family and child readily discuss concerns and ask appropriate questions
Help child adjust to potential loss	Allow child time and opportunity to go through grief process Allow for expression of feelings regarding limb loss and undesirable effects of chemotherapy Assist child to cope with side effects Encourage independence	Child expresses feelings regarding impending alteration in life style

Continued.

Nursing Care Summary: The Child with Cancer—cont'd

NURSING GOALS	NURSING INTERVENTIONS	EXPECTED PATIENT/FAMILY OUTCOMES
RRP	**Family process, alteration in**	
	Etiology: situational crisis (child with a life-threatening disease)	
Support family	Help family plan for future, especially toward helping child live a normal life	Family discusses feelings and concerns
	Encourage family to discuss feelings regarding child's course prior to diagnosis and his prospects for survival	
	Discuss with family how they will tell child about outcome of surgery and need for additional treatment (if appropriate)	
	Advise family of expected therapy side effects vs toxicities; clarify which demand medical evaluation (mucosal ulceration, hemorrhagic cystitis, peripheral neuropathy, evidence of infection or dehydration)	Family demonstrates understanding of consequences of therapies
	Reassure family that such reactions are not caused by return of cancer cells	
	Interpret prognostic statistics carefully, realizing family's temporary need to interpret them as they see necessary	
	Refer to local chapter of American Cancer Society, Leukemia Society of America, Inc. or other organizations	
	See also The hospitalized child, p. 1075; Family of the hospitalized child, p. 1081	
Prepare family for diagnostic/therapeutic procedures	Explain reason for each test (fingersticks, venipunctures, bone marrow aspirations, lumbar punctures, x-ray treatments)	Family demonstrates understanding of procedures (specify learnings and manner of demonstration)
	Explain basic elements of blood to provide foundational information for tests and therapies	
	Encourage older children and parents to learn meaning of various blood values	
	Explain bone marrow aspiration and lumbar puncture with step-by-step approach and point out those few procedures that are painful	
	Use recall of each step as method of distraction	
	Whenever possible, make use of procedures that minimize discomfort, such as Broviac catheter, heparin lock, or Ommaya reservoir	
	Explain reason for radiotherapy	
	Explain responsibility of child, e.g., need to remain motionless during test and/or radiotherapy	
	Explain operative procedure honestly (if appropriate)	
	Avoid overpreparation	
	Avoid overemphasis on benefits, which may not be evident for several days postoperatively	
	Arrange for child and parents to visit special intensive care unit where he will be postoperatively	Child and family visit ICU
	Explain to child what he will experience after surgery	Child and family demonstrate understanding of information presented (specify information and manner of demonstration)
	See also Preparation for procedures, p. 1104	
Prepare child's scalp for surgery for brain tumor	Prepare child and parents for head shaving	Head is shaved with minimum of distress to child and family
	Provide absolute privacy	
	Save long hair by braiding it first	
	Allow child to look into mirror at different stages to lessen shock of total baldness	

Nursing Care Summary: The Child with Cancer—cont'd

NURSING GOALS	NURSING INTERVENTIONS	EXPECTED PATIENT/FAMILY OUTCOMES
Prepare child's scalp for surgery for brain tumor—cont'd	Provide attractive covering (lacy nightcap or baseball cap) Shave head carefully to prevent skin cuts, which can become infected Cleanse scalp as prescribed Prepare child and parents for large dressing; may help to show picture or wrap gauze around doll's head	
Prepare family for mood changes	Prepare family for expected mood changes from steroids Interpret mood changes based on drugs or reactions to disease/treatment	Family demonstrates understanding of behavior changes
Support child during treatment for myelosuppression	Explain reason for antibiotics and/or transfusions, particularly why platelets are reserved for acute, uncontrolled bleeding episodes Anticipate need for crossmatched platelets and white blood cell count; encourage family to locate potential donors Observe for signs of transfusion reaction; a febrile reaction is common with leukocyte transfusion and is *not* a contraindication for its use Record approximate time for hemostasis to occur after administration of platelets	Child demonstrates understanding of procedures and tests (specify method and learnings)
Prepare for discharge	Answer questions regarding posthospital care Teach parents skills and give information necessary for home care Teach stump care, if appropriate, to parents and child, if child is old enough to assume some responsibility Assess home for environmental barriers (such as stairs), accessibility of school, if necessary	Child and family demonstrate skills needed for home care (specify)
	Arrange for and emphasize importance of maintaining therapy regimen Arrange for acquisition of needed supplies if appropriate Encourage family to allow child to live as normal a life as possible, especially resumption of school	Child and family demonstrate understanding of therapeutic regimen
	Help child prepare for questions from peers regarding "brain surgery," hair loss, or moon face Refer to appropriate agencies and groups to facilitate care and adjustment, such as American Cancer Society, parent groups Maintain contact with family	Child attends school with reasonable regularity (specify) Family receives continuing support (specify type and amount)

Nursing Interventions Related to Medical Management

Assist in establishing diagnosis
  Assist with diagnostic procedures and tests
  Collect specimens as indicated
Eradicate malignancy
  Administer antimetabolites as prescribed
  Assist with radiotherapy as ordered
Prevent infection
  Administer antibiotics
Prevent hemorrhage
  Administer platelets
Relieve pain
  Administer analgesics as prescribed
  Avoid aspirin or any of its compounds
  Administer drugs on preventive schedule
  Monitor effectiveness of therapy on pain assessment
    record (p. 1072)

Manage problems of radiotherapy and drug toxicity
  Give antiemetic prior to onset of nausea and vomiting
  Give drug before bedtime and/or on empty stomach
    whenever possible
Position postoperatively
  Consult with surgeon regarding positioning, which
    may differ from the following:
  Infratentorial—position child flat and on either
    side, not on back; neck is usually slightly ex-
    tended to prevent strain on sutures
  Supratentorial—elevate head, usually above level
    of heart; do not lower head unless ordered by
    physician
  Post sign above bed noting exact position of head

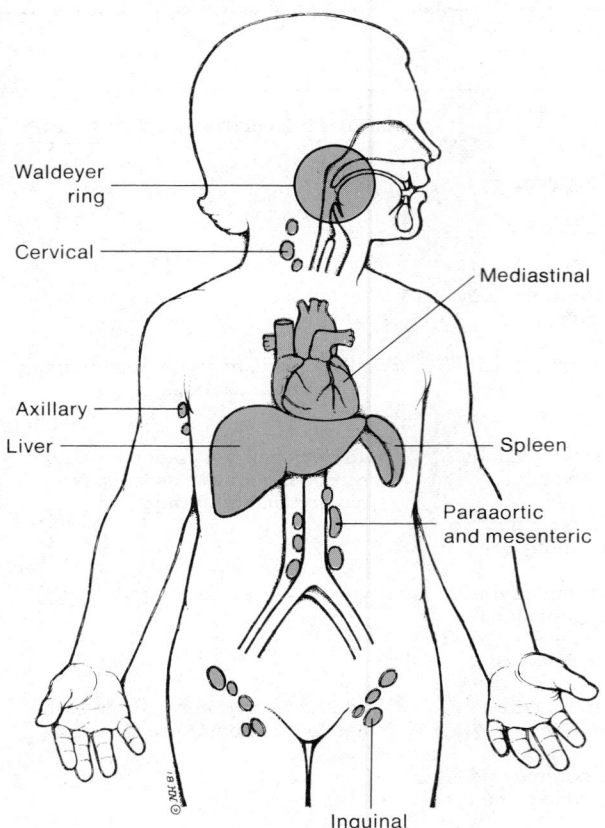

Fig. 36-2. Main areas of lymphadenopathy and organ involvement in Hodgkin disease.

LYMPHOMAS

The lymphomas are a group of neoplastic diseases that arise from the lymphoid and reticuloendothelial systems. They are usually divided into the Hodgkin and non-Hodgkin lymphomas (NHL) and subdivided according to tissue type and extent of disease (staging). In children non-Hodgkin lymphoma, which has been called lymphosarcoma, reticulum cell sarcoma, and giant follicular lymphoma, is more common than Hodgkin disease. Although Hodgkin disease is extremely rare before 5 years of age, there is a striking increase in children 15 to 19 years, when it occurs with almost the same frequency as leukemia.

HODGKIN DISEASE

Hodgkin disease or lymphoma affects about 5 per million children, mostly adolescents. The malignancy originates in the lymphoid system and primarily involves the lymph nodes. It predictably metastasizes to nonnodal or extralymphatic sites, especially the spleen, liver, bone marrow, and lungs, although no tissue is exempt from involvement (Fig. 36-2). It is classified according to four histologic types: (1) lymphocytic predominance, (2) nodular sclerosis, (3) mixed cellularity, and (4) lymphocytic depletion. With present treatment protocols, the histologic stage of the disease has less prognostic significance than previously, although children with the lymphocyte-depleted histology are likely to do poorly (Tan and Chan, 1983).

Clinical Staging and Prognosis

Accurate staging of the extent of disease is the basis for treatment protocols and expected prognoses. Stages include the following:

Stage I: Lesions are limited to one lymph node area or only one additional extralymphatic site (IE), such as the liver, lungs, kidney, or intestines.

Stage II: Two or more lymph node regions on the same side of the diaphragm or one additional extralymphatic site or organ (IIE) on the same side of the diaphragm is involved.

Stage III: Lymph node regions on both sides of the diaphragm are involved, or one extralymphatic site (IIIE), spleen (IIIS), or both (IIISE).

Stage IV: Cancer has metastasized diffusely throughout the body to one or more extralymphatic sites with or without involvement of associated lymph nodes.

Each stage is further subdivided into A or B. *A* denotes absence of associated general symptoms. *B* indicates presence of symptoms such as night sweats, fever, or weight loss of 10% or more during the preceding 6 months. In stages II and III, subtype B has a significantly poorer prognosis than subtype A.

Prognosis for patients with Hodgkin disease has improved dramatically in the past few years, largely as a result of the systematic staging procedure and improved treatment protocols. The prognosis is excellent in children with localized disease, and even in those with disseminated disease, long-term remissions are possible in more than half of the patients. For example, in one study 81% of children in stage I, 76% in stage II, 74% in stage III, and 69% in stage IV were without evidence of disease 5 years after diagnosis (Tan and Chan, 1983). Unfortunately, a number of children may have late recurrences of the original disease or develop a second malignancy, especially osteosarcoma, soft tissue sarcoma, thyroid carcinoma, or leukemia.

Clinical Manifestations

Hodgkin disease is characterized by painless enlargement of lymph nodes. The most common finding is enlarged, firm, nontender, movable nodes in the cervical area. In children the ''sentinel'' node located near the left clavicle may be the first enlarged node. Enlargement of axillary and inguinal lymph nodes is less frequent.

Other signs and symptoms depend on the extent and location of involvement. Mediastinal lymphadenopathy may cause a persistent nonproductive cough. Enlarged retroperitoneal nodes may produce unexplained abdominal pain. Systemic symptoms include low-grade and/or intermittent fever (Pel-Ebstein disease), anorexia, nausea, weight loss, night sweats, or pruritus. Generally such symptoms indicate advanced lymph node and extralymphatic involvement.

Diagnostic Evaluation

The history and physical examination often yield important clues to the disease, such as fevers, night sweats, or weight loss, and enlarged lymph nodes, spleen, or liver. Because of the multiple organs that can become involved, diagnosis consists of several tests to confirm the presence of Hodgkin disease and to assess the extent of involvement for accurate staging. Tests include complete blood count, uric acid levels, liver function tests, urinalysis, and erythrocyte sedimentation rate. Computerized axial tomography of the chest, liver, spleen, and bone is done to detect metastasis.

With the advent of computerized tomography, a special procedure, lymphangiography, may not be needed, although elimination is controversial. A lymphangiogram involves the intradermal injection of a dye (usually alphazurine) in the first interdigital space of each foot for visualization of the lymphatic vessels. One or more vessels are then chosen for catheterization, and a radiopaque medium, usually ethiodized oil (Ethiodol), is injected under pressure to visualize the entire lymphatic chain in the lower extremities, groin, iliopelvic and abdominal-aortic regions, and the thoracic duct. If the axillary, periclavicular, and supraclavicular lymph nodes must be examined, the same procedure is performed in the hands.

Biopsy is essential to diagnosis and staging. The enlarged lymph node is excised and analyzed for histologic type and evidence of the *Sternberg-Reed cell,* a giant cell with a dark-staining nucleolus. Although the cell is considered diagnostic of Hodgkin disease because it is absent in the other lymphomas, it may occur in infectious mononucleosis. A bone marrow aspiration or biopsy is also usually performed. A laparotomy is recommended for definitive pathologic staging and the spleen is removed, although it remains a controversial practice because of the risk of overwhelming infections from asplenia. During this procedure the entire abdomen is examined for evidence of disease; samples of the liver are taken for microscopic study. Biopsies of any involved lymph nodes and the spleen are performed. During surgery, metal clips are placed to outline margins of involved sites for irradiation and to monitor any disease progression. The ovaries may be moved out of the radiation field (oophoropexy) to protect them from irradiation damage.

Therapeutic Management

The primary modalities of therapy are radiation and chemotherapy. Each may be used alone or in combination. The decision is based on the clinical staging. The goal of treatment is obviously a cure; however, aggressive therapy increases the chances of complications in the disease-free state and can seriously compromise the quality of life. Consequently, numerous research studies are presently investigating treatment options to minimize long-term sequelae. Based on the diversity of approaches to treatment, the following is an overview of general principles that may or may not apply to all children. One of the major concerns with combined radiation and antineoplastic drug therapy is the serious late effects in children with an excellent prognosis.

Children with favorable stage I disease may receive only involved field (IF) radiation. Those with stage II or III disease are candidates for extended field (EF) radiation (involved areas plus adjacent nodes) or total nodal irradiation (TNI) (the entire axial lymph node system). Chemotherapy is usually combined with radiation. In stage IV, chemotherapy is the primary form of treatment, although limited radiation may be given to areas of bulky disease. The most widely used drug regimen is MOPP (mechlorethamine [Mustargen], vincristine [Oncovin], prednisone, and procarbazine). Several other drug combinations may be used, such as adriamycin, bleomycin, vinblastine, and dacarbazine (ABVD).

Follow-up care of children off therapy is essential to identify relapse. In children with asplenia, prophylactic antibiotics are administered for an indefinite period and immunizations against pneumococci, meningococci, and *Haemophilus influenzae* are recommended (see pp. 529-530).

Nursing Considerations

Nursing care involves the same objectives as for patients with other types of cancer, namely, (1) preparation for diagnostic and operative procedures, (2) explanation of treatment side effects, and (3) family support (see Chapters 22 and 23). The nurse bases the specific care plan on the clinical stage of the disease. Since this is most often a disease of adolescents and young adults, the nurse must have an appreciation of their psychologic needs and reactions during the diagnostic and treatment phases.

Prepare the family for diagnostic/operative procedures. Once the child is hospitalized for suspected Hodgkin disease, a battery of diagnostic tests is ordered. The family needs an explanation of why each test is performed, since many of them, such as bone marrow aspiration (see p. 1565), are not routine. If lymphangiography is performed, the child needs to be prepared for the test, and particularly told that the length of the procedure is anywhere from 2 to 10 hours and frequently averages 4 to 5 hours. Although the feet are anesthetized, the initial injections are painful. Immobilization of the feet during lymphatic vessel catheterization may be uncomfortable and tiresome, especially since the child must remain still for long periods. Whenever possible the child is encouraged to sleep or diversions should be provided, such as listening to music, reading, or talking. Ideally a family member should be allowed to accompany the child. Fluids and food are not necessarily restricted. If allowed, provisions are made for the child to have a favorite drink or snack.

The procedure is not without complications, the most serious of which is pulmonary embolism from the oil-based dye ethiodized oil (Ethiodol). Fine pulmonary emboli produce symptoms of slight fever, chills, pleuritic pain, mild dyspnea, and a dry cough. Aspirin is helpful to reduce the fever and relieve the pain. The symptoms usually subside within 24 to 48 hours.

Severe oil embolism may occur after dye has been infused too rapidly. Signs of this complication include cyanosis, distended neck veins, hypotension, liver tenderness, and edema in the lower extremities from increased venous resistance. Emergency medical treatment usually involves supplemental oxygen and antihypotensive drugs. The child may become very apprehensive and need considerable reassurance. Usually sedation is avoided, because it may depress the respiratory center.

Expected reactions to the dye include abnormal taste sensations, retrosternal burning, headache, sleeplessness, diarrhea, and elevated temperature. The alphazurine turns the urine and skin of the feet and/or hands bluish green. Although the urine clears rapidly, the discoloration of skin may last for months. Adolescents may be very self-conscious about the staining, especially in the hands.

Since a cutdown procedure is done for vessel catheterization, a pressure bandage may be in place. The area(s) is observed for signs of bleeding and subsequent infection. Sutures are usually removed in 7 to 10 days. Ordinarily the child has no restrictions on activity after the test. However, he is cautioned to keep the wound clean and to avoid excessive irritation from shoes.

Preparation for a laparotomy is similar to that for any other surgery. One special area of concern for families is the effects of the splenectomy on bodily functions. Although not a vital organ, the spleen does have an important role in resisting infection, particularly in young children. The family needs to be aware of the benefits of the procedure in terms of staging and potential risks. Compliance is a major issue with indefinite administration of antibiotics, and every effort should be made to employ strategies that enhance compliance (see p. 1110).

Explain treatments and side effects. Explanations of chemotherapeutic reactions vary with the specific drug regimen. Drugs commonly used are outlined in Table 36-3, and the most common side effects, such as nausea and vomiting, body image changes, neuropathy, and mucosal ulceration, are discussed under Leukemias.

Involved field radiation results in few side effects, sometimes consisting only of a mild skin reaction. With extended field radiation to the chest and abdomen, nausea and vomiting, weight loss, and mucosal ulceration (esophagitis, gastric ulcers) are common side effects. The usual measures for providing relief have been discussed on p. 1582 and are outlined in Table 36-4.

The most common side effect of extensive radiation is malaise, which may result from damage to the thyroid gland, causing hypothyroidism. Lack of energy is particularly difficult for adolescents, because it prevents them from keeping up with their peers. Sometimes the adolescent will push himself to the point of physical exhaustion rather than admit fatigue and succumb to the decreased activity tolerance. The nurse cautions parents to observe for such behavior, such as extreme fatigue at the end of the day, falling asleep at the dinner table, inability to concentrate on homework, or an increased susceptibility to infection. Regular bedtimes and periodic rest times are important for these children, especially during chemotherapy when myelosuppression increases the risk of infection and debilitation. Before discharge the nurse should discuss a feasible school schedule with the parents and child. If alterations are necessary, such as elimination of strenuous physical education, they are discussed with the teacher, nurse, and principal. Follow-up care is essential to diagnose hypothyroidism early and institute thyroid replacement.

An area of concern for adolescents is the high risk of sterility from irradiation and chemotherapy. Both irradiation to the gonads and drugs, particularly procarbazine and alkylating agents, may lead to infertility. Younger patients with a greater complement of oocytes are more likely to retain ovarian function (Horning and others, 1981).

Although sexual function is not altered, the appearance of secondary sexual characteristics and menstruation may be delayed in the pubescent child. Adolescents should be informed of these side effects early in the course of the diagnosis and treatment. Delayed sexual maturation may be an extremely sensitive and painful area for children (see Chapter 20). It is important for the nurse to respect their concern and refrain from casually placating them with expressions such as, "You'll catch up someday."

NON-HODGKIN LYMPHOMA

Non-Hodgkin lymphoma (NHL) occurs in between 7 and 8 per million children under age 15, about one and one-half times the incidence of Hodgkin disease. Childhood NHL is strikingly different from Hodgkin disease and adult NHL in several respects (Gardner and Graham-Pole, 1983):

1. The disease is usually diffuse rather than nodular
2. The cell type is either undifferentiated or poorly differentiated
3. Dissemination occurs earlier, more often, and more rapidly
4. Mediastinal involvement and invasion of meninges are common.

Staging and Prognosis

NHL is heterogeneous, exhibiting a variety of morphologic, cytochemical, and immunologic features, not unlike the diversity seen in leukemia. Classification is based on the pattern of histologic presentation, namely, nodular (circumscribed) or diffuse (spread out). Immunologically these cells are also classified as T-cells, B-cells, an example of which is Burkitt lymphoma, or null cells, which lack specific immunologic properties.

The clinical staging system used in Hodgkin disease is of little value in NHL, although that system has been modified for NHL and other systems have been developed. Favorable prognosis is defined by (1) lymph node involvement only and limited to one or two adjacent lymphatic regions (excluding the mediastinum); (2) an extranodal site in the nasopharynx, oropharynx, or other isolated extranodal site, with or without regional lymphadenopathy; or (3) gastrointestinal involvement, with or without regional lymphadenopathy, limited to the mesentery (White and Siegel, 1984).

The use of aggressive combination chemotherapy has had a major impact on the survival rates of children with NHL. Overall survival statistics range from 50% to 80% depending on the extensiveness of the disease. Children with disease localized to one or two nodes on the same side of the diaphragm demonstrate an 80% to 100% 2-year disease-free survival; survival rates for disseminated disease drop to 76% to 52% (Gardner and Graham-Pole, 1983). Since relapse after 2 years is rare, survival after 24 months is considered a cure.

Clinical Manifestations

Clinical manifestations depend on the anatomic site and extent of involvement. Many of those seen in Hodgkin disease may be present in NHL, although rarely does a single symptom give rise to the diagnosis. Rather, metastasis to the bone marrow or central nervous system may produce signs and symptoms typical of leukemia. Lymphoid tumors compressing various organs may cause intestinal or airway obstruction, cranial nerve palsies, or spinal paralysis.

The exception to the usual presentation of NHL is Burkitt lymphoma, a type of cancer that is rare in the United States but endemic in parts of Africa. It is a rapidly growing neoplasm that is most commonly seen as a mass in the jaw, abdomen, or orbit. However, no anatomic site appears exempt from involvement. Peripheral lymphadenopathy, hepatosplenomegaly, or signs of conversion to leukemia are rarely seen.

Diagnostic Evaluation

Since widespread disease exists in most children with NHL at presentation, thorough pathologic staging is unnecessary. Current recommendations for staging include a surgical biopsy for histopathologic confirmation of disease with cytochemical and immunologic evaluation, bone marrow aspiration, radiologic studies, especially computerized tomograms of the lungs and gastrointestinal organs, and lumbar puncture.

Therapeutic Management

The present treatment protocols for NHL include an aggressive approach using irradiation and chemotherapy. Similar to leukemic therapy, the protocols include induction, consolidation, and maintenance phases, some with intrathecal methotrexate and/or cranial irradiation. Several drug protocols exist, and most of them contain several antineoplastic agents. One of the most commonly used regimens, known as the LSA_2-L_2 protocol, includes cyclophosphamide, vincristine, intrathecal methotrexate, prednisone, daunomycin, 6-thioguanine, cytosine arabinoside, BCNU, and L-asparaginase with or without radiotherapy. Another drug combination is cyclophosphamide, vincristine (Oncovin), intrathecal and intravenous methotrexate, and prednisone (COMP).

These multi-agent regimens are administered for 6 to 24 months (Link, 1985).

Nursing Considerations

Nursing care of the child with NHL is very similar to the care required for children with leukemia. Many of the same drugs are employed, although the schedules differ. Because of the intensive chemotherapy protocol, nursing care is primarily directed toward managing the side effects of these agents. The reader is encouraged to apply the principles of care discussed under Leukemias and in the Nursing care summary to the care of the child with NHL.

Nervous System Tumors

Two major forms of childhood cancer are derived from neural tissue. Brain tumors are the most common solid tumors that occur in children and are second only to leukemia as a form of cancer. Neuroblastomas are the most common malignant tumors of infancy and are second only to brain tumors as the type of solid malignancy seen during the first 10 years (Lopez-Ibor and Schwartz, 1985). Both of these tumors have presented difficulties in identifying successful modes of treatment and have not demonstrated the dramatic improvements in survival that many other forms of cancer have enjoyed.

BRAIN TUMORS

Tumors of the central nervous system account for about 20% of all childhood cancers and have an annual incidence of 2.4 per 100,000 children under 15 years. The majority of tumors (about 60%) are *infratentorial* (below the tentorium cerebelli), which means that they occur in the posterior third of the brain, primarily in the cerebellum or brain stem. This anatomic distribution accounts for the frequency of symptoms resulting from increased intracranial pressure. A smaller number are *supratentorial,* or within the anterior two thirds of the brain, mainly the cerebrum. In adults the majority of tumors are of the latter type.

Classification

Because the neoplasms can arise from any cell within the cranium, it is possible to have tumors originating from the nerve cells, neuroepithelium, glia, cranial nerves, blood vessels, pineal gland, and hypophysis. Within each of these structures, specific cells may be involved to provide a histologic classification of the major tumors found in children. The major infratentorial tumors of childhood are listed in the box. *Gliomas,* arising from glial cells, the supporting structures of the brain, are the most common brain tumors in children.

Clinical Manifestations

The signs and symptoms of brain tumors are directly related to their anatomic location and size and to some extent the

MAJOR BRAIN TUMORS OF CHILDHOOD

Medulloblastoma
Most common tumor (20% of brain tumors)
Fast growing, highly malignant
Characteristic presenting signs include headache, vomiting, ataxia
Improved survival rates with irradiation and excision of most or all of tumor
Overall survival rate of approximately 77%

Cerebellar astrocytoma
Accounts for about 17% of brain tumors
Benign, cystic, and slow growing
Characteristic presenting signs include clumsiness (usually one hand), awkward gait (stumbling to one side), headache, vomiting
Surgical excision associated with high rate of cure (94%) in well-differentiated-type tumors but low rate (38%) in diffuse type

Brain stem glioma
Accounts for about 10% to 15% of brain tumors
Often grows to a very large size before causing symptoms
Characteristic presenting signs include diplopia, facial weakness, and difficulty walking (headache and vomiting are uncommon)
Surgical excision is very difficult because of tumor location in vital brain centers; removal is attempted whenever possible
Palliative therapy with irradiation shrinks tumor to prolong survival
Overall 5-year survival rate is 20% to 30%

Ependymomas
Accounts for about 9% of brain tumors
Demonstrates varying rates of growth
Most invade ventricles, obstructing flow of cerebro-spinal fluid
Characteristic presenting signs include headache, vomiting, and ataxia
Goal of surgery is gross total resection
Role of a radiotherapy and chemotherapy is controversial
Overall 5-year survival rate is 25%

Data from Walker, R., and Allen, J.: Pediatric brain tumors, Pediatr. Ann. 12(5):383-391, 1983.

age of the child. In infants, whose sutures are still open, virtually no early detectable symptoms develop. It is not until spinal fluid obstruction causes markedly increased head size that a lesion may be suspected. Because the tumor typically grows to a large size before being diagnosed, prognosis in infants is generally poorer than in older children (Ertel, 1980).

Even in older children, clinical manifestations are nonspecific. However, the most common symptoms are headache, especially upon awakening, and vomiting that is not related to feeding and is attributable to increased intracranial pressure. The common presenting symptoms of brain tumors are presented in Table 36-7.

Diagnostic Evaluation

Diagnosis of a brain tumor is based subjectively on presenting clinical signs and objectively on neurologic tests. Be-

cause the signs and symptoms are vague and easily overlooked, early diagnosis necessitates a high index of suspicion during history taking. A number of tests may be employed in the neurologic evaluation (see Table 37-4), but the most common diagnostic procedure is computerized tomography (CT). It permits direct visualization of the brain parenchyma, ventricles, and surrounding subarachnoid space. By the intravenous injection of radiographic contrast agents, intracranial blood vasculature can be demonstrated (Hershey and Zimmerman, 1985). The use of magnetic resonance imaging in diagnosing is in its infancy but is thought to be a promising noninvasive technique that avoids the hazards of radiation (Kulkarni and others, 1985). When a positive CT scan is obtained, angiography may be done to provide information about the tumor's blood supply and degree of vascularity, which may assist the surgeon in planning the operative approach. Other tests (e.g. electroencephalography or lumbar puncture) may be performed, although the latter is dangerous in the presence of increased intracranial pressure.

Definitive diagnosis is based on tissue specimens obtained during surgery. Occasionally special techniques are required for determining the cell type. This period of waiting is one of anxiety for the family, who are aware of its relevance to prognosis.

Therapeutic Management

Treatment may involve the use of surgery, radiotherapy, and chemotherapy. All three may or may not be used, depending on the type of tumor. The treatment of choice is total extirpation of the tumor without residual neurologic damage. Patients with the most complete tumor removal have the greatest chance of survival. Radiotherapy is used to treat most tumors and to shrink the size of the tumor prior to attempting surgical removal. The use of chemotherapy is controversial and has not demonstrated significant improvement in survival. The drugs most commonly used are nitrosoureas (CCNU), vincristine, methotrexate, and cisplatinum (Walker and Allen, 1983). In addition, other drugs, such as corticosteroids, may be needed to manage complications, such as brain edema.

The problems of treatment and relatively poor prognosis are compounded by the serious late effects of all three modes of therapy. Surgery may cause injury to important areas of the brain, especially when attempting to remove invasive tumors. Radiation has serious long-term consequences, including radiation somnolence syndrome (see p. 1583), brain necrosis, endocrine dysfunction, and behavioral/intellectual deficits. Chemotherapy is also not without its deleterious effects (see Table 36-5).

Nursing Considerations

Nursing care of the child with a brain tumor involves (1) observing for signs and symptoms related to the tumor, (2) preparing the child and parents for the diagnostic tests and operative procedure, (3) preventing postoperative complications, (4) planning for discharge, and (5) promoting a return to optimum functioning. The principles of care are similar

Table 36-7 Clinical manifestations and assessment of brain tumors	
SIGNS AND SYMPTOMS	**ASSESSMENT**
Headache	
Recurrent and progressive	Record location, severity, and duration
In frontal or occipital areas	Use pain rating scale to assess severity of pain (p. 1070)
Worse on arising, less during day	Note changes in relation to time of day and activity
Intensified by lowering head and straining, such as during bowel movement, coughing, sneezing	Observe changes in behavior in infants (persistent irritability, crying, and head rolling)
Vomiting	
With or without nausea or feeding	Record time, amount, and relationship to feeding,
Progressively more projectile	nausea, and activity
More severe in morning	
Relieved by moving about and changing position	
Neuromuscular changes	
Incoordination or clumsiness	Test muscle strength, gait, coordination and reflexes
Loss of balance (use of wide-based stance, falling, tripping, banging into objects)	(see pp. 277-281)
Poor fine motor control	
Weakness	
Hyporeflexia or hyperreflexia	
Positive Babinski sign	
Spasticity	
Paralysis	
Behavioral changes	
Irritability	Observe behavior regularly
Decreased appetite	Compare observations with parental reports of normal
Failure to thrive	behavioral patterns
Fatigue (frequent naps)	Monitor growth and food intake
Lethargy	Monitor activity and sleep
Coma	
Cranial nerve neuropathy	
Cranial nerve involvement varies according to tumor location	Assess cranial nerves, especially VII (facial), IX (glossopharyngeal), X (vagus), V (trigeminal, sensory roots), and VI (abducens) (see p. 282)
Most common signs	Assess visual acuity, binocularity, and peripheral vision
Head tilt	(see pp. 245-249)
Visual defects (nystagmus, diplopia, strabismus, episodic "greying out" of vision, and visual field defects)	
Vital sign disturbances	
Decreased pulse and respiration	Measure vital signs frequently
Increased blood pressure	Monitor pulse and respirations for 1 full minute
Decreased pulse pressure	Record pulse pressure (difference between systolic and
Hypothermia or hyperthermia	diastolic blood pressure)
Other signs	
Seizures	Record seizure activity (see p. 1666)
*Cranial enlargement	Measure head circumference daily (infant and young
*Tense, bulging fontanel at rest	child)
Nuchal ridigity	Perform funduscopic examination if skilled in procedure
Papilledema (edema of optic nerve)	

*Present only in infants and young children.

regardless of the type of intracranial lesion. Since a brain tumor is a potentially fatal diagnosis, the reader is urged to incorporate the psychologic interventions discussed in Chapter 23 with those elaborated on in this section.

Observe for signs and symptoms. A child admitted to the hospital with neurologic dysfunction is often suspected of having a brain tumor, although the actual diagnosis is as yet unconfirmed. Establishing a baseline of data on which to compare preoperative and postoperative changes is an essential step toward planning physical care and preventing complications. It also allows the nurse to assess the degree of physical incapacity and the family's emotional reaction to the diagnosis. For example, children with cerebellar astrocytoma may have displayed vague cerebellar symptoms for several years before a tumor is suspected. For these parents the revelation of a neoplasm may be more of a shock than for those who have witnessed a rapid deterioration in their child's abilities. Common presenting signs and assessment procedures to document significant changes in the child's condition are summarized in Table 36-7.

Prepare the family for diagnostic/operative procedures. The suspected diagnosis of a brain tumor is always a crisis event. Despite the fact that some tumors are removed with excellent results, the physician can rarely give definitive answers regarding prognosis until after surgery. Therefore parents and older children require much emotional support to face the diagnostic procedures and a craniotomy.

How the child is prepared for the diagnostic tests depends on his age and previous experience. Since most of the tests involve x-ray equipment, the child may be familiar with the procedure. Preparing children for a CT scan is discussed on p. 1629 and preparation for a lumbar puncture on p. 1565. Once surgery is scheduled, the child needs an explanation of what to expect. By the time most children are late preschoolers, they know that the head and brain are important parts of their body. It may be helpful to have a child draw his concept of the brain in order to clarify misconceptions and base the explanation on his level of understanding.

Although the temptation is to justify the need for surgery by stating that removing the tumor will take away various symptoms, the nurse should refrain from emphasizing this point too strenuously. Postsurgery headaches and cerebellar symptoms, such as ataxia, may be aggravated rather than improved. Surgery may not improve vision. With optic gliomas the child will be blind in one eye. Finally, surgical removal of the mass may be impossible, and after surgery there may be temporary deterioration of functioning. Being honest before surgery most often makes honesty after the operation easier because no false hopes were created.

Honesty does not negate instilling hope. A truthful explanation regarding the operation is: "The physician will see exactly where the tumor is. If it is small and in one place, it will be removed. If it is large, as much of it as possible will be removed so that some of your symptoms will go away." It is best to deliver information in small amounts to let the child pursue additional answers. For example, some children will ask about what happens when part of the tumor is left in. An honest reply is that, after surgery, the physician will try to shrink the tumor with a special radiation machine and/or drugs. A further explanation of radiation or drug side effects is unwarranted, since the child will be bombarded with information before it is relevant.

Usually the night before surgery the child's head is shaved. This can be traumatic to the child and parents. However, it can be approached in a sensitive, positive way. If the child's hair is long, it should be braided so that the long swatch can be saved. Showing the child how he looks at different stages of the process helps him prepare for the final appearance.

Once the hair is clipped very short or shaved, the child can be given a cap or scarf to wear in order to camouflage the baldness. Every precaution is taken to protect the child from teasing or ridicule by other children before surgery. It is also emphasized that the hair will regrow shortly after the operation. Depending on the child's immediate adjustment to the hair loss, the nurse may introduce the idea of wearing a wig until the hair is grown in, particularly if additional irradiation or chemotherapy is anticipated.

In some hospitals a special technician shaves the scalp to minimize the risk of skin cuts. Sometimes the shaving is done in the operating room with the child under anesthesia. The scalp is shampooed before surgery. During these procedures the child is afforded maximum privacy.

The child is also told about the size of the dressing. Usually the entire scalp is covered to maintain a tight wound closure, even if a small incision is made. Infratentorial head dressings may be attached to the upper back and around toward the neck in order to maintain slight extension and alignment as a precaution against wound rupture. Applying a similar dressing or "special hat" to a doll is often a less traumatic way of demonstrating the physical appearance.

The child also needs a brief explanation of how he will feel after surgery and where he will be. Ordinarily he will return to a special intensive care unit, which he may visit beforehand depending on hospital policy. He should be aware that he may be sleepy for some time after surgery and that a headache is likely, although it should last only a few days.

Parents need similar explanations before surgery, especially in terms of special equipment used in the intensive care unit, dressings, and their child's behavior. For example, they should know that it is not unusual for the child to be comatose or lethargic for a few days after surgery. The nurse may wish to encourage less frequent visiting during this period so that parents can rest and be able to support their child when he awakens.

It is also advisable for the nurse to participate in preoperative conferences with the physician and parents. The nurse needs to know what information the parents have been given in order to be able to give further explanations or emotional support when necessary.

Prevent postoperative complications. Usually the surgeon will prescribe specific orders for vital signs, positioning, fluid regulation, and medication. These vary somewhat, depending on the location of the craniotomy. The following are general principles of care for infratentorial or supratentorial surgery. Additional aspects of care are discussed in Chapter 37, such as care of the child with seizures and care of the unconscious child in terms of respiratory status and neurologic assessment.

Observation. Vital signs are taken as frequently as every 15 to 30 minutes until stable. Temperatures taken via rectal or axillary routes are particularly important because of hyperthermia resulting from surgical intervention in the hypothalamus or brain stem and from some types of general anesthesia. To prepare for this reaction, a cooling blanket should be placed on the bed *before* the child returns to the unit so that it is ready for use when needed. Since the temperature control centers are affected, the nurse monitors body temperature often when any cooling measures are employed, because hypothermia can occur suddenly.

When temperature is elevated, an infectious process must always be suspected, particularly if the febrile state occurs 1 to 2 days after surgery. The most likely types of infection are meningitis and respiratory infection. The probable cause of meningitis is wound contamination. Signs of meningitis, such as opisthotonos, Kernig and Brudzinski signs (pp. 281 and 282), and nuchal rigidity (see also Chapter 37), are very similar to those of increased intracranial pressure and must be carefully evaluated to determine whether they indicate an infection.

There is an especially high risk of respiratory infections because of the imposed immobility, danger of aspiration, and possible depression from the brain stem, and the usual precautions in terms of coughing, deep breathing, and turning as allowed are instituted. Regular pulmonary assessments should be performed to identify adventitious sounds or any areas of diminished or absent breath sounds. Blood pressure is also taken at frequent intervals. The deflated cuff is left on the arm between readings to allow for the least movement and disturbance of the child. Ocular signs are recorded at least every hour. Sluggish, dilated, or unequal pupils are reported to the physician, since they may indicate increased pressure.

Observations for function are not instituted until the child regains consciousness. However, as soon as possible the nurse should begin testing reflexes, handgrip, and functioning of the cranial nerves. Muscle strength is usually less after surgery from general weakness but should improve daily. Ataxia may be significantly worse with cerebellar intervention, but it will slowly improve. Edema near the cranial nerves may depress important functions such as the gag, blink, or swallowing reflex.

The nurse records behavior at regular intervals, noting sleep patterns, response to stimuli, and level of consciousness. Although a child may be comatose for a few days, once he regains consciousness there should be a steady increase in alertness. Regression to a lethargic, irritable state indicates increasing pressure, possibly caused by meningitis.

Dressings are observed for evidence of drainage. If a drain is in place, the physician specifies this, since drainage frequently soaks through the dressing. If soiled, the dressing is not removed but reinforced with dry sterile gauze. The approximate amount of drainage is estimated and recorded. To keep an accurate account of drainage, the soiled area is circled with a pen every hour or so. In this way continuous bleeding is easily recognized. If a colorless drainage is noted, this is reported immediately, since it most likely is cerebrospinal fluid from the incisional area. A foul odor from the dressing may indicate an infection. Such a finding is reported, and a culture is taken.

Once the child is alert, his arms may need to be restrained to prevent him from removing the dressing. Even a child who has been cooperative before surgery must be closely supervised during the initial stages of regaining consciousness, when disorientation and restlessness are common. Elbow restraints are satisfactory to prevent the hands

from reaching the head, although additional restraint may be necessary to preserve an infusion line and maintain a side-lying position.

Positioning. Correct positioning after surgery is critical to prevent pressure against the operative site, reduce intracranial pressure, and avoid the danger of aspiration. If a large tumor was removed, the child is not placed on the operative site, since the brain may suddenly shift to that cavity, causing trauma to the blood vessels, linings, and the brain itself. The nurse confers with the surgeon to be certain of the correct position, including degree of neck flexion. The first 24 to 48 hours after brain surgery are critical. If position is restricted, notice of this is posted above the head of the bed. When the child is turned, every precaution is used to prevent jarring or malalignment in order to prevent undue strain on the sutures. Two nurses, one supporting the head and the other the body, are needed. The use of a turning sheet may facilitate turning of a heavy child.

The child with an infratentorial operation is usually positioned flat and on either side. Pillows should be placed against his back, not his head, to maintain the desired position. Ordinarily the head and neck are kept in midline with the body and slightly extended. In a supratentorial craniotomy the head is usually elevated above the heart to facilitate cerebrospinal fluid drainage and decrease excessive blood flow to the brain to prevent hemorrhage. Trendelenburg position is contraindicated in both types of surgeries because it increases intracranial pressure and the risk of hemorrhage. If shock is impending, the physician is notified immediately, before the head is lowered.

Fluid regulation. With an infratentorial craniotomy the child is allowed nothing by mouth for at least 24 hours and longer if the gag and swallowing reflexes are depressed or he is comatose. With a supratentorial operation, feeding may be resumed soon after the child is alert, sometimes within 24 hours. Clear water is always started first, because of the danger of aspiration. If the child vomits, oral liquids are stopped. Vomiting not only predisposes to aspiration but also increases intracranial pressure and incisional rupture.

Intravenous fluids are continued until fluids are well tolerated. Because of the cerebral edema postoperatively and danger of increased intracranial pressure, fluids are carefully monitored. If drugs, such as prophylactic antibiotics, are given intravenously, the medication amount is calculated as part of the intravenous fluid. For example, if the child is to receive 20 ml per hour and the diluted drug is 5 ml, the intravenous solution is reduced to 15 ml for that hour. When small amounts are infused, the intravenous drip should be electronically monitored for greater accuracy.

A hypertonic solution such as mannitol or dextrose may be necessary to remove excess fluid. These drugs cause rapid diuresis. After surgery the child may have a Foley catheter. Urine output is monitored after administration of these drugs to evaluate their effectiveness.

When the child is able to take fluids, he should be fed to conserve strength and minimize movement. If there is any sign of facial paralysis, the child is fed slowly to prevent choking or aspiration. Scrupulous mouth care is essential to prevent oral infection. Sometimes gavage feeding is necessary when bodily functions are too depressed to permit safe oral feedings or the child refuses to eat or drink. In the latter instance the nurse should employ every measure to encourage acceptance of fluids or solids. (See p. 1115 for nursing interventions.)

Comfort measures. Although used after most other types of surgery, postoperative analgesics may not be routinely prescribed, because they may mask signs of altered consciousness or body functioning. However, this varies and if analgesics are ordered they should be used effectively, preferably on a preventive basis and in sufficient doses (see p. 1070).

Headache may be severe and is largely the result of cerebral edema. Measures to relieve some of the discomfort include providing a quiet, dimly lit environment, restricting visitors to a minimum, preventing any sudden jarring movement, such as banging into the bed, and preventing an increase in intracranial pressure. The last is most effectively achieved by proper positioning and prevention of straining, such as during coughing, vomiting, or defecating. Bowel movements are monitored to prevent constipation. Stool softeners may be given as soon as liquids are tolerated to facilitate easy passage of stool. Placing an ice bag on the forehead may also provide some headache relief, especially if facial edema is severe.

Brain edema may also severely depress the gag reflex, necessitating suctioning of oral secretions. Facial edema may also be present, necessitating eye care if the lids remain partially open. Ice compresses applied to the eyes for short periods help in relieving the edema. A depressed blink reflex also predisposes to corneal ulceration. Irrigating the eyes with saline drops and covering them with eye dressings are important steps in preventing this complication.

Support the family. The emotional needs of the family are great when the diagnosis is a brain tumor, and feelings are influenced by the extent of surgery, any neurologic deficits, expected prognosis, and additional therapy. Since few definitive answers can be given before surgery, the surgeon's report is a significant finding that can vary from a completely benign, resected neoplasm to a highly malignant, invasive, and only partially removed tumor. Although parents try to prepare themselves for a potentially fatal diagnosis, it is a shock for them.

Ideally a nurse should be with the family when the physician visits with them to discuss with parents the expected prognosis and plan of therapy. Although parents may hear only a fraction of what they are told, they can begin to put the future into perspective. While some children will be cured, those with residual tumor may die within a relatively short period of time or live for several years. Regardless of the future prospects, the parents' thinking must be directed toward helping the child recover and resume a normal life to his fullest potential.

It is also a time to encourage parents to verbalize their feelings about the diagnosis. Often they express tremendous guilt for attributing the insidious onset of symptoms, such as ataxia, visual difficulty, or headache, to minor "complaints" by the child. Parents may have punished their child for clumsiness, thinking he was being careless. The nurse listens to such statements, emphasizing the normalcy of the parents' reactions. Sometimes it may be helpful to precipitate such a discussion with a statement such as, "It is difficult to know when a child's complaints are significant, because so often they are caused by minor ailments." Any comments that insinuate that the parents should have sought medical advice sooner are not offered, since such remarks only add to the parents' guilt feelings.

During this period the nurse should also discuss with parents what they plan to tell the child. If he was prepared honestly as described previously, the diagnosis can be expressed in a similar manner, such as, "The physician removed most of the tumor, and the rest will be treated with special drugs and x-ray treatments." As the child improves, he will need additional explanation about the treatment (similar to that discussed for leukemia) as well as the reason for residual neurologic effects, such as ataxia or blindness. Since the hair was shaved before surgery, hair loss is less of a concern from treatment, although its regrowth will be delayed by 3 to 6 months, depending on length of therapy. At this point it is advisable to reinforce the idea of a wig.

Promote return to optimum functioning. The ultimate goal is a cured child who has maximum functioning. As soon as possible the child should resume his usual activities within his limits, especially returning to school.* Until the skull is completely healed, the child may need to wear a helmet if he engages in any active sport. The school nurse and teacher should confer with the parents to discuss activity restrictions, such as physical education, and the reactions of schoolmates to the child's appearance. Since children often equate brain surgery with "going crazy," it is important to prepare the child for possible remarks to this effect. As one child told a classmate, "It's *your* head they should have fixed, because you're crazy. Can't you see that I'm all better?"

After discharge the family needs continuing medical and emotional support from health personnel. Even with children who are long-term survivors after treatment for a brain tumor, residual disabilities, such as growth retardation, cranial nerve palsies, sensory defects, motor abnormalities, especially ataxia, intellectual deficits, dysphagia, dysgraphia, and behavioral problems, are not uncommon (Hirsch and others, 1979). It is difficult to assess the exact cause of the nonphysical disabilities, since numerous variables influence the total rehabilitation of the child. However, the high frequency of late effects attests to the tremendous need for follow-up care despite successful treatment of the tumor.

The realm of possible consequences following the diagnosis of a brain tumor is vast. They are not discussed here.

---

*Excellent publications, including the pamphlet *When your child is ready to return to school*, are available from the Association for Brain Tumor Research, Suite 200, 6232 N. Pulaski Rd., Chicago, IL 60646.

Rather, the reader is urged to refer to other sections of the text that deal with possible outcomes, such as the paralyzed, visually impaired, or unconscious child or the care of a child with a ventricular shunt, seizure disorder, or meningitis. Numerous physical problems can occur with progression of the tumor that may necessitate additional procedures. For example, frequent vomiting, anorexia, and nausea may require nonoral routes of feeding, such as gastrostomy or parenteral alimentation. Trials with chemotherapy may necessitate the use of central venous access devices. Whenever these procedures are instituted, the nurse may be responsible for teaching the family appropriate home care to allow the child the highest quality of life for the longest period of time. (See discussion of home care in Chapter 26.)

NEUROBLASTOMA

Neuroblastoma occurs in about 1 in 10,000 live births, with a slightly higher incidence in males. About half the cases occur in children under 2 years of age, and another fourth occur in children under age 4. These tumors originate from embryonic neural crest cells that normally give rise to the adrenal medulla and the sympathetic ganglia. Consequently, the majority of the tumors arise from the adrenal gland or from the retroperitoneal sympathetic chain. Therefore the primary site is within the abdomen. Other sites may be within the head, neck, chest, or pelvis.

Staging and Prognosis

In recent years there has been an attempt to classify tumors according to stages in order to establish improved criteria for treatment and prognosis at the time of diagnosis and surgery. Neuroblastoma has been classified into five different stages:

Stage I: The tumor is confined to the organ or structure of origin.

Stage II: The tumor extends in continuity beyond the primary site but does not cross the midline; regional lymph node involvement on the same side may be present.

Stage III: The tumor extends in continuity beyond the midline; bilateral regional lymph node involvement may be present.

Stage IV: There is remote disease involving the skeleton, parenchymal organs, soft tissue, or distant lymph nodes.

Stage IV-S (special stage): Stage I or II with remote disease confined to one or more sites, either the liver, skin, or bone marrow, without roentgenographic evidence of skeletal metastasis.

Neuroblastoma is a "silent" tumor. In more than 70% of cases, diagnosis is made after metastasis occurs, with the first signs caused by involvement in the nonprimary site, usually the lymph nodes, bone marrow, skeletal system, skin, or liver. Because of the frequency of invasiveness, prognosis for neuroblastoma is poor.

The age of the child and the stage of the disease at diagnosis are important prognostic factors. Survival is inversely correlated with age. If all stages are grouped together, the survival rates are 72% for birth to age 11 months, 28% for ages 12 to 23 months, and 12% for ages 2 years or more. This marked difference in survival rates by age is partly accounted for by the larger proportion of very young children with stage I, II, or IV-S disease (Evans, 1980). However, survival expectancy improves again for children over 6 years of age. Infants who remain free of disease for 1 year after treatment are usually cured, but older children have experienced relapses several years after cessation of treatment (Lopez-Ibor and Schwartz, 1985). Neuroblastoma is one of the few tumors that demonstrate spontaneous regression (especially stage IV-S), possibly as a result of maturity of the embryonic cell or the development of an active immune system.

Clinical Manifestations

The signs and symptoms of neuroblastoma depend on the location and stage of the disease. Most presenting signs are caused by compression of adjacent structures. With abdominal tumors the most common presenting sign is a firm, nontender, irregular mass in the abdomen that crosses the midline (in contrast to Wilms tumor, which is usually confined to one side). Compression of the kidney, ureter, or bladder may cause urinary frequency or retention.

Distant metastasis frequently causes supraorbital ecchymosis, periorbital edema, and proptosis (exophthalmos) from invasion of retrobulbar soft tissue (Fig. 36-3). Lymphadenopathy, especially in the cervical and supraclavicular areas, may also be an early presenting sign. Bone pain may

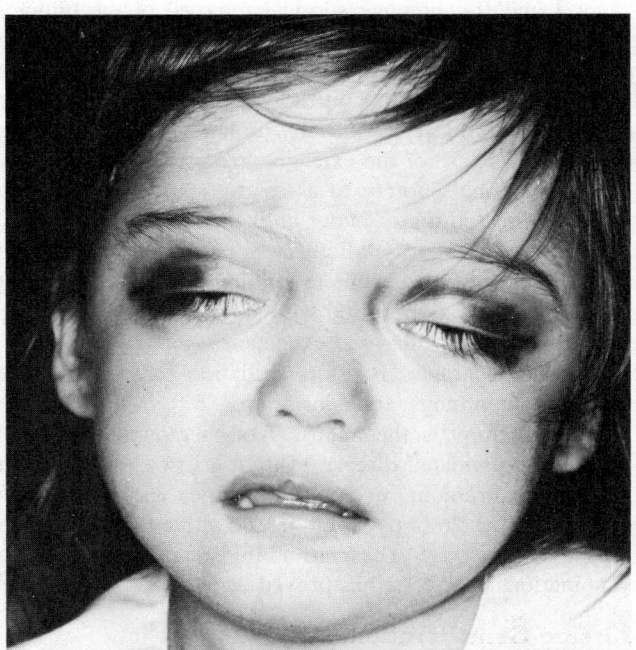

Fig. 36-3. Supraorbital ecchymoses associated with periorbital metastases.
Courtesy Howard A. Britton. From Sutow, W.W., Vietti, T.J., and Fernbach, D.J., editors: Clinical pediatric oncology, ed. 2, St. Louis, 1977, The C.V. Mosby Co.

or may not be present with skeletal involvement. Vague symptoms of widespread metastasis include pallor, weakness, irritability, anorexia, and weight loss.

Other primary tumors may cause significant clinical effects, such as neurologic impairment from an intracranial lesion, respiratory obstruction from a thoracic mass, or varying degrees of paralysis from compression of the spinal cord. Infrequently a child may have symptoms of increased catecholamine excretion, such as flushing, hypertension, tachycardia, and diaphoresis.

Diagnostic Evaluation

Diagnostic evaluation is aimed at locating the primary site and areas of metastasis. Skull, neck, chest, abdominal, and bone computerized tomographs and a bone marrow test are used to locate a tumor mass and/or metastasis. With an adrenal neuroblastoma an intravenous pyelogram often demonstrates a downward displacement of the affected kidney but normal renal function. Neuroblastomas, particularly those arising on the adrenal glands or from a sympathetic chain, excrete the catecholamines epinephrine and norepinephrine. Analyzing the breakdown products that are normally excreted in the urine, namely, vanillylmandelic acid (VMA), homovanillic acid (HVA), dopamine, and norepinephrine, permits detection of a suspected tumor both before and after medical/surgical intervention.

Therapeutic Management

Accurate clinical staging is important for establishing initial treatment. Therefore surgery is employed both to remove as much of the tumor as possible and to obtain biopsies. In stages I and II, complete surgical removal of the tumor is the treatment of choice. If the tumors are large, partial resection is attempted, with a course of irradiation postoperatively to shrink the tumor in the hope of complete removal at a later date. Surgery is usually limited to biopsy in stages III and IV because of the extensive metastasis, although the use of additional surgery to assess tumor regression or remove a regressed tumor is not unlikely.

The precise role of radiotherapy is unclear. It does not appear to be of any benefit in children with stage I and II disease; it is commonly used with stage III disease although it may not improve survival expectancy; and it may make a large tumor operable. It offers palliation for metastatic lesions in bones, lungs, liver, or brain.

Chemotherapy is the mainstay of therapy for extensive local or disseminated disease. The drugs of choice are vincristine, doxorubicin, cyclophosphamide, adriamycin, cisplatin, and VM-26 (a podophyllin derivative that works similarly to vincristine). They are administered in a variety of combinations, but none has proved superior.

Nursing Considerations

Nursing considerations are similar to those discussed previously for leukemia and brain tumors, including psychologic and physical preparation for diagnostic and operative procedures, prevention of postoperative complications for abdominal, thoracic, or cranial surgery, and explanation of chemotherapy and radiotherapy and their side effects (see Tables 36-3 and 36-4).

Since this tumor carries a poor prognosis for many children, every consideration must be given the family in terms of coping with a life-threatening illness (see Chapter 23). Because of the high degree of metastasis at the time of diagnosis, many parents suffer much guilt for not having recognized signs earlier. Often the guilt is expressed as anger toward professionals for not diagnosing it sooner. Parents need much support in dealing with these feelings and expressing them to the appropriate people.

Bone Tumors

Malignant bone tumors represent less than 1% of all malignant neoplasms but are more common in children than adults. The peak ages during childhood are 15 to 19 years. The sexes are affected equally until puberty, at which time the ratio approaches 2:1 in favor of males. This propensity for males with a peak incidence during adolescence is thought to be because of the accelerated growth rate of osseous tissue.

GENERAL CONSIDERATIONS

Neoplastic disease can arise from any tissues involved in bone growth, such as osteoid matrix, bone marrow elements, fat, blood and lymph vessels, nerve sheath, and cartilage. In children the two types that account for 85% of all primary malignant bone tumors are osteogenic sarcoma and Ewing sarcoma. They have several characteristics in common, which are discussed below. Specific information about each tumor is then elaborated on further.

Clinical Manifestations

Most malignant bone tumors produce localized pain in the affected site, which may be severe or dull and in most cases is attributable to trauma or the vague complaint of "growing pains." It is often relieved by a flexed position, which relaxes the muscles overlying the stretched periosteum. Frequently it draws attention when the child limps, curtails his own physical activity, or is unable to hold heavy objects.

Diagnostic Evaluation

Diagnosis begins with a thorough history and physical examination. A primary objective is to rule out causes such as trauma or infection. Careful questioning regarding pain is essential in attempting to determine the duration and rate of tumor growth. Physical assessment focuses on functional status of the affected area, signs of inflammation, size of the mass, involvement of regional lymph nodes, and any systemic indication of generalized malignancy, such as anemia, weight loss, frequent infection, and so on.

Definitive diagnosis is based on radiologic studies, particularly computerized tomography, to determine the extent of the lesion; radioisotope bone scans to evaluate metastasis; and either needle or surgical bone biopsy to determine the histologic pattern. Radiologic findings are characteristic for each type of tumor. In osteogenic sarcoma, needlelike new bone formation growing at right angles to the diaphysis (shaft) produces a "sunburst" appearance. In Ewing sarcoma, the deposits of new bone in layers under the periosteum produce an "onionskin" appearance. In both types of bone tumors, soft tissue infiltration may be apparent.

At present there is no reliable biochemical test for bone cancers. Elevated alkaline phosphatase levels may occur in osteoid tumors. Several tests may be done for differential diagnosis in terms of secondary bone metastasis from Wilms tumor, neuroblastoma, retinoblastoma, rhabdomyosarcoma, lymphoma, or leukemia. Lung tomography is usually a standard procedure, since pulmonary metastasis is the most common complication of primary bone tumors. Bone marrow aspiration is helpful in diagnosing Ewing sarcoma.

Prognosis

A better understanding of the biology of neoplastic growth has resulted in more aggressive treatment and improved prognosis. The natural history of osteogenic sarcoma and Ewing sarcoma suggests that multiple submicroscopic foci of metastatic disease are present at the time of diagnosis despite clinical evidence of localized involvement. Before the use of aggressive multimodal therapy, pulmonary metastasis invariably appeared in 6 to 24 months in patients with osteogenic sarcoma who were treated with surgical excision of the tumor. Now, with surgery for osteosarcoma or intensive radiotherapy for Ewing sarcoma combined with chemotherapy, survival statistics are improving for both types of bone cancer. Survival rates differ according to the specific treatment protocols and are influenced by a number of factors, such as site of primary tumor, especially in Ewing sarcoma, and the presence or absence of metastatic disease at diagnosis. However, approximately 50% of children with either type of bone cancer can be expected to be long-term survivors, and various cancer centers are reporting higher figures (Ettinger, 1983).

OSTEOGENIC SARCOMA

Osteogenic sarcoma (osteosarcoma) is the most frequently encountered malignant bone cancer in children. Its peak incidence is between 10 and 25 years of age. It presumably arises from bone-forming mesenchyme, which gives rise to malignant osteoid tissue. Most primary tumor sites are in the diaphysis of long bones, especially in the lower extremities. More than half occur in the femur, particularly the distal portion, with the rest involving the humerus, tibia, pelvis, jaw, and phalanges.

Therapeutic Management

Optimum treatment of osteosarcoma is controversial. The traditional approach has consisted of radical surgical resection or amputation of the affected area followed by intensive chemotherapy. Depending on the tumor site, surgery includes amputation of the affected extremity at least 7.5 cm (3 inches) above the proximal tumor margin or above the joint proximal to the involved bone. With tumors of the distal femur, preservation of the hip joint may be possible. Other procedures include an above-the-knee amputation for tumors of the tibia or fibula, a hemipelvectomy for tumors of the innominate (hip) bone, and a forequarter amputation (removal of arm, scapula, and portion of the clavicle on the affected side) for tumors of the upper humerus. Another surgical approach for selected patients is the limb salvage procedures, which involve en bloc resection of the primary tumor with prosthetic replacement of the involved bone. For example, with osteosarcoma of the distal femur, a total femur and joint replacement is performed. When pulmonary metastasis is found, thoracotomies have resulted in prolonged survival and potential cure (Ettinger, 1983).

Chemotherapy now plays a vital role in treatment. Antineoplastic drugs, such as methotrexate with citrovorum factor rescue, adriamycin, bleomycin, actinomycin, cyclophosphamide, and cisplatin, may be administered singly or in combination and may be employed both before and after surgery. These combined-modality approaches have significantly improved the prognosis in osteosarcoma.

Nursing Considerations

Nursing care depends on the type of surgical approach. Obviously, the family may have more difficulty adjusting to an amputation than a limb salvage procedure. In either instance, preparation of the child and family is critical. Straightforward honesty is essential in gaining the cooperation and trust of the child. The diagnosis of cancer should not be disguised with falsehoods such as "infection." For the child to gradually accept the need for radical surgery, he must be aware of the lack of alternatives for treatment. While the responsibility of telling the child is generally left to the physician, the nurse should be present at the discussion or be aware of exactly what is said to the child. The child should be told a few days before surgery to allow him time to think about the diagnosis and consequent treatment and to ask questions.

Sometimes children have many questions about the prosthesis, limitations on physical ability, and prognosis in terms of cure. At other times they react with silence or with a calm manner that belies their concern and fear. Either response must be accepted, because it is part of the grieving process of a loss. For those who wish information, it may be helpful to introduce them to another amputee before surgery or to show them pictures of the prosthesis.* However,

---

*A source of information is the National Amputation Foundation, Inc., 12-45 150th St., Whitestone, NY 11357.

the nurse must be careful not to overwhelm children with information. A sound approach is to answer their questions without offering additional information. For those who do not pursue additional information, the nurse expresses a willingness to talk, with such expressions as, "Anytime you would like to talk or ask questions about the surgery, tell me." The nurse should not push the topic unless the child initiates the conversation. Silence does not always mean nonacceptance.

The child is also informed of the need for chemotherapy. Although it is best to introduce this subject before surgery, since treatment begins as soon as possible postoperatively, caution must be exercised in offering too much information at one time. It is wise to discuss hair loss with emphasis on positive aspects, such as wearing a wig. Since bone tumors affect adolescents and young adults, it is not unusual for them to become angry over all the radical body alterations. One child remarked, "By the time you are done with me, I will be more false than real." Sensing a feeling of powerlessness, the nurse encouraged the child to discuss his thoughts about surgery and chemotherapy, focusing on what alternatives there were available to him. The child finally stated, "I know there is no other way, but I don't have to like it." The nurse agreed, supporting the child's legitimate right to such feelings.

If an amputation is performed, the child is usually fitted with a temporary prosthesis immediately after surgery, which permits early functioning and fosters psychologic adjustment. If this is not done, the child requires stump care, which is the same as for any amputee. A permanent prosthesis is usually fitted within 6 to 8 weeks. During hospitalization the child begins physical therapy to become proficient in the use and care of the device.

Discharge planning must begin early during the postoperative period. Once the child has begun physical therapy, the nurse should consult with the therapist and physician to evaluate the child's physical and emotional readiness to reenter school. It is an opportune time to involve a community nurse in the home care of the child. Every effort is made to promote normalcy and gradual resumption of realistic preamputation activities.* Role playing in anticipation of such experiences is very beneficial in preparing the child for the inevitable confrontation by others. Environmental barriers, such as stairs, are assessed in terms of the accessibility of the school and/or home, especially since the child may need to use crutches or a wheelchair before complete healing and prosthetic competency are achieved.

The nurse encourages the child to select clothing that best camouflages the prosthesis, such as pants or long-sleeved shirts. Well-fitted prostheses are so natural looking that girls can usually wear sheer stockings without revealing the device. Emphasizing feminine or masculine apparel helps the child regain his feeling of self-identity. Even during the

postoperative period, encouraging the child to wear blue jeans and a shirt may distract his attention from the deformity and focus it on familiar aspects of appearance.

The family and child need a great deal of support in adjusting not only to a life-threatening diagnosis but also to alteration in body form and function. Since loss of a limb constitutes a grieving process, those caring for the child need to recognize that the reactions of anger and depression are normal and necessary. Often parents view the anger as a direct affront to them for allowing the amputation to occur, or they see the depression as rejection. On the contrary, these are not interpersonal attacks but self-attempts to cope with a loss.

EWING SARCOMA

Ewing sarcoma arises in the marrow spaces of the bone rather than from osseous tissue. The tumor originates in the shaft of long and trunk bones, most often affecting the femur, tibia, fibula, humerus, ulna, vertebra, scapula, ribs, pelvic bones, and skull. It occurs almost exclusively in individuals under age 30, with the majority between 4 and 25 years of age.

Therapeutic Management

Surgical amputation is not routinely recommended but may be considered when the results of radiotherapy render the extremity useless or deformed (such as from retarded growth in young children) or the tumor appears resectable. The treatment of choice is intensive irradiation of the involved bone combined with chemotherapy. A widely used drug regimen includes vincristine, actinomycin D, cyclophosphamide, and adriamycin (often referred to as VACA).

Nursing Considerations

The psychologic adjustment to Ewing sarcoma is typically less traumatic than to osteogenic sarcoma because of the preservation of the affected limb. Many families accept the diagnosis with a sense of relief in knowing that this type of bone cancer does not necessitate amputation, and initially they may not be aware of the deleterious effects on the irradiated site. Consequently, they need preparation for the various diagnostic tests, including bone marrow aspiration and surgical biopsy, and adequate explanation of the treatment regimen. High-dose radiotherapy often causes a skin reaction of dry or moist desquamation followed by hyperpigmentation. The nurse advises the child to wear loose-fitting clothes over the irradiated area to minimize additional skin irritation. Because of increased sensitivity, the area is protected from sunlight and sudden changes in temperature, such as from heating pads or ice packs. The child is encouraged to use the extremity as tolerated. Occasionally an active exercise program may be planned by the physical therapist to preserve maximum function.

The child needs the same considerations for adjusting to the effects of chemotherapy as any other cancer patient. The

---

*Information about special programs for children with amputations such as "Sunshine Skiers," is available from the Candlelighters Foundation, 2025 Eye St., N.W., Washington, DC 20006.

drug regimen usually results in hair loss, severe nausea and vomiting, peripheral neuropathy, and possibly cardiotoxicity. Every effort should be made to outline a treatment plan that allows the child maximum resumption of a normal lifestyle and activities.

Other Solid Tumors

In addition to the cancers already discussed, several other types of solid tumors may occur in children. Wilms tumor, rhabdomyosarcoma, and retinoblastoma are unique in that they tend to be diagnosed early, typically before 5 years of age. Wilms tumor and retinoblastoma are also unusual in that they are among the few types of cancer that may occur in both hereditary and nonhereditary forms.

WILMS TUMOR

Wilms tumor, or nephroblastoma, is the most frequent intraabdominal tumor of childhood and the most common type of renal cancer. Its frequency is estimated to be 1 per 200,000 to 250,000 children. The peak incidence is at 3 years of age. Wilms tumor is one of the childhood cancers that show an increased incidence among siblings and identical twins, reflecting evidence of genetic inheritance. The mode of inheritance in familial cases, which accounts for less than 2% of all Wilms tumors, is autosomal dominant with variable penetrance (estimated at 63%) and expressivity. Thus gene carriers may develop no tumors (37%), unilateral tumors (48%), or bilateral tumors (15%). All bilateral cases and 15% of unilateral cases are probably hereditary (Strong, 1984). Unfortunately, there is no method of identification of gene carriers.

Wilms tumor is also associated with several congenital anomalies; the most common are aniridia, hemihypertrophy, and genitourinary anomalies, such as hypospadias, cryptorchidism, and ambiguous genitalia. Other less common anomalies are microcephaly, pigmented and vascular nevi, pinna deformities, and mental and growth retardation.

Staging and Prognosis

Wilms tumor probably arises from a malignant, undifferentiated metanephrogenic blastoma (a cluster of primordial cells capable of initiating the regeneration of an abnormal structure). Its occurrence slightly favors the left kidney, which is advantageous because surgically this kidney is easier to manipulate and remove. Although the tumor may become quite large, it remains encapsulated for an extended period. During surgery the tumor is staged to maximize the effectiveness of treatment protocols. The following abbreviated criteria for staging are most commonly used:

Stage I: Tumor is limited to kidney and completely resected.

Stage II: Tumor extends beyond kidney but is completely resected.

Stage III: Residual nonhematogenous tumor is confined to abdomen.

Stage IV: Hematogenous metastases; deposits beyond stage III, namely, to lung, liver, bone, and brain.

Stage V: Bilateral renal involvement is present at diagnosis.

The histology of the tumor cells is also identified and classified according to two groups: favorable histology (FH) and unfavorable histology (UH). Only about 12% of Wilms tumors demonstrate unfavorable histology, which is associated with a poorer prognosis and demands a more aggressive treatment protocol, regardless of the clinical stage.

Survival rates for Wilms tumor are the highest among all childhood cancers. Children with localized tumor (stages I and II) have a 90% chance of cure with multimodal therapy. In children with metastasis, survival rates are approximately 85% (Baum and Morgan, 1983).

Clinical Manifestations

The most common presenting sign is a swelling or mass within the abdomen. The mass is characteristically firm, nontender, confined to the midline, and deep within the flank. If it is on the right side, it may be difficult to distinguish from the liver, although, unlike that organ, it does not move with respiration. Parents usually discover the mass during routine bathing or dressing of the child.

Other clinical manifestations are the result of compression from the tumor mass, metabolic alterations secondary to the tumor, or metastasis. Hematuria occurs in less than one fourth of children with Wilms tumor. Anemia, usually secondary to hemorrhage within the tumor, results in pallor, anorexia, and lethargy. Hypertension, probably caused by secretion of excess amounts of renin by the tumor, occurs occasionally. Other effects of malignancy include weight loss and fever. If metastasis has occurred, symptoms of lung involvement, such as dyspnea, cough, shortness of breath, and pain in the chest, may be evident.

Diagnostic Evaluation

In a child suspected of having Wilms tumor, special emphasis is placed on the history and physical examination for presence of congenital anomalies, family history of cancer, and signs of malignancy, such as weight loss, size of liver and spleen, indications of anemia, and lymphadenopathy. Specific tests include radiographic studies, including intravenous pyelogram, computerized tomography, hematologic studies (polycythemia is sometimes present if the tumor secretes excess erythropoietin), biochemical studies, and urinalysis. Studies to demonstrate the relationship of the tumor to the ipsilateral kidney and the presence of a normal functioning kidney on the contralateral side are essential. If a large tumor is present, an inferior venacavagram is necessary to demonstrate possible tumor involvement adjacent to the vena cava. A bone marrow aspiration is electively performed to rule out metastasis.

Therapeutic Management

The remarkable survival rates for children with Wilms tumor have been the result of a cooperative group of specialists who formed the National Wilms Tumor Study (NWTS) to systematically investigate optimum treatment protocols, including surgery, radiation, and chemotherapy. Combined treatment of surgery and chemotherapy with or without radiation is based on the clinical stage and histologic pattern.

Surgery is scheduled as soon as possible after confirmation of a renal mass, usually within 24 to 48 hours after admission. A large transabdominal incision is performed for optimum visualization of the abdominal cavity. The tumor, affected kidney, and adjacent adrenal gland are removed. Great care is taken to keep the encapsulated tumor intact, since rupture can seed cancer cells throughout the abdomen, lymph channel, and bloodstream. The contralateral kidney is carefully inspected for evidence of disease or dysfunction. Regional lymph nodes are inspected and a biopsy is performed when indicated. Any involved structures, such as part of the colon, diaphragm, or vena cava, are removed. Metal clips are placed around the tumor site for exact marking during radiotherapy.

If both kidneys are involved, a partial nephrectomy is performed on the less affected kidney, with a total nephrectomy on the opposite side, and the child is treated with radiotherapy and chemotherapy. When a transplant is feasible, such as from a twin, sibling, or parent, bilateral nephrectomy is considered.

Postoperative radiotherapy is indicated for all children with Wilms tumor except those with stage I disease and favorable histology. Chemotherapy is indicated for all stages. The most effective agents for treating Wilms tumor are actinomycin D and vincristine, sometimes combined with adriamycin. Duration of therapy varies, ranging from 6 to 15 months.

Nursing Considerations

The nursing care of the child with Wilms tumor is similar to that of other cancers treated with surgery, irradiation, and chemotherapy. However, there are some significant differences discussed for each phase of nursing intervention.

Preoperative care. As with many of the other cancers, the diagnosis of Wilms tumor is a shock. Frequently the child has no physical indication of the seriousness of the disorder other than a palpable abdominal mass. Since in the majority of instances it is the parents who discover the mass, the nurse needs to take into account their feelings regarding the diagnosis. Whereas some parents are grateful for their detection of the tumor, others feel guilty for not finding it sooner or anger toward the physician for missing it on earlier examinations.

The preoperative period is one of swift diagnosis. Typically surgery is scheduled within 24 to 48 hours of admission. The nurse is faced with the challenge of preparing the child and parents for all laboratory and operative procedures. Because of the little time available, explanations should be kept simple and repeated often with attention to what the child will experience. Besides usual preoperative observations, blood pressure is monitored, since hyperten-

sion from excess renin production is a possibility.

There are several special preoperative concerns, the most important of which is that the tumor is not palpated unless absolutely necessary because manipulation of the mass may cause dissemination of cancer cells to adjacent and distant sites. In teaching hospitals in which many medical and nursing students are assigned to one patient, it may be necessary to post a sign on the bed that reads "DO NOT PALPATE ABDOMEN." This same precaution is extended to parents as soon as Wilms tumor is suspected. Careful bathing and handling are also important in preventing trauma to the tumor site.

Since radiotherapy and chemotherapy are usually begun immediately after surgery, parents need an explanation of what to expect, such as major benefits and side effects, although the timing of the information should be considered to avoid overwhelming the family. Ideally the nurse should be present during physician- parent conferences in order to answer questions as they arise. It is usually better to reserve telling the child about these side effects until after surgery. Alopecia, usually of most concern to older children, does not occur until 2 weeks after the initial treatment regimen. Therefore the child can be prepared for the hair loss postoperatively.

Postoperative care. Despite the extensive surgical intervention necessary in many children with Wilms tumor, the recovery period is usually rapid. The major nursing responsibilities are those following any abdominal surgery (see Nursing care summary on p. 1421). Since these children are at risk for intestinal obstruction from vincristine-induced adynamic ileus, radiation-induced edema, and postsurgical adhesion formation, gastrointestinal activity, such as bowel movements, bowel sounds, distention and vomiting, is monitored. Other considerations are frequent evaluation of blood pressure and observation for signs of infection, especially during chemotherapy. Because of the myelosuppression from the drugs, pulmonary hygiene measures are instituted in the immediate postoperative period to prevent complications.

Support the family. The postoperative period is frequently difficult for parents. The shock of seeing their child immediately after surgery may be the first realization of the seriousness of the diagnosis. It also marks the confirmation of the stage of the tumor. During this period the nurse should again be with parents to assure them of the child's recovery after surgery and to assess their understanding of the pathology report.

Older children need an opportunity to deal with their feelings concerning the many procedures to which they have been subjected in rapid succession. Play therapy with dolls, puppets, or drawing can be extremely beneficial in helping them adjust to the surgery and hair loss. It is not unusual for children to feel betrayed because they were not adequately prepared for the extent of surgery, the need for additional therapy, or the seriousness of the disorder.

Because the child is left with only one kidney, certain

precautions are recommended to prevent injury to the organ, such as avoiding contact sports or any other activity that has a high risk potential. Urinary tract infections should be prevented with good hygiene, especially in girls, and adequate fluid intake. Prompt detection and treatment of any genitourinary signs or symptoms is mandatory.

RHABDOMYOSARCOMA

Soft tissue sarcomas are the fourth most common type of solid tumors in children. These malignant neoplasms originate from undifferentiated mesenchymal cells in muscles, tendons, bursae, and fascia, or fibrous, connective, lymphatic, or vascular tissue. They derive their name from the specific tissue(s) of origin, such as myosarcoma (*myo*—muscle). Rhabdomyosarcoma (*rhabdo*—striated) is the most common soft tissue sarcoma in children. Because striated (skeletal) muscle is found almost anywhere in the body, these tumors occur in many sites, the most common of which are the head and neck, especially the orbit. The disease occurs in children in all age-groups but most commonly in children younger than 5 years of age. Its incidence is approximately 4.4 per million for white children under age 15, but only 1.3 per million for black children in this age-group.

Rhabdomyosarcoma arises from embryonic mesenchyme. Four subtypes are recognized:

1. **Embryonal**—most common type; most frequently found in the head, neck, abdomen, and genitourinary tract
2. **Alveolar**—second most common type; most often seen in deep tissues of the extremities and trunk
3. **Botryoid**—third most common type; appears as multiple grapelike clusters or polyps, usually found in cavities such as the vagina, urinary bladder, ear, and nasopharynx
4. **Pleomorphic**—rare in children (adult form); most often occurs in soft parts of extremities and trunk

Staging and Prognosis

Careful staging is extremely important for planning treatment and determining prognosis. The Intergroup Rhabdomyosarcoma Study has established the following clinical staging (Maurer, 1979):

Group I: Localized disease; tumor completely resected and regional nodes not involved
Group II: Localized disease with microscopic residual, or regional disease with no residual or with microscopic residual
Group III: Incomplete resection or biopsy with gross residual disease
Group IV: Metastatic disease present at diagnosis

With the change in treatment from radical surgery or radiotherapy to a multimodal approach, survival rates for all stages have increased considerably. The 2-year survival rate approximates 70% overall, with specific 3-year survival rates varying for each clinical stage: 85% for group I, 76% for group II, 75% for group III, and 38% for group IV. Data

Table 36-8 Clinical manifestations of rhabdomyosarcoma according to tumor site

LOCATION	SIGNS AND SYMPTOMS
Orbit	Rapidly developing unilateral proptosis Ecchymosis of conjunctiva Loss of extraocular movements (strabismus)
Nasopharynx	Stuffy nose (earliest sign) Nasal obstruction—dysphagia, nasal voice (obstruction of posterior nasal conchae), serous otitis media (obstruction of eustachian tube) Pain (sore throat and ear) Epistaxis Palpable neck nodes Visible mass in oropharynx (late sign)
Paranasal sinuses	Nasal obstruction Local pain Discharge Sinusitis Swelling
Middle ear	Signs of chronic serous otitis media Pain Sanguinopurulent drainage Facial nerve palsy
Retroperitoneal area (usually a "silent" tumor)	Abdominal mass Pain Signs of intestinal or genitourinary obstruction
Perineum	Visible superficial mass Bowel or bladder dysfunction (from tumor compression)

suggest that children who remain disease free for 2 years are probably cured; however, if relapse occurs, the prognosis for long-term survival is extremely poor (Miser and Pizzo, 1985).

Clinical Manifestations

The initial signs and symptoms are related to the site of the tumor and compression of adjacent organs (Table 36-8). Some tumor locations, particularly the orbit, produce symptoms early in the course of the illness and contribute to rapid diagnosis and improved prognosis. Other tumors, such as those of the retroperitoneal area, produce no symptoms until they are large, invasive, and widely metastasized. In some instances a primary tumor site is never identified.

Diagnostic Evaluation

Unfortunately, many of the signs and symptoms attributable to rhabdomyosarcoma are vague and frequently suggest a common childhood illness, such as "earache" or "runny nose." However, diagnosis begins with a careful examination of the head and neck area, particularly palpation of a nontender, firm, hard mass. The nasopharynx and oropharynx are inspected for any evidence of a visible mass.

Roentgenographic studies to isolate a tumor site are performed, accompanied by chest x-ray examinations, lung tomograms, bone surveys, and bone marrow aspiration to rule out metastasis. A lumbar puncture is indicated for head and neck tumors. An excisional biopsy is done to confirm histologic type.

Therapeutic Management

Since this tumor is highly malignant, with metastasis frequently occurring at time of diagnosis, aggressive multimodal therapy is recommended. In the past, radical surgical removal of the tumor was the treatment of choice, but with improved survival from combined chemotherapy and radiation, surgery plays a lesser role. Complete removal of the primary tumor is advocated whenever possible. However, biopsy only is required in certain tumor locations, such as those of the orbit when followed by radiation and chemotherapy. This is a fortunate change, because it avoids the devastating effects of enucleation, amputation, or pelvic exenteration.

High-dose irradiation to the primary tumor is recommended, except in group I tumors. Chemotherapy plays a major role in treatment of all groups. Drugs that are cytotoxic for rhabdomyosarcoma are vincristine, actinomycin D, and cyclophosphamide (collectively known as VAC), with or without adriamycin.

Nursing Considerations

The nursing responsibilities are similar to those for other types of cancer, especially the solid tumors when surgery is employed. Specific objectives include (1) careful assessment for signs of the tumor, especially during well-child examinations; (2) preparation of the child and family for the multiple diagnostic tests (see pp. 1565 and 1580); and (3) supportive care during each stage of multimodal therapy. The reader is urged to review Nursing considerations for leukemia and Chapter 23 for emotional support of the family in the event of a poor prognosis.

RETINOBLASTOMA

Retinoblastoma is a congenital malignant tumor arising from the retina. It is a relatively rare tumor in the United States and occurs less frequently than any of the cancers previously discussed with an incidence of 3.4 per million in children under 15 years. Like Wilms tumor it can be inherited, and it may be present at birth or may arise in the retina during the first 2 years of life. The average age of the child at the time of diagnosis is 17 months; it is usually diagnosed earlier in hereditary cases and later in nonhereditary types.

Retinoblastoma may be caused by (1) a somatic mutation, (2) a germinal mutation, or (3) a chromosomal aberration. *Somatic mutations* (those occurring in the general body cells, as opposed to the germ cells or gametes) are a sporadic event and consequently are nonhereditary. They

are always unilateral. *Germinal mutations* are passed to future generations. All bilateral retinoblastomas are considered hereditary. Hereditary retinoblastomas are transmitted as an autosomal-dominant trait, with an 80% penetrance. Consequently, 20% of gene carriers remain unaffected.

Retinoblastoma has also been associated with partial deletion of the long arm of a group D chromosome (number 13) and chromosomal polyploidy (excessive numbers of chromosomes), such as trisomy 21. In children who have chromosomal aberrations and retinoblastoma, there is often an increased incidence of mental retardation and congenital malformations, although the vast majority of children with retinoblastomas apparently have normal chromosomes and intelligence.

Staging and Prognosis

Staging of retinoblastomas is done under indirect ophthalmoscopy before surgery to accurately determine tumor size (measured in disc diameters—DD) and location (according to an imaginary line called the equator drawn on the midplane of the eye). The following classification by Reese-Ellsworth is commonly used:

> **Group I:** Very favorable
> Solitary tumor, less than 4 DD, at or behind the equator
> Multiple tumors, none greater than 4 DD, all at or behind the equator
> **Group II:** Favorable
> Solitary tumors, 4 to 10 DD, at or behind the equator
> Multiple tumors, 4 to 10 DD, behind the equator
> **Group III:** Doubtful
> Any lesion anterior to the equator
> Solitary tumors larger than 10 DD behind the equator
> **Group IV:** Unfavorable
> Multiple tumors, some larger than 10 DD
> Any lesion extending anteriorly to the ora serrata
> **Group V:** Very unfavorable
> Massive tumors involving more than half the retina
> Vitreous seeding

The classification system has been used to define cure in terms of numbers of years free of disease and in terms of preservation of useful vision in the affected eye (favorable, doubtful, or unfavorable). Cure rates for survival are much better than for retention of useful vision. The overall 5-year survival rate is 86.5% for unilateral tumors and 88% for bilateral tumors; most of the deaths occur in children with group V disease (Tapley, Strong, and Sutow, 1984). Retinoblastoma is one of the tumors that may spontaneously regress.

Of major concern in long-term survivors is the development of secondary tumors, especially osteogenic sarcoma. Children with bilateral disease (hereditary form) are more likely to develop secondary cancers than children with unilateral disease. It is thought that these individuals are predisposed to developing cancer, and radiation increases their risk.

Clinical Manifestations

Retinoblastoma has few grossly obvious signs. Typically it is the parent who first observes a whitish "glow" in the pupil, known as the *cat's eye reflex* or *leukokoria*. The reflex represents visualization of the tumor as the light momentarily falls on the mass (Fig. 36-4). When a tumor arises in the macular region (area directly at the back of the retina when the eye is focused straight ahead), a white reflex may be seen when the tumor is quite small. It is best observed when a bright light is shining toward the child as he looks forward. It is sometimes accidentally discovered by parents when taking a photograph of their child using a flash attachment.

When the tumor arises in the periphery of the retina, it must grow to a considerably large size before light can strike it sufficiently to produce the cat's eye reflex. In this situation it is seen only when the child looks in certain directions (sideways) or if the observer stands at an oblique angle to the child's face as the child looks straight ahead. The fleeting nature of the reflex often results in a delayed diagnosis, because health professionals fail to appreciate the ominous significance of the parents' findings.

The next most common sign is strabismus resulting from poor fixation of the visually impaired eye, particularly if the tumor develops in the macula, the area of sharpest visual acuity. Blindness is usually a late sign, but it frequently is not obvious unless the parent consciously observes for behaviors indicative of loss of sight, such as bumping into objects, slowed motor development, or turning of the head to see objects lateral to the affected eye.

Another common presenting sign is a red, painful eye, often accompanied by glaucoma. Other common clinical manifestations include orbital cellulitis, unilateral mydriasis, a change in the color of the iris, hyphema, white spots on the iris, nystagmus, and complaints indicative of systemic metastasis, such as weight loss, poor appetite, or fatigue.

Diagnostic Evaluation

The first step in diagnosis is carefully listening to and recognizing the significance of reports from family members regarding suspected abnormalities within the eye. Parental remarks that in any way suggest the presence of such findings must be taken seriously and further investigated. For example, if the parent indicates that the child has a strange expression or an unusual glow in his eye, every attempt is made to duplicate the circumstances necessary to observe these changes. Children suspected of having this disorder are referred to an ophthalmologist. Definitive diagnosis is usually based on indirect ophthalmoscopy employing scleral indentation, which is done under general anesthesia with maximum dilation of the pupils.

A potentially useful test is catecholamine excretion by measuring vanillylmandelic or homovanillic acid in the urine. These substances are excreted by some retinoblastomas as well as by neuroblastomas. If distant metastasis is suspected, a bone marrow aspiration, bone survey, and lumbar puncture may be performed.

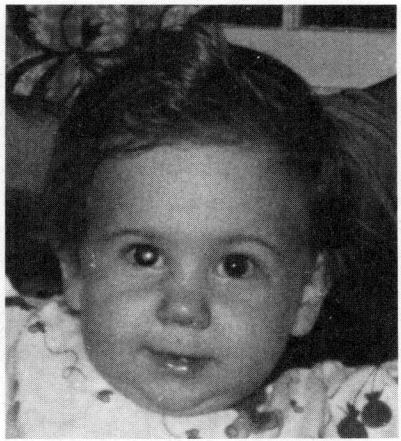

Fig. 36-4. Cat's eye reflex. Whitish appearance of lens is produced as light falls on tumor mass in right eye.

Therapeutic Management

Treatment of retinoblastoma depends chiefly on the stage of the tumor at diagnosis. In general, unilateral retinoblastomas in stages I, II, and III are treated with irradiation. The aim of radiotherapy is to preserve useful vision in the affected eye and eradicate the tumor.

Other approaches toward treating small, localized tumors involve (1) cobalt plaque applicators (surgical implantation of a cobalt 60 applicator on the sclera until the maximum radiation dose has been delivered to the tumor), (2) light coagulation (use of a laser beam to destroy retinal blood vessels that supply nutrition to the tumor), and (3) cryotherapy (freezing of the tumor, which destroys the microcirculation to the tumor and the cells themselves through microcrystal formation). One of the reasons for investigating treatments other than radiotherapy is to minimize the risk of radiation-induced malignancies later in life.

With advanced tumor growth, especially optic nerve involvement, enucleation of the affected eye is the treatment of choice. The use of chemotherapy in advanced disease, even in group V, is controversial and has not shown improved survival. Drugs that may be used in the treatment of metastatic disease include vincristine, cyclophosphamide, actinomycin, and adriamycin. In the case of central nervous system disease, intrathecal methotrexate, or a combination of methotrexate, cytosine arabinoside, and hydrocortisone may be administered (Tapley, Strong, and Sutow, 1984).

With bilateral disease, every attempt is made to preserve useful vision in the less affected eye with enucleation of the severely diseased eye. When bilateral tumors are found very early, enucleation may be prevented with only the use of radiotherapy to both eyes.

Nursing Considerations

The care of the child with retinoblastoma involves much attention to individual aspects of diagnosis, treatment protocols, and possible hereditary factors. Nursing objectives include (1) identifying signs of retinoblastoma, (2) prepar-

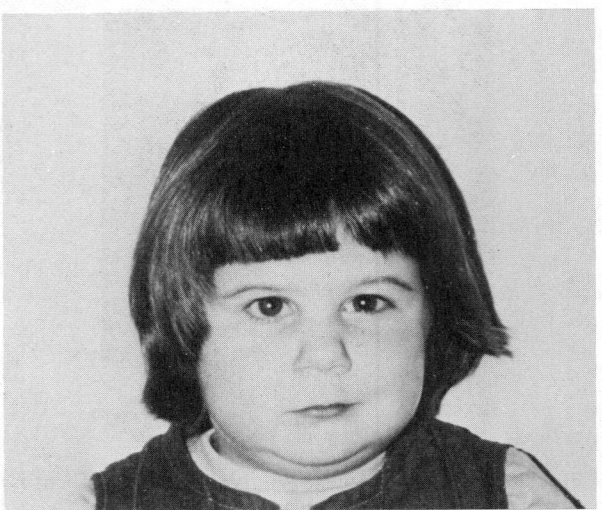

Fig. 36-5. Preschooler with right prosthetic eye.

ing the family for diagnostic/therapeutic procedures and home care, and (3) providing emotional support. The importance of recognizing possible early signs and appreciating their significance has already been discussed.

Prepare the family for diagnostic/therapeutic procedures and home care. Since the tumor is usually diagnosed in infants or very young children, most of the preparation for diagnostic tests and treatment involves parents. After indirect ophthalmoscopy the child may not see very clearly, or his eyes may be sensitive to light because of pupillary dilation. Parents are made aware of these normal reactions before the procedure.

Once the disease is staged, the physician confers with the parents regarding treatment. Unless the diagnosis is made very early, an enucleation is performed. Parents are told about the procedure as well as about the benefits of a prosthesis. Parents often believe the operation is bloody and mutilating, envisioning that the eye is "ripped out of its socket." Actually, the surgery is very similar to scooping a nut out of its shell. All the adnexal structures of the eye, such as the lids, lashes, and tear glands, are left undisturbed.

Showing parents pictures of another child with an artificial eye may be very helpful in their adjustment to the thought of disfigurement (Fig. 36-5). Although the idea of loss of vision is a very distressing one, most parents seem to realize that there is no alternative. The facts that the unaffected eye retains normal vision and that the affected eye is probably already blind are particularly helpful in promoting acceptance of the imposed impairment and should be emphasized.

After surgery, the parents need to be prepared for the child's facial appearance. An eye patch is in place, and the child's face may be edematous or ecchymotic. Parents often fear seeing the surgical site because they imagine a cavity in the skull. On the contrary, the lids are usually closed, and the area does not appear sunken because a surgically implanted sphere (Fig. 36-6, A) maintains the shape of the

eyeball. The implant is covered with conjunctiva, and when the lids are open, the exposed area resembles the mucosal lining of the mouth. Once the child is fitted for a prosthesis (Fig. 36-6, B), usually within 3 weeks, the facial appearance returns to normal.

After an uneventful recovery from enucleation, plans can be made for discharge from the hospital, usually within 3 to 4 days postoperatively. Parents need instruction regarding care of the surgical site and preparation for any additional therapy. They should be given the opportunity to see the socket as soon after surgery as possible. A good time to do this without unduly pressuring them is during dressing changes. They should then be encouraged to participate in the dressing changes.

Care of the socket is minimal and easily accomplished. The wound itself is clean and has little or no drainage. If an antibiotic ointment is prescribed, it is applied in a thin line on the surface of the tissues of the socket. To cleanse the site, an irrigating solution may be ordered and is instilled daily or more frequently if necessary, *before* application of the antibiotic ointment. The dressing consists of an eye pad taped over the surgical site with nonirritating tape; it is changed daily. Self-adhesive eye pads can also be used as dressings. They require less manipulation for application and are available at most surgical supply stores and pharmacies. Once the socket has healed completely, a dressing is no longer necessary, although there are several reasons for continuing to have the child wear the eye patch. Infants

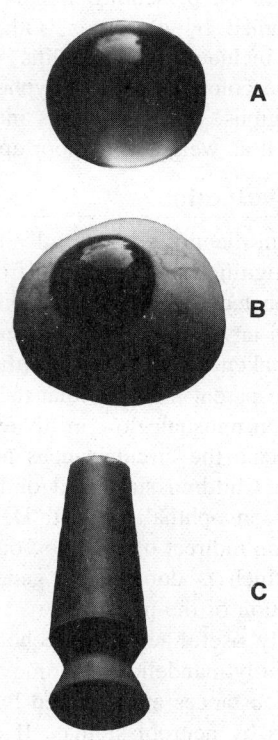

Fig. 36-6. Prosthetic eye devices. **A,** Spherical implant; **B,** prosthetic eye; and **C,** rubber plunger.

and toddlers explore their environment with their hands, and the socket is available to exploring fingers without an eye patch in place. Although there is little danger of the child injuring the socket, parents may feel more secure with the socket covered. This also helps prevent infection.

Initial instructions for care of the prosthesis are given by the ocularist, who fits and manufactures the device. Once in place, the prosthesis need not be removed unless cleaning is necessary, in which case it is taken out by gently pulling down on the lower lid, which frees the lower edge of the prosthesis, and applying pressure to the upper lid. If the child resists by forcing the lids shut, a small rubber instrument resembling a plunger (Fig, 36-6, *C*) can be used to facilitate removal and reinsertion. The end of the plunger is moistened and placed on top of the prosthetic iris. The lower eyelid is retracted, and the prosthesis is pulled out with a downward motion.

The prosthesis is cleaned by placing it in hot water and soaking it for several minutes. Reinsertion is easier if the prosthesis remains wet. To reinsert the prosthesis, the lids are separated, and with the prosthesis held in the correct position (it should be marked to indicate the nasal side), it is pushed up under the upper lid, allowing the lower lid to cover its lower edge.

Because the prosthesis is easily removed, the child may accidentally cause it to dislodge. Reactions of children vary from fear that they have ''lost'' their eye to matter-of-fact acceptance. The first time can be disturbing to both parents and child, but it is just one part of the child's adjusted lifestyle. If the child is old enough to understand, the parent can explain that he has a ''special'' eye that can accidentally fall out but that can also be quickly put back in place.

Safety is a major concern to prevent damage to the unaffected eye. Safety measures such as those presented in Table 25-5 should be practiced at all times, and rough contact sports should be avoided or protective eye wear worn during such activity.

Support the family. The diagnosis of retinoblastoma presents some special concerns in addition to those created by any type of cancer. Families with a history of the disorder may feel great guilt for transmitting the defect to their offspring, especially if they knowingly ''played the odds'' and parented an affected child. Conversely, when parents are aware of the probability and have an affected child, early treatment results in such favorable outcomes that parental adjustment may be rapid. In families with no history of retinoblastoma, the discovery of the diagnosis is a shock, frequently complicated by guilt for not having found it sooner. Since parents frequently are the first to observe the cat's eye reflex, they may feel angry at themselves or others, especially professionals, for delaying a more thorough examination. Each of these variables needs to be considered in offering supportive care to the family.

Other concerns are also related to the hereditary aspects of the disease. Of great importance to parents is the recurrence risk of retinoblastoma in their subsequent offspring and in the offspring of the surviving affected child (Table 36-9). With improving prognosis for these children, the necessity of genetic counseling to prevent transmission of the disease is assuming greater importance. (See p. 172 for a discussion of the nurse's role in genetic counseling.) In addition, these families are encouraged to seek regular follow-up care for the affected child to detect secondary tumors, and all subsequent offspring of unaffected parents and survivors should undergo regular periodic indirect ophthalmoscopy under anesthesia to detect retinoblastoma at its earliest stage.

Table 36-9 Recurrence risks of retinoblastoma in families with an affected child

TYPE OF TUMOR	RISK TO SUBSEQUENT SIBLINGS	RISK TO AFFECTED CHILD'S OFFSPRING
Unilateral*	1%-5%	7%-15%
Bilateral†	10%	50%

Compiled from a variety of sources and personal communication with Dr. Ellsworth (1979).
*Refers only to families with negative family history.
†Regardless of family history.

CONCEPT SUMMARIES

- Criteria used to determine cure of cancer include cessation of therapy, continuous freedom from clinical and laboratory evidence of cancer, and minimal or no risk of relapse as determined by previous experience with disease.

- Although the cure rate for most types of childhood cancer has improved, the late effects of treatment are of increasing concern.

- Determination of malignancy and metastasis is made by history and physical examination, laboratory tests, imaging techniques, and biopsy.

- The major modes of cancer therapy are surgery, chemotherapy, radiotherapy, immunotherapy, and bone marrow transplantation.

- Chemotherapeutic agents are classified according to their cytotoxic action: alkylating agents, antimetabolites, plant alkaloids, antitumor antibiotics, and hormones.

- Types of bone marrow transplants are allogeneic, autologous, and syngeneic.

- Treatment of leukemia follows four phases: remission induction, sanctuary therapy, maintenance therapy, and reinduction.

- Nursing goals in the care of the child with leukemia are to prepare the family for diagnostic and therapeutic procedures, prevent complications of myelosuppression (infection, hemorrhage, anemia), manage problems of irradiation and drug toxicity (nausea and vomiting, anorexia, mucosal ulceration, neuropathy, hemorrhagic cystitis, alopecia, moon face, mood changes), and provide continued emotional support.

- The lymphomas include Hodgkin and non-Hodgkin lymphoma; Hodgkin disease affects primarily adolescents.

- Nursing care of the child with a brain tumor includes to observe for signs and symptoms related to the tumor, prepare the child and family for diagnostic tests and operative procedures, prevent postoperative complications, plan for discharge, and promote a return to optimum health.

- The traditional approach to treatment of osteosarcoma has been radical surgical resection or amputation; however, chemotherapy is now playing an increasing role.

- Wilms tumor shows an increased incidence among siblings and identical twins, demonstrating a hereditary predisposition.

- Rhabdomyosarcoma may occur almost anywhere in the body, but the most common sites are the head and neck.

- Common presenting signs in retinoblastoma are cat's eye reflex, strabismus, and red, painful eye.

REFERENCES

ASHP: Technical assistance bulletin on handling cytotoxic drugs in hospitals, Am. J. Hosp. Pharm. 42(1):131-137, 1985.

Allegretta, G.J., Weisman, S.J., and Altman, A.J.: Oncologic emergencies II: hematologic and infectious complications of cancer and cancer treatment, Pediatr. Clin. North Am. 32(3):613-624, 1985.

American Academy of Pediatrics, Committee on Infectious Diseases: Report of the committee on infectious diseases, ed. 20, Elk Grove Village, IL, 1986, American Academy of Pediatrics.

Askin, F.B., and others: Occult testicular leukemia: testicular biopsy at three years continuous complete remission of childhood leukemia; a Southwest Oncology Group Study, Cancer 47:470-475, 1981.

Baum, E., and Morgan, E.: Wilms' tumor, Pediatr. Ann. 12(5):357-363, 1983.

Bergemann, D.A.: Handling antineoplastic agents, Am. J. Intravenous Therapy 10(1):13-17, 1983.

Bernstein, I., and others: Immunodiagnosis and immunotherapy of childhood malignancies, Pediatr. Clin. North Am. 32(3):575-600, 1985.

Bernstein, I.L., Webster, M.M., and Bernstein, I.D.: Food aversions in children receiving chemotherapy for cancer, Cancer 50(12):2961-2963, 1982.

Bleyer, W.A.: Acute lymphoid leukemia, Pediatr. Ann. 12(4):277-292, 1983.

Bleyer, W.A.: Cancer chemotherapy in infants and children, Pediatr. Clin. North Am. 32(3):557-574, 1985.

Cancer facts and figures, 1986, New York, 1986, American Cancer Society.

Ch'ien, L.T., and others: Long-term neurological implications of somnolence syndrome in children with acute lymphocytic leukemia, Ann. Neurol. 8(3):273-277, 1980.

Cimprich, B.: Symptom management: constipation, Cancer Nurs. 8(1)suppl.:39-43, 1985.

Cohen, F.: Clinical genetics in nursing practice, Philadelphia, 1984, J.B. Lippincott Co.

Daeffler, R.: Oral hygiene measures for patients with cancer, II, Cancer Nurs. 3(6):427-432, 1980.

Dolgin, M.J., and others: Anticipatory nausea and vomiting in pediatric cancer patients, Pediatrics 75(3):547-552, 1985.

Ertel, I.J.: Brain tumors in children, CA 30(6):306-321, 1980.

Esseltine, D.W., and others: Significance of a (4;11) translocation in acute lymphoblastic leukemia, Cancer 50(3):503-506, 1982.

Ettinger, L.J.: Osteosarcoma, Pediatr. Ann. 12(5):374-382, 1983.

Evans, A.E.: Staging and treatment of neuroblastoma, Cancer 45:1799-1802, 1980.

Fernbach, D.J.: The role of the family physician in the care of the child with cancer, CA 35(5):258-270, 1985.

Feusner, J.: The use of platelet transfusions, Am. J. Pediatr. Hematol. Oncol. 6(3):255-260, 1984.

Flaherty, A.M.: Symptom management: nausea and vomiting, Cancer Nurs. 8(1)suppl.:36, 1985.

Friedman, R.J., Rigel, D.S., and Kopf, A.W.: Early detection of malignant melanoma: the role of physician examination and self-examination of the skin, CA 35(3):130-151, 1985.

Gallo, R.C.: The virus-cancer story, Hosp. Pract. 18(6):79-89, 1983.

Gardner, R.V., and Graham-Pole, J.: Non-Hodgkin's lymphoma, Pediatr. Ann. 12(4):322-335, 1983.

Gershon, A.A., and others: Live attenuated varicella vaccine: efficacy for children with leukemia in remission, JAMA 252(3):355-362, 1984.

Grier, H.E., and Weinstein, H.J.: Acute nonlymphocytic leukemia, Pediatr. Clin. North Am. 32(3):653-668, 1985.

Harvey, E.B., and others: Prenatal x-ray exposure and childhood cancer in twins, N. Engl. J. Med. 312(9):541-545, 1985.

Hazra, T.A., and Shipman, B.: Dental problems in pediatric patients with head and neck tumors undergoing multiple modality therapy, Med. Pediatr. Oncol. 10(1):91-95, 1982.

Henschel, L.: Fever patterns in the neutropenic patient, Cancer Nurs. 8(6):301-305, 1985.

Hershey, B.L., and Zimmerman, R.A.: Pediatric brain computed tomography, Pediatr. Clin. North Am. 32(6):1477-1508, 1985.

Hirsch, J.F., and others: Medulloblastoma in childhood: survival and functional results, Acta Neurochir. 48(1,2):1-15, 1979.

Hockenberry, M.J., and Cotanch, P.H.: Hypnosis as adjuvant antiemetic therapy in childhood cancer, Nurs. Clin. North Am. 20(1):105-108, 1985.

Holland, J.C.: Why patients seek unproven cancer remedies: a psychological perspective, CA 32(1):10-14, 1982.

Holmes, H., and Holmes, F.: After ten years, what are the handicaps and life styles of children treated for cancer? Clin. Pediatr. 14(9):819-823, 1975.

Holmes, W.: SQ chemotherapy at home, Am. J. Nurs. 85(2):168-169, 1985.

Horning, S.J., and others: Female reproductive potential after treatment for Hodgkin's disease, N. Engl. J. Med. 304(23):1377-1382, 1981.

Katz, E.R., Kellerman, J., and Siegel, S.E.: Behavioral distress in children with cancer undergoing medical procedures: developmental considerations, J. Consult. Clin. Psychol. 48(3):356-365, 1980.

Koocher, G.P., and O'Malley, J.E.: The Damocles syndrome: psychosocial consequences of surviving childhood cancer, New York, 1981, McGraw-Hill Book Co.

Kovatch, A.L., and others: Oral trimethoprim/sulfamethoxazole for prevention of bacterial infection during the induction phase of cancer chemotherapy in children, Pediatrics 76(5):754-760, 1985.

Krontiris, T.G.: The emerging genetics of human cancer, N. Engl. J. Med. 309(7):404-409, 1983.

Kulkarni, M.V., and others: Magnetic resonance imaging in pediatrics, Pediatr. Clin. North Am. 32(6):1509-1522, 1985.

Lansky, S.B., and others: Late effects: psychosocial, Clin. Oncol. 4(2):239-246, 1985.

Link, M.P.: Non-Hodgkin's lymphoma in children, Pediatr. Clin. North Am. 32(3):699-720, 1985.

Lopez-Ibor, B., and Schwartz, A.D.: Neuroblastoma, Pediatr. Clin. North Am. 32(3):755-778, 1985.

Lukens, J.N.: The use of nutritional therapy, Am. J. Pediatr. Hematol. Oncol. 6(3):261-265, 1984.

Maurer, H.: Rhabdomyosarcoma, Pediatr. Ann. 8(1):17-35, 1979.

McCalla, J.L.: Nursing implications of diagnostic and staging procedures. In Fochtman, D., and Foley, G.V.: Nursing care of the child with cancer, Boston, 1982, Little, Brown & Co.

Melzack, R., Guite, S., and Gonshor, A.: Relief of dental pain by ice massage of the hand, Can. Med. Assoc. J. 122:189-191, 1980.

Miser, J., and Pizzo, P.: Soft tissue sarcomas in childhood, Pediatr. Clin. North Am. **32**(3):779-800, 1985.

Moldawer, N.P., and Murray, J.L.: The clinical uses of monoclonal antibodies in cancer research, Cancer Nurs. **8**(4):207-213, 1985.

Morrow, G.R., and Morrell, C.: Behavioral treatment for the anticipatory nausea and vomiting induced by cancer chemotherapy, N. Engl. J. Med. **307**(24):1476-1480, 1982.

Musgrave, S., Dickerman, J.D., and Land, V.J.: Second or subsequent remission with a disease-free survival of 5 years or longer in acute lymphocytic leukemia of childhood: results of a national survey, Pediatrics **77**(5):765-769, 1986.

Nauseef, W.M., and Maki, D.G.: A study of the value of simple protective isolation in patients with granulocytopenia, N. Engl. J. Med. **304**(8):448-453, 1981.

O'Malley, J., and others: Psychiatric sequelae of surviving childhood cancer, Am. J. Orthopsychiatry **49**(4):606-616, 1979.

O'Malley, J., and others: Visible physical impairment and psychological adjustment among pediatric cancer survivors, Am. J. Psychiatry **137**(1):94-96, 1980.

Perin, G., and Frase, D.: Development of a program using general anesthesia for invasive procedures in a pediatric outpatient setting, J. Assoc. Pediatr. Oncol. Nurs. **3**(4):8-10, 1985.

Pinkel, D.: Cure of the child with cancer—definition and prospective. In Proceedings of the National Conference on the Care of the Child with Cancer, New York, 1979, American Cancer Society.

Pochedly, C.: "Guinea pigs" get the best treatment, Pediatr. Nurs. **9**(5):64-67, 1978.

Poplack, D.G.: Acute lymphoblastic leukemia in childhood, Pediatr. Clin. North Am. **32**(3):669-697, 1985.

Pratt, C.B.: Some aspects of childhood cancer epidemiology, Pediatr. Clin. North Am. **32**(3):541-556, 1985.

Quinn, J.J.: Bone marrow transplantation in the management of childhood cancer, Pediatr. Clin. North Am. **32**(3):811-834, 1985.

Rahr, V.: Giving intrathecal drugs, Am. J. Nurs. **86**(7):829-831, 1986.

Rivard, C.E., and others: Maintenance chemotherapy for childhood acute lymphoblastic leukaemia: better in the evening, Lancet **2**(8467):1264-1266, 1985.

Robison, L.L., and others: Down syndrome and acute leukemia in children: a 10-year retrospective survey from Children's Cancer Study Group, J. Pediatr. **105**(2):235-242, 1984.

Ruccione, K.: The role of nurses in late effects evaluations, Clin. Oncol. **4**(2):205-221, 1985.

Ruccione, K.: Acute leukemia in children: current perspectives, Issues Compr. Pediatr. Nurs. **6**(5-6):329-362, 1983.

Shulman, S.T.: Acyclovir treatment of disseminated varicella in childhood malignant neoplasms, Am. J. Dis. Child. **139**(2):137-140, 1985.

Simone, J.V., and Rivera, G.: Management of acute leukemia. In Sutow, W.W., Fernbach, D.J., and Vietti, T.J., editors: Clinical pediatric oncology, ed. 3, St. Louis, 1984, The C.V. Mosby Co.

Stolar, M.H., Power, L.A., and Veile, C.S.: Recommendations for handling cytotoxic drugs in hospitals, Am. J. Hosp. Pharm. **40**(7):1163-1171, 1983.

Strauss, R.G.: The role of granulocyte transfusions, Am. J. Pediatr. Hematol. Oncol. **6**(3):247-253, 1984.

Strong, L.C.: Genetics, etiology, and epidemiology of childhood cancer. In Sutow, W.W., Fernbach, D.J., and Vietti, T.J., editors: Clinical pediatric oncology, ed. 3, St. Louis, 1984, The C.V. Mosby Co.

Sutow, W.W.: General aspects of childhood cancer. In Sutow, W.W., Fernbach, D.J., and Vietti, T.J., editors: Clinical pediatric oncology, ed. 3, St. Louis, 1984, The C.V. Mosby Co.

Tan, C.T.C., and Chan, K.W.: Hodgkin's disease, Pediatr. Ann. **12**(4):306-321, 1983.

Tapley, N.D., Strong, L.C., and Sutow, W.W.: Retinoblastoma. In Sutow, W.W., Fernbach, D.J., and Vietti, T.J., editors: Clinical pediatric oncology, ed. 3, St. Louis, 1984, The C.V. Mosby Co.

Terrin, B.N., McWilliams, N.B., and Maurer, H.M.: Side effects of metoclopramide as an antiemetic in childhood cancer chemotherapy, J. Pediatr. **104**(1):138-140, 1984.

van Eys, J., editor: The truly cured child: the new challenge in pediatric cancer care, Baltimore, 1977, University Park Press.

Walker, R.W., and Allen, J.C.: Pediatric brain tumors, Pediatr. Ann. **12**(5):383-391, 1983.

Welbury, R.R., and others: Dental health of survivors of malignant disease, Arch. Dis. Child. **59**(12):1186-1187, 1984.

White, L., and Siegel, S.E.: Non-Hodgkin's lymphoma in childhood. In Sutow, W.W., Fernbach, D.J., and Vietti, T.J., editors: Clinical pediatric oncology, ed. 3, St. Louis, 1984, The C.V. Mosby Co.

Wiley, F.M., and DeCuir-Whalley, S.: Allogeneic bone marrow transplantation for children with acute leukemia, Oncol. Nurs. Forum **10**(3):49-53, 1983.

Wolff, L.J.: Use of prophylactic antibiotics, Am. J. Pediatr. Hematol. Oncol. **6**(3):267-276, 1984.

Woods, W.G.: Prevention of graft-vs.-host disease, Am. J. Pediatr. Hematol. Oncol. **6**(3):283-286, 1984.

Yasko, J.M.: Holistic management of nausea and vomiting caused by chemotherapy, Topics Clin. Nurs. **7**(1):26-38, 1985.

Zelter, L., and others: Psychologic effects of illness in adolescence. II. Impact of illness in adolescence—crucial issues, J. Pediatr. **97**(1):132-138, 1980.

BIBLIOGRAPHY
Cancer in Children

Baker, H.W.: Classics in oncology: needle aspiration biopsy; an introduction, CA **36**(2):69-70, 1986.

Fergusson, J., and Hobbie, W.: Home visits for the child with cancer, Nurs. Clin. North Am. **20**(1):109-116, 1985.

Fochtman, D., and Foley, G.V., editors: Nursing care of the child with cancer, Boston, 1982, Little, Brown & Co.

Frank-Stromborg, M., and others: Carcinogens: are some risks acceptable?, Am. J. Nurs. **86**(7):814-817, 1986.

Fraser, M.C., and McGuire, D.B.: Skin cancer's early warning system, Am. J. Nurs. **84**(10):1232-1236, 1984.

Hockenberry, M.J., and Bologna-Vaughn, S.: Preparation for intrusive procedures using noninvasive techniques in children with cancer: state of the art versus new trends, Cancer Nurs. **8**(2):97-102, 1985.

Labson, L.H.: Interpreting clues to childhood cancer, Patient Care **16**(3):19-63, 1982.

Littlefield, J.W.: Genes, chromosomes, and cancer, J. Pediatr. **104**(4):489-494, 1984.

Love, R.R., and Olsen, S.J.: An agenda for cancer prevention in nursing practice, Cancer Nurs. **8**(6):329-338, 1985.

Marchette, L., and Holloman, F.: A first-hand report on the new body scanners, RN **48**(11):28-31, 1985.

Martin, H.E., and Ellis, E.B.: Classics in oncology: biopsy by needle puncture and aspiration, CA **36**(2):71-82, 1986.

Miller, L.P., and Miller, D.R.: The pediatrician's role in caring for the child with cancer, Pediatr. Clin. North Am. **31**(1):119-130, 1984.

Napolitano, L.V.: What about cancer 'epidemics' in children?, Patient Care **16**(3):39, Feb. 1982.

Napolitano, L.V.: When cancer threatens a child, Patient Care **16**(3):14-63, Feb. 1982.

Pavlovsky, S.: The human T cell leukemia/lymphoma virus etiologically linked to lymphomas and leukemias of T origin, Cancer Therapy Update **III**(5):2-5, 1983.

Silverberg, E.: Cancer statistics, 1986, CA **36**(1):32-42, 1986.

Sutow, W.W., Fernbach, D.J., and Vietti, T.J., editors: Clinical pediatric oncology, ed. 3, St. Louis, 1984, The C.V. Mosby Co.

Thorne, S.: The family cancer experience, Cancer Nurs. **8**(5):285-291, 1985.

Waskerwitz, M.J., and Ruccione, K.: An overview of cancer in children in the 1980s, Nurs. Clin. North Am. **20**(1):5-30, 1985.

Welch-McCaffrey, D.: Cancer, anxiety, and quality of life, Cancer Nurs. **8**(3):151-158, 1985.

Modes of Cancer Therapy (General)

Brown, A.E.: Management in the febrile, neutropenic patient with cancer: therapeutic considerations, J. Pediatr. **106**(6):1035-1041, 1985.

Burkhalter, P.K.: Cancer quackery, Am. J. Nurs. **77**(3):451-453, 1977.

Cameron, C.O., and Wallace, N.: Having a bone marrow test: a child's perspective, Child. Health Care **12**(1):41-42, 1983.

Crosley, M.A.: Watch out for nutritional complications of cancer, RN **48**(3):22-27, 1985.

Golden, W.: Routine protective isolation: worth the trouble in neutropenic patients?, JAMA **242**(19):2045, 1979.

Holland, J.C.: Why patients seek unproven cancer remedies: a psychological perspective, CA **32**(1):10-14, 1982.

Krakoff, I.H.: Cancer chemotherapeutic agents, CA **31**(3):130-140, 1981.

Kramer, R.F.: *Pneumocystis carinii* pneumonia: a problem revisited, J. Assoc. Pediatr. Oncol. Nurs. **1**(3):16-23, 1984.

Labson, L.H.: Approaching a child's cancer treatment, Patient Care **16**(7):115-147, 1982.

Labson, L.H.: Giving acute care in childhood cancer, Patient Care **16**(7):151-195, 1982.

Lansky, S.B.: Impediments to treatment and rehabilitation of the childhood cancer patient, CA **35**(5):302-308, 1985.

Lichtiger, B., and Huh, Y.O.: Transfusion therapy for patients with cancer, CA **35**(5):311-316, 1985.

Luban, N.L.C.: Transfusion therapy with platelets and leukocytes, Pediatr. Ann. **12**(6):437-441, 1983.

Napolitano, L.V.: Referring children to cancer centers, Patient Care **16**(3):67-93, 1982.

Ostchega, Y., and Culnane, M.: Tumor markers: key pieces to your cancer patient's clinical picture, Nursing 85 **15**(9):48-51, 1985.

Petton, S.: Your role in radiation therapy, RN **48**(2):32-37, 1985.

Pizzo, P.A.: Granulocytopenia and cancer therapy: past problems, current solutions, future challenges, Cancer **54**(11):2649-2661, 1984.

Pizzo, P.A., and others: Oral antibiotic prophylaxis in patients with cancer: a double-blind randomized placebo-controlled trial, J. Pediatr. **102**(1):125-133, 1983.

Pizzo, P.A., and others: Fever in the pediatric and young adult patient with cancer: a prospective study of 1001 episodes, Medicine **61**(3):153-165, 1982.

Potter, S.: Critical infections in the pediatric oncologic patient, Nurs. Clin. North Am. **16**(4):699-706, 1981.

Smith, S.D., and others: Total care: recent advances in the treatment of children with cancer, J. Kans. Med. Soc. **80**(3):113-140, 1979.

Sontesgard, L., and others: A way to minimize side effects from radiation therapy, Am. J. Maternal Child Nurs. **1**(1):27-31, 1976.

Unproven methods of cancer management: O. Carl Simonton, M.D., CA **32**(1):58-61, 1982.

Veninga, K.S.: Improving nutrition in children with cancer, Pediatr. Nurs. **11**(1):18-20, 1985.

Whitley, R.J., and Crist, W.M.: Management of infections, Pediatr. Ann. **12**(6):445, 1983.

Chemotherapy

Anderson, M., and Faulkner, N.: Amphotericin B: effective management of adverse reactions, Cancer Nurs. **5**(6):461-464, 1982.

Association of Pediatric Oncology Nurses: Cancer chemotherapy, Newport Beach, CA, 1985, Association of Pediatric Oncology Nurses.

Berg, S.: Pharmacology: dexamethasone's new use in cancer treatment, J. Assoc. Pediatr. Oncol. Nurs. **2**(2):46-48, 1985.

Berg, S.: Pharmacology: cytarabine (ara-C)—a drug profile, J. Assoc. Pediatr. Oncol. Nurs. **1**(2):30-32, 1984.

Bersani, G., and Carl, W.: Oral care for cancer patients, Am. J. Nurs. **83**(4):533-536, 1983.

Chan, M.K.: Pharmacology: cyclophosphamide—a drug profile, J. Assoc. Pediatr. Oncol. Nurs. **1**(3):30-33, 1984.

Daeffler, R.: Oral hygiene measures for patients with cancer, III, Cancer Nurs. **4**(1):29-35, 1981.

Dodd, M.J.: Self-care for side effects in cancer chemotherapy: an assessment of nursing interventions, part 2, Cancer Nurs. **6**(1):63-67, 1983.

Dodd, M.J., and Mood, D.W.: Chemotherapy: helping patients to know the drugs they are receiving and their possible side effects, Cancer Nurs. **4**(4):311-318, 1981.

Durant, J.R.: The problem of nausea and vomiting in modern cancer chemotherapy, CA **34**(1):2-6, 1984.

Fischer, R.G.: Handling antineoplastic drugs, Pediatr. Nurs. **12**(1):59, 1986.

Geltman, R.L., and Paige, R.L.: Symptom management in hospice care, Am. J. Nurs. **83**(1):78-85, 1983.

Gralla, R.J., and others: Antiemetic efficacy of high-dose metoclopramide: randomized trials with placebo and prochlorperazine in patients with chemotherapy-induced nausea and vomiting, N. Engl. J. Med. **305**:905-909, 1981.

Griffiths, S.S.: Changes in body image caused by antineoplastic drugs, Issues Compr. Pediatr. Nurs. **4**(1):17-27, 1980.

Hart, C.N., and others: Patient care evaluation: a comparison of current practice and nursing literature for oral care of persons receiving chemotherapy, Oncol. Nurs. Forum **9**(2):22-27, 1982.

Hughes, C.B.: Giving cancer drugs: IV: some guidelines, Am. J. Nurs. **86**(1):34-38, 1986.

Hunt, J.M., Anderson, J.E., and Smith, I.E.: Scalp hypothermia to prevent Adriamycin-induced hair loss, Cancer Nurs. **5**(1):25-31, 1982.

Iannacci, L., and Piomelli, S.: Use of venous access lines, Am. J. Pediatr. Hematol. Oncol. **6**(3):277-281, 1984.

Jacobs, A., Clifford, P., and Kay, H.E.M.: The Ommaya reservoir in chemotherapy for malignant disease in the CNS, Clin. Oncol. **7**:123-129, 1981.

Jones, R.B., Frank, R., and Mass, T.: Safe handling of chemotherapeutic agents: a report from the Mount Sinai Medical Center, CA **33**(5):258-263, 1983.

Klopovich, P.M., and Trueworthy, R.C.: Adherence to chemotherapy regimens among children with cancer, Topics Clin. Nurs. **7**(1):19-25, 1985.

Krahe, E.M.: You can't be too careful with cytotoxic drugs, RN **48**(2):71-72, 1985.

Levitt, D.Z.: Cancer chemotherapy: those dreaded side effects and what to do about them. Part 1, RN **43**(6):53-56, 1980.

Levitt, D.Z.: Cancer chemotherapy: those dreaded side effects and what to do about them. Part 2, RN **43**(8):57-60, 1980.

Levitt, D.Z.: Cancer chemotherapy: those dreaded side effects and what to do about them. Part 3, RN **43**(9):51-60, 1980.

Levitt, D.Z.: Cancer chemotherapy: those dreaded side effects and what to do about them. Part 4, RN **43**(12):33-56, 1980.

Levitt, D.Z.: Cancer chemotherapy: those dreaded side effects and what to do about them. Part 5, RN **44**(2):56-59, 1981.

Maxwell, M.B.: Reexamining the dietary restrictions with procarbazine (an MAOI), Cancer Nurs. **3**(6):451-457, 1980.

Nursing implications of cancer chemotherapy, Nursing 83 **13**(7):56a-56b, 1983.

Petton, S.: Easing the complications of chemotherapy: a matter of little victories, Nursing 84 **14**(2):58-63, 1984.

Satterwhite, B.A., Pryor, A.S., and Harris, M.B.: Development and evaluation of chemotherapy fact sheets, Cancer Nurs. **3**(4):277-283, 1980.

Schnipper, I.M.: Symptom management: anorexia, Cancer Nurs. **8**(1)suppl.:33-35, 1985.

Smith, S.D., and others: A reliable method for evaluating drug compliance in children with cancer, Cancer **43**:169-173, 1979.

Speciale, J.L., and Kaalaas, J.: Infuse-a-port: new path for I.V. chemotherapy, Nursing 85 **15**(10):40-43, 1985.

Troutman, J.: Step-by-step guide to trouble-free IV chemotherapy, RN **28**(9):32-34, 1985.

Vogel, T.C., and McSkimming, S.A.: Teaching parents to give indwelling C.V. catheter care, Nursing 83 **13**(1):55-56, 1983.

Wagner, L., and Gorely, M.: Body image and patients experiencing alopecia as a result of cancer chemotherapy, Cancer Nurs. **2**(5):365-369, 1979.

Waskerwitz, M.J.: Special nursing care for children receiving chemotherapy, J. Assoc. Pediatr. Oncol. Nurs. **1**(1):16-25, 1984.

Yasko, J.M.: Holistic management of nausea and vomiting caused by chemotherapy, Topics Clin. Nurs. **7**(1):26-38, 1985.

Bone Marrow Transplantation

Bone marrow transplantation in childhood cancer, The Candlelighters Childhood Cancer Foundation Progress Reports **V**(special issue):1-24, 1985.

Cogliana-Shutta, N.A., Broda, E.J., and Gress, J.S.: Bone marrow transplantation: an overview and comparison of autologous, syngeneic, and allogeneic treatment modalities, Nurs. Clin. North Am. **20**(1):49-66, 1985.

Engelhard, D., Marks, M.I., and Good, R.A.: Infections in bone marrow transplant recipients, J. Pediatr. **108**(3):335-346, 1986.

Hutchison, M.M., editor: Symposia on bone marrow transplantation, Nurs. Clin. North Am. **18**(3):509-610, 1983.

Kamani, N.: Marrow transplantation in pediatric hematologic disorders, Pediatr. Ann. **14**(9):661-670, 1985.

Lenarsky, C., and Feig, S.A.: Bone marrow transplantation for children with cancer, Pediatr. Ann. **12**(6):428-435, 1983.

Marshall, D.: Care of the pediatric oncology patient in a laminar air flow setting: a conceptual framework for nursing practice, Nurs. Clin. North Am. **20**(1):67-82, 1985.

McGlave, P.B.: The status of bone marrow transplantation for leukemia, Hosp. Pract. **20**(11):97-110, 1985.

Patenaude, A.F., Szymanski, L., and Rappeport, J.: Psychological costs of bone marrow transplantation in children, Am. J. Orthopsychiatry **49**(3):409-422, 1979.

Pfefferbaum, B., Lindamood, M., and Wiley, F.M.: Stages in pediatric bone marrow transplantation, Pediatrics **61**(4):625-628, 1978.

Nuscher, R., and others: Bone marrow transplantation: a lifesaving option, Am. J. Nurs. **84**(6):764-772, 1984.

Sanders, J.E., and others: Marrow transplantation for children in first remission of acute nonlymphoblastic leukemia: an update, Blood **66**(2):460-462, 1985.

Sondel, P., and others: Pediatric bone marrow transplantation: current progress and future prospects, Pediatrics **72**(6):818-822, 1983.

Storb, R.: Bone marrow transplantation: progress and problems, J. Pediatr. **105**(3):414-418, 1984.

Wiley, F.M., Lindamood, M.M., and Pfefferbaum-Levine, B.: Donor-patient relationship in pediatric bone marrow transplantation, J. Assoc. Pediatr. Oncol. Nurs. **1**(3):8-14, 1984.

Long-Term Sequelae of Treatment

Aisenberg, A.: Acute nonlymphocytic leukemia after treatment for Hodgkin's disease, Am. J. Med. **75**:449-454, 1983.

Blatt, J., and others: Testicular function in boys after chemotherapy for acute lymphoblastic leukemia, N. Engl. J. Med. **304**:1121-1124, 1981.

Brouwers, P., and others: Long-term neuropsychologic sequelae of childhood leukemia: correlation with CT brain scan abnormalities, J. Pediatr. **106**(5):723-728, 1985.

Byrd, R.: Late effects of treatment of cancer in children, Pediatr. Clin. North Am. **32**(3):835-857, 1985.

Carl, W.: Oral complications in cancer patients, Am. Fam. Physician **27**(2):161-170, 1983.

Copeland, D.R., and others: Neuropsychological sequelae of childhood cancer in long-term survivors, Pediatrics **75**(4):745-753, 1985.

Eiser, C.: Psychological development of the child with leukemia: a review, J. Behav. Med. **2**(2):141-157, 1979.

Gilman, P.A., and Miller, R.W.: Cancer after acute lymphocytic leukemia, Am. J. Dis. Child. **135**:311-312, 1981.

Gogan, J.L., and others: Pediatric cancer survival and marriage: issues affecting adult adjustment, Am. J. Orthopsychiatry **19**(3):423-430, 1979.

Greene, P.E., and Fergusson, J.H.: Nursing care in childhood cancer, late effects of therapy, Am. J. Nurs. **82**(3):443-446, 1982.

Hickey, A.J., and others: Survey of oral/dental needs of patients receiving chemotherapy for malignant disease, Compendium of Continuing Education **II**(2):92-95, 1981.

Hutter, J.: Late effects in children with cancer, Am. J. Dis. Child. **140**(1):17-19, 1986.

Jaffe, N., and others: Dental and maxillofacial abnormalities in long-term survivors of childhood cancer: effects of treatment with chemotherapy and radiation to the head and neck, Pediatrics **73**(6):816-823, 1984.

Koocher, G.P., and others: Psychological adjustment among pediatric cancer survivors, J. Child Psychol. Psychiatry **21**(2):163-173, 1980.

McCalla, J.L.: A multidisciplinary approach to identification and remedial intervention for adverse late effects of cancer therapy, Nurs. Clin. North Am. **20**(1):117-130, 1985.

McHaney, V.A., and others: Hearing loss in children receiving cisplatin chemotherapy, J. Pediatr. **102**(2):314-318, 1983.

Meadows, A.T., and Silber, J.: Delayed consequences of therapy for childhood cancer, CA **35**(5):271, 1985.

Oberfield, S.E., and others: Long-term endocrine sequelae after treatment of medulloblastoma: prospective study of growth and thyroid function, J. Pediatr. **108**(2):219-223, 1986.

Peterson, D.E., and Sonis, S.T.: Oral complications of cancer chemotherapy: present status and future studies, Cancer Treatment Reports **66**(6):1251-1256, 1982.

Reimer, R.R.: Risk of a second malignancy related to the use of cytotoxic chemotherapy, CA **32**(5):286-292, 1982.

Robison, L.L., and others: Factors associated with IQ scores in long-term survivors of childhood acute lymphoblastic leukemia, Am. J. Pediatr. Hematol. Oncol. **6**:115-121, 1984.

Ruccione, K., and Fergusson, J.: Late effects of childhood cancer and its treatment, Oncol. Nurs. Forum **11**(5):54-64, 1984.

Takaue, Y., and others: Second malignant neoplasm in treated Hodgkin's disease, Am. J. Dis. Child. **140**(1):49-51, 1986.

Wells, R.J., and others: The impact of cranial irradiation on the growth of children with acute lymphocytic leukemia, Am. J. Dis. Child. **137**(1):37-39, 1983.

Leukemias/Lymphomas

Ablin, A.R.: Managing the problem of hyperleukocytosis in acute leukemia, Am. J. Pediatr. Hematol. Oncol. **6**(3):287-290, 1984.

American Academy of Pediatrics, Committee on Infectious Diseases: Expanded guidelines for use of varicella-zoster immune globulin, Pediatrics **72**(6):886-887, 1983.

Brunell, P.A., and others: Risk of herpes zoster in children with leukemia: varicella vaccine compared with history of chickenpox, Pediatrics **77**(1):53-56, 1986.

Canellos, G.P.: Hodgkin's disease, Pediatr. Rev. **6**(1):3-9, 1984.

Dampier, C., and Chilcote, R.R.: Acute non-lymphoid leukemia, Pediatr. Ann. **12**(4):293-305, 1983.

Devney, R.B., and others: Serial thyroid function measurements in children with Hodgkin disease, J. Pediatr. **105**(2):223-227, 1984.

Dunn, N.L., and Maurer, H.M.: The role of the practitioner in the care of children with acute leukemia, Pediatr. Rev. **5**(3):81-87, 1983.

Gilchrist, G.S., and Evans, R.G.: Contemporary issues in pediatric Hodgkin's disease, Pediatr. Clin. North Am. **32**(3):721-734, 1985.

Hays, D.M., and others: Complications related to 234 staging laparotomies performed in the intergroup Hodgkin's disease in childhood study, Surgery **96**:471-478, 1984.

Houlihan, N.G.: Leukemia: the leukemia process, Cancer Nurs. **4**(2):149-160, 1981.

Houlihan, N.G.: Leukemia: nursing management, Cancer Nurs. **4**(5):397-405, 1981.

Houlihan, N.G., and Feeley, A.M.: Leukemia: the acute and chronic leukemias, Cancer Nurs. **4**(4):323-338, 1981.

Houlihan, N.G., and Flaherty, A.M.: Leukemia: a hematology review, Cancer Nurs. **4**(1):61-71, 1981.

Lacher, M.J.: Hodgkin's disease: historical perspective, current status, and future directions, CA **35**(2):88-94, 1985.

Steinhorn, S.C.: Improved survival among children with acute leukemia diagnosed in the 1970s, Cancer Treat. Rep. **68**:953-958, 1984.

Tafuro, P., and Gurevich, I.: Prevention and management of varicella in high-risk individuals, Am. J. Maternal Child Nurs. **9**(5):314-317, 1984.

Ultmann, J.E., and Jacobs, R.H.: The non-Hodgkin's lymphomas, CA **35**(2):66-87, 1985.

Weisman, S.J., Berkow, R.L., and Baehner, R.L.: Chronic leukemia of childhood, Pediatr. Rev. **6**(1):26-30, 1984.

Nervous System Tumors

Allen, J.C.: Childhood brain tumors: current status of clinical trials in newly diagnosed and recurrent disease, Pediatr. Clin. North Am. **32**(3):633-652, 1985.

Cleaveland, M.J.: Nursing care in childhood cancer: brain tumor, Am. J. Nurs. **82**(3):422-425, 1982.

Duffner, P.K., Cohen, M.E., and Freeman, A.I.: Pediatric brain tumors: an overview, CA **35**(5):287-301, 1985.

Flores, L., and others: Delay in the diagnosis of pediatric brain tumors, Am. J. Dis. Child. **140**(7):684-686, 1986.

Graus, F., Walker, R.W., and Allen, J.C.: Brain metastases in children, J. Pediatr. **103**(4):558-561, 1983.

Hayes, F.A., and Green, A.A.: Neuroblastoma, Pediatr. Ann. **12**(5):366-372, 1983.

Maul, S.K.: Childhood brain tumors: a special nursing challenge, Am. J. Maternal Child Nurs. **9**(2):123-129, 1984.

Tuchman, M., and others: Value of random urinary homovanillic acid and vanillylmandelic acid levels in the diagnosis and management of patients with neuroblastoma: comparison with 24-hour urine collections, Pediatrics **75**(2):324-328, 1985.

Bone Tumors

Boren, H.A., and Meell, H.: Adolescent amputee ski rehabilitation program, J. Assoc. Pediatr. Oncol. Nurs. **2**(1):16-23, 1985.

Bourne, B.A., and Kutcher, J.L.: Amputation: helping a patient face loss of a limb, RN **48**(2):38-45, 1985.

Gandy, E.D., and Veigh, G.: Help the amputee stand on his own again, Nursing 84 **14**(7):46-49, 1984.

Jaffe, N.: Advances in the management of malignant bone tumors in children and adolescents, Pediatr. Clin. North Am. **32**(3):801-810, 1985.

Jaffe, N., and others: Control of primary osteosarcoma with chemotherapy, Cancer **56**(3):461-466, 1985.

Kutcher, J., and Bourne, B.: Postop needs of the amputee, RN **48**(2):46-47, 1985.

Ritchie, J.A.: Nursing the child undergoing limb amputation, Am. J. Maternal Child Nurs. **5**(2):114-120, 1980.

Taylor, W.F., and others: Trends and variability in survival among patients with osteosarcoma: a 7-year update, Mayo Clin. Proc. **60**:91-104, 1985.

Walters, J.: Coping with a leg amputation, Am. J. Nurs. **81**(7):1349-1352, 1981.

Solid Tumors

Asch, M.J., and others: Prognostic factors and outcome in bilateral Wilms' tumor, Cancer **56**(10):2524-2529, 1985.

Baum, E.S., and Morgan, E.R.: Wilms' tumor, Pediatr. Ann. **12**(5):357-363, 1983.

Becton, D.L., and Friedman, H.S.: Management of solid tumors in children, Compr. Therapy **10**(11):58-66, 1984.

Belasco, J., and D'Angio, G.J.: Wilms' tumor, CA **31**(5):258-270, 1981.

Bishop, J.O.: Retinoblastoma, Pediatr. Ann. **8**(1):12-33, 1979.

Catalano, J.D.: Leukokoria—the differential diagnosis of a white pupil, Pediatr. Ann. **12**(7):498-505, 1983.

Clouse, J.W., and others: The changing management of Wilms' tumor over a 30-year period: 1949-1978, Cancer **56**(10):1484-1489, 1985.

D'Angio, G.J.: Wilms' tumor and neuroblastoma in children, Pediatr. Rev. **6**(1):10-19, 1984.

D'Angio, G.J., and others: Wilms' tumor: an update, Cancer **45**:1791-1798, 1980.

De Graff, S.S.N., and others: Unexpected cure in metastatic rhabdomyosarcoma, Arch. Dis. Child. **60**(5):482-484, 1985.

Friedman, A.L.: Wilms' tumor detection in patients with sporadic aniridia, Am. J. Dis. Child. **140**(2):173-174, 1986.

Ghavimi, F.: Rhabdomyosarcoma, Pediatr. Ann. **12**(5):395-401, 1983.

Green, D.M.: The diagnosis and management of Wilms' tumor, Pediatr. Clin. North Am. **32**(3):735-754, 1985.

Jenkin, D., and Sonley, M.: Soft-tissue sarcomas in the young, Cancer **46**:621-629, 1980.

King, D.R., and Clatworthy, W., Jr.: The pediatric patient with sarcoma, Semin. Oncol. **8**(2):215-221, 1981.

Miser, J.S., and Pizzo, P.A.: Soft tissue sarcomas in childhood, Pediatr. Clin. North Am. **32**(3):779-800, 1985.

Rubin, C.M., and others: Intraocular retinoblastoma group V: an analysis of prognostic factors, J. Clin. Oncol. **3**(5):680-685, 1985.

Wong, D.L., and Dornan, L.R.: Nursing care in childhood cancer—retinoblastoma, Am. J. Nurs. **82**(3):425-431, 1982.

Chapter 37

The Child with a Cerebral Dysfunction

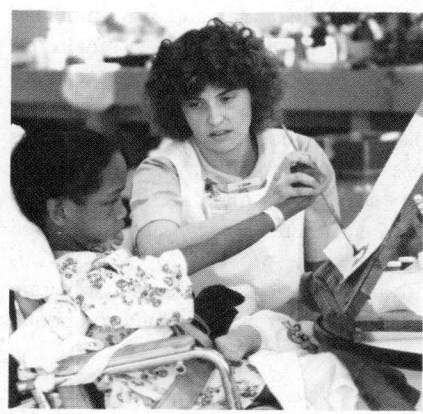

Cerebral Structure and Function
Development of the neurologic system
Central nervous system
Brain coverings
The brain
Increased intracranial pressure

Evaluation of Neurologic Status
Assessment: general aspects
History
Physical examination
Altered states of consciousness
Etiology
Level of consciousness
Coma assessment
Neurologic examination
Vital signs
Skin
Eyes
Motor function
Posturing
Reflexes
Special diagnostic procedures

The Child with Cerebral Compromise
Nursing the unconscious child
Respiratory management
Neurologic assessment
Increased intracranial pressure monitoring
Nutrition and hydration
Medications
Elimination
Hygienic care
Positioning and exercise
Stimulation
Family support
Head injury
Etiology
Pathophysiology
Complications
Diagnostic evaluation
Therapeutic management
Nursing considerations
Near-drowning
Pathophysiology
Clinical manifestations
Therapeutic management
Nursing considerations

Intracranial Infections
Bacterial meningitis
Etiology
Pathophysiology
Clinical manifestations
Diagnostic evaluation
Therapeutic management
Nursing considerations
Nonbacterial (aseptic) meningitis
Brain abscess
Encephalitis
Etiology
Clinical manifestations
Diagnostic evaluation
Therapeutic management
Nursing considerations
Rabies
Therapeutic management
Nursing considerations

Reye syndrome
Etiology
Pathophysiology
Clinical manifestations
Diagnostic evaluation
Therapeutic management
Nursing considerations

Seizure Disorders
Epilepsy: general concepts
Etiology
Pathophysiology
Clinical manifestations
Epilepsy: classification
Partial seizures
Generalized seizures
Epilepsy: therapeutic management and nursing care
Diagnostic evaluation
Therapeutic management
Nursing considerations
Febrile seizures
Breath-holding spells
Migraine

Neural control of body function is made possible by a complex communication network, and, within this network, control makes integration possible. Any disturbance in this central communication system can produce alterations in the way in which the system receives, integrates, and responds to stimuli entering the system. These disturbances are reflected in a variety of clinical manifestations, depending on the focus of the disturbance and the integrity of the conducting mechanism. This chapter is concerned primarily with alterations in consciousness caused by seizure activity, infectious processes, and trauma.

Cerebral Structure and Function

The nervous system is composed of three intimately connected and functioning parts: (1) the central nervous system, composed of two cerebral hemispheres, the brain stem, the cerebellum, and the spinal cord; (2) the peripheral nervous system, which consists of the cranial nerves that arise from or travel to the brain stem and the spinal nerves that travel to or from the spinal cord, which may be motor (efferent) or sensory (afferent); and (3) the autonomic nervous system, composed of the sympathetic and parasympathetic systems that provide automatic control of vital functions.

Since this chapter is concerned primarily with disturbances of the brain, the major emphasis will be placed on this system. The structure and function of the spinal cord and autonomic system are elaborated in Chapters 39 and 40.

DEVELOPMENT OF THE NEUROLOGIC SYSTEM

In contrast to other body tissues, which grow rapidly after birth, the nervous system grows proportionately more rapidly before birth. Two periods of rapid brain cell growth occur during fetal life. There is a dramatic increase in the number of neurons between 15 and 20 weeks of gestation, and another increase in rate begins at 30 weeks of gestation and extends to 1 year of age. This rapid growth during infancy continues during early childhood, then slows to a more gradual rate during later childhood and adolescence. Brain volume is readily reflected in head circumference, which increases six times as much during the first year as in the second year of life. One half of the postnatal brain growth is achieved by age 1 year, 75% by age 3, and 90% by age 6.

The brain growth and final form depend on the development and multiplication of neurons. Creation of new cells is believed to occur only during the first 100 days of gestation. During the remainder of gestation cells divide and multiply at the astonishing rate of 250,000 per minute (Restak, 1984). It is believed that no new nerve cells appear after the sixth month of fetal life. Postnatal growth consists of increasing the amount of cytoplasm around the nuclei of the ten billion existing cells, increasing the number and intricacy of communications with other cells, and advancing their peripheral axons to keep pace with expanding body dimensions.

The brain comprises 12% of the body weight at birth. It doubles this weight in the first year, and by age 5 or 6 years its weight at birth has tripled. Thereafter growth slows until in adulthood the brain is only about 2% of the total body weight. The surface configuration also changes with development. The early embryonic brain surface is smooth, but with advancing development the sulci deepen. This process continues throughout childhood. At birth the cortex is only about one half of its adult thickness, although all the major surface features are present. There is very little cortical control over body movements at birth with the movements guided principally by primitive reflexes (see p. 314). With advancing development and maturation, the brain, through association pathways, exercises increasing control over much of the reflex activity. This allows the growing child to perform progressively complex tasks requiring coordinated movements. Persistence of primitive reflexes may suggest defective cortical development.

Cortical control is closely associated with the acquisition of a myelin coating on the nerves. Although nerve fibers are able to conduct impulses without this myelin sheath, the impulses travel at a slower rate and with more likelihood of diffusion. Myelinization of the various nerve tracts in the central nervous system, which allows progressive neuromotor function, follows the cephalocaudal and proximodistal sequence. It appears first with the fibers of the spinal cord and cranial nerves, then in the brain stem and corticospinal tracts. The rate of myelogenesis accelerates rapidly after birth. In general, the pathways concerned with sensation are myelinated early, before the motor pathways. The acquisition of motor skills depends on the maturation and myelination of the nervous system, and no amount of special training or practice will hasten the process. Most of the advancing performance in an infant is a direct result of brain development and only depends indirectly on environmental stimuli.

CENTRAL NERVOUS SYSTEM

The bony skull forms the strongest covering and provides the primary protection to the brain. It is an expansible structure in the infant and young child but becomes rigid in the older child and adolescent. Blood is supplied to the dura mater by the middle meningeal artery, a branch of the external carotid artery. It enters the skull at a point inferior to the temporal bone, then branches over the surface of the dura, usually encased in a groove in the temporal and parietal bones. Damage to this artery or its branches is a frequent cause of an epidural hematoma.

Brain Coverings

Within the skull the brain is covered and protected further by three membranes, the *meninges*—the dura mater, arachnoid membrane, and pia mater (Fig. 37-1). The tough outer membrane, the *dura mater,* is a double layer that serves as the outer meningeal layer and the inner periosteum of the cranial bones separated by the *epidural space.* The dura is closely attached to the skull in infancy, causing slower spread of blood in epidural hemorrhage. This adherence explains why epidural hemorrhages are uncommon in the first 2 years of life.

Between these layers of dura inside the skull lie large venous sinuses. Sheets of the dura mater also extend downward and inward to form partitions within the cranium. Projecting downward into the longitudinal fissure is the sheet of dura called the *falx cerebri,* separating the cerebral hemispheres, and the *falx cerebelli,* separating the cerebellar hemispheres. Another segment is a tentlike structure, the

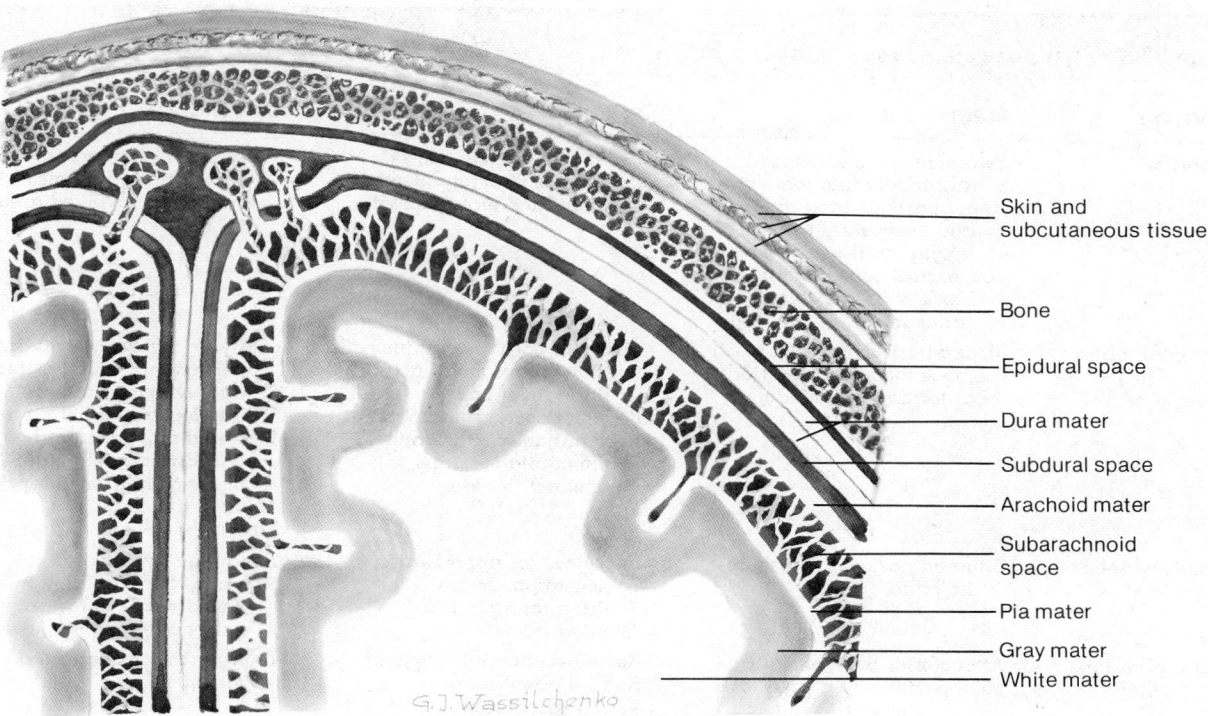

Skin and
subcutaneous tissue

Bone

Epidural space

Dura mater

Subdural space

Arachoid mater

Subarachnoid
space

Pia mater

Gray mater
White mater

G.J.Wassilchenko

Fig. 37-1. Protective coverings of the brain.

tentorium, which separates the cerebellum from the occipital lobe of the cerebrum. The large gap through which the brain stem passes is the tentorial hiatus, the site of herniation in untreated intracranial pressure.

The middle meningeal layer, the *arachnoid membrane,* is a delicate, avascular, weblike structure that loosely surrounds the brain. Between the arachnoid and the dura mater lies the subdural area, a potential space that normally contains only enough fluid to prevent adhesion between the two membranes. However, during cerebral trauma, the fine blood vessels that bridge the subdural space are stretched and ruptured, causing venous blood to escape where it spreads freely.

The innermost covering layer, the *pia mater,* is a delicate transparent membrane that, unlike the other coverings, adheres closely to the outer surface of the brain, conforming to the folds (gyri) and furrows (sulci). Within the pial layer lie the arteries and veins of the brain. Between the pia mater and the arachnoid membrane is the *subarachnoid space.* Cerebrospinal fluid (CSF) fills the entire subarachnoid space surrounding the brain and spinal cord, which acts as a protective cushion for the brain tissue. Further protection is provided by fibrous filaments known as *arachnoid trabeculae,* which help anchor the brain. When the head receives a blow, these attachments allow the arachnoid to slide on the dura, preventing excessive movement.

The Brain

The brain can be divided into six major divisions, each of which plays a vital role in regulation and control of body function. Each hemisphere is artificially divided into lobes.

Pressure on or damage to these lobes produces observable signs or symptoms directly related to the area of pathology, which provides clues to the location of the damage. The major structures of the brain and their functions are briefly outlined in Table 37-1.

The two large cerebral hemispheres that occupy the anterior and medial fossae of the skull are separated in the upper part by the *longitudinal fissure.* This separation is complete anteriorly and posteriorly, but centrally the hemispheres are joined by the block of fibers known as the *corpus callosum,* the largest fiber bundle in the brain. These fibers interconnect cortical areas of the right and left hemispheres. Destruction of the corpus callosum causes hemispheric independence or "split brain."

Situated deeply within each hemisphere and on each side of the midline are the *basal ganglia* (or cerebral nuclei), which serve as vital sorting areas for messages passing to and from the hemispheres. Connected to the hemispheres by thick bunches of nerve fibers is the *brain stem,* through which all the nerve fibers traverse as they pass from the hemispheres to the cerebellum and spinal cord. The brain stem extends from the base of the hemispheres through the foramen magnum, where it is continuous with the spinal cord. Within the cranium and behind the brain stem is the cerebellum. Any pressure exerted on the intracranial structures can cause compression of the brain stem and prolapse of the cerebellum through the foramen magnum.

Cerebral blood flow. The blood supply to the brain tissue is carried by the internal carotid arteries, which branch to supply the various brain segments. The volume of blood to the brain, which constitutes only 17% of the car-

Table 37-1 Structure and function of the brain

STRUCTURE	DESCRIPTION	FUNCTION	DYSFUNCTION
Cerebrum	Two hemispheres divided (artificially into lobes) Upper parts divided anteriorly and posteriorly by longitudinal fissure Lower parts joined centrally by block of fibers, corpus callosum	Center for consciousness, thought, memory, sensory input, and motor activity	Pressure or damage produces signs and symptoms specific to involved areas
Frontal lobes	Most anteriorly located of all lobes that end posteriorly at fissure of Rolando	Posterior portion contains cells that control motor activity throughout body Basis for social interaction Recognition of cause and effect relationships, abstract thinking	Injury or damage to anterior portion may cause personality changes, altered intellectual functioning Impaired movement of body part directly related to motor center for that part Memory deficits Language deficits
Parietal lobes	Situated posterior to fissure of Rolando	Important for appreciation of sensation, somatic interpretation and integration	Language dysfunction Aphasia, apraxia, motor, and sensory loss to lower extremities, atopognosia
Occipital lobe	At posterior base of skull Most posteriorly placed lobe	Receives stimuli for vision Spatial orientation Visual recognition	Injury produces impaired vision
Temporal lobes	Situated anterior to occipital lobe and inferior to parietal lobes	Receives and interprets stimuli for taste, vision, sound, and smell Converts crude visual impressions into recognizable images	Injury or destruction causes inability to interpret meanings of sensory experiences
	Point where temporal, parietal, and occipital lobes converge	Primary interpretive area	Impairment causes inability to interpret sensory stimuli; difficulty in understanding higher levels of meaning of body sensory experiences
	Point where temporal, parietal, and frontal lobes converge	Center for speech, hearing	Impairment produces aphasia Hearing dysfunction
Cerebellum	Located just below posterior part of cerebrum and separated from it by tentorium Contains two lateral lobes joined by midline portion, vermis	Necessary for refinement and coordination of all muscle movements, including walking, talking, and control of muscle tone and balance	Dysmetria, ataxia, dysarthria, hypotonia, nystagmus, dystonia Rest tremor
Basal ganglia	Situated deeply within cerebral hemispheres on either side of midline	Unconscious or automatic control of lower motor centers Excitation causes inhibition of muscle tone throughout body	Chorea, athetosis Dystonia Rest tremor
Diencephalon	Situated between cerebrum and mesencephalon	Contains diffuse fibers that compose reticular activating system	Stupor
Thalamus	Rounded mass forms most of lateral wall of third ventricle and part of floor of lateral ventricles	Major relay station for sensory impulses to cerebral cortex Activates cerebral cortex	Impaired consciousness

Table 37-1 Structure and function of the brain—cont'd

STRUCTURE	DESCRIPTION	FUNCTION	DYSFUNCTION
Hypothalamus	Lies beneath thalamus Forms floor of third ventricle	Vital control center for involuntary functions (e.g., blood pressure, satiety, hunger, rage, feeding, water conservation, temperature, sleep regulation, libido) Controls secretion of tropic hormones	Impairment causes alterations in vegetative functions Somnolence; coma Anorexia, loss of weight, fever, diabetes insipidus, loss of libido Endocrine disorders
Brain stem	Extends from cerebral hemisphere to spinal cord	All cranial nerves (except I) arise from brain stem	Stupor, coma
Mesencephalon (midbrain)	Lies below inferior surface of cerebellum and above pons Ventral portion composed of cerebral peduncles	Main connection between forebrain and hindbrain Contains nuclei for third, fourth, and part of fifth cranial nerves Control of eye movement	Impaired consciousness No independent movement or verbal response Decerebrate posturing Neurologic hyperventilation Impaired function of muscles supplied by these nerves
Pons	Located just above medulla oblongata	Contains pneumotaxic center—control of respiration Cranial nerves V through VIII	Deep, rapid, or periodic breathing Impaired function of muscles supplied by these nerves
Medulla	Forms attachment of brain to spinal cord Separated from pons by horizontal groove	Contains vital centers, including respiratory and vasomotor cranial nerves IX, X, XI, XII	Impaired vital functions No response to any stimuli Ataxic (biot) breathing Flaccid muscle tone Deep tendon, gag, corneal reflexes absent

diac output, supplies the brain with 20% of the body oxygen. The brain, an "inactive" organ, uses 10 times the oxygen used by the body as a whole. Only the heart uses more oxygen per gram of tissue.

Cerebral blood flow (CBF) is the result of two opposing forces—cerebral blood pressure (the difference between systemic arterial pressure and cerebral venous pressure) and cerebral vascular resistance. At blood pressures between 50 and 150 mm Hg, CBF remains constant. Since cerebral venous pressure is usually very low and relatively constant, the cerebral blood pressure is determined mainly by systemic arterial pressure.

Autoregulation. One of the most important factors in the control of CBF is *autoregulation,* the unique ability of cerebral arterial vessels to change their diameter in response to fluctuating CPP. Consequently, cerebral vessels maintain a constant blood flow during alterations in blood pressure and perfusion caused by body posture, increased intracranial pressure, decreased cardiac output, or narrowing or occlusion in the major blood vessels of the neck. Autoregulation fails when the limits of cerebral vascular dilatation are reached; then CBF decreases, causing clinical symptoms of ischemia (nausea, fainting, dizziness, and dim vision). Conversely, increased MAP leads to "breakthrough of autoregulation," with increased CBF leading to microhemorrhages

and cerebral edema (Mueller and others, 1982). Autoregulation may be impaired locally or globally as a result of trauma and/or ischemia.

Changes in PaO_2 or $PaCO_2$ have a profound effect on autoregulation. Hypercapnia ($PaCO_2$ over 40 mm Hg) or increased levels of lactic acid have a pronounced dilating effect on cerebral arterioles that increases cerebral blood flow (CBF) and thus cerebral volume. Hypocapnia ($PaCO_2$ 25 to 30 mm Hg) constricts cerebral arterioles and decreases CBF. Changes in PaO_2 between 70 and 100 mm Hg have little effect on the cerebral vascular system. However, profound hypoxia (PaO_2 below 50 mm Hg) dramatically increases CBF. Consequently, maintenance of the airway and effective ventilation are of primary importance in the initial management of the neurologically impaired patient.

Oxygen. Metabolic requirements for oxygen by the brain are not affected by rest or sleep, although they are reduced by narcosis and coma and altered by changes in temperature. CBF is not altered when body temperature is maintained between 35° C and 40° C. Oxygen consumption of the brain is increased by hyperthermia and decreased by hypothermia. The brain depends on a constant supply of oxygen-rich blood, and since the oxygen need of the brain is great in relation to the volume of blood supplied, it extracts more oxygen from each unit of circulating blood.

SIGNS OF INCREASED INTRACRANIAL PRESSURE (ICP) IN INFANTS AND CHILDREN

Infants
Tense, bulging fontanel; lack of normal pulsations
Separated cranial sutures
Macewen (cracked-pot) sign
Irritability
High-pitched cry
Increased occipital-frontal circumference (OFC)
Distended scalp veins
Changes in feeding
Cries when held or rocked
"Setting sun" sign

Children
Headache
Nausea
Vomiting—often without nausea
Diplopia, blurred vision
Seizures

Personality and behavior signs
Irritability (toddlers), restlessness
Indifference, drowsiness, or lack of interest
Decline in school performance
Diminished physical activity and motor performance
Increased complaints of fatigue, tiredness; increased time devoted to sleep
Significant weight loss possible from anorexia and vomiting
Memory loss if pressure is markedly increased
Inability to follow simple commands
Progression to lethargy and drowsiness

Late signs
Lowered level of consciousness
Decreased motor response to command
Decreased sensory response to painful stimuli
Alterations in pupil size and reactivity
Sometimes decerebrate or decorticate posturing
Cheyne-Stokes respirations
Papilledema

Oxygen supply to the brain is compromised when the supply is inadequate as a result of impaired respiration, hypotension, increased intracranial pressure, or vascular damage, spasm, or compression. Neurons are highly susceptible to elevated $PaCO_2$, and the metabolic damage to brain tissue caused by an inadequate supply of well-oxygenated blood can often exceed the effects of trauma. Respiratory acidosis resulting from increased $PaCO_2$ levels can produce symptoms indistinguishable from those of head injury.

Blood-brain barrier. The blood-brain barrier (BBB) is an anatomic-physiologic feature of the brain that separates the brain parenchyma from the blood. Cerebral capillaries, unlike those in other parts of the body, have no fenestrations or pores. The tight junctions of the vascular endothelium are thought to be responsible for the selective nature of the BBB. The mature BBB allows facilitated diffusion of glucose and passive diffusion of water and carbon dioxide but is impermeable to protein and does not permit passage of many active substances. However, the BBB of the fetus and

newborn is normally indiscriminately permeable, allowing protein and other large and small molecules to pass freely between the cerebral vessels and the brain. Conditions that cause cerebral vascular dilatation (hypertension, hypercapnia, hypoxia, and acidosis) disrupt the BBB, as do hyperosmotic fluids, which cause shrinkage of vascular endothelium and widen the vascular junctions (Mueller and others, 1982).

INCREASED INTRACRANIAL PRESSURE

The brain, tightly enclosed in the solid bony cranium, is well protected but highly vulnerable to pressure that may accumulate within the enclosure. Its total volume—brain, CSF, and blood—must remain approximately the same at all times. A change in the proportional volume of one of these components (e.g., increase or decrease in intracranial blood) must be accompanied by a compensatory change in another (e.g., decrease or increase in CSF)—the Monro-Kellie doctrine. In this way the volume and pressure normally remain constant. Examples of compensatory changes are reduction in blood volume, decrease in production of CSF, increase in CSF absorption, or shrinkage of brain mass by displacement of intracellular and extracellular fluid.

In children with open fontanels, compensation may take place by skull expansion and widened sutures. However, at any age the capacity for spatial compensation is limited. An increase in intracranial pressure (ICP) may be caused by tumors or other space-occupying lesions, accumulation of fluid within the ventricular system, bleeding, or edema of cerebral tissues. Once compensation is exhausted, any further increase in volume will result in a rapid rise in ICP.

Early signs and symptoms of increased ICP are often subtle and assume many patterns, such as personality changes, irritability, and fatigue (see accompanying box). In older children subjective symptoms are headache, especially when lying flat (e.g., on awakening in the morning) or when coughing, sneezing, or bending over, and nausea and vomiting. The child may complain of double vision or blurred vision with movement of the head. Seizures are not uncommon. In children whose cranial sutures have not closed, there is an increase in the head circumference and bulging fontanels. As pressure increases, pupils become progressively sluggish in reaction, eventually to become fixed and dilated, sometimes referred to as "blown." The level of consciousness progressively deteriorates from drowsiness to eventual coma. Problems related to increased ICP are discussed in relation to congenital malformations, brain tumor, and head injuries.

Physiologic and biochemical changes within the cerebral vasculature serve to complicate the primary causes of increased ICP. Initially, especially in cases of trauma, there is often increased blood flow as a result of venous congestion or vasomotor paralysis. If cerebral hypoxia is associated with the cerebral dysfunction, the compensatory vasodilation caused by oxygen deficiency will tend to increase the cerebral flow. However, as ICP progressively increases, blood flow is reduced with diminished blood supply to the brain tissues. The classic responses observed in adults (widening pulse pressure and increased blood pressure) are rarely seen in children and, if so, are a very late sign. Breathing characterized by periods of hyperpnea that alternate with apnea (Cheyne-Stokes respirations) is seen in brain stem damage.

Evaluation of Neurologic Status

Dysfunction of the central nervous system (CNS) can be manifest in almost any system in the body and may be the result of a number of causes. Methods used to evaluate neurologic function have been discussed in relation to numerous aspects of child care. The neurologic examination is an integral part of the health assessment (see p. 278), assessment of gestational age (see p. 303), and the newborn assessment (see p. 313). Some of the tests used to differentiate neuromuscular disorders are discussed in Chapter 39. The assessment tools and examinations in this chapter are primarily those used to assess intracranial integrity. An overall discussion of some factors that influence assessment is followed by some general observations. More specific techniques are discussed in relation to assessment of level of consciousness.

ASSESSMENT: GENERAL ASPECTS

Children younger than 2 years are difficult to evaluate neurologically. Early infant neurologic responses are primarily reflexive; these responses are gradually replaced by meaningful movement in the characteristic cephalocaudal direction of development. This evidence of progressive maturation reflects more extensive myelinization and changes in neurochemical and electrophysiologic properties. Furthermore, children younger than age 2 are unable to respond to directions designed to elicit specific responses.

Most information about infants and small children is gained through observation of their spontaneous and elicited reflex responses, by their development of increasingly complex locomotor and fine motor skills, and by eliciting progressively sophisticated communicative and adaptive behaviors. The presence of a primitive reflex beyond the time it would normally disappear is an important clue to neurologic dysfunction. In evaluating the infant or young child it is also important to obtain the pregnancy and delivery history to determine the possible effect of intrauterine environmental influences known to affect the orderly maturation of the central nervous system. These influences include maternal infections, chemicals, trauma, and metabolic insults.

History

A family history can sometimes offer clues regarding possible genetic disorders with neurologic manifestations. An inventory of family members often identifies conditions that might otherwise be overlooked, especially siblings who

have died or relatives whose conditions have been hidden from memory. Questions regarding specific neurologic problems are mentioned, such as mental retardation, deafness, epilepsy, blindness, unusual movements, weakness, ataxia, and progressive mental deterioration.

A history is very important because it provides valuable clues regarding the cause of unconsciousness. There may have been an injury or short febrile illness, or the child may be known to have diabetes. A history of any event that led to the health care assessment is probed, especially when it involves injury, encounter with an animal or insect, ingestion of neurotoxic substances, inhalation of chemicals, or past illness. Sudden or progressive alterations in movement or mental abilities may provide clues for investigation.

Physical Examination

Physical evaluation includes observation of the size and shape of the head, spontaneous activity and postural reflex activity, and sensory responses. The attitude is observed. It is noted whether the infant assumes a normal flexed posture or one of extreme extension, opisthotonos, or hypotonia. Extremities are observed for symmetry of movement. Excessive tremulousness or frequent twitching movements may be significant signs indicating the onset of a seizure disorder. Seizure activity is suspected if holding the extremity snugly does not stop the activity. An abnormal respiratory cycle such as prolonged apnea, ataxic breathing, paradoxic chest movement, and hyperventilation (central neurogenic) may be the result of a neurologic problem.

Skin and hair texture may be important factors in detecting certain neurologic diseases. Facial features may suggest a specific syndrome, and a high-pitched, piercing cry is associated with central nervous system disorders. Abnormal eye movements, inability to suck or swallow, lip smacking, asymmetric contraction of facial muscles, and yawning may indicate cranial nerve involvement.

Older children can be evaluated by the usual methods employed in a neurologic examination. In addition, an estimation of the level of development provides essential information about neurologic function. These accomplishments are discussed throughout the book in relation to evaluation for specific disorders such as mental retardation, failure to thrive, attention deficit disorder, cerebral palsy, cerebral tumors, and other physical or behavioral problems. The Denver Developmental Screening Test (Appendix B) serves as an excellent screening tool for assessing developmental progress in the young child.

Muscular activity. Muscular activity and coordination, including ocular movements and gait, are valuable sources of information. Ocular movements, pupillary response, facial movements, and mouth functions provide clues regarding cranial nerve involvement or impingement (see p. 282 for testing cranial nerves). Testing reflexes (p. 279), strength, coordination, and presence and location of tremors, twitching, tics, or other unusual movements (Table 37-2) are also aspects of the neurologic assessment. Abnormalities of gait that indicate cerebral dysfunction include:

Table 37-2 Description of abnormal involuntary muscular movements

TERM	DESCRIPTION
Ataxia	Gross incoordination that may become worse with the eyes closed
Spasm	Involuntary contraction of a muscle mass; cramp (if painful), convulsion (if violent)
Spasticity	Prolonged and steady contraction of a muscle characterized by clonus (alternating relaxation and contraction of the muscle) and exaggerated reflexes
Rigidity	Inability to flex a joint
Tremors	Constant small involuntary movements
Twitching	Spasmodic movements of short duration
Tic	Involuntary, compulsive, stereotyped movement of an associated group of muscles
Choreiform movements	Quick, jerky, grossly incoordinated, irregular movements that may disappear on relaxation
Athetosis	Slow, writhing, wormlike, constant, grossly incoordinated movements that increase on voluntary activity and decrease on relaxation
Dystonia	Slow twisting movements of limbs or trunk
Associated movements	Voluntary movement of one muscle accompanied by involuntary movement of another muscle
Mirroring movements	Same as associated movements except with symmetric muscle groups

Ataxia—impaired ability to coordinate movements; staggering gait and postural imbalance.

Spastic paraplegic gait—narrow based with a tendency to walk on the toes, along with flexion at the knees and hips, and shuffling. Thighs adducted, and knees may strike each other with each step; in younger children a "scissoring" position results when lower limbs cross because of increased adductor tone. Patients walk stiffly and take slow, deliberate steps. Increased difficulty when attempting to walk on heels or run.

Spastic hemiplegic gait—involved leg extended, circumducted, plantar flexed, and does not swing naturally at the knee or hip.

Cerebellar gait—staggering, irregularity, unsteadiness, wide-based lurching movement in any direction, and tendency to veer in one lateral direction (hemispheric lesion).

Extrapyramidal gait—rigidity, paucity of automatic movements, and bradykinesia (slowness of all movements) with associated bending of trunk and head, arms adducted at shoulders and flexed at elbows and wrists, fingers extended; festination (upper body moves forward in advance of lower part) causing more rapid steps and risk of falling.

ALTERED STATES OF CONSCIOUSNESS

Consciousness implies awareness—the ability to respond to sensory stimuli and have subjective experiences. There are two components of consciousness: *alertness,* an arousal-waking state including the ability to respond to stimuli, and *cognitive power,* including the ability to process stimuli and produce verbal and motor responses (Millikan, 1981).

An altered state of consciousness usually refers to varying states of unconsciousness that may be momentary or may last for hours, days, or indefinitely. *Unconsciousness* is depressed cerebral function—the inability to respond to sensory stimuli and have subjective experiences. *Coma* is defined as a state of unconsciousness from which the patient cannot be aroused even with powerful stimuli.

The seat of consciousness or *alerting area* of the brain is in the reticular formation—the central core of the brain stem. The reticular formation extends from the midbrain to the medulla. The *reticular activating system* (RAS) receives collaterals from and is stimulated by *every* major somatic and special sensory pathway in the brain. Disturbances of consciousness may occur when any part of the reticular, thalamic, hypothalamic, and cortical circuits is sufficiently impaired. However, the effects may vary according to the areas involved. For example, small lesions of the reticular or hypothalamic regions will produce a profound effect, whereas extensive impairment of the cortex is required to produce quantitatively similar results.

Etiology

An altered state of consciousness may be the outcome of several processes that affect the central nervous system. Some, such as the diffuse changes seen in encephalitis, are directly related to cerebral insult; others are the result of dysfunction to other organs or processes manifest by central nervous system signs. For example, biochemical changes can impair neurologic function without morphologic findings, as in hypoglycemia.

Level of Consciousness

Various terms are used to describe alterations in level of consciousness (LOC), and since they have not been standardized, they are subject to a wide range of interpretation. Level of consciousness is determined by observations of the patient's responses to his environment. Other diagnostic tests such as motor activity, reflexes, and vital signs are more variable and do not necessarily directly parallel the depth of the comatose state. The most consistently used terms are described in the following segments.

Sleep. Sleep, or normal unconsciousness, is a cyclic (regularly recurring) physiologic state characterized by absence of alertness, cognition, and voluntary movement that is readily reversible by an auditory, visual, or tactile stimulus. The posture is immobile, body processes are partially suspended, and there is intermittent dreaming that the person may be able to recall.

Table 37-3 Pediatric coma scale

	SCORE	OVER 1 YEAR	LESS THAN 1 YEAR
Eyes opening	4	Spontaneously	Spontaneously
	3	To verbal command	To shout
	2	To pain	To pain
	1	No response	No response
		OVER 1 YEAR	**LESS THAN 1 YEAR**
Best motor response	6	Obeys	
	5	Localizes pain	Localizes pain
	4	Flexion withdrawal	Flexion withdrawal
	3	Flexion—abnormal (decorticate rigidity)	Flexion—abnormal (decorticate rigidity)
	2	Extension (decerebrate rigidity)	Extension (decerebrate rigidity)
	1	No response	No response
		OVER 5 YEARS	**2-5 YEARS**
Best verbal response	5	Oriented and converses	Appropriate words and phrases
	4	Disoriented and converses	Inappropriate words
	3	Inappropriate words	Cries and/or screams
	2	Incomprehensible sounds	Grunts
	1	No response	No response
TOTAL	3-15		

Modification of Glasgow Coma Scale.

GLASGOW COMA SCALE (VERBAL RESPONSE, INFANTS)

One month
1. None
2. Crying to stimuli
3. Crying spontaneously
4. Blinks when eyelashes touched
5. Throaty noises

Two months
1. None
2. Crying to stimuli
3. Shuts eyes to light
4. Smiles when caressing
5. Babbles—single vowel sounds

Three months
1. None
2. Crying to stimuli (moans)
3. Stares to response and looks at environment
4. Smiles to sound stimulation
5. Coos, chuckles, *vowels* in a prolonged way

Four months
1. None
2. Crying to stimuli (moans)
3. Turns head to sound
4. Smiles spontaneously or when stimulated, laughs when socially stimulated
5. Modulating voice and perfect vocalization of vowels

Five and six months
1. None
2. Crying to stimuli (moans)
3. Localizes general direction of sound
4. Discrimination family members
5. Babbles to people, toys

Seven and eight months
1. None
2. Crying to stimuli (moans)
3. Recognizes familiar voices and family
4. Babbles
5. "Ba," "Ma," "Da"

Nine and ten months
1. None
2. Crying to stimuli (moans)
3. Recognizes (smiles or laughs)
4. Babbles
5. "MaMa," "DaDa"

Eleven and twelve months
1. None
2. Crying to stimuli (moans)
3. Recognizes—smiles
4. Babbles
5. Words (specifically "Mama" and "Dada")

Courtesy Dr. Kenneth Shapiro, Department of Neurosurgery, Albert Einstein College of Medicine, New York, New York. From Zimmerman, S.S., and Gildea, J.H.: Critical care pediatrics, Philadelphia, 1985, W.B. Saunders Co.

Confusion. The responses of confused patients demonstrate a failure to comprehend their surroundings. They appear to lose their proper bearings. They are unable to estimate direction or location, are apt to be disoriented in time, and may misidentify people. They have a short attention span, have difficulty in following even simple directions, and tend to misinterpret events. They may be hyperactive or apathetic and immobile. They are usually able to give relevant answers to simple questions about their age or the location of pain, but will give irrelevant and inaccurate answers to more complex questions. However, they are alert and their arousal responses are intact.

Delirium. Delirium is a state characterized by confusion, disorientation, fear, irritability, agitation, and hyperactivity. It is marked by illusions (false interpretation of sensory perceptions), hallucinations (false sensory perceptions), and delusions (false ideas). Patients are commonly loud, talkative, suspicious, and agitated. Delirium is often associated with high fever, toxic substances, and shock states. Physical signs often include tremulousness and sweating, and the person frequently responds with a ''startle'' reaction to unexpected stimuli.

Pseudowakeful states. In pseudowakeful states, also known as akinetic mutism or apallic syndrome, the patient sits or lies with eyes open but fails to follow objects or lights, does not turn his eyes toward a noise, and does not speak. In less developed states the patient may follow objects or persons with his eyes, turn slowly toward a sound and appear about to speak, but remain silent. This is sometimes described as a ''reptilian stare.'' Response to external stimuli is similar to that of a patient in stupor or light coma. Some of these patients are restless and hyperkinetic; others remain motionless and speechless. These pseudowakeful states may be observed in coma of toxic origin or in focal lesions involving the diencephalon either primarily or secondarily by pressure.

Comatose states. Diminished alertness as a result of pathologic conditions occurs as a continuum and is designated as the *comatose state,* which extends from somnolence on one end to deep coma at the other. To produce coma the following must occur: (1) extensive, diffuse, *bilateral* cerebral hemispheric destruction (the brain stem may be intact), (2) a lesion in the diencephalon (Table 37-1), or (3) destruction of the brain stem down to the level of the lower pons.

Coma Assessment

Several scales have been devised in an attempt to standardize the description and interpretation of the degree of depressed consciousness. The most popular of these is the Glasgow Coma Scale (GCS), which consists of a three-part assessment: eye opening, verbal response, and motor response. Since the usefulness of the original scale with very young children is limited, the scale with variations adapted to the young patient is provided in Table 37-3 and the accompanying box. When assessing level of consciousness in young children, it is often useful to have a parent present to help elicit a desired response. An infant or child may not respond in an unfamiliar environment or to unfamiliar voices.

Numerical values, 1 to 5, are assigned to the levels of response in each category. The sum of these numerical values provides an objective measure of the patient's level of consciousness. The lower the score, the deeper the coma. A normal person would score the highest, 15; a score of 7 or below is generally accepted as a definition of coma; the lowest score, 3, indicates deep coma.

The GCS in itself is not sufficient to determine the responses of all children. For example, a quadriplegic child can score very low but be cerebrally all right because the child cannot respond to commands physically. However, it provides a more objective method for evaluating the state of consciousness in the majority of cases.

Irreversible coma. There is no precise diagnosis for clinical death. Different tissues undergo permanent damage after varying periods of exposure to an ongoing insult; therefore the brain (especially the cerebrum) has become the tissue of most importance in determining the time of death. The current concept of dying is one of a process that takes place over a finite interval of time, rather than an event that occurs spontaneously. The patient who meets the criteria for brain death will eventually suffer cardiovascular collapse (usually within hours).

Organ transplantation has created a need to subdivide the process of death in order to obtain viable tissues at a time when the brain is already dead. The clinical criteria for brain death must be so constituted that there is *no error.* Although the legal status of the concept of death varies among individual states and communities in the United

---

DEFINITION OF IRREVERSIBLE COMA, AD HOC COMMITTEE OF THE HARVARD MEDICAL SCHOOL

1. Unreceptivity and unresponsivity—intensely painful stimuli evoke no response, including change in respiration.
2. No movement or breathing—observed for at least 1 hour by physicians. Respirator may be turned off for 3 minutes if PCO_2 is normal at beginning of trial and patient has been breathing room air for 10 minutes.
3. No reflexes—including pupillary, vestibular, other brainstem postural; also includes deep tendon reflexes and plantar response.
4. Flat electroencephalogram—increased gains for at least part of run; noncephalic electrode and electrocardiogram obtained simultaneously.
5. All tests are to be repeated at least 24 hours later with no change.
6. The cause of coma is not hypothermia (temperature below 32.2° C) or central nervous system depressants.

From Swaiman, K.F., and Wright, F.S.: The practice of pediatric neurology, ed. 2, St. Louis, 1982, The C.V. Mosby Co., p. 152. Based on data from Beecher, H.K.: JAMA **205:**337, 1968.

States, the most frequently used criteria for establishing irreversible coma or a nonfunctioning brain are the Harvard Criteria (see box). See also Tissue donation (p. 968).

NEUROLOGIC EXAMINATION

The purpose of the neurologic examination is to establish an accurate, objective baseline of neurologic function. Therefore it is essential that the neurologic examination be documented in a fashion that is *reproducible*. In this way a comparison of baseline, previous, and current findings allows the observer to detect subtle changes in the neurologic status that might not be evident otherwise. Descriptions of behaviors should be simple, objective, and easily interpreted: "Drowsy but awake and conversationally rational/oriented," "Sleepy but arousable with vigorous physical stimuli. Pressure to nail base of right hand results in upper extremity flexion/lower extremity extension."

Vital signs, observation of posture and movement (both spontaneous and elicited), eye examination, and reflex testing all provide valuable clues regarding the level of consciousness, the site of involvement, and the probable cause, although they do not necessarily parallel the depth of a comatose state.

Vital Signs

Pulse, respiration, and blood pressure provide information regarding the adequacy of circulation and the possible underlying cause of altered consciousness. Autonomic activity is most intensively disturbed in deep coma and in brain stem lesions. Body temperature is often elevated, and sometimes the elevation may be extreme. Coma of a toxic origin may produce hypothermia. High temperature is most frequently a sign of an acute infectious process or heat stroke but may be caused by ingestion of some drugs (especially salicylates, alcohol, and barbiturates) or intracranial bleeding. A fever sometimes follows a cerebral seizure.

The pulse is variable and may be rapid, slow and bounding, or feeble. Blood pressure may be normal, elevated, or at shock levels. The Cushing reflex or pressor response that causes a slowing of the pulse and an increase in blood pressure is uncommon in children; when it occurs, it is a very late sign. Vital signs are also affected by medications. For assessment purposes *changes* in pulse and blood pressure are more important than the direction.

Respirations are more often slow, deep, and irregular. Slow and deep breathing is often seen in the heavy sleep caused by sedatives, after seizures, or in cerebral infections. Slow, shallow breathing may result from sedatives or narcotics. Hyperventilation (deep and rapid respirations) is usually the result of metabolic acidosis or abnormal stimulation of the respiratory center in the medulla caused by salicylate poisoning, hepatic coma, or Reye syndrome.

Breathing patterns have been described with a number of terms (e.g., apneustic, cluster, ataxic, Cheyne-Stokes). However, it is better to describe what is being observed rather than placing a label on it. The terms are often used and interpreted incorrectly. Periodic and irregular breathing are signs of brain stem (especially medullary) dysfunction. This is an ominous sign that often precedes complete apnea. The odor of the breath may provide additional clues, for example, the fruity, acetone odor of ketosis, the foul odor of uremia, the fetid odor of hepatic failure, or the odor of alcohol.

Skin

The skin may offer clues to the cause of unconsciousness. The body surface should be examined for the presence of injury, needle marks, petechiae, bites, and ticks. Evidence of toxic substances may be found on the hands, face, mouth, and clothing—especially in small children.

Eyes

Pupil size and reactivity are assessed (Fig. 37-2). Pinpoint pupils are commonly observed in poisoning, such as opiate or barbiturate poisoning, or in brain stem dysfunction. Widely dilated and reactive pupils are often seen after seizures and may involve only one side. Dilated pupils may also be caused by eye trauma. Widely dilated and fixed pupils suggest paralysis of cranial nerve III secondary to pressure from herniation of the brain through the tentorium. A unilateral fixed pupil usually suggests a lesion on the same side. Bilateral fixed pupils usually imply brain stem damage if present for more than 5 minutes. Dilated and unreactive pupils are also seen in hypothermia, anoxia, ischemia, poisoning with atropine-like substances, or prior instillation of mydriatic drugs. The sudden appearance of a fixed and dilated pupil is a neurosurgical emergency.

Some of the therapies used (e.g., barbiturates) can alter pupil size and reaction. The description of eye movements should indicate whether one or both eyes are involved and how the reaction was elicited. The parents should be asked if the child has a strabismus. A preexisting strabismus will cause the eyes to appear normal under compromise.

Blinking observed at rest or in response to a sudden loud noise or bright light implies that the pontine reticular formation is intact. The corneal reflex, blinking of the eyelids when the cornea is touched with a wisp of cotton or a camel hair pencil, is used to test the integrity of the ophthalmic division of cranial nerve V.

Eye movements are assessed by the doll's head maneuver, in which the child's head is rotated quickly to one side and then to the other. When brain stem centers for eye movement are intact, there is conjugate (paired or working together) movement of the eyes in the direction opposite to the head rotation. Absence of this response suggests dysfunction of the brain stem or oculomotor nerve (cranial nerve III). Downward or lateral deviation is frequently observed in association with pupillary dilation in dysfunction of cranial nerve III because of tentorial herniation. This assessment is not attempted until after cervical spine injury

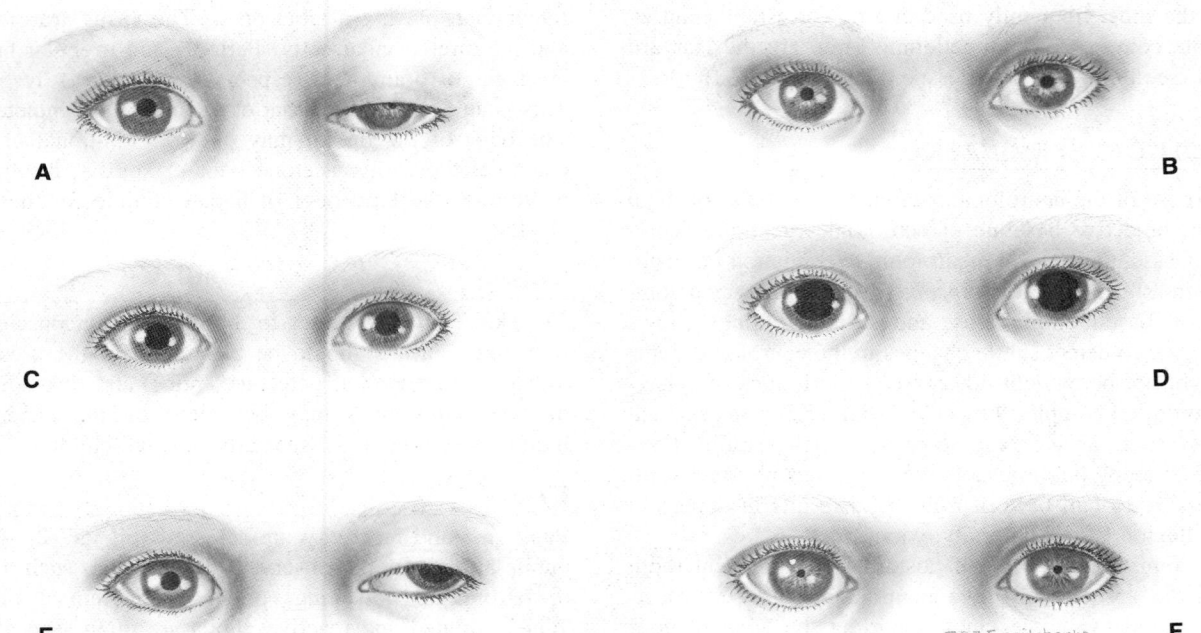

Fig. 37-2. Variations in pupil size with altered states of consciousness. **A,** Ipsilateral pupillary constriction with slight ptosis. **B,** Bilateral small pupils. **C,** Midposition, light fixed to all stimuli. **D,** Bilateral dilated and fixed pupils. **E,** Dilated pupil, left eye abducted with ptosis. **F,** Pinpoint pupils.

has been ruled out for the child who is suspected of or has sustained a traumatic injury.

The caloric test, or oculovestibular response, is elicited by irrigating the external auditory canal with ice water. This normally causes conjugate movement of the eyes toward the side of stimulation. This is lost when the pontine centers are impaired, thus providing important information in assessment of the comatose patient.

Funduscopic examination reveals additional clues. Papilledema, if it develops at all, will not be evident early in the course of unconsciousness because papilledema takes 24 to 48 hours to develop. The presence of preretinal (subhyaloid) hemorrhages in children is almost invariably the result of acute trauma with intracranial bleeding, usually subarachnoid or subdural hemorrhage.

Motor Function

Observation of spontaneous activity, posture, and response to painful stimuli provides clues to the location and extent of cerebral dysfunction. Even subtle movements (e.g., the out-turning of a hip) should be noted and the child observed for other signs. Asymmetric movements of the limbs or absence of movement suggests paralysis. In hemiplegia the affected limb lies in external rotation and will fall uncontrollably when lifted and allowed to drop. These observations should be described rather than labeled. In the deeper comatose states there is little or no spontaneous movement and the musculature tends to be flaccid. There is considerable variability in the motor behavior in lesser degrees of coma. For example, the child may be relatively immobile or rest-

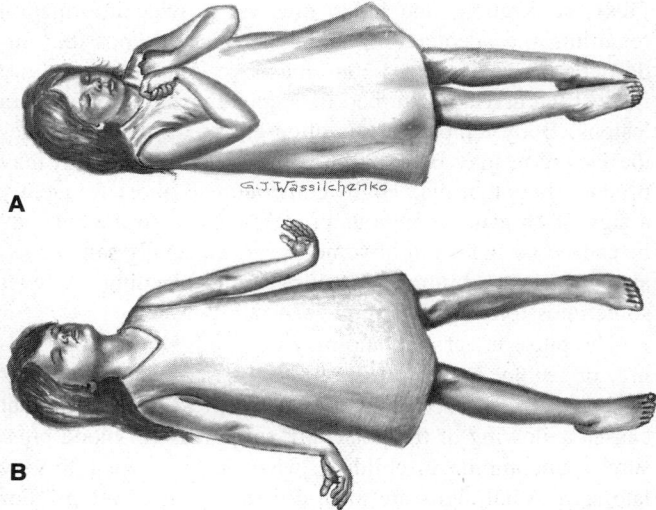

Fig. 37-3. A, Decorticate posturing. **B,** Decerebrate posturing.

less and hyperkinetic; muscle tone may be increased or decreased. Tremors, twitching, and spasms of muscles are common observations. The patient may display purposeless plucking or tossing movements. Combative or negativistic behavior is not uncommon. Hyperactivity is more common in acute febrile and toxic states than in cases of increased intracranial pressure. Convulsions are common in children and may be present in coma as a result of any cause. Any repetitive or convulsive movements should be described.

Posturing

As cortical control over motor function is lost in brain dysfunction, primitive postural reflexes emerge. These are evident in posturing and motor movements directly related to the area of the brain involved. Posturing reflects a balance between the lower exciting and the higher inhibiting influences, and strong muscles overcome weaker ones. *Decorticate posturing* (Fig. 37-3, *A*) is seen when there is severe dysfunction of the cerebral cortex. Typical decorticate posturing includes adduction of arms at the shoulders, the arms being flexed on the chest with the wrists flexed and the hands fisted, and the lower extremities being extended and adducted. *Decerebrate posturing* (Fig. 37-3, *B*), a sign of dysfunction at the level of the midbrain, is characterized by rigid extension and pronation of the arms and legs. Unilateral decerebrate posturing is often caused by tentorial herniation.

The posturing may not be evident when the child is quiet but can usually be elicited by applying painful stimuli, such as a blunt object pressed on the base of the nail. Nurses should avoid applying thumb pressure to the supraorbital region of the frontal bone (risk of orbital damage) or knuckle pressure to the sternum (risk of bruising). Noxious stimuli, such as suctioning, will elicit a response, as may turning or touching. When describing posturing, the stimulus needed to provoke the response is as important as the reaction.

Reflexes

Testing of some reflexes may be of limited value. In general, the corneal, pupillary, muscle-stretch, superficial, and plantar reflexes tend to be absent in deep coma. The state of reflexes is variable in lighter grades of unconsciousness and depends on the underlying pathologic process and the location of the lesion. The doll's eye reflex maneuver, described previously, reflects paralysis of cranial nerve III. Absence of corneal reflexes and presence of a tonic neck reflex are associated with severe brain damage. Babinski reflex, in which the lateral portion of the foot is stroked, may be of value if it is found to be present consistently in children older than 1 year. A positive Babinski reflex is significant in assessment of pyramidal tract lesions when it is unilateral and associated with other pyramidal signs. A fluctuating Babinski reflex is often observed after seizures (see Fig. 8-10, *B*).

SPECIAL DIAGNOSTIC PROCEDURES

Numerous diagnostic procedures are used for assessment of cerebral function. Laboratory tests that may help to delineate the cause of unconsciousness include blood glucose, urea nitrogen, electrolyte (pH, sodium, potassium, chloride, calcium, and bicarbonate) tests; clotting studies, hematocrit, and a complete blood count; liver function tests; blood cultures if there is fever; and sometimes studies to detect lead or other toxic substances, such as drugs.

An electroencephalogram may provide important information. For example, generalized random slow activity suggests suppressed cortical function; localized slow activity suggests a focal lesion, such as a mass; and generalized projected patterns suggest brain stem involvement. A flat tracing is one of the criteria used as evidence of brain death. Examination of spinal fluid is carried out when toxic encephalopathy or infection is suspected. Lumbar puncture is ordinarily delayed if intracranial hemorrhage is suspected and is contraindicated in the presence of ICP.

Auditory and visual evoked potentials are sometimes used in neurologic diagnosis of very young children. Visual evoked potential testing is used to determine the functional integrity of the visual system, to test retinal function, and to detect lesions of the visual cortex (Mizrahi and Dorfman, 1980). Brain stem auditory evoked potentials are useful for evaluating the continuity of brain stem auditory tracts and are particularly useful for detecting demyelinating disease and neoplasms of the brain stem and distinguishing between brain stem and cortical lesions. For example, a normal evoked potential in a comatose patient suggests involvement of the cerebral hemispheres.

Highly sophisticated tests are carried out with specialized equipment by skilled personnel. Most of these tests are outlined in Table 37-4. Because such tests can be threatening to children, a child will need preparation for, and support and reassurance during, the tests. (See also Preparation for procedures, p. 1104).

Children who are old enough to understand require careful explanation of the procedure, why it is being done, what they will experience, and how they can help. School-age children usually appreciate a more detailed description of why contrast material is injected. The importance of lying still for tests, particularly tomography, needs to be stressed. Children unfamiliar with the machines can be shown a picture beforehand. Although radiographic examinations are not painful, the machinery is often so frightening in appearance that the child protests because of anxiety.

This is especially true of tomography, which requires that the child's head be placed within a special immobilizing device, although for only about 5 minutes. Chin and cheek pads are sometimes used to prevent the slightest head movement, and straps are applied to the body to prevent a slight change in body position. The nurse can explain these events to a frightened child by comparing them to an astronaut's preparation for a space flight. It is very important to emphasize to the child that at no time is the procedure painful.

It is helpful for nurses to become acquainted with the equipment and the general environment in which the test will take place so that they can better explain the procedure to the child at his level of understanding. Equipment is often strange and ominous to a child and may be perceived as a frightening monster. It is especially frightening to young children to experience a large mechanical device coming toward them as if to crush or devour them. They need

Table 37-4 Diagnostic procedures

TEST	DESCRIPTION	PURPOSE	COMMENTS
Lumbar puncture (LP)	Long needle is inserted between L3 and L4 vertebrae into subarachnoid space; cerebrospinal fluid (CSF) pressure is measured, and sample is collected for examination	Diagnostic—measures spinal fluid pressure, obtains CSF for visualization and laboratory analysis Therapeutic—injection of medication, spinal anesthesia	Contraindicated in patients with increased intracranial pressure or infected skin over puncture site
Subdural tap	Needle is inserted into anterior fontanel or coronal suture	Helps rule out subdural effusions Relieves intracranial pressure	Requires shaving scalp Infant placed in semierect position after subdural tap to minimize leakage from site; avoid crying if possible Check site frequently for evidence of leakage
Ventricular puncture	Needle is inserted into lateral ventricle via anterior fontanel	Removes CSF to relieve pressure	Used if LP unsuccessful or contraindicated Risk of intracerebral or ventricular hemorrhage
Electroencephalography	Records changes in electric potential of brain Electrodes are placed at various points on scalp and amplified Impulses are recorded by electromagnetic pen	Measures electric activity of cerebral cortex Detects electric abnormalities—diagnosis of seizures Used to determine brain death	Patient should rest quietly during procedure May require sedation Reduce external stimuli to a minimum during procedure
Computed tomography (CT scan)	Pinpoint x-ray beam is directed on horizontal or vertical plane to provide series of "cuts" or "slices" that are fed into computer and assembled in image displayed on videoscreen and transferred to permanent record	Visualized horizontal and vertical cross section of brain at any axis Distinguishes density of various intracranial tissues and structures—congenital abnormalities hemorrhage, tumors, and demyelinating and inflammatory processes	Noninvasive procedure Requires sedation Can be done on outpatient basis Rapid, relatively safe and accurate
Nuclear brain scan	Intravenous injection of radioactive material that is counted and recorded after fixed time interval	Test material accumulates in areas where blood-brain barrier is defective Identifies focal brain lesions (e.g., tumors, abscesses) Positive uptake of material with encephalitis and subdural hematoma Visualizes CSF pathways	Requires sedation in young or uncooperative children and intravenous infusion In normal children or noncommunicating hydrocephalus there is no retrograde filling of ventricles Areas of concentrated uptake of material are termed "hot spots"
Transillumination	Flashlight with rubber adapter is held snugly against infant's head in totally darkened room	Varying degrees of localized glowing may be seen in abnormal fluid accumulation in various areas of head	Normally in full-term infant, a halo of light extends 1 to 2 cm from rim of light source
Echoencephalography	Pulses of ultrasonic waves are beamed through head; echoes from reflecting surfaces are recorded graphically	Identifies shifts in midline structures from their normal positions as a result of intracranial lesions May show ventricular dilation	Simple, safe, rapid procedure

Table 37-4 Diagnostic procedures—cont'd

TEST	DESCRIPTION	PURPOSE	COMMENTS
Radiography	Skull films are taken from several projections—lateral, posterolateral, axial (submentoventrical), half-axial	Shows fractures, dislocations, spreading suture lines, and craniostenosis Shows degenerative changes, bone erosion, and calcifications	Simple, noninvasive procedure
Magnetic resonance imaging (MRI) or nuclear magnetic resonance (NMR)	Produces radiofrequency emissions from elements (e.g., hydrogen, phosphorus), which are converted to visual images by computer	Permits visualization of morphologic features of target structures Permits tissue discrimination unavailable with many techniques	Noninvasive Require heavy sedation for lengthy immobilization Parent or attendant can remain in room with child Does not visualize bone detail or calcifications
Positron emission transaxial tomography (PETT)	IV injection of positron-emitting radionucleotide; local concentrations are detected and transformed into a visual display by computer	Detects and measures blood volume and flow in brain, metabolic activity, and biochemical changes within tissues, etc.	Requires lengthy period of immobility Minimum exposure to radiation
Real time ultrasonography (RTUS)	Similar to CT but uses ultrasound instead of ionizing radiation	Allows high-resolution anatomic visualization in variety of imaging planes	Produces images similar to CT scan Especially useful in neonatal CNS problems
Digital subtraction angiography (DSA)	Contrast dye injected IV; computer "subtracts" all tissues without contrast medium, leaving clear image of contrast medium in vessels studied	Visualizes vasculature of target tissue Visualizes finite vascular abnormalities	Safe alternative to angiography Patient must remain still during procedure

constant reassurance from a trusted companion (Fig. 37-4).

Physical preparation may involve administration of a sedative. If so, the child should be helped through the preparation and administration and assured that someone will remain with him (if this is possible). The child will need continual support and reinforcement during the procedures in which he remains conscious. The child's vital signs and physiologic response to the procedure are monitored throughout. Care after the test depends on the nature of the procedure.

Children who have undergone a procedure with general anesthesia require postanesthesia care, including positioning to prevent aspiration of secretions and frequent assessment of vital signs and level of consciousness. In addition, other neurologic functions, such as pupillary responses, motor strength, and movement, are tested at regular intervals. Any surgical wound resulting from the test is checked for bleeding, cerebrospinal fluid leakage, and other complications. Children who undergo repeated subdural taps should have their hematocrit measured daily to detect any blood loss from the procedure.

The child's emotional reaction to the procedure is also considered. He should be allowed to express his feelings about the experience through verbal expression and the use of therapeutic play.

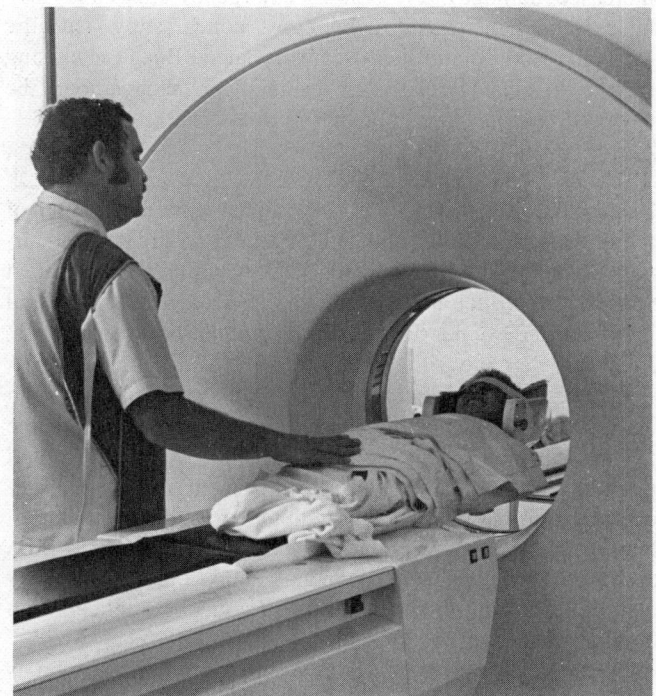

Fig. 37-4. This child reflects the stress and feeling of powerlessness during tomography even when accompanied by a kind and supportive person.

The Child with Cerebral Compromise

The child who has sustained some manner of cerebral compromise as a result of physical injury, infection, near-drowning, or toxic injury is usually in varying states of consciousness. No matter what the etiology, the nursing efforts are directed primarily toward detection of possible alterations in condition and preventing further damage to the various systems and tissues. Care of the unconscious child is almost the same no matter what the cause of the condition.

NURSING THE UNCONSCIOUS CHILD

The unconscious child requires continuous nursing attendance with observation, recording, and evaluation of changes in objective signs. These observations provide valuable information regarding the patient's progress. Often they serve as a guide to diagnosis and treatment. Therefore careful and detailed observations are essential for the patient's welfare. In addition, vital functions must be maintained and complications prevented through conscientious and meticulous nursing care. The outcome of unconsciousness may be early and complete recovery, death within a few hours or days, persistent and permanent unconsciousness, or recovery with varying degrees of residual mental and/or physical disability.

Emergency measures are directed toward assuming a patent airway, treatment of shock, and reduction of intracranial pressure (if present). Delayed treatment often leads to increased damage. As soon as emergency measures have been implemented—in many cases concurrently—specific therapies for specific causes are initiated. Because nursing care is so closely related to the medical management, the two will be considered together here.

Respiratory Management

Respiratory effectiveness is the primary concern in care of the unconscious child, and establishment of an adequate airway is *always* the first priority. Carbon dioxide has a potent vasodilating effect and will increase CBF and ICP. Cerebral hypoxia that extends longer than 4 minutes causes irreversible brain damage.

Children in lighter stages of coma may be able to cough and swallow, but those in deeper states of coma are unable to handle secretions, which tend to pool in the throat and pharynx. The child is positioned to prevent aspiration of secretions, and the stomach is emptied to reduce the likelihood of vomiting. In infants, blockage of air passages from secretions can happen in seconds. In addition, upper airway obstruction from laryngospasm is a frequent complication in comatose children.

A temporary airway can be used for the child who is suffering a temporary loss of consciousness, such as after a seizure or anesthesia. For children who remain unconscious for a period of time, a nasotracheal or orotracheal tube is inserted to maintain the open airway and facilitate removal of secretions. A tracheostomy is performed in cases in which laryngoscopy for introduction of an endotracheal tube would be difficult or dangerous. Suctioning is used as often as needed to clear the airway. Respiratory status is observed and evaluated regularly. Signs of respiratory embarrassment may be an indication for ventilatory assistance.

When the respiratory center is involved, mechanical ventilation is usually indicated (see p. 1322). Blood gas analysis is performed regularly, and oxygen is administered when indicated. Moderately severe hypoxia and respiratory acidosis are often present but not always evident from clinical manifestations. Hyperventilation frequently accompanies unconsciousness and may lead to respiratory alkalosis, or it may represent the body's attempt to compensate for metabolic acidosis. Therefore blood gas and pH determinations are essential guides for electrolyte therapy. Chest physiotherapy is carried out on a regular basis, and the child's position is changed at least every 2 hours to prevent pulmonary complications.

Neurologic Assessment

Continual observation of vital signs, pupillary reaction, and level of consciousness is essential to management of central nervous system disorders. Regular assessment of neurologic signs is a vital part of nursing comatose children. Vital signs are taken and recorded regularly. The frequency depends on the cause of coma, the status, and the progression of cerebral involvement. Intervals may be as frequent as every 15 minutes or as long as every 2 hours. Significant alterations are reported immediately. Temperature is taken every 2 to 4 hours, depending on the patient's condition.

An elevated temperature is not uncommon in children with central nervous system dysfunction; therefore a light covering is sufficient. Vigorous efforts are needed, such as tepid sponge baths or application of a hypothermia blanket, to prevent brain damage.

The level of consciousness is assessed periodically, including size, equality, and reaction of pupils to light; signs of meningeal irritation, such as nuchal rigidity; and level of consciousness. This includes response to vocal commands, spontaneous behavior, resistance to care, and response to painful stimuli; motions of any kind, changes in muscle tone or strength, and body position are noted. Seizure activity is described according to type and length of seizure and body areas involved (see p. 1666).

Sedatives are usually avoided but may be indicated when marked agitation or restlessness may result in further damage. If so, chloral hydrate or diphenhydramine (Benadryl), and occasionally Haldol, are preferred. These drugs are less likely to produce respiratory depression. However, favorable results are achieved with the administration of codeine. Sometimes a large initial dose of phenobarbital is administered, even to the extent that short-term respiratory support is required. Anticonvulsants, primarily phenytoin (Dilantin), are ordered for control of seizure activity.

Increased Intracranial Pressure Monitoring

Prompt intervention is lifesaving in the comatose patient who has evidence of marked increase in ICP. When increased ICP is the result of accumulation of cerebrospinal fluid from obstruction of cerebrospinal fluid flow, a ventricular tap will provide relief quickly and effectively. Evacuation of a hematoma reduces pressure from this source. Indications for inserting an ICP monitor are (1) Glasgow Coma Scale evaluation of less than 6, (2) Glasgow Coma Scale evaluation of less than 8 with respiratory assistance, (3) deterioration of condition, and (4) subjective judgment regarding clinical appearance and response.

ICP is monitored directly by means of a hollow subarachnoid bolt (Richmond screw) or an intraventricular catheter with fibroscopic sensors that are attached to a monitoring system. In the bolt method the end of the bolt is placed into the subarachnoid space. In children over 3 years of age this is accomplished through a bur hole. The bolt is stabilized with dressings, but these are not changed or disturbed, even to check the site. The placement of the bolt is not adjusted by anyone except the neurosurgeon who placed the device. Irrigation and nursing management are the same as for any other line (e.g., arterial or central venous pressure). The neurosurgeon is notified if a satisfactory wave form is not observed.

The catheter method involves introduction of a catheter into the lateral ventricle on the nondominant side, if known, or placement in the subdural space. In infants a fontanel transducer can be used to detect impulses from a pressure sensor and convert them to electrical energy (Fig. 37-5). The electrical energy is then converted to visible waves or numerical readings on an oscilloscope. The catheter has the advantage of providing a means of extraventricular (or continuous) drainage to reduce pressure. A drainage bag attached to the system is kept at the level of the ventricles and can be lowered to decrease ICP. Antibiotics are usually instilled into the ventricle once daily, and fluid is obtained for culture.

Nurses caring for patients with intracranial monitoring devices must be acquainted with the system, assist with insertion, interpret the monitor readings, and be able to distinguish between danger signals and mechanical dysfunction.

For increased ICP resulting from cerebral edema, several medical measures are available. Osmotic diuretics may provide rapid relief in emergency situations. Although their effect is transient, lasting only about 6 hours, they can be lifesaving in emergencies. These substances are rapidly excreted by the kidneys and carry with them large quantities of sodium and water. Mannitol (or sometimes urea) administered intravenously is the drug most frequently employed for rapid reduction. The infusion is generally given slowly

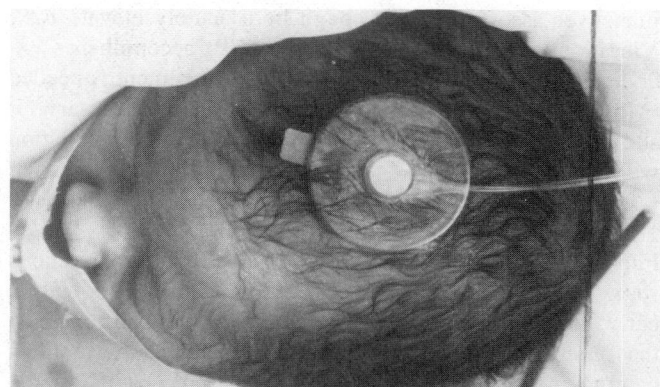

Fig. 37-5. Infant with intracranial pressure monitor.
Photography by Jo Barr, San Jose, CA.

but may be pushed rapidly if there is herniation or impending herniation. Because of the profound diuretic effect of the drug, an indwelling catheter is inserted to ensure bladder emptying. Adrenal corticosteroids are sometimes given to reduce cerebral edema, although their use is controversial. The effect is less rapid than that of the osmotic diuretics, but high doses can be used over an extended period for prolonged control. Assisted ventilation also helps to reduce ICP by causing vasoconstriction of cerebral arteries. Hyperventilation serves to decrease the $Paco^2$.

Nursing activities. In cases of high levels of increased ICP, nursing procedures tend to trigger reactive pressure waves in many patients. For example, increased intrathoracic or abdominal pressure will be transmitted to the cranium. Particular care should be taken in positioning these patients to avoid neck vein compression, which may further increase ICP by interfering with venous return. The head of the bed is elevated 15 to 30 degrees and the child positioned so that the head is maintained in a midline to facilitate venous drainage and avoid jugular compression. Turning side to side is contraindicated because of the risk of jugular compression. The child can be propped to one side or the other; and the use of an alternating pressure or egg-carton mattress reduces the chance of prolonged pressure to vulnerable areas.

Therefore it is important to avoid activities that cause pain, emotional stress, or crying or those that might trigger a convulsive seizure. Gentle range of motion exercises can be carried out but should not be performed vigorously. Nontherapeutic touch can cause an increase in ICP. Any disturbing procedures to be performed should be scheduled to take advantage of therapies that reduce ICP, such as osmotherapy and sedation. Efforts are taken to minimize or eliminate environmental noise. Sudden, loud noises cause peripheral vasoconstriction, increased mean arterial pressure, and contribute to increased ICP (Smith, 1983).

Suctioning. Suctioning and percussion are poorly tolerated and are therefore contraindicated unless there are concurrent respiratory problems. Hypoxia and the Valsalva maneuver associated with cough both acutely elevate ICP. Vibration, which does not increase ICP, accomplishes excellent results and should be tried first if treatment is needed (Morriss and Cook, 1984). If suctioning is necessary, it should be used judiciously and preceded by hyperventilation with 100% oxygen.

Nutrition and Hydration

Fluids and calories are supplied initially by the intravenous route (see Chapter 28). An intravenous infusion is started early, and the type of fluid administered is determined by the general condition of the patient. Fluid therapy requires careful monitoring and adjustment based on neurologic signs and electrolyte determinations. Often comatose children are unable to cope with the same amounts of fluid they could handle at other times, and overhydration must be avoided to prevent fatal cerebral edema.

Later, nutrition is provided in a balanced formula given by nasogastric or gastrostomy tube. The nasogastric tube is usually taped in place with care to prevent pressure on the nares. Most children have continuous feedings, but if bolus feedings are used, the tube is rinsed with water after each feeding. Tubes are replaced according to unit policy. Nostrils are alternated with each replacement to prevent nasal irritation and pressure. Overfeeding should be avoided to prevent vomiting with its attendant danger of aspiration. Stomach contents are aspirated and measured before feeding to ascertain the amount remaining in the stomach. If the residual volume is excessive (depending on the size of the child), the dietitian and physician should be consulted regarding alteration of the formula composition to provide the needed calories and nutrients in a smaller volume. The aspirated contents should always be refed.

Hydration is maintained in the same manner. When cerebral edema is a threat, fluids may be restricted to reduce the chance of fluid overload. Skin and mucous membranes are examined for signs of dehydration. Observation for signs of altered fluid balance related to abnormal pituitary secretions is a part of nursing care.

Altered pituitary secretion. An altered ability to handle fluid loads is attributed in part to the inappropriate secretion of antidiuretic hormone (ISADH) and diabetes insipidus (DI) resulting from hypothalamic dysfunction (see p. 1686 and p. 1685). ISADH frequently accompanies central nervous system diseases such as head injury, meningitis, encephalitis, brain abscess, brain tumor, and subarachnoid hemorrhage. In the patient with ISADH, scant quantities of urine are excreted, electrolyte analysis reveals hyponatremia and hyposmolality, and manifestations of overhydration are evident. It is important to evaluate all parameters, since the reduced urine output might be erroneously interpreted as a sign of dehydration. The treatment of ISADH consists of restriction of fluids until serum electrolytes and osmolality return to normal levels. Since ISADH frequently occurs with meningitis in children, fluid restriction is often prescribed.

Likewise DI is not uncommon following intracranial trauma. There is increased urine volume and the accompanying danger of dehydration. Adequate replacement of fluids is essential, and observation of electrolyte balance is necessary to detect signs of hypernatremia and hyperosmolality. Exogenous vasopressin may be administered.

Medications

The cause of unconsciousness determines specific drug therapies. Children with infectious processes are given antibiotics appropriate to the disease and the infecting organism, and corticosteroids are prescribed for inflammatory conditions and edema. Cerebral edema is an indication for osmotherapy with osmotic diuretics (e.g., mannitol), diuretics (e.g., furosemide), and/or hypertonic glucose solution. Sedatives are often indicated for extreme restlessness, agitation, and hyperresponsiveness to stimuli. Sedatives or anticonvulsants are prescribed for seizure activity.

Deep coma may be induced by administration of barbiturates to diminish activities that might contribute to increased intracranial pressure. Barbiturate coma requires extensive monitoring, cardiovascular and respiratory support, and ICP monitoring to assess response to therapy. Paralyzing agents, such as pancuronium (Pavulon) also may be needed to aid in performing diagnostic tests, improving effectiveness of therapy, and reducing risks of secondary complications. Elevation of ICP and/or heart rate of patients who are being given paralyzing agents or are under sedation may indicate the need for another dose of either or both medications.

Thermoregulation. Fever often accompanies cerebral dysfunction, and if fever is present, measures are implemented to reduce the temperature to prevent brain damage from hyperthermia and to reduce metabolic demands generated by the increased body temperature. Antipyretics are the method of choice for fever reduction; cooling devices are used for hyperthermia. Laboratory tests and other methods are used to attempt to determine the cause, if any, of the hyperthermia.

Hypothermia may be used in conjunction with barbiturate coma to reduce cerebral metabolic demands and minimize cerebral injury. However, most institutions have abandoned the use of this form of therapy because of increased risk of complications, such as arrhythmias and changes in electrolyes.

Elimination

A retention catheter is usually inserted in the older child, and a plastic collection bag is placed on the infant or small child. Long-term use of collection bags creates excoriation problems, however. The child who formerly had bowel and bladder control is generally incontinent. The collecting devices help keep the skin clean and provide a means for obtaining an accurate intake and output measurement. If the child remains comatose for a long period, the indwelling catheter may be removed and periodic bladder emptying accomplished by intermittent catheterization or, sometimes, pressure applied over the suprapubic area (Credé). Stool softeners are usually sufficient to maintain bowel function, but suppositories or enemas may be needed occasionally for adequate elimination.

Hygienic Care

Routine measures for cleansing and maintaining skin integrity are an integral part of nursing care of the unconscious child. Skin folds require special attention to prevent excoriation. The child who is unable to move is prone to develop tissue breakdown and pressure necrosis; therefore the child is placed on a sheepskin, egg-carton pad, or other resilient appliance (alternating mattresses and water-filled mattresses are also used) to prevent pressure on prominent areas of the body. The goal is prevention by regular change of position and inspection of vulnerable areas, such as the ankle, trochanter, and shoulder. Since supine positioning is seldom employed, the occiput and sacrum are less likely to be involved. Bed linen and any clothing are kept dry and free of wrinkles. Rubbing the back and extremities with lotion or other lubricating preparation stimulates circulation and helps prevent drying of the skin.

Mouth care is performed at least twice daily, since the mouth tends to become dry or coated with mucus. The teeth are carefully brushed with a soft toothbrush or cleaned with gauze saturated with saline. Commercially prepared cleansing devices, such as Toothettes, are convenient for cleansing the mouth and teeth. Lips are coated with ointment, glycerine, or other preparations to protect them from drying, cracking, or blistering.

The deeply comatose child is also prone to eye irritation. The corneal reflexes are absent; therefore the eyes are easily irritated or damaged by linen, dust, or other substances that may come in contact with them. There is excessive dryness as a result of decreased secretions, especially if the child is undergoing osmotherapy to reduce or prevent brain edema, and incomplete closure of the eyes. The eyes should be examined regularly and carefully for early signs of irritation or inflammation. Artificial tears (methylcellulose) are placed in the eyes every 1 to 2 hours. Sometimes eye dressings may be needed to protect the eyes from possible damage.

The hair is combed and styled neatly. Long hair is usually braided and secured with rubber bands. The scalp should be kept clean with dry or wet shampoos as needed. The child's head may be shaved for tests or surgical procedures. If so, the hair is saved if possible and given to the family.

Positioning and Exercise

The unconscious child is positioned to prevent aspiration of saliva, nasogastric secretions, and vomitus and to minimize intracranial pressure. The head of the bed is elevated, and the child is placed on the side or in a semiprone position. A small, firm pillow is placed under the head, and the uppermost limbs are flexed and supported with pillows. The weight of the body should not rest on the dependent arm. In the semiprone position the child lies with the dependent arm at the side behind the body and the opposite side supported on pillows with the uppermost arm and leg flexed and resting on the pillows. This position prevents undue pressure on the dependent extremities. The dependent position of the face encourages drainage of secretions and prevents the flaccid tongue from obstructing the airway.

Normal range of motion exercises help to maintain function and prevent contractures of joints. Exercises should be done gently and with full range of motion. A small rolled pad can be placed in the palms to help maintain proper position of fingers; footboards or boots can be used to help prevent footdrop; splinting may be needed to prevent severe contractures of wrist, knee, or ankle in decerebrate children.

Stimulation

Sensory stimulation is important in the care of the unconscious child, just as it is in the care of the alert child. For the temporarily unconscious or semiconscious child, sensory stimulation helps to arouse the child to the conscious state and orient him in terms of time and place. Auditory and tactile stimulation are especially valuable. Tactile stimulation is not appropriate for the child in whom it may elicit an undesirable response. However, for other children tactile contact often has a relaxing and calming effect. When the child's condition permits, holding or rocking the child has a soothing effect and provides the body contact needed by young children.

The auditory sense is often present in a state of coma. Hearing is the last sense to be lost and the first one to be regained; therefore the child should be spoken to as any other child. Conversation around the child should not include thoughtless or derogatory remarks. A radio playing soft music, a music box, or a record player is frequently used to provide auditory stimulation. Singing the child's favorite songs or reading a favorite story within his hearing is a tactic used to maintain his contact with a familiar world. Having parents tape songs or stories provides a continuous source of familiar stimulation. Above all, it is important to remember that this is a child who has all the needs of any ill child.

Family Support

Dealing with the parents of an unconscious child is especially difficult. They may demonstrate all the guilt, fear, hostility, and anxiety of any parent of a seriously ill child (see Chapter 22). In addition, these parents are faced with the uncertain outcome of the cerebral dysfunction. The fear of death, mental retardation, or other permanent disability is present. Nursing intervention with parents depends on the nature of the pathologic condition, the personality of the parents, and the parent-child relationship before injury or illness.

The child may regain consciousness within a short time. If there is little or no residual effect, the child will be dismissed to home care fairly soon. The parents need the most intensive nursing intervention during the period of crisis and uncertainty. During the recovery phase they are given information, information is clarified, and they are encouraged to become involved in the child's care. Often the child's hospitalization is brief; however, some children require extended hospitalization for intensive therapy and rehabilitation.

The parents of children who die within hours or days require the support and guidance that the parents of any dying child would need in coping with the reality and resolving their grief (see Chapter 23).

Probably the most difficult situations are those that involve children who are unconscious permanently or for an indefinite period. Unlike parents who lose a child through death, the finality is lacking for these parents, often leaving them in a state of suspended grief. The presence of the child renders the parents unable to resolve the loss. Like parents of dying children, parents of the comatose child search for any signs of hope. Well-meaning friends and relatives relate instances of miraculous recoveries. The parents seek confirmation and support for such possibilities and assign erroneous meanings to any sign in the child, such as muscle contractions, that might be interpreted as evidence of recovery.

Like parents who lose a child through death, the parents of the child lost to their world attempt to reconstitute a representation of the child. They bring items that belong to the child, such as favorite toys, music, and other objects cherished by the child. This is interpreted as an attempt to provide stimulation for the child in the hope of eliciting a response, to let the hospital staff know the child as the unique individual he was so that the parents' distress can be better appreciated, and to reconstitute an image of the child "lost" to them and for whom they mourn. An awareness of these behaviors and coping mechanisms provides nurses with the understanding that helps them support the parents in their grief process.

Superimposed on the process of grieving for the "lost" child, parents may be faced with difficult decisions. First,

there is the child whose brain is so severely damaged that his vital functions must be maintained by artificial means. The parents must make the final decision to remove life-support systems. Since the decision is so difficult for parents, the physician is frequently placed in a position of making the decision indirectly. After providing the parents with all the information, the physician will suggest that the child be removed from the life support to "see if he can make it on his own." The approach relieves the parents of the decision and can be effective, but it is based on evaluation of the intellectual level and emotional state of the parents. Sometimes parents may even choose to refuse treatment if they believe it to be best for the child and the family (informed dissent).

Second, there is the child who has survived the illness or injury that produced the brain damage but is left unconscious permanently. In such a situation the parents must decide whether to place the child in a chronic care facility or make arrangements to care for the child at home. During these decisions the nurse can listen to the parents' discussions regarding alternatives, provide information where appropriate, and support the family in their decision. The nurse can help the family prepare for the transfer of the child and make referrals to persons or agencies that can provide additional assistance.

There is also the child who survived the cerebral insult, who is not comatose, but whose physical and/or mental capacity is limited, either minimally or severely. Families of such children must cope with the long and tedious rehabilitation process and uncertain outcome. The drain on financial, emotional, and social resources can be enormous.

For parents who choose to care for their child at home, planning for home care begins early in the process of recovery. The family should become involved with the care of the child as soon as they indicate an interest and ability to do so. They will need education and support in learning to care for the child, regular follow-up observation and assessment of the home management, and planning for some respite care of the child. Parents need to understand that it is important to plan for periodic relief from the continual care of the child. (see Discharge planning and home care, p. 1094).

Nursing Care Summary: The Unconscious Child

NURSING GOALS	NURSING INTERVENTIONS	EXPECTED PATIENT/FAMILY OUTCOMES
H-HMP	**Injury; potential for tissue damage**	
	Risk factors: physical immobility, depressed sensorium	

Assess neurologic status	Monitor vital signs
	Check pupillary reaction for size, reaction to light and accommodation, equality of responses
	Note and describe
	   Voluntary movements of extremities (e.g., purposeful, random)
	   Changes in muscular tone
	   Changes in position of body and/or head
	   Tremor, twitching
	   Seizure activity (e.g., generalized or local)
	   Signs of meningeal irritation (e.g., nuchal rigidity, opisthotonos)
	Measure occipital-frontal circumference of infants
	   Assess status of fontanel—full or sunken, tense or soft
		*Signs of neurologic alterations are detected early

Prevent respiratory complications	Position for optimum ventilation Turn frequently—at least every 2 hours Avoid contact with persons with upper respiratory infection Maintain patent airway Remove accumulated secretions promptly Provide good oral hygiene	Child exhibits no evidence of lung dysfunction
Prevent corneal irritation	Patch eyes if indicated Keep lids completely closed	Corneas remain clear and moist
Detect early signs of cerebral hypoxia	Monitor vital signs Observe changes in color of face, lips, extremities Observe for changes in responsiveness Observe for seizure activity Monitor intracranial pressure	*Signs of cerebral hypoxia are detected early
Protect from physical injury	Keep side rails up Pad hard surfaces that may injure extremities during spontaneous or involuntary movement	Child remains free of physical injury
H-HMP	**Injury: potential for increased intracranial pressure**	
	Risk factors: cerebral edema, space occupying lesion, hemorrhage, inflammation, increased cerebral spinal fluid volume	
Prevent cerebral edema	Elevate head of bed to 15 to 45 degrees Monitor vital signs and neurologic signs to detect early indications of increased intracranial pressure Monitor fluid intake and output Observe for signs of impending overhydration	Child exhibits no signs of increased intracranial pressure *Early signs are detected and appropriate action initiated

Minimize intracranial pressure	Elevate head of the bed 15 to 45 degrees
	Avoid positions or activities that increase
	   intracranial pressure
	   Pressure on neck veins
	   Flexion or extension of neck
	   Head rotation
	   Valsalva maneuver
	   Painful stimuli
	   Respiratory procedures (especially suctioning)
	Prevent constipation
	Provide
	   Quiet, subdued environment
	   Pleasant auditory experiences
	   Therapeutic touch
	Avoid emotionally stressful conversation (e.g., about pain, condition, prognosis)
		Intracranial pressure remains within safe limits
		Child shows no evidence of increased intracranial pressure

*Nursing outcome.

Continued.

Nursing Care Summary: The Unconscious Child—cont'd

NURSING GOALS	NURSING INTERVENTIONS	EXPECTED PATIENT/FAMILY OUTCOMES
N-MP **Fluid volume deficit, potential** **Risk factors: self-care deficit, immobility, altered sensorium**		
Prevent dehydration	Provide fluids as needed	Child exhibits no evidence of dehydration
N-MP **Oral mucous membrane, alteration in** **Etiology: mouth breathing, NPO**		
Prevent drying and caking	Provide meticulous mouth care	Mucous membranes remain clean, moist, and free of irritation
N-MP **Hyperthermia** **Etiology: altered temperature control**		
Prevent or control hyperthermia	Assess temperature regularly to detect elevation Remove excess coverings	Body temperature remains within safe limits
N-MP **Skin integrity, impairment of: potential** **Risk factors: immobility, body secretions**		
Maintain skin integrity	Place child on sheepskin, egg-carton pad, or other resilient surface Change position frequently unless contraindicated by increased ICP Protect pressure points (e.g., trochanter, sacrum, ankle, shoulder, occiput) Inspect skin surfaces regularly for signs of irritation, redness, evidence of pressure Cleanse skin regularly, at least once daily Protect skin folds and surfaces that rub together Keep clothing and linen clean and dry Carry out good perineal care under urine collection device Stimulate circulation by gentle rubbing with lotion or other lubricating substance Protect lips with cream or ointment	Skin remains clean and intact
EP **Bowel elimination, alteration in: constipation** **Etiology: physical inactivity, immobility**		
Ensure adequate elimination	Provide sufficient liquid intake, unless contraindicated by cerebral edema or if over-hydration is a threat	Bowel is evacuated daily
A-EP **Airway clearance, ineffective** **Etiology: perceptual and cognitive impairment**		
Maintain patent airway	Position to prevent aspiration Semiprone position Side-lying position Aspirate airway as needed Insert oral airway if indicated Avoid neck hyperextension	Child breathes easily; respirations are within normal limits
A-EP **Mobility, impaired physical** **Etiology: perceptual and cognitive impairment**		
Maintain limb flexibility and functions	Perform passive range of motion exercises Position to reduce contractures—splint contracting joints if needed	Joints remain flexible and retain full range of motion

Nursing Care Summary: The Unconscious Child—cont'd

NURSING GOALS	NURSING INTERVENTIONS	EXPECTED PATIENT/FAMILY OUTCOMES
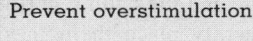 **A-EP**	**Self-care deficit: feeding, bathing/hygiene, dressing/grooming, toileting (level 4)** **Etiology: perceptual and cognitive impairment**	
Ensure adequate nutritional intake	Provide nourishment in manner suitable to child's condition	Child obtains sufficient nourishment
Provide hygienic care	Bathe daily or more often, if indicated Dress appropriately Keep hair combed and styled	Child appears clean and as well groomed as possible within limitations of his condition
Provide toileting	Diaper as needed Use collection appliances, if feasible Clean skin well after each elimination	Child's diaper area remains clean and free of irritation
CPP	**Sensory-perceptual alteration: visual, auditory, kinesthetic, gustatory, tactile, olfactory** **Etiology: central nervous system depression, bed rest**	
Assess level of consciousness	Observe and record Change in spontaneous behavior Resistance to care Response to verbal commands Response to noxious stimuli Type of verbalization or crying	Consciousness level is determined
Provide sensory stimulation	Provide tactile stimulation (if it does not wake undesirable muscle response, e.g., seizures) Provide auditory stimulation by voice, radio, music box, etc. Provide visual stimuli appropriate for age Provide proprioceptive stimulation by rocking, cuddling, etc.	Child is provided with sensory stimulation appropriate to his age and condition
Prevent overstimulation	Avoid stimulation that precipitates undesirable responses Space nursing activities for minimal disturbance	Child exhibits no seizure activity or undue restlessness and agitation
RRP	**Family process, alteration in** **Etiology: situational crisis (child with a serious illness)**	
Support family	Explain therapies; clarify and reinforce information given to family by physician Interpret child's behaviors and responses Allow expression of feelings and concerns Accept aggressive behavior	Family demonstrates an understanding of child's behaviors, therapies, and probable outcome
Assist in child placement, if indicated	Provide needed information Answer family's questions; encourage expression of feelings Refer to persons or agencies for further information and clarification Support parent's decisions	Family verbalizes feelings and concerns
Arrange for discharge and follow-up care	Teach family techniques and procedures needed in care of child Arrange for follow-up visit by appropriate persons (e.g., public health nurse)	Family demonstrates skills and procedures for child's care

Nursing Interventions Related to Medical Management

Maintain patent airway
  Administer care of endotracheal tube or tracheostomy if appropriate; have equipment available for emergency insertion if indicated for respiratory distress
Ensure adequate respiration
  Assist with insertion of endotracheal tube
  Monitor artificial ventilation

Ensure adequate circulation
  Assist with establishment of intravenous infusion
  Monitor intravenous infusion
  Administer intravenous fluids as prescribed
Assist with diagnostic tests
  Collect specimens as ordered
  Carry out examinations as indicated or ordered, such as urine specific gravity, blood samples

Continued.

Nursing Interventions Related to Medical Management—cont'd

Assist with diagnostic tests—cont'd
Prepare for and assist with diagnostic procedures, such as lumbar puncture, x-ray examination
Interpret and report results of tests

Provide nutrition and hydration
Monitor intravenous feedings when ordered
Feed prescribed formula by means of nasogastric or gastrostomy tube

Prevent increased intracranial pressure
Administer paralyzing agents if prescribed

Prevent cerebral hypoxia
Maintain patent airway
Provide oxygen as indicated by objective signs or as ordered
If on mechanical ventilation:
Monitor for correct settings, proper functioning
Prepare to provide artificial ventilation in case of ventilatory failure; have AmBU bag at hand
Administer medications as ordered to prevent cerebral edema and improve cerebral circulation

Prevent cerebral edema
Monitor intravenous fluids carefully
Administer hyperosmolar fluids as prescribed

Administer corticosteroids as ordered
Weigh daily or as ordered to detect fluid accumulation or reduction
Monitor intracranial pressure

Prevent hyperthermia
Administer antipyretics, if prescribed
Apply and monitor hypothermia blanket if indicated or ordered; administer antishivering agents if ordered

Prevent seizures
Administer sedatives or anticonvulsants as prescribed

Ensure adequate elimination
Administer stool softener
Administer suppositories or enema as indicated
Apply urine collecting device or insert indwelling catheter (if ordered)
Provide proper care of catheter

Prevent respiratory complications
Perform percussion, vibration, and suctioning every 3-4 hours

Prevent corneal irritation
Instill "artificial tears"

HEAD INJURY

Head injury can be defined as any pathologic process involving the scalp, skull, meninges, or brain as the result of mechanical force. Accidental injury is the major single cause of death in the pediatric age-group, and although it cannot be stated with certainty, most of these injuries are probably the result of central nervous system trauma. Rarely does a child attain adulthood without having sustained a significant bump or blow to the head. Most do not require hospitalization, but it is estimated that 200,000 children are admitted to hospitals each year for evaluation and treatment of head injury. Of these, approximately 5% to 10% exhibit neurologic signs (DeVivo and Dodge, 1977).

Etiology

Falls are the leading cause of head injury. Motor vehicle–related accidents are the major cause of severe and fatal head injury at all ages. Child abuse is a cause of severe head injury in children less than 1 year of age. Vigorous shaking of an infant can cause central nervous system damage, especially a whiplash type of injury and subdural hematoma. Short falls are also common in this age-group. Unrestrained children from age 2 to 10 years sustain head injuries in motor vehicles. Unhelmeted children on bicycles and impact injuries in sports are the causes of a significant number of injuries in children over 12 years of age. Adolescents are most often injured in motor vehicle accidents.

The exposed nature of the head renders it particularly vulnerable to external violence, and many of the physical characteristics of children predispose them to craniocerebral trauma. For example, infants are frequently left unattended on beds, in high chairs, and in other places from which they can fall. Because the head of an infant or toddler is proportionately large and heavy in relation to other body parts, it is the most likely to be injured. Incomplete motor development contributes to falls at all ages, and the natural curiosity and exuberance of children frequently place them in situations in which they are likely to incur an injury.

Pathophysiology

The skull forms such an excellent protection for the brain that, although nervous tissue is delicate, it usually requires a severe blow to cause significant damage. However, the protective mechanisms vary between individuals and are also influenced by age. For example, a small child's resilient skull may withstand a blow that would be severely damaging to an aged individual. The elastic, pliable skulls of infants and young children absorb much of the direct energy of physical impact to the head and afford some protection to intracranial structures.

Physical forces act on the head through *acceleration, deceleration,* or *deformation.* Injury occurs by way of compression, tearing, or shearing, either singly, in combination, or in succession. Acceleration or deceleration is more descriptive of the circumstances responsible for most head injuries. When the stationary head receives a blow, the sudden acceleration causes deformation of the skull and mass movement of the brain. Continued movement of the intracranial contents allows the brain to strike parts of the skull (e.g., the sharp edges of the sphenoid or the irregular surface of the anterior fossa) or the edges of the tentorium.

Although the brain volume remains unchanged, significant distortion and cavitation take place as the brain changes shape in response to the force transmitted from the impact

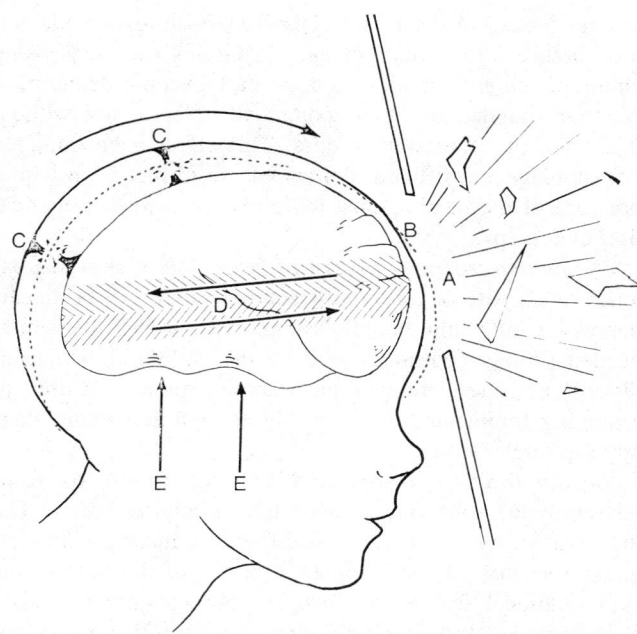

Fig. 37-6. Mechanical distortion of cranium during closed head injury. **A,** Preinjury contour of skull. **B,** Immediate postinjury contour of skull. **C,** Torn subdural vessels. **D,** Shearing forces. **E,** Trauma from contact with floor of cranium.

Redrawn from Grubb, R.L., and Coxe, W.S.: Central nervous system trauma: cranial. In Eliasson, S.G., Presky, A.L., and Hardin, W.B., Jr., editors: Neurological pathophysiology, New York, 1974, Oxford University Press.

to the skull. This deformation can cause bruising at the point of impact (*coup*) and/or at a distance as the brain collides with the unyielding surfaces far removed from the point of impact (*contrecoup*) (Fig. 37-6). Some of the changes related to this phenomenon may be a result of a momentary increased pressure that produces a temporary negative pressure with cavitation and vaporization contralaterally. Thus a blow to the occipital region can cause severe injury to the frontal and temporal areas of the brain. Sudden deceleration, as takes place during a fall, causes the greatest cerebral injury at the point of impact.

Another effect of brain movement is shearing stresses, which are caused by unequal movement or different rates of acceleration at various levels of the brain. A shearing force may tear small arteries that travel from the cerebral surfaces through the meninges to the dural sinuses to cause subdural hemorrhages. Shearing or stretching effects can also be transmitted to nerve fibers. Maximum stress from the shearing force occurs at the interface between structures of different density so that the gray matter (cell body) rapidly accelerates while the white matter (axions) tends to lag behind. Although shearing forces are maximum at the cerebral surface and extend toward the center of rotation within the brain, the most serious effects are frequently in the area of the brain stem.

Another source of damage occurs when severe compression of the skull causes the brain to be forced through the tentorial opening. This can produce irreparable damage to the brain stem (see Fig. 37-7). Since the uncus of the temporal lobe is the presenting part, this complication is usually referred to as uncal herniation.

As a whole, head injuries can be regarded as localized or generalized. In localized injuries the force is spent on a local area of both skull and underlying tissues; in generalized injuries the force is transmitted to the entire skull, causing widespread movement, distortion, and damage. Local injuries frequently cause hemorrhage and infection, but generalized trauma is associated with a higher mortality. Many head injuries involve both localized and generalized disorders. The physical processes cause numerous pathologic changes that produce several clinical syndromes.

Concussion. The most common head injury is concussion, a transient and reversible neuronal dysfunction with instantaneous loss of awareness and responsiveness from trauma to the head that persists for a relatively short time, usually minutes or hours. It is generally followed by amnesia for the moment of the injury and a variable period before the injury. This posttraumatic amnesia is characteristic and reflects the extent and severity of injury to the brain after blunt trauma. Posttraumatic amnesia consists of two parts: (1) retrograde amnesia, the period of time before impact for which the patient has no memory, and (2) anterograde amnesia, the period of memory loss after injury. Amnesia in both of these periods tends to lessen with time, although there is some permanent amnesia.

The pathogenesis of concussion is still unclear but may be a result of shearing forces that cause stretching, compression, and tearing of nerve fibers, particularly in the area of the central brain stem, the seat of the reticular activating system. It has also been suggested that the anatomic alterations of nerve fibers cause the release of large quantities of acetylcholine into the cerebrospinal fluid and a reduction in oxygen consumption with increased lactate production.

Contusion and laceration. The terms *contusion* and *laceration* are used to describe visible bruising and tearing of cerebral tissue. Contusions represent petechial hemorrhages along the superficial aspects of the brain at the site of impact (*coup* injury) and/or a lesion remote from the site of direct trauma (*contrecoup* injury). In serious accidents there may be multiple sites of injury.

The more common points of injury are the poles and undersurfaces of frontal and temporal lobes. Contusions may cause focal disturbances in strength, sensation, or visual awareness. The degree of brain damage in the contused areas varies according to the extent of vascular injury. Signs will vary from mild, transient weakness of a limb to prolonged unconsciousness and paralysis. However, the signs and symptoms may be clinically indistinguishable from concussion. As a rule, contusions are less common in infants and young children than in adults with comparable trauma, and contrecoup injuries are relatively rare in infants.

Cerebral lacerations are generally associated with penetrating or depressed skull fractures. However, they may occur without fracture in small children. When brain tissue is actually torn, with bleeding into and around the tear, usually

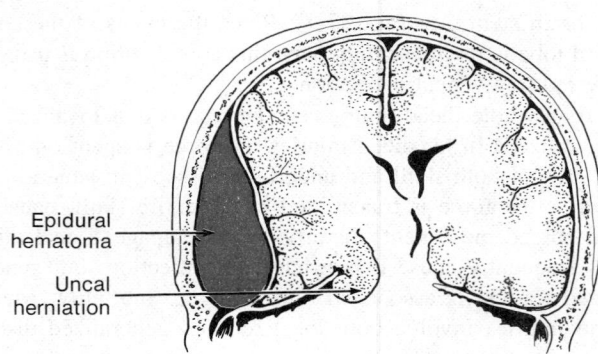

Fig. 37-7. Epidural (extradural) hematoma and compression of temporal lobe through tentorial hiatus.

more severe and prolonged unconsciousness and paralysis occur, leaving permanent scarring and some degree of disability.

Fractures. The immature skull, because of its flexibility, is able to sustain a greater degree of deformation than the adult skull before it incurs a fracture. It requires a great deal of force to produce a fracture in the skull of an infant. A fracture may occur with little or no brain damage, or severe and fatal brain injury can take place without fracture. The undersurface of the skull contains grooves in which the meningeal arteries lie. A fracture that runs through one of these grooves may tear the artery and produce severe and damaging hemorrhage. The types of fractures that occur are linear, depressed, compound, basilar, and diastatic. As a rule, the faster the blow, the greater the likelihood of a depressed fracture; a low-velocity impact tends to produce a linear fracture.

Linear fractures comprise about 75% of childhood skull fractures (Rosman and Herskowitz, 1982). The lines of the fracture are predetermined by the site and velocity of the impact as well as the strength of the bone. Linear fractures are often asymptomatic in older children and heal in 3 to 4 months without special treatment, unless they involve a blood vessel, enter the paranasal sinuses, or impinge on the brain stem or cranial nerves. The location of the fracture often provides clues to the possibility of such complications. For example, a fracture that extends through the squamous portion of the temporal bone is more apt to be associated with laceration of the middle meningeal artery, and fractures extending through the base of the skull may cause leakage of cerebrospinal fluid and/or blood into either the auditory or nasal passages. In infants the uneven ossification and the absence of buttresses cause fracture lines to be irregular, following no predictable pattern.

Depressed fractures are those in which the bone is locally broken, usually into several irregular fragments that are pushed inward, causing pressure on the brain. The inner portion of the bone is more extensively fragmented than the outer portion, which almost invariably produces tears in the dura. Both linear and comminuted (fracture consisting of

several breaks in the bone) depressed fractures are uncommon before 2 to 3 years of age. In infants and very young children, the soft, malleable bone may become dented in a peculiar rounded or ''ping-pong ball'' depression without laceration of either skin or dura. This effect is encountered occasionally in difficult deliveries, resulting from either pressure of the head against the pelvis or incorrect application of forceps.

Compound fractures consist of laceration of skin that extends to the site of the bony fracture, which can be linear, depressed, or comminuted. Prompt surgical debridement is needed (unless contraindicated by the child's clinical condition), as is reduction of the fracture, either elevating or removing fragmented bone. Antibiotic and antitetanus therapy are implemented.

Basilar fractures involve the basilar portion of the frontal, ethmoid, sphenoid, temporal, or occipital bones. The diagnosis of basilar fractures is difficult to make from radiographs because of the complex structure of the base of the skull. Clinical features include hemorrhage into the nose, nasopharynx, or middle ear (hemotympanum if it occurs behind the ear drum). Effusion of blood is seen on the posterior neck, and under and posterior to the ear (Battle sign). Anterior basal fracture produces the characteristic hemorrhage about the eyes (''raccoon eyes''). Cranial nerve palsies may occur involving primarily nerves I, VIII, and VII in order of decreasing frequency.

Diastatic fractures are traumatic separation of cranial sutures. These most frequently affect the lambdoid suture and are rarely seen beyond the first 4 years of life. They require no specific treatment.

Complications

The major complications of trauma to the head are hemorrhage, infection, edema, and herniation through the tentorium. Infection is always a hazard in open injuries, and edema is related to tissue trauma. Vascular rupture may occur even in minor head injuries, causing hemorrhage between the skull and cerebral surfaces. Compression of the underlying brain produces effects that can be rapidly fatal or insidiously progressive.

Epidural hemorrhage. Epidural (extradural) hemorrhage is usually secondary to rupture of the middle meningeal artery, most often as a result of skull fracture that penetrates the groove in the skull occupied by the artery. However, a child's skull can be indented with sufficient force to tear the middle meningeal artery and then rebound intact without causing a fracture. Hemorrhage can also derive from dural veins or the dural sinuses, especially in infants and small children, in whom fracture is less likely to occur. In 20% to 40% of children a skull fracture is not detectable.

The blood accumulates between the dura and the skull to form a hematoma, which, because of the difficulty with which dura is stripped from bone, forces the underlying brain contents downward and inward as it expands (Fig. 37-7). Since bleeding is generally arterial, brain compression

Table 37-5 Comparison of acute epidural and acute subdural hematomas

VARIABLE	EPIDURAL HEMATOMA	SUBDURAL HEMATOMA
Location	More often infratentorial	More often supratentorial
Fracture:		
Supratentorial	75%	30%
Infratentorial	Almost always	Frequent
Source of blood:		
Supratentorial	More likely arterial	Venous
Infratentorial	Venous	Venous
Age	Over 2 years	Less than 2 years
Laterality	Usually unilateral	Usually bilateral
Seizures	Less than 25%	75%
Preretinal and retinal hemorrhages	Less than 25%	75%
Increased ICP	Present	Present
CT configuration	Lentiform	Crescentic
Mortality	25%	Less than 25%
Morbidity	Low	High

occurs rapidly. Most often the expanding hematoma is located in the parietotemporal region, forcing the medial portion of the temporal lobe under the edge of the tentorium, where it causes pressure on nerves and blood vessels. Pressure on the arterial supply and venous return to the reticular formation causes loss of consciousness; pressure on cranial nerve III (oculomotor nerve) produces dilation and (later) fixation of the ipsilateral pupil. Pressure on the fibers of the pyramidal tract is evidenced by contralateral weakness or paralysis and increased deep tendon reflexes. Extreme pressure may extend to the brain stem to cause decerebrate signs and disturbances in the respiratory and other vegetative centers.

The classic clinical picture of epidural hemorrhage (momentary unconsciousness followed by a normal period, then lethargy or coma) is seldom evident in children. The period of impaired consciousness is frequently lacking, and the symptom-free period is atypical because of nonspecific complaints such as irritability, headache, and vomiting. The symptom-free period frequently lasts longer than 48 hours. Clinically significant epidural hematomas are uncommon in children younger than 4 years of age. These differences may be caused by the decreased tendency of the resilient skull to fracture; the ability of blood to escape through widened sutures, an open fontanel, or a fracture; bleeding from smaller vessels with less rapid and massive bleeding; lower systolic blood pressure in children; and possibly the brain being less susceptible to pressure changes in children. See Table 37-5 for a comparison between epidural and subdural hematomas.

Subdural hemorrhage. A subdural hemorrhage is bleeding between the dura and the cerebrum, usually as a result of rupture of cortical veins that bridge the subdural space (Fig. 37-8). Unlike epidural hemorrhage, which develops inwardly, subdural hemorrhage tends to develop more slowly and spreads thinly and widely until it is limited

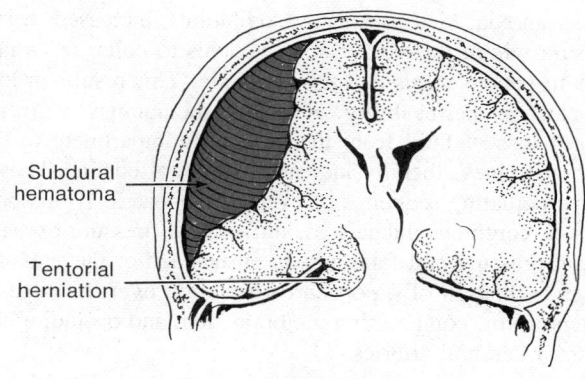

Fig. 37-8. Subdural hematoma.

by the dural barriers—the falx and tentorium. Subdural hematoma is fairly common in infants, frequently as the result of birth trauma.

Subdural hemorrhage can cause either acute or chronic subdural hematoma. Acute subdural hematoma may be associated with contusions or lacerations. It develops within minutes or hours of injury and is associated with a high mortality and poor prognosis. Chronic subdural hematoma is more common. The clinical course and manifestations are variable and depend on the damage sustained by the brain substance and the age of the child. Delayed symptoms are common in children with open fontanels and sutures. The most common presenting manifestations in children are seizures, vomiting, and irritability, drowsiness, or other personality changes. Older children may complain of headache. Less common signs are developmental retardation and failure to thrive.

Presenting signs of acute hematoma include evidence of ICP, such as increased head size and bulging fontanels (in the infant), retinal hemorrhages, extraocular palsies (especially cranial nerve VI), hemiparesis, quadriplegia, and sometimes elevated temperature. Older children may display an unsteady gait, and papilledema is usually present. Since papilledema is a late sign of increased intracranial pressure, it constitutes an emergency. In infants the bleeding may be extensive enough to lower the hematocrit significantly and may be observed before any change in level of consciousness in fast-expanding lesions.

Repeated subdural taps often provide relief in the infant. Surgical evacuation of the hematoma is the treatment of choice in the older child and is frequently required in infants.

Other hemorrhagic lesions. Subarachnoid and intracerebral hemorrhages may occur as the result of head injury. Seizures, nuchal rigidity, and altered consciousness are features of subarachnoid hemorrhage. Manifestations of intracranial bleeding depend on the size and location of the resulting hematoma.

Cerebral edema. Some degree of brain edema is expected after craniocerebral trauma and often accompanies any of the previous disorders. Cerebral edema caused by direct cellular injury or vascular injury induces vascular stasis, anoxia, and further vasodilation. Increased tissue pressure within the skull causes venules to collapse, which leads to venous stasis and tissue anoxia. This results in loss of selective permeability of tissue membranes with increased loss of fluid from the vascular compartment to the cerebral tissues, thereby increasing cerebral edema. Thus a self-perpetuating sequence of events is repeated. If this progression continues unchecked, intracranial pressure exceeds arterial pressure and fatal anoxia ensues and/or the pressure causes herniation of a portion of the brain over the edge of the tentorium, compressing the brain stem and occluding the posterior cerebral arteries.

Posttraumatic syndromes. Postconcussion syndrome is a common sequela to brain injury, and the manifestations vary with the age of the child. Most often there are behavioral disturbances (such as aggressiveness, withdrawal, and regression), sleep disturbances, phobias, emotional lability, irritability, and alterations in school performance.

The syndrome occurs very frequently in children under 1 year of age. Within minutes to an hour after a minimum head injury a child becomes pale, sweating, irritable, and sleepy and may vomit. The syndrome requires no treatment. In children beyond 1 year of age the syndrome may progress to coma with pupillary changes, apnea, and even death (Bruce, 1984).

The adolescent syndrome, similar to that of adults, includes headache, dizziness, irritability, and impaired concentration. The symptoms are self-limited and relatively mild. Postconcussion syndrome in children is unique. It consists of behavior changes that may include aggression, disobedience, regressive behavior, and anxiety. The duration of manifestations can vary from several days to several months (Rosman and Herskowitz, 1982).

Posttraumatic seizures occur in a number of children who survive a head injury. They are more common in young children and in those who sustain cerebral lacerations. The onset may be in the first 24 hours, usually within the first year, and in most cases within 2 years after the injury.

Structural complications may occur as the result of head injuries. Hydrocephalus is seen when there has been subarachnoid hemorrhage or infection. Focal deficits, including optic atrophy, cranial nerve palsies, motor deficits, diabetes insipidus, or aphasia, may be seen. The type of residual effect depends on the location and nature of the trauma. True mental retardation occurs only after severe injuries.

Some children younger than 3 years develop a fluid-filled cyst, or cephalhydrocele, after a linear fracture. This occurs as a result of a tear in the dura and arachnoid or because a piece of arachnoid is entrapped between bone fragments, causing cerebrospinal fluid to accumulate beneath the scalp.

Diagnostic Evaluation

A detailed history, both past and present, is essential in evaluating the child with craniocerebral trauma. It is important to know whether the child suffers from disorders such as drug allergies, hemophilia, diabetes mellitus, or epilepsy; such information may assist in diagnosis. In addition, events surrounding the injury often supply significant data. For example, if a child stumbles and falls while running and strikes his head on the sidewalk, it is usually safe to assume that the neurologic manifestations are a direct result of the injury. However, if a child sinks to the sidewalk and in doing so strikes his head, there may be other causes that contributed to the injury. Sometimes a traumatic injury, even a minor one, will aggravate a preexisting disease process, thereby producing neurologic signs out of proportion to the injury.

Whether or not the infant or child exhibited alterations in consciousness must be determined. Usually this information is easily elicited from older children, but in young children it may be difficult to differentiate between a breath-holding spell and a seizure. The parents of infants are asked if the infant cried immediately after the injury. After a minor injury, initial unconsciousness (if present) is brief and the child will ordinarily exhibit a transient period of confusion, somnolence, and listlessness, most often accompanied by irritability, pallor, and one or more episodes of vomiting.

A severe head injury, such as one sustained in a fall from a significant height or a motor vehicle accident, requires prompt evaluation and treatment. Since head injuries are frequently accompanied by injuries in other areas (spine, viscera, extremities), the examination is performed with care to avoid further damage.

Initial assessment. The initial assessment of the child with a head injury is carried out quickly in relation to vital signs, level of consciousness, and ocular signs. It is not uncommon for excited and irritable children to have a rapid pulse, hyperventilate, appear pale, and feel clammy shortly after an injury. However, deep, rapid, periodic, or intermittent and gasping respirations, wide fluctuations or noticeable slowing of the pulse, and widening pulse pressure or marked fluctuations in blood pressure are signs of brain stem involvement. It is important to note that marked hypotension may represent internal injuries.

Ocular signs such as fixed and dilated pupils, fixed and constricted pupils, and pupils that are poorly reactive or unreactive to light and accommodation indicate increased intracranial pressure or brain stem involvement. It is important to remain with the patient who demonstrates fixed and dilated pupils, since these are ominous signs with the probability of respiratory arrest. Ophthalmic examination may reveal retinal changes. Dilated, nonpulsating blood vessels indicate increased ICP before the appearance of papilledema. Retinal hemorrhages are seen in acute head injuries.

Less urgent but important additional assessments include examination of the scalp for lacerations and palpation for depressed skull fractures, widely separated sutures, and the size and tension of fontanels, which indicate intracranial hemorrhage or rapidly developing cerebral edema. However, a significant amount of blood loss can occur from scalp lacerations. Bleeding from the nose or ears (although uncommon in children) needs further evaluation, and a watery discharge from the nose (rhinorrhea) that is positive for glucose (as tested with Dextrostix) suggests leaking of cerebrospinal fluid from a skull fracture.

Injury to the skin, extremities, and abdomen is not uncommon after severe blunt head trauma and must be ruled out by sensory examination in children with altered motor function. Testing reflexes provides information about cerebral and pyramidal involvement, although transient abnormalities of the abdominal reflexes and Babinski sign may be present in children with mild head trauma. Conscious, cooperative children are examined for cerebellar signs such as ataxia. However, it is not uncommon for children to display unsteadiness, clumsiness, and tremor on intentional movement after head injury.

Temperature may be moderately elevated for a day or two following an initial mild hypothermia after injury. A persistent fever may indicate subarachnoid hemorrhage or infection.

An accurate assessment of these various clinical signs provides baseline information. Serial evaluations, preferably by a single observer, help to detect changes in the neurologic status. Alterations in mental status, evidenced by increased difficulty in rousing the child, mounting agitation, development of focal lateral neurologic signs, or marked changes in vital signs, usually indicate extension or progression of the basic pathologic process.

Special tests. After a thorough clinical examination, a variety of diagnostic tests are helpful in providing a more definitive diagnosis of the type and extent of the trauma. Where available, computed tomography (CT) is especially valuable in diagnosis of neurologic trauma and usually makes other diagnostic procedures unnecessary. It is easily carried out, is noninvasive, and can be repeated serially for reassessment in the patient who remains unconscious or shows progressive neurologic deterioration.

Where available, magnetic resonance imaging has replaced cerebral angiography. Skull films and other radiographic tests may be indicated. Echoencephalography may

contribute to diagnosis and management. Electroencephalography is not particularly helpful for early diagnosis but is useful for defining seizure activity or focal destructive lesions after the acute phase of illness. Lumbar puncture is rarely employed in craniocerebral trauma and is contraindicated in the presence of increased intracranial pressure.

In the infant or small child a subdural tap through a fontanel or coronal suture may establish the diagnosis of subdural or epidural hemorrhage. In some centers monitoring intracranial pressure is part of the assessment.

Therapeutic Management

The majority of children with mild to moderate concussion who have not lost consciousness can be cared for and observed at home after careful examination reveals no serious intracranial injury. The parents are instructed to check the child every 2 hours to determine any changes in responsiveness. The sleeping child should be wakened to see if he can be roused normally. Parents are advised to maintain contact with the attending physician, who usually wishes to examine the child again in 1 or 2 days. The manifestations of epidural hematoma in children do not generally appear until 24 hours or more after injury. Maintaining contact for continued observation and reevaluation, when indicated, facilitates early diagnosis and treatment of possible complications such as hematoma, hydrocephalus, cysts, and posttraumatic seizures. Children with minor injuries who live a significant distance from medical facilities or whose parents or caregiver is not deemed reliable in observing their condition are generally hospitalized for 24 to 48 hours for observation.

Children with severe injuries, those who have lost consciousness for more than a few minutes, and those with prolonged and continued seizures or other focal or diffuse neurologic signs must be hospitalized until their condition is stable and their neurologic signs have diminished.

The child is maintained on nothing by mouth or restricted to clear liquids, if able to take fluids by mouth, until it is determined that vomiting will not occur. Intravenous fluids are indicated in the child who is comatose or displays dulled sensorium and/or in the child with persistent vomiting. The volume of intravenous fluid is carefully monitored to avoid aggravating any cerebral edema and to minimize the possibility of overhydration in case of inappropriate secretions of antidiuretic hormone. However, damage to the hypothalamus or pituitary may produce diabetes insipidus with its accompanying hypertonicity and dehydration. Fluid balance is closely monitored by daily weight, accurate intake and output measurement, and serum osmolality to detect early signs of water retention, excessive dehydration, and states of hypertonicity or hypotonicity.

Restlessness can be satisfactorily managed, if necessary, with diphenhydramine (Benadryl) or chloral hydrate, and headache is usually controlled with acetaminophen (Tylenol). Anticonvulsants are used for seizure control and frequently in cases of suspected contusion or laceration. Antibiotics are administered if there are lacerations, cerebrospinal fluid leakage, or excessive cerebral tissue damage. Prophylactic tetanus toxoid is given as appropriate (see p. 529). Cerebral edema is managed as described for the unconscious child. Hyperthermia is controlled with tepid sponges or a hypothermia blanket.

Surgical therapy. Scalp lacerations are sutured after careful examination of underlying bone. Depressed fractures require surgical reduction and removal of bone fragments. Torn dura is sutured. "Ping-pong ball" skull fractures in very young infants ordinarily correct themselves within a few weeks and do not require specific treatment, although they can be reduced by pressure against the bone.

Prognosis. The outcome of craniocerebral trauma depends on the extent of injury and complications. However, the outlook is generally more favorable for children than for adults. Over 90% of children with concussions or simple linear fractures recover without symptoms after the initial period. The incidence of fatalities and neurologic sequelae is lower in children, even in those with severe head injuries. The prognosis for recovery is primarily related to the duration of coma rather than to the degree of injury (Eiben and others, 1984; Mahoney and others, 1983).

The concern regarding outcome is increasingly focused on cognitive, emotional, and/or mental problems. Recent studies indicate that children experience a higher frequency of psychologic disturbances following head injury, whereas adults are more prone to complaints of a physical nature. Children who suffer even minor head injuries exhibit unacceptable behavior, poor attention span, impaired self-control, difficulty managing stress or frustration, oversensitivity, irritability, mental inconsistency, personality changes, headaches, and memory impairment (Boll, 1985; Jacobson and others, 1986; Rutter, 1981).

Nursing Considerations

The hospitalized child requires careful neurologic assessment and evaluation, including vital signs, repeated at frequent intervals provide information needed to establish a correct diagnosis, observe for signs and symptoms of increased ICP, determine clinical management, and prevent many complications.

The child is placed on bed rest, usually with the head of the bed elevated slightly, and appropriate safety measures, such as side rails kept up for older children and seizure precautions for children of all ages, are implemented. The extremely restless child may require that hard surfaces be padded and restraint used to prevent the possibility of further injury. Care is individualized according to the specific needs of the child. The unconscious child is managed as described in the previous section, but most childhood head injuries are those causing momentary stunning or temporary unconsciousness. The child may be restless and irritable, but more often his reaction is to fall asleep when left undisturbed. A quiet environment helps reduce the restlessness and irritability. Bright lights shining directly into the child's face are irritating. This often makes checking the ocular responses more difficult to perform and more aggravating to the child.

Frequent examinations of vital signs, neurologic signs, and level of consciousness are extremely important nursing observations. When possible they should be performed by a single observer in order to better detect subtle changes that may indicate worsening of neurologic status. Pupils are checked for size, equality, reaction to light, and accommodation. After the initial elevations usually seen after injury, the vital signs generally return to normal unless there is brain stem involvement. An axillary temperature is the safest method of measuring temperature, since seizures are not uncommon and vomiting is a frequent response in children, especially when the child is disturbed.

Probably the most important nursing observation is assessment of the child's level of consciousness. Alterations in consciousness appear earlier in the progression of an injury than alterations of vital signs or focal neurologic signs (see p. 1624) for evaluation of responsiveness). Some expected responses may be misinterpreted as deviations from the normal. Frequent examinations of alertness are fatiguing to the child; therefore the child often desires to fall asleep, which may be confused with depressed consciousness. When left alone, the child promptly dozes. It is not uncommon to observe ocular divergence through the partially closed eyelids.

Observations of position and movement provide additional information. Any abnormal posturing is noted as well as whether or not it occurs continuously or intermittently. Are the child's hand grips strong and equal in strength? Are there any signs of decerebrate or decorticate posturing? What is the child's response to stimulation? Is movement purposeful, random, or absent? Are movement and/or sensation equal on both sides or restricted to one side only?

The child may complain of headache or other discomfort. The child who is too young to describe a headache will be fussy and resist being handled. The child who suffers from vertigo will often assume a position and vigorously resist efforts to move him. Forcible movement causes the child to vomit and display spontaneous nystagmus. Seizures, relatively common in children with craniocerebral trauma, may be of any type but are more often generalized regardless of the type of injury. Any seizure activity should be carefully observed and described in detail (see p. 1666).

Drainage from any orifice is noted. Bleeding from the ear suggests the possibility of a basal skull fracture. The amount and characteristics of the drainage are observed, and since the auditory canal may be a source of infection, dry, sterile cotton can be placed loosely at the orifice and changed when soiled. Suctioning through the nares is contraindicated, since there is a high risk of secondary infection and the probability of the catheter entering the brain substance through the fracture.

Head trauma is frequently accompanied by other undetected injuries; therefore any bruises, lacerations, or evidence of internal injuries or fractures of the extremities are noted and reported. Associated injuries are evaluated and treated appropriately.

The child with normal level of consciousness is usually allowed clear liquids unless fluid is restricted. If the child has an intravenous infusion, it is maintained as prescribed. The diet is advanced to that appropriate for the child's age as soon as his condition permits. Intake and output are measured and recorded, and any incontinence of bowel or bladder is noted in the child who has been toilet trained.

The child should be observed for any unusual behavior, but interpretation of behavior should be made in relation to the child's normal behavior. For example, urinary incontinence during sleep would be of no consequence in a child who routinely wets the bed but would be highly significant for one who is always dry. In addition, a child who is subject to nightmares might cry out and demonstrate agitated behavior at night. Parents are valuable resources in evaluating objective behaviors of their children. Information obtained from parents at or shortly after admission is helpful in evaluating the child's behavior, for example, the ease with which the child is roused normally, his usual sleeping position, how much he sleeps during the day, motor activity of which he is capable (rolling over, sitting up, climbing), hearing and visual acuity, appetite, and manner of eating (spoon, bottle, cup). There would be less concern about a child who falls asleep several times during the day if this particular type of behavior is consistent with his usual behavior.

When the child is discharged, the parents are advised of probable posttraumatic symptoms that may be expected, such as behavioral changes, sleep disturbances, phobias, and seizures. They should understand observations that should be made and how to contact the physician, nurse, or health facility in case the child develops any unusual signs or symptoms. The importance of follow-up evaluation should be emphasized, and it is often advisable to refer the family to a public health agency for home follow-through to be certain that the child receives posthospital evaluation.

The rehabilitation and management of the child with permanent brain injury are beyond the scope of this discussion, but it is an important aspect of care. Rehabilitation of brain-injured children is begun as soon as feasible and usually involves the family and a rehabilitation team. Careful assessment of the child's capabilities, limitations, and probable potential is made as early as possible and appropriate interventions implemented to maximize the residual capacities. The **National Head Injury Foundation*** ''arose from the mutual frustration and sense of hopelessness experienced by families in their search for appropriate facilities and support to return head-injured loved ones to their maximum functioning potential.'' It provides information and listings of rehabilitation services and support groups throughout the country.

*P.O. Box 567, Framingham, MA 01701-0196.

Emergency Treatment: *Head Injury*

1. Assess child
2. Clean any abrasions with soap and water
    Apply clean dressing
        If bleeding, apply ice for 1 hour to relieve pain and swelling
3. Give only clear liquids until no vomiting for at least 6 hours
4. Give no analgesics
5. Check pupil reaction every 4 hours (including twice during night) for 48 hours
6. Awaken two times during night
7. Have someone sleep in same room as child for two nights
8. Should be seen by physician if there is any of the following:
Injury sustained
    —at high speed (e.g., auto)
    —fall from a significant distance (e.g., roof, tree)
    —from great force (e.g., baseball bat)
    —under suspicious circumstances
Child less than 6 months of age
Unconscious over 5 seconds
Discomfort (crying) more than 10 minutes after injury
Headache that is severe, worsening, interferes with sleep
Vomiting three or more times
Swelling in front or above earlobe
Child is confused or not behaving normally
Difficult to rouse from sleep
Difficulty with speaking
Blurring of vision or seeing double
Unsteady gait
Difficulty using upper extremities
Neck pain
Pupils dilated or fixed

NEAR-DROWNING

Drowning is not an uncommon accident in childhood. It ranks second as a cause of accidental death in children. About 85% of these children are male and the majority are between ages 10 and 19 years (Spyker, 1985). However, a significant number are infants under age 3. Most cases are accidental, usually involving children who are helpless in water, such as inadequately attended children in or near swimming pools or infants in bathtubs; small children who fall into ponds, streams, and flooded excavations, usually near home; occupants of pleasure boats who fail to wear life preservers; children who have diving accidents; and children who are able to swim but overestimate their endurance.

Drowning can take place in any body of water, including such unlikely places as a pail of water. Top-heavy toddlers fall head first into a pail of water, their arms become trapped, and they are unable to free themselves (Scott and Eigen, 1980). Hot tubs and whirlpool spas have been implicated in childhood drowning injury. The suction created at the outlet is strong enough to trap even larger children underwater (Monroe, 1982), and rapidly proliferating *Pseudomonas aeruginosa* have been reported as complicating hot tub submersion injury (Tron, Baldwin, and Price, 1985).

With expeditious treatment many children can and are being saved. For purposes of this discussion, several terms need clarification:

drowning Death from asphyxia while submerged, regardless of whether fluid has entered the lungs.

near-drowning Survival at least 24 hours after submersion in a fluid medium.

These can be further described as:

drowning without aspiration Death from respiratory obstruction and asphyxia while submerged, usually as a result of prolonged laryngospasm. This is also called *dry drowning* (approximately 10% of drownings).

drowning with aspiration Death from the combined effects of asphyxia and changes secondary to fluid aspiration while submerged.

near-drowning without aspiration Survival, at least temporarily, following asphyxia after submersion in a fluid medium.

near-drowning with aspiration Survival, at least temporarily, following aspiration of fluid while submerged.

delayed death caused by drowning Death as the result of complications subsequent to successful resuscitation following submersion.

Pathophysiology

The major pulmonary changes that occur in drowning are directly related to the length of submersion (regardless of the type and amount of fluid aspirated), the physiologic response of the victim, and the development and degree of immersion hypothermia. In addition, cerebral recovery depends on the effectiveness of initial resuscitation and subsequent critical care measures to support cerebral salvage.

Physiologic factors that influence the extent of damage from immersion include resistance to asphyxia and anoxia, which shows some individual variation. There is greater resistance with diminishing age; young children can withstand longer periods of submersion. More important is the drowning, or diving, reflex. This neurologic response is triggered by immersion of the face in cold water. Blood is shunted away from the periphery, and the flow is concentrated to the brain and heart predominantly. There is a profound bradycardia, but the diminishing supply of oxygen is delivered to these essential organs. Consequently, although the brain may appear to be severely damaged, it has the potential for recovery even after lengthy submersion.

Submerged children struggle initially. There is laryngospasm, and they swallow water and frequently vomit. This is followed by terminal gasping and aspiration. Cardiopulmonary arrest is secondary to asphyxia after about 4 to 6 minutes of complete submersion. The problems created by near-drowning are (1) hypoxia and asphyxiation; (2) aspiration, and (3) hypothermia (except near-drowning in hot tubs).

Hypoxia is the primary problem because it results in global cell damage, and different cells tolerate variable lengths of anoxia. Neurons, especially cerebral cells, sustain irreversible damage after 4 to 6 minutes of submersion. The heart and lungs can survive up to 30 minutes. Regardless of the amount of water aspirated, there is arterial hypoxemia (resulting from atelectasis with shunting of blood through the nonventilated alveoli) and a combined respiratory acidosis (resulting from retained carbon dioxide) and metabolic acidosis (caused by buildup of acid metabolites due to anaerobic metabolism). Although electrolyte imbalances are contributing factors, they are not the major causes of morbidity and mortality, as had been previously thought. The pathologic events are directly related to the duration of submersion. The major difficulty is acute ventilatory insufficiency. Approximately 10% of drowning victims die without aspirating fluid but succumb from acute asphyxia as a result of prolonged reflex laryngospasm.

Aspiration of fluid occurs in the majority of drownings. The aspirated fluid results in pulmonary edema, atelectasis, airway spasm, and pneumonitis, which aggravates the hypoxia. It was previously thought that submersion in salt water and fresh water altered the physiologic response to near-drowning. However, there is no clinically significant difference in human survivors and it does not alter the therapy or outcome.

Immersion in cold water (at or less than 20° C, or 68° F) produces a significant and slow fall in body temperature; but in very cold water (at below 5° C, or 41° F) body temperature falls at an incredibly rapid rate as a result of cutaneous capillary paralysis and accelerated heat loss (Keatinge, as cited in Conn, Edmonds, and Barker, 1979). Hypothermia occurs rapidly in infants and children partly because of their large surface area relative to size and partly as a result of the cold water itself. Water is an excellent heat conductor and the contact with the skin is increased by struggling. Hypothermia may make resumption or maintenance of cardiac function possible if body temperature is less than 30° C. Profound hypothermia is usually evidence of lengthy submersion.

Clinical Manifestations

Clinical manifestations are directly related to the degree of consciousness following rescue and resuscitation. These are categorized as follows:

Category A: Awake. Minimum injury.
　　　　　Fully conscious. May have mild hypothermia, mild chest radiograph changes, mild arterial blood gas abnormalities.
Category B: Blunted sensorium. Moderate injury.
　　　　　Obtund, stuporous, purposeful response to painful stimuli, mild to moderate hypothermia, frequently respiratory distress, chest radiographs abnormal, arterial blood gas abnormalities
Category C: Comatose. Severe anoxia.
　　　　　Patient unarousable, abnormal response to pain, abnormal respiratory pattern, seizures, shock, marked arterial blood gas abnormalities, abnormal chest radiographs, arrhythmias, metabolic acidosis, hyperkalemia, hyperglycemia, disseminated intravascular coagulation,

C1: Decorticate, Cheyne-Stokes respirations
C2: Decerebrate, central hyperventilation
C3: Flaccid, apneustic or cluster breathing
C4: Flaccid, apneic no detectable circulation

Therapeutic Management

Resuscitative measures should begin at the scene of a drowning and the victim transported to the hospital with maximum ventilatory and circulatory support. Many victims need care for some time after aspiration of fluid. In the hospital, intensive pulmonary care is implemented and continued according to the needs of the patient.

In general, the management of the near-drowning victim is based on the degree of cerebral insult. The first priority is to restore oxygen delivery to the cells and prevent further hypoxic damage. A spontaneously breathing child will do well in an oxygen-enriched atmosphere; the more severely affected child will require endotracheal intubation and mechanical ventilation. Blood gases and pH are monitored frequently as a guide to oxygen, fluid, and electrolyte therapies.

Category A patients are managed symptomatically with oxygen administration, warming, and symptomatic treatment. Laboratory assessment of electrolytes provides a guide to needed therapy. These children are usually well enough to be discharged in 12 to 24 hours.

Category B patients are admitted to the hospital and treated symptomatically as Category A patients, with regular monitoring of neurologic and respiratory status. The respiratory symptoms predominate and are managed with oxygen therapy, correction of acidosis, and furosemide to stimulate diuresis.

Category C patients require invasive life-support measures. These children do best if they are mechanically ventilated, at least for 12 to 24 hours. Unassisted respiration consumes too much energy, which is best directed to the needs of the brain. More severely affected children are managed as any other unconscious child (see p. 1632). Increased ICP is usually not a problem in children who do well, but when present (even with treatment) is associated with death or significant neurologic damage.

Because of the frequency of complications after near-drowning, any patient should be hospitalized for 12 to 48 hours for observation. If the victim is one of the 10% who do not aspirate water, is rescued and resuscitated before circulatory arrest, and does not suffer damage to the central nervous system, recovery should be complete. The outcome for near-drowning is excellent for most category C1 and C2 patients if they are resuscitated and receive intensive care. The poorest outlook is for children in category C4, especially when associated with complications such as disseminated intravascular coagulation, intestinal sloughing, shock, and arrhythmias.

Aspiration pneumonia is a frequent complication that occurs about 48 to 72 hours after the episode. Bronchospasm, alveolar-capillary membrane damage, atelectasis, abscess formation, and hyaline membrane disease are other complications that occur after aspiration of fluid.

Nursing Considerations

Nursing care depends on whether the child is a near-drowning or a drowning victim. If the child survives, he may need intensive respiratory nursing care with attention to vital signs, mechanical ventilation and/or tracheostomy, blood gas determination, chest therapy, and intravenous infusion. Frequently the child is comatose for an indefinite period and requires the same care as an unconscious child.

Probably the most difficult aspect in the care of the child victim of near-drowning is dealing with the parents, whose guilt reactions are severe. The magnitude of the event is so great that efforts to provide comfort and support are of only limited success. Parents need to hear that everything possible is being done to treat the child, and this message needs to be repeated often.

Most drownings, particularly of infants or small children, could have been prevented with adequate supervision. If the child dies, the sudden, unexpected nature of the death and the particular circumstances of the accident, especially in terms of guilt for not preventing it, compound the grief for these individuals (see Chapter 23). The parents of the child who is saved from death are faced with the anxiety of not knowing what the outcome will be and sometimes wish for the death of the child. Because their situation generates such intense feelings of loneliness, it is important for families to know that they are not alone. They need to be reminded frequently that there are caring people to assist them both during the crisis and later. Additional sources of support that can be recommended are psychiatric and social work consultants, community services, and religious support. Self-help groups are excellent if these are available in the community.

Nurses often have difficulty relating to the parents if obvious neglect has precipitated the accident and subsequent problems; therefore it is important for those who care for these children and their families to assess their own feelings about the situation as well as the coping abilities and resources of the family. Caring for near-drowning victims and their families requires the nurse to be sensitive to the needs of the child and the family and to recognize his or her own reactions and emotions.

Prevention. All children should be taught to handle themselves in the water. Even very young children can learn to do so sufficiently to avoid panic and propel themselves to safety until they can be removed from the water. The American Academy of Pediatrics supports the recommendations of the YMCA regarding guidelines for swimming instruction for children less than 3 years of age. The programs recommended for older infants and toddlers are not those that promise to ''waterproof'' or ''drownproof'' the child, which can lead to complacency on the part of parents who believe the child can ''swim.'' Those that offer water enrichment and emphasize water familiarization, water fun, and stress water safety and parent participation are best for very young children. These programs train both parent and child in swimming instruction, safety precautions, and risk awareness.

Water safety and survival training should be required for all school-age children, and nurses can be active advocates in their communities. Nurses are also in a position to emphasize the importance of adequate adult supervision when children are in the water. Young children should never be left unattended when in the water.

Intracranial Infections

The nervous system and its coverings are subject to infection by the same organisms that affect other organs of the body. However, the nervous system is limited in the ways in which it responds to injury. Infectious processes share virtually the same clinical and pathologic features. They differ primarily in the growth and virulence of the specific organism. It is generally difficult to distinguish between the various etiologic agents from clinical manifestations. Laboratory studies are needed to identify the causative agent. The inflammatory process can affect the meninges (*meningitis*), brain (*encephalitis*), or spinal cord (*myelitis*).

The most common infection of the central nervous system is meningitis, which can be caused by a variety of organisms, but the three main types are:

1. **Bacterial,** or pyogenic, caused by pus-forming bacteria, especially the meningococcus, pneumococcus, and influenza bacillus
2. **Tuberculous,** caused by the tubercle bacillus
3. **Viral,** or aseptic, caused by a wide variety of viral agents

Encephalitis is usually caused by a virus, and the discussion is limited to viral encephalitis. Myelitis is not discussed.

BACTERIAL MENINGITIS

Bacterial meningitis is a potentially fatal disease, and although the advent of antimicrobial therapy has had a marked effect on the course and prognosis, it remains a significant cause of illness in the pediatric age-groups. Its importance lies primarily in the frequency with which it occurs in infancy and childhood and the unnecessarily high death rates and residual damage caused by undiagnosed and untreated or inadequately treated cases. Ninety percent of cases occur in children between the ages of 1 month and 5 years; infants aged 6 to 12 months are at greatest risk (Krugman and others, 1985).

Etiology

Bacterial meningitis can be caused by any of a variety of bacterial agents. *Haemophilus influenzae* (type B), *Streptococcus pneumoniae,* and *Neisseria meningitidis* (meningococcus) organisms are responsible for bacterial meningitis in 95% of children older than 2 months. *H. influenzae* is the predominant organism in children 3 months to 3 years of age but is rare in the infant younger than 3 months, who is apparently protected by passively acquired bactericidal substances, and in children older than 5 years of age, who are beginning to acquire this protection (Krugman and others, 1985; Bell and others, 1982).

Other organisms are the β-hemolytic streptococcus, *Staphylococcus aureus,* and *Escherichia coli*. The leading causes of neonatal meningitis are the group B streptococci and *E. coli* organisms. *E. coli* infection is seldom seen beyond infancy. Meningococcic (epidemic cerebrospinal) meningitis occurs in epidemic form and is the only type readily transmitted by droplet infection from nasopharyngeal secretions. Although this condition may develop at any age, the risk of meningococcal infection increases with the number of contacts; therefore it occurs predominantly in school-age children and adolescents.

There appear to be some seasonal variations. Meningitis caused by *H. influenzae* is a disease that primarily occurs in autumn or early winter. Pneumococcal and meningococcal infections can occur at any time but are more common in later winter or early spring. The increased incidence of *H. influenzae* in certain ethnic groups and in families suggests that there may be a genetic susceptibility to the disease (Hill, 1983).

Several factors may predispose the child to the development of bacterial meningitis. Males are affected more often than females, and this is somewhat more pronounced in the neonatal period. The highest incidence of meningitis occurs between ages 6 and 12 months, and the greatest morbidity after meningitis appears to involve children who were afflicted between birth and 4 years of age. Maternal factors, such as premature rupture of fetal membranes and maternal infection during the last week of pregnancy, are major causes of neonatal meningitis.

Deficiencies in the immune mechanisms and decreased leukocyte activity may influence the incidence in newborns, children with immunoglobulin deficiencies, and children receiving immunosuppressant drugs. Meningitis appears to occur as an extension of a variety of bacterial infections, probably as a result of the lack of acquired resistance to the various etiologic organisms. The presence of preexisting central nervous system anomalies, neurosurgical procedures or injuries, sickle cell anemia, or primary infections elsewhere in the body are factors related to an increased susceptibility.

Pathophysiology

The most common route of infection is vascular dissemination from a focus of infection elsewhere. For example, organisms from the nasopharynx invade the underlying blood vessels and enter the cerebral blood supply or form local thromboemboli that release septic emboli into the bloodstream. Invasion by direct extension from infections in the paranasal and mastoid sinuses is less common. Organisms also gain entry by direct implantation after penetrating wounds, skull fractures that provide an opening into the skin or sinuses, lumbar puncture or surgical procedures, and anatomic abnormalities such as spina bifida or foreign bodies such as a ventricular shunt. Once implanted, the organisms spread into the cerebrospinal fluid, by which the infection spreads throughout the subarachnoid space.

The infective process is that seen in any bacterial infection—inflammation, exudation, white blood cell accumulation, and varying degrees of tissue damage. The brain becomes hyperemic and edematous, and the entire surface of the brain is covered with a layer of purulent exudate, which varies with the type of organism. For example, meningococcal exudate is most marked over the parietal, occipital, and cerebellar regions; the thick, fibrinous exudate of pneumococcal infection is confined chiefly to the surface of the brain, particularly the anterior lobes; and the exudate of streptococcal infections is similar to that of pneumococcal infections, but thinner.

Clinical Manifestations

The clinical manifestations of acute bacterial meningitis depend to a large extent on the age of the child. The picture is also influenced to some degree by the type of organism, the effectiveness of therapy for antecedent illness, and whether it occurs as an isolated entity or as a complication of another illness or injury.

Children and adolescents. The illness is likely to be abrupt, with fever, chills, headache, and vomiting that are associated with or quickly followed by alterations in sensorium. Often the initial sign is a seizure, which may recur as the disease progresses. The child is extremely irritable and agitated and may develop photophobia, delirium, hallucinations, aggressive or maniacal behavior, or drowsiness, stupor, and coma. Sometimes the onset is slower, frequently preceded by several days of respiratory or gastrointestinal symptoms. Occasionally a prior infection treated with antibiotics masks or delays the signs of meningitis.

The child resists flexion of the neck, and as the disease progresses, the neck stiffness becomes marked until the head is drawn into extreme overextension (opisthotonos). Kernig and Brudzinski signs are positive. Reflex responses are variable, although they show hyperactivity. The skin may be cold and cyanotic with poor peripheral perfusion.

Other signs and symptoms may appear that are peculiar to individual organisms. Petechial or purpuric rashes usually indicate a meningococcal infection, especially when the eruption is associated with a shocklike state. Joint involvement is seen in meningococcic and *H. influenzae* infection. A chronically draining ear commonly accompanies pneumococcal meningitis. *E. coli* infection may be associated with a congenital dermal sinus that communicates with the subarachnoid space.

Infants and young children. The classic picture of meningitis is rarely seen in children between 3 months and 2 years of age. The illness is characterized by fever, poor feeding, vomiting, marked irritability, and frequent seizures, which are often accompanied by a high-pitched cry. A bulging fontanel is the most significant finding, and nuchal rigidity may or may not be present. Brudzinski and Kernig signs are not usually helpful in diagnosis, since they are difficult to elicit and evaluate in children in this age-group.

Neonatal. Meningitis in newborn and premature infants is extremely difficult to diagnose. The vague and nonspecific manifestations, characteristic of all neonatal sepsis, bear little resemblance to the findings in older children. These infants are usually well at birth but within a few days begin to look and behave poorly. They refuse feedings, have poor sucking ability, and may vomit or have diarrhea. They display poor tone, lack of movement, and a poor cry. Other nonspecific signs that may be present include hypothermia or fever (depending on the maturity of the infant), jaundice, irritability, drowsiness, seizures, respiratory irregularities or apnea, cyanosis, and weight loss. The full, tense, and bulging fontanel may or may not be present until late in the course of the illness, and the neck is usually supple. Untreated, the child's condition will decline to cardiovascular collapse, seizures, and apnea.

Complications. The incidence of complications from acute bacterial meningitis has been significantly reduced with early diagnosis and vigorous antimicrobial therapy. If infection extends to the ventricles, thick pus, fibrin, or adhesions may occlude the narrow passages, thereby obstructing the flow of cerebrospinal fluid to cause obstructive hydrocephalus. Subdural effusions occur frequently, and thrombosis may occur in meningeal veins or venous sinuses. Destructive changes may take place in the cerebral cortex, and brain abscesses may form by direct extension of the infection or by vascular dissemination. Extension of the infection to the areas of the cranial nerves or compression necrosis from increased pressure may cause deafness, blindness, or weakness or paralysis of facial or other muscles of the head and neck.

One of the most dramatic and serious complications usually associated with meningococcal infections is peripheral circulatory collapse, known as the Waterhouse-Friderichsen syndrome, which if untreated is rapidly fatal. Extensive and diffuse intravascular coagulation with marked thrombocytopenia occurs with any form but is most common in meningococcic (epidemic cerebrospinal) meningitis.

Other acute complications of meningitis include the syndrome of inappropriate secretion of antidiuretic hormone (ISADH) (p. 1686), subdural effusions, seizures, cerebral edema and herniation, and hydrocephalus. Obstruction to the flow of cerebrospinal fluid occurs in the acute phase of illness by clumping of purulent material in the drainage channels and in the chronic phase by adhesive arachnoiditis or fibrotic obstruction through any of the ventricular foramina.

Extension of the inflammation to cranial nerves or compression and destruction of the nerves from intracranial pressure can produce permanent impairment of vision or hearing and other nerve palsies. Auditory nerve damage is usually followed by permanent deafness. Other long-term complications include cerebral palsy, mental retardation, seizures, learning disorder, and attention deficit disorder.

Hemiparesis and quadriparesis may result from damage caused by arteritis and/or thrombosis or other mechanisms. Behavioral changes are noted in some children, and there is evidence to indicate that psychometric and behavioral defects may be a significant concomitant sign of meningitis in childhood, although it is difficult to determine the degree to which meningitis affects the intelligence quotient of children.

Diagnostic Evaluation

A diagnosis of acute bacterial meningitis cannot be made on the basis of clinical manifestations. A definitive diagnosis is made only by examination of the cerebrospinal fluid by means of a lumbar puncture. The fluid pressure is measured and samples are obtained for culture, Gram stain, blood cell count, and determination of glucose and protein content. The findings are usually diagnostic. Culture and stain are needed to identify the causative organism. Spinal fluid pressure is usually elevated, but interpretation is often difficult when the child is crying.

There is generally an elevated white blood cell count, predominantly polymorphonuclear leukocytes, but it may be extremely variable. The glucose level is reduced, generally in proportion to the duration and severity of the infection. The relationship between the cerebrospinal fluid glucose and serum glucose levels is important in evaluating the glucose content of cerebrospinal fluid; therefore a serum glucose sample is drawn approximately ½ hour before the lumbar puncture. Protein concentration is usually increased.

A blood culture is advisable for all children suspected of meningitis and occasionally proves positive when cerebrospinal fluid culture is negative. Nose and throat cultures may provide helpful information in some cases.

Several newer techniques for diagnosing or differentiating bacterial meningitis are available. Detection of bacterial capsular antigens in cerebrospinal fluid (CSF), serum, or urine is accomplished by counterimmunoelectrophoresis (CIE), enzyme-linked immunosorbent assays (ELISA), or latex particle agglutination (LPA). LPA is a rapid test (5 to 10 minutes) and more sensitive than CIE. Even more sensitive is ELISA, which is usually reserved for diagnosis of partially treated meningitis when CSF culture and LPA are negative. C-reactive protein (CRP) levels appear to be reliable in differentiating between bacterial and aseptic meningitis. Levels are usually high in bacterial disease, and persistently elevated or increased levels of serum CRP indicate a complication of bacterial meningitis or presence of a bacterial infection in a previously diagnosed viral meningitis (Yogev, 1985).

Therapeutic Management

Acute bacterial meningitis is a medical emergency that requires early recognition and immediate institution of therapy to prevent death and avoid residual disabilities. The initial therapeutic management includes:

Isolation
Initiation of antimicrobial therapy
Maintenance of optimum hydration
Maintenance of ventilation
Reduction of increased intracranial pressure
Management of bacterial shock
Control of seizures
Control of extremes of temperature
Correction of anemia
Treatment of complications

The child is isolated from other children, usually in an intensive care unit for close observation. An intravenous infusion is started as soon as the lumbar puncture has been completed in order to facilitate the administration of antimicrobial agents, fluids, anticonvulsive drugs, and blood if needed. The child is placed on a cardiac monitor.

Drugs. Until the causative organism is identified, the choice of antibiotic is based on the known sensitivity of the organism most likely to be the infective agent in any given situation and the probable interactions with the specific patient. Except under special circumstances, the drugs are administered intravenously throughout the course of treatment. The drugs are given in large doses, and the period of therapy is determined by CSF findings and the child's clinical condition.

The drug of choice in older infants and children is the broad-spectrum antibiotic ampicillin, which is effective against the usual causative organisms and is associated with very low toxicity. In areas in which *H. influenzae* has become resistant to ampicillin or in children with well-documented sensitivity to penicillin, chloramphenicol may be the drug of choice for initial treatment. For most organisms ampicillin (often in association with chloramphenicol) or penicillin is continued. Cefotaxime may be substituted for the previous drugs in some children with *H. influenzae* infection. For some organisms other drugs may be employed, usually in conjunction with ampicillin, for example, gentamycin and/or kanamycin for *E. coli*.

Nonspecific measures. Maintaining hydration is a prime concern, and intravenous fluids and the type and amount of fluid are determined by the patient's condition. The optimum hydration involves correction of any fluid deficits followed by low maintenance levels to prevent cerebral edema. If indicated, measures are employed to reduce intracranial pressure as described previously (see p. 1633).

Complications are treated appropriately, such as aspiration of subdural effusion in infants and heparin therapy for children who develop disseminated intravascular coagulation syndrome. Shock, if it occurs in the child, is managed by restoration of blood volume and maintenance of electrolyte balance. Seizures occur in about 30% of affected children during the first few days of treatment (Feigin and Neglia, 1986). These are controlled with appropriate anticonvulsants.

Lumbar puncture is carried out as needed to determine the effectiveness of therapy. The patient is evaluated neurologically during the convalescent period and at regular intervals during the succeeding year.

Prognosis. The age of the child, the rapidity of diagnosis after onset, and the adequacy of therapy are important in the prognosis of bacterial meningitis. The mortality of neonatal meningitis is approximately 50%, although late-onset B streptococcal meningitis carries a 15% to 20% case fatality. With *H. influenzae* disease and meningococcal meningitis, the mortality rate is 5% to 10%, and with pneumococcal meningitis in infancy and childhood, about 20%.

Sequelae of bacterial meningitis are most frequently seen when the disease occurs in the first 2 months of life and least often found in children with meningococcal meningitis. The residual deficits in infants are primarily a result of communicating hydrocephalus and the greater effects of cerebritis on the immature brain. In older children the residual effects are related to the inflammatory process itself or result from vasculitis associated with the disease.

Prevention. Vaccines are now available for types A, C, Y, and W-135 meningococci and *H. influenzae* type B. At the present time type A is effective in children aged 3 months and older; the other three types are effective in those aged 2 years and older (Feigin and Neglia, 1986). Meningoccal vaccine is recommended for household, nursery school, and hospital staff contacts of a primary case caused by type A or type C meningitis. Household contacts may also be treated prophylactically with rifampin. *H. influenzae* type B vaccine is recommended for all children at 24 months of age (p. 529).

Nursing Considerations

The first priority of nursing care of a child suspected of having meningitis is to administer the antibiotic as soon as it is ordered. The child is also placed on respiratory isolation for at least 24 hours after implementation of antimicrobial therapy. Nurses should take necessary precautions to protect themselves and others from possible infection. Parents are taught the proper protective procedures and supervised in their application.

The room should be kept as quiet as possible and environmental stimuli kept at a minimum, since most affected children are sensitive to noise, bright lights, and other external stimuli. Most children are more comfortable without a pillow and with the head of the bed slightly elevated. A side-lying position is more often assumed because of nuchal rigidity. The nurse should avoid actions, such as lifting the child's head, that cause pain or increase discomfort. Measures are employed to ensure safety, since the child is often restless and subject to seizures.

The nursing care of the child with meningitis is determined by the child's symptoms and treatment. Observation of vital signs, neurologic signs, level of consciousness, urine output, and other pertinent data is carried out at frequent intervals. The child who is unconscious is managed as described previously (see p. 1632), and all children are observed carefully for signs of complications just described, especially signs of increased intracranial pressure, shock, or respiratory distress.

Fluids and nourishment are determined by the child's status. The child with dulled sensorium is usually given nothing by mouth. Other children are allowed clear liquids initially and progressed to a diet suitable for their age. Careful monitoring and recording of intake and output are needed to determine deviations that might indicate impending shock or increasing fluid accumulation, such as cerebral edema or subdural effusion.

One of the most difficult problems in nursing care of children with meningitis is maintaining the intravenous infusion for the length of time needed to provide adequate antimicrobial therapy. Older infants and small children require restraining devices to maintain the integrity of the infusion site. These children should be released from the restraints as often as possible to reduce the ill effects of long-term immobilization. The children should be allowed ambulation and other normal activities as soon as the condition allows and as often as feasible. In some children, especially older ones, a heparin-lock device can be employed to allow for more freedom of movement. The infusion site is monitored for signs of inflammation as well as for patency. Some medications are highly irritating to veins and may tend to produce phlebitis if continued in the same site over a prolonged time. These children are particularly in need of attendance and opportunities for play.

NONBACTERIAL (ASEPTIC) MENINGITIS

Aseptic meningitis is a benign syndrome caused by a number of agents, principally viruses, and is frequently associated with other diseases, such as measles, mumps, herpes, and leukemia. Enteroviruses and mumps viruses account for a large number of cases.

The onset may be abrupt or gradual. The initial manifestations are headache, fever, malaise, gastrointestinal symptoms, and signs of meningeal irritation that develop a day or two after the onset of illness. Abdominal pain and nausea and vomiting are common; back and leg pain, sore throat, chest pain, and generalized muscular aches or pains are found occasionally. There may be a maculopapular rash. These symptoms usually subside spontaneously and rapidly, and the child is well in 3 to 10 days with no residual effects.

Diagnosis is based on clinical features and cerebrospinal fluid findings, which include increased lymphocytes, predominantly mononuclear cells. It is important to differentiate this benign disorder from the more serious form of meningitis and to diagnose and treat any disease of which it is a manifestation.

Treatment is primarily symptomatic, such as aspirin for headache, moist heat for muscle aches and pains, and positioning for comfort. Antimicrobial agents may be administered and isolation enforced until a definitive diagnosis is made as a precaution against the possibility that the disease might be of bacterial origin.

BRAIN ABSCESS

Localized suppuration in the central nervous system, as elsewhere in the body, constitutes an abscess. Brain abscesses may be multiple or single and are identified less often in infancy than in later childhood. They are two to three times more common in boys than in girls (Strauss, 1986).

Abscesses result from a variety of infections. They may be caused by hematogenous spread of organisms from foci of infection in other areas of the body. Intracerebral abscesses form when pyogenic organisms gain access to neural tissue by way of the bloodstream from foci of infection or from direct inoculation of organisms from meningitis, penetrating trauma, or surgical procedures. Cerebral abscesses are often caused by venous extension from purulent middle ear infection and mobilization of septic thrombi in children with right-to-left cardiac shunts (especially tetralogy of Fallot), but they can occur secondary to pulmonary suppuration, such as bronchiectasis or pulmonary abscess.

The most common sites of intracerebral abscesses are the temporal and frontal lobes, and the most frequently demonstrated organisms are the streptococci, pneumococci, and staphylococci. Early signs of the disease are vague, and the insidious onset often includes vomiting, lethargy, fever, and progression to coma. Specific neurologic signs are related to the area invaded by the infectious process and, as this area enlarges, resemble those produced by an intracranial tumor. Cerebellar abscesses produce signs associated with any posterior fossa mass (see Brain tumors, p. 1595).

During abscess formation, antibiotic therapy is effective. Fully established abscesses may require surgical management, either by needle aspiration or, if well-encapsulated and in a safe area of the brain, by surgical excision. The child is treated symptomatically with frequent CT scans to monitor the progress of the abscess. Where possible, the source of the infection is eradicated.

ENCEPHALITIS

Encephalitis is an inflammatory process of the central nervous system producing altered function of various portions of the brain and spinal cord. Encephalitis can be caused by a variety of organisms, including bacteria, spirochetes, fungi, protozoa, helminths, and viruses. Most infections are associated with viruses, and this discussion is limited to these etiologic agents.

Etiology

Encephalitis can occur as the result of (1) direct invasion of the central nervous system by a virus or (2) postinfectious involvement of the central nervous system after a viral disease. Often the specific type of encephalitis in a particular patient may not be identified for some time or not at all. The cause of over half the cases reported in the United States is unknown. The majority of cases of known etiology are associated with the childhood diseases of measles, mumps, varicella, and rubella and, less often, the enteroviruses and herpes viruses.

The multiplicity of causes of viral encephalitis makes diagnosis difficult. Most are those involved with arthropod vectors (togaviruses and bunyaviruses) and those associated with hemorrhagic fevers (arenaviruses, filoviruses, Hantaan viruses). The vector reservoir for most agents pathogenic for

humans and detected in the United States is the mosquito; therefore most cases of encephalitis appear during the hot summer months and subside during the autumn. One type found along the United States–Canadian border is carried by ticks.

Clinical Manifestations

The clinical features of encephalitis are similar regardless of the agent involved. Manifestations can range from a mild benign form that resembles aseptic meningitis, lasting a few days and being followed by rapid and complete recovery, to a fulminating encephalitis with severe central nervous system involvement. The onset may be sudden or gradual with malaise, fever, headache, dizziness, apathy, stiffness of the neck, nausea and vomiting, ataxia, tremors, hyperactivity, and speech difficulties. In severe cases there is high fever, stupor, seizures, disorientation, spasticity, and coma that may proceed to death. Ocular palsies and paralysis also may occur.

Diagnostic Evaluation

The diagnosis is made on the basis of clinical findings, circumstances associated with the disease, and, where possible, identification of the specific virus. Togaviruses (some of which were formerly labeled arboviruses) are rarely detected in the blood or spinal fluid, but viruses of herpes, mumps, measles, and enteroviruses may be found in cerebrospinal fluid. Serologic diagnosis may be reached by means of a variety of antibody tests. The first should be drawn as soon after onset as possible and the second 2 or 3 weeks later.

Therapeutic Management

Patients suspected of having encephalitis are hospitalized promptly for skilled nursing care and observation. Treatment is primarily supportive, including conscientious nursing care, control of cerebral manifestations, and adequate nutrition and hydration, with observations and management as for other disorders involving cerebral injury. Follow-up care with periodic reevaluation and rehabilitation are important for survivors with residual effects of the disease.

Nursing Considerations

Nursing care of the child with encephalitis is the same as for any unconscious child and for the child with meningitis. Neurologic monitoring, administration of medications, and support of the child and parents are the major aspects of care.

RABIES

Rabies is an acute infection of the nervous system caused by a virus that is almost invariably fatal. It is transmitted to humans by the saliva of an infected mammal introduced through a bite or skin abrasion. Over 75% of animals reported as rabid have been raccoons, although no human rabies case has ever been known to result from a raccoon bite. Other animals in order of frequency are skunks, bats, foxes, and groundhogs (Morbidity and Mortality Weekly Report, 1982). The domestic dog, formerly considered a prime source, is relatively well controlled by rabies vaccination programs. Wild animals, with more than 85% of reported animal rabies, now represent the greatest rabies exposure hazard for man in the United States (Wehrle, 1986). Unusual behavior in an animal is cause for suspicion; children should be warned to beware of wild animals that appear to be friendly.

The disease is uncommon in humans, but the highest incidence occurs in children under 15 years. The incubation period usually ranges from 1 to 3 months but may be as short as 10 days or as long as 8 months. Only 10% to 15% of persons bitten develop the disease, but once symptoms are present, rabies progresses inexorably to a fatal outcome. The disease is characterized by a period of general malaise, fever, and sore throat followed by a phase of excitement featuring by hypersensitivity and increased reaction to external stimuli, convulsions, maniacal behavior, and choking. Attempts at swallowing may cause such severe spasm of respiratory muscles that apnea, cyanosis, and anoxia are produced—the characteristics from which the term *hydrophobia* was derived. Diagnosis is made on the basis of history and clinical features. Once symptoms appear, treatment is of little avail, but the long incubation period allows time for induction of active and passive immunity before the onset of illness.

Therapeutic Management

Two types of immunizing products are available for use in humans: (1) the inactivated rabies vaccines, which induce inactive immune response, and (2) the globulins, which contain preformed antibodies. The two types of products should be used concurrently for rabies postexposure treatment when prophylaxis is indicated.

The current therapy for a rabid animal bite consists of thorough cleansing of the wound and passive immunization with human rabies immune globulin (RIG) or hyperimmune antirabies serum (ARS) as soon as possible after exposure to provide rapid, short-term passive immunity. RIG is the preferred treatment, since many persons are sensitive to horse serum, from which ARS is derived.

Postexposure active immunity is conferred by administration of the recently developed human diploid cell rabies vaccine (HDCV). The first dose of the vaccine is given at the same time as the immune globulin and followed by injections at 3, 7, 14, and 21 days after exposure. An additional dose in 90 days is recommended by the World Health Organization.

Nursing Considerations

Parents as well as children are frightened by the urgency and seriousness of the situation. They need anticipatory guidance for the therapy and support and reassurance re-

garding the efficacy of the preventive measures for this dreaded disease. The vaccine is well tolerated by children, but mass immunization is unnecessary and unlikely to be implemented. In areas in which rabies is rare the schedule given is sufficient. However, certain circumstances may warrant vaccination, such as when a child is being taken to an area of the world where rabies in stray dogs is still a problem.

REYE SYNDROME

Reye syndrome (RS) is a disorder defined as toxic encephalopathy associated with other characteristic organ involvement. It is being identified with increasing frequency and characterized by fever, profoundly impaired consciousness, and disordered hepatic function. The ages of affected children range from 2 months to adolescence, with peak incidences occurring at 6 and 11 years. This syndrome is one of the most common causes of encephalopathy in children.

Etiology

The etiology of the disorder is obscure, but most cases of Reye syndrome follow a common viral illness, most frequently influenza or varicella. The association is emphasized by reporting of cases and increased incidence of influenza B and A. There have also been reports of an association between the ingestion of aspirin during the prodromal illness and the occurrence of Reye syndrome. Consequently, the Committee on Infectious Diseases of the American Academy of Pediatrics (1982) has recommended that aspirin should not be prescribed under usual circumstances for children with varicella or those suspected of having influenza. Recent studies lend support to this observation (Remington and others, 1986; Hurwitz and others, 1985). Conclusions of these studies are that "recent changes in the patterns of aspirin given for viral illnesses among children and teenagers in the United States could explain some of the observed changes in the epidemiology of Reye syndrome" (Barrett and others, 1986).

It has also been observed that children who developed Reye syndrome had a more severe prodromal illness than sick control subjects and that fever may play a role (Wilson and Brown, 1982). Various other theories are also being proposed and examined.

Pathophysiology

The liver of a patient with Reye syndrome appears yellow or reddish yellow with a considerable amount of fat distributed in small droplets throughout—a diagnostic characteristic of the disease. Electron microscopy reveals abnormally large and swollen mitochondria in liver and brain cells, which suggests the probability that the primary defect is some form of mitochondrial failure. There is a reduction in the enzymes that convert ammonia to urea, which is reflected in a hyperammonemia. Brain dysfunction and death are the result of swollen or damaged cells.

STAGING CRITERIA FOR REYE SYNDROME

Stage I Vomiting, lethargy, and drowsiness; liver dysfunction; Type I EEG, follows commands, pupillary reaction brisk

Stage II Disorientation, combativeness, delirium, hyperventilation, hyperactive reflexes, appropriate responses to painful stimuli; evidence of liver dysfunction; Type I EEG, pupillary reaction sluggish

Stage III Obtunded, coma, hyperventilation, decorticate rigidity, preservation of pupillary light reaction and oculovestibular reflexes (although sluggish); Type II EEG

Stage IV Deepening coma, decerebrate rigidity, loss of oculocephalic reflexes, large and fixed pupils, loss of doll's eye reflex, loss of corneal reflexes; minimum liver dysfunction; Type III or IV EEG, evidence of brain stem dysfunction

Stage V Seizures, loss of deep tendon reflexes, respiratory arrest, flaccidity; Type IV EEG; usually no evidence of liver dysfunction

---

Clinical Manifestations

The onset of the disease is preceded in most cases by prodromal symptoms, including malaise, cough, rhinorrhea, or sore throat. The child appears to be recovering but then develops recurrent, intractable vomiting and central nervous system dysfunction. As the child's condition progressively deteriorates, cerebral signs and symptoms appear, accompanied by various physiologic changes. Clinically, liver involvement is limited to mild hepatomegaly.

Various staging criteria have been developed that help to objectively evaluate the patient's progress, to predict a probable outcome, and to evaluate the efficacy of therapies. The staging that is used most frequently involves five stages. The manifestations of the various clinical stages are outlined in the accompanying box.

The clinical course of the disease is rapid, and mortality is high (40%), particularly in children younger than 2 years and if convulsions are part of the clinical picture. Fortunately recovery is rapid and complete in those who survive, and residual disability is uncommon.

Diagnostic Evaluation

Evidence of liver dysfunction is reflected by elevated serum glutamic-oxaloacetic transaminase (SGOT), serum glutamic-pyruvic transaminase (SGPT), and lactic dehydrogenase (LDH) levels. Liver-dependent clotting factors, such as prothrombin, are diminished. Serum bilirubin and alkaline phosphatase levels are usually unaffected. Elevated ammonia levels establish the diagnosis and tend to correlate with the clinical manifestations and prognosis. In the majority of children blood sugar levels fall to below 50 mg/dl, with reduced insulin levels and diminished glucagon response. There is a combined respiratory alkalosis and metabolic acidosis. Cerebrospinal fluid is normal, if examined. Definitive diagnosis is established by liver biopsy.

Therapeutic Management

The most important aspect of successful management of the child with Reye syndrome is early diagnosis and aggressive therapy in an effort to prevent progression of the disease. It is determined by the clinical stage of the disease and the rapidity with which it progresses. For children at stage I, treatment is primarily supportive and directed toward restoring blood sugar levels, controlling cerebral edema, correcting acid-base imbalances, and eliminating factors known to increase intracranial pressure. Intravenous administration of hypertonic (10%) glucose solution with added insulin helps to replace glycogen stores, but it is controlled to avoid overhydration. The pH and electrolyte levels are monitored and replaced according to regular assessments. Sometimes corticosteroids are useful. Noninvasive monitoring is adequate to assess status and progress.

Stages II through V require more aggressive measures. The child is admitted to an intensive care unit where invasive support and monitoring are implemented to supplement supportive measures. The objectives of therapy are to normalize organ function and to prevent irreversible brain damage. Since increased ICP kills, the major efforts are directed toward preventing and/or reducing cerebral edema. Those designed to lower intracranial pressure involve significant risk and require intensive care and observation. ICP monitoring is begun, and intravenous mannitol, urea, or glycol and hypertonic solutions are administered to elevate blood osmolality, which causes fluid to move out of edematous tissues. Tracheal intubation, preferably nasotracheal, is performed as soon as possible, and the child is placed on controlled hyperventilation to decrease carbon dioxide levels. Children who are able to breathe spontaneously tend to hypoventilate.

A standard approach is curarization and sedation. Skeletal muscles are paralyzed with administration of d-tubocurarine or pancuronium (Pavulon) to prevent any activity, especially coughing, that might increase ICP. Curarization does not affect sensory input; therefore the child's anxiety may be sufficient to cause cerebral hypertension. Exchange transfusions or peritoneal dialysis has been used in some cases to reduce elevated blood ammonia levels.

Nursing Considerations

The child who is acutely ill with Reye syndrome requires continuous and intensive nursing care. On admission to the hospital numerous procedures and observations must be carried out as quickly as possible. In addition to an appraisal of vital functions and neurologic status, the nurse assists with a lumbar puncture, obtaining blood for laboratory examination, and insertion of various intravenous lines such as peripheral, arterial, and central venous pressure. A retention catheter and a nasogastric tube are inserted, and when respirations are compromised, an endotracheal tube is inserted and attached to a respirator for controlled respirations. If equipment is available, a pressure monitoring device is inserted for continuous monitoring of intracranial pressure.

Care and observations are implemented as for any child with an altered state of consciousness (p. 1632) and increasing ICP. Accurate and frequent monitoring of intake and output is essential for adjusting fluid volumes to prevent both dehydration and cerebral edema. The child paralyzed and in a drug-induced coma is totally dependent on the caregivers, and meticulous vigilance and attention to all biologic needs are mandatory. Since hypovolemic shock is a constant danger in children with controlled fluid intake and osmotic diuresis, vital signs, including central venous pressure and/or cardiac output (Swan-Ganz catheter), are monitored frequently. Laboratory analysis of serum electrolytes, pH, blood urea nitrogen, glucose, osmolality, and blood gases serves as a guide for therapy, and arranging for their collection is a nursing responsibility. Because of related liver dysfunction, the nurse must observe for signs of impaired coagulation such as prolonged bleeding and petechiae.

Recovery from Reye syndrome is rapid, usually without sequelae if there has been early diagnosis and implementation of therapy. However, in her studies Weeks (1976) has observed a trend in the behaviors when children waken from the unconscious state. The stress and anxiety they appear to feel in a strange and unfamiliar environment are consistently expressed in silent and withdrawn behavior. The children respond to basic questioning but do not display their prehospitalization personality and social behavior until they are transferred from the critical care area.

The children awaken disoriented, with no recollection of events that took place during the critical phase of their illness. Strange equipment being used in their care that was started while they were unconscious requires explanation. The appearance of other ill children is puzzling and frightening, increasing their anxiety and stress concerning their own situation. They are powerless to control what is happening to them. Nurses can help these children deal with their stress by orienting them to where they are and the circumstances of their being there, describing what is expected of them, and giving them a sense of control whenever possible. Encouraging parents to visit and providing other items associated with home, such as a favorite toy, a photograph, or other item, help them maintain a link with their lives outside the confines of the critical care environment. Understanding and individualized care help children to weather the stresses and tension of this period of crisis.

Family support. Parents of children with Reye syndrome need a great deal of emotional support. They are usually frightened by the child's appearance, the treatment, and the life-threatening severity and suddenness of the illness. Their distress is increased if they believe that their actions may have contributed to a delay in diagnosis. Parents are encouraged to verbalize their guilt feelings and are provided with reassurance that they did not contribute to the child's condition, that the development of the disease cannot be an-

ticipated, and that their care was proper under the circumstances. They need to be kept informed regarding the child's progress, to have diagnostic procedures and therapeutic management explained, and to be given concerned and sympathetic support.

The **National Reye's Syndrome Foundation*** has been established by the parents of a child who died from this disease in hope of encouraging research on the disease and of educating parents and health professionals.

Seizure Disorders

Convulsive phenomena are among the most frequently observed neurologic dysfunctions in children and can occur with a wide variety of conditions involving the central nervous system. Generally a *convulsion* is defined as involuntary muscular contractions and relaxation; a *seizure* is a sudden attack. Persons who have a tendency to experience seizures are said to have *epilepsy*. The words are all used synonymously. More specifically, seizure phenomena are characterized by a single attack or recurrent transient attacks of involuntary loss of consciousness, altered motor activity and/or autonomic function, disturbed feelings or behavior associated with excessive neuronal discharges. These discharges may be focal or diffuse, and the sites of the discharges determine the clinical manifestations observed during the attack.

EPILEPSY: GENERAL CONCEPTS

Seizures result from paroxysmal discharges in cortical neurons and are symptoms of abnormal brain function. They are considered to be a symptom of an underlying disease process.

Etiology

Seizure disorders have numerous and varied causes. Most seizures are *idiopathic*. Although the cause of idiopathic epilepsy is unknown, it may indicate genetic factors that in some way alter the seizure threshold to influence neuronal discharge. Congenital defects and some genetic disorders (such as tuberous sclerosis) have seizures as a manifestation. Febrile and breath-holding seizures are related to a lowered seizure threshold that tends to have a higher incidence in certain families. Hereditary electroencephalographic abnormalities have been detected in some families, and there is a higher incidence of seizures among relatives of children with idiopathic convulsive disorders.

A seizure disorder also can be *acquired* as a result of brain injury during prenatal, perinatal, or postnatal periods. This injury may be caused by trauma, hypoxia, infections, exogenous or endogenous toxins, and a variety of other factors. Biochemical events (e.g., hypoglycemia, hypocal-

---

*P.O. Box RS, Benzonia, MI 49616.

ETIOLOGY OF SEIZURES IN CHILDREN

NONRECURRENT (ACUTE)	RECURRENT (CHRONIC)
Febrile episodes	Idiopathic epilepsy
Intracranial infection	Epilepsy—secondary to prior
Intracranial hemorrhage	Trauma
Space-occupying lesions (cyst, tumor)	Hemorrhage
Acute cerebral edema	Anoxia
Anoxia	Infections
Toxins	Toxins
Drugs	Degenerative phenomena
Tetanus	Congenital defects
Lead encephalopathy	Parasitic brain disease
Shigella, Salmonella	Hypoglycemia injury
Metabolic alterations	Epilepsy—sensory stimulus
Hypocalcemia	Epilepsy-stimulating states
Hypoglycemia	Narcolepsy and catalepsy
Hyponatremia or hypernatremia	Psychogenic
Hypomagnesemia	Tetany from hypocalcemia, alkalosis
Alkalosis	Hypoglycemia states
Disorders of amino acid metabolism	Hyperinsulinism
Deficiency states	Hypopituitarism
Hyperbilirubinemia	Adrenocortical insufficiency
	Hepatic disorders
	Uremia
	Allergy
	Cardiovascular dysfunction or syncopal episodes
	Migraine

cemia, and certain nutritional deficiencies) produce seizure activity. A partial list of causative factors is shown in the boxed material.

The incidence of causative factors associated with childhood seizures is frequently related to the age of the child. Seizures are more common during the first 2 years of life than during any other period of childhood. In very young infants the most frequent causes are birth injuries, that is, intracranial trauma, hemorrhage, or anoxia, and congenital defects of the brain. Acute infections are a frequent cause of seizures in late infancy and early childhood but become an infrequent cause in middle childhood. In children older than 3 years of age the most common factor is idiopathic epilepsy.

Other contributing factors are fatigue, undue excitement, and stressful situations at home or school. Excessive fluid intake or fluid retention, such as occurs during premenstrual tension, produces alterations in the serum (and brain) concentrations of sodium, potassium, and water, which may precipitate seizures. There appear to be periods of functional instability of the brain, normally when falling asleep or awakening from sleep. At these times seizures are more likely to occur. The hormonal and metabolic changes associated with adolescence can alter the convulsive threshold. Photogenic stimulation by such commonplace things as television, rays of the sun, or certain kinds of music in susceptible children have been implicated in precipitating seizures in some instances.

Pathophysiology

Regardless of the etiologic factor or the type of seizure, the basic mechanism is the same. There are electric discharges that (1) may arise from central areas in the brain that affect consciousness immediately, (2) may be restricted to one area of the cerebral cortex, producing manifestations characteristic of that particular anatomic focus, or (3) may begin in a localized area of the cortex and spread to other portions of the brain, which, if sufficiently extensive, produce generalized neurologic manifestations.

Seizure activity is believed to be caused by spontaneous electric discharge initiated by a group of hyperexcitable cells referred to as the *epileptogenic focus*. These cells display increased electric excitability but may remain quiescent over a period of time while discharging intermittently as evidenced on electroencephalographic tracings. Normally these discharges are restrained from spreading beyond the focal area by normal inhibitory mechanisms.

In response to any of a variety of physiologic stimuli, such as cellular dehydration, abnormal blood sugar levels, electrolyte imbalance, fatigue, emotional stress, and endocrine changes, these hyperexcitable cells activate normal cells in surrounding areas and in distant, synaptically related cells. When the neuronal excitation from the epileptogenic focus spreads to the brain stem, particularly the midbrain and reticular formation, a generalized seizure develops. These centers within the brain stem, known as the centrencephalic system, are responsible for the spread of the epileptic potentials. The discharges can originate spontaneously in the centrencephalic system or be triggered by a focal area in the cortex. Seizures are designated as focal, focal with rapid generalization, and generalized, on the basis of these characteristic neuronal discharges, as recorded by electroencephalography. In a large proportion of children focal seizures spread to other areas, ultimately becoming generalized with loss of consciousness.

Clinical Manifestations

There are a number of observations that provide information that can help identify the type of seizure and the area of the brain where the neuronal discharges originate. Some of these clues that distinguish epileptic seizures from other seizure episodes are: abrupt onset, genuine loss of awareness, brief duration, rapid recovery, and stereotypic episodes. Some examples are migraine, toxic effects of drugs, syncope, and hyperventilation, and transient ischemic attacks, and breath-holding spells in infants.

A seizure is a finite event and consists of a limited number of clinical manifestations. In most cases these can be reduced to commonalities. Generalized seizures without a focal onset may occur at any age and at any time, day or night. The interval between attacks may be minutes, weeks, or even years. Children, compared to adults, seldom report an aura or warning.

There are several features that may be observed during various seizures. A clear description of these phenomena is a valuable aid in localizing the area involved and frequently suggests the underlying pathology. The initial event may provide the best clue for assessing the type of seizure and its localization. These include sensory-hallucinatory phenomena, motor effects, sensorimotor effects, and loss of consciousness. The duration of a seizure is determined by separating the active portion of the seizure from the manifestations following it.

Sensory-hallucinatory phenomena. An *aura* is the peculiar sensation experienced by some persons just before the onset of a seizure. The aura serves two useful purposes. It warns the person of the impending attack so that he is able to seek privacy and a safe place to lie down before the seizure begins. The nature of the sensation can also provide the most reliable clue to help localize the origin of the discharge. The most common epileptic aura is a sensation of dizziness or an unusual feeling of ascending abdominal discomfort. Other sensations are those described as sensorimotor.

Motor effects. Sometimes there will be only minimum effects with little interference with activity; single groups of muscles may be activated; there can be complex reactive movement patterns, or repetitive, stereotyped movements described as automatisms (e.g., lip-smacking, swallowing, or chewing). *Eye movement* provides clues to the focus of the seizure. Discharges in the cortex of one hemisphere tend to cause the eyes to deviate to the opposite side. Bilateral discharges tend to cause the eyes to move upward or straight ahead. However, after the seizure, the eyes will often deviate in the opposite direction. When the child's eyes are closed during the attack, a gentle attempt to open them may provide valuable information.

Muscle contraction during the seizure can be one of three types: *clonic, tonic,* or *jacksonian*. Clonic contractions are those in which opposing muscles contract and relax alternately, producing rhythmic movements. Tonic contractions are those in which all the muscles are maintained in a contraction for a time, causing the person to become rigid. Jacksonian contractions are those in which muscular twitchings begin in one area and spread to another.

Laterality of seizure activity is an important observation. Motor activity may involve the entire body, one side, or one or more body parts. The body part or side involved implies an electric discharge in the corresponding area of the opposite cerebral cortex. *Complex motor activity* is observed in some types of seizures. Seizures may begin with or consist of complex, stereotyped, or repetitive activities. These are often associated with lesions in the temporal lobe.

Sensorimotor effects. Various sensorimotor sensations may accompany a seizure; these may include a tingling or prickling sensation, hallucinations or light flashes, tastes, smells, or sounds. The focal areas implicated are visual hallucinations (occipital or temporal lobe), verbal phenomena (the dominant hemisphere), unusual tastes, odors, visceral sensations, or dreamy feelings (temporal lobe). Autonomic activity may include pallor, sweating, flushing, piloerection, and pupillary dilatation.

Alteration of consciousness. Consciousness may be unaffected, lost completely, or altered but not lost. Persons who do not lose consciousness usually have some degree of reactivity and may even talk, but activity is incomplete, inappropriate, bizarre, or automatic with impaired memory for the event.

Loss of consciousness causes amnesia for the attack and indifference to the environment with no response to stimuli. Loss of consciousness commonly accompanies a seizure and indicates generalized cortical or centrencephalic involvement. The loss of consciousness is frequently shown by various manifestations such as incontinence or injury.

Other observations. In addition to the initial event, which helps localize the cerebral site of origin and is usually stereotyped for a given patient, the circumstances that precipitated the attack or in which the attack occurred are important. The *postictal state,* the period following a seizure, may be varied. The child may be drowsy, be uncoordinated, have transient aphasia, confusion, and display some sensory or motor impairment. Weakness, hypotonia, or inactivity of a body part may be an indication of an epileptogenic focus in the contralateral corresponding cortical region.

EPILEPSY: CLASSIFICATION

There are many different types of epileptic seizures and each has unique characteristics. The onset of a seizure is abrupt, paroxysmal, and transitory, and signs are highly variable as evidenced by the previous discussion. The International Classification of Epileptic Seizures divides seizures into two major categories: partial seizures and generalized seizures (see box).

Partial Seizures

Partial seizures are caused by abnormal electric discharges from epileptogenic foci limited to a more or less circumscribed region of the cerebral cortex. There is usually evidence that the irritating focus of the seizure is secondary to an underlying condition that causes damage to brain tissue. Focal lesions include scars from previous craniocerebral trauma, atrophy, malformations, or tumors. Focal seizures may arise from any area of the cerebral cortex, but the frontal, temporal, and parietal lobes are the ones most often affected. The area of cerebral involvement is reflected by clinical manifestations.

Partial seizures are categorized as (1) those with elementary or simple symptoms, (2) those with associated impairment of consciousness, and (3) those with impaired consciousness and that spread to become generalized. All have their onset in a specific area of the brain.

Simple partial seizures. Focal seizures are characterized by localized motor symptoms; somatosensory, psychic, autonomic symptoms; or a combination of these. The abnormal discharges remain unilateral. The most common motor seizure in children is the aversive seizure, in which the eye or eyes and head turn away from the side of the focus.

INTERNATIONAL CLASSIFICATION OF EPILEPTIC SEIZURES

I. Partial Seizures (seizures beginning locally)
  A. Simple partial seizures (with elementary symptomatology; consciousness unimpaired)
    1. with motor symptoms
    2. with somatosensory or special sensory symptoms
    3. with autonomic symptoms
    4. compound forms (with psychic symptoms)
  B. Complex partial symptomatology (temporal lobe or psychomotor seizures; generally with impaired consciousness)
    1. with impairment of consciousness only
    2. with cognitive symptomatology
    3. with affective symptomatology
    4. with psychosensory symptomatology
    5. with psychomotor symptomatology
    6. compound forms
  C. Partial seizures, secondarily generalized
II. Generalized seizures (bilaterally symmetrical; without local onset; with impairment of consciousness)
    1. tonic-clonic (grand mal) seizures
    2. tonic seizures
    3. clonic seizures
    4. absence (petit mal) seizures
    5. atonic seizures
    6. myoclonic seizures
    7. infantile spasms
    8. akinetic seizures
III. Unilateral seizures (those involving one hemisphere)
IV. Unclassified epileptic seizures (due to incomplete data)

Modified from Commission on Classification and Terminology of the International League Against Epilepsy: Proposal for revised clinical and electroencephalographic classification of epileptic seizures, Epilepsia **22**:489-501, 1981.

In some children the upper extremity toward which the head turns is abducted and extended and the fingers are clenched, giving the impression that the child is looking at the closed fist. The child may be aware of the movement or lose consciousness simultaneously with assuming the position.

A common form is the sylvian seizure, in which there are tonic-clonic movements involving the face, salivation, and arrested speech. These are most common during sleep. On rare occasions children display the *jacksonian* march, an orderly, sequential progression of clonic movements that begin in a foot, hand, or face and, as electric impulses spread from the irritable focus to continuous regions of the cortex, move or "march" body parts activated by these cerebral regions. Motor seizures are particularly common in hemiplegic children. The movements, which are usually clonic, begin in the hemiplegic hand, spread to the entire affected side and, in many cases, become generalized seizures. Postictal weakness is common after this type of seizure.

Special sensory seizures are characterized by various sensations, including numbness, tingling, prickling, paresthesia, or pain that originates in one area (e.g., face or extremities) and spreads to other parts of the body. Visual sensations or formed images may be manifestations. Motor phenomena such as posturing or hypertonia may accompany sensory seizures. Special sensory seizures are uncommon in children under 8 years of age.

Complex partial seizures. Partial seizures with complex symptoms are the most difficult to recognize and are among those most difficult to control. Because they involve more organized and higher level cerebral function as well as sensory and motor function, they have been termed *psychomotor seizures.* The attack is characterized by a period of altered behavior for which the individual is amnesic and during which he is unable to respond to his environment. Although the child does not lose consciousness during an attack, he has no recollection of his behavior during the seizure. Drowsiness or sleep usually follows the seizure. Confusion and amnesia may be prolonged.

Psychomotor seizures are observed more often in children from 3 years of age through adolescence and are more common in adults than in children. The seizures are most characteristically associated with focal lesions of the temporal lobe and are sometimes referred to as temporal lobe seizures.

Complex sensory phenomena associated with the beginning of a seizure reflect the complicated connections and integrative functions of that area of the brain. The most frequent sensation is a strange feeling in the pit of the stomach that rises toward the throat. This feeling is often accompanied by odd or unpleasant odors or tastes, complex auditory or visual hallucinations, or ill-defined feelings of elation or strangeness (e.g., *déjà vu*, a feeling of familiarity in a strange environment). Small children may emit a cry or attempt to run for help as a manifestation of an aura. Strong feelings of fear and anxiety and a distorted sense of time and self may be mental symptoms associated with an episode.

A variety of patterns of motor behavior may be observed during a psychomotor attack. The attacks are usually stereotypic and recur in a similar manner with each subsequent seizure. It is sometimes difficult to determine whether the manifestations are related to a seizure disorder or to a nonconvulsive behavioral disturbance. The child may suddenly cease his activity, appear dazed, stare into space, become confused and apathetic, and become limp, stiff, or display some form of posturing. The primary feature may be confusion, and the child may perform purposeless, complicated activities in a repetitive manner (automatisms), such as walking, running, kicking, laughing, or speaking incoherently, most often followed by postictal confusion or sleep. The predominant observations may be oropharyngeal activities, such as smacking, chewing, drooling, swallowing, and nausea or abdominal pain followed by stiffness, a fall, and postictal sleep. Rarely children manifest auras such as rage or temper tantrums, and aggressive acts are uncommon during a seizure.

Generalized Seizures

Generalized seizures without a focal onset appear to arise in the reticular formation and the clinical observations indicate that the initial involvement is from both hemispheres. Loss of consciousness occurs and is the initial clinical manifestation. Unlike partial seizures that become generalized, there is no aura. Attacks occur at any time, day or night, and the interval between attacks may be minutes, hours, weeks, or even years. Most affected persons first experience seizures in childhood, and children whose seizures begin before age 4 years have mental retardation and behavioral and learning problems more frequently than those whose seizures begin after age 4.

Tonic-clonic seizures. The generalized tonic-clonic seizure, traditionally known as *grand mal,* is the most common and most dramatic of all seizure manifestations of childhood. The seizure usually occurs without warning. There is a rolling of the eyes upward and immediate loss of consciousness. If the child is standing, he falls to the floor or ground. The child stiffens in a generalized and symmetric tonic contraction of the entire body musculature. The arms usually flex, whereas the legs, head, and neck extend. The child may utter a peculiar piercing cry produced as the jaws clap shut and the thoracic and abdominal muscles contract, forcing air through tightly closed vocal cords. This tonic phase lasts approximately 10 to 20 seconds, during which the child is apneic and may become cyanotic. Autonomic stimulation causes increased salivation.

The tonic rigidity is replaced by violent jerking movements as the trunk and extremities undergo rhythmic contraction and relaxation of the clonic phase. During this time the child may foam at the mouth and be incontinent of urine and feces. As the attack ends, the movements become less intense and occur at longer intervals until they cease entirely. The clonic phase generally lasts about 30 seconds but can vary from only a few seconds to a half hour or longer. A series of seizures at intervals too brief to allow the child to regain consciousness between the time one attack ends and the next begins is known as *status epilepticus.* This requires emergency intervention. A succession of interrupted seizures can lead to exhaustion, respiratory failure, and death.

In the postictal state the child appears to relax but may remain semiconscious and difficult to rouse. He may awaken in a few minutes but remains confused for several hours. The child is poorly coordinated with mild impairment of fine motor movements. He may have visual and speech difficulties and may vomit or complain of severe headache. When left alone, the child usually sleeps for several hours. On awakening he is fully conscious but usually feels tired and complains of sore muscles and headache but has no recollection of the entire event.

Absence seizures. Absence seizures, traditionally called *petit mal* or *lapses,* are characterized by a brief loss of consciousness with minimal or no alteration in muscle tone and may go unrecognized because the child's behavior is changed very little. Attacks almost always first appear during childhood. In most instances the onset occurs between 4 and 12 years of age. Attacks are rarely detected before age 5, usually cease at puberty, but may be seen in adults. They are more common in girls than in boys.

The onset of absence seizures is abrupt, and the child suddenly develops 20 or more attacks daily. Characteristically the brief loss of consciousness appears without warning or aura and usually lasts about 5 to 10 seconds. Slight loss of muscle tone may cause the child to drop objects, but he is able to maintain postural control and seldom falls. There are frequently minor movements such as lip-smacking, twitching of eyelids or face, or slight hand movements. The sudden arrest of activity and consciousness is not accompanied by incontinence, and the child is amnesic for the episode but may need to reorient himself to the previous activity. An attack is often mistaken for inattentiveness or daydreaming. Frequent attacks can result in slowed intellectual processes and deterioration in schoolwork and behavior, which is sometimes the first indication of the problem. Attacks can be precipitated by hyperventilation, hypoglycemia, stresses (emotional and physiologic), fatigue, or sleeplessness. See Table 37-6 for a comparison of simple partial, complex partial, and absence seizures.

Atonic and akinetic seizures. Akinetic and atonic seizures are manifest as a sudden, momentary loss of muscle tone and postural control. *Atonic* refers to loss of muscle tone; *akinetic* is loss of movement. The onset is usually between 2 and 5 years of age. The sudden loss of postural tone and reflexes causes the child to fall to the floor violently. The child is unable to break the fall by putting out his hand and may incur a serious injury to the face, head, or shoulder. Loss of consciousness is only momentary. Akinetic attacks recur frequently during the day, particularly in the morning hours and shortly after the child awakens. Atonic seizures are also known as *drop attacks.*

Myoclonic seizures. Myoclonic seizures include a variety of convulsive episodes characterized by sudden, brief contractures of a muscle or group of muscles, occurring singly or repetitively without loss of consciousness or postictal state. The seizure may or may not be symmetric and may be isolated as benign essential myoclonus or may occur in association with other seizure forms. Myoclonus frequently appears normally in the course of falling asleep or is observed as a nonspecific symptom in many diseases of the nervous system, such as viral encephalitis, uremic encephalopathy, and degenerative diseases of the cerebrum.

Infantile spasms. Infantile myoclonus, massive spasms, hypsarrhythmia, salaam attacks, or infantile myoclonic spasms most commonly occur between 3 and 12 months of age. They are twice as common in males as in females. In infants who are able to sit but not stand, the seizure is observed as a sudden dropping forward of the head and neck with trunk flexed forward and knees drawn up—the "salaam" or "jackknife" seizure. The attack may consist of a series of sudden, brief, symmetric, muscular contractions by which the head is flexed, the arms are extended, and the legs are drawn up. The eyes may roll upward or inward, and the seizure may be preceded or followed by a cry or giggling. There may or may not be loss of consciousness, and the infant will sometimes flush, turn

Table 37-6 Comparison of simple partial, complex partial, and absence seizures

CLINICAL MANIFESTATIONS	SIMPLE PARTIAL	COMPLEX PARTIAL	ABSENCE
Age of onset	Any age	Uncommon before age 3 years	Uncommon before age 3 years
Frequency (per day)	Variable	Rarely over 1-2 times	Multiple
Duration	Usually less than 30 seconds	Usually over 60 seconds, rarely less than 10 seconds	Usually less than 15 seconds, rarely more than 30 seconds
Aura	May be sole manifestation of seizure	Frequently	Never
Impaired consciousness	Never	Always	Always, but may be brief
Automatisms	No	Frequently	Frequently
Clonic movements	Frequently	Occasionally	Occasionally
Postictal impairment	Occasionally	Frequently	Never
Mental	Frequently	Common	Unusual

pale, or become cyanotic. The child may have numerous seizures during the day without postictal drowsiness or sleep.

Less often, alternate clinical forms are observed and include extensor spasms rather than flexion of arms, legs, and trunk and head-nodding. Lightning attacks, which involve a single, momentary, shocklike contraction of the entire body, are another variant.

Infantile spasms are frequently associated with cerebral abnormalities, such as structural malformations, severe anoxic brain damage, phenylketonuria, and degenerative changes. Microcephaly, choreoathetoid or tonic posture, and abnormal movements are frequently present. There may be a history of maternal infection, prematurity, or birth injury, and development is retarded before the onset of seizures. The outlook for normal intelligence is poor.

EPILEPSY: THERAPEUTIC MANAGEMENT AND NURSING CARE

The management of epilepsy requires a well-organized approach. It involves diagnosis, therapy, and monitoring of progress to ensure the efficacy of therapy. Parental involvement is absolutely essential and education and support are vital to the success of any therapeutic plan.

Diagnostic Evaluation

Establishing a diagnosis is critical. The process of diagnosis in a child with a convulsive disorder has two major foci: (1) to ascertain the type of seizure the child has experienced, and (2) to attempt to understand the cause of the attacks. The assessment and diagnosis rely heavily on a thorough history, skilled observation, and employment of several diagnostic tests.

It is especially important to differentiate epilepsy from other brief alterations in consciousness and/or behavior. Epilepsy results from a wide range of etiologies. It is unusual to observe the child during a seizure in the assessment process. A complete, accurate, and detailed history should be obtained from a reliable and knowledgeable informant. This history involves prenatal, perinatal, and neonatal periods, including any instances of infection, apnea, colic, or poor feeding, and information regarding any previous accidents or serious illnesses.

History of the seizure(s) should be equally detailed, including the type of seizure or description of the child's behavior during the attack(s), the age at onset, and the time at which the seizure occurs (i.e., early morning, before meals, while awake, or during sleep). Any factors that may have precipitated the seizure are important, including fever, infection, falls that may have caused trauma to the head, anxiety, fatigue, and activity (e.g., hyperventilation or exposure to strong stimuli such as bright flashing lights or loud noises). If the child can describe any sensory phenomena, these are recorded. The duration and progression of the seizure (if any) and the postictal feelings and behavior, such as confusion, inability to speak, amnesia, headache, and sleep, are recorded.

A complete physical and neurologic examination, including developmental assessment of language, learning, behavior, and motor abilities, often provides clues to neurologic disturbances. A family history can offer clues to paroxysmal disorders such as migraine, breath-holding spells, febrile convulsions, or neurologic diseases that may be related to the convulsive disorder.

Laboratory studies that may prove to be of value include a complete blood cell count (for evidence of lead poisoning) and white blood cell count for signs of infection. Blood and cerebrospinal fluid glucose may give evidence of hypoglycemic episodes, and serum electrolytes, blood urea nitrogen, calcium, and other blood studies might indicate metabolic disturbances. Lumbar puncture can confirm a suspected diagnosis of cerebrospinal infection or trauma.

Skull radiographs, computed tomography, echoencephalograms, brain scans, and other studies help to identify skull abnormalities, separation of sutures, and intracranial calcifications. Invasive techniques are rarely indicated.

The electroencephalogram (EEG) is obtained for all children with convulsive manifestations and is the most useful tool for evaluating seizure disorders. The electroencephalogram is carried out under varying conditions—with the child asleep, awake, awake with provocative stimulation (flashing lights, noise), and hyperventilating. Stimulation elicits abnormal electric activity, which is recorded on the electroencephalogram. Various seizure types produce characteristic electroencephalographic patterns—high-voltage spike discharges are seen in grand mal seizures with abnormal patterns in the intervals between seizures; a 3-per-second spike and wave pattern is observed in a petit mal seizure; and absence of electrical activity in an area suggests a large lesion, such as an abscess or subdural collection of fluid.

Variations of the EEG are video recordings of the patient during waking and/or sleeping. The full body image is displayed on half of the video screen, the facial image is shown on one fourth, and selected EEG channels are displayed on the remaining one fourth. Split-screen capabilities allow modification and arrangement of a larger number of channels and images. Polygraph equipment is also used to monitor physiologic data such as respiratory effort, eye movements, heart rate, and systemic blood pressure. These techniques can be used concurrently and are especially valuable in differentiating epileptic activity from paroxysmal behavior or nonepileptic motor events.

Therapeutic Management

The objective of treatment of convulsive disorders is to control the seizures or to reduce their frequency, discover and correct the cause when possible, and help the child who has recurrent seizures to live as normal a life as possible. Seizures of a recurrent nature are treated as soon as the diagnosis is established. If the seizure activity is a manifestation of an infectious, traumatic, or metabolic process, the seizure therapy is instituted as a part of the general therapeutic regimen.

Drug therapy. It is known that persons predisposed to epilepsy have seizures when their basal level of neuronal excitability exceeds a critical point or threshold; no attack occurs if the excitability is maintained below this threshold. The administration of anticonvulsive drugs serves to raise this threshold and prevent seizures. Consequently the primary therapy for convulsive disorders is the administration of the appropriate anticonvulsant drug or combination of drugs in a dosage that provides the desired effect without causing undesirable side effects or toxic reactions. Anticonvulsant (antiepileptic) drugs are believed to exert their effect primarily by reducing the responsiveness of normal neurons to the sudden, high-frequency nerve impulses that arise in the epileptogenic focus. Thus the convulsive seizure is effectively suppressed; the abnormal brain waves may or may not be altered. Complete control can be achieved in only 50% to 75% of epileptics, however, even with careful atten-

tion to details of therapy. The anticonvulsant, or antiepileptic, drugs used for control of seizures are outlined in Table 37-7. Some success has been achieved in treating infantile spasms with adrenocorticotropic hormone (ACTH).

Therapy is begun with a single drug known to be effective for the child's particular type of seizure, and the dosage is gradually increased until the seizures are controlled or the child develops signs of toxicity. If the drug is effective but does not sufficiently control the seizures, a second drug is added in gradually increasing doses. Once seizures are controlled, the drug or drugs are continued for a prolonged time.

Periodic reevaluation of the drug is important to assess the continued effectiveness and to alter the dosage if indicated. The dosage will need to be increased as the child grows. Blood levels often prove valuable in determination of optimum dosage levels. Blood cell counts, urinalysis, and liver function tests are obtained at frequent intervals in children receiving particular anticonvulsant medications. Repeat electroencephalograms are generally obtained every 1½ to 2 years.

When a medication is discontinued, the dosage should be reduced gradually over 1 to 2 weeks. Sudden withdrawal of a drug can cause an increase in the number and severity of seizures, often precipitating status epilepticus. If the time for reducing the medication coincides with puberty or, in younger children, occurs during periods when the child is subject to frequent infections, the drug is continued for a longer period.

Complications of drug therapy. Side effects of continued use of anticonvulsant medications are sometimes distressing to the child and the family. It is also important to be aware that phenytoin (Dilantin) causes gingival hyperplasia that can be cosmetically undesirable. Frequent gum massage and careful attention to good oral hygiene are recommended. Application of steroid cream is effective in some instances, but in severe cases of overgrowth surgical removal of excess gingiva may be required. Ataxia and rashes often disappear when drug dosages are reduced, and drowsiness from some drugs can sometimes be counteracted by judicious use of dextroamphetamine (Dexedrine). Depression, which has been reported in children with epilepsy who are taking barbiturate anticonvulsants, can be relieved by changing drugs (Ferrari, Barabas, and Matthews, 1983).

A different brand of the same medication, particularly phenytoin, may not be equivalent in composition and bioavailability; therefore if a change in the phenytoin product or dosage form is needed, serum drug levels are monitored until the therapeutic dosage is achieved (Raebel, 1983). More troublesome, however; is the accumulating evidence indicating that anticonvulsant therapy may have detrimental effects on behavior and mental function (Ellenberg and others, 1984). A statement to this effect has been issued by the Committee on Drugs of the American Academy of Pediatrics (1985), who stress that physicians prescribe the appropriate drug and be alert to reports of side effects in addition to encouraging development of screening tests of subtle in-

Table 37-7 Major drugs used for control of seizures

DRUG	COMMENTS	SIDE EFFECTS
Partial seizures and/or generalized tonic-clonic seizures		
Primary agents		
Carbamazepine (Tegretol)	Relatively free from unwanted side effects; fewer sedative properties	Side effects: blurred vision, diplopia, drowsiness, vertigo, and headache
Phenytoin (Dilantin)	Generally effective and safe May cause behavioral disturbances in children May aggravate absence and myoclonic seizures May induce folate deficiency	Side effects: gum hyperplasia, hirsutism, ataxia, nystagmus, diplopia, anorexia, nausea, nervousness
Mephenytoin	Effective anticonvulsant Regular monitoring of blood count	Side effects: rash, drowsiness, ataxia Severe toxicity: aplastic anemia; granulocytosis
Secondary agents		
Clorazepate (Tranxene)	Few side effects	Some drowsiness
Primidone* (Mysoline)	Effective with phenobarbital in mixed-type seizure patterns	Side effects: drowsiness, ataxia, diplopia
Phenobarbital (Luminal)	Safest overall drug Most useful in combination with other drugs May interfere with concentration and motor speed May cause vitamin D and folic acid deficiencies	Side effects: drowsiness, irritability, hyperactivity, skin rash, mild ataxia, hyperpyrexia
Valproic acid (Depakene)	Relatively free from unwanted effects Frequently given in association with other anticonvulsants Potentiates action of phenobarbital and phenytoin Excessively sweet taste may aggravate nausea; give with food	Side effects: anorexia, nausea, drowsiness
Ethosuximide (Zarontin)	Occasionally aggravates generalized seizures Administer with food	Side effects: nausea, gastric discomfort, anorexia, headache, drowsiness
Methsuximide (Celontin)	May induce folate deficiency	Side effects: drowsiness, nausea, headache, vertigo
Phensuximide	Less effective than others; used when others fail Slightly nephrotoxicity; monthly urinalysis	Side effects: drowsiness, headache, vertigo, nausea
Ancillary agents		
Dextroamphetamine (Dexadrine)	Given to counteract drowsiness and lethargy	
Acetozolamide (Diamox)	Given to reduce fluid accumulation	
Absence seizures		
Primary agents	Drug of choice for absences	
Ethosuximide	See above	
Valproic acid	See above	
Methsuximide	See above	
Phenobarbital	See above	
Clonazepam (Clonopin)	Usually given as adjunct to other anticonvulsants	Side effects: lethargy, ataxia, hyperactivity, agitation, nystagmus, slurred speech, rhinorrhea
Trimethadione (Tridione)	May aggravate generalized seizures Monthly blood counts and urinalysis	Side effects: rash, photophobia, nausea, irritability, drowsiness Severe toxicity: leukopenia, agranulocytosis, nephrosis

*May be used as a primary agent.

Table 37-7   Major drugs used for control of seizures—cont'd

DRUG	COMMENTS	SIDE EFFECTS
Ancillary agents	See facing page.	
Atonic, akinetic, and myoclonic seizures Combinations of agents in I and II		
Status epilepticus (convulsive)		
Diazepam (Valium)	Administer intravenously Rapid onset of action but short duration; unless followed by longer-acting anticonvulsant seizures usually recur in 20 to 30 minutes	
Lorazepam (Ativan)	Longer acting than diazepam	
Phenytoin (Dilantin)	Longer-acting drug; little additional hypnotic effect Effective in controlling tonic-clonic status	
Phenobarbital (Luminal)	Slowly absorbed by brain parenchyma; requires 10 to 20 minutes for antiepileptic effect	
Paraldehyde	Use is controversial Used if other drugs are ineffective	
General anesthesia	Used if anticonvulsants are ineffective	

tellectual and behavioral side effects and performing studies to evaluate and compare the effects of anticonvulsant therapy.

Status epilepticus. Status epilepticus is managed by supportive measures, including maintaining an adequate airway, administration of oxygen, and hydration, and by the intravenous administration of either diazepam or phenobarbital. Most physicians prefer diazepam for its dramatic effect on persistent seizures. The child must be closely monitored during administration to detect early alterations in vital signs that may indicate impending cardiac arrest or respiratory depression. When diazepam is ineffective, phenobarbital, often in extremely high levels that may require respiratory support, is given (intravenously) as the initial medication. Occasionally paraldehyde is administered (intramuscularly or rectally). Cases that do not respond to drug therapy may require the use of intravenous lidocaine, general anesthesia, or a potent skeletal muscle relaxant such as curare. This should be administered by an anesthesiologist.

Surgical therapy. When seizure activity is determined to be caused by a hematoma, tumor, or other progressive cerebral lesion, surgical removal is the treatment. When medication is unsuccessful and accumulated evidence indicates a single, distinct epileptogenic focus in a surgically removable and functionally silent area of the brain, excision of the involved tissue is sometimes considered. With children, surgery is reserved for those who suffer from repetitive, incapacitating seizures that are caused by a focal brain abnormality. Resection of the focus is done only if its removal does not result in significant loss of vital functions, such as speech and movement (Mills, 1982). Surgical excision of the epileptogenic focus does not eliminate the need for continuation of drug therapy. Drug administration is re-

started as soon as the patient regains consciousness and is continued until he is free of seizures for at least 4 years.

Nursing Considerations

Nursing care of the child with a convulsive disorder involves both acute care during a seizure and long-term management, including support of the child and the family and education of the child, family, and community regarding the disorder.

Acute care. Nurses, when they first witness a child in a generalized cerebral seizure, are often frightened, puzzled, and immobilized. These reactions are normal but can reduce the effectiveness of care for the child and interfere with observations of the event. The child must be protected from injury during the seizure, and nursing observations made during the attack provide valuable information for diagnosis and management of the disorder.

It is impossible to halt a seizure once it has begun, and no attempt should be made to do so. The nurse must remain calm, stay with the child, and prevent him from sustaining any harm during the attack. If possible, the child should be isolated from the view of others by closing a door or pulling screens around him. A seizure can be very upsetting to visitors and to other children and their families. If other persons are present, they should be assured that the affected child is in no danger, and after the attack they can be provided with a simple explanation to meet their needs.

The convulsing child should not be moved or forcefully restrained, and force should not be exerted in an attempt to place a solid object between his teeth. If the child is standing and the nurse is able to reach him in time, or if the child is seated in a chair (including a wheelchair), he should be eased to the floor immediately. After the attack the child should be placed on his side in his bed or a similar place to

Observations: The Child During a Generalized Convulsive Seizure

OBSERVE SEIZURE

Describe
- Only what is actually observed
- Order of events
- Duration of seizure

Onset
- Significant preseizure events—bright lights, noise, excitement, emotional outbursts
- Behavior
  - Change in facial expression, such as of fear
  - Cry or other sound
  - Stereotyped or automatous movements
  - Random activity
- Position of head, body, extremities
  - Unilateral or bilateral posturing of one or more extremities
  - Body deviation to side
- Time of onset

Movement
- Change of position, if any
- Site of commencement—hand, thumb, mouth, generalized
- Tonic phase, if present—length, parts of body involved
- Clonic phase—twitching or jerking movements, parts of body involved, sequence of parts involved, generalized, change in character of movements
- Lack of movement of any extremity

Face
- Color change—pallor, cyanosis, flushing
- Perspiration
- Mouth—position, deviating to one side, teeth clenched, tongue bitten, frothing at mouth, flecks of blood or bleeding

Eyes
- Position—straight ahead, deviation upward, deviation outward, conjugate or divergent
- Pupils (if able to assess)—change in size, equality, reaction to light and accommodation

Respiratory effort
- Presence and length of apnea
- Presence of stertor

Other
- Involuntary urination
- Involuntary defecation

OBSERVE POSTICTALLY

Method of termination

State of consciousness—unresponsiveness, drowsiness, confusion

Orientation to time, place, persons, and so on

Sleeping but able to be aroused

Motor ability
- Any change in motor power
- Ability to move all extremities
- Any paresis or weakness
- Ability to whistle (if appropriate to age)

Speech—changes, peculiarities, type and extent of any difficulties

Sensations
- Complaint of discomfort or pain
- Any sensory impairment of hearing, vision
- Recollection of preseizure sensations, warning of attack
- Awareness that attack was beginning

Promote rest
- Make child comfortable
- Allow child to rest after seizure
- Reduce sensory stimuli
- Record length of postictal sleep
- Notify physician if seizure is followed by other seizures in rapid succession or if duration of seizure is excessive

Reduce anxiety
- Provide calm, relaxed atmosphere

---

allow him to sleep until he awakens. If the child is at school or away from his home, the parents should be contacted so that he can be taken home to rest.

A child who is known to have convulsive attacks or one who is under observation for seizures will require special precautions. The extent of these measures will depend on the type and frequency of the seizure. The child who is subject to daily seizures should not be permitted to engage in activities in which he might be injured, such as climbing, swimming, or handling sharp implements, and most of these children are advised to wear lightweight protective helmets. Such helmets can be purchased at bicycle shops. These children should have side rails on beds with the hard surfaces padded if there is danger that they could hurt themselves.

A child who has infrequent seizures or who is relatively free of seizures will have few restrictions on his activities. When the child is hospitalized, appropriate precautions should be implemented, such as side rails kept up when the child is sleeping or resting, especially if the seizures are of the grand mal variety, since many of these children are sub-

ject to nocturnal attacks. The bed should be protected with a waterproof mattress or sheeting.

An important nursing function during a convulsion is to observe the seizure and describe its pertinent features. This includes the child's behavior before, during, and after the attack. Grand mal seizures and other seizures with dramatic manifestations are easily detected, but petit mal episodes may be more difficult to detect. They are easily misinterpreted as inattention. Any unusual behavior, even seemingly inconsequential behavior such as a momentary interruption of activity, staring, or mental blankness, should be described. The more detailed these descriptions, the more valuable they are for assessment. The nurse notes the time that the seizure began and times the length of the seizure. This is especially important if the child becomes cyanotic.

Long-term care. Care of the child with a recurrent convulsive disorder involves the physical care and instruction regarding the importance of the drug therapy and, probably more significant, the problems related to the emotional aspects of the disorder. There are few diseases that generate as much anxiety among relatives as epilepsy. Fears and misconceptions about the disease and its treatment abound in the lay person's mind. For many it represents the archetype of severe hereditary affliction. Therefore the foci of nursing care are directed toward helping the child and the family to deal with the psychologic and sociologic problems related to the disorder and to educate the child, his family, his peers, and the public in general toward a more realistic and liberal view of the disease.

Physical aspects. Children subject to seizures are placed on some type of drug therapy. The nurse can help the parents plan the administration of the medication at convenient times in order to disrupt the family routine as little as possible. Once a sufficient blood level of the drug has been achieved, the daily dosage can be given at less frequent intervals to reduce the interruptions in the parents' and the child's daily activities. This also increases the likelihood of compliance. The most convenient times for administration seem to be with meals or at bedtime. Although the anticonvulsant drugs are available in liquid extracts or emulsions, the tablet form is preferred by neurologists. The unequal distribution of the drug in the solute and the increased likelihood of inaccurate measurements make liquid medication less desirable. For small children the tablet of the proper dosage can be crushed and administered in syrup, jelly, or other palatable substances. Children taking phenobarbital and/or phenytoin should receive adequate vitamin D and folic acid, since deficiencies of both have been associated with these anticonvulsants.

It is important to impress on the family the necessity of continuing the medication regularly without interruption for as long as required. This is usually 2 to 3 years after the last seizure, at which point the drug is discontinued slowly over a period of weeks to avoid the possibility of precipitating a seizure. Planning ahead to replace a nearly empty bottle will prevent the risk of running out of the medication. It is sometimes easy to skip doses or omit them for any of a variety of reasons, especially when the child is free of seizures most of the time. This is particularly so when the child is older and assumes the responsibility for his medication. Omitting medication is the most frequent cause of status epilepticus.

The parents and the child will need to know the side effects of the drug prescribed. They should understand the common side effects so that they can report any unusual observations that might indicate unfavorable reactions. These should be known in detail. Parents should understand that the child needs periodic physical assessment and laboratory studies if he is taking phenytoin, primidone, ethosuximide, or methsuximide. Possible adverse effects on the hematopoietic system, liver, and kidneys may be reflected in symptoms such as fever, sore throat, enlarged lymph nodes, jaundice, and bleeding manifestations such as easy bruising, petechiae, ecchymoses, and epistaxis.

Parents need to be warned of possible behavioral changes as the convulsions are controlled in children taking primi-

---

Emergency Treatment: *Seizure*

Do not attempt to restrain child or use force
Protect child during seizure
If child is standing or sitting in wheelchair at beginning of attack, ease child down so that he will not fall; when possible, place cushion or blanket under child
Do not put anything in child's mouth
Loosen restrictive clothing
Prevent child from hitting hard or sharp objects that might cause injury during uncontrolled movements
Remove object(s)
Pad object(s)
Move furniture out of way
Allow seizure to end without interference
When seizure has stopped, check for breathing
If not present, use mouth-to-mouth resuscitation
Check around mouth for evidence of burns or suspicious substances that might indicate poisoning
Remain with child
When child is able to move, seek help

---

done, phenobarbital, or phenytoin. Changes in personality, indifference to school activities and family, hyperactivity, or even psychotic behavior may sometimes be observed.

The degree to which activities are restricted is individualized for each child and depends on the type, frequency, and severity of the seizures, the child's response to therapy, and the length of time the seizures have been controlled. Normal healthy activities are encouraged for children, and participation in competitive sports is determined on an individual basis. With encouragement most older children can accept the restrictions placed on activities. Contact sports such as football, karate, or wrestling are to be avoided, but basketball, baseball, and tennis are allowed. Climbing trees or apparatuses from which the child might fall and be seriously injured is not usually permitted. The well-controlled epileptic child can ride a bicycle or swim if accompanied by a companion.

Because the child is encouraged to attend school, camp, and other normal activities, the school nurse and the teacher should be made aware of the child's condition and his therapy. They can help to ensure regularity of medication and any special care the child might need. The child's teacher should be instructed regarding care of the child during a seizure so that he or she can act in a calm manner for the welfare of the child and to influence the attitude of the child's classmates.

Parents of the epileptic child. Parental attitudes and management of a child with a convulsive disorder are as varied as those of other parents of children with a chronic disorder, and they are subject to the same long-term problems (see Chapter 22). Whether the seizures result from illness, injury, or unknown etiology, the parents may feel guilt, anxiety, and often humiliation. In the past, epilepsy has had a derogatory connotation. The parents want to know if it will affect the child's mental capacities. To many persons epilepsy is erroneously associated with mental deficiency. Seizures do frequently accompany other manifestations of severe brain damage from disease or injury, but the majority of children with seizures, like any population of healthy children, display a wide range of intelligence.

Parents also wonder how the illness will affect the child's future and need reassurance that the illness will not shorten the life of the child and that he can attend school, marry, and have the right to elect to have children. The child will need vocational guidance, and the parents will need to become familiar with the laws in their state regarding any limitations that might be imposed on the child because of the disorder. It should be emphasized that the seizures can be controlled or greatly reduced in the large majority of affected children and that new studies hold the promise of progress in treatment in the future. Parents need reassurance that in this enlightened day and age there is less stigma attached to the disease than there has been in the past.

It is important to encourage a healthy attitude toward the child and his disease and to help the parents feel competent in their ability to meet their responsibilities to the child. The child should be reared as any normal child with natural concern tempered by the understanding of his need not to be overprotected. Many parents refrain from correcting or punishing the child, especially if they have had the experience of such an emotional stress precipitating an attack. The child must not be made to feel that he is different. Parents should be encouraged to be honest and open about the disorder with the child and to others. Some parents are tempted to try to conceal the nature of the child's illness because of their belief that the disorder is shameful or a disgrace to the family.

Restrictions on the child's activities will be necessary for safety, but this area can be approached in a positive way in terms of what the child *can* do rather than what he cannot do. Sometimes parents curtail the child's activities more than necessary. The child needs to experience the maturing influences of play and work. The **Epilepsy Foundation of America***is a national organization that works toward and for the welfare of epileptic persons and their families, helps with employment and legal problems, and provides education to patients, families, and communities.

The epileptic child. The child who is provided the security of a loving family, rewards and punishments no different from those of other children, and support in acquiring self-esteem is more apt to have a positive attitude toward his disease. Development of normal emotional maturity is inhibited by parental overprotection, indulgence, and restrictions. Maladaptation and a negative self-image are stimulated by peer and family rejection, embarrassment and humiliation, teasing by playmates, and social segregation.

The child derives his self-concept and self-esteem from his observations of others' reactions to him and his own perception of his capabilities. When others consider the child to be different, inferior, or an object of ridicule, he comes to view himself as different, inferior, and incapable. The child may become frustrated because his activities are limited or because he is excluded from activities in which he feels capable of participating but is segregated from them by others, including his family. Such children are encouraged in dependency.

Behavioral problems are common in children with epilepsy and can become a more serious problem than the seizures. Much of the behavior difficulty, especially aggressive or delinquent behaviors, has been attributed to the child's reaction to parental rejection. Feelings of guilt, frustration, depression, and self-negation can contribute to antisocial behaviors.

The suddenness and unpredictability of the attacks and the reactions of others further influence his feelings. The child needs to learn about his disease and the role that the medication plays in contributing to his prolonged wellbeing. As soon as he is old enough, the child should assume responsibility for taking his own medication. He should be advised to carry a card or a Medic Alert bracelet with pertinent information about his condition. Planning activities with the child and emphasizing those in which he can engage rather than those in which he cannot participate help the child to succeed and to gain satisfaction in his achievements. The child should be offered opportunities and encouraged to exercise judgment in his daily life.

The adolescent period may prove to be a trying time for the epileptic child. The normal changes and emotional responses may be confused with symptoms of the disease. Normal rebellious attitudes and behavior may cause the more insecure adolescent, angry at being different, to stop taking medication. Sudden withdrawal of the drug together with the accelerated metabolic needs and the increased stress of this period of life will often cause a resumption of, or an increase in, seizures. Normally the adolescent with a convulsive disorder will need his dosage increased to meet the new growth needs. Limits imposed on the young person's activities at a time when he desires freedom and independence may bring his handicap into sharp focus. For example, some states do not allow epileptic persons to obtain a driver's license, even when the disease is controlled; in others there are restrictions on employment, insurance, and, in a few isolated instances, a marriage license.

Epilepsy should not be a severe handicap to most youngsters, and the nurse, by assuming the role of patient advocate, helping to educate the public regarding the disease, working toward making opportunities available to persons with the disorder, and lobbying for legislation that recognizes the needs of the individual with a seizure disorder, can help to erase the stigma that still remains regarding the disease.

*4351 Garden City Dr., Landover, MD 20785.

Nursing Care Summary: The Child with a Convulsive Disorder

NURSING GOALS	NURSING INTERVENTIONS	EXPECTED PATIENT/FAMILY OUTCOMES
HP-HMP Injury: potential for trauma **Risk factors: subject to sudden seizure**		
Protect from injury during seizure	See emergency treatment: seizure Educate parents and child regarding appropriate activities for child Age-appropriate Avoid contact sports Avoid situations that pose danger during a seizure (climbing trees, play apparatus) Provide companionship during permissible activities such as swimming, bicycling Educate teachers and other persons associated with child regarding correct behavior during a seizure Encourage wearing of light-weight helment (seizures not well controlled)	Child exhibits no evidence of physical injury Child wears helmet
Prevent seizures	Emphasize importance of compliance with anticonvulsant medications Avoid situations known to precipitate a seizure (e.g., blinking lights, emotional stress, video games)	Child takes medication as prescribed Child remains free of seizure activity
Prevent complications from medication	Be aware of and teach family to recognize unfavorable reactions to medications Encourage periodic physical and laboratory assessment to determine possible deviations from normal findings	Child and family demonstrate understanding of possible unfavorable responses to medications and appropriate intervention (specify)
SP-SCP Self-concept, disturbance in: body image, self-esteem, personal identity **Etiology: perception of disability (self and others)**		
Develop a positive self-concept	Encourage child to express feelings and concerns about the disease and its implications Encourage child to discuss how he thinks others feel about his disorder Help child assess his strengths and assets Emphasize strengths Help child set realistic goals	Child expresses feelings and concerns Child describes his strengths Child expresses realistic expectations
RRP Family process, alteration in **Etiology: situational crisis (birth of a child with a chronic illness)**		
Support parents	Allow for expression of feelings regarding child's disorder and its ramifications Refer to organizations such as the Epilepsy Foundation of America for assistance and education Be available to families	Family expresses feelings and concerns Family contacts agency(ies)
Understand the disease	Assist family in understanding the disorder, its therapies, and possible implications Help family to achieve realistic view of child and his capabilities	Family demonstrates understanding of the disorder, its therapy, and implications
Prepare family for home management	Teach family the administration of medications Stress importance of complying with therapeutic regimen Teach seizure prevention and management	Family complies with instructions; child is seizure-free Family demonstrates proper management of child during a seizure (specify means of demonstration)

Continued.

Nursing Interventions Related to Medical Management

Assist with diagnosis
Prepare child and family for diagnostic procedures
Assist with diagnostic tests
Observe and accurately describe child's behavior before, during, and after a seizure (see box, p. 1666)

Control seizure activity
Administer anticonvulsants

FEBRILE SEIZURES

Febrile convulsions are transient disorders of children that occur in association with a fever. They are one of the most common neurologic disorders of childhood, affecting 3% to 5% of children. Most febrile convulsions occur after 6 months of age and usually before age 3 years, with increased frequency in children younger than 18 months. They are unusual after 5 years of age. Boys are affected about twice as often as girls, and there appears to be an increased susceptibility in families, indicating a possible genetic predisposition.

The cause of febrile seizures is still uncertain. In most children the height and rapidity of the temperature elevation seem to be factors. The fever usually exceeds 38.8° C (101.8° F) and occurs during the temperature rise rather than after a prolonged elevation. Sometimes it constitutes the dramatic beginning of an illness. Febrile seizures usually accompany an upper respiratory or gastrointestinal infection, and 25% of children with simple febrile seizures have a recurrence of the seizure with subsequent infections. Since fevers are almost impossible to prevent in children, efforts are directed toward preventing an increase in the temperature.

Treatment consists of controlling the seizure with phenobarbital or diazepam (Valium) in appropriate dosage, reducing the temperature by administration of aspirin or acetaminophen (Tylenol). Whether or not to implement continuous prophylactic anticonvulsant therapy in children who have experienced their initial febrile convulsion is still controversial. At present, anticonvulsant therapy is recommended for those children with febrile seizures who are at increased risk for developing sequelae.

In children who exhibit febrile seizures, there is an increased risk of epilepsy with the increase in the number of seizures. As the number of seizures increases, the severity of the seizures also increases. The chance of developing chronic seizure disorder is increased in children who have a prolonged convulsion, those with focal seizures, those who have a near relative who experiences convulsions, and those with an abnormal electroencephalogram. Recurrences are more likely when the first seizure occurs in the first year of life. Seventy-five percent of recurrences take place within 1 year of the first febrile seizure and almost 90% within 2 years of onset.

BREATH-HOLDING SPELLS

Breath-holding spells (reflex hypoxic crisis) are readily recognized and follow a distinct clinical pattern. Not a true convulsive disorder, the typical attack has its onset in infants between the ages of 6 and 18 months and may occur up to 4 years of age. The episode is characterized by violent crying and cessation of breathing that is precipitated by fright, frustration, or anger. The breath is usually held on expiration, and the child becomes cyanotic, loses consciousness, and may display a few clonic convulsions of the extremities. The episode ends with a gasp and the color returns promptly. The frequency of attacks varies considerably, but they almost always disappear by 5 to 6 years of age.

Breath-holding spells are a benign entity, and drug therapy is generally not indicated. Family therapy may be beneficial, since many children appear to use an attack or the threat of an attack to assert themselves and to express anger. Parents need reassurance that the attacks do not represent a danger to the child, and this knowledge may even help to decrease or eliminate the incidence of attacks.

MIGRAINE

Migraine is the most common paroxysmal disorder that affects the brain. It is characterized by chronic recurrent headache, often preceded by visual disturbances and accompanied by nausea and vomiting. The cause is unknown, although attacks may be precipitated by stress, fatigue, stroboscopic stimulation, anxiety, conflict, or certain foods. Emotional factors may play a part.

There are two phases in the pathologic development of migraine, both caused by a functional disturbance of intracerebral circulation. Initially there is a prodromal phase caused by vasoconstriction of intracranial vessels followed by dilation of the extracranial vessels, which produces a throbbing, pulsating, and pounding headache.

A family history of migraine is elicited in over 50% of the patients, and some observers have noted that children often display a characteristic personality. They tend to be meticulous, compulsive, unusually mature for their age, and high achievers in school and strive to please the family at home. They have difficulty in expressing anger or rage. Boys are affected twice as often as girls.

The diagnosis is seldom made until the child is old enough to relate his symptoms, although one in five children has his first attack before age 5 years. Early in life the symptoms are nonspecific, such as recurrent abdominal pain, car sickness, and restlessness, and the child may display head-banging or sudden alterations in personality. The typical attack of migraine begins early in the day, often awakening the child. The prodromal symptoms, induced by vasoconstriction, consist of transient visual disturbances or other neurologic disabilities. In a few minutes or sometimes a few hours, the aura is followed by throbbing unilateral head pain accompanied by nausea and vomiting. Sleep ordinarily terminates an attack.

Treatment is symptomatic. For most patients the vasoconstrictor ergotamine tartrate taken at the onset of symptoms provides relief. Simple analgesics such as aspirin or acetaminophen may be effective and are usually the preferred medication. The outlook for the child with migraine is good, but the child and his parents should be informed that the predisposition to the headaches is lifelong, although benign, and should not interfere with normal activities.

- Encephalitis may result from direct invasion of the CNS by a virus or from postinfectious involvement of the CNS after viral disease.

- There has been a strong association between ingestion of aspirin during prodromal illness and Reye syndrome.

- Seizure disorders may exhibit sensory-hallucinatory phenomena, motor effects, sensorimotor effects, and loss of consciousness.

- Partial seizures are categorized as simple, with associated impairment of consciousness and those with impaired consciousness and that spread to become generalized.

- Generalized seizures are categorized as tonic-clonic, absence, atonic and akinetic, myoclonic, and infantile spasms.

- Long-term care of the child with recurrent convulsive disorders includes physical care and education regarding the importance of drug therapy and problems related to emotional aspects of the disorder.

CONCEPT SUMMARIES

- The nervous system is composed of the central nervous system, peripheral nervous system, and autonomic nervous system.

- Gait abnormalities that may indicate cerebral dysfunction include ataxia, spastic paraplegic gait, spastic hemiplegic gait, cerebellar gait, and extrapyramidal gait.

- Levels of consciousness include sleep, confusion, delirium, pseudo-wakeful states, and comatose states.

- Complete neurologic examination takes into account vital signs, posture and movement, eye examination, and reflex testing.

- Nursing care of the unconscious child focuses on respiratory management, neurologic assessment, increased intracranial pressure monitoring, supplying adequate nutrition and hydration, drug therapy, promoting elimination, hygienic care, positioning and exercise, stimulation, and family support.

- Fractures resulting from head injuries may be classified as depressed, compound, basilar, and diastatic.

- Complications of head trauma include epidural and subdural hemorrhage, cerebral edema, posttraumatic syndromes, and infections.

- Problems resulting from near-drowning include hypoxia and asphyxiation, aspiration, and hypothermia.

- Nursing care of the child with meningitis includes administration of antibiotics, prevention of self-infection, removal of environmental stimuli, correct positioning, vital signs monitoring, IV therapy, and promoting fluid and nutritional status.

REFERENCES

Barrett, M.J., and others: Changing epidemiology of Reye syndrome in the United States, Pediatrics **77:**598-602, 1986.

Bell, W.E., and others: Infections of the brain and spinal cord. In Swaiman, K.F., and Wright, F.S.: The practice of pediatric neurology, ed. 2, St. Louis, 1982, The C.V. Mosby Co.

Boll, T.: Minor head injury in children, out of sight but not out of mind, J. Clin. Child Psychol. **12:**74-80, 1985.

Bruce, D.A.: Delayed deterioration of consciousness after trivial head injury in children, Brit. Med. J. **289:**715-716, 1984.

Committee on Drugs, American Academy of Pediatrics: Behavioral and cognitive effects of anticonvulsant therapy, Pediatrics **76:**644-647, 1985.

Committee on Infectious Diseases, American Academy of Pediatrics: Aspirin and Reye syndrome, Pediatrics **69:**810-812, 1982.

Conn, A.W., Edmonds, J.F., and Barker, G.A.: Cerebral resuscitation in near-drowning, Pediatr. Clin. North Am. **26:**691-701, 1979.

De Vivo, D.C., and Dodge, P.R.: Diagnosis and management of head injury. In Smith, C.A., editor, The critically ill child, ed. 3, Philadelphia, 1985, W.B. Saunders Co.

Eiben, C.F., and others: Functional outcome of closed head injury in children and young adults, Arch. Phys. Med. Rehabil. **65:**168-170, 1984.

Ellenberg, J.H., Hirtz, D.G., and Nelson, K.B.: Age at onset of seizures in young children, Ann. Neurol. **15:**127-134, 1984.

Feigin, R.D., and Neglia, J.P.: Bacterial meningitis and septicemia beyond the neonatal period. In Gellis, S.S., and Kagan, B.M.: Current pediatric therapy 12, Philadelphia, 1986, W.B. Saunders Co.

Ferrari, M., Barabas, G., and Matthews, W.: Psychologic and behavioral disturbance among epileptic children treated with barbiturate anticonvulsants, Am. J. Psychiatry **140:**112-113, 1983.

Hill, J.C.: Summary of a workshop on *Haemophilus influenzae* type B vaccines, J. Infect. Dis. **148:**167-175, 1983.

Hurwitz, E.S., and others: Public Health Service study on Reye's syndrome and medications, N. Engl. J. Med. **313:**849-857, 1985.

Jacobson, M.S., and others: Follow-up of adolescent trauma victims: a new model of care, Pediatrics **77:**236-241, 1986.

Krugman, S., and others: Infectious diseases of children, ed. 8, St. Louis, 1985, The C.V. Mosby Co.

Mahoney, W.J., and others: Long-term outcome of children with severe head trauma and prolonged coma, Pediatrics **71**:756-762, 1983.

Millikan, C.H.: Evaluating depth of consciousness, Patient Care **15**(16):127-141, 1981.

Mills, M.: When a child has surgery for focal epilepsy, J. Maternal Child Nurs. **7**:304-308, 1982.

Mizrahi, E.M., and Dorfman, L.J.: Sensory evoked potentials: clinical applications in pediatrics, J. Pediatr. **97**:1-5, 1980.

Monroe, B.: Immersion accidents in hot tubs and whirlpool spas, Pediatrics **69**:805-807, 1982.

Morbidity and Mortality Weekly Report **31**:592-593, 1982.

Morriss, F.C., and Cook, J.D.: Increased intracranial pressure. In Levin, D.L., Morriss, F.C., and Moore, G.C., editors: A practical guide to pediatric intensive care, ed. 2, St. Louis, 1984, The C.V. Mosby Co.

Mueller, S.M., and others: Vascular diseases of the brain and spinal cord. In Swaiman, K.F., and Wright, F.S.: The practice of pediatric neurology, ed. 2, vol. 2, St. Louis, 1982, The C.V. Mosby Co.

Raebel, M.: Nonequivalence of phenytoin capsules and tablets, N. Engl. J. Med. **309**:925, 1983.

Remington, P.L., and others: Decreasing trends in Reye syndrome and aspirin use in Michigan, 1979 to 1984, Pediatrics **77**:93-98, 1986.

Restak, R.M.: The brain, New York, 1984, Bantam Books.

Rutter, M.: Psychological sequelae of brain damage in children, Am. J. Psychiatry **138**:1533-1544, 1981.

Scott, P.H., and Eigen, H.: Immersion accidents involving pails of water in the home, J. Pediatr. **96**:282-284, 1980.

Smith, S.L.: Continuous intracranial pressure monitoring: implications and applications for critical care, Crit. Care Nurse **3**(4):42-51, 1983.

Spyker, D.A.: Submersion injury: epidemiology, prevention, and management, Pediatr. Clin. North Am. **32**:113-125, 1985.

Strauss, R.H.: Brain abscess. In Gellis, S.S., and Kagan, B.M.: Current pediatric therapy 12, Philadelphia, 1986, W.B. Saunders Co.

Tron, V.A., Baldwin, V.J., and Price, G.E.: Hot tub drownings, Pediatrics **75**:789-790, 1985.

Weeks, H.: What every ICU nurse should know about Reye's syndrome, Am. J. Maternal Child Nurs. **1**:231-238, 1976.

Wilson, J.T., and Brown, R.D.: Reye syndrome and aspirin use: the role of prodromal illness severity in the assessment of relative risk, Pediatrics **69**:822-825, 1982.

Yogev, R.: Advances in diagnosis and treatment of childhood meningitis, Pediatr. Infect. Dis. **4**:321-325, 1985.

BIBLIOGRAPHY
General

Coffey, R.J.: Pediatric neurological emergencies. In Pierog, J.E., and Pierog, L.J., editors: Pediatric critical illness and injury, Rockville, MD, 1984, Aspen Systems Corporation.

Conway, B.L.: Carini and Owens' neurological and neurosurgical nursing, ed. 8, St. Louis, 1982, The C.V. Mosby Co.

Gever, L.N.: Mannitol: the osmotic diuretic of choice, Nursing 85 **15**(7):64, 1985.

Hicks, D.A.: Cerebral edema. In Pierog, J.E., and Pierog, L.J., editors: Pediatric critical illness and injury, Rockville, MD, 1984, Aspen Systems Corporation.

James, H.E.: Neurologic evaluation and support in the child with an acute brain insult, Pediatr. Ann. **15**:16-22, 1986.

Mauss-Clum, N.: Bringing the unconscious patient back safely: nursing makes the critcal difference, Nursing 82 **12**(8):34-42, 1982.

Rimar, J.M.: Pancuronium bromide, J. Maternal Child Nurs. **10**:65, 1985.

Scherer, P.: Assessment: the logic of coma, Am. J. Nurs. **86**:541-550, 1986.

Stolarik, A.: What the comatose patient can tell you, RN **48**(4):26-33, 1985.

Diagnostic Procedures

Engler, M.B., and Engler, M.M.: The hazards of magnetic resonance imaging, Am. J. Nurs. **86**:650, 1986.

Ferry, P.C.: Computed cranial tomography in children, J. Pediatr. **96**:961-967, 1980.

Gooding, C.A., and others: Nuclear magnetic resonance imaging of the brain in children, J. Pediatr. **104**:509-515, 1984.

Hanigan, W.C., Wright, S.M., and Wright, R.M.: Clinical utility of magnetic resonance imaging in pediatric neurosurgical patients, J. Pediatr. **108**:522-529, 1986.

Hershey, B.L., and Zimmerman, R.A.: Pediatric brain computed tomography, Pediatr. Clin. North Am. **32**:1477-1508, 1985.

Jackson, P.L.: Assessing increased intracranial pressure in infants and young children, Crit. Care Update **10**(9):8-15, 1983.

King, R.C.: Checking the patient's neurological status, RN **45**(12):57-632, 1982.

Leonard, J.C., and others: Nuclear magnetic resonance: an overview of its spectroscopic and imaging applications in pediatric patients, J. Pediatr. **106**:757-761, 1985.

Marchette, L., and Holloman, F.: A first-hand report on the new body scanners, RN **48**(11):28-31, 1985.

McManus, J.C., and Hausman, K.A.: Deciphering diagnostic studies: cerebrospinal fluid analysis, Nursing 82 **12**(8):43-47, 1982.

Mills, G.C.: Preparing children and parents for cerebral computed tomography, Am. J. Maternal Child Nurs. **5**:403-407, 1980.

Mizrahi, E.M., and Kellaway, P.: Cerebral concussion in children: assessment of injury by electroencephalography, Pediatrics **73**:419-425, 1984.

Slota, M.C.: Neurological assessment of the infant and toddler, Crit. Care Nurse **3**(5):87-92, 1983.

Slota, M.C.: Pediatric neurological assessment, Crit. Care Nurse **3**(6):106-112, 1983.

Increased Intracranial Pressure

Boortz-Marx, R.: Factors affecting intracranial pressure: a descriptive study, J. Neurosurg. Nurs. **17**:89-94, 1985.

Burgess, K.A.: Increased I.C.P., NursingLife **5**(2):33-48, 1985.

Committee on Drugs, Section on Anesthesiology: Guidelines for the elective use of conscious sedation, deep sedation, and general anesthesia in pediatric patients, Pediatrics **77**:754, 1986.

Hausman, K.A.: Critical care of the child with increased intracranial pressure, Nurs. Clin. North Am. **16**:647-656, 1981.

Hinkle, J.L.: Treating traumatic coma, Am. J. Nurs. **86**:551-556, 1986.

Jackson, P.L.: Increased intracranial pressure in infants and young children, Crit. Care Q. **3**:47-59, 1981.

Kaktis, J.V.: An introduction to monitoring intracranial pressure in critically ill children. In Pierog, J.E., and Pierog, L.J., editors: Pediatric critical illness and injury, Rockville, MD, 1984, Aspen Systems Corporation.

McNamara, M., and Quinn, C.: Epidural intracranial pressure monitoring: theory and clinical application, J. Neurosurg. Med. **13**:267-281, 1981.

Mitchell, P.H.: Intracranial hypertension: implications of research for nursing care, J. Neurosurg. Nurs. **12**:145-154, 1980.

Mitchell, P.H., Ozuna, J., and Lipe, H.P.: Moving the patient in bed: effects on intracranial pressure, Nurs. Research **30**:212-218, 1981.

Robinet, K.: Increased intracranial pressure: management with an intraventricular catheter, J. Neurosurg. Nurs. **17**:95-104, 1985.

Stuart, G.G., and others: Severe head injury managed without intracranial pressure monitoring, J. Neurosurg. **59**:601-605, 1983.

Brain Death

Elliott, J., and Smith, D.R.: Meeting family needs following severe head injury: a multidisciplinary approach, J. Neurosurg. Nurs. **17**:111-113, 1985.

Joynt, R.J.: A new look at death, JAMA **252**:680-682, 1984.

Murphy, P.: When a non-death death occurs, Nursing 86 **16**(7):34-39, 1986.

Outwater, K., and Rockoff, M.: Apnea testing to confirm brain death in children, Crit. Care Med. **12**:357-358, 1984.

Rowland, T.W., Donnelly, J.H., and Jackson, A.H.: Apnea documentation for determination of brain death in children, Pediatrics **74**:505-508, 1984.

Head Injury

Billmire, M.E., and Myers, P.A.: Serious head injury in infants: accident or abuse? Pediatrics **75**:340-342, 1985.

Bowers, S.A., and Marshall, L.F.: Severe head injury: current treatment and research, J. Neurosurg. Nurs. **14**:210-218, 1982.

Brink, J.D., Imbus, C., and Woo-Sam, J.: Physical recovery after severe closed head trauma in children and adolescents, J. Pediatr. **97**:721-727, 1980.

Dershewitz, R.A., Kaye, B.A., and Swisher, C.N.: Treatment of children with posttraumatic transient loss of consciousness, Pediatrics **72**:602-607, 1983.

Hahn, J.F.: Cerebral edema and neurointensive care, Pediatr. Clin. North Am. **27**:587-592, 1980.

Lipe, H.P.: Prevention of nervous system trauma from travel in motor vehicles, J. Neurosurg. Nurs. **17**:77-82, 1985.

Meier, E.M.: Evaluating head trauma in infants and children, J. Maternal Child Nurs. **8**:54-57, 1983.

Mirr, M.P., Jankowski, K., and Taylon, M.A.: Nursing management for barbiturate therapy in acute head injuries, Heart Lung **12**:52-59, 1983.

Spielman, G.: Metabolic complications associated with severe diffuse brain injury, J. Neurosurg. Nurs. **17**:83-88, 1985.

Stevens, M.: Post-concussion syndrome, J. Neurosurg. Nurs. **14**:239-244, 1982.

Near-Drowning

Blauer, R.E.: Emergency: dealing with drownings ... you can help keep the near-drowning victim alive, RN **48**(5):41-42, 1985.

Frewen, T.C., and others: Cerebral resuscitation therapy in pediatric near-drowning, J. Pediatr. **106**:615-617, 1985.

Laughlin, J.J., and Eigen, H.: Pulmonary function abnormalities in survivors of near drowning, J. Pediatr. **100**:26-30, 1982.

Moore, G.C.: Near-drowning. In Levin, D.L., Morriss, F.C., and Moore, G.C., editors: A practical guide to pediatric intensive care, ed. 2, St. Louis, 1984, The C.V. Mosby Co.

Pearn, J.: Drowning. In Dickerman, J.D., and Lucey, J.F.: The critically ill child: diagnosis and management, ed. 3, Philadelphia, 1985, W.B. Saunders Co.

Rogers, M.C.: Near-drowning: cold water or a hot topic? J. Pediatr. **106**:603-604, 1985.

Stickler, J.F., and Shawman, T.: A child drowns: a nursing perspective, Am. J. Maternal Child Nurs. **6**:324-328, 1981.

Intracranial Infections

Devriendt, J., and others: Fatal encephalitis apparently due to rabies. Occurrence after treatment with human diploid cell vaccine but not rabies immune globulin, JAMA **248**:2304-2306, 1982.

Edwards, M.S., and Baker, C.J.: Complications and sequelae of meningococcal infections in children, J. Pediatr. **99**:540-545, 1981.

Edwards, M.S., and others: Long-term sequelae of group B streptococcal meningitis in infants, J. Pediatr. **106**:717-722, 1985.

Ferguson, C.K., and Roll, L.J.: Human rabies, Am. J. Nurs. **81**:1175-1179, 1981.

Ferguson, C.K., and Roll, L.J.: Rabies in humans, Crit. Care Nurs. **10**(7):11-16, 1983.

Goitein, K.J., and Tamir, I.: Cerebral perfusion pressure in central nervous system infections of infancy and childhood, J. Pediatr. **103**:40-43, 1983.

Gray, B.M., and others: Quantitative levels of C-reactive protein in cerebrospinal fluid in patients with bacterial meningitis and other conditions, J. Pediatr. **108**:665-670, 1986.

Hieber, J.P.: Encephalitis/meningitis. In Levin, D.L., Morriss, F.C., and Moore, G.C., editors: A practical guide to pediatric intensive care, ed. 2, St. Louis, 1984, The C.V. Mosby Co.

Immunization Practices Advisory Committee: Rabies prevention, Morbid. Mortal. Weekly Rep. **29**:278, 1980.

Jadavji, T., Humphreys, R.P., and Prober, C.G.: Brain abscesses in infants and children, Pediatr. Infect. Dis. **4**:394-398, 1985.

Kaplan, S.L., and Feigin, R.D.: Treatment of meningitis in children, Pediatr. Clin. North Am. **30**:259-269, 1983.

Kaplan, S.L., and others: Onset of hearing loss in children with bacterial meningitis, Pediatrics **73**:575-578, 1984.

Nebens, I.A., and Jackson, B.S.: A case of acute fulminating meningococcemia, Am. J. Nurs. **82**:1390-1393, 1982.

Plotkin, S.A.: New rabies vaccine (commentary), Pediatrics **68**:131-132, 1981.

Rimar, J.M., and Goschke, B.: Fulminant meningococcemia in children, Heart Lung **14**:385-390, 1985.

Sell, S.H.: Long term sequelae of bacterial meningitis in children, Pediatr. Infect. Dis. **2**:90-93, 1983.

Taylor, H.G., and others: Intellectual, neuropsychological, and achievement outcomes in children six to eight years after recovery from *Haemophilus influenzae* meningitis, Pediatrics **74**:198-205, 1984.

Wald, E.R., and others: Long-term outcome of group B streptococcal meningitis, Pediatrics **77**:217-221, 1986.

Wink, D.: Bacterial meningitis in children, Am. J. Nurs. **84**:456-460, 1984.

Yogev, R.: Cerebrospinal fluid shunt infections: a personal view, Pediatr. Infect. Dis. **4**:113-118, 1985.

Reye Syndrome

Belkengren, R.P., and Sapala, S.: Reye syndrome: clinical guidelines for practitioners in ambulatory care, Pediatr. Nurs. **7**(2):26-28, 1981.

Boutros, A.R., and others: Reye syndrome: a predictably curable disease, Pediatr. Clin. North Am. **27**:539-552, 1980.

Budd, R.A., and Rothwell, R.: Spotting Reye's syndrome while there's still time, RN **46**(12):38-42, 1983.

Dalgas, P.: Reye's syndrome update, J. Maternal Child Nurs. **8**:345-349, 1983.

El-Mallakh, R.S.: Temperature, mitochondria, and Reye's syndrome (letter), Pediatrics **71**:985, 1983.

Hansen, J.R., and others: Reye syndrome associated with aspirin therapy for systemic lupus erythematosis, Pediatrics **76**:202-205, 1985.

Lopez, T., Oleri, L., and Redican, W.: Reye's syndrome: a review of research studies, J. Sch. Health **52**:206-210, 1982.

Martelli, M.E.: Teaching parents about Reye's syndrome, Am. J. Nurs. **82**:260-263, 1982.

Miller, J., and Arsenault, L.: Reye's syndrome, Neurosurg. Nurs. **15**(3):154-164, 1983.

Reitman, M.A., and others: Motor disorders of voice and speech in Reye's syndrome survivors, Am. J. Dis. Child. **138**:1129-1131, 1984.

Rennebohm, R.M., and others: Reye syndrome in children receiving salicylate therapy for connective tissue disease, J. Pediatr. **107**:877-880, 1985.

Rogers, M.F., and others: National Reye syndrome surveillance, 1982, Pediatrics **75**:260-264, 1985.

Sullivan-Boylai, J., and others: Reye syndrome in children less than 1 year old: some epidemiologic observations, Pediatrics **65**:627, 1980.

Seizure Disorders

Anas, N.G., and others: Ventilatory chemosensitivity in subjects with a history of childhood cyanotic breath-holding spells, Pediatrics **75**:76-79, 1985.

Austin, J.K., McBride, A.B., and Davis, H.W.: Parental attitude and adjustment to childhood epilepsy, Nurs. Res. **33:**92-96, 1984.

Baumer, J.H., and others: Many parents think their child is dying when having a first febrile convulsion, Dev. Med. Child Neurol. **23:**462-464, 1981.

Coulter, D.L.: The psychosocial impact of epilepsy in childhood, Child. Health Care **11:**48-53, 1982.

Dahlquist, N.R., Mellinger, J.F., and Klass, D.W.: Hazard of video games in patients with light-sensitive epilepsy, JAMA **249:**776-777, 1983.

Daneshmend, T.K., and Campbell, M.J.: Dark Warrior epilepsy, Br. Med. J. **284:**1751-1752, 1982.

Emerson, R., and others: Stopping medication in children with epilepsy, N. Engl. J. Med. **304:**19, 1981.

Gever, L.N.: Anticonvulsants, Nursing 84 **14:**41, 1984.

Holmes, G.L.: Partial seizures in children, Pediatrics **77:**725-731, 1986.

Knudsen, F.U.: Effective short-term diazepam prophylaxis in febrile convulsions, J. Pediatr. **106:**487-490, 1985.

Lerman, P., and Kivity, S.: The efficacy of corticotropin in primary infantile spasms, J. Pediatr. **101:**294-296, 1982.

McGrath, D.M.: Nursing management of the child in status epilepticus, Issues Compr. Pediatr. Nurs. **5:**273-277, 1981.

McGrath, D.M.: Video recording seizure activity in children, J. Maternal Child Nurs. **8:**218-220, 1983.

McLain, L.W., Martin, J.T., and Allen, J.H.: Cerebellar degeneration due to chronic phenytoin therapy, Ann. Neurol. **7:**18-25, 1980.

Mizrahi, E.M.: Electroencephalographic/polygraphic/video monitoring in childhood epilepsy, J. Pediatr. **105:**1-9, 1984.

Morriss, F.C., and Cook, J.D.: Status epilepticus. In Levin, D.L., Morriss, F.C., and Moore, G.C., editors: A practical guide to pediatric intensive care, ed. 2, St. Louis, 1984, The C.V. Mosby Co.

Muehl, J.N.: Seizure disorders in children: prevention and care, Am. J. Maternal Child Nurs. **4:**154-160, 1979.

Norman, S.E.: Surgical treatment of epilepsy, Am. J. Nurs. **81:**994-996, 1981.

Norman, S.E., and Browne, T.R.: Seizure disorders, Am. J. Nurs. **81:**985-994, 1981.

Ojemann, L.M., and Ojemann, G.A.: Treatment of epilepsy, Am. Fam. Physician **30**(2):113-128, 1984.

O'Neill, S.: Dealing with seizures, RN **47**(9):39-41, 1984.

Parrish, M.A.: A comparison of behavioral side effects related to commonly used anticonvulsants, Pediatr. Nurs. **10:**149-152, 1984.

Rothner, A.D., and Erenberg, G.: Status epilepticus, Pediatr. Clin. North Am. **27:**593-602, 1980.

Santilli, N., and Tonelson, S.: Screening for seizures, Pediatr. Nurs. **7**(2):11-15, 1981.

Sasso, S.S.: Phenytoin for seizure disorders, J. Maternal Child Nurs. **9:**279, 1984.

Singer, W.D., Rabe, E.F., and Haller, J.S.: The effect of ACTH therapy upon infantile spasms, part 1, J. Pediatr. **96:**485-489, 1980.

Tucker, C.A.: Complex partial seizures, Am. J. Nurs. **81:**996-1000, 1981.

Vining, E.P.G., and Freeman, J.M.: Classification and evaluation of seizures, Pediatr. Ann. **14:**711–723, 1985.

Vining, E.P.G., and Freeman, J.M.: Discussion and explanation of seizures to the parents and child, Pediatr. Ann. **14:**737-739, 1985.

Vining, E.P.G., and Freeman, J.M.: Paroxysmal events which are not seizures, Pediatr. Ann. **14:**726-727, 1985.

Vining, E.P.G., and Freeman, J.M.: Status epilepticus, Pediatr. Ann. **14:**764-770, 1985.

Walson, P.D., and others: Once daily doses of phenobarbital in children, J. Pediatr. **97:**303-305, 1980.

Williams, A., Swisher, C., and Bremer, H.L.: Critical care of seizures, Crit. Care Update **8**(7):22-25, 1981.

Wright, F.S.: Epilepsy in childhood, Pediatr. Clin. North Am. **31:**177-188, 1984.

Febrile Seizures

Berkowitz, C.D., and Jones, C.R.: The PNP's role in evaluation and management of febrile seizures, Pediatr. Nurs. **9:**432-434, 1983.

Bindler, R.M., and Howrey, L.B.: Nursing care of children with febrile seizures, Am. J. Maternal Child Nurs. **3:**270-273, 1978.

Camfield, P.R., and others: The first febrile seizure—antipyretic instruction plus either phenobarbital or placebo to prevent recurrence, J. Pediatr. **97:**16-21, 1980.

Fishman, M.A.: Febrile seizures: the treatment controversy, J. Pediatr. **94:**177-184, 1979.

Fishman, M.A.: The consensus development conference on febrile seizures (commentary), J. Pediatr. **97:**933, 1980.

Nelson, K.B., and Ellenberg, J.H.: Prognosis in children with febrile seizures, Pediatrics **61:**720-727, 1978.

Vining, E.P.G., and Freeman, J.M.: Discussion and explanation of seizures to the parents and child, Pediatr. Ann. **14:**737-739, 1985.

Migraine

Gascon, G.G.: Chronic and recurrent headaches in children and adolescents, Pediatr. Clin. North Am. **31:**1027-1051, 1984.

McCarthy, A.M.: Chronic headaches in children, Pediatr. Nurs. **8:**88-93, 1982.

McCarthy, A.M., and Mehegan, J.: Migraine headaches in children: treatment, Pediatr. Nurs. **8:**173-176, 1982.

Monro, J., and others: Food allergy in migraine, Lancet, July 5, 1980, pp. 1-4.

Paulson, G.W.: Migraine headaches in children, Pediatr. Nurs. **6**(4):41-42, 1980.

Rothner, A.D.: Headaches in children: current guidelines to diagnosis and therapy, Pediatr. Consult. **1**(6):1-8, 1980.

Shinnar, S., and D'Souza, B.: Migraine in children and adolescents, Pediatr. Rev. **3:**257-262, 1982.

Thompson, J.A.: Diagnosis and treatment of headache in the pediatric patient, Curr. Probl. Pediatr. **10:**8-24, 1980.

Chapter 38

The Child with Endocrine Dysfunction

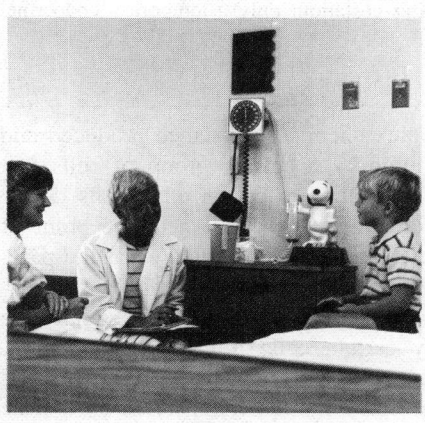

The major chemical regulators of the body are internal secretions and their secreting cells, which are collectively known as the endocrine system. The function of the endocrine system is to secrete intracellularly synthesized hormones into the circulation where they are transported to nearby or distant sites to stimulate, catalyze, or serve as pacemaker substances for metabolic processes. Together with the closely related but more rapidly reacting nervous system, the endocrine system serves to integrate the various physiologic functions of the organism in adjusting to external and internal environmental demands. Endocrine substances even in extremely small concentrations are effective in modifying metabolism, behavior, and development.

This chapter is primarily concerned with problems associated with oversecretion or undersecretion of the major hormones or defective responses in those organs and tissues sensitive to these hormones. The initial discussion is devoted to disorders of the large, interrelated neuroendocrine system. The most common endocrine disturbance in childhood, diabetes mellitus—caused by defective pancreatic hormone (insulin) secretion—is discussed at length.

The Endocrine System

The endocrine system consists of three components: (1) the cell, which sends a chemical message by means of a hormone; (2) the target cells, or end organs, which receive the chemical message; and (3) the environment through which the chemical is transported (blood, lymph, extracellular fluids) from the site of synthesis to the sites of cellular action. The endocrine system controls or regulates metabolic processes governing energy production, growth, fluid and electrolyte balance, response to stress, and sexual reproduction.

The endocrine glands are distributed throughout the body:

pituitary gland (hypophysis cerebi) A pea-sized gland that lies within a deep bony depression at the base of the cranium, the sella turcica, and is attached to the hypothalamus on the undersurface of the brain by a slender infundibulum or pituitary stalk

thyroid gland Two large lateral lobes and a connecting portion, the isthmus, situated on the anterior aspect of the neck just below the larynx

parathyroid glands Four or five (there may be more or less) small round bodies attached to the posterior surfaces of the lateral lobes of the thyroid gland

adrenal glands Pyramid-shaped glands situated atop the kidneys, fitting like caps over these organs

ovaries Glands located in the female pelvis on each side of the uterus at the fimbriated end of the fallopian tubes

testes Oval-shaped glands situated within the male scrotum

islands of Langerhans Small clusters of endocrine cells within the pancreas situated between the acinar or exocrine-secreting portions of the gland

Several additional structures may also be considered as endocrine glands, although they are not usually included:

pineal body (epiphysis cerebri) A gland located in the cranial cavity behind the midbrain and third ventricle, the functions of which are largely speculative

thymus A gland situated behind the sternum and below the thyroid gland; plays an important role in immunity but only during fetal life and early childhood

gastrointestinal glands Mucosal lining of the gastrointestinal tract containing cells that produce hormones that play important roles in controlling and coordinating secretory and motor activities of digestion

placenta A body that secretes ovarian hormones and chorionic gonadotropin during gestation; only a temporary endocrine gland

HORMONES

A hormone is a complex chemical substance produced and secreted into body fluids by a cell or group of cells that exerts a physiologic controlling effect on other cells. Some are *local hormones* creating their effect near the point of secretion. For example, acetylcholine, released at the parasympathetic and skeletal nerve endings, mediates the synaptic activity of the nervous system; secretin, a digestive hormone secreted by certain cells lining the duodenum, stimulates the pancreas to release a watery secretion; and, the prostaglandins, or tissue hormones, secreted by a wide variety of organs (including the seminal vesicles, kidneys, lungs, iris, brain, and thymus), usually diffuse only a short distance to integrate activities of neighboring cells.

General hormones are produced in one organ or part of the body and are carried through the bloodstream to a distant part, or parts, of the body where they initiate or regu-

Fig. 38-1. Anterior pituitary hormones and their target organs and tissues. See text for discussion.

From Anthony, C.P., and Thibodeau, G.A.: Textbook of anatomy and physiology, ed. 10, St. Louis, 1979, The C.V. Mosby Co.

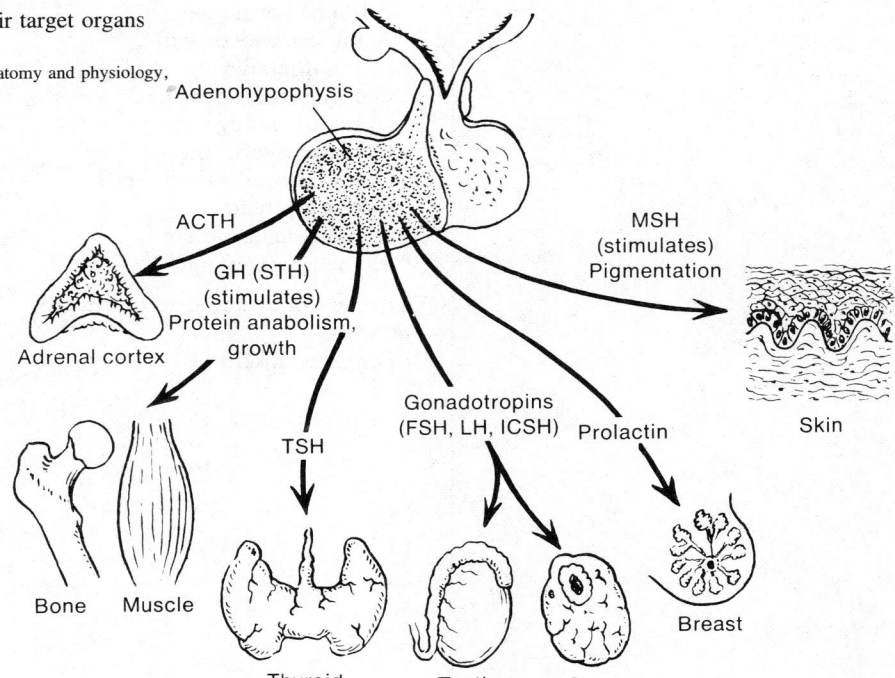

late physiologic activity of an organ or group of cells. Some of these hormones (such as thyroid hormone and growth hormone) affect most cells of the body, whereas others (such as the tropic hormones) produce their effects on specific tissues. The tissues affected by this specific action are called *target tissues*. For example, the pituitary hormones stimulate the adrenal glands and the thyroid gland to secrete adrenocorticotropin and thyrotropic hormone, respectively.

Control of Hormone Secretion

Hormones are released by endocrine glands into the bloodstream, where they are carried to responsive tissues. These responsive, or target, tissues may be another endocrine gland, an organ, or tissue. Regulation of hormonal secretion is based on negative feedback. As a general rule, endocrine glands have a tendency to oversecrete their particular hormones. However, once the physiologic effect of the hormone has been achieved, this information is transmitted to the producing gland, either directly or indirectly, to inhibit further secretion. If the gland undersecretes, the inhibition is relieved and the gland increases production of the hormone. As a result, the hormone is secreted according to the amount needed. This is the primary function of the tropic hormones.

The endocrine gland primarily responsible for stimulation and inhibition of target glandular secretions is the anterior pituitary, or "master gland." Tropic (which literally means "turning") hormones secreted by the anterior pituitary regulate the secretion of hormones from various target organs (Fig. 38-1). As blood concentrations of the target hormones reach normal levels, a negative message is sent to the anterior pituitary to inhibit release of the tropic hormone. For example, thyroid-stimulating hormone (TSH) responds to low levels of circulating thyroid hormone (TH). As blood levels of thyroid hormone reach normal concentrations, a negative feedback message is sent to the anterior pituitary, resulting in diminished release of thyroid-stimulating hormone.

The pituitary gland is, in turn, controlled by either hormonal or neuronal signals from the hypothalamus. Two types of substances are secreted from the hypothalamus: (1) releasing hormones and (2) inhibitory hormones, which are secreted within the hypothalamus and transported by way of the pituitary portal system to the anterior pituitary, where they stimulate the secretion of tropic hormones. An example of this is the secretion of corticotropin-releasing factor (CRF) by the hypothalamus, which stimulates the pituitary to secrete adrenocorticotropic hormone (ACTH). In this instance the anterior pituitary is the target of the hypothalamus and secondarily effects a response from another target gland, the adrenals. The adrenals in turn secrete glucocorticoids, which have multiple target sites throughout the body. Pituitary hormones that lack feedback control from the product of a target tissue (growth hormone, prolactin, and me-

lanocyte-stimulating hormone) require hypothalamic inhibitors and stimulators for their control.

Not all hormones depend on other hormones for their release. For example, insulin is secreted in response to blood glucose concentrations. Other glandular hormones that are not under the control of the pituitary gland are glucagon, parathyroid hormone (PTH), antidiuretic hormone (ADH), and aldosterone. The major endocrine glands, the hormones they secrete, as well as their effects are described in Table 38-1.

NEUROENDOCRINE INTERRELATIONSHIPS

Homeostasis is maintained by two regulatory systems: the endocrine and the autonomic nervous systems (collectively known as the neuroendocrine system). The autonomic nervous system consists of the sympathetic and parasympathetic systems that control nonvoluntary functions, specifically of smooth muscle, myocardium, and glands. The parasympathetic system, in particular, is primarily involved in regulating digestive processes, whereas the sympathetic system functions to maintain homeostasis during stress.

The higher autonomic centers, located in the hypothalamus and limbic system, help control the functioning of both autonomic systems. Both the sympathetic and parasympathetic nerve fibers secrete neurotransmitting substances—acetylcholine, released by cholinergic fibers, and norepinephrine, released by adrenergic fibers. Neural release of norepinephrine into the plasma produces the same effects as secretion of this substance by the adrenal medulla. This similarity in chemical activity demonstrates the interrelatedness between the two systems.

The neuroendocrine system acts by synthesizing and releasing various chemical substances that regulate body functions. Information is carried by means of neural impulses in the autonomic system and by the blood in the endocrine system. In general, neural responses are more rapid and localized; endocrine responses are more lasting and widespread. The two systems function synergistically because neural impulses transmitted to the central nervous system stimulate the hypothalamus to manufacture and release several releasing or inhibiting factors.

Because of the interdependent relationship of these glands, a malfunction in one gland produces effects elsewhere in the body. Endocrine dysfunction may result because of an intrinsic defect in the target gland (primary) or because of a diminished or elevated level of tropic hormones (secondary). Endocrine problems occur from hypofunction or hyperfunction of the glands. Primary hypofunction is usually associated with a more profound deficiency of the target gland hormone because little or no hormone is secreted. In secondary dysfunction the target glands secrete some of their hormones but in smaller amounts and less rapidly.

Hyperfunction or hypofunction may also be the result of

Table 38-1 Summary of the endocrine system

GLAND/HORMONE	EFFECT	HYPOFUNCTION	HYPERFUNCTION
Adenohypophysis (anterior pituitary)*			
Somatotropic hormone (STH) or growth hormone (GH) Target tissue: bones	Promotes growth of bone and soft tissues Has main effect on linear growth Maintains a normal rate of protein synthesis Conserves carbohydrate utilization and promotes fat mobilization Is essential for proliferation of cartilage cells at epiphyseal plate Is ineffective after epiphyseal closure Has hyperglycemic effect (antiinsulin action)	Epiphyseal fusion with cessation of growth Prepubertal dwarfism Pituitary cachexia (Simonds disease) Generalized growth retardation Hypoglycemia	Prepubertal gigantism Achromegaly (after full growth is attained) Diabetes mellitus Postpubertal hypoproteinemia
Thyrotropin (thyroid-stimulating hormone [TSH]) Target tissue: thyroid gland	Promotes and maintains growth and development of thyroid gland Stimulates thyroid hormone secretion	Hypothyroidism Marked delay of puberty Juvenile myxedema	Hyperthyroidism Thyrotoxicosis Graves disease
Adrenocorticotropic hormone (ACTH) Target tissue: adrenal cortex	Promotes and maintains growth and development of adrenal cortex Stimulates adrenal cortex to secrete glucocorticoids and androgens	Acute adrenocortical insufficiency (Addison disease) Hypoglycemia Increased skin pigmentation	Cushing syndrome
Gonadotropins Target tissue: gonads	Stimulate gonads to mature and produce sex hormones and germ cells	Absent or incomplete spontaneous puberty	Precocious puberty
Follicle-stimulating hormone (FSH) Target tissue: ovaries, testes	Male: Stimulates development of seminiferous tubules Initiates spermatogenesis Female: Stimulates graafian follicles to mature and secrete estrogen	Hypogonadism, Sterility Loss of secondary sex characteristics Amenorrhea	Precocious puberty Primary gonadal failure Hirsutism Polycystic ovary
Luteinizing hormone (LH)† Target tissue: ovaries, testes	Male: Stimulates differentiation of Leydig cells, which secrete androgens, principally testosterone Female: Produces rupture of follicle with discharge of mature ova Stimulates secretion of progesterone by corpus luteum	Hypogonadism Sterility Impotence Loss of secondary sex characteristics Ovarian failure Eunuchism	Precocious puberty Primary gonadal failure Hirsutism Polycystic ovary
Prolactin (luteotropic hormone) Target tissue: ovaries, breasts	Stimulates milk secretion Maintains corpus luteum and progesterone secretion during pregnancy	Inability to lactate Amenorrhea	Galactorrhea Functional hypogonadism
Melanocyte-stimulating hormone (MSH) Target tissue: skin	Promotes pigmentation of skin	Diminished or absent skin pigmentation	Increased skin pigmentation

*For each anterior pituitary hormone there is a corresponding hypothalamic releasing factor. A deficiency in these factors caused by inhibiting anterior pituitary hormone synthesis produces the same effects (see text for more detailed information).
†In the male, LH is sometimes known as interstitial cell–stimulating hormone (ICSH).

Table 38-1 Summary of the endocrine system—cont'd

GLAND/HORMONE	EFFECT	HYPOFUNCTION	HYPERFUNCTION
Neurohypophysis (posterior pituitary)			
Antidiuretic hormone (ADH) (vasopressin) Target tissue: renal tubules	Acts on distal and collecting tubules, making them more permeable to water, thus increasing reabsorption and decreasing excretion of urine	Diabetes insipidus	Syndrome of inappropriate secretion of ADH Fluid retention Hyponatremia
Oxytocin Target tissue: uterus, breasts	Stimulates powerful contractions of uterus Causes ejection of milk from alveoli into breast ducts (letdown reflex)		
Thyroid			
Thyroxine (T_4) and triiodothyronine (T_3)	Regulates metabolic rate; controls rate of growth of body cells Especially important for growth of bones, teeth, and brain Promotes mobilization of fats and gluconeogenesis	Hypothyroidism Myxedema Hashimoto thyroiditis General growth is greatly reduced; extent depends on age at which deficiency occurs	Exophthalmic goiter (Graves disease) Accelerated linear growth Early epiphyseal closure
Thyrocalcitonin	Regulates calcium and phosphorus metabolism Influences ossification and development of bone		
Parathyroid glands			
Parathyroid hormone (PTH)	Promotes calcium reabsorption from blood, bone, and intestines Promotes excretion of phosphorus in kidney tubules	Hypocalcemia (tetany)	Hypercalcemia (bone demineralization) Hypophosphatemia
Adrenal cortex			
Mineralocorticoids Aldosterone	Simulate renal tubules to reabsorb sodium, thus promoting water retention but potassium loss	Adrenocortical insufficiency	Electrolyte imbalance Hyperaldosteronism
Sex hormones (androgens, estrogens, progesterone)	Influence development of bone, reproductive organs, and secondary sexual characteristics	Male feminization	Adrenogenital syndrome
Glucocorticoids Cortisol (hydrocortisone and compound F) Corticosterone (compound B)	Promote normal fat, protein, and carbohydrate metabolism In excess, tend to accelerate gluconeogenesis and protein and fat catabolism Mobilize body defenses during period of stress Suppress inflammatory reaction	Addison disease Acute adrenocortical insufficiency Impaired growth and sexual function	Cushing syndrome Severe impairment of growth with slowing of skeletal maturation
Adrenal medulla			
Epinephrine (Adrenalin), norepinephrine (noradrenalin)	Produces vasoconstriction of heart and smooth muscles (raises blood pressure) Increases blood sugar via glycolysis Inhibits gastrointestinal activity Activates sweat glands		Hyperfunction caused by: Pheochromocytoma Neuroblastoma Ganglioneuroma

Continued.

Table 38-1 Summary of the endocrine system—cont'd

GLAND/HORMONE	EFFECT	HYPOFUNCTION	HYPERFUNCTION
Islands of Langerhans of pancreas			
Insulin (β-cells)	Promotes glucose transport into the cells Increases glucose utilization glycogenesis, and glycolysis Promotes fatty acid transport into cells and lipogenesis Promotes amino acid transport into cells and protein synthesis	Diabetes mellitus	Hyperinsulinism
Glucagon (α-cells)	Acts as antagonist to insulin, thereby increasing blood glucose concentration by accelerating glycogenolysis Able to inhibit secretion of both insulin and glucagon		Hyperglycemia
Somatostatin (δ-cells)	Able to inhibit secretion of both insulin and glucagon		
Ovaries			
Estrogen	Accelerates growth of epithelial cells, especially in uterus following menses Promotes protein anabolism Promotes epiphyseal closure of bones Promotes breast development during puberty and pregnancy Plays role in sexual function Stimulates water and sodium reabsorption in renal tubules Stimulates ripening of ova	Lack of or repression of sexual development	Precocious puberty, early epiphyseal closure
Progesterone	Prepares uterus for nidation of fertilized ovum and aids in maintenance of pregnancy Aids in development of alveolar system of breasts during pregnancy Inhibits myometrial contractions Has effect on protein catabolism Promotes salt and water retention, especially in endometrium		
Testes			
Testosterone	Accelerates protein anabolism for growth Promotes epiphyseal closure Promotes development of secondary sex characteristics Plays role in sexual function Stimulates testes to produce spermatozoa	Delayed sexual development or eunuchoidism	Precocious puberty, early epiphyseal closure

an increase or a decrease in secretion of the tropic hormones (primary) with a consequent increase in the target gland hormones (secondary) or a hypersecretion or hyposecretion of the target glands. A summary of the endocrine glands, their functions, and the primary effects of oversecretion or undersecretion is given in Table 38-1.

Disorders of Pituitary Function

Deficiencies of the anterior pituitary hormones may be the result of organic defects or of idiopathic etiology and may occur as a single hormonal problem or in combination with other hormonal deficiencies. The clinical manifestations depend on the hormones involved and the age of onset. If the tropic hormones are involved, the resulting disorder reflects the altered stimulus to the target gland. For example, if thyroid-stimulating hormone is deficient, thyroid hormone is also deficient and the child displays the manifestations of hypothyroidism.

An overproduction of the anterior pituitary hormones can result in gigantism (caused by excess growth hormone production during childhood), hyperthyroidism, hypercortisolism (Cushing syndrome), and precocious puberty from excessive gonadotropins. Overproduction is thought to be caused by hyperplasia of the pituitary cells—which may eventually progress to a tumor (adenoma)—or a primary hypothalamic defect that results in excess of the hormone's respective releasing factor. Although the initial clinical manifestations are a result of pituitary hypersecretion, eventually pituitary insufficiency occurs and the signs of panhypopituitarism become evident.

HYPOPITUITARISM

Hypopituitarism is diminished or deficient secretion of pituitary hormones. The consequences of the condition depend on the degree of dysfunction and lead to gonadotropin deficiency with absence or regression of secondary sex char-

---

EFFECTS OF PANHYPOPITUITARISM

Growth hormone (GH)
Short stature but proportional height and weight
Delayed epiphyseal closure
Retarded bone age proportional to height
Premature aging
Increased insulin sensitivity

Thyroid-stimulating hormone (TSH)
Short stature with infantile proportions
Dry, coarse skin, yellow discoloration, pallor
Cold intolerance
Constipation
Somnolence
Bradycardia
Dyspnea on exertion
Delayed dentition, loss of teeth

Gonadotropins
Absence of sexual maturation or loss of secondary sex characteristics
Atrophy of genitalia, prostate gland, breasts
Amenorrhea without menopausal symptoms
Decreased spermatogenesis

Adrenocorticotropic hormone (ACTH)
Severe anorexia, weight loss
Hypoglycemia
Hypotension
Hyponatremia, hyperkalemia
Adrenal apoplexy, especially in response to stress
Circulatory collapse

Antidiuretic hormone (ADH)
Polyuria
Polydipsia
Dehydration

Melanocyte-stimulating hormone (MSH)
Decreased pigmentation

---

acteristics; somatotropin deficiency, in which children display retarded somatic growth; thyrotropin deficiency that produces hypothyroidism (p. 1691); and corticotropin deficiency, which results in manifestations of adrenal hypofunction (p. 1694). Hypopituitarism can result from any of the conditions listed in the accompanying box.

The most common organic cause of pituitary hyposecretion is tumors in the pituitary or hypothalamic region, especially the craniopharyngiomas. These tumors usually invade the anterior and posterior pituitary lobes and the hypothalamus causing panhypopituitarism, a generalized disorder involving multiple systems (see box above). The child may evidence growth retardation for quite some time before developing any symptoms or signs of increased intracranial pressure, local compression, or the destructive effects of the tumor. Other causes of panhypopituitarism sometimes include encephalitis, head trauma (rarely), and congenital hypoplasia of the hypothalamic area.

Idiopathic hypopituitarism is usually related to growth hormone (GH) deficiency, which inhibits somatic growth in all cells of the body. Although children with hypopituitarism are normal at birth, they show growth patterns that pro-

---

ETIOLOGY OF HYPOPITUITARISM

Aplasia or hypoplasia
   Developmental defects
   Idiopathic—sporadic; genetic
Destructive lesions
   Trauma—perinatal; child abuse; basal skull fracture
   Infiltrative lesions—tumors; tuberculosis; toxoplasmosis; hemochromatosis; sarcoidosis
   Irradiation—CNS; eye; middle ear
   Autoimmune hypophysitis
   Surgery—removal of pharyngeal pituitary; ablation of craniopharyngioma or other tumor
   Vascular—aneurysm; infarct
Functional deficiency
   Psychosocial dwarfism
   Anorexia nervosa

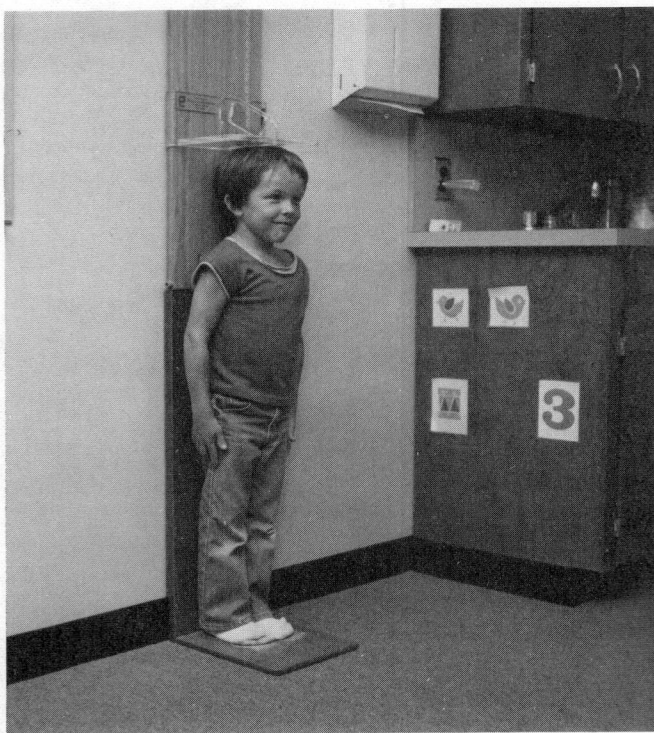

Fig. 38-2. Ten-year-old child with growth hormone deficiency. Height is 42.5 inches.

Photography by John Roy, Saint Francis Hospital. On location at Children's Medical Center, Tulsa, OK.

gressively deviate from the normal growth rate, often beginning in infancy. The chief complaint in most instances is short stature. Of those who seek help, boys outnumber girls three to one. The extent of idiopathic GH deficiency may be complete or partial, but the cause is unknown. It is frequently associated with other pituitary hormone deficiencies, such as deficiencies of thyroid-stimulating hormone (TSH) and adrenocorticotropic hormone (ACTH); thus it is theorized that the disorder is probably secondary to hypothalamic deficiency. It has also been observed that there is a higher than average frequency in some families, which indicates a possible genetic etiology in a number of instances.

Clinical Manifestations

The usual presenting complaint with dwarfism is short stature. These children generally grow normally during the first year and then follow a slowed growth curve that is below the third percentile. In children with a partial GH deficiency, the growth retardation is less marked than in children with complete GH deficiency. Height may be retarded more than weight because with good nutrition these children can become overweight or even obese. Their well-nourished appearance is an important diagnostic clue to differentiation from other disorders such as failure to thrive.

Skeletal proportions are normal for the age, but these

children appear younger than their chronologic age (Fig. 38-2). However, later in life premature aging is common. The appearance of fine wrinkles about the eyes and mouth gives these children a peculiar impression of immaturity combined with presenility. They tend to be relatively inactive and are less apt to participate in aggressive, sporting-type activities. Bone age is nearly always retarded but is closely related to height age—the degree of retardation depends on the duration and extent of the hormonal deficiency. Children with diminished function of recent onset may show little retardation in skeletal age, whereas children with a long-standing deficiency may evidence a skeletal age only 40% to 50% of their chronologic age. It is difficult to predict their eventual height. Because the period of growth is prolonged past adolescence into the third or fourth decade, many of them reach a permanent height of 4 to 5 feet.

Usually primary teeth appear at the expected age, but the eruption of the permanent teeth is delayed. Because of the underdeveloped jaw, the teeth are overcrowded and malpositioned. Sexual development is usually delayed but is otherwise normal. Even without growth hormone replacement, dwarf adults are able to reproduce normal offspring. However, if the gonadotropins are deficient, sexual maturation is absent.

Most of these children have normal intelligence. In fact, during early childhood they often appear precocious in their learning because their ability seems to exceed their small size. However, emotional problems are not uncommon, especially as they near puberty when their smallness becomes increasingly apparent compared to their peers.

Diagnostic Evaluation

Only a small number of children with delayed growth or short stature have hypopituitary dwarfism. In the majority of instances the cause is constitutional delay (see p. 853). Diagnostic evaluation is aimed at isolating organic causes, which in addition to GH deficiency may include hypothyroidism, hypersecretion of cortisol, gonadal aplasia, chronic illness, or nutritional inadequacy.

A complete diagnostic evaluation should include a family history, a history of the child's growth patterns and previous health status, physical examination, radiographic surveys, and endocrine studies.

Family history. A family history is of utmost importance in relating short stature to genetic background. Children with constitutional delays frequently are the products of parents who experienced similar slow growth patterns and delayed sexual maturation. A small percentage of those with hypopituitarism demonstrate an autosomal-recessive inheritance pattern. Height and weight of siblings should be compared to the child's growth patterns at comparable age periods.

Child's history. The child's history should include a thorough prenatal history to rule out maternal disorders that may have influenced growth, such as malnutrition. Birth height and weight should be compared to gestational age.

Children with hypopituitarism are usually of normal size and gestational age at birth.

The child's past health history is investigated for evidence of chronic illness that may have influenced growth patterns, although a chronic illness, such as congenital heart disease, malabsorptive disorders, severe anemia, or neurologic impairments, usually has been identified long before the growth problem becomes a concern. Signs and symptoms suggesting a tumor, such as visual disturbances, headache, and signs of increasing intracranial pressure, are important. Such symptoms often precede retarded growth but may not have been regarded as significant. With lesions involving the hypothalamus, the history may also reveal characteristic manifestations of dysfunction such as somnolence, thermodysregulation, epilepsy, and hyperphagia, resulting in obesity. Since a craniopharyngioma can affect the secretion of any of the pituitary hormones, assessment for hypothyroidism, hypoadrenalism, and hypoaldosteronism should also be included.

Whenever possible, the child's growth patterns since birth should be evaluated. Age of onset of short stature provides a significant diagnostic clue. Progressive retardation in height and weight since early childhood suggests idiopathic hypopituitary dwarfism, whereas a recent change from normal growth is more characteristic of a tumor. In addition, these children are usually well nourished, ruling out other causes of growth failure.

Physical examination. Accurate measurement of height and weight and comparison to standard growth charts are essential. Other measurements may include crown-to-pubis and pubis-to-heel length to compare body proportions, and sexual development should be assessed and compared to age-appropriate development. Observation of general appearance yields valuable clues, especially signs of premature aging and infantile facial features. A funduscopic examination and testing for visual acuity should be performed to detect evidence of ocular damage from a tumor.

Radiographic surveys. Radiographic examination of the wrist for centers of ossification is important in evaluating growth. Epiphyseal maturation is retarded in hypopituitarism but consistent with retardation in height. This is in contrast to hypothyroidism, in which bone maturation is greatly retarded, or gonadal dysplasia, such as Turner syndrome, in which bone age is near normal. Radiographic studies should also include a skull series, which is most helpful in identifying abnormalities such as an abnormally small sella turcica or evidence of a space-occupying lesion such as craniopharyngioma. Computed tomography, radionuclide scans, or carotid angiograms may be needed to establish diagnosis and localization of lesions.

Endocrine studies. Definitive diagnosis is based on absent or subnormal reserves of pituitary GH. Since GH levels are normally so low in children that differentiation from abnormal concentrations is unreliable, growth hormone secretion should be stimulated followed by measurement of blood levels. Exercise is a natural and benign stimulus for GH release and elevated levels can be detected after 20 minutes of strenuous exercise in normal children. Also GH levels are elevated 45 to 90 minutes following the onset of sleep.

If physiologic methods are inconclusive, GH release can be stimulated pharmacologically, which is a method employed to identify children who do not respond to treatment with GH. Agents used to provoke GH are L-dopa, insulin-arginine, and glucagon, and tests with each may be required. GH levels below 5 ng/ml after two provocative tests establish the diagnosis. Somatomedin-C levels, compared with age- and sex-matched controls, are also used to detect GH deficiency. Levels are very low in GH-deficient children but, in most cases, rise significantly within 16 to 28 hours of human GH administration (DiGeorge, 1983).

Since retarded growth may be caused by other endocrine disorders (such as hypothyroidism or gonadotropic deficiency), Turner syndrome, or emotional deprivation, or may be associated with other forms of delayed growth (such as tissue unresponsiveness to GH or primordial dwarfism), tests for these conditions are often performed.

Therapeutic Management

Treatment of GH deficiency caused by organic lesions is directed toward correction of the underlying disease process, e.g., surgical removal or irradiation of a tumor. The definitive treatment of GH deficiency is replacement of GH and is successful in 80% of affected children. Unfortunately the supplies of human GH (hGH) are limited because they must be obtained from human cadavers. Also human GH has caused half the treated patients to develop circulating antibodies to hGH that inhibit its activity. Biosynthetic GH prepared by recombinant DNA technology is expected to be approved for use at an early date.

Children who respond to the therapy typically increase their growth rate from 3.5 to 4 cm/year before treatment to 8 to 10 cm/year during the first year of therapy. Young children usually respond better than adolescents, obese children better than thin children, and severely GH-deficient children better than those with partial deficiencies (Underwood, 1986).

Children with other hormone deficiencies require replacement therapy to correct the specific disorders. This may involve administration of thyroid extract, cortisone, testosterone, or estrogens and progesterone. The sex hormones are usually begun during adolescence to promote normal sexual maturation.

Nursing Considerations

The principal nursing consideration is identification of children with growth problems. Despite the fact that the majority of growth problems are not a result of organic causes, any delay in normal growth and sexual development poses special emotional adjustments for these children.

The nurse may be a key person in helping to establish a diagnosis. For example, if serial height and weight records are not available, the nurse can question parents about the child's growth in comparison to that of siblings, peers, or relatives. Investigating clothing sizes is often helpful in determining growth at different ages. Parents of these children frequently comment that the child wore out clothes before he grew out of them or that, if the clothing fit the body, it often was too long in the sleeves or legs.

Because the behavioral or physical changes that suggest a tumor are insidious, they are frequently overlooked. It is important to correlate the onset of any positive findings with the initial evidence of growth retardation. For example, visual problems and headache are not uncommon in school-age children and can coincidentally occur after a growth problem is recognized. If fact, headache may represent the emotional trauma caused by short stature rather than be a symptom of a tumor. This line of questioning should be pursued cautiously to avoid unduly alarming parents about the possibility of a brain tumor.

Part of a nurse's role in helping establish a diagnosis is assisting with diagnostic tests. Preparation of child and family is especially important if a number of tests are being performed, and the child will require particular attention during provocative testing. For example, children have difficulty overcoming hypoglycemia generated by tests with insulin so they must be observed carefully for signs of hypoglycemia. Thin children under 5 years of age are at particular risk, especially those with low fasting-glucose levels (DiGeorge, 1983). Children receiving GH therapy need to be prepared for the required injections three times per week (see Preparation for procedures in Chapter 27).

Child and family support. Once a diagnosis confirming an organic cause of the problem is made, the parents and child need an opportunity to express their thoughts and feelings. Not infrequently a growth problem that was present since birth is missed until adolescence, at which time the child's difference in body development becomes dramatically evident when compared to peers. Family members may feel anger and resentment toward members of the health staff for not detecting the problem sooner. Parents may experience guilt for not seeking medical attention earlier, especially if the child had been miserable from experiencing ridicule and criticism from associates. Each family member needs a sympathetic listener who is aware of his needs and realizes the importance of remaining objective and not defensive or overly apologetic. Appropriate emotional support from the nurse can include an affirmation of each person's justified feelings, such as anger or guilt, and emphasis on the treatment plan and prospects for improvement in the future.

Children require additional support because even when hormone replacement is successful, their eventual adult height is attained at a slower rate than that of their peers. They need assistance in setting realistic expectations regarding improvement. For example, increases in height of 3 to 5 inches are common during the first year of therapy, but increases are less dramatic during subsequent years. Both sexes, but especially males, need guidance toward appropri-

ate vocational goals. For example, children with aspirations for athletic sports such as basketball would be better advised to explore other activities not so dependent on excessive height.

Since these children appear younger than their chronologic age, others frequently relate to them in infantile or childish ways. Parents and teachers benefit from guidance directed toward setting realistic expectations for the child based on age and abilities. For example, in the home such children should have the same age-appropriate responsibilities as their siblings. As they approach adolescence they should be encouraged to participate in group activities with their peers. They should wear styles that accentuate their actual age and not size. If abilities and strengths are emphasized rather than physical size, such children are more likely to develop a positive self-image (see also p. 854.)

PITUITARY HYPERFUNCTION

Excess growth hormone before closure of the epiphyseal shafts results in proportional overgrowth of long bones, until the individual reaches a height of 8 feet or more. Vertical growth is accompanied by rapid and increased development of muscles and viscera. Weight is increased but is usually in proportion to height. Proportional enlargement of head circumference also occurs and may result in delayed closure of the fontanels. Children with a pituitary secreting tumor may also demonstrate signs of increasing intracranial pressure, especially headache.

If hypersecretion of GH occurs after epiphyseal closure, growth is in the transverse direction, producing a condition known as *acromegaly*. Typical facial features include overgrowth of head, lips, nose, tongue, jaw, and paranasal and mastoid sinuses; separation and malocclusion of the teeth in the enlarged jaw; disproportion of the face to the cerebral division of the skull; increased facial hair; and thickened, deeply creased skin.

Diagnostic Evaluation

Diagnosis is based on a history of excessive growth during childhood and evidence of increased levels of GH. Radiographic studies may reveal a tumor in an enlarged sella turcica, normal bone age, enlargement of bones (such as the paranasal sinuses) and evidence of joint changes. Endocrine studies to confirm excess of other hormones, specifically thyroid, cortisol, and sex hormones, should also be included in the differential diagnosis.

Therapeutic Management

If a lesion is present, surgical treatment by cryosurgery or hypophysectomy is performed to remove the tumor whenever feasible. Other therapies aimed at destroying pituitary tissue include external irradiation and radioactive implants. Depending on the extent of surgical extirpation and the degree of pituitary insufficiency, hormone replacement with thyroid extract, cortisone, and sex hormones may be necessary.

Nursing Considerations

The primary nursing consideration is early identification of children with excessive growth rates. Although medical management is unable to reduce growth already attained, height can be retarded, and the earlier the treatment, the more control there is in predetermining a normal adult height. Nurses in ambulatory settings who are frequently involved in growth screening should refer children who demonstrate excessive linear growth for a medical evaluation. They should also observe for signs of a tumor, especially headache, and evidence of concurrent hormonal excesses, particularly the gonadotropins, which cause sexual precocity.

These children require the same emotional support as those with short stature. However, girls may suffer from the effects of excessive height much more than boys (see Tall stature on p. 854). In fact, males may find the tallness an asset when pursuing sports such as basketball. Children and their parents need an opportunity to express their thoughts. A compassionate nurse can be very supportive to these children, especially before adolescence when they are larger than their peers. The nurse can emphasize to a tall girl that as boys grow older they become taller and that she will not always be looking down at them. Since early adolescence is a time of idol worship, the nurse can point out marriages of celebrities in which the woman is taller than the man to help the girl gain a perspective that not all heterosexual relationships must follow stereotypic models.

PRECOCIOUS PUBERTY

Normally the hypothalamic-releasing factors stimulate secretion of the gonadotropic hormones from the anterior pituitary at the time of puberty. In the male, interstitial cell–stimulating hormone stimulates Leydig cells of the testes to secrete testosterone; in the female follicle-stimulating hormone and luteinizing hormone stimulate the ovarian follicles to secrete estrogens. This sequence of events is known as the hypothalamic-pituitary-gonadal axis. If for some reason there is premature activation of this cycle, the child will display evidence of advanced or precocious puberty (see also Precocious puberty, p. 855).

In most cases the cause is unknown and treatment chiefly involves psychologic support to the child and family. Despite the early sexual development, maturation of the gonads and the appearance of secondary sexual characteristics proceed normally. The most difficult time for the child is usually the school years before adolescence. After puberty physical differences from peers are no longer present.

Although the child's heterosexual behavior is appropriate for the chronologic age, the nurse should emphasize to parents that the child is fertile. Usually no form of contraception is necessary, unless the child is sexually active. In this situation proper counseling is important because forms of birth control such as estrogen pills will prematurely initiate epiphyseal closure, resulting in stunted linear growth.

DIABETES INSIPIDUS

The principal disorder of posterior pituitary hypofunction is diabetes insipidus (DI) (sometimes called neurogenic DI) resulting from hyposecretion of antidiuretic hormone (ADH), or vasopressin, and producing a state of uncontrolled diuresis. This disorder is not to be confused with nephrogenic diabetes insipidus, a rare hereditary disorder affecting primarily males, caused by unresponsiveness of the renal tubules to the hormone (see p. 1274).

Neurogenic diabetes insipidus may result from a number of different causes. Primary causes are familial or idiopathic and, of the total groups, approximately 45% to 50% are idiopathic. Secondary causes include trauma (accidental or surgical), tumors, granulomatous disease, infections (meningitis or encephalitis), or vascular anomalies (aneurysm). Certain drugs, such as alcohol or phenytoin diphenylhydantoin, can cause a transient polyuria.

Clinical Manifestations

The cardinal signs of diabetes insipidus are polyuria and polydipsia. In the older child excessive urination accompanied by a compensatory insatiable thirst may be so intense that the child does little than go to the toilet and drink fluids. Not infrequently the first sign is enuresis. In the infant the initial symptom is irritability that is relieved with feedings of water but not milk. The infant is also prone to dehydration, electrolyte imbalance, hyperthermia, azotemia, and potential circulatory collapse.

Dehydration is usually not a serious problem in older children who are able to drink larger quantities of water. However any period of unconsciousness, such as after trauma or anesthesia, may be life threatening because the voluntary demand for fluid is absent. During such instances careful monitoring of urine volumes and blood concentration and intravenous fluid replacement are essential to prevent dehydration.

Diagnostic Evaluation

The simplest test used to diagnose this condition is restriction of oral fluids and observation of consequent changes in urine volume and concentration. Normally reducing fluids results in concentrated urine and diminished volume. In diabetes insipidus fluid restriction has little or no effect on urine formation but causes weight loss from dehydration. Accurate results from this procedure require strict monitoring of fluid intake, urine output, measurement of urine concentration (specific gravity or osmolality), and frequent weight checks. A weight loss between 3% and 5% indicates moderate dehydration and requires termination of the fluid restriction.

If this test is positive, the child should be given a test dose of injected aqueous vasopressin (Pitressin), which should alleviate the polyuria and polydipsia. Unresponsiveness to exogenous vasopressin usually indicates nephrogenic diabetes insipidus.

An important diagnostic consideration is to differentiate DI from other causes of polyuria and polydipsia, especially diabetes mellitus. Other tests employed in the diagnostic evaluation include a skull x-ray film to detect a tumor, kidney function tests and blood electrolyte levels to assess renal failure, and specific endocrine studies to isolate associated problems. In rare instances a psychologic consultation may be warranted to confirm the possibility of compulsive water drinking because of psychogenic causes.

Therapeutic Management

The usual treatment is hormone replacement, either with an intramuscular or subcutaneous injection of vasopressin tannate in peanut oil or nasal sprays of aqueous lysine vasopressin. The injectable form has the advantage of lasting for 48 to 72 hours, which affords the child a full night's sleep. However it has the disadvantages of requiring frequent injections as well as proper preparation of the drug. To be effective the active material must be thoroughly resuspended in the oil by being held under warm running water for 10 to 15 minutes and shaken vigorously before being drawn into the syringe. If this is not done, the oil is injected minus the antidiuretic hormone. Small brown particles, which indicate drug dispersion, must be seen in the suspension.

The nasal spray has the benefit of being a simple, painless route of administration. However, applications must be repeated every 2 to 6 hours to prevent recurrence of symptoms. To provide longer relief during the night, a cotton pledget moistened with the spray can be inserted into the nostril. However, mucous membrane irritation caused by a cold or allergy renders this route unreliable. Although the vaginal and buccal mucosa are substitute routes for the spray, they can be inconvenient. A new, long-acting analog of arginine vasopressin is available as a nasal spray that can be administered twice daily to achieve adequate control. It is also available for parenteral use.

Nursing Considerations

The initial objective is identification of the disorder. Since an early sign may be sudden enuresis in a child who is toilet trained, excessive thirst with bed-wetting is an indication for further investigation. Another clue is persistent irritability and crying in an infant that is relieved only by bottle-feedings of water. Following head trauma or certain neurosurgical procedures, the development of DI can be anticipated; therefore these patients must be closely monitored for signs of the disorder. Observations include body weight, serum electrolytes, blood urea nitrogen, hematocrit, and urine specific gravity taken before surgery and every other day following the procedure. Fluid intake and output should be carefully measured and recorded. The alert patient is able to adjust intake to urine losses, but the unconscious or very young patient will require closer fluid observation. In children who are not toilet trained, collection of urine specimens may necessitate bagging the child with a urine-collecting device.

After confirmation of the diagnosis, parents need a thorough explanation regarding the condition with specific clarification that diabetes insipidus is a different condition from diabetes mellitus. They must realize that treatment is lifelong. If the child is to receive the injectable vasopressin (Pitressin), ideally both parents should be taught the correct procedure for preparation and administration of the drug. Once the child is old enough, he should be encouraged to assume full responsibility for his care. (See the discussion of diabetes mellitus on p. 1714 for ways to help the child learn to give his own injections.)

For emergency purposes these children should wear Medic Alert tags. Older children should carry the nasal spray with them for temporary relief of symptoms. School personnel need to be aware of the problem in order that they can grant the child unrestricted use of the lavatory. Failure to permit this may result in embarrassing accidents that often result in the child's unwillingness to attend school.

INAPPROPRIATE SECRETION OF ANTIDIURETIC HORMONE

The disorder that results from hypersecretion of the posterior pituitary hormone, or antidiuretic hormone (ADH, vasopressin), is known as the *syndrome of inappropriate secretion of ADH (SIADH)*. SIADH is observed with increased frequency in a variety of conditions, especially those involving infections, tumors, or other central nervous system disease and trauma to the central nervous system.

The manifestations are directly related to fluid retention and hypotonicity. Serum osmolality is low, and urine osmolality is inappropriately elevated. When serum sodium levels are diminished to 110 mEq/L, the child displays anorexia, nausea (and sometimes vomiting), irritability, and personality changes. With progressive reduction in sodium, other neurologic signs, stupor, and convulsions may be evident. The symptoms usually disappear when the underlying disorder is corrected.

The immediate management consists of restricting fluids. Subsequent management depends on the cause and severity. Fluids continue to be restricted to one-fourth to one-half maintenance. When there are no fluid abnormalities but SIADH can be anticipated, fluids are often restricted expectantly at two-thirds to three-fourths maintenance.

Nursing Considerations

The first goal of nursing management is recognizing the presence of SIADH from symptoms described in patients at risk. When children display the signs of the disorder, careful measurements similar to those implemented for neurogenic diabetes insipidus should be carried out.

Disorders of Thyroid Function

The thyroid gland secretes two types of hormones: thyroid hormone, which consists of two hormones, thyroxine (T_4) and triiodothyronine (T_3), and thyrocalcitonin. The secretion of thyroid hormones is controlled by thyroid-stimulating hormone (TSH) from the anterior pituitary, which in turn is regulated by the thyrotropin-releasing factor (TRF) from the hypothalamus as a negative feedback response. Consequently hypothyroidism or hyperthyroidism may result from a defect in the target gland or from a disturbance in the secretion of TSH or TRF. Since the functions of T_3 and T_4 are qualitatively the same, the term "thyroid hormone" (TH) will be used throughout the discussion.

The synthesis of thyroid hormones depends on available sources of dietary iodine and tyrosine. The thyroid is the only endocrine gland capable of storing excess amounts of hormones for release as needed. During circulation in the bloodstream, thyroxine and triiodothyronine are bound to carrier proteins (thyroxine-binding globulin [TBG]). They must be unbound before they are able to exert their metabolic effect.

The main physiologic action of thyroid hormone is to regulate the basal metabolic rate and thereby control the processes of growth and tissue differentiation, as outlined in the accompanying box. Unlike somatotropin, thyroid hormone is involved in many more diverse activities influencing the growth and development of body tissues. Therefore a deficiency of thyroid hormone exerts a more profound effect on growth than that seen in hypopituitarism.

Thyrocalcitonin helps maintain blood calcium levels by decreasing the calcium concentration. Its effect is opposite that of parathormone, in that it inhibits skeletal demineralization and promotes calcium deposition in the bone.

PHYSIOLOGIC EFFECTS OF THYROID HORMONE

Regulates metabolic rate of all cells; protein, fat, and carbohydrate catabolism; and nitrogen excretion

Regulates body heat production and heat-dissipating mechanisms

Regulates protein synthesis and catabolism, amino acid incorporation into protein, and transcription of messenger RNA

Increases gluconeogenesis and peripheral utilization of glucose

Maintains appetite and secretion of gastrointestinal substances

Maintains calcium mobilization

Stimulates cholesterol synthesis and hepatic mechanisms that remove cholesterol from the circulation; stimulates lipid turnover and free fatty acid release

Regulates hepatic conversion of carotene to vitamin A

Maintains growth hormone secretion, skeletal maturation, and tissue differentiation

Is necessary for muscle tone and vigor and normal skin constituents

Maintains cardiac rate, force, and output

Affects respiratory rate, depth of oxygen utilization, and carbon dioxide formation

Affects central nervous system development and cerebration during first 2 to 3 years

Affects milk production during lactation and menstrual cycle fertility

Maintains sensitivity to insulin and insulin degradation

Affects red cell production

Affects cortisol secretion, probably caused by direct effect on adrenal glands and by increaseing ACTH secretion

---

HYPOTHYROIDISM

Hypothyroidism is one of the most common endocrine problems of childhood. It may be either congenital or acquired and represents a deficiency in secretion of thyroid hormones. Hypothyroidism from dietary insufficiency of iodine is now rare in the United States because the use of iodized salt has permitted a readily available source of the nutrient.

Congenital Hypothyroidism

Screening programs for detecting hypothyroidism in the newborn period have significantly altered the adverse effects of this disorder. Most infants, but not all, are detected within the first month of life and evaluated so that therapy with L-thyroxine can be implemented without delay. Therapy is initiated before definitive diagnosis is established by thyroid image testing. TSH levels remain elevated for 1 to 2 weeks after initiation of therapy; therefore the test can be performed up to 5 to 7 days after treatment is begun. The test is important for a definitive diagnosis in order to plan long-term therapy and parent counseling.

Infants with thyroid dysgenesis will have permanent, sporadically recurring disease but will need no further testing, whereas those with congenital athyrosis may have transient disease as a result of transplacentally acquired maternal blocking antibodies (Foley, 1986). Parents of infants with hereditary (autosomal recessive) hypothyroidism will need genetic counseling and the disease explained in order that subsequent infants can be evaluated at birth for presence of the disease. (See p. 358 for a discussion of congenital hypothyroidism.)

Juvenile Hypothyroidism

Beyond infancy primary hypothyroidism may be caused by a number of defects. For example, a congenital hypoplastic thyroid gland may provide sufficient amounts of TH during the first year or two but be inadequate when rapid body growth increases demands on the gland. Partial or complete thyroidectomy for cancer or thyrotoxicosis can leave insufficient thyroid tissue to furnish hormones for body requirements. Irradiation for Hodgkin disease or other malignancies causes thyroid dysfunction in approximately one third of children and adolescents (DiGeorge, 1983). Infectious processes may be a cause of hypothyroidism. It can also occur when dietary iodine is deficient.

Clinical manifestations depend on the extent of dysfunction and the age of the child at the onset. The presenting symptoms are decelerated growth from chronic deprivation of thyroid hormone or thyromegaly. Impaired growth and development are less when hypothyroidism is acquired at later age and, since brain growth is virtually complete by 2 to 3 years of age, mental retardation or neurologic sequelae are not associated with juvenile hypothyroidism. Other manifestations are myxedematous skin changes (dry skin, puffiness around the eyes, sparse hair) constipation, sleepiness, and mental decline.

Therapy is thyroid hormone replacement, the same as hypothyroidism in the infant, although the prompt treatment needed in the infant is not required in the child. In children with severe symptoms, the restoration of euthyroidism is achieved more gradually with administration of increasing amounts of L-thyroxine over 4 to 8 weeks to avoid symptoms of hyperthyroidism that can occur with treatment of chronic hypothyroidism.

Nursing Considerations

The importance of early recognition in the infant has already been discussed in Chapter 9. Cessation or retardation in growth in a child whose growth has previously been normal should alert the observer to the possibility of hypothyroidism. Following diagnosis and implementation of thyroxine therapy, the importance of compliance and periodic monitoring of response to therapy should be stressed to parents. The child should learn to take responsibility for his own health as soon as he is old enough.

GOITER

A goiter is an enlargement or hypertrophy of the thyroid gland. It may occur in deficient (hypothyroid), excessive (hyperthyroid), or normal (euthyroid) thyroid hormone secretion. It can be congenital, usually as a result of maternal administration of antithyroid drugs and/or iodides during pregnancy, or acquired. The acquired disease can result from increased secretion of pituitary thyrotropic hormone in response to decreased circulating levels of thyroid hormones or from infiltrative neoplastic or inflammatory processes. In areas where dietary iodine (essential for TH production) is deficient, goiter can be endemic.

Enlargement of the thyroid gland can be mild and noticeable only when there is an increased demand for TH, e.g., during periods of rapid growth. Where iodine deficiency is severe, a large percentage of the population display goiters. Enlargement of the thyroid at birth can be sufficient to cause severe respiratory distress. Sporadic goiter is usually caused by lymphocytic thyroiditis and intrinsic biochemical defects in synthesis of the hormones are associated with goiters. Thyroid hormone replacement is necessary to treat the hypothyroidism and reverse the thyroid-stimulating hormone effect on the gland.

Nursing Considerations

Identification of large goiters is facilitated by their obvious appearance. Smaller nodules may be evident only on palpation. Nurses in ambulatory settings need to be aware of the possibility of goiters and report such findings to a physician. Benign enlargement of the thyroid gland may occur during adolescence and should not be confused with patho-

logic states. Nodules rarely are caused by a cancerous tumor but always require evaluation. Since they are frequently associated with a history of exposure to irradiation of the neck or upper thorax, inquiry about this possibility is part of the assessment.

If an infant is born with a goiter, immediate precautions are instituted for emergency ventilation, such as supplemental oxygen and a tracheostomy set. Positioning the child with the neck hyperextended often facilitates breathing. Immediate surgery to remove part of the gland may be lifesaving.

When thyroid replacement is necessary, parents have the same needs regarding its administration as discussed for the parents of children who have hypothyroidism (Chapter 9).

LYMPHOCYTIC THYROIDITIS

Lymphocytic thyroiditis (Hashimoto disease, juvenile autoimmune thyroiditis) is the most common cause of thyroid disease in children and adolescents and accounts for the largest percentage of juvenile hypothyroidism. It accounts for many of the enlarged thyroid glands formerly designated as thyroid hyperplasia of adolescence or "adolescent goiter." The disease is four to seven times more common in girls than in boys and four times more common in white than in black persons (Fink and Beall, 1982). Although it can occur during the first 3 years of life, it more frequently appears after age 6. It reaches a peak incidence at adolescence (DiGeorge, 1983), and there is evidence that the disease is self-limited (Mäenpää and others, 1981).

Pathophysiology

There is a strong genetic predisposition to the development of autoimmune thyroiditis, although no mode of inheritance has been delineated and the basic stimulus or autoimmune defect is unknown. There is a close relationship between this disease and other thyroid disorders (Graves disease, idiopathic hypothyroidism, idiopathic myxedema) and autoimmune disorders (pernicious anemia, Addison disease, type I diabetes mellitus, and hypoparathyroidism) in families. An increased incidence of the histocompatibility antigens HLA-DR3 and HLA-DR5 has been observed in patients with autoimmune thyroiditis (Sack and others, 1983).

The disease is characterized by lymphocytic infiltration of the gland, germinal-center inflammation, and, in many patients, replacement with fibrous tissue. In the early stages there may be only hyperplasia. A defect in autoregulation allows the persistence of a T-cell clone, which induces a cell-mediated immune response. Several antithyroid antibodies have been recognized in patients with thyroiditis.

Clinical Manifestations

The presence of the enlarged thyroid gland is usually detected by the physician or pediatric nurse practitioner during a routine examination, although it may be noted by parents when the youngster swallows. In most children the entire gland is enlarged symmetrically (but may be asymmetric), firm, freely movable, and nontender. There may be manifestations of moderate tracheal compression (sense of fullness, hoarseness, and dysphagia), but it is extremely rare for nontoxic diffuse goiter to enlarge to the extent that its size causes mechanical obstruction. Most children are euthyroid but some display symptoms of hypothyroidism. Others have signs suggestive of hyperthyroidism, such as nervousness, irritability, increased sweating, or hyperactivity.

Diagnostic Evaluation

Thyroid function tests are usually normal although TSH levels may be slightly or moderately elevated. With progressive disease the T_4 decreases followed by a decrease in T_3 levels and an increase in TSH. A variety of abnormalities in radioactive iodine uptake may be noted. The majority of children have serum antibody titers to thyroid antigens, but fewer children have a positive red blood cell hemagglutination test. When both tests are used almost all children with thyroid autoimmunity are detected. However, levels in children are lower than in adults; therefore repeated measurements may be needed in doubtful cases because titers may increase later in the disease (DiGeorge, 1983).

Therapeutic Management

In many cases the goiter is transient and asymptomatic and regresses spontaneously within a year or two. Therapy of nontoxic diffuse goiter is usually simple, uncomplicated, and effective. Oral administration of thyroid hormone will decrease the size of the gland significantly. It provides the feedback needed to suppress thyroid-stimulating hormone stimulation, and the hyperplastic thyroid gland gradually regresses in size. Surgery is contraindicated in this disorder. Untreated patients should be evaluated periodically.

Nursing Considerations

Nursing care consists of identifying the youngster with thyroid enlargement, reassuring the child that the condition is probably only temporary, and reinforcing instructions for thyroid therapy.

HYPERTHYROIDISM

The largest percentage of hyperthyroidism in childhood is caused by Graves disease, usually associated with an enlarged thyroid gland and exophthalmos. The peak incidence of the disease occurs between 12 and 14 years of age but may be present at birth in children of thyrotoxic mothers. The incidence is five times higher in girls than in boys.

The hyperthyroidism of Graves disease is apparently caused by a serum thyroid-stimulating immunoglobulin but no specific etiology has been identified. There is definitive evidence for familial association with a high concordance incidence in twins. A large number of persons (approximately 80%) with the disease possess the histocompatibility antigens HLA-B8.

Clinical Manifestations

The development of manifestations is highly variable. Manifestations develop gradually with an interval between onset and diagnosis of approximately 6 to 12 months. The principal clinical features are excessive motion—irritability, hyperactivity, short attention span, tremors, insomnia, and emotional lability. Gradual weight loss despite a voracious appetite is common. Linear growth and bone age are usually accelerated. Muscle weakness often occurs. Hyperactivity of the gastrointestinal tract may cause vomiting and frequent stooling. Cardiac manifestations include a rapid pounding pulse even during sleep, widened pulse pressure, systolic murmurs, and cardiomegaly. During slight exertion, such as climbing stairs, dyspnea occurs. The skin is warm, flushed, and moist. Heat intolerance may be severe and is accompanied by diaphoresis. The hair is unusually fine and unable to hold a wave.

Exophthalmos (protruding eyeballs), observed in many children, is accompanied by a wide-eyed staring expression, increased blinking, lid lag, lack of convergence, and absence of wrinkling of the forehead when looking upward. As protrusion of the eyeball increases, the child may not be able to completely cover the cornea with the lid. Visual disturbances may include blurred vision and loss of visual acuity.

Diagnostic Evaluation

Presence of a thyroid mass in a child requires a thorough history including inquiry into prior irradiation to the head and neck and exposure to a goiterogen (Reiter and others, 1981). Diagnosis is established on the basis of increased levels of T_4 and T_3. Thyrotropin (TSH) is suppressed to unmeasurable levels. Other tests are rarely indicated.

Therapeutic Management

Therapy for hyperthyroidism is controversial, but all methods are directed toward retarding the rate of hormone secretion. The three acceptable modes available are (1) the antithyroid drugs, which interfere with the biosynthesis of thyroid hormone, including propylthiouracil (PTU) and methimazole (MTZ, Tapazole); (2) subtotal thyroidectomy, and (3) ablation with radioiodine (^{131}I-iodide). Each is effective but each has advantages and disadvantages (Foley, 1986).

Drug therapy. Most centers favor drugs as an initial therapy. An effective response to these drugs occurs after a latent period, since they inhibit production of additional thyroid hormone but do not retard secretion of stored supplies. Generally some improvement is noted within the first 2 weeks, with evidence of decreased nervousness, less fatigue, increased strength, a lowered pulse, and weight gain. In many children an initial treatment course of 1 to 2 years will be followed by a complete remission of the disorder. Those who relapse may benefit from a second course of therapy but may also be candidates for surgical intervention.

Disadvantages include toxic drug reactions requiring alternate therapy, chronic dependency on the drug, and failure to produce remission in a large number of patients. The most serious side effect of these antithyroid drugs is agranulocytosis (pronounced leukopenia), which generally occurs within the initial weeks or months of therapy. It is usually accompanied by a sore throat and fever. Treatment involves immediate discontinuation of the drug, isolation of the child, and administration of antibiotics and glucocorticoids.

Thyroidectomy. Surgical treatment involves surgical ablation of the thyroid (thyroidectomy). Although this approach has the advantage of being a long-lasting form of therapy without the need for multiple-dose drug therapy, it has a number of serious disadvantages including the increased incidence of hypothyroidism and the need for thyroxine therapy, infrequent recurrent laryngeal nerve palsy and permanent hypoparathyroidism, keloid formation of the anterior cervical scar in susceptible individuals, and (rarely) surgical mortality. Therefore surgery in most centers is reserved for children who do not respond to or comply with the use of antithyroid drugs or who are prone to recurrences.

Radioiodine therapy. Radioiodine therapy is not recommended for children because of the increased risk of subsequent carcinoma of the thyroid and the possibility of genetic damage.

Thyrotoxicosis. Thyrotoxicosis (thyroid "crisis" or thyroid "storm") may occur from sudden release of the hormone. Although unusual in children, a crisis can be life-threatening. These "storms" are evidenced by acute onset of severe irritability and restlessness, vomiting, diarrhea, hyperthermia, hypertension, severe tachycardia, and prostration. There may be rapid progression to delirium, coma, and even death. A crisis may be precipitated by acute infection, surgical emergencies, or discontinuation of antithyroid therapy. Treatment in addition to antithyroid drugs is administration of beta-adrenergic blocking agents (propranolol), which provide relief from the adrenergic hyperresponsiveness that produces the disturbing side effects of the reaction. Therapy is usually required for 2 to 3 weeks.

Nursing Considerations

The initial nursing objective is identification of children with hyperthyroidism. Since the clinical manifestations often appear gradually, the goiter and ophthalmic changes may not be noticed and the excessive activity may be attributed to behavioral problems. Nurses in ambulatory settings, particularly those caring for children in school, need to be alert to signs that suggest this disorder, especially weight loss together with an excellent appetite, academic difficulties resulting from short attention span and inability to sit still, unexplained fatigue and sleeplessness, and difficulty with fine motor skills, such as writing.

Much of a child's care is related to treating physical symptoms before a response to drug therapy is achieved. The child needs a quiet, unstimulated environment that is conducive to rest. Sometimes hospitalization is necessary during the immediate treatment phase to remove the child from a troubled home. A regular routine is beneficial in providing frequent rest periods, minimizing the stress of coping with unexpected demands, and meeting the child's needs promptly.

Since the nervous manifestations often interfere with schoolwork, a consultation with the child's teachers is important in advising them of the medical reason for the problem and suggesting ways of helping the child adjust. For example, he may benefit from a shortened school day or at least study periods in a quiet area. Limiting demands on the child, such as reciting in class or participating in extracurricular activities, may help conserve strength for academic studies. Despite the excessive activity of these children, they tire easily, experience muscle weakness, and are unable to relax to recoup their strength.

Emotional lability is often manifest by sudden episodes of crying or elation. Such behavior, coupled with irritability, disrupts interpersonal relationships, creating difficulties within and outside the home. Parents need help in understanding the uncontrollable nature of these outbursts and ways of minimizing them through decreased environmental stimulation, stress, and frustration. The child should be encouraged to express feelings about his behavior and the effect that it has on others. The nurse can encourage the child to concentrate on friendships with one special peer rather than a group until such time as the condition is stabilized.

Heat intolerance may produce considerable family conflict. Since the child prefers a cooler environment than others, he is likely to open windows, complain about the heat, wear minimal clothing, and kick off blankets while sleeping. Although the child should dress in accordance with climatic conditions, the use of light cotton clothing in the home, good ventilation, frequent baths, and adequate hydration is helpful in providing comfort. Hygiene should be stressed because of excessive sweating.

Dietary requirements should be adjusted to meet the child's increased metabolic rate. Although the need for calories is increased, these should be provided in wholesome foods rather than "junk" foods. The child may require vitamin supplements to meet the daily requirement. Rather than three large meals, the child's appetite may be better satisfied by five or six moderate meals throughout the day. Family members should refrain from making remarks about the child's appetite since he may voluntarily restrict his eating to avoid such attention.

Once therapy is instituted, the drug regimen is explained, emphasizing the importance of observing for side effects of antithyroid drugs. Untoward effects of propylthiouracil and related compounds include urticarial rash, fever, arthritis, or arthralgia. There may be enlargement of the salivary and cervical lymph glands, diminished sense of taste, hepatitis, and edema of the lower extremities. Since sore throat and fever accompany the grave complication of leukopenia, these children should be seen by a physician if these occur. Parents should also be aware of the signs of hypothyroidism, which can occur from overdose of the drugs. The most common indications are lethargy and somnolence.

Psychologic preparation of the child for thyroidectomy is similar to that for any other surgical procedure (see Chapter

27). However, of special consideration is the site of the incision. The fear of having the throat cut is very real and in older children is associated with death. The nurse should explain that the throat is not cut, only the skin, to allow for removal of the gland. Showing the child a picture of the anatomic location of the thyroid around the trachea is often helpful. The child should be prepared for the dressing around the neck and the possibility of an endotracheal or "breathing" tube after surgery.

Postoperative care involves positioning with the neck slightly flexed to avoid strain on the sutures and observation for bleeding and complications. Damage to the recurrent laryngeal nerve is evidenced by severe stridor and/or hoarseness. Earliest indication of hypoparathyroidism may be anxiety and mental depression, followed by paresthesia and evidence of heightened neuromuscular excitability, such as Chvostek and Trousseau signs and carpopedal spasm (tetany).

Disorders of Parathyroid Function

The parathyroid glands secrete parathormone (PTH), whose main function, along with vitamin D and calcitonin, is homeostasis of serum calcium concentration. The effect of PTH on calcium is opposite that of thyrocalcitonin. The principal effects of PTH on its target sites include:

Bones—increases osteoclastic activity and causing phosphate-producing bone demineralization
Kidneys—increases absorption of calcium and excretion of phosphate
Gastrointestinal tract—promotes calcium absorption

The net result of the integrated action of PTH and vitamin D is maintenance of serum calcium levels within a narrow normal range and the mineralization of bone. Secretion of PTH is controlled by a negative feedback system involving the serum calcium ion concentration. Low ionized calcium levels stimulate PTH secretion, causing absorption of calcium by the target tissues; high ionized calcium concentrations suppress PTH.

HYPOPARATHYROIDISM

There are two classic forms of hypoparathyroidism that are observed during childhood: *idiopathic hypoparathyroidism,* in which there is deficient production of PTH, and *pseudohypoparathyroidism,* in which production of PTH is increased but end-organ responsiveness to the hormone is deficient. The presenting signs or symptoms are similar.

Idiopathic hypoparathyroidism may occur as a component of multi-glandular failure, possibly related to autoimmune phenomena, or from parathyroidectomy. Familial hypoparathyroidism is inherited as an X-linked recessive trait, with early onset in male infants, usually in the first month of life. Pseudohypoparathyroidism is also thought to be inherited as an X-linked dominant trait with variable expressivity.

Hypoparathyroidism can also occur secondary to other causes. Postoperative hypoparathyroidism may follow thyroidectomy with acute or gradual onset and be transient or permanent. Two forms of transient hypoparathyroidism may be present in the newborn, both of which are the result of a relative PTH deficiency. One type is caused by maternal hyperparathyroidism or maternal diabetes mellitus. A more common later form appears almost exclusively in infants fed a milk formula with a high phosphate to calcium ratio (see p. 357).

Clinical Manifestations

Children with pseudohypoparathyroidism are short with round faces, short thick necks, and short and stubby fingers and toes with dimpling of the skin over the knuckles. None of these are observed in hypoparathyroidism. In both types the skin can be dry, scaly, and coarse with skin eruptions, the hair is often brittle, and the nails are thin and brittle with characteristic transverse grooves. Subcutaneous soft tissue calcifications appear in pseudohypoparathyroidism but not in idiopathic hypoparathyroidism. Dental and enamel hypoplasia occurs in both types.

Tetany, convulsions (grand mal, petit mal, or focal seizures), carpopedal spasm, muscle cramps and twitching, paresthesias, and laryngeal stridor are often the initial symptoms in both types. Mental retardation is a prominent feature of pseudohypoparathyroidism and may also occur in idiopathic hypoparathyroidism but is less frequent in later onset disease and early diagnosis and treatment. Swings of emotion, loss of memory, depression, and confusion can occur. Papilledema may be seen in the idiopathic disease but is rare in pseudohypoparathyroidism. Since hypoparathyroidism results in decreased bone resorption and inactive osteoclastic activity, skeletal growth is retarded.

Diagnostic Evaluation

The diagnosis of hypoparathyroidism is made on the basis of clinical manifestations associated with decreased serum calcium and increased serum phosphorus. Levels of plasma PTH are low in idiopathic hypoparathyroidism but high in pseudohypoparathyroidism. End-organ responsiveness is tested by the administration of PTH with measurement of urinary cyclic AMP. Kidney function tests are included in the differential diagnosis to rule out renal insufficiency. Although bone radiographs are usually normal, they may demonstrate increased bone density and suppressed growth.

Therapeutic Management

The objective of treatment is to maintain normal serum calcium and phosphate levels with minimum complications. Acute or severe tetany is corrected immediately by intravenous and oral administration of calcium gluconate and follow-up daily doses to achieve normal levels. Twice daily serum calcium measurements are taken to monitor the efficacy of therapy and prevent hypercalcemia. When diagnosis is confirmed, vitamin D therapy is begun. Vitamin D therapy is somewhat difficult to regulate because the drug has a prolonged onset and a long half-life. Some advocate beginning with a lower dose with stepwise increases and careful monitoring of serum calcium until stable levels are achieved. Others prefer rapid induction with higher doses and rapid reduction to lower maintenance levels.

Long-term management consists of administration of massive doses of vitamin D, and oral calcium supplementation may be useful in maintaining adequate serum calcium levels, although it is not essential. Frequent monitoring of blood calcium and phosphorus is done until the levels have stabilized, then monitoring is done monthly and less often until the child is seen at 6-month intervals. Renal function, blood pressure, and serum vitamin D levels are measured every 6 months. Serum magnesium levels are measured every 3 to 6 months to permit detection of hypomagnesemia, which may raise the requirement for vitamin D.

Vitamin D toxicity is a constant concern and a serious complication of therapy, which can occur even after prolonged stabilization of serum calcium. This is possibly related to resolution of bone disease (Tsang, Noguchi, and Steichen, 1979).

Nursing Considerations

The initial objective is recognition of hypocalcemia. Unexplained convulsions, irritability (especially to external stimuli), gastrointestinal symptoms, and positive signs of tetany should lead the nurse to suspect this disorder. Much of the initial nursing care is related to the physical manifestations and includes institution of seizure and safety precautions, reduction of environmental stimuli, and observation for signs of laryngospasm, such as stridor, hoarseness, and a feeling of tightness in the throat. A tracheostomy set and injectable calcium gluconate should be placed near the bedside for emergency use. The administration of calcium gluconate requires precautions against extravasation of the drug.

After initiation of treatment, the nurse discusses with the parents the need for continuous daily administration of calcium salts and vitamin D. Because vitamin D toxicity can be a serious consequence of therapy parents are advised to watch for signs which include weakness, fatigue, lassitude, headache, nausea, vomiting, and diarrhea. Early renal impairment is manifest by polyuria, polydipsia, and nocturia.

HYPERPARATHYROIDISM

Hyperparathyroidism is rare in childhood but can be be primary or secondary. The most common cause of primary hyperparathyroidism is adenoma of the gland. The most common causes of secondary hyperparathyroidism are chronic renal disease, renal rickets, and congenital anomalies of the urinary tract. The common factor is hypercalcemia.

Clinical Manifestations

The manifestations of primary hyperparathyroidism are conveniently grouped according to the system involved.

Gastrointestinal—nausea, vomiting, abdominal discomfort, and constipation
Central nervous system—delusions, confusion, hallucinations, impaired memory, lack of interest and initiative, depression, and varying levels of consciousness
Neuromuscular—weakness, easy fatigability, muscle atrophy (especially proximal muscles of the lower limbs), twitching of the tongue, paresthesias in extremities
Skeletal—vague bone pain, subperiosteal resorption of phalanges, spontaneous fractures, and absence of lamina dura around the teeth
Renal—polyuria and polydipsia, renal colic, and hypertension

Diagnostic Evaluation

Blood studies to confirm the presence of elevated calcium and lowered phosphorus levels are routinely performed. Measurement of PTH, as well as several tests to isolate the cause of the hypercalcemia, such as renal function studies, should be included. Other procedures employed to substantiate the physiologic consequences of the disorder include electrocardiography and radiographic bone surveys.

Therapeutic Management

Treatment depends on the cause of hyperparathyroidism. The treatment of primary hyperparathyroidism is surgical removal of the tumor or hyperplastic tissue. Treatment of secondary hyperparathyroidism is directed at the underlying contributing cause, which subsequently restores the serum calcium balance. However, in some instances the underlying disorder is irreversible, such as in chronic renal failure. In this instance treatment is aimed at raising serum calcium levels in order to inhibit the stimulatory effect of low levels on the parathyroids. This includes oral administration of calcium salts, high doses of vitamin D to enhance calcium absorption, a low-phosphorus diet, and administration of a phosphorus-mobilizing aluminum hydroxide to reduce phosphate absorption.

Nursing Considerations

The initial nursing objective is recognition of the disorder. Since secondary hyperparathyroidism is a consequence of chronic renal failure, the nurse is always alert to signs suggestive of this complication, especially bone pain and fractures. Since urinary symptoms are the earliest indication, assessment of other body systems for evidence of high calcium levels is indicated when polyuria and polydipsia coexist. Change in behavior, especially inactivity, unexplained gastrointestinal symptoms, and cardiac irregularities should provide clues to the possibility of hyperparathyroidism.

Much of the initial nursing care is related to the physical symptoms and prevention of complications. To minimize renal calculi formation, hydration is essential. Fruit juices that maintain a low urinary pH, such as cranberry or apple juice, are encouraged, since acidity of body fluids promotes calcium absorption. All urine should be strained for evidence of renal casts.

Safety precautions, such as side rails in place at all times and assistance with ambulation, are instituted because of the tendency toward fractures and muscular weakness. Children with renal rickets (osteodystrophy) may wear braces to minimize skeletal deformities. These should be worn as prescribed. If the child is confined to bed, the nurse should consult with the physical therapist regarding proper use of orthopedic appliances.

Vital signs should be taken frequently and the pulse counted for 1 full minute to detect irregularities. A decrease in pulse rate should be reported, since it may signal severe bradycardia and cardiac arrest. The diet needs supervision to ensure compliance with low-phosphate foods, particularly dairy products. The nurse should instruct parents regarding foods that need to be avoided and the necessity of administering calcium and vitamin D.

If surgery is anticipated, care is similar to that discussed for the child with hyperthyroidism (p. 1691). Since hypocalcemia is a potential complication, observation for signs of tetany, institution of seizure precautions, and having calcium gluconate available for emergency use are part of the nursing plan.

Disorders of Adrenal Function

The adrenal glands consist of two distinct portions: the cortex, or outer section, and the medulla, or inner core, each of which produces different hormones.

ADRENAL HORMONES

The adrenal cortex secretes the hormones, collectively known as steroids, that are essential to life. The medulla produces the catecholamines, epinephrine and norepinephrine. Since these chemicals are also produced by the sympathetic nervous system, absence of the adrenal supply is not incompatible with life.

Adrenal Cortex

The cortex secretes three groups of hormones that are classified according to their biologic activity: (1) glucocorticoids (cortisol, corticosterone), (2) mineralocorticoids (aldosterone), and (3) sex steroids (androgens, estrogens, and progestins). The glucocorticoids and mineralocorticoids influence metabolic regulation and stress adaptation. The sex steroids influence sexual development but are not essential because the gonads secrete the major supply of these hormones.

Glucocorticoids. The most important glucocorticoids in humans are cortisol and corticosterone whose principal effects are outlined in the accompanying box. The secretion of the glucocorticoids is controlled by adrenocorticotropic hormone (ACTH) from the anterior pituitary. That means a decrease in circulating levels of cortisol results in an increased secretion of adrenocorticotropic hormone, which

---

PHYSIOLOGIC EFFECTS OF GLUCOCORTICOIDS

Stimulation of gluconeogenesis by the liver (a hyperglycemic effect)
Increased protein catabolism with resulting reduction in protein stores (except in the liver)
Increased mobilization and utilization of fatty acids for energy
Increased storage of adipose tissue in certain sites
Decreased inflammatory and allergic actions
Regulation of fluid and electrolytes by promoting sodium retention and potassium excretion by the kidneys and by water diuresis through direct antagonistic action against antidiuretic hormone
Increased gastric acid and pepsin production
Suppression of lymphocytes, eosinophils, and basophils but elevation of neutrophils, erythrocytes, and thrombocytes

---

stimulates the adrenal cortex to secrete additional glucocorticoids.

In times of stress the anterior pituitary is stimulated by corticotropin-releasing factor from the hypothalamus, which causes the release of increased amounts of ACTH. Stressful stimuli capable of provoking this response include trauma, anesthesia, surgical intervention, sepsis, acute anoxia, hypothermia, hypoglycemia, and emotional states, especially panic, anxiety, or anger.

Secretion of the glucocorticoids is also regulated by body rhythms. Blood levels of cortisol demonstrate a typical diurnal or circadian pattern. In individuals who follow a regular routine of nighttime sleeping, cortisol levels are highest in the early morning hours after arising and lowest in the evening hours before bedtime. Major actions of glucocorticoids are outlined in the accompanying box.

Mineralocorticoids. The most important mineralocorticoid is aldosterone. Like cortisol, it promotes sodium retention, as do the anions, chloride and bicarbonate, and potassium excretion in the renal tubules. However, its effect is many times more potent than that of the glucocorticoids in maintaining extracellular fluid volume, acid-base balance, and normal potassium levels.

Aldosterone secretion is primarily under control of the renin-angiotensin system. The juxtaglomerular cells of the kidney respond to decreased arterial pressure and/or blood volume and to decreased sodium concentrations by secreting the enzyme renin into the blood. Renin in turn converts angiotensinogen to angiotensin I and then to angiotensin II. Increased levels of angiotensin stimulate the adrenal cortex to secrete aldosterone, which preserves sodium, thereby retaining water. The renin-angiotensin mechanism also results in increased blood pressure.

Sex steroids. Except for the first few days of life, the sex hormones are normally secreted in only minimum amounts until adolescence, at which time they play a role in pubertal changes. Their actions are the same as those of the

PHYSIOLOGIC EFFECTS OF CATECHOLAMINES

Increased cardiac activity
Vasoconstriction of blood vessels (elevation of blood pressure)
Increased rate and depth of respirations
Bronchial dilation
Inhibition of gastrointestinal activity
Increased muscular contraction
Pupillary dilation
Increased metabolic rate
Heightened sensory awareness
Diaphoresis

gonadal hormones on internal and external sexual structures and skeletal growth.

Adrenal Medulla

The adrenal medulla secretes the catecholamines, epinephrine and norepinephrine. Both hormones have essentially the same effects on different organs as those caused by direct sympathetic stimulation, except that the hormonal effects last several times longer. Their major actions are outlined in the accompanying box.

Although the catecholamines evoke similar responses from target sites, there are some important differences. Epinephrine has a greater effect on cardiac activity than norepinephrine, but it causes only weak constriction of the blood vessels of muscles in comparison to the effect of norepinephrine. As a result, norepinephrine elevates blood pressure, whereas epinephrine increases cardiac output. Another important difference is their effect on metabolism. Epinephrine increases the metabolic rate to a much greater extent than norepinephrine. These differences in action have been attributed to the catecholamines' effects on α- or β-adrenergic receptors. Supposedly norepinephrine can only affect those effector cells that contain α-receptors, which are mostly excitatory in nature (constriction and contraction). Epinephrine, however, can affect both α- and β- receptors, and β-receptors are mostly inhibitory (dilation and relaxation).

Control of secretion of catecholamines, primarily in response to physiologic or emotional stress, is through the hypothalamus. Also, stimulation of the sympathetic nervous system results in the release of epinephrine and norepinephrine from the sympathetic nerves and adrenal medulla. Both systems support each other, and one can be substituted for the other. For this reason there is no condition attributable to hypofunction of the adrenal medulla. Even in bilateral adrenalectomy, catecholamine replacement is not necessary because the sympathetic release of these chemicals is sufficient to meet all the physiologic functions required to cope with stressful events.

Catecholamine-secreting tumors are the primary cause of adrenal medullary hyperfunction. In children the most com-

mon neoplasms of this type are pheochromocytoma, neuroblastoma, and ganglioneuroma. Ganglioneuromas are thought to be neuroblastomas that have undergone maturation into a benign tumor composed of ganglion cells. These tumors are associated with less abnormal catecholamine secretion than the other two types, but persons with ganglioneuromas may have a clinical picture of chronic diarrhea, failure to thrive, skin rash, hypokalemia, persistent cough, and abdominal distention. The exact reason for these symptoms is unknown, although they are attributable to the tumor because they disappear after surgical extirpation of the mass.

ACUTE ADRENOCORTICAL INSUFFICIENCY

The acute form of adrenocortical insufficiency (adrenal crisis) may result from a number of causes during childhood. Although a rare disorder, some of the more common etiologic factors include hemorrhage into the gland from trauma, which may be caused by a prolonged, difficult labor; fulminating infections, such meningococcemia, which result in hemorrhage and necrosis (Waterhouse-Friderichsen syndrome); abrupt withdrawal of exogenous sources of cortisone or failure to increase exogenous supplies during stress; or as a result of congenital adrenogenital hyperplasia of the salt-losing type.

Clinical Manifestations

Early symptoms of adrenocortical insufficiency include increased irritability, headache, diffuse abdominal pain, weakness, nausea and vomiting, and diarrhea. Generalized hemorrhagic manifestations are present in the Waterhouse-Friderichsen syndrome. Fever increases as the condition worsens and is accompanied by signs of central nervous system involvement, such as nuchal rigidity, convulsions, stupor, and coma. The child is in a shocklike state with a weak, rapid pulse, decreased blood pressure, shallow respirations, cold clammy skin, and cyanosis. Circulatory collapse is the terminal event.

In the newborn, adrenal crisis is accompanied by extreme hyperpyrexia, tachypnea, cyanosis, and convulsions. Usually there is no evidence of infection or purpura. However, hemorrhage into the adrenal gland may be evident as a palpable retroperitoneal mass.

Diagnostic Evaluation

There is no rapid, definitive test for confirmation of acute adrenocortical insufficiency. Routine procedures such as measurement of plasma cortisol levels are too time-consuming to be practical. Therefore diagnosis is usually made based on clinical presentation, especially when a fulminating sepsis is accompanied by hemorrhagic manifestations and signs of circulatory collapse despite adequate antibiotic therapy. Since there is no real danger in administering a cortisol preparation for a short period, treatment should be instituted immediately. Improvement with this therapy confirms the diagnosis.

Therapeutic Management

Treatment involves replacement of cortisol, replacement of body fluids to combat dehydration and hypovolemia, administration of glucose solutions to correct hypoglycemia, and specific antibiotic therapy in the presence of infection. Initially intravenous hydrocortisone (Solu-Cortef) is administered. Normal saline containing 5% glucose is given parenterally to replace lost fluid, electrolytes, and glucose. If hemorrhage has been severe, whole blood may be replaced. In the event that these measures do not reverse the circulatory collapse, vasopressors such as phenylephrine (Neo-Synephrine), levarterenol (Levophed), or metaraminol (Aramine) are used for immediate vasoconstriction and elevation of blood pressure.

Once the child's condition is stabilized, oral doses of cortisone, fluids, and salt are given, similar to the regimen used for chronic adrenal insufficiency. To maintain sodium retention, aldosterone is replaced by synthetic salt-retaining steroids, such as fluhydrocortisone (Florinef) or desoxycorticosterone acetate (DOCA acetate).

Nursing Considerations

Because of the abrupt onset and potentially fatal outcome of this condition, prompt recognition is essential. Vital signs and blood pressure are taken every 15 minutes to monitor the hyperpyrexia and shocklike state. Seizure precautions are instituted, since convulsions from the elevated temperature are not uncommon. As soon as therapy is instituted, the nurse should monitor the child's response to fluid and cortisol replacement. Too rapid administration of fluids can precipitate cardiac failure, whereas overdosage with cortisol produces hypotension and a sudden fall in temperature. The nurse should regulate intravenous infusions carefully to guard against too rapid administration of drugs. Intake and urinary output should be recorded.

Once the acute phase is over and the hypovolemia is corrected, the child is started on oral fluids, such as small quantities of ginger ale, fruit juice, or salted broth. Too rapid ingestion of oral fluids may induce vomiting, which increases dehydration. Therefore the nurse should plan a gradual schedule for reintroducing liquids. For children who refuse to drink, the prospect of having the intravenous infusion removed once oral fluids are increased is often a motivating factor.

An ascending flaccid paralysis may occur on the second to third day of treatment because of an abnormally low serum potassium level secondary to overtreatment with cortisol and sodium chloride. The nurse should observe for signs of hypokalemia, such as cardiac irregularities and poor muscle control, and should evaluate serum electrolyte levels. The condition is rapidly corrected with intravenous and oral potassium replacement. When the oral preparation is given, it should be mixed with a small amount of strongly flavored fruit juice to disguise its bitter taste.

The sudden, severe nature of this disorder necessitates a great deal of emotional support for the child and family. The child may be placed in an intensive care unit where the surroundings are strange and frightening. Despite the need for emergency intervention, the nurse must be sensitive to the family's psychologic needs and prepare them for each procedure, even if this is as brief as a statement, such as, ''The intravenous infusion is necessary to replace fluid that the child is losing.'' Since recovery within 24 hours is often dramatic, the nurse should keep the parents apprised of the child's condition, emphasizing signs of improvement such as a lowered temperature and elevated blood pressure. If paralysis occurs, the nurse should assure them that this condition is temporary and quickly reversed.

If treatment needs to be continued past the acute stage, parents require the same preparation as those of children with chronic adrenal insufficiency. Preparation for discharge should begin as soon as possible after the child's condition has stabilized.

CHRONIC ADRENOCORTICAL INSUFFICIENCY

Chronic adrenocortical insufficiency (Addison disease) is rare in children. When it does occur, it is usually caused by a destructive lesion of the adrenal glands, neoplasms, or an idiopathic cause. At one time generalized tuberculosis was the leading cause of adrenal gland destruction.

Evidence of this disorder is usually gradual in onset, since 90% of adrenal tissue must be nonfunctional before signs of insufficiency are manifest. However, during periods of stress when demands for additional cortisol are increased, symptoms of acute insufficiency may appear in a previously well child. The cardinal signs and symptoms are:

  Muscular weakness and mental fatigue, which are aggravated by slight additional exertion or minor illness

  Pigmentary changes of previous scars, palmar creases, mucous membranes, and hair; hyperpigmentation over pressure points (elbows, knees, or waist); or, less frequently, loss of pigmentation (vitiligo)

  Weight loss resulting from dehydration and anorexia from impaired gastrointestinal functioning (decreased hydrochloric acid)

  Hypotension and small heart size, which predispose to dizziness and syncopal (fainting) attacks

  Irritability, apathy, and negativism

  Signs of hypoglycemia, such as headache, hunger, weakness, trembling, and sweating; other signs seen in some children are recurrent unexplained convulsions, an intense craving for salt, and acute abdominal pain

Definitive diagnosis is based on measurements of functional cortisol reserve. The cortisol and urinary 17-hydroxycorticosteroid levels are low and fail to rise while plasma ACTH levels are elevated with corticotropin (ACTH) stimulation, the definitive test for the disease.

Therapeutic Management

Treatment involves replacement of glucocorticoids (cortisol) and mineralocorticoids (aldosterone). Some children are able to be maintained solely on oral supplements of cortisol (cortisone or hydrocortisone preparations) with a liberal intake of salt. During stressful situations, such as infection, emotional upset, or surgery, the dosage must be tripled to accommodate the body's increased need for glucocorticoids. Failure to meet this requirement will precipitate an acute crisis. Overdosage produces appearance of cushingoid signs.

Children with more severe states of chronic adrenal insufficiency require mineralocorticoid replacement to maintain fluid and electrolyte balance. Other forms of therapy include monthly injections of desoxycorticosterone acetate or implantation of desoxycorticosterone acetate pellets subcutaneously every 9 to 12 months.

Nursing Considerations

Once the disorder is diagnosed, parents need guidance concerning drug therapy. They must be aware of the continuous need for cortisol replacement. Sudden termination of the drug because of inadequate supplies or inability to ingest the oral form because of vomiting places the child in danger of an acute adrenal crisis. Therefore parents should always have a spare supply of the medication in the home. Ideally they should have a prefilled syringe of hydrocortisone in the home and be instructed in proper technique for intramuscular administration of the drug in case of a crisis. As was mentioned earlier, unnecessary administration of cortisone will not harm the child but, if needed, may be lifesaving. Any evidence of acute insufficiency should be reported to the physician immediately.

Parents also need to be aware of side effects of the drugs. Undesirable side effects of cortisone include gastric irritation, which is minimized by ingestion with food or the use of an antacid, increased excitability and sleeplessness, weight gain that may require dietary management to prevent obesity, and, rarely, behavioral changes, including depression or euphoria. Parents should be aware of signs of overdose (see Table 38-2) and report these to the physician. In addition, the drug has a very bitter taste, which creates a challenge for nurses and parents in its administration.

The side effects of mineralocorticoids are primarily caused by overdosage and include generalized edema, which is first noticed around the eyes; hypertension, which may cause headaches; cardiac arrhythmias; and signs of hypokalemia. Ideally the child should be evaluated periodically for evidence of excessive medication. Emphasizing the importance of routine follow-up care is a significant nursing responsibility.

Since the body cannot supply endogenous sources of cortical hormones during times of stress, the home environment should be stable and relatively unstressful. Parents need to be aware that during periods of emotional or physical crisis the child requires additional hormone replacement. The child should wear a Medic Alert tag to permit medical personnel to adjust his requirements during emergency care.

CUSHING SYNDROME

Cushing syndrome is a characteristic group of manifestations caused by excessive circulating free cortisol. It can result from a variety of etiologies, which generally fall into one of four categories:

1. Pituitary Cushing syndrome with adrenal hyperplasia, usually attributed to an excess of ACTH
2. Adrenal Cushing syndrome with hypersecretion of glucocorticoids, generally the result of adrenocortical neoplasms
3. Ectopic Cushing syndrome with autonomous secretion of ACTH, most often caused by extrapituitary neoplasms
4. Iatrogenic Cushing syndrome, frequently the result of administration of large amounts of exogenous corticosteroids

Cushing syndrome is uncommon in children and when seen is often caused by excessive or prolonged steroid therapy that produces a cushingoid appearance. This condition is reversible once the steroids are gradually discontinued. Abrupt withdrawal will precipitate acute adrenal insufficiency. Gradual withdrawal of exogenous supplies is necessary to allow the anterior pituitary an opportunity to secrete increasing amounts of adrenocorticotropic hormone to stimulate the adrenals to produce cortisol.

Clinical Manifestations

Because the actions of cortisol are widespread, clinical manifestations are equally profound and diverse (Table 38-2 and Fig. 38-3). Those symptoms that produce changes in physical appearance occur early in the disorder and are of considerable concern to older children. The physiologic disturbances, such as hyperglycemia, susceptibility to infection, hypertension, and hypokalemia, may have life-threatening consequences unless recognized early and treated successfully.

Diagnostic Evaluation

Several tests are helpful in confirming excess cortisol levels, such as fasting blood glucose levels for hyperglycemia, serum electrolyte levels for hypokalemia and alkalosis, 24-hour urinary levels of elevated 17-hydroxycorticoids and 17-ketosteroids, and radiographic studies of bone for evidence of osteoporosis and of the skull for enlargement of the sella turcica. Another procedure used to establish a more definitive diagnosis is the dexamethasone (cortisone) suppression test. Administration of an exogenous supply of cortisone normally suppresses adrenocorticotropic hormone production. However, in individuals with Cushing syndrome, cortisol levels remain elevated. This test is helpful in differentiating between children who are obese and those who appear to have cushingoid features.

Therapeutic Management

Treatment depends on the cause. In most cases surgical intervention involves bilateral adrenalectomy and postoperative replacement of the cortical hormones (the therapy for this is the same as that outlined for chronic adrenal insufficiency). If a pituitary tumor is found, surgical extirpation or irradiation may be chosen. In either of these instances, treatment of panhypopituitarism with replacement of growth hormone, thyroid extract, antidiuretic hormone, gonadotropins, and steroids may be necessary for an indefinite period.

Nursing Considerations

Nursing care also depends on the cause. When cushingoid features are caused by steroid therapy, the effects may be lessened with administration of the drug early in the morning and on an alternate-day basis. Giving the drug early in the day maintains the normal diurnal pattern of cortisol secretion. If given during the evening, it is more likely to produce symptoms because endogenous cortisol levels are already low and the additional supply exerts more pronounced effects. An alternate-day schedule allows the anterior pituitary an opportunity to maintain more normal hypothalamic-pituitary-adrenal control mechanisms.

If an organic cause is found, nursing care is related to the treatment regimen. Although a bilateral adrenalectomy permanently solves one condition, it reciprocally produces another syndrome. Before surgery parents need to be adequately informed of the operative benefits and disadvantages. Postoperative teaching regarding drug replacement is the same as discussed in the previous section.

Postoperative complications of adrenalectomy are related to the sudden withdrawal of cortisol. The nurse should observe for signs of a shocklike state, especially hypotension and hyperpyrexia. Anorexia and nausea and vomiting are very common and may be improved with the use of nasogastric compression. Muscle joint pain may be severe, requiring use of analgesics. The psychologic depression can be profound and may not improve for months. Parents should be aware of the physiologic reasons behind these symptoms in order to be supportive of the child. Facial changes that occur rapidly often help to improve family members' disposition but may not affect the child's behavior until his physiologic state is stabilized.

Table 38-2   Clinical manifestations of Cushing syndrome

SIGNS/SYMPTOMS	PHYSIOLOGIC CAUSE	SIGNS/SYMPTOMS	PHYSIOLOGIC CAUSE

Centripetal fat distribution
  Truncal obesity
  Supraclavicular fat pads
  Fat pads on neck and
    back ("buffalo hump")
Rounded or "moon" face
	Increased appetite and deposition of fat	Osteoporosis
		  Compression fractures of
		    vertebrae
		  Kyphosis
		  Backache
		  Retarded linear growth
			Increased glomerular filtration rate and excretion of calcium and decreased absorption of calcium from intestinal tract

Muscular wasting
  Thin extremities
  Pendulous abdomen
  Muscle weakness
Thin skin and subcutaneous tissue
Poor wound healing
	Increased protein catabolism resulting in negative nitrogen balance	Hypercalciuria—renal calculi	

		Psychoses
		  Irritability
		  Insomnia
		  Euphoria
		  Depression
		  Frank psychoses
			Cause unknown

Increased susceptibility to infection Decreased inflammatory response	Decreased production and circulating levels of antibodies by lysis of fixed plasma cells and lymphocytes	Peptic ulcer	Increased production of hydrochloric acid and pepsin and decreased gastric mucous production
Excessive bruising Petechial hemorrhages	Capillary weakness resulting from loss of protein	Hyperglycemia Glycosuria	Increased gluconeogenesis by liver and decreased rate of glucose utilization by cells
Facial plethora ("red cheeks") Reddish purple abdominal striae	Thin skin that allows capillary blood to be visible, increased color from polycythemia	Latent or overt diabetes	Overstimulation of Islands of Langerhans

Hypertension— arteriosclerosis	Increased salt and water retention (hypervolemia)	Virilization
		  Hirsutism
		  Acne
		  Deepening of voice
		  Clitoral enlargement
		  Tendency toward male
		    physique in female
		  Amenorrhea
		  Impotence
			Excess production of androgens

Hypokalemia Alkalosis	Increased excretion of potassium and hydrogen ions		

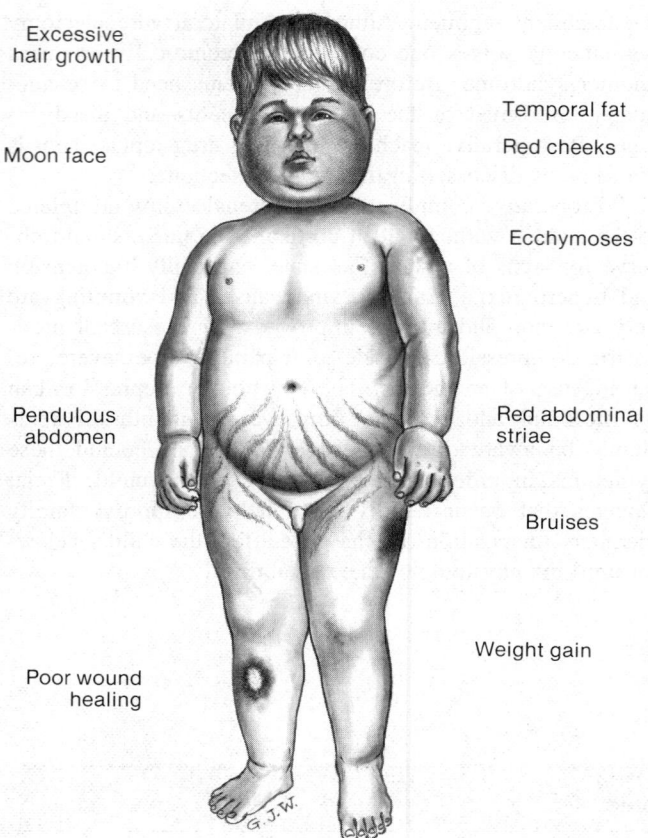

Excessive hair growth

Moon face

Temporal fat

Red cheeks

Ecchymoses

Pendulous abdomen

Red abdominal striae

Bruises

Weight gain

Poor wound healing

Fig. 38-3. Characteristics of Cushing syndrome.

CONGENITAL ADRENOGENITAL HYPERPLASIA

Disorders caused by excessive secretion of androgens by the adrenal cortex are known variously as *congenital adrenogenital hyperplasia (CAH), adrenocortical hyperplasia (ACH), adrenogenital syndrome (AGS),* and *congenital adrenocortical hyperplasia (CAH).* Although hyperfunction of the adrenal gland can occur from a number of causes, such as a virilizing adrenal tumor, in children the most common cause is congenital adrenogenital hyperplasia, an inborn deficiency of various enzymes necessary for the biosynthesis of cortisol. Congenital adrenogenital hyperplasia is inherited as an autosomal-recessive disorder or may be result from a tumor or maternal ingestion of steroids.

Pathophysiology

Interference in the biosynthesis of cortisol during fetal life results in an increased production of adrenocorticotropic hormone, which stimulates hyperplasia of the adrenal gland. Depending on the enzymatic defect, increased quantities of cortisol precursors and androgens are secreted. There are six major types of biochemical defects. The most common is partial or complete *21-hydroxylase deficiency.* With partial deficiency, enough aldosterone is produced to preserve sodium and adequate cortisol is produced to prevent signs of adrenocortical insufficiency.

In the complete or salt-losing form, insufficient amounts of aldosterone and cortisol are produced, so that circulatory collapse occurs without immediate replacement of the mineralocorticoids and glucocorticoids. In *11-hydroxylase deficiency* there is an increase in the mineralocorticoid 11-desoxycorticosterone, which leads to hypertension. In each of these types there is excess production of androgens, which causes in females ambiguous female genitalia and precocious genital development in males. Other forms of congenital adrenogenital hyperplasia do not result in excess production of androgens but cause various degrees of hypoaldosteronism or hyperaldosteronism.

Clinical Manifestations

Excessive androgens cause masculinization of the urogenital system during the twelfth and twentieth weeks of fetal development. The most pronounced abnormalities occur in the female, who is born with varying degrees of ambiguous genitalia (pseudohermaphroditism). Masculinization of external genitalia causes the clitoris to enlarge so that it appears as a small phallus. Fusion of the labia produces a sac-like structure resembling the scrotum without testes. However, no abnormal changes occur in the internal sexual organs, although the vaginal orifice is usually closed by the fused labia (see also p. 482).

In the male, enlargement of the genitals (macrogenitosomia precox) and frequent erections are the principal signs. When androgen production is not excessive, virilizing effects in the female may be minimal or absent and the male may have evidence of pseudohermaphroditism, such as microphallus, hypospadias, and incompletely fused scrotum.

Untreated congenital adrenogenital hyperplasia results in early sexual maturation, with enlargement of the external sexual organs; development of axillary, pubic, and facial hair; deepening of the voice; acne; and marked increase in musculature with changes toward an adult male physique. However, in contrast to precocious puberty, breasts do not develop in the female, and she remains amenorrheic and infertile. In the male the testes remain small and spermatogenesis does not occur. In both sexes linear growth is accelerated and epiphyseal closure is premature, resulting in short stature by the end of puberty.

Diagnostic Evaluation

Clinical diagnosis is initially based on congenital abnormalities that lead to difficulty in assigning sex to the newborn and on signs and symptoms of adrenal insufficiency or hypertension. Definitive diagnosis is confirmed by evidence of increased 17-ketosteroid levels in most types of congenital adrenogenital hyperplasia. Usually the level of 17-hydroxycorticoids is low or near normal. In complete 21-hydroxylase deficiency, blood electrolytes demonstrate loss of sodium and chloride and elevation of potassium. In older children bone age is advanced and linear growth is increased. A buccal smear for positive sex determination should always be done in any case of ambiguous genitalia.

Another test that can be used to visualize the presence of pelvic structures is ultrasonography, a noninvasive, painless imaging technique that does not require anesthesia or sedation. It is especially useful in congenital adrenogenital hyperplasia because it readily identifies the absence or presence of female reproductive organs in a newborn or child with ambiguous genitalia. Because it yields immediate results, it has the advantage of determining the child's gender long before the more complex laboratory results for chromosomal analysis or steroid levels are available.

Therapeutic Management

The initial medical objective is to confirm the diagnosis and assign a sex to the child, usually according to the genotype. In both sexes cortisone is administered to suppress the abnormally high secretions of adrenocorticotropic hormone, and, if begun early enough, is very effective. Cortisone depresses the secretion of adrenocorticotropic hormone by the adenohypophysis, which in turn inhibits the secretion of adrenocorticosteroids, which stems the progressive virilization. The signs and symptoms of masculinization in the female gradually disappear and excessive early linear growth is slowed. Puberty occurs normally at the appropriate age.

The recommended oral dosage is 15 to 20 mg/m^2 of body surface in divided doses to simulate the normal diurnal pattern of adrenocorticotropic hormone secretion (Burnett, 1980). Since these children are unable to produce cortisol in response to stress, it is necessary to increase the dosage during episodes of infection, fever, or other stresses. Acute emergencies require immediate intravenous or intramuscular administration. Emergency situations include bacterial and viral infections, surgery, fractures, major injuries, and sometimes insect stings. For those children with the salt-losing type of congenital adrenogenital hyperplasia, the replacement of aldosterone as outlined under chronic adrenal insufficiency is instituted, and they should be provided with supplementary dietary salt.

Depending on the degree of masculinization in the female, reconstructive surgery may be required to reduce the size of the clitoris, separate the labia, and create a vaginal orifice. This should be done after the infant is physically able to withstand the procedure and before she is old enough to be aware of the abnormal genitalia. Plastic surgery is generally done in stages and yields excellent cosmetic results. Reports concerning sexual satisfaction after partial clitoridectomy indicate that the capacity for orgasm and sexual gratification is not necessarily impaired.

Unfortunately not all children with congenital adrenogenital hyperplasia are diagnosed at birth and raised in accordance with their genetic sex. Particularly in the case of affected females, masculinization of the external genitalia may have led to sex assignment as a male. In males diagnosis is usually delayed until early childhood, when signs of virilism appear. In these situations it is advisable to continue rearing the child as a male in accordance with assigned sex and phenotype. Hormonal replacement may be required

to permit linear growth and to initiate male pubertal changes. Surgery is usually indicated to remove the female organs and reconstruct the phallus for satisfactory sexual relations. Obviously these individuals are not fertile.

Nursing Considerations

Of major importance is recognition of ambiguous genitalia in newborns. If there is any question regarding assignment of sex, the parents need to be told immediately to prevent the embarrassing situation of informing family members of the child's sex and then having to change the announcement. As with any congenital defect, the parents require an adequate explanation of the condition and a period of time to grieve for the loss of perfection. In this instance they may also need to grieve for the loss of the desired sex child. For example, the birth of a phenotypically male infant may fulfill their wish for a son. Knowledge of the child's actual sex may leave them disappointed. Such situations may also lead them to discuss the possibility of raising the child as a male despite the actual sex. This is a difficult question that requires thoughtful discussion among the parents and members of the health team.

In general, rearing the genetically female child as a female is preferred because of the success of surgical intervention and the satisfactory results with hormones in reversing virilism and providing a prospect of normal puberty and the ability to conceive. This is in contrast to the choice of rearing the child as a male, in which case the child is sterile and may never be able to function satisfactorily in heterosexual relationships. If the parents persist in their decision to assign a male sex to a genetically female child, a psychologic consultation should be requested to explore their motivations and ensure their understanding of the child's future consequences.

Parents need an explanation regarding this disorder that facilitates their explaining it to others. Before confirmation of the diagnosis and sex of the child, the nurse should refer to the infant as "child" or "baby" rather than by the pronouns "he" or "she" and definitely not "it." When referring to the external genitalia, it is preferable to refer to them as sex organs and to emphasize the similarity between the penis/clitoris and scrotum/labia during fetal development. In this way it can be explained that the sex organs were overdeveloped because of too much male hormone secretion. Using a correct vocabulary allows parents to explain the abnormalities to others in a straightforward manner, just as if the defect involved the heart or an extremity.

It is also important to stress that sex assignment and rearing depend on psychosocial influences, not on genetic sex hormonal influences during fetal life. Parents often fear that the infant will retain "male behavioral characteristics" because of prenatal masculinization and will not be able to develop "feminism." Using the word "hermaphrodite" often confuses parents because they interpret this term to mean that the child is "half male–half female." Since the prognosis for normal sexual development is excellent after early treatment, the nurse should foster identification with the child as one sex only. It is also beneficial to mention that ambiguous genitalia have no relationship with homosexual or bisexual activity later in life.

As soon as the sex is determined, parents should be informed of the findings and encouraged to choose an appropriate name, and the child should be identified as a male or female, with no reference to ambiguous sex. If the appearance of the enlarged genitalia in a female child concerns the parents, they should be encouraged to discuss their feelings. Suggesting ways to avoid questioning remarks from visitors, such as diapering the child in a separate room, is also helpful. If surgery is anticipated, before and after photographs of reconstruction help to reinforce the expected cosmetic benefits.

Nursing considerations regarding cortisol and aldosterone replacement are the same as those that are discussed for chronic adrenocortical insufficiency. However, since parents may be overwhelmed with the diagnosis and obvious abnormalities at the time of birth, they may not hear all the discharge instructions regarding the medication schedule. A follow-up visit by a public health nurse is ideal to ensure that parents understand and comply with the treatment regimen. Likewise, nurses in well-child facilities should assume responsibility for guidance and supervision regarding this aspect of care during each visit.

Since infants are especially prone to dehydration and salt-losing crises, parents need to be aware of signs of dehydration and the urgency of immediate medical intervention to stabilize the child's condition. Parents, and later the child, need to understand that the medical regimen must be a lifelong commitment; therefore, they should be provided with the education and counseling that will ensure informed and willing compliance (Winter, 1980). They also need to know that growth retardation that may have occurred before therapy cannot be overcome and that normal stature is not a realistic expectation, even though growth velocity may improve with medication.

In the unfortunate situation in which sex is erroneously assigned and later diagnosed, parents need a great deal of help in understanding the reason for the incorrect sex identification and the options for sex reassignment and/or medical/surgical intervention. Since children become aware of their sexual identity by 18 months to 2 years of age, it is believed that any reassignment after this period can cause tremendous psychologic conflicts in the child. Therefore sex rearing should be continued as previously established with medical/surgical intervention as required.

A dilemma often arises, however, regarding what the child should know about his condition, especially gender identification. Because the knowledge that one has been reared opposite his genetic gender can initiate profound psychologic problems, it is recommended that the child not be told this fact but rather be given an explanation regarding his physical disabilities, such as infertility, and the need for hormone replacement and plastic surgery. Parents, in turn, must believe that the child has been raised according to his

"true sex," which is absolutely honest, since sex is not solely a biologic entity but an expression of multiple environmental influences.

Since the hereditary form of adrenogenital hyperplasia is an autosomal-recessive disorder, parents should be referred for genetic counseling before conceiving another child. The nurse's role is to ensure that parents understand the probability of transmitting the trait or disorder with each pregnancy. Affected offspring also require genetic counseling since both sexes are generally able to reproduce. (See Chapter 5 for recurrence risks and genetic counseling.)

HYPERALDOSTERONISM

Excessive secretion of aldosterone may be caused by an adrenal tumor or, in some types of adrenogenital syndromes, may be the result of enzymatic deficiency. The signs and symptoms are caused by increased sodium levels, water retention, and potassium loss. Hypervolemia causes hypertension and resultant headaches. Paradoxically, funduscopic changes resulting from increased blood pressure and edema from water retention are minimal. Hypokalemia results in muscular weakness, paresthesia, episodes of paralysis, and tetany and may be responsible for polyuria and consequent polydipsia.

The clinical diagnosis is suspected when there are findings of hypertension, hypokalemia, and polyuria that fail to respond to antidiuretic hormone administration. Renin and angiotensin titers are abnormally low. Urinary levels of 17-hydroxycorticosteroids and 17-ketosteroids are normal in primary hyperaldosteronism caused by of an aldosterone-secreting tumor but are usually abnormal in adrenogenital syndrome.

Therapeutic Management

Temporary treatment of the disorder involves replacement of potassium and administration of spironolactone (Aldactone), a diuretic that blocks the effects of aldosterone, thereby promoting excretion of sodium and water while preserving potassium. Definitive treatment is similar to that for chronic adrenocortical insufficiency.

Nursing Considerations

An important nursing consideration is recognition of the syndrome, particularly in children who demonstrate high blood pressure. Other clues include bed-wetting, excessive thirst, and unexplained weakness. After the diagnosis, nursing care should be related to the treatment regimen. If diuretics are used, they should be administered in the morning to avoid accidents during the night. Children need unrestricted lavatory privileges at school. Potassium supplements should be mixed with fruit juice to increase their acceptability, and potassium-rich foods should be encouraged. The parents need to be aware of the signs of hypokalemia and hyperkalemia.

After an adrenalectomy, nursing care is similar to that for chronic adrenocortical insufficiency.

PHEOCHROMOCYTOMA

Pheochromocytomas most commonly arise from the chromaffin cells of the adrenal medulla but may occur wherever these cells are found, such as along the paraganglia of the aorta or thoracolumbar sympathetic chain. Approximately 10% of these tumors are located in extraadrenal sites. In children they are frequently bilateral or multiple and are generally benign. Often there is a familial transmission of the condition as an autosomal-dominant trait that tends to favor males.

Clinical Manifestations

The clinical manifestations of pheochromocytoma are caused by an increased production of catecholamines, producing hypertension, tachycardia, headache, decreased gastrointestinal activity with resultant constipation, increased metabolism with anorexia, weight loss, hyperglycemia, polyuria, polydipsia, hyperventilation, nervousness, and diaphoresis. In severe cases signs of congestive heart failure are evident.

Diagnostic Evaluation

The clinical manifestations mimic those of other disorders, such as hyperthyroidism, diabetes mellitus, or functional hyperventilation. Therefore several tests specific to these conditions may be performed as part of the differential diagnosis. In only a small number of instances is a palpable tumor suggestive of the diagnosis. Definitive tests include measurement of urinary levels of the catecholamine metabolites, especially vanillylmandelic acid (VMA); histamine stimulation, which will provoke a hypertensive attack from sudden release of large amounts of catecholamines; and alpha-blocking agents (phentolamine [Regitine]), which will produce a hypotensive episode by inhibiting the action of circulating catecholamines.

Therapeutic Management

Definitive treatment consists of surgical removal of the tumor. In children the tumors may be bilateral requiring a bilateral adrenalectomy and life-long glucocorticoid and mineralocorticoid therapy. The major complications that can occur during surgery are severe hypertension, tachyarrhythmias, and hypotension. The first two are caused by excessive release of catecholamines during manipulation of the tumor and the latter from catecholamine withdrawal and hypovolemic shock (New, Levine, and Temeck, 1986).

Preoperative preparation is implemented beginning 1 to 3 weeks before surgery to prevent these complications. This consists of medication to inhibit the effects of catecholamines. The major group of drugs used is the alpha-adrenergic blocking agents with or without beta-adrenergic blocking agents. The most commonly used alpha-adrenergic blocker is phenoxybenzamine (Dibenzyline), a longer-acting medication given orally every 12 hours. The shorter-acting phentolamine (Regitine) is equally effective but less satisfactory for long-term use, although it is useful for acute hypertension. To control catecholamine release when alpha-adrenergic blocking agents are inadequate, the child is given beta-adrenergic blocking agents, usually propranolol (Inderal) or metyrosine (Demser).

Success of therapy is judged by lowering of blood pressure to normal, absence of hypertensive attacks (flushing or blanching, fainting, headache, palpitations, tachycardia, nausea and vomiting, profuse sweating), decrease in perspiration, and disappearance of hyperglycemia. A disadvantage of these drugs is their inability to block the effects of catecholamines on beta-receptors.

Nursing Considerations

An initial nursing objective is identification of children with this disorder. Outstanding clues are hypertension and hypertensive attacks. Because of behavioral changes (nervousness, excitability, overactivity, even psychosis), increased cardiac and respiratory activity may appear to be related to an acute anxiety attack. Therefore a careful history of the onset of symptoms and association with stressful events is helpful in distinguishing between an organic and a psychologic cause for the symptoms.

Preoperative nursing care involves frequent monitoring of vital signs and observing for evidence of hypertensive attacks and congestive heart failure. Therapeutic effects are evidenced by normal vital signs and absence of glycosuria. Urine should be tested at least daily for sugar and acetone. Any signs of hyperglycemia should be noted and reported immediately.

The environment should be conducive to rest and free of emotional stress. This requires adequate preparation during hospital admission and before surgery. Parents should be encouraged to room-in with their child and to participate in his care. Play activities need to be tailored to the child's energy level but should not be overly strenuous or challenging, since these can increase metabolic rate and promote frustration and anxiety.

After surgery the child should be observed for signs of shock from removal of excess catecholamines. If a bilateral adrenalectomy was performed, the nursing interventions are those discussed for chronic adrenocortical insufficiency.

Disorders of Pancreatic Hormone Secretion

The islets of Langerhans of the pancreas have three major functioning cells: the alpha cells, which produce glucagon, the beta cells, which produce insulin, and the delta cells, which produce somatostatin. Glucagon causes an increase in the blood glucose by stimulating the liver and other cells to release stored glucose (glucogenolysis). Glucagon acts as an emergency supplier of glucose whenever the blood glucose falls too low and is believed to function more independently when insulin is lacking. Somatostatin, although secreted by the islet cells, is found in greater supply in the hypothalamus, where it prevents the release of growth hormone. In the islets of Langerhans somatostatin is believed to regulate the release of insulin and glucagon. This discussion of disorders of pancreatic hormone secretion is limited to diabetes mellitus.

DIABETES MELLITUS

Diabetes mellitus (DM) is a disease of metabolism characterized by a deficiency (relative or absolute) of the hormone insulin. It is the most common metabolic disease, affecting approximately 10 to 12 million persons in the United States, and is now believed to be a syndrome, that is, a group of diseases of differing etiologies with common signs and symptoms (Guthrie and Guthrie, 1983). The overall result is a metabolic adjustment or physiologic change in almost all areas of the body.

DM affects approximately 1:600 school-age children. The disease is rarely diagnosed in infancy and children younger than school age have a lower incidence of the disease than school-age children. The peak incidence is reached during early adolescence and then declines through the remainder of adolescence. It can be manifest at any age, but over 80% of diagnosed cases are in the adult population; therefore, the older the individual, the greater the chance of developing some type of diabetes.

The disease is more prominent in Caucasians and rare in African blacks, Asians, Native Americans, and Eskimos. The incidence in black Americans corresponds with the percentage of Caucasian genes in the black population (MacDonald, 1983).

Classification

Diabetes mellitus can be classified as idiopathic and secondary. Secondary DM can be precipitated by exogenous factors and is usually (but not always) reversible when the primary disorder is treated. These include pancreatic trauma, disease (cystic fibrosis, carcinoma), or resection; hormones (Cushing syndrome, primary aldosteronism, pheochromocytoma), drugs or chemicals (some diuretics, hormones, psychoactive agents, catecholamines, antineoplastic agents); insulin receptor abnormalities; and, a variety of genetic syndromes that are associated with glucose intolerance or frank diabetes.

Gestational diabetes is the appearance of DM or abnormalities of glucose tolerance for the first time during pregnancy. The metabolic and hormonal changes of pregnancy are diabetogenic, and the disorder occurs in 1% to 2% of all pregnancies. Gestational diabetes can appear during the second trimester but usually occurs during the third trimester. The glucose tolerance most often returns to normal soon after delivery, although up to 50% of these women may be expected to develop non-insulin-dependent diabetes within 10 years. It is important to identify the condition because it is associated with a significant increase in perinatal morbidity and mortality. Therefore early detection and aggressive treatment should be implemented to prevent newborn complications (see Infant of the diabetic mother, p. 417).

Idiopathic DM can be classified into two major groups and one newly described type:

Insulin-dependent (IDDM), or type I—characterized by catabolism and the development of ketosis in the absence of insulin replacement therapy; onset is typically in childhood and adolescence but can be at any age

Non-insulin-dependent (NIDDM), or type II—appears to involve resistance to insulin action and defective glucose-mediated insulin secretion; onset is usually after age 40 and there appears to be considerable heterogeneity; affected persons may or may not require daily insulin injections

Maturity-onset diabetes of youth (MODY)—transmitted as an autosomal dominant disorder in which there is formation of structurally abnormal insulin that has decreased biologic activity

Characteristics of IDDM and NIDDM are outlined in Table 38-3. Because DM of childhood is, with few exceptions, the IDDM, or type I form, the remainder of the discussion will be devoted to this important cause of long-term health problems. However, NIDDM will be included as appropriate for comparison throughout.

Etiology

The clinical syndrome of DM results from a large variety of etiologic and pathogenic mechanisms. IDDM is now believed to be an autoimmune disease that arises when a person with a genetic predisposition is exposed to a precipitating event, such as a viral infection. NIDDM is more likely to be influenced by stronger, but as yet unknown, genetic factors.

Genetic factors. IDDM is not inherited but heredity is unquestioned as a prominent factor in the etiology. A variety of genetic mechanisms have been proposed but most favor a multifactorial inheritance or a recessive gene somehow linked to the human lymphocyte antigen (HLA) on the number 6 chromosome at the loci designated A, B, C, and D. From 8 to 30 possible antigens are coded for each locus and some have alternate types (e.g., D and DR) or subtypes (e.g., A1, A2). The D and DR antigens are more strongly related to IDDM than the A, B, and C. Persons with IDDM almost always have the DR3 and DR4 HLA antigens; 75% possess the Dw4 subtype. However many persons with DR3 or DR4 never develop diabetes. Also, in populations such as the Japanese and African blacks, the frequency of the D8 allele is low and IDDM is rare. It is also interesting that D2 and DR2 are rarely found in patients with IDDM. These and the B7 alleles are believed to exert a protective effect against the development of IDDM (Cohen, 1984).

The various combinations (haplotypes) of HLA have been associated with IDDM, and each combination is associated with different disease features. Certain combinations are related to features such as high response to insulin antibodies, age of onset, seasonal variation, and association with autoimmune endocrine disorders. No matter what combination of haplotypes appears in the individual, three basic types of IDDM have been identified relative to HLA types: (1) those that are B8 and DR3 positive, (2) those that are B15 and DR4 positive, and (3) those that are positive for all four antigens (Guthrie and Guthrie, 1983). In excess of 90%

Table 38-3 Comparison of characteristics of type I and type II diabetes mellitus

CHARACTERISTIC	TYPE I (IDDM)	TYPE II (NIDDM)
Age on onset	Less than 20 years	Over 40 years
Type of onset	Abrupt	Gradual
Sex ratio	No sex difference	Females outnumber males
Percentage of population	5%-8%	85%-90%
Heredity:		
Family history	Sometimes	Frequently
HLA	Associations	No associations
Twin concordance	25-50%	90-100%
Ethnic distribution	Primarily caucasians	Common to all
Presenting symptoms	Three Ps* common	May be none
Nutritional status	Underweight	Overweight
Insulin (natural):		
Pancreatic content	Usually 0	Over 50% normal
Serum insulin	Low to absent	High or low
Primary resistence	Minimum	Marked
Islet-cell antibodies	85%	Less than 5%
Metabolic control	Difficult	Usually easy
Stability	Unstable	Stable
Therapy:		
Insulin	Always	20-30% of patients
Oral agents	Ineffective	Often effective
Diet only	Ineffective	Often effective
Chronic complications	Greater than 80%	Variable
Ketoacidosis	Common	Infrequent

*Three Ps = polyuria, polydipsia, and polyphagia.

of all patients with IDDM carry either HLA DR3, DR4, or both (Drash, 1983).

The genetic influence in NIDDM and IDDM appears to differ in several ways. Nearly 100% of offspring of parents who both have NIDDM develop that type of diabetes, but only 45% to 60% of the offspring of both parents who have IDDM will develop the disease. The incidence doubles with every 20% of excess weight, and this figure applies to the young as well as to the older diabetic person.

Autoimmune mechanisms. It is now accepted that an autoimmune process is involved in the great majority of persons who develop IDDM. Pancreatic islet cell antibodies (ICAs) are found in about 80% of patients newly diagnosed with IDDM. The antibodies disappear by 1 year after diagnosis in most persons, but in some they may persist for years. The current theory is that the presence of the HLA genes causes a defect in the immune system that renders the possessor susceptible to viral infections. In DR3-positive persons the virus invades the beta cells and initiates an autoimmune process that gradually destroys them. Without beta cells no insulin can be produced. It is unclear whether the ICAs are the result of the inflammatory process or a significant aspect of the beta cell destruction. Controversy exists regarding whether the autoimmune response is primarily mediated by the lymphocyte response, the humoral (antibody) response, or is a result of the two (Drash, 1983).

There is a strong association between IDDM and other autoimmune endocrine disorders. An increased incidence of other autoimmune endocrine disorders, such as thyroiditis and Addison disease, has been found in families of children with DR3-associated IDDM.

It has also been found that anti-islet cell antibodies are detected in a number of unaffected first-degree relatives of children with IDDM. Over a 3-year period more than 10% of these people developed diabetes (Rabinowe and Eisenbarth, 1984) and 30% of siblings of diabetic children who are positive for ICA may develop diabetes within 5 years. These findings offer hope of identifying persons at risk for diabetes with the eventual possibility of screening and implementation of immunotherapy. Immunosuppression therapy is controversial and has been attempted only in controlled situations with selected persons. The effects of life-long immunosuppression must be carefully weighed against the life-long effects of diabetes.

Viruses. Viruses have been implicated in the etiology of diabetes. Islet cells appear to be particularly susceptible to either direct viral damage or chemical insult. The body reacts to this damaged or changed tissue in an autoimmune phenomenon. Therefore the virus serves as a precipitating factor or "trigger." The Coxsackie group of viruses (especially the Coxsackie B4 virus) has created the most interest, but mumps, cytomegalovirus, Epstein-Barr virus, and infectious hepatitis viruses have all been implicated. However, no specific virus has been clearly documented as the precipitating factor (Drash, 1983).

Also a seasonal variation has been noted in the onset of DM. Although this seasonal variation is not evident in children under 5 years of age, the marked increase in older children during the winter months strongly suggest an infectious disease relationship in either the etiology or expression of diabetes in children (Fishbein and others, 1982; Cahill and McDevitt, 1981).

Type II diabetes. Although IDDM is the predominant form of diabetes in the pediatric age-group, NIDDM, or type II diabetes, can also occur in children. NIDDM can be further classified as obese and nonobese, which are also subgrouped into those who require insulin and those who do not. The disturbed carbohydrate metabolism of NIDDM may be a result of a sluggish or insensitive secretory response in the pancreas or a defect in body tissues that requires unusual amounts of insulin, or it may be the case that the insulin secreted is rapidly destroyed, inhibited, or inactivated in affected persons.

Many persons with NIDDM can be managed on diet alone; others need oral hypoglycemic agents to stimulate insulin production. Some may need insulin to prevent hypoglycemia but, unlike those with IDDM, they do not depend on insulin to sustain life (Guthrie and Guthrie, 1983).

Pathophysiology

Insulin is needed to support the metabolism of carbohydrates, fats, and proteins, primarily by facilitating the entry of these substances into the cell. Insulin is needed for the entry of glucose into the muscle and fat cells, prevention of mobilization of fats from fat cells, and storage of glucose as glycogen in the cells of liver and muscle. Insulin is not needed for the entry of glucose into nerve cells or vascular tissue. The chemical composition and molecular structure of insulin are such that it fits into receptor sites on the cell membrane. Here it initiates a sequence of poorly defined chemical reactions that alter the cell membrane to facilitate the entry of glucose into the cell and stimulate enzymatic systems outside the cell that metabolize the glucose for energy production.

With a deficiency of insulin, glucose is unable to enter the cell and its concentration in the bloodstream increases. The increased concentration of glucose *(hyperglycemia)* produces an osmotic gradient that causes the movement of body fluid from the intracellular space to the extracellular space and into the glomerular filtrate in order to "dilute" the hyperosmolar filtrate. Normally the renal tubular capacity to transport glucose is adequate to reabsorb all the glucose in the glomerular filtrate. When the glucose concentration in the glomerular filtrate exceeds the threshold (180 mg/dl), glucose "spills" into the urine along with an osmotic diversion of water *(polyuria)*, a cardinal sign of diabetes. The urinary fluid losses cause the excessive thirst *(polydipsia)* observed in diabetes. As might be expected, this water

washout results in a depletion of other essential chemicals.

Protein is also wasted during insulin deficiency. Since glucose is unable to enter the cells, protein is broken down and converted to glucose by the liver (glucogenesis); this glucose then contributes to the hyperglycemia. These mechanisms are similar to those seen in starvation when substrate (glucose) is absent. The body is actually in a state of starvation during insulin deficiency. Without the use of carbohydrates for energy, fat and protein stores are depleted as the body attempts to meet its energy needs. The hunger mechanism is triggered, but the increased food intake *(polyphagia)* enhances the problem by further elevating the blood glucose (Fig. 38-4).

Ketoacidosis. When insulin is absent, glucose is unavailable for cellular metabolism and the body chooses alternate sources of energy, principally fat. Consequently fats break down into fatty acids, and glycerol in the fat cells and in the liver is converted to ketone bodies (β-hydroxybutyric acid, acetoacetic acid, acetone). The ketone bodies can be used as an alternative source of fuel to glucose but are utilized in the cells at a limited rate. Any excess is eliminated in the urine (ketonuria) or the lungs (acetone breath). The ketone bodies are strong acids that lower serum pH, producing *ketoacidosis*.

Ketones are organic acids that readily produce excessive quantities of free hydrogen ions, causing a fall in plasma pH. Then chemical buffers in the plasma, principally bicarbonate, combine with the hydrogen ions to form carbonic acid, which readily dissociates into water and carbon dioxide. The respiratory system attempts to eliminate the excess carbon dioxide by increased depth and rate—Kussmaul respirations, or the hyperventilation characteristic of metabolic acidosis. The ketones are buffered by sodium and potassium in the plasma. The kidney attempts to compensate for the increased pH by increasing tubular secretion of hydrogen and ammonium ions in exchange for fixed base, thus depleting the base buffer concentration.

Potassium levels are also a problem and were once the cause of unexplained deaths shortly after insulin therapy was instituted. With cellular death, potassium is released from the cell into the bloodstream and excreted by the kidney where the loss is accelerated by the osmotic diuresis. The total body potassium is then decreased, even though the serum potassium level may be elevated as a result of the decreased fluid volume in which it circulates. Alteration in serum and tissue potassium can make cardiac arrest a potential problem.

If these conditions are not reversed by insulin therapy in combination with correction of the fluid deficiency and electrolyte imbalance, progressive deterioration occurs with dehydration, electrolyte imbalance, acidosis, coma, and death. Diabetic ketoacidosis should be diagnosed promptly in a seriously ill patient and therapy instituted.

Long-term complications. Long-term complications of diabetes involve the microvasculature and macrovasculature. The principal microvascular complications are nephro-

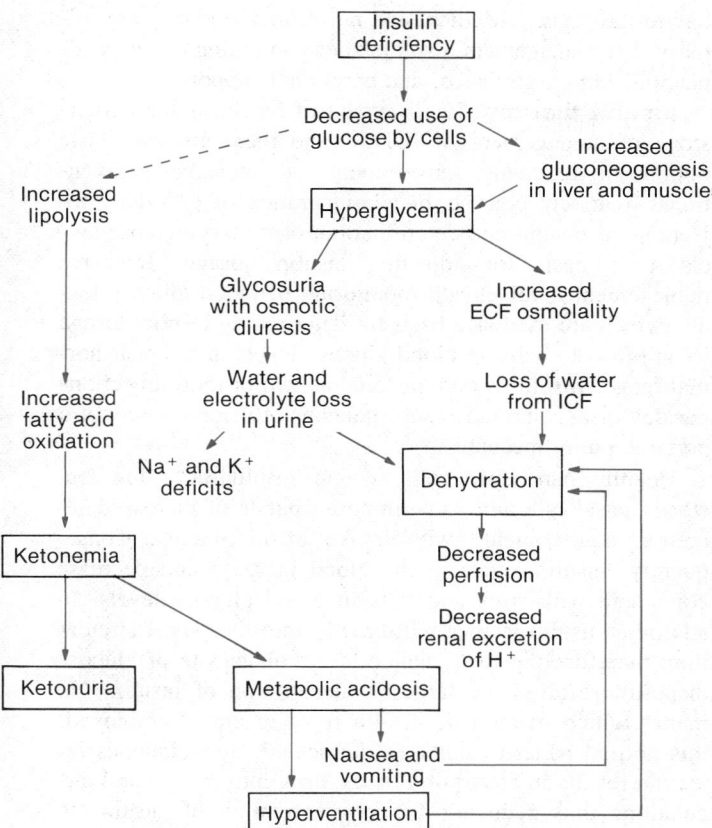

Fig. 38-4. Pathophysiology of acidosis in diabetes mellitus.

pathy, retinopathy, and neuropathy. Life expectancy for persons developing diabetes under 20 years of age is reduced by approximately one third, and the most frequent cause of death is nephropathy, with diabetic retinopathy as one of the leading causes of blindness. Retinopathy appears more frequently in teenage females with IDDM who have both HLA DR3 and DR4 (Malone and others, 1984). Microvascular disease develops in the first 30 years of diabetes, beginning in the first 10 to 15 years with renal involvement evidenced by proteinuria and clinically apparent retinopathy. Persons appear to be free of these complications if they have not been manifested in the first 30 years (Rosenbloom, 1983).

With poor diabetic control, vascular changes appear as early as 2½ to 3 years after diagnosis; however, with good to excellent control, changes have been postponed for 20 or more years. Changes before puberty are uncommon, but after puberty the poorer the control, the more rapid the vascular changes. The process appears to be one of *glycosylation*, wherein proteins from the blood become deposited in the walls of small vessels (e.g., glomeruli) where they become trapped by "sticky" glucose compounds (glycosyl radicals). The build-up of these substances over time causes narrowing of the vessels with subsequent interference with microcirculation to the affected areas (Rosenbloom, 1984; Starkman and others, 1986). Macrovascular disease devel-

ops after 25 years of diabetes and creates the predominant problems in patients with NIDDM.

Other complications have been observed in diabetic children. Hyperglycemia appears to influence thyroid function, and altered function is frequently observed at the time of diagnosis as well as in poorly controlled diabetics. Limited mobility of small joints of the hand occurs in 30% of 7- to 18-year-old children with IDDM and appears to be related to changes in the skin and soft tissues surrounding the joint as a result of glycosylation.

Clinical Manifestations

The symptomatology of diabetes is more readily recognizable in children than in adults, so it is surprising that the diagnosis may sometimes be missed or delayed. Diabetes is a great imitator; influenza, gastroenteritis, and appendicitis are the conditions most often diagnosed, only to find that the disease was really diabetes. Diabetes should be suspected in those families with a strong family history of diabetes, especially if there is one child in the family with diabetes.

The sequence of chemical events described previously results in hyperglycemia and acidosis, which in turn produce weight loss and the three "polys" of diabetes—polyphagia, polydipsia, and polyuria—the cardinal symptoms of the disease. In NIDDM diabetes (which has also been found in older children), the insulin values are found to be elevated, 80% to 90% of this population have been found to be overweight, and there is often fatigue and frequent infections (such as monilial infections in females).

The IDDM diabetic has markedly decreased insulin levels and, as diabetes becomes complete, there is no demonstrable insulin at all. The child may start wetting the bed, become irritable and "not himself," or act overly tired. Abdominal discomfort is common. Weight loss, though quite observable on the charts, may be a less frequent presenting complaint because of the fact that the family might not have noticed the change. Another outstanding feature of diabetes is thirst. One couple reported that their child, during a trip from California to Kansas, drank the contents of a gallon jug of water between each gas station stop. At a certain point in the illness the child may actually refuse fluid and food, adding to the increasing state of dehydration and malnutrition. Other symptoms include dry skin, blurred vision, and sores that are slow to heal. More commonly in children, fatigue and bed-wetting are the chief complaints that prompt parents to take their child for evaluation.

The child may be *hyperglycemic,* with elevated blood glucose levels and glucose in the urine; may be in *diabetic ketosis,* with ketones as well as glucose in the urine but not be noticeably dehydrated; or may be suffering from *diabetic ketoacidosis,* with dehydration, electrolyte imbalance, and acidosis.

Mild diabetes. Although most childhood diabetes is recognized during the rapid initial deterioration in carbohydrate metabolism, others with more benign disease are being identified with increasing frequency. A few are detected accidentally by urinalysis before overt symptoms are observed. Maturity-onset diabetes of youth (MODY) is sometimes seen in an obese teenager. This type, like NIDDM, can often be controlled with diet restriction.

Diagnostic Evaluation

Three groups of children who should be considered as possibly diabetic are (1) children who have glycosuria, polyuria, and a history of weight loss or failure to gain despite a voracious appetite; (2) those with transient or persistent glycosuria; and (3) those who display manifestations of metabolic acidosis, with or without stupor or coma. In every case diabetes must be considered if there is glycosuria, with or without ketonuria, in association with otherwise unexplained hyperglycemia (Sperling, 1983).

Glycosuria by itself is not diagnostic of diabetes. Other sugars, such as galactose, can produce a positive Clinitest and other conditions may cause a mild degree of glycosuria. These are infection, trauma, emotional or physical stress, hyperalimentation, and some renal or endocrine diseases. Tests used to determine glycosuria are the glucose oxidase tapes (Tes-Tape and Clinistix) or Clinitest tablets.

A fasting blood sugar greater than 120 mg/dl is almost certain to be caused by diabetes. Postprandial blood glucose determinations and the traditional oral glucose tolerance tests have yielded low detection rates in children and are not usually necessary for establishing a diagnosis. Serum insulin levels may be normal or moderately elevated at the onset of diabetes; delayed insulin response to glucose indicates the presence of prediabetes.

Ketoacidosis must be differentiated from other causes of acidosis or coma including hypoglycemia, uremia, gastroenteritis with metabolic acidosis, salicylate intoxication, encephalitis, and other intracranial lesions. Diabetic ketoacidosis is determined by the presence of hyperglycemia (blood glucose measurement equal to or greater than 300 mg/dl), ketonemia (strongly positive), acidosis (pH less than 7.30 and bicarbonate less than 15 mEq/L), glycosuria, and ketonuria.

Therapeutic Management

The management of the child with IDDM consists of a multidisciplinary approach involving the family, the child (when appropriate), and professionals including a pediatrician, diabetes nurse educator, nutritionist, and sometimes a psychologic support service from a mental health professional. Communication between the team members is essential and extends to other individuals in the child's life, such as teachers, the school nurse, school guidance counselor, and coach.

The definitive treatment is replacement of insulin that the child is unable to produce. However insulin needs are also affected by nutritional intake, activity, and other life events, such as illnesses. The complexity of the disease and its management requires that the child and family adjust their life-style to meet the changes that the disease imposes on day-to-day living. Medical and nutritional guidance are primary, but management also includes continuing diabetes education, family guidance, and emotional support.

Insulin therapy. Replacement of insulin is the cornerstone of management of IDDM, and there are two basic options in treatment: conventional and intensive. Conventional treatment consists of administration of two daily injections of insulin and determination of urinary glucose levels as a basis for adjusting insulin dosage. Intensive management involves self-monitoring of blood glucose levels, which are used as a basis for determining insulin dosage in an effort to achieve blood glucose levels in the near-normal range. Insulin is administered as two or more injections per day or as continuous subcutaneous infusion by way of a portable pump mechanism.

Healthy pancreatic cells secrete insulin at a low but steady basal rate with superimposed bursts of increased secretion that coincide with intake of nutriments. Consequently, insulin levels in the blood increase and decrease coincident with rises and falls in blood glucose levels. In addition, insulin is secreted directly into the portal circulation; therefore the liver, which is the major site of glucose disposal, receives the largest concentration of insulin. No matter which method of insulin replacement is employed, this normal pattern cannot be duplicated. Subcutaneous injection results in absorption of the drug into the general circulation, thus reducing the concentrations of insulin to which the liver is exposed.

Insulin preparations. Insulin is available in highly purified beef, pork, or beef-pork preparations, and in the newer human insulin manufactured by gene-splicing techniques. Human and pork varieties are less allergenic than beef preparations, and the animal insulins are less expensive than the synthetic human insulins.

Insulin is available in rapid-, intermediate-, and long-acting preparations, and all are packaged in the strength of 100 units/ml. Other dosages are available for situations where extraordinarily large or small dosages are required.

Dosage. Most children can be controlled satisfactorily with a twice daily insulin regimen consisting of a combination of rapid-acting (regular) and intermediate-acting (NPH or Lente) insulin drawn up into the same syringe and injected before breakfast and before the evening meal. The amount of regular insulin needed before breakfast is determined by late morning and early afternoon blood glucose measurements, and the evening dose by the bedtime measurement. If bedtime measurements are high, regular insulin is added to the presupper injection. When regular insulin is not needed in the afternoon presupper dose, better control is achieved when the second intermediate-acting insulin is given at bedtime instead of presupper (Wolfsdorf, 1986).

Regular insulin is best given at least 30 minutes before meals. This allows sufficient optimum time for absorption and a significantly less rise in blood glucose following the meal than when the meal is eaten immediately following the insulin injection. Some authorities advocate multiple injections throughout the day rather than the twice daily regimen, that is, a once daily dose of long-acting (Ultralente) insulin to simulate the basal insulin secretion and injections of rapid-acting insulin before each meal. A multiple daily injection (MDI) program is particularly suitable for the difficult-to-control diabetic child.

The precise dose of insulin needed cannot be predicted. Therefore regimen of total dosage and percentage of regular to intermediate-acting insulin should be determined empirically for each child. Usually 60% to 75% of the total daily dose is given before breakfast and the remainder before the evening meal. Furthermore insulin requirements do not remain constant but change continuously during growth and development, and the need varies according to the child's activity level. For example, less insulin is required during the active spring and summer months. Illness also alters insulin requirements.

Methods of administration. Daily insulin is administered subcutaneously by twice daily injections, by multiple dose injections, or by means of a portable pump. The pump is an electromechanical device designed to deliver fixed amounts of a dilute solution of regular insulin continuously, thereby more closely imitating the release of the hormone by the islet cells.

There are two types of insulin pumps: closed-loop systems and open-loop systems. The closed-loop system is self-contained and designed to detect and respond to changing blood glucose levels. Unfortunately this type of system is very large and requires a venous access. It is used only in the hospital situation where close glucose monitoring is needed, e.g., for the patient during surgery, during labor, in ketoacidosis, or for insulin readjustment.

An open-loop system continuously infuses very small amounts of insulin subcutaneously at basal levels and delivers larger doses, or boluses, of insulin as set by the wearer, usually 30 minutes before meals. Approximately half the daily dose is infused in basal doses and half in bolus doses. The system consists of a syringe to hold the insulin, a plunger, and a mechanism to drive the plunger. The insulin flows from the syringe through a catheter to a needle inserted into subcutaneous tissue (the abdomen or thigh) and the lightweight device is worn on a belt or a shoulder holster. The needle and catheter are changed every 48 hours by the child or parent, using aseptic technique, and taped in place.

The device can be adjusted to deliver a larger amount of insulin before meals. The amount of insulin is based on capillary blood sugar measurements, which the child or parent tests by means of a drop of blood on a chemically treated test strip (Dextrostix, Chemstrip bG) with the aid of a color chart or a glucose monitor (Dextrometer or Glucometer).

Although the pump provides more even insulin release, it has certain disadvantages. It cannot be removed for more than 1 hour, which limits some activities, such as bathing and swimming (it is damaged by water) and like any other mechanical device, it is subject to malfunction. However, the pumps are equipped with alarms that signal problems that may arise such as rundown batteries, blocked needle or tubing, or a malfunction that allows uncontrollable insulin delivery.

Researchers are experimenting with a new approach to insulin administration—intranasal. When insulin is combined with bile salts the mixture can be administered by way of an aerosol pump. The insulin is able to cross the nasal mucosa to increase serum levels. The duration of action is not long enough to be a total replacement for injections but may be of value as insulin supplementation at mealtime. Patients are cautioned not to attempt to inhale standard insulin because it is not absorbed through the mucosa without an appropriate transport medium.

Monitoring. Monitoring the effectiveness of insulin therapy is a vital part of management. It is the only way in which to determine the amount of insulin needed by a child at any given time. Several measurements are used to evaluate the glucose levels as a basis for insulin administration and regulation.

Urine. Urine testing has been a mainstay of diabetic management in the past but urine tests for glucose have many limitations. There is poor correlation between simultaneous glycosuria and blood glucose concentration. Even the double-voided specimens may not accurately reflect the concurrent level of blood glucose. Glucose does not appear in the urine until the blood glucose concentration is well above the optimum range. However, urine testing can be carried out periodically to detect evidence of ketonuria. It is recommended that urine always be tested during an illness and whenever blood glucose is 250 mg/dl or higher when measured twice in a row 4 to 6 hours apart.

Blood glucose. Home blood glucose monitoring (HBGM) has improved diabetes management and is used successfully by children from the onset of their diabetes. By testing their own blood, children are able to change their insulin regimen to maintain their glucose level in the euglycemic range of 80 to 120 mg/dl. Diabetes management depends to a great extent on home glucose monitoring. In general, children tolerate the testing well.

Glycosylated hemoglobin. The measurement of glycosylated hemoglobin (hemoglobin A_{1c}) levels is a satisfactory method for assessing the control of the difficult-to-control diabetic patient. As red blood cells circulate in the bloodstream, glucose molecules gradually attach to the hemoglobin A molecules and remain there for the lifetime of the red blood cell, approximately 120 days. The attachment is not reversible; therefore this glycosylated hemoglobin serves as a reflection of the average blood glucose levels that have taken place during the previous 1 to 3 months. The test is of value in assessing long-term glucose control, detecting incorrect testing, monitoring effectiveness of changes in treatment, defining patients' goals, and detecting noncompliance in the diabetic child who is suspected of "cheating" regularly.

Nutrition. Essentially the nutritional needs of children with diabetes are no different from those of healthy children. They need no special foods or supplements. They need sufficient calories to balance daily expenditure for en-

NUTRITIONAL PRINCIPLES IN TYPE I DIABETES

1. Develop a basic daily meal plan that is relatively consistent in terms of:
   Total energy (calorie) intake
   Balance of energy-yielding nutrients (carbohydrates, fats, and proteins)
2. Provide for compensatory changes for nonbasal circumstances:
   Extra food for extra activity
   Extra insulin or activity for extra food
3. Avoid hyperglycemia by:
   Omitting rapidly absorbed simple sugars from regular meal planning
4. Avoid hypoglycemia by:
   Reasonably consistent meal timing
   Provision of snacks

From Skyler, J.S.: Dietary planning in insulin-dependent diabetes mellitus, Pediatr. Ann. 12:652-657, 1983.

ergy and to satisfy the requirement for growth and development. Unlike the healthy child whose insulin is secreted in response to food intake, insulin injected subcutaneously has a relatively predictable time of onset, peak effect, duration of action, and absorption rate depending on the type of insulin used. Consequently the timing of food consumption must be regulated to correspond to the time and action of the insulin prescribed.

Meals and snacks must be eaten at the same times each day and the total number of calories and proportions of basic nutrients must be consistent from day to day. The constant release of insulin into the circulation makes the child prone to hypoglycemia between the three daily meals unless a snack is provided between meals and at bedtime. The distribution of calories should be calculated to fit the activity pattern of each child. For example, a child who is more active in the afternoon will need the larger snack at that time. This larger snack might also be split to allow some food at school and some food after school. Alterations in food intake should be made so that food, insulin, and exercise are balanced. Extra food is needed for extra activity.

The food intake may be planned in a variety of ways but is based on a balanced diet that incorporates six basic food groups: milk, meat, vegetables, fat, fruit, and bread. The family may follow the exchange system approved by the American Diabetes Association (ADA) or the point system, based on 75 kcal equaling 1 point. The exchange system indicates the amount (portion size) of each food by volume or weight and is prescribed in terms of the number of exchanges from each food group that constitutes each meal and snack. This ensures day-to-day consistency in total calories, protein, fat, and carbohydrate while allowing a choice from a wide variety of foods.

Concentrated sweets are eliminated and, because of the increased risk for atherosclerosis in diabetics, fat is reduced to 30% of the total caloric requirement. Dietary fiber has become increasingly important in dietary planning because of its influence on digestion, absorption, and metabolism of many nutrients. It has been found to diminish the rise in blood sugar after meals.

Correctly used, the diet allows for flexibility and the incorporation of preferred foods in most instances. In the diabetic child, food restriction should never be used for diabetic control, although some restrictions may be imposed for weight control if the child is overweight. In general the child's appetite should be the guide for the amount of calories needed with the total calorie intake adjusted to appetite and activity. Basic principles of diet management are outlined in the accompanying box.

Exercise. Exercise is encouraged and never restricted unless indicated by other health conditions. Exercise lowers blood sugar levels, depending on the intensity and duration of the activity. Consequently exercise should be included as part of diabetic management and the type and amount of exercise should be planned around the child's interests and capabilities. However, in most instances children's activities are unplanned, and the resulting decrease in blood sugar can be compensated for by providing extra snacks before (and if prolonged during) the activity. Insulin should not be reduced unless the needed increase in food cannot be tolerated. In addition to a feeling of well-being, regular exercise aids in utilization of food and often requires less insulin.

Physical training tends to increase tissue sensitivity to insulin, even in the resting state. Consequently it is especially important to understand the relationship between the activity and the diabetic regimen. Vigorous muscular contraction increases regional blood flow and accelerates the absorption and circulation of insulin that is injected into the area, which can contribute to development of hypoglycemia. If exercise involving leg muscles is planned, it is recommended that nonexercised sites (arm or abdomen) should be used for insulin injection. This practice may replace the need for further increased carbohydrate intake or reduced insulin dose (or both) to avoid exercise-induced hypoglycemia.

Children with poorly controlled diabetes are particularly at risk for hypoglycemia with exercise or may actually stimulate ketoacid production. Therefore the child who has marked hyperglycemia and ketonuria should be discouraged from strenuous physical activity until satisfactory control of the diabetes is achieved by appropriate adjustments of insulin and diet (Wolfsdorf, 1986).

Athletes and those youngsters who regularly participate in organized sports are advised to adjust their insulin dosage in anticipation of sustained physical activity during the part of the day devoted to strenuous exercise. For example, the morning dose of intermediate-acting insulin may need to be reduced to compensate for after-school sports activity. Optimum adjustments for each child are determined primarily by trial and error. Nutritional needs of the athlete are subject to those dietary needs discussed for sports participation in Chapter 20 as well as the diabetic dietary management.

Hypoglycemia. Occasional episodes of hypoglycemia are an integral part of insulin therapy, and an objective of diabetic management is to achieve the best possible glycemic control while minimizing the frequency and severity of hypoglycemia. Even well-controlled children may experience mild symptoms of hypoglycemia almost daily, but if the signs and symptoms are recognized early and promptly relieved by appropriate therapy, the child's activity should be interrupted for no more than a few minutes.

The most common causes of hypoglycemia are bursts of physical activity without additional food, or delayed, omitted, or incompletely consumed meals. Sometimes the reaction from sustained exercise may occur several hours after the exercise. Occasionally hypogylcemic reactions occur unexpectedly and without apparent cause. They may be the result of an inadvertent or deliberate error in insulin administration.

Gastroenteritis, in which there is a gastric stasis, may impede the absorption of food even though the child is eating reasonably well. It can also occur when the blood glucose level is so low it causes stasis. Then the child may eat a meal or snack and still have an insulin reaction. Continued feeding does not seem to alter the blood glucose level, because the simple glucose or sugar remains in the stomach.

The signs and symptoms of hypoglycemia are caused by both increased adrenergic activity and impaired brain function. The increased adrenergic nervous system activity plus increased secretion of catecholamines produce nervousness, pallor, tremulousness, palpitations, sweating, and hunger. Weakness, dizziness, headache, drowsiness, irritability, loss of coordination, convulsions, and coma are more severe responses and reflect central nervous system glucose deprivation and the body's attempts to elevate the serum glucose levels (Fig. 38-5).

It is often difficult to distinguish between hyperglycemia and a hypoglycemic reaction (Table 38-4). Since the symptoms are similar and usually begin with changes in behavior, the simplest way to differentiate between the two is to test the blood glucose level. Blood glucose is low in hypoglycemia while in hyperglycemia the glucose content will

Table 38-4 Comparison of manifestations of hypoglycemia and hyperglycemia

VARIABLE	HYPOGLYCEMIA	HYPERGLYCEMIA
Onset	Rapid (minutes)	Gradual (days)
Mood	Labile, irritable, nervous, weepy,	Lethargic
Mental status	Difficulty concentrating speaking, focusing, coordinating	Dulled sensorium Confused
Inward feeling	Shaky feeling, hunger Headache Dizziness	Thirst Weakness Nausea/vomiting Abdominal pain
Skin	Pallor Sweating	Flushed Signs of dehydration
Mucous membranes	Normal	Dry, crusty
Respirations	Shallow	Deep, rapid (Kussmaul)
Pulse	Tachycardia	Less rapid, weak
Breath odor	Normal	Fruity, acetone
Urine	Diminished output	Frequent urination
Neurologic	Tremors Late: hyperflexia dilated pupils, convulsion	Diminished reflexes Paresthesia
Ominous signs	Shock, coma	Acidosis, coma
Blood:		
Glucose	Low: below 60 mg/dl	High: 250 mg/dl or more
Ketones	Negative	High/large
Osmolarity	Normal	High
pH	Normal	Low (7.25 or less)
Hematocrit	Normal	High
HCO$_3$	Normal	Less than 20 mEq/l
Urine:		
Output	Normal	Polyuria (early) to oliguria (late)
Sugar	Negative	High
Acetone	Negative	High

be significantly elevated. In doubtful situations it is safer to give the child some simple sugar. This will help alleviate the symptoms in the case of hypoglycemia but will do little harm if the child is hyperglycemic.

Children are usually able to detect the onset of hypoglycemia, but some are too young to implement treatment. Parents should become adept at recognizing the onset of symptoms—for example, a change in a child's behavior such as tearfulness or euphoria. In the majority of cases, simple concentrated sugar, such as honey, that can be held in the mouth for a short time will elevate the blood glucose level and alleviate the symptoms. The simpler the carbohydrate the more rapidly it will be absorbed. For a mild reaction milk is a good food to use in children. It supplies them with

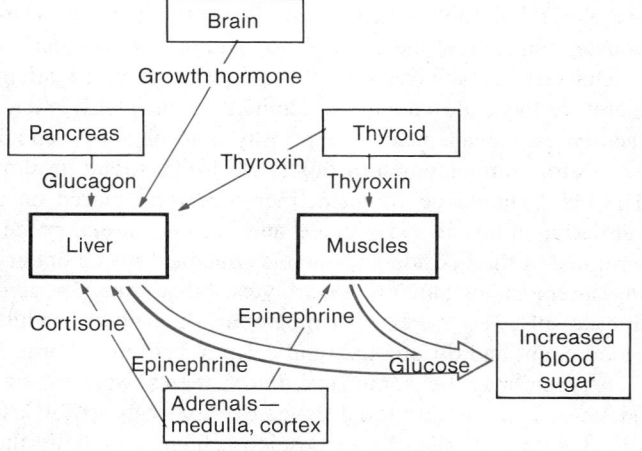

Fig. 38-5. Body systems respond to hypoglycemia in various ways to increase blood sugar level.

lactose or milk sugar as well as a more prolonged action from the protein and fat (aids in decreased absorption). All children with diabetes should carry with them sugar-containing candy, such as Life Savers or Charms, or some sugar cubes.

It is better to overtreat than to undertreat, but overtreatment should be kept to a minimum whenever possible. The treatment may be repeated in 10 to 15 minutes if the initial response is not satisfactory. With good response to the simple sugar, the pulse rate should show a noticeable change in 2 to 3 minutes. Rest and the addition of food should be part of the plan.

An insulin reaction is often the most feared aspect of diabetes, since severe brain symptoms may develop. In a severe reaction the various areas of the brain respond in sequence: the forebrain with increased drowsiness and perspiration, the hypothalamus and thalamus with tachycardia and loss of consciousness, the midbrain with seizure activity that may be started from stimulation initially from the hypothalamus, and finally the hindbrain with responses of deeper coma and decreasing reflexes. The treatment of choice for hypoglycemia is 50% glucose administered intravenously.

Glucagon is sometimes prescribed for home treatment of hypoglycemia. It is available as a tablet to be mixed with diluting fluid from its accompanying bottle and is administered intramuscularly or subcutaneously. It functions by releasing stored glycogen from the liver and requires about 15 to 20 minutes to elevate the blood glucose level. Once the child is responsive, the lost glycogen stores are replaced by small amounts of sugar-containing fluid administered frequently until the child feels comfortable about trying solid foods.

Somogyi effect. Somogyi effect should be recognized as a separate response and can be a cause of poor glycemic control. This phenomenon is a physiologic reflex response to a decreased blood glucose level, which results in release of counterregulatory hormones (epinephrine, growth hormone, and corticosteroids) and a rebound hyperglycemia. The condition should be suspected in children whose blood or urine glucose levels are high and who are receiving a relatively large dose of insulin. More frequent blood monitoring (especially at times of anticipated peak insulin action) will usually identify this condition. Treatment consists of increasing the amount of food eaten and/or decreasing the insulin. Hyperglycemia and glycosuria will subside as hypoglycemia and the counterregulatory hormonal response subside.

Illness management. Illness alters diabetes management and maintaining control is usually related to the seriousness of the illness. In the well-controlled child an illness will run its course as it does in the nondiabetic child. The goal is to maintain some glycosuria but to keep the urine free of acetone. Some glycosuria and ketonuria is expected in most illness, even with diminished food intake, and is an indication for increased insulin. Because a decreased appetite occurs during illness, a 20% decrease in caloric intake (simpler foods along with fluids and simple sugars) may reduce the need for insulin.

New data support the concept that life expectancy in the diabetic child is lengthened if the body is maintained in as normal a physiologic state as possible. Promotion of good health, a balance of adequate rest and exercise, and good nutrition along with close management of the disease will allow the person with diabetes to live as long as if not longer than the nondiabetic person, who may not develop health and nutrition habits as good as those of the properly managed diabetic person.

Surgery. The physiologic and emotional stresses related to surgery require careful adjustment of insulin. Since the child receives intravenous glucose during surgery and the stress of the surgery itself will also raise the blood glucose level, the risk of an insulin reaction is very slight. Regular insulin should be continued until the child is able to tolerate oral feedings and a return to the routine pattern of insulin administration.

Islet cell transplantation. There has been some experimentation with islet cell transplants. Viable insulin-producing cells are injected into the portal vein where they take root in the liver and eventually produce up to two thirds of the needed insulin. Some persons have received whole pancreas transplants and need no insulin supplementation. However, because it is an allograft, persons receiving islet cell transplants require immunosuppression, which in itself is a risk factor. The major use of transplants has been in persons who have serious complications, particularly those whose deteriorating kidneys have required renal transplants and who are necessarily on immunosuppression. Islet transplants may eventually be made more effective and possible without the need for powerful immunosuppressants.

Therapeutic Management: Diabetic Ketoacidosis

Diabetic ketoacidosis (DKA), the most complete state of insulin deficiency, is a life-threatening situation. Management consisting of rapid assessment, adequate insulin to reduce the elevated blood glucose, fluids to overcome dehydration, and electrolyte replacement (especially potassium and bicarbonate) can reverse the ketoacidosis within a few hours.

Diabetic ketoacidosis constitutes an emergency situation; therefore the child should be admitted to an intensive care facility for management. The priority is to obtain a venous access for administration of fluids, electrolytes, and insulin. The child should be weighed, measured, and placed on a cardiac monitor. Blood glucose and acetone levels are determined at the bedside and samples obtained for laboratory measurements of glucose, electrolytes, blood urea nitrogen, arterial pH, PO_2, PCO_2, hemoglobin, hematocrit, white blood count and differential, and calcium and phosphorus.

Oxygen may be administered to patients who are cyanotic and in whom arterial oxygen is less than 80%. Gastric suction is applied to unconscious children to avoid the possibility of pulmonary aspiration. Antibiotics may be administered to febrile children after appropriate specimens are obtained for culture. A Foley catheter may or may not be inserted for urine samples and measurement. Unless the child is unconscious, a collection bag is usually sufficient for accurate assessments.

Fluid and electrolyte therapy. All patients with diabetic ketoacidosis suffer from dehydration (10% of total body weight in severe ketoacidosis) due to the osmotic diuresis, accompanied by depletion of electrolytes, sodium, potassium, chloride, phosphate, and magnesium. Serum pH and bicarbonate reflect the degree of acidosis. Prompt and adequate fluid therapy restores tissue perfusion and suppresses the elevated levels of stress hormones.

The initial hydrating solution is isotonic saline solution. Even normal saline is hypotonic relative to the patient's serum hyperosmolality; therefore a gradual decline in osmolality is desirable because too rapid reduction in osmolality predisposes the child to cerebral edema, the most serious complication of therapy (Sperling, 1984). The intravenous saline is followed by 5% dextrose when blood glucose levels are sufficiently reduced. Present evidence indicates that sodium bicarbonate neither hastens resolution of acidosis nor improves survival (Lever and Jaspan, 1983). However, it may be given to improve cardiac contractility and enhance peripheral vascular responsiveness to catecholamines (Wolfsdorf, 1986).

Serum potassium levels may be normal on admission, but following fluid and insulin administration the rapid return of potassium to the cells can seriously deplete serum levels with the attendant risk of cardiac arrhythmias. As soon as the child has voided and insulin has been given, vigorous potassium replacement is implemented. The cardiac monitor is employed as a guide to therapy and configuration of T waves should be followed every 30 to 60 minutes to determine changes that might indicate alterations in potassium concentration (widening of the QT interval and the appearance of a U wave following a flattened T wave indicate hypokalemia; an elevated and spreading T wave and shortening of the QT interval indicate hyperkalemia).

Insulin. The preferred method for administering insulin to the child with ketoacidosis is a continuous infusion of low-dose insulin consisting of a 0.1 U/kg priming dose followed by 0.1 U/kg/hr. This appears to be an efficient, simple, and physiologically sound form of therapy (Sperling, 1984). The insulin is added to 0.5% normal saline and some of the mixture is run through the intravenous tubing to saturate the insulin binding sites that exist on the plastic tubing. It has been found that plastic tubing and in-line filters can chemically bind to significant amounts of insulin, thereby reducing the amount of the medication reaching the bloodstream (Butler, Munson, and DeLuca, 1980; Turco, 1982). The dose is controlled at a rate to lower the blood glucose about 100 mg/dl/hr to obtain a blood glucose level of approximately 200 mg/dl, then continued until the pH and serum bicarbonate are normal. Subcutaneous insulin is then instituted.

Nursing Considerations: General Care

Education is the cornerstone of diabetes management and the major responsibility in diabetes nursing care. This includes education and reinforcement of information for the family and the child who is old enough to participate in self-management of the disease. With a diabetic child, parents must supervise and manage the child's therapeutic program, but the child should assume responsibility for self-management as soon as he is capable. Children can begin to test their own urine at a relatively young age, and most should be able to administer their own insulin at about 9 years of age. In situations in which the parents are inconsistent and/or unreliable, the child should be taught self-care at an earlier age. It must be understood, however, that education programs cannot be conducted as one-time activities with the expectation that they will achieve permanent behavior changes. Education is a long-term nursing activity as family and patient needs change and new findings are applied.

Concepts of child and family education. Children and their families vary in educational background and the capacity to learn and understand the various aspects of the therapeutic program. Some families respond best to very simple explanations and directions, whereas others expect thorough, in-depth information about the physiologic processes and responses associated with the disease and its therapy. All the principles of teaching and learning are applied in the educational process; therefore, before beginning, the nurse must determine the optimum time, place, method, and content to be taught. Self-management, the ultimate goal for the diabetic child, is more likely to occur when the child understands the disease and the care it requires. Properly educated, any family should be able to follow a program of regulated control satisfactorily.

When to teach a diabetic family is best judged by the psychologic state of the family and/or the child and the time of initial diagnosis. If a child is newly diagnosed, the psychologic adjustment to the disease can block the learning process completely—for example, members of the family may in a follow-up visit state that it is the first time that they have heard a certain bit of information when, in reality, the specific material had been covered several times in the course of teaching.

Certainly the first 3 or 4 days after diagnosis is not an optimum time for learning. In fact, the later the more complex material is presented, the better. For example, one successful program teaches only essential, or survival, information first and intense information a month later. Another program advocates as a choice of time for teaching 1 week after diagnosis followed by a review of survival techniques 2 weeks after discharge. Probably the most inopportune and ineffective time for teaching is the day or so after diagnosis when the education must be compressed into a few hours or days so that the child can be discharged early. Whether teaching is conducted on an outpatient basis or in a preparatory, in-depth manner on an inpatient basis, the ability of the individuals involved to learn must be accurately assessed. This includes assessment of the educational back-ground and emotional stability of the individual(s) involved and the use of appropriate measurement tools, such as a pretest or an objective assessment of the learner's educational level.

The setting for the educational process can facilitate the learning process. An environment that is too hot or too cold or one in which there is too much noise will distract the learner. Bedside education may be necessary in some cases, but the coming and going of a number of people are distracting. There are times in the educational process when individual instruction is needed, but contact with other children and/or parents can assist in adjustment to the reality of the disease and the implications of having a chronic condition. Supplementary material such as audiovisual aids enhances the learning process and promotes retention of information.

A child learns best when sessions are kept short, no more than 15 to 20 minutes. The parents do best in periods of 45 to 60 minutes and often longer if they are inquisitive. Education should involve all the senses, and, although visual aids are valuable tools, participation is the most effective method for learning. For example, to teach urine testing, the technique is explained, the procedure is demonstrated, and the learner is allowed to perform the procedure followed by a review of the material by visual aids, with learning validated by some testing method that includes a feedback. A variety of teaching methods and teaching aids can be employed. Some visual aids may be beautifully illustrated but miss a major point; therefore materials should be previewed for accuracy and appropriateness. Varying the presentation with a variety of audiovisual materials, including films, slide-tape programs, and books, stimulates the senses and helps the individual to learn.

Several organizations are prepared to assist with education and dissemination of knowledge. The **American Diabetes Association, Inc.,*** **Canadian Diabetes Association,**† **Juvenile Diabetes Foundation International,**‡ and **Juvenile Diabetes Foundation International—Canada**§ are valuable resources for a wide variety of educational materials. The **National Diabetes Information Clearinghouse**‖ publishes a number of comprehensive annotated bibliographies including "Educational Materials for and about Young People with Diabetes," a compilation of resource materials for children, siblings, parents, teachers, and health professionals, and "Sports and Exercise for People with Diabetes."

The content of the educational course must include all aspects of the disease as they specifically relate to the individual child. There are many aspects of the disease that may not be covered in an initial educational course but can be postponed until subsequent office or clinic visits or can be done through referral sources such as the American Diabetes Association. The minimal information needed is that which will help the family manage from one day to the next; expanded information helps the individual with the biopsychosocial adjustment basic to in-depth knowledge about the disease. The more the family understands about the disease in relation to body needs, the better they are able to maintain a high degree of control. Important content needed for minimum management is discussed briefly in the following segments.

Identification. One of the first things that should be called to the attention of the parents is the need for the child to wear some means of medical identification. Usually recommended is the Medic Alert identification, a stainless steel, silver, or gold-plated identification bracelet or necklace that is visible and immediately recognizable. It contains a collect telephone number that medical personnel can call around the clock for medical records and personal information.

Nature of diabetes. The better the parents understand the pathophysiology of diabetes and the function and action of insulin and glucagon in relation to calorie intake, the better will be their understanding of the disease and its effect on the child. Parents need answers to a number of questions (voiced or unvoiced) that can provide them an increased feeling of security in coping with the disease. For example, they may want to know about the various procedures performed on their child and treatment rationale, such as what is being put in the intravenous bottle and the expected effect.

Meal planning. Normal nutrition is a major aspect of the family education program. Diet instruction is usually conducted by the nutritionist with reinforcement and guidance from the nurse (Fig. 38-6). The family is taught how the meal plan relates to the requirements of growth and development, the disease process, and the insulin regimen. Meals and snacks are modified around the child and his present food menu, preserving cultural patterns and preferences as much as possible. Extensive exchange lists are available that include foods that are compatible with most life-styles.

Learning about foods within specific food groups helps in making choices. Weights and measures of foods are used as eye-training devices for defining food volumes and should be practiced for about 3 months, with gradual progression to estimation of food portions. Even when the child and/or family become competent in estimating food volumes, reassessment should take place weekly or monthly and when there is any change of brands. Members of the family should also be guided in reading labels for the nutritional value of foods and food contents.

Family members should also become familiar with the concept of calories. Calorie changes may be necessary in case a food is not available in sufficient quantity or if they wish to eat foods that may be more difficult to calculate, such as pizza or other fast-food items. Discussion includes situations the child might encounter in the classroom and the

*2 Park Ave., New York, NY 10010.
†123 Edward St., Suite 601, Toronto, Ontario, Canada M5G 1E2.
‡23 E. 26th St., New York, NY 10010.
§4632 Yonge St., Suite 201, Willowdale, Ontario, Canada M2N 5M1.
‖Box NDIC, Bethesda, MD 20205.

school cafeteria. For example, the kindergarten or first-grade student might like to have a special box from which to select sugar-free items for occasions when treats containing excess sugar are brought to the classroom by others. Parents can supply substitute treats for the child who is invited to attend a birthday party or other outing.

Role-playing and discussion help the teenager to choose foods when out on dates, with friends in their homes, or on a food break after school. The young diabetic can even join

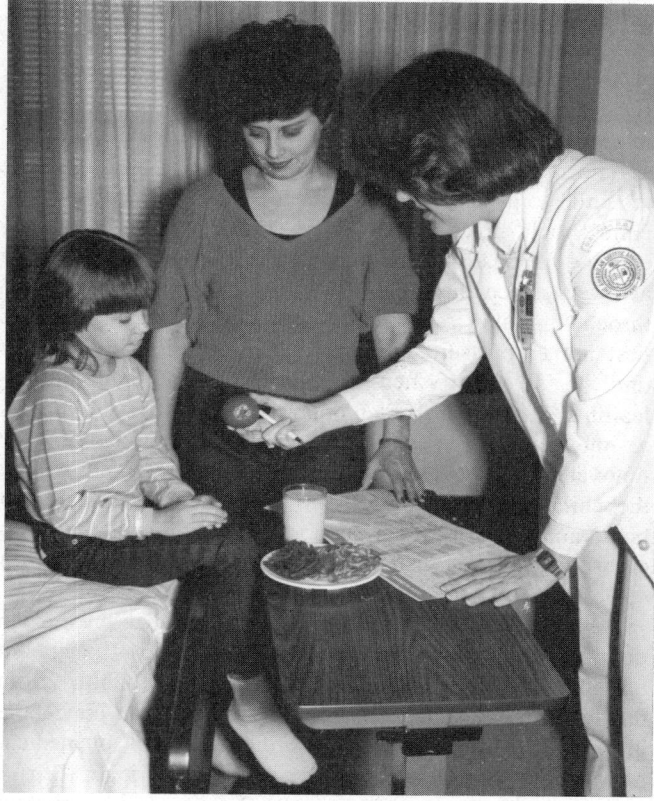

Fig. 38-6. Nutritionist instructs child and family using food models to explain food exchanges.

the gang for fast food on occasion. Lists of popular fast-food items and items served at the major fast-food chains can be obtained from the American Diabetic Association (ADA) to help guide food selections. It is important that the child know the nutritional value of these items (the major chains are remarkably uniform), but he should be cautioned to avoid high-fat and high-sugar items, for example, choosing a plain hamburger instead of a double cheeseburger. (See Table 38-5 for a small sample of some popular fast-food items.)

Children should be advised to use sugar substitutes with moderation in items such as soft drinks. Artificial sweeteners have been shown to be safe but if there is any question about amounts the physician, dietitian, or nurse specialist can provide guidelines based on body weight. "Sugar-free" chewing gum and candies made with sorbitol are not usually recommended for diabetic children. Although sorbitol is less cariogenic than other varieties, it is an alcohol sugar that is metabolized to fructose and then to glucose. Furthermore large amounts can cause an osmotic diarrhea. Most dietetic foods contain sorbitol also. They are more expensive and, when labels are read carefully, it is found that the caloric content is equal to or even greater than the regular varieties.

Traveling requires advance planning, especially when a trip involves crossing time zones. A number of tips are included in pamphlets available free of charge from the local chapter of the ADA or the publishers.* Suggestions for traveling include what will be needed from the doctor before leaving, what and how much to take along, planning for needs in transit, what to consider at the destination, and when the child returns home. Planning is needed no matter what type of travel is considered—automobile, plane, bus, or train. The ADA also has a computer service that can provide a vacation schedule of insulin and meals based on the accustomed regimen and the anticipated changes.

*Vacations, travel, and diabetes: Becton Dickson and Company, Rochelle Park, NJ 07662. Vacationing with Diabetes: E.R. Squibb, P.O. Box 4000, Princeton, NJ 08540.

Table 38-5 Exchange equivalents for selected fast-food items

FOOD	EXCHANGE EQUIVALENTS			
	LEAN-MED. MEAT	BREAD	FAT	VEGETABLE
Arby's roast beef sandwich (regular)	2½	2	½	—
Burger King "Whopper"	3	3	3½	1
Kentucky Fried				
Original dinner (2 pieces chicken, potatoes, gravy, cole slaw, roll)	3½	3	3	2
McDonald's "Big Mac"	3	2	3	2
Pizza Hut cheese pizza (½ of 10")	2	3	1	2
Taco Bell				
Taco	2	1	1	—
Beef burrito	3	2	1	2
Wendy's cheeseburger (single)	4	2	2	—

Insulin. Families need to understand the treatment method and the insulin prescribed, including the effective duration, onset, and peak action. They also need to know the characteristics of the various types of insulins, the proper mixing and dilution of insulins, and how to substitute another type when their usual brand is not available. Insulin need not be refrigerated but should be maintained at a temperature below 29.4° C (85° F). An extra supply can be kept in the refrigerator.

Injection procedure. Learning to give the insulin injections is a source of anxiety for both the parents and the child. It is helpful for the learner to know that this important aspect of care will become as routine as brushing the teeth. First, the basic injection technique is taught using an orange or similar item and sterile normal saline for practice.* To gain the child's confidence, the nurse can demonstrate the technique by giving a skillful injection to the parent and then have the parent return the demonstration by giving the nurse an injection. With practice and confidence the parents soon are able to give the insulin injection to the child and he will trust them. Another effective strategy is to instruct the child, then have the child teach the technique to his parents while the nurse observes. Both parents should participate, and as little time as possible should elapse between instruction and the actual injection, especially with parents and the teenage learner.

Insulin can be injected into any area in which there is skin over muscle with fatty tissue between. Usually the smaller the child, the thinner the skin. The length and angle of the needle are altered according to the thickness of the skin. The pinch technique is the most effective method for obtaining skin tightness to allow easy entrance of the needle to subcutaneous tissues in children. The site selected will sometimes depend on whether the child or parent administers the insulin. The arms, thighs, hips, and abdomen are usual injection sites for insulin. The child can reach the thighs, abdomen, and part of the hip and arm easily but may require help to inject other sites. For example, a parent can pinch a loose fold of skin of the arm while the child injects the insulin.

The parents and child are helped to work out a rotation pattern to various areas of the body to enhance absorption, since insulin absorption is slowed by the fat pads that develop in overused injection areas (Young and others, 1984). The most efficient rotation plan involves giving about 4 to 6 injections in one area (each injection about 1 inch [2.5 cm) apart or the diameter of the insulin vial from the previous injection] and then moving to another area.

It is important to remember that the absorption rate varies in different parts of the body. Absorption has been demonstrated to be more rapid in the arm, less rapid in the abdomen, and slowest when injected into the thigh (Binder and others, 1984; Galloway and others, 1981; Berger and oth-

ers, 1982; Koivisto and Felig, 1980). The methodical use of one anatomic area and then moving to another (as described in the previous paragraph) minimizes variation in absorption rates. However, absorption is also altered by vigorous exercise, which enhances absorption from exercised muscles. Therefore it is recommended that excess exercise be avoided during the time the insulin is expected to peak (Thatcher, 1985). It has also been found that massaging the site following injection facilitates absorption (Dillon, 1983).

Injection sites for an entire month can be determined in advance on a simple chart. For example, the body outline described on p. 223 can be constructed and insulin sites marked by the child. After injection the child places the date on the appropriate site. In order to keep in practice, it is a good idea for the parent to give a 2 or 3 injections a week in the areas that are difficult for the child to reach.

The same basic methodology is employed when teaching the child to give his own insulin injections (Fig. 38-7). The child should practice first on an orange or a doll, building courage gradually. The first attempt will undoubtedly be awkward since the child tends to slowly push the needle through the skin rather than using a quick approach. It is best not to pressure him into assuming this responsibility until he is ready. When the child participates in a group-learning situation or has an opportunity to observe his peers giving their own injections, he may become more strongly motivated. The parents should be warned that at some time the child will give himself an uncomfortable injection at home and will need their support and encouragement. Otherwise he may not wish to give himself another injection for some time.

Teaching includes the proper way to equalize pressure in the bottle by injecting an amount of air equal to the amount of solution withdrawn and how to remove air bubbles from the syringe. When insulin dosages are small, an air bubble in the syringe can displace a significant amount of medication. Since the introduction of the low-dose syringe, the risk of incorrect dosage has diminished. Patients who have small doses of mixed insulins should be advised and instructed to use these syringes. Insulin syringes should be compared for accuracy, comfort, strength, and the family and/or child should be able to choose both "their" insulin and "their" syringe from a variety of samples. Use of the same syringe (even during hospitalization) is recommended to prevent errors in dosage caused by varying amounts of dead space among syringes (Wong, 1982).

When the child's dosage requires the injection of both short- and intermediate-acting insulin at the same time, most families prefer to mix the two and use a single injection. Regular insulin is used to cover the blood sugar rise from breakfast; the slower-acting insulin helps control blood sugar later in the day. Therefore the mixture accomplishes two purposes with one injection. There are some problems that can arise from this accepted practice, and the family should understand what happens when insulins are mixed.

The longer-acting insulins contain ingredients (protamine in NPH, zinc in lente) that bind to the insulin allowing for

---

*Highly recommended is home care instructions on subcutaneous injection available in Wong, D.L., and Whaley, L.F.: Clinical handbook of pediatric nursing, St. Louis, 1986, The C.V. Mosby Co.

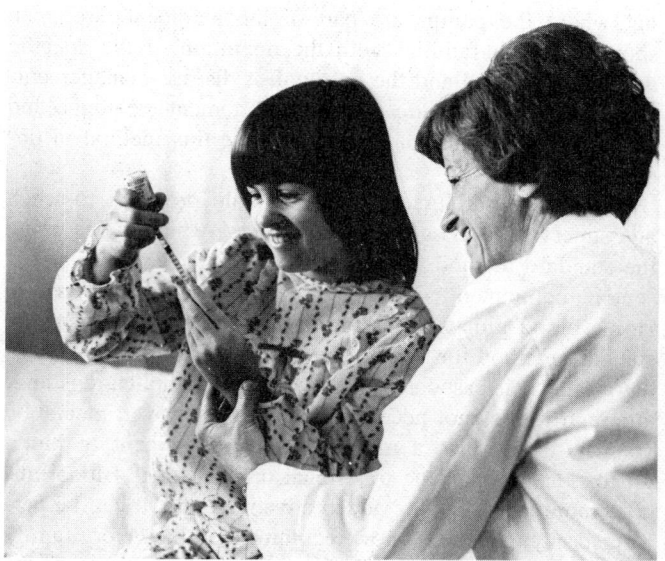 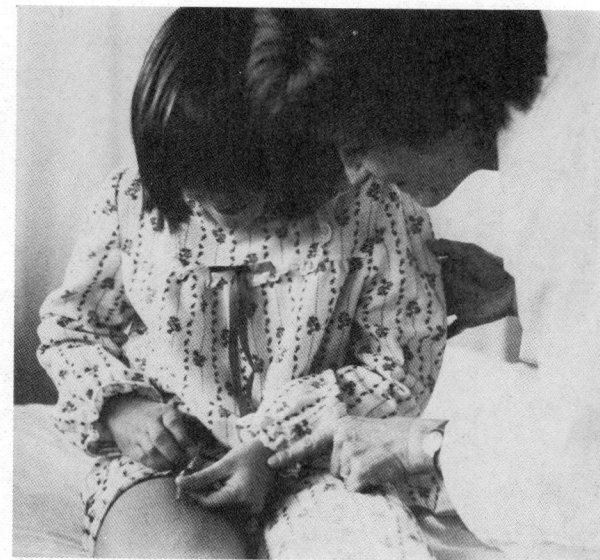

Fig. 38-7. School-age children are able to administer their own insulin.

gradual release after injection, and some brands contain extra binding compounds. When short-acting (regular) insulin is mixed with longer-acting insulin (NPH or lente) a portion of the short-acting insulin can bind with the surplus protamine or zinc and convert to the longer-acting type, altering the effect on blood sugar. For example, blood sugar may be unusually high after breakfast and unusually low after the mid-day meal. The degree of alteration depends on the type of longer-acting insulin, the ratio of short- to long-acting insulin, and how long the mixture is allowed to stand before injection.

To obtain the maximum benefit from mixing insulins the recommended practice is to (1) inject the measured amount of air (equivalent to the dosage) into the longer-acting insulin, (2) inject the measured amount of air into the regular insulin and, without removing the needle, (3) withdraw the regular insulin, and (4) insert the needle (already containing the regular insulin) into the longer-acting insulin and withdraw the desired amount. The mixture should be injected immediately—in less than 5 minutes after mixing (Jenkins and Molitch, 1986).

It has become acceptable practice to reuse disposable needles and syringes up to 7 days. Research has shown that no infection has resulted and there is a considerable saving (Collins and others, 1983; Aziz, 1984; Borders, Bingham, and Riddle, 1984). If this method is approved it is important to stress the importance of vigorous handwashing before handling any equipment and capping the syringe immediately after use and storing it in the refrigerator to decrease the possibility of infection. The nurse should also teach proper disposal of equipment after use. Needles should be broken off if possible and the plunger of low-dose syringes broken. An excellent means for disposal is in an opaque container such as an empty coffee can, bleach bottle, or milk carton, any of which can be discarded with other household trash.

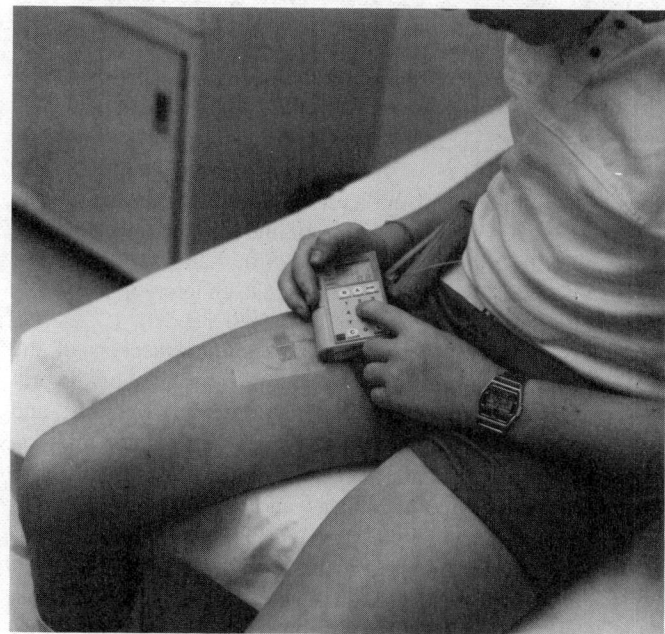

Fig. 38-8. Child programming insulin pump. Note insertion site on anterior thigh.
Photography by John Roy, Saint Francis Hospital. On location at Children's Medical Center, Tulsa, OK.

Continuous subcutaneous insulin infusion. Some children are considered candidates for use of a portable insulin pump, and even some young children with unsatisfactory metabolic control can benefit from its use (Fig. 38-8). The child and the parents are taught to operate the device, including the mechanics of the pump, battery changes, and alarm systems. There are a number of devices available on the market that vary in the basal rates they are able to de-

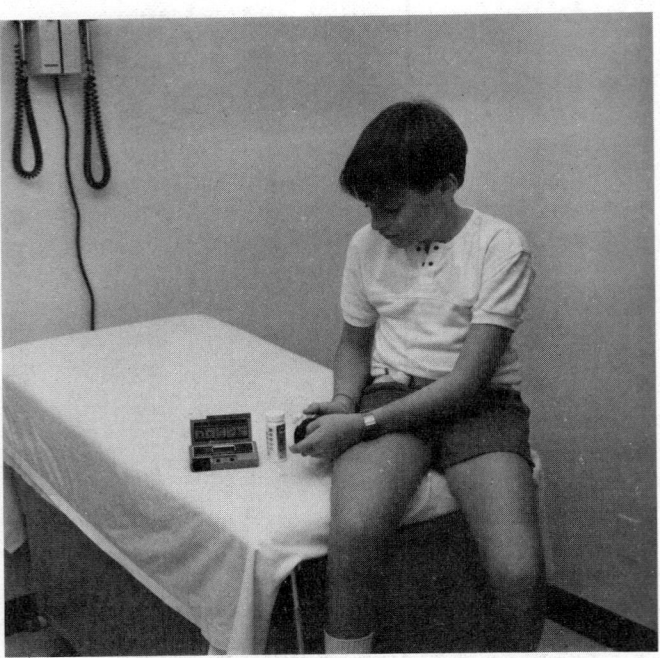

Fig. 38-9. Child using Autolet to obtain blood sample. Glucometer and reagent strips at hand.

Photography by John Roy, Saint Francis Hospital. On location at Children's Medical Center, Tulsa, OK.

liver and in the cost of the equipment. Most children can be adequately controlled with one of the simpler models (Rosenstock, Strowig, and Raskin, 1985). Families can investigate the various devices at the local chapter of the ADA and select the model that best suits their needs.

Parents and child learn (1) the technical aspects of the pump and self-monitoring of blood glucose; (2) how to prevent and treat hyperglycemia, sick-day management, and diet planning; (3) effects of exercise, stress, and diet on blood glucose levels; and (4) decision-making strategies to evaluate blood glucose patterns and how to make adjustments in all aspects of the regimen. The child may be hospitalized for regulation and instruction.

Since numerous blood glucose measurements (at least four times per day) are an essential part of infusion pump use, families must acquire a monitor and learn its use if this has not been a part of their regular management. Intensive education and supervision are critical to obtaining maximum efficiency and control. This is particularly important if the family has been accustomed to a fixed insulin regimen. They must realize that simply wearing the pump will not normalize blood glucose. It is merely a tool for using the information from self blood-glucose monitoring as a guide for adjusting the insulin delivery.

The major problem with the use of the insulin pump is inflammation from an allergic reaction or infection at the insertion site. The site should be cleaned thoroughly before the needle is inserted, then covered with a transparent dressing. The site is changed and rotated every 48 hours (this may vary) or at the first sign of inflammation. Nurses work-

ing where the pumps are part of the therapeutic regimen should become familiar with the operation of the specific device being used and the protocol of disease management. Others should be aware of this management technique and be prepared to assist patients who have this method in operation.

Monitoring. Nurses should also be prepared to teach and supervise blood glucose monitoring, which is becoming the standard method for assessing glucose levels and an essential component of insulin infusion pump treatment. Home blood glucose monitoring (HBGM) is becoming the standard method for monitoring glucose control on a day-to-day basis. It is associated with very few complications and, although it does not necessarily lead to improved metabolic control, it provides a more accurate assessment of blood glucose levels than the traditional urine testing. Blood glucose monitoring has the added advantage that it can be performed anywhere. It is now recommended that every family with a type I diabetic child have equipment available for HBGM (Chase, 1983).

Blood for testing can be obtained by two different methods: manually or with a mechanical bloodletting device. A mechanical device is recommended for children although the child and family should learn to use both methods in the event of mechanical failure (Fig. 38-9). Several lancet devices are available from which to choose and each provides a means for obtaining a large drop of blood for testing on a reagent strip. Children are cautioned not to allow anyone else to use their lancet because of the danger of contracting hepatitis or other blood-borne diseases.

The blood is applied to the reagent strip and after the appropriate time interval is read by comparison with a color scale to obtain the blood glucose reading. The family should investigate the various mechanical devices and reagent strips available and, in collaboration with their health professional, select one for consistent use based on ease of operation, cost, and availability. For children or families who are color blind or have difficulty distinguishing colors on the scale, a meter with a readout may be a safer method of assessment.

The cost of reagent strips is considerably more than the testing material for urine testing. An expense-saving strategy that is suggested by some professionals is splitting the strips in half lengthwise to provide two readings instead of one from each strip. This is not recommended by all professionals, however. Although expensive, a glucose monitor offers the greatest accuracy in assessing blood glucose levels, but the initial expense may be a deterrent. Information on monitoring products can be obtained from the ADA or from local representatives of the major suppliers.

Urine testing. Urine testing is easily taught and should include all methods, not just the test to be used for the particular child. Urine testing for glucose and acetone is carried out as instructed by the health professional. First-voided specimens are more practical for home urine testing, but many physicians prefer second-voided specimens, especially in the hospital setting. To obtain a second-voided specimen, the child is instructed to void and the sample is discarded (tested or untested according to the individual physician). One-half hour later the child again voids and the sample is tested. The results reflect the amount of glucose "spilling" into the urine at that particular time rather than the glucose accumulated since the previous test.

Testing for acetone is usually recommended during times of illness or when there are high glucose readings. Since moisture will cause changes to take place in both glucose and acetone reagent tablets, families are instructed to discard tablets that are discolored, that have been open for a specified time, or after an expiration date. The potentially toxic tablets should also be stored in a safe place away from small children.

Shopping. Families are advised to investigate all sources of obtaining supplies for managing the disease. Prices are often lower when supplies are purchased in volume; however, it is not advisable to buy bulk items that are unfamiliar or untried since the new items may not satisfactory for the individual child. Costs vary considerably among pharmacies and other suppliers, including the numerous discount mail-order establishments. When buying by mail it is important to find one that responds to the family's satisfaction and that allows the family ample time for delivery to avoid running out of supplies. Parents are also cautioned not to substitute insulins or the type of insulin syringe (e.g., a 1 ml syringe for the customary low-dose type) simply to save money. Parent groups and the local ADA can offer some suggestions for investigation.

Hyperglycemia. Severe hyperglycemia is most often caused by illness, growth, or emotional upset. With careful glucose monitoring any elevation can be managed by adjustment of insulin or food intake. Parents should understand how to adjust food, activity, and insulin at the time of illness or when the child is treated for an illness with a medication known to raise the blood glucose level. The hyperglycemia is managed by increasing insulin soon after the increased glucose is noted.

Hypoglycemia. Hypoglycemia is caused by imbalances of food intake, insulin, and activity. Ideally hypoglycemia should be prevented and parents need to be prepared to prevent, recognize, and treat the problem. They should be familiar with the signs of hypoglycemia and instructed in treatment, including care of the child with seizures (see p. 1666). Hypoglycemia can be managed effectively as outlined in the emergency treatment box.

It is advisable for parents to plan for anticipated extra excitement or exercise. In addition, gastroenteritis will often decrease insulin slightly if vomiting and/or diarrhea occur or if the appetite is depressed from nausea. If the urine is negative for glucose but acetone is present, the family should be aware of the increased need for simple sugar.

Hygiene. All aspects of personal hygiene should be emphasized for the child with diabetes. The child has not had time to develop the blood vessel disease that causes a decrease in peripheral circulation; therefore, foot care is not as important in the child as it is in the adult with diabetes.

Emergency Treatment: *Hypoglycemia*

Mild reaction:
Give child food
Milk, crackers, fruit

Moderate reactions:
Give child simple sugar
Life saver, sugar cube
Follow with food

Severe reaction:
Administer glucagon
Follow in 15 to 20 minutes with simple sugar

However the child should be cautioned against walking barefoot, and the correct method of nail and extremity care instituted for each particular child (with the guidance of a podiatrist) will begin health practices that last a lifetime. Eyes should be checked once a year unless the child wears glasses and then as directed by the ophthalmologist. Regular dental care is emphasized, and cuts and scratches should be treated with plain soap and water unless otherwise indicated.

Exercise. Exercise should be planned, as may be necessary for the sedentary teenager, or observed, as is found in most active children. If the child is more active at one time of the day than at another, food and/or insulin can be altered to meet the activity pattern of the individual child. Food should be increased in the summer when children tend to be more active. Decreased activity on return to school may require a decrease in food intake. The child who is active in team sports will need an increase in food intake on the days of activity, and races or other competition may call for a slightly higher food intake than practice times.

Food will usually need to be repeated for prolonged activity periods, often as frequently as every 45 minutes to 1 hour. Families should be informed that if increased food is not tolerated, decreased insulin is the next course of action. If the timing of the exercise is changed so that the supper meal is delayed, the insulin in the second or third dose of the day may be moved back to precede the mealtime. Sugar may sometimes be needed during exercise periods for quick response. Parents should be aware that if sugar is seen in the urine after extreme activity it may represent the Somogyi reflex (see p. 1710).

Record-keeping. Keeping information about food, insulin, blood sugar measurements, and glucosuria is useful to the physician as well as to the family. The record should contain information on insulin doses and variations in urine tests that include as many urine tests as possible. Urine, glucose, acetone, and blood glucose should be recorded, especially during illness. Insulin reactions should be noted, including the time, severity, treatment, and response to treatment. Dietary variations are noted so that an increased glucose level can be analyzed in relation to insulin dose, food intake, and activity level. The record should contain types and variations in activity that are markedly above or below the expected activity levels, dietary variations, and illnesses. If lapses in management occur (such as eating a candy bar), the child should be encouraged to note it and not be condemned for the transgression.

Complications. It is debatable whether or not knowledge of potential hazards of poor control should be shared with the family and child. If so, the implications of the disease should be presented in a tactful, clear, and nonfearful manner. Knowledge of the complications of diabetes and their relationship to control provides a basis for knowledgeable decision-making. Eye and kidney disease are the greatest threats, with neurologic complications close behind. Clear explanations of these problems clarify false information often given by well-meaning friends. By this time the nurse has developed a rapport with the patient and family and knows at what level and how openly the problem can be discussed. The information should include discussion of research so that the family is left with the positive impression that others are concerned about finding answers and preventing complications. It also gives them hope that somehow, some way, a prevention and/or cure is possible.

Self-management. Self-management is the key to close control. Being able to make changes at the time they are needed rather than waiting until the next contact with health professionals is important for self-management and gives the individual and family the feeling that they have control over the disease. Psychologically this helps the family members feel that they are useful and participating members of the team. Learning to look at records objectively gives the child support. As children grow and assume more and more responsibility for self-management, they develop confidence in their ability to manage their disease and in themselves as persons. They grow to respond to the disease and to make more accurate interpretations and changes in self-management when they become adults.

Self-management techniques to be mastered are the testing and adjustment of insulin and diet with alterations in day-to-day activities and unusual occurrences. However, limitations should be set regarding how many alterations can be made without consulting with the health professionals. The degree of control before the illness is a determining factor in seeking medical help during illness. In an individual with poor control it takes but a few hours before the trouble is severe, whereas if control is good before the illness several days may elapse before help is needed. Patients and families are cautioned to seek assistance if there are elevated glucose levels and urine has not become free of acetone after 24 hours of self-management.

Nursing Considerations: Acute Care

Diabetic children may be admitted to the hospital at the time of their initial diagnosis, during illness or surgery, or for episodes of ketoacidosis, which may be precipitated by any of a variety of factors. Most diabetic children are able to keep the disease under control with periodic assessment and adjustment of insulin, diet, and activity as needed under the supervision of a physician. Under most circumstances these children can be managed very well at home and require hospitalization only for a serious illness or upset.

However there are a small number of diabetic children who exhibit a degree of metabolic lability and who have repeated episodes of diabetic ketoacidosis that require hospitalization, which interferes with education and social development. These children appear to display a characteristic personality structure. They tend to be unusually passive and nonassertive and to come from families that are inclined to smooth over conflicts without resolution. Children in this type of setting experience emotional arousal with little, if any, opportunity or ability to bring about its termination. Other children from psychosocially dysfunctional families display behavioral and personality problems. This emotional stress causes an increased production of endogenous catecholamines, which stimulates fat breakdown leading to ketonemia and ketonuria.

Loving discipline is a supportive measure for any child; however, children with poorer diabetic control come from predominantly disruptive family units with little or no discipline as part of the family life-style. Lack of control is psychologically harmful. Since many of the psychosocial problems are not immediately apparent, psychosocial assessment and involvement by professionals are required together with ongoing emotional support and counseling to reverse the patterns of ketoacidosis (White and others, 1984).

Hospital management. The child with diabetic ketoacidosis requires intensive nursing care. Vital signs should be observed and recorded frequently. Hypotension caused by the contracted blood volume of the dehydrated state may cause decreased peripheral blood flow, which can be particularly hazardous to the heart, lungs, and kidneys. An elevated temperature may indicate the presence of infection and should be reported so that treatment can be implemented immediately.

Careful and accurate records should be maintained, including vital signs (pulse, respiration, temperature, blood pressure), intravenous fluids, electrolytes, insulin, blood glucose level, and intake and output. A urine collection device or retention catheter is used to obtain the urine measurements, which include volume, specific gravity, and glucose and acetone values. The volume relative to the glucose content is important, since 5% glucose in a 300 ml sample is a significantly greater amount than a similar reading from a 75 ml sample. A diabetic flow sheet maintained at the bedside provides an ongoing record of the vital signs, urine and blood tests, amount of insulin given, and intake and output of the patient. The level of consciousness is assessed and recorded at frequent intervals. The comatose child generally regains consciousness fairly soon after initiation of therapy but is managed as any unconscious child during that time.

When the critical period is over, the task of regulating insulin dosage to diet and activity is begun. The same meticulous records of intake and output, urine glucose and acetone levels, and insulin administration are maintained. The capable child should be actively involved in his own care and is given responsibility for keeping the intake and output record, testing the urine, and, when appropriate, administering his own insulin—all under the supervision and guidance of the nurse.

Nursing Considerations: Psychosocial Adjustment

The parents and other family members of the child with newly diagnosed diabetes mellitus experience various emotional responses to the crises just as the physiologic responses affect the child. Care in the acute setting is short but may create fears and frustrations. The prospect of a chronic illness in their child engenders all the feeling and concerns that are faced by parents of children with other chronic illnesses (see Chapter 22). The threat of complications and death is always present as well as the continuing drain on emotional and financial resources.

Certain fears may develop as a result of past experiences with the disease. A severe insulin reaction with seizures is certainly one experience that contributes to fear of repetition. Once parents experience a seizure or the adolescent has one in a public place, the desire to maintain better control is reinforced. They must understand how to prevent problems and how to handle problems calmly and coolly if they occur and understand the complexities of the body, the disease, and its complications. Young children usually adjust well to problems related to the disease. With toddlers and preschoolers, insulin injections and glucose testing may be difficult at first. However, they usually accept the procedures when the parents use a matter-of-fact approach without calling attention to a "hurt" and treat the procedure as any other routine part of a child's life. Following the injection, time with some special and positive attention such as reading, talking, or other pleasant activity is one way to convert children who initially refuse injections to those who accept them.

Children in the years before adolescence probably accept their condition most easily. They are able to understand the basic concepts related to their disease and its treatment. They are able to test blood glucose and urine, recognize food groups, give injections, keep records, and distinguish between feelings of fear, excitement, and hypoglycemia. They understand how to recognize, prevent, and treat hypoglycemia. However, they still need considerable parental involvement.

Adolescents appear to have most difficulty in adjusting. Adolescence is a time when there is much stress toward being perfect and being like their peers and, no matter what others say, having diabetes is being different. If children can accept the difference as a part of life, in other words, that each person has something different about him, then with adequate parental support they should be able to adjust well.

Problems of adjustment to diabetes are especially difficult for the youngster whose disease is diagnosed in adolescence. Denial is sometimes expressed by omitting insulin, not performing tests, and eating incorrectly although denial of the disease usually diminishes during this period as the diabetic youngster begins to feel competent and worthy. This is the age when greatest falsification of records occurs. Diabetes is a defect that emphasizes vulnerability and imperfection when the search for identity is the foremost developmental task.

Camping and other special groups are very useful. In the camp for children with diabetes, these children learn that they are not alone. As a result, they become more independent and resourceful in the nondiabetic camp setting, especially if they have had experience in a diabetic camp. Useful information about such camps and organizations can be obtained from the American Diabetes Association (ADA). A free list of accredited camps specifically for children and teens with diabetes is also available.*

Inaccurate doses of insulin may occur inadvertently or, if done frequently, as an attention-seeking device, or in a number of cases, as a subconscious but socially accepted method of suicide. Inaccurate intake of food leads to overweight, which may also represent a subconscious death wish. Psychiatric counseling may be needed if suicidal tendencies are amplified by the diabetes.

Rehospitalizations are most often related to poor control of the disease, although it is also possible that they are indirectly related to noncoping and a method of avoiding the pressures caused by family and peers. The hospital may represent an environment that is peaceful and free of stress. The goal for this problem is to determine the cause of the hospitalization. It may be because of poor control or poor self-management or the need for better supportive management at home. Evaluation should be based on both the physiologic as well as the psychologic adjustment of the child and the family.

Parents. Parents develop guilt feelings when they have a child with any chronic disease, especially one with a hereditary component. They cope with these feelings in a number of ways. For example, they may be overprotective or neglectful. Guilt-ridden parents may blame themselves for the disease, consciously or subconsciously. Nevertheless, they must come to realize through education and counseling that there was nothing they could have done to prevent the disease and that it was not their fault, since environmental as well as hereditary factors may be involved in the development of the disease.

Parents who are overprotective suffer from feelings of guilt as well as fear of the unknown. Overprotection is a

---

*Camp Directory, 1660 Duke St., Alexandria, VA 22314.

mechanism that alters the guilt responses to justify their own needs—for example, ''If the child is in my sight, nothing worse will happen than has already happened by the child getting diabetes. Therefore, I am going to watch this child every single minute so that nothing further can happen to him.'' The overprotective parent becomes the smothering parent, one that hampers the growth, development, and maturation of the affected child.

The neglectful parent, on the other hand, has a different problem. This response is a mechanism developed to block feelings that give pain and provide relief from feelings of guilt—''This is your disease and I have no responsibilities related to your disease; therefore if anything bad happens to you as a result of you having this disease, it is not my fault.'' The neglectful parent assigns responsibilities to the child before he is mature enough to accept a more adult role.

Threatened parents look at the disease as a way to keep the child tied to them. If the child learns to be independent, as is expected of the child in a camping experience, the parent may feel threatened and place obstacles in the child's path to independent development. Problems in the parental response provide a challenge for the nurse to assist by counseling or, if severe enough, to appropriately refer the parents to resources designed to help them alter their behavior.

Children who are sufficiently mature may be seen alone by the health professional, although the parents should not be made to feel that they are being left out. Times should be set aside during the child's health visit or afterward to meet the needs of the parents. They should also be included in special sessions to keep them abreast of the child's management, to help them continue to participate in the child's care, and to provide them with an opportunity to express their own feelings concerning their own or their child's adjustment to the disease. The amount of information that they offer at this time can give clues to their level of support of the child and help assist in decisions concerning the therapeutic management of the child. This helps guide the child through the most disruptive time of life—the teenage years.

Health professionals must be aware of parents who voice support and appear to be supporting the child to the optimum level but who, upon deeper interview techniques, are found to be supporting the child in word but not by action. These parents seldom see the need for following through from verbalizing to fulfilling the real needs of the child and unknowingly place obstacles in the child's path. They may be assisting the child in growing up too fast and therefore insecurely. Counseling is urgently needed for these parents who need to realize how their behavior affects the child. The classroom experience, group therapy, or parenting programs can help guide the parents' relationships with their children. All parents should be made to recognize that as children grow and develop they are children first and children with diabetes second. The ultimate goal for these parents is to be supportive to their children, to communicate more effectively, and to help their children develop in a more acceptable manner.

Nursing Care Summary: The Child with Diabetes Mellitus

NURSING GOALS	NURSING INTERVENTIONS	EXPECTED PATIENT/FAMILY OUTCOMES
HP-HMP Injury: Potential for tissue damage (ketoacidosis) **Risk factors: Dehydration, cerebral dysfunction**		
Recognize diabetic ketoacidosis	Be alert to signs of acidosis, especially in children with known diabetes melitus Observe for evidence of precipitating factors such as infection, stress, or omission of insulin injections	*Signs of ketoacidosis are detected and appropriate actions initiated
Treat associated problems	Carry out therapeutic regimen as prescribed for infection if present Implement appropriate care for the child who is unconscious	*Signs of associated problems are detected early and appropriate actions implemented
Detect alterations in status	Maintain meticulous records Assess vital signs frequently Observe for signs of complications such as cerebral edema, hyperkalemia, or hypokalemia	*Signs of altered status are detected early and appropriate actions initiated
Ensure adequate hydration	Assess state of hydration Monitor fluid intake and output	Child exhibits evidence of good hydration

*Nursing outcome.

Nursing Care Summary: The Child with Diabetes Mellitus—cont'd

NURSING GOALS	NURSING INTERVENTIONS	EXPECTED PATIENT/FAMILY OUTCOMES
HP-HMP Injury: Potential for tissue damage (hypoglycemia) **Risk factors: Metabolic imbalance**		
Recognize signs of hypoglycemia early	Be particularly alert at times when blood glucose levels are lowest Observe for lability of mood, irritability, seizures, and indications of subjective symptoms such as shaky feeling, headache, hunger, and impaired vision (p. 1709) Test for glucose	*Signs of hypoglycemia are recognized
Elevate blood glucose level	Offer readily absorbed carbohydrates such as orange juice, hard candy, or milk	Child ingests an appropriate carbohydrate Child displays no evidence of hypoglycemia
A-EP Diversional activity deficit **Etiology: Hospitalization**		
Provide for exercise and diversion	Provide activities in and around hospital unit Arrange for occupational therapy program that includes physical activity	Child engages in regular scheduled exercise
CPP Knowledge deficit (diabetic management) **Etiology: Newly diagnosed diabetic**		
Determine the educational needs of child and/or family	Assess the understanding and level of intelligence of the learners Select methods, vocabulary, and content appropriate to the level of the learner	*Appropriate teaching tools are assembled for teaching child and family

Educate child and/or regarding diabetic management	Allow 3 or 4 days for family and child to begin to adjust to the initial impact of the diagnosis
	 Select an environment conducive to learning
	 Allow ample time for the education process
	 Restrict length of teaching sessions
	     Child—15-20 minutes
	     Parents—45-60 minutes
	 Involve all senses and employ a variety of teaching strategies
	 Provide pamphlets or other supplementary materials
		Child and/or family display attitudes conducive to learning

Nature of the disease	Provide information regarding the pathophysiology of diabetes and the function and actions of insulin and glucagon in relation to caloric intake Answer questions and clarify misconceptions Explain function and expected effects of procedures and tests	Child and/or family demonstrate(s) an understanding of the disease and its therapy (specify indicators)
Meal planning	Enlist the services of a dietitian Emphasize the relationship between normal nutritional needs and the disease Become familiar with the family's food preferences Teach or reinforce the learners' understanding of the basic food groups	Child and/or family demonstrates an understanding of diet planning and food selection (specify indicators)

*Nursing outcome.

Continued.

Nursing Care Summary: The Child with Diabetes Mellitus—cont'd

NURSING GOALS	NURSING INTERVENTIONS	EXPECTED PATIENT/FAMILY OUTCOMES
Meal planning—cont'd	Help the child and family estimate food weights by volume Suggest low-carbohydrate snack items Guide family in assessing the labels of food products Teach or reinforce an understanding of the concept of calories Relate caloric equivalents to familiar foods Retain cultural patterns and family preferences as much as possible	
Medication	Teach child and family the characteristics of the insulins prescribed for the child Teach the proper mixing of insulins and acceptable substitutions (when the familiar brand is unavailable)	Child and/or family demonstrates an understanding of insulin, its various forms, and action (specify indicators)
Injection procedure	Impress upon the learners that the procedure will be a routine part of the child's life Involve caregivers and the child, if old enough Teach basic techniques using an orange or similar item Use demonstration and return demonstration techniques on another before injecting the child Help families and child work out a set rotational pattern Teach proper care of insulin and equipment	Child and/or family demonstrates injection technique correctly Child and/or family develop a rotation plan

Continuous infusion pump	Teach:
	  Basic pump mechanism
	  Preparing and loading syringe
	  Programming
	  Preparation, injection, and care of injection site
		Child and/or family demonstrate correct use of pump and care of injection site

Blood glucose testing	Teach: blood glucose monitoring and/or use of equipment selected for use Interpretation of results Care and maintenance of equipment	Child and/or family demonstrate the correct use of the glucose monitoring equipment
Urine testing	Teach: all methods of urine testing and interpretation of results Proper care of test materials and equipment	Child and/or family demonstrate urine testing and interpretation
Hygiene	Emphasize the importance of personal hygiene Encourage regular dental care and yearly ophthalmologic examinations Teach proper care of cuts and scratches Teach proper foot care	Family demonstrates an understanding of the importance of proper hygiene
Exercise	Help plan an exercise program Reiterate physician's instructions regarding adjustment of food and/or insulin to meet the child's activity pattern	Family helps child outline and carry out a regular exercise program
Hyperglycemia and hypoglycemia	Instruct learners regarding prevention of hyperglycemia or hypoglycemia Instruct them in how to recognize signs of hyperglycemia and hypoglycemia (especially hypoglycemia) Explain the relationship of insulin needs to illness, activity, and emotional upset Teach how to adjust food, activity and insulin at times of illness and during other situations that alter blood sugar levels Suggest carrying source of carbohydrate such as sugar cubes or hard candy in pocket or handbag Instruct parents and child in how to treat hypoglycemia with food, simple sugars, or glucagon	Family demonstrates an understanding of the signs and management of a hypoglycemic reaction (specify)

Nursing Care Summary: The Child with Diabetes Mellitus—cont'd

NURSING GOALS	NURSING INTERVENTIONS	EXPECTED PATIENT/FAMILY OUTCOMES
Identification	Encourage the acquisition of a means of identification, such as an identification bracelet, and explanation of the child's condition in case of emergency	Family acquires and child wears identification bracelet
General health status	Avoid exposure to infections	Child exhibits no signs of infection

Record keeping	Help child and family to design a form for keeping records of
	    Insulin administered
	    Blood and urine tests
	    Food intake
	    Marked variation in exercise
	    Illness
		Family and child keep an accurate record of insulin administration, glucose testing, etc.

Self-management	Encourage honesty in recording, such as eating a forbidden candy bar Encourage independence in applying the concepts learned in teaching sessions Instruct when to seek assistance from medical personnel	Child takes responsibility for management of his disease comensurate with age and capabilities

SP-SCP   **Self-concept, disturbance in: Body image**
Etiology: Biologic changes (insulin dependency)

Promote positive self-esteem	Encourage child to express feelings and concerns Determine assets and strengths Help devise coping strategies for managing areas of concern	Child verbalizes his feelings and concerns Child maintains pre-diagnosis activities and relationships
Promote positive adjustment to the disease	Assist child and family in solving problems associated with each of the child's developmental stages Encourage the child to maintain normal activity pattern Encourage interpersonal relationships with peers Suggest involvement with special groups and facilities for diabetic children Be alert to signs that may indicate rebellion against the disease, such as noncompliance or other forms of acting-out Be available for consultation when needed	Child interacts with other children according to developmental level Child becomes involved with special group activities

RRP   **Family process, alteration in**
Etiology: situational crisis (child with a chronic disorder)

Support family	All for expression of feelings Encourage family in efforts to adjust to the child's disease and its effect on the family life-style Assist family in problem solving Assess interpersonal relationships within the family, especially behaviors that reflect family attitudes toward the affected child Provide anticipatory guidance regarding expectations as child progresses through developmental stages Intervene where behaviors indicate rejection or overprotection Refer family to the American Diabetes Association, the Juvenile Diabetes Foundation, and other agencies and services that help meet their special needs	Family incorporates the needs of the child into the family lifestyle Family verbalizes feelings and concerns regarding the special needs of the child and their effect on the family process Family copes with developmental and situational crises with minimum family disruption

Continued.

Nursing Interventions Related to Medical Management

Assist with diagnosis
Check blood glucose as ordered
Obtain and check urine specimen for glucose, acetone, and specific gravity as ordered
Collect 24-hour urine specimen for glucose if ordered
Order or obtain blood for analysis
Assist with glucose tolerance test

Replace insulin deficit
Understand the action of insulin
Understand the differences in composition, time of onset, and duration of action for the various insulin preparations
Employ correct techniques when preparing and administering insulin
Subcutaneous injection
Rotation of sites

Assess status
General
Maintain beside flow sheet, including vital signs, intake, output, blood glucose, copper reduction test (Clinitest), acetone test (Acetest), and insulin administered (varies according to institution)

Vital signs
Measure vital signs as ordered, usually every 4 hours
Urine
Measure intake and output
Test for glucose, acetone, and specific gravity
Time measurement, as ordered
Preprandial and bedtime
Double-voided specimens
Every 4 hours
Perform Clinitest using one-, two-, or five-drop method and Acetest as ordered
Blood glucose
Order fasting blood sugar (FBS) daily or as requested
Withhold breakfast and insulin until after blood is drawn for test
Obtain blood glucose measurements as prescribed

Treat hypoglycemia
Administer glucagon, if ordered

Ketoacidosis
Replace fluid and electrolyte losses
Monitor intravenous infusion
Correct hyperglycemia
Administer insulin intravenously and subcutaneously as prescribed
Monitor blood glucose levels every 1-2 hours as ordered
Monitor urine glucose and acetone every 1-2 hours if ordered

Assess status
Monitor mental status, level of consciousness
Monitor serum electrolytes, pH, glucose, and blood gases
Monitor urine glucose, acetone, specific gravity, and volume frequently
Attach to cardiac monitor

CONCEPT SUMMARIES

- The endocrine system has three components: the cell, which sends a chemical message via a hormone; target cells, which receive the message; and the environment through which the chemical is transported from the site of synthesis to the sites of cellular action.

- Pituitary dysfunction is manifest primarily by growth disturbance.

- The main physiologic action of thyroid hormone is to regulate the basal metabolic rate and control the processes of growth and tissue differentiation.

- Disorders of thyroid function include hypothyroidism, autoimmune thyroiditis, goiter, and hyperthyroidism.

- Therapy for hyperthyroidism is directed at retarding the rate of hormone secretion and may include drug therapy, thyroidectomy, or radioiodine therapy.

- Classic forms of hypoparathyroidism in childhood are idiopathic—deficient production of PTH—and pseudohypoparathyroidism—increased PTH production with end organ unresponsiveness to PTH.

- The adrenal cortex secretes three important groups of hormones: glucocorticoids, mineralocorticoids, and sex steroids.

- Disorders of adrenal function include acute adrenocortical insufficiency, chronic adrenocortical insufficiency, Cushing syndrome, congenital adrenogenital hyperplasia, and hyperaldosteronism.

- Four categories of Cushing syndrome are pituitary, adrenal, ectopic, and iatrogenic.

- Management of congenital adrenogenital hyperplasia includes assignation of a sex according to genotype, administration of cortisone, and, possibly, reconstructive surgery.

- Childhood diabetes mellitus is categorized as insulin-dependent, non-insulin-dependent, and maturity-onset diabetes of youth.

- The focus of diabetes management is insulin replacement, diet, and exercise.

- Education of families includes explanation of diabetes, meal planning, administering insulin injection, monitoring, general hygienic practices, promoting exercise, record-keeping, and observing for complications.

REFERENCES

Aziz, S.: Recurrent use of disposable syringe-needle units in diabetic children, Diabetes Care **7:**118-120, 1984.

Berger, M., and others: Absorption kinetics and biologic effects of subcutaneous insulin preparations, Diabetes Care **5:**77-91, 1982.

Binder, C., and others: Insulin pharmacokinetics, Diabetes Care **7:**188-199, 1984.

Borders, L., Bingham, P., and Riddle, M.: Traditional insulin-use practices and the incidence of bacterial contamination and infection, Diabetes Care **7:**121, 1984.

Burnett, J.: Congenital adrenocortical hyperplasia, Am. J. Nurs. **80:**1304-1308, 1980.

Butler, L.D., Munson, J.M., and DeLuca, P.P.: Effect of inline filtration on the potency of low-dose drugs, Am. J. Hosp. Pharm. **37:**935, 1980.

Cahill, G.F., and McDevitt, H.O.: Insulin-dependent diabetes mellitus: the initial lesion, N. Engl. J. Med. **304:**1454-1465, 1981.

Chase, H.P.: Monitoring glucose control and use of a diabetes control index in insulin-dependent diabetes mellitus, Pediatr. Ann. **12:**643-650, 1983.

Cohen, F.L.: Clinical genetics in nursing practice, Philadelphia, 1984, J.B. Lippincott Co.

Collins, B.J., and others: Safety of reusing disposable plastic insulin syringes, Lancet **1:**559-561, 1983.

DiGeorge, A.M.: The endocrine system. In Behrman, R.E., and Vaughan, V.C., III: Textbook of pediatrics, ed. 12, Philadelphia, 1983, W.B. Saunders Co.

Dillon, R.: Improved serum insulin profiles in diabetic individuals who massaged their insulin injection sites, Diabetes Care **6:**399-401, 1983.

Drash, A.L.: The epidemiology of diabetes mellitus in children and adolescents, Pediatr. Ann. **12:**629-635, 1983.

Fink, J.N., and Beall, G.N.: Immunologic aspects of endocrine diseases, JAMA **248:**2696-2700, 1982.

Fishbein, H.A., and others: The diabetes type I (insulin-dependent diabetes mellitus registry: seasonal incidence, Diabetologia **23:**83-89, 1982.

Foley, T.P.: Thyroid disease. In Gellis, S.S., and Kagan, B.M.: Current pediatric therapy 12, Philadelphia, 1986, W.B. Saunders Co.

Galloway, J.A., and others: Factors influencing the absorption, serum insulin concentration and blood glucose responses after injections of regular insulin and various insulin mixtures, Diabetes Care **4:**366-376, 1981.

Guthrie, D.W., and Guthrie, R.A.: The disease process of diabetes mellitus, Nurs. Clin. North Am. **18:**617-630, 1983.

Jenkins, C.A., and Molitch, M.E.: Get the most out of mixing insulin, Diabetes Forecast **39**(1):13-14, 1986.

Koivisto, V.A., and Felig, P.: Alterations in insulin absorption and in blood glucose control associated with varying insulin injection sites in diabetic patients, Ann. Intern. Med. **92:**59-65, 1980.

Lever, E., and Jaspan, J.: Sodium bicarbonate therapy in severe diabetic ketoacidosis, Am. J. Med. **75:**263-268, 1983.

MacDonald, M.J.: Etiology and classification of diabetes in children, Primary Care **10:**531-551, 1983.

Mäenpää, J., and others: Natural course of juvenile autoimmune thyroiditis, Pediatr. **107:**898-904, 1985.

Malone, J.I., and others: Risk factors for diabetic retinopathy in youth, Pediatrics **73:**756-761, 1984.

New, M.I., Levine, L.S., and Temeck, J.W.: Disorders of the adrenal gland. In Gellis, S.S., and Kagan, B.M.: Current pediatric therapy 12, Philadelphia, 1986, W.B. Saunders Co.

Rabinowe, S.L., and Eisenbarth, G.S.: Type I diabetes mellitus: a chronic autoimmune disease? Pediatr. Clin. North Am. **31:**531-543, 1984.

Reiter, E.O., and others: Childhood thyromegaly: recent developments, J. Pediatr. **99:**507-518, 1981.

Rosenbloom, A.L.: Long-term complications of type I (insulin-dependent) diabetes mellitus, Pediatr. Ann. **12:**665-685, 1983.

Rosenbloom, A.L.: Skeletal and joint manifestations of diabetes mellitus, Pediatr. Clin. North Am. **31:**569-589, 1984.

Rosenstock, J., Strowig, S., and Raskin, P.: Insulin pump therapy: a realistic appraisal, Clin. Diabetes **3:**1, 27- 30, 1985.

Sack, J., and others: Association of autoimimmune thyroiditis and HLA-DR5 in multiple family members, J. Pediatr. **103:**758-760, 1983.

Sperling, M.A.: Diabetes mellitus. In Behrman, R.E., and Vaughan, V.C., III: Textbook of pediatrics, ed. 12, Philadelphia, 1983, W.B. Saunders Co.

Sperling, M.A.: Diabetic ketoacidosis, Pediatr. Clin. North Am. **31:**591-610, 1984.

Starkman, H., and others: Limited joint mobility (LJM) of the hand in patients with diabetes mellitus: relation to chronic complications, Ann. Rheum. Dis. **4:**130-151, 1986.

Thatcher, G.: Insulin injections: the case against random rotation, Am. J. Nurs. **85:**690-692, 1985.

Tsang, R.C., Noguchi, A., and Steichen, J.J.: Pediatric parathyroid disorders, Pediatr. Clin. North Am. **26:**223-249, 1979.

Turco, S.J.: Adsorption of insulin in infusion containers and tubing, Am. J. Intrav. Ther. Nutr. **9:**44, 1982.

Underwood, L.E.: Endocrine system. In Gellis, S.S., and Kagan, B.M.: Current pediatric therapy 12, Philadelphia, 1986, W.B. Saunders Co.

White, K., and others: Unstable diabetes and unstable families: a psychosocial evaluation of diabetic children with recurrent ketoacidosis, Pediatrics **73:**749-755, 1984.

Winter, J.S.D.: Marginal comment: current approaches to the treatment of congenital adrenal hyperplasia, J. Pediatr. **97:**81-82, 1980.

Wolfsdorf, J.I.: Diabetes mellitus. In Gellis, S.S., and Kagan, B.M.: Current pediatric therapy 12, Philadelphia, 1986, W.B. Saunders Co.

Wong, D.L.: The significance of dead space in syringes, Am. J. Nurs. **82:**1237, 1982.

Young, R.J., and others: Diabetic lipohypertrophy delays insulin absorption, Diabetes Care **7:**479-480, 1984.

BIBLIOGRAPHY

Pituitary Dysfunction

August, G.P., and others: Hypopituitarism and the CHARGE association, J. Pediatr. **103:**424-425, 1983.

Fairchild, R.S.: Diabetes insipidus: a review, Crit. Care Q. **3**(3):111-118, 1980.

McElroy, D.B., and Davis, G.T.: SIADH and the acutely ill child, Am. J. Maternal Child Nurs. **11:**193-196, 1986.

Shore, R.M., and others: Bone mineral status in growth hormone deficiency, J. Pediatr. **96:**393-396, 1980.

Solomon, B.L.: The hypothalamus and the pituitary gland: an overview, Nurs. Clin. North Am. **15:**435-451, 1980.

Stern, M., and Zaiken, H.: Assessing the child with short stature, Pediatr. Nurs. **11:**106-110, 1985.

Stewarts, M.L.K.: When patient has the "other" diabetes, RN **48**(5):54-58, 1985.

Zucker, A.R., and Chernow, B.: Diabetes insipidus and the syndrome of inappropriate antidiuretic hormone release, Crit. Care Q. **6**(3):63-74, 1983.

Disorders of Thyroid Function/Disorders of the Parathyroid Gland

Arcangelo, V.P.: Simple goiter, Nursing 83 **13**(3):47, 1983.

Bachrach, L.K., and others: Use of ultrasound in childhood thyroid disorders, J. Pediatr. **103:**547-552, 1983.

Brown, A.L., and others: Racial differences in the incidence of congenital hypothyroidism, J. Pediatr. **9:**934-936, 1981.

Honigman, R.E.: Thyroid function tests, Nursing 82 **12**(4):68-71, 1982.

Sharkey, P.L., and Myer, S.A.: Hyperthyroidism, Crit. Care Update **8**(5):12-24, 1981.

Adrenal Dysfunction

Camunas, C.: Surviving pheochromocytoma, Am. J. Nurs. **83:**887-891, 1983.

Darland, N.W.: Congenital adrenocortical hyperplasia: supportive nursing interventions, J. Pediatr. Nurs. **1**(2):117-123, 1986.

Larson, C.A.: The critical path of adrenocortical insufficiency, Nursing 84 **14**(10):66-69, 1984.

Lee, P.D.K., Winter, R.J., and Green, O.C.: Virilizing adrenocortical tumors in childhood: eight cases and a review of the literature, Pediatrics **76:**437-444, 1985.

New, M.I., and Levine, L.S.: New developments in congenital adrenal hyperplasia, Pediatr. Ann. **10:**346-355, 1981.

Sanford, S.J.: Dysfunction of the adrenal gland: physiologic considerations and nursing problems, Nurs. Clin. North Am. **15:**481-498, 1980.

Diabetes Mellitus: General

Brouhard, B.H.: Control and monitoring for the child with insulin-dependent diabetes mellitus, Am. J. Dis. Child. **137:**787-794, 1983.

Brouhard, B.H.: Management of the very young diabetic, Am. J. Dis. Child. **139:**446-447, 1985.

Christensen, K.S.: Self-management in diabetic children, Diabetes Care **6:**552-555, 1983.

Cunningham, L.: Sports nutrition for the serious athlete, Diabetes Forecast **39**(1):63-64, 1986.

Daneman, D., Becker, D.J., and Drash, A.L.: Factors affecting glycosylated hemoglobin values in children with insulin-dependent diabetes, J. Pediatr. **99:**847-853, 1981.

DiFlorio, I.A., and Duncan, P.: Design for successful patient teaching, J. Matern. Child Nurs. **11:**246-249, 1986.

Donohue-Porter, P.: Insulin-dependent diabetes mellitus, Nurs. Clin. North Am. **20:**191-198, 1985.

Ellis, D., and others: Proteinuria in children with insulin-dependent diabetes: relationship to duration of disease, metabolic control, and retinal changes, J. Pediatr. **102:**673-680, 1983.

Faro, B.: Maintaining good control in children with diabetes, Pediatr. Nurs. **9:**368-373, 1983.

Gale, E.A.M., and others: In search of the Somogyi effect, Lancet **2**(8189):279-282, 1980.

Guthrie, D.: Helping the diabetic manage his self-care, Nursing 80 **10**(2):57-64, 1980.

Guthrie, D.W., and Guthrie, R.A., editors: Nursing management of diabetes mellitus, ed. 2, St. Louis, 1982, The C.V. Mosby Co.

Ingersoll, G.M., and others: Cognitive maturity and self-management among adolescents with insulin-dependent diabetes mellitus, J. Pediatr. **108:**620-623, 1986.

Jackson, R.L.: Education of the parents of a child with diabetes, Nutr. Today **15**(3):30-34, 1980.

Jackson, R.L.: Growth and maturation of children with insulin-dependent diabetes mellitus, Pediatr. Clin. North Am. **31:**545-567, 1984.

Lebovitz, H.E.: Etiology and pathogenesis of diabetes mellitus, Pediatr. Clin. North Am. **31:**521-530, 1984.

Leslie, N.D., and Sperling, M.A.: Relation of metabolic control to complications in diabetes mellitus, J. Pediatr. **108:**491-497, 1986.

Lobo, M.L.: Nursing implications in camps for children with diabetes. In Chinn, P.L., and Leonard, K.B., editors: Current practice in pediatric nursing, vol. 3, St. Louis, 1980, The C.V. Mosby Co.

Maclaren, N.K., and Henson, V.: The genetics of insulin-dependent diabetes, Growth Genetics & Hormones **2**(1):1-4, 1986.

Miller, B.K., and White, N.E.: Diabetes assessment guide, Am. J. Nurs. **80:**1314-1316, 1980.

Ory, M.G., and Dronenfeld, J.J.: Living with juvenile diabetes mellitus, Pediatr. Nurs. **6**(5):47-50, 1980.

Pelczynski, L., and Reilly, A.: Helping your diabetic patients help themselves, Nursing 81 **11**(5):76-81, 1981.

Pond, H.: Parental attitudes toward children with a chronic medical disorder: special reference to diabetes mellitus, Diabetes Care **2:**425-431, 1979.

Rainwater, N.: Adherence to the diabetes medical regimen: assessment and treatment strategies, Pediatr. Ann. **12:**658-661, 1983.

Robertson, C.: Clear the exercise hurdles for your diabetic patient, Nursing 84 **14**(10):58-63, 1984.

Rosenbloom, A.L.: Primary and subspeciality care of diabetes mellitus in children and youth, Pediatr. Clin. North Am. **31:**107-117, 1984.

Rosenbloom, A.L., Kohrman, A., and Sperling, M.: Classification and diagnosis of diabetes mellitus in children and adolescents, J. Pediatr. **98:**320-323, 1981.

Rotter, J., and others: HLA genotype study of insulin dependent diabetes, Diabetes **32:**169-174, 1983.

Rowland, T.W., and others: Glycemic control with physical training in insulin-dependent diabetes mellitus, Am. J. Dis. Child. **139:**307-309, 1985.

Schiffrin, A., and others: Feasibility of strict diabetes control in insulin-dependent diabetic adolescents, J. Pediatr. **103:**522-527, 1983.

Schneider, A.J.: Starting insulin therapy in children with newly diagnosed diabetes, Am. J. Dis. Child. **137:**782-786, 1983.

Sims, D.F., editor: Diabetes: reach for health and freedom, St. Louis, 1984, The C.V. Mosby Co.

Stein, R., and others: Exercise and the patient with type I diabetes mellitus, Pediatr. Clin. North Am. **31:**665-673, 1984.

Stucky, V.: The meal plan. In Guthrie, D.W., and Guthrie, R.A., editors: Nursing management of diabetes mellitus, ed. 2, St. Louis, 1982, The C.V. Mosby Co.

Sutherland, D.E.R., and others: Pancreas transplantation, Pediatr. Clin. North Am. **31:**735-750, 1984.

Tamborlane, W.V., and Sherwin, R.S.: Diabetes control and complications: new strategies and insights, J. Pediatr. **102:**805-813, 1983.

Diabetes Mellitus: Insulin Administration

Bougnères, P.F., and others: Insulin pump therapy in young children with type I diabetes, J. Pediatr. **105:**212-217, 1984.

Childs, B.P.: Insulin infusion pumps, Nursing 83 **13**(11):55-57, 1983.

Dexter, D.M.: The new insulins, Am. J. Nurs. **81:**146-148, 1981.

Fendya, D.G., and Flynn, K.: Nursing care for children with hypoglycemia due to hyperinsulinism, Am. J. Maternal Child Nurs. **6:**100-105, 1981.

Fredholm, N.Z.: The insulin pump: new method of insulin delivery, Am. J. Nurs. **81:**2024-2026, 1981.

Kaye, R.: Research and practice in the treatment of insulin-dependent diabetes: a survey of 53 pediatric diabetologists, Pediatrics **74:**1079-1085, 1984.

Knott, S.P., and Herget, M.J.: Teaching self-injection to diabetics: an easier and more effective way, Nursing 84 **14**(1):57, 1984.

Langdon, D.R., Frederick, D.J., and Sperling, M.A.: Comparison of single- and split-dose insulin regimens with 24-hour monitoring, J. Pediatr. **99:**854-861, 1981.

Menchik, R.: The new insulin pumps: tight control—at a price, RN **46**(5):52-59, 1983.

Nathan, D.M.: The importance of intensive supervision in determining the efficacy of insulin pump therapy, Diabetes Care **6:**295-297, 1983.

Noto, R.A., and others: Improved management of brittle-psychosocial diabetes by use of a portable insulin infusion pump, J. Pediatr. **107:**100-102, 1985.

Slama, G., and others: Multiple use of disposable insulin syringe-needle units, JAMA **244:**266-267, 1980.

Tamborlane, W.V., and Press, C.M.: Insulin infusion pump treatment of type I diabetes, Pediatr. Clin. North Am. **31:**721-734, 1984.

Witt, M.F., White, N.H., and Santiago, J.V.: Roles of site and timing of the morning insulin injection in type I diabetes, J. Pediatr. **103:**528-533, 1983.

Diabetes Mellitus: Testing and Monitoring

Aziz, S., and Hsiang, Y.-H.: Comparative study of home blood glucose monitoring devices: visidex, chemstrip bG, glucometer, and accu-chek bG, Diabetes Care **6:**529-532, 1983.

Bergman, M., and Felig, P.: Self-monitoring of blood glucose levels in diabetes: principles and practice, Arch. Intern. Med. **144**:2029-2034, 1984.

Canfield, M.E., Kemp, S.F., and Hoff, C.P.: Assessment of a new blood glucose strip: comparison of visidex, visidex II, and chemstrip bG with gluocse analyzer determination of blood glucose, Diabetes Care **8**:77-82, 1985.

Clarson, C., and others: Self-monitoring of blood glucose: how accurate are children with diabetes at reading chemstrip bG? Diabetes Care **8**:354-358, 1985.

Connors, M.H.: Blood glucose monitoring in childhood diabetes, Nurse Pract. **9**:30-32, 62, 1984.

Daneman, D., and others: The role of self-monitoring of blood glucose in the routine management of children with insulin-dependent diabetes mellitus, Diabetes Care **8**:1-4, 1985.

Fow, S.M.: Home blood glucose monitoring in children with insulin-dependent diabetes mellitus, Pediatr. Nurs. **9**:439-442, 1983.

Joyce, M.A., Kuzich, C.M., and Murphy, D.M.: Those new blood glucose tests, RN **46**(4):46-52, 1983.

King, G., Steggles, D., and Harrop, J.S.: Performance and storage of reagent strips for measuring blood glucose, Br. Med. J. **285**:1165, 1982.

Loman, D., and Galgani, C.: Monitoring diabetic children's blood-glucose levels at home, J. Matern. Child Nurs. **9**:192-196, 1984.

Lombrail, P., and others: Abnormal color vision and reliable self-monitoring of blood glucose, Diabetes Care **7**:318-321, 1984.

MacDonald, M.J.: Personal blood glucose testing in children, Primary Care **10**:565-581, 1983.

Metzger, M.J.: A new test for blood sugar, Am. J. Nurs. **83**:763-764, 1983.

Miller, V.G.: Diabetes: let's stop testing urine, Am. J. Nurs. **86**:54, 1986.

Nelson, J.D., Woelk, M.A., and Sheps, S.: Self glucose monitoring: a comparison of the glucometer, glucoscan and hypocount B, Diabetes Care **6**:262-267, 1983.

Plasse, N.J.: Monitoring blood glucose at home: a comparison of three products, Am. J. Nurs. **81**:2028-2029, 1981.

Robertson, C.: How to teach patients to monitor blood glucose, RN **48**(12):24-25, 1985.

Silverstein, J.H., and others: Accuracy of two systems for blood glucose monitoring without a meter (chemstrip/visidex), Diabetes Care **6**:533-535, 1983.

Stevens, A.D.: Monitoring blood glucose at home: who should do it, Am. J. Nurs. **81**:2026-2027, 1981.

Surr, C.W.: Teaching patients to use the new blood-glucose monitoring products, Part I, Nursing 83 **13**(1):42-45, 1983.

Surr, C.W.: Teaching patients to use the new blood-glucose monitoring products, Part II, Nursing 83 **13**(2):58-62, 1983.

Villeneuve, M.E., Murphy, J., and Mazze, R.S.: Evaluating blood glucose monitors, Am. J. Nurs. **85**:1258-1259, 1985.

White, N.E., and Miller, B.K.: Glycohemoglobin: a new test to help the diabetic stay in control, Nursing 83 **13**(8):55-57, 1983.

Diabetes Mellitus: Nutrition

Alli, C.R., and Crapo, P.A.: Sweetener safety: the bitter debate, Diabetes Forecast **38**(3):34-37, 1985.

Arky, R.A.: Nutrition therapy for the child and adolescent with type I diabetes mellitus, Pediatr. Clin. North Am. **31**:711-719, 1984.

Chait, A.: Dietary management of diabetes mellitus, Contemp. Nutr. **9**(2):1-2, 1984.

Franz, M.J.: Fast food: where's the nutrition? Diabetes Forecast **38**(6):31-34, 1985.

Heins, J.M.: Dietary management in diabetes mellitus, Nurs. Clin. North Am. **18**:631-643, 1983.

Lorenz, R.A., Christensen, N.K., and Pichert, J.W.: Diet-related knowledge, skill, and adherence among children with insulin-dependent diabetes mellitus, Pediatrics **75**:872-876, 1985.

Mayniuk, M.D.: Fighting fat at college, Diabetes Forecast **38**(5):52, 1985.

Skyler, J.S.: Dietary planning in insulin-dependent diabetes mellitus, Pediatr. Ann. **12**:652-657, 1983.

Diabetes Mellitus: Complications

Chipman, J.J., and Marks, J.F.: Diabetic ketoacidosis. In Levin, D.L., Morriss, F.C., and Moore, G.C., editors: A practical guide to pediatric intensive care, ed. 2, St. Louis, 1984, The C.V. Mosby Co.

Fort, P., Waters, S.M., and Lifshitz, F.: Low-dose insulin infusion in the treatment of diabetic ketoacidosis: bolus versus no bolus, J. Pediatr. **96**:36-40, 1980.

Gill, G.V., and Alberti, K.G.G.M.: The ups and downs of brittle diabetes, Diabetes Forecast **39**(1):45-46, 50, 1986.

Golden, M.P., Herrold, A.J., and Orr, D.P.: An approach to prevention of recurrent diabetic ketoacidosis in the pediatric population, J. Pediatr. **107**:195-200, 1985.

Hansen, K.A., and Duck, S.C.: Teledyne sleep sentry: evaluation in pediatric patients for detection of nocturnal hypoglycemia, Diabetes Care **6**:597-600, 1983.

Kyner, J.L.: Diabetic ketoacidosis, Crit. Care Q. **3**(2):65-75, 1980.

Lavine, R.L.: How to recognize ... and what to do about ... hypoglycemia, Nursing 79 **9**(4):52-55, 1979.

Lillo, R., and Masteller, D.: Outpatient management of children in diabetic ketoacidosis, Pediatr. Nurs. **8**:383-385, 1982.

Narins, B.: Products to help with insulin reactions, Diabetes Forecast **39**(5):26, 1986.

Stock, P.L.: Action stat! insulin shock, Nursing 85 **15**(4):53, 1985.

Stock-Barkman, P.: Confusing concepts: is it diabetic shock or diabetic coma? Nursing 83 **13**(6):33-41, 1983.

Diabetes Mellitus: Psychosocial

Ahlfield, J.E., Soler, N.G., and Marcus, S.D.: Adolescent diabetes mellitus: parent/child perspectives of the effect of the disease on family and social interactions, Diabetes Care **6**:393-398, 1983.

Banion, C.R., Miles, M.S., and Carter, M.C.: Problems of mothers in management of children with diabetes, Diabetes Care **6**:548-551, 1983.

Bobrow, E.S., AvRuskin, T.W., and Siller, J.: Mother-daughter interaction and adherence to diabetes regimens, Diabetes Care **8**:146-151, 1985.

Brown, A.J.: School-age children with diabetes: knowledge and management of the disease, and adequacy of self-concept, J. Matern. Child Nurs. **14**(1):47-61, 1985.

Cerreto, M.C., and Travis, L.B.: Implications of psychological and family factors in the treatment of diabetes, Pediatr. Clin. North Am. **31**:689-710, 1984.

Etzwiler, D.D.: Education and participation of patients and their families, Pediatr. Ann. **12**:638-642, 1983.

Hoette, S.J.: The adolescent with diabetes mellitus, Nurs. Clin. North Am. **18**:763-776, 1983.

King, C.R., Jr.: Family issues in diabetes. In Azarnoff, P., and Hardgrove, C., editors: The family in child healthcare, New York, 1981, John Wiley & Sons.

Kovacs, M., and others: Initial coping response and psychosocial characteristics of children with insulin-dependent diabetes mellitus, J. Pediatr. **106**:827-834, 1985.

Krauser, K.L., and Madden, P.B.: The child with diabetes mellitus, Nurs. Clin. North Am. **18**:749-762, 1983.

Lindsey, N.M.: Insights into interventions for coping with diabetes, Nursing 83 **13**(3):48-49, 1983.

Lowe, E., and Arsham, G.: "I know how you feel," Diabetes Forecast **38**(11):56-62, 1985.

Moffatt, M.E.K., and Pless, I.B.: Locus of control in juvenile diabetic campers: changes during camp, and relationship to camp staff assessments, J. Pediatr. **103**:146-150, 1983.

Moran, M.M.: Diabetes camps: management guidelines, Pediatr. Nurs. **11**:183-186, 1985.

Ryan, C., Vega, A., and Drash, A.: Cognitive deficits in adolescents who developed diabetes early in life, Pediatrics **75**:921-927, 1985.

Saucier, C.P.: Self concept and self-care management in school-age children with diabetes, Pediatr. Nurs. **10**:135-138, 1984.

Unit Fourteen

The Child with a Problem that Interferes with Locomotion

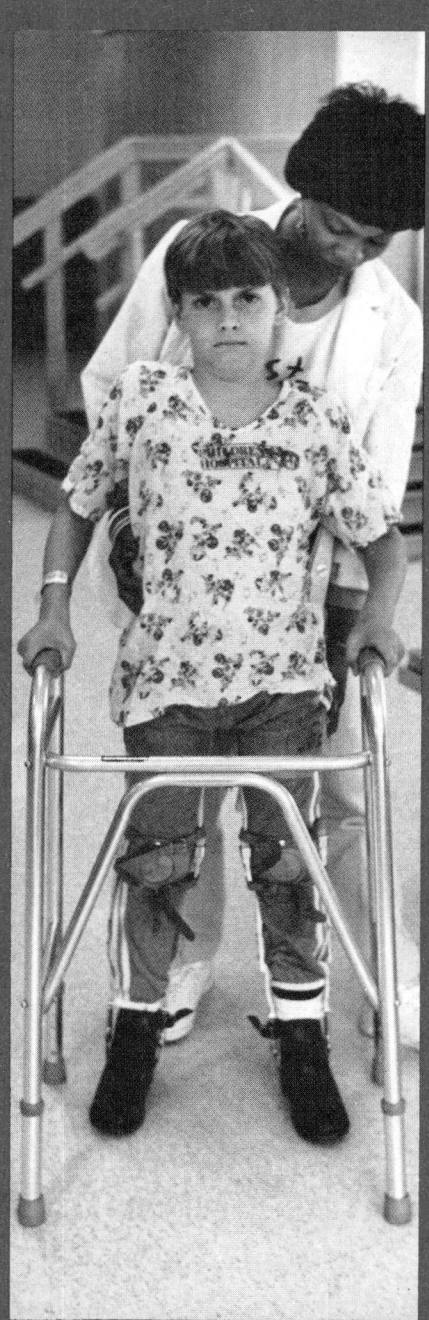

Childhood is the age of onset for a variety of physically disabling conditions of hereditary, infectious, or traumatic etiologies. Many disorders that interfere with locomotion are present at birth; a few of these have been discussed previously, including congenital defects such as myelomeningocele, dislocation of the hip, and foot deformities (see Chapter 11). Others appear later in childhood. Of these, some can occur at any age, such as fractures; others make their appearance at ages characteristic for the specific condition, such as muscular dystrophy during early childhood and slipped epiphysis at puberty.

Some locomotor disabilities are acquired in an instant, such as amputation or spinal cord injury, whereas others develop over an extended period, like tuberculosis or progressive muscular atrophy. Some, like fractures, need only short-term therapy; others, such as spinal cord injuries and cerebral palsy, require long-term therapy and a longer period of adjustment and involve the whole problem of daily living activities.

The physical limitations may involve only temporary inconvenience, or they may be permanent with the need to substitute an alternative form of locomotion. Some are helped by specific treatments; for others therapy is merely supportive. A large number of these disabilities require a health team approach with contributions from a variety of specialists. Concomitant problems associated with permanent disabilities, particularly those acquired in later childhood, are emotional adjustment and alterations in self-image.

Chapter 39, *The Child with Neuromuscular, Musculoskeletal, or Articular Dysfunction*, is concerned primarily with congenital and acquired disorders involving neurologic, muscular, skeletal, and articular systems, whereas Chapter 40, *The Immobilized or Traumatically Injured Child*, deals with the consequences of traumatic injury. The coverage is by no means comprehensive, but representative examples are used to illustrate specific problems.

Chapter 39

The Child with Neuromuscular, Musculoskeletal, or Articular Dysfunction

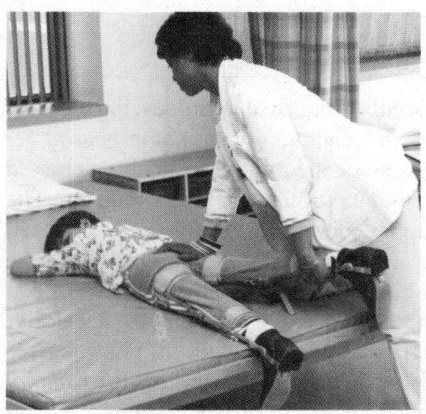

Defects in locomotion can be associated with diseases or deficits in the supporting structures (the skeleton), the movement-producing structures (muscles or their innervation), or the articulating structures (joints) of the body. Defects in bones are readily identified in most instances, but disorders involving muscular function offer more difficult problems of diagnosis. All interfere in some way with adequate locomotion. The first part of this chapter is devoted to the child with neuromuscular dysfunction; the second part deals with defects primarily caused by musculoskeletal and articular disorders.

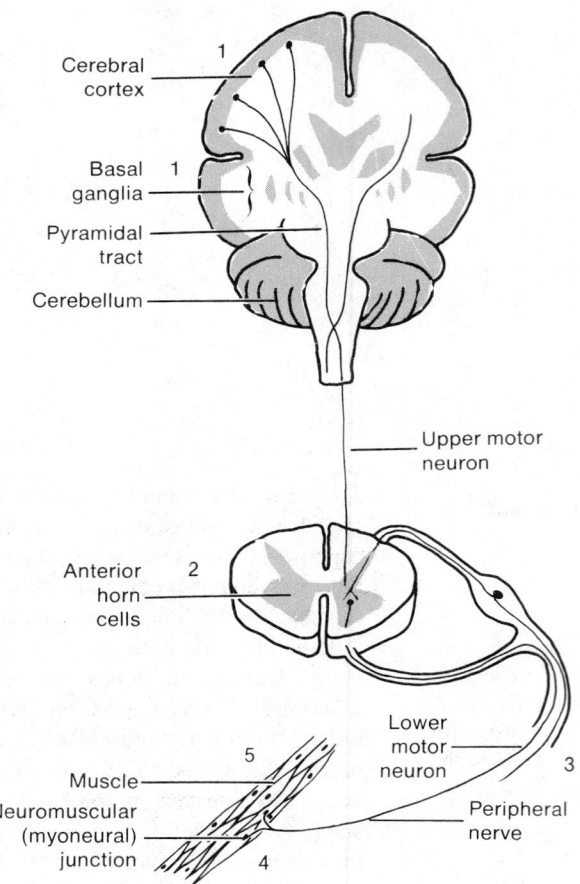

Cerebral cortex — 1

Basal ganglia — 1

Pyramidal tract

Cerebellum

Upper motor neuron

Anterior horn cells — 2

Lower motor neuron

Muscle — 5

Neuromuscular (myoneural) junction — 4

Peripheral nerve — 3

Fig. 39-1. Site of origin for neuromuscular disorders. *1,* Cerebral palsy. *2,* Poliomyelitis, spinal muscular atrophy. *3,* Mononeuropathies, polyneuropathies. *4,* Myasthenia gravis, neurotoxic disorders. *5,* Muscular dystrophies.

Neuromuscular Dysfunction

Weakness or abnormal performance of skeletal muscle may represent a defect in the muscle itself or reflect a pathologic disorder at some point along the neural pathway from the cortex of the brain to the neuromuscular junction. The identification of the source of muscle dysfunction includes not only the testing of muscle function but also the systematic elimination of possible disorders of neural structures on which muscle function depends for its stimulus. In a few disorders muscle disease may be accompanied by a neural disorder.

Some clinical features are shared by muscle disease (myopathy), which differs in many ways from muscle dysfunction resulting from disorders of neuronal structures—brain, cranial nerve nuclei, long nerve tracts, anterior horn cells of the spinal cord, and peripheral nerves. Motor function is accomplished by means of the simple reflex arcs or by way of impulses transmitted from the cerebral cortex and other centers in the brain through the various nerve pathways of the central nervous system. The upper motor neurons con-

sist of cells that lie in the cerebral cortex and fibers that traverse the brain stem and spinal cord to terminate at their synapses with the anterior horn cells. The anterior horn cells, axons, and peripheral nerve branches constitute the lower motor neurons. The motor unit consists of the lower motor neuron, the neuromuscular junction, and the muscle fibers it supplies (Fig. 39-1). The upper motor neuronal pathways from the cerebrum to the lower motor neuron are described as (1) pyramidal—those whose fibers extend from the cortex, come together in the medulla, cross from one side to the other, then extend down the cord to synapse with anterior horn motor neurons; and (2) extrapyramidal—a complex network of motor neurons that comprise relays between motor areas of the cortex, basal ganglia, thalamus, cerebellum, and brain stem.

CLASSIFICATION AND DIAGNOSIS

The site of pathologic disturbance determines the type of muscular dysfunction. In general, *upper motor neuron* lesions produce weakness associated with spasticity, increased deep tendon reflexes, and abnormal superficial reflexes. The primary disorder of upper motor neuron dysfunction is cerebral palsy. Lesions of *lower motor neurons* interrupt the reflex arc, causing weakness and atrophy of the skeletal muscles involved with associated hypotonia or flaccidity, which eventually progress to atrophy with varying degrees of contracture deformity. A disorder of the *extrapyramidal pathway* and the cerebellum rarely produces muscle weakness.

Lower motor neuron involvement is usually symmetric (except that of poliomyelitis and single peripheral nerve disease), whereas disorders of the pyramidal tract are more often asymmetric. Muscle wasting is characteristic of lower motor neuron lesions and more marked than in diseases of muscles. Deep tendon reflexes are briskly active in upper motor neuron disease, are diminished or absent in lower motor neuron disease, and depend on the progress of muscle degeneration in the myopathies.

These disorders can also be categorized according to onset: those in which there is acute onset of flaccid paralysis and those with more gradual onset and progressive degeneration. In most instances the sudden appearance of flaccid paralysis in a previously healthy child can be attributed to an infectious process. Neurotoxins (e.g., botulism, tick paralysis, or heavy metal poisoning), pressure on the spinal cord from tumors or abscesses, and spinal cord injury are less likely causes. Hereditary factors and metabolic disease are more often responsible for muscular weakness and atrophy of gradual onset.

Classification

The most useful classification of neuromuscular disorders is one that defines the source of the pathologic lesion: the anterior horn cells of the spinal cord, the peripheral nerves, the myoneural junction, and the muscles.

Diseases of anterior horn cells. Diseases and disorders that affect the anterior horn cells are the result of destruction or atrophy of the anterior horn of the spinal column with the inability to transfer impulses from sensory neurons to motor neurons. Enteroviruses, which have a worldwide distribution, are prominent etiologic agents that selectively affect anterior horn cells. These include the polioviruses, of which there are three types: coxsackieviruses, groups A and B, and the ECHO viruses. Degeneration of the anterior horn cells is caused by inherited disorders, primarily the spinal muscular atrophies.

Neuropathies. Disorders affecting peripheral nerves may be *mononeuropathies,* involving a single nerve and the muscles it innervates, or *polyneuropathies,* which involve multiple nerves and the muscles they supply. Neuropathies are caused by a number of hereditary diseases, traumatic injury, infections, poisons, and (secondarily) some metabolic diseases. Polyneuropathy can be restricted to specific areas (as in diabetes mellitus); some hereditary diseases involve skeletal muscles extensively. Usually distal limbs (feet and hands) are affected first, with gait disturbance and footdrop as early manifestations. The involvement gradually progresses medially as the disorder becomes more severe.

In some polyneuropathies there is segmented or patchy loss of the myelin sheath of nerve fibers; in others the primary process appears to be progressive degeneration of nerve fibers. Examples of acute and chronic polyneuropathies are infectious polyneuritis and peroneal atrophy, respectively.

Neuromuscular junction disease. Disorders involving a neurohormonal deficiency interfere with transmission of nerve impulses to muscles at the neuromuscular junction. Normally nerve impulses are transmitted to skeletal muscles across the neuromuscular junction by acetylcholine. This is accomplished in three steps: (1) acetylcholine is released from vesicles in the terminal nerve endings; (2) it then diffuses across the junction and contacts receptor sites in the muscle membrane, stimulating the muscle to contract; and (3) it is removed by the action of cholinesterase. Interference at any of these three steps will block transmission of nerve impulses and prevent muscular contraction.

Several toxic substances act at the myoneural junction to inhibit nerve impulses to the skeletal muscles. Examples of toxins that prevent release of acetylcholine are those that produce the paralysis of botulism and tick paralysis. Action at receptor sites is blocked by the drug curare. Paralysis resulting from inhibition of cholinesterase release is caused by poisoning with organic phosphate insecticides.

Diseases of muscles. Disorders that affect the muscles directly may be a result of inflammatory, degenerative, or metabolic causes. Chief among these are the muscular dystrophies.

Diagnostic Tools

To aid in differentiating between diseases with similar manifestations, several general diagnostic tools are employed. In addition, a number of more definitive tests are used to establish a specific diagnosis. The neurologic examination is a basic test that helps to assess the extent of motor and sensory responses.

The *electromyogram* (EMG) measures the electric potentials generated in individual muscles. A small metal disk is placed on the skin overlying the muscle to be tested, or a sterile needle electrode is inserted directly into the muscle. The electric activity generated in the skeletal muscles is measured at rest, with slight voluntary contraction, and with maximal contraction. The electric activity is amplified and displayed on a cathode ray oscilloscope. Needle electrodes are sensitive enough to pick up the activity of a single muscle fiber, and so this is usually the method of choice.

Nerve conduction velocity, the velocity of electric impulse conduction along motor or sensory nerves, is frequently measured in conjunction with electromyography. Certain diseases affect the peripheral nerves, prolonging the conduction time from the point of stimulation of the nerve to the muscle and increasing the duration of the evoked potential of the muscle.

Muscle biopsy is the most useful laboratory examination to confirm and classify muscle disorders. *Serum enzyme measurements* are helpful in diagnosis and monitoring the course of muscular disease. These include:

Creatine phosphokinase (CPK): found in skeletal muscle and a few other organs and elevated in skeletal muscle disease; the most specific test

Aldolase: present in skeletal and heart muscle and significantly elevated in muscle damage

Serum glutamic-oxaloacetic transaminase (SGOT): elevated in muscle disease but has wider distribution in organs

Lactic dehydrogenase (LDH): elevated in muscle disease but has wider distribution

HYPOTONIA

Decreased muscle tone in an infant is not an unusual observation in the newborn nursery and is one of the most common presenting symptoms in neuromuscular disorders. It may also indicate a variety of systemic conditions. Frequent causes are cerebral trauma or hypoxia at birth, but most neuromuscular disorders with hypotonia as the presenting symptom are genetically determined, especially Down syndrome and infantile spinal muscular atrophy.

Clinical Manifestations

Hypotonia, sometimes called the *floppy infant syndrome,* is marked by diminished muscle tone and weakness in response to both spontaneous and passive motion and to reflex testing. The infant, when placed in a supine position, assumes a characteristic "frog posture" or lies in some other unusual position at rest. Normally, the young infant who is held in ventral suspension (i.e., with the examiner's hand supporting the infant under the chest) will respond by slightly raising his head with his back relatively straight, arms flexed and slightly abducted, and knees partly flexed. The hypotonic infant droops over the supporting hand with head and extremities hanging loosely, resembling an in-

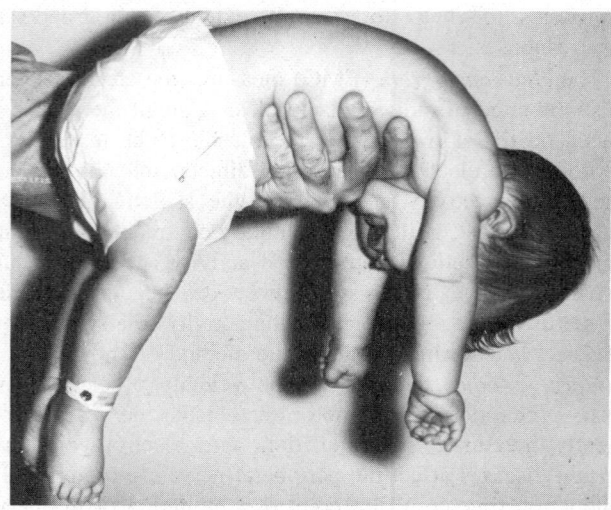

Fig. 39-2. Hypotonicity demonstrated by horizontal suspension in an infant with Werdnig-Hoffman disease.

From Swaiman, K.F., and Wright, F.S.: The practice of pediatric neurology, ed. 2, St. Louis, 1982, The C.V. Mosby Co.

verted U (Fig. 39-2). The muscles feel flabby when palpated and there is marked head lag when the infant is pulled to a sitting position. Poor sucking may be noted.

Therapeutic Management and Nursing Considerations

The management of these infants is determined on the basis of the cause of the hypotonia. It is a nursing responsibility to record and report findings that suggest hypotonia in an infant so that further evaluation can be carried out and therapeutic measures implemented if indicated.

CEREBRAL PALSY

Cerebral palsy (CP) is a nonspecific term applied to impaired muscular control resulting from a nonprogressive abnormality in the pyramidal motor system (motor cortex, basal ganglia, cerebellum). The etiology, clinical features, and course are variable, characterized by abnormal muscle tone and coordination as the primary disturbances. It is the most common permanent physical disability of childhood, and although the incidence is not known, various studies suggest that it varies from 1.5:1000 to 5:1000 live births.

Etiology

A variety of prenatal, perinatal, and postnatal factors contribute to the etiology of cerebral palsy, singly or multifactorially (see box). The dominant mechanism of damage is ischemia and/or asphyxia, and the preterm/low-birth-weight infant is particularly vulnerable. Next in frequency are those infants who experience severe perinatal asphyxia. Congenital infections, metabolic conditions, and intrauterine ischemic events are implicated less often, and genetic factors as such rarely cause CP (Paneth, 1986). The multifactorial implication is exemplified by the preterm infant of low birth weight who suffers perinatal asphyxia, infection, or a metabolic condition.

Pathophysiology

It is difficult to establish a precise location of neurologic lesions based on etiology or clinical signs because there is no characteristic pathologic picture. In some cases there are gross malformations of the brain. In others there may be evidence of vascular occlusion, atrophy, loss of neurons, and laminar degeneration that produce narrower gyri, wider sulci, and low brain weight. Anoxia plays the most significant role in the pathologic state of brain damage, which is frequently secondary to other causative mechanisms.

There are a few exceptions. In some cases the manifestations or etiology can be related to anatomic areas. For example, cerebral palsy associated with prematurity is usually spastic diplegia caused by hypoxic infarction or hemorrhage in the area adjacent to the lateral ventricles. In the athetoid type of cerebral palsy caused by kernicterus and hemolytic disease of the newborn, there are pigment deposits in the basal ganglia and some cranial nerve nuclei. Hemiparetic cerebral palsy is frequently associated with mechanical trauma to the cortex or cerebrovascular accident of the middle cerebral artery. Cerebral hypoplasia and sometimes neonatal hypoglycemia are related to ataxic cerebral palsy. Generalized cortical and cerebral atrophy have been shown to cause severe quadriparesis with mental retardation and microcephaly.

Clinical Manifestations

The alert observer may be suspicious of CP when a child demonstrates some of the following groups of manifestations.

Delayed gross motor development. This is a universal manifestation of cerebral palsy. The child shows a delay in all motor accomplishments, and the discrepancy between motor ability and expected achievement tends to increase with successive developmental milestones as growth

---

APPROXIMATE DISTRIBUTION OF CAUSES IN CEREBRAL PALSY

1. Low birth weight, preterm birth	35% to 40%
2. Perinatal asphyxia in term infants	25% to 30%
3. Congenital and perinatal infections (CMV, rubella, toxoplasma, neonatal meningitis)	5% to 10%
4. Intrauterine ischemic events	5% to 10%
5. Congenital brain anomalies not evident on clinical examination	5% to 10%
6. Perinatal metabolic conditions other than asphyxia (hyperbilirubinemia, hypoglycemia, hyperosmolarity, amino acid disorders)	5%
7. Genetic origin	2% to 5%

From Paneth, N.: Etiologic factors in cerebral palsy, Pediatr. Ann. 15:191, 194-201, 1986.

advances. It is especially significant if other developmental behavior, such as language and personal-social achievement, is normal.

Abnormal motor performance. Neuromotor dysfunction is particularly evident in motor performance. An early sign is preferential unilateral hand use that may be apparent at about 6 months of age. Hand dominance does not normally develop until the preschool years. Abnormal crawl with progression by hand movements only and with lower extremities and hips hiked along, much like a "bunny hop," is seen in diplegia. Children with hemiplegia use an asymmetric crawl using the unaffected arm and leg to propel themselves on either the buttocks or the abdomen. Spasticity may cause the child to stand or walk on the toes. Uncoordinated or involuntary movements are characteristic of dyskinetic cerebral palsy, and facial grimacing and writhing movements of the tongue, fingers, and toes are signs of athetosis. Other significant signs of motor dysfunction are poor sucking and feeding difficulties with persistent tongue thrust. Head staggering, tremor on reaching, and truncal ataxia may be observed as well.

Alterations of muscle tone. Increased or decreased resistance to passive movements is a sign of abnormal muscle tone. The child may exhibit opisthotonic postures (exaggerated arching of the back), he may feel stiff on handling or dressing, and there is difficulty in diapering him because of spasticity of hip adductor muscles and lower extremities. When the child is pulled to a sitting position, he may extend the entire body, rigid and unbending at the hip and knee joints. This is an early sign of spasticity.

Abnormal postures. Children with spastic cerebral palsy assume abnormal postures at rest or when their position is changed. From an early age a child lying in a prone position will maintain the hips higher than the trunk with the legs and arms flexed or drawn under the body. In the supine position spasticity is evident by scissoring and extension of legs and with the feet plantar flexed. This posture is exaggerated when the child is suspended vertically or when others try to make him bear weight. Spasticity may be mild or severe depending on the degree of impairment. A persistent infantile resting and sleeping posture, (i.e., arms abducted at shoulders, elbows flexed, and hands fisted) is a sign of spasticity when it remains constant after 4 to 5 months of age. The hemiparetic child may rest with the affected arm adducted and held against the torso with the elbow pronated and slightly flexed and the hand closed.

Reflex abnormalities. Persistence of primitive infantile reflexes is one of the earliest clues to cerebral palsy, for example, obligatory tonic neck reflex at any age or nonobligatory persistence beyond 6 months of age and the persistence or even hyperactivity of the Moro, plantar, and palmar grasp reflexes. Hyperreflexia, ankle clonus, and stretch reflexes can be elicited from many muscle groups on fast passive movements, for example, resistance to passive abduction when hips are suddenly separated (adductor catch).

Associated disabilities. Some of the disabilities associated with cerebral palsy are subnormal learning and rea-

soning capacity (mental retardation), impaired behavioral and interpersonal relationships (attention deficit disorder), seizures, and impairment of special senses.

Mental retardation. The most serious disability is mental retardation. One third of the children with cerebral palsy have normal intelligence (fewer have high normal or superior intelligence compared with the normal population); one third are mildly retarded; and one third are moderately retarded or below (low-grade deficiency is more common in persons with cerebral palsy than in the general population). As a group children with athetosis and ataxia are intellectually superior to those with other types of cerebral palsy. Incidence of severe or profound retardation is highest in rigid, atonic, and quadriparetic cerebral palsy.

Seizures. Seizures are more apt to accompany postnatally acquired hemiplegia. They are an unusual finding in athetosis and diplegia. The most common type is grand mal seizures, and the peak incidence of commencement is between 2 and 6 years of age. Approximately 50% of children with cerebral palsy have some type of seizure (Molnar and Taft, 1977).

Attention deficit disorder. The manifestations of attention deficit disorder may occur in children with cerebral palsy. The primary presenting symptoms are poor attention span, marked distractibility, hyperactive behavior, and defects of integration (see p. 786).

Sensory impairment. Abnormalities of vision occur more often in cerebral palsy, and hearing loss is frequently an associated disability. Strabismus is much higher in spastic children, and hearing loss is often seen in athetosis.

Clinical Classification

Cerebral palsy has been classified in several ways, but the most useful classification is based on the nature and distribution of neuromuscular dysfunction.

Spastic cerebral palsy. The most common clinical type, spastic cerebral palsy, represents an upper motor neuron type of muscular weakness. The reflex arc is intact and the characteristic physical signs are increased stretch reflexes, increased muscle tone, and (often) weakness. Early neurologic manifestations are usually generalized hypotonia or decreased tone that lasts for a few weeks or may extend for months or even as long as a year. The clinical features of spastic CP are outlined in the box on p. 1736.

Dyskinetic cerebral palsy. Dyskinesis implies abnormal involuntary movements. These movements originate in the basal ganglia, especially the globus pallidus, and the nuclei of cranial nerve VIII and of other cranial nerves. Movements disappear in sleep and are aggravated by stress. The major manifestation is athetosis, characterized by slow, wormlike, writhing movements that usually involve all extremities, the trunk, neck, facial muscles, and tongue. Dyskinetic movements of tongue and other pharyngeal, laryngeal, and oral muscles cause drooling and dysarthria (imperfect speech articulation), which makes it difficult to understand what the child is saying. There is often high-frequency hearing loss or deafness and conjugate upward gaze palsy, in which the eyes are converged toward the midline and displaced upward.

Involuntary movements may take on choreiform (involuntary, irregular, jerking movements) and dystonic (disordered muscle tone) manifestations that increase in intensity under emotional stress and during adolescence. Deformities rarely develop as a result of continuous uncontrollable movements that maintain joint mobility.

Ataxic cerebral palsy. The least common type of cerebral palsy, ataxia, is caused by a defect in the cerebellum or its pathways and is characterized by nonprogressive failure of muscle coordination and irregular muscle action. Affected children have a wide-based gait and perform rapid repetitive movements poorly. There is disintegration of movements of the upper extremities when the child reaches for objects. Cerebellar coordination tends to improve as the child grows, but there is very slow development in the first 3 to 5 years of life.

Mixed-type cerebral palsy. A combination of spasticity and athetosis is described as mixed-type cerebral palsy. Many affected children are severely disabled. This combination is sometimes observed after traumatic postnatal head injury.

Rigid, tremor, and atonic types. These types are uncommon. Both rigid and atonic types have a poor prognosis, with deformities and lack of active movement. Tremors as a leading manifestation in cerebral palsy are rare. The tremor is seen at rest and on movement, but motor accomplishments are favorable and musculoskeletal complications do not occur.

Diagnostic Evaluation

Infants at risk based on known etiologic factors associated with cerebral palsy warrant careful assessment during early infancy in order to identify signs of muscular dysfunction as early as possible. Careful assessment of the low-birthweight or preterm infant, the infant with a low Apgar score at 5 minutes, and the infant who demonstrated other perinatal or neonatal abnormalities such as seizures, intracranial hemorrhage, or metabolic disturbances should be carried out. Early recognition is made more difficult by lack of reliable neonatal neurologic signs. Cortical control of movement does not occur until later in infancy; therefore motor impairment associated with voluntary control is usually not apparent until after 2 to 4 months of age at the earliest. More often the likelihood of a diagnosis cannot be confirmed until the second half of the first year. Motor dysfunction in some mildly affected infants may be overlooked until they exhibit delay or abnormality of some advanced motor skills such as standing or walking.

Persistence of primitive reflexes may be of value, and two offer assistance in diagnosis: the asymmetric tonic neck reflex and the crossed extensor reflex. The tonic neck reflex normally disappears between 4 and 6 months of age. An "obligatory" response is considered abnormal. This is elicited by turning the infant's head to one side, holding it there for 20 seconds. When a crying infant is unable to move from the asymmetric posturing of the tonic neck reflex when crying, it is considered to be "obligatory" and an abnormal response. The crossed extensor reflex, which normally disappears by 4 months, is elicited by applying a noxious stimulus to the sole of one extremity with the knee extended. Normally the contralateral foot will respond with extensor, abduction, and then adduction movements. Finding these reflexes after the age when they should have disappeared suggests the possibility of CP (Taft, 1984).

The neurologic examination and history are the primary modalities for diagnosis. A thorough knowledge of normal variations of motor development is required for detecting abnormal progress, and a careful history is elicited to detect possible etiologic factors. The child's spontaneous movements and behavior are observed, including posture, attitude, and muscle size, function, and tone.

Supplemental diagnostic tests may be employed, such as electroencephalography, tomography, screening for metabolic defects, and serum electrolyte values. The possibility of slowly progressive degenerative disease and early onset, slowly growing brain tumors must be ruled out.

Therapeutic Management: General Concepts

The goals of therapy for children with cerebral palsy are early recognition and promotion of an optimum developmental course in order that the child may realize his potential within the limits of his brain dysfunction. The disorder is permanent, and therapy is chiefly symptomatic and preventive. To be effective it requires the services of an organized team of health professionals that considers (1) the nature of the physical disability, (2) defects associated with the disorder, and (3) the interpersonal and social influences encountered by the affected child.

The beneficial influences of a habilitation program on both child and family are based on recognition of the disability as early as possible and implementation of treatment. Parents are essential to a treatment program, and their cooperation and confidence are considered in all aspects of management. With early diagnosis parents can begin to provide sensorimotor experiences that are essential for cognitive development, since central nervous system structures depend on stimulation and use to maintain their functional integrity.

The broad aims of therapy are (1) to establish locomotion, communication, and self-help; (2) to gain optimum appearance and integration of motor functions; (3) to correct associated defects as effectively as possible; and (4) to provide educational opportunities adapted to the needs and capabilities of the individual child. Each child is evaluated and managed on an individual basis. The plan of therapy may involve a variety of settings, facilities, and specially trained persons, including the parents. The scope of the child's needs may require, in addition to the pediatrician and nurse, such professionals as a psychologist and/or psychiatrist, orthopedist, physical therapist, teacher, social worker, speech pathologist and/or therapist, neurologist, orthotist, audiologist, and occupational therapist.

Mobilizing devices. Braces and other devices are often used to help prevent or reduce deformity. Braces can increase the energy efficiency of gait, control joint alignment, or both. Most bracing is poorly tolerated by young children, and children with functioning upper extremities often remove a lower extremity brace.

Some of the more commonly used mobility devices include wheeled scooter boards that allow the child to propel himself while his abdomen or total body is supported and legs positioned with wedges to prevent scissoring. Wheeled go-carts provide good sitting balance and serve as an early "wheelchair" experience for young children (see Fig. 40-8). Strollers can be equipped with custom seats for depen-

dent mobilization. Special devices for independent mobilization that allow the upper extremities to remain free are particularly valuable for children with lower extremity involvement (Fig. 39-3). A number of wheelchairs can be customized to meet the needs and preferences of older children (see Mobilizing devices, Chapter 40).

The use of infant walkers is discouraged. They have been found to pose a risk of injury to normal children and are especially hazardous for children with CP. It has been observed that infant walkers bring out and exaggerate abnormal motor patterns, prevent integration of primitive reflexes, and delay development of normal balance and protective responses in children with CP (Holm, Harthun-Smith, and Tada, 1983).

Surgery. Orthopedic surgery may be required to decrease or abolish spastic muscle imbalance. This includes tendon lengthening procedures (especially heel-cord lengthening), release of spastic wrist flexor muscles, and correction of hip and adductor muscle spasticity or contracture to improve locomotion. Surgical intervention is usually reserved for the child who does not respond to the more conservative measures but is also indicated for the child whose spasticity causes progressive deformities. Surgery is primarily used to improve function rather than for cosmetic purposes and is followed by physical therapy. Neurosurgical procedures are used only in selected cases.

Medication. Drugs to decrease spasticity have little usefulness in improving function in cerebral palsy. Antianxiety agents have been used to some extent to relieve excessive motion and tension, particularly in the athetoid child.

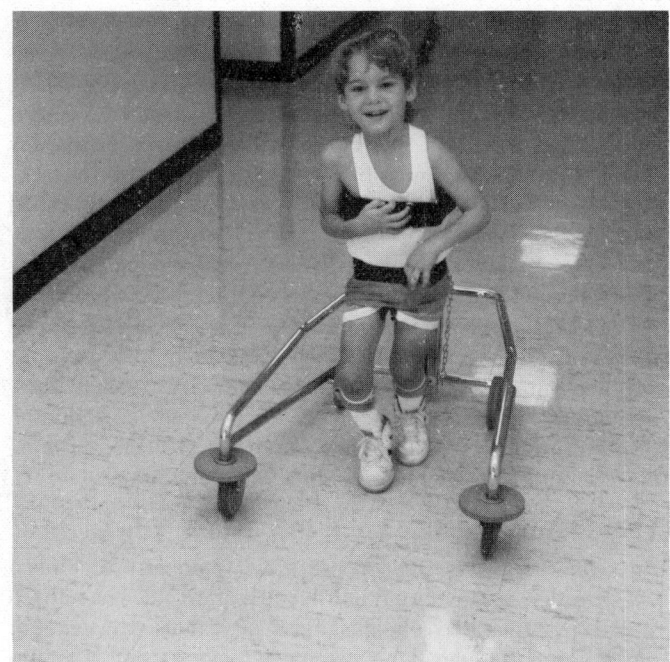

Fig. 39-3. Child in ambulation device that allows arm freedom.
Photography by John Roy, Saint Francis Hospital, on location at Children's Medical Center, Tulsa, OK.

Skeletal muscle relaxants, such as dantrolene (Dantrium), baclofen, and methocarbamol (Robaxin), may be used on a short-term basis for older children and adolescents. Diazepam (Valium) is used frequently but should be restricted to older children and adolescents (Sternfeld, 1986). The drugs have been successful in relieving stiffness and thus facilitating ease of motion. Local nerve block to motor points of a muscle with a neurolytic agent such as phenol solution reduces spasticity temporarily.

Anticonvulsant medications are used routinely for children who have seizures. Generally phenobarbital and phenytoin are most widely prescribed and appear to be effective in most instances. Other anticonvulsants or combinations are needed in special situations. Regular periodic monitoring of blood levels is required to obtain the desired anticonvulsant effect with the smallest possible dosage. Hyperactive, dyskinetic children perform better when given dextroamphetamine or other drugs used for the child with attention deficit disorder.

Technical aids. A wide variety of technical aids are available to improve the functioning of children with CP. For example, specially designed electromechanical toys that employ the concept of biofeedback operate from a head unit. The toy is manipulated only when the head and trunk are in correct alignment. Eye-hand coordination can also be enhanced by appropriately designed toys and games.

The most numerous devices are those which facilitate nonvocal communication. Microcomputers combined with voice synthesizers aid children with speech difficulties to "speak." These and others print messages onto screen monitors and paper. These devices have made it apparent that some children have been erroneously considered to be mentally retarded (Sternfeld, 1986).

Many other electronic devices allow independent functioning. Sensors can be activated and deactivated by using a head-stick, tongue, or other voluntary muscle movement over which the child has control. The application of this technology makes it possible for persons with CP to eventually function in their own apartments and can be extended into the workplace.

Other considerations. Care of visual and auditory deficits requires the attention of appropriate specialists, and speech therapy involves the services of a speech therapist (see Chapter 25). Dental care is especially important for children with CP and is all too frequently overlooked. Regular visits to the dentist and dental prophylaxis, including brushing, fluoride, and flossing (after several teeth are present), should be instituted as soon as the teeth erupt.

Therapeutic Management: Physical Therapy

Physical therapy is one of the most frequently employed conservative treatment modalities. It requires the specialized skills of a qualified therapist with an extensive repertoire of exercise methods who can design a program to stimulate each child to achieve his functional goals. In general, physical therapy is directed toward good skeletal alignment for the spastic child; training in purposeful acts, even in the face of involuntary motion, for the athetoid child; and maximum development of proprioceptive sense in ataxia.

An active therapy program involves the family, the physical therapist, and often other members of the health team, especially the nurse. The major approach employs traditional types of therapeutic exercises that consist of stretching, passive, active, and resisted movements applied to specific muscle groups or joints to maintain or increase range of motion, strength, or endurance. Another approach is one of "patterning," which attempts to alter abnormal tone and posture and elicit desired movements through positional manipulation or other means of modifying or augmenting sensory output. These programs require intensive daily manipulation and a legion of volunteers to carry out the program. The American Academy of Pediatrics (1982) has issued a strong statement against this form of treatment for neurologically disabled children. Therefore this option will not be discussed further.

No therapeutic approach is able to achieve spectacular changes in the ultimate outcome of motor disability. Therefore the most practical approach is to select a mode of intervention that is most appropriate for the specific problem and that best suits the need of the individual child at any given time. Early efforts are focused on alleviating abnormal postures by positioning and range of motion exercises. For example, rather than pulling a spastic infant to a sitting position by the arms, which stimulates hypertonic extensor muscles of the back, he is slowly pushed forward by hands placed posteriorly on his trunk. Extensor spasticity and scissoring of legs can be avoided if the infant straddles a thigh or hip when carried in the sitting position.

Passive range of motion exercises, stretching, and elongation exercises are valuable at any age, even at early ages when the child is unable to cooperate. They are of particular value for postural abnormalities around various joints. For example, stretching of the gastrocnemius muscle and its tendon helps to prevent tightness and spasticity that leads to toe walking and equinus position of the ankle. When the child is old enough to cooperate, some active extension can be performed with passive motion applied to complete joint extension. Prevention of contracture deformity is a prime function of physical therapy.

Functional and adaptive training (occupational therapy). Training in manual skills and activities of daily living proceeds along developmental lines and according to the child's functional level. Sitting, balance, crawling, and walking are encouraged at appropriate ages, accompanied by stimulation of protective extension and equilibrium reactions. When standing is attempted, therapy may be needed to strengthen and improve balance, which is sometimes facilitated by the use of braces, especially to control plantar flexion and less often to prevent knee flexion caused by hamstring muscle spasticity and inadequate control of hip and knee extensor muscles. Walking, using reciprocal leg motion, should be attempted at the appropriate age even if the child requires considerable assistance from braces and other persons, and the child should be encouraged to progress to parallel bars or other ambulatory aids as soon as possible (see Fig. 40-4).

Hand activities are begun early to improve motor function and provide the child with sensory experiences and information about his environment. Use of extremities requires some stability of the trunk; therefore a gross motor position in which the child has some active control is selected. Objects and toys are chosen to provide needed sensory input, using a variety of shapes, forms, and textures. The child will electively use the less affected or unaffected hand as the dominant one, and there are differing opinions about whether or not the child should be therapeutically encouraged to use the deficient extremity. Undue insistence often provokes an adverse emotional reaction. Play that encourages the use of hands for unimanual and bimanual activities is initiated early. Large balls, a doll carriage to push, or other toys that require some manner of manipulation are accepted without resistance and promote assistive use of both hands. Play is a valuable tool in a therapeutic program and is selected to combine therapy with the child's ability and interest. This often requires a great deal of ingenuity and inventiveness on the part of those involved in the child's care.

The child may need considerable help (and patience) in learning to feed, dress, and care for his personal hygiene needs, the most important and earliest tasks on which to concentrate. Children should be fed in the normal eating position. When they have difficulty with sucking and swallowing, it is a temptation to hold them in a semireclining posture to make use of gravity flow. This method does not promote active swallowing, however, and the neck hyperextension may even interfere with swallowing. A more flexed sitting position with arms brought forward to decrease the tendency toward back and neck extension is more natural during bottle- or spoon-feeding and encourages active swallowing.

As the child progresses from simple feeding and self-care activities, training is extended to include other tasks that are within his developmental and functional capabilities, such as cooking or typing. It should be remembered that a child should not be expected to learn a task until he is at the developmental stage at which it would normally be accomplished. In all activities of daily living it is important to capitalize on the child's assets and compensate for his liabilities. For example, a child with visual-motor dysfunction would be helped by substituting an electric typewriter for the laborious task of handwriting. Learning one-handed tying of shoelaces would be needed by a hemiparetic child. The level of expected independence is related to both gross and fine motor manipulation, and even when complete independence in a specific activity is not realistic, the child should learn any part of the task that he can master. However, motor function is not the sole purpose of learning as

much independence as possible. Any accomplishment promotes self-reliance and self-esteem for healthier personality development.

Speech training under the supervision of a speech therapist is begun early, before the child learns poor habits of communication. Parents and others can help by following the directions of the speech therapist and by talking to the child slowly and using pictures or handling objects about which the adult is speaking. Feeding techniques, such as forcing the child to use his lips and tongue in eating, help to facilitate speech—for example, placing food at the side of the tongue, first one side then the other; making the child use his lips to take food from a spoon rather than placing it directly on his tongue; and avoiding using the teeth to remove the food from the utensil. If severe dysarthria prevents articulate speech and the child has reasonable intelligence, nonverbal communication is taught.

Education. As in all aspects of care, educational requirements are determined by the child's needs and potential. This includes the severity of the child's disease and the presence and degree of associated conditions that affect learning and participation, such as learning impairment, abnormal actions or behavior, impaired vision and/or hearing, and seizures. Children with mild physical disability, normal intelligence, and no associated learning disability should attend regular school, although this is sometimes difficult because of the physical structure of the school. When attendance at regular school is not appropriate for the child, special classes or school facilities designed to meet the special needs of disabled children are available in most larger communities. For those who are unable to benefit from formal education, a training program may be appropriate. At adolescence prevocational and vocational counseling and guidance are arranged. At any phase or in any setting, education is geared toward the child's assets.

Recreation. Recreational activities are also a necessary part of growing up. Recreational outlets and after-school activities should be considered for the child who is unable to participate in the regular athletic and other peer activities. Some can compete in athletic and artistic endeavors, and there are many games and pasttimes that are suited to their capabilities. Sports, physical fitness, and recreation programs are encouraged for children with CP, and young children should be exposed to all physical activities available to nondisabled children.

There are numerous developmental centers that have facilities for indoor and outdoor activities designed to appeal to children of all ages. If these are not available, they should be instigated. Such programs require adequate supervision to avoid any harmful effects, however. Recreational activities serve to stimulate children's interest and curiosity, help them adjust to their disability, improve their functional abilities, and build self-esteem. Competitive sports are also becoming increasingly available to disabled children and offer an added dimension to physical activities. Information on training programs and competition on local, state, regional, and national levels can be obtained from the **National Association of Sports for Cerebral Palsy.***

Nursing Considerations

Nurses in a community setting, especially those in public health, in physicians' offices and clinics, and in schools, are more likely to become involved with a family in which there is a child with cerebral palsy. Both the child and the family need the help, support, and encouragement that nurses are prepared to offer, and nurses can be involved in all aspects of the child's management. Nurses who know the family and their special needs and problems are in the best position to provide guidance and support.

Early recognition of cerebral palsy is often a result of alert observation by the nurse. Detection begins at birth, and the nurse should be especially observant for signs in an infant who has a history that includes any of the prenatal and perinatal conditions that predispose to brain damage. Unusual manifestations in a newborn can be signs of a variety of conditions, but an infant who displays poor feeding, rigidity, tenseness, or hypotonia merits closer scrutiny. A history of these unexplained signs is cause for repeated assessment. The disorder is not readily identifiable in the early months of life; often evidence is not apparent until the child begins to walk.

Delayed attainment of developmental milestones is one of the most valuable clues to recognizing CP; therefore slow development in a child offers one of the earliest indications of neurologic impairment. Nurses working with children need to be well acquainted with normal child growth and development and the tools of assessment. The earlier any deviation from normal is detected, the better the outlook for optimum developmental attainment. It is also important that the child receive appropriate therapy from persons or agencies qualified to provide such services. Parents are sometimes tempted to follow advice from unreliable sources. Nurses who are acquainted with services and facilities can refer the family to qualified practitioners.

Nurses who work directly with the child in the home or in the therapeutic setting are members of the health team who plan and carry out a program of therapy. Since children are being treated at an earlier age, parents are participating earlier in treatment programs for their disabled child. They are taught the proper handling and home care of young children with cerebral palsy. Parents need carefully programmed steps so that their change of role from parent to therapist can be melded into the already established relationship. The nurse or therapist needs to have documented data about the parent-child relationship before teaching the parent how to facilitate the child's posture or inhibit certain reflex patterns.

Parents learn how to posture children, how to introduce and carry out appropriate exercises, and how to place children in appropriate positions for play, dressing, eating, bathing, toileting, and other daily activities. Nurses are acquainted with the special needs of the child and the physical therapy objectives and modalities; thus they are able to reinforce the plan and assist the family in devising and modifying equipment and activities to follow through and reinforce the therapy program in the home, for example, modifying eating utensils by building up spoon handles for easier grasp and modifying clothes to facilitate self-help (see also Chapter 24).

Because children with CP expend so much energy in their efforts to accomplish activities of daily living, more frequent rest periods should be arranged to avoid fatigue that may aggravate their limited capabilities. The diet should include extra calories to help meet these extra energy demands. Safety precautions are implemented, such as the child wearing a bicycle helmet if he is subject to falls or there is a chance of injuring his head on hard objects. Furniture should be upholstered or sharp edges padded to protect the child from injury. Because their respiratory muscles are less efficient, these children are more susceptible to common upper respiratory infections and should avoid contact with infected persons. Dental problems are more frequent in children with cerebral palsy, which creates a need for meticulous attention to all aspects of dental care.

Parents are sometimes very preoccupied with their ability to perform activities such as positioning the child; as a result, the child's personal comfort and satisfaction may be overlooked. They often perceive their child's inability to perform or behave to be a direct result of their own inadequacy in working with the child. The parents are so intent on achieving a desired goal, such as flexing the child's knees, that they repeatedly remind the child of his errors but fail to acknowledge or support his less-than-successful efforts to comply, even though he is willing. Nurses can help parents integrate therapy into play activities in more natural and less frustrating ways.

Some children have difficulty in keeping their heads upright. Because of this they cannot explore much of their environment and process the information. Parents need to be complimented on their efforts to provide a stimulating environment for these children. These infants are "at risk" for delayed development in holding up their heads, righting their shoulders and trunks for stable posture, sitting, pulling, standing, and crawling. Most parents of children with impaired movements benefit from support and practical suggestions for feeding, moving, holding, and encouraging the infant to explore his hands and feet and to begin to play.

Although practical advice is important, the nurse or physical therapist should offer suggestions at a pace that can be absorbed by the parents to avoid making them feel inadequate in their parenting abilities. The parents are encouraged to define their concern, acknowledge the concern as genuine, and ask the parents how long they have tried a certain approach. In this way the nurse is able to find out what works, what does not work, and *what the parents* would

---

*United Cerebral Palsy Association, Inc., 66 East 34th St., New York, NY 10016.

like to try next. The parents are given positive feedback for their observations of the infant, the progress *they* note, and how *they* differentiate the child's needs. Sometimes parents need support simply because the demands made on them are very fatiguing. It is probably better for parents of young children with cerebral palsy to reduce the *quantity* of involvement with their child, rather than reduce the *quality* of the interactions. As the normal preschool child acquires autonomous skills, language, and mobility, he spends less time with his parents and is less dependent.

Probably the nursing interventions most valuable to the family are support and help in coping with the emotional aspects of the disorder, many of which are discussed in relation to the disabled child (Chapter 22). Initially the parents need supportive counseling directed toward understanding the implications of the diagnosis and all the feelings that it engenders. Later they need clarification regarding what they can expect from the child and from health professionals. Having a child with cerebral palsy implies numerous problems of daily management and changes in family life.

There are constant demands with few rewards, and the day-by-day changelessness of these demands is trying to parents. Many find that their child with cerebral palsy gives them little pleasure. The nurse needs to support the parents in their frustration, their problem solving, their concerns, their approaches to helping the child, and their lack of gratification, as well as the positive approaches they use. All of these aspects must be explored and discussed. Parents as well as other members of the family require a great deal of support and counseling. Siblings of a child with a disability are affected and may respond to the presence of the child with overt or less evident behavioral problems. The family needs a relationship with nurses who can provide continued contact, support, and encouragement through the long process of habilitation.

Parents can also find help and solace from parent groups with whom they can share problems and concerns and from whom they can derive comfort and practical information. The national organization, **United Cerebral Palsy Association,*** has branches in most communities. The address of the nearest branch can be obtained from a local telephone directory, local agency directory, or a local health department or by writing to the national headquarters. The association provides a variety of services for children and families. There are also a number of excellent books available to serve as guides for parents and nurses who work with the cerebral palsied child.†

Hospitalized child. Cerebral palsy is not a disorder that requires hospitalization; therefore when children with cerebral palsy are hospitalized they are usually admitted for another reason or for corrective surgery. Consequently many nurses are not accustomed to handling these children. Nurses who have never been associated with a child with cerebral palsy may react in a variety of ways, including fear, revulsion, or overwhelming pity. The basic concept to keep in mind when caring for these children is that they are, first of all, children who happen to be afflicted with a disorder that limits their capacities in performing some activities of daily living and, for some, communicating with others. They should be approached and treated the same as any child in the hospital. The nurse's actions should convey acceptance, affection, and friendliness and promote a feeling of trust and dependability in the child. This is especially true with older children who have normal intelligence but who may have communication problems. Frequently nurses tend to "talk down" to these children and do things for them that they are perfectly capable, although not as adeptly, of doing for themselves. This is especially humiliating to a teenager who values independence and self-esteem.

To facilitate the care and management of the child, the therapy program should be continued, insofar as his condition allows, during the time he is hospitalized. This should be incorporated into his nursing care plan and every effort expended to make certain that the ground that has been so laboriously gained is not lost. Encouraging the parents to room-in and actively participate in the child's care facilitates a continuation of the home therapy program and helps the child adjust to an unfamiliar environment.

The child with cerebral palsy frequently displays behavioral problems. In some of these children the emotional disturbance is probably a reflection of the brain lesion. However, in most cases the behavioral problem is the result of conscious or unconscious rejection by others, particularly the parents. This is not surprising, since this condition is often frightening and unpleasant to others. These children may be viewed by some as being socially unacceptable, which may cause a parent to reject the child. When parents are helped to accept the child, the behavioral problems are significantly reduced.

PROGRESSIVE INFANTILE SPINAL MUSCULAR ATROPHY (WERDNIG-HOFFMANN DISEASE)

Progressive infantile spinal muscular atrophy (Werdnig-Hoffmann disease) is a disorder characterized by progressive weakness and wasting of skeletal muscles caused by degeneration of anterior horn cells. It is inherited as an autosomal-recessive trait and is the most common paralytic form of the "floppy infant syndrome." The site of the pathologic condition is the anterior horn cells of the spinal cord and the motor nuclei of the brain stem, but the primary effect is atrophy of skeletal muscles.

Clinical Manifestations

The age of onset is variable, but the earlier the onset the more fulminating the course and the more disseminated and

---

*66 E. 34th St., New York, NY 10016.
†Especially recommended are Levy, J.: The baby exercise book, New York, 1975, Random House; and Finnie, N.R.: Handling the young cerebral palsied child at home, New York, E.P. Dutton & Co.

Nursing Care Summary: The Child with Cerebral Palsy

NURSING GOALS	NURSING INTERVENTIONS	EXPECTED PATIENT/FAMILY OUTCOMES
HP-HMP	**Injury: potential for trauma** **Risk factors: physiologic disability, neuromuscular impairment**	
Detect infants at risk	Take careful history of prenatal factors and circumstances surrounding birth that predispose to fetal anoxia	*Affected infants are detected early
Recognize disorder early	Be alert for evidence of motor dysfunction in infant Be alert for associated disabilities Presence of seizures Sensory impairment such as hearing loss, strabismus Hyperactive behavior, marked distractibility, etc.	
Prevent deformity	Apply and correctly use braces Carry out and teach family to perform stretching exercises Employ appropriate range of motion exercises Perform preoperative and postoperative care for child who requires corrective surgery	Child benefits from appropriate preventive measures (specify measures and child's expected response)
Prevent physical injury	Provide safe physical environment Padded furniture Side rails on bed Sturdy furniture that does not slip Avoid scatter rugs and polished floors Select toys appropriate to age and physical limitations Encourage sufficient rest Use restraints when child is in chair or vehicle Provide child who is prone to falls with protective helmet and enforce its use Institute seizure precautions for susceptible child	Family provides a safe environment for the child (specify)
N-MP	**Nutrition, alteration in: less than body requirements** **Etiology: greater than normal energy expenditure**	
Ensure balanced diet	Provide extra calories to meet extra energy demands of increased muscle activity Monitor weight gain Provide vitamin, mineral, and/or protein supplements if eating habits are poor	Child eats a balanced diet Weight remains within acceptable limits (specify)
A-EP	**Activity intolerance** **Etiology: decreased energy and fatigue, perceptual/cognitive impairment**	
Promote relaxation	Maintain a well-regulated schedule that allows for adequate rest and sleep periods Be alert for evidence of fatigue, which tends to aggravate symptoms	Child is sufficiently rested
Promote general health	Ensure regular routine health maintenance Physical assessment Dental care Immunizations	Child receives regular health assessments (specify schedule) Child receives appropriate immunizations (specify) and dental care (specify)

*Nursing outcome.

Nursing Care Summary: The Child with Cerebral Palsy—cont'd

NURSING GOALS	NURSING INTERVENTIONS	EXPECTED PATIENT/FAMILY OUTCOMES
A-EP Mobility, impaired physical **Etiology: neuromuscular impairment**		
Establish locomotion	Encourage sitting, crawling, and walking at appropriate ages Carry out therapies that strengthen and improve control Assist child in using reciprocal leg motion when learning to walk Provide incentives to locomotion Ensure adequate rest before attempting locomotion activities Incorporate play that encourages desired behavior Employ aids that facilitate locomotion such as parallel bars, crutches, etc. Prepare child and family for surgical procedures if indicated	Child acquires locomotion within his capabilities (specify)
 **A-EP Self-care deficit: feeding, bathing/hygiene, dressing/grooming, toileting (specify level)** **Etiology: neuromuscular impairment**		
Promote self-help	Encourage child to assist in his care as age and capabilities permit Select toys and activities that allow maximum participation by child and that improve motor function and sensory input Avoid undue persistence to accomplish a goal Encourage activities that require both unimanual and bimanual activities Adapt utensils, foods, and clothing to facilitate self-help, e.g., large-bowled spoon with padded handle, finger foods and foods that adhere to, rather than slip from, utensil, and clothing that opens from front with Velcro closings rather than buttons Assist parents in toilet training the child	Child engages in self-help activities commensurate with his capabilities
RRP Communication, impaired: verbal **Etiology: neuromuscular impairment**		
Facilitate communication	Enlist services of a speech therapist early Talk to child slowly Use articles and pictures to reinforce speech Employ feeding techniques that help facilitate speech such as using lips, teeth, and various tongue movements Teach and use nonverbal communication methods to dysarthritic child who would benefit, e.g., Blissymbols	Child is able to communicate his needs to caregivers (specify desired communication and means of accomplishment)

Continued.

Nursing Care Summary: The Child with Cerebral Palsy—cont'd

NURSING GOALS	NURSING INTERVENTIONS	EXPECTED PATIENT/FAMILY OUTCOMES
SP-SCP	**Self-concept, disturbance in: body image, self-esteem** **Etiology: physical disability, appearance**	

Promote a positive self-image	Capitalize on child's assets and provide compensation for his liabilities
	 Praise child for accomplishments and "near" accomplishments such as partial completion of a task
	 Set realistic goals for child
	 Encourage an appealing physical appearance
	     Good body hygiene, clean straight teeth, and good grooming
	     Stylish clothing
	     Makeup for teenage girls
	 Encourage recreational outlets and after-school activities appropriate to child's capabilities
	 Allow child to discuss himself, his disorder, and how he thinks others feel about him
	 Encourage him to become involved with children who have similar problems
	 Encourage attendance at schools with facilities that meet child's special needs
	 Talk to child at his mental level
		Child exhibits behaviors that indicate elevated self-esteem (specify)
		
		 Child is clean, well groomed, and wears age-appropriate, attractive clothing
		 Child discusses feelings and concerns
		 Child attends school regularly

Prepare for tests and procedures	Prepare child and family for needed surgical procedures Arrange for hearing and visual tests; assist parents in acquiring corrective devices	Child with correctable defects receives appropriate therapy (specify)
RRP	**Family process, alteration in** **Etiology: birth of a child with a disability**	
Support family	Allow for expression of feelings regarding child, family's own guilt regarding causes of disorder, impact disorder has on family Help family explore frustrations and concerns Assist family in problem solving	Family discusses feelings and concerns regarding the child's capabilities and family's ability to cope with his needs
Promote optimum family functioning	Assist family in carrying out prescribed treatment regimen and assuming responsibility at its own pace and readiness Encourage early and consistent participation in treatment programs Provide praise and encouragement for compliance and innovation Help family achieve realistic view of child's capabilities and outlook for future Help family to view child rather than defects Support siblings and help them to understand affected child, his special needs, and the impact this has on their lives Refer to counseling services (as appropriate), parent groups, and organizations with special services, e.g., United Cerebral Palsy Association Maintain contact with family	Family understands and carries out prescribed therapeutic programs Family participates with support groups Family contacts health agency(ies)

Nursing Intervention Related to Medical Management

Prevent convulsions in seizure-prone child
    Administer anticonvulsant drugs

severe the motor weakness. The disorder may be manifest early, often at birth, frequently in utero, and almost always before 2 years of age. The manifestations and prognosis are categorized according to age of onset.

Group 1. This group comprises the infants who acquire the disease in utero or during the first 2 months of life. Inactivity is the most prominent feature. The infant lies in the frog position with legs externally rotated, abducted, and flexed at the hips. There is weakness and limited movements of the shoulder and arm muscles, but active movement is usually limited to fingers and toes. Breathing is diaphragmatic with sternal retractions caused by intercostal muscle paralysis. The cry and cough are weak, and secretions tend to pool in the pharynx. The facies are alert, and sensation and intellect are normal. These infants do not progress to sit alone, roll over, or walk. Early death (usually by 3 years of age) from respiratory failure or infection is usual. The most common complication is pneumonia.

Group 2. The infants in this group manifest the disease between 2 and 12 months of age. The symptoms are less devastating than in group 1 (Fig. 39-4). The weakness is confined to the arms and legs at first but later becomes generalized. The legs are usually involved to a greater extent than the arms. Pectus excavatum is prominent and is the result of unopposed diaphragmatic breathing. Movements are absent during complete relaxation or sleep. Some of these infants are able to sit if placed in position and in rare instances can stand holding onto furniture. The life span varies from 7 to 84 months.

Group 3. Children in this group experience onset of symptoms in the second year of life. They have normal head control and sit unassisted by 6 to 8 months of age. Thigh and hip muscles are weak but those who manage to walk have lumbar lordosis, waddling gait, genu recurvatum, and protuberant abdomen. Ambulation becomes increasingly difficult; children are confined to a wheelchair by the second decade. Deep tendon reflexes may be present early but disappear. It is often difficult to distinguish between these children and those with juvenile spinal muscular atrophy.

Therapeutic Management

The diagnosis is established from electromyography demonstrating a denervation pattern and is confirmed by muscle biopsy. Treatment is symptomatic and preventive, primarily prevention of infection and treating orthopedic problems, the most serious of which is scoliosis. Many children benefit from powered chairs, lifts, special mattresses, and accessible environmental controls. Vigorous antibiotic therapy and pulmonary physical therapy are implemented during upper respiratory infections.

Nursing Considerations

The infant or small child with extensive paralysis requires frequent change of position to prevent physical injury and complications, especially pneumonia. The pharynx requires

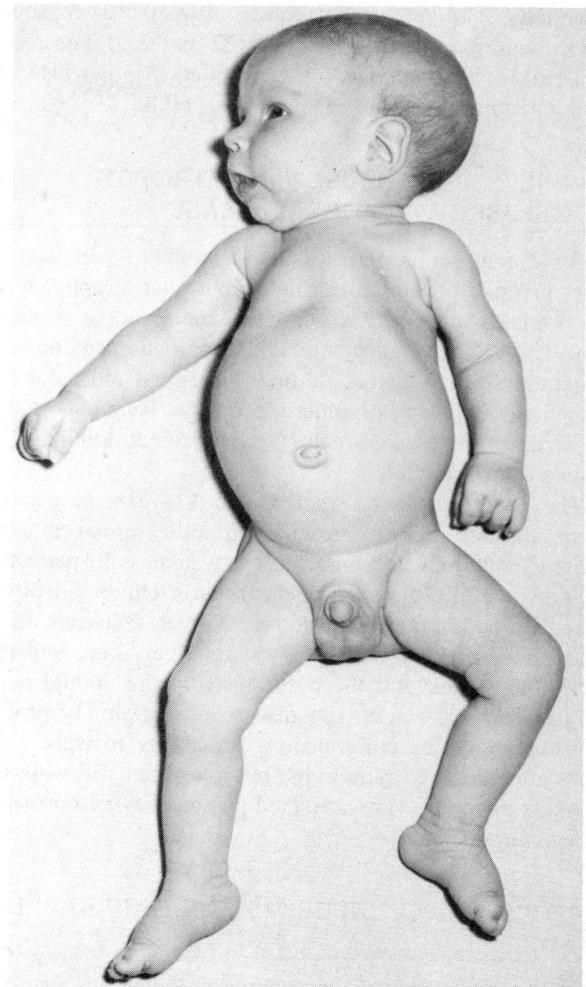

Fig. 39-4. Patient with group 1 Werdnig-Hoffman disease lying in typical posture of abduction of legs at hips and flexion of knees. Arms are flexed slightly with little movement at shoulders. Movements of fingers and toes are present. Pectus excavatum deformity of chest is common and is result of unopposed diaphragmatic breathing.

From Swaiman, K.F., and Wright, F.S.: The practice of pediatric neurology, ed. 2, St. Louis, 1982, The C.V. Mosby Co.

frequent suctioning to remove secretions, and feeding must be carried out slowly and carefully to prevent aspiration. Since these children are intellectually normal, verbal, tactile, and auditory stimulation are important aspects of care. Supporting them so that they can see the activities around them and transporting them in a buggy for a change of environment provide stimulation and a broader scope of contacts.

Children who are able to sit require proper support and attention to alignment to prevent deformities and other complications. The child with group 3 disease will need attention to education needs and opportunities for social interaction with other children. Parents of a chronically ill or potentially fatally ill child require a great deal of support and encouragement (see Chapters 22 and 23). The parents of a child with a genetically transmitted disorder also need to be encouraged to seek genetic counseling.

JUVENILE SPINAL MUSCULAR ATROPHY (KUGELBERG-WELANDER DISEASE)

Juvenile spinal muscular atrophy (Kugelberg-Welander disease, juvenile proximal hereditary muscular atrophy) is also the result of anterior horn cell and motor nerve degeneration. The disease is characterized by a pattern of muscular weakness similar to that of infantile spinal muscular atrophy. Several modes of inheritance have been reported for the disease—autosomal-recessive, autosomal-dominant, and X-linked recessive.

The onset occurs between 2 and 17 years of age with symptoms resembling group 3 infantile spinal muscular atrophy, although proximal muscle weakness (especially of the pelvic girdle) appears later, in early childhood or adolescence, and the progression is slower. Muscles of the lower arms and legs are involved relatively late, and muscles of the trunk and those supplied by the cranial nerves are usually unaffected. The disease runs a slowly progressive course. Some children lose the ability to walk 8 to 9 years after onset of symptoms, but many can still walk after 20 years or more. Many affected persons have a normal life expectancy.

INFECTIOUS POLYNEURITIS (GUILLAIN-BARRÉ SYNDROME)

Infectious polyneuritis, also known as infectious neuronitis or Guillain-Barré syndrome, is probably the most common form of polyneuritis and may occur at any age. It is an acute polyneuropathy in which motor dysfunction predominates over sensory disturbance; there is bilateral facial paresis or paralysis and occasionally weakness of the bulbar and respiratory musculature. Although children are less often affected than adults, the incidence in the pediatric age-group appears to be increasing, with higher susceptibility in children between ages 4 and 10 years. Both sexes are affected with equal frequency.

The precise etiologic agent is unknown. Since the disease has been associated with a number of viral infections or the administration of vaccines, it has been suggested that it may be a toxic sequela of an original infection, an activated latent virus, or a manifestation of an acute infection. Among illnesses that have been associated with the disease are infectious mononucleosis, measles, mumps, and a glandular feverlike syndrome. It may also be associated with *Mycoplasma* and *Pneumocystis* infections or gram-negative organisms. There has been an association with a vaccination process (the swine flu immunization of 1976). Some believe that it may represent a cell-mediated immunologic response directed at the peripheral nerves.

Pathophysiology

Pathologic changes in spinal and cranial nerves consist of inflammation and edema with rapid, segmented demyelination and compression of nerve roots within the dural sheath. Nerve conduction is impaired, producing ascending partial or complete paralysis of muscles innervated by the involved nerves.

Clinical Manifestations

The paralytic manifestations are usually preceded by a mild influenza-like illness or sore throat. The onset can be rapid, reaching peak activity within 24 hours, or gradual progression of symptoms over days or weeks. Neurologic symptoms initially involve muscle tenderness, sometimes accompanied by paresthesia and cramps. Proximal muscle weakness progressing to paralysis usually occurs before distal weakness and there is a tendency toward symmetric involvement. In most patients paralysis ascends from the lower extremities, frequently involving the muscles of the trunk, upper extremities, and those supplied by cranial nerves. The seventh (facial) cranial nerve is almost universally affected.

Tendon reflexes are depressed or absent, and paralysis is flaccid and may include variable degrees of sensory impairment. Paralysis may involve facial, extraocular, labial, lingual, pharyngeal, and laryngeal muscles. Evidence of intercostal and phrenic nerve involvement includes breathlessness in vocalizations and shallow, irregular respirations. Most patients complain of muscle tenderness or sensitivity to slight pressure. Urinary incontinence or retention and constipation are frequently present.

Course. The general health of the child and the extent of paralysis influence the outcome of the illness. Almost all deaths are caused by respiratory failure; therefore early diagnosis and access to respiratory support are especially important. Muscle function begins to return 2 days to 2 weeks after the onset of symptoms, and recovery is complete in most cases. The rate of recovery is usually related to the degree of involvement, which may extend from a few weeks to months. The greater the degree of paralysis, the longer the recovery phase.

Diagnostic Evaluation

Criteria established by the Ad Hoc NINCDS Committee (1978) include the following:

1. The paralysis may follow a nonspecific infection, but an illness known to be associated with polyradiculoneuropathy, such as herpes zoster or diphtheria, should not be present.
2. Findings should include multiple or diffuse lower motor unit paralysis that is rapid or gradual in onset, symmetric involvement, progressive weakness, and areflexia.
3. Sensory involvement may be present but generally is less severe than the motor weakness.
4. Cerebrospinal fluid examination should contain fewer than 10 white cells/mm^3.
5. Cerebrospinal fluid protein concentration should equal or exceed 60 mg/dl.

Therapeutic Management

Treatment of Guillain-Barré syndrome is symptomatic. Corticosteroid therapy has been of benefit in the early stages. Respiratory and pharyngeal involvement requires assisted ventilation, frequently with tracheostomy.

Nursing Considerations

Nursing care is essentially supportive and is the same as that required for quadriplegia from any cause. Since the care of the quadriplegic child is discussed in Chapter 40, it will not be considered at length here. The emphasis of care is on close observation to assess the extent of paralysis and prevention of complications.

During the acute phase of the disease the child's condition should be carefully observed for possible difficulty in swallowing and respiratory involvement. There should be a respirator on standby, with a cardiac monitor attached, and suction apparatus, tracheostomy tray, and vasoconstrictor drugs available at the bedside. Vital signs and level of consciousness are monitored frequently. For the child who develops respiratory dysfunction, the care is the same as that of any child with respiratory distress requiring mechanical ventilation (see p. 1322 and care of the child with tetanus who is given muscle relaxant drugs).

Throughout the recovery phase special emphasis is placed on prevention of complications, including good postural alignment, frequent change of position, and passive range of motion exercises. Children with oral and pharyngeal involvement are usually fed via a nasogastric tube to ensure adequate feeding. Bowel and bladder care is needed to avoid constipation and urine retention. Sensory impairment makes the child susceptible to burns and trophic ulcers.

Physical therapy is limited to passive range of motion exercises during the evolving phase of the disease. Later, as the disease stabilizes and recovery begins, an active physical therapy program is implemented to prevent contracture deformities and facilitate muscle recovery. This may include active exercise, gait training, and bracing.

Throughout the course of the illness child and parent support is paramount. The usual rapidity of the paralysis and the long period of recovery tax the emotional reserves of all family members greatly. The parents and child benefit from repeated reassurance that recovery is occurring and from realistic information regarding the possibility of permanent disability. In the event of a residual disability, the family needs assistance in accepting and adjusting to the loss of function (see Chapter 22).

TETANUS

Tetanus, or lockjaw, is an acute, preventable, and often fatal disease caused by an exotoxin produced by the anaerobic spore-forming, gram-positive bacillus *Clostridium tetani*. It is characterized by painful muscular rigidity primarily involving the masseter and neck muscles. There are four requirements for the development of tetanus: (1) presence of tetanus spores or vegetative forms of the bacillus, (2) injury to the tissues, (3) wound conditions that encourage multiplication of the organism, and (4) a susceptible host.

Tetanus spores are found in soil, dust, and the intestinal tracts of humans and animals, especially herbivorous animals. The organisms are more prevalent in rural areas but are readily carried to urban areas by the wind. The organisms are not invasive but enter the body by way of wounds, particularly a puncture wound, burn, or crushed area. They may enter through a very minor, unnoticed break in the skin such as a thorn or needle prick, bee sting, or scratch. In the newborn infection may occur through the umbilical cord, usually in situations in which infants are delivered in contaminated surroundings. The disease has the greatest incidence in months when persons are more involved in outdoor activities. Drug addicts are especially susceptible from poor injection technique and the use of street heroin, which is often mixed with quinine, a protoplasmic poison that favors the growth of the organism.

Pathophysiology

When conditions are favorable, the organisms proliferate and elaborate two exotoxins: (1) tetanospasmin, a potent toxin that affects the central nervous system to produce the clinical manifestations of the disease, and (2) tetanolysin, which appears to have no significance. The ideal conditions for growth of the organisms are devitalized tissues without access to air, such as wounds that have not been washed or kept clean and those that have crusted over, trapping pus beneath. The exotoxin appears to reach the central nervous system by way of either the neuron axons or the vascular system. The toxin becomes fixed on nerve cells of the anterior horn of the spinal cord and the brain stem. The toxin acts at the myoneural junction to produce the muscular stiffness and lower the threshold for reflex excitability.

The incubation period for tetanus varies from 1 to 54 days but is generally less than 14 days. The more extensive the injury, the shorter the incubation period and the more severe the symptoms.

Clinical Manifestations

There are several forms of the disease. *Local tetanus* is a less severe form characterized by persistent rigidity of muscles near the inoculation site, which may persist for weeks or months, but some cases resolve without sequelae. *Otogenous tetanus* is generalized or local tetanus that follows chronic otitis media where *C. tetani* is a secondary invader, surviving in purulent discharge. *Cephalic tetanus,* a rare form, follows infection of the head or face and can occur as a complication of acne or otitis media. This form is often limited to cranial nerves III, IV, VII, IX, X, and XII but may progress to generalized tetanus.

Generalized tetanus is the most common and dangerous form of the disease. The manner of onset varies, but the initial symptoms are usually a progressive stiffness and tenderness of the muscles in the neck and jaw. The characteristic difficulty in opening the mouth (trismus), caused by sustained contraction of the jaw-closing muscles, is evident early and gives the disease its common name, lockjaw. Spasm of facial muscles produces the so-called sardonic smile *(risus sardonicus)*. Progressive involvement of the trunk muscles causes opisthotonos and a boardlike rigidity of abdominal and limb muscles. There is difficulty in swallowing, and the patient is highly sensitive to external stimuli. The slightest noise, a gentle touch, or bright light will trigger convulsive muscular contractions that last seconds to minutes. The paroxysmal contractions recur with increased frequency until they become almost continuous.

Mentation is unaffected; the patient remains alert and pain and distress are reflected in rapid pulse, sweating, and an anxious expression. Laryngospasm and tetany of respiratory muscles and accumulated secretions predispose to respiratory arrest, atelectasis, and pneumonia. Fever is usually absent or only mild; presence of fever generally indicates a poor prognosis. As the child recovers from the disease, the paroxysms become less and less frequent and gradually subside. Survival beyond 4 days usually indicates recovery, but complete recovery may require weeks.

The mortality rate is about 30%, but the disease is almost invariably fatal in the newborn. The incubation period is short with the appearance of symptoms 3 to 10 days following exposure. The first symptom is difficulty sucking, which progresses to total inability to suck, excessive crying, irritability, and nuchal rigidity.

Therapeutic Management: Prevention

Preventive measures are based on the immune status of the affected child and the nature of the injury. Specific prophylactic therapy after trauma is administration of either tetanus toxoid or tetanus antitoxin. Children who have completed the immunization series (see p. 529) are given a tetanus toxoid booster prophylactically if none has been given in the prior 10 years for a clean minor wound or, if there is a heavily contaminated wound, if none has been given in the previous 5 years. Protective levels of antibody are maintained for at least 10 years; therefore antitoxin is not indicated for the fully immunized child. (See also Table 12-9.)

The unprotected or inadequately immunized child who sustains a "tetanus-prone" wound (for example, contaminated soil, crush injury, burn, compound fracture, retained foreign body, or a wound unattended for 24 hours) should receive human tetanus immune globulin (TIG). Human tetanus immune globulin is preferred to tetanus antitoxin (TAT) because of its absence of sensitivity reactions and longer half-life. Once the toxin has bound to central nervous system tissue, antitoxin has no effect, but if the binding has taken place only peripherally, administration of human tetanus immune globulin or bovine or horse tetanus antitoxin will prevent binding in the central areas. Concurrent administration of both human tetanus immune globulin and toxoid at separate sites is recommended both to provide protection

and to initiate the active immune process. Completion of active immunization is carried out according to the usual pattern.

Proper surgical cleansing and débridement of contaminated wounds reduce the chance of infection.

Therapeutic Management: Treatment

The affected child is best treated in an intensive care facility where close and constant observation and equipment for monitoring and respiratory support are readily available. A quiet environment is preferred to reduce external stimuli. Neonates are placed in an open unit or Isolette in which a constant environmental temperature can be maintained and oxygen supplied.

General supportive care, including maintenance of adequate fluid and electrolyte balance and caloric intake, is indicated. Indwelling oral or nasogastric feedings are used whenever possible, but severe laryngospasm may necessitate intravenous alimentation or gastrostomy feeding. Recurrent laryngospasm or excessive accumulation of secretions may require endotracheal intubation.

Antitoxin therapy to neutralize toxins not yet bound to nervous tissue is the most specific therapy for tetanus. Human tetanus immune globulin is preferred, but, if unavailable, tetanus antitoxin is given. Antibiotics are administered to control the proliferation of the vegetative forms of the organism at the site of infection. When the child recovers, active immunization should take place, since the disease does not confer a permanent immunity.

Local care of the wound by surgical debridement and cleansing helps reduce the numbers of proliferating organisms at the site of injury. An antibacterial agent such as pHisoHex or povidone-iodine (Betadine) followed by a dilute solution of hydrogen peroxide has proved effective. The cleansing should be repeated several times during the first 48 hours, and deep infected lacerations are usually exposed and débrided.

Sedatives or muscle relaxants are administered to help reduce muscle spasm and prevent convulsions. The most widely used is diazepam (Valium), but phenobarbital, chloral hydrate, the phenothiazines, and paraldehyde may be employed. Patients with severe tetanus and those who do not respond to other sedatives may require the administration of a neuromuscular blocking agent, usually pancuronium bromide (Pavulon) or δ-tubocurarine. Because of their paralytic effect on respiratory muscles, use of these drugs requires mechanical ventilation and constant attendance by trained personnel until muscle spasms are controlled.

Tracheostomy is often indicated and should be performed before severe respiratory distress develops. Administration of corticosteroids has met with success in some instances.

Nursing Considerations

In caring for the child with tetanus, every effort should be made to control or eliminate stimulation from sound, light, and touch. Although a darkened room is ideal, sufficient light is essential in order that the child can be carefully observed; light appears to be less irritating than vibratory or auditory stimuli. The infant or child is handled as little as possible, and extra effort is expended to avoid any sudden and/or loud noise.

Medications are administered as prescribed, and vital signs are observed and recorded at frequent intervals. The location and extent of muscle spasms and assessment of their severity are important nursing observations. Respiratory status is carefully evaluated for any signs of embarrassment, and appropriate emergency equipment is kept available at all times. Muscle relaxants and sedatives that may be prescribed can also cause respiratory depression; therefore the child must be assessed for excessive central nervous system depression. Blood gases are obtained frequently to evaluate the respiratory status. Attention to hydration and nutrition may involve monitoring an intravenous infusion, monitoring nasogastric or gastrostomy feedings, and suctioning oropharyngeal secretions when indicated.

If a potent muscle relaxant such as pancuronium bromide (Pavulon) is used, the total paralysis makes oral communication impossible. Therefore all the child's needs must be anticipated and procedures carefully explained beforehand. As the dose of medication is decreased, the child regains movement of the eyelids and facial muscles, which gives him some opportunity to express emotions and indicate choices through a signal system, for example, blinking the lids to indicate "yes" or "no."

Although most affected children are neonates and receive the nursing care and assessment of any high-risk infant (Chapter 10), the older child may acquire a tetanus infection. Since the child's mental status is clear, he is aware of what is happening to him and is often in a state of terror. He should not be left alone, and all efforts should be made to reduce his anxiety, which can contribute to muscular spasms. A calm and reassuring manner and sympathetic understanding can help immeasurably in getting the child through this crisis situation.

BOTULISM

Botulism is a serious food poisoning that results from ingestion of the preformed toxin produced by the anaerobic bacillus *Clostridium botulinum*. The most common source of the toxin is improperly sterilized home-canned foods. Nervous system symptoms appear abruptly about 12 to 36 hours after ingestion of contaminated food and may or may not have been preceded by acute digestive disturbance. There is weakness, dizziness, headache, difficulty in talking and speaking, diplopia, and vomiting. Progressive respiratory paralysis is life threatening.

Treatment consists of intravenous administration of botulism antitoxin and general supportive measures. Toxins vary in protein-binding capacity. Some have a relatively short half-life and do not bind to tissues firmly; therefore

therapy is continued until paralysis abates. Others toxins appear to bind irreversibly to nerve endings and are therefore not amenable to neutralization (Polin and Brown, 1979). Respiratory support is often needed and should be available at the bedside ready for use if indicated.

Infant Botulism

Infant botulism, unlike the disease in older persons, is caused by ingestion of spores or vegetative cells of *C. botulinum* and the subsequent release of the toxin from organisms colonizing the gastrointestinal tract. There appears to be no common food or drug source of the organisms; however, the *C. botulinum* organisms have been found in honey fed to affected infants.

There is wide variation in the severity of the disease, from mild constipation to progressive sequential loss of neurologic function and respiratory failure. Botulism toxin exerts its effect by inhibiting the release of acetylcholine at the myoneural junction, thereby impairing motor activity of muscles innervated by affected nerves.

The affected infant is usually well before the onset of symptoms. Constipation is a common presenting symptom, and almost all infants exhibit generalized weakness and a decrease in spontaneous movements. Deep tendon reflexes are usually diminished or absent; cranial nerve deficits are common (especially CN VII, IX, X, and XI), as evidenced by loss of head control, difficulty in feeding, weak cry, and reduced gag reflex. The most frequently recognized form of thedisease is consistent with the "floppy infant syndrome."

Two common practices that tend to aggravate the condition and contribute to respiratory arrest include the administration of aminoglycosides and neck flexion during positioning for lumbar puncture or computed tomography scans (Johnson, Clay, and Arnon, 1979). Aminoglycosides decrease acetylcholine release and thus potentiate the neurologic deficit, especially in the nerve terminals innervating the diaphragm. When the soft tissue obstruction to the airway is relieved following positioning for procedures, additional stress is placed on the myoneural junction as the infant attempts to regain respiratory efficiency through rapid, repetitive muscle activity of the intrinsic muscles of the pharynx and the neck muscles.

Diagnosis is made on the basis of history, physical examination, and laboratory detection of fecal toxin. Treatment consists of supportive measures, primarily respiratory and nutritional. Botulinal antitoxin, used in adults and older children, is not administered to infants. Evidence indicates that the infants recover without it and its therapeutic efficacy is lacking. Furthermore, since the antitoxin is made from horse serum, it may cause serum sickness or anaphylaxis and may induce a life-long hypersensitivity (Arnon, 1986).

Nursing Considerations

Nursing responsibilities include observing for and reporting signs of muscle impairment and providing intensive nursing care when the infant is hospitalized (see Nursing care of the high-risk infant, Chapter 10). Parental support and reassurance are important. Most infants recover when the disorder is recognized and therapy implemented. Parents should be aware that during recovery patients fatigue easily when muscular action is sustained. This has important implications for timing the resumption of feedings because of the risk of aspiration. They should also be advised that normal bowel action may not return for several weeks; therefore a stool softener can be beneficial. Cathartics and enemas are not advised.

Home supervision of the outpatient and education regarding possible modes of infection (such as use of honey as formula sweetener) are nursing responsibilities. An infant who is recovering from botulism must avoid contact with other infants for about 3 months or until excretion of organisms has ceased.

MYASTHENIA GRAVIS

Myasthenia gravis (MG) is relatively uncommon in childhood but may appear in two forms: neonatal and juvenile. The precise mechanism has not been determined, but the abnormality is associated with altered function of cholinesterase on the acetylcholine released at the neuromuscular junction.

Neonatal Myasthenia Gravis

A *transient* form of myasthenia gravis occurs in approximately 15% of infants born to mothers with myasthenia gravis who may not be aware that they have the disease. The muscular weakness results from transplacentally acquired maternal acetylcholine receptor antibodies. These infants display generalized weakness and hypotonia at birth with a depressed Moro reflex, ptosis, ineffective sucking and swallowing reflexes, and weak cry. There is no evidence of neurologic damage. In this form the symptoms usually disappear within 2 to 4 weeks.

Persistent neonatal myasthenia gravis is a familial abnormality of neuromuscular transmission that is not immunologically mediated. It appears indistinguishable from the transient form, but the mother usually does not have the disease. The disease persists throughout life, and more than one sibling may be affected, which suggests a genetic etiology. Sex distribution is equal. The disorder is relatively resistant to drug therapy, and the eyelid and extraocular muscles seem to be the muscles most severely affected.

Juvenile Myasthenia Gravis

Juvenile myasthenia gravis appears to be identical to that seen in adults and usually has its onset after age 10 years, but it may appear as early as age 2 years. Girls are affected six times as often as boys. The disorder results from an acquired immunologically mediated dysfunction of the neuromuscular postsynaptic acetylcholine receptor (Seybold and Lindstrom, 1981).

The most common symptoms are general paralysis of the optic muscles with ptosis and diplopia. Difficulty in swallowing, chewing, and speaking are also prominent, accompanied by weakness and paralysis of all skeletal muscles. The signs and symptoms are more pronounced in the late afternoon and evening. They are relieved by rest and made worse by exercise.

Diagnostic Evaluation

The diagnosis is made on the basis of the characteristic distribution of muscle weakness and the progressive weakness on repeated or sustained muscular contraction. The diagnosis is established by observation of the response to the anticholinesterase drugs. Intravenous administration of a small test dose of edrophonium (Tensilon) produces a beneficial effect in 1 minute but lasts for less than 5 minutes. Electromyography is helpful in diagnosis and reveals high amplitude muscle responses followed by contractions of rapidly diminishing amplitude.

Although the pathologic mechanism for transient neonatal, persistent neonatal, and juvenile MG are different, it is sometimes difficult to distinguish the three types clinically. Juvenile MG is frequently associated with anti-acetylcholine antibodies, whereas this finding is absent in persistent neonatal MG.

Therapeutic Management

Treatment consists of the oral administration of anticholinesterase drugs, the least toxic of which is pyridostigmine (Mestinon). The initial dose is 30 mg every 4 hours in the older child and 5 mg every 4 hours in the infant. The dosage is gradually increased until a satisfactory result is obtained. The child must be observed for signs of parasympathetic stimulation from overmedication. These include lacrimation, salivation, abdominal cramps, sweating, diarrhea, vomiting, bradycardia, and weakness of respiratory muscles.

Nursing Considerations

These children need continuous medical and nursing supervision. The parents are taught the importance of accurate administration of medications, with special emphasis on recognizing side effects with the dangers of choking, aspiration, and respiratory distress.

Parents are counseled regarding promoting a life-style that minimizes stress and maximizes relaxation. Strenuous activity is discouraged. They are also warned of the possibility of a sudden exacerbation of symptoms during times of physical or emotional stress (myasthenia crisis) that requires immediate medical attention. They should receive instruction in providing respiratory assistance until help arrives or the child can be transported to medical aid.

The prognosis in persistent congenital myasthenia gravis is usually good. Although there is gradual worsening of symptoms with age, the life span is not affected significantly. A high percentage of persons with childhood-onset (juvenile) myasthenia gravis become resistant or unresponsive to medication, with the danger of exacerbation and respiratory failure. Spontaneous remissions are infrequent.

Muscular Dysfunction

As skeletal development is responsible for linear growth, muscle growth accounts for a significant portion of the increase in body weight. The number of muscle fibers is established by the fourth or fifth month of fetal life and remains constant throughout life. Differences in muscle size between individuals and differences in one person at various times during a lifetime are a result of the ability of the separate muscle fibers to increase in size. The increase in muscle fiber length that accompanies growth is also associated with an increase in the number of nuclei in the fibers. This increase is most apparent during the adolescent growth spurt. At this time the increase in secretion of growth hormone and adrenal androgens stimulates the growth of muscle fibers in both sexes, but the growth in boys is further stimulated by the secretion of testosterone.

At about 6 months of prenatal life, muscle mass constitutes approximately one sixth of the body weight; at birth, about one fourth, and at adolescence, one third. The variability in size and strength of muscle is influenced by genetic constitution, nutrition, and exercise. At all ages muscles increase in size with use and shrink with inactivity. Consequently maintaining muscle tone to minimize the amount of atrophy in skeletal muscle through active or passive range of motion exercises is an important protective nursing function.

Skeletal muscles are subject to a large number of disorders that cause degeneration of muscle fibers with subsequent loss of function. In most instances there is fibrous connective tissue replacement of muscle fibers, proximal muscles are affected more severely than distal ones, and the lower extremities are affected to a greater extent than the upper extremities. Children with muscle disease characteristically develop a waddling gait and have difficulty in running, climbing, and rising from a sitting position. Innervation is not affected.

Diseases of skeletal muscles can be inflammatory (such as polymyositis), the result of endocrine dysfunction (such as hypothyroidism and hyperthyroidism), or caused by congenital defects (such as absence of muscle, periodic paralysis, and the various muscular dystrophies and myotonias). Inflammation occurs in a number of infectious illnesses such as trichinosis, toxoplasmosis, and those caused by coxsackievirus and is seen in collagen diseases, including lupus erythematosus, periarteritis nodosa, dermatomyositis, rheumatoid arthritis, and polymyositis.

In addition to the electromyogram, measurement of serum enzyme activity, especially creatine phosphokinase, is often helpful in differential diagnosis of muscle disease. The intracellular enzyme creatine phosphokinase is present in muscle tissues and very few other organs and is released in large amounts in some diseases of muscles such as muscular dystrophy. Creatine phosphokinase is not elevated in neurogenic disease. Although the treatment in a large number of muscle disorders is palliative and symptomatic rather than curative, an accurate diagnosis is essential for purposes of rehabilitation, counseling, and treatment in those amenable to specific therapy.

JUVENILE DERMATOMYOSITIS

Dermatomyositis is a multisystem inflammatory disorder of unknown etiology and often difficult to distinguish from muscular dystrophy. There is proximal limb and trunk muscle weakness and loss of reflexes. Neck muscles are frequently affected, and the child may have difficulty in lifting the head or supporting it in an upright position. Muscles tend to be stiff and sore. Distal muscle strength and reflex response remain unaffected. Dermatomyositis, frequently classified as a collagen disease, is characterized by red, indurated skin lesions over the malar areas and nose and a violet discoloration of the eyelids. The skin over extensor muscle surfaces may be erythematous, scaly, and atopic.

Dermatomyositis responds to corticosteroid therapy, and with early and vigorous treatment most affected children recover. Physical therapy is essential to prevent contracture deformity and to rebuild muscle strength. Bracing or splinting may be needed.

MUSCULAR DYSTROPHIES

The muscular dystrophies (MD) constitute the largest and most important single group of muscle diseases of childhood. They all have a genetic origin in which there is gradual degeneration of muscle fibers and are characterized by progressive weakness and wasting of symmetric groups of skeletal muscles with increasing disability and deformity. In all forms of muscular dystrophy there is insidious loss of strength, but each differs in regard to muscle groups affected, age of onset, rate of progression, and inheritance patterns.

The basic defect in muscular dystrophy is unknown, although it appears to be caused by a metabolic disturbance unrelated to the nervous system. Serum creatine phosphokinase is consistently increased in affected individuals, which assists in diagnosis and affords a means for early detection of the disorder in asymptomatic children in families at risk.

Treatment of the muscular dystrophies consists mainly of providing supportive measures, including physical therapy, orthopedic procedures to minimize deformity, and assisting the affected child in meeting the demands of daily living.

The various forms of muscular dystrophy are summarized in Table 39-1, and the initial sites of muscle involvement in the major types are illustrated in Fig. 39-5.

Table 39-1 Summary of primary myopathies with onset in childhood

PRIMARY MYOPATHY/ INHERITANCE PATTERN	AGE OF ONSET	INITIAL MANIFESTATIONS	PROGRESSION	THERAPY
Muscular dystrophies Pseudohypertrophic (Duchenne) X-linked recessive; sporadic	Early childhood; age 1-3 years	Lordosis Waddling gait Difficulty in rising from floor and climbing stairs Fat deposits replace wasted gastrocnemius muscles	Rapid Ultimately involves all voluntary muscles Death usually occurs between ages 15 and 25 years	Supportive Physical therapy to prevent disuse atrophy of unaffected muscles
(Becker) X-linked recessive	Middle childhood; age 2½-21 years, mean age 11	Pseudohypertrophy of calves, atrophy of thighs	Slow Wheelchair bound 20-30 years after onset Life expectancy slightly decreased; usually between 23 and 63 years	Supportive
Limb-girdle Autosomal recessive (usually)	Late childhood or during adolescence; over age 8 years	Weakness of proximal muscles of both pelvic and shoulder girdles	Variable but usually slow Most become incapacitated within 20 years of onset, in some, disability may remain slight	Supportive Physical therapy to prevent disuse atrophy of unaffected muscles
Facioscapulohumeral (Landouzy-Déjerine) Autosomal dominant	Early adolescence; over age 8 years	Lack of facial mobility Difficulty in raising arms over head Forward slope of shoulders	Very slow May be intervals with no progression Considerable disability in time but life span unaffected	Supportive
Congenital dystrophy Unknown but familial tendency	At birth	Small, weak muscles May be multiple contracture deformities	Rapid Death in early infancy	None
Ocular myopathy (ophthalmoplegia) Autosomal dominant	Late childhood; over age 10 years	Weakness of extraocular muscles, causing ptosis Gradually spreads to pharyngeal muscles with difficulty in swallowing and speaking	Slow	Corticosteroids may be useful Plastic surgery to correct ptosis
Myotonic dystrophies Myotonia congenita (Thomsen disease) Autosomal dominant	Early childhood	Difficulty in relaxing muscles after contraction Aggravated by cold and emotional excitement	None Mild, lifelong disability	Drug therapy— phenytoin
Myotonic dystrophy (Steinert disease) Autosomal dominant	Adolescence or older May manifest at birth	Weakening of hand and forearm muscles Inability to relax hand grip Eye, tongue, and masseter muscles often affected In infants, difficulty in nursing and proximal muscle weakness Aggravated by cold	Variable Reaches severe stage of disability 15-20 years after onset Normal life span rarely attained	Symptoms may be relieved by drugs— procainamide orally three times daily or phenytoin

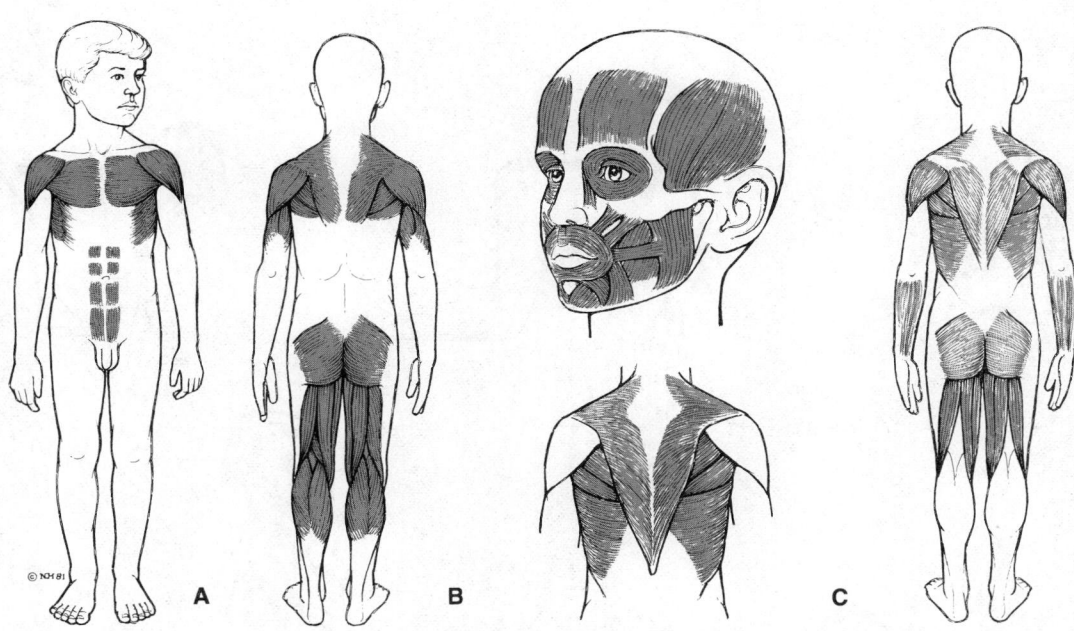

Fig. 39-5. Initial muscle groups involved in muscular dystrophies. **A,** Pseudohypertrophic; **B,** fascioscapulohumeral; **C,** limb-girdle.

PSEUDOHYPERTROPHIC (DUCHENNE) MUSCULAR DYSTROPHY

The most severe and the most common muscular dystrophy of childhood is pseudohypertrophic MD. An X-linked inheritance pattern is identified in 50% of cases; the remainder appear as sporadic cases and probably represent fresh mutations. As in all X-linked disorders, males are affected almost exclusively. The incidence is 1:3000 to 1:5000 male births (Cohen, 1984).

The clinical course is characteristic:

1. Early onset, usually between 3 and 5 years of age
2. Progressive muscular weakness, wasting, and contractures
3. Calf muscle hypertrophy in most cases
4. Loss of independent ambulation by 9 to 11 years of age
5. Slowly progressive generalized weakness during teenage years
6. Relentless progression until death from respiratory or cardiac failure

Clinical Manifestations

Evidence of muscle weakness usually appears during the third year, although there may have been a history of delay in motor development, particularly walking. Difficulty in running, riding a bicycle, and climbing stairs are usually the first symptoms noted. Later abnormal gait on a level surface becomes apparent. In the early years rapid developmental gains may mask the progression of the disease. Questioning of parents may reveal that the child has difficulty in rising from a sitting or supine position. Occasionally enlarged calves may be noticed by parents.

Typically the affected male has a waddling gait and lordosis, falls frequently, and develops a characteristic manner of rising from a squatting or sitting position on the floor (Gowers sign) (Fig. 39-6)—he turns onto his side or abdomen, flexes his knees to assume a kneeling position, then with knees extended gradually pushes his torso to an upright position by "walking" his hands up his legs. The muscles, especially of the thighs and upper arms, become enlarged from fatty infiltration and feel unusually firm or woody on palpation. The name *pseudohypertrophy* is derived from this muscular enlargement. Profound muscular atrophy occurs in later stages, and as the disease progresses, contractures and deformities involving large and small joints are common complications. Ambulation usually becomes impossible by 12 years of age. Facial, oropharyngeal, and respiratory muscles are spared until the terminal stages of the disease. Ultimately the disease process involves the diaphragm and auxiliary muscles of respiration, and cardiomegaly is common. The cause of death is usually respiratory tract infection or cardiac failure.

Mild mental retardation is commonly associated with muscular dystrophy. The mean intelligence quotient is about 20 points below the normal, and frank mental deficit is present in 25% of these children.

Complications. The major complications of muscular dystrophy include contractures, disuse atrophy, infections, obesity, and cardiopulmonary problems.

Contracture deformities of hips, knees, and ankles occur from early selective muscle involvement and often exaggerate the weakness. Passive range of motion exercises,

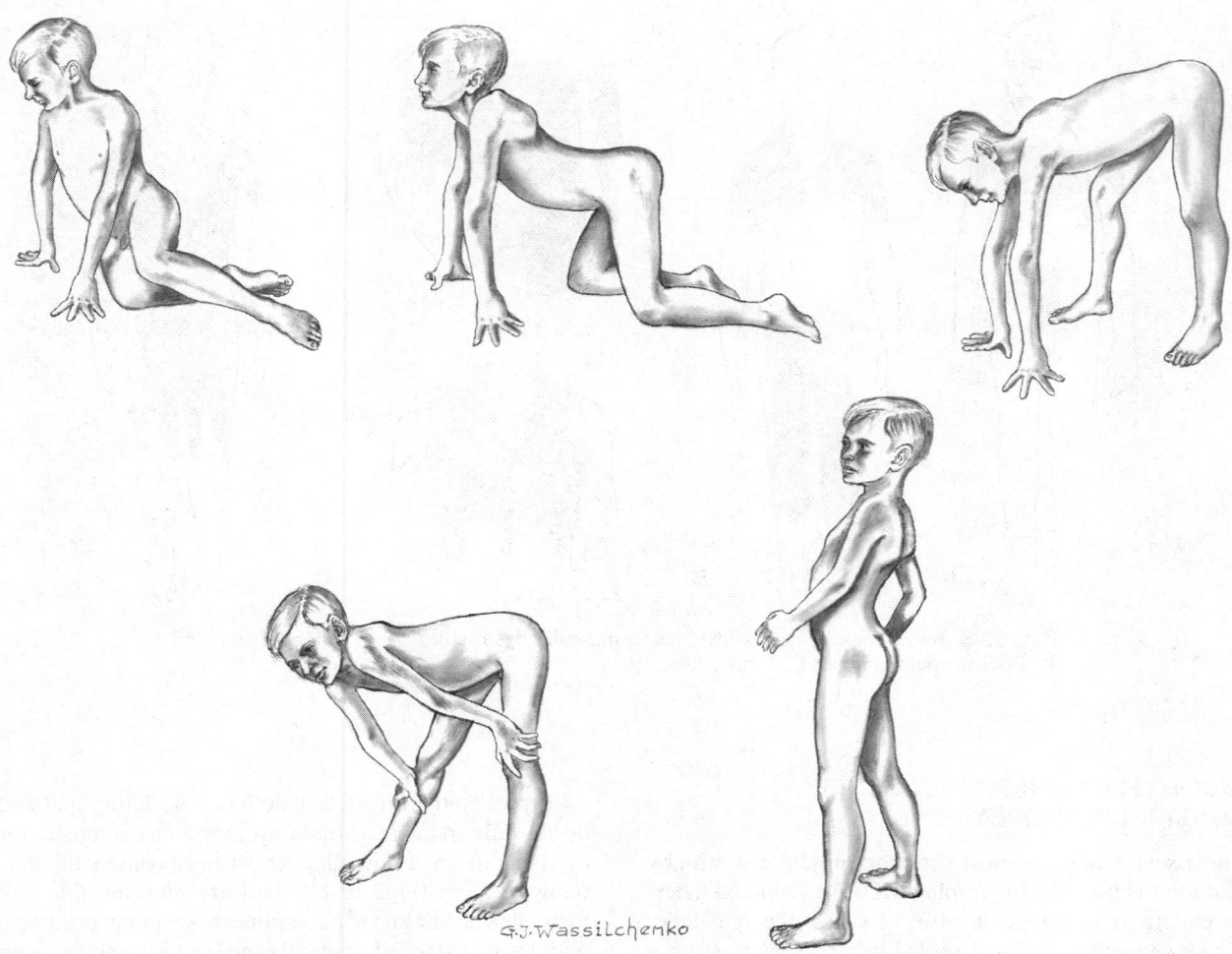

Fig. 39-6. Child with Duchenne muscular dystrophy attains standing posture by assuming a kneeling position, then gradually pushing his torso upright (with knees straight) by ''walking'' his hands up his legs (Gower sign). Note marked lordosis in upright position.

stretching, and active exercises under the supervision of a physical therapist are effective in treating reducible contractures. Nonreducible contractures require wedge casting or surgical reduction. Scoliosis caused by muscle imbalance is common and tends to progress even when the child becomes dependent on a wheelchair. Bracing with a rigid corset may be needed for support, although it may interfere with mobility. Frequent rest periods in the recumbent position are often beneficial. For correction of deformities it is essential to select a procedure that immobilizes the child for as short a period as possible to minimize the chances of developing disease atrophy.

Atrophy of disuse from prolonged inactivity occurs readily when the child is immobilized or confined to bed with illness, injury, or surgery. To minimize this complication, physical therapy should be implemented if bed rest extends beyond a few days. A daily goal for the well child should be at least 3 hours of ambulation when disability is moderate to maintain muscle strength.

Infections become increasingly frequent as the dystrophic process produces a progressive decrease in vital capacity resulting from weakness of primary, secondary, and associated muscles of respiration. Consequently even minor upper respiratory infections may become serious problems in these children. Prompt and vigorous antibiotic therapy supplemented by postural drainage and intermittent respiratory therapy are effective. Because these children are unable to cough, secretions collect easily.

Obesity is a frequent complication that contributes to premature loss of ambulation. Children with restricted opportunity for physical activity and who suffer from boredom easily consume calories in excess of their needs. This is compounded by overfeeding by well-meaning family and friends. Proper dietary intake and a diversified recreational program help reduce the likelihood of obesity and enable the child to maintain ambulation and functional independence for a longer time.

Cardiac manifestations are usually late events but may occur in the ambulatory child. Most significant of these, cardiac failure, is difficult to correct in advanced cases, but treatment with digoxin and diuretics is often beneficial in the early stages of the disease.

Diagnostic Evaluation

The disease is confirmed by serum enzyme measurement, muscle biopsy, and electromyography. The serum creatine phosphokinase, aldolase, and serum glutamic-oxaloacetic transaminase levels are extremely high in the first 2 years of life before onset of clinical weakness. They diminish with muscle deterioration but do not reach normal levels until severe muscle wasting and incapacitation have occurred. Muscle biopsy reveals degeneration of muscle fibers with fibrosis and fatty tissue replacement. Electromyography shows decrease in amplitude and duration of motor unit potentials. Diagnosis poses few problems in children 2 to 7 years of age, but in older children the similarity of symptoms to those of limb-girdle muscular dystrophy and some other myopathies confuses the diagnosis.

Therapeutic Management

There is no effective treatment for childhood muscular dystrophy. Maintaining function in unaffected muscles for as long as possible is the primary goal. It has been found that children who remain as active as possible are able to avoid wheelchair confinement for a longer period. Early recourse to a wheelchair accelerates deconditioning and promotes the development of lower extremity contractures. Maintenance of function often includes range of motion exercises, surgery to release contracture deformities, bracing, and performance of activities of daily living (ADL). Genetic counseling is recommended for parents, female siblings, and maternal aunts and their female offspring (see Chapter 5).

Nursing Considerations

The care and management of a child with muscular dystrophy involve the combined efforts of a comprehensive health team, and nurses can help clarify the roles of these health professionals to family and others. The major emphasis of nursing care is to assist the child and his family to cope with the progressive, incapacitating, and fatal nature of the disease, to help design a program that will afford a greater degree of independence and reduce the predictable and preventable disabilities associated with the disorder, and to assist them to deal constructively with the limitations the disease imposes on their daily lives.

Working closely with other team members, nurses help the family in developing the child's self-help skills to give the child the satisfaction of being as independent as possible for as long as possible. It is tempting for parents to overprotect their affected children. Children derive pleasure and build self-esteem from performing actions that produce visible pleasure in their parents. Even the physical weakness that prevents the child from physical competition with other children has little effect on the child as long as it does not affect the parents' attitude toward him as an individual. Therefore parents must be helped to develop a balance between limiting the child's activity because of muscular

weakness and allowing him to accomplish things by himself. This requires continual evaluation of the child's capabilities, which are often difficult to assess. It is not always possible to know when the child seeks parental assistance because he wants a little extra attention or because his muscles are overtired. Fortunately most children with muscular dystrophy instinctively recognize this need to be as independent as possible and strive to do so.

Practical difficulties faced by families are physical limitations of housing and mobility. Families often live in houses or apartments that are unsuited to wheelchairs—no street-level entrance, upstairs bedrooms and bathrooms, no tub. Many of these families have no independent means of transportation. Assisting with these problems involves team problem solving. Parents also need help in buying and modifying clothing for their disabled child. It is difficult to find clothing and footwear to wear comfortably in a wheelchair, to fit over contracted limbs, and to fit an obese child. Parents' social activities are also restricted, and the family's activities must be continually modified to the needs of the affected child (see Chapter 22). The child cannot be left with an ordinary teenage baby-sitter but requires a specially trained person, such as a student nurse. Consequently parents, too, tend to lead more isolated lives. When the child becomes increasingly helpless, the family may consider a skilled nursing facility to provide the care needed. Nurses can assist with decision making and support the family in the decision.

Each child's therapy program is tailored to his individual needs and capabilities, and families should be active participants. Parents need assistance with the physical therapy program and education regarding a home regimen of exercises and activity. Many parents erroneously believe that if the child expends himself sufficiently this will overcome the weakness and prevent progression of the disease process. They should also be advised to notify the nurse or other designated person when the child becomes even temporarily bedridden so that the exercise program can be continued, although modified, during this time.

Children with muscular dystrophy are typically passive, frequently withdrawn, and emotionally immature. As their physical condition deteriorates to the point that they can no longer keep up with friends and classmates, they tend to become socially isolated. Their physical capabilities diminish, and their dependency increases at the ages when most children are expanding their range of interests and relationships. To gain associations, they often learn behaviors that bring them the rewards of other children's company. These friends are often children who have been rejected by more able-bodied classmates.

No matter how successful the program and how well the family adapts to the disorder, superimposed on the physical and emotional problems associated with a child with a long-term disability is the constant presence of the ultimate outcome of the disease. All the manifestations seen in the child with a fatal illness are encountered in these families (see Chapter 23). The guilt feelings of the mother may be particularly pronounced in this disorder because of the mother-to-son transmission of the defective gene.

Nurses are especially valuable health professionals as they come to know the family and the family's problems. Nurses can be alert to problems and needs of the families and make necessary referrals when supplementary services are indicated. The **Muscular Dystrophy Association of America, Inc.*** has branches in most communities to provide assistance to families in which there is a member with muscular dystrophy.

Musculoskeletal Dysfunction

The disorders affecting the skeletal structures and associated musculature are primarily congenital, traumatic, secondary to metabolic dysfunction, or idiopathic in origin. Some appear at any age, such as fractures, whereas others have a predilection for a different stage of the childhood span of growth and development. There are those detected at birth or shortly after, such as congenital foot and hip deformities (see Chapter 11); Legg-Calvé-Perthes disease affects children in middle childhood; and slipped femoral capital epiphysis and scoliosis are more characteristic of late childhood and adolescence.

TORTICOLLIS

Torticollis (wry neck) is a congenital or acquired condition of limited neck motion in which the neck is flexed and turned to the affected side as a result of shortening of the sternocleidomastoid muscle. In early infancy a firm, nontender mass may be felt in the midportion of the muscle. The mass regresses and is replaced by fibrous tissue. If the condition remains untreated, there is permanent limitation of neck movement and the head and face become asymmetric, probably related to impaired blood supply to the depressed side of the head.

Treatment consists of gentle stretching exercises. The face is turned toward the affected muscle while the head is tilted in the opposite direction with the neck extended. The position is held for a count of 5 and repeated 10 times, twice daily (Watts and Kirkpatrick, 1983). The exercises are best performed by two persons—one to control the torso and one to manipulate the head. If stretching exercises are unsuccessful, surgical release of the sternocleidomastoid muscle may be needed.

Nursing Considerations

Nurses are alert to the possibility of torticollis in infants with limited head movement. After diagnosis it is frequently a nursing responsibility to teach and supervise the family in performing the exercises. The exercise requires very explicit instructions to the family and compliance is mandatory. The

nurse also suggests that the child be placed in the crib or playpen in a way that encourages turning the head away from the deformity in order to observe activities and interesting items. Feeding and play with the child can be used to encourage turning the head in the direction desired for correction.

LEGG-CALVÉ-PERTHES DISEASE (COXA PLANA)

Legg-Calvé-Perthes disease (LCPD), sometimes called coxa plana or osteochondritis deformans juvenilis, is a self-limited disorder in which there is aseptic necrosis of the femoral head. The disease affects children 3 to 12 years, but most cases occur in males between 4 and 8 years as an isolated event. In approximately 10% to 15% of cases the involvement is bilateral; most of the affected children have a skeletal age significantly below their chronologic age. The male/female ratio is 4:1 or 5:1; white children are affected 10 times more frequently than black children.

Pathophysiology

The cause of the disease is unknown, but there is a disturbance of circulation to the femoral capital epiphysis that produces an ischemic aseptic necrosis of the femoral head. During middle circulation to the femoral epiphysis is more tenuous than at other ages, being supplied almost entirely by lateral retinacular vessels. These can become obstructed by trauma, inflammation, coagulation defects, and a variety of other causes (Staheli, 1986). This circulatory impairment appears to extend to the epiphysis and acetabulum as well. The pathologic events seem to take place in four stages:

Stage I: Septic necrosis or infarction of the femoral capital epiphysis with degenerative changes producing flattening of the upper surface of the femoral head—the *avascular stage*.

Stage II: Capital bone absorption and revascularization with fragmentation (vascular resorption of the epiphysis) that gives a mottled appearance on radiograms—the *fragmentation*, or *revascularization*, *stage*.

Stage III: New bone formation, which is represented on radiographs as calcification and ossification or increased density in the areas of radiolucency; this filling-in process appears to take place from the periphery of the head centrally—the *reparative stage*.

Stage IV: Gradual reformation of the head of the femur without radiolucency and (hopefully) to a spherical form—the *regenerative stage*.

The entire process may encompass as little as 18 months or continue for several years. The reformed femoral head may be severely altered or appear entirely normal.

Clinical Manifestations

The onset is insidious and the history may reveal only intermittent appearance of a limp on the affected side or a symptom complex including hip soreness, ache, or stiffness that can be constant or intermittent. The pain may be experienced

*810 Seventh Ave., New York, NY 10019.

in the hip, along the entire thigh, or in the vicinity of the knee joint. The pain and limp are usually most evident on arising and at the end of a long day of activities. The pain is usually accompanied by joint dysfunction and limited range of motion. There may be a vague history of trauma. The diagnosis is established by radiographic examination.

Therapeutic Management

Since deformity occurs early in the disease process, the aim of treatment is to keep the head of the femur "contained" in the acetabulum, which serves as a mold to preserve the spherical shape of the head and to maintain a full range of motion. Activity causes microfractures of the soft, ischemic epiphysis, which tend to induce synovitis, stiffness, and adductor contracture (Staheli, 1986). The initial therapy is rest, which helps reduce inflammation and restore motion. Active motion is encouraged. In some cases traction is applied to stretch tight adductor muscles.

Containment can be accomplished by non-weight-bearing devices such as an abduction brace, leg casts, or a leather harness sling that prevents weight bearing on the affected limb; by various weight-bearing appliances such as abduction-ambulation braces or casts after a period of bed rest and traction; and surgical reconstructive and containment procedures. Conservative therapy must be continued for 2 to 4 years, although braces constructed from lightweight materials allow the child to maintain a nearly normal activity level. Surgical correction, although a relatively recent advance and subject to additional risks (such as anesthesia, infection, and blood transfusion), returns the child to normal activities in 3 to 4 months.

The disease is self-limited, but the ultimate outcome of therapy depends on early and efficient treatment and the age of onset of the disorder. Younger children, whose epiphyses are more cartilagenous, have the brightest prognosis for complete recovery. The later the diagnosis is made, the more damage has occurred before treatment is implemented. In most cases, with good patient compliance, the prognosis is excellent.

Nursing Considerations

Nurses are often the first health professionals to identify affected children and to refer them for medical evaluation. They are also persons on whom the child and his family can rely to help them to understand and adjust to the therapeutic measures. Since most care of the child is conducted on an outpatient basis, the major emphasis of nursing care is teaching the family the care and management of the corrective appliance selected for therapy. The family needs to learn the purpose, function, application, and care of the corrective device and the importance of compliance in order to achieve the desired outcome.

One of the most difficult aspects associated with the disorder is coping with a normally active child who feels well but must remain relatively inactive. Suitable activities must be devised to meet the needs of the child in the process of developing a sense of initiative or industry. Activities that meet the creative urges are well received. This is also an opportune time to encourage the child to begin a hobby such as collections, model building, or crafts.

SLIPPED FEMORAL CAPITAL EPIPHYSIS

Slipped femoral capital epiphysis (SFCE), or coxa vara, refers to the spontaneous displacement of the proximal femoral epiphysis in a posterior and inferior direction. It develops most frequently shortly before or during accelerated growth and the onset of puberty (children between the ages of 10 and 16 years—median age, 13 for boys, 11 for girls) and is most frequently observed in obese children. Bilateral involvement has been reported variously as 16% to 40%.

Pathophysiology

The cause of SFCE is unknown, but it occurs most often in "overlarge" youngsters or very tall, thin, rapidly growing children. There has been some evidence to implicate hormonal factors; for example, resistance of the growth plate to shear stress is decreased by growth hormone and increased by sex hormone, suggesting that the disorder may be related to excess sex hormone in the tall child and decreased sex hormone in the obese child. It has also been associated with endocrine abnormalities, renal osteodystrophy, and growth hormone therapy. SFCE has been reported to precede the diagnosis of hypothyroidism in an impressive number of cases (Puri and others, 1985).

The pathologic processes as seen in x-ray films involve first a rarefaction of bone on the lower femoral side of the epiphysis with widening of the growth plate. After trauma or slight injury the femoral portion of the epiphysis slides upward but remains attached by the thick, continuous periosteum. As slipping increases, the epiphyseal displacement becomes posterior and inferior. The slipping produces deformity of the femoral head and stretches the blood vessels to the epiphysis.

Clinical Manifestations

The following different varieties of clinical behavior have been observed: (1) an episode of trauma in which the epiphysis is acutely displaced in a previously functional joint; (2) gradual displacement without definite injury with progressively increased hip disability; (3) intermittent bouts of displacement alternating with periods of well-being with gradual appearance of symptoms associated with ambulation (such as external rotation); and (4) a combined gradual and traumatic displacement, in which there is gradual slippage with further displacement caused by injury.

Slipped femoral epiphysis is suspected when an adolescent or preadolescent youngster, especially one who is obese or tall and lanky, begins to limp and complains of pain in the hip continuously or intermittently. The pain is frequently referred to the groin, anteromedial aspect of the thigh, or knee. Physical examination reveals early restriction of internal rotation on adduction and external rotation deformity with loss of abduction and internal rotation as the severity increases. The diagnosis is confirmed by radiographic examination.

Therapeutic Management

The treatment varies with the degree of displacement but involves surgical stabilization and correction of deformity. In mild cases simple pin fixation is sufficient. More extensive displacement requires skeletal traction followed by pin fixation or osteotomy. The prognosis depends on the degree of deformity and the occurrence of complications, such as avascular necrosis and cartilaginous necrosis. As in other disorders, early diagnosis and implementation of therapy increase the likelihood of a satisfactory cure.

Nursing Considerations

Nursing care is the same as that for a child in a cast or a child in traction, discussed in Chapter 40.

KYPHOSIS AND LORDOSIS

The spine, consisting of numerous segments, can acquire deformation curves of three types: kyphosis, lordosis, and scoliosis (Fig. 39-7).

Kyphosis

Kyphosis is an abnormally increased convex angulation in the curvature of the thoracic spine (Fig. 39-7, *B*). It can occur secondary to disease processes such as tuberculosis, chronic arthritis, osteodystrophy, or compression fractures of the thoracic spine. The most common form of kyphosis is "postural." Children, especially during the time when skeletal growth outpaces growth of muscle, are prone to exaggeration of a tendency toward kyphosis. They assume bizarre sitting and standing positions. This is particularly common in self-conscious adolescent girls who assume a round-shouldered slouching posture in the attempt to hide their developing breasts.

Postural kyphosis is almost always accompanied by a compensatory postural lordosis, an abnormally exaggerated concave lumbar curvature. Treatment consists of postural exercises to strengthen shoulder and abdominal muscles and bracing for more marked deformity. Unfortunately treatment is difficult because of the nature of the adolescent personality. The normal rebellious tendencies of the adolescent together with continual parental nagging to "stand up straight" often interfere with compliance to a therapeutic regimen. The best approach is to emphasize the cosmetic value of corrective therapy and to place the responsibility on the adolescent for carrying out an exercise program at home with regular visits to and assessments by a therapist. Most adolescents respond well to selected sports as a supplement to regular exercise. Boys prefer weight lifting (preferably performed from a prone or supine position on a bench) and track sports. Girls respond well to dancing classes (ballet or modern dancing). Swimming is excellent and has the added

advantages of exercising all muscles, eliminating gravity, and teaching breath control.

Lordosis

Lordosis is an accentuation of the cervical or lumbar curvature beyond physiologic limits (Fig. 39-7, *C*). It may be a secondary complication of a disease process, the result of trauma, or idiopathic. It is often seen in association with flexion contractures of the hip, obesity, congenital dislocated hip, and slipped femoral capital epiphysis. During the pubertal growth spurt lordosis of varying degrees is observed in teenagers, especially girls. In obese children the weight of the abdominal fat alters the center of gravity, causing a compensatory lordosis. Unlike kyphosis, severe lordosis is usually accompanied by pain.

Treatment involves management of the predisposing cause when possible, such as weight loss and correction of deformities. Postural exercises and/or support garments are helpful in relieving symptoms in some cases; however, these do not usually affect a permanent cure.

SCOLIOSIS

Scoliosis, the most common spinal deformity, is a lateral curvature of the spine usually associated with a rotary deformity that eventually causes cosmetic and physiologic alterations in the spine, chest, and pelvis. It can appear at any age but is more frequent in adolescent girls.

Etiology

Scoliosis can be caused by a number of etiologic agents and may occur spontaneously or in association with other diseases or deformities. Scoliosis can be *structural* or *functional*. Functional, postural, or nonstructural scoliosis is caused by some other deformity, such as unequal leg length. The curve is flexible and corrects by bending. The curve may be postural with a slight curve that disappears when the child lies down or tries to compensate for a leg-length discrepancy. A transient scoliosis may be produced by pressure on a nerve root or inflammation. Functional scoliosis can be corrected by treating the underlying problem.

Structural scoliosis is characterized by changes in the spine and its supporting structures that causes loss of flexibility and noncorrectable deformity. The spine fails to straighten on side-bending, and a truly structural deformity displays a rotational deformity not observed in functional curvatures. Structural scoliosis may be congenital or a secondary defect associated with other disorders, especially neuromuscular disease or paralysis. In 70% of cases it is "idiopathic" without apparent cause; however, evidence indicates that it is probably genetic and transmitted as an autosomal-dominant trait with incomplete penetrance or is multifactorial. The various causes of structural scoliosis are outlined in the accompanying box.

Recent evidence has implicated neurologic deficits in the etiology of idiopathic scoliosis, although the site of damage is not apparent (Barrack and others, 1984). The primary def-

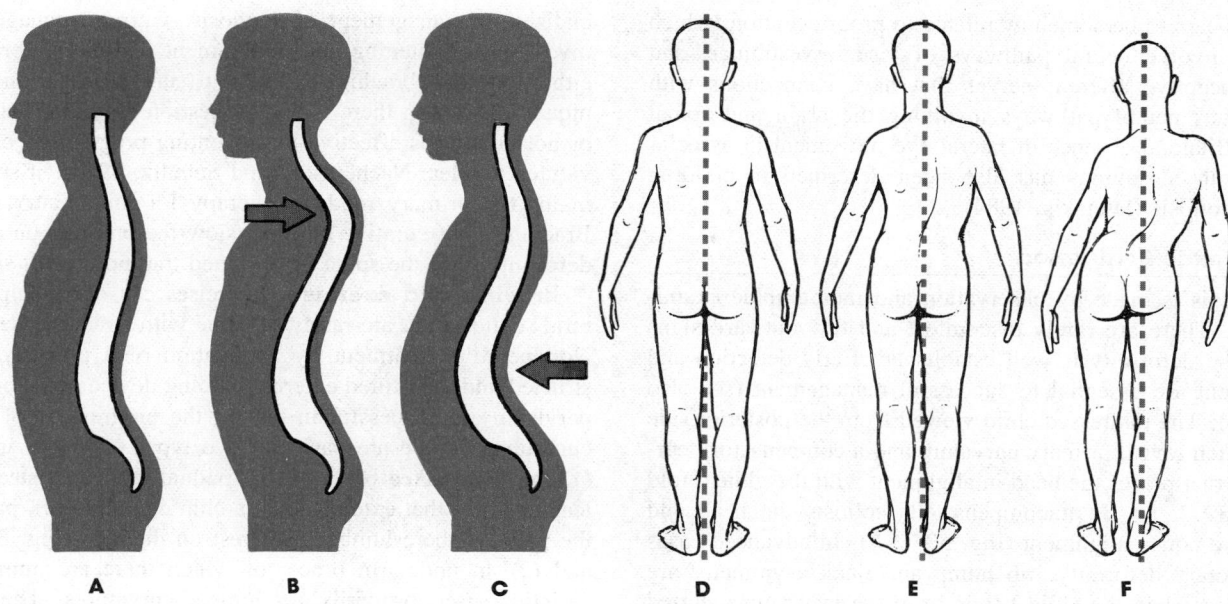

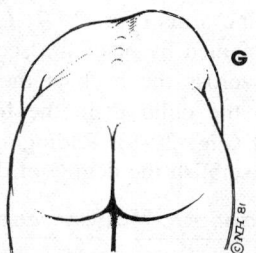

Fig. 39-7. Defects of spinal column. **A,** Normal spine. **B,** Kyphosis. **C,** Lordosis. **D,** Normal spine in balance. **E,** Mild scoliosis in balance. **F,** Severe scoliosis not in balance. **G,** Rib hump and flank asymmetry seen in flexion due to rotary component.
Redrawn from Hilt, N.E., and Schmitt, E.W.: Pediatric orthopedic nursing, St. Louis, 1975, The C.V. Mosby Co.

CAUSES OF STRUCTURAL SCOLIOSIS

Idiopathic (genetic) scoliosis
Infantile
    Age of onset—birth to 3 years of age
    More common in males
    Usually left thoracic curve
    Poor prognosis
Juvenile
    Age of onset—4 to 10 years of age
    More equal distribution between sexes
    Usually right thoracic curve
    Severity increases with growth
Adolescent
    Age of onset—10 years of age to skeletal maturity
    Predominant in females, about 7:1
    Right thoracic and thoracolumbar curves more common

Congenital scoliosis
Associated with meningomyelocele or other dysrhaphism
Hemivertebrae

Neuromuscular (paralytic) scoliosis
Caused by muscular imbalance
Neurogenic
    Lower motor neuron disease such as poliomyelitis, spinal muscular atrophy
    Upper motor neuron disease such as cerebral palsy
Myogenic
    Progressive disease such as muscular dystrophy
    Static disease such as amyotonia congenita
Mixed—weakness and overpull by stronger trunk muscles such as Friedreich ataxia

Neurofibromatosis
Short sharp thoracic curve often associated with kyphosis

Traumatic
Thoracogenic—result of thoracotomy and thoracoplasty with rib resection
Spinal trauma
    Irradiation such as tumor therapy
    Fractures

Spinal irritation
Spinal cord tumor
Nerve root irritation

Miscellaneous
Secondary to irritation
    Tumor
    Inflammation
Nutritional—rickets
Metabolic—renal osteodystrophy

Mesenchymal disease
Congenital disorders
    Dwarfism
    Disease of connective tissue such as arachnodactyly, arthrogryposis multiplex congenita
    Disease of bone such as osteogenesis imperfecta
Acquired disorders—rheumatoid arthritis

icit appears to be somehow related to proprioception, which could involve neural pathways of visual, vestibular, and proprioceptive afferent nerves that have connections with numerous neural pathways involving the brain and spinal cord. Bilateral absence of lateral eye movement in association with nystagmus has also been described in children with scoliosis (Dretakis, 1984).

Diagnostic Evaluation

Diagnosis is made by observation and radiographic examination. There are rarely discomfort and few outward signs until the deformity is well established. Early detection and treatment are essential to successful management (see also p. 276). The undressed child viewed from the posterior side will often reveal primary curvature and a compensatory curvature that places the head in alignment with the gluteal fold (Fig. 39-7, *E*). In uncompensated scoliosis the head and hips are not in alignment (Fig. 39-7, *F*). In advanced cases with rotary deformity, rib hump and flank asymmetry are observed when the child bends from the waist unsupported with the arms (Fig. 39-7, *G*). A clinical deformity can be documented by placing a scoliometer, a modified inclinometer, across the back at the point of maximum deformity while the child is in the forward-bent position (Bunnell, 1984) (Fig. 39-8). Radiographs taken in the standing position establish the degree of deformity.

Therapeutic Management: Nonoperative

A thorough examination, history, and assessment of the child are carried out in order to evaluate the status of the deformity, factors contributing to the defect, and factors that may influence the outcome of therapy. Treatment is best undertaken in a center in which a team is available that spe-

cializes in management of scoliosis. Current management involves straightening and realignment of the vertebrae by either external (bracing) or internal (surgical) fixation techniques. Although there is some question regarding whether or not bracing is effective in preventing progression of curvatures (Miller, Nachemson, and Schultz, 1984), it still remains the primary mode of therapy for minor curvatures. Bracing is not curative but may slow the progression of the deformity until the spine has reached the more adult size.

Bracing and exercise. Exercises can often help postural scoliosis but are rarely of value with structural defects. Nonoperative treatment by application of a properly constructed and well-fitted external bracing device and close supervision are successful in halting the progression of most curvatures. There are basically two types of braces in use: (1) the Milwaukee brace, an individually adapted steel and leather brace that extends from a chin cup and neck pads to the pelvis, where lumbar pads rest on the hips (Fig. 39-9), and (2) an underarm brace, of which there are numerous varieties, used primarily for lumbar curvatures. The Milwaukee brace is suitable for virtually all curves and is the benchmark of current orthotic treatment (Renshaw, 1985). The brace is used for minimum curvatures and is worn 23 hours a day but offers little interference with normal activity.

Supplemental exercises are employed daily both in and out of the brace to prevent atrophy of spinal and abdominal muscles. The brace is adjusted at regular trimonthly intervals and, when radiographic examinations reveal bone maturity, the child is gradually weaned from the brace over a 1- to 2-year period. The brace is then worn only at night until the spine is absolutely mature. An underarm modification of the Milwaukee brace has been designed that is

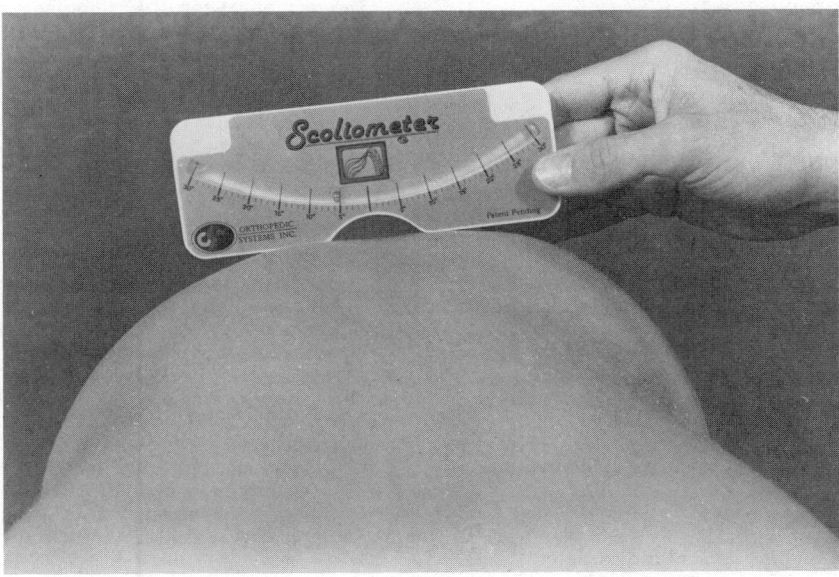

Fig. 39-8. Scoliometer used to document clinical deformity seen in patients with scoliosis.

From Bunnell, W.P.: Nonoperative treatment of spinal deformity: the case for observation. In AAOS: Instructional course lectures, vol. 36, St. Louis, 1985, The C.V. Mosby Co., p. 108.

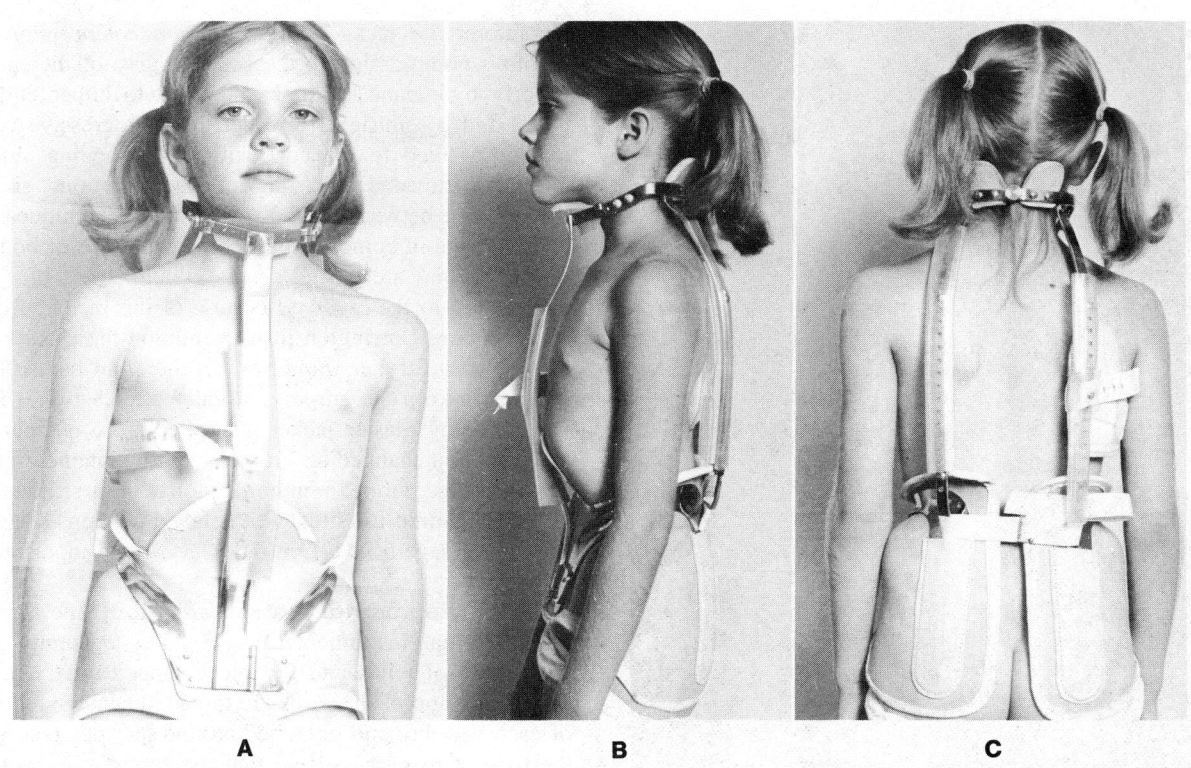

Fig. 39-9. Milwaukee brace. **A,** Front view; **B,** side view; **C,** rear view.
From Blount, W.P. and Mueller, K.H.: Praxis **8:**139-149, June 1972.

receiving greater patient acceptance. An orthoplast jacket is molded with specific built-in corrective forces for each patient. However, its use is limited to patients with low curvatures.

Electrical stimulation. Many young patients with mild to moderate curvatures have an alternative to bracing in the form of electrical stimulation. An electrical stimulator generates an electrical pulse that is transmitted to muscles on the convex side of the curvature. The electrical stimulation causes the muscles to contract at regular and frequent intervals, straightening the spine. Stimulators currently available involve either electrodes taped to the skin surface over standard electrode gel and attached to a battery-operated mechanism or surgically implanted receiver and leads coupled to an external transmitter by an external antenna. The devices are worn at night, allowing unrestricted activity during waking hours.

The stimulation, although not painful, may be associated with an uncomfortable sensation, and transient sleep problems are usual during the first month of treatment. Surface stimulators are poorly tolerated by children under 10 years of age. The cost of surface stimulation compares favorably with the cost of bracing, but the implanted option is considerably higher and involves hospitalization for the implant procedure.

Reports indicate that stimulation prevents progression of scoliosis in the majority of patients. There are advantages and disadvantages to the treatment, however. Skin irritation is a common complication of surface stimulation, and the implant stimulators require two surgical procedures—one for placement and one for removal (McCollough, 1985).

Therapeutic Management: Operative

Surgical intervention may be required for correction. The indications for surgery are:

Physiologic: Pulmonary function is diminished considerably, approximately 50%
Functional: Children with neurologic disabilities have difficulty sitting or walking because of imbalance
Cosmetic: Some children whose curvature is amenable to bracing are unable to use that therapy because of a self-image problem
Pain: Although rare in children, some older youngsters may have chronic discomfort from sitting on one buttock continually; pressure sores become a problem

With few exceptions the techniques consist of spinal realignment and straightening by way of external or internal fixation and instrumentation combined with bony fusion (arthrodesis) of the realigned spine. The degree of curvature and the cause determine the decision for surgery. Bracing and exercise have been universally disappointing in curves greater than 40 degrees, and paralytic and congenital curves, which will eventually progress, are best treated with early surgical stabilization. Age of the child and location of the curvature influence the decision for surgery, and any curve that does not respond to more conservative measures requires surgical correction.

For the most severe scoliotic curvatures, traction is often

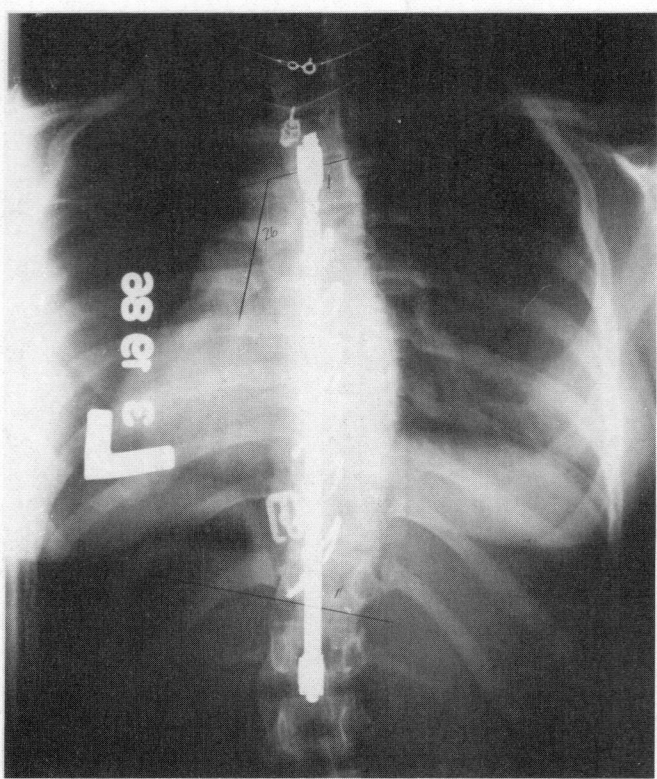

Fig. 39-10. Harrington rod with Luque wires.
Courtesy Dr. Mark Capehart, Tulsa, OK.

needed for a time before spinal fusion to provide partial correction and more flexibility. Methods incorporating either continuous or intermittent traction are employed. One type consists of a leather head halter and pelvic girdle attached to a system of ropes and pulleys that can be manipulated by the patient. More rigid deformities are best managed by skeletal traction techniques.

The traction is applied to the spine by way of a metal ring, or halo, attached to the skull and pins inserted into either the distal femur or the iliac wings of the pelvis. With halo-femoral traction the child is placed on a special Stryker frame, and progressive traction is applied by weight in twice daily increments. Halo-pelvic traction is applied by means of turnbuckles, and the child can remain ambulatory. Another alternative is halo-wheelchair traction, applied by means of a pulley system and weights suspended from behind the chair, using the weight of the child's upright body for countertraction. The halo is used both preoperatively and postoperatively. Casting is used by some orthopedists, but success with these techniques is variable.

Harrington instrumentation. The most frequently performed operative techniques for correction of the deformity involve the implantation of a rigid metal appliance. The *Harrington distraction* system consists of a metal rod applied to the *concave* side of the scoliotic curve, with cannulated hooks attached to the vertebra at each end of the curve. The spine is straightened by progressive distraction between the hooks in a manner similar to the mechanism of

an automobile jack. The *Harrington compression* system employs compression to the *convex* curve of the spine posteriorly by means of hooks attached to either end of the curve and a semirigid, threaded rod. Progressive compression is applied to the convexity by advancing small nuts along the threaded rod from opposite directions, shortening the distance between the hooks. The two techniques are frequently used in combination. Chips and strips of bone (from ilium or tibia) are placed across prepared vertebrae to provide fusion to the involved portion of the vertebral column.

Following Harrington instrumentation the child is immobilized on a Stryker frame. When the child has sufficiently recovered from the surgery, usually after 8 to 12 days, an immobilizing plaster jacket is applied from occiput to pelvis, which is changed at 3 months and maintained for a total of 6 months. Further immobilization with a removable cast may be required for sites with delayed healing. Regular follow-up management is continued at 3- to 6-month intervals for 3 to 5 years.

Luque segmental instrumentation. The Luque segmental spinal instrumentation provides segmental stability by the use of wires and flexible L-shaped rods. By way of a posterior approach, wires are threaded beneath the laminae of each vertebra and tightened around the rods resting along the transverse processes so that the spinal column is stabilized by transverse traction on each vertebra. After the rods are wired in place, the anesthesia is lightened and the patient requested to wiggle the toes to ensure no spinal cord involvement. The patient is reanesthetized and the spine fused with a bone graft taken from the iliac crest. The advantage to this procedure is that the patient can walk within a few days and no postoperative immobilization is required. The disadvantage is a possibility of spinal nerve damage.

Dwyer instrumentation. The Dwyer instrumentation and fusion technique involves transfixing cannulated screws to each vertebra in the curvature, then threading a titanium cable through the cannulae of the screw heads. When satisfactory correction is achieved, the screw heads are crimped to the cable, and bone chips (obtained from the iliac bone) are placed between adjacent vertebral bodies to facilitate fusion. Tension is then applied to the cable to maintain alignment. This procedure requires an anterior approach, but because the cable does not provide rigid fixation, a supplemental fusion via a posterior approach is needed. The Dwyer procedure is performed less frequently in children with idiopathic scoliosis but is well suited to treatment of spina bifida. Children with Dwyer instrumentation are cared for in bed.

Other. Other surgical procedures have been tried and proved successful in selected cases. Many of the current procedures combine the features of the methods previously described. Various modifications of the Harrington procedure are used. One that is used infrequently combines the Harrington and Dwyer (Zielke) procedures. A newer approach uses the distraction force of the Harrington rods plus the strength of Luque segmentation (Cotrel-Dubdousset procedure) (Fig. 39-10).

Nursing Considerations

Treatment for scoliosis extends over a significant portion of the affected child's period of growth. In adolescents this period is the one in which their identity, physical and psychologic, is formed. For some youngsters much of this time is spent in the hospital setting immobilized in complex, unattractive appliances. For those treated on an outpatient basis it means a modified life-style and being "different" from their peers, even though they are usually able to engage in many activities enjoyed by other youngsters.

When the child first faces the prospect of a prolonged period in a brace, cast, or other device, the therapy program and the nature of the device must be explained thoroughly to the child and parents so that they will have an understanding of the anticipated results, how the appliance corrects the defect, the freedoms and constraints imposed by the device, and what they can do to help achieve the desired goal. The management involves the skills and services of a team of specialists, including the orthopedist, physical therapist, orthotist (a specialist in fitting orthopedic braces), nurse, social worker, and sometimes a pulmonary specialist.

It is difficult for a child to be restricted at any phase of development, but the teenager needs continual positive reinforcement, encouragement, and as much independence as can be safely assumed during this time. Although adolescents cope well for the first year or two after casting, problems may arise as the time extends. Nurses need to be aware of this and be prepared to provide support and encouragement if problems arise (Davis and Lewis, 1984). Guidance and assistance regarding anticipated problems, such as selection of clothing and participation in social activities, are appreciated by adolescent youngsters. Socialization with peers should be encouraged and every effort expended to help the adolescent feel attractive and worthwhile.

Since many persons view any disability as deviant, the child will need help in learning how to deal with reactions of others to the appliance. Preparation for such responses places the child at an advantage. The best approach is usually to initiate the interaction by mentioning the device and its purpose. This alleviates the ambiguity surrounding the appliance and its purpose and reduces the anxiety on the part of the child and the other person. Most importantly the child should be helped to view the condition and appliance in a positive way and avoid seeing them as a stigma. There are youngsters who have the education and peer counseling and support who find positive aspects to wearing a brace in addition to improved posture and relief of symptoms. They enjoy the increased attention from peers and the experience of "being different" (Gratz and Papalia-Finlay, 1984).

Preoperative care. The child hospitalized for surgical management requires preparation for the procedures involved, which are puzzling and often frightening to the very young patient. They need to know what is going to happen, especially during the traction procedures, and a full explanation of why the procedure is necessary (one child thought that the traction was applied to "break" the bones) and of the potential outcome of the surgery.

During the progressive traction application the patient needs to be observed carefully for signs of neurologic impairment. Assessments of neurologic function are performed regularly and include assessment of the nerves both distally and proximally to the curvature. Particular attention should be paid to the cranial nerves and deep tendon reflexes in the extremities. Loss of lateral gaze and the inability to follow a moving object is an early sign of excessive neurologic traction. Other early signs include hyperreflexia of the lower extremities and dysesthesia in a glove and stocking distribution (Micheli, Magin, and Rouvales, 1979). (See Nursing care of the child in traction, p. 1811, for care of specific management and care.)

Postoperative care. Postoperatively patients are monitored in an intensive care unit. They are placed on an egg-carton mattress to prevent pressure areas, and the child with Harrington instrumentation will be placed on a Stryker frame, which facilitates care and lessens the possibility of damage to the fusion and indwelling instruments from twisting the spine and the possibility of "popping out" the rods. Nurses who work with these appliances should become familiar with their mechanism before assuming responsibility for patient care. The child who is not on a Stryker frame must be carefully logrolled when turned.

In addition to the usual postoperative assessments—of wound, circulation, and vital signs—the neurologic status of the patient requires special attention, especially that of the extremities. Prompt recognition of any neurologic impairment is imperative because delayed paralysis may develop that requires removal of the instrumentation. The patient is encouraged to exercise by contracting and relaxing the thigh and calf muscles periodically.

There is usually some degree of paralytic ileus following the procedure; therefore nursing includes care of the nasogastric intubation and assessment for returning bowel function. Urinary retention is common and often requires insertion of an indwelling catheter. Because of the extensive blood loss during the surgical procedure and renal hypoperfusion, observation of urinary output is especially important.

The child usually has considerable pain for the first few days following surgery and requires frequent administration of pain medication (see p. 1068). Because of the anterior approach, patients with Dwyer instrumentation also require thoracotomy care in addition to the care related to the fusion and realignment procedures.

Children with a Luque procedure are kept flat for 12 hours before logrolling is begun. The head of the bed can be elevated on the second day and range of motion exercises begun. Activity is begun by instructing the patient to roll from a side-lying position to a sitting position. Next walking slowly with the aid of a safety belt and walker is allowed, and finally unassisted ambulation, which is usually achieved by the sixth day.

All patients are started on physiotherapy as soon as they are able, beginning with range of motion exercises and many of the activities of daily living. Self-care such as washing and eating is always encouraged. Some simple physical therapy may be begun during this acute stage. Throughout the hospitalization diversionary activities and contact with family and friends are an important part of nursing care and planning.

The family is encouraged to become involved with the patient's care to facilitate the transition from hospital to home management. Family members learn to apply and care for the brace or learn cast care, with special attention to jagged edges on the cast, padding of the appliance, and daily skin checks for reddened areas, especially in areas such as under the arms or over the hips. They may need assistance in modifying the environment for limited ambulation and acquiring needed home care items such as an egg-crate mattress, straight-backed chair, and a raised toilet seat. The child and family need to learn efficient ways to move and carry out various activities of daily living. The diet may require modification. Overeating and constipation can be problems related to limited activity.

Detection. One of the major functions of nurses is to learn to detect the presence of scoliosis. Screening procedures are simple and require only a 30-second observation. Unfortunately, studies have indicated that current screening procedures are less than ideal (Morais and others, 1985; Viviani and others, 1984), and too many children are exposed to radiographs in the attempt to rule out scoliosis in normal children. Methods of improving the effectiveness of screening and the application to all school children should be a goal of nursing.

Several organizations provide education and services to both families and professionals. The **National Scoliosis Foundation, Inc.** * is devoted to awareness and action for early detection and prevention of spinal deformity. They offer educational support materials for parents, schools, and health care providers. A lists of books, pamphlets, and other materials are available on request. The **Scoliosis Association,** † a national self-help group, has a number of chapters throughout the United States, and The **Scoliosis Research Society,** ‡ an organization of physicians and scientists, has published an excellent book, "Scoliosis: A Handbook for Patients."

---

*P.O. Box 547, Belmont, MA 02178.
†1 Penn Plaza, New York, NY 10119.
‡ 444 North Michigan Ave., Chicago, IL 60611. The book can be purchased by sending $1.00 to the organization.

Nursing Care Summary: The Child with Mild Structural Scoliosis

NURSING GOALS	NURSING INTERVENTIONS	EXPECTED PATIENT/FAMILY OUTCOMES
HP-HMP Injury: potential for trauma **Risk factors: unaccustomed brace**		
Prevent injury	Assess environment for hazards Teach safety precautions such as using handrail on stairways and avoiding slippery surfaces Help develop safe methods of mobilization	Child remains free of accidents related to wearing brace
Help child adjust to restricted movement	Demonstrate alternative modes of accomplishing tasks such as getting in and out of bed, dressing Help devise alternatives for restricted activities and coping with awkwardness	Child demonstrates appropriate adaptation to corrective device (specify)
N-MP Skin integrity, impairment of: potential **Risk factors: brace**		
Prevent skin irritation and breakdown	Examine skin surfaces in contact with brace for signs of irritation Implement corrective action to treat or prevent skin breakdown	Skin remains clean with no evidence of irritation
SP-SCP Self-concept, disturbance in: body image **Etiology: perception of defect in body structure**		
Assist in physical adjustment to appliance	Assess brace and its fit Attempt to determine source of any discomfort Refer to orthotist for needed adjustment and service Assist with plan for personal hygiene Help in selection of appropriate apparel to wear over brace and footwear to maintain proper balance	Brace fits well and produces no discomfort Child complies with directions for wear and care of brace Child is well groomed and wears attractive attire

Nursing Care Summary: The Child with Mild Structural Scoliosis —cont'd

NURSING GOALS	NURSING INTERVENTIONS	EXPECTED PATIENT/FAMILY OUTCOMES
	Reinforce teaching regarding removal and reapplication of appliance	
	Investigate any complaints of discomfort	
Promote positive self-concept	Encourage child to discuss feelings about wearing brace	Child verbalizes feelings and concerns
	Emphasize positive aspects and eventual outcome	Child plans in terms of long-range goals as well as short-range ones

RRP **Family process, alteration in**
Etiology: situational crisis (child with a structural defect)

Prepare for application of brace	Reinforce and clarify explanations provided by orthopedist—explanations of Appliance Plan of care Activities allowed/restricted Child's and family's responsibilities in therapy Prepare child and family for surgery if indicated	Child and family demonstrate an understanding of teaching (specify learning and method of demonstration)
Continue ongoing evaluation	Be alert to comments by child or family members that indicate possible problems Recommend screening for other family members	Problems are dealt with early
Encourage compliance to regimen	Establish communication with child and family Assess understanding of plan of care Instruct child and family in various aspects of therapy and care as needed Provide feedback and praise for positive behavior Provide assistance and encouragement when needed Arrange appointments Assist family with transportation to appointments Identify goals with achievable outcomes Include family in setting goals Allow to express discouragement at what appears to be slow progress and interference with activities	Child and family comply with directions regarding corrective device
Promote normal growth and development	Encourage independence where appropriate Allow for dependence when needed Involve in scheduling appointments and other aspects of care Encourage school attendance and socialization with peers Encourage involvement in activities compatible with limitations	Child assumes responsibility for self-care and management of corrective device
Help child develop positive self-image	Accentuate positive aspects of appearance Motivate to develop good habits of personal hygiene Encourage to wear attractive clothes and hairstyle Emphasize positive long-term outcome Help devise positive ways to deal with reactions of others	Child engages in age-appropriate activities
Provide for supportive services	Refer to social services for financial assistance, transportation, etc., if needed Refer to specialized agencies for information and education Determine if referrals were utilized	Family members avail themselves of assistance when needed

Orthopedic Infections

Infections of bones and joints are not uncommon and often pose a problem of diagnosis because of their similarity of symptoms. The most frequently observed infection is osteomyelitis, and in populations where tuberculosis is endemic, this disease is encountered increasingly in nursing practice.

OSTEOMYELITIS

Osteomyelitis, an infectious process of bone, can occur at any age but occurs most frequently between ages 5 and 14. It is twice as common in boys as in girls.

Etiology

Any organism can cause osteomyelitis, and there is some relationship between the age of the child and the type of organism responsible. In older children staphylococci are the most common organisms, approximately 80% of which are *Staphylococcus aureus;* in younger children other organisms predominate, especially *Haemophilus influenzae.* A recent report describes *Pseudomonas aeruginosa* osteomyelitis acquired from puncture wounds. The organism was present in the soles of the sneakers the children were wearing (Fisher, Goldsmith, and Gilligan, 1985). In children with sickle cell anemia *Salmonella* organisms are frequently responsible for osteomyelitis.

Osteomyelitis can be acquired from *exogenous* or *hematogenous* sources. Exogenous osteomyelitis is acquired by invasion of the bone by direct extension from the outside as a result of a penetrating wound, open fracture, contamination during surgery, or secondary extension from an overlying abscess or burn.

Hematogenous spread of organisms from a preexisting focus is the most common source of infection. Common sources of foci include furuncles, skin abrasions, impetigo, upper respiratory tract infection, acute otitis media, tonsillitis, abscessed teeth, pyelonephritis, or infected burns. Other factors that predispose to development of osteomyelitis are poor physical condition, poor nutrition, and surroundings that are not hygienic.

Pathophysiology

Infective emboli from the focus of infection travel to the small end arteries in the bone metaphysis, where they set up an infectious process. The infection does not spread to the epiphysis, since it has a blood supply separate from the metaphysis. The infectious process leads to local bone destruction and abscess formation. The abscess with its collected necrotic debris exerts pressure within the rigid, unyielding bone and ruptures into the subperiosteal space, where the pressure lifts and strips the periosteum. The infection spreads beneath the periosteum, causing thrombosis of vessels and adding further to the bony necrosis.

In infants and very young children the elevated periosteum attempts to wall off the infection by forming new bone—*involucrum.* Underneath, the cortex, deprived of blood supply, dies and the necrotic bone that cannot be absorbed continues to produce more intraosseous tension and necrosis. Granulation forms around the dead bone, or *sequestrum.* Sinuses may form between the sequestra and the skin surface or into a joint to create a suppurative arthritis. Small areas of sequestrum may be absorbed, but larger areas surrounded by dense bone become honeycombed with sinuses that retain infective material and cause exacerbations for years (the chronic stage of osteomyelitis).

Clinical Manifestations

Signs and symptoms of *acute* hematogenous osteomyelitis begin abruptly and build up to a maximum intensity during the first few days of the disease, usually less than 1 week. There is frequently a history of trauma to the affected bone.

The child with acute osteomyelitis appears very ill. He is irritable and restless with elevated temperature, rapid pulse, and dehydration. There is usually localized tenderness, increased warmth, and diffuse swelling over the involved bone. The extremity is painful, especially on movement. The child holds it in semiflexion, and the surrounding muscles are tense and resist passive movement. Most cases involve the femur or tibia and to a lesser extent the humerus and hip. In infants the diagnosis is more difficult because of lack of systemic symptoms. The disorder may involve multiple bones or joints because of the difficulty in confining an infectious process in children in this age-group.

In *subacute* hematogenous osteomyelitis symptoms have been present for a longer period and the child sometimes has been treated with antibiotics, often for another infection, which modify the clinical symptoms. In some instances the infection may produce a walled-off abscess rather than a spreading infection.

Diagnostic Evaluation

In acute osteomyelitis there is marked leukocytosis and an elevated erythrocyte sedimentation rate. Blood culture is usually positive during the early stage, but radiographic findings are often negative or show only soft tissue swelling for 10 to 14 days. After this time the radiographic findings reveal new bone formation. Tomography may reveal bone changes at an early stage, and scintigraphy reveals a greater uptake of radionucleotides in osteomyelitic bone than in normal bone.

Similar symptoms are observed in rheumatic fever, rheumatoid arthritis, leukemia and other malignant lesions, cellulitis, erysipelas, and scurvy. Sometimes the osteomyelitis may be unrecognized if it occurs as a complication of a severe toxic and debilitating illness.

Therapeutic Management

As soon as blood cultures have been drawn, prompt and vigorous intravenous antibiotic therapy is initiated. The choice is influenced by age, and the dosage determined is sufficient to ensure high blood and tissue levels. Since most cases of osteomyelitis are caused by staphylococci, large doses of penicillin G are administered and supplemented by methicillin or oxacillin. In children younger than 3 years of age, the infectious agents are more apt to be penicillin-resistant staphylococci or gram-negative organisms; therefore the agents of choice are usually methicillin, nafcillin, or clindamycin in conjunction with ampicillin. Neonates in whom coliform organisms are likely to be involved are given kanamycin or gentamicin, either intramuscularly or *slowly* intravenously in addition to intravenously administered ampicillin.

When the infective agent is identified, the appropriate antibiotic is usually continued for at least 3 to 4 weeks, but the length of therapy is determined by the duration of symptoms, the initial response to treatment, and the sensitivity of the organism in the specific case. Because of prolonged high-dose therapy, it is important to monitor hematologic, renal, hepatic, and other organ systems that might be adversely affected by the drugs.

Antibiotic therapy is accompanied by local treatment. The child is placed on complete bed rest, and immobilization of the affected extremity, which may require a splint or bivalved cast, is continued throughout therapy to limit the spread of infection and, when it is a complication of a fracture, to maintain alignment of bone fragments. Weight bearing on the nonfractured leg is prohibited to avoid the possibility of pathologic fracture.

Opinions differ regarding surgical intervention, but many advocate sequestrectomy and surgical drainage to decompress the metaphyseal space before pus erupts and spreads to the subperiosteal space to form abscesses that strip the periosteum from bone or form draining sinuses. When these complications occur, a chronic infection usually persists. When surgical drainage is carried out, polyethylene tubes are placed in the wound—one tube instills an antibiotic solution directly into the infected area by gravity, and the other, connected to a suction apparatus, provides drainage.

Nursing Considerations

During the acute phase of illness any movement of the affected limb will cause discomfort to the child; therefore he should be positioned comfortably with the affected limb supported. Moving and turning are carried out carefully and gently to minimize discomfort. The child may require pain medication or sedation. Vital signs are taken and recorded frequently, and measures are implemented to reduce a significant temperature elevation.

Antibiotic therapy requires careful observation and monitoring of the intravenous equipment and site. Since more than one antibiotic is usually administered, the compatibility of the drugs must be determined and care taken to avoid mixing noncompatible drugs. A double, or piggyback, setup is safest so that there is less opportunity for the two drugs to come in contact with each other. The stability of the drugs and their toxic nature are also considered when deter-

mining the rate of administration. The needle must be well situated in the vein to ensure that the drug does not infiltrate into surrounding tissues where it may produce tissue damage. For this type of long-term antibiotic therapy, the heparin lock is the preferred method of intravenous administration.

The child with an open wound is placed on complete or wound isolation precautions, depending on the policies of the institution. The wound is managed according to the directions of the physician. Antibiotic solution administered directly into the wound is most efficiently accomplished with a regular intravenous infusion setup that is prepared and regulated as any intravenous infusion. The drainage tubes are connected to low Gomco or wall suction for continuous removal. Intake and output are measured and recorded, and the character of the wound drainage is noted. The amount and character of drainage on wound dressing are also noted.

Casts are sometimes employed for immobilization, and, if so, routine cast care is carried out. The extremity is examined for sensation, circulation, and pain, and the area over the inflammation is usually left open for observation. The affected area, casted or uncasted, is assessed for color, swelling, heat, and tenderness.

The child usually has a poor appetite and may be subject to vomiting. Nourishment in the form of high-calorie liquids such as fruit juices, gelatin, and juice bars should be encouraged until the child begins to feel better. The appetite returns as the acute symptoms subside. During convalescence adequate nutrition must be maintained to aid healing and reconstitution of new bone.

When the acute stage subsides, the child begins to feel better, his appetite improves, and he becomes interested in his surroundings and relationships. He wishes to move about in bed and is allowed to do so. However, weight bearing on the affected limb is not permitted until healing is well under way in order to avoid pathologic fractures. Diversional and constructive activities become important nursing interventions. The child is usually confined to bed for some time after the acute phase but may be allowed to move about the unit on a gurney or in a wheelchair when isolation and bed rest are no longer necessary. At this stage the continuous intravenous infusion may be replaced by a heparin lock to allow greater freedom.

As the infection subsides, physical therapy is instituted to ensure restoration of optimum function. The child is usually discharged with oral antibiotics, and his progress is followed closely for some time.

SEPTIC (SUPPURATIVE, PYOGENIC, PURULENT) ARTHRITIS

The source of infection of the joints, like infection of bone, is usually by hematogenous dissemination and spread from another focus. Occasionally it may result from direct extension of a soft tissue infection. The infection occurs predominantly in males, especially in the adolescent age-group. In infancy the age distribution is more nearly equal. Any joint may be involved, but the hip, knee, shoulder, and other large joints are more commonly affected. It usually affects only one joint.

The signs and symptoms of suppurative arthritis, unlike osteomyelitis, are usually characteristic. The presence of a warm and tender joint, painful on even gentle pressure, is sufficient to differentiate it from osteomyelitis, in which gentle passive motion is tolerated. When superficial joints are involved, they are exquisitely painful and swollen; deep-seated joints show little superficial evidence. In most instances there is history of a traumatic injury to the affected joint. Fever, leukocytosis, and increased erythrocyte sedimentation rate are present but may not be demonstrated in affected infants.

The most common pathogens are *Staphylococcus aureus,* group A streptococci, and *Haemophilus influenzae.* Diagnosis is made from blood culture, joint fluid aspirate, and radiograms.

Therapeutic Management and Nursing Considerations

Treatment consists of open surgical drainage of hip and shoulder joint disease and repeated needle aspirations of the joint space in other joints. The goals are (1) to cleanse the joint to avoid destruction of articular cartilage, (2) to decompress the joint to avoid interference with the blood supply to the epiphysis, (3) to eradicate the infection with adequate antibiotic therapy, and (4) to prevent secondary bone infection and hematogenous spread. Therapy is similar to that for osteomyelitis: intravenous antibiotic therapy, relief of pain, immobilization of the joint, and prohibition of weight bearing until healing is complete. Nursing care is the same as that for osteomyelitis.

TUBERCULOSIS

Tubercular infection of the bones is acquired by hematogenous dissemination from a primary tubercular focus. The most common sites in infants and small children are the carpals and phalanges and corresponding bones of the feet. One or several bones may be involved, with spindle-shaped swelling and tenderness as soft tissues are affected. The process, relatively painless, persists with intermittent symptoms for several months and may leave a permanent deformity. Affected areas are immobilized with a splint or cast.

Tuberculosis of Spine (Tuberculous Spondylitis)

In older children the infection attacks the body of one or more vertebrae, destroying the bone, and spreads to all the articular tissues, producing a kyphotic deformity. The lower thoracic spine is most frequently affected. Symptoms are insidious. The child will be irritable and complain of persistent or intermittent pain over the areas innervated by spinal nerves that arise adjacent to the affected vertebrae. There is muscle splinting and pain when increased pressure is placed on the child's head. The child assumes a position that best eases the weight on the diseased vertebrae, such as avoiding bending and walking stiffly and carefully on the toes, and prefers to rest on the abdomen or across a chair or a lap.

Treatment is immobilization with extension on a Bradford frame or plaster body cast until there is no evidence of active infection followed by spinal fusion. Antimicrobial therapy and drainage of tubercular abscess are standard therapies. The reparative process is slow, but in most instances recovery takes place with little or no deformity. Nursing care is similar to care of the child with scoliosis.

Tuberculosis of Hip

The hip is the joint most commonly affected by tuberculosis, but the process usually begins in the epiphysis of the femoral head and then erupts into the joint capsule. The initial manifestation is a limp that occurs intermittently, most often on arising in the morning or after exercise. There is progressive destruction of the femoral head with symptoms of pain, and the thigh gradually becomes fixed and adducted with internal rotation. There may be swelling around the hip and abscess formation.

Treatment involves bed rest, traction to reduce muscle spasm, and appropriate drug therapy. Hip fusion may be necessary in severe cases.

Skeletal and Articular Dysfunction

There are a variety of disorders involving bones. Fractures of bones are relatively common in childhood (see Chapter 40). Rickets is less common but is still a preventable disease in most instances, and uncommon disorders of bone and connective tissue such as arachnodactyly (Marfan syndrome) and achondroplasia do not cause immobilization. Bone tumors (see Chapter 36) are dreaded diseases, and bone infections are responsible for significant morbidity. There are other rare disorders, but only one—osteogenesis imperfecta— is elaborated further.

The most prominent articular disorder in children is rheumatoid arthritis. Although usually classified as a collagen disease, lupus erythematosus is also considered in this section because a frequent symptom is joint discomfort.

OSTEOGENESIS IMPERFECTA

Osteogenesis imperfecta (OI) is a group of heterogenous inherited disorders of connective tissue and characterized by connective tissue and bone defects including one or more of the following: varying degrees of bone fragility leading to fractures, blue sclerae, progressive bone deformities, presenile hearing loss, and dentinogenesis, hypoplastic teeth with an opalescent blue or brown discoloration of teeth (Cohen, 1984). The inheritance pattern is autosomal-dominant in the majority of cases, although the most severe form demonstrates autosomal-recessive inheritance.

Persons with OI appear to have abnormal precollagen type I that prevents the formation of collagen, the major component of connective tissue. The precollagen remains relatively inert and unable to undergo final transformation into collagen. Consequently, bone of these patients consists of large areas of osseous tissues devoid of an organized trabecular pattern and increased numbers of large osteoblasts. Lamellae, when present, are very thin. The more severe the degree of OI, the greater the number of osteocytes and the greater the disruption of the normal architectural patterns of the bone.

At present OI is believed to consist of four different variations as outlined in Table 39-2. Type II, the most severe form of OI, is characterized by multiple intrauterine or perinatal fractures and severe deformity and, often, early death. The brittle nature of the bones renders them easily fractured by the slightest trauma.

The diseases of later onset run a milder course. The tendency to fracture appears later (at variable ages) and disappears after puberty. During childhood the shafts of long bones are slender with reduced cortical thickness resulting from defective periosteal bone formation. In addition to the features already described, the child with OI has thin skin, hyperextensibility of ligaments, a tendency to recurrent epistaxis, excess diaphoresis, tendency to bruise easily, and mild hyperpyrexia. The disease shows variable expressivity, that is, the number and extent of pathologic features appear in any individual range, from severe to minimal involvement. The incidence of fractures decreases at puberty when the body's production of hormones helps strengthen bones.

The treatment is primarily supportive. Several drugs have been tried but appear to be of limited benefit. Lightweight braces and splints help support limbs, prevent fractures, and aid in ambulation. Physical therapy helps avoid disuse osteoporosis and strengthens muscles, which in turn improves bone density. Exercises are usually simple ones against light resistance or water exercises with swimming. Patients with milder disease are encouraged to participate in sports. Exercise also gives the child a sense of well-being and confidence in his body (Root, 1984).

Surgery is sometimes used to help treat the manifestations of the disease. Surgical techniques are used to correct deformities that interfere with bracing, standing, or walking. For the child with recurrent fractures, inserting an intermedullary rod provides stability to bones. Unfortunately the rods must be replaced as the child grows, otherwise fractures may occur through the unprotected portion of the bone.

Nursing Considerations

Infants and children with this disorder require careful handling to prevent fractures. They must be supported when turning, positioning, moving, and fondling. Even changing a diaper may cause a fracture in severely affected infants. These children should never be held by the ankles when diapering but gently lifted by the buttocks.

Both parents and the affected child need education re-

Table 39-2 Classification of osteogenesis imperfecta

TYPE		CHARACTERISTICS
I*	A	Mild bone fragility, blue sclerae, normal teeth, presenile deafness (age 20-30 years); autosomal-dominant inheritance
	B	Same as A except dentinogenesis imperfecta instead of normal teeth
	C	Same as B; no bone fragility
II		Lethal; stillborn or die in early infancy; severe bone fragility, multiple fractures at birth; 10% of OI cases; autosomal-recessive inheritance
III		Severe bone fragility leads to severe progressive deformities; normal sclerae; marked growth failure; most autosomal-recessive; few autosomal-dominant
IV	A	Mild to moderate bone fragility; normal sclerae; short stature; variable deformity; autosomal-dominant
	B	Same as A except dentinogenesis imperfecta instead of normal teeth; approximately 6% of OI cases

*Two thirds of cases are type I.

garding the child's limitations and guidelines in planning suitable activities that promote optimum development as well as protect him from harm. Realistic occupational planning and genetic counseling are part of the long-term goals of care. Educational materials and information can be obtained from the **Osteogenesis Imperfecta Foundation, Inc.*** and from the **American Brittle Bone Society.†** These organizations also have a network that can put a family in contact with other families with a similar problem.

JUVENILE ARTHRITIS

Clinically and pathologically juvenile arthritis (JA), juvenile rheumatoid arthritis (JRA), or juvenile chronic polyarthritis (CJA) is an inflammatory disease with an unknown inciting agent and a slight tendency to occur in families. Both infectious and autoimmune theories have been presented, but there is no convincing evidence to establish either one as an etiologic agent. There are two peak ages of onset: between 2 and 5 years of age and between 9 and 12 years of age. Females are affected somewhat more frequently than males. In many instances the disease remains undiagnosed for years.

Juvenile arthritis is, in many ways, similar to the adult disease, but there are many features that are quite distinct. A distinguishing feature is its tendency to occur in the prepubertal child. Characteristics of JA include negative results in the latex fixation test in 90% of cases: classic symptoms

*P.O. Box 838, Manchester, NH 03105.

†1256 Merrill Drive, Marshallton, West Chester, PA 19380.

of spiking fever, skin rash, or pericarditis in 5% to 10% of cases; tendency to be very mild in 70% of cases, with few joints involved; development of iridocyclitis as a complication in 8% to 20% of milder forms; and "burning itself out" over 2 to 3 years in milder forms and over 8 to 10 years in most other forms.

Pathophysiology

The rheumatic process is characterized by a chronic inflammation of the synovium with joint effusion and eventual erosion, destruction, and fibrosis of the articular cartilage. Adhesions between joint surfaces and ankylosis of joints occur if the process persists long enough.

Clinical Manifestations

Whether a single joint or multiple joints are involved, stiffness, swelling, and loss of motion develop in the affected joints. They are swollen and warm to the touch but seldom red. The swelling results from edema, joint effusion, and synovial thickening. The affected joints may be tender and painful to the touch or relatively painless. The limited motion, early in the disease, is the result of muscle spasm and joint inflammation; later it is caused by ankylosis or soft tissue contracture. Morning stiffness or "gelling" of the joint(s) is characteristic and present on arising in the morning or after inactivity. Infections, injuries, or operations often precipitate a flare-up of the arthritis; therefore prompt recognition and treatment of infections are necessary.

Growth may be retarded during periods of active disease, usually with growth spurts during remissions. In severe long-standing cases growth is significantly retarded. Corticosteroid therapy is also a contributing factor. There may be growth disturbances, either overgrowth or undergrowth, adjacent to the inflamed joints—for example, altered leg length after knee involvement and micrognathia (receding chin) from temporomandibular arthritis.

JA is a variable disease and is now recognized to pursue three major disease courses: *systemic onset, monoarticular* or *pauciarticular* (involving few joints, usually less than five), and *polyarticular* (simultaneous involvement of four or more joints). These groups, including subgroups, and the manifestations associated with each are outlined in Table 39-3.

Course. The outcome and sources of morbidity are variable and unpredictable in any individual patient. The disease, even in severe forms, is rarely life-threatening. Chronic joint pain is characteristic of polyarticular and systemic disease; the major morbidity in type I patients is chronic iridocyclitis (inflammation of the iris and ciliary body) and spondyloarthropathy in type II disease. There may be exacerbations and remissions or the symptoms may continue for years. The symptoms may cause little disability or (less commonly) are severe with joint destruction and permanent deformity. Although the disease usually remits at puberty, some patients continue to have active arthritis into adulthood.

The overall prognosis for children with JA is good. At least 75% eventually enter long remissions without signifi-

cant residual deformity or impaired function. The poorest prognosis is associated with rheumatoid factor–positive polyarthritis and systemic-onset disease. The most debilitating complications are severe hip disease and loss of vision from iridocyclitis (Schaller and Wedgwood, 1983).

Diagnostic Evaluation

The diagnosis of JA is one of exclusion, that is, differentiation from a variety of disorders with similar manifestations at the onset of the disease. Radiographic findings are variable, but the earliest manifestations are widening joint spaces followed by gradual evidence of fusion and articular destruction. There may be evidence of soft tissue swelling, osteoporosis, and periostitis around affected joints.

There are no specific diagnostic tests for JA. The erythrocyte sedimentation rate may or may not be elevated, depending on the degree of inflammation present. Leukocytosis is generally present in the early stages of classic systemic disease. The latex fixation test, the most common test used to detect the presence of rheumatoid factor in adults, is negative in 90% of juvenile cases. Rheumatoid factors are found in some children, usually those with disease of later onset. Antinuclear antibodies are found in three fourths of rheumatoid factor–positive and one fourth of rheumatoid factor–negative children and in pauciarticular type I diseases, but not in children with systemic onset or pauciarticular type II disease. There is a strong relationship between the presence of antinuclear antibodies and chronic iridocyclitis but no relationship to the severity of the disease.

Therapeutic Management

There is no specific cure for juvenile rheumatoid arthritis. The major goals of therapy are to preserve joint function, prevent physical deformities, and relieve symptoms without iatrogenic harm. This involves both initial and long-term planning, parent and patient education and counseling, physical and occupational therapy, good health and nutritional education and management, specific drug therapy, orthopedic consultation, and periodic eye examination (Brewer, 1986).

Whenever possible, the child is treated at home under the supervision of the health team, and intermittent treatment by qualified professionals is administered. Hospitalization may be needed during severe exacerbations or when intercurrent illness warrants. Iridocyclitis, which is unique to JA, is a not uncommon complication that requires the attention of an ophthalmologist.

Drugs. A variety of antirheumatic drugs are available, and most are effective in suppressing the inflammatory process and relieving pain. The drugs may be given alone or in combination. The most frequently prescribed drugs are the nonsteroidal antiinflammatory drugs.

NSAIDs. The primary group of drugs prescribed for JA are the nonsteroidal antiinflammatory drugs (NSAIDs). These include aspirin, tolmetin sodium, ibuprofen, and naproxen, among others. All these drugs act in a similar manner, and none is superior to the other in producing the de-

Table 39-3 Characteristics of juvenile arthritis related to mode of onset

	SYSTEMIC ONSET	PAUCIARTICULAR (TWO SUBTYPES)	POLYARTICULAR (TWO SUBTYPES)
Percentage of patients	30%	45%	25%
Age at onset	Bimodal distribution 1-3 years of age 8-10 years of age	Type I: Less than 10 years Type II: over 10 years	Throughout childhood and adolescence
Sex ratio (F:M)	1.5:1	Type I: almost all F Type II: 1:9	Mostly female
Joints involved	Any Only 20% have joint involvement at time of diagnosis	Usually confined to lower extremities—knee, ankle, and eventually sacroiliac; sometimes elbow	Any joints: usually symmetric involvement of small joints Hip involvement in 50% Spine involved in 50%
Extraarticular manifestations	Fever, malaise, myalgia, rash, pleuritis or pericarditis, adenomegaly, splenomegaly, hepatomegaly	Type I: chronic iridocyclitis; mucocutaneous lesions Type II: acute iridocyclitis; sacroiliitis common; eventual ankylosing spondylitis in many Type III: arthritis only	Systemic signs minimal Possible low-grade fever, malaise, weight loss, rheumatoid nodules, and/or vasculitis
Laboratory tests	Elevated ESR; RF negative; ANA rarely positive; anemia; leukocytosis	Elevated ESR; ANA positive Type I: HLA-DRW5 positive Type II: HLA-B27 positive Type III: HLA-TMo positive	Elevated ESR Type I: RF positive Type II: RF negative
Long-term prognosis	Mortality—1%-2% of all JA patients Joint destruction in 40%	Continuous disease; eventual remission in 60% Type I: ocular damage; functional blindness in 10% Type II: ankylosing spondylitis Type III: best outlook for recovery	Longer duration; more crippling; remission in 25% Type I: high incidence of disabling arthritis Type II: outlook good

sired effects—analgesic, antipyretic, and antiinflammatory. Reduction in fever takes place in hours, relief of pain occurs in a matter of hours or days (more often in weeks, however), but the antiinflammatory effect (reductions in swelling, pain on motion, tenderness, and limitation of motion of involved joints) does not occur for 30 to 37 days (Brewer, 1986). Consequently, these drugs should not be discontinued without an adequate trial period. Sometimes several drugs are tried before one or two are found that are effective and safe for any given child.

Since there is a narrow margin between effective and toxic doses, the levels are monitored regularly until the dosage is sufficient to maintain the optimum level and a satisfactory clinical response. The total daily dose is divided into four doses to be administered with each meal and at bedtime. Some find better compliance when the drug is given only twice daily.

SAARDs. The second group of drugs used to treat JA are the slower acting antirheumatic drugs (SAARDs). These include gold, D-penicillamine, and hydroxychloroquine. SAARD drugs may be added to the regimen when one or two NSAIDs have been ineffective. Injectable gold is the initial SAARD used. The weekly injections can be a problem with young children, but cooperation is important. An oral gold preparation is available but not yet approved for use in children. Hydroxychloroquine, an antimalarial drug that requires a longer period of time to effect a response, is seldom used in the United States.

Other drugs. Cytotoxic drugs such as cyclophosphamide, azathioprine, chlorambucil, and methotrexate are reserved for patients with severe debilitating disease and who have responded poorly to NSAIDs and SAARDs.

Corticosteroids are the most potent antiinflammatory agents available. However, they do not cure the disease or prevent joint damage, and their chronic side effects are undesirable. They are administered in the lowest effective dose, given on alternate days rather than daily, and used for the shortest period possible. Indications for daily corticosteroid (prednisone) therapy are life-threatening disease (such as pericarditis), incapacitating systemic disease unresponsive to other antiinflammatory therapy, and iridocyclitis.

Physical management. Programs of physical management are individualized for each child and designed to reach the ultimate goal—preservation of function and/or preventing deformity. Physical therapy is directed toward specific joints, focusing on strengthening muscles, mobilizing restricted joint motion, and preventing or correcting deformities; occupational therapy assumes responsibility for generalized mobility and performance of activities of daily living.

General treatment or maintenance programs vary; physiotherapists may be involved several times weekly to monthly in management of a home program (ideally in association with the child's school), or their visits may be limited to infrequent review of the home program for compliance, effectiveness, and need. Strength is frequently lost around the involved joints, and inactivity leads to generalized weakness. However, normal activities of daily living and the child's natural tendencies to be active are usually sufficient to maintain muscle strength and joint mobility. Exercising in a pool is excellent, since it allows freedom of movement with support and minimal gravitational pull. When joints are inflamed, heavy resistance aggravates the pain, and, at these times, simple isometric or tensing exercises that do not involve joint movement are generally tolerated and should be encouraged. Range of motion exercises are an important aspect of therapy and are continued after evidence of disease has disappeared in order to detect any signs of recurrence.

Most physicians recommend splinting and positioning during rest to help minimize pain and prevent or reduce flexion deformity. Joints most frequently splinted are knees, wrists, and hands. Positioning during rest is also important. The children rest on a firm mattress with no pillow or a very low one and have no support under the knee. Loss of extension in the knee, hip, and wrist causes special problems and requires vigilance to detect the earliest signs of involvement and vigorous attention to prevent deformity with specialized passive stretching, positioning, and resting splints.

Surgery. The benefits of synovectomy, an established preventive and therapeutic procedure in adults, are questionable in the child with rheumatoid arthritis. It is used primarily in pauciarticular disease. Joint replacement is proving successful in older children but is reserved until the child is fully grown. The cooperation of the child is imperative. Joint fusion is sometimes used.

Nursing Considerations

The child with JA presents a challenge to himself and his family and to the professionals who help them cope with this prototype of chronic illness. The effects of the disease are felt in every aspect of the child's life—in physical activities, social experiences, and personality development. Much of the child's adjustment to the stresses and demands of the disease and the level of functioning he achieves are directly related to the reaction and support he receives from his family and the health professionals concerned with his care and management.

Promote general health. The general health of the child and siblings must be considered and is frequently overlooked as parents and health personnel concentrate on the disease. A well-balanced diet and assessment of nutri-

tional status are integral parts of health supervision. The discomfort and increased need for rest may create problems of weight control. Excess weight causes additional strain on inflamed joints, especially those of the lower extremities. Excessive fatigue and overexertion should be avoided by regular periods of rest, especially during acute flare-ups of arthritis. Symptoms may exacerbate during a viral illness.

Posture and body mechanics are important for the child with juvenile rheumatoid arthritis, both when he is at rest and when he is active. He must have a firm mattress to maintain good alignment of spine, hips, and knees and no pillow or a very thin one. The child who is confined to bed either at home or in the hospital may require supports or splints to maintain positioning. Waterbeds or an electric blanket (or electric sheet) placed under the bottom sheet provides comforting warmth. Lying in the prone position is encouraged to straighten hips and knees, such as during rest periods or television viewing. The family is instructed in the principles and purposes of splints so that they can use them judiciously.

School-age children are allowed to attend school, even on days when there may be some pain or discomfort. The aid of the school nurse is enlisted so that the child is permitted to take the prescribed medication at school and to arrange for rest in the nurse's office during the day. Split days or half days may help a child remain involved in school. Permitting the child to come to school late allows time to gain joint movement and reduce the time at school to avoid exhaustion. It is important that the child attend school to learn skills and engage in social interaction, especially if the JA continues to limit physical skills.

Facilitate compliance. The child and family are involved in the therapeutic plan. They need to know the purpose and correct use of any splints and appliances and the medication regimen. The family is instructed regarding administration of medications as well as the value of a regular schedule of administration to maintain a satisfactory drug level in the body. They need to know that aspirin should not be given on an empty stomach and to be alert for signs of aspirin toxicity, which include hyperventilation as a sign of acidosis, bleeding from decreased clotting capacity, tinnitus (ringing in the ears) as a sign of cranial nerve VIII involvement, and undue drowsiness that may indicate central nervous system depression. If evidence of drug toxicity is noted, they are instructed to stop the medication and notify the health professional.

Encourage heat and exercise. Heat has been shown to be beneficial to children with arthritis. Moist heat is best for relieving pain and stiffness, and the most efficient and practical method is in the bathtub. The temperature and duration of the bath are specified by the therapist but usually do not exceed 10 minutes at 37.8° C (100° F). Sometimes a daily whirlpool bath, paraffin bath, or hot packs may be used as needed for temporary relief of acute swelling and pain. Hot packs are easily applied at home using a Turkish towel wrung out after being immersed in hot water or heated in a microwave oven, applied to the area, and covered with plastic for 20 minutes. Painful hands or feet can be immersed in a pan of water for 10 minutes two or three times daily in addition to tub baths.

Pool therapy is the easiest method for exercising a large number of joints. Swimming activities strengthen muscles and maintain mobility in larger joints. Most children have access to a therapy pool, although transportation may be a problem for some families. Very small children who are frightened of the water can carry out their exercises in the bathtub. Small children love to splash, kick, and throw things in the water.

Activities of daily living provide satisfactory exercise for older children to maintain maximum mobility with minimum pain. They should be encouraged in their efforts and patiently allowed to dress and groom themselves, to assume daily tasks, and to care for their belongings. It is often difficult for stiff fingers to manipulate buttons, comb or brush hair, and turn faucets, but parents and other caregivers should refrain from assisting them. In addition, the child should learn and understand why others do not help him. Many helpful devices, such as Velcro fasteners, tongs for manipulating difficult items, and grab bars installed in bathrooms for safety, can be employed to facilitate tasks. A raised toilet seat often makes the difference between dependent and independent toileting, since weak quadriceps muscles and sore knees inhibit the ability to raise the body from a low sitting position.

A child's natural affinity for play offers many opportunities for incorporating therapeutic exercises. Throwing or kicking a ball, hanging from monkey bars, and riding a tricycle (with seat raised to achieve maximum leg extension) are excellent moving and stretching exercises for a very young child whose daily living activities are physically limited.

An effective approach to beginning the day's activities is to awaken the child early to give him the medication and then to allow him to sleep for an hour. On arising, the child takes a hot bath (or shower) and carries out a simple ritual of limbering-up exercises, after which he commences the activities of the day, such as going to school; exercise, heat, and rest are spaced throughout the remainder of the day according to individual needs and schedules. Parents are instructed in exercises that fit the needs of the child.

The **Arthritis Foundation*** and the **Juvenile Arthritis Foundation*** provide services for both parents and professionals, and nurses should refer families to these agencies as an added resource. Information can also be obtained from the **Arthritis Information Clearing House.**†

The child. Juvenile arthritis affects every aspect of the child's daily life. The physical pain and limitations interfere with performance of normal tasks and provision of self-care. Even simple tasks, such as dressing, hair combing, use of the bathroom, cutting food, climbing stairs, manipulating doors and faucets, and using public transportation, are difficult or impossible. There may be school difficulties related to transportation to and from school, stairs, and loss of time as a result of exacerbations and hospitalization. Physical limitations interfere with participation in many activities, both curricular and extracurricular, which limits peer contacts and interaction and increases social isolation. These problems are especially critical for adolescents, for whom peer acceptance and relationships are so vital to personality development. These children increasingly turn to solitary activities and to the family at a time when they are expected to move into greater independence and relationships with peers (see p. 697).

Changes in personality usually accompany JA, as with any chronic illness. These changes may be temporary, such as demanding, irritable behavior, or may be manifest in a more permanent way, such as passive hostility, uncommunicativeness, and manipulativeness. Efforts should be made to break through the child's defenses and to identify his anxieties, concerns, and conflicts in order to intervene early to prevent the development of permanent personality problems. (See Chapter 22 for problems of the child with chronic illness.)

Families. The beginning of the disease is often sudden and frightening, and its variable course with cycles of remissions and exacerbations is discouraging. Many parents become susceptible to unorthodox cures advanced by well-meaning friends and advertisers. These should be carefully evaluated. Obviously harmless measures such as wearing a copper bracelet need not be discouraged, but parents must be dissuaded from questionable or conspicuously harmful practices such as active exercising of swollen, feverish joints. Parents' understanding of the disease and their attitude toward the child are the key to the success or failure of a treatment program, and major foci of nursing intervention are parental education and support.

Nurses are alert to cues that signal undue anxiety and guilt that may lead to an unhealthy degree of overprotection, such as preoccupation with causative factors, constant analysis of effects of various therapies, experimenting with diets, and continually searching for a magical cure. The dangers of parental overprotection and overindulgence can be especially detrimental to the progress of the child with rheumatoid arthritis. Sometimes parents are hesitant to give prescribed medications, keep the child home from school unnecessarily, restrict interaction with age-mates, exhibit reluctance to discipline the child, and assume self-care activities that are best performed by the child.

Most of the reactions, problems, and concerns of families of a child with juvenile rheumatoid arthritis are those of any parents of a chronically ill and/or handicapped child. The impact of the diagnosis is felt most acutely by the parents, who demonstrate anxiety, guilt, and all the manifestations of the grief process. The problems and needs of these families are discussed extensively in Chapter 22, and the reader is directed to this chapter for additional guidance in planning care.

---

*1314 Spring Street, N.W., Atlanta, GA 30309.
†P.O Box 9782, Arlington, VA 22209.

Nursing Care Summary: The Child with Juvenile Arthritis

NURSING GOALS	NURSING INTERVENTIONS	EXPECTED PATIENT/FAMILY OUTCOMES
HP-HMP	**Injury: potential for infection, tissue damage**	
	Risk factors: musculoskeletal impairment, impaired mobility	
Preserve joint function	Carry out or supervise physical therapy regimen Muscle-strengthening exercises Joint mobilization exercises Apply splints, sandbags, if needed, to maintain position and reduce flexion deformity Lie flat in bed with joints extended Use prone position frequently with no pillow, or a very thin one	Joint flexibility improves in relation to baseline findings Child develops no contractures
Prevent other complications	Avoid exposure to infections Stress importance of regular ophthalmologic examination for early detection of possible eye complications Carry out frequent assessments for evidence of improvement, exacerbation, or complications, especially iridocyclitis (blurred vision, pain, and/or redness in eyes) Seek medical treatment promptly for upper respiratory tract (or other) infections	Child exhibits no evidence of infection Signs of complications are detected early and appropriate action is taken
N-MP	**Nutrition, alteration in: potential for more than body requirement**	
	Etiology: decreased mobility	
Maintain nutritional status	Ensure well-balanced diet that does not produce excessive weight gain Schedule regular exercise program appropriate to child's age, interests, and capabilities, but avoid overexertion or fatigue	Child consumes sufficient nourishment without weight gain Child exercises regularly
A-EP	**Diversional activity, deficit**	
	Etiology: discomfort, decreased mobility	
Provide diversion	Incorporate therapeutic exercises in play activities Swimming Throwing a ball Hanging from monkey bar Riding tricycle or bicycle Supervise and encourage activities of daily living Encourage child's natural tendency to be active Encourage interaction with family and peers Include child in planning and scheduling care	Child engages in activities suitable to his interests, capabilities, and developmental level
A-EP	**Self-care deficit: feeding, bathing/hygiene, dressing/grooming, toileting (specify level)**	
	Etiology: musculoskeletal impairment	
Carry out activities of daily living	Encourage maximum independence Provide and/or help devise methods to facilitate independent functioning Select clothes for convenience in putting on and fastening Modify utensils (spoons, toothbrush, comb, etc.) for easier grasp Elevate toilet seat, if needed Install handrails for convenience and safety (hallways, bathroom) Teach application of splints (when able) and encourage responsibility for their use	Child is involved in self-help to his maximum capabilities
Conserve energy	Schedule regular periods for sleep and rest, especially during acute flare-ups	Child engages in appropriate activities without undue fatigue

Nursing Care Summary: The Child with Juvenile Arthritis—cont'd

NURSING GOALS	NURSING INTERVENTIONS	EXPECTED PATIENT/FAMILY OUTCOMES
CPP	**Comfort, alteration in: pain** **Etiology: musculoskeletal impairment**	

Reduce discomfort	Assess need for pain medication
	 Carry out appropriate nonpharmacologic pain reduction techniques
	 Provide heat to painful joints by way of
	    Tub baths, including whirlpool
	    Paraffin baths
	    Warm moist packs
	    Soaks
	 Maintain preventive schedule of drug administration
	 Avoid overexercising painful, swollen joints
		Child is able to move without discomfort

SP-SCP	**Self-concept, disturbance in: body image** **Etiology: perception of disability**	
Help adjust to chronic illness	Plan schedule of activities that includes exercise and rest Promote independence Encourage regular school attendance Enlist aid of school nurse regarding medication schedule and rest periods Discourage activities that increase isolation from others	Child discusses his disease and his feelings about his disability Child engages in appropriate activities with peers

Promote self-esteem	Explore child's feelings regarding his disability
	    Limitations
	    Stress of being "different"
	    Difficulty competing
	    Relationships with peers
	    Self-image
	 Help child to learn about his disease and its therapies
		Child demonstrates an understanding of his disease and its therapy

RRP	**Family process, alteration in** **Etiology: situational crisis (child with a chronic illness)**	

Support family	Reinforce explanation of disease
	 Explore attitude toward child and his disease
	 Allow for expression of feelings
	 Be alert for cues that signal undue anxiety and guilt
	    Preoccupation with causative factors
	    Constant analysis of effects of therapies
	    Experimentation with diets and folk remedies
	    Seeking of magical cures
	 Be alert for overprotective behaviors
	    Assuming self-care activities for child
	    Restricting child's activities and interaction with peers
	 Refer to parent support groups
	 Refer to agencies that provide special services, for example, Arthritis Foundation, Arthritis Information Clearing House
		Family demonstrates an understanding of the child's disease and its therapies
		 Family verbalizes feelings and concerns
		 Family members avail themselves of services

Prepare family for home management	Instruct in administration of prescribed medications
	    Help plan regular schedule of administration
	    Instruct regarding special precautions of administration
	    Instruct regarding signs of toxicity
	 Educate regarding carrying out physical therapies
	 Impress importance of compliance with medication and exercise regimen
		Family demonstrates skills needed for home management

Continued.

Nursing Interventions Related to Medical Management

Assist with diagnosis
  Assist with laboratory tests such as erythrocyte sedimentation rate, latex fixation
  Assist with radiographic tests

Assist with joint aspiration
Reduce inflammation
  Administer antiinflammatory drugs

LUPUS ERYTHEMATOSUS

Lupus erythematosus (LE), which literally means "red wolf" because of the characteristic butterfly rash on the face of some affected individuals, is a chronic inflammatory disease of the collagen or supporting tissues of the body. It characteristically follows a course of remissions and exacerbations. Because connective tissue is found practically everywhere, almost any organ or structure can be affected.

LE in childhood consists of two basic types: a transient neonatal disease apparently related to maternal pathology and a group of chronic diseases that usually have their onset after infancy. These diseases correspond to systemic LE (SLE), discoid LE, disseminated LE, subacute cutaneous LE, or lupus panniculitis in adults. The major portion of the discussion will be limited to SLE.

Etiology

The cause of LE is not known. The theory generally accepted, which is based on response to steroids and immunosuppressant agents, is autoimmunity. It is believed that some inciting event such as stress, infection, extreme fatigue, or exposure to various chemicals, drugs, or excessive sunburn triggers a reaction that alters the body's immune response to its own tissues. The supporting evidence for this finding is that (1) many individuals report such events before onset of symptoms and (2) such events enhance an exacerbation of known lupus disease.

Technically LE is not an inherited disease, although it demonstrates a tendency to occur within families. In addition, family members without actual disease may have findings suggestive of lupus, such as LE cells, abnormal sensitivity to sun, a history of arthritis or allergies, or unusual drug reactions. It is well documented that some individuals develop a lupuslike reaction to drugs such as isoniazid, penicillin, tetracycline, sulfa preparations, phenothiazines, and phenytoin (Dilantin).

Clinical Manifestations

Because SLE can affect almost any tissue, the clinical manifestations are variable. The onset is usually insidious, with vague signs such as low-grade fever, arthritis or arthralgia, generalized aching, and rash. However, rapid involvement of vital organs, primarily the kidneys, can herald an accelerated course with minimum or absent involvement of other sites. The following is a discussion of manifestations related to various tissues involved.

Cutaneous lesions. The majority of children (approximately 90%) with LE have cutaneous involvement at some time during their illness (Schaller, 1982), and about one third of children have skin disease as the chief complaint. A "butterfly rash," an erythematous blush or scaly erythematous patches, appears over the bridge of the nose and symmetrically extending to each cheek and may extend to the scalp, neck, chest, and extremities. Sometimes they are pruritic, look like severe sunburn or hives, or may become bullous. They have a tendency to scar and are aggravated by exposure to ultraviolet rays.

Some patients experience sensitivity to cold (Raynaud phenomenon), especially in the hands and feet. Cyanosis may be present and ulcers often develop in dry and cracked skin. Patchy areas of alopecia may occur, although during remission the hair usually regrows.

Musculoskeletal system. The most common symptom is generalized weakness, usually accompanied by arthritis, myalgia, joint swelling, and stiffness. Usually the joint involvement is not severe enough to cause deformity, although it may result in temporary disability from pain.

Central nervous system. Evidence of neurologic involvement varies from forgetfulness, excitability, and headache to seizures and frank psychosis. Idiopathic epileptic seizures may be an early sign of beginning, yet undiagnosed, SLE. Any of the cranial nerves can be affected, and paralysis from spinal cord involvement may occur.

Heart and lungs. The serous linings of the lungs and heart may become inflamed, resulting in pleurisy or pericarditis, respectively. Both complications are usually reversible with rest. However, renal involvement within a few weeks or months may follow an attack of pleurisy.

Kidneys. The glomerulus is the usual site of destruction. Presumably antigen-antibody complexes are deposited primarily in the glomerular basement membrane, initiating an inflammatory response that results in tissue damage. An early sign of renal involvement is proteinuria. The gravest prognostic sign in SLE is renal involvement and consequent kidney failure. Although supportive approaches, such as hemodialysis and kidney transplant, have improved the outlook for these patients, tissue damage in other vital organs, especially the heart and lungs, may foreshorten the benefits derived from life-supporting techniques.

Blood. Anemia from decreased erythrocytes is common, although the exact reason is unclear. In females amenorrhea may be secondary to the anemia. The platelets and plasma proteins may also be affected.

Lymphoid system. Sometimes the spleen and often the cervical, axillary, and inguinal lymph nodes are enlarged. A type of LE hepatitis may develop during the course of the disease.

Gastrointestinal tract. Nausea and vomiting, diarrhea, and abdominal pain may be present and at times may falsely suggest conditions such as appendicitis.

Diagnostic Evaluation

SLE has been called the "great imitator," since its clinical manifestations may point to a variety of unrelated conditions. The diagnosis of LE is established by the demonstration of any four of eleven diagnostic criteria (see box).

A neurologic examination should be done to provide baseline data for evaluating subtle changes in behavior and function. Sometimes a psychiatric evaluation may also be warranted, since personality alterations caused by steroids and renal damage are difficult to distinguish from those resulting from central nervous system involvement.

Therapeutic Management

The objectives of medical treatment are (1) to reverse the autoimmune and inflammatory processes and (2) to prevent exacerbations and complications. Therapy involves the use of specific and supportive medications and regulation of activity and diet.

Drugs. The principal drugs used to control inflammation are the corticosteroids. They are administered in doses sufficient to suppress symptoms, then tapered to the lowest suppressive dose. During periods of exacerbation a large dose may be given for variable periods of time; if given for prolonged periods, they subject the child to all the side effects of steroid therapy. One alternative of administration is the "pulse" method, the administration of a large dose of steroids intravenously over a 20- to 30-minute period on 3 consecutive days. Large doses may be needed to treat seizures and other central nervous system manifestations. Sometimes the immunosuppressive agent azathioprine (Imuran) helps reduce the amount of steroids needed.

Another group of drugs effective in relieving the dermatologic, arthritic, and renal symptoms of the disease are antimalarial preparations, such as hydroxychloroquine (Plaquenil) and chloroquine (Aralen). Although the exact action of these drugs on LE is not known, often they permit a continued remission with a lowered dose of steroids.

Nonsteroidal antiinflammatory agents, such as aspirin, play an important role by relieving muscle and joint pains and reducing tissue inflammation. Drugs used to control various complications include anticonvulsants, antihypertensives, and antibiotics. The selection of appropriate medication in each of these categories is essential, since many of them greatly aggravate the disease process.

Regulation of activity and diet. The goal of restricted activity is to prevent a recurrence of the disease. Although the exact relationship is unclear, fatigue, stress, or sudden exertion brings about a relapse of symptoms. An effective schedule must provide for gradual resumption of pre–lupus erythematosus activity and maximal rest periods, usually 8 to 10 hours of sleep a night and one or two rest times during the day.

Diet may be restricted depending on weight gain and/or fluid retention from steroids and renal damage. The most frequently prescribed diet modification is moderate or low salt. Low-protein diets may be necessary to prevent elevated nitrogen levels. Weight reduction may help preserve maximum joint function and conserve energy.

Nursing Considerations

The principal nursing goal is to help the child and family adjust to the limitations and treatments of the disease and to prevent exacerbations and complications. Since older female adolescents are the most likely group to be affected, the nurse must have an awareness of their special needs, such as body image changes, present and future vocational activities, social relationships, and emerging sexuality. Although this is a potentially fatal disorder, nurses are encouraged to apply those principles of adjusting to a chronic illness that are discussed in Chapter 22.

Assist family in adjusting to disease and its treatment. SLE is a complex disease. Although much is known about its effect on connective tissues and appropriate types of treatment, few concrete facts are available. However, family members need an understanding of the disease process to gain an appreciation of the necessity of regular,

---

CRITERIA FOR DIAGNOSIS OF SYSTEMIC LUPUS ERYTHEMATOSUS

1. Butterfly rash
2. Discoid rash
3. Photosensitivity
4. Oral ulcers
5. Arthritis
6. Serositis
7. Renal disorder
8. Neurologic disorder(s) (psychosis, coma, seizures, paresis)
9. Hematologic disorder(s) (anemia, thrombocytopenia, leukopenia)
10. Immunologic disorder(s) (anti-DNA, LE prep, Anti-SM, STS)
11. Antinuclear antibody

uninterrupted drug administration, moderate activity, and dietary modifications. Usually diagnostic tests are performed during hospitalization, which allows the nurse an opportunity to help the family learn about the disease.

Several organizations have been formed to help children and families learn about and adjust to the disease. These include the **National Lupus Erythematosus Foundation,*** the **Lupus Foundation of America,†** and **Leanon (Lupus Erythematosus Anonymous).‡** The nurse should be aware of what information the family is receiving, because learning about joint deformity, sudden bouts of pain and disability, a disfiguring rash, and the possibility of renal failure can be overwhelming. Nurses should also be aware of advertised nonmedical approaches to treatment, since quackery abounds when no known cure exists.

The nurse has the responsibility of helping the adolescent adjust to drug therapy. The side effects of steroids and immunosuppressant drugs are discussed under leukemia and outlined in Table 36-3. Most of the antimalarial drugs have few side effects. However, hydroxychloroquine and chloroquine can cause irreversible retinal damage; therefore frequent ophthalmic examinations are necessary. In addition, after exposure to the sun, the skin may tan less and become more erythematous and the hair may lighten.

Body image changes from both the disease and the drugs are a major concern. Each of these should be approached in a positive manner by discussing the use of cosmetics and wigs. Sometimes health professionals fail to adequately assess the child's adjustment reactions and regard the depression and withdrawal as effects of the disease rather than a response to body image changes.

Restricted activity imposes many hardships for these children. Unlike other diseases that may require a long convalescent period with ultimate resumption of normal activity, this disease warrants lifelong activity restrictions, although the child may be able to continue to participate in moderation. The child and family need to weigh the consequences of activity against the pleasures. For example, a day of skiing, with proper sun precautions, may be worth the achiness for the following day or even week. This provides the youngster with some sense of control over his life. The severity of the disease is also a factor if the risk of irreversible damage is great.

Whenever dietary restrictions are necessary, the nurse works with the child and parents, focusing on the family member who regularly prepares meals. Several commercial cookbooks are available with salt-restricted recipes. Since there are so many hidden sources of sodium, besides what is added at the table, families need a written list of restricted and allowed foods. The nurse also takes into account "adolescent" snacks outside the home that are high in sodium, such as pizza, hamburgers, frankfurters, and most baked goods. Unfortunately there are few well-accepted "fast-food" substitutions. However, compromising by eating a hamburger without cheese, ketchup, or pickles and French fried potatoes without added salt may be acceptable.

Prevent exacerbations and complications. The list of "don't's" for these individuals is long. The importance of adequate rest has already been stressed. The necessity of adhering to the medication schedule is paramount. Some adolescents, in an attempt to lessen the side effects of steroids, may elect to skip a few doses. The nurse emphasizes that steroids not only are essential to maintaining a remission but must be taken daily (or as prescribed) to prevent sudden withdrawal from the drug, which may precipitate a serious physiologic crisis. Affected persons are also advised to seek medical attention during periods of stress, illness, or before elective surgical procedures, such as dental extraction, since the body may require larger amounts of the drug. They should carry an identification card or Medic Alert tag emphasizing their dependence on steroids.

To prevent flare-up of the disease from drugs, the patient should keep a drug record to identify any prescription that may be contraindicated. For example, a physician unfamiliar with the patient may prescribe penicillin by using one of its trade names and the patient may unknowingly develop a reaction. If the family frequents one pharmacist, this person should be aware of restricted drugs.

Skin care is important. In those individuals who are sensitive to the sun, exposure to it must be avoided. It is important to stress that reflected sun through clouds, on snow, on water, or on white cement can cause a severe reaction. Although clothes can protect most areas of the body, special sunscreening agents are necessary for the face (see p. 776). Parents should be encouraged to purchase sunscreens with the highest sun protective factor (PF) rating available. A large-brimmed hat helps in partially shading the face.

Sometimes patients are requested to routinely check their urine for protein by using a reagent strip that changes color when protein is present. Just as in diabetic testing, the nurse assesses the adolescent's understanding of the test. The patient should report any evidence of proteinuria or of advanced renal diseases, such as fluid retention, azotemia (e.g., ammonia odor on breath), irritability, and exhaustion.

The youngster with kidney involvement is subject to long-term management that may entail hemodialysis and/or kidney transplant. Nursing considerations for each procedure are discussed in Chapter 30.

---

*5430 Van Nuys Ave., Van Nuys, CA 91401.
†11673 Holly Springs Dr., St. Louis, MO 63141.
‡P.O. Box 10243, Corpus Christi, TX 78410.

CONCEPT SUMMARIES

- Upper motor neuron lesions produce weakness associated with spasticity, increased deep tendon reflexes, and abnormal superficial reflexes; lower motor neuron lesions interrupt the reflex arc, causing weakness and atrophy of the skeletal muscles.

- The most useful classification of neuromuscular disorders defines the source of the lesion: anterior horn cells of the spinal cord, peripheral nerves, myoneural junction, and muscles.

- Clinical manifestations of cerebral palsy include delayed gross motor development, abnormal motor performance, alterations of muscle tone, abnormal postures, reflex abnormalities, and associated disabilities such as mental retardation, seizures, attention deficit disorder, and sensory impairment.

- Therapy for cerebral palsy takes into account the nature of the physical disability, defects associated with the disorder, and interpersonal and social influences encountered by the affected child.

- Werdnig-Hoffman disease, is characterized by progressive weakness and wasting of skeletal muscles caused by degeneration of anterior horn cells.

- Nursing care of the child with Guillain-Barré syndrome is aimed at vital sign monitoring, ensuring alignment and positioning, physical therapy, and support of the family.

- Tetanus occurs tetanus spores or vegetative bacilli enter a wound and multiply in a susceptible host.

- Infant botulism results from the release of toxins from *C. botulinum* colonizing the GI tract.

- Primary management of myasthenia gravis is oral administration of anticholinesterase drugs.

- Muscular dystrophies are the largest and most important group of muscular dysfunctions in childhood.

- Major complications of Duchenne muscular dystrophy include contractures, disuse atrophy, infections, obesity, and cardiopulmonary problems.

- Common musculoskeletal dysfunctions in childhood include torticolli, Legg-Calvé-Perthes syndrome, slipped femoral capital epiphyses, kyphosis and lorosis, and scoliosis.

- Nonoperative management of scoliosis includes bracing, exercise, and electrical stimulation.

- Nursing care of the child with osteomyelitis is directed at positioning, careful monitoring of vital signs, drugs, IV equipment and site, and nutrition.

- Osteomyelitis is acquired by direct or secondary invasion or hematogenous spread of infectious organisms.

- Goals of therapy for juvenile arthritis are to preserve joint function, prevent physical deformities, and relieve symptoms without iatrogenic harm.

- Nursing care of juvenile arthritis involves promoting general health, facilitating compliance, and encouraging heat and exercise.

- Objectives of therapy for lupus erythematosus are to reverse autoimmune and inflammatory processes and to prevent exacerbations and complications.

REFERENCES

Ad Hoc NINCDS Committee: Criteria for diagnosis of Guillain-Barré syndrome, Ann. Neurol. **3**:565-568, 1978.

American Academy of Pediatrics Policy Statement: The Doman-Delacato treatment of neurologically handicapped children, Pediatrics **70**:810-812, 1982.

Arnon, S.S.: Infant botulism. In Gellis, S.S., and Kagan, B.M.: Current pediatric therapy 12, Philadelphia, 1986, W.B. Saunders Co.

Barrack, R.L., and others: Proprioception in idiopathic scoliosis, Spine **9**:681-685, 1984.

Brewer, E.J.: Collagen vascular disease. In Gellis, S.S., and Kagan, B.M.: Current pediatric therapy 12, Philadelphia, 1986, W.B. Saunders Co.

Bunnell, W.P.: An objective criterion for scoliosis screening, J. Bone Joint Surg. **66-A**:1381-1385, 1984.

Cohen, F.L.: Clinical genetics in nursing practice, Philadelphia, 1984, J.B. Lippincott Co.

Davis, S.E., and Lewis, S.A.: Managing scoliosis: fashions for the body and mind, Am. J. Maternal Child Nurs. **9**:186-187, 1984.

Dretakis, E.K.: Scoliosis associated with congenital brain-stem abnormalities: a report of eight cases, Int. Orthop. **8**:37, 1984.

Dubowitz, V.: Evaluation and differential diagnosis of the hypotonic infant, Pediatr. Rev. **6**:237-243, 1985.

Fisher, M.C., Goldsmith, J.F., and Gilligan, P.H.: Sneakers as a source of *Pseudomonas aeruginosa* in children with osteomyelitis following puncture wounds, J. Pediatr. **106**:607-609, 1985.

Gratz, R.R., and Papalia-Finlay, D.: Psychosocial adaptation to wearing the Milwaukee brace for scoliosis: a pilot study of adolescent females and their mothers, J. Adolesc. Health Care **5**:237-242, 1984.

Holm, V.A., Harthun-Smith, L., and Tada, W.L.: Infant walkers and cerebral palsy, Am. J. Dis. Child. **137**:1189-1190, 1983.

Johnson, R.O., Clay, S.A., and Arnon, S.S.: Diagnosis and management of infant botulism, Am. J. Dis. Child. **132**:586-588, 1979.

McCollough, N.C., III: Electrical stimulation in management of idiopathic scoliosis. In Stauffer, E.S., editor: Instructional course lectures, vol. 36, St. Louis, 1985, The C.V. Mosby Co.

Micheli, L.J., Magin, M.A., and Rouvales, R.: The patient with scoliosis: surgical management and nursing care, Am. J. Nurs. **79**:1599-1607, 1979.

Miller, J.A.A., Nachemson, A.L., and Schultz, A.B.: Effectiveness of braces in mild idiopathic scoliosis, Spine **9**:632-635, 1984.

Molnar, G.E., and Taft, L.T.: Pediatric rehabilitation: cerebral palsy and spinal cord injuries. Part I, Curr. Probl. Pediatr. **7**(3):6-46, 1977.

Morais, T., and others: Age- and sex-specific prevalence of scoliosis and the value of school screening programs, Am. J. Public Health **75**:1377-1380, 1985.

Paneth, N.: Etiologic factors in cerebral palsy, Pediatr. Ann. **15**:191, 194-201, 1986.

Polin, R.A., and Brown, L.W.: Infant botulism, Pediatr. Clin. North Am. **26**:345-354, 1979.

Puri, R., and others: Slipped upper femoral epiphysis and primary juvenile hypothyroidism, J. Bone Joint Surg. **67-B**:14-20, 1985.

Renshaw, T.S.: Orthotic treatment of idiopathic scoliosis and kyphosis. In Stauffer, E.S., editor: Instructional course lectures, vol. 36, St. Louis, 1985, The C.V. Mosby Co.

Root, L.: The treatment of osteogenesis imperfecta, Orthop. Clin. North Am. **15**:775-790, 1984.

Schaller, J.: Lupus in childhood, Clin. Rheum. Dis. **8**:219-228, 1982.

Schaller, J.G., and Wedgwood, R.J.: Rheumatic and connective tissue diseases of childhood. In Behrman, R.E., and Vaughan, V.C., III: Textbook of pediatrics, ed. 12, Philadelphia, 1983, W.B. Saunders Co.

Seybold, M.E., and Lindstrom, J.M.: Myasthenia gravis in infancy, Neurology **31**:476-480, 1981.

Staheli, L.T.: The hip. In Gellis, S.S., and Kagan, B.M.: Current pediatric therapy 12, Philadelphia, 1986, W.B. Saunders Co.

Sternfeld, L.: Cerebral palsy. In Gellis, S.S., and Kagan, B.M.: Current pediatric therapy 12, Philadelphia, 1986, W.B. Saunders Co.

Taft, L.T.: Cerebral palsy, Pediatr. Rev. 6:35-44, 1984.

Viviani, G.R., and others: Assessment of accuracy of the scoliosis school screening examination, Am. J. Public Health, 74:497-498, 1984.

Watts, H.G., and Kirkpatrick, L.J., Jr.: Orthopedic problems. In Behrman, R.E., and Vaughan, V.C., III: Textbook of pediatrics, ed. 12, Philadelphia, 1983, W.B. Saunders Co.

BIBLIOGRAPHY

General

Bernard, B., and others: Exercise for children with physical disabilities, Issues Compr. Pediatr. Nurs. 5:99-107, 1981.

Conway-Rutkowski, B.L.: Carini and Owens' neurological and neurosurgical nursing, ed. 8, St. Louis, 1982, The C.V. Mosby Co.

Downey, J.A., and Low, N.L., editors: The child with disabling illness, ed. 2, Philadelphia, 1984, W.B. Saunders Co.

Kempe, C.H., Silver, H.K., and O'Brien, D., editors: Current pediatric diagnosis and treatment, ed. 9, Los Altos, CA, 1986, Lange Medical Publications.

Lenox, A.C.: When motor nerves die, Am. J. Nurs. 83:540-546, 1983.

Schade, J., and Passo, S.: Needs assessment of parents in pediatric ambulatory care, J. Ambul. Care Man. 4:23-32, 1981.

Swaiman, K.F., and Wright, F.S.: The practice of pediatric neurology, vol. 2, St. Louis, 1982, The C.V. Mosby Co.

Cerebral Palsy

Barabas, G., and Taft, L.T.: The early signs and differential diagnosis of cerebral palsy, Pediatr. Ann. 15:203-214, 1986.

Coffman, S.P.: Parents' perceptions of needs for themselves and their children in a cerebral palsy clinic, Issues Compr. Pediatr. Nurs. 6:67-77, 1983.

Diamond, M.: Rehabilitation strategies for the child with cerebral palsy, Pediatr. Ann. 15:230-236, 1986.

Pilon, B.H., and Smith, K.A.: A parent group for the Hispanic parents of children with severe cerebral palsy, Child. Health Care 14:96-102, 1985.

Steele, S.: Young children with cerebral palsy: practical guidelines for care, Pediatr. Nurs. 11:259-267, 1985.

Task Force on Joint Assessment of Prenatal and Perinatal Factors Associated with Brain Disorders: National Institutes of Health report on causes of mental retardation and cerebral palsy, Pediatrics 76:457-458, 1985.

Wolraich, M.L.: Counseling families of children with cerebral palsy, Pediatr. Ann. 15:239-244, 1986.

Neuropathies/Diseases of Neuromuscular Junction

Barry, L.: The patient with myasthenia gravis really needs you, Nursing 82 12(7):50-53, 1982.

Brand, D., and others: Adequacy of antitetanus prophylaxis in six hospital emergency rooms, N. Engl. J. Med. 309:636-640, 1983.

Brown, L.: Commentary: infant botulism and the honey connection, J. Pediatr. 94:337-338, 1979.

Dezfulian, M., Yolken, R., and Bartlett, J.: Rapid diagnosis of a case of infant botulism by enzyme immunoassay, Pediatr. Infect. Dis. 4:399-401, 1985.

Engel, A.G.: Myasthenia gravis and myasthenic syndromes, Ann. Neurol. 16:519-523, 1984.

Fink, J.N., and Arnason, B.G.W.: Immunologic aspects of neurological and neuromuscular diseases, JAMA 248:2710-2715, 1982.

Jemison-Smith, P., and Hubbell, H.: Guillain-Barré syndrome, Crit. Care Update 10(6):12-16, 1983.

Kess, R.: Suddenly in crisis: unpredictable myasthenia, Am. J. Nurs. 84:994-998, 1984.

Lefvert, A.K., and Osterman, P.O.: Newborn infants to myasthenic mothers: a clinical study and an investigation of acetylcholine receptor antibodies in 17 children, Neurology 33:133-138, 1983.

L'Hommedieu, C.L., and Polin, R.A.: Progression of clinical signs in severe infant botulism, Clin. Pediatr. 20:90-95, 1980.

Miller, D.K.: The challenge of infant botulism, Am. J. Maternal Child Nurs. 7:180-183, 1982.

Mills, N., and Plasterer, H.H.: Guillain-Barré syndrome: a framework for nursing care, Nurs. Clin. North Am. 15:257-264, 1980.

Pasternak, J.F., and others: Exchange transfusion in neonatal myasthenia, J. Pediatr. 99:644-646, 1981.

Research Review: Tetanus: controlled, but still hazardous, Immunol. Update 2(1):2-4, 1980.

Roach, E.S., and others: Early-onset myasthenia gravis, J. Pediatr. 108:193-197, 1986.

Roderick, M.A.: Botulism, Nursing 82 12(6):59, 1982.

Roderick, M.A.: Tetanus, Nursing 82 12(7):63, 1982.

Sebilia, A.J.: "When was your last tetanus shot?" RN 47(8):18-24, 1985.

Snead, O.C., III, and others: Juvenile myasthenia gravis, Neurology 30:732-737, 1980.

Muscular Dysfunction

Brady, M.H.: Lifelong care of the child with Duchenne muscular dystrophy, Am. J. Maternal Child Nurs. 4:227-230, 1979.

Carroll, J.E.: Diagnosis and management of Duchenne muscular dystrophy, Pediatr. Rev. 6:195-200, 1985.

Firth, M., and others: Interview with parents of boys suffering from Duchenne muscular dystrophy, Dev. Med. Child Neurol. 25:466-471, 1983.

Flynn, I., Schwetz, K., and Williams, D.: Muscular dystrophy: comprehensive nursing care, Nurs. Clin. North Am. 14:123-132, 1979.

Nursing Grand Rounds: Muscular dystrophy: a nursing point of view, Nursing 80 10(1):456-459, 1980.

Spencer, C.H., and others: Course of treated juvenile dermatomyositis, J. Pediatr. 105:399-408, 1984.

Thompson, C.E.: Diagnosis of proximal muscle weakness in childhood, Pediatr. Basics 31:4-8, 1981.

Vaughan, S.M., and Whittle, E.: Caring for the child with dermatomyositis, Issues Compr. Pediatr. Nurs. 7:255-267, 1984.

Zatz, M.: Diagnosis, carrier detection, and genetic counseling in the muscular dystrophies, Pediatr. Clin. North Am. 25:557-573, 1978.

Musculoskeletal Disorders

Benchot, R.J.: The adolescent with slipped capital femoral epiphysis, Point of View 19:6-9, 1982.

Bunnell, W.P.: Back pain in children, Orthop. Clin. North Am. 13:587-603, 1982.

Colter, J.M.: Office management in Legg-Calvé-Perthes syndrome, Orthop. Clin. North Am. 13:619-627, 1982.

Hussey, C.G.: Surviving a handicap in everyday life: how to help, Am. J. Maternal Child Nurs. 4:46-50, 1979.

Malkiewicz, J.: A pragmatic approach to musculoskeletal assessment, RN 45(11):57-62, 1982.

Scoliosis

Allard, J.L., and Dibble, S.L.: Scoliosis surgery: a look at Luque rods, Am. J. Nurs. 84:609-611, 1984.

Anderson, B.: The patient with scoliosis: Carole, a girl treated with bracing, Am. J. Nurs. 79:1592-1597, 1979.

Axelgaard, J., and Brown, J.C.: Lateral electrical surface stimulation for the treatment of progressive idiopathic scoliosis, Spine 8:242-260, 1983.

Czeizel, A., and others: Genetics of adolescent idiopathic scoliosis, J. Med. Genet. 15:424-427, 1978.

deToledo, C.H.: The patient with scoliosis: the defect: classification and detection, Am. J. Nurs. **79**:1588-1591, 1979.

Eckerson, L.F., and Axelgaard, J.: Lateral electrical surface stimulation as an alternative to bracing the treatment of idiopathic scoliosis; treatment protocol and patient acceptance, Phys. Ther. **64**:483-490, 1984.

Ferguson, R.L., and Allen, B.L.: Segmental spinal instrumentation for routine scoliotic curve, Contemp. Orthop. **2**:450-454, 1980.

Fitz, C.R.: Diagnostic imaging in children with spinal disorders, Pediatr. Clin. North Am. **32**:1537-1558, 1985.

Hall, J.E.: Preoperative assessment of the patient with a spinal deformity. In Stauffer, E.S., editor: Instructional course lectures, vol. 36, St. Louis, 1985, The C.V. Mosby Co.

Jones, M.C.: Clinical approach to the child with scoliosis, Pediatr. Rev. **6**:219-222, 1985.

Karlin, L.I.: Disorders of the spine and shoulder girdle. In Gellis, S.S., and Kagan, B.M.: Current pediatric therapy 12, Philadelphia, 1986, W.B. Saunders Co.

Luque, E.R.: Segmental spinal instrumentation for correction scoliosis, Clin. Orthop. **163**:192-198, 1982.

Rutechi, B., and Seligson, D.: Caring for the patient in a halo apparatus, Nursing 80 **10**(10):73-77, 1980.

Schatzinger, L.H., Brower, E.M., and Nash, C.L., Jr.: The patient with scoliosis: spinal fusion: emotional stress and adjustment, Am. J. Nurs. **79**:1608-1612, 1979.

Thomassen, P.F.: Helping your scoliosis patient walk tall, RN **47**(2):34-37, 1984.

Wenger, D.R., Carollo, J.J., and Wilkerson, J.A.: Biomechanics of scoliosis correction by segmental spinal instrumentation, Spine **7**:260-264, 1982.

Wenger, D.R., and others: Laboratory testing of segmental spinal instrumentation versus traditional Harrington instrumentation for scoliosis treatment, Spine **7**:265-269, 1982.

Orthopedic Infections

Aronoff, S.C., and Scoles, P.V.: Treatment of childhood skeletal infections, Pediatr. Clin. North Am. **30**:271-280, 1983.

Kilcoyne, R.F., and Plumly, T.F.: Infections of bones and joints, Nurs. Pract. **8**(3):12, 63, 66, 1983.

Volberg, F.M., and others: Unreliability of radiographic diagnosis of septic hip in children, Pediatrics **73**:118-120, 1984.

Osteogenesis Imperfecta

Guerrein, A.T.: Osteogenesis imperfecta: a disorder that breaks more than our hearts, Am J. Maternal Child Nurs. **7**:315-318, 1982.

Sillence, D.: Osteogenesis imperfecta: an expanding panorama of variants, Clin. Orthop. **159**:11, 1981.

Varni, M.A., and Jaffe, M.: Osteogenesis imperfecta: the basics, Pediatr. Nurs. **10**:29-33, 1984.

Wynne-Davies, R., and Gormley, J.: Clinical and genetic patterns in osteogenesis imperfecta, Clin. Orthop. **159**:26, 1981.

Juvenile Arthritis

Baum, J.: Treatment of juvenile arthritis, Am. Family Phys. **27**:133-139, 1983.

Brewer, E.J., and others: Plasma exchange in selected patients with juvenile rheumatoid arthritis, J. Pediatr. **98**:194-200, 1981.

Fink, C.W.: Predicting the outcome of JRA, Consultant **19**:40-46, 1979.

Giannini, E.H., Brewer, E.J., and Person, D.A.: Auranofin in the treatment of juvenile rheumatoid arthritis, J. Pediatr. **102**:138-141, 1983.

Gorman, T.K., and Marsh, M.E.: Arthritis at an early age, Am. J. Nurs. **84**:1472-1477, 1984.

Hollister, J.R.: Delay in motor development as a presentation of juvenile rheumatoid arthritis, J. Pediatr. **98**:581-583, 1981.

Jacobs, J.C., Berdon, W.E., and Johnston, A.D.: HLA-B27-associated spondyloarthritis and enthesopathy in childhood: clinical, pathologic, and radiographic observations in 58 patients, J. Pediatr. **100**:521-528, 1982.

Lindsley, C.B.: The child with arthritis, Issues Compr. Pediatr. Nurs. **2**(4):23-32, 1977.

Manners, P.J., and Ansell, B.M.: Slow-acting antirheumatic drug use in systemic onset juvenile chronic arthritis, Pediatrics **77**:99-103, 1986.

McCarthy, P.L., and others: Evaluation of arthritis and arthralgia in children, Clin. Pediatr. **19**:183-190, 1980.

Rennebohm, R., and Correll, J.K.: Comprehensive management of juvenile rheumatoid arthritis, Nurs. Clin. North Am. **19**:647-662, 1984.

Spruck, M.: Gold therapy, Am. J. Nurs. **79**:1246-1248, 1979.

Wortmann, D.W., and others: Renal papillary necrosis in juvenile rheumatoid arthritis, J. Pediatr. **97**:37-40, 1980.

Systemic Lupus Erythematosus (SLE)

Ascheim, J.H.: The adolescent and systemic lupus erythematosus: a developmental and educational approach, Issues Compr. Pediatr. Nurs. **5**:293-307, 1981.

Englund, J.A., and Lucas, R.V.: Cardiac complications in children with systemic lupus erythematosus, Pediatrics **72**:724-730, 1983.

Lee, L.A., and Weston, W.L.: Lupus erythematosus in childhood, Dermatol. Clin. **4**:151-160, 1986.

Phadke, K., and others: Acute renal failure as the initial manifestation of systemic lupus erythematosus in children, J. Pediatr. **105**:38-41, 1984.

White, J.F., and Ziegler, G.L.: Patient management of systemic lupus erythematosus, Crit. Care Update **7**(8):5-15, 1980.

Chapter 40

The Immobilized or Traumatically Injured Child

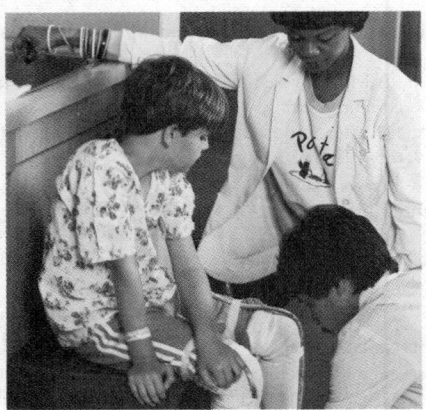

The Immobilized Child
Immobilization
Etiology of immobilization
Physiologic effects of immobilization
Psychologic effects of immobilization
Nursing considerations
Mobilization devices
Braces
Crutches and canes
Special beds
Wheelchairs

The Child and Trauma
Trauma management
Etiology of trauma
Prevention of injuries
Assessment of trauma
Dislocations
Patella
Radial head

Fractures
Etiology
Pathophysiology
Clinical manifestations
Diagnostic evaluation
Therapeutic management
Bone healing and remodeling
The child in a cast
The cast
Nursing considerations
The child in traction
Purposes of traction
Types of traction (general)
Upper extremity traction
Lower extremity traction
Cervical traction
Nursing considerations
Fracture complications
Circulatory impairment
Nerve compression syndromes
Compartmental syndromes
Epiphyseal damage
Nonunion
Malunion
Infection
Kidney stones
Pulmonary emboli
Amputation
Nursing considerations
Spinal cord injuries
Review of essential neuromuscular physiology
Etiology
Pathophysiology
Clinical manifestations
Diagnostic evaluation
Therapeutic management
Nursing considerations
Physical rehabilitation
Psychosocial rehabilitation
Sexuality
Summary

Traumatic injuries are common in childhood. Most are relatively minor and cause little disruption in the daily life of the child and produce only minor discomfort. However, accidents are the leading cause of death in the pediatric age-group. Every year thousands of children die and many thousands more are permanently disabled as a result of trauma. Some injuries, such as those involving the musculoskeletal system, heal in a short time, whereas others, such as fractured femurs and spinal cord injuries, require long-term care and a rehabilitative team approach throughout the acute and restorative stages of the child's care.

The Immobilized Child

Immobilization is a major therapy for injuries to soft tissues, long bones, ligaments, vertebrae, and joints. Restriction of motion for a period of time at the site at which muscle or bone integrity has been disrupted allows tissue and bone to heal. However, prolonged immobilization, whether for therapy or because of disability, can produce severe complications, many of which are preventable. The nurse's awareness and implementation of appropriate actions during this restrictive state can significantly reduce the adverse effects of immobilization. Thus nursing care plans must focus not only on tissue and bone healing but also on regaining functional use of the injured part to the greatest extent possible.

Some aspects of musculoskeletal trauma were discussed in relation to sports injuries in Chapter 20. This chapter is concerned with skeletal trauma and some of its complications and nursing responsibilities. The related problems of multiple trauma, which include cardiovascular and pulmonary collapse, rupture of internal organs, and head injury, although frequently associated with trauma, will not be included in this chapter. The last section of this chapter will deal with the complex problems of spinal cord disorders.

IMMOBILIZATION

One of the most difficult aspects of illness is the immobility it often imposes on a child. Children's natural tendency to be mobile influences all elements of growth and development—physical, social, psychologic, and emotional. It is also important for expression and for dealing with anxiety and frustration. For these reasons children are immobilized only when necessary and for the shortest time possible.

Etiology of Immobilization

The usual reason for immobilizing or restricting the activity of a child is illness or injury. Bed rest or mechanical restraining devices are frequently prescribed to aid in the healing and restorative processes. When children are ill, they are content to remain quiet, and most of them instinctively reduce their activity. It is children who are forced to remain inactive because of physical limitations or therapy who display the multiple effects of restricted movement. The most frequent reasons for immobility are congenital defects (e.g., spina bifida), degenerative disorders (e.g., muscular dystrophy), and infections or accidents that impair the integumentary system (severe burns), the musculoskeletal system (fractures or osteomyelitis), or the neurologic system (spinal cord injury, polyneuritis, or head injury). Sometimes therapies, such as traction and spinal fusion, are responsible for prolonged immobilization.

Physiologic Effects of Immobilization

Although the bulk of information about the effects of immobility has been obtained from studies on adults, it is assumed that similar results occur in children. Many clinical studies, including space program research, have documented predictable consequences that occur following immobilization and the absence of gravitational force. Functional and metabolic responses to restricted movement can be noted in most of the body systems, all of which have a direct influence on the child's growth and development, because homeostatic mechanisms thrive on normal use and need feedback to maintain dynamic equilibrium. Inactivity leads to a decrease in the functional capabilities of the whole body as dramatically as the lack of physical exercise leads to muscle weakness.

Most of the pathologic changes that take place during immobilization arise from decreased muscle strength and mass, decreased metabolism, and bone demineralization, which are closely interrelated with one change leading to or affecting another. Some results of immobilization are primary and produce a direct effect; other pathophysiologic consequences occur frequently but seem to be more indirect and are therefore secondary effects. Many pathophysiologic changes affect more than one body system, with the primary or secondary effect being demonstrated in both systems.

Children who are confined to bed during a disease process or who are immobilized with an injury are usually restricted in movement for a relatively short time or are sufficiently active to avoid the physical consequences of immobility. Most physical and biologic effects of immobilization are the result of complete immobility, usually as a result of paralysis caused by nervous system infection (e.g., poliomyelitis, encephalitis, or polyneuritis) or trauma to the brain or spinal cord. Partial paralysis or weakness may be caused by birth defects (usually meningomyelocele), trauma, infection, or degenerative disease, such as muscular dystrophy or muscular atrophy.

The major effects of immobilization (Fig. 40-1) are related directly or indirectly to decreased muscle activity, which produces numerous primary changes in both muscular and bone structures with secondary alterations in the cardiovascular, respiratory, metabolic, and renal systems. The major consequences are:

1. Significant loss of muscle strength, endurance, and muscle mass (atrophy)
2. Bone demineralization leading to osteoporosis
3. Loss of joint mobility and contractures

The larger the portion of the body immobilized and the longer the immobilization, the greater the hazards of immobility.

Muscular system. Inactive muscle loses strength at the rate of 3% per day and, in instances without primary neuromuscular deficit, sometimes requires several weeks or months to regain function. A stretching can occur as muscle loses its tone or as excessive strain is put on weakened muscle, for example, stretching by tight bed covers or poor body position that produces wristdrop or footdrop experienced by debilitated children. The disuse leads to tissue

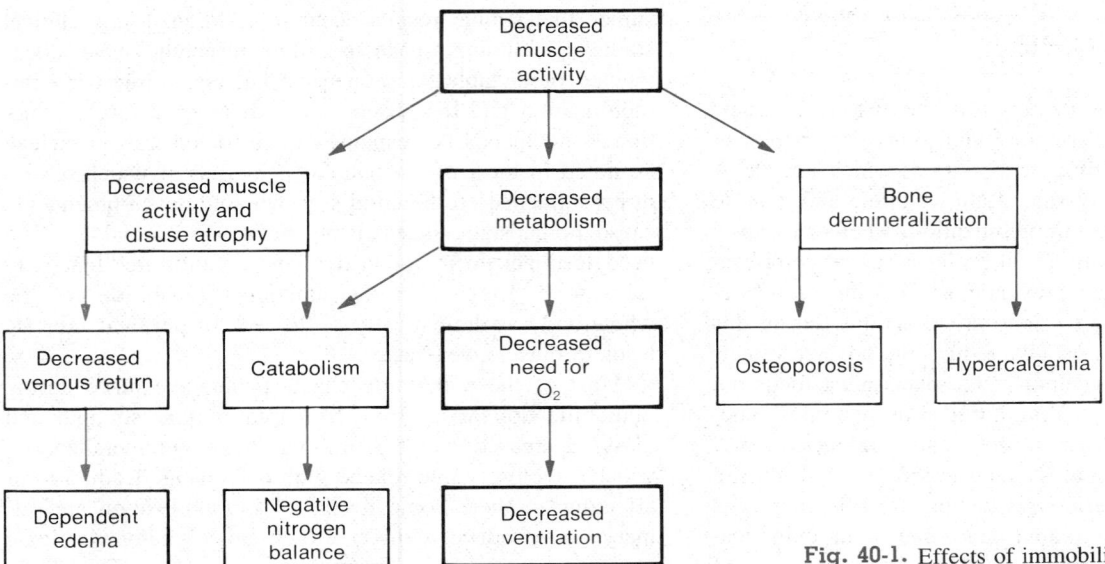

Fig. 40-1. Effects of immobilization.

breakdown and loss of the muscle mass (atrophy). The chief intracellular muscle enzyme, creatine, is released into the serum as the muscle atrophies; therefore serum levels provide an indication of the amount of muscle mass undergoing degeneration. Inactive muscle also affects the cardiovascular system by decreasing venous return and cardiac output.

Skeletal system. The daily stresses on bone created by motion and weight bearing maintain the balance between bone formation (osteoblastic activity) and bone resorption (osteoclastic activity). When these stresses are diminished, bone formation ceases, whereas the bone destruction continues, thus disrupting the state of equilibrium. Calcium becomes severely depleted, and there is increased secretion of phosphorus and nitrogen. This demineralization of the bone (osteoporosis) makes the skeletal structures prone to pathologic fractures.

In children who are unable to move, such as the child who is unconscious or paralyzed or the child with rheumatoid arthritis, joint mobility becomes restricted because, in the absence of normal structural stretching, collagen fibers generating within the joint become fibrotic and further limit movement. This tissue fibrosis creates a shortening of the muscles and a contracture of the joint. Any decrease in circulation to the joint by edema, inflammation, or restrictive positioning will contribute to further fibrotic changes. The problem rapidly becomes cyclic as the contracture leads to muscle fatigue and pain, which causes the child to splint the site, thus leading to more fibrosis. This process is further exaggerated because body flexor muscles are stronger than the extensor muscles, and unless range of motion is instituted within 3 to 7 days, contractures will develop. Frequent disabling contractures are hip flexion, knee flexion, shoulder stiffness, and plantar flexion of the feet.

Cardiovascular system. There are three major cardiovascular consequences of immobility: orthostatic hypotension, increased workload of the heart, and thrombus formation. During movement, muscle contraction causes

pressure on peripheral veins, which in turn causes the venous valves to close, thus assisting return of the blood to the heart when the individual is in an upright position. In the absence of this assistance blood tends to pool in the dependent areas, reducing the blood supply to trunk and brain. In addition, direct reflex stimulation to the splanchnic and peripheral vessels causes them to constrict when a person is upright. Impairment of this neurovascular orthostatic reflex activity from lack of motion causes further interference with venous return. The individual displays signs of excessive autonomic activity, that is, pallor, sweating, and restlessness that is frequently followed by fainting. The child with a spinal cord injury has unique problems with orthostatic hypotension, which is discussed later in this chapter.

Changes in vascular resistance caused by the horizontal position and immobility alter the distribution of blood within the body. The reduction in gravity pressure to the extremities causes much of the total blood volume to be redistributed from the lower extremities to other parts of the body. Consequently there is an increase in the venous return and the volume of blood to be handled by the heart, which is reflected in an elevated blood pressure. Therefore the cardiac output and stroke volume are increased as well as a progressive increase in heart rate. When immobilization extends over a period of time, there is a compensatory decrease in blood volume and a decrease in heart rate and blood pressure.

Without muscle contraction the venous stasis and increased intravascular pressure in the extremities lead to dependent edema. If undue pressure is exerted on the major veins by positioning or mechanical devices, the likelihood of interstitial edema is increased. Most frequently this situation is seen when the child is placed on his side with one leg resting on the other or when the youngster is permitted to sit for a long time with pressure on the large veins behind the knee and in the groin. Edematous tissue is prone to infection and trauma, especially tissue located over an area that receives much of the body's weight.

Circulatory stasis combined with hypercoagulability of the blood resulting from factors such as increased serum calcium or damage to the inner walls of blood vessels by trauma or infection can lead to thrombus and embolus formation. Bed rest alone will not produce the blood-clotting problems, but debilitated persons often have one or more of these other contributing factors. Sudden chest pain and dyspnea, the symptoms of pulmonary edema, or pain and swelling in the lower extremities, which indicate deep vein thrombosis, are constant concerns of the nurse.

The deconditioned state of cardiac function, caused by skeletal muscle inactivity, can produce a variety of secondary problems in other systems. However, the major clinical manifestation is increased pulse and heart rate in response to an active exercise program. After prolonged immobility the child should build up his activity tolerance slowly to allow the heart to regain its optimum capabilities.

Respiratory system. Initially the effects of immobilization are compensatory or adaptive. The basal metabolic rate is decreased because with reduced expenditure of energy the cells require less oxygen and produce less carbon dioxide. Lessened demand for oxygen–carbon dioxide exchange causes the respirations to become slower and more shallow. Chest expansion may be limited by the supine posture; by abdominal distention caused by accumulation of feces, gas, or fluid; and by mechanical restriction such as a body cast, brace, or tight binders. Reduced muscle power and coordination secondary to altered innervation can also hinder respiratory movement. More effort is required to expand the lungs in the supine position (see Fig. 31-3).

Prolonged immobility also reduces the normal movement of secretions from the tracheobronchial tree, particularly in the presence of impaired muscle function and positional changes that normally facilitate removal of secretions. A weak and ineffectual cough reflex contributes to stasis of secretions and the possibility of airway obstruction. Shallow respirations and obstruction of the airway with thick mucus contribute to the development of secondary complications such as atelectasis, hypostatic pneumonia, and respiratory acidosis.

Gastrointestinal system. Prolonged immobility produces a state of negative nitrogen balance resulting from the increased catabolic activity related to muscle atrophy. This and the reduced energy requirements contribute to a diminished appetite and a resulting decrease in ingestion of nutrients. The mechanisms of eating and feeding become more difficult with immobility, and the risk of aspiration is increased. Intake is further influenced by associated psychologic factors.

The process of elimination depends on the integration of smooth and skeletal muscle activity and on visceral reflex patterns. Immobility may interfere with these mechanisms as well as with the gravitational effect on stool passing through the intestines. Slowing of stool in the colon causes the feces to become hard, and the bowel wall is not stimulated to further its peristaltic movement down the tract to the rectum. Weakened muscles used in defecation (diaphragmatic and abdominal muscles) are unable to produce the intra-abdominal pressure needed for elimination. Sometimes embarrassment in using the bedpan may be the cause of not responding to the urge to defecate.

Urinary system. The structure of the urinary system is designed to function in an upright posture. When the gravitational force is altered by the reclining position, the peristaltic contractions of the ureters are insufficient to overcome gravitational resistance. Consequently there may be stasis of urine in the kidney pelves, and any particulate matter that settles in the calyces may serve as nuclei for calculi formation or as foci for infection.

In the horizontal position the individual has difficulty in relaxing the perineal musculature and external sphincter sufficiently to initiate the integrated reflex micturition mechanism that involves the external sphincter, the internal sphincter, and the detrusor muscle of the bladder wall. If adequate intra-abdominal pressure is exerted, voiding can occur, but if the individual does not respond to the sensation to void, bladder distention leads to stasis and its complications add to overflow incontinence, a source of embarrassment. In time reflex and back pressure may impair renal function, and urinary tract infection is always a hazard with urine retention.

Normally the kidney is able to handle the increased metabolites from protein breakdown and bone demineralization. However, the increased level of calcium excreted may predispose to the formation of calculi. Calculi formation is further favored by urinary stasis, infection, and an alkaline urine caused by the decreased production of the acid by-products of metabolism. Painless hematuria may be the only clue to diagnosis.

Metabolism. Immobility or severe restriction of activity is often accompanied by decreased or inappropriate nutritional intake that frequently leads to decreased basal metabolic rate, a negative nitrogen balance associated with catabolism, and a high calcium serum level.

All body systems are influenced by a decrease in metabolism. The altered energy level leads to further fatigue and lack of motivation for moving. Although less of a problem in children, immobilized persons often feel sluggish and have a poor appetite, particularly for protein foods. The protein breakdown in the body related to a loss of muscle and other tissues is more apt to be severe after injury or surgery. Protein breakdown produces nitrogenous wastes, and on the fifth or sixth day of catabolic protein metabolism, an increase in urinary nitrogen develops that contributes to anemia and delayed healing.

Another metabolic problem is hypercalcemia associated with bone catabolism. Completely immobilized youngsters are especially prone to hypercalcemia. Symptoms include nausea and vomiting, polydipsia, polyuria, and lethargy that usually appears 4 to 8 weeks after immobilization. In quadriplegia it may occur within 10 days and last for as long as 6 months. The accelerated rates of bone metabolism in youngsters make the bone demineralization a greater hazard.

Fig. 40-2. Sequence of events in tissue breakdown.

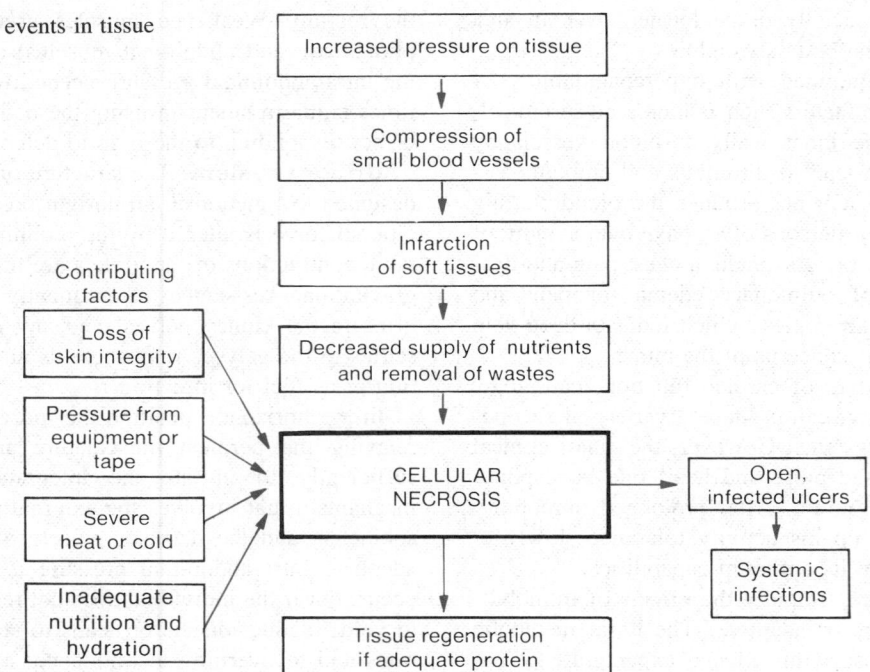

Larger amounts of calcium are released into the blood than the kidney can excrete, and calcium continues to accumulate in the serum. High levels of serum calcium decrease neuronal permeability that can lead to a depression of the central and peripheral nervous systems. Symptoms including smooth and skeletal muscle fatigue, diminished reflexes, and atony of the gastrointestinal tract are the result of the depressed nervous system.

Medical treatment for hypercalcemia consists of restricting dietary calcium, increasing weight bearing when this is possible, and most importantly vigorous hydration (e.g., 3000 to 4000 ml/day of fluid for a teenager). Electrolyte imbalances are corrected, and diuretics are administered to promote removal of calcium. Sometimes pharmacologic agents, such as corticosteroids, oral phosphates, and thyrocalcitonin, may be used to lower serum calcium levels. Any urinary tract infection is treated.

A child with bone demineralization may not develop hypercalcemia, but the excess amount of calcium that his kidneys are required to excrete may produce a negative calcium balance with more calcium than citric acid lost in the urine. This imbalance causes the urine to become alkaline with the potential danger of renal calculi, especially if there is an accompanying retention of urine.

Integumentary system. Circulation to the skin is reduced during inactivity and may be further impeded by dependent edema. Circulation is especially compromised in places where the bone surface is near the skin, such as areas over the sacrum, occiput, trochanter, and ankle, and continued impairment causes rapid necrosis with ulcer formation. Mechanical irritation from appliances, such as straps, rods, and ropes, and the friction of bedclothes during turning or other movement can produce skin breakdown. Healing ca-

pacity is also impaired by poor circulation, negative nitrogen balance, and anemia. Immobilization often makes it difficult to carry out adequate cleansing and hygienic measures, which may also contribute to tissue breakdown in areas that are difficult to reach. Children with neurologic deficit should be guarded against extremes of heat and cold in direct contact with the skin.

Cellular breakdown caused by prolonged pressure can be identified by several characteristics. Normally when pressure is applied to the skin, the skin appears pale but becomes very red, or hyperemic, after pressure is removed. This reactive hyperemia should disappear within 5 to 15 minutes. Prolonged redness (over 30 minutes) indicates that a pressure area is developing and treatment should be instituted. Other manifestations of tissue ischemia include an increase in temperature in the area, blistering, swelling, or dark purple or black areas. The pressure area may be limited to the skin and subcutaneous layers or may be deeper and more extensive. The skin changes observed may represent the top of a cone-shaped area with widespread tissue destruction, beneath which tissue rapidly ulcerates and creates a large hole that sometimes extends to the bone. The skin may be broken or even accompanied by a purulent drainage. Fig. 40-2 illustrates the sequence of events in tissue breakdown.

Neurosensory system. Studies indicate that immobilization does not produce neurosensory consequences directly; however, two occurrences—loss of innervation and sensory and perceptual deprivation—are common.

Peripheral nerves, in contrast to skeletal muscles, do not degenerate with disuse, but loss of innervation takes place if nerves are damaged by pressure or if their blood supply is disrupted. Improper body positioning or poorly applied casts or restraints can place unwarranted pressure on nerves and blood vessels that can lead to ischemia and nerve degeneration. Frequent sites of this compression phenomenon are pressure on the peroneal nerve, resulting in footdrop or on the radial nerve, leading to wristdrop. These complications significantly interfere with attempts to regain functional use of extremities, but they can be prevented by conscientious nursing assessment and intervention. Preventing pressure on vulnerable areas and avoiding unnatural positions of flexion and extension that apply inappropriate pressure on nerves and blood vessels reduce the likelihood of compression injury. Periodic plantar flexion and dorsiflexion of the feet and hands will stimulate circulation and keep nerves from becoming pinched. Numbness and tingling are symptoms of neurologic impairment and should be evaluated immediately.

Psychologic Effects of Immobilization

For children one of the most difficult aspects of illness is immobilization. Throughout childhood physical activity is an integral part of daily life and is essential for physical growth and development. It also serves children as an instrument for communication and expression and as a means for learning about and understanding their world. It helps them deal with a variety of feelings and impulses and provides a mechanism by which they can exert control over inner tensions. Children respond to anxiety with increased activity. Removal of this power deprives them of necessary input and a natural outlet for their feelings and fantasies. Through movement children also gain sensory input that provides an essential element for developing and maintaining a body image.

In daily life children's activity is restricted in many ways: limits are set on behavior and expression, activity is restricted by physical and verbal barriers, and neuromuscular function is affected directly by disease or injury. The child perceives restraint by persons or inanimate objects as either comforting or stressful. Adult controls on behavior often provide the child with a sense of security in frightening situations or when he fears loss of control. On the other hand, forced inactivity deprives him of one of his most valuable means for dealing with stress. A child who is confined to bed may become a victim of his fears and fantasies without the physical means for stress reduction. Sometimes a child will impose restrictions on himself, particularly in interaction with others, by confining himself to his bed with blankets pulled about him or by retreating into sleep in the presence of stimulation.

The active child has many opportunities for input from a wide variety of settings. When he is immobilized by disease or as a part of a treatment regimen, he experiences diminished environmental stimuli with a loss of tactile input and an altered perception of himself and his environment. Sudden or gradual immobilization narrows the amount and variety of environmental stimuli he receives by means of all of his senses: touch, sight, hearing, taste, smell, and proprioception—a feeling of where he is in his environment.

This sensory deprivation frequently leads to a feeling of isolation, boredom, and being forgotten, especially by his peers.

Sensorimotor activity is a predominant mode of activity in infants; even newborns respond with rage when they are physically restrained. Physical interference with the activity of infants and young children gives them a feeling of helplessness. It has also been found that speech and language skills require sensorimotor activity and experience. There appears to be a significant relationship between physical restraint and the incidence of language problems. Children who are restrained by casts, splints, or straps during the first 3 years of life have more difficulty with language than children whose activities were unrestricted. Language delay is even more marked in children with neurologic impairment (Sibinga and Freedman, 1971).

Observations of children's behavior during restraint indicate some differences between infants and older children. Initially infants temporarily freed from physical restraint remain immobile and then submit without protest to restoration of restraint. However, with subsequent release, their activity level progressively increases, as does their protesting behavior after reapplication of restraints. In contrast, toddlers and preschool children show a decrease in protest with each subsequent removal and restoration of restraint. It is uncertain whether this diminished protest in these children reflects inhibitions developed as a result of frustration or a development of trust that the nurse will return to release the restraints.

The struggle for independence is thwarted by imposed immobility. For the toddler, exploration and imitative behaviors are essential to developing a sense of autonomy; the preschooler's expression of initiative is evidenced by his penchant for vigorous physical activity; the school-age child's development is strongly influenced by physical achievement and competition; and the adolescent relies on mobility to achieve independence. The quest for mastery at every stage of development is related to mobility. To the child the inability to move is threatening to self-preservation and reactivates the struggle between activity and passivity and between dependence and independence.

Behavioral changes are noted when a child experiences prolonged sensory deprivation. These behaviors are demonstrated by a higher than normal level of anxiety: restlessness, difficulty in problem solving, inability to concentrate on activities, and egocentrism. The monotony of the situation can lead to sluggish intellectual and psychomotor responses, decreased communication skills, increased fantasizing, and even hallucinations and disorientation. The child is likely to become depressed over his loss of ability to function or the marked changes in his body image. His significant others are apt to notice regressive behavior and a greater reliance on them for tasks he is able to perform; He seeks their attention by reverting to earlier developmental behaviors, such as wanting to be fed, bed-wetting, and baby talk. In many ways the immobilized child is realistically dependent on others; therefore intelligent and sensitive care is required to prevent major growth and developmental regressions during the period of immobility.

Limbs in casts or traction transmit less than normal sensory data. The presence of sensory impairment may be a concomitant problem of the involved part. Numbness or loss of feeling markedly alters proprioception. A child who has limited ability to feel others touching him not only experiences less tactile stimuli in a physical sense but is also deprived of warm, loving feelings that arise from being touched. The loss of feeling derived from touch can further add to his sense of being isolated and unwanted.

The type and extent of immobilization influence the emotional response. When children are able to see the reason for their restraint (e.g., a cast or intravenous infusion), they are less likely to be resistant. The child whose activity is restricted because of a nonvisible disorder (e.g., rheumatic fever) finds it difficult to understand the reason for adult restrictions on activity, imagines the worst, and may react with noncompliance and overactivity when unobserved. Children may react to immobility by active protest, anger, and aggressive behavior, or they may become quiet, passive, and submissive. Often children believe that the immobilization is a justified punishment for misbehavior. Children should be allowed to discharge their anger, but it should be within the limits of safety to their self-esteem and not damaging to the integrity of others. For example, providing an object to attack rather than a person or a valued possession is safe and therapeutic.

Unfortunately most adults resent and find it difficult to deal with the acting-out behavior of children. Too often this behavior is considered ''bad'' even when it is obviously a release of tension. In some cases, such as the paralyzed child, nurses may feel inadequate to cope with the child's profound distress and feelings of hopelessness, and the professional help of a psychologist or psychiatrist is needed.

The most difficult situations are those involving major injuries and diseases that produce a disfigurement or a severe loss of function that directly affects a child's self-image, such as burns, amputation, or the sudden catastrophic effects of an accident that leaves a healthy, athletic child paralyzed for life. Feelings of anger and hostility are difficult for the child to express when he is at the mercy of his environment. He dares not speak out against or defy the authorities on whom he depends so completely. Consequently his aggression may be masked by cheerfulness or rigidity. When he is unable to express his anger, the aggression is often displayed inappropriately through regressive behavior and outbursts of crying or temper tantrums over insignificant irritations, such as warm milk, a wrinkled collar, or a delay in routine.

Effect on families. Brief periods of immobilization have few effects on the family; however, catastrophic illness or disability severely taxes the resources of the family. In general, emotionally mature families with financial resources and satisfactory problem-solving skills handle the crises well. Their needs are often very specific, primarily in the areas of instruction concerning medical and nursing care, community resources to contact, and emotional support as they go through the grief process. However, many families are unstable, are already plagued by unmet needs, operate from crisis to crisis, and are often unable to use outside help appropriately. For these families the new situation can disrupt the entire family; therefore the rehabilitation team must help the family members identify unmet needs and actively help in the family's problem-solving process. The following are commonly occurring problems:

1. Financial strains may decrease or totally eliminate the family's resources.
2. The focus of attention is placed, at least temporarily, on the affected member; therefore other members of the family may feel neglected or their needs may not be met.
3. The family may have difficulty in accepting the child's altered body image.
4. Individual family members may be unable to express their feelings and become immobilized in the face of the crisis.

The family's needs can often be met by the physician and nurse but may also require the services of other professionals, such as a social worker, psychiatrist, or marriage counselor. In preparation for discharge, home visits are advisable and home management is frequently planned weeks in advance of the actual discharge, including special considerations for economic, physical, and psychologic needs. A severely disabled child is very dependent, and caregivers need rest periods to revitalize themselves. Individual and group counseling is beneficial for preproblem-solving situations and provides an emotional support system. Parent groups are also helpful and often allow nonthreatening social contact. The families of permanently disabled children need long-term resources, since some of the most difficult problems arise as they try to sustain high-quality care for many years (see Chapter 22).

Nursing Considerations

The effects of immobilization can be minimized and in many instances prevented by conscientious nursing care. The major goals in care of the immobilized child are to prevent the pathophysiologies associated with immobility and to use measures for regaining function and remobilization within the limitations of the therapeutic regimen or the physical disabilities of the child.

Frequent position changes help to prevent dependent edema and fluid movement and to stimulate circulation, respiratory function, gastrointestinal motility, and neurologic sensations. When the child's condition allows, the child can periodically assume the upright position on a tilt table or similar device to stimulate gastrointestinal and renal function and increase the stress on bones.

Each metabolic disturbance is treated specifically. Metabolism is increased by activity within the limitations of the disability and capabilities of the child. High-protein, high-calorie foods are encouraged for correction of negative nitrogen balance. This may be difficult to correct by diet, especially if anorexia is present. Stimulating the appetite with small servings of attractively arranged preferred foods may be sufficient. Sometimes supplementary nasogastric feedings or hyperalimentation may be needed.

Diet modification for the child with increased serum calcium presents problems, because the dairy foods that children often desire are high in this mineral. Acid ash foods such as cereals, meats, poultry, fish, and cranberry or apple juice are encouraged. Lying in a prone position may precipitate problems with swallowing or self-feeding. Therefore offering small bites, controlling swallowing with semisolid food, and using a straw for fluids are nursing behaviors that will prevent choking. A suction machine should be in the vicinity for emergencies. The primary nursing measure for hypercalcemia is conscientious hydration and active remobilization as soon as possible.

Adequate hydration promotes bowel and kidney function and helps prevent complications in these systems. A knowledge of the child's previous bowel habits and of a method to get him to a commode helps promote elimination and will be valuable data if needed for a bowel program. Embarrassment can be avoided by a mutually satisfactory communication system. Whenever possible, the child should be helped into a sitting position so that he can use a fracture urinal or a bedpan. Providing privacy for toileting and encouraging the child to participate in solving toileting problems will increase the chances of a successful program.

Children should be encouraged to be as active as their condition and restrictive devices allow. This poses few problems for children, whose innate ingenuity and natural inclination toward mobility provide them with the impetus for physical activity. They need the opportunity, the materials or objects to stimulate activity, and the encouragement and participation of others. Those who are unable to move will need passive exercise and movement.

Whenever possible, transporting the child by stretcher, stroller, or wagon outside the confines of his room will increase environmental stimuli and provide social contact with others. While hospitalized, the child will benefit from frequent visitors, clocks and calendars, and a program of diversional therapy, which will help him to function in a more normal way. As soon as possible he should wear "street clothes" and resume school and preinjury hobbies. Play is the most useful tool of nursing (see Chapter 26), and activities, which are selected on the basis of interest, ability, and limitations, should include some form of physical activity that encourages the use of uninvolved muscles and joints. Any activity that is tolerated (e.g., turning in bed or changing position of a bed in the room) helps to alter the monotony of immobilization and dissipates tension and frustration.

Using dolls to illustrate and explain the restraining method is a valuable tool for small children. Placing a cast, tubing, or other restraining equipment on the doll offers the child a nonthreatening opportunity to express, through the doll, his feelings concerning the restrictions and the nurse and provides a means for anticipatory teaching and explanation of needed restraining devices.

One of the most useful interventions to help children cope with immobility is participation in their own care. Self-care to the maximum extent is usually well received by children. They can help plan their daily routine, select their diet (when possible), and choose the clothes they are to wear, including innovative adornment, such as a baseball cap, brightly colored stockings, or other items of apparel that express each child's autonomy and individuality. They should be encouraged to do as much for themselves as they are able in order to keep muscles active and their interest alive. If feasible, they should be placed where they can benefit from the company of other children who are immobilized which assures them that they are not singled out for this treatment.

It is important for the child to understand behavioral limitations or rules, and his questions should be answered. For example, he needs to know the reasons for medical, nursing, occupational, and physical therapy and to know that schedules are necessary. In some areas he has a choice; in others he does not. He may or may not be permitted to sleep late, but he can choose his own clothing. Most of a child's activity of daily living is play; therefore therapies that incorporate this concept are more apt to gain his cooperation.

Visits from significant persons, such as family and friends, offer occasions for emotional support and also provide opportunities for learning the child's care. A severely disabled child's needs can be very complex, and family members require time to assimilate the teachings and demonstrations needed to understand his situation and care.

Some privacy is needed, particularly by the teenager, and most long-term health care facilities recognize that rooms shared by two to four youngsters are better environments for habilitation or rehabilitation. When roommates are selected according to age and companionship, a chance is available to safely test out thoughts and feelings with others. If a traumatic incident caused the child's disability, guilt feelings may be displayed overtly or masked behind regressive or aggressive behavior. The feeling that "I must have been bad to receive this fate" is common, and honest feedback stating "It just happened—it was an accident" needs repeating many times. Additional aspects of grieving are involved if there was a loss of another in the accident. All of these feelings need to be brought out and dealt with. In addition, professional persons working with the severely disabled child must not baby or overprotect him but help him to cope with his altered body image and reestablish his self-esteem.

For a child with greatly restricted movement, for example, the quadriplegic child or the child with a large bilateral hip spica cast, nursing care is a challenge. These situations require long-term care either in the hospital or at home, but, wherever the care occurs, consistent planning and coordination of activities with professionals and significant others are vital. Nursing assessment includes psychosocial data as well as physical manifestations, since long-term immobilization has a profound effect on the child and the family. Nursing approaches are evaluated frequently and continued, discontinued, or modified to meet the changing problems and goals. Physical effects of immobilization and appropriate nursing considerations are summarized in Table 40-1.

Table 40-1 Summary of physical effects of immobilization with nursing interventions*

PRIMARY EFFECTS	SECONDARY EFFECTS	NURSING CONSIDERATIONS
Muscular system		
Decreased muscle strength, tone, and endurance	Decreased venous return and decreased cardiac output	Use elastic stockings or wrap legs with Ace bandages to promote venous return
	Decreased metabolism and need for oxygen	
	Decreased exercise tolerance	
	Bone demineralization	Place in upright posture when possible
Disuse atrophy and loss of muscle mass	Catabolism	Perform range of motion, active, passive, and stretching exercises
	Loss of strength	
Loss of joint mobility	Contractures, ankylosis of joints	Maintain correct body alignment
		Use joint splints as indicated to prevent further deformity
Weak back muscles	Secondary spinal deformities	Maintain body alignment
Weak abdominal muscles	Impaired respiration	See nursing considerations for respiratory system
Skeletal system		
Bone demineralization— osteoporosis, hypercalcemia	Negative calcium balance	In paralysis, use upright posture on tilt table
	Pathologic fractures	
	Calcium deposits	Handle extremities carefully when turning and positioning
	Extraosseous bone formation, especially at hip, knee, elbow, and shoulder	Administer calcium-mobilizing drugs (diphosphonates) if ordered
	Renal calculi	Ensure adequate intake of fluid
		Acidify urine
		Promptly treat urinary tract infections
Negative calcium balance	Life-threatening electrolyte imbalance	Monitor blood levels of calcium electrolytes
		Provide electrolyte replacement as indicated
Metabolism		
Decreased metabolic rate	Slowing of all systems	Mobilize as soon as possible
	Decreased food intake	Perform active and passive resistive and deep breathing exercises
		Ensure adequate food intake
		Provide a high-protein diet
Negative nitrogen balance	Decline in nutritional state	Encourage small, frequent feedings with protein and preferred foods
	Impaired healing	Prevent pressure areas
Hypercalcemia	Electrolyte imbalance	See nursing considerations for skeletal system
Decreased production of stress hormones	Decreased physical and emotional coping capacity	Identify etiologies of stress
		Implement appropriate interventions to lower physical and psychosocial stresses
Cardiovascular system		
Decreased efficiency of orthostatic neurovascular reflexes	Inability to adapt readily to upright position	Monitor peripheral pulses and skin temperature changes
	Pooling of blood in extremities in upright posture	Wrap legs in elastic bandage or stockings to decrease pooling when upright
Diminished vasopressor mechanism	Orthostatic hypotension with syncope— hypotension, decreased cerebral blood flow, tachycardia	Provide abdominal support
		In severe cases, use antigravitational suit
		Administer peripheral sympathetic stimulating agents such as ephedrine if ordered
		Position horizontally
Altered distribution of blood volume	Decreased cardiac work load	Monitor hydration and urine output
	Decreased exercise tolerance	

*Use measures that apply. Not all problems will be applicable in every situation.

Table 40-1 Summary of physical effects of immobilization with nursing interventions—cont'd

PRIMARY EFFECTS	SECONDARY EFFECTS	NURSING CONSIDERATIONS
Venous stasis	Pulmonary emboli and/or thrombi	Have frequent position changes Elevate extremities without knee flexion Ensure adequate fluid intake Perform active or passive exercises or movement, if ordered Prescribe routine wearing of antiembolic stockings or wrap lower extremities from metatarsus to gluteal folds Measure circumference of extremities periodically Give anticoagulant drugs if ordered until mobilization possible Promptly intervene to maintain adequate oxygen if signs and symptoms of pulmonary emboli
Dependent edema	Tissue breakdown and susceptibility to infection	Administer good skin care Turn every 2 hours Monitor skin color, temperature, and integrity
Respiratory system Decreased need for oxygen	Altered oxygen–carbon dioxide exchange and metabolism	Exercise as tolerated Use position for chest expansion
Decreased chest expansion and diminished vital capacity	Diminished oxygen intake Dyspnea and inadequate arterial oxygen saturation; acidosis	Use prone positioning without pressure on abdomen to allow gravity to aid in diaphragm excursion When sitting, be certain of good alignment to prevent pressure on respiratory mechanism
Poor abdominal tone and distention	Interference with diaphragmatic excursion	Avoid restriction of chest and abdominal musculature Supply torso support to promote chest expansion
Mechanical or biochemical secretion retention	Hypostatic pneumonia Bacterial and viral pneumonia Atelectasis	Change position frequently Carry out percussion, vibration, and drainage (or suctioning) as necessary
Loss of respiratory muscle strength	Poor cough	Encourage coughing and deep breathing Support chest wall when coughing Use special devices such as a rocking bed, Ambu bag, incentive spirometers, intermittent positive-pressure breathing Observe for signs of acute respiratory distress with blood gas levels measured as necessary
	Upper respiratory infection	Avoid contact with infected persons Provide adequate hydration
Gastrointestinal system Distention caused by poor abdominal muscle tone	Interference with respiratory movements	Use abdominal binder if indicated Monitor bowel sounds Encourage small, frequent feedings
	Difficulty in feeding in prone position	Sit in upright position if possible

Continued.

Table 40-1 Summary of physical effects of immobilization with nursing interventions—cont'd

PRIMARY EFFECTS	SECONDARY EFFECTS	NURSING CONSIDERATIONS
No specific primary effect	Gravitation effect on feces through ascending colon or weakened smooth muscle tone may cause constipation	Carry out bowel training program with hydration, stool softeners, and mild laxatives if necessary
	Anorexia	Stimulate appetite with favored foods
Urinary system Alteration of gravitational force	Difficulty in voiding in prone position	Position as upright as possible to void
Impaired ureteral peristalsis	Urinary retention in calyces and bladder	Hydrate to ensure adequate urinary output for age
	Infection	Collect specimens as needed
	Renal calculi	Stimulate bladder emptying with warm water, running water, striking suprapubic area
		Catheterize only for severe retention
		Administer urinary tract antiseptics as indicated
Integumentary system No specific primary effect	Decreased circulation and pressure leading to tissue injury	Turn and position at least every 2 hours
	Difficulty with personal hygiene	Frequently inspect total skin surface
		Eliminate mechanical factors causing pressure, friction, or irritation
		Assess ability to perform hygienic care and assist with bathing, grooming, and toileting as needed

*Use measures that apply. Not all problems will be applicable in every situation.

MOBILIZATION DEVICES

Children usually respond well to mobilization and require little encouragement, but they need instruction in correct use of appliances, their operation, and precautions for their safe usage.

Braces

Paralyzed or markedly weakened extremities can sometimes be stabilized by metal braces that facilitate walking. Some are designed to stabilize the extremities and offer support during ambulation. Special joint hinges permit the hip, knee, and ankle to flex during sitting, whereas the leg is held rigid during ambulation. Meticulous skin care and the wearing of protective clothing under the brace are necessary. Well-fitted braces promote ambulation, whereas ill-fitting braces are dangerous to the balance of the child and frequently cause muscle stress and tissue breakdown. Braces for the growing child will need frequent adjusting and replacement by the orthotist if long-term use is necessary.

The Jewett-Taylor brace is frequently used to support the spine and trunk during ambulation in conditions such as scoliosis and spinal cord injury. The brace must fit each body curvature to avoid undue pressure on tissues and imbalance between muscle groups. Bony prominences where the brace has contact, such as along the spine, chin, and iliac crests, are observed closely for pressure or irritation and are padded as necessary. A corset with metal stays may provide the needed torso support, especially for a paraplegic child. Generally the corset is more comfortable than the metal and leather brace and presents fewer problems with dressing. A specialized brace that can be used to provide upright mobility in the small child with lower limb paralysis is the parapodium. With these devices the child shifts body weight to achieve locomotion.

Parallel bars. Parallel bars provide secure hand rails on both sides of the child as he learns to walk again with or without braces. As he becomes more proficient, a walker with or without wheels is substituted for the bars and the child is no longer confined to a limited territory. He then progresses to crutches.

Crutches and Canes

Crutches are used when a child is not allowed to bear weight or can only place part of his body weight on an extremity, such as most lower leg injuries. A variety of crutches can be employed, and the selection is determined

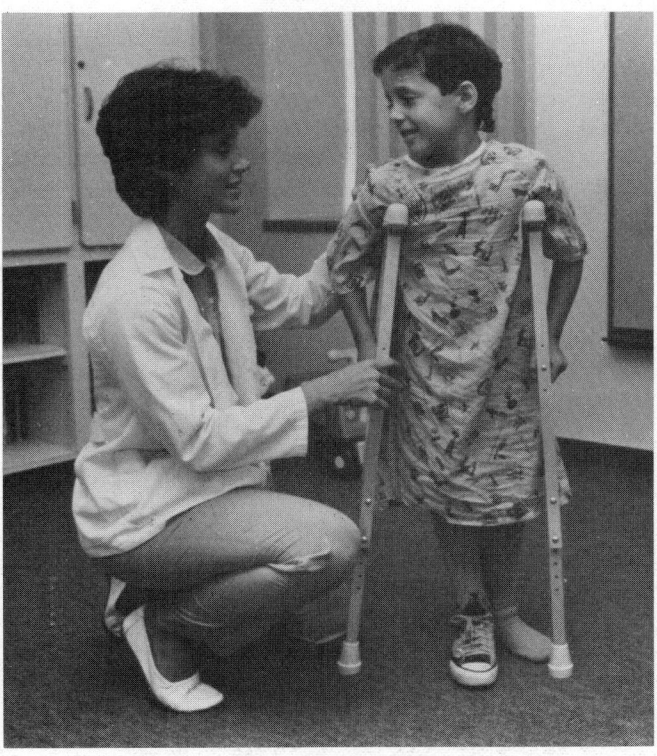

Fig. 40-3. Child learning to walk with crutches.
Photography by John Roy, Saint Francis Hospital, Tulsa, OK.

by the individual needs of the child. *Axillary* crutches are used most frequently as temporary assistance. *Forearm* crutches are the usual selection for children who anticipate permanent use, such as the paraplegic child who is able to use braces. For children with limited hand and arm strength or function, *trough* crutches allow the weight to be assumed by the elbow. For habilitating small children who have not yet learned to walk or who are unsteady, special crutches stabilized with three or four legs provide needed stability for the child to maintain an upright position and learn to walk.

The child must be properly fitted for the crutch or cane to prevent poor posture and crutch pressure on the axilla during ambulation. Teaching crutch and cane use is usually assumed by the physical therapist in most institutions but is also the responsibility of nurses, especially those in physicians' offices, outpatient departments, and schools. Nurses are the persons who supervise the use of crutches in pediatric units and in the home (Fig. 40-3). The type of crutch gait taught to the child depends on his degree of stability, whether or not the knees can be flexed, and the specific goal established for the child.

Bed exercises for strengthening arms and shoulders are important if immobilization has been prolonged. The youngster gains confidence in ambulating by wearing a safety belt held onto by the therapist. The types of gaits used and instructions to the child are similar to those given adults. They are conveyed with language the child understands and with demonstration. Most children grasp the techniques readily.

Special Beds

Older quadriplegic children often require a special bed to immobilize the head and spine during the early phases of spinal cord injury care. Some rehabilitation units use a regular bed for the patient in cervical traction, whereas others use a Stryker frame or one of the Roto-Rest beds. Whatever special bed is used, the success of its use is greatly influenced by the preparation of the child. Explanations of how the bed works and, when possible, showing the child someone being turned in the bed, are needed. Nursing personnel need in-service practice in the operation of these beds to ensure the safe handling of the equipment.

A Stryker frame employs two frames, one anterior and one posterior, to turn the child horizontally. The Stryker wedge frame was designed to allow prone-supine turning by one person. Cervical traction can easily be attached to the stationary frame and presents no discomfort when turning as long as the weights are prevented from swinging. Before turning, the child's arms and legs are aligned within the frame and straps are wrapped around the entire ''sandwich'' of frames. All of the skin areas should be checked with each turning.

The Roto-Rest bed operates electrically; with the person's entire body securely immobilized by firm bolsters, he is slowly and constantly rotated from side to side. Traction can be attached to this bed, and various parts can be removed to permit care and physical therapy. The continuous changes of position decrease the problems of pressure areas and promote venous circulation. The bed has a major advantage over a Stryker frame for teenagers with tracheostomies or other conditions that do not allow placing them in the prone position. The bed is made in an adult size and is suited only for large children.

Wheelchairs

Wheelchairs are used temporarily or permanently as a means of transportation. For temporary use, a wheelchair should fit the child and contain any adaptations needed, such as an elevating leg rest or reclining back. The child is taught how to transfer in and out of the chair and how to propel it safely. Prescribing a wheelchair for permanent use is the joint responsibility of physician and therapist after an assessment of home and surroundings. A wheelchair should be neither too small nor too large, preferably one that can be adapted to the child's growth needs. Detachable or rotating armrests, which permit easy transfer in and out, are needed for children with spinal cord injuries.

Other desirable features are detachable and swing-away footrests and detachable desk arms. Elevating leg rests are required for children who are prone to contractures, and a reclining back rest is needed for those who may have poor trunk balance. A proper cushion with adequate padding should be provided for the child who has decreased sensation. Hand rim and brake lever projections are helpful for the child with upper extremity weakness. The paraplegic child will require upper arm strengthening exercises and in-

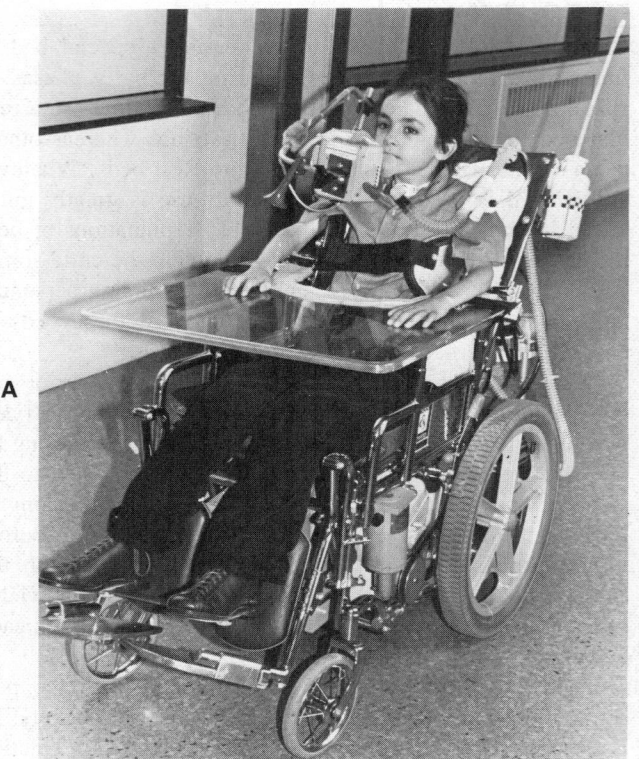 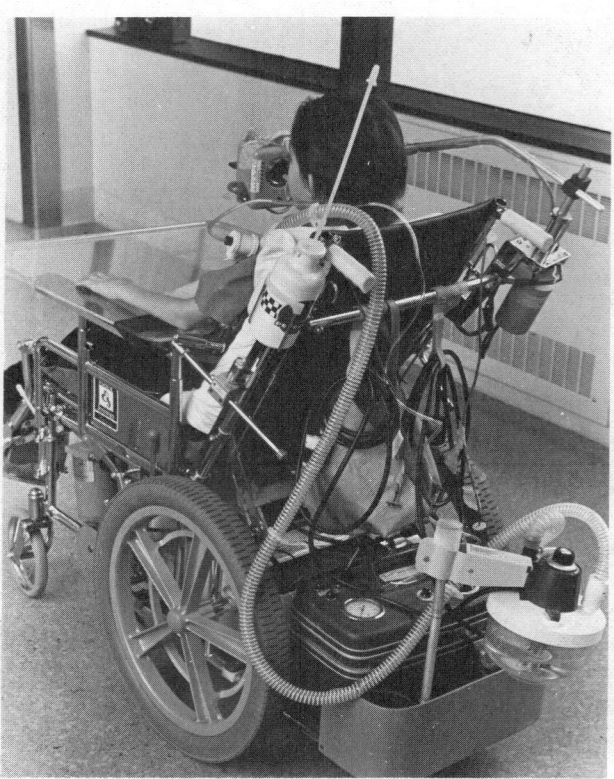

Fig. 40-4. Motorized wheelchair for quadriplegic child. **A,** Front view. **B,** Back view. Note portable respirator.

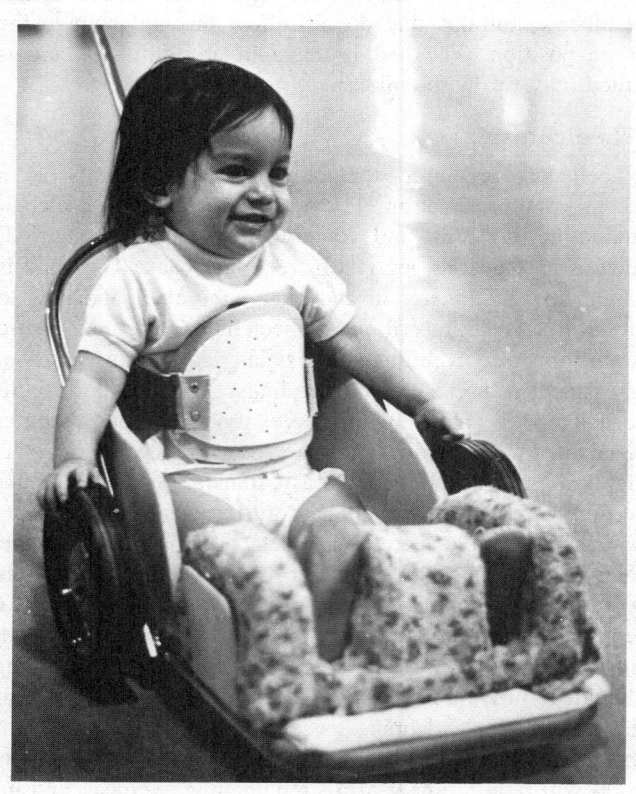

Fig. 40-5. Mobilization device for toddler.

struction on transfer techniques before wheelchair mobilization. Often a tilt table must be used to overcome the problems of orthostatic hypotension before wheelchair sitting can be tolerated.

Various motorized chairs are available for marked upper extremity weakness, and mouth- or cheek-operated models are available for children who do not have the use of upper extremities so that children can operate them independently (Fig. 40-4). Very small children who have permanent paralysis of lower extremities are provided with specially designed units that allow independent mobility (Fig. 40-5). A detachable handle on these units permits their conversion to strollers.

The Child and Trauma

Trauma is the leading cause of death in children over age 1 year (see Chapter 1) and an important cause of disability during childhood and adolescence. A variety of structures constitute the musculoskeletal system. Each component part of the musculoskeletal system is essential for the mobility needed to perform activities of daily living, such as walking, feeding, dressing, and playing. The skeleton or bony framework provides the support; the muscles, tendons, ligaments, and joints allow for active movement. Muscles are attached to bones by tendons, and strong, fibrous bands (ligaments) attach the bone ends to an articulated joint. Muscles are innervated by sensory and motor fibers from the central nervous system. Any or all of these structures can be involved in a traumatic injury and may alter the course of healing in certain situations.

TRAUMA MANAGEMENT

In order to provide optimum care for trauma victims, community resources for children must be available and appropriately organized for rapid transit, skilled care, and specialized facilities. With such a system of care for pediatric patients, the mortality and morbidity can be minimized (Ramenofsky and Morse, 1983).

Etiology of Trauma

In many ways childhood trauma differs little from trauma in adults. However, many aspects of injury are affected by the developmental stage of the child in both the type of injury that is incurred and the physiologic response to injury.

Accidental injury. Among the leading causes of morbidity in children are medical problems resulting from traumatic injury at home, at school, in an automobile, or associated with recreational activities. Children's everyday activities include vigorous play, such as climbing, falling, running into immovable objects, and receiving blows to any part of their bodies. All of these activities make them prone to injury. Adolescents are vulnerable to multiple and severe trauma because they are mobile on bikes and motorcycles and active in sports. Speed and congested surroundings often intensify the chance of injury. Young children and teenagers usually do not calculate risks as they learn to manipulate their environment and achieve developmental goals. Therefore accidents are a part of most childhood experiences. Fortunately, when children fall or are hit, their body resilience protects them from incurring serious damage to soft tissue, the musculoskeletal system, or other body organs. Their bones are more flexible and therefore do not resist the external forces that are likely to cause fractures.

Child abuse injury. Unfortunately careless handling of an infant or child, in some instances intentional physical abuse, is not uncommon in our society. A multitude of different types of bone and soft tissue injuries are inflicted on children by adults (see p. 681), and smaller children who are unable to protect themselves are most vulnerable. It is estimated that perhaps 25% of fractures in children under 3 years of age are the result of child abuse. Emergency room and pediatric office personnel should be alert to situations in which the child's injuries are not congruent with the parent's description of the incident; in which the child's behavior, such as lack of crying or fearful mannerisms are not the expected ones; or in which x-ray films show multiple healed fractures. For example, toddlers do not readily fall and break bones or catch a leg in the crib and break it. Reporting these incidents will aid in securing help for the child and parents. A traumatic incident that produces physical injury to an infant or child may be the outcome of an accident

Emergency Treatment: Trauma

1. Make certain that the child and rescuer are not in immediate danger of additional trauma
   Do not move child unless absolutely necessary
   Keep child flat unless injury or symptoms specifically indicate otherwise:
   Head injury—elevate head slightly
   Vomiting—carefully turn head to side
2. Apply ABCs of emergency management
   Airway—ensure open airway
   Breathing—promote breathing; if not breathing, begin pulmonary resuscitation (see p. 1328)
   Circulation—check pulse; if no pulse, begin chest compression (see p. 1329)
3. Assess for extent of injury
4. Stop bleeding with direct pressure to the wound or at appropriate bleeding point(s)
   Elevate injured part
   Apply sterile or clean dressing
   Use tourniquets only when bleeding cannot be stopped by any other means
   Release tourniquet pressure every 15 to 20 minutes
   Notify person(s) taking over care of the child of the presence of tourniquet(s)
   Do not remove tourniquet until a physician is present
5. Assess for further injury
6. Determine state of consciousness
   Talk to child
   Observe child's behavior
7. Check for evidence of decreased motor or sensory function in extremities
   Infant and young child—observe spontaneous movement in extremities
   Older child—ask if able to wiggle extremities
8. Evaluate pain—present, absent; severe, mild
   Attempt to alleviate with nonpharmacologic techniques
9. Assess pulses in extremity distal to the injury
   Check color and temperature of extremities
10. Manage any injuries appropriately, e.g., splint fractures, (see p. 1805)
11. Identify child
12. Get information regarding the injury from witnesses, if any
13. Call EMR or transport to nearest facility

NOTE: If spinal cord injury is suspected, do not move child unless absolutely necessary for the child's safety.

that was no one's fault or may be associated with child abuse. A well-documented history is essential to determine the cause of the injury.

Birth injuries. During the birth process, fractures, dislocations, and/or nerve damage may be sustained. These injuries most often occur when the baby is large, when the presentation is breech, or when forceful extraction is used because of fetal distress. The two most common types of musculoskeletal injuries incurred during birth are fractured clavicle and brachial plexus injury. The presence of a qualified person at delivery will aid in reducing the complications of a difficult delivery. Complete postdelivery assessment of the newborn is essential for early detection of neurologic and/or musculoskeletal problems. Birth injuries are discussed on p. 341.

Prevention of Injuries

Hazardous environmental factors play a major role in the number of serious accidents incurred by children. Stairways without hand rails or a gate at the top, cluttered walkways, waxed floors, or throw rugs can contribute to a severe fall. Playground equipment should be checked periodically for hazards, and play areas should be supervised. Adults in charge of sports activities are encouraged to promote the use of safety-tested equipment and to follow game rules to prevent trauma and overplaying of a young athlete whose immature musculoskeletal system and lack of coordination cannot tolerate excessive abuse.

Musculoskeletal trauma is most likely to occur in contact sports, with sprains being common. Certain contact sports, such as football, tend to produce joint damage, especially knee injuries. Severe hyperflexion of the neck from diving, trampoline activities, or football produces spinal cord injury and quadriplegia. Protective head and shoulder gear is helpful, but youngsters usually do not consistently wear appropriate protection unless they are well supervised (see Sports injuries p. 844).

For children riding in a car, an effective infant or child car seat is a must to avoid their being thrown during a sudden stop or collision (see pp. 538 and 618). If this practice is begun when the child is an infant, the young child will be more likely to develop the habit of securing safety belts before the engine is started. In their everyday life observant nurses are a valuable community resource in giving suggestions to parents and schools that might prevent at least some very serious injuries. (See also injury prevention segments in Health promotion sections devoted to children of various age-groups.)

Assessment of Trauma

The site of the injury usually influences the order of priority interventions when instituting emergency care. The safety of both the victim and his "Good Samaritan" rescuers must be considered in order to prevent further injury. For example, removing a child from a burning building or the bottom of a swimming pool is the obvious action to the logically thinking person, but an anxious rescuer may not consider his safety to be of prime importance. The major reason for thinking through steps to be taken in an emergency before the actual incident occurs is to have a mental repertory of preplanned actions available at a stimulus-response level.

Emergency management. The priorities for care of the child at the scene of the injury are outlined in the accompanying box. The first concerns are always for airway, breathing, and circulation after which other injuries are managed as indicated by the assessment. Severe bleeding is treated by removing gross debris from the wound, such as glass, but not if a large object is impaled in the victim. In this situation the wound is covered with a sterile or clean dressing and direct pressure is applied over the wound or at appropriate pressure points. Possible sprains are treated by elevation, compression, and application of cold if possible (see p. 846).

Assessment of the child involves observation from head to toes because infants and young children are unable to communicate except by crying and other behaviors. Therefore pinpointing areas of pain is very difficult. To check for any motor or sensory dysfunction in extremities, the nurse should note any spontaneous movement, which provides the best clue in infants and young children. Older children are able to follow directions for wiggling toes or fingers. The child is not encouraged to move all extremities until after it is determined that no spinal injury is present.

A spinal cord injury is suspected if there is loss of sensation or motor function. In this case the child is moved only if remaining in his present position is a threat to his safety, if so, he is carried in log fashion with the head and neck held firmly in a neutral position. No attempt should be made to transport the child until adequate help can be obtained to keep the body in straight alignment throughout and after the repositioning. Pain at the level of the injury, local muscle spasms, and sensorimotor loss are the outstanding features of this type of injury.

The child should be identified as soon as feasible by anyone who knows the child. It is important to determine if the child has any existing health problems that might have implications for the circumstances of the injury and for therapeutic management. Any witnesses are asked for details about the incident to aid in assessment of the child's emotional responses.

In situations of severe injury the emergency medical team will be needed to treat for shock and to transport the child adequately to the nearest emergency facility. Hospital emergency departments have protocols for managing injuries, including establishing an intravenous line, ventilatory assistance, and monitoring vital signs as well as radiography, laboratory, and other diagnostic services.

Systematic assessment. There are several factors that can affect a child's response to trauma. An undetected congenital anomaly can contribute to a complicated injury. Acute gastric distension is a frequent occurrence in children because of the crying and screaming that accompanies an injury. The temperature of young children is unstable because of their large surface area related to body mass, and temperature maintenance is critical in trauma management. Children also experience rapid metabolic changes. When they are ill, children are really ill; but, as they recover, they change very rapidly. In addition, children have a small amount of blood volume in the absolute sense. Whereas blood volume is 60% of total body weight in the adult, it is 70% to 85% in the child.

The first priority on admission to an emergency facility is rapid assessment of the ABC status (airway, breathing, and circulation). Since the overwhelming majority of childhood injuries are the result of blunt-impact trauma, multiple organ involvement is a common finding; therefore it is essential to perform a systematic assessment of the trauma victim. The most efficient method consists of a head to toe assessment:

Head

Observe for level of consciousness

Feel the head—palpate for depression or swelling over the cranium; feel the facial bones for depression or pain

Observe for bruises, petechiae of skin and conjunctiva, singed hair, extraocular movement, pupil size and reactivity

Observe the palate and mobility of the maxilla if child is cooperative

Neck

Observe status of neck veins (distended with chest injury), swelling, bruising, deformity of thyroid cartilage, penetrating wounds

Palpate cervical spine (maintaining traction and neutral position), thyroid for tenderness, position of trachea, evidence of subcutaneous emphysema, carotid pulses

Auscultate for bruits

Chest

Observe symmetry of respiratory movement, flail segment, bruising, penetrating wounds

Palpate clavicles, sternum, thoracic spine, subcutaneous emphysema; compress rib cage for local tenderness

Auscultate for diminished breath sounds (hemothorax or pneumothorax), shifted or muffled heart sounds, pericardial rub

Abdomen

Observe for distention, bruising, penetrating wounds, blood at the meatus or perineum

While patient is quiet, palpate the bladder gently; compress the pelvic brim

Auscultate for diminished bowel sounds, bruits

Extremities

Observe for perfusion, gross deformity, spontaneous movement

Palpate pulses at ankles, wrists, groin; palpate for local bone tenderness and sensation

It must be remembered in the process of assessment that coma can be caused by disorders other than cerebral trauma, for example, hypoxia and shock. Neurologic emergencies are relatively uncommon, except for epidural hematoma; therefore time can be used for a thorough assessment. Any detected injuries are managed as appropriate for the particular injury sustained.

DISLOCATIONS

Dislocations are less common in children than in older persons, but some types are peculiar to the younger age-groups. Before final closure of the epiphyses, injuries to the joints are more likely to cause epiphyseal separation than dislocation. For example, shoulder dislocation occurs most often in older adolescents, and dislocation unaccompanied by fracture is rare. Dislocation of the phalanges is the most common type seen in children, followed by elbow dislocations. Injury to the hip causes dislocation more frequently than femoral neck fracture (often experienced by persons in the older age-groups). In children younger than 5 years of age the hip is usually dislocated by a fall, but trauma is minimum because of the largely cartilaginous acetabulum and general joint laxity. Children with naturally lax joints, such as children with Down syndrome, are more prone to recurrent dislocation of the hip. (See also Dislocations, p. 846.)

Patella

Dislocation of the patella is a recurrent episode in some children; in others it is the result of injury. It is common among adolescent girls. The patella is always dislocated laterally. Most dislocations are reduced either spontaneously or by a companion before the child is seen by a physician. Therapy is immobilization for 3 to 4 weeks. Surgery may be needed for recurrent dislocations.

Radial Head

The most common dislocation injury, often handled by a pediatrician, is subluxation of the head of the radius in the elbow that occurs when a child between ages 1 and 4 years stumbles or is pulled along while holding onto the hand of an adult. The child is jerked upward by the adult while his arm is in a position of extension. The child has an anxious expression, whines, and complains of pain in the elbow and wrist, refuses to move the arm, and holds it with the opposite hand and in a slightly flexed and pronated position.

The physician manipulates the arm by applying firm finger pressure to the head of the radius and then supinates and flexes the forearm to return the bone structures to normal alignment. A click is heard, and functional use of the arm returns within 30 minutes. However, the longer the subluxation is present, the longer it takes for the child to recover mobility after treatment.

FRACTURES

The musculoskeletal system, like all the body systems of the newborn, is immature, and the specific functions of the system develop slowly so that the muscles, bones, tendons, and ligaments can function in an integrated fashion to perform complex tasks. The process of ossification, the gradual conversion of precursor substances (namely cartilage) to bony structures, begins in the embryo and continues until the child is 18 to 21 years of age. In long bones this process progresses outwardly from the diaphysis, the hard shaftlike portion that constitutes the major portion of the bone. Within this hard, compact shaft is the hollow medullary canal composed of the bone marrow. The epiphysis, located at the ends of long bones, consists of layers of cartilage, subchondral bone, and spongelike cancellous bone. Situated between the diaphysis and epiphysis is the epiphyseal plate, which plays a major role in the longitudinal growth of the developing child. The periosteum, the thin, tough membrane covering all bones, contains blood vessels that nourish the living bone (Fig. 40-6). Damage to this thin membrane can be a major problem in bone growth and healing.

Bones fracture when the resistance of the bone against the stress being exerted yields to the stress force. Fractures are a common injury at any age but are more likely to occur in children and aged persons. The natural tendency toward active mobility and their limited gross motor coordination make children more susceptible to physical injury.

Etiology

The causes of fracture injuries in children are those just described for general traumatic injuries in childhood. Fractures in infancy are more often the result of birth trauma, injury, or child abuse. Aside from motor vehicle accidents, true accidents rarely occur in infancy; therefore injury in children in that age-group warrants further investigation. In any small child radiographic evidence of fractures at various stages of healing are, with few exceptions, the result of physical abuse. Most often early bone trauma in infants consists of periosteal bleeding in the long bones of arms and legs, usually caused by rough handling, twisting, and pulling, which is not evident on radiographic examination until 3 to 6 weeks after the injury.

Fractures of the forearm are common bone injuries in childhood and are usually caused when the child extends the palm of the hand to break a fall. The force resulting from a fall on the outstretched hand progresses up the length of the extremity with the possibility of injury to finger, wrist, elbow, shoulder, and/or clavicle (Fig. 40-7). The clavicle is probably the bone most frequently broken in children; approximately half of clavicle fractures occur in children under 10 years of age. Hip fractures are rare in children and require a great deal of violence to produce. A femoral neck fracture may be sustained in children 6 or 7 years of age as a result of pedestrian-automobile accidents because their hip height is on the same level as an automobile bumper. In older children the femur is the most likely target, in adolescents knee injuries are common.

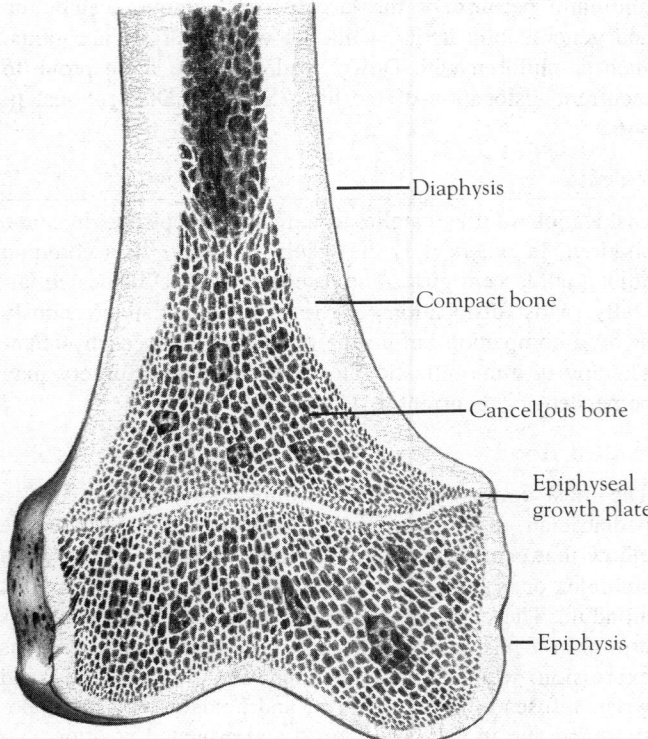

Fig. 40-6. Bone showing relationships of compact and cancellous bone, epiphysis, epiphyseal plate, and diaphysis.

From Thompson, J.M., and others: Clinical nursing, St. Louis, 1986, The C.V. Mosby Co., p. 428.

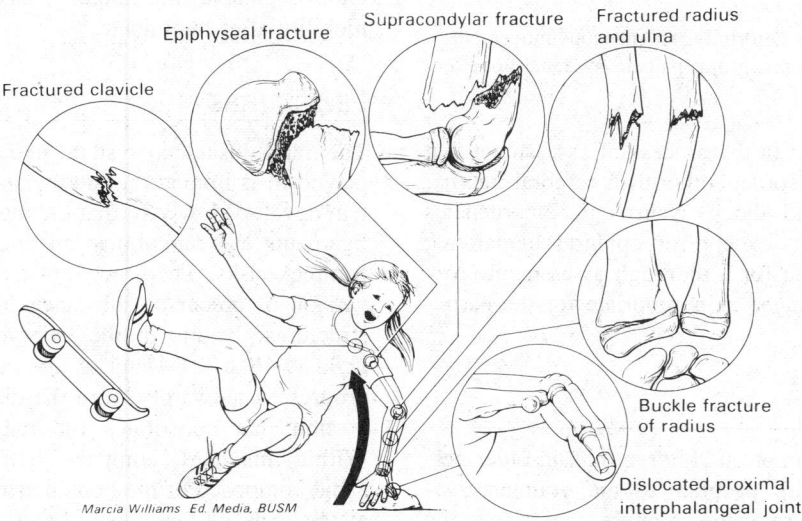

Fig. 40-7. Trauma resulting from progression of force in fall on outstretched hand.
From Segal, D.: Pediatr. Clin. North Am. **26:**793-802, 1979.

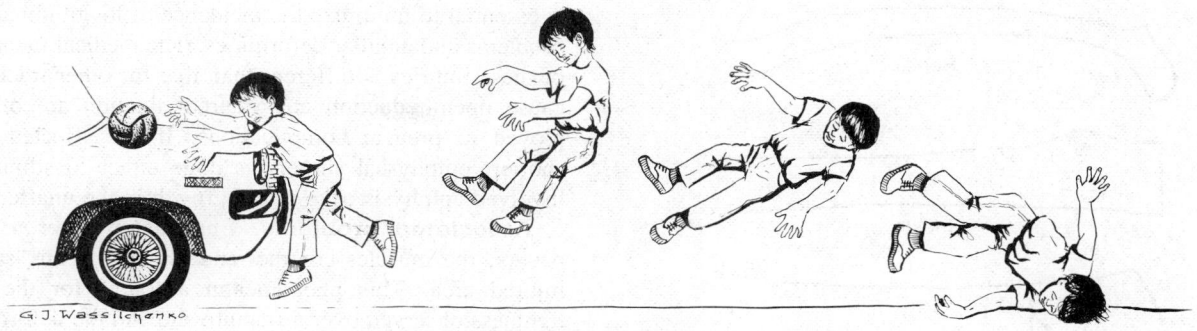

Fig. 40-8. Triad of injuries sustained when a child is struck by automobile.

Children fall from heights (e.g., trees, roofs) as their insatiable curiosity and immature judgment lure them to places of danger. Fractures in school-age children are often the result of bicycle-automobile accidents or skateboard injury. At all ages motor vehicle accidents are a frequent cause of bone injury. Most children who are hit by an automobile are between 4 and 7 years of age and sustain a triad of injuries, which must be kept in mind when making an assessment of injuries: (1) the child's femur, which is at the level of the bumper, is fractured, (2) the hood of the automobile produces injuries to the child's trunk, and (3) a contralateral head injury is usually sustained when the child is thrown to the ground by the impact (Fig 40-8). Therefore a child with any of these injuries who was struck by an automobile should be examined for evidence of the other two.

Pathophysiology

The anatomic, biomechanical, and physiologic nature of children's skeletons causes differences in the pattern of fractures, the problems of diagnosis, and the methods of treatment. The bones of the adult are strong and require a violent traumatic force to fracture and are accompanied by massive injury to surrounding soft tissues. In children the bones are more easily injured and may result from minor falls or twists and thus are likely to be accompanied by damage. As a result, features of children's fractures not observed in the adult include the following:

1. The growth plate, a thick, elastic portion of bone where growth takes place, serves to absorb shock and protect joint surfaces from injury and is the means by which the limb is able to grow and to straighten itself. Growth is stimulated by a fracture in the diaphysis, whereas damage to the growth plate can cause shortening and often a progressive angular deformity.
2. The periosteum of a child's bone is thicker, stronger, and has more active osteogenic potential compared with the adult.
3. The pliable bones of growing children are more porous than those of the adult, which allows them to bend, buckle, and break in a "greenstick" manner. The greater porosity increases the flexibility of the bone and dissipates and absorbs a significant amount of the force upon impact.

4. Healing is more rapid in children, and the rapidity is inversely related to the age of the child. The younger the child, the more rapid the healing process. Nonunion of bone fragments is almost unknown in children.
5. Stiffness is unusual and, unlike adults, an uninjured joint in a child can be immobilized for a long period without producing stiffness that lasts longer than a few minutes. Injured joints do become stiff, however, and the current trend is toward early mobilization and active range of motion exercises as preventive measures.
6. Children only complain when something is wrong. Unreasonable crying, restlessness, and calling for the parents are usually indications that something is amiss and require investigation.

Types of fractures. A fractured bone consists of fragments—the fragment closer to the midline, or the proximal fragment, and the fragment farthest from the midline, or the distal fragment. When fracture fragments are separated, the fracture is *complete;* when fragments remain attached, it is said to be *incomplete.* The fracture line can be:

transverse Crosswise, at right angles to the long axis of the bone.
oblique Slanting but straight, between a horizontal and a perpendicular direction.
spiral Slanting and circular, twisting around the bone shaft.

All fractures affect the entire cross-section of the bone. The twisting of an extremity while the bone is breaking results in the spiral break. If the fracture does not produce a break in the skin, it is a *simple,* or *closed,* fracture. *Open,* or *compound,* fractures are those with an open wound through which the bone is or has protruded. If the bone fragments cause damage to other organs or tissues (e.g., the lung or bladder), the injury is said to be *complicated.* When small fragments of bone are broken from the fractured shaft and lie in the surrounding tissue, the fracture is called *comminuted.* This type of fracture is rare in children. The types of fractures that occur most often in children are shown in Fig. 40-9.

bends A child's flexible bone can be bent 45 degrees or more before breaking. However, if bent, the bone will straighten slowly, but not completely, to produce some deformity but without the angulation that exists when the bone breaks.

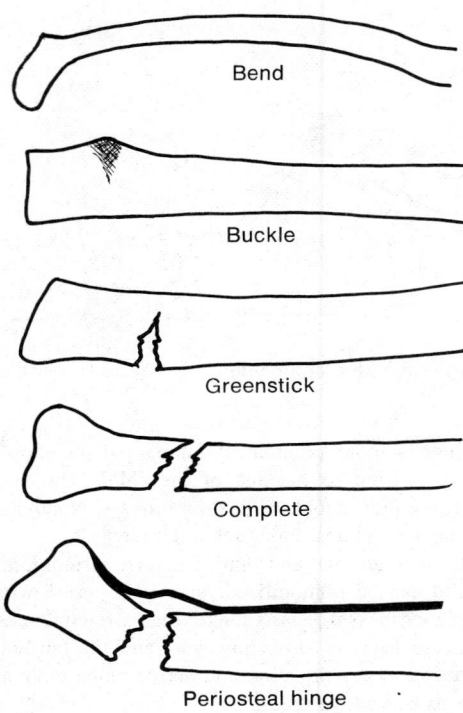

Fig. 40-9. Types of fractures in children.

Bends occur more commonly in the ulna and fibula, often associated with fractures of the radius and tibia.

buckle fracture Compression of the porous bone produces a *buckle,* or *torus,* fracture. This appears as a raised or bulging projection at the fracture site. Torus fractures occur in the most porous portion of the bone near the metaphysis (the portion of the bone shaft adjacent to the epiphysis) and are more common in young children.

greenstick fracture Occurs when a bone is angulated beyond the limits of bending. The compressed side bends and the tension side fails, causing an incomplete fracture similar to the break observed when a green stick is broken.

complete fracture Divides the bone fragments. They often remain attached by a periosteal hinge, which can aid or hinder reduction.

Epiphyseal injuries. The weakest point of long bones is the cartilage growth plate or epiphyseal plate. Consequently this is a frequent site of damage during trauma. Under most conditions, fractures in this area proceed along the zone of degenerating cartilage cells, before the cartilage begins to ossify, without damage to the growth plate, thus causing little damage. Healing is usually prompt. When fracture lines deviate from a transverse direction through the degenerating cells, more serious damage to the epiphysis and the plate may occur. Fig. 40-10 illustrates the types of epiphyseal injuries in order of increasing risk of permanent epiphyseal damage and possible growth disturbance.

Detection of epiphyseal injuries is sometimes difficult, and they may be mistaken for dislocations or ligamentous injuries. Fractures involving the epiphysis or epiphyseal plate present special problems in determining whether or not bone growth will be affected. Early and correct assessment

is essential to minimize the incidence of longitudinal growth problems and angular deformities. The medical management of these injuries is different than that for other fractures because open reduction and internal fixation are often employed to prevent complications. If the affected limb is shorter, epiphyseal surgery is done either to stimulate the involved epiphysis or to retard growth in the unaffected leg.

Associated problems. Immediately after a fracture occurs, the muscles contract and physiologically splint the injured area. This phenomenon accounts for the muscle tightness observed over a fracture site and the deformity that is produced as the muscles pull the bone ends out of alignment. This muscle response must be overcome by traction or complete muscle relaxation, that is, anesthesia, in order to realign the distal bone fragment to the proximal bone fragment.

Contusions of the soft tissues frequently accompany fractures, especially of femurs, and severe hemorrhage into the tissues is not uncommon. Both the bleeding and pain are major contributors to shock associated with this injury; therefore suspected musculoskeletal injury should be treated as a fracture until radiographic confirmation can be made. The surrounding tissue will be swollen, and a hematoma is usually present. The soft tissue injury must be treated as any contusion. Since the injury may cause damage to essential structures, the circulatory and neurologic status of tissues distal to the fracture are carefully assessed; especially for femoral and supracondylar fractures of the elbow.

Clinical Manifestations

Children demonstrate the usual signs of injury—generalized swelling, pain or tenderness, and diminished functional use of the affected part. There may be bruising, severe muscular rigidity, and sometimes crepitus (a grating sensation at the fracture site), which are also frequent signs in adults. More often the fracture is remarkably stable because of the usually intact periosteum. The child may even be able to use an affected arm or walk on a fractured leg. However, a fracture should be strongly suspected in a small child who refuses to walk.

Although neurologic and vascular damage is much less frequent in children than in adult patients, the integrity of these structures must be accurately assessed. This is often

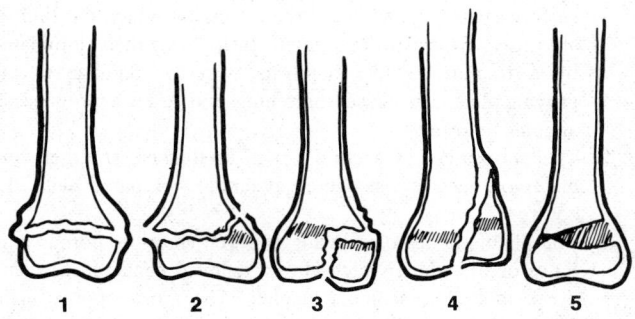

Fig. 40-10. Types of epiphyseal injuries in order of increasing risk.

difficult in infants and young children who are unable to cooperate. Vascular injury is most likely to occur with supracondylar fractures of the humerus and femur. Femoral and popliteal vessels and the sciatic nerve are prone to trauma in femoral fractures; humeral fractures may cause damage to the medial, ulnar, or radial nerves and to the brachial artery. The three ''Ps'' of ischemia from a vascular injury—*pain, pulselessness, and paralysis*—should be kept in mind when making an assessment.

Diagnostic Evaluation

A medical history is often lacking for childhood injuries. Infants are unable to communicate, and older children are unreliable informants and seldom volunteer information (even under direct questioning) when the injury occurred during forbidden activities. Unless they are witnesses to the injury, parents may misinterpret what the child is trying to say. In cases of child abuse parents may give false information deliberately in order to protect themselves.

Radiography. Radiographic examination is the most useful diagnostic tool for assessing skeletal trauma. The calcium deposits in bone make the entire structure radiopaque. However, in normal growth and development bony structures ossify from precursor substances, usually cartilage, to form true bone from the shaft or diaphysis toward the epiphysis. This ossification process begins in the embryo and continues until bone formation is completed by 18 to 21 years of age. Ossification centers alter the appearance of the bone, and much of the skeleton of infants and young children is composed of radiolucent growth cartilage that does not appear on radiograms. In addition, the epiphyseal cartilage and undisplaced separations of the epiphysis, which often occur, are not easily detected on x-ray films. Many physicians obtain a film of the uninjured limb for a direct comparison to help identify minor alterations in alignment and configuration of the epiphysis and associated injuries that might be missed. Radiographic films are taken after fracture reduction and in some situations may be taken during the healing process to determine satisfactory progress.

Blood studies. Severe soft tissue, muscle, and bone injury often results in a destruction of red blood cells with a rise in bilirubin and a fall in the hemoglobin or hematocrit reading. The child's homeostatic mechanisms are activated to correct the problem, and generally only supportive therapy with high-protein diet and iron replacement is needed. When muscle integrity is disrupted, enzymes normally contained within muscles are released into the bloodstream. Serum levels of creatine, alkaline phosphatase, serum glutamicoxaloacetic transaminase (SGOT), and lactic dehydrogenase (LDH) may increase in proportion to the amount of muscle damage.

A normal physiologic response to tissue injury is the inflammatory process with a slight elevation of white blood cells, especially neutrophils. When infection occurs, the rise in leukocytes is anticipated and the accompanying symptoms of fever and lethargy develop.

Therapeutic Management

The majority of children's fractures heal well, and nonunion is rare. Most are readily reduced by simple traction and immobilization until healing takes place. The goals of fracture management are:

1. To regain alignment and length of the bony fragments (reduction)
2. To retain alignment and length (immobilization)
3. To restore function to the injured parts

In children the bone fragments are usually realigned and immobilized by traction or by closed manipulation and casting until adequate callus is formed. Weight bearing and active movement for the purpose of regaining function can begin after the fracture site is stable. The child's natural tendency to be active is usually sufficient to restore normal mobility, and physical therapy is rarely needed. Open reduction is seldom required and is limited to fractures that cannot be maintained by conservative methods and when there is interposed tissue or injury to arteries or nerves. However, surgical reductions are more apt to delay normal healing and often predispose to nonunion. In the majority of cases children's fractures can be managed by closed reduction and plaster immobilization, which is often provided on an outpatient basis with reevaluation in 7 to 10 days.

Children are most frequently hospitalized for fractures of the femur and the supracondylar area of the distal humerus. If simple reductions cannot be achieved or a neurovascular problem is detected after injury, observation in a hospital unit is indicated. Severe contusions with profound swelling cannot be treated with a cast, which would act as a tourniquet on the extremity, and badly malaligned fractures require traction for a time before a cast is applied.

The method of fracture reduction is determined by:

Age of child
Degree of displacement
Amount of overriding
Degree of edema
Condition of skin and soft tissue
Sensation and circulation distal to fracture

Some problems that are associated with fracture injury and involve both the physician and nurse in their care are:

Control of pain, hemorrhage, and edema
Relief of muscle spasms
Realignment of fracture fragments
Promotion of bone healing
Immobilization of fracture until adequate healing has begun
Prevention of secondary complications
Limitation of disuse syndrome
Restoration of function

The specific interventions and nursing responsibilities in the general management directed toward restoring bone integrity and functional use are discussed in relation to the major modalities of fracture immobilization—casting and traction.

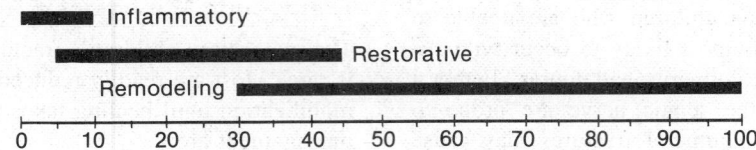

Fig. 40-11. Approximate time devoted to inflammatory, restorative, and remodeling phases of bone healing. Scale indicates percent of healing time.

BONE HEALING PROCESS*

Time†	Physiologic events
Impact	Fracture Injury to soft tissue enveloping site Periosteal tissue torn Vessels rupture
3-5 minutes	Bone and tissue bleeding after injury *Hematoma forms and clots;* fibrin assists in clotting periosteal membrane, which aids in repair Osteoblastic activity stimulated
After 24 hours	Blood supply increases, bringing available calcium, phosphate, and fibroblasts, which convert to osteoblasts (bone-forming cells)
Next few days	Hematoma becomes *granulation tissue;* forms framework for deposition of bone-forming substances Bulging growth of tissue as osteoblasts produce intercellular substance or matrix in which calcium and phosphate is deposited (beginning of callus)
2-3 days	*Halisteresis* (softening of bone ends) ⅛-¼ inch absorption of bone cells
6-10 days	*Provisional callus develops;* holds bone fragments together but will not support body weight
14-21 days	*True callus* develops; seen on x-ray; usually more than needed but with remodeling, excess callus absorbs; gradual weight bearing
3-10 weeks	*Callus to bone,* which grows beneath periosteum of fragments; fuses defect by ossification; no intermedullary canal
Over 9-month period	Bone marrow cavity restored; fracture line can always be seen on x-ray film

*Total healing time depends on age, type of bone, and complications.
†Process in infants and young children is more rapid.

Surgical intervention. When surgical intervention is necessary to realign a fracture, the child needs physical and psychologic preparation. The preoperative teaching is the same as for any other surgical procedure, except that orthopedic surgery uses a variety of rods, screws, and plates and the child needs to know about these unfamiliar things and how they will appear when he returns from the operation. The fixating devices are made of substances that do not act as foreign proteins to the body and therefore are not rejected. Usually the rods are driven down the shaft of the long bones, whereas screws and plates are attached to the side of the bone shaft. Postoperatively the bone healing proceeds as a new fracture with the callus formation process. Generally the child with an internal fixation device sit in a chair and walk with a walker or crutches within a few hours or days. The most common postoperative complications are infections and slippage of the fixation device. The nurse's responsibility includes close monitoring of neurovascular changes in the involved extremity and the prevention of postanesthesia problems.

Bone Healing and Remodeling

Bone healing follows a patterned sequence of events (see box) and consists of three phases: inflammatory, restorative, and remodeling (Fig. 40-11). When the bone breaks, the envelope of subcutaneous tissue, muscle, and periosteal tissue surrounding the site is torn, blood vessels rupture, and a hematoma forms. The ends of the fractured bone segments, deprived of circulation, die as far back as the nearest collateral circulation. Necrotic tissue accumulates, and an inflammatory response takes place at the site with its characteristic vasodilation, plasma exudation, and edema. The organization and resorption of the hematoma proceeds, and the reparative phase begins with the reestablishment of local circulation. Repair requires an adequate blood supply and immobilization of the fracture fragments.

When there is a break in the continuity of bone, the periosteal and intraosseous osteoblasts are in some way stimulated to maximum activity. New osteoblasts are formed in immense numbers almost immediately after the injury and begin building a bridge, as evidenced by a bulging growth of osteoblastic tissue and new bone matrix between the fractured bone fragments. This is followed by deposition of calcium salts to form a *callus,* which provides stability (Fig. 40-12).

Bone healing is characteristically rapid in children because of the thickened periosteum and generous blood supply. In the young child, for example, there is frequently a solid union of the femoral shaft in 3 to 4 weeks, whereas in the adult, callus sufficient to avoid deformities from con-

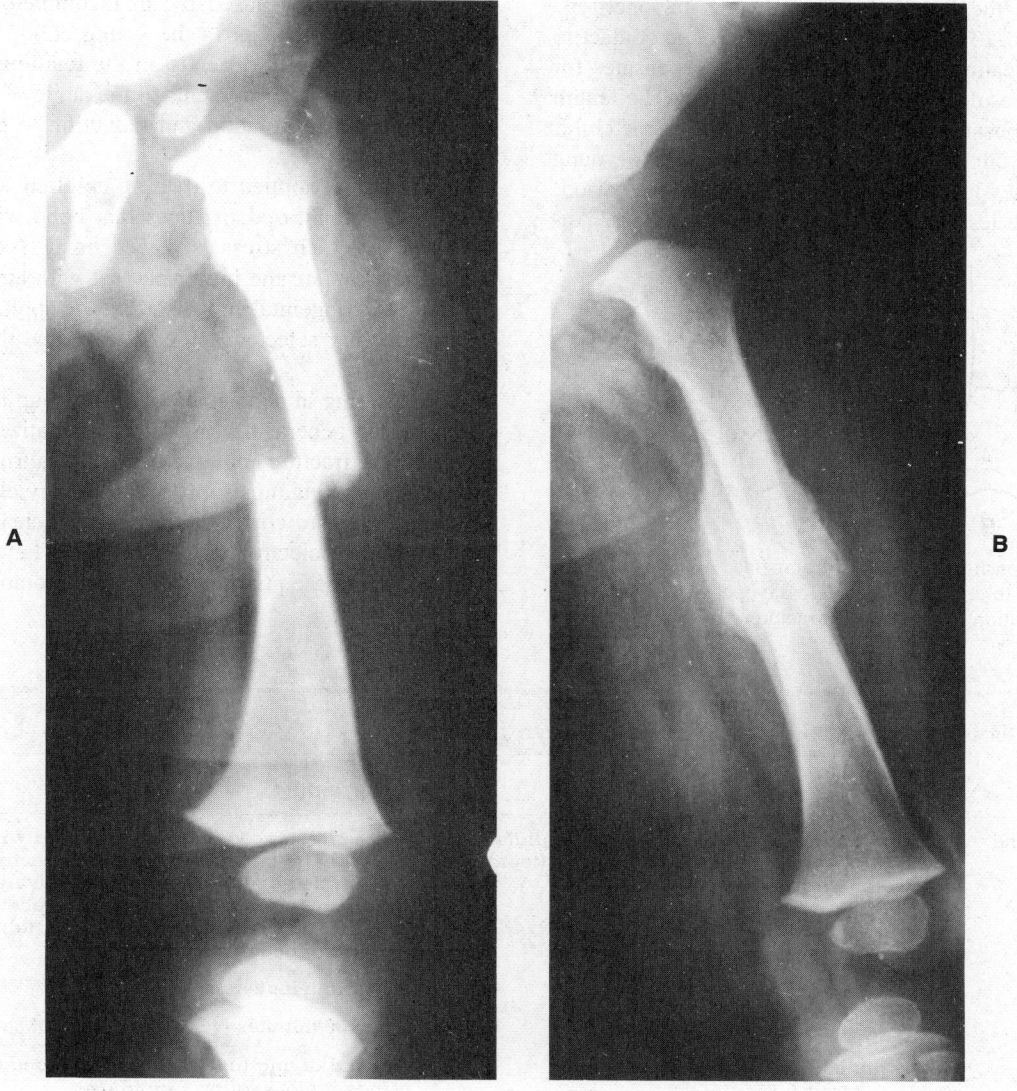

Fig. 40-12. Fractured femur. Most fractured femurs in childhood are of piral type shown here. Note comparison of original x-ray films. **A,** with 6-month postfracture film. **B,** showing callus formation.

Courtesy Henrietta Egleston Hospital for Children, Atlanta, GA. From Hilt, N.E., and Schmitt, E.W.: Pediatric orthopedic nursing, St. Louis, 1975, The C.V. Mosby Co.

stant muscle contraction associated with movement may not take place in less than 10 to 16 weeks. The approximate healing times for a femoral shaft are:

Neonatal period—2 to 3 weeks
Early childhood—4 weeks
Later childhood—6 weeks
Adolescence—8 to 10 weeks

Remodeling is a unique process that occurs in the healing of fractures of long bone before epiphyseal closure. When a bone remodels, the irregularities produced by the fracture become indistinct, as hollows are filled in and angles are rounded off in the healing process, which gives the bone a straighter appearance. It does not alter the alignment of the bone. The buildup of new bone or callus will restore a portion of the normal bone structure in most cases despite ob-

servable malalignment. The younger the child and the closer the proximity of the fracture to the growth plate, the more likely it is that spontaneous correction will take place. In some instances a 90-degree angle will straighten in a year, but rotational deformities do not correct themselves. Various factors such as the type and location of the fracture, the age of the child, and the amount of fragment angulation or rotation will influence the degree of correction in alignment that can be obtained by remodeling.

The position of the bone fragments in relation to one another influences the rapidity of healing and the residual deformity. A gap between fragments delays (or prevents) healing (Fig. 40-13, *A*). Healing is prompt and complete with end-to-end apposition (Fig. 40-13, *B*), but the fracture stimulates accelerated growth of the neighboring epiphysis, which causes bony overgrowth and increased length of the extremity. When the fragments overlap in a bayonet-type reduction (Fig. 40-13, *C*), there is sufficient bone contact to allow for rapid healing and the lost length compensates for overgrowth as a result of epiphyseal stimulation. The length that can be compensated for depends on the age of the child. Approximately 1 cm of overlap can be allowed in a young child, but in child who is near the end of the growth period, correction will be less; therefore overlap must be less. An-

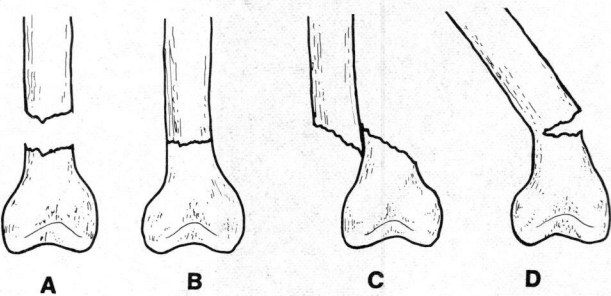

Fig. 40-13. Relationships of fracture fragments. **A,** Gap between fragments. **B,** End-to-end apposition. **C,** Bayonet apposition or overlap. **D,** Angulation of incomplete fracture.

gulation deformity caused by an incomplete fracture (Fig. 40-13, *D*) may remodel in the young child, but the degree of residual deformity depends on the relationship of the angulation of the bone fragments to the angle of the joint. This requires careful evaluation and reduction to prevent permanent deformity.

Wolff law is applied to treating children with orthopedic problems. Paraphrased, it states that bone will grow in the direction in which stress is placed on it. Examples of the use of this law are the hip spica cast with an abduction bar for treating congenital hip disorders or application of casts or traction at a selected angle to influence the direction of bone healing.

Bone healing in persons of any age-group is greatly influenced by the general health of the traumatized person. The child with a fracture requires adequate nutrition, including supplementary vitamins. No special dietary changes need to be made except to correct nutritional deficiencies. Monitoring of fluid and electrolyte balance, renal function, and possible anemia are equally important to promote wellness of the child.

Table 40-2 Comparison of plaster of Paris and synthetic cast

	PLASTER OF PARIS	SYNTHETIC
Composition and preparation	Cotton tape permeated with calcium sulfate crystals that interlock as tape dries (tepid water-activated)	1. Polyester/cotton tape permeated with polyurethane resin (cool water-activated) 2. Knitted fiberglass tape with polyurethane resin (tepid water-activated or photoactivated) 3. Knitted thermoplastic polyester fabric (hot water-activated)
Setting time	3 to 8 minutes	3 to 15 minutes
Drying time	10 to 72 hours (varies with cast size)	5 to 30 minutes (varies with kind of cast
Indentations	Slow drying time increases possibility	Rapid drying time reduces likelihood of indentations; allows rapid use
Weight	Relatively heavy; bulky; difficulty wearing regular clothing	Lightweight; less bulky; can wear with regular clothing; allows for greater range of activity
Conformity	Molds readily to body part	Does not mold easily to body parts; unsuitable for small children or severely displaced fractures
Surface	Smooth exterior; does not scratch clothing or furniture	Rough exterior; can snag clothing or furniture; abrasive to skin
Cost	Relatively inexpensive; an advantage if cast changes anticipated	Expensive; cost three to seven times that of plaster casts
Stability	Relatively stable; must keep cast dry; clean with damp cloth and a dry, low-abrasive cleanser	May get cast wet or immerse in water with permission from doctor (with use of nonabsorbent synthetic lining); clean with small amount of mild soap and water; dry with towel followed by blow dryer on cool or warm setting
Miscellaneous	Child may feel uncomfortable warming or burning under cast while drying (chemical reaction) Skin under cast may become irritated Cast must be protected when around water (bathing)	Special aids may be required for application or removal of some types Increased activity may displace fracture Skin under cast may become macerated from inadequate drying after water immersion

Data from Lane, P. L., and Leem M.M.: Special care for special casts, Nursing 83 **13**(7):50, 1983; Wise, L.B.: A comparison of orthopedic casts: breaking the mold, Am. J. Maternal Child Nurs. **11**:174-176, 1986.

THE CHILD IN A CAST

Nurses are frequently in a position where they must make the initial assessment of a child with a suspected fracture (see Emergency treatment box). The child and the parents are frightened and upset, the child is in pain, and, since most fractures are obvious, the parents and frequently the child are already convinced of the diagnosis. Therefore if the child is alert and there is no evidence of hemorrhage, the initial nursing interventions are directed toward calming and reassuring the child and his parents so that an extensive assessment can be more easily accomplished.

Maintaining a calm manner and speaking in a quiet voice, the nurse can ask the parents to describe what happened and how they feel about it. Since the child usually arrives with the limb supported in some manner, this minute or two does not delay or endanger the treatment. It is best not to touch the child initially but to ask him to point to the painful area and to wiggle his fingers or toes. By this time he usually feels relatively safe and will allow someone to gently touch him just enough to feel the pulse and test for sensation. A child's anxiety is greatly influenced by previous experiences with injury and health personnel. However, the child needs to be told what will happen and what he can do to help. The affected limb need not be palpated and should not be moved unless properly splinted. If the child is at home or if the physician is not present to examine the child, some type of splint should be applied carefully for transport to the hospital and to the radiography department and cast room.

The Cast

The completeness of the fracture, the type of bone involved, and the amount of weight that can be placed on the limb influence how much of the extremity must be included in the cast to immobilize the fracture site completely. In most situations the joints above and below the fracture are immobilized to eliminate the possibility of movement that might cause displacement at the fracture site. Four major categories of casts are used for immobilization of fractures: *upper extremity* to immobilize wrist and/or elbow, *lower extremity* to immobilize ankle and/or knee, *spinal and cervical* for immobilization of the spine, and *spica casts* to immobilize the hip and knee.

Casting materials. Most casts are constructed from gauze strips and bandage impregnated with plaster of Paris. Other lighter weight and water-resistant materials (e.g., fiberglass and polyurethane resin) are also being used with increasing frequency in casts for selected types of fractures. The light-weight casts are satisfactory for arms and hip spicas on infants and very young children; plaster is better for large hip spicas and legs. Table 40-2 compares the relative merits of plaster and synthetic casts.

Cast application. When a cast is being applied by a physician, it is often the nurse's role to set up the cast materials and hold the extremity in alignment, Fig. 40-14. Special cast tables that hold the child's body are used for applying large hip spica casts. If possible, the child should be

Emergency Treatment: *Fracture*

1. Assess extent of injury—5 "Ps"
   Pain and point of tenderness
   Pulse—distal to the fracture site
   Pallor
   Paresthesia—sensation distal to the fracture site
   Paralysis—movement distal to the fracture site
2. Determine the mechanism of injury
3. Move injured part as little as possible
   Cover open wounds with sterile or clean dressing
4. Immobilize the limb, including joints above and below fracture site; do not attempt to reduce fracture or push protruding bone under the skin
   Soft splint (pillow or folded towel)
   Rigid splint (rolled newspaper or magazine)
   Uninjured leg can serve as splint for leg fracture if no splint available
5. Reassess neurovascular status
6. Apply traction if circulatory compromise is present
7. Elevate the injured limb if possible
8. Apply cold to the injured area
9. Call EMT or transport to medical facility

allowed to play with a small doll that has a cast so that he understands what will be done. Before the cast is applied the extremities are checked for the presence of rings or other items that might cause constriction from swelling, and these are removed. Identification bands are placed on a noninjured extremity if hospitalization is anticipated.

A tube of stockinette is stretched over the area to be casted, and bony prominences are padded with soft cotton sheeting. Dry rolls of gauze impregnated with plaster of Paris are immersed in a pail of cold water with the open end of the roll downward to allow soaking of the bandage. The wet plaster rolls are put on in a bandage fashion and molded to the extremity. A heat-producing chemical reaction occurs between the plaster and water as the plaster becomes a crystalline gypsum. During application of the cast the underlying stockinette is pulled over the raw edges of the cast and secured with a layer of wet plaster ½ to 1 inch below the rim to form a smooth padded edge to protect the skin.

If the physician does not form such a protective edge with stockinette, the raw edges of the cast can be protected by a "petaled" edge. Small pieces approximately 2 to 3 inches long are cut from 1- or 1½-inch wide adhesive tape. The edges are rounded with scissors, and each of these "petals" is placed over the edge of the cast, each petal slightly overlapping the previous petal to form a smooth, neat edge. It is easier to apply the petal to the underside of the cast first and then bring the unadhered edge to the front, pressing firmly so that the edges remain securely attached. Band-Aids can be used instead of the tape petals for quicker preparation and a slightly padded cast edge.

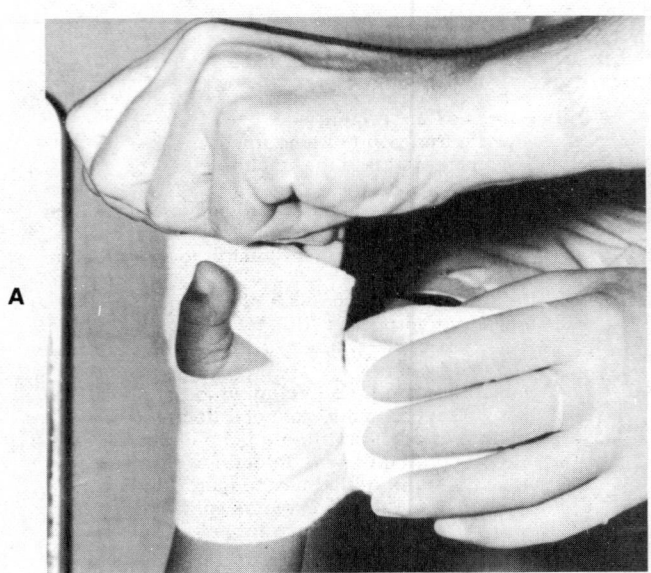

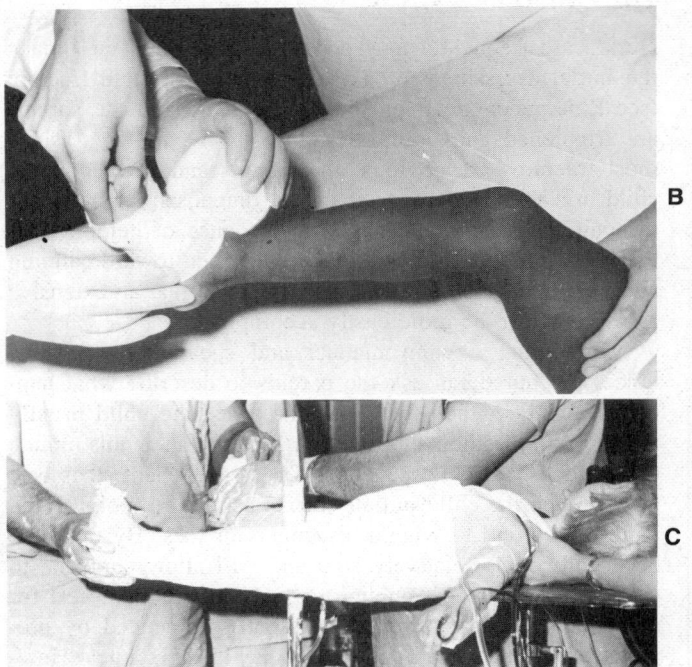

Fig. 40-14. Proper methods of holding child for cast application. **A,** Arm cast: arm should be held by fingers (and upper arm, if necessary) and off side of table or bed to permit exposure of entire arm. **B,** Leg cast: foot and toes are grasped with one hand as shown, and upper thigh with other hand; maintaining knee in flexion will discourage kicking. **C,** Hip spica cast: one individual maintains desired leg position; another individual pushes child at shoulder level toward perineal post, child's shoulders and pelvis should remain level.

From Hilt, N.E., and Schmitt, E.W.: Pediatric orthopedic nursing, St. Louis, 1975, The C.V. Mosby Co.

Nursing Considerations

The complete evaporation of the water from the hip spica cast can take 24 to 48 hours when traditional types of plaster materials are used. Drying occurs within 8 to 10 hours with new quick-drying substances. Turning the child at least every 2 hours will help to dry the cast evenly. The cast must remain uncovered to allow the cast to dry from the inside out. A regular fan to circulate air may be helpful during high-humidity weather. Heated fans or dryers should not be used because they cause the cast to dry on the outside and remain wet beneath and can cause burns from heat conduction by way of the cast to the underlying tissue.

A wet cast should be supported by a pillow covered with plastic and handled by the palms of the hands to prevent indenting the cast and creating pressure areas. A dry plaster of Paris cast produces a hollow sound when tapped with the finger. If "hot spots" are felt on the cast surface (usually indicating infection beneath the area), this should be reported so a window can be made in the cast to observe the site.

During the first few hours after a cast is applied, the chief concern is that the extremity may continue to swell to the extent that the cast becomes a tourniquet, shutting off circulation and producing neurovascular complications. A measure for reducing the likelihood of this potential problem is to elevate the body part, thereby increasing venous return. If edema is excessive, casts are bivalved, that is, cut

to make an anterior and a posterior half that are held together with an elastic bandage. The cast and the involved extremity are observed frequently for neurovascular integrity, and any signs of compromise, such as pain, swelling, discoloration (pallor or cyanosis) of the exposed portions, lack of pulsation and warmth, or the inability to move the exposed part(s), are reported immediately.

When casting an extremity that has sustained an open fracture, a window is often left over the wound area to allow for observation and for dressing of the wound. A surgical reduction is usually casted as for a closed fracture. For the first few hours after surgery there may be substantial bleeding that will soak through the cast. Periodically the circumscribed blood-stained area should be outlined with a ball-point pen or pencil and the time indicated to provide a guide for assessing the amount of bleeding.

Cutting the cast to remove it or to relieve tightness is frequently a frightening experience for a child. He fears the sound of the cast cutter and is terrified that his flesh as well as the cast will be cut. Since it works by vibration, a cast cutter cuts only the hard surface of the cast. This can be demonstrated on the nurse or person removing the cast. However, the vibration generates heat that may be felt by the child, and this should be explained. Preparation for the procedure will help reduce his anxiety, especially if a trusting relationship has been established between the child and the nurse. Many young children come to regard the cast as part of themselves, which intensifies their fear of removal. Using the analogy of having fingernails or hair cut sometimes helps reduce their anxiety. They need continual reassurance that all is going well and that their behavior is accepted.

Nursing Care Summary: The Child in a Cast

NURSING GOALS	NURSING INTERVENTIONS	EXPECTED PATIENT/FAMILY OUTCOMES
HP-HMP	**Injury: potential for tissue damage** **Risk factors: edema, limited respiratory excursion (spica cast)**	

Maintain optimum temperature	Check temperature; imbalance can be produced by
	    Chemical reaction in cast drying process, which generates heat
	    Water evaporation, which causes heat loss
		Body temperature remains less than 38°C (100.4° F)

Maintain cast integrity	Do not allow weight bearing until cast is completely dry—even if weight-bearing device is attached Change position of child in body cast or hip spica cast periodically; small child can be managed easily; adolescent may require one or two persons; eventually children become very adept at moving themselves Do *not* use abduction stabilizer bar between legs of hip spica as handle for turning Position with buttocks lower than shoulders during toileting to prevent urine from flowing under cast at the back; body can be supported on pillows	Cast dries evenly
	Protect rim of cast around perineal area of body cast with plastic film or Saran Wrap to prevent soiling during toileting Use plastic-backed disposable diaper with edges tucked underneath rim of cast for infants and small children who are not toilet trained or who are prone to "accicents"; a sanitary napkin can also be used if waterproof material is placed between pad and cast Caution against activities that might cause physical damage to cast Remove soiled areas of cast with damp cloth and small amount of white, low-abrasive cleanser	Cast remains clean and intact
Prevent circulatory impairment	Elevate casted extremity Place leg cast on pillows, making certain that leg is well supported and that there is no pressure on heel Elevate arm on pillows or support in stockinette sling suspended from intravenous infusion pole—either in bed or during ambulation; triangular arm sling is adequate for lesser elevation and support	Toes/fingers are warm, pink, sensitive, and evidence good capillary filling

	Monitor cardiovascular status
	    Monitor peripheral pulses
	    Blanch skin on extremity distal to fracture to ascertain adequate circulation to the part
	Feel cast for tightness; cast should allow insertion of fingers between skin and cast after it has dried
	Assess for increase in
	    Pain
	    Swelling
	    Coldness
	    Cyanosis
	Assess finger or toe movement and sensation
	    Request child to move fingers or toes
	    Report signs of impending circulatory impairment immediately
	    Instruct child to report any feelings of numbness or tingling
		Pulse is palpable in affected extremity, and pulses are equal bilaterally
		Child moves extremity when instructed to do so

Continued.

Nursing Care Summary: The Child in a Cast—cont'd

NURSING GOALS	NURSING INTERVENTIONS	EXPECTED PATIENT/FAMILY OUTCOMES
Observe for signs of infection	Smell cast for foul odor Be alert to increased temperature, lethargy, and discomfort	Cast remains clean, with no odor Child exhibits no evidence of infection
Observe for respiratory impairment	Assess child's chest expansion Observe respiratory rate Observe color and behavior	Respiratory efforts remain within normal limits (see inside front cover for normal variations)

N-MP   Skin integrity, impairment of: potential
Risk factors: presence of cast

Prevent skin from becoming irritated	Make certain that all edges are smooth and free from irritating projections; trim and/or pad as necessary; petal cast edges if needed Keep crumbs and other items from getting between cast and skin Inspect skin for irritation or pressure areas Inspect inside cast for items that a small child may place there Caution older children not to place items under cast Keep exposed skin clean and free of irritants	Skin remains clean with no evidence of irritation

A-EP   Diversional activity deficit
Etiology: immobility

Provide diversion	Involve the child in planning his care to the extent of his capabilities Arrange for and encourage interaction with others as feasible	Child becomes involved in planning his care and activities Child interacts with family and other children
Promote growth and development	Provide diversional activities appropriate to the child's condition, physical limitations, and developmental level	Child engages in activities appropriate to developmental level and interests

A-EP   Mobility, impaired physical
Etiology: musculoskeletal impairment

Maintain muscle use of unaffected areas	Encourage to ambulate as soon as possible Support casted arm in sling Teach use of mobilizing devices such as crutches for casted leg (walking device is applied when weight bearing allowed) Encourage child with an ambulation device to walk as soon as general condition allows Provide and encourage use of muscles in play activities and diversions Carry out range of motion exercises of unaffected limbs if paralyzed	Unaffected extremities maintain good muscle tone Child engages in activities appropriate to his age and condition

A-EP   Self-care deficit: feeding, bathing/hygiene, dressing/grooming, toileting (specify level)
Etiology: musculoskeletal impairment

Provide nourishment	Assist with feeding Facilitate self-help	Child eats with minimum assistance
Maintain hygiene	Assist with bathing, dressing, grooming	Child is clean and well-groomed
Facilitate toileting	Provide utensils needed for toileting Instruct child in use of utensils Modify utensils when indicated Provide for privacy	Toileting is carried out with a minimum of distress to child

Nursing Care Summary: The Child in a Cast—cont'd

NURSING GOALS	NURSING INTERVENTIONS	EXPECTED PATIENT/FAMILY OUTCOMES
CPP **Comfort, alteration in: pain** **Etiology: fracture, presence of cast**		
Provide comfort	Assess need for pain medication (p. 1068) Implement appropriate nonpharmacologic pain reduction techniques (p. 1071) Position for comfort; use pillows to support dependent areas Alleviate itching underneath cast by alcohol swabs; cool air blown from Asepto syringe, fan, or hair dryer (on low or cool setting); or scratching or rubbing the unaffected extremity Avoid using powder or lotion under cast, since these substances have tendency to "ball" and produce irritation	Child exhibits no evidence of discomfort Minor discomforts are eased

SP-SCP **Fear** **Etiology: perception of cast removal**		
Support child during cast removal	Explain procedure Demonstrate safety of equipment Provide reassurance	Child cooperates throughout procedure Child displays interest in procedure

RRP **Family process, alteration in** **Etiology: situational crisis (injured child)**		
Educate family	Teach cast care and support of casted part Make certain that parents understand signs of circulatory impairment and infection	Family demonstrates cast care
Support family	Help family plan suitable activities Help family in problem solving of modification of clothing to fit over casted area Help family devise supportive devices and modification of furniture for positioning (e.g., pillows, pads) Help family in problem solving of means of transporting child See also The child in the hospital, p. 1075; Family of the hospitalized child, p. 1081	Family provides appropriate care of cast and seek assistance when needed Family positions child comfortably and safely Family transports child with appropriate safety (specify)

Nursing Intervention Related to Medical Management

Alleviate pain
  Administer analgesics as prescribed
  Use a pain assessment record to monitor effectiveness of analgesics

Frequently the child will be discharged to home care after a cast is applied in the emergency room or clinic. Parents need instructions on drying and caring for the cast and checking for signs and symptoms that indicate that the cast is too tight (see box, p. 1810). They should also be told to take the child to the health professional for attention if the cast becomes too loose, since a loose cast no longer serves its purpose. A cast is a badge of honor for the child and serves as visible evidence of an otherwise invisible injury (Fig. 40-15).

After the cast is removed, the skin surface will be caked with desquamated skin and sebaceous secretions. Simple soaking in a bathtub is usually sufficient for its removal but may require a period of several days to eliminate the accumulation completely. Application of olive oil or lotion may provide comfort. Parents and child should be instructed not to pull or forcibly remove this material with vigorous scrubbing because it may cause excoriation and bleeding.

Keep the casted extremity elevated on pillows or similar support for the first day, or as directed by the physician.

Avoid indenting the cast until it is thoroughly dry.

Observe the extremities (fingers or toes) for any evidence of swelling or discoloration (darker or lighter than a comparable extremity) and contact the health professional if noted.

Check movement of the visible extremities frequently.

Follow physician's orders regarding any restriction of activities.

Restrict strenuous activities for the first few days.

　Engage in quiet activities but encourage use of muscles.

　Move the joints above and below the cast on the affected extremity.

Encourage frequent rest for a few days keeping the injured extremity elevated while resting.

Avoid allowing the affected limb to hang down for any length of time.

　Keep an injured upper extremity elevated (e.g., in a sling) while upright.

　Elevate a lower limb when sitting and avoid standing for too long.

Do not allow the child to put anything inside the cast.

　Keep small items away from small children that might be placed inside the cast.

Keep a clear path for ambulation.

　Remove toys, hazardous floor rugs, pets, or other items over which the child might stumble.

Use crutches appropriately if lower limb fracture.

　The crutches should fit properly, have a soft rubber tip to prevent slipping, and be well padded at the axilla.

tions, the object either changes its state of rest or motion or remains in equilibrium. The use of traction in the management of fractures is the direct application of these forces to produce equilibrium at the fracture site. A forward force (traction) is produced by attaching weight to the distal bone fragment, which is balanced by the backward force of the muscle pull (countertraction) and the frictional force between the patient and the bed. Thus the three essential components of traction management are traction, countertraction, and friction (Fig. 40-16).

To reduce or realign a fracture site, traction is provided by weights applied to the distal bone fragment; body weight provides countertraction. By adjusting the line of pull upward or downward or by adducting or abducting the extremity, the physician uses these forces to align the distal and proximal bone fragments. To attain equilibrium, the amount of forward force is adjusted by adding weight to or subtracting weight from the traction, and/or countertraction can be increased by elevating the foot of the bed to create a greater gravitational pull to the backward force. A bed board placed under the mattress of heavy children prevents sagging which might otherwise change the direction of the forces applied to the fracture.

The three primary purposes of traction for reduction of fractures are:

1. To fatigue the involved muscle and reduce muscle spasm so that bones can be realigned
2. To position the distal and proximal bone ends in desired realignment to promote satisfactory bone healing
3. To immobilize the fracture site until realignment has been achieved and sufficient healing has taken place to permit casting or splinting

THE CHILD IN TRACTION

Bone fragments that cannot be aligned initially by simple traction and stabilization with a cast require the extended pulling force offered by continuous traction. Traction may be used for other purposes also:

To provide rest for an extremity
To help prevent or improve contracture deformity
To correct a deformity
To treat a dislocation
To allow preoperative or postoperative positioning and alignment
To provide immobilization of specific areas of of the body
To reduce muscle spasms (rare in children)

In most of these cases the traction is often applied at night and intermittently during the day. Muscle relaxants may be administered for muscle spasms.

Purposes of Traction

When forces having both direction and magnitude act on an object at the same point simultaneously from opposite direc-

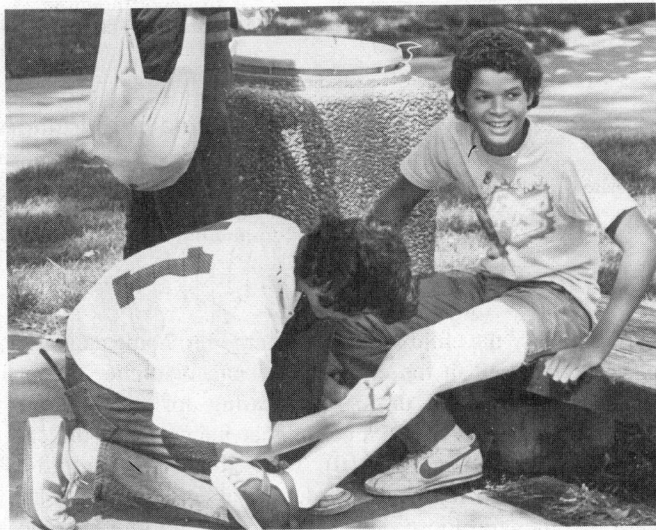

Fig. 40-15. A cast serves as an excellent medium for collecting autographs and assorted graffiti.
Photography by Garibaldi, San Lorenzo, CA.

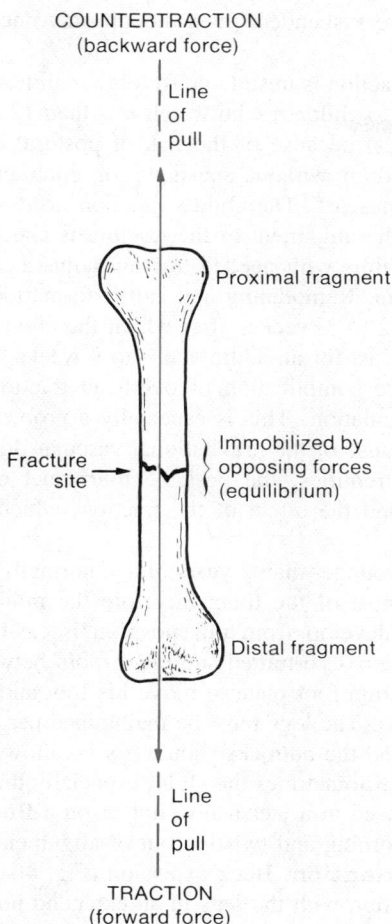

COUNTERTRACTION
(backward force)

Line
of
pull

Proximal fragment

Fracture
site

Immobilized by
opposing forces
(equilibrium)

Distal fragment

Line
of
pull

TRACTION
(forward force)

Fig. 40-16. Application of traction for maintaining equilibrium.

Fatiguing of a muscle is accomplished by applying constant stress to the muscle so that the buildup of lactic acid will produce muscle relaxation. The all-or-none law, characteristic of muscle contractability, influences the complete relaxation. When muscle is stretched, muscle spasm ceases and permits the realignment of the bone ends. The continuous maintenance of traction is important during this phase because releasing the traction allows the muscle's normal contracting ability to again cause a malpositioning of the bone ends.

The realignment of the fragments is a gradual process that is achieved more rapidly in infants, who have limited muscle tone, than in muscular teenagers. The desired line of pull and callus formation are checked periodically by radiographic examination. The traction pull to some degree immobilizes the fracture site; however, adjunctive immobilizing devices such as splints or casts are sometimes used with skeletal traction. In injuries in which there is severe soft tissue swelling or vascular and nerve damage, it is customary to use traction until these complications have been resolved and it is safe to apply a cast. Immobilization with

traction will be maintained until the bone ends are in satisfactory realignment, after which a less-confining type of immobilization, usually a cast, will be applied.

Types of Traction (General)

The pull needed for traction can be applied to the distal bone fragment in several ways:

manual traction Traction applied to the body part by the hand placed distally to the fracture site. Nurses frequently provide manual traction during cast application.

skin traction Pull applied directly to the skin surface and indirectly to the skeletal structures. The pulling mechanism is attached to the skin with adhesive material or an elastic bandage. Both types are applied over soft foam-backed traction straps to distribute the traction pull.

skeletal traction Pull applied directly to the skeletal structure by a pin, wire, or tongs inserted into or through the diameter of the bone distal to the fracture.

Manual traction is used by the physician in uncomplicated arm or leg fractures in which there is little overriding of the bones and minimum muscle pull to overcome. Manual traction is used to realign bone fragments for immediate cast application. Skin traction is applied when there is minimum displacement and little muscle spasticity but is contraindicated when there is associated skin damage. Skin traction has specific limits of weight that it can pull without causing tissue breakdown. Skeletal traction is employed when significant traction pull must be applied in order to achieve realignment and immobilization. By inserting a pin or wire into the bone, the stress is placed on the bone and not on the surrounding tissue.

The type of traction applied is determined primarily by the age of the child, the condition of the soft tissues, and the type and degree of displacement of the fracture. Fractures most commonly treated by application of traction are those involving the humerus, femur, and vertebrae. The major types of traction for specific fractures are discussed in the following section.

Upper Extremity Traction

Treatment of fractures of the humerus by traction is accomplished either by overhead suspension, in which the arm, bent at the elbow, is suspended vertically by skin or skeletal attachment and traction is applied to the distal end of the humerus, or by Dunlop traction.

Dunlop traction. With Dunlop traction (Fig. 40-17) the arm is suspended horizontally, using either skin or skeletal attachment. When skin traction is used, straps are placed on the lower and upper arm with the arm flexed to accomplish pull in two directions: one along the longitudinal direction of the upper arm and one to maintain alignment of the lower arm. In instances such as supracondylar fractures, the amount of traction pull needed to align the site more critically necessitates that the Dunlop traction have a skeletal wire placed in the upper arm to allow the additional weight.

Fractures of the humerus, which are usually the result of a fall with the arm in extension, frequently involve the supracondylar portion. There are three major complications associated with this injury: Volkmann contractures (p. 1818), traumatic injury to the median, ulnar, or radial nerves, and angulation deformities. The fracture must be carefully reduced, sometimes under anesthesia, and because of the danger of complications, children with closed reduction of supracondylar fractures are often hospitalized for observation. In severely malaligned fractures closed reduction under anesthesia is followed by application of skeletal traction for 2 to 3 weeks, after which a long arm cast is applied for an additional 2 to 3 weeks.

Lower Extremity Traction

The frequent site for a femoral fracture is in the middle one third of the shaft as pictured by the x-ray film in Fig. 40-12. With this fracture there is significant overriding but minimum displacement. In a fracture in the lower one third of the shaft, the pull of the gastrocnemius muscle causes the distal fragment to become downwardly displaced. The severity of the fracturing force and the ability of the muscles to hold the fracture out of alignment will determine the fracture type and the amount of overriding of the fragments. The periosteum may remain intact, but a spiral fracture with much displacement often occurs.

Fractures of the femur can often be reduced with immediate application of a hip spica cast in young children. When traction is required, several types may be employed, based on the initial assessment.

Bryant traction. When a traction pulls only in one direction, it is called *running traction*. Bryant traction is this type of traction (Fig. 40-18). Adhesive traction strips are applied to the child's legs and secured with elastic bandages wrapped from the foot to the groin. Both of the child's hips are flexed at a 90-degree angle with the knees in extension and the legs suspended by pulleys and weights. The child's weight supplies the countertraction; therefore the buttocks are slightly elevated off the bed. By applying the same amount of traction to both legs and restraining the torso, the pelvis and hips are prevented from rotating and equal stress is placed on the growing extremities. The ankle bones are protected with stockinette or cotton wadding. This type of traction is used for children younger than 2 years of age whose weight is not sufficient to provide adequate countertraction without the additional gravitational force.

Both legs are suspended, even though only one may be involved.

Bryant traction is unsuitable for older children and is usually limited to children who weigh less than 12 to 14 kg (26 to 30 pounds) because of the risk of postural hypertension and to children without spasticity or contractures of the hamstring muscles. The child's position needs to be monitored, and the alignment of the fracture is checked by periodic x-ray films with needed traction adjustments made by the physician. Remodeling and callus formation occur rapidly within 2 to 3 weeks, after which the child is placed in a hip spica cast for an additional 3 to 9 weeks.

A specific complication of overhead traction is impairment of circulation. This is especially a problem in Bryant traction because of the gravitational vascular draining of the elevated extremities, the possible tourniquet effect of the bandages, and the effect of the traction, which can trigger vasospasms.

A child younger than 2 years of age normally has his hips in flexion most of the time; therefore the mild contracture that might develop from this position is easily corrected. The youngster is permitted sufficient room between his foot and the traction foot plate to move his foot and prevent ankle problems. The legs must be maintained perpendicular to the trunk, and the buttocks should not be allowed to rest on the mattress. Sometimes the child, especially the very active child, is placed in a jacket restraint or on a Bradford frame to prevent turning and twisting out of alignment.

Buck extension. Buck extension (Fig. 40-19) is a type of skin traction with the legs in an extended position, but it differs from Bryant traction in that the hips are not flexed. The postural hypertension that could develop as a result of Bryant traction is avoided, and this traction allows for greater mobility. Turning from side to side is permitted with care to maintain the involved leg in alignment. Buck extension is used primarily for short-term immobilization or frequently for correcting contracture or bone deformities such as Legg-Calvé-Perthes disease.

Russell traction. Russell traction (Fig. 40-20) uses skin traction on the lower leg and a padded sling under the knee. Two lines of pull, one along the longitudinal line of the lower leg and one perpendicular to the leg, are produced. This combination of pulls allows realignment of the lower extremity and immobilizes the hip and knee in a flexed position. The hip flexion must be kept at the prescribed angle to prevent fracture malalignment, since there is no direct support under the fracture and the skin traction may slip. Because the traction is set up to have two ropes

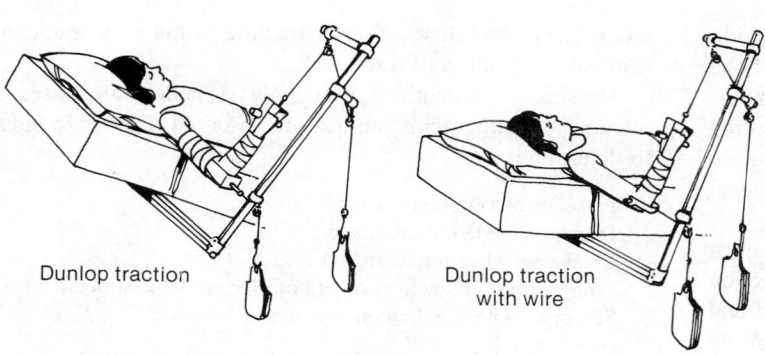

Dunlop traction

Dunlop traction
with wire

Fig. 40-17. Dunlop traction.

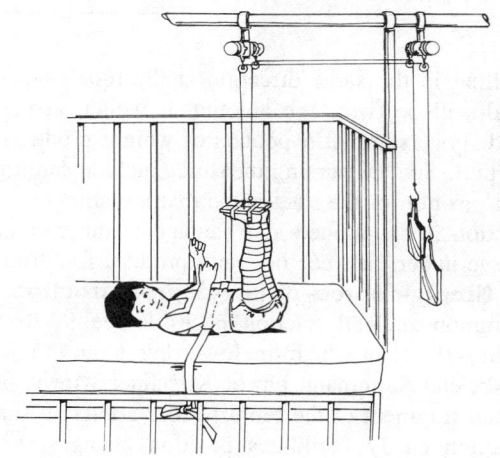

Fig. 40-18. Bryant traction.

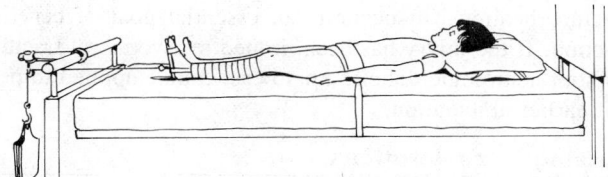

Fig. 40-19. Buck extension traction.

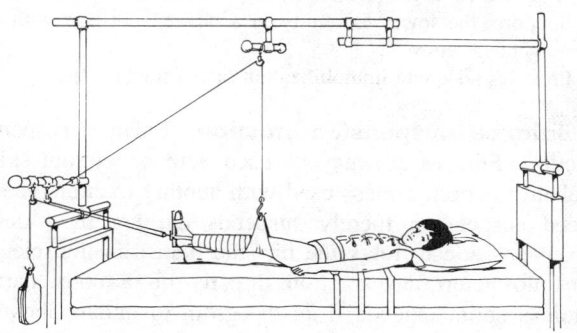

Fig. 40-20. Russell traction.

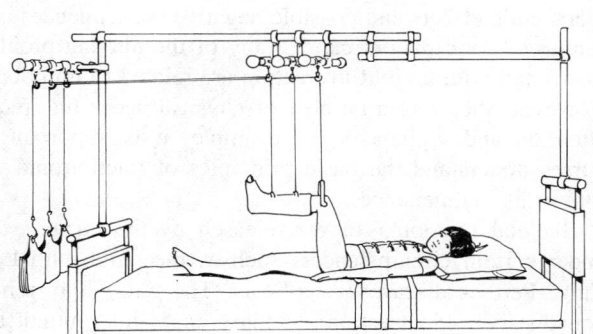

Fig. 40-21. Ninety-degree-90-degree traction.

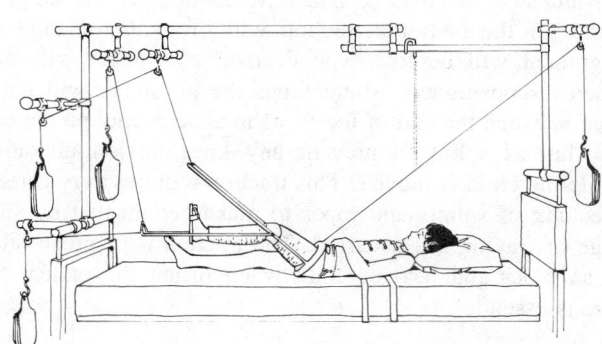

Fig. 40-22. Balance suspension with Thomas ring splint and Pearson attachment.

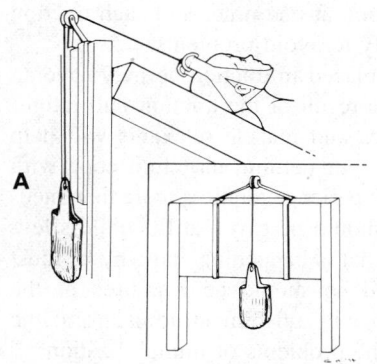

A

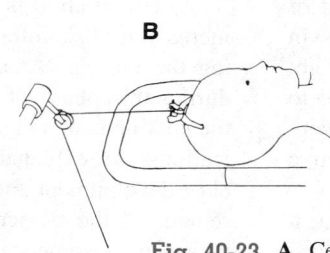

B

Fig. 40-23. A, Cervical traction. **B,** Crutchfield tong traction.

Figs. 40-17 to 40-23 from Hilt, N.E., and Schmitt, E.W.: Pediatric orthopedic nursing, St. Louis, 1975, The C. V. Mosby Co.

pulling in the same direction at the foot plate, the traction pull will be twice the amount of weight at the end of the bed. For example, 5 pounds of weight produces 10 pounds of pull. Special nursing measures include carefully checking the position of the traction so that the amount of desired hip flexion is maintained and damage to the common peroneal nerve under the knee does not produce footdrop.

Ninety-degree–ninety-degree traction. The most common skeletal traction is 90-degree–90-degree traction (Fig. 40-21) in which the lower leg is put in a boot cast and a skeletal Steinmann pin or Kirschner wire is placed in the distal fragment of the femur. From a nursing standpoint this traction easily facilitates position changes, toileting, and prevention of traction complications. This traction:

Achieves the desired line of pull for reducing the fracture by means of the skeletal traction
Allows a 90-degree flexion of both the hip and knee
Supports the lower extremity in a desired position with good venous return
Provides adequate immobilization of the fracture site

Balance suspension traction. Balance suspension traction (Fig. 40-22) may be used with or without skin or skeletal traction. Unless used with another traction, the balanced suspension merely suspends the leg in a desired flexed position to relax the hip and hamstring muscles and does not exert any traction directly on a body part. A Thomas splint extends from the groin to midair above the foot and a Pearson attachment supports the lower leg. Towels or pieces of felt covered with stockinette are clipped or pinned to the splints for leg support. Note that the ropes are attached to create a balanced traction. If the child is lifted off the bed, the traction will lift with him and no alignment will be lost. The Pearson attachment will stay wherever positioned. Many times the physician will put a rope between the end of the Pearson attachment and the end of Thomas splint to prevent any knee flexion alteration while the child is moved. This traction requires very careful checking of splints and ropes to make certain that no slippage or fraying has occurred. The traction is of great value in an older and heavier child when lifting the patient for care is essential.

Cervical Traction

The cervical area is a vulnerable site for flexion or extension injuries to muscle, vertebrae, and/or the spinal cord. Cervical muscle trauma without other complications is treated with a cervical soft or hard collar to relieve the weight of the head from the fracture site. Intermittent cervical skin traction might be employed with a child halter and weight to decrease muscle spasms (Fig. 40-23). Injuries limited to cervical muscles can be very uncomfortable but, with prompt medical care, usually resolve with conservative treatment.

When a child displaces or fractures a cervical vertebra, it is necessary to reduce and immobilize the site with cervical skeletal traction. The spinal cord runs through the intraver-

tebral canal, and dislocation or fracture of the vertebrae can also cause spinal cord trauma.

Physical examination, especially a neurologic assessment, and radiographic studies are essential diagnostic aids to determine:

Presence of vertebral fracture
Degree of vertebral dislocation
Displacement of intravertebral disc
Compression of spinal cord and other neurologic structures
Sensory, motor, and autonomic nerve deficits

Cervical traction is usually accomplished by making bur holes in the skull and inserting Crutchfield or Barton tongs. The head is placed in a hyperextended position, and, as the neck muscles fatigue with constant traction pull, the vertebral bodies gradually are pulled apart and the cord is no longer pinched between the vertebrae. Immobilization until fracture healing can occur is an essential goal of cervical traction. If the injury has been limited to a vertebral fracture without neurologic deficit, a halo cast can be applied to permit earlier ambulation.

Nursing Considerations

Traction is a valuable therapy if the purposes for the traction are achieved without complications. Generally the child in traction is hospitalized under the direct care of nurses who develop individualized nursing care plans based on an understanding of correct traction management. Evaluating the therapeutic effects and possible negative consequences is essential to good patient care. Many of the nursing problems associated with a child in traction are related to immobility. However, there are a number of physical needs that require attention and vigilance. For example, it is important that nurses understand the basic principles of traction and their role in its maintenance.

Skeletal traction is never released by the nurse, except under certain circumstances, such as the child with Legg-Calvé-Perthes disease or scoliosis. The nurse may remove nonadhesive skin traction. In these cases intermittent traction is periodically released and reapplied as ordered. When skin traction must be constantly maintained, such as in fractures, nurses may occasionally remove and reapply the Ace bandage if this is approved by the attending physician, provided that *someone manually maintains the traction during the rewrapping process*. It is not uncommon for a child to have several types of traction at one time, and each traction must be assessed separately to avoid problems.

When the child is first placed in traction he may have an increase in discomfort as a result of the traction pull fatiguing the muscle. Analgesics and muscle relaxants will help during this phase of care, but helping the child cope with the confinement and new experience requires more than medications. An explanation should be given at the child's level of development about what is happening and why he must remain in the device, and he should be reassured of the presence of someone who will aid him in adjusting to the traction and coping with the problems of immobilization.

Nursing Care Summary: The Child in Traction

NURSING GOALS	NURSING INTERVENTIONS	EXPECTED PATIENT/FAMILY OUTCOMES
HP-HMP **Injury: potential for damage** **Risk factors: immobility, presence of traction**		

Prevent complications	Assess circular dressings for excessive tightness
	 Assess restraining devices
	   Make certain that they are not too loose or too tight
	   Remove periodically and check for pressure areas
	 Encourage deep breathing frequently with maximum inspiratory chest expansion
	 Note any neurovascular changes, such as
	   Color in skin and nail beds
	   Alterations in sensation
	   Alterations in motor ability
	 Take immediate action to correct problem or report to physician if neurovascular changes are found
	 Record findings of neurovascular changes
	 Carry out passive, active, or active-with-resistance exercises of uninvolved joints
	 Note if any tightness, weakness, or contractures are developing in uninvolved joints and muscles
	 Take measures to correct or prevent further development of weakness, such as applying foot plate to prevent footdrop
		Circulation in extremities remains satisfactory: movement, good color, sensation present
		 Child exhibits no signs of complications

N-MP **Skin integrity, impairment of: potential** **Risk factors: immobility**		
Prevent skin breakdown	Provide sheepskin or alternating pressure mattress underneath hips and back Make total body skin checks for redness or breakdown, especially over areas that receive greatest pressure Wash and dry skin at least twice daily Stimulate circulation with gentle massage over pressure areas Change position at least every 2 hours to relieve pressure	Skin remains clean and intact with no evidence of irritation
A-EP **Diversional activity, deficit** **Etiology: immobility**		
Provide diversion	Involve the child in planning his care to the extent of his capabilities Arrange and encourage interaction with others as feasible	Child helps plan care and schedule Child interacts with family and other children
Promote growth and development	Provide diversional activities appropriate to the child's limitations and developmental level	Child engages in activities appropriate to condition and developmental level (specify)
A-EP **Mobility, impaired physical** **Etiology: musculoskeletal impairment**		
Maintain limb function	Provide apparatus and encourage child in activities that provide exercise for uninvolved muscles and joints	Joints remain flexible; muscles retain tone

Continued.

Nursing Care Summary: The Child in Traction—cont'd

NURSING GOALS	NURSING INTERVENTIONS	EXPECTED PATIENT/FAMILY OUTCOMES

**A-EP   Self-care deficit: feeding, bathing/hygiene, dressing/grooming, toileting (specify level)
Etiology: musculoskeletal impairment**

NURSING GOALS	NURSING INTERVENTIONS	EXPECTED PATIENT/FAMILY OUTCOMES
Provide adequate nutrition and hydration	Encourage fluid intake so child stays well hydrated Provide nourishing, nonconstipating diet with preferred foods when possible and foods that child can manage unassisted Make certain that child ingests sufficient amount of calcium-rich foods	Child is well nourished and hydrated
Promote maximum self-help	Devise means to facilitate self-help in daily activities Assist with self-care activities where needed, for example, bathe inaccessible parts, make food easy to eat without assistance, provide grooming	Child assists with self-care activities—feeds self, washes reachable areas, attends to grooming within his capabilities (specify)
Facilitate elimination	Use fracture pan for bowel movements and voiding for females Check frequency and consistency of bowel movements Adjust fluid and food intake according to stools, for example, increase fluids, fruits, grains for constipation	Elimination is managed with minimum difficulty Child has regular bowel movements

**SP-SCP   Fear
Etiology: discomfort, knowledge deficit**

NURSING GOALS	NURSING INTERVENTIONS	EXPECTED PATIENT/FAMILY OUTCOMES
Decrease anxiety and gain cooperation	Explain traction apparatus to child Explain to child what his nursing care will be Determine with child how he can participate in his care Make certain that child knows how to call for help Assure child that he will not be left totally helpless	Child cooperates throughout procedure
Relieve pain and discomfort	Use pads, pillows, and rolls to position for comfort Assess child's behavior to determine if traction causes pain or discomfort (see p. 1068) Apply nonpharmacologic pain-reduction techniques (see p. 1071)	Child plays and interacts readily Child exhibits no signs of discomfort

**RRP   Family process, alteration in
Etiology: situational crisis (injured child)**

NURSING GOALS	NURSING INTERVENTIONS	EXPECTED PATIENT/FAMILY OUTCOMES
Support parents	Explain traction and its desired effects Allow parents to ask questions and express concerns Assist with needed services; make appropriate referrals when indicated See also The child in the hospital, p. 1075; Family of the hospitalized child, p. 1081	Parents ask questions regarding their concerns Parents demonstrate an understanding of child's condition and therapies Parents acquire needed services

Nursing Interventions Related to Medical Management

Maintain traction
Understand purpose of traction
Understand function of traction in each specific situation
Check desired line of pull and relationship of distal fragment to proximal fragment
    Check whether fragment is being directed upward, adducted, or abducted
Check function of each component
    Position of bandages, frames, splints
    Ropes
        In center tract of pulley
        Taut
        No fraying
        Knots tied securely
    Pulleys
        In original position on attachment bar; have not slid from original site
        Wheels freely movable
    Weights
        Correct amount of weight
        Hanging freely
        In safe location
Check bed position—head or foot elevated as directed for desired amount of pull and countertraction
Do not remove skeletal traction or adhesive traction straps on skin traction
Skin traction
    Replace nonadhesive straps and/or Ace bandage on skin traction when permitted and/or absolutely necessary, but make certain that traction on limb is maintained by someone during procedure

Assess bandages to ascertain if they are correctly applied (diagonal or spiral), not too loose or too tight, which could cause slippage and malalignment of traction
Skeletal traction
    Check pin sites frequently for signs of bleeding, inflammation, or infection
    Cleanse and dress pin sites as ordered
    Apply topical antiseptic or antibiotic daily as ordered
    Cover ends of pins with protective cord or padding to prevent child's being scratched by pin
    Note pull of traction on pin; pull should be even
    Check pin screws to be certain that screws are tight in metal clamp that attaches traction apparatus to pin
Relieve pain
Administer pain medication as needed
Administer muscle relaxants if ordered
Maintain alignment
Observe for correct body alignment with emphasis on alignment of shoulder, hip, and leg
Check after child has moved
Apply restraints when indicated
Maintain correct angles at joints
Prevent constipation
Administer stool softeners as indicated
Administer rectal suppository or mild laxative if indicated

The specific nursing responsibilities for the patient in cervical traction include:

1. Watching for any changes in neurologic signs and symptoms that indicate that traction is benefitting or causing more problems.
2. Carrying out meticulous skin care around the tong sites. The nursing protocol is to clean the sites several times a day with saline solution or hydrogen peroxide and then apply a topical antiseptic such as povidone-iodine (Betadine). Sloughing of the pin site and osteomyelitis of the skull bone are potential dangers.
3. Use of the guidelines in the Nursing care summary: the child in traction.
4. Log rolling the child's body without flexion of neck or spine at least every 2 hours. Stryker frames are often used with cervical traction to facilitate maintaining alignment.
5. Placing supporting pillows beside the neck before turning and having necessary pillows available to support the back, arms, and legs.
6. Use of nursing approaches for persons with spinal cord injuries as elaborated later in this chapter.

FRACTURE COMPLICATIONS

Complications associated with fractures and immobilization are varied and have some problems in common. In addition to problems related to immobilization, the major complications of fractures include the following areas.

Circulatory Impairment

If the trauma or immobilizing device restricts veins or arteries in the affected extremity, bone healing will be seriously impaired. Careful assessment of the pulses, skin color, and temperature is an important nursing responsibility. After injury, swelling of tissues occurs more rapidly in the child than in the adult. In the upper extremity, brachial, radial, ulnar, and digital pulses are felt. In the leg, femoral, popliteal, posterior tibial, and dorsalis pedis pulses are checked. When circulatory impairment is evident (absence of pulse, discoloration, swelling, pain), the nurse takes quick action to relieve the problem by reporting the situation immediately. If the physician is unable to come and release the pressure, the nurse must be able to cut the cast in half to form a bivalve cast or make a large window in it to decrease the pressure.

Closely associated with an inadequate blood supply is a low hematocrit value, which can result from the initial blood loss or surgically induced anemia. Although the blood flow may be adequate, a lowered amount of hemoglobin will not provide a sufficient supply of oxygen for tissue repair.

Nerve Compression Syndromes

Nerve damage can take place at the time of injury, develop in the process of realignment, or be a complication of an immobilizing apparatus. The syndromes are classified according to the anatomic area affected and can involve the median (carpal tunnel syndrome), ulnar (at wrist or elbow), radial, posterior tibial (tarsal tunnel syndrome), common peroneal, or sciatic nerves. Peroneal nerve damage can result in footdrop, and radial nerve impairment produces wristdrop. Both of these disabilities can significantly interfere with activities of daily living. Sensory testing with touch and pinprick and evaluating motor strength by asking the child to move the unaffected joint distal to the injury are common means of determining neurologic involvement. Subjective symptoms are pain or discomfort, muscular weakness, a burning sensation, limitation of motion, and altered sensation. Treatment is alleviation of pressure on the nerve. The physician determines whether correcting the alignment will alleviate pressure on the nerve or if surgical intervention is necessary. At times sensory or motor changes indicate ischemia and the treatment is correction of the vascular disturbance.

Compartmental Syndromes

A *compartment* is a group of muscles surrounded by tough, inelastic fascial tissue. The compartment syndrome occurs when increased pressure within this closed space rises and compromises circulation to the muscles and nerves within the space. Muscles and nerves of both upper and lower extremities are enclosed within such compartments. The most frequent causes of compartment syndrome are tight dressings or casts, hemorrhage, trauma, burns, and surgery.

Signs and symptoms of compartment syndrome reflect a deficit or deterioration of neuromuscular status in the anatomic area surrounding the involved structures. These include motor weakness and pain or discomfort, and tenseness may be noted on palpation of the area. Because early detection is important in preventing permanent damage to tissues, specialists recommend continuous monitoring of compartment pressures by way of a small slit tip catheter inserted into the compartment. Treatment of compartment syndrome is immediate relief of pressure, which sometimes requires fasciotomy.

Volkmann contracture. Volkmann contracture (ischemic muscular atrophy) is a serious, persistent flexion contraction of the forearm and hand caused by massive infarction of muscle. Pressure from a cast or tight bandage in the area of the elbow begins with arterial occlusion and then progresses to muscle anoxia and reflex vasospasms. Finally the lack of blood supply leads to muscle necrosis and replacement with fibrous tissue, which produces paralysis and a clawlike hand contracture. Any fracture that requires excessive traction can be complicated by Volkmann contracture, however, it occurs most often in the elbow.

The neuromuscular symptoms are severe pain (although pain is not always a manifestation), pallor or cyanosis, edema, absence of pulses in the extremity, and loss of sensitivity. Unrelieved, the occlusive hypoxic process can cause some contracture if ischemia lasts as little as 6 hours. A great deal of muscle damage occurs after 12 to 24 hours; 48 hours of ischemia produces severe deformity with muscle fibrosis and contractures in 5 to 10 days. If not treated, the contracture leads to severe deformity and paralysis.

The immediate treatment is to remove any mechanically obstructive materials, such as tight bandages, and extend the joint to free blood vessels. If the symptoms do not improve within a few hours, arteriography is done in anticipation that surgery may be needed to decrease arterial spasms and to improve the blood supply by separation of the fascial sheaths of the involved muscles.

Epiphyseal Damage

Growth of bone originates from the epiphyseal plate, and damage to this structure could result in an unequal extremity length. Surgical intervention to the epiphysis on the affected extremity or to the epiphyseal line on the opposite extremity is the usual treatment.

Nonunion

Bone healing and callus formation can span and repair only a limited space between fragments. When inadequate reduction, poor immobilization, or a damaged or softened cast cannot maintain the bone fragments in correct alignment for repair, bone healing is impaired. Based on the physiologic needs for bone healing, the factors most likely to interfere with bone healing and cause delayed union or nonunion are:

Separation of bone fragments at fracture site
Loss of hematoma
Interposition of tissue between bone fragments
Loss of bone tissue, especially from necrosis
Infection
Poor nutrition
Interruption of blood supply
Diseases that influence calcium metabolism (e.g., thyroid disorder)
Cancer of bone
Administration of steroids

The hematoma, which becomes the matrix for bone deposition in the break, must be free of infection or bits of adipose or connective tissue. The constant supply of nutrients and bone-forming cells brought to the area by way of the bloodstream provides the vital ingredients for repair.

Sometimes artificial means are employed to facilitate bone healing. Bone grafting becomes necessary when bone nonunion occurs. The donor sites are usually the tibia or the iliac crest. Bleeding of bone ends may need to be artificially stimulated, and at times holes are drilled near the bone ends in an attempt to increase circulation. Postsurgical immobilization of the recipient area is crucial to a successful graft.

Malunion

Malunion is fracture union with increased angulation or deformity at the fracture site. It can be detected at any stage in the healing process or after complete healing. Unsatisfactory reduction is the usual reason for malunion. A cast or splint that allows fracture movement will also likely result in malunion. Periodic radiographic examinations will help detect this complication and avoid its becoming a major problem over a long period.

Excessive deformity can be corrected during the healing process through realignment and reimmobilization. However, attempts at correction may cause delayed union or nonunion; therefore the degree of deformity is carefully evaluated in light of these complications and the probability of sufficient spontaneous alignment that occurs with growth and continuation of the healing process is considered. Correction of the malunion when healing is near completion requires surgical intervention.

Infection

Osteomyelitis, infection of the bone, is often secondary to a bloodstream infection but is a potential problem in open fractures or when bone surgery has been performed. Any bacterial organism can cause this infectious process; however, *Staphylococcus aureus* is the most frequent pathogen. (See p. 1766 for a discussion of osteomyelitis.)

Kidney Stones

Although uncommon in children, renal calculi are a potential risk whenever the child has a limb that is is non–weight bearing for a long time, especially if the circumstances also produce urinary stasis. Preventative measures for renal calculi are to maintain good hydration, to mobilize the child as much as possible, and to check closely the amount and characteristics of urinary output. Any urinary tract infection should be treated promptly with appropriate antimicrobials and urine acidification because the nucleus of the calculi is often composed of bacterial debris or calcium and the buildup of stone is precipitated by alkaline urine. An associated problem, hypercalcemia, is reviewed under problems of the immobilized child.

Pulmonary Emboli

Blood, air, or fat emboli can be a hazard to the child with a fracture. As postinjury bleeding and clotting occur, a small piece of the clot can travel to vital organs, such as the lung, heart, or brain, and produce a life-threatening vascular obstruction and ischemia. Generally the pulmonary system is the most frequent site for emboli deposition, but it may not occur until 6 to 8 weeks after the injury.

Fat emboli are the greatest threat to an individual with multiple fractures, particularly in fractures of the long bones such as the femur. Fat droplets from the marrow are transferred to the general circulation by means of venous-arterial route, where they can be transported to the lung or brain. This type of emboli phenomenon occurs within the first 24 hours, generally in the second 12 hours after the injury occurs.

Emboli in the vital organs produce the classic symptoms of shock. Petechial hemorrhages of the chest and shoulders are the outstanding signs that differentiate this condition from other kinds of shock. In the immobilized child who suddenly develops chest pain and dyspnea when turned, pulmonary embolism should be suspected. The severe dyspnea must be treated immediately by elevating the head when possible and administering oxygen by means of mask, cannula, or hood. Deep breathing, coughing, and mechanical respiratory assistance are important to maintain adequate alveolar gas exchange. An intravenous infusion is established to treat the shock and administer medications such as heparin and corticosteroids.

AMPUTATION

A child may be born with the congenital absence of a body part, have a traumatic loss of an extremity, or need a surgical amputation for a pathologic condition such as osteogenic sarcoma. With today's surgical technology and the quick thinking of bystanders who save a traumatically amputated body part, some children have had fingers and arms sewn back on with variable degrees of functional use regained. A severed part should be wrapped in a clean cloth or placed in saline if possible and taken to the hospital with the victim.

An operative amputation or the surgical repair of a permanently severed limb focuses on constructing an adequately nourished stump. A smooth, healthy, padded stump, free of nerve endings, is important in prothesis fitting and subsequent ambulation. In some situations in which there is no vascular or neurologic deficit, a cast is applied to the stump immediately after the operation and a pylon, metal extension, and artificial foot are attached so that the patient can walk on the temporary prothesis within a few hours.

Nursing Considerations

Stump shaping is done postoperatively with special elastic bandaging using a figure-of-8 bandage, which applies pressure in a cone-shaped fashion. This technique decreases stump edema, controls hemorrhage, and aids in developing desired contours so that the child will bear weight on the posterior aspect of the skin flap rather than on the end of the stump. Stump elevation may be used during the first 24 hours, but after this time the extremity should not be left in this position because contractures in the proximal joint will develop and seriously hamper ambulation. Monitoring proper body alignment will further decrease the risk of flexion contractures.

For older children and adolescents, arm exercises and bed pushups, as well as parallel bars, which are used in prothesis-training programs, help to build up the arm muscles necessary for walking with crutches. Full range of motion exercises of joints above the amputation must be performed several times daily, using active and isotonic exercises. Young children are spontaneously active and require little encouragement.

Depending on the child's age, he or his parents will need to learn stump hygiene with careful soap and water washing every day and checking for skin irritation, breakdown, or infection. A tube of stockinette or talcum powder is used to slide the prosthesis on more easily. A careful skin check must be done every time the prosthesis is removed, and prosthesis tolerance time must be adjusted to prevent skin breakdown.

For the child who has had an amputation, phantom limb sensation is an expected experience because the nerve-brain connections are still present. Gradually these sensations fade. Preoperative discussion of this phenomenon will aid the child in understanding his "unusual feelings" and not hide his experiences from others. Limb pain, especially pain that increases with ambulation, should be evaluated for the possibility of a neuroma at the free nerve endings in the stump. Psychogenic phantom limb pain is a complex problem involving the child's response to the altered body image and the coping mechanisms he uses to handle the new experience. The problems of amputation, particularly the psychologic aspects, are discussed on p. 1603.

SPINAL CORD INJURIES

Spinal cord injuries with major neurologic involvement are not a common cause of physical handicap in childhood. However, there are a sufficient number of children with these injuries admitted to major medical centers, and because of the increased survival as the result of improved management, nurses are more likely to become involved with such children. In addition, the catastrophic nature of spinal cord injury with its serious sequelae and the importance of preventive and functional rehabilitation justify a discussion of the topic. The principles of management and nursing care apply to all spinal cord lesions regardless of etiology, particularly myelomeningocele, the most common cause of paraplegia in the pediatric age-group.

No comprehensive studies are available to indicate the incidence of spinal cord injury in children. Isolated reports show the highest incidence to be in young adults, whereas major rehabilitation centers report from two to four new cases per year in children.

However, it is not rare to have a number of teenagers with spinal cord injuries in the population of rehabilitation centers, and their care is complex, since it involves nursing activities associated with vertebral fracture healing, immobilization for a prolonged period of time, psychosocial disruption of the child and the family, and a neurologic deficit.

The first part of this chapter focused on musculoskeletal trauma and care of the immobilized child, which is applicable to the child with damage to the spinal cord. The child with a spinal cord injury presents additional problems, specifically complications related to the neuropathology of the central and autonomic nervous systems. The following definitions are used to describe the neurologic deficit:

paraplegia Paralysis of two extremities, usually the lower limbs.

quadriplegia, or **tetraplegia** Functional disuse in all four extremities.

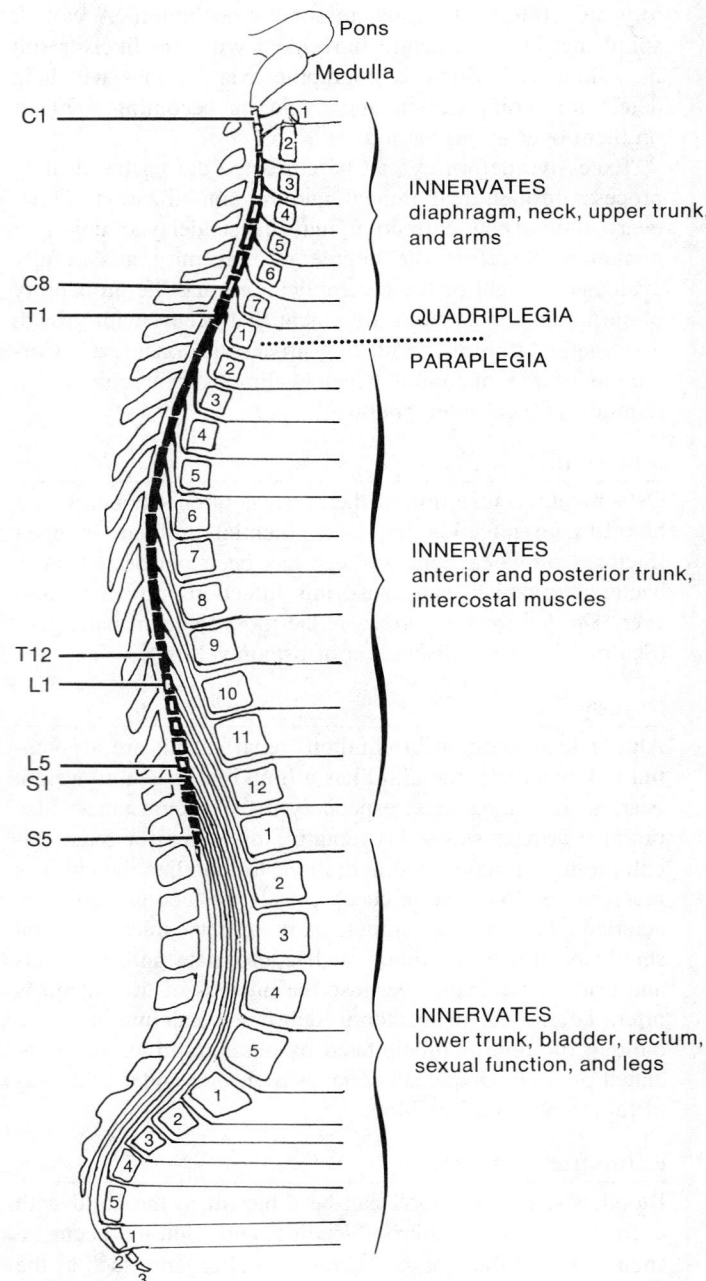

Fig. 40-24. Relationships of spinal cord segments and spinal nerves to vertebral bodies. Cervical nerves exit through intervertebral foramina above their respective vertebral bodies (seven cervical vertebrae and eight cervical nerves). Spinal cord ends at L1 and L2 vertebral level.

Modified from Mayo Clinic: Clinical examinations in neurology, Philadelphia, 1971, W.B. Saunders, Co.

A high level of paraplegia may create major problems in being able to sit upright without support, whereas paraplegic children with lower level injuries can walk with minimum assistance. The extent of paralysis is determined by both neurologic and clinical assessment. Although the majority of children with spinal cord injuries are paraplegic, many

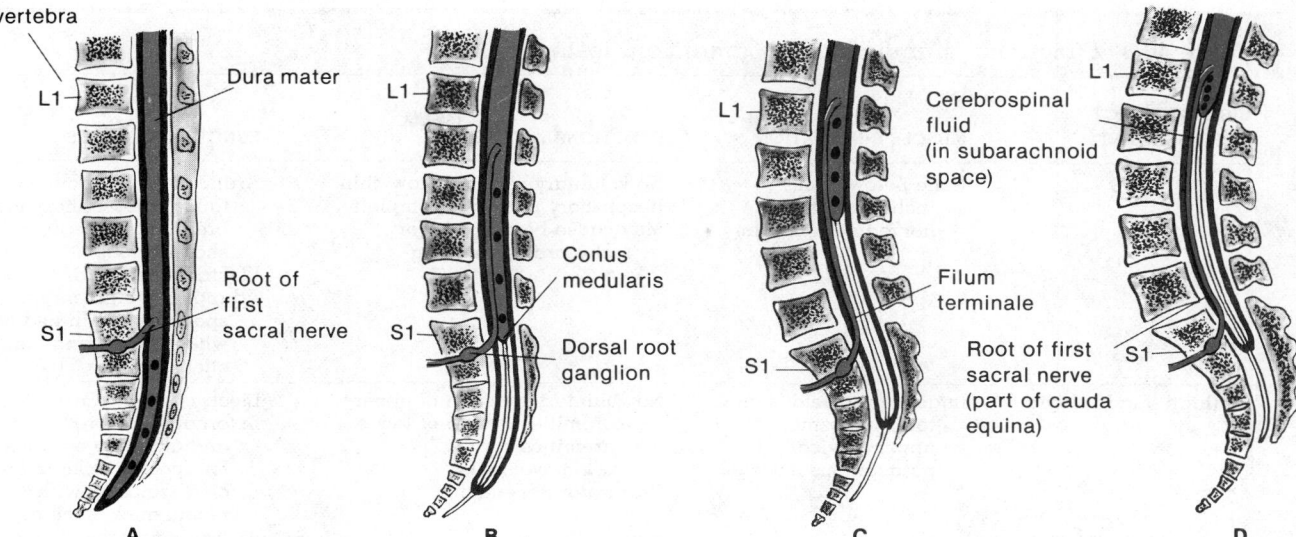

Body of vertebra

L1

Dura mater

S1

Root of
first
sacral nerve

L1

S1

Conus
medularis

Dorsal root
ganglion

L1

S1

Cerebrospinal
fluid
(in subarachnoid
space)

Filum
terminale

Root of first
sacral nerve
(part of cauda
equina)

L1

S1

A   B   C   D

Fig. 40-25. Diagrams showing position of caudal end of spinal cord in relation to vertebral column and meninges at various stages of development. Increasing inclination of root of first sacral nerve is also illustrated. **A,** Eight weeks. **B,** 24 weeks. **C,** Newborn. **D,** Adult. *L1,* First lumbar vertebra; *S1,* first sacral vertebra.

are quadriplegic. Some quadriplegic children are able to move only their face and neck muscles, whereas others are able to lift and bend their arms but are unable to perform fine hand movements. Almost every physiologic system is disrupted in a child with high-level quadriplegia. Not only are the central and peripheral nerves impaired, but there is also autonomic nervous system dysfunction. Vital structures such as blood vessels, lungs, bladder, and bowel are affected. Therefore an understanding of neuromuscular physiology is essential to effectively care for the child with damage or injury to the spinal cord.

Review of Essential Neuromuscular Physiology

The spinal cord extends from the medulla oblongata to the lower border of the first lumbar vertebra and contains millions of nerve fibers (Fig. 40-24). However, because of its protected location, a considerable amount of direct trauma is required to cause injury. Posteriorly the cord is protected by the spinous processes, which are stabilized by related ligaments and muscles. It is further protected by the spinal fluid, which surrounds it and absorbs some of the shock.

Development of the spinal cord. The spinal cord demonstrates alterations relative to the vertebral column during prenatal and early postnatal growth. In the embryo the spinal cord extends the full length of the vertebral canal, but because the bony vertebral column and the cord have different growth rates, the cord in the newborn ends at the level of the third and fourth lumbar vertebrae. In the adult it ends higher at the level of the first lumbar vertebra (Fig. 40-25). The disparity in growth rates also involves the spinal nerves attached to the cord. In the early developing embryo the spinal nerves are directed nearly horizontal to

the intervertebral foramina, through which they emerge from the spinal column. At full growth the upper cervical nerves are still directed nearly horizontally, but the lower nerves project more and more obliquely downward toward their intervertebral foramina. The sacral and coccygeal nerves are arranged in relation to one another with their direction nearly vertical in such a way that they resemble the arrangement of hairs in a horse's tail, hence the term *cauda equina.*

Spinal nerves. The 31 nerves of the spinal cord are divided into five segments—*cervical* (eight), *thoracic* (twelve), *lumbar* (five), *sacral* (five), and *coccygeal* (one). The eight cervical cord segments lie within the first seven vertebrae, and the remaining cord segments extend from the first thoracic vertebra to the lower level of the first lumbar vertebra; therefore the cord segments do not anatomically match by number the 30 associated vertebrae. However, nerves that arise from the cord segments exit from the spinal column at the numerically corresponding vertebrae. In describing injuries to the spinal cord, the highest point at which there is normal function is referred to in relation to these segments, for example, an intact cord at the sixth cervical segment is designated as a C6 injury.

Certain areas of the curved vertebral column are less stable and more prone to damage from severe flexion and twisting. These sites are the cervical area and the junction of the thoracic and lumbar regions. The cervical vertebrae are fractured most frequently, and this high level of injury causes extensive paralysis and many associated neurologic problems (see Table 40-3).

The spinal cord is nourished by branches of the vertebral and radicular arteries. Traumatic tearing or embolic occlu-

Table 40-3 Functional significance of spinal cord lesions

HIGHEST INTACT CORD SEGMENT	MUSCLE INNERVATION	FUNCTIONAL CAPACITY	FUNCTIONAL GOALS
C1-3	None below chin, including phrenic nerve to diaphragm	No voluntary control below chin Respiratory paralysis complete May cause bradycardia or tachycardia, vomiting	Artificial respiration; can be taught glossopharyngeal breathing to be used for short periods Electric wheelchair Adaptive equipment for special tasks in bed or wheelchair using mouth stick
C4 (high quadriplegia)	Intact sternocleidomastoid, trapezius, upper cervical paraspinous muscles	No voluntary function of upper extremities, trunk, or lower extremities All neck movements Respirator dependent	Electric wheelchair Externally powered devices and adaptive equipment for special tasks in bed or wheelchair with mouth stick, such as turning pages, using electric typewriter Totally dependent for activities of daily living
C5	Partial deltoid, biceps, major muscles of rotator cuffs of shoulders Diaphragm	Abduction, flexion, and extension of arm Flexion and extension of forearm Unable to roll over or attain sitting position Abdominal respiration Poor respiratory reserve	Electric wheelchair Requires attendant to assist in moving and transfer to wheelchair Adaptive devices for self-feeding, grooming, using electric typewriter Vocational potential with adaptive devices
C6	Pectoralis major, serratus anterior, latissimus dorsi muscles Complete deltoid and brachioradialis muscles Partial triceps muscle	Significant increase in function over that with lesion at C5 level Adduction and medial rotation of arm Wrist extension Good elbow flexion	Cuff strapped to hand permits use of implements for self-care and other activities Able to assist in dressing and transfer Hand rim extension permits independence in wheelchair
C7	Triceps and finger flexor and extensor muscle Shoulder depressor muscles Still nerve disruption to intercostal muscles	With elbow stabilized in extension and intact shoulder depressor muscles able to lift body weight Grasp and release still weak; dexterity lacking	Almost complete independence within limitations of wheelchair Requires some assistance in transfer and lower extremity dressing Hand splints helpful Can roll over in bed, sit up in bed, and eat independently Homebound employment possible Outside work usually not feasible
T1-10 (high paraplegia)	Full innervation of upper extremity muscles	Full use of upper extremities, including intrinsic muscles of hand Trunk balance poor May have difficulty in lifting sufficiently to put on lower extremity clothing Considerable energy expenditure to put on long leg braces with extensive attachments	Completely wheelchair dependent Trunk balance benefits from training Able to drive automobile with hand controls May be braced for standing May hold job away from home Cannot manage public transportation

Table 40-3 Functional significance of spinal cord lesions—cont'd

HIGHEST INTACT CORD SEGMENT	MUSCLE INNERVATION	FUNCTIONAL CAPACITY	FUNCTIONAL GOALS
T10-L2	Full abdominal and upper back muscle control	Good trunk balance Good respiratory reserve Can accomplish moderate hiphiking using external oblique and latissimus dorsi muscles	Ambulation with bilateral long braces using four-point or swing-through crutch gait Usually able to negotiate curbs Some able to use public transportation Few vocational limitations as long as does not require much walking or standing
L3 or below	Quadriceps muscle Partial gluteus and hamstring muscles	May be lumbar lordosis Floppy ankles	Ambulates well, often with short leg braces with or without cane Difficulty in getting out of wheelchair May never require wheelchair

sion of these vessels can markedly jeopardize the cord tissue. When this rich blood supply is impaired, the result frequently is severe neurologic deficit, extending even to complete loss of cord function at that level.

Cell bodies of interneurons and motor neurons within the spinal cord are identified as H-shaped gray matter surrounded by columns of white myelinated nerve fibers, each column serving as a route for a specific type of impulse, such as touch, vibration, pain, and temperature (Fig. 40-26). Nerve pathways in the spinal cord transmit sensory and motor impulses between peripheral receptors and the brain, conduct impulses through the reflex arc, and convey sympathetic and parasympathetic nerve impulses from the brain to peripheral structures. (See also Fig. 39-1.)

Sensory transmission begins in the peripheral receptors where sensory receptors pick up a wide variety of stimuli and transfer the impulses, by means of peripheral nerves, to the spinal nerves where they make ganglionic connections and enter the cord posteriorly. At this point the impulses

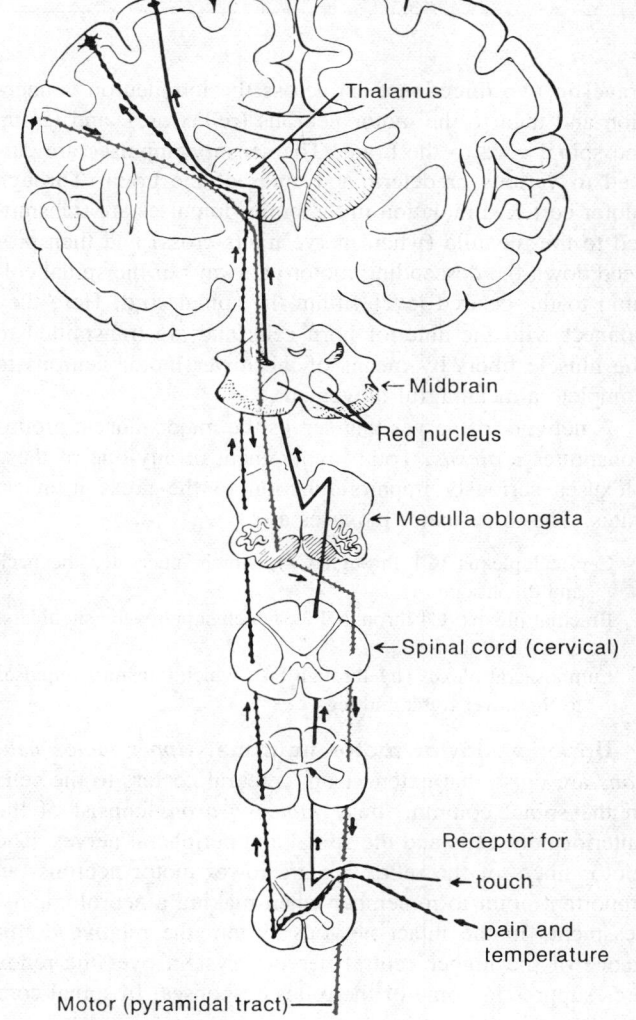

Fig. 40-26. Diagram of main motor and sensory pathways. Perception of touch, passive motion, position, and vibration is transmitted through posterior tract in spinal cord through medical lemniscus in brain stem to thalamus and through internal capsule to cortex (this pathway is represented by solid line). Pain and temperature sensations are transmitted through anterolateral tract and lateral lemniscus to thalamus, then through internal capsule to cortex *(irregular line)*. Motor impulses are transmitted by pyramidal tract, descending from cerebral cortex, crossing in medulla to opposite side, and continuing to anterior horns of spinal cord *(red line)*.

From Conway, B.L.: Carini and Owens' neurological and neurosurgical nursing, ed. 7, St. Louis, 1978, The C.V. Mosby Co.

DIFFERENCES IN CLINICAL MANIFESTATIONS BETWEEN UPPER AND LOWER MOTOR NEURON SYNDROMES

Upper motor neuron syndrome	Lower motor neuron syndrome
Spastic paralysis in muscle groups below lesion (reflex arcs below lesion are intact)	Flaccid paralysis caused by muscle atonia (reflex arcs are permanently damaged)
Hyperreflexia with tendon reflexes exaggerated, Babinski reflex present	Reflex with associated muscle response absent
No wasting of muscle mass because of increased muscle tone	Marked atrophy of atonic muscle
Flexion contractures and spasms of muscle groups below lesion level common	Fasciculations(localtwitching of muscle groups) common No flexor spasms
No skin or tissue changes	Loss of hair Skin and tissue changes Cornified nails

travel in two directions: (1) across the intraneuron connection and then to the motor neurons (reflex arc), and (2) up the spinal cord to the brain. The sensory impulses are carried to various predetermined areas of the brain. Through motor cortex stimulation in the brain, impulses are transmitted to the medulla (where nerve tracts cross) and then proceed down the descending motor pathways of the spinal column to the desired level within the spinal cord. Here they connect with the anterior horn cells and are transmitted to the muscle fibers by means of the lower motor neurons to complete a meaningful movement.

A network of nerves that serves the major muscle groups constitutes a *plexus.* Total involvement of any one of these plexuses seriously impairs function to the areas it innervates. The three major plexuses are:

Cervical plexus (C1 through C4), which innervates the neck and diaphragm
Brachial plexus (C4 through T1), which supplies the shoulders, chest, and arms
Lumbosacral plexus (L1 through S4), which transmits impulses to the lower trunk and legs

Upper vs lower motor neurons. *Upper motor neurons* are those that extend from cerebral centers to the cells in the spinal column; *lower motor neurons* consist of the anterior horn cells and the spinal and peripheral nerves. The motor fibers of the reflex arc are lower motor neurons, an important point to remember when making a neurologic assessment. In the intact nervous system the relative dominance of the higher central nervous system over the reflex arcs suppresses some of the reflex responses. In spinal cord

injury when the higher centers no longer exert an influence, spastic responses are observed in muscles innervated by the intact lower motor neurons. Most persons with spinal cord injuries have upper motor neuron injuries; children born with spinal cord defects have primarily lower motor neuron deficits. The box at left illustrates the differences between upper and lower motor neuron syndromes.

Effect on sensory and motor tracts. Voluntary muscle control is lost when complete transection of the cord occurs. In partial transection function is altered in varying degrees, depending on the areas innervated by the nerves involved. Because of the crossing of the motor tracts at various levels, it is possible for an injured person to have motor paralysis in one leg but retain pain and temperature sensation to that leg while losing these sensations in the opposite leg, which retains its motor function.

Although a transected cord injury leads to sensory loss, it is not uncommon for the injured person to have pain experiences. Smooth or skeletal muscle spasms, destruction of the myelin sheath (with impulses crossing over to adjacent nerves), and scar formation or irritation of nerve endings may cause pain. The pain suffered by a quadriplegic or paraplegic person is often intensified because of the loss of sensation in other parts. Narcotics should be used with discretion, and when possible, tranquilizers (which are good muscle relaxants) such as diazepam (Valium) are preferred. Severe and prolonged pain should be medically evaluated for treatable pathology.

Effect on autonomic system. The sympathetic and parasympathetic systems receive both excitatory and inhibitory stimuli from the autonomic centers in the cerebral cortex, limbic system, and hypothalamus. These stimuli are transmitted by means of the cord with a feedback mechanism within the ascending fibers of the cord that normally controls descending input. Axons of the many central nervous system neurons synapse with the autonomic preganglionic fibers and thus are able to alter their patterned responses. The most significant effects of autonomic disruption are:

1. Decreased muscle tone and impairment of vasoconstrictive effects of sympathetic innervation that cause venous pooling, diminished venous return to the heart, decreased cardiac output, and hypotension, especially orthostatic hypotension
2. Disruption between the thermoregulatory center in the hypothalamus and the skin receptors—blood vessels remain dilated during the initial stage, the child is unable to sweat in response to increased environmental temperature, and body temperature can elevate rapidly
3. Loss of voluntary control of bowel and bladder function because of damage to L1, L2, and L3 levels and parasympathetic fibers from S2, S3, and S4 levels, which innervate these organs
4. Altered sexual function, such as lack of erection, ejaculation, and orgasm resulting from interference with numerous nerve fibers and plexuses of sympathetic and parasympathetic nerves

Etiology

The most common cause of serious spinal cord damage in children is congenital defects of the spinal cord. Postnatal causes are primarily accidental injury, especially motor vehicle accidents (including automobile-bicycle and all-terrain vehicle accidents), sports injuries (especially from diving, trampoline activities, and football), and birth trauma.

The majority of the approximately 7000 spinal cord injuries involving aquatic accidents cause permanent paralysis. In fact, diving, surfing, and water skiing accounted for 77% of all spinal injuries in a 10 year study (Morbidity and Mortality Weekly Report, 1982), and those from diving alone exceed the total reported from all other sports. The large majority of diving accidents (60% to 100%) occur outside organized organized sports programs (Bruce, Schut, and Sutton, 1984).

Transverse myelitis (inflammation of the spinal cord) has also been reported to develop from inadvertent intra-arterial administration of long-acting penicillin when injected into the buttocks. Damage can be extensive enough to result in paraplegia or even lower limb amputation (Schanzer and Jacobson, 1985; Stoller and Losey, 1985).

Mechanisms of injury. In automobile accidents most spinal cord injuries in children are the result of indirect trauma caused by sudden hyperflexion or hyperextension of the neck, often combined with a rotational force. Trauma to the spinal cord without evidence of vertebral fracture or dislocation is particularly apt to occur in motor vehicle accidents when proper restraints are not used. An unrestrained child becomes a projectile during sudden deceleration and is subject to injury from contact with a variety of objects inside and outside the automobile.

Falling from heights occurs less often in children than in adults, but vertebral compression of the spine from blows to the head or buttocks occurs in water sports (diving and surfing) or falls from horses or other athletic injuries. Birth injuries may occur in breech delivery from traction force on the cord during delivery of the head and shoulders. A number of teenagers receive cord injuries when they are accidentally shot or stabbed in the back. Infants sustain cervical cord damage (as well as brain and eye damage, mental retardation, and death) when they are shaken. Infants have very weak neck muscles, and during vigorous shaking their heavy heads wobble rapidly back and forth.

Injuries in children tend to occur higher up in the cervical spine than they do in adults, typically levels C3 through C5. Most adult injuries occur below C5 (Dean, 1982). Common sites of injury in children are C1 and C2, C5 and C6, and T12 and L1. Fracture dislocation is the most frequent immediate cause of spinal cord injury, particularly in the lower cervical region, because of the marked mobility of the neck. Spinal cord injury without fracture, although unusual in adults, is not uncommon in the child whose spine is suppler, weaker, and more mobile than that of the adult, so the force is more easily dissipated over a larger number of segments. In children the vertebral column, composed of cartilaginous rings, is capable of considerable elongation, whereas the cord itself, its meninges, and its vascular supply are unable to withstand the same degree of traction.

Pathophysiology

The severity of the force, the mechanisms of the injury, and the degree of the individual's muscular relaxation at the time of the injury greatly influence the extensiveness of the trauma. Compression, contusion, laceration, or anatomic transection are the basic types of cord injuries and usually involve the following four interrelated pathologic changes:

1. Cellular damage to cord tissue
2. Hemorrhage and vascular damage
3. Structural changes of white and gray matter related to vascular disruption, inflammation, and edema
4. Local biochemical response to trauma

These changes are interrelated in that one can lead to the other. For example, an acute injury produces a decreased blood supply to the cord tissue with resulting ischemia that can lead to cellular necrosis. Acid metabolites accumulate during the hypoxic state and can contribute to further cellular damage. A concurrent inflammatory process produces cord edema above and below the traumatized segment, which further decreases the blood supply. Research on spinal cord trauma indicates that the neurotransmitters norepinephrine and dopamine can be markedly altered in the first few hours after injury, which causes further development of hemorrhagic necrosis in the central gray matter.

Clinical Manifestations

As a result of these pathologic responses to the initial trauma, spinal cord injury causes three stages of response; therefore the extent and severity of damage cannot be determined at first. Immediate loss of function is caused by both anatomic and impaired physiologic function, and improved function may not be evident for weeks or even months.

First stage. Manifestations of the initial response to acute injury is flaccid paralysis below the level of the damage. This stage is known as diaschisis or *spinal shock syndrome* and is caused by the sudden disruption of central and autonomic pathways. The local effects of cord edema and ischemia produce a physiologic transection with or without an anatomic severance. The signs and symptoms will depend on the location and severity of the cord damage, but most children with a spinal cord injury experience some spinal shock. These symptoms are:

Absence of reflexes at or below the cord lesion, resulting in flaccidity or limpness of the involved muscles
Loss of sensation and motor function
Autonomic dysfunction with symptoms of hypotension, low or high body temperatures, loss of bladder and bowel control, and autonomic dysreflexia (p. 1830)

These symptoms occur soon after the injury and last 1 to 6 weeks with much autonomic reflex cord function returning in about 3 weeks. The length of this stage is to some degree indicative of the extent of later recovery. In general, the shorter the duration of spinal shock, the more neurologic return can be anticipated. In children with cauda equina injuries at or below level L1, flaccid paralysis persists unless there is subsequent recovery. It may also remain in cases in which there is extensive damage below the level of injury because of severe vascular compromise.

The problems related to this first stage are the serious consequences of prolonged immobility: atrophy of both paralyzed and noninvolved muscles caused by inactivity; negative nitrogen balance resulting from loss of appetite, partially as a result of depression; calcium loss from bone caused by lack of weight bearing with subsequent urinary calculi; urinary retention; risk of decubiti from prolonged pressure; reduced cardiac output and plasma volume; atonic bladder with urinary retention; and respiratory compromise, especially in children with high-level involvement. Autonomic paralysis also affects thermoregulatory functions. Afferent impulses from the skin temperature receptors are not integrated; therefore the patient is subject to alterations in the environmental temperature. Body temperature rises or falls as the ambient temperature changes; thus hyperthermia can result from excessive ambient temperature, such as too many covers.

Second stage. Except in the situations previously mentioned, flaccid paralysis is replaced by spinal reflex activity and increasing spasticity or, in partial lesions, greater or lesser degree of neurologic recovery. At this stage diagnosis may be confused in infants. Spinal reflexes that occur in paralyzed limbs may be misinterpreted as the normal movements in the infant. Even minor stimuli, such as rubbing the mattress, are sufficient to elicit spinal reflexes. Concurrent crying may also lead to the erroneous impression that sensation is intact. Absence of spontaneous leg movement of the extremities when the infant is held vertically suspended under the axilla is highly suggestive of paralysis. Reflex withdrawal or extension of the limb after tactile or pinprick stimulus confirms a diagnosis.

Spasticity leads to different problems than those associated with flaccid paralysis. Spasticity predisposes to contractures, especially of the hip adductor and hip and knee flexor muscles and the heel cords. Frequent contraction of muscles in spastic paralysis plus increased activity and assisted weight bearing reduce the progress of bone demineralization and nitrogen loss. The previously flaccid, atonic bladder now becomes hypertonic, and, instead of continuous dribbling, the urine is expelled involuntarily at intervals by reflex action.

The paralytic nature of autonomic function is replaced by *autonomic dysreflexia,* especially when the lesions are above the midthoracic level. With disturbed central inhibitory control, sensory stimuli may produce a sudden generalized increase in sympathetic activity manifested by flushing of the face, sweating of the forehead, pupillary constriction, marked hypertension, headache, and bradycardia. The precipitating stimulus may be merely a full bladder or rectum or other internal or external sensory input. It can be a catastrophic event; therefore nurses must be alert to this possibility and take immediate action to eliminate the stimulus.

Third stage. In the final stage of response to spinal cord injury the neurologic signs are stabilized regarding loss and recovery of function. The major emphasis is on rehabilitation.

A problem unique to injury in childhood is progressive spinal deformity that is usually not seen in adults or in adolescents near the end of the growth period. Scoliosis develops in a high percentage of children with high thoracic and cervical lesions and is almost certain to occur in the quadriplegic child whose injury occurred in infancy or early childhood. Consequently affected infants and children are placed in a carefully constructed trunk support. Kyphosis usually appears locally at the site of the initial injury, especially when it is resulting from hyperflexion-type injuries. Proper immobilization during vertebral healing helps to prevent progressive deformity. Increasing lordosis occurs with the development of hip contracture caused by spasticity or by prolonged sitting in the nonambulatory child.

Diagnostic Evaluation

A history is a vital part of diagnostic evaluation of all accidental injuries and is the basis of any assessment. The nature of the injury gives valuable clues regarding the possible type of damage incurred and provides direction for proceeding with further assessment without the risk of additional damage.

A complete neurologic examination is performed on any child suspected of having a spinal cord injury to determine if damage was incurred and, if so, the level and extent of any impairment in the central and autonomic nervous systems.

In order for a neurologic unit of the central nervous system to be considered normal, it must be determined that:

1. The reflex arcs are functioning.
2. The sensory tracts are intact when each dermatome is examined separately.
3. The voluntary motor response demonstrates ability to move a body part against gravity on command.

Testing of a reflex arc is done by stimulating the peripheral receptors at a specific site, such as eliciting the patellar reflex. Symmetric testing is performed to ascertain whether the neurologic deficit involves the cord bilaterally or unilaterally. A sufficient number of reflexes are tested to test motor function thoroughly. Sensory tracts are tested with the blunt end of a safety pin to assess pressure sensitivity and with the sharp point to elicit pain. Hot and cold water, a tuning fork, and cotton may also be used to determine specific sensory loss, for example, temperature, vibration, and light touch.

The body surface has delineated zones, or dermatomes, that accurately correspond to the spinal cord segment receiving the sensory input from the peripheral nerves in that zone. Systematically pinpricking the body surface in each

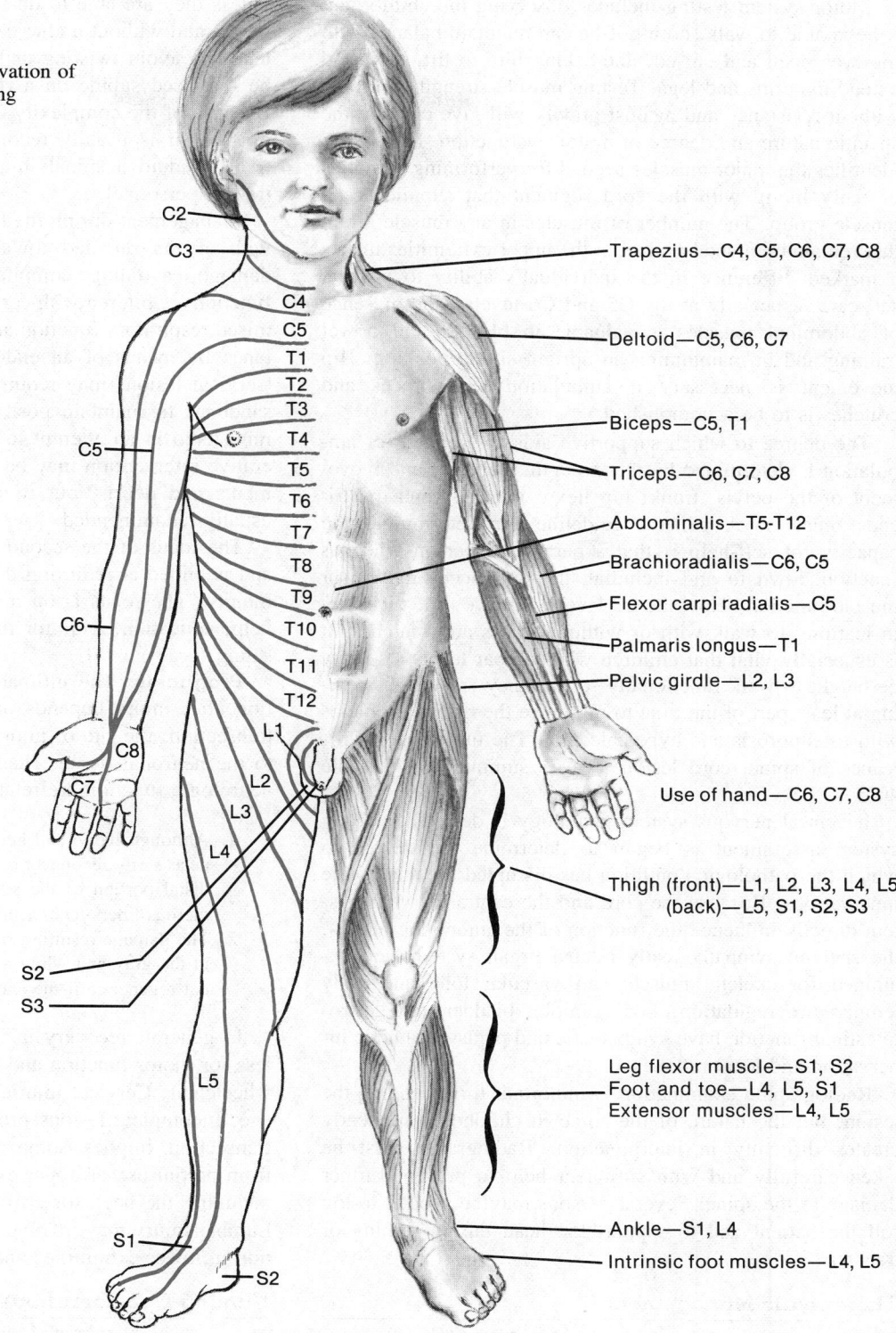

Fig. 40-27. Dermatomes and innervation of major muscles needed for performing activities of daily living.

Trapezius—C4, C5, C6, C7, C8

Deltoid—C5, C6, C7

Biceps—C5, T1

Triceps—C6, C7, C8

Abdominalis—T5-T12

Brachioradialis—C6, C5

Flexor carpi radialis—C5

Palmaris longus—T1

Pelvic girdle—L2, L3

Use of hand—C6, C7, C8

Thigh (front)—L1, L2, L3, L4, L5
(back)—L5, S1, S2, S3

Leg flexor muscle—S1, S2
Foot and toe—L4, L5, S1
Extensor muscles—L4, L5

Ankle—S1, L4

Intrinsic foot muscles—L4, L5

zone can determine if the sensory pathways are intact. Fig. 40-27 shows the zones and the spinal cord segments they represent. The examiner tests for each specific sensory fiber in the dermatome areas in which there is a suspected neurologic deficit. Proprioception, or knowing where one's extremities are, is a very vital sense for ambulating safely.

Matching cord level to vertebra is more difficult in in-

fants and young children than it is in older children and adults because the sacral and several lower lumbar cord segments lie at a lower position, especially during the first 2 years of life (see Fig. 40-25). The spinal anatomy approaches adult configuration by the time the child reaches 7 or 8 years; by late adolescence the conus medullaris has usually reached the level of L1.

Motor system testing includes observing the child's gait if he is able to walk, noting if he can maintain balance with his eyes open and closed, and asking him to lift, flex, and extend his arms and legs. Testing muscle strength with and without resistance and against gravity will give clues to the specific nature and degree of motor dysfunction. Fig. 40-27 identifies the major muscles needed for performing activities of daily living with the cord segment that supplies each muscle group. The number of muscles in any muscle group that remain completely intact in the upper extremities makes a marked difference in the individual's ability to provide self-care, especially at the C5 and C6 levels. The presence of abdominal muscles is valuable in bladder and bowel training and in maintaining an upright sitting position. Hip movement is necessary if ambulation with braces and crutches is to be accomplished.

The degree to which supportive aids are needed for ambulation is determined by the strength, stability, and movement of the pelvis, trunk, hip flexor muscles, and quadriceps muscles. A general guideline for determining the capacity for self-help is that a paraplegic person who has function down to and including the quadriceps muscle or muscle function below the L3 level will have little difficulty in learning to walk with or without braces and crutches. It is especially vital that children with lumbar levels of injury be taught to walk functionally so that they are weight bearing at least part of the time to minimize the risk of problems with osteoporosis and hypercalcemia. The functional significance of spinal cord lesion level is summarized in Table 40-3.

If central nervous system pathology is detected, a body system assessment is begun to determine the degree to which the pathologic condition has disrupted the autonomic innervations. Because the cord and the central nervous system directly influence the function of the autonomic nerves, the specific sympathetically related organ systems are examined for skeletal muscle and vascular tone and body temperature regulation. For example, bladder and gastrointestinal function have sympathetic and parasympathetic innervation and local reflexes.

Radiographic examination is important for localizing the lesion, but the nature of the spine in childhood frequently creates difficulty in interpretation. Radiograms must be taken carefully and with sufficient help to prevent further damage to the spine. Several persons may be needed to log roll the patient and to support the head during turning or transfer.

Therapeutic Management

The management of the child with spinal cord injury is complex and controversial. Initial care begins at the scene of the accident; therefore education and training of rescue personnel in stabilization and transfer techniques to prevent or reduce the severity of injury are of utmost importance. In any situation in which spinal cord injury is suspected or a possibility, the child should be calmed, reassured, and advised not to move, and no one should be allowed to move him unless they are able to do so carefully. He should be lifted gently and without undue haste (preferably by a coordinated team) to avoid twisting or bending the spine. If conscious, he is placed supine on a rigid surface to prevent sagging. Because of the complexity and relative infrequency of these injuries, it is usually recommended that these persons be transferred to a spinal injury center for care by specially trained personnel.

Management during the first stage is primarily supportive with efforts directed toward preventing further neuronal damage, avoiding complications, and maintaining vital functions. Children with cervical lesions often have compromised respiratory function and may require ventilatory assistance by means of an endotracheal tube or tracheostomy. Cervical lesions may require halter or skeletal traction and sandbags to maintain position, and corticosteroids are administered in an attempt to prevent destructive edema. Operative intervention may be necessary to remove bone fragments and debris, but routine surgical exploration is not usually recommended.

The focus of the second phase is primarily rehabilitative and is aimed at returning the patient to the home and community. The focus is on maximizing the potential for self-help, education, and, for the older child, vocational counseling.

Prognosis. The ultimate outlook for spinal cord function after injury depends on the completeness of the cord transection, the site of injury, and the complicating damage to the neuronal tissue. Healing of the injury and return of neurologic function are related to two factors:

1. Although individual nerve fibers do regenerate, they do not necessarily reconnect or make synaptic connections with the distal portion of the severed fibers, and the chance of numerous fibers reconnecting is highly unlikely.
2. The damage resulting from cord ischemia produces necrosis in the gray and white matter of the cord tissue, which does not regenerate if the axon cylinder is not intact.

In general, recovery in thoracic lesions is usually hopeless for motor function and victims are relegated to life in a wheelchair. Cervical injuries are variable in extent of damage. Incomplete lesions produce hemiplegia, and complete transection implies some involvement of all extremities from partial use of upper extremities to complete paralysis, including the need for artificial maintenance of respiration. Lumbar injury may involve partial or complete loss of function in lower extremities and bladder.

Nursing Considerations

The nursing care of the paraplegic or quadriplegic child is complex and challenging. As a member of the acute care and the rehabilitation teams, the nurse is involved in all aspects of care. Ideally, initial care takes place in a special intensive care unit with personnel trained to handle spinal cord injuries, and nursing management is concerned primarily with prevention of complications and maintenance of functions.

Once the acute period is over, the lesion is usually static and nonprogressive, regardless of whether the paralysis is secondary to trauma, congenital defects, infection, treated tumor, or surgery. In treatment of children with spinal cord injuries, the nurse is a member of a team of specialists including physicians from a number of speciality areas, physical and occupational therapists, psychologists, social workers, teachers, and vocational counselors. Each team member has a unique contribution to make, and mutual agreement for specific areas of responsibility is determined during regularly scheduled team conferences. Periodic evaluation of the team's progress is discussed in subsequent conferences.

Although care of the child with a spinal cord injury is, in most aspects, the same as that of any immobilized child, there are some important differences.

Respiratory care. The child with a high-level injury (quadriplegia) will require continuous respiratory assistance. In most instances a tracheostomy is the method of choice for greater ease in clearing secretions and for less trauma to tissues for long-term respirator dependence. Respiratory therapy personnel are responsible for establishing and maintaining the equipment, but the nurse must understand how it works and recognize deviations from the prescribed rate and volume and mechanical malfunction. In case of malfunction the nurse must be prepared for maintaining respirations manually with a ventilation bag. In some youngsters breathing pacemaker devices (phrenic nerve stimulators) are implanted to stimulate the phrenic nerve and produce diaphragmatic contractions and lung expansion without a ventilator. If the child has a pacemaker, part of the nursing function is understanding its function and operation.

Children with lesions below the C4 level are seldom dependent on respirators, but their vital capacity is significantly reduced. They should be positioned for optimum chest expansion, and a variety of breathing exercises and assistive devices are employed to stimulate deep breathing. Intermittent positive-pressure breathing by machine may be needed, and vital capacity and blood gases are monitored periodically. Percussion and vibration, with suction as necessary, are performed several times daily, and nebulized oxygen may be needed occasionally. Regular routine monitoring of breath sounds to assess for adequate ventilation in all lobes is part of routine care.

The cough reflex is markedly diminished and, together with weak intercostal muscles, the youngster may have difficulty with secretions. Increasing the elastic qualities of the lung by exercise will help to achieve a productive cough.

Temperature regulation. Vital signs and other general assessments are carried out periodically, with particular attention to alterations that might indicate adverse autonomic responses. Temperature regulation usually creates few problems, although environmental conditions can influence body temperature. During the spinal shock stage the dilated capillaries conducting body heat to the subcutaneous tissues cause heat loss to the environment. In hot weather, without the capacity to sweat, the body retains heat. Consequently clothing and blankets are added or removed ac-cording to the body temperature. An elevated temperature that cannot be corrected by environmental measures should be evaluated for urinary tract or upper respiratory infection. However, excessive perspiration observed in sentient areas usually indicates an elevated ambient temperature.

Skin care. In cases in which spinal cord injury is associated with vertebral fracture, cervical traction with Crutchfield tongs is maintained for several weeks until there is sufficient evidence of bone healing. Initially the child is turned every 2 hours around the clock by specially trained personnel. An alternating pressure mattress, egg carton mattress, or sheepskin is kept underneath the child, and the skin is thoroughly inspected at least once a day for signs of pressure, especially over bony prominences. Prevention of decubiti is much easier than treatment. A number of factors contribute to the risk of skin breakdown in these children: decreased sensation, poor nutrition from negative nitrogen balance, low hemoglobin level, spasticity, and improper positioning.

The areas most apt to be affected are the sacrum, scapulae, heels, and occiput when the child is in a supine position; the trochanters and the lateral aspect of the ankles, heels, and knees when in a side-lying position; and the ischial tuberosities when in a sitting position. The common type of pressure lesion begins in deeper tissues and is only visible on the surface at a later stage; therefore areas that feel firm, irregular, warm, or appear to be only slightly reddened require careful evaluation. Keeping the skin clean and dry is particularly important in these children, especially those who are incontinent. Treatment of pressure areas or decubiti is instituted early, according to the protocol of the institution.

Physical therapy. Physical therapy is a vital part of nursing care. Maintaining good body alignment, preventing pressure from bed linen, providing proper support, and applying splints as ordered and padded booties to hold the feet in correct position are important in daily care. Range of motion, passive, and active exercises are carried out under the guidance of a physical therapist. In children with upper motor neuron involvement, the spasticity that develops may require administration of an antispasmodic, usually diazepam. Decreasing stimuli to the muscles also helps reduce spasticity. For example, tight clothing and bed linen should be avoided, and extremities should be handled by the joints rather than by the belly of the muscle. Anticipating the possibility of spasms when the child is moved and providing the necessary safety precautions prevent possible injury during transport.

During the period of immobilization, unless there are contraindications, exercises are aimed at maintaining and increasing strength of the child's intact musculature. Upper extremity strengthening is especially important to the paraplegic child who must rely on these muscle groups for turning, transferring, dressing, crutch walking, and other activities. Children are usually eager to use their muscles and respond to interesting and innovative activities.

Neurogenic bladder. When the bladder is denervated,

as in the acute stage of spinal shock syndrome or after lower motor neuron damage, the bladder wall is flaccid. The danger in this type of neurogenic bladder is overextension. This lack of tone causes a deficiency in the ability of the bladder to respond to changes in passive pressure. That is, if the bladder is filled, emptied, and filled again, the pressure observed the second time will be less than the pressure noted after the first filling. Therefore it is important to prevent overdistention by periodic emptying, even though there may be dribbling between emptying. In contrast, the upper motor neuron lesion causes an increase in tone and bladder contractions that often includes the urinary sphincter. Thus even though the bladder empties periodically by reflex action, complete emptying is prevented, resulting in urinary retention and ureteral reflux. Administration of antispasmodics such as dicyclomine (Bentyl) relaxes bladder musculature and promotes increased bladder capacity and more adequate emptying.

The intervals of urination depend on many factors, including patterns of fluid intake and perspiration. Most children require some type of external collecting device. This is relatively simple in males, but no satisfactory device is available for females, who usually must rely on diapers and incontinent pants. As early as possible attempts are made to keep the child relatively dry by regulating fluid intake and output and periodically emptying the bladder by manual expression by applying downward pressure on the bladder (Credé maneuver), intermittent catheterization, or both. External pressure on the bladder is a relatively safe procedure in females. Pressure will be released via the urethra with the possibility of some reflux. However, males have a peculiar muscle arrangement around the urethra at the base of the bladder that causes a reflex contraction on stimulation and poses the danger of a ruptured bladder or significant ureteral reflux. The older paraplegic child can be taught to express urine manually and to perform self-catheterization.* Bladder-training programs usually begin with intermittent bladder emptying at regular intervals, which are gradually increased. Periodic urine cultures and, in manual emptying, periodic catheterization for residual volume are performed until the child achieves regular, complete emptying.

The urine is kept acidic to decrease the likelihood of stone formation and to inhibit bacterial growth. Ascorbic acid, 1 to 4 g daily, is most effective. The traditional cranberry juice may also be advised. Oral antimicrobials are frequently administered prophylactically. Maintenance of bladder dynamics and control of urinary tract infections are of utmost importance. Pyelonephritis and renal failure are the most significant causes of death in long-standing paraplegia.

Bowel training. Successful bowel training is easier to institute than bladder management. The aim is to control defecation until an appropriate time and place are found. A diet with sufficient roughage for adequate stool bulk and

insertion of a glycerin or bisacodyl (Dulcolax) suppository at a convenient time, either morning or evening, are often all that are necessary to induce a bowel movement within a short time. The probability of an accident between times is diminished once the bowel is completely evacuated. Stool softeners, such as dioctyl sodium sulfonsuccinate (Colace), are usually prescribed, and manual anal stimulation may help initiate evacuation, especially in spastic paraplegia. Sometimes an oral laxative such as bisacodyl may be necessary. Once an appropriate regimen is established, little modification is required.

Autonomic dysreflexia. Children with high-level lesions are very susceptible to the development of autonomic dysreflexia, which requires prompt action to prevent encephalopathy and shock. As soon as a quick assessment has ruled out other causes, such as orthostatic hypertension, someone should take the blood pressure while the bladder is checked for distention (the usual precipitating cause). The bladder is drained slowly, and if symptoms are not relieved, any tight clothing is loosened and the bowel is checked for the pressure of impacted feces. If removal of the causative agent is unsuccessful in controlling the syndrome, intravenous administration of an antihypertensive drug is indicated followed by oral maintenance doses. Antispasmodics may also be administered.

The specific neurogenic problems related to spinal cord lesions are listed in Table 40-4 with the associated nursing interventions.

Remobilization. As soon as his condition warrants, the child is moved from a reclining to an erect position. Cardiovascular deconditioning and impaired autonomic responses below the level of injury will cause pooling of blood in the extremities because of peripheral vasodilation, a drop in blood pressure, and a feeling of light-headedness, dizziness, or fainting on sudden assumption of an upright posture. Therefore an upright position must be accomplished gradually by first placing the child on a tilt table and securing him by passive restraint, after which the table is slowly elevated from a horizontal to a 30-degree semireclining position (Fig. 40-28). This is performed twice daily for 20 to 30 minutes, gradually increasing the angle until the vertical angle is reached.

During the procedure vital signs are monitored and behavior is observed for subjective symptoms of syncope. Elastic hose or wrapping the lower extremities with elastic bandage from instep to groin and applying an abdominal binder reduce the pooling of blood. The process of achieving upright posture may require several weeks. After tolerance is achieved, the child will be ready to begin to use a wheelchair. Each time the child gets up this should be accomplished slowly by gradually elevating the bed over 20 to 30 minutes before placing him in the wheelchair, then gradually lowering the legs after he has been in the chair a short time.

All adaptive devices help children increase their mobility, function, and endurance. The paraplegic child with

---

*Home care instructions for self-catheterization can be found in Wong, D.L., and Whaley, L.F.: Clinical handbook of pediatric nursing, ed. 2, St. Louis, 1986, The C.V. Mosby Co.

Table 40-4 Specific neurogenic problems related to spinal cord lesions with associated interventions

PROBLEM	STRUCTURAL INNERVATIONS	SPECIFIC PROBLEM	INTERVENTION
Neurogenic bowel	Parasympathetic (mostly vagal)—increases smooth muscle mobility, tone, and secretions Sympathetic—decreases gastrointestinal motility Voluntary central nervous system control—control of external sphincter and timing of defecation	Atony of gastric and upper intestinal segment—paralytic ileus Development of stress ulcer from excessive vagal stimulation Fecal incontinence or constipation	Nothing given by mouth; decompression with nasogastric tube Antacids; diet control Bowel training program with diet regulation, suppositories, mild laxative, stool softeners, manual evacuation
Neurogenic bladder	Parasympathetic—contraction of bladder wall to facilitate emptying of bladder, relaxing of sphincter muscle Sympathetic—maintains internal sphincter tone and relaxes wall of bladder	Lower motor neuron damage or spinal shock—urinary retention with overflow incontinence Upper motor neuron damage after shock—bladder spasms, external sphincter paralysis, internal sphincter spasm	Evaluation of kidney function Use of Foley catheter if necessary Intermittent catheterization program Administration of antispasmodic dicyclomine (Bentyl)
Autonomic dysreflexia	Visceral distention or irritation, particularly bowel or bladder, triggers sensory impulses, which travel to cord lesion and are blocked to activate excessive sympathetic reflex reaction; not controlled by higher centers Usually occurs in persons with a lesion at T4 level or above	Hypertension (basoconstriction below lesion) Occipital pounding headache Flushed face (vasodilatation above lesion) Tachycardia, bradycardia Sweating below lesion levels Can lead to cerebrovascular accident or epilepsy	Bowel or bladder emptied gently Topical anesthetic (tetracaine [Pontocaine]) instilled in bladder or rectum to reduce irritability (prophylactic) Parasympatholytic drugs (methantheline [Banthine]) given, as well as drugs to lower blood pressure and prevent seizures
Orthostatic hypotension	Sympathetic—stimulates vascular tone to maintain blood pressure	Pooling of blood in dependent areas Syncope when head elevated or body in upright position	Ambulating activities performed *slowly* Sitting tolerance time recorded and gradually increased Antistasis support with elastic stocking or Ace bandage wraps Head lowered if orthostatic episode occurs
Thermoregulation	Hypothalamic and autonomic regulation to control peripheral sweating and evaporative heat loss	Faulty adaptation to changes in environmental temperatures	Frequent monitoring of body temperature Environmental temperature adjusted by raising or lowering, especially cooling ambient temperature Clothing suitable for environment High temperatures lowered slowly with cool sponges
Sexual dysfunction	Nerves at S2 to S4 levels innervate sensory and motor components of genitalia	Inability to feel sexual stimuli Inability to have and maintain an erection and/or ejaculation, particularly in lower motor neuron damage	Touch approach Alternative methods for sexual gratification Referral to qualified sex therapist for long-term sexual adjustment

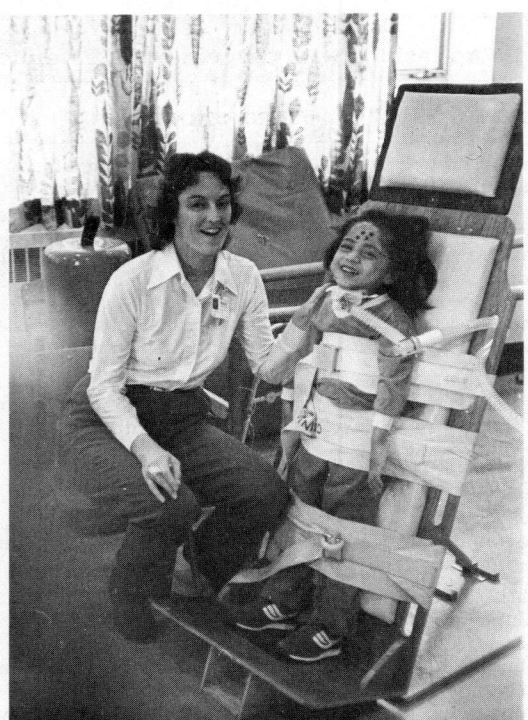

Fig. 40-28. Child on tilt table with physical therapist.

some lower extremity function progresses to parallel bars and then to a walker; the quadriplegic child learns to use a wheelchair. The wheelchair is among the most valuable aids available to the child with a spinal cord injury, and its selection should be made carefully in relation to where it will be used, architectural barriers, and the functional capacity of the child. For lower extremity paralysis the wheelchair described earlier is applicable. For children with severe upper extremity paralysis, a variety of motorized wheelchairs are used, but the more complex they are, the greater their cost, weight, and tendency to break down (see Fig. 40-4). Wheelchair tolerance is gained over a period of time accompanied by measures to prevent orthostatic hypotension and pressure sores.

A variety of braces and other appliances can be adapted for use by many children with spinal cord injuries. The primary purpose of lower extremity bracing in the child with a spinal cord injury is for ambulation, although correction of deformities may be attempted. However, the efficacy is limited because of the tendency to develop pressure lesions over insensate areas. The higher the lesion, the more support required, with the accompanying difficulties of getting into the brace and the greater energy expended in using the appliance. The energy required in ambulating with crutches and braces is two to four times greater than that required for normal walking.

Children with their natural and overwhelming propensity for mobility usually attain, or may even surpass, the maximum expectation in ambulation. However, as they approach

adulthood, the increasing weight and energy cost usually cause them to resort to predominant use of the wheelchair for mobility and the pursuit of more intellectual and vocational interests. Wheelchair mobility has the advantage in that it requires no more energy than normal walking and allows the paraplegic person to maintain the speed of other pedestrians on level ground.

Physical Rehabilitation

Physical rehabilitation has been briefly described in the foregoing segments, and the major aims are to prepare the child and family to resume life at home and in the community. Members of the rehabilitation team work collaboratively to identify the child's problems and to plan realistic interventions. This is one of the more complex health teams, and the integration of activities is coordinated by one team member, most often the physician who is a specialist in physical medicine and rehabilitation. Through mutual trust, good communication, professional respect, and sincere interest in the child and the family, members of the team attempt to achieve their collaborative goals. Training in the rehabilitation center involves achieving the maximum expected accomplishments commensurate with the physical capacities. Instruction for home routine is stressed and includes all the precautions and management implemented in the hospital, that is, skin care, nutrition, bladder and bowel training, and an exercise program.

The overall goals of rehabilitation of the child with an acquired spinal injury and habilitation of the child with a congenital defect are:

Maximizing function and minimizing the disabling effects of the pathology
Assisting the child and family in setting realistic goals for the child, learning to be good problem solvers, and using the assets he has
Helping the child to cope with the stigma of being different and to build a valued self-concept

Physical rehabilitation of the quadriplegic child takes approximately 6 months; a paraplegic child can achieve these goals in 1 to 3 months, but he requires constant vigilance to avoid complications. Emotional adjustments take longer, especially in the older child and adolescent. In most children the outlook is favorable unless life-threatening consequences of urinary pathology are severe or emotional adjustment is poor.

A restorative program is begun as soon as possible after injury. Frequent changes in body position while in bed are essential, using positioning aids such as splints and pillows to support body parts after turning. One of the primary goals is to use interventions for regaining function and remobilization within the limitations of the therapeutic regimen and the child's physical disabilities. An overhead trapeze bar and side rails aid a larger child with upper extremity use to move about in bed. Exercises to develop his ability to bend the elbow and raise the lower arm may need additional therapies to enable him to perform self-feeding or self-dressing. The child is encouraged to become involved in activities appropriate to his developmental level and physical capabilities.

Exercise therapy is the focal point of all restorative interventions. It is important to maintain the movement, tone, and strength in uninvolved joints and muscles and to exercise affected musculoskeletal structures as soon as possible. There are many types of exercises with various purposes, and the guiding principle is that the child should perform the type of exercise that will accomplish the major goal of active movement against resistance. Exercise programs must be scheduled at least two times each day with approximately 10 repetitive movements during each exercise. A complete exercise program takes time, since each major joint and muscle group requires several movements to accomplish full range of motion and strengthening.

The child will be more enthusiastic if toys and play strategies can be incorporated into the therapy. Exercises can be a part of other nursing care such as hygienic procedures and dressing. To perform an activity of daily living such as bathing, feeding, or dressing, the child may require an adaptive device to compensate for functional loss. Velcro straps replace zippers and buttons, a spoon handle is enlarged when the grip is poor, or a hand splint is provided with a strap to hold the utensil. Environmental adaptations include ramps, lowered furniture, or special hydraulic lifts for transferring larger children. Most adaptive aids do not encourage muscle strengthening but assist the child in the functional use of whatever movement remains.

Psychosocial Rehabilitation

Early acquired or congenital disability is usually more readily accepted by the child than paralysis that appears later in childhood. Rehabilitation includes not only the child's emotional responses but also those of the persons who maintain the closest contacts with the child. It involves intensive education so that members of the family understand the nature of the disability, the therapeutic regimen, and complications so that they are able to provide the physical and emotional support needed by the child. As with any disability, the child should be treated as normally as possible and encouraged in developmental tasks at the age at which he would normally be expected to acquire abilities and perform activities. However, goals must be realistic, and the child should not be forced beyond his capabilities. The child's and the family's routines and the parents' childrearing practices will be significantly altered.

As he becomes aware of the impact of the disability and its implications, the youngster may become self-effacing and begin to think of himself as very different, ugly, undesirable to others, less than human, or a useless cripple. When his appearance and physical capacity have changed markedly, the responses of peers, family, professionals, and even strangers who come in contact with him influence his perception of himself and can significantly alter his self-con-

cept. Any loss related to his preinjury state is a severe threat to the development of a positive identity. All disabled youngsters grieve their losses, and the way in which they are able to weather the crisis and adjust to their new physical state depends on the way in which they deal with adversity and the help they receive from others. Satisfactory adjustment is not necessarily related to the extent of the disability. Sometimes children with marked impairment make a better adjustment than those with only minimum disability. All must go through the process of grieving this loss. The typical sequence in the grief process is:

1. Preshock or unawareness of what has happened or is happening to him—his perception of reality is fuzzy, his responses may be "automatic" or inappropriate, and he seems somewhat detached.
2. Shock and disbelief—experienced as he becomes more aware of his losses and feels the threat to his being. Panic and anxiety are common feelings coupled with thoughts such as "It didn't really happen."
3. Some form of denial—often resorted to when normal coping mechanisms are inadequate to handle the situation. Attitudes associated with denial include "I'm not really unable to move," or "I'll be okay in a short time." The denial may include withdrawal behaviors such as sleeping a great deal or by focusing on less threatening concerns such as toys or food.
4. Confrontations of the reality of the situation—have an impact on the child, and he begins to acknowledge what is occurring. This usually provokes anger and depression.

Severe depression can be emotionally and intellectually immobilizing, but it indicates that the child is no longer hiding behind denial. It is desirable in a child's rehabilitation for him to begin to express his negative feelings toward the situation, since these feelings, redirected by efforts of the rehabilitation team, are the ones that will motivate him toward learning a new way of life.

The multiple problems related to altered self-image, especially in the older child and adolescent, have been discussed in relation to the disabled child (Chapter 22). The severely disabled child may need to alter some concepts about self and social roles. If he describes an adult as someone with complete control over his body and the ability to do what he wants when he wants to, he will need to develop a more realistic definition of interdependent adult living. The needs of the permanently disabled youngster must be reevaluated periodically by the total rehabilitation team, including the youngster and his family. As a young adult the disabled teenager may not be financially independent, which alters his choice of occupation or profession. Vocational rehabilitation involves not only helping the permanently disabled teenager find meaningful work activities but also to assist him in enrolling in formal educational programs.

Sexuality

The problems of self-concept are particularly marked when the child with a spinal cord injury reaches puberty and are likely to be even more intense if the disability occurs during adolescence. Sexual development and awareness and changing perceptions of body image are prominent aspects of adolescence, and a loss in these areas is a severe blow to the youngster. Development of secondary sex characteristics does not seem to be altered by spinal cord injury, and it is now believed that, with comprehensive rehabilitation, well-motivated young people can look forward to successful participation in marital and family activities.

In females, if the injury occurs after the onset of menstruation, there is usually a temporary cessation and irregularity of menstrual flow, but in the majority of menstruation usually resumes. Ovulation and conception are possible, but females will not experience vulval or clitoral orgasms, although they can learn to use other errogenous zones for a sexual experience. This is important to emphasize in sex education, because many females have the misconception that because they lack sensation, they are unable to conceive. Also, the pregnant paraplegic or quadriplegic may be unaware that she is in labor, and those with a high-level injury are subject to autonomic hyperreflexia during labor.

As soon as the adolescent male becomes aware of his functional loss, he will be concerned about his sexual capacities regardless of the type of sexual experiences he had before the spinal cord injury. The physician and/or psychologist will provide him with information about what he can expect regarding erection, ejaculation, and other sexual experiences. The health professional should take the initiative in discussing sexuality with the child and his family. Parents of younger children will want to know about their child's sexual and reproductive potential. As his interest and understanding increase, the child needs to know the specifics of physiology, prognosis, and sexual techniques related to his particular problems.

A male with an upper motor neuron lesion may be capable of reflex erections and, with penile stimulation, may maintain erection for a time. However, ejaculation is possible only with intact innervation at S2, S3, and S4 levels, which is seldom present. Erection is usually absent in lower motor neuron dysfunction. Only a small percentage of males with complete lesions have children because of loss of ejaculation and decreased incidence of successful intercourse.

Erection can be achieved psychogenically or reflexogenically. Psychogenic stimulation can be visual, olfactory, somatesthetic, and/or auditory with subsequent integration of the sensory input and autonomic nerve response. An individual must have a functional cervicothoracolumbar cord to have a psychogenic erection. Reflexogenic erections occur when the lower motor neuron reflexes in the sacral region are intact and local skin or penal stimulation produces an erection. In general, the male with an incomplete upper motor neuron injury will be very successful in having psychogenic and reflexogenic erections and coitus. Those with complete upper motor neuron injuries are usually able to have reflexogenic erections; males with complete lower motor neuron injuries or damage are least likely to have erections and coitus.

A knowledgeable rehabilitation team will be valuable to the child as he experiences loss as a sexual being. This is especially true of the paraplegic or quadriplegic teenager. Most sexual counseling for the adolescent with a spinal cord injury focuses on developing the idea that sex means different things to individuals, and the youngster is encouraged to discuss his ideas. Most rehabilitation teams have an active program in sexual counseling to help the child learn intimacy and how to function sexually within his limitations. Through individual and group counseling he gains new attitudes concerning his sexuality. Knowledge that sexual gratification comes from giving and sharing assists him to look at alternative ways to achieve sexual gratification for himself and his partner. For example, he learns the value of masturbation as a means to determine if he can have and sustain an erection. As he adjusts to trials and successes, he develops his own ways of achieving sexual experiences exclusive or inclusive of intercourse.

While in the hospital the teenage youngster may display aggressive sexual behavior toward the nurses. Flirtatious behavior is a way of checking out with others his or her acceptance as a sexual being. This behavior can be handled easily by setting behavioral limits. Approaches that help nurses cope with the youngster with the prospect of altered sexual roles include:

1. Exploring their own attitudes toward sex and being aware of their abilities and limitations in relating with the youngster on this topic.
2. Use of resource people to answer questions that they are unable to answer or feel uncomfortable in handling.
3. Respecting another's attitudes and sexual behaviors, unless they are self-destructive, and trying to be nonjudgmental while maintaining their own attitudes and beliefs.
4. Reinforcing that sexual roles are learned and that there is more to sex than functioning in a ''prescribed'' physical manner.

Summary

The outlook for children with spinal cord injury is favorable for integration into society. Increased awareness of the needs of persons with disabilities has removed many structural and occupational barriers. The success of a rehabilitation program is not judged by how well the child manages within the rehabilitation setting but by how well he functions on the outside. In addition to agencies that offer assistance to children with disabilities in general, some agencies provide specific assistance to paralyzed persons, including children. Some of these are the **National Spinal Cord Injury Association,** * the **Spinal Cord Society,** † the **National Wheelchair Athletic Associastion,** ‡ and the **National Handicapped Sports and Recreation Association.** § Other sources of information and assistance are listed in Appendix E.

---

*149 California St., Newton, MA 02158.
†2410 Lakeview Dr., Fergus Falls, ME 56537.
‡2107 Templeton Gap Rd., Colorado Springs, CO 80907.
§P.O. Box 33141, Farragut Station, Washington, DC 20033.

CONCEPT SUMMARIES

- Immobility has a profound effect on all elements of growth and development.

- The major consequences of immobilization are loss of muscle strength, endurance, and muscle mass; bone demineralization leading to osteoporosis; loss of joint mobility; and contractures.

- In the care of the immobilized child, nurses are concerned with position changes, adequate dietary intake, adequate hydration, promotion of activity, and involvement of child in self-care.

- Trauma is the leading cause of death in children and is caused by accidental injury, child abuse injury, and birth injuries.

- Dislocation in children commonly involves the patella and radial head.

- Features of children's fractures not observed in the adult include presence of growth plate, thicker and stronger periosteum, porosity of bone, more rapid healing, and less stiffness.

- Types of fractures seen in children are bends, buckle, greenstick, and complete.

- Goals of fracture management in children are to regain alignment and length of the bony fragments, retain alignment and length, and restore function to injured parts.

- The method of fracture reduction is determined by the age of the child, degree of displacement, amount of overriding, amount of edema, condition of skin and soft tissues, sensation, and circulation distal to fracture.

- The primary purposes of traction are to fatigue involved muscle and reduce muscle spasm, to position bone ends in desired realignment, and to immobilize fracture site until realignment has been achieved to permit casting or splinting.

- Complications of fractures are circulatory impairment, nerve compression syndromes, compartmental syndromes, epiphyseal damage, nonunion, malunion, infection, kidney stones, and pulmonary emboli.

- Spinal cord injuries usually involve the following four interrelated pathologic changes: cellular damage to cord tissue, hemorrhage and vascular damage, structural changes of white and gray matter related to vascular disruption, inflammation and edema, and local biochemical response to trauma.

- Therapeutic management of spinal cord injury is directed toward preventing further neuronal damage, avoiding complications, and maintaining vital functions.

- Goals of rehabilitation in spinal cord injury are to maximize function, assist the child and family in realistic goal setting, and help child cope with stigma and build his self-concept.

REFERENCES

Bruce, D.A., Schut, L., and Sutton, L.N.: Brasin and cervical spine injuries occurring during organized sports activities in children and adolescents, Primary Care **11**:175-194, 1984.

Dean, D.F.: The child with possible spinal cord injury, Emerg. Med. **14**:122-127, 1982.

Perspectives in disease prevention and health promotion, Morbid. Mortal. Weekly Rep. **31**:417-419, 1982.

Ramenofsky, M.L., and Morse, T.S.: Standards of care for the critically injured pediatric patient, J. Trauma **22**:921-933, 1983.

Schanzer, H., and Jacobson, J.H.: Tissue damage caused by the intramuscular injection of long-acting penicillin, Pediatrics **75**:741-744, 1985.

Sibinga, M.S., and Freedman, C.J.: Restraint and speech, Pediatrics **48**:116-122, 1971.

Stoller, K.P., and Losey, R.: Inadvertent intra-arterial injection of penicillin: an unseen danger, Pediatrics **75**:785-786, 1985.

BIBLIOGRAPHY

General

Asher, R.A.J.: The dangers of going to bed, Crit. Care Update **6**(9):4-49, 1983.

Drehobl, P.: Quadriceps contracture, Am. J. Nurs. **80**:1650-1651, 1980.

Feins, N.R.: Multiple trauma, Pediatr. Clin. North Am. **26**:759-772, 1979.

Hilt, N.E., and Cogburn, S.B.: Manual of orthopedics, St. Louis, 1980, The C.V. Mosby Co.

Lentz, M.: Selected aspects of deconditioning secondary to immobilization, Nurs. Clin. North Am. **16**:729-737, 1981.

Love-Mignogna, S.: Taping and splinting: seven common problems and how to solve them, Nursing 80 **10**(4):88-92, 1980.

Quan, L., and Marcuse, E.K.: The epidemiology and treatment of radial head sublaxation, Am. J. Dis. Child. **139**:1194-1197, 1985.

Sigmon, H.D.: Helping your long-term trauma patient travel the road to recovery, Nursing 84 **14**(1):58-63, 1984.

Turner, M.C., and others: Blood pressure elevation in children with orthopedic immobilization, J. Pediatr. **95**:989-992, 1979.

Trauma

Campbell, P.M.: Transportation of the critially ill and injured child, Crit. Care Q. **8**(1):1-12, 1985.

Crawford, A.H., and Cionni, A.S.: Management of pediatric orthopedic injuries by the emergency medicine specialist. In Pierog, J.E., and Pierog, L.J., editors: Pediatric critical illness and injury, Rockville, MD, 1984, Aspen Systems Corp.

Haller, J.A., and others: Organization and function of a regional pediatric trama center: does a system of management improve outcome? J. Trauma **23**:691-696, 1983.

Harris, B.H.: Management of multiple trauma, Pediatr. Clin. North Am. **32**:175-181, 1985.

King, D.R.: Trauma in infancy and childhood: initial evaluation and management, Pediatr. Clin. North Am. **32**:1299-1310, 1985.

King, R.C.: Dealing with abrasions and lacerations, RN **47**(6):53-56, 1984.

Ludwig, S., and Fleisher, G.: Textbook of pediatric emergency medicine, Baltimore, MD, 1983, Williams & Wilkins.

Lyon, S.H.: Critical care of the child with multi-trauma, Nurs. Clin. North Am. **16**:657-670, 1981.

Morse, T.S.: The child with multiple injuries, Emerg. Med. Clin. North Am. **1**:175-185, 1983.

Pashley, J., and Wahlstrom, M.L.: Polytrauma: the patient, the family, the nurse, and the health team, Nurs. Clin. North Am. **16**:721-727, 1981.

Ragiel, C.A.: The impact of critical injury on patient, family, and clinical systems, Crit. Care Q. **7**(3):73-78, 1984.

Stevens, W.S., Rodgers, B.M., and Newman, B.M.: Pediatric trauma associated with all-terrain vehicles, J. Pediatr. **109**:25-29, 1986.

Thomas, D.O.: The ABCs of pediatric emergencies, RN **47**(3):34-41, 1984.

Veise-Berry, S.W.: Nursing considerations during radiologic examination of the massively injured trauma patient, Crit. Care Q. **6**(1):55-63, 1983.

Fractures

Bailey, M.: Emergency! First aid for fractures, Nursing 82 **12**(11):72-81, 1982.

Cassels, C.J.: Fundamentals of long bone traction, Part I, Crit. Care Update **10**(3):36-39, 1983.

Cassels, C.J.: Fundamentals of long bone traction, Part II, Crit. Care Update **10**(4):26-31, 1983.

Cassels, C.J.: Fundamentals of long bone traction, Part III, Crit. Care Update **10**(5):38-39, 1983.

Evers, J.A., and Werpachowski, D.: Dealing with fractures, RN **47**(11):53-57, 1984.

Hamdan, J.A., Taleb, Y.A., and Ahmed, M.S.: Traction induced hypertension in chidlren, Clin. Orthop. **185**:87-89, 1984.

Howard, M., and Corbo-Pelaia, S.A.: Psychological after effects of halo traction . . . a review of acute care, Am. J. Nurs. **82**:1839-1843, 1982.

Ibrahim, K.: An overview of childhood fractures, Pediatr. Nurs. **10**:57-65, 1984.

Lane, P.L, and Lee, M.M.: New synthetic casts: what nurses need to know, Orthop. Nurs. **1**(6):13-20, 1982.

Lane, P.L., and Lee, M.M.: Synthetic materials have changed casts and cast care, Nursing 83 **13**(7):50-51, 1983.

Linshaw, M.A., and others: Traction-related hypertension in children, J. Pediatr. **95**:994-996, 1979.

Robinson, J.E., and Marx, L.O.: A nail-safe method, Am. J. Nurs. **85**:158-161, 1985.

Stout, J.A., and Gibbs, K.R.: The child undergoing a leg-lengthening procedure, Am. J. Nurs. **81**:1152-1155, 1981.

Swanson, V.M.: The school-age traction patient: toward better behavior patterns, J. Assoc. Care Child. Health **9**(1):12-14, 1980.

Wise, L.B.: A comparison of orthopedic casts: breaking the mold, J. Maternal Child Nurs. **11**:174-176, 1986.

Spinal Cord Injuries

Andberg, M.M., Rudolph, A., and Anderson, T.P.: Improving skin care through patient and family training, Top. Clin. Nurs. **5**(2):45-54, 1983.

Anderson, J.M., and Schutt, A.M.: Spinal injury in children, a review of 156 cases seen from 1950 to 1978, Mayo Clin. Proc. **55**:499-504, 1980.

Birdsall, C.: How do you teach female self-catheterization? Am. J. Nurs. **85**:1226-1227, 1985.

Brouillette, R.T., Ilbawi, M.N., and Hunt, C.E.: Phrenic nerve pacing in infants and children: a review of experience and report on the usefulness of phrenic nerve stimulation studies, J. Pediatr. **102**:32-39, 1983.

Buchanan, L.E.: Emergency! First aid for spinal cord injury, Nursing 82 **12**(8):68-75, 1982.

Chui, L., and Bhatt, K.: Automatic dysreflexia, Rehab. Nurs. **8**(2):16-19, 1983.

Coffman, S.: Description of nursing diagnosis: alteration in bowel elimination related to neurogenic bowel in children with myelomeningocele, Issues Compr. Pediatr. Nurs. **9**:179-191, 1986.

D'Agnostino, J.: Nursing rehabilitation of the quadriplegic adolescent, J. Assoc. Care Child. Health **9**(3):87-91, 1981.

DeJong, G., and others: Independent living outcomes in spinal cord injury: multivariate analysis, Arch. Phys. Med. Rehabil. **65**:66-72, 1984.

Ehrlich, W., and Brem, A.S.: A prospective comparison of urinary tract infections in patients treated with either clean intermittent catheterization or urinary diversion, Pediatrics **70**:665-669, 1982.

Eliminating suppositories in bowel training, Am. J. Nurs. **86**:522-523, 1986.

Garber, S.L., and others: Trochanteric pressure in spinal cord injury, Arch. Phys. Med. Rehab. **63**:549-552, 1982.

Goldberg, R.T.: Toward an understanding of the rehabilitation of the disabled adolescent, Rehabil. Lit. **42**:66-74, 1981.

Johnson, J.H.: Rehabilitative aspects of neurologic bladder dysfunction, Nurs. Clin. North Am. **15**:293-307, 1980.

King, R.B., and Dudas, S.: Rehabilitation of the patient with a spinal cord injury, Nurs. Clin. North Am. **15**:225-243, 1980.

Manning, L.S., and Young, D.J.: Teaching is a two-way street, Nursing 81 **11**(9):58-60, 1981.

McConnaughey, L.J.: Spinal cord injury in children, Point of View **21**(3):6-7, 1984.

Preston, K., and Couglin, R.: Phrenic nerve stimulators, Rehabil. Nurs. **9**:17-22, 1984.

Sneed, R.C., Stover, L.S., and Fine, P.R.: Spinal cord injury associated with all-terrain vehicle accidents, Pediatrics **77**:271-274, 1986.

Sullivan-Bolyai, S., Swanson, M., and Shurtleff, D.B.: Toilet training the child with neurogenic impairment of bowel and bladder function, Issues Compr. Pediatr. Nurs. **7**:33-43, 1984.

Torg, J.S., and Das, M.: Trampoline-related quadriplegia: review of the literature and reflections on the American Academy of Pediatrics' position statement, Pediatrics **74**:804-812, 1984.

Tortorelli, B.A., Church, J., Garis, V.: Intermittent self-catheterization: a learning packet, Rehabil. Nurs. 31-32, 1984.

Troth, L.L.: Spasticity management in spinal cord injury, Rehabil. Nurs. **8**(1):14-17, 1983.

Uehling, D.T., and others: Impact of an intermittent catheterization program on children with myelomeningocele, Pediatrics **76**:892-895, 1985.

Versluys, H.P.: Physical rehabilitation and family dynamics, Rehab. Literature **41**:58-65, 1980.

Weinberg, J.S.: Human sexuality and spinal cord injury, Nurs. Clin. North Am. **17**:407-419, 1982.

Wright, B.A.: Developing constructive views of life with a disability, Rehabil. Lit. **41**:274-279, 1980.

Appendix A   Family Assessment

Family APGAR Questionnaire

PART I

The following questions have been designed to help us better understand you and your family. You should feel free to ask questions about any item in the questionnaire.

The space for comments should be used when you wish to give additional information or if you wish to discuss the way the question is applied to your family. Please try to answer all questions.

Family is defined as the individual(s) with whom you usually live. If you live alone, your "family" consists of persons with whom you now have the strongest emotional ties.

For each question, check only one box

	Almost always	Some of the time	Hardly ever
I am satisfied that I can turn to my family for help when something is troubling me. Comments: _____	☐	☐	☐
I am satisfied with the way my family talks over things with me and shares problems with me. Comments: _____	☐	☐	☐
I am satisfied that my family accepts and supports my wishes to take on new activities or directions. Comments: _____	☐	☐	☐
I am satisfied with the way my family expresses affection and responds to my emotions, such as anger, sorrow, and love. Comments: _____	☐	☐	☐
I am satisfied with the way my family and I share time together. Comments: _____	☐	☐	☐

Scoring: The patient checks one of three choices which are scored as follows: 'Almost always' (2 points), 'Some of the time' (1) point, or 'Hardly ever' (0). The scores for each of the five questions are then totaled. A score of 7 to 10 suggests a highly functional family. A score of 4 to 6 suggests a moderately dysfunctional family. A score of 0 to 3 suggests a severely dysfunctional family.
*According to which member of the family is being interviewed the nurse may substitute for the word 'family' either spouse, significant other, parents, or children.

Fig. A-1. Family APGAR questionnaire. **A,** Part I.
Adapted from Smilkstein, G.: The Family APGAR: a proposal for a family function test and its use by physicians, J. Fam. Pract. **6**(6):1231-1239, 1978.

Family APGAR Questionnaire

PART II

Who lives in your home?* List the persons according to their relationship to you (for example, spouse, significant other,† child, or friend).

Check the column that best describes how you now get along with each member of the family listed.

RELATIONSHIP	AGE	SEX

WELL	FAIRLY	POORLY

B

If you don't live with your own family, list the persons to whom you turn for help most frequently. List according to relationship (for example, family member, friend, associate at work, or neighbor).

Check the column that best describes how you now get along with each person listed.

RELATIONSHIP	AGE	SEX

WELL	FAIRLY	POORLY

*If you have established your own family, consider your "home" as the place where you live with your spouse, children, or "significant other" (see next footnote for definition): otherwise, consider home as your place of origin, for example, the place where your parents or those who raised you live.
†Significant other is the partner you live with in a physically and emotionally nurturing relationship but to whom you are not married.

Fig. A-1, cont'd. B, Part II.

HOME Inventory for Families of Infants and Toddlers

Family name _____ Date _____ Visitor _____

Child's name _____ Birthdate _____ Age _____ Sex _____

Caregiver for visit _____ Relationship to child _____

Family composition _____
(Persons living in household, including sex and age of children)

Family   Language   Maternal   Paternal
ethnicity _____ spoken _____ education _____ education _____

Is mother employed? _____ Type of work when employed _____

Is father employed? _____ Type of work when employed _____

Address _____

Current child care arrangements _____

Summarize past
year's arrangements _____

Caregiver for visit _____ Other persons present _____

Comments _____

_____

SUMMARY

Subscale	Score	Lowest middle	Middle half	Upper fourth
I. Emotional and verbal RESPONSIVITY of parent		0-6	7-9	10-11
II. ACCEPTANCE of child's behavior		0-4	5-6	7-8
III. ORGANIZATION of physical and temporal environment		0-3	4-5	6
IV. Provision of appropriate PLAY MATERIALS		0-4	5-7	8-9
V. Parent INVOLVEMENT with child		0-2	3-4	5-6
VI. Opportunities for VARIETY in daily stimulation		0-1	2-3	4-5
TOTAL SCORE		0-25	26-36	37-45

For rapid profiling of a family, place an X in the box that corresponds to the raw score on each subscale and the total score.

Fig. A-2. HOME Inventory for Families of Infants and Toddlers.
From Caldwell, B., and Bradley, R.: Manual of home observation for measurement of the environment, rev. ed., 1984, Little Rock, AR.

AUTHOR'S NOTE: HOME inventories for families and preschoolers (3 to 6 years) and elementary age children (6 to 10 years) are available from Bureau of Educational Research (see p. 211 for address).

HOME Inventory

Place a plus (+) or minus (−) in the box alongside each item if the behavior is observed during the visit or if the parent reports that the conditions or events are characteristic of the home environment. Enter the subtotal and the total on the front side of the Record Sheet.

I. Emotional and verbal RESPONSIVITY

1. Parent spontaneously vocalizes to child twice.	
2. Parent responds verbally to child's verbalizations.	
3. Parent tells child name of object or person during visit.	
4. Parent's speech is distinct and audible.	
5. Parent initiates verbal exchanges with visitor.	
6. Parent converses freely and easily.	
7. Parent permits child to engage in "messy" play.	
8. Parent spontaneously praises child at least twice.	
9. Parent's voice conveys positive feelings toward child.	
10. Parent caresses or kisses child at least once.	
11. Parent responds positively to praise of child offered by visitor.	
Subtotal	

II. ACCEPTANCE of child's behavior

12. Parent does not shout at child.	
13. Parent does not express annoyance with or hostility to child.	
14. Parent neither slaps nor spanks child during visit.	
15. No more than one instance of physical punishment during past week.	
16. Parent does not scold or criticize child during visit.	
17. Parent does not interfere or restrict child more than three times.	
18. At least ten books are present and visible.	
19. Family has a pet.	
Subtotal	

III. ORGANIZATION of environment

20. Substitute care is provided by one of three regular substitutes.	
21. Child is taken to grocery store at least once/week.	
22. Child gets out of house at least four times/week.	
23. Child is taken regularly to doctor's office or clinic.	
24. Child has a special place for toys and treasures.	
25. Child's play environment is safe.	
Subtotal	

IV. Provision of PLAY MATERIALS

26. Muscle activity toys or equipment.	
27. Push or pull toy.	
28. Stroller or walker, kiddie car, scooter, or tricycle.	
29. Parent provides toys for child during visit.	
30. Learning equipment appropriate to age—cuddly toys or role-playing toys.	
31. Learning facilitators—mobile, table and chairs, high chair, play pen.	
32. Simple eye-hand coordination toys.	
33. Complex eye-hand coordination toys (those permitting combination).	
34. Toys for literature and music.	
Subtotal	

V. Parental INVOLVEMENT with child

35. Parent keeps child in visual range, looks at often.	
36. Parent talks to child while doing household work.	
37. Parent consciously encourages developmental advance.	
38. Parent invests maturing toys with value via personal attention.	
39. Parent structures child's play periods.	
40. Parent provides toys that challenge child to develop new skills.	
Subtotal	

VI. Opportunities for VARIETY

41. Father provides some care daily.	
42. Parent reads stories to child at least three times weekly.	
43. Child eats at least one meal per day with mother and father.	
44. Family visits relatives or receives visits once a month or so.	
45. Child has three or more books of his/her own.	
Subtotal	

TOTAL SCORE	

Fig. A-2, cont'd. HOME Inventory.

Appendix B   Developmental Assessment

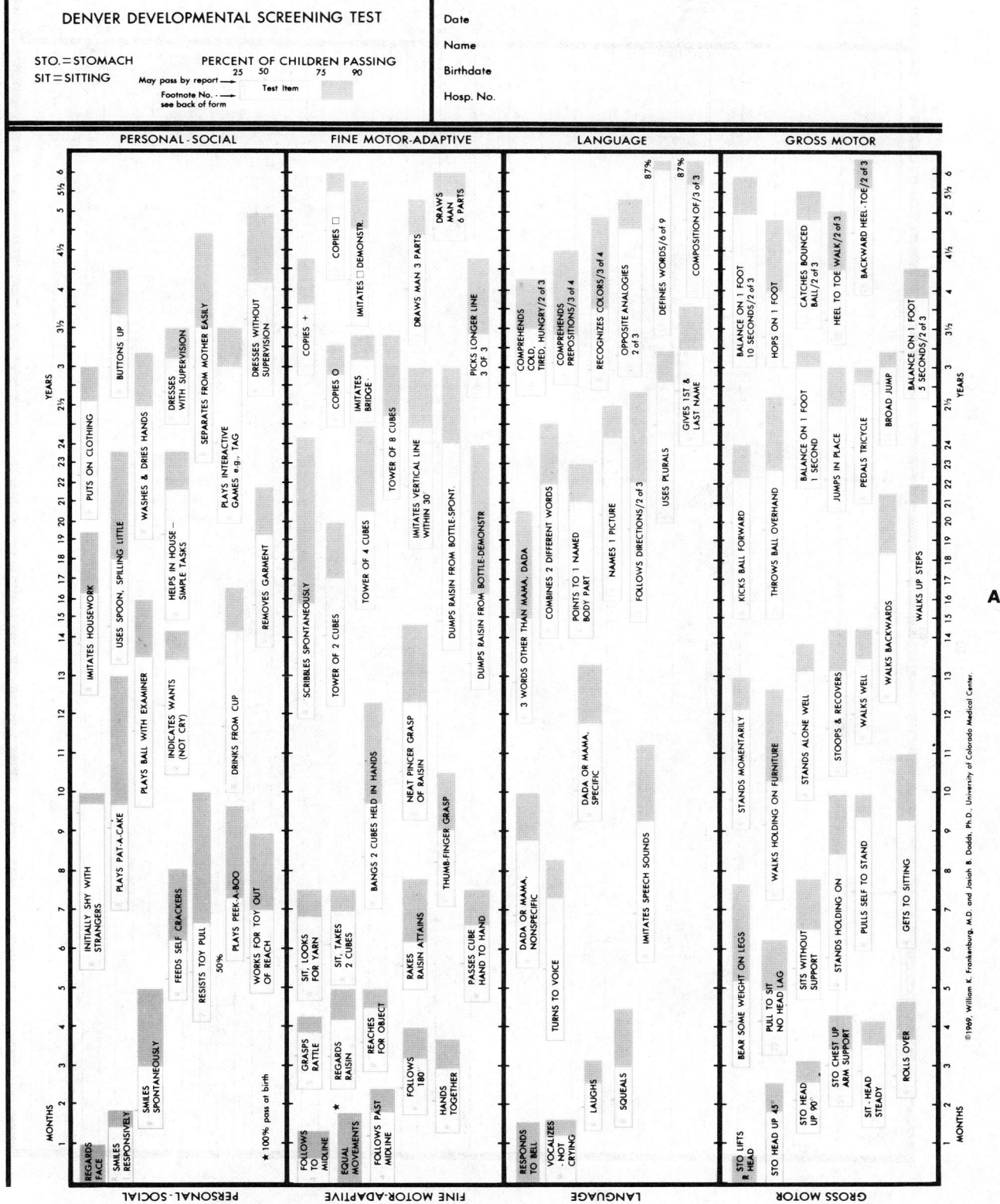

Fig. B-1. A, Denver Developmental Screening Test.
From W.K. Frankenburg and J.B. Dodds, University of Colorado Medical Center, 1969.

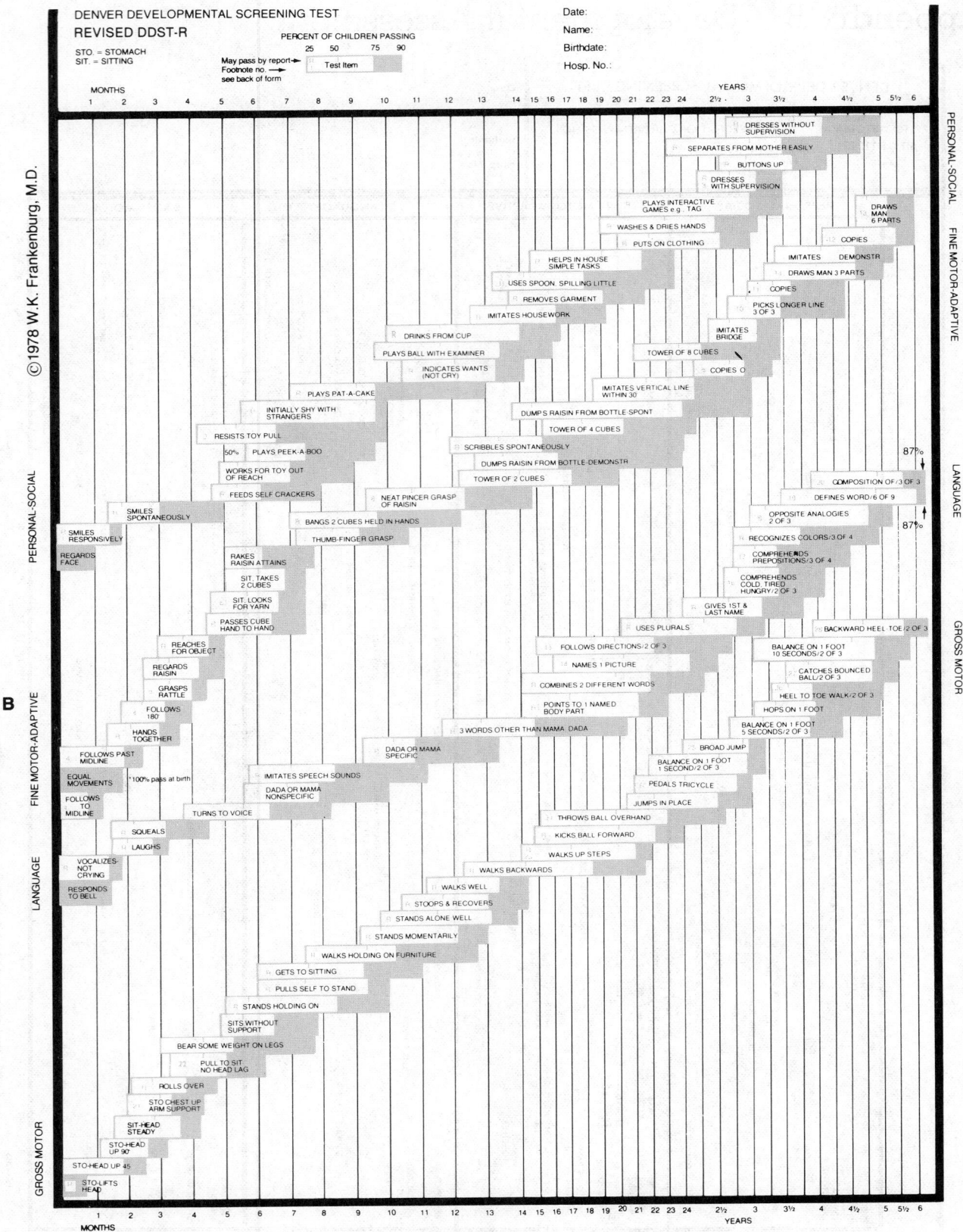

Fig. B-1, cont'd. B, DDST revised (DDST-R). Resembling a growth curve, this form places items at lowest age level starting at bottom left and progresses upward to right with increasing age.
B from Frankenburg, W.K., Sciarillo, W., and Burgess, D.: The newly abbreviated and revised Denver Developmental Screening Test, J. Pediatr. **99**(6):995-999, 1981.

DIRECTIONS

DATE:

NAME:

BIRTHDATE:

HOSP. NO.:

1. Try to get child to smile by smiling, talking or waving to him. Do not touch him.
2. When child is playing with toy, pull it away from him. Pass if he resists.
3. Child does not have to be able to tie shoes or button in the back.
4. Move yarn slowly in an arc from one side to the other, about 6" above child's face.
   Pass if eyes follow 90° to midline. (Past midline; 180°)
5. Pass if child grasps rattle when it is touched to the backs or tips of fingers.
6. Pass if child continues to look where yarn disappeared or tries to see where it went. Yarn
   should be dropped quickly from sight from tester's hand without arm movement.
7. Pass if child picks up raisin with any part of thumb and a finger.
8. Pass if child picks up raisin with the ends of thumb and index finger using an over hand
   approach.

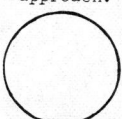 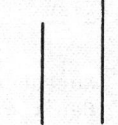 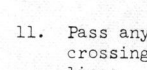 

9. Pass any en-   10. Which line is longer?   11. Pass any   12. Have child copy
   closed form.   (Not bigger.) Turn   crossing   first. If failed,
   Fail continuous   paper upside down and   lines.   demonstrate
   round motions.   repeat. (3/3 or 5/6)

When giving items 9, 11 and 12, do not name the forms. Do not demonstrate 9 and 11.

13. When scoring, each pair (2 arms, 2 legs, etc.) counts as one part.
14. Point to picture and have child name it. (No credit is given for sounds only.)

C

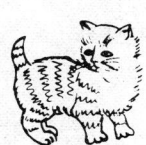 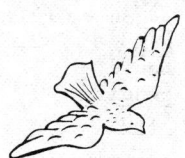 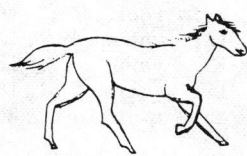 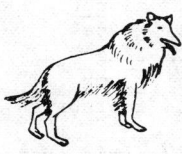 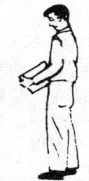

15. Tell child to: Give block to Mommie; put block on table; put block on floor. Pass 2 of 3.
    (Do not help child by pointing, moving head or eyes.)
16. Ask child: What do you do when you are cold? ..hungry? ..tired? Pass 2 of 3.
17. Tell child to: Put block on table; under table; in front of chair, behind chair.
    Pass 3 of 4. (Do not help child by pointing, moving head or eyes.)
18. Ask child: If fire is hot, ice is ?; Mother is a woman, Dad is a ?; a horse is big, a
    mouse is ?. Pass 2 of 3.
19. Ask child: What is a ball? ..lake? ..desk? ..house? ..banana? ..curtain? ..ceiling?
    ..hedge? ..pavement? Pass if defined in terms of use, shape, what it is made of or general
    category (such as banana is fruit, not just yellow). Pass 6 of 9.
20. Ask child: What is a spoon made of? ..a shoe made of? ..a door made of? (No other objects
    may be substituted.) Pass 3 of 3.
21. When placed on stomach, child lifts chest off table with support of forearms and/or hands.
22. When child is on back, grasp his hands and pull him to sitting. Pass if head does not hang back.
23. Child may use wall or rail only, not person. May not crawl.
24. Child must throw ball overhand 3 feet to within arm's reach of tester.
25. Child must perform standing broad jump over width of test sheet. (8-1/2 inches)
26. Tell child to walk forward, ⮾⮾⮾⮾→ heel within 1 inch of toe.
    Tester may demonstrate. Child must walk 4 consecutive steps, 2 out of 3 trials.
27. Bounce ball to child who should stand 3 feet away from tester. Child must catch ball with
    hands, not arms, 2 out of 3 trials.
28. Tell child to walk backward, ←⮾⮾⮾⮾ toe within 1 inch of heel.
    Tester may demonstrate. Child must walk 4 consecutive steps, 2 out of 3 trials.

DATE AND BEHAVIORAL OBSERVATIONS (how child feels at time of test, relation to tester, attention
span, verbal behavior, self-confidence, etc,):

Fig. B-1, cont'd. C, Directions for numbered items on testing form.
C from W.K. Frankenburg and J.B. Dobbs, University of Colorado Medical Center, 1969.

DENVER ARTICULATION SCREENING EXAM
for children 2½ to 6 years of age

Instructions: Have child repeat each word after
you. Circle the underlined sounds that he pronounces correctly. Total correct sounds is the
Raw Score. Use charts on reverse side to score
results.

Name:

Hosp. No.:

Address:_____

_____

Date: _____   Child's age: _____   Examiner: _____   Raw score: ____
Percentile: _____   Intelligibility: _____   Result: _____

1. table   6. zipper   11. sock   16. wagon   21. leaf
2. shirt   7. grapes   12. vacuum   17. gum   22. carrot
3. door   8. flag   13. yarn   18. house
4. trunk   9. thumb   14. mother   19. pencil
5. jumping   10. toothbrush 15. twinkle   20. fish

Intelligibility: (circle one)
   1. Easy to understand   3. Not understandable
   2. Understandable ½ the time   4. Can't evaluate

Comments:

A

Date: _____   Child's age: _____   Examiner: _____   Raw score: ____
Percentile: _____   Intelligibility: _____   Result: _____

1. table   6. zipper   11. sock   16. wagon   21. leaf
2. shirt   7. grapes   12. vacuum   17. gum   22. carrot
3. door   8. flag   13. yarn   18. house
4. trunk   9. thumb   14. mother   19. pencil
5. jumping   10. toothbrush 15. twinkle   20. fish

Intelligibility: (circle one)
   1. Easy to understand   3. Not understandable
   2. Understandable ½ the time   4. Can't evaluate

Comments:

Date: _____   Child's age: _____   Examiner: _____   Raw score ____
Percentile: _____   Intelligibility: _____   Result: _____

1. table   6. zipper   11. sock   16. wagon   21. leaf
2. shirt   7. grapes   12. vacuum   17. gum   22. carrot
3. door   8. flag   13. yarn   18. house
4. trunk   9. thumb   14. mother   19. pencil
5. jumping   10. toothbrush 15. twinkle   20. fish

Intelligibility: (circle one)
   1. Easy to understand   3. Not understandable
   2. Understandable ½ the time   4. Can't evaluate

Fig. B-2. A, Denver Articulation Screening Examination for Children 2½ to 6 years of age.
From A.F. Drumwright, University of Colorado Medical Center, 1971.

To score DASE words: Note raw score for child's performance. Match raw score line (extreme left of chart) with column representing child's age (to the closest previous age group). Where raw score line and age column meet number in that square denotes percentile rank of child's performance when compared to other children that age. Percentiles above heavy line are ABNORMAL percentiles, below heavy line are NORMAL.

PERCENTILE RANK

Raw Score	2.5 yr.	3.0	3.5	4.0	4.5	5.0	5.5	6 years
2	1							
3	2							
4	5							
5	9							
6	16							
7	23							
8	31	2						
9	37	4	1					
10	42	6	2					
11	48	7	4					
12	54	9	6	1	1			
13	58	12	9	2	3	1	1	
14	62	17	11	5	4	2	2	
15	68	23	15	9	5	3	2	
16	75	31	19	12	5	4	3	
17	79	38	25	15	6	6	4	
18	83	46	31	19	8	7	4	
19	86	51	38	24	10	9	5	1
20	89	58	45	30	12	11	7	3
21	92	65	52	36	15	15	9	4
22	94	72	58	43	18	19	12	5
23	96	77	63	50	22	24	15	7
24	97	82	70	58	29	29	20	15
25	99	87	78	66	36	34	26	17
26	99	91	84	75	46	43	34	24
27		94	89	82	57	54	44	34
28		96	94	88	70	68	59	47
29		98	98	94	84	84	77	68
30		100	100	100	100	100	100	100

B

To score intelligibility:	NORMAL	ABNORMAL
2½ years	Understandable ½ the time, or, "easy"	Not understandable
3 years and older	Easy to understand	Understandable ½ time Not understandable

Test result: 1. NORMAL on Dase and Intelligibility = NORMAL

2. ABNORMAL on Dase and/or Intelligibility = ABNORMAL

*If abnormal on initial screening rescreen within 2 weeks.
If abnormal again child should be referred for complete speech evaluation.

Fig. B-2, cont'd. B, Percentile rank.

Lit. 217

DENVER EYE SCREENING TEST

Name:
Hospital No.:
Ward:
Address:

1ST SCREENING: DATE: ____ Date: ____

Vision Tests	Right Eye Normal	Right Eye Abnormal	Right Eye Untestable	Left Eye Normal	Left Eye Abnormal	Left Eye Untestable
1. "E" (3 years and above—3 to 5 trials)	3P	3F	U	3P	3F	U
2. Picture card (2 1/2 - 2 11/12 yrs.—3 to 5 trials)	3P	3F	U	3P	3F	U
3. Fixation (6 months - 2 5/12 years)	P	F	U	P	F	U
4. Squinting		yes			yes	

Tests for Non-Straight Eyes	Normal	Abnormal	Untestable
1. Do your child's eyes turn in or out, or are they ever not straight?	NO	YES	
2. Cover Test	P	F	
3. Pupillary Light Reflex	P	F	U

Total Test Rating (Both Eyes): Normal / Abnormal / Untestable

RESCREENING: DATE: ____ Date: ____

Vision Tests	Right Eye Normal	Right Eye Abnormal	Right Eye Untestable	Left Eye Normal	Left Eye Abnormal	Left Eye Untestable
1. "E" (3 years and above—3 to 5 trials)	3P	3F	U	3P	3F	U
2. Picture card (2 1/2 - 2 11/12 yrs.—3 to 5 trials)	3P	3F	U	3P	3F	U
3. Fixation (6 months - 2 5/12 years)	P	F	U	P	F	U
4. Squinting		yes			yes	

Tests for Non-Straight Eyes	Normal	Abnormal	Untestable
1. Do your child's eyes turn in or out, or are they ever not straight?	NO	YES	
2. Cover Test	P	F	
3. Pupillary Light Reflex	P	F	U

Total Test Rating (Both Eyes): Normal / Abnormal / Untestable

Normal (passed vision test plus no squint, plus passed 2/3 tests for non-straight eyes)

Abnormal (abnormal on any vision test, squinting or 2 of 3 procedures for non-straight eyes)

Untestable (untestable on any vision test or untestable on 2/3 tests for non-straight eyes)

Future Rescreening Appointment for Total Test Rating (Abnormal or Untestable)

Fig. B-3. Denver Eye Screening Test.
From W.K. Frankenburg and J.B. Dobbs, University of Colorado Medical Center, 1969.

Appendix C Growth Measurements

Height and Weight Measurements for Boys

AGER*	HEIGHT BY PERCENTILES						WEIGHT BY PERCENTILES					
	5		50		95		5		50		95	
	CM	INCHES	CM	INCHES	CM	INCHES	KG	LB	KG	LB	KG	LB
Birth	46.4	18¼	50.5	20	54.4	21½	2.54	5½	3.27	7¼	4.15	9¼
3 months	56.7	22¼	61.1	24	65.4	25¾	4.43	9¾	5.98	13¼	7.37	16¼
6 months	63.4	25	67.8	26¾	72.3	28½	6.20	13¾	7.85	17¼	9.46	20¾
9 months	68.0	26¾	72.3	28½	77.1	30¼	7.52	16½	9.18	20¼	10.93	24
1	71.7	28¼	76.1	30	81.2	32	8.43	18½	10.15	22½	11.99	26½
1½	77.5	30½	82.4	32½	88.1	34¾	9.59	21¼	11.47	25¼	13.44	29½
2†	82.5	32½	86.8	34¼	94.4	37¼	10.49	23¼	12.34	27¼	15.50	34¼
2½†	85.4	33½	90.4	35½	97.8	38½	11.27	24¾	13.52	29¾	16.61	36½
3	89.0	35	94.9	37¼	102.0	40¼	12.05	26½	14.62	32¼	17.77	39¼
3½	92.5	36½	99.1	39	106.1	41¾	12.84	28¼	15.68	34½	18.98	41¾
4	95.8	37¾	102.9	40½	109.9	43¼	13.64	30	16.69	36¾	20.27	44¾
4½	98.9	39	106.6	42	113.5	44¾	14.45	31¾	17.69	39	21.63	47¾
5	102.0	40¼	109.9	43¼	117.0	46	15.27	33¾	18.67	41¼	23.09	51
6	107.7	42½	116.1	45¾	123.5	48½	16.93	37¼	20.69	45½	26.34	58
7	113.0	44½	121.7	48	129.7	51	18.64	41	22.85	50¼	30.12	66½
8	118.1	46½	127.0	50	135.7	53½	20.40	45	25.30	55¾	34.51	76
9	122.9	48½	132.2	52	141.8	55¾	22.25	49	28.13	62	39.58	87¼
10	127.7	50¼	137.5	54¼	148.1	58¼	24.33	53¾	31.44	69¼	45.27	99¾
11	132.6	52¼	143.3	56½	154.9	61	26.80	59	35.30	77¾	51.47	113½
12	137.6	54¼	149.7	59	162.3	64	29.85	65¾	39.78	87¾	58.09	128
13	142.9	56¼	156.5	61½	169.8	66¾	33.64	74¼	44.95	99	65.02	143¼
14	148.8	58½	163.1	64¼	176.7	69½	38.22	84¼	50.77	112	72.13	159
15	155.2	61	169.0	66½	181.9	71½	43.11	95	56.71	125	79.12	174½
16	161.1	63½	173.5	68¼	185.4	73	47.74	105¼	62.10	137	85.62	188¾
17	164.9	65	176.2	69¼	187.3	73¾	51.50	113½	66.31	146¼	91.31	201¼
18	165.7	65¼	176.8	69½	187.6	73¾	53.97	119	68.88	151¾	95.76	211

Adapted from National Center for Health Statistics (NCHS), Health Resources Administration, Department of Health, Education and Welfare, Hyattsville, MD. Conversion of metric data to approximate inches and pounds by Ross Laboratories.
*Years unless otherwise indicated.
†Height data include some recumbent length measurements, which make values slightly higher than if all measurements had been of stature (standing height).

Height and Weight Measurements for Girls

AGE*	HEIGHT BY PERCENTILES						WEIGHT BY PERCENTILES					
	5		50		95		5		50		95	
	CM	INCHES	CM	INCHES	CM	INCHES	KG	LB	KG	LB	KG	LB
Birth	45.4	17¾	49.9	19¾	52.9	20¾	2.36	5¼	3.23	7	3.81	8½
3 months	55.4	21¾	59.5	23½	63.4	25	4.18	9¼	5.4	12	6.74	14¾
6 months	61.8	24¼	65.9	26	70.2	27¾	5.79	12¾	7.21	16	8.73	19¼
9 months	66.1	26	70.4	27¾	75.0	29½	7.0	15½	8.56	18¾	10.17	22½
1	69.8	27½	74.3	29¼	79.1	31¼	7.84	17¼	9.53	21	11.24	24¾
1½	76.0	30	80.9	31¾	86.1	34	8.92	19¾	10.82	23¾	12.76	28¼
2†	81.6	32¼	86.8	34¼	93.6	36¾	9.95	22	11.8	26	14.15	31¼
2½†	84.6	33¼	90.0	35½	96.6	38	10.8	23¾	13.03	28¾	15.76	34¾
3	88.3	34¾	94.1	37	100.6	39½	11.61	25½	14.1	31	17.22	38
3½	91.7	36	97.9	38½	104.5	41¼	12.37	27¼	15.07	33¼	18.59	41
4	95.0	37½	101.6	40	108.3	42¾	13.11	29	15.96	35¼	19.91	44
4½	98.1	38½	105.0	41¼	112.0	44	13.83	30½	16.81	37	21.24	46¾
5	101.1	39¾	108.4	42¾	115.6	45½	14.55	32	17.66	39	22.62	49¾
6	106.6	42	114.6	45	122.7	48¼	16.05	35½	19.52	43	25.75	56¾
7	111.8	44	120.6	47½	129.5	51	17.71	39	21.84	48¼	29.68	65½
8	116.9	46	126.4	49¾	136.2	53½	19.62	43¼	24.84	54¾	34.71	76½
9	122.1	48	132.2	52	142.9	56¼	21.82	48	28.46	62¾	40.64	89½
10	127.5	50¼	138.3	54½	149.5	58¾	24.36	53¾	32.55	71¾	47.17	104
11	133.5	52½	144.8	57	156.2	61½	27.24	60	36.95	81½	54.0	119
12	139.8	55	151.5	59¾	162.7	64	30.52	67¼	41.53	91½	60.81	134
13	145.2	57¼	157.1	61¾	168.1	66¼	34.14	75¼	46.1	101¾	67.3	148¼
14	148.7	58½	160.4	63¼	171.3	67½	37.76	83¼	50.28	110¾	73.08	161
15	150.5	59¼	161.8	63¾	172.8	68	40.99	90¼	53.68	118¼	77.78	171½
16	151.6	59¾	162.4	64	173.3	68¼	43.41	95¾	55.89	123¼	80.99	178½
17	152.7	60	163.1	64¼	173.5	68¼	44.74	98¾	56.69	125	82.46	181¾
18	153.6	60½	163.7	64½	173.6	68¼	45.26	99¾	56.62	124¾	82.47	181¾

Adapted from National Center for Health Statistics, Health Resources Administration, Department of Health, Education and Welfare, Hyattsville, MD. Conversion of metric data to approximate inches and pounds by Ross Laboratories.
*Years unless otherwise indicated.
†Height data include some recumbent length measurements, which make values slightly higher than if all measurements had been of stature.

Growth Standards of Healthy Chinese Children and Adolescents (Urban)*

AGE (MONTHS OR YEARS)	BOYS				GIRLS			
	WEIGHT (KG)	HEIGHT (CM)	HEAD CIRCUMFERENCE (CM)	CHEST CIRCUMFERENCE (CM)	WEIGHT (KG)	HEIGHT (CM)	HEAD CIRCUMFERENCE (CM)	CHEST CIRCUMFERENCE (CM)
Birth	3.27	50.6	34.3	32.8	3.17	50.0	33.7	32.6
1 mo	4.97	56.5	38.1	37.9	4.64	55.5	37.3	36.9
2 mo	5.95	59.6	39.7	40.0	5.49	58.4	38.7	38.9
3 mo	6.73	62.3	41.0	41.3	6.23	60.9	40.0	40.3
4 mo	7.32	64.4	42.0	42.3	6.69	62.9	41.0	41.1
5 mo	7.70	65.9	42.9	42.9	7.19	64.5	41.9	41.9
6 mo	8.22	68.1	43.9	43.8	7.62	66.7	42.8	42.7
8 mo	8.71	70.6	44.9	44.7	8.14	69.0	43.7	43.4
10 mo	9.14	72.9	45.7	45.4	8.57	71.4	44.5	44.2
12 mo	9.66	75.6	46.3	46.1	9.04	74.1	45.2	45.0
15 mo	10.15	78.3	46.8	46.8	9.54	76.9	45.6	45.8
18 mo	10.67	80.7	47.3	47.6	10.08	79.4	46.2	46.6
21 mo	11.18	83.0	47.8	48.3	10.56	81.7	46.7	47.3
24 mo	11.95	86.5	48.2	49.2	11.37	85.3	47.1	48.2
2½ yr	12.84	90.4	48.8	50.2	12.28	89.3	47.7	49.0
3 yr	13.63	93.8	49.1	50.8	13.1	92.8	48.1	49.8
3½ yr	14.45	97.2	49.4	51.5	14.0	96.3	48.5	50.5
4 yr	15.26	100.8	49.7	52.2	14.89	100.1	48.9	51.2
4½ yr	16.07	103.9	50.0	53.0	15.63	103.1	49.1	51.8
5 yr	16.88	107.2	50.2	53.6	16.46	106.5	49.4	52.5
5½ yr	17.65	110.1	50.5	54.4	17.18	109.2	49.6	53.0
6 yr	19.25	114.7	50.8	55.6	18.67	113.9	50.0	54.2
7 yr	21.01	120.6	51.1	57.1	20.35	119.3	50.2	55.5
8 yr	23.08	125.3	51.4	58.8	22.43	124.6	50.6	57.1
9 yr	25.33	130.6	51.7	60.8	24.57	129.5	50.9	58.6
10 yr	27.15	134.4	51.9	62.0	27.05	134.8	51.3	60.7
11 yr	30.13	139.2	52.3	64.3	30.51	140.6	51.7	63.5
12 yr	33.05	144.2	52.7	66.5	34.82	146.6	52.3	67.2
13 yr	36.90	149.3	53.0	68.9	38.52	150.7	52.8	70.3
14 yr	42.03	156.5	53.5	72.4	42.26	153.7	53.1	73.3
15 yr	46.91	162.0	54.3	76.0	45.37	155.5	53.4	75.6
16 yr	50.90	165.6	54.9	78.8	47.43	156.8	53.8	76.6
17 yr	53.11	167.7	55.2	80.8	48.57	157.4	53.9	77.9

Adapted from Practical Pediatrics; edited by Peking Children's Hospital, 1979.

*Measurements of rural Chinese children are slightly lower.

NOTE: A comparison of the average growth of American and Chinese children demonstrates that on the standard NCHS growth charts the mean height and weight for Chinese children fall in the 10th percentile, as compared to the mean growth measurements for American children, which comprise the 50th percentile.

Head Circumference Charts

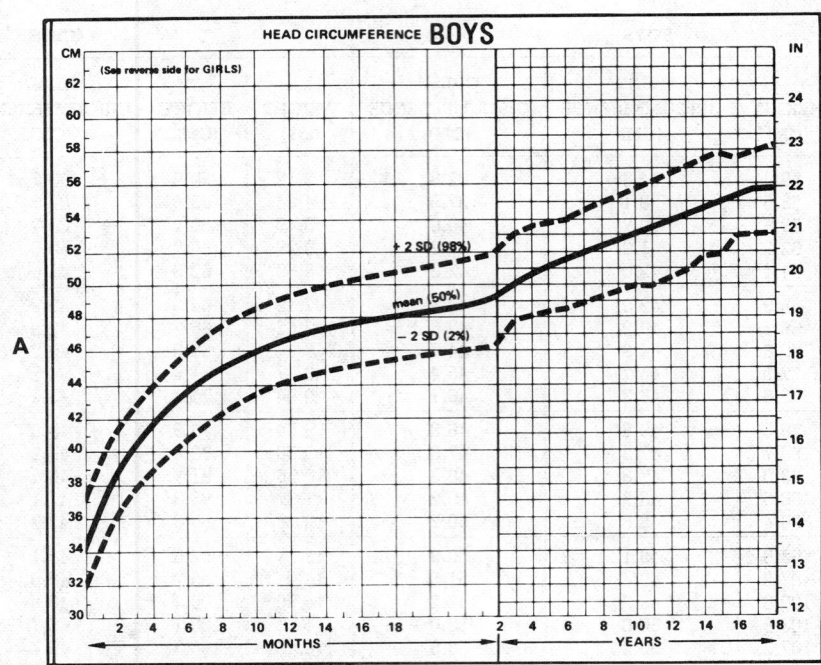

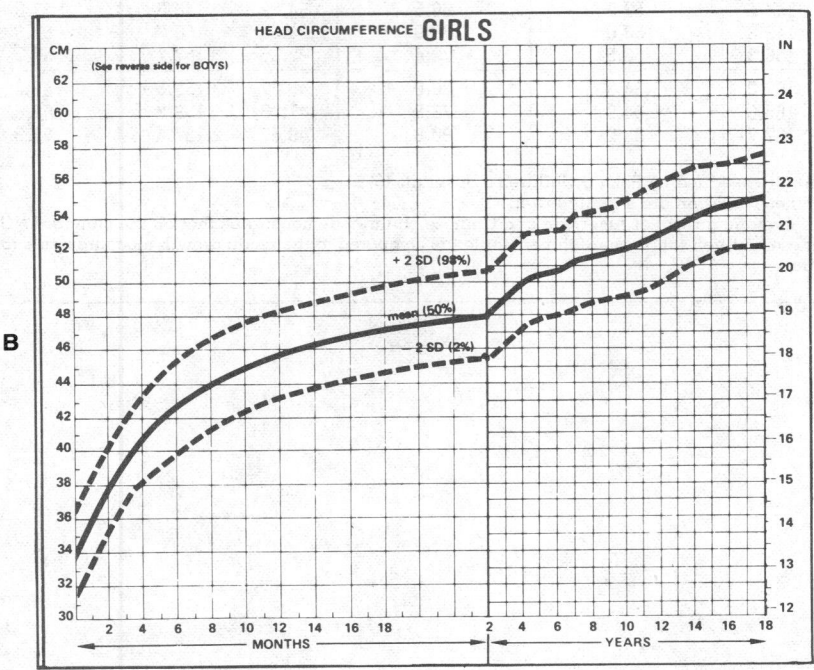

Fig. C-1. Head circumference charts. **A,** Boys; **B,** girls.

From Nellhaus, G.: Composite international and interracial graphs, Pediatrics **41**:106, 1968. Reprinted by permission.
Copyright American Academy of Pediatrics, 1968.

Percentiles for Triceps Skinfold

| AGE GROUP (YEARS) | TRICEPS SKINFOLD PERCENTILES (mm²) | | | | | | | | | |
| | MALES | | | | | FEMALES | | | | |
	5	25	50	75	95	5	25	50	75	95
1-1.9	6	8	10	12	16	6	8	10	12	16
2-2.9	6	8	10	12	15	6	9	10	12	16
3-3.9	6	8	10	11	15	7	9	11	12	15
4-4.9	6	8	9	11	14	7	8	10	12	16
5-5.9	6	8	9	11	15	6	8	10	12	18
6-6.9	5	7	8	10	16	6	8	10	12	16
7-7.9	5	7	9	12	17	6	9	11	13	18
8-8.9	5	7	8	10	16	6	9	12	15	24
9-9.9	6	7	10	13	18	8	10	13	16	22
10-10.9	6	8	10	14	21	7	10	12	17	27
11-11.9	6	8	11	16	24	7	10	13	18	28
12-12.9	6	8	11	14	28	8	11	14	18	27
13-13.9	5	7	10	14	26	8	12	15	21	30
14-14.9	4	7	9	14	24	9	13	16	21	28
15-15.9	4	6	8	11	24	8	12	17	21	32
16-16.9	4	6	8	12	22	10	15	18	22	31
17-17.9	5	6	8	12	19	10	13	19	24	37
18-18.9	4	6	9	13	24	10	15	18	22	30
19-24.9	4	7	10	15	22	10	14	18	24	34

From Frisancho, A.: New norms of upper limb fat and muscle areas for assessment of nutritional status, Am. J. Clin. Nutr. **34:**2540-2545, 1981.

Percentiles of Upper Arm Circumference

| AGE GROUP (YEARS) | ARM CIRCUMFERENCE PERCENTILES (mm) | | | | | | | | | |
| | MALES | | | | | FEMALES | | | | |
	5	25	50	75	95	5	25	50	75	95
1-1.9	142	150	159	170	183	138	148	156	164	177
2-2.9	141	153	162	170	185	142	152	160	167	184
3-3.9	150	160	167	175	190	143	158	167	175	189
4-4.9	149	162	171	180	192	149	160	169	177	191
5-5.9	153	167	175	185	204	153	165	175	185	211
6-6.9	155	167	179	188	228	156	170	176	187	211
7-7.9	162	177	187	201	230	164	174	183	199	231
8-8.9	162	177	190	202	245	168	183	195	214	261
9-9.9	175	187	200	217	257	178	194	211	224	260
10-10.9	181	196	210	231	274	174	193	210	228	265
11-11.9	186	202	223	244	280	185	208	224	248	303
12-12.9	193	214	232	254	303	194	216	237	256	294
13-13.9	194	228	247	263	301	202	223	243	271	338
14-14.9	220	237	253	283	322	214	237	252	272	322
15-15.9	222	244	264	284	320	208	239	254	279	322
16-16.9	244	262	278	303	343	218	241	258	283	334
17-17.9	246	267	285	308	347	220	241	264	295	350
18-18.9	245	276	297	321	379	222	241	258	281	325
19-24.9	262	288	308	331	372	221	247	265	290	345

From Frisancho, A.: New norms of upper limb fat and muscle areas for assessment of nutritional status, Am. J. Clin. Nutr. **34:**2540-2545, 1981.

Appendix D   Common Laboratory Tests

TEST	SPECIMEN	AGE/SEX	NORMAL VALUE
Ammonia nitrogen	Plasma or serum	Newborn	90-150 µg/dL
		0-2 weeks	79-129
		>1 month	29-70
		Thereafter	15-45
	Urine, 24 hr		1.3-7.0 mg/d
Amphetamine	Serum, plasma	Therap. conc.	20-30 ng/ml
		Toxic conc.	>200
Amylase	Serum	Newborn	5-65 U/L
Bechman; BMD	Urine, 24 hr	<1 yr	25-125
		1-17 yr	23-85
Anti-deoxyribonu-clease B titer (Anti-DNAse titer)	Serum		≤170 units

			Plasma mOsmol/kg	Plasma ADH pg/ml
Antidiuretic hormone (hADH, vasopressin)	Plasma		270-280:	<1.5
			280-285:	<2.5
			285-290:	1-5
			290-295:	2-7
			295-300:	4-12

TEST	SPECIMEN	AGE/SEX	NORMAL VALUE
Antistreptolysin O titer (ASO)	Serum		
Normal			<166 Todd units
Recent streptococcal infection			200-2500 Todd units
Base excess	Whole blood	Newborn	(−10)-(−2) mmol/L
		Infant	(−7)-(−1)
		Child	(−4)-(+2)
		Thereafter	(−3)-(+3)
Bicarbonate (HCO₃)	Serum	Arterial	21-28 mmol/L
		Venous	22-29
Bile acids, total	Serum, fasting		0.3-2.3 µg/ml
	Serum, 2 hr postprandial		1.8-3.2
	Feces		120-225 µg/ml

			Premature	Full-term
Bilirubin, total	Serum	Cord	<2.0 mg/dL	<2.0 mg/dL
		0-1 day	<8.0	<6.0
		1-2 days	<12.0	<8.0
		2-5 days	<16.0	<12.0
		Thereafter	<2	0.2-1.0

TEST	SPECIMEN	AGE/SEX	NORMAL VALUE
Bilirubin, direct (conjugated)			0.0-0.2 mg/dL
Bleeding time (Ivy)	Skin puncture	Normal	2-7 min
		Borderline	7-11
(Simplate)			2.75-8
Blood urea nitrogen (BUN) (see urea nitrogen)			
Blood volume	Whole blood	Male	52-83 mL/kg
		Female	50-75
C-reactive protein (CRP)	Serum	Cord	10-350 ng/mL
		Adult	68-8200 ng/mL
Calcitonin (hCT)	Serum or plasma	Newborn	
		Term, cord	30-240 pg/mL
		48 hr	91-580
		7 days	77-293
		Premature, cord	30-265
		48 hr	108-670
		7 days	79-570
		Adult: Male	<100
		Female	4 times lower (increases in pregnancy)

Modified from Behrman, R.E., and Vaughan, V.C., III: Nelson textbook of pediatrics, ed. 12, Philadelphia, 1983, W.B. Saunders Co.

TEST	SPECIMEN	AGE/SEX	NORMAL VALUE
Calcium, ionized	Serum, plasma, or whole blood	Cord	5.5 ± 0.3 mg/dL
		Newborn	4.3-5.1
		24-48 hr	4.0-4.7
		Thereafter	4.48-4.92 or 2.24-2.46 mEq/L
Calcium, total	Serum	Cord	9.0-11.5 mg/dL
		Newborn, 3-24 hr	9.0-10.6
		24-48 hr	7.0-12.0
		4-7 days	9.0-10.9
		Child	8.8-10.8
		Thereafter	8.4-10.2
	Urine, 24 hr	Ca-free diet	5-40 mg/d
		Low to average Ca in diet	50-150
		Average	100-300
	CSF		4.2-5.4 mg/dL or 2.1-2.7 mEq/L
	Feces	Average	0.64 g/d
Carbamazepine	Serum, plasma	Therap. conc.	8-12 μg/mL
		Toxic conc.	>15
Carbon dioxide, partial pressure (PCO_2)	Whole blood, arterial	Newborn	27-40 mm Hg
		Infant	27-41
		Thereafter: Male	35-48
		Female	32-45
Carbon dioxide (total CO_2)	Serum or plasma	Cord	14-22 mmol/L
		Premature (1 week)	14-27
		Newborn	13-22
		Infant	20-28
		Child	20-28
		Thereafter	23-30
β-Carotene	Serum	Infant	20-70 μg/dL
		Child	40-130
		Thereafter	60-200
Catecholamines, fractionated	Plasma	Norepinephrine	
		Supine	100-400 pg/mL
		Standing	300-900
		Epinephrine	
		Supine	<70 pg/mL
		Standing	<100
		Dopamine	
		(no postural change)	<30 pg/mL
	Urine, 24 hr	Norepinephrine	
		0-1 yr	0-10 μg/d
		1-2 yr	0-17
		2-4 yr	4-29
		4-7 yr	8-45
		7-10 yr	13-65
		Thereafter	15-80
		Epinephrine	
		0-1 yr	0-2.5 μg/d
		1-2 yr	0-3.5
		2-4 yr	0-6.0
		4-7 yr	0.2-10
		7-10 yr	0.5-14
		Thereafter	0.5-20
		Dopamine	
		0-1 yr	0-85 μ/d
		1-2 yr	10-140
		2-4 yr	40-260
		Thereafter	65-400
Catecholamines, total	Urine, 24 hr	2-3 mo	12.2 ± 4 to 19.6 ± 14.5 μg/m^2/d
		4-10 mo	19.2 ± 18 to 29.9 ± 21.3 μg/m^2/d
		12-18 mo	19.3 ± 14.3 to 33.5 ± 14.4 μg/m^2/d
		Adult	<280 μg/d
Cerebrospinal fluid pressure	CSF		70-180 mm water

Continued.

Common Laboratory Tests—cont'd

TEST	SPECIMEN	AGE/SEX	NORMAL VALUE
Cerebrospinal fluid volume	CSF	Child	60-100 mL
		Adult	100-160
Chloral hydrate	Serum	As trichloroethanol	
		Therap. conc.	2-12 µg/mL
		Toxic conc.	>20
Chloride	Serum or plasma	Cord	96-104 mmol/L
		Newborn	97-110
		Thereafter	98-106
	CSF		118-132
	Urine, 24 hr	Infant	2-10 mmol/d (diet-dependent)
		Child	15-40
		Thereafter	110-250
	Sweat	Normal homozygote	0-35 mmol/L
		Marginal (e.g., asthma, Addison disease, malnutrition)	30-60
		Cystic fibrosis	60-200 mmol/L
Cholesterol, total	Serum or plasma	Cord	45-100 mg/dL
		Newborn	53-135
		Infant	70-175
		Child	120-200
		Adolescent	120-210
		Thereafter	140-310
Clotting time (Lee-White)	Whole blood		5-8 min (glass tubes)
			5-15 min (room temp)
Coagulation factor assays	Plasma (citrate)		
Factor I, see fibrinogen			
Factor II			0.5-1.5 U/mL or
			60%-150% of normal
Factor IV, see calcium			
Factor V			0.5-2.0 U/mL or
			60%-150% of normal
Factor VII			65%-135% of normal
Factor VIII			60%-145% of normal
Factor VIII antigen			50%-200% of normal
Factor IX			60%-140% of normal
Factor X			60%-130% of normal
Factor XI			65%-135% of normal
Factor XII			65%-150% of normal
Factor XIII (fibrin stabilizing factor, FSF)	Whole blood (citrate or oxalate)	Minimum hemostatic level	0.02-0.05 U/mL or 1%-2% of normal
Complement components			
Total hemolytic complement activity	Plasma		75-160 U/mL or >33% of plasma CH_{50}
Total complement decay rate (functional)	Plasma		~10%-20%
		Deficiency	>50%
Copper	Serum	Birth-6 mo	20-70 µg/dL
		6 yr	90-190 µg/dL
		12 yr	80-160 µg/dL
		Adult: Male	70-140 µg/dL
		Female	80-155 µg/dL
Coproporphyrin	Urine, 24 hr		34-234 µg/d
	Feces, 24 hr		<30 µg/g dry wt
			400-1200 µg/d
Cortisol	Serum or plasma	Newborn	1-24 µg/dL
		0800 hr	5-23 µg/dL
		1600 hr	3-15
		2000 hr	≤50% of 0800 hr
Cortisol, free	Urine, 24 hr	Child	2-27 µg/d
		Adolescent	5-55
		Adult	10-100

TEST	SPECIMEN	AGE/SEX	NORMAL VALUE
Creatine kinase (CK, CPK)	Serum	Newborn	68-580 U/L
		Adult: Male	12-70
		Female	10-55
		Ambulatory: Male	25-90
		Female	10-70
		Higher after exercise	
Creatinine	Serum	Cord	0.6-1.2 mg/dL
		Newborn	0.3-1.0
		Infant	0.2-0.4
		Child	0.3-0.7
		Adolescent	0.5-1.0
		Adult: Male	0.6-1.2
		Female	0.5-1.1
	Urine, 24 hr	Infant	8-20 mg/kg/d
		Child	8-22
		Adolescent	8-30
		Adult	14-26
Creatinine clearance (endogenous)	Serum or plasma and urine	Newborn	40-65 ml/min/1.73 m^2
		<40 yr: Male	97-137 ml/min/1.73m^2
		Female	88-128 ml/min/1.73m^2
Diazepam	Serum, plasma	Therap. conc.	100-1000 ng/mL
		Toxic conc.	>5000
Differential count, see leukocyte differential count			
Digoxin	Serum, plasma	Therap. conc.	
		CHF	0.8-1.5 ng/mL
		Arrhythmias	1.5-2.0
		Toxic conc.	
		Child	>2.5
		Adult	>3.0
Dihydrotestosterone (DHT)	Serum	Prepubertal	<3.5 ng/dL
		Pubertal	**M** **F**
		stage I:	<10 <10
		II:	<20 <15
		III:	<35 <25
		IV-V:	<75 <25
		Adult:	60-300 10-40
Eosinophil count	Whole blood, capillary blood		50-350 cells/mm^3 (μL)
Erythrocyte (RBC) count	Whole blood	Cord	3.9-5.5 million/mm^3
		1-3 days	4.0-6.6
		1 wk	3.9-6.3
		2 wk	3.0-5.4
		2 mo	2.7-4.9
		3-6 mo	3.1-4.5
		0.5-2 yr	3.7-5.3
		2-6 yr	3.9-5.3
		6-12 yr	4.0-5.2
		12-18 yr: Male	4.5-5.3
		Female	4.1-5.1
Erythrocyte sedimentation rate (ESR)	Whole blood		
Westergren (modified)		Child	0-10 mm/hr
		<50 yr: Male	0-15
		Female	0-20
Wintrobe		Child	0-13
		Adult: Male	0-9
		Female	0-20
ZETA			41%-54%

Continued.

Common Laboratory Tests—cont'd

TEST	SPECIMEN	AGE/SEX	NORMAL VALUE
Erythropoietin			
RIA	Serum		<5-20 mU/mL
Hemagglutination			25-125
Bioassay			5-18
Estradiol	Serum or	Male, pubertal	
	plasma	stage I:	2-8 pg/mL
	(heparin or	II:	11
	EDTA)	III:	>20
		Adult, Male	8-36
		Female, pubertal	
		stage I:	0-23
		II:	0-66
		III:	0-105
		IV:	20-300
		Follicular	10-90
		Midcycle	100-500
		Luteal	50-240
		Urine, 24 hr	0-6 µg/d
		Adult, Male	
		Female	
		Follicular:	0-3
		Ovulatory peak:	4-14
		Luteal:	4-10
Estrogens, total	Serum	Child:	<30 pg/ml
		Male	40-115
		Female, cycle—days	
		1-10 days	61-394
		11-20 days	122-437
		21-30 days	156-350
		Prepubertal	≤40
	Urine, 24 hr	Child	1.0 (mean) µg/d
		Male, pubertal	
		Stage I:	2.5 (mean) µ/d
		II:	5.9 (mean)
		III:	6.2 (mean)
		Adult, Male:	5-25
		Female, Preovulation	5-25
		Ovulation	28-100
		Luteal peak	22-80
		Pregnancy	<45,000
Ethanol	Whole blood	Toxic conc.	50-100 mg/dL
	(oxalate),	Depression of CNS	>100
	serum		
Ethosuximide	Serum, plasma	Therap. conc.	40-100 µg/mL
		Toxic conc.	>150
Fat, fecal	Feces (72 hr)	Infant, breast-fed	<1 g/d
		0-6 yr	<2
		Adult	<7
Fatty acids, free	Serum or	Adult	8-25 mg/dL
	plasma	Children and obese adults	<31
Fetal hemoglobin, see hemoglobin F			
α_1-Fetoprotein	Serum	Adult	<40 ng/mL
		Mean	2.6 ± 1.6 (1 SD) ng/mL
		Fetal	peak of 200-400 mg/dL in first trimester
		1 yr.	<30 ng/mL
			±2

TEST	SPECIMEN	AGE/SEX	NORMAL VALUE	
α_1-Fetoprotein (cont'd)		weeks	median mg/dL	log SD
	Amniotic fluid	11-12	24	10-50
		13-14	23	13-41
		15-16	18	9-35
		17-18	15	6-33
		19-20	10	5-25
		21-25	7	4-14
		26-30	6	3-10
		31-35	2	0.5-7
		36-40	1	0.2-3
Fibrinogen	Plasma	Newborn	125-300 mg/dL	
		Thereafter	200-400	
Folate	Serum	Newborn	7.0-32 ng/mL	
		Thereafter	1.8-9	
	Erythrocytes		150-450 ng/mL cells	
Follicle stimulating hormone (hFSH)	Serum or plasma (heparin)	Birth-1 yr, Male	(IRP-2-hMG)	
		Female	<1-12 mU/mL	
		1-8 yr, Male	<1-20	
		Female	<1-6	
		9-10 yr, Male	<1-4	
		Female	<1-10	
		11-12 yr, Male	2-8	
		Female	2-12	
		13-14 yr, Male	3-11	
		Female	3-15	
		Adult, Male	3-15	
		Female	4-25 mU/mL	
		Premenopausal:	4-30	
		Midcycle peak:	10-90	
		Pregnancy:	Low to undetectable	
Galactose	Serum	Newborn	0-20 mg/dL	
		Thereafter	<5	
	Urine	Newborn	≤60 mg/dL	
		Thereafter	<14	
Glucose	Serum	Cord	45-96 mg/dL	
		Premature	20-60	
		Neonate	30-60	
		Newborn, 1 day	40-60	
		Newborn, >1 day	50-90	
		Child	60-100	
		Thereafter	70-105	
	Blood	Thereafter	65-95 mg/dL	
	CSF	Adult	40-70 mg/dL	
	Urine (quantitative)		<0.5 g/d	
	(qualitative)		Negative	
Glucose, 2 hr postprandial	Serum		<120 mg/dL	
			Diabetes: see glucose tolerance test, oral	
Glucose tolerance test (GTT, oral)	Serum	Dosages Adult: 75 g		
		Child: 1.75 g/kg of ideal weight up to maximum of 75 g		

Time	Normal	Diabetic
Fasting	70-105	>115
60 min	120-170	≥200
90 min	100-140	≥200
120 min	70-120	≥140

Continued.

Common Laboratory Tests—cont'd

TEST	SPECIMEN	AGE/SEX	NORMAL VALUE
Growth hormone (hGH, Somatotropin)	Plasma Fasting, at rest	Cord Newborn Child Adult: Male Female	10-50 ng/mL 10-40 <5 <5 <8
Hematocrit (HCT, Hct)	Whole blood	1 day (cap) 2 days 3 days 2 mo 6-12 yr 12-18 yr: Male Female	48%-69% 48%-75% 44%-72% 28%-42% 35%-45% 37%-49% 36%-46%
Hemoglobin (Hb)	Whole blood	1-3 days (cap) 2 mo 6-12 yr 12-18 yr: Male Female	14.5-22.5 g/dL 9.0-14.0 11.5-15.5 13.0-16.0 12.0-16.0
Hemoglobin A	Whole blood		>95% of total
Hemoglobin F	Whole blood	1 day 5 days 3 wk 6-9 wk 3-4 mo 6 mo Adult	77.0% ± 7.3% HbF 76.8% ± 5.8% 70.0% ± 7.3% 52.9% ± 11.0% 23.2% ± 16.0% 4.7% ± 2.2% <2.0%
17-Hydroxycorticosteroids (17-OHCS)	Urine, 24 hr	0-1 yr Child Adult, Male Female	0.5-1.0 mg/d 1.0-5.6 3.0-10.0 2.0-8.0 or: 3-7 mg/g creatinine
17-Hydroxyprogesterone (17-OHP)	Serum	Male Pubertal stage I: Adult: Female Pubertal stage I: Follicular: Luteal: Postmenopausal:	 0.1-0.3 ng/mL 0.2-1.8 0.2-0.5 0.2-0.8 0.8-3.0 0.04-0.5
Immunoglobulin A (IgA)	Serum	Cord Newborn 1/2-6 mo 6 mo-2 yr 2-6 yr 6-12 yr 12-16 yr Thereafter	0-5 mg/dL 0-2.2 3-82 14-108 23-190 29-270 81-232 60-380
Immunoglobulin D (IgD)	Serum	Newborn Thereafter	None detected 0-8 mg/dL
Immunoglobulin E (IgE)	Serum	Male Female	0-230 IU/mL 0-170
Immunoglobulin G (IgG)	Serum	Cord Newborn 1/2-6 mo 6 mo-2 yr 2-6 yr 6-12 yr 12-16 yr Adults (higher in Blacks)	760-1700 mg/dL 700-1480 300-1000 500-1200 500-1300 700-1650 700-1550 600-1600
Immunoglobulin M (IgM)	Serum	Cord Newborn 1/2-6 mo 6 mo-2 yr	4-24 mg/dL 5-30 15-109 43-239

TEST	SPECIMEN	AGE/SEX	NORMAL VALUE
Immunoglobulin M (IgM) (cont'd)		2-6 yr	50-199 mg/dL
		6-12 yr	50-260
		12-16 yr	45-240
		Thereafter	40-345
		Results vary with std. preparation	
Insulin (12 hr fasting)	Serum or plasma (no anti-coagulant)	Newborn	3-20 μU/mL
		Thereafter	7-24
Iron	Serum	Newborn	100-250 μg/dL
		Infant	40-100
		Child	50-120
		Thereafter: Male	50-160
		Female	40-150
		Intoxicated child	280-2550
		Fatally poisoned child	>1800
Iron-binding capacity, total (TIBC)	Serum	Infant	100-400 μg/dL
		Thereafter	250-400
17-Ketogenic steroids (17-KGS)	Urine, 24 hr	0-1 yr	<1.0 mg/d
		1-10 yr	<5
		11-14 yr	<12
		Thereafter, Male	5-23
		Female	3-15
Ketone bodies			
Qualitative	Serum		Negative
	Urine, random		Negative
Quantitative	Serum		0.5-3.0 mg/dL
17-Ketosteroids (17-KS), total Zimmerman reaction	Urine, 24 hr	14 days-2 yr	<1 mg/d
		2-6 yr	<2
		6-10 yr	1-4
		10-12 yr	1-6
		12-14 yr	3-10
		14-16 yr	5-12
		Thereafter	
		Male, 18-30 yr	9-22
		Male, >30 yr	8-20
		Female	6-15
			Decreases with age
Chromatography	Urine, 24 hr	Adult, Male	5.0-12.0
		Female	3.0-10.0
Lactate	Whole blood (heparin)	Venous	0.5-2.2 mmol/L
		Arterial	0.5-1.6
		Inpatients,	
		Venous	0.9-1.7
		Arterial	<1.25
Lead	Whole blood	Child	<30 μg/dL
		Adult	<40
		Acceptable for industrial exposure	<60
		Toxic	≥100
	Urine, 24 hr		<80 μg/L
Leukocyte count (WBC)	Whole blood		× **1000 cell/mm³ (μL)**
		Birth	9.0-30.0
		24 hr	9.4-34.0
		1 mo	5.0-19.5
		1-3 yr	6.0-17.5
		4-7 yr	5.5-15.5
		8-13 yr	4.5-13.5
		Adult	4.5-11.0
	CSF		× **1000 cells/mm³ (μL)**
		Premature	0-25 mononuclear
			0-100 polymorphonuclear
			0-1000 RBC

Continued.

Common Laboratory Tests—cont'd

TEST	SPECIMEN	AGE/SEX		NORMAL VALUE	
Leukocyte count (WBC) (cont'd.)		Newborn		0-20 mononuclear 0-70 polymorphonuclear 0-800 RBC	
		Neonate		0-5 mononuclear 0-25 polymorphonuclear 0-50 RBC	
		Thereafter		0-5 mononuclear	
Leukocyte differential count	Whole blood	Myelocytes	0%	0	Cells/mm^3 (μL)
		Neutrophils—"bands"	3%-5%	150-400	
		Neutrophils—"segs"	54%-62%	3000-5800	
		Lymphocytes	25%-33%	1500-3000	
		Monocytes	3%-7%	285-500	
		Eosinophils	1%-3%	50-250	
		Basophils	0.075%	15-50	
Lysergic acid diethylamine	Plasma Urine	After hallucinogenic dose:		0.005-0.009 μg/mL 0.001-0.050	
Magnesium	Serum	Newborn, 2-4 days		1.2-1.8 mEq/L	
		5 mo-6 yr		1.65 $\pm$ 0.23 (2 SD)	
		6-12 yr		1.56 $\pm$ 0.18	
		12-20 yr		1.56 $\pm$ 0.21	
		Adult		1.3-2.1 (Higher in females during menses)	
Mean corpuscular hemoglobin (MCH)	Whole blood	Birth		31-37 pg/cell	
		1-3 days (cap)		31-37	
		1 wk-1 mo		28-40	
		2 mo		26-34	
		3-6 mo		25-35	
		0.5-2 yr		23-31	
		2-6 yr		24-30	
		6-12 yr		25-33	
		12-18 yr		25-35	
		18-49 yr		26-34	
Mean corpuscular hemoglobin concentration (MCHC)	Whole blood	Birth		30%-36% Hb/cell or g Hb/dL RBC	
		1-3 days (cap)		29%-37%	
		1-2 wk		28%-38%	
		1-2 mo		29%-37%	
		3 mo-2 yr		30%-36%	
		2-18 yr		31%-37%	
		>18 yr		31%-37%	
Mean corpuscular volume (MCV)	Whole blood	1-3 days (cap)		95-121 μm^3	
		0.5-2 yr		70-86	
		6-12 yr		77-95	
		12-18 yr: Male		78-98	
		Female		78-102	
Methemoglobin (MetHb)	Whole blood			0.06-0.24 g/dL or 0.78% $\pm$ 0.37% of total Hb	
Myoglobin	Serum Urine, random			6-85 ng/mL Negative	
Niacin (nicotinic acid)	Urine, 24 hr			0.3-1.5 mg/d	
Occult blood	Feces, random			Negative (<2 mL blood/d in ~100-200 g stool)	
	Urine, random			Negative	
Osmolality	Serum Urine, random	Child, Adult		275-295 mOsmol/kg H_2O 50-1400 mOsmol/kg H_2O, depending on fluid intake. After 12 hr fluid restriction: >850 mOsmol/kg H_2O	
	Urine, 24 hr			$\simeq$300-900 mOsmol/kg H_2O	
Oxygen, partial pressure (Po$_2$)	Whole blood, arterial	Birth		8-24 mm Hg	
		5-10 min		33-75	
		30 min		31-85	
		>1 hr		55-80	
		1 day		45-95	
		Thereafter (Decreased with age)		83-108	

TEST	SPECIMEN	AGE/SEX	NORMAL VALUE
Oxygen saturation	Whole blood, arterial	Newborn	40%-90%
		Thereafter	95%-99%
Paraldehyde	Serum, plasma	Therap. conc.	
		Sedation	10-100 μg/mL
		Anesthesia	>200
		Toxic conc.	20-40
		Lethal conc.	>50
Partial thromboplastin time (PTT)	Whole blood (Na citrate)		
Nonactivated			60-85 s (Platelin)
Activated			25-35 s (differs with method)
pH	Whole blood, arterial	Premature (48 hr)	7.35-7.50
		Birth, full term	7.11-7.36
		5-10 min	7.09-7.30
		30 min	7.21-7.38
		>1 hr	7.26-7.49
		1 day	7.29-7.45
		Thereafter	7.35-7.45
		Must be corrected for body temperature	
	Urine, random	Newborn/neonate	5-7
		Thereafter (average≃6)	4.5-8
	Stool		7.0-7.5
Phenacetin	Plasma	Therap. conc.	1-20 μg/mL
		Toxic conc.	50-250
Phenobarbital	Serum, plasma	Therap. conc.	15-40 μg/mL
		Toxic conc.	
		Slowness, ataxia, nystagmus	35-80
		Coma with reflexes	65-117
		Coma without reflexes	>100
Phenylalanine	Serum	Premature	2.0-7.5 mg/dL
		Newborn	1.2-3.4
		Thereafter	0.8-1.8
	Urine, 24 hr	10 days-2 wk	1-2 mg/d
		3-12 yr	4-18 mg/d
		Thereafter	trace-17 mg/d or: 6 ± 2 mg/g creatinine
Phenylpyruvic acid, qualitative	Urine, fresh random		Negative by FeCl$_3$ test
Phenytoin	Serum, plasma (heparin, EDTA); collect at steady-state trough conc.	Therap. conc.	10-20 μg/mL
		Toxic conc.	>20
Phospholipids, total	Serum or plasma (EDTA)	Newborn	75-170 mg/dL
		Infant	100-275
		Child	180-295
		Adult	125-275
Phosphorus, inorganic	Serum	Cord	3.7-8.1 mg/dL
		Premature (1 wk)	5.4-10.9
		Newborn	4.3-9.3
		Child	4.5-6.5
		Thereafter	3.0-4.5
Plasma volume	Plasma	Male	25-43 mL/kg
		Female	28-45

Continued.

Common Laboratory Tests—cont'd

TEST	SPECIMEN	AGE/SEX	NORMAL VALUE
Platelet count (thrombocyte count)	Whole blood (EDTA)	Newborn (After 1 wk, same as adult)	$84\text{-}478 \times 10^3/mm^3$ (μL)
		Adult	$150\text{-}400 \times 10^3 mm^3$ (μL)
Potassium	Serum	Newborn	3.9-5.9 mmol/L
		Infant	4.1-5.3
		Child	3.4-4.7
		Thereafter	3.5-5.1
	Plasma (heparin)		3.5-4.5
	Urine, 24 hr		2.5-125 mmol/d varies with diet
Primidone	Serum, plasma (heparin)	Therap. conc.	5-12 μg/mL
		Toxic conc.	>15
Progesterone	Serum	Male	
		Pubertal stage I:	0.11-0.26 ng/mL
		Adult:	0.12-0.3
		Female	
		Pubertal stage I:	0-0.3
		II:	0-0.46
		III:	0-0.6
		IV:	0.05-13.0
		Follicular:	0.02-0.9
		Luteal:	6.0-30.0
Protein			
Total	Serum	Premature	4.3-7.6 g/dL
		Newborn	4.6-7.4
		Child	6.2-8.0
		Adult, recumbent	6.0-7.8
			~0.5 g higher in ambulatory patients

Electrophoresis

	g/dL Albumin	α_1-Globulin	α_2-Globulin	β-Globulin	γ-Globulin
Premature	3.0-4.2	0.1-0.5	0.3-0.7	0.3-1.2	0.3-1.4
Newborn	3.6-5.4	0.1-0.3	0.3-0.5	0.2-0.6	0.2-1.0
Infant	4.0-5.0	0.2-0.4	0.5-0.8	0.5-0.8	0.3-1.2
Thereafter	3.5-5.0	0.2-0.3	0.4-1.0	0.5-1.1	0.7-1.2
					Higher in blacks

TEST	SPECIMEN	AGE/SEX	NORMAL VALUE
Total	Urine, 24 hr		1-14 mg/dL
			50-80 mg/d (at rest)
			<250 mg/d after intense exercise
Total	CSF		Lumbar: 8-32 mg/dL
Prothrombin (PT)			
One-stage (Quick)	Whole blood (Na citrate)	In general	11-15 s (varies with type of thromboplastin)
		Newborn	Prolonged by 2-3 sec
Two-stage modifier (Ware and Seegers)	Whole blood (Na citrate)		18-22 sec
RBC count, see erythrocyte count			
Red cell volume	Whole blood	Male	20-36 mL/kg
		Female	19-31 mL/kg
Renin (renin activity, plasma; PRA)	Plasma	2-4 yr	2.37 ± 0.57 (1 SE) ng/mL/H
		5-6 yr	1.48 ± 0.17
		7-9 yr	2.13 ± 0.44
		10-11 yr	1.96 ± 0.36
		14-15 yr	1.18 ± 0.28
		16-17 yr	1.08 ± 0.25
		Normal sodium diet:	
		Supine:	1.6 ± 1.5
		Standing (4 hr):	4.5 ± 2.9
		Low sodium:	
		Supine:	3.2 ± 1.1
		Standing (4 hr):	9.9 ± 4.3

TEST	SPECIMEN	AGE/SEX	NORMAL VALUE	
Reticulocyte count	Whole blood	Adults	0.5%-1.5% of erythrocytes or 25,000-75,000/mm³ (μL)	
	Capillary	1 day	3.2% ± 1.4%	
		7 days	0.5% ± 0.4%	
		1-4 wk	0.6% ± 0.3%	
		5-6 wk	1.0% ± 0.7%	
		7-8 wk	1.5% ± 0.7%	
		9-10 wk	1.2% ± 0.7%	
		11-12 wk	0.7% ± 0.3%	
Riboflavin (vitamin B₂)	Urine, random, fasting	1-3 yr	500-900 μg/g creatinine	
		4-6 yr	300-600	
		7-9 yr	270-500	
		10-15 yr	200-400	
		Adult	80-269	
Salicylates	Serum, plasma	Therap. conc.	15-30 mg/dL	
		Toxic conc.	>30	
Sediment	Urine, fresh random			
Casts		Hyaline	Occasional (0-1) casts/hpf	
		RBC	Not seen	
		WBC	Not seen	
		Tubular epithelial	Not seen	
		Transitional and squamous epithelial	Not seen	
Cells		RBC	0-2/hpf	
		WBC		
		Males	0-3/hpf	
		Females and children	0-5/hpf	
		Epithelial	Few; more frequent in newborn	
		Bacterial, unspun spun	No organisms/oil immersion field <20 organisms/hpf	
Sedimentation rate, see erythrocyte sedimentation rate				
Sodium	Serum or plasma	Newborn	136-146 mmol/L	
		Infant	139-146	
		Child	138-145	
		Thereafter	136-146 40-220 (diet-dependent)	
	Urine, 24 hr		10-40 mmol/L	
	Sweat	Cystic fibrosis	>70	

			M	F
Somatomedin C	Plasma	Vary with laboratory, e.g., Nichols Institute		
		0-2 yr	0.10-0.72	0.10-1.7 × 1000 U/mL
		3-5 yr	0.12-1.5	0.15-2.3
		6-10 yr	0.19-2.2	0.44-3.6
		11-12 yr	0.22-3.6	1.50-6.9
		13-14 yr	0.79-5.5	0.81-7.4
		15-17 yr	0.76-3.3	0.59-3.1
		18-64 yr	0.34-1.9	0.45-2.2
		Endocrine Sciences		
		Cord	0.25-0.66	
		0-1 yr	0.17-0.62	
		1-5 yr	0.14-0.94	
		6-12 yr	0.87-2.06	
		13-17 yr	1.35-3.00	
		18-25 yr	0.92-2.06	
		Thereafter	0.70-2.04	

Continued.

Common Laboratory Tests—cont'd

TEST	SPECIMEN	AGE/SEX	NORMAL VALUE
Specific gravity	Urine, random	Adult	1.002-1.030
		After 12 hr fluid restriction	>1.025
	Urine, 24 hr		1.015-1.025
Testosterone, total	Serum	Prepubertal	
		Male	6.6 ± 2.5 ng/dL
		Female	6.6 ± 2.5
		Adult	
		Male	572 ± 135
		Female	37 ± 10
Theophylline	Serum, plasma (heparin, EDTA)	Therap. conc.	
		Bronchodilator	8-20 μg/mL
		Prem. apnea	6-13
		Toxic. conc.	>20
Thiamin (vitamin B₁)	Serum	0-2.0 μg/dL	
	Urine, acidify with HCl	1-3 yr	176-200 μg/g creatinine
		4-6 yr	121-400
		7-9 yr	181-350
		10-12 yr	181-300
		13-15 yr	151-250
		Thereafter	66-129
Thrombin time	Whole blood (Na citrate)		Control time ± 2 sec when control is 9-13 sec
Thyroxine, total (T₄)	Serum	Cord	8-13 μg/dL
		Newborn	11.5-24 (lower in low-birth-weight infants)
		Neonate	9-18
		Infant	7-15
		1-5 yr	7.3-15
		5-10 yr	6.4-13.3
		Thereafter	5-12
		Newborn screen (filter paper)	6.2-22
Tourniquet test (capillary fragility)			<5-10 petechiae in 2.5 cm circle on forearm (halfway between systolic and diastolic pressure for 5 min); 0.8 petechiae in 6 cm circle (50 torr for 15 min); 10-20 petechiae in 5 cm circle (80 mm Hg)

TEST	SPECIMEN	AGE/SEX	M	F
Triglycerides (TG)	Serum, after ≥ 12 hr fast	Cord blood	10-98	10-98 mg/dL
		0-5 yr	30-86	32-99
		6-11 yr	31-108	35-114
		12-15 yr	36-138	41-138
		16-19 yr	40-163	40-128

TEST	SPECIMEN	AGE/SEX	NORMAL VALUE
Triiodothyronine, free	Serum	Cord	130 ± 10(SE) mean pg/dL
		1-3 days	410 ± 20
		6 wk	400 ± 20
		Adults (20-50 yr)	230-660 pg/dL
Triiodothyronine, total (T₃-RIA)	Serum	Cord	30-70 ng/dL
		Newborn	75-260
		1-5 yr	100-260
		5-10 yr	90-240
		10-15 yr	80-210
		Thereafter	115-190
Urea nitrogen	Serum, plasma	Cord	21-40 mg/dL
		Premature (1 wk)	3-25
		Newborn	3-12
		Infant/child	5-18
		Thereafter	7-18

TEST	SPECIMEN	AGE/SEX	NORMAL VALUE
Uric acid			
Phosphotungstate	Serum	Newborn	2.0-6.2 mg/dL
		Adults: Male	4.5-8.2
		Female	3.0-6.5
Uricase		Child	2.0-5.5 mg/dL
		Adults: Male	3.5-7.2
		Female	2.6-6.0
Urine volume	Urine, 24 hr	Newborn	50-300 mL/d
		Infant	350-550
		Child	500-1000
		Adolescent	700-1400
		Thereafter: Male	800-1800
		Female	600-1600
			(varies with intake and other factors)
Valproic acid	Serum, plasma	Therap. conc.	50-100 μg/mL
		Toxic conc.	>100
Vanillylmandelic acid	Urine, 24 hr	Newborn	<1.0 mg/d
(Vanilmandelic acid)		Infant	<2.0
		Child	1-3
		Adolescent	1-5
		Thereafter	2-7
		or: 1.5-7 μg/mg	
		creatinine	
Vitamin A	Serum	Newborn	35-75 μg/dL
		Child	30-80
		Thereafter	30-65
WBC, see leukocyte			

Appendix E   Resources for Families and Health Care Professionals

GENERAL RESOURCES: CHILD HEALTH AND SPECIAL SERVICES*

American Academy of Pediatrics
Publications Dept.
P.O. Box 927
141 Northwest Point Rd.
Elk Grove Village, IL 60007

American Dietetic Association
430 N. Michigan Ave.
Chicago, IL 60611

American Hospital Association
Dept. of Order Processing
840 N. Lakeshore Dr.
Chicago, IL 60611

American Institute of Family Relations
4942 Vineland Ave.
North Hollywood, CA 91601

Association of Birth Defects in Children
3201 E. Crystal Lake Ave.
Orlando, FL 32806

Association for the Care of Children's Health
3615 Wisconsin Ave., N.W.
Washington, DC 20016

Association for Children with Syndromes, Inc.
2612 Martin Ave.
Bellmore, NY 11710

The Association for Neurometabolic Disease
2707 Cheltenham Rd.
Toledo, OH 43606

Boys Town
Communications & Public Service Division
Father Flanagan's Boys' Home
Boys Town, NE 68010

Canadian Institute of Child Health
17 York St.
Ottawa, Ontario K1N 5S7

Centering Corp.
P.O. Box 3367
Omaha, NE 68103-0367

Children's Defense Fund
122 C St., N.W., Suite 400
Washington, DC 20001

Children in Hospitals
31 Wilshire Park
Needham, MA 02192

Child Welfare League of America
440 First St., N.W.
Washington, DC 20001
    or
67 Irving Pl.
New York, NY 10003

Closer Look/Parents Campaign for
    Handicapped Children and Youth
1201 16th St., N.W.
Washington, DC 20036

Federation for Children with Special Needs, Inc.
120 Boylston St., Suite 338
Boston, MA 02116

Government Printing Office
Superintendent of Documents
Washington, DC 20402

Hereditary Disease Foundation
9701 Wilshire Blvd.
Beverly Hills, CA 90212

Human Resources Center
I. V. Willets Rd.
Albertson, NY 11507

March of Dimes Birth Defects Foundation
1275 Mamaroneck Ave.
White Plains, NY 10605

Mead Johnson
Nutritional Division
2404 W. Pennsylvania St.
Evansville, IN 46285

Medic-Alert Foundation
P.O. Box 1009
Turlock, CA 95380

Medic-Alert Foundation International
2323 Colorado Ave.
Turlock, CA 95380

National Center for Education in
    Maternal and Child Health
3520 Prospect St., N.W.
Washington, DC 20057

National Center for Health Statistics
Dept. of Health and Human Services
Public Health Service
3700 East-West Highway
Hyattsville, MD 20782

National Child Nutrition Project
101 N. 33rd St.
Philadelphia, PA 19104

National Dairy Council
6300 N. River Rd.
Rosemont, IL 60018-4233

National Easter Seal Society for Crippled Children
2023 W. Ogden Ave.
Chicago, IL 60612

National Foundation for Jewish Genetic Diseases, Inc.
250 Park Ave., Suite 1000
New York, NY 10177

National Genetics Foundation
555 W. 57th St.
New York, NY 10019

*Organizations serving the needs of children and families with specific disorders are listed as appropriate throughout the text.

National Health Safety Awareness Center
333 N. Michigan Ave.
Chicago, IL 60601

The National Information System for
    Health Related Services
University of South Carolina
1244 Blossom St.
Columbia, SC 29208

National Institutes of Child Health and
    Human Development
Building 31, Room 2A-32
9000 Rockville Pike
Bethesda, MD 20205

National Institutes of Marriage & Family Relations
6116 Rolling Rd., Suite 316
Springfield, VA 22152

National Mental Health Association
1021 Prince St.
Alexandria, VA 22341-2971

National Rehabilitation Association
633 S. Washington St.
Alexandria, VA 22314

National Safety Council
444 N. Michigan Ave.
Chicago, IL 60611

Nutrition Action–Center for Service
    in the Public Interest
1755 S St., N.W.
Washington, DC 20009

Office of Consumer Information
1009 Premier Building
Washington, DC 20201

Office of Disease Prevention and Health Promotion
300 Seventh St., N.W., Room 613
Washington, DC 20201

Office of Human Development Services
HDS/OPA Printing and Distribution Management Branch
Hubert H. Humphrey Building, Room 350 G
220 Independence Ave., S.W.
Washington, DC 20201

Pediatric Projects
P.O. Box 1880
Santa Monica, CA 90406

"Plain Talk" and "Caring about Kids" Series
U.S. Dept. of Health and Human Services
Public Health Service
Alcohol, Drug Abuse, and Mental Health Administration
5600 Fishers Lane
Rockville, MD 20857

Public Affairs Pamphlets
381 Park Ave. S.
New York, NY 10016

Reaching Out: A Directory of Voluntary Organizations in
    Maternal and Child Health
National Center for Education in Maternal and Child Health
38th and R Sts., N.W.
Washington, DC 20057

Ross Laboratories
Division Abbott Laboratories
Creative Services and Information
625 N. Cleveland Ave.
Columbus, OH 43216

Sarah K. Davidson Family–Patient Health Education Library
Strong Children's Medical Center
University of Rochester Medical Center
P.O. Box 777
601 Elmwood Ave.
Rochester, NY 14642

SKIP (Sick Kids need Involved People)
216 Newport Dr.
Severna Park, MD 21146

Source Book Publications
(National directory of products/services for disabled)
P.O. Box 1586
Winter Park, FL 32789

U.S. Consumer Product Safety Commission
1111 18th St., N.W.
Washington, DC 20207

U.S. Department of Agriculture
Office of Public Information
Food and Nutrition Service
3101 Park Center Dr.
Alexandria, VA 22302

U.S. House of Representatives
Select Committee on Children, Youth, and Families
H2-385, House Office Building Annex 2
Washington, DC 20515

Wyeth Laboratories
P.O. Box 8299
Philadelphia, PA 19101

NATIONAL CLEARINGHOUSES

Arthritis Information Clearinghouse
P.O. Box 9782
Arlington, VA 22209

Cancer Information Clearinghouse
National Cancer Institute
Office of Cancer Communications
Building 31, Room 10A-18
9000 Rockville Pike
Bethesda, MD 20892

Clearinghouse on Child Abuse and Neglect
P.O. Box 1182
Washington, DC 20013

Clearinghouse on the Handicapped
Switzer Building, Room 3132
330 C St., S.W.
Washington, DC 20202

Consumer Information Center
P.O. Box 100
Pueblo, CO 81002

Food and Drug Administration
Office of Consumer Affairs
5600 Fishers Lane
Rockville, MD 20857

Food and Nutrition Information Center
National Agricultural Library Building, Room 304
Beltsville, MD 20705

Health Information Resources
National Health Information Clearinghouse
P.O. Box 1133
Washington, DC 20013

High Blood Pressure Information Center
120/80 National Institutes of Health
Bethesda, MD 20892

National Clearinghouse for Alcohol Information
P.O. Box 2345
Rockville, MD 20857

National Clearinghouse for Drug Abuse Information
P.O. Box 416
Kensington, MD 20795

National Clearinghouse for Family Planning Information
P.O. Box 12921
Arlington, VA 22209

National Health Information Clearinghouse ''Healthfinder''
P.O. Box 1133
Washington, DC 20013-1133

National Clearinghouse for Mental Health Information
Public Inquiries Section
5600 Fishers Lane, Room 15C-17
Rockville, MD 20857

National Diabetes Information Clearinghouse
Box NDIC
Bethesda, MD 20892

National Digestive Diseases Education and
    Information Clearinghouse
1255 23rd St., N.W., Suite 275
Washington, DC 20037

National Health Information Clearinghouse
P.O. Box 1133
Washington, DC 20013-1133

National Highway Traffic Safety Administration
NES-11 HL
U.S. Department of Transportation
400 7th St., S.W.
Washington, DC 20590

National Information Center for Handicapped
    Children and Youth
P.O. Box 1492
Washington, DC 20013

National Injury Information Clearinghouse
5401 Westbard Ave., Room 625
Washington, DC 20207

National Institute of Mental Health
Public Inquiries Branch
Parklawn Building, Room 15C-05
5600 Fishers Lane
Rockville, MD 20857

National Library Service for the
    Blind and Physically Handicapped
Library of Congress
Washington, DC 20542

National Maternal and Child Health Clearinghouse
3520 Prospect St., N.W., Ground Floor
Washington, DC 20057

National Rehabilitation Information Center
4407 8th St., N.E.
Washington, DC 20017

National Self-Help Clearinghouse
33 W. 42nd St., Room 1210
New York, NY 10036

Office of Cancer Communications
National Cancer Institute
Cancer Information Service
Building 31, Room 10A-18
9000 Rockville Pike
Bethesda, MD 20892

Office on Smoking and Health
Technical Information Center
Park Building, Room 1-10
5600 Fishers Lane
Rockville, MD 20857

President's Council on Physical Fitness and Sports
450 5th St., N.W., Suite 7103
Washington, DC 20001

Self-Help Center
1600 Dodge Ave., Suite S-122
Evanston, IL 60201

Sudden Infant Death Syndrome Clearinghouse
8201 Greensboro Dr., Suite 600
McLean, VA 22102

Westchester Self-Help Clearinghouse
Westchester Community College
75 Grosslands Rd.
Valhalla, NY 10595

Index

School experience, 716-717, 730
  adolescent and, 819; *see also* Adolescent
School health, 729-731
School history, 204
School nursing services, 742-743
School phobia, 793-794
  child with special needs and, 949
School vision, definition of, 1025
School-age child, 703-801
  age profiles of, 718-729
  altered body image in, 971
  anticipatory guidance of family of, 746-747
  attention deficit disorder and, 786-790
  behavioral disorders of, 786-798
  biologic development of, 704-706
  body image development of, 709-710
  burn hazards and, 1217
  child with special needs and, 949-950
  chronic illness or disability and, 935-936
  cognitive development of, 708-709
  communication and, 194
  concerns related to normal growth and
      development of, 716-733
  conversion reaction and, 795-796
  death and, 958
  dental health and, 738-740
  dental problems and, 752-755
  depression in, 796-797
  divorce and, 86
  encopresis and, 792-793
  enuresis and, 790-792
  health behavior and, 734-735
  height and weight gain of, 105
  injury prevention and, 743-746
  Kohlberg moral development of, 710
  Lyme disease and, 785-786
  malocclusion and, 754
  neurofibromatosis of, 784-785
  nutrition and, 735
  peptic ulcer in, 1435
  periodontal disease and, 753-754
  physical activity and, 736-738
  physical examination of, 221
  preparing for procedure of, 1106
  promoting optimum growth and
      development of, 704-733
  promoting optimum health for, 733-747
  psychosocial development of, 706-708
  recurrent abdominal pain and, 794-795
  resting heart rates of, 1505
  schizophrenia and, 797
  school health and, 741-743
  school phobia and, 793-794
    child with special needs and, 949
  separation anxiety and, 1056
  sex education and, 740-741
  skin disorders of, 755-767
    animal bites and, 782-784
    bacterial, 767-768
    cat scratch disease and, 784
    chemical or physical contacts in, 771-777
    clinical manifestations of, 758-761
    cold injury and, 776-777
    congenital, 786
    contact dermatitis in, 773-775
    dermatophytoses in, 768-771
    diagnosis of, 761
    drug reactions in, 775
    foreign bodies in, 777
    fungal infection of, 768-771
    human bites and, 784
    infections in, 767-771
    insect and animal contacts in, 777-784
    insect stings in, 780-782
    nursing considerations in, 762-767
    pathophysiology of, 758

School-age child—continued
  skin disorders of—continued
    pediculosis capitis and, 778-780
    poison ivy, oak, and sumac, 774-775
    rickettsial, 771, 773
    scabies, 778
    structure and function of skin in, 756-758
    sunburn, 775-776
    therapy for, 761-762
    trauma in, 777
    viral, 768, 769
  sleep and rest and, 735-738
  social development of, 711-716
  specific learning disability and, 790
  spiritual development of, 710-711
  stress and, 1054
  summary of growth and development in,
      716, 718-729
  systemic mycotic infections and, 771-772
  temperament of, 716
  trauma to teeth and, 755
Sclera, 242
Scolding, toddler and, 608
Scoliosis, 260, 276, 1758-1766
  nursing care summary of, 1764-1765
  surgery and, 1763
Scoliosis Association, 1764
Scoliosis Research Society, 1764
Scorpions, 782
Scout film, 1254
Scratches, 777
Screening
  for disease, 170, 273, 320
  for epidemiologic information, 171
  genetic, 170-172
  for metabolic disease in newborn, 320
  for reproductive information, 170
  of school children for scoliosis, 1764
Scrotum, 273
  adolescence and disorders of, 861
  hernia and, 270
Scurvy, 551-552
Seasonal allergic rhinitis, 1375
Seat restraints, 538, 618, 1796
Sebaceous glands, 242, 296, 757, 809, 836
Seborrheic dermatitis, 574
Sebum, 757
Secobarbital, 912
Second heart sound, 266, 267, 311
Secondary amenorrhea, 863
Secondary circular reaction, 504
Secondary group, culture and, 27
Secondary sex characteristics, 804, 808, 809, 813
Second-degree burn, 1218-1219, 1220
Second-voided specimens, 1716-1717
Secretion
  of antidiuretic hormone, inappropriate,
      1634, 1686
  renal, 1249
Secretory cell, 1408
Security, need for, 138
Sedation
  Crohn disease and, 1434
  dosage of, 1130
  hazard of, asthma and, 1387
  rectal administration of, 1139
  Reye syndrome and, 1656
  tomography and, 1631
Seductiveness, 691
Seesaw respirations, 263
Seizure, 1657-1671
  absence, 1661
  acute renal failure and, 1282
  atonic and akinetic, 1661
  bacterial meningitis and, 1651
  breath-holding spells in, 1670

Seizure—continued
  cerebral palsy and, 1735
  comparison of partial, complex partial, and
      absence of, 1662
  complex partial, 1660
  epilepsy, 1657-1670
    classification of, 1659-1662
    general concepts of, 1657-1659
    nursing care of, 1662-1670
    therapeutic management and nursing care
        of, 1662-1670
  etiology of, 1658
  febrile, 231, 1670
  generalized, 1660-1662
  head injury and, 1644
  high-risk newborn and, 415-417
  history of, 1662
  migraine, 1670-1671
  myoclonic, 1661
  neonatal, causes of, 416
  nursing care summary in, 1669-1670
  observations during, 1666
  partial, 1659-1660
  simple partial, 1659-1660
  tonic-clonic, 1661
Seizure activity, 1623
Selenium, 557, 770
Self-care
  cognitive impairment and, 990-996
  determining capacity for paraplegic, 1828
  dressing and, 994, 995-996
  feeding and, 524, 990, 991, 992
  immobilization and, 1789
  muscular dystrophy and, 1755
  promotion of, 1066-1067
  visual impairment and, 1036
Self Help for Hard of Hearing People, 1019
Self-accusation, 928
Self-awareness
  nurse reaction to fatally ill child and,
      979-980
  play and, 134-135
Self-catheterization, 437
Self-concept, 26, 139
  content of, 120
  definition of, 120
  development of, 120-121
  obesity and, 892
  role models and, 28
Self-confidence, 33
Self-consciousness, 712
Self-dressing program, 994, 995
Self-esteem, 121, 139
  definition of, 121
  of family, chronic illness or disability
      and, 929
  immobilization and, 1789
  school-age child and, 707-708
Self-evaluation, 707
Self-feeding
  activities for, 991, 992
  infant and, 524
Self-grooming, 995-996
Self-help aids for feeding, 990, 991
Self-Help Clearinghouse, 944-945
Self-help skills; *see* Self-care
Self-image, epileptic child and, 1668; *see also*
      Body image; Self-concept; Self-
      esteem
Self-quieting abilities of infant, 327
Self-reporting, medication compliance
      and, 1110
Self-sacrifice of family, 929
Self-stimulatory behavior, 997, 1029
Sella turcica
  enlargement of, 1696

Conversion Tables

Conversion of Pounds to Kilograms for Pediatric Weights

Pounds →

↓	0	1	2	3	4	5	6	7	8	9
0	0.00	0.45	0.90	1.36	1.81	2.26	2.72	3.17	3.62	4.08
10	4.53	4.98	5.44	5.89	6.35	6.80	7.35	7.71	8.16	8.61
20	9.07	9.52	9.97	10.43	10.88	11.34	11.79	12.24	12.70	13.15
30	13.60	14.06	14.51	14.96	15.42	15.87	16.32	16.78	17.23	17.69
40	18.14	18.59	19.05	19.50	19.95	20.41	20.86	21.31	21.77	22.22
50	22.68	23.13	23.58	24.04	24.49	24.94	25.40	25.85	26.30	26.76
60	27.21	27.66	28.22	28.57	29.03	29.48	29.93	30.39	30.84	31.29
70	31.75	32.20	32.65	33.11	33.56	34.02	34.47	34.92	35.38	35.83
80	36.28	36.74	37.19	37.64	38.10	38.55	39.00	39.46	39.93	40.37
90	40.82	41.27	41.73	42.18	42.63	43.09	43.54	43.99	44.45	44.90
100	45.36	45.81	46.26	46.72	47.17	47.62	48.08	48.53	48.98	49.44
110	49.89	50.34	50.80	51.25	51.71	52.16	52.61	53.07	53.52	53.97
120	54.43	54.88	55.33	55.79	56.24	56.70	57.15	57.60	58.06	58.51
130	58.96	59.42	59.87	60.32	60.78	61.23	61.68	62.14	62.59	63.05
140	63.50	63.95	64.41	64.86	65.31	65.77	66.22	66.67	67.13	67.58
150	68.04	68.49	68.94	69.40	69.85	70.30	70.76	71.21	71.66	72.12
160	72.57	73.02	73.48	73.93	74.39	74.84	75.29	75.75	76.20	76.65
170	77.11	77.56	78.01	78.47	78.92	79.38	79.83	80.28	80.74	81.19
180	81.64	82.10	82.55	83.00	83.46	83.91	84.36	84.82	85.27	85.73
190	86.18	86.68	87.09	87.54	87.99	88.45	88.90	89.35	89.81	90.26
200	90.72	91.17	91.62	92.08	92.53	92.98	93.44	93.89	94.34	94.80

Conversion of Pounds and Ounces to Grams for Pediatric Weights

Pounds	Kilograms	Pounds	Kilograms	Ounces	Kilograms	Ounces	Kilograms
1	0.454	9	4.082	1	0.028	9	0.255
2	0.907	10	4.536	2	0.057	10	0.283
3	1.361	11	4.990	3	0.085	11	0.312
4	1.814	12	5.443	4	0.113	12	0.340
5	2.268	13	5.897	5	0.142	13	0.369
6	2.722			6	0.170	14	0.397
7	3.175			7	0.198	15	0.425
8	3.629			8	0.227		

Conversion Factors for Temperature*

Celsius	Fahrenheit	Celsius	Fahrenheit	Celsius	Fahrenheit	Celsius	Fahrenheit
34.0	93.2	36.4	97.5	38.6	101.5	41.0	105.9
34.2	93.6	36.6	97.9	38.8	101.8	41.2	106.1
34.4	93.9	36.8	98.2	39.0	102.2	41.4	106.5
34.6	94.3	37.0	98.6	39.2	102.6	41.6	106.8
34.8	94.6	37.2	99.0	39.4	102.9	41.8	107.2
35.0	95.0	37.4	99.3	39.6	103.3	42.0	107.6
35.2	95.4	37.6	99.7	39.8	103.6	42.2	108.0
35.4	95.7	37.8	100.0	40.0	104.0	42.4	108.3
35.6	96.1	38.0	100.4	40.2	104.4	42.6	108.7
35.8	96.4	38.2	100.8	40.4	104.7	42.8	109.0
36.0	96.8	38.4	101.1	40.6	105.2	43.0	109.4
36.2	97.2			40.8	105.4		

*$(°C) \times (9/5) + 32 = °F$
$(°F - 32) \times (5/9) = °C$
°C = temperature in Celsius (centigrade) degrees
°F = temperature in Fahrenheit degrees